KEEP THIS BOOK!

WHEN YOU PURCHASED

Physical Rehabilitation, you didn't just buy a required text for your course, you invested in a curriculum-spanning resource that will guide you from your first class to preparing for the NPTE.

WHEN YOU START YOUR CAREER

Physical Rehabilitation will be your most trusted reference for client/patient care in whichever setting you work.

WHEN YOU THINK ABOUT SELLING

Physical Rehabilitation at the end of the semester for a few dollars, don't. Use it as you grow from a rookie to a seasoned clinician.

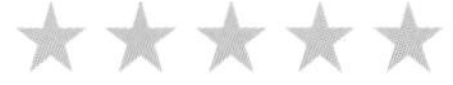

A Classic and a must in your shelf of PT books. "I have had this book ever since I was in college and it has proven to be valuable to me now that I am in my 11th year of practice as it was when I was still in my budding internship."

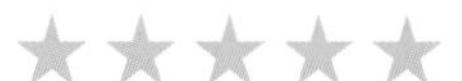

Five Stars. "This book is very comprehensive and contains almost everything you need to know for the NPTE exam."

This book is every Physical Therapy Students Bible. "...if you purchase this book during your first semester of PT school, it will help you immensely! Don't wait until Neuro PT to purchase this book. Use this book as a guide for every PT class from Integumentary to Pediatrics to Neuroanatomy!"

—Amazon Reviewers

Physical Rehabilitation

SEVENTH EDITION

Physical Rehabilitation

SEVENTH EDITION

Susan B. O'Sullivan, PT, EdD
Professor Emerita
Department of Physical Therapy
School of Health and Environment
University of Massachusetts Lowell
Lowell, Massachusetts

Thomas J. Schmitz, PT, PhD
Professor Emeritus
Division of Physical Therapy
School of Health Professions
Long Island University
Brooklyn Campus
Brooklyn, New York

George Fulk, PT, PhD
Professor, Chair
Department of Physical Therapy Education
College of Health Professions
SUNY Upstate Medical University
Syracuse, NY

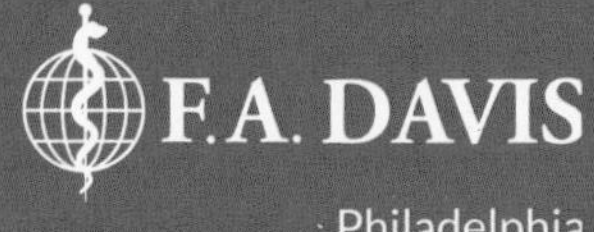

F.A. DAVIS
Philadelphia

F. A. Davis Company
1915 Arch Street
Philadelphia, PA 19103
www.fadavis.com

Printed in the United States of America

Last digit indicates print number: 10 9 8 7 6 5 4 3 2

Senior Acquisitions Editor: Melissa Duffield
Director of Content Development: George W. Lang
Senior Developmental Editor: Jennifer A. Pine
Content Project Manager: Julie Chase
Art and Design Manager: Carolyn O'Brien

Library of Congress Cataloging-in-Publication Data

Names: O'Sullivan, Susan B., editor. | Schmitz, Thomas J., editor. | Fulk, George D., editor.
Title: Physical rehabilitation / [edited by] Susan B. O'Sullivan, Thomas J. Schmitz, George Fulk.
Description: Seventh edition. | Philadelphia: F.A. Davis Company, [2019]
Identifiers: LCCN 2018036884 (print) | LCCN 2018037477 (ebook) | ISBN 9780803694644 | ISBN 9780803661622 (hard cover)
Subjects: | MESH: Physical Therapy Modalities | Physical Examination | Disability Evaluation | Orthopedic Equipment
Classification: LCC RM700 (ebook) | LCC RM700 (print) | NLM WB 460 | DDC 615.8/2—dc23
LC record available at https://lccn.loc.gov/2018036884

PREFACE

With the seventh edition of *Physical Rehabilitation,* we continue a tradition of striving for excellence that began more than 35 years ago. We are gratified by the continuing wide acceptance of *Physical Rehabilitation* by faculty, students, and clinicians.

The text is designed to provide a comprehensive approach to the rehabilitation management of adult patients. As such, it is intended to serve as a primary textbook for professional-level physical therapy students and as an important resource for practicing therapists as well as for other rehabilitation professionals. The seventh edition recognizes the continuing evolution of the profession and integrates basic and applied research to guide and inform evidence-based practice. It also integrates principles of patient/client management (examination, evaluation, diagnosis, prognosis, intervention, and outcomes) presented in the American Physical Therapy Association's *Guide to Physical Therapist Practice* and terminology from the World Health Organization's *International Classification of Functioning, Disability, and Health* (ICF).

Physical Rehabilitation is organized into three sections. Section One (Chapters 1–9) includes chapters on clinical decision making and examination of basic systems as well as examination of function and the environment. Section Two (Chapters 10–29) addresses many of the diseases, disorders, and health conditions commonly seen in the rehabilitation setting. Appropriate examination and intervention strategies are discussed for related body structure/function impairments, activity limitations, and participation restrictions in societal interactions. Health promotion and wellness strategies are also considered. Emphasis is placed on parameters of learning critical to ensuring the patient/client can achieve identified goals and expected outcomes. The final section, Section Three (Chapters 30–32), includes orthotics, prosthetics, and seating and wheeled mobility.

A central element of the text is a strong pedagogical format designed to facilitate and reinforce the learning of key concepts. Each chapter of *Physical Rehabilitation* includes an initial content outline, learning objectives, an introduction and summary, questions for review (self-assessment), and extensive references. Web-based resources for clinicians and patients/families are also provided. Application of important concepts is promoted through end-of-chapter case studies, which include guiding questions designed to enhance clinical decision-making skills. Many health condition–focused chapters contain *Tables of Outcome Measures* emphasizing tests and measures commonly used in clinical practice, and *tables* that summarize and critically appraise research relevant to the chapter content. Our hope is that these tables may provide a model for readers to continue to critically examine clinical practice using high-quality research findings. We also hope it will inspire enthusiasm about the importance of continuous, lifelong, self-directed learning.

The visuals have been enhanced with the addition of new illustrations and photographs. Design changes and a full-color format provide a reader-friendly environment and augment understanding of content. Valuable resources for the seventh edition include 14 online case studies with accompanying video segments illustrating aspects of the initial examination, interventions, and outcomes for patients undergoing active rehabilitation. The cases were authored by practicing therapists from various parts of the country who were directly involved in the care of the case study patient participant. The knowledge and clinical skills of these dedicated case study contributors are well represented in the online materials. The case studies include patients with chronic obstructive pulmonary disease and respiratory distress syndrome, burns, amputation, spinal cord injury, Parkinson's disease, traumatic brain injury, stroke, vestibular dysfunction, and multiple sclerosis. Questions are posed that address key elements in developing the plan of care for each patient. All case study materials (patient history, examination data, video segments, answers to guiding questions for student feedback) are available online at Davis*Plus*. Suggested answers to the end-of-chapter case study *Guiding Questions* and *Questions for Review* (self-assessment) are also available online.

Online resources also include sample examination questions consistent with the format of the National Physical Therapy Examination. In separate files, also available at Davis*Plus,* answers to the questions are provided for student feedback.

As we have gratefully noted with previous editions, our greatest asset and inspiration in preparing the seventh edition of *Physical Rehabilitation* has been an extraordinary group of contributing authors. We are most fortunate to have this group of talented individuals whose breadth and scope of professional knowledge and experience seems unparalleled. These individuals are recognized experts from a variety of specialty areas who have graciously shared their knowledge and clinical practice expertise by providing relevant, up-to-date, and practical information within their respective content areas.

The seventh edition has also benefited from the input of numerous individuals engaged in both academic and clinical practice settings who have used and reviewed the content. We are grateful for their constructive feedback and have instituted many of their suggestions and changes. As always, we welcome suggestions for improvements from our colleagues and students.

As physical therapists continue to take on more and greater professional responsibilities and challenges, the very nature of this text makes it a perpetual "work in progress." We are grateful for the opportunity to contribute to the academic literature in physical therapy, as well as to the professional development of those preparing to enter a career devoted to improving the quality of life of those we serve.

We acknowledge the very important contributions that physical therapists make in the lives of their patients. This book is dedicated to those therapists—past, present, and future—who guide and challenge their patients to lead a successful and independent life and who work toward building a community to improve the health of society.

—Susan B. O'Sullivan
Thomas J. Schmitz
George D. Fulk

CONTRIBUTING EDITORS

Edward W. Bezkor, PT, DPT, OCS, MTC, CAFS
Case Study and Multimedia Editor

Evangelos Pappas, PT, PhD, OCS
Test Bank Coordinator

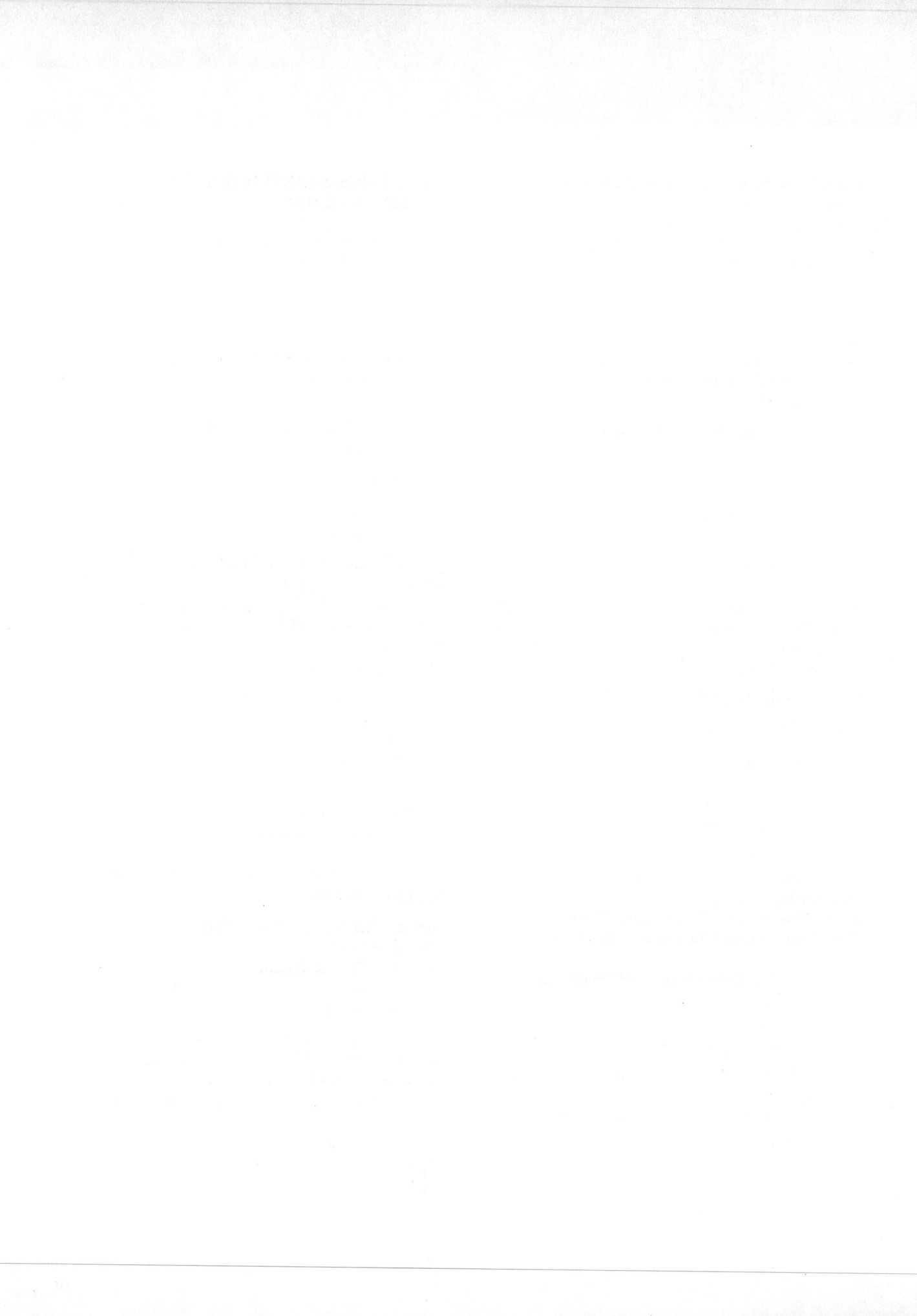

CONTRIBUTING AUTHORS

Andrea L. Behrman, PT, PhD, FAPTA
Professor
Department of Neurological Surgery
Kentucky Spinal Cord Injury Research Center
University of Louisville
Louisville, Kentucky

Edward W. Bezkor, PT, DPT, OCS, CAFS
Assistant Professor
University of St. Augustine for Health Sciences
Doctor of Physical Therapy Program
San Marcos, California

Janet R. Bezner, PT, DPT, PhD, FAPTA
Associate Professor
Texas State University
College of Health Professions
Department of Physical Therapy
San Marcos, Texas

Beth Black, PT, DSc
Associate Professor
Physical Therapy Program
School of Health Sciences
Oakland University
Rochester, Michigan

Mark Bowden, PhD, PT
Associate Professor and Director, Division of Physical Therapy
Department of Health Professions
College of Health Professions
Medical University of South Carolina
Charleston, South Carolina

Judith M. Burnfield, PT, PhD
Director, Institute for Rehabilitation Science and Engineering
Director, Movement and Neurosciences Center
Clifton Chair in Physical Therapy and Movement Science
Institute for Rehabilitation Science and Engineering
Madonna Rehabilitation Hospitals
Lincoln, Nebraska

Guilherme M. Cesar, PT, PhD
Assistant Research Director, Movement and Neurosciences Center
Institute for Rehabilitation Science and Engineering
Madonna Rehabilitation Hospitals
Lincoln, Nebraska

Kevin K. Chui, PT, DPT, PhD, GCS, OCS, CEEAA, FAAOMPT
Director and Professor
School of Physical Therapy and Athletic Training
College of Health Professions
Pacific University
Hillsboro, Oregon

Laura J. Cohen, PT, PhD, ATP/SMS
Principal, Rehabilitation and Technology Consultants, LLC
Arlington, Virginia

Vanina Dal Bello-Haas, PT, PhD
Associate Professor
Assistant Dean, Physiotherapy Program
School of Rehabilitation Science
McMaster University
Hamilton, Ontario, Canada

Judith E. Deutsch, PT, PhD, FAPTA
Professor and Director Rivers Lab
Department of Rehabilitation and Movement Sciences
Rutgers Biomedical and Health Sciences
Rutgers University
Newark, New Jersey

Konrad J. Dias, PT, DPT, PhD, CCS
Professor
Program in Physical Therapy
Maryville University
St Louis, Missouri

Lee Dibble, PT, PhD, ATC
Professor and Associate Chair
University of Utah
Department of Physical Therapy and Athletic Training
Salt Lake City, Utah

Joan E. Edelstein, PT, MA, FISPO
Special Lecturer
Program in Physical Therapy
Columbia University
New York, New York

Nora E. Fritz, PT, DPT, PhD, NCS
Assistant Professor, Physical Therapy and Neurology
Department of Health Care Sciences
Eugene Applebaum College of Pharmacy and Health Sciences
Wayne State University
Detroit, Michigan

George Fulk, PT, PhD
Professor and Chair
Department of Physical Therapy Education
College of Health Professions
SUNY Upstate Medical University
Syracuse, New York

Jessica Galgano, PhD, CCC-SLP
Adjunct Instructor
Department of Rehabilitation Medicine
School of Medicine
New York University
New York, New York

Maura Daly Iversen, PT, DPT, SD, MPH, FNAP, FAPTA
Associate Dean, Clinical Education, Rehabilitation and New Initiatives, Bouvé College of Health Sciences
Professor, Department of Physical Therapy, Movement and Rehabilitation Sciences
School of Health Professions, Bouvé College of Health Sciences
Affiliated Professor, College of Engineering
Northeastern University
Boston, Massachusetts

Deborah G. Kelly, PT, DPT, MSEd
Associate Professor
Division of Physical Therapy
Department of Rehabilitation Sciences
College of Health Sciences
University of Kentucky
Lexington, Kentucky

Margery A. Lockard, PT, PhD
Clinical Professor
Health Sciences Department
Physical Therapy and Rehabilitation Sciences Department
College of Nursing and Health Professions
Drexel University
Philadelphia, Pennsylvania

Bella J. May, PT, EdD, FAPTA, CEEAA (1930–2016)
Formerly Professor Emerita
Georgia Health Science University
Augusta, Georgia
Adjunct Professor of Physical Therapy
California State University Sacramento
Sacramento, California

Tara L. McIsaac, PT, PhD
Associate Professor
Department of Physical Therapy
Arizona School of Health Sciences
A.T. Still University
Mesa, Arizona

Richard J. McKibben, PT, DSc, ECS
Faculty, Doctor of Science in Health Science
Rocky Mountain University of Health Professions
Provo, Utah
Owner/Electromyographer
Integrity Rehab Management, LLC
Hamilton, Georgia

Coby D. Nirider, PT, DPT, CBIS
Chief Clinical Officer
Brookhaven Hospital
Neurologic Rehabilitation Institute
Tulsa, Oklahoma

Cynthia C. Norkin, PT, EdD
Associate Professor Emerita
Founding Director
Division of of Physical Therapy
School of Rehabilitation and Communications Studies
Ohio University
Athens, Ohio

Susan B. O'Sullivan, PT, EdD
Professor Emerita
Department of Physical Therapy
University of Massachusetts Lowell
School of Health and Environment
Lowell, Massachusetts

Evangelos Pappas, PT, PhD, OCS
Associate Professor
Faculty of Health Sciences
Discipline of Physiotherapy
University of Sydney
Lidcombe, New South Wales, Australia

Ingrid S. Parry, PT, MS
Rehabilitation Research Therapist
Shriners Hospital for Children, Northern California
University of California, Davis
Sacramento, California

Leslie G. Portney, PT, DPT, PhD, FAPTA
Professor Emerita, Department of Physical Therapy
MGH Institute of Health Professions
Boston, Massachusetts

Pat Precin, PhD, PsyD, NCPsyA, LP, OTR/L, FAOTA
Associate Professor
Programs in Occupational Therapy
Columbia University
New York, New York

Reginald L. Richard, PT, MS (retired)
Formerly Clinical Research Coordinator Burn Rehabilitation
U.S. Army Institute of Surgical Research
Fort Sam Houston, Texas

Leslie N. Russek, PT, DPT, PhD, OCS
Associate Professor
Department of Physical Therapy
Clarkson University
Potsdam, New York

Martha Taylor Sarno, MA, MD (hon)
Research Professor
Department of Rehabilitation Medicine
School of Medicine
New York University
New York, New York

Faith Saftler Savage, PT, ATP
Seating Specialist
The Boston Home
Boston, Massachusetts

David A. Scalzitti, PT, PhD
Assistant Professor
Program in Physical Therapy
School of Medicine and Health Sciences
George Washington University
Washington, District of Columbia

Thomas J. Schmitz, PT, PhD
Professor Emeritus
Department of Physical Therapy
School of Health Professions
Long Island University
Brooklyn, New York

Michael C. Schubert, PT, PhD
Associate Professor
Laboratory of Vestibular NeuroAdaptation
Department of Otolaryngology Head and Neck Surgery and Physical Medicine and Rehabilitation
School of Medicine
Johns Hopkins University
Baltimore, Maryland

Julie Ann Starr, PT, DPT, CCS
Clinical Associate Professor
Department of Physical Therapy
College of Health and Rehabilitation Sciences: Sargent College
Boston University
Boston, Massachusetts

Carolyn A. Unsworth, OTR, PhD
Professor, Discipline of Occupational Therapy
Central Queensland University
Melbourne Campus
Melbourne, Victoria, Australia

R. Scott Ward, PT, PhD, FAPTA
Professor and Chair
Department of Physical Therapy and Athletic Training
College of Health
University of Utah
Salt Lake City, Utah

Marie Westby, PT, PhD
Physical Therapy Teaching Supervisor
Mary Pack Arthritis Program
Vancouver Coastal Health
Vancouver, British Columbia, Canada

D. Joyce White, PT, DSc, MS
Associate Professor Emerita
Department of Physical Therapy
University of Massachusetts Lowell
Lowell, Massachusetts

Christopher Kevin Wong, PT, PhD, OCS
Associate Director, Program in Physical Therapy
Associate Professor of Rehabilitation and Regenerative Medicine
Columbia University Medical Center
Program in Physical Therapy
New York, New York

Sheng-Che Yen, PT, PhD
Assistant Professor
Department of Physical Therapy, Movement and Rehabilitation Sciences
Bouvé College of Health Sciences
Northeastern University
Boston, Massachusetts

ACKNOWLEDGMENTS

The ongoing development of *Physical Rehabilitation* has been in all aspects a collaborative venture. Its fruition has been made possible only through the expertise and gracious contributions of many talented individuals. Our appreciation is considerable.

Heartfelt thanks are extended to our contributing authors. Each has brought a unique body of knowledge, as well as distinct clinical practice expertise, to his and her respective chapters. Their commitment to physical therapist education is collectively displayed in content presentations that carefully reflect the scope of knowledge and skills required of a dynamic, evolving physical therapy practice environment. We are extremely grateful to each of our contributors and heartened by the excellence they bring to the seventh edition.

Heartfelt thanks are also extended to the practicing clinicians who prepared the case studies and video segments. Their contributions expertly move text content to clinical practice and significantly add to the development of clinical reasoning skills of our readers. We would like to thank Edward W. Bezkor, who served tirelessly as Case Study and Multimedia Editor and effectively coordinated case study contributions as well as many production elements. Thanks also to Yvonne Gillam, Freelance Editor and Media Consultant, and Liz Schaeffer, Developmental Editor/Electronic Products Coordinator, for their work in editing the patient videos.

A note of special thanks is extended to the following individuals for their assistance with filming the online video case studies: Jan BenDor, Producer and Videographer; Christine Flynn, New York College of Osteopathic Medicine of New York Institute of Technology; Don Packard, University of Michigan Hospital; Robert Price, University of Washington Medical Center; Sarah Ohiorhenuan, California Rehabilitation Institute; and Evan T. Cohen, Rutgers, The State University of New Jersey, School of Health Professions.

Many of the new patient photographs were possible owing to the efforts of Edward W. Bezkor and Robert J. Schreyer and the photography expertise of Jason Torres, J. Torres Photography, and Christopher Lenney. We thank also those individuals and companies who contributed new photographs to the individual chapters and to those patients/clients who allowed their photographs to be used throughout the text.

We would like to thank Evangelos Pappas, Test Bank Editor, for his expertise and efforts in developing guidelines for questions consistent with the National Physical Therapy Examination format and soliciting expert item writers for the test bank of examination questions. Our hope is that the test bank will become a valuable resource for both faculty and students who use our book.

Our appreciation goes to the dedicated professionals at F.A. Davis Company: Margaret M. Biblis, Editor-in-Chief; Melissa Duffield, Senior Acquisitions Editor; Jennifer A. Pine, Senior Developmental Editor; Amelia Blevins, Developmental Editor, Digital Products; Julie Chase, Content Project Manager; Sharon Lee, Production Manager; and Paul Marone, Marketing Manager. These individuals are recognized for their continued support, encouragement, and unwavering commitment to excellence. Thanks also are extended to Lynn Lusk, Project Manager, Progressive Publishing Services.

We wish to thank the numerous students, faculty, and clinicians who over the years have used *Physical Rehabilitation* and provided us with meaningful and constructive comments that have greatly enhanced this edition. It is our sincere hope that this feedback will continue.

Finally, we are grateful for our continuing strong and productive working relationship that has allowed us to complete a project of this scope through seven editions.

—Susan B. O'Sullivan
Thomas J. Schmitz
George D. Fulk

ABOUT THE AUTHORS

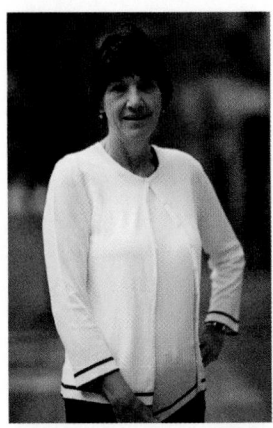

Dr. Susan B. O'Sullivan is Professor Emerita, Department of Physical Therapy, University of Massachusetts Lowell. She is co-editor and contributing author of *Physical Rehabilitation, Improving Functional Outcomes in Physical Rehabilitation,* and Therapy Ed's *National Physical Therapy Examination Review and Study Guide.* She holds an EdD in Human Development from the School of Education and Master of Science and Bachelor of Science degrees from Sargent College at Boston University. Dr. O'Sullivan's research, teaching, and clinical experience is in the area of adult neurological rehabilitation. She has also held academic appointments at Boston University. In 2012 the APTA Neurology Section honored Dr. O'Sullivan with the Award for Excellence in Neurologic Education. She is also the recipient of the University of Massachusetts Lowell Award for Teaching Excellence.

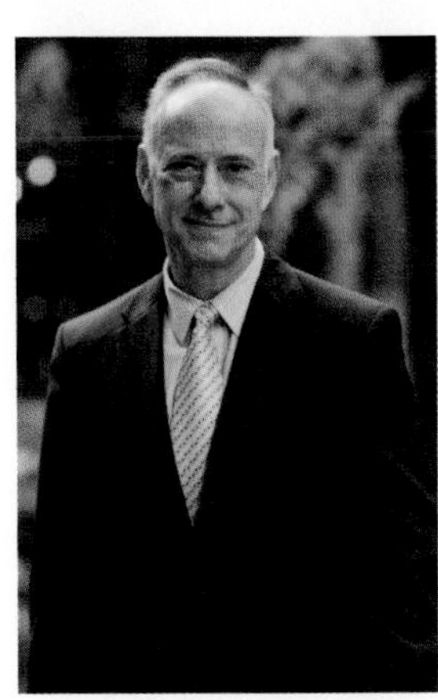

Dr. Thomas J. Schmitz is Professor Emeritus, Department of Physical Therapy, Long Island University. He is co-editor and contributing author of *Physical Rehabilitation* and *Improving Functional Outcomes in Physical Rehabilitation.* He holds a PhD from New York University, a Master of Science degree from Boston University, and a Bachelor of Science degree from SUNY at Buffalo. His primary clinical experience is in the area of adult neurological rehabilitation. Dr. Schmitz is the recipient of Long Island University's David Newton Award for Excellence in Teaching and the Trustees Award for Scholarly Achievement. He has also held academic appointments at Boston University, Sargent College, and Columbia University, College of Physicians and Surgeons.

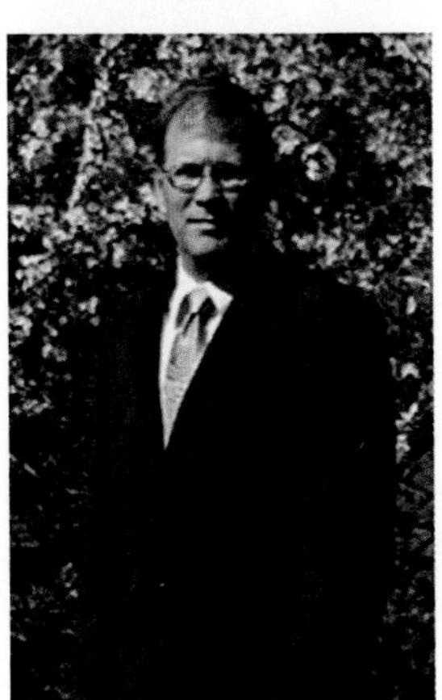

Dr. George D. Fulk is Professor and Chair, Department of Physical Therapy Education in the College of Health Professions at SUNY Upstate Medical University. He is co-editor and contributing author of *Physical Rehabilitation*, and contributing author of *Improving Functional Outcomes in Physical Rehabilitation.* He received his entry-level physical therapy degree from the University of Massachusetts at Lowell and his PhD from Nova Southeastern University. Dr. Fulk's research, teaching, and clinical expertise are in the areas of enhancing motor recovery and quality of life in people with neurological health conditions. He has also held faculty appointments at Clarkson University in Potsdam, New York, and Notre Dame College in Manchester, New Hampshire.

Dr. Fulk's research has focused on measuring and improving locomotor capability in people with stroke. He has authored numerous journal articles, conference papers, and textbook chapters in these areas. He is also the Digital Media Editor and an Associate Editor for the *Journal of Neurological Physical Therapy*, and serves as a reviewer for many peer-reviewed journals.

CONTENTS

VIDEO CASE STUDIES

Fourteen video case studies are available online at Davis*Plus*. Each includes a narrative presentation and three accompanying video segments (examination, intervention, and outcomes) together with guiding questions designed to challenge clinical decision-making skills. Student feedback is provided via suggested answers to the guiding questions posted in a separate online file.

CASE STUDY 1: Critical Care Patient in the Intensive Care Unit

(applicable to Chapters 1, 2, 12, and 13)

James Tompkins, PT, DPT
Department of Physical Medicine and Rehabilitation
Mayo Clinic Hospital
Phoenix, Arizona

Joseph L. Verheijde, PhD, MBA, PT
Department of Physical Medicine and Rehabilitation
Mayo Clinic Hospital
Scottsdale, Arizona

Bhavesh M. Patel, MD, FRCPC
Departments of Critical Care and Respiratory Care
Mayo Clinic Hospital
Phoenix, Arizona

CASE STUDY 2: Patient With Burns

(applicable to Chapter 24)

Jill Quarles, PT, MS • Sophie Manning, PT, BSc
Michigan Medicine
Ann Arbor, Michigan

CASE STUDY 3: Patient With a Below Knee Amputation

(applicable to Chapter 22)

Kim Stover Rosso, PT, MSPT • Laura Pink-Baker, PT, DPT
Michigan Medicine
Ann Arbor, Michigan

CASE STUDY 4: Patient With Spinal Cord Injury

(applicable to Chapter 20)

Alex Eubank, PT, DPT
Dodd Hall Rehabilitation Services
Ohio State University Wexner Medical Center
Columbus Ohio

CASE STUDY 5: Patient With Spinal Cord Injury

(applicable to Chapter 20)

Sally Taylor, PT
Shirley Ryan AbilityLab
(Formerly the Rehabilitation Institute of Chicago)
Chicago, Illinois
Assistant Professor
Department of Physical Therapy and Human Movement Sciences
Northwestern University, Feinberg School of Medicine
Chicago, Illinois

CASE STUDY 6: Patient With Parkinson's disease

(applicable to Chapter 18)

Edward W. Bezkor, PT, DPT, OCS, MTC, CAFS
Assistant Professor
University of St. Augustine for Health Sciences
Doctor of Physical Therapy Program
San Marcos, California

Michelle Farella-Accurso, PT, DPT
New York College of Osteopathic Medicine of New York Institute of Technology
Adele Smithers Parkinson's Disease Research and Treatment Center
Department of Physical Therapy
Old Westbury, New York

CASE STUDY 7: Patient With Traumatic Brain Injury and Shoulder Amputation

(applicable to Chapters 19 and 22)

Faye Bronstein PT, DPT, NCS
NYU Langone Health
Rusk Rehabilitation
New York, New York

CASE STUDY 8: Patient With Traumatic Brain Injury

(applicable to Chapter 19)

Victoria Stevens, PT, NCS • *Kate Rough, PT, DPT, NCS*
University of Washington Medical Center
Rehabilitation Medicine
Seattle, Washington

CASE STUDY 9: Patient With Right Hemorrhagic CVA

(applicable to Chapter 15)

Alicia Esposito O'Hara, PT, DPT, NCS
NYU Langone Health
Rusk Rehabilitation
New York, New York

CASE STUDY 10: Patient With Left Ischemic CVA

(applicable to Chapter 15)
Greg Hartley, PT, DPT, GCS • Gemma Longfellow, PT, MSPT, GCS • Karen J. Lagares, PT, DPT, GCS
St. Catherine's Rehabilitation Hospital
North Miami, Florida

CASE STUDY 11: Patient With Right Thalamic Ischemic Infarct and Left Lateral Medullary Ischemia

(applicable to Chapter 15)
Hendrika Lietz, PT, DPT, NCS
University of Michigan Hospital
Ann Arbor, Michigan

CASE STUDY 12: Patient With Right Basal Ganglia Intraparenchymal Hemorrhage

(applicable to Chapter 15)
Patricia Laverty, PT, DPT • Maria Julia Vila, PT, MPT
New York University Langone Medical Center
Rusk Institute of Rehabilitation Medicine
New York, New York

CASE STUDY 13: Patient With Vestibular Disorder

(applicable to Chapter 21)
Bryan Hujsak, PT, DPT, NCS
The New York Eye and Ear Infirmary
Vestibular Rehabilitation
New York, New York

CASE STUDY 14: Patient With Multiple Sclerosis

(applicable to Chapter 16)
Maria Rundell, PT, DPT, NCS, MSCS
Outpatient Lead Therapist
HealthSouth Rehabilitation Hospital of Colorado Springs
Colorado Springs, Colorado

SECTION ONE

Clinical Decision Making and Examination

Clinical Decision Making

Susan B. O'Sullivan, PT, EdD

Chapter 1

LEARNING OBJECTIVES

1. Define clinical reasoning and identify factors that affect clinical decision making.
2. Identify the components of the International Classification of Functioning, Disability, and Health.
3. Describe the key steps in the patient/client management process.
4. Define the major responsibilities of the physical therapist in planning effective treatments.
5. Identify potential problems that could adversely affect the physical therapist's clinical reasoning.
6. Discuss strategies to ensure patient participation in developing the plan of care (POC).
7. Identify key elements of physical therapy documentation.
8. Discuss the importance of evidence-based practice in developing the POC.
9. Discuss the importance of clinical practice guidelines (CPGs).
10. Analyze and interpret patient /client data, formulate realistic goals and outcomes, and develop a POC when presented with a clinical case study.

CHAPTER OUTLINE

■ CLINICAL REASONING/ CLINICAL DECISION MAKING

Clinical reasoning is a multidimensional, non-linear cognitive process that involves synthesis of information and collaboration with the patient, caregivers, and health care team. The clinician integrates information about the patient, the task, and the setting in order to reach decisions and determine actions in accordance with best available evidence. Clinical decisions are the outcomes of the iterative clinical reasoning process and form the basis of patient/client management. Numerous factors influence decision making, including the clinician's goals, knowledge base and expertise, psychosocial skills, problem-solving strategies, and procedural skills. Decision making is also influenced by patient/client characteristics, including goals, values, and beliefs; physical, psychosocial, educational, and cultural factors; and overall resources, time, and level of financial and social support.

Frameworks and models may be used to organize the clinical reasoning process. Those frameworks may change over time based on the evolution of the field of physical therapy or the conceptualization of health by the World Health Organization (WHO). For example, the WHO used a disablement model (the International Classification of Impairments, Disabilities, and Handicaps [ICIDH]) that evolved into an enablement model called the International Classification of Functioning and Health (ICF). Frameworks can be specific to the profession. In physical therapist practice, the *Guide to Physical Therapist Practice* is organized using the patient management system and more recently incorporating the ICF.

Physical therapists practice in a variety of clinical environments, including acute, rehabilitation, and chronic care facilities. Therapists have many different roles in these settings, including direct patient care and case management as a member of a collaborative team, with referral to and consultation with other providers and supervision of personnel (e.g., physical therapist assistants, other support staff). Decision making is influenced by interaction and involvement of other providers,[1] as depicted in Figure 1.1. Decision making is also influenced by the clinical practice environment. In *primary care,* therapists provide integrated, accessible health care services that address a large majority of personal health care needs, develop a sustained partnership with patients, and practice within the context of family and community. Primary care is also provided in school, industrial, or workplace settings.

Secondary care is provided to patients who are initially treated by other practitioners and then referred to physical therapists.

Tertiary care is provided to patients in highly specialized, complex, and technology-based settings (e.g., burn units) or in response to requests from other health care practitioners for consultation and specialized services (e.g., for individuals with spinal cord lesions). Therapists also have active roles in *prevention* and health promotion, wellness, and fitness with a wide variety of populations.

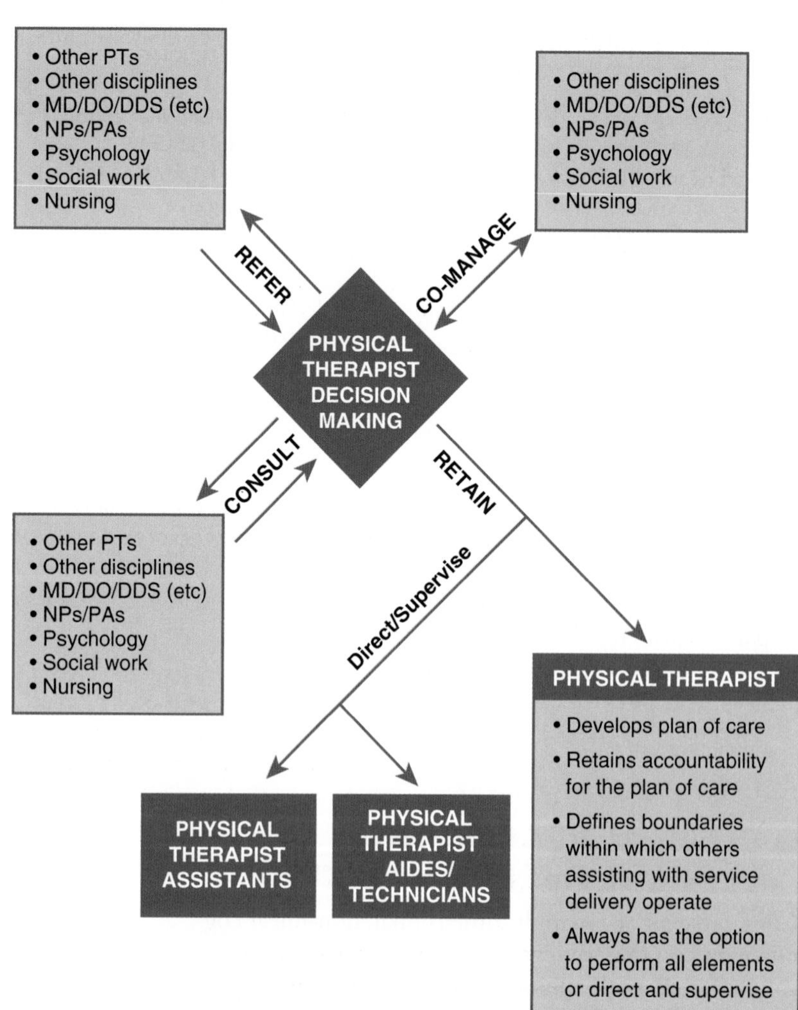

Figure 1.1 Physical therapist decision making related to the involvement of other providers. *(Introduction to the Guide to Physical Therapist Practice.* Guide to Physical Therapist Practice 3.0. *Alexandria, VA: American Physical Therapy Association; 2014. Available at: http://guidetoptpractice.apta.org/content/1/SEC1.body. Accessed December 1, 2017.)*

Box 1.1 provides a summary of the terminology used to define clinical practice environments.[1]

Physical therapists today practice as primary care providers in complex environments and are called upon to reach increasingly complex decisions under significant practice constraints. For example, a therapist may be required to complete the examination and determine a plan of care (POC) for the complicated patient with multiple co-morbidities within 24 to 48 hours of admission to a rehabilitation facility. Limited insurance coverage with high co-pays and limited allocation of physical therapy treatment sessions also complicate the decision making process. Novice practitioners can easily become overwhelmed. This chapter presents a framework for clinical decision making and patient/client management that can assist in organizing and prioritizing data and in planning effective treatments compatible with the needs and goals of the patient/client and members of the health care team.

INTERNATIONAL CLASSIFICATION OF FUNCTIONING, DISABILITY, AND HEALTH

The WHO's International Classification of Functioning, Disability, and Health (ICF) model provides an important framework for understanding and categorizing health conditions and patient problems by clearly defining the complex interaction among health condition, impairment, activity limitation, participation restriction, and contextual factors.[2] The American Physical Therapy Association (APTA) has joined WHO, the World Confederation for Physical Therapy (WCPT),

Box 1.1 Clinical Practice Environments Terminology[1]

Prevention is the avoidance, minimization, or delay of the onset of impairment, activity limitation, and/or participation restrictions. Includes primary, secondary, and tertiary prevention initiatives for individuals as well as selective intervention initiatives for subsets of the population at risk for impairments, activity limitations, and/or participation restrictions.

- **Primary prevention** prevents a target condition in a susceptible or potentially susceptible population through specific measures such as general health efforts.
- **Secondary prevention** decreases the duration of illness, severity of disease, and number of sequelae through early diagnosis and prompt intervention.
- **Tertiary prevention** limits the degree of disability and promotes rehabilitation and restoration of function in patients with chronic and irreversible diseases.

Primary care is defined as the provision of integrated, accessible health care services by clinicians who are accountable for addressing a large majority of personal health care needs, developing a sustained partnership with patients, and practicing within the context of family and community.

Secondary care is the care provided to patients who are initially treated by other practitioners and then referred to physical therapists.

Tertiary care is the care provided to patients in highly specialized, complex, and technology-based settings (e.g., burn units) or in response to requests of other health care practitioners for consultation and specialized services (e.g., for individuals with spinal cord lesions).

Acute care involves the care of individuals with severe symptoms, illnesses, or life- or limb-threatening health conditions, regardless of their cause. It generally serves as an entry-point to health care, is short-term, and encompasses preventive and primary care.

Rehabilitation includes health care services that help an individual keep, restore, or improve skills and functioning for daily living that have been lost or impaired because a person was sick, hurt, or disabled. These services may include physical therapy, occupational therapy, speech-language pathology, and psychiatric rehabilitation services in a variety of inpatient and outpatient settings.

Chronic care addresses preexisting or long-term illness and involves a continuum of integrated care over time and delivered in a variety of settings. It addresses loss of functional abilities and assists in helping individuals maintain independence and a high level of functioning. Chronic care encompasses medical care, rehabilitative care, and supportive services.

Health promotion is any effort taken to allow an individual, group, or community to achieve awareness of—and empowerment to pursue—prevention and wellness. Services include identifying risk factors and implementing services to reduce risk factors, preventing or slowing the functional decline and disability, and enhancing activity, participation, wellness, and fitness.

Wellness is a state of being that incorporates all facets and dimensions of human existence, including physical health, emotional health, spirituality, and social connectivity.

and other international professional organizations in endorsing the ICF classification. Figure 1.2 presents the structure of the ICF model.[1]

The ICF provides descriptions of health, health conditions, functioning, and disabilities that are associated with a health condition and contextual factors that can influence outcomes.[3] *Health* is defined as a state of complete physical, mental, and social well-being and not merely the absence of disease or infirmity. *Health condition* is an umbrella term for disease, disorder, injury, or trauma and may include other circumstances, such as aging, stress, congenital anomaly, or genetic predisposition. It may also include information about pathogeneses and/or etiology. *Body functions* are physiological functions of body systems (including psychological functions). *Body structures* are anatomical parts of the body such as organs, limbs, and their components.

Impairments are the problems an individual may have in body function (physiological functions of body systems) or structure (anatomical parts of the body). The resulting significant deviation or loss is the direct result of the health condition. For example, a patient with stroke may present with sensory loss, paresis, dyspraxia, and hemianopsia (direct impairments). Impairments may be mild, moderate, severe, or complete and may be permanent, resolve as recovery progresses, or become progressively worse, as may be the case in a neurodegenerative disease such as Parkinson's disease. Impairments may also be indirect (secondary), the sequelae or complications that originate from other systems. They can result from preexisting impairments or the expanding multisystem dysfunction that occurs with prolonged bedrest and inactivity, an ineffective POC, or lack of rehabilitation intervention. Examples of indirect impairments include decreased vital capacity and cardiovascular endurance, disuse atrophy and weakness, contractures, decubitus ulcers, deep vein thrombosis, renal calculi, urinary tract infections, pneumonia, and depression.

Activity is the execution of a task or action by an individual. *Activity limitations* are difficulties an individual may have in executing tasks or actions. These can include limitations in the performance of cognitive and learning skills; communication skills; *functional mobility skills* such as transfers, walking, lifting, or carrying objects; and *activities of daily living* (ADL). *Basic activities of daily living* (BADL) include self-care activities of toileting, maintaining hygiene, bathing, dressing, eating, drinking, and having social (interpersonal) interactions. The person with stroke may demonstrate difficulties in all of the above areas and be unable to perform the actions, tasks, and activities that constitute the "usual activities" for this individual.

Participation is an individual's involvement in a life situation, the societal perspective of functioning. *Participation restrictions* are problems an individual may experience with involvement in daily life situations and societal interactions. Categories of life roles include home management, work (job/school/play), and community/leisure. These include *instrumental activities of daily living* (IADL) such as housecleaning, preparing meals, shopping, telephoning

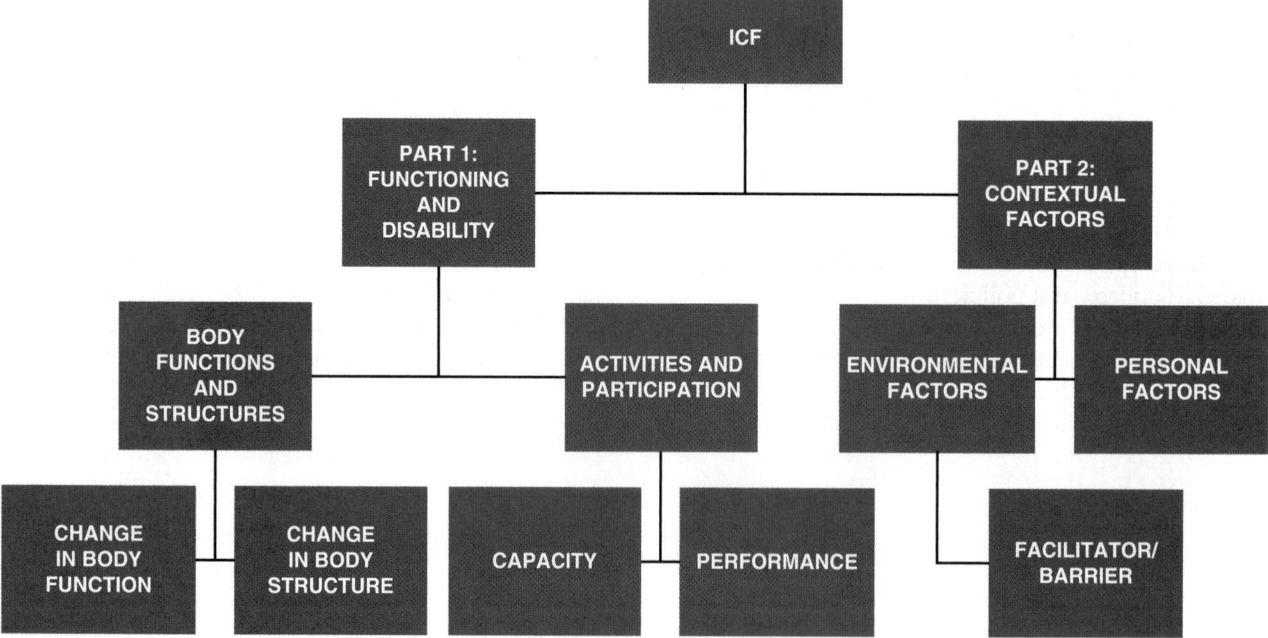

Figure 1.2 Structure of the International Classification of Functioning, Disability and Health (ICF) model of functioning and disability. *(Introduction to the Guide to Physical Therapist Practice.* Guide to Physical Therapist Practice 3.0. *Alexandria, VA: American Physical Therapy Association; 2014. Available at: http://guidetoptpractice.apta.org/content/1/SEC1.body. Accessed December 1, 2017.)*

or other modes of communication, and managing finances, as well as work and leisure activities (e.g., sports, recreation, travel). Thus, the individual with stroke is unable to resume societal roles and activities such as working, parenting, attending church, or playing golf.

Performance describes what an individual does in his or her current environment, which includes use of assistive devices or personal assistance, whenever the individual uses them to perform actions or tasks. *Performance qualifiers* indicate the extent of participation restriction (difficulty) in performing tasks or actions in an individual's current real-life environment. All aspects of the physical, social, and attitudinal world constitute the environment. Difficulty can range from mild to moderate to severe.

Capacity describes an individual's ability to execute a task or an action (highest probable level of functioning in a given domain at a given moment). *Capacity qualifiers* indicate the extent of activity limitation and are used to describe an individual's highest probable level of functioning (ability to do the task or action). Qualifiers can range from the assistance of a device (e.g., adaptive equipment) or another person (minimal to moderate to maximal assistance) or environmental modification (home, workplace). Thus, the patient with stroke may demonstrate moderate difficulty in locomotion in the home environment (performance qualifiers) and require the use of an ankle-foot orthosis, small-based quad cane, and moderate assistance of one (capacity qualifiers).

Contextual factors represent the entire background of an individual's life and living situation. These include both environmental factors and personal factors. *Environmental factors* make up the physical, social, and attitudinal environment in which people live and conduct their lives. Factors range from products and technology (for personal use in daily living, mobility and transportation, communication) and physical factors (home environment, terrain, climate) to social support and relationships (family, friends, personal care providers), attitudes (individual and societal), and institutions and laws (housing, communication, transportation, legal, financial services, and policies).

Personal factors are the particular background of an individual's life, including gender, age, coping styles, social background, education, profession, past and current experience, overall behavior pattern, character, and other factors that influence how disability is experienced by an individual. Qualifiers include factors that serve as barriers or facilitators. *Barriers* (disablement risk factors) are factors within an individual's environment that, through their absence or presence, limit functioning and create disability. *Facilitators* (assets) are factors in an individual's environment that, through their absence or presence, improve functioning and disability. Both can range from mild to moderate to strong in their influence on functioning. Box 1.2 summarizes ICF terminology on functioning, disability, and health.[3]

The ICF Checklist is a practical tool to elicit and record information on functioning and disability of an individual.[4] The WHO also has CORE sets, which provide a list of body structure/functions, activities, and participation that are commonly seen with certain health conditions. These can be helpful for novice therapists when first learning the ICF and about a certain health condition (www.icf-research-branch.org/icf-core-sets-projects2).

■ PATIENT/CLIENT MANAGEMENT

Steps in patient/client management include (1) examination of the patient; (2) evaluation of the data and identification of problems; (3) determination of the physical therapy diagnosis and prognosis; (4) determination of the POC; (5) intervention; and (6) reexamination and evaluation of treatment outcomes (Fig. 1.3). Physical therapists are uniquely qualified to focus on the *movement system,* defined in APTA's vision statement as "a collection of systems (cardiovascular, pulmonary, endocrine, integumentary, nervous, and musculoskeletal) that interact to move the body or its component parts" (www.apta.org/MovementSystem/). Thus, the overall focus is on optimizing functional performance and participation across the life span using movement-related interventions.

Examination

Examination involves identifying and defining the patient's impairments, activity limitations, and restrictions in participation and the resources available to determine appropriate intervention. It consists of the following components: the patient history, systems review, tests and measures, and task analysis. Examination begins with patient referral or initial entry (direct access) and continues as an ongoing process throughout the episode of care. Ongoing reexamination allows the therapist to evaluate progress and modify interventions as appropriate.

History

Information about the patient's history and current health status is obtained from review of the medical record and interviews (patient, family, caregivers). The medical record provides detailed reports from members of the health care team; processing these reports requires an understanding of disease and injury, medical terminology, differential diagnosis, laboratory and other diagnostic tests, and medical management. The use of resource material or professional consultation can assist the novice clinician.

The initial interview is an important tool used to obtain information from the patient, including learning patient goals, establishing rapport and mutual trust, ensuring open communication lines, and enhancing motivation. Communication skills and questioning techniques are used to focus on current health condition, past medical history, personal context, and emotional context. Several factors are key to ensuring effective patient involvement,

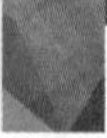

Box 1.2 International Classification of Functioning, Disability, and Health (ICF) Terminology[2,3]

Body functions are physiological functions of body systems (including psychological functions).
Body structures are anatomical parts of the body such as organs, limbs, and their components.
Health is a state of complete physical, mental, and social well-being and not merely the absence of disease or infirmity.
Health condition is an umbrella term for disease, disorder, injury, or trauma and may also include other circumstances, such as aging, stress, congenital anomaly, or genetic predisposition. It may also include information about pathogeneses and/or etiology.
Impairments are problems in body function or structure such as a significant deviation or loss.
Activity is the execution of a task or action by an individual.
Activity limitations are difficulties an individual may have in executing activities.
Capacity describes an individual's ability to execute a task or an action (highest probable level of functioning in a given domain at a given moment).
Contextual factors represent the entire background of an individual's life and living situation.

- **Personal factors** are the particular background of an individual's life, including gender, age, coping styles, social background, education, profession, past and current experience, overall behavior pattern, character, and other factors that influence how disability is experienced by an individual.
- **Environmental factors** make up the physical, social, and attitudinal environment in which people live and conduct their lives, including social attitudes, architectural characteristics, and legal and social structures.
- **Barriers** are factors within an individual's environment that, through their absence or presence, limit functioning and create disability.
- **Facilitators** are factors in an individual's environment that, through their absence or presence, improve functioning and disability.

Disability is an umbrella term for impairments, activity limitations, and participation restrictions. It denotes the negative aspects of the interaction between an individual (with a health condition) and that individual's contextual factors (environmental and personal factors).
Functioning encompasses all body functions and structures, activities, and participation.
Participation is an individual's involvement in a life situation; societal perspective of functioning.
Participation restrictions are problems an individual may experience in involvement in life situations. Participation restriction is determined by comparing an individual's participation to that which is expected from an individual without a disability in a particular culture or society.
Performance describes what an individual does in his or her current environment. The current environment includes assistive devices or personal assistance, whenever the individual uses them to perform actions or tasks.
Performance qualifiers indicate the extent of participation restriction (difficulty) in performing tasks or actions in an individual's current real-life environment.

including active listening, empathy, building rapport, asking appropriate questions, summarizing and validating patient responses, and effectively using non-verbal communication cues. During the interview, the therapist should listen carefully to what the patient says and ask key questions that allow the patient to express feelings (e.g., What are you most concerned about?) and ideas (e.g., What are your thoughts or ideas about what may have caused this?). What do you expect or hope for? What would be important for us to include in your plan of care? Empathy is best relayed to the patient by recognizing the patient's feelings and demonstrating understanding of the patient's unique individual experiences (e.g., Can you help me understand how you see or experience your health condition?). Building good rapport allows the patient to feel comfortable and opens the lines of communication. The therapist's communication (e.g., tone of voice, choice of language) and non-verbal communication (e.g., facial expressions, gestures, eye contact) influences the patient's level of comfort with the interviewer and the overall outcome.

Conversely, the therapist should observe the patient for any physical manifestations that reveal emotional context, such as slumped body posture, grimacing, and poor eye contact. The therapist should be sensitive to differences in culture and ethnicity that can influence how the patient or family member responds during the interview or examination process. Biases, prejudices, preconceptions, and judgments on the part of the therapist can interfere with active listening and in processing what the patient is saying. Ensuring effective communication with the patient promotes cooperation and serves to make the therapist's observations more valid, which is crucial to the success of the POC.[5-7]

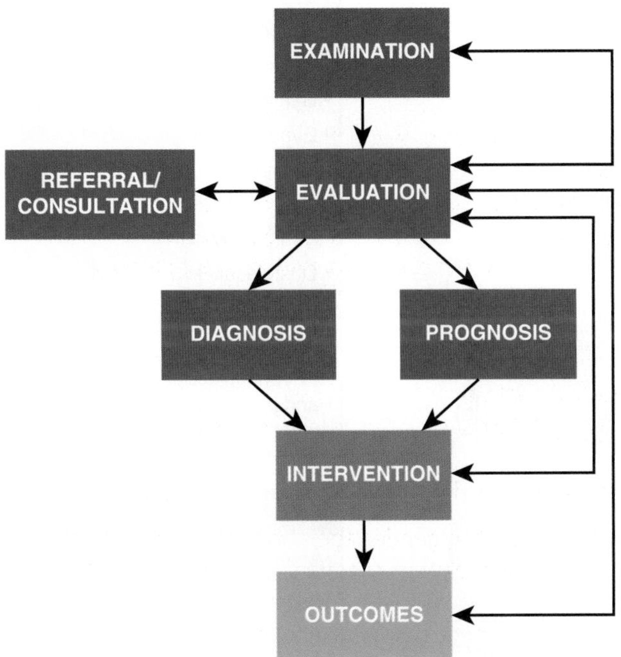

Figure 1.3 The process of physical therapist patient and client management. *(Principles of Physical Therapist Patient and Client Management.* Guide to Physical Therapist Practice 3.0. *Alexandria, VA: American Physical Therapy Association; 2014. Available at: http://guidetoptpractice.apta.org/content/1/SEC2.body. Accessed December 1, 2017.)*

During the interview, the therapist asks the patient a series of questions, using both open-ended and closed-ended questions. Open-ended questions require more than a simple yes/no response (e.g., What symptoms are you currently experiencing?) while closed-ended questions limit the patient's responses to a yes/no answer or a nod (e.g., Do you have any pain today?). Questions are posed regarding the history of the present illness or condition. Specifically, the patient is asked to describe current problems, chief complaint (reason for seeking physical therapy), and chronological account leading up to the episode of care. Questions then explore location, quality, and severity of the symptoms or problems as well as timing (occurrence), factors that aggravate or relieve them, and associated manifestations (other symptoms or problems) that may be occurring. Questions are posed regarding functioning (e.g., How has your health condition affected your daily life? What have you had to give up because of your health condition?). The patient will often describe his or her difficulties in terms of activity limitations or participation restrictions (what he or she can or cannot do). General questions about functional activities and participation should be directed toward delineating the difference between capacity and performance. For example, "Since your stroke, how much difficulty do you have walking long distances?" "How does this compare to before you had the stroke?" (capacity). Questions directed toward examining performance can include "What problem(s) do you have when walking?" "Is this problem with walking made worse or better with the use of an assistive device?" Questions are also posed regarding the patient's past medical history, health habits (e.g., smoking history, alcohol use), family history, and personal and social history. Information about physical environment, vocation, recreational interests, exercise likes and dislikes, and type, frequency, and intensity of regular activity should be obtained.[5-8] The types of data that may be generated from a patient history are presented in Figure 1.4.[1] Sample interview questions are included in Box 1.3.

Pertinent information can also be obtained from the patient's family or caregiver. For example, patients with central nervous system (CNS) involvement and severe cognitive and/or communication impairments and younger pediatric patients will be unable to accurately communicate their existing problems. The family member/caregiver then assumes the primary role of assisting the therapist in identifying problems and providing relevant aspects of the history. The perceived needs of the family member or caregiver can also be determined during the interview.

Systems Review

The use of a screening examination (brief systems review) allows the therapist to quickly scan the patient's body systems and determine areas of intact function and dysfunction. These systems include[1]:

- *Musculoskeletal:* assessment of gross symmetry, gross range of motion, gross strength, height and weight
- *Neuromuscular:* assessment of gross coordinated movement (e.g., balance, gait, locomotion, transfers, and transitions) and motor function (motor control and motor learning)
- *Cardiovascular/pulmonary:* assessment of heart rate, respiratory rate, blood pressure, and edema
- *Integumentary:* assessment of skin integrity, pliability (texture), presence of scar formation, and skin color
- *Communication ability, affect, and language*: assessment of the ability to produce and understand speech, and communicate thoughts and feelings
- *Cognitive ability:* assessment of consciousness, orientation (person, place, and time), expected emotional/behavioral responses, and learning preferences (e.g., learning barriers, education needs)

Information is also obtained about other major body systems (e.g., endocrine, gastrointestinal, genitourinary) to determine if referral for additional medical evaluation is needed. Areas of deficit together with an accurate knowledge of the main health condition (disorder or disease) (1) confirm the need for further or more detailed examination; (2) rule out or differentiate specific system involvement; (3) determine if referral to another health care professional is warranted; and (4) focus the search of the origin of symptoms to a specific location or body

ACTIVITIES AND PARTICIPATION

- Current and prior role functions (eg, self-care and domestic, education, work, community, social, and civic life)

CURRENT CONDITION(S)

- Concerns that led the patient or client to seek the services of a physical therapist
- Concerns or needs of the patient or client who requires the services of a physical therapist
- Current therapeutic interventions
- Mechanisms of injury or disease, including date of onset and course of events
- Onset and pattern of symptoms
- Patient or client, family, significant other, and caregiver expectations and goals for the therapeutic intervention
- Patient or client, family, significant other, and caregiver perceptions of patient's or client's emotional response to the current clinical situation
- Previous occurrence of current condition(s)
- Prior therapeutic interventions

GENERAL DEMOGRAPHICS

- Age
- Education
- Primary language
- Race/ethnicity
- Sex

FAMILY HISTORY

- Familial health risks

GENERAL HEALTH STATUS (SELF-REPORT, FAMILY REPORT, CAREGIVER REPORT)

- General health perceptions
- Mental functions (eg, memory, reasoning ability, depression, anxiety)
- Physical function (eg, mobility, sleep patterns, restricted bed days)

GROWTH AND DEVELOPMENT

- Developmental history
- Hand dominance

LIVING ENVIRONMENT

- Assistive technology (eg, aids for locomotion, orthotic devices, prosthetic requirements, seating and positioning technology)
- Living environment and community characteristics
- Projected destination at conclusion of care

MEDICAL/SURGICAL HISTORY

- Cardiovascular
- Endocrine/metabolic
- Gastrointestinal
- Genitourinary
- Gynecological
- Integumentary
- Musculoskeletal
- Neuromuscular
- Obstetrical
- Psychological
- Pulmonary
- Prior hospitalizations, surgeries, and preexisting medical and other health-related conditions

MEDICATIONS

- Medications for current condition
- Medications previously taken for current condition
- Medications for other conditions

OTHER CLINICAL TESTS

- Laboratory and diagnostic tests
- Review of available records (eg, medical, education, surgical)
- Review of other clinical findings (eg, nutrition and hydration)

REVIEW OF SYSTEMS

- Cardiovascular/pulmonary systems
- Endocrine system
- Eyes, ears, nose, or throat
- Gastrointestinal system
- Genitourinary/reproductive systems
- Hematologic/lymphatic systems
- Integumentary system
- Neurologic/musculoskeletal systems

SOCIAL/HEALTH HABITS (PAST AND CURRENT)

- Behavioral health risks (eg, tobacco use, drug abuse)
- Level of physical fitness

SOCIAL HISTORY

- Cultural beliefs and behaviors
- Family and caregiver resources
- Social interactions, social activities, and support systems

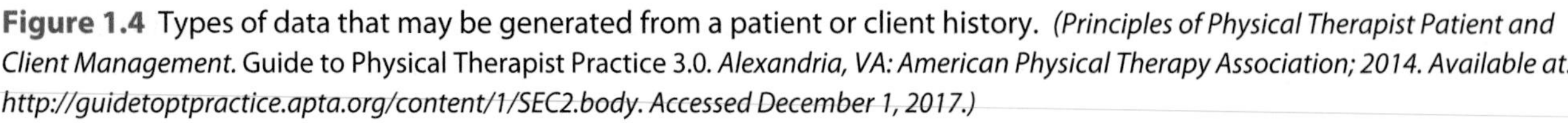

Figure 1.4 Types of data that may be generated from a patient or client history. *(Principles of Physical Therapist Patient and Client Management.* Guide to Physical Therapist Practice 3.0. *Alexandria, VA: American Physical Therapy Association; 2014. Available at: http://guidetoptpractice.apta.org/content/1/SEC2.body. Accessed December 1, 2017.)*

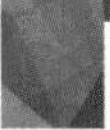

Box 1.3 Sample Interview Questions[7,8]

1. **Interview questions designed to identify the nature and history of the current problem(s):**
   What problem(s) brings you to therapy?
   When did the problem(s) begin?
   What happened to precipitate the problem(s)?
   How long has the problem(s) existed?
   How are you taking care of the problem(s)?
   What makes the problem(s) better?
   What makes the problem(s) worse?
   Are you seeing anyone else for the problem(s)?
2. **Interview questions designed to engage the patient in treatment planning:**
   What specific concerns or fears do you have? What is your greatest concern?
   What are your thoughts or ideas about what may have caused this?
   How has this affected you emotionally?
   Help me understand how you see or experience your illness or condition?
   What are your goals?
   What are your expectations about what might happen with your illness or condition?
   What would make you feel that you are making progress in dealing with your chief concern?
   What do you hope this treatment can do for you?
   What would be important to include in your plan of care?
   What questions do you have?
3. **Interview questions designed to identify desired outcomes in terms of essential functional activities:**
   How has this illness/condition affected your daily life?
   What activities or experiences are important to you?
   What activities do you normally do at home/work/school?
   What activities do you have difficulty with? How is this different than before your illness or condition (i.e., extra time, extra effort, different strategy)?
   What activities have you had to give up because of your illness or condition?
   What activities do you need help to perform that you would rather do yourself?
   How can I help you be more independent?
4. **Interview questions designed to identify environmental conditions in which patient activities typically occur:**
   Describe your home/school/work environment.
   How do you move around/access areas in the home (i.e., bathroom, bedroom, entering and exiting the home)? How safe do you feel?
   How do you move around/access areas in the community (i.e., workplace, school, grocery store, shopping center, community center, stairs, curbs, ramps)? How safe do you feel?
   How can I help you be more independent?
5. **Interview questions designed to identify available social supports:**
   Who do you turn to for help in difficult situations?
   Who lives with you?
   Who assists in your care (i.e., BADL, IADL)?
   Who helps you with the activities you want to do (i.e., walking, stairs, transfers)?
   Are there activities you have difficulty with that would benefit from additional assistance?
6. **Interview questions designed to identify the patient's knowledge of potential disablement risk factors:**
   What problems might be anticipated in the future?
   What can you do to eliminate or reduce the likelihood of that happening?

part. An important starting point for identification of areas to be examined is consideration of all potential (possible) factors contributing to an observed activity limitation or participation restriction. Consultation is appropriate if the needs of the patient/client are outside the scope of the expertise of the therapist assigned to the case. For example, a patient recovering from stroke is referred to a dysphagia clinic for a detailed examination of swallowing function by a dysphagia specialist (speech-language pathologist).

Screening examinations are also used for healthy populations. For example, the physical therapist can screen individuals to identify risk factors for disease such as decreased activity levels, stress, and obesity. Screening is also conducted for specific populations such as pediatric clients (e.g., for scoliosis), geriatric clients (e.g., to identify fall risk factors), athletes (e.g., pre-performance examinations), and working adults to identify the risk of musculoskeletal injuries in the workplace (e.g., ergonomic examinations). These screens may involve observation, oral history, and/or a brief examination. Additional screening examinations may be mandated by institutional settings. For example, in a long-term care facility, the therapist may be asked to review the chart or briefly examine a patient for indications of changes in functional status. The therapist then determines the need for further physical therapy services based on completing a screening examination.

Tests and Measures

More definitive tests and measures are used to provide objective data to accurately determine the degree of impairments and specific level of function and dysfunction. They are used to support the therapist's clinical judgments about the diagnosis, prognosis, and POC.[1] Examination may begin at the level of body structure/function to identify potential impairments; for example, diminished muscle strength (e.g., manual muscle test [MMT]) and impaired range of motion (ROM) (e.g., goniometric measurements), and progresses to an examination of function (activity limitations and participation restrictions) (e.g., 6-minute Walk Test, Timed Up and Go). Alternatively, the therapist may begin with an examination of functional performance, during which the therapist analyzes the differences between the patient's performance and the "typical" or expected performance of a task (task analysis). For example, the patient with stroke is asked to transfer from bed to wheelchair. The therapist observes the performance and determines that the patient lacks postural support (stability), adequate lower-extremity extensor strength to reach the full upright position, and adequate ROM in ankle dorsiflexors. The therapist then progresses to a detailed examination of body structures/functions, which leads to the identification of potential impairments. The decision as to which approach to use is based on the results of the screening examination and the therapist's knowledge of the health condition. Key information to obtain during an examination of function is the level of independence or dependence, as well as the need for physical assistance, external devices, or environmental modifications.

Selection of specific tests and measures and depth of the examination is dependent upon several factors, including the patient's health condition (severity and complexity of the problem), stage of recovery (acute, subacute, chronic), phase of rehabilitation (early, middle, or late), cognition and behavior (level of arousal, communication ability, ability to participate in the examination), and setting (hospital, home, community, work). Adequate training and skill in performing specific tests and measures are crucial in ensuring both validity and reliability of the tests. Failure to correctly perform an examination procedure can lead to the gathering of inaccurate data and the formation of an inappropriate POC. The use of disability-specific standardized instruments (e.g., the Fugl-Meyer Assessment of Physical Performance for individuals with stroke) can facilitate the examination process but may not always be appropriate for each individual patient.

The therapist needs to carefully review the unique problems of the patient to determine the appropriateness and sensitivity of an instrument. Box 1.4 presents categories for tests and measures identified in the *Guide to Physical Therapist Practice, 3.0.*[1] The remaining chapters in Section 1 focus on specific tests and measures. Several websites also provide rich resources for information on tests and measures. For example, readers can access the Rehabilitation Measures Database developed at the Rehabilitation Institute of Chicago at www.rehabmeasures@sralab.org. This site provides a comprehensive description and review of literature on a large number of tests and measures with online links to access the instrument directly (e.g., the Berg Balance Scale). The APTA maintains a

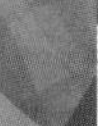

Box 1.4 Categories for Tests and Measures[1]

- Aerobic capacity/endurance
- Anthropometric characteristics
- Assistive technology
- Balance
- Circulation (arterial, venous, lymphatic)
- Community, social, and civic life
- Cranial and peripheral nerve integrity
- Education life
- Environmental factors
- Gait
- Integumentary integrity
- Joint integrity and mobility
- Mental functions
- Mobility (including locomotion)
- Motor function
- Muscle performance (including strength, power, endurance, and length)
- Neuromotor development and sensory processing
- Pain
- Posture
- Range of motion
- Reflex integrity
- Self-care and domestic life
- Sensory integrity
- Skeletal integrity
- Ventilation and respiration
- Work life

From *Guide to Physical Therapist Practice 3.0.* American Physical Therapy Association; 2014, with permission. Available at: http://guidetoptpractice.apta.org/. Accessed May 10, 2016.

website, www.ptnow.org, that can also be accessed to search for tests and measures as well as clinical practice guidelines (CPGs) developed by the professional association.

Novice therapists should resist the tendency to gather excessive and extraneous data in the mistaken belief that more information is better. Unnecessary data will only confuse the picture, rendering clinical decision making more difficult and unnecessarily raising the cost of care. If problems arise that are not initially identified in the history or systems review, or if the data obtained are inconsistent, additional tests and measures may be indicated. Consultation with an experienced clinician can provide an important means of clarifying inconsistencies and determining the appropriateness of specific tests and measures.

Evaluation

Data gathered from the initial examination must then be organized and analyzed. The therapist identifies and prioritizes the patient's impairments, activity limitations, and participation restrictions and develops a *problem list.* It is important to accurately recognize those clinical problems associated with the primary disorder and those associated with co-morbid conditions. Table 1.1 presents a sample problem list.

Impairments, activity limitations, and participation restrictions must be analyzed to identify causal relationships. For example, shoulder pain in the patient with hemiplegia may be due to several factors, including hypotonicity and loss of voluntary movement, which are direct impairments, or soft tissue damage/trauma from improper transfers, which is an indirect impairment resulting from an activity. Determining the causative factors is a difficult yet critical step in determining appropriate treatment interventions and resolving the patient's problem. The skilled clinician is also able to identify the impact of barriers and facilitators in the patient's environment to incorporate strategies to minimize or maximize these factors within

Table 1.1 Sample Prioritized Problem List for a Patient With Stroke

Direct Impairments	Indirect Impairments	Activity Limitations	Participation Restrictions
R hemiparesis RUE > RLE	R shoulder subluxation	Dep bed mobility: minA	
Hypotonicity RUE	Dec ROM R shoulder	Dep BADL: min/mod A	IADL: unable
Spasticity RLE		Dep transfers: modA X 1	Dec ability to perform social roles: spouse
Synergy Patterns: RLE > RUE		Dep locomotion: modA X 1	Dec home and community mobility
Gait Deficits		Stairs: unable	
Balance Deficits: Standing > Sitting	Kyphosis, forward head	Inc fall risk	
Dec Endurance			
Mild Dysarthria			Dec communication
Mild Cognitive Deficits: Dec STM			Dec problem-solving
Dec Motor Planning Ability			
CO-MORBIDITIES:	Diabetic Peripheral Neuropathy		
Dec Sensation Both Feet	Inc risk skin lesions	Inc fall risk	
Small Ulcer L Foot (5th Toe)			

Contextual factors: physical, social, attitudinal
One-level ranch house; entry with 2 steps, no handrails
Highly motivated
Personal factors: individual's life and living situation
Spouse is primary caregiver; has osteoporosis and decreased vision (bilateral cataracts).
Has 2 involved sons living within 30-mile radius.
Key: BADL: basic activities of daily living; Dec: decreased; Dep: dependent; IADL: instrumental activities of daily living; Inc: increased; minA: minimal assistance; modA: moderate assistance; R: right; RLE: right lower extremity; RUE: right upper extremity; STM: short-term memory.

the POC. A POC that emphasizes and reinforces facilitators enhances function and the patient's ability to experience success. Improved motivation and engagement are the natural outcomes of reinforcement of facilitators.

Accurate collection and interpretation of data allows the therapist to determine a diagnosis and prognosis and to develop a POC. It is important to note that examination and evaluation are ongoing processes that continue throughout the episode of care and are essential in determining success toward reaching stated goals and outcomes and responses to selected interventions.[1]

Diagnosis

The diagnostic process (differential diagnosis) requires the clinician to collect, evaluate, and categorize data according to a classification scheme relevant to the clinician and to determine whether the patient's presenting problems are amenable to physical therapy intervention. It guides the prognosis and selection of interventions during the development of the POC. The *diagnosis* includes descriptors that are used to "identify the impact of a condition on function at the level of the system (especially the movement system) and at the level of the whole person."[1:Ch2] Thus, the diagnosis is a reflection of the professional body of knowledge, the expertise and clinical reasoning of the physical therapist, and the boundaries placed on the profession by the law and health care agencies. The diagnosis typically includes the level of impairment, activity limitation, and participation restrictions. In contrast, the *medical diagnosis* refers to the identification of a disease, disorder, or condition (pathology/pathophysiology) primarily at the cellular, tissue, or organ level. Examples include:

Physical therapy diagnosis: Impaired motor function and sensory integrity affecting the left non-dominant side with dependent functional mobility and ADL.
Medical diagnosis: Cerebrovascular accident
Physical therapy diagnosis: Impaired motor function, peripheral nerve integrity, and sensory integrity associated with a complete thoracic spinal cord lesion resulting in dependent functional mobility and ADL.
Medical diagnosis: Spinal cord injury (SCI)

The use of diagnostic categories specific to physical therapy (1) allows for successful communication with colleagues and patients/caregivers about the conditions that require the physical therapist's expertise, (2) provides an appropriate classification for establishing standards of examination and treatment, and (3) directs examination of treatment effectiveness, thereby enhancing evidence-based practice. Physical therapy diagnostic categories also facilitate successful reimbursement when linked to functional outcomes and enhance direct access of physical therapy services.[9]

The APTA's revised and adapted *preferred practice patterns* can be reviewed as a possible way to assist students and novice physical therapists with clinical decision making.[10] The patterns represent the collaborative effort of experienced physical therapists who have detailed the broad categories of problems commonly seen by physical therapists within the scope of their knowledge, experience, and expertise. It includes four main categories of conditions: musculoskeletal (Patterns 4A–4J), neuromuscular (Patterns 5A–5I), cardiovascular/pulmonary (Patterns 6A–6J), and integumentary (Patterns 7A–7E). Each pattern includes the following elements: (1) risk factors or consequences of pathology along with possible impairments, activity limitations, or participation restrictions, (2) tests and measures, (3) factors that may require a new or modify an existing episode of care, and (4) categories of interventions.

Prognosis

The term *prognosis* refers to the predicted optimal level of improvement in function and amount of time needed to reach that level.[1] An accurate prognosis may be determined at the onset of treatment for some patients. For other patients with more complicated conditions such as severe traumatic brain injury (TBI) accompanied by extensive disability and multisystem involvement, a prognosis or prediction of level of improvement can be determined only at various increments during the course of rehabilitation. Knowledge of recovery patterns can be useful to guide decision making.

Therapists also need to compare levels of habitual performance (what a person currently does) to highest level an individual is capable of (what a person could potentially do) to arrive at realistic outcomes. The amount of time needed to reach optimal recovery is an important determination, one that is required by Medicare and many other insurance providers. Predicting optimal levels of recovery and time frames can be a challenging process for the novice therapist. Use of experienced clinicians as resources and mentors as well as referring to the literature can facilitate this step in the decision making process. In rehabilitation settings, the POC also includes a statement regarding the patient's overall *rehabilitation potential.* This is typically expressed in one word: *excellent, good, fair,* or *poor.*

Plan of Care

The POC outlines anticipated patient management. The therapist evaluates and integrates data obtained from the patient/client history, the systems review, and tests and measures. The therapist must consider multiple factors when determining the POC, such as the patient's current condition (stability, chronicity, or severity of the condition; level of impairment and physical function), co-morbidities (premorbid conditions, complications, secondary impairments), age, overall health status, resources (psychosocial, economic), living environment, and potential discharge placement (e.g., home or another health care facility).

Multisystem involvement, severe impairment and functional loss, extended time of involvement (chronicity), and multiple co-morbid conditions are parameters that significantly increase the complexity of the decision making process. Professional consultation with expert clinicians and mentors is an effective means of helping the novice sort through the complex issues involved in decision making, especially when complicating factors intervene.[11] There is an accumulating body of evidence on expertise in physical therapy practice, spearheaded by the pivotal work of Jenson and colleagues.[12-15] These researchers have shown that the knowledge, skills, and decision making abilities used by expert clinicians can be identified, nurtured, and taught. The novice therapist may benefit from a period of active mentoring by expert clinicians early in clinical practice (e.g., clinical residency program).

Respecting patient values and incorporating patient preferences and needs into the POC is a key element in successful outcomes. *Patient-centered care* is defined by the Institute of Medicine as "providing care that is respectful of and responsive to individual patient preferences, needs, values and ensuring that patient values guide all clinical decisions."[16] The patient is viewed as an active participant and collaborative partner who participates in the goal-setting process, makes informed choices, and assumes responsibility for his or her own health care. Therapists who place strong emphasis on communicating effectively; educating their patients, families, and caregivers; and teaching self-management skills can successfully empower patients. The natural outcomes of this approach are improved satisfaction with care, improved therapy outcomes, and improved adherence to suggested lifestyle changes. Some rehabilitation plans have failed miserably simply because the therapist did not fully involve the patient in the planning process, producing goals or outcomes that were not meaningful to the patient (e.g., independent wheelchair mobility for the patient with incomplete SCI). That same patient may have established a very different set of personal goals and expectations (e.g., return to walking). For many patients for whom complete recovery is not expected, the overall "goal of any rehabilitation program must be to increase the ability of individuals to manage their lives in the context of ongoing disability, to the greatest extent possible."[7, p. 11] This cannot be effectively done if the therapist assumes the role of expert and sole planner, establishing the rules, regulations, and instructions for rehabilitation. Rather, it is critical to engage the patient in problem-solving and promote lifelong skills in health management.

The patient's ability and motivation to participate in planning can vary. The more ill the patient, the more anxiety and the less likely that he or she will want to be actively involved in planning. As the illness resolves and the patient begins to improve, the more likely he or she will want to be engaged in planning the treatment. Also, the more difficult the problems encountered, the more likely patients are to put their trust in "the experts" and the less likely they are to trust their own abilities to reach effective decisions. The therapist needs to guard against promoting dependence on the expert (the "my therapist syndrome") to the exclusion of the patient's listening to his or her own thoughts and feelings and participating in problem-solving. In this instance, the patient's feelings of perceived helplessness are increased while the patient's ability to utilize his or her own decision making abilities is delayed or restricted.[7,17] See Box 1.3 for sample questions designed to engage the patient in the treatment planning process.

A major focus of the POC is producing meaningful changes in function at the personal/social level by reducing activity limitations and participation restrictions. Achieving independence in locomotion or in ADL, return to work, or participation in recreational activities is important to the patient/client in terms of improving quality of life (QOL). QOL is defined as the sense of total well-being that encompasses both physical and psychosocial aspects of the patient's life. Finally, not all impairments can be remedied by physical therapy. Some impairments are permanent or progressive, the direct result of unrelenting pathology such as amyotrophic lateral sclerosis. In this example, a primary emphasis on reducing the number and severity of indirect impairments and activity limitations is appropriate.

Essential components of the POC include (1) goals and expected outcomes; (2) the prognosis; (3) a general statement of the interventions to be used, including proposed duration and frequency required to reach the goals; and (4) anticipated discharge plans.

Goals and Outcomes

An important first step in the development of the POC is determining *goals* (the intended impact on functioning) and *outcomes* (the predicted level of optimal functioning at the conclusion of the episode of care). Goals are the interim steps necessary to achieve expected outcomes. They address patient-identified problems (PIP), non-patient-identified problems (NPIP), and predicted changes in impairments, activity limitations, and participation restrictions. They also address predicted changes in overall health, risk reduction and prevention, wellness and fitness, and optimization of patient/client satisfaction.

Goal statements should be measurable, functionally driven, and time limited. They also involve a negotiated process of reconciling goals related to PIP and NPIP. There are four essential elements:

- *Individual:* Who will perform the specific behavior or activity required or aspect of care? Goals and outcomes are focused on the *patient/client.* This includes individuals who receive direct-care physical therapy services and/or individuals who benefit from consultation and advice, or services focused on promoting, health, wellness, and fitness. Goals can also be focused on family members or caregivers; for example, the parent of a child with a developmental disability.

- *Behavior/activity:* What is the specific behavior or activity the patient/client will demonstrate? This includes changes in impairments (e.g., ROM, strength, balance), changes in activity limitations (e.g., transfers, ambulation, ADL), and changes in participation restrictions (e.g., community mobility, return to school or work).
- *Condition:* What are the conditions under which the patient/client's behavior is measured? The statement specifies the specific conditions or measures required for successful achievement; for example, distance achieved, required time to perform the activity, the specific number of successful attempts out of a specific number of trials. Statements focused on functional changes should include a description of the conditions required for acceptable performance. For example, the functional levels of performance in the Functional Independence Measure (FIM) are used in the majority of rehabilitation facilities in the United States. This instrument grades levels from No Helper/Independence (grade 7) to No Helper/Modified Independence (grade 6; device), to Helper/Modified Dependence (grades 5, 4, and 3; supervision, minimal, moderate, assistance), to Helper/Complete Dependence (grades 2 and 1; maximal, total assistance) (see Chapter 8, Examination of Function) for a complete description of this instrument).[18] The type of environment required for a successful outcome of the behavior should also be specified: clinic environment (e.g., quiet room, level floor surface, physical therapy gym), home (e.g., one flight of eight stairs, carpeted surfaces), and community (e.g., uneven grassy surfaces, curbs, ramps).
- *Time:* How long will it take to achieve the stated goal? Goals can be *short-term* (generally considered to be 2 to 3 weeks) and *long-term* (longer than 3 weeks).

Outcomes describe the predicted level of optimal improvement attained at the end of the episode of care or rehabilitation stay. Outcome statements should also be measurable, functionally driven, time limited, and with the same four essential elements. In instances of severe disability and incomplete recovery, for example, the patient with TBI, the therapist, and team members may have difficulty determining the expected outcomes at the beginning of rehabilitation. Long-term goals can be used that focus on the expectations for a specific time period or stage of recovery (e.g., in TBI, minimally conscious states, confusional states).

Each POC has multiple goals and outcomes. Goals may be linked to the successful attainment of more than one outcome. For example, attaining ROM in dorsiflexion is critical to the functional outcomes of independence in transfers and locomotion. The successful attainment of an outcome is also dependent on achieving many different goals. For instance, independent locomotion with an assistive device in home and community environments (the outcome) is dependent on increasing strength, ROM, and balance skills (the goals). In formulating a POC, the therapist accurately identifies the relationship between and among goals and then sequences them appropriately. Goals and outcomes are modified following a significant change in patient status. Box 1.5 presents examples of outcome and goal statements.

Interventions

The next step is to determine the intervention, defined as the purposeful interaction of the physical therapist with the patient/client and, when appropriate, other individuals involved in his or her care. Interventions include various physical therapy procedures and techniques to produce changes in the condition that are consistent with the diagnosis and prognosis.[1] Components of physical therapy intervention also include patient or client instruction. Box 1.6 presents the APTA's list of intervention categories.

Patient/Client Related Instruction

In an era of managed care and shorter time allocations for an episode of care, effective patient/client-related instruction is critical to ensuring optimal care and successful rehabilitation. Communication strategies are developed within the context of the patient/client's age, cultural background, language skills, and educational level, and the presence of specific communication or cognition impairments. Therapists may provide direct one-on-one instruction to a variety of individuals, including patients/clients, families, caregivers, and other interested persons. Additional strategies can include group discussions or classes, or instruction through printed or audiovisual materials. Educational interventions are directed toward ensuring an understanding of the patient's condition, training in specific activities and exercises, addressing the relevance of interventions to improve function, and achieving an expected outcome. In addition, educational interventions are directed toward ensuring a successful transition to the home environment (instruction in home exercise programs [HEP]), returning to work (ergonomic instruction), or resuming social activities in the community (environmental access). It is important to document what was taught, who participated, when the instruction occurred, and overall effectiveness. The need for repetition and reinforcement of educational content should also be documented in the medical record.

Procedural Interventions

Skilled physical therapy includes a wide variety of procedural interventions, which can be broadly classified into

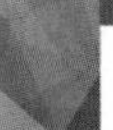

Box 1.5 Examples of Outcome and Goal Statements

The following are examples of expected outcomes, all to be achieved within the anticipated rehab stay:

The patient will be independent and safe in ambulation using an ankle-foot orthosis and a quad cane on level surfaces for unlimited community distances and for all daily activities within 8 weeks.

The patient will demonstrate modified dependence with close supervision in wheelchair propulsion for limited household distances (up to 50 feet) within 8 weeks.

The patient will demonstrate modified dependence with minimum assistance of one person for all transfer activities in the home environment within 6 weeks.

The patient will demonstrate independence in BADL with minimal setup and equipment (use of a reacher) within 6 weeks.

The patient and family will demonstrate enhanced decision making skills regarding the health of the patient and use of health care resources within 6 weeks.

The following are examples of anticipated goals with variable time frames:

Short-Term Goals

The patient will increase strength in shoulder depressor muscles and elbow extensor muscles in both upper extremities from good to normal within 3 weeks.

The patient will increase ROM 10 degrees in knee extension bilaterally to within normal limits within 3 weeks.

The patient will be independent in the application of lower-extremity orthoses within 1 week.

The patient and family will recognize personal and environmental factors associated with falls during ambulation within 2 weeks.

The patient will attend to task for 5 min out of a 30-min treatment session within 3 weeks.

Long-Term Goals

The patient will independently perform transfers from wheelchair to car within 4 weeks.

The patient will ambulate with bilateral knee-ankle-foot orthoses and crutches using a swing-through gait and close supervision for 50 feet within 5 weeks.

The patient will maintain static balance in sitting with centered, symmetrical weight-bearing and no upper-extremity support or loss of balance for up to 5 minutes within 4 weeks.

The patient will sequence a three- to five-step routine task with minimum assistance within 5 weeks.

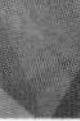

Box 1.6 Intervention Categories[1]

- Patient or client instruction
- Airway clearance techniques
- Assistive technology: prescription, application, and, as appropriate, fabrication or modification
- Biophysical agents
- Functional training in self-care and in domestic, education, work, community, social, and civic life
- Integumentary repair and protection techniques
- Manual therapy techniques
- Motor function training
- Therapeutic exercise

From *Guide to Physical Therapist Practice 3.0*. American Physical Therapy Association; 2014, with permission. Available at: http://guidetoptpractice.apta.org/. Accessed May 10, 2016.

three main groups: restorative, compensatory, and preventative. *Restorative interventions* are directed toward remediating or improving the patient's status in terms of impairments, activity limitations, participation restrictions, and recovery of function. The involved extremities and/or trunk exhibiting movement deficiencies are targeted for intervention. This approach assumes an existing potential for change (e.g., neural plasticity of brain and spinal cord function; potential for muscle strengthening or improving aerobic endurance). For example, the patient with incomplete SCI undergoes locomotor training using body weight support and a treadmill. Patients with chronic progressive pathology (e.g., those with Parkinson's disease) may not respond to restorative interventions aimed at resolving direct impairments; interventions aimed at restoring or optimizing function and modifying indirect impairments can, however, have a positive outcome.

Compensatory interventions are directed toward promoting optimal function using new motor patterns. These can result from the adaptation of remaining motor elements (using involved segments) or substitution. In substitution, functions are taken over or replaced by different body segments using different motor patterns. The activity (task) can be adapted (changed) in order to achieve function. In substitution, the uninvolved or less involved extremities are targeted for intervention. For example, the patient with left hemiplegia learns to eat or dress using the less involved right upper extremity (UE); the patient with complete T1 paraplegia learns to roll using UEs and momentum. Environmental adaptations are also used to facilitate relearning of functional skills and optimal performance. For example, the patient with TBI can dress by selecting clothing from color-coded drawers. Compensatory/substitution interventions can be used in conjunction with restorative interventions to maximize function or when restorative interventions are unrealistic or unsuccessful (e.g., the patient with severe impairment, declining health condition, and multiple co-morbidities).

Preventative interventions are directed toward minimizing potential problems (e.g., anticipated indirect impairments, activity limitations, and participation restrictions) and maintaining health. For example, early resumption of upright standing using a tilt table minimizes the risk of pneumonia, bone loss, and renal calculi in the patient with SCI. A successful educational program for frequent skin inspection can prevent the development of pressure ulcers in that same patient.

Interventions are chosen based on the examination and evaluation of the patient, the physical therapy diagnosis, the prognosis, and the goals and expected outcomes. The therapist relies on knowledge of foundational science and interventions (e.g., principles of motor learning, motor control, muscle performance, task-specific training, and cardiovascular endurance) to determine those interventions that are likely to achieve successful outcomes. A list of intervention categories and specific interventions within each category can be found in APTA's *Guide to Physical Therapist Practice 3.0.*[1] It is important to identify all possible interventions early in the process, to carefully weigh those alternatives, and then to decide on the interventions that have the best probability of success. Narrowly adhering to one treatment approach reduces the available options and may limit or preclude successful outcomes. Use of a protocol (e.g., predetermined exercises for the patient with hip fracture) standardizes aspects of care but may not meet the individual needs of the patient. Protocols can foster a separation of examination/evaluation findings from the selection of interventions.

A general outline of the POC is constructed. Schema can be used to present a framework for approaching a specific aspect of treatment and assist the therapist in organizing essential intervention elements of the plan. One such commonly used schema for exercise intervention is the *FITT (frequency, intensity, time, type) equation*, presented in Box 1.7.

The therapist should choose interventions that accomplish more than one goal and are linked to the expected outcomes. The interventions should be effectively sequenced to address key impairments first and to achieve optimum motivational effect, interspacing the more difficult or uncomfortable procedures with easier ones. The therapist should include tasks that motivate the patient and ensure success during the treatment session. Whenever possible, the therapist should end each treatment session on a positive note. This helps the patient retain a positive feeling of success and look forward to the next treatment.

Coordination and Communication

Case management requires therapists to be able to communicate effectively with all members of the rehabilitation team, directly or indirectly. For example, the therapist communicates directly with other professionals at case conferences, team meetings, or rounds or indirectly through documentation in the medical record. Effective communication enhances collaboration and understanding.

Therapists are also responsible for coordinating care at many different levels. The therapist delegates appropriate aspects of treatment to physical therapy assistants and oversees the responsibilities of physical therapy aides. The therapist coordinates care with other professionals, family, or caregivers regarding specific interventions and times. For example, for early transfer training to be effective, consistency in how everyone transfers the patient is important. The therapist also coordinates discharge planning with the patient and family and other team members. Therapists may be involved in providing POC recommendations to other facilities such as long-term care facilities.

Discharge Planning

Discharge planning is initiated early in the rehabilitation process during the data collection phase and intensifies as goals and expected outcomes are close to being reached. Discharge planning may also be initiated if the patient refuses further treatment or becomes medically or psychologically unstable. If the patient is discharged before outcomes are reached, the reasons for discontinuation of services must be carefully documented.

In the discharge summary, the therapist should include current physical/functional status, degree of goals/outcomes achieved, reasons for goals/outcomes not being achieved, and the *discharge prognosis*. This is typically a one-word response such as *excellent, good, fair,* or *poor*. It reflects the therapist's judgment of the patient's ability to

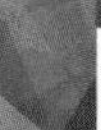

Box 1.7 The FITT Equation for Exercise Intervention

***Frequency:* How Often will the Patient Receive Skilled Care?**

This is typically defined in terms of the number of times per week treatment will be given (e.g., daily or three times per week), or the number of visits before a specific date.

***Intensity:* What is the Prescribed Intensity of Exercises or Activity Training?**

For example, the POC includes sit-to-stand repetitions, 3 sets of 5 reps each, progressing from high seat to low.

***Time (duration):* How Long will the Patient Receive Skilled Care?**

This is typically defined in terms of days or weeks (e.g., three times per week for 6 weeks). The duration of an anticipated individual treatment session should also be defined (e.g., 30- or 60-min sessions).

***Type of intervention:* What are the Specific Exercise Strategies or Procedural Interventions Used?**

Necessary components that should be identified include the following:

- **Posture and activity:** A description of the specific posture and activity the patient must perform (e.g., sitting, weight shifting or standing, modified plantigrade, reaching).
- **Techniques used:** Mode of therapist action or intervention used (e.g., guided, active-assisted, or resisted movement) or specific technique (e.g., rhythmic stabilization, dynamic reversals).
- **Motor learning strategies used:** Strategies specific to type of feedback (e.g., knowledge of results, knowledge of performance) and scheduling of feedback (e.g., constant or variable), practice schedule (e.g., blocked, serial, or random order), and environment (e.g., closed/structured or open/variable).
- **Additional required elements:** Those elements necessary to assist the patient in the exercise or activity (e.g., verbal cues, manual contacts) or equipment (e.g., elastic band resistance, therapy ball, body weight support system with motorized treadmill).

maintain the level of function achieved at the end of rehabilitation without continued skilled intervention. Elements of an effective discharge plan are included in Box 1.8.

Implementation of the Plan of Care

The therapist must consider many factors in structuring an effective treatment session. The patient's involvement, comfort, motivation, and optimal performance should be a priority along with safety and privacy during the treatment session. The environment should be structured appropriately to reduce distractions and improve motor learning. See Chapter 10, Strategies to Improve Motor Control for more information on interventions to enhance motor function.

The patient's immediate pretreatment level of function or initial state should be carefully examined. General state organization of the CNS and homeostatic balance of the somatic and autonomic nervous systems are important determinants of how a patient may respond to intervention. A wide range of influences, from emotional to cognitive to organic, may affect how a patient reacts to a particular treatment. Some patients who are overly stressed may demonstrate altered homeostatic responses. For example, the patient with TBI who presents with high arousal and agitated behaviors can be expected to react to treatment in unpredictable ways, frequently demonstrating "fight or flight" responses. Similarly, patients with TBI who are lethargic may be difficult to arouse and demonstrate limited ability to participate in therapy sessions. Changes in patient/client status and responses to individual treatment sessions should be carefully monitored and documented.

Expert clinicians develop the "art of clinical practice" by learning to adjust their input (e.g., verbal commands and manual contacts) based on patient response. Treatment thus becomes a dynamic and interactive process between patient and therapist. Shaping of behavior can be further enhanced by careful orientation to the purpose of the tasks and how they meet the patient's needs and the plan for subsequent sessions. This helps to engage the patient and ensure optimal cooperation and motivation.

Reexamination of the Patient and Evaluation of Expected Outcomes

This step is ongoing and involves continuous reexamination of the patient and a determination of the efficacy of treatment. Data are evaluated within the context of the patient's progress toward goals and expected outcomes set forth in the POC. A determination is made whether the goals and outcomes are reasonable given the patient's diagnosis and progress. If the patient attains the desired level of competence for the stated goals, revisions in the POC are indicated. If the patient attains the desired level of competence for the expected outcomes, discharge is considered. If the patient fails to achieve the stated goals or outcomes, the therapist must determine why. Were the goals and outcomes realistic given the clinical problems and database? Were the interventions

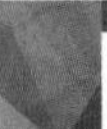

Box 1.8 Elements of the Discharge Plan

Patient, family, or caregiver education—instruction includes information regarding the following:

- Current condition (pathology), impairments, activity limitations, and participation restrictions
- Ways to reduce risk factors for recurrence of condition and developing complications, indirect impairments, activity limitations, and participation restrictions
- Ways to maintain/enhance performance and functional independence
- Ways to foster healthy habits, wellness, and prevention
- Ways to assist in transition to a new setting (e.g., home, skilled nursing facility)
- Ways to assist in transition to new roles

Plans for follow-up care or referral to another agency: patient and caregiver are provided with the following:

- Information regarding follow-up physical therapy care or referral for additional services to another agency (e.g., home care agency, outpatient facility) as needed
- Information regarding community support group and community fitness center as appropriate

Instruction in a home exercise plan: patient/caregiver instruction regarding the following:

- Home exercises, activity training, ADL training
- Use of assistive technology (e.g., assistive devices, orthoses, prosthetics, wheelchairs) provided

Evaluation/modification of the home environment:

- Planning regarding the home environment and modifications needed to assist the patient in the home (e.g., installation of ramps and rails, bathroom equipment such as tub seats, raised toilet seats, bathroom rails, furniture rearrangement or removal to ease functional mobility)
- All essential equipment and renovations should be in place before discharge

selected at an appropriate level to challenge the patient, or were they too easy or too difficult? Were facilitators appropriately identified and the patient sufficiently motivated? Were intervening and constraining factors (barriers) identified? If the interventions were not appropriate, additional information is sought, goals modified, and different treatment interventions selected. Revision in the POC is also indicated if the patient progresses more rapidly or slowly than expected. Each modification must be evaluated in terms of its overall impact on the POC. Thus, the plan becomes a fluid statement of how the patient is progressing and what goals and outcomes are achievable. Its overall success depends on the therapist's ongoing clinical decision making skills and on engaging the patient's cooperation and motivation.

■ DOCUMENTATION

Documentation is an essential requirement that serves as a record of patient/client care, including patient/client status, physical therapy management, and outcome of physical therapy intervention. Importantly, it demonstrates appropriate utilization of services for timely reimbursement from third-party payers. It also provides a mechanism for communication among the rehabilitation team members and may be used for policy or research purposes and outcomes analysis.[1] Written documentation is formally done at the time of admission and discharge, and at periodic intervals during the course of rehabilitation (interim or progress notes). Many clinical settings require documentation for every treatment session. The format and timing of notes will vary according to the regulatory requirements specified by institutional policy, Medicare and third-party payers, state law, and specific accreditation organization (i.e., The Joint Commission, Commission on the Accreditation of Rehabilitation Facilities [CARF], and so forth). Data included in the medical record should be meaningful (important, not just nice to have), complete and accurate (valid and reliable), timely (recorded promptly), and systematic (regularly recorded). Patient involvement in the development and monitoring of the POC should be carefully documented. A description of specific interventions, any modifications needed, and communication/collaboration with other providers/patient/family/caregivers should also be included. Defensible Documentation for Patient/Client Management is a comprehensive series of documents available from APTA that includes Documentation Elements, General Guidelines, Current Concerns, Improving Your Clinical Documentation, and a Documentation Review Sample Checklist. These documents can be accessed at www.practice-dept@apta.org.[19]

In the United States, all health care facilities must comply with Medicare coding and billing using the *ICD-10-CM Official Guidelines for Coding and Reporting*. These codes are developed by the Centers for Medicare and Medicaid Services (CMS) and the National Center for Health Statistics (NCHS). Adherence to these guidelines is required under the Health Insurance Portability and Accountability Act (HIPAA). Thus, therapists need to be informed about current coding and include pertinent information consisting of the medical diagnosis code (e.g., G460 Middle cerebral artery syndrome) and the reason the patient/client is being seen (e.g., G8194 Hemiplegia, unspecified affecting left non-dominant side). For current ICD-10 coding resources, visit the Provider Resources section of the CMS ICD-10 website.[20] APTA maintains an affordable cloud-based tool that enables physical therapy providers, coders, and administrators to rapidly identify the most specific ICD-10 codes for timely, accurate billing.[21]

Electronic documentation systems have gained expanded use in physical therapy and provide a fully integrated and completely paperless workflow for managing patient care. This includes managing referrals, initial intake data, progress and discharge notes, scheduling, and billing. Advantages of electronic documentation include standardization of data entry, increased speed of access to data, and integration of data that can be used for a wide variety of applications (e.g., clinical management of patients, quality control, clinical research). Information about the patient and his or her medical history is readily available from any computer or electronic device with Internet access. Therapists also can receive notification of when the patient arrives or checks in, as well as notice of scheduled evaluations and required POC updates. Software programs typically do not allow notes be filed unless all the required elements are completed. Thus, overall efficiency of practice management is increased with decreased errors in documentation and improved accuracy of reimbursements. Many different companies provide software programs for physical therapy that focus on specific practice settings (e.g., outpatient rehabilitation, home care, private practice). Therapists using documentation software for electronic entry of patient data should ensure that programs comply with appropriate provisions for security and confidentiality.

■ EVIDENCE-BASED PRACTICE

Improved patient outcomes can be achieved by *evidence-based practice* (EBP), defined as "the integration of best research evidence with our clinical expertise and our patient's unique values and circumstances."[22] Therapists should utilize tests and measures and interventions that have undergone rigorous scientific examination while resisting use of interventions simply because they are in widespread clinical use. Numerous resources are available to assist the therapist in this process. The APTA has published a *Clinical Research Agenda* designed to support, explain, and enhance physical therapy clinical practice.[23,24] EBP tools are available on the APTA's evidence-based web portal PTNow. This site allows easy access to journals, clinical summaries, tests and measures, CPGs, Cochrane Reviews, and the Rehabilitation Reference Center.[25] Several texts are available that summarize valuable information regarding principles of EBP.[26-29] Key articles that discuss relevant issues in EBP include the works of Scalzitti,[30] Jette, D et al.,[31] Maher et al.,[32] Goldstein et al.,[33] and Jette, A.[34] Components of EBP are summarized in Figure 1.5.

The essential steps of EBP[22] are as follows:

Step 1: A clinical problem is identified and an answerable question is formulated.
Step 2: A systematic literature review is conducted and evidence collected.
Step 3: The research evidence is critically analyzed for its validity (closeness to the truth), impact (size of the effect), and applicability (usefulness in clinical practice).
Step 4: The critical appraisal is synthesized and integrated with the clinician's expertise and the patient's unique values and circumstances.
Step 5: The effectiveness and efficiency of the steps in the evidence-based process are evaluated.

A well-constructed clinical question contains four elements: (1) the patient/client or population and clinical characteristics, (2) the specific intervention to be studied, (3) the comparison to an alternative intervention, and (4) the outcome achieved. This is represented by the acronym PICO—patient, intervention, comparison, outcome. For example, one study examined patients with low back pain (P) and compared specific interventions (I, C) (therapeutic exercise, transcutaneous electrical nerve stimulation, thermotherapy, ultrasound, massage, E-stim system, and traction). Outcomes (O) identified as being important to the patient (pain, function, patient global assessment, QOL, and return to

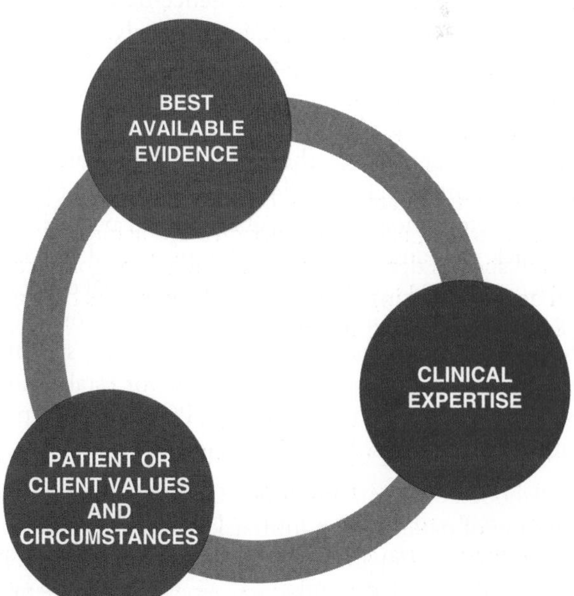

Figure 1.5 Components of evidence-based practice. (*Introduction to the Guide to Physical Therapist Practice.* Guide to Physical Therapist Practice 3.0. *Alexandria, VA: American Physical Therapy Association; 2014. Available at: http://guidetoptpractice.apta.org/content/1/SEC1.body. Accessed December 1, 2017.)*

work) were examined.[35] Questions about diagnosis or prognosis require modification of this model. For example, for a patient with low back pain (P), the specific tests utilized to reach the diagnosis are examined (T), and the outcome (O) determined (how sensitive and specific was the test in diagnosing the problem).[28]

Using Evidence to Guide Clinical Decisions

A hierarchy of evidence should be considered. At the top of the hierarchy are *clinical practice guidelines* and systematic reviews (e.g., *Cochrane Database of Systematic Reviews, Physiotherapy Evidence Database*[36]). Next is a consideration of individual randomized controlled trials (RCTs) followed by other less rigorous research designs (e.g., cohort design, case-control designs, single-subject design, qualitative design).

Evidence-based clinical practice guidelines (EBCPGs) are defined as systematically developed statements to guide clinicians in using the best available evidence in patient care. They are developed through a combination of (1) expert consensus; (2) systematic reviews and meta-analysis; and (3) analysis of patient preferences combined with outcome-based guidelines. CPGs include an evaluation of the quality of relevant scientific literature and recommendations for treatment likely to be effective and beneficial as well as those likely to be ineffective or harmful. For example, the *Philadelphia Panel* is a multidisciplinary, international panel of rehabilitation experts comprising a group of clinical specialty experts from the United States and the Ottawa Methods Group from Canada. This panel uses a structured and rigorous methodology to formulate evidence-based practice guidelines. In one example, the panel analyzed the evidence of selected interventions for low back pain. The evidence was then translated into EBCPGs by reviewing key outcomes and deciding whether the intervention had clinical benefit. In the low back pain study, the panel recommended the following: (1) the use of therapeutic exercises for chronic, subacute, and post-surgery low back pain and (2) continuation of normal activities for acute low back pain. The panel found lack of evidence regarding efficacy for the use of other interventions (e.g., thermotherapy, ultrasound, massage, electrical stimulation).[37] APTA has endorsed a process for establishing CPGs and has published a number CPGs in conjunction with APTA sections. Examples include:

- Orthopedic section: published CPGs for the rehabilitation of patients with low back pain,[38] hip pain and mobility impairments,[39,40] knee pain and mobility impairments,[41,42] ankle stability and movement coordination impairments,[43,44] heel pain,[44] neck pain,[45] and shoulder impairments.[46]
- Cardiovascular and pulmonary and acute care sections: published CPG on the management of individuals at risk for or diagnosed with venous thromboembolism.[47]
- Academy of Geriatric Physical Therapy: published CPG on the management of falls in community-dwelling older adults.[48]
- Academy of Neurologic Physical Therapy: published CPGs on vestibular rehabilitation for peripheral vestibular hypofunction.[49]

According to Rothstein, these studies are clinically important in that they "are not telling us what is known and what is not known, but what is supported by evidence and what is not supported by evidence."[50, p. 1620] It is also important to consider the overall quality of the CPG document and to consider the methodology used. The Appraisal of Guidelines for Research and Evaluation Enterprise (AGREE) was developed to contribute to the science and advancement of practice guidelines through various programs of research and international collaborations. CPGs can be evaluated using the AGREE II Instrument.[51] This is used by the APTA for its resources, including PTNow and *Physical Therapy* (journal of the APTA). This process helps to ensure that published guidelines are trustworthy. CPGs provide a summation of best possible evidence for use in clinical practice. They should be viewed as general recommendations and do not provide detail regarding specific recommendations (e.g., aerobic exercise is recommended but the specifics of frequency, intensity, and time are not).

A *systematic review* (SR) is a comprehensive examination and analysis of the literature using critical appraisal skills. The researcher determines key resources to provide the evidence. These include peer-reviewed and evidence-based journals, electronic medical databases, and online search engines (e.g., PubMed). Table 1.2 includes commonly used electronic databases in physical therapy. Specific criteria are developed for the inclusion and exclusion of the research studies selected for review. Studies employing different designs may be analyzed individually or compared qualitatively; studies of similar design may be combined quantitatively (e.g., meta-analysis).

Critical analysis of research findings involves detailed examination of methodology, results, and conclusions. The clinician should be able to answer the following questions: (1) What is the level of evidence? (2) Is the evidence valid? and (3) Are the results important and clinically relevant? The Physiotherapy Evidence Database (PEDro) scale was developed by physiotherapists at the University of Sydney to assist clinicians in evaluating the quality of rehabilitation literature.[36] Interpretation and synthesis of the evidence must be considered within the context of the specific patient/client problem. Examination begins with the purpose of the study, which should be clearly stated, and the review of literature, which should be relevant in terms of the specific question asked. The methods/design should be closely examined. Research design varies and can be evaluated in terms of levels of evidence and grades of recommendation in order of most to least rigorous (Table 1.3).

Table 1.2 Commonly Used Electronic Databases in Physical Therapy

Database or Search Engine	Website
MEDLINE—U.S. National Library of Medicine: search service to Medline and Pre-Medline (database of medical and biomedical research), free public access	www.ncbi.nlm.nih.gov
PTNow (replaces Open Door and Hooked on Evidence): APTA maintained search engine of evidence-based physical therapy practice, including tests and measures, clinical summaries, clinical practice guidelines, and Cochrane Reviews; members only	www.ptnow.org
PEDro, Physiotherapy Evidence Database: Includes abstracts, systematic reviews, and clinical practice guidelines in physiotherapy. PEDro is produced by the Centre for Evidence-Based Physiotherapy (CEBP) at the George Institute for Global Health, University of Sydney.	www.pedro.org.au
Physiotherapy Choices: An initiative of the CEBP, this database is designed for use by consumers of physiotherapy services, including patients, their friends and families, health service managers, and insurers.	www.physiotherapychoices.org.au
Cochrane Central Register of Controlled Trials (CCTR): A bibliographic database of definitive clinical trials Cochrane Database of Systematic Reviews: Abstracts and topic reviews	www.cochrane.org
National Rehabilitation Information Center (NARIC) citations and abstracts of research articles and books on all aspects of rehabilitation	www.naric.com
Clinical Trials Registry, National Institutes of Health: Provides information about ongoing clinical trials	www.clinicaltrials.gov
Database of Abstracts of Reviews of Effects (DARE): Reviews of evidence based medicine including abstracts of systematic reviews	www.york.ac.uk/inst/crd
Cumulative Index to Nursing and Allied Health Literature (CINAHL): Includes abstracts and bibliographies	www.ebscohost.com
Health Information Research Unit, McMaster University: Evidence-Based Health Informatics: Includes the Canadian Cochrane database	http://hiru.mcmaster.ca
Center for International Rehabilitation Research Information and Exchange: Maintains a database of rehabilitation research	www.cirrie.buffalo.edu
Rehabilitation Measures Database, Shirley Ryan Ability Lab, was developed by the Rehabilitation Institute of Chicago: Maintains a comprehensive database of rehabilitation tests and measures	www.rehabmeasures@.sralab.org
GoogleScholar: Search engine that references several disciplines, including physical therapy; includes citations, abstracts, and articles	www.scholar.google.com

Although an RCT provides the most rigorous design, there are times when other designs are indicated. For example, there may be ethical issues involving control groups that receive no treatment when treatment is clearly beneficial. In addition, when outcomes are not clearly understood or defined (e.g., QOL issues), designs such as single-case studies may be indicated. See Chapter 8, Examination of Function for additional discussion.

CLINICAL DECISION MAKING FRAMEWORKS

Hypothesis-Oriented Algorithm

Decision making frameworks, such as algorithms, have been developed by experienced practitioners to guide clinicians in their decision making. For example, Rothstein and Echternach developed the *hypothesis-oriented algorithm for clinicians* (HOAC).[52,53] An algorithm is a graphically represented step-by-step guide designed to assist clinicians in problem-solving by considering several possible solutions. It is based on specific clinical problems and identifies the decision steps and possible choices for evaluation and treatment planning. Hypotheses are generated about why the patient's problems exist and criteria are generated to test the hypotheses. A series of questions are posed, typically in a branching program of yes/no choices, addressing whether the measurements met testing criteria, the hypotheses generated were viable, goals were met, strategies were appropriate, and tactics were implemented correctly. A "no" response

Table 1.3 Levels of Evidence and Grades of Recommendation

Level	Intervention	Grade of Recommendation
1	**a.** Systematic review (SR)[a] of randomized control trials (RCT)[b] **b.** Individual RCT with narrow confidence interval	A: Strong evidence
2	**a.** SR of Cohort studies[c] **b.** Individual Cohort study or individual low-quality RCT	B: Moderate evidence
3	**a.** SR of case-control studies[d] **b.** Individual case-control study	B: Moderate evidence
4	Case-series,[e] cohort or poor-quality cohort and case-control studies	C: Weak evidence
5	Expert opinion or bench research	D: Theoretical/foundational None or conflicting evidence

[a]SR, systematic review: A review in which the primary studies are summarized, critically appraised, and statistically combined; usually quantitative in nature with specific inclusion/exclusion criteria.

[b]RCT, randomized controlled trial: An experimental study in which participants are randomly assigned to either an experimental or control group to receive different interventions or a placebo; the most rigorous study design.

[c]Cohort study: A prospective (forward-in-time) study; a group of participants (cohort) with a similar condition receives an intervention and is followed over time and outcome evaluated; comparison is made to a matched group who do receive the intervention (quasi-experimental with no randomization).

[d]Case-control study: A retrospective study in which a group of subjects with a condition of interest are identified for research after outcomes are achieved (e.g., studying the impact of an intervention on level of participation); a comparison group is used.

[e]Case series: Clinical outcomes are evaluated of a single group of patients with a similar condition.

Adapted from Oxford Centre for Evidence-Based Medicine: Levels of Evidence. May 2001. Retrieved September 10, 2016, from www.cebm.net

to any of the questions posed in an algorithm is an indication for reevaluation of the viability of the hypotheses generated and reconsideration of the decisions made. In using HOAC as framework for clinical decision making, the therapist also distinguishes between existing problems and anticipated problems, defined as deficits that are likely to occur if an intervention is not used for prevention. The value of an algorithm is that it guides the therapist's decisions and provides an outline of the decisions made. See Chapter 17, Amyotrophic Lateral Sclerosis for examples of hypothesis-oriented algorithms.

Integrated Framework for Decision Making

The integrated framework for clinical decision making unifies multiple models for clinical reasoning (Fig. 1.6).[54] The framework is patient-centered and is anchored by the patient/client management of the *Guide to Physical Therapist Practice 3.0.* In every step of the integrated model, the clinician poses a hypothesis and then proceeds to collect information to either support or refute that hypothesis. This process is described in the HOAC for clinical decision making. Specific emphasis is placed on interviewing to gather the patient- and non-patient-identified problems.

The integrated model uses motor learning theory to inform clinical reasoning. This includes setting up the environment, creating a practice schedule, and dosing appropriately. The task is the basic unit of analysis and the plan of care. Task assessment is informed by Gentile's taxonomy[55] as well as the Hedman model.[56] Biomechanics are used to assess tasks such as sit-to-stand and gait.

The integrated model can be used in a sequential or non-sequential manner. A novice clinician may follow the steps of the patient client management model in order, but a more experienced clinician may jump several steps. The use of the model is illustrated in Chapter 15, Stroke.

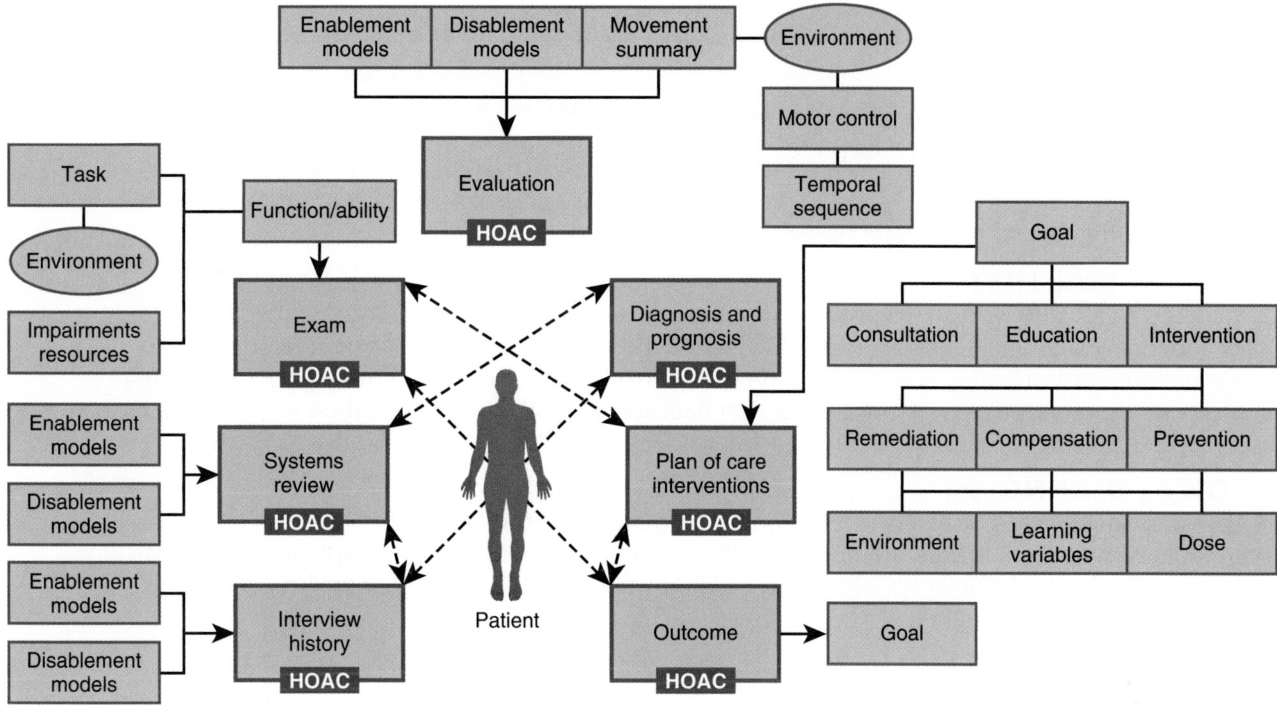

Figure 1.6 Integrated Framework. *(Schenkman, M, Deutsch, JE, and Gill-Body, K: An integrated framework for decision making in neurologic physical therapy practice. Phys Ther 86(12):1682, 2006.)*

SUMMARY

An organized process of clinical decision making allows the therapist to systematically plan effective treatments. The steps identified in the patient/client management process are (1) examine the patient, and collect data through history, systems review, and tests and measures; (2) evaluate the data and identify problems; (3) determine the diagnosis and prognosis; (4) determine the POC; (5) implement the POC; and (6) reexamine the patient and evaluate treatment outcomes. Patient participation in planning is essential in ensuring successful outcomes. Evidence-based practice allows the therapist to select interventions that have been shown to provide meaningful change in patients' lives. Inherent to the therapist's success in this process are an appropriate knowledge base and experience, critical thinking and decision making skills, and communication and teaching skills. Documentation is an essential requirement for effective communication among the rehabilitation team members and for timely reimbursement of services.

Note: The author gratefully acknowledges the contributions of Judith Deutsch, PT, PhD, FAPTA, and George D. Fulk, PT, PhD, to this chapter.

Questions for Review

1. What are the key steps in patient /client management?
2. Differentiate between impairments, activity limitations, and participation restrictions. Define and give an example of each.
3. What are the essential elements of goal and outcome statements? Write two examples of each.
4. Differentiate between restorative and compensatory interventions. Give an example of each.
5. What is the FITT equation? Give an example of how is it used in formulating interventions for a POC.
6. What are the essential steps in evidence-based practice?
7. In evidence-based practice, what are the elements of a well-constructed clinical question? Give an example.
8. What is the highest level of evidence available for evidence-based clinical practice guidelines?

CASE STUDY

PRESENT HISTORY

The patient is a 78-year-old woman who tripped and fell at home ascending the stairs outside the front door. She was admitted to the hospital after sustaining a transcervical, intracapsular fracture of the right femur. The patient had an open reduction and internal fixation (ORIF) procedure of the right lower extremity (RLE) to reduce and pin the fracture. After 2 weeks of acute hospital admission, the patient is at home and referred for home care physical therapy.

PAST MEDICAL HISTORY

Patient is a very thin woman (98 pounds) with long-standing problems with osteoporosis (on medication for 5 years). She has a history of falls, three in the last year alone. Approximately 3 years ago she had a myocardial infarction and presented with third-degree heart block, requiring implantation of a permanent pacemaker. She underwent cataract surgery with lens implantation in the right eye 2 years ago; the left eye is scheduled for similar surgery within the next few months.

MEDICAL DIAGNOSES

Coronary artery disease (CAD), hypertension (HTN), mitral valve prolapse, s/p permanent heart pacer, s/p right cataract with implant, osteoporosis (moderate to severe in the spine, hips, and pelvis), osteoarthritis with mild pain in right knee, s/p left elbow fracture (1 year ago), left ankle fracture (2 years ago), urinary stress incontinence.

MEDICATIONS

Fosamax 70 mg weekly
Atenolol 24 mg PO daily
MVI (multivitamin concentrate) with Fe tab PO daily
Metamucil 1 tb prn PO daily, Colace 100 mg PO bid
Tylenol No. 3 tab prn/mild pain

SOCIAL SUPPORT/ENVIRONMENT

The patient is a retired schoolteacher who was recently widowed after 48 years of marriage. She has two sons, one daughter, and four grandchildren; all live within an hour's driving distance. One of her children visits every weekend. She has a rambunctious black Labrador puppy that is 8 months old and was given to her "for company" at the time her husband died. She was walking the dog at the time of the accident. She is an active participant in a garden club, which meets twice a month, and in weekly events at the local senior center. Previously she was driving her car for all community activities.

She lives alone in a large old New England farmhouse. Her home has an entry with four stairs and no rail. Inside there are 14 rooms on two floors. The downstairs living area has a step down into the family room with no rail. There are 14 stairs to the second floor, with rails on either side. The upstairs sleeping area is cluttered with large, heavy furniture. The second-floor bathroom is small, with a high claw-foot tub with pedestal feet and a lip. There is no added equipment.

PHYSICAL THERAPY EXAMINATION

1. Mental status
   Alert and oriented ×3
   Pleasant, cooperative, articulate
   No apparent memory deficits
   Good problem-solving and safety awareness about hip precautions
2. Cardiopulmonary status
   Pulse 74; BP 110/75
   Endurance: good; min SOB with 20 min of activity
3. Sensation
   Vision: wears glasses; cloudy vision L eye; impaired depth perception
   Hearing: WFL
   Sensation: BLEs intact
4. Skin
   Incision is healed and well approximated
   Wears bilateral TEDs q a.m. × 6 wk

5. ROM
   LLE, BUEs: WFL
   Right hip:
   Flex: 0° to 85°
   Ext: NT (not tested)
   Abd: 0° to 20°
   Add: NT
   IR, ER: NT
   Right knee and ankle: WFL
6. Strength (MMT)
   LLE, BUEs: WFL
   RLE:
      Hip flex NT
      Hip ext NT
      Hip abd NT
      Knee ext: 4/5
      Ankle: DF 4/5, PF 4/5
7. Posture
   Flexed, stooped posture: moderate kyphosis, flexed hips and knees
   Half-inch leg length shortening on RLE
   Mild resting head tremor
8. Balance
   Sitting balance: WFL
   Standing balance:
      Berg Balance Test: Total Score: 42/56
      Item 2 Standing, unsupported, EO: 4—able to stand safely for 2 minutes
      Item 6 Standing unsupported EC: 3—able to stand for 10 sec with supervision
      Item 7 Standing unsupported feet together: 1—needs help, can stand for 15 sec
      Item 8 Forward reach: 3—can safely reach 5 in (12 cm)
      Item 13 (tandem stance) and Item 14 (stand on one leg): 0—unable
9. Gait
   Ambulates with standard walker and supervision approximately 200 feet on level surfaces, partial weight-bearing
   Walks with increased flexion of both hips and knees, dorsal spine
   Requires shoe insert to level pelvis
   Stairs: modified dependence—one flight of stairs with rail, SBQC and supervision
   Gait speed: not tested at this time
10. Functional status (patient was completely independent [I] before her fall)
   I bed mobility
   Modified I in sit to stand and stand to sit transfers
   Uses 2-inch foam cushions to elevate seat of kitchen chair and living room chair to assist in standing up
   Unable to do tub transfers at present
   I dressing—upper
   Modified I dressing—lower, uses reacher device
   Bathing, minimal assist (MinA) of home health aide for sponge baths
   IADL: requires moderate assistance (ModA) of home health aide for homemaker activities
11. Patient is highly motivated. "I want to get my life back together, get my dog home again so I can take care of him."

PRIMARY INSURANCE

Medicare with supplemental policy

Guiding Questions

1. Develop a prioritized problem list for this patient's POC. Identify and categorize the patient's impairments (direct, indirect, composite). Identify her activity limitations and participation restrictions.

2. What information is available about her functional status within the home in terms of performance versus capacity qualifiers?
3. What is her rehabilitation prognosis?
4. Write two expected outcome and two goal statements to direct her POC.
5. Identify two treatment interventions for her POC.
6. What precautions should be observed?
7. What tests and measures can be used to determine successful attainment of outcomes?

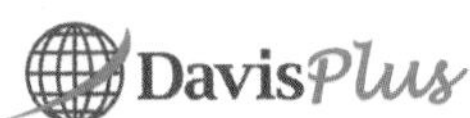

For additional resources, including answers to the questions for review and case study guiding questions, please visit **http://davisplus.fadavis.com.**

References

1. *Guide to Physical Therapist Practice 3.0.* Alexandria, VA: American Physical Therapy Association; 2014. Available at: http://guidetoptpractice.apta.org/. Accessed April 10, 2016.
2. World Health Organization (WHO): International Classification of Functioning, Disability and Health: ICF. WHO, Geneva, Switzerland, 2001. Available at: www.who.int/classifications/icf/en/. Accessed September 10, 2016.
3. World Health Organization (WHO): Towards a Common Language for Functioning, Disability and Health: ICF. WHO, Geneva, Switzerland, 2002. Retrieved September 10, 2016, from www.who.int/classifications/icf/training/icfbeginnersguide.pdf.
4. World Health Organization (WHO): ICF Checklist, Version 2.1a, Clinician Form for International Classification of Functioning, Disability and Health. WHO, Geneva, Switzerland, 2003. Retrieved September 10, 2016, from www.who.int/classifications/icf/training/icfchecklist.pdf.
5. Fortin, AH, et al: Smith's Patient Centered Interviewing: An Evidence-Based Method, ed 3. McGraw Hill, New York, 2012.
6. Lyles, J, et al: Evidence-based patient-centered interviewing. JCOM 8(7):28, 2001.
7. Ozer, M, Payton, O, and Nelson, C: Treatment Planning for Rehabilitation—A Patient-Centered Approach. McGraw-Hill, New York, 2000.
8. Randall, KE, and McEwen, IR: Writing patient-centered functional goals. Phys Ther 80:1197, 2000.
9. Sarhman, SA: Diagnosis by the physical therapist—a special communication. Phys Ther 68:1703, 1988.
10. Adapted practice patterns. *Guide to Physical Therapist Practice 3.0.* Alexandria, VA: American Physical Therapy Association; 2014. Available at: www.apta.org. Accessed April 10, 2016.
11. Jensen, GM, et al: Expertise in Physical Therapy Practice, ed 2. Saunders Elsevier, St. Louis, MO, 2006.
12. Jensen, GM, Shepard, KF, and Hack, LM: The novice versus the experienced clinician: Insights into the work of the physical therapist. Phys Ther 70:314, 1990.
13. Jensen, GM, et al: Expert practice in physical therapy. Phys Ther 80:28–51, 2000.
14. Resnik, L, and Jensen, G: Using clinical outcomes to explore the theory of expert practice in physical therapy. Phys Ther 83:1090, 2003.
15. Shephard, K, et al: Describing expert practice in physical therapy. Qual Health Res 9:746–758, 1999.
16. Institute of Medicine: Crossing the Quality Chasm: A New Health System for the 21st Century. Washington, DC: National Academies Press, 2001, p 6. doi:10.17226/10027.
17. Epstein, R, and Street, R: The values and value of patient-centered care. Ann Fam Med 9(2):100, 2011.
18. Guide for the Uniform Data Set for Medical Rehabilitation (including the FIM instrument), Version 5.0. State University of New York, Buffalo, 1996.
19. American Physical Therapy Association Board of Directors: Guidelines: Physical Therapy Documentation of Patient/Client Management (BOD G03-05-16-41). Retrieved February 28, 2016, from www.apta.org/uploadedFiles/APTAorg/About_Us/Policies/Practice/DocumentationPatientClientManagement.pdf.
20. Centers for Medicare and Medicaid Services: CMS Medicare Coding. Retrieved September 13, 2016, from www.cms.gov/Medicare/Coding/ICD10/2017-ICD-10-CM-and-GEMs.html.
21. American Physical Therapy Association: Identifying the Correct Codes for ICD-10. Retrieved September 13, 2016, from www.apta.org.
22. Staus, S, et al: Evidence-Based Medicine: How to Practice and Teach EBM, ed 4. Churchill-Livingstone-Elsevier, New York, 2011.
23. Guccione, A, Goldstein, M, and Elliott, S: Clinical research agenda for physical therapy. Phys Ther 80:499–513, 2000.
24. Goldstein, M, et al: The revised research agenda for physical therapy. Phys Ther 91:165–174, 2015.
25. American Physical Therapy Association: Evidence-based practice & research. Retrieved September 10, 2016, from www.apta.org.
26. Law, M, and MacDermid, J (eds): Evidence-Based Rehabilitation, ed 3. Slack Inc., Thorofare, NJ, 2014.
27. Jewell, D: Guide to Evidence-Based Physical Therapy Practice, ed 3. Jones & Bartlett, Boston, 2015.
28. Fetters, L, and Tilson, J: Evidence-Based Physical Therapy. F.A. Davis, Philadelphia, 2012.
29. Portney, L, and Watkins, M: Foundations of Clinical Research, ed 3. F.A. Davis, Philadelphia, 2015.
30. Scalzitti, D: Evidence-based guidelines: Application to clinical practice. Phys There 81(10), 1622, 2001.
31. Jette, D, et al: Evidence-based practice: Beliefs, attitudes, knowledge, and behaviors of physical therapists. Phys Ther 83(9): 786, 2003.
32. Maher, CG, et al: Challenges for evidence-based physical therapy: Accessing and interpreting high-quality evidence on therapy. Phys Ther 84(7):644, 2004.
33. Goldstein, M, et al: Vitalizing practice through research and research through practice: The outcomes of a conference to enhance delivery of care. Phys Ther 91(8): 1275, 2011.
34. Jette, A: 43rd Mary McMillan Lecture: Face into the storm. Phys Ther 96: 1, 2012.
35. Philadelphia Panel: Evidence-based clinical practice guidelines on selected rehabilitation interventions: Overview and methodology. Phys Ther 81:1629, 2001.
36. Physiotherapy Evidence Database: The Pedro scale. Retrieved September 10, 2016, from pedro.org.au.
37. Philadelphia Panel: Evidence-based clinical practice guidelines on selected rehabilitation interventions for low back pain. Phys Ther 81:1641, 2001.
38. Orthopedic section, APTA: Low back pain: Clinical practice guidelines linked to the International Classification of Functioning, Disability, and Health. JOSPT 42(4):A44, 2012.
39. Orthopedic section, APTA: Hip pain and mobility impairments: Hip osteoarthritis: Clinical practice guidelines linked to the International Classification of Functioning, Disability, and Health. JOSPT 39(4):A18, 2009.
40. Orthopedic section, APTA: Nonarthritic hip joint pain: Clinical practice guidelines linked to the International Classification of Functioning, Disability, and Health. JOSPT 39(4):A18, 2009.

41. Orthopedic section, APTA: Knee pain and mobility impairments: Meniscal and articular cartilage lesions clinical practice guidelines linked to the International Classification of Functioning, Disability, and Health. JOSPT 40(6):A30, 2010.
42. Orthopedic section, APTA: Knee ligament sprains: Clinical practice guidelines linked to the International Classification of Functioning, Disability, and Health. JOSPT 40(6):A31, 2010.
43. Orthopedic section, APTA: Ankle stability and movement coordination impairments, ankle ligament sprains: Clinical practice guidelines linked to the International Classification of Functioning, Disability, and Health. JOSPT 43(9):A29, 2013.
44. Orthopedic section, APTA: Heel pain—plantar fasciitis: Clinical practice guidelines linked to the International Classification of Functioning, Disability, and Health. JOSPT 40(6):A30, 2010.
45. Orthopedic section, APTA: Neck pain: Clinical practice guidelines linked to the International Classification of Functioning, Disability, and Health. JOSPT 40(6):A30, 2010.
46. Orthopedic section, APTA: Adhesive capsulitis: Clinical practice guidelines linked to the International Classification of Functioning, Disability, and Health. JOSPT 43(5):A26, 2013.
47. Hillegass, E, et al: Role of physical therapists in the management of individuals at risk for or diagnosed with venous thromboembolism: Evidence-based clinical practice guideline. Phys Ther 96(2):143, 2016.
48. Avin, K, et al: Management of falls in community-dwelling older adults: Clinical guidance from the Academy of Geriatric Physical Therapy of the American Physical Therapy Association. Phys Ther 95(6):815, 2015.
49. Hall, CD, et al: Vestibular rehabilitation for peripheral vestibular hypofunction: An evidence-based clinical practice guideline. J Neurol Phys Ther 40(2):124, 2016.
50. Rothstein, J: Autonomous practice or autonomous ignorance? Phys Ther 81:1620, 2001.
51. AGREE Next Steps Consortium: The AGREE II Instrument (Electronic version), 2013 update. Retrieved September 9, 2016, from www.agreetrust.org.
52. Rothstein, J, and Echternach, J: Hypothesis-oriented algorithm for clinicians. Phys Ther 66(9):1388.
53. Rothstein, JM, Echternach, JL, and Riddle, DL: The hypothesis-oriented algorithm for clinicians II (HOAC II): A guide for patient management. Phys Ther 83:455, 2003.
54. Schenkman, M, Deutsch, JE, and Gill-Body, K: An integrated framework for decision making in neurologic physical therapy practice. Phys Ther. 86(12): 1682, 2006.
55. Gentile, AM: Skill acquisition: Action, movement, and neuromotor processes. In Carr, JH, Shepherd, RB, Gordon, J, Gentile, AM, and Held, JM (eds): Movement Science. Foundations for Physical Therapy in Rehabilitation. Aspen Publishers, Maryland, 1987.
56. Hedman, L, Rogers, M, and Hanke, T: Neurologic professional education: Linking the foundation science of motor control with physical therapy interventions for movement dysfunction. JNPT 20(1):9, 1996.

Chapter 2

Examination of Vital Signs

Thomas J. Schmitz, PT, PhD

LEARNING OBJECTIVES

1. Discuss the rationale for including vital sign measures in the patient examination.
2. Explain the relevance of vital signs data to developing a diagnosis, determining the prognosis, and establishing a plan of care.
3. Recognize the importance of vital signs data in determining physiological response to treatment and evaluating patient progress.
4. Describe the procedure for monitoring temperature, pulse, respiration, blood pressure, and oxygenation saturation (pulse oximetry).
5. Differentiate between normal and abnormal values or ranges for each vital sign.
6. Identify the normative variations in vital signs and the factors that influence these changes.
7. Explain the rationale for using pulse oximetry in the presence of unstable oxygen saturation levels.
8. Describe the recommended elements for documentation of vital signs data.

CHAPTER OUTLINE

Examination of body temperature, heart rate (HR), respiratory rate (RR), and blood pressure (BP) provides the physical therapist with important data about the status of the cardiovascular/pulmonary system. Owing to their importance as indicators of the body's physiological status and response to physical activity, environmental conditions, and emotional stressors, they are collectively referred to as vital signs. Because many important clinical decisions are based in part on these measures, accuracy is essential.

The *Guide to Physical Therapist Practice* includes examination of vital signs (HR, RR, and BP) in the cardiovascular/pulmonary systems review and among the tests and measures used to characterize or quantify aerobic capacity/endurance, circulation (arterial, venous, lymphatic), and ventilation and respiration. Pulse oximetry is included among the tests and measures used for examination of ventilation and respiration and aerobic capacity/endurance.[1] Although not considered a primary vital sign, pulse oximetry is an important related measure that provides information on arterial blood (hemoglobin) oxygen saturation levels. Pulse oximetry data allow the therapist to screen and monitor for *hypoxemia*—decreased oxygen concentrations of arterial blood. Hypoxemia is often associated with pulmonary disorders that impair ventilation of the lungs (e.g., pneumonia, chronic obstructive pulmonary disease [COPD], anemia, respiratory muscle weakness, and circulatory impairments).

Also referred to as *cardinal signs,* vital signs provide quantitative measures of the status of the cardiovascular/pulmonary system and reflect the function of internal organs. Variations in vital signs are a clear indicator that some change in the patient's physiological status has occurred. Taken at rest and during and after exercise, these measures also provide important data on aerobic capacity and endurance. Together with other examination data, vital sign measures assist the physical therapist in making clinical judgments to do the following[1]:

1. Determine the patient's baseline status.
2. Identify potential risk factors, suspected pathology, and impairments of body functions and structures.
3. Develop the diagnosis, prognosis, and plan of care (POC).
4. Periodically re-examine the patient throughout the episode of care to determine if outcome expectations are being met.
5. Evaluate the effectiveness of interventions in achieving goals (intended impact on functioning) and outcomes (results of implementing POC that indicate the impact on functioning).
6. Determine if a referral, or consultation with, another practitioner is needed.

The physical therapist's clinical decision-making will determine which vital signs should be measured and the frequency of measurement for an individual patient within a specific context (e.g., self-paced ambulation on level surfaces vs. stair climbing). Although taking vital sign measures may be delegated to a physical therapist assistant (PTA), the physical therapist will evaluate and determine the significance of the data.

■ NORMATIVE VITAL SIGN DATA

Many resources provide vital signs values across age groups. Normative data are typically presented as averages or as a range of values for the age group from which they were derived; using a range reflects the variability of values designated as normal. Table 2.1 provides examples of normative vital signs data presented by age using ranges, and Table 2.2 provides a combination of averages and ranges.[2,3]

Table 2.1 Comparison of Normal Vital Signs for Various Ages Reported as Ranges

Age	Temperature °F (°C)	Pulse Rate	Respiratory Rate	Blood Pressure (mm Hg)
Newborn	98.6–99.8 (37–37.7)	120–160	30–80	Systolic: 50–52 Diastolic: 25–30 Mean: 35–40
3 yr	98.5–99.5 (36.9–37.5)	80–125	20–30	Systolic: 78–114 Diastolic: 46–78
10 yr	97.5–98.6 (36.3–37)	70–110	16–22	Systolic: 90–132 Diastolic: 5–86
16 yr	97.6–98.8 (36.4–37.1)	55–100	15–20	Systolic: 104–108 Diastolic: 60–92
Adult	96.8–99.5 (36–37.5)	60–100	12–20	Systolic: <120 Diastolic: <80
Older adult	96.5–97.5 (35.9–36.3)	60–100	15–25	Systolic: <120 Diastolic: <80

From Dillon,[2] with permission.

Table 2.2 Comparison of Normal Vital Signs for Various Ages Reported Using a Combination of Averages and Ranges

Age	Temperature Average* °F (°C)	Pulse Average (Range) Beats per Min	Respirations Range Breaths per Min	Blood Pressure Average mm Hg
Newborn	98.2 (36.8) axillary	130 (80–180)	30–60	80/40
1 to 3 years	99.9 (37.7) rectal	110 (80–150)	20–40	98/64
6 to 8 years	98.6 (37) oral	95 (75–115)	20–25	120/56
10 years	98.6 (37) oral	90 (70–100)	17–22	110/58
Teen	98.6 (37) oral	80 (55–105)	15–20	110/70
Adult	98 (36.7) oral	80 (60–100)	12–20	<120/80
Adult over 70 years	95–96.8 (35–36) oral	80 (60–100)	12–20	120/80, up to 160/95

*Averages with the exception of "Adult over 70 years" reported as a range.
From Wilkinson, et al,[3] with permission.

Clinical Note: Normative vital sign data provides the physical therapist with a *general reference* for comparison during evaluation of clinical findings. Values included in normative tables should be considered cautiously because discrepancies and inconsistencies exist among sources. In addition, these tables typically do not include information about sample size or data collection strategies. As discussed later in this chapter, another consideration in using these data is that vital sign values are specific to the individual (may typically run slightly higher or lower) and are influenced by multiple factors, such as normal diurnal patterns, environmental temperature, physical activity, and emotions. Accurate interpretation requires knowledge of an individual's baseline measures as well as existing influencing factors at the time measures are taken.

The National Health and Nutrition Examination Survey (NHANES) provides some of the most recent and comprehensive normative data published for BP and HR values. NHANES is a research program conducted by the National Center for Health Statistics, Division of Health and Nutrition Examination Surveys, part of the Centers for Disease Control and Prevention (CDC). NHANES was originally conducted periodically between 1971 and 1994 and became annual in 1999. The surveys address different topics that focus on the health and nutritional status of adults and children in the United States. Data collection combines both interviews and physical examinations conducted in a mobile examination center.[4] As identified on the CDC website, the major objectives of the NHANES are to:

- Estimate the number and percentage of persons in the U.S. population and in designated subgroups with selected diseases and risk factors.
- Monitor trends in the prevalence, awareness, treatment, and control of selected diseases.
- Monitor trends in risk behaviors and environmental exposures.
- Study the relationship between diet, nutrition, and health.
- Explore emerging public health issues and new technologies.
- Provide baseline health characteristics that can be linked to mortality data from the National Death Index or other administrative records (e.g., enrollment and claims data from the Centers for Medicare and Medicaid Services).[4]

The NHANES survey includes data on mean BP for 19, 921 adults aged 18 and over.[5] Means of systolic blood pressure (SBP) and diastolic blood pressure (DBP) were reported for adults by multiple variables, including sex and hypertension status (normal, treated, and untreated). Data on mean BP values from this analysis are presented in Figure 2.1 for males and in Figure 2.2 for females. Mean resting HR values are also available, reported by several variables, including sex and age using a sample of 35,302 people.[6] These resting pulse rate estimates are presented in Table 2.3 for males and in Table 2.4 for females.

"Normal" resting vital sign measures are specific to the individual and referred to as *baseline values.* Some people typically display baseline values different from those represented by normative data. For example, aerobically trained individuals often have resting HRs of less than 60 beats per minute (bpm), with some reports of values in the low 30s.[7] Such variation underscores the importance of knowing baseline measures and of monitoring vital signs as a sequential process for each individual. Vital sign measurements yield the most useful information when performed and recorded at *periodic intervals over time* as opposed to a single measurement taken at a given point in time. Serial recording allows changes in patient status or response to treatment to be monitored over time and can indicate an acute change in physiological status at a specific point in time (e.g., response to an exercise test).

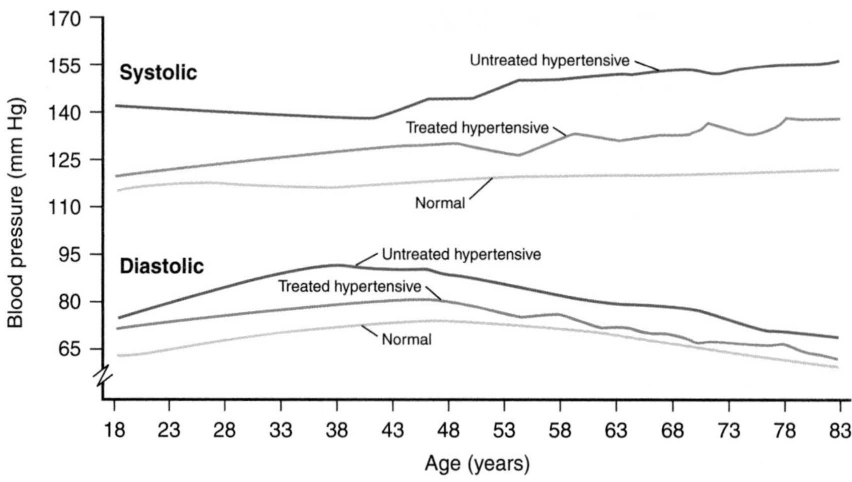

Figure 2.1 Mean systolic and diastolic pressure for men aged 18 years and over, by age and hypertension status. *(From Wright et al.[5])*

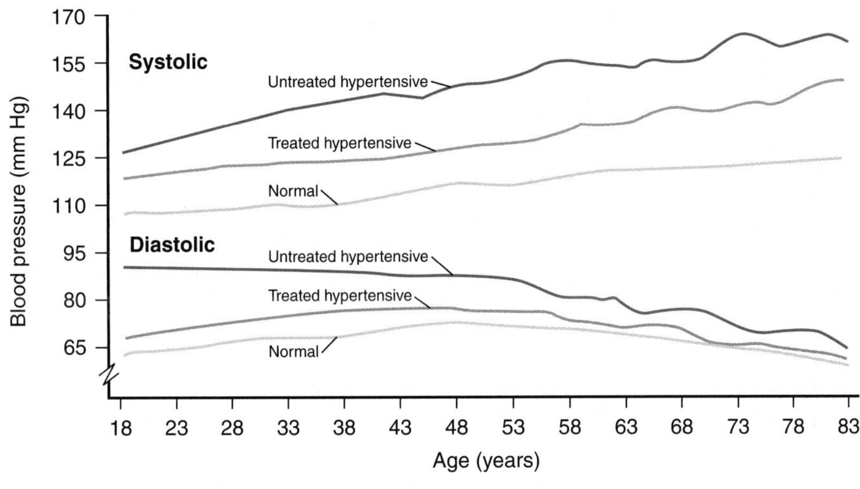

Figure 2.2 Mean systolic and diastolic pressure for women aged 18 years and over, by age and hypertension status. *(From Wright et al.[5])*

On examination, initial vital sign measures may be well within normal ranges. In these circumstances, Wilkinson et al suggest that one should "not become complacent when a client's vital signs are within normal limits. Although stable vital signs *indicate* physiologic well-being, they do not *guarantee* it. Vital signs alone are limited in detecting some important physiologic changes; for example, vital signs may sometimes remain stable in the presence of moderately large blood loss. Evaluate the vital signs in the context of your overall assessment of the client."[8, p. 421]

At times, an abnormally high or low value for a vital sign may be obtained. In such situations, it is important to maintain a calm, professional demeanor and not adversely react to the information. As discussed later in this chapter, multiple factors can alter vital sign values, including those that are patient related (e.g., emotion, stress, excessive caffeine ingestion) and/or practitioner related (e.g., faulty positioning and measurement, incorrect blood pressure cuff size). Any abnormal values should be investigated and, if deemed appropriate, repeated to confirm accuracy.

Table 2.3 Resting Pulse Rate Estimates for U.S. Males, by Age Group National Health and Nutrition Examination Survey, 1999–2008

Age Group (years)	*n*	Mean	SE Mean
Under 1	972	128	1.1
1	712	116	0.8
2–3	1,148	106	0.4
4–5	864	94	0.6
6–8	1,212	86	0.5
9–11	1,130	80	0.5
12–15	2,190	77	0.4
16–19	2,411	72	0.4
20–39	3,445	71	0.3
40–59	2,559	71	0.3
60–79	1,147	70	0.5
80 and over	197	71	1.1

n = sample size for each age category; SE: standard error. Data exclude persons with a current medical condition or medication use that would affect the resting pulse rate.

Table 2.4 Resting Pulse Rate Estimates for U.S. Females, by Age Group National Health and Nutrition Examination Survey, 1999–2008

Age Group (years)	*n*	Mean	SE Mean
Under 1	931	130	1
1	633	119	0.8
2–3	1,107	108	0.5
4–5	900	97	0.6
6–8	1,264	88	0.5
9–11	1,236	85	0.5
12–15	2,310	80	0.4
16–19	2,082	79	0.4
20–39	3,061	76	0.3
40–59	2,409	73	0.3
60–79	1,163	73	0.4
80 and over	219	73	0.9

n = sample size for each age category; SE: standard error. Data exclude persons with a current medical condition or medication use that would affect the resting pulse rate.

If repeated measures are required, calmly explain to the patient that you want to verify the values obtained. Alfaro-LeFevre[9, p. 75] offers the following guidelines for validating questionable data:

- Double-check information that is extremely abnormal or inconsistent with patient cues.
- Double-check that equipment is functioning correctly.
- Recheck data obtained (e.g., take BP in opposite arm or 10 minutes later).
- Examine for factors that may alter accuracy (e.g., determine if someone with an elevated temperature and no other symptoms has just had a hot cup of coffee).
- When uncertain, ask a more experienced therapist to recheck a vital sign measure.
- Make a comparison of subjective and objective data to determine if what the patient *states* is consistent with *data obtained* (e.g., compare actual pulse rate with the patient's subjective perceptions of a "racing heart").

ALTERATIONS IN VITAL SIGN VALUES: OVERVIEW OF INFLUENTIAL VARIABLES

Lifestyle Patterns and Patient Characteristics

Several lifestyle patterns (modifiable) and patient characteristics (non-modifiable) influence vital sign measures. Lifestyle patterns include, but are not limited to, caffeine intake, tobacco use, diet, alcohol consumption, response to stress, obesity, physical activity level, medications, and use of illegal drugs. Patient characteristics include hormonal status, age, sex, and family history. Other variables that affect vital sign measures include time of day, time of the month (menstrual cycle), general health status, emotional distress, and pain. Information about lifestyle patterns and patient characteristics is gathered from the patient history, the systems review, and tests and measures. Factors identified as modifiable become the focus of patient-related instruction (e.g., current condition, risk factor reduction) and/or health promotion and wellness strategies. Specific factors influencing each vital sign are addressed in greater detail later in the chapter.

Culture and Ethnicity

As with any physical therapy test or measure, the influence of culture and ethnicity on vital sign measures can vary from subtle to marked. For example, a patient who appears anxious or hostile during examination of vital signs may be displaying a response to stress typically shared by others who have a deep-seated distrust of American health care practices. Another example might be a Muslim female patient who exhibits a stress reaction to being examined by a male therapist. These situations can clearly affect the accuracy of the vital sign measures. *Culture* refers to an integration of learned behaviors (not biologically inherited), norms, and symbols characteristic of a society that are passed from generation to generation.[10] It is a set of shared behavioral standards that includes fundamental values, beliefs, attitudes, and customs, including those related to health care and illness.[11-13] *Ethnicity* is defined as an affiliation with a group of people who share a common cultural origin or background, or common racial, national, religious, linguistic, or cultural characteristics.[12] Culture and ethnicity directly affect the attitudes held by an individual toward health care.[14]

Cultural competency in health care can be defined as having the appropriate knowledge and skills to deliver care consistent with a patient's cultural beliefs and practices.[13] Emphasizing the overarching importance of cultural competence, Leavitt proposes that "for physical therapy practitioners, cultural competence is an essential element in making effective and efficient examination, evaluation, diagnosis, prognosis, and intervention possible. Developing rapport, collecting and synthesizing patient data, recognizing personal functional concerns, and developing the plan of care for a particular patient requires cultural competence."[10, p. 4]

Recent demographic changes in the United States have created greater societal diversity and have heightened the need for culturally competent physical therapists. Data from the 2010 Census (conducted every 10 years) demonstrate the evolving diversity of cultures and ethnicities that comprise the U.S. population.[15] Several salient elements of the data report include the following:

- All major race groups increased in population size between 2000 and 2010, but they grew at different rates.
- The Asian population grew faster than any other major race group between 2000 and 2010.
- More than half the growth in the total population of the United States between 2000 and 2010 was due to an increase in the Hispanic population.
- The only major race group to experience a decrease in its proportion of the total population was the "white alone" population (i.e., those reporting only one race). This group's share of the total population fell from 75% in 2000 to 72% in 2010.

Reflective of the importance of cultural competence in understanding and responding effectively to the cultural needs of patients in health care settings, the U.S. Department of Health and Human Service's Office of Minority Health published *National Standards for Culturally and Linguistically Appropriate Services in Health Care* with input from a national advisory committee. The proposed standards are offered as guidelines for providers, policymakers, accreditation and credentialing agencies, purchasers of health benefits (including labor unions), patients, and advocates (e.g., local and national ethnic, immigrant, and other community-focused organizations), as well as educators and other members of the health care community.[16]

The World Confederation for Physical Therapy (WCPT) includes cultural competence in the WCPT Guideline for Standards of Physical Therapy Practice.[17] The American Physical Therapy Association (APTA) has taken a prominent role in promoting cultural competence. The APTA website (APTA.org) is a rich resource on the topic and includes a variety of important documents, videos, articles, courses, and educator resources. Cultural competence is cited in all major APTA documents.[18] The Commission on Accreditation in Physical Therapy Education includes cultural competence in the evaluative criteria for accreditation of education programs for the preparation of physical therapists[19] and physical therapist assistants.[20] It is also included in *A Normative Model of Physical Therapist Professional Education*[21] and *A Normative Model of Physical Therapist Assistant Education.*[22]

Burton and May Ludwig offer the following suggestions for interaction with a culturally diverse population[23]:

- Address the patient using his or her surname with appropriate title (Mr., Mrs., Ms., or Miss). First names should be used only with the patient's invitation to do so.
- Respect the individual's beliefs and attitudes regarding health care, traditions, and religion.
- Use common proper English; slang terms should be avoided.
- If a language barrier exists, an interpreter should be used (preferably not a family member).
- Eye contact should be used cautiously; some cultures perceive eye contact as disrespectful or a challenge to authority.
- Direct attention to the patient's facial expressions and nonverbal communication, because this may provide clues that your communication is not being understood.
- Seek clarification if you do not understand something that the patient has said.

Cultural competency is addressed in an expanding body of literature. For further examination of cultural diversity in health care, the reader is referred to the work of Leavitt,[10] Spector,[14] Purnell,[24] Perez and Luquis,[25] Jeffreys,[26] and Ritter and Graham.[27]

PATIENT OBSERVATION

Observation refers to the deliberate use of the senses (vision, hearing, smell) to gather information about the patient.[8,9] Observation alone will not provide definitive diagnostic information, nor will it allow one to draw conclusions or inferences;[23] however, observation may provide clues to underlying problems,[2] inform development of well-structured impairment-specific or activity limitation–specific questions during history taking, guide selection of screening examinations, and assist with prioritizing tests and measurements.[28]

Using a logical, consistent sequence will create a systematic approach to observation (e.g., first facial expression and overall appearance, then any immediate signs of pain or distress, skin condition). This will improve efficiency, conserve time, and help ensure that no areas are overlooked. The following are examples of the types of information and/or clues to underlying problems that may be gathered via observation:

- Signs of immediate patient distress or discomfort (e.g., pain, grimacing, difficulty breathing) are typically evident by observation of facial expressions, use of accessory muscles for breathing, an irregular or labored breathing pattern, and frequent positional changes. Use of accessory muscles of breathing may be indicative of cardiac or pulmonary impairments.
- Obesity or the presence of cachexia, a state of malnutrition or wasting associated with many chronic diseases, may indicate clues about nutritional status. Central obesity (trunk and face) and fat pads near the collarbone and the back of the neck may be associated with Cushing's syndrome.
- *Diaphoresis* (profuse perspiration) may indicate that the body is working to compensate for a reduced cardiac output. It is associated with a variety of potential causes, including myocardial infarct, hypotension, and shock; it may also be associated with hyperthermia (e.g., faulty thermoregulation), thyroid hyperactivity, anxiety, and overactive sweat glands. Excessive sweating may also be related to environmental conditions or patient participation in strenuous physical activity prior to visit. The term *hyperhidrosis* also refers to abnormally increased perspiration.
- A disagreeable body odor may suggest poor hygiene (e.g., impaired self-care abilities or lack of resources) or the presence of a wound (e.g., infected drainage) or underlying disease;[8] a fruity breath smell may be suggestive of high blood glucose or diabetic ketoacidosis.[28]
- Various sounds of respiration may be heard, such as wheezing, crackles, or sighs (discussed later in this chapter and in Chapter 12, Chronic Pulmonary Dysfunction). Potential considerations include a narrowed airway (e.g., asthma, congestive heart failure [CHF], tracheal stenosis), COPD, presence of foreign object, or secretions partially blocking an airway.
- The presence of a cough may be caused by a relatively benign airway irritant (e.g., dust particles) or may indicate the presence of a disease such as asthma, bronchitis, COPD, lung cancer, or pneumonia. An acute cough typically resolves within 3 weeks or less (e.g., upper respiratory tract infection). A chronic or persistent cough is typically defined as lasting more than 8 weeks.

- Asymmetry of body parts at rest and during movement, incoordination or abnormal movements may suggest atrophy, hypertrophy, impaired motor function, or underlying disease (e.g., cerebral vascular accident). Facial features should also be observed for symmetry.
- The skin is the largest organ of the body; observation of skin color provides important preliminary data about the efficiency of the cardiovascular/pulmonary system and may be an indicator of disease, inflammation, and infection.[23,28] Cyanosis is a bluish discoloration associated with inadequate oxygenation of arterial blood (i.e., hemoglobin does not contain normal levels of oxygen). Central cyanosis causes diffuse skin color changes in "central" aspects of the body (e.g., trunk, head) as well as color changes in the oral mucosa.[29] These membranes are normally pink and shiny regardless of skin color. Central cyanosis indicates marked arterial desaturation and occurs when oxygen saturation is less than 80% (normal is 95% to 100%).[2] It is associated with diseases of the cardiovascular/pulmonary system and carbon monoxide poisoning. Peripheral cyanosis causes color changes in the nail beds and lips owing to decreased cardiac output, exposure to cold (vasoconstriction), or arterial or venous obstruction. It is frequently transient and is often relieved by warming the area. Common skin color changes with associated causes are presented in Box 2.1.
- The skin should also be observed for changes in texture and hair growth. Patients with diabetes mellitus or atherosclerosis typically lack hair growth on the legs and display thickening of the nails of the fingers and toes. Skin texture also varies with age and poor nutritional status. Skin lesions may be indicative of pathological changes or trauma.
- The color and appearance of fingernails should be noted. With normal circulation and oxygen supply, they should be pink (or light brown in dark-skinned individuals) and free of irregularities. Examples of pathological changes in nails include the following:
    - *Beau's lines:* are deep grooved (indented) transverse lines across the nail resulting from disruption of nail growth caused by trauma or disorders such as Raynaud's disease (decreased blood flow to fingers), psoriasis, or infection around the nail plate.
    - *Black nails* are caused by blood under the nail; usually the result of trauma.

Box 2.1 Common Skin Color Changes

- **Cyanosis:** Bluish-gray discoloration of the skin and mucous membranes.
- **Central cyanosis:** Caused by hypoxia and results in color changes in central aspects of body and mucous membranes; associated with diseases of the cardiovascular and pulmonary system and central nervous system disorders that impair respiration.
- **Peripheral cyanosis:** Caused by hypoxia with color changes in the nail beds and lips; associated with decreased cardiac output, exposure to cold (extreme vasoconstriction), and arterial (peripheral vascular disease) or venous obstruction (deep vein thrombosis).
- **Acute cyanosis:** Caused by hypoxia from a blocked airway (asphyxiation or choking) with rapid onset of skin color changes initially in the face, lips, and nail beds.
- **Ecchymosis:** Caused by bruising (bleeding under the skin) and may be seen anywhere on the body; new bruises appear *bluish purple* while older bruises are *greenish yellow*; often caused by trauma (e.g., falls, sports injury, physical abuse); patients on blood thinning agents (e.g., Coumadin) tend to bruise more easily.
- **Erythema:** Reddened area of skin caused by increased blood flow (hyperemia); associated with skin irritation or injury, infection, and inflammation; redness over a bony prominence warns of the potential development of a decubitus ulcer.
- **Flushing:** Diffuse redness of face; may involve other body areas; related to emotions (embarrassment, anger), physical exertion, fever, and increased temperature of environment.
- **Jaundice:** Caused by impaired liver function (e.g., hepatitis, liver cancer), the skin takes on a yellow-orange hue; it is best observed in the sclera, mucous membranes, and palm of hands and sole of the feet.
- **Pallor (pale):** The skin takes on a lighter tone (more white with decreased pink hue) than normal for the individual (a normally "fair" skin color should be ruled out); for darker skin, pallor is apparent by loss of red tones; associated with anemia (low hemoglobin) and impaired circulation; observed in the face, palms, mucous membranes, and nail beds.
- **Petechiae:** Tiny red or purple hemorrhagic spots caused by capillary bleeding with subsequent leakage of blood into the skin; tend to appear in clusters and often seen on the ankles and feet but can occur anywhere on body; may be a sign of thrombocytopenia (low platelet count); as platelets play a critical role in clotting, reduced counts impair clotting and increase the risk of bleeding; low platelet counts are associated with a variety of medications (e.g., anticoagulants, aspirin, steroids, and chemotherapy drugs) and disorders (e.g., acute and chronic infections, leukemia, systemic lupus erythematosus, and scleroderma).

- *Clubbing* is a bulbous swelling of fingertips secondary to proliferation of connective tissue between the nail matrix and distal phalanx[30] accompanied by a loss of the normal angle between the nail bed and the skin (Fig. 2.3); nails appear bluish gray (cyanotic) and become soft and boggy (spongy). Clubbing develops gradually over time and is associated with diagnoses that involve long-standing hypoxia, such as congenital heart defects and cardiopulmonary diseases.
- *Half-and-half nails* (also called *Lindsay's nails*) are seen with renal failure; the distal portion of the nail turns red, pink, or brown; there is a distinct line of demarcation between the two halves.
- *Onycholysis* is detachment of the nail from the nail bed; associated with trauma, fungal infections, psoriasis, and overactive thyroid gland.
- *Mee's lines* are transverse white lines across the breadth of the nail associated with systemic diseases such as renal failure, Hodgkin's disease, malaria, and sickle cell anemia; classically associated with arsenic poisoning.
- *Pitting* is characterized by tiny punctate depressions in the nail caused by systemic diseases such as Reiter's syndrome, psoriasis, and eczema.
- *Splinter hemorrhages* are tiny hemorrhages creating reddish lines of blood under the nail (appears as if a "splinter" is lodged under nail) associated with bacterial endocarditis and trauma.

- Abnormal posture may be suggestive of pain or structural abnormalities of the pelvis (pelvic obliquity), pectoral, or vertebral regions that may also interfere with respiratory patterns.
- Edema may be associated with CHF, liver failure, lymphedema, or venous insufficiency; localized edema may result from varicose veins, thrombophlebitis, or trauma.

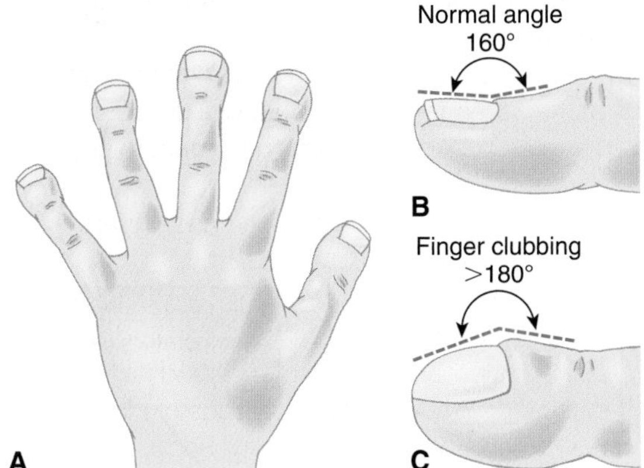

Figure 2.3 (A) Clubbing of fingertips is associated with long-term hypoxic states; (B) normal nail plate angle of 160°; (C) a nail plate angle of 180° or more occurs with clubbing.

TEMPERATURE

Body temperature represents a balance between the heat produced or acquired by the body and the amount lost. Because humans are warm-blooded, or *homoiothermic,* body temperature remains relatively constant despite changes in the external environment. This is in contrast to cold-blooded, or *poikilothermic,* animals (such as reptiles), in which body temperature varies with that of their environment.

Thermoregulatory System

The purpose of the thermoregulatory system is to maintain a relatively constant internal body temperature. This system monitors and acts to maintain temperatures that are optimal for normal cellular and vital organ function. The thermoregulatory system consists of three primary components: the thermoreceptors, the regulating center, and the effector organs.[31,32]

Thermoreceptors

The thermoreceptors provide input to the temperature-regulating center located in the hypothalamus. The regulating center is dependent on information from thermoreceptors to achieve constant temperatures. Once this information reaches the regulatory center, it is compared with a "set point" standard or optimal temperature value. Depending on the contrast between the "set" value and incoming information, mechanisms may be activated to either conserve or dissipate heat.[33]

Peripheral and central thermoreceptors provide afferent temperature input to the regulating center. The peripheral receptors (skin temperature), composed primarily of free nerve endings, have a high distribution in the skin. Central thermoreceptors (core temperature) are located in the deep tissues (e.g., abdominal organs), nervous system, and the hypothalamus.[33,34] The thermoreceptors located in the hypothalamus are sensitive to temperature changes in blood perfusing the hypothalamus. These cells also can initiate responses to either conserve or dissipate heat. They are particularly sensitive to core temperature changes and monitoring body warmth.[31] The thermoreceptors permit *feed forward* responses to expected changes in core temperature (e.g., change in environmental temperature).

The cutaneous peripheral thermoreceptors demonstrate a larger distribution of cold receptors than warmth receptors and are sensitive to rapid changes in temperature.[31] Signals from these receptors enter the spinal cord through afferent nerves and travel to the hypothalamus via the lateral spinothalamic tract.

Regulating Center

The temperature-regulating center of the body is located in the hypothalamus. The hypothalamus coordinates the heat production and loss processes, much like a thermostat, ensuring an essentially constant, stable body temperature. By influencing the effector organs, the hypothalamus achieves a relatively precise balance between heat production and heat loss. In a healthy individual, the hypothalamic thermostat is set and carefully maintained at 98.6° ± 1.8°F (37° ± 1°C).[31] In situations in which input from thermoreceptors indicates a drop in temperature below the "set" value, mechanisms are activated to conserve heat. Conversely, a rise in temperature will activate mechanisms to dissipate heat. Mechanisms to dissipate heat are particularly important during strenuous exercise. Figure 2.4 summarizes the primary physiological adjustments to exercise or increases in environmental temperature that occur during heat acclimation (physiological adaptations to dissipate and improve tolerance to heat). These responses are activated through hypothalamic control of the effector organs. Input to the effector organs is transmitted through pathways of both the somatic and autonomic nervous systems.[31,32,35,36]

Effector Organs

The effector organs respond to both increases and decreases in temperature. The primary effector systems include vascular, metabolic, skeletal muscle (shivering), and sweating. These effector systems function either to increase or to dissipate body heat.

Conservation and Production of Body Heat

When body temperature is lowered, mechanisms are activated to conserve heat and increase heat production. The following are descriptions of heat conservation and production mechanisms:

- *Vasoconstriction of blood vessels:* The hypothalamus activates sympathetic nerves, an action that results in vasoconstriction of cutaneous vessels throughout the body. This significantly reduces the lumen of the vessels and decreases blood flow near the surface of the skin, where the blood would normally be cooled. Thus, the amount of heat lost to the environment is decreased.
- *Decrease (or absence) of sweat gland activity:* To reduce or to prevent heat loss by evaporation, sweat gland activity is diminished. Sweating is totally abolished with cooling of the hypothalamic thermostat below approximately 98.6°F (37°C).[31]
- *Cutis anserina or piloerection*: Also a response to cooling of the hypothalamus, this heat conservation mechanism is commonly described as "gooseflesh." The term *piloerection* means "hairs standing on end." Although of less significance in humans, this mechanism functions to trap a layer of insulating air near the skin and decrease heat loss in lower mammals with greater hair covering.

The body also responds to decreased temperature with several mechanisms, including shivering and hormonal regulation, designed to produce heat. These mechanisms are activated when body temperature falls below a critical temperature level.[32] The primary motor center for shivering is located in the posterior hypothalamus. This area

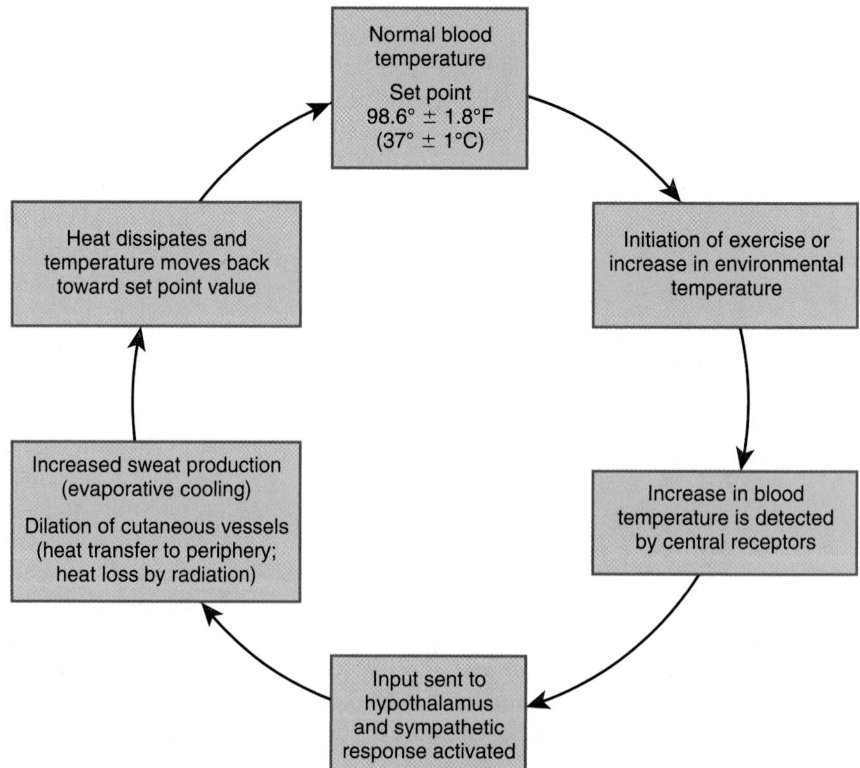

Figure 2.4 Thermoregulatory response during heat acclimation. Increased body temperature activates heat (loss) dissipation to maintain normal body temperature.

is activated by cold signals from the skin and spinal cord. In response to cold, impulses from the hypothalamus activate the efferent somatic nervous system, causing increased tone of skeletal muscles. As the tone gradually increases to a certain threshold level, *shivering* (involuntary muscle contraction) is initiated, and heat is produced. This shivering reflex can be at least partially suppressed through conscious cortical control and voluntary muscle activity.[37]

The function of hormonal influence in thermal regulation is to increase cellular metabolism, which subsequently increases body heat. Increased metabolism occurs through circulation of two hormones from the adrenal medulla: *norepinephrine* and *epinephrine*. This is called *chemical thermogenesis*. Circulating levels of these hormones, however, are of greater significance in maintaining body temperature in infants than in adults. Heat production by these hormones can be increased in an infant by as much as 100%, as opposed to 10% to 15% in an adult.[32]

A second form of hormonal regulation involves increased output of *thyroxine* by the thyroid gland. Thyroxine increases the rate of cellular metabolism throughout the body. This response, however, occurs only as a result of prolonged cooling, and heat production is not immediate.[31] The thyroid gland requires several weeks to hypertrophy before increased demands for thyroxine can be achieved.

Loss of Body Heat

Excess heat is dissipated from the body through four primary methods: radiation, conduction, convection, and evaporation.

- *Radiation:* The transfer of heat by electromagnetic waves from one object to another is accomplished by radiation. This heat transfer occurs through the air between objects that are not in direct contact. Heat is lost to surrounding objects that are colder than the body (e.g., a wall or surrounding objects in the room).
- *Conduction:* The transfer of heat from one object to another through a liquid, solid, or gas takes place by conduction. This type of heat transfer requires direct molecular contact between two objects, as when a person is sitting on a cold surface, or when heat is lost in a cool swimming pool. Heat is also lost by conduction to air.
- *Convection:* The transfer of heat by movement of air or liquid (water) is achieved by convection. This form of heat loss is accomplished secondary to conduction. Once the heat is conducted to the air, the air is then moved away from the body by convection currents. Use of a fan or a cool breeze provides convection currents. Heat loss by convection is most effective when the air or liquid surrounding the body is continually moved away and replaced.
- *Evaporation:* Dissipation of body heat by the conversion of a liquid to a vapor occurs by evaporation. This form of heat loss occurs on a continual basis through the respiratory tract and through perspiration from the skin. Evaporation provides the major mechanism of heat loss during heavy exercise. Profuse sweating provides a significant cooling effect on the skin as it evaporates. In addition, this cooling of the skin functions to further cool the blood as it is shunted from internal structures to cutaneous areas. Figure 2.5 illustrates the mechanisms of heat loss from the body.

Abnormalities in Body Temperature

Increased Body Temperature

Pyrexia is the elevation of normal body temperature, more commonly referred to as fever. Fever is part of the body's natural defense against infectious disease (invading pathogens). Increasing internal temperatures creates an environment less favorable for viruses and bacteria to replicate. Fever occurs when the "set" value of the hypothalamic thermostat is triggered to rise by circulating pyrogens (fever-producing substances) secreted primarily

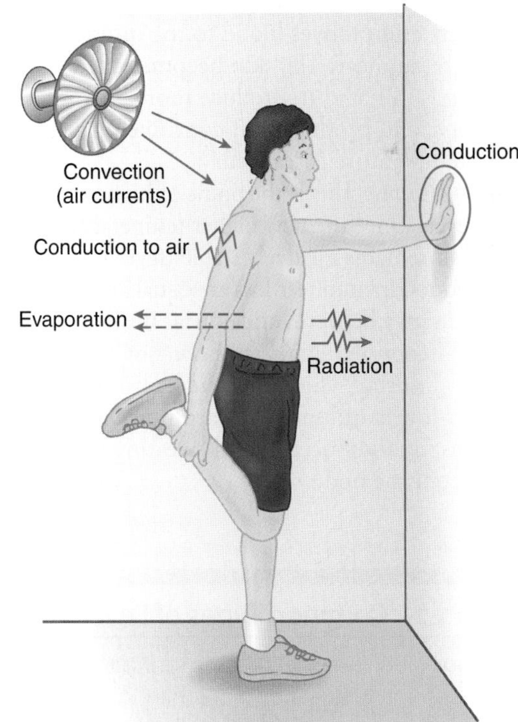

Figure 2.5 Mechanisms of heat loss from body. *Conduction* is the transfer of heat by direct contact between two objects (hand on wall); *radiation* occurs through electromagnetic waves between objects not in direct contact with each other (subject's body and wall); heat loss by *convection* is accomplished via air currents (wall fan) after the heat is conducted to air; *evaporation* converts liquid (perspiration) to a vapor.

from toxic bacteria, viruses, or injured body tissue. The effects of these pyrogens result in fever during illness. As a result of the new, higher thermostat value, the body responds by activating its heat conservation and production mechanisms. These mechanisms raise body temperature to the new, higher value over a period of several hours. Thus a fever, or febrile state, is produced.

The clinical signs and symptoms of a fever vary with the level of disturbance of the thermoregulatory center and with the phase of the fever. These signs and symptoms may include general malaise, headache, increased pulse and respiratory rate, chills, piloerection, shivering, loss of appetite (anorexia), pale skin that later becomes flushed and hot to the touch, nausea, irritability, restlessness, constipation, sweating, thirst, coated tongue, decreased urinary output, weakness, and insomnia.[23,38]

The *prodromal* period of fever occurs just prior to onset; nonspecific symptoms may be experienced, such as a slight headache, muscle aches, general malaise, or loss of appetite. Three phases (stages) have been identified to describe a fever:

- *Phase 1—Onset:* This is the period from either gradual or sudden rise until the maximum temperature is reached; symptoms include chills, shivering, and pale appearance of skin. As body temperature is raised (e.g., in response to infection), cutaneous vasoconstriction moves blood to the interior of the body to retain heat. The skin becomes cool, and shivering is initiated to produce more heat. Attempts to preserve and produce heat continue until a new, higher temperature is reached.
- *Phase 2—Course:* This is the point of highest elevation of the fever. Once the new higher temperature is reached, it remains relatively stable (fever is sustained); heat production and heat loss are equal and shivering stops; skin may be warm and appear flushed.
- *Phase 3—Termination (defervescence* or *crisis):* This is the period during which the fever subsides and temperatures lower and move toward normal. Cutaneous vasodilation occurs, and sweating is initiated to help cool the body.

Several types of fevers present unique characteristics that are named based on their distinguishing clinical feature: *continuous, intermittent, relapsing,* or *remittent* (Box 2.2).

An unusually high fever above 106.7°F (41.5°C) is called *hyperpyrexia.* Hyperthermia is an uncontrolled increase in body temperature with an unchanged setting of the thermoregulatory center. Excessively high body temperatures are caused by an inability of the thermoregulatory system to lose heat fast enough to balance excessive heat production or high environmental temperatures. Examples of hyperthermia include heat exhaustion and heat stroke. *Heat exhaustion* is associated with exercise and physical exertion in high environmental temperatures where the cardiovascular system cannot meet the demands of blood flow to the skin (thermoregulation) and to the muscles (metabolic exercise requirements). Symptoms include profuse sweating, fatigue, faintness, dizziness, weak and rapid pulse, nausea, headache, and vomiting. Treatment typically includes stopping physical activity, moving to a cooler environment, drinking fluid, removing tight clothing, assuming a supine position with legs elevated, and applying available cooling methods such as fans or ice packs or towels. *Heat stroke* is a more severe form of hyperthermia in which the thermoregulatory system essentially fails. It can be life-threatening and requires immediate emergency medical attention to rapidly reduce body temperature (ice water immersion, ice packs). Symptoms include rapid and shallow breathing; mental status changes (confusion, delirium); strong, rapid pulse; lack of sweating; faintness; throbbing headache; and eventually loss of consciousness or death.[8,32,40-43]

Decreased Body Temperature

Exposure to extreme cold produces a lowered body temperature called *hypothermia.* With prolonged exposure to cold, there is a decrease in metabolic rate, and body temperature gradually falls. As cooling of the brain occurs, there is a depression of the thermoregulatory center. The function of the thermoregulatory center becomes seriously impaired when body temperature falls

Box 2.2 Common Types of Fever

Continuous (also known as *constant* or *sustained*): Body temperature is constantly elevated above normal throughout day but does not fluctuate by more than 1.8°F (1°C) in 24 hours; seen in uncomplicated minor infection, urinary tract infection, lobar pneumonia, typhoid (foodborne illness), infective endocarditis, and typhus (flea-borne disease).

Intermittent: Body temperature alternates between periods of fever for some hours of the day with return to normal temperatures for the remaining hours; seen in malaria and septicemia.

Relapsing (also known as *recurrent* or *periodic*): Periods of fever are interspersed with normal temperatures; each last at least one day; seen in non-infectious inflammatory diseases such as rheumatoid arthritis and Crohn's disease, recurrent infections, malignancy (neoplastic fever), and infections caused by certain species of Borrelia spirochetes (ticks and lice).[39]

Remittent: Elevated body temperature throughout day that fluctuates more than 3.6°F (2°C) within a 24-hour period but never returns to normal; seen in infective endocarditis and typhoid infection.

below approximately 94°F (34.4°C) and is completely lost with temperatures below 85°F (29.4°C).[33] Therefore, the body's heat regulatory and protection mechanism is lost. Symptoms of hypothermia include decreased HR and RR, cold and pale skin, cyanosis, decreased cutaneous sensation, depression of mental and muscular responses, and drowsiness, which may eventually lead to coma. If hypothermia is left untreated, the progression of these symptoms may lead to death.

Factors Influencing Body Temperature

A statistical average or normal temperature of 98.6°F (37°C) taken orally has been established for body temperature in an adult population. However, a range of values is more representative of normal body temperature because certain everyday circumstances (e.g., time of day) or activities (e.g., exercise) influence the body's temperature. In addition, some individuals typically run a *slightly higher* or *lower* body temperature than the statistical average. Therefore, deviations from the average will be apparent from individual to individual, as well as between measures taken from the same person under varying circumstances.

Time of Day

The term *circadian rhythm* describes a 24-hour cycle of normal variations in body temperature. Certain predictable and regular changes in temperature occur on a daily basis. Body temperature tends to be lowest between 4:00 and 6:00 a.m. and highest between 4:00 and 8:00 p.m. Digestive processes and the level of skeletal muscle activity significantly influence these regular changes in body temperature. For individuals who work at night, this pattern is usually inverted.[31,33]

Age

Compared with adults, infants demonstrate a higher normal temperature owing to the immaturity of the thermoregulatory system. Infants are particularly susceptible to environmental temperature changes, and their body temperature will fluctuate accordingly. Young children also average higher normal temperatures because of the heat production associated with increased metabolic rate and high physical activity levels. Elderly populations tend to demonstrate lower than average body temperatures, owing to a variety of factors, including lower metabolic rates, decreased subcutaneous tissue mass (which normally insulates the body against heat loss), decreased physical activity levels, and inadequate diet.

Emotions/Stress

Stimulation of the sympathetic nervous system causes increased production of epinephrine and norepinephrine with a subsequent increase in metabolic rate.

Exercise

The effects of exercise on body temperature are an important consideration for physical therapists. Strenuous exercise significantly increases body temperature because of an increase in metabolic rate. Active muscle contractions are an important and potent source of heat production. During exercise, body temperature increases are proportional to the relative intensity of the workload. Vigorous exercise can increase the metabolic rate by as much as 20 to 25 times that of the basal level.[31]

Menstrual Cycle

Increased levels of progesterone during ovulation cause body temperature to rise 0.5°F to 0.9°F (0.3°C to 0.5°C). This slight elevation is maintained until just prior to the initiation of menstruation, at which time it returns to normal levels.

Pregnancy

Because of increased metabolic activity, body temperature remains elevated by approximately 0.9°F (0.5°C). Temperature returns to normal after parturition.

External Environment

Generally, warm weather tends to increase body temperature, and cold weather decreases body temperature. Environmental conditions influence the body's ability to maintain constant temperatures. For example, in hot, humid environments, the effectiveness of evaporative cooling is severely diminished because the air is already heavily moisture laden. Other forms of heat dissipation are also dependent on environmental factors such as movement of air currents (convection). Clothing also can be an important external consideration because it can function either to conserve or to facilitate release of body heat. The amount and type of clothing is important. To dissipate heat, absorbent, loose-fitting, light-colored clothing is most effective. To conserve heat, several layers of lightweight clothing to trap air and to insulate the body are recommended.

Measurement Site

Body temperatures vary among body parts. Rectal and tympanic (ear) membrane temperatures are from 0.5°F to 0.9°F (0.3°C to 0.5°C) higher than oral temperatures; axillary temperatures are approximately 1.1°F (0.6°C) lower than oral temperatures. Oral temperature in a healthy adult population is generally considered to be 98.6°F (37°C), and for rectal and tympanic membrane temperatures the value is 99.5°F (37.5°C). Being an external measure, the axillary value is somewhat lower at 97.6°F (36.5°C).

Ingestion of Warm or Cold Foods

Oral temperatures will be affected by oral intake, including smoking. Patients should refrain from smoking or eating for at least 15 minutes (preferably 30 minutes) prior to an oral temperature reading.

Figure 2.6 presents a comparison of Fahrenheit and centigrade temperature values with ranges of normal and altered body temperature. If a situation occurs that requires changing a temperature reading from one scale to the other, a conversion formula can be used. To convert centigrade into Fahrenheit, multiply the centigrade value by 9/5 and add 32 ($F = [9/5 \times C°] + 32°$). To change from Fahrenheit into centigrade, subtract 32 from the Fahrenheit value and multiply by 5/9 ($C = [F - 32°] \times 5/9$).

Types of Thermometers

Glass Mercury Thermometers

For many years, temperatures had been taken using a glass thermometer, which consists of a glass tube with a bulbous tip filled with mercury. Once the bulb is in contact with body heat, the mercury expands and rises in the glass column to register body temperature. A narrowing of the base prevented reflux of mercury down the tube. The device had to be shaken vigorously to return the mercury to the bulb before the next use. Owing to the highly poisonous nature of mercury and breakability of glass, automated thermometers have largely replaced their use in patient care settings. The World Health Organization (WHO),[44] the U.S. Environmental Protection Agency,[45] and the National Institute of Standards and Technology[46] warn against using mercury thermometers and encourage replacement with non-mercury-containing devices whenever possible. Some states have laws restricting the manufacture and sale of mercury thermometers. Many areas also offer collection/exchange programs for mercury-containing devices.[45]

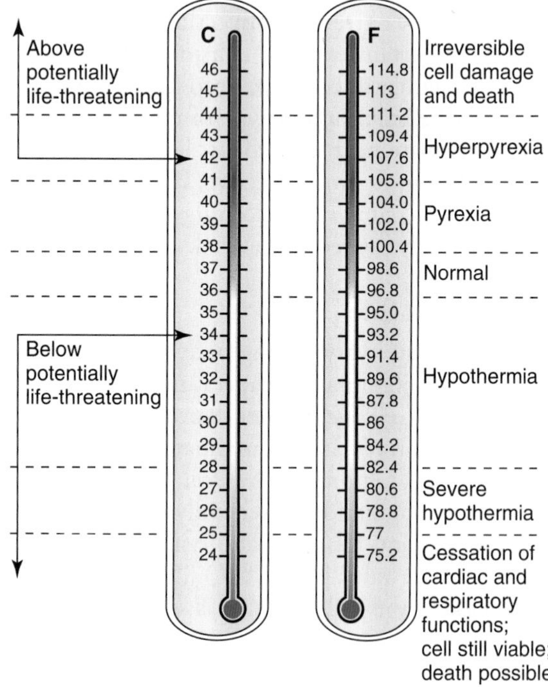

Figure 2.6 Comparison of Fahrenheit and centigrade scales indicating ranges of normal and altered body temperature. *(Adapted from Wilkinson, et al,[8, p. 423] with permission.)*

Clinical Note: Glass thermometers containing mercury may still be found in the home care setting. Their continued use should be discouraged whenever possible. Replacement with an automated thermometer should be encouraged.

Automated Thermometers

Automated thermometers are widely used in patient care settings. They provide a rapid (several seconds), highly accurate measure of body temperature, displayed digitally. Standard clinical automated thermometers consist of a portable battery-operated unit, an attached probe, and plastic disposable probe covers (Fig. 2.7A). An important advantage of these thermometers is the low chance of cross-infection, so long as the probe covers are used only once. Other automated devices are designed to monitor more than one vital sign and interface directly with the electronic health record (EHR). By scanning the patient's hospital identification bracelet, two-way wireless communication links ID numbers to patient names for positive identification at the bedside. The device reduces time required and potential errors of manual documentation as data are relayed directly to the EHR. Data (e.g., respiratory rate, pain level) may also be entered manually (Fig. 2.7B).

Oral Thermometers

Handheld automated oral (digital "stick") thermometers are readily available commercially. These units are typically about 5 inches in length with a tapered design (Fig. 2.8). One end of the device has a narrow tip and serves as the probe; in some models the tip is flexible. The opposite end is broad and houses the battery. These thermometers also provide a flashed, digital display of body temperature; most models have memory capabilities. Typically, these devices are used for a single patient; however, they can also be used with disposable probe covers.

Temporal Artery Thermometer

Noninvasive temporal artery thermometers measure body temperature by sliding a probe, held flat against the skin,[47] in a straight line from the center of the forehead, across the temporal artery area to the hairline (Fig. 2.9). The probe is then lifted from the forehead, centered on the mastoid process behind the ear, and slid down to the soft depression behind the earlobe (this helps eliminate the possibility of a false low

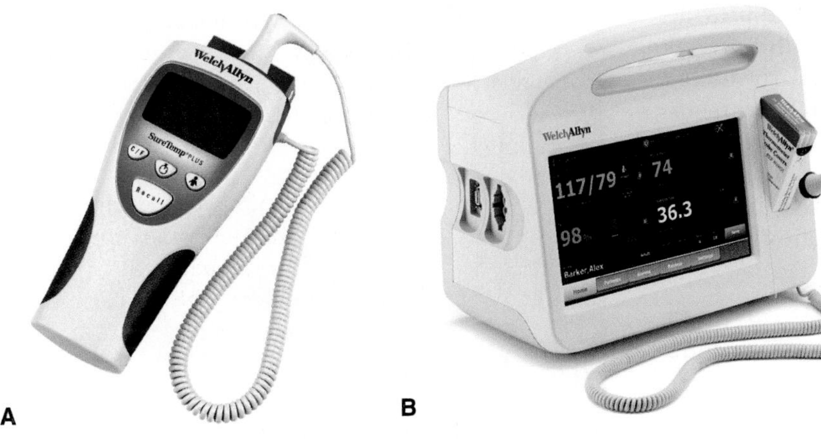

Figure 2.7 (A) Handheld electronic thermometer with disposable probe covers reduces the risk of cross-contamination. (B) This device interfaces with the electronic health record (EHR). The unit measures temperature, blood pressure, and oxygen saturation levels (pulse oximetry). *(Courtesy of Welch Allyn, Skaneateles Falls, NY 13153-0220.)*

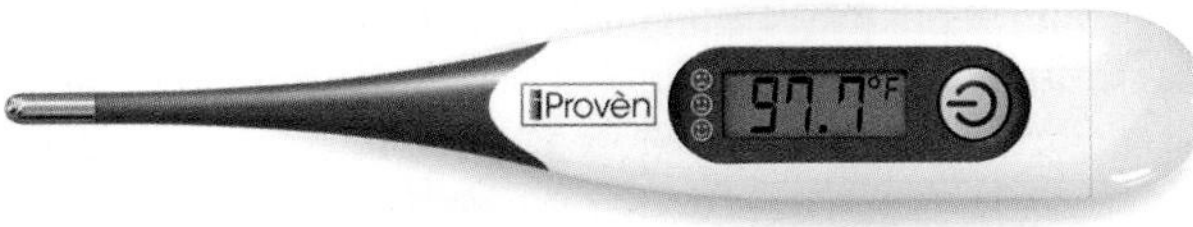

Figure 2.8 Handheld automated oral thermometers are self-contained with an internal battery; the proximal end houses the digital display and battery, and the distal end serves as the temperature probe. *(Courtesy of iProvèn, Netherlands.)*

temperature caused by evaporative cooling in the presence of forehead perspiration). The thermometer detects heat emitting from the skin surface over the temporal artery. The probe can be cleaned with an alcohol swab or used with disposable probe caps. For patients in isolation, tubular sheaths that cover the entire unit are available for optimum infection control. As a measurement site, the temporal artery is easily accessible and poses low risk of injury as there is no contact with mucous membranes.

Note: Depending on the manufacturer, a variety of features may be available on automated thermometers such as memory recall of previous recording(s), the ability to toggle between F and C values, timers (e.g., pulse measures), and auto shutoff.

Tympanic Thermometer

Tympanic (ear) infrared thermometers measure body temperature through a sensor probe placed in the ear that detects infrared (thermal) radiation from the tympanic membrane. This location provides an important reflection of core temperature because the tympanic membrane receives its blood supply from a tributary of the internal carotid artery, which supplies the hypothalamus (temperature-regulating center). These handheld portable thermometers include an ear probe

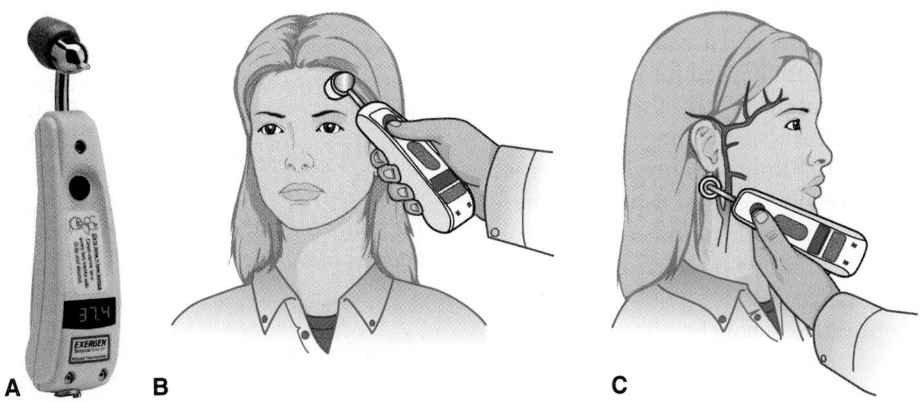

Figure 2.9 (A) Temporal artery thermometer. *(Courtesy of Exergen Corporation, Watertown, MA 02472.)* (B) The probe is moved in a straight line laterally from center of forehead toward hairline. (C) The probe is then centered on the mastoid process behind the ear and slid down to the soft depression behind the earlobe. *(Adapted from Wilkinson, JM, et al,[47, p. 188] with permission.)*

(used with a single-use disposable cover) and provide a digital display of body temperature within several seconds (Fig. 2.10A). They are particularly useful when oral monitoring is contraindicated, for patients not capable of cooperating or following directions, in emergency situations where rapid temperature values are required, and for children who may have difficulty remaining still during other types of monitoring.

Noncontact Forehead Thermometers

Noncontact infrared thermometers measure temperature using the surface area of the forehead (Fig. 2.10B). Because these thermometers do not touch the patient, there is no risk of contamination. Based on manufacturer's specifications, the thermometers are held a specified distance from the center of the forehead. If the forehead is perspiring, temperature can be measured over other surface areas (e.g., neck, axilla). As they are noncontact, they are practical for large-scale screenings (e.g., emergency department entry, epidemic infectious disease control), can be used while the patient is sleeping, and potentially cause less distress compared to more conventional methods. Noncontact thermometers are also available with connectivity to a smartphone using a dedicated application (app) that allows tracking of temperature readings (Fig. 2.10C).

Disposable Single-Use Oral and Skin Surface Thermometers

Single-use oral thermometers are placed under the tongue. They consist of a thin plastic strip with a series of raised calibrated dots impregnated with a temperature-sensitive chemical (Fig. 2.11). The dots change color to indicate the temperature. After the thermometer is removed from the mouth, the dots are examined for color changes to determine the temperature reading (Fig 2.12). They are available in both Fahrenheit and Celsius scales and are disposed of after use. Although most commonly used for oral temperatures, disposable thermometers can also be used to obtain axillary temperatures, and some are available with covers (sheaths) containing semirigid stays that allow use for rectal measurements. Disposable thermometers play an important role in infection control, as they reduce the potential for transfer of infectious agents from reusable equipment.

Skin surface thermometers consist of heat-sensitive strips (tape, patches, or disks) that provide a general measure of body surface temperature. They also respond to body temperature by changing color and are more frequently used with children. They must be applied to dry skin. The forehead and abdomen are common placement sites. The temperature readings are nonspecific and are usually confirmed with a more precise measuring instrument if deviations are noted.

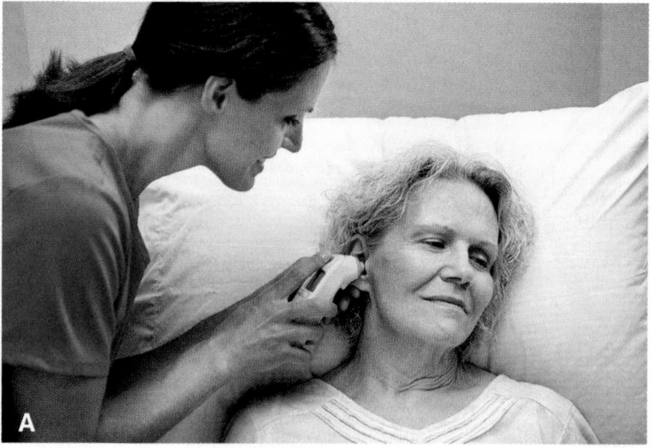

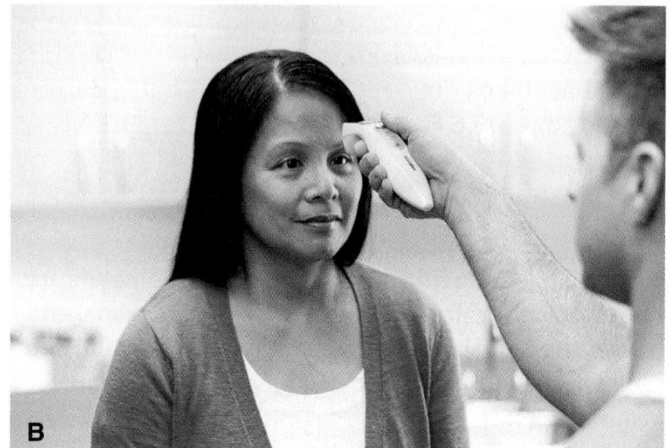

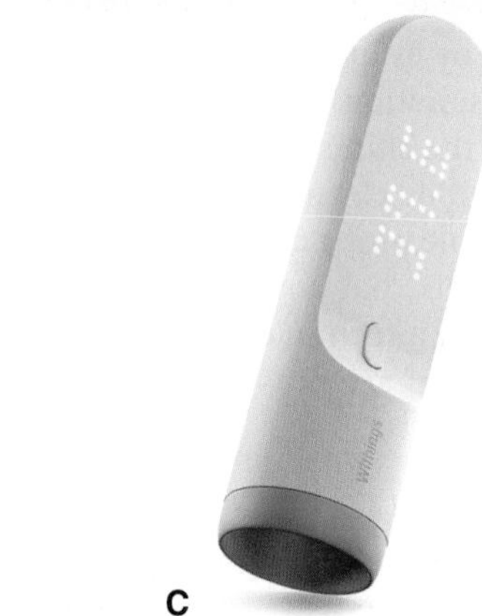

Figure 2.10 (A) Tympanic (ear) thermometer. (B) Noncontact forehead thermometer. *(Courtesy of Welch Allyn, Skaneateles Falls, NY 13153-0220.)* (C) Noncontact forehead thermometer with connectivity to a smartphone. *(Courtesy of Withings, Cambridge, MA 02142.)*

Clinical Note: Automated handheld infrared thermographic scanners are available for detecting subtle skin temperature changes (e.g., patients with altered vascular perfusion).

Hand Hygiene

Although addressed here as a precursor to examining vital signs, hand hygiene is a paramount consideration

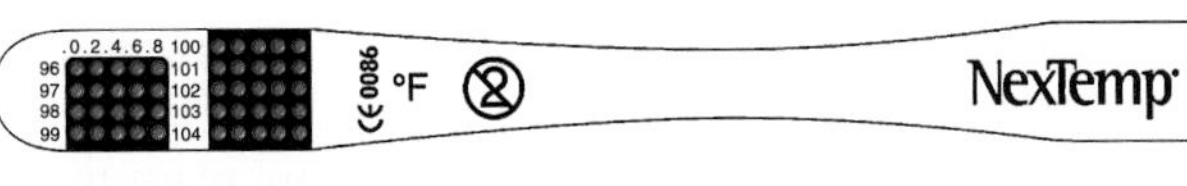

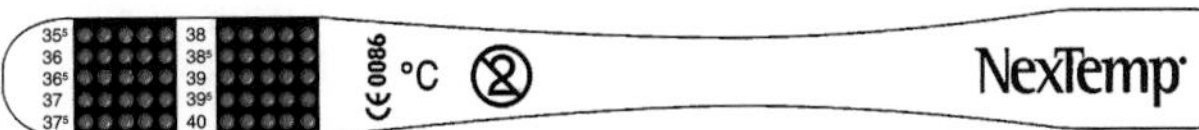

Figure 2.11 Disposable single-use thermometer in Fahrenheit *(top)* and centigrade *(bottom)* scales. *(Courtesy of Medical Indicators, Inc., Pennington, NJ 08534.)*

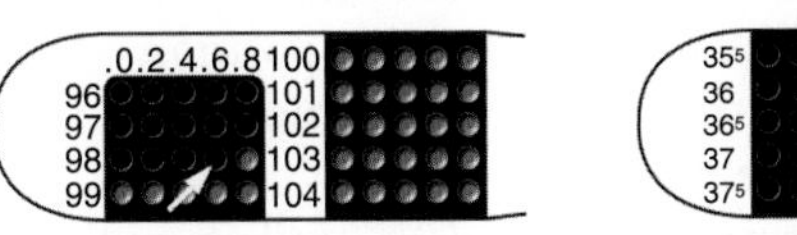

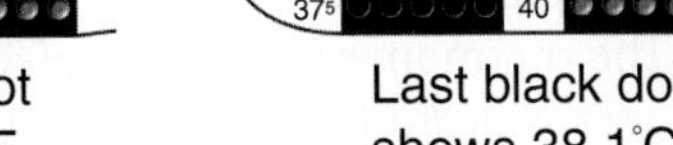

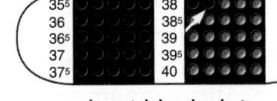

Figure 2.12 The chemical dots on the disposable single-use thermometers change color from green to black to reflect the temperature (Fahrenheit, *left,* and centigrade, *right*). The green dots turn black from left to right. The last dot to turn black indicates the temperature. Note there are two grids of dots on each scale (*left* and *right*). Values that fall in the right grid indicate fever is present. In the example on the right, 100.5°F (38.1°C) represents fever. *(Courtesy of Medical Indicators, Inc., Pennington, NJ 08534.)*

with all aspects of patient care, as it plays a critical role in preventing transmission of pathogens in health care settings. According to WHO, *health care–associated infection* (HCAI) represents a major patient safety concern, and its prevention should be a top priority in all patient care settings and institutions. The WHO states, "The impact of HCAI implies prolonged hospital stay, long-term disability, increased resistance of microorganisms to antimicrobials, massive additional financial burden, high costs for patients and their families, and excess deaths."[48, p. 6]

Hand hygiene is accomplished by washing hands with soap and water or by rubbing hands with an alcohol-based formula. Alcohol-based hand rubs are an efficient and effective way to inactivate a broad spectrum of microorganisms from the hands.[48] The factors on which WHO has based its recommendations for hand rubs are presented in Box 2.3. When using an alcohol-based hand rub, enough product should be used to cover all hand surfaces. The hands are then rubbed together until dry. The hand rubbing technique is illustrated in Appendix 2.A.

When using soap and water, enough product should be used to cover all hand surfaces. Clean running water assists with removing microorganisms, and a warm temperature removes less protective oil from the hands than hot water. The force of the water should not cause splashing, which can promote the transfer of microorganisms.

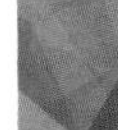

Box 2.3 Factors Considered by WHO in Recommending Hand Rubs

WHO recommends alcohol-based hand rubs based on the following factors:

1. Evidence-based, intrinsic advantages of fast-acting and broad-spectrum microbicidal activity with a minimal risk of generating resistance to antimicrobial agents
2. Suitability for use in resource-limited or remote areas with lack of accessibility to sinks or other facilities for hand hygiene (including clean water, towels, and so forth)
3. Capacity to promote improved compliance with hand hygiene by making the process faster and more convenient
4. Economic benefit by reducing annual costs for hand hygiene, representing approximately 1% of extra costs generated by health care–associated infection (HCAI)
5. Minimization of risks from adverse events because of increased safety associated with better acceptability and tolerance than other products

From WHO,[48, p. 57,] with permission.

Care should be taken not to lean against the sink to avoid contact with a potentially contaminated area. The technique for hand washing is presented in Appendix 2.B.

To draw attention to the indications for hand hygiene and its practical application, WHO has developed "My Five Moments for Hand Hygiene": (1) before touching the patient; (2) before a clean/aseptic procedure; (3) after body fluid exposure risk; (4) after touching a patient; and (5) after touching patient surroundings.[48]

Clinical Note: As with all physical therapy examinations, before a vital sign measure is taken, the procedure and its rationale should be explained in terms appropriate to the patient's understanding and confirmation made of patient safety, privacy, modesty, comfort, and understanding.

Measuring Body Temperature

For purposes of establishing baseline data and determining response to treatment, physical therapists generally use oral monitoring. Oral temperatures are contraindicated for patients with *dyspnea* or who are mouth breathers, have had oral surgery, or have a history of epilepsy or are prone to seizures. They also should not be used with infants or small children or patients who are irrational, unconscious, or uncooperative. In situations in which oral temperatures may be contraindicated and an automated unit with an alternative sensor is unavailable, an axillary measurement may be substituted.

Measuring Oral Temperature: Automated Thermometer

A. Assemble equipment: An automated thermometer with disposable probe covers or sheaths.
B. Wash hands.
C. Procedure:
  1. Turn on the power.
  2. Grasp the proximal aspect of the thermometer with the thumb and forefinger and attach the disposable cover over the distal probe tip until it snaps or locks in place. (Some units have a proximal button that releases the probe cover after temperature reading is complete.) For a small handheld automated unit, the probe covers are designed as a plastic sheath.
  3. Ask patient to open his or her mouth, and place the covered probe at the posterior base of the tongue to the right or left of the frenulum in the sublingual pocket. This placement positions the tip of the thermometer over superficial blood vessels that reflect core body temperature. Instruct the patient to close the lips (not teeth) around the thermometer. Continue to hold the probe in place, because the weight of the probe may displace it from the sublingual pocket.
  4. Hold the probe in the sublingual pocket until an audible beep is heard (several seconds). The beep indicates maximum temperature has been reached. Remove the probe from the patient's mouth and note the temperature reading on the digital display for recording.
  5. Remove the probe cover over a waste receptacle for disposal. If available on the unit, use the probe release mechanism; if a plastic sheath cover is used, use a clean paper towel for removal. (Cover sheath with paper towel, place thumb and forefinger proximally on probe over paper towel, and slide fingers distally.)
  6. Return thermometer to appropriate storage cradle.
  7. Wash hands.

Measuring Axillary Temperature: Automated Thermometer

A. Assemble equipment: An automated thermometer with disposable probe covers or sheaths and a towel or gauze pads to dry axillary region. (Moisture will conduct heat.)
B. Wash hands.
C. Procedure:
  1. Expose the axilla, and ensure that area is dry. If any moisture is present, the area should be gently towel dried with a patting motion. (Vigorous rubbing will increase temperature of the area.)
  2. Turn on the power.
  3. Grasp the proximal aspect of the thermometer with the thumb and forefinger, and attach the disposable cover or sheath over the distal probe tip.
  4. With the patient in a supine position, place the tip of the thermometer in the center of the axillary region between the trunk and upper arm (Fig. 2.13) The patient's upper extremity (UE) should be placed tightly across the chest to keep the thermometer in place. (Asking the patient to move the hand toward the opposite shoulder is often a useful direction.) If the patient is disoriented or very young, the thermometer must be held in place. Axillary temperature can also be taken in a sitting position, but this carries the risk of the thermometer dropping to the floor.
  5. The thermometer is left in place until an audible beep is heard (several seconds). The beep indicates that maximum temperature has been reached. Remove the probe from the patient's axilla, and note the temperature reading on the digital display for recording.
  6. Remove the probe cover or sheath over a waste receptacle for disposal.
  7. Return thermometer to appropriate storage cradle.
  8. Wash hands.

Note: Generally, a temperature reading is assumed to be an oral measure unless otherwise noted. Documentation software typically includes entry labels for temperature source (e.g., oral, axillary, rectal). If documenting manually, axillary values are designated by a circled A after the temperature or the designation "AT" for *axillary temperature* (e.g., 95°F AT). Similarly, the designation "RT" (*rectal temperature*) or a circled *R* after the value indicates a rectal measure (e.g., 99°F ®).

Measuring Tympanic Membrane Temperature: Automated Tympanic Thermometer

A. Assemble equipment: Tympanic (infrared) thermometer and disposable probe covers.
B. Wash hands.
C. Procedure:
  1. Attach the disposable cover to the probe, holding the edges with the thumb and forefinger. (Ensure that the firm circular collar of the cover engages with the base by gently pushing it down to snap it into place; do not touch the plastic film of the probe cover.)
  2. Turn the patient's head to one side. Follow the manufacturer's recommendation for insertion and positioning of the ear. Some tympanic thermometers require straightening of the ear canal before insertion by pulling the ear up and back

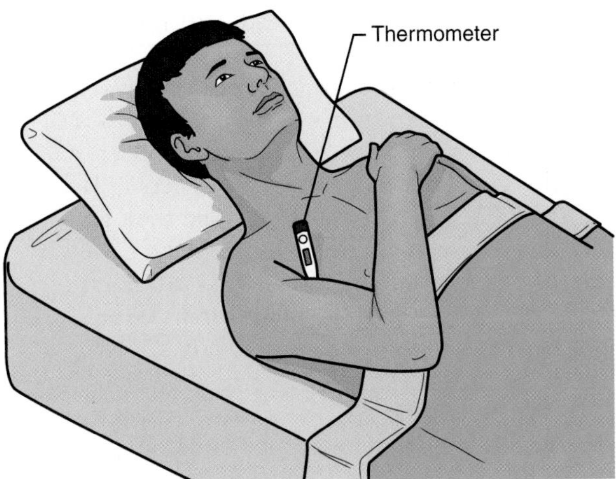

Figure 2.13 Positioning for monitoring axillary temperature. Placing the patient's arm across the chest forces cool air out of the axilla that could potentially result in a lower temperature value. This positioning also places the probe near the vascular supply to the axilla. The proximal portion of the thermometer should be angled toward the patient's head.

for adults and pulling down and back for a child.[47,49]

3. Insert the probe snugly into the ear canal. Use a firm, gentle pressure; avoid forcing the probe too deeply. The probe should seal the opening of the ear canal. To ensure accurate reading, the probe should be angled anteriorly toward the jawline, as if approaching the patient from behind.
4. Press the button that activates the thermometer. The temperature is displayed within several seconds. An audible beep or flashing light will signal when the maximum temperature is reached.
5. Gently remove the probe from the ear. Eject or remove the probe cover over a waste receptacle for disposal. For manual removal of the probe cover, use a clean paper towel or tissue.
6. Return tympanic thermometer to protective case or storage base. Most units include a protective cap that fits over the probe tip.
7. Wash hands.

■ PULSE

The *pulse* is the wave of blood in the artery created by contraction of the left ventricle during a cardiac cycle (one complete cycle of cardiac muscle contraction and relaxation). With each contraction, blood is pumped into an already full aorta. The inherent elasticity of the aortic walls allows expansion and acceptance of the new supply. The blood is then forced out and surges through the systemic arteries. It is this wave or surge of blood that is felt as the pulse. The strength or amplitude of the pulse reflects the amount of blood ejected with each myocardial contraction, or *stroke volume* (SV).

Peripheral pulses are those located in the periphery of the body that can be felt by palpating an artery over a bony prominence or other firm surface. Examples of peripheral pulses include the radial, carotid, and popliteal pulses. The *apical pulse* is a central pulse located at the apex of the heart that is monitored using a stethoscope.

Pressure changes in the large arteries during the cardiac cycle are reflected in the relatively smooth and rounded appearance of the normal arterial waveform (Fig. 2.14 [top]). The lowest point of pressure occurs during ventricular diastole, while the highest point occurs during ventricular systole (peak ejection). The notch on the descending slope of the pulse wave represents closure of the aortic valve and is not palpable. A healthy adult heart beats an average of 70 times per minute, a rate that provides continuous circulation of approximately 5 to 6 liters of blood through the body. The pulse can be palpated wherever a superficial artery can be stabilized over an underlying surface. In monitoring the pulse, specific attention is directed toward determining three parameters: *rate, rhythm,* and *quality.*

Rate

The HR is the number of pulsations (peripheral pulse waves) or frequency per minute. Bradycardia is an abnormally slow HR, less than 60 bpm. Tachycardia is an excessively high HR, greater than 100 bpm. *Palpitation* refers to the sensation of a rapid or irregular HR perceived by the patient without actually palpating a peripheral pulse. Multiple factors influence the HR, including age, sex, emotional status, stress, and physical activity level. Body size and stature also influence HR. Tall, thin individuals generally have a slower HR than those who are obese or have stout frames.

Rhythm

The pulse *rhythm* is the pattern of pulsations and the intervals between them. In a healthy individual, the rhythm is regular and indicates that the time intervals between pulse beats are essentially equal. *Arrhythmia* or *dysrhythmia* refers to an irregular rhythm in which pulses are not evenly spaced. An irregular rhythm may present as premature, late, or missed pulse beats, or random, irregular beats in either a predictable or an unpredictable pattern.[50] Irregular rhythms are often associated with conduction abnormalities or an impulse originating from a site other than the sinoatrial node.

Quality

The *quality* (force, volume) of the pulse refers to the amount of force created by the ejected blood volume against the arterial wall during each ventricular contraction. In examining the quality of the pulse, the therapist is determining the feel of the blood as it passes through a vessel. The quantity (volume) of blood within the vessel produces the force of the pulse. Normally, the pulse volume of each beat is the same. The

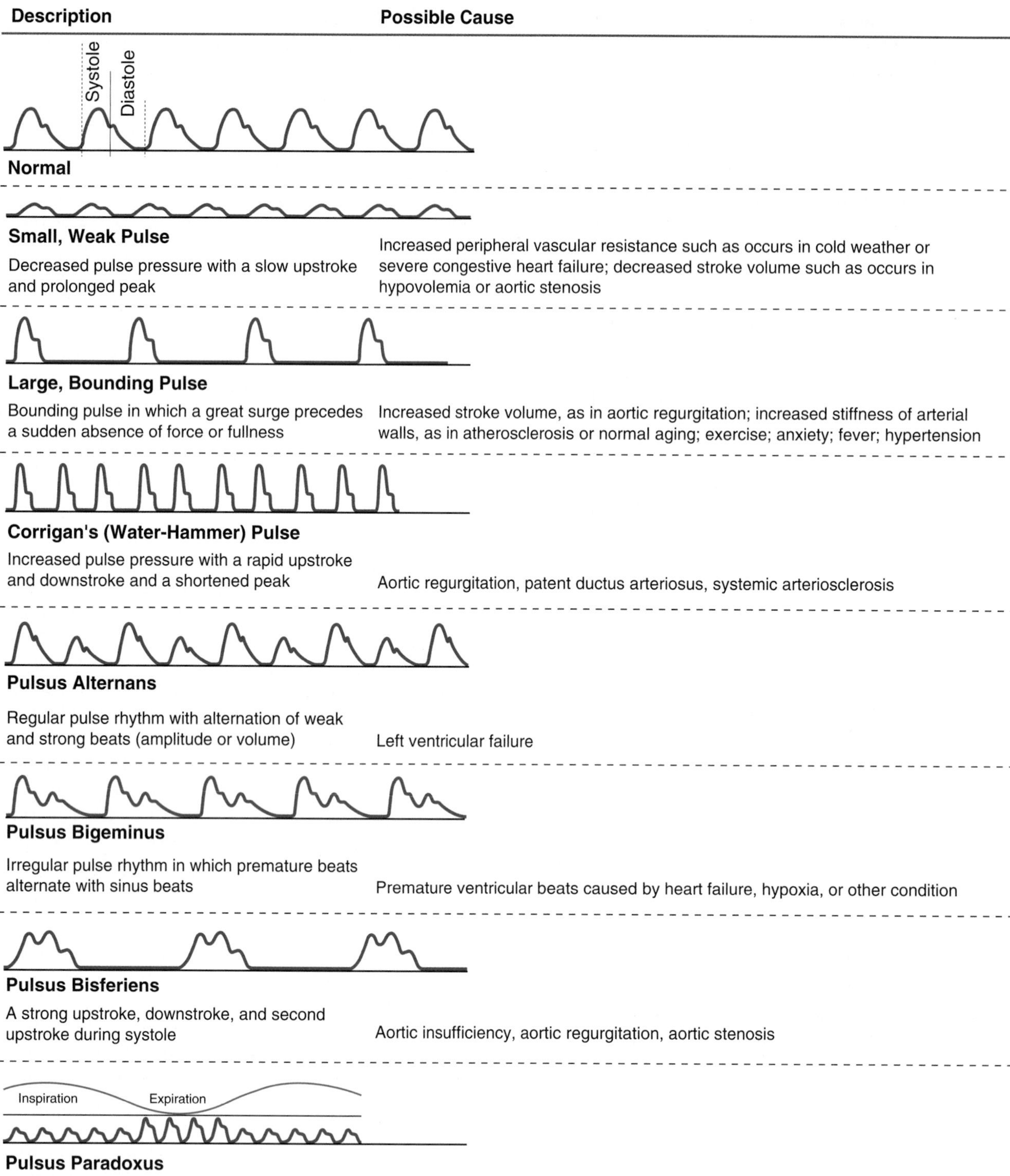

Description
Possible Cause
Systole
Diastole
Normal
Small, Weak Pulse
Decreased pulse pressure with a slow upstroke and prolonged peak
Increased peripheral vascular resistance such as occurs in cold weather or severe congestive heart failure; decreased stroke volume such as occurs in hypovolemia or aortic stenosis
Large, Bounding Pulse
Bounding pulse in which a great surge precedes a sudden absence of force or fullness
Increased stroke volume, as in aortic regurgitation; increased stiffness of arterial walls, as in atherosclerosis or normal aging; exercise; anxiety; fever; hypertension
Corrigan's (Water-Hammer) Pulse
Increased pulse pressure with a rapid upstroke and downstroke and a shortened peak
Aortic regurgitation, patent ductus arteriosus, systemic arteriosclerosis
Pulsus Alternans
Regular pulse rhythm with alternation of weak and strong beats (amplitude or volume)
Left ventricular failure
Pulsus Bigeminus
Irregular pulse rhythm in which premature beats alternate with sinus beats
Premature ventricular beats caused by heart failure, hypoxia, or other condition
Pulsus Bisferiens
A strong upstroke, downstroke, and second upstroke during systole
Aortic insufficiency, aortic regurgitation, aortic stenosis
Inspiration
Expiration
Pulsus Paradoxus
Pulse with a markedly decreased amplitude during inspiration
Constrictive pericarditis, pericardial tamponade, advanced heart failure, severe lung disease

Figure 2.14 Normal (*top*) and abnormal pulses, as reflected in arterial waveforms. *(From Dillon,[2, p. 477] with permission.)*

force of the pulse is greater with a higher blood volume and weaker with a lower blood volume. The volume is examined by noting how easily the pulse can be obliterated. A normal pulse is described as full or strong and can be palpated using moderate pressure of the fingers over a bony landmark. With lower volumes, the pulse is small, is easily obliterated, and is termed *weak* or *thready*. With increased volume, the pulse is large, is difficult to obliterate, and is termed a *bounding* (or *full*) pulse; a feeling of high tension is noted. A numerical scale is often used to document the quality (strength) of the pulse (Table 2.5).

In addition to rate, rhythm, and quality, the feel of the arterial wall under the examiner's fingertips should be determined. Normally, a vessel will feel smooth, elastic, soft, flexible, and relatively straight. With advancing age, vessels may demonstrate sclerotic changes. These changes frequently cause the vessels to feel twisted, hard, or cordlike, with decreased elasticity and smoothness.

Several other important terms are used to describe variations in pulse. The term *bigeminal* is used to describe an abnormality in pulse rhythm where two beats occur in rapid succession (double systolic peak). *Pulsus alternans* (alternating pulse) is marked by a fluctuation in amplitude between beats (a strong and a weak), with minimal change in overall rhythm. A normal pulse beat is followed by a premature beat of diminished amplitude. A *paradoxical* pulse (pulsus paradoxus) is decreased amplitude of the pressure wave detected during quiet inspiration with a return to full amplitude on expiration; it is often associated with obstructive lung disease. See Figure 2.14 for a schematic illustration of normal (top) and common alterations in arterial pulse waveforms. See Chapter 13, Heart Disease for a thorough discussion of cardiac pathologies and the cardiac examination.

Factors Influencing Heart Rate

Essentially, any factor that alters the metabolic rate will also influence HR. Several factors are of particular importance when considering HR.

Age

Fetal HR averages 120 to 160 bpm. The HR for a newborn ranges between 70 and 170, with an average of 120 bpm. HR gradually decreases with age until it stabilizes in adulthood (see Tables 2.1 and 2.2). The adult HR range is generally considered to be between 60 and 100 beats per minute; however, in highly trained athletes, the resting value may be considerably lower. This lowered resting value occurs because the effectiveness of each cardiac contraction is 40% to 50% greater in the trained versus untrained individual.[32]

Sex

Men and boys typically have slightly lower HR than women and girls.

Emotions/Stress

Responses to a variety of emotions (e.g., grief, fear, anger, excitement, anxiety) activate the sympathetic nervous system, with a resultant increase in HR. The stress-inducing effects of moderate to severe pain will also elevate HR.

Exercise

Oxygen demands of skeletal muscles are significantly increased during physical activity. At rest, only 20% to 25% of the available muscle capillaries are open.[31,33] During vigorous exercise, extensive vasodilation causes all capillaries to open. The HR increases to provide additional blood flow to muscles and to meet the increased oxygen requirement. For physical therapists, monitoring a patient's HR is an important method of evaluating response to exercise. Typically, HR will increase as a function of the activity's intensity (termed *chronotropic competence*).

A linear relationship exists between HR and intensity of workload. To use the HR effectively to prescribe exercise, both the patient's resting and predicted maximal HRs must be determined. Maximum HR values can be determined by a maximal graded exercise test, whenever possible, or by using various published formulas. Common formulas are the age-adjusted HR formula (maximum HR [HR_{max}] = 220 minus age) and the Karvonen formula (target HR = $[(HR_{max} - HR_{rest}) \times \%\ \text{intensity}] + HR_{rest}$). For moderate-intensity exercise, the CDC recommends that the target HR be 50% to 70% of predicted HR maximum and for vigorous-intensity exercise, it should be 70% to 85%.[51] Lower exercise intensities are indicated for individuals with low fitness levels.

In examining HR response to exercise, level of aerobic fitness also must be considered. Both resting HR and submaximal exercise HR are typically lower in trained individuals. In response to identical exercise intensity, a sedentary person's HR will demonstrate greater acceleration when compared with a trained individual. Although the metabolic requirements of an activity are the same, the lower HR response in a trained individual occurs as a result of a more efficient (increased) SV owing to greater cardiac strength and efficiency. The linear relationship between HR and workload exists for both trained and untrained individuals. However, the rate of rise will differ. When compared with a sedentary person, the trained individual will achieve a higher work output

Table 2.5 Numerical Scale for Grading Pulse Quality (Strength)

Grade	Pulse	Description
0	Absent	No perceptible pulse even with maximum pressure
1+	Thready	Barely perceptible; easily obliterated with slight pressure; fades in and out
2+	Weak	Difficult to palpate; slightly stronger than thready; can be obliterated with light pressure
3+	Normal	Easy to palpate; requires moderate pressure to obliterate
4+	Bounding	Very strong; hyperactive; is not obliterated with moderate pressure

and greater oxygen consumption before reaching a specified submaximal HR.

Medications

The impact of medications on HR is particularly important for patients with cardiac disease or hypertension. Beta blockers (beta-adrenergic blocking agents) are a category of drugs that block the sympathetic beta receptors and decrease both resting HR and HR response to exercise.[31] They are commonly used in the treatment of angina pectoris, arrhythmias, hypertension, and the acute phase of myocardial infarction. Examples of prescribed beta blockers include acebutolol, atenolol, bisoprolol, metoprolol, nadolol, nebivolol, and propranolol. Patients taking beta blockers typically experience early fatigue with exercise; an alternative to HR monitoring, such as Ratings of Perceived Exertion scale, should be considered to monitor exercise intensity.[52] See additional discussion in Chapter 13, Heart Disease.

Systemic or Local Heat

During periods of fever, HR will increase. The body will attempt to dissipate heat by vasodilation of peripheral vessels. HR will increase to shunt blood flow to cutaneous areas for cooling. Local applications of thermal modalities (such as a hot pack) may also elevate HR to increase blood flow to cutaneous areas secondary to arteriolar and capillary dilation.

Pulse Sites

A peripheral pulse can be monitored at a variety of sites on the body (Fig. 2.15). A superficial artery located over a bone or underlying firm surface is easiest to palpate. Box 2.4 identifies the peripheral pulse locations, provides example indications for their use, and shows palpation sites.[47,50,53]

The apical (central) pulse is considered the most accurate because it measures the actual sounds of the heart values opening and closing. It is monitored by auscultation (listening), using a stethoscope directly over the apex (lower portion pointing to the left) of the heart. Apical pulses are used when peripheral pulses are weak or imperceptible, when other sites are either inaccessible (e.g., surgery) or difficult to palpate (e.g., infants), and when the effects of cardiac medications designed to alter HR and rhythm need to be monitored.

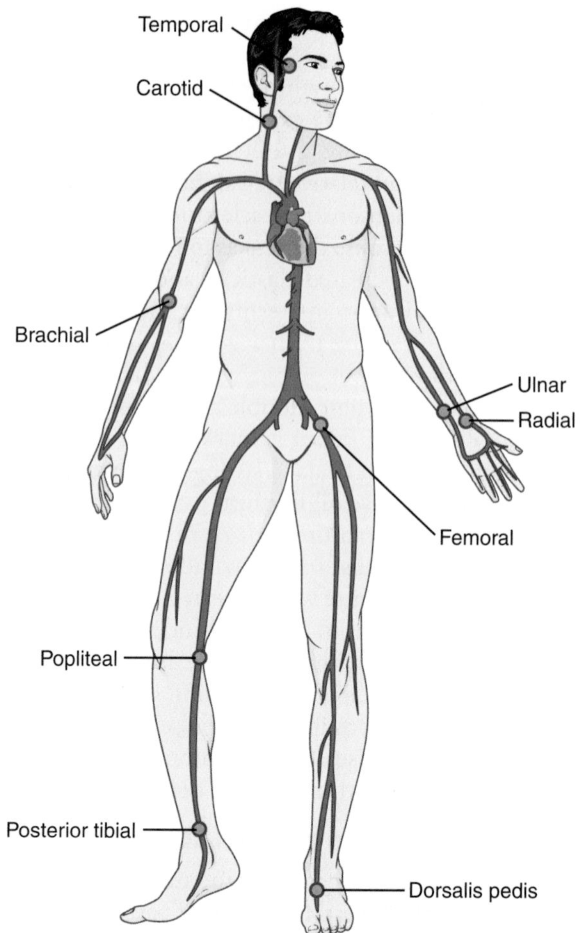

Figure 2.15 Common sites for monitoring peripheral pulses.

Monitoring Pulse

Peripheral pulses are monitored by palpation using the index and third finger of one hand. The thumb should not be used because it has its own pulse, which will interfere with monitoring. Generally, a light pressure is used initially to locate the pulse, and then more firm pressure is used when determining the rate, rhythm, and quality. The fingertips should be moved gently over the selected site until the strongest pulsation is found. To monitor resting values, the patient should be resting quietly for at least 5 minutes prior to the pulse measurement.

The radial artery is the most common site for measuring the pulse. With few modifications, the same procedure can be followed for monitoring at other pulse sites.

Measuring Radial Pulse

A. Assemble equipment: Watch with a second hand.
B. Wash hands.
C. Procedure:
  1. Explain procedure and rationale in terms appropriate to the patient's understanding.
  2. Ensure patient understanding, modesty, safety, and comfort.
  3. Place the patient's wrist in a neutral position relative to flexion and extension, and support the forearm. If measuring from supine, the forearm can be supported across the patient's chest or at his or her side with partial flexion of the elbow. From a sitting position, the forearm can rest across the patient's thigh, supported by a pillow or the therapist's arm. This relaxed positioning of the UE generally facilitates artery palpation.

Box 2.4 Pulse Location, Indications for Use, and Palpation Sites

Pulse Location and Indications for Use	Palpation Sites
Temporal: Over temporal bone; superior and lateral to the eye. Used with infants, when radial pulse inaccessible, and by anesthesiologists for monitoring during surgery.	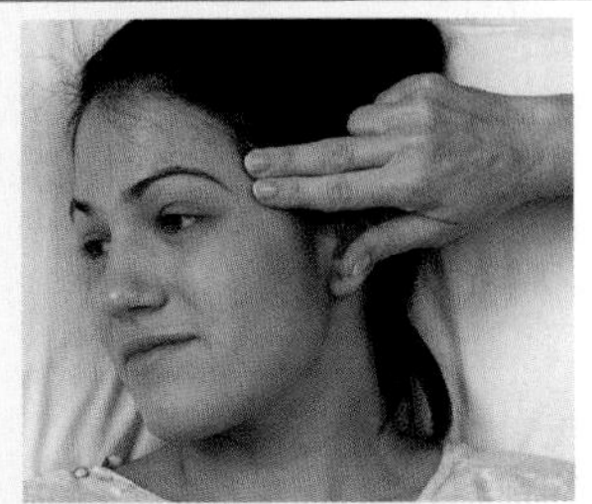
Carotid: On either side of the lower neck, below the jaw, fingers over thyroid cartilage between the trachea and medial border of sternocleidomastoid. Used with infants, during shock or cardiac arrest, to monitor cranial circulation; easily accessible if other peripheral pulses difficult or too weak to locate.[i]	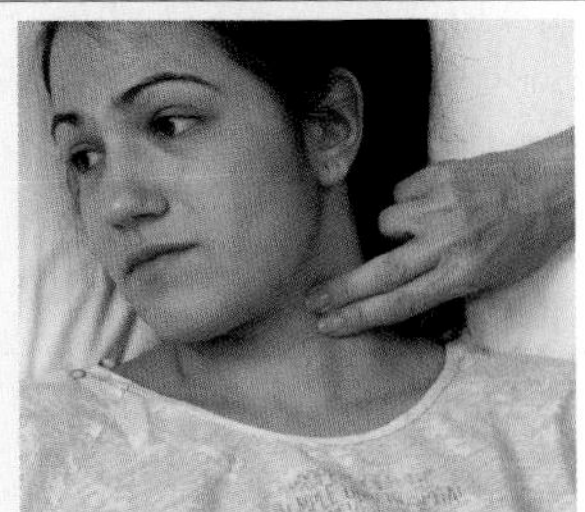
Brachial: Medial aspect of antecubital fossa, elbow should be slightly flexed and supported to avoid contraction of biceps. Used to monitor blood pressure and during cardiac arrest.	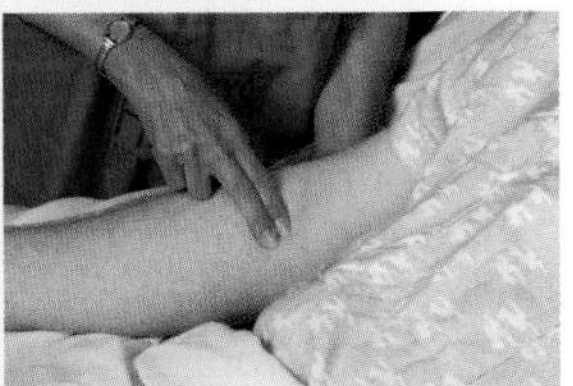
Radial: Distal radius at base of the thumb, lateral to tendon of the flexor carpi radialis. Most common site for peripheral pulse monitoring; easy to locate and easily accessible.	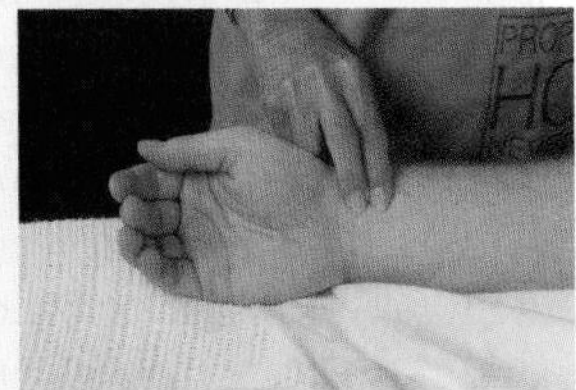
Femoral: Inferior to the inguinal ligament, midway between the anterior superior iliac spine and the symphysis pubis; typically monitored in supine. Used to monitor lower extremity circulation and during cardiac arrest.	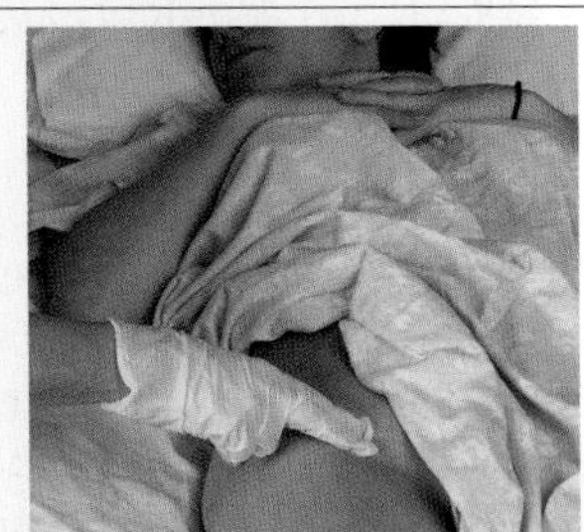
Popliteal: Inferior aspect of popliteal fossa; popliteal artery is deep and at times may be difficult to palpate; typically monitored in prone position with knee flexed to relax hamstrings and popliteal fascia; can also be accomplished in supine position. Used to monitor thigh blood pressure and lower extremity circulation; weak or absent popliteal pulse may indicate impaired flow or blockage in femoral artery.	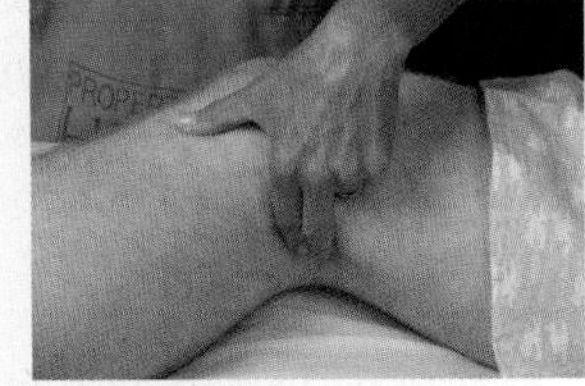

Continued

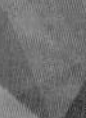

Box 2.4 Pulse Location, Indications for Use, and Palpation Sites—cont'd

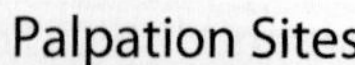

Pulse Location and Indications for Use	Palpation Sites
Pedal (dorsalis pedis): Dorsal, medial aspect of foot, lateral to the tendon of the extensor hallicus longus; ankle should be slightly dorsiflexed; some individuals have congenitally nonpalpable pedal pulses. Used to monitor circulation to feet.	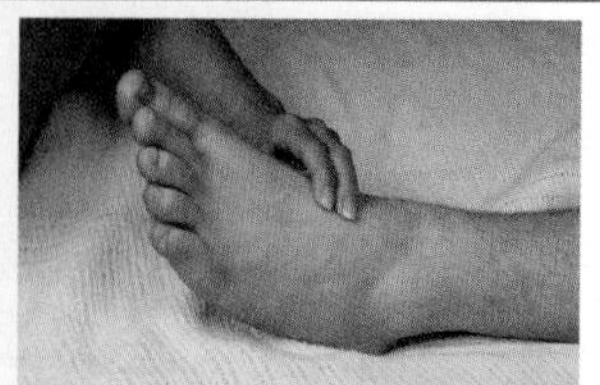
Posterior tibial: Posterior and inferior to the medial malleolus. Used to monitor circulation to feet; weak or absent pulse may be indicative of arterial disease (e.g., atherosclerosis) or occlusion.	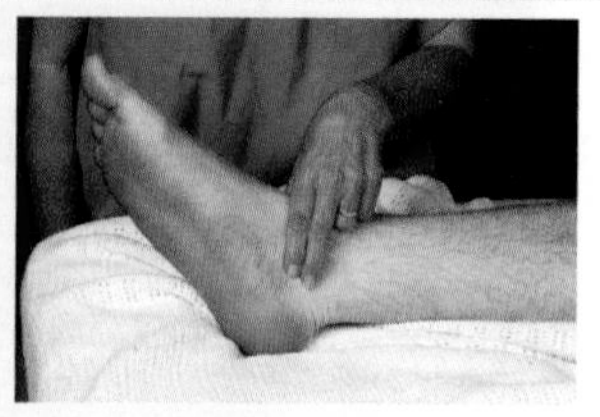

Images from Wilkinson, JM, et al,[47, pp. 191–194] with permission.

[i] ***Precaution:*** Pressure should never be applied bilaterally over carotid arteries or high on the neck to avoid stimulation of the carotid sinus and a subsequent reflex drop in pulse rate and blood pressure.

4. Place the fingers squarely and firmly over the radial pulse; use only enough pressure to feel the pulse accurately. If the pressure is too great, it will occlude the artery.
5. Once the strongest pulsation is located, note the position of the second hand on the watch. The first pulsation should be counted as zero to avoid overestimating. Determine the *rate* (number of beats per minute) by counting the pulse for 30 seconds and multiplying by 2; if any irregularities are noted, a full 60-second count should be taken to improve accuracy. Note the *rhythm* (time intervals between pulse beats) and the *quality* (force) of the pulse.
6. Wash hands.

Measuring Apical Pulse

A. Assemble equipment: Watch with a second hand, stethoscope, and antiseptic wipes for cleaning earpieces and diaphragm of stethoscope before and after use.
B. Wash hands.
C. Procedure:
  1. Explain the procedure and rationale in terms appropriate to the patient's level of understanding. Indicate that there will be a request to remain quiet during monitoring to avoid interference with auscultation.
  2. Ensure patient understanding, modesty, safety, and comfort. Apical pulses are typically monitored with the patient either supine or sitting.
  3. Use an antiseptic wipe to clean the earpieces and diaphragm of the stethoscope.
  4. Expose the sternum and chest.
  5. Locate the site where pulse will be monitored; the apical pulse is located approximately 3.5 inches (8.9 cm) to the left of the midsternum, in the fifth intercostal space, within an inch of the midclavicular line drawn parallel to the sternum (Fig. 2.16). These landmarks are guides to locating the apical pulse. In some individuals, a stronger pulse may be noted by altering placement of the stethoscope (e.g., placement in the fourth or sixth intercostal space).
  6. Place the earpieces of the stethoscope (tilting slightly forward) into the ears. The tubes of the stethoscope should not be crossed and should hang freely.
  7. Place the flat disk diaphragm of the stethoscope over the apex of the heart and locate the point where the apical pulse is heard most clearly. This is called the *point of maximal impulse*. If the rhythm is regular, count the pulse for 30 seconds and multiply by 2. If any irregularities are noted, take a full 60-second count. The pulse will be heard as a *lub-dub*. The first heart sound (S1 ["lub"]) is caused by closure of the atrioventricular (tricuspid and mitral) valves at the beginning of systole. The second heart sound (S2 ["dub"]) is caused by closure of the semilunar (aortic and pulmonic) valves at the end of systole.
  8. Wash hands and clean the stethoscope. If the same examiner is using the stethoscope again, it is not necessary to clean the earpieces; the diaphragm should always be cleaned.

Measuring Apical–Radial Pulse

Monitoring the apical–radial pulse involves two examiners simultaneously measuring the pulse at two separate locations: (1) the apical pulse at the apex of the heart; and (2) the radial pulse at the wrist. The values from the

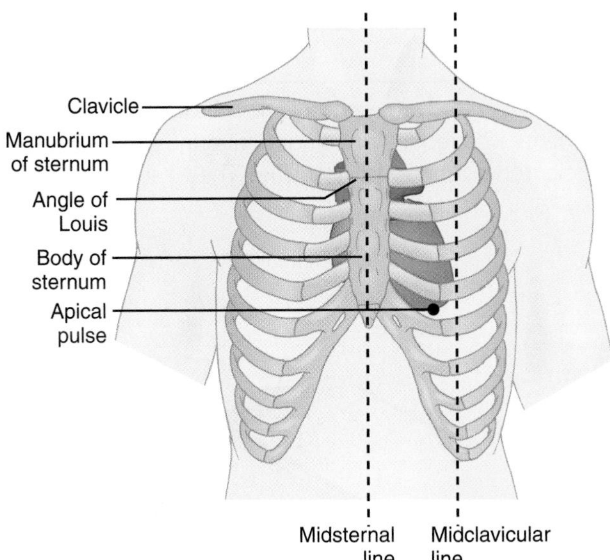

Figure 2.16 The apical pulse is located approximately 3.5 inches to the left of the midsternum, in the fifth intercostal space.

two different sites are then compared. Typically, the apical and radial pulse values are the same. However, in some situations (e.g., variations in SV or vascular occlusion), blood pumped from the heart may not be reaching the distal site, causing a weak or imperceptible radial pulse. For example, if the heart contracts prematurely, the ventricles have insufficient time to fill, resulting in a diminished SV and creating an imperceptible pulse in the radial artery.[32] On the other hand, SV may be normal with a weak or imperceptible radial pulse, suggesting a more peripheral problem such as impaired flow or blockage within a vessel. In either situation, there is a deficit in the number of radial pulses when compared with the number of apical pulses.[32] This is called a *pulse deficit,* defined as the difference between the rate of radial and apical pulses. The value of this measure is that it provides important information about the cardiovascular system's ability to perfuse the body.

Automated Heart Rate Monitoring

Advances are continual in the design, features, accuracy, waterproofing, information storage capacity, and Bluetooth capabilities of heart rate monitors (HRMs). In addition to monitoring HR, some HRMs provide data on HR variability (calculation of the time between pulses), real-time display of percentage of maximum HR, and estimates of maximal oxygen uptake (Vo_{2max}). Many HRMs allow data to be downloaded wirelessly to a computer (e.g., tablet, smartphone, watch) for analysis and storage using software programs and apps such as MOCAheart (MOCACARE, Palo Alto, CA 94303) and Health Mate (Withings, Cambridge, MA 02142). This provides a permanent record and sequential data on exercise performance. Most models allow programming of a prescribed exercise HR range with an audible and/or visible warning when the HR is outside the predetermined range. Some models include a talking feature that "speaks" HR information. Memory capabilities allow storage of exercise information over a variable number of exercise sessions.

HRMs consist of two basic elements: (1) a sensor that transmits data; and (2) a monitor that incorporates a receiver, microprocessor, and display. Wireless HRMs employ technology (Bluetooth, Bluetooth SMART, or ANT+) to allow information transfer between electronic devices while others include a lead wire with a distal sensor (e.g., earlobe clip, fingertip cover, or finger sleeve). Some monitors integrate sensors into a chest strap that provides wireless transmission of signals to a monitor worn as a wristwatch. Another style replaces the chest strap with fingertip sensors directly on the wristwatch. HR data are recorded when a fingertip is placed in contact with the sensor. Some HRMs are equipped with more than one type of sensor. This feature allows selection of the sensor that is most appropriate for the activity and the user.

HRMs are frequently used in prescribed exercise and training programs because they provide a practical, accurate method of pulse monitoring and are lightweight, comfortable, and easy to use. Many types of exercise training devices (e.g., treadmills, stair climbers, stationary bicycles, elliptical machines) incorporate HRMs directly into the unit by means of a metal handgrip sensor device.

Other HRM features are available and differ with the model and manufacturer. Among the more common features are multi-function wrist monitors (consisting of a watch, stopwatch, alarm clock, lap timer, calendar, and data storage), illuminated and large-number LCD displays (some with a zoom feature that doubles the size of information on the screen), visual graphics (e.g., "time in zone graph"), memory displays of previous training sessions, estimates of calories burned and energy expended during exercise, and HR statistics (average, minimum, maximum). Some units combine the ability to monitor HR with measures of blood oxygenation (oximetry). Several examples of personal vital signs monitors that include HRMs are presented in Box 2.5. As advances occur rapidly, manufacturer websites are a rich source of information about the most recent enhancements in features and technology.

Doppler Ultrasound

Doppler ultrasound (DUS) is a noninvasive instrument used to examine pulses that are extremely weak or faint or that are obliterated by even slight pressure or when arterial flow is severely compromised (e.g., deep vein thrombosis, superficial thrombophlebitis, arteriosclerosis, thromboangiitis obliterans, vascular tumors of the extremities). DUS is based on the principle that high-frequency ultrasound waves directed

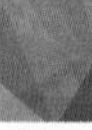

Box 2.5 Personal Vital Sign Monitors

Presented here are examples of personal vital sign monitors that connect wirelessly to electronic devices that display, analyze, and store data. These devices are an important accessory for patients who require ongoing monitoring of vital signs. They are relatively compact, easy to use, and can remain with the patient throughout daily activities. These monitors also indicate if data fall within normative or target (e.g., HR) ranges.

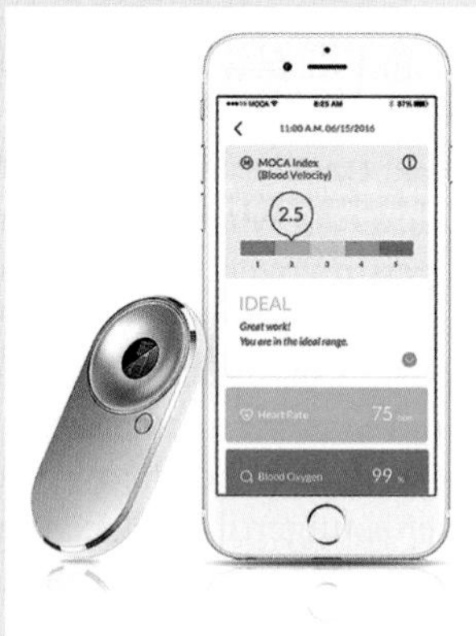

(A) This device measures heart rate, pulse wave velocity, and oxygen saturation (oximetry) *(Courtesy of MocaCare, Palo Alto, CA 94303.)*

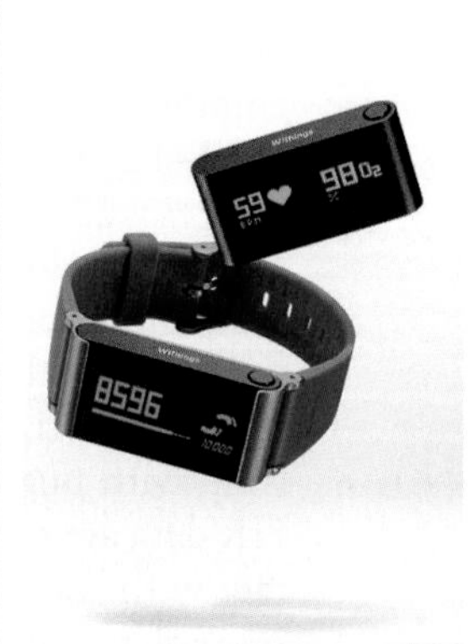

(B) Activity tracker, HR monitor, and pulse oximeter (used with wristband or clip) *(Courtesy of Withings, Cambridge, MA 02142.)*

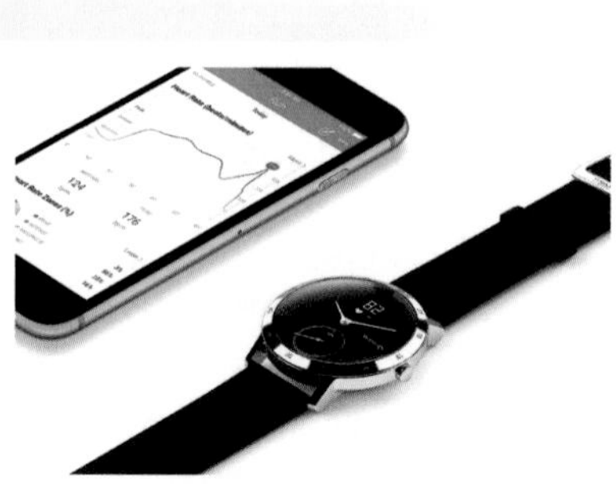

(C) Activity tracker and heart rate monitor *(Courtesy of Withings, Cambridge, MA 02142.)*

at a moving interface (i.e., blood flowing through a vessel) will cause a change in the wave frequency reflective of the velocity of the moving interface (called the *Doppler effect*). In essence, the DUS measures how sound waves are reflected off moving blood cells. The resultant frequency change caused by the movement alters the pitch of the sound waves as they are reflected back to the examiner; the pulse is heard as a swooshing sound.[54] The change in pitch heard by the examiner provides important information about the blood flow through a vessel.

The essential elements of a DUS device include the ultrasound unit, a handheld probe (piezoelectric crystal) that transmits and receives sound waves, and earpieces that look similar to those on a stethoscope or a small speaker to amplify the sound. Passed gently over the skin surface above an artery using ample coupling gel, the probe transmits high-frequency sound waves to an artery. The waves are disturbed by movement of the red blood cells, reflected back to the probe, and transformed into an amplified audible sound.[55]

The audible sound represents the difference in frequency between the waves directed at the vessel and those reflected back by motion of blood cells; the frequency is proportional to the velocity of the moving red blood cells. The absence of an audible sound indicates no detection of movement and, subsequently, no perfusion.[54] Using a computer interface, the flow measures can be graphically displayed and stored. It should be noted that although the specific characteristics of the reflected sounds are not diagnostic, they can assist in identifying abnormal flow.[56]

Pulse Oximetry

Pulse oximetry provides a measure of arterial blood oxygenation that is updated with each pulse wave. Oxygen is carried in the blood in two forms: (1) dissolved in arterial plasma; and (2) combined with hemoglobin.[31] Arterial plasma transports only about 3% of the oxygen in blood and is measured as Pao_2 (partial pressure of oxygen). The greater amount of oxygen (approximately 97%) is carried by hemoglobin and measured as Sao_2 (arterial hemoglobin oxygen saturation). Pulse oximetry measures arterial blood oxygen saturation as a noninvasive intervention.[57] Oxygen saturation via pulse oximetry is reported as Spo_2[58] and can be measured at any adequately perfused peripheral pulse.

Normal oxygen saturation levels are between 96% and 100%. In general, saturation levels below 90% are considered significant and warrant additional testing beyond the data provided by pulse oximetry (e.g., arterial blood gas analysis), as well as marking the potential need for administration of supplemental oxygen.[59] *Hypoxemia* is a term used to describe deficient oxygenation of the blood. *Hypoxia* is a diminished supply of oxygen available to body tissues, and *anoxia* is the complete lack of oxygen,[33] a condition that can be sustained for only a very brief period.

Alterations in heart function (e.g., heart attack, heart failure, arrhythmias) typically reduce cardiac output and the amount of oxygen delivered to tissues. Lung conditions also affect oxygen saturation levels and impair ability of the lungs to oxygenate blood. These include anemia (reduction in number of hemoglobin molecules available to carry oxygen), hypoventilation (e.g., COPD, bronchitis, emphysema, pneumonia, asthma), and diffusion impairments that affect blood-gas exchange (e.g., alveolar fibrosis, interstitial fluid).

The pulse oximeter provides data on the percent of oxygen that is combined with hemoglobin (Spo_2). In hospital settings, pulse oximeters are typically included in units designed to gather multiple measures such as pulse, temperature, and BP (see Fig 2.7B). Portable units are relatively small (Fig. 2.17), are easy to use and transport, and provide the therapist with immediate information about the patient's saturation levels. (Personal vital sign monitors also frequently include pulse oximetry [see Box 2.5].) The display provides a digital percentage of the amount of hemoglobin saturated with oxygen and a pulsatile waveform and pulse rate, with an audible signal indicating each pulsation. The patient interface is provided by a lead wire and sensor that attaches to the unit. The sensor is placed over a pulsating arteriolar vascular bed.[58] Several types of sensors are available, including fingertip sleeves, adhesive designs for use on fingertips and forehead (temporal artery), as well as nasal, earlobe, and foot styles. Others are self-contained and clip over the distal finger. The sensors contain two light sources (red and infrared) and a photodetector. The dual light source is used because oxygenated and deoxygenated hemoglobin have different patterns of light absorption.[60] The ratio of the amount of each light absorbed during systole and diastole allows quantification of an oxygen saturation measurement (Spo_2).[58-60]

Pulse oximetry contributes to (1) early identification of hypoxemia; (2) monitoring patient tolerance to activity; and (3) evaluating patient response to treatment. Pulse oximetry measures may be done continuously, intermittently to generate a series of values over time, or as a single measure at a given point in time (e.g., as an initial screening tool). The measurement pattern will be determined within the context of the patient history and examination findings. Telemetry oximetry monitoring allows continuous communication of Spo_2 data from remote locations.[58]

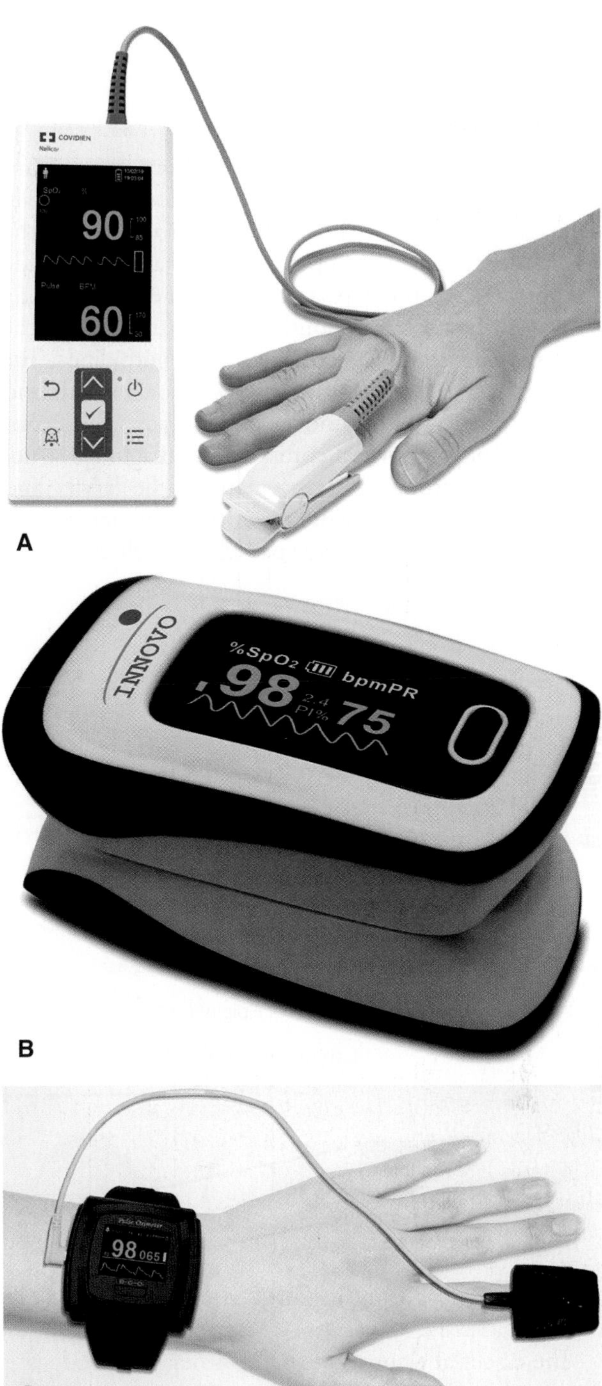

Figure 2.17 Pulse oximeters provide data on arterial blood oxygen saturation as well as pulse rate. (A) Hand-held unit with fingertip sensor. *(A, Courtesy of Medtronic, Boulder, CO 80301.)* (B) Fingertip clip design. (C) Wrist unit with finger sleeve. *(B, C, Courtesy of Innovo Medical, Stafford, TX, 77477.)*

RESPIRATION

The primary function of respiration (movement of air into and out of the lungs) is to supply the body with oxygen for metabolic activity and to remove carbon dioxide. The respiratory system consists of a series of branching tubes and brings atmospheric oxygen into contact with the gas exchange membrane of the lungs in the alveoli. Oxygen is then transported throughout the body via the cardiovascular system. *External respiration* is the exchange of oxygen and carbon dioxide between the lungs and the environment. *Internal respiration* is the exchange of oxygen and carbon dioxide between the circulating blood and body tissues.

Respiratory System

The entire pathway that transports air from the environment extends from the mouth and nose down to the alveolar sacs. Figure 2.18 illustrates the structures of the respiratory system. The upper respiratory airways include the nose, mouth, pharynx, and larynx. Air enters the body by way of the nose and mouth and is then moved to the pharynx, where it is warmed, filtered, and humidified. The pharynx serves as a common pathway for both air and food. Inspired air is then moved to the larynx, which contains the epiglottis, vocal cords, and cartilaginous structures. The anatomical arrangement of the larynx and pharyngeal muscles provides the critical function of protecting the lungs from foreign particles, as well as assisting with phonation (production of vocal sounds) and coughing, which is the primary physiological mechanism for clearing the airways. The *laryngopharynx* is the area where solid and liquid food intake is separated from inspired air. It is also the site of bifurcation into the larynx and esophagus. The pharyngeal muscles close the glottis during swallowing to protect the lungs from aspiration. If a foreign body passes the glottis and enters the tracheobronchial tree, the cough reflex is initiated to clear the air passage. Immediately below the thyroid cartilage of the larynx (i.e., the Adam's apple) is the site for emergency opening to the tracheal air pathway (*tracheostomy*).[33,61,62]

The trachea is approximately 4 to 5 inches (11 to 13 cm) long and continues from the cartilaginous structures of the neck into the thorax. At the level of the carina, the trachea divides into two mainstem bronchi. The carina contains the majority of cough receptors and is located

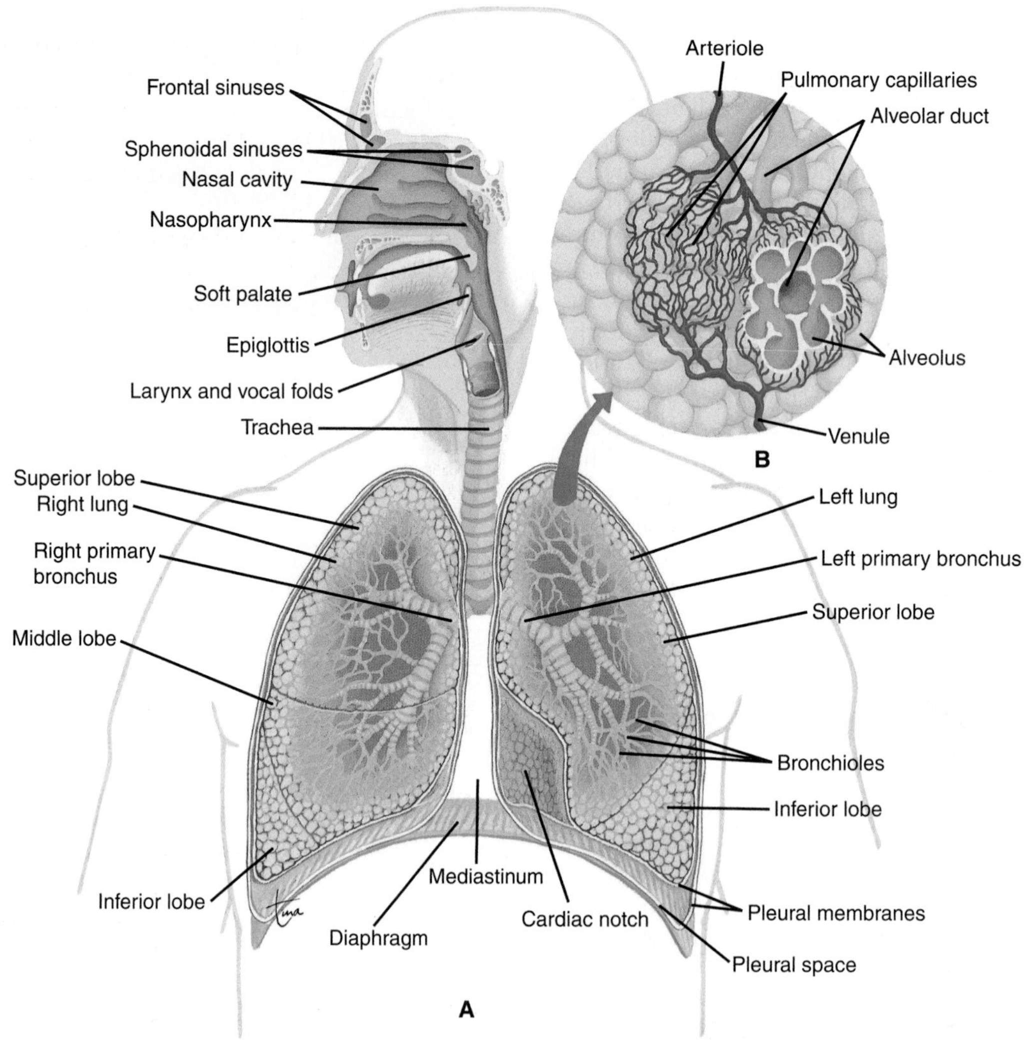

Figure 2.18 Structures of the respiratory system. (A) Anterior view of the upper and lower respiratory tracts. (B) Microscopic view of alveoli and pulmonary capillaries. (The colors represent the vessels, not the oxygen content of the blood within the vessels.) *(From Scanlon and Sanders,[61, p. 386] with permission.)*

approximately between the sternum and manubrium at the second intercostal space. The right and left mainstem bronchi are asymmetrical in size and shape and continue into the lower respiratory tract, further subdividing into the respiratory bronchioles, where gas exchange begins. However, gas exchange primarily occurs in the alveolar ducts and the large surface area provided by the alveoli. The respiratory bronchioles, alveolar ducts, and alveoli (alveolar sacs) comprise the *respiratory zone* for gas exchange (Fig. 2.19). The *conductive zone* (trachea, bronchi, and terminal bronchioles) provides for continuous movement of air into and out of the lungs; these areas do not contribute to gas exchange.[33,60-63]

Inspiration is initiated by contraction of the diaphragm and intercostal muscles. During contraction of these muscles, the diaphragm moves downward and the intercostals lift the ribs and sternum up and outward. The thoracic cavity is thus increased in size and allows for lung expansion. Normal inspiration lasts 1 to 1.5 seconds. During relaxed breathing, expiration is essentially a passive process. Once the respiratory muscles relax, the thorax returns to its resting position, and the lungs recoil. This ability to recoil occurs because of the inherent elastic properties of the lungs. Normal expiration lasts 2 to 3 seconds.[50]

Regulatory Mechanisms

Regulation of respiratory function involves multiple components of both neural and chemical control and is closely integrated with the cardiovascular system. Breathing is controlled by the respiratory center, which lies bilaterally in the pons and medulla. Motor nerves whose cell bodies are located in this area control the respiratory muscles. The respiratory center provides control of both the *rate* and the *depth* of breathing in response to the metabolic needs of the body.[64]

Both *central* and *peripheral* chemoreceptors influence respiration. *Central* chemoreceptors are located in the respiratory center and are sensitive to changes in either carbon dioxide or hydrogen ion levels of arterial blood. An increase in either carbon dioxide levels or hydrogen ions will stimulate breathing.[32] *Peripheral* chemoreceptors are located at the bifurcation of the carotid arteries (carotid bodies) and in the arch of the aorta (aortic bodies). These receptors are sensitive to the partial pressure of oxygen (PaO_2) in the arterial blood. When PaO_2 levels in arterial blood drop, afferent impulses carry this information to the respiratory center. Motor neurons to the respiratory muscles are stimulated to increase tidal volume (amount of air exchanged with each breath) or, with very low oxygen levels, to increase the respiratory rate as well. These peripheral chemoreceptors cause an increase in respiration only when PaO_2 levels fall to approximately 60 mm Hg (from a normal level of about 90 to 100 mm Hg). This is because the receptors are sensitive only to PaO_2 levels in plasma and not to the total oxygen in blood.[32,64]

Respiration also is influenced by a protective stretch mechanism called the *Hering-Breuer reflex*. Pulmonary stretch receptors throughout the walls of the lungs detect

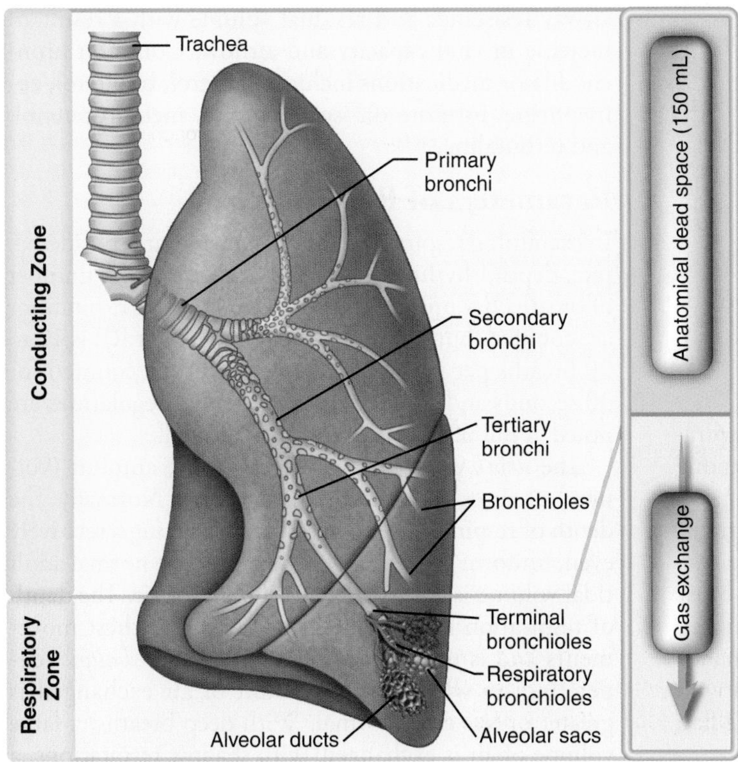

Figure 2.19 Primary components of the conducting and respiratory zones. The conducting zone transports inhaled air to and from the respiratory zone where air exchange takes place. The air exchange occurs in progressively increasing increments in the respiratory bronchioles, alveolar ducts, and alveolar sacs. *(Adapted from Van Guilder and Janot,[62, p. 132] with permission.)*

the amount of stretch imposed by entering air. When overstretched, these receptors send impulses to the respiratory center to inhibit further inspiration and increase the duration of expiration. Impulses stop at the end of expiration so that another inspiration can be initiated. In adults, this reflex is rarely demonstrated and would likely not be activated until tidal volume reached higher than 1.5 liters.[32] Respiration is also stimulated by vigorous movements of joints and muscle (exercise) and is strongly influenced by voluntary cortical control.

Factors Influencing Respiration

Multiple factors can alter normal, relaxed, effortless respiration. As with temperature and pulse, any influence that increases the metabolic rate also will increase RR. Increased metabolism and subsequent demand for oxygen will stimulate increased respiration. Conversely, as metabolic demands diminish, respirations also will decrease. Several influencing factors are of particular importance when examining respiration. These include age, body size, stature, exercise, and body position.

Age

The RR of a newborn is between 30 and 90 breaths per minute. The rate gradually slows until adulthood, when it ranges between 12 and 20 breaths per minute. In elderly individuals, the RR increases owing to decreased elasticity of the lungs and decreased efficiency of gas exchange. Other factors associated with normal aging that affect respiratory function include weakening of respiratory muscles, deterioration of alveolar walls, decreased thoracic mobility, and decreased lung volumes.[65]

Body Size and Stature

Men generally have a larger vital capacity than women, adults larger than adolescents, and children. Tall, thin individuals generally have a larger vital capacity than stout or obese individuals. With larger lung capacity there is also a lower RR.

Exercise

Respiratory rate and depth will increase with exercise as a result of increased oxygen demand and carbon dioxide production.

Body Position

The recumbent position can significantly affect respiration and predispose the patient to stasis of fluids. Among the influential factors that limit normal lung expansion when lying down are compression of the chest against the supporting surface and pressure from abdominal organs against the diaphragm. Both of these factors cause increased resistance to breathing. Difficult recumbent breathing is common during the late stages of pregnancy as the fetus shifts the diaphragm upward. Patients with CHF also experience labored breathing when lying flat, which improves when standing or sitting up.

Environment

Exposure to pollutants such as gas and particle emissions, asbestos, chemical waste products, or coal dust can diminish the ability to transport oxygen. Other common offending pollutants include high ozone concentrations, sulfur dioxide, and carbon monoxide.[36] These respiratory irritants typically increase mucus production. High altitudes also affect the respiratory system owing to reduced air mass (i.e., the partial pressure of oxygen in inspired air is low). This means fewer oxygen molecules per liter of air, reducing arterial blood oxygen levels and triggering shortness of breath (*dyspnea*) and reduced tolerance to activity. Hyperventilation, tachycardia, and pulmonary edema (accumulation of fluid in alveolar walls) can also occur at high altitudes.[36,66,67]

Emotions/Stress

Stress and emotions can cause an increased rate and depth of respirations owing to stimulation of the sympathetic nervous system.

Pharmacological Agents

Essentially any drug that depresses central nervous system (CNS) function will result in respiratory depression. Narcotic agents (e.g., opioids, meperidine hydrochloride) will decrease the rate and depth of respirations. Other categories of CNS depressant agents include barbiturates (e.g., phenobarbital, secobarbital), benzodiazepines (e.g., lorazepam, midazolam, diazepam), neuroleptics (e.g., chlorpromazine, haloperidol, clozapine), muscle relaxants, tricyclic antidepressants, and anticonvulsants. Conversely, bronchodilators decrease airway resistance and residual volume with a resultant increase in vital capacity and airflow. Common bronchodilator medications include albuterol, bitolterol, epinephrine, formoterol, isoproterenol, metaproterenol, and terbutaline.[68,69]

Parameters of Respiration

In examining respiration, four parameters are considered: rate, depth, rhythm, and sound. The *rate* is the number of breaths per minute. Either inspirations or expirations are counted, but not both. The normal adult RR is 12 to 20 breaths per minute. The rate should be counted for 30 seconds and multiplied by 2. If any irregularities are noted, a full 60-second count is indicated.

The *depth* of respiration refers to the amount (volume) of air exchanged with each breath. Normally, the depth of respirations is consistent, producing a relatively even, uniform movement of the chest. The normal adult tidal volume is approximately 500 mL of air. The depth of respiration is determined by observing chest movements and is usually described as *deep* or *shallow,* depending on whether the amount of air exchanged is greater or less than normal. With deep breaths, a large volume of air is exchanged; with shallow respirations, a small amount of air is exchanged, typically with minimal lung expansion or chest wall movement.

The *rhythm* refers to the regularity of inspirations and expirations. Normally, there is an even time interval between respirations. The respiratory rhythm is described as *regular* (normal) or *irregular* (abnormal).

The *sound* of respirations refers to deviations from normal, quiet, effortless breathing. Although some respiratory sounds are audible, accurate identification requires auscultation (listening with a stethoscope placed directly against the chest wall). Normal (*vesicular*) breath sounds are heard primarily during inspiration and sound relatively smooth and soft.[60] Common abnormal (*adventitious*) sounds of breathing include the following:

- **Wheeze (Wheezing):** A continuous whistling sound produced by air passing through a narrowed airway such as a bronchi or bronchiole. This is often compared to the whistling produced when stretching the neck of a balloon and allowing air to escape slowly through the narrowed passageway. It may be heard on both inspiration and expiration but is more prominent on expiration. Wheezing is a common symptom of asthma and is also seen in CHF. It can also result from an airway obstruction.
- **Stridor:** A harsh, high-pitched crowing sound that occurs with upper airway obstructions resulting in narrowing of the glottis or trachea. It is apparent in patients with tracheal stenosis or presence of a foreign object.
- **Crackles (rales):** Rattling or bubbling sounds caused by secretions in the air passages of the respiratory tract. The sound is often compared to that of rustling a cellophane bag. Crackles may be heard with the ear but are most accurately determined using a stethoscope. Crackles are apparent in patients with CHF.
- **Sigh:** A deep inspiration followed by a prolonged, audible expiration. Occasional sighs are normal and function to expand alveoli; frequent sighs are abnormal and may be indicative of emotional stress.
- **Stertor:** A snoring sound owing to partial obstruction (e.g., secretions) in the upper airway (e.g., trachea, large bronchi).

Patterns of Respiration

Examination of the rate, rhythm, and depth allows the therapist to determine the pattern of respiration. Not all patients will present with a distinct pattern of respiration. However, several patterns occur with sufficient frequency that uniform terminology has been developed for their identification. Common respiratory patterns are presented in Figure 2.20.

Eupnea is the term used to describe a normal breathing pattern of 12 to 20 times per minute in an adult. Hyperventilation is an abnormally fast rate and depth of respiration often associated with anxiety, emotional stress, and panic disorders. A common response to an acute episode is to have the patient rebreathe into a paper bag, which replaces some of the lost carbon dioxide (hypocapnia). CNS or pulmonary disorders may cause prolonged hyperventilation. Hypoventilation is a reduction in the rate and depth of respirations. This decrease in the amount of air entering the lungs causes an increase in arterial carbon dioxide levels.

Difficult or labored breathing is called *dyspnea*. Patients with dyspnea require increased, noticeable effort to breathe and often appear as if struggling to get air into the lungs. In an effort to increase effectiveness of respiration, accessory muscles such as the intercostals and abdominals are often active. The intercostals assist in raising the ribs to expand the thoracic cavity; the abdominals assist function of the diaphragm. Additional muscles that may provide accessory functions in respiration are the sternocleidomastoid, pectoralis major and minor, scalenes, and subclavius. Use of accessory muscles to breathe is referred to as costal or thoracic breathing. Pain and nasal flaring sometimes accompany dyspnea (to bring in more oxygen). Acute episodes may be brought on by blockage of an air passage, infection of the respiratory tract, or trauma to the thorax. Long-standing dyspnea is a hallmark of COPD, such as asthma or bronchitis.

Orthopnea is difficult or labored breathing (dyspnea) when the patient is lying down that is relieved by sitting or standing. The change in positioning causes gravity to lower the abdominal organs, allowing increased room for chest expansion. Orthopnea is a characteristic symptom of CHF and also may be seen with asthma, advanced emphysema, and pulmonary edema. *Tachypnea* is an abnormally fast RR, usually greater than 24 breaths per minute. This pattern is seen with respiratory insufficiency and fever as the body attempts to rid itself of excess heat. *Bradypnea* is an abnormally slow RR, usually 10 breaths or fewer per minute. Bradypnea is associated with impairment of the respiratory control center, as may occur with increased intracranial pressure (tumor), drug intake (narcotics), or metabolic disorder. *Apnea* is the absence of respirations and is usually transient. If sustained for longer than several minutes, brain damage and death may occur. Cheyne-Stokes respiration is characterized by a period of apnea lasting 10 to 60 seconds, followed by gradually increasing depth and frequency of respirations (hyperventilation). It occurs with depression of the cerebral hemispheres (e.g., coma), in basal ganglia disease, and occasionally in CHF.

Respiratory Examination

Because respiration is under both voluntary (cortical) and involuntary control, it is important that the patient is unaware that respiration is being examined. Once aware of the examination, characteristics of the breathing pattern will likely be altered. This is a normal reaction to being observed. It is often recommended that respirations be observed immediately after taking the pulse. After monitoring the pulse, the fingers can remain in place at the

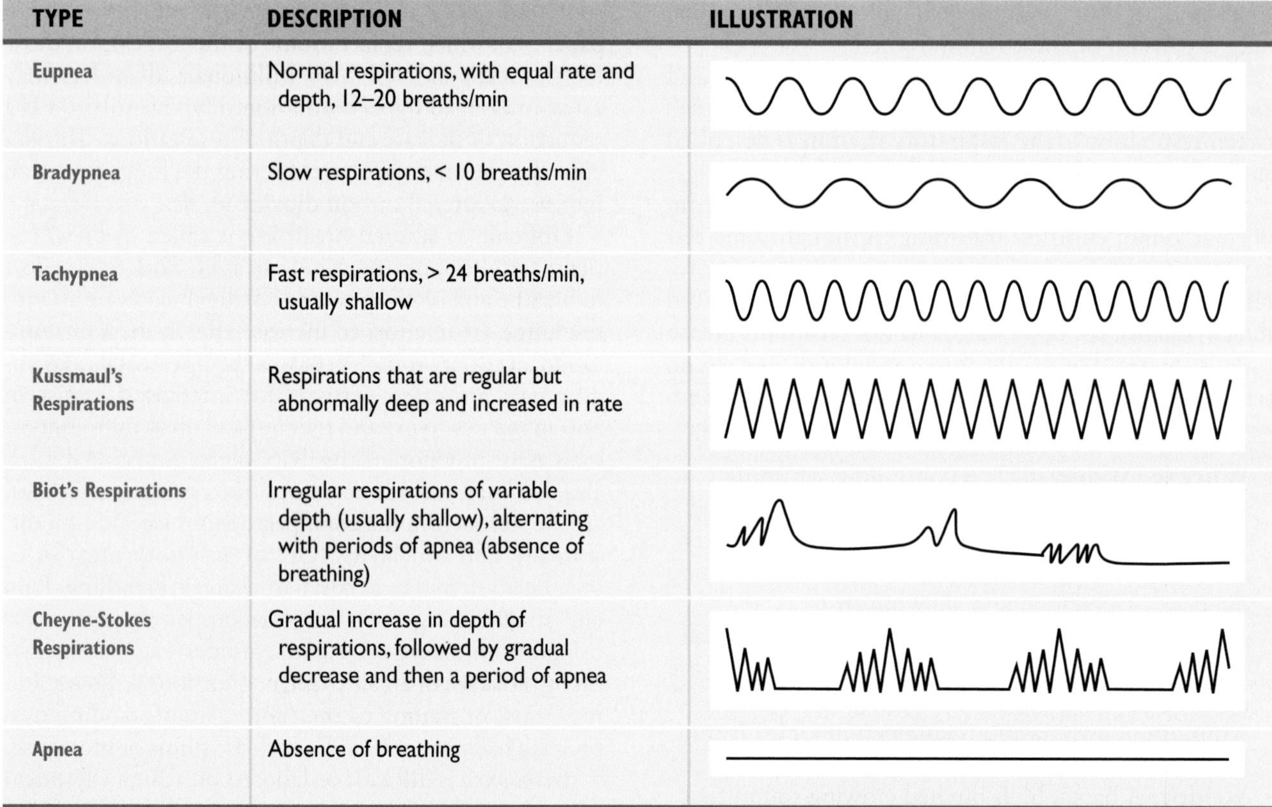

TYPE	DESCRIPTION	ILLUSTRATION
Eupnea	Normal respirations, with equal rate and depth, 12–20 breaths/min	
Bradypnea	Slow respirations, < 10 breaths/min	
Tachypnea	Fast respirations, > 24 breaths/min, usually shallow	
Kussmaul's Respirations	Respirations that are regular but abnormally deep and increased in rate	
Biot's Respirations	Irregular respirations of variable depth (usually shallow), alternating with periods of apnea (absence of breathing)	
Cheyne-Stokes Respirations	Gradual increase in depth of respirations, followed by gradual decrease and then a period of apnea	
Apnea	Absence of breathing	

Figure 2.20 Normal (eupnea) and abnormal respiratory patterns. *(From Wilkinson, et al,[8, p. 444] with permission.)*

pulse site, and respirations can be monitored without drawing the patient's conscious attention to his or her breathing pattern. Ideally, respiration should be examined with the chest exposed. If this is not possible, or if respirations cannot be easily observed through clothing, maintain fingers on the radial pulse site and place the patient's forearm across the chest. This will allow limited palpation without drawing conscious input from the patient. Chapter 12, Chronic Pulmonary Dysfunction, provides a more thorough discussion of the respiratory examination.

Monitoring Respiration

A. Assemble equipment: Watch with a second hand.

B. Wash hands.

C. Procedure:

1. Ensure patient understanding, safety, modesty, and comfort. Respirations are typically monitored with the patient either supine or sitting. *Note:* The patient should be in a quiet resting position for at least 5 minutes prior to monitoring respirations.
2. Expose chest area; if area cannot be exposed and respirations are not readily observable, place patient's forearm across chest and keep fingers positioned as if continuing to monitor the radial pulse.
3. As the patient breathes, observe the rise and fall of the chest; note the amount of effort required or audible sounds produced during breathing. (Normally, respiration is effortless and silent.)
4. Using the second hand of a watch, determine the rate by counting respirations (either inspirations or expirations, but not both) for 30 seconds and multiply by 2.
5. Identify the rhythm (regularity of inspirations and expirations); note deviations from normal uninterrupted, even spacing. If any irregularities are noted, count for a full 60 seconds to accommodate the fluctuations and ensure an accurate count.
6. Observe the depth of respiration; determine if a small, large, or approximately normal volume of air is inspired. Observe involvement of accessory muscles, which suggests weakness in the primary muscles of breathing (diaphragm and external intercostal muscles); if difficult to observe, palpation of chest wall excursion can be used to identify depth of respiration. Record as shallow, deep, or normal.

   Note: Chest wall excursion can also be determined by circumferential chest measures using a tape measure at three specific bony landmarks: (1) the sternal angle of Luis; (2) the xiphoid

process; and (3) midway between the xiphoid process and the umbilicus.
7. If indicated, determine the sound of breathing using a stethoscope.
8. Return clothing if chest has been exposed.
9. Wash hands.

BLOOD PRESSURE

Blood pressure refers to the force the blood exerts against a vessel wall. It is measured in millimeters of mercury (mm Hg) and recorded in the form of a fraction (e.g., 119/79). The top number indicates systolic pressure, and the bottom indicates diastolic pressure. Because liquid flows only from a higher to a lower pressure, the pressure is highest in the arteries, lower in the capillaries, and lowest in veins.[31,33]

Inasmuch as the heart is an intermittent pulsatile pump, pressure is measured at both the highest and lowest points of the pulse. These points represent the systolic (ventricular contraction) and diastolic (ventricular relaxation) pressures. The systolic pressure is the highest pressure exerted by the blood against the arterial walls. The diastolic pressure (which is constantly present) is the lowest pressure. The elastic properties of the arterial walls allow for expansion and recoil in response to the changing volume of circulating blood during the cardiac cycle. The mathematical difference between the systolic and diastolic pressures is called the *pulse pressure*. For example, a systolic pressure of 119 mm Hg and a diastolic pressure of 79 mm Hg result in a pulse pressure of 40 mm Hg.

BP is a function of two primary elements: (1) cardiac output (amount of blood flow, CO); and (2) peripheral resistance (impediment to blood flow within a vessel, R) that the heart must overcome. The relationship between BP, CO, and R is expressed in the equation: $BP = CO \times R$. Additional factors that contribute to this relationship include the diameter and elasticity of vessel walls, blood volume, and blood viscosity.

Blood Pressure Regulation

The *vasomotor center* is located bilaterally in the lower pons and upper medulla. It transmits impulses through sympathetic nerves to all vessels of the body. The vasomotor center is tonically active, producing a slow, continual firing in all vasoconstrictor nerve fibers. It is this slow, continual firing that maintains a partial state of contraction of the blood vessels and provides normal *vasomotor tone*.[35] The vasomotor center assists in providing the stable arterial pressure required to maintain blood flow to body tissue and organs. This occurs because of its close connection to the cardiac controlling center in the medulla (because changes in cardiac output will influence BP). In addition, the vasomotor and cardiac controlling centers require input from afferent receptors.

Afferent input regarding BP is provided primarily by *baroreceptors* and *chemoreceptors*. The *baroreceptors* (pressoreceptors) are stimulated by the stretch of the vessel wall from alterations in pressure. These receptors have a high concentration in the walls of the internal carotid arteries above the carotid bifurcation and in the walls of the aortic arch. Baroreceptors located in the *carotid sinuses* of the carotid arteries monitor BP to the brain. Baroreceptors in the *aortic sinuses* of the aortic arch are responsible for monitoring BP throughout the body.

In response to an increase in BP, the baroreceptor input to the vasomotor center results in an inhibition of the vasoconstrictor center of the medulla and excitation of the vagal center.[33] This results in a decreased HR, decreased force of cardiac contraction, and vasodilation, with a subsequent drop in BP. The baroreceptor input during a lowering of BP would produce the opposite effects.

The *chemoreceptors* are stimulated by reduced arterial oxygen concentrations, increases in carbon dioxide tension, and increased hydrogen ion concentrations. These receptors lie close to the baroreceptors. Those located in the carotid artery are called *carotid bodies,* and on the aortic arch they are termed *aortic bodies*. Impulses from these receptors travel to the brain (cardioregulatory and vasomotor centers) via afferent pathways in the vagus and glossopharyngeal nerves. Efferent impulses from these centers, in response to alterations in BP, will alter HR, strength of cardiac contractions, and size of blood vessels.[32]

Factors Influencing Blood Pressure

Many factors influence pressure. As with all vital signs, BP is represented by a range of normal values and will yield the most useful data when monitored over a period of time. Important influences to be considered when examining BP include blood volume, diameter and elasticity of arteries, cardiac output, age, exercise, and arm position.

Blood Volume

The amount of circulating blood in the body directly affects pressure. Blood loss (e.g., hemorrhage) will cause pressure to drop and can result in hypovolemic shock from inadequate tissue perfusion. Conversely, an increase in the amount of circulating blood (e.g., blood transfusion) will cause the pressure to rise. Reduced fluid volume, as may occur with diarrhea or inadequate oral intake (dehydration), will also lower BP; excess fluid, as occurs with CHF, will increase pressure. Essentially, any situation causing a shift (increase or decrease) in body fluids (intravascular, interstitial, or intracellular) will alter BP. Bladder distention can also contribute to BP elevation.

Diameter and Elasticity of Arteries

The diameter (size) of the vessel lumen will provide either *increased peripheral resistance* (vasoconstriction) or *decreased resistance* (vasodilation) to cardiac output. The elasticity of the vessel wall also influences resistance. Normally, the expansion and recoil properties of the arterial walls provide a continuous, smooth flow of blood into the capillaries and veins between heartbeats. With age, these properties are diminished; arterial stiffness decreases vessel wall compliance. Thus, there is a higher resistance to blood flow with resultant *increase* in BP.

A characteristic feature of arteriosclerosis is reduced vessel wall compliance in response to fluctuations in pressure. For older adults, elevated BP is often associated with the degenerative effects of arteriosclerosis. As the disease progresses, small arteries and arterioles lose elasticity, the walls become thick and hard and unable to yield to pressure exerted by blood flow, and the lumen gradually narrows and may eventually become blocked. Multiple factors can contribute to hypertension in elders (e.g., smoking, activity level, obesity, diet, comorbidities such as cardiac or vascular disease). In her extensive literature review, Pinto suggests that "The increase in BP with age is most likely due to complex and varied factors moulded [molded] and influenced by the individual environment and lifestyle."[70, p. 110]

Cardiac Output

When increased amounts of blood are pumped into the arteries, the walls of the vessels distend, resulting in a higher BP. With lower cardiac output, less blood is pushed into the vessel, and there is a subsequent drop in pressure.

Age

BP varies with age. It normally rises gradually after birth and reaches a peak during puberty. By late adolescence (18 to 19 years), adult BP is reached. For many years, the normal adult BP was considered 120/80 mm Hg. A BP value of 119/79 mm Hg or below is now the normal adult standard.[71,72] Table 2.6 presents new categories of BP from a recent report by the American College of Cardiology (ACC) and the American Heart Association (AHA) titled *Guideline for the Prevention, Detection, Evaluation, and Management of High Blood Pressure in Adults*.[71] The new guideline is an update of *The Seventh Report of the Joint National Committee on Prevention, Detection, Evaluation, and Treatment of High Blood Pressure*.[72]

The ACC/AHA guideline recognizes the high prevalence of hypertension that affects millions of individuals in the United States and worldwide and provides comprehensive information addressing its prevention and treatment. Hypertension is an important risk factor for many disorders, including myocardial infarct, heart failure, stroke, and kidney disease. The new ACC/AHA guideline[71] classifies normal adult BP as below 120/80 mm Hg, elevated BP as 120–129/80 mm Hg, hypertension stage 1 as 130–139/80–89 mm Hg, and hypertension stage 2 as 140/90 mm Hg or higher (see Table 2.6). The ACC/AHA "guideline is intended to be a resource for the clinical and public health practice communities. It is designed to be comprehensive but succinct and practical in providing guidance for prevention, detection, evaluation, and management of high BP."[71, p. 12]

Table 2.6 Adult Blood Pressure Categories[71]

BP Category	Systolic BP (mm Hg)	Diastolic BP (mm Hg)
Normal	<120	<80
Elevated	120–129	<80
Hypertension		
Stage 1	130–139	80–89
Stage 2	≥140	≥90

Clinical Note: Seen more frequently with elders is *white coat hypertension* or *nonsustained hypertension*. This occurs in individuals whose blood pressure is higher in a clinical setting than outside the clinic; it is believed to be associated with the stress and anxiety of seeing a health care professional (the "white coat").

Exercise

Physical activity increases cardiac output. In response to the intensity of the workload, there is a progressive increase in SBP, no change or a slight increase in DBP, and a widening of pulse pressure. Greater increases are noted in systolic pressure owing to proportional changes in pressure gradient of peripheral vessels. This means that although cardiac output during exercise is high, vasodilation reduces peripheral resistance to maintain a relatively lower diastolic pressure. A drop in SBP of 10 mm Hg or more with increasing exercise intensity or failure of SBP to increase with heightened workload is considered an abnormal response and is indication for stopping exercise.[43]

Valsalva Maneuver

The Valsalva maneuver is an attempt to exhale forcibly with the glottis, nose, and mouth closed. It causes an increase in intrathoracic pressure with an accompanying collapse of the veins of the chest wall. There is a subsequent decrease in blood flow to the heart, a decreased venous return, and a drop in BP. This maneuver serves to internally stabilize the abdominal and chest wall during periods of rapid and maximum exertion such as lifting a heavy object. When the breath is released, the intrathoracic pressure decreases, and venous return is suddenly reestablished as an "overshoot" mechanism to compensate for the drop in BP. In turn, there is a marked increase in HR and BP. This rapid rise in arterial pressure causes vagal slowing of the HR (bradycardia). Although the Valsalva maneuver can temporarily enhance muscle function via internal stabilization, it has an indirect undesirable effect of increasing BP and should be avoided by individuals with cardiac impairment and hypertension.[31,35]

Clinical Note: A common misconception concerning the Valsalva maneuver is that it directly increases HR and BP. As described earlier, it is the body's recovery mechanism of suddenly increasing venous return that causes this increase. The subsequent drop in BP due to the Valsalva maneuver may result in seeing "black dots" and the feeling of dizziness that often accompanies straining while lifting a heavy object.

Orthostatic Hypotension

Associated with prolonged immobility and periods of bedrest, orthostatic or postural hypotension is a sudden drop in BP that occurs when movement to upright postures (sitting or standing) is initiated. The positional change causes gravitational blood pooling in the lower extremity (LE) veins. Venous return and cardiac outputs are reduced, with resultant cerebral hypoperfusion. This can trigger an episode of light-headedness, dizziness, or even loss of consciousness (syncope). In response to positional changes under normal circumstances, BP is maintained by reflex vasoconstriction (via baroreceptors), which increases HR. After a period of inactivity, postural hypotension should be anticipated; it requires a gradual acclimation to the upright position until normal reflex control returns.

Other predisposing factors for postural hypotension include exercise, drugs such as antihypertensives and vasodilators, reduction in baroreceptor response with aging, the Valsalva maneuver, and hypovolemia (abnormally low volume of circulating blood).[73,74] Patients with CNS involvement of the autonomic nervous system (e.g., patients with acute cervical spinal cord injury or Parkinson's disease) typically exhibit episodes of orthostatic hypotension with position changes. As a useful precaution, any patient restricted to a recumbent position for even short periods should be considered at risk for postural hypotension. These events can be minimized by use of external pressure supports such as abdominal binders and support or full-length elastic stockings (elastic bandages can also be used effectively) and a very gradual acclimation to upright postures. Should postural hypotension occur during the examination, the patient should be moved to a sitting position from standing or a reclined position from sitting with the legs elevated.

Orthostatic hypotension is examined by first taking initial HR and BP with the patient in supine, at rest for 5 minutes. The patient is then moved directly to the standing position; HR and BP are repeated immediately and again at 3 minutes. A patient is orthostatic if SBP drops more than 20 mm Hg or if DBP drops more than 10 mm Hg, or if experiencing light-headedness or dizziness.[75]

Arm Position

BP may vary as much as 20 mm Hg by altering arm position. For consistency of measurements, the patient should be sitting with the arm in a horizontal, supported position at heart level. If patient condition or the type of activity precludes these positions, alterations should be carefully documented. As with other vital signs, factors such as fear, anxiety, or emotional stress also will cause an increase in BP.

Risk Factors

High BP is also associated with many risk factors, including high sodium intake, obesity and being overweight, a sedentary lifestyle, heavy alcohol consumption, pregnancy, sex, and age. In the United States, approximately 77.9 million (1 out of every 3) adults have high BP.[76] Projections suggest that by 2030, 41.4% of U.S. adults will have hypertension. Until age 45 years, a greater percentage of men than women have high BP; between 45 and 64 years of age, the percentage of men and women is comparable; and after that a much higher percentage of women than men have high BP.[76] African Americans are at greater risk for high BP than Caucasians. The rate of hypertension among this group is 44%, among the highest in the world.[77] Heredity (parental history of high BP) also places the individual at greater risk. Globally, the WHO estimates that more than 1 in 5 adults worldwide have high BP with related complications accounting for 9.4 million deaths worldwide per year.[78]

In addition, some medications can either increase BP or interfere with anti-hypertensive drugs. These drugs include steroids, NSAIDs, diet pills, cyclosporine, erythropoietin, tricyclic anti-depressants, monoamine oxidase inhibitors, and some oral contraceptives.

Equipment Requirements

A non-invasive or *indirect* measure of BP is used by physical therapists. In critical care settings, invasive or *direct* measures of BP are obtained by placing a thin catheter directly into an artery. The equipment required for taking BP using the more common noninvasive auscultatory (listening) method includes a *sphygmomanometer* and a *stethoscope*. The sphygmomanometer (frequently referred to as a *blood pressure cuff*) consists of a flat, airtight, inflatable latex bladder. The bladder is covered with a cotton or nylon sleeve that extends beyond the length of the bladder. There are two tubes that extend from the cuff. One is attached to a rubber bulb that has a valve to maintain or to release air from the cuff. The second tube is attached to a pressure manometer (portion of sphygmomanometer that registers the pressure reading). In patient care settings, sphygmomanometers may be wall mounted or placed on a mobile stand with a wheeled base.

BP cuffs are typically secured on the patient's extremity by a hook and loop closure. They come in a variety of sizes. In adults, the width of the bladder should be approximately 40% of the arm circumference, and bladder length should be enough to encircle at least 80% of arm circumference. Obtaining a cuff of appropriate size is important. Cuffs that are too narrow will show inaccurately high readings; cuffs that are too wide will show inaccurately low readings.[72]

The manometer registers the BP reading. Manometers are either *aneroid* or *mercury* with a 300 mm Hg scale marked in 2-mm increments. The mercury manometer registers BP on a mercury-filled calibrated cylinder (Box 2.6A). At the uppermost portion of the mercury column is a convex curve called the *meniscus*. A reading is obtained by viewing the meniscus at *eye level*. If not observed directly at eye level, an inaccurate reading will be obtained. The aneroid manometer registers BP by way of a circular calibrated dial and needle (Box 2.6B and C); automated BP units provide a digital LCD (Box 2.6D and E) or use an app to connect wireless to an electronic device (Box 2.6F). Owing to health and environmental concerns, aneroid manometers and automated displays have largely replaced mercury manometers in patient care settings.

Automated sphygmomanometers are self-inflating battery (rechargeable) or electrically powered units; many battery-powered models are also equipped with an AC adapter. Some include the "average mode" feature that performs two or three readings and then averages the total. Devices designed for clinical use often include several cuff sizes (e.g., small, medium, large, and extra-large). In hospital settings, BP is often included in units designed to measure multiple vital signs (see Fig. 2.7B). Automated sphygmomanometers designed for home use are described in Box 2.6 (D, E, F).

To monitor BP with a mercury or aneroid sphygmomanometer, an acoustic stethoscope is used to listen to the sounds over the artery as pressure is released from the cuff. By a combination of listening through the stethoscope and watching the manometer, the BP reading is obtained. A stethoscope amplifies and carries body sounds to the examiner's ears. Proximally, it consists of two rubber or plastic earpieces attached to narrow metal tubing that projects laterally from the earpieces about 1 inch (2.5 cm) and then downward about 6 inches (15 cm). The tubes are connected by a flexible, semi-circular metal spring mechanism that is often rubber-coated. These metal tubes are referred to as *binaurals* (designed for use in both ears). The semi-circular spring provides tension to maintain the position of the earpieces in the examiner's ears during use. The metal tubes then insert into fork-shaped rubber or plastic tubing that joins to form a single lumen and attach to the head distally (Fig. 2.21). Some stethoscopes (e.g., Sprague Rappaport–type stethoscope) are designed with two separate tubes that do not join and lead individually directly to the head of the stethoscope (the two tubes are held together with small metal clasps).

There are two types of distal sensing microphones on stethoscopes: a *bell shape* and a *flat-disk diaphragm*. Stethoscopes may have only one type of head; others have a combination design with one side bell shaped and the other a flat disk (see Fig. 2.21). The bell shape amplifies low-frequency sounds such as those produced in blood vessels; this type is generally recommended for determining BP. The flat-disk diaphragm is more useful for high-frequency sounds such as heart and lung sounds. However, Kantola and colleagues[79] found that either side of the stethoscope head could be used for reliable measurement of BP.

Another type of sensor incorporates both high- and low-frequency capabilities of the two shapes into a single-sided unit that eliminates the need to turn the head over. To hear low-frequency sound (bell shape), lighter pressure of the examiner's fingers is used; firmer pressure allows high-frequency sounds to be heard.

Battery-powered stethoscopes provide higher levels of amplification with volume control and dual-frequency sound filtering; some are available with interchangeable removable heads. A design variation for emergency medical service personnel provides higher amplification levels by replacing the earpieces with a headset designed to block out noise in a moving ambulance. Disposable stethoscopes are also available for use in high-risk settings where minimizing the risk of cross-infection is essential.

Korotkoff's Sounds

When measuring BP, a series of sounds called Korotkoff's sounds are heard through the stethoscope. The bell side of the stethoscope is generally recommended for auscultation because Korotkoff's sounds are low frequency. Initially when pressure is applied through the cuff around the patient's arm, the blood flow is occluded and no sound is heard through the stethoscope. As the pressure is gradually released, a series of five phases of sounds can be identified.

The therapist should be alert for the presence of an auscultatory gap, especially in patients with BP above normal values (hypertension). An auscultatory gap is the temporary disappearance of sound normally heard over the brachial artery between phases 1 and 2 and may cover a range of as much as 40 mm Hg. Not identifying this gap may lead to an underestimation of systolic pressure and overestimation of diastolic pressure.

Phase I: The first clear, faint, rhythmic tapping sound, which gradually increases in intensity, is heard. The period when blood initially flows through the artery is recorded as *systolic pressure.* This represents the highest pressure in the arterial system during ventricular contraction. *Be alert for an auscultatory gap.*

Phase II: A murmur or swishing sound is heard as the artery widens and more blood flows through it.

Phase III: Sounds become crisp, more intense, and louder; blood is now flowing relatively unobstructed.

Box 2.6 Examples of Sphygmomanometers

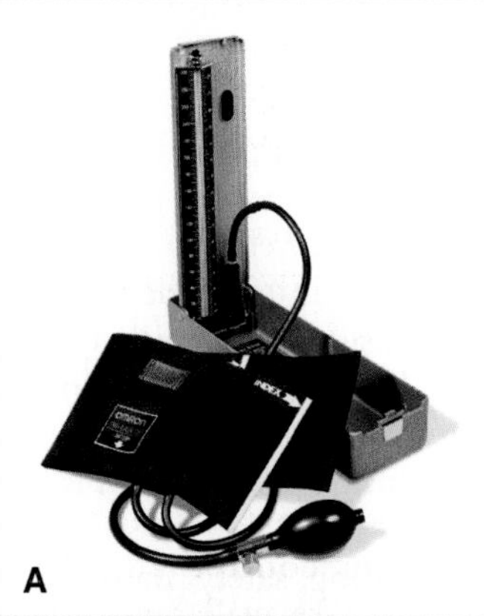

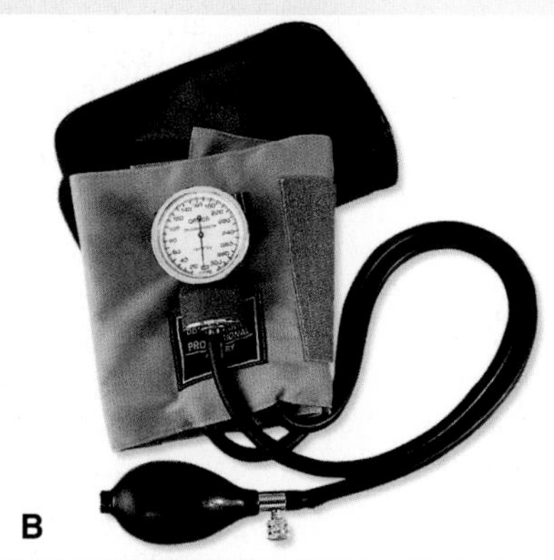

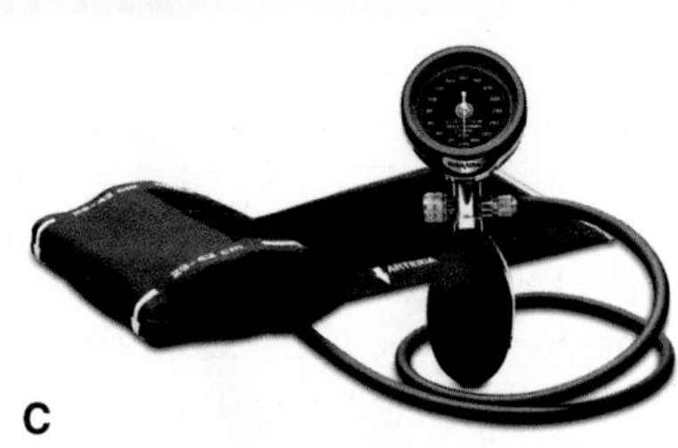

Manual sphygmomanometers (A, B, and C) have traditionally been used to monitor BP. Air is manually pumped into the inflatable cuff. As pressure is slowly released, heart sounds are monitored using a stethoscope. (A) Mercury gauge manometer—no longer in general use due to mercury toxicity. (B) Aneroid manometer with dial that clips to cuff. (C) Aneroid manometer with handheld dial.

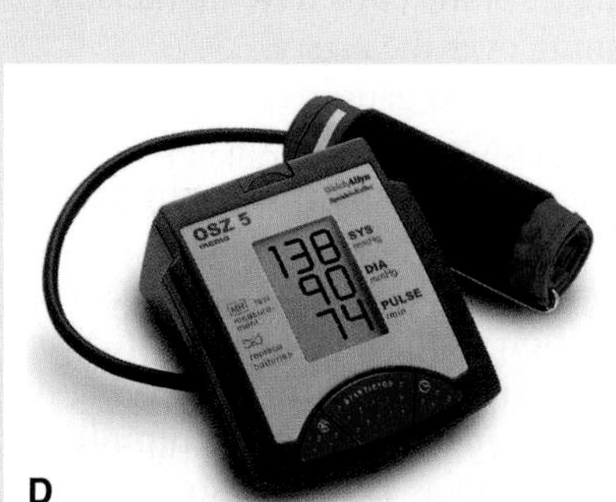

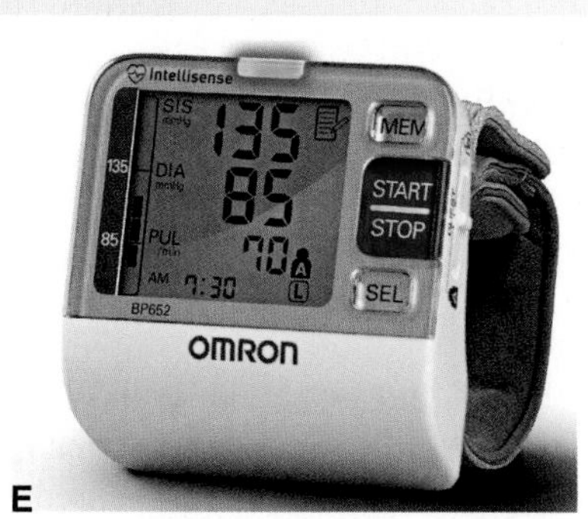

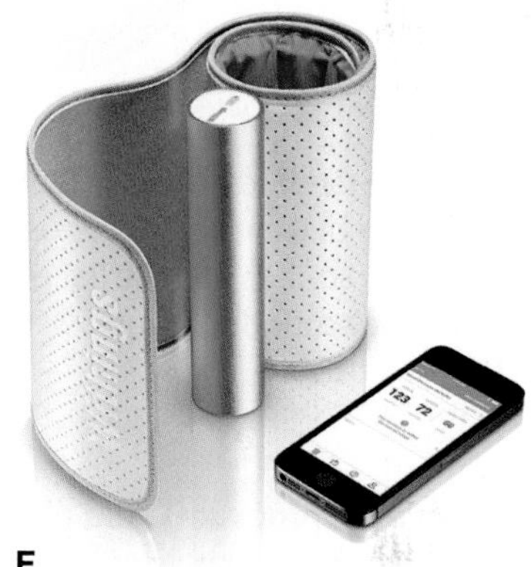

Automated sphygmomanometers (D, E, and F) designed for home use are convenient and practical for patients requiring frequent self-monitoring. They provide a rapid digital display, monitor pulse (in most cases), allow data storage, and are easy to use (place cuff and activate start button). Automated sphygmomanometers do not require a stethoscope; during automated inflation and deflation, the diastolic and systolic pressures are recorded. These devices monitor BP at the traditional arm location (D) or at the wrist (E). Some units provide wireless connectivity (F). For both arm and wrist cuffs, patients should be instructed that the UE should be relaxed and supported at heart level. *(A, B, and E courtesy of Omron, Inc., Lake Forest, IL 60045; C and D courtesy of Welch Allyn, Skaneateles Falls, NY 13153-0220; F courtesy of Withings, Cambridge, MA 02142.)*

Phase IV: Sound is distinct, with abrupt muffling; soft blowing quality.

Phase V: Last sound is heard; recorded as *diastolic pressure* in adults.

A BP reading with a systolic pressure of 117 and a second diastolic reading of 76 would be recorded as 117/76. An important consideration in determining BP is that it should be done in a minimal amount of time. The BP cuff acts as a tourniquet. As such, venous pooling and considerable discomfort to the patient will occur if the cuff is left in place too long. The brachial artery is the most common site for BP monitoring. A description for monitoring LE BP is also presented.

Measuring Brachial Blood Pressure

A. Assemble equipment:
   1. A stethoscope.
   2. A sphygmomanometer with a bladder size appropriate for the arm. In adults, the width of the bladder should be about 40% of the arm circumference (measurement can be made using a tape measure midway between the acromion and

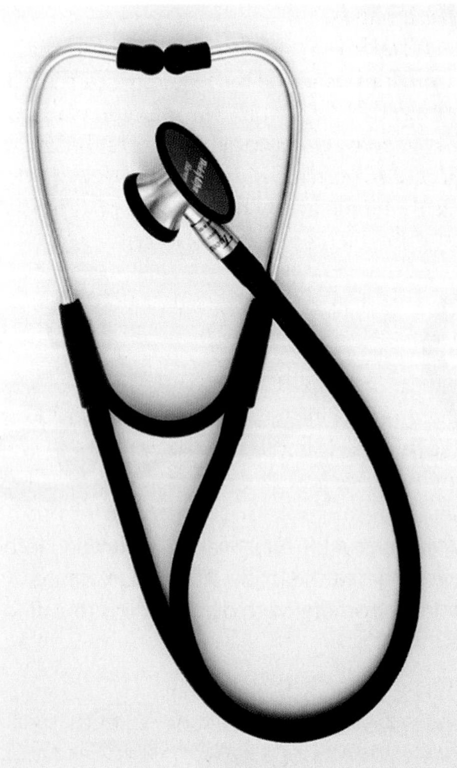

Figure 2.21 Standard acoustic stethoscope with dual head. The bell-shaped side is used to auscultate low-frequency sounds and the flat disk side is used for high-frequency sounds. *(Courtesy of Welch Allyn, Skaneateles Falls, NY 13153-0220.)*

olecranon processes), and bladder length should be enough to encircle at least 80% of arm circumference. In children, the bladder should be long enough to completely encircle the entire arm.

Note: These measurements refer to the internal bladder size and not the external encasing cuff.

3. Antiseptic wipes for cleaning earpieces and the head of the stethoscope before and after use.

B. Wash hands.

C. Procedure:

1. Explain procedure and rationale in terms appropriate to the patient's understanding. Indicate that there will be a request to remain quiet during monitoring to avoid interference with auscultation.

   Note: As with other vital sign measures, BP is monitored after the patient has been in a relaxed quiet setting for a period of time because activity or physical exertion will cause an elevation in measurements.

2. Guide the patient to the desired position. The sitting position is recommended with the back supported, the legs uncrossed, and feet flat on floor. Placing the chair next to a treatment table will facilitate UE positioning. The UE should be free of clothing. (Rolling up a garment sleeve is not acceptable owing to the tourniquet effect produced and interference with cuff positioning.) The midpoint of the arm should be at heart level with the elbow slightly flexed and the palm up. This can be effectively accomplished by supporting the UE on a treatment table. (If needed, pillows can be used to further adjust height.)

   Note: If a supine position is used, the arm should be at the patient's side and slightly elevated to the middle of the trunk. If measuring BP in a standing position (e.g., monitoring postural hypotension), ensure that the arm is supported at heart level.

3. Ensure patient understanding, safety, modesty, and comfort.
4. Use antiseptic wipes to clean the earpieces and head of stethoscope.
5. Wrap the deflated cuff snugly and evenly around the patient's bare arm approximately 1 inch (2.5 cm) above the antecubital fossa; the center of the cuff should be in line with the brachial artery (Fig. 2.22). Some cuffs have markers to guide positioning over the artery.
6. Ensure that the aneroid gauge is easily visible. (A mercury manometer must be on a level surface at eye level.) Check that the sphygmomanometer registers zero.

   Note: The first time a patient's BP is measured, an estimation of the systolic pressure should be made. This will ensure that during the actual measure, an adequate level of cuff inflation is used. The procedure is as follows:

   a. Locate and palpate the radial artery on the distal forearm of the cuffed arm.
   b. Close the valve of the BP cuff (turn clockwise).
   c. While continuing to monitor the pulse, rapidly inflate the BP cuff to 30 mm Hg above the level at which the radial pulse is extinguished.
   d. Note the pressure value on the gauge. (This is the estimate of maximum pressure required to measure systolic pressure for the individual patient.)
   e. Allow air to release quickly.

7. Place the earpieces of the stethoscope (tilting slightly forward) into the ear canals; the tubes of the stethoscope should not be crossed or in contact with each other and should hang freely.
8. Locate and palpate the brachial artery slightly above and medial to the antecubital fossa. Place the head of the stethoscope firmly over the brachial pulse point at the lower border of the BP cuff. Sufficient pressure should be used to avoid gapping between the circumference of the stethoscope head and the skin.

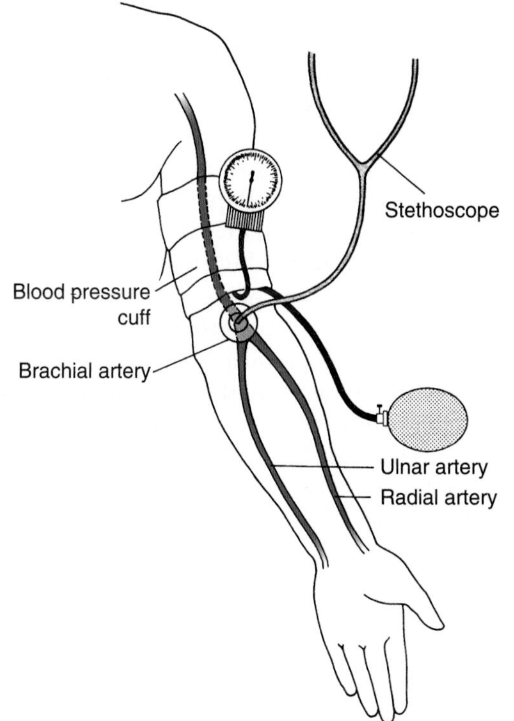

Figure 2.22 Placement of blood pressure cuff and stethoscope for monitoring brachial artery blood pressure.

9. Close the valve of the BP cuff (turn clockwise), and rapidly and steadily inflate the cuff to approximately 30 mm Hg above the estimated systolic pressure.
10. Release the thumb valve carefully, allowing air out slowly; air should be released at a rate of 2 mm Hg per heartbeat. Listen for the appearance of Korotkoff's sounds.
11. Watch the manometer closely and note the point at which the first rhythmic tapping sound is heard (a mercury manometer must be viewed at eye level); this is the point when blood first begins to flow through the artery and represents the systolic pressure (Korotkoff phase 1). Deflections in the dial or column of mercury will now be noted.
12. Continue to release air carefully at a rate of 2 mm Hg per heartbeat. Note when the sound first becomes muffled (Korotkoff phase 4) because quickly thereafter the sound will disappear (Korotkoff phase 5); this is recorded as the diastolic pressure.
13. Allow remainder of air to release quickly.
14. Clean the head and earpieces of the stethoscope with antiseptic wipes. If the same examiner is using the stethoscope again, it is not necessary to clean the earpieces. However, the head of the stethoscope should always be cleaned between patients.
15. Wash hands.

    Note: It is generally recommended that at least two BP measurements be taken and the values averaged.[70] At least a 1-minute interval should elapse between repeated measures. In its examination of hypertension, the ACC/AHA guideline recommends use of BP averages of at least 2 readings obtained on at least 2 occasions.[71]

Measuring Popliteal (Thigh) Blood Pressure

Measurement of popliteal BP is indicated in situations in which comparisons between the UE and LE are warranted, such as peripheral vascular disease. They also are used when UE pressures are contraindicated, such as after trauma or surgery. In comparison to the brachial artery, the popliteal artery normally yields a higher systolic pressure; diastolic values are approximately the same. Essentially, the procedure is the same as that for determining pressure at the brachial artery, with the following variations:

1. The patient is in a prone position; alternatively, the supine position may be used. Expose the LE using appropriate draping procedures.
2. Locate the pulse by palpation in the popliteal fossa. Flexing the knee slightly facilitates pulse location, as the artery is deep within the posterior knee. Knee flexion also facilitates stethoscope placement. Because the popliteal pulse is deep, it is often useful to initially palpate it using the first two or three fingers of each hand on either side of the posterior knee. Once a pulse is perceived, attention is then directed to locating the strongest pulse point.
3. Wrap the deflated cuff snugly and evenly around the patient's midthigh. (A wide cuff is used; use guidelines for cuff size described for brachial BP.) The center of the bladder should be directly over the popliteal artery.

    Note: As described for brachial BP, an estimate of maximum pressure required to measure systolic pressure can be made using the popliteal or dorsalis pedis artery.
4. Proceed with auscultating the pressure as for the brachial artery.

Recording Results

The nursing section of the EHR is an important source of vital sign data and should be checked regularly. Here, data are typically provided in numeric and/or graph form, with time represented on the horizontal axis and the measured values on the vertical axis. Many software programs automatically create graphs from numerical data entries. The visual record allows easy identification of data trends reflective of normal variations or a response to disease or therapeutic intervention. For the therapist practicing in facilities where such forms are used, familiarity with the specific recording system is important. For manual documentation, several methods are used to differentiate vital sign entry; they generally include both numeric entries and graphs using some variation of open and closed circles, connecting lines, color codes, or other symbols to discriminate among temperature, HR, RR, and BP data.

For purposes of physical therapy documentation, vital signs data entry points are often included in documentation software. Alternatively, vital sign data may be included directly within the narrative portion of the note. An important element in recording this information is that it allows easy comparison from one entry to the next. The date, time of day, patient position, examiner's name, and equipment used should all be clearly indicated. Any deviations from standard BP measurement protocol should be documented.

RESOURCES

Multiple Internet resources are available to enhance patient understanding of the implications of altered vital sign values and the importance of maintaining values within normal ranges, in addition to presenting strategies to prevent, detect, and obtain treatment for the precipitating causes. Many organizations provide a rich source of online information and education for patients and families as well as clinical guidelines and resource materials for health professionals. Several examples are provided in Appendix C.

SUMMARY

Examination of vital signs is an important component of the review of systems. Vital sign measures provide information about the patient's physiological status, may identify potential risk factors, and can serve as a screening tool for undiagnosed problems. Establishing and maintaining a database of values for an individual patient informs clinical decisions for determining the diagnosis and prognosis, designing the POC, and monitoring response to treatment.

The procedure for measuring each vital sign has been presented. Because multiple factors influence vital signs, the most useful data are obtained when measures are taken at periodic intervals rather than as a single measure in time. Sequential measures allow changes in patient status or response to treatment (e.g., exercise prescription) to be monitored over time, as well as indicating an acute change in status at a specific point in time.

Questions for Review

1. In monitoring a patient's blood pressure, you obtain values that are markedly higher from those documented by another therapist yesterday. How would you respond to this situation?
2. Prior to a vital signs examination, what preliminary data can be obtained by a careful systematic observation of the patient?
3. Together with other examination data, vital sign measures assist the physical therapist in making clinical decisions about what aspects of patient care?
4. Provide examples of lifestyle patterns (modifiable) and patient characteristics (nonmodifiable) that may influence vital sign measures.
5. What are the mechanisms by which the body conserves and produces heat?
6. What methods are used to dissipate excess heat from the body? Provide a description of each.
7. Hand hygiene plays a critical role in preventing transmission of pathogens. What are the five moments of hand hygiene developed by WHO to draw attention to its importance and practical application?
8. What is the procedure for measuring oral temperature using a handheld battery-powered thermometer?
9. What three pulse parameters (characteristics) are considered during monitoring? Describe each.
10. Where is the stethoscope placed to monitor apical pulse?
11. What is a pulse deficit and how is it derived?
12. What medical conditions would alert the therapist to the potential need for monitoring oxygen saturation levels using pulse oximetry?
13. What parameters (characteristics) are considered in examining respiration? Describe each.
14. What is the procedure for measuring brachial blood pressure using a stethoscope and aneroid sphygmomanometer?

CASE STUDY

EMERGENCY ROOM ADMISSION

A 24-year-old man was separated from his skiing group due to an unexpected and violent snowstorm. His being in an unfamiliar area without electronic communication complicated the situation. A 2-day helicopter search located him after approximately 48 hours of exposure to temperatures that ranged between 10°F and 20°F (–12.22°C and –6.67°C). The emergency team initiated intravenous fluid replacement (to help restore fluid and electrolyte balance) en route to the hospital.

HISTORY

As reported by his parents, medical history is unremarkable except for the usual childhood diseases. He had recently relocated to the area in the hopes of becoming a competitive skier (an activity he has enjoyed all his life). He works as an accountant for a local investment firm.

ADMITTING DIAGNOSIS

Hypothermia and frostbite of the toes, thumb, and index and middle fingers, bilaterally.

- **Blood pressure:** Systolic pressure is 45 mm Hg; diastolic not perceptible.
- **Pulse:** Decreased rate, small, weak carotid pulse (12 bpm); peripheral pulses not perceptible.
- **Respiratory rate:** 6 breaths per minute; respirations barely perceptible.
- **Temperature:** 82°F (27.78°C) (rectal).
- **Cognition:** Depressed, unresponsive.
- **Deep tendon reflexes:** Absent.
- **Motor function:** No spontaneous movement.
- **Cutaneous sensation:** Unresponsive to all sensory modalities, including pain.
- **Integument:** Pale, cold on palpation; bluish gray appearance of nail beds and lips.

PHYSICAL THERAPY

The patient is now in the intensive care unit and a referral has been made to physical therapy requesting "examination and treatment."

GUIDING QUESTIONS

1. Describe the body system responses to hypothermia.
2. What symptoms of hypothermia are presented by the patient?
3. During the early portion of the patient being stranded, input from thermoreceptors would have indicated a drop in temperature below the "set" temperature value. What mechanisms would have been activated to conserve heat?
4. Considering this patient is unresponsive and cyanotic, what is the most appropriate pulse to monitor? Why?

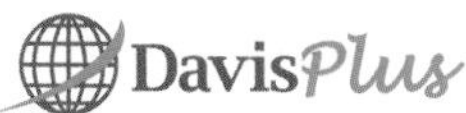

For additional resources, including answers to the questions for review and case study guiding questions, please visit **http://davisplus.fadavis.com.**

References

1. *Guide to Physical Therapist Practice 3.0.* Alexandria, VA: American Physical Therapy Association; 2014. Available at: http://guidetoptpractice.apta.org/. Accessed July 14, 2018.
2. Dillon, PM: Nursing Health Assessment, ed 2. FA Davis, Philadelphia, 2007.
3. Wilkinson, JM, et al: Fundamentals of Nursing, ed 3. Electronic Study Guide. FA Davis, Philadelphia, 2016.
4. Centers for Disease Control and Prevention (CDC): National Health and Nutrition Examination Survey. CDC, Atlanta, GA. Retrieved August 4, 2018, from www.cdc.gov/nchs/nhanes/index.htm.
5. Wright, JD, et al: Mean Systolic and Diastolic Blood Pressure in Adults Aged 18 and Over in the United States, 2001–2008, National Health Statistics Reports; Number 35. National Center for Health Statistics, Hyattsville, MD, 2011. Retrieved August 1, 2016, from www.cdc.gov/nchs/products/nhsr.htm.
6. Ostchega, Y, et al: Resting pulse rate reference data for children, adolescents, and adults: United States, 1999–2008, National Health Statistics Reports; Number 41. National Center for Health Statistics, Hyattsville, MD, 2011. Retrieved August 1, 2016, from www.cdc.gov/nchs/products/nhsr.htm.
7. Guilder, GP, and Janot, JM: Acute and chronic cardiorespiratory responses to exercise. In Porcari, J, Bryant, C, and Comana, F (eds): Exercise Physiology. FA Davis, Philadelphia, 2015, p 196.
8. Wilkinson, JM, et al: Fundamentals of Nursing, ed 3, vol 1. FA Davis, Philadelphia, 2016.
9. Alfaro-LeFevre, R: Applying Nursing Process: A Tool for Critical Thinking, ed 7. Wolters Kluwer/Lippincott Williams and Wilkins, Philadelphia, 2010.
10. Leavitt, R (ed): Cultural Competence: A Lifelong Journey to Cultural Proficiency. Slack, Thorofare, NJ, 2010.
11. Tripp-Reimer, T, Johnson, R, and Sorofman, B: Cultural dimensions. In Stanley, M, Blair, KA, and Beare, PG (eds): Gerontological Nursing: Promoting Successful Aging with Older Adults, ed 3. FA Davis, Philadelphia, 2005, p 25.

12. Tseng, W, and Streltzer, J: Cultural Competence in Health Care: A Guide for Professionals. Springer Science and Business Media, New York, 2008.
13. Purnell, LD: Transcultural diversity and health care. In Purnell, LD (ed): Transcultural Health Care: A Culturally Competent Approach, ed 4. FA Davis, Philadelphia, 2013, p 3.
14. Spector, RE: Cultural Diversity in Health and Illness, ed 9. Pearson, New York, 2017.
15. US Census Bureau: Overview of Race and Hispanic Origin: 2010 Census Briefs. US Department of Commerce, Economics and Statistics Administration, Washington, DC, 2011. Retrieved August 4, 2016, from www.census.gov/prod/cen2010/briefs/c2010br-02.pdf.
16. US Department of Health and Human Services (USDHHS) Office of Minority Health (OMH): National Standards for Culturally and Linguistically Appropriate Services in Health Care. USDHHS (OMH), Washington, DC, 2001. Retrieved August 4, 2016 from http://minorityhealth.hhs.gov/assets/pdf/checked/finalreport.pdf.
17. World Confederation for Physical Therapy (WCPT): WCPT Guideline for Standards of Physical Therapy Practice, WCPT, London, UK, 2011. Retrieved August 12, 2016 from www.wcpt.org/sites/wcpt.org/files/files/Guideline_standards_practice_complete.pdf.
18. American Physical Therapy Association (APTA): Blueprint for Teaching Cultural Competence in Physical Therapy Education. APTA, Alexandria, VA, Updated 2014. Retrieved July 14, 2018 from www.apta.org/Educators/Curriculum/APTA/Cultural Competence/.
19. Commission on Accreditation in Physical Therapy Education (CAPTE): Evaluative Criteria for Accreditation of PT Programs. APTA, Alexandria, VA, 2014. Retrieved August 4, 2016, from www.capteonline.org/AccreditationHandbook/.
20. Commission on Accreditation in Physical Therapy Education (CAPTE): Evaluative Criteria for Accreditation of PTA Programs. APTA, Alexandria, VA, 2013. Retrieved August 4, 2016, from www.capteonline.org/AccreditationHandbook/.
21. American Physical Therapy Association (APTA): A Normative Model of Physical Therapist Professional Education: Version 2004. APTA, Alexandria, VA, 2004.
22. American Physical Therapy Association (APTA): A Normative Model of Physical Therapist Assistant Education: Version 2007. APTA, Alexandria, VA, 2007.
23. Burton, M, and May Ludwig, LJ: Fundamentals of Nursing Care. FA Davis, Philadelphia, 2011.
24. Purnell, LD: Guide to Culturally Competent Health Care, ed 3. FA Davis, Philadelphia, 2013.
25. Perez, MA, and Luquis, RR (eds): Cultural Competence in Health Education and Health Promotion, ed 2. Jossey-Bass/A Wiley Brand, San Francisco, 2014.
26. Jeffreys, M (ed): Teaching Cultural Competence in Nursing and Health Care: Inquiry, Action, and Innovation, ed 3. Springer, New York, 2016.
27. Ritter, LA, and Graham, DH: Multicultural Health, ed 2. Jones & Bartlett Learning, Burlington, MA, 2017.
28. Campbell, L, Gilbert, MA, and Laustsen, GR: Clinical Coach for Nursing Excellence. FA Davis, Philadelphia, 2010.
29. Denunzio, C, and Heuer, AJ: Fundamentals of physical examination. In Heuer, AJ, and Scanlan, CL (eds): Wilkins' Clinical Assessment in Respiratory Care, ed 7. Elsevier, Maryland Heights, MO, 2014, p 73.
30. McCarthy, M, and Shelledy, DC: Physical assessment. In Shelledy, DC, and Peters, JI: Respiratory Care Patient Assessment and Care Plan Development. Jones and Bartlett Learning, Burlington, MA, 2016, p 137.
31. McArdle, WD, Katch, FI, and Katch, VL: Exercise Physiology: Nutrition, Energy, and Human Performance, ed 8. Wolters Kluwer Health, Baltimore, MD, 2015.
32. Hall, JE: Guyton and Hall Textbook of Medical Physiology, ed 13. Elsevier, Philadelphia, 2016.
33. Barrett, KE, et al: Ganong's Review of Medical Physiology, ed 24. McGraw Hill/Lange, New York, 2012.
34. Sherwood, L: Human Physiology: From Cells to Systems, ed 8. Brooks/Cole (Cengage Learning), Belmont, CA, 2013.
35. McArdle, WD, Katch, FI, and Katch, VL: Essentials of Exercise Physiology, ed 5. Wolters Kluwer/Lippincott Williams and Wilkins, Philadelphia, 2016.
36. Powers, SK, and Howley, ET: Exercise Physiology: Theory and Application to Fitness and Performance, ed 9. McGraw-Hill, New York, 2015.
37. Witzmann, FA: Regulation of body temperature. In Rhoades, RA, and Bell, DR (eds): Medical Physiology: Principles for Clinical Medicine, ed 4. Wolters Kluwer/Lippincott Williams and Wilkins, Philadelphia, 2013, p 550.
38. Levenhagen, K, and Peterson, C: Infectious disease. In Cavallaro Goodman, CC, and Fuller, KS (eds): Pathology: Implications for the Physical Therapist, ed 4. Elsevier/Saunders, St. Louis, MO, 2015, p 318.
39. Centers for Disease Control and Prevention (CDC): Tick-Borne Relapsing Fever (TBRF). CDC, Atlanta, GA. Retrieved September 2, 2016, from www.cdc.gov/relapsing-fever/.
40. Dinarello, CA, and Porat, R: Fever. In Kasper, DL, et al (eds): Harrison's Principles of Internal Medicine, ed 19. McGraw Hill, New York, 2015, p. 123.
41. Comana, F: Thermoregulatory system and thermoregulatory responses to exercise. In Porcari, J, Bryant, C, and Comana, F (eds): Exercise Physiology. FA Davis, Philadelphia, 2015, p 302.
42. National Institutes of Health (NIH): Hyperthermia: Too Hot for Your Health, NIH, U.S. Department of Health and Human Services, Bethesda, MD, 2012. Retrieved September 14, 2016 from www.nih.gov/news-events/news-releases/hyperthermia-too-hot-your-health-1.
43. American College of Sports Medicine: ACSM's Guidelines for Exercise Testing and Prescription, ed. 9. Wolters Kluwer/Lippincott Williams and Wilkins, Philadelphia, 2014.
44. World Health Organization (WHO): Developing National Strategies for Phasing Out Mercury-Containing Thermometers and Sphygmomanometers in Health Care, Including in the Context of the Minamata Convention on Mercury. WHO, Geneva, Switzerland, 2015. Retrieved October 1, 2016 from www.who.int/ipcs/assessment/public_health/WHOGuidanceReporton Mercury2015.pdf.
45. United States Environmental Protection Agency (EPA): Thermometers. EPA, Washington, DC, 2016. Retrieved October 1, 2016, from www.epa.gov/mercury/mercury-thermometers.
46. National Institute of Standards and Technology (NIST): Mercury Thermometer Alternatives. NIST, Gaithersburg, MD, 20899. Retrieved November 1, 2016, from www.nist.gov/pml/mercury-thermometer-alternatives.
47. Wilkinson, JM, et al: Fundamentals of Nursing, ed 3, vol 2. FA Davis, Philadelphia, 2016.
48. World Health Organization (WHO): WHO Guidelines on Hand Hygiene in Health Care. WHO, Geneva, Switzerland, 2009. Retrieved November 6, 2016, from http://whqlibdoc.who.int/publications/2009/9789241597906_eng.pdf.
49. Smith, SF, et al: Clinical Nursing Skills: Basic to Advanced Skills, ed 9. Pearson, Hoboken, NJ, 2017.
50. Berman, AT, Snyder, S, and Frandsen, G: Kozier and Erb's Fundamentals of Nursing: Concepts, Process, and Practice, ed 10. Pearson, Hoboken, NJ, 2016.
51. Centers for Disease Control and Prevention (CDC): Target Heart Rate and Estimated Maximum Heart Rate. CDC, Atlanta, GA. Retrieved November 8, 2016, from www.cdc.gov/physicalactivity/basics/measuring/heartrate.htm.
52. Sipe, C: Older adults. In Porcari, J, Bryant, C, and Comana, F (eds): Exercise Physiology. FA Davis, Philadelphia, 2015, p 710.
53. Moore, KL, Dalley, AF, and Agur, AMR: Clinically Oriented Anatomy, ed 7. Wolters Kluwer/Lippincott Williams & Wilkins, Philadelphia, 2014.
54. Myers, BA: Wound Management: Principles and Practice, ed 3. Prentice Hall, Upper Saddle River, NJ, 2012.
55. Patterson, GK: Vascular evaluation. In Sussman, C, and Bates-Jensen, BM (eds): Wound Care: A Collaborative Practice Manual for Health Professionals, ed 4. Wolters Kluwer/Lippincott Williams & Wilkins, Philadelphia, 2012, p 173.
56. Rees, S: Vascular assessment. In Merriman, LM, and Turner, W (eds): Merriman's Assessment of the Lower Limb, ed 3. Churchill Livingstone/Elsevier, Philadelphia, 2009, p 75.
57. Vines, DL: Respiratory monitoring in critical care. In Heuer, AJ, and Scanlon, CL (eds): Wilkins' Clinical Assessment in Respiratory Care, ed 7. Mosby/Elsevier, Maryland Heights, MO, 2014, p 314.

58. Clinical Monograph: Monitoring Oxygen Saturation with Pulse Oximetry. Nellcor, Pleasanton, CA, 2001. Retrieved November 10, 2016 from http://macomb-rspt.com/FILES/RSPT1050/MODULE%20G/Pulse_Oximetry_Monograph.pdf.
59. Cahalin, LP, and Buck, LA: Physical therapy associated with cardiovascular pump dysfunction and failure. In DeTurk, WE, and Cahalin, LP (eds): Cardiovascular and Pulmonary Physical Therapy: An Evidence-Based Approach, ed 2. McGraw-Hill, New York, 2011, p 529.
60. Weinberger, SE, Cockrill, BA, and Mandel, J: Principles of Pulmonary Medicine, ed 6. Elsevier/Saunders, Philadelphia, 2014.
61. Scanlon, VC, and Sanders, T: Essentials of Anatomy and Physiology, ed 7. FA Davis, Philadelphia, 2015.
62. Van Guilder, GP, and Janot, JM: Respiratory System. In Porcari, J, Bryant, C, and Comana, F (eds): Exercise Physiology. FA Davis, Philadelphia, 2015, p 128.
63. Collins, SM, and Cocanour, B: Anatomy of the cardiopulmonary system. In DeTurk, WE, and Cahalin, LP (eds): Cardiovascular and Pulmonary Physical Therapy: An Evidence-Based Approach, ed 2. McGraw-Hill, New York, 2011, p 85.
64. Packel, L: The respiratory system. In Cavallaro Goodman, C, and Fuller, KS (eds): Pathology: Implications for the Physical Therapist, ed 4. Elsevier/Saunders, St Louis, MO, 2015, p 772.
65. Certo, C: Cardiopulmonary Rehabilitation of the Geriatric Patient and Client. In Lewis, CB: Aging: The Health-Care Challenge, ed 4. FA Davis, Philadelphia, 2002, p 143.
66. Prentice, WE: Arnheim's Principles of Athletic Training: A Competency-Based Approach, ed 15. McGraw-Hill, New York, 2014.
67. Porcari, J, and Drum, S: Altitude, pollution, and underwater diving: Effects on exercise capacity. In Porcari, J, Bryant, C, and Comana, F (eds): Exercise Physiology. FA Davis, Philadelphia, 2015, p 802.
68. Woo, TM: Drugs Affecting the Respiratory System. In Woo, TM, and Wynne, AL: Pharmacotherapeutics for Nurse Practitioner Prescribers, ed 3. FA Davis, Philadelphia, 2011, p 381.
69. Ciccone, CD: Medications. In DeTurk, WE, and Cahalin, LP (eds): Cardiovascular and Pulmonary Physical Therapy: An Evidence-Based Approach, ed 2. McGraw-Hill, New York, 2011, p 209.
70. Pinto, E: Blood pressure and ageing. Postgrad Med J 83:109, 2007. Retrieved November 12, 2016, from www.ncbi.nlm.nih.gov/pmc/articles/PMC2805932/pdf/109.pdf.
71. Whelton PK, et al: 2017 ACC/AHA/AAPA/ABC/ACPM/AGS/APhA/ASH/ASPC/NMA/PCNA guideline for the prevention, detection, evaluation, and management of high blood pressure in adults: A report of the American College of Cardiology/American Heart Association Task Force on Clinical Practice Guidelines. J Am Coll Cardiol 71(19):e127-e248. Retrieved July 14, 2018 from http://hyper.ahajournals.org/content/early/2017/11/10/HYP.0000000000000065
72. Chobanian, AV, Bakris GL, Black HR, et al: Seventh report of the Joint National Committee on Prevention, Detection, Evaluation, and Treatment of High Blood Pressure: The JNC 7 report. JAMA 289(19):2560, 2003.
73. Smirnova, IV: The cardiovascular system. In Cavallaro Goodman, C, and Fuller, KS (eds): Pathology: Implications for the Physical Therapist, ed 4. Elsevier/Saunders, St Louis, MO, 2015, p 538.
74. VanMeter, KC, and Hubert, RJ: Gould's Pathophysiology for the Health Professions, ed 5. Saunders/Elsevier, St Louis, MO, 2014.
75. Centers for Disease Control and Prevention (CDC): Measuring orthostatic blood pressure. CDC, Atlanta, GA. Retrieved August 4, 2018 from www.cdc.gov/steadi/pdf/Measuring_Orthostatic_Blood_Pressure-print.pdf
76. American Heart Association: High blood pressure statistical fact sheet—2014 update. American Heart Association, Dallas, TX. Retrieved November 12, 2016, from www.heart.org/idc/groups/heart-public/@wcm/@sop/@smd/documents/downloadable/ucm_462020.pdf
77. American Heart Association: Heart disease and stroke statistics—2012 update. American Heart Association, Dallas, TX. Retrieved November 12, 2016, from circ.ahajournals.org/content/early/2011/12/15/CIR.0b013e31823ac046.
78. World Health Organization (WHO): Q & As on hypertension. WHO, Geneva, Switzerland, 2015. Retrieved November 12, 2016, from www.who.int/features/qa/82/en/.
79. Kantola, I: Bell or diaphragm in the measurement of blood pressure? J Hypertens 23(3):499, 2005.

Supplemental Readings

Boatin AA, et al: Wireless Vital Sign Monitoring in Pregnant Women: A Functionality and Acceptability Study. Telemed J E Health 22(7):564, 2016.

Cardona-Morrell, M, et al: Effectiveness of continuous or intermittent vital signs monitoring in preventing adverse events on general wards: A systematic review and meta-analysis. Int J Clin Pract 70(10):806, 2016.

Cardoso, CR, and Salles, GF: Prognostic importance of ambulatory blood pressure monitoring in resistant hypertension: Is it all that matters? Curr Hypertens Rep 18(12):85, 2016.

Granholm, A, et al: Respiratory rates measured by a standardised clinical approach, ward staff, and a wireless device. Acta Anaesthesiol Scand 60(10):1444, 2016.

Kiekkas, P, et al: Agreement of infrared temporal artery thermometry with other thermometry methods in adults: Systematic review. J Clin Nurs 25(7–8):894, 2016.

Liu, C, et al: Comparison of stethoscope bell and diaphragm, and of stethoscope tube length, for clinical blood pressure measurement. Blood Press Monit 21(3):178, 2016.

Lakhe A, et al: Development of digital stethoscope for telemedicine. J Med Eng Technol 40(1):20, 2016.

Mizuno, T, et al: Pharmacist blood pressure management programs using telemonitoring systems are useful for monitoring side effects of antihypertensive drugs in a community pharmacy. Clin Case Rep 4(11):1041, 2016.

Niven, DJ, et al: Accuracy of peripheral thermometers for estimating temperature: A systematic review and meta-analysis. Ann Intern Med 163(10):768, 2015.

Ostchega, Y, et al: Blood pressure cuff comparability study. Blood Press Monit 21(6):345, 2016.

appendix

2.A Hand-Rubbing Technique

Hand Hygiene Technique With Alcohol-Based Formulation

Duration of the entire procedure: 20–30 seconds

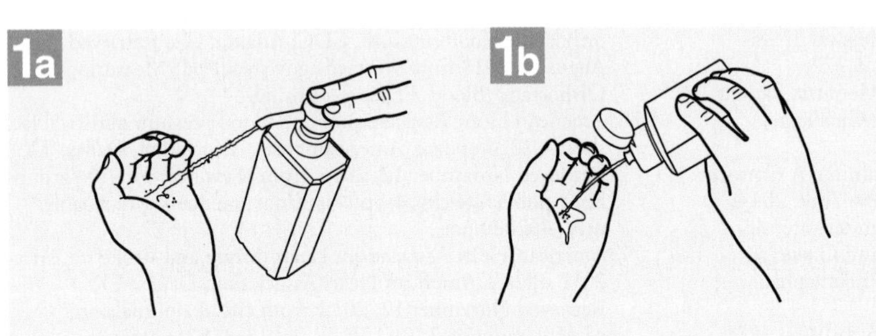

Apply a palmful of the product in a cupped hand, covering all surfaces.

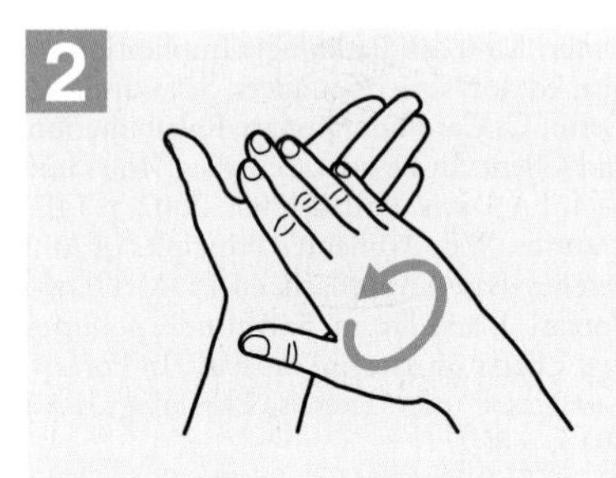

Rub hands palm to palm.

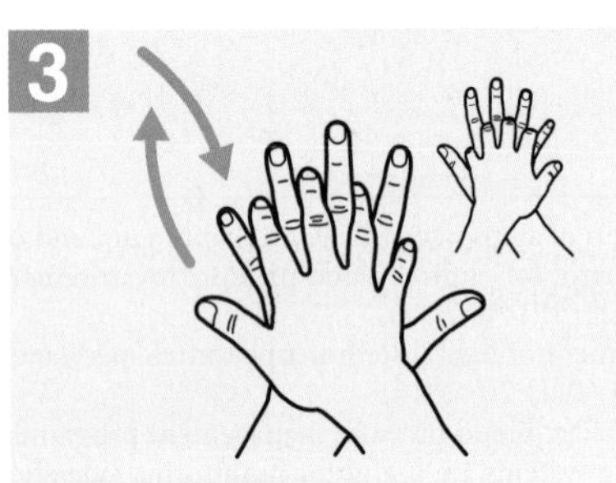

Right palm over left dorsum with interlaced fingers and vice versa.

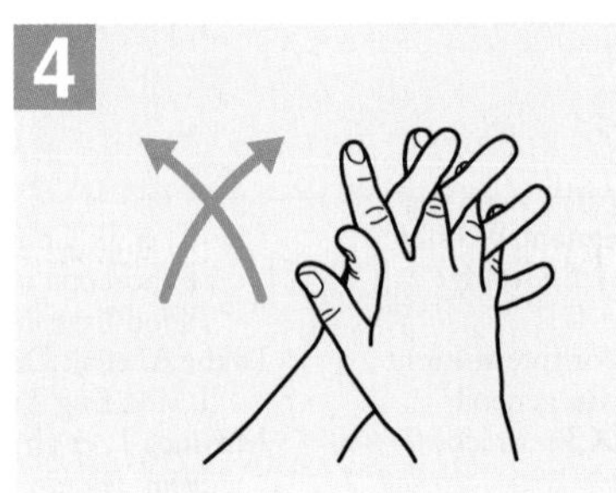

Palm to palm with fingers interlaced.

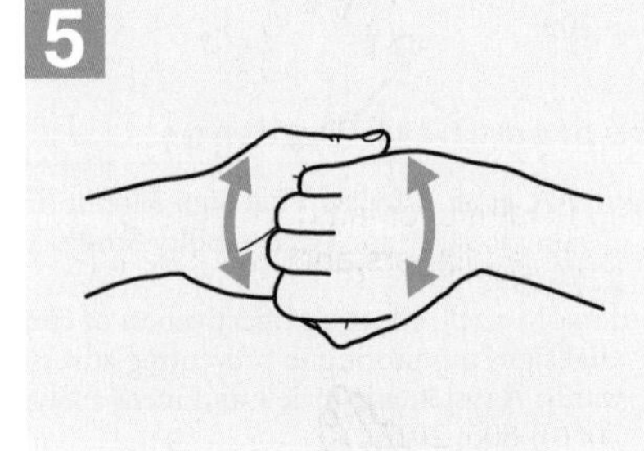

Backs of fingers to opposing palms with fingers interlocked.

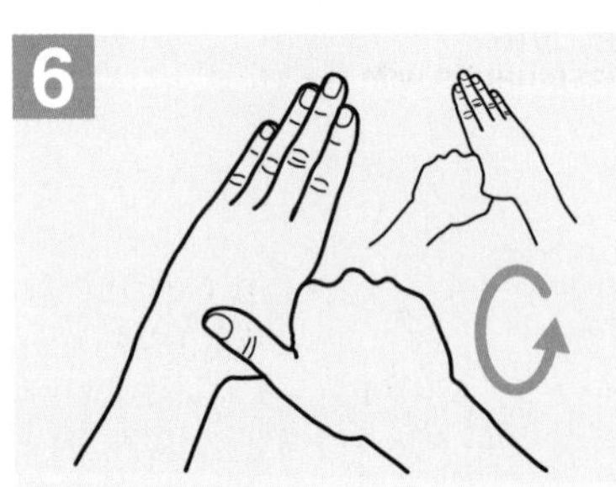

Rotational rubbing of left thumb clasped in right palm and vice versa.

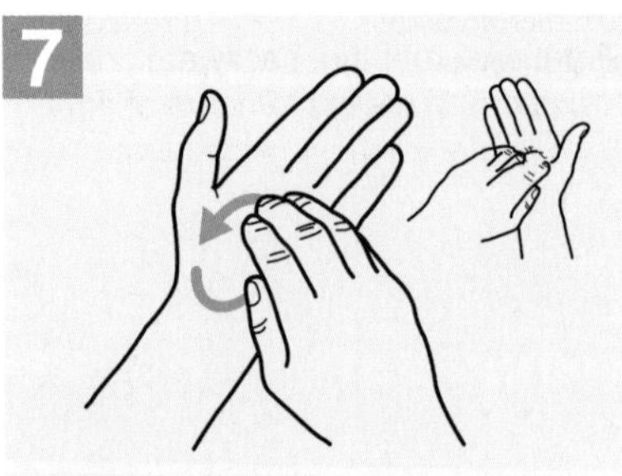

Rotational rubbing, backward and forward with clasped fingers of right hand in left palm and vice versa.

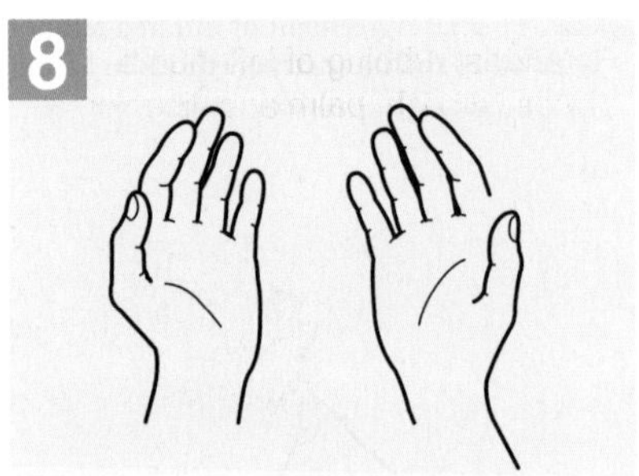

Once dry, your hands are safe.

(From WHO[48, p. 155] with permission.)

appendix 2.B

Hand-Washing Technique

Hand Hygiene Technique With Soap and Water

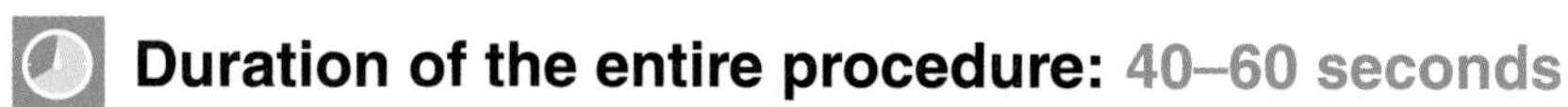

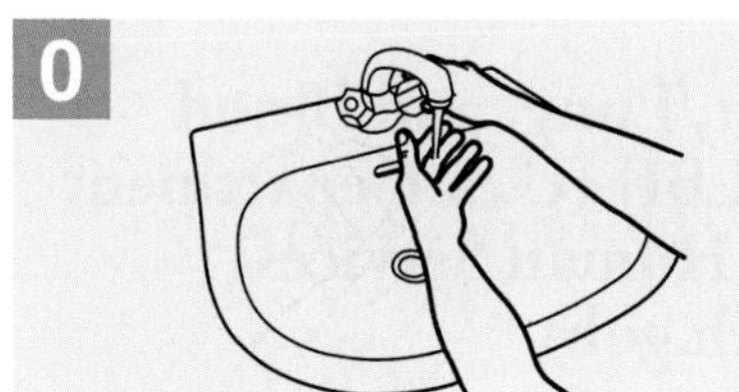

Wet hands with water.

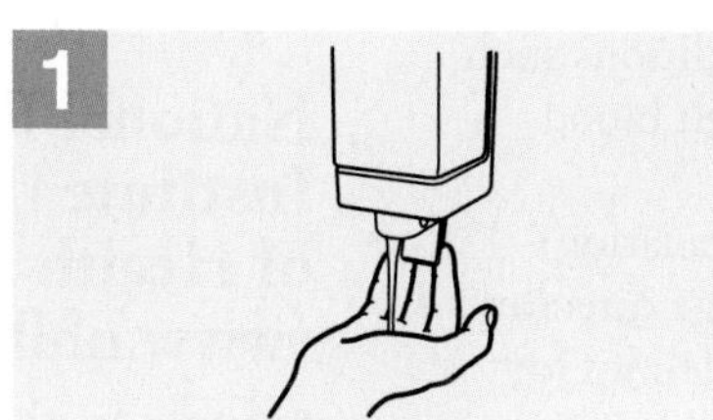

Apply enough soap to cover all hand surfaces.

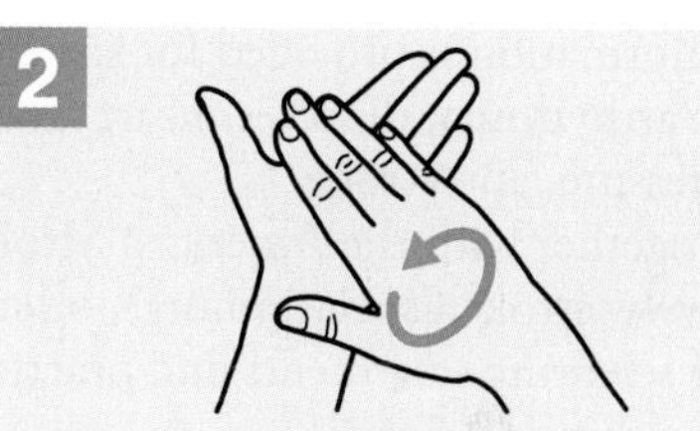

Rub hands palm to palm.

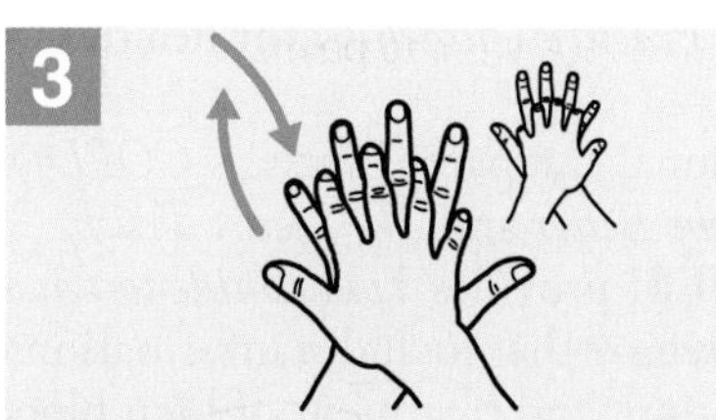

Right palm over left dorsum with interlaced fingers and vice versa.

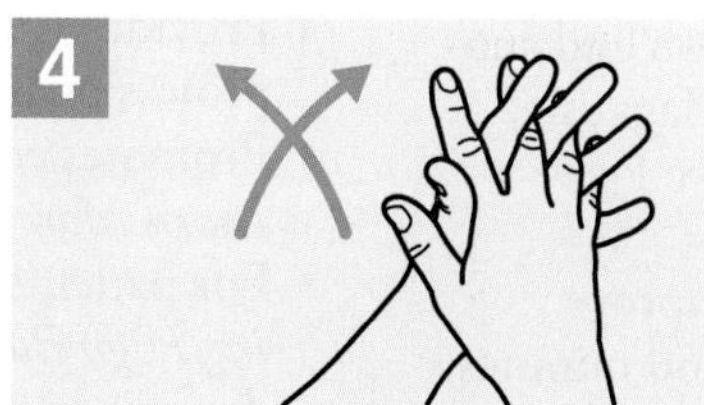

Palm to palm with fingers interlaced.

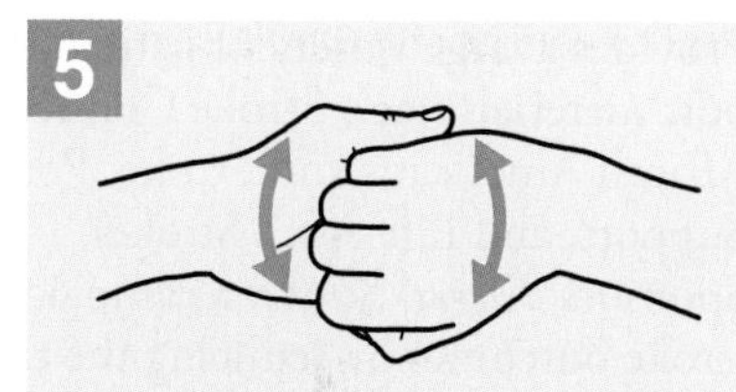

Backs of fingers to opposing palms with fingers interlocked.

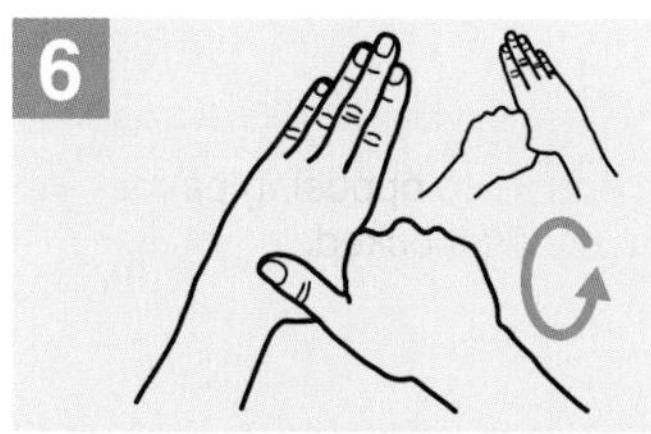

Rotational rubbing of left thumb clasped in right palm and vice versa.

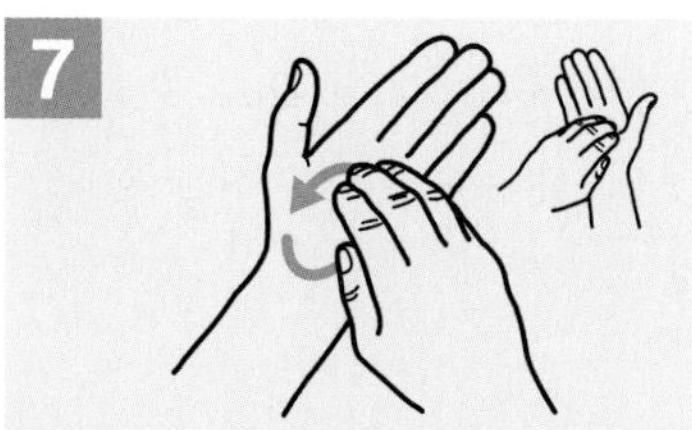

Rotational rubbing, backward and forward with clasped fingers of right hand in left palm and vice versa.

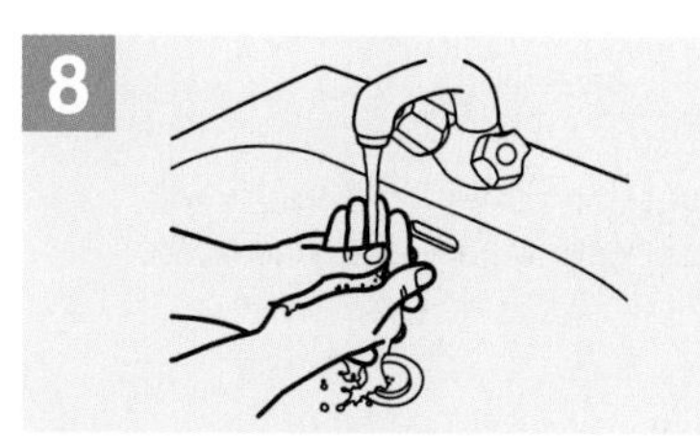

Rinse hands with water.

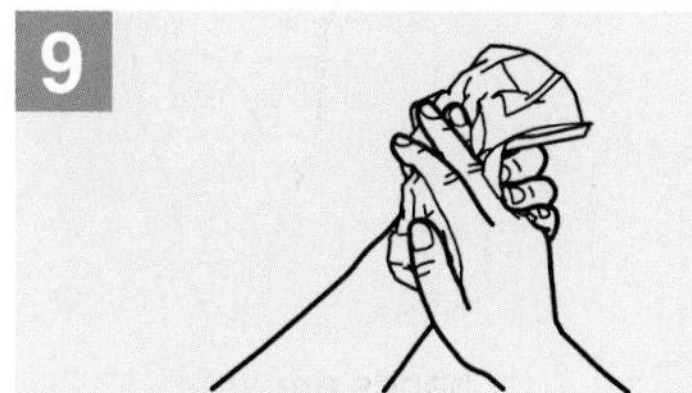

Dry hands thoroughly with a single use towel.

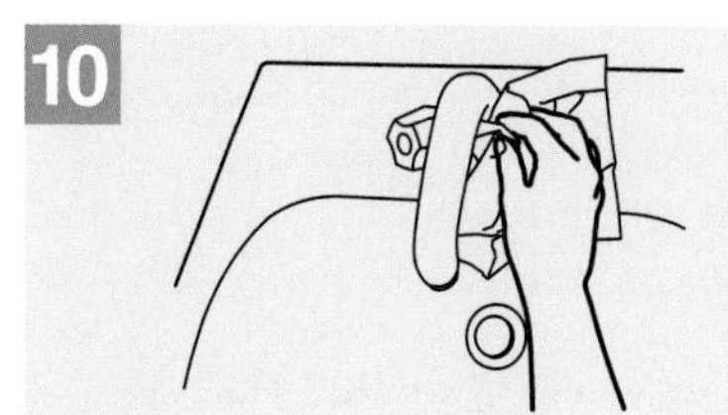

Use towel to turn off faucet.

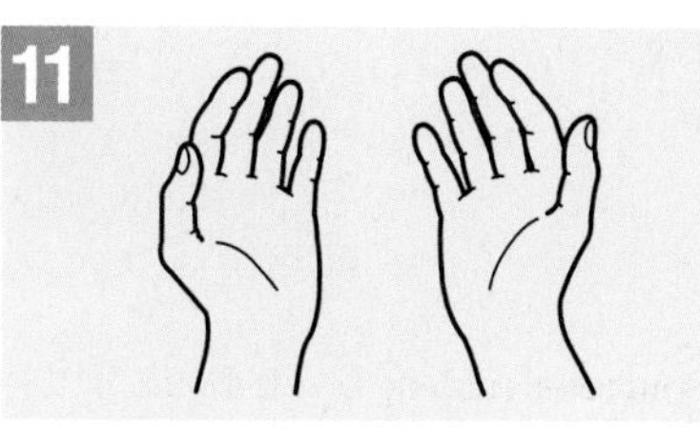

Your hands are now safe.

(From WHO[48, p. 156] with permission.)

appendix 2.C

Resources for Patients, Families, and Clinicians

American Heart Association (www.heart.org/HEARTORG)

- Provides patient information on multiple health topics, including nutrition, physical activity, weight, and stress management and smoking cessation.
- Information is provided for specific conditions such as arrhythmia, diabetes, heart attack, high blood pressure, and stroke.
- Together with the American Stroke Association (www.strokeassociation.org), offers a large directory of scientific statements and practice guidelines for health professionals.

American Stroke Association (www.strokeassociation.org)

- Provides a large variety of patient education and support materials (e.g., Stroke Connection Magazine, African Americans and Stroke, Post-Stroke Peer Support, and Life After Stroke).
- Sponsors *Target: Stroke*, a campaign to improve stroke outcomes by reducing the time to 60 minutes or less between onset of stroke and initiation of intravenous thrombolysis. Support includes publications, patient education, and clinical tools. www.strokeassociation.org/STROKEORG/Professionals/Target-Stroke_UCM_314495_SubHomePage.jsp
- Makes available a directory of stroke statements and guidelines.

National Heart, Lung, and Blood Institute [NHLBI] (U.S. Department of Health and Human Services) (www.nhlbi.nih.gob)

- Sponsors the *National High Blood Pressure Education Program*. The goal of the program is to reduce deaths and disability associated with high blood pressure through education.
- Provides *Clinical Practice Guidelines* for health professionals.
- Promotes educational campaigns such as *COPD: Learn More Breathe Better* and *The Heart Truth.*
- For patients, NHLBI provides *Your Guide to Lowering High Blood Pressure* that includes information on detection, prevention, and treatment of high blood pressure.

Examination of Sensory Function

Kevin K. Chui, PT, DPT, PhD, GCS, OCS, CEEAA, FAAOMPT
Sheng-Che Yen, PT, PhD
Thomas J. Schmitz, PT, PhD

Chapter 3

LEARNING OBJECTIVES

1. Understand the purpose(s) of performing a sensory examination.
2. Understand the relationship between preliminary mental status screening and tests for sensory function.
3. Describe the classification and function of the receptor mechanisms involved in the perception of sensation.
4. Identify the spinal pathways that mediate sensation.
5. Understand the guidelines for administering an examination of sensory function.
6. Describe the testing protocol for each sensory modality.
7. Using the case study example, apply clinical decision making skills to application of sensory examination data.

CHAPTER OUTLINE

SENSORY INTEGRATION

"If all of the sensory stimuli which enter the central nervous system were allowed to bombard the higher centers of the brain, the individual would be rendered utterly ineffective. It is the brain's task to filter, organize, and integrate a mass of sensory information so that it can be used for the development and execution of the brain's functions."
—A. Jean Ayers, PhD[1, p. 25]

The human system is continually inundated with sensory information from a variety of environmental inputs as well as from movement, touch, awareness of the body in space, sight, sound, and smell. "In all higher order motor behaviors, the brain must correlate sensory inputs with motor outputs to accurately assess and control the body's interaction with the environment."[2, p. 32] Sensory integration is the ability of the brain to organize, interpret, and use sensory information. This integration provides an internal representation of the environment that informs and guides motor responses.[2] These sensory representations provide the foundation on which motor programs for purposeful movements are planned, coordinated, and implemented.[3] Ayers defined *sensory integration* as "the neurological process that organizes sensation from one's own body and from the environment and makes it possible to use the body effectively within the environment."[4, p. 11] In an intact system, sensory integration occurs automatically without conscious effort.

Sensory integration is a theory developed by A. Jean Ayers (1920–1989), an occupational therapist whose work focused on examining the manner in which sensory integration develops, identifying patterns of dysfunction in children with learning disorders, and developing intervention strategies to improve processing of sensory information. Mailloux and Miller-Kuhaneck recently summarized the evidenced-based approach that Ayers used to develop this theory for clinical application.[5] The theory purports that disordered sensory integration directly affects both motor and cognitive learning and that interventions designed to enhance sensory integration will improve learning.[1] Bundy and Murray[6] suggest the value of the theory lies in its usefulness in (1) explaining behaviors of individuals with impaired sensory integration functions, (2) establishing a plan of care (POC) to address specific impairments, and (3) predicting expected outcomes of the selected interventions. A review article by Schaaf and colleagues[7] summarized sensory integration research on children with autism spectrum disorder and proposes a three-pillar road map to guide future research consisting of practice, advocacy, and education.

■ SENSATION AND MOVEMENT

Motor learning and motor performance are inextricably linked to sensation. As a motor task is practiced, the individual learns to anticipate and correct or modify movements based on sensory input organized and integrated by the central nervous system (CNS). The CNS uses this information to influence movement by both feedback and feedforward control. *Feedback control* uses sensory information received *during the movement* to monitor and adjust output. *Feedforward control* is a proactive strategy that uses sensory information obtained from experience. Signals are sent in *advance of movement,* allowing for anticipatory adjustments in postural control or movement.[3,8] The primary role of sensation in movement is to (1) guide selection of motor responses for effective interaction with the environment and (2) adapt movements and shape motor programs through feedback for corrective action. Sensation also provides the important function of protecting the organism from injury. See Chapter 5, Examination of Motor Function: Motor Control and Motor Learning, for a more detailed discussion of CNS control of motor function.

■ SENSORY INTEGRITY

The term *somatosensation* (somatosensory) refers to sensation received from the skin and musculoskeletal system, as opposed to that from specialized senses such as sight or hearing. Examination of sensory function involves testing *sensory integrity* by determining the patient's ability to interpret and discriminate among incoming sensory information. The sensory examination is based on the premise that within the intact human system, sensory information is taken in from the body and the environment; the CNS then processes and integrates the information for use in planning and organizing behavior. This premise is more aptly termed a *theoretical construct* (a concept that represents an *unobservable* event). We cannot *directly* observe CNS processing, integration of sensory information, or the motor planning process. However, our current knowledge of CNS function and motor behavior provides evidence that these unobservable events do occur. We *can* observe impairments in motor behavior, but can only *hypothesize* that they truly result from faulty sensory integration mechanisms.[6]

The *Guide to Physical Therapist Practice 3.0* defines *sensory integrity* as "the soundness of cortical sensory processing, including proprioception, vibration sense, stereognosis, and cutaneous sensation."[9] Sensory integrity is included among the list of 26 categories of tests and measures that may be used by physical therapists during a patient initial examination or during subsequent visits as part of a reexamination.

This chapter focuses primarily on examination of somatosensory integrity of the trunk and extremities as well as screening for cranial nerve integrity; testing approaches for examining *cranial nerve integrity* and *reflex testing* are addressed in Chapter 5, Examination of Motor Function: Motor Control and Motor Learning. As the CNS analyzes and uses all sensory input to identify movement errors and initiate corrective responses, examination of sensory function typically precedes examination of motor function. This sequence assists the physical therapist in differentiating the impact of sensory impairments on motor function.

■ CLINICAL INDICATIONS

Indications for examination of sensory function are based on the history and systems review. Data from the history and systems review include family, social, medical, and surgical history; demographics; general health status; activities and participation; current condition(s); growth and development; living environment; social/health habits; medications; and status of body systems (e.g., cardiovascular, pulmonary, integumentary).[9] These data may indicate the existence of pathology or health condition resulting in sensory function changes. Box 3.1 presents examples of risk factors, health, wellness, and fitness needs, together with pathologies, impairments of body functions and

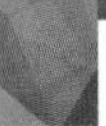

Box 3.1 Examination of Sensory Integrity: Examples of Clinical Indications

The physical therapist uses the results of tests and measures to determine the integrity of an individual's sensory, perceptual, and somatosensory processes. Responses monitored at rest, during activity, and after activity may indicate the presence or severity of an impairment, activity limitation, or participation restriction.

Examples of Clinical Indications

Risk factors for impaired sensory integrity
- Lack of safety awareness in all environments
- Risk-prone behaviors (e.g., working without protective gloves)
- Substance abuse

Health, wellness, and fitness needs
- Fitness, including physical performance (e.g., inadequate balance, limited perception of arms and legs in space)
- Health and wellness (e.g., inadequate understanding of role of proprioception in balance)

Pathology or health condition
- Cardiovascular (e.g., lymphedema, peripheral vascular disease)
- Integumentary (e.g., burn, frostbite)
- Musculoskeletal (e.g., derangement of joint; disorders of bursa, synovia, and tendon)
- Neuromuscular (e.g., cerebral palsy, stroke, developmental delay, spinal cord injury, traumatic brain injury)
- Pulmonary (e.g., ventilatory pump failure)
- Multisystem (e.g., AIDS, Guillain-Barré syndrome, trauma)

Impairments of body functions and structures
- Circulation (e.g., numb feet)
- Integumentary integrity (e.g., redness under orthosis)
- Muscle performance (e.g., decreased grip strength)
- Posture (e.g., asymmetrical alignment)

Activity limitations and participation restrictions
- Self-care (e.g., inability to put on trousers while standing due to foot numbness)
- Domestic life (e.g., difficulty with sorting laundry due to hand numbness)
- Education (e.g., inability to sit for full classes due to sensory loss in trunk and lower extremities)
- Work life (e.g., inability to operate cash register due to clumsiness)
- Community, social, and civic life (e.g., inability to drive car due to loss of spatial awareness, inability to play guitar due to hyperesthesia)

Adapted from *Guide to Physical Therapist Practice 3.0*,[9] with permission of the American Physical Therapy Association.

structures, activity limitations, and participation restrictions associated with changes in sensory integrity.

Sensory dysfunction may be associated with any pathology or injury affecting either the peripheral nervous system (PNS), the CNS, or both. Deficits may occur at any point within the system, including the sensory receptors, peripheral nerves, spinal nerves, spinal cord nuclei and tracts, brain stem, thalamus, and sensory cortex.[10] Examples of conditions that generally demonstrate some level of sensory impairment include pathology, disease, or injury to the peripheral nerves such as trauma (e.g., fracture) that can sever, crush, or damage a nerve; metabolic disturbances (e.g., diabetes, hypothyroidism, alcoholism); infections (e.g., Lyme disease, leprosy, HIV); impingement or compression (e.g., arthritis, carpal tunnel syndrome); burns; toxins (e.g., lead, mercury, chemotherapy); and nutritional deficits (e.g., vitamin B_{12}). Sensory impairments are also associated with injury to nerve roots or spinal cord, cerebral vascular accident (CVA), transient ischemic attack, tumors, multiple sclerosis (MS), and brain injury or disease. These examples, which are not all inclusive, indicate the wide spectrum of injuries, diseases, and pathologies that may present with some element of sensory deficit.

Pattern (Distribution) of Sensory Impairment

Examination of sensory function contributes critical information to establishing a physical therapy diagnosis and prognosis, identifying goals and expected outcomes, and developing a POC. A seminal feature of the examination involves determining the *pattern* (specific boundaries) of sensory involvement. Pattern identification is accomplished using knowledge of skin segment innervation by the dorsal roots and peripheral nerves (Figs. 3.1 and 3.2). The term *dermatome* (or *skin segment*) refers to the skin area supplied by one dorsal root.[11] The graphic illustration of skin segment innervation as presented in Figures 3.1 and 3.2 is referred to as a *dermatome map*. There exist some discrepancies among published dermatome maps

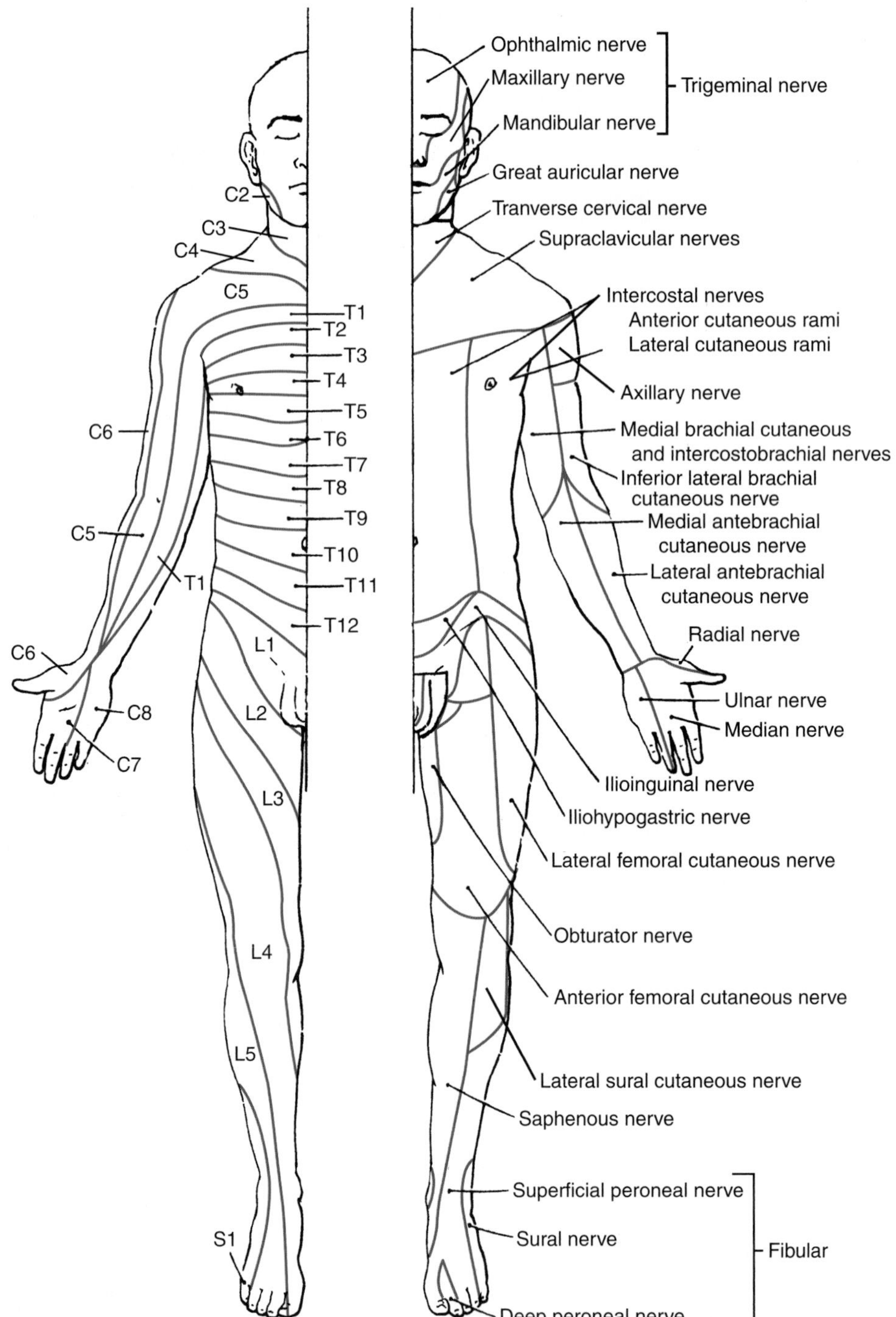

Figure 3.1 Anterior view of skin segment innervation by dorsal roots (*left*) and peripheral nerves (*right*). *(From Gilman and Newman,[11, p. 43] with permission.)*

based on the methodologies used to identify skin segment innervation. In a clinical commentary, Downs and Laporte[12] discuss the history of dermatome mapping, including the variations in methodologies employed and the inconsistencies in the dermatome maps used in education and practice. In a similar review article by Apok and colleagues, inconsistencies in dermatome pattern distribution and overlap are discussed.[13] A recent study by Ladak and colleagues presents preliminary findings, based on a synthesis of literature, of a refined dermatome map that incorporates physical neural connections.[14] As new technology allows for more precise identification of nerve distribution, cutaneous spinal nerve distribution will likely continue to be reevaluated.

Clinical Note: Considerable variation exists in the clinical presentation of sensory impairments. This variability is typically associated with the nervous system involved (CNS vs. PNS), the type of injury, pathology, or disease, as well as the severity, extent, and duration of involvement.

During the review of systems, asking the patient to carefully describe the pattern or distribution of sensory

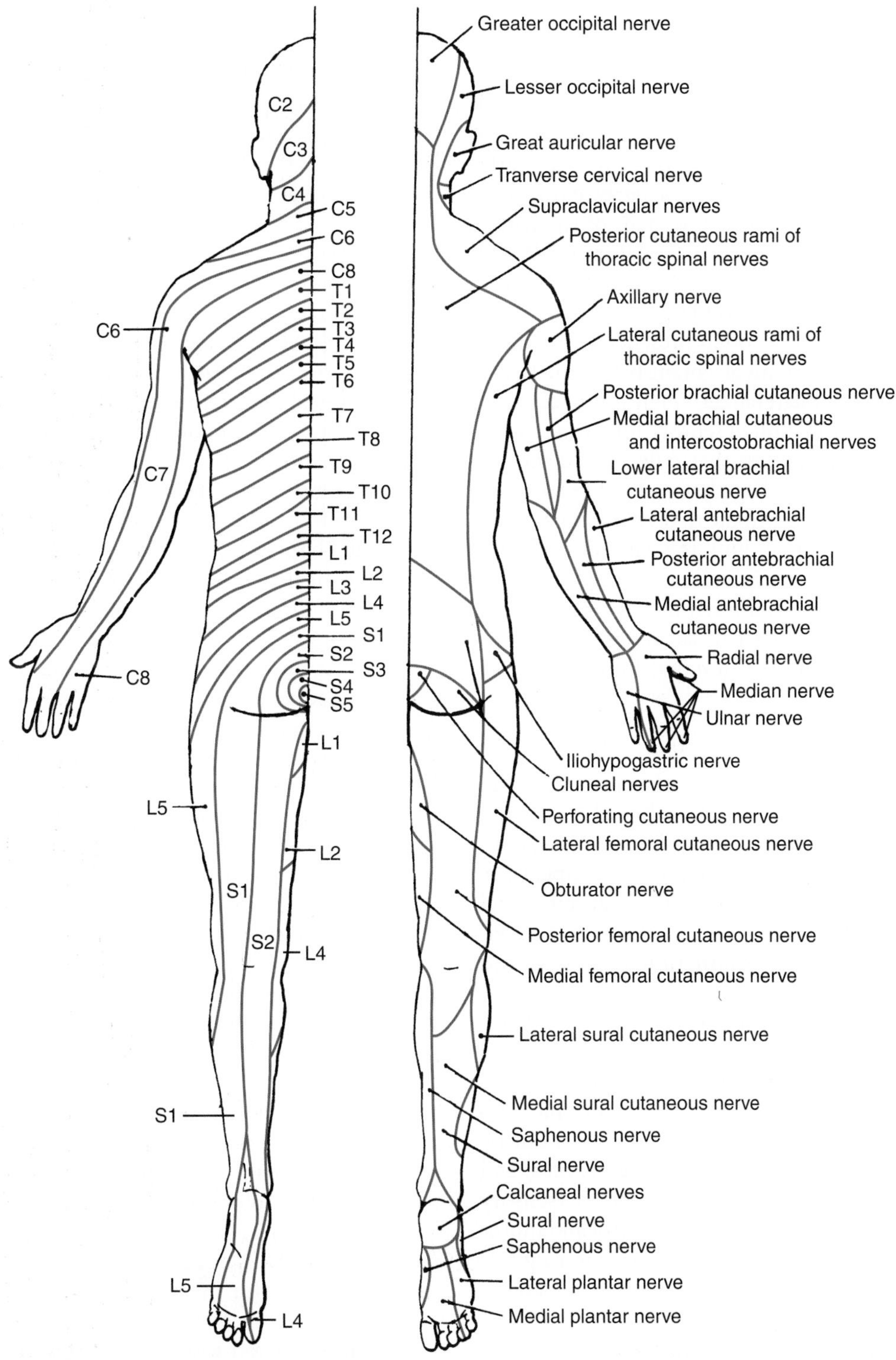

Figure 3.2 Posterior view of skin segment innervation by dorsal roots (*left*) and peripheral nerves (*right*). *(From Gilman and Newman,[11, p. 44] with permission.)*

symptoms (e.g., tingling, numbness, diminished, or absent sensation) provides the therapist with preliminary information to help guide the examination and to assist in identifying the dermatome(s) and nerve(s) involved. Peripheral nerve injuries generally present sensory impairments that parallel the distribution of the involved nerve and correspond to its pattern of innervation. For example, if a patient presents with complaints of numbness on the ulnar half of the ring finger, the little finger, and the ulnar side of the hand, the therapist would be alerted to carefully address ulnar nerve (C8 and T1) integrity during the sensory examination.[15] Complaints of sensory disturbances on the palmar surface of the thumb and the palmar and distal dorsal aspects of the index, middle, and the radial half of the ring finger would be indicative of median nerve (C6–8 and T1) involvement.

Other patterns of sensory loss may be associated with specific pathology. For example, with peripheral neuropathy (e.g., diabetes), sensory loss is often an early symptom and presents in a *glove and stocking* distribution (referring to the typical involvement of the hands and feet that spreads proximally).[16] In contrast, MS frequently presents with an unpredictable or scattered pattern of sensory or motor involvement.[17]

Spinal cord injury (SCI) often presents with a more diffuse pattern of sensory involvement below the lesion level that is typically bilateral, although not necessarily symmetrical.[18] Examination of sensory function following SCI provides critical data that reflect the degree of neurological impairment. Together with other tests and measures, sensory data contribute to determining the relative completeness of the injury, the existence of *zones of partial preservation* (areas distal to a complete lesion that retain partial innervation), symmetry or asymmetry of the lesion, and the presence of sacral sensation below the neurological level of the lesion (a defining feature of an incomplete lesion).

Spinal Cord Tracts

Examination of sensory function also provides data that reflect the integrity of the spinal cord tracts that carry somatosensory information.[18] For example, contralateral loss or impairment of pain and temperature perception is suggestive of lesions in the anterolateral tracts. Deficits in discriminative sensations such as vibration and two-point discrimination suggest lesions of the dorsal column.

Evidence of both sensory and motor loss is usually indicative of nerve root involvement (recall that the dorsal and ventral roots converge to form the spinal nerves). CNS lesions (e.g., CVA, brain injury) may produce significant sensory impairments characterized by a diffuse pattern of involvement (e.g., head, trunk, and limbs) and can result in significant motor dysfunction (sensory ataxia) and impairment of fine motor control and motor learning. These impairments can also present a significant threat of injury to anesthetic limbs (e.g., an inability to determine the temperature of bathwater).

■ AGE-RELATED SENSORY CHANGES

Alterations in sensory function occur with normal aging and should be clearly differentiated from those associated with specific illness, disease, or pathology. In recent years, there has been a gradual expansion of interest in and information about the causes and consequences of age-related sensory changes. This has been evident through the large and expanding body of literature devoted to the neuroscience of aging and its impact on function and quality of life of older adults.[19-31] The topics addressed are specific age-related changes in vision, hearing, and the somatosensory system; treatment, prevalence, and risk factor information; as well as the role of public policy and public health in addressing age-related sensory loss. *Healthy People 2020,*[32] published by the U.S. Department of Health and Human Services, presents a comprehensive health promotion and wellness agenda for the second decade of the 21st century. The overarching goals of *Healthy People 2020* are to (1) attain high-quality, longer lives free of preventable disease, disability, injury, and premature death; (2) achieve health equity, eliminate disparities, and improve the health of all groups; (3) create social and physical environments that promote good health for all; and (4) promote quality of life, healthy development, and healthy behaviors across all life stages. The first goal draws national attention to an expanding population of older adults and the impact of age (including changes in sensation such as vision and hearing) on health improvement and health promotion strategies. Decreased acuity of many sensations occurs and is considered a characteristic finding with aging.[33] The exact morphology of diminished sensation with age has not been completely established. However, several neurological changes have been identified and suggest potential explanations.

Over the life span, neurons are replaced at a declining rate and this may account for the decline of the brain's average weight with aging. Although a feature of Alzheimer's disease, normal aging does not produce a significant loss in the number of cortical neurons.[34] Other changes in the brain include degeneration of neurons with the presence of replacement gliosis, lipid accumulation in the neurons, loss of myelin, and development of neurofibrils (masses of small, tangled fibrils) and plaques on the cells.[34,35] There is also a decrease in the number of enzymes responsible for synthesis of dopamine, norepinephrine, and to a lesser degree acetylcholine, as well as depletion of the neuronal dendrites in the aging brain.[36,37]

Electrophysiological studies have identified a gradual reduction in conduction velocity of sensory nerves with advancing age, and this may reflect degenerative changes in myelin sheaths or loss or reduction in size of sensory axons.[38-41] Evoked potentials provide a quantitative measure of sensory function and have been found to decrease in amplitude with age.[42] A reduction in the number of Meissner's corpuscles[43] has also been identified. These corpuscles, responsible for touch detection, are limited to hairless areas and become sparse, take on an irregular distribution, and vary in size and shape with age. Age-related changes in morphology and decreased concentrations of Pacinian corpuscles, responsive to rapid tissue movement (e.g., vibration), have also been reported.[44]

Degenerative changes in myelin have been documented in both the central and peripheral nervous systems.[45] In a review of the literature on the effects of normal aging on myelin and nerve fibers, Peters[46] suggests that (1) age-associated cognitive decline is more likely due to widespread damage to myelin sheaths of cortical neuron axons than to actual loss of these neurons and (2) the resulting changes in conduction velocity alter the normal timing of neuronal circuits.

In the PNS, a decrease in the distance between the nodes of Ranvier has been associated with advancing age.[47] This finding may be related to a slowing of saltatory conduction identified by some authors.[34,38] Destruction of myelin sheaths has been linked to a reduced expression of primary myelin proteins and axonal atrophy and to a reduced expression and axonal transport of cytoskeletal proteins.[48] As compared to younger subjects, lower sensory nerve conduction velocities have been documented in older adults.[40,41]

Although not an exhaustive list, other documented age-related sensory changes include altered postural stability and control,[49-51] diminished response to tactile stimuli,[52-53] reduced vibratory[54,55] and proprioceptive acuity,[56,57] decreased cutaneous temperature thresholds,[58-61] and diminished two-point discrimination.[62,63]

These changes frequently appear in the presence of age-related visual or hearing losses that impair compensatory capabilities. In addition, some medications may further influence the distortion of sensory input. This combination of sensory impairments may pose a variety of activity limitations for an older adult such as postural instability, exaggerated body sway, balance problems, wide-based gait, diminished fine motor coordination, tendency to drop items held in the hand, and difficulty in recognizing body positions in space. Table 3.1 Evidence Summary provides an overview of research exploring age-related sensory changes.

Clinical Note: In addition to age-related sensory changes, activity limitations may be exacerbated by muscle weakness associated with a reduction in the number and size of skeletal muscle fibers and overall cross-sectional area of muscle.

■ PRELIMINARY CONSIDERATIONS

Accuracy of data from examination of sensory function relies on the patient's ability to respond to application of multiple somatosensory stimuli. Use of several easily administered preliminary tests will provide sufficient data to determine the patient's ability to concentrate on, and respond to, the battery of sensory test items. The two general categories of preliminary tests include the patient's (1) arousal level, attention span, orientation, and cognition,[64] and (2) memory, hearing, and visual acuity. These preliminary tests are typically considered with sensory involvement associated with CNS lesions.

Arousal, Attention, Orientation, and Cognition

A necessary first step is to determine the patient's arousal level for participation in the test protocol. *Arousal* is the state of responsiveness of the human system to sensory stimulation. It is described by using traditionally accepted key terms and definitions to identify the patient's level of consciousness. These terms include *alert, lethargic, obtunded, stupor,* and *coma* and represent a continuum of physiological readiness for activity. They are defined as follows:[64]

- *Alert.* The patient is awake and attentive to normal levels of stimulation. Interactions with the therapist are normal and appropriate.
- *Lethargic.* The patient appears drowsy and may fall asleep if not stimulated in some way. Interactions with the therapist may get diverted. Patient may have difficulty in focusing or maintaining attention on a question or task.
- *Obtunded.* The patient is difficult to arouse from a somnolent state and is frequently confused when awake. Repeated stimulation is required to maintain consciousness. Interactions with the therapist may be largely unproductive.
- *Stupor* (semicoma). The patient responds only to strong, generally noxious stimuli and returns to the unconscious state when stimulation is stopped. When aroused, the patient is unable to interact with the therapist.
- *Coma* (deep coma). The patient cannot be aroused by any type of stimulation. Reflex motor responses may or may not be seen.

Reliable information about the integrity of the somatosensory system can be obtained from patients who are alert. Reliability is proportionally reduced in patients with lethargy and nonexistent in patients who are obtunded, stuporous, or comatose.

Attention is selective awareness of the environment or responsiveness to a stimulus or task without being distracted by other stimuli.[8,11,65] Attention can be examined by asking the patient to repeat items on a progressively more challenging list. These repetition tasks can begin with two or three items and gradually progress to longer lists. For example, the patient might be asked to count by fives or sevens or to spell words backward (e.g., book, fork, bottle, garden).[66] Spelling words backward can be made more challenging by using progressively longer words (e.g., computer, telephone, automobile). Individuals with a high attention span will be able to perform the task. In contrast, attention deficits will be apparent when the order of letters is confused.

Orientation refers to the patient's awareness of time, person, and place (or space). In medical record documentation, the results of this mental status screening are

Table 3.1 Evidence Summary Research Exploring Age-Related Changes in Sensory Function

Reference	Method(s)	Subjects/Design	Results	Conclusions/ Comments
Senthikumari et al[41]	Examined age-related differences in nerve conduction velocity of the median nerve. Median motor and sensory conduction velocity was measured.	Included 103 individuals without a history of neurological illness, divided into three groups: group I (ages 15–30, n = 40); group II (ages 31–45, n = 31); and group III (ages 46–60, n = 32). Groups were not significantly different for gender or BMI.	Significant differences found in median motor/sensory conduction velocity between groups: group I = 59.5±3.3/64.4±6.8; group II = 56.7±1.1/60.2±5.7; group III = 52.8±4.3/54.5±7.5. The correlation between age and median motor (−0.41) and sensory (−0.54) was significant and negative.	There was a significant decrease in median motor and sensory nerve conduction velocity with age. Furthermore, there was a significant inverse relationship between median nerve conduction velocity and age. Age can affect the conduction velocity of the median nerve. This study is limited by its cross-sectional design.
Alanazy et al[54]	Vibration threshold was tested at the distal interphalangeal joint (index finger) and interphalangeal joint (great toe) using a conventional tuning fork (CTF) and a Rydel-Seiffer tuning fork (RSTF).	The vibration threshold of normal healthy adults (n = 281) was examined using a CTF and RSTF.	Associations between the CTF and RSTF were moderate for finger and toe measures (Spearman's correlation coefficient = 0.59 and 0.64, respectively). As a covariate, only age had a significant negative effect on vibration threshold. Reference values for vibration thresholds are also provided.	The CTF and RSTF provided comparable results. Among the possible covariates, only age had an effect (negative) on vibration thresholds. Reference values stratified by age are also provided for each instrument and each body part.
Ko et al[56]	Examined ankle proprioception in aging men and women using passive motion detection (threshold) and movement tracking.	Examined 289 aging adults (ages 51–95) without severe lower limb pain or limited ankle mobility (i.e., < 10 degrees of plantarflexion or dorsiflexion). Women (n = 131) were significantly younger, shorter, and weighed less when compared to males (n = 158).	When adjusting for height and weight, there were several significant findings suggesting an age-associated reduction in proprioception. Age-associated differences in proprioception were also found between genders: men at slower speeds and females at faster speeds.	Proprioception of men and women, as measured by threshold and tracking, decreased with increasing age. The paradigm used in this study should be replicated using a longitudinal design.

often abbreviated "oriented × 3," referring to the three parameters of time, person, and place. If a patient is not fully oriented to one or more domains, the notation would read "oriented × 2 (time)" or "oriented × 1 (time, place)." With partial orientation entries, it is customary to include the *domains of disorientation* within parentheses. Box 3.2 presents sample questions for examining orientation.[11,64,65]

Cognition is defined as the process of knowing and includes both awareness and judgment.[8] Nolan[64] suggests three areas for testing cognition-dependent functions: (1) fund of knowledge, (2) calculation ability, and (3) proverb interpretation. *Fund of knowledge* is defined as the sum of an individual's learning and experience in life, which will be highly variable and different for each patient. Detailed information about

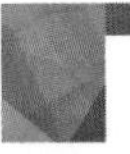

Box 3.2 Sample Questions for Examining Orientation

A series of simple questions is posed to the patient. The questions are designed to determine the patient's understanding of recognition of who he or she is; the location, including the present facility (the name of hospital or clinic); the present time; and the passage of time.

Person

- What is your name?
- Do you have a middle name?
- How old are you?
- When were you born?

Place

- Do you know where you are right now?
- What kind of a place is this?
- Do you know what city and state we are in?
- What city or town do you live in?
- What is your address at home?

Time

- What is today's date?
- What day of the week is it?
- What time is it?
- Is it morning or afternoon?
- What season is it?
- What year is it?
- How long have you been here?

From Nolan,[64, p. 26] with permission.

premorbid knowledge base is often not available. However, a number of general categories of information can be used to test this cognitive function. Sample questions might include the following:[64]

- Who became president after Kennedy was shot?
- Who is the current vice president of the United States?
- Which is more—a gallon or a liter?
- In what country is the Great Pyramid?
- What would you add to your food to make it sweeter?
- In what state would you find the city of Boston?
- What are the elements that make up water and salt?
- Can you name a car made by General Motors?
- Who is Charles Dickens?

Calculation ability examines foundational mathematical abilities.[64,65] Two associated terms are *acalculia* (inability to calculate) and *dyscalculia* (difficulty in accomplishing calculations).[64] This cognitive screening can be administered either verbally or in written format. The patient is asked to mentally perform a series of calculations when provided with mathematical problems. The test should be initiated with simple problems and progress to the more difficult. Adding and subtracting are generally easier than multiplication and division. An alternative approach is to provide written mathematical problems and ask the patient to fill in the answer: $4 + 4 =$ ____; $10 + 22 =$ ____; $46 \times 8 =$ ____; $13 \times 7 =$ ____; $4 \times 3 =$ ____; $6 \times 6 =$ ____; and so forth.

Proverb interpretation examines the patient's ability to interpret use of words outside of their usual context or meaning. This is a sophisticated cognitive function. During the screening, the patient should be asked to describe the meaning of the proverb. Sample proverbs include the following:[64,65]

- People who live in glass houses shouldn't throw stones.
- A rolling stone gathers no moss.
- A stitch in time saves nine.
- The early bird catches the worm.
- The dog that trots about finds the bone.
- The empty wagon makes the most noise.
- Every cloud has a silver lining.
- Grass doesn't grow on a busy street.

Memory, Hearing, and Visual Acuity

Also related to the ability to respond during sensory testing is the status of the patient's memory and hearing function as well as visual acuity.

Memory

Both long- and short-term memory should be examined. Impairments of short-term memory will be the most disruptive to collecting sensory information owing to patient difficulties in remembering and following directions. *Long-term (remote) memory* can be examined by requesting information on date and place of birth, parents' names, number of siblings, date of marriage, schools attended, or other historical facts such as "Where were you on September 11, 2001?"[66] *Short-term memory* can be addressed by verbally providing the patient with a series of words or numbers. For example, ask the patient to repeat a series of three words (e.g., *car, book, cup*) immediately and again in 5 minutes. Individuals with normal memory function should be able to recall the list 5 minutes[11] later and at least two of the items from the list after 30 minutes.[64] Use of numbers could include a seven-digit list; a short sentence could also be used to test short-term memory. To ensure understanding of the task, the patient should repeat the sequence immediately.

Hearing

Observing the patient's response to conversation can provide a gross assessment of hearing. Note should be made of how alterations in voice volume and tone influence patient response. Whispering 40 inches (1 m) from each ear can be used to compare hearing on both sides.

A vibratory tuning fork can be used to examine and compare air conduction hearing to bone conduction hearing. *Air conduction hearing* involves signals transmitted through air to the inner ear and is examined by placing a vibrating tuning fork near the pinna. *Bone conduction hearing* refers to sounds transmitted through bone and is tested by placing a vibrating tuning fork on the mastoid process.[67,68]

Visual Acuity

A basic visual examination[68] can be made using a standard Snellen chart mounted on the wall or visual acuity cards for use at bedside. A Snellen chart (standard eye chart) includes a series of uppercase letters that gradually decrease in size as the viewer moves down the chart. If the patient uses corrective lenses, they should be worn during testing and should be clean. Visual acuity is typically recorded at 20 feet (6 m) from the Snellen chart. This distance is then placed over the size of the printed letter the individual is able to read comfortably. For example, on a continuum of visual acuity, 20/20 is considered excellent and 20/200 is considered poor acuity.[11]

Clinical Note: Some diagnoses or comorbidities directly affect vision such as MS, hypertension, and diabetes. Examining the cranial nerves (CNs) will provide additional information about vision. For example, the oculomotor nerve (CN III) is often affected by diabetes (oculomotor nerve palsy).

Peripheral field vision can be examined by sitting directly in front of the patient with outstretched arms. The index fingers should be extended and gradually brought toward the midline of the patient's face. The patient is asked to identify when the therapist's approaching finger is first seen. Differences between right and left visual field should be noted carefully. Depth perception may be grossly checked by holding two pencils or fingers (one behind the other) directly in front of the patient. The patient is asked to touch or grasp the foreground object.

Because tests of sensory integrity require a verbal response to the stimulus, patients with arousal, attention, orientation, cognitive, or short-term memory impairments generally cannot be accurately tested. However, impairments in vision, hearing, or speech will not adversely affect test results if appropriate adaptations are made in providing instructions and indicating responses (e.g., signaling with either one or two fingers during tests for two-point discrimination, pointing to an area of stimulus contact, mimicking joint position sense or awareness of movement with the contralateral extremity, or object identification by selecting from a group of items during tests for stereognosis).

CLASSIFICATION OF THE SENSORY SYSTEM

Several different schemes have been proposed for categorizing the sensory system. Among the more common is classification by the type (or location) of *receptors* and the *spinal pathway* mediating information to higher centers.

Sensory Receptors

Sensory receptors (sensory nerve endings) are located at the distal end of an afferent nerve fiber. Once stimulated, they give rise to perception of a specific sensation. Sensory receptors are highly sensitive to the type of stimulus for which they were designed (termed *receptor specificity*). This specificity of nerve fiber sensitivity to a single modality of sensation is called the *labeled line principle.*[69] This means that individual tactile sensations are perceived when specific types of receptors are stimulated. For example, in response to touch, selective activation of Merkel's discs and Ruffini endings generate the sensation of steady pressure in the cutaneous area above the active receptors.[70]

It should be noted that the term *modality* has a specific meaning within the context of sensation. Modality "defines a general class of stimulus, determined by the type of energy transmitted by the stimulus and the receptors specialized to sense that energy."[70, p. 413] Each type of sensation perceived (e.g., vision, hearing, taste, touch, smell, pain, temperature, proprioception) is referred to as a *modality of sensation.*

The three divisions of sensory receptors include those that mediate the (1) superficial, (2) deep, and (3) combined (cortical) sensations.[11]

Superficial Sensation

Exteroceptors are responsible for the superficial sensations.[71] They receive stimuli from the external environment via the skin and subcutaneous tissue. Exteroceptors are responsible for the perception of pain, temperature, light touch, and pressure.[11,71]

Deep Sensation

Proprioceptors are responsible for the deep sensations. These receptors receive stimuli from muscles, tendons, ligaments, joints, and fascia[65] and are responsible for position sense[72] and awareness of joints at rest, movement awareness (kinesthesia), and vibration.

Combined Cortical Sensations

The combination of both the superficial and deep sensory mechanisms makes up the third category of combined sensations. These sensations require information from both exteroceptive and proprioceptive receptors, as well as intact function of cortical sensory association areas. The cortical combined sensations include stereognosis, two-point discrimination, barognosis, graphesthesia, tactile localization, recognition of texture, and double simultaneous stimulation.

Spinal Pathways

Sensations also have been classified according to the system by which they are mediated to higher centers. Sensations are mediated by either the *anterolateral spinothalamic system* or the *dorsal column-medial lemniscal system.*[34,71,73]

Anterolateral Spinothalamic

This system initiates self-protective reactions and responds to stimuli that are potentially harmful in nature. It contains slow-conducting fibers of small diameter, some of which are unmyelinated. The system is concerned with transmission of thermal and nociceptive information, and mediates pain, temperature, crudely localized touch, tickle, itch, and sexual sensations.

Dorsal Column–Medial Lemniscal System

The dorsal column is the system involved with responses to more discriminative sensations. It contains fast-conducting fibers of large diameter with greater myelination. This system mediates the sensations of discriminative touch and pressure sensations, vibration, movement, position sense, and awareness of joints at rest. The two systems are interdependent and integrated so as to function together.

TYPES OF SENSORY RECEPTORS

The sensory receptors frequently are divided according to their structural design and the type of stimulus to which they preferentially respond. These divisions include (1) *mechanoreceptors,* which respond to mechanical deformation of the receptor or surrounding area; (2) *thermoreceptors,* which respond to changes in temperature; (3) *nociceptors,* which respond to noxious stimuli and result in the perception of pain; (4) *chemoreceptors,* which respond to chemical substances and are responsible for taste, smell, oxygen levels in arterial blood, carbon dioxide concentration, and osmolality (concentration gradient) of body fluids; and (5) *photic (electromagnetic) receptors,* which respond to light within the visible spectrum.[10,11,71,74]

The perception of pain is not limited to stimuli received from nociceptors, because other types of receptors and nerve fibers contribute to this sensation. High intensities of stimuli to any type of receptor may be perceived as pain (e.g., extreme heat or cold and high-intensity mechanical deformation).

The general classification of sensory receptors is presented in Box 3.3.[65,69,75] Note that this list also includes the receptors responsible for electromagnetic (visual) and chemical stimuli.

Cutaneous Receptors

Cutaneous sensory receptors are located at the terminal portion of the afferent fiber. These include free nerve endings, hair follicle endings, Merkel's discs, Ruffini endings, Krause's end-bulbs, Meissner's corpuscles, and Pacinian corpuscles. The density of these sensory receptors varies for different areas of the body. For example, there are many more tactile receptors in the fingertips than in the back. These areas of higher receptor density correspondingly display a higher cortical representation in somatic sensory area I. Receptor density is a particularly important consideration in interpreting the results of a sensory

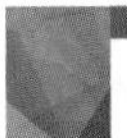

Box 3.3 Classification of Sensory Receptors

I. Mechanoreceptors
  A. Cutaneous sensory receptors
    1. Free nerve endings
    2. Hair follicle endings
    3. Merkel's discs
    4. Ruffini endings
    5. Krause's end-bulbs
    6. Meissner's corpuscles
    7. Pacinian corpuscles
II. Deep Sensory Receptors
  A. Muscle receptors
    1. Muscle spindles
    2. Golgi tendon organs
    3. Free nerve endings
    4. Pacinian corpuscles
  B. Joint receptors
    1. Golgi-type endings
    2. Free nerve endings
    3. Ruffini endings
    4. Paciniform endings
III. Thermoreceptors
  A. Cold
    1. Cold receptors
  B. Warmth
    1. Warmth receptors
IV. Nociceptors
  A. Pain
    1. Free nerve endings
    2. Extremes of stimuli*
V. Electromagnetic Receptors
  B. Vision
    1. Rods
    2. Cones
VI. Chemoreceptors
  A. Taste
    1. Receptors of taste buds
  B. Smell
    1. Receptors of olfactory nerves in olfactory epithelium
  C. Arterial oxygen
    1. Receptors of aortic and carotid bodies
  D. Osmolality
    1. Probably neurons of supraoptic nuclei
  E. Blood CO_2
    1. Receptors in or on surface of medulla and in aortic and carotid bodies
  F. Blood glucose, amino acids, fatty acids
    1. Receptors in hypothalamus

*Extremes of stimuli to other sensory receptors will be perceived as pain.

Adapted from Waxman,[65] Hall,[69] and Mtui et al.[75]

examination for a given body surface. Figure 3.3 illustrates the cutaneous sensory receptors and their respective locations within the various layers of skin.

Free Nerve Endings

These receptors are found throughout the body. Stimulation of free nerve endings results in the perception of pain, temperature, touch, pressure, tickle, and itch sensations.[10,65]

Hair Follicle Endings (Hair End-Organs)

At the base of each hair follicle, a free nerve ending is entwined. The combination of the hair follicle and its nerve provides a sensitive receptor. These receptors are sensitive to mechanical movement and touch.[76,77]

Merkel's Discs

These touch receptors are located below the epidermis in hairless smooth (glabrous) skin with a high density in the fingertips. They are sensitive to low-intensity touch, as well as to the velocity of touch, and respond to constant indentation of the skin (pressure). They provide for the ability to perceive continuous contact of objects against the skin and are believed to play an important role in both two-point discrimination and localization of touch.[71,77] Merkel's discs are also believed to contribute to the recognition of texture.

Ruffini Endings

Located in the deeper layers of the dermis, these encapsulated endings are involved with the perception of touch and pressure. They are slowly adapting and particularly important in signaling continuous skin deformation such as tension or stretch; they are also found in joint capsules and assist with joint position sense.[69,77]

Krause's End-Bulb

The function of these bulbous encapsulated nerve endings is not clearly understood. They are located in the dermis and conjunctiva of the eye. They are believed to be low-threshold mechanical receptors that may play a contributing role in the perception of touch and pressure.

Meissner's Corpuscles

Located in the dermis, these encapsulated nerve endings contain many branching nerve filaments within the capsule. They are low-threshold, rapidly adapting and in high concentration in the fingertips, lips, and toes, areas that require high levels of discrimination. These receptors play an important role in discriminative touch (e.g., recognition of texture) and movement of objects over skin.[34,69,77]

Pacinian Corpuscles

These receptors are located in the subcutaneous tissue layer of the skin and in deep tissues of the body (including tendons and soft tissues around joints). They are stimulated by rapid movement of tissue and are quickly adapting. They play a significant role in the perception of deep touch and vibration.[77,78]

Deep Sensory Receptors

The deep sensory receptors are located in muscles, tendons, and joints[65,69,73] and include both muscle and joint receptors. They are concerned primarily with posture, position sense, proprioception, muscle tone, and speed and direction of movement. The deep sensory receptors include the muscle spindle, Golgi tendon organs, free nerve endings, Pacinian corpuscles, and joint receptors.

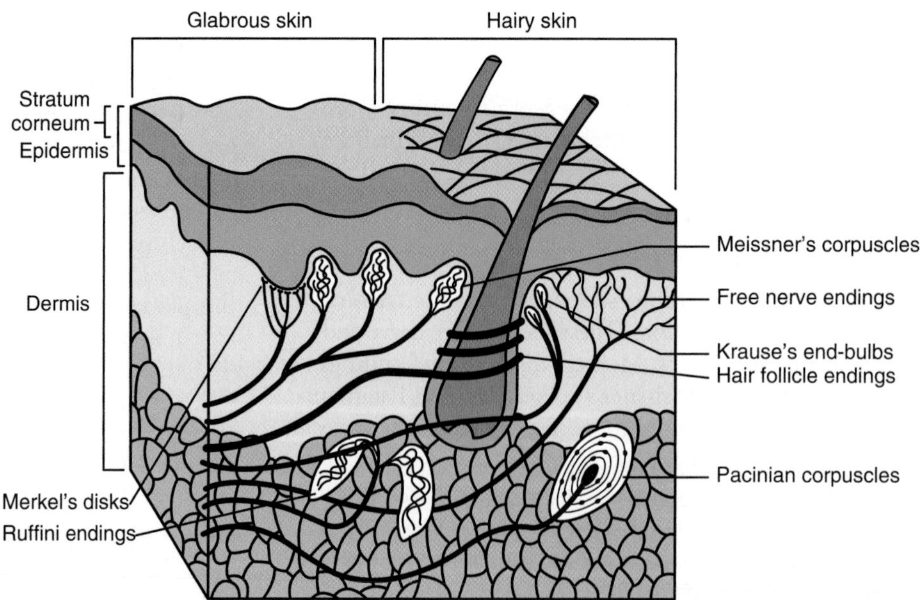

Figure 3.3 The cutaneous sensory receptors and their respective locations within the various layers of skin (epidermis, dermis, and the subcutaneous layer).

Muscle Receptors

Muscle Spindles

The muscle spindle fibers (intrafusal fibers) lie in a parallel arrangement to the muscle fibers (extrafusal fibers). They monitor changes in muscle length (Ia and II spindle afferent endings) as well as velocity (Ia ending) of these changes. The muscle spindle plays a vital role in position and movement sense and in motor learning.

Golgi Tendon Organs

These receptors are located in a series at both the proximal and distal tendinous insertions of the muscle. The Golgi tendon organs function to monitor tension within the muscle. They also provide a protective mechanism by preventing structural damage to the muscle in situations of extreme tension. This is accomplished by inhibition of the contracting muscle and facilitation of the antagonist.

Free Nerve Endings

These receptors are within the fascia of the muscle. They are believed to respond to pain and pressure.

Pacinian Corpuscles

Located within the fascia of the muscle, these receptors respond to vibratory stimuli and deep pressure.

Joint Receptors

Golgi-Type Endings

These receptors are located in the ligaments and function to detect the rate of joint movement.

Free Nerve Endings

Found in the joint capsule and ligaments, these receptors are believed to respond to pain and crude awareness of joint motion.

Ruffini Endings

Located in the joint capsule and ligaments, Ruffini endings are responsible for the direction and velocity of joint movement.

Paciniform Endings

These receptors are found in the joint capsule and primarily monitor rapid joint movements.

■ PATHWAYS FOR TRANSMISSION OF SOMATIC SENSORY SIGNALS

Somatic sensory information enters the spinal cord through the dorsal roots. Sensory signals are then carried to higher centers via ascending pathways from one of two systems: the *anterolateral spinothalamic system* or the *dorsal column–medial lemniscal system*.[79,80]

Anterolateral Spinothalamic Pathway

The spinothalamic tracts are diffuse pathways concerned with nondiscriminative sensations such as pain, temperature, tickle, itch, and sexual sensations.[65,79,80] This system is activated primarily by mechanoreceptors, thermoreceptors, and nociceptors and is composed of afferent fibers that are small diameter and slowly conducting. Sensory signals transmitted by this system do not require discrete localization of signal source or precise gradations in intensity.

After originating in the dorsal roots, the fibers of the spinothalamic pathway immediately cross and ascend up the spinal cord through the medulla, pons, and midbrain to the ventroposterolateral (VPL) nucleus of the thalamus (Fig. 3.4). Axons of the VPL neurons project to the somatosensory cortex via the internal capsule.[34,78]

Compared with the dorsal column–medial lemniscal system, the anterolateral spinothalamic pathways make up a cruder, more primitive system. The spinothalamic tracts are capable of transmitting a wide variety of sensory modalities. However, their diffuse pattern of termination results in only crude abilities to localize the source of a stimulus on the body surface and in poor intensity discrimination.[65] The three major tracts of the spinothalamic system are the (1) *anterior (ventral) spinothalamic tract,* which carries the sensations of crudely localized, light touch and pressure; (2) the *lateral spinothalamic tract,* which carries pain and temperature; and (3) the *spinoreticular tract,* which is involved with pain sensations, especially diffuse, deep, and chronic pain.[65,79,80]

Dorsal Column–Medial Lemniscal Pathway

This system is responsible for the transmission of discriminative sensations received from specialized mechanoreceptors.[65,79,80] Sensory modalities that require fine gradations of intensity and precise localization on the body surface are mediated by this system. Sensations transmitted by the dorsal column–medial lemniscal pathway include discriminative touch, stereognosis, tactile pressure, barognosis, graphesthesia, recognition of texture, kinesthesia, two-point discrimination, proprioception, and vibration.

This system is composed of large, myelinated, rapidly conducting fibers. After entering the dorsal column, the fibers ascend to the medulla and synapse with the dorsal column nuclei (nuclei gracilis and cuneatus). From here they cross to the opposite side and pass up to the thalamus through bilateral pathways called the *medial lemnisci.* Each medial lemniscus terminates in the ventral posterolateral thalamus. From the thalamus, third-order neurons project to the somatic sensory cortex. Projection to sensory association areas in the cortex allows for the perception and interpretation of the combined cortical sensations (Fig. 3.5).[65,69,71,78] Table 3.2 presents a comparison of the most salient features of each ascending pathway.

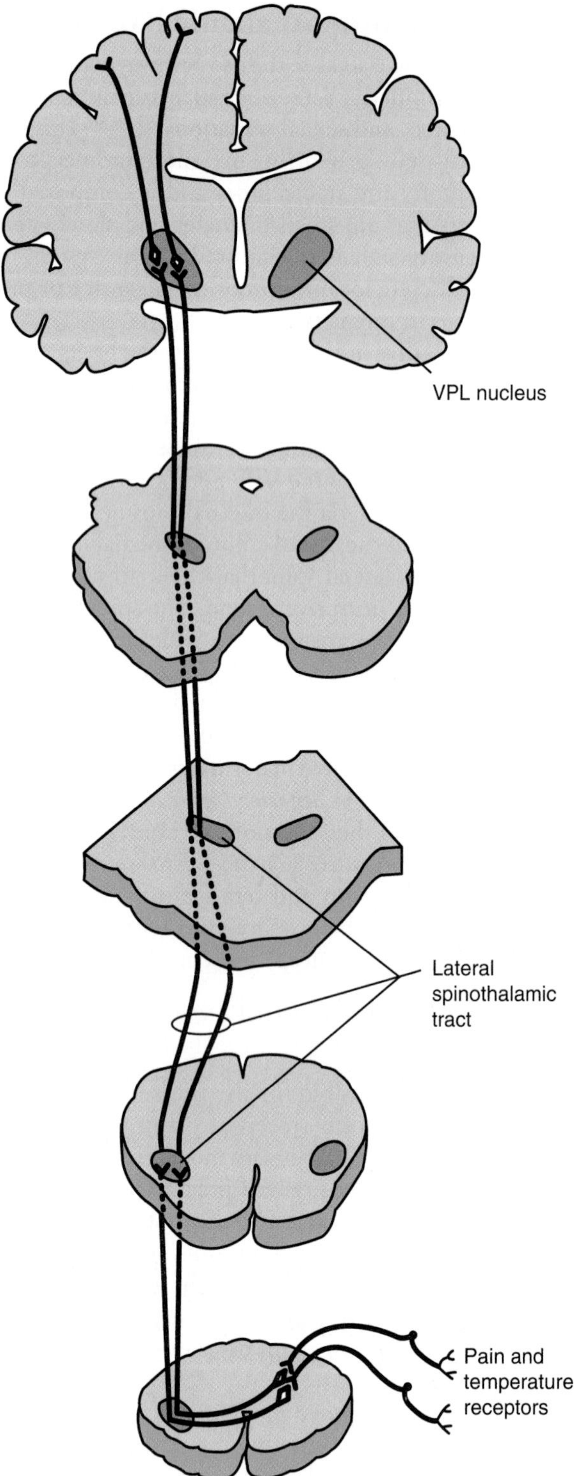

Figure 3.4 Anterolateral spinothalamic tract carrying pain and temperature.

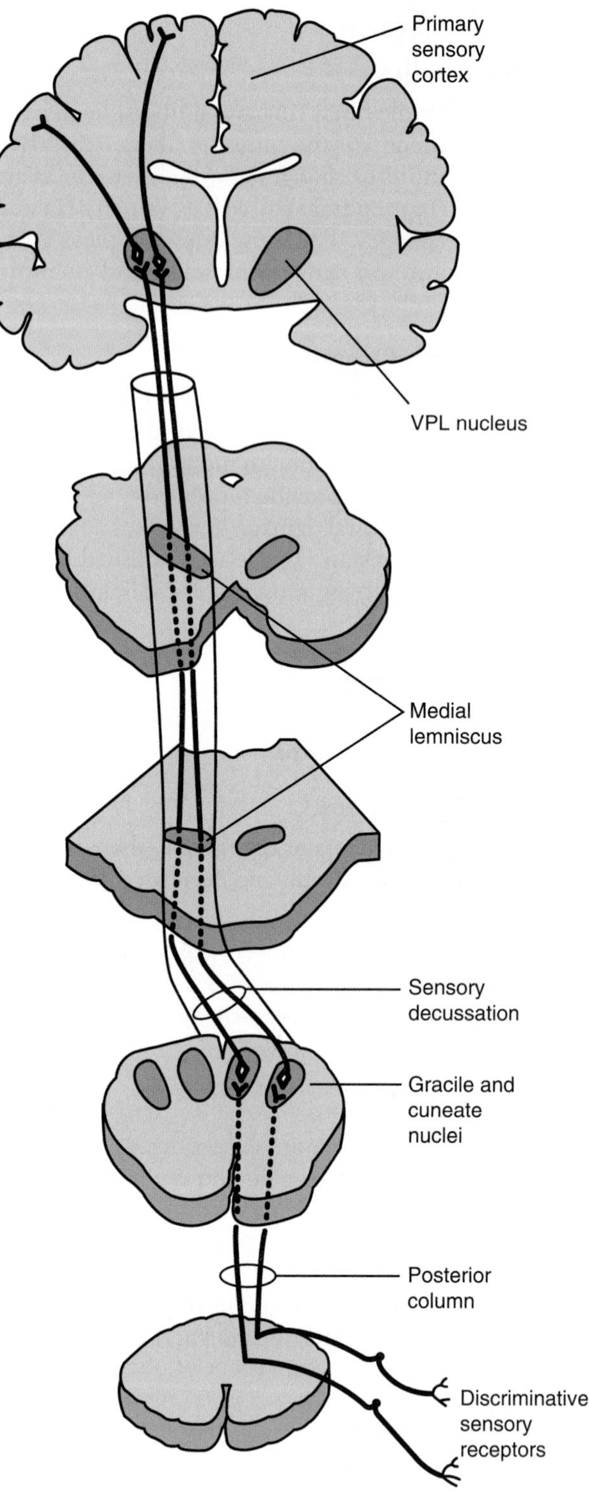

Figure 3.5 Dorsal column–medial lemniscal tract carrying discriminative sensations such as kinesthesia and touch.

■ SOMATOSENSORY CORTEX

The most complex processing of sensory information occurs in the somatosensory cortex, which is divided into three main divisions: primary somatosensory cortex (S-I), secondary somatosensory cortex (S-II), and posterior parietal cortex (Fig. 3.6A). The primary somatosensory (S-I) area occupies a lateral strip called the *postcentral gyrus* (posterior to the central sulcus) and includes four distinct areas: Brodmann's areas 3a, 3b, 1, and 2. S-I neurons identify the location of stimuli as well as discern the size, shape, and texture of objects. At the superior aspect of the lateral sulcus is the secondary somatosensory cortex (S-II),

Table 3.2 Features of Pathways for Transmission of Somatic Sensory Signals

Pathway	Type of Sensation	Afferent Fibers	Origin	Projection
Anterolateral spinothalamic	Nondiscriminative (e.g., pain, temperature); broad spectrum of sensory modalities; crude localization; poor intensity discrimination; poor spatial orientation relative to origin of stimulus	Small diameter, slowly conducting	Skin: mechanoreceptors, thermoreceptors, nociceptors	From dorsal roots of spinal nerves, synapse at dorsal horns; fibers cross and move up spinal cord, through medulla, pons, and midbrain to the ventroposterolateral nucleus of thalamus
Dorsal column–medial lemniscal	Discriminative (e.g., stereognosis, two-point discrimination); precise localization; fine intensity gradations; high degree of spatial orientation relative to origin of stimulus	Large, rapidly conducting	Skin, joints, tendons: specialized mechanoreceptors	From dorsal roots of spinal nerves, ascend to medulla, synapse with dorsal column nuclei, cross to contralateral side and ascend to thalamus; then project to sensory cortex

which is innervated by neurons from S-I. S-II projects to the insular cortex, which innervates the temporal lobe, believed important in tactile memory. The posterior parietal lobe is behind S-I and consists of areas 5 and 7. Area 5 integrates tactile input from mechanoreceptors of the skin with proprioceptive input from muscles and joints. Area 7 integrates stereognostic and visual information from visual, tactile, and proprioceptive input.[73,78,81,82] These processing areas analyze and integrate somatosensory information and contribute to motor performance by (1) determining the initial position required before a movement occurs, (2) error detection as movement occurs, and (3) identification of movement outcomes, which helps to shape learning.

Animal models have provided considerable insight into the function of the cortical association areas. Complete removal of area S-I of the somatosensory system produces deficits in position sense and the ability to determine the size, texture, and shape of objects. Temperature and pain perception are diminished but not abolished. Owing to reliance on input from S-I, removal of S-II results in severe impairment of the perception of both shape and texture of objects. Animal models have also shown reduced ability to learn new discriminative tasks, which are based on the shape of an object. Insult to the posterior parietal cortex presents profound impairments in attending to sensory input from the contralateral side of the body.[81]

The sensory homunculus (somatotopic map) represents a cross-sectional view through the postcentral gyrus and identifies the relative size of the cortex devoted to specific body parts (Fig. 3.6B). Note that certain areas of the body are exaggerated such as the hand, face, and mouth, owing to greater innervation density of the skin. The relative size of body parts represents both the *density* of sensory input from the body region as well as the *importance* of sensory information from the area as it relates to function.[78,81] For example, the relative size of the foot is reflective of its importance in locomotion; the relative size of the index finger reflects its role in fine motor skills. In contrast, cortical areas for the trunk and back are small, implying a lower receptor density and reduced role in sensory perception related to function.

Using two-point discrimination as an example, Bear et al[83] provide an extraordinary illustration of how our ability to perceive a stimulus varies remarkably across the body:

> *Two-point discrimination varies at least twentyfold across the body. Fingertips have the highest resolution. The dots of Braille are 1 mm high and 2.5 mm apart; up to six dots make a letter. An experienced Braille reader can scan an index finger across a page of raised dots and read about 600 letters per minute, which is roughly as fast as someone reading aloud. Several reasons explain why the fingertip is so much better than, say, the elbow for Braille reading: (1) There is a much higher density of mechanoreceptors in the skin of the fingertip than on other parts of the body; (2) the fingertips are enriched in receptor types that have small receptive fields; (3) there is more brain tissue (and thus more raw computing power) devoted to the sensory information of each square millimeter of fingertip than elsewhere; and (4) there may be special neural mechanisms devoted to high-resolution discriminations.*[83, p. 392]

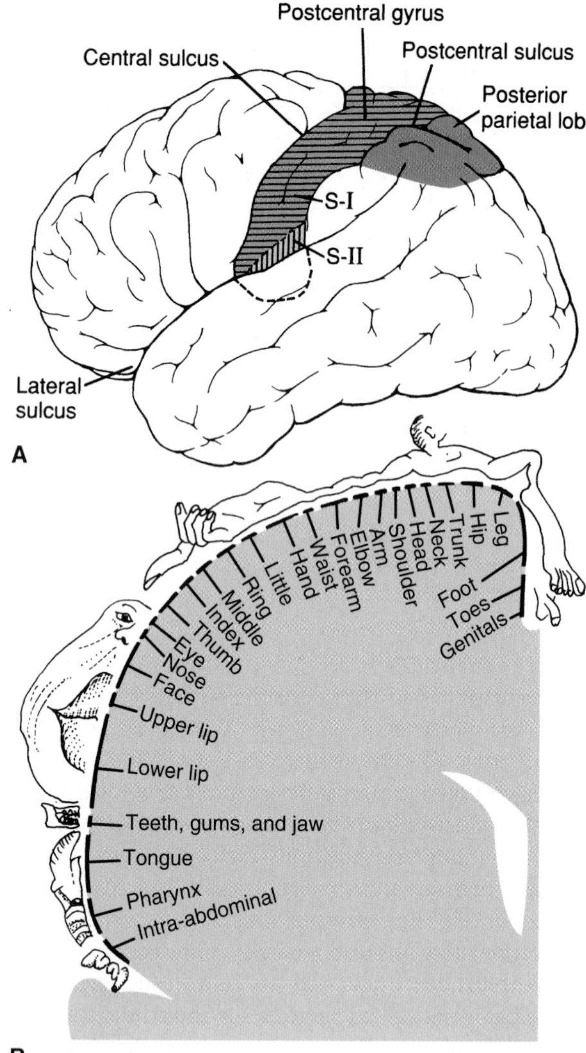

Figure 3.6 (A) The somatosensory cortex has three main divisions: The primary (S-I) and secondary (S-II) areas and the posterior parietal lobe. (B) The sensory homunculus. Areas of the body used for tactile discrimination (e.g., lips, tongue, and fingers) are represented by large areas of cortical tissue. Areas with reduced cortical representation, such as the trunk, are reflective of body parts with lesser roles in sensory perception. *(From Kandel, ER, and Jessell, TM: Touch. In Kandel, ER, Schwartz, JH and Jessell, TM: Principles of Neural Science, ed 3. Appleton and Lange, Norwalk, CT, 1991, pp. 368 [A] and 372[B], with permission.)*

PREPARATION FOR ADMINISTERING THE SENSORY EXAMINATION

Before initiating the examination of sensory function, the testing environment should be identified and prepared, needed equipment gathered, and consideration given to patient preparation (i.e., what information and instruction will be provided).[67,68,84,85]

Testing Environment

The sensory examination should be administered in a quiet, well-lit area. Depending on the number of body areas to be tested, either a sitting or recumbent position may be used. If full-body testing is indicated, both prone and supine positions will be required and use of a treatment table is recommended to allow examination of each side of the body.

Equipment

To perform a sensory examination, the following equipment and materials are used:

1. *Pain.* A large-headed safety pin or a large paper clip that has one segment bent open (providing one *sharp* and one *dull* end). The sharp end of the instrument should not be sharp enough to risk puncturing the skin. If a large-headed safety pin is used, the sharp end may be further blunted by light sanding. Commercially available single-use protected neurological pins are recommended (Fig. 3.7).

Clinical Note: The Tip Therm® is an early detection tool for identification of changes in thermal perception designed for monitoring polyneuropathy associated with diabetes (Fig. 3.8).[86] It provides a method for patients to test temperature sensitivity of their feet independently. It provides only a gross estimate of temperature perception; however, its convenience, low cost, and patients' ability to use it are important characteristics. The tool can be used many times, requires no energy, and uses the special characteristics of synthetic material and metal. One end is metal and the opposite side is synthetic material. Both materials are essentially at room temperature; however, the metal end takes more heat from the body (metal has a higher conductivity than the synthetic end). As a result, the metal end is perceived as warmer and the synthetic end as cooler.

2. *Temperature.* Two standard laboratory test tubes with stoppers.
3. *Light touch.* A camel-hair brush, a piece of cotton, or a tissue.
4. *Vibration.* Tuning fork and earphones (if available, to reduce auditory clues). Tuning forks are made of steel or magnesium alloy and grossly resemble a two-pronged fork. When the tines are stuck against a surface (usually the palm of the examiner's hand), the fork resonates at a specific pitch (e.g., 128, 256, or 512 Hz), determined by the length of the two U-shaped prongs (tines).
5. *Stereognosis (object recognition).* A variety of small, commonly used articles such as a comb, fork, paper clip, key, marble, coin, pencil, and so forth.
6. *Two-point discrimination.* Several instruments are available to measure two-point discrimination. A

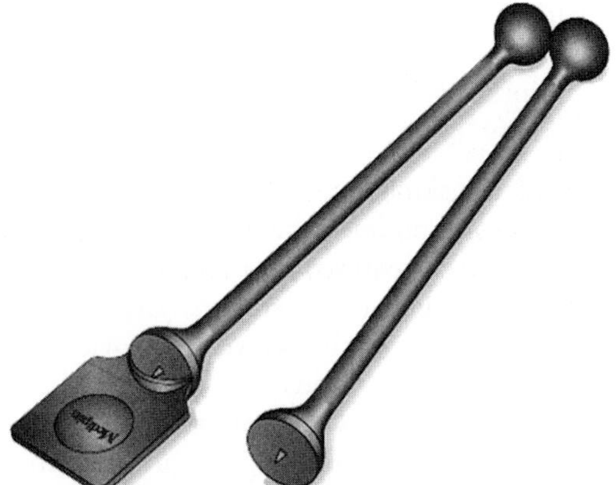

Figure 3.7 Single use protected neurological pin. The image on the *left* shows the pin prior to use with the protective cap intact (although schematically presented to allow visualization of pin location). On the *right,* the protective cap is removed and the pin exposed. On the opposite end of the pin is a smooth rounded surface used to randomly intersperse application of a dull stimulus. After use, the point is destroyed by compressing it against a hard surface and disposed of in a biohazard receptacle. *(Courtesy of US Neurologicals, Kirkland, WA 98033.)*

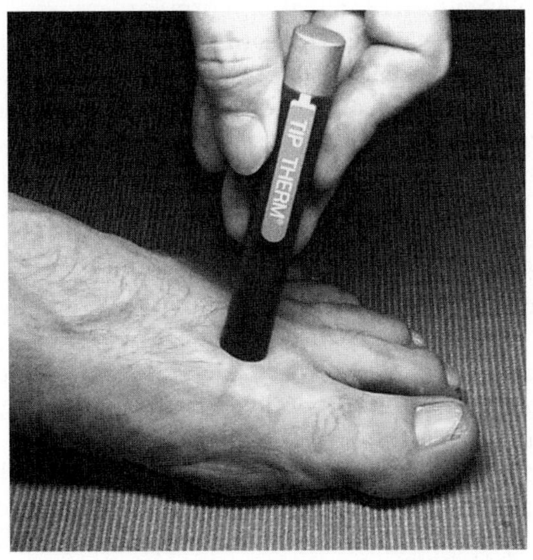

Figure 3.8 The Tip Therm® is a thermal instrument designed for patient monitoring of gross temperature perception of the feet. The instrument is 4 inches (100 mm) long with a .59-inch (15 mm) diameter. *(Courtesy of Tip-Therm® GmbH, Düsseldorf, Germany.)*

two-point discrimination aesthesiometer (Fig. 3.9) is a small handheld instrument designed to measure the shortest distance that two points of contact on the skin can be distinguished. It consists of a small ruler with one stationary and one moveable (sliding) tip coated with vinyl. The vinyl coverings help to minimize the impact of temperature on perception of contact. Some instruments also have a third tip, allowing ease of alternating from two points to a single point

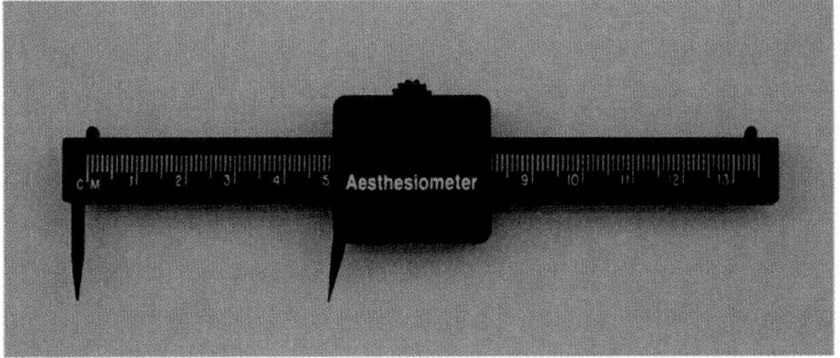

Figure 3.9 A handheld aesthesiometer provides a quantitative measure of two-point discrimination. The two-point threshold is determined by gradually bringing the tips closer together as it is sequentially applied to the patient's skin. The scale is calibrated to the nearest 0.1 cm and measures up to 14 cm.

of contact during testing. If used on an uneven body surface, care should be taken not to allow the "ruler" portion of the instrument to make contact with the skin. *Note:* The term *aesthesiometer* is not specific to this instrument; it is used to describe any number of instruments designed to examine touch perception.

For finer gradations in measurement (e.g., fingertips), small circular disks can be used to measure two-point discrimination (Fig. 3.10). These instruments typically allow quantification of two-point discrimination from 1 to 25 mm.

7. *Recognition of texture.* Samples of fabrics of various texture such as cotton, wool, burlap, or silk (approximately 4 × 4 inches [10 × 10 cm]).

Patient Preparation

A full explanation of the purpose of the testing should be provided. The patient also should be informed that cooperation is necessary to obtain accurate test results. It is of considerable importance that the patient be requested *not to guess* if uncertain of the correct response.

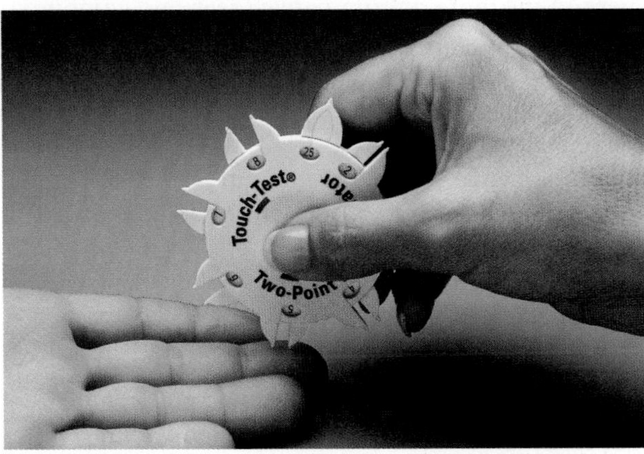

Figure 3.10 This circular two-point discrimination instrument consists of two joined plastic rotating disks with rounded tips placed at standard testing intervals. *(Courtesy of North Coast Medical, Inc., Morgan Hill, CA 95037.)*

During the examination, the patient should be in a comfortable, relaxed position. Preferably, the tests should be performed when the patient is well rested. Considering the high level of concentration required, it is not surprising that fatigue has been noted to adversely affect results of some sensory tests.[87]

Note: A "trial run" or demonstration of each test should be performed just prior to actual administration. This will orient the patient to the sensation being tested, what to anticipate, and what type of response is required. The importance of this initial trial should not be underestimated. If a practice trial is inadequately or not performed, what appears to be a sensory impairment may in reality only be a reflection of the patient's lack of understanding of the testing protocol or how to respond to a stimulus.

Some method of occluding the patient's vision during the testing should be used (vision should not be occluded during the explanation and demonstration). Visual input is prevented because it may allow for compensation of a sensory deficit and thus decrease the accuracy of test results. The traditional methods of occluding vision include a fabric blindfold (such as those worn by travelers to sleep on an airplane), a small folded towel, or by asking the patient to keep the eyes closed. These methods are practical in most instances. However, in situations of CNS dysfunction, a patient may become anxious or disoriented if vision is occluded for a long period of time. In these situations, a small screen or folder may be preferable as a visual barrier. Whatever method is used, it should be removed between the tests while directions and demonstrations are provided.

THE SENSORY EXAMINATION

The superficial (exteroceptive) sensations are usually examined first, inasmuch as they consist of more primitive responses, followed by the deep (proprioceptive), and then the combined cortical sensations. If a test indicates impairment of the superficial responses, some impairment of the more discriminative (deep and combined) sensations also will be noted and is a contraindication to further testing (e.g., lack of touch sensation would be a contraindication for testing stereognosis). That is, the primary modality of sensation (touch) must be sufficiently intact to permit meaningful testing of cortical sensory function (ability to identify objects placed in the hand).

For each sensory test, the following data will be generated:

- The modality tested
- The quantity of involvement or body surface areas affected (pattern identification)
- The degree or severity of involvement (e.g., absent, impaired, or delayed responses)
- Localization of the exact boundaries of the sensory impairment
- The patient's subjective feelings about changes in sensation
- The potential impact of sensory loss on function (i.e., activity limitation, disability)

Knowledge of skin segment (dermatome) innervation by the dorsal roots and peripheral nerve innervation (see Figs. 3.1 and 3.2) is required for making sound, accurate diagnostic and prognostic judgments. They serve as critical references during testing as well as provide a framework for documenting results.

Sensory tests are typically performed in a distal to proximal direction. This progression will conserve time, particularly when dealing with localized lesions involving a single extremity, where deficits tend to be more severe distally. It is generally not necessary to test every segment of each dermatome; testing general body areas is sufficient. However, once a deficit area is noted, testing must become more discrete and the exact boundaries of the impairment should be identified. A skin pencil may be useful to mark the boundaries of sensory change directly. This information should be transferred later to a sensory examination form, graphically presented on a dermatome chart, and peripheral nerve involvement identified. Figure 3.11 presents a sample Sensory Examination Form.

A single documentation form applicable to the variety of patients seen in different practice settings does not exist. Specialized centers or organizations have developed specific forms to examine sensory function (e.g., the American Spinal Injury Association Standard Neurological Classification of Spinal Cord Injury, described in Chapter 20, Traumatic Spinal Cord Injury). However, the following are common elements of sensory examination forms: (1) a dermatome chart to graphically display findings; (2) a grading scale (e.g., 0 = absent; 1 = impaired; 2 = normal; NT = not testable; and so forth) to score patient perception of individual modalities; and (3) a section for narrative comments.

Most often the dermatome charts are completed using a color code (i.e., each color represents a different sensory modality). The colors used to plot each sensation are then coded by the examiner directly on the form (see Fig. 3.11). In many instances hatch marks of varying density are used to represent gradations in sensory impairment (i.e., the closer together, the greater the sensory impairment). With this method, a completely colored-in area indicates no response to a given sensation. With varied or "spotty" sensory loss, it is not uncommon that more than one dermatome chart is required to completely depict all test findings. With use of several dermatome charts, the sensation(s) represented should appear in bold print at the top of each page.

The form presented in Figure 3.11 provides the foundational elements of documentation typically included for sensory examinations. It should be modified or expanded to meet the needs of a given population or

This form provides a record of the type, severity, and location of sensory impairments. It should be used in conjunction with additional dermatome sheets, if needed, to graphically outline the exact boundaries of the impairment. The designations P and D may be added to the grading key to indicate either a proximal (P) or a distal (D) location of the impairment on a limb or body part. The dermatome chart should be color coded and filled in using varying density hatch marks (higher density for more severe areas of impairment). Indicate the color used for documentation in the box titled Color Code (a different color should be used for each sensation). Separate notation should be made for examination of the face and identification of peripheral nerve involvement. Abnormal responses should be briefly described in the comments section.

Patient Name: ______________________ Date: __________

Examiner: ______________________

Sensations	Upper Extremity		Lower Extremity		Trunk		Comments
	Right	Left	Right	Left	Right	Left	
Pain							
Temperature							
Touch							
Vibration							
Two-Point Disc							
Kinesthesia							
Proprioception							
Stereognosis							

Note: Areas shaded indicate sensation not typically tested for corresponding body part.

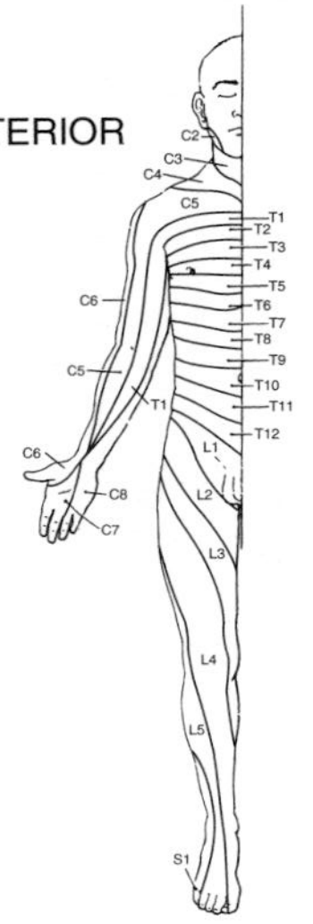

Key to Grading
0 = Absent, no response
1 = Decreased, delayed response
2 = Increased, exaggerated response
3 = Inconsistent response
4 = Intact, normal response
NT = unable to test
P = proximal; D = distal

Color Code

Color	Sensation

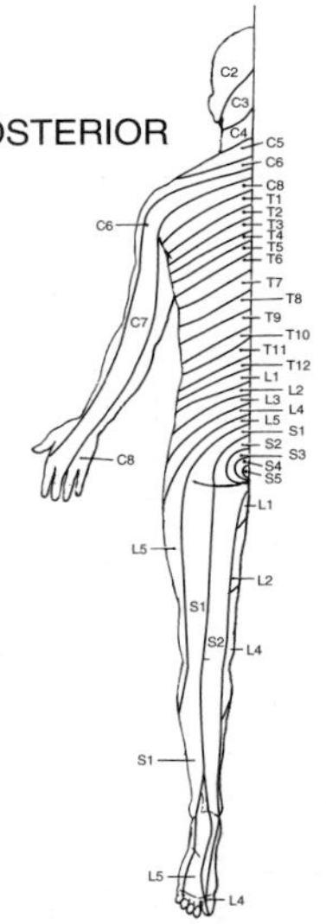

Indicate Peripheral Nerve Involvement:

ANTERIOR

POSTERIOR

Figure 3.11 Sample Sensory Examination Form.

facility. It is also not uncommon for therapists to include sensory testing data within the body of a narrative or progress report.

Clinical Note: Physical therapy electronic documentation software for the sensory examination typically include some variation of the elements presented in Figure 3.11. If greater detail is warranted, additional dermatome charts may be scanned into the system.

During testing, the application of stimuli should be applied in a random, unpredictable manner with variation in timing. This will improve accuracy of the test results by avoiding a consistent pattern of application, which might provide the patient with "clues" to the correct response. During application of stimuli, consideration must be given also to skin condition. Scar tissue or calloused areas are generally less sensitive and will demonstrate a diminished response to sensory stimuli. Recall that a trial test is performed to instruct the patient in what to expect and how to respond to application of the specific stimuli. Remember, too, that patient vision is occluded during testing.

The following sections present the individual sensory tests. The tests are subdivided for superficial, deep, and combined cortical sensations. Table 3.3 presents terminology used to describe common sensory impairments.

Clinical Note: Hands should always be washed prior to and after patient contact. "Hand hygiene is a major component of standard precautions and one of the most effective methods to prevent transmission of pathogens associated with health care."[88, p. 1] The World Health Organization (WHO) recommends hand washing with soap and water for 40 to 60 seconds and hand rubbing using an alcohol-based hand rub for 20 to 30 seconds.[89] See "Hand Hygiene" in Chapter 2 , Examination of Vital Signs for a more detailed discussion and figures illustrating hand hygiene techniques using soap and water and an alcohol-based hand rub.

Superficial Sensations

Pain Perception

This test is also referred to as *sharp/dull discrimination* and indicates function of protective sensation. To test

Table 3.3 Terminology Describing Common Sensory Impairments

Abarognosis	Inability to recognize weight
Allesthesia	Sensation experienced at a site remote from point of stimulation
Allodynia	Pain produced by a non-noxious stimulus
Analgesia	Complete loss of pain sensitivity
Astereognosis	Inability to recognize the form and shape of objects by touch (synonym: *tactile agnosia*)
Atopognosia	Inability to localize a sensation
Causalgia	Painful, burning sensations, usually along the distribution of a nerve
Dysesthesia	Touch sensation experienced as pain
Hypalgesia	Decreased sensitivity to pain
Hyperalgesia	Increased sensitivity to pain
Hyperesthesia	Increased sensitivity to sensory stimuli
Hypoesthesia	Decreased sensitivity to sensory stimuli
Pallanesthesia	Loss or absence of sensibility to vibration
Paresthesia	Abnormal sensation such as numbness, prickling, or tingling, without apparent cause
Thalamic syndrome	Vascular lesion of the thalamus resulting in sensory disturbances and partial or complete paralysis of one side of the body, associated with severe, boring-type pain; sensory stimuli may produce an exaggerated, prolonged, or painful response
Thermanalgesia	Inability to perceive heat
Thermanesthesia	Inability to perceive sensations of heat and cold
Thermhyperesthesia	Increased sensitivity to temperature
Thermhypoesthesia	Decreased temperature sensibility
Thigmanesthesia	Loss of light touch sensibility

pain awareness, the sharp and dull ends of a large-headed safety pin, a reshaped paper clip (the segment pulled away from the body of the paper clip provides a sharp end), or a single-use protected neurological pin (see Fig. 3.7) are used. The instrument should be carefully cleaned before administering the test and disposed of immediately afterward (owing to the protective cap on the neurological pin, cleaning is not required). The sharp and dull ends of the instrument are randomly applied perpendicularly to the skin. To avoid summation of impulses, the stimuli should not be applied too close to each other or in too rapid a succession. To maintain a uniform pressure with each successive application of stimuli, the safety pin, reshaped paper clip, or protected neurological pin should be held firmly and the fingers allowed to "slide" down the instrument once in contact with the skin. This will avoid the chance of gradually increasing pressure during application. The instrument used to test pain perception should be sharp enough to deflect the skin but not puncture it.

Response

The patient is asked to verbally indicate *sharp* or *dull* when a stimulus is felt. All areas of the body may be tested.

Temperature Awareness

This test determines the ability to distinguish between warm and cool stimuli. Two test tubes with stoppers are required for this examination; one should be filled with warm water and the other with crushed ice. Ideal temperatures for cold are between 41°F (5°C) and 50°F (10°C) and for warmth, between 104°F (40°C) and 113°F (45°C). Caution should be exercised to remain within these ranges, because exceeding these temperatures may elicit a pain response and consequently inaccurate test results. The side of the test tube should be placed in contact with the skin (as opposed to only the distal end). This technique provides sufficient surface area contact to determine the temperature. The test tubes are randomly placed in contact with the skin area to be tested. All skin surfaces should be tested.

Response

The patient is asked to reply *hot* or *cold* after each stimulus application.

> **Clinical Note:** The clinical usefulness of thermal testing may be problematic. Nolan[87] points out that the tests are extremely difficult to duplicate on a day-to-day basis, owing to rapid changes in temperature once the test tubes are exposed to room air. Although it is a simple test to perform, determining changes over time is not practical unless a method of monitoring the temperature of the test tubes is used.[87]

Touch Awareness

This test determines perception of tactile touch input. A camel-hair brush, piece of cotton (ball or swab), or tissue is used. The area to be tested is lightly touched or stroked. Examination of finer gradations of light touch can be quantified using monofilaments (see the "Quantitative Sensory Testing and Specialized Testing Instruments" section).

Response

The patient is asked to indicate when he or she recognizes that a stimulus has been applied by responding "yes" or "now."

Note: A quantitative score for pain perception, temperature, and light touch awareness can be obtained by dividing the number of *correct responses* by the *number of stimuli* applied (normal response would be 100%).[90] Also, inability to verbally communicate does not necessary preclude obtaining accurate data. For example, having the patient hold up one or two fingers might be used for dichotomous responses (yes/no; hot/cold). Other options might include nodding, pointing to index cards containing printed responses, or using hand gestures to indicate recognition of a stimulus.

Pressure Perception

The therapist's fingertip or a double-tipped cotton swab is used to apply a firm pressure on the skin surface. This pressure should be firm enough to indent the skin and to stimulate the deep receptors. This test can also be administered using the thumb and fingers to squeeze the Achilles tendon.[87]

Response

The patient is asked to indicate when an applied stimulus is recognized by responding "yes" or "now."

Deep Sensations

The deep sensations include *kinesthesia, proprioception,* and *vibration.* Kinesthesia is the awareness of movement. Proprioception includes position sense and the awareness of joints at rest. *Vibration* refers to the ability to perceive rapidly oscillating or vibratory stimuli. Although these sensations are closely related, they are examined individually.

Kinesthesia Awareness

This test examines *awareness of movement.* The extremity or joint(s) is moved passively through a relatively small range of motion (ROM). Small increments in ROM are used as joint receptors fire at specific points throughout the range. The therapist should identify the range of movement being examined (e.g., initial, mid-, or terminal range). As discussed, a trial run or demonstration of the procedure should be performed prior to actual testing. This will ensure that the patient and the therapist agree on terms to describe the direction of movements.

Response

The patient is asked to describe verbally the direction (up, down, in, out, and so forth) and range of movement in terms previously discussed with the therapist while the extremity is *in motion.* The patient may also respond by simultaneously duplicating the movement with the contralateral extremity. This second approach, however, is impractical with proximal lower extremity joints, owing to potential stress on the low back. During testing, movement of larger joints is usually discerned more quickly than that of smaller joints. The therapist's grip should remain constant and minimal (fingertip grip over bony prominences) to reduce tactile stimulation.

Proprioceptive Awareness

This test examines *joint position sense* and the *awareness of joints at rest.* The extremity or joint(s) is moved through a ROM and held in a static position. Again, small increments of range are used. The words selected to identify the range of movement examined should be identified to the patient during the practice trial (e.g., initial, mid-, or terminal range). As with kinesthesia, caution should be used with hand placements to avoid excessive tactile stimulation.

Response

While the extremity or joint(s) is held in a static position by the therapist, the patient is asked to describe the position verbally or to duplicate the position of the extremity or joint(s) with the contralateral extremity (position matching). This test may also be performed unilaterally using the same extremity or joint(s); first held in position by the examiner, then returned to resting position, followed by active duplication of position by patient using the same limb.

Clinical Note: Based on a series of position matching studies conducted in the Motor Control Laboratory at the University of Michigan, Goble[91] presents several important factors to assist clinicians in making informed decisions about proprioceptive matching test outcomes:

- For position matching tests, there are different memory influences and different interhemispheric communication requirements between use of the ipsilateral extremity (same arm positioned by examiner is used to actively replicate the joint angle[s]) versus contralateral limb (patient moves opposite extremity from that used by examiner).
- Likely owing to the enhanced role of the right hemisphere in proprioceptive feedback processing, the left arm appears to have an advantage in matching tasks.
- The magnitude of the reference joint angle (larger magnitudes associated with greater error) and how reference positions are established (fewer errors noted when active movement used to establish position versus passive movement by examiner) will influence performance.
- Proprioceptive acuity must be considered within the context of anticipated changes occurring over the life span or that are diagnosis specific (e.g., stroke).
- Task workspace (area in which activities of daily living are typically performed) appears to influence joint position matching performance. During position matching experiments, greater performance occurred to the left of body midline with the fewest errors in the far left of the workspace.

Vibration Perception

This test requires a tuning fork that vibrates at 128 Hz.[87] The ability to perceive a vibratory stimulus is tested by placing the base of a vibrating tuning fork on a bony prominence (such as the sternum, elbow, or ankle). The tuning fork base (the "handle" of the fork) is held between the examiner's thumb and index finger without making contact with the tines. The tines are then briskly hit against the open palm of the examiner's opposite hand to initiate the vibration. Care must be taken not to touch the tines, as this will stop the vibration. The base of the fork is then placed over a bony prominence. If vibration sensation is intact, the patient will perceive the vibration. If there is impairment, the patient will be unable to distinguish between a vibrating and non-vibrating tuning fork. Therefore, there should be a random application of vibrating and non-vibrating stimuli.

Auditory clues can pose a challenge in obtaining accurate test results. Typically, it is easy to hear the sound of the tines making vigorous contact with the examiner's hand to initiate the vibration. If the sound is not heard, it provides an easy indicator to the patient that the next application will be non-vibrating. To minimize this effect, the vibration can be initiated for *every* stimulus application; however, when a non-vibrating stimulus is desired, brief contact of the therapist's fingers on the tines will stop the vibration prior to placement on the skin. This, though, does not solve the problem of the auditory cues generated during application of a vibrating stimulus. The best solution is use of sound-occlusive earphones (the type worn by airport ground workers). Unfortunately, such earphones are seldom available in a clinic setting.

Response

The patient is asked to respond by verbally identifying or otherwise indicating if the stimulus is vibrating or non-vibrating each time the fork makes contact.

Combined Cortical Sensations

Stereognosis Perception

This test determines the ability to recognize the form of objects by touch (stereognosis). A variety of small, easily obtainable, and culturally familiar objects of differing size and shape are required (e.g., keys, button, ring, coins,[92] and so forth). A single object is placed in the hand, the patient manipulates the object, and then he or she identifies the item verbally. The patient should be allowed to handle several sample test items during the explanation and demonstration of the procedure.

Response

The patient is asked to name the object verbally. For patients with speech impairments, sensory testing shields can be used (Fig. 3.12). Alternatively, the item manipulated can be identified from a group of images presented after each test.

Tactile Localization

This test determines the ability to localize touch sensation on the skin (topognosis). The patient is asked to identify the specific point of application of a touch stimulus (e.g., tip of ring finger, lateral malleus, and so forth) and not simply the perception of being touched. Tactile localization is typically not tested in isolation and frequently examined in combination with similar tests such as pressure perception or touch awareness. Using a cotton swap or fingertip, the therapist touches different skin surfaces. After each application of a stimulus, the patient is given time to respond.

Response

The patient is asked to identify the location of the stimuli by pointing to the area or by verbal description. The patient's eyes may be open during the response component of this test. The distance between the application of the stimulus and the site indicated by the patient can be measured and recorded. Accuracy of localization over various parts of the body may be compared to determine the relative sensitivity of different areas.

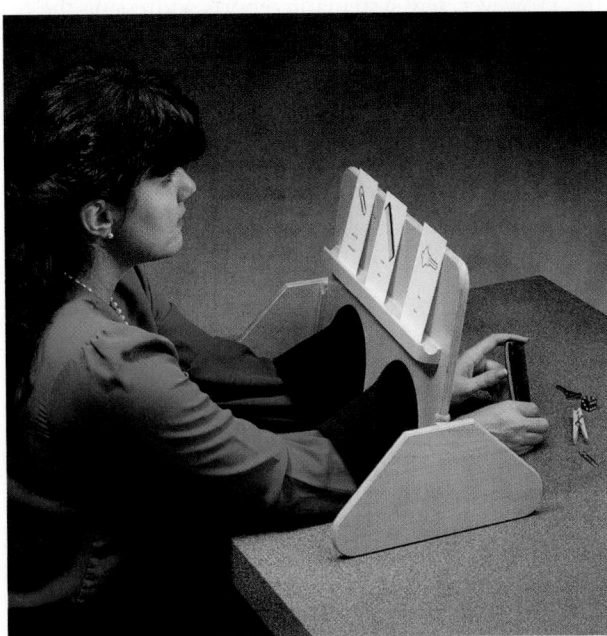

Figure 3.12 A sensory testing shield can be used for examining stereognosis in the presence of speech or language impairments. In this simulation, the subject manipulates the object without the use of visual input. Following manipulation, the subject points to the matching object pictured on the ledge of the testing shield. *(Courtesy of North Coast Medical, Inc., Morgan Hill, CA 95037.)*

Two-Point Discrimination

This test determines the ability to perceive two points applied to the skin simultaneously. It is a measure of the smallest distance between two stimuli (applied simultaneously and with equal pressure) that can still be perceived as two distinct stimuli. Two-point discrimination values vary for different individuals and by gender and body parts, and may be negatively influenced by fatigue.[93] As this sensory function is most refined in the distal upper extremities, this is the typical site for testing. It is believed to contribute to precision grip movements and instrumental activities of daily living (IADL).[94]

Two-point discrimination is among the most practical and easily duplicated tests for cutaneous sensation. Some years ago, a series of classic two-point discrimination studies were conducted by Nolan.[95-97] The purpose of his research was to establish normative data on two-point discrimination for young adults. His sample consisted of 43 college students ranging in age from 20 to 24 years. Values from Nolan's studies for the upper and lower extremities as well as the face and trunk are presented in Appendix 3.A. The results from these studies should be used cautiously, inasmuch as they relate to a specific population. They should not be generalized for interpreting data from older or younger patients. Normative data for two-point discrimination have been documented by several authors, including van Nes et al,[98] Kaneko et al,[99] Vriens and van der Glas,[100] and Koo et al.[101]

As mentioned earlier, the aesthesiometer (see Fig. 3.9) and the circular two-point discriminator (see Fig. 3.10) are among the most common devices used for measurement. Two reshaped paper clips can also be used; however, this requires the assistance of a second examiner to measure the distance between the two points using a small ruler. During the test procedure, the two tips of the instrument are applied to the skin simultaneously with tips spread apart. To increase the validity of the test, it is appropriate to alternate the application of two stimuli with the random application of only a single stimulus (the purpose of the third tip on some aesthesiometers). With each successive application, the two tips are gradually brought closer together until the stimuli are perceived as one. The smallest distance between the stimuli that is still perceived as two distinct points is measured.

Response

The patient is asked to identify the perception of "one" or "two" stimuli.

Double Simultaneous Stimulation

This test determines the ability to perceive simultaneous touch stimuli (double simultaneous stimulation). The therapist simultaneously (and with equal pressure) touches (1) identical locations on opposite sides of the body, (2) proximally and distally on opposite sides of the body, and/or (3) proximal and distal locations on the same side of the body. The term *extinction phenomenon* is used to describe a situation in which only the proximal stimulus is perceived, with "extinction" of the distal.

Response

The patient verbally states when a touch stimulus is perceived and the number of stimuli felt.

Described below are several additional tests for the combined (cortical) sensations including graphesthesia (traced finger identification), recognition of texture, and barognosis (recognition of weight). However, these tests are usually not performed if stereognosis and two-point discrimination are found to be intact.

Graphesthesia (Traced Figure Identification)

This test determines the ability to recognize letters, numbers, or designs "written" on the skin. Using a fingertip or the eraser end of a pencil, a series of letters, numbers, or shapes is traced on the palm of the patient's hand. During the practice trial, agreement should be reached about the orientation of the tracings (e.g., the bottom of the traced figures will always be oriented toward the base of the patient's hand [wrist].) Between each separate drawing, the palm should be gently wiped with a soft cloth to clearly indicate a change in figures to the patient. This test is a useful substitute for stereognosis when paralysis prevents grasping an object. Talmasov and Ropper[102] recently described an interesting case report of a patient with a right parietal lesion resulting in isolated agraphesthesia for numbers and letters.

Response

The patient is asked to verbally identify the figures drawn on the skin. For patients with speech or language impairments, the figures can be selected (pointed to) from a series of line drawings.

Recognition of Texture

This test determines the ability to differentiate among various textures. Suitable textures may include cotton, wool, burlap, or silk. The items are placed individually in the patient's hand, and he or she is allowed to manipulate the sample texture.

Response

The patient is asked to identify the individual textures as they are placed in the hand. They may be identified by name (e.g., silk, cotton) or by texture (e.g., rough, smooth).

Barognosis (Recognition of Weight)

This test determines the ability to recognize different weights. A set of discrimination weights consisting of small objects of the same size and shape but of graduated weight is used (Fig. 3.13). The therapist may choose to place a series of different weights in the same hand one at a time, place a different weight in each hand simultaneously, or ask the patient to use a fingertip grip to pick up each weight.

Response

The patient is asked to identify the comparative weight of objects in a series (i.e., to compare the relative weight of the object with the previous one), or when the objects are placed (or picked up) in both hands simultaneously, the patient is asked to compare the weight of the two objects. The patient responds by indicating that the object is "heavier" or "lighter."

Clinical Note: Impaired sensation is a contraindication to or precaution for use of some physical agents because the end range of intensity or duration is frequently associated with the patient's subjective report of how the intervention feels (i.e., patient tolerance).

RELIABILITY

Reliability is an important parameter of any test or measure. However, few systematic reports addressing the reliability of traditional sensory tests appear in the literature. This is likely due to the inability to accurately quantify test results. In an important early reliability study by Kent,[103] the upper limbs of 50 adult patients

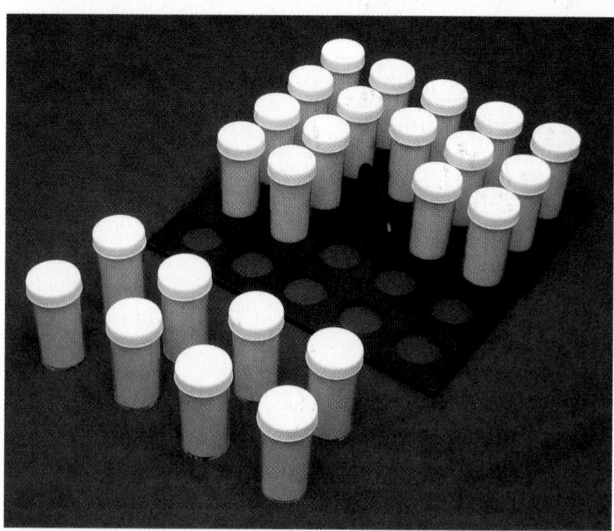

Figure 3.13 Discrimination weights are identical in size, shape, and texture. The only distinguishing feature is their variation in weight. *(Courtesy of Lafayette Instruments, Lafayette, IN 47903.)*

with hemiplegia were tested for sensory and motor deficits. Three sensory tests were administered and then repeated by the same examiner within 1 to 7 days. Results revealed a high reliability for both stereognosis (r = 0.97) and position sense (r = 0.90). A lower reliability was reported for two-point discrimination, with correlation coefficients ranging from 0.59 to 0.82, depending on the body area tested.

More recently, Moloney et al[104] examined the interrater reliability of thermal quantitative sensory testing in young healthy adults. The interrater reliability for cold detection threshold (ICC = 0.27–0.55), warm detection threshold (ICC = 0.38–0.69), cold pain threshold (ICC = 0.88–0.94), and heat pain threshold (ICC = 0.52–0.86) ranged from poor to high. Wu and Li[105] examined proprioception using an arm position-matching paradigm. Without visual or auditory cues, healthy older adults were tested in three different joints and positions. Moderate interrater reliability was reported for each position: shoulder flexion at 60 degrees (ICC = 0.49), elbow flexion at 40 degrees (ICC = 0.47), and wrist extension at 50 degrees (ICC = 0.64). Tyros et al[106] examined vibration disappearance thresholds of the median nerve, using a 128 Hz tuning fork, on patients with chronic whiplash associated disorder. Both intra- (ICC = 0.955) and interrater (0.983) reliability were excellent. Meirte et al[107] examined the reliability of touch pressure threshold within burn scars and healthy controls using the Semmes Weinstein monofilament test. Interrater reliability was excellent for burn scars (ICC = 0.908) and fair for the control group (ICC = 0.731). Intrarater reliability was high for burn scars (ICC = 0.822) as well as for the control group (ICC = 0.807). Reidy et al[92] examined stereognosis in younger and older adults using a house key, button, ring, and coin. When using their dominant hand, there was no significant difference between younger (95% to 100% correct) and older adults (87.5% to 100% correct) in accurately discriminating individual objects. However, when using the nondominant hand, there was a significant difference between the ability of younger (97.5% correct) and older (75% correct) adults to identify the button.

Although limited published data are available related to reliability measures, several approaches can be used to improve this aspect of the tests, including (1) use of consistent guidelines for completing the tests; (2) administration of the tests by trained, skillful examiners; and (3) subsequent retests performed by the same individual. It also should be noted that the patient's understanding of the test procedure and the patient's ability to communicate results further influence the reliability of sensory tests. As developing advances in technology (see discussion below) provide tools for quantitative sensory testing, greater emphasis on reliability will follow. Additional research related to standardization of testing protocols and identification of normative data for various age groups will improve the overall reliability and interpretation of test results.

QUANTITATIVE SENSORY TESTING AND SPECIALIZED TESTING INSTRUMENTS

With the expanding availability of specialized testing systems and instruments, quantitative sensory testing (QST) has gained considerable clinical and research interest. This is clearly evident from the expanding body of literature on this topic.[108-115] QST allows quantification of the level of stimuli required for perception of a sensory modality. Although sufficient data are not available to predict the ultimate integration of QST instrumentation into clinical practice, preliminary information suggests its potential usefulness. This section provides a brief overview of selected QST devices and is certainly not all-inclusive. The Internet provides a rich source of information on this developing technology and instrumentation.

TSA-II NeuroSensory Analyzer + VSA 3000 Vibratory Sensory Analyzer (Medoc, Ltd., Durham, NC)

This computer-controlled system (Fig. 3.14) is capable of generating and recording a response to repeatable vibratory and thermal stimuli (i.e., warmth, cold, heat- or cold-induced pain). For testing thermal sensation, a "thermode" capable of heating or cooling is placed on the patient's skin (Fig. 3.15). The patient is asked to respond to the stimulus by pushing a response button. A sensory threshold is recorded and a computer comparison

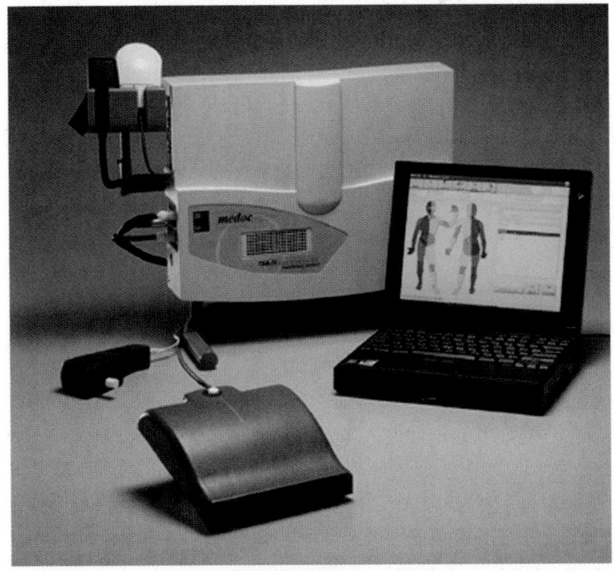

Figure 3.14 TSA-II NeuroSensory Analyzer + VSA 3000 Vibratory Sensory Analyzer. This system provides quantitative measures of both thermal and vibratory stimuli using a variety of patient interfaces. Note the small handheld vibratory device on the far left. *(Courtesy of Medoc, Ltd., Durham, NC 27707.)*

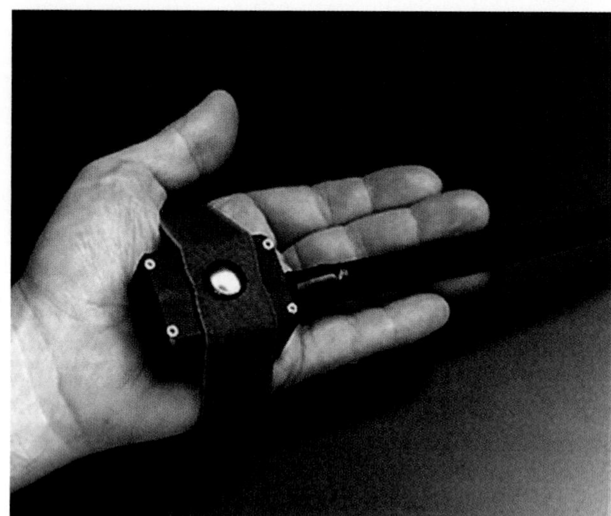

Figure 3.15 Thermode placed in hand for measuring perception of thermal stimuli. *(Courtesy of Medoc, Ltd., Durham, NC 27707.)*

to age-matched normative data is generated. The system includes hand and foot (Fig. 3.16) support vibratory stimulators as well as a handheld vibrating device (see Fig 3.14, far left). A variety of report formats can be generated; a sample is presented in Figure 3.17. Several examples of clinical applications include neuropathies (e.g., diabetic, metabolic, cancer), compression injuries, and pharmacological trials.

von Frey Aesthesiometer II (Somedic AB, Hörby, Sweden)

Monofilaments are not new to examination of sensory function and are actually considered a classic tool for measuring touch-evoked potentials (Fig. 3.18). They are designed to detect very small changes in touch threshold. The filaments are available as sets, in various sizes (i.e., thicknesses from 0.128 to 0.508 mm), with each

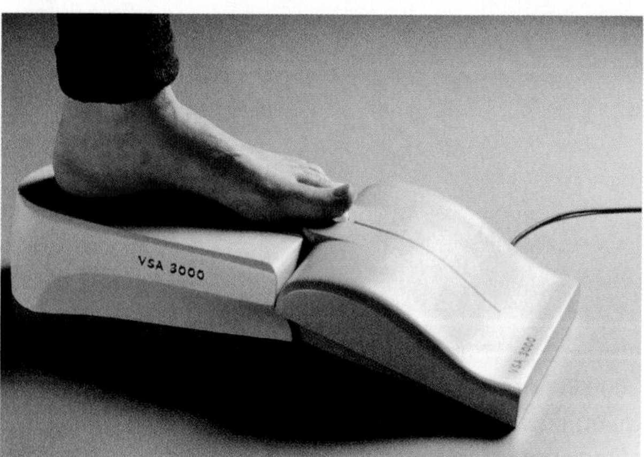

Figure 3.16 Foot support vibratory stimulator. *(Courtesy of Medoc, Ltd., Durham, NC 27707.)*

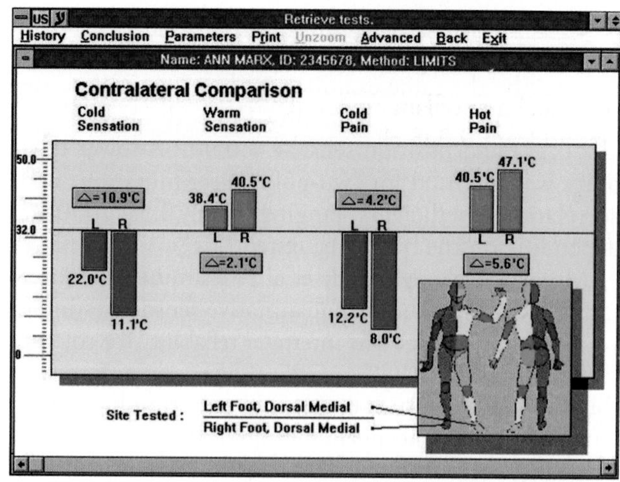

Figure 3.17 Computer-generated data from thermal testing that presents a comparison between the two sides of the body. Note the data for the right foot presents consistently higher threshold values than that of the left. Values are generated for each foot as well as the total difference between the feet. All values are in Celsius. Conversions for the temperature scale on the left border are 32°C = 89.6°F and 50°C = 122°F. *(Courtesy of Medoc, Ltd., Durham, NC 27707.)*

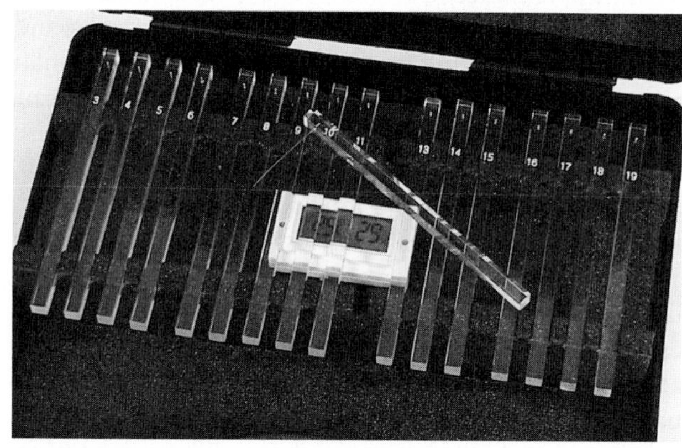

Figure 3.18 von Frey aesthesiometer. This set contains a series of monofilaments mounted on Plexiglas handles. *(Courtesy of Somedic AB, Hörby, Sweden.)*

mounted on a handle. The nominal force required for bending the monofilament increases from 0.026 g for the first handle to 100 g for the last (pressure range of between 5 g/mm^2 and 178 g/mm^2). The filaments are applied individually to the patient's skin until it bends; each filament provides a specific amount of force (thicker filaments are used if the thinner are not perceived). With vision occluded, the patient responds "yes" when a stimulus is felt. The filaments are held perpendicular to the skin, and application is usually repeated three times at each testing site.[90] Monofilaments are frequently used in hand-rehabilitation clinics; other examples of clinical applications include neuropathies (e.g., diabetic) and peripheral nerve injuries.

Touch Test Sensory Evaluator (North Coast Medical, Inc., Morgan Hill, CA)

Individual monofilaments are also available in increments ranging from 0.008 to 300 g (Fig. 3.19). These instruments are convenient and can be carried in a pocket. The handle opens to a 90° angle for testing; when folded, it protects the monofilament when not in use.

Rydel-Seiffer 64/128 Hz Graduated Tuning Fork (US Neurologicals, Kirkland, WA)

This quantitative tuning fork contains small scaled weights on the distal ends of the two prongs, converting it from 128 to 64 Hz (Fig. 3.20). The two triangles move closer together and their intersection moves upward as the intensity of vibration decreases. The intensity where the patient no longer perceives the vibration is recorded as the number adjacent to the intersection of the triangles. This instrument allows more sensitive and specific testing for detecting sensory changes as compared to qualitative tuning forks and has demonstrated high intertester and intratester reliability.[116]

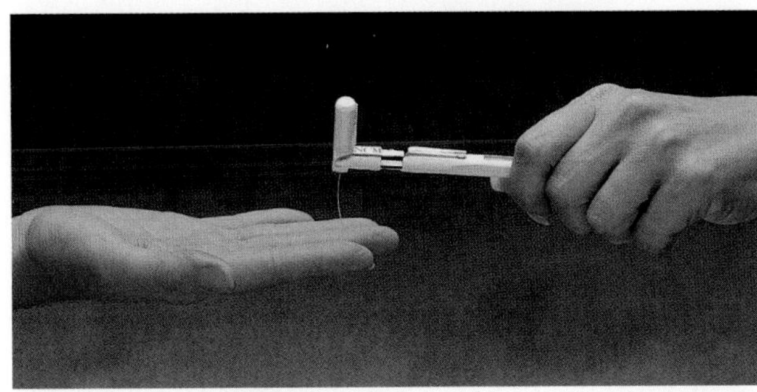

Figure 3.19 Individual monofilament. *(Courtesy of North Coast Medical, Inc., Morgan Hill, CA 95037.)*

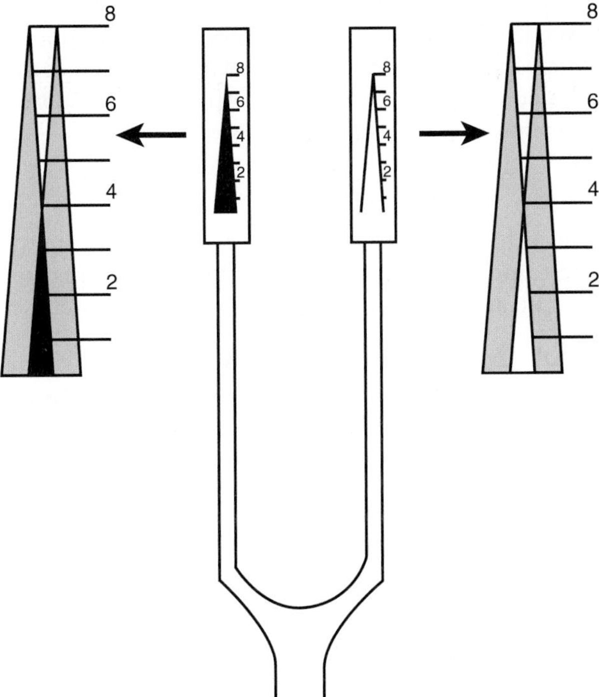

Figure 3.20 Schematic illustration of the Rydel-Seiffer tuning fork. *(Courtesy of US Neurologicals, Kirkland, WA, 98033.)*

Rolltemp II (Somedic Sales AB, Hörby, Sweden)

This instrument is used as a screening tool for determining changes in perception of thermal sensation (Fig. 3.21). The rollers are housed in a storage unit to maintain temperature. The individual rollers are placed in contact with the skin to provide a gross estimate of temperature perception.

Bio-Thesiometer (Bio-Medical Instrument Co, Newbury, OH)

This instrument is designed to quantitatively measure threshold perception of a vibratory stimulus (Fig. 3.22). The stimulus is applied using a handheld device applied to the skin. Intensity of stimulation can be preset or gradually increased until the threshold is reached (or gradually lowered until no longer felt).

Vibrameter (Somedic Sales AB, Hörby, Sweden)

The Vibrameter also quantitatively measures the perception of vibration (Fig 3.23). Standardized test points have been identified for use with this instrument.

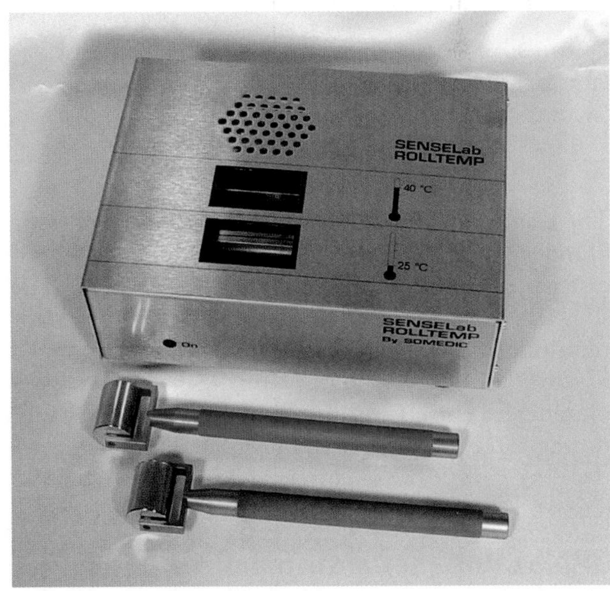

Figure 3.21 The Rolltemp provides a quick screening tool for thermal sensation. The rollers are mounted on handles and stored upright in the two square insertion points on the storage unit. One roller is maintained at 40°C (104°F); the other at 25°C (77°F). *(Courtesy of Somedic Sales AB, Hörby, Sweden.)*

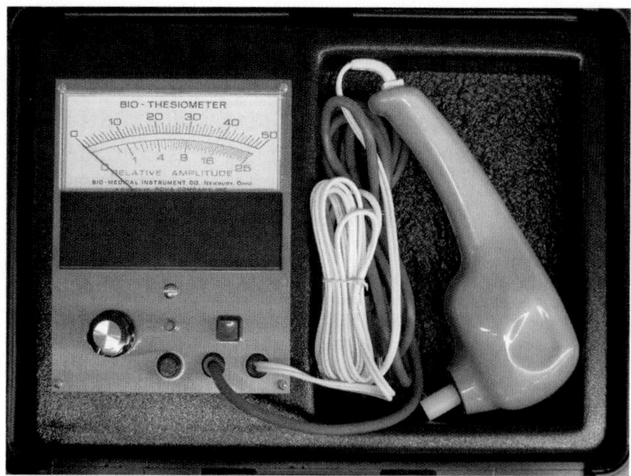

Figure 3.22 Bio-Thesiometer for measuring perception of vibratory stimulus. *(Courtesy of Bio-Medical Instrument Co., Newbury, OH, 44065.)*

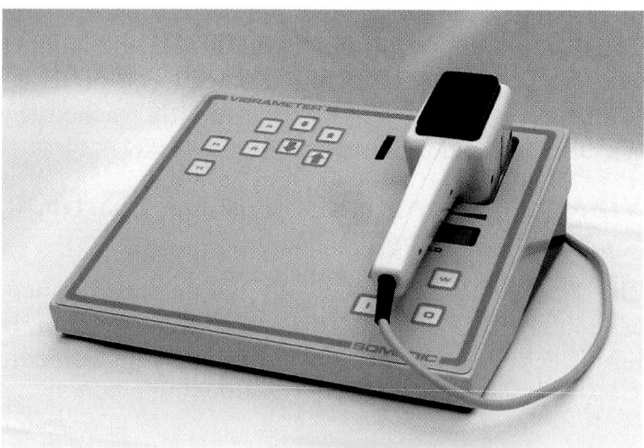

Figure 3.23 Vibrameter for measuring perception of vibratory stimulus *(Courtesy of Somedic Sales AB, Hörby, Sweden.)*

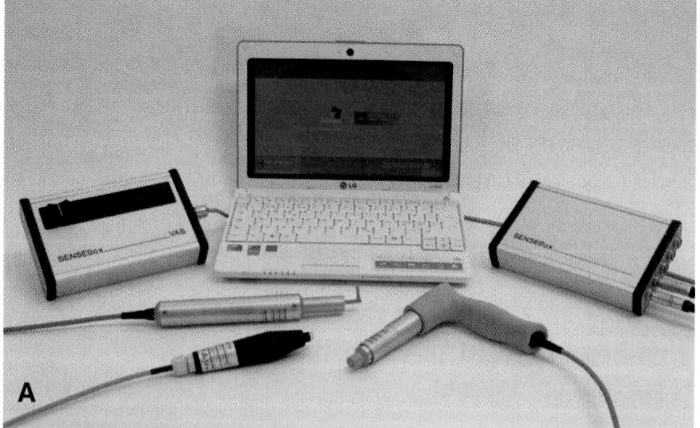

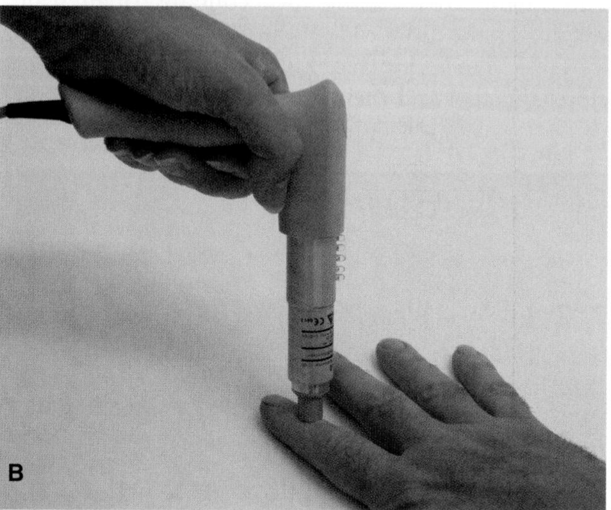

Figure 3.24 (A) SENSEBox. Viewing counterclockwise, to the left of computer is the electronic patient response visual analog scale, von Frey transducer for touch evoked potentials, pushbutton patient response device, algometer transducer for measuring sensitivity to pain, and data collection unit. (B) Algometer transducer for SENSEBox. *(Courtesy of Somedic Sales AB, Hörby, Sweden.)*

The test points (e.g., dorsum of the metacarpal bone of index finger, first metatarsal, and on tibia) allow for ease of comparison and interpretation of results. The sites also represent relatively long neural pathways for transmission to the CNS. Stimulus is applied using the handheld device. A study by Conaire et al[117] reported a moderate correlation between the Vibrameter and tuning fork (manufacturer and model number specified) as evidence of concurrent validity (ICC = 0.515–0.634).

SENSEBox (Somedic Sales AB, Hörby, Sweden)

This instrument measures pain thresholds (algometer) and touch-evoked potentials (von Frey transducer). It determines the relationship between the intensity of controlled mechanical stimuli and patient response. Handheld transducers are used to apply the stimuli (Fig. 3.24A and B). Patient responses are recorded using a handheld push-button device or a continuous electronic visual analog scale. During examination, data are automatically stored in a computer database.

MSA (Modular Sensory Analyzer) Thermotest (Somedic Sales AB, Hörby, Sweden)

The MSA Thermotest (Fig. 3.25) measures response to thermal (warm and cold) stimuli. Thermodes of different sizes allow testing of various anatomical locations. A computer interfaces using SenseLab software that sets up and runs the Thermotest and allows for analysis and storage of data. Temperatures range from 41°F to 125.6°F (5°C to 52°C).

CRANIAL NERVE FUNCTION

An examination of cranial nerves provides information about their individual function as well as insight into the location of intracranial lesions.[118,119] Data generated

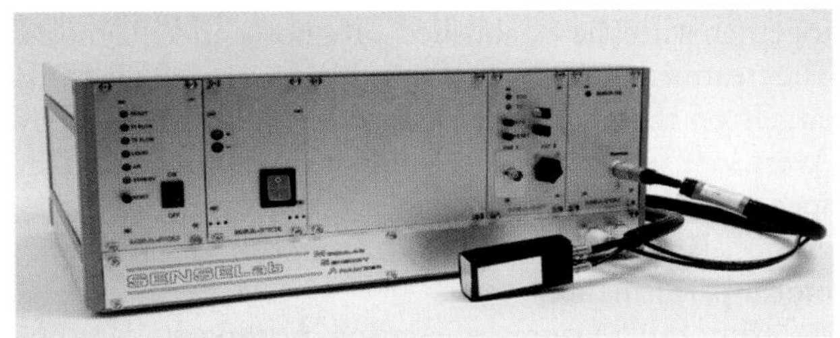

Figure 3.25 MSA Thermotest. In the right foreground is a 1 x 2 inch (25 x 50 mm) standard thermode for application of thermal stimuli.

may include function of muscles innervated by the cranial nerves; visual, auditory, sensory, and gag reflex integrity; perception of taste; swallowing characteristics; eye movements; and constriction and dilation patterns of the pupils.

Table 3.4 provides a summary of the functional components of the cranial nerves. Box 3.4 presents examples of tests appropriate for each cranial nerve. Impairments noted during initial testing may indicate that a more comprehensive examination is warranted. See Chapter 5, Examination of Motor Function: Motor

Table 3.4 Functional Components of the Cranial Nerves

Number	Name	Components	Function
I	Olfactory	Afferent	Olfaction (smell)
II	Optic	Afferent	Vision
III	Oculomotor	Efferent	
		Somatic	Elevates eyelid
			Turns eye up, down, in
		Visceral	Constricts pupil
			Accommodates lens
IV	Trochlear	Efferent (somatic)	Turns the adducted eye down and causes intorsion (inward rotation) of eye
V	Trigeminal	Mixed	
		Afferent	Sensation from face
			Sensation from cornea
			Sensation from anterior tongue
		Efferent	Muscles of mastication
			Dampens sound (tensor tympani)
VI	Abducens	Efferent (somatic)	Turns eye out
VII	Facial	Mixed	
		Afferent	Taste from anterior tongue
		Efferent (somatic)	Muscles of facial expression
			Dampens sound (stapedius)
		Efferent (visceral)	Tearing (lacrimal gland)
			Salivation (submandibular and sublingual glands)
VIII	Vestibulocochlear	Afferent	Balance (semicircular canals, utricle, saccule)
			Hearing (organ of Corti)
IX	Glossopharyngeal	Mixed	
		Afferent	Taste from posterior tongue
			Sensation from posterior tongue
			Sensation from oropharynx
		Efferent	Salivation (parotid gland)
X	Vagus	Mixed	
		Afferent	Thoracic and abdominal viscera
		Efferent	Muscles of larynx and pharynx
			Decreases heart rate
			Increases GI motility
XI	Spinal accessory	Efferent	Head movements (sternocleidomastoid and trapezius)
XII	Hypoglossal	Efferent	Tongue movements and shape

GI = gastrointestinal.
From Nolan[64, p. 44] with permission.

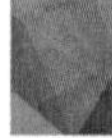

Box 3.4 Tests for Cranial Nerve Function[11,64]

Cranial nerve I: Examine olfactory acuity using non-noxious odors such as lemon oil, coffee, cloves, or tobacco.
Cranial nerve II: Examine visual acuity using a Snellen chart; both central and peripheral vision is tested.
Cranial nerves III, IV, and VI: Determine equality and size of pupils; reaction to light; presence of strabismus (loss of ocular alignment); ability of eyes to follow a moving target without head movement; presence of ptosis of eyelid.
Cranial nerve V: Sensory tests of face (sharp/dull discrimination, light touch); open and close jaw against resistance; jaw jerk reflex.
Cranial nerve VII: Examine any asymmetry of face at rest and during voluntary contraction.
Cranial nerve VIII: Test auditory acuity using a vibrating tuning fork (Weber test) placed on vertex of skull or forehead; patient indicates on which side the tone is louder. Rub fingers together at a distance and gradually bring toward patient; note distance when first heard. Alter volume of conversation. Rinne test (conductive hearing loss), vibrating tuning fork placed on mastoid process, then near external ear canal; note hearing acuity.
Cranial nerve IX: Examine taste on posterior one-third of tongue; examine gag reflex.
Cranial nerve X: Examine swallowing; observe uvula and soft palate for any asymmetry (tongue depressor).
Cranial nerve XI: Examine strength of the sternocleidomastoid and trapezius muscles.
Cranial nerve XII: With tongue protruded, examine ability to move tongue rapidly from side to side.

Control and Motor Learning, for additional information on cranial nerve examination.

SENSORY INTEGRITY WITHIN THE CONTEXT OF TREATMENT

Learning a motor behavior is dependent on the patient's ability to take in sensory information from the body and the environment (sensory intake), process it (sensory integration), and use it to plan and organize behavior (output). When patients experience impairment in processing sensory intake, deficits typically occur in planning and organizing behavior. This produces behaviors that may interfere with successful motor learning and motor function.

The POC designed for a patient with impaired sensation is typically guided by one of two approaches, the *Sensory Integration Approach* and the *Compensatory Approach*. The selection of a treatment model is based on a complete data set of information from all examinations together with the established prognosis and diagnosis. The treatment approach depicted in Figure 3.26 is based largely on the Sensory Integration Model developed by Ayers.[1,120-124] The basic premise of this approach is that specific treatment techniques can enhance sensory integration (CNS processing) with a resultant change in motor performance.

Using the Sensory Integration Approach, data obtained from the examination of sensory function informs development of a POC to enhance opportunities for *controlled* sensory intake within a framework of meaningful functional skills. During treatment, the patient is provided guided practice in planning and organizing motor behaviors using both *intrinsic* feedback (from the movement itself) and *augmented* feedback (cues planned

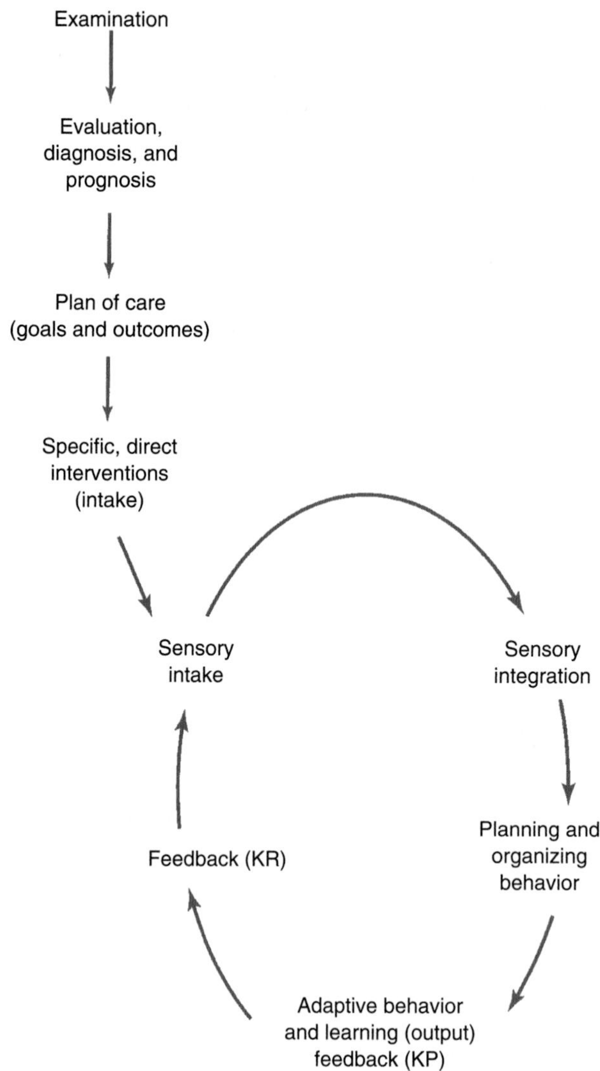

Figure 3.26 Elements of patient management for sensory impairment. KP refers to knowledge of performance (feedback about the quality of movement produced) and KR refers to knowledge of result (feedback about the end result or outcome of the movement). *(Adapted from Bundy and Murray.[6, p. 5])*

by the therapist). This approach is designed to improve the ability of the CNS to process and integrate information and promote motor learning. The reader is referred to the work of Ayers[1,120-124] and Bundy and Murray[6] for a detailed presentation of both the theory and practice of the Sensory Integration Model.

The Compensatory Approach is a more traditional intervention that focuses on patient education to accommodate the limitations imposed by the sensory deficit. The therapist's role is to assist the patient in achieving optimum functional capacity, minimizing activity limitations, protecting anesthetic limbs, and creating appropriate environmental adaptations to enhance safety and function. Guided by this approach, the therapist instructs the patient in practical strategies such as testing bathwater with a thermometer or body part with intact sensation before entering; not going barefoot; regularly checking insensitive skin areas for cuts or bruises (particularly important for patients with diabetes); adaptations ("compensations" for the sensory loss) that can include substituting vision for absent tactile cues when carrying objects; wearing heat-resistant gloves when working in the kitchen; using a rolling cart in the kitchen or other work space to transport items from one area to another; and arranging kitchen supplies to eliminate need for access to storage areas directly over the stove.

SUMMARY

Examination of sensory function provides important information about the integrity of the somatosensory system. Findings from the examination assist in making clinical judgments about diagnosis, prognosis, goals and expected outcomes, as well as establishing the POC. Periodic reexamination provides critical data on changes in patient status and in determining progress toward goals and outcomes. Individual tests for each sensory modality have been presented. Reliability of these test procedures can be improved by careful adherence to consistent guidelines, administration of tests by trained individuals, and subsequent retests performed by the same examiner. Documentation of test results should address the type(s) of sensation affected, the quantity, the degree of involvement, and the localization of the exact boundaries of the sensory deficits. Finally, it should be emphasized that additional research related to sensory testing is warranted. Further development of QST techniques, standardized protocols, valid and reliability measures, and additional normative data will significantly improve the clinical applications of data obtained from the examination of sensory function.

Questions for Review

1. Define a *dermatome* and describe a precaution with using published dermatome maps.
2. Identify six pathologies or health conditions that would warrant (or indicate the need for) examination of sensory function.
3. Describe the five terms used to document a patient's level of consciousness.
4. Which type of sensory receptor is responsible for position sense and awareness of joints at rest, during movement, and vibration? How would you comprehensively examine this sensory receptor?
5. Which type of muscle receptor senses tension, and how does it affect the muscle when under extreme tension?
6. For a suspected localized lesion, in which direction would you conduct your examination of sensory function? Why?
7. Describe four purposes of screening the sensory system.
8. Describe how the data from the examination of sensory function is used by the physical therapist.
9. Describe equipment (items) that can be used to assess stereognosis.
10. What type of findings from an examination of sensory function would indicate that a referral is warranted?
11. Explain why impaired sensation is a contraindication to or precaution for use of some physical agents.
12. What information would you provide to the patient prior to administration of sensory tests to obtain informed consent?
13. Which muscles would you test to assess the spinal accessory cranial nerve?
14. Describe the variables you would use to record the results of sensory testing.

CASE STUDY

A 68-year-old woman presents for outpatient physical therapy with an improperly fitted cane. You escort her to the examination room while observing her gait pattern, which is characterized by a slower self-selected walking speed, wide base of support, increased time spent in double limb support, and increased step variability. She has a long-standing history of hypertension (15 years), hypercholesterolemia (10 years), and poorly controlled diabetes (25 years). In addition to reporting several falls in the past 6 months, none of which resulted in injury serious enough to be hospitalized, the patient describes increasing pain in her lower extremities that is deep, sharp, and burning; that is symmetrical; and that occasionally wakes her up at night. The patient lives alone in a one-bedroom apartment in a building with an elevator and level entrance to the lobby.

GUIDING QUESTIONS

1. Of all the senses, which one is most often affected by the patient's medical conditions, and how would you assess it?
2. Given her history of falls, which sensory systems should you examine? Why? How?
3. How would you examine pain sensation, and what findings would you expect given the long-standing history of diabetes? Why is it important to examine pain sensation?
4. How would you quantitatively measure touch awareness (touch-evoked potentials) in this patient?
5. The test findings indicate mild loss of proprioception and vibration in the lower extremities (distal more than proximal). What receptors are responsible for these sensory modalities? Where are the receptors located? Identify the ascending pathway that mediates proprioception and vibration.

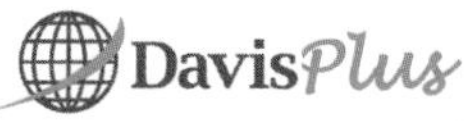

For additional resources, including answers to the questions for review and case study guiding questions, please visit **http://davisplus.fadavis.com**

References

1. Ayers, JA: Sensory Integration and Learning Disorders. Western Psychological Services, Los Angeles, 1972.
2. Byl, NN: Multisensory control of upper extremity function. Neurology Report 26(1):32, 2002.
3. Wolpert, DM, Pearson, KG, and Ghez, C: The organization and planning of movement. In Kandel, ER, et al: Principles of Neural Science, ed 5. McGraw-Hill, New York, 2013, p. 743.
4. Ayers, AJ: Sensory Integration and Praxis Tests (SIPT Manual). Western Psychological Services, Los Angeles, 1989.
5. Mailloux, Z, and Miller-Kuhaneck, H: Evolution of a theory: How measurement has shaped Ayres Sensory Integration. Am J Occup Ther 68(5):495, 2014.
6. Bundy, AC, and Murray, EA: Sensory integration: A. Jean Ayres' theory revisited. In Bundy, AC, Lane, SJ, and Murray, EA: Sensory Integration: Theory and Practice, ed 2. FA Davis, Philadelphia, 2002, p. 3.
7. Schaaf, RC, et al: State of the science: A roadmap for research in sensory integration. Am J Occup Ther 69(6):1, 2015.
8. Cooper, C, and Canyock, JD: Evaluation of sensation and intervention for sensory dysfunction. In Pendleton, HM, and Schultz-Krohn, W (eds): Pedretti's Occupational Therapy: Practice Skills for Physical Dysfunction, ed 7. Elsevier/Mosby, St. Louis, 2013, p. 575.
9. Guide to Physical Therapist Practice 3.0. Alexandria, VA: American Physical Therapy Association; 2014. Available at: http://guidetoptpractice.apta.org/. Accessed August 9, 2017.
10. Aminoff, MJ, Greenberg, DA, and Simon, RP: Clinical Neurology, ed 9. Lange Medical Books/McGraw-Hill, New York, 2015.
11. Gilman, S, and Newman, SW: Manter and Gatz's Essentials of Clinical Neuroanatomy and Neurophysiology, ed 10. FA Davis, Philadelphia, 2003.
12. Downs, MB, and Laporte C: Conflicting dermatome maps: Educational and clinical implications. J Orthop Sports Phys Ther 41(6):427, 2011.
13. Apok, V, et al: Dermatomes and dogma. Pract Neurol 11:100, 2011.
14. Ladak, A, Tubbs, RS, and Spinner, RJ: Mapping sensory nerve communications between peripheral nerve territories. Clin Anat 27:681, 2014.
15. Dong, Q, et al: Entrapment neuropathies in the upper and lower limbs: Anatomy and MRI features. Radiol Res Pract 2012:1, 2012.
16. Callaghan, BC, et al: Diabetic neuropathy: Clinical manifestations and current treatment. Lancet Neurol 11(6): 521, 2012.
17. Garg, N, and Smith, TW: An update on iummunopathogenesis, diagnosis, and treatment of multiple sclerosis. Brain and Behav 5(9): 1, 2015.
18. Diaz, E, and Morales, H: Spinal cord anatomy and clinical syndromes. Sem Ultrasound CT MR 37(5): 360, 2016.
19. Schott, JM: The neurology of ageing: What is normal. Pract Neurol 0:1, 2017.
20. Chang, CM, Young, YH, and Cheng, PW: Age-related changes in ocular vestibular evoked potentials via galvanic vestibular stimulation and bone conducted vibration modes. Acta Otolaryngol 132(12):1295, 2012.
21. Cortese, G, and Burger, C: Neuroinflammatory challenges compromise neural function in the aging brain: Postoperative cognitive delirium and Alzheimer's disease. Behav Brain Res 322(Pt B):269, 2017.
22. Damoiseaux, JS: Effects of aging on functional and structural brain connectivity. Neuroimage, 2017 [Epub ahead of print] PMID: 28159687; DOI: 10.1016/j.neuroimage.2017.01.077
23. Dushanova, J, and Christov, M: The effect of aging on EEG brain oscillations related to sensory and sensorimotor functions. Adv Med Sci 59:61, 2014.
24. Sorond, F, et al: Aging, the central nervous system, and mobility in older adults: Neural mechanisms of mobility impairment. J Gerontol A Biol Sci Med Sci 70(12):1526, 2015.
25. Humes, L: Age-related changes in cognitive and sensory processing: Focus on middle-aged adults. Am J Audiol 24(2):94, 2015.
26. Kohama, S, Rosene, D, and Sherman, S: Age-related changes in human and non-human primate white matter: From myelination disturbances to cognitive decline. Age (Dordr) 34(5):1093, 2012.

27. Kuba, M, et al: Aging effect in pattern, motion, and cognitive visual evoked potentials. Vision Res 62:9, 2012.
28. Ho, MC, et al: Age-related changes of task-specific brain activity in normal aging. Neurosci Lett 507(1):78, 2012.
29. Li, S, et al: Age-related changes in the surface morphology of the central sulcus. Neuroimage 58(2):381, 2011.
30. Halewyck, FA, et al: Factors underlying age-related changes in discrete aiming. Exp Brain Res 233:1733, 2015.
31. Woytowicz, E, Whitall, J, and Westlake, KP: Age-related changes in bilateral upper extremity coordination. Curr Geriatr Rep 5(3): 191, 2016.
32. US Department of Health and Human Services, Office of Disease Prevention and Health Promotion: Healthy People 2020. Washington, DC. Retrieved April 5, 2017, from www.healthypeople.gov/.
33. Shumway-Cook, A, and Woollacott, MH: Motor Control: Translating Research into Clinical Practice, ed 5. Wolters Kluwer/Lippincott Williams & Wilkins, Philadelphia, 2017.
34. Ropper, AH, Samuels, MA, and Klein, JP: Adams and Victor's Principles of Neurology, ed 10. McGraw-Hill, New York, 2014.
35. Gould, BE, and Dyer, RM: Pathophysiology for the Health Related Professions, ed 4. Saunders/Elsevier, Philadelphia, 2011.
36. Sanes, JR, and Jessell, TM: The aging brain. In Kandel, ER, et al: Principles of Neural Science, ed 5. McGraw-Hill, New York, 2013, p. 1328.
37. Shankar, SK: Biology of aging brain. Indian J Pathol Microbiol 53(4):595, 2010.
38. Lewis, CB, and Bottomley, JM: Geriatric Physical Therapy: A Clinical Approach, ed 3. Pearson Education, Upper Saddle River, NJ, 2008.
39. Fuller, KS: Introduction to central nervous system disorders. In Goodman, CC, and Fuller, KS: Pathology: Implications for the Physical Therapist, ed 4. Saunders/Elsevier, St. Louis, 2015, p 1371.
40. Jagga, ML, and Verma, SK: Effect of aging and anthropometric measurements on nerve conduction properties—a review. JESP 7(1):1, 2011.
41. Senthilkumari, KR, Umamaheswari, K, and Bhaskaran, M: A study on median nerve conduction velocity in different age groups. Int J Res Med Sci 3(11):3313, 2015.
42. Onofri, M, et al: Age-related changes in evoked potentials. Neurophysiol Clin 31(2):83, 2001.
43. Matsuoka, S, et al: Quantitative and qualitative studies of Meissner's corpuscles in human skin, with special reference to alterations caused by aging. J Dermatol 10(3):205, 1983.
44. Stuart M, et al: Effects of aging on vibration detection thresholds at various body regions. BMC Geriatr 3:1, 2003.
45. Bartzokis, G, et al: Lifespan trajectory of myelin integrity and maximum motor speed. Neurobiol Aging 31(9):1554, 2010.
46. Peters, A: The effects of normal aging on myelin and nerve fibers: A review. J Neurocytol 31:581, 2002.
47. Lascelles, RG, and Thomas, PK: Changes due to age in internodal length in the sural nerve of man. J Neurol Neurosurg Psychiatry 29:40, 1966.
48. Verdu, E, et al: Influence of aging on peripheral nerve function and regeneration. J Peripher Nerv Syst 5(4):191, 2000.
49. Toledo, D, and Barela, J: Age-related differences in postural control: Effects of the complexity of visual manipulation and sensorimotor contribution to postural performance. Exp Brain Res 232:493, 2014.
50. Yeh, TT, et al: Age-related changes in postural control to the demands of a precision task. Hum Mov Sci 44:134, 2015.
51. Tsai, YC, Hsieh, LF, and Yang, S: Age-related changes in posture response under a continuous and unexpected perturbation. J Biomech 47(2):482, 2014.
52. Brodoehl, S, et al: Age-related changes in somatosensory processing of tactile stimulation—an fMRI study. Behav Brain Res 238:259, 2013.
53. Decorps, J, et al: Effect of ageing on tactile transduction processes. Ageing Research Reviews 13:90, 2014.
54. Alanazy, MH, et al: The conventional tuning fork as a quantitative tool for vibration threshold. Muscle Nerve 55(5):1, 2017.
55. Venkatesan, L, Barlow, SM, and Kieweg D: Age- and sex-related changes in vibrotactile sensitivity of hand and face in neurotypical adults. Somatos Mot Res 32(1):44, 2014.
56. Ko, SU, et al: Sex-specific age associations of ankle proprioception test performance in the older adults: Results from the Baltimore Longitudinal Study of Aging. Age Ageing 44(3):485, 2015.
57. Ingemanson, ML, et al: Use of a robotic device to measure age-related decline in finger proprioception. Exp Brain Res 234:83, 2016.
58. Guergova, S, and Dufour, A: Thermal sensitivity in the elderly: A review. Ageing Res Rev 10(1):80, 2011.
59. Kemp, J, et al: Age-related decline in thermal adaptation capacities: An evoked potentials study. Psychophysiology 51(6):539, 2014.
60. Inoue, Y, et al: Sex differences in age-related changes on peripheral warm and cold innocuous thermal sensitivity. Physiol Behav 164(Pt A):86, 2016.
61. Tseng, MT, et al: Effect of aging on the cerebral processing of thermal pain in the human brain. Pain 154(10):2120, 2013.
62. Bowden, J, and McNulty, P: Age-related changes in cutaneous sensation in the healthy human hand. Age (Dordr)35(4):1077, 2013.
63. Franco, P, Santos, K, and Rodacki, A: Joint positioning sense, perceived force level, and two-point discrimination tests of young and active elderly adults. Braz J Phys Ther 19(4):304, 2015.
64. Nolan, MF: Introduction to the Neurologic Examination. FA Davis, Philadelphia, 1996.
65. Waxman, SG: Clinical Neuroanatomy, ed 28. Lange Medical Books/McGraw-Hill, New York, 2017.
66. Norris, D, Clark, M, and Shipley, S: The Mental Status Examination. Am Fam Physician 94(8):635, 2016.
67. Wills, A: How to perform a neurological examination. Medicine 40(8):409, 2012.
68. Wills A: How to perform a basic neurological exam. Medicine 44(8):464, 2016.
69. Hall, JE: Guyton and Hall Textbook of Medical Physiology, ed 13. Saunders/Elsevier, Philadelphia, 2016.
70. Gardner, EP, and Johnson KO: Sensory coding. In Kandel, ER, et al: Principles of Neural Science, ed 5. McGraw-Hill, New York, 2013, p. 449.
71. Kiernan, JA, and Rajakumar, N: Barr's The Human Nervous System: An Anatomical Viewpoint, ed 10. Wolters Kluwer/Lippincott Williams & Wilkins, Philadelphia, 2014.
72. Schmidt, RA, and Lee, TD: Motor Control and Learning: A Behavioral Emphasis, ed 5. Human Kinetics, Champaign, IL, 2011.
73. Lundy-Ekman, L: Neuroscience: Fundamentals for Rehabilitation, ed 4. Saunders/Elsevier, St. Louis, 2013.
74. Gardner, EP, and Johnson, KO: The somatosensory system: Receptors and central pathways. In Kandel, ER, et al: Principles of Neural Science, ed 5. McGraw-Hill, New York, 2013, p. 475.
75. Mtui, E, Gruener, G, and Dockery, P: Fitzgerald's Clinical Neuroanatomy and Neuroscience, ed 5. Elsevier, Philadelphia, 2016.
76. O'Connor, A, and McCreesh, K: Function and dysfunction of joint. In Petty, NJ (ed): Principles of Neuromusculoskeletal Treatment and Management: A Guide for Therapists. Churchill Livingstone/Elsevier, New York, 2011, p. 3.
77. Siegel, A, and Sapru, HN: Essential Neuroscience, ed 3. Wolters Kluwer/Lippincott Williams & Wilkins, Philadelphia, 2015.
78. Bear, MF, Connors, BW, and Paradiso, MA: Neuroscience: Exploring the Brain, ed 4. Wolters Kluwer/Lippincott Williams & Wilkins, Philadelphia, 2016.
79. Bican, O, Minager, A, and Pruitt, A: The spinal cord: A review of functional neuroanatomy. Neurol Clin 31(1):1, 2013.
80. Diaz, E, and Morales, H: Spinal cord anatomy and clinical syndromes. Semin Ultrasound CT MR 37(5):360, 2016.
81. Gardner, EP, and Johnson KO: Touch. In Kandel, ER, et al: Principles of Neural Science, ed 5. McGraw-Hill, New York, 2013, p. 498.
82. Borich, MR, et al: Understanding the role of the primary somatosensory cortex: Opportunities for rehabilitation. Neuropsychologia 79:246, 2015.
83. Bear, MF, Connors, BW, and Paradiso, MA: Neuroscience: Exploring the Brain, ed 3. Wolters Kluwer/Lippincott Williams & Wilkins, Philadelphia, 2007.
84. Williams, D, et al: Reviewing the evidence base for the peripheral sensory examination. Int J Clin Pract 68(6):756, 2014.
85. Zasler, ND: Validity assessment and the neurological physical examination. NeuroRehabilitation 36(4):401, 2015.

86. Gefen, A: Technologies for detecting loss of multiple sensory modalities in diabetic foot neuropathy. Diabetes Manage 2(2):149, 2012.
87. Nolan, MF: Clinical assessment of cutaneous sensory function. Clin Manage Phys Ther 4:26, 1984.
88. World Health Organization (WHO): Standard precautions in health care. WHO, Geneva, Switzerland, 2007. Retrieved June 1, 2017, from www.who.int/csr/resources/publications/EPR_AM2_E7.pdf.
89. World Health Organization (WHO): WHO Guidelines on Hand Hygiene in Health Care. WHO, Geneva, Switzerland, 2009. Retrieved June 1, 2017, from http://whqlibdoc.who.int/publications/2009/9789241597906_eng.pdf.
90. Theis, JL: Assessing abilities and capacities: Sensation. In Vining Radomski, M, and Trombly Latham, CA (eds): Occupational Therapy for Physical Dysfunction, ed 7. Wolters Kluwer/Lippincott Williams & Wilkins, Philadelphia, 2013.
91. Goble, DJ: Proprioceptive acuity assessment via joint position matching: From basic science to general practice. Phys Ther 90(8):1176, 2010.
92. Reidy, M, et al: Cold, hard cash: Clinical assessment of stereognosis using common objects and coins in older subjects. Eur Geriatr Med 7(2):180, 2016.
93. Han, J, et al: Comparisons of changes in the two-point discrimination test following muscle fatigue in healthy adults. J Phys Ther Sci 17:551, 2015.
94. Gutman, SA, and Schonfeld, AB: Screening Adult Neurologic Populations: A Step-by-Step Instruction Manual, ed 2. AOTA Press, Bethesda, MD, 2009.
95. Nolan, MF: Limits of two-point discrimination ability in the lower limb in young adult men and women. Phys Ther 63:1424, 1983.
96. Nolan, MF: Quantitative measure of cutaneous sensation: Two-point discrimination values for the face and trunk. Phys Ther 65:181, 1985.
97. Nolan, MF: Two-point discrimination assessment in the upper limb in young adult men and women. Phys Ther 62:965, 1982.
98. van Nes, SI, et al: Revising two-point discrimination assessment in normal aging and in patients with polyneuropathies. J Neurol Neurosurg Psychiatry 79(7):832, 2008.
99. Kaneko, A, Asai, N, and Kanda, T: The influence of age on pressure perception of static and moving two-point discrimination in normal subjects. J Hand Ther 18(4):421, 2005.
100. Vriens, JP, and van der Glas, HW: Extension of normal values on sensory function for facial areas using clinical tests on touch and two-point discrimination. Int J Oral Maxillofac Surg 38(11):1154, 2009.
101. Koo, JP, et al: Two-point discrimination of the upper extremities of healthy Koreans in their 20's. J Phys Ther Sci 28(3):870, 2016.
102. Talmasov, D, and Ropper, AH: Tactile asymbolia. J Clin Neurosci 26:164, 2016.
103. Kent, BE: Sensory-motor testing: The upper limb of adult patients with hemiplegia. J Am Phys Ther Assoc 45:550, 1965.
104. Moloney, NA, et al: Reliability of thermal quantitative sensory testing of the hand in a cohort of young, healthy adults. Muscle Nerve 44(4):547, 2011.
105. Wu, YH, and Li, KY: The inter-rater reliability of manually performed arm position matching test. Physiotherapy 101(Supplement 1):e1665, 2015.
106. Tyros, I, Soundy, A, and Heneghan, NR: Vibration sensibility of the median nerve in a population with chronic whiplash associated disorder: Intra- and interrater reliability study. Man Ther 25:81, 2016.
107. Meirte, J, et al: Interrater and intrarater reliability of the Semmes-Weinstein aesthesiometer to assess touch pressure threshold in burn scars. Burns 41:1261, 2015.
108. Blumenstiel, K, et al: Quantitative sensory testing profiles in chronic back pain are distinct from those in fibromyalgia. Clin J Pain 27(8):682, 2011.
109. Geletka, BJ, O'Hearn, MA, and Courtney, CA: Quantitative sensory testing changes in the successful management of chronic low back pain. J Manual Manipulative Ther 20(1):16, 2012.
110. Gröne, E, et al: Test order of quantitative sensory testing facilitates mechanical hyperalgesia in healthy volunteers. J Pain 13(1):73, 2012.
111. Gerber, C, et al: Test-retest and interobserver reliability of quantitative sensory testing according to the protocol of the German Research Network on Neuropathic Pain (DFNS): A multi-centre study. Pain 152(3):548, 2011.
112. Grone, E, et al: Test order of quantitative sensory testing facilitates mechanical hyperalgesia in healthy volunteers. J Pain 13(1):73, 2012.
113. Moeller-Bertram, T, et al: Sensory small fiber function differentially assed with diode laser quantitative sensory testing in painful neuropathy. Pain Med 14(3):417, 2013.
114. Backonja, MM, et al: Value of quantitative sensory testing in neurological and pain disorders: NeuPSIG consensus. Pain 154(9):1807, 2013.
115. Knutti, IA, Suter, MR, and Opsommer, E: Test-retest reliability of thermal quantitative sensory testing on two sites within the L5 dermatome of the lumbar spine and lower extremity. Neurosci Lett 579:157, 2014.
116. Pestronk, A, et al: Sensory exam with a quantitative tuning fork: Rapid, sensitive and predictive of SNAP amplitude. Neurology 62(3):461, 2004.
117. Conaire, E, Rushton, A, and Wright, C: The assessment of vibration sense in the musculoskeletal examination: Moving towards a valid and reliable quantitative approach to vibration testing in clinical practice. Man Ther 16:296, 2011.
118. Mahadevan, V: Anatomy of the cranial nerves. Surgery 30(3):95, 2012.
119. Damodaran, O, et al: Cranial nerve assessment: A concise guide to clinical examination. Clin Anat 27(1):25, 2014.
120. Ayers, JA: Tactile functions: Their relation to hyperactive and perceptual motor behavior. Am J Occup Ther 18:83, 1964.
121. Ayers, JA: Interrelations among perceptual-motor abilities in a group of normal children. Am J Occup Ther 20:288, 1966.
122. Ayers, JA: Improving academic scores through sensory integration. J Learn Disabil 5:338, 1972.
123. Ayers, JA: Cluster analysis of measures of sensory integration. Am J Occup Ther 31:362, 1977.
124. Ayers, JA: Sensory Integration and the Child. Western Psychological Services, Los Angeles, 1979.

Supplemental Readings

Abraira, VE, and Ginty, DD: The sensory neurons of touch. Neuron 79(4):618, 2013.

Kistemaker, DA, et al: Control of position and movement is simplified by combined muscle spindle and Golgi tendon organ feedback. J Neurophysiol 109(4):1126, 2013.

Owens, DM, and Lumpkin, EA: Diversification and specialization of touch receptors in skin. Cold Spring Harb Perspect Med 4(6):1, 2014.

Pleger, B, and Villringer, A: The human somatosensory system: From perception to decision making. Prog Neurobiol 103:76, 2013.

Prochazka, A, and Ellaway, P: Sensory systems in the control of movement. Compr Physiol 2(4):2615, 2012.

Raji, P, et al: Relationship between Semmes-Weinstein Monofilaments perception test and sensory nerve conduction studies in carpal tunnel syndrome. NeuroRehabilitation 35(3):543, 2014.

Suokas, AK, et al: Quantitative sensory testing in painful osteoarthritis: A systematic review and meta-analysis. Osteoarthritis Cartilage 20(10):1075, 2012.

Uddin, Z, and MacDermid, JC: Quantitative sensory testing in chronic musculoskeletal pain. Pain Med 17(9):1694, 2016.

Two-Point Discrimination Values for Healthy Subjects 20 to 24 Years of Age

appendix **3.A**

Two-Point Discrimination Values for the Upper Extremities of Healthy Subjects 20 to 24 Years of Age ($N = 43$)

Skin Region	X (mm)	S
Upper—lateral arm	42.4	14.0
Lower—lateral arm	37.8	13.1
Mid—medial arm	45.4	15.5
Mid—posterior arm	39.8	12.3
Mid—lateral forearm	35.9	11.6
Mid—medial forearm	31.5	8.9
Mid—posterior forearm	30.7	8.2
Over first dorsal interosseous muscle	21.0	5.6
Palmar surface—distal phalanx, thumb	2.6	0.6
Palmar surface—distal phalanx, long finger	2.6	0.7
Palmar surface—distal phalanx, little finger	2.5	0.7

Two-Point Discrimination Values for the Lower Extremities of Healthy Subjects 20 to 24 Years of Age ($N = 43$)

Skin Region	X (mm)	S
Proximal—anterior thigh	40.1	14.7
Distal—anterior thigh	23.2	9.3
Mid—lateral thigh	42.5	15.9
Mid—medial thigh	38.5	12.4
Mid—posterior thigh	42.2	15.9
Proximal—lateral leg	37.7	13.0
Distal—lateral leg[a]	41.6	13.0
Medial leg	43.6	13.5
Tip of great toe	6.6	1.8
Over 1–2 metatarsal interspace	23.9	6.3
Over 5th metatarsal	22.2	8.6

[a] $n = 41$

Two-Point Discrimination Values for the Face and Trunk of Healthy Subjects 20 to 24 Years of Age (*N* = 43)

Skin Region	*X* (mm)	S
Over eyebrow	14.9	4.2
Cheek	11.9	3.2
Over lateral mandible	10.4	2.2
Lateral neck	35.2	9.8
Medial to acromion process	51.1	14.0
Lateral to nipple	45.7	12.7[a]
Lateral to umbilicus	36.4	7.3[b]
Over iliac crest	44.9	10.1[c]
Lateral to C7 spine	55.4	20.0[b]
Over inferior angle of scapula	52.2	12.6[b]
Lateral to L3 spine	49.9	12.7[b]

[a] *n* = 26
[b] *n* = 42
[c] *n* = 33
From Nolan,[95-97] with permission of the American Physical Therapy Association.

Musculoskeletal Examination

Evangelos Pappas PT, PhD, OCS
D. Joyce White, PT, DSc, MS

Chapter 4

LEARNING OBJECTIVES

1. Identify the purposes of performing a musculoskeletal examination.
2. Discuss the components of a musculoskeletal examination.
3. Identify questions that should be included in a patient interview.
4. Describe the procedures used to selectively test specific tissue types in a musculoskeletal examination.
5. Identify additional procedures that often complement a musculoskeletal examination.
6. Using the case study examples, apply clinical decision making skills in evaluating musculoskeletal examination data.

CHAPTER OUTLINE

The musculoskeletal system includes bones; muscles with their related tendons and synovial sheaths; bursa; and joint structures such as cartilage, menisci, capsules, and ligaments. Acute injuries or chronic conditions of the musculoskeletal system can greatly affect function by causing direct impairments such as pain, inflammation, swelling, structural deformity, restricted joint movement, joint instability, and muscle weakness. Examples of diagnoses that result in direct impairment of the musculoskeletal system include fracture, rheumatoid arthritis (RA) and other systemic diseases, osteoarthritis, (OA), joint dislocation, tendinitis, bursitis, muscle strain/rupture, and ligament sprain/rupture. Importantly, musculoskeletal disorders are the second most common cause of disability worldwide, measured by years lived with disability, with low back pain being the most frequent condition.[1] In addition to primary musculoskeletal impairments, many pathological conditions that initially affect other body systems such as the neurological, cardiovascular, or pulmonary systems, can result in secondary or indirect impairment of the musculoskeletal system. Both direct and indirect musculoskeletal impairments can contribute to activity limitations, participation restrictions, and disability that affect a patient's ability to perform certain tasks and roles in society. Thus, performing a systematic, evidence-based, and thorough evaluation is an important skill for health care professionals who encounter patients with musculoskeletal disorders (e.g., physical therapists, athletic trainers, general practitioners, orthopedic surgeons), as it will form the foundation for an effective treatment plan. In addition to clinical competence, the clinician should demonstrate respect, interest, and empathy toward patients, who frequently feel vulnerable and lost within the health care system.

This chapter discusses the purposes of, and provides a general framework for, conducting a musculoskeletal examination. Other resources are available that provide detailed musculoskeletal testing procedures of specific body regions.[2-4]

PURPOSES OF THE MUSCULOSKELETAL EXAMINATION

Evaluation of data from the musculoskeletal examination contributes to establishing a diagnosis and prognosis, setting anticipated goals and expected outcomes, and developing and implementing a plan of care (POC). A musculoskeletal examination is also an important component of evaluating treatment outcomes both periodically during the treatment process and at the conclusion of the episode of care. The purposes of performing a musculoskeletal examination include the following:

1. To determine the presence and extent of impairments, activity limitations, and disability involving muscles, bones, and related joint structures.
2. To identify the specific tissues and pathology causing/contributing to the impairment, activity limitation, or disability when possible.
3. To establish objective baseline status that will be used to measure progress.
4. To formulate appropriate goals, expected outcomes, and plan of care in consultation with the patient.
5. To evaluate the effectiveness of rehabilitation or medical or surgical management.
6. To identify risk factors associated with the development or worsening of impairments, activity limitations, or disabilities.
7. To determine the need for orthotic and adaptive equipment necessary for functional performance of activities of daily living (ADL) and occupational and/or recreational activities.
8. To assess and address psychosocial issues that may interfere with recovery and motivate the patient.

EXAMINATION PROCEDURES

Patient History and Interview

Before Beginning the Examination

Before beginning the physical examination, it is important to gain as much information as possible about the patient's current condition and past medical history. This information will help to direct and focus the physical examination to an area and system of the body. Information on symptoms and functional ability will help to establish a baseline against which treatment effectiveness can be judged. It will also help ensure that the examination and subsequent treatment are conducted safely and efficiently.

Typically, most of this information is obtained while interviewing the patient. However, utilizing other information sources can be very efficient and provide objectivity and details to supplement interview data. If the patient is hospitalized in an acute care or rehabilitation setting, the medical records—including admission reports, progress notes, medication sheets, surgical summaries, imaging reports, and laboratory test results—should be available and sought out. Referral summaries from previous medical care settings that review prior treatment approaches and discuss functional status may also be included. Other members of the health care team can be consulted for their input.

Medical History Questionnaires

Outpatient clients often arrive with only a general diagnosis from a referring physician, or they may be self-referred. In such cases, it will be helpful to ask the patient to complete a medical history questionnaire before the examination process. This should include space for the patient to note the chief problem and date of onset; diagnostic tests performed for the problem; name and date of all surgeries; all medications currently being taken; past or current treatment for the problem (including those initiated by patient); a checklist of common medical conditions the patient may have experienced; previous surgeries; brief family medical history; and questions regarding patient's age, occupation, and lifestyle, such as smoking, alcohol use, and exercise. Figure 4.1 provides an example of a medical history questionnaire. The *Guide to Physical Therapy Practice 3.0* also includes a detailed template for a patient self-administered health questionnaire.[5]

A thorough understanding of the patient's medical background is critical for selection and safe application of examination and treatment procedures. For example, a family history of heart disease or risk factors such as obesity and smoking should prompt the therapist to further investigate symptoms that may indicate cardiovascular system involvement and make appropriate referral if necessary. A history of diabetes mellitus should prompt the therapist to suspect and test for potentially compromised peripheral vascular and peripheral nervous systems, and to possibly avoid the use of heat modalities during treatment.

A brief history should be obtained concerning medical problems and prior surgeries involving other body regions and systems. Conditions involving the cardiac, respiratory, neurological, vascular, metabolic, endocrine, gastrointestinal, genital urinary, visual, and dermatological systems should be noted. Having a patient complete a medical history questionnaire before the examination is an efficient means of obtaining this information, but the information should also be verified during the interview. Therapists need to be aware of other conditions that mimic signs and symptoms often attributable to the musculoskeletal system. For example, inflammation of the gallbladder (cholecystitis) may result in right shoulder pain. However, shoulder pain related to cholecystitis typically is not mechanical—that is, it will not increase with shoulder movements or testing of shoulder musculature, as would typically occur in the presence of musculoskeletal conditions. Patients with cholecystitis would likely have additional symptoms such as upper abdominal discomfort, bloating, belching, nausea, and intolerance of fried foods. Knowledge of systemic human pathology allows the therapist to recognize conditions requiring additional physician evaluation and intervention.

Indications that the patient may have serious pathology that requires urgent medical care and is outside the scope of physical therapy are frequently termed *red flags*. Physical therapists should be very proficient in recognizing these red flags and acting accordingly. Physical therapists, especially those with orthopedic board certification, demonstrate very high levels of competence in making correct decisions for medical referral.[6]

The purpose of this questionnaire is to assist us in providing you with quality care by obtaining a better understanding of your total health status. This questionnaire is part of your confidential medical record.

NAME: ______________________ DATE: __________

CHIEF PROBLEM OR COMPLAINT: ______________________

REFERRING MD: ______________________ DATE OF NEXT MD VISIT: __________

MEDICATIONS: Please list *all* medications currently being taken, along with the dosage, if known, and frequency.

1. ______________________ 4. ______________________

2. ______________________ 5. ______________________

3. ______________________ 6. ______________________

SURGERY: Please list *all* surgeries and approximate date.

1. ______________________ DATE: __________

2. ______________________ DATE: __________

3. ______________________ DATE: __________

4. ______________________ DATE: __________

DIAGNOSTIC TESTS: Please check tests for current problem only.

X-rays: __________ CT Scan: __________ MRI: __________ Bone Scan: __________

EMG: __________ Blood Test: __________ Myelogram: __________ Others: __________

OCCUPATION: ______________________

LIFE STYLE: Non Smoker: ____ Smoke ____/day

No Alcohol: ____ Alcohol ____/day or ____/week

No Exercise: ____ Exercise ____/day or ____/week

FAMILY HISTORY: Mother, Father, siblings: Alive and healthy: __________

If deceased, cause of death: ______________________

Figure 4.1 An example of a medical history recording form. *(Courtesy of North Andover Physical Therapy Associates, North Andover, MA.)*

DO YOU HAVE, OR HAVE YOU HAD, ANY OF THE FOLLOWING: Please check *all* that apply.

___ High blood pressure
___ Heart problems
___ Heart palpitations, murmur
___ Chest pain

___ Shortness of breath
___ Coughing

___ Difficulty sleeping lying flat
___ Lung problems
___ Asthma
___ Allergies

___ Ulcers
___ Recent weight gain or loss
___ Nausea, vomiting
___ Bowel or bladder changes
___ Loss of appetite

___ Sexual dysfunction
___ Abnormal or painful menstruation
___ Pelvic inflammatory disease
___ Currently pregnant
___ Date of last mammogram:_____

___ Blood in urine
___ Incontinence

___ Seizures
___ Head trauma
___ Paralysis
___ Loss of consciousness
___ Headaches

___ Numbness or tingling
___ Dizziness
___ Balance problems

___ Arthritis

___ Hot or cold intolerance
___ Diabetes
___ Low blood sugar
___ Thyroid problems

___ Tumors ___ Cancer
___ Bleeding or bruising
___ Dialysis
___ Blood transfusion

___ Rashes
___ Scars
___ Changes in hair or nails

___ Wear eye glasses, contacts
___ Changes in vision
___ Blurred or double vision

___ Difficulty swallowing
___ Ear pain
___ Vocal changes
___ Ringing in ears

___ Dentures
___ Major dental work
___ Difficulty eating

___ Varicose veins
___ Muscle cramps
___ Joint or muscle pain

___ Psychiatric or psychological care

___ Fractures (broken bones)
Where?______________________
___ Problem requiring orthopedic shoes
___ Hip or ankle problem
___ Unusual illness as child

Please check if you have ever been in a motor vehicle accident ______

Figure 4.1—cont'd

Patient self-administered health questionnaires have been shown to be generally accurate.[7] It is important for the therapist to review and clarify the information with the patient. Sometimes important medical background and medication data are inadvertently forgotten as the patient focuses on current problems. Verbally reviewing the information with the patient may jog his or her memory. The validity of red flags has been taken at face value in the medical community for several decades. Recent research has determined that despite the widespread endorsement of red flag checklists for patients with low back pain, there is limited evidence for most items.[8] For example, previous history of malignancy increases the likelihood of spinal malignancy, while older age, prolonged corticosteroid use, severe trauma, and presence of a contusion or abrasion increases the likelihood of spinal fracture.[8] Coordinated efforts in recent years to create more evidence-based red flag screening tools are promising and may result in more accurate identification of patients with serious pathology.[9]

Other Questionnaires

A good practice that allows the therapist to establish the extent of impairments at baseline is the use of condition- or body region–specific questionnaires. These questionnaires are time-efficient, as they can be completed by the patient and reviewed by the therapist prior to patient interview. They also provide valuable information regarding the tasks that the patient has difficulty with and can serve as excellent tools to measure progress considering that the psychometric properties (e.g., minimal detectable change) of many of these questionnaires have been investigated. Examples of such questionnaires include:

- Western Ontario and McMaster Universities Osteoarthritis Index (WOMAC) for knee and hip osteoarthritis (www.physio-pedia.com/WOMAC_Osteoarthritis_Index)
- Neck Disability Index (NDI) for neck pain (www.physio-pedia.com/Neck_Disability_Index)
- Oswestry Disability Index for low back pain (https://en.wikipedia.org/wiki/Oswestry_Disability_Index)
- Disabilities of the Arm, Shoulder and Hand questionnaire (DASH) for upper extremity disorders (www.physio-pedia.com/DASH_Outcome_Measure)
- Knee injury and Osteoarthritis Outcome Score (www.koos.nu/)
- Fear-Avoidance Beliefs Questionnaire (FABQ) (www.physio-pedia.com/Fear%E2%80%90Avoidance_Belief_Questionnaire)
- Tampa Scale of Kinesiophobia (TSK) (www.novopsych.com/tsk-2.html)

Clinicians are strongly encouraged to identify appropriate questionnaires for their patient population and routinely use them at the initial examination and during reexamination sessions. The location, intensity, and quality of pain are frequently assessed with a body diagram that is completed by the patient (Fig. 4.2). The McGill Pain Questionnaire[10] can clarify symptoms further (Fig. 4.3).

Initial Observation

Frequently, the therapist will meet patients in the waiting area and escort them to the treatment room. There are two primary goals that are important to achieve during the initial observation. The first goal is to introduce yourself to the patients and make a good first impression. Be polite and courteous and establish rapport. Let the patients know that you are available to them and that they have your attention. The second goal is to observe them in an unobtrusive manner as they move. Note the quality of motion as they rise from the chair and walk. Observe their facial expression for signs of pain or discomfort.

Patient Interview

After reviewing the information gained from medical records, other health care providers, and the patient-completed questionnaires, the therapist is ready to begin the patient interview. It is important to listen carefully and allow the patient enough time to provide relevant details. Quite frequently, the most likely diagnoses will emerge from a thorough history taking. Ideally, the patient interview should be conducted in a quiet, well-lit room that offers a measure of privacy. To encourage good communication, the therapist and patient should be at a similar eye level, facing each other, with a comfortable space between them of about 3 feet (1 m). The patient should have the therapist's undivided attention; telephone calls and other interruptions should be avoided. The therapist may wish to have paper and pen

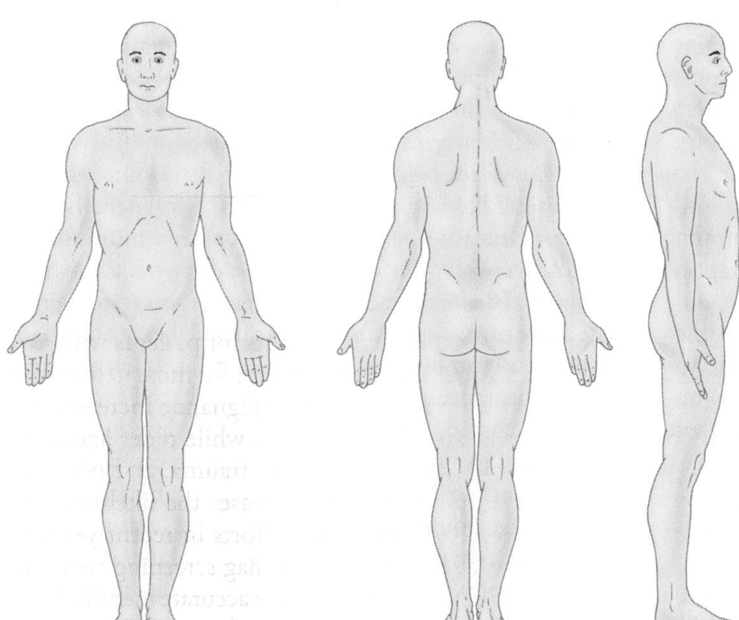

Figure 4.2 This body chart can supplement the patient's verbal description of the location of the pain.

Look carefully at the twenty groups of words. If any word in any group applies to *your* pain, please circle that word – but do not circle more than *one word in any one group* – so you must choose the *most suitable word* in that group.

In groups that do not apply to your pain, there is no need to circle *any* word – just leave them as they are.

Group 1	*Group 2*	*Group 3*	*Group 4*	*Group 5*
Flickering Quivering Pulsing Throbbing Beating Pounding	Jumping Flashing Shooting	Pricking Boring Drilling Stabbing Lancinating	Sharp Gritting Lacerating	Pinching Pressing Gnawing Cramping Crushing
Group 6	*Group 7*	*Group 8*	*Group 9*	*Group 10*
Tugging Pulling Wrenching	Hot Burning Scalding Searing	Tingling Itching Smarting Stinging	Dull Sore Hurting Aching Heavy	Tender Taut Rasping Splitting
Group 11	*Group 12*	*Group 13*	*Group 14*	*Group 15*
Tiring Exhausting	Sickening Suffocating	Fearful Frightful Terrifying	Punishing Gruelling Cruel Vicious Killing	Wretched Blinding
Group 16	*Group 17*	*Group 18*	*Group 19*	*Group 20*
Annoying Troublesome Miserable Intense Unbearable	Spreading Radiating Penetrating Piercing	Tight Numb Drawing Squeezing Tearing	Cool Cold Freezing	Nagging Nauseating Agonizing Dreadful Torturing

Figure 4.3 The McGill Pain Questionnaire. The first 10 groups of words are somatic (describing what the pain feels like), 11–15 are affective, 16 is evaluative, and 17–20 miscellaneous. *(From Melzack[10].)*

or tablet available to record particular dates and information that is easily forgotten, but the interview should flow as an active conversation, not a dictation session. If the therapist uses an electronic device to document the interview, this should be explained to the patient in advance to avoid misunderstandings. Repeated practice greatly improves the therapist's ability to listen, direct the interview, and establish a positive working relationship with the patient. Several physical therapy education programs provide students with the opportunity to interview standardized patients, which helps them develop interview skills.

Over the course of the interview, the therapist gains information about the patient's current complaints, including onset, location, type and behavior of symptoms, current medications, previous treatments, secondary medical problems, medical history, and goals for the physical therapy episode of care. The patient's age and sex should be noted; some conditions are more common in particular demographics. Often, detailed information about a patient's occupation, recreational activities, and social/living situation are required to understand the cause of the impairments and activity limitations and to develop a relevant plan of care (POC) that focuses on the patient's goals. Open-ended, objective questions that do not promote biased answers should be used. For example, instead of asking "Is your right knee painful?" the therapist should ask, "Where are your symptoms located?"

The therapist should carefully guide the interview to keep it focused on pertinent information and conclude in a timely manner. All questions should use conversational language rather than medical terminology so the patient easily understands the questions. The therapist should ask one question at a time and obtain a response before proceeding to other questions. Follow-up inquiries may be needed to clarify initial answers. It is important for the therapist to keep an open mind during the interview and not rush to conclusions about the patient's symptoms and diagnosis. The therapist should keep in mind that one of the goals of the assessment is to decide whether the pathology falls within the scope of physical therapy practice. In this respect, the therapist should carefully explore the possibility of red flags that may require urgent surgical or medical treatment or referral to a different health care practitioner.

The following sequence is suggested as a way of organizing the interview. Similar information on general patient interviewing can be found in other texts.[3,4] The interview should begin with a general question such as "What brings you to physical therapy today?" or "What seems to be the problem?" If the patient is hospitalized, the question may need to be rephrased to avoid having the patient retell the medical history to every health care provider. "I see from your medical chart that you fractured your hip and underwent a surgical repair yesterday. Is that what happened?" The patient should be given the opportunity to present the story. The therapist should ask follow-up questions to differentiate between pain and loss of function, identify the first occurrence of the symptoms (even if it was several years ago), get a detailed account of the mechanism of injury (if relevant), understand the change in symptoms over time and their behavior during the day, identify factors that alleviate or aggravate the symptoms, and establish the type and effectiveness of previous treatments. In the conclusion of this phase of the interview, it is important to understand the goals that your patient has from physical therapy. This will provide some initial information that should be used at the end of the assessment to discuss and determine mutually agreed upon goals and expected outcomes. The therapist should not presume to know what issues are important to the patient. Answers to these questions help the therapist to determine whether the patient has realistic expectations or will need further patient education concerning his or her condition and typical recovery. For example, an elderly patient who is hospitalized after a fractured hip may expect to remain in the acute care hospital for 2 weeks before being able to independently ambulate and resume self-care. Given current health insurance practices, more realistic goals may need to be discussed, such as discharge from the hospital in 3 or 4 days to a rehabilitation or extended care facility for further nursing care, physical and occupational therapy, or discharge home with home health aides, visiting nurses, and home care physical and occupational therapists.

Finally, it is a good habit for the therapist to conclude the interview by asking the patients if they have something else to add and allow enough time for a response. The information elicited with the questions discussed above may be supplemented with additional questions based on the specific region of the body being examined and suspected etiologies. The physical therapist's knowledge of anatomy, kinesiology, pathokinesiology, physiology, and pathophysiology, as well as the physical presentation and progression of musculoskeletal conditions, provide the appropriate background on which to base and develop patient interview questions.

Medications

The type, frequency, dose, and effect of medications the patient is taking should be noted. The use of analgesic or anti-inflammatory medications may reduce the intensity of symptoms at the time of the examination. Changes in the use of these medications may make it difficult to determine the effects of physical therapy treatment. The secondary effects of some medications may necessitate the modification of examination and treatment techniques. For example, prolonged use of corticosteroids is associated with *osteopenia* (reduced bone mass) and reduced tensile strength of ligaments. The therapist may need to limit manual force applied through the lever of long bones to prevent fracture or ligament tear. The use of anticoagulants may make the patient susceptible to contusions and *hemarthrosis* and require close monitoring for bruising and joint swelling. The amount of force used in exercise and manual therapies may need to be reduced. Medications that affect balance and motor coordination may make the prescription of certain exercises risky. Therapists should investigate the potential side effects of medications that patients are using and make appropriate modifications to the POC. Finally, patients are frequently asking therapists about whether they should use certain medications. Therapists are encouraged to obtain a thorough understanding of the physical therapy practice act within their state and ensure that they stay within its limits when they answer questions regarding medications.

Social History and Occupational, Recreational, and Functional Status

Questions in this area might include the following: "What type of work do you do in and outside of the home? How has this problem affected your ability to perform your job? Care for your children? Play golf? Dress? Bathe?" Certain occupational and recreational activities may contribute to the problem or interfere with recovery. Strategies such as joint preservation techniques and use of assistive devices may need to be considered to allow performance of necessary tasks. Medical insurance companies often make treatment reimbursement decisions based on a patient's functional status as related to the medical problem. In addition to the questionnaires that have been presented earlier and that can provide important information on the type of functional activities patients are having difficulty performing, there are specific questionnaires that assess health-related quality of life, such as the Medical Outcomes Study Short Form 36 (SF-36) (www.rehabmeasures@sralab.org) and Short Form 12 (SF12). See Chapter 8, Examination of Function, for additional information.

"Do you have to climb stairs to get into your house? To reach the bedroom? Bathroom?" Characteristics of the home environment may determine whether a patient who uses an ambulatory assistive device requires instruction in stair activities before returning home. The condition of floors, size of halls and doorways, placement of furniture, and ease of use of the bathroom will need to be considered for a patient using a wheelchair. A more detailed discussion of examination of the environment including the home, workplace, and community can be found in Chapter 9, Examination of the Environment.

"Do you live alone?" It is helpful to understand the patient's living situation to determine if others are available to assist with exercise programs, ambulation, and transfer activities. Some patients have responsibility for the care of children, elderly parents, or a disabled spouse or sibling. These responsibilities may need to be restructured to allow time for rest and recovery.

"Do you use tobacco products? Alcohol? Recreational drugs?" Cigarette smoking has been associated with decreased bone density, delayed bone healing after fractures, greater spinal disk degeneration, increased low back pain, and increased upper extremity (UE) and lower extremity (LE) musculoskeletal disorders. Use of alcohol and recreational drugs can lead to risk-taking behaviors resulting in increased incidence of injuries or difficulty in safely performing functional activities and home exercise programs (HEPs). Therapists may wish to advise a patient to reduce the use of these substances and refer him or her to the appropriate social services or self-help organizations for counseling.

Systems Review

Depending on the previous medical history and findings of the interview, the therapist may decide to selectively review certain systems. It is impractical to perform a thorough systems review on every patient. However, in patients who have a history of heart disease or symptoms that may be consistent with cardiovascular pathology, it would be wise to perform a review of the cardiovascular system. This would include assessment of heart rate, blood pressure, respiratory rate, and edema. Patients who are getting out of bed for the first time following recent surgery or prolonged bedrest should routinely have vital signs taken to establish baseline values before movement. The therapist may decide to assess body temperature if infection is suspected or inspect the integumentary system for systemic disorders. *Cyanosis* (a blue discoloration of the skin) in the hands and feet may indicate serious pathology of the cardiopulmonary system. *Clubbing,* in which the distal finger and nail become rounded (bulbous), is believed to be caused by chronic hypoxemia and is typically associated with cardiovascular and respiratory diseases or neurovascular abnormalities.[11] Yellow skin tone may be due to increased carotene intake or liver disease. Brown, highly pigmented, hairy areas sometimes overlay bony defects such as spina bifida. Open wounds should be measured and diagrammed in patient records. New scars will be red, and older scars will be white in color. Skin tissue thickenings such as *calluses* can indicate chronic overloading and stress. Thin, glossy skin with decreased elasticity and hair loss is often found with peripheral nerve lesions or neurovascular disorders.

Communication and cognitive ability such as orientation to person, place, and time, as well as general arousal state is assessed during the interview. If deficits in these areas are present, the examination may need to be modified to gain accurate information. The use of simple words, concise instructions, and task demonstrations may be helpful. Distractions in the environment should be kept to a minimum. Communication difficulties may be overcome through the use of foreign language interpreters, gestures, drawings, and language boards. Changes in medications, upright positioning, and access to natural light via windows and skylights may improve patient arousal and orientation to time. Depending on the type of deficit, the patient may benefit from an evaluation by a neurologist, neuropsychologist, speech-language pathologist, and/or occupational therapist. Detailed information for assessing other systems is provided elsewhere in this textbook. However, it is crucial for the physical therapist to consider whether a systems review is indicated and decide at this stage whether it is appropriate to proceed with further examination or refer the patient to the physician.

Screening Examination

The musculoskeletal physical therapist will frequently encounter patients who report symptoms that could be arising from different body regions. For example, patients who report neck and upper extremity symptoms may have pathology in the neck, in the upper extremity, or in both regions. A screening examination (similar to the systems review) is situation-dependent and assesses gross range of motion (ROM) and strength. For example if cervical ROM is full, symmetrical, and painless, it is unlikely that the neck is the source of the symptoms. If, on the other hand, cervical motion causes change in peripheral symptoms, a more thorough cervical examination is required. In summary, the musculoskeletal screening examination allows the therapist to identify the region that requires a more detailed investigation.

Scanning Examination

A scanning examination is used when the therapist suspects that the patient may experience symptom referral due to radiculopathy or other similar neurological pathology. There are two scanning exams, one for the upper quadrant and one for the lower quadrant. The scanning examination should not take more than a few minutes to perform, and its findings frequently allow the therapist to determine the source of the pathology (e.g., radiculopathy, peripheral neuropathy, contractile tissue pathology). The scanning exam consists of strength, sensation, and reflex testing. A detailed knowledge of myotomes and dermatomes is required to identify the spinal level that causes the symptoms (Fig. 4.4); however, the clinician is cautioned that there are large variations in dermatomal maps in different textbooks. Considering that many dermatomal maps that are currently in use were created in the late 19th and early 20th centuries and utilize different methodologies, it is important to understand that the exact dermatomal distribution is currently under debate.[12]

Observation/Inspection

Observation begins with the therapist's first contact with the patient, whether at bedside in the case of hospitalized patients, or in the waiting room for outpatients. The patient's general posture and ability to perform functional activities—change bed position, transfer from sitting to standing, ambulate to the examining room—provides information about the severity of symptoms, willingness to move, available ROM, and muscle strength. This information, although preliminary, helps to focus and individualize the physical examination. For example, a patient with a shoulder disorder who uses the UE to push off from a chair during transfers, stands with level bilateral shoulder height, and has an alternating arm swing during gait would be expected to have milder symptoms, tolerate a more extensive examination, and have greater mobility and muscle strength than a patient who stands with an elevated scapula and protectively cradles the UE during transfers and gait. If functional difficulties and gait abnormalities were noted, detailed functional status and gait examinations would be performed later.

To perform the physical examination and inspect specific areas of the body, the patient must be suitably dressed. Observation of the shoulders, elbows, or spine will require males to remove their shirt and females to wear only a bra or loose hospital gown that can be draped to expose the UE and back. To observe the LEs, patients should undress from the waist down, wearing only undergarments or shorts.

Once the patient is in the privacy of an examining room and appropriately disrobed, the therapist begins a careful inspection of the body region implicated in the interview and the biomechanically related areas. The therapist should be aware of the limitations of the naked human eye in identifying postural problems; even experienced therapists commonly disagree on whether asymmetries are present. One way to standardize the postural assessment is by consistently using the dominant eye to assess posture. To find out which eye is your dominant eye, hold your palms away from you, creating a "frame"

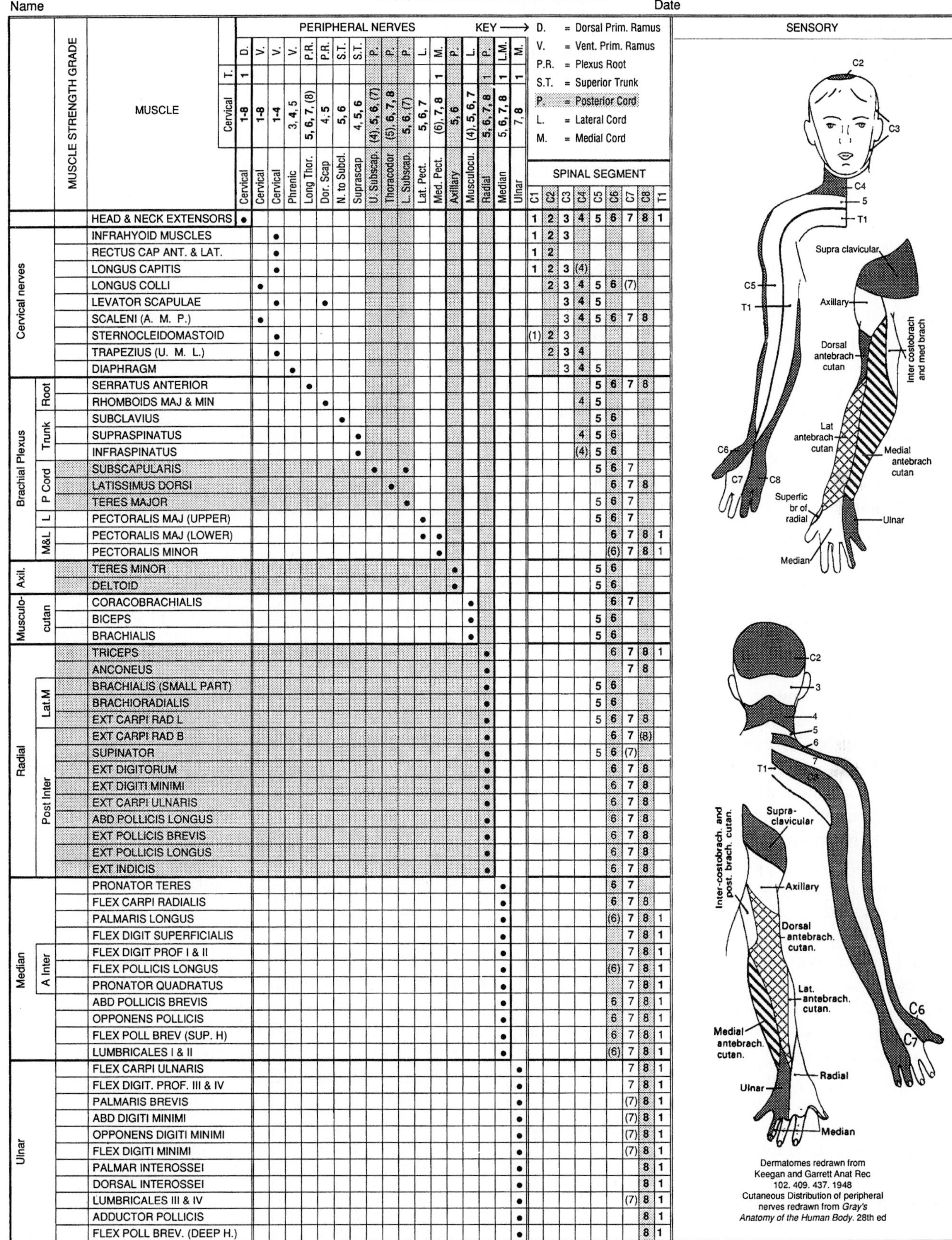

SPINAL NERVE AND MUSCLE CHART

NECK, DIAPHRAGM AND UPPER EXTREMITY

Name Date

KEY → D. = Dorsal Prim. Ramus; V. = Vent. Prim. Ramus; P.R. = Plexus Root; S.T. = Superior Trunk; P. = Posterior Cord; L. = Lateral Cord; M. = Medial Cord

PERIPHERAL NERVES

Group	Muscle	Muscle Strength Grade	Cervical (D. Cervical 1-8, T. 1)	Cervical (V. 1-8)	Cervical (V. 1-4)	Phrenic (V. 3, 4, 5)	Long Thor. (P.R. 5, 6, 7, (8))	Dor. Scap (P.R. 4, 5)	N. to Subcl. (S.T. 5, 6)	Suprascap (S.T. 4, 5, 6)	U. Subscap. (P. (4), 5, 6, (7))	Thoracodor (P. (5), 6, 7, 8)	L. Subscap. (P. 5, 6, (7))	Lat. Pect. (L. 5, 6, 7)	Med. Pect. (M. (6), 7, 8, T. 1)	Axillary (P. 5, 6)	Musculocu. (L. (4), 5, 6, 7)	Radial (P. 5, 6, 7, 8, T. 1)	Median (L.M. 5, 6, 7, 8, T. 1)	Ulnar (M. 7, 8, T. 1)
	HEAD & NECK EXTENSORS		●																	
Cervical nerves	INFRAHYOID MUSCLES				●															
	RECTUS CAP ANT. & LAT.				●															
	LONGUS CAPITIS				●															
	LONGUS COLLI			●																
	LEVATOR SCAPULAE				●			●												
	SCALENI (A. M. P.)			●																
	STERNOCLEIDOMASTOID				●															
	TRAPEZIUS (U. M. L.)				●															
	DIAPHRAGM					●														
Brachial Plexus – Root	SERRATUS ANTERIOR						●													
	RHOMBOIDS MAJ & MIN							●												
Brachial Plexus – Trunk	SUBCLAVIUS								●											
	SUPRASPINATUS									●										
	INFRASPINATUS									●										
Brachial Plexus – P Cord	SUBSCAPULARIS										●		●							
	LATISSIMUS DORSI											●								
	TERES MAJOR												●							
Brachial Plexus – L	PECTORALIS MAJ (UPPER)													●						
Brachial Plexus – M&L	PECTORALIS MAJ (LOWER)													●	●					
	PECTORALIS MINOR														●					
Axil.	TERES MINOR															●				
	DELTOID															●				
Musculo-cutan	CORACOBRACHIALIS																●			
	BICEPS																●			
	BRACHIALIS																●			
Radial	TRICEPS																	●		
	ANCONEUS																	●		
Radial – Lat.M	BRACHIALIS (SMALL PART)																	●		
	BRACHIORADIALIS																	●		
	EXT CARPI RAD L																	●		
Radial – Post Inter	EXT CARPI RAD B																	●		
	SUPINATOR																	●		
	EXT DIGITORUM																	●		
	EXT DIGITI MINIMI																	●		
	EXT CARPI ULNARIS																	●		
	ABD POLLICIS LONGUS																	●		
	EXT POLLICIS BREVIS																	●		
	EXT POLLICIS LONGUS																	●		
	EXT INDICIS																	●		
Median	PRONATOR TERES																		●	
	FLEX CARPI RADIALIS																		●	
	PALMARIS LONGUS																		●	
	FLEX DIGIT SUPERFICIALIS																		●	
Median – A Inter	FLEX DIGIT PROF I & II																		●	
	FLEX POLLICIS LONGUS																		●	
	PRONATOR QUADRATUS																		●	
Median	ABD POLLICIS BREVIS																		●	
	OPPONENS POLLICIS																		●	
	FLEX POLL BREV (SUP. H)																		●	
	LUMBRICALES I & II																		●	
Ulnar	FLEX CARPI ULNARIS																			●
	FLEX DIGIT. PROF. III & IV																			●
	PALMARIS BREVIS																			●
	ABD DIGITI MINIMI																			●
	OPPONENS DIGITI MINIMI																			●
	FLEX DIGITI MINIMI																			●
	PALMAR INTEROSSEI																			●
	DORSAL INTEROSSEI																			●
	LUMBRICALES III & IV																			●
	ADDUCTOR POLLICIS																			●
	FLEX POLL BREV. (DEEP H.)																			●

SPINAL SEGMENT

Muscle	C1	C2	C3	C4	C5	C6	C7	C8	T1
HEAD & NECK EXTENSORS	1	2	3	4	5	6	7	8	1
INFRAHYOID MUSCLES	1	2	3						
RECTUS CAP ANT. & LAT.	1	2							
LONGUS CAPITIS	1	2	3	(4)					
LONGUS COLLI		2	3	4	5	6	(7)		
LEVATOR SCAPULAE			3	4	5				
SCALENI (A. M. P.)			3	4	5	6	7	8	
STERNOCLEIDOMASTOID	(1)	2	3						
TRAPEZIUS (U. M. L.)		2	3	4					
DIAPHRAGM			3	4	5				
SERRATUS ANTERIOR					5	6	7	8	
RHOMBOIDS MAJ & MIN				4	5				
SUBCLAVIUS					5	6			
SUPRASPINATUS				4	5	6			
INFRASPINATUS				(4)	5	6			
SUBSCAPULARIS					5	6	7		
LATISSIMUS DORSI						6	7	8	
TERES MAJOR					5	6	7		
PECTORALIS MAJ (UPPER)					5	6	7		
PECTORALIS MAJ (LOWER)						6	7	8	1
PECTORALIS MINOR						(6)	7	8	1
TERES MINOR					5	6			
DELTOID					5	6			
CORACOBRACHIALIS						6	7		
BICEPS					5	6			
BRACHIALIS					5	6			
TRICEPS						6	7	8	1
ANCONEUS							7	8	
BRACHIALIS (SMALL PART)					5	6			
BRACHIORADIALIS					5	6			
EXT CARPI RAD L					5	6	7	8	
EXT CARPI RAD B						6	7	(8)	
SUPINATOR					5	6	(7)		
EXT DIGITORUM						6	7	8	
EXT DIGITI MINIMI						6	7	8	
EXT CARPI ULNARIS						6	7	8	
ABD POLLICIS LONGUS						6	7	8	
EXT POLLICIS BREVIS						6	7	8	
EXT POLLICIS LONGUS						6	7	8	
EXT INDICIS						6	7	8	
PRONATOR TERES						6	7		
FLEX CARPI RADIALIS						6	7	8	
PALMARIS LONGUS						(6)	7	8	1
FLEX DIGIT SUPERFICIALIS							7	8	1
FLEX DIGIT PROF I & II							7	8	1
FLEX POLLICIS LONGUS						(6)	7	8	1
PRONATOR QUADRATUS							7	8	1
ABD POLLICIS BREVIS						6	7	8	1
OPPONENS POLLICIS						6	7	8	1
FLEX POLL BREV (SUP. H)						6	7	8	1
LUMBRICALES I & II						(6)	7	8	1
FLEX CARPI ULNARIS							7	8	1
FLEX DIGIT. PROF. III & IV							7	8	1
PALMARIS BREVIS							(7)	8	1
ABD DIGITI MINIMI							(7)	8	1
OPPONENS DIGITI MINIMI							(7)	8	1
FLEX DIGITI MINIMI							(7)	8	1
PALMAR INTEROSSEI								8	1
DORSAL INTEROSSEI								8	1
LUMBRICALES III & IV							(7)	8	1
ADDUCTOR POLLICIS								8	1
FLEX POLL BREV. (DEEP H.)								8	1

SENSORY

Dermatomes redrawn from Keegan and Garrett Anat Rec 102. 409. 437. 1948
Cutaneous Distribution of peripheral nerves redrawn from *Gray's Anatomy of the Human Body*. 28th ed

Figure 4.4 Manual muscle testing recording forms that aid in determining the site or level of a nerve lesion. *(From Kendall et al,[43] with permission.)*

with your index fingers and thumbs. Place the frame with a focal point in the distance in its center. Close one eye. If you can still see the focal point, the eye that is open is your dominant eye (https://en.wikipedia.org/wiki/Ocular_dominance).

Another way to improve postural assessment is to use smartphones or tablets, which utilize integrated digital cameras. This may decrease the influence of some of the factors that contribute to postural assessment error and may potentially produce better measurements. Freely available software tools such as *Image J (https://imagej.nih.gov/ij/) that has been developed by the National Institutes of Health* can be used to objectively measure alignment. Finally, recent efforts to standardize postural assessment and validate it with the use of objective biomechanical tools may result in better evidence in this area.[13]

The LEs and lumbar region, being intricately involved in weight-bearing activities, should be inspected as a functional unit. Likewise, conditions involving the shoulder require the examination of the cervical and thoracic regions, and vice versa. Visual inspection should focus on bone, soft tissue structures, skin, and nails. The therapist should view the body region anteriorly, posteriorly, and laterally. Often palpation, which is discussed in the next section, is combined with observation.

Bone shafts and joints are judged against normative models for symmetry, comparing one side of the body to the other. Contour and alignment should be considered. Common causes of changes in bone contour include acute fractures, callus formation or bone angulation owing to healed fractures, congenital variations, bone hyperplasia at tendon insertions, and arthritis. Alignment differences can be due to the above conditions as well as muscle and soft tissue tightness, muscle weakness, muscle and ligament laxity, and joint dislocation.

For patients with musculoskeletal involvement, an examination for postural alignment is often indicated. From an *anterior* view, both eyes, shoulders (acromion processes), iliac crests, anterior superior iliac spines, greater trochanters of the femur, patellae, and ankle medial malleoli should be horizontally level. Waist angles should be symmetrical. Patellae and feet should face anteriorly. *Laterally,* the line of gravity should bisect the external auditory meatus, acromion process, and greater trochanter, and lie just posterior to the patella and anteriorly to the lateral malleolus (Fig. 4.5).[14]

The cervical and lumbar spine should exhibit normal lordotic curves, and the thoracic spine a normal kyphotic curve. From a *posterior* view, the earlobes, shoulders, inferior angles of the scapula, iliac crests, posterior superior iliac spines, greater trochanters, buttock and knee creases, and malleoli should be level. The spine should be straight, with the medial borders of the scapulae equidistant from the spine. Varus, valgus, and hyperextension knee deformities and pes planus/cavus should be noted. The therapist should be aware of the mixed evidence regarding the association between posture and pain/pathology and avoid the temptation to change small postural deviations that cannot be reasonably linked to patients' impairments. For example, even though increased thoracic kyphosis can restrict shoulder ROM, there is currently no evidence that it predisposes people to shoulder pain.[15] On the other hand, there is more evidence that a pronated foot posture is linked to the development of lower extremity overuse injuries.[16] Postural assessment remains an important aspect of physical therapy assessment and should be measured with objective tools when possible as one of the factors that may contribute to the development of pain.[17]

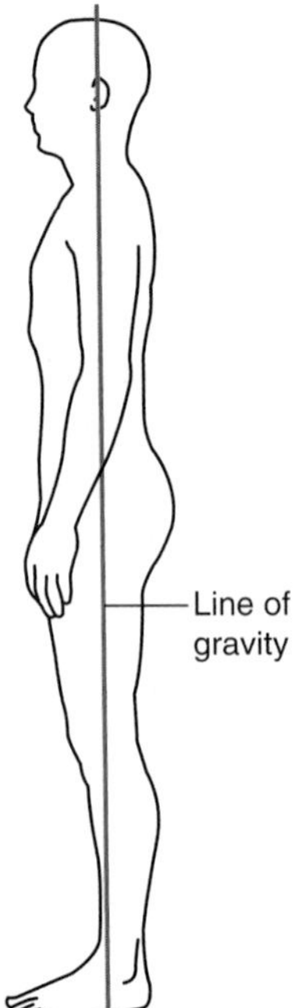

Figure 4.5 The location of the line of gravity from the lateral view. *(From Levangie and Norkin,[14] with permission.)*

The size and contour of soft tissue structures should be inspected and compared bilaterally. An increase in size may indicate soft tissue edema, joint effusion, or muscle hypertrophy. A decrease in size often indicates muscle atrophy. A loss of soft tissue continuity can suggest a muscle rupture. Cysts, rheumatoid nodules, ganglia, and gouty tophi can all change soft tissue contour.

Abnormalities noted during observation may be further documented with objective anthropometric measurements. Using a flexible plastic tape measure, limb lengths are measured between bony landmarks and compared bilaterally. For example, leg length is commonly measured from the anterior superior iliac spine to the medial malleolus. Circumferential measurements help substantiate joint effusion, edema, and muscle hypertrophy and atrophy. Typically, these measurements are taken at specified distances above or below a bony landmark so they can be reliably reproduced during subsequent measurements. For example, circumference measurements of the upper arm should be taken at noted distances distal to the acromion process or proximal to the olecranon process. If measurements are needed of the hands or feet, volumetric measurements can be taken by submerging the distal extremity in a container of water and noting the volume of water that is displaced.

Palpation

Palpation is an important physical therapy skill that can provide valuable information. It can be done after observation or later in the examination (especially if there is a risk that palpation can produce high levels of pain, which may then affect proper baseline measures for ROM or strength). Palpation requires detailed knowledge of anatomy and a systematic approach. All structures on one body surface should be systematically palpated before proceeding to another surface. For example, all structures on the patient's anterior surface should be palpated before beginning to palpate structures on the posterior surface. The uninvolved side is palpated first to acquaint the patient with the procedure and, in some cases, to serve as a normative model for comparison. The therapist should develop a system of moving from superior to inferior structures, medial to lateral, or superior and then inferior from a joint line. Which direction the therapist moves is not important, but the palpation process should be consistent and thorough.

Palpation of bone, soft tissue structures, and the skin is performed by varying the therapist's tactile pressure and using various parts of the hands. Light tactile pressure allows palpation of superficial tissues like the skin, whereas more pressure is needed to palpate deeper structures such as bone. Usually the fingertips are used for palpation, but large, deeper structures such as the greater trochanter of the femur or borders of the scapula are easier to locate using the entire surface of the hand. Rolling the skin and soft tissue between the fingertips and thumb helps the therapist judge myofascial mobility. Changes in skin temperature may be easier to detect using the posterior surface of the therapist's hand. When moving from one area to another, the therapist's hand should stay in firm contact with the skin whenever possible to prevent a tickling sensation. The fingers should not "crawl" or "walk" across the skin.

During palpation, the therapist seeks feedback from the patient to help localize painful structures. Some lesions in deep or proximal structures will refer symptoms to other body areas, but localized tenderness often helps to implicate particular structures. Localized skin temperature should be noted: cool temperatures suggest reduced circulation, whereas warmth indicates increased circulation and often inflammation. Skin and soft tissue density and extensibility should be considered. Often muscle spasms and adhesions in skin and connective tissue can be found with palpation. The quality (amplitude) of peripheral pulses will provide gross information on arterial blood supply. Bilateral edema in the ankles and legs that forms pits with tactile pressure (termed *pitting edema*) can indicate cardiac failure or liver or renal conditions. Unilateral pitting edema is typically associated with obstruction of returning circulation.

Range of Motion

Joints and their related structures are examined by performing active and passive joint motions. Joint motion is a necessary component of functional tasks. Numerous studies have identified the ROM needed in the LE during gait[18] and when climbing stairs,[19] rising from a chair,[20] and squatting, kneeling, and sitting cross-legged.[21,22] The ROM needed in the UE to eat with a spoon[23] and perform many UE activities[24] has been examined. Careful examination of joint movement for ROM, end-feel, effect on symptoms, and pattern of restriction helps identify and quantify impairments causing activity limitations and determines which structures need treatment.

Active Range of Motion

The examination of joint motion begins by testing *active range of motion* (AROM). The patient is asked to move a body part through the osteokinematic motions at the involved and other biomechanically related joints. *Osteokinematics* refers to the gross angular motions of the shafts of bones. These motions are described as occurring in the three cardinal planes of the body: flexion and extension in the sagittal plane, abduction and adduction in the frontal plane, and medial and lateral rotation in the transverse plane. For example, in an examination of the hip, the patient would be asked to move the hip into flexion, extension, abduction, adduction, and medial and lateral rotation. Often flexion and extension of the knee, as well as flexion, extension, rotation, and lateral flexion of the lumbar spine, are tested, because knee and spine motions can affect hip function. Some therapists prefer to have the patient move in functional, combined motions rather than in straight plane motions. For example, a patient would be asked to reach a hand behind the head to test shoulder abduction and medial rotation simultaneously rather than perform isolated, individual motions.

Active motion is a good musculoskeletal screening procedure to further focus the physical examination. The amount, quality, and pattern of motion, as well as the occurrence of pain and crepitus, should be noted. For purposes of musculoskeletal screening, AROM can be visually estimated to determine if motion is within functional limits; however, objective and accurate measurements are needed to establish a pathological baseline and to evaluate treatment response. In addition to goniometers, inclinometers and smartphone apps can be used in this regard, as they have excellent psychometric properties.[25,26] Normal ROM varies among individuals and is influenced by factors such as age and sex,[27] as well as measurement methods.[28] Restricted movement can be determined by comparing to the opposite, uninvolved extremity, if possible, or to normative values by age and sex.[29] Complete and painless AROM frequently suggests that further passive testing of that motion is unnecessary unless the therapist needs to assess the end-feel. If, however, the amount of active motion is less than normal, the therapist will not be able to isolate the cause without further testing. Capsule, ligament, muscle, and soft tissue tightness; joint surface abnormalities; and muscle weakness are all capable of causing limitations in AROM. Pain during AROM may be due to the contracting, stretching, or pinching of contractile tissues such as muscles, tendons, and their attachments to bone, or it may be due to the stretching or pinching of non-contractile tissues such as ligaments, joint capsules, and bursa. Variations in the quality and pattern of active motion can result from central and peripheral nervous system disorders and metabolic conditions, in addition to disorders involving musculoskeletal structures. So, although active motion is an effective screening procedure, positive findings require further tests to identify the underlying etiology and thus enable effective treatment.

Passive Range of Motion

Passive motions are movements performed by the therapist without the assistance of the patient. The term *passive range of motion* (PROM) typically refers to the amount of osteokinematic motion available when the patient's joint is moved without the patient's assistance. Normally, PROM is slightly greater than AROM because joints have a small amount of motion at the end of the range that is not under voluntary control. PROM is examined not only for amount of motion, but also for the motion's effect on symptoms, the type of tissue resistance felt by the therapist at the end of the motion (end-feel), and the pattern of limitation.

Passive range of osteokinematic motions depends on the integrity of joint surfaces and the extensibility of the joint capsule, ligaments, muscles, tendons, and soft tissue. Limitations in PROM may be due to bone or joint abnormalities or shortening of soft tissue structures. Because the therapist provides the muscle force needed to perform PROM, rather than the patient, PROM (unlike AROM) does not depend on the patient's muscle strength and coordination.

Pain during PROM is often due to moving, lengthening, or pinching of non-contractile structures. Pain occurring at the end of PROM may be due to lengthening contractile structures and non-contractile structures. Pain during PROM is not due to the active shortening (contracting) of muscle and the resulting pull on tendon and bone attachments. By comparing active and passive motions that cause pain, and noting the location of the pain, the therapist gains important information about which injured tissues are involved.

For example, on examination, a patient is found to have limited and painful active knee flexion. This pain and limitation may be coming from the contraction of the hamstring muscles, the lengthening of the quadriceps muscle, and the approximation of the tibiofemoral and patellofemoral joint surfaces, menisci, joint capsule, ligaments, or bursae. If the symptoms are eliminated during PROM, the hamstring muscles are likely the source of the symptoms (as they do not contract during PROM). The performance of resisted isometric knee flexion would be used to confirm the presence of a lesion in the hamstring muscles.

Both the beginning and the end of the motion are measured to identify the "range" of movement and are recorded using both the start and end values (e.g., 0° to 110°). Using the most common notation system, the 0° to 180° system, all motions except rotation begin in anatomical position at 0° and progress toward 180°. For example, a motion that begins at 0° and ends at 135° would be recorded as 0°–135°. A ROM that does not start with 0° or ends prematurely indicates joint *hypomobility*. Joint *hypermobility* at the beginning of the range is noted by the inclusion of a zero (the normal starting position) between the starting and ending measurements. For example, if the elbow joint has 5° of hypermobility in extension and 140° of flexion, it would be recorded as 5°–0°–140°. Hypermobility at the end of the ROM is denoted by an ending value higher than normal. Measurement results are incorporated into narrative reports or recorded on specialized forms. Specialized ROM recording forms typically have joints and motions listed centrally, with multiple columns on the left and right sides to record the date, examiner's initials, and ROM values of serial measurements (Fig. 4.6). These forms readily allow comparison of serial measurements to assess patient progress.

A systematic review of the reliability of PROM of the UE found 22 relevant studies of usually poor methodological quality. Using an instrument (goniometer or inclinometer) to measure PROM demonstrated higher reliability than eyeballing. Most studies reported acceptable reliability when an inclinometer or a goniometer were used.[30] Lower reliability was found for the LE; however, knee flexion demonstrated acceptable reliability more consistently than other directions of motion.[31] In an often cited study, Boone et al found the average standard deviation between measurements made on the same subjects by different testers to be 4.2° for UE motions and 5.2° for LE motions.[32] These issues with reliability have been attributed to difficulties in measuring complex versus simple hinged joints, in palpating bony landmarks, and in moving heavy body parts.[32] The use of standardized positions, stabilization of the body part proximal to the joint being tested, use of bony landmarks to align the goniometer, and repeated testing conducted by the same therapist (rather than multiple therapists) all help to improve the validity and reliability of goniometric measurements.[33]

End-Feel

The end of each motion at each joint is limited from further movement by particular anatomical structures. The type of structure that limits a joint motion has a

Range of Motion—Lower Extremity

Patient's Name ______________________________ Date of Birth ____________

Left				Right		
			Date			
			Examiner's Initials			
			Hip			
			Flexion			
			Extension			
			Abduction			
			Medial Rotation			
			Lateral Rotation			
			Knee			
			Flexion			
			Ankle			
			Dorsiflexion			
			Plantarflexion			
			Inversion—Tarsal			
			Eversion—Tarsal			
			Inversion—Subtalar			
			Eversion—Subtalar			
			Inversion—Midtarsal			
			Eversion—Midtarsal			
			Great Toe			
			MTP Flexion			
			MTP Extension			
			MTP Abduction			
			IP Flexion			
			Toe			
			MTP Flexion			
			MTP Extension			
			MTP Abduction			
			PIP Flexion			
			DIP Flexion			
			DIP Extension			
			Comments:			

Figure 4.6 Range of motion recording form for the lower extremity. The multiple columns on either side of the centrally listed joints and motions are used to record the date, examiner's initials, and ROM values from serial measurements. *(From Norkin and White,[29] with permission.)*

characteristic feel, which may be detected by the therapist performing the passive ROM. This feeling, which is experienced by the therapist as resistance, or a barrier to further motion, is called the *end-feel.* Cyriax and Cyriax,[34] Kaltenborn,[35] and Paris[36] have described a variety of normal (physiological) and abnormal (pathological) end-feels. Normal end-feels are generally described as *hard* (bony), *soft* (soft tissue approximation), *elastic* (elongation of musculotendinous structures), or *capsular* (elongation of capsule or ligaments). Elbow extension that is limited by the contact between the olecranon and the olecranon fossa is an example of a bony end-feel; elbow flexion that is limited by the contact between the biceps and anterior forearm soft tissues is an example of a soft end-feel; hip flexion with the knee straight that is limited by the elongation of the hamstrings is an example of an elastic end-feel; and wrist flexion that is limited by the elongation of the dorsal capsule and ligaments is an example of a capsular end-feel.

End-feels are considered to be abnormal when they occur sooner or later in the ROM than is typical, or if they are not the type of end-feel that is normally found for that joint motion. Abnormal end-feels have been associated with more pain than normal end-feels.[37] Abnormal, pathological end-feels can be categorized as variations of soft, firm, and hard end-feels. For example, assuming a motion that has a normal capsular end-feel, the presence of a soft, boggy end-feel may indicate edema while a hard end-feel may indicate a loose intra-articular body fragment. An abnormal end-feel is the *empty end-feel.* This term describes the inability of the therapist to detect any anatomical barrier to the end of the ROM. Rather, the patient through verbal or nonverbal cues indicates that no further motion should occur, usually because of pain.

The ability to determine the type of end-feel is important in helping the therapist identify the limiting structures and choose a focused and effective treatment. Developing this ability takes practice and sensitivity. PROM, particularly toward the end of the motion, must be performed slowly and carefully. Secure stabilization of the bone proximal to the joint being tested is critical in preventing multiple joints and structures from moving and interfering with determination of the end-feel.[38, 39]

Capsular and Non-Capsular Patterns of Restricted Motion

Cyriax and Cyriax[34] initially described characteristic patterns of restricted joint ROM due to diffuse, intra-articular inflammation involving the entire joint capsule. These patterns of restricted motion, which usually involve multiple motions at a joint, are called *capsular patterns* and are typically associated with osteoarthritis. The restrictions do not involve the loss of a fixed number of degrees, but rather the loss of a proportion of one motion relative to another. Capsular patterns vary from joint to joint. Table 4.1 presents common capsular patterns. Although therapists have been using capsular patterns in clinical decision making for many years, research demonstrates that the patterns of ROM restriction in the presence of osteoarthritis are complex and difficult to summarize.[40] Restricted

Table 4.1 Capsular Patterns of Extremity Joints

Joint	Capsular Pattern
Shoulder (Glenohumeral Joint)	Maximum loss of external rotation Moderate loss of abduction Minimum loss of internal rotation
Elbow Complex	Flexion loss is greater than extension loss
Forearm	Equally restricted in pronation and supination
Wrist	Equal restrictions in flexion and extension
Carpometacarpal Joint I *Carpometacarpal Joints II–V*	Abduction and extension restriction Equally restricted in all directions
Finger Interphalangeal	Flexion loss is greater than extension loss
Hip	Maximum loss of internal rotation, flexion, abduction Minimal loss of extension
Knee (Tibiofemoral Joint)	Flexion loss is greater than extension loss
Ankle (Talocrural Joint)	Plantarflexion loss is greater than extension loss
Subtalar Joint	Restricted varus motion
Midtarsal Joint	Restricted dorsiflexion, plantarflexion, abduction, and medial rotation
Metatarsophalangeal Joint I *Metatarsophalangeal Joints II–V* *Interphalangeal Joints*	Extension loss is greater than flexion Variable, tend toward flexion restriction Tend toward extension restriction

Capsular patterns are from Cyriax and Cyriax[34] and Kaltenborn.[40]

passive ROM that is not proportioned similarly to a capsular pattern is called a *non-capsular pattern* of restricted motion.[34] Non-capsular patterns are caused by conditions involving structures other than the entire joint capsule. For example, shortness of the iliopsoas muscle will result in the non-capsular pattern of limited passive hip extension; the passive range of other hip motions will not be affected. This is in contrast to the capsular pattern of the hip caused by diffuse joint effusion or capsular fibrosis, in which there is loss of passive internal rotation, flexion, and abduction.

The sole recognition of a capsular or non-capsular pattern is not enough to direct appropriate treatment. Information gained from the patient history, observation, palpation, active and passive ROM, end-feels, resisted isometric muscle tests, joint mobility tests, and special tests must be integrated to determine the most likely cause of the symptoms.

Accessory Joint Motions

If passive ROM is found to be limited or painful, an examination of arthrokinematic motions in indicated. *Arthrokinematics* refers to the motion of joint surfaces. These motions, often called *accessory* or *joint play motions,* are used to determine joint mobility and integrity. Accessory joint motions are typically described as glides (or slides), spins, and rolls. A *glide* (*slide*) is a linear motion of one surface sliding over another (Fig. 4.7). A *roll* is a rotary motion similar to the bottom of a rocking chair rolling over the floor or a tire rolling over a road (Fig. 4.8). A *spin* is a rotary motion around a fixed point or axis (Fig. 4.9).

Accessory motions usually occur in combination with each other and result in angular movement of the bone shaft, or osteokinematic motion. Kaltenborn[35] refers to the combination of translatory glide and the rotary motion of rolling as *roll-gliding*. The combination of a roll and glide allows for increased ROM by recentering the moving surface on the stable surface. The direction of the rolling and gliding components of roll-gliding depends on whether a concave or convex joint surface is moving. If a concave joint surface is moving, the gliding component occurs in the same direction as the rolling or angular movement of the bone's shaft (Fig. 4.10). For example, during flexion of the knee with the femur fixed, the shaft of the tibia rolls posteriorly while the tibia's joint surface (concave) also glides posteriorly. If a convex joint surface is moving, the gliding component occurs in the direction opposite to the rolling or angular movement of the bone's shaft. For example, during abduction

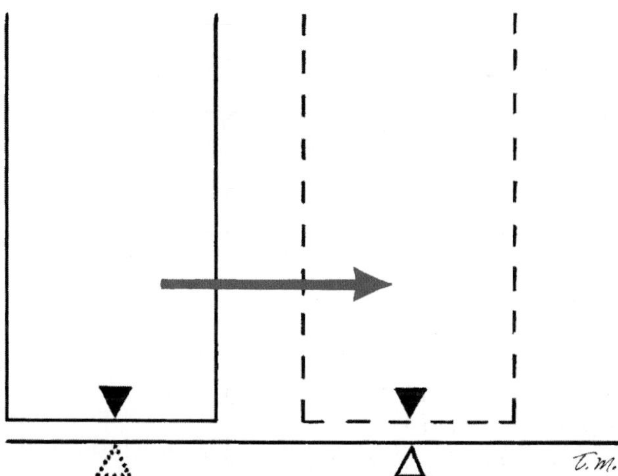

Figure 4.7 A glide (slide) is a type of linear accessory joint motion in which points on a moving joint surface comes in contact with new points on the opposing joint surface. *(From Norkin and White,[29] with permission.)*

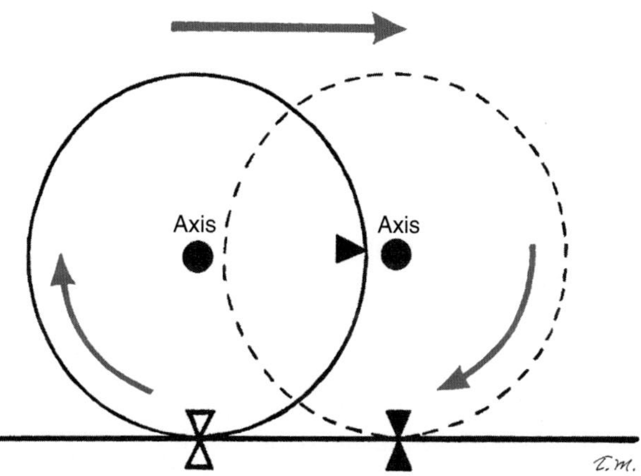

Figure 4.8 During a roll, new points on the moving joint surface come in contact with new points on the opposing surface. The axis of rotation also moves, in this case to the right. *(From Norkin and White,[29] with permission.)*

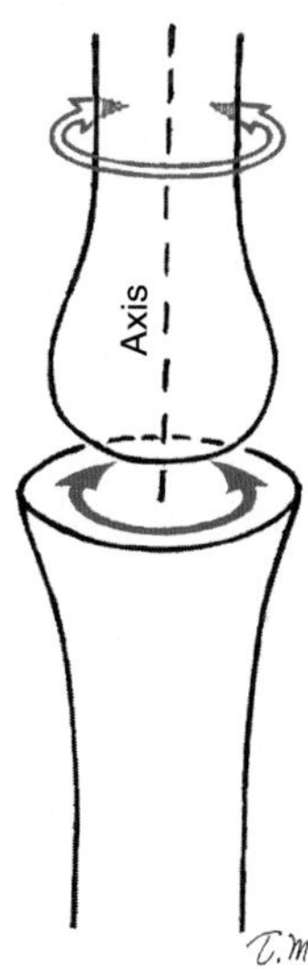

Figure 4.9 A spin is an accessory joint motion in which all the points on the moving surface rotate around a fixed axis. *(From Norkin and White,[29] with permission.)*

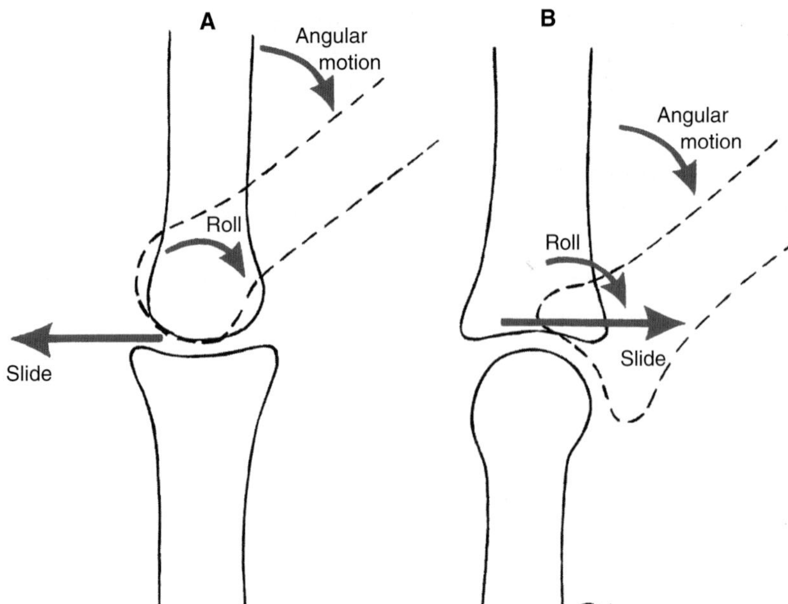

Figure 4.10 Diagrammatic representation of the concave-convex rule. (A) If the joint surface of the moving bone is convex, gliding is in the opposite direction of the angular movement of the bone. (B) If the joint surface of the moving bone is concave, gliding is in the same direction as the angular movement of the bone. *(From Norkin and White,[29] with permission.)*

of the glenohumeral joint, the shaft and humeral head (convex) roll cranially, while the contacting articular surface of the humeral head glides caudally. In the human body, roll-gliding is by far the most frequently occurring arthrokinematic motion, although there are several instances of pure spin motions. An example of a spin joint motion would be supination and pronation of the radius at the humeroradial joint.

Normal arthrokinematic (accessory) motions are necessary for full and symptom-free osteokinematic motions. The careful examination of accessory motions helps to more specifically locate and treat the source of impaired osteokinematic motions. The patient cannot perform accessory motions actively because these motions are not under voluntary control. Rather, the therapist tests them passively. The accessory motions most commonly tested are translatory: glides that are parallel to the joint surfaces, and *distractions* and *compressions* that are perpendicular to the joint surfaces. Kaltenborn,[35] and Hertling and Kessler[4] describe specific testing and treatment techniques that focus on accessory motions—usually under the topic of *joint mobilization.* Careful attention must be given to general patient positioning, specific joint positioning, relaxation of surrounding muscles, stabilization of one joint surface, and mobilization of the other joint surface.

Accessory joint motions are examined for amount of motion, effect on symptoms, and end-feel. The ranges of accessory motions are very small and cannot be measured with goniometers or standard rulers. Rather, they are typically compared to the same motion on the contralateral side of the patient's body, or compared to the therapist's past experience in testing people of similar age and sex as the patient. The testing accessory motions put stress on specific anatomical structures. A change in symptoms during the performance of an accessory motion helps to implicate particular structures. Distraction stresses the entire joint capsule and numerous ligaments surrounding and supporting the joint. Glides stress a specific part of the joint capsule and particular ligaments, depending on the direction of the glide and joint. Compression applies force to intracapsular structures such as meniscus, bone, cartilage, and projections of the synovial lining of the joint capsule into the joint space. Accessory motions are of such a small magnitude that they do not stress surrounding muscles. Angular changes in joint position that typically occur during osteokinematic ROM movements more effectively change the length of muscle tissue. Normal and abnormal end-feels noted during passive accessory motions are characterized as soft, firm, and hard. Similar to end-feels noted during passive osteokinematic motions, they help determine the limiting structures and guide treatment planning. As with other manual assessment techniques, the clinician is cautioned against overreliance on their findings due to questionable reliability.[41]

Muscle Performance

Muscle performance is the ability of a muscle to do work in terms of strength, power, and endurance. *Muscle strength,* as described in the *Guide to Physical Therapist Practice 3.0,*[5] is the force exerted by a muscle or group of muscles to overcome a resistance in one maximal effort. Clinical methods of determining muscle strength include manual muscle testing (MMT), handheld dynamometry, and isokinetic dynamometry. Depending on the patient, other characteristics related to muscle performance may also be tested. *Muscle power* is work produced per unit of time, or the product of strength and speed. *Muscle endurance* is the ability of the muscle to contract repeatedly over time. In addition to these quantitative measures, the patient's qualitative response in terms of changes in pain during resisted isometric testing is important in identifying musculotendinous lesions.

Resisted Isometric Testing

When a lesion in contractile tissues such as muscle or tendons and their insertions into bone, resisted isometric testing can be used to further clarify which type of tissue, contractile or inert, is involved. *Increased pain* during a resisted isometric contraction, caused by shortening of the muscle and pulling on the tendon, helps to confirm the involvement of contractile tissues. Sometimes more pain is felt when the contraction is released and lengthening occurs; this would still be considered a positive finding for a lesion in contractile tissues. The *lack of pain* during resisted isometric testing, pain noted with limited accessory joint motions, a capsular pattern of joint restriction, or particular end-feels during PROM and accessory joint motions help to confirm the involvement of inert tissues. For example, bicipital tendinopathy would be painful during resisted isometric testing of elbow flexion and shoulder flexion. An adhesive capsulitis of the glenohumeral joint would be painless during these same resisted isometric maneuvers.

Resisted isometric testing must be performed carefully to stress particular contractile tissue while avoiding stress to surrounding inert tissue. The therapist should place the patient's joint in a position midway through the ROM, so that minimal tension is put on inert structures. The body part proximal to the joint being tested must be well stabilized by the therapist to minimize extraneous muscle substitutions. The patient is then asked to hold the position while the therapist gradually applies resistance. Joint movement is strictly avoided. Although some compression of articular surfaces will occur during the isometric contraction, this does not usually present a problem in interpreting the results.

In addition to determining the absence or presence of pain during the resisted isometric testing, the therapist should also note the strength of the muscle contraction. If weakness is found, more extensive testing of muscle strength should be performed using MMT or dynamometers. Muscle weakness may be due to many causes, including pathologies involving upper motor neurons, peripheral nerves, neuromuscular junctions, muscles, and tendons. Pain, fatigue, and disuse atrophy can also cause weakness. The pattern of muscle weakness will help to identify the site of the pathology and direct treatment.

Several authors have suggested using the results of resisted isometric testing to determine the type of pathology. The strength of the muscle contraction (strong or weak) and the presence or absence of pain (painful or painless) are used to implicate possible pathologies (Table 4.2). A resisted isometric test finding of "weak and painful" warrants expansion to include not only serious pathologies, but also relatively minor muscle damage and inflammation such as that induced by eccentric isokinetic exercise. Intra-tester and inter-tester reliability of resisted isometric testing of the knee and shoulder has been examined and found not acceptable in general; however, it was better for the knee compared to the shoulder.[42]

Table 4.2 Results of Resisted Isometric Testing

Findings	Possible Pathologies
Strong and painless	There is no lesion or neurological deficit involving the tested muscle and tendon.
Strong and painful	There is a minor lesion of the tested muscle or tendon.
Weak and painless	There is a disorder of the nervous system, neuromuscular junction, a complete rupture of the tested muscle or tendon, or disuse atrophy.
Weak and painful	There is a serious, painful pathology such as a fracture or neoplasm. Other possibilities include an acute inflammatory process that inhibits muscle contraction, exercise induced muscle damage or a partial rupture of the tested muscle or tendon.

Manual Muscle Testing

Manual muscle testing involves manually applied resistance by the therapist to test and determine muscle grades. Generally, the patient is positioned so that the muscle or muscle group being tested has to move or hold against the resistance of gravity. If this is well tolerated, the therapist applies manual resistance gradually to the distal end of the body part in which the muscle inserts and in a direction opposite to the torque produced by the muscle(s) being tested in the form of a *break test* in which the patient holds a joint position until the therapist gradually overpowers the patient and an eccentric contraction begins to occur. The break test is performed at the end of the ROM when testing one-joint muscles and at mid-range when testing two-joint muscles.[43] In addition, many therapists apply manual resistance while the patient moves through the ROM, in what is called a *make test*, or an *active resistance test*, so that the muscle's ability to contact concentrically against maximal resistance can also be determined. In the case of weaker muscles that cannot hold or move well against gravity, the patient is repositioned and attempts to move the body part through a gravity-minimized (horizontal) plane of motion. During all testing, stabilization of the body part on which the muscle originates and careful avoidance of substitution by other muscle groups are emphasized. A grading system is used with categories of Normal (grade 5), Good (grade 4), Fair (grade 3), Poor (grade 2), Trace (grade 1), and Zero (Table 4.3).[44]

It is important to note that this numerical scale indicates ordinal data, because the intervals between the numbers do not represent equal units of measure. The MMT grades of *Good* and *Normal* typically encompass a large range of muscle strength, whereas the grades of *Fair, Poor,* and *Trace* include a much narrower range. Sharrard,[45] counting alpha motor neurons in spinal cords of individuals with poliomyelitis at the time of autopsy, found that muscles previously receiving a grade of *Good* had 50% of their innervated motor neurons, whereas muscles graded as *Fair* had only 15% of their motor neurons. Beasley[46] noted that patients with poliomyelitis were graded as having *Good, Fair,* and *Poor* knee extension when they had on average only 43%, 9%, and 3% of the knee extension force of normal subjects, respectively. Andres et al,[47] in a study of four muscle groups in patients with amyotrophic lateral sclerosis, found that the muscles were often graded as *Normal* until up to 50% of strength was lost. Overall, the reliability and validity of MMT is within acceptable limits.[48] However, a wide range of strength values within an MMT grade and an overlap in strength values between adjacent MMT grades has been observed.[49] Global strength scores that average MMT results from multiple muscle groups also resulted in higher reliability.[50]

Although more costly and time-consuming than MMT, handheld dynamometry can be used to improve objectivity and sensitivity as needed. When muscles are strong enough to move against gravity and the dynamometer's lever arm, isokinetic dynamometry may also be used.

Grade definitions modified from Kendall et al[43] and Hislop et al[44] are presented in Table 4.3 with additional criteria as to the amount of motion completed by the

Table 4.3 Manual Muscle Testing Grades

Grades	Grade Abbreviations	0–5 Scale	0–10 Scale	Criteria
Normal	N	5	10	Full available ROM, against gravity, strong manual resistance
Good plus	G+	4+	9	Full available ROM, against gravity, nearly strong manual resistance
Good	G	4	8	Full available ROM, against gravity, moderate manual resistance
Good minus	G–	4–	7	Full available ROM, against gravity, nearly moderate manual resistance
Fair plus	F+	3+	6	Full available ROM, against gravity, slight manual resistance
Fair	F	3	5	Full available ROM, against gravity, no resistance
Fair minus	F–	3–	4	At least 50% but not full ROM, against gravity, no resistance
Poor plus	P+	2+	3	Full available ROM, gravity minimized, slight manual resistance
Poor	P	2	2	Full available ROM, gravity minimized, no resistance
Poor minus	P–	2–	1	At least 50% but not full ROM, gravity minimized, no resistance
Trace plus	T+	1+		Minimal observable motion (less than 50% ROM), gravity minimized, no resistance
Trace	T	1	T	No observable motion, palpable muscle contraction, no resistance
Zero	0	0	0	No observable or palpable muscle contraction

patient to delineate the grades of *Fair minus, Poor minus,* and *Trace plus.* The grades *Fair plus* through *Normal* depend on the therapist's interpretation of what is minimal, moderate, and maximal resistance. A *Normal* grade is typically equated with the normal strength for that muscle given the patient's age, sex, and body size. It should be noted that there is considerable variability in the amount of resistance that *Normal* muscles can be expected to hold against. For example, large muscles in the LE will normally hold against considerable force and be difficult to overpower during a break test, while small muscles of the hand will normally hold against less force and be easily overpowered during a break test. The application of resistance throughout the arc of motion (make test or active resistance test) in addition to resistance at only one point in the arc of motion (break test) may help in accurately judging a muscle's strength.

Handheld Dynamometry

Handheld dynamometers (HHDs) are portable devices, placed between the therapist's hand and the patient's body, that measure mechanical force at the point of application (Fig. 4.11). Patients are typically asked to push against resistance in a maximal isometric contraction (make test) or hold a position until the resistance overpowers the muscle producing an eccentric contraction (break test). The force measured by the dynamometer will vary depending on the method of applying the resistance (make or break test), the patient's body position in relationship to gravity, the joint angle, the dynamometer placement on the patient (lever arm), the stabilization to prevent muscle substitution, and the therapist's strength.[51] Although force values determined with make and break tests are highly correlated, break tests usually result in greater force values than make tests,[52] so they should not be used interchangeably.

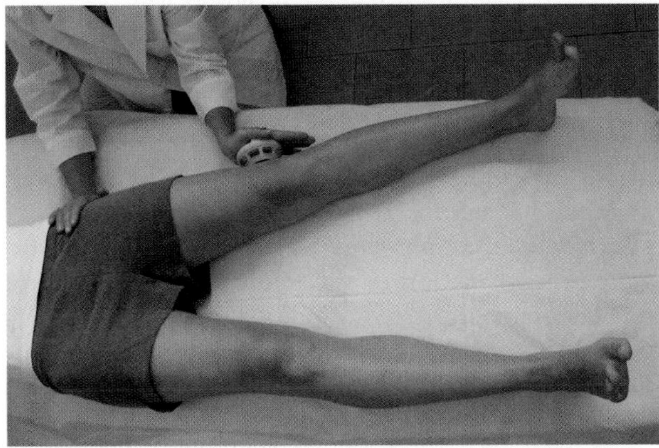

Figure 4.11 Measurement of the strength of the left hip abductors with a handheld dynamometer. The handheld dynamometer measures force at the point of application, which should be converted to torque by multiplying the force by the distance from the joint axis.

To reduce the effect of moving a body segment's weight on force measurements, it is recommended that muscle groups be tested in gravity-minimized positions. For example, to test the strength of the hip abductors, the patient would be positioned supine so that the muscle action would pull in a horizontal plane relative to the ground (see Fig. 4.11). The joint should also be positioned at an easily reproducible angle so that muscle length remains constant. The dynamometer is applied perpendicular to the body segment at an established location on the patient's body. When muscles contract, they produce *torque* that creates angular joint motion. The therapist must apply sufficient resistance to oppose the patient's torque to ensure an isometric (make test) or an eccentric contraction (break test). To provide greater resistance than what can be achieved manually, the dynamometer can be attached to a fixed surface or an isokinetic dynamometer can be used in the isometric setting.

Normative force values for particular muscle groups by age and sex have been reported;[53] however, attention must be directed to replicating methods used in the normative studies to ensure appropriate comparisons. Some authors have also included regression equations to take into account body weight and height.[53] For patients with unilateral conditions, it may be helpful to compare results to that of the uninvolved extremity. In general, it is expected that side-to-side differences are less than 11%.[53,54]

Muscle forces measured with HHD have been compared to forces measured with isokinetic dynamometers to evaluate concurrent validity with good results.[55-57] Reliability seems to be better when testing the UEs than when testing the LEs and trunk.[58-60] Agre et al[61] found the standard deviation of the repeated measurements expressed as a percentage of the mean force measurements (coefficient of variation of replication) to be 5.1% to 8.3% for the UE muscle groups and 11.3% to 17.8% for the LE muscle groups. Researchers believe some of the error in using HHDs is due to off-center loading of the dynamometer, difficulties in positioning and stabilization, and limitations in the strength and experience of the examiners.

Isokinetic Dynamometry

Isokinetic dynamometers are stationary, electromechanical devices that control the velocity of a moving body segment by resisting and measuring the patient's effort so that the body segment cannot accelerate beyond the preset angular velocity (Fig. 4.12). Isokinetic dynamometers can be used to measure the torque produced during isometric, concentric, and eccentric contractions. Isokinetic dynamometers, although expensive and cumbersome, are especially helpful in examining the performance of large, strong muscle groups. In such situations, MMT and HHDs are often insensitive to muscle performance abnormalities.[51] Muscle groups acting at the knee, shoulder, back, and to a lesser extent the elbow and ankle are those most frequently tested with isokinetic devices.

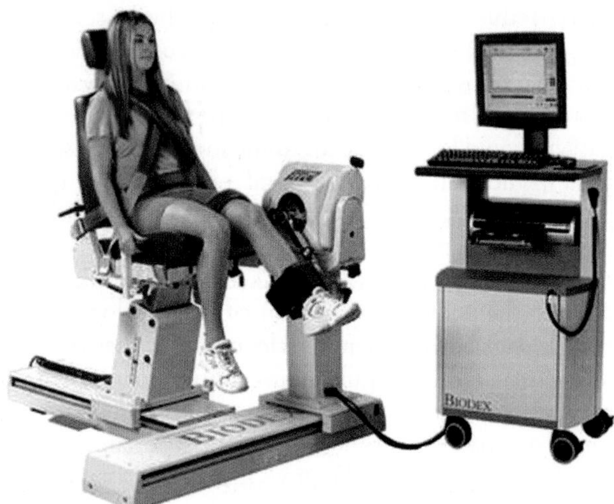

Figure 4.12 An isokinetic dynamometer is being used to measure muscle performance characteristics of the right knee extensors (quadriceps). Peak torque is the most frequently noted characteristic. *(Courtesy of Biodex Medical Systems, Inc., Shirley, NY 11967.)*

Isokinetic dynamometers measure torque and ROM as a function of time. Muscle performance characteristics most often noted are peak (maximal) torque, peak torque/body weight (Nm/kg), and average torque. Work measurements can be derived from the angular displacement and torque values. Power, which is work per unit time, also can be determined. Endurance (muscle fatigue) can be assessed by measuring the time required for peak torque to decrease by a certain percentage. Many factors such as patient pain, fear, or fatigue; damp settings; preload forces; mechanical artifact; and acceleration and deceleration ramping can affect the variability of torque measurements.

Special Tests

After completing the patient interview, observation, palpation, and examination of ROM, accessory motions, and muscle performance, the therapist may suspect the nature of the pathology. Special tests, designed to focus on specific conditions in a particular region of the body, may be helpful in confirming the diagnosis. A therapist would ordinarily choose to perform only those tests indicated by previous findings that are relevant to the area of the body being examined and the pathology that is part of the working hypotheses. False-positive and false-negative results are common. However, a positive test finding in conjunction with other aspects of the examination would be highly suggestive of pathology. A detailed presentation of the many special tests that are used in orthopedic assessment is beyond the scope of this chapter and can be found elsewhere.[2] Prior to performing a special test, the clinician should have a good sense of the pre-test probability of the pathology that the special test is designed to assess. Based on the outcome of the special test(s), the clinician should calculate the post-test probability of the pathology. For special tests to be helpful, they need to have good diagnostic properties (sensitivity and specificity). Because special tests frequently have poor diagnostic properties, researchers have used clusters of tests that frequently provide more clinically relevant information and assistance in the diagnostic process.[62] The reader is referred to specialized textbooks that discuss these important concepts in further detail.[63]

One category of special tests is used to determine the integrity of ligaments. The therapist performs these *ligamentous instability tests,* also called *ligament stress tests,* on a relaxed, passive joint. These maneuvers are often similar to tests of accessory or joint play motions. If possible, results should be compared with those from the uninvolved, contralateral joint. Examples of ligamentous instability tests include the *Lachman test,* which examines injury to the anterior cruciate ligament; the *posterior drawer test,* which examines damage to the posterior cruciate ligament of the knee; and the *varus and valgus stress tests,* which examine the integrity of collateral ligaments at the elbow and knee.

In addition to ligament instability tests, there are more general tests that examine joint laxity. These tests are often called *apprehension tests* because the patient is placed in a vulnerable joint position while being monitored for apprehension. For example, to test for anterior subluxation or dislocation of the glenohumeral joint, the shoulder is positioned in 90° of abduction and moved toward external rotation. These provocative tests are considered positive and should be stopped if they begin to elicit patient discomfort.

The length of muscles that cross and act at one joint can usually be examined in the process of testing PROM. However, some muscles cross and act at two or more joints. Some special tests examine the length of these multi-joint muscles. The *Thomas test,* which examines the length of hip flexors, and the *Ober test,* which focuses on the length of the tensor fascia lata, are examples of special muscle length tests.[43]

Numerous special tests address common conditions affecting the integrity of muscle and tendon structures. These tests typically stretch or contract the inflamed or injured structure, resulting in pain if the tests are positive. For example, the *Finkelstein test*[2] is used to examine inflammation of the tendons of the abductor pollicis longus and extensor pollicis brevis by stretching these structures over the wrist and thumb. Often the therapist will have previously noted pain, limitation, and possibly weakness during tests for ROM and muscle performance; special tests are used to clarify these earlier findings.

Another category of special tests reproduces the symptoms caused by irritation, compression, or restricted mobility of peripheral nerves. For example, the *Tinel test,* which involves manual tapping over superficial nerve sites, is positive for nerve irritation when pain, numbness, burning, or tingling sensations are elicited. The *Phalen and reverse Phalen tests* for carpal tunnel syndrome place the wrist in full flexion and extension, respectively, for 60 to 90 seconds to reproduce pain and paresthesia of the median nerve. *Neurodynamic tests* utilize sequential positioning of two or more joints to lengthen and mobilize neural tissue independent from surrounding non-neural structures.[64] The ability to complete the sequence of joint positions is compared to the uninvolved side. Once symptoms are provoked, the examiner moves one of the joints out of the nerve lengthening position to determine if the symptoms are relieved and confirm the involvement of neural tissue. However, before conducting neurodynamic testing, all joints in the sequence should be tested and cleared for joint and non-neural soft tissue limitations so as not to confound the results.[65] An example of a neurodynamic test is the *slump test,* which requires the sequential motions of thoracic, lumbar, and cervical spine flexion, hip flexion, ankle dorsiflexion, and knee extension to assess the mechanosensitivity of the spinal cord, cervical and lumbar nerve roots, and sciatic nerve.[65]

Functional Movement Analysis

Physical therapists are experts in the evaluation of motion. The conclusion of the physical examination represents an excellent opportunity to assess the quantity and quality of functional motion, focusing on the motions that are painful, difficult, or relevant to the patient's occupation or recreational activities. In the musculoskeletal setting, these activities typically include activities of daily living such as gait (see Chapter 7, Examination of Gait) or standing from a chair, athletic activities (e.g., squatting, jumping, throwing a ball), or occupational activities (e.g., lifting boxes). The motion should be viewed from different angles and assessed systematically. Recent technological advances allow the recording of functional activities with smartphones, tablets, or digital cameras and the careful analysis of angles at different parts of the task. Motions can be slowed down and relevant frames can be analyzed in detail. For the patients whose job involves the use of a computer and their symptoms exacerbate later in the day, an office *ergonomic evaluation* may provide unique insight into the source of the symptoms and the implementation of simple yet effective solutions.

Additional Tests and Measurements

Depending on findings, other tests and measurements may be indicated. Many of these additional examination procedures are discussed in detail in other chapters of this book. For example, patient complaints of paresthesia or difficulty in muscle performance often indicate neurological involvement that calls for testing of superficial, deep, and proprioceptive sensations (see Chapter 3, Examination of Sensory Function), reflexes and motor tone (see Chapter 5, Examination of Motor Function: Motor Control and Motor Learning), and coordination and balance (see Chapter 6, Examination of Coordination and Balance). Data from these tests together with muscle performance results help to identify conditions affecting peripheral nerves, spinal nerve roots, and the CNS. Therapists must distinguish peripheral nerve versus nerve root patterns of sensory and motor innervation. Figure 4.4 presents muscle testing recording forms that are helpful in recognizing impaired innervation patterns. Myotomes that are often included as parts of a musculoskeletal examination are shown in Table 4.4, and deep tendon reflexes are presented in Chapter 5. Upper motor neuron lesions usually result in hyperreflexia, whereas lower motor neuron lesions involving the spinal nerve root or peripheral nerves usually cause hyporeflexia of deep tendon reflexes. When pain sensitization is suspected, the therapist should utilize appropriate tests that assess relevant properties (e.g., pressure hyperalgesia, thermal hyperalgesia, temporal summation).[66] For more details on the assessment of pain, see Chapter 25, Chronic Pain.

Impairments in ROM, accessory joint motions, and motor performance may affect activities of daily living (ADL) and occupational and recreational activities. In such cases, the examination of functional abilities (see Chapter 8, Examination of Function) and environmental surroundings (see Chapter 9, Examination of the Environment) is often appropriate. Sometimes findings indicate the need for additional testing by other health professionals such as physician specialists, psychologists, speech-language pathologists, and occupational therapists.

Imaging and Other Medical Information

Due to direct access and changes in physical therapy education, therapists are increasingly becoming the primary care musculoskeletal specialists of choice. As part of this evolving role, they are frequently provided with the opportunity to incorporate the findings of imaging and other medical information into the musculoskeletal assessment. Many physical therapy programs have either dedicated courses or large aspects of courses focusing on imaging. Similarly, dedicated textbooks provide therapists with the necessary expertise to incorporate the findings of imaging studies in the diagnostic process.[67] The clinician is cautioned to avoid the temptation of starting the assessment by reviewing imaging studies and reserve this for last to confirm or refute the working hypotheses. Incidental findings in imaging studies are common[68] and can frequently complicate the process of arriving to the correct diagnosis.

■ EVALUATION OF EXAMINATION FINDINGS

At the conclusion of the musculoskeletal examination, all pertinent historical, subjective, and physical findings are evaluated to establish a physical therapy diagnosis on

Table 4.4 Myotomes[2]

Level	Upper Quarter Myotomes	
	Action to Be Tested	*Muscle*
C5	Shoulder abduction, shoulder flexion	Deltoid
C5, C6	Elbow flexion	Biceps
	Wrist extension	Extensor carpi radialis longus Extensor carpi radialis brevis
C7	Elbow extension	Triceps
	Wrist flexion	Flexor carpi radialis Flexor carpi ulnaris
C8	Ulnar deviation	Flexor carpi ulnaris Extensor carpi ulnaris
T1	Digit abduction/adduction	Interossei
Level	**Lower Quarter Myotomes**	
	Action to Be Tested	*Muscle*
L2, L3	Hip flexion	Iliopsoas
L2, L3, L4	Knee extension	Quadriceps
L4	Ankle dorsiflexion	Anterior tibialis
L5	Extension of great toe	Extensor hallucis longus
S1	Plantarflexion	Gastrocnemius
	Ankle eversion	Peroneus longus Peroneus brevis

which treatment is based. A *diagnosis* has been defined as a label encompassing a cluster of signs and symptoms, syndromes, or categories.[5] The specific tissues causing the impairments should be identified when possible so that treatment can be focused and effective. The therapist should be aware that frequently identifying the exact tissue pathology is not possible, particularly for certain categories such as low back pain.[68] The therapist must have a thorough understanding of the pathologies commonly affecting the body segment under consideration. The symptoms and clinical manifestations of these pathologies are compared to the current examination findings to establish a diagnosis. The American Physical Therapy Association's (APTA's) revised and adapted *Musculoskeletal Preferred Practice Patterns* can assist students and novice physical therapists in categorizing diagnoses into common clusters. Information is provided on risk factors, examination, evaluation/diagnosis/prognosis, interventions, and outcomes (available at: www.apta.org/Guide/PracticePatterns).

Sometimes the evaluation process does not yield a clearly identifiable diagnosis. In such cases, a provisional diagnosis and the alleviation of symptoms and impairments become the basis for treatment. In other instances, the evaluation may indicate the presence of two or more conditions. The therapist should then prioritize and focus initially on the condition causing the most serious impairments, activity limitations, and disability.

The evaluation should clearly determine the baseline for the patient's symptoms, impairments, activity limitations, and participation restrictions. This information becomes the basis of the clinical problem list and guides development of anticipated goals and expected outcomes. The results of future examinations can be compared to this baseline to evaluate the effectiveness of treatment.

In addition to establishing a diagnosis and baseline data, the evaluation of findings should ascertain etiological factors. Unless the underlying causes of the condition are recognized and treated, chronic problems can be expected. The therapist must not only direct attention to the specifically involved tissues, but must also think more broadly of physiological units of function and biomechanics. For example, a patient with a sprain of the medial collateral ligament of the knee may initially respond well to treatment consisting of compression elastic wrapping, ice, elevation, reduced activity, and a protective non-weight-bearing crutch gait. However, if the condition is partially due to abnormal foot mechanics, the resumption of normal weight-bearing activities may cause reinjury unless the alignment of the foot and leg is improved with orthotics. Similarly, a patient with supraspinatus tendinopathy may react well to rest and gentle glenohumeral ROM exercises, but often also requires eventual strengthening of the rotator cuff, scapulothoracic musculature, and restoration of normal scapulohumeral rhythm.

Other information that affects the prognosis and course of treatment should be determined during the evaluation process. The mode and mechanism of onset must be established. Was the onset sudden, gradually acquired, or congenital? Generally, the prognosis is better for a condition caused by a well-defined event than for a congenital condition or one with an insidious, gradual onset. The mode and mechanism of onset also provide clues to help develop strategies for prevention of reoccurring episodes of the injury or condition.

Finally, an analysis of the examination findings should establish the stage of the patient's condition. The stage, whether acute, subacute, or chronic, can indicate how well the patient will tolerate mechanical loads such as those imposed by daily activities or by a therapist during treatment. The *acute stage* is usually defined as occurring up to the first 48 to 72 hours after onset. The *subacute stage* may continue up to 2 weeks to several months after onset. Typically, conditions are considered in the *chronic stage* after 3 to 6 months. Another way of defining the stages, which is probably more relevant to treatment planning, focuses on tissue inflammation and the repair process. Conditions in an *acute inflammation stage* will show signs and symptoms of inflammation associated with hyperemia, increased capillary permeability with protein and plasma leakage, and an influx of granulocytes and other defensive cells. These signs and symptoms include swelling, elevated skin temperature at the lesion site, and pain at rest that worsens with ROM and resisted isometric contractions that even minimally stress the involved tissues. The *chronic inflammation stage* produces signs and symptoms associated with attempts at tissue repair, including an increase in the number of fibrocytes and the presence of granulation tissue; the patient will now have minimal or no swelling and elevated temperature at the lesion site. Pain tends to occur only at the extremes of ROM when the end-feel is reached, or with a moderate to maximal amount of isometric resistance. Tissues in an acute stage will often not tolerate mechanical loading from daily, recreational, occupational, or therapeutic activities. The force, frequency, and duration of treatment procedures must be monitored closely so as not to increase inflammation and worsen the condition. In contrast, tissues in the chronic stage will usually tolerate and require treatment procedures involving more mechanical loading, frequency, and duration to effect positive changes in the tissues. The stage of the condition also adds prognostic information. Typically, an acute condition will show more spontaneous improvement over a shorter period of time than a chronic condition. A chronic condition usually requires a longer period of treatment to promote a smaller improvement in status.

SUMMARY

The musculoskeletal examination provides important information concerning the status of bones, articular cartilage, joint capsules, ligaments, and muscles. The examination process begins with a review of the patient's medical records and a detailed interview. Careful observation, palpation, and ROM, accessory joint motion, and muscle performance tests are typically performed. Depending on the findings, special tests particular to the body region under examination may need to be included. Examination of the peripheral and central nervous systems, gait, functional ability, and the environment is often required. At the conclusion of this process, all findings must be evaluated to determine the diagnosis, baseline status, etiological factors, mode of onset, and stage (acute, subacute, or chronic) of the condition. At this point, the prognosis, goals, expected outcomes, and POC can be developed.

Questions for Review

1. What are the purposes of a musculoskeletal examination?
2. What information about the patient's symptoms should be obtained during a patient interview?
3. What are the types of normal end-feels? What types of tissue contribute to these end-feels?
4. Compare capsular versus noncapsular patterns of restricted motion.
5. Give at least three examples of osteokinematic and arthrokinematic motions. How do arthrokinematic motions combine to produce osteokinematic motion in a typical synovial joint in which the moving joint surface is concave? Convex?

6. Distinguish between muscle strength, endurance, and power.
7. Discuss the implications of a weak and painful finding during the performance of resisted isometric testing.
8. What factors are important in determining manual muscle testing grades? What would be the criteria for manual muscle testing grades of *Good, Fair,* and *Poor*?
9. What are the advantages and disadvantages of using manual muscle testing, handheld dynamometers, and isokinetic dynamometers to determine muscle strength?
10. What would a positive finding on a glenohumeral apprehension test indicate?

CASE STUDY 1

A 45-year-old man enters the outpatient physical therapy department with a complaint of right shoulder pain of 1 week's duration. The pain began Monday morning following a weekend of scraping and painting his house. The patient describes his pain as aching and troublesome; his pain is a 6 on a pain scale of 0 to 10. He reports that he is married and is having difficulty in home maintenance activities such as lawn mowing. He is able to perform only 30% of his normal home and recreational activities. The therapist decides to conduct a musculoskeletal examination.

While palpating the shoulder region, increased tenderness in the region of the bicipital groove of the right anterior shoulder is noted. AROM of the right shoulder reveals increased pain and some limitations during shoulder flexion, abduction, and extension; all other active motions are pain free and within normal ROM limits. Passive shoulder motions are pain free with normal ROM, except for shoulder extension, which is limited and causes an increase in pain toward the end of motion.

GUIDING QUESTIONS

1. What additional information should be gathered during the interview?
2. What is a capsular pattern of limitation? Does this patient have a capsular pattern of limitation for the glenohumeral joint?
3. The therapist suspects the presence of bicipital tendinopathy. Do the findings during testing of active and passive ROM support this diagnosis? Explain.
4. What additional tests should be performed to selectively examine contractile tissue and help to support or repudiate the diagnosis of bicipital tendinopathy? Provide a rationale for your selection.

CASE STUDY 2

A 14-year-old girl is referred for outpatient physical therapy 12 weeks after sustaining midshaft fractures of her left tibia and fibula from a bicycle accident. Her long leg cast was removed yesterday. The fracture is well healed. The patient reports her left knee and ankle are stiff and painful when she tries to move them. She also describes her left leg as weak. At this time she is ambulating with two crutches, weight-bearing as tolerated, with hopes of progressing off the crutches as soon as possible.

GUIDING QUESTIONS

1. On observation, the patient's left thigh and calf appear to be thinner than the right. How can this observation be objectively measured and documented? Why might the patient's left leg be thinner than the right?
2. Passive ROM for left knee flexion is 10° to 70°. The end-feel for left knee flexion is firm. What is the normal end-feel for knee flexion?
3. What accessory joint motion should be examined considering the limitation in passive knee flexion ROM? Apply the concave–convex rules for determining the direction of the glide given the shape of the joint surfaces.
4. In addition to observing, palpating, and testing active ROM, passive ROM, accessory joint motions, and muscle performance, what other testing procedures would be important to include in the examination of this patient?

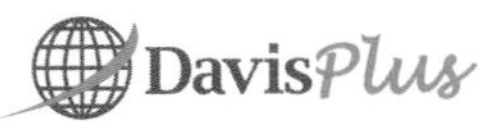

For additional resources, including answers to the questions for review and case study guiding questions, please visit **http://davisplus.fadavis.com.**

References

1. Vos, T, et al: Years lived with disability (YLDs) for 1160 sequelae of 289 diseases and injuries 1990-2010: A systematic analysis for the Global Burden of Disease Study 2010. Lancet 380(9859): 2163–2196, 2012.
2. Magee, D: Orthopaedic Physical Assessment, ed 6. Elsevier Saunders, St. Louis, 2014.
3. Dutton, M: Dutton's Orthopaedic Examination, Evaluation, and Intervention, ed 3. McGraw Hill, New York, 2012.
4. Hertling, D, and Kessler, RM: Management of Common Musculoskeletal Disorders, Physical Therapy Principles and Methods, ed 4. Lippincott Williams & Wilkins, Philadelphia, 2006.
5. *Guide to Physical Therapist Practice 3.0*. Alexandria, VA: American Physical Therapy Association; 2014. Available at: www.guidetoptpractice.apta.org. Accessed March 10, 2016.
6. Jette, D, et al: Decision-making ability of physical therapists: Physical therapy intervention or medical referral. Phys Ther, 86(12):1619–1629, 2007.
7. Boissonnault, W, and Badke, M: Collecting health history information: The accuracy of a patient self-administered questionnaire in an orthopedic outpatient setting. Phys Ther 85(6):531–543, 2005.
8. Downie, A, et al: Red flags to screen for malignancy and fracture in patients with low back pain: systematic review. Br Med J 347, 2013.
9. George, SZ, et al: Development of a review-of-systems screening tool for orthopaedic physical therapists: Results from the Optimal Screening for Prediction of Referral and Outcome (OSPRO) Cohort. J Orthop Sports Phys Ther 45(7):512–526, 2015.
10. Melzack, R: The McGill Pain Questionnaire: Major properties and scoring methods. Pain 1(3):277–299, 1975.
11. Talley, N, and O'Connor, S: Clinical Examination: A Guide to Physical Diagnosis, ed 4. Williams & Wilkins, Baltimore, 2001.
12. Downs, MB, and Laporte, C: Conflicting dermatome maps: Educational and clinical implications. J Orthop Sports Phys Ther 41(6):427–434, 2011.
13. Collins, CK, et al: The reliability and validity of the Saliba Postural Classification System. J Man Manip Ther 24(3):174–181, 2016.
14. Levangie, P, and Norkin, C: Joint Structure and Function: A Comprehensive Analysis, ed 5. FA Davis, Philadelphia, 2011.
15. Barrett, E, et al: Is thoracic spine posture associated with shoulder pain, range of motion and function? A systematic review. Man Ther 26:38–46, 2016.
16. Neal, BS, et al: Foot posture as a risk factor for lower limb overuse injury: A systematic review and meta-analysis. J Foot Ankle Res 7(1):55, 2014.
17. Sahrmann, SA: Does postural assessment contribute to patient care? J Orthop Sports Phys Ther 32(8):376–379, 2002.
18. Rowe, PJ, et al: Knee joint kinematics in gait and other functional activities measured using flexible electrogoniometry: How much knee motion is sufficient for normal daily life? Gait Post 12(2): 143–155, 2000.
19. Protopapadaki, A, et al: Hip, knee, ankle kinematics and kinetics during stair ascent and descent in healthy young individuals. Clin Biomech 22(2):203–210, 2007.
20. Janssen, WG, Bussmann, HB, and Stam, HJ: Determinants of the sit-to-stand movement: A review. Phys Ther 82(9):866–879, 2002.
21. Hemmerich, A, et al: Hip, knee, and ankle kinematics of high range of motion activities of daily living. J Orthop Res 24(4): 770–781, 2006.
22. Mulholland, SJ, and Wyss, UP: Activities of daily living in non-Western cultures: Range of motion requirements for hip and knee joint implants. Int J Rehabil Res 24(3):191–198, 2001.
23. Packer, TL, et al: Examining the elbow during functional activities. OTJR 10(6):323–333, 1990.
24. Ryu, J, et al: Functional ranges of motion of the wrist joint. J Hand Surg 16(3):409–419, 1991.
25. Vohralik, SL, et al: Reliability and validity of a smartphone app to measure joint range. Am J Phys Med Rehabil 94(4):325–330, 2015.
26. Milani, P, et al: Mobile smartphone applications for body position measurement in rehabilitation: A review of goniometric tools. PM&R 6(11):1038–1043, 2014.
27. Chen, J, et al: Meta-analysis of normative cervical motion. Spine 24(15):1571, 1999.
28. Boon, AJ, and Smith, J: Manual scapular stabilization: Its effect on shoulder rotational range of motion. Arch Phys Med Rehabil 81(7):978–983, 2000.
29. Norkin, C, and White, D: Measurement of Joint Motion: A Guide to Goniometry, ed 5. FA Davis, Philadelphia, 2016.
30. van de Pol, RJ, van Trijffel, E, and Lucas, C: Inter-rater reliability for measurement of passive physiological range of motion of upper extremity joints is better if instruments are used: A systematic review. J Physiother 56(1):7–17, 2010.
31. van Trijffel, E, et al: Inter-rater reliability for measurement of passive physiological movements in lower extremity joints is generally low: A systematic review. J Physiother 56(4):223–235, 2010.
32. Boone, DC, and Azen, SP: Normal range of motion of joints in male subjects. J Bone Joint Surg (Am) 61(5):756–759, 1979.
33. Mohsin, F, McGarry, A, and Bowers, RJ: Factors influencing the reliability of the universal goniometer in measurement of lower-limb range of motion: A literature review. J Prosthet Orthot 27(4):140–148, 2015.
34. Cyriax, J, and Cyriax, P: Illustrated Manual of Orthopaedic Medicine. Butterworth, London, 1983.
35. Kaltenborn, F: Manual Mobilization of the Joints: The Extremities, ed 5. Oslo: Olaf Norlis Bokhandel, 1999.
36. Paris, S: Extremity Dysfunction and Mobilization. Institute Press, Atlanta, 1980.
37. Petersen, CM, and Hayes, KW: Construct validity of Cyriax's selective tension examination: Association of end-feels with pain at the knee and shoulder. J Orthop Sports Phys Ther 30(9):512–527, 2000.
38. Chesworth, BM, et al: Movement diagram and "end-feel" reliability when measuring passive lateral rotation of the shoulder in patients with shoulder pathology. Phys Ther 78(6):593–601, 1998.
39. Hayes, KW, and Petersen, CM: Reliability of assessing end-feel and pain and resistance sequence in subjects with painful shoulders and knees. J Orthop Sports Phys Ther 31(8):432–445, 2001.
40. Klässbo, M, Harms-Ringdahl, K, and Larsson, G: Examination of passive ROM and capsular patterns in the hip. Physiother Res Int 8(1):1–12, 2003.
41. Ellenbecker, TS, et al: Intrarater and interrater reliability of a manual technique to assess anterior humeral head translation of the glenohumeral joint. J Shoulder Elbow Surg 11(5):470–475, 2002.
42. Hayes, KW, and Petersen, CM: Reliability of classifications derived from Cyriax's resisted testing in subjects with painful shoulders and knees. J Orthop Sports Phys Ther 33(5):235–246, 2003.
43. Kendall, F, McCreary, E, and Provance, P: Muscles: Testing and Function. Williams & Wilkins, Baltimore, 1993.
44. Hislop, H, Avers, D and Brown,M: Daniels and Worthingham's Muscle Testing, ed 9. Elsevier, Philadelphia, 2014.
45. Sharrard, WJW: Muscle recovery in poliomyelitis. J Bone Joint Surg (Br) 37-B(1):63–79, 1955.
46. Beasley, W: Quantitative muscle testing: Principles and application to research and clinical services. Arch Phys Med Rehabil 42: 398–425, 1961.
47. Andres, PL, et al: A comparison of three measures of disease progression in ALS. J Neurol Sci 139:64–70, 1996.

48. Cuthbert, SC, and Goodheart, GJ: On the reliability and validity of manual muscle testing: A literature review. Chiropr Osteopat 15(1):4, 2007.
49. Bohannon, RW: Measuring knee extensor muscle strength. Am J Phys Med Rehabil 80(1):13–18, 2001.
50. Escolar, DM, et al: Clinical evaluator reliability for quantitative and manual muscle testing measures of strength in children. Muscle Nerve 24(6):787–793, 2001.
51. Mulroy, SJ, et al: The ability of male and female clinicians to effectively test knee extension strength using manual muscle testing. J Orthop Sports Phys Ther 26(4):192–199, 1997.
52. Bohannon, RW: Make tests and break tests of elbow flexor muscle strength. Phys Ther 68(2):193–194, 1988.
53. Phillips, BA, Lo, SK, and Mastaglia, FL: Muscle force measured using "break" testing with a hand-held myometer in normal subjects aged 20 to 69 years. Arch Phys Med Rehabil 81(5):653–661, 2000.
54. Andrews, AW, Thomas, MW, and Bohannon, RW: Normative values for isometric muscle force measurements obtained with hand-held dynamometers. Phys Ther 76(3):248–259, 1996.
55. Bohannon, RW: Hand-held compared with isokinetic dynamometry for measurement of static knee extension torque (parallel reliability of dynamometers). Clin Phys Physiol Meas 11(3):217–222, 1990.
56. Brinkrnann, JR: Comparison of a hand-held and fixed dynamometer in measuring strength of patients with neuromuscular disease. J Orthop Sports Phys Ther 19(2):100–104, 1994.
57. Visser, J, et al: Comparison of maximal voluntary isometric contraction and hand-held dynamometry in measuring muscle strength of patients with progressive lower motor neuron syndrome. Neuromuscul Disord 13(9):744–750, 2003.
58. Bohannon, RW, and Andrews, AW: Interrater reliability of hand-held dynamometry. Phys Ther 67(6):931–933, 1987.
59. Moreland, J, et al: Interrater reliability of six tests of trunk muscle function and endurance. J Orthop Sports Phys Ther 26(4): 200–208, 1997.
60. Riddle, DL, et al: Intrasession and intersession reliability of hand-held dynamometer measurements taken on brain-damaged patients. Phys Ther 69(3):182–189, 1989.
61. Agre, JC, et al: Strength testing with a portable dynamometer: Reliability for upper and lower extremities. Arch Phys Med Rehabil 68(7):454–458, 1987.
62. Hegedus, EJ, et al: Combining orthopedic special tests to improve diagnosis of shoulder pathology. Phys Ther Sport 16(2):87–92, 2015.
63. Cleland, J, Koppenhaver, S, and Su, J: Netter's Orthopaedic Clinical Examination: An Evidence-Based Approach. Elsevier, Philadelphia, 2016.
64. Butler, D: Mobilisation of the Nervous System. Churchill Livingstone, Melbourne, 1991.
65. Coppieters, MW, et al: Addition of test components during neurodynamic testing: Effect on range of motion and sensory responses. J Orthop Sports Phys Ther 31(5): 226–237, 2001.
66. Fingleton, C, et al: Pain sensitization in people with knee osteoarthritis: A systematic review and meta-analysis. Osteoarthr Cart 23(7):1043–1056, 2015.
67. McKinnis, L: Fundamentals of Musculoskeletal Imaging, ed 4. FA Davis, Philadelphia, 2014.
68. Chou, R, et al: Diagnosis and treatment of low back pain: A joint clinical practice guideline from the American college of physicians and the American pain society. Ann Intern Med 147(7):478–491, 2007.

Examination of Motor Function: Motor Control and Motor Learning

Susan B. O'Sullivan, PT, EdD
Richard J. McKibben, PT, DSc, ECS
Leslie G. Portney, PT, DPT, PhD, FAPTA

Chapter 5

LEARNING OBJECTIVES

1. Identify the purposes and components of the examination of motor function: motor control and motor learning.
2. Describe the examination process and specific tests and measures of various components of motor function.
3. Discuss the implications of common deficits associated with disorders of motor function for examination and treatment planning.
4. Discuss factors that influence the complexity of the motor examination and evaluation process.
5. Describe the instrumentations systems and general methodology of electrodiagnosis in the performance of electromyography (EMG) and nerve conduction study (NCS) examinations.
6. Describe the characteristics of normal and abnormal EMG and NCS findings.
7. Discuss the implications of clinical EMG and NCS findings for goal setting and treatment planning.
8. Discuss factors that influence determination of the physical therapy diagnosis with disorders of motor function.
9. Analyze and interpret patient data, formulate realistic goals and expected outcomes, and identify appropriate interventions when presented with a clinical case study.

CHAPTER OUTLINE

OVERVIEW OF MOTOR FUNCTION

Motor control evolves from a complex set of neural, physical, and behavioral processes that govern posture and movement. Some movements have a genetic basis and emerge through processes of normal growth and development. Examples of these include the largely reactive reflex patterns that predominate during much of early life and in some patients with brain damage. Other movements, termed *motor skills,* are learned through interaction and exploration of the environment. Practice and feedback are important variables in defining motor learning and motor skill development. Sensory information about movement is used to guide and shape the development of motor programs. A *motor program* is defined as "an abstract representation that, when initiated, results in the production of a coordinated movement sequence."[1, p. 497] Examples include the complex neural circuitry in the spinal cord known as *central pattern generators* that control locomotion and gait.

Higher-level motor programs can be viewed as abstract rules or code for coordinated actions that are stored (*generalized motor programs* [GMPs]). GMPs contain information about the order of events, the timing of events (temporal structure), the overall force of contractions, and the muscle(s) or limb(s) used in the movements. Sensory feedback from the responding limbs, as well as from the environment, modifies the resulting movements. A *motor plan* (*complex motor program*) is an idea or plan for purposeful movement that is made up of several component motor programs. *Motor memory* (*procedural memory*) involves the recall of motor programs or subroutines and includes information on (1) initial movement conditions; (2) sensory parameters (how the movement felt, looked, and sounded); (3) specific movement performance parameters (*knowledge of performance*); and (4) outcome of the movement (*knowledge of results*).

The cooperative actions of multiple systems allow for accommodation of movement to match the specific demands of the task and the environment. This is defined by *systems theory,* a distributed model of motor control. The central concept is that many systems interact to produce coordinated movement, not just the nervous system. For example, mechanical factors of the musculoskeletal system (body mass, inertia, and gravity) contribute to the overall quality of the movement produced. Cognition (attention, memory, learning, judgment, and decision making) and perception (interpretation of sensation) are also critical. Impairments in any of these interacting systems can significantly alter the quality of the movement produced and the level of function achieved.[2] Another concept is that units of the central nervous system (CNS) are organized around specific task demands (termed *task systems*). The entire CNS may be necessary for complex tasks, whereas only small portions may be needed for simple tasks. Command levels vary depending on the specific task executed. Thus, the highest level of command may not be required in the execution of some simple movements.[2,3] Lateral pathways are involved in voluntary movements of distal musculature and are under direct cortical control (i.e., corticospinal and rubrospinal tracts). Ventromedial pathways are involved in control of posture and locomotion and are under brain stem control (i.e., vestibulospinal tracts, tectospinal tract, and pontine and medullary reticulospinal tracts). The neurons of the ventral horn of the spinal cord are the final common pathway to engage the peripheral muscles for function.

Motor skills are acquired and modified by actions of the CNS through processes of motor learning. *Motor learning* is defined as "a set of internal processes associated with practice or experience leading to relatively permanent changes in the capability for skilled behavior."[1, p. 497] The CNS organizes and integrates vast amounts of sensory information. *Feedback* is response-produced information received during or after the movement and is used to monitor output for corrective actions. *Feedforward,* the sending of signals in advance of movement to ready the sensorimotor systems, allows for anticipatory adjustments in postural activity. Processing of information by the CNS is both serial and parallel, leading to the production of coordinated movement. *Coordination* is the ability to execute smooth, accurate, and controlled motor responses. *Coordinative structures* (synergies) are the functionally linked muscles that are constrained by the nervous system to act cooperatively to produce an intended movement.[1]

Recovery is the reacquisition of the ability to perform movement in the same manner as it was performed prior to injury (i.e., same body segments). Function is restored in neural tissue that was initially lost after injury. Task performance is similar to that used by nondisabled individuals. *Compensation* refers to the performance of movement in a new manner. Alternative movements can result from (1) the *adaptation* of remaining motor elements or (2) *substitution* of movements using different motor elements or body segments. Neural tissue acquires a new function, and tasks are accomplished using alternate muscles or limbs. For example, the patient with stroke dresses using the less involved upper extremity (UE). A determination needs to be made as to whether the movements demonstrate recovery or compensation. If compensatory movements are present, are they of sufficient quality and efficiency to permit return of function?[4]

Neural plasticity refers to the adaptive capacity of the CNS to change and repair itself. The brain changes in both structure and function as it encodes experiences and learns new behaviors (i.e., experience-dependent neural plasticity). Learning involves both short-term changes (e.g., increases in the strength of synaptic connections) and long-term changes (e.g., changes in genes, neurons, and neuronal networks within specific brain regions).[5] As learning progresses, there is a shift from short-term to long-term processes. Motor (procedural) memory allows for continued access of this information for repeat performance or modification of existing patterns of movement. Thus the patient with brain damage (e.g., traumatic brain injury [TBI], stroke) can progress and improve in motor function with an effective rehabilitation plan of care. The therapist needs to ensure the examination accurately identifies all elements of the patient's motor function. Box 5.1 summarizes terminology related to motor control. See additional discussion in Chapter 10, Strategies to Improve Motor Function.

Damage to the CNS interferes with motor function processes. Lesions affecting areas of the CNS can produce

Box 5.1 Terminology: Motor Control

Coordinative structures (synergies): Functionally linked muscles that are constrained by the CNS to act cooperatively to produce an intended movement.

Motor ability: A genetically predetermined characteristic or trait of a person that underlies performance of certain motor skills.

Motor control: The underlying substrates of neural, physical, and behavioral aspects of movement.

- **Reactive motor control:** Movements are adapted in response to ongoing feedback (e.g., muscle stretch causes an increase in muscle contraction in response to a forward weight shift).
- **Proactive (anticipatory) motor control:** Movements are adapted in advance of ongoing movements via feedforward mechanisms (e.g., the postural adjustments made in preparation for catching a heavy, large ball).

Motor plan: An idea or plan for purposeful movement that is made up of component motor programs.

Motor program: An abstract representation that, when initiated, results in the production of a coordinated movement sequence.[1, p. 497]

Motor learning: A set of internal processes associated with feedback or practice leading to relatively permanent changes in the capability for motor skill.[1, p. 497]

Motor skill: An action or task that has a goal to achieve; acquisition of skill is dependent on practice and experience and is not genetically defined. *Alternative definition*: An indicator of the quality of performance.

Motor recovery: The reappearance of motor patterns present prior to central nervous system injury performed in the same manner as prior to injury; tasks are accomplished similar to nondisabled individuals.

Motor compensation: The appearance of new motor patterns resulting from changes in the central nervous system involving (1) *adaptation* of the remaining motor elements of the involved limbs or body segments (tasks are accomplished using alternative movement patterns) or (2) *substitution* (tasks are accomplished using alternate limbs or body segments).

Motor control and the environment: Movements are shaped to the specific environments in which they occur.

Anticipation-timing (time-to-contact): The ability to time movements to a target or an event (e.g., an obstacle) in the environment, requiring precise control of movements (e.g., running to kick a soccer ball).

Regulatory conditions: Those features of the environment to which movement must be molded to be successful (e.g., stepping on a moving walkway or into a revolving door).

- **Closed skills:** Movements performed in a stable or fixed environment (e.g., activities practiced in a quiet room).
- **Open skills:** Movements performed in a changing or variable environment (e.g., activities practiced in a busy gym).
- **Self-paced skills:** Movements that are initiated at will and whose timing is controlled or modified by the person (e.g., walking).
- **Externally paced skills:** Movements that are initiated and paced by dictates of the external environment (e.g., walking in time with a metronome).

specific, recognizable deficits that are relatively consistent among patients (e.g., patients with upper motor neuron syndrome). Individual differences in neural plasticity, recovery, and functional outcomes can be expected. In conditions with widespread damage to the CNS (e.g., TBI) the resultant problems in motor function are numerous, complex, and difficult to delineate. An accurate picture of the scope of deficits may not be readily apparent on initial examination. A process of reexamination over time will generally yield an understanding of the patient's performance capabilities and deficits. The comprehensive examination focuses on delineation of impairments, activity limitations, and participation restrictions. Those impairments that directly affect motor function should be clearly identified. Goals, expected outcomes, and a plan of care (POC) can then be effectively developed.

This chapter will review essential components of examination, factors that may constrain the motor function examination (preliminary examinations), and elements of the motor function examination (with the exception of the examination of coordination and balance, which is discussed in Chapter 6, Examination of Coordination and Balance). Required elements of motor learning and examination are also discussed. Finally, instrumentation systems and general methodology used to perform an electromyography (EMG) and nerve conduction velocity (NCV) examination are discussed along with the characteristics of normal and abnormal EMG and NCV findings.

COMPONENTS OF THE EXAMINATION

The examination of motor function involves three components: (1) patient history, (2) a review of relevant systems, and (3) specific tests and measures that allow formulation of the diagnosis, prognosis, and POC.[6]

Patient History

During the patient/client history, information is gathered on (1) general demographics, (2) social history, (3) employment/work (job/school/play), (4) living environment, (5) general health status, (6) social/health habits, (7) family history, (8) medical/surgical history, (9) current condition(s)/chief complaint(s), (10) functional status and activity level, (11) medications, and (12) other clinical tests. Information is obtained from the patient and other interested persons (e.g., family members, significant others, and caregivers). If the patient is unable to communicate accurate and meaningful information, as is frequently the case with injury to the brain, data must be gathered from other sources (e.g., family members, caregivers). A review of the medical record can be used to verify and triangulate data obtained from personal communications. Often, the medical record of a patient with pronounced deficits in motor function (e.g., the patient with TBI) contains a large amount of data that can be unwieldy and difficult to sort through. The therapist can benefit from the application of a framework to identify and classify problems. The International Classification of Functioning, Disability and Health (ICF) model[7] focuses on impairments, activity limitations, and participation restrictions, and provides a useful framework. It is discussed fully in Chapter 1, Clinical Decision Making.

Systems Review

A systems review serves the purpose of a screening examination; that is, a brief or limited examination of body systems. The physical therapist can then use this information to identify potential problems that will require more extensive testing. For example, screening examinations for posture and tone may reveal significant impairments. More detailed tests and measures are then required to delineate the exact nature of the problems uncovered. Sometimes screening examinations reveal problems in communication and/or cognition that preclude further testing. For example, a patient with stroke and severe communication and cognitive impairments will be unable to follow directions and cooperate with many individual tests of physical function. The therapist will document this in the medical record as *unable to test at the present time due to severe communication/cognitive deficits.*

Tests and Measures

Therapists should select standardized methods and instruments with established validity and reliability whenever possible, consistent with the American Physical Therapy Association's (APTA) goal of *evidence-based practice.*[6] Examination of motor function is a multifaceted process that typically requires a number of different tests and measures. Information should be obtained about specific impairments (i.e., body functions and structure) and their impact on movement and function (i.e., activity limitations and participation restrictions). Instruments can be general (providing an overall measure of health) or specific (providing condition-specific, body-region specific, or individual-specific data). Instruments can be self-report or performance-based with a focus on qualitative or quantitative aspects of movement.[6] Many different instruments focusing on motor function are discussed in later chapters in this text. The Rehabilitation Measures Database developed by the Rehabilitation Institute of Chicago, Center for Rehabilitation Outcomes Research (www.rehabmeasures.org), provides a valuable source of information on specific tests and measures, as does the Academy of Neurologic Physical Therapy EDGE Taskforce Outcome Measures (www.neuropt.org).

Qualitative assessment of motor function requires insights and understanding of patterns of normal movement or postures. The therapist uses inductive reasoning processes (formulating generalizations from specific observations). The experienced therapist or expert clinician is far more efficient in reaching decisions about qualitative performance than the novice therapist. Quantitative instruments use objective measurement as a way of examining performance. Documentation requirements imposed by the health care system and third-party payers increasingly emphasize objective instruments as evidence of the need for, as well as the effectiveness, of services. However, many aspects of motor function are not easily measured, especially in the patient with neurological insult or injury. For example, motor learning is not directly measurable but rather is inferred from measures of performance, retention, generalizability, and adaptability. Thus, these constructs are used to infer changes in the CNS that occur with learning. The therapist must be sensitive to the nature of the variables being examined and identify appropriate measures that provide a meaningful analysis of patient function. It is not likely that any one measure will provide all of the data needed for the examination of motor function.

Reexamination is performed to determine if goals and outcomes are being met and if the patient is benefiting from the POC. If goals and expected outcomes are not being met, modifications in the POC are needed. The patient who has reached a plateau and does not show continued progress over time should be considered for discharge. Many patients with deficits in motor function typically undergo multiple episodes of rehabilitation as recovery occurs (e.g., TBI or stroke). Patients with chronic progressive conditions (e.g., Parkinson's disease, multiple sclerosis) also typically experience multiple episodes of rehabilitation when deterioration with loss of function occurs.

■ FACTORS THAT MAY CONSTRAIN THE MOTOR FUNCTION EXAMINATION

Patients who sustain brain damage either through trauma or disease may present with a number of cognitive, emotional, perceptual, or communication deficits that can significantly affect how they experience the environment and interact with others. Impairments in sensation and sensory integrity can also profoundly influence a patient's movement responses. It is important to understand how the examination of motor function can be influenced by these factors. Using tests and directions that confuse a patient during an examination or are clearly beyond the capabilities of the patient will only yield inaccurate information about a patient's movements.

Consciousness and Arousal

Examination of consciousness and arousal is important in determining the degree to which an individual is able to respond. The *ascending reticular activating system* includes core neurons in the brain stem, the locus coeruleus, and raphe nuclei that synapse directly on the thalamus, cortex, and other brain regions. It functions to arouse and awaken the brain and control sleep–wake cycles. High levels of activity are associated with extreme excitement (high arousal), whereas lesions in the brain stem are associated with sleep and coma. The *descending reticular activating system* is composed of the pontine and medullary reticulospinal tracts. The pontine (medial) reticulospinal tract enhances spinal cord antigravity reflexes and extensor tone of lower limbs. The medullary (lateral) reticulospinal tract has the opposite effect, reducing antigravity control.[8]

Five different levels of consciousness have been identified. *Consciousness* refers to a state of arousal accompanied by awareness of one's environment. A conscious patient is awake, alert, and oriented to his or her surroundings. *Lethargy* refers to altered consciousness in which a person's level of arousal is diminished. The lethargic patient appears drowsy but when questioned can open the eyes and respond briefly. The patient easily falls asleep if not continually stimulated and does not fully appreciate the environment. Attempts to communicate with the patient are difficult, owing to deficits in maintaining focus. The therapist should speak in a loud voice while calling the patient's name. Questions should be simple and directed toward the individual (e.g., How are you feeling?).

Obtunded state refers to diminished arousal and awareness. The obtunded patient is difficult to arouse from sleeping and once aroused, appears confused. Attempts to interact with the patient are generally nonproductive. The patient responds slowly and demonstrates little interest in or awareness of the environment. The therapist should shake the patient gently as if awakening someone from sleep and again use simple questions. *Stupor* refers to a state of altered mental status and responsiveness to one's environment. The patient can be aroused only with vigorous or unpleasant stimuli (e.g., painful stimuli such as flexion of the great toe, sharp pressure or pinch, or rolling a pencil across the nail bed). The patient demonstrates little in the way of voluntary verbal or motor responses. Mass movement responses may be observed in response to painful stimuli or loud noises. The unconscious patient is said to be in a *coma* and cannot be aroused. The eyes remain closed and there are no sleep–wake cycles. The patient does not respond to repeated painful stimuli and may be ventilator dependent. Reflex reactions may or may not be seen, depending on the location of the lesion(s) within the CNS.[9]

Clinically, the patient can progress from one level of consciousness to another. For example, with an intracranial bleed, the swelling and mass effect compresses the brain, resulting in decreasing levels of consciousness. The patient progresses from consciousness, to lethargy, to stupor, and finally to coma. If medical interventions are successful, recovery is evidenced by a reverse progression. True coma is generally time limited. Patients emerge into a *minimally conscious (vegetative) state,* characterized by return of irregular sleep–wake cycles and normalization of the so-called vegetative functions—respiration, digestion, and blood pressure control. The patient may be aroused but remains unaware of his or her environment. There is no purposeful attention or cognitive responsiveness. The term *persistent vegetative state* is used to describe individuals who remain in a vegetative state 1 year or longer after TBI and 3 months or more for anoxic brain injury. This state is caused by severe brain injury.

The *Glasgow Coma Scale* (GCS) is a gold standard instrument used to document level of consciousness in acute brain injury. Three areas of function are examined: eye opening, best motor response, and verbal response. Total GCS scores range from a low of 3 to a high of 15. A total score of 8 or less is indicative of severe brain injury and coma, a score between 9 and 12 is indicative of moderate brain injury, and a score between 13 and 15 is indicative of mild brain injury.[10] The *Rancho Los Amigos Levels of Cognitive Function* is widely used in rehabilitation facilities to examine the return of the person with brain injury from coma (Level I, no response) to consciousness (Level VIII, purposeful–appropriate). Different levels of behavioral function are described (e.g., confused states, automatic states).[11] See Chapter 19, Traumatic Brain Injury, for a complete discussion of both these instruments.

Examination of the pupillary size and reaction can also reveal important information about the unconscious patient. Pupils that are bilaterally small may be indicative of damage to the sympathetic pathways in the hypothalamus or metabolic encephalopathy. Pinpoint pupils are suggestive of a hemorrhagic pontine lesion or narcotic overdose (e.g., morphine, heroin). Pupils that are fixed in mid-position and slightly dilated are suggestive of midbrain damage, whereas large bilaterally fixed and dilated pupils suggest severe anoxia or drug toxicity (e.g., tricyclic antidepressants). If only one pupil is fixed and dilated, temporal lobe herniation with compression of the oculomotor nerve and midbrain is likely.[8]

Whereas an appropriate level of arousal allows for optimal motor performance, very low or high levels of arousal can cause deterioration in motor performance.

This is referred to as the *inverted-U principle* (Yerkes–Dodson law).[12,13] Patients at either end of the arousal continuum (either very high or very low) may not respond at all or may respond in an unpredictable manner. This phenomenon may explain the reactions of patients with brain damage who are labile and lack homeostatic controls for normal function. Under conditions of severe stress, performance can become severely disrupted.

Therapists need to examine *autonomic nervous system* (ANS) responses. The actions of the ANS are typically widespread with multiple systems engaged. The ANS has two main divisions: the sympathetic nervous system (SNS) and the parasympathetic nervous system (PNS) (Table 5.1). The SNS allows actions to be initiated to protect the individual during conditions of stress (*the alarm system*). Motor systems become engaged in carrying out defensive commands, producing *fight or flight responses* (e.g., the aroused patient with TBI may hit or bite). The PNS is activated continuously to maintain *homeostasis*. It shuts down when the SNS is activated and works to restore homeostasis afterward.

Critical components for baseline examination include (1) a representative sampling of ANS responses, including heart rate (HR), blood pressure (BP), respiratory rate (RR), pupil dilation, and sweating; (2) a determination of patient reactivity, including the degree and rate of response to stimulation; and (3) a determination of physiological stressors (e.g., environmental factors). Careful monitoring during a motor performance examination assists in defining homeostatic stability. Specific guidelines for the examination of vital functions can be found in Chapter 2, Examination of Vital Signs.

Autonomic dysregulation is characteristic of certain diseases and conditions and can be seen in patients with TBI, Parkinson's disease, multiple sclerosis (MS), and spinal cord injury (SCI) (particularly injury above T5). Examination of baseline ANS parameters should, therefore, precede other elements of the motor examination in the patient suspected of autonomic instability. Ongoing monitoring is also critical to ensuring that accurate data are collected and to safeguard the patient.

Table 5.1 Effects of Autonomic Nervous System Stimulation

SNS Stimulation	PNS Stimulation
Fight or Flight Response	*Maintains Homeostasis*
Hypervigilance; increased awareness of environment	Decreased awareness of environment
Pupils dilate	Pupils constrict
Heart rate (HR) increases	Heart rate slows
Blood pressure (BP) increases	Blood pressure slows
Respiration increases and quickens	Respiration slows, becomes shallow
Blood flow to muscles increases; blood flow to skin and gastrointestinal track decreases	Blood flow returns to viscera/GI tract
Digestion slows; release of insulin and digestive enzymes slows	Digestion returns
Glucose production and release increases	
Activation of mass muscles	Relaxation of most muscle groups
Sweating increases	Sweating ceases

PNS = parasympathetic nervous system; SNS = sympathetic nervous system.

Cognition

A screening examination of cognitive abilities should include orientation, attention, memory, and executive or higher-order cognition (e.g., calculating abilities, abstract thinking, constructional ability). Abnormalities can occur with neurological disease (e.g., frontal lobe disease, TBI) or psychiatric illness (e.g., panic attacks, depression following stroke). Impaired cognitive function deficits can range from orientation and memory deficits to poor judgment; distractibility; and difficulties in information processing, abstract reasoning, and learning, to name just a few. Patients with deficits across many or all areas of cognitive function demonstrate diffuse or multifocal pathology (e.g., Alzheimer's disease, chronic brain syndrome). Patients with deficits in only one or a few areas of testing typically demonstrate focal deficits (e.g., stroke).[14] The physical therapist may be one of the first professionals to interact with the patient and should be able to screen for cognitive deficits and initiate appropriate referrals. Consultation with an occupational therapist or neuropsychologist is necessary to obtain an accurate picture of these deficits and to help structure the examination of motor function. The reader is referred to Chapter 27, Cognitive and Perceptual Dysfunction.

Orientation

Orientation is the ability to comprehend and to adjust oneself with regard to time, location, and identity of persons. It is examined with respect to (1) *time* (What day/month/season/year is it? What is the time of day?); (2) *place* (Where are you? What city/state are we in? What is the name of this place?); and (3) *person* (What is your name? How old are you? Where were you born? What is the name of your wife/husband?). The therapist records the accuracy of the patient's responses. Findings are documented in the medical record as follows: Patient is alert and oriented ×3 (time, person, place) or ×2 (person, place), depending on the domains correctly identified.

An additional domain that can be examined is *circumstance* (What happened to you? What kind of a place is this? Why do people come here?). To answer these last questions correctly, the individual must be able to take in, store, and recall new information. This may be severely disrupted in the patient with TBI. Disorientation is also common in the patient with delirium or advanced dementia.

Attention

Attention is the directing of consciousness to a person, thing, perception, or thought. It is dependent on the capacity of the brain to process information from the environment or from long-term memory. An individual with intact *selective attention* is able to screen and process relevant sensory information about both the task and the environment while screening out irrelevant information. The complexity and familiarity of the task determine the degree of attention required. If new or complex information is presented, concentration and effort are increased. Patients who are inattentive will have difficulty concentrating. Attention deficits are typically seen in individuals with delirium, brain injury, dementia, mental retardation, or performance anxiety.

Selective attention can be examined by asking the patient to attend to a particular task. For example, the therapist asks the patient to repeat a short list of numbers forward or backward (*digit span test*). The therapist documents the number of digits the patients is able to recall. Normally individuals can recall seven forward and five backward numbers. For patients with communication impairments, the therapist can read a list of items while the patient is asked to identify or signal each time a particular item is mentioned. *Sustained attention* (or vigilance) is examined by determining how long the patient is able to maintain attention on a particular task (time on task). *Alternating attention* (attention flexibility) is examined by requesting the patient to alternate back and forth between two different tasks (e.g., add the first two pairs of numbers, then subtract the next two pairs of numbers). Requesting the patient to perform two tasks simultaneously is used to determine *divided attention.* For example, the patient talks while walking (*Talks While Walking Test*), or walks while locating an object placed to the side (simulated grocery shopping). Documentation should include the specific component of attention examined, timed responses of slowness or hesitation in the response (latency), the duration and frequency of episodes of inattention, the environmental conditions that contribute to or hinder attention abilities, and the amount of required redirection (verbal cueing) to the task.

Memory

Memory is the process of registration, retention, and recall of past experience, knowledge, and ideas. *Declarative (explicit) memory* involves the conscious recollection of facts, past events, experiences, and places. *Motor (procedural or implicit) memory* involves recall of movements or motor information and storage of motor programs, subroutines, or schema as well as perceptual and cognitive skills. Patients with brain injury and deficits in the medial temporal lobe areas and hippocampus demonstrate profound deficits in declarative memory while they may retain elements of motor memory, which is more broadly distributed in the CNS motor areas (striatum, cerebellum, premotor cortex).

The length of time required from initial acquisition into memory also distinguishes types of memory. *Immediate memory* (immediate recall) refers to the immediate registration and recall of information after an interval of a few seconds (e.g., "Repeat these three items after me"). *Short-term memory* (STM) (recent memory) refers to the capability to remember current, day-to-day events (e.g., what was eaten for breakfast, the date), learn new material, and retrieve material after an interval of minutes, hours, or days. *Long-term memory* (LTM) (remote memory) refers to the recall of facts or events that occurred years before (e.g., birthdays, anniversary, historic facts). It includes items an individual would be expected to know.

A simple test for memory involves presenting a short list of words of unrelated objects (e.g., pony, coin, pencil) and asking the patient to repeat those words immediately after presentation (immediate recall) and again 5 minutes after presentation (STM). LTM can be determined by having the patient recall events or persons from his or her past (Where were you born? Where did you go to school? Where do/did you work?). The patient's fund of general knowledge can also be examined (Who is the president? Who was president during World War II?). The questions selected should represent sensitivity to the cultural and educational background of the patient. It is important to consider that memory may be influenced by attention, motivation, rehearsal, fatigue, and other factors. The *Mini-Mental Status Examination* (MMSE) provides a valid and reliable quick screen of cognitive function.[15]

Patients with *amnesia* experience partial or total, permanent or transient loss of memory. *Anterograde amnesia (post-traumatic amnesia)* refers to the inability to learn new material acquired after a brain insult. *Retrograde amnesia* refers to the inability to remember previous learning acquired before the occurrence of a brain insult. Patients with *delirium (acute confusional state)* typically demonstrate impairments in immediate memory and STM along with confusion, agitation, disorientation, and usually illusions or hallucinations. Patients with *dementia* demonstrate broad-based memory and learning impairments. Significant memory deficits are also seen in patients with diffuse encephalopathies, bilateral temporal lesions, and Korsakoff's psychosis (thiamine deficiency). Certain drugs can improve memory (e.g., CNS stimulates, cholinergic agents), whereas other drugs can degrade memory (e.g., benzodiazepines, anticholinergic drugs).

Patients who demonstrate difficulty in retrieving information will often relate that the information is on the "tip of their tongue" (the *tip of the tongue phenomenon*). Various different strategies can be used to facilitate recall of information (e.g., prompting, rehearsal, and repetition). If attention and memory are impaired, instructions during the examination should be kept simple and brief (one-level commands vs. two- or three-level commands). The therapist should structure or choose an environment in which distractions are reduced (i.e., a closed environment) to ensure maximum performance during the examination. Demonstration and positive feedback can assist the patient to understand what is expected and can be used to motivate and improve performance. Use of any memory-enhancing strategies during an examination should be carefully documented in the patient's record. It is also important to remember that diffuse declarative memory deficits can persist while procedural memory for well-learned motor tasks can be retained (e.g., the patient with brain injury remembers how to pedal a bicycle). Documentation should include delineation of declarative versus procedural memory deficits.

Executive Functions

Executive functions (higher cognitive functions) include abstract thinking, problem-solving, judgment, reasoning, and so forth. They represent advanced cognitive function and are dependent on the presence and interaction of basic cognitive functions (i.e., attention, memory, language). The patient with brain injury may demonstrate an inability to manipulate information, initiate and terminate activities, recognize errors, problem-solve, and think abstractly. Insight (the ability to understand either oneself or an external situation) and judgment (the ability to form an opinion, reach a decision, or plan an action after analyzing a problem and comparing choices) are also affected by brain injury.[14] The presence of any of these deficits can significantly impact the examination of motor function, as well as learning and performance. Referral to an occupational therapist and/or neuropsychologist is indicated for comprehensive examination and evaluation (see Chapter 27, Cognitive and Perceptual Dysfunction). Recognition and understanding of these deficits can improve the validity of the motor function examination and the effectiveness of the rehabilitation POC. Collaboration and consistency of team members is paramount in order to reduce potential frustrations and inappropriate expectations.

Communication

The patient's grasp of information and ability to communicate should be ascertained. The physical therapist should listen carefully to spontaneous speech during the initial examination sessions. The patient's understanding of spoken language can be determined using simple tests. Word comprehension can be determined by varying the difficulty of commands, from one- to two- or three-stage commands (e.g., Point to your nose; Point to your right hand and lift your left hand). Repetition and naming can be tested (Repeat after me; name the parts of a watch). Problems with articulation (*dysarthria*) are evidenced by speech errors, such as difficulties with timing, vocal quality, pitch, volume, and breath control. Problems of *fluency*, word flow without pauses or breaks, should be noted. Speech that flows smoothly but contains errors, neologisms (nonsense words), misuse of words, and circumlocutions (word substitution) is indicative of *fluent aphasia* (e.g., Wernicke's aphasia, sensory or receptive aphasia). The patient typically demonstrates deficits in auditory comprehension with well-articulated speech marked by word substitutions.

Speech that is slow and hesitant with limited vocabulary and impaired syntax is indicative of *nonfluent aphasia* (e.g., Broca's aphasia). Articulation is labored and word-finding difficulties are apparent. In some settings, especially the acute hospital setting, the physical therapist may be the first to become aware of communication deficits. Referral to a speech language pathologist is indicated for comprehensive examination and evaluation (see Chapter 28, Neurogenic Disorders of Speech and Language). Recognition and understanding of these deficits can improve the validity of the motor function examination and the effectiveness of the POC. This may include simplifying instructions, using written instructions, or using alternative forms of communication such as gestures, pantomime, or communication boards. A common error is to assume that the patient understands the task at hand when he or she really has no idea what is expected. To ensure accuracy of testing, frequent checks for comprehension should be performed throughout the examination. For example, the use of message discrepancies (saying one thing and gesturing another) can be used to test the patient's level of understanding.

Sensory Integrity and Integration

Sensory information is a critical component of motor function. It provides the necessary feedback for determination of initial position before a movement, error detection during the movement, and movement outcomes necessary to shape further learning. A *closed-loop system* of motor control is defined as "a control system that employs feedback, a reference of correctness, computation of error, and subsequent correction in order to maintain a desired state."[1, p. 462] A variety of feedback sources are used to monitor movement, including visual, vestibular, proprioceptive, and tactile inputs. The term *somatosensation* (or *somatosensory inputs*) is sometimes used to refer to sensory information received from the skin and musculoskeletal systems. The CNS analyzes all available movement information, determines error, and institutes appropriate corrective actions as necessary. Thus, a thorough sensory examination of each of these systems is an important first step in the examination of motor function. See Chapter 3, Examination of Sensory

Function, for a complete discussion of this topic. The primary role of closed-loop systems in motor control appears to be the monitoring of constant states such as posture and balance, and the control of slow movements, or those requiring a high degree of precision or accuracy.

Feedback information is also essential during learning of new motor skills. Patients who have deficits in any movement-monitoring sensory system may be able to compensate with other sensory systems. For example, the patient with major proprioceptive losses can use vision as an error-correcting system to maintain a stable posture. When vision is also impaired (e.g. the patient with diabetic neuropathy and retinopathy), however, postural instability becomes readily apparent. Significant sensory losses and inadequate compensatory shifts to other sensory systems may result in severely disordered movement responses. The patient with proprioceptive losses and severe visual disturbances such as diplopia (commonly seen in the patient with MS) may be unable to maintain a stable posture. An accurate examination, therefore, requires that the therapist not only look at each individual sensory system but also at the overall sensory interaction and integration and the adequacy of compensatory adjustments. Postural tasks, balance, slow (ramp) movements, tracking tasks, or new motor tasks provide the ideal challenge in which to test feedback control mechanisms and closed-loop processes. See discussion in Chapter 6, Examination of Coordination and Balance.

An *open-loop system* of motor control is a "control system with preprogrammed instructions to a set of an effectors; it does not use feedback information and error-detection processes."[1, p. 497] Movements emerge from learned motor schema that contain "a rule, concept, or relationship formed on the basis of experience."[1, p. 499] Rapid and skilled movement sequences or well-learned movements can thus be completed without the benefit of sensory feedback. In reality, most movements have elements of both closed- and open-loop control processes (hybrid control system).

■ ELEMENTS OF THE MOTOR FUNCTION EXAMINATION

Tone

Tone is defined as the resistance of muscle to passive elongation or stretch. It represents a state of slight residual contraction in normally innervated, resting muscle, or steady-state contraction. Tone is influenced by a number of factors, including (1) physical inertia, (2) intrinsic mechanical-elastic stiffness of muscle and connective tissues, and (3) spinal reflex muscle contraction (tonic stretch reflexes). It excludes resistance to passive stretch from fixed soft tissue contracture. Because muscles rarely work in isolation, the term *postural tone* is preferred by some clinicians to describe a pattern of muscular tension that exists throughout the body and affects groups of muscles. Tonal abnormalities are categorized as *hypertonia* (increased above normal resting levels), *hypotonia* (decreased below normal resting levels), or *dystonia* (impaired or disordered tonicity).

Hypertonia

Spasticity

Spasticity is a motor disorder characterized by a velocity-dependent increase in muscle tone with increased resistance to stretch; the larger and quicker the stretch, the stronger the resistance of the spastic muscle. During rapid movement, initial high resistance (spastic catch) may be followed by a sudden inhibition or letting go of the limb (relaxation) in response to a stretch stimulus, termed *clasp-knife response.* Chronic spasticity is associated with contracture, abnormal posturing and deformity, functional limitations, and disability.

Spasticity arises from injury to descending motor pathways from the cortex (pyramidal tracts) or brain stem (medial and lateral vestibulospinal tracts, dorsal reticulospinal tract), producing disinhibition of spinal reflexes with hyperactive tonic stretch reflexes or a failure of reciprocal inhibition. The result is hyperexcitability of the alpha motor neuron pool. It occurs as part of *upper motor neuron (UMN) syndrome.* See Table 5.2 for a review of both the negative and positive features of UMN syndrome. Typical patterns of spasticity that influence both resting posture and movement are seen in UMN syndrome (Table 5.3). In addition, the patient with UMN syndrome will also typically present with spasms, spastic co-contraction, associated reactions, clonus, and the Babinski sign. *Associated reactions* are defined as involuntary movements resulting from activity occurring in other parts of the body (e.g., sneezing, yawning, squeezing the hand). *Clonus* is characterized by cyclical, spasmodic alternation of muscular contraction and relaxation in response to sustained stretch of a spastic muscle. Clonus is common in the plantarflexors but may also occur in other areas of the body such as the jaw or wrist. The *Babinski sign* is dorsiflexion of the great toe with fanning of the other toes on stimulation of the lateral sole of the foot.[16-18]

Rigidity

Rigidity is a hypertonic state characterized by stiffness and resistance to movement that is independent of the velocity of movement. It is associated with lesions of the basal ganglia and is seen in Parkinson's disease. Rigidity is the result of excessive supraspinal drive (upper motor neuron facilitation) acting on alpha motor neurons; spinal reflex mechanisms are typically normal. *Leadpipe rigidity* refers to a constant increase in muscular tone and stiffness of affected muscles. *Cogwheel rigidity* refers to the coexistence of rigidity with tremor producing stiffness and a ratchet-like jerkiness when a body part is manipulated. It is commonly seen in UE movements (e.g., wrist or

Table 5.2 Positive and Negative Features of Upper Motor Neuron Syndrome

Negative Features	Positive Features
Paresis and paralysis	Spasticity
Loss of dexterity	Stereotyped movement synergies; spastic dystonia
Fatigue	Spasms (flexor, extensor/adductor)
	Spastic co-contraction
	Extensor plantar response (Babinski sign)
	Clonus
	Exaggerated deep tendon reflexes (DTR)
	Associated reactions
	Disturbances in movement efficiency and speed; mass movements

elbow flexion and extension). Tremor, bradykinesia, and loss of postural stability are also associated motor deficits in patients with Parkinson's disease.

Decorticate and Decerebrate Rigidity

Severe brain injury can result in coma with decorticate or decerebrate rigidity. *Decorticate rigidity* refers to sustained contraction and posturing of the upper limbs in flexion and the lower limbs in extension. The elbows, wrists, and fingers are held in flexion with shoulders adducted tightly to the sides while the lower extremities (LEs) are held in extension, internal rotation, and plantarflexion. *Decerebrate rigidity* (abnormal extensor response) refers to sustained contraction and posturing of the trunk and limbs in a position of full extension. The elbows are extended with shoulders adducted, forearms pronated, and wrists and fingers flexed. The LEs are held in stiff extension with plantarflexion. Decorticate rigidity is indicative of a corticospinal tract lesion at the level of the diencephalon (above the superior colliculus), whereas decerebrate rigidity indicates a corticospinal lesion in the brain stem between the superior colliculus and vestibular nucleus. *Opisthotonus* is characterized by strong and sustained contraction of the extensor muscles of the neck and trunk, resulting in a rigid, hyperextended posture. Extensor muscles of the proximal limbs may also be involved. These postures are considered exaggerated and severe forms of spasticity.

Dystonia

Dystonia is a prolonged involuntary movement disorder characterized by twisting or writhing repetitive movements and increased muscular tone. *Dystonic posturing* refers to sustained abnormal postures caused by co-contraction of muscles that may last for several minutes or hours, or may be permanent. Dystonia results from a CNS lesion commonly in the basal ganglia and can be inherited (primary idiopathic dystonia), associated with neurodegenerative disorders (Wilson's disease, Parkinson's disease on excessive L-dopa therapy), or metabolic disorders (amino acid or lipid disorders). Dystonia can affect only one part of the body (*focal dystonia*) as seen in spasmodic torticollis (wry neck) or isolated writer's cramp. *Segmental dystonia* affects two or more adjacent areas (e.g., torticollis and dystonic posturing of the UE).[17]

Hypotonia

Hypotonia and *flaccidity* are terms used to define abnormally low tone or absent muscular tone. Resistance to passive movement is diminished, stretch reflexes are dampened or absent, and limbs are easily moved (floppy). Hyperextensibility of joints is common. *Lower motor neuron (LMN) syndrome* results from lesions that affect the anterior horn cell and peripheral nerve (e.g., peripheral neuropathy, cauda equina lesion, radiculopathy). It produces symptoms of decreased or absent tone, decreased or absent reflexes, paresis, muscle fasciculations and fibrillations with denervation, and neurogenic atrophy. Mild decreases in tone along with asthenia (weakness) can also be seen in cerebellar lesions. Acute UMN lesions (e.g., hemiplegia, tetraplegia, paraplegia) can produce temporary hypotonia, termed *spinal shock* or *cerebral shock,* depending on the location of the lesion. The duration of CNS depression and hypotonia that occurs with shock is highly variable, lasting days or weeks. It is typically followed by the development of spasticity and UMN signs.

Examination of Tone

An examination of tone consists of (1) initial observation of resting posture, (2) passive motion testing, and (3) active motion testing. Variability of tone is common. For example, spasticity can vary in presentation from morning to afternoon, day to day, or even hour to hour, depending on a number of factors, including (1) volitional effort and movement, (2) anxiety and pain, (3) position and interaction of tonic reflexes, (4) medications, (5) general health, (6) ambient temperature, and (7) state of CNS arousal or alertness. In addition, urinary bladder status (full or empty), fever and infection, and metabolic and/or electrolyte imbalance can also influence tone. The therapist should therefore consider the impact of each of these factors in determining tone. Repeat (serial) testing and a consistent approach to examination is necessary to improve the accuracy and reliability of test results.[17]

Initial observation of the patient can reveal abnormal posturing of the limbs or body. Careful inspection should be made regarding the position of the limbs, trunk, and head. With spasticity, posturing in fixed, antigravity positions is common; for example, a spastic

Table 5.3 Typical Patterns of Spasticity in Upper Motor Neuron Syndrome

Upper Limbs	Actions	Muscles Affected
Scapula	Retraction, downward rotation	Rhomboids
Shoulder	Adduction and internal rotation, depression	Pectoralis major, latissimus dorsi, teres major, subscapularis
Elbow	Flexion	Biceps, brachialis, brachioradialis
Forearm	Pronation	Pronator teres, pronator quadratus
Wrist	Flexion, adduction	Flexor carpi radialis
Hand	Finger flexion, clenched fist thumb, adducted in palm	Flexor digitorum profundus/sublimis, adductor pollicis brevis, flexor pollicis brevis
Lower Limbs	**Actions**	**Muscles Affected**
Pelvis	Retraction (hip hiking)	Quadratus lumborum
Hip	Adduction (scissoring) Internal rotation Extension	Adductor longus/brevis Adductor magnus, gracilis Gluteus maximus
Knee	Extension	Quadriceps
Foot and ankle	Plantarflexion Inversion Equinovarus Toes claw (tarsometatarsal extension, metatarsophalangeal flexion) Toes curl (tarso- and metatarsophalangeal flexion)	Gastrocnemius/soleus Tibialis posterior Long toe flexors Extensor hallucis longus Peroneus longus
Hip and knee (prolonged sitting posture)	Flexion Sacral sitting	Iliopsoas Rectus femoris, pectineus Hamstrings
Trunk	Lateral flexion with concavity Rotation	Rotators Internal/external obliques
Posture forward (prolonged sitting posture)	Excessive forward flexion Forward head	Rectus abdominis, external obliques Psoas minor

The form and intensity of spasticity may vary greatly, depending on the CNS lesion site and extent of damage. The degree of spasticity can fluctuate within each individual (i.e., due to body position, level of excitation, sensory stimulation, and voluntary effort). Spasticity predominates in antigravity muscles (i.e., the flexors of the upper extremity and the extensors of the lower extremity). If left untreated, spasticity can result in movement deficiencies, subsequent contractures, degenerative joint changes, and deformity.
MP: meta

Adapted from Mayer.[19]

UE is typically held fixed against the body with the shoulder adducted, elbow flexed, forearm supinated with wrist/fingers flexed. In the supine position, the LEs are typically held in extension, adduction with plantarflexion, and inversion (see Table 5.3).[19] Limbs that appear floppy and lifeless (e.g., LE rolled out to the side in external rotation) may indicate hypotonicity. *Palpation* of the muscle belly may yield additional information about the resting state of muscle. Consistency, firmness, and turgor should all be examined. Hypotonic muscles will feel soft and flabby, whereas hypertonic muscles will feel taut and harder than normal.

Passive motion testing reveals information about the responsiveness of muscles to stretch. Because these responses should be examined in the absence of voluntary control, the patient is instructed to relax, letting the therapist support and move the limb. During a passive motion test, the therapist should maintain firm and constant manual contact, moving the limb in all motions. When tone is normal, the limb moves easily and the therapist is able to alter direction and speed without feeling abnormal resistance. The limb is responsive and feels light. Hypertonic limbs generally feel stiff and resistant to movement, whereas flaccid limbs feel heavy and unresponsive. Many older individuals may find it difficult to relax during passive movements (termed *paratonia*); their stiffness should not be mistaken for hypertonicity. Varying the speed of movement is an important determinant of spasticity. In a spastic limb, resistance may be near normal when the limb is moved at a slow velocity. Faster movements intensify the resistance to passive motion. It is also important to remember that muscle stiffness with spasticity will offer the greatest resistance during the first stretch and that with each successive stretch resistance can be reduced by as much as 20% to 60%.[17] In the patient with rigidity, resistance is constant and not responsive to increasing the velocity of passive motion.

Clonus, spasmodic alteration of antagonistic muscle contractions, is examined using a quick stretch stimulus that is then maintained. For example, ankle clonus is tested by sudden dorsiflexion of the foot and maintaining the foot in dorsiflexion. Clasp-knife phenomenon, increased muscle resistance to passive movement followed by a sudden release of the muscle, is examined by passive motion testing. All limbs and body segments are examined, with particular attention given to those identified as problematic in the initial observation. Comparisons should be made between upper and lower limbs and right and left extremities. Asymmetrical tonal abnormalities are typically indicative of neurological dysfunction.

Modified Ashworth Scale

The *Modified Ashworth Scale* (MAS) is the gold standard used to assess muscle spasticity in patients with lesions of the CNS and is commonly used in many rehabilitation facilities (Table 5.4). The original *Ashworth Scale* (AS), a 5-point ordinal scale, was developed as a simple clinical tool to test the efficacy of an antispastic drug in patients with MS.[20] Bohannon and Smith[21] modified the instrument scale by adding an additional 1+ grade to increase the sensitivity of the instrument, making it a 6-point scale. In both versions, the examiner uses passive motion to assess resistance to passive motion due to spasticity. There is a lack of operational definitions as to how fast to move the limb. Thus the MAS measures muscle tone at one, unspecified velocity, which can result in variation in overall reliability. For example, the MAS has been shown to have moderate to good intrarater reliability but only poor to moderate interrater reliability. Reliability has also been shown to vary with the muscles being tested.[22] Limitations with use of the scale include (1) inability to detect small changes, (2) inability to distinguish between soft tissue viscoelastic and neural changes, and (3) problems with psychometric properties (unequal distances of scores). The lower MAS ratings of 1, 1+, and 2 are most problematic. Training is suggested to improve interrater reliability between examiners.[23-29]

Table 5.4 Modified Ashworth Scale for Grading Spasticity

Grade	Description
0	No increase in muscle tone.
1	Slight increase in muscle tone, manifested by a catch and release or by minimal resistance at the end of the ROM when the affected part(s) is moved in flexion or extension.
1+	Slight increase in muscle tone, manifested by a catch, followed by minimal resistance throughout the remainder (less than half) of the ROM.
2	More marked increase in muscle tone through most of the ROM, but affected part(s) easily moved.
3	Considerable increase in muscle tone, passive movement difficult.
4	Affected part(s) rigid in flexion or extension.

From Bohannon and Smith,[21, p. 207] with permission.

Tardieu/Modified Tardieu Scale

The *Tardieu Scale* for assessing spasticity is a performance-based test of the quality of muscle tone during three different velocities: slow-velocity stretch (V1, as slow as possible), the speed of the limb falling under gravity (V2), and fast-velocity stretch (V3, moving as fast as possible).[30,31] The quality of muscle reaction is measured using an ordinal scale (0–5), where 0 is no spasticity, 4 is severe spasticity, and 5 is joint immobility. The *Modified Tardieu Scale* uses an additional measurement of joint angles. One goniometric measurement (R1) is taken at the onset of resistance (catch or clonus) to quick stretch (V3). The second measurement (R2) is taken at the full PROM, taken at very slow speed (V1). The difference between the two measures, R2–R1, represents the velocity-dependent tone component of the muscle. Intrarater reliability is adequate to excellent and varies with muscles tested and training.[32,33] For example, in patients with severe brain injury, reliability ranged from 0.64 to 0.87.[33] Interrater reliabilities are lower and also vary with training.[34-36]

Documentation of Tone Abnormalities

Documentation of tone abnormalities should include a determination of the specific body segments demonstrating abnormal tone, the type of abnormality present (e.g., spasticity, rigidity), whether the changes are symmetrical or asymmetrical, resting postures and associated signs (e.g., UMN syndrome), and factors that modify (increase or diminish) tone. It is important to remember that measurement of tone in one position does not mean that tone will be the same in other positions or during functional activities. A change in position such as sitting up or standing up can substantially alter the requirements for postural tone. Of great importance is a description of the effects of tone on active movements, posture, and function.

Reflex Integrity

Deep Tendon Reflexes

A *reflex* is an involuntary, predictable, and specific response to a stimulus that is dependent on an intact reflex arc (sensory receptor, afferent neurons, efferent neurons, and responding muscles or gland). The *deep tendon reflex* (DTR) results from stimulation of the stretch-sensitive IA afferents of the neuromuscular spindle, producing muscle contraction via a monosynaptic pathway. DTRs are tested by tapping sharply over the muscle tendon with a standard reflex hammer or with the tips of the therapist's fingers. To ensure adequate response, the muscle is positioned in midrange and the patient is instructed to relax. Stimulation can result in observable movement of the joint (brisk or strong responses). Weak responses may be evident only with palpation (slight or sluggish responses with little or no joint movement). The quality and magnitude of responses should be carefully documented. Reflexes are graded on a 0 to 5+ scale:

0 Absent, no response
1+ Low normal, diminished
2+ Normal
3+ Brisker or more reflexive than normal
4+ Very brisk, hyperreflexive, with clonus
5+ Sustained clonus

Table 5.5 presents an overview of the examination of DTRs.

If DTRs are difficult to elicit, responses can be enhanced by specific reinforcement maneuvers. In the *Jendrassik maneuver,* the patient hooks the fingers of both hands together and strongly pulls them apart. While this pressure is maintained, LE reflexes are tested. Maneuvers that can be used to reinforce responses in the

Table 5.5 Examination of Deep Tendon Reflexes

Myostatic Reflexes (Stretch)	Stimulus	Response
Jaw (CN V)	Patient is sitting, with jaw relaxed and slightly open. Place finger on top of chin; tap downward on top of finger in a direction that causes the jaw to open.	Jaw rebounds and closes
Biceps Musculocutaneous nerve (C5, C6)	Patient is sitting with arm flexed and supported. Place thumb over the biceps tendon in the cubital fossa, stretching it slightly. Tap thumb or directly on tendon.	Slight contraction of elbow flexors
Brachioradialis (supinator) Radial nerve (C5, C6)	Patient is sitting with arm flexed onto the abdomen. Place finger on the radial tuberosity and tap finger with hammer.	Slight contraction of elbow flexors, slight wrist extension or radial deviation
Triceps Radial nerve (C6, C7)	Patient is sitting with arm supported in abduction, elbow flexed. Palpate triceps tendon just above olecranon. Tap directly on tendon.	Slight contraction of elbow extensors
Finger flexors Median nerve (C6–T1)	Hold hand in neutral position. Place finger across palmar surface of distal phalanges of four fingers and tap.	Slight contraction of finger flexors
Hamstrings Tibial branch, sciatic nerve (L5, S1, S2)	Patient is prone with knee semiflexed and supported. Palpate tendon at the knee. Tap on finger or directly on tendon.	Slight contraction of knee flexors
Quadriceps (patellar, knee jerk) Femoral nerve (L2, L3, L4)	Patient is sitting with knee flexed, foot unsupported. Tap tendon of quadriceps muscle between the patella and tibial tuberosity.	Slight contraction of knee extensors
Achilles (ankle jerk) Tibial (S1–S2)	Patient is prone with foot over the end of the plinth or sitting with knee flexed and foot held in slight dorsiflexion. Tap tendon just above its insertion on the calcaneus. Maintaining slight tension on the gastrocnemius-soleus group improves the response.	Slight contraction of plantarflexors

upper extremities (UEs) include squeezing the knees together, clenching the teeth, or making a fist with the contralateral extremity. The use of any reinforcing maneuvers to elicit responses in patients with hyporeflexia should be carefully documented.

DTRs are increased in UMN syndrome (e.g., stroke) and decreased in LMN syndrome (e.g., peripheral neuropathy, nerve root compression), cerebellar syndrome, and muscle disease. *Reflex spread* (the extension of the response beyond the muscle normally expected to contract) is indicative of UMN syndrome. Because each DTR arises from specific spinal segments, an absent reflex can be used to identify the level of a spinal lesion (e.g., radiculopathy).

Superficial Cutaneous Reflexes

Superficial cutaneous reflexes are elicited with a light stroke applied to the skin. The expected response is brief contraction of muscles innervated by the same spinal segments receiving the afferent inputs from the cutaneous receptors. A stimulus that is strong may produce irradiation of cutaneous signals with activation of protective withdrawal reflexes. Cutaneous reflexes include the plantar reflex, confirming toe signs (Chaddock), and abdominal reflexes. The *plantar reflex* (S1, S2) is tested by applying a stroking stimulus on the sole of the foot along the lateral border and up across the ball of the foot. A normal response consists of flexion of the big toe; sometimes the other toes will demonstrate a downgoing (flexion) response or no response at all. An abnormal response (*positive Babinski sign*) consists of extension (upgoing) of the big toe, with fanning of the lateral four toes. It is indicative of a corticospinal (UMN) lesion. The *Chaddock's sign* is elicited by stroking around the lateral ankle and up the lateral dorsal aspect of the foot. It also produces extension of the big toe and is considered a confirmatory toe sign. The *abdominal reflex* is elicited with brisk, light strokes over the skin of the abdominal muscles. A localized contraction under the stimulus is produced, with a resultant deviation of the umbilicus toward the area stimulated. Each of the four quadrants should be tested in a diagonal direction. Umbilical deviation in a superior/lateral direction indicates integrity of spinal segments T8 to T9. Umbilical deviation in an inferior/lateral direction indicates integrity of spinal segments T10 to T12. Loss of response is abnormal and indicative of pathology (e.g., thoracic spinal cord injury). Asymmetry from side to side is highly significant with respect to neurological disease. Abdominal reflexes may be absent in patients with obesity or abdominal surgeries. Table 5.6 presents an overview of the examination of superficial cutaneous reflexes.

Primitive and Tonic Reflexes

Primitive and *tonic reflexes* are present during infancy as a stage in normal development and become integrated by the CNS at an early age. Once integrated, these reflexes are not generally recognizable in adults in their pure form. They may continue, however, as adaptive fragments of behavior, underlying normal motor control. Persistent reflexes (sometimes termed *obligatory reflexes*) beyond the expected age of development or appearing in adult patients following brain injury are always indicative of neurological involvement. Patients who exhibit these reflexes typically present with extensive brain damage (e.g., stroke, TBI) and other UMN signs.

Reflexes important to examine in the patient suspected of abnormal reflex activity include flexor withdrawal, traction, grasp, tonic neck, tonic labyrinthine, positive support, and associated reactions. *Flexor withdrawal reflex*

Table 5.6 Examination of Superficial Cutaneous Reflexes

Superficial Reflexes (Cutaneous)	Stimulus	Response
Plantar (S1, S2)	With blunt object (key or wooden end of applicator stick), stroke the lateral aspect of the sole, moving from the heel to the ball of the foot, curving medially across the ball of the foot. Alternate stimuli for plantar (for sensitive feet): • Chaddock: stroke lateral ankle and lateral aspect of foot. • Oppenheim: stroke down tibial crest	Normal response is flexion (plantarflexion) of the great toe and sometimes the other toes (negative Babinski sign). Abnormal response, termed a *positive Babinski sign,* is extension (dorsiflexion) of the great toe with fanning of the four other toes (indicates UMN lesions). Same as for plantar.
Abdominal reflexes Above umbilicus = T8–T10 Below umbilicus = T10–T12	Position patient in supine, relaxed. Make brisk, light stroke over each quadrant of the abdominals from the periphery to the umbilicus.	Localized contraction under the stimulus, causing the umbilicus to move toward the stimulus. Note: can be masked by obesity.

is generally the simplest to observe and is judged by appearance of an overt movement response. *Tonic neck reflexes,* on the other hand, bias the musculature and may not be visible through overt movement responses. In fact, movement is rarely produced but rather posture is typically influenced through tonal adjustments. Thus, the term *tuning reflexes* is an appropriate description of their function. Abnormal postures should be examined for their reflex dependence (e.g., the patient with brain injury exhibits excessive extensor tone in supine but not in sidelying). To obtain an accurate examination, the therapist must be concerned with several factors. The patient must be positioned appropriately to allow for the expected response. An adequate test stimulus is essential, including both an adequate magnitude and duration of stimulation. Keen observation skills are needed to detect what may be subtle movement changes and abnormal responses. Palpation skills can assist in identifying tonal changes not readily apparent to the eye. Primitive and tonic reflexes are graded using a 0 to 4+ scale[37]:

- 0+ Absent
- 1+ Tone change: slight, transient with no movement of the extremities
- 2+ Visible movement of extremities
- 3+ Exaggerated, full movement of extremities
- 4+ Obligatory and sustained movement, lasting for more than 30 seconds

Table 5.7 presents an overview of the examination of primitive and tonic reflexes.

Documentation of Reflex Integrity

Documentation of reflex abnormalities should include a determination of (1) specific reflexes tested; (2) findings, including degree of abnormality found (specific deficits); (3) associated signs (e.g., UMN syndrome); and (4) factors that influence or modify reflexes. Of great importance is a description of the effects of abnormal reflex behavior on active movements, posture, and function.

Cranial Nerve Integrity

There are 12 pairs of cranial nerves (CNs), all distributed to the head and neck with the exception of CN X (vagus), which is distributed to the thorax and abdomen. CNs I, II, and VIII are purely sensory and carry the special senses of smell, vision, hearing, and equilibrium. Cranial nerves III, IV, and VI are purely motor and control pupillary constriction and eye movements. Cranial nerves XI and XII are also purely motor, innervating the sternocleidomastoid, trapezius, and tongue muscles. Cranial nerves V, VII, IX, and X are mixed, containing both motor and sensory fibers. Motor functions include chewing (V), facial expression (VII), swallowing (IX, X), and vocal sounds (X). Sensations are carried from the face and head (V, VII, IX), alimentary tract, heart, vessels, lungs (IX, X), and tongue, mouth, and palate (VII, IX, X). Parasympathetic secretomotor fibers (ANS) are carried by CN III for control of smooth muscles in the eyeball, VII for control of salivary and lacrimal glands, IX to the parotid salivary gland, and X to the heart, lungs, and most of the digestive system.

An examination of CN function should be performed with suspected lesions of the brain, brain stem, and cervical spine. Deficits in olfactory function (CN I) should be suspected with lesions of the nasal cavity and anterior/inferior cerebrum. Lesions of the optic pathways (optic nerve [CN II], optic chiasma, optic tract, lateral geniculate body, superior colliculus) and visual cortex may produce visual deficits. Midbrain (mesencephalic) lesions may result in deficits of CNs III and IV (oculomotor, trochlear). Pontine lesions may involve several CNs, including V (ophthalmic, maxillary, and mandibular branches) and VI (abducens). Nuclei of CNs VII (facial) and VIII (vestibular and cochlear branches) are located at the junction of the pons and medulla. Lesions affecting the medulla may involve CNs IX (glossopharyngeal), X (vagus), XI (spinal accessory), and XII (hypoglossal). The spinal root of XI is found in the upper five cervical segments. The CNs, their function, clinical tests, and possible abnormal findings are presented in Table 5.8.

Documentation of Cranial Nerve Integrity

Documentation of an examination of CN integrity should include a determination of (1) specific cranial nerves tested; (2) findings, including the degree of abnormality observed (specific deficits); and (3) the effects of abnormal cranial nerve integrity on function. The patient's perceptions of loss of function should also be identified.

Musculoskeletal Integrity

Examination of the musculoskeletal system is essential and should occur early in the examination of motor function. Important elements include joint integrity and mobility, as well as muscle performance, including strength, power, endurance, and length. See discussion in Chapter 6, Musculoskeletal Examination.

Postural Alignment, Joint Integrity, and Mobility

Joint limitations restrict the normal coordinated action of muscles and alter the biomechanical alignment of body segments and posture. Long-standing immobilization results in contracture (a fixed resistance resulting from fibrosis of tissues surrounding a joint) and restricted movement. The resultant compensatory movement patterns are frequently dysfunctional, producing additional stresses and strains on the musculoskeletal system. They are also more energy costly and can significantly limit motor and functional performance. For example, shortening of the gastrocnemius muscles results in a toe-walking gait pattern; tightness of the hip adductors results in a scissoring gait pattern. Changes in alignment secondary

Table 5.7 Examination of Primitive and Tonic Reflexes

Primitive/Spinal Reflexes	Stimulus	Response
Flexor withdrawal	Noxious stimulus (pinprick) to sole of foot. Tested in supine or sitting position.	Toes extend, foot dorsiflexes, entire LE flexes uncontrollably. Onset: 28 weeks of gestation. Integrated: 1–2 months.
Crossed extension	Noxious stimulus to ball of foot of LE fixed in extension; tested in supine position.	Opposite LE flexes, then adducts and extends. Onset: 28 weeks' gestation. Integrated: 1–2 months.
Traction	Grasp forearm and pull up from supine into sitting position.	Grasp and total flexion of the UE. Onset: 28 weeks' gestation. Integrated: 2–5 months.
Moro	Sudden change in position of head in relation to trunk; drop patient backward from sitting position.	Extension, abduction of UEs, hand opening, and crying followed by flexion, adduction of arms across chest. Onset: 28 weeks' gestation. Integrated: 5–6 months.
Startle	Sudden loud or harsh noise.	Sudden extension or abduction of UEs, crying. Onset: birth. Integrated: persists.
Grasp	Maintained pressure to palm of hand (palmar grasp) or to ball of foot under toes (plantar grasp).	Maintained flexion of fingers or toes. Onset: palmar, birth; plantar, 28 weeks' gestation. Integrated: palmer, 4–6 months; plantar, 9 months.
Tonic/brain stem reflexes	Stimulus	Response
Asymmetrical tonic neck (ATNR)	Rotation of the head to one side.	Flexion of skull limbs, extension of the jaw limbs, "bow and arrow" or "fencing" posture. Onset: birth. Integrated: 4–6 months.
Symmetrical tonic neck (STNR)	Flexion or extension of the head.	With head flexion: flexion of UEs, extension of LEs; with head extension: extension of UEs, flexion of LEs. Onset: 4–6 months. Integrated: 8–12 months.
Symmetrical tonic labyrinthine (TLR or STLR)	Prone or supine position.	With prone position: increased flexor tone/flexion of all limbs; with supine: increased extensor tone/extension of all limbs. Onset: birth. Integrated: 6 months.
Positive supporting	Contact to the ball of the foot in upright standing position.	Rigid extension (co-contraction) of the LEs. Onset: birth. Integrated: 6 months.
Associated reactions	Resisted voluntary movement in any part of the body.	Involuntary movement in a resting extremity. Onset: birth–3 months. Integrated: 8–9 years.

LE = lower extremity; UE = upper extremity.

Table 5.8 Examination of Cranial Nerve Integrity

Cranial Nerve	Function	Test	Possible Abnormal Findings
I **Olfactory**	Olfaction (Smell)	Test sense of smell on each side (close off other nostril): use common, nonirritating odors.	Anosmia (inability to detect smells), seen with frontal lobe lesions.
II **Optic**	Vision	Visual acuity test: uses Snellen eye chart; test each eye separately (covering other eye); test at distance of 20 ft. Visual field test: test temporal and vertical peripheral vision (visual fields) by confrontation.	Blindness, myopia (impaired far vision), presbyopia (impaired near vision) Field defects: homonymous hemianopsia.
III **Oculomotor**	Pupillary reflex Accommodation Convergence	Shine light in eye: pupil constricts Eye accommodates to light Pupils move medially when viewing object at close range	Absence of pupillary constriction Lateral strabismus (Exotropia) Anisocoria (unequal pupils) Horner's syndrome, CN III paralysis
III, IV, VI **Oculomotor, trochlear, and abducens** (tested simultaneously)	Extraocular movements CN III: turns eye up, down, in; elevates eyelid CN IV: turns eye down when adducted CN VI: turns eye out	Test saccadic movements: ask patient to look up, down, medial, and lateral Test pursuit eye movements: ask patient to follow moving finger Test one eye at a time; other eye occluded	Lateral strabismus: eyeball turns lateral; can cause diplopia or nystagmus Impaired eye movements Ptosis Medial strabismus: eyeball turns inward; can cause diplopia or nystagmus
V **Trigeminal: ophthalmic, maxillary, mandibular divisions**	Sensory function: face Sensory: cornea Motor function: muscles of mastication	Test pain, light touch sensations: forehead, cheeks, inner oral cavity (occlude vision). Test corneal reflex: touch lightly with wisp of cotton. Palpate temporal and masseter muscles. Observe spontaneous movements. Have patient open mouth, move jaw side to side. Bite down on tongue depressor, hold against resistance	Loss of facial sensations, numbness with CN V lesion Trigger area with trigeminal neuralgia Loss of corneal reflex ipsilaterally (blinking in response to corneal touch) Weakness, wasting of muscles When opened, deviation of jaw to ipsilateral side Asymmetry of jaw movement Asymmetry of jaw strength

Continued

Table 5.8 Examination of Cranial Nerve Integrity—cont'd

Cranial Nerve	Function	Test	Possible Abnormal Findings
VII Facial	Motor function: facial muscles	Test strength and symmetry of facial muscles: have patient elevate eyebrows and forehead; wrinkle forehead, smile, frown, and pucker lips, close eyes tightly, puff out both cheeks.	Paralysis: Inability to close eye, drooping corner of mouth, difficulty with speech articulation Unilateral LMN: Bell's palsy (PNI) Bilateral LMN: Guillain-Barré Unilateral UMN: stroke
	Sensory function: taste to anterior two thirds of tongue	Apply sweet, salty, and sour solutions to outer and lateral portions of anterior tongue using a cotton swab (occlude vision).	Incorrectly identifies solution Decreased taste
VIII Vestibulocochlear	Vestibular function	Test balance and protective functions: vestibulospinal function (VSR) Test eye–head coordination: vestibular ocular reflex (VOR)	Vertigo, decreased balance, decreased protective responses (disequilibrium) Gaze instability with head rotations, nystagmus (constant, involuntary cyclical movement of the eyeball)
	Cochlear function	Test auditory acuity Weber test for lateralization: place vibrating tuning fork on top of head, mid-position; check if sound heard in one ear, or equally in both Rinne test: Compares air and bone conduction, place vibrating tuning fork on mastoid bone, then close to ear canal; sound heard longer through air than bone	Deafness, impaired hearing, tinnitus Unilateral conductive loss: sound lateralized to impaired ear Sensorineural loss: sound heard in good ear Conductive loss: sound heard through bone is equal to or longer than air Sensorineural loss: sound heard longer through air
IX Glossopharyngeal	Sensory function: posterior one-third of tongue, pharynx, middle ear	Apply sweet, salty, and sour solutions to posterior tongue	Incorrectly identifies solution, loss of taste on posterior tongue
IX, X Glossopharyngeal and Vagus (tested simultaneously)	Phonation	Listen to voice quality	Dysphonia: hoarse voice; denotes vocal cord weakness; nasal quality denotes palatal weakness
	Swallowing	Examine for difficulty in swallowing: glass of water, different consistencies of food	Dysphagia: difficulty swallowing; loss of swallowing reflexes
	Palatal, pharynx control	Have patient say "ah"; observe motion of soft palate (elevates) and position of uvula (remains midline).	Dysarthria: difficulty articulating words clearly, slurs words Palate fails to elevate, (lesion of CN X); asymmetrical elevation with unilateral paralysis
	Gag reflex	Stimulate back of throat lightly on each side.	Loss of gag reflex: lesion of CN IX; possibly CN X

Table 5.8 Examination of Cranial Nerve Integrity—cont'd

Cranial Nerve	Function	Test	Possible Abnormal Findings
XI Accessory	Motor function Spinal nerve root Trapezius muscle	Examine bulk, strength. In sitting, ask patient to elevate the shoulder upward against resistance applied in the direction of depression.	LMN: atrophy, fasciculations, weakness Weakness, inability to approximate the acromion and the occiput
	Sternocleidomastoid	In supine, ask patient to flex head anterolaterally and rotate head to opposite side; resistance is applied in an obliquely posterior direction.	Weakness, inability to flex head laterally and forward, rotate head to contralateral side
	Cranial nerve root:	Examine laryngeal elevation by placing index and middle fingers over patient's Adam's apple (laryngeal muscles); ask patient to swallow	Dysphagia due to decreased laryngeal elevation
XII Hypoglossal	Motor function: tongue movements	Listen to patient's articulation.	Dysarthria (seen with lesions of CN X or CN XII, also V, VII)
		Examine resting position of tongue.	Atrophy or fasciculations of tongue (LMN, ALS)
		Ask patient to protrude tongue, move tongue side to side	Impaired movements with deviation of tongue to weak side UMN lesion: tongue deviates away from side of cortical lesion Check for tongue tremors or involuntary tongue movements

to muscle tightness alter postural control. For example, in standing, anterior pelvic tilting and flexion of the hips and knees are typically the result of hip flexor tightness. In sitting, posterior pelvic tilting is associated with kyphosis and forward head position and is typically the result of hamstring tightness. Abnormalities in alignment that alter the center of mass (COM) within the base of support (BOS) place increased demands on the postural control system. For example, the patient with chronic stroke will demonstrate altered postural alignment in standing with more weight distributed over the less affected limb and away from the more affected limb. This patient also typically demonstrates a more forward leaning posture with greater anterior pelvic tilt, resulting in limitations in balance and postural control.[38]

Muscle Atrophy

Atrophy, the loss of muscle bulk (wasting), occurs when functional mobility is lost (disuse atrophy) and from LMN disease (neurogenic atrophy) or protein–calorie malnutrition. *Disuse atrophy* is evident after periods of inactivity, developing in weeks or months. It is generally widespread and affects antigravity muscles to a greater extent. Strength can be negatively influenced by disuse atrophy. The lack of resistive load on muscle reduces the overall number of sarcomeres and results in diminished capacity of muscle for developing torque (contractile strength). It also results in reduced passive tension of muscle with loss of joint stability and increased risk for postural abnormality.[39] *Neurogenic atrophy* accompanies LMN injury (e.g., peripheral nerve injury, spinal root injury) and occurs rapidly, generally within 2 to 3 weeks. Atrophy is also accompanied by other signs of LMN injury (e.g., decreased or absent tone, decreased or absent DTRs, fasciculations, weak or absent voluntary movements). Distribution is limited to a segmental or focal pattern (nerve root).

Examination of Muscle Atrophy

During the examination of muscle atrophy, the therapist should visually inspect the muscle symmetry and shapes, comparing and contrasting their size and contour. Muscles that look flat or concave are indicative of atrophy. Comparisons should be made between and within limbs. Is the atrophy unilateral or bilateral? Are multiple limbs involved? Is the atrophy more proximal, or distal, or both? Limb girth measurements can be used to compare a limb undergoing neurogenic atrophy with the corresponding normal limb. Palpation at rest and during muscle contraction is used to determine muscle tension.

Girth measurements or volumetric displacement measures (e.g., hands or feet) can be used to confirm visual inspection findings.

Strength and Power

Muscle performance is the capacity of muscle(s) to generate forces while *muscle strength* is the force exerted by muscle(s) to overcome a resistance.[6] Isotonic contractions involve active shortening of muscles, and eccentric contractions involve active lengthening of muscles. Isometric contractions produce high levels of tension for holding contractions without overt movement. *Muscle power* is defined as the work produced per unit of time or the product of strength and speed.[6] Muscle performance depends on a number of interrelated factors, including length–tension characteristics, viscoelasticity, velocity, and metabolic adequacy (i.e., fuel storage and delivery). Of equal importance are the integrated actions of the CNS (neuromuscular control factors) acting on motor units, including (1) the number of motor units recruited, (2) the type of motor units recruited, and (3) the discharge rate and continuing modulation of motor units. The CNS controls the recruitment order and timing of muscles. Synergistic movements and postural adjustments are also dependent on the integrity of the peripheral nerves and on the muscle fibers.

Patients with impairments in motor function and neurological injury pose unique challenges for the examination of muscle performance. *Weakness* is the inability to generate sufficient levels of force and can vary from *paresis* (partial weakness) to *plegia* (absence of muscle strength). Weakness is seen in patients with UMN syndrome, along with other UMN signs (e.g., spasticity, hyperreflexia). Patients may present with *hemiplegia* (one-sided paralysis), *paraplegia* (LE paralysis), or *tetraplegia* (quadriplegia). Weakness also appears in patients with LMN lesions.

Patients with stroke demonstrate significant changes in muscle performance, including altered recruitment patterns, abnormal times to achieve force, and decreased motor unit firing rates.[40] They also demonstrate up to a 50% decrease in motor units of affected extremities within 2 months after insult with greater losses of Type II (fast twitch) fibers.[41] Muscle performance in patients with stroke is influenced by the presence of other UMN impairments, including spasticity, disordered synergistic activity/mass patterns of movements, abnormal muscle co-contraction, and/or profound sensory deficit.[42-44] Strength losses are typically greater in the distal extremity than the proximal. Strength losses have also been found on the "supposedly normal" extremities.[45,46] The bilateral effects of an ipsilateral cortical lesion is evidence of the small percentage (estimated 10%) of corticospinal tract fibers that remain uncrossed. Possible other unidentified factors may also exist. This information has prompted use of terms such as *less involved* or *less affected* in place of more traditional terms such as *unaffected, uninvolved, sound, normal,* or *good* side. This also casts doubt as to the validity of using the contralateral uninvolved side as a reference for normal muscle strength in patients with hemiplegia.

In patients with peripheral sensorimotor neuropathy (e.g., chronic diabetic neuropathy) or acute motor neuropathy (e.g., Guillain-Barré), strength losses are typically greater in distal segments (i.e., foot and ankle) than proximal with involvement of more proximal segments as the disease progresses. In neuropathy, the progression is slow (months or years), whereas in Guillain-Barré the progression is rapid (days or weeks) and more complete, involving not just the proximal LEs but also the trunk, UEs, and in some cases the lower CN nerves. Patients with primary muscle disease (e.g., myopathies) typically experience proximal weakness, whereas patients with myasthenia gravis experience decremental strength losses. Thus, the first contraction of a muscle may start out strong and then each succeeding contraction gets weaker and weaker.

Examination of Muscle Strength and Power

The clinical examination of muscle strength and power utilizes standardized methods and protocols (e.g., manual muscle testing [MMT], handheld dynamometers, instrumented isokinetic systems). See Chapter 4, Musculoskeletal Examination, for a thorough discussion of this topic. Analysis of muscle timing, including amplitude, duration, waveform, and frequency can be obtained using EMG (see later section in this chapter on EMG examination). Activity analysis of functional performance also yields important data about muscle performance.

Strength testing measures (MMT) were originally developed to examine motor function in patients with polio (an LMN disease). There are validity issues when used in the clinical examination of patients with UMN lesions.[47,48] Strength testing using standardized protocols may be inappropriate for some patients with UMN syndrome. Appropriate criteria are therefore critical in determining whether the standards of validity and reliability of MMT are met. First and foremost, the therapist must consider the patient's movement capabilities. Individual isolated joint movements, mandated by standardized MMT procedures and isokinetic protocols, may not be possible in the presence of UMN lesion where stereotypical abnormal movement patterns (obligatory synergies) are present. The presence of abnormal co-activation, spasticity, and abnormal posturing may preclude the patient's ability to perform isolated joint movements. These barriers to normal movement are termed *active restraint.* The prescribed test positions may also be precluded by the presence of abnormal reflex activity (e.g., supine testing influenced by presence of the tonic labyrinthine reflex). Muscle and soft tissue changes in viscoelasticity (e.g., contracture) offer a form of *passive restraint* and may also preclude the use of standardized testing. In these instances, the decision should be made *not* to use standardized MMT procedures. An estimation of strength can be made from observations of active movements during performance of functional activities. For example, shallow knee bends or sit-to-stand transfers can be used to examine the strength of hip extensors and knee extensors. Standing heel-rises or toe-rises can be used to examine the strength of foot–ankle muscles (dorsiflexors, plantarflexors). Documentation should clearly indicate that UMN involvement precluded use of standardized MMT procedures. Estimates of strength can be made based on observations during active functional movements. Inability to move or support the body against gravity should receive a poor grade. The ability to move the body against gravity should receive a fair grade, while the ability to move the body against gravity and resistance should receive a good grade. When using functional tasks, it is important to remember that muscle performance is graded using the synergistic actions of muscles acting together and not the isolated actions of individual muscles as required in the MMT.

If MMT is used, therapists should utilize standardized positions whenever possible. If a modified position is required (e.g., the patient lacks full range of motion [ROM] or adequate stabilization), it should be carefully documented. *Substitutions* (muscle actions that compensate for specific muscle weakness) should be identified, eliminated whenever possible, and carefully documented. For example, the patient with SCI typically presents with common muscle substitutions (e.g., wrist extensors are used to close the fingers using tenodesis grasp). Knowledge of common substitutions is very helpful when working with this patient group.

Isokinetic testing is an important part of a comprehensive examination of patients with disorders of motor function. It allows the therapist to monitor many important parameters of motor function, including a muscle's ability to generate force throughout the range, peak torques, and ability to generate torques at changing velocities (velocity-spectrum testing). Rate of tension development (time to peak torque) and shape of the torque curve can also be determined. Concentric, isometric, and eccentric contractions and reciprocal agonist/antagonist relationships can be analyzed. Testing results yield important information for understanding functional performance.[49-52] Validity and reliability of isokinetic testing is well established.[53-57]

Patients with stroke typically demonstrate a variety of deficits when tested with an isokinetic dynamometer, including (1) decreased torque overall in the more affected limb when compared to the less affected limb; (2) decreased torque with increasing movement speeds; (3) decreased limb excursion; (4) extended times to peak torque development and the duration time peak torque is held; and (5) increased time intervals between reciprocal contractions. For example, many patients with stroke are unable to develop tension above 70° to 80° per second. When this value is compared to the speed needed for normal walking (100° per second), reasons for gait difficulties become readily apparent. Normative data, when available, can provide an appropriate reference for evaluating and interpreting patient data.[59,60]

Documentation of Strength and Power

Documentation of strength and power changes should include a determination of the specific muscles and body segments tested and tests used; the type and degree of changes present (e.g., paresis, paralysis); whether the changes are symmetrical or asymmetrical, distal or proximal; presence of associated signs (e.g., UMN or LMN); presence of atrophy; and factors that modify muscle performance. A description of the effects of muscle weakness on active movements, posture, and function should be included. When examining functional performance, it is important to remember that strength estimates taken in one position do not necessarily generalize to other positions (e.g., ability to move while supporting full body weight in upright standing).

Muscle Endurance and Fatigue

Muscle endurance allows the muscle to sustain forces or to generate forces repeatedly over time.[6] An examination of muscle endurance is important in determining functional capacity. Fatigue is an overwhelming sustained sense of exhaustion and decreased capacity for physical and mental work at the usual level. Fatigue can be the result of excessive activity caused by an accumulation of metabolic waste products (e.g., lactic acid); malnutrition (i.e., deficiency of nutrients); cardiorespiratory disturbances (i.e., inadequate oxygen and nutrients to the tissues); emotional stress; and other factors. Although fatigue is protective and serves a useful function in guarding against overwork and injury, it is a serious problem for some individuals. For example, patients with postpolio syndrome or chronic fatigue syndrome may experience significant restrictions in their functional activities and work as a result of debilitating fatigue. Other groups of individuals who may also experience significant limitations as a result of fatigue include those with MS, Parkinson's disease (PD), amyotrophic lateral sclerosis (ALS), Duchenne muscular dystrophy, and Guillain-Barré syndrome. Additional factors that can influence fatigue include health status, environmental context (e.g., stressful environment), and temperature (e.g., heat stress in the patient with MS).[61]

Exhaustion is defined as the limit of endurance, beyond which no further performance is possible. Most patients can report with great accuracy the point at which exhaustion is reached. Of concern with some patients is *overwork weakness (injury),* defined as "a prolonged decrease in absolute strength and endurance due to excessive activity of partially denervated muscle."[62, p. 22] For example, patients with postpolio syndrome may experience weakness following strenuous activity that is not recovered with ordinary rest. They report having to spend the entire next day or two in bed following an exhaustive exercise session. It is therefore important to document the type, length, and effectiveness of rest attempts. *Delayed onset muscle soreness* is prolonged in patients with overwork weakness, peaking between 1 and 5 days after activity.

Examination of Fatigue

An examination of fatigue begins with the initial interview. The patient is asked to identify those activities that are fatiguing, the frequency and severity of fatigue episodes, and the circumstances surrounding the onset of fatigue. It is important to identify the *fatigue threshold,* which is that level of exercise that cannot be sustained.[63] In most cases, the onset of fatigue is gradual, not abrupt, and dependent on the intensity and duration of the activity attempted. Precipitating activities should be identified within the context of habitual daily activity. The patient is asked to identify any solutions used to overcome debilitating fatigue and how successful they are.

Self-assessment questionnaires are particularly useful for the patient with significant fatigue. The *Modified Fatigue Impact Scale* (MFIS) is an instrument initially developed to assess quality-of-life problems related to fatigue in patients with MS. The scale has 21 items that focus on three areas of function. It uses a 5-point Likert scale, with 0 = Never to 4 = Almost always. The total score is 0 to 84, with subscales for physical (0–36), cognitive (0–40), and psychosocial (0–8) functioning.[64,65] It has excellent test-retest reliability (ICC = 0.85) when used with patients with MS.[66] The *Fatigue Severity Scale* is a 9-item questionnaire with questions that focus on the severity of fatigue and how it interferes with activity levels and lifestyle. The items are scored on a 7-point scale, with 1 = strongly disagree and 7= strongly agree. It has been used with multiple populations, including those with MS, PD, and post-polio syndrome, and has been shown to be a good screening tool in PD.[67-71]

The examination can then proceed with specific performance-based testing. As this is likely to be fatiguing to the patient, performance testing should focus on those key functional activities important to the patient's daily life that were identified in the earlier interview or questionnaire. The therapist should carefully document the patient's reported level of fatigue during performance testing. The level of independence, modified independence (device required), or level of assistance required (minimal, moderate, or maximal) should also be documented. The grading criteria for the *Functional Independence Measure* (FIM) provides a useful scoring key, and the functional activities tested (e.g., transfers, locomotion) are basic to independent living.[72] During performance testing, perceived level of fatigue can also be documented using the *Borg Scale for Rating of Perceived Exertion.*[73] In order to better determine the level of muscle fatigue, the therapist should ask the patient to identify two separate scores, one for the level of muscular fatigue and one for the level of central fatigue (breathlessness). Timed performance on functional tasks (e.g., timed self-care tasks, time to walk, 6-minute walk test) also provides objective and reproducible measures of levels of muscle fatigue.

Documentation

Documentation of muscle endurance and fatigue should include a determination of (1) activities that result in debilitating fatigue, including onset, duration, and recovery; (2) level of assistance or assistive devices required; (3) the time on task; (4) the frequency and effectiveness of rest attempts; (5) any compensatory strategies adopted and their effectiveness; and (6) perceived impact on quality of life. Results of specific questionnaires and tests are documented. Social and environmental stressors should also be described along with the patient's emotional/psychological responses (e.g., degree of depression or anxiety).

Voluntary Movements

Synergies are functionally linked muscles that are constrained by the CNS to act cooperatively to produce an intended motor action. They are used to simplify control, reduce or constrain the degrees of freedom, and initiate coordinated patterns of movement. *Degrees of freedom* refers to the number of separate independent dimensions of movement that must be controlled by engaging these cooperative units of muscle action.[1] Synergistic movements are defined by precise spatial and temporal organization that requires a high degree of coordination involving control of speed, distance, direction, rhythm, and levels of muscle tension. In individuals with normal motor control, voluntary movement patterns are functional, task specific, and highly variable, depending on the task purpose and environment. The CNS controls patterns of (1) single-limb and multiple-limb movements, (2) bilateral (bimanual) symmetrical and asymmetrical movements, (3) reciprocal movements, and (4) patterns of proximal stabilization and postural support. Movements are also appropriately timed with events in the environment (*coincident timing*).

Abnormal Patterns of Movement

Organization of movement is typically disturbed with pathology of the CNS. Lesions of the cerebellum produce significant deficits in coordination (i.e., dyssynergia, dysmetria, dysdiadochokinesia, tremor, dysarthria, gait ataxia), tone (i.e., hypotonia), and strength (i.e., asthenia). Lesions of the basal ganglia produce significant deficits in tone and movement (i.e., rigidity, tremor, akinesia, bradykinesia, dystonia, chorea, hemiballismus). See Chapter 6, Examination of Coordination and Balance, for a complete discussion.

Lesions of the corticospinal tracts (e.g., stroke, TBI) can produce atypical movement patterns or abnormal *obligatory synergies,* defined as movements that are primitive and highly stereotyped. Voluntary movements are limited with loss of ability to adapt movements to changing demands. Selective movement control (isolated joint movements) is severely disordered or disappears completely. Patients with stroke typically demonstrate obligatory flexion and extension synergies (see Chapter 15, Stroke). Abnormal synergies are highly predictable and characteristic of the middle stages of recovery from stroke.[74,75]

The examination of obligatory synergistic patterns is both qualitative and quantitative. The therapist observes whether voluntary movement can be initiated, whether it can be completed, and how the movement is carried out. If movement is stereotypic and obligatory, what muscle groups are linked together? How strong are the linkages between muscle groups? Are there linkages between upper and lower limbs or one side to another (associated reactions)? Are the movements influenced by other components of UMN syndrome, such as primitive reflexes, spasticity, paresis, or position? For example, does elbow, wrist, and finger flexion always occur when shoulder flexion is initiated? Is head turning used to initiate or reinforce UE flexion (asymmetric tonic neck reflex [ATNR])? Therapists also need to identify when these patterns occur, under what circumstances, and what variations are possible. In patients with brain lesions, lessening of abnormal synergy dominance and emergence of selective movement control are evidence of recovery. Disability-specific measures such as the *Fugl-Meyer Post-Stroke Assessment of Physical Performance* have been developed to provide an objective and quantifiable measure of obligatory synergies and recovery after stroke[76] (see Chapter 15, Stroke). Many of the available standardized tests and measures to assess abnormal movement patterns and control are discussed in later chapters. For example, tests and measures used to assess voluntary movement control include *Motor Assessment Scale,*[77] *Rivermead Mobility Index,*[78] *Wolf Motor Function Test,*[79] *Motor Activity Log,*[80] *Arm Motor Ability Test.*[81]

Abnormal Postural Patterns

Postural patterns and control of the trunk are also typically disturbed in patients with brain lesions. Primary impairments seen in patients with stroke or TBI (i.e., changes in strength, tone, muscle activation and timing, and sensation) all contribute to disordered postural control. The therapist needs to closely examine the patient's postural patterns and movement control during changes in position that require greater and greater levels of control. For example, the patient is asked to move from supine to side-lying to sitting and finally to standing. Disordered postural control and loss of balance typically becomes evident as the patient moves into the higher postures characterized by a reduced base of support (BOS) and higher center of gravity (COG) (e.g., moving from sitting to standing). Examples of the standardized tests and measures used to assess postural control include the *Trunk Control Test,*[82] *Trunk Impairment Scale,*[83] *Function in Sitting Test,*[84] and the *Postural Assessment Scale for Stroke Patients.*[85]

Documentation

Documentation of abnormal movements should include a determination of (1) what abnormal movements are present and where; (2) what is the nature of the abnormal movement pattern (e.g., obligatory synergies); (3) what are the elements or components; (4) what influences the abnormal movements (e.g., spasticity and hyperreflexia coexist with obligatory synergies); (5) what variations or adaptive movements are possible, if any; and (6) what is the effect of abnormal movements on function.

Table 5.9 presents a summary of the differential diagnosis summary comparing UMN and LMN syndromes. Table 5.10 compares the major types of CNS disorders by location of lesion/motor control disorders.

■ TASK ANALYSIS

Task analysis is the process of breaking a specific activity down into its component parts to understand and evaluate the demands of the task and the underlying characteristics of the performance demonstrated. *Task organization* refers to how the components of the task are interdependent. Tasks can demonstrate *low organization* in which the task components are relatively independent (e.g., dressing). *High organization* refers to task components that are highly interrelated (e.g., walking). The process begins with an understanding of normal movements and normal kinesiology associated with the task. The therapist examines and evaluates the patient's performance and analyzes the differences compared to "typical" or expected performance. Critical skills in this process include accurate observation and recognition of barriers or obstacles to moving in the correct pattern. Interpretations are made about the nature of the motor performance and the possible links between documented impairments and performance difficulties. For example, the patient who is unable to transfer from bed to wheelchair may lack postural trunk support (stability), adequate LE extensor control (strength), and ability to maintain control while moving from one surface to the other (dynamic control). Or the patient with acute stroke sits up from supine using the less affected UE for support and propulsion. The more affected extremities lag behind, not well integrated into the movement pattern. The final sitting position is asymmetrical with most of the weight borne on the less affected side and the more affected UE held in an abnormally flexed and adducted position. A determination of how the environment affects performance must also be made. For example, the patient with TBI is highly distractible with poor attention in the busy clinic environment, resulting in an inability to complete a transfer task. It is important

Table 5.9 Differential Diagnosis: Comparison of Upper Motor Neuron (UMN) and Lower Motor Neuron (LMN) Syndromes

	UMN Lesion	LMN Lesion
Location of lesion, Structures involved	Central nervous system cortex, brain stem, corticospinal tracts, spinal cord	Cranial nerve nuclei/nerves Spinal cord: anterior horn cell, spinal roots Peripheral nerve
Diagnosis/ pathology	Stroke, traumatic brain injury, spinal cord injury	Polio, Guillain-Barré Peripheral nerve injury Peripheral neuropathy Radiculopathy
Tone	Increased: hypertonia Velocity dependent	Decreased or absent: hypotonia, flaccidity Not velocity dependent
Reflexes	Increased: hyperreflexia, clonus Exaggerated cutaneous and autonomic reflexes, +Babinski	Decreased or absent: hyporeflexia Cutaneous reflexes decreased or absent
Involuntary movements	Muscle spasms: flexor or extensor	With denervation: fasciculations
Strength	Weakness or paralysis: ipsilateral (stroke) or bilateral (SCI) Corticospinal: contralateral if above decussation in medulla; ipsilateral if below Distribution: never focal	Ipsilateral weakness or paralysis Limited distribution: segmental or focal pattern, root-innervated pattern
Muscle bulk	Disuse atrophy: variable, widespread distribution, especially of antigravity muscles	Neurogenic atrophy: rapid, focal distribution, severe wasting
Voluntary movements	Impaired or absent: dyssynergic patterns, obligatory mass synergies	Weak or absent if nerve interrupted

From O'Sullivan and Siegelman,[123, p. 153] with permission.

to document these qualitative findings, as they provide valuable information necessary for developing an effective POC to improve motor function. The term *activity demands* refers to the requirements imbedded in each step of the activity. The term *environmental demands* (constraints) refers to the physical characteristics of the environment or features required for successful performance of movement (regulatory conditions). Questions posed in Box 5.2 can be used as a guide for movement/ task analysis.

Functional Tasks

Tasks are commonly grouped into functional categories. *Activities of daily living* (ADL) refer to those daily living skills necessary for an adult to manage life. *Basic ADL* (BADL) include grooming skills (e.g., oral hygiene, showering or bathing, dressing), toilet hygiene, feeding, and personal device care. Instrumental ADL (IADL) include money management, functional communication and socialization, functional and community mobility, and health maintenance. *Functional mobility skills* (FMS) refer to those skills involved in bed mobility transfers, walking, and stair climbing.[86-90] See Chapter 8, Examination of Function, for a complete discussion.

Motor Skills

Motor skills can be categorized by different classification schemes.[91] One widely used classification scheme in physical therapy categorizes tasks by either mobility or stability functions. *Mobility* tasks require the individual to move the body from one posture to another in a controlled manner. Both the base of support (BOS) and center of mass (COM) are moving. *Stability* (*static postural control*) tasks require the individual to maintain posture in a stable, unchanging position with the COM over the BOS. Stability can be further divided into static versus dynamic postural control. During *dynamic postural control,* stability is adjusted and maintained while parts of the body (UE or LE) are moving. See Table 5.11 for characteristics, examples of movement tasks, and potential impairments.

Table 5.10 Differential Diagnosis: Comparison of Major Types of Central Nervous System Disorders

Location of Lesion	Cerebral Cortex Corticospinal Tracts	Basal Ganglia	Cerebellum	Spinal Cord
Diagnosis / pathology	Stroke	Parkinson's disease	Tumor, stroke	Trauma, tumor, vascular insult: complete, incomplete SCI
Sensation	Impaired or absent: depends on lesion location; contralateral sensory loss	Not affected	Not affected	Impaired or absent below the level of lesion
Tone	Hypertonia/spasticity velocity-dependent; clasp-knife Initial flaccidity: cerebral shock	Lead-pipe rigidity: increased, uniform resistance Cogwheel rigidity: increased, ratchet-like resistance	Normal or may be decreased	Hypertonia/spasticity below the level of the lesion Initial flaccidity: spinal shock
Reflexes	Hyperreflexia	Normal or may be decreased	Normal or may be decreased	Hyperreflexia
Strength	Contralateral weakness or paralysis: hemiplegia or hemiparesis Disuse weakness in chronic stage	Disuse weakness in chronic stage	Normal or weak: asthenia	Impaired or absent below the level of the lesion: paraplegia or paraparesis; tetraplegia or tetraparesis
Muscle bulk	Normal during acute stage; disuse atrophy in chronic stage	Normal or disuse atrophy	Normal	Disuse atrophy
Involuntary movements	Spasms	Resting tremor	None	Spasms
Voluntary movements	Dyssynergic: abnormal timing, co-activation, fatigability	Bradykinesia: slowness of movement Akinesia: absence of movement	Ataxia: intention tremor dysdiadochokinesia dysmetria dyssynergia nystagmus	Above level of lesion: intact (normal) Below level of lesion: impaired or absent
Postural control	Impaired or absent, depends on lesion location Impaired balance	Impaired: stooped (flexed) Impaired balance	Impaired: truncal ataxia Impaired balance	Impaired below level of lesion Impaired balance
Gait	Impaired: gait deficits due to abnormal weakness, synergies, spasticity, timing deficits	Impaired: shuffling, festinating gait	Impaired: ataxic gait deficits, wide-based, unsteady	Impaired or absent: depends on level of lesion

From O'Sullivan and Siegelman,[123, p. 152] with permission.
SCI = spinal cord injury.

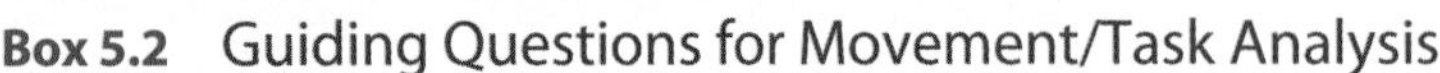

Box 5.2 Guiding Questions for Movement/Task Analysis

Movement/task analysis requires an understanding of normal human movement. By providing a basis for comparison, this information informs evaluation of a patient's task performance. Critical skills include accurate observation, recognition, and interpretation of movement deficiencies; determination of how underlying impairments relate to the movement deficiencies observed; and determination of what needs be altered and how. The following questions can be used as a guide for task analysis.

A. What are the normal requirements of the functional task being observed?

1. What are the musculoskeletal components (ROM, muscle length, muscle strength) required for successful completion of the task?
2. What are the cognitive and sensory/perceptual components required for successful completion of the task?
3. What are the elements of motor control required for successful completion of the task? Mobility, stability, dynamic stability, skill?
4. What are the initial conditions (starting position, alignment, base of support) required?
5. How and where is the movement initiated?
6. What is the overall sequence of movements (motor plan) required?
7. What are the requirements for timing, force, and direction of movements?
8. What are the requirements for postural control and balance?
9. How is the movement terminated (ending base of support, ending alignment)?
10. What are the motor learning factors that must be considered?

B. How successful is the patient's overall movement in terms of intended outcome?

1. Was the overall movement sequence successfully completed?
2. How well was the movement performed? Quality, efficiency, and economy of movement?
3. What components of the patient's movements are normal? Almost normal?
4. What components of the patient's movements are abnormal ? Missing or delayed?
5. Are compensatory movements evident? Are they functional or non-functional?
6. What are the underlying impairments that constrain or impair the movements?
7. Do movement errors increase over time? Is fatigue a constraining factor?
8. Are the required motor control elements met? Mobility, stability, dynamic stability, or skill?
9. Are the requirements for postural control and balance met? Is patient safety evident throughout the task?
10. Can the patient successfully adapt to changing task demands?
11. What difficulties do you expect this patient will have with other functional tasks?
12. Is adaptive equipment required? What is the level of success in using the equipment?
13. How successful were the motor learning strategies? Practice schedule? Feedback?

C. What environmental factors must be considered?

1. What environmental factors constrain or impair the movements?
2. Can the patient adapt successfully to changing environmental demands?
3. What difficulties do you expect this patient will have in other environments?
4. Are there any sociocultural factors that influence performance?

Adapted from *A Compendium for Teaching Professional Level Neurologic Content*, Academy of Neurologic Physical Therapy, American Physical Therapy Association, 2016.

During the examination of tasks requiring *mobility,* key elements the therapist should observe and document include:

- The ability to initiate movements.
- Strategies utilized and overall control of movement.
- The ability to terminate movement.
- The level and type of assistance required (e.g., manual cues, verbal cues, guided movements).
- Environmental constraints that may influence performance.

During examination of tasks requiring *static postural control,* key elements the therapist should observe and document include:

- The position and stability of the BOS.
- The position and stability of the COM within the BOS.
- The length of time the posture can be maintained.
- Postural steadiness (degree of postural sway and direction of instability).
- The number of episodes and direction of loss of balance (LOB) and fall safety risk.

Table 5.11 Motor Skills: Mobility and Stability Functions

Categories	Characteristics	Examples	Impairments in Motor Control
Mobility	Ability to move and change position; requires dynamic postural control, reactive and proactive balance	Bed mobility, transfers, sit-to-stand, supine-to-stand, walking, stair-climbing; moving around the environment	Failure to initiate or control movements; poor control of posture and balance; inability to adapt to changing environment
Stability/static postural control	Ability to maintain postural stability and orientation with the COM over the BOS; both BOS and body (COM) are fixed	Holding steady in antigravity postures: prone-on-elbows, quadruped, sitting, kneeling, half-kneeling, modified plantigrade, or standing	Failure to maintain a steady posture; excessive postural sway; wide BOS; high guard arm position or handhold; loss of balance (COM exceeds BOS)
Stability/dynamic postural control	Ability to maintain postural stability and orientation with the COM over the BOS; BOS is fixed while UEs or LEs are in motion	Weight shifting; UE reaching in any of the above antigravity postures; LE stepping in modified plantigrade or standing	Failure to maintain or control posture during dynamic extremity movements; increased sway or loss of balance

BOS = base of support; COM = center of mass; LE = lower extremity; UE = upper extremity.

- The degree of added stabilization required from UEs or LEs (e.g., handhold, hooked legs).
- The level and type of assistance required (manual, verbal).
- Environmental constraints that may influence performance.

During examination of tasks requiring *dynamic postural control,* key elements the therapist should observe and document include:

- The ability of the patient to modify the BOS to accommodate changing COM during extremity movements.
- The degree of postural stability maintained by the weight-bearing segments using above stability criteria.
- The range and degree of control of extremity movements.
- Environmental constraints that may influence performance.

Documentation

During an analysis of motor skills, key elements the therapist should observe and document include (1) the type of skill being demonstrated; (2) the ability to organize and control movements; (3) the overall quality, efficiency, and economy of movement; (4) the success in attaining the action-goal (outcome); (5) the ability to easily and successfully adapt to changing task demands; (6) the ability to easily and successfully adapt to changing environmental demands; and (7) verbal cues and assistance, if any, required.

The qualitative analysis of motor skills can be enhanced by filming patient performance. Patient responses are recorded, providing a permanent record of motor performance that allows the therapist the opportunity to compare responses over time. Recordings made at 3 or 6 weeks of recovery can be compared easily without reliance on the therapist's memory or written notes. Accuracy of observations can be improved. A therapist who is closely involved in assisting or guarding during performance may not be attentive enough to observe all movement parameters (e.g., when assisting the patient with TBI with severe ataxia). Films can be viewed on a computer repeatedly at different speeds to determine control during different tasks and at different body segments. Two visuals can also be viewed side by side (simultaneously) for comparison. For example, a patient's performance in a task such as sitting up from supine can be observed first at regular speeds, then at slow-motion speeds. Stop-action or freezing a frame can be used to isolate a problematic point in the movement sequence. This may be helpful, particularly for the inexperienced therapist, in improving both the quality and reliability of observations. Repeat trials on a functional performance test may needlessly tire the patient while yielding a decrease in performance. Sequential recordings over the course of rehabilitation provide visual documentation of patient progress and can be an important motivational and educational tool in therapy for use with the patient and family.

Reliability of recordings for intersession comparisons can be improved by the following measures. Placement of equipment should be planned in advance to achieve the best location and should be consistently placed over subsequent sessions. Use of a tripod can improve the stability of the recording. Using the voice-over function, verbal descriptions of the performance during each trial can be added to the visuals and can be documented in a written summary.[92] Examples of recorded case studies accompanying this text can be viewed online at http://davisplus.fadavis.com.

MOTOR LEARNING

Motor learning is a complex process that requires spatial, temporal, and hierarchical organization within the CNS, leading to relatively permanent changes in the capability for motor skill.[1] As mentioned earlier, changes in the CNS are not directly observable, but rather are inferred from improvement in performance as a result of practice or experience. Individual differences in learning are expected and influence both the rate and degree of learning possible. Motor learning abilities among individuals vary across three main foundational categories of abilities: cognitive abilities, perceptual speed ability, and psychomotor ability.[93] Differences occur as a result of both genetics and experience. The therapist should be sensitive to such factors as alertness, anxiety, memory, speed of processing information, speed and accuracy of movements, and uniqueness of the setting. In addition, recovering patients may vary in their learning potential according to the pathology present, the number and type of impairments, recovery potential and general health status, and comorbidities. Although most skills can be learned through practice or experience, the therapist should be sensitive to the patient's underlying capabilities (abilities) that support certain skills. For example, some patients with SCI may not be able to learn to manage curbs using "wheelies" because of the difficulty of the task, their residual abilities, and their general health status.

Stages of Motor Learning

Fitts and Posner[94] described three main stages in learning a motor skill: (1) the cognitive stage, (2) the associative stage, and (3) the autonomous stage of learning. Their model provides a useful framework for examining and developing strategies to improve motor learning and is used in this chapter as well as in Chapter 10, Strategies to Improve Motor Function. A three-stage process was later supported by the work of Anderson.[95,96] It is important to remember that these stages are not fixed or discrete but rather are overlapping.[1]

In the early *cognitive stage,* the learner develops an understanding of task. During practice, *cognitive mapping* allows the learner to assess abilities and task demands, identify relevant and important stimuli, and develop an initial movement strategy (motor program) based on explicit memory of prior movement experiences. The learner performs initial practice of the task, retaining some strategies while discarding others in order to develop an initial movement strategy. During successive practice trials, the learner modifies and refines the movements. During this stage, there is considerable cognitive activity and each movement requires a high degree of conscious attention and thought. Most learners are highly dependent on the use of visual feedback to shape movements. Performance is initially inconsistent, with large gains occurring as the patient progresses to the next stage. The basic "What to do?" decision is answered.

The second and middle stage is the *associated stage* of motor learning. During this stage, the learner practices and refines the motor patterns, making subtle adjustments. Spatial and temporal organization increases while errors and extraneous movements decrease. Performance becomes more consistent and cognitive activity decreases. The learner is less dependent on visual feedback while use of proprioceptive feedback increases. Thus, the learner begins to learn the "feel" of the movement. This stage can persist, depending on the learner and the level of practice. The "How to do?" decision is answered.

The third and final stage is the *autonomous phase* of motor learning. The learner continues to practice and refine motor patterns. The spatial and temporal components of movement become highly organized over time with extensive periods of practice (e.g., weeks, months or years). Performance is at a very high level (e.g., skilled gymnast). At this stage of learning, movements are largely error-free and automatic with only a minimal level of cognitive monitoring and attention. The learner is now free to concentrate on other things such as a secondary task (dual-task performance) or on other aspects of the environment (e.g., sports competition). The "How to succeed?" decision has been answered.

Patients with brain injury admitted to active rehabilitation often have to relearn basic motor skills using entirely different motor control mechanisms and strategies. Activities and movements that were easily done before now become unfamiliar and challenging. These patients can persist in the cognitive learning stage for some time before they develop the idea of a movement skill. Impairments in motor control can influence performance and learning during the associated stage, which can also be prolonged. Many times patients are discharged from rehabilitation before the skills become refined and learning completed. Many patients fail to reach the third stage of learning evidenced by highly skilled performance.

Measures of Motor Learning

Performance Observations

Traditionally, changes in performance during practice have been used to assess motor learning. However, it is possible to improve performance during the initial practice session (acquisition phase) while not retaining the skill. For example, the patient with stroke demonstrates improved sitting posture and balance at the end of a therapy session but on return the next day continues to demonstrate prior poor sitting posture and loss of balance. This is indicative of temporary changes associated with practice versus true motor learning (retained motor skills), which may only become evident with repeat practice sessions. In addition, factors such as fatigue, anxiety, poor motivation, boredom, or drugs can cause performance to deteriorate during practice while learning may still be occurring. For example, the patient with MS who is fatigued and stressed performs very poorly during scheduled treatment but returns after the weekend rested and calm and is able to perform the task with ease.

Performance is best used as a measure of motor learning during a retention test or a transfer test (discussed later in this section). Table 5.12 presents some possible measures of motor performance. For example, an individual recovering from stroke is able to demonstrate functional independence in transfers after a series of training sessions. Improvement in functional scores (e.g., FIM scores) documents changes in the level of assistance needed. Qualitative changes in performance compared to the criterion skill can also be used to document motor

Table 5.12 Measures of Motor Performance

Category	Examples of Measures	Performance Examples
Outcome Measures	**Movement Time (MT):** The time interval between the initiation of a movement and completion of a movement, in seconds or minutes	10-Meter Walk Test (10-MWT) Time to complete a functional task (e.g., transfer wheelchair to mat) Minnesota Rate of Manipulation Test
	Reaction Time (RT): The time interval between the presentation of a stimulus and the initiation of a response, in seconds or minutes	Time to initiate a functional task after cueing is provided (e.g., supine-to-sit or sit-to-stand transfers)
	Distance: The total distance completed, in meters or feet	6- or 12-Minute Walk Test
	Observational Performance Changes: Observation of deviations of performance with respect to target behaviors	Observational gait analysis: Systematic examination of movement patterns of body segments at each point in the gait cycle
	Changes in Performance Scores using a standardized outcome measure	Changes in scores on the Functional Independence Measure, Barthel Index, Berg Balance Scale, or Purdue Pegboard Test
	Errors in Performance using a criterion task	*Error in program selection*: Patient with stroke incorrectly transfers to the less affected side when asked to transfer to the more affected side. *Error in program execution*: Patient with TBI becomes distracted and is unable to complete a transfer.
	Constant Error (CE): The average error of a set of scores from a target value; a measure of average bias	Patient exhibits an average distance on a Functional Reach Test of 6 inches on 3 trials; mean for age (72 years, women; ≥13.8 inches)
	Variable Error (VE): The SD of a set of scores about the subject's own average score; a measure of movement consistency	Patient exhibits an average SD on a Functional Reach Test of 3 inches on 3 trials
	Number of Successful Attempts: During practice of an activity compared to total number of attempts **Percentage of Successful Attempts**	Patient performs an independent sit-to-stand transfer 4 out of 10 attempts Patient performs an independent sit-to-stand transfer 40% of attempts
	Time on Target, compared to total time of the activity, in sec or min	Patient is able to maintain independent stability in sitting (or standing) for 2 min during a 5-min trial

Continued

Table 5.12 Measures of Motor Performance—cont'd

Category	Examples of Measures	Performance Examples
	Time in Balance	Number of seconds patient is able to maintain BOS within COM while standing on foam
	Trials to Completion: Number of trials required until correct response obtained	10 practice trials required for patient to be independent in wheelchair to mat transfers
Instrumental Response Measures	**Limb displacement, trajectory**	Distance limb(s) traveled to produce response during instrumental motion analysis, kinematic gait analysis
	Velocity	Speed limb(s) moved while performing response during instrumental motion analysis or isokinetic dynamometry
	Acceleration/deceleration	Acceleration/deceleration pattern while moving during instrumental motion analysis or isokinetic dynamometry
	Joint angle	Angle of each joint during instrumental motion analysis, or using electrogoniometry
	Muscle activity/electromyography (EMG) testing: The electrical activity of muscle based on motor unit activity	Patterns and timing of muscle activity at rest and during contraction compared to normative muscle activity values (e.g., amplitude, duration, shape, sound, and frequency); correlated with clinical findings of muscle weakness and performance
	Nerve conduction velocity (NCV) testing: The conduction time (speed) with which a peripheral motor or sensory nerve conducts an impulse.	Direct stimulation to a nerve with recording of the evoked potential at a different point, compared to normative NCV values (e.g., evoked potentials, elapsed time); correlated with clinical findings of muscle weakness and sensory changes

BOS = base of support; COM = center of mass; min = minutes; SD = standard deviation; sec = seconds; TBI = traumatic brain injury.

learning. Thus, the movement is performed with improved motor control, indicative of changes in spatial and temporal organization. Error scores can be used to document accuracy of movement. Therefore, therapists can report the number and type of errors (constant, variable) that occur within a given practice session and across practice attempts. A decrease in the frequency of error provides indirect evidence of improvements in learning. One common measurement problem in skill learning is the *speed–accuracy trade-off.* Typically, initial practice sessions are characterized by slowed performance in order to improve movement accuracy. As learning progresses, performance speed is increased once accuracy demands are satisfied. The therapist documents the time it takes to complete the activity along with the number of errors. Reduced effort and concentration are indicative of improved performance and should be documented. A high degree of cognitive monitoring is necessary in early learning (cognitive stage). In contrast, performance across the associative and autonomous stages of motor learning is characterized by a reduced level of cognitive monitoring and increased automaticity.[93] As learning progresses, performance is increasingly characterized by consistency and accuracy. Thus, the acquired skills are observed for variability within and across practice sessions, which can be expected to decrease.

Performance plateaus, defined as a leveling off of performance after a period of steady improvement, characterize normal practice and can be expected. During plateaus, learning may still be going on, whereas performance is not changing. Problems can also occur with the measurement instruments selected. Failure to demonstrate improved performance can be the result of *ceiling effects,* defined as a high level of performance in which further improvement cannot be detected owing to limitations in the performance measure. Conversely, *floor effects* are a low level of performance in which further decreases cannot be detected by limitations in the performance measure. They can affect a determination of negative learning.

Retention Tests

Reliable inferences about motor learning can be made through the use of retention tests and transfer tests. *Retention* refers to the ability of the learner to demonstrate the skill over time and after a period of no practice (*retention interval*). A *retention test* is defined as "a performance test administered after a retention interval for the purposes of assessing learning."[1, p. 499] Retention intervals can be of varying lengths. For example, a patient who is seen only once a week in an outpatient clinic is asked to demonstrate a skill practiced the previous week. Performance after the retention interval is compared to performance on the initial practice session. A *difference score* can be determined and documented—that is, the difference in performance scores from the end of the original acquisition phase and the beginning of the retention phase. Performance may show a slight initial decrease but should return to original performance levels within relatively few practice trials after the retention interval if learning has occurred (termed *warm-up decrement*). It is important not to provide any verbal cueing or knowledge of results during the retention trial. This same patient may have been given a home exercise program (HEP) that includes daily practice of the desired skill. If, on return to the clinic some weeks later, performance of the desired skill has not been maintained or has deteriorated, the therapist might reasonably conclude that the patient has not been diligent with the HEP and learning has not been retained.

Transfer Tests

Transfer of learning refers to the gain (or loss) in the capability for performance in one task as a result of practice or experience on some other task.[1, p. 465] Learning obtained from the criterion task enhances (*positive transfer*) or detracts from (*negative transfer*) learning on other tasks. For example, the patient with stroke practices feeding skills using the less affected UE. The feeding task is then practiced using the more affected UE. During a transfer test, the therapist observes and documents the effectiveness of task performance on the second task (e.g., number and frequency of practice trials, time, effort) and compares it with the performance on the first criterion task. Transfer of learning is greatest when tasks have similar stimuli and similar responses.

Adaptation of Motor Skills

Adaptation of motor skills refers to the ability to modify (adapt) how movements are performed in response to changing task and environmental demands.[1] *Adaptation of skills* (transfer of skills) refers to the ability of the individual to apply a learned motor skill to the learning of other similar or related skills. For example, individuals who learn to transfer from wheelchair to platform mat can apply that learning to other variations of transfers (e.g., wheelchair to car, wheelchair to bathtub). The therapist observes and documents how successful the patient was in learning the variation of the skill (i.e., number of practice trials, time, and effort required to perform these new types of transfers). These parameters are typically reduced from that required to learn the initial skill.

Adaptation of context (changing environmental demands) is also an important measure of learning. This is the adaptability required to perform a learned motor skill in altered environmental situations. Thus, an individual who has learned a skill (e.g., walking with a cane in the physical therapy clinic) should be able to apply that learning to new and variable environments (e.g., walking at home, outdoors, or on a busy street). The therapist observes and documents how successful the patient is in performing the skill in the new and varied environments. The patient who is able to perform the skill in only one type of environment—for example, the patient with TBI who is only able to function within a tightly controlled, clinic environment (*closed environment*)—demonstrates limited and largely nonfunctional skills in other more *open environments*. This patient is not likely to return home independent in the community environment and will likely require placement in an more structured, assisted living setting.

Problem-Solving Skills

The patient who is able to engage in active introspection and self-evaluation of performance and reach decisions independently about how to improve performance demonstrates an important element of learning. Some physical therapists overemphasize guided movements and errorless practice. Although this may be important for safety reasons, lack of exposure to performance errors may preclude the patient from developing capabilities for self-evaluation. In an era of fiscal responsibility and limitations on the amount of physical therapy sessions allowed, many patients are able to learn only the very basic skills while in active rehabilitation. Much of the necessary learning of functional skills occurs after discharge and during outpatient episodes of care. The therapist cannot possibly structure practice sessions to meet all of the functional challenges the patient may face. The acquisition of independent problem-solving/decision making skills ensures that the final goal of rehabilitation—independent function—can be achieved. The therapist needs to promote, observe, and document this very important function, including the patient's self-perceptions of how effective the decisions reached are.

Motivation

Motivational factors include personal sense of self-determination (i.e., choice and collaboration), self-efficacy (i.e., confidence in one's capabilities), and focused attention. They are important factors in ensuring active participation, learning, and retention of motor skills.[97] Highly motivated individuals devote greater effort to learning a task and are willing to devote more focused time to practice. Individuals who are not motivated to learn are not engaged and limit their effort and practice. Therapists need to explore with the patient their own perceptions about their disability or injury, their personal goals, their feelings about competence, and perceptions for success in achieving their goals. Equally important is an assessment of the patient's understanding of the relevance of the learning activity or skill to their daily life. A rehabilitation POC that focuses on involved decision making, active participation, and self-direction is critical in ensuring that the patient will be able to continue practice once discharged and retain learned motor skills. Self-determination and self-management are key elements in ensuring success in real-world environments. Assessment of these factors should be an ongoing process throughout the rehabilitation episode of care. It is important to remember that the patient will experience a number of motivational "ups and downs." The therapist who accurately identifies and reacts to these changes can provide effective intervention, including encouragement and positive reinforcement. Continuing documentation of the patient's motivational and emotional status is key.

Memory and Learning Styles

Learning is the acquisition of knowledge or ability. In *declarative (explicit) learning,* individuals acquire specific knowledge about the world they live in through conscious processes (i.e., attention, awareness, memorization). *Procedural (implicit or motor) memory* refers to the acquisition or modification of movement.[2] During rehabilitation, patients are called upon to use both types of learning. For example, declarative memory is used to learn the sequence of events in a transfer while procedural memory is used to perform the motor skill. Individuals vary in their *learning style,* defined as their characteristic mode of acquiring, processing, and storing knowledge. Learning styles differ according to a number of factors, including personality characteristics, reasoning styles (inductive or deductive), and initiative (active or passive). Some individuals utilize an *analytical/objective* learning style. They process information in a step-by-step order and learn best with factual information and structure. Other individuals are more *intuitive/global* learners. They tend to process information all at once and learn best when information is personalized and presented within the context of practical, real-life examples. They may have difficulty in ordering steps and comprehending details. Some individuals rely heavily on visual processing and demonstration to learn a task. Others depend more on auditory processing, talking themselves through a task. Individual characteristics and preferences are best determined by talking with the patient and family, using careful listening and observation skills. The medical record may also provide information concerning relevant premorbid history (e.g., educational level, occupation, interests). A thorough understanding of each of these factors allows the therapist to appropriately structure the learning environment and therapist–patient interactions.

■ ELECTROPHYSIOLOGICAL INTEGRITY OF MUSCLE AND NERVE

In the evaluation of muscle performance and motor control, we are concerned with the integrity of both central and peripheral mechanisms. The assessment of electrophysiological properties of nerve and muscle provides essential information to understand and assist in the diagnosis of neuromuscular disease or trauma, identify the location of a lesion within the PNS, and establish reasonable prognosis or rate of healing or decay. In order to appreciate deficiencies in peripheral neuromuscular function, clinicians must have a basic understanding of the anatomy and physiology of the nerve and muscle cells. Requirements for peripheral motor response include the successful ability to create an action potential at the lower motor neuron, transmit that signal down the motor neuron and across the neuromuscular junction and result in subsequent muscle contraction. There is a potential for failure in each of these "phases" of neuromuscular transmission due to pathology. Such disorders can result in weakness or lack of motor coordination in movement, resulting in disruption to feedback and motor control mechanisms. These conditions may be related to disorders or disease processes affecting the peripheral nerve (sensory and motor), muscle, or the neuromuscular junction.[98,99]

Electrodiagnosis (EDX) of muscle and nerve is a specialization applied to evaluate the scope of a neuromuscular disorder through assessment of muscle and nerve activity using EMG and NCS. EMG assesses muscle function at rest and during activity, and NCS determines the speed and strength with which a peripheral motor or sensory nerve conducts an impulse. Together, data from EMG and NCS tests assist with establishing goals and expected outcomes for patients with musculoskeletal and neuromuscular disorders. Practitioners providing EDX should have thorough knowledge of anatomy and physiology of muscle and nerve, the biophysical understanding of the instruments used to collect signals, and an understanding of the pathophysiology of nerve and muscle disorders. EDX is only part of a complete patient examination, which will include a thorough understanding of the patient's history and clinical findings. For example, the therapist would also examine muscle strength, pain, reflexes, fatigue, sensory function, and the presence of atrophy, as well as functional abilities and special tests related to the suspected condition. The findings from the clinical examination will suggest which muscles and/or nerves will be tested with EMG and NCS. EDX findings are not diagnostic in isolation and must be considered in relation to other clinical findings and findings from other physical therapy, medical, and physiological tests and measurements.[99]

Neuromuscular Transmission, Injury, and Repair

Neuromuscular Transmission

Nerve cells (neurons) communicate with one another and to other organs, such as muscle and sensory organs, in order to transmit signals that allow motor and sensory function. Neurons are small in diameter, usually much smaller than a hair, and can be as long as the distance from your back to the tip of your toe! A *motor unit* is composed of one anterior horn cell, one axon, its neuromuscular junction, and all the muscle fibers innervated by that axon (Fig. 5.1). The cell body or nucleus of the neuron is the location of many protein particles and organelles that provide critical neuron function to keep the cell alive and allow repair. Without communication with the cell body, a peripheral nerve will die. This process is called *Wallerian degeneration.* Dendrites are proximal terminals that receive input from other cells. The axons project away from the cell bodies and carry electrical signals toward targeted organs such as muscles.

Nerves are comprised of groups of neurons that can provide sensory, motor, or autonomic signals to and from other nerves and transmitting organs. Peripheral nerves (Fig 5.2) are typically surrounded by myelin, which is made of water, fat, and protein and provides electrical insulation to the neurons; this allows for neurons to conduct impulses at increased speed. The main cell of myelin in the peripheral nervous system is called the *Schwann cell,* and spaces between the cells are called the *nodes of Ranvier.* Nerves are like coated cables that are comprised of bundles of neurons. Each bundle is called a *fascicle,* and the nerve trunk is a collection of fascicles. Connective tissue structures assist in the organization and protection of neurons and are known as the *endoneurium, perineurium,* and *epineurium.* The endoneurium surrounds individual axons and provides a conduit for nerves to grow and travel. Perineurium envelopes the fascicles and epineurium surrounds the entire nerve trunk.[100]

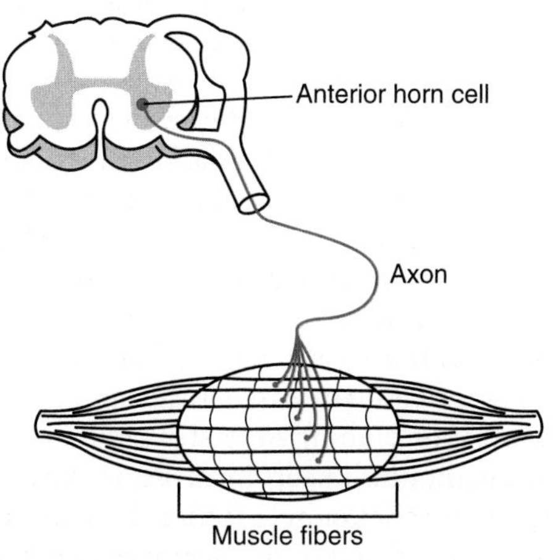

Figure 5.1 The motor unit.

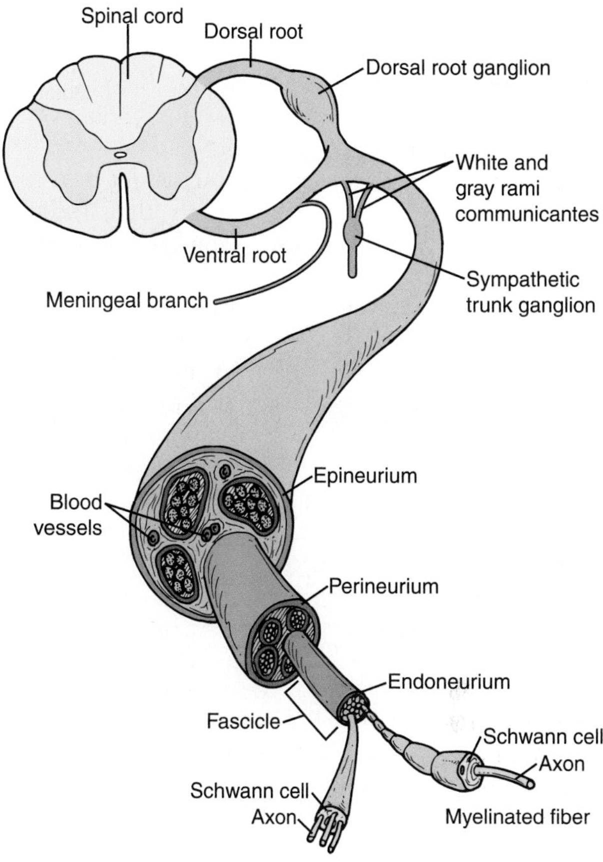

Figure 5.2 Peripheral nerve.

The Neuromuscular Junction

The *neuromuscular junction* (NMJ) (Fig. 5.3) is the location of electrical transmission from the nerve to the muscle cell and is comprised of three distinct parts. The *synaptic terminal* is the end bulb of the lower motor neuron. Within the synaptic terminal are large numbers of synaptic vesicles that contain acetylcholine (ACH), which is a substance necessary for electrical neurotransmission. The *motor end plate* is the part of the muscle cell in closest proximity to the synaptic terminal, where there is a high concentration of post-synaptic terminals. These terminals are arranged in folds of muscle membrane and increase the area to which ACH can bind. The space between the synaptic terminal and motor end plate is known as the *synaptic cleft.*[100]

The Muscle Cell

Striated skeletal muscle cell is comprised of bundles of elongated myofibrils (actin and myosin) surrounded by a cellular membrane known as the *sarcolemma.* The

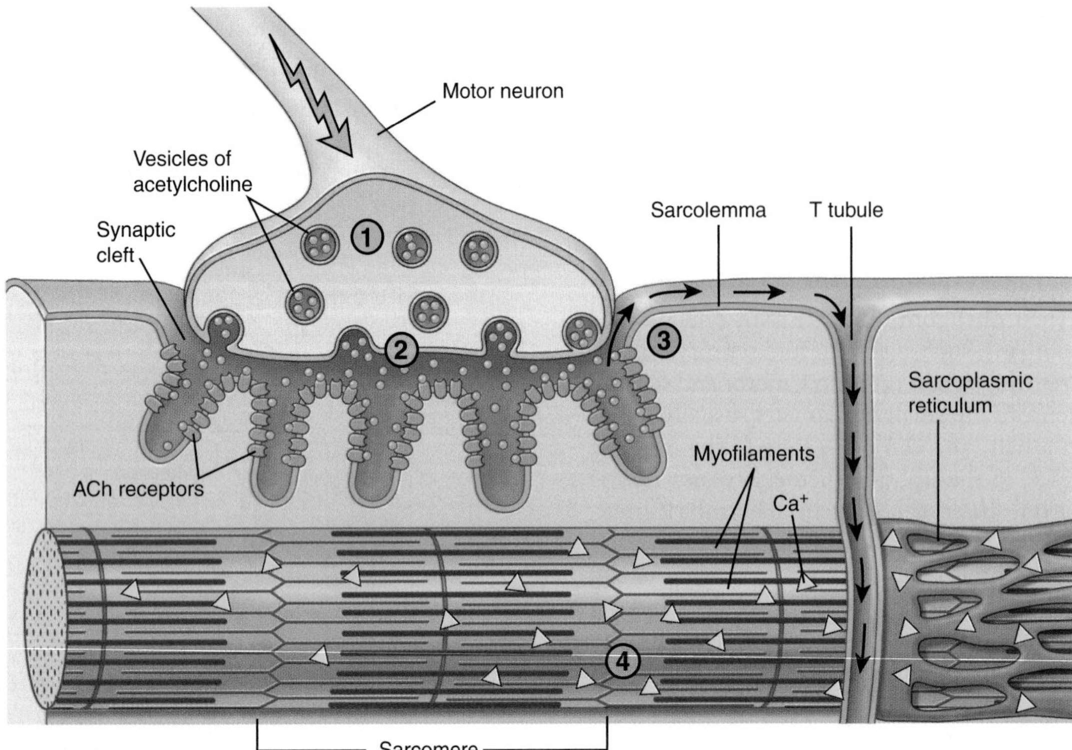

Figure 5.3 The neuromuscular junction and muscle cell.

sarcolemma is enveloped in capillaries, t-tubules, nuclei, and sarcoplasmic reticulum, which collectively comprise the muscle fiber. Muscle fibers are covered in a connective tissue matrix known as *endomysium* and are bundled similarly to peripheral nerve in a cable-like fashion of fascicles. The connective tissue surrounding individual fascicles is known as *perimysium*. The epimysium surrounds the total bundle of many fascicles. These connective tissue structures continue beyond the contractile structures of the muscle cell as the tendons, which then attach onto the bone[100] (see Fig 5.3).

The Action Potential

When descending/ascending electrical input reaches an axon, there is a disruption in the resting membrane potential, which is a balance of sodium and potassium concentrations within and outside the cell. Resting membrane potential is variable, from –90 to –70 mV. When descending electrical input reaches the lower motor neuron, voltage-gated sodium channels open and there is an exchange where sodium can rush into the cell in an attempt to balance the concentrations of these ions. Smaller positively charged potassium ions are subsequently forced out the cell, and the resting membrane polarity becomes more positive. If the electrical potential reaches a threshold for depolarization (approximately 20 mV), an action potential is created and an impulse travels down the axon. The speed and success of the action potential conduction is dependent on the thickness of the axon and the presence of myelin. Action potentials travel down the myelinated axons through *saltatory conduction,* in which the action potential jumps from one node of Ranvier to the next, where there are high concentrations of sodium/potassium channels.[100] When myelin or axon thickness is disrupted in certain pathologies, the ability of the axon to transmit at normal speeds and strengths can be affected and can lead to abnormal motor or sensory function. When nerve injury affects myelin, it is considered demyelination, and when there is Wallerian degeneration of the axon, it is considered axonal loss. Collectively, injury or disease to the nerve itself is called neuropathy and can occur in individual nerves, isolated areas, or more widespread throughout the peripheral nerves.[99]

Neuromuscular Transmission

When the nerve action potential reaches the terminal axon, calcium channels open and acetylcholine (ACH) is released into the NMJ. ACH binds to ACH receptors on the motor end plate, and an action potential is generated; this causes the release of calcium ions and finally triggers contraction of the muscle cell. Certain disease processes affecting the release of calcium at the presynaptic terminal or binding of ACH at the post-synaptic terminal can diminish neuromuscular transmission and subsequently impair muscle function. A condition affecting neuromuscular transmission would be considered a neuromuscular junction disorder.[100]

Muscle Contraction

During muscle contraction, proteins and structural cells slide over one another to create a shortening of the muscle. Calcium released from the "sarcoplasmic reticulum" at the motor end plate opens binding sites on actin filaments, which bind to myosin. Myosin heads undergo a pivoting action to shorten the cell and then detaches when adenosine triphosphate (ATP) binds to the myosin.[100] The muscle cell is secured to the extracellular matrix through a series of protein molecules, including dystrophin, which allows for mechanical stability and provides a reasonable anchor for contraction. In certain disease or inflammatory processes, such as the muscular dystrophies or myositis, the muscle cell loses structural integrity and leads to poor muscle performance. This destructive muscle condition leads to variability of muscle fiber size and infiltration of fibrous connective tissue. This is considered a *myopathy.*

Nerve Injury and Repair

Nerve injury is generally characterized by demyelination or axon loss and can be partial or complete. Demyelination can result from inflammation, immune disorders, genetic predisposition, or exposure to toxic chemicals and/or mechanical forces such as compression or shearing. Disturbance of the myelin can reduce myelin thickness or invagination that leads to a widening of the nodes of Ranvier with sodium channel redistribution. This can occur focally, segmentally, or uniformly along a nerve. When this occurs, saltatory conduction is altered and results in slowing, altered shapes of nerve potentials and/or blocking of nerve transmission altogether (conduction block).[99]

When an axon loses continuity with its cell body, Wallerian degeneration occurs. Also known as *axon loss,* this process begins immediately with one or two nodes of Ranvier dying back and with progressive degeneration distally along the neuron. This degenerative process typically requires 5 to 7 days to complete in motor neurons and 7 to 10 days in sensory neurons. As long as the cell body has continuity with its terminal nerve branch, the branch will remain alive. For example, if an upper motor neuron is damaged due to stroke, the lower motor neuron (whose cell body lies within the anterior horn of the spinal cord) remains intact, as does the remainder of the lower motor neuron. Even though the patient cannot fire the nerve because of the central damage in the brain, the lower motor neuron remains alive and can carry information normally. Similarly, imagine a patient with cervical radiculopathy who has weakness and sensory changes in a specific nerve root distribution. There may be weakness and Wallerian degeneration involving the lower motor neuron but not in the sensory neurons because the primary sensory neuron cell bodies reside in the dorsal root ganglia, which are distal to the typical site of nerve root compression in cervical radiculopathy. Injury to nerve proximal to the dorsal root ganglia is often called a *preganglionic lesion.* This is a very important concept in understanding EDX, evaluating data, and formulating a reasonable diagnostic impression.[99]

In an attempt to organize nerve structure and progression of injury, an early publication by Seddon[101] proposed classifications of nerve injury, which was later expanded by Sunderland[102] to highlight involvement of the connective tissue support system of the axon. Seddon's classification of nerve injury by *neuropraxia, axonotmesis,* and *neurotmesis* and Sunderland's first- to fifth-degree injury classification have become common methods of describing nerve damage (Fig 5.4). It is important to recognize that neuropraxia and first-degree injury involve demyelination and more specifically conduction block. Axonotmesis/neurotmesis and second- to fifth-degree injury involve axon loss with gradual loss of supportive connective tissue elements in the nerve. Ability of a nerve to recover is largely dependent on the preservation of a regenerating neuron's connective tissue support structure, specifically preservation of the endoneurium. In axonotmesis and second-degree injuries, the endoneurium remains intact and serves as a conduit for the regenerating axon, which improves the likelihood of nerve recovery. In contrast, with neurotmesis or third- to fifth-degree injuries, the endoneurium, perineurium, or epineurium is lost, and no conduit exists for neuron regeneration.

Nerve healing occurs through either remyelination or reinnervation by way of axonal sprouting or axonal regeneration (Fig 5.5). In remyelination and with optimal conditions of nutrition, removal or control of disease, and/or cessation of compression, Schwann cells produce new myelin, and action potential speeds and strengths will improve and can even return to normal. Reinnervation due to collateral axon sprouting requires the presence of uninjured axons within the injured nerve bundle. Similar to surviving branches on a tree that has been pruned, uninjured neurons will sprout new branches to reinnervate the target organs of the injured neurons. Earliest collateral sprouts require 6 to 8 weeks to be documented. It is generally agreed that a nerve will require about 20% to 25% of uninjured axons to achieve recovery without residual functional weakness. This occurs from collateral axon sprouting, as each terminal neuron branch can grow up to five collateral sprouts. This means that a peripheral nerve can lose quite a large percentage of axons and still recover well. Reinnervation owing to axonal regeneration is a slower process, and under optimal conditions, the injured nerve bulb can regenerate along an intact endoneurium at a rate of about 1 mm per day, or 1 inch (25.4 mm) per month. Age, other disease processes, and distance to the target organ significantly influence a neuron's successful regeneration. EDX can assist in identifying nerve injury through localization, determining the extent of injury and involvement of myelin versus axon loss, and assessing reinnervation by way of collateral axon sprouting versus axon regeneration.[99]

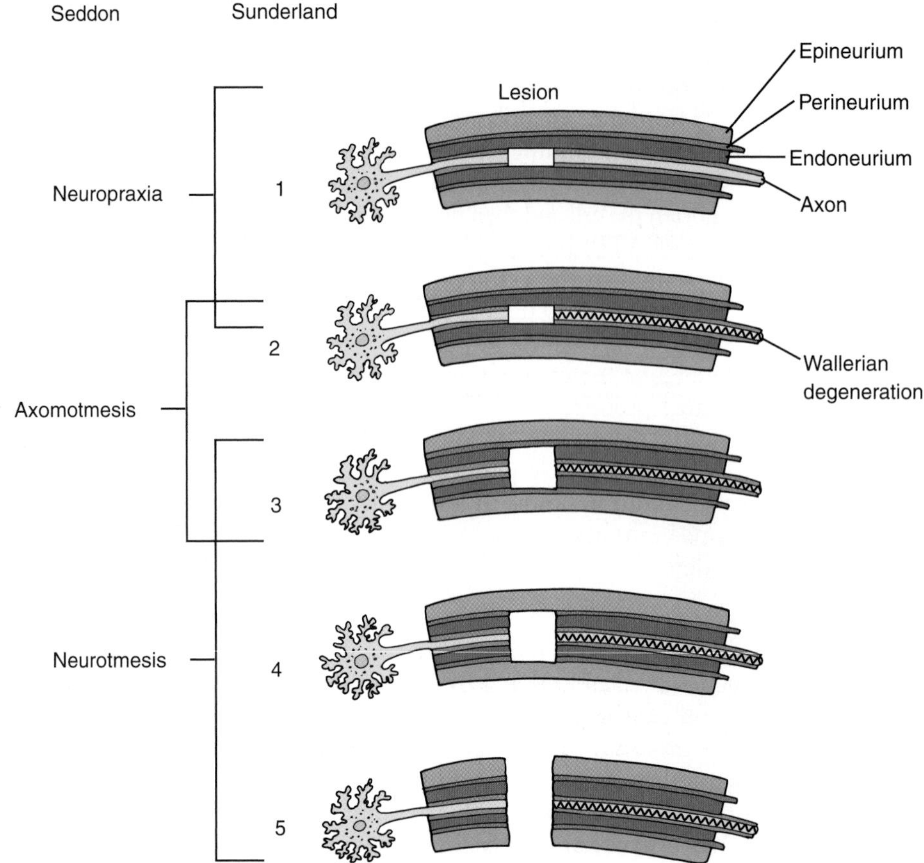

Figure 5.4 Seddon and Sunderland classification of nerve injury.

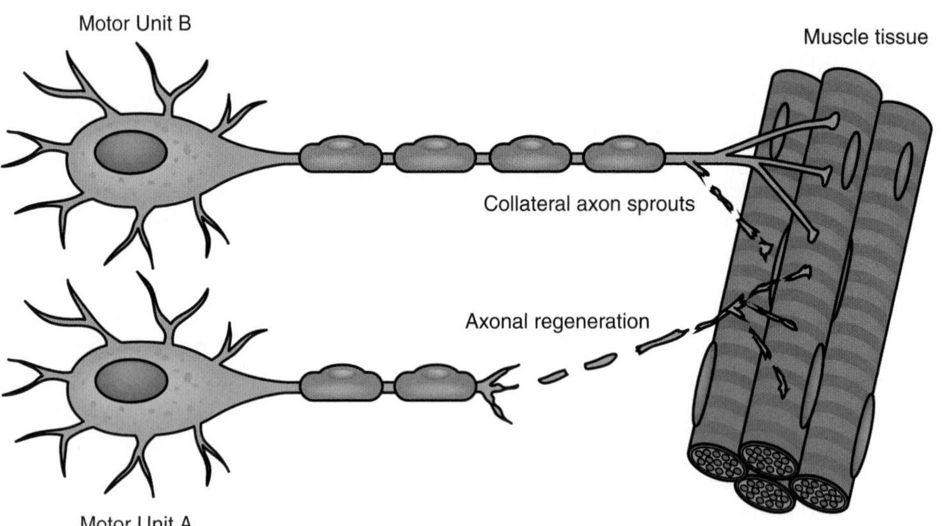

Figure 5.5 Remyelination and reinnervation.

Concepts of Electrodiagnosis

Both EMG and NCS recordings are made using biomedical equipment that can record and store evoked potential data elicited from the stimulation of nerves and electrical activity from within the muscle (Fig 5.6A). Electrodes are placed on, in, or near muscle or nerve to record bioelectric charges. Recordings are transported to an amplifier for signal processing. Following amplification, the equipment filters ambient noise that would otherwise distort the intended bioelectric charges, and the digitized analog signal is displayed on an oscilloscope for analysis. Audio amplification with speakers also permits acoustic monitoring of these nerve and muscle potentials.

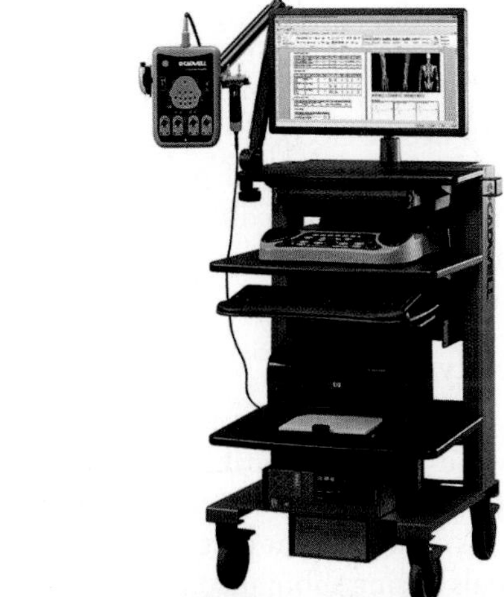

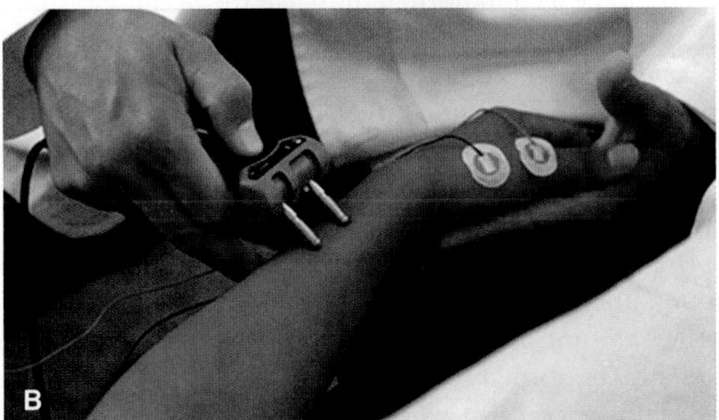

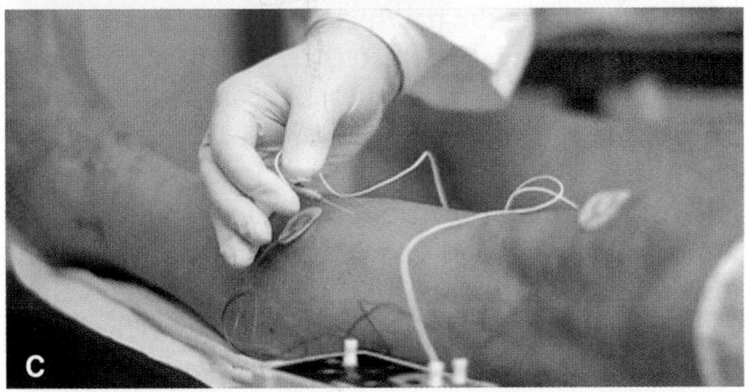

Figure 5.6 EMG machine, EMG, and NCS setup. (A) EMG machine. *(Courtesy of Cadwell Laboratories, Kennewick, WA.)* (B) Sensory NCS of the superficial radial nerve. (C) Needle EMG of the anterior tibialis.

A stimulator is used in NCS and is electronically synchronized with the oscilloscope to fire the nerve. Intensity of the stimulator is dependent upon the voltage, amperage, and pulse duration of the stimulus.

There are three types of electrodes used for recordings. A *ground electrode* serves as a zero voltage reference and reduces extraneous electrical noise and interference. The *recording electrode* (pickup electrode) records the intended potential and extraneous signals, and the *reference electrode* records extraneous signals and different aspects of the intended potential.

In NCS, small surface electrodes are usually used to record the evoked potential from the test muscle or directly from the nerve under study. NCS recordings can also be made using intramuscular or subcutaneous needles. The *recording electrode* is placed over the belly of the test muscle and a reference electrode is taped over the tendon of the muscle (see Fig 5.6B).

For EMG, the most common types of needle electrodes are bipolar and monopolar. A *bipolar electrode* is a hypodermic needle, through which a single wire made of platinum or silver is threaded. The cannula shaft and wire are insulated from each other, and only their tips are exposed. The wire and the needle cannula act as recording and reference electrodes, and the difference in potential between them is recorded in volts. A *monopolar needle electrode* is composed of a single fine needle, insulated except at the tip. A second surface electrode placed on the skin near the site of insertion serves as the reference electrode. These electrodes are generally less painful than bipolar electrodes because they are smaller in diameter and do not have a cutting edge (see Fig. 5.6C).

Bioelectric potentials travel through body fluids in all directions, not just in the direction of the recording electrode. Fibrous tissue, fat, and blood vessels act as insulators in this process. Therefore, the actual pattern of the flow of electrical activity is not predictable. The signals that do reach the electrode are transmitted to an amplifier. The activity produced by all the individual fibers of nerve or muscle at any one time is summated, reaching the electrode almost simultaneously. Electrodes only record potentials they pick up, without differentiating their origin. Therefore, if two motor units contract at the same time, from the same or adjacent muscles, the activity from fibers of both units will be summated and recorded as one large potential.

The size and shape of the evoked potentials can be affected by several variables. The proximity of the electrodes to the nerve and muscle that are firing will affect the amplitude and duration of the recorded potential. Targets that are farther away will contribute less to the recorded potential. The number and size of the muscle fibers or neurons will influence the evoked potential size. Finally, the distance between the fibers will affect the output, because if the fibers are very spread out, less of their total activity is likely to reach the electrodes.

In addition to these variables, many excess signals, or *artifacts,* can be recorded and processed simultaneously with the EMG signal. An artifact is any unwanted electrical activity that arises outside of the tissues being examined. These artifacts can be of sufficient voltage to distort the output signal markedly, such as those coming from other electrical equipment or fluorescent lights. Electromyographers will usually observe the output signal on an oscilloscope or computer screen to monitor artifacts, then employ troubleshooting techniques to minimize unwanted noise.

The EMG Examination

EMG is the recording of the electrical activity of muscle while at rest and during motor unit activation. Data are visualized on an oscilloscope with audio feedback that allows the examiner to distinguish between normal and abnormal activity.

Insertional Activity

Initially, the patient is asked to relax the muscle to be examined during insertion of the needle electrode. Insertion into a contracting muscle is uncomfortable but tolerable. At this time, the electromyographer will observe a spontaneous burst of potentials, called *insertional activity,* which is possibly caused by the needle breaking through muscle fiber membranes. This normally lasts less than 300 milliseconds (msec).[103] Insertional activity can be described as normal, reduced, absent or increased (Fig 5.7). *Increased insertional activity* is representative of muscle membrane instability and is frequently seen in nerve injury or muscle degeneration. Reduced insertional activities generally represent chronic neuropathy or myopathy in which there has been significant atrophy of muscle and/or infiltration of fat and connective tissue within the muscle. *Decreased insertional activity* implies non-viable muscle tissue, and the examiner may feel increased resistance when advancing the needle. The needle electrode will be moved to different areas and depths of each muscle. This is necessary because of the small area from which a needle electrode will pick up electrical activity and because the effects of pathology may vary within a single muscle. Up to 25 different points within a single muscle may be examined by moving and redirecting the needle electrode.

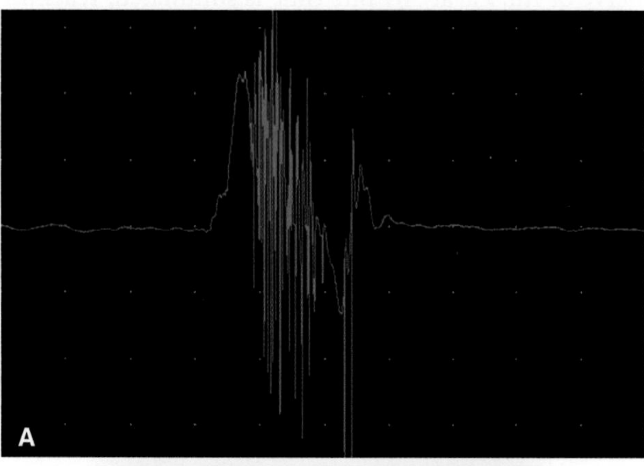

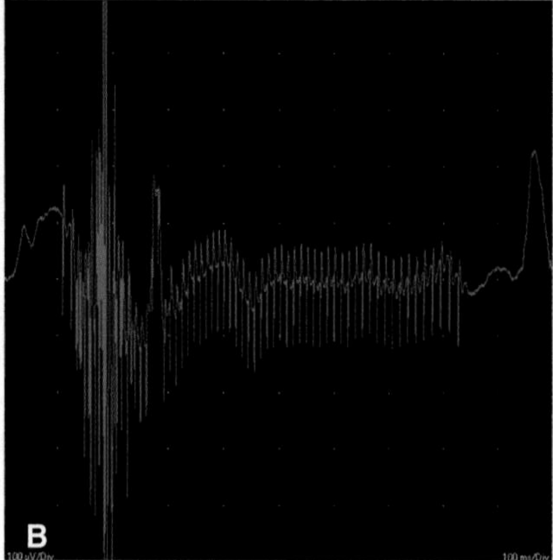

Figure 5.7 Insertional activity. (A) Normal insertional activity. (B) Increased insertional activity.

Resting Activity

Following cessation of insertional activity, a normal relaxed muscle will exhibit electrical silence, which is the absence of electrical potentials. Observation of silence in the relaxed state is an important part of the EMG examination. Potentials arising spontaneously during this period can be seen in normal muscle if the needle electrode is close to a neuromuscular junction. *Miniature end plate potentials* are thought to represent small releases of ACH at a NMJ that are not sufficient to propagate a muscle fiber action potential, and *end plate spikes/end plate potentials* represent sufficient release of ACH at the NMJ to cause depolarization of individual muscle fibers. End plate potentials are irregular in their firing rates and are often uncomfortable to the patient when encountered.[99] They are not indicative of pathology and are seen frequently in normal muscle. When encountered, it is important to confirm what they are and then move the needle away from the painful area (Fig. 5.8A,B).

There are several characteristic potentials observed during the relaxed state that are considered abnormal. *Fibrillation potentials* are believed to arise from spontaneous depolarization of a single muscle fiber. They are not visible through the skin. Fibrillation potentials are biphasic spikes and are indicative of muscle membrane instability. They are seen in neuropathic disorders, such as peripheral nerve lesions, anterior horn cell disease, radiculopathies, and polyneuropathies with axonal degeneration (see Fig 5.8C). They are also found in muscle degenerative conditions such as muscular dystrophy, dermatomyositis, polymyositis, and less frequently in myasthenia gravis. Their sound is a high-pitched click, which has been likened to the sound of rain falling on a roof or rhythmic wrinkling tissue paper. *Positive sharp waves* have been observed in denervated muscle at rest, often accompanied by fibrillation potentials, and they, too, are reported in primary muscle disease, especially muscular dystrophy and polymyositis. The waves are typically biphasic, with a sharp initial positive deflection (below baseline) followed by a slow negative phase. The negative phase is of much lower amplitude than the positive phase and of much longer duration, sometimes up to 100 msec. The peak-to-peak amplitude may be variable, with voltages from 50 microvolts (uV) to 2 millivolts (mV). The sound has been described as a dull thud (see Fig. 5.8D). While morphology (shape) is different in positive sharp waves and fibrillations, it is thought that they represent the same phenomena of

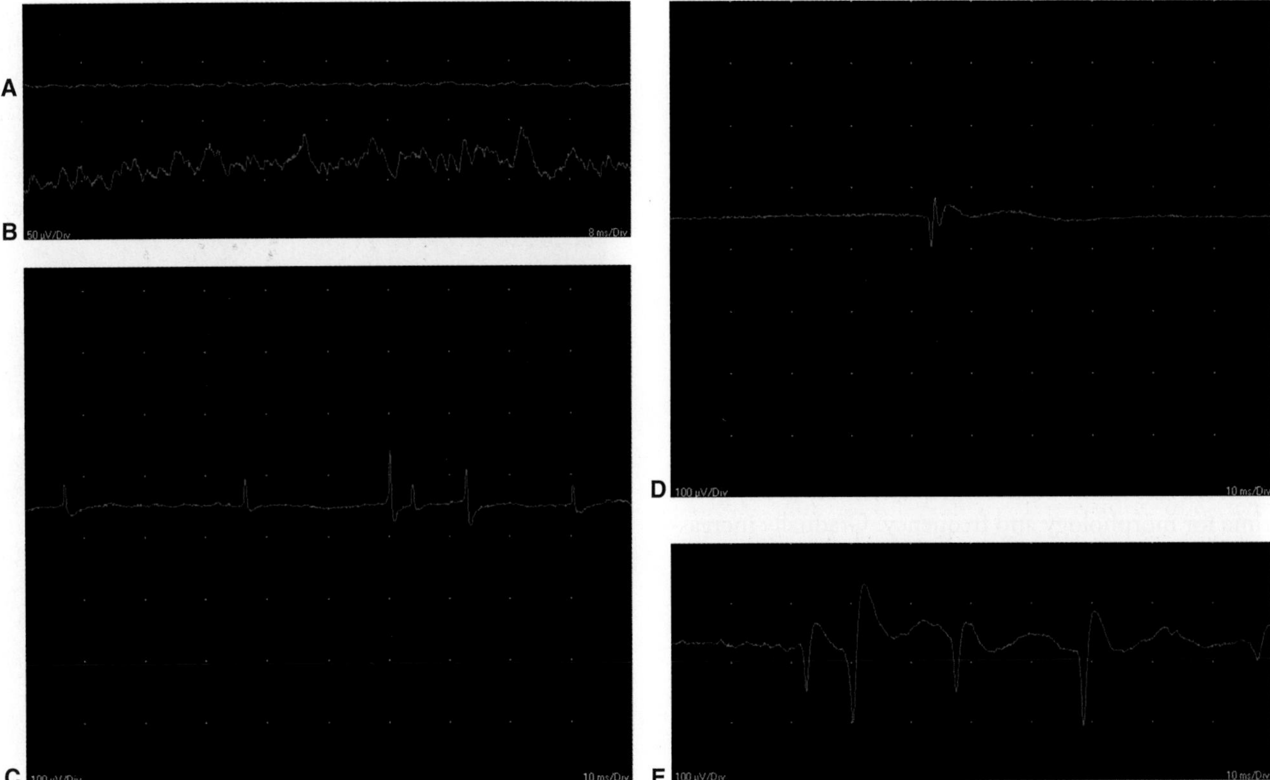

Figure 5.8 Resting activity. (A) Normal resting activity. (B) End plate potentials. (C) End plate spikes. (D) Fibrillation potentials. (E) Positive sharp waves.

spontaneous discharge of a muscle fiber but look differently due to the orientation of the needle electrode with respect to the discharging muscle fiber.[99] In fact, it is common to see a fibrillation or positive sharp wave morph from one to the other during the examination. Fibrillations and positive sharp waves can be observed in EMG within a week, particularly in proximal muscles, but require up to 3 weeks following axon loss injury to become more widespread.

Complex repetitive discharges may be seen with lesions of the anterior horn cell and peripheral nerves and with myopathies. The discharge is characterized by an extended train of potentials with the same or nearly the same waveform. The feature that distinguishes these discharges from other spontaneous potentials is their regular and repetitive waveform. The frequency usually ranges from 5 to 100 impulses per second. *Myotonic discharges* are repetitive potentials that increase and decrease in amplitude in a waxing and waning fashion. They are found in myotonic disorders such as myotonic dystrophy, as well as other myopathies. The sound is highly characteristic and sounds like a dive-bomber. High-frequency discharges are probably triggered by movement of the needle electrode within unstable muscle fibers or by volitional activity.[99]

Fasciculations are spontaneous *motor unit action potentials* (MUAPs) seen with irritation or degeneration of the anterior horn cell, chronic peripheral nerve lesions, nerve root compression, and muscle spasms or cramps. They are believed to represent the involuntary asynchronous firing of motor units. Their sound has been described as a low-pitched thump. Fasciculations are often visible through the skin and can be seen as a small twitch. They are not by themselves a definitive abnormal finding, as they are often seen in normal individuals, particularly in muscles of the calves, eyes, hands, and feet.[104] *Myokymia* also represents spontaneous bursts of motor unit firing that is more uniform and can fire fast at rates from 2 Hz to 60 Hz.[99] Like fasciculations, myokymic potentials are not by themselves indicative of pathology and may be seen in normal or fatigued muscle.

Motor Unit Morphology and Recruitment

After observing the muscle at rest, the patient is asked to contract the muscle minimally. When a muscle is contracted to produce force, a single axon conducts an impulse to all its muscle fibers, causing them to depolarize at relatively the same time. This depolarization produces electrical activity that is manifested as a MUAP and can be recorded and displayed graphically. A MUAP is actually the summation of electrical potentials from all the fibers of that unit close enough to the electrodes to be recorded. The amplitude (voltage) is affected by the number of fibers involved or by the motor unit territory. The duration and shape are functions of the distance of the fibers from the recording electrodes, the more distant fibers contributing to terminal phases of the potential. Because of these variables, each motor unit will have a distinctive shape and vary in amplitude and number of phases, where a *phase* represents a section of a potential crossing above or below the baseline. MUAPs are examined with respect to morphology (amplitude, duration, shape) and frequency of firing. These parameters are the essential characteristics that distinguish normal from abnormal potentials. Initially, a type I MUAP is recruited at approximately 5 Hz. As resistance is increased, that first MUAP increases frequency until it reaches approximately 10 Hz, when another type I MUAP is recruited. The pattern of increasing frequency and addition of more MUAPs continues until type II MUAPs are recruited. Typically, only one to three MUAPs can visibly be assessed qualitatively at any given time for morphology and frequency. Gradually increasing the force of contraction will allow the electromyographer to observe the pattern of recruitment in the muscle but not qualitatively assess morphology. With greater effort, the increased numbers of potentials are summated and can no longer be recognized, but an overall *interference pattern* can be estimated. The characteristics of the MUAP will change when there is damage to either the nerve or muscle. EMG equipment has improved over the years and most models have features to provide quantitative MUAP analysis that can improve the objective assessment of MUAP characteristics. In normal muscle, the peak-to-peak amplitude of typical MUAP may range from 150 microvolts uV to 5 millivolts mV. The duration of the potential is a measure of time from onset to cessation of the electrical potential, typically from 2 to 14 msec[105] (Fig 5.9A). The typical shape of a MUAP is biphasic or triphasic and generally not displaying greater than four phases.

Polyphasic potentials, which are MUAPs having five or more phases, are generally considered abnormal when seen in large numbers (see Fig 5.9B). It is normal to observe small numbers of *polyphasic potentials*; however, when polyphasic potentials represent approximately 20% or more of a muscle's output, it may be an abnormal finding. However, caution is warranted in identifying pathology based solely on the presence of polyphasic MUAPs, as some authors have reported their appearance in greater than 30% of normal subjects.[99] Polyphasic potentials may also be seen during degeneration and after regeneration of a peripheral nerve. Polyphasic potentials with longer than normal durations are considered a sign of motor neuropathy and may be a result of the asynchronous firing of muscle fibers within a MUAP that is undergoing reinnervation owing to collateral sprouting. This phenomenon is probably due to the difference in the length of the terminal branches and maturity of myelin in the sprouting axons extending to each muscle fiber. As some muscle fibers become reinnervated by collateral sprouts, they will generate action potentials along with the other muscle fibers within that motor unit. The

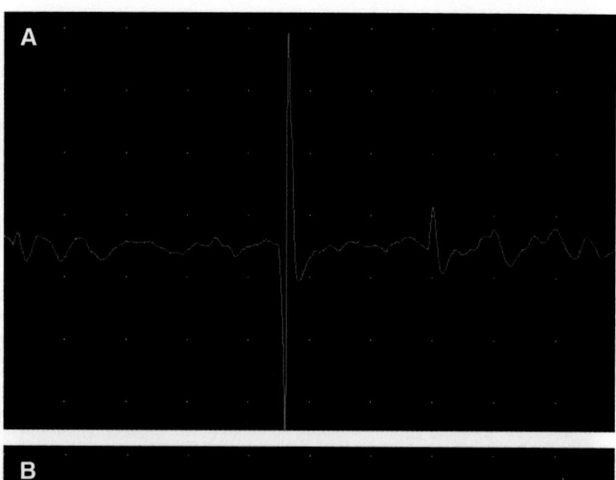

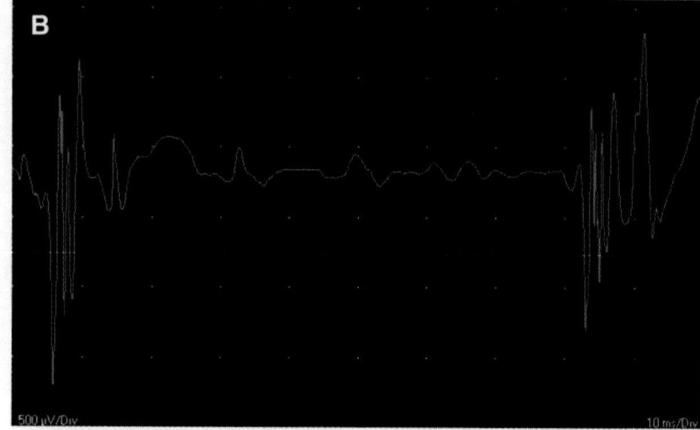

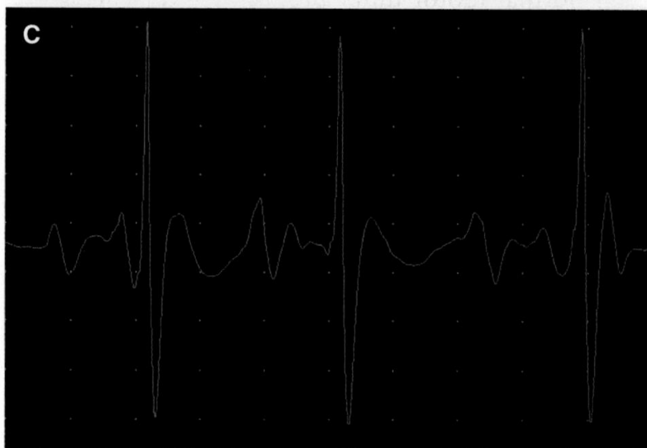

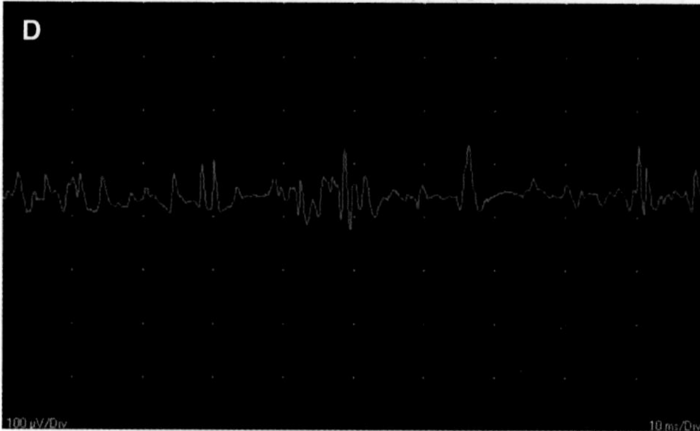

Figure 5.9 Motor unit morphology and recruitment. (A) Normal motor unit. (B) Polyphasic motor unit. (C) Larger than normal amplitude motor unit with neuropathic recruitment. (D) Short duration, low amplitude motor units with myopathic recruitment.

result is a normal amplitude MUAP with larger number of phases and longer duration than a normal motor unit.

Following axonal degeneration, collateral sprouts mature. Successfully reinnervated muscle fibers typically demonstrate *larger than normal amplitude MUAP,* also known as a *Giant MUAP* (see Fig 5.9C). Generally, MUAPs exceeding 5 mV are considered larger than normal. These potentials may be seen in post-polio syndrome and other neuropathic conditions such as chronic radiculopathy or focal nerve entrapments like carpal tunnel syndrome.[106-108]

In a complete axon loss nerve injury, reinnervation can occur due to axonal regeneration. Recall that the presence of an endoneurial tube is critical for successful axonal regeneration. As the first regenerating axons reach their intended muscle fibers, the potential will look very similar to a fibrillation potential, and as more terminal branches reach muscle fibers, the MUAP will be small in amplitude and highly polyphasic. Early MUAPs representing axonal regeneration have been termed *nascent motor units.* As these MUAPs mature, the number of phases will decrease and the morphology and duration will become more normal.

In primary muscle disease (myopathies), polyphasic potentials are seen but are generally of smaller amplitude than normal motor units and are typically of shorter duration. These multiphasic changes occur because of a decrease in the number of active muscle fibers within the individual motor units due to pathology. Although the entire unit will fire during voluntary contraction, fewer fibers are available in each unit to contribute to the total voltage and the duration of the potential. The result is a MUAP of lower than normal amplitude and potentially shorter duration (see Fig. 5.9D).

Firing frequencies of any given MUAP are generally less than 12 Hz to 15 Hz if only one to three MUAPs are isolated on an oscilloscope. In a condition of motor axon loss where there are less available MUAPs for recruitment to produce force, firing frequencies may be seen in excess of 15 Hz and can be accompanied by a less than full interference pattern. The MUAP morphological changes consisting of long duration polyphasia or larger than normal amplitudes with overall reduced and fast firing frequencies is consistent with *neuropathic recruitment* (see Fig 5.9C). Conversely and as discussed in primary muscle generation, motor unit morphology can show MUAPs with shorter duration and low amplitude polyphasia. The total availability of motor units remains normal, so overall interference patterns will be normal; however, muscle degeneration will result in less viable muscle tissue producing resistance to demanded force during the EMG. The resulting interference pattern will occur sooner than anticipated and is considered *early recruitment.* The combination of MUAP morphology changes consisting of low amplitude, short-duration polyphasia with early recruitment is consistent with *myopathic recruitment* (see Fig 5.9D).

Nerve Conduction Studies

Nerve conduction studies (NCS) involve direct stimulation to initiate an impulse in motor or sensory nerves. The *conduction time* is measured by recording the *evoked potential* either from the muscle innervated by the motor nerve or from the sensory nerve itself. NCS can be tested on any peripheral nerve that is superficial enough to be stimulated through the skin at two different points. The most commonly tested motor nerves are the ulnar, median, fibular (peroneal), tibial, radial, femoral, and sciatic nerves. Commonly tested sensory nerves include the median, ulnar, radial, sural, and superficial fibular nerves, but this is not at all a comprehensive list of available nerves to examine. Complete guidelines for performing NCS tests are available in comprehensive references.[99,103,105,109,110]

Motor Nerve Conduction Studies

Because a peripheral nerve trunk houses both sensory and motor fibers, recording potentials directly from a peripheral nerve makes monitoring of purely sensory or motor nerves impossible. Therefore, to isolate the potentials conducted by motor axons of a mixed nerve, the evoked potential is recorded from a distal muscle innervated by the nerve under study. Although the stimulation of the nerve will evoke sensory and motor impulses, only the motor fibers contribute to the contraction of the muscle. For example, to test the ulnar nerve, the test muscle is typically the abductor digiti minimi. Other examples are the following: for the median nerve, the abductor pollicis brevis; for the fibular nerve, the extensor digitorum brevis; and for the tibial nerve, the abductor hallucis. Of course, motor evoked potentials can be recorded from any muscle if its target nerve can be stimulated and a recording electrode can be properly placed on or within the muscle.

For the purposes of illustration, the test procedure for the motor NCV of the median nerve will be described (Fig. 5.10). The technique is basically the same for all nerves, except for the sites of stimulation and placement of the electrodes. For this example, the recording electrode is taped over the abductor pollicis brevis. The stimulating electrode is placed over the median nerve at multiple sites, including the palm, wrist, elbow, and axilla, and a recording is made at each site. At the moment the stimulus is produced, the *stimulus artifact* is seen at the left of the oscilloscope screen. A trigger mechanism controls this and it will, therefore, always appear in the same spot on the screen, facilitating consistent measurements. This spike is purely mechanical and does not represent any muscle activity. The stimulus intensity starts out low and is slowly increased until the evoked potential is clearly observed. When the stimulating electrode is properly placed over the nerve, all muscles innervated distal to that point will contract and the patient will see and feel the hand jump. The intensity is then increased until the evoked response no longer increases in size. At

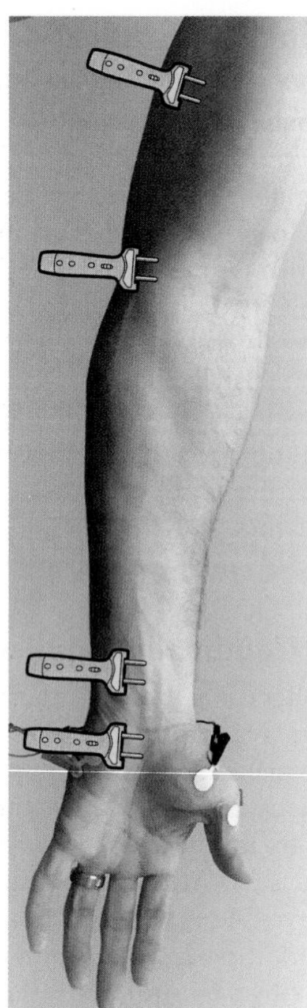

Figure 5.10 Sites of stimulation for median motor nerve conduction.

that time, the intensity is increased further to be sure that the stimulus is *supramaximal.* Because the intensity must be sufficient to reach the threshold of all motor fibers in the nerve, a supramaximal stimulus is required. It is also essential that the stimulator be properly placed over the nerve trunk so that the stimulus reaches all the motor axons.

As in the EMG signal, the potentials seen on the screen represent the electrical activity detected by the recording electrode. The signal will represent the difference in electrical potential between the recording and reference electrodes. When the supramaximal stimulus is applied to the median nerve at the wrist, all the axons in the nerve will depolarize and begin conducting an impulse, transmitting the signal across the motor end plate, initiating depolarization of the muscle fibers. During these events, the recording electrodes do not record a difference in potential because no activity is taking place beneath the electrodes. When the muscle fibers begin to depolarize, the electrical potentials are transmitted to the electrodes, and a deflection is seen on the oscilloscope. This is the evoked potential, which is called the *M wave.* The M wave is also referred to as the *motor action potential* (MAP) or *compound motor action potential* (CMAP). The CMAP represents the summated activity of all motor units in the muscle that responded to stimulation of the nerve trunk. The amplitude of this potential is, therefore, a function of the total voltage produced by the contracting motor units. The initial deflection of the CMAP is the negative portion of the wave, above the baseline. Conduction parameters of interest include latency, nerve conduction velocity, amplitude, and morphology.[99,103]

Calculation of Motor Nerve Conduction Velocity

The point at which the CMAP leaves the baseline indicates the time elapsed from the initial propagation of the nerve impulse to the depolarization of the muscle fibers beneath the electrodes. This is called the *response latency.* The latency is measured in milliseconds from the stimulus artifact to the onset of the CMAP. This time alone is not a valid measurement of nerve conduction because it incorporates time related to other events besides pure nerve conduction—namely, transmission across the NMJ and generation of the muscle action potential. Therefore, these extraneous factors must be eliminated from the calculation of the motor NCV, so that the measurement reflects only the speed of conduction within the nerve trunk.

To account for these distal variables, the nerve is stimulated at a second, more proximal point. This will produce a response similar to that seen with distal stimulation. The stimulus artifact will appear in the same spot on the screen, but the CMAP will originate in a different place because the time for the impulses to reach the muscle would, obviously, be longer. Subtraction of the *distal latency* from the *proximal latency* will determine the conduction time for the nerve trunk segment between the two points of stimulation. *Nerve conduction velocity* (NCV) is determined by dividing the distance between the two points of stimulation (measured along the surface) by the difference between the two latencies (velocity = distance/time).

NCV = Conduction distance/(Proximal latency – Distal latency).

NCV is always expressed in meters per second (m/s), although distance is usually measured in centimeters and latencies in milliseconds. These units must be converted during calculation. To compute the motor NCV, the latencies are determined for each stimulation site along the nerve by measuring the time from the stimulus artifact to the initial CMAP deflection. The segment conduction time is calculated by taking the difference between latencies of adjacent stimulation sites. *Conduction distance* is then determined by measuring the length of the nerve between the two points of stimulation. For example in Figure 5.11:

Wrist latency: 3.1 msec
Elbow latency: 6.7 msec
Conduction distance: 220 mm or 22 cm
CV = 220 mm / (6.7 msec – 3.1 msec) = 220 mm/ 3.6 msec = 61 m/s

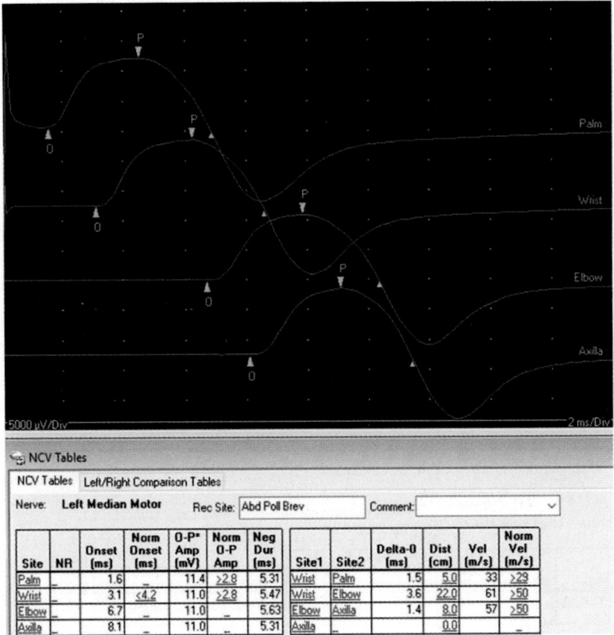

Site	NR	Onset (ms)	Norm Onset (ms)	0-P* Amp (mV)	Norm 0-P Amp	Neg Dur (ms)
Palm	_	1.6	_	11.4	≥2.8	5.31
Wrist	_	3.1	≤4.2	11.0	≥2.8	5.47
Elbow	_	6.7	_	11.0	_	5.63
Axilla	_	8.1	_	11.0	_	5.31

Site1	Site2	Delta-0 (ms)	Dist (cm)	Vel (m/s)	Norm Vel (m/s)
Wrist	Palm	1.5	5.0	33	≥29
Wrist	Elbow	3.6	22.0	61	≥50
Elbow	Axilla	1.4	8.0	57	≥50
Axilla	_		0.0		_

Figure 5.11 Median motor nerve conduction.

Interpretation of the motor NCV is made in relation to normal values, which are usually expressed as mean values, standard deviations, and ranges. Many investigators in different laboratories have determined normal values.[110] Even so, average values seem to be fairly consistent. The motor NCV for the UE has a fairly wide range, with values reported from 50 to 70 m/s. The average normal value is about 60 m/s. For the LE, the average value is about 50 m/s. Distal latencies and average normal amplitudes of CMAPs are also available in such tables, but these must be viewed with caution, because technique, electrode setup, instrumentation, and patient size can affect these values. Age and temperature can also influence NCS measurements, decreasing after age 35 and with lower temperature.[98] The reader is referred to more comprehensive discussions for complete details about techniques for studying various nerves and for tables of normal values.[105,109,110]

It is important to note that the value calculated as the conduction velocity is actually a reflection of the speed of the fastest axons in the nerve. Although all axons are stimulated at the same point in time, and supposedly fire at the same time, their conduction rates vary with their size. Not all motor units will contract at the same time; some receive their nerve impulse later than others. Therefore, the initial CMAP deflection represents the contraction of the motor unit, or units, with the fastest conduction velocity. The curved shape of the CMAP is reflective of the progressively slower axons reaching their motor units at a later time. Figure 5.12A demonstrates slower than normal wrist to palm conduction velocity and slower wrist to abductor pollicis latency in a patient with carpal tunnel syndrome.

The CMAP can also provide useful information about the integrity of the nerve or muscle. The shape and configuration of the CMAP should be examined along the course of the nerve tested and changes duly noted. *Temporal dispersion* is a phenomenon representing asynchronous recording of muscle fibers contributing to the CMAP due to varying speeds of individual motor neurons. While increasing the length of a segment will accentuate some disparity among neuron speed, demyelinating conditions often cause significant temporal dispersion in CMAPs.[99,103] Figure 5.12B demonstrates temporal dispersion in the tibial motor CMAP of a patient with diabetes-related peripheral polyneuropathy. Notice that the distal latency and leg velocity measures fall just outside of normal limits, but the CMAP morphology is longer in duration with smaller amplitude when comparing the knee to ankle CMAPs.

In instances of *partial neuropraxia or conduction block,* distal CMAP amplitude is normal, but stimulation proximal to the lesion is comparatively reduced without significant temporal dispersion. Figure 5.12C shows slowing with partial conduction block of just over 30% occurring at or just distal to the medial epicondyle in the ulnar motor NCS of a patient with cubital tunnel syndrome. To identify a conduction block, stimulation must occur distally and proximally to the nerve lesion. However, there are scenarios where this is not possible. For example, in assessing a brachial plexus disorder, difficulty may be experienced stimulating the axillary nerve distal to the clavicle. In contrast, stimulating the radial nerve is generally easily accessible both distally and proximally. This is an important concept, particularly when recognizing the improved prognostic implications of a neuropathy demonstrating conduction block as opposed to axon loss.

In motor axon loss, the CMAP distal to the lesion is expected to reflect lower than normal CMAP amplitude. Figure 5.12D depicts the motor NCS in a patient with severe carpal tunnel syndrome. In addition to slowed latency from wrist to the abductor pollicis brevis and slowed NCV from wrist to palm, the amplitude of the CMAP is well below the lower limit of normal. These parameters reflect the summated voltage over time produced by all the contracting motor units within the test muscle. Therefore, as this muscle is partially denervated, fewer motor units are contracting after nerve stimulation. This will cause the CMAP amplitude to decrease. Temporal dispersion may accentuate, depending on the conduction velocity of the intact units. Similar changes may also be evident in myopathic conditions, in which all motor units are intact but fewer fibers of variable size are available in each motor unit.

The shape of the CMAP can also be variable. Deviation from a smooth curve need not be abnormal, and it is often useful to compare the proximal and distal CMAPs with each other as well as with the contralateral side if indicated. They should be similar. In abnormal conditions,

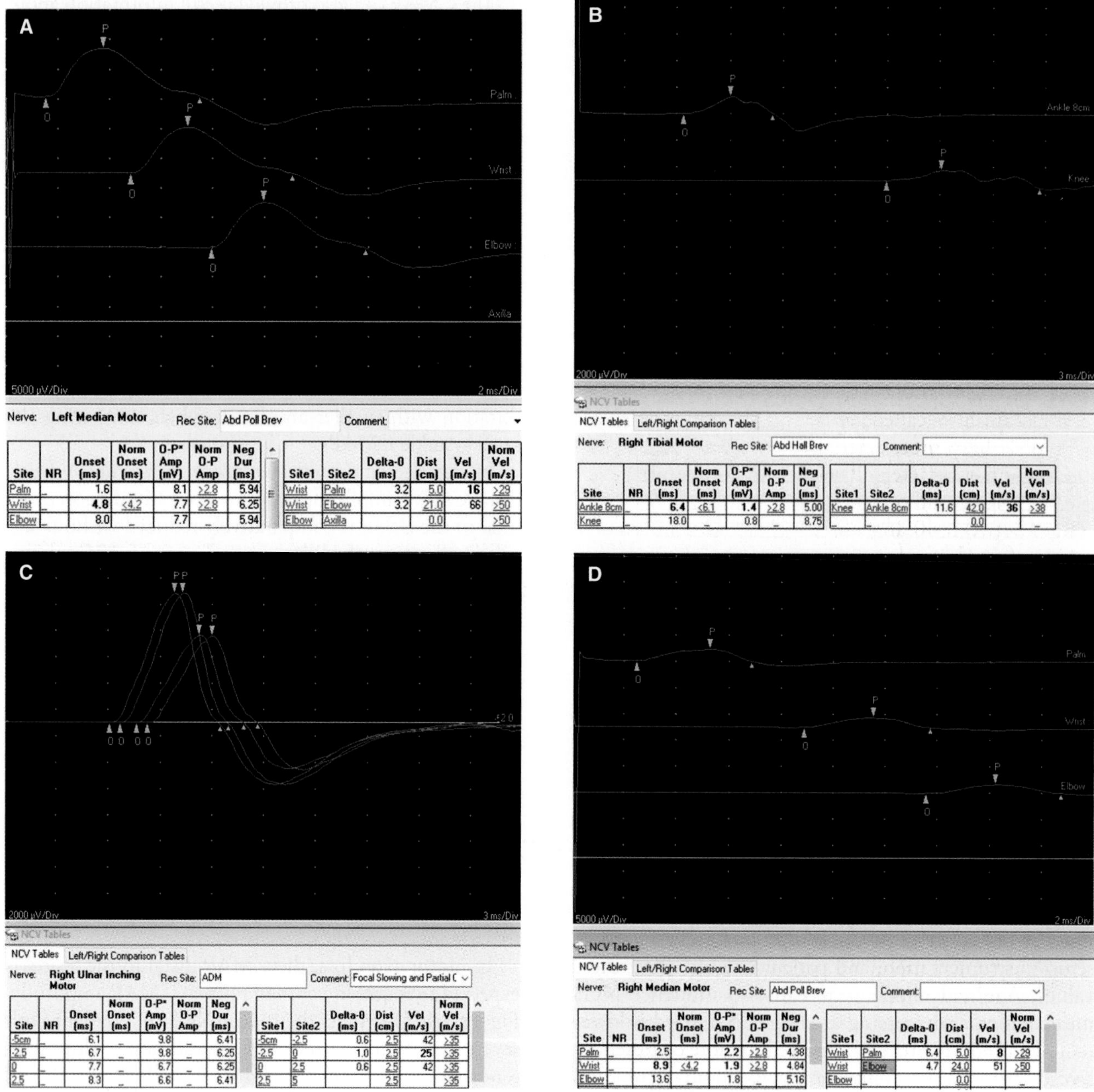

Figure 5.12 Abnormal motor nerve conduction studies. (A) Mild median slowing focally across the wrist. (B) Temporal dispersion of tibial motor nerve. (C) Partial motor conduction block of ulnar nerve at elbow. (D) Severe median slowing across the wrist with partial axon loss.

changes in shape may be the result of a significant slowing of conduction in some axons, repetitive firing, or asynchronous firing of axons after a single stimulus. Anatomic variations in innervation of muscle can also influence distal to proximal CMAP morphology, so it is important that EDX providers have a thorough understanding of neuromuscular anatomy and physiology.

Sensory Nerve Conduction Studies

Sensory neurons demonstrate the same physiological properties as motor neurons, and NCV can be measured in a similar way. However, some differences in technique are necessary to differentiate between sensory and motor axons. Although sensory fibers can be tested using *orthodromic conduction* (physiological direction) or *antidromic conduction* (opposite to normal conduction), antidromic measurements appear to be more common. For the same reason that motor axons are examined by recording over muscle, sensory axons are either stimulated or recorded from digital sensory nerves. This minimizes the activity of the motor axons from the recorded potentials.

The stimulating electrode used for sensory NCS tests is typically provided by ring, surface, or needle electrodes placed around the base of the digit innervated by the nerve, directly over or subcutaneously near the anatomic location of the nerve. Again, a comprehensive understanding of surface anatomy is paramount. Sensory potentials for the median and ulnar nerves can be recorded antidromically by stimulating at the wrist, elbow, and upper arm. Typically the sensory study of these nerves is limited to stimulation at the wrist. Other sensory nerves can be studied in the UEs and include the superficial radial, medial antebrachial cutaneous, lateral antebrachial cutaneous, and the dorsal cutaneous branch of the ulnar nerve. In the LEs, the sensory nerves most commonly studied are the sural nerve and the superficial fibular (peroneal) nerves. Other nerves that have been studied include the lateral femoral cutaneous, saphenous, and deep fibular (peroneal). Sensory evoked potentials are also called *sensory nerve action potentials* (SNAPs). Like motor nerve conduction, the sensory conduction parameters of interest include latency, amplitude, NCV, and morphology. Normal sensory NCV ranges between 40 and 75 m/s. Amplitude, measured with surface electrodes, are variable and can range from 2 uV to 120 uV, and duration should be short, generally less than 2 msec. Sensory evoked potentials are usually sharp, not rounded like the CMAP. Sensory NCVs are slightly faster than motor NCVs because of the uniformly larger diameter of sensory nerves contributing to the SNAP.[99,103] Figure 5.13A depicts normal antidromic sensory NCS of a median nerve to digit III. In this figure, latency is measured to the negative peak of the potential and SNAP amplitude from baseline to negative peak. Figure 5.13B depicts abnormal sensory NCS from the median nerve of a patient with mild carpal tunnel syndrome.

H Reflex

The *H reflex* is a useful diagnostic measure for radiculopathy and peripheral neuropathy. Its most common application is in testing the integrity of the sensory and motor monosynaptic pathways of S1 nerve roots via the tibial nerve and to a lesser extent at C6–C7 and L3–4 via the median or femoral nerves.[111] In traditional testing, a submaximal stimulus is applied to the tibial nerve at the popliteal fossa, and a motor response is recorded from the medial portion of the soleus muscle. The action potentials travel along the IA afferent neurons toward the spinal cord, synapsing onto interneurons at the level of the spinal cord, then alpha motor neurons within the anterior horn. The consequent activation of the motor neuron leads to an impulse traveling peripherally to the soleus muscle, resulting in a muscle contraction. Because the stimulus causes impulses to travel both distally and proximally within a mixed motor and sensory neuron, the latency of this response comprises a measure of the integrity of both sensory and motor fibers (Fig. 5.14A).

An average tibial H reflex latency is around 30 msec but is affected by limb length, age, and temperature.[112]

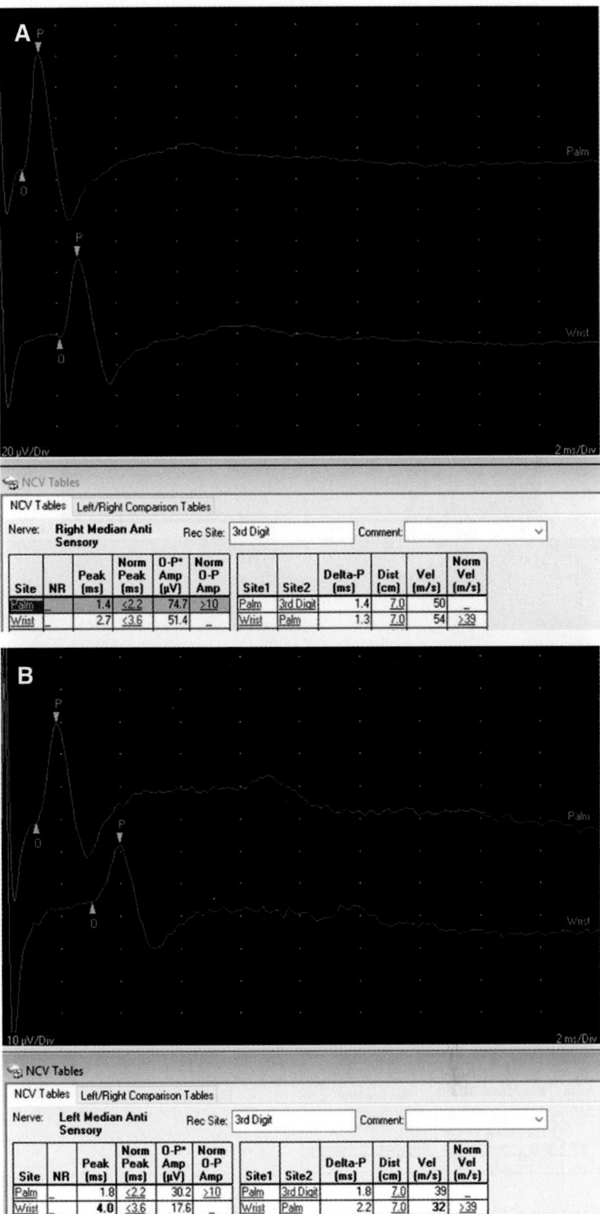

Site	NR	Peak (ms)	Norm Peak (ms)	O-P* Amp (µV)	Norm O-P Amp
Palm	_	1.4	<2.2	74.7	>10
Wrist	_	2.7	<3.6	51.4	_

Site1	Site2	Delta-P (ms)	Dist (cm)	Vel (m/s)	Norm Vel (m/s)
Palm	3rd Digit	1.4	7.0	50	_
Wrist	Palm	1.3	7.0	54	>39

Site	NR	Peak (ms)	Norm Peak (ms)	O-P* Amp (µV)	Norm O-P Amp
Palm	_	1.8	<2.2	30.2	>10
Wrist	_	4.0	<3.6	17.6	_

Site1	Site2	Delta-P (ms)	Dist (cm)	Vel (m/s)	Norm Vel (m/s)
Palm	3rd Digit	1.8	7.0	39	_
Wrist	Palm	2.2	7.0	32	>39

Figure 5.13 Sensory nerve conduction study. (A) Normal median sensory nerve conduction study. (B) Mild focal slowing of median sensory nerve at wrist.

A slowed latency with otherwise normal distal NCS parameters is indicative of abnormal proximal function, often from a herniated disc or other nerve root impingement. Because of more proximal involvement, the peripheral motor and sensory NCS would not be affected. This latency may also identify nerve root compression before obvious EMG changes occur.

The F wave

F waves are a form of NCS test that allows for study of proximal nerve segments that would otherwise be inaccessible to routine nerve conduction studies. F wave abnormalities can be an indicator of peripheral nerve

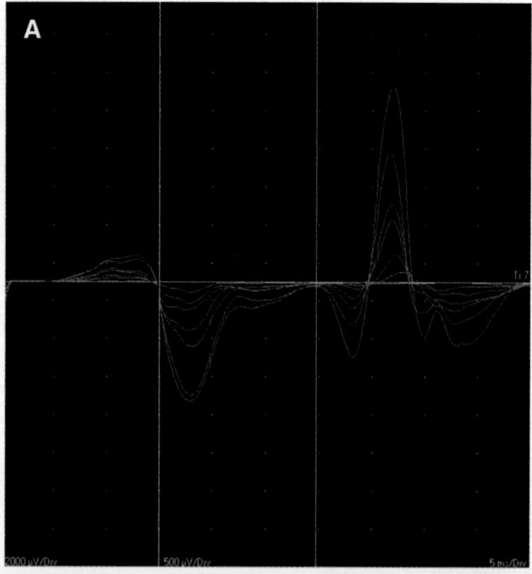

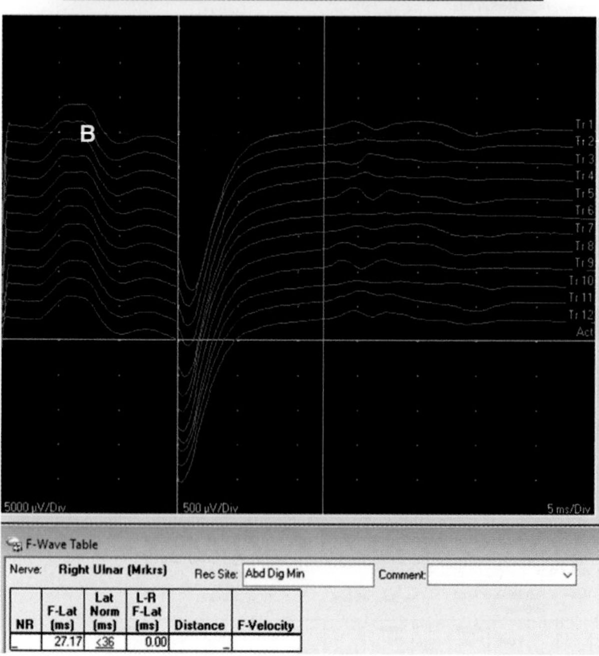

NR	F-Lat (ms)	Lat Norm (ms)	L-R F-Lat (ms)	Distance	F-Velocity
_	27.17	<36	0.00	_	

Figure 5.14 Late responses. (A) Reflex of tibial nerve. (B) Waves of ulnar nerve.

pathology or demyelination. The F wave ratio compares the conduction in the proximal half of the total pathway with the distal and may be used to determine the site of conduction slowing—for example, to distinguish a root lesion from a distal generalized neuropathy.[113] The F wave is elicited by the supramaximal stimulus of a peripheral nerve at a distal site, leading to propagation of impulses in both directions. While the orthodromic impulse travels to the distal muscle, the antidromic response travels to the anterior horn cell, depolarizing the axon hillock, leading to depolarization of dendrites, which in turn depolarizes the axon hillock once again, generating an orthodromic volley back to the muscle. No synapse is involved, so the F wave is not considered a reflex, but rather a measure of motor neuron conduction (see Fig 5.14B).

The F wave has some merit to assist other nerve conduction and EMG measures and is most helpful in the diagnosis of conditions where the most proximal portion of the axon is involved, such as Guillain-Barré syndrome, thoracic outlet syndrome, brachial plexus injuries, and radiculopathies with more than one nerve root involved.[105] The latency of the F wave is generally about 30 seconds in the upper limb and less than 60 seconds in the lower limb and is influenced by age and limb length. Only a small percent of motor neurons actually participate in the F response.[99] Because it is an inconsistent response, it must be calculated on the basis of at least 10 successive trials.[103]

Repetitive Nerve Stimulation

Repetitive nerve stimulation (RNS) is a technique used to evaluate for suspected NMJ disorders. RNS requires technical proficiency, attention to electrode placement, immobilization of the limb, and temperature control.[114-117] A baseline CMAP is recorded from a target muscle (preferably one that is clinically weak). Then a protocol of repetitive supramaximal stimulations is delivered in a train of 5 to 10 CMAPs at a low rate of stimulus frequency, around 2 Hz to 5 Hz. Comparisons of amplitude are made typically between the first and fourth or first and fifth CMAPs. If there is an amplitude decrement greater than 10%, it is considered abnormal. Following the first train of stimuli, a protocol series of exercise and periods of rest are performed between trains of stimuli. If there is decrement at low rates of stimulation, either fast RNS (20–50 Hz) or brief isometric contraction (to mimic tetany) is performed followed by another train of stimuli. In NMJ disorders, the response to slow and fast RNS can help determine pre- versus post-synaptic NMJ disorders (Fig. 5.15)

Disorders of Peripheral Nerve

Electrophysiological findings usually correlate with clinical signs in patients with neuropathic or myopathic involvement. As discussed, lesions of peripheral nerve fall into two categories, *demyelination* and *axonal loss*. Lesions involving peripheral nerve can occur focally, diffusely, segmentally or along a specific nerve root distribution. They can also involve motor nerves sparing sensory nerves or sensory nerve sparing motor nerves. A skilled

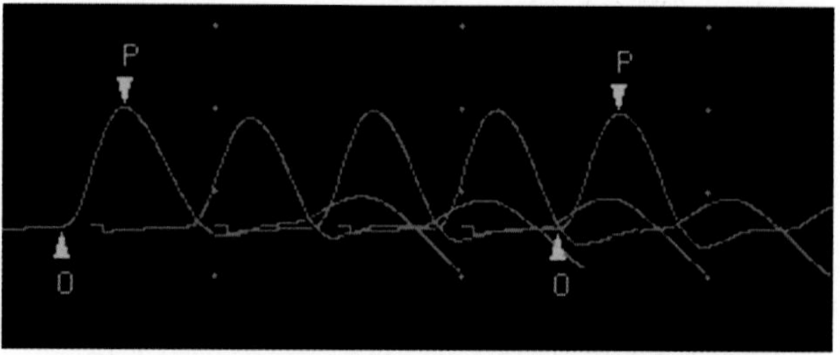

Figure 5.15 Repetitive nerve stimulation of ulnar nerve.

electrodiagnostician should have the capabilities to perform and interpret findings from the EMG and NCS in order to concisely convey an impression of the neurophysiological state of a patient's condition.

In focal neuropathy, NCS tests can detect evidence of degeneration and slowing of fibers across the site of compression but may be normal above and below that site. For example, patients with carpal tunnel syndrome may have abnormal motor and sensory NCS findings across the wrist with normal findings in the median nerve proximal to the carpal tunnel and in other nerves of the same limb. EMG abnormalities of increased insertion, fibrillations, and positive sharp waves may be noted in the thenar muscles but not in proximal median innervated muscles or other muscles of the same limb. Recruitment in the thenar muscles may show reduced interference pattern with fast-firing, long-duration polyphasic and/or larger than normal amplitude MUAPs.

Radiculopathy may involve sensory and motor abnormalities on clinical examination, but generally, the motor and sensory NCS is fairly normal unless motor axon loss is severe, at which point low amplitude CMAPs may be evident. SNAP amplitudes are generally preserved, despite the patient complaining of altered sensation, as most nerve root compression due to radiculopathy occurs proximal to the dorsal root ganglia and the cell body is in continuity with the distal axon. This is considered a *preganglionic lesion* and is an important distinguishing EDX characteristic in radiculopathy. H reflexes or F waves could be absent or delayed in the nerves supplied by the involvement spinal root level. EMG may show evidence of neuropathy with insertion, rest, and volitional testing in the distribution of the radiculopathy with sparing of muscles supplied by other nerve root levels.

Plexopathy refers to neuropathy involving components of the brachial, cervical, lumbar, or lumbosacral plexuses. It can be related to a number of different causes, including trauma, immune-mediated inflammation, birth-related injury, tumors, surgical complications, and unknown etiology (idiopathic). Plexopathy can occur in isolated trunks, divisions, or cords with or without extension of the injury distal into the terminal nerve branches. Isolated lesions involving a single trunk, division, or cord is rare. Slowed NCV across the plexus can be recognized. SNAP amplitudes with EMG changes in the distribution of the plexus components involved are the most sensitive indicators of sensory and motor axon loss in plexopathy.[118,119] Sparing of EMG changes in the paraspinal muscles helps rule out nerve root pathology.

Polyneuropathy affects multiple nerves and typically results in sensory changes, distal weakness, and hyporeflexia. It can be related to medical conditions, such as diabetes, alcoholism, or renal disease, as well as secondary complications related to cancer and its treatments.[99,103] These conditions manifest as axonal damage and/or demyelination and sensory and/or motor nerve involvement. Polyneuropathy can occur diffusely, segmentally, or peripherally. While EMG/NCS findings are not specific to a single diagnosis, the pattern of involvement can assist with narrowing the cause of the polyneuropathy.[120]

Motor Neuron Disorders

Motor neuron disorders typically involve degeneration of the anterior horn cell, such as in poliomyelitis, or diseases that involve both UMNs and LMNs, such as ALS. Abnormal resting potentials are classically seen with these disorders, as well as reduced recruitment, allowing single motor unit potentials to be visible even with an interference pattern. CMAPs may be reduced in amplitude. Motor NCV can be slightly slowed, depending on the distribution of degeneration and propensity for larger, faster fibers to undergo loss earlier in the disease. EMG will show neuropathic patterns with normal sensory NCS findings.

Myopathies

In *myopathy,* such as the muscular dystrophies and inflammatory myopathies (e.g., myositis, polymyositis, dermatomyositis), the motor unit remains intact, but degeneration of muscle fibers is evident. Motor latencies and NCVs should be normal, although the CMAP amplitudes can be reduced in more weak and involved muscles. Sensory NCS will also be normal. In early stages, EMG will show prolonged insertion activity, fibrillations, and positive sharp waves at rest and often complex repetitive discharges. Recruitment will show full interference patterns with minimal recruitment (early recruitment) with motor unit morphology demonstrating short-duration, low-amplitude polyphasic potentials with voluntary activity. In advanced stages, insertional activity becomes reduced with increased resistance to needle advancement with little electrical activity due to fibrosis of muscle tissue.

Neuromuscular Junction Disorders

In NMJ disorders, such as botulism toxicity, myasthenia gravis (MG), and Lambert-Eaton myasthenic syndrome (LEMS), there is a disturbance of neuromuscular transmission occurring at the NMJ at either the pre- or post-synaptic terminals. EDX abnormalities are most commonly seen using repetitive nerve stimulation and with observed CMAP changes to brief exercise. In post-synaptic NMJ disorders such as MG, baseline CMAPs are generally normal with no change following brief contraction. In slow RNS of 2 Hz to 5 Hz, a decrement may be seen.[116] With fast RNS of 20 Hz to 30 Hz, decrements persist or do not change. In LEMS, baseline CMAPs are generally low with significant improvement following brief exercise. Slow RNS shows decrement, but fast RNS demonstrates significant increase in CMAP amplitude.[115] Sensory NCS and EMG is generally normal in NMJ disorders, although there may be some MUAP amplitude variability. In LEMS, one could expect reduced recruitment.[114]

Assessing Severity and Estimating Prognosis in Neuropathy

Seddon and Sunderland offer a reasonable concept of nerve injury classification and lay the foundation for the progression of nerve injury from demyelination to axon loss.[101,102] Table 5.13 illustrates a proposed alternative classification of injury-predicted recovery.[99,121,122] It identifies severity of nerve injury from very mild to complete. Characteristics of the EDX in both the EMG and NCS can assist in determining if an injury involves predominantly myelin, axons, or both. Typically, more mild cases of neuropathy involve myelin and are characterized by slowing of motor/sensory latencies and NCV with possible conduction block. Nerve injury is considered more severe as axonal loss occurs. Axonal loss is recognized in the NCS as decrements in SNAP and CMAP amplitudes, and in the EMG with abnormal resting potentials, reduced recruitment, and motor unit morphological changes representing evidence of collateral axonal sprouting. Preservation of motor axons is essential for muscle function and is therefore a critical characteristic of interest. When there is significant loss of motor axons, the timing required for healing can be protracted with the possibility of residual deficit that can be influenced by age, other illnesses, and distance from the injury to the target muscles.

■ EVALUATION

Evaluation refers to the clinical judgments therapists make based on the data gathered from the examination. Numerous factors influence the judgments therapists make when working with patients with impairments of motor function, including complexity and understanding of the nervous system, clinical findings, psychosocial considerations, and overall physical function and health. Therapists evaluate data in terms of severity of problems (impairments, activity limitations, participation restrictions) and level of recovery or chronicity. Therapists must also consider the consequences of failure to intervene appropriately when the patient is at risk for additional impairments or prolonged activity limitation. Potential discharge placement and resources also influence evaluation of the data and development of the POC. There is a clear need for the therapist to focus on those problems

Table 5.13 Alternative Classification of Nerve Injury Progression and Prognosis

Severity	Type of Injury	EDX Findings	Recovery	Time to Recover	Prognosis
Very Mild	Mild Demyelination	Mild slow NCV/ latencies Preserved SNAPs/ CMAPs Normal EMG	Remyelination	2–12 weeks	Excellent
Mild	Advanced Demyelination	Advanced slow NCV/Latencies Partial CB, preserved SNAP/CMAP Normal EMG	Remyelination	2–12 weeks	Excellent
Moderate	Demyelination/ Mild Axon Loss	Reduced SNAP, Preserved CMAPs CB, mild EMG changes	Remyelination Collateral Sprouts	2–6 months	Excellent
Severe	Moderate Axon Loss	Absent SNAP, Low CMAP Advanced EMG changes	Collateral Sprouts	2–6 months	Good
Profound	Severe Axon Loss	CMAP 80%–100% reduced Advanced EMG changes	Collateral Sprouts Axon Regeneration	up to 18 months	Guarded/Fair
Complete	Severed Nerve	No Recordable NCS No MUAPs Advanced EMG changes	Surgery required	Protracted	Guarded at Best

that directly affect function and can be successfully remediated.

DIAGNOSIS

The *physical therapy diagnosis* is determined from evaluation of examination findings and is based on the results of both qualitative and quantitative assessments. Level of impairments, activity limitations, and participation restrictions are identified. Information is used to determine the diagnosis, which describes the impact of the condition on function at the level of the movement system and the whole person. It serves to direct the physical therapy intervention.[6] See discussion in Chapter 1, Clinical Decision Making. The therapist must also consider the results of an examination of skills in motor learning and problem-solving, motivation and emotional status, and learning styles. Typically the patient with brain insult or injury demonstrates profound deficits in motor function. Novice therapists can gain understanding and insights into the complex examination and practice issues facing therapists who work with these patients from experienced, senior therapists.

SUMMARY

Examination of motor function is a challenging process that requires the physical therapist to accurately determine and categorize findings. An understanding of normal motor control and motor learning is essential to this process. Determining the causative factors responsible for abnormal movement patterns and behaviors is based on comparison of expected or normal responses (norm-referenced behaviors) with the patient's abnormal ones. This can best be achieved by a systematic and thorough approach to examination. Emphasis should be on the use of valid, reliable, and responsive measurement tools. The assessment of electrophysiological properties of nerve and muscle provides essential information to understand neuromuscular disease or trauma, the location of a lesion in the PNS, and prognosis or rate of healing or decay.

Examination of systems yields valuable information about the integrity of individual components (e.g., neuromuscular, musculoskeletal, cognitive). It is important to recall that normal motor control and motor learning is achieved through the integrated action of the CNS. The therapist must therefore also focus on integrated function evidenced through an examination at the functional level. Success in rehabilitation is also dependent on our ability to understand the motivation and learning abilities of the patient and potential training strategies important for cognitive engagement and practice. Our theoretical understanding of the CNS, motor control, and motor learning processes is both incomplete and imperfect. Therapists must, therefore, be constantly aware of the changing knowledge base in neuroscience and in neurological rehabilitation to incorporate new ideas into their examination and intervention plan.

Note: The authors gratefully acknowledge the contributions of Mark Brooks, PT, DSc, ECS, OCS to this chapter.

Questions for Review

1. Differentiate between recovery of function and compensation.
2. Describe the examination of consciousness and arousal. How can the levels of consciousness and arousal influence the motor function examination?
3. Differentiate between selective attention and alternating attention. How should each be examined?
4. Differentiate between spasticity and rigidity. How should each be examined?
5. Describe the examination of a hyperactive patellar deep tendon reflex. What scores are used to document an increased DTR?
6. A patient with stroke exhibits abnormal control of eye muscles and is unable to move the eyes smoothly in all directions. Cranial nerve testing should include which nerves and tests?
7. What are the issues of validity for using manual muscle testing as part of the examination of a patient with UMN syndrome (stroke) who exhibits strong spasticity and strong obligatory synergies?
8. A patient with multiple sclerosis reports fatigue as the number one symptom that impairs functional independence in the home environment. How should this patient's fatigue be examined and documented?
9. Define *stability*. How should it be examined?
10. Differentiate between the use of performance observations and retention tests in providing evidence of motor learning.

11. Differentiate EMG from NCS and how each can be utilized to assess nerve and muscle integrity.
12. Differentiate EMG from NCS and how each can be utilized to assess nerve and muscle integrity.
13. Describe how the EMG and NCS can estimate severity of nerve injury and prognosis for recovery.
14. What is a fibrillation potential on EMG? What is it indicative of?
15. How is nerve conduction velocity calculated?

CASE STUDY

The patient is a 17-year-old female who is 6 months post–motor vehicle accident (MVA). At the time of admission to the hospital, she was comatose and decerebrate. CT scan revealed intracranial bleeding into the right occipital horn. She received a tracheostomy and a gastrostomy. Two months post-MVA, she was transferred to a *long-term care facility* specializing in TBI.

On initial admission she was able to open her eyes to verbal and tactile stimuli but was unable to visually track. She withdrew her upper and lower extremities in response to stimulation but was not able to move them on command. She was alert but confused, and was unable to carry on a conversation. ROM was within normal limits (WNL) except for right elbow flexion (20° to 100°) and right knee flexion (10° to 110°). She demonstrated increased tone in her left upper extremity (LUE), 3 on Modified Ashworth Scale, 4 on MAS in her right upper extremity (RUE), and 4 in both lower extremities (BLEs). She exhibited 4+ bilateral ankle clonus. She was unable to sit unsupported. During supported sitting in the wheelchair, her head and trunk control was poor, with persistent posturing to the left side.

She is now 6 months post-MVA and is currently being examined for transfer to active rehabilitation status.

PHYSICAL THERAPY EXAMINATION FINDINGS

Consciousness/Arousal

Fully awake; responds appropriately to varying stimuli.
Oriented to person; some confusion with orientation to place and time.
Can become agitated with minimal stimulation, especially when tired.

Cognition/Behavior

Demonstrates difficulty with concentration and attention.
Able to follow simple instructions (one-level commands) but occasionally forgets what is asked of her.
Reaction time is slowed as the number of choices is increased.
Easily forgets what she is doing.

Sensory Integrity

Aware of sensory input (pinprick, vibration, light touch) to all extremities.
Unable to discern common objects placed in either hand for stereognosis discrimination.

Joint Integrity and Mobility

RLE: plantarflexion contracture (40° to 50°); flexion contractures at the hip (10° to 120°) and knee (10° to 120°).
RUE: flexor contracture at the elbow (10° to 110°).
Full passive ROM in the LUE and LLE.

Tone

Increased bilaterally (R > L).
On Modified Ashworth Scale: RUE and RLE 3; LUE and LLE 2.

Reflex Integrity

Hyperactive, 3+ DTRs RUE, RLE.
3+ bilateral ankle clonus.

Cranial Nerve Integrity

Dysphagia and dysphonia are present.

Muscle Performance

Strength is decreased in the RUE, RLE, and trunk (unable to test with MMT).
She is unable to sustain R knee extension during standing.

Voluntary Movement Patterns

RUE moves in partial range, obligatory mass flexor synergy pattern only.

RLE moves in flexor and extensor synergy patterns with no variation.

LUE and LLE demonstrate full voluntary control with isolated joint movements. Coordination is decreased. Unable to reach directly to an object that is held out to her and demonstrates foot placement problems with the LLE in sitting or in standing.

Demonstrates problems with coordinating limb and trunk movements.

Postural Control and Balance

Demonstrates good head control in all positions.

Sitting: can sit independently for up to 5 minutes. Demonstrates difficulty in maintaining weight equally on both buttocks. Tends to list to the right side while placing weight primarily on her left buttock. Able to reach to the left and forward; demonstrates loss of balance (LOB) with minimal reaching to right.

Standing: able to stand in parallel bars with minimal assistance of 1 (Min A x 1) for up to 2 minutes. Has to be reminded to place weight on RLE. Tends to lose her balance easily if she moves quickly; associated with brief episodes of dizziness and vertigo.

Functional Mobility Skills

Rolling: requires supervision and occasional Min A x1 with rolling to the right; she requires maximal assist (Max A x 1) when rolling to the left.

Supine-to-sit: able to come to sitting by rolling to the L side and pushing up with her LUE; requires Min A x 1.

Transfers: able to perform stand pivot transfers with Min A x 1.

Gait: does not initiate ambulation on her own. Can ambulate the length of the parallel bars (2 m or 6 ft) with maximal assistance of two persons. Requires posterior splint to stabilize R knee.

Propels wheelchair by using the LUE and both feet for pushing; requires supervision for safety.

Motor Learning

Demonstrates profound deficits in short-term memory; unable to remember new information presented during therapy. Her memory for events and learning that occurred before the MVA is good.

GUIDING QUESTIONS

Based on your evaluation of the data presented in the case history and the physical therapy examination, answer the following questions:

1. How has this patient's level of consciousness/arousal changed from admission to the long-term care facility to the current evaluation? How might this influence the examination of motor function?
2. Develop a physical therapy problem list. Categorize the patient's problems in terms of (1) direct impairments, (2) indirect impairments, and (3) functional limitations.
3. Prioritize the problems in terms of this patient's needs for the POC.
4. Determine the physical therapy diagnosis for this patient.

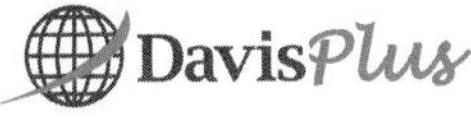

For additional resources, including answers to the questions for review and case study guiding questions, please visit **http://davisplus.fadavis.com.**

References

1. Schmidt, R, and Lee, T: Motor Control and Learning, ed 5. Human Kinetics, Champaign, IL, 2011.
2. Shumway-Cook, A, and Woollacott, M: Motor Control: Theory and Practical Applications, ed 5. Lippincott Williams & Williams/Wolters Kluwer, Philadelphia, 2017.
3. Bernstein, N: The Coordination and Regulation of Movements. Pergamon Press, New York, 1967.
4. Kleim, J, and Jones, T: Principles of experience-dependent neural plasticity: Implications for rehabilitation after brain damage. J Speech Lang Hear Res 51(1):S225, 2008.
5. Levin, M, Kleim, J, and Wolf, S: What do motor "recovery" and "compensation" mean in patients following stroke? Neurorehabil Neural Repair 23:313, 2009.
6. *Guide to Physical Therapist Practice 3.0.* Alexandria, VA: American Physical Therapy Association; 2014. Available at: http://guidetoptpractice.apta.org/.Accessed 9.10.15
7. World Health Organization (WHO): ICF: Towards a Common Language for Functioning, Disability, and Health. Geneva, Switzerland, 2002. Retrieved March 4, 2017, from www.who.int/classifications/en.

8. Bear, M, Connors, B, and Paradiso, M: Neuroscience: Exploring the Brain, ed 4. Lippincott Williams & Wilkins/Wolters Kluwer, Philadelphia, 2016.
9. Bickley, LS, and Szilagyi, P: Bates' Guide to Physical Examination and History Taking, ed 11. Lippincott Williams & Wilkins/Wolters Kluwer, Philadelphia, 2013.
10. Jennett, B, and Bond, M: Assessment of outcome after severe head injury: A practical scale. Lancet 1:480, 1975.
11. Rancho Los Amigos Hospital: Rehabilitation of the Head Injured Adult. Professional Staff Association, Downey, CA, 1979.
12. Duffy, E: Activation and Behavior. Wiley, New York, 1962.
13. Yerkes, R, and Dodson, J: The relation of strength of stimulus to rapidity of habit-formation. J Comp Neurol Psychol 18(5):459, 1908.
14. Strub, R, and Black, F: The Mental Status Examination in Neurology, ed 4. FA Davis, Philadelphia, 2000.
15. Folstein, M: Mini-mental state: A practical method for grading the cognitive state of patients for the clinician. J Psychiatr Res 12:189, 1975.
16. Shean, G, and McGuire, R: Spastic hypertonia and movement disorders: Pathophysiology, clinical presentation, and quantification. PM & R 1:9, 2009.
17. Gracies, JM: Pathophysiology of spastic paresis. I: Paresis and soft tissue changes. Muscle Nerve 31:535, 2005.
18. Gracies, JM: Pathophysiology of spastic paresis. II: Emergence of muscle overactivity. Muscle Nerve 31:552, 2005.
19. Mayer, NH, Esqquenazi, A, and Childers, MK: Common patterns of clinical motor dysfunction. Muscle Nerve:21, 1997.
20. Ashworth, B: Preliminary trial of carisoprodol in multiple sclerosis. Practitioner 192:540, 1964.
21. Bohannon, R, and Smith, M: Interrater reliability of a modified Ashworth scale of muscle spasticity. Phys Ther 67:206, 1987.
22. Gregson, JM, et al: Reliability of measurements of muscle tone and muscle power in stroke patients. Age Ageing 29:223, 2000.
23. Ghotbi, N, et al: Measurement of lower-limb muscle spasticity: Intrareliability of Modified Ashworth Scale. JRRD 48(1):83, 2011.
24. Craven, BC, and Morris, AR: Modified Ashworth Scale reliability for measurement of lower extremity spasticity among patients with SCI. Spinal Cord 48:207, 2010.
25. Ansari, NN, et al: The interrater and intrarater reliability of the Modified Ashworth Scale in the assessment of muscle spasticity: Limb and muscle group effect. Neuro Rehabil 23:231, 2008.
26. Mehrholz, J, et al: Reliability of the Modified Tardieu Scale and the Modified Ashworth Scale in adult patients with severe brain injury: A comparison study. Clin Rehabil 19:751, 2005.
27. Blackburn, M, et al: Reliability of measurements obtained with the Modified Ashworth Scale in the lower extremities of people with stroke. Phys Ther 82:25, 2002.
28. Pandyan, AD, et al: A review of the properties and limitations of the Ashworth and Modified Ashworth Scales as measures of spasticity. Clin Rehabil 1:373, 1999.
29. Pandyan, AD, et al: A biomechanical investigation into the validity of the Modified Ashworth Scale as a measure of elbow spasticity. Clin Rehabil 17:290, 2003.
30. Tardieu, G, Shentoub, S, and Delaure, R: [Research on a technic for measurement of spasticity.]. Rev Neurol (Paris) 91(2):143, 1954.
31. Haugh, AB, Pandyan, A, and Johnson, G: A systematic review of the Tardieu Scale for the measurement of spasticity. Disabil Rehab 28(15):899, 2006.
32. Gracies, JM, et al: Reliability of the Tardieu Scale for assessing spasticity in children with cerebral palsy. Arch Phys Med Rehabil 91(3):421, 2010.
33. Mehrholz, J, et al: Reliability of the Modified Tardieu Scale and the Modified Ashworth Scale in adult patients with severe brain injury: A comparison study. Clin Rehabil 19(7):751, 2005.
34. Singh, P, et al: Intra-rater reliability of the modified Tardieu scale to quantify spasticity in elbow flexors and ankle plantar flexors in adult stroke subjects. Ann Indian Acad Neurol 14(1):23, 2011.
35. Ansari, et al: The Modified Tardieu Scale for the measurement of elbow flexor spasticity in adult patients with hemiplegia. Brain Injury 22:1007m, 2008.
36. Patrick, E, and Ada, L: The Tardieu Scale differentiates contracture from spasticity whereas the Ashworth Scale is confounded by it. Clin Rehabil 20(2):173, 2006.
37. Capute, A, et al: Primitive reflex profile: A pilot study. Phys Ther 58:1061, 1978.
38. Verheyden, G, et al. Postural alignment is altered in people with chronic stroke and related to motor and functional performance. JNPT 38:239, 2014.
39. Sahrmann, S: Diagnosis and Treatment of Movement Impairment Syndromes. Mosby, St. Louis, 2002.
40. Kokotilo, K, Eng, JJ, and Boyd, L: Reorganization of brain function during force production after stroke. JNPT 33:45, 2009.
41. Frascarelli, M, Mastrogregori, L, and Conforti, L: Initial motor unit recruitment in patients with spastic hemiplegia. Electromyogr Clin Neurophysiol 38:267, 1998.
42. Noskin, O, et al: Ipsilateral motor dysfunction from unilateral stroke: Implications for the functional neuroanatomy of hemiparesis. J Neurol Neurosurg Psychiatry 79:401, 2008.
43. Chae, J, et al: Muscle weakness and cocontraction in upper limb hemiparesis: Relationship to motor impairment and physical disability. Neurorehabil Neural Repair 16:241, 2002.
44. Hacmon, RR, et al: Deficits in intersegmental trunk coordination during walking are related to clinical balance and gait function in chronic stroke. JNPT 36(4):173, 2012.
45. Andrews, AW, and Bohannon, RW: Distribution of muscle strength impairments following stroke. Clin Rehabil 14:79, 2000.
46. Marque, P, et al: Impairment and recovery of left motor function in patients with right hemiplegia. J Neurol Neurosurg Psychiatry 62:77, 1997.
47. Rothstein, J, et al: Commentary. Is the measurement of muscle strength appropriate in patients with brain lesions? Phys Ther 69:230, 1989.
48. Bohannon, R: Is the measurement of muscle strength appropriate in patients with brain lesions? Phys Ther 69:225, 1989.
49. Rothstein, J, et al: Clinical uses of isokinetic measurements. Phys Ther 67:1840, 1987.
50. Perrin, DH: Isokinetic Exercise and Assessment. Human Kinetics, Champaign, IL, 1993.
51. Brown, LE: Isokinetics in Human Performance. Human Kinetics, Champaign, IL, 2000.
52. Mhandi, E, and Bethoux, F: Isokinetic testing in patients with neuromuscular diseases: A focused review. Am J Phys Med Rehabil 92(2):163, 2013.
53. Barbee, J, and Landis, D: Reliability of Cybex computer measures. Phys Ther. 68:737, 1984.
54. Johnson, J, and Siegel, D: Reliability of an isokinetic movement of the knee extensors. Res Q 49:88–90, 1978.
55. Mawdsley, RH, and Knapik, J: Comparison of isokinetic measurements with test repetitions. Phys Ther 62:169–172, 1982.
56. Perrin, DH: Reliability of isokinetic measures. J Athl Train 23:319–321, 1986.
57. Timm, KE, et al: The mechanical and physiological performance reliability of selected isokinetic dynamometers. Isokinet Exerc Sci. 2:182–190, 1992.
58. Pohl, P, et al: Reliability of lower extremity isokinetic strength testing in adults with stroke. Clinical Rehabil 14:601, 2000.
59. Kim, C, et al: Reliability of dynamic muscle performance in hemiparetic upper limb. JNPT 29:1, 2005.
60. Curtis, C, and Weir, J: Overview of exercise responses in healthy and impaired states. Neurology Report 20:13, 1996.
61. American College of Sports Medicine: ACSM's Exercise Management for Persons with Chronic Disease and Disabilities, ed 3. Human Kinetics, Champaign, IL, 2009.
62. Bennett, R, and Knowlton, G: Overwork weakness in partially denervated skeletal muscle. Clin Orthop 12:22, 1958.
63. Bigland-Richie, B, and Woods, J: Changes in muscle contractile properties and neural control during human muscular fatigue. Muscle Nerve 7:691, 1984.
64. Fisk, J, et al: The impact of fatigue on patients with multiple sclerosis. J Can Sci Neurol 21:9, 1994.
65. Fisk, J, et al: Measuring the functional impact of fatigue: Initial validation of the fatigue impact scale. Clin Infect Dis 18 Suppl 1:S79, 1994.
66. Rietberg, M, et al: Measuring fatigue in patients with multiple sclerosis: Reproducibility, responsiveness and concurrent validity of three Dutch self-report questionnaires. Disabil Rehabil 32(22):1870, 2010.

67. Learmonth, YC, et al: Psychometric properties of the Fatigue Severity Scale and the Modified Fatigue Impact Scale. J Neurol Sci 331:102, 2013.
68. Grace, J, et al: A comparison of fatigue measures in Parkinson's disease. Parkinsonism Relat Disord 13(7):443, 2007.
69. Hagell, P, et al: Measuring fatigue in Parkinson's disease: A psychometric study of two brief generic fatigue questionnaires. J Pain Symptom Manage 32(5):420, 2006.
70. Koopman, FS, et al: Measuring fatigue in polio survivors: Content comparison and reliability of the fatigue severity scale and the checklist individual strength. J Rehabil Med 46(8):761, 2014.
71. Krupp, L, et al: The fatigue severity scale. Application to patients with multiple sclerosis and systemic lupus erythematosus. Arch Neurol 46(10):1121, 1989.
72. Guide for the Uniform Data Set for Medical Rehabilitation (including the FIM instrument), Version 5.0 State University of Buffalo, 1996.
73. Borg, G: Borg's Perceived Exertion and Pain Scales. Human Kinetics, Champaign, IL, 1998.
74. Brunnstrom, S: Movement Therapy in Hemiplegia. Harper & Row, New York, 1970.
75. Twitchell, T: The restoration of motor function following hemiplegia in man. Brain 74:443, 1951.
76. Fugl-Meyer, A: The post-stroke hemiplegic patient. I: A method for evaluation of physical performance. Scand J Rehabil Med 7:13, 1975.
77. Carr, JH, et al: Investigation of a new motor assessment scale for stroke patients. Phys Ther 65: 175, 1985.
78. Hsieh, C, et al: Validity and responsiveness of the Rivermead Mobility Index in stroke patients. Scand J Rehab Med 32(3):140, 2000.
79. Wolf, S, et al: Assessing Wolf Motor Function Test as outcome measure for research in patients after stroke. Stroke 32:1635, 2001.
80. Uswatte, G, et al: The Motor Activity Log-28 assessing daily use of the hemiparetic arm after stroke. Neurol 67(7):1189, 2006.
81. Kopp, B, et al: The Arm Motor Ability Test: Reliability, validity, and sensitivity to change of an instrument for assessing disabilities in activities of daily living. Arch Phys Med Rehabil 78(6):615, 1997.
82. Collin, C, and Wade, D: Assessing motor impairment after stroke: A pilot reliability study. J Neurol Neurosurg Psych 53(7):576, 1990.
83. Verheyden, G, et al: The Trunk Impairment Scale: A new tool to measure motor impairment of the trunk after stroke. Clin Rehab 18(3):326, 2004.
84. Gorman, SL, et al: Development and validation of the function in sitting test in adults with acute stroke. JNPT 34(3):150, 2010.
85. Benaim, C, et al: Validation of a standardized assessment of postural control in stroke patients: The Postural Assessment Scale for Stroke Patients (PASS). Stroke 30(9):1862, 1999.
86. VanSant, A: Life span development in functional tasks. Phys Ther 70:788, 1990.
87. Shenkman, M, et al: Whole-body movements during rising to standing from sitting. Phys Ther 70:638, 1990.
88. VanSant, A: Rising from a supine position to erect stance: Description of adult movement and a developmental hypothesis. Phys Ther 68:185, 1988.
89. Green, L, and Williams, K: Differences in developmental movement patterns used by active vs sedentary middle-aged adults coming from a supine position to erect stance. Phys Ther 72:560, 1992.
90. Richter, R, et al: Description of adult rolling movements and hypothesis of developmental sequences. Phys Ther 69:63, 1989.
91. Gentile, A: Skill acquisition: Action, movement and neuromotor processes. In Carr, JH, et al (eds): Movement Science: Foundations for Physical Therapy in Rehabilitation, ed 2. Aspen, Gaithersburg, MD, 2000, p. 111.
92. Lewis, A: Documentation of movement patterns used in the performance of functional tasks. Neurol Rep 16:13, 1992.
93. Ackerman, P: Individual differences in skill learning: An integration of psychometric and information processing perspectives. Psychol Bull 102:3, 1988.
94. Fitts, P, and Posner, M: Human Performance. Brooks/Cole, Belmont, CA, 1969.
95. Anderson, JR: Acquisition of cognitive skill. Psychol Rev 89:369, 1982.
96. Anderson, JR: Learning and memory: An Integrated Approach. Wiley, New York, 1995.
97. Winstein, C, et al: Infusing motor learning research into neurorehabilitation practice: A historical perspective with case exemplar from the Accelerated Skill Acquisition Program. JNPT 38: 190, 2014.
98. Lynch, MC, and Cohen, JA: A primer on electrophysiologic studies in myopathy. Rheum Dis Clin North Am 37(2):253, vii, 2011.
99. Dumitru, D, Amato, AA, and Zwarts, M: Electrodiagnostic Medicine, ed 2, Hanley & Belfus, Philadelphia, 2002.
100. Kandel, ER, et al: Principles of Neural Science, ed 5, McGraw-Hill, New York, 2012.
101. Seddon, H: Three types of nerve injury. Brain 66:237, 1943.
102. Sunderland, S, et al: A classification of peripheral nerve injuries producing loss of function. Brain 74:491, 1951.
103. Kimura, J: Electrodiagnosis in Diseases of Nerve and Muscle: Principles and Practice, ed 4. Oxford University Press, New York, 2013.
104. Van der Heijden, A, Spaans, F, and Reulen, J: Fasciculation potentials in foot and leg muscles of healthy young adults. Electroencephalogr Clin Neurophysiol 93:163, 1994.
105. Echternach, JL: Introduction to Electromyography and Nerve Conduction Testing, ed 2. Slack, Thorofare, NJ, 2002.
106. Rodriguez, AA, et al: Electromyographic and neuromuscular variables in post-polio subjects. Arch Phys Med Rehabil 76:989, 1995.
107. Roeleveld, K, et al: Motor unit size estimation of enlarged motor units with surface electromyography. Muscle Nerve 21:878, 1998.
108. Stalberg, E, and Grimby, G: Dynamic electromyography and muscle biopsy changes in a 4-year follow-up: Study of patients with a history of polio. Muscle Nerve 18:699, 1995.
109. Pease, WS, Lew, HL, and Johnson, EW: Johnson's Practical Electromyography, ed 4. Lippincott Williams & Wilkins, Philadelphia, 2006.
110. Kumbhare, D, Robinson, L, and Buschbacher, R: Buschbacher's Manual of Nerve Conduction Studies, ed 3. Springer, New York, 2015.
111. Gersh, MR: Electrotherapy in Rehabilitation. FA Davis, Philadelphia, 1992.
112. Misiaszek, JE: The H-reflex as a tool in neurophysiology: Its limitations and uses in understanding nervous system function. Muscle Nerve 28:144, 2003.
113. Mallik, A, and Weir, AI: Nerve conduction studies: Essentials and pitfalls in practice. J Neurol Neurosurg Phys 76 (Suppl 2):23, 2005.
114. Harvey, AM, and Masland, RL: The electromyogram in myasthenia gravis. Bull Johns Hopkins Hosp 69:1, 1941.
115. Tim, RW, Massey, JM, and Sanders, DB: Lambert-Eaton myasthenic syndrome (LEMS): Clinical and electrophysiologic features and response to therapy of 59 patients. Ann NY Acad Sci 841:823, 1998.
116. Mayer, RF, and Williams, IR: Incrementing responses in myasthenia gravis. Arch Neurol 31:24, 1974.
117. Oh, SJ, et al: Electrophysiological and clinical correlation in myasthenia gravis. Ann Neurol 12:348, 1982.
118. Ferrante, MA: Brachial plexopathies: Classification, causes and consequences. Muscle Nerve 30:547, 2004.
119. Ferrante, MA, and Wilbourn, A: The utility of various sensory nerve conduction responses assessing brachial plexopathies. Muscle Nerve 18:879, 1995.
120. Donofrio, PD, and Albers, JW: AAEM minimonograph #34: polyneuropathy: Classification by nerve conduction studies and electromyography. Muscle Nerve 13:889, 1990.
121. Bland, J: A neurophysiological grading scale for carpal tunnel syndrome. Muscle Nerve 23:1280, 2000.
122. Greathouse, DG, et al: GEHS neurophysiological classification system for patients with carpal tunnel syndrome. US Army Med Dep J 60, 2016.
123. O'Sullivan, S, and Siegelman, R: National Physical Therapy Examination Review & Study Guide. Therapy Ed, Evanston, IL, 2018.

Chapter 6 Examination of Coordination and Balance

Thomas J. Schmitz, PT, PhD
Susan B. O'Sullivan, PT, EdD

LEARNING OBJECTIVES

1. Understand the purposes of performing an examination of coordination and balance.
2. List the types of data generated from the examination.
3. Describe the common coordination and balance impairments associated with lesions of the central nervous system.
4. Explain the primary age-associated changes that affect coordination and balance.
5. Provide a rationale for the preliminary patient observation before performing an examination.
6. Identify the motor task requirements and movement capabilities addressed during an examination of coordination and balance.
7. Differentiate between tests used to examine coordination and balance.
8. Using the case study example, apply clinical decision making skills to application of coordination and balance examination data.

CHAPTER OUTLINE

EXAMINATION OF COORDINATION

A key component of motor function, coordination is the ability to execute smooth, accurate, controlled movement. "Coordinated movement involves multiple joints and muscles that are activated at the appropriate time and with the correct amount of force so that smooth, efficient, and accurate movement occurs. Thus, the essence of coordination is the sequencing, timing, and grading of the activation of multiple muscles groups."[1, p. 121]

The ability to produce these responses is dependent on sensory information from the body and environment, visual and vestibular input, and a fully intact musculoskeletal and neuromuscular system. Coordinated movements are characterized by appropriate speed, distance, direction, timing, and muscular tension. In addition, they involve appropriate synergistic influences (muscle recruitment), easy reversal between opposing muscle groups (appropriate sequencing of contraction and relaxation), and proximal fixation to allow distal motion or maintenance of a posture.[2] Schmidt and Lee define coordination as the "behavior of two or more degrees of freedom in relation to each other to produce skilled activity."[3, p. 494] Awkward, extraneous, uneven, or inaccurate movements characterize *coordination impairments*.

Two terms often associated with coordination are *dexterity* and *agility*.[4] *Dexterity* refers to skillful use of the fingers during fine motor tasks.[5] *Agility* refers to the ability to rapidly and smoothly initiate, stop, or modify movements while maintaining postural control.

There are several general types of coordination. *Intralimb* coordination refers to movements occurring within a single limb[6-9] (e.g., alternately flexing or extending the elbow; use of one upper extremity [UE] to brush the hair; or motor performance of a single lower extremity [LE] during a gait cycle). *Interlimb* (bimanual) coordination refers to the integrated performance of two or more limbs working together[10-16] (e.g., alternately flexing one elbow while extending the other; bilateral UE tasks as required during transfers or dressing activities; or between limb movements of the LEs and/or UEs during walking). *Visual motor* coordination[17-21] refers to the ability to integrate both visual and motor abilities with the environmental context to accomplish a goal (e.g., tracing over a zigzag line, writing a letter, riding a bicycle, or driving an automobile). A subcategory of visual motor coordination with important implications for activities of daily living (ADL) is *eye–hand coordination*,[22-26] such as required for using eating utensils, personal hygiene, or reaching for a visual target (e.g., a book from a shelf). Eye–hand coordination is perhaps more aptly termed *eye–hand–head coordination* because movement of the head is typically required for the eyes to fixate on a target or object.

Physical therapists are frequently involved in the management of patients with coordination impairments. Data from the examination of coordination inform the therapist about existing impairments. These impairments are often associated with activity limitations that are related to, and indicative of, the type, extent, and location of central nervous system (CNS) pathology. Some CNS lesions present very classic and stereotypical impairments, but others are much less predictable. Diagnoses associated with coordination impairments include traumatic brain injury, Parkinson's disease, multiple sclerosis, Huntington's disease, cerebral palsy, Sydenham's chorea, cerebellar tumors, vestibular pathology, and some learning disabilities.

In the Test and Measure Categories, the *Guide to Physical Therapist Practice 3.0*[4] includes impaired coordination among the examples of clinical indications for mobility (including locomotion), gait, balance, motor function, and cranial and peripheral nerve injury. Measurement of dexterity, coordination, and agility is indicated to characterize or quantify motor function as well as neuromotor development and sensory processing. Coordination exercises are included among the therapeutic exercises performed by physical therapists.

The purposes of performing a coordination examination are presented in Figure 6.1. In addition, data from the coordination examination assist the therapist with establishing the diagnosis of underlying impairments, activity limitations, and participation restrictions (disability); assist with establishing goals to remediate impairments and formulating expected outcomes that encompass remediation of activity limitations and participation restrictions; and support decision making in establishing a prognosis and determining specific, direct interventions.

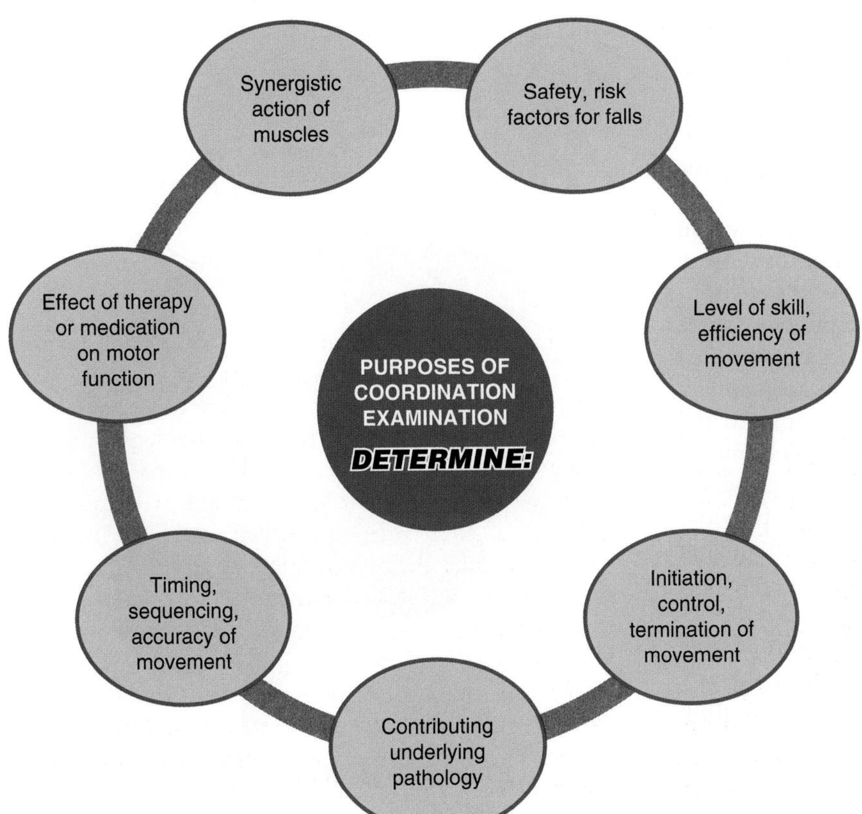

Figure 6.1 Purposes of performing a coordination examination.

OVERVIEW OF THE MOTOR SYSTEM

The motor system can be grossly divided into *peripheral* and *central* elements. The peripheral somatic motor system includes muscles, joints, and their sensory and motor innervation.[27] The central elements can be divided into three hierarchical levels to assist understanding their organization as well as delineating the contribution of each neuroanatomical structure. However, this does not imply a strictly top-down control of coordinated movement, as each level of the nervous system can influence other levels (above and below) depending on task demands (i.e., flexible hierarchical theory). Bear et al[27] provide a practical description of the three hierarchical levels relative to their functional contributions to motor control: "The highest level, represented by the association areas of the neocortex and basal ganglia of the forebrain, is concerned with *strategy:* the goal of the movement and the movement strategy that best achieve[s] the goal. The middle level, represented by the motor cortex and cerebellum, is concerned with *tactics:* the sequences of muscle contractions, arranged in space and time, required to smoothly and accurately achieve the strategic goal. The lowest level, represented by the brain stem and spinal cord, is concerned with *execution:* activation of the motor neuron and interneuron pools that generate the goal-directed movement and make any necessary adjustments of posture."[27, p. 452]

The motor system can also be viewed as having a *parallel arrangement*. For example, information is conveyed not only from the motor cortex to the spinal cord but also directly from premotor areas. Although the cerebellum and basal ganglion are involved in movement, they have no direct output to the spinal cord. Instead, their effect on movement is provided via connections to the motor cortex.[28]

The critical role of sensory input on the motor system cannot be overemphasized. The integration of sensory input provides an internal representation of the environment that informs and guides motor responses.[2] These sensory representations provide the foundation on which motor programs for purposeful movements are planned, coordinated, and implemented. Sensory input to the motor system guides selection and adaptation of motor responses and shapes motor programs for corrective action. For example, the somatosensory system provides the needed information to adjust walking when moving from a smooth surface to an uneven terrain; to maintain standing balance on a moving bus; or to make the required adjustments when throwing a ball from a stable sitting surface (chair) versus an unstable one (therapy ball). To rule out sensory impairments as a contributing factor to coordination impairments, examination of sensory function (see Chapter 3, Examination of Sensory Function) should *precede* the coordination examination.

The Motor Cortex

The principal brain area involved in motor function is the motor cortex, which comprises cortical (Brodmann's) areas 4 and 6, located in a demarcated area of the frontal lobe called the *precentral gyrus* (Fig. 6.2). However, planning coordinated movement to accomplish a task involves many areas of the neocortex as it requires knowledge of the body's position in space, the location of the intended target, selection of an optimum movement strategy (i.e., which joints, muscles, or body segments will be used), memory storage until time of execution, and specific instructions to implement the movement strategy selected (where to move or what to do).[28,29]

Brodmann's area 4 is designated the *primary motor cortex*, as it is the most specific cortical motor area containing the largest concentration of corticospinal neurons.[30] This area is electrically excitable, and stimuli of low intensity evoke a motor response. It lies anterior to the central sulcus on the precentral gyrus and controls contralateral voluntary movements. Brodmann's area 6 is also electrically excitable but requires stimuli of higher intensities to cause a motor response.[31] It lies just anterior to area 4 and is subdivided into the superiorly placed *supplementary motor area* (SMA) and the inferiorly positioned *premotor area* (PMA).[31]

The SMA gives rise to axons that directly innervate motor units involved in initiation of movement, simultaneous bilateral grasping movements, sequential tasks, and orientation of the eyes and head. The PMA provides input to the reticulospinal neurons innervating motor units that control trunk and proximal limb movements

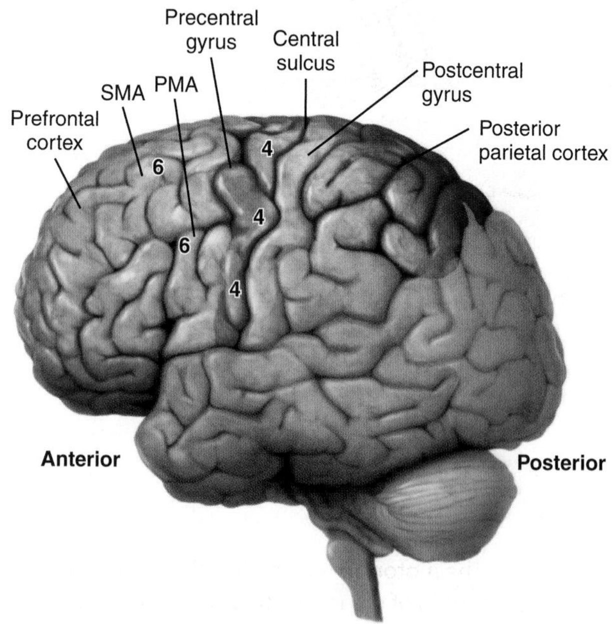

Figure 6.2 Primary areas of the cortex involved in coordinated movement.

and contributes to anticipatory postural changes.[27,32] Stimulation of area 4 typically results in uncomplicated movements of a single joint whereas stimulation to the premotor areas (area 6) evokes more intricate coordinated movements involving multiple joints.[29]

The somatotopic organization of the motor cortex is very similar to the sensory cortex. The motor homunculus schematically illustrates the amount of cortical area devoted to motor control of a given body part or region (Fig. 6.3). Beginning on the lateral aspect of the homunculus, the mouth and face areas are represented; moving upward are areas devoted to the hands, trunk, LEs, and feet. Note that areas requiring finer gradations of control such as the fingers, hand, and face (including muscles of speech) occupy a disproportionately larger representation (approximately half) in the motor cortex. The SMA and PMA are similarly somatotopically organized.

The motor cortex receives information from three primary sources: the *somatosensory cortex* (peripheral receptive fields), the *cerebellum,* and the *basal ganglia.* Somatosensory input is relayed directly to the primary motor cortex from the thalamus (e.g., cutaneous tactile sensations, joint and muscle receptors). The thalamus also relays information to the motor areas from the cerebellum and the basal ganglia. These connections allow for integration of motor control functions of the motor cortex, cerebellum, and basal ganglia (i.e., to carry out the appropriate course of motor action).[33]

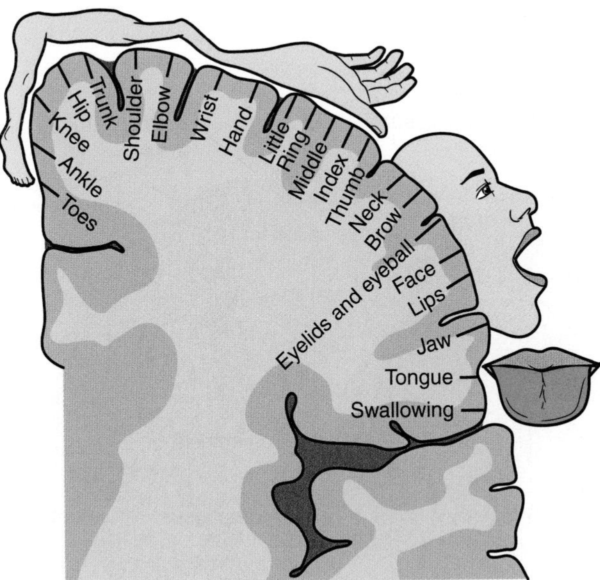

Figure 6.3 The motor homunculus indicates the somatotopic organization of the motor cortex. The relative greater size of some body parts such as the hand, fingers, face (lips and tongue) reflects the large proportion of the motor cortex devoted to controlling these areas.

Descending Motor Pathways

The most important descending pathway of the motor system is the corticospinal (pyramidal) tract that transmits signals from the motor cortex directly to the spinal cord. It is among the longest and largest CNS tracts. It originates primarily in areas 4 and 6 and passes through the internal capsule and the brainstem. A majority of fibers then cross to the opposite side in the medulla and descend through the lateral corticospinal tracts of the spinal cord. The fibers that do not cross at the medulla form the ventral corticospinal tracts, but a majority of these eventually cross to the opposite side in the cervical or upper thoracic regions. All fibers of the corticospinal tract terminate on the interneurons of the cord gray matter. The corticospinal tract is concerned with skilled, fine motor control, especially of the distal limbs.[33] The other major descending motor pathways that control neurons innervating muscle include the following:

- Corticobulbar tract: Some fibers project directly to motor cranial nerve (CN) nuclei (e.g., trigeminal, facial, hypoglossal), and others to the reticular formation before reaching CN nuclei.
- Tectospinal tract: This relatively small tract projects to motor neurons in the cervical cord; fibers influence neurons innervating neck muscles, as well as the spinal accessory nucleus (CN XI); important in guiding head movements during visual motor tasks.
- Reticulospinal tract (medial and lateral): Projects to the anterior horn of the spinal cord; important influence on muscle tone and reflex activity via influence on muscle spindle activity (increasing or decreasing sensitivity); the pontine (medial) reticulospinal tract facilitates extension of the LEs (excitation of extensor motor neurons) augmenting antigravity reflexes of the spinal cord; important influence on posture and gait. The medullary (lateral) reticulospinal tract has the reverse effect (excitation of flexor motor neurons).
- Vestibulospinal tracts (medial and lateral): The lateral vestibulospinal tract descends to all levels of the spinal cord; important contributions to postural control and movements of the head (facilitates axial extensors; inhibits axial flexors). The medial vestibulospinal tract projects primarily to the ipsilateral cervical spinal cord which is also involved in coordinated head and eye movements.
- Rubrospinal tract: This tract merges with the corticospinal tract in the cervical region. Its role in human motor control is considered insignificant. It is believed that during primate evolution the role of this tract was completely taken over by the corticospinal tract.

Cerebellum

The primary function of the cerebellum is regulation of movement, postural control, and muscle tone. Although all of the mechanisms of cerebellar function are not clearly understood, lesions have been noted to produce typical patterns of impaired motor function and balance and decreased muscle tone (see the "Cerebellar Pathology" section).

Several theories of function of the cerebellum in motor activity have been established. Among the more widely held is that the cerebellum functions as a *comparator* and *error-correcting mechanism.*[29,34] The cerebellum compares the commands for the *intended* movement transmitted from the motor cortex with the *actual* motor performance of the body segment. This occurs by a comparison of information received from the cortex with that obtained from peripheral feedback mechanisms (termed *feedforward control*). The motor cortex and brain stem motor structures provide the commands for the intended motor response (internal feedback).[34] Peripheral feedback during the motor response is provided by muscle spindles, Golgi tendon organs, joint and cutaneous receptors, the vestibular apparatus, and the eyes and ears (external feedback). This feedback provides continual input regarding posture and balance, as well as position, rate, rhythm, and force of slow movements of peripheral body segments. If the input from the feedback systems does not compare appropriately (i.e., movements deviate from the intended command), the cerebellum supplies a corrective influence. This effect is achieved by corrective signals sent to the cortex, which, via motor pathways, modifies or corrects the ongoing movement (e.g., increasing or decreasing the level of activity of specific muscles). The cerebellum also functions to modify cortical commands for subsequent movements.[34]

This CNS analysis of movement information, determination of level of accuracy, and provision for error correction is referred to as a closed-loop system. Schmidt and Lee define this model as "a control system employing feedback, a reference for correctness, a computation of error, and subsequent correction in order to maintain a desired state."[3, p. 493] It should be noted that not all movements are controlled by this system. Stereotypical movements (e.g., gait activities) and rapid, short-duration movements, which do not allow sufficient time for feedback to occur, are theorized to be controlled by an open-loop system, defined as "a control system with preprogrammed instructions to a set of effectors; it does not use feedback information and error-detection processes."[3, p. 497] In this system, it is believed that control originates centrally from a motor program, which is a memory or preprogrammed pattern of information for coordinated movement. The motor system then follows the established pattern largely independent of feedback or error-detection mechanisms. Motor programs can be called up in their entirety, modified, or reassembled in a new order. They provide the important function of freeing higher executive levels from attending to all aspects of a motor response. See Chapter 10: Strategies to Improve Motor Function, for a more thorough discussion of motor control and motor learning.

Basal Ganglia

The basal ganglia are a group of nuclei located at the base of the cerebral cortex (Fig. 6.4). The three main nuclei of the basal ganglia are the *caudate nucleus,* the *putamen,* and the *globus pallidus.* These nuclei have close

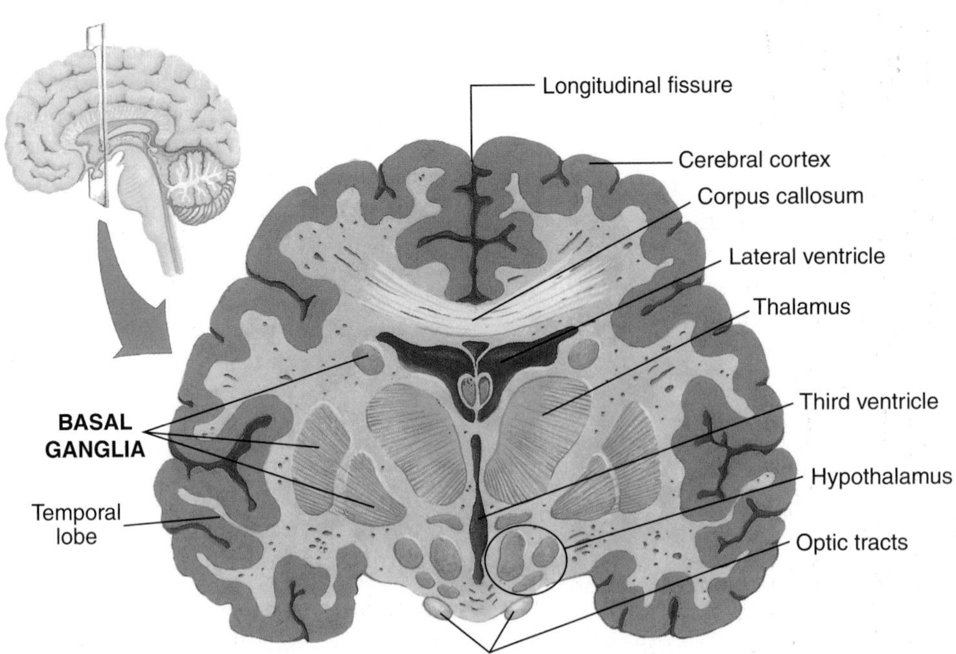

Figure 6.4 Frontal section of the brain in anterior view showing location of the basal ganglion within the cerebral cortex. *(Adapted from Scanlon and Sanders[35, p. 199] with permission.)*

anatomical and functional connections with two other subcortical nuclei that are also frequently considered as part of the basal ganglia: the *subthalamic nucleus* and the *substantia nigra*.[28]

Although the influences of the basal ganglia on movement are not understood as clearly as those of the cerebellum, there is evidence that the basal ganglia play an important role in several complex aspects of movement and postural control. These include the initiation and regulation of gross intentional movements, planning and execution of complex motor responses, facilitation of desired motor responses while selectively inhibiting others, and the ability to accomplish automatic movements and postural adjustments.[33,35,36] In addition, the basal ganglia play an important role in maintaining normal background muscle tone. This is accomplished by the inhibitory effect of the basal ganglia on both the motor cortex and lower brainstem. The basal ganglia also are believed to influence some aspects of both perceptual and cognitive functions.[36]

The motor portion of the basal ganglia assumes a somatotopic organization. The anatomical positioning of the basal ganglia provides insight into its contribution to motor performance. The areas of the brain associated with movement (primary motor cortex, supplementary motor area, premotor area, and the somatosensory cortex) form dense projections to the motor portion of the putamen. Output of this pathway forms the *motor circuit* of the basal ganglia, which is directed back to the supplementary motor area and the premotor area. These two areas and the primary motor cortex are all interconnected, and each has descending projections to the brain stem motor centers and spinal cord. This anatomical arrangement indicates that the influence of the basal ganglia on motor function is indirect and mediated by descending projections from the cortical motor areas.[36,37]

Dorsal (Posterior) Column–Medial Lemniscal Pathway

Regulation of movement is dependent on sensory afferent information. Peripheral somatosensory receptors and pathways provide information about the status of the environment, the status of the body, and the status of the body in relation to the environment.[3] This information is encoded and conveyed to various parts of the CNS. The data are processed based on peripheral feedback and memory, which leads to selection (or modification) of a movement strategy appropriate to the task demands and environmental conditions.

The dorsal column–medial lemniscal pathway is particularly important to coordinated movement, as it is responsible for the afferent transmission of discriminative sensations. Sensory modalities that require fine gradations of intensity and precise localization on the body surface are mediated by this system. Sensations transmitted by the dorsal column–medial lemniscal pathway include discriminative touch, stereognosis, tactile pressure, barognosis, graphesthesia, recognition of texture, kinesthesia, two-point discrimination, proprioception, and vibration.

This system is composed of large, myelinated, rapidly conducting fibers. After entering the dorsal column, the fibers ascend to the medulla and synapse with the dorsal column nuclei (nuclei gracilis and cuneatus). From here they cross to the opposite side and pass up to the thalamus through bilateral pathways called the *medial lemnisci*. Each medial lemniscus terminates in the ventral posterolateral thalamus. From the thalamus, third-order neurons project to the somatic sensory cortex.

■ FEATURES OF COORDINATION IMPAIRMENTS

As the cerebellum, basal ganglia, and dorsal column–medial lemniscal pathway provide input to, and act together with, the cortex in the production of coordinated movement, lesions in any of these areas affect higher-level processing and execution of coordinated motor responses. Although it is incorrect to assign all problems of incoordination to one of these sites, lesions in these areas are responsible for many characteristic motor deficits seen in adult populations. The following sections present an overview of common clinical features associated with lesions in each of these areas.

Cerebellar Pathology

A number of specific motor impairments that affect coordinated movement are associated with cerebellar pathology.[38-42] Many of these impairments either directly or indirectly influence the patient's ability to execute accurate, smooth, controlled movements. The motor deficits identified emphasize the crucial influence of the cerebellum on equilibrium, posture, muscle tone, and initiation and force of movement. *Ataxia* is perhaps the most common term used to describe motor impairments of cerebellar origin. Cerebellar ataxia is a general, comprehensive term used to describe loss of muscle coordination as a result of cerebellar pathology. Ataxia may affect gait, posture, and patterns of movement and is linked to difficulty initiating movement, as well as errors in the rate, rhythm, and timing of responses.

Perlman[43] provides an adept summary of the motor impairments associated with each of the major anatomic regions of the cerebellum as follows: "The cerebellum has three anatomic divisions that account for the three types of dysfunction commonly seen: (1) the midline (vermis, paleocerebellum), which underlies titubation, truncal ataxia, orthostatic tremor, and gait imbalance; (2) the hemispheres (neocerebellum—right controlling the right side of the body and left controlling the left side), which contribute to limb ataxia (e.g., dysdiadochokinesia, dysmetria, and kinetic tremor), dysarthria, and hypotonia; and (3) the posterior (flocculonodular lobe, archicerebellum), which also influences posture and gait as well as causing eye movement disorders (e.g., nystagmus, vestibulo-ocular reflex disruption)."[43, p. 216]

The following motor impairments are manifestations of cerebellar pathology:

- *Asthenia* is generalized muscle weakness associated with cerebellar lesions.
- *Dysarthria* is a disorder of the motor component of speech articulation. The characteristics of cerebellar dysarthria are referred to as scanning speech (often described as having a *one-word-at-a-time* quality or words may be broken into separate syllables). This speech pattern is typically slow and may be slurred, hesitant, with prolonged syllables and inappropriate pauses. Word use, selection, and grammar remain intact, but the melodic quality of speech is altered.[34,39,44]
- *Dysdiadochokinesia* is an impaired ability to perform rapid alternating movements. This deficit is observed in movements such as rapid alternation between pronation and supination of the forearm. Movements are irregular, with a rapid loss of range and rhythm especially as speed is increased.[39]
- *Dysmetria* is an inability to judge the distance or range of a movement. It may be manifested by an overestimation (hypermetria) or an underestimation (hypometria) of the required range needed to reach an object or goal.
- *Dyssynergia (movement decomposition)* describes a movement performed in a sequence of component parts rather than as a single, smooth activity. For example, when asked to touch the index finger to the nose, the patient might first flex the elbow, and then adjust the position of the wrist and fingers, further flex the elbow, and finally flex the shoulder.
- *Asynergia* is the loss of ability to associate muscles together for complex movements.
- *Gait ataxia* involves ambulatory patterns that typically demonstrate a broad base of support (BOS). Upright stance stability is often poor and the arms may be held away from the body to improve balance (high guard position). Stepping patterns are irregular in direction and distance. Initiation of forward progression of a LE may start slowly, and then the extremity may unexpectedly be flung rapidly and forcefully forward and audibly hit the floor.[45] Gait patterns tend to be generally unsteady (postural instability), irregular, and staggering, with deviations from an intended forward line of progression (veering to one side; swaying or pitching in different directions).
- *Hypotonia* is a decrease in muscle tone. It is believed to be related to the disruption of afferent input from stretch receptors and/or lack of the cerebellum's facilitatory efferent influence on the fusimotor system. A diminished resistance to passive movement will be noted, and muscles may feel abnormally soft and flaccid. Diminished deep tendon reflexes also may be noted.[34] *Note:* After testing the patellar tendon jerk with a reflex hammer in a normal subject, the knee typically returns immediately to the resting state. With cerebellar pathology, the knee may oscillate six to eight times before returning to rest.[34]
- *Nystagmus* is a rhythmic, quick, oscillatory, back-and-forth movement of the eyes. It is typically apparent as the eyes move away from midline to fix on an object in either the medial or lateral field (i.e., extremes of temporal or nasal vision).[46] The patient has difficulty holding the gaze on the object in the peripheral field. An involuntary drift back to midline with immediate return to the object may be observed.[47] Nystagmus causes difficulty with accurate fixation and vision and is believed linked to the cerebellum's influence on synergy and tone of the extraocular muscles.
- *Rebound phenomenon*, originally described by Holmes, is the loss of the check reflex,[45] or check factor, which functions to halt forceful active movements when resistance is eliminated. Normally, when application of resistance to an isometric contraction is suddenly removed, the limb will remain in approximately the same position by action of the opposing muscle(s). For example, in applying resistance to an isometric contraction in the middle range of elbow flexion and then releasing it without warning, the intact subject will "check" or stop the motion quickly through activation of the opposing triceps, as well as feedback regarding joint position and force required to prevent further motion. With cerebellar involvement, the patient is unable to stop the motion, and the limb will move suddenly when resistance is released. The patient may strike himself or herself or other objects when the resistance is removed.
- *Tremor* is an involuntary oscillatory movement resulting from alternate contractions of opposing muscle groups. Different types of tremors are associated with cerebellar lesions. An intention tremor, or kinetic tremor, occurs during voluntary motion of a limb and tends to increase as the limb nears its intended goal or when speed is increased.[34] Intention tremors are diminished or absent at rest. Postural (static) tremor may be evident by back-and-forth oscillatory movements of the body while the patient maintains a standing posture. Postural tremors also may be observed as up-and-down oscillatory movements of a limb when it is held against gravity. *Titubation* typically refers to rhythmic oscillations of the head (side-to-side or forward-and-backward movements, or the movements may have a rotary component); however, the term is also less frequently used to refer to axial involvement of the trunk.

In addition to these characteristic clinical features of cerebellar involvement, a greater length of time may also be required to initiate voluntary movements (delayed reaction time). Difficulty may also be observed in stopping or changing the force, speed, or direction of movement, prolonging movement time.[28] Motor learning will also be affected. Recall that the cerebellum compares the intended movement (internal feedback) with the actual movement (external feedback). For subsequent movements, the cerebellum generates corrective signals to reduce the errors (feedforward control). Lack of this feedforward control is responsible for deficits in motor learning and coordination.

Basal Ganglia Pathology

Patients with lesions of the basal ganglia typically demonstrate several characteristic motor deficits. These include (1) poverty and slowness of movement; (2) involuntary, extraneous movement; and (3) alterations in posture and muscle tone.[32,37] Thus, patients with basal ganglia involvement present on a continuum of motor behavior from severely diminished as seen in advanced Parkinson's disease to excessive extraneous movements apparent with Huntington's disease.[37]

The following motor impairments are manifestations of basal ganglia pathology:

- *Akinesia* is an inability to initiate movement and is seen in the late stages of Parkinson's disease. This deficit is associated with assumption and maintenance of fixed postures (freezing episodes). A tremendous amount of mental concentration and effort is required to perform even the simplest motor activity.
- *Athetosis* is characterized by slow, involuntary, writhing, twisting, "wormlike" movements. Frequently, greater involvement in the distal UEs is noted;[48] this may include fluctuations between hyperextension of the wrist and fingers and a return to a flexed position, combined with rotary movements of the extremities. Many other areas of the body may be involved, including the neck, face, tongue, and trunk. The phenomena are also referred to as *athetoid movements*. Pure athetosis is relatively uncommon and most often presents in combination with spasticity, tonic spasms, or chorea. Athetosis can be a clinical feature of some forms of cerebral palsy.
- *Bradykinesia* is a decreased amplitude and velocity of voluntary movement.[49] It may be demonstrated in a variety of ways, such as a decreased arm swing; slow, shuffling gait; difficulty initiating or changing direction of movement; lack of facial expression; or difficulty stopping a movement once begun. Bradykinesia is characteristic of Parkinson's disease.
- *Chorea* is characterized by involuntary, rapid, irregular, and jerky movements involving multiple joints. Choreiform movements demonstrate irregular timing, are most apparent in the UEs and cannot be voluntarily inhibited; it is associated with Huntington's disease.[50,51]
- *Choreoathetosis* is a term used to describe a movement disorder with features of both chorea and athetosis.
- *Dystonia* (dystonic movements) involves sustained involuntary contractions of agonist and antagonist muscles,[37,51] causing abnormal posturing (*dystonic posture*) or twisting movements. Most common in trunk and extremity musculature but also may affect the neck, face, and vocal cords. Torsion spasms also are considered a form of dystonia, with spasmodic torticollis being the most common.[45]
- *Hemiballismus* involves large-amplitude sudden, violent, flailing motions of the arm and leg of one side of the body. Primary involvement is in the axial and proximal musculature of the limb. Hemiballismus results from a lesion of the contralateral subthalamic nucleus.[28,31]
- *Hyperkinesis* is abnormally increased muscle activity or movement; *hypokinesis* is a decreased motor response especially to a specific stimulus.
- *Rigidity* is an increase in muscle tone causing greater resistance to passive movement. It tends to be more pronounced in the flexor muscles of the trunk and extremities, causing activity limitations in such areas as dressing, transfers, speech, eating, and postural control.[1] Two types of rigidity may be seen: *lead-pipe* and *cogwheel*. Lead-pipe rigidity is a uniform, constant resistance felt by the examiner as the extremity is moved through a range of motion (ROM). Cogwheel rigidity is considered a combination of the lead-pipe type with tremor. It is characterized by a series of brief relaxations or "catches" as the extremity is passively moved.
- *Tremor* is an involuntary, rhythmic, oscillatory movement observed at rest (resting tremor).[52] Resting tremors typically disappear or decrease with purposeful movement but may increase with emotional stress. Tremors associated with basal ganglia lesions (e.g., Parkinson's disease) are frequently noted in the distal UEs in the form of a "pill-rolling" movement, where it looks as if a pill is being rolled between the first two fingers and the thumb. Motion of the wrist, and pronation and supination of the forearm, may be evident. Tremors also may be apparent at other body parts as well, such as the jaw; this is characteristic of Parkinson's disease. Table 6.1 provides a summary of common coordination impairments associated with pathology of the cerebellum and basal ganglia.

Dorsal (Posterior) Column–Medial Lemniscal Pathology

Coordination impairments associated with dorsal column–medial lemniscal (DCML) lesions are somewhat less characteristic than those produced by either cerebellar or basal ganglia pathology. Lesions of the DCML

Table 6.1 Common Coordination Impairments Associated With Pathology of the Cerebellum and Basal Ganglia

	Cerebellar Pathology
Asthenia	Generalized muscle weakness
Asynergia	Loss of ability to associate muscles together for complex movements
Delayed reaction time	Increased time required to initiate voluntary movement
Dysarthria	Disorder of the motor component of speech articulation
Dysdiadochokinesia	Impaired ability to perform rapid alternating movements
Dysmetria	Inability to judge the distance or range of a movement
Dyssynergia	Movement performed in a sequence of component parts rather than as a single, smooth activity; decomposition
Gait disorders	Ataxic pattern; broad base of support; postural instability; high-guard position of UEs
Hypotonia	Decrease in muscle tone
Hypermetria	Overestimation of distance or range needed to accomplish a movement
Hypometria	Underestimation of distance or range needed to accomplish a movement
Nystagmus	Rhythmic, quick, oscillatory, back-and-forth movement of the eyes
Rebound phenomenon	Inability to halt forceful movements after resistive stimulus removed; patient unable to stop sudden limb motion
Tremor	Involuntary oscillatory movement resulting from alternate contractions of opposing muscle groups
• Intention (kinetic)	Oscillatory movement during voluntary motion; increases as the limb nears target; diminished or absent at rest
• Postural (static)	Exaggerated oscillatory movement of the body in standing posture or of a limb held against gravity
Titubation	Rhythmic oscillations of the head; axial involvement of the trunk
	Basal Ganglia Pathology
Akinesia	Inability to initiate movement; associated with fixed postures
Athetosis	Slow, involuntary, writhing, twisting, "wormlike" movements; frequently greater involvement in distal UEs
Bradykinesia	Decreased amplitude and velocity of voluntary movement
Chorea	Involuntary, rapid, irregular, jerky movements involving multiple joints; most apparent in UEs
Choreoathetosis	Movement disorder with features of both chorea and athetosis
Dystonia (dystonic movements)	Sustained involuntary contractions of agonist and antagonist muscles
Hemiballismus	Large-amplitude sudden, violent, flailing motions of the arm and leg of one side of the body
Hyperkinesis	Abnormally increased muscle activity or movement
Hypokinesis	Decreased motor response especially to a specific stimulus
Rigidity	Increase in muscle tone causing greater resistance to passive movement; greater in flexor muscles
• Lead-pipe	Uniform, constant resistance as limb is moved
• Cogwheel	Series of brief relaxations or "catches" as limb is passively moved
Tremor (resting)	Involuntary, rhythmic, oscillatory movement observed at rest

UEs = upper extremities.

typically result in coordination and equilibrium impairments related to the patient's lack of joint position sense and awareness of movement and impaired localized touch sensation. Recall that this ascending pathway carries the peripheral (external) feedback required for feedforward control. It mediates sensations critical to coordinated movement such as proprioception, kinesthesia, and discriminative touch.

Disturbances of gait are a common finding with DCML pathology. The gait pattern is usually wide-based and swaying, with uneven step lengths and excessive lateral displacement. The advancing leg may be lifted too high and then dropped abruptly with an audible impact. Watching the feet during locomotion is typical and is indicative of a proprioceptive loss. Another common deficit seen with DCML pathology is dysmetria. As mentioned, this is an impaired ability to judge the required distance or range of movement and may be noted in both the UEs and LEs. It is manifested by the inability to place an extremity accurately or to reach a target object. For example, in attempting to lock a wheelchair brake, the patient may inaccurately judge (overestimate or underestimate) the required movement needed to reach the brake handle. Fine motor skills may also be impaired owing to alterations in discriminative tactile and object recognition abilities.

Because vision can assist in guiding movements and maintaining balance, as well as improve accuracy of discriminative tasks, visual feedback can be an effective mechanism to compensate partially for DCML pathology. Thus, coordination and/or balance problems will be exaggerated when vision is occluded or when the patient's eyes are closed. The inability to maintain standing balance with the feet together when the eyes are closed is termed a positive *Romberg sign* and is usually indicative of proprioceptive loss. Visual guidance will also reduce the manifestations of dysmetria and diminished tactile perception. However, some noticeable slowing of movements may be observed as visually guided motions are generally more accurate when speed of movement is reduced.

■ AGE-RELATED CHANGES AFFECTING COORDINATED MOVEMENT

Alterations in the ability to execute smooth, accurate, controlled motor responses occur with aging. The importance of understanding the basis of these changes is reflected in the large body of literature devoted to examining various aspects of motor performance in older adults.[53-71] This section presents an overview of the most salient age-associated changes affecting coordinated movement. For a more comprehensive perspective on the physiological, neurological, and musculoskeletal changes associated with aging, the reader is referred to the work of Guccione, Wong, and Avers;[69] Saxon, Etten, and Perkins;[70] and Robnett and Chop.[71]

Decreased strength. Diminished strength is a well-documented finding in older adults.[55,60,62,63,72] *Sarcopenia* refers to an age-associated loss of skeletal muscle mass (decreased cross-sectional area), as well as changes in the ability of muscle tissue to regenerate.[65-68] This loss has a direct impact on strength, endurance, mobility, and the ability to perform smooth controlled motor responses. A combination of factors is believed to contribute to this loss of muscle mass, including nutritional deficiencies, decreased ability to synthesize protein, neurological decline, altered endocrine function, lack of exercise (inactivity), and the presence of a chronic disease (comorbidity). Other contributing factors to decreased strength include a loss of alpha motor neurons (decreased number of functional motor units), loss or atrophy of fast-twitch fibers (most notably type IIb), reduced number and diameter of muscle fibers,[73] diminished oxidative capacity of exercising muscle, and a subsequent reduction in ability to produce torque.[72,74] In general, there is greater loss of strength in antigravity muscles of the back and LEs (e.g., latissimus dorsi, hip extensors, quadriceps) as compared to the UE and greater loss in proximal than distal muscles.

Slowed reaction time. Older adults typically move more slowly. This is particularly evident for tasks that require both speed and accuracy; speed will decrease to ensure greater accuracy (speed–accuracy trade-off).[75] In general, the time interval between application of a stimulus and initiation of movement is increased.[3] This finding is also linked to degenerative changes in the motor unit. In addition, *premotor reaction time* (time interval between onset of a stimulus and initiation of a response) and *movement time* (time interval between the initiation of movement and the completion of movement) are lengthened with normal aging.[64] Evidence also suggests that greater cognitive resources are required to accomplish a task, especially those involving fine motor skills and dual-task performance.[76]

Decreased range of motion. Investigations examining subjects from various age groups have found reduced ROM in older adults. Decreases in ROM with advancing age have been found for multiple joints, including the ankle;[77,78] elbow, forearm, shoulder, hip;[72,78] and knee.[78] James and Parker[79] found consistent declines in both active and passive ROM for 10 LE joints in a population of 80 healthy adults older than 70 years of age. Increased joint tightness tends to be most evident toward the end of ROM and may affect the overall skill in performing coordinated movements. Decreased ROM has been linked to biological aging of joint surfaces,[79] degenerative changes in collagen fibers, decreased strength, dietary deficiencies, and sedentary lifestyle.

Postural changes. A straight-line projecting through the ear, acromion, greater trochanter, posterior patella, and lateral malleolus represents the lateral view of normal postural alignment. Examples of common postural changes seen with aging include forward head, rounded shoulders (kyphosis), altered lordotic curve (either flattened or exaggerated), and a slight increase in hip and knee flexion. The trunk may be held anterior to the hips with a widened BOS. Neurological and musculoskeletal decline (e.g., diminished disc height, decreased strength and ROM), as well as inactivity and prolonged sitting, may contribute to poor postural alignment. The presence of comorbidities (e.g., osteoporosis, arthritis) often exacerbate these postural changes. Of particular importance is the potential loss of ability to fully accomplish preparatory postural adjustments before execution of a movement.

Changes affecting coordinated movement in the older adult may be accentuated further by decreased balance and increased postural sway (oscillating movements of body over feet),[80,81] a reduction in postural limits of stability (LOS), degenerative joint changes, reduced flexibility, alterations in sensation (see Chapter 3, Examination of Sensory Function), perceptual impairments (see Chapter 27, Cognitive and Perceptual Dysfunction), and diminished vision and hearing acuity. Knowledge of these anticipated age-related changes improves the therapist's ability to establish effective communication to optimize patient performance, as well as assist with interpretation of test results. The potential presence of these changes has important implications for how the therapist communicates with, and provides directions to, the patient during the coordination examination. Sensitive and accurate communication that enhances the therapeutic interaction is central to the role of the physical therapist. This involves conveying information in a language or context that is meaningful and intelligible to the patient and communicates trust, respect, and compassion.

Changes in skilled motor performance are a predictable aspect of normal aging. However, this information should not negate or undermine the importance of treatment strategies to improve functional performance and quality of life. An important consideration in treatment planning is that the aging neuromuscular system maintains its physiological adaptive response to training stimuli.[82] Physical therapy intervention is highly effective in promoting and sustaining a more successful approach to aging. This is an important consideration as the population ages. It is estimated that by the year 2030, 20% of U.S. residents will be aged 65 and over, as compared with 13% in 2010 and 9.8% in 1970.[83]

COORDINATION TESTS

Coordination tests generally can be divided into two main categories: gross motor movements and fine motor movements. *Gross motor movements* include body posture, balance, and extremity movements involving large muscle groups. Examples of gross motor activities include reaching, crawling, kneeling, standing, walking, and running. *Fine motor movements* involve utilization of small muscle groups that allow skillful, controlled manipulation of objects. Examples of fine motor activities include finger dexterity tasks such as buttoning a shirt, turning pages, typing, and writing.

Clinical Note: During the systems review, examination of ROM, strength, and sensation typically precede the coordination examination because impairments in any of these areas may influence the ability to produce smooth, accurate, controlled motor responses. However, it is also important to note that coordination impairments may occur in the presence of normal ROM, strength, and intact sensation. As with all examination procedures, knowledge of the patient's cognition, language, and communication ability is prerequisite.

Coordination tests focuses on movement capabilities in the following key areas:

- *Reciprocal motion,* which is the ability to reverse movement between opposing muscle groups
- *Movement composition,* or synergy, which involves movement control achieved by synergistic muscle groups acting together
- *Movement accuracy,* which is the ability to gauge or judge distance and speed of voluntary movement
- *Fixation or limb holding,* which addresses the ability to hold the position of an individual limb or limb segment

Coordination and balance (discussed in the following section) tests address capabilities in four basic areas of functional task requirements: transitional mobility, stability (static postural control), dynamic postural control (controlled mobility), and skill. See discussion in Chapter 5, Examination of Motor Function: Motor Control and Motor Learning, and Table 5.12, Measures of Motor Performance.

Coordination tests are ordered based on increasing challenge to the patient and typically utilizes the following sequence: (1) unilateral tasks, (2) bilateral symmetrical tasks, (3) bilateral asymmetrical tasks, and (4) multilimb tasks (these constitute the highest level of difficulty).

ADMINISTERING THE COORDINATION EXAMINATION

Before initiating the coordination examination, the testing environment should be identified and prepared, needed equipment gathered, and patient considerations addressed. Preliminary patient observation will provide valuable insight into motor function and inform test selection.

Preparation

Testing Environment/Equipment

The coordination examination should be administered in a quiet, well-lit treatment area. Ideally, the room should be equipped with two standard chairs and a mat or treatment table. A watch or timer should be available for timed components of the examination, as well as a method of occluding vision.

Patient Considerations

The coordination examination should be administered when the patient is well rested. A full explanation of the purpose of the testing should be provided. Each coordination test is described and demonstrated individually by the therapist before actual testing. Such demonstrations should be attended to carefully, as lack of clarity will negatively affect motor responses. Because testing procedures require mental concentration and some physical activity, fatigue, apprehension, or fear may adversely influence test results.

Preliminary Observation

Observation is an essential skill in clinical decision making. Accurate and careful patient observation provides a rich source of preliminary information before performing a coordination examination. Inasmuch as treatment intervention will be directed, at least in part, toward improving functional performance and activity levels, initial observations should logically focus here. Depending on the practice environment, the patient might be observed performing any number of functional activities. In an outpatient setting, the patient might be observed walking to a treatment area, unbuttoning and removing an outer garment, maintaining a standing position, moving from standing to sitting, maintaining a sitting posture, writing, and so forth. In an inpatient setting, observation may also include bed mobility, self-care activities, transfers, handling eating utensils, changing position from lying or sitting to standing, and so forth. Use of appropriate patient guarding techniques is indicated during observations. Careful observation will provide insight into areas of impairment and provide the following general information:

- Overall level of skill in each activity and amount of assistance or assistive devices required
- The occurrence of extraneous limb movements, oscillations; specific extremities involved
- Postural sway or unsteadiness
- Distribution: proximal and/or distal musculature, unilateral or bilateral
- Situations or occurrences that alter (increase or decrease) impairments
- Amount of time required to perform an activity
- Level of safety, fall risk

Examination

Guided by information from the preliminary observation of functional activities, tests should be selected to address the required movement capabilities of interest for the individual patient.

Table 6.2 presents sample coordination tests performed in sitting and supine. Although multiple tests are presented, a single test is often appropriate to examine several different movement capabilities simultaneously to conserve time. For example, the finger-to-nose test can be used to examine reciprocal motion, movement composition, as well as the presence of intention tremor. The tests presented are intended as examples and are not all-inclusive. Other activities may be developed that are equally effective in examining a particular impairment and may be more appropriate for an individual patient; one such example is shown in Figure 6.5. As noted, performance in any variety of functional skills (e.g., ADL, wheelchair skills, transfers, locomotion) is also an effective means of examining many aspects of movement capabilities. Table 6.3 includes selected impairments and suggested tests appropriate for the clinical problem.

Table 6.2 Coordination Tests*

1. Finger-to-nose	The shoulder is abducted to 90° with the elbow extended. The patient is asked to bring the tip of the index finger to the tip of his or her nose. Alterations may be made in the initial starting position to observe performance from different planes of motion.
2. Finger-to-therapist's finger	The patient and therapist sit opposite each other. The therapist's index finger is held in front of the patient. The patient is asked to touch the tip of his or her index finger to the therapist's index finger. The position of the therapist's finger may be altered during testing to observe ability to change distance, direction, and force of movement.
3. Finger-to-finger	Both shoulders are abducted to 90° with the elbows extended. The patient is asked to bring both hands toward the midline and approximate the index fingers from opposing hands.

Continued

Table 6.2 Coordination Tests*—cont'd

4. Alternate nose-to-finger	The patient alternately touches the tip of his or her nose and the tip of the therapist's finger with the index finger. The position of the therapist's finger may be altered during testing to observe ability to change distance, direction, and force of movement.
5. Finger opposition	The patient touches the tip of the thumb to the tip of each finger in sequence. Speed may be gradually increased.
6. Mass grasp	An alternation is made between opening and closing fist (from finger flexion to full extension). Speed may be gradually increased.
7. Pronation/supination	With elbows flexed to 90° and held close to body, the patient alternately turns the palms up and down. This test also may be performed with shoulders flexed to 90° and elbows extended. Speed may be gradually increased. The ability to reverse movements between opposing muscle groups can be examined at many joints. Examples include active alternation between flexion and extension of the knee, ankle, elbow, or fingers.
8. Rebound test	The patient is positioned with the elbow flexed. The therapist applies sufficient manual resistance to produce an isometric contraction of biceps. Resistance is suddenly released. Normally, the opposing muscle group (triceps) will contract and "check" movement of the limb. Many other muscle groups can be tested for this phenomenon, such as the shoulder abductors or flexors and the elbow extensors.
9. Tapping (hand)	With the elbow flexed and the forearm pronated, the patient is asked to "tap" the hand on the knee.
10. Tapping (foot)	The patient is asked to "tap" the ball of one foot on the floor without raising the knee; heel maintains contact with floor.
11. Pointing and past pointing	The patient and therapist are opposite each other. Both patient and therapist bring shoulders to 90° of flexion with elbows extended and index fingers of both hands extended. The therapist's and patient's index fingers are lightly touching. The patient is asked to fully flex the shoulder (fingers will be pointing toward ceiling) and then return to the horizontal position and "point" (lightly touch) the therapist's index finger (target) (see Fig.6.5). A normal response consists of an accurate return to the starting position. In an abnormal response, there is typically a "past pointing," or movement beyond the target. Several variations to this test include movements in other directions such as toward 90° of shoulder abduction or toward 0° of shoulder flexion (finger will point toward floor). After each movement, the patient is asked to return to the initial horizontal starting position and "point" to the target.
12. Alternate heel-to-knee; heel-to-toe	From a supine position, the patient is asked to touch the knee and big toe alternately with the heel of the opposite extremity.
13. Toe-to-examiner's finger	From a supine position, the patient is instructed to touch the great toe to the examiner's finger. The position of finger may be altered during testing to observe ability to change distance, direction, and force of movement (to stabilize lower back, the opposite hip and knee may be flexed).
14. Heel-on-shin	From a supine position, the heel of one foot is slid up and down the shin of the opposite LE.
15. Drawing a circle	The patient draws an imaginary circle in the air with either UE or LE (a table or the floor also may be used). This also may be done using a figure-eight pattern. This test may be performed in the supine position for the LE.
16. Fixation or position holding	UE: The patient holds arms horizontally in front (sitting or standing). LE: The patient is asked to hold the knee in an extended position (sitting).

*Tests should be performed first with eyes open and then with eyes closed. Abnormal responses include a gradual deviation from the "holding" position and/or a diminished quality of response with vision occluded. Unless otherwise indicated, tests are performed with the patient in a sitting position.

LE = Lower extremity; UE = upper extremity

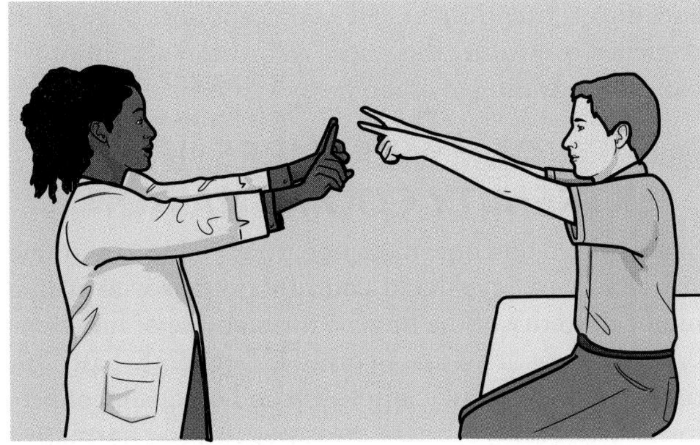

Figure 6.5 Coordination test for pointing and past pointing. From bilateral shoulder flexion, the patient is returning to the start position to "point" (lightly touch) the therapist's index fingers (target). Both arms should be tested, either separately or simultaneously. The test can be performed in either sitting or standing.

Table 6.3 Sample Tests for Selected Coordination Impairments

Impairment	Sample Test
Dysdiadochokinesia	Finger-to-nose Alternate nose-to-finger Pronation/supination Knee flexion/extension Walking, alter speed or direction
Dysmetria	Pointing and past pointing Drawing a circle or figure eight Heel on shin Placing feet on floor markers; sitting, standing
Dyssynergia	Finger-to-nose Finger-to-therapist's finger Alternate heel-to-knee Toe-to-examiner's finger
Hypotonia	Passive movement Deep tendon reflexes
Tremor (intention)	Observation during functional activities (tremor will typically increase as target is approached or movement speed increased) Alternate nose-to-finger Finger-to-finger Finger-to-therapist's finger Toe-to-examiner's finger
Tremor (resting)	Observation of patient at rest; limb or jaw movements Observation during functional activities (tremor will diminish significantly or disappear with movement)
Tremor (postural)	Observation of steadiness of normal posture; sitting, standing
Asthenia	Fixation or position holding (upper and lower extremity) Application of manual resistance to determine ability to hold
Rigidity	Passive movement Observation during functional activities Observation of resting posture(s)
Bradykinesia	Walking, observation of arm swing and trunk motions Walking, alter speed and direction Request that a movement or gait activity be stopped abruptly Observation of functional activities: timed tests
Disturbances of posture	Fixation or position holding (upper and lower extremity) Displace balance unexpectedly in sitting or standing (perturbation) Standing, alter base of support (e.g., one foot directly in front of the other; standing on one foot)
Disturbances of gait	Walk along a straight line Walk sideways, backward March in place Alter speed and direction of ambulatory activities Walk in a circle

Attention should be directed to carefully guarding the patient during testing. During testing, the following questions can be used to help direct the therapist's observations:

- Are movements direct, precise, and easily reversed?
- Do movements occur within a reasonable or normal amount of time?
- Does increased speed of performance affect quality of motor activity (speed-accuracy trade-off)?
- Can continuous and appropriate motor adjustments be made if speed and direction are changed?
- Can a position or posture of the body or specific extremity be maintained without swaying, oscillations, or extraneous movements?
- Are placing movements of both UEs and LEs accurate?
- Does occluding vision alter the quality of motor activity?
- Is there greater involvement proximally or distally?

- Is there greater involvement on one side of body versus the other?
- Does the patient fatigue rapidly?
- Is there a consistency of motor response over time?

Documentation

Approaches to documentation of examination data vary among institutions and individual therapists. The format for recording also varies among electronic software programs. Within the section on motor function, some programs include entries for coordination and dexterity and/or hand function. Others include check box options for specific coordination impairments based on body segment location while others provide sections for narrative descriptions of motor function. Alternatively, an observational examination form can be used to record findings and subsequently scanned into the electronic health record.

An observational examination form is useful in providing a composite picture of coordination impairments. An example is provided in Appendix 6.A. These forms are often developed within clinical settings. They may be general, or they may be specific to a given group of patients, such as those with brain injuries. They typically include a rating scale in which level of performance is weighted using a numeric scale with descriptors for each score. A comments section allows for additional narrative descriptions of patient performance. In general, these forms are *not standardized* and *lack reliability testing*. However, they do provide a systematic method of data collection and documentation. In addition, use of the same form for periodic reexamination facilitates ease of comparison of changes over time.

Measuring the length of time required to complete a motor or functional task provides an important quantitative measure of movement capability. Because accomplishing an activity in a reasonable amount of time is an important criterion of performance, the length of time required to accomplish certain tasks has important implications for both function and safety. For example, assume a patient with a spinal cord injury who uses a wheelchair plans to return to school but requires 2.5 hours to complete dressing activities. The time element here would not be considered functional, especially if attempting to make an early morning class. Consider also an ambulatory patient with an ataxic gait unable to cross a street in the allotted time provided by the traffic signal. This time requirement presents a considerable patient safety issue and, as such, would also not be considered functional. Many standardized measurements, such as the Timed Up and Go (TUG) Test,[84,85] include time as a measure of patient performance.

Periodic video recording of patient performance can be used effectively to document coordination impairments and monitor progress over time. For some patients, such recordings can provide the basis for suggestions about altering movement strategies to improve function and direct attention to safety precautions. Viewed in sequence over time, the visual record can also improve patient motivation to attain further gains.

OUTCOME MEASURES: UPPER EXTREMITY COORDINATION

Standardized outcome measures are available to examine arm–hand and eye–hand coordination, as well as fine motor dexterity of the fingers, through use of function-based tasks or activities. Scoring is frequently based on time required for task completion and on quality of performance. Many of these measures include normative data to assist with interpretation of test results.

The examining therapist should be knowledgeable about testing guidelines and interpretation of results. Adherence to the prescribed method of administration is particularly important. Any deviations from the established protocol will affect the validity and reliability of the measures and subsequently make comparisons with published norms invalid. Importantly, standardized tests provide objective measures of patient progress over time.

Table 6.4 [86-111] includes examples of outcome measures designed to examine arm, hand, and finger coordination. Additional examples are visually depicted in Box 6.1.[112-121] Many other standardized and commercially distributed tests are available. Selection of outcome measures should be based on the strength of available data addressing: *reliability* (e.g., test-retest, intra-rater, and interrater), *validity* (concurrent, criterion-related, and predictive) and *sensitivity to change* (responsiveness, minimally detectable change [MDC], and minimal clinically important difference [MCID]). Additional considerations in selection include the availability of normative data, the type of impairments the instrument was designed to measure, and the intended population (general application or diagnosis-specific).

OVERVIEW OF POSTURAL CONTROL AND BALANCE

Postural control involves maintained orientation of the relative positions of body parts with respect to each other and gravity. Balance is the condition in which all the forces acting on the body are balanced such that the *center of mass* (COM) is within the stability limits, the boundaries of the *base of support* (BOS). The overall goals of the postural control system, stability and function, are achieved through integrated CNS systems of control. *Reactive postural control* occurs in response to external forces acting on the body (e.g., perturbations) displacing the COM or moving the BOS (e.g., moveable platform, therapy ball). Feedback systems provide the sensory inputs required to initiate corrective responses. *Proactive (anticipatory) postural control* occurs in anticipation of internally generated, destabilizing forces imposed on the body's own movements (e.g., catching a weighted ball). An individual's

Table 6.4 Outcome Measures: Arm, Hand, and Finger Coordination

Outcome Measure (OM) and ICF Category (ICF)	Description	Scoring	Minimally Detectable Change (MDC); Minimal Clinically Important Difference (MCID)
OM: Box and Blocks Test (BBT)[86-93] **ICF:** 1	Examines manual dexterity. A rectangular box with a central divider creates two compartments. One compartment contains 150 colored wooden blocks. As many blocks as possible are moved, one at a time, from one compartment to the other in 60 seconds.	The number of blocks transferred are counted. Higher scores indicate better manual dexterity. Normative values are available based on sex and age.[90]	For a 2-week training program, MDC = 4 blocks per minute; 6-month follow-up MDC = 6 blocks per minute (patients with chronic stroke, n = 17).[93] MDC: 5.5 blocks per minute (change: 18%) (patients with acute and chronic stroke, n = 62).[87]
OM: Wolf Motor Function Test (WMFT)[94-99] **ICF:** 1	Examines upper extremity (UE) motor ability using 15 function-based tasks and two strength items.	Scores based on performance time (WMFT-TIME) and Functional Ability Scale (WMFT-FAS) using a 6-point ordinal scale (0 = does not attempt with the involved arm, to 5 = arm does participate; movement appears to be normal). Maximum time to complete an item is 120 seconds. Maximum score is 75. Normative data are available based on age.[98]	MDC95: 0.7 seconds (average WMFT) MDC95: 0.1 points (average for WMFT-FAS (patients with hemiplegia, n = 96).[94] MDC90: 4.36 seconds for WMFT MDC90: 0.37 points for WMFT-FAS MCID: 1.5–2 seconds for WMFT MCID: 0.2–0.4 points for WMFT-FAS (patients with stroke, n = 57).[95]
OM: Action Research Arm Test (ARAT)[97,100-105] **ICF:** 1	Examines UE function using a 19-item measure divided into four subscales: grasp, grip, pinch, and gross arm movement.	Scores are based on a 4-point ordinal scale (0 = can perform no part of test to 3 = performs test normally).	MCID: 5.7 points (10% of total range of the scale) (patients with chronic stroke, n = 20).[104]
OM: Nine-Hole Peg Test (9HPT)[87,100,106-108] **ICF:** 1, 2	Measure of finger dexterity. One at a time, pegs are moved from a container and placed, as quickly as possible, into holes on a board. Pegs are then individually removed from holes and returned to container.	Score based on time (seconds) required to complete the task. Alternatively, the number of pegs placed within 50 or 100 seconds is counted and recorded as pegs placed/second. Normative values are available.[107]	MDC: 32.8 seconds (change: 54%) (patients with acute and chronic stroke, n = 62)[87] MDC: 2.6 seconds (dominant hand) MDC: 1.3 seconds (nondominant hand) (patients with Parkinson's disease, n = 262)[106] Minimum detectable change of 2.6 sec for the dominant hand and 1.3 sec for the nondominant hand Minimum detectable change of 2.6 sec for the dominant hand and 1.3 sec for the nondominant hand

Continued

Table 6.4 Outcome Measures: Arm, Hand, and Finger Coordination—cont'd

Outcome Measure (OM) and ICF Category (ICF)	Description	Scoring	Minimally Detectable Change (MDC); Minimal Clinically Important Difference (MCID)
OM: Sollerman Hand Function Test (SHFT)[109-111] **ICF**: 1, 2, 3	Examines hand grips while performing 20 tasks using common items encountered in ADL (e.g., coins, buttons, pen, cup, screwdriver, telephone) within 60 seconds.	Performance is timed; scored on a 5-point scale from 0 = task cannot be performed at all to 4 = task is completed without any difficulty within 20 seconds and the prescribed hand-grip of normal quality. The 20 sub-test task scores are added for a total maximum score of 80.	MDC: 6.7–6.9 (patients with hand burns, n = 21)[110]

ICF CATEGORY: 1 = Body structure/function; 2 = Activity; 3 = Participation
ADL = Activities of daily living

Box 6.1 Examples of Outcome Measures: Upper Extremity Coordination

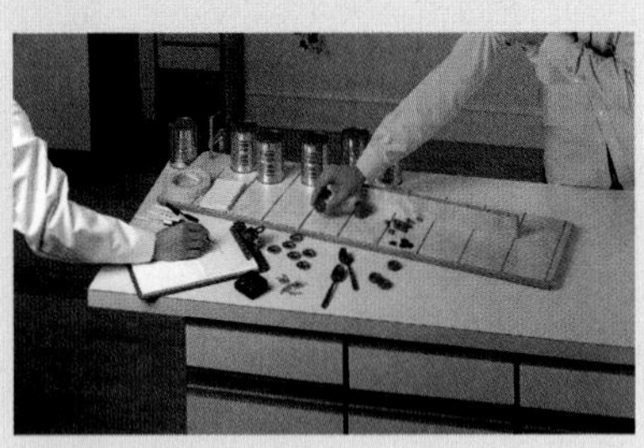

The *Jebsen-Taylor Hand Function Test* (Fig. A) examines hand and finger coordination using seven subtests of functional skills (e.g., writing, card turning, picking up small objects, simulated eating, stacking). Scored on time required to complete task. Normative data are available based on age, sex, maximum time, and hand dominance.[106,112-114] *(Courtesy of Sammons Preston Rolyan, Bolingbrook, IL 60440-3593.)*

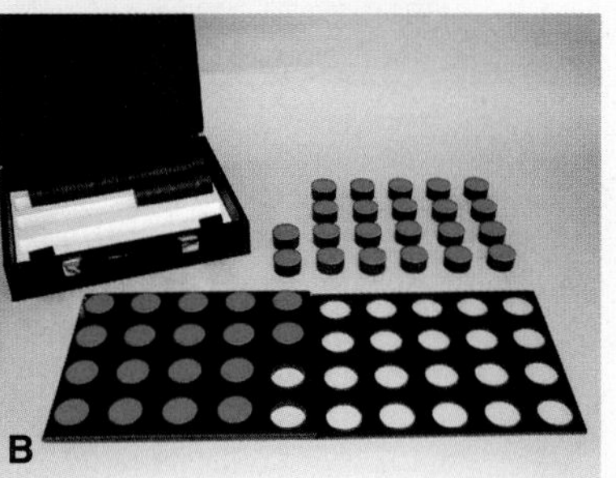

Minnesota Manual Dexterity Test (Fig. B) consists of two operations, *placing* and *turning* and requires use of a board with wells and round disks. After a practice trial, scores are based on the time required to complete each of four trials for each operation. Normative data are available. An expanded variation of this test is the Minnesota Rate of Manipulation Test, which includes five operations: placing, turning, displacing, one-hand turning and placing, and two-hand turning and placing.[115-117]

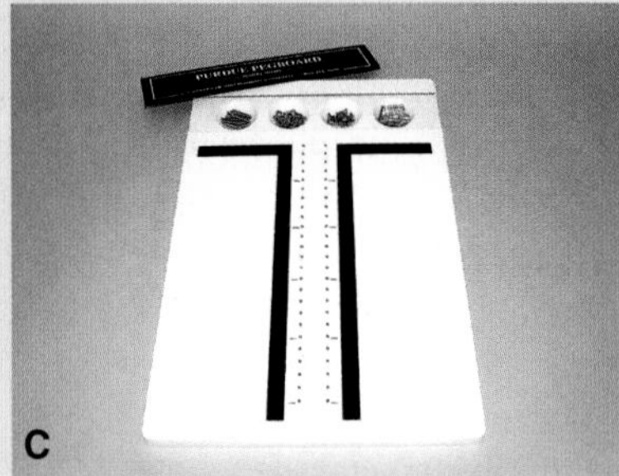

The *Purdue Pegboard Test* (Fig. C) examines coordination of the arm/hand/fingers by placement of pins, collars, and/or washes on a pegboard. There are several categories of subtests, including right-hand prehension, left-hand

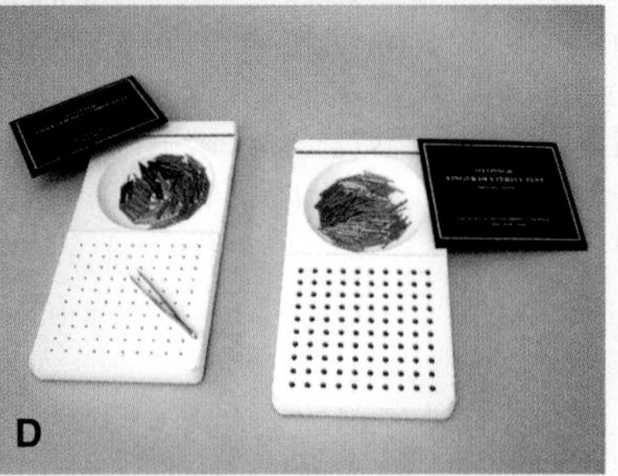

The *O'Connor Tweezer Test* (Fig. D, *left*) and the *Finger Dexterity Test* (Fig. D, *right*) examine the ability to rapidly manipulate small objects. The Tweezer Test emphasizes eye–hand and fine motor dexterity using tweezers to

Box 6.1 Examples of Outcome Measures: Upper Extremity Coordination—cont'd

prehension, prehension test with both hands, and assembly. Scores are based on the number of assemblies completed within either a 30- or 60-second period. Normative values are available.[118-121]

place a single pin in each 1/16th-inch-diameter hole. The Finger Dexterity Test also addresses fine motor dexterity through manual placement of three pins per hole. Scoring is based on time required to complete task.

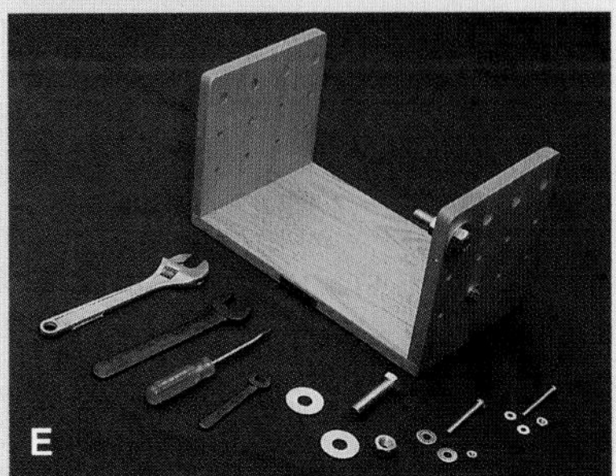

The *Hand Tool Dexterity Test* (Fig. E) utilizes ordinary tools to examine coordinated movement of arm/hand/fingers during a functional task. The test frame consists of a flat board to which two side uprights are attached. The test requires disassembly of the nuts and bolts on one upright using the appropriate tools and reassembling them on the opposite upright. The test is timed and normative data are available. *(Courtesy of Lafayette Instrument Co., Lafayette, IN 47903.)*

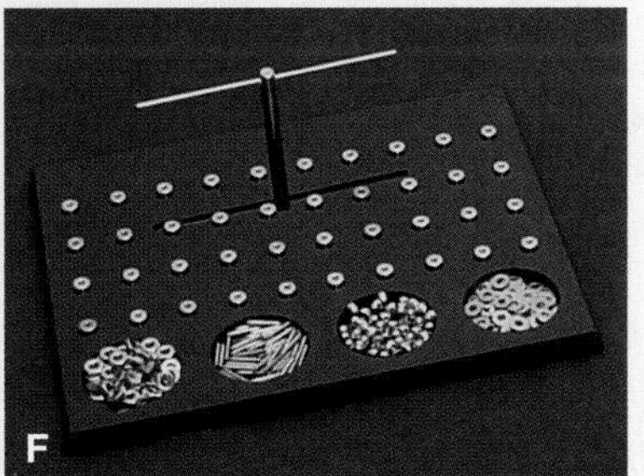

The *Roeder Manipulative Aptitude Test* (Fig. F) examines arm/hand/finger coordination as well as eye–hand coordination. Test materials consist of a high-density plastic board with four wells for washers, rods, caps, and nuts; a T-bar for placement of washer–nut assemblies; and rows of sockets for installing nuts. The test includes four timed operations: dominant hand rod–cap assembly and T-bar washer–nut assembly using both hands, right hand, and left hand. Normative data are available. *(Courtesy of Lafayette Instrument Co., Lafayette, IN 47903.)*

prior experiences allow the various elements of the postural control system to be pretuned or readied for upcoming movements using feedforward mechanisms. Postural requirements vary depending on the characteristics of the task and the environment. *Adaptive postural control* allows the individual to modify postural responses to changing task and environmental demands. Balance emerges from a complex interaction of (1) sensory systems responsible for the detection of body position and motion, (2) motor systems responsible for organization and execution of motor synergies, and (3) higher-level CNS processes responsible for integration and action plans. An examination of balance must therefore focus on each of these three areas.

Postural Alignment and Weight Distribution

Normal postural alignment in standing can be examined by observing skeletal alignment using a plumb line (or posture grid). More sophisticated analysis can be achieved using motion analysis systems with light-emitting signals, photography, and electromyography. In standing, the COM occurs at a point about two-thirds of the body height above the BOS. Static posture in standing is examined by positioning the patient with the feet apart, normal stance width. When viewed from the side (sagittal plane alignment), the plumb line is positioned just in front of the lateral malleolus. The vertical *line of gravity* is expected to fall close to most joint axes: slightly anterior to the ankle and knee joints, at or slightly posterior to the hip joint, through midline of the trunk, just anterior to the shoulder joint, and through the external auditory meatus (Fig. 6.6).

Natural spinal curves are present but flattened in upright stance, depending on the level of postural tone, lumbar and cervical lordosis, and thoracic or dorsal kyphosis. The pelvis is held in neutral position, with no anterior or posterior tilt. When viewed from the front or back (frontal plane analysis), the feet are positioned equidistant from the plumb line. The examiner looks for equal weight distribution between feet and symmetry of the trunk and extremities. Normal alignment minimizes the need for active muscle contraction during standing. Muscles that are tonically active at low levels during quiet stance include tibialis anterior and gastrocnemius-soleus; tensor fascia latae, gluteus medius, and iliopsoas; and abdominals and erector spinae.[122]

In sitting when viewed from the side, head and trunk are vertical. Natural spinal curves are present and the pelvis is maintained in a neutral position (Fig. 6.7). When viewed from the front or back, the

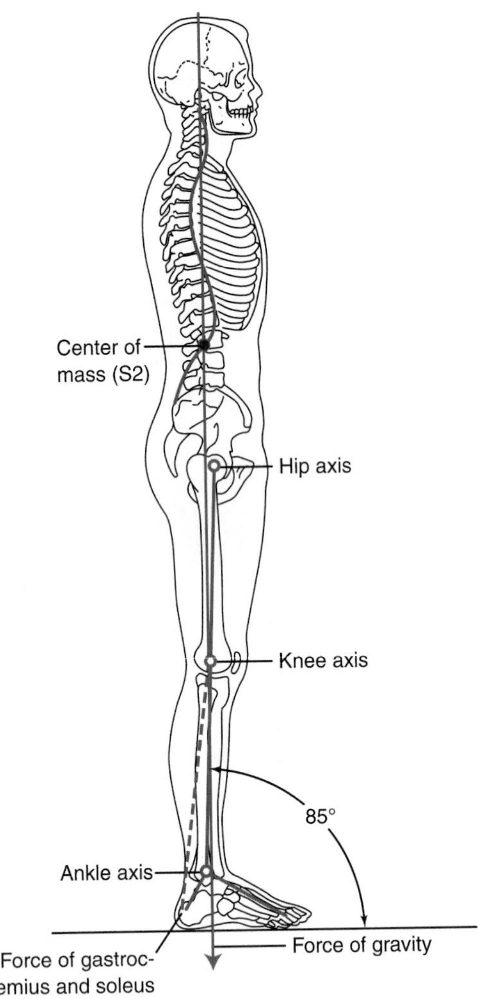

Figure 6.6 Normal postural standing alignment in sagittal plane. In optimal alignment, the line of gravity passes through the identified anatomical structures.

trunk and head are held in a midline orientation with symmetrical weight-bearing on both LEs (buttocks, thighs, and feet).[122]

Limits of stability (LOS) are defined as the maximum distance an individual is able or willing to lean in any direction without loss of balance or changing the BOS. Thus, in standing, an individual can shift forward and backward or side to side without losing balance or taking a step. LOS is influenced by a number of factors, including individual characteristics such as height and foot length for anterior/posterior (AP) LOS and distance between the feet and height for medial/lateral (ML) LOS.[123] Both COM position and movement (velocity and displacement) influence LOS.[124] The midpoint of LOS is termed the *COM alignment. Steadiness* refers to the ability to maintain a given posture with minimum movement (sway).[125] During standing, an individual normally exhibits small range postural shifts (*postural sway*), cycling intermittently from side to side and from heel to toe. *Sway envelope* refers to the path of the body's movement during standing. During walking, there are minimal COM movements up and down and side to side, resulting in a smooth sinusoidal curve. In sitting, the BOS is larger and COM lower (just above the support base), resulting in greater LOS.

Examination of Postural Alignment

Postural alignment and sway can be examined using visual inspection with the patient standing against a postural grid.[126] More sophisticated instrumentation, dynamic posturography, utilizes force plates to measure and quantify ground reaction forces, either center of force (COF) measures or center of pressure (COP) measures. COF is calculated using only vertical forces, and COP is calculated using both vertical and horizontal shear forces. The weight of each foot is determined, forces calculated, and converted into a visual image (Fig. 6.8). Software analysis provides data on initial stance position (center of alignment), mean sway path, total sway excursion (LOS), and the zone of stability. These findings are valid and reliable measures of postural control.[127,128]

Using this information, the therapist can objectively determine the patient's postural symmetry, which is a reflection of the amount of weight placed on each foot. Patients with asymmetry may present with the COP positioned away from midline. For example, the patient with stroke typically stands with most of the weight on the less affected limb. Steadiness can be determined by using postural sway measures. A large sway path is evidence of postural unsteadiness. Another example is the patient with ataxia who typically demonstrates hypermetric responses, with excessive sway, uncoordinated movements, and limited postural steadiness. The patient with Parkinson's disease presents with the opposite problem, hypometric responses with diminished sway and excessive stabilization.[129,130] Limits of stability are determined by asking the patient to actively shift weight in any direction as far as possible without losing balance or taking a step. Patients with deficits in motor control typically have reduced LOS (reduced COP excursion). For example, the patient with stroke demonstrates reduced stability limits to the more affected side. The patient with Parkinson's disease typically demonstrates reduced LOS overall with significant anterior stability limits if a stooped posture is evident. LOS and COM alignment are also typically altered in other pathological states (e.g., muscle weakness, skeletal deformity, and tonal abnormalities). Reexamination after training using force platform biofeedback has been used to document recovery of postural control following stroke.[131,132] It has also been used to demonstrate the effectiveness of training using biofeedback force platform training devices.[125,130,133]

Sensory Strategies for Balance

The sensory systems (vision, somatosensory, and vestibular) provide the CNS with important information about postural control and balance, including information

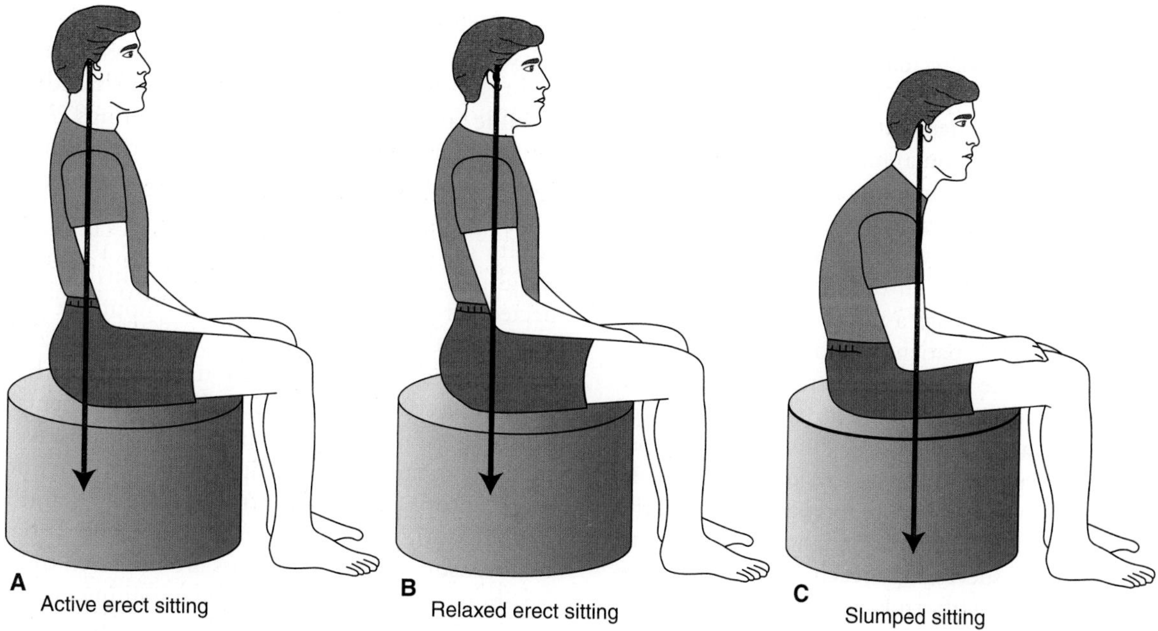

Figure 6.7 Normal sagittal plane postural alignment in sitting: (A) In optimal alignment, the line of gravity passes close to the axes of rotation of the head and neck, and trunk. (B) During relaxed sitting, the line of gravity changes very little, remaining close to those axes. (C) During slumped sitting, the line of gravity is well forward of the spine and hips. *(From O'Sullivan, SB, and Schmitz, TJ.* Improving Functional Outcomes in Physical Rehabilitation, ed 2. *FA Davis, Philadelphia, 2016.)*

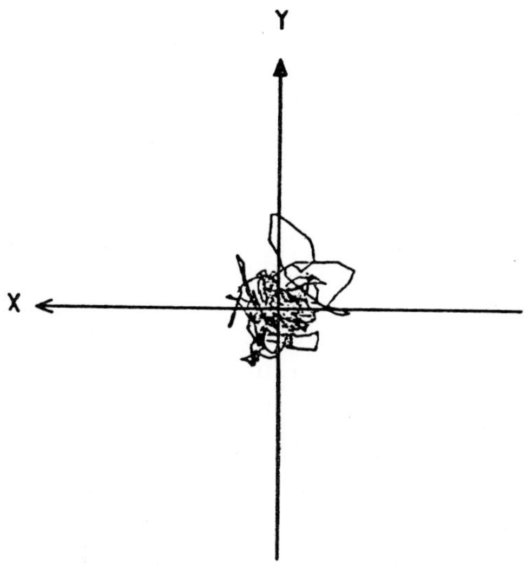

Figure 6.8 Postural sway. Recording of the movement of the center of pressure for 60 seconds in a subject standing on a balance platform. Values: mean amplitude of sway path in inches = .13 × .15; length of path = 32.2; and velocity = .45 in/sec. *(From Smith, L, et al: Brunnstrom's Clinical Kinesiology, ed 5. FA Davis, Philadelphia, 1996, p. 406, with permission.)*

about the results of our own actions and the surrounding environment. The CNS integrates these inputs and initiates both goal-directed conscious actions and automatic, unconscious adjustments in posture and movements. Each individual sensory system provides unique and important information, and no one system provides all the information needed.

The visual system serves as an important source of information for the ability to perceive movements and detect the relative orientation of body segments and orientation of the body in space. This ability has been termed *visual proprioception.*[134] Two separate functional visual systems have been identified. Various different names have been used: (1) *focal vision* (cognitive or explicit vision) and (2) *ambient vision* (sensorimotor or implicit vision). Focal vision plays a major role in localizing features in the environment and in our conscious reaction to visual events. In contrast, ambient vision utilizes the entire visual field to provide information on the localizing features about the environment and to guide movements using largely nonconscious awareness.[3] Thus, each visual system has a unique functional significance. For example, the patient with brain injury who has a condition called *optic ataxia* can recognize an object using focal vision but cannot use visual information to accurately guide the hand to reach and grasp an object in the environment (impaired ambient vision). The opposite occurs in a patient with stroke experiencing *visual agnosia.* The patient cannot recognize common objects or people but can use the ambient visual system to navigate the environment. Vision also contributes to righting reactions of the head, trunk, and limbs (optical righting reactions).

Visual acuity (focal vision) can be examined using a Snellen eye chart. A distance acuity poorer than 20/50 will have a significant effect on postural stability.[135]

Whereas focal vision is detected by the central retina only, ambient vision is detected by the entire visual field (central and peripheral vision). Patients with loss of peripheral vision (e.g., a patient with stroke and hemianopsia or a patient with glaucoma) may demonstrate deficits in visual proprioception and functional performance. Peripheral vision can be examined using the *confrontation method.* The patient sits in front of the therapist and is instructed to focus gaze on the therapist's nose. The therapist then slowly brings a target (moving finger or pencil) slowly into the patient's field of view from the right or left side. The patient is instructed to indicate (point or declare) when and where the target is detected. Ambient vision can be examined by instructing the patient to navigate across the busy physical therapy gym. The abilities to navigate safely, to localize features in the environment, and to anticipate changes necessary to avoid obstacles and successfully reach the target area are determined. Patients with stroke who exhibit *topographical disorientation* will have difficulty navigating their environment and understanding the relationship of one place to another.

Somatosensory inputs include the cutaneous and pressure sensations from the body segments in contact with the support surface (e.g., the feet in standing, the buttocks, thighs, and feet in sitting) and muscle and joint proprioception throughout the body. Light touch contact from the hands on a stable surface is also a form of somatosensory input used as a balance aid.[136] This provides information about the relative orientation and movement of the body in relation to the support surface. Cutaneous sensation (touch and pressure) of the feet/ankles and proprioception of the feet/ankles and hips are particularly important in maintaining upright standing balance. Sensory examination of the extremities and trunk is therefore essential (see Chapter 3, Examination of Sensory Function).

The vestibular system is an important source of information for postural control and balance. The semicircular canals (SCCs) detect angular acceleration and deceleration forces acting on the head, whereas the otolith organs detect linear acceleration and orientation of the head with reference to gravity. The SCCs are sensitive to fast (phasic) movements of the head, and the otoliths respond to slow head movements and positional change referenced to gravity. The vestibular system functions to stabilize gaze during head movements via the *vestibulo-ocular reflex (VOR),* and to assist in the regulation of postural tone and postural muscle activation via the vestibulo-spinal reflexes (VSR). Tests for vestibular function include positional and movement testing. The patient is observed for symptoms of vestibular dysfunction (e.g., dizziness, vertigo, nystagmus).[137] See Chapter 21, Vestibular Disorders, for a complete discussion of this topic.

During stance, all sensory inputs contribute to the maintenance of posture. Sensory weighting theory specifies that the CNS weights the various sensory inputs depending on the specific sensory environment and task.[138-141] *Quiet stance* is defined as standing with a stable support surface and surroundings. *Perturbed stance* is defined as standing during a brief displacement of the support surface (moving surface) or displacement of the COM over BOS (perturbation). In intact adults during quiet stance, the CNS places greater weight on somatosensory inputs. During an unexpected perturbation, somatosensory inputs are activated quicker and provide much of the early restabilizing control, whereas vision and vestibular inputs with slower processing speeds contribute to later components of the postural restabilizing response.[142] If somatosensory inputs are impaired (e.g., peripheral neuropathy) or if somatosensory conflict is introduced (e.g., standing on dense foam), vision assumes a greater role. If both somatosensory and visual inputs are impaired or absent, vestibular inputs are critical to maintaining posture and resolving sensory conflict. CNS use of sensory inputs is flexible. Balance responses are task and context dependent and are triggered by CNS weighting based on availability, timing, and accuracy of specific sensory inputs.

Because sensory inputs are redundant, stable balance can be maintained with significant impairment, on unstable surfaces, or in sensory conflict situations. However, if more than one sensory system is deficient, substantial deficiencies in balance control will be evident.[143] For example, the patient with chronic diabetes who has significant diabetic neuropathy (loss of somatosensory inputs from the feet and ankles) and significant diabetic retinopathy (impaired vision) will demonstrate significant postural instability and increased fall risk. In addition, the cognitive system plays an important role in attending to and interpreting the information for CNS planning of effective postural responses. Attentional demands vary depending on the task (new learning versus familiar response) and the environment (open versus closed or dual-tasking). Patients with impairments in cognition or attention demonstrate increased fall risk, especially for those activities with high stability demands.

Examination of Sensory Strategies

Romberg Test

The *Romberg test* is one of the oldest tests to assess sensorimotor control and was developed to diagnose tabes dorsalis.[144] During the test, the patient is instructed to stand with feet together (touching each other), eyes open (EO), unaided for 20 to 30 seconds. If the patient demonstrates significant sway or instability with EO, the test is over. The patient is then asked to stand with eyes closed (EC). The test is negative if the patient is stable and well balanced with either EO or EC. The test is positive if the patient is able to stand with EO but demonstrates significant instability (significant postural sway or loss of balance) with EC. During testing, it is important to tell the patient you are prepared to catch him or her in the event of a fall. The patient should not be given any clues to help orient and stabilize posture. A positive Romberg test is indicative of severe loss of proprioception (e.g., *sensory ataxia*) that occurs with posterior column lesions in the spinal cord (e.g., cervical spondylosis, tumor, degenerative spinal cord disease, tabes dorsalis). Patients with a mild vestibular or midline cerebellar lesions can usually compensate with the use of vision (EO). With severe lesions, truncal instability and loss of balance occur with EO (e.g., the patient with cerebellar ataxia). In the sharpened Romberg test, the feet are placed in tandem (heel-to-toe position) and the EO to EC conditions imposed. Individuals who are older or obese may have increased difficulty with the sharpened Romberg test. The findings of the Romberg test are qualitative, and as such it has more value as a screening tool than as a definitive test.

Sensory Organization Test

The *Sensory Organization Test* (SOT) is based on the work of Nashner[138,139] and is used to assess the sensory contributions to postural control and balance. It examines body sway during quiet standing under six different sensory test conditions (Fig. 6.9). Dynamic posturography equipment is used to provide a moving platform that introduces mechanical perturbations (sliding or tilting movements). A moving visual surround screen is sway referenced and introduces visual conflict. Both the surround and force plate are referenced to the patient by means of hydraulic mechanisms. Test condition 1 provides accurate somatosensory, visual, and vestibular information and is the baseline reference. Each of the other five conditions systematically varies sensory inputs, increasing the level of sensory conflict and postural difficulty (Table 6.5).

Conditions 1 to 3 are all performed with the patient standing on a stable support surface, feet shoulder width apart, providing accurate somatosensory inputs. Visual inputs are varied: condition 1 uses EO (baseline condition), and condition 2 uses EC. Condition 3 uses a moving visual surround (screen) referenced to body sway, thus providing inaccurate visual information. Conditions 4 through 6 repeat the visual conditions but with an altered support surface (moving platform) that provides inaccurate somatosensory information. In conditions 5 and 6, maintenance of posture depends on availability and accuracy of vestibular inputs with the reduction of both vision and somatosensory inputs. The patient is asked to maintain each position for 20 seconds; three trials are used for each condition.

Dynamic posturography equipment (standing on a forceplate) provides objective measurement of postural sway and COP. Composite equilibrium scores and weighted averages of scores are computed for each of the six conditions. The *Equilibrium Score* quantifies how well the patient performed during each of the six conditions in terms of sway or postural stability. Ratios comparing

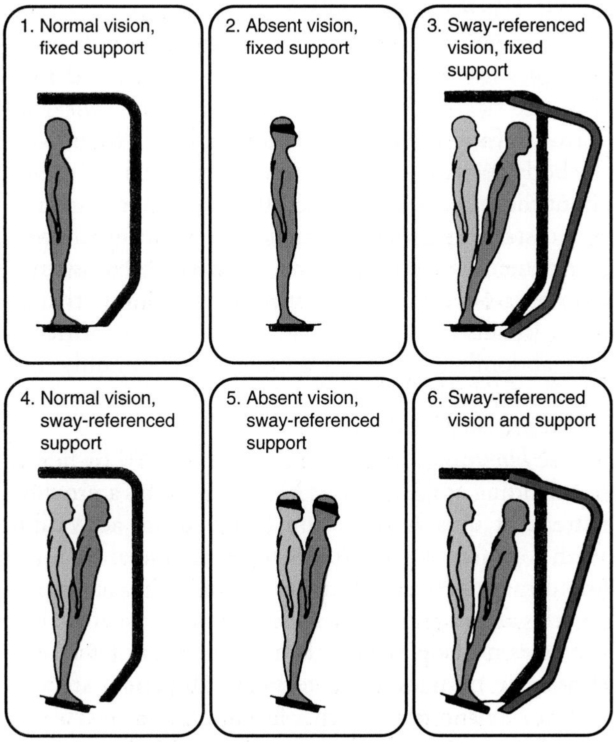

1. Normal vision, fixed support
2. Absent vision, fixed support
3. Sway-referenced vision, fixed support
4. Normal vision, sway-referenced support
5. Absent vision, sway-referenced support
6. Sway-referenced vision and support

Figure 6.9 The Sensory Organization Test.

Table 6.5 Test Conditions: Sensory Organization Test/Clinical Test of Sensory Interaction and Balance

Condition	Sensory Input
Condition 1 Eyes Open, Stable Surface (EOSS)	All sensory systems available, unaltered (baseline condition)
Condition 2 Eyes Closed, Stable Surface (ECSS)	Vision absent Somatosensory unaltered Vestibular intact
Condition 3* Visual Conflict, Stable Surface (VCSS)	Vision altered Somatosensory unaltered Vestibular intact
Condition 4 Eyes Open, Moving Surface (EOMS)	Vision unaltered Somatosensory altered Vestibular intact
Condition 5 Eyes Closed, Moving Surface (ECMS)	Vision absent Somatosensory altered Vestibular intact
Condition 6* Visual Conflict, Moving Surface (VCMS)	Vision altered Somatosensory altered Vestibular intact

*Conditions omitted in the mCTSIB

one condition to another provides information regarding reliance on one sensory system over another. Center of gravity (COG) is computed for its position relative to the center of the BOS. Additional analyses of motor coordination using electromyography (EMG) can be used to provide information about the relative level of individual muscle activity, as well as overall muscle recruitment patterns during each of the test positions. As in all testing of postural control and balance, patient safety is an important consideration. During posturography, the patient wears an overhead safety harness to prevent falls. Upper extremity support is not allowed during the test. However, the equipment includes hand rails that can be used as an additional element of safety.

Clinical Test of Sensory Interaction and Balance

In the absence of sophisticated and expensive posturography equipment, a modified version has been developed that can be performed in clinical settings. The *Clinical Test of Sensory Interaction and Balance* (CTSIB) is a low-tech version of the SOT developed by Shumway-Cook and Horak.[145] It utilizes medium-density foam to substitute for a moving platform and a visual conflict dome affixed to the subject's head to substitute for a moving visual surrounding. Six sensory conditions are tested, similar to the SOT (see Table 6.5).[146] The patient is asked to stand with shoes removed, feet together, and arms folded across chest with hands touching shoulders. Each test position is maintained for 30 seconds. Time (in seconds) is documented. If the patient is unable to maintain the 30 seconds, a second trial and, if needed, a third trial is given and scores across the three trials averaged. Increased sway is documented using the following scale: 1 = minimal sway; 2 = mild sway; 3 = moderate sway; and 4 = fall. Sway can also be documented using a postural grid. Subjective patient complaints (e.g., nausea, dizziness) are also documented. The test is stopped if the patient alters the posture (widens or moves feet, moves arms from original position, opens eyes during EC trial) or loses balance, requiring manual assistance. Time to administer is 10 to 20 minutes. A shorter modified CTSIB (mCTSIB) is available that uses four of the six original sensory conditions. Conditions 3 and 6 are omitted (see Table 6.6).[147] Time to administer is less than 10 minutes.

Interpreting the Results of SOT and CTSIB

Interpreting the results of the SOT and CTSIB requires an understanding of how the sensory conditions are manipulated (see Table 6.5). Patients who are visually dependent for postural control will demonstrate instability in conditions 2, 3, 5, and 6 (EC or visual conflict). Patients who are surface/somatosensory dependent will demonstrate instability in conditions 4, 5, and 6 (standing on a moving platform [SOT] or foam [CTSIB]). Patients with vestibular dysfunction will demonstrate instability in conditions 5 and 6 (inability to rely on vision or somatosensory inputs). Patients who demonstrate sensory selection problems present with abnormal findings in conditions 3 through 6.

A number of research studies have examined sensory interaction and balance with different populations. For example, studies have investigated the responses of community dwelling adults with a history of falls[148,149] and patients with stroke,[150,151] Alzheimer's disease,[152] Parkinson's disease,[153,154] vestibular dysfunction,[155-157] and traumatic brain injury.[158]

Motor Strategies for Balance

In observational studies of infants and young children and lesioned animals (decerebration experiments), righting and equilibrium reactions comprise the *postural reflex mechanism.* Automatic *righting reactions* (RR) orient the head in space (optical RR, labyrinthine RR, body-on-head RR) and the body in relation to the head and support surface (neck-on-body RR, body-on-body RR). *Equilibrium reactions* include tilting reactions and parachute or protective reactions. In normal adults, however, postural adjustments are far more complex and demonstrate a high degree of adaptability in response to both task and environmental context demands. Postural adjustments vary from the simple stretch reflex responses to the activation of specific movement strategies (synergistic patterns). Muscles closest to the BOS are particularly important to the maintenance of balance. As the LOS is reached with a COM disturbance, the magnitude of the postural response is increased.

Fixed Support Strategies

The term *fixed-support strategies* refers to those movement strategies used to control the COM over a fixed BOS (in-place strategies). In standing, the *ankle strategy* involves shifting the COM forward and back by moving the body (legs and trunk) as a relatively fixed pendulum about the ankle joints (Fig. 6.10). Muscles are activated in a distal-to-proximal sequence. With forward sway, gastrocnemius is activated first, followed by hamstrings, then paraspinal muscles. With backward sway, the anterior tibialis is activated first, followed by quadriceps, then abdominals. The ankle strategy is commonly used when sway frequencies are low and disturbances of the COM are small and well within the LOS.

The *hip strategy* involves shifts in the COM by flexing or extending at the hips (see Fig. 6.10). It has a proximal pattern of muscle activation before distal activation. With forward sway, abdominals are activated first, followed by quadriceps. With backward sway, paraspinal muscles are activated first, followed by hamstrings. Hip strategies provide primary control for mediolateral stability. Hip muscles (abductors and adductors) are activated to control lateral sway. The hip strategy is typically recruited with faster sway frequencies (greater than 1 Hz) and larger disturbances of the COM or when the

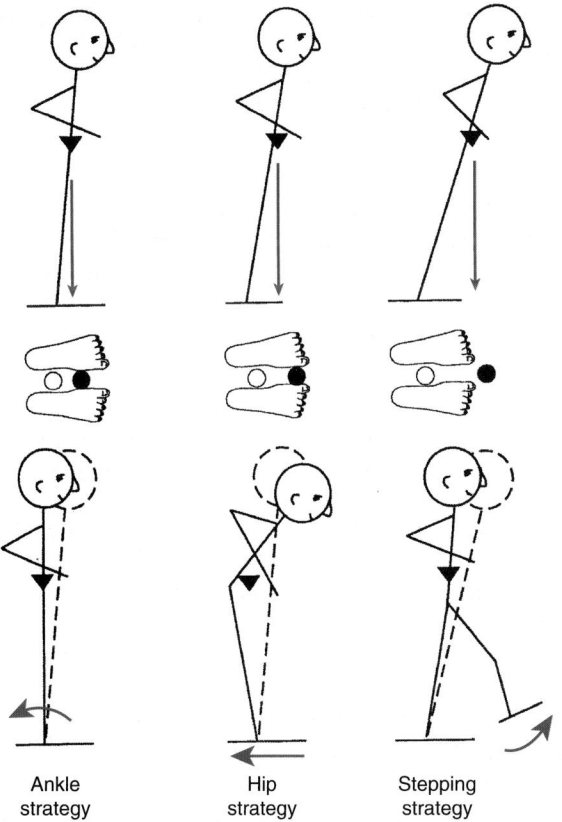

Figure 6.10 Strategies for correcting balance perturbations.

support surface is small (less than the size of the feet) or compliant (e.g., standing on foam).[159,160]

Change-in-Support Strategies

Change-in-support strategies are defined as movements of the lower or upper limbs to make a new contact with the support surface. The *stepping strategy* realigns the BOS under the COM by using rapid steps or hops in the direction of the displacing force; for example, forward or backward steps. In instances of lateral destabilization, the individual takes a side step or a cross step to bring the BOS back under the COM. The stepping strategies are typically recruited in response to fast, large postural perturbations when ankle and hip strategies are not adequate to recover balance (e.g., when the COM exceeds the BOS) (see Fig. 6.10). Change-in-support movements of the upper limbs (reach or grasp) can also assist in stabilizing the COM over the BOS and serve as a protective function in absorbing impact and protecting the head in a fall event. *Reaching movements* assist in extending the BOS and stabilizing posture. These reactions were found to be prevalent in destabilization situations, occurring in 85% of trials. Stepping strategies were also frequent, leading researchers to suggest that change-in-support strategies should not be viewed just as strategies of last resort. They are often initiated well before the COM nears or exceeds the LOS, contrary to the traditional view.[160-162]

Although these movement strategies have been investigated individually as distinct movement patterns, research has also shown that during normal balance combinations of strategies are used.[159] Control of movement strategies should be viewed on a continuum. The CNS quickly moves between patterns, depending on the control demands of the activity and environment. Thus, a destabilizing force may yield an initial ankle strategy that progresses quickly to a hip strategy as increased control is warranted to recover balance. When the displacement is large and ankle and hip strategies prove inadequate, a stepping strategy may be necessary to prevent a fall.[163] The CNS uses continuous sensory feedback monitoring to achieve flexibility and adaptability of movement strategies for multidirectional postural control.

Strategies in Sitting

In sitting, the BOS is comprised of the thighs and buttocks and the feet if in contact with the support surface. Postural strategies in sitting to maintain balance include movement of the trunk about the hips. Backward sway elicits primary responses in hip flexors along with activity of the abdominals and neck flexors. In forward sway, extensor muscles of the hips are activated along with the extensors of the neck and trunk. If the feet are in contact with the floor, tibialis anterior is recruited during forward reaching movements of the arm and the gastrocnemius is recruited to brake forward movements and return the body to erect sitting.[164] Somatosensory inputs from backward rotation of the pelvis may have an important role in triggering postural strategies in sitting.[165] In frontal plane movements, activity of the hip abductors and adductors along with the quadratus lumborum is important for providing mediolateral stability.

Examination of Movement Strategies

Standing Control

An examination of movement strategies should begin with biomechanical and musculoskeletal elements (ROM, postural tone, and strength). Weakness and limited ROM in the ankles will influence successful use of an ankle strategy, whereas weakness and limited ROM about the hips will influence the hip strategy. Limitations of neck ROM can be expected in patients with primary vestibular disorders. Available movement strategies in response to AP and ML destabilizations should be determined.

Dynamic posturography provides an effective way to study movement patterns during standing. The *Movement Coordination Test,* developed by Nashner,[160] provides information about postural responses to control the COM when the platform moves, including symmetry of weight-bearing and forces generated, latency of postural responses, amplitude of response in relation to the stimulus size, and strategy utilized (ankle or hip). EMG monitoring can reveal specific muscle activation patterns and latencies. The main disadvantage of this equipment is limited use in the clinic due to expense and lack of portability (e.g., it is typically found in specialized balance or vestibular dysfunction clinics). Correlation with performance during functional tasks (e.g., walking) is also lacking.

During perturbed stance, the direction of perturbations can be varied (AP and ML). The movement strategies utilized and success of restabilization efforts should be examined and documented. Specific directional instability may be evident. Patients may demonstrate an absence or decreased use of one strategy with increased dependence on another. For example, older adults with somatosensory loss in the feet and ankles typically forgo the ankle strategy and utilize an early hip strategy. The sequencing of movement synergies should be examined and a determination of the pattern of activation made. For example, the ascending pattern of activation (distal–proximal) may be absent in patients with strong spasticity. The therapist is likely to see a proximal-to-distal activation pattern with strong co-activation of spastic muscles in the hips and knees.

Seated Control

Seated postural control and balance should be examined. During quiet sitting, the degree and direction of sway should be determined. During perturbed unsupported sitting, the available movement strategies to prevent destabilization should be examined and documented.[165] Grasp strategies (holding on to the edge of the seat) or LE hooking strategies (the foot and leg hook around the platform mat leg) are common strategies in the presence of significant instability. Seated instability is common in many patients with neurological dysfunction. For example, patients with stroke may demonstrate increased sway, problems activating trunk muscles (e.g., voluntary trunk flexion and extension), limited extent and direction of reaching, and altered postural alignment with greater weight placed on the less affected side.

For both standing and seated control, the therapist determines and documents if the movement strategies are (1) present and normal, (2) present but limited or delayed, (3) present but inappropriate for the particular context or situation, (4) abnormal, or (5) absent. The ability to modify postural strategies and adapt movements to changing task conditions should also be documented. For example, the patient can be asked to stand first with normal stance width, then with a narrowed BOS (feet together, in tandem, or single leg stance). Table 6.6 presents criteria that can be used to document functional balance with descriptors that define both static and dynamic control in sitting and standing. Time in balance is a frequent measurement parameter (e.g., patient is able to maintain steady balance in sitting without handheld support for up to 5 minutes).

Table 6.6 Documenting Functional Balance

Normal	Patient able to maintain steady balance without handhold support (static). Patient accepts maximal challenge and can shift weight easily within full range of LOS in all directions (dynamic).
Good	Patient able to maintain balance without handhold support, limited postural sway (static). Patient accepts moderate challenge; able to maintain balance while picking up object off floor (dynamic).
Fair	Patient able to maintain balance with handhold support; may require occasional minimal assistance (static). Patient accepts minimal challenge; able to maintain balance while turning head/trunk (dynamic).
Poor	Patient requires handhold support and moderate to maximal assistance to maintain position (static). Patient unable to accept challenge or move without loss of balance (dynamic).
Absent	Patient unable to maintain balance.

LOS = limits of stability

Anticipatory postural control

Anticipatory postural control, the ability to activate postural adjustments in advance of destabilizing voluntary movements, should be examined. For example, the therapist asks the patient while standing or sitting to raise both arms overhead or catch a weighted ball. Changes in postural stability control are examined and documented during the performance of the voluntary activity. Impaired anticipatory postural control is found in many individuals with impairments in motor function, including patients with stroke,[166,167] Parkinson's disease,[168] and brain injury.[169]

Dual-Task Control

Dual-task control should be examined. This is the ability to perform a secondary task (motor or cognitive) while maintaining standing or seated control. For example, while standing, the patient is asked to count backward from 100 by 7 (simultaneous verbal-cognitive task) or to pour water into a glass (secondary motor task). Patients with Parkinson's disease have been shown to demonstrate significant impairment in dual-task control.[170,171] Patients with traumatic brain injury and stroke have also been shown to demonstrate problems with dual-task control.[172,173]

OUTCOME MEASURES: POSTURAL CONTROL AND BALANCE

This section reviews selected postural control and balance outcome measures in common use. Individual tests can utilize a number of different postures (e.g., sitting, standing) and activities (e.g., sit-to-stand, walking, stair climbing) that challenge control. Tests typically include items that challenge both static or steady-state control and dynamic control. Asking the patient to maintain a steady posture in sitting or standing without handheld support tests static control. Test items can vary the BOS (e.g., the patient is asked to stand with double-limb support, single-limb support, tandem standing). Superimposing movement tests dynamic control (e.g., sit-to-stand, UE reach, stepping, step-ups). Walking test items challenge dynamic control and can include items of changing directions (e.g., forward, backward, sideward, pivoting) walking with head turns, or walking around obstacles. Before using, the clinician should analyze each test to determine what aspects of postural control and balance are being examined (e.g., static or dynamic control, proactive or reactive control, sensory interaction). The patient's unique impairments and activity limitations will help determine which test is the most appropriate to use in terms of postures and activities included. Some tests are diagnosis-specific and developed for a specific population. For example, the Berg Balance Scale was initially developed for use with patients with stroke.[174] Others were developed with a more generalized purpose. For example, the Tinetti Performance Oriented Mobility Assessment was developed to examine the frail elderly, especially nursing home residents, with a propensity to fall.[175] Oftentimes these instruments have been generalized for use with different populations and in different settings.

The patient should be instructed that a variety of functional activities will be used during testing. Some activities will be more difficult than others and may result in instability. The patient should be assured that the therapist will at all times protect him or her from a fall. During testing, all safety precautions should be observed, including close or contact guarding and use of a safety belt as indicated.

Scoring systems vary and can include an ordinal scale (e.g., 4-point or 5-point) as well as timed components. Some scale items are anchored with specific performance and time criteria (e.g., for single-leg stance, able to lift leg independently and hold for greater than 10 seconds) while others use more general terms (e.g., unable or loses balance, unsteady, or steady). Tests and measures also vary in the time required to administer. Some are relatively short (e.g., 5 to 10 minutes) while others are quite comprehensive and lengthy (e.g., 30 to 40 minutes). In observing patient performance, the clinician may determine additional qualitative comments are necessary. These comments can address patient safety/fall risk, extraneous movements, excessive time requirements, alterations in speed, need for verbal cueing and assistive devices, and impact of the environment on test results.

Table 6.7 includes examples of outcome measures designed to examine postural control and balance. Many other standardized tests are available. Selection of outcome measures should be based on the strength of available data addressing: *reliability* (e.g., test-retest, intra-rater, and interrater), *validity* (concurrent, criterion-related, and predictive) and *sensitivity to change* (responsiveness, minimally detectable change [MDC], and minimal clinically important difference [MCID]). Additional considerations in selection include the availability of normative data, the type of impairments the instrument was designed to measure, and the intended population. The reader is referred to the *Rehabilitation Measures Database* (www.rehabmeasures@sralab.org) and APTA's *Academy of Neurologic Physical Therapy Outcome Measures*, Edge files (www.neuropt.org) for additional information.

Performance-Based Measures

Berg Balance Scale

The *Berg Balance Scale* (BBS) developed by Berg, et al,[174,176] is an objective measure of static and dynamic balance abilities in sitting, sit-to-stand, and standing. There are six static balance items and eight dynamic balance items, with the first six items considered a measure of basic balance ability. The test is scored using a 5-point ordinal scale (0–4) with detailed descriptors for each score. Some items are timed. Average time to administer is 14 to 20 minutes. Test-retest and interrater/intrarater reliability is excellent as is predictive and concurrent validity.[177,178] BBS scores have been shown to be useful in predicting falls in the elderly and in evaluating changes in patients with stroke.[179,180] Scores of 45 or below are associated with high risk of falls with significant increase below a score of 40.[181,182] Using individual item analysis, data from community-dwelling elders and those with chronic stroke revealed that selected BBS items may have greater accuracy than the total BBS in identifying individuals with high fall risk. These items include picking an object up off the floor and standing on one leg, as well as turning 360°, placing alternate foot on stool, and tandem stance.[183] Minimal detectable change of the BBS has been reported for elderly people.[184-187]

Tinetti Performance-Oriented Mobility Assessment

The *Performance-Oriented Mobility Assessment* (POMA), developed by Tinetti et al,[175,188] provides a measure of both static and dynamic balance. It was developed for use with the frail elderly, especially nursing home residents with a propensity to fall. Items are organized into two subtests of balance and gait. Balance test items

Table 6.7 Outcome Measures: Examination of Balance

Outcome Measure and ICF Category	Description	Scoring	MDC and MCID
Clinical Test of Sensory Interaction and Balance (CTSIB)[145] **ICF: 1, 2** **Modified CTSIB**	Performance-based test: examines postural control and balance under 6 different sensory conditions Uses 4 conditions	Time in balance is measured during a 30-sec trial. Sway/loss of balance is documented using a 4-point scale (1–4): 1 = minimal sway to 4 = fall	MDC: mCTSIB: AD = 0.34[152] MCID: NA
Berg Balance Scale (BBS)[174,176,177] **ICF: 2**	Mulitask performance test (14 items): examines static and dynamic balance using 6 static and 8 dynamic tasks; items 1–5 = tests of basic balance ability Excellent test-retest and interrater reliability (ICC); predictive/concurrent validity	Uses 5-point ordinal scale (0–4) with specific task criteria; 0 = unable to perform and 4 = independent; some items timed Max score = 56 points Predictive: scores of 45 or below = high risk for falls in elderly	MDC: OA = 4.6–3.3 points depending on initial scores[184] Acute stroke = 6.9 points[185] Chronic stroke = 4.66 points[186] PD = 5 points[187] MCID: NA
Tinetti Performance Oriented Mobility Assessment (POMA)[188,189] **ICF: 2**	Multitask performance test (16 items): 9 balance (POMA-B): 4 static, 5 dynamic 7 gait (POMA-G) Excellent test-retest and interrater reliability (ICC); predictive/concurrent validity	Scoring: some items use a 3 point ordinal scale (0–2) while some items use a 2-point scale timed (0,1); some items are timed (15 ft [4.57 m] walk) Max score = 28 points Predictive: scores of 18 and below = high risk of falls in the elderly	MDC: OA = 4.2, 4 points[190] Stroke = 6 points[191] MCID: NA
Functional Reach Test (FRT)[196,197] **ICF: 2** **Multidirectional Reach Test (mFRT)[197]** **Modified Functional Reach (mFRT)[198,199]**	Single task performance test: examines postural stability (LOS) during standing forward reach; requires adequate shoulder ROM Excellent test-retest and interrater reliability (ICC); content validity Examines postural stability during multidirectional reach Examines postural stability during a multidirectional sitting reach test	Scoring + maximum distance of a forward reach; uses a yard stick Uses 2 practice trials and 3 test trials Normative data are available based on age[196]	MDC: PD = 7.32 cm[199] Stroke = 6.79[203] SCI = 5.16–4.10[204] MCID: NA
Timed Up and Go (TUG)[207] **ICF: 2** **Dual-Task Variations:** **TUG Manual** **TUG Cognitive[215]**	Multitask performance test: examines functional mobility during stand up, walk 3 m, turn, walk back, and sit down Excellent test-retest and interrater reliability (ICC); Predictive/concurrent validity	Scoring: test is timed Uses 1 practice/3 trials for average score Predictive: Scores 11–20 typical for frail elderly >30 sec = high risk for falls	MDC: NA MCID: NA

Table 6.7 Outcome Measures: Examination of Balance—cont'd

Outcome Measure and ICF Category	Description	Scoring	MDC and MCID
Balance Evaluation Systems Test (BESTest)[216] **ICF: 1,2**	Multitask performance test (36 items) across 6 systems: mechanical constraints, LOS, APAs, postural responses, sensory orientation, and stability in gait Excellent test-retest and interrater reliability (ICC); predictive/concurrent validity	Scoring: uses 4-point ordinal scale (0–3) with 0 = severe impairment to 3 = no impairment; some items timed Total score = 108 points	MDC: CD adults= 8.9 points[222] PD = 6.5 points[217] Subacute stroke = 7.81 points[220] MCID: NA
Mini-BESTest[221]	Includes 14 items across 4 systems	Uses 3-point ordinal scale (0–2)	
Dynamic Gait Index (DGI)[182] **ICF: 2**	Multitask performance test: examines walking (20 ft/ 6.1 m walkway) steady state, changing speeds, with head turns, stepping over and around obstacles, pivoting, and stair climbing Excellent test-retest and interrater reliability (ICC); predictive/concurrent validity	Scoring: uses a 4-point ordinal scale (0–3) with 0 = severe impairment to 3 = no gait dysfunction Max score of 24 points	MDC: CD elderly = 2.9 points[226] Chronic stroke = 2.6 points[224] Stroke = 4 points[227] MS = 4.19–5.54 points[228] PD = 2.9 points[229] Vestibular = 3.2 points[222] MCID CD elderly = 1.90[230]
Walking While Talking Test (WTT)[231] **ICF: 2, 3**	A dual-task performance test that examines divided attention and balance/ falls while walking; uses a distance of 20 ft, turn, and return (40 ft total) Cognitive tasks can be used: reciting alphabet (WWT-simple), reciting every other letter (WWT-complex) Adequate interrater reliability; test-retest NA Predictive/concurrent validity	Scoring: time needed to complete the distance Predictive: time of 20 sec or longer WWT-simple = high risk for falls; Time of 33 sec or longer WWT-complex = high risk for falls	MDC: NA MDC: NA MCID: NA
Function in Sitting Test (FIST)[248] **ICF: 2**	Multitask performance test (14 items): examines sitting balance including sensory, motor, proactive, reactive, and steady state balance Patient sits on edge of bed with hips and knees at 90°, feet flat on floor, hands on lap unless needed for support	Scoring: uses 5-point ordinal scale (0–4) with 0 = complete assistance and 4 = independent	MDC: Acute stroke = 5.63[248] Adults with sitting balance dysfunction = 5.63[250] MCID > 6.5[250]

Continued

Table 6.7 Outcome Measures: Examination of Balance—cont'd

Outcome Measure and ICF Category	Description	Scoring	MDC and MCID
	Excellent test-retest, intrarater reliability Good to excellent predictive/concurrent validity		
Activities-Specific Balance Confidence (ABC)[251]	16-item self-report measure; patients rate their balance confidence for different daily activities including reaching/picking up objects, walking/stairs in the home and in the community (parking lot, crowded mall, escalator, icy sidewalks) Excellent test-retest reliability Interrater/intrarater NA Predictive/concurrent validity	Scoring: items are rated from 0–100, with 0 = no confidence and 100 = complete confidence Overall score calculated by adding item scores and dividing by total number of items Scores less than 67: 69% predictive of recurrent falls	MDC: PD = 13,[254] 11.12[255] MCID: NA
Tinetti Falls Efficacy Scale (FES)[256] **ICF: 2,3**	10-item self-report measure: patients assess their level of confidence and fear of falling during common daily activities Excellent test-retest reliability; interrater/intrarater NA Predictive/concurrent validity	Scoring: items are rated from 1 = very confident to 10 = not confident at all Total score: ranges from 10 = best possible to 100 = worst possible	MDC = NA MCID = NA

ICF CATEGORY: 1 = Body structure/function; 2 = Activity; 3 = Participation

AD = Alzheimer's disease; APA = Anticipatory postural adjustments; CD adults = community dwelling; LOS = Limits of stability; MCID = Minimal clinically important difference; MDC = Minimal detectable change; NA = Not available (not established); OA = Older adults; PD = Parkinson's disease; MS = multiple sclerosis; SCI = Spinal cord injury

For additional information, see Rehabilitation Measures Database at www.rehabmeasures@sralab.org

include static sitting balance, sit-to-stand and stand-to-sit, standing balance (static, with sternal nudge, EC), and dynamic standing balance (turning 360°). Gait test items include initiation of gait, path, missed step (trip or loss of balance), turning, and timed walk. Some items are scored on a 2-point scale (0 or 1) and some on a 3-point (0 to 2) scale. Average time to administer is 10 to 15 minutes. The POMA scale has a total possible score of 28. Test-retest and interrater/intrarater reliability is excellent, as is predictive and concurrent validity.[189-191] Patients who score less than 19 are considered at high risk for falls, and those who score between 19 and 24 are at moderate risk for falls. Studies have looked at its ability to detect change in individuals with stroke,[191] Parkinson's disease,[192,193] and amyotrophic lateral sclerosis.[194] A revised form, the POMA Ia, includes five additional items and was designed for use as a predictor of falls among community-dwelling elderly (with a total possible score of 40).[195]

Functional Reach Test

The *Functional Reach Test* (FRT) is a single-item test developed by Duncan et al[196,197] to provide a quick screen of balance problems in older adults. It has been shown a marker of physical frailty.[198] Functional reach is the maximal distance one can reach forward beyond arm's length while maintaining a fixed BOS in the standing position. The test uses a level yardstick mounted on the wall and positioned at the height of the patient's acromion. The patient stands sideward next to the wall (without touching), feet normal stance width and weight equally distributed on both feet.

The shoulder is flexed to 90° and elbow extended with the hand fisted. An initial measurement is made of the position of the third metacarpal along the yardstick. For forward reach, the patient is instructed to lean as far forward as possible without losing balance or taking a step. A second measurement is then taken using the third metacarpal for reference. This measurement is then subtracted from the initial measurement. See Table 6.8 for normative values of FRT. Time to administer is 5 minutes. Several studies have examined the ability of the FRT to detect change in patients with Parkinson's disease.[199-201]

The *Multidirectional Reach Test (MDFRT),* developed by Newton,[202] evolved from the earlier FRT and measures how far an individual can reach in the forward, backward, and lateral directions. For backward reach, the test position is the same as FR with the yardstick position reversed to detect posterior movements. For lateral reach, the patient faces away from the wall and reaches sideways to the right (and then to the left) as far as possible. One practice trial is allowed before the start of three test trials. The therapist records functional reach in inches for all three trials and then averages the three trials. The amount of reach is influenced by several factors, including the size and height of the individual, sex, age, and health. The movement strategy used during a reach test should be documented (i.e., ankle or hip strategy, trunk rotation, scapular protraction). See Table 6.9 for normative values of MDRT for older adults. Reliability and ability to detect change has been studied in Parkinson's disease.[199-202] The *modified Functional Reach Test (mFRT)* incorporates forward and lateral reach to each side in sitting has been shown to be a reliable measure.[203-205]

Table 6.8 Functional Reach (FR) Reference Values (NORMS) by Age

Age	Men (inches)	Women (inches)
20–40	16.7 (± 1.9)	14.6 (± 2.2)
41–69	14.9 (± 2.2)	13.8 (± 2.2)
70–87	13.2 (± 1.6)	10.5 (± 3.5)

From Duncan et al.[196]

Timed Up and Go Test

The *Get Up and Go (GUG) test* was developed by Mathias et al[206] as a quick measure of dynamic balance and mobility. The patient is seated comfortably in a firm chair with arms and back resting against the chair. The patient is then instructed to rise and walk as quickly and safely as possible 3 m (10 ft), cross a line marked on floor, turn around, walk back, and sit down. The patient is allowed to use an assistive device typically used but must complete the test without manual assistance. Time to administer is less than 5 minutes. Performance on the original GUG test used a 5-point ordinal scale ranging from 1, Normal (no risk of falls) to 5, Severely Abnormal (high risk of falls). The subjective nature of the grades yielded only limited reliability.

Efforts by Podsiadlo and Richardson[207] to improve the objectivity and reliability resulted in the *Timed Up and Go Test* (TUG), which is widely used today. Timing with a stopwatch begins when the patient is instructed with "go" and ends when the patient returns to the start position seated in the chair. Healthy adults are able to complete the test in less than 10 seconds. Older adults (ages 60 to 80) have also been shown to average scores less than 10 (mean of 8).[207-209] Scores of 11 to 20 seconds are considered typical for frail elderly or individuals with a mild disability; scores over 30 seconds are indicative of impaired mobility and high fall risk. The TUG has been used to examine functional mobility deficits in patients with stroke[210,211] and Parkinson's disease.[212,213] Minimal detectable changes have been reported for people with Parkinson's disease.[214] Variations of the TUG include the *TUG cognitive* (TUGcog) in which the individual is asked to perform a simultaneous cognitive task (e.g., count backward from 100 by 3s) or *TUG manual* (TUGman) in which the individual performs a simultaneous manual task (e.g., holds a cup filled with water). Researchers found mean scores for dual-tasking on the TUG can be expected to increase slightly (e.g., TUG 8.4, TUG man 9.7, TUGcog 9.7) for community-dwelling adults.[215]

Balance Evaluation Systems Test

The *Balance Evaluation Systems Test* (BESTest) was developed by Horak and colleagues[216] as a comprehensive assessment of postural control and balance. It includes

Table 6.9 Multidirectional Reach Test (MDRT) Reference Values

REACH–MDRT	Mean (Inches) Standard Deviation Mean Age, 74	Above Average (inches)	Below Average (inches)
Forward	8.9 ± 3.4	>12.2	<5.6
Backward	4.6 ± 3.1	>7.6	<1.6
Right lateral	6.2 ± 3	>9.4	<3.8
Left lateral	6.6 ± 2.8	>9.4	<3.8

From Newton.[202]

36 items that examine six subsystem categories of postural control: biomechanical constraints (5 items), stability limits/verticality (3 items), transitions/anticipatory postural responses (5 items), reactive postural responses (5 items), sensory orientation (2 items), and stability in gait (7 items). Table 6.10 summarizes the subsystem categories and test items. It incorporates some items from earlier tests (i.e., functional reach, modified CTSIB, Timed Up and Go, Dynamic Gait Index). The BESTest uses a 4-point ordinal scale (0–3) with 0 = severe impairment to 3 = no impairments and specific descriptors for each score. The total score is 108 points with subscores available in each of the above categories. A percent score is also calculated. Some items are measured (functional reach), and some are timed (TUG). Time to administer is 30 minutes. Training is required (training manual, workshops, online resources available). Subjects are tested wearing flat-heeled shoes or with shoes and socks off. They are allowed to use an assistive device if needed but are scored 1 point lower for that item; if they require physical assistance, they receive a score of 0 for that item. Test-retest and interrater/intrarater reliability are excellent, as is predictive/concurrent and construct validity.[217] Minimal detectable change has been reported for community-dwelling adults with and without balance dysfunction[216] and for patients with Parkinson's disease[217-219] and subacute stroke.[220] A shortened version of this test is available, the Mini-BESTest. This version contains 14 items grouped into four categories: anticipatory postural adjustments (3 items), reactive postural control (3 items), sensory orientation (3 items), and dynamic gait (5 items).[221] Time to administer is 10 to 15 minutes.

Table 6.10 Components of the Balance Evaluation Systems Test (BESTest)[216]

Subsystem Categories	Test Items
Biomechanical Constraints	Base of support Center of mass alignment Ankle strength and range Hip and lateral trunk strength Sit on floor and stand up
Stability Limits/ Verticality	Sit, vertical and lateral lean, L and R Functional reach forward Functional reach lateral, L and R
Transitions/ Anticipatory Postural Adjustment	Sit to stand* Rise to toes* Stand on one leg L and R* Alternate stair touching Standing arm raise
Reactive Postural Control	In-place response—forward In-place response—backward Compensatory stepping—forward* Compensatory stepping—backward* Compensatory stepping—lateral, L and R*
Sensory Orientation (mCTSIB)	Standing, EO, firm surface* Standing, EC, firm surface Standing, EO, on foam Standing, EC, on foam* Standing, EC, on incline*
Stability in Gait	Walk, level surface Walk with change in gait speed* Walk with horizontal head turns* Walk with pivot turns* Walk and step over obstacles* Timed Up and Go Timed Up and Go—cognitive*

*Items included on the Mini-BESTest.[221]
EC = eyes closed; EO = eyes open; L = left; R = right
Complete BESTest copies and training materials, available at www.bestest.us.

Dynamic Gait Index

The *Dynamic Gait Index* (DGI) developed by Shumway-Cook et al,[182] examines a patient's ability to perform steady state walking and variations on command. Items include changing speed, walk with head turns (look right or left, look up or down), walk and pivot turn, walk while stepping over or around obstacles, and stair climbing (up and down). A 4-point scale (0–3) includes specific descriptors of normal control: 3 = no gait dysfunction, 2 = minimal impairment, 1 = moderate impairment, and 0 = severe impairment, with a maximum possible score of 24. Time to administer is less than 10 minutes. The DGI appears to be sensitive in predicting likelihood for falls with older adults (a score below 19 is indicative of increased fall risk).[182] Test-retest and interrater/intrarater reliability are excellent, as are predictive/concurrent and construct validity.[222-225] Minimal detectable change has been established for community-dwelling elderly[226,227] and individuals with stroke,[224,228] multiple sclerosis,[229] Parkinson's disease,[230] and vestibular disorders.[222]

Walking While Talking Test

The *Walking While Talking Test (WWT)* is a dual-task measure that can be used to determine the effects of divided attention by introducing a secondary task, talking while walking.[231] The patient walks at a self-selected comfortable speed for a distance of 20 ft (6 m), turns, and returns (total distance of 40 ft [12 m]). Cognitive tasks are superimposed on the motor activity. The patient is asked to recite the alphabet (WWT-simple) or recite every other letter (WWT-complex). The time required to complete the test is recorded. This test is predictive for falls in community-dwelling elderly.[231] Individuals who require a time of 20 seconds or longer (WT-simple) or a time of 33 seconds or longer (WWT-complex) are at high risk for falls. Performance changes can be documented, including hesitations or stops, postural instability, and increased walking variability (steps off path). Cognitive changes (number of errors, mental slowing) can also be documented. Patients with impaired attention and automatic postural control can be expected to demonstrate difficulty on this test.[232] Dual-task performance impairments have been found in individuals with stroke,[233,234] traumatic brain injury,[235,236] multiple sclerosis,[237] Parkinson's disease,[238-241] and in older adults at risk for falls.[232,242-244] Alternate forms of this test exist.[245] For example, the Stops Walking While Talking Test (SWWT) includes initiating a conversation while the patient is walking. The test is positive if the individual stops walking while talking.[246,247]

Function in Sitting

The *Function in Sitting Test* (FIST) developed by Gorman et al[248] is a 14-item test that examines a person's ability to maintain sitting balance during static sitting (hands in lap) with eyes open and eyes closed, as well as during dynamic challenges to balance. Reactive challenges include nudges (anterior, posterior, and lateral). Anticipatory challenges include moving the head side to side, lifting the foot, turning and picking an object up from behind, performing a forward and lateral reach, picking up an object from the floor, and scooting (anterior, posterior, and lateral). The FIST is scored on a 5-point ordinal scale: 0 = complete assistance, 1 = needs assistance to complete task, 2 = upper extremity support required to complete the task, 3 = verbal or tactile cues or extra time required to complete task, and 4 = independent. Descriptors accompany each of the scores. Time to administer is less than 15 minutes. The FIST was developed by a panel of experts and tested on adults with acute stroke (within 3 months of insult). It demonstrates excellent reliability (test-retest, interrater/intrarater) and good to excellent predictive/concurrent validity.[249,250] Researchers have reported minimal detectable change for patients with acute stroke and adults with sitting balance dysfunction.[250]

Self-Report Measures

Activities-Specific Balance Confidence Scale

The *Activities-Specific Balance Confidence (ABC)* scale developed by Powell and Meyers[251] is a 16-item self-report measure that asks individuals to rate their overall level of self-confidence in performing both household and community activities. Household activities include walking around the house, walking up and down stairs, picking up a slipper off the floor, and several reaching activities (reach at eye level, reach on tiptoes, stand on chair to reach). Community activities include walking to a car, getting in and out of a car, walking on various surfaces (parking lot, ramp) and environments (crowded mall, icy sidewalk), and riding an escalator. The individual is asked to rate his or her confidence on a scale from 100% (complete confidence) to 0% (no confidence). Overall score is calculated by adding all scores and dividing by 16 (total number of items). Length of test is 30 minutes or less. Test-retest reliability is excellent.[252-255] Researchers have identified the minimal detectable change for patients with Parkinson's disease.[254,255]

Tinetti Falls Efficacy Scale

The *Falls Efficacy Scale* developed by Tinetti et al[256] is a self-report measure that examines how confident an individual feels to perform 10 activities of daily living (ADL) without falling. The items on the test include both basic ADL (getting dressed and undressed, taking a bath or shower) and instrumental ADL (cleaning house, preparing simple meals, simple shopping). The functional mobility items include getting in and out of a car, going up and down stairs, walking around the neighborhood, reaching, and hurrying to answer the phone. The individual is asked to rate his or her confidence level on a 1 (very confident) to 10 (not confident at all) scale. Total scores can range from 10 (best possible) to the highest score 100 (not confident at all). Length of test is 10 to 15 minutes. Test-retest reliability is moderate to excellent.[256,257]

SUMMARY

An examination of coordination and balance provides important information about motor and sensory function. Evaluation of examination data allows the therapist to establish the diagnosis and identify underlying impairments, activity limitations, and participation restricts. The therapist then formulates the POC including goals, prognosis, interventions, and expected outcomes.

A variety of outcome measures for coordination and balance have been identified. Selection should be based on the strength of available data addressing their *reliability*, *validity*, and *sensitivity to change*. Additional considerations in selection include the availability of normative data, the type of impairments the instrument was designed to measure, and the intended population (general application or diagnosis-specific).

Documentation should include the type, severity, and location of the impairments, as well as factors that alter the quality of performance. Emphasis has been placed on the variety of influences that affect movement capabilities. As such, evaluation of test results must be considered with respect to findings from other examinations such as sensation, ROM, muscle strength, muscle tone, and functional status.

Questions for Review

1. What are the purposes of performing a coordination examination of motor function?
2. What are the contributions (functions) of the cerebellum to coordinated movement?
3. How is peripheral feedback provided during a motor response?
4. Differentiate between motor impairments associated with cerebellar pathology and basal ganglion pathology. Provide at least five characteristic impairments for each area.
5. What predictable aspects of normal aging may affect coordinated movement?
6. Accurate and careful patient observation is an important source of preliminary information before performing a coordination examination. What type of activities would you select for the observation? What information will the observation provide?
7. Assume you are about to initiate a coordination examination. What screenings would be appropriate?
8. Identify three upper extremity and three lower extremity coordination tests that could be used to examine a patient with severe ataxia as a result of traumatic brain injury.
9. Differentiate between coordination tests for intention tremor and postural tremor.
10. What are the sensory conditions examined in the Clinical Test for Sensory Interaction in Balance (CTSIB)? How should the results be interpreted?
11. Differentiate between the Berg Balance Scale and the Performance-Oriented Mobility Test (Tinetti) in terms of aspects of balance tested.
12. The Balance Evaluation Systems Test (BESTest) was developed to examine multiple aspects of postural control and balance. What are the six systems that items are grouped into? How is it scored?

CASE STUDY

The patient is a 62-year-old man with a 5-year history of Parkinson's disease. Since the time of the diagnosis, he reports a progressive decline in functional activity level. With encouragement from his wife and children, he took an early retirement 3 years ago from his career as a commercial airline pilot. He lives with his wife of 38 years in a one-level suburban home. His four adult children all live in neighboring communities. The patient takes Sinemet (a combination of L-dopa/carbidopa). The physical therapy referral is for examination to document baseline function before beginning outpatient rehabilitation.

Initial examination reveals the following:

- Movements are decreased and slowed.
- A uniform, constant resistance is felt as the extremities are moved passively; patient reports an overall feeling of stiffness that is worse during medication "off" times.
- Involuntary, rhythmic, oscillatory movements of the distal upper extremities are observed at rest (pill rolling).
- Patient has difficulty with distal upper extremity (UE) movements required for buttoning shirts, using eating utensils, and writing.
- Patient has difficulty initiating movement transitions and is unable to stand up from a chair or roll from prone to supine without difficulty.
- Patient stands with a flexed, stooped posture, positioned at the forward limits of the BOS.
- Standing balance is easily displaced with tendency to fall stiffly.
- Patient has difficulty changing direction of movement or stopping while walking.
- Reports regular falls (two to three times per week).
- Berg Balance Scale score: 38 out of 56.

GUIDING QUESTIONS

1. Describe this patient's motor impairments and activity limitations.
2. Explain the clinical manifestations of bradykinesia.
3. Select the coordination tests you would use to examine the patient's movement capabilities in performing alternating distal UE movements.

4. What are the requirements for documentation?
5. What standardized tests for postural control and balance test might yield the best evidence in terms of this patient's limitations?
6. What does a Berg Balance Test score of 38 indicate?

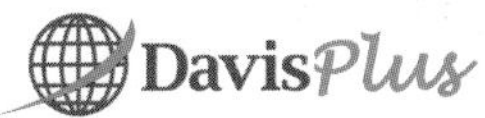

For additional resources, including answers to the questions for review and case study guiding questions, please visit **http://davisplus.fadavis.com.**

References

1. Shumway-Cook, A, and Woollacott, MH: Motor Control: Translating Research into Clinical Practice, ed 5. Wolters Kluwer, Philadelphia, 2017.
2. Byl, NN: Multisensory control of upper extremity function. Neurology Report (now JNPT) 26(1):32, 2002.
3. Schmidt, RA, and Lee, TD: Motor Control and Learning: A Behavioral Emphasis, ed 5. Human Kinetics, Champaign, IL, 2011.
4. *Guide to Physical Therapist Practice 3.0.* Alexandria, VA: American Physical Therapy Association; 2014. Available at: http://guidetoptpractice.apta.org/. Accessed August 25, 2018.
5. Wiesendanger, M, and Serrien, DJ: Toward a physiological understanding of human dexterity. News Physiol Sci 16:228, 2001.
6. Asmussen, MJ, Przysucha, E, and Zerpa, C: Intralimb coordination in children with and without developmental coordination disorder in one-handed catching. J Mot Behav 46(6):445, 2014.
7. Ohmura, Y, et al: Developmental changes in intralimb coordination during spontaneous movements of human infants from 2 to 3 months of age. Exp Brain Res 234(8), 2016.
8. Rinaldi, LA, and Monaco, V: Spatio-temporal parameters and intralimb coordination patterns describing hemiparetic locomotion at controlled speed. JNER 10(1):1, 2013.
9. Romanazzi, M, Galante, D, and Sforza, C: Intralimb joint coordination of the lower extremities in resistance training exercises. J Electromyogr Kinesiol 25(1):61, 2015.
10. Krasovsky, T, et al: Effects of walking speed on gait stability and interlimb coordination in younger and older adults. Gait Posture 39(1):378, 2014.
11. Tkachenko, P, and Bobyntsev, I: Relationship between amplitude parameters of stimulation myography and bimanual coordination in men and women during performance of motor tasks of different complexity. Bull Exp Biol Med 158(6):711, 2015.
12. Sakurada, T, Ito, K, and Gomi, H: Bimanual motor coordination controlled by cooperative interactions in intrinsic and extrinsic coordinates. Eur J Neurosci 43(1):120, 2016.
13. Lafe, C, Pacheco, M, and Newell, K: Bimanual coordination and the intermittency of visual information in isometric force tracking. Exp Brain Res 234(7):2025, 2016.
14. Zelic, G, Mottet, D, and Lagarde, J: Perceptuo-motor compatibility governs multisensory integration in bimanual coordination dynamics. Exp Brain Res 234(2):463, 2016.
15. Kantak, S, McGrath, R, and Zahedi, N: Goal conceptualization and symmetry of arm movements affect bimanual coordination in individuals after stroke. Neurosci Lett 626:86, 2016.
16. Kennedy, D, Rhee, J, and Shea, C: Symmetrical and asymmetrical influences on force production in 1:2 and 2:1 bimanual force coordination tasks. Exp Brain Res 234(1):287, 2016.
17. Sun, Q, et al: Assessing drivers' visual-motor coordination using eye tracking, GNSS and GIS: A spatial turn in driving psychology. J Spat Sci 61(2):299, 2016.
18. Parmar, PN, Huang, FC, and Patton JL: Simultaneous coordinate representations are influenced by visual feedback in a motor learning task. Conf Proc IEEE Eng Med Biol Soc (Aug):6762, 2011.
19. Sarpeshkar, V, and Mann, DL: Biomechanics and visual-motor control: How it has, is, and will be used to reveal the secrets of hitting a cricket ball. Sports Biomech 10(4):306, 2011.
20. Coats, RO, and Wann, JP: The reliance on visual feedback control by older adults is highlighted in tasks requiring precise endpoint placement and precision grip. Exp Brain Res 214(1):139, 2011.
21. Wang, J, et al: Aging reduces asymmetries in interlimb transfer of visuomotor adaptation. Exp Brain Res 210(2):283, 2011.
22. Lee, K, Hui-Chen, C, and Tsang, W: The effects of practicing sitting Tai Chi on balance control and eye-hand coordination in the older adults: A randomized controlled trial. Disabil Rehabil 37(9):790, 2015.
23. Gopal, A, and Murthy, A: Eye-hand coordination during a double-step task: Evidence for a common stochastic accumulator. J Neurophysiol 114(3):1438, 2015.
24. Hiraoka, K, et al: Interaction between the premotor processes of eye and hand movements: Possible mechanism underlying eye-hand coordination. Somatosens Mot Res 31(1):49, 2014.
25. Gao, KL, et al: Eye-hand coordination and its relationship with sensori-motor impairments in stroke survivors. J Rehabil Med 42(4):368, 2010.
26. Srinivasan, D, and Martin, BJ: Eye-hand coordination of symmetric bimanual reaching tasks: Temporal aspects. Exp Brain Res 203(2):391, 2010.
27. Bear, MF, Connors, BW, and Paradiso, MA: Neuroscience: Exploring the Brain, ed 3. Lippincott Williams & Wilkins/Wolters Kluwer, Philadelphia, 2007.
28. Vanderah, TW, and Gould, DJ: Nolte's The Human Brain: An Introduction to Its Functional Anatomy, ed 7. Elsevier, St. Louis, 2016.
29. Rizzolatti, G, and Kalaska, JF: Voluntary movement: The parietal and premotor cortex. In Kandel, ER, et al (eds): Principles of Neural Science, ed 5. McGraw-Hill, New York, 2013, p. 865.
30. Mihailoff, GA, and Haines, DE: Motor system II: Corticofugal systems and the control of movement. In Haines, DE (ed): Fundamental Neuroscience for Basic and Clinical Applications, ed 4. Churchill Livingstone/Elsevier, New York, 2013, p. 338.
31. Ropper, AH, Samuels, MA, and Klein, JP: Adams and Victor's Principles of Neurology, ed 10. McGraw-Hill Education, New York, 2014.
32. Lundy-Ekman, L: Neuroscience: Fundamentals for Rehabilitation, ed 4. Elsevier, Philadelphia, 2013.
33. Hall, JE: Guyton and Hall Textbook of Medical Physiology, ed 13. Elsevier, Philadelphia, 2016.
34. Lisberger, SG, and Thach, WT: The cerebellum. In Kandel, ER, et al (eds): Principles of Neural Science, ed 5. McGraw-Hill, New York, 2013, p. 960.
35. Scanlon, VC, and Sanders, T: Essentials of Anatomy and Physiology, ed 7. FA Davis, Philadelphia, 2015.
36. Melnick, ME: Basal ganglia disorders. In Umphred, DA, et al (eds): Umphred's Neurological Rehabilitation, ed 6. Elsevier, St. Louis, 2013, p. 601.
37. Wichmann, T, and DeLong, MR: The basal ganglia. In Kandel, ER, et al (eds): Principles of Neural Science, ed 5. McGraw-Hill, New York, 2013, p. 982.
38. Younger, DS: Correlative neuroanatomy. In Younger, DS (ed): Motor Disorders, ed 3. Rothstein Publishing, Brookfield, CT, 2015, p 3.
39. Morton, SM, and Bastian, AJ: Movement dysfunction associated with cerebellar damage. In Umphred, DA, et al (eds): Umphred's Neurological Rehabilitation, ed 6. Elsevier, St. Louis, 2013, p. 631.
40. Marsden, J, and Harris, C: Cerebellar ataxia: Pathophysiology and rehabilitation. Clin Rehabil 25:195, 2011.
41. Mattson Porth, C: Essentials of Pathophysiology, ed 4. Wolters Kluwer, Philadelphia, 2015.
42. Grimaldi, G: Deficits of limb movements. In Gruol, DL, et al (eds): Essentials of Cerebellum and Cerebellar Disorders: A Primer for Graduate Students. Springer International, Switzerland, 2016, p. 481.

43. Perlman, SL: Cerebellar ataxia. Curr Treat Options Neurol 2(3):215, 2000.
44. Silveri, MC: Speech deficits. In Gruol, DL, et al (eds): Essentials of Cerebellum and Cerebellar Disorders: A Primer for Graduate Students. Springer International, Switzerland, 2016, p. 477.
45. Waxman, SG: Clinical Neuroanatomy, ed 27. McGraw-Hill, New York, 2013.
46. Gutman, SA: Quick Reference Neuroscience for Rehabilitation Professionals: The Essential Neurologic Principles Underlying Rehabilitation Practice, ed 3. Slack, NJ, 2017.
47. Fuller, KS: Introduction to central nervous system disorders. In Goodman, CC, and Fuller, KS (eds): Pathology: Implications for the Physical Therapist, ed 4. Elsevier, St Louis, MO, 2015, p. 1371.
48. Ma, TP: The basal nuclei. In Haines, DE (ed): Fundamental Neuroscience for Basic and Clinical Applications, ed 4. Elsevier, Philadelphia, 2013, p. 354.
49. Palacio, R: The body language of movement disorders. In Fernandez, HH, Machado, AG, and Pandya, M (eds): A Practical Approach to Movement Disorders: Diagnosis and Management, ed 2. Demos Medical, New York, 2015, p. 3.
50. Kiernan, JA, and Rajakumar, N: Barr's The Human Nervous System: An Anatomical Viewpoint, ed 10. Wolters Kluwer, Philadelphia, 2014.
51. Fuller, KS, Demarch, E, and Winkler, PA: Degenerative diseases of the central nervous system. In Goodman, CC, and Fuller, KS (eds): Pathology: Implications for the Physical Therapist, ed 4. Elsevier, St Louis, MO, 2015, p. 1455.
52. Ahmed, A: Tremors. In Fernandez, HH, Machado, AG, and Pandya, M (eds): A Practical Approach to Movement Disorders: Diagnosis and Management, ed 2. Demos Medical, New York, 2015, p. 27.
53. Kiyama, S, et al: Distant functional connectivity for bimanual finger coordination declines with aging: An fMRI and SEM exploration. Front Hum Neurosci 8(Apr 25):251, 2014.
54. Loehrer, PA, et al: Ageing changes effective connectivity of motor networks during bimanual finger coordination. NeuroImage 143(Dec):325, 2016.
55. Lin, C: Influence of aging on bimanual coordination control. Exp Gerontol 53(May):40, 2014.
56. Ruitenbeek, P, et al: Cortical grey matter content is associated with both age and bimanual performance, but is not observed to mediate age-related behavioural decline. Brain Struct Funct 222(1):437, 2017.
57. Shetty, K, Vinutha Shankar, MS, and Annamalai, N: Bimanual coordination: Influence of age and gender. J Clin Diagn Res 8(2):15, 2014.
58. Fujiyama, H, et al: Age-related changes in frontal network structural and functional connectivity in relation to bimanual movement control. J Neurosci 36(6):1808, 2016.
59. Maike, H, et al: Switching between hands in a serial reaction time task: A comparison between young and old adults. Front Aging Neurosci 7(Sep):176, 2015.
60. Roberts, H, et al: Grip strength and its determinants among older people in different healthcare settings. Age Aging 43(2):241, 2014.
61. Schrack, JA: The role of energetic cost in the age-related slowing of gait speed. J Am Geriatr Soc 60(10):1811, 2012.
62. Yorke, AM, et al: Grip strength values stratified by age, gender, and chronic disease status in adults aged 50 years and older. J Geriatr Phys Ther 38(3):115, 2015.
63. Demura, T, et al: Examination of factors affecting gait properties in healthy older adults: Focusing on knee extension strength, visual acuity, and knee joint pain. J Geriatr Phys Ther 37(2):52, 2014.
64. Ihira, H, et al: Age-related differences in postural control and attentional cost during tasks performed in a one-legged standing posture. J Geriatr Phys Ther 39(4):159, 2016.
65. Studenski, SA, et al: The FNIH Sarcopenia Project: Rationale, study description, conference recommendations, and final estimates. J Gerontol A Biol Sci Med Sci 69(5):547, 2014.
66. McLean, RR, and Kiel, DP: Developing consensus criteria for sarcopenia: An update. J Bone Miner Res 30(4):588, 2015.
67. Correa-de-Araujo, R, and Hadley, E: Skeletal muscle function deficit: A new terminology to embrace the evolving concepts of sarcopenia and age-related muscle dysfunction. J Gerontol A Biol Sci Med Sci 69(5):591, 2014.
68. McLean, RR, et al: Criteria for clinically relevant weakness and low lean mass and their longitudinal association with incident mobility impairment and mortality: The Foundation for the National Institutes of Health (FNIH) Sarcopenia Project. J Gerontol A Biol Sci Med Sci 69(5):576, 2014.
69. Guccione, AA, Wong, RA, and Avers, D: Geriatric Physical Therapy, ed 3. Elsevier/Mosby, St. Louis, 2012.
70. Saxon, SV, Etten, MJ, and Perkins, EA: Physical Change and Aging: A Guide for the Helping Professions, ed 6. Springer, New York, 2015.
71. Robnett, RH, and Chop, W (eds): Gerontology for the Health Care Professional. Jones and Bartlett, Burlington, MA, 2015.
72. Anderson, DE, and Madigan, ML: Healthy older adults have insufficient hip range of motion and plantar flexor strength to walk like healthy young adults. J Biomech 47(5):1104, 2014.
73. Verdijk, LB, et al: Characteristics of muscle fiber type are predictive of skeletal muscle mass and strength in elderly men. JAGS 58(11):2069, 2010.
74. King, GW, et al: Effects of age and localized muscle fatigue on ankle plantar flexor torque development. J Geriatr Phys Ther 35(1):8, 2012.
75. Forstmann, BU, et al: The speed-accuracy tradeoff in the elderly brain: A structural model-based approach. J Neurosci 31(47):17242, 2011.
76. Fraser, SA, Li, KZ, and Penhune, VB: Dual-task performance reveals increased involvement of executive control in fine motor sequencing in healthy aging. J Gerontol B Psychol Sci Soc Sci 65(5):526, 2010.
77. Kumar, S, et al: Normal range of motion of hip and ankle in Indian population. Acta Orthop Traumatol Turc 45(6):421, 2011.
78. Soucie, JM, et al: Range of motion measurements: Reference values and a database for comparison studies. Haemophilia 17(3):500, 2011.
79. James, B, and Parker, AW: Active and passive mobility of lower limb joints in elderly men and women. Am J Phys Med Rehabil 68(4):162, 1989.
80. Kouzak, M, and Masani, K: Postural sway during quiet standing is related to physiological tremor and muscle volume in young and elderly adults. Gait Posture 35(1):11, 2012.
81. Kouzaki, M, and Shinohara, M: Steadiness in plantar flexor muscles and its relation to postural sway in young and elderly adults. Muscle Nerve 42(1):78, 2010.
82. Vandervoort, AA: Aging of the human neuromuscular system. Muscle Nerve 25(1):17, 2002.
83. Colby, SL, and Ortman, JM: The Baby Boom Cohort in the United States: 2012 to 2060. U.S. Department of Commerce, Economics and Statistics Administration, U.S. Census Bureau, 2014. Retrieved January 23, 2017 from www.census.gov/prod/2014pubs/p25-1141.pdf.
84. Hermana, T, Giladia, N, and Hausdorffa, JM: Properties of the "Timed Up and Go" Test: More than meets the eye. Gerontology 57(3):203, 2011.
85. Yuksel, E, et al: Assessing minimal detectable changes and test-retest reliability of the Timed Up and Go Test and the 2-Minute Walk Test in patients with total knee arthroplasty. J Arthroplasty 32(2):426, 2017.
86. Canny, ML, et al: Reliability of the box and block test of manual dexterity for use with patients with fibromyalgia. Am J Occup Ther 63(4):506, 2009.
87. Chen, HM, et al: Test-retest reproducibility and smallest real difference of 5 hand function tests in patients with stroke. Neurorehabil Neural Repair 23(5):435, 2009.
88. Desrosiers, J, et al: Validation of the Box and Block Test as a measure of dexterity of elderly people: Reliability, validity, and norms studies. Arch Phys Med Rehabil 75:751, 1994.
89. Goodkin, DE, et al: Comparing the ability of various compositive outcomes to discriminate treatment effects in MS clinical trials. The Multiple Sclerosis Collaborative Research Group (MSCRG). Mult Scler 4(6):480, 1998.
90. Mathiowetz, V, et al: Adult norms for the Box and Block Test of manual dexterity. Am J Occup Ther 39(6):386, 1985.
91. Paltamaa, J, et al: Measuring deterioration in international classification of functioning domains of people with multiple sclerosis who are ambulatory. Phys Ther 88(2):176, 2008.

92. Platz, T, et al: Reliability and validity of arm function assessment with standardized guidelines for the Fugl-Meyer Test, Action Research Arm Test and Box and Block Test: A multicentre study. Clin Rehabil 19(4):404, 2005.
93. Siebers, A, et al: The effect of modified constraint-induced movement therapy on spasticity and motor function of the affected arm in patients with chronic stroke. Physiother Can 62(4):388, 2010.
94. Fritz, SL, et al: Minimal detectable change scores for the Wolf Motor Function Test. Neurorehabil Neural Repair 23:662, 2009.
95. Lin, K, et al: Minimal detectable change and clinically important difference of the Wolf Motor Function Test in stroke patients. Neurorehab Neural Repair 23:429, 2009.
96. Morris, DM, et al: The reliability of the Wolf Motor Function Test for assessing upper extremity function after stroke. Arch Phys Med Rehabil 82:750, 2001.
97. Nijland, R, et al: A comparison of two validated tests for upper limb function after stroke: The Wolf Motor Function Test and the Action Research Arm Test. J Rehabil Med 42(7):694, 2010.
98. Wolf, SL, et al: Pilot normative database for the Wolf Motor Function Test. Arch Phys Med Rehabil 87(3):443, 2006.
99. Wolf, SL, et al: Assessing Wolf Motor Function Test as outcome measure for research in patients after stroke. Stroke 32:1635, 2001.
100. Beebe, JA, and Lang, CE: Relationships and responsiveness of six upper extremity function tests during the first six months of recovery after stroke. JNPT 33(2):96, 2009.
101. Lang, C, et al: Estimating minimal clinically important differences of upper extremity measures early after stroke. Arch Phys Med Rehabil 89(9):1693, 2008.
102. Lin, JH, et al: Psychometric comparisons of 4 measures for assessing upper-extremity function in people with stroke. Phys Ther 89:840, 2009.
103. van der Lee, JH, et al: The responsiveness of the Action Research Arm Test and the Fugl-Meyer Assessment scale in chronic stroke patients. J Rehabil Med 33(3):110, 2001.
104. van der Lee, JH, et al: The intra- and interrater reliability of the Action Research Arm Test: A practical test of upper extremity function in patients with stroke. Arch Phys Med Rehabil 82(1):14, 2001.
105. van der Lee, JH, et al: Improving the Action Research Arm Test: A unidimensional hierarchical scale. Clin Rehabil 16(6):646, 2002.
106. Earhart, G, et al: The 9-Hole Peg Test of upper extremity function: Average values, test-retest reliability, and factors contributing to performance in people with Parkinson disease. JNPT 35(4):157, 2011.
107. Oxford Grice, K, et al. (2003). Adult norms for a commercially available Nine Hole Peg Test for finger dexterity. Am J Occup Ther 57(5):570, 2003.
108. Wang, Y, et al: Assessing dexterity function: A comparison of two alternatives for the NIH toolbox. J Hand Ther (4):313, 2011.
109. Sollerman, C, and Ejeskar, A: Sollerman hand function test: A standardised method and its use in tetraplegic patients. Scand J Plast Reconstr Surg Hand Surg 29(2):167, 1995.
110. Weng, LY, et al: Excellent reliability of the Sollerman hand function test for patients with burned hands. J Burn Care Res 31(6):904, 2010.
111. Singh, HP, Diaz, JJ, and Thompson, JR: Timed Sollerman Hand Function Test for analysis of hand function in normal volunteers. J Hand Surg Eur Vol 40(3):298, 2015.
112. Mak, MK, et al: Use of Jebsen Taylor Hand Function Test in evaluating the hand dexterity in people with Parkinson's disease. J Hand Ther 28(4):389, 2015.
113. Davis Sears, E, and Chung, KC: Validity and responsiveness of the Jebsen-Taylor Hand Function Test. J Hand Surg Am 35(1):30, 2010.
114. Asher, IE (ed): Asher's Occupational Therapy Assessment Tools: An Annotated Index, ed 4. American Occupational Therapy Association, Bethesda, MD, 2014.
115. Tesio, L, et al: Bimanual dexterity assessment: Validation of a revised form of the turning subtest from the Minnesota Dexterity Test. Int J Rehabil Res 39(1):57, 2016.
116. Lourenção MIP, et al: Analysis of the results of functional electrical stimulation on hemiplegic patients' upper extremities using the Minnesota manual dexterity test. Int J Rehabil Res 28(1):25, 2005.
117. Surrey, LR, et al: A comparison of performance outcomes between the Minnesota Rate of Manipulation Test and the Minnesota Manual Dexterity Test. Work 20(2):97, 2003.
118. Muller, MD, et al: Test-retest reliability of Purdue Pegboard performance in thermoneutral and cold ambient conditions. Ergonomics 54(11):1081, 2011.
119. Shin, S, Demura, S, and Aoki, H: Effects of prior use of chopsticks on two different types of dexterity tests: Moving Beans Test and Purdue Pegboard. Percept Motor Skills 108(2):392, 2009.
120. Darweesh, SK, et al: Simple test of manual dexterity can help to identify persons at high risk for neurodegenerative diseases in the community. J Gerontol A Biol Sci Med Sci 72(1):75, 2017.
121. Rodriguez-Aranda, C, Mittner, M, and Vasylenko, O: Association between executive functions, working memory, and manual dexterity in young and healthy older adults: An exploratory study. Percept Mot Skills 122(1):165, 2016.
122. Levangie, P, and Norkin, C: Joint Structure and Function: A Comprehensive Analysis, ed 5. FA Davis, Philadelphia, 2011.
123. Nashner, L: Sensory, neuromuscular, and biomechanical contributions to human balance. In Duncan, P (ed): Balance. American Physical Therapy Association, Alexandria, VA, 1990, p. 5.
124. Pai, Y, et al: Thresholds for step initiation induced by support-surface translation: A dynamic center-of-mass model provides much better prediction than a static model. J Biomech 33:387, 2000.
125. Nichols, D: Balance retraining after stroke using force platform biofeedback. Phys Ther 77:553, 1997.
126. Horak, F: Clinical measurement of postural control in adults. Phys Ther 67:1881, 1987.
127. Goldie, P, et al: Force platform measures for evaluating postural control: Reliability and validity. Arch Phys Med Rehabil 70:510, 1989.
128. Liston, R, and Brouwer, B: Reliability and validity of measures obtained from stroke patients using the Balance Master. Arch Phys Med Rehabil 77:425, 1996.
129. Horak, F, et al: Postural perturbations: New insights for treatment of balance disorders. Phys Ther 77:517, 1997.
130. Dettman, M, et al: Relationships among walking performance, postural stability, and functional assessments of the hemiplegic patient. Am J Phys Med 66:77, 1987.
131. De Haart, M, et al: Recovery of standing balance in postacute stroke patients: A rehabilitation cohort study. Arch Phys Med Rehabil 85:886, 2004.
132. Geurts, A, et al: A review of standing balance recovery from stroke. Gait Posture 22:267, 2005.
133. Dickstein, R, et al: Foot-ground pressure pattern of standing hemiplegic patients: Major characteristics and patterns of movement. Phys Ther 64:19, 1984.
134. Lee, DN, and Lishman, JR: Visual proprioceptive control of stance. J Hum Mov Stud 1:87, 1975.
135. Brandt, T, et al: Visual acuity, visual field and visual scene characteristics affect postural balance. In Igarash, M, and Black, F (eds): Vestibular and Visual Control on Posture and Locomotor Equilibrium, Karger, Basel, 1985.
136. Jeka, J: Light touch contact as a balance aid. Phys Ther 77:249, 1997.
137. Herdman, S: Vestibular Rehabilitation, ed 4. FA Davis, Philadelphia, 2014.
138. Nashner, L: Adaptive reflexes controlling human posture. Exp Brain Res 26:59, 1976.
139. Nashner, L, and McCollum, G: The organization of human postural movements: A formal basis and experimental synthesis. Behav Brain Sci 9:135, 1985.
140. Kuo, A, et al: Effect of altered sensory conditions on multivariate descriptors of human postural sway. Exp Brain Res 122:15, 1998.
141. Peterka, R: Sensorimotor integration in human postural control. J Neurophysiol 88:1097, 2002.
142. Horak, F, Earhart, G, and Dietz, V: Postural responses to combinations of head and body displacements: Vestibular and somatosensory interactions. Exp Brain Res 141:410, 2001.
143. Horak, F, et al: Postural strategies associated with somatosensory and vestibular loss. Exp Brain Res 82:167, 1990.
144. Romberg, M: Manual of Nervous Diseases of Man. London, Sydenham Society, 1853.

145. Shumway-Cook, A, and Horak, F: Assessing the influence of sensory interaction on balance: Suggestion from the field. Phys Ther 66:1548, 1986.
146. Cohen, H, et al: A study of the clinical test of sensory interaction and balance. Phys Ther 73(6):346, 1993.
147. Whitney, SL, and Wrisley, DM: The influence of footwear on timed balance scores of the modified clinical test of sensory interaction and balance. Arch Phys Med Rehabil 85:439, 2004.
148. Ricci, NA, et al: Sensory interaction on static balance: a comparison concerning the history of falls of community-dwelling elderly. Geriatr Gerontol Int 9(2):165, 2009.
149. Boulgarides, LK, et al: Use of clinical and impairment-based tests to predict falls by community-dwelling older adults. Phys Ther 83(4):328, 2003.
150. Liston, RA, and Brouwer, BJ: Reliability and validity of measures obtained from stroke patients using the Balance Master. Arch Phys Med Rehabil 77(5):425, 1996.
151. Bernhardt, J, et al: Changes in balance and locomotion measures during rehabilitation following stroke. Physiother Res Int 3(2):109, 1998.
152. Chong, RK, et al: Sensory organization for balance: specific deficits in Alzheimer's but not in Parkinson's disease. J Gerontol Series A: Biolog Sci and Med Sci 54(3):M122, 1999.
153. Colnat-Coulbois, S, et al: Management of postural sensory conflict and dynamic balance control in late-stage Parkinson's disease. Neurosci 193:363, 2011.
154. Frenklach, A, et al: Excessive postural sway and the risk of falls at different stages of Parkinson's disease. Mov Disord 24(3):377, 2009.
155. Basta, D, et al: Stance performance under different sensorimotor conditions in patients with post-traumatic otolith disorders. J Vestib Res 17(1):25, 2007.
156. Cohen, HS, and Kimball, KT: Usefulness of some current balance tests for identifying individuals with disequilibrium due to vestibular impairments. J Vestib Res 18(5):295, 2008.
157. Pedalini, ME, et al: Sensory organization test in elderly patients with and without vestibular dysfunction. Acta Otolaryngol 129(9):962, 2009.
158. Kaufman, KR, et al: Comparison of subjective and objective measurements of balance disorders following traumatic brain injury. Med Eng Phys 28(3):234, 2006.
159. Horak, F, and Nashner, L: Central programming of postural movements: Adaptation to altered support-surface configuration. J Neurophysiol 55:1369, 1986.
160. Nashner, L: Fixed patterns of rapid postural responses among leg muscles during stance. Exp Brain Res 30:13, 1977.
161. Maki, B, and McIlron, W: The role of limb movements in maintaining upright stance: The "change-in-support" strategy. Phys Ther 77:488, 1977.
162. Brown, L, Shumway-Cook, A, and Woollacott, M: Attentional demands and postural recovery: The effects of aging. J Gerontol 54A:M165–M171, 1999.
163. Creath, R, et al: A unified view of quiet and perturbed stance: Simultaneous co-existing excitable modes. Neurosci Lett 377:75, 2005.
164. Dean, C, and Shepherd, R: Task-related training improves performance of seated reaching tasks following stroke: A randomized controlled trial. Stroke 28:722, 1997.
165. Forssberg, H, and Hirschfeld, H: Postural adjustments in sitting humans following external perturbations: Muscle activity and kinematics. Exp Brain Res 97:515, 1994.
166. Horak, F, et al: The effects of movement velocity, mass displaced and task certainty on associated postural adjustments made by normal and hemiplegic individuals. J Neurol Neurosurg Psychiatry 47:1020, 1984.
167. Slijper, H, et al: Task-specific modulation of anticipatory postural adjustments in individuals with hemiparesis. Clin Neurophysiol 113:642, 2002.
168. Latash, M, et al: Anticipatory postural adjustments during self-inflicted and predictable perturbations in Parkinson's disease. J Neurol Neurosurg Psychiatry 58:326, 1995.
169. Arce, F, Katz, N, and Sugarman, H: The scaling of postural adjustments during bimanual load-lifting in traumatic brain-injured adults. Hum Move Sci 22:749, 2004.
170. Morris, M, et al: Postural instability in Parkinson's disease: A comparison with and without a concurrent task. Gait Posture 12:205, 2000.
171. Ashburn, A, and Stack, E: Fallers and non-fallers with Parkinson's disease (PD): The influence of a dual task on standing balance. Mov Disord 15(Suppl 3):78, 2000.
172. Brauer, S, et al: Simplest tasks have greatest dual task interference with balance in brain injured adults. Hum Move Sci 23:489, 2004.
173. Hyndman, D, and Ashburn, A: "Stops Walking When Talking" as a predictor of falls in people with stroke living in the community. J Neurol Neurosurg Psychiatry 75:994, 2004.
174. Berg, K, et al: Measuring balance in the elderly: Preliminary development of an instrument. Physiother Can 41:304, 1989.
175. Tinetti, M, et al: A fall risk index for elderly patients based on number of chronic disabilities. Am J Med 80:429, 1986.
176. Berg, K, et al: A comparison of clinical and laboratory measures of postural balance in an elderly population. Arch Phys Med Rehabil 73:1073, 1992.
177. Berg, K, et al: Measuring balance in the elderly: Validation of an instrument. Can J Public Health 83(Suppl 2):S7, 1992.
178. Berg, K, et al: The Balance Scale: Reliability assessment for elderly residents and patients with an acute stroke. Scand J Rehabil Med 27:27, 1995.
179. Thorbahn, L, and Newton, R: Use of the Berg Balance Test to predict falls in elderly persons. Phys Ther 76:576, 1996.
180. Blum, L, and Korner-Bitensky, N: Usefulness of the Berg Balance Scale in stroke rehabilitation: A systematic review. Phys Ther 88:559, 2008.
181. Muir, SW, et al: Use of the Berg Balance Scale for predicting multiple falls in community-dwelling elderly people: A prospective study. Phys Ther 88:449, 2008.
182. Shumway-Cook, A, et al: Predicting the probability of falls in community dwelling older adults. Phys Ther 77:812, 1997.
183. Alzayer, L, Beninato, M, and Portney, L: The accuracy of individual Berg Balance Scale items compared with the total Berg score for classifying people with chronic stroke according to fall history. JNPT 33:136, 2009.
184. Donoghue, D, and Stokes, E: How much change is true change? The minimum detectable change of the Berg Balance Scale in elderly people. J Rehabil Med 41:343, 2009.
185. Stevenson, TJ: Detecting change in patients with stroke using the Berg Balance Scale. Aust J Physiother 47(1):29, 2001.
186. Hiengkaew, V, et al: Minimal detectable changes of the Berg Balance Scale, Fugl-Meyer Assessment Scale, Timed "Up & Go" Test, gait speeds, and 2-minute walk test in individuals with chronic stroke with different degrees of ankle plantarflexor tone. Arch Phys Med Rehabil 93(7):1201, 2012.
187. Steffen, TM, et al: Age- and gender-related test performance in community-dwelling elderly people: Six-Minute Walk Test, Berg Balance Scale, Timed Up & Go Test, and gait speeds. Phys Ther 82(2):128, 2002.
188. Tinetti, M, and Ginter, S: Identifying mobility dysfunctions in elderly patients: Standard neuromuscular examination or direct assessment? JAMA 259:1190, 1988.
189. Cipriany-Dacko, L, et al: Interrater reliability of the Tinetti Balance Scores in novice and experienced physical therapy clinicians. Arch Phys Med and Rehabil 78(10):1160, 1997.
190. Faber, MJ, Bosscher, RJ, and van Wieringen, PC: Clinimetric properties of the Performance-Oriented Mobility Assessment. Phys Ther 86(7):944, 2006.
191. Canbek, J, et al: Test-retest reliability and construct validity of the Tinetti Performance-Oriented Mobility Assessment in people with stroke. JNPT, 37(1):14, 2013.
192. Behrman, AL, et al: Sensitivity of the Tinetti Gait Assessment for detecting change in individuals with Parkinson's disease. Clin Rehabil 16(4):399, 2002.
193. Kegelmeyer, DA, et al: Reliability and validity of the Tinetti Mobility Test for individuals with Parkinson disease. Phys Ther 87(10):1369, 2007.
194. Kloos, AD, et al: Interrater and intrarater reliability of the Tinetti Balance Test for individuals with amyotrophic lateral sclerosis. JNPT 28(1):12, 2004.
195. Tinetti, M, et al: Risk factors for falls among elderly persons living in the community. N Engl J Med 319:1701, 1993.
196. Duncan, P, et al: Functional reach: A new clinical measure of balance. J Gerontol 45:M192, 1990.
197. Duncan, P, et al: Functional reach: Predictive validity in a sample of elderly male veterans. J Gerontol 47:M93, 1992.

198. Weiner, D, et al: Functional reach: A marker of physical frailty. J Am Geriatr Soc 40:203, 1992.
199. Schenkman, M, et al: Reliability of impairment and physical performance measures for persons with Parkinson's disease. Phys Ther 77(1):19, 1997.
200. Smithson, F, et al: Performance on clinical tests of balance in Parkinson's disease. Phys Ther 78(6):577, 1998.
201. Steffen, T, and Seney, M: Test-retest reliability and minimal detectable change on balance and ambulation tests, the 36-item short-form health survey, and the unified Parkinson disease rating scale in people with parkinsonism. Phys Ther 88(6):733, 2008.
202. Newton, R: Validity of the multi-directional reach test: A practical measure for limits of stability in older adults. J Gerontol Med Sci 56A:M248, 2001.
203. Katz-Leurer, M, et al: Reliability and validity of the modified functional reach test at the sub-acute stage post-stroke. Disabil Rehabil 31(3):243, 2009.
204. Lynch, S, Leahy, P, and Barker, S: Reliability of measurements obtained with a modified functional reach test in subjects with spinal cord injury. Phys Ther 78:1128, 1998.
205. Thompson, M, and Medley, A: Forward and lateral sitting functional reach in younger, middle-aged, and older adults. J Geriatr Phys Ther 30(2):43, 2007.
206. Mathias, S, et al: Balance in elderly patients: The "Get Up and Go" test. Arch Phys Med Rehabil 67:387, 1986.
207. Podsiadlo, D, and Richardson, S: The timed "Up and Go": A test of basic mobility for frail elderly persons. J Am Geriatr Soc 39:142, 1991.
208. Isles, R, et al: Normal values of balance tests in women aged 20–80. J Am Geriatr Soc 52:1367, 2004.
209. Pondal, M, and del Ser, T: Normative data and determinants for the timed "Up and Go" test in a population-based sample of elderly individuals without gait disturbances. J Geriatr Phys Ther 31(2):7, 2008.
210. Faria, C, Teixeira-Salmela, L, and Nadeau, S: Effects of the direction of turning on the timed Up and Go test with stroke patients. Top Stroke Rehabil 16:196, 2009.
211. Ng, S, and Hui-Chan, C: The timed Up and Go test: Its reliability and association with lower-limb impairments and locomotor capacities in people with chronic stroke. Arch Phys Med Rehabil 86:1641, 2005.
212. Campbell, C, et al: The effect of attentional demands on the timed Up and Go test in older adults with and without Parkinson's disease. Neurol Rep 3:2, 2003.
213. Dibble, L, and Lange, M: Predicting falls in individuals with Parkinson's disease: A reconsideration of clinical balance measures. JNPT 30:60, 2006.
214. Haug, SL, et al: Minimal detectable change of the timed "up and go" test and the dynamic gait index in people with Parkinson disease. Phys Ther 91(1):114, 2010.
215. Shumway-Cook, A, et al: Predicting the probability for falls in community-dwelling older adults using the Timed Up & Go Test. Phys Ther 80(9):896, 2000.
216. Horak, FB, et al: The Balance Evaluation Systems Test (BESTest) to differentiate balance deficits. PhysTher 89(5):484, 2009.
217. Leddy, AL, et al: Functional gait assessment and balance evaluation system test: Reliability, validity, sensitivity, and specificity for identifying individuals with Parkinson disease who fall. Phys Ther 91(1):102, 2011.
218. Leddy, AL, et al: Utility of the Mini-BESTest, BESTest, and BESTest sections for balance assessments in individuals with Parkinson disease. JNPT 35(2):90, 2011.
219. Duncan, RP, et al: Comparative utility of the BESTest, Mini-BESTest, and Brief-BESTest for predicting falls in individuals with Parkinson disease: a cohort study. Phys Ther 93(4):542, 2013.
220. Chinsongkram, B, et. al: Reliability and validity of the Balance Evaluation Systems Test (BESTest) in people with subacute stroke. Phys Ther 94(11):1632, 2014.
221. Franchignoni, F, et al: Using psychometric techniques to improve the Balance Evaluation System's Test: The mini-BESTest. J Rehabil Med 42(4):323, 2010.
222. Hall, CD, and Herdman, SJ: Reliability of clinical measures used to assess patient with peripheral vestibular disorders. JNPT 30:74, 2006.
223. Wrisley, DM, et al: Reliability of the Dynamic Gait Index in people with vestibular disorders. Arch Phys Med Rehabil 84:1528, 2003.
224. Jonsdottir, J, and Cattaneo, D: Reliability and validity of the Dynamic Gait Index in persons with chronic stroke. Arch Phys Med Rehabil 88:1410, 2007.
225. McConvey, J, and Bennett, SE: Reliability of the Dynamic Gait Index in individuals with multiple sclerosis. Arch Phys Med Rehabil 86:130, 2005.
226. Romero, S, et al: Minimum detectable change of the Berg Balance Scale and Dynamic Gait Index in older persons at risk for falling. J Geriatric Phys Ther 34(3):131, 2011.
227. Pardasaney, PK, et al: Sensitivity to change and responsiveness of four balance measures for community-dwelling older adults. Phys Ther 92(3):388, 2012.
228. Lin, JH, et al: Psychometric comparisons of 3 functional ambulation measures for patients with stroke. Stroke 41(9):2021, 2010.
229. Cattaneo, D, et al: Reliability of four scales on balance disorders in persons with multiple sclerosis. Disabil Rehabil 29(24):1920, 2007.
230. Huang, SL, et al: Minimal detectable change of the timed "up & go" test and the dynamic gait index in people with Parkinson disease. Phys Ther 91(1):114, 2011.
231. Verghese, J, et al: Validity of divided attention tasks in predicting falls in older individuals: A preliminary study. J Am Geriatr Soc 50(9):1572, 2002.
232. Verghese, J, et al: Mobility stress test approach to predicting frailty, disability, and mortality in high-functioning older adults. J Am Geriatr Soc 60(10):1901, 2012.
233. Bowen, A, et al: Dual-task effects of talking while walking on velocity and balance following a stroke. Age Ageing 30:319, 2001.
234. Pohl, PS, et al: Older adults with and without stroke reduce cadence to meet the demands of talking. J Geriatr Phys Ther 34(1):35, 2011.
235. Park, NW, Moscovitch, M, and Robertson, IH: Divided attention impairments after traumatic brain injury. Neuropsychologia 37:1119, 1999.
236. McCulloch, K: Attention and dual-task conditions: Physical therapy implications for individuals with acquired brain injury. JNPT 31:104, 2007.
237. Penner, I, et al: Analysis of impairment related functional architecture in MS patients during performance of different attention tasks. J Neurol 250:461, 2003.
238. Rochester, L, et al: Attending to the task: Interference effects of functional tasks on walking in Parkinson's disease and the roles of cognition, depression, fatigue and balance. Arch Phys Med Rehabil 85:1578, 2004.
239. Camicioli, R, et al: Verbal fluency task affects gait in Parkinson's disease with motor freezing. J Geriatric Psych Neurol 11(4):181, 1997.
240. O'Shea, S, et al: Dual task interference during gait in people with Parkinson disease: Effects of motor versus cognitive secondary tasks. Phys Ther 82(9):888, 2002.
241. LaPointe, L, et al: Talking while walking: Cognitive loading and injurious falls in Parkinson's disease. Int J Speech Lang Pathol 12(5):455, 2010.
242. Verghese, J, et al: Walking while talking: Effect of task prioritization in the elderly. Arch Phys Med Rehabil 88(1):50, 2007.
243. Deshpande, N, et al: Gait speed under varied challenges and cognitive decline in older persons: A prospective study. Age Ageing 38(5):509, 2009.
244. Hall, CD, et al: Cognitive and motor mechanisms underlying older adults' ability to divide attention while walking. Phys Ther 91(7):1039, 2011.
245. Brandler, TC, et al: Walking while talking: Investigation of alternate forms. Gait Posture 35(1):164, 2012.
246. Lundin-Olsson, L, et al: "Stops walking when talking" as a predictor of falls in elderly people. Lancet 349:617, 1997.
247. de Hoon, EW, et al: Quantitative assessment of the stops walking while talking test in the elderly. Arch Phys Med Rehabil 84(6):838, 2003.
248. Gorman, S, et al: Development and validation of the Function in Sitting Test in adults with acute stroke. JNPT 34:150, 2010.
249. Gorman, SL, Rivera, M, and McCarthy, L: Reliability of the Function in Sitting Test (FIST). Rehabil Res Pract 2014:593280, 2014.

250. Gorman, SL, et al: Examining the function in sitting test for validity, responsiveness, and minimal clinically important difference in inpatient rehabilitation. Arch Phys Med Rehabil 95(12):2304, 2014.
251. Powell, L, and Meyers, A: The Activities-specific Balance Confidence (ABC) Scale. J Gerontol Med Sci 50A(1):M28–M34, 1995.
252. Powell, LE, and Myers, AM: The Activities-specific Balance Confidence (ABC) Scale. J Gerontol. Series A, Biological Sciences and Medical Sciences 50A(1):M28–34, 1995.
253. Botner, EM, et al: Measurement properties of the Activities-specific Balance Confidence Scale among individuals with stroke. Disab Rehabil 27(4):156, 2005.
254. Steffen, T, and Seney, M: Test-retest reliability and minimal detectable change on balance and ambulation tests, the 36-item short-form health survey, and the unified Parkinson disease rating scale in people with parkinsonism. Phys Ther 88(6):733, 2008.
255. Dal Bello-Haas, V, et al: Psychometric properties of activity, self-efficacy, and quality-of-life measures in individuals with Parkinson disease. Physiother Can 63(1):47, 2011.
256. Tinetti, M, Richman, D, and Powell, L: Falls efficacy as a measure of fear of falling. J Gerontol 45:P239–P243, 1990.
257. Hellstrom, K, and Lindmark, B: Fear of falling in patients with stroke: A reliability study. Clinic Rehabil 13(6):509, 1999.

Coordination Examination Form

appendix **6.A**

Patient Name:____________________ Examiner:____________________
Date: _______

Coordination Tests: Performed in Sitting and Supine

Key to Grading

4 Normal Performance
3 Minimal Impairment: Able to accomplish activity; slightly less than normal control, speed, and steadiness
2 Moderate Impairment: Able to accomplish activity; movements are slow, awkward, and unsteady
1 Severe impairment: Able only to initiate activity without completion; movements are slow with significant unsteadiness, oscillations, and/or extraneous movements
0 Activity Impossible

Notations should be made under comments section if:

- Lack of visual input renders activity impossible or alters quality of performance
- Verbal cuing is required to accomplish activity
- Alterations in speed affect quality of performance
- Excessive amount of time required to complete activity
- Changes in arm position alters sitting balance
- Postural instability is evident: unsteadiness, oscillations, extraneous movements
- Fatigue alters consistency of response
- Performance affects patient safety; requires contact guarding

LEFT	TEST	RIGHT	COMMENTS
	Finger-to-nose		
	Finger-to-therapist's finger		
	Finger-to-finger		
	Alternate nose-to-finger		
	Finger opposition		
	Mass grasp		
	Pronation/supination		
	Rebound phenomenon		
	Tapping (hand)		
	Tapping (foot)		
	Pointing and past-pointing		
	Alternate heel-to-knee; heel-to-toe		
	Toe-to-examiner's finger		
	Heel-on-shin		
	Drawing a circle (hand)		
	Drawing a circle (foot)		
	Fixation/position holding (UE)		
	Fixation/position holding (LE)		

Chapter 7

Examination of Gait

Judith M. Burnfield, PT, PhD
Guilherme M. Cesar, PhD
Cynthia C. Norkin, PT, EdD

LEARNING OBJECTIVES

1. Define the terms used to describe normal gait.
2. Describe the variables that are examined in each of the following types of gait analyses: kinematic qualitative analysis, kinematic quantitative analysis, and kinetic analysis.
3. Describe and provide examples of some of the most commonly used types of gait profiles.
4. Compare and contrast the advantages and disadvantages of kinematic qualitative and kinematic quantitative gait analyses.
5. Using the case study example, apply clinical decision making skills in evaluating gait analysis data.

CHAPTER OUTLINE

One of the major purposes of rehabilitation is to help patients achieve the highest level of function given their specific impairments so they can participate optimally in activities of interest. Human ambulation, or gait, is one of the basic components of independent function commonly affected by either disease or injury. Consequently, the desired outcome of many physical therapy interventions is to restore or improve a patient's ambulatory status. *Gait,* defined as the manner in which a person walks (e.g., cadence, step length, stride length, speed and rhythm) differs from *locomotion,* which refers to an individual's capacity to move from one place to another.[1] Although there are many specific reasons for performing a gait analysis, all of them require some information about the walking capacity of either an individual or a group of people with a particular disability. Because there are multiple approaches to gait analysis, ranging from very simple to extremely complex, the therapist must carefully consider how information obtained from a gait analysis is to be used. General as well as specific clinical indications for conducting a gait analysis may be found in the *Guide to Physical Therapist Practice 3.0,* some of which are included below.[1]

PURPOSES OF GAIT ANALYSIS

1. To assist with understanding the gait characteristics of a particular disorder. This includes the following:
   - Obtaining accurate descriptions of gait patterns and gait variables typical of different conditions
   - Identifying and describing gait deviations present, or typically present, in specific disorders
   - Determining balance, endurance, energy expenditure, and safety
   - Determining the functional ambulation capabilities of the patient in relation to functional ambulation demands of the home, community, and work environments
   - Classifying the severity of disability
   - Predicting a patient's future status
2. To assist with movement diagnosis by:
   - Identifying and describing gait deviations and describing the differences between a patient's performance and the parameters of normal gait
   - Analyzing gait deviations and identifying the mechanisms responsible for producing them
   - Examining balance, endurance, energy expenditure, and safety and determining their impact on gait

3. To inform selection of intervention(s) by guiding the therapist in:
   - Proposing appropriate treatment of impairments that may improve gait performance
   - Determining the need for adaptive, assistive, orthotic, prosthetic, protective, or supportive devices or equipment
4. To evaluate the effectiveness of treatment and guide the therapist in:
   - Determining how interventions such as therapeutic exercise, endurance activities, developmental activities, strengthening or stretching, electrical stimulation, balance training, surgical procedures, and medication will affect gait
   - Determining the effectiveness and fit of devices or equipment selected in providing joint protection and support, correcting deviations and dysfunctions, reducing energy expenditure, and promoting safe locomotive function

Many examples illustrating these purposes are found in the literature: descriptions of the differences between a patient's performance and the parameters of normal gait;[2-12] identification of the mechanisms causing dysfunction;[13,14] determination of either the need for, or the effectiveness of, a prosthetic device;[13,15] comparison of the effects of different types of assistive devices;[16,17] determination of either the need for, or the effectiveness of, an orthotic device;[18-22] determination of the effects of treatment interventions;[23-25] determination of energy expenditure;[15,16,26] and prediction of future status.[27-29]

SELECTION OF APPROACH TO GAIT ANALYSIS

The type of gait analysis that is selected depends on the purpose of the analysis, the type of equipment available, and the experience, knowledge, and skills of the therapist. The equipment necessary for performing a specific type of gait analysis, in turn, depends on the purpose of the analysis, equipment availability, and the amount of time the therapist can expend. Equipment used in a gait analysis may be either as simple as a pencil, paper, and stopwatch[30] or as complex as an electronic imaging system with force plates embedded in the floor and electromyography electrodes placed on the client.[31-34] To select the appropriate method, the therapist must be aware of the types of analyses available and be able to determine which methods are reliable and valid. Much of the information about gait characteristics of particular disorders, as well as the mechanisms responsible for producing them, has been achieved in clinical research settings using complex instrumentation often not available for general patient use. However, given a firm understanding of the biomechanics of normal gait, including characteristic joint motions and muscle demands, a therapist can use less complex methods to identify variations in movement patterns from normal and problem-solve likely causes. Efficacious treatment approaches can then be employed to address underlying causes.

Regardless of the method, a gait analysis of individual patients should provide reliable and valid data that can be used as a basis for describing present status (performance limitations and strengths), planning and implementing interventions, evaluating effectiveness and progress over time, evaluating outcomes, and in some instances, predicting future status.

GAIT TERMINOLOGY

The Gait Cycle

The fundamental unit of walking is the *gait cycle,* which has both spatial (distance) and temporal (time) parameters. In normal walking, a gait cycle begins when the heel of the reference extremity contacts the supporting surface and ends when the heel of the same extremity contacts the ground again. In some abnormal gaits, the heel may not be the first part of the foot to contact the ground, so the gait cycle may be considered to begin when some other portion of the reference limb contacts the ground. The cycle ends with the next ipsilateral contact of that same portion of the foot with the ground.

The gait cycle is divided into two periods, *stance* and *swing* (Fig. 7.1). In normal gait at a comfortable walking speed, *stance* constitutes approximately 60% of the gait cycle and is defined as the interval in which the reference foot is in contact with the ground. *Swing* comprises approximately 40% of the gait cycle and occurs when the reference limb is not in contact with the ground. A single gait cycle includes periods of stance and swing for both the right and left limbs. During gait, body weight is smoothly transferred from one limb to the next during two intervals of double limb stance in the gait cycle when both limbs are in contact with the ground at the same time. *Initial double limb stance* occurs at the beginning of the gait cycle as weight transfers onto the outstretched reference limb from the trailing limb. *Terminal double limb stance* occurs at the end of stance as body weight transfers from the trailing reference limb to the lead limb. Initial double limb stance on the reference limb corresponds with the contralateral limb's terminal double limb stance. *Single limb support,* arising between the two double limb stance periods, is the portion of the gait cycle where only one limb supports body weight. The duration of each of these variables may be measured; for example, *cycle time, stance time* (right and left), *swing time* (right and left), initial *double limb stance time, terminal double limb stance time,* and *single limb support time.*

Two steps, a right step and a left step, form a *stride,* and a stride is equal to a gait cycle. Step and stride may be defined in two dimensions: distance and time. *Step*

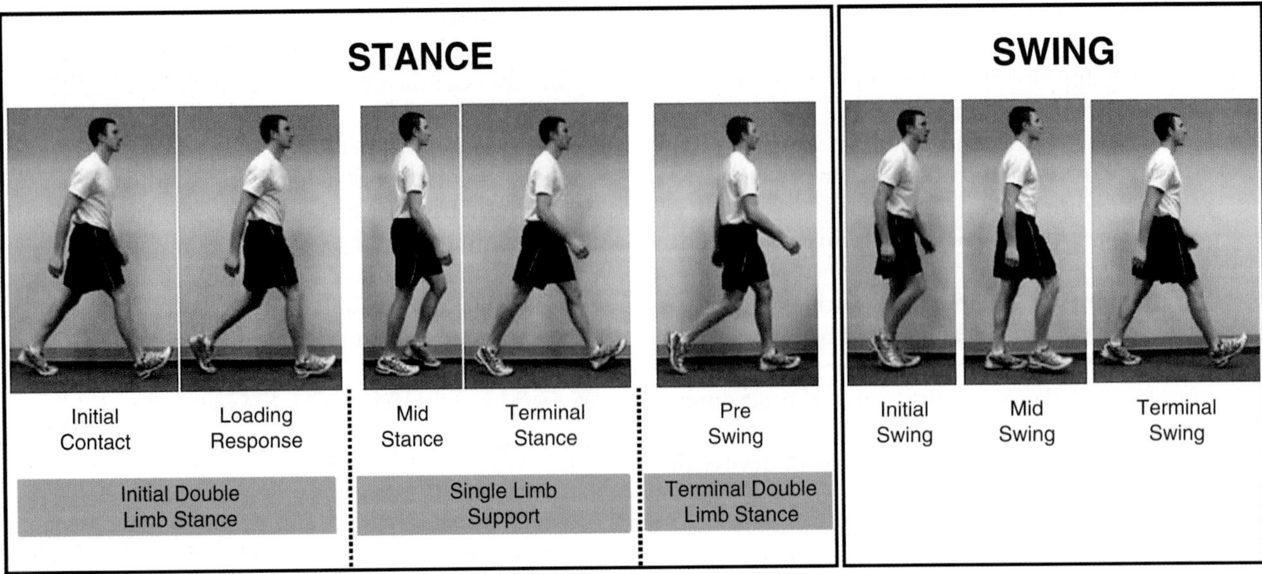

Figure 7.1 The eight phases of the gait cycle. Stance, the period when the reference limb is in contact with the ground, is comprised of the following five phases: initial contact, loading response, mid stance, terminal stance, and pre-swing. Swing, the period when the limb is off the ground, is comprised of the following three phases: initial swing, mid swing, and terminal swing. In addition, there are two periods in gait when both limbs are in contact with the ground: initial double limb stance (initial contact and loading response) and terminal double limb stance (pre-swing). Also, there is one period, single limb support, in which only one limb is in contact with the ground. Single limb support includes the phases of mid stance and terminal stance. Note that the contralateral limb is in swing during the reference limb's single limb support. *(Courtesy of Movement and Neurosciences Center, Institute for Rehabilitation Science and Engineering, Madonna Rehabilitation Hospitals, Lincoln, NE 68506).*

length is the distance from the point of heel strike of one extremity to the point of heel strike of the opposite extremity, whereas stride length is the distance from the point of heel strike of one extremity to the next point of heel strike of the same extremity. An alternative portion of the foot that consistently contacts the ground can be used as a reference point if the heel is not the first point of contact, as with some abnormal gait patterns. *Stride time* and *step time* refer to the length of time required to complete a step and a stride, respectively (Fig. 7.2).

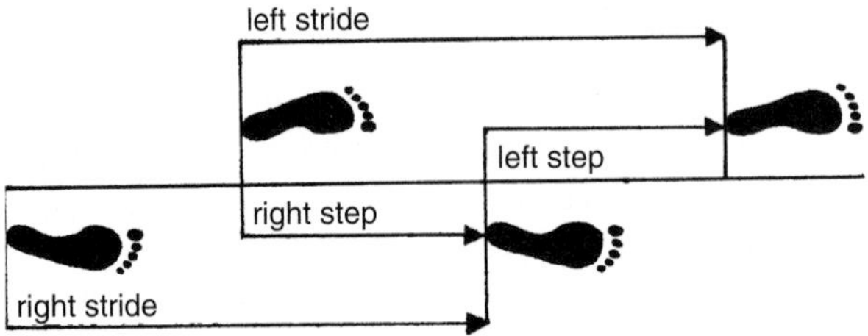

Figure 7.2 A right stride and a left stride. Right stride length is the distance between the point of contact of the right heel (at the lower left corner of the diagram) and the next contact of the right heel. Left stride length is the distance between the point of contact of the left heel (at the top left of the diagram) to the point of contact at the next left heel. Each stride contains two steps, but only both steps in the left stride are labeled. The left stride contains a right step and a left step. The right step length (shown in the middle of the diagram) is the distance between the left heel contact to the point of the right heel contact. Left step length is the distance between the right heel contact and the next left heel contact. Step and stride times refer to the amount of time required to complete a step and to complete stride, respectively.

Phases of Gait

Early terminology describing the phases of gait included descriptors for both stance (i.e., heel strike, footflat, midstance, heel-off, and toe off) and swing (i.e., acceleration, mid swing, and deceleration). Though useful for describing normal gait, the terminology is sometimes confusing in the presence of pathology. For example, many individuals with pretibial weakness or severe plantarflexion contractures lack a heel-first contact at "heel strike." Some individuals with plantarflexor spasticity maintain their heel off the ground throughout stance, not just during heel-off. Others with profound plantarflexor weakness may fail to achieve a period of heel-off and instead lift the full foot from the ground at the end of stance.

To avoid the confusions associated with earlier terminology, Perry and colleagues from Rancho Los Amigos National Rehabilitation Center developed a generic terminology to describe the eight functional phases of gait.[34,35] The first five phases constitute stance: initial contact, loading response, mid stance, terminal stance, and pre-swing. The latter three comprise swing: initial swing, mid swing, and terminal swing. The similarities and differences between the two terminologies are presented in Table 7.1.

The first stance phase, *initial contact,* represents the moment in time when the outstretched limb first hits the ground. During the next phase, *loading response,* body weight is rapidly accepted onto the outstretched limb. A small wave of knee flexion helps dissipate the impact forces associated with body weight loading onto the limb. Initial contact and loading response are the two phases that constitute *initial double limb stance,* which is sometimes referred to as *weight acceptance.*[34] Initial double limb stance ends when the foot opposite the reference limb lifts from the ground for swing.

During the next two phases, *mid stance* and *terminal stance,* body weight progresses forward over a single stable limb. By terminal stance, the heel rises from the ground, the leg achieves a "trailing limb" posture, and the trunk advances well in front of the reference foot. Another term for the combined phases of mid stance and terminal stance is *single limb support,* reflective of only one limb being in contact with the ground.[34]

Pre-swing, the last phase of stance, is sometimes referred to as *terminal double limb stance* or *push-off.* During pre-swing, body weight transfers from the trailing limb to the contralateral lead limb, which is experiencing initial contact and loading response. As the proportion of body weight supported by the trailing limb diminishes, residual energy stored in the Achilles tendon during mid and terminal stance rapidly plantarflexes the ankle despite a lack of significant plantarflexor muscle activity.[34,36-38] The knee flexes to 40°, over half of the 60° required for foot clearance during the subsequent phase.

Table 7.1 Comparison of Gait Terminology

	Rancho Los Amigos[34,35]	Traditional
Stance	*Initial Contact:* Beginning of stance when heel or some other portion of foot contacts ground. Component of initial double limb stance.	*Heel Strike:* Beginning of stance when heel first contacts ground.
	Loading Response: Body weight rapidly loads onto lead limb from trailing limb. Hip remains stable, knee flexes to absorb shock, and forefoot lowers to ground. Immediately follows initial contact and is final component of initial double limb stance. Ends when opposite limb lifts from ground for swing.	*Foot Flat:* Immediately follows heel strike when sole of foot contacts floor.
	Mid Stance: Trunk progresses from behind to in front of ankle over single stable limb. First half of single limb support. Starts when contralateral foot lifts from ground for swing.	*Midstance:* Point at which body passes directly over reference extremity.
	Terminal Stance: Trunk continues forward progression relative to foot. Heel rises from ground and limb achieves trailing limb posture. Second half of single limb support. Ends with contralateral initial contact.	*Heel Off:* Point following midstance when reference limb's heel leaves ground.
Swing	*Pre-swing:* Body weight rapidly unloads from reference limb and reference limb prepares for swing during this terminal double limb stance period. Starts with contralateral initial contact and ends at ipsilateral limb toe off.	*Toe Off:* Point following heel off when only the reference limb's toe is contacting ground.
	Initial Swing: Starts when reference foot lifts from ground. Hip, knee, and ankle rapidly flex for clearance and advancement during this initial 1/3 of swing.	*Acceleration:* Beginning portion of swing from reference limb toe off to point when reference limb is directly under the body.
	Mid Swing: Thigh continues advancing, knee begins to extend, and ankle achieves neutral posture during this middle 1/3 of swing.	*Midswing:* Portion of swing when reference limb passes directly below body. Extends from the end of acceleration to beginning of deceleration.
	Terminal Swing: During this final 1/3 of swing, knee achieves maximal extension and ankle remains at neutral in preparation for heel first initial contact. Ends when foot contacts ground.	*Deceleration:* Portion of swing when reference limb is decelerating in preparation for heel strike.

Lifting of the foot from the ground reflects the onset of the first phase of swing, *initial swing.* Rapid flexion of the knee and hip ensue. During *mid swing,* the thigh continues to advance into flexion, achieving a peak of approximately 25° relative to vertical. The knee begins to extend and the tibia achieves a characteristic vertical position by the end of mid swing. The ankle reaches neutral (0° dorsiflexion). During *terminal swing,* further thigh flexion is curtailed; however, the knee continues to extend until it observationally appears neutral. The ankle remains at neutral in preparation for a heel-first initial contact.

Characteristic features of normal gait are presented in Tables 7.2, 7.3, and 7.4. The gait phases, as well as normative values for joint motions, internal moments of force, and muscle activity, are presented in the first four columns of these tables. Familiarity with the normal motion patterns provides the therapist with a basis of comparison to identify deviations from standard. The internal moments (or torques) at each joint reflect the forces generated by muscles' contractile and noncontractile components, as well as ligaments and joint capsules. Internal moments counterbalance the external moments that are created by forces such as gravity and inertia acting on the body segments. In the current chapter, we will describe internal joint moments, as this appears to be the more common reference point used in published literature. However, knowledge of the external moments (and thus the internal moments) is helpful for interpreting the characteristic patterns of muscle activation that contribute to stability, forward progression, shock absorption, and limb clearance throughout the gait cycle. For example, during the single-limb support period of normal gait, a progressively increasing external dorsiflexion moment occurs as body weight progresses anterior to the ankle joint. Without a counteracting force from the plantarflexors, the ankle would collapse into dorsiflexion. The force generated by the plantarflexors contributes to an internal plantarflexor moment that prevents tibial collapse while simultaneously allowing controlled forward progression. Thus, the internal plantarflexor moment generated by the plantarflexors resists the external dorsiflexion moment created in large part by the force of gravity on the body.

Abnormalities in timing (e.g., activity that is premature or delayed) and amplitude (either too much or too little) can disrupt normal gait patterns. Familiarity with the muscle activity and function associated with normal gait allows therapists to identify potential causes of deviations. The last two columns of Tables 7.2, 7.3, and 7.4 present the possible effects of muscle weakness and potential compensations. The purpose of the tables is to identify components of normal gait that must be considered when observing gait and to provide an example of how to analyze the causes of an atypical gait pattern or particular deviation.

TYPES OF GAIT ANALYSES

The types of analyses in use today can be classified under two broad categories: *kinematic* and *kinetic.* Kinematic gait analysis is used to describe movement patterns without regard for the forces involved in producing the movement. A kinematic gait analysis consists of a description of movement of the body as a whole and/or body segments in relation to each other during gait. Kinematic gait analysis can be either *qualitative* or *quantitative.* Kinetic gait analysis is used to determine the forces involved in gait. In some instances, both kinematic and kinetic gait variables may be examined in one analysis. In addition to examining kinematic and kinetic variables, physiological variables such as heart rate, oxygen consumption, energy cost, and muscular activation patterns (electromyography) may be considered.

Kinematic Qualitative Gait Analysis

The most common method used in clinical settings is a *qualitative gait analysis.* This method usually requires only a small amount of equipment and a minimal amount of time. The primary variable examined in a qualitative kinematic analysis is *displacement,* which includes a description of patterns of movement, deviations from normal body postures, and joint angles at specific points in the gait cycle.

Observational Gait Analysis

Few clinical settings have the resources (space, money, or time) required to complete an instrumented gait analysis on every patient. As a result, observational gait analysis (OGA) often serves as an essential component of many physical therapy examinations. The results of an OGA are used to identify structural and activity limitations and to plan an intervention and assess the outcomes. While physical therapists seek an easy-to-administer tool to identify gait abnormalities, guide treatment approaches (e.g., need for orthotic devices), and assess progress,[39] the validity and reliability of existing scales remains less than optimal. This section highlights tools/approaches that clinicians may consider using.

The *Rancho Los Amigos Observational Gait Analysis* system is probably the most common OGA system used by physical therapists.[34,35] The Rancho Los Amigos OGA method involves a systematic examination of the movement patterns of key body segments (foot, ankle, knee, hip, pelvis, and trunk) during each phase of the gait cycle. The system uses a recording form comprising 45 descriptors of common gait deviations such as toe drag, excess plantarflexion and dorsiflexion, excess knee varus or valgus, pelvic hiking, and forward or backward trunk leans (Fig. 7.3). The observing therapist must determine whether or not a deviation is present and note the occurrence and timing of the deviation on the special form.[35]

Considerable training and practice are necessary to develop the observational skills needed for performing any OGA. Therapists who wish to learn the Rancho method can study the *Rancho Los Amigos Observational Gait Analysis Handbook.*[35] Practice gait videos, useful for developing and improving one's observational skills and

Table 7.2 Ankle and Foot: Normative Sagittal Plane Data and Impact of Weakness[34,35]

Phase	Characteristic Joint Position	Internal Joint Moment	Normative Muscle Activity	Effect(s) of Weakness	Possible Compensation(s)
Initial Contact	Neutral (0° dorsiflexion)	Dorsiflexor moment achieves peak during loading response	Pretibial muscles (tibialis anterior, extensor digitorum longus, extensor hallucis longus) decelerate forefoot lowering and draw tibia forward following initial contact.	Borderline weakness (3+/5) may be accompanied by a foot slap following a heel first initial contact. Profound weakness (2+/5 or less) may result in foot flat or forefoot initial contact if pretibial strength is insufficient for achieving neutral ankle.	With borderline weakness, may slow gait to decrease demands on pretibial muscles during loading response. Alternatively, may contact ground with excess plantarflexion to decrease demands on pretibial muscles.
Loading Response	5° plantarflexion				
Mid Stance	5° dorsiflexion	Plantarflexor moment reaches peak during terminal stance	Plantarflexors (gastrocnemius, soleus, flexor digitorum longus, flexor hallucis longus, tibialis posterior, peroneus longus, and peroneus brevis) progressively increase activity throughout two phases to allow controlled forward progression of tibia. Elastic energy stored in Achilles tendon.	Excess dorsiflexion, uncontrolled tibial advancement, delayed or absent heel-off. However, if vastii are weak (vastus intermedius, vastus lateralis, vastus medialis longus, and oblique), may avoid excess dorsiflexion as it would contribute to excess knee flexion and high demand on weakened vastii.	Shortened step length and slower velocity to reduce demands on calf muscles.
Terminal Stance	10° dorsiflexion				
Pre-Swing	15° plantarflexion		Calf muscles cease in early pre-swing. Stored elastic energy in Achilles tendon contributes to rapid plantarflexion as limb unloads.	Low or no heel-off and lack of rapid plantarflexion.	Use of more proximal muscles to prepare limb for advancement and clearance.
Initial Swing	5° plantarflexion	Low dorsiflexor moment	Pretibial muscles elevate foot to neutral by mid swing and then maintain in that posture.	Excess plantarflexion and foot drag, particularly in mid swing. Poor posture for subsequent initial contact.	Hip hike, excess hip flexion or abduction to assist with limb clearance, or contralateral vault (excessive plantarflexion) to facilitate reference limb clearance.
Mid Swing	Neutral				
Terminal Swing	Neutral				

Table 7.3 Knee: Normative Sagittal Plane Data and Impact of Weakness[34,35]

Phase	Characteristic Joint Position	Internal Joint Moment	Normative Muscle Activity	Effect(s) of Weakness	Possible Compensation(s)
Initial Contact	Appears fully extended	Brief flexor moment	Low amplitude hamstring activity (semimembranosus, semitendinosus, biceps femoris [long head]) resists knee hyperextension.	Reliance on posterior capsule to stabilize joint and to prevent hyperextension.	*Shading represents column heading information not applicable to the identified phase of gait.*
Loading Response	20° flexion	Extensor moment	Eccentric vastii activity (vastus intermedius, vastus lateralis, vastus medialis longus, and oblique) allows knee flexion for shock absorption but prevents collapse.	Unable to stabilize knee during flexion leading to limb collapse.	Avoid knee flexion (as flexion increases vastii demand) by use of (1) excess plantarflexion or (2) forward trunk lean to lessen knee extensor moment.
Mid Stance	Appears fully extended	Extensor moment transitions to flexor moment	Vastii activity ceases by middle of mid stance.		
Terminal Stance	Appears fully extended	Flexor moment			
Pre-Swing	40° flexion	Extensor moment	Rectus femoris modulates rate of knee flexion.		
Initial Swing	60° flexion		Biceps femoris (short head), gracilis, and sartorius contribute to knee flexion.	Limited knee flexion for foot clearance.	Compensatory hip hike, excess hip flexion, or abduction to assist clearance.
Mid Swing	25° flexion	Flexor moment	Hamstrings modulate rate of knee extension (and thigh advancement).		
Terminal Swing	Appears fully extended		Hamstrings continue activity and vastii become active in preparation for demands of initial double limb stance.	With profound vastii weakness (less than 2+/5) may see inadequate knee extension in terminal swing.	Past retract of thigh or extension thrust of knee to ensure full knee extension.

for learning how to use the recording forms, may be obtained by visiting the Rancho Research Institute website (www.ranchoresearch.org/education/materials) or by writing to Rancho Research Institute at Rancho Los Amigos National Rehabilitation Center, 7601 East Imperial Highway, Downey, CA 90242.

Podiatrists have developed their own unique OGA system.[40] A biomechanical gait analysis form for podiatrists was described by Southerland.[40] This form is used in conjunction with a static quantitative analysis that includes measurements of range of motion (ROM) of all joints from the hip to the toes and measurements of limb

Table 7.4 Hip: Normative Sagittal Plane Data and Impact of Weakness[34,35]

Phase	Characteristic Joint Position (Thigh Relative to Vertical)	Internal Joint Moment	Normative Muscle Activity	Effect(s) of Weakness	Possible Compensation(s)
Initial Contact	20° flexion	Extensor moment	Single joint hip extensors and abductors contract vigorously to stabilize pelvis and trunk over femur. Hamstring activity diminishing.	Difficulty stabilizing pelvis and hip joint, leading to anterior tilt and increased hip flexion in sagittal plane. If abductors weak, contralateral pelvic drop may occur.	Decrease terminal swing hip flexion to limit demands on weak hip extensors during initial contact and loading response. Posterior trunk lean to reduce extensor moment. For weak abductors, may lean trunk laterally toward stance limb to reduce abductor demands.
Loading Response	20° flexion				
Mid Stance	Neutral	Extensor moment transitions to flexor moment	Residual hamstring activity assists with hip extension at beginning of phase. Low-level abductor activity stabilizes pelvis.	Contralateral pelvic drop.	May lean trunk laterally toward stance limb to reduce abductor demands.
Terminal Stance	20° apparent hyperextension (anatomical hip joint does not allow 20° extension, but hip appears to be extended 20° due to the combined impact of hip extension, backward pelvic rotation, and anterior pelvic tilt on thigh angulation relative to vertical).	Increasing flexor moment	Low amplitude tensor fascia lata activity.	Contralateral pelvic drop.	May lean trunk laterally toward stance limb to reduce abductor demands.
Pre-Swing	10° apparent hyperextension	Flexor moment	Rectus femoris assists with early thigh advancement.		
Initial Swing	15° flexion	Flexor moment	Iliacus, adductor longus, gracilis, and sartorius actively advance thigh.	With profound hip flexor weakness (less than 2/5), may exhibit limited hip flexion, thigh advancement, and foot clearance.	To facilitate limb clearance, may compensate with ipsilateral hip hiking, excess hip abduction, or contralateral limb vaulting (excessive plantarflexion).

Continued

Table 7.4 Hip: Normative Sagittal Plane Data and Impact of Weakness[34,35]—cont'd

Phase	Characteristic Joint Position (Thigh Relative to Vertical)	Internal Joint Moment	Normative Muscle Activity	Effect(s) of Weakness	Possible Compensation(s)
Mid Swing	25° flexion	Extensor moment	Increasing hamstring activity at end of phase restrains further thigh advancement.		
Terminal Swing	20° flexion	Extensor moment	Hamstrings continue to control thigh posture, while single joint hip extensors and abductors rapidly increase activity in preparation for demands of next phase of gait.	Failure to achieve optimum limb position prior to initial contact.	Alter speed.

length. Detailed information is also collected on both the dorsal and plantar surfaces of the feet such as callus formation and corns. The examiner is expected to document abnormalities such as hallux valgus and hammer toes. The dynamic qualitative component of the analysis uses a shorthand system for recording the details of the OGA. The acronym GHORT (*G*ait, *H*omunculus, *O*bserved, *R*elational, and *T*abulator) is used to assist in recording information gathered from the observational analysis. Following completion of the dynamic portion, the rater's qualitative impressions of the patient's gait are compared with the results of the static analysis to verify the accuracy of the findings and determine the causes of abnormal function. The author states that after the first five analyses, a new rater's results are the same as or similar to those of other raters; however, the author did not reference any reliability and/or validity studies.[40] In general, these observational protocols provide the therapist with a systematic approach to OGA by directing the observer's attention to a specific joint or body segment during a given point in the gait cycle.

The advantages of OGAs are that they require little or no instrumentation, are inexpensive to use, and can yield general descriptions of gait variables. The disadvantages are that the observational method, being dependent on both the therapist's training and observational skills, is subjective and has only low to moderate reliability,[41] and validity has not been demonstrated.[42] Difficulties involved in observing and making accurate judgments about motions occurring simultaneously at numerous body segments, and inadequate training in OGA methods are thought to contribute to the low reliability. Also, therapists differ in their observational skills. A drawback to using the Rancho Los Amigos OGA technique is that reliability and validity of the method have not been published.

Digital Video Recording

If therapists decide to use an OGA method, they should consider using a digital video recorder (DVR) that has the capability of slowing or stopping motion. A visual record is especially important when using the Rancho Los Amigos format because of the time involved in examining a large number of variables at six body parts. Most patients cannot walk continuously for the length of time required to complete a detailed, full-body observational analysis. Furthermore, the observers cannot rate or score a large number of variables while a subject is walking. Digital records of a patient's initial performance that can be replayed in slow motion allow therapists the time needed to make judgments about gait events. Activating the DVR pause feature, a goniometer, aligned with body segments displayed on the video monitor, can be used to assess (validate) joint angles during critical phases. This may also help refine the therapist's observational skills.

Although the use of DVRs may provide an opportunity for observers to determine the reliability of their scoring, reliability will probably remain low to moderate[43-46] unless therapists are knowledgeable about normal gait parameters and variables and are adequately trained to use the measuring instrument. Russell et al[47] found that when observers were trained in the scoring of a Gross Motor Function Measure, a significant improvement occurred following training compared

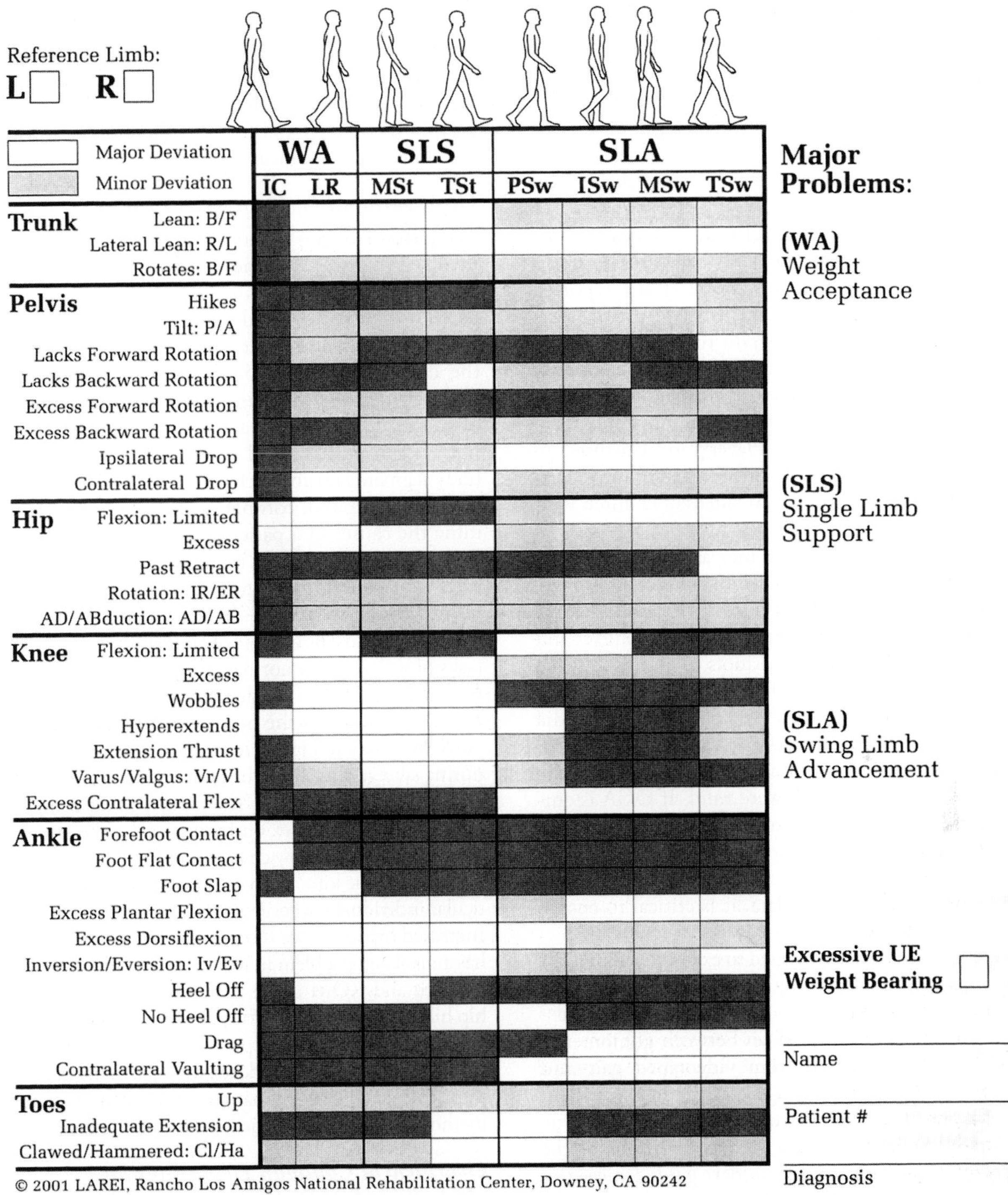

GAIT ANALYSIS: FULL BODY

RANCHO LOS AMIGOS NATIONAL REHABILITATION CENTER PHYSICAL THERAPY DEPARTMENT

Reference Limb:

L☐ R☐

☐ Major Deviation

☐ Minor Deviation

		WA		SLS		SLA			
		IC	LR	MSt	TSt	PSw	ISw	MSw	TSw
Trunk	Lean: B/F								
	Lateral Lean: R/L								
	Rotates: B/F								
Pelvis	Hikes								
	Tilt: P/A								
	Lacks Forward Rotation								
	Lacks Backward Rotation								
	Excess Forward Rotation								
	Excess Backward Rotation								
	Ipsilateral Drop								
	Contralateral Drop								
Hip	Flexion: Limited								
	Excess								
	Past Retract								
	Rotation: IR/ER								
	AD/ABduction: AD/AB								
Knee	Flexion: Limited								
	Excess								
	Wobbles								
	Hyperextends								
	Extension Thrust								
	Varus/Valgus: Vr/Vl								
	Excess Contralateral Flex								
Ankle	Forefoot Contact								
	Foot Flat Contact								
	Foot Slap								
	Excess Plantar Flexion								
	Excess Dorsiflexion								
	Inversion/Eversion: Iv/Ev								
	Heel Off								
	No Heel Off								
	Drag								
	Contralateral Vaulting								
Toes	Up								
	Inadequate Extension								
	Clawed/Hammered: Cl/Ha								

Major Problems:

(WA) Weight Acceptance

(SLS) Single Limb Support

(SLA) Swing Limb Advancement

Excessive UE Weight Bearing ☐

Name

Patient #

Diagnosis

Figure 7.3 Full Body Gait Analysis Form. *(From Observational Gait Analysis Handbook,[35] with permission.)*

with the observers' pretraining scoring of the videotape. Brunnekreef and colleagues[48] identified higher interrater reliability among expert raters of orthopedic gait disorders (intraclass correlation coefficient [ICC] = 0.54) when using a form developed by the experts than the values documented for experienced (ICC = 0.42) and inexperienced (ICC = 0.40) raters using the same form. On the other hand, Eastlack et al[49] found only low to moderate interrater reliability among 54 practicing physical therapists who rated 10 gait variables while observing the videotaped gait of three patients. These therapists had reported that they were comfortable performing observational gait analyses. The lack of agreement among raters found in this study, as well as the raters' lack of knowledge of normal gait parameters and terminology, has serious implications for patient treatments based on the results of observational gait analyses.[49] Krebs[50] argues that OGA is impossible to perform in a clinical setting. However, in a study using OGA, physical therapists were able to make accurate and reliable judgments of scored push-off power in the videotaped gait of subjects following stroke. This study suggests that focused analysis on specific gait parameters may be more reliable than general analyses.[51]

Specialized video analysis software may improve interrater reliability of gait measures compared to traditional video viewing methods. Borel et al[52] reported increased measurement agreement between two raters when using Dartfish®, a program that allows users to measure joint angles, distance, and time variables directly from digital videos. (*Note*: For this chapter, all manufacturer contact information is presented in Appendix 7.C.) Raters used Windows Media Player® and Dartfish® to perform the measurements required to determine Observational Gait Scale scores for 20 videos of children with cerebral palsy (CP).

Interrater agreement values increased for select variables (knee position midstance, foot contact midstance, timing of heel rise, hindfoot midstance, and the composite total score) when using the digital goniometer and the line drawing and temporal tools of Dartfish®. One potential negative was that it took longer to complete the analysis using Dartfish® than Windows Media Player (18 versus 10 minutes per video, respectively). Additionally, this study did not determine whether the more consistent values also were valid. If OGA is employed, it should be used in conjunction with quantitative measures. Digital video recordings or videotape can provide a permanent record of the patient's gait. However, as with other patient data, it is critical to ensure confidential storage of images.

Videography may also be used to examine joint ROM at the hip, knee, and ankle by taking goniometric measurements directly from the paused screen. Stuberg et al[53] found no significant differences between goniometric measurements calculated from videotaped gait and measurements generated using a digitizer in 10 children with CP and 9 typically developing children. Six blue markers, placed over key anatomical locations of the lower extremity (LE) and shoulder, guided measurements. The use of markers to guide measurements emphasizes the importance of ensuring that joints (or apparent axes of rotation) are clearly visible to facilitate measurements with the eye or a goniometer.

Mobile Device Software Applications

More recently, program applications (apps) for mobile devices such as *smartphones* and *tablets* have emerged that are being used in health care and athletic settings to assess gait. Coaches Eye® and Spark Motion® are two examples of apps used for movement assessment. Videos recorded with these apps can be watched in slow-motion. The clinician also has the option to overlay prior videos, integrate grids and drawings to assist with visual analysis, and calculate approximate joint angles on the videos/images for subsequent comparison.[54] Although clinically appealing, the validity and reliability of these apps have not been fully explored and further validation with patients is still needed for clinical application.[55]

Observational Gait Analysis Process

The purpose of this section is to introduce the process involved in an OGA. The first step in the process involves the identification and accurate description of the patient's gait pattern and any existing deviations. The second step involves a determination of the causes of the deviations. To properly identify and describe a patient's gait, the therapist must have good knowledge of gait terminology and an accurate mental picture of normal gait postures and normal displacements of the body segments during each gait phase and in each plane of analysis (sagittal, coronal, and transverse). To determine the causes of a patient's gait pattern and specific deviations, the therapist must understand the normal roles and functions of muscles during gait and the normal forces involved.[34,35,56,57]

Deviations occur because of an inability to perform the tasks of walking in a normal fashion. For example, a patient with paralysis of the dorsiflexors (which causes a foot drop) cannot attain the normal neutral position of the ankle necessary to complete the task of clearing the floor during swing. Therefore, the patient must use some other method to clear the floor. The patient could compensate for inadequate dorsiflexion by increasing the amount of hip and knee flexion, by circumduction of the entire limb, or by hiking the hip. The type of compensation that a particular individual selects depends on the specific disability. Increased hip and knee flexion may be used if the patient has an isolated problem in the ankle and adequate muscle strength and ROM in the extremity. Circumduction or hip hiking may be used if the patient has either a stiff knee or extensor thrust, which prevents use of increased knee flexion to raise the plantarflexed foot above the floor.[7] The therapist must be aware that patients may use a variety of methods to compensate for joint or muscle deficits.

Overview of Common Deviations and Underlying Causes

Tables 7.5 to 7.8 present common gait deviations and possible causes for the deviations. Given that muscle demands vary across phases of gait, the causes of a specific deviation also frequently vary based on the phase. For example, a common cause of excess plantarflexion during swing is weak pretibial muscles. However, this is not a common cause of excess plantarflexion during mid stance and terminal stance, as the pretibial muscles are

Table 7.5 Common Ankle and Foot Deviations[34,35]

Deviation	Phase(s)	Description	Possible Causes	Analysis
Toes or forefoot contact	Initial contact	Toes or forefoot are first point of contact with ground instead of heel.	Leg length discrepancy; plantarflexion contracture or spasticity; profound dorsiflexor weakness; painful heel; excessive knee flexion when combined with any impairment that limits ability to achieve neutral ankle.	Examine range of motion (ROM) and leg lengths and for hip and/or knee flexion contractures and/or ankle plantarflexion contractures. Examine muscle tone and timing of activity in plantarflexors. Examine pretibial strength and for heel pain.
Foot flat contact	Initial contact	Entire foot simultaneously touches ground at initial contact.	Plantarflexion contracture; weak dorsiflexors; knee flexion contracture that prevents optimal tibial alignment prior to initial contact.	Examine ROM at ankle and knee and strength of pretibial muscles.
Foot slap	Loading response	Forefoot "slaps" the ground following a heel first initial contact.	Weak dorsiflexors or reciprocal inhibition of dorsiflexors.	Examine strength. Evaluate muscle activation timing of pretibial muscles.
Excess plantarflexion	Mid stance and/or terminal stance	Ankle fails to achieve 5° dorsiflexion at mid stance and/or 10° dorsiflexion at terminal stance.	Plantarflexion contracture; overactivity or spasticity of the plantarflexors; could be intentional to avoid ankle and knee collapse if plantarflexors and vastii are weak.	Examine ROM and tone for plantarflexion contracture and plantarflexor tone (spasticity); examine strength of calf muscles and vastii. Evaluate if deviation may be intentional due to dual areas of weakness.
Excess dorsiflexion	Mid stance and/or terminal stance	Ankle collapses into more than 5° dorsiflexion at mid stance and/or more than 10° dorsiflexion at terminal stance.	Inability of plantarflexors to control tibial advance. Knee flexion or hip flexion contractures.	Examine ROM and plantarflexor strength and for hip and knee flexion contractures.
Early heel rise	Mid stance	Heel comes off ground in mid stance.	Spasticity or contracture of plantarflexors.	Examine ROM and tone for plantarflexor spasticity and contractures.
No heel off	Terminal stance and/or pre-swing	Heel fails to elevate from ground appropriately during terminal stance.	Weak plantarflexors; weak invertors that fail to lock midfoot in terminal stance; inadequate toe extension ROM; painful forefoot or toes.	Examine strength of plantarflexors and tibialis posterior; toe extension ROM, particularly the first metatarsal phalangeal joint; and for forefoot pain.
Toe clawing	Stance	Toes flex and "grab" floor	Spasticity of toe flexors; excessive activation of toe flexors to compensate for weakness of the gastrocnemius and soleus; plantar grasp reflex that is only partially integrated; positive supporting reflex.	Examine tone of toe flexors, strength of plantarflexors, and presence of primitive reflexes.

Continued

Table 7.5 Common Ankle and Foot Deviations[34,35]—cont'd

Deviation	Phase(s)	Description	Possible Causes	Analysis
Excess inversion or eversion	Stance or swing	Subtalar joint is excessively inverted or everted in contrast to expected position.	Excessive inversion: overactivity or contracture of invertors; reduced activity of evertors; primitive extensor pattern. Excessive eversion: overactivity or contracture of evertors; reduced activity or strength of invertors; primitive flexor pattern.	Examine strength and timing of lower extremity (LE) movements and tone; and for contractures.
Drag	Swing	Some portion of reference foot contacts ground during swing	Pretibial muscle weakness; plantarflexor spasticity or contractures; inadequate knee or hip flexion.	Examine ROM of ankle, knee and hip; strength of muscles critical for limb clearance.

Table 7.6 Common Knee Deviations[34,35]

Deviation	Phase	Description	Possible Causes	Analysis
Excess knee flexion	All phases	Knee is in greater flexion than expected for the given phase.	Knee flexor spasticity or contracture that exceeds position required for given phase; painful or effused knee; proprioceptive loss at knee; shorter LE on contralateral side. In addition, consider weak calf or hip flexion contracture if it occurs during single limb support.	Examine tone, spasticity, and ROM (contractures); and for pain, effusion, and proprioceptive loss at knee; leg length discrepancy.
Limited knee flexion	Loading response	Knee achieves less than expected 20° flexion.	May be intentional to decrease demands on weak quadriceps; secondary to plantarflexor or quadriceps tone, spasticity, or contracture; or proprioceptive impairment at knee.	Examine strength, tone, spasticity, of plantarflexors and quadriceps; plantarflexion and knee extension ROM; knee proprioception.
	Pre-swing and initial swing	Knee achieves less than expected flexion for given phase (i.e., 40° and 60° flexion, respectively).	May be secondary to plantarflexor tone, spasticity, or contracture that limits forward tibial progression in terminal stance; quadriceps tone, spasticity; proprioceptive impairment at knee; knee pain or effusion; calf weakness or hip flexion contracture that limits ability to achieve the trailing limb posture in terminal stance (a critical precursor to rapid knee flexion during pre-swing and initial swing). During initial swing, weakness of knee flexors also may contribute.	Examine tone and spasticity of plantarflexors, vastii, and rectus femoris; ROM and knee proprioception. Examine for pain and effusion. Examine plantarflexor strength and for hip flexion contracture. Evaluate if these factors may be inhibiting achievement of optimum limb posture.

Table 7.6 Common Knee Deviations[34,35]—cont'd

Deviation	Phase	Description	Possible Causes	Analysis
Knee hyperextension	Stance	Extension of knee beyond anatomical neutral	Structural abnormality; may develop over time in presence of flaccid/weak quadriceps, which is compensated for by excess plantarflexion and/or posterior pull on thigh by gluteus maximus; quadriceps spasticity, accommodation to a fixed plantarflexion deformity, or impaired proprioception can contribute to hyperextension if knee is exposed to deforming forces for extended duration.	Examine strength of vastii; tone, spasticity of plantarflexors and quadriceps; ROM and knee proprioception.
Wobble	Stance	Alternating flexion and extension at knee joint	Consider proprioceptive impairments or alternating spasticity of knee flexors and extensors.	Examine knee for proprioceptive impairments and spasticity.

Table 7.7 Common Hip Deviations[34,35]

Deviation	Phase(s)	Description	Possible Causes	Analysis
Excess flexion	Initial contact and loading response	Hip positioned in greater flexion (thigh relative to vertical) than expected for given phase.	Single joint hip extensor weakness (gluteus maximus, adductor magnus) with compensation by hamstrings; severe hip and/or knee flexion contractures; hypertonicity of hip or knee flexors.	Examine single joint hip extensor and hamstring strength; hip and knee flexion ROM, tone, and spasticity.
	Mid stance through pre-swing		Hip flexion or knee flexion contractures or spasticity; weak plantarflexors failing to control excess tibial advancement; painful or effused hip; may be	Examine tone and spasticity of hip and knee flexors; ROM of hip and knee; strength of plantarflexors and hip for joint pain.
	Swing		compensatory to assist with limb clearance if limb is functionally too long; flexion synergy during swing resulting in too much flexion.	Examine for compensation, determine if ankle and knee of reference limb are achieving correct joint positions. Examine contralateral limb to determine if deviations are occurring on opposite side (e.g., excess stance dorsiflexion); could contribute to clearance problems on reference side.
Limited flexion	Initial contact, loading response, initial swing, mid swing, terminal swing	Hip positioned in less flexion (thigh relative to vertical) than expected for given phase.	May be intentional to limit demand on weak hip extensors during loading response; weak hip flexors, or single joint hip extensor; hamstring spasticity or contracture limiting terminal swing advancement prior to initial contact.	Examine strength of hip flexors and extensors; ROM of hip and for spasticity of hip extensors and hamstrings.

Continued

Table 7.7 Common Hip Deviations[34,35]—cont'd

Deviation	Phase(s)	Description	Possible Causes	Analysis
Circumduction	Swing	Lateral circular movement of limb consisting initially of abduction, external rotation, followed by adduction and internal rotation in latter portion of swing.	Compensation for weak hip flexors or for inability to shorten leg for limb clearance.	Examine strength of hip flexors, knee flexors, and ankle dorsiflexors; ROM in hip and knee flexion, and ankle dorsiflexion and for abnormal extensor pattern.
Internal rotation	All phases	Internal rotation of femur.	Spasticity or contractures of internal rotators; weakness of external rotators; excessive forward rotation of contralateral pelvis.	Examine tone, internal rotation ROM, and strength of external rotators.
External rotation	All phases	External rotation of femur.	Spasticity or contractures of external rotators; weakness of internal rotators.	Examine tone, external rotation ROM, and strength of internal rotators.
Abduction	All phases	Abducted position of femur relative to vertical.	Contracture of the gluteus medius or iliotibial band; during swing, could be used to assist with foot clearance.	Examine hip abductor range of motion and for any factors that would necessitate compensatory assistance with clearance.
Adduction	All phases	Adducted position of femur relative to vertical	Hip adductor spasticity/ contracture. Excess contralateral pelvic drop.	Examine tone of hip flexors and adductors; muscle strength of hip abductors.

Table 7.8 Common Pelvic and Trunk Deviations[34,35]

Deviation	Phase(s)	Description	Possible Causes	Analysis
Backward trunk lean	Stance or swing	Posterior lean of the trunk relative to vertical	Purposeful to reduce demands on weakened stance limb gluteus maximus or to assist with limb advancement when hip flexion capability is limited.	Examine hip extensor and flexor strength.
Forward trunk lean	Primarily stance	Anterior lean of trunk relative to vertical	Compensation for quadriceps weakness. Forward lean reduces knee extensor moment and thus demand on vastii. May also be used to accommodate hip or knee flexion contractures.	Examine quadriceps strength and hip and knee for contractures.
Ipsilateral trunk lean	Most commonly occurs during reference limb stance	Lateral trunk lean toward reference extremity	Most commonly occurs during reference limb stance. Compensation for ipsilateral hip abductor weakness, hip joint pain, iliotibial band tightness or scoliosis.	Examine ipsilateral gluteus medius strength; hip pain and ipsilateral iliotibial band tightness and for trunk ROM.
Contralateral trunk lean	Most commonly occurs during reference limb swing	Lateral trunk lean toward opposite extremity	May be used to assist with pelvic elevation to ensure foot clearance if reference limb is functionally too long (owing to deviations or leg length discrepancy).	Examine contralateral gluteus medius strength, hip pain and for iliotibial band tightness and for trunk ROM. Examine for factors contributing to swing limb

Table 7.8 Common Pelvic and Trunk Deviations[34,35]—cont'd

Deviation	Phase(s)	Description	Possible Causes	Analysis
			Compensation for contralateral hip abductor weakness, hip joint pain, iliotibial band tightness, or scoliosis.	being too long (e.g., limited knee flexion or excess plantarflexion during initial swing or a leg length discrepancy).
Contralateral pelvic drop	Stance	Drop of contralateral iliac crest below ipsilateral iliac crest	Ipsilateral hip abductor weakness, hip adductor spasticity, or hip adduction contracture.	Examine strength, flexibility, and tone of ipsilateral hip abductors and adductors.
Ipsilateral pelvic drop	Swing	Drop of ipsilateral iliac crest below contralateral iliac crest	Contralateral hip abductor weakness, hip adductor spasticity, or hip adduction contracture.	Examine strength, flexibility, and tone of contralateral hip abductors and adductors.
Pelvic hike	Swing	Elevation of ipsilateral iliac crest above contralateral iliac crest	Action of quadratus lumborum to assist with limb clearance when hip flexion, knee flexion, and/or ankle dorsiflexion are inadequate for limb clearance.	Examine strength and ROM at knee, hip, and ankle; examine muscle tone at knee and ankle.

not normally active during this period. Instead, excess plantarflexion during mid and terminal stance would more likely arise from the influence of plantarflexor spasticity or contractures on joint motion during this period. Thus, detective work is required to link the observed gait deviations with the specific demands of a phase in order to determine the most likely cause(s). Accurate determination of the impairments leading to the gait deviation is essential for guiding treatment interventions.

Appendix 7.A, Recording Form for Observational Gait Analysis, provides a sample gait analysis recording form. Check marks (√) are used to indicate observation of a specific deviation. The two columns on the far right are used to record possible causes and findings from the clinical analyses. To guide the OGA process, note that the form presented in Appendix 7.A has been formatted similarly to Tables 7.5 through 7.8. If the reader decides to use the gait analysis recording forms presented in this text, reliability tests should be conducted because these forms are presented only as guides and have not been evaluated.

Guidelines for Performing an OGA

Guidelines for performing an OGA are presented below.

1. Select the area in which the patient will walk and measure the distance that you want the patient to traverse.
2. Position yourself to allow an unobstructed view of the subject. If digitally recording, the cameras should be positioned to view the patient's entire body (LEs as well as the head and trunk) from both the sagittal and coronal perspectives. To avoid errors in estimating the amplitude of joint angles due to angle parallax,[34,53] it is important to perform measurements on paused digital images only when the patient's LEs or body is in the same plane as the image view. Out-of-plane views can lead to distorted angle measurements.
3. Select the joint or body segment to be observed first (e.g., ankle and foot), and mentally review the normative joint positions and muscle activity for the phase of the gait period being observed (e.g., initial contact).
4. Select the plane of observation that will be used first, either the sagittal plane (view from the side) or the coronal plane (view from the front and/or back) and which side of the patient's body (either right or left) will be observed first.
5. Observe the selected body segment at a specific phase (e.g., initial contact) and make a decision about the segment's joint position. Note any deviations from normal.
6. Observe either the same body segment during the next phase or another segment at the same phase (e.g., initial contact) of the gait period. As described in number 5, again make a decision about the segment's joint position. Note any deviations from normal.
7. Repeat the process described in number 6 until you have completed an observation of all segments across all phases of the gait cycle in both the sagittal and coronal planes. Remember to concentrate on one body segment or joint at a time during one phase of the gait cycle. Do not jump from one segment to another or from one phase to another.
8. Always perform observations on both sides (right and left). Although only one side may be involved pathologically, the other side of the body may be affected.

9. Hypothesize likely causes of gait deviations (e.g., impairments in strength, ROM, or spasticity).
10. Confirm likely causes of gait deviations based on physical therapy clinical evaluation.
11. Develop and implement a treatment plan to address key underlying causes of gait dysfunction.
12. Periodically use OGA to reassess the patient's gait and determine response to treatment.

OGA in Neuromuscular Disorders

The gait patterns of individuals with neuromuscular deficits are influenced primarily by impaired motor function and motor control, weakness, abnormalities in muscle tone and synergistic organization, influences of nonintegrated early reflexes, diminished influence of righting and balance reactions, and dissociation among body parts. If proximal stability (e.g., co-contraction of the postural muscles of the trunk) is threatened by atypically low, high, or fluctuating muscle tone, controlled mobility is lost. In gait, a loss of control over the sequential timing of muscular activity may result in asymmetrical step and stride lengths. In addition, deviations may occur such as forward or backward trunk leaning, excessive or decreased hip or knee flexion, or altered dorsiflexion or plantarflexion.

In the presence of multiple muscle involvement or neurological deficits that affect balance, coordination, and muscle tone, the deviations observed and the analysis of these deviations will be more complex than indicated in the tables. Examples of gait patterns associated with impaired motor function, spasticity, and hypotonus follow.

An individual with spasticity (e.g., an individual with diplegic CP) may have a posteriorly tilted pelvis, forward flexion of the upper trunk, protracted scapulae, and somewhat excessive neck extension. Excessive hip flexion, with adduction and internal rotation (scissoring) may be observed during stance and may be accompanied by either excessive knee flexion or hyperextension. During late stance, plantarflexor weakness may allow the ankle to collapse into excess dorsiflexion and the knee into excess flexion. Alternatively, the ankle may be positioned in excess dorsiflexion in late stance as a means of accommodating a knee flexion contracture or hamstring tightness/spasticity.

In other individuals with hypertonia, hyperextension at the knee occurs in stance and may be accompanied by plantarflexion and inversion at the ankle and foot. Electromyographic (EMG) recordings may show prolonged activity in the quadriceps and in the gastrocnemius-soleus muscle group. The hamstring, gluteal, and dorsiflexor muscle groups may be reciprocally inhibited.

In individuals with low muscle tone (hypotonia) in the trunk, core stability (tonic extension and co-contraction of axial muscles) is diminished. The pelvis may be anteriorly tilted so that the upper trunk is slightly extended. The scapulae may be retracted and the head may be forward. During stance, the hip may be flexed and the knee may be hyperextended, accompanied by ankle plantarflexion. The foot may be pronated with the majority of body weight borne on the medial border. Frequently, these individuals show diminished longitudinal trunk rotation and sluggish trunk balance reactions. They tend to rely on protective extension reactions of the limbs to maintain balance. The staggering or stepping reactions of the LEs may be pronounced, stride length and step length may be uneven, and gait may be wide based and unsteady.

Although neurological gait patterns may be complex and an analysis of the causes may be difficult, a detailed OGA can provide valuable data. Generally, to analyze gait patterns in persons who have sustained neurological damage, the following preliminary questions must be asked:

1. What is the influence of abnormal tone (hypertonicity, hypotonicity, fluctuating tone) on joint position and movement?
2. How does the position of the head influence muscle tone, position, and movement?
3. How does weight-bearing influence muscle tone, position, and movement?
4. What is the influence of abnormal (obligatory) synergistic activity on position and movement?
5. What is the impact of weakness (paresis) on position and movement?
6. How do coordination impairments affect position and movement?
7. What is the influence of impaired balance reactions on position and movement?
8. How do contractures alter position and movement?
9. What is the impact of sensory loss (e.g., proprioceptive, visual, vestibular) on position and movement?
10. How do medications impact muscle tone and weakness throughout the day?
11. What is the impact of inappropriately timed activation of a muscle on walking (e.g., how does premature onset of the tibialis anterior or delayed cessation of the gastrocnemius impact foot clearance and forward progression during gait)?

Ambulation Profiles and Scales

Profiles and rating scales constitute types of gait analyses that often include both qualitative (observational) and quantitative (spatial and temporal) measures. Profiles and scales are used for a variety of reasons, such as examination of ambulation skills,[58,59] determination of the patient's need for assistance, identification of a change in a patient's status,[59] screening for identification of the patient's need for physical therapy,[60] and identification of individuals (e.g., older adults) who are at risk for falling.[27,28] Gait analyses of one type or another may be either the sole focus of a profile, or the gait analysis may constitute only a small portion of a broad examination profile that includes balance skills and other functional activities. One particular advantage of some of these profiles is that subordinate gait skills such as standing balance may be examined in individuals who may be unable to walk independently. Since many of these profiles were developed for use with specific populations, comparative data may be available to the therapist.

The following profiles have been selected for review in this chapter because they are in current use and have been examined for reliability and/or validity: the Functional Ambulation Profile;[58] the Emory Functional Ambulation Profile[61] and the Modified Emory Functional Ambulation Profile;[62] the Iowa Level of Assistance Score;[63] the Functional Independence Measure;[64] the Functional Independence Measure plus the Functional Assessment Measure;[65,66] the Community Balance and Mobility Scale;[59,67,68] the Gait Abnormality Rating Scale (GARS)[69] and the Modified GARS;[27] the Dynamic Gait Index;[70-72] the Functional Gait Assessment;[73-77] the High-Level Mobility Assessment Tool;[78-83] the Fast Evaluation of Mobility, Balance, and Fear;[84] the Figure-of-8 Walk Test;[85] the Tinetti Performance Oriented Mobility Assessment;[86] and the Walking Index for Spinal Cord Injury II.[87,88] Thresholds for clinical importance, including the minimal clinically important difference (MCID; i.e., the smallest change in an outcome considered important by a patient/clinician) and the minimal detectable change (MDC; i.e., the smallest level of change within a measure that corresponds with a change in ability) for many of these assessments are provided in Table 7.9.

Functional Ambulation Profile and Modifications

The *Functional Ambulation Profile* (FAP), developed by Arthur J. Nelson, PT, PhD, FAPTA, is designed to examine gait skills on a continuum from standing balance in the parallel bars to independent ambulation.[58] A stopwatch is used to measure the amount of time required either to maintain a position or perform a task. The test consists of three phases. In the first phase, the patient is asked to perform three tasks in the parallel bars: bilateral stance, uninvolved leg stance, and involved leg stance. In the second phase, the patient is asked to transfer weight from one LE to the other as rapidly as possible. In the third phase, the patient is asked to walk 20 ft (6 m) in the parallel bars, with an assistive device, and, if possible, independently. Wolf et al[61] evaluated the tool's reliability and validity in a study of 56 adults (28 with stroke and 28 without). The authors reported high interrater reliability (≥0.997) between two examiners who rated subjects' test performance. Construct validity was supported based on the test's ability to distinguish between those with and those without a stroke. Concurrent validity was demonstrated by strong correlations with participants' outcomes on the Timed 10-Meter Walk Test and the Berg Balance Scale.

A more recent version of the FAP developed at Emory University is called the *Emory Functional Ambulation Profile* (EFAP).[61] This profile differs from the original FAP in that five environmental challenges have been added. The individual may negotiate the environmental challenges with or without the use of orthotics or assistive devices.

The *Modified Emory Functional Ambulation Profile*[62] (mEFAP) incorporates manual assistance into the EFAP. Subtasks include 16.4-ft (5 m) walking on a hard floor and on a carpeted floor, rising from a chair, completing a 9.8-ft (3 m) walk and sitting back down, negotiating a standardized obstacle course, and ascending and descending five stairs. Liaw et al[89] evaluated the psychometric properties of the mEFAP in 40 individuals during the early phase of stroke recovery and 20 individuals with chronic strokes. The authors concluded that the mEFAP had good reliability, validity, and responsiveness for assessing walking function in patients with stroke undergoing rehabilitation.

Iowa Level of Assistance Scale

The *Iowa Level of Assistance Scale* (ILAS)[63] examines four functional tasks: getting out of bed, standing from bed, ambulating 15 ft (4.57 m), and walking up and down three steps. The patient's performance on the tasks is rated according to the following seven levels: (1) not tested for safety reasons; (2) activity attempted but not completed; (3) maximum assistance (therapist applies three or more points of contact); (4) moderate assistance (therapist applies two points of contact); (5) minimal assistance (therapist provides one point of contact); (6) standby assistance (no therapist contact but therapist not comfortable leaving patient); and (7) independence (therapist comfortable leaving room). Shields et al[63] examined the reliability, validity, and responsiveness of the ILAS in 86 inpatients recovering from total hip or knee replacements and reported good intratester (k = 0.79 to 0.90) and moderate intertester (k = 0.48 to 0.78) reliability. Scores on the tool correlated highly with Harris Hip Rating Scale scores (r = –.86).

Functional Independence Measure

The *Functional Independence Measure (FIM)* was created as part of a project funded by the National Institute of Handicapped Research, designed to develop the Guide for a Uniform Data Set for Medical Rehabilitation.[90] The FIM is an 18-item measure that examines elements of a patient's physical, psychosocial, and social function. The FIM is now proprietary and is the trademark of the Uniform Data System for Medical Rehabilitation, a division of the University of Buffalo Foundation Activities (see Chapter 8 for further discussion of the FIM). The FIM Locomotion: Walk/Wheelchair Guide is the portion of the document titled *The FIM System Clinical Guide, Version 5.2* related to gait and includes a seven-point level of assistance rating scale ranging from complete independence to total assistance (Table 7.10). A study designed to evaluate the accuracy of clinical judgments of patient functioning

(Text continued on page 253)

Table 7.9 Outcome Measures: Select Functional Assessments of Gait Capability

Outcome Measure and ICF Category	Description	Scoring	MCID/MDC
Timed Up and Go (TUG) **ICF: 2 (Activity)**	Test evaluates time (in seconds) required for individuals to rise from chair, walk 3 meters, turn around, walk back to the chair, and sit down. Test is completed with individuals wearing regular footwear and any assistive device normally used for ambulation.	NA	***Alzheimer's Disease***[277] Average age 81 (9) years; mild to severe Alzheimer's disease. MDC: 4.09 seconds ***Children with Down Syndrome***[278] MDC: 1.26 seconds ***Children with Cerebral Palsy***[279] Age range: 3–10 years. *By motor function* MCD, GMFCS I: 1.4 seconds MCD, GMFCS II: 2.87 seconds MCD, GMFCS III: 8.74 seconds MCID, GMFCS I: 1.12 seconds MCID, GMFCS III: 4.65 seconds *By age* MCD, 3–5 years old: 1.59 seconds MCD, 6–10 years old: 0.95 seconds ***Chronic Stroke***[158] Average age 58 (6) years; 6–46 months post-stroke. MDC: 2.9 seconds Smallest Real Difference (SRD): 23%[158] ***Parkinson's Disease***[97,280,281] Average age 65 (8) years (range 40–80 years); Hoehn-Yahr stages I to III. MDC: 4.85 seconds[280] Average age 68 (12) years; Hoehn-Yahr stages I to III. MDC: 3.5 seconds[97] Average age 71 (12) years; Hoehn-Yahr stages I to IV; mean disease duration 14 (6) years. MDC: 11 seconds[281] ***Pregnant Women with Pelvic Girdle Pain***[282] Average age 31 (2) years; week of pregnancy 28.7 (7.4). MDC: 1.16 seconds ***Spinal Cord Injury***[108,283] Acute traumatic or ischemic SCI; American Spinal Injury Association (ASIA) classification level A, B, C, D; C2–L1. MDC: 10.8 seconds or 30%
10-Meter Walk Test (10MWT) **ICF: 2 (Activity)**	Test evaluates walking speed as individuals walk 10 meters (32.8 feet) without assistance. Time is measured only in middle 6 meters to allow for acceleration and deceleration. Alternatively,	NA	***Geriatrics***[284] Average age 78 (8) years. MCID: Small meaningful change: 0.05 m/s Substantial meaningful change: 0.10 m/s ***Hip Fracture***[285] Average age 79 (8) years (range 64–95 years). MDC: 0.17 m/s

Table 7.9 Outcome Measures: Select Functional Assessments of Gait Capability—cont'd

Outcome Measure and ICF Category	Description	Scoring	MCID/MDC
	individuals can traverse 14 meters with middle 10 meters timed. Speed calculated by dividing distance covered by time required for individual to walk given distance. Test can be performed at preferred walking speed or at fastest possible speed. Assistive devices may be used if normally required for ambulation.		***Parkinson's Disease***[281] Average age 71 (12) years; Hoehn-Yahr stages I to IV; mean disease duration 14 (6) years. MDC, comfortable gait speed: 0.18 m/s MDC, fastest gait speed: 0.25 m/s ***Pregnant Women with Pelvic Girdle Pain***[282] Average age 31 (2) years; week of pregnancy 28.7 (7.4). MDC: 0.47 seconds ***Spinal Cord Injury***[108,283,286-288] Incomplete SCI (<12 months post-injury); C2–L1. MDC: 0.13 m/s[108,283,286,287] Chronic motor incomplete SCI (greater than 6 months post-injury); average age 42 years. MCID: 0.06 m/s[288] ***Stroke***[289,290] Acute stroke (≤45 days); average age 64 (13) years. MCID, comfortable gait speed: 0.16 m/s[289] Acute stroke (average of 35 [18] days post-stroke); average age 67 (14) years MDC: All participants: 0.30 m/sec[290] Those who required physical assistance to walk: 0.07 m/sec[290] Those who could walk without assistance: 0.36 m/sec[290] *speed measured over middle 5 meters of a 9-meter walk at comfortable pace Subacute stroke; average age 70 (10) years. MCID: Small meaningful change: 0.06 m/s[284] Substantial meaningful change: 0.14 m/s[284] ***Traumatic Brain Injury***[291,292] Median age 23 years (range 15–50 years). MDC: 0.05 m/s [291] MCID, comfortable gait speed: 0.15 m/s [292] MCID, fastest gait speed: 0.25 m/s[292]

Continued

Table 7.9 Outcome Measures: Select Functional Assessments of Gait Capability—cont'd

Outcome Measure and ICF Category	Description	Scoring	MCID/MDC
6-Minute Walk Test (6MWT) **ICF: 2 (Activity)**	Test evaluates walking endurance and aerobic capacity as individuals cover as far a distance as possible over 6 minutes. Assistive devices may be used if normally required for ambulation.	NA	***Alzheimer's Disease***[277] Average age 81 (9) years; mild to severe Alzheimer's disease. MDC: 33.5 m (109.9 ft) ***Chronic Obstructive Pulmonary Disease (COPD)***[293,294] Average age 67 years MDC and MCID: 54 m (177.2 ft) ***Geriatrics***[284] Three groups of older adults with average age 78 (8), 74 (6), and 70 (10), last group comprised of stroke patients. MDC: 50 m (164 ft) ***Osteoarthritis, Hip or Knee***[295] Average age 64 (11) years MDC: 61.3 m (201.1 ft) ***Parkinson's Disease***[281] Average age 71 (12) years; Hoehn-Yahr stages I to IV; mean disease duration 14 (6) years. MDC: 82 m (269 ft) ***Spinal Cord Injury***[283,286,287] Incomplete SCI (<12 months post-injury); C2–L1. MDC: 45.8 m (150 ft) or 22% change ***Chronic Stroke***[158,296] Average age 67 (10) years; average time since onset 1.8 (0.9) years. MCID: 34.4 m (112.9 ft)[296] Average age 58 (6) years; average time since onset 6–46 months. MDC: 36.6 m (120 ft) or 13% change[158]
2-Minute Walk Test (2MWT) **ICF: 2 (Activity)**	Test evaluates walking endurance and aerobic capacity as individuals walk as far as possible in 2 minutes. Assistive devices may be used if normally required for ambulation.	NA	***Adults with Neurological Disorders***[297] Average age 47 (13) years; time since onset of disease 6 (7) years; 12 different diagnoses, including myelopathy, stroke, tumor, Huntington's disease, and head injury. MDC: 16.4 m (53.8 ft) ***Children with Disabilities***[298] Children aged 6–12 years with neuromuscular disorders, including cerebral palsy and muscular dystrophy. MCID: Entire group: 23.2 m (76.12 ft) Children walking with aids: 15.7 m (51.51 ft) Children walking independently: 16.6 m (54.46 ft) ***General Population***[299] Average age 46 (18) years (range 18–85 years).

Table 7.9 Outcome Measures: Select Functional Assessments of Gait Capability—cont'd

Outcome Measure and ICF Category	Description	Scoring	MCID/MDC
			MDC: Men and women combined: 42.5 m (139.44 ft) Men only: 47.2 (154.86 ft) Women only: 33.4 m (109.58 ft) ***Geriatrics***[300] Average age 87 (6) years (range 76–95 years); long-term care residents. MDC: 12.2 m to 14.7 m (40 ft to 48.2 ft) ***Lower-Extremity Amputation***[301] Average age 66 (13) years; individuals > 2 years post-unilateral amputation. MDC: 34.3 meters (112.5 ft) ***Multiple Sclerosis***[302] Average age 66 (13) years; Expanded Disability Status Scale 1.5 to 6.5. MDC: 19.2 m (63 ft) ***Stroke***[303] Chronic stroke, average time since onset 40.2 (34.3) months, range from 6–145 months; average age 63.5 (10) years. MDC: 13.4 m (44 ft) *Ankle Plantarflexor Tone* Modified Ashworth Scale 0: 14.1 m (46.26 ft) Modified Ashworth Scale 1 to 1+: 13.4 m (43.96 ft) Modified Ashworth Scale ≥2: 13.1 m (42.98 ft)
Dynamic Gait Index (DGI) **ICF: 2 (Activity)**	Test evaluates gait ability and dynamic balance. Individuals perform 8 walking tests. Tasks include: **1.** Walk at steady state. **2.** Walk and change speeds. **3.** Walk with horizontal head turns. **4.** Walk with vertical head turns. **5.** Walk and pivot turn. **6.** Walk and step over obstacles. **7.** Walk and step around obstacles. **8.** Climb stairs. Assistive devices may be used if normally required for ambulation.	A 4-point ordinal scale, ranging from 0–3, is used to rate each task; 0 indicates lowest level of function. Total Score = 24 Interpretation < 19/24 = predictive of falls in the elderly > 22/24 = safe ambulators	***Community-Dwelling Elderly***[304,305] Average age 76 years (range 59–88 years); history of falls or near falls in previous 12 months. MDC: 2.9 points[304] Average age 76 (7) years. MCID: Total sample: 1.90 points[305] Those with initial scores < 21/24: 1.80 points[305] Those with initial scores ≥ 21/24: 0.60 points[305] ***Multiple Sclerosis***[98] Average age 42 (13) years; time since onset of disease 8.7 (8.8) years. MDC: 4.19–5.54 points ***Parkinson's Disease***[97] Average age 67.5 (11.6) years; Hoehn-Yahr stages I to III; disease duration between 2 months and 15 years. MDC: 2.9 points or 13.3%

Continued

Table 7.9 Outcome Measures: Select Functional Assessments of Gait Capability—cont'd

Outcome Measure and ICF Category	Description	Scoring	MCID/MDC
			***Stroke*[77]** Average age 61 (13) years; median time since stroke onset of 9 months (range 3–36 months). MDC: 4 points or 16.6% ***Chronic Stroke*[71]** Average age 62 (13) years; mean time since stroke onset of 4 (8) years (range 0.5–35 years). MDC: 2.6 points ***Vestibular Disorders*[306,307]** Average age 52 (13) years; time since onset of disease 28 (59) months; peripheral vestibular disorders. MDC: 3.2 points[306] *MDC calculated from information provided in the article. Average age 60 (18) years (range 18–95 years); balance and vestibular disorders. MDC: 4 points[307]
Modified Dynamic Gait Index (mDGI) **ICF: 2 (Activity)**	Test evaluates gait ability and dynamic balance. Individuals perform 8 walking tests. Tasks include: **1.** Walk at steady state. **2.** Walk and change speeds. **3.** Walk with horizontal head turns. **4.** Walk with vertical head turns. **5.** Walk and pivot turn. **6.** Walk and step over obstacles. **7.** Walk and step around obstacles. **8.** Climb stairs. Assistive devices may be used if normally required for ambulation.	A 4-point ordinal scale (ranging from 0–3) is used to rate gait pattern and time required to complete task, and a 3-point ordinal scale (ranging from 0–2) is used to rate level of assistance. The score 0 indicates lowest level of function. Total Score = 64	***Gait Abnormality*[308]** Average age 80 years (range 52–94 years). MDC, total score: 6.3 points MDC, gait pattern: 3.9 points MDC, time: 2.8 points MDC, level of assistance: 2 points ***Individuals without Disabilities*[308]** Average age 66 years (range 20–99 years). MDC, total score: 5.5 points MDC, gait pattern: 3.2 points MDC, time: 2.5 points MDC, level of assistance: 1.9 points ***Parkinson's Disease*[308]** Average age 71 years (range 41–88 years). MDC, total score: 6.8 points MDC, gait pattern: 3.7 points MDC, time: 3 points MDC, level of assistance: 1.5 points ***Stroke*[308]** Average age 64 years (range 24–93 years). MDC, total score: 7.4 points MDC, gait pattern: 3.8 points MDC, time: 3.4 points MDC, level of assistance: 2.8 points ***Traumatic Brain Injury*[308]** Average age 54 years (range 15–91 years). MDC, total score: 7.4 points

Table 7.9 Outcome Measures: Select Functional Assessments of Gait Capability—cont'd

Outcome Measure and ICF Category	Description	Scoring	MCID/MDC
			MDC, gait pattern: 4.1 points MDC, time: 3.4 points MDC, level of assistance: 2.7 points ***Vestibular Disorders***[308] Average age 67 years (range 23–94 years). MDC, total score: 7.2 points MDC, gait pattern: 3.9 points MDC, time: 3.6 points MDC, level of assistance: 2.3 points
Functional Gait Assessment (FGA) **ICF: 2 (Activity)**	This modification of DGI also evaluates gait ability and dynamic balance. Individuals perform 10 walking tests. Tasks include: **1.** Walk at steady state. **2.** Walk and change speeds. **3.** Walk with horizontal head turns. **4.** Walk with vertical head turns. **5.** Walk and pivot turn. **6.** Walk and step over obstacles. **7.** Walk with narrow base of support. **8.** Walk with eyes closed. **9.** Walk backward. **10.** Climb stairs. Assistive devices may be used if normally required for ambulation.	A 4-point ordinal scale, ranging from 0–3, is used to rate each task; 0 indicates lowest level of function. Total Score = 30	***Geriatrics***[309] Community-dwelling adults referred to physical therapy for balance training; average age 79 (7) years (range 60–96 years). MCID: 4 points ***Parkinson's Disease***[310] Average age 72 (9) years; Hoehn-Yahr stages I to III; average falls reported over 6 months 1.4 (1.5). MDC: 4 points ***Stroke***[77] Average age 61 (13) years; median time since stroke onset of 9 months (range 3–36 months). MDC: 4.2 points or 14.1%; clinically: 5 points ***Vestibular Disorders***[307] Average age 60 (18) years (range 18–95 years); balance and vestibular disorders. MDC: 6 points
Tinetti Performance Oriented Mobility Assessment (Tinetti; TMT; POMA) **ICF: 2 (Activity)**	Test evaluates gait and balance ability. It composes a 9-item balance portion and a 7-item gait portion. Gait tasks include assessment of walk initiation; step characteristics (e.g., length, height, symmetry, and continuity); walking path; trunk motion and posture; and walking stance. Assistive devices may be used if normally required for ambulation.	Items assessed using 3-point (0–2) or 2-point (0–1) scale; highest score indicates independence with each test item. Total assessment score = 28; Gait assessment score = 12	***Knee Osteoarthritis***[311] Average age 51 (6) years; onset of disease 3.7 (2.4) years. MDC, total assessment: 0.97 points MDC, balance portion: 0.75 points MDC, gait portion: 0.63 points ***Older Adults***[312] Average age 83 (7) years; individuals residing in long-term self-care and nursing care facilities. MDC, individual assessment: 4–4.2 points MDC, group assessment: 0.7–0.8 points ***Stroke***[102] Acute stroke (average of 8 [5] days post-stroke); average age 75 (11) years. MDC: 6 points

Continued

Table 7.9 Outcome Measures: Select Functional Assessments of Gait Capability—cont'd

Outcome Measure and ICF Category	Description	Scoring	MCID/MDC
Walking Index for Spinal Cord Injury (WISCI II) **ICF: 2 (Activity)**	Index measures walking function of individuals with acute or chronic spinal cord injury by scoring ability to walk 10 meters.	Index ranges from 0–20, where 0 represents most severe impairment. Scores increase as individuals are able to walk with a combination of independence from use of unilateral or bilateral orthotics, 1 or 2 assistive devices, and physical assistance from 1 or 2 helpers.	***Chronic Spinal Cord Injury***[106] Average age 43 (14) years; time since injury 6 (6) years MDC: 1 point

Table 7.10 The FIM® Instrument Seven-Level Scoring System for Locomotion—Version 5.2

LOCOMOTION: WALK/WHEELCHAIR: Includes walking, once in a standing position, or if using a wheelchair, once in a seated position, on a level surface. Performs safely. Indicate the most frequent mode of locomotion (Walk or Wheelchair). If both are used about equally, code: "Both."

NO HELPER

7 Complete Independence—Subject *walks* a minimum of *150* ft (50 m) without assistive devices. Does not use a wheelchair. Performs safely.

6 Modified Independence—Subject *walks* a minimum of *150* ft (50 m) but uses a brace (orthosis) or prosthesis on leg, special adaptive shoes, cane, crutches, or walkerette; takes more than reasonable time or there are safety considerations. *If not walking,* subject operates manual or motorized wheelchair independently for a minimum of *150* ft (50 m); turns around; maneuvers the chair to a table, bed, toilet; negotiates at least a 3% grade; maneuvers on rugs and over door sills.

5 Exception (Household Ambulation)—Subject walks only short distances (a minimum of *50* ft or 17 m) *independently* with or without a device. Takes more than reasonable time, or there are safety considerations, or operates a manual or motorized wheelchair independently only short distances (a minimum of *50* ft or 17 m).

HELPER

5 Supervision

If walking, subject requires standby supervision, cueing, or coaxing to go a minimum of *150* ft (50 m).

If not walking, requires standby supervision, cueing, or coaxing to go a minimum of *150* ft (50 m) in wheelchair.

4 Minimal Contact Assistance—Subject performs 75% or more of locomotion effort to go a minimum of *150* ft (50 m).

3 Moderate Assistance—Subject performs 50% to 74% of locomotion effort to go a minimum of *150* ft (50 m).

2 Maximal Assistance—Subject performs 25% to 49% of locomotion effort to go a minimum of *50* ft (17 m). Requires assistance of one person only.

1 Total Assistance—Subject performs less than 25% of effort, or requires assistance of two people, or does not walk or wheel a minimum of *50* ft (17 m).

Comment: If the subject requires an assistive device for locomotion: wheelchair, prosthesis, walker, cane, AFO, adapted shoe, etc., the Walk/Wheelchair score can never be higher than level 6. The mode of locomotion (Walk or Wheelchair) must be the same on admission and discharge. If the subject changes mode of locomotion from admission to discharge (usually wheelchair to walking), record the admission mode and scores based on the *more frequent mode of locomotion at discharge.*

found that bias and poor judgment of a patient's functional level played a significant role in 50 rehabilitation professionals' ratings of patient functioning. The authors of the study suggested that blind ratings of the FIM and training in eliminating bias would improve accuracy.[91]

Functional Assessment Measure

The 12-item *Functional Assessment Measure (FAM)* was developed by a multidisciplinary group of clinicians at Santa Clara Valley Medical Center, San Jose, California,[65,92] to provide a measure of disability that reflected the communication, psychosocial adjustment, and cognitive functions of populations of individuals who sustained traumatic brain injury (TBI) and stroke. The 12 items are: swallowing, car transfer, community access, reading, writing, speech intelligibility, emotional status, adjustment to limitations, employability, orientation, attention, and safety judgment. The FAM uses a 7-point rating scale modeled after the FIM to examine the individual's level or degree of independence, amount of assistance required, use of adaptive or assistive devices, and percentage of tasks completed successfully.[65,92]

The 12 items of the FAM have been combined with the 18-item FIM to produce the FIM + FAM with the intent of providing more detailed data for TBI[66] and stroke populations. The FIM and FIM + FAM total scales are psychometrically similar measures of global disability, whereas the Barthel Index, FIM, and FIM + FAM motor scales are similar measures of physical disability.[93] However, in a study of 376 patients with stroke in Canadian inpatient rehabilitation units who were concurrently given the FIM and the FAM, the results of a Rasch analysis showed that in the motor domain, only the FAM community access item was more difficult for subjects to accomplish than the FIM items. In the cognitive domain, the only FAM item that extended the range of the FIM was the one assessing employability. In light of the results, Linn et al[94] concluded that adding the FAM items to the FIM reduced test efficiency and provided only minimal protection against ceiling effects of the FIM.

Community Balance and Mobility Scale

The *Community Balance and Mobility Scale*[59] was developed to evaluate balance and mobility skills in individuals who have experienced mild to moderate TBI. The scale consists of 13 items that include opportunities to assess multitasking (e.g., walking and looking at a target placed to the right or left), sequencing of movements (crouching to pick up an object from the floor and then continuing to walk), and complex motor skills (laterally and rapidly moving sideways by crossing one foot over the other and having to respond to unexpected commands to change direction). Six items are performed on both the right and left side, each of which is rated on a 6-point scale from 0 (poorest performance) to 5 (best performance).[59,67] Although the tool was developed specifically to assess individuals who have sustained mild to moderate TBI, it also has been used to measure balance and mobility in community-dwelling individuals following a stroke and in those with varying severity of chronic obstructive pulmonary disease.[59,67,68]

Gait Abnormality Rating Scale and Modifications

The *Gait Abnormality Rating Scale* (GARS)[69] was designed to distinguish nursing home residents with a recent history of two or more falls from a control group of residents without a recent fall history. The test developers selected 16 features of the gait cycle and a scoring system, in which the features are scored on a 0 to 3 rating scale (0 = normal, 1 = mildly impaired, 2 = moderately impaired, and 3 = severely impaired). Among the 16 features rated, arm-swing amplitude, upper extremity (UE) and LE synchrony, and guardedness best distinguished fallers from other subjects. The distinguishing features could be used to identify residents at risk for falling. Time, space, and resources are often very limited in nursing homes, and the only expenses involved in administering the GARS include purchase of a digital video recorder, recording media, and the therapist's time to film, review, and rate the digital recordings. However, the GARS does not provide information regarding the type of falls (trips, slips, losing balance) sustained by this population.[69] Therefore, it is not helpful in determining the cause of falls.

The *Modified GARS (GARS-M)* is a seven-item version of the GARS and contains the following variables: (1) variability, (2) guardedness, (3) staggering, (4) foot contact, (5) hip ROM, (6) shoulder extension, and (7) arm–heel strike synchrony. These variables were selected for inclusion because they were found to be the most reliable in the original GARS. Scoring is the sum of the seven items; the total score represents a rank ordering for risk of falling based on the number of gait abnormalities recognized and the severity of any abnormality identified. A higher score is associated with a more abnormal gait. Similar to the GARS, the GARS-M scores distinguished between older adults with a history of falling and those individuals who had no fall history. The GARS-M has been deemed a good predictor for persons at risk for falls.[27]

Dynamic Gait Index

The *Dynamic Gait Index* (DGI) was designed to examine the ability to adapt gait to changes in task demands. The tool was initially developed for use in community-dwelling older adults with balance and vestibular disorders[95] but has since been used across a variety of ages and patient populations.[96] The DGI uses a 0 (severe impairment) to 3 (normal) scale to rate performance on eight items, including gait on even surfaces, gait while changing speeds, gait and head turns in a vertical or horizontal direction, stepping over obstacles, and gait with pivot turns and steps. Whitney et al[95] evaluated DGI scores and fall history in adults with vestibular disorders and reported that the odds of falling within the past 6 months were 2.58 fold higher with DGI scores of 19 or lower.[95] The tool has since been used to evaluate dynamic gait and balance in a variety of patient populations, including individuals with Parkinson's disease,[97] stroke,[71] and multiple sclerosis.[98]

The DGI was further revised to enhance measurement capability. The modified DGI includes the same eight tasks as the DGI but integrates an evaluation of three facets of performance for each task: gait pattern (24 total points), level of assistance (16 total points), and time required to complete each task (24 total points). This modification enables monitoring of changes in any of the three facets of walking performance, in contrast to the original scoring system based on gait pattern alone. The three facets can also be combined into a single total modified DGI score. Shumway-Cook et al reported that the modified DGI score explained approximately 80% of the total variance in walking performance in a large population of patients with impaired mobility due to varied neurological disorders and also individuals without known disabilities.[99]

The *Four-Item Dynamic Gait Index* consists of only half of the original eight DGI items (i.e., gait on level surfaces, changes in gait speed, and horizontal and vertical head turn activities).[72] It is faster to administer and displays adequate capacity to differentiate between individuals with and without balance and vestibular disease.

Functional Gait Assessment

The *Functional Gait Assessment* (FGA) is another modification of the original eight-item DGI. It was developed to address some of the ceiling effect attributes of the DGI when used with individuals with vestibular disorders and to clarify instructions and operational definitions associated with administering the tool.[76] Seven of the eight original DGI tasks were preserved, and three new items were added: gait with a narrow base of support, ambulating backward, and gait with eyes closed. In a study assessing age-referenced norms for FGA performance in independently living adults between the ages of 40 and 89 years, the tool was found to have excellent interrater reliability (ICC = 0.93).[75] In addition, intrarater and interrater reliability were deemed adequate given seven physical therapists' and three physical therapist students' repeated ratings of six patients with vestibular disorders (total FGA score reliability: intrarater = 0.83; interrater = 0.84).[76] Use of a threshold FGA score of 20/30 or less correctly predicted the unexplained falls experienced by six participants during a 6-month follow-up period in a study of community-dwelling 60- to 90-year-olds.[74] However, the authors recommend use of a threshold score of 22/30 or less as a more conservative criterion for those at risk for falls. The FGA has been used in studies of specific patient populations, including Parkinson's disease[73] and stroke.[77]

High-Level Mobility Assessment Tool

The *High-Level Mobility Assessment Tool* (HiMAT) was designed to measure high-level mobility skills required for employment and social roles, as well as for leisure and sporting activities for younger adults recovering from a TBI.[80] The tool consists of 13 items and requires only a stopwatch, a 14-step staircase, inked moleskin markers, a brick-sized object, and a tape measure to complete.[78,100] Tasks assessed include walking (forward, backward, on toes, over an obstacle, in a figure 8), running, a run stop, skipping, hopping forward, bounding (affected and non-affected), and going up and down stairs with and without a railing. All items are marked on a 5-point scale (0 = unable to perform to 4 = performing item normally) except for two stair items that are rated on a 6-point scale (0 to 5). The maximum achievable score is 54. The tool is only appropriate for patients who can ambulate independently for at least 20 meters without an assistive device. Thus it is most appropriate for higher functioning patients, such as those in the latter stages of an inpatient rehabilitation program or already living in the community. Interrater reliability and test-retest reliability are high (both ICCs = 0.99).[81] Between-day testing scores demonstrated a small improvement over the 24 hours (1 point), which is suggestive of improved performance with test familiarity. This highlights the importance of allowing patients an opportunity to practice the test at least once before scoring.

The original 13-item HiMAT has been revised to a shorter, faster-to-administer version that includes only eight items: walk (forward, backward, toes, obstacle), run, skip, hop, and bound on the nonaffected LE.[83] One key difference between the two versions is that stair items were eliminated. This addresses a challenge clinicians experience when trying to administer the 13-item HiMAT test in environments lacking a 14-step staircase. Because it was the easiest item on the original scale, elimination of stairs is not expected to influence assessment of high-level mobility skills. However, it is possible that the tool may be more susceptible to a floor effect because it is less able to distinguish between abilities of more severely disabled individuals.

Fast Evaluation of Mobility Balance and Fear

The *Fast Evaluation of Mobility, Balance, and Fear* (FEMBAF) is another instrument designed to identify risk factors, functional performance, and factors that hinder mobility.[84] It consists of a 22-item risk factor questionnaire and an 18-item performance component, which includes, among other measures, stair ascent and descent, stepping over an obstacle, and one-legged standing. Di Fabio and Seay[84] reported that the FEMBAF served as a valid and reliable measurement of risk factors, functional performance, and factors that hinder mobility in their study of 35 community-dwelling older adults.

Figure-of-8 Walk Test

Many measures of overground walking focus primarily on gait performed along a straight path (e.g., the 5-meter walk test). In contrast, the Figure-of-8 Walk Test (F8W)[85] was developed to assess both curved and straight path walking in older adults with walking difficulties. The number of steps, total time, and smoothness of movement are examined as an individual completes a single figure-of-8 walk around two cones spaced 5 ft apart (Fig. 7.4). In a study of performance on the F8W in 51 older community-dwelling adults with walking difficulty, Hess et al[85] reported significant correlations between the time to complete the F8W and overground gait speed, the GARS-M score, select physical function and efficacy measures, step length and width variability, and measures of executive function (i.e., the Trail Making Test B, Trails B). The number of steps required to complete the F8W correlated significantly with gait speed, select physical function and efficacy measures, step width variability, and performance on the Trails B. Movement smoothness correlated significantly only with step width variability.

Tinetti Performance Oriented Mobility Assessment

The Tinetti Performance Oriented Mobility Assessment (POMA) was initially developed to be administered to older adults but has since been used with different patient populations, such as those with Parkinson's disease[101] and stroke.[102] The test consists of gait and balance items and takes approximately 15 minutes to administer. The gait assessment evaluates body posture (i.e., trunk motion), step characteristics, and walking initiation, path, and stance while individuals walk across the examination room or a hallway at a self-selected pace and also at a faster speed using usual assistive devices/orthoses.

Walking Index for Spinal Cord Injury II

The Walking Index for Spinal Cord Injury II (WISCI II) is a valid and reliable tool that was created to evaluate walking ability of adults and children with spinal cord injury (paraplegia and tetraplegia) based on the extent and nature of assistance (combination of orthoses, assistive devices, and physical assistance) required to walk 10 meters at self-selected speed.[103-108] The test takes up to about 15 minutes to administer, depending on the individual's capacity and the need to don orthoses. The WISCI II is generally used in conjunction with other measures (e.g., 10-Meter Walk Test) to provide a more comprehensive quantification of walking function in individuals with SCI.[109-111]

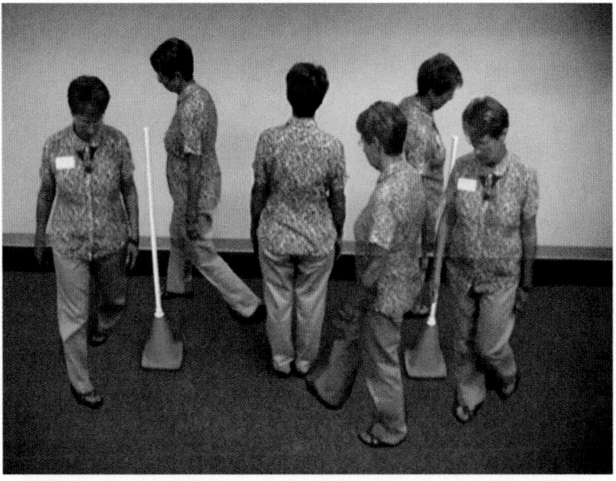

Figure 7.4 Individual performing the Figure-of-8 Walk Test, a tool developed to quantify walking ability in older adults with mobility disorders. Time to complete, number of steps, and smoothness of movement are used to score an individual's walking performance of a single figure-of-8 path around two cones spaced 5 feet apart.

Kinematic Quantitative Gait Analysis

Kinematic quantitative gait analysis is used to obtain information on spatial and temporal gait variables, as well as motion patterns. The data obtained through these analyses are quantifiable and therefore provide the therapist with baseline data that can be used to plan treatment programs and evaluate progress toward goals or goal attainment. The fact that the data are quantifiable is important because third-party payers are demanding that therapists use measurable parameters when examining patient function, establishing treatment strategies, and documenting outcomes.

Spatial and temporal measures may be critical factors in determining a patient's independence in ambulation. For example, in a study by Graham et al[112] of 174 ambulatory adults aged 65 years and older who were admitted to a medical-surgical unit, a walking velocity (69 ft/min [21 m/min]) was identified as a meaningful threshold to differentiate those capable of independent ambulation in a hospital setting from those requiring assistance. When considering community environments, an individual may need to attain a certain gait speed to cross a local street within the time allotted by a crossing light or may need to walk a certain distance to shop in the local supermarket.

In a study of walking capability of individuals greater than 3 months post-stroke, Perry et al[113] established that walking speed was a valid predictor of community walking status. Speeds of less than 79 ft/min (24 m/min) predicted household walking, and speeds between 79 and 157 ft/min (24 and 48 m/min) predicted limited community walking status. The ability to walk faster than 157 ft/min (48 m/min) predicted unlimited community walking. It is interesting to note that the mean velocity of the community ambulators was only 60% of the 262 ft/min (80 m/min) average velocity of typical, nondisabled adults.[34] This slower velocity is sufficient for many typical activities that individuals recovering from a stroke may need to perform, yet is less than the normal capacity required to cross a wide commercial street within the traffic signal time.[114] More recent research by Fulk et al[115] demonstrated that the gait speed values developed by Perry et al may overestimate actual walking activity in the home and community. The authors reported that for stroke survivors, a comfortable gait speed of 96 ft/min (29 m/min) discriminated between home and community ambulators, and a comfortable gait speed of 183 ft/min (56 m/min) discriminated between limited community and full community ambulators.[115]

Therapists need to survey the community to determine the distance and time requirements for accessing stores and public buildings before making a judgment about a patient's functional ambulation status. Considering the large footprints of many supermarkets, club warehouses, and hardware stores, individuals should be able to ambulate for a minimum of about 2,000 ft (600 m) without sitting down in order to independently ambulate in the community.[116] Robinett and Vondran[117] found that target goals on a sample of gait analysis forms were low compared to distance and velocity requirements for crossing the street found in a community survey. Walsh et al[118] reported that individuals 1 year after total knee arthroplasty achieved more than 80% of the normal walking speeds of their age- and gender-matched counterparts. However, for 62% of the females and 25% of the males, the normal walking speed attained would not be sufficient to cross a street intersection safely.

Spatial and Temporal Variables

The variables measured in a quantitative gait analysis are listed and described in Table 7.11. Because spatial and temporal variables are affected by a number of factors such as age,[119-123] gender,[124,125] height and weight,[126,127] level of physical activity,[128,129] and level of maturation,[130] attempts have been made to take some of these factors into account. Ratios, such as stride-length divided by functional leg length, may be used to normalize for differences in patients' leg lengths. Step length divided by the subject's height is a method sometimes used to normalize differences among patients' heights. In an attempt to control for both height and weight, body weight is divided by standing height to yield the body mass index. Other ratios are used to assess symmetry, for example, right swing time divided by left swing time and swing time divided by stance time. Sutherland et al[130] listed the ratio of pelvic span to ankle spread as one way to determine development of mature gait in children.

Measurement of Spatial and Temporal Variables

The techniques and equipment required for measurement of spatial and temporal variables range from simple to complex. The time requirements also vary, and the therapist must be familiar with different methods of examining these variables in order to select the method most appropriate to each situation. Before selecting a measurement method, the therapist must understand the variable in question and how that variable is related to the patient's gait.

Simple Methods of Measuring Spatial and Temporal Variables

Measurement of spatial variables such as degree of foot angle, width of base of support (BOS), step length, and stride length can be determined simply and inexpensively by recording the patient's footprints during gait. Simple methods of recording footprints include either the application of paints, ink, or chalk to the bottom of the patient's foot or shoe. For example, ink-soaked patches[131] and felt-tipped markers[132] have been attached to the bottom or back of patient's shoes to measure variables such as step length, stride length, step width, and foot angle.

Another way of obtaining step length and stride length data is by placing a grid pattern on the floor.[133] Masking tape is placed on the floor to create a straight-line grid pattern about 1 ft (30 cm) wide and 32 ft (10 m) long. The tape is marked off in 1-in (3-cm) increments for its entire length, and the segments are numbered consecutively so that the patient's heel strikes can be identified. The therapist then calls out the heel strike locations from the numbers on the grid pattern into a tape recorder.

Many variables, such as velocity, stride length, step length, and cadence, may be calculated by using a stopwatch to measure the elapsed time required for a patient to walk a known distance and recording the number of right and left steps during that same period (see Table 7.11). If assessing variables across a short distance (e.g., 20 or 30 ft [6 or 10 m]), patients are often positioned a few steps before the "start line" so that they can achieve a steady state for the data collection.[82,131] They are also encouraged to walk a few steps beyond the "finish line." The "rolling start and finish" mitigates the influence of slow velocities at the initiation and termination of a walk on overall values compared to the "standing start and finish."[82]

Todd et al[123] tested 84 typically developing children (41 girls and 43 boys) aged 13 months to 12 years, and analyzed data from more than 200 other children aged 11 months to 16 years. A two-dimensional gait graph was developed that provides a visual record of a child's walking performance. Although the gait graph is similar in appearance to graphs used for height and weight, it shows norms for gait dimensions of cadence and stride length adjusted by height.

Two relatively simple and standardized methods that have been used to quantify walking speed in the clinical setting are the *6-Minute Walk Test* (6MWT) and the *10-Meter Walk Test* (10MWT). A stopwatch and tape measure are the tools required to complete the tests. A form for recording temporal and spatial gait parameters is presented in Appendix 7.B.

6-Minute Walk Test

In the 6MWT,[134,135] the distance covered walking for 6 minutes is determined. Whereas the tool was initially used as a measure of endurance and exercise capacity for individuals with cardiac and pulmonary pathology,[134,135] it has since been used to assess walking endurance in clients with a variety of underlying conditions, including Parkinson's disease,[136] acquired brain injury,[137] stroke,[138] and cerebral palsy.[139] One protocol for performing the 6MWT includes asking clients to walk as far as they can at their usual pace for 6 minutes

Table 7.11 Gait Variables: Quantitative Gait Analysis

Variable	Description
Speed	A scalar quantity that has magnitude but not direction.
Free speed	A person's normal walking speed.
Slow speed	A speed slower than a person's normal speed.
Fast speed	A rate faster than normal.
Cadence	The number of steps taken per unit of time (e.g., steps/minute). $$\text{Cadence} = \frac{\text{number of steps}}{\text{time}}$$ A simple method of measuring cadence is by counting the number of steps taken in a given amount of time. The only equipment necessary is a stopwatch, paper, and pencil. The average cadence of adult women (117 steps/min) is slightly higher than of adult men (111 steps/min).[34]
Velocity	A measure of a body's motion in a given direction.
Linear velocity	The rate at which a body moves in a straight line.
Angular velocity	The rate of rotation of a body segment around an axis.
Walking velocity	The rate of linear forward motion of the body. This is measured in either centimeters per second or meters per minute. To obtain a person's walking velocity, divide the distance traversed by the time required to complete the distance. $$\text{Walking velocity} = \frac{\text{distance}}{\text{time}}$$ Walking velocity may be affected by age, level of maturation, height, gender, type of footwear, and weight. Also, velocity may affect cadence, step, stride length, and foot angle as well as other gait variables. The average self-selected walking velocity of 20- to 85-year-old males (86 m/min) is slightly faster than similar aged females (77 m/min).[34]
Acceleration	The rate of change of velocity with respect to time. Body acceleration has been defined by Smidt and Mommens[313] as the rate of change of velocity of a point posterior to the sacrum. Acceleration is usually measured in meters per second per second (m/s^2).
Angular acceleration	The rate of change of the angular velocity of a body with respect to time. Angular acceleration is usually measured in radians per second per second ($radians/s^2$).
Stride time	The amount of time that elapses during one stride; that is, from one foot contact (heel strike if possible) until the next contact of the same foot (heel strike). Both stride times should be measured. Measurement is usually in seconds.
Step time	The amount of time that elapses between consecutive right and left foot contacts (heel strikes). Both right and left step times should be measured. Measurement is in seconds.
Stride length	The linear distance between two successive points of contact of the same foot. It is measured in centimeters or meters. The average stride length for normal adult males is 1.46 meters.[34] The average stride length for adult females is 1.28 meters.[34]
Swing time	The amount of time during the gait cycle that one foot is off the ground. Swing time should be measured separately for right and left extremities. Measurement is in seconds.
Double support time	The amount of time spent in the gait cycle when both lower extremities are in contact with the supporting surface. Measured in seconds.
Cycle time (stride time)	The amount of time required to complete a gait cycle. Measured in seconds.
Step length	The linear distance between two successive points of contact of the right and left lower extremities. Usually a measurement is taken from the point of heel contact at initial contact of one extremity to the point of heel contact of the opposite extremity. If a patient does not have a heel strike on one or both sides, the measurement can be taken from the heads of the first metatarsals. Measured in centimeters or meters.

Continued

Table 7.11 Gait Variables: Quantitative Gait Analysis—cont'd

Variable	Description
Width of walking base (step width)	The width of the walking base (base of support) is the linear distance (in the frontal plane) between one foot and the opposite foot. Measured in centimeters or meters.
Foot angle (degree of toe out or toe in)	The angle of foot placement with respect to the line of progression. Measured in degrees.
Bilateral stance time (for the FAP)	The length of time up to 30 seconds that a person can stand upright in the parallel bars bearing weight on both lower extremities.
Uninvolved stance time (for the FAP)	The length of time up to 30 seconds that an individual can stand in the parallel bars while bearing weight on the uninvolved lower extremity (involved extremity is raised off the supporting surface).
Involved stance time (for the FAP)	The length of time up to 30 seconds that an individual can stand in the parallel bars on the involved lower extremity (uninvolved lower extremity is raised off the supporting surface).
Dynamic weight transfer rate (for the FAP)	The rate at which an individual standing in the parallel bars can transfer weight from one extremity to another. Measured in seconds from the first lift-off to the last lift-off.
Parallel bar ambulation (for the FAP)	Length of time required for an individual to walk the length of the parallel bars as rapidly as possible. Two trials are averaged to obtain this measurement. Measurement is in seconds.

FAP = Functional Ambulation Profile.

while using their customary assistive devices and orthotics.[140] Clients walk in a tight oval path around two chairs spaced 18 meters apart, facilitating calculation of the overall distance traveled. Another protocol, used by the American Thoracic Society, emphasizes walking "as far as possible" while clients walk on a straight line and pivot around cones placed 30 meters apart.[141] Participants stop and rest as needed, but the stopwatch continues. Standardized encouragement is provided periodically. The final distance walked (in meters) is divided by either 6 to determine average velocity in m/min or by 360 if reporting as m/sec.

This simple test, used in combination with other physical performance and impairment measures (e.g., ROM and muscle strength), can either monitor decline or evaluate improvement associated with treatment interventions. Mossberg[137] found that the 6MWT was a reliable measure of functional ambulation (distance walked) for patients with acquired brain injury. Fulk et al[138] identified that the 6MWT score served as a significant predictor of the average number of steps taken per day by community-dwelling individuals with chronic stroke, accounting for 46% of the variance in community walking activity.

Numerous prediction equations have been developed to estimate the expected 6-minute walk distance based on factors such as height, age, weight, and heart rate; however, these equations have accounted for only 20% to 78% of the variance in 6MWT distances in individuals without known disability.[142-149] Variations in the procedures used across studies, as well as variability in the ages studied, likely contributed to differences in predicted outcomes for the distance walked in 6 minutes. Factors that appear to improve reliability between testing sessions include standardizing the instructions given to the patient, the type and amount of verbal encouragement, and the location of testing (e.g., a long corridor or a circular track).[82,142,150] These factors, as well as other patient characteristics such as age, height, weight, and even ethnicity,[142,146,149] should be considered when comparing a patient's value to normative data.

Fulk et al[115] reported that distance traversed during the 6MWT was the strongest predictor of home versus community ambulation capacity, and limited versus full/unlimited community ambulation status in a secondary analysis of walking activity data from two stroke trials. A 6MWT distance of at least 205 m discriminated between home and community ambulators, while the capacity to walk farther than at least 288 m differentiated between limited and unlimited community ambulators.

Alternative tests for individuals with limited endurance include the *1-Minute Walk Test*,[151-153] the *2-Minute Walk Test*,[154,155] and the *3-Minute Walk Test*.[70] A *12-Minute Walk Test* also is available for individuals with greater endurance.[135,154]

Timed Walk Tests (5 m, 10 m, and 30 m)

Timed walked tests measure how long it takes to walk a specified distance and then use these data to calculate an average walking speed. Different distances have been used, including 5 m,[156,157] 10 m,[155,158-160] and 30 m.[160] One common protocol for performing a 10-m timed walk test is to have the client ambulate across a 14-m walkway using his/her traditional assistive and LE orthotic devices.[140] The time (seconds) required to traverse the middle 10 m of the walkway is recorded with a stopwatch. Two repetitions are completed at the client's preferred comfortable speed and at a fast pace. Speed (m/sec) is calculated by dividing 10 m by the time (in seconds) required to traverse the path. To determine speed in m/min, the previously calculated speed is multiplied by 60. Average cadence and stride length also can be calculated by recording the number of steps required to traverse the 10 m. Physiological responses (e.g., heart rate, blood pressure, respiratory rate) can be monitored immediately before and after the walking trial.

Despite efforts to standardize the test, some variability still is evident in the published literature, including the path taken (i.e., straight line versus a turn), use of assistive devices, speed (self-selected comfortable versus fast), and use of a rolling start and finish (i.e., capacity to take a few steps before and after start and finish lines, respectively) versus a standing start and finish.[82] Thus, when comparing a patient's speed to published normative data, consideration should be given to procedures used.

Low-Cost Instrumentation for Quantifying Spatial and Temporal Variables

Accelerometers During walking, the body generates forces that can be measured using an accelerometer. These data can then be used to calculate spatial and temporal gait features such as cadence, step symmetry, step duration, and stride duration. The methods for measuring the acceleration forces vary widely (e.g., strain gauge, piezoresistive, capacitive, and piezoelectric), but in general, many of these devices provide an affordable, noninvasive, easy-to-apply means for quantifying select gait characteristics over extended periods (days to weeks) in the home and community.[161]

Triaxial accelerometers have been attached to the trunk in order to measure mean acceleration, cadences, and step and stride lengths.[162-166] Accelerometers have also been attached to the head and pelvis to determine acceleration patterns of these anatomical regions while subjects walked on different surfaces.[167] Simultaneous use of multiple accelerometers has enabled successful differentiation of locomotor activities. For example, one system used five accelerometers (one on each foot and thigh and one on the sternum) to differentiate walking speeds (slow, medium, and fast) and types of activities (e.g., walking, stair negotiation, running, and jumping) with a high level of accuracy (greater than 94%) in 69 participants free of any known impairments of the locomotor system.[168]

The accuracy of accelerometer data can be impacted by many factors.[161,168,169] Devices need to be oriented correctly in relation to the manufacturer's specifications; otherwise the acceleration signals may not correspond correctly with the direction of movement, and interpretation will be confounded. Significant adipose tissue, upper extremity (UE) movement to use assistive devices, or excessively loose mounting of the device can introduce movement artifact into the signal, again confounding interpretation. Finally, in patient populations, the acceleration signals may be altered if pathology disrupts normal foot-floor contact patterns or contributes to abnormal alignment of body parts (e.g., the impact of a persistent forward trunk lean on a trunk-mounted accelerometer in an individual with Parkinson's disease).[161]

The StepWatch Activity Monitor™ (SAM) is one example of a commercially available accelerometer.[170-174] It records the number of strides taken in 1-minute intervals during daily activities for up to 15 consecutive days. The SAM includes a sensor (custom accelerometer) that measures 0.30 × 2 × 0.80 in (7.5 × 50 × 20 mm) and weighs approximately 1.3 oz (37 g) (Fig. 7.5). The battery provides up to 4 to 5 years of continual use.[175] The case is contoured to fit just above the lateral malleolus and is attached by an elastic strap. A personal computer is used to set up the SAM for monitoring and also for downloading data to a computer. Michael et al[171] used the SAM to evaluate the walking capacity of adults in the chronic phase of stroke recovery and identified significantly reduced step frequency (mean = 2,837 steps/day) compared to sedentary older adults (5,000 to 6,000 steps/day).

A growing number of consumer-oriented activity monitors are available commercially, and preliminary research suggests that some devices may be useful for characterizing stepping capacity in select clinical populations. For example, Fitbit activity monitors have been used with a variety of populations to evaluate step count in laboratory environments and real-world environments.[176-182] Steps counted using the Fitbit (One and Zip) demonstrated excellent agreement (ICC = 0.88) with the number of visually counted steps during a 2-Minute Walk Test in a study of 32 community-dwelling older adults without known pathology.[183] Fulk et al[184] compared steps recorded during a 2-Minute Walk Test using the Fitbit Ultra to those documented from videotaped recordings of the same test and reported that in high-functioning people with chronic stroke and TBI, the Fitbit Ultra might provide a low-cost alternative for measuring step activity compared to other, more expensive, activity monitoring devices. Although the Fitbit Ultra's step count accuracy (ICC [2,1] = 0.73) exceeded those of other consumer-oriented activity monitors tested, including the Yamax Digi-Walker SW-701 (ICC [2,1] = 0.42) and the Nike+ FuelBand (ICC [2,1] = 0.20), the accuracy was below that of the SAM (ICC [2,1] = 0.97). On average, all devices (including the SAM) underestimated the actual number of steps taken.

Gyroscopes *Gyroscopes* are another type of instrument that may be used to estimate spatial and temporal gait parameters. The gyroscope measures the Coriolis acceleration of a vibrating triangular prism. The signal from the prism is proportional to the angular velocity. The instruments are light, portable, and relatively inexpensive.

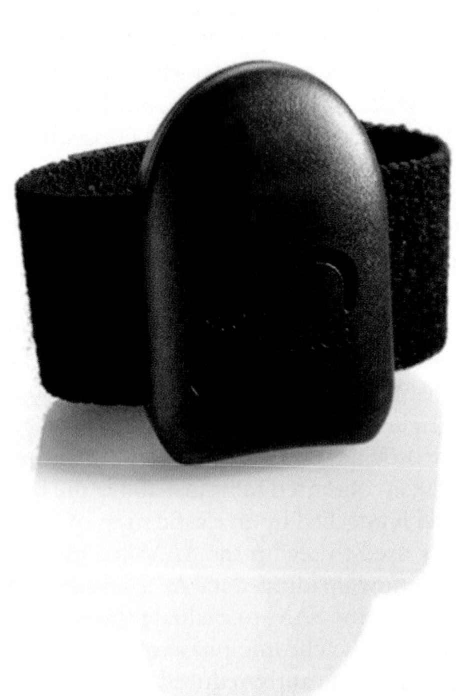

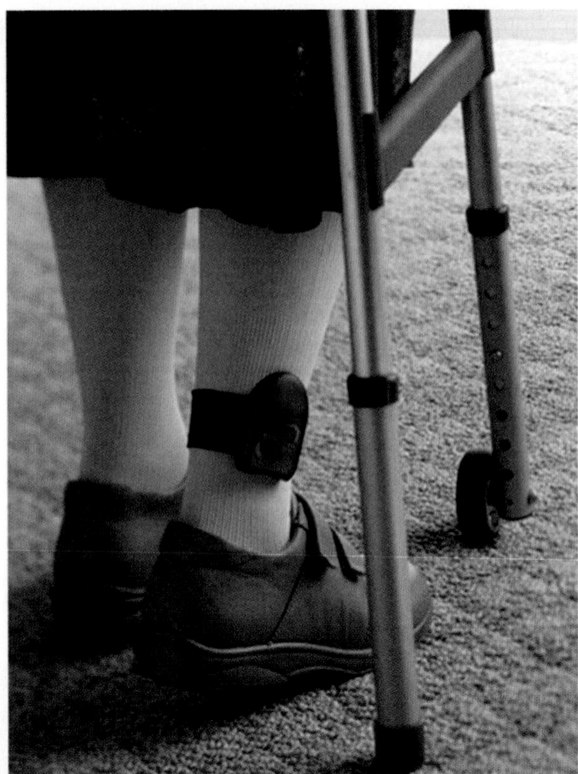

Figure 7.5 The Step Watch Activity Monitor 3® (SAM) is a pager-sized instrument worn at the ankle for long-term monitoring of gait function. *(Courtesy of Modus Health, Edmonds, WA 98020.)*

A single uniaxial gyroscope attached on the skin surface of the lower leg can provide data for calculating cadence, determining number of steps, and estimating stride length and walking speed.[185]

Kotiadis et al[186] developed an integrated system that included accelerometers, gyroscopes, and customized inertial algorithms to replace the footswitches often used to trigger drop foot stimulators. Testing and refinement was performed for an individual after stroke who used a footswitch-driven drop foot stimulator. The combination of accelerometer and gyroscope data was sufficient for defining gait phases and controlling the drop foot stimulator during walking and stair-negotiation activities.

Instrumented Systems for Determining Spatial and Temporal Gait Parameters

Commercially available walkways (e.g., GAITRite®, Strideway™, Zeno™) and footswitch systems (e.g., Krusen Limb Monitor, Stride Analyzer) can be used to measure spatial and temporal gait variables. Manufacturer contact information for select equipment is presented in Appendix 7.C.

Walkways Compared to more complex systems that require cameras and footswitches, instrumented walkways provide a reliable, valid, and relatively affordable means for rapidly quantifying spatial and temporal gait parameters.[187-193] These portable devices are used by clinics and research facilities to help classify and quantify the severity of a patient's disability and to guide and assess the effectiveness of treatment interventions. Two walkways widely available are the GAITRite® and the Zeno™ Walkway.

The GAITRite® is one example of a commercially available walkway system (Fig. 7.6). The 1/8-inch-thick, 2-foot wide, 16-foot-long portable walkway in this system contains 18,482 sensors embedded between a sheet of vinyl and a layer of rubber. Spatial and temporal parameters can be measured, as well as dynamic pressure mapping of footprints during walking. The pressure parameters measured include peak pressure, pressure time, and sectional integrated pressure over time. The walkway system can be used with or without shoes, orthoses, or walking aids, and the GAITRite software is capable of calculating spatial and temporal parameters and displaying them in graphs and tables.

In general, the GAITRite® provides a valid means for reliably documenting many gait-related temporal and spatial parameters.[189,190,192] Bilney et al[192] reported high correlations between values recorded on the GAITRite® mat and those recorded using the Clinical Stride Analyzer® for walking speed (0.99), stride length (0.99), and cadence (0.99) for 25 healthy adults walking at three speeds (self-selected, slow, and fast). The reliability of repeated measures appears better at self-selected and fast speeds, compared to slower speeds.[192] Decreased consistency across measurements was documented for BOS[190,191] and toe in and toe

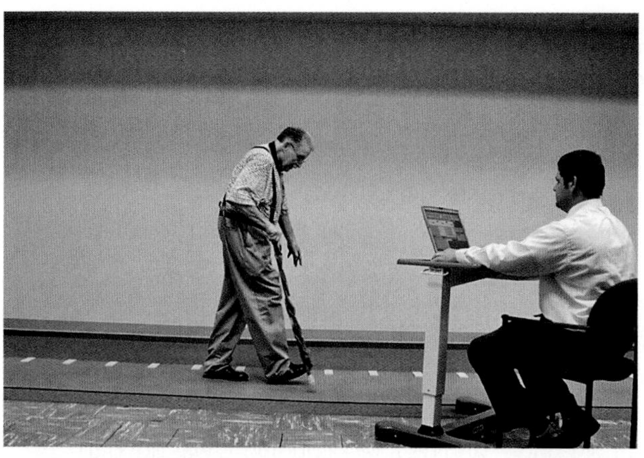

Figure 7.6 Individual with Parkinson's disease walking across the GAITRite® mat while temporal and spatial gait characteristics are recorded, including walking velocity, stride length and duration, cadence, and step length and duration. *(Courtesy of Movement and Neurosciences Center, Institute for Rehabilitation Science and Engineering, Madonna Rehabilitation Hospitals, Lincoln, NE 68506.)*

out variables,[190,191] particularly in older adults.[191] Strong concurrent validity also has been reported for temporal and spatial gait measures recorded in outpatients recovering from strokes, even when the UE was engaged in using an assistive device.[188] The Evidence Summary Table (Table 7.12) provides an overview of selected reliability and validity studies performed using the GAITRite® mat.

The portable Zeno™ Walkway system (Fig. 7.7) is available in 8- to 52-foot lengths and varying widths (2, 3, or 4 feet). One key feature relative to other commercially available instrumented walkways is the availability of wider mats that allow use with gait tests requiring turning maneuvers. The Zeno™ walkway integrates 16 levels of pressure sensors (each 1 cm in diameter) to detect gait characteristics. Spatial (e.g., step length, step width, toe in/out angle) and temporal (e.g., velocity, single limb, and double limb support time) parameters can be displayed side by side with videos and images from an integrated video camera system. The software can also be used to calculate an estimated center of mass and to detect pressure applied through an assistive device (e.g., walker or cane).

Table 7.12 Evidence Summary Table

Studies assessing the reliability and validity of the GAITRite® System's measurement of temporal and spatial gait variables

	Graser et al (2016)[314]
Design	Cross-sectional
Level of Evidence	IV
Subjects	Children aged 13 ± 3.6 years (9 girls, 21 boys) with gait disorders who were participating in inpatient rehabilitation. Diagnoses included cerebral palsy, stroke, traumatic brain injury, demyelination of central nervous system, astrocytoma, postinfectious encephalopathy, medulla blastoma, transverse myelopathy, and ataxia.
Intervention	Children performed the 10MWT (preferred and maximum speeds) and the 6MWT during two separate sessions while GAITRite® was used to record stride characteristics simultaneously (i.e., velocity, cadence, double support [percentage of the gait cycle], step length, normalized velocity [ratio of velocity and leg length], step-extremity-ratio [ratio of leg- and step-length], and step time).
Results	The median Intraclass Correlation Coefficient (ICC) value calculated from all GAITRite® variables was 0.93. The lowest ICC values occurred for step length (less affected side) during 10MWT max speed (0.61) and for step time (more affected side) and extremity-step-ratio (for the less affected side) during 10MWT preferred speed (0.81). The highest ICC values occurred for step length symmetry during 10MWT preferred speed (0.95) and for step length (most affected side and left side) during 6MWT (0.97).
Comments	The authors concluded that timed walking tests as well as temporal and spatial gait parameters obtained from the GAITRite® system appeared reliable in children with neurological gait disorders
	Cho et al (2014)[315]
Design	Cross-sectional (single-group repeated-measures)
Level of Evidence	IV
Subjects	43 chronic stroke patients (23 female, 20 male) with average age of 52 ± 4 years, approximately 7 ± 0.9 months post stroke.

Continued

Table 7.12 Evidence Summary Table—cont'd

	Cho et al (2014)[315]
Intervention	Individuals walked at a self-selected comfortable speed on two separate days (up to 48 hours apart) while spatial and temporal gait parameters (speed, cadence, step and stride length, and single limb support period) were measured with GAITRite® under two conditions: walking alone (single task) and walking while counting backward (dual task). Participants were allowed to use assistive devices usually required for ambulation.
Results	During single-task condition, all ICC values were high (0.99) with the lowest ICC value recorded for stride length, paretic leg (0.98). During the dual-task condition, ICC values ranged from 0.69 (cadence) to 0.90 (step length, paretic leg).
Comments	The authors concluded that the test–retest reliability of the GAITRite® system for measurement of spatial and temporal gait parameters under single- and dual-task conditions was good to very good.
	Peters et al (2014)[316]
Design	Cross-sectional
Level of Evidence	IV
Subjects	62 adults with unilateral, chronic stroke (>6 months), divided into three groups: (1) household ambulators (HA: n=12, 4 females; self-selected walking speed of <0.4 m/s); (2) limited community ambulators (LCA: n=24, 4 females; self-selected walking speed of 0.4–0.8 m/s); and (3) community ambulators (CA: n=26, 11 females; self-selected walking speed of >0.8 m/s).
Intervention	Participants walked across GAITRite® at self-selected speed as speed was measured along with the time (measured with a stopwatch) required to traverse the middle 3 meters of the walkway (3-meter walk test, 3MWT).
Results	Average walking speed differed between GAITRite® and 3MWT for all groups: HA group: GAITRite® 0.25 (0.11) m/s, 3MWT 0.27 (0.11) m/s LCA group: GAITRite® 0.56 (0.11) m/s, 3MWT 0.52 (0.10) m/s CA group: GAITRite® 1.03 (0.16) m/s, 3MWT 0.89 (0.15) m/s Both walking measurements had excellent within-session reliability. For GAITRite®, ICC values for HA, LCA, and CA groups were 0.97, 0.89, and 0.93, respectively; for the 3MWT, ICC values were 0.97, 0.91, and 0.85, respectively.
Comments	The authors concluded that although both the 3MWT and the GAITRite® produced highly reliable measures of walking speed for individuals with chronic stroke, the two measures did not demonstrate concurrent validity; therefore, these tests should not be used interchangeably in this population.
	Wong et al (2014)[317]
Design	Retrospective
Level of Evidence	III
Subjects	46 adults randomly selected from a pool of 195 inpatients post-stroke.
Intervention	Patients walked at self-selected speed across the GAITRite® 2–4 times, with a gait aid when needed. Five raters independently processed gait data, including velocity, step time, step length, and step width. Three raters re-processed the data after a delay of at least 1 month.
Results	Inter-rater reliability displayed high mean ICC values (0.94 to 0.99), with lowest values recorded for left (0.81) and right (0.84) step width. Intrarater reliability ICC values were highest for velocity and right step length (0.99 to >0.99), with the largest range of ICC values observed for step width, from 0.74 to 0.97 (left step) and 0.96 (right step).
Comments	The authors concluded that GAITRite® is a reliable gait assessment tool to quantify spatial and temporal characteristics of gait in individuals attending inpatient stroke rehabilitation. Further recommendation involves the same rater processing all GAITRite® data when possible.

Table 7.12 Evidence Summary Table—cont'd

Stokic et al (2009)[188]	
Design	Cross-sectional
Level of Evidence	IV
Subjects	52 healthy adults (29 males, 23 females; mean age = 47 years, range = 23–87 years) and 20 individuals with chronic stroke (11 males, 9 females; mean age = 58 years, range = 16–90 years).
Intervention	Gait characteristics (velocity, stride time and length, step length, percent single support, percent total support) were recorded simultaneously by the GAITRite® and an eight-camera motion analysis system as participants performed multiple walks at a self-selected speed.
Results	Mean differences in calculated values between the two methods were ≤1.5% of the mean values calculated for each group.
Comments	The authors concluded that the GAITRite® and motion analysis system provided comparable temporal and spatial measures in healthy adults and those recovering from a stroke.
Webster et al (2005)[318]	
Design	Cross-sectional
Level of Evidence	IV
Subjects	5 males and 5 females (mean age = 66.5 years, range = 54–83 years) at least 121 months post unicompartmental knee replacement surgery.
Intervention	Individual step and averaged spatial and temporal variables obtained with the GAITRite® system were compared with the same variables recorded with the Vicon-512 three-dimensional motion analysis system.
Results	Walking speed, cadence, step length, and step time variables averaged across one walk for both systems showed an excellent level of agreement between systems. No significant systematic differences were found between step length and step time values between the two systems.
Comments	The authors concluded that the GAITRite® is a valid tool for measuring both averaged and individual step gait variables. The small number of subjects is one drawback of this study plus the fact that all subjects walked without any problems that were linked to their surgery.
Bilney et al (2003)[192]	
Design	Cross-sectional
Level of Evidence	IV
Subjects	25 healthy adults (13 males, 12 females; mean age = 40.5 years, range = 21–71 years) without neurological, orthopedic, cardiac, or respiratory condition that affected their gait.
Intervention	The gait variables measured by the GAITRite® were compared with the same variables obtained with the Clinical Stride Analyzer (speed, cadence, stride length, right and left single leg support time, and double support as a percentage of the gait cycle).
Results	ICCs for speed, cadence, and step length showed excellent agreement between the two systems for each speed condition (slow, preferred, and fast). Double support showed the largest mean difference between the two systems. Correlations between the two systems for single leg support time were moderate to high.
Comments	The authors concluded that the GAITRite® had strong concurrent validity and test-retest reliability for selected spatial and temporal variables in normal adults.
McDonough et al (2001)[189]	
Design	Cross-sectional
Level of Evidence	IV
Subjects	One healthy female with equal leg lengths
Intervention	

Continued

Table 7.12 Evidence Summary Table—cont'd

	McDonough et al (2001)[189]
Results	Excellent paper-and-pencil and GAITRite® spatial measure correlations (ICC > 0.95) and video-based and GAITRite® temporal correlations (ICC > 0.93) were reported.
Comments	The authors concluded that the GAITRite® was a valid and reliable tool for measuring selected spatial and temporal gait variables.
	Menz et al (2004)[191]
Design	Cross-sectional
Level of Evidence	IV
Subjects	30 younger adults (12 males, 18 females; mean age = 28.5 years, range 22–40 years) and 31 older adults (13 males, 18 females; mean age = 80.8 years, range 76–87 years) without known pathology.
Intervention	Test-retest reliability of temporal and spatial gait parameters was measured using the GAITRite® as subjects walked at a self-selected comfortable speed three times in one session and then repeated the process approximately 2 weeks later. ICCs and coefficients of variation (CV) were calculated.
Results	Reliability of walking speed, cadence, and step length was excellent for younger and older adults (ICCs: 0.82–0.92; CVs: 1.4%–3.5%). Base of support and toe in/out angles also demonstrated high ICCs (0.49–0.94); however, CVs were higher in younger (CVs: 8.3% to17.7%) and older adults (CVs: 14.3%–33%).
Comments	The authors concluded that the GAITRite® displayed excellent reliability for most temporal and spatial gait parameters in both study groups, but that base of support and toe in/out angles should be interpreted cautiously, particularly in older adults.
	Van Uden and Besser (2004)[190]
Design	Cross-sectional
Level of Evidence	IV
Subjects	21 adults (12 men, 9 women; mean age = 34 years, range: 19–59 years) without known lower extremity orthopedic disorders or pain that would affect their gait.
Intervention	Test-retest reliability of GAITRite® temporal and spatial gait measures were recorded at participants' self-selected free and fast speeds on two occasions 1 week apart. Factors evaluated included walking speed, step length, stride length, base of support, step time, stride time, swing time, stance time, single and double support times, and toe in/toe out angle.
Results	At the self-selected walking speed, all measurements had ICCs ≥0.92 except base of support (ICC = 0.80). At the fast speed, all measurements had ICCs >0.89 except base of support (ICC = 0.79).
Comments	The authors concluded that spatial-temporal gait measurements demonstrated good to excellent test-retest reliability over the 1-week period.

Humphrey et al[194] reported moderate to high ICC values of spatial and temporal variables recorded between the Zeno™ Walkway and the GAITRite® with 30 older adults (average age 75 ± 6 years) without known disabilities walking across both systems at self-selected comfortable (e.g., step length ICC = 0.892; stride length ICC = 0.899; single support % ICC = 0.835) and fast speeds (step length ICC = 0.921; stride length ICC = 0.919; single support % ICC = 0.877). The Zeno system/software has been used across a variety of patient populations, including studies focused on freezing of gait in Parkinson's disease,[195] as well as gait initiation[196] and termination[197,198] in individuals with multiple sclerosis.

Footswitches and Footswitch Systems Footswitches are pressure-sensitive switches placed either on the patient's feet or the inside or outside of the shoes. The switches do not require a walkway, but the patient usually has to carry or wear a data collection device. Footswitches consist of transducers and a semiconductor and are used to signal such events as the heel contacting the ground.

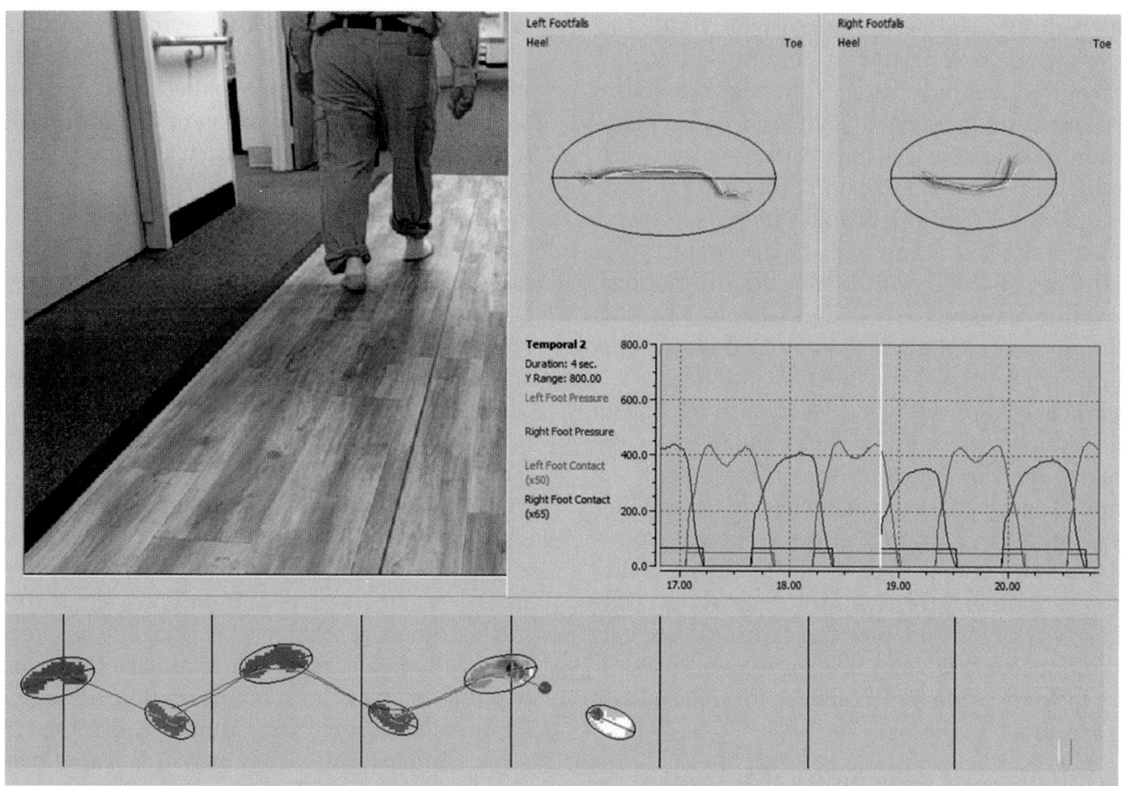

Figure 7.7 Example of data generated with ProtoKinetics software following walking trial performed on Zeno Walkway™ by individual with deformity of right foot and ankle. Right top graph indicates center of pressure excursion under each foot with red line representing the average excursion. Note the shortened excursion under the right foot. Middle graph displays pressure pattern over time for three successive complete left footfalls (red line) and three right footfalls (blue line). The rate and amplitude of loading is diminished under right foot (blue line) compared to left foot (red line). Bottom graph displays pressure pattern and relative foot angle across successive steps. *(Courtesy of ProtoKinetics, 60 Garlor Dr, Havertown, PA 19083.)*

One type of footswitch device used to examine both temporal and loading variables is the *Krusen Limb Load Monitor*.[199] This device consists of a pressure-sensitive force plate that can be worn in a patient's shoe. It can be connected to a strip chart recorder to yield a permanent record of temporal and spatial gait variables.[199]

The *Stride Analyzer* is a footswitch system with special insoles containing four pressure-sensitive switches placed under the heel, the heads of the first and fifth metatarsals, and the great toe. The parameters measured by this system include stride length, velocity, cadence, cycle time, single and double limb support time, swing time, and stance time. These measurements are recorded automatically, and the information is transmitted to a computer that analyzes the data. The computer can also provide graphic displays of foot–floor contact patterns. Times are presented in seconds and as a percentage of the gait cycle. The computer analysis also includes a percentage of normal using a built-in database (Appendix 7.D). The advantages of the Stride Analyzer system are that measurements from both feet are available, the system is easy to move from place to place, and normative data comparisons are available because it has been used by a large number of physical therapists with different populations.[14-16,21,60,200-208]

The Stride Analyzer is suitable for use with various age groups as well as for patients with neurological or orthopedic involvement. For example, in a study by Mulroy et al,[19] footswitches were taped to the shoe bottoms of 30 individuals recovering from a stroke to assess the effects of three ankle-foot orthosis (AFO) designs on walking and to determine whether an ankle plantarflexion contracture influenced response to the orthoses. The conditions assessed included walking with usual footwear using three different AFOs, each with unique settings: (1) dorsiflexion assist with a dorsiflexion stop; (2) plantarflexion stop with free dorsiflexion; and (3) a rigid (solid) ankle. The footswitches were used to compare stride characteristics across conditions and to help define gait phases for subsequent analysis of joint kinematics and muscle activation patterns (electromyography [EMG]). Gait parameters were compared across the orthotic conditions and between participants with and without moderate ankle plantarflexion contractures. The authors reported that individuals without a contracture benefited from AFO designs that allowed stance phase dorsiflexion mobility (e.g., the plantarflexion stop with free dorsiflexion or the dorsiflexion assist with a dorsiflexion stop), as the rigid (solid) ankle inhibited forward progression of the tibia. Those with quadriceps weakness benefited from an AFO with plantarflexion mobility during loading response (i.e., the dorsiflexion assist with a dorsiflexion stop), as knee flexion motion was diminished compared to the other two AFO conditions.

Powers et al[200] used the Stride Analyzer in an analysis of 22 individuals with transtibial amputations to determine the relationship between isometric muscle force and temporal and spatial gait parameters. Mean walking speed was limited to only 59% of normal, owing to reductions in both cadence (83% normal) and stride length (69% normal). Hip extensor torque of the residual limb served as the only predictor for both free and fast walking speeds. Hip abductor torque of the sound limb was the only predictor of cadence for free and fast walking speeds.

Evaluation of Joint Kinematics (Motion)

Electrogoniometers

Joint displacement can be measured relatively simply by using an electrogoniometer. Early electrogoniometer designs included two rigid links connected by a potentiometer that converted movement into an electrical signal that was proportional to the degree of movement. The rigid links or arms of the electrogoniometer were attached to the proximal and distal limb segments. More recent designs use a flexible shaft and two small end blocks that are affixed to the proximal and distal segments of the joint. The new design allows electrogoniometers to be worn under clothing for extended periods of recording time. Biometrics produces a wide variety of electrogoniometers, including twin-axis designs that simultaneously measure joint motion in multiple planes. Lam et al[209] used these devices to study hip (abduction/adduction) and knee (flexion/extension) during corrective stumbling responses to mechanical perturbations applied to the foot of healthy infants during treadmill stepping. The authors reported that perturbations to the dorsum of the foot during swing resulted in an increase in flexor EMG activity and an increase in knee flexion during swing. Electrogoniometers provide an affordable means of measuring joint motion during walking.[34]

Video-Based Motion Analysis Systems

Two-dimensional (2D) and three-dimensional (3D) video-based motion analysis systems are available for gait analysis; however, their use is limited due to challenges with providing accurate data. Two-dimensional video-based systems use a single digital video camcorder to track subject motion. Computer software programs then assist with identifying points of reference. Unfortunately, joint angles that are out of plane (either because of rotation of the limb or due to the position of the individual relative to the camera) will not be calculated accurately. Three-dimensional video-based motion analysis systems use two or more digital video camcorders to gather 3D coordinate data. Hardware is used to synchronize data recorded from the various cameras, and postprocessing is used to identify points of reference either automatically or manually. Markers can be affixed to the skin to help identify anatomical landmarks. Though portable in nature, the accuracy of 2D and 3D video-based systems is a limitation.

Optical Motion Analysis Systems

Imaging-based systems are the most sophisticated and expensive methods of determining joint displacement and patterns of motion. In computerized motion analysis systems, markers placed on body segments such as the hip, knee, and ankle are tracked by automated systems. Motion analysis systems primarily use either *active* or *passive* markers for tracking motion.[33] *Active markers* are usually light-emitting diodes (LEDs) that flash at given frequencies.[210] Each marker is placed over a prespecified location and its individual frequency is used to identify the marker as it moves across space at each instant in time. To power the LED, the participant is either tethered by cable to a central power source or wears a power pack. Fine cables then extend between each LED and the power unit. LEDs are relatively expensive and the thin cables can break. One challenge to the automated labeling of active markers is that reflections from shiny floor surfaces can confound marker identification, particularly for markers located on the feet. Codamotion, Qualisys, PhaseSpace, and Phoenix Technologies are manufacturers that produce systems that use active markers.

Passive markers (Fig. 7.8) require an external source of illumination that may be provided by external light sources or a ring of infrared-emitting diodes located around the camera lens. In the latter case, the diodes on the camera pick up the infrared light reflected by the markers that they can "see," which means that a large number of cameras are necessary for obtaining unrestricted views of markers. Qualisys, Vicon, and Motion Analysis are three manufacturers that produce systems that use passive markers.

When the systems were first developed, visualization of passive markers was problematic, but now markers are automatically tracked and a computer performs thousands of computations. However, passive marker systems require many cameras, are expensive, and require training to operate the hardware and software. Figure 7.9 provides an example of a computer-generated display of kinematic data recorded using passive markers (Qualisys Motion Analysis System) as well as signals recorded from EMG sensors. In Figure 7.10, the degrees of motion for the

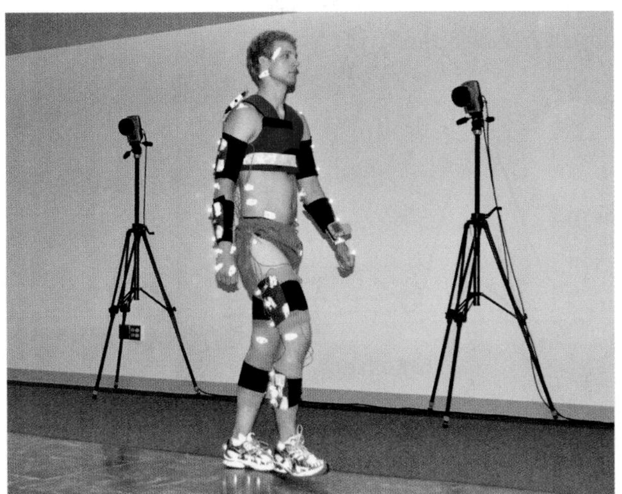

Figure 7.8 Qualisys Oqus Series-3 cameras track motion of passive reflective markers placed over known anatomical landmarks and in clusters on body segments as the subject walks along a 6-meter walkway. Marker data will be used to reconstruct joint motions of the upper extremities, trunk, and lower extremities throughout the gait cycle. *(Courtesy of Movement and Neurosciences Center, Institute for Rehabilitation Science and Engineering, Madonna Rehabilitation Hospitals, Lincoln, NE 68506.)*

knee and ankle are plotted against time (A) and are plotted as a percentage of a time-normalized gait cycle (B), where 0% corresponds to initial contact of the reference limb and 100% represents the next ipsilateral limb initial contact. In Figure 7.11, stick figures are shown with accompanying knee angles.

A number of important problems still exist with the use of both active and passive marker systems. Obstruction of markers by body segments, skin/soft tissue motion, marker vibration, and improper placement of markers in relation to the joint center of motion can introduce potential errors. Determining the location of the hip joint center is particularly problematic. The ball-and-socket anatomy means that the center of the hip joint is located in the center of the femoral head. Difficulty palpating the femoral head makes accurate marker placement elusive. Radiographic studies have been performed to develop and refine algorithms that can be used to calculate the hip joint center relative to palpable landmarks (e.g., the anterior superior iliac spine, pubic tubercle).[211] Finally, inconsistencies in marker placement have been identified as one of the leading sources of variability in kinematic findings.[212] Following implementation of a standardized protocol for marker placement, Gorton et al[212] reported a 20% average

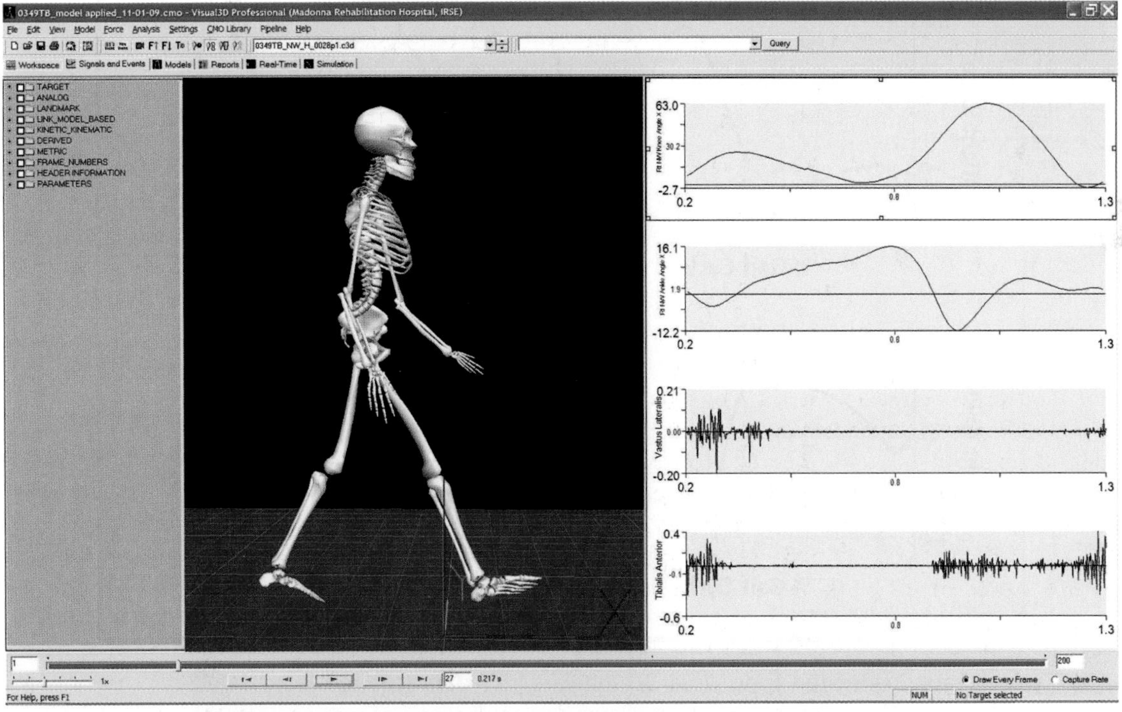

Figure 7.9 Visual 3D computer display of kinematic data recorded using the Qualisys Motion Analysis System and surface electromyographic data recorded using the MA-300 EMG system during overground gait for a 31-year-old male. Reflective markers, applied over known locations, provided the anatomical reference for displayed skeleton and for subsequent analysis of joint motions. To the right of the skeleton, sagittal plane joint motions for the knee and ankle are displayed in the top two rows while surface EMG data for the vastus lateralis and tibialis anterior are displayed in the bottom two rows. *(Courtesy of Dr. Yu Shu, Movement and Neurosciences Center, Institute for Rehabilitation Science and Engineering, Madonna Rehabilitation Hospitals, Lincoln, NE 68506.)*

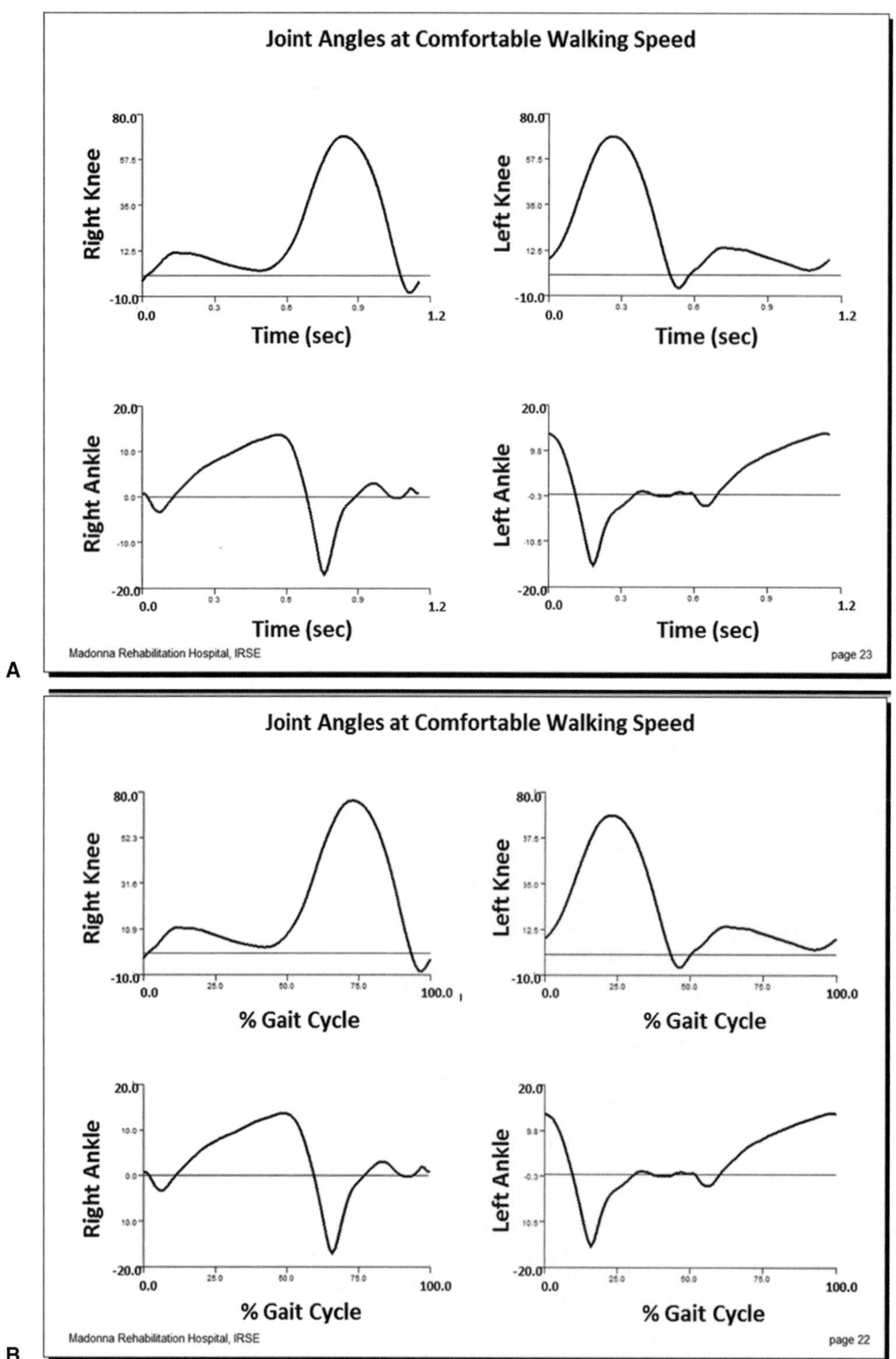

Figure 7.10 Typical graphs generated using Visual 3D software from data acquired using a Qualisys motion analysis system. The graphs show bilateral knee and ankle range-of-motion patterns recorded during a full right lower extremity gait cycle plotted against time (A) and as a percentage of the gait cycle (B). Note that left foot's initial contact occurred at approximately 0.6 seconds (approximately 50% gait cycle). *(Courtesy of Thad Buster, Movement and Neurosciences Center, Institute for Rehabilitation Science and Engineering, Madonna Rehabilitation Hospitals, Lincoln, NE 68506.)*

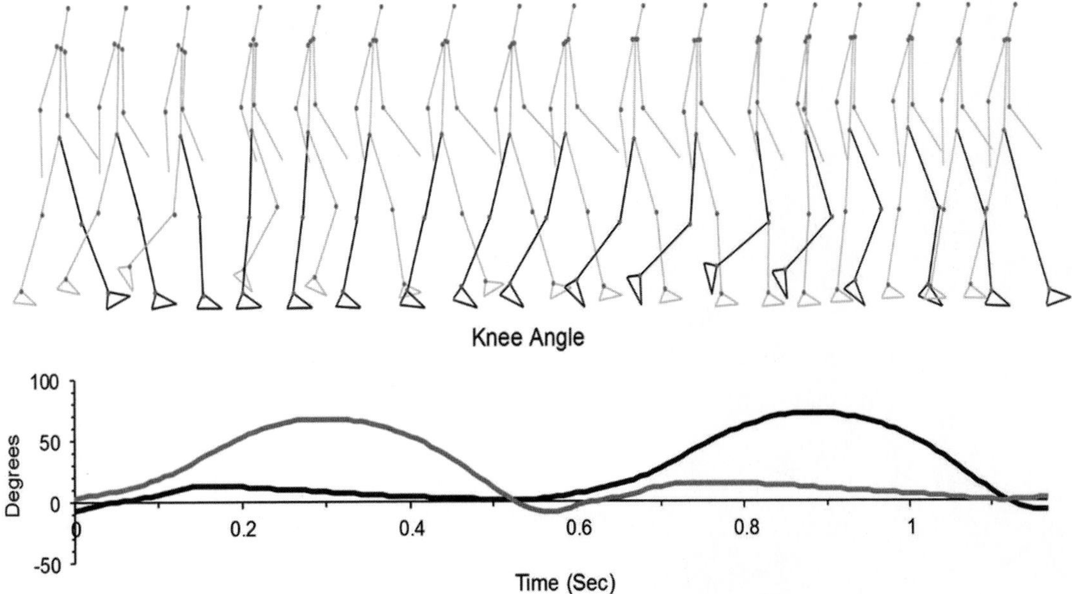

Figure 7.11 Another format for presentation of the data from a motion-analysis system is computer-generated stick figure representations of one complete gait cycle. In this particular case, the pattern of knee motion is graphically presented below the stick figures. Note that the right knee (darker lower extremity in top figure and darker line in lower figure) is hyperextended at initial contact. *(Courtesy of Movement and Neurosciences Center, Institute for Rehabilitation Science and Engineering, Madonna Rehabilitation Hospitals, Lincoln, NE 68506.)*

decrease in the standard deviation of 7 of 9 kinematic measures recorded by 24 examiners in 12 motion analysis laboratories using two different camera systems.

As affordable computer processing and storage capabilities rapidly expand, the varying motion analysis products on the market also are evolving. Many video-based systems currently available are able to track markers to within 0.04 in (1 mm) of accuracy, enabling relatively precise tracking of the markers.[213] Most systems have the capacity to integrate with other technology, enabling simultaneous acquisition of relevant gait data such as footswitches to identify foot-floor contact patterns and stride characteristics, EMG systems to examine muscle activation patterns, and force plates to determine ground reaction forces. EMG, when recorded simultaneously with stride characteristics data, can be used to identify the particular portion of the gait cycle in which the muscle activity occurs. Figure 7.12 depicts how EMG and kinematic data can be used to explore factors contributing to abnormal gait patterns. The person depicted experienced difficulty with foot clearance during swing owing, in part, to excess plantarflexion during mid and terminal swing. Out-of-phase activity of the gastrocnemius during late swing contributed to the excess plantarflexion and foot clearance challenge. In addition, the individual walked with a "stiff-legged" gait pattern with the knee excessively extended throughout much of the gait cycle compared to the anticipated motion profile. Inappropriately timed activity of the vastus lateralis contributed, in part, to the observed knee deviations. Refer to Chapter 5, Examination of Motor Function: Motor Control and Motor Learning, for a more detailed discussion of EMG.

Key differentiating features among motion analysis systems include price, marker system options (e.g., active, passive, or both active and passive), and the capabilities and efficiency of postprocessing software. A number of systems provide manufacturer-generated analysis software that is relatively easy to learn; however, it may be difficult to modify/customize the software to meet the needs of more elaborate studies. Report-generating capabilities differ notably across systems as well and should be considered, depending on the expectations of the laboratory or clinic (e.g., need to produce rapid, easily interpretable reports for inclusion in patient charts versus export of data for statistical analysis for research purposes). Appendix 7.C includes a list of gait analysis software and hardware manufacturers and their contact information. Given the evolving nature of technology, the reader is encouraged to visit the websites provided for the most up-to-date information about the capabilities of different systems.

Electromagnetic Motion Analysis System

One challenge with optical tracking systems is that the motion analysis cameras need to be able to "see" the markers to track their position and subsequently calculate kinematic data. This can be difficult when clients use multiple assistive devices or require substantial physical assistance from one or more therapists to navigate the walkway. An alternative motion analysis technology

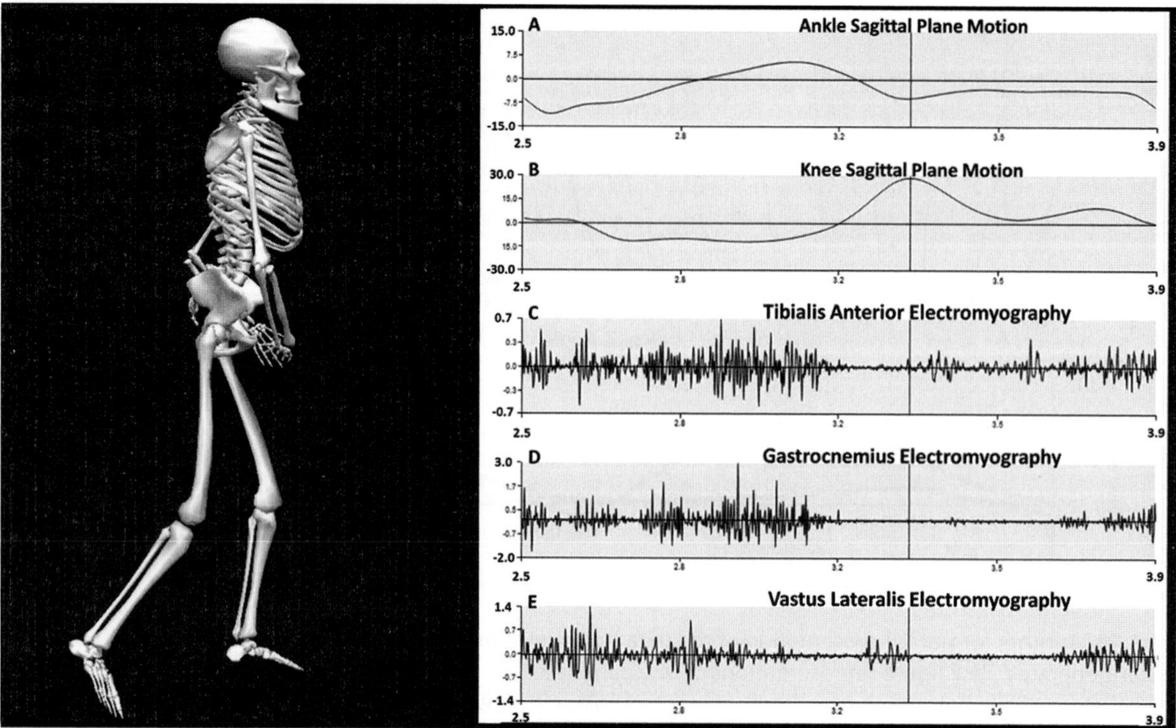

Figure 7.12 Skeleton image of individual post–brain injury walking. Graphs display data from a single right lower extremity stride (i.e., right initial contact to next ipsilateral initial contact), including sagittal plane motion of ankle (A) and knee (B), as well as corresponding EMG from right gastrocnemius (C) and vastus lateralis (D). Right ankle demonstrates excess plantarflexion during mid and terminal swing and at initial contact. Premature out-of-phase activity of the right gastrocnemius from mid swing through loading response contributed to the excess plantarflexion, despite tibialis anterior activity during swing. Individual does not achieve normal 60° of knee flexion during initial swing, resulting in challenges with limb clearance. Loading response knee flexion is also curtailed, leading to reduced shock absorption. The knee is postured in hyperextension throughout single limb support. Out-of-phase activity of vastus lateralis during pre-swing contributed to limited knee flexion during pre-swing and initial swing. Foot flat initial contact arising from premature activity of gastrocnemius during swing reduced heel rocker and contributed to limited knee flexion during loading response. Prolonged vastus lateralis activity during single limb support contributed to sustained knee hyperextension. Prolonged activity of tibialis anterior throughout single limb support contributed to frontal plane instability of subtalar joint. *(Courtesy of Thad Buster, Movement and Neurosciences Center, Institute for Rehabilitation Science and Engineering, Madonna Rehabilitation Hospitals, Lincoln, NE 68506.)*

employs electromagnetic tracking capabilities to determine the 3D coordinates of location and angulation of each sensor. Flock of Birds®, Nest of Birds®, and MotionStar® (all manufactured by Ascension Technology), and FASTRAK® (manufactured by Polhemus) are examples of electromagnetic motion analysis technology. MotionStar® allows tracking of up to 120 sensors simultaneously and thus can perform motion analysis on more than one subject simultaneously. To date, a small number of studies have been published that used electromagnetic motion analysis technology to study gait-related activities.[214-218] The equipment has garnered a following in the virtual-reality environments and animation industry.

Kinetic Gait Analysis

Kinetic Variables

Kinetic gait analyses are directed toward determination and analysis of the forces involved in gait, including ground (floor) reaction forces (GRFs), joint torques, center of pressure (COP), center of mass (COM), mechanical energy, moments of force, power, support moments, work, joint reaction forces, and intrinsic foot pressure (Table 7.13). Although in the past kinetic gait analyses have been used primarily for research purposes, at the present time they are being used clinically as well. Given the risk of foot pressure injuries arising from high

Table 7.13 Gait Variables: Kinetic Gait Analysis

Ground reaction forces	Vertical, anterior-posterior, and medial-lateral forces created as a result of foot contact with the supporting surface. These forces are equal in magnitude and opposite in direction to the force applied by the foot to the ground. Ground reaction forces are measured with force platforms in newtons (N) or pound force.
Pressure	Pressure = force per unit area. In gait analysis, the parameters that are usually measured include the peak pressure, the pressure-time integral, and the overall pattern of pressure distribution under the foot.
Center of Pressure (COP)	The point of application of the resultant force. Movement of the COP as a function of time is used as a measure of stability of a subject who is either standing or walking on a force plate.
Torque (Moment of Force)	The turning or rotational effect produced by the application of a force. The greater the perpendicular distance from the point of application of a force from the axis of rotation, the greater the turning effect, or torque, produced. Torque is calculated by multiplying the force by the perpendicular distance from the point of application of the force and the axis of rotation. Torque = force × perpendicular distance or moment arm.

plantar pressures in individuals with diabetic sensory neuropathy, some clinicians are using special pressure mapping insoles to determine if clients may be at risk for developing a pressure injury. A patient walks while wearing the special insoles and the pressures are recorded. If high pressures are identified on the bottom of the foot, patients may be referred to have special orthotics and/or shoes fabricated to help redistribute the pressures.

The instrumentation required to examine kinetic variables is complex and expensive, because derivation of kinetics requires knowledge of all forces acting on the body part being analyzed (e.g., the foot or the thigh). The analysis usually starts with the forces being applied to the foot, which is determined by a force plate embedded in the floor. These plates contain load transducers that measure the COP, COM, and GRFs during gait. Typically, the force plates are based on either strain gage or piezoelectric technology.

Calculation of kinetic variables at the ankle requires knowledge of the forces acting on the foot, body mass, and location of the COM (derived from standard anthropometric tables), as well as knowledge about the acceleration of the COM. Once this knowledge is obtained, equations can be developed to calculate the net forces and net moments occurring at the ankle, at that particular instant in time, in order for the foot to have moved with those particular accelerations. Once forces and moments at the ankle are determined, similar equations can be applied to the adjacent proximal segment (lower leg). One then knows, for each instant in time, whether the dominant internal moment is being caused by the dorsiflexors or the plantarflexors. If the internal moment for each instant in time is multiplied by the net angular velocity between the ankle and the lower leg, the result is knowledge of the net power being produced by the muscles across the ankle. Concentric contractions add power to the limb (power generation), and eccentric contractions reduce power (power absorption). Variations in expected patterns of power generation and absorption are particularly useful in identifying deficiencies and in determining treatment goals. Unfortunately, a detailed explanation of the calculation of COM, COP, and moments and power is beyond the scope of the current chapter. Readers interested in learning more about these concepts are referred to a book written by David Winter included on the supplemental reading list.

The GRF is defined as the net vertical and shear (or horizontal) forces acting between the foot and the supporting surface. The force is three-dimensional and can be resolved into three components: vertical, anterior–posterior, and medial–lateral (Fig. 7.13). Each component varies throughout the gait cycle and is affected by velocity, cadence, and body mass. The averaged waveforms of the vertical and anterior–posterior force components, presented as a percentage of body weight, show consistent patterns across individuals without pathology for loading rate, peak force, average force, and unloading rate. The vertical force waveform shows a characteristic double hump. The anterior–posterior force has a characteristic negative phase (representing deceleration of the body's mass after the foot hits the ground) followed by a positive phase (reflecting acceleration as body mass moves forward in late stance). In the frontal plane, an initial laterally directed GRF peaks shortly after initial contact. This is most commonly followed by an extended medially directed GRF.

Friction is required while walking and acts in the opposite direction of the desired motion. For example, during loading response, the foot imparts forward (anterior) shear force onto the floor as body weight loads onto the

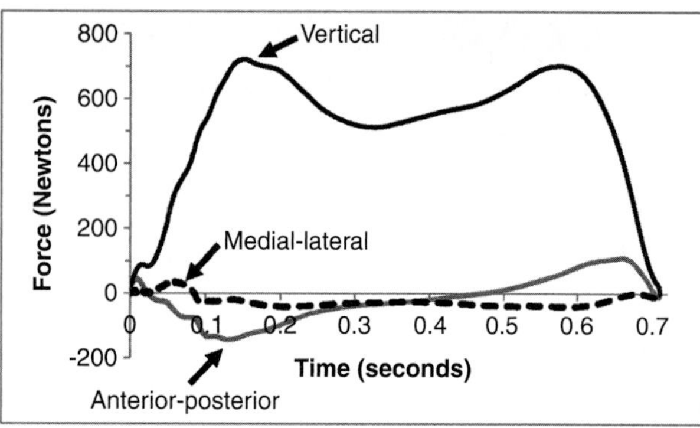

Figure 7.13 Computer-generated graph of the vertical, anterior-posterior and medial-lateral components of the ground-reaction force obtained as an adult walks across an AMTI force plate. *(Courtesy of Movement and Neurosciences Center, Institute for Rehabilitation Science and Engineering, Madonna Rehabilitation Hospitals, Lincoln, NE 68506.)*

limb. Friction resists the tendency of the foot to slip forward. An individual's friction needs during walking, sometimes referred to as *utilized* or *required friction,* can be measured as an individual walks across a force plate. It is calculated as the ratio of the individual's shear (resultant of the anterior–posterior and medial–lateral forces) and vertical GRF components. When an individual's walking friction needs exceed the friction available at the foot-floor interface, a slip is likely to occur.[12,29,219] A tribometer is a device used to measure the friction available on different floor surfaces and in the presence of contaminants (e.g., water or oil). Some floor manufacturers will report on the slip resistance of the surfaces they distribute (e.g., different types of tile). Floor surfaces with a higher available friction (as measured by a tribometer) are generally more slip resistant.

Instruments for Measuring Kinetic Variables

Force Plate Technology

Force plates, such as those produced by both Kistler Instrument Corp. and Advanced Mechanical Technology, Inc. (AMTI), are capable of measuring the GRF, as well as calculating the COM, acceleration, velocity, *displacement, power,* and *work.* A graphic display is possible showing the waveforms of the GRF. Kistler Instrument Corp. also markets a treadmill called the Gaitway. The treadmill is capable of measuring the GRF and COP during both walking and running. In addition to graphical presentation and statistical functions, the treadmill system can calculate temporal and spatial parameters.

Cook et al[11] used a force plate to investigate the effect of a knee flexion restriction (using a brace) and walking speed on the GRF. The authors concluded that the application of a brace to restrict knee flexion for the purpose of protection after injury, or while surgically repaired structures were healing, may actually increase the stress on both the braced and unbraced limbs.

Hesse et al[220] compared the trajectories of the COP and the COM in 10 healthy individuals and 14 subjects with hemiparesis. They found that the healthy subjects showed no differences in the behavior of the COP, COM, temporal parameters, and step length when initiating gait with either the right or left extremity. In comparison, patients with hemiparesis showed pronounced asymmetric behavior depending on which limb was the starting limb (affected vs. less affected). Whereas patients who initiated gait with the affected limb were similar to healthy subjects, patients who started gait with the less-affected limb showed inconsistent movement of the COP and were incapable of producing directional movement of the body's COM. This suggests therapists should be cautious about promoting that type of gait initiation because the affected leg may be too weak to support starting gait with the less affected leg. Rossi et al[8] investigated the COM, COP, and GRF in a study of gait initiation in patients with transtibial amputations. These authors found that the patients consistently loaded the intact limb more than the prosthetic limb regardless of which limb initiated gait.[8]

Force plates may be used either as part of, or in combination with, motion analysis systems, and temporal and spatial analysis systems, as well as in conjunction with EMG and electrogoniometry, for a comprehensive analysis of kinematic and kinetic gait variables. Perry et al[14] incorporated simultaneous recording of GRFs, joint motions, and LE muscle activation patterns to explore an apparent paradox related to the efficiency of toe walking and potential need for therapeutic intervention. Previous researchers identified a lower internal plantarflexor moment during toe walking compared to traditional heel-toe gait and suggested that the plantarflexed foot provided a potential compensatory advantage by reducing the need for plantarflexor strength.[221] However, the earlier researchers had not included measurements of muscle activation (EMG) in their study. The inclusion of EMG into Perry et al's follow-up study[14] as well as subsequent modeling studies[222,223] of the biomechanical demands of toe walking, highlighted the source of the apparent paradox. Although the internal moments were lower,[14] plantarflexor muscle activation (mean and peak) actually increased because of the biomechanically inefficient position associated with maintaining a plantarflexed foot (less than optimal length–tension of the plantarflexors).[222] The plantarflexed foot also created the need for compensatory adjustments in muscle activation at more proximal joints.[223] This series of studies highlights a potential limitation of using only kinematic and kinetic data to interpret muscle activation patterns; that is, various patterns of muscle co-activation can create the same internal moment. In addition, when a muscle is at an inefficient position on the length–tension curve, it may require greater activation to generate the same internal moment compared to the demands when more optimally aligned.

Plantar Pressure Measurement Systems

Pressure measurement systems may also be used with force plates. Pressure is equal to force divided by area and is measured by pressure sensors. Therefore, pressure is equal to the force on the sensor divided by the area of the sensor. Plantar pressure measurements are used most commonly in gait analysis to determine the pressure distribution under the foot: foot-to-ground contact, foot-to-shoe contact, and shoe-to-ground contact. Pressure measurements may be used to determine orthotic efficacy, pressure injury risk in diabetes, and for regulating weight-bearing following surgery. Many different types of measurement techniques have been developed for measuring contact pressures.

Novel Electronics' pedar® and emed® pressure mapping systems provide a means for examining pressures. The pedar® system consists of insoles (in a variety of lengths and widths) that can be placed inside shoes to measure plantar pressures. Each pressure insole consists of a 0.08-in (2-mm) thick array of 99 capacitive pressure sensors used to calculate a variety of measures, including peak pressures, mean pressures, contact area, and pressure-time integral. An example of the type of information obtained from the pedar® system is presented in Figure 7.14.

The pedar® insoles can also be used to measure barefoot pressures by securing them to the foot with a thin pair of nylon stockings.[224] Burnfield et al[224] used the pedar® system to study plantar pressures patterns in older adults while walking barefoot and with shoes at three predetermined velocities (187, 262, and 295 ft/min [57, 80, and 97 m/min]). Compared to slower speeds, fast walking was associated with higher peak pressures under the heel, central and medial metatarsals, and toes, whereas walking barefoot was associated with greater peak pressures under the heel and central metatarsals compared to walking with shoes (Fig. 7.15). These findings suggest that when protection of the plantar surface of the heel and forefoot is important (e.g., with diabetic sensory neuropathy), patients should be encouraged to use shoes and avoid walking at fast speeds for prolonged periods. Subsequent work comparing barefoot walking and wearing shoes, examined plantar pressures while walking on grass, carpet, and concrete and identified particularly high pressures when walking barefoot on concrete.[225] Burnfield et al[226] focused on understanding how plantar pressures in young and middle-aged adults vary across common forms of cardiovascular exercise, including treadmill walking, treadmill running, elliptical training, stair stepping, and recumbent cycling. The authors concluded that when protection of the forefoot is important (e.g., diabetic foot neuropathies), biking and stair climbing offer optimal pressure reductions; however, in situations where protection of the heels from high pressures

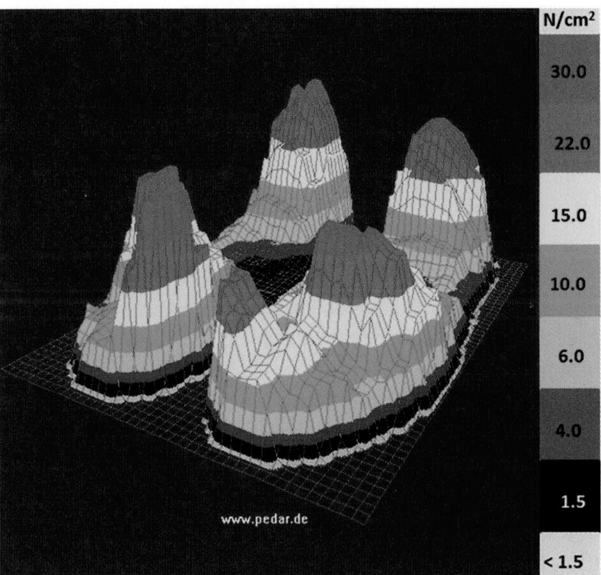

Figure 7.14 Magnitude and location of peak pressure during a left and right step of a young adult without disability walking overground with shoes at self-selected comfortable speed. Images from both feet are placed side by side for comparison. The highest pressures (displayed in pink) occurred under the heel, metatarsal heads, and right great toe. Relatively low pressures (displayed in black, blue, and teal) were documented under the midfoot regions. *(Courtesy of Thad Buster, Movement and Neurosciences Center, Institute for Rehabilitation Science and Engineering, Madonna Rehabilitation Hospitals, Lincoln, NE 68506.)*

and forces is warranted, recumbent biking, stair climbing, and elliptical training provide greater relief.[226]

The emed® pedography platform is a portable device used to record and evaluate pressure distribution under the foot in static and dynamic conditions. Semple et al[227] used the emed® system to examine COP progression as individuals with rheumatoid arthritis (RA) and individuals without known foot pathology walked. Clients with RA displayed reduced loading of painful regions of the foot as evidenced by delaying progression of the COP across the less painful midfoot followed by rapid progression of the COP across the deformed and painful forefoot.

Tekscan has a system called the *F-Scan® Bipedal In-Shoe Plantar Pressure/Force Measurement System* that measures bipedal plantar pressures using paper-thin disposable pressure sensors placed in a patient's shoes. The sensor is ultrathin, flexible, and can be trimmed to fit; it includes 960 sensing locations distributed across the entire plantar surface. Reliability of the F-Scan system was determined by Randolph et al[228] to be sufficient for the purpose of designing corrective measures to relieve excessive pressures on the foot. Another system produced by Tekscan is called *Mat-Scan System®*, which is a pressure-sensing floor mat that allows the clinician to identify barefoot

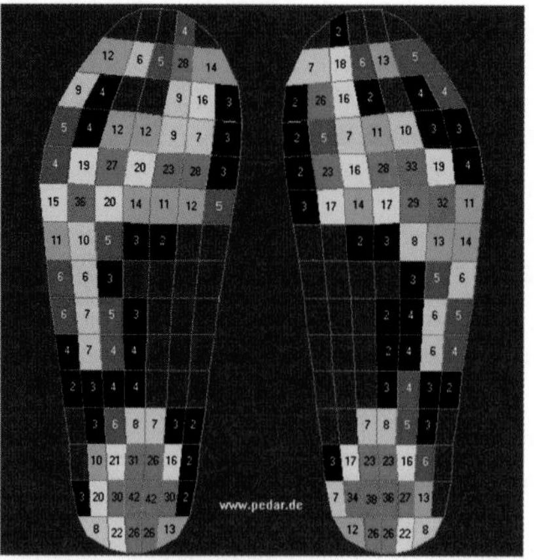

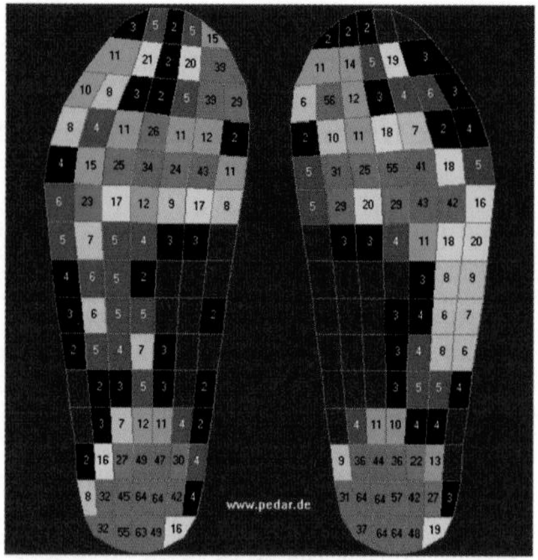

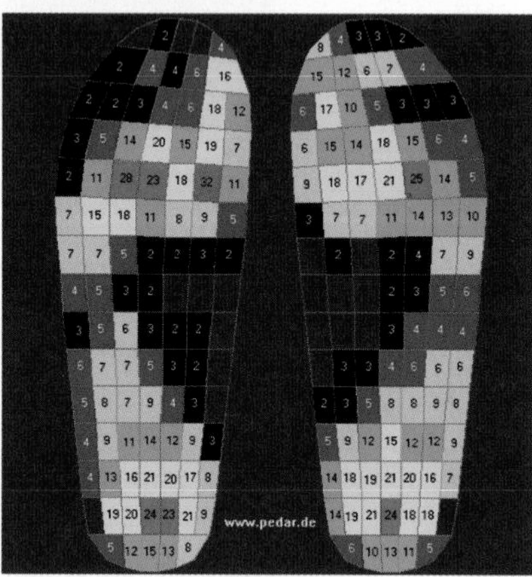

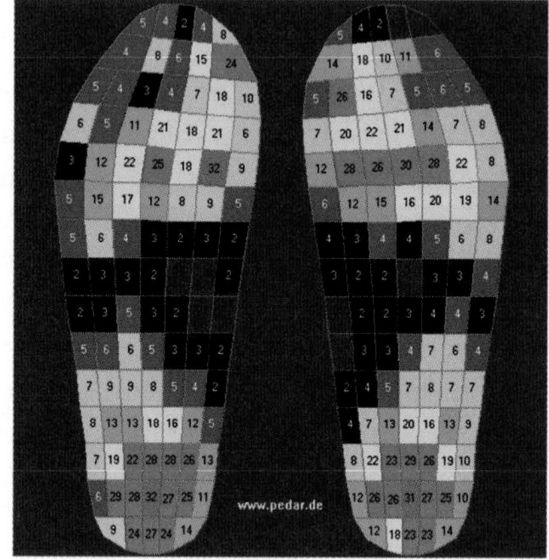

Figure 7.15 Pedar (Novel, Inc.) pressure mapping while walking barefoot (top row) and in shoes (bottom row) at self-selected comfortable (left column) and fast (right column) speeds for a 29-year-old male revealed higher pressures under the heel, metatarsal heads, and great toe during barefoot walking at a fast speed compared to the relatively low pressures while walking in shoes at a comfortable speed. Numbers within each square represent the peak pressure (N/cm^2) experienced during the walking trial. *(Courtesy of Adam Taylor, Movement and Neurosciences Center, Institute for Rehabilitation Science and Engineering, Madonna Rehabilitation Hospitals, Lincoln, NE 68506.)*

pressures. Mueller et al[229] used the *F-Scan System* to determine how footwear design impacted plantar pressures in 30 individuals with transmetatarsal amputations who were at risk for additional amputations owing to a history of diabetes. Though all footwear designs reduced plantar pressures under the distal portion of the residual foot compared to traditional footwear with a toe-filler, the most effective design included a full-length shoe with a total contact custom-molded Plastazote insert and a rigid rocker bottom sole. This work has important clinical implications given the high incidence of additional amputations in those with diabetes who have already lost a portion of one limb.[230] Armstrong et al[231] found that patients who have high plantar pressures and wounds greater than 3.12 in. (8 cm) took significantly longer to heal than other patients.

Isokinetic and Isometric Torque Measurement Systems

Simple handheld dynamometers and isokinetic dynamometer systems can be used to obtain static and dynamic peak torques before obtaining temporal and spatial measures. Connelly and Vandervoort[129] found that decreases in isometric and dynamic quadriceps strength led to significant decreases in fast-paced and self-selected speed in older women. In a study examining the relationship between sagittal plane LE isokinetic muscle torques and stride characteristics for a group of elderly ambulatory men, maximal isokinetic hip extensor torque was identified as the only significant independent predictor of stride length, cadence, and free walking velocity.[232] These latter findings highlight the importance of maintaining hip extensor strength in older sedentary males.

Software for Processing, Analyzing, and Displaying Kinematic and Kinetic Data

The Visual 3D, innovative software for biomechanical analysis and modeling, is used to process a variety of gait analysis data (e.g., kinematics, EMG, force plates, gyroscopes). It works with nearly all motion-capture systems and has an integrated report generator. It allows users to expand beyond manufacturer predetermined marker sets and analysis rules. However, to fully appreciate the versatility and robustness of the Visual 3D software, it is beneficial to have access to someone with programming skills.

Summary of Kinematic and Kinetic Gait Analysis

Based on the history of gait analysis, one may expect that many gait analysis systems will continue to evolve and more innovative methods of quantifying human gait will be created. However, the most important issues for physical therapists is how reliable and valid the information is, and how information can be used to fulfill the four purposes for gait analysis (presented in the "Purposes of Gait Analysis" section of this chapter) as described in the *Guide for Physical Therapist Practice 3.0*.[233] In brief, these purposes are to assist with understanding the gait characteristics of a particular disorder, to assist with movement diagnosis, to inform selection of intervention(s), and to evaluate the effectiveness of treatment.

The primary advantages of temporal and spatial measures are that they can be determined simply and inexpensively and that they yield objective and reliable baseline data that can be used to formulate anticipated goals and expected outcomes and to evaluate the patient's progress. For example, gait patterns displayed by patients with arthritis often are characterized by a reduced rate and range of knee motion and a slower gait velocity compared to subjects without known pathology. Brinkmann and Perry[234] found that following joint replacement for arthritis, the rate and range of knee motion and gait velocity increased above preoperative levels but did not reach normal levels.

Usually, increases in measures such as cadence and velocity indicate improvement in a patient's gait. However, comparisons with normal standards are appropriate only if the goal of treatment is to restore a normal gait pattern (e.g., for a patient recovering from a meniscectomy). Comparison with normative standards may not be appropriate for a patient who has had a cerebral vascular accident. The appropriate norms for examining the gait of a patient with hemiplegia may be either a population of patients with hemiplegia who are of similar age, gender, and involvement or the patient's pretreatment gait.

Therapists must be cautious when selecting a norm or standard by which to measure patient progress. Significant age, gender, weight, and activity level–related differences have been found in both temporal and spatial measures.[235-237] Himann et al[236] found that an older group (63 to 102 years) of 289 subjects had a significantly slower self-selected walking speed and smaller step length in comparison to a younger group. Age was a significant determinant of walking speed after age 62, but height was a significant determinant before age 62. Step length has been found to be significantly shorter and the double limb support stance period significantly increased in an elderly sample compared to a database of young adults.[119] Cho et al[238] found a number of gender differences in kinematic and kinetic gait variables. For example, females had shorter stride lengths and narrower step widths, a more anteriorly tilted pelvis, greater hip flexion and internal rotation, greater knee valgus, and smaller ankle joint moment compared to males. Some of these changes were attributed to the anatomically wider female pelvis.[238]

Few disadvantages exist regarding kinematic quantitative gait analysis, except for the possible expense involved in instrumentation, the time required to apply the markers accurately to ensure valid and reliable data, and the fact that a certain amount of uncertainty exists about how to normalize for leg length, height, age, gender, weight, level of maturation, and disability. The interpretation of motion patterns obtained through motion analysis systems usually involves comparisons of an individual's data with a mean curve for normal subjects using one standard deviation (SD) for boundaries. Sutherland et al[239] suggest that motion patterns cannot be fully analyzed without consideration of all points along the curve. They propose the use of prediction regions (multiples of the SD above and below the mean curve of data for each point in the gait cycle). Within a prediction region (Fig. 7.16), if any point along the curve of joint motion falls outside of the defined region, the patient's gait is considered to be abnormal.

Gait Pattern Classification

Identification of gait parameters that deviate widely from a norm is a fairly simple outcome of gait analysis. However, identification of groups or clusters of gait deviations that characterize a known disorder is more complicated and represents one of the very urgent needs in gait analysis. In an attempt to classify gait disorders, a number of statistical techniques are being used for both kinematic and kinetic gait variables. The bootstrap technique[240] is used to establish the boundaries (prediction regions) about the mean curve for healthy control subjects in order to establish the limits of normal variability. *Discriminant analysis* is used to recognize gait patterns of healthy people and persons with gait deviations. *Principal components analysis* is useful to reduce the large quantities of data acquired in a gait analysis to a set of features that accurately describe gait patterns. *Cluster analysis* is used to place subjects in homogeneous groups, or clusters, based on specified input parameters.

Normalcy Index

Principal components analysis was used to develop the *Normalcy Index* (NI), which was able to quantify the amount of deviation in a subject's gait compared to the gait of an average unimpaired person.[241] The NI is sensitive enough to distinguish unimpaired subjects from idiopathic toe walkers and to distinguish between involved and less involved limbs of subjects following stroke. However, the gait pathology of non-independent walkers was not well categorized. The authors suggested that perhaps the inclusion of kinetic variables along with kinematic variables might be helpful.

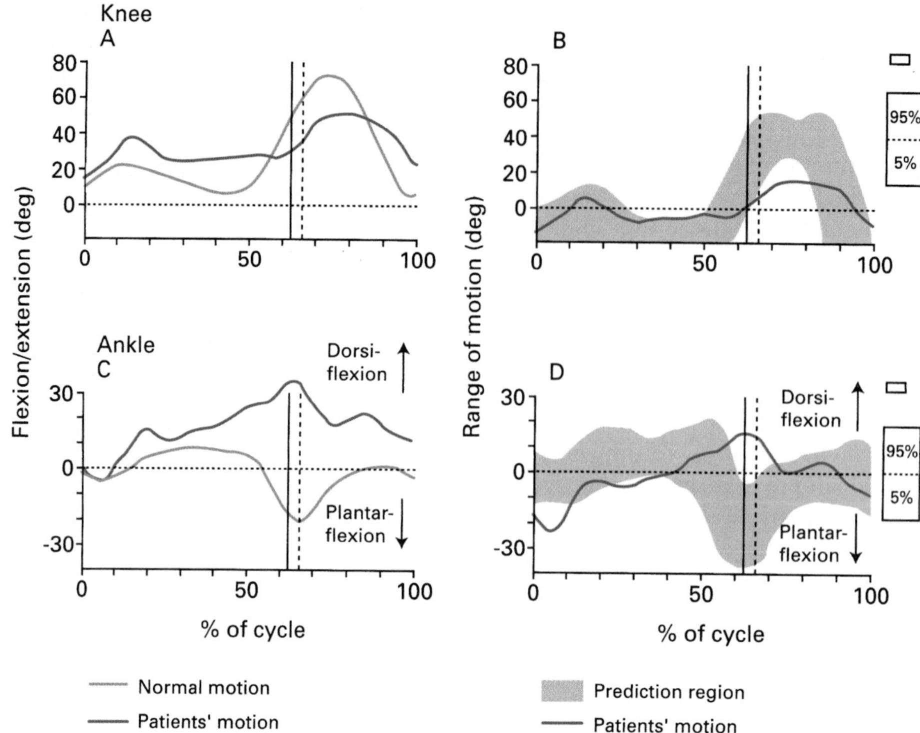

Figure 7.16 Prediction regions. *(Sutherland et al,[239] with permission.)*

The principal components method derived the NI by assigning weighted factors inversely proportional to the amount of variation exhibited by each gait measure in the unimpaired population. However, since the data come from a motion analysis system, they are subject to sources of error such as soft tissue artifacts and marker misplacement.[241]

Cluster Analysis

Cluster analysis is a commonly used statistical technique in the social sciences that has also been used to create an objective classification system of gait patterns. Cluster analysis has been used to classify gait patterns of patients with stroke based on temporal and spatial parameters for each phase of the gait cycle. Four clusters of gait patterns were identified: *fast, moderate, flexed,* and *extended.*[242] The authors suggested that clinicians use critical parameters to categorize patients with stroke so that intervention programs could be more specifically targeted to underlying impairments.

Energy Cost Analysis During Gait

Walking at constant speed is a cyclical activity that requires the body to add energy by means of concentric contractions and to absorb energy by means of eccentric contractions. These energy transfers and exchanges are cleverly designed to make walking efficient.[26] Generally, conditions that affect either the motor control of gait and posture or conditions that affect joint and muscle structure and function will increase the energy cost of gait.[15,243-247] The type of footwear,[248] use of assistive devices, and speed of gait affect energy expenditure as well.[249] Energy expenditure is an important consideration in gait analyses, particularly in neurological conditions in which muscular resources may be low. There are three general approaches in determining energy costs: *physiological measurement, mechanical energy analysis,* and *heart rate data.* The selection of a particular approach should be done for the purpose of taking the measure and the relative importance of test characteristics outlined in the "Types of Gait Analyses" section of this chapter.

Physiological Energy Cost Measures

Physiological cost measures estimate the heat (energy) produced by a subject at rest and during exercise by indirect calorimetry, based on the assumption that all energy-using reactions of the body depend on oxygen uptake. The most common method of measuring oxygen uptake during walking is open-loop spirometry in which exhaled air is sampled and analyzed for its oxygen content, classically using the Douglas bag method.[26] Stationary or moving metabolic carts or lightweight portable devices perform breath-by-breath oxygen and carbon dioxide analysis.

Two parameters of prime interest are *oxygen cost* and *oxygen rate.* One may be interested in the oxygen cost or energy expenditure per unit of distance walked (in mL/kg/m), which relates to the physiological work involved in the task and reflects gait efficiency. Alternatively, the oxygen rate, or energy expenditure per unit of time (in mL/kg/min), reflects the power of walking and is interpreted using knowledge of walking speed.[244,250] Perry et al[15] used a modified Douglas bag assembly to compare the energy expenditure required for an individual with bilateral transfemoral amputations and bilateral transradial (below elbow) amputations to walk at a self-selected speed using different prosthetic devices. When wearing the microprocessor-controlled C-Leg prostheses, the subject walked the farthest and fastest compared to the traditional non-microprocessor-controlled articulating prostheses and stubbies (nonarticulating, short prosthetic limbs). The overall rate of oxygen consumption and oxygen cost was lower while using the C-Legs compared with walking with either of the other prostheses.

Physiological cost analysis methods are most useful for comparing the energy cost of walking with normal values or an individual's maximum capacity and for determining the effects on energy costs of interventions such as the use of orthoses, prostheses, or assistive devices. Physiological cost analyses reflect overall costs of walking with respect to time or distance, but they cannot discern the possible causes. If insight into the particular movements is needed, mechanical energy analysis can be helpful.

Mechanical Energy Cost Determination

There are two methods of obtaining mechanical energy costs. In the first method, kinematic data alone are required, using estimates of masses of body parts and of COM locations of these parts. By employing a spatial motion analysis system with basic equations of motion and anthropometric constants for masses of body parts, the potential energy and translational and rotational kinetic energy levels of each body part can be calculated. The differences between values obtained at each time increment indicate energy cost. Various equations are used to combine the costs across body parts to yield the total body cost. The large head-arms-and-trunk segment shows excellent exchanges between kinetic and potential energy types, providing the body with energy efficiency. When the body is at its highest position (mid stance), it is also moving most slowly, but as the head-arms-and-trunk "roll down the hill" into initial contact of the foot, this potential energy is changed into kinetic energy, and the head-arms-and-trunk picks up speed. In this way, a great deal of energy is saved and the movement is efficient. However, if the person walks very slowly or very quickly, or has a stiff knee and has to lift one side of the body excessively to clear the floor, the energies are no longer complementary in size and/or shape; less energy exchange can take place.[251] These modes of walking are less efficient than normal walking.

The second method of obtaining mechanical energy costs uses a kinetic approach. Briefly stated, the energy changes in a body part between subsequent instants in time are calculated (1) from the product of the forces on each end of the joint and the velocity of the point of application and (2) from the muscle powers, which are the product of each muscle moment and the angular velocity of the body part. In some cases, the muscle is adding energy to the part (generation), and, in other cases, it is absorbing energy. There are a number of different methods of handling the calculations of mechanical energy, exchanges, and transfers, but a sound approach is described by McGibbon et al.[252]

Heart Rate Data

A third general approach to determining the relative energy cost of gait is by measuring the heart rate (HR) during ambulation. Relative energy consumption has been found to be highly correlated with HR, and absolute level of energy consumption has been found to be highly correlated with HR and maximum walking speed. The most accurate way to determine HR is to use a telemetry system that produces beat-by-beat information as well as electrocardiographic activity. Many inexpensive HR monitors are also available and some are designed to download stored information to a computer (see Chapter 2, Examination of Vital Signs). HR responses to ambulation can also be determined by palpation of the radial or carotid arteries, though somewhat more error may be present.

HR measures have been shown to be adequately sensitive for some applications. For example, simple measures of HR and maximum ambulatory velocity allowed accurate prediction ($r = 0.89$) of energy consumption in children with myelomeningocele based on measures recorded from 21 children treadmill walking, 8 children using wheelchairs, and 5 children using both modes.[253] However, Herbert et al[245] found no difference in HR between children with transtibial amputations and those with intact LEs even though energy consumption was 15% higher in the children with amputations. Perhaps because the conditions were more disparate, Waters et al[243] found that in patients with hip arthrodesis, oxygen consumption was 32% greater than normal and that HR was significantly greater than normal.

An energy index based on HR called the *Physiological Cost Index (PCI)* was developed specifically to determine the relative costs of walking per unit of distance walked.[254] Calculated as the difference between the walking HR and the resting HR divided by the average speed, it is expressed in beats per meter. The reliability of PCI has been investigated in individuals without known pathology,[255-257] children with CP,[258] as well as people with spinal cord[257,259] and brain injuries.[137] The index has been used to quantify improvements following an intervention in individuals with spinal cord injury (SCI),[260,261] RA,[262] and stroke.[263-265] For example, PCI was used as a key outcome measure in a study assessing the effects of a 12-week intervention that combined functional electrical stimulation with conventional rehabilitation to manage dropfoot in individuals recovering from a stroke.[265] While walking speed increased 38.7% between the initiation and end of the trial, PCI decreased 34.6%, suggesting improved function and efficiency.

The relationship between PCI and oxygen consumption has been studied across a variety of populations, including individuals with amputations,[266] individuals with SCIs,[259] and individuals without known disabilities.[255] Some researchers have found oxygen uptake measures to be more repeatable and less variable than PCI.[256,259,267,268] One concern that has been raised is that HR measures may be affected by altered vagal or sympathetic regulation due to brain injury[269-272] or medication.[273]

The *Total Heart Beat Index* provides an alternative approach for determining the relative energy efficiency of walking. It is calculated by dividing the total (cumulative) number of heartbeats during exercise by the total distance traveled in a given time period.[257] It has been used to study walking efficiency in individuals with diabetic foot pressure injuries and amputations,[274] chronic incomplete SCIs,[275] and intellectual and developmental disabilities.[276] Reliable and valid use of the measure with populations with blunted HR responses requires study.

SUMMARY

This chapter has provided an overview of select methods for kinematic and kinetic gait analyses. Many of the common variables examined in gait analyses have been defined and described, and examples of studies using gait analyses have been presented. OGA and temporal and spatial variables have been emphasized because they appear to be the most common types of analyses used in the clinical setting. A brief overview of some of the motion analysis systems has been provided. Readers are encouraged to investigate the capabilities of individual motion analysis systems and to consult the gait literature for reliability and validity studies regarding these systems. The ability to perform a gait analysis that accurately describes a patient's gait will provide important quantifiable information necessary for optimal treatment planning and outcomes assessment.

Questions for Review

1. Describe the three different types of gait analyses (kinematic qualitative, kinematic quantitative, and kinetic), and list the variables examined in each type. Identify at least one variable from each type of analysis and describe a technique/technology that could be used to examine the variable.
2. Compare the advantages and disadvantages of a kinematic qualitative gait analysis with the advantages and disadvantages of a kinematic quantitative analysis.
3. Describe how a therapist would determine the concurrent validity of temporal and spatial gait measures recorded using the Zeno™ instrumented mat with values calculated using the Stride Analyzer.
4. A new client is referred to physical therapy with gait dysfunction arising from severe diabetic sensory and motor neuropathy. The patient has a history of recurrent pressure injuries, bilaterally, under his first metatarsal heads that have impaired his ability to stand/walk at work for prolonged periods of time. He recently received a new pair of custom molded orthotic shoe inserts and was instructed to use them in his shoes to help reduce plantar pressures. Unfortunately, he is unable to feel whether they are fitting or not, secondary to the sensory neuropathy. What technology could be used to assess the effectiveness of the inserts at reducing plantar pressures? What activities should be assessed and why?
5. A person walks with excessive dorsiflexion, no heel-off and limited toe extension in terminal stance. Hip and knee analysis reveals excess flexion during stance with absence of the normal "trailing limb" posture characteristic of terminal stance. Identify potential causes for these deviations. What additional tests or measures should be performed?
6. A person reports falling two to three times per week since a recent exacerbation of her multiple sclerosis. Observational gait analysis reveals excess hip flexion, knee flexion, and ankle plantarflexion in mid swing. The individual uses a past retract pattern to diminish hip and knee flexion in late swing but plantarflexion remains excessive. Following a foot flat initial contact, the ankle remains excessively plantarflexed and knee flexion is limited. Identify potential causes for these deviations. What additional tests or measures should be performed?
7. Identify methods that can be used to determine the energy costs that a patient incurs while walking.
8. How could a gait analysis of temporal parameters be used to demonstrate a patient's progress or lack of progress?

CASE STUDY

HISTORY

This 65-year-old woman is 5 days post–right total hip arthroplasty. The surgery was performed following a femoral neck fracture incurred during a fall on the ice in front of her home. She has had daily bedside physical therapy for the past 3 days and now is independent in transfers. However, she needs to be independent in walking before she goes home.

She has a past history of diabetes mellitus (onset age 50), which is controlled with daily insulin injections. She has a recurrent history of foot pressure injuries and has been hospitalized on two occasions to manage infected foot pressure injuries. She denies any history of "heart problems." She does not participate in any regular exercise program and spends a great deal of time sitting during her work as a seamstress. She is alert and oriented to time and place and has a pleasant demeanor. She is 5 feet 3 inches tall, and weighs 160 pounds.

Goniometric Examination of Passive Range of Motion (Degrees)

Lower Extremities

Joint	Motion	Left	Right
Hip	Flexion	WFL	15–40*
	Extension	WFL	0–10*
	Abduction	WFL	0–20*
	Adduction	WFL	0–10*
	Medial rotation	WFL	Not tested*
	Lateral rotation	WFL	0–20*
Knee	Flexion	WFL	0–120
Ankle	Dorsiflexion	WFL	0–15
	Plantarflexion	WFL	0–45
	Inversion	WFL	0–5
	Eversion	WFL	0–20

*Painful with movement.
WFL = within functional limits.
Upper extremities: All ROM measurements are WFL.

Manual Muscle Test (MMT)

Lower Extremities

Joint	Movement	Left	Right
Hip	Flexion	G	F
	Extension	G	P
	Abduction	G	P
	Adduction	G	F+
	Lateral rotation	G	F+
	Medial rotation	G	F+
Knee	Flexion	G	F+
	Extension	G	F+
Ankle	Dorsiflexion	F	P
	Plantarflexion	F	F
	Inversion	F	F
	Eversion	F+	F
Toes	Flexion	F	F
	Extension	P	P

Upper extremities: All muscle grades are within the G to G– range.

Sensory Examination		
	Plantar Aspect Left Foot	Plantar Aspect Right Foot
Sharp/dull	5	5
Light touch	5	5
Temperature	5	5
Proprioceptive sensation	4	4

NUMERIC VALUES REFER TO THE SENSATION SCALE BELOW.

SENSATION SCALE

1. Intact: normal, accurate
2. Decreased: delayed response
3. Exaggerated: increased sensitivity
4. Inaccurate: inappropriate perception of stimuli
5. Absent: no response
6. Inconsistent or ambiguous

INSPECTION

Patient has a pressure injury on the medial aspect of the right plantar surface that is 0.7 × 6.0 cm in diameter and 1.5 mm deep.

FUNCTIONAL EXAMINATION

Locomotion

FIM level = 5

Transfers

FIM level = 7

Activities of Daily Living

Eating: FIM = 7
Bathing: FIM = 7
Dressing: FIM = 7

GUIDING QUESTIONS

1. Develop a physical therapy problem list.
2. Complete the sample OGA form for the right lower extremity based on the information presented (see Appendix 7.A). What deviations would you expect to see for the right lower extremity, and why? How might gait change if the client is instructed to not bear weight on the right forefoot secondary to the plantar pressure injury?
3. Present your recommendations for physical therapy intervention.

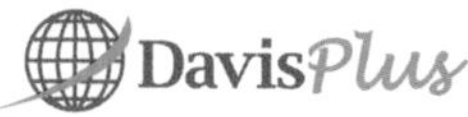

For additional resources, including answers to the questions for review and case study guiding questions, please visit **http://davisplus.fadavis.com.**

References

1. *Guide to Physical Therapist Practice 3.0.* Alexandria, VA: American Physical Therapy Association; 2014. Available at http://guidetoptpractice.apta.org/. Accessed April 26, 2017.
2. Buster, TW, et al: Lower extremity kinematics during walking and elliptical training in individuals with and without traumatic brain injury. J Neurol Phys Ther 37(4):176–186, 2013.
3. Mueller, MJ, et al: Differences in the gait characteristics of patients with diabetes and peripheral neuropathy compared with age-matched controls. Phys Ther 74:299–313, 1994.
4. Von Schroeder, HP, et al: Gait parameters following stroke: A practical assessment. J Rehabil Res Dev 32(1):25, 1995.
5. Walker, S, Helm, P, and Lavery L: Gait pattern alteration by functional sensory substitution in healthy subjects and in diabetic subjects with peripheral neuropathy. Arch Phys Med Rehabil. 78:853–857, 1997.
6. Hesse, S, et al: Asymmetry of gait initiation in hemiparetic stroke subjects. Arch Phys Med Rehabil 78(7):719–724, 1997.
7. De Quervain, IA, et al: Gait pattern in the early recovery period after stroke. J Bone Joint Surg Am 78(10):1506–1514, 1996.
8. Rossi, SA, Doyle, W, and Skinner, HB. Gait initiation of persons with below-knee amputation: The characterization and comparison of force profiles. J Rehabil Res Dev 32(2):120–127, 1995.

9. Roth, EJ, et al: Hemiplegic gait. Relationships between walking speed and other temporal parameters. Am J Phys Med Rehabil 76(2):128–133, 1997.
10. Al-Zahrani, KS, and Bakheit, AMO. A study of the gait characteristics of patients with chronic osteoarthritis of the knee. Disabil Rehabil 24(5):275–280, 2002.
11. Cook, TM, et al: Effects of restricted knee flexion and walking speed on the vertical ground reaction force during gait. J Orthop Sports Phys Ther 25(4):236–244, 1997.
12. Burnfield, JM, Tsai, YJ, and Powers, CM. Comparison of utilized coefficient of friction during different walking tasks in persons with and without a disability. Gait Posture 22(1):82–88, 2005.
13. Postema, K, et al: Energy storage and release of prosthetic feet. Part 1: Biomechanical analysis related to user benefits. *Prosthet Orthot Int* 21(1):17–27, 1997.
14. Perry, J, et al: Toe walking: Muscular demands at the ankle and knee. Arch Phys Med Rehabil 84(1):7–16, 2003.
15. Perry, J, et al: Energy expenditure and gait characteristics of a bilateral amputee walking with C-Leg prostheses compared with stubby and conventional articulating prostheses. Arch Phys Med Rehabil 85(10):1711–1717, 2004.
16. Park, ES, Park, CI, and Kim JY: Comparison of anterior and posterior walkers with respect to gait parameters and energy expenditure of children with spastic diplegic cerebral palsy. Yonsei Med J 42(2):180–184, 2001.
17. Haubert, LL, et al: A comparison of shoulder joint forces during ambulation with crutches versus a walker in persons with incomplete spinal cord injury. Arch Phys Med Rehabil 87(1):63–70, 2006.
18. Self, BP, Greenwald, RM, and Pflaster DS: A biomechanical analysis of a medial unloading brace for osteoarthritis in the knee. Arthritis Care Res 13(4):191–197, 2000.
19. Mulroy, SJ, et al: Effect of AFO design on walking after stroke: Impact of ankle plantar flexion contracture. Prosthet Orthot Int 34(3):277–292, 2010.
20. Gok, H, et al: Effects of ankle-foot orthoses on hemiparetic gait. Clin Rehabil 17(2):137–139, 2003.
21. Radtka, SA, et al: A comparison of gait with solid, dynamic, and no ankle-foot orthoses in children with spastic cerebral palsy. Phys Ther 77:395–409, 1997.
22. Eng, JJ, and Pierrynowski, MR: The effect of soft foot orthotics on three-dimensional lower-limb kinematics during walking and running. Phys Ther 74(9):836–844, 1994.
23. Irons, SL, et al: Novel motor-assisted elliptical training intervention improves Six-Minute Walk Test and oxygen cost for an individual with progressive supranuclear palsy. Cardiopulm Phys Ther J 26(2):36–41, 2015.
24. Granata, KP, Abel, MF, and Damiano, DL: Joint angular velocity in spastic gait and the influence of muscle-tendon lengthening. J Bone Joint Surg Am 82(2):174–186, 2000.
25. Damiano, DL, Kelly, LE, and Vaughn, CL: Effects of quadriceps femoris muscle strengthening on crouch gait in children with spastic diplegia. Phys Ther 75:658–671, 1995.
26. Waters, RL, and Mulroy, SJ: The energy expenditure of normal and pathological gait. Gait Posture 9(3):207–231, 1999.
27. Van Swearingen, JM, et al: The modified Gait Abnormality Rating Scale for recognizing the risk of recurrent falls in community-dwelling elderly adults. Phys Ther 76(9):994–1002, 1996.
28. Shumway-Cook, A, et al: Predicting the probability for falls in community-dwelling older adults. Phys Ther 77(8):812–819, 1997.
29. Burnfield, JM, and Powers, CM. Prediction of slips: An evaluation of utilized coefficient of friction and available slip resistance. Ergonomics 49(10):982–995, 2006.
30. Wall, JC, and Scarbrough, J. Use of a multimemory stopwatch to measure the temporal gait parameters. J Orthop Sports Phys Ther 25(4):277–281, 1997.
31. Sutherland, DH: The evolution of clinical gait analysis part III—kinetics and energy assessment. Gait Posture 21(4):447–461, 2005.
32. Sutherland, DH: The evolution of clinical gait analysis part 1: Kinesiological EMG. Gait Posture 14:61–70, 2001.
33. Sutherland, DH: The evolution of clinical gait analysis part II: Kinematics. Gait Posture 16(2):159–179, 2002.
34. Perry, J, and Burnfield, JM: Gait Analysis: Normal and Pathological Function. Slack Incorporated, Thorofare, NJ, 2010.
35. Pathokinesiology Service and Physical Therapy Department. Observational Gait Analysis, ed 4. Los Amigos Research and Education Institute, Inc., Rancho Los Amigos National Rehabilitation Center, Downey, CA, 2001.
36. Ishikawa, M, et al: Muscle-tendon interaction and elastic energy usage in human walking. J Appl Physiol 99(2):603–608, 2005.
37. Maganaris, CN, and Paul, JP: Tensile properties of the in vivo human gastrocnemius tendon. J Biomech 35(12):1639–1646, 2002.
38. Fukunaga, T, et al: In vivo behavior of human muscle tendon during walking. Proc R Soc Lond B 268:229–233, 2001.
39. Toro, B, Nester, CJ, and Farren PC: The status of gait assessment among physiotherapists in the United Kingdom. Arch Phys Med Rehabil 84:1878–1884, 2003.
40. Southerland, CC: Gait evaluation. In Valmassy, RL (ed): Clinical Biomechanics of the Lower Extremities. Mosby-Yearbook, St. Louis, MO, 1996, pp. 149–177.
41. Krebs, DE, Edelstein, JE, and Fishman, S: Reliability of observational kinematic gait analysis. Phys Ther 65(7):1027–1033, 1985.
42. Bernhardt, J, Bate, PJ, and Matyas, TA: Accuracy of observational kinematic assessment of upper-limb movements. Phys Ther 78(3):259–270, 1998.
43. Gilbertson, TJ, et al: Clinical gait measures for ambulatory children with cerebral palsy: A review. J Prosthet Orthot 28(1): 2–12, 2016.
44. Rathinam, C, et al: Observational gait assessment tools in paediatrics—a systematic review. Gait Posture 40(2):279–285, 2014.
45. Del Pilar Duque Orozco, M, et al: Reliability and validity of Edinburgh visual gait score as an evaluation tool for children with cerebral palsy. Gait Posture 49:14–18, 2016.
46. Tas, S, et al: A comparison of results of 3-dimensional gait analysis and observational gait analysis in patients with knee osteoarthritis. Acta Orthop Traumatol Turc 49(2):151–159, 2015.
47. Russell, DJ, et al: Training users in the gross motor function measure: Methodological and practical issues. Phys Ther 74(7): 630–636, 1994.
48. Brunnekreef, JJ, et al: Reliability of videotaped observational gait analysis in patients with orthopedic impairments. BMC Musculoskelet Disord 6:17–26, 2005.
49. Eastlack, ME, et al: Interrater reliability of videotaped observational gait-analysis assessments. Phys Ther 71(6):465–472, 1991.
50. Krebs, DE: Interpretation standards in locomotor studies. In Craik, R, and Oatis, C (eds): Gait Analysis: Theory and Application. Mosby-Yearbook, St. Louis, MO, 1995, pp. 334–354.
51. McGinley, JL, et al: Accuracy and reliability of observational gait analysis data: Judgments of push-off in gait after stroke. Phys Ther 83(2):146–160, 2003.
52. Borel, S, Schneider, P, and Newman CJ: Video analysis software increases the interrater reliability of video gait assessments in children with cerebral palsy. Gait Posture 33(4):727–729, 2011.
53. Stuberg, WA, et al: Comparison of a clinical gait analysis method using videography and temporal-distance measures with 16-mm cinematography. Phys Ther 68(8):1221–1225, 1988.
54. Mills, K: Motion analysis in the clinic: There's an app for that. J Physiother 61(1):49–50, 2015.
55. Sánchez Rodríguez, MT, et al: Neurorehabilitation and apps: A systematic review of mobile applications (English Edition). Neurologia 2016.
56. Levangie, PK, and Norkin, CC: Joint Structure and Function: A Comprehensive Analysis, ed 5. FA Davis, Philadelphia, 2011.
57. Craik, RL, and Otis, CA: Gait assessment in the clinic: Issues and approaches. In Rothstein JM (ed): Measurement in Physical Therapy. Churchill Livingstone, London, 1985, pp. 169–205.
58. Nelson, AJ: Functional ambulation profile. Phys Ther 54(10): 1059-1065, 1974.
59. Howe, JA, et al: The Community Balance and Mobility Scale—a balance measure for individuals with traumatic brain injury. Clin Rehabil 20(10):885–895, 2006.
60. Harada, N, et al: Screening for balance and mobility impairment in elderly individuals living in residential care facilities. Phys Ther 75(6):462–469, 1995.
61. Wolf, SL, Catlin, PA, and Gage, K: Establishing the reliability and validity of measurements of walking time using the Emory Functional Ambulation Profile. Phys Ther 79(12):1122–1133, 1999.
62. Baer, HR, and Wolf, SL: Modified Emory Functional Ambulation Profile: An outcome measure for the rehabilitation of poststroke gait dysfunction. Stroke 32(4):973–979, 2001.

63. Shields, RK, et al: Reliability, validity, and responsiveness of functional tests in patients with total joint replacement. Phys Ther 75(3):169–176, 1995.
64. *Uniform Data System for Medical Rehabilitation. 1997–2009. The FIM System Clinical Guide Version 5.2.* Buffalo, UDSMR.
65. Santa Clara Valley Medical Center. Introduction to the Functional Assessment Measure. The Center for Outcome Measurements in Brain Injury (COMBI). 2017. Retrieved April 28, 2017, from http://tbims.org/combi/FAM/index.html.
66. Hawley, CA, et al: Use of the functional assessment measure (FIM+FAM) in head injury rehabilitation: A psychometric analysis. J Neurol Neurosurg Psychiatry 67(6):749–754, 1999.
67. Butcher, SJ, Meshke, JM, and Sheppard, MS: Reductions in functional balance, coordination, and mobility measures among patients with stable chronic obstructive pulmonary disease. J Cardiopulm Rehabil 24(4):274–280, 2004.
68. Knorr, S, Brouwer, B, and Garland, SJ: Validity of the Community Balance and Mobility Scale in community-dwelling persons after stroke. Arch Phys Med Rehabil 91(6):890–896, 2010.
69. Woollacott, MH, and Tang, PF: Balance control during walking in the older adult: Research and its implications. Phys Ther 77(6):646–660, 1997.
70. Shumway-Cook, A, and Woollacott, WJ: Motor Control: Translating Research Into Clinical Practice, ed 4. Williams and Wilkins, Baltimore, 2011.
71. Jonsdottir, J, and Cattaneo, D: Reliability and validity of the Dynamic Gait Index in persons with chronic stroke. Arch Phys Med Rehabil 88(11):1410–1415, 2007.
72. Marchetti, GF, and Whitney, SL: Construction and validation of the 4-Item Dynamic Gait Index. Phys Ther 86(12):1651–1660, 2006.
73. Leddy, AL, Crowner, BE, and Earhart, GM: Functional Gait Assessment and Balance Evaluation System Test: Reliability, validity, sensitivity, and specificity for identifying individuals with Parkinson disease who fall. Phys Ther 91(1):102–113, 2011.
74. Wrisley, DM, and Kumar, NA: Functional gait assessment: Concurrent, discriminative, and predictive validity in community-dwelling older adults. Phys Ther 90(5):761–773, 2010.
75. Walker, ML, et al: Reference group data for the Functional Gait Assessment. Phys Ther 87(11):1468–1477, 2007.
76. Wrisley, DM, et al: Reliability, internal consistency, and validity of data obtained with the Functional Gait Assessment. Phys Ther 84(10):906–918, 2004.
77. Lin, JH, et al: Psychometric comparisons of 3 functional ambulation measures for patients with stroke. Stroke 41(9):2021–2025, 2010.
78. Williams, G, et al: The high-level mobility assessment tool (HiMAT) for traumatic brain injury. Part 1: Item generation. Brain Inj 19(11):925–932, 2005.
79. Williams, GP, et al: The high-level mobility assessment tool (HiMAT) for traumatic brain injury. Part 2: Content validity and discriminability. Brain Inj 19(10):833–843, 2005.
80. Williams, G, et al: The concurrent validity and responsiveness of the High-level Mobility Assessment Tool for measuring the mobility limitations of people with traumatic brain injury. Arch Phys Med Rehabil 87(3):437–442, 2006.
81. Williams, GP, et al: High-Level Mobility Assessment Tool (HiMAT): Interrater reliability, retest reliability, and internal consistency. Phys Ther 86(3):395–400, 2006.
82. Tyson, S, and Connell, L: The psychometric properties and clinical utility of measures of walking and mobility in neurological conditions: A systematic review. Clin Rehabil 23(11):1018–1033, 2009.
83. Williams, G, Pallant, J, and Greenwood, K: Further development of the High-level Mobility Assessment Tool (HiMAT). Brain Inj 24(7):1027–1031, 2010.
84. Di Fabio, RP, and Seay, R: Use of the "Fast Evaluation of Mobility, Balance, and Fear" in elderly community dwellers: Validity and reliability. Phys Ther 77(9):904–917, 1997.
85. Hess, RJ, et al: Walking skill can be assessed in older adults: Validity of the Figure-of-8 Walk Test. Phys Ther 90(1):89–99, 2010.
86. Tinetti, ME: Performance-oriented assessment of mobility problems in elderly patients. J Am Geriatr Soc 34:119–126, 1986.
87. Dittuno, PL, and Ditunno, JF, Jr. Walking index for spinal cord injury (WISCI II): Scale revision. Spinal Cord 39(12):654–656, 2001.
88. Ditunno, Jr JF, et al: The Walking Index for Spinal Cord Injury (WISCI/WISCI II): nature, metric properties, use and misuse. Spinal Cord 51:346-355, 2013.
89. Liaw, LJ, et al: Psychometric properties of the modified Emory Functional Ambulation Profile in stroke patients. Clin Rehabil 20(5):429–437, 2006.
90. Morton T: Uniform data system for rehab begins: First tool measures dependent level. Progress Report, American Physical Therapy Association, 1986.
91. Wolfson, AM, Doctor, JN, and Burns, SP: Clinician judgments of functional outcomes: How bias and perceived accuracy affect rating. Arch Phys Med Rehabil 81(12):1567–1574, 2000.
92. Gurka, JA, et al: Utility of the Functional Assessment Measure after discharge from inpatient rehabilitation. J Head Trauma Rehabil 14(3):247–256, 1999.
93. Hobart, JC, et al: Evidence-based measurement: Which disability scale for neurologic rehabilitation? Neurology 57(4):639–644, 2001.
94. Linn, RT, et al: Does the Functional Assessment Measure (FAM) extend the Functional Independence Measure (FIM) instrument? A rasch analysis of stroke inpatients. J Outcome Meas 3(4): 339–359, 1999.
95. Whitney, SL, Hudak, MT, and Marchetti, GF: The Dynamic Gait Index relates to self-reported fall history in individuals with vestibular dysfunction. J Vestib Res 10(2):99–105, 2000.
96. Brown, KE, et al: Physical therapy outcomes for persons with bilateral vestibular loss. Laryngoscope 111:1812–1817, 2001.
97. Huang, SL, et al: Minimal detectable change of the Timed "Up & Go" test and the Dynamic Gait Index in people with Parkinson disease. Phys Ther 91(1):114–121, 2011.
98. Cattaneo, D, Jonsdottir, J, and Repetti S: Reliability of four scales on balance disorders in persons with multiple sclerosis. Disabil Rehabil 29(24):1920, 2007.
99. Shumway-Cook, A, et al: Expanding the scoring system for the Dynamic Gait Index. Phys Ther 93(11):1493–1506, 2013.
100. Williams, EN, et al: Investigation of the Timed "Up & Go" Test in children. Dev Med Child Neurol 47(8):518–524, 2005.
101. Kegelmeyer, DA, et al: Reliability and validity of the Tinetti Mobility Test for individuals with Parkinson disease. Phys Ther 87(10):1369–1378, 2007.
102. Canbek, J, et al: Test-retest reliability and construct validity of the tinetti performance-oriented mobility assessment in people with stroke. J Neurol Phys Ther 37(1):14–19, 2013.
103. Ditunno, PL, and Ditunno, JF: Walking Index for Spinal Cord Injury (WISCI II): Scale revision. Spinal Cord 39:654–656, 2001.
104. Scivoletto, G, et al: Walking Index for Spinal Cord Injury version II in acute spinal cord injury: Reliability and reproducibility. Spinal Cord 52(1):65-69, 2014.
105. Thielen, CC, et al: Evaluation of the Walking Index for Spinal Cord Injury II (WISCI-II) in children with Spinal Cord Injury (SCI). Spinal Cord, 2016.
106. Burns, AS, et al: The reproducibility and convergent validity of the walking index for spinal cord injury (WISCI) in chronic spinal cord injury. Neurorehabil Neural Repair 25(2):149–157, 2011.
107. Ditunno, JF, et al: Validity of the walking scale for spinal cord injury and other domains of function in a multicenter clinical trial. Neurorehabil Neural Repair 21:539–550, 2007.
108. van Hedel, HJ, Wirz, M, and Dietz, V: Assessing walking ability in subjects with spinal cord injury: Validity and reliability of 3 walking tests. Arch Phys Med Rehabil 86(2):190–196, 2005.
109. Steeves, JD, et al: Guidelines for the conduct of clinical trials for spinal cord injury (SCI) as developed by the ICCP panel: Clinical trial outcome measures. Spinal Cord 45(3):206–221, 2007.
110. Jackson, AB, et al: Outcome measures for gait and ambulation in the spinal cord injury population. J Spinal Cord Med 31(5): 487–499, 2008.
111. Labruyere, R, Agarwala, A, and Curt, A: Rehabilitation in spine and spinal cord trauma. Spine 35(21 Suppl):S259–262, 2010.
112. Graham, JE, et al: Walking speed threshold for classifying walking independence in hospitalized older adults. Phys Ther 90(11):1591–1597, 2010.
113. Perry, J, et al: Classification of walking handicap in the stroke population. Stroke 26(6):982–989, 1995.
114. Lerner-Frankiel, MB, et al: Functional community ambulation: What are your criteria? Clin Manag Phys Ther 6(2):12–15, 1986.
115. Fulk, GD, et al: Predicting home and community walking activity poststroke. Stroke 48(2):406–411, 2017.

116. Andrews, AW, et al: Update on distance and velocity requirements for community ambulation. J Geriatr Phys Ther 33(3):128–134, 2010.
117. Robinett, CS, and Vondran, MA: Functional ambulation velocity and distance requirements in rural and urban communities. A clinical report. Phys Ther 68(9):1371–1373, 1988.
118. Walsh, M, et al: Physical impairments and functional limitations: A comparison of individuals 1 year after total knee arthroplasty with control subjects. Phys Ther 78(3):248–258, 1998.
119. Winter, DA, et al: Biomechanical walking pattern changes in the fit and healthy elderly. Phys Ther 70:340–347, 1990.
120. Blanke, D, and Hageman, PA: Comparison of gait of young men and elderly men. Phys Ther 69:144–148, 1989.
121. Bohannon, R: Walking speed: reference values and correlates for older adults. J Orthop Sports Phys Ther 24:86–90, 1996.
122. Ostrosky, KM, et al: A comparison of gait characteristics in young and older subjects. Phys Ther 74(7):637–646, 1994.
123. Todd, F, et al: Variations in the gait of normal children. A graph applicable to the documentation of abnormalities. J Bone Joint Surg Am 71(2):196–204, 1989.
124. Murray, MP, Drought, AB, and Kory, RC. Walking patterns of normal men. J Bone Joint Surg Am 46A:335–360, 1964.
125. Murray, MP, Kory, RC, and Sepic, SB. Walking patterns of normal women. Arch Phys Med Rehabil 51:637–650, 1970.
126. Spyropoulos, P, et al: Biomechanical gait analysis in obese men. Arch Phys Med Rehabil 72(13):1065–1070, 1991.
127. Hills, AP, and Parker, AW. Gait characteristics of obese children. Arch Phys Med Rehabil 72(6):403–407, 1991.
128. McGibbon, CA, and Krebs, DE: Discriminating age and disability effects in locomotion: Neuromuscular adaptations in musculoskeletal pathology. J Appl Physiol 96(1):149–160, 2004.
129. Connelly, DM, and Vandervoort, AA: Effects of detraining on knee extensor strength and functional mobility in a group of elderly women. J Orthop Sports Phys Ther 26(6):340–346, 1997.
130. Sutherland, D: The development of mature gait. Gait Posture 6:163–170, 1997.
131. Holden, MK, et al: Clinical gait assessment in the neurologically impaired: Reliability and meaningfulness. Phys Ther 64(1): 35–40, 1984.
132. van Loo, MA, et al: Inter-rater reliability and concurrent validity of step length and step width measurement after traumatic brain injury. Disabil Rehabil 25(21):1195–1200, 2003.
133. Robinson, JL, and Smidt, GL: Quantitative gait evaluation in the clinic. Phys Ther 61(3):351–353, 1981.
134. Guyatt, GH, et al: The 6-minute walk: A new measure of exercise capacity in patients with chronic heart failure. Can Med Assoc J 132(8):919–923, 1985.
135. Butland, RJ, et al: Two-, six-, and 12-minute walking tests in respiratory disease. Br Med J (Clin Res Ed) 284(6329):1607–1608, 1982.
136. Schenkman, M, et al: Reliability of impairment and physical performance measures for persons with Parkinson's disease. Phys Ther 77(1):19–27, 1997.
137. Mossberg, KA: Reliability of a timed walk test in persons with acquired brain injury. Am J Phys Med Rehabil 82(5):385–390, 2003.
138. Fulk, GD, et al: Predicting home and community walking activity in people with stroke. Arch Phys Med Rehabil 91(10): 1582–1586, 2010.
139. Fitzgerald, D, et al: Six-minute walk test in children with spastic cerebral palsy and children developing typically. Pediatr Phys Ther 28(2):192–199, 2016.
140. Sullivan, KJ, et al: Effects of task-specific locomotor and strength training in adults who were ambulatory after stroke: Results of the STEPS randomized clinical trial. Phys Ther 87(12):1580–1602, 2007.
141. American Thoracic Society. Committee on Proficiency Standards for Clinical Pulmonary Function Laboratories. ATS statement: Guidelines for the six-minute walk test. Am J Respir Crit Care Med 166(1):111–117, 2002.
142. Jenkins, S, et al: Regression equations to predict 6-minute walk distance in middle-aged and elderly adults. Physiother Theory Pract 25(7):516–522, 2009.
143. Geiger, R, et al: Six-Minute Walk Test in children and adolescents. J Pediatr 150(4):395–399.e392, 2007.
144. Chetta, A, et al: Reference values for the 6-min walk test in healthy subjects 20-50 years old. Respir Med 100(9):1573–1578, 2006.
145. Camarri, B, et al: Six minute walk distance in healthy subjects aged 55-75 years. Respir Med 100(4):658–665, 2006.
146. Casanova, C, et al: The 6-min walk distance in healthy subjects: Reference standards from seven countries. Eur Respir J 37(1):150–156, 2011.
147. Priesnitz, CV, et al: Reference values for the 6-min walk test in healthy children aged 6-12 years. Pediatr Pulmonol 44(12): 1174–1179, 2009.
148. Troosters, T, Gosselink, R, and Decramer, M: Six minute walking distance in healthy elderly subjects. Eur Respir J 14(2): 270–274, 1999.
149. Poh, H, et al: Six-minute walk distance in healthy Singaporean adults cannot be predicted using reference equations derived from Caucasian populations. Respirology 11(2):211–216, 2006.
150. Bohannon, RW: Six-minute Walk Test: A meta-analysis of data from apparently healthy elders. Top Geriatr Rehabil 23(2): 155–160, 2007.
151. Kerr, C, McDowell, BC, and Cosgrove A: Oxygen cost versus a 1-minute walk test in a population of children with bilateral spastic cerebral palsy. J Pediatr Orthop 27(3):283–287, 2007.
152. McDowell, BC, et al: Test-retest reliability of a 1-min walk test in children with bilateral spastic cerebral palsy (BSCP). Gait Posture 29(2):267–269, 2009.
153. McDowell, BC, et al: Validity of a 1 minute walk test for children with cerebral palsy. Dev Med Child Neurol 47(11):744–748, 2005.
154. Kosak, M, and Smith, T: Comparison of the 2-, 6-, and 12-minute walk tests in patients with stroke. J Rehabil Res Dev 42(1):103–107, 2005.
155. Rossier, P, and Wade, DT: Validity and reliability comparison of 4 mobility measures in patients presenting with neurologic impairment. Arch Phys Med Rehabil 82(1):9–13, 2001.
156. English, CK, et al: The sensitivity of three commonly used outcome measures to detect change amongst patients receiving inpatient rehabilitation following stroke. Clin Rehabil 20(1):52–55, 2006.
157. Askim, T, et al: Effects of a community-based intensive motor training program combined with early supported discharge after treatment in a comprehensive stroke unit: A randomized, controlled trial. Stroke 41(8):1697–1703, 2010.
158. Flansbjer, U-B, et al: Reliability of gait performance tests in men and women with hemiparesis after stroke. J Rehabil Med 37(2):75–82, 2005.
159. Hollman, JH, et al: Minimum detectable change in gait velocity during acute rehabilitation following hip fracture. J Geriatr Phys Ther 31(2):53–56, 2008.
160. Nilsagard, Y, et al: Clinical relevance using timed walk tests and "Timed Up and Go" testing in persons with multiple sclerosis. Physiother Res Int 12(2):105–114, 2007.
161. Kavanagh, JJ, and Menz, HB: Accelerometry: A technique for quantifying movement patterns during walking. Gait Posture 28(1):1–15, 2008.
162. Moe-Nilssen, R: Test-retest reliability of trunk accelerometry during standing and walking. Arch Phys Med Rehabil 79(11): 1377–1385, 1998.
163. Moe-Nilssen, R, and Helbostad, JL: Estimation of gait cycle characteristics by trunk accelerometry. J Biomech 37(1): 121–126, 2004.
164. Henriksen, M, et al: Test-retest reliability of trunk accelerometric gait analysis. Gait Posture 19(3):288–297, 2004.
165. Levine, JA, Baukol, PA, and Westerterp, KR: Validation of the Tracmor triaxial accelerometer system for walking. Med Sci Sports Exerc 33:1593–1597, 2001.
166. Hartmann, A, et al: Reproducibility of spatio-temporal gait parameters under different conditions in older adults using a trunk tri-axial accelerometer system. Gait Posture 30(3):351–355, 2009.
167. Menz, HB, Lord, SR, and Fitzpatrick, RC: Acceleration patterns of the head and pelvis when walking on level and irregular surfaces. Gait Posture 18(1):35–46, 2003.
168. Zhang, K, et al: Measurement of human daily physical activity. Obes Res 11(1):33–40, 2003.
169. Foerster, F, Smeja, M, and Fahrenberg, J: Detection of posture and motion by accelerometry: A validation study in ambulatory monitoring. Comput Human Behav 15(5):571–583, 1999.
170. Macko, RF, et al: Microprocessor-based ambulatory activity monitoring in stroke patients. Med Sci Sports Exerc 34(3):394–399, 2002.

171. Michael, KM, Allen, JK, and Macko, RF: Reduced ambulatory activity after stroke: The role of balance, gait, and cardiovascular fitness. Arch Phys Med Rehabil 86(8):1552–1556, 2005.
172. Gebruers, N, et al: Monitoring of physical activity after stroke: A systematic review of accelerometry-based measures. Arch Phys Med Rehabil 91(2):288–297, 2010.
173. Hartsell, H, et al: Accuracy of a custom-designed activity monitor: Implications for diabetic foot ulcer healing. J Rehabil Res Dev 39(3):395–400, 2002.
174. Brandes, M, and Rosenbaum, D: Correlations between the step activity monitor and the DynaPort ADL-monitor. Clin Biomech (Bristol, Avon) 19(1):91–94, 2004.
175. Coleman, KL, et al: Step activity monitor: Long-term, continuous recording of ambulatory function. J Rehabil Res Dev 36(1):8–18, 1999.
176. Balto, JM, Kinnett-Hopkins, DL, and Motl, RW: Accuracy and precision of smartphone applications and commercially available motion sensors in multiple sclerosis. Mult Scler J Exp Transl Clin 2, 2016.
177. McIninch, J, Datta, S, and DasMahapatra, P: Remote tracking of walking activity in MS patients in a real-world setting. Neurology 84(14):P3.209, 2015.
178. Singh, AK, et al: Accuracy of the FitBit at walking speeds and cadences relevant to clinical rehabilitation populations. Disabil Health J 9(2):320–323, 2016.
179. Ferguson, T, et al: The validity of consumer-level, activity monitors in healthy adults worn in free-living conditions: A cross-sectional study. Int J Behav Nutr Phys Act 12(1):42, 2015.
180. Simpson, LA, et al: Capturing step counts at slow walking speeds in older adults: Comparison of ankle and waist placement of measuring device. J Rehabil Med 47(9):830–835, 2015.
181. Klassen, TD, et al: "Stepping Up" activity poststroke: Ankle-positioned accelerometer can accurately record steps during slow walking. Phys Ther 2015.
182. Sullivan, JE, et al: Feasibility and outcomes of a community-based, pedometer-monitored walking program in chronic stroke: a pilot study. Top Stroke Rehabil 21(2):101–110, 2014.
183. Paul, SS, et al: Validity of the Fitbit activity tracker for measuring steps in community-dwelling older adults. BMJ Open Sport Exerc Med 1(1):e000013, 2015.
184. Fulk, GD, et al: Accuracy of 2 activity monitors in detecting steps in people with stroke and traumatic brain injury. Phys Ther 94(2):222–229, 2014.
185. Aminian, K, et al: Spatio-temporal parameters of gait measured by an ambulatory system using miniature gyroscopes. J Biomech 35(5):689–699, 2002.
186. Kotiadis, AD, Hermensa, HJ, and Veltinka, PH: Inertial gait phase detection for control of a drop foot stimulator: Inertial sensing for gait phase detection. Med Eng Phys 32(4):287–297, 2010.
187. Barker, S, et al: Accuracy, reliability, and validity of a spatiotemporal gait analysis system. Med Eng Phys 28(5):460–467, 2006.
188. Stokic, DS, et al: Agreement between temporospatial gait parameters of an electronic walkway and a motion capture system in healthy and chronic stroke populations. Am J Phys Med Rehabil 88(6):437–444, 2009.
189. McDonough, AL, et al: The validity and reliability of the GAITRite system's measurements: A preliminary evaluation. Arch Phys Med Rehabil 82(3):419–425, 2001.
190. van Uden, C, and Besser, M: Test-retest reliability of temporal and spatial gait characteristics measured with an instrumented walkway system (GAITRite®). BMC Musculoskelet Disord 5(1):13, 2004.
191. Menz, HB, et al: Reliability of the GAITRite® walkway system for the quantification of temporo-spatial parameters of gait in young and older people. Gait Posture 20(1):20–25, 2004.
192. Bilney, B, Morris, M, and Webster, K: Concurrent related validity of the GAITRite® walkway system for quantification of the spatial and temporal parameters of gait. Gait Posture 17(1): 68–74, 2003.
193. Titianova, EB, et al: Gait characteristics and functional ambulation profile in patients with chronic unilateral stroke. Am J Phys Med Rehabil 82(10):778, 2003.
194. Humphrey, S, et al: Concurrent validity of Zeno and GAITRite walkway systems in healthy older adults. Proceedings of the American College of Sports Medicine 2016.
195. Beck, EN, Ehgoetz Martens, KA, and Almeida, QJ: Freezing of gait in Parkinson's disease: An overload problem? PLoS One 10(12):e0144986, 2015.
196. Wajda, DA, et al: Preliminary investigation of gait initiation and falls in multiple sclerosis. Arch Phys Med Rehabil 96(6): 1098–1102, 2015.
197. Roeing, KL, et al: Gait termination in individuals with multiple sclerosis. Gait Posture 42(3):335–339, 2015.
198. Roeing, KL, Moon, Y, and Sosnoff, JJ: Unplanned gait termination in individuals with multiple sclerosis. Gait Posture 53: 168–172, 2017.
199. Wolf, SL, and Binder-Macleod, SA: Use of the Krusen Limb Load Monitor to quantify temporal and loading measurements of gait. Phys Ther 62(7):976–984, 1982.
200. Powers, CM, et al: The influence of lower extremity muscle force on gait characteristics in individuals with below-knee amputations secondary to vascular disease. Phys Ther 76(4):369–377, 1996.
201. Burnfield, JM, et al: Similarity of joint kinematics and muscle demands between elliptical training and walking: Implications for practice. Phys Ther 90(2):289–305, 2010.
202. Morris, ME, et al: Changes in gait and fatigue from morning to afternoon in people with multiple sclerosis. J Neurol Neurosurg Psychiatry 72(3):361–365, 2002.
203. Powers, CM, et al: The effects of patellar taping on stride characteristics and joint motion in subjects with patellofemoral pain. J Orthop Sports Phys Ther 26(6):286–291, 1997.
204. O'Shea, S, Morris, ME, and Iansek, R: Dual task interference during gait in people with Parkinson disease: Effects of motor versus cognitive secondary tasks. Phys Ther 82(9):888–897, 2002.
205. Evans, MD, Goldie, PA, and Hill, KA: Systematic and random error in repeated measurements of temporal and distance parameters of gait after stroke. Arch Phys Med Rehabil 78(7):725–729, 1997.
206. Maurer, BT, et al: Quantitative identification of ankle equinus with applications for treatment assessment. Gait Posture 3(1): 19–28, 1995.
207. Teixeira-Salmela, LF, et al: Effects of muscle strengthening and physical conditioning training on temporal, kinematic and kinetic variables during gait in chronic stroke survivors. J Rehabil Med 33(2):53–60, 2001.
208. Schwartz, MH, et al: Comprehensive treatment of ambulatory children with cerebral palsy: An outcome assessment. J Pediatr Orthop 24(1):45–53, 2004.
209. Lam, T, et al: Stumbling corrective responses during treadmill-elicited stepping in human infants. J Physiol 553(1):319–331, 2003.
210. Woltring, HJ, and Marsolais, EB: Optoelectric (Selspot) gait measurement in two- and three-dimensional space, a preliminary report. Bull Prosthet Res 17:46–52, 1980.
211. Bell, A, Pedersen, D, and Brand, R: A comparison of the accuracy of several hip center location prediction models. J Biomech 23(6):617–621, 1990.
212. Gorton, GE, Hebert, DA, and Gannotti, ME: Assessment of the kinematic variability among 12 motion analysis laboratories. Gait Posture 29(3):398–402, 2009.
213. Richards, JG: The measurement of human motion: A comparison of commercially available systems. Hum Mov Sci 18:589–602, 1999.
214. Childs, JD, et al: Alterations in lower extremity movement and muscle activation patterns in individuals with knee osteoarthritis. Clin Biomech (Bristol, Avon) 19(1):44–49, 2004.
215. de Bengoa Vallejo, RB, Gómez, RS, and Iglesias, MEL: Clinical improvement in functional hallux limitus using a cut-out orthosis. Prosthet Orthot Int 40(2):215–223, 2016.
216. Klous, M, et al: Differences in kinetics and coordination between walking barefoot and walking in rocker bottom shoes. J Sports Res 2(3):77–88, 2015.
217. Cornwall, MW, and McPoil, TG: Motion of the calcaneus, navicular, and first metatarsal during the stance phase of walking. J Am Podiatr Med Assoc 92(2):67–76, 2002.
218. Fishco, WD, and Cornwall, MW: Gait analysis after talonavicular joint fusion: 2 case reports. J Foot Ankle Surg 43(4):241247, 2004.
219. Burnfield, JM, and Powers CM. Influence of age and gender of utilized coefficient of friction during walking at different speeds. In Marpet, MI, and Sapienza, MA (eds): Metrology of Pedestrian Locomotion and Slip Resistance. ASTM International, West Conshohocken, PA, 2003, pp 3–16.

220. Hesse, S, et al: Treadmill training with partial body weight support: influence of body weight release on the gait of hemiparetic patients. J Neurol Rehabil 11:15–20, 1997.
221. Kerrigan, DC, et al: Compensatory advantages of toe walking. Arch Phys Med Rehabil 81(1):38–44, 2000.
222. Neptune, RR, Burnfield, JM, and Mulroy, SJ. The neuromuscular demands of toe walking: A forward dynamics simulation analysis. J Biomech 40(6):1293–1300, 2007.
223. Sasaki, K, et al. Muscle compensatory mechanisms during able-bodied toe walking. Gait Posture 27:440–446, 2008.
224. Burnfield, JM, et al: The influence of walking speed and footwear on plantar pressures in older adults. Clin Biomech (Bristol, Avon) 19(1):78–84, 2004.
225. Mohamed, O, et al: Effect of terrain on foot pressure during walking. Foot Ankle Int 26(10):859–869, 2005.
226. Burnfield, JM, et al: Variations in plantar pressure variables across five cardiovascular exercises. Med Sci Sports Exerc 39(11): 2012–2020, 2007.
227. Semple, R, et al: Regionalised centre of pressure analysis in patients with rheumatoid arthritis. Clin Biomech (Bristol, Avon) 22(1):127–129, 2007.
228. Randolph, AL, et al: Reliability of measurements of pressures applied on the foot during walking by a computerized insole sensor system. Arch Phys Med Rehabil 81(5):573, 2000.
229. Mueller, MJ, Strube, MJ, and Allen, BT: Therapeutic footwear can reduce plantar pressure in patients with diabetes and transmetatarsal amputation. Diabetes Care 20(4):637–641, 1997.
230. Mueller, MJ, Allen, BT, and Sinacore, DR: Incidence of skin breakdown and higher amputation after transmetatarsal amputation: Implications for rehabilitation. Arch Phys Med Rehabil 76: 50–54, 1995.
231. Armstrong, DG, Lavery, LA, and Bushman, TR: Peak foot pressures influence the healing time of diabetic foot ulcers treated with total contact casts. J Rehabil Res Dev 35(1):1–5, 1998.
232. Burnfield, JM, et al: The influence of lower extremity joint torque on gait characteristics in elderly men. Arch Phys Med Rehabil 81(9):1153–1157, 2000.
233. American Physical Therapy Association. *Guide to Physical Therapist Practice,* ed 3. American Physical Therapy Association, Alexandria, VA, 2016.
234. Brinkmann, JR, and Perry, J: Rate and range of knee motion during ambulation in healthy and arthritic subjects. Phys Ther 65:1055–1060, 1985.
235. Winter, DA, et al: Biomechanical walking pattern changes in the fit and healthy elderly. Phys Ther 70(6):340–347, 1990.
236. Himann, JE, et al: Age-related changes in speed of walking. Med Sci Sports Exerc 20(2):161–166, 1988.
237. Hageman, PA, and Blanke, DJ: Comparison of gait of young women and elderly women. Phys Ther 66(9):1382–1387, 1986.
238. Cho, SH, Park, JM, and Kwon, OY: Gender differences in three dimensional gait analysis data from 98 healthy Korean adults. Clinical Biomechanics (Bristol) 19(2):145–152, 2004.
239. Sutherland, D, et al: Clinical use of prediction regions for motion analysis. Dev Med Child Neurol 38(9):773–781, 1996.
240. Chester, VL, Tingley, M, and Biden, EN: Comparison of two normative paediatric gait databases. Dyn Med 6:8, 2007.
241. Romei, M, et al: Use of the Normalcy Index for the evaluation of gait pathology. Gait Posture 19(1):85–90, 2004.
242. Mulroy, S, et al: Use of cluster analysis for gait pattern classification of patients in the early and late recovery phases following stroke. Gait Posture 18(1):114–125, 2003.
243. Waters, RL, et al: Energy expenditure following hip and ankle arthrodesis. J Bone Joint Surg Am 70:1032, 1988.
244. Marsolais, EB, and Edwards, BG: Energy costs of walking and standing with functional neuromuscular stimulation and long leg braces. Arch Phys Med Rehabil 69(4):243–249, 1988.
245. Herbert, LM, et al: A comparison of oxygen consumption during walking between children with and without below-knee amputations. Phys Ther 74(10):943–950, 1994.
246. Davies, MJ, and Dalsky, GP: Economy of mobility in older adults. J Orthop Sports Phys Ther 26(2):69–72, 1997.
247. Torburn, L, et al: Energy expenditure during ambulation in dysvascular and traumatic below-knee amputees: A comparison of five prosthetic feet. J Rehabil Res Dev 32(2):111–119, 1995.
248. Ebbeling, CJ, Hamill, J, and Crussemeyer, JA: Lower extremity mechanics and energy cost of walking in high-heeled shoes. J Orthop Sports Phys Ther 19(4):190–196, 1994.
249. Waters, RL, et al: Energy-speed relationship of walking: Standard tables. J Orthop Res 6(2):215–222, 1988.
250. Olgiati, R, Burgunder, JM, and Mumenthaler, M. Increased energy cost of walking in multiple sclerosis: Effect of spasticity, ataxia, and weakness. Arch Phys Med Rehabil 69(10):846–849, 1988.
251. Olney, SJ, Monga, TN, and Costigan, PA: Mechanical energy of walking of stroke patients. Arch Phys Med Rehabil 67:92–98, 1986.
252. McGibbon, CA, Krebs, DE, and Puniello, MS: Mechanical energy analysis identifies compensatory strategies in disabled elders' gait. J Biomech 34(4):481–490, 2001.
253. Findley, TW, and Agre, JC: Ambulation in the adolescent with spina bifida. II. Oxygen cost of mobility. Arch Phys Med Rehabil 69(10):855–861, 1988.
254. MacGregor, J: The objective measurement of physical performance with Long-Term Ambulatory Physiological Surveillance Equipment (LAPSE). Proceedings of the 3rd International Symposium on Ambulatory Monitoring, London, pp. 29–39, 1979.
255. Graham, RC, Smith, NM, and White, CM: The reliability and validity of the Physiological Cost Index in healthy subjects while walking on 2 different tracks. Arch Phys Med Rehabil 86: 2041–2046, 2005.
256. Boyd, R, et al: High- or low-technology measurements of energy expenditure in clinical gait analysis? Dev Med Child Neurol 41(10):676–682, 1999.
257. Hood, VL, et al: A new method of using heart rate to represent energy expenditure: The Total Heart Beat Index. Arch Phys Med Rehabil 83(9):1266–1273, 2002.
258. Raja, K, et al: Physiological cost index in cerebral palsy: its role in evaluating the efficiency of ambulation. J Pediatr Orthop 27(2):130–136, 2007.
259. Ijzerman, MJ, et al: Validity and reproducibility of crutch force and heart rate measurements to assess energy expenditure of paraplegic gait. Arch Phys Med Rehabil 80(9):1017–1023, 1999.
260. Winchester, P, et al: A comparison of paraplegic gait performance using two types of reciprocating gait orthoses. Prosthet Orthot Int 17(2):101–106, 1993.
261. Harvey, LA, et al: Energy expenditure during gait using the walkabout and isocentric reciprocal gait orthoses in persons with paraplegia. Arch Phys Med Rehabil 79:945–949, 1998.
262. Steven, MM, et al: The physiological cost of gait (PCG): A new technique for evaluating nonsteroidal anti-inflammatory drugs in rheumatoid arthritis. Br J Rheumatol 22:141–145, 1983.
263. Olney, SJ, et al: A randomized controlled trial of supervised versus unsupervised exercise programs for ambulatory stroke survivors. Stroke 37:476–481, 2006.
264. Stein, RB, et al: A multicenter trial of a footdrop stimulator controlled by a tilt sensor. Neurorehabil Neural Repair 20(3): 371–379, 2006.
265. Sabut, SK, et al: Effect of functional electrical stimulation on the effort and walking speed, surface electromyography activity, and metabolic responses in stroke subjects. J Electromyogr Kinesiol 20(6):1170–1177, 2010.
266. Chin, T, et al: The efficacy of Physiological Cost Index (PCI) measurement of a subject walking with an intelligent prosthesis. Prosthet Orthot Int 23(1):45–49, 1999.
267. Bowen, TR, et al: Variability of energy-consumption measures in children with cerebral palsy. J Pediatr Orthop 18(6):738–742, 1998.
268. Danielsson, A, Willén, C, and Sunnerhagen, KS: Measurement of energy cost by the Physiological Cost Index in walking after stroke. Arch Phys Med Rehabil 88:1298–1303, 2007.
269. Naver, HK, Blomstrand, C, and Wallin, BG: Reduced heart rate variability after right-sided stroke. Stroke 27(2):247–251, 1996.
270. Colivicchi, F, et al: Cardiac autonomic derangement and arrhythmias in right-sided stroke with insular involvement. Stroke 35(9):2094–2098, 2004.
271. Korpelainen, JT, et al: Dynamic behavior of heart rate in ischemic stroke. Stroke 30(5):1008–1013, 1999.

272. Lakusic, N, Mahovic, D, and Babic, T: Gradual recovery of impaired cardiac autonomic balance within first six months after ischemic cerebral stroke. Acta Neurol Belg 105(1):39–42, 2005.
273. Gordon, N, et al: Physical activity and exercise recommendations for stroke survivors. An American Heart Association scientific statement from the Council on Clinical Cardiology, Subcommittee on Exercise, Cardiac Rehabilitation, and Prevention; the Council on Cardiovascular Nursing; the Council on Nutrition, Physical Activity, and Metabolism; and the Stroke Council. Circulation 109:2031–2041, 2004.
274. Kanade, R, et al: Walking performance in people with diabetic neuropathy: Benefits and threats. Diabetologia 49(8):1747–1754, 2006.
275. Kim, MO, et al: The assessment of walking capacity using the Walking Index for Spinal Cord Injury: Self-selected versus maximal levels. Arch Phys Med Rehabil 88(6):762–767, 2007.
276. Lotan, M, Yalon-Chamovitz, S, and Weiss, PL: Improving physical fitness of individuals with intellectual and developmental disability through a Virtual Reality Intervention Program. Res Dev Disabil 30(2):229–239, 2009.
277. Ries, JD, et al: Test-retest reliability and minimal detectable change scores for the timed "up & go" test, the six-minute walk test, and gait speed in people with Alzheimer disease. Phys Ther 89(6):569–579, 2009.
278. Martin, K, et al: Minimal detectable change for TUG and TUDS tests for children with Down syndrome. Pediatr Phys Ther 29(1):77–82, 2017.
279. Carey, H, et al: Reliability and responsiveness of the timed up and go test in children with cerebral palsy. Pediatr Phys Ther 28(4):401–408, 2016.
280. Dal Bello-Haas, V, et al: Psychometric properties of activity, self-efficacy, and quality-of-life measures in individuals with Parkinson disease. Physiother Can 63(1):47–57, 2011.
281. Steffen, T, and Seney, M: Test-retest reliability and minimal detectable change on balance and ambulation tests, the 36-item short-form health survey, and the unified Parkinson disease rating scale in people with parkinsonism. Phys Ther 88(6):733–746, 2008.
282. Evensen, NM, Kvale, A, and Braekken, IH: Reliability of the timed up and go test and ten-metre timed walk test in pregnant women with pelvic girdle pain. Physiother Res Int 20(3): 158–165, 2015.
283. Lam, T, Noonan, VK, and Eng, JJ: A systematic review of functional ambulation outcome measures in spinal cord injury. Spinal Cord 46(4):246–254, 2008.
284. Perera, S, et al: Meaningful change and responsiveness in common physical performance measures in older adults. J Am Geriatr Soc 54(5):743–749, 2006.
285. Latham, NK, et al: Performance-based or self-report measures of physical function: Which should be used in clinical trials of hip fracture patients? Arch Phys Med Rehabil 89(11):2146–2155, 2008.
286. van Hedel, HJ, Dietz, V, and Curt, A: Assessment of walking speed and distance in subjects with an incomplete spinal cord injury. Neurorehabil Neural Repair 21(4):295–301, 2007.
287. Van Hedel, HJ, Wirz, M, and Curt A. Improving walking assessment in subjects with an incomplete spinal cord injury: responsiveness. Spinal Cord 44(6):352–356, 2006.
288. Musselman, K: Clinical significance testing in rehabilitation research: What, why, and how? Phys Ther Rev 12(4):287–296, 2007.
289. Tilson, JK, et al: Meaningful gait speed improvement during the first 60 days poststroke: Minimal clinically important difference. Phys Ther 90(2):196–208, 2010.
290. Fulk GD, Echternach JL. Test-retest reliability and minimal detectable change of gait speed in individuals undergoing rehabilitation after stroke. *Journal of Neurologic Physical Therapy.* 2008; 32(1):8–13.
291. Watson, MJ: Refining the ten-metre walking test for use with neurologically impaired people. Physiotherapy 88(7):386–397, 2002.
292. van Loo, MA, et al: Test-re-test reliability of walking speed, step length and step width measurement after traumatic brain injury: a pilot study. Brain Inj 18(10):1041–1048, 2004.
293. Rasekaba, T, et al: The six-minute walk test: a useful metric for the cardiopulmonary patient. Intern Med J 39(8):495–501, 2009.
294. Redelmeier, DA, et al: Interpreting small differences in functional status: the Six Minute Walk test in chronic lung disease patients. Am J Respir Crit Care Med 155(4): 1278–1282, 1997.
295. Kennedy, DM, et al: Assessing stability and change of four performance measures: A longitudinal study evaluating outcome following total hip and knee arthroplasty. BMC Musculoskelet Disord 6:3, 2005.
296. Tang, A, Eng, JJ, and Rand, D: Relationship between perceived and measured changes in walking after stroke. J Neurol Phys Ther 36(3):115–121, 2012.
297. Rossier, P, and Wade, DT: Validity and reliability comparison of 4 mobility measures in patients presenting with neurologic impairment. Arch Phys Med Rehabil 82(1):9–13, 2001.
298. Pin, TW, and Choi, HL: Reliability, validity, and norms of the 2-min walk test in children with and without neuromuscular disorders aged 6–12. Disabil Rehabil 1–7, 2017.
299. Bohannon, RW, Wang, YC, and Gershon, RC: Two-minute walk test performance by adults 18 to 85 years: Normative values, reliability, and responsiveness. Arch Phys Med Rehabil 96(3): 472–477, 2015.
300. Connelly, DM, et al: Clinical utility of the 2-minute walk test for older adults living in long-term care. Physiother Can 61(2): 78–87, 2009.
301. Resnik, L, and Borgia, M: Reliability of outcome measures for people with lower-limb amputations: Distinguishing true change from statistical error. Phys Ther 91(4):555–565, 2011.
302. Gijbels, D, et al: Predicting habitual walking performance in multiple sclerosis: Relevance of capacity and self-report measures. Mult Scler 16(5):618–626, 2010.
303. Hiengkaew, V, Jitaree, K, and Chaiyawat, P: Minimal detectable changes of the Berg Balance Scale, Fugl-Meyer Assessment Scale, Timed "Up & Go" Test, gait speeds, and 2-minute walk test in individuals with chronic stroke with different degrees of ankle plantarflexor tone. Arch Phys Med Rehabil 93(7):1201–1208, 2012.
304. Romero, S, et al: Minimum detectable change of the Berg Balance Scale and Dynamic Gait Index in older persons at risk for falling. J Geriatr Phys Ther 34(3):131–137, 2011.
305. Pardasaney, PK, et al: Sensitivity to change and responsiveness of four balance measures for community-dwelling older adults. Phys Ther 92(3):388–397, 2012.
306. Hall, CD, and Herdman, SJ: Reliability of clinical measures used to assess patients with peripheral vestibular disorders. J Neurol Phys Ther 30(2):74–81, 2006.
307. Marchetti, GF, et al: Responsiveness and minimal detectable change of the dynamic gait index and functional gait index in persons with balance and vestibular disorders. J Neurol Phys Ther 38(2):119–124, 2014.
308. Matsuda, PN, Taylor, CS, and Shumway-Cook, A: Evidence for the validity of the modified dynamic gait index across diagnostic groups. Phys Ther 94(7):996–1004, 2014.
309. Beninato, M, Fernandes, A, and Plummer, LS: Minimal clinically important difference of the functional gait assessment in older adults. Phys Ther 94(11):1594–1603, 2014.
310. Petersen, C, et al: Reliability and minimal detectable change for sit-to-stand tests and the functional gait assessment for individuals with Parkinson disease. J Geriatr Phys Ther 2017.
311. Parveen, H, and Noohu, MM: Evaluation of psychometric properties of Tinetti performance-oriented mobility assessment scale in subjects with knee osteoarthritis. Hong Kong Physiother J 36:25–32, 2017.
312. Faber, MJ, Bosscher, RJ, and van Wieringen, PC: Clinimetric properties of the performance-oriented mobility assessment. Phys Ther 86(7):944–954, 2006.
313. Smidt, GL, and Mommens, MA: System of reporting and comparing influence of ambulatory aids on gait. Phys Ther 60(5):551–558, 1980.
314. Graser, JV, Letsch, C, and van Hedel, HJ: Reliability of timed walking tests and temporo-spatial gait parameters in youths with neurological gait disorders. BMC Neurol 16:15, 2016.

315. Cho, KH, Lee, HJ, and Lee, WH: Test-retest reliability of the GAITRite walkway system for the spatio-temporal gait parameters while dual-tasking in post-stroke patients. Disabil Rehabil 37(6):512–516, 2015.
316. Peters, DM, et al: Concurrent validity of walking speed values calculated via the GAITRite electronic walkway and 3 meter walk test in the chronic stroke population. Physiother Theory Pract 30(3):183–188, 2014.
317. Wong, JS, et al: Inter- and intra-rater reliability of the GAITRite system among individuals with sub-acute stroke. Gait Posture 40(1):259–261, 2014.
318. Webster, KE, Wittwer, JE, and Feller, JA: Validity of the GAITRite walkway system for the measurement of averaged and individual step parameters of gait. Gait Posture 22(4): 317–321, 2005.

Supplemental Readings

Brach, JS, et al: Diabetes mellitus and gait dysfunction and possible explanatory factors. Phys Ther 88:1365–1374, 2008.
Hergenroeder, AL, et al: Association of Body Mass Index with self-report and performance-based measures of balance and mobility. Phys Ther 91:1223–1234, 2011.
Winter, DA: Biomechanics and Motor Control of Human Movement, ed 4. John Wiley and Sons, New York, 2009.

appendix 7.A

Recording Form for Observational Gait Analysis

Patient's name ____________ Age ____ Gender ____ Height ______ Weight ______

Diagnosis ____________

Footwear ____________ Assistive devices ____________

Date ____________ Therapist ____________

DIRECTIONS: Place a check (√) in the space opposite the deviation if the deviation is observed.

Body Segment/ Plane Observed	Deviation	Stance										Swing						Possible Cause(s)	Analysis
		IC		LR		MSt		TSt		PSw		ISw		MSw		TSw			
Ankle and foot	None	R	L	R	L	R	L	R	L	R	L	R	L	R	L	R	L		
Sagittal plane observations	Foot flat																		
	Foot slap																		
	Heel off																		
	No heel off																		
	Excessive plantarflexion																		
	Excessive dorsiflexion																		
	Toe drag																		
	Toe clawing																		
	Contralateral vaulting																		
Frontal plane observations	Varus																		
	Valgus																		
Knee	None																		
Sagittal plane observations	Excessive flexion																		
	Limited flexion																		
	No flexion																		
	Hyperextension																		
	Genu recurvatum																		
	Diminished extension																		

Body Segment/ Plane Observed	Deviation	Stance					Swing			Possible Cause(s)	Analysis
		IC	LR	MSt	TSt	PSw	ISw	MSw	TSw		
Frontal plane observations	Varus										
	Valgus										
Hip	None										
Sagittal plane observations	Excessive flexion										
	Limited flexion										
	No flexion										
	Diminished extension										
Frontal plane observations	Abduction										
	Adduction										
	External rotation										
	Internal rotation										
	Circumduction										
	Hiking										
Pelvis	None										
Sagittal plane observations	Anterior tilt										
	Posterior tilt										
	Increased backward rotation										
	Increased forward rotation										
	Limited backward rotation										
	Limited forward rotation										
	Drops on contralateral side										
Trunk	None										
Frontal plane observations	Backward rotation										
	Lateral lean										
	Forward rotation										
	Backward lean										
	Forward lean										

Key: IC = Initial Contact; LR = Loading Response; MSt = Mid Stance; TSt = Terminal Stance; PSw = Pre-swing; ISw = Initial Swing; MSw = Mid Swing; TSw = Terminal Swing

appendix

7.B Temporal and Spatial Measures Gait Analysis Form

Patient's name____________________________ Age______ Gender _____ Height____________ Weight_________

Diagnosis ____

Ambulatory aids: Yes _________ No _________

Type: Crutch(es) _________________________ Cane(s): R____________ Walker: ________________________

L____________

Other: _________________________

Instructions: Distance walked, elapsed time, and walking velocity can be calculated for a single walking trial or averaged across multiple walking trials if the patient's endurance permits. Therapist should provide an average value (calculated across multiple complete steps/strides) for the stride and step lengths, width of walking base, and foot angles.

Date	
Therapist's initials	
Distance walked (distance from first to last heel strike)	
Elapsed time (time from first to last heel strike)	
Walking velocity (distance walked divided by elapsed time)	
Left stride length (distance between two consecutive left heel strikes)	
Right stride length (distance between two consecutive right heel strikes)	
Left step length (distance between a right heel strike and the next consecutive left heel strike)	
Right step length (distance between a left heel strike and the next consecutive right heel strike)	
Step length difference (difference between right and left step lengths)	
Cadence (total number of steps taken divided by the elapsed time)	
Width of walking base (perpendicular distance between right and left heel strike)	
Left foot angle (angle formed between a line bisecting the left foot and the line of progression)	
Right foot angle (angle formed between a line bisecting the right foot and the line of progression)	
Right stride length to right lower extremity length (right stride length divided by right lower extremity length)	
Left stride length to left lower extremity length (left stride length divided by left lower extremity length)	

Manufacturer Contact Information for Gait Analysis Hardware and Software

appendix **7.C**

Manufacturer	Address	Gait Analysis Product(s)	Website
Advanced Medical Technology, Inc (AMTI)	176 Waltham Street Watertown, MA 02472	Forceplates and sensors	http://www.amti.biz
Ariel Performance Analysis System	Ariel Dynamics 6 Alicante St. Trabuco Canyon, CA 92679	Gait and motion analysis hardware and software	www.arielnet.com
Ascension Technology Corporation	P.O. Box 527 Burlington, VT 05402	Flock of Birds motion analysis hardware and software	www.ascension-tech.com
B and L Engineering	1901 Carnegie Ave. Suite Q Santa Ana, CA 92705	Stride Analyzer and EMG hardware and software	www.bleng.com
Bioengineering Technology Systems (BTS)	147 Prince Street Suite 10 Brooklyn, NY 11201	Integrated gait systems	www.btsbioengineering.com/
Biometrics Ltd.	PO Box 340 Ladysmith, VA 22501	Electrogoniometers	www.biometricsltd.com/gonio.htm
Charnwood Dynamics Ltd.	Fowke Street Rothley, Leicestershire LE7 7PJ United Kingdom	Coda motion analysis hardware and software	www.codamotion.com
C-Motion, Inc.	20030 Century Blvd Suite 104A Germantown, MD 20874	Visual 3D software for analyzing biomechanical data	www.c-motion.com/index.php
Coach's Eye	2405 Woodlake Drive Okemos, Michigan 48864-5910	Movement analysis application	www.coachseye.com/
Modus Health	123 Second Avenue South, Suite 220 Edmonds, WA 98020	StepWatch Activity Monitor 3™	https://modushealth.com/
Dartfish	6505 Shiloh Rd. Suite 110-B Alpharetta, GA 30005	Movement analysis software	www.dartfish.com
GAITRite®	CIR Systems, Inc 60 Garlor Drive Havertown, PA 19083	Instrumented gait mat	www.gaitrite.com
Kistler Instrument Corporation	75 John Glenn Dr. Amherst, NY 14228-2171	GaitWay Treadmill®, force plates, accelerometers	www.kistler.com

Continued

Manufacturer	Address	Gait Analysis Product(s)	Website
Motion Analysis Corporation	3617 Westwind Blvd Santa Rosa, CA 95403	Gait and motion analysis hardware and software	www.motionanalysis.com
Northern Digital Inc.	103 Randall Drive Waterloo, Ontario Canada N2V 1C5	Optotrak and 3D Investigator Motion Capture Systems	www.ndigital.com/
Novel Electronics, Inc	964 Grand Ave St. Paul, MN 55105	emed®, pedar®, and pliance® pressure mapping hardware and software	www.novelusa.com
Phoenix Technologies Incorporated	4302 Norfolk St. Burnaby, BC Canada V5G 4J9	Motion analysis hardware and software	www.ptiphoenix.com/index.php
Polhemus	40 Hercules Drive P.O. Box 560 Colchester, VT 05446	Motion analysis hardware and software	www.polhemus.com
ProtoKinetics	60 Garlor Drive Havertown, PA 19083	Zeno Walkway instrumented gait mat	www.protokinetics.com/zeno-walkway/
Qualisys AB	Packhusgatan 6 S-411 13 Gothenburg, Sweden	Gait and motion analysis hardware and software	www.qualisys.com
Spark Motion	5420 Butler Road, Suite 204 Bethesda, Maryland 20816	Movement analysis application	www.sparkmotion.com/
Tekscan, Inc.	307 W. First St. South Boston, MA 02127	F-Scan®, MatScan®, and Strideway™ pressure and force mapping hardware and software	www.tekscan.com
Vicon Motion Analysis System	Vicon Colorado 7388 S. Revere Parkway Suite 901 Centennial, CO 80112	Gait and motion analysis hardware and software	www.vicon.com/
Windows Media Player®	Microsoft Corporation Redmond, WA 98052	Video player for viewing video recordings of gait	https://www.microsoft.com/en-us/download/windows-media-player-details.aspx
Xsens North America Inc.	2684 Lacy Street Suite 205 Los Angeles, CA 90031	Motion tracking hardware and software	www.xsens.com/

Sample Report from Stride Analyzer System

appendix **7.D**

STRIDE CHARACTERISTICS AND FOOT-FLOOR CONTACT PATTERNS

LABORATORY

INSTITUTION

Patient Name:	Jane Doe	**Trial:**	004
Patient ID #:	9999	**Strides:**	6
Test Date:	10/25/2018	**Sex:**	F
Diagnosis:	(R) Hemiparesis	**Age (years):**	30

STRIDE CHARACTERISTICS: Self-selected walking speed without assistive device

	Absolute	**% Normal**
Velocity (m/min):	30.4	37.5
Cadence (steps/min):	77.1	65.4
Stride Length (m):	0.79	57.6
Gait Cycle (sec):	1.55	152
	Right	**Left**
Single Limb Support (% Normal):	55	61
Single Limb Support (% GC):	26.5	29
Swing (% GC):	29	26.5
Stance (% GC):	71	73.5
Initial Double Limb Support (%GC):	15.7	28.6
Terminal Double Limb Support (%GC):	28.6	15.7

Left Foot (stance = 73.5% GC)	
Heel:	Normal contact (0.0% GC) Delayed cessation (53.9% GC)
Fifth Metatarsal:	Premature contact (5.7% GC) Appropriate cessation (70.9% GC)
First Metatarsal:	Appropriate contact (18% GC) Appropriate cessation (71.5% GC)
Toe:	Appropriate contact (47.5% GC) Appropriate cessation (73.5% GC)
Right Foot (stance = 71% GC)	
Heel:	Normal contact (0.0% GC) Delayed cessation (52.3% GC)
Fifth Metatarsal:	Premature contact (0.8% GC) Appropriate cessation (71% GC)
First Metatarsal:	Appropriate contact (14.4% GC) Premature cessation (57.9% GC)
Toe:	Appropriate contact (44.4% GC) Premature cessation (59.5% GC)

Chapter 8 Examination of Function

David A. Scalzitti, PT, PhD

LEARNING OBJECTIVES

1. Discuss the concepts of health, function, activity, participation, disability, impairment, activity limitations, and participation restrictions.
2. Define *function* and discuss the purposes and components of the examination of function.
3. Select activities and roles appropriate to an individual's particular characteristics and condition to guide examination of function.
4. Compare and contrast characteristics of various tests of function, including performance measures and self-report measures.
5. Identify factors to consider in the selection of instruments for testing function.
6. Compare and contrast various scoring methods used in instruments to measure function.
7. Discuss the issues of reliability, validity, and responsiveness as they relate to the measurement of function.
8. Using the case study example, apply clinical decision making skills in evaluating data from the examination of function.

CHAPTER OUTLINE

A clinician needs to consider the purposes of obtaining the measurement in deciding which measure of function to use. For example, is the measure to describe a specific activity limitation or describe an individual's overall level of function? Will the measure be used to measure an individual's current status or to assess the outcomes of an episode of care? Will the measure be used to determine the destination at discharge, to obtain reimbursement, to meet regulatory requirements, or some combination of these reasons? As function may incorporate performance at the level of body systems, the person, and society, or a combination of these, the clinician should be cognizant of the ability of the measure to capture the applicable information.

The ultimate objective of any rehabilitation program is to return the individual to a lifestyle that is as close to their previous level of function as possible or, alternatively, to maximize the current potential for function and maintain it. For an otherwise healthy person with a fractured arm, this may be a reasonably simple process: improving range of motion, strength, and impairments in body function will generally correlate with the reestablishment of skills related to the performance of activities, such as dressing and feeding. However, considering the person with a stroke, the task is much more complex because the problems are much more extensive, complicated, and interwoven. The two cases, however, are broadly similar. In both instances, the therapist begins by describing the problem in functional terms obtained from the history, performing a review of body systems and detailed examination using selected tests and measures, evaluating the data, establishing a diagnosis and prognosis, implementing interventions to reduce or to eliminate the problems identified, and documenting the progress toward the desired functional outcome.[1]

Every individual values the ability to live independently. The construct of function encompasses all those tasks, activities, and roles that identify a person as an independent adult or as a child progressing toward adult independence. These activities require the integration of both cognitive and affective abilities with motor skills. Functional activity is a patient-referenced concept and is dependent on what the individual self-identifies as essential to support physical and psychological well-being, as well as to create a personal sense of meaningful living. Function is not totally individualistic, however; there are certain categories of activities that are common to everyone. Eating, sleeping, elimination, and hygiene are major components of survival and protection common to all animals. Particular to humans are the evolutionary advancements of bipedal locomotion and complex hand activities, which permit independence in the personal environment. Participation in work and recreational activities by humans are examples of functional activities in a social context.

This chapter presents a conceptual framework for examining functional status based on the International Classification of Functioning, Disability, and Health (ICF) (see also Chapter 1, Clinical Decision Making). It presents an overview of the purposes of the examination of function and the range and rigor of formal test instruments currently available to clinicians and researchers. Considerations in test selection and principles of administration are also presented.

A CONCEPTUAL FRAMEWORK

Chronically ill and disabled persons represent a large segment of the population in the United States. In 2014, approximately 43 million Americans (13%) were considered to have a disability (limited in their usual activities due to one or more chronic conditions).[2] Traditionally, persons with disabilities may have been categorized or classified according to their medical diseases or conditions. Medical procedures such as physical examination and laboratory tests are the primary tools to delineate the problems created by disease. Strict focus on a biomedical model, with its emphasis on the characteristics of *disease* (etiology, pathology, and clinical manifestations), may contribute to reducing patients to the *medical labeling* of these individuals; for example, referring to people as amputees, paraplegics, or arthritics rather than as individuals with these conditions. This model virtually ignores the equally important psychological, social, and behavioral dimensions of the illness, which accompanies the disease. *Illness* refers to the personal behaviors that emerge when the reality of having a disease is internalized and experienced by an individual. Factors related to illness often play a key role in determining the success or failure of rehabilitation efforts well beyond the nature of the medical condition that prompted a patient's referral to physical therapy. In helping the individual with a disease, physical therapists come to understand each person's illness as well.

A broad conceptual framework is necessary to fully understand the concept of health and its relationship to function and disability. Terms such as *well-being, health-related quality of life,* and *functional status* are often used interchangeably to describe health status. The most global definition of health has been provided by the World Health Organization (WHO), which defined health as "a state of complete physical, mental, and social well-being, and not merely the absence of diseases and infirmity."[3, p. 459] Although such global definitions are useful as philosophical statements, they lack the precision necessary for measurement by clinicians or researchers.

In order to describe the components of health and provide a unified and standard language and framework for the description of health and health-related states, the ICF *International Classification of Functioning, Disability, and Health (ICF)* was developed.[4] The ICF complements other classifications of the WHO such as the *International Classification of Diseases,* 10th revision (ICD-10).[5] Whereas the ICD-10 is a classification of diseases, disorders, and other health conditions, the ICF attempts to provide a meaningful description of the components of health and its relationship to a person with the health condition. *Function* in the ICF is an umbrella term encompassing all body functions and structures, activities, and participation, whereas *disability* is a term that encompasses impairments in body functions and structures, activity limitations, and participation restrictions. Both function and disability are represented in the ICF, to provide for the description of a continuum of the components of health from positive aspects to items an individual is not able to perform or perform in a limited manner or with assistance.

The ICF framework consists of two parts. The first part describes components of function and disability in the context of health, whereas the second part describes contextual factors, which may interact with the components of the first part (Fig. 8.1). These components of the ICF do not model a process of disablement; rather, the ICF provides an approach to classification of function and disability from multiple perspectives. The relationship between components and parts of the ICF does not imply causality. Bidirectional arrows are used in Figure 8.1 to represent a complex relationship. For example, a health condition such as angina may influence aspects of mobility such as gait, whereas at the same time increasing one's mobility by performing a regular walking program may influence the management of the health condition. In addition, a limitation in one component of the framework does not imply limitations in other components.

Body functions are defined by the ICF as the physiological functions of body systems, and body structures are parts of the body such as organs, limbs, and their components. *Impairment* is the term used to refer to problems in body function or structure. Although body functions and structures are classified in separate sections of the ICF, the classifications are designed to be used

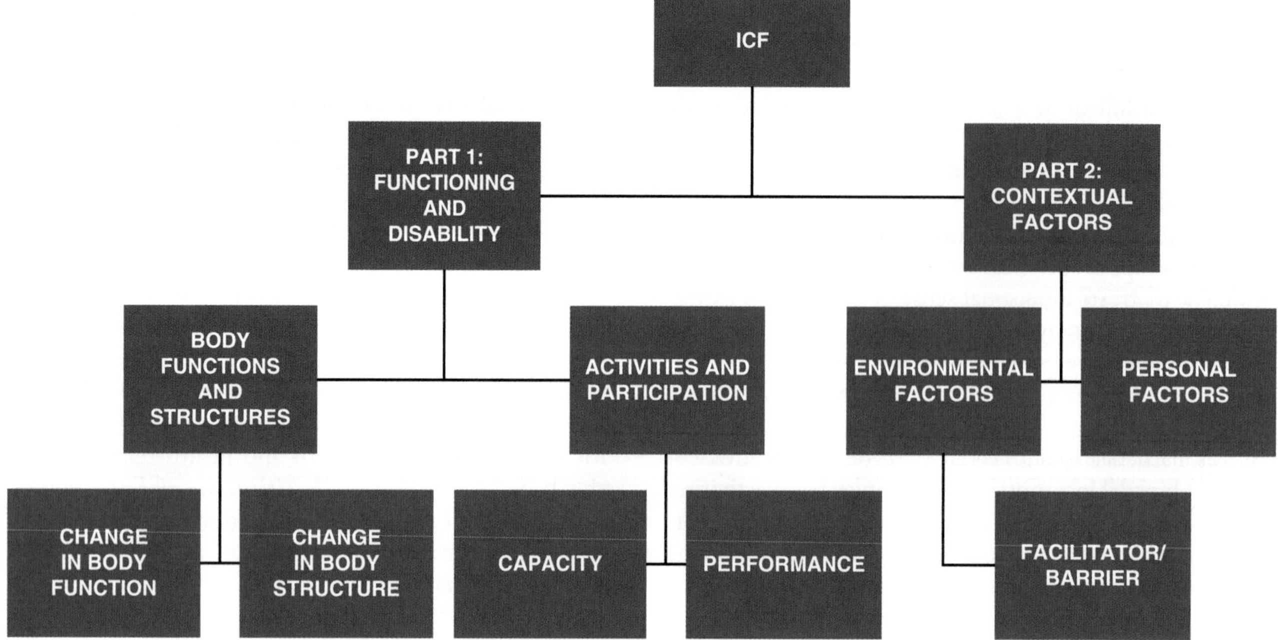

Figure 8.1 Structure of the International Classification of Functioning, Disability and Health (ICF) model of functioning and disability from *Guide to Physical Therapist Practice 3.0*. *(Introduction to the Guide to Physical Therapist Practice 3.0. Alexandria, VA: American Physical Therapy Association; 2014. Available at: http://guidetoptpractice.apta.org/content/1/SEC1.body. Accessed December 1, 2017.)*

together. For example, the chapter titled "Neuromuscular and Movement-Related Functions" in the body functions classification corresponds with the chapter titled "Structures Related to Movement" in the body structures classification. Hence, for a person with rheumatoid arthritis, a clinician may use aspects of the body functions classification to describe range of motion of the interphalangeal joints and muscle performance of the hand intrinsic muscles and the body structures classification to describe the integrity of the joints of the hand. The headings for the chapters in the ICF classification of body functions and structures are in Table 8.1.

The ICF defines activity as the execution of a task or action by an individual and participation as involvement in a life situation. The terms used to describe problems in these domains are *activity limitations* and *participation restrictions*. Through the definitions of activity and participation, an attempt is made to differentiate what a person can do because of characteristics of the individual and those of society. In the ICF, however, a single list covers both activity and participation. Instead of separate lists, the ICF allows users to differentiate activities and participation. Possible operational definitions suggested in the ICF include (1) designating some domains as activities and others as participation with no overlap, (2) designating some domains as activities and others as participation allowing for overlap, (3) designating all detailed domains as activities and the broad categories as participation, and (4) using all domains as both activities and participation.[4, pp. 234-237] To date, no standard exists for the distinction of the classification of activity and participation, and physical therapists should be aware of the potential uses of the classification for practice and research.[6]

The headings for the nine chapters in the ICF classification of activities and participation and examples of classification within a chapter are presented in Figure 8.2. The chapters are considered the first level of classification and can be used to categorize positive and negative aspects of function. The second level of classification includes categories of different actions, tasks, and activities. Subcategories provide additional detail for the main categories. For example, moving around is a category within the mobility domain of the ICF, and crawling is a subcategory of the moving around category. These subcategories allow for more specific description of the categories (third-level and fourth-level classification).

Contextual factors are included in the ICF model to represent the complete background of an individual's life. These factors may interact as facilitators or barriers to the health condition and to the components of function. The consideration of each contextual factor as either a *barrier* or a *facilitator* is made from the perspective of the individual whose situation is being described. Contextual factors have two components: *environmental factors*, which are external to the individual and can have

Table 8.1 ICF Classification of Body Functions and Body Structures

Body Functions	Body Structures
Mental functions	Structures of the nervous system
Sensory functions and pain	The eye, ear, and related structures
Voice and speech functions	Structures involved in voice and speech
Functions of the cardiovascular, hematological, immunological, and respiratory systems	Structures of the cardiovascular, immunological, and respiratory systems
Functions of the digestive, metabolic, and endocrine systems	Structures related to the digestive, metabolic, and endocrine systems
Genitourinary and reproductive functions	Structures related to the genitourinary and reproductive systems
Neuromusculoskeletal and movement-related functions	Structures related to movement
Functions of the skin and related structures	Skin and related structures

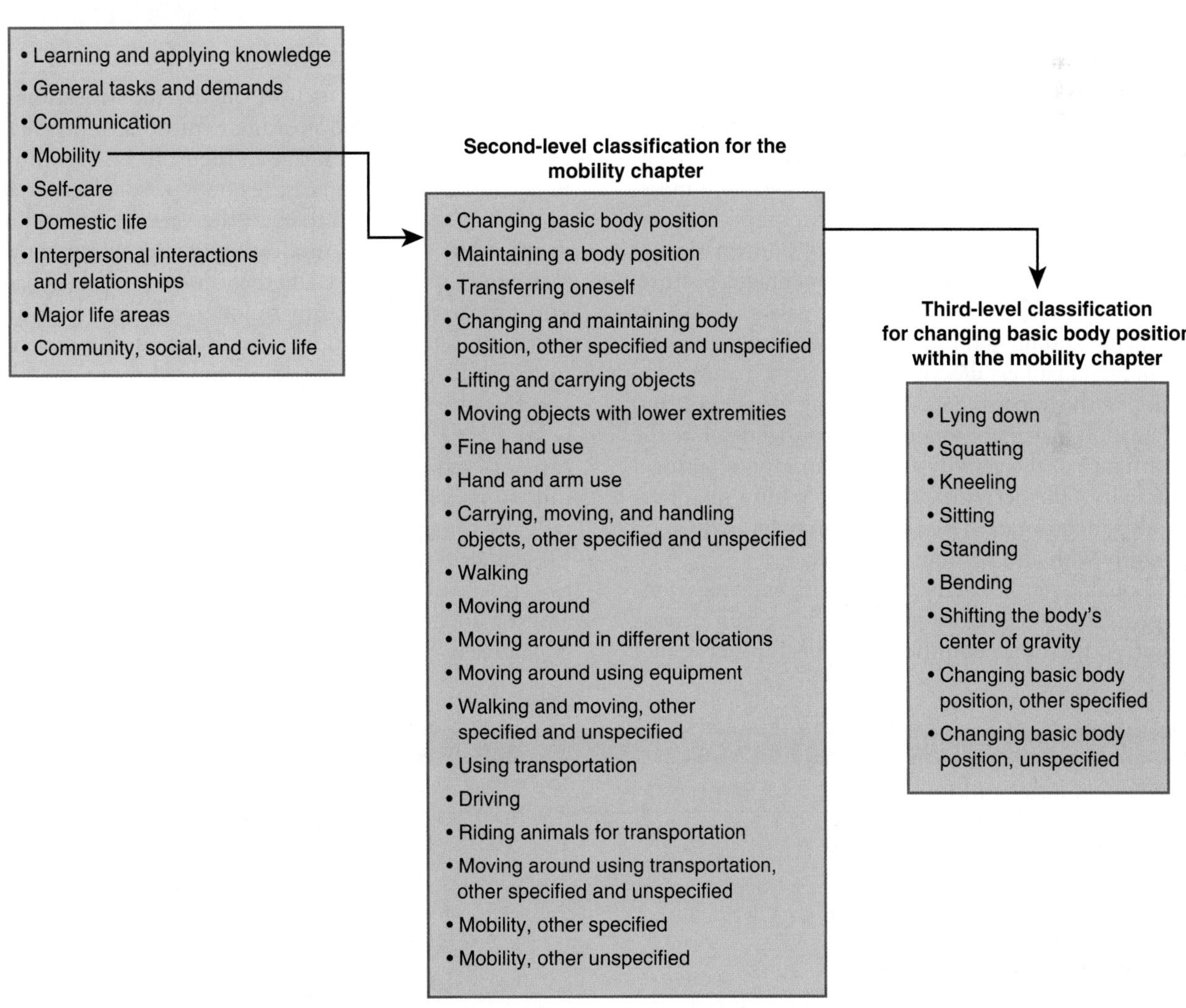

Figure 8.2 ICF Classification of Activities and Participation. *(From Brandt EN, Jr, and Pope AM,[7, p. 9] with permission.)*

positive or negative influence on performance, and *personal factors,* which are features of the individual such as age, gender, and race that are not part of a health condition or health state. Due to the bidirectional nature of the ICF framework, contextual factors may also be modified by the components of part 1. Environmental factors are classified by the ICF; however, a classification of personal factors is notably omitted (Table 8.2).

The ICF emphasizes the interaction between the person and the environment as critical to understanding functioning and disability. Physical therapists can help change discriminatory social attitudes and environmental restrictions such as architectural barriers that stigmatize individuals and restrict participation in all aspects of society. The modification of factors that are barriers and incorporation of factors that are facilitators is as important to functioning as the amelioration of activity limitations.[7]

In addition to providing a framework for the classification of function, the ICF provides a classification scheme for coding, which, although not in widespread use by physical therapists, may be particularly intriguing in its delineation of actions, tasks, and activities in an implicit hierarchy of functioning. Within this hierarchy, actions (e.g., rolling, bending, sitting, standing, lifting, and reaching) are constituents of tasks and activities (e.g., bathing, dressing, and grooming). Tests and measures of actions are particularly relevant to physical therapist practice, as they capture the complex integration of systems that permits an individual to maintain a posture, transition to other postures, or sustain safe and efficient movement. Coding of body functions and structures may incorporate qualifiers describing the extent, nature, and location of the impairments. The coding of activities and participation may incorporate qualifiers that describe the performance of the activity and the capacity to perform the activity. The activities and participation qualifiers may also incorporate how the task may be performed differently with and without assistance.

Although typical patterns of deficits in body functions and problems in activities may exist in certain disease categories, the exact empirical relationship between a particular set of impairments in body functions and structure and activity limitations is not yet known.[8] The cause-and-effect relationship between an impairment and an activity limitation is most often inferred in the clinic from empirical evidence. For example, physical therapists may assume that the reason a patient cannot transfer independently is causally linked to the fact that the individual has lost enough lower extremity range of motion at the hip (e.g., hip flexion contractures) to prevent balancing in a fully upright posture. The return of activity following remediation of the impairment of joint mobility is then considered clinical evidence of a relationship between the impairment and the limitation. One should be aware, however, that activity may be restored without complete resolution of the impairments of body function and structures and vice versa. Therefore, it is important that the physical therapist measure all of the appropriate components of an individual's function.

EXAMINATION OF FUNCTION

Purpose of Examination of Function

Analysis of function focuses on the identification of pertinent activities and measurement of an individual's ability to successfully engage in them. In essence, functional testing is used to measure how a person does certain tasks or fulfills certain roles in the various dimensions described by the ICF. Application of selected functional tests and measures yield data that can be used as (1) baseline information for setting function-oriented goals and outcomes of intervention; (2) indicators of a patient's initial abilities and progression toward more complex functional levels; (3) criteria for placement decisions (e.g., the need for inpatient rehabilitation, extended care, or community services); (4) manifestations of an individual's level of safety in performing a particular task and the risk of injury with continued performance; (5) evidence of the effectiveness of a specific intervention (medical, surgical, or rehabilitative) on function; and (6) documentation to support payer requirements of change in functional status during an episode of care.

Table 8.2 Environmental Factors in the ICF

First-Level Classification	Examples
Products and technology	Medications, clothes, prosthetics, walking devices, scooters, hearing aids, ramps, assets
Natural environment and human-made changes to environment	Geography, climate, light, air quality
Support and relationships	Immediate family, extended family, friends, persons in positions of authority, personal assistants, domesticated animals, health professionals
Attitudes	Individual attitudes of immediate family members, individual attitudes of health professionals, societal attitudes
Services, systems, and policies	Housing, transportation, legal, associations, health, education, political

General Considerations

Physical therapists possess a unique body of knowledge related to the identification, remediation, and prevention of movement dysfunction. Thus, they have traditionally been involved in the examination of physical function. Other members of the rehabilitation team, including the occupational therapist, nurse, rehabilitation counselor, and recreational therapist, are also typically involved in administering and interpreting functional tests. Some formal instruments were designed to be completed collectively by the team. Other tests are compiled in separate sections by specific health professionals and housed together in the patient's chart. Where teams exist, physical therapists are typically responsible for the testing of aspects of function related to mobility, such as bed mobility, transfers, and locomotion (wheelchair mobility, ambulation, negotiation of stairs and graded elevations, walking for longer distances in the community, and so forth). Instruments to measure activities of daily living (ADL) may be administered by a physical therapist alone or cooperatively with other health professionals. When overlap among team members exists–for example, the performance of toilet transfers–the data may be collected by the physical therapist, an occupational therapist, or a nurse. In these instances, testing should be coordinated to reduce duplication and unnecessary patient stress. In noninstitutional settings or where there is no team, the physical therapist is often responsible for determining all aspects of these instruments.

Testing Perspectives

Function tests can utilize two highly divergent perspectives on what is to be tested or measured by the physical therapist. It is extremely important that the therapist determine in advance whether data are needed to describe the *habitual level* of a patient's ability to do certain tasks and activities or to identify the patient's *capacity* to perform certain tasks and activities, whether the patient habitually performs up to that level or not, or even performs them at all. These perspectives are incorporated within the ICF by the constructs of performance and capacity and the ICF allows for the separate coding of both constructs.

These divergent viewpoints directly affect what types of tests and measures should be chosen and what parameters of measurement are appropriate to yield data useful to making clinical judgments. For example, the focus on capacity or performance may influence the selection of either a self-report measure or performance-based measure. Most important, physical therapists must consider the differences between capacity for function and habitual function in determining the prognosis for rehabilitation and estimating the likelihood of the success of an intervention. Patients accept a therapist's recommendations regarding the anticipated goals of treatment only if there is the perceived need and motivation to function habitually at the highest level of ability. Understanding the difference between what a person actually does or would be willing to do and what that person potentially could do is an essential component of designing realistic, and achievable, functional goals. For example, even though a person might have the capacity to climb stairs, there may not be any willingness or opportunity to do so. Ultimately, physical therapists must abide by each patient's own decision regarding which tasks and activities will be incorporated into a daily routine and what is a meaningful level of function, regardless of the therapist's professional opinion.

Regardless of the particular instrument used, there are several basic considerations to keep in mind. The setting chosen must be conducive to the type of testing and free of distractions. Instructions should be precise and unambiguous. Testing may be biased by fatigue. If a patient performs best in the morning but tires by afternoon, an accurate determination of functional ability must consider the variation in the patient's performance. Therapists should be aware of patients whose energy fluctuates during the day and interpret the data accordingly. In general, information related to body functions and body structure, activities, and participation, as well as personal and environmental factors, should be generated during the initial examination (or as soon as feasible) so the information may be considered together to develop a picture of a patient's function. Retesting should occur at regular intervals during treatment to document progress and before discharge from the episode of care. As an example, Medicare G-codes for physical therapy outpatients requires inclusion of functional limitation reporting at the initial visit, at least every 10 visits, and at discharge.[9]

Types of Instruments

Performance-Based Tests

A performance-based test involves observing the patient performing an activity. Generally, the therapist who chooses a performance-based test is searching for an indication of what a person can do under a specific set of circumstances, which may or may not be similar to their natural environment. If a performance-based test is chosen with the intention of making inferences about how the patient will perform at home, the conditions and setting should be as similar as possible to the actual environment in which the patient usually performs the tasks and activities. This is an important distinction between assessments of the capacity to function at home as compared to their ability to perform the tasks at home. A performance-based approach may be used either to describe the patient's current level of function or to identify the maximum level of function possible.

During the administration of the test, each task is presented and the patient is asked to perform it. For example, to examine current level of function in wheelchair mobility, a patient would receive this instruction: "Push your wheelchair over to that red chair and stop." To determine the patient's maximum level of function in this activity, the instruction might specify a particular manner of performance: "Push your wheelchair over to that red chair *as quickly as you can* and stop." Understanding the difference between these two commands, even though both are observation-based performance of wheelchair mobility, is essential to sound clinical decision making. Data from the first example identify only what the patient can do under specific circumstances but does not support the inference that the patient will be able to wheel across a busy intersection in the short time span allotted at a typical crosswalk. The form of the instruction determines whether an inference can be made about the patient's maximal level of function in formulating the goals for intervention and the plan of care.

In either case, a patient is given no additional instructions or assistance unless he or she is unable or unsure of how to perform. Then only as much direction or assistance as is needed is given and documented. Appropriate safety precautions should be taken during the session so that the patient does not attempt tasks that are potentially dangerous.

Many tests have been considered as functional performance measures, including the *6-Minute Walk Test*,[10] the *Physical Performance and Mobility Examination*,[11] the *Functional Reach Test*,[12,13] the *Get Up and Go Test*,[14] the *Timed Up and Go Test*,[15] and the Short *Physical Performance Battery*.[16] A performance instrument of this sort typically measures either a complex integration of impairments, the performance of actions, or a combination of both by direct observation. Overall, the tests do provide some insight into the individual's capabilities to maintain a posture, transition to other postures, or sustain safe and efficient movement. The data from such a test, gathered under controlled conditions, characterize a person's performance limitations as a result of impairments, and may purport to predict the success or failure of an individual in performing goal-directed tasks or activities under natural conditions, using a score that summates the combined effects of impairments throughout and across systems on movement dysfunction. Each of these tests can contribute to an understanding of an aspect of a person's function, but they should not be used to represent all aspects of function. Although these tests employ the method of direct observation of performance, they most often do not measure the task or activity as it might be accomplished in the "real" world of the patient, which is also influenced by motivation and habit.

Self-Reports

In contrast to the method of direct observation, useful data on how a person functions may also be gathered by *self-report,* in which the patient is asked directly either by the therapist or a trained interviewer (*interviewer report*) or via a *self-administered report* instrument. The self-administered report may be administered in a paper-and-pencil format or in an electronic version. These reports may be completed during the therapy visit, or the patient may be asked to complete the report before or after the treatment session. The critical issue for a self-report to capture function correctly and completely lies in providing clearly worded questions without language bias, concise directions on completing the questions, and a format that encourages accurate reporting of answers to all questions. Self-report is a valid method of determining function and may be preferable to performance-based methods in some circumstances.[17] Self-reports should be designed so that questions are asked in a standard format and answers are recorded as specified by the predetermined choices. For example, a paper-and-pencil test may be difficult for those with upper extremity impairments to complete.

Clinical personnel who act as interviewers must be trained to administer a questionnaire. Interviewers should practice until they have reached a high degree of agreement with expert examiners of the same cases. Periodic retraining may be necessary if interviewers do not have frequent practice administering the instrument. The interview should be scheduled with the patient in advance and conducted in an environment conducive to complete concentration. Interviews may be conducted by phone or in person, but the mode of administration should be kept consistent if comparisons of the data are to be made. Ad lib prompting by the interviewer or caregivers for answers is discouraged because these intrusions into the patient's self-report tend to bias results. If the patient has had help in filling out a form or responding to questions, this should be noted. Similarly, if a spouse, family member, or caregiver has provided the data, this should be documented as well.

The distinction in perspectives on function that was discussed regarding performance-based measures of function also holds for self-reports. It is extremely important to distinguish between questions that indicate a person's habitual performance (e.g., "*Do* you cook your own meals?") and those that identify a person's perceived capacity to perform a task (e.g., "If you had to, *could* you cook your own meals?"). It may also be important to distinguish between an individual's performance of an activity and his or her confidence in performing an activity. For example, confidence and performance for 21 items are measured in separate scales in APTA's *Outpatient Physical Therapy Improvement in Movement Assessment Log (OPTIMAL)*.[18]

The time frame reference of self-reporting is also a relevant consideration. A therapist should decide in advance if the relevant "window" on a person's functional level is the past 24 hours, last week, last month, or the previous year. One can easily imagine how the same person might respond differently regarding the same functional activity depending on frame of reference. Instruments that examine only short-term objectives may not relate well to the long-term objectives of a rehabilitation program.

Instrument Parameters and Formats

Performance-based and self-report instruments grade performance on a number of different criteria in a variety of formats. There is no one parameter or format that is perfect for every type of clinical encounter or research need. It is particularly important that documentation of a patient's progress not be blunted by *floor* or *ceiling* effects. For example, if a therapist wishes to measure changes in function among generally well elderly patients and the most advanced functional activity on an instrument measures "independent ambulation on level surfaces," there would be no room to demonstrate either progression or decline except around ambulation on level surfaces. Similarly, a patient who was severely debilitated might improve in transfers from needing the maximum assistance of two persons to maximum assistance of one. If the instrument only measures change from "maximum assistance" to "moderate assistance," this patient's real improvement will not be recorded.

Descriptive Parameters

Therapists should use descriptive terms that are well defined and unambiguous. Meanings of descriptive terms should be clear to all others using the medical record. Box 8.1 provides a sample set of acceptable terms and definitions. Please note that although in widespread clinical usage, there is little empirical evidence for the definitions provided for terms such as *minimal assistance* or *moderate assistance*. The definitions presented here are at best one operational definition to describe these terms. Additional terms used to qualify function include *dependence* and *difficulty*. Most often, the term *independent* refers to the complete absence of a need for human or mechanical assistance to accomplish a task, but some scoring systems consider reliance on devices and aids as a modified form of independence when used without the help of another person. The use of equipment during the performance of a functional task should be explicitly noted; for example, "independent in ambulation with axillary crutches" or "independent in dressing with adapted clothing and a long-handled shoe horn."

Difficulty is a hybrid term that suggests an activity poses an extra burden for the patient, regardless of dependence level. It is unclear whether it is a measure of overall perceptual-motor skill, coordination, endurance, efficiency, or a combination of measures. Difficulty can be measured in two ways. One approach assumes that difficulty is likely to be present and quantifies the degree of difficulty that the individual experiences while performing the activity (e.g., "How much difficulty do you have while doing household chores? None, some, or a great deal?"). The other approach quantifies the frequency that the difficulty is encountered (e.g., "How often do you have difficulty putting on your shoes? Never, sometimes, very often, or always?").

Often it is helpful to qualify a person's performance by linking observations with nonspecific indicators of impairments such as the energy consumption required to complete the functional task and the degree to which patients must exert themselves to engage in the activity. Simple measurements of a patient's physiological response to activity generally include heart rate, respiratory rate, blood pressure, and oxygen saturation, obtained at rest (baseline measurements), during (as possible), or immediately after completion of the most stressful elements of the activity. For example, "Heart rate increased to 100 beats per minute with independent ambulation on stairs; no increase in respiratory rate." In addition, the patient's perceived fatigue, rating of perceived exertion, and overt signs of physiological stress, such as shortness of breath, also should be noted. These notations may assist the therapist in a quick identification of some obvious impairments that limit function, which should be followed by more specific tests and measures of impairment.

Additional descriptors frequently used to qualify functional performance further include (1) pain, (2) fluctuations according to the time of day, (3) medication level, and (4) environmental influences. Any factors that modify a patient's function should be carefully noted and considered by the physical therapist evaluating examination data.

Quantitative Parameters

The time it takes to complete a series of activities is often used to enhance a therapist's quantification of function when a given speed of performance is required or an improvement in performance speed is expected. A common example of timed functional skills is found in premedication and postmedication performance of individuals with Parkinson disease who are placed on L-dopa therapy. Examples of activities that may be timed include (1) walking a set distance, (2) writing one's signature, (3) donning an article of clothing, and (4) crossing a street during the time of a "Walk" light. Scores of timed tests should not be taken as absolute, but rather as one dimension of performance. Although the ability to complete a particular activity in a specified period of time does provide one kind of important data on a patient's overall ability, it may not always be correct to conclude that what is being measured as "quicker" can be interpreted as "better." For example, the patient may get dressed quickly (within seconds), but do so with poorly coordinated movements and a haphazard outcome. When the task is slowed down, the movements may become more coordinated, with a more satisfactory functional outcome, even though the time taken to do the task increases. Similarly, certain medical conditions that affect energy expenditure may require that the patient properly pace a functional activity to complete it successfully. Thus, time scores alone do not always yield the complete functional picture. When interpreted in light of other aspects of the patient's clinical presentation, they do provide an added dimension to

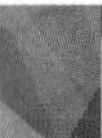

Box 8.1 Functional Examination and Impairment Terminology

Definitions

1. **Independent (I):** Patient is able consistently to perform skill safety with no one present.
2. **Supervision (S):** Patient requires someone within arm's reach as a precaution; low probability of patient having a problem requiring assistance.
3. **Close guarding (CloseG):** Person assisting is positioned as if to assist, with hands raised but not touching patient; full attention on patient; fair probability of patient requiring assistance.
4. **Contact guarding (ContactG):** Therapist is positioned as with close guarding, with hands on patient but not giving any assistance; high probability of patient requiring assistance.
5. **Minimum assistance (MinA):** Patient is able to complete majority of the activity without assistance.
6. **Moderate assistance (ModA):** Patient is able to complete part of the activity without assistance.
7. **Maximum assistance (MaxA):** Patient is unable to assist in any part of the activity.

Descriptive Terminology

A. Bed Mobility
1. Independent–no cuing* is given
2. Supervision
3. Minimum assistance
4. Moderate assistance
5. Maximum assistance

(2–5: may require cues)

B. Transfers, Ambulation
1. Independent–no cuing is given
2. Supervision
3. Close guarding
4. Contact guarding
5. Minimum assistance
6. Moderate assistance
7. Maximum assistance

(2–7: may require cues)

C. Functional Balance Grades

1. Normal	Patient able to maintain steady balance without support (static). Accepts maximal challenge and can shift weight easily and within full range in all directions (dynamic).
2. Good	Patient able to maintain balance without support, limited postural sway (static). Accepts moderate challenge; able to maintain balance while picking object off floor (dynamic).
3. Fair	Patient able to maintain balance with handhold support; may require occasional minimal assistance (static). Accepts minimal challenge; able to maintain balance while turning head/trunk (dynamic).
4. Poor	Patient requires handhold and moderate to maximal assistance to maintain posture (static). Unable to accept challenge or move without loss of balance (dynamic).
5. No balance	

*Types of cues: verbal, visual, or tactile. In some instances (e.g., a person with a memory deficit, short attention, learning disability, visual loss), a decrease in the number of cues may represent treatment progress, even though the level of dependence remains the same. Interim progress notes can denote these changes by citing frequencies (e.g., two out of three tries) or an arbitrarily defined rank order scale (e.g., always/occasionally/rarely).

the evaluation of data collected during examination of a function.

Response Formats

Function can be measured with tests that report data as nominal, ordinal, interval, and ratio measures. The clinician should consider the uses of the measure when deciding which format to use. In cases where the clinical decision is nominal, such as is the patient ready for discharge to home, a nominal measure such as whether the patient can or cannot independently ascend 10 stairs may be adequate. When a numeric value is obtained, such as the score from the Berg Balance scale,[19] the clinician may interpret the score as a dichotomous measure related to the decision (e.g., Does the patient have or not have adequate balance for discharge to home?). In cases where the clinical decision is more complex, such as the amount of assistance a patient needs with activities, nominal measures cannot be used and the measure should reflect the type and amount of information needed for the decision.

Nominal Measures

One of the simplest formats in functional tests uses a nominal level of measurement by presenting a checklist of various functional tasks on which the patient is simply scored as able to do/not able to do, independent/dependent, completed/incomplete, or the like. The results are not particularly descriptive of the exact nature of an individual's limitations and usually require further examination before interpretation. Nominal measures, however, may be helpful in making dichotomous decisions. For example, knowledge of the ability to perform ADL skills by themselves is important in deciding if a patient can be discharged to living independently at home.

Ordinal Measures

A few tests use descriptive scales that describe a range of performance or the degree to which a person can perform the task. Most commonly, the scales are ordinal or rank-order scales; for example, "no difficulty," "some difficulty," or "unable to do"; or "always," "sometimes," "rarely," or "never." (For additional examples, consider the scales in Box 8.1). Scales may be graded in ascending or descending order. The primary drawback in using such a system to score function is that these grades do not define categories that are separated by equal intervals. For example, it is not possible to tell whether the patient who went from maximal assistance to moderate assistance changed as much as a patient who also went one level between moderate assistance and minimal assistance.

Summary or additive measures grade a specific series of skills, award points for part or full performance, and sum the subscores as a proportion of the total possible points, such as 60/100 or 40/56. These summary measures may be considered as interval measures if the scores on the scale represent equal intervals; otherwise these measures may be considered as ordinal measures. One method to determine if the points on the scale represent equal intervals is through the use of Rasch analysis.[20] Although these summative scales typically may include a score of zero, this value represents a floor effect of the scale and not necessarily the absence of the construct. An example of a summary measure, which may be used to measure functional mobility and activities of self-care, is the Barthel Index.[21]

Some formal, standardized instruments for testing function summarize detailed information about a complex area of function into an overall index score. Use of these instruments facilitates the interpretation of complex data and enables the clinician to perform cross-disease, cross-program, and cross-population comparisons of function. Caution must be exercised in considering only summated scores, however, because potentially important individual differences in functional ability can be masked.[22] A patient who is limited in only a few of the many tasks covered on a functional test will most likely score well, despite what could be substantial limitations in discrete functional activities that are pertinent to the physical therapist's anticipated goals of treatment. Similarly, two patients with the same numeric score might be quite different in their functional deficits, having gained (or lost) their points on different activities. Although these measures yield a "hard number," which is regarded statistically as an interval level of measurement, the degree to which "points" are truly equal intervals or only ordinal should be carefully scrutinized.

Interval/Ratio Measures

Visual analog scales attempt to represent measurement quantities in terms of a straight line placed horizontally or vertically on paper (Fig. 8.3). The endpoints of the line are labeled with descriptive or numeric terms to anchor the extremes of the scale and provide a frame of reference for any point in the continuum between them. Some scales will also use descriptors or numeric intervals between the endpoints to assist the individual in grading responses. Commonly a visual analog line of 10 centimeters (100 millimeters) is used. The patient is asked to bisect the line at a point representing self-reported position on the scale. The patient's score is then obtained by measuring from the zero mark to the mark bisecting the scale.

Examples of the use of visual analog scales in rehabilitation settings may be to measure pain, dyspnea, function, or satisfaction with care. Since visual analog scales include a true zero and equal intervals (e.g., mm) they may be analyzed as ratio measures. In contrast, some clinicians may use a numeric rating scale (e.g., rate your function on a scale from 0 to 10) to measure similar impairments. Although providing a numeric rating may be quicker to obtain in clinical settings, scores obtained may not represent interval or ratio data, as the reporting of a numeric value may not represent equal intervals. For example, a 4 reported by one patient may not represent twice as much function as a 2 reported by another patient. This is due to the nature of interval and ratio scales because a ratio scale allows for the comparison of scores using addition,

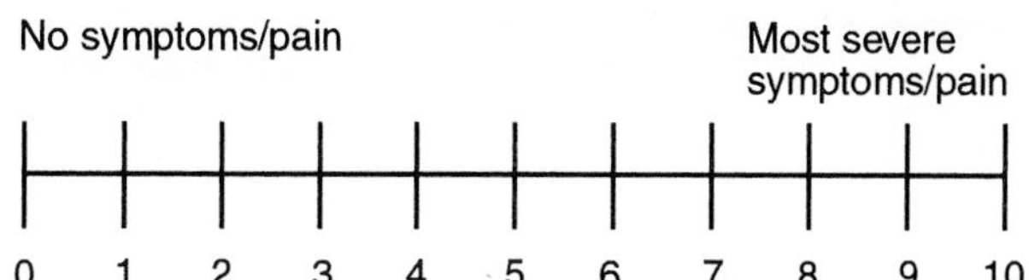

Figure 8.3 A visual analog scale for measuring pain or other symptoms. The patient is instructed to mark the line at the point that corresponds to the degree of pain or severity of symptoms that are experienced. From the Uniform Data System for Medical Rehabilitation, a division of UB Foundation Activities, Inc. (UDSMRSM). *(Guide for the Uniform Data Set for Medical Rehabilitation [including the FIMTM instrument], Version 5.1. Buffalo, NY 14214: State University of New York at Buffalo; 1997, with permission.)*

subtraction, multiplication, or division, and an interval scale allows for the comparison of scores using addition or subtraction. These mathematical functions cannot be performed with ordinal or nominal scores.

Knowledge of the level of measurement is important in analyzing data from groups of patients, such as a rehabilitation unit wishing to summarize the functional status of patients admitted during a specified time period. For interval and ratio measures, means and standard deviations may be calculated (assuming the data follow a normal distribution). For ordinal measures, medians and interquartile ranges are appropriate, whereas nominal measures may be represented by modes or by frequency counts. The distinction in the level of measurement is also important in the decision to use either parametric or nonparametric statistics to analyze data obtained from groups of patients.

INTERPRETING TEST RESULTS

Clearly, the single most important consideration in examining functional status is using the test results correctly to establish and revise the anticipated goals and expected outcomes of intervention and the plan of care. The therapist should carefully delineate the contributing factors that result in the functional deficit. When diminished ability is evident, the therapist must attempt to ascertain the cause of the problem. Some important questions to ask include the following:

1. What are the normal movements necessary to perform the task?
2. Which impairments inhibit performance or completion of the task? For example, do factors such as poor motor planning and execution, decreased strength, decreased range of motion, or altered joint integrity impede function? Does fatigue hamper functional ability?
3. Are the patient's functional deficits the result of impaired communication, perception, vision, hearing, or cognition?

Examples of the kinds of questions a therapist must pose to assess function and integrate findings into a comprehensive treatment program are found using the case vignettes in Table 8.3.

Although the activity limitation in each case is identical, the contributing factors, goals and outcomes, and the interventions would be markedly different. In case A, the patient's inability to transfer can reasonably be attributed to decreased strength. When ameliorated, it is likely that the patient will go on to achieve an outcome of independent ambulation with a prosthesis. The patient in case B has factors that cannot be addressed solely through physical therapy. In addition, it may be difficult to determine whether it is the paralysis or the aphasia that compromises efforts to assess and improve function. Although a similar goal of independence in wheelchair mobility and transfers may be proposed, reexamination throughout the episode of care may demonstrate that functional deficits persist, despite improvement in motor function. In that case, the impairments in comprehension and language function may be the more important factors contributing to functional limitation. Thus, the design of rehabilitation programs is based on the impairments that presumably underlie the functional deficits. If remediation of the impairment does not solve the functional problem, the therapist needs to reexamine the initial clinical impression by looking for other potentially causative factors.

Some functional tasks may need to be analyzed more precisely. Activities can be broken down into subordinate parts, or subroutines. A *subordinate part* is defined as an element of movement without which the task cannot proceed safely or efficiently. For example, bed mobility includes the following subordinate parts: (1) scooting in bed (changing position for comfort or skin care and getting to the edge), (2) rolling onto the side, (3) lowering the legs, (4) sitting up, and (5) balancing at the edge of the bed. A functional loss of independent bed mobility may result from an inability to perform any or all of these subroutines. These are not only checkpoints for examining

Table 8.3 Sample Case Vignettes

Case A	Case B
36-year-old male construction worker	72-year-old female homemaker
Dx: traumatic right transtibial amputation; following fracture left femur	Dx: CVA with right hemiplegia with global aphasia
Partial Examination Findings	
Motor Control and Muscle Performance	
Decreased in all extremities following prolonged immobilization	Flaccid paralysis right extremities
Activity Limitations	
Unable to transfer from bed to wheelchair	Unable to transfer from bed to wheelchair

Dx = diagnosis.

patients, but they also later represent the anticipated goals of various interventions. The more involved the patient, the slower the learner, or complex the task, the more the functional task may need to be broken down into subordinate parts.

Determining the Quality of Instruments

Within the rehabilitation setting, many tools exist for the measurement of function or its components. A number of excellent sources are available on the Internet to learn about the psychometric properties of functional measures (Box 8.2). In many cases, the sources include links to the instruments or information in how to perform or obtain the measures. In deciding which measure to use the instrument's *reliability, validity,* and *responsiveness* should be considered. If the reliability and validity of an instrument have not been established, little faith can be put in the results obtained or in the conclusions drawn from the results. Responsiveness of an instrument is important in determining if the change in a patient's score on two different occasions truly represents a change in their function. In light of the fact that the viability of physical therapy as a reimbursable service rests on the demonstration of functional outcomes, the importance of these concepts to functional testing becomes clear. In accordance with APTA's Standards of Measurement, physical therapists should use only those instruments whose reliability and validity are known.[23] Although no instrument will have perfect psychometric properties, therapists must be able to gauge the certainty of their data and the appropriate scope of inferences drawn from the data.

Reliability

A reliable instrument measures a phenomenon dependably, time after time, accurately, predictably, and without variation. If a functional test is not reliable, the patient's initial baseline status or the true effect of treatment can be concealed. An instrument with acceptable *test–retest reliability* is stable and will not indicate change when none has occurred. Tests performed by the same therapist of the same performance should be highly correlated (*intrarater reliability*). Instruments should also have strong *interrater reliability,* or agreement among multiple observers of the same event. If a patient is examined by several therapists in the course of treatment, or reexamined over time to determine long-term change, the reliability of these measurements must be known. To use functional tests with maximum accuracy, (1) scoring criteria must be defined clearly and must be mutually exclusive; (2) criteria must be strictly applied to each clinical situation; and (3) all therapists in a facility must be retrained periodically in the use of the instrument to ensure similarity.

Values for reliability coefficients have been provided; however, disclaimers are generally added that these should not be considered absolute cutoffs. For example, Portney and Watkins suggest less than 0.50 as poor reliability, 0.50 to 0.75 as moderate reliability, and greater than 0.75 as good reliability.[24, p. 82] In interpreting these values, the clinician needs to consider the precision of the measurement and how the results of the test will be applied in practice. A clinician should only use these values as guidelines, and not as absolutes, in determining the accuracy of the measurement and needs to consider the purpose of using the instrument. If high precision is needed in the instrument for clinical decision making, values of a reliability coefficient higher than the minimal threshold for "good" reliability should be used. In addition to the value of the reliability coefficient, the clinician should consider the variability of the measurement that may be expressed through values such as a standard deviation (SD) or confidence interval (CI).

Box 8.2 Internet Resources for Functional Measures

Rehabilitation Measures Database	www.rehabmeasures@sralab.org
PTNow	www.ptnow.org
EDGE task force	www.neuropt.org/professional-resources/neurology-section-outcome-measures-recommendations

EDGE = Evaluation Database to Guide Effectiveness

Validity

Validity is a multifaceted concept and established in many different ways. Questions regarding an instrument's validity attempt to determine (1) whether an instrument designed to measure function truly does just that, (2) what the appropriate applications of the instrument are, and (3) how the data should be interpreted. First, the valid instrument should, on the face of it, appear to measure what it purports to measure (*face validity*).[23,24] For example, an instrument claiming to measure balance should appear to measure some aspect of balance. Another critical dimension is whether the assessment instrument measures all the important or specified dimensions of function (*content validity*). If there were a gold standard (an unimpeachable measure of a phenomenon, such as a laboratory test with normative values), then a new instrument could be tested against the results of this standard (*criterion-related validity*). Such a gold standard does not exist for functional instruments. New functional measurement tools can, however, be compared to existing ones that are accepted measures of the same functional activities. The degree to which the two instruments agree helps to establish *concurrent validity*. Concurrent validity can also be demonstrated by showing that an instrument corresponds appropriately to measures of other phenomena. This method is particularly relevant for self-report instruments. The concurrent validity of some self-report instruments has been determined by comparison with clinician ratings and other clinical findings; for example, a person's level of function as indicated by an instrument correlates directly with clinician's ratings of improvement and inversely with the patient's reports of pain.

In the comparison of a test of function to a gold standard or to another existing instrument one should be concerned with the ability of the measure to make an accurate classification. *Sensitivity* of a test refers to the proportion of individuals with a limitation in function (as identified by the gold standard or existing instrument) who are correctly classified. In other words, sensitivity is an indication of how well a test identifies persons who should have a positive finding on the test. In contrast, *specificity* of a test refers to the proportion of individuals who do not have a limitation in function who are correctly classified. Additional properties of a test are the positive predictive value and the negative predictive value. The *positive predictive value* is the proportion of people who have a positive finding on a test who actually have a limitation in function as classified by the comparison test; the *negative predictive value* is the proportion of people who have a negative finding on a test who do not have a limitation in function.

Both sensitivity and specificity are expressed as values between 0 and 1. Ideally, both sensitivity and specificity should be as close to 1 as possible, but this is very rare in reality. Different tests, however, will be better at identifying those with the condition and others will be better at identifying those without the condition. This will be reflected in the magnitude of their sensitivity and specificity scores. When values of sensitivity or specificity are very close to 1, the SpPIn and SnNOut acronyms may help with interpretation.[25,26] The acronym SpPIn (specific test when positive, rules IN disease) refers to tests that have very high specificity: a positive finding helps to rule in the condition. SnNOut (specific test when negative, rules OUT disease), on the other hand, refers to tests that have very high sensitivity: a negative finding helps to rule out the condition. In general to apply these acronyms, sensitivity and specificity values greater than 0.95 may be considered very high.

Sensitivity and specificity values may be combined to obtain a likelihood ratio (LR) with the equations in Box 8.3. The calculation of likelihood ratios may be helpful in determining how much the test result influences the identification of a patient's condition or identification of a limitation in function. This is especially helpful in cases when sensitivity and specificity are not high enough to apply the SpPIn and SnNOut rules.

The larger the value of a positive likelihood ratio, the more helpful the finding of a positive test is in identifying the condition. Likewise, the smaller the value of a negative likelihood ratio (e.g., close to zero), the more helpful the finding of a negative test is in ruling out the condition. In contrast, a positive or negative likelihood ratio close to 1 is not helpful in identifying the condition. Likelihood ratios can be helpful in determination of posttest odds through their application in Bayes' theorem (i.e., the pretest odds x the likelihood ratio = the posttest odds).[25,26]

Box 8.3 Formulas to Determine Likelihood Ratios From Sensitivity and Specificity Values

Positive Likelihood Ratio = (Sensitivity)/(1 - Specificity)
Negative Likelihood Ratio = (1 - Sensitivity)/(Specificity)

where Sensitivity = Number of True Positives/(Number of True Positives Plus the Number of False Negatives)
and Specificity = Number of True Negatives/(Number of True Negatives Plus the Number of False Positives)

There is also the *predictive validity* of a test or measure, which indicates the likelihood of a subsequent phenomenon or event (e.g., return to work) on the basis of a prior phenomenon (e.g., a baseline measure of function). Finally, the degree to which an instrument measures abstract concepts such as physical mobility or social interaction can be established over time (*construct validity*). Construct validation, using a variety of statistical procedures, is a never-ending process as our understanding of the construct is further refined as instruments are developed to measure it.

Responsiveness

In addition to reliability and validity, a measure of functional status should be sufficiently sensitive to reflect *responsiveness* or a meaningful change in a patient's status. The change should exceed the *minimal detectable change* (MDC) of the instrument and a *minimal clinical important difference* (MCID). The MDC can be described as the smallest amount of change in a measurement that exceeds the measurement error of the instrument.[24,27] A physical therapist should be aware of published MDC values for the instruments used to measure function. A sample of MDC values for the 6-Minute Walk Test, the Timed Up and Go Test, and gait speed are presented in Table 8.4. As illustrated by the table, it is important to keep in mind that MDC values are specific for the patient population in whom the instrument was investigated.

In cases where MDC values may not exist in the literature, values may be calculated if the reliability coefficient, such as an intraclass correlation coefficient (ICC), and a measure of its variability is known, such as the SD. Box 8.4 provides equations that present the relationship

Table 8.4 Examples of Minimal Detectable Change Values for the 6-Minute Walk Test, the Timed-Up-and-Go Test, and Gait Speed in Different Clinical Populations

Test	Population of Interest	MDC	Reference
6MWT	Total hip and knee arthroplasty	61.34 m	Kennedy et al, 2005[28]
	Older adults	65 m	Mangione et al, 2010[29]
	Alzheimer disease	33.5 m	Ries et al, 2009[30]
	Stroke (inpatient rehabilitation)	54.1 m	Fulk et al, 2008[31]
	Multiple sclerosis	88 m*	Learnmouth et al, 2013[32]
TUG	Total hip and knee arthroplasty	2.49 sec	Kennedy et al, 2005[28]
	Older adults	4 sec	Mangione et al, 2010[29]
	Alzheimer disease	4.09 sec	Ries et al, 2009[30]
	Stroke (outpatient)	7.84 sec*	Hiengkaew et al, 2012[33]
	Multiple sclerosis	10.6 sec*	Learnmouth et al, 2012[34]
Gait speed	Total hip and knee arthroplasty (tested as fast self-paced walk time to complete 40 meters)	4.04 sec	Kennedy et al, 2005[28]
	Older adults	0.19 m/s	Mangione et al, 2010[29]
	Alzheimer disease	0.094 m/s	Ries et al, 2009[30]
	Stroke (outpatient)	0.18 m/s*	Hiengkaew et al, 2012[33]
	Multiple sclerosis	0.26 m/s*	Paltamaa et al, 2008[35]

m = meters; MDC = minimal detectable change; m/s = meters per second; 6MWT = 6-Minute Walk Test; sec = seconds; TUG = Timed-Up-And-Go Test

* Note these values are MDC_{95}, whereas all other values are MDC_{90}.

Box 8.4 Formulas to Determine Minimal Detectable Change From a Reliability Coefficient

$$MDC_{95} = 1.96 \times SEM \times SEM \times \sqrt{2}$$

$$\textit{Where } SEM = SD \times \sqrt{1 - ICC}$$

between the MDC_{95} (the amount of change with 95% confidence beyond measurement error) and the standard error of the measurement (SEM). The second equation can be used to determine the SEM if the value of the reliability coefficient and the standard deviation (SD) from one of the groups used to determine reliability is known. Note that because the ICC and the SD are from a specific sample, the calculated SEM and MDC_{95} are only generalizable to persons with similar conditions.

For example, if a study of persons after total knee arthroplasty reported an ICC of 0.75 for knee flexion with an SD of 5 degrees, the SEM is equal to 2.5 degrees. Using this value in the first equation, the MDC_{95} is 6.925 degrees. In other words, the measure of knee flexion would need to change more than 7 degrees to have 95% confidence that this change was due to something other than measurement error.

The MCID is the smallest difference in a measured variable that signifies an important rather than a trivial difference in the patient's condition.[24,27] The value of the MCID should exceed the value of the MDC; in other words, the MCID needs to exceed the measurement error. For example, a 50-meter change in distance on the 6-Minute Walk Test may be beyond measurement error; however, is the ability to walk 50 meters within 6 minutes meaningful to an individual patient's function? A number of different ways have been suggested to determine values for the MCID.[24, pp. 646–652] No universal method exists. Controversies exist among the strategies to determine MCID based on the perspective of what is meaningful, as well as issues related to measurement.[36,37] The clinician should consult the literature for recommended values of the MCID for measures of function. Like the interpretation of the MDC, in consulting published values for the MCID for a measure of function, the clinician needs to consider the sample for which the values were established.

Considerations in Selection of Instruments

A large number of instruments have been developed to assess and to classify function. Given the plethora of instruments that currently exist, it is quite reasonable to ask how these instruments compare with one another.

It is important to remember that no instrument is perfect for all patients or in all situations. No instrument can measure all the items potentially relevant to a particular individual and provide the perfect composite picture. For example, one instrument may provide an extensive measure of ADL, but not deal with psychological or social dimensions of function. Another instrument may investigate social functioning while omitting some ADL tasks. Many items overlap from instrument to instrument. For example, a question on the ability to ambulate is a common item found in most physical function instruments. Although instruments may cover the same kind of activity, the questions posed about the performance of the same activity may be quite different. For example, one instrument may investigate the degree of difficulty and of human assistance required to "dress yourself, including handling of closures, buttons, zippers, snaps." Another may ask, "How much help do you need in getting dressed?" As discussed, differences also may exist in the time frames sampled in the various instruments. Critical questions to ask in selecting an instrument are presented in Box 8.5.

Extrapolating items from a variety of instruments may provide the kind of data desired but should be considered with extreme caution inasmuch as this process changes reliability or validity of the measurements. Factors such as the theoretic orientation of the user, the purpose for using the instrument, and the relevance of particular functional items to certain patient populations all enter into the decision making process. In the final analysis, the choice of instrument may be dictated by practical considerations. For example, self-report instruments, which rely on information from the patient, are limited in use to mentally competent individuals. Time and resources for administration also may influence test selection, or some rehabilitation facilities may adopt the use of a specific instrument for all patients (e.g., the Functional Independence Measure [FIM]). In any case, many suitable instruments are available for assessing functional status, some of which are commonly used by clinicians as well as researchers.

Box 8.5 Critical Questions to Ask in Selecting an Instrument

1. What are the domains or categories that the assessment instrument focuses on?
2. How adequately does the instrument measure the domain or domains being sampled?
3. What areas of physical function are included? Does the instrument measure ADL? Does the instrument measure instrumental activities of daily living (IADL); for example, more advanced skills such as managing personal affairs, cooking, and driving? Mobility skills?
4. What aspect of function is being measured? Is the level of dependence–independence considered? What is the length of time required to complete the functional task? Degree of difficulty? Influence of pain?
5. What is the time frame sampled in the instrument?
6. What is the mode of administration?
7. What type of scoring system is used?
8. Are multiple instruments necessary to provide a more complete picture of functional status?
9. Who completes the instrument–the clinician, the patient (self-report), or family member (proxy)?
10. How long does the instrument take to complete?

SINGLE DIMENSION VERSUS MULTIDIMENSIONAL MEASURES OF FUNCTION

Among the factors to consider in selecting a measure of function is whether a single dimension measure or a multidimensional measure should be used. For example, *single dimension measures* may include a specific construct such as balance, gait, or reaching; whereas multidimensional measures would include a combination of these constructs or may have items from different domains of the ICF (e.g., impairments, activity limitations, and participation restrictions). As an example of a single test, gait speed may be used to represent function. This test may frequently be used in clinical settings because it requires a minimal amount of time to perform and little equipment other than a stopwatch and a hallway free of obstructions. For the test, the time for the patient to ambulate a specified distance, such as 10 meters, is recorded and speed is calculated as distance divided by time and frequently reported as meters per second. Although this is a test of a specific mobility item (walking), one might make inferences to a patient's function based on this test. The clinician, however, is responsible to check with the literature to determine if the inferences are supported by evidence, because there are some specific populations where gait speed may be representative of a patient's ability to function. For example, in a study of persons after hip arthroplasty it was demonstrated that gait speed was more representative of the capacity to ambulate than performance because when the patients were tested in real-world environments, their gait speed was slower than in the clinic. However, in this case the measure of capacity versus performance was highly correlated ($\rho = 0.440$).[38] Recent evidence among older persons also suggests that the measure of gait speed is highly related to overall health.[39] For populations that have not been tested, however, a clinician should be cautious in using gait speed to make inferences regarding function.

Other tests may use multiple items to measure a single dimension, such as the 14 items in the Berg Balance Scale to calculate a balance score. A clinician is justified using these instruments to describe the dimension of interest related to the patient's problem. However, unless data exist, they should not be used to make inferences regarding other impairments, activity limitations, or participation restrictions. Other instruments specific to those dimensions should be used as appropriate to the patient's presentation.

Alternatively, a clinician may take an approach to understand a patient's health status in all its domains. Further instrument development has resulted in the emergence of *multidimensional health status instruments* to measure the spectrum of health status more comprehensively. Used in conjunction with traditional clinical methods of examining signs and symptoms, multidimensional functional status instruments can add an important comprehensive view of a patient's function to the overall health status. In this respect, they add a crucial, and previously missing, component in evaluating the health of individuals.

Many comprehensive instruments are being developed to measure multiple dimensions of the ICF to present an overall view of a person's function. Specifically, several *ICF Core Sets* are being developed for specific patient conditions, such as stroke,[40] or by settings such as postacute rehabilitation settings.[41] Each core set includes items related to body functions, body structures, activities, participation, and contextual factors important to the specific condition or setting. These core sets are being developed using expert opinion and are being empirically tested to determine if representative items are included.[42,43] These core sets potentially may allow a clinician to focus on the most relevant items from the myriad of specific items in the ICF classification.

The final section of this chapter briefly presents three multidimensional instruments a physical therapist may use in practice. In addition, a fourth instrument, the Patient-Specific Functioning Scale, is included to represent a measure of aspects of function important to an individual patient. Many other instruments exist, some of which were mentioned previously in this chapter and some of which are included in other chapters. For additional measures, please review the websites in Box 8.2.

For the purposes of illustration, three multidimensional instruments, the *Functional Independence Measure* (FIM), the *Outcome and Assessment Information Set* (OASIS), and the *Short Form* (36) *Health Survey* (SF-36) are presented. Choice of a multidimensional instrument carries the same caveats mentioned for instruments a single dimension.[44] No instrument measures all potentially relevant items. In addition, depending on how an item is worded, items that may appear to measure the same aspect of function may be measuring different aspects of performance.[45] Table 8.5 presents a comparison of items covered. In the area of physical function, questions on the ability to ambulate are the only items these instruments have in common. Aspects of physical function not covered in any of these instruments include bed mobility and dexterity. The FIM and the OASIS include more ADL items than the SF-36. The SF-36 investigates work performance, whereas the FIM and the OASIS do not. This is not surprising, given that the FIM was originally developed as a tool for the inpatient rehabilitation setting and the OASIS was expressly designed for home health agencies, both generally serving older patients. In contrast, the development of the SF-36 was focused on younger adult populations in ambulatory care. Anxiety and depression are addressed as areas of psychological function in the SF-36 and the OASIS, but not in the FIM. The OASIS does not explore social function, in contrast to the other two. Finally, only the SF-36 records general health perceptions.

Table 8.5 Items Covered in Selected Multidimensional Functional Assessment Instruments

	FIM	SF-36	OASIS
Symptoms	–	+	+
Physical function			
Transfers	+	–	+
Ambulation	+	+	+
ADL			
Bathing	+	+	+
Grooming	+	–	+
Dressing	+	+	+
Feeding	+	–	+
Toileting	+	–	+
IADL			
Indoor home	–	+	+chores
Outdoor home	–	+	+chores/ shopping
Community	–	+	+travel/ drive car
Work/school	–	+	–
Affective function			
Communication	+	–	+
Cognition	+	–	+
Anxiety	–	+	+
Depression	–	+	+
Social function			
Interaction	+	+	–
Activity/leisure	–	+	–
General health	–	+	–perceptions

■ SAMPLE INSTRUMENTS TO ASSESS FUNCTION

The Functional Independence Measure

The FIM[46,47] is an 18-item measure of physical, psychological, and social function that is part of the Uniform Data System for Medical Rehabilitation (UDSMR)[48]

(Table 8.6). The UDSMR collects data from participating rehabilitation facilities and issues summary reports of the records that have been entered into the UDSMR database. The FIM uses the level of assistance an individual needs to grade functional status from total independence to total assistance. A person may be regarded as independent if a device is used, but this is recorded separately from "complete" independence. A 7-point scale is used based on the percentage of active participation from the patient. Complete independence for an item is scored as a 7 and a 1 is defined as total assistance required to perform the activity or the item is not testable. Precise definitions are provided for each level of assistance. The instrument lists six self-care activities: feeding, grooming, bathing, upper body dressing, lower body dressing, and toileting. Bowel and bladder control, aspects of which some may consider as impairments rather than function, are categorized separately. Functional mobility is tested through three items on transfers. Under the category of locomotion, walking and using a wheelchair are listed equivalently, whereas stairs are considered separately. The FIM also includes two items on communication and three on social cognition.

The FIM measures what the individual does, not what that person could do under certain circumstances. The interrater reliability of the FIM has been established at an acceptable level of psychometric performance (ICCs ranging from 0.86 to 0.88).[47] The face and content validity of the FIM, as well as its ability to capture change in a patient's level of function, have also been determined. Any clinical worker can administer the FIM after appropriate training in using the response set for each item.

Rasch analysis has been applied to the scale scores of the FIM, which are ordinal measures, in order to create interval scale measurements.[49] In addition, the *WeeFIM*, an 18-item instrument based on the FIM, has been developed for use for children between the ages of 6 months and 18 years.[50]

Table 8.6 Categories and Items of the Functional Independence Measure (FIM)

Self-Care	A. Eating B. Grooming C. Bathing D. Dressing–Upper E. Dressing–Lower F. Toileting
Sphincter Control	G. Bladder H. Bowel
Transfers	I. Bed, Chair, Wheelchair J. Toilet K. Tub, Shower
Locomotion	L. Walk/Wheelchair M. Stairs
Communication	N. Comprehension O. Expression
Social Cognition	P. Social Interaction Q. Problem Solving R. Memory

Additional information on the FIM is available from www.udsmr.org/WebModules/FIM/Fim_About.aspx.

The Outcome and Assessment Information Set

The OASIS was designed to ensure the collection of pertinent data on the adult patient in the home care setting that would allow home health agencies to assess the quality of care by measuring the outcomes of care.[51,52] Since 1999, home health agencies have been mandated to use the OASIS as a *Condition of Participation in the Medicare program* by the Health Care Financing Administration. The current version of OASIS, known as OASIS-C, contains core items covering sociodemographic characteristics, environmental factors, social support, health status, and functional status.[53] This version of the instrument was approved in 2009 and represents a substantial change from preceding versions. OASIS is not designed to be a comprehensive examination of a patient or an "add-on" measurement. OASIS items are meant to be integrated into the clinical record to highlight various aspects of a patient's status that identify particular needs for care on admission to the home health service, at follow-up every 60 days, and at discharge. The OASIS was intended to be a discipline-neutral record, administered by any health professional, including physical therapists.

Ease of administration increases with familiarity with the instrument. Unlike most other instruments, the response sets that accompany each item are specifically matched to the item. Some response sets have only two possible descriptions of behavior, whereas others have as many as nine possible descriptions of behavior. Therefore, the user must be familiar with the possible response set to each item and anticipate that comfort level in using this instrument will increase over a learning curve. Items from the ADL/instrumental ADL (IADL) section are listed in Table 8.7.

The SF-36

The *SF-36* contains 36 items based on questions used in the RAND Health Insurance Study. These 36 items were culled from the 113 questions used by RAND in the *Medical Outcomes Study* (MOS) to explore the relationship between physician practice styles and patient outcomes.[54] Thus, it was named the SF-36, because it was a short form of the MOS instrument with only 36 questions. The MOS provided important data on the functional status of adults with specific chronic conditions[55] and

Table 8.7 Outcome and Assessment Information Set (OASIS): Items From the ADLs/IADLs Section

Grooming
Current Ability to Dress Lower Body
Current Ability to Dress Upper Body
Bathing
Toilet Transferring
Toileting Hygiene
Transferring
Ambulation/Locomotion
Feeding or Eating
Current Ability to Plan and Prepare Light Meals
Ability to Use Telephone
Prior Functioning ADL/IADL
Multifactorial Falls Risk Assessment

Additional information on the OASIS is available from www.cms.gov/Medicare/Quality-Initiatives-Patient-Assessment-Instruments/OASIS/index.html.

Table 8.8 Domains of the Short Form 36 (SF-36)

Physical Functioning
Role Limitations due to Physical Problems
General Health Perceptions
Vitality
Social Functioning
Role Limitations due to Emotional Problems
General Mental Health
Health Transition

Additional information on the SF-36 is available from www.rand.org/health/surveys_tools/mos/36-item-short-form.html.
Information regarding licensing fees for the Short Form Health Surveys is available from https://campaign.optum.com/sf36

the well-being of patients experiencing depression compared to subjects with a chronic medical condition.[56] The SF-36 demonstrated high reliability and validity (correlation coefficients ranging from 0.81 to 0.88).[57-60] Normative data for these self-report items have been collected.[61]

All but one of the 36 questions of the SF-36 are used to form eight different scales: vitality, physical functioning, bodily pain, general health perceptions, physical role functioning, emotional role functioning, social role functioning, and mental health (Table 8.8). Items are scored on nominal (yes/no) or ordinal scales. Each possible response to an item on a scale is assigned a number of points. The total points for all items within a scale are then added and transformed mathematically to yield a percentage score, with 100% representing optimal health. The SF-36 has been used in a number of studies that describe the health status and physical functioning of patients with a variety of impairments receiving physical therapy services.[62-68]

A shortened version has been developed that uses a subset of items from the SF-36.[69] This version, known as *SF-12,* includes items from each of the eight concepts represented in the SF-36 and allows for the calculation of physical and mental subscale scores. An advantage to using fewer questions is that less time is required to complete the survey. This, however, may be at the expense of having a less precise score that may not be as sensitive to change for an individual patient.[70] The development of the SF-36 stands as the premier example, to date, of a complete and published exploration of the psychometric properties of an instrument as an essential part of its development, and a testament to the responsibility of its creators in verifying the quality of the SF-36 as a scientific tool.

The Patient-Specific Functional Scale

A number of measures have been developed to measure aspects of function for patients seen in outpatient settings. Among the measures that are in common use and have been validated among specific patient groups are the *Neck Disability Index,*[71] the *Oswestry Low Back Pain Questionnaire,*[72] the *Disabilities of the Arm, Shoulder and Hand* (DASH),[73] the *Lower Extremity Functional Scale* (LEFS),[74] and the *Foot and Ankle Ability Measure* (FAAM).[75] These measures include items for common functional tasks specific to certain patient groups. For example, the LEFS includes items related to the use of the lower extremities such as walking, going up and down stairs, and running. These items represent common functional items for most patients with similar conditions.

In contrast to the use of functional measures that use a list of standardized items, a clinician may be interested in assessing specific functional items that are most important to each individual patient and the patient's goals. The *Patient-Specific Functional Scale* (PSFS) can be used by a patient to identify the three most important activities to them, quantify the limitation, and measure change on follow-up visits.[76] Specifically, the patient is asked to identify up to three important activities they are unable to perform at their previous level due to their health condition. Each of the activities is given a score on a 0 to 10 scale, where 0 represents being unable to perform the activity and 10 represents the ability to perform the activity at the same level before the onset of the condition. The total score on the PSFS is obtained by adding each activity score and dividing by the number of activities. For example, a college student who sprained an ankle playing intramural basketball may identify the following three activities as limited: walking to class with crutches, standing for chemistry labs, and running. This student may provide initial scores for these three items as 5, 3, and 0, respectively, which results in a total PSFS score of 2.7 [(5 + 3 + 0)/3]. On follow-up visits, a patient is asked to score the same three activities in order to assess the change in his functional status. In the example provided, the student may no longer require crutches for walking and reports this item as a 10. However, he still has pain with prolonged standing, which he scores a 7, and he has not resumed running for playing basketball, so he scores this a 5. This results in a total score of 7.3 (22/3). This value exceeds the published value for the MDC_{90} for the PSFS of 2 points.[76] Note, however, that this value for the MDC was determined in a sample of persons with low back pain.

Another benefit of the PSFS is that it can be used with patients with different musculoskeletal conditions, making it a useful tool for practice. Populations tested include those with low back pain, cervical dysfunction, knee conditions, upper extremity problems, joint replacement, and lower-limb amputations.[77-80] In addition to use with individual patients, the validity of the PSFS has been shown for group data, which supports its use in clinical research.[81]

SUMMARY

This chapter has presented a conceptual framework for understanding function and for the examination of functional status. The traditional medical model, with its narrow focus on disease and its symptoms, fails to consider the impact of the condition on the person, as well as the broader social, psychological, and behavioral dimensions of illness. All these factors have an impact on an individual's activity and participation. Although individual aspects of function may be assessed, examination of functional status must be viewed as a broad, multidimensional process. Finally, specific aspects of functional examination have been discussed, including purpose, selection of instruments, aspects of test administration, interpretation of test results, and determination of instrument quality.

Questions for Review

1. How does the measurement of function relate to health?
2. Your rehabilitation facility uses the FIM. How can the instrument be administered to ensure that the results can be used with confidence in both treatment planning and research?
3. What criteria can be used in the selection of a functional instrument?
4. Discuss the uses, advantages, and disadvantages of performance-based instruments, interviewer reports, and self-administered reports.
5. Explain how environment, fatigue, and other related issues affect measurement of function. Suggest ways to control these factors in the clinic.
6. Identify the major types of scoring systems used in functional instruments. What are some common errors in interpretation of testing results?
7. Review Tables 8.6, 8.7, and 8.8. Hypothesize a caseload in a particular setting and indicate how and when you could use each of these instruments with the proposed population. Describe the advantages and disadvantages of each. Imagine that you are looking to follow the progress of these same patients to another setting. Which instruments would you choose?
8. Using one of the instruments, develop a set of results and use them to identify treatment goals and outcomes and to formulate a plan of care.
9. For each of the following, identify particular physical tasks relevant to that individual's functional status:
   - A 22-year-old female file clerk
   - A 31-year-old male physical therapist assistant
   - A 39-year-old female homemaker with children
   - A 45-year-old male construction worker
   - A 56-year-old female school teacher
   - A 65-year-old male journalist
10. Discuss the relationship among disease, body structures, body functions, activity, participation, environmental factors, and personal factors.

CASE STUDY

A 78-year-old woman with a diagnosis of osteoarthritis was admitted for a right total hip replacement. The patient reported a long-standing history of discomfort. She described the hip pain as radiating posteriorly to the buttock and low back and exacerbated by weight-bearing and stair climbing. Over the past 12 months she has experienced a very marked increase in pain and stiffness. Radiographic findings demonstrated degenerative changes of both the acetabulum and femoral head consistent with osteoarthritis. The surgical intervention replaced the right femoral head and neck with a metallic prosthesis and the acetabulum was resurfaced with a plastic cup. Past medical history is unremarkable.

SOCIAL HISTORY

The patient is a retired manager of a small accounting firm that she and her husband established. Her husband is deceased. She has three grown children who all live in neighboring communities. Before the functional limitations imposed by the hip pain, the patient had been independent in all ADL and IADL. She also volunteered her accounting services 1 day per week to a local charity that provides meals to homebound individuals. She was a regular participant in family outings; enjoyed going to the theater, concerts, and special museum events; and was an active member of the community's historical preservation society. Recently, these activities had to be curtailed owing to the increased hip discomfort. She essentially had no activities outside the home for 3 months before admission and used a walker to minimize weight-bearing and reduce pain. She also required the assistance of a home care aide 4 hours a day two times per week (primarily for shopping, errands, and some household management tasks). She expressed considerable distress at being unable to take a bath and having to rely on the assistance of another person for some basic care activities. She had been using aspirin for its analgesic and anti-inflammatory effects. However, the pain experienced in recent months was not alleviated by the aspirin and other conservative measures. She has been instructed to use local applications of heat, periodic rest intervals, and gentle range-of-motion (ROM) exercises. The patient has extensive medical insurance coverage and is without financial concerns.

POSTSURGICAL RIGHT HIP PRECAUTIONS

No hip flexion beyond 90°.
Avoid crossing one leg or ankle over the other.
Avoid internal rotation of right lower extremity.

REVIEW OF SYSTEMS

Communication, Affect, Cognition, Learning Style: Fully communicative and oriented ×3. Cooperative and motivated. Hearing intact. Wears corrective lens; experiences "night blindness," which she describes as seeing poorly in dim light and her eyes take several seconds longer than normal to adjust from brightness to dimness.

Cardiopulmonary: Heart rate (HR) = 84 beats/minute; blood pressure (BP) = 130/78 mm Hg; respiratory rate (RR) = 16 breaths/minute; no appreciable increases with activity.

Integumentary: Surgical wound healing well; staples removed.

Strength: Upper extremity gross ROM is within normal limits (WNL). Gross strength generally good to normal, except hands. Left hip, knee, and ankle at least good on break test. Partial weight-bearing on right lower extremity.

Joint Integrity and Mobility: Patient reports some sporadic episodes of wrist and finger stiffness on awakening in the morning and after periods of immobility. Crepitus noted in right knee. Heberden's nodes noted at the distal interphalangeal (DIP) and proximal interphalangeal (PIP) joints of the left index finger.

Range of Motion: Right knee and ankle within functional limits; right hip not tested.

Muscle Performance: Grip strength is reduced bilaterally.

Pain: Patient denies pain in wrist or fingers, or right hip.

Gait, Locomotion, and Balance: The patient is ambulating on level surfaces with supervision using bilateral standard aluminum axillary crutches with partial weight-bearing on the right lower extremity. Stair climbing also requires minimal assistance. It is anticipated that the patient will be independent with ambulation on level surfaces at time of discharge from the hospital.

Functional Status: Impaired bed mobility (modified independence device), sit-to-stand, transfers (minimum assistance).

Home Environment: The patient lives alone in a fifth-floor apartment in a building with an elevator. The living space is a one-bedroom apartment on a single level.

Patient Goals: The patient is extremely motivated to once again be an independent manager of her personal care and household management needs. The prosthetic replacement has successfully relieved much of the pain experienced in the hip before surgery (most of her current discomfort is described as minor and associated with the surgical incision). She would also like to return to her family, volunteer, social, and leisure activities. She is very determined to discontinue the home care assistance as soon as possible.

GUIDING QUESTIONS

1. Based on the findings of the initial examination, discuss the links between the condition, impairments in body structures and body functions, activity limitations, participation restrictions, and contextual factors using the ICF model.
2. Identify the specific ADL and IADL skills that would need to be examined to return this patient to the highest level of function and achieve the patient's goals for rehabilitation. Discuss the appropriateness of the instruments presented in this chapter for measuring her function and documenting the outcomes of patient management.

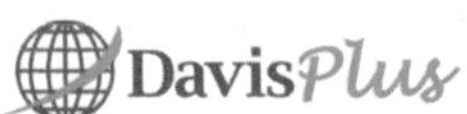

For additional resources, including answers to the questions for review and case study guiding questions, please visit **http://davisplus.fadavis.com.**

References

1. *Guide to Physical Therapist Practice 3.0.* Alexandria, VA: American Physical Therapy Association; 2014. Available at: www.guidetoptpractice.apta.org. Accessed February 1, 2017.
2. Lucas, JW, and Benson, V: Tables of Summary Health Statistics for the U.S. Population: 2015 National Health Interview Survey. National Center for Health Statistics. 2017. Retrieved February 1, 2017, from www.cdc.gov/nchs/nhis/SHS/tables.htm.
3. World Health Organization (WHO): The First Ten Years of the World Health Organization. World Health Organization, Geneva, 1958.
4. World Health Organization (WHO): International Classification of Functioning, Disability and Health. World Health Organization, Geneva, 2001.
5. World Health Organization (WHO): ICD 10: International Statistical Classification of Diseases and Related Health Problems, Tenth Revision, Volume 1. World Health Organization, Geneva, 1992.
6. Jette, AM, Haley, SM, and Kooyoomjian, JT: Are the ICF activity and participation dimensions distinct? J Rehabil Med 35(3):145, 2003.
7. Brandt, EN, Jr, and Pope, AM (eds): Enabling America: Assessing the Role of Rehabilitation Science and Engineering. National Academy Press, Washington, DC, 1997.
8. Jette, AM, and Keysor, JJ: Disability models: Implications for arthritis exercise and physical activity interventions. Arthritis Rheum 49:114, 2003.
9. Functional Limitation Reporting Under Medicare. American Physical Therapy Association. Retrieved February 1, 2017, from www.apta.org/Payment/Medicare/CodingBilling/FunctionalLimitation/.
10. Guyatt, GH, et al: The 6-minute walk: A new measure of exercise capacity in patients with chronic heart failure. Can Med Assoc J 132:923, 1985.
11. Winograd, CH, et al: Development of a physical performance and mobility examination. J Am Geriatr Soc 42:743, 1994.
12. Duncan, PW, et al: Functional reach: A new clinical measure of balance. J Gerontol 45:192, 1990.
13. Duncan, PW, et al: Functional reach: Predictive validity in a sample of elderly male veterans. J Gerontol 47:93, 1992.
14. Mathias, S, et al: Balance in elderly patients: The "Get Up and Go" test. Arch Phys Med Rehabil 67:387, 1986.
15. Podsiadlo, D, and Richardson, S: The timed "Up and Go": A test of basic functional mobility for frail elderly persons. J Am Geriatr Soc 39:142, 1991.
16. Guralnik, JM, et al: A short physical performance battery assessing lower extremity function: Association with self-reported disability and prediction of mortality and nursing home admission. J Gerontol 49:85, 1994.
17. Tager, IB, et al: Reliability of physical performance and self-reported functional measures in an older population. J Gerontol 53:295, 1998.
18. Guccione, AA, et al: Development and testing of a self-report instrument to measure actions: Outpatient Physical Therapy Improvement in Movement Assessment Log (OPTIMAL). Phys Ther 85:515, 2005.
19. Berg, KO, et al: Measuring balance in the elderly: validation of an instrument. Can J Public Health 83 Suppl 2:S7, 1992.
20. Wright, BD, et al: FIM measurement properties and Rasch model details. Scand J Rehabil Med 29:267, 1997.
21. Mahoney, F, and Barthel, D: Functional evaluation: The Barthel Index. Md Med J 14:61, 1965.
22. Guccione, AA, et al: Defining arthritis and measuring functional status in elders: Methodological issues in the study of disease and disability. Am J Public Health 80:949, 1990.
23. Standards for Tests and Measurements in Physical Therapy Practice. Phys Ther 71:589, 1991.
24. Portney, LG, and Watkins, MP: Foundations of Clinical Research: Applications to Practice, ed 3. FA Davis, Philadelphia, PA, 2015.
25. Straus, SE, et al: Evidence-Based Medicine: How to Practice and Teach It, ed 4. Churchill Livingstone, Edinburgh, 2011.
26. Fetters, L, and Tilson, J: Evidence Based Physical Therapy. FA Davis, Philadelphia, PA, 2012.
27. Riddle, D, and Stratford, P: Is This Change Real? Interpreting Patient Outcomes in Physical Therapy. FA Davis, Philadelphia, PA, 2013.
28. Kennedy, DM, et al: Assessing stability and change of four performance measures: A longitudinal study evaluating outcome following total hip and knee arthroplasty. BMC Musculoskelet Disord 28(6):3, 2005.
29. Mangione, KK, et al: Detectable changes in physical performance measures in elderly African Americans. Phys Ther 90:921, 2010.
30. Ries, JD, et al: Test-retest reliability and minimal detectable change scores for the timed "up and go" test, the six-minute walk test, and gait speed in people with Alzheimer disease. Phys Ther 89:569, 2009.
31. Fulk, GD, et al: Clinometric properties of the six-minute walk test in individuals undergoing rehabilitation poststroke. Physiother Theory Pract 24:195–204, 2008.
32. Learnmouth, YC, et al: The reliability, precision, and clinically meaningful change of walking assessments in multiple sclerosis. MSJ 19:1784, 2013.
33. Hiengkaew, V, Jitaree K, and Chaiyawat, P: Minimal detectable changes of the Berg Balance Scale, Fugl-Meyer Assessment Scale, Timed "Up & Go" Test, gait speeds, and 2-Minute Walk Test in individuals with chronic stroke with different degrees of ankle plantarflexor tone. Arch Phys Med Rehabil 93:1201, 2012.

34. Learnmouth, YC, et al: Reliability and clinical significance of mobility and balance assessments in multiple sclerosis. Int J Rehabil Res 35:69, 2012.
35. Paltamaa, J, et al: Measuring deterioration in International Classification of Functioning domains of people with multiple sclerosis who are ambulatory. Phys Ther 88:176, 2008.
36. Gatchel, RJ, and Mayer, TG: Testing minimal clinically important difference: Consensus or conundrum? Spine J 10(4):321, 2010.
37. Rennard, SI: Minimal clinically important difference, clinical perspective: An opinion. COPD 2(1):51, 2005.
38. Foucher, KC, et al: Differences in preferred walking speeds in a gait laboratory compared with the real world after total hip replacement. Arch Phys Med Rehabil 91(9):1390–1395, 2010.
39. Studenski, S, et al: Gait speed and survival in older adults. JAMA 305(1):50–58, 2011.
40. Geyh, S, et al: ICF Core Sets for stroke. J Rehabil Med 44(Suppl): 135–141, 2004.
41. Grill, E, et al: ICF Core Sets for early post-acute rehabilitation facilities. J Rehabil Med 43(2):131–138, 2011.
42. Starrost, K, et al: Interrater reliability of the extended ICF core set for stroke applied by physical therapists. Phys Ther 88(7): 841, 2008.
43. Algurén, B, Lundgren-Nilsson, A, and Sunnerhagen, KS: Functioning of stroke survivors–A validation of the ICF core set for stroke in Sweden. Disabil Rehabil 32(7):551, 2010.
44. Guccione, AA, and Jette, AM: Multidimensional assessment of functional limitations in patients with arthritis. Arthrit Care Res 3:44, 1990.
45. Guccione, AA, and Jette, AM: Assessing limitations in physical function in persons with arthritis. Arthr Care Res 1:170, 1988.
46. Granger, CV, et al: Advances in functional assessment for medical rehabilitation. Top Geriatr Rehabil 1:59, 1986.
47. Granger, CV, et al: Functional assessment scales: A study of persons with multiple sclerosis. Arch Phys Med Rehabil 71:870, 1990.
48. Guide for the Uniform Data Set for Medical Rehabilitation (Adult FIM), Version 4.0. Buffalo, Uniform Data System for Medical Rehabilitation, UB Foundation Activities, Inc, 1993.
49. Heinemann, AW, et al: Relationships between impairment and physical disability as measured by the Functional Independence Measure. Arch Phys Med Rehabil 74:566, 1993.
50. Ottenbacher, KJ, et al: Measuring developmental and functional status in children with disabilities. Dev Med Child Neurol 41:186, 1999.
51. Krisler, KS, et al: OASIS Basics: Beginning to Use the Outcome and Assessment Information Set. Center for Health Services and Policy Research, Denver, 1997.
52. Shaughnessy, PW, and Crisler, KS: Outcome-based Quality Improvement. A Manual for Home Care Agencies on How to Use Outcomes. National Association for Home Care, Washington, DC, 1995.
53. Deitz, D, et al: OASIS-C: Development, testing, and release. An overview for home healthcare clinicians, administrators, and policy makers. Home Health Nurse 28(6):353–362, quiz 363–364, 2010.
54. Tarlov, AR, et al: The Medical Outcomes Study: An application of methods for monitoring the results of medical care. JAMA 262: 925, 1989.
55. Stewart, AL, et al: Functional status and well-being of patients with chronic conditions: Results from the Medical Outcomes Study. JAMA 262:907, 1989.
56. Wells, KB, et al: The functioning and well-being of depressed patients: Results from the Medical Outcomes Study. JAMA 262:914, 1989.
57. Stewart, AL, et al: The MOS short general health survey: Reliability and validity in a patient population. Med Care 26:724, 1988.
58. Ware, JE, and Sherbourne, CD: The MOS 36-item short form health survey (SF-36): I. Conceptual framework and item selection. Med Care 30:473, 1992.
59. McHorney, CA, et al: The MOS 36-item short form health survey (SF-36): II. Psychometric and clinical tests of validity in measuring physical and mental health constructs. Med Care 31:247, 1993.
60. McHorney, CA, et al: The MOS 36-item short form health survey (SF-36): III. Tests of data quality, scaling assumptions, and reliability across diverse patient groups. Med Care 32:40, 1994.
61. Ware, JE, et al: SF-36 Health Survey: Manual and Interpretation Guide. Boston, the Health Institute, New England Medical Center, 1993.
62. Mossberg, KA, and McFarland, C: Initial health status of patients at outpatient physical therapy clinics. Phys Ther 75:1043, 1995.
63. Jette, DU, and Downing, J: Health status of individuals entering a cardiac rehabilitation program as measured by the Medical Outcomes Study 36-item short form survey (SF-36). Phys Ther 74:521, 1994.
64. Jette, DU, and Downing, J: The relationship of cardiovascular and psychological impairments to the health status of patients enrolled in cardiac rehabilitation programs. Phys Ther 76:130, 1996.
65. Jette, DU, and Jette, AM: Physical therapy and health outcomes in patients with spinal impairments. Phys Ther 76:930, 1996.
66. Jette, DU, and Jette, AM: Physical therapy and health outcomes in patients with knee impairments. Phys Ther 76:1178, 1996.
67. Jette, DU, et al: The disablement process in patients with pulmonary disease. Phys Ther 77:385, 1997.
68. Ware, J, Kosinski, M, and Keller, SD: A 12-item short-form health survey: Construction of scales and preliminary tests of reliability and validity. Med Care 34:220, 1996.
69. Riddle, DL, Lee, KT, and Stratford, PW: Use of SF-36 and SF-12 health status measures: A quantitative comparison for groups versus individual patients. Med Care 39:867, 2001.
70. Zhang, Y, Zhou, and Sun, Y: Assessment of health-related quality of life using the SF-36 in Chinese cervical spondylotic myelopathy patients after surgery and its consistency with neurological function assessment: a cohort study. Health Qual Life Outcomes 13: 1, 2015.
71. Vernon, H, and Mior, S: The Neck Disability Index: A study of reliability and validity. J Manipulative Physiol Ther 14: 409, 1992.
72. Fairbank, JC, Couper, J, and Davies, JB: The Oswestry Low Back Pain Questionnaire. Physiotherapy 66: 271, 1980.
73. Hudak, PL, Amadio, PC, and Bombardier, D: Development of an upper extremity outcome measure: the DASH (disabilities of the arm, shoulder, and hand). The Upper Extremity Collaborative Group (UECG). Am J Ind Med 30: 372, 1996.
74. Binkley, JM, et al: The Lower Extremity Functional Scale: Scale development, measurement properties, and clinical application. North American Orthopaedic Rehabilitation Research Network. Phys Ther 79: 371, 1999.
75. Martin, RL, et al: Evidence of validity for the Foot and Ankle Ability Measure (FAAM). Foot Ankle Int 26: 968, 2005.
76. Stratford, P, et al: Assessing disability and change on individual patients: A report of a patient specific measure. Physiotherapy Canada 47:258, 1995.
77. Horn, KK, et al. The Patient-Specific Functional Scale: psychometrics, clinimetrics, and application as a clinical outcome measure. J Orthop Sports Phys Ther 42:30, 2012.
78. Hefford, C, et al. The Patient-Specific Functional Scale: Validity, reliability and responsiveness in patients with upper extremity musculoskeletal problems. J Orthop Sports Phys Ther 42:56, 2012.
79. Resnik, L, and Borgia, M: Reliability of outcome measures for people with lower-limb amputations: Distinguishing true change from statistical error. Phys Ther 91:555, 2011.
80. Chatman, AB, et al: The Patient-Specific Functional Scale: Measurement properties in patients with knee dysfunction. Phys Ther 77: 820, 1997.
81. Abbott, JH, and Schmitt, JS: The Patient-Specific Functional Scale was valid for group-level change comparisons and between-group discrimination. J Clin Epid 67:681, 2014.

Supplemental Readings

Escorpizo, R, et al: Creating an interface between the International Classification of Functioning, Disability and Health and physical therapist practice. Phys Ther 90:1053, 2010.

Field, MJ, and Jette, AM (eds): The Future of Disability in America. Institute of Medicine Committee on Disability in America. National Academies Press, Washington, DC, 2007.

Jette, AM: Physical disablement concepts for physical therapy research and practice. Phys Ther 74(5):380, 1994.

Nagi, S: Disability concepts revisited. In Pope, AM, and Tarlov, AR (eds): Disability in America: Toward a National Agenda for Prevention. National Academy Press, Washington, DC, 1991, p. 309.

World Health Organization (WHO): International Classification of Impairments, Disabilities, and Handicaps. World Health Organization, Geneva, 1980.

Chapter 9 Examination and Modification of the Environment

Thomas J. Schmitz, PT, PhD

LEARNING OBJECTIVES

1. Identify the role of the physical therapist in examination of the physical environment.
2. Understand the importance of environmental accessibility in optimizing patient function.
3. Identify common home, work life, and community environmental factors that affect patient function.
4. Describe strategies used to examine environmental impact on patient function.
5. Identify the general categories of tests and measures, tools used for gathering data, and data used in documenting examination of environmental factors.
6. Identify strategies to improve patient function through environmental modifications.
7. Describe the scope of adaptive equipment and assistive technology available for individuals with disability.
8. Recognize the importance of an examination of the environment within the context of a comprehensive rehabilitation plan of care.

CHAPTER OUTLINE

For individuals undergoing rehabilitation, addressing the environment in which he or she will live and function is an essential component of physical therapy intervention. A well-developed plan of care (POC) that achieves independence in all activities of daily living (ADL) for a full-time wheelchair user will fall short if entrance to the home is precluded by stairs or if the bathroom is inaccessible. As such, the patient's planned living environment warrants early and consistent consideration during the course of rehabilitation. For most patients, returning home and to a familiar community is a high priority. This is particularly true for elders who function better in familiar surroundings and have strong bonds to a cherished home associated with a lifetime of important events.

Disability or disease places new emotional, care-related, and financial demands on the family. While adjusting to these demands, the unexpected challenge of addressing needed modifications to a beloved home is often overwhelming. A critical role for the physical therapist in this area is that of advocate for the patient and family by providing the needed education, counsel, environmental analysis, and recommendations to assist with successful transition to the discharge setting. With collaborative input from other disciplines (e.g., occupational therapy, speech-language pathology) and knowledge of environmental barriers and their potential solution, availability of community resources, and needed assistive and/or adaptive equipment, as well as information about the patient's functional capabilities, cultural background, characteristics of the home environment, and financial resources, the physical therapist is in a unique position to guide the patient and family in optimizing accessibility. For most patients, the environmental examination extends beyond the home to the community and the availability of appropriate transportation; for others, it will include examination of the workplace, school, or higher education setting.

This chapter considers key environmental design concepts and common barriers impacting access. It addresses strategies to examine various aspects of the physical environment including the home, workplace, and community. Also included are approaches to modifying the environment to improve accessibility as well as legislation stipulating access requirements for public buildings and transportation.

PHYSICAL ENVIRONMENT

A variety of both built and natural objects comprise the *physical environment* in which an individual functions. Built objects refer to buildings and structures created by humans; natural objects include other humans, as well as geographical objects such as vegetation, mountains, rivers, uneven terrain, and so forth.[1] The environment encompasses a substantial range of components that affect human function and includes the individual's home, neighborhood, community, and method(s) of transportation, in addition to the individual's educational, workplace, entertainment, commercial, and natural settings.[2]

Barriers are environmental factors that, through their presence or absence, prevent optimal function and create disability.[3] Included among the identified risk factors for barriers encountered in routine daily environments is diminished access to home, school, work, or community.[3] *Accessibility* is the degree to which an environment affords use of its resources with respect to an individual's level of function. *Accessible design* typically refers to structures that meet prescribed standards for accessibility. In the United States, these standards are available from the American National Standard Institute,[4] the Fair Housing Amendments Act of 1988, and the Uniform Federal Accessibility Standards. Requirements for public and commercial buildings are regulated by the guidelines of the Americans with Disabilities Act (ADA) Standards for Accessible Design.[5] The World Health Organization's (WHO's) *International Classification of Functioning, Disability and Health* (ICF) recognizes disability and functioning as an outcome of the dynamic interaction between health conditions and contextual factors (environmental and personal). *Environmental factors* include the physical, social, and attitudinal environment in which the person lives and functions. Examples of *personal factors* include sex, age, coping styles, and other characteristics that may influence how an individual experiences disability.[6] The ICF is discussed in Chapter 1.

UNIVERSAL DESIGN

Universal design (UD) refers to the design of environments and products that can be used by all people to the greatest extent possible regardless of age, ability, or disability. This design concept emphasizes social inclusion by creating products and environments that are usable by a wide range of individuals of different ages, statures, sizes, and abilities, and it addresses the changing needs of human beings across the life span. Other terms associated with this design concept include *inclusive design, accessible design, life span design, aging-in-place design,* and *sustainable design.*

Universal design has been identified as an outgrowth of the disability rights movement in the 1960s, although some earlier recognition of the concepts has been identified. Its foundational elements of ensuring equal opportunity and eliminating discrimination based on disability has been embraced in many parts of the world.[7,8] The design principles provide a human-centered framework for creating spaces, furniture, landscapes, products, and services that can seamlessly accommodate diverse ability levels across generations.[9]

Evidence-based design (EBD) supports and informs UD. EBD is defined by the Center for Health Design "as the process of basing decisions about the built environment on credible research to achieve the best possible outcomes."[10, p. 2] It emphasizes use of research to influence the design process and evaluate design innovations. Traditionally associated with health care architecture, EBD now supports design decisions for many structures in the built environment, including schools, office spaces, performance centers, restaurants, museums, and prisons.[11]

Although UD is both accessible and free of barriers, it is not the same as bringing existing buildings or structures into compliance with the ADA Standards for Accessible Design[5] or other building codes or laws. Applying such standards to existing structures often results in important but selective accessibility. In contrast, UD is applied from the *inception* of a building design plan (new construction) versus eliminating barriers in existing structures. For example, the need to retrofit an existing structure with a ramp or accessible bathrooms would not be needed had the original design plan considered the needs of all users.

Incorporated into initial planning, UD elements are essentially "invisible" as compared to adaptations or add-ons made to existing structures. They apply to all features and spaces of a dwelling. Several examples of UD elements include stepless entrances, wide hallways and doorways, level transitions between rooms (no doorway thresholds), use of nonslip floors, lever door handles, rocker light switches, single-handle sink faucets, and no-step shower access. Reinforced walls capable of supporting handrails or grab bars and large closets aligned from floor-to-floor suitable for housing a residential elevator are examples of UD elements intended to meet the future needs of residents.

Principles of Universal Design

The Principles of Universal Design (Appendix 9.A) were developed at the Center for Universal Design (CUD) at North Carolina State University by a group of experts that included architects, product designers, engineers, and environmental design researchers. The principles provide guidance for the design of products and environments. They are also intended to educate designers and consumers about characteristics that increase usability for everyone.[12] Key elements of the principles include the following:

- *Equitable use.* The design is useful and marketable to people with diverse abilities.
- *Flexibility in use.* The design accommodates a wide range of individual preferences and abilities.
- *Simple and intuitive.* Use of the design is easy to understand, regardless of the user's experience, knowledge, language skills, or current concentration level.
- *Perceptible information.* The design communicates necessary information effectively to the user, regardless of ambient conditions or the user's sensory abilities.
- *Tolerance for error.* The design minimizes hazards and the adverse consequences of accidental or unintended actions.
- *Low physical effort.* The design can be used efficiently, comfortably, and with a minimum of fatigue.
- *Size and space for approach and use.* Appropriate size and space is provided for approach, reach, manipulation, and use regardless of the user's body size, posture, or mobility.

DISABILITY ACCESS SYMBOLS

Reflective of the importance of *environmental accessibility*, an internationally recognized *wheelchair symbol* identifies buildings accessible to individuals with a disability. The Rehabilitation Act of 1973 (Sections 503 and 504) requires that all organizations receiving federal funding provide accessible programs and activities. The Americans with Disabilities Act (1990) expanded accessibility to the private sector to improve employment opportunities, as well as environmental access to retail businesses, cultural events, movie theaters, restaurants, travel, and so forth. Other access symbols identify the availability of assistive listening devices, telephones with interactive text capabilities (TTY), which allow the user to communicate using a keyboard and visual display, volume-controlled telephones, availability of sign language interpretation, and so forth. The Disability Access Symbols are presented in Figure 9.1. These symbols are prominently displayed to identify and make public the availability of accessible services.

PURPOSE OF EXAMINATION

A primary outcome of rehabilitation is for the patient to be fully functional in a former environment and lifestyle. To achieve this outcome, continuity of accessibility must exist within the individual's environmental context. With full accessibility as a goal, examination of the environment addresses the *patient–environment relationship* relative to accessibility, safety, usability, and function. The purposes of an environmental examination are multiple and serve to:

1. Determine the degree of patient safety and level of function in the physical environment.
2. Identify barriers that may affect usability or compromise performance of customary tasks or activities.
3. Make realistic recommendations regarding accessibility, barriers, modifications, and safety to the patient and family as needed, to the employer, to government agencies or other potential funding sources, and to third-party payers.
4. Determine the need for adaptive equipment or assistive technology to support and promote function.
5. Assist in preparing the patient and family for the patient's return to a former environment and to help determine whether further services may be required (e.g., outpatient treatment, home care services, and so forth).

EXAMINATION STRATEGIES

Physical therapists use a variety of tests and measures to examine physical impediments (e.g., safety hazards, access problems, design barriers) affecting the patient–environment relationship. The data generated are used to recommend modifications to the environment, guide selection of adaptive equipment and assistive technology, and/or propose alternative approaches to performing a task or activity (e.g., improve safety, conserve energy) to promote optimum function. The *Guide to Physical Therapist Practice 3.0*[3] includes Environmental Factors among test and measure categories used by physical therapists. Table 9.1 presents examples of the tests and measures used, data-gathering tools, and types of data generated.

Depending on the nature of the patient's disability, data collection tools used for examination of the environmental may include (1) interviews, (2) self-reports (checklists, questionnaires) and performance-based measures (observation) of function, (3) measures of environmental impact on function, (4) visual depictions (photographs, video recordings) and dimensions of physical space (structural specifications), (5) viewing the environment from a remote site, and (6) on-site visits.

A combination of two or more of these strategies may be warranted to generate all needed data. Cost containment has placed restrictions on time and travel allocations for on-site visits. In such situations, several data collection alternatives (e.g., interview, self-report, performance-based measures and simulations, use of photographs and/or diagrams [floor plan with dimensions] of the physical space) can be implemented to achieve the goals of the environmental examination.

Telehealth (telecommunication technology) offers considerable potential to view an environment at a remote

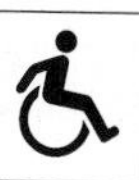

Symbol for Accessibility

The wheelchair symbol should only be used to indicate access for individuals with limited mobility including wheelchair users. For example, the symbol is used to indicate an accessible entrance, bathroom or that a phone is lowered for wheelchair users. Remember that a ramped entrance is not completely accessible if there are no curb cuts, and an elevator is not accessible if it can only be reached via steps.

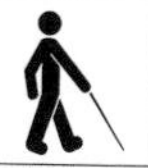

Access (Other Than Print or Braille) for Individuals Who Are Blind or Have Low Vision

This symbol may be used to indicate access for people who are blind or have low vision, including: a guided tour, a path to a nature trail or a scent garden in a park; and a tactile tour or a museum exhibition that may be touched.

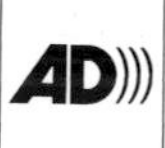

Audio Description

A service for persons who are blind or have low vision that makes the performing arts, visual arts, television, video, and film more accessible. Description of visual elements is provided by a trained Audio Describer through the Secondary Audio Program (SAP) of televisions and monitors equipped with stereo sound. An adapter for non-stereo TVs is available through the American Foundation for the Blind, (800) 829-0500. For live Audio Description, a trained Audio Describer offers live commentary or narration (via headphones and a small transmitter) consisting of concise, objective descriptions of visual elements (e.g., a theater performance or a visual arts exhibition).

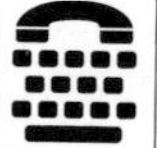

Telephone Typewriter (TTY)

This device is also known as a text telephone (TT), or telecommunications device for the deaf (TDD). TTY indicates a device used with the telephone for communication with and between deaf, hard of hearing, speech impaired and/or hearing persons.

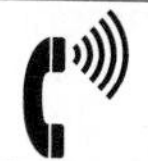

Volume Control Telephone

This symbol indicates the location of telephones that have handsets with amplified sound and/or adjustable volume controls.

Assistive Listening Systems

These systems transmit amplified sound via hearing aids, headsets or other devices. They include infrared, loop and FM systems. Portable systems may be available from the same audiovisual equipment suppliers that service conferences and meetings.

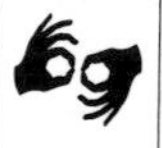

Sign Language Interpretation

The symbol indicates that Sign Language Interpretation is provided for a lecture, tour, film, performance, conference or other program.

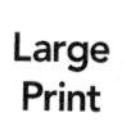

Accessible Print (18 pt. or Larger)

The symbol for large print is "Large Print" printed in 18 pt. or larger text. In addition to indicating that large print versions of books, pamphlets, museum guides and theater programs are available, you may use the symbol on conference or membership forms to indicate that print materials may be provided in large print. Sans serif or modified serif print with good contrast is important, and special attention should be paid to letter and word spacing.

The Information Symbol

The most valuable commodity of today's society is information; to a person with a disability it is essential. For example, the symbol may be used on signage or on a floor plan to indicate the location of the information or security desk, where there is more specific information or materials concerning access accommodations and services such as "LARGE PRINT" materials, audio cassette recordings of materials, or sign interpreted tours.

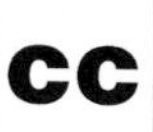

Closed Captioning (CC)

This symbol indicates a choice for whether or not to display captions for a television program or videotape. TV sets that have a built-in or a separate decoder are equipped to display dialogue for programs that are captioned when selected by the viewer. The Television Decoder Circuitry Act of 1990 requires TV sets (with screens 13" or larger) to have built-in decoders as of July, 1993. Also, videos that are part of exhibitions may be closed captioned using the symbol with instruction to press a button for captioning.

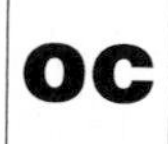

Opened Captioning (OC)

This symbol indicates that captions, which translate dialogue and other sounds in print, are always displayed on the videotape, movie or television program. Open Captioning is preferred by many including deaf and hard-of-hearing individuals, and people whose second language is English. In addition, it is helpful in teaching children how to read and in keeping sound levels to a minimum in museums and restaurants.

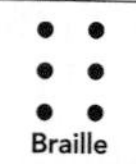

Braille Symbol

This symbol indicates that printed material is available in Braille, including exhibition labeling, publications, and signage.

The Disability Access Symbols were produced by the Graphic Artists Guild Foundation with support and technical assistance from the Office for Special Constituencies, National Endowment for the Arts. Special thanks to the National Endowment for the Arts. Graphic design assistance by the Society of Environmental Graphic Design. Consultant: Jacqueline Ann Clipsham, with permission.

Figure 9.1 Disability access symbols.

site using a voice-over-Internet protocol service and software application (e.g., Skype, Linphone) or other videoconferencing protocol. A large and expanding body of literature addresses the extensive application of telehealth in providing health care services,[13-23] including physical therapy.[24-29] In a document titled *Telehealth—Definitions and Guidelines,* the Board of Directors of the American Physical Therapy Association (APTA) defines telehealth as "the use of electronic communications to provide and deliver a host of health-related information and health care services, including, but not limited to, physical therapy–related information and services, over large and small

Table 9.1 Examination of the Environment: Examples of Tests and Measures, Data-Gathering Tools, and Data Used in Documentation.

The physical therapist uses tests and measures to determine whether the individual's environment is adequate to enable optimal participation in his or her various roles. Responses monitored at rest, during activity, and after activity may indicate the presence or severity of an impairment, activity limitation, or participation restriction.

Tests and Measures	Data-Gathering Tools	Documentation
Assistive technology needs (e.g., observations, questionnaires, videographic assessments) Caregiver capacity (e.g., assessment of caregiver and caregiver resources) Current and potential barriers (e.g., checklists, interviews, observations, questionnaires, safety assessment) Physical space and environments routinely encountered (e.g., accessibility survey, observations, photographic assessments, questionnaires, videographic assessments) Quality of life (e.g., scales, surveys)	Cameras and photographs Equipment trial and simulation Structural specifications (e.g., blueprints or building plans) Tape measures Universal design criteria Video cameras and video recordings	Clinical rationale to justify need for appropriate assistive technology or reasonable accommodations Description of environmental factors that create barriers to activity and participation (e.g., lack of access to workplace due to long distance from parking area to main entrance) Description of features of home, work, school, or community physical environments Descriptions of physical space, including doorway widths, floor surfaces, distances of required travel, maneuvering space, and accessibility of bathrooms Level of compliance with regulatory standards (e.g., compliance of public buildings with Americans with Disabilities Act)

From *Guide to Physical Therapist Practice 3.0*,[3] with permission. APTA is not responsible for the translation from English.

distances. Telehealth encompasses a variety of health care and health promotion activities, including, but not limited to, education, advice, reminders, interventions, and monitoring of interventions."[30, p. 1]

Sanford et al[31] reported on an early application of telehealth to examination of the home environment. The authors compared data from an actual on-site home examination with those obtained from remote videoconferencing technology. The data suggested that videoconferencing has the potential for enabling therapists to examine the patient's environment regardless of distance or location. The data from the remote examination identified 51 of the 59 problems (86.4%) documented from the on-site visit and 54 of the 60 quantitative measures (90%) obtained from the on-site visit.

Interview

Exploration of the environment is typically initiated by interviewing the patient and family. If the patient's impairments and activity limitations affect only isolated tasks or activities or if accessibility issues involve limited physical environmental factors, an interview may be all that is needed to identify the barriers and provide recommendations and suggestions to improve performance and resolve access problems. In the presence of more formidable disability, the interview may be the first of several strategies used to collect data about the patient's environment. The interview can be used to establish the general characteristics of the environment (number of levels, stairs, railings, and so forth), identify any special problems previously encountered by the patient, alert the therapist to potential safety hazards, and determine the need for further tests and measures to obtain essential information. The interview process also provides the therapist an opportunity to gain knowledge of family/caregiver characteristics, including (1) attitude toward the patient; (2) the extent of their desire to have the patient return to his or her environment; (3) their caregiving goals and capabilities; and (4) attitude toward rehabilitation team members, which may influence receptivity to suggested environmental modifications.

Self-Report and Performance-Based Measures of Function

Self-reports involve asking the patient to provide information about the ability to perform certain tasks and activities in specific environments (see Appendix 9.B). Administration can be either in a paper-and-pencil format or by way of an interview conducted by the therapist. An inherent shortcoming of self-report instruments is that an individual may overestimate performance capabilities or underestimate the impact of barriers. Accuracy of reporting can be improved by requesting that the patient (1) focus the performance information on a recent time interval (e.g., *within* the previous week) and (2) distinguish between actual performance of an activity (e.g., *daily* use of shower for bathing) versus perceived ability in the absence of consistent execution of the task.

Performance-based measures address classification of functional abilities and identification of activity limitations and participation restrictions. The therapist administers these measures while observing patient performance of an activity. A variety of instruments are available that include quantitative scoring systems. Examples of instruments used to examine balance, mobility, and fall risk include the *Functional Reach* (FR) *Test*[32-34] and *Multidirectional Reach Test* (MDFR),[35,36] *Timed Up and Go* (TUG) *Test*,[37] *Performance-Oriented Mobility Assessment* (POMA),[38-40] and the *Berg Balance Scale* (BBS).[41-44] These tests are presented in Chapter 6, Examination of Coordination and Balance (see also Table 6.7). Interpretation of results is typically guided by comparison to normative data. These measures yield important information about the impact of impairments on function and help predict patient performance within his or her natural environment. Performance-based tests and self-reports of function are discussed in Chapter 8, Examination of Function.

Environmental Factors Outcome Measures

The environment directly affects the ability to perform tasks and activities that support physical, social, and psychological well-being. Environmental factors can either *constrain* or *promote* patients' abilities to perform customary actions within their social/cultural contexts. A variety of instruments have been developed that address the impact of environmental determinants on function and participation. Table 9.2 includes examples

Table 9.2 Outcome Measures: Examination of Environmental Factors

OUTCOME MEASURE and ICF Category	DESCRIPTION	SCORING	MDC and MCID
Home and Community Environment (HACE)[45] ICF: 3	Examines environmental barriers and facilitators in the following domains: home and community mobility, basic mobility and communication devices, transportation factors, and attitudes.	Self-report instrument used to identify features of the home or community that may affect community participation. Instrument available in the work of Keysor, et al[46] and online.[47]	**NA**
Craig Handicap Assessment and Reporting Technique (CHART)[48] ICF: 2, 3	Designed to examine an individual's function within his or her societal context using six domains of function: physical independence, cognitive independence, mobility, occupation, social integration, and economic self-sufficiency.	Each area is scored based on a range of 0–100 points (600 points maximum) with greater levels of participation receiving higher scores. The CHART Short Form (CHART-SF)[49,50] is a 19-item shortened version of the CHART. Available online.[51]	**NA**
Craig Hospital Inventory of Environmental Factors (CHIEF)[52,53] ICF: 3	Rates frequency and impact of 25 items across 5 domains that prevent functioning within the home and community; also includes social, attitudinal, and policy barriers; response items carry numeric values. A CHIEF short form (CHIEF-SF) contains 12 items from the original inventory.[54]	Scores calculated by multiplying frequency of occurrence (0 = never to 4 = daily) by magnitude (big problem = 2 or little problem = 1) to provide an *impact score*. Higher scores indicate greater impact of environmental factors. Available online.[55]	**NA**
***Facilitator and Barriers Survey* of environmental influences on participation among people with lower limb *Mobility* impairments and limitations (FABS/M)**[56] ICF: 2, 3	Self-report examining environmental facilitators and barriers to participation for individuals with mobility impairments; includes 61 questions, 133 items.	Scores based on frequency of encounter and magnitude of impact on participation within six domains: mobility device, built features of homes, built/natural features in community, community destination access, community facilities access, and community support network. Available in the work of Gray et al.[56]	**NA**

ICF CATEGORY: 1 = Body Structure/Function, 2 = Activity, 3 = Participation
MCID = Minimal clinically important difference
MDC = Minimal detectable change
NA = Not available (not established)

of outcome measures designed to examine environmental factors.[45-56] Additional sources of outcome measures include the Academy of Neurologic Physical Therapy EDGE Taskforce Outcome Measures Recommendations (www.neuropt.org) and the Rehabilitation Measures Database (www.rehabmeasures.org/default.aspx).

Description of Physical Environment

The therapist may request that family members provide a description of the physical environment. This can effectively be accomplished via visual depictions (e.g., streaming video using a computer, smartphone, or tablet, photographs, videotapes, diagrams, floor plans) in combination with actual dimensions (structural specifications obtained with a tape measure) of the setting in which the patient is expected to function.

Suggestions for modifications can be made from the visual representations and measured dimensions of the patient's environment. Such environmental information will allow the therapist to simulate aspects of the patient's surroundings (before discharge) for practicing tasks while directing attention to maximizing safety and function. This will also assist the therapist to determine the need for assistive or adaptive equipment.

On-Site Visits

On-site visits require that one or more rehabilitation team members together with the patient travel to the physical location where the patient will be required to function (home, community, and/or work or school). A major advantage of the on-site visit is that it allows observation of performance in the actual environment in which the activities must be accomplished. On-site visits are often useful in reducing patient, family, caregiver, and/or employer apprehension concerning the patient's ability to function within the environment. The on-site visit also provides an important opportunity for the therapist to identify safety hazards and make recommendations regarding specific environmental barriers. During the visit, patient activity should be interspersed with adequate rest intervals to ensure that fatigue is not an influencing factor.

Whichever examination strategy or combination of strategies are applied, the scope and breadth of the information gathered will be enhanced by involvement of patient and family members. Because it is usually not feasible for the therapist to examine all aspects of the patient's total environment, involvement of other individuals can be instrumental in ensuring that the goal of maximum accessibility, function, and participation is met. This is particularly important for addressing community access. The therapist can direct and guide an investigation of community recreational, educational, and commercial facilities, as well as availability of public transportation. Guidance can also be provided in the essential role of exploring funding sources for needed modifications (potential funding sources are addressed later in this chapter).

Data from an examination of the environment are used to evaluate the need for specific recommendations and interventions. Corcoran and Gitlin[1] identify five major areas of intervention strategies: (1) *assistive* or *adaptive devices* such as grab bars, long-handled reachers, adapted eating utensils (e.g., rocker knife), canes, or walkers; (2) *safety devices,* such as lighting, smoke detectors, or sensing devices; (3) *structural alterations,* which include widening doors, installing railings or ramps, or removing a doorway threshold; (4) *modification* or *altered location of environmental objects,* such as disabling a stove, using extension levers on door handles, removing throw rugs, or moving furniture; and (5) *task modification,* such as use of visual, auditory, or other sensory cueing, work simplification, and energy conservation or joint preservation techniques.

The following sections offer suggestions for examination and modification of the home and workplace environment. The information presented is neither exhaustive nor inclusive of the needs of every patient. The environmental considerations are intended to direct attention to some of the more common access, usability, and safety concerns.

■ EXAMINATION OF THE HOME

Preparation for On-Site Visit

Before an on-site visit to the patient's home, occupational and physical therapy treatment sessions should be scheduled that will include participation from family and caregivers. These visits serve several functions. They provide an opportunity to become familiar with the patient's capabilities and activity limitations. They give the family/caregivers time to learn safe methods (e.g., proper body mechanics, guarding techniques) for assisting with locomotion, transfers, exercise, and/or functional activities. During these sessions, the occupational and physical therapists will have an opportunity to provide instruction in the use of assistive devices, adaptive equipment, and/or assistive technology. The time spent in family and caregiver education is often pivotal in facilitating the patient's successful return to the home, community, and/or work or school environments.

Clinical Note: Although often restricted by reimbursement issues, when feasible, a day or weekend patient visit to his or her home should be encouraged and arranged before the on-site visit. An advantage of such visits is that problems not previously anticipated by the therapist, patient, or family may be uncovered. Following the visit, the patient's immediate assessment of his or her ability to function within the environment should be obtained. This can be accomplished using a self-report instrument designed to gather perceptions about environment features that either constrain or promote activity performance (see Appendix 9.B). Emphasis can then be placed on initial development of a plan to resolve identified problems before the on-site visit and the patient's actual return to the environment.

Preceding the on-site visit, information should be gathered about several important areas that will influence both the preparation for and the types of recommendations made during the visit. This information includes the following:

- Information about the patient's present level of function (e.g., communication skills, bed mobility, transfers, locomotion, and so forth); data should be gathered from all involved disciplines (occupational therapist, physical therapist, speech-language pathologist, and so forth).
- Knowledge of physical assistance or verbal cueing required for performance of functional activities.
- Characteristics and dimensions of required adaptive or assistive devices and equipment (e.g., walker, crutches, raised toilet seat, commode, hospital bed).
- Information about predicted level of function or improvement (expected outcomes).
- Nature of the activity limitations or participation restrictions (i.e., static or progressive).
- Insurance coverage, financial resources, and availability of potential funding sources (in terms of capacity to modify environment or obtain needed adaptive and assistive devices or assistive technology).
- Knowledge of the patient's future plans (household management, family care, employment outside the home, school, vocational training, and so forth).
- Knowledge of whether the house or apartment is owned or rented; the type and ownership of the home can affect or even preclude the type of modifications the patient may require. However, it should be noted that the Fair Housing Act requires landlords to allow individuals with disabilities to make reasonable access modifications to both personal living space and common space such as entryways.
- Information about the relative permanence of the dwelling; if the patient has plans to move in the near future, it will influence the type of modifications recommended (e.g., installing permanent ramps versus removable ones or paving a gravel driveway).

This information can be obtained from a variety of sources, including the patient, rehabilitation team conferences, patient/family and caregiver conferences or interviews, health record documentation from all disciplines involved, and social service interviews. Once this information is gathered, decisions can be made concerning what adaptive or assistive devices will be needed and the appropriate team members to accompany the patient on the visit.

Clinical Note: Although social workers are key members of the team throughout the rehabilitation process, they play a particularly important role in planning for transition to home and community. Discharge plans are enhanced and facilitated by the social worker's collaborative role as patient advocate and knowledge of community resources such as referral sources (home care, medical follow-up, legal assistance), accessible housing, available transportation, and potential financial assistance or funding resources.

Ideally, given their complementary expertise and skills, both the physical and occupational therapist accompany the patient on the home visit. They assume shared responsibility for examining the patient–environment interface. Depending on the specific needs of the patient and family, a speech-language pathologist, social worker, or nurse also may be among the rehabilitation team members visiting the home. For purposes of organization and structure, home visits are often divided into two global elements: (1) accessibility of the dwelling's *exterior* and (2) examination of the home's *interior*. Photographs are useful for providing images of environmental factors posing barriers to accompany letters of justification for needed modifications. A tape measure and home examination form are also important tools during the visit. Many rehabilitation departments develop their own home examination forms to meet the particular needs of their patient population. The forms (or checklists) help to organize the visit and are useful in directing attention to all necessary details. An example of a Home Examination Form is provided in Appendix 9.C. This form can be expanded or modified, depending on the specific needs of the individual or patient population. Some caution must be used in interpreting data from home examination forms that have not been standardized or examined for reliability.

On-Site Visit

On arrival at the home for the on-site visit, the patient may need to rest for a short while before beginning the home examination. This is an important consideration, because patients may become very excited or emotional when returning to a home environment after a lengthy absence. This may be true even if a day or weekend visit occurred before the formal home visit.

One method of gathering data about the interior of the home is to begin with the patient in bed as though it were morning. Simulation of all daily tasks and activities, including dressing, grooming, bathroom activities, and preparation of meals, can ensue. The patient should attempt to perform all transfer, exercise, locomotion, self-care, and homemaking activities as independently as possible. This will provide an additional opportunity to teach the family and caregivers how and when to assist the patient.

Exterior Accessibility

Route of Entry

1. If there is more than one entry to the dwelling, the most accessible should be selected (closest to driveway, most level walking surface, fewest stairs, available handrails, and so forth).
2. Ideally, the driveway should be a smooth, level surface with easy access to the home. Walking surfaces to the entrance should be carefully examined. Cracked and uneven surfaces should be repaired or an alternate route selected.
3. The route to entrance should be level and well lit and provide adequate cover from adverse weather conditions. Package shelves near the entrance are useful for freeing hands to unlock and/or open doors.
4. The height, number, and condition of stairs should be noted. Ideally, steps should not be greater than 7 in. (180 mm) high with a minimum depth of 11 in. (280 mm).[4] *Nosings,* also referred to as "lips," are the 0.5 in. (13 mm) curved overhangs on the front edge of stairs. These overhangs are often problematic because they can cause a patient's toe to catch and prevent smooth transition to the next step. Nosings should be removed or reduced, if possible. Installing small wood bevels under the overhangs that taper down toward the lower step and provide a smoother contour can minimize nosing (Fig. 9.2A). The steps also should have a nonslip surface to improve traction. This can be accomplished by adding abrasive strips (Fig. 9.2B).
5. Handrails should be installed, if needed. In general, handrail height should measure between a minimum of 34 in. (865 mm) and a maximum of 38 in. (965 mm) high for stairs (Fig. 9.3A), ramps, and level walking surfaces. This range in handrail height allows for modifications to accommodate needs of particularly tall or short individuals. At least one handrail should extend a minimum of 12 in. (305 mm) beyond the foot and top of the stairs (Fig. 9.3B). Outside, cross-sectional diameter of circular handrails should be between a minimum of 1.25 in. (32 mm) and a maximum of 2 in. (51 mm). If mounted adjacent to a wall, clearance between the handrail and wall should be a minimum of 1.5 in. (38 mm).[4,5]
6. Installation of a ramp requires adequate space. Materials used to construct large ramps include durable steel, wood, wood alternative composite decking materials (combination of wood and plastic), and concrete; smaller ramps can be made from aluminum or fiberglass. The minimum ramp grade (incline or slope) for a wheelchair ramp is that for every inch of threshold height there is a corresponding 12 in. (305 mm) of ramp length (a running slope of 1:12).[4] Outdoor ramps exposed to inclement weather such as snow or ice formation require a more gradual running slope of approximately 1:20. Ramps should be a minimum of 36 in. (915 mm) wide, with a nonslip surface. The overall rise of any ramp should be no greater than 30 in. (760 mm). Handrails also should be included on the ramp with a minimum height of 34 in. (865 mm) and a maximum height of 38 in. (965 mm) and extend 12 in. (305 mm) beyond the top and bottom of the ramp (Fig. 9.3C).[4,5] Small, commercially available ramps can be used for traversing curbs and small step heights.
7. Vertical platform lifts and stairway lifts are commercially available and may be a consideration when inadequate space is available for a ramp. *Vertical platform lifts* (Fig. 9.4) travel approximately 8 ft (243.84 cm) straight up and down. Both open and enclosed models are available. Platform lifts are often installed adjacent to stairs with an upper landing and are available in a variety of dimensions, with lengths ranging from 54 to 60 in. (137.16 to 152.4 cm) and widths ranging from 34 to 42 in. (86.36 to 106.68 cm). The lift brings the wheelchair user from the ground level to the landing level to access the entrance to the home (these lifts can be used indoors as well). *Stairway lifts* are installed directly onto existing outdoor stairways; however, they are more frequently used indoors. The stairway lifts are mounted on runners that traverse the length of the stairs and slightly beyond. Many models allow the platform to fold up against an adjacent wall to allow free stair access for others entering the home (see below Interior Accessibility: General Considerations, *Stairs*).

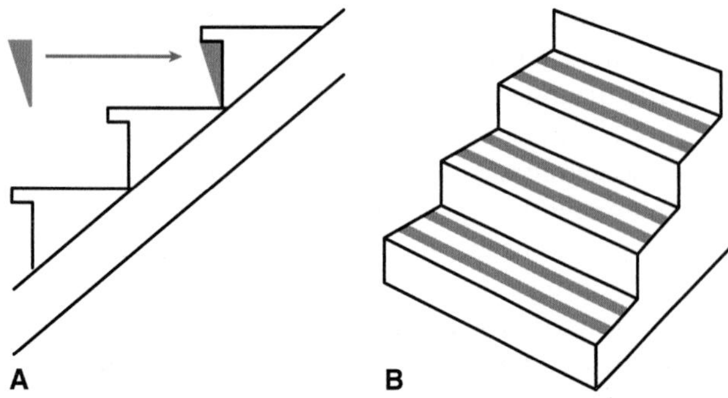

Figure 9.2 (A) Wood bevels placed under nosings minimize the danger of "toe-catching" during transition to the next step. (B) Abrasive strips of a contrasting color improve traction and depth perception.

Entrance

1. For individuals using a wheelchair, the entrance should have a platform large enough to allow the patient to rest and to prepare for entry. This platform area is particularly important when a ramp is

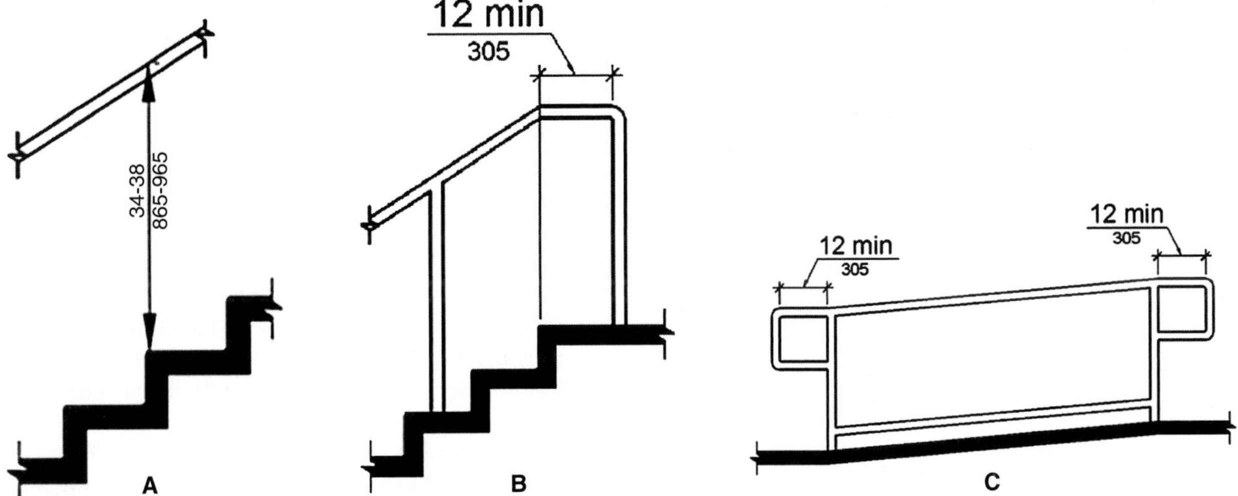

Figure 9.3 (A) Handrail height for stairs. (B) Handrail extension at top of stairs. A similar handrail extension of 12 in. (305 mm) is placed at bottom of stairs; (C) Handrail extensions should run a minimum of 12 in. (305 mm) beyond the top and bottom edge of ramp. *(From 2010 ADA Standards for Accessible Design[5] [A, p. 154; B, p. 157; C, p. 175].)*

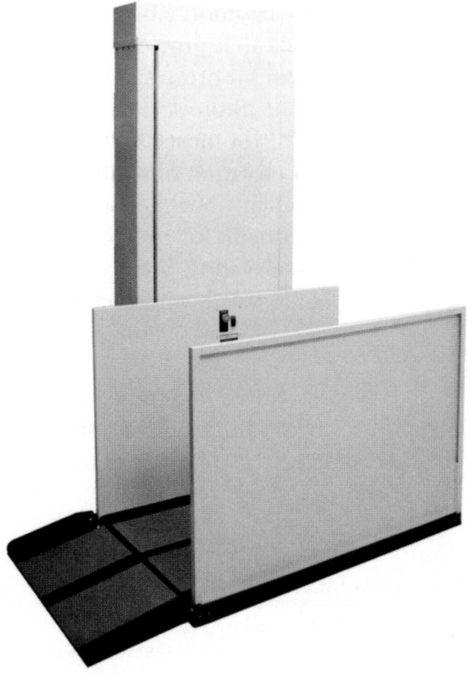

Figure 9.4 Powered residential vertical lift. This lift has a 600-lb weight capacity. The platform measures approximately 36 in. wide and 48 in. deep (91.44 × 121.92 cm). *(Courtesy of AmeriGlide, Inc., Raleigh, NC 27610.)*

in use. It provides for safe transit from the inclined surface to the level surface. If an individual using a wheelchair is required to open a door that swings out, this area should be at least 5 × 5 ft (153 × 153 cm). If the door swings in and away from the patient, a space at least 3 ft (91.5 cm) deep and 5 ft (153 cm) wide is required.

2. The door locks should be accessible to the patient. The height of the locks should be determined, as well as the amount of force required to turn the key. Alternative lock systems (e.g., voice- or card-activated locks, remote control locks, keypad electronic security systems, push-button padlocks) may be an important consideration for some patients. Particular attention should be directed toward ensuring that the locking mechanism on the door is sufficiently illuminated.
3. The door handle should be turned easily by the patient. Rubber doorknob covers (that stretch over a round doorknob and provide a textured grip) or lever-type handles are often easier to use for patients with limited grip strength. Lever handles do not require the same strength or range of motion (ROM) needed for traditional round doorknobs.[7]
4. The door should open and close in a direction that is functional for the patient. A long canvas "door strap" may be attached to the outside of the door (or around the door handle) to help an individual using a wheelchair close the door when leaving. A long, sturdy belt can also be used as a door strap.
5. Remote control automatic door openers are available that attach to existing doors that can open, close, and lock the door; some are equipped with customized "stay-open" features to accommodate the time required to enter or exit. A handheld remote control or a touch pad can be used to activate these devices.
6. Installation of an intercom system allows the patient to see and/or hear who is at the door. Many allow remote control opening of a door from any location in the home.

7. If there is a raised threshold in the doorway, it should be removed. If removal is not possible, the threshold should be lowered to no greater than 1/2 in. (13 mm) in height, with beveled edges;[4] alternatively, a threshold ramp may be installed (see Interior Accessibility: General Considerations, *Doors*). If needed, weather-stripping the door will help prevent drafts.
8. The doorway width should be measured. Generally, 32 to 34 in. (81 to 86 cm) is an acceptable doorway width to accommodate most wheelchairs. Bariatric chairs require increased width.
9. If the door is weighted to aid in closing, the pressure should not exceed 8 lb (3.6 kg) to be functional for the patient.
10. A kick plate (metal guard) may be added to doors frequently entered by individuals using a wheelchair or ambulatory assistive devices. The kick plate should measure 12 in. (30 cm) in height from the bottom of the door.

Clinical Note: Several distinct considerations are required to address the environmental needs of patients who are overweight or obese, generally defined and classified using body mass index (BMI)[57] (Table 9.3). Data from the most recent National Health and Nutrition Examination Survey indicated that greater than one-third of adults and almost 17% of youth were obese.[58] An overview of the unique environmental needs of this population are presented in Box 9.1.

Interior Accessibility: General Considerations

Furniture Arrangement and Features

1. Sufficient room should be made available for maneuvering a wheelchair or ambulating with an assistive device. An initial strategy is to move as much furniture as possible against the walls to increase clearance and stability (i.e., prevent sliding of furniture during movement transitions). Further stability can be achieved by placing rubber cups (floor guards) under the legs of sofas and chairs. Items such as coffee tables, footstools, or electrical wires should not obstruct access to furniture.
2. Clear passage must be allowed from one room to the next.
3. Typically, overstuffed sofas and chairs do not provide the needed support for sit-to-stand movement transitions. Although generally not the case, ideally living room chairs should have double armrests, a firm seating surface, and an upright back. Sometimes a suitable chair can be found in a different location within the home and moved to the living room. Another option is to modify the current furniture by placing a fitted wooden board under the seat cushion and behind the seat back (if removable). If a new chair is to be purchased, recommended features of the chair should be provided to the patient and family (e.g., the height of the seat should allow the knees to flex approximately 90° with the feet flat on the floor, a firm cushioned seat, a firm cushioned back that provides adequate upright support, and double armrests).
4. Use of any unstable furniture such as rocking chairs should be discouraged for most patients. Chairs that provide mechanized elevation of the back of the seat are commercially available but should be used with caution. It may be difficult for a patient to stabilize the feet as the seat is elevating. This causes the feet (and pelvis) to slide forward, with potential for a fall.

Electrical Controls

1. Unrestricted access should be provided to wall switches and electrical outlets. Power strips (surge protectors) can be used to increase the number of

Table 9.3 Classification of Overweight and Obesity by BMI, Waist Circumference, and Associated Disease Risks

			Disease Risk* Relative to Normal Weight and Waist Circumference	
	BMI (kg/m²)	Obesity Class	Men 102 cm (40 in.) or less Women 88 cm (35 in.) or less	Men > 102 cm (40 in.) Women > 88 cm (35 in.)
Underweight	< 18.5		-	-
Normal	18.5–24.9		-	-
Overweight	25–29.9		Increased	High
Obesity	30–34.9	I	High	Very High
	35–39.9	II	Very High	Very High
Extreme Obesity	40+	III	Extremely High	Extremely High

* Disease risk for type 2 diabetes, hypertension, and CVD.
\+ Increased waist circumference also can be a marker for increased risk, even in persons of normal weight.
From *National Institutes of Health*.[57]

Box 9.1 Bariatric Considerations

Patients who are obese often require specialized equipment for being lifted, moved, transferred, or transported. Bariatric equipment is space consuming; this is often exacerbated by older homes designed and built when the statistical averages for adult height and weight were less than today. The following are environmental considerations specific to this population.

- ***Patient, Family, and Caregiver Training:*** Specific training in the use of bariatric equipment and patient handling is critical. Patients who are obese often require assistance throughout the day for many routine activities (e.g., positional changes, supine-to-sit, sit-to-stand, bathing, toileting, and dressing). These care requirements emphasize the need for highly trained caregivers able to promote safety and injury prevention for both patient and themselves. When possible, the patient should be encouraged to assume the lead in directing those responsible for care.
- ***Physical Assistance:*** More than one individual may be required to assist the patient. There may be situations where as many as three or four people are needed for patient handling. Third-party payers challenge reimbursement for more than one support person in the home simultaneously (duplication of services). This may require involvement from extended family members and/or require the patient and family to seek creative funding sources to meet this need (see section titled "Funding Sources").
- ***Bariatric Equipment:*** Inherent to its purpose, bariatric equipment is oversized, is designed for increased weight capacity, and is generally heavier and costlier than its standard adult equivalent. Bariatric equipment is extensive and includes beds (some with built-in scales), bariatric mattresses with high weight capacities, bedside commodes, standard and overhead lifts, reclining chairs, steel-framed chairs, powered lift chairs with a 1,000-lb (453.59-kg) weight capacity, bathroom equipment, adaptive equipment, wheelchairs (widths up to 48 in. [121.92 cm]), scooters, and ambulatory assistive devices. Providers of durable medical equipment typically offer patient, family, and caregiver in-home instruction. Some provide ongoing support should additional caregivers require training.
- ***Risk of Ulceration:*** Patients who are obese are at increased risk for developing pressure ulcers secondary to their size and immobility. They may be unable to effectively change positions, creating excess pressure on susceptible areas for long periods. This may require use of a specialized mattress (e.g., low air loss with alternating pressure). Moisture or perspiration may contribute to ulcer formation.
- ***Care Environment:*** Large beds (e.g., 42 to 54 in. [106.68 to 137.16 cm] wide, 80 to 90 in. [203.2 to 228.6 cm] long, and up to 1,000-lb [453.59-kg] weight capacity), lifts, and other large bariatric equipment require larger room dimensions. Passage of bariatric equipment generally requires a door width of 60 in. (152.4 cm). A large window may need to be temporarily removed to allow passage of oversized items. Ample floor space is also needed for caregivers to interface with the patient in and around the equipment. Five feet of clear floor space is recommended on each side and at the foot of the bed. The floor surface and support structures beneath need to be carefully examined. They must be able to support a patient weight ranging from 500 to 1,000 lb (226.8 to 453.59 kg) together with all needed equipment and supplies. Often space is made available on the first level of a dwelling (versus navigating patient and equipment up a narrow staircase to a small second-floor bedroom). This may require conversion of the living room to a patient care area. An environmental control unit is an important consideration.
- ***Bathroom:*** Space is a primary concern in gaining access to a standard residential bathroom. Sufficient door width is needed to accommodate patient size, an assistive device, and/or the individual(s) guarding the patient. A 60-in. (152.4-cm) door width and turning radius is recommended. To place a bariatric commode with armrests over a toilet or allow a two-person assist, ample space of 24 in. (60.96 cm) is needed on each side with a 44-in. (111.76-cm) front clearance. A bidet may be recommended to assist cleansing. The toilet and sink should be floor mounted with a 1,000-lb (543.59-kg) weight capacity. Longer than typical grab bars with a 1,000-lb (543.59-kg) weight capacity should be installed on reinforced walls. The shower stall should be a minimum of 4 × 6 ft (1.22 × 1.83 m) and include a level entrance, a bariatric shower seat, a shower hand sprayer, and grab bars with a 1,000-lb (543.59-kg) weight capacity. The use of shower curtains is recommended over solid doors to facilitate caregiver assistance.

outlets, as well as improve access. Outlets may need to be raised and wall switches lowered. For individuals using a wheelchair, use of pull cord extensions may allow control of high electrical switches.

2. Some patients may benefit from replacement of standard toggle wall switches controlling overhead lights or fans with rocker switches that require less fine motor skill and can be activated with a fisted hand, lateral aspect of hand, or distal forearm. Rocker switches are available with illuminated surfaces and with occupancy (motion) sensor devices that automatically turn on or off. The plates surrounding wall switches come in a variety of colors and will be easier to see if they contrast with the existing wall color. For example, in rooms with light-colored walls (white, off-white, beige), darker

electrical outlet and light-switch plates can be selected. Voice- and noise-activated (clapping) lighting controls are also available. A ground fault circuit interrupter (GFCI) should be installed in wet locations such as bathrooms to prevent against electrical shock. A GFCI outlet acts as a monitor for current imbalance between the hot and neutral wires and breaks the circuit if that situation occurs (e.g., faulty appliances, worn cords, or appliance contact with water). In new home construction, GFCI installation is now required; they must be retrofitted in older homes.

3. For some patients, vision may be enhanced by use of higher wattage bulbs, fluorescent lighting, full-spectrum bulbs, daylight bulbs, or high-intensity halogen lamps. Long-life, energy-efficient LED lightbulbs reduce the frequency of required bulb changes.
4. Inexpensive, programmable electrical timers can be used to regularly turn lights on and off throughout the day and night.
5. Inexpensive night-lights can be placed in strategic locations to provide additional illumination. Some are available with motion sensors.
6. Dimmer switches with touch pads (or small sliding levers) can be used to activate lamps. The dimmer module is plugged into a wall outlet and the lamp attached to the module. The lamp can be turned on or off and the level of brightness changed by touching the pad or moving the lever. Voice-activated dimmers are also available.
7. Inexpensive remote control units can be used in any room of the home to control lights or small appliances. The simplest designs of these remote-control units send signals through existing wires (receiver modules are plugged into existing outlets and appliances are plugged into the receiver and controlled by a handheld remote); others are wireless. Receiver modules can also be wired directly into the electrical system of the dwelling. Remote control units are available with large-print buttons and numbers.

Clinical Note: Many cellular phone apps are available to remotely control an expanding variety of smart appliances such as thermostats, televisions, fans, smoke/carbon monoxide alarms, garage doors, home theater systems, water heaters, door locks, and lighting and security systems.

Floors

1. Floors should be nonslip and level; hardwood floors are ideal. When carpeting is used, a dense, low pile (0.25 to 0.5 in. [0.64 to 1.27 cm]), low-level loop generally provides for easiest movement of a wheelchair or ambulatory assistive device. Industrial-style or indoor/outdoor carpeting typically meet these requirements. High pile carpeting and carpet padding increases roll resistance (e.g., wheelchair, rolling walker); firmer carpeting decreases roll resistance. Carpeting with bold patterns of mixed colors may be visually confusing and impair judgment of spatial distances.[59] Padding under carpet is generally not recommended; if used, it should be very firm.[5] Floor coverings may need to be secured to the floor to prevent bunching or rippling under wheelchair use.
2. Floors should be examined for uneven or unlevel areas. This may be particularly problematic with older wooden floors. Joints in wood flooring should be shallow and no more than 0.25 to 0.5 in. (0.64 to 1.27 cm) wide. Deep joints wider than 0.75 in. (1.9 cm) will cause wheelchair casters to turn and lodge, blocking movement.[59] Optimally, problem areas should be repaired or replaced. If restoration is not possible, several other solutions might be recommended: (1) establish a path of movement for the patient that eliminates use of the problematic area, (2) place a piece of furniture over the offending area, or (3) place brightly colored tape along the borders of the area to continually remind the patient to avoid this area of potential danger.
3. Scatter rugs should be removed; larger area rugs can be secured with a good-quality carpet tape. Use of nonskid waxes should be encouraged.
4. If flooring is to be replaced, matte finishes should be recommended to reduce glare. Patients with visual impairments will benefit from a contrasting colored border along the perimeter of the room to help mark the boundaries of the space. Wide, colored tape can also be used effectively.

Doors

1. Raised thresholds should be removed to provide a flush, level surface. If structural elements prevent removal, small threshold ramps ("transition wedges") can be easily installed (Fig. 9.5).
2. Doorways may need to be widened (if less than 32 in. [815 mm] wide) to allow clearance for a wheelchair or assistive device. Doors may have to be removed, reversed (e.g., to open outward for easier exit, especially in the case of an emergency), or replaced with folding doors. Several other options are available to increase door clearance:
   - Pocket doors, which slide into the adjacent wall when not in use, are an option for new construction. However, they cannot be easily installed in existing structures. Some sliding doors allow installation on the outside of the door frame and wall to minimize structural changes.
   - Removal of the wood strips on the inside of a door frame will add approximately 0.75 to 1 in. (2 to 2.5 cm) of clearance.

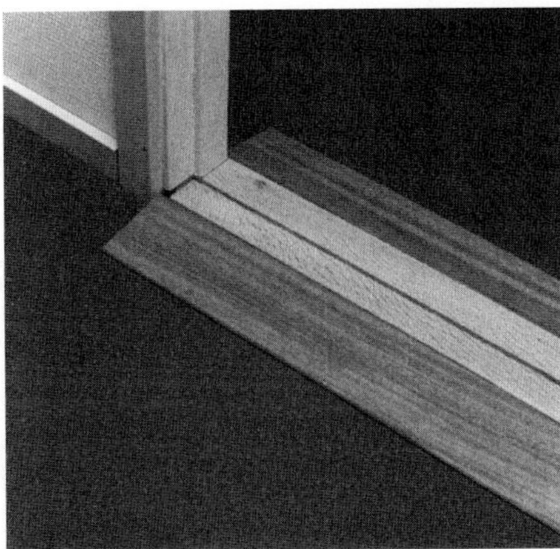

Figure 9.5 Common materials used for threshold ramps are wood (shown) and aluminum with a lacquered non-slip surface. They can be used between rooms, if threshold cannot be removed. *(Courtesy of Guldmann, Inc., Tampa, FL 33634.)*

- Use of *offset* hinges (also called *swing-clear hinges*), which swing the open door clear of the frame provide approximately 2 additional inches (5 cm) of space.
- Removal of the door with installation of a curtain (inexpensive spring-loaded curtain rods and a fabric or plastic shower curtain can be used); if used for a bathroom door, this option is less than optimal because it compromises privacy.

3. As mentioned in regard to exterior doors, handles inside the home should also be examined. Rubber doorknob covers or lever-type handles may be important considerations. Placed over a standard doorknob, extenders can be used to create a lever handle (Fig. 9.6). Knurled (roughened) surface door handles are used on interiors of buildings and dwellings when frequented by persons with visual impairments. These abrasive, knurled surfaces provide tactile clues that the door leads to a hazardous area and alerts the individual to danger. (Note: Brightly colored roughened areas are also used on flooring to indicate potential danger; for example, the edge of a train or subway platform.)

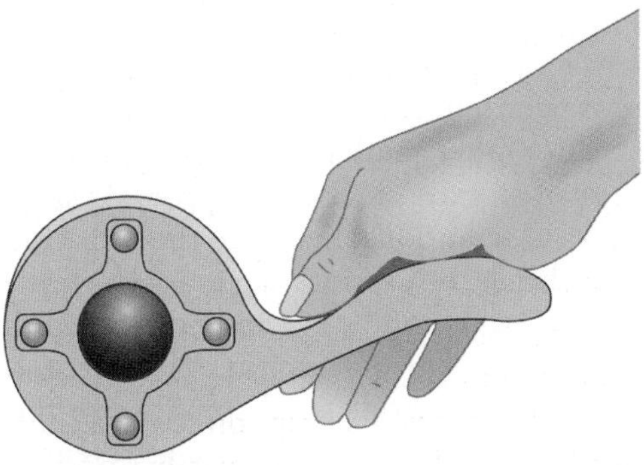

Figure 9.6 Doorknob extender.

Windows

1. To reduce glare, window films can be installed; frosted films are effective at diffusing light without appreciably reducing ambient light.
2. Heavy draperies or shades can also be used with the added benefit of absorbing internal background noise to improve hearing and conversation.
3. Remote control systems for closing or opening window coverings either partially or fully are commercially available.
4. Although not frequently seen in older dwellings, casement windows provide several important features for individuals using a wheelchair or for patients with limited upper extremity function. Casement windows open using a crank-style handle and can be locked with a single lever locking mechanism located near the bottom of the window. Automatic openers are available on these windows.

Stairs

1. All indoor stairwells should have handrails and should be well lighted. Ideally, handrails should extend a minimum of 12 in. (305 mm) past the top and bottom of the stairs for added safety[4,5] (see Fig. 9.3A). Battery-operated touch lamps are a practical supplement where electrical light sources are unavailable. Inexpensive track lighting provides multiple adjustable lamps and requires only a single electrical source. Lighting should be bright with glare and reflection minimized. Motion detection lights that automatically turn on when the patient approaches the stairs (or other area of the home) can also be an important safety consideration.
2. Stairs should be free of clutter. Rather than climbing the stairs to move a single item to the next level, patients sometimes "store" or collect items on the stairs. This creates several safety hazards: (1) initially bending over to pick up the items before stair climbing can alter postural stability; (2) negotiating stairs holding several objects can impair balance and limit use of the handrail; and (3) other household members may not see the item(s), precipitating a fall. As an alternative, a chair or small table placed near the stairs can be used to hold a canvas sling bag or small 'stair basket' with handles (that can be held in one hand) to collect items until the patient is ready to move to another floor level.
3. For individuals with decreased visual acuity or age-related visual changes, adhesive, light-reflective *tactile warning strips* provide contrasting textures on the surface of the top and bottom stair(s) to alert them that the end of the stairwell is near. They can also be used on each step to identify its edge. Circular bands of tape also can be placed at the top and bottom of the handrail for the same purpose. Tactile warning strips placed on the floor can be used to signal a change in level of the walking surface or entrance to another area or room of the dwelling.

4. Many patients with visual impairment will benefit also from bright, contrasting color tape on the border of each stair. Warm colors (reds, oranges, and yellows) are generally easier to see than cool colors (blues, greens, and violets).
5. For patients unable to negotiate stairs who require access to the second floor of a dwelling, a motorized stairlift may be an option (Fig. 9.7). These units are available with a variety of options such as swing-away arms for wheelchair transfers, wide adjustable seat width (22.5 to 25.5 in. [57 cm to 64 cm]), and wireless call/send controls. Outdoor models are also available, as well as units to accommodate curves or turns in the stairwell. Residential elevators are another, more costly option; they require construction of an enclosed shaft. If the residence has "stacked" closets (same position on different floors), these closet spaces can be combined to form an elevator shaft.

Heating Units

1. All radiators, heating vents, and hot water pipes should be appropriately screened off or insulated with pipe covers to prevent burns, especially for patients who have sensory impairments. Adaptations may be required to allow patient access to heat controls (e.g., remote thermostat control, use of reachers or enlarged, extended, or adapted handles on heat control valves).
2. The heating source should be clear of combustible material and clutter. Use of space heaters should be discouraged.

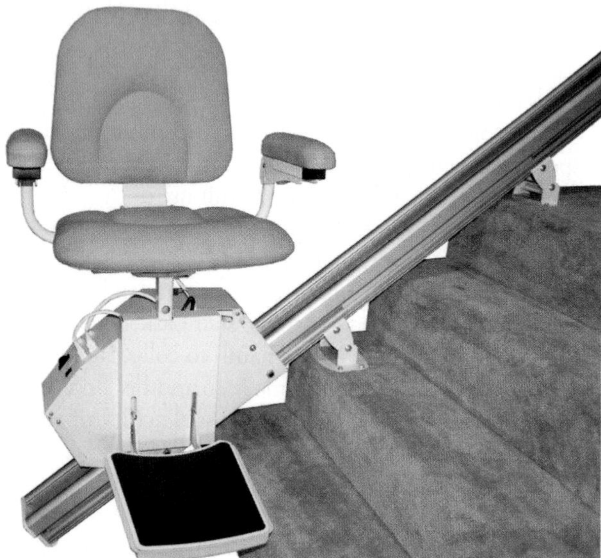

Figure 9.7 Powered stairlift. When not in use, the stairlift folds up against wall. It has a rack-and-pinion drive system that can safely transport up to 350 lb. The seat measures 19 in. (48.26 cm) wide and 14 in. (35.56 cm) deep. *(Courtesy of AmeriGlide, Inc., Raleigh, NC 27610).*

Smoke and Carbon Monoxide Alarms

Smoke and carbon monoxide alarms should be in the home and checked regularly. Many models include voice warning announcements ("Fire" or "Low Battery") and allow testing the alarm using a remote control or cell phone app. At least one alarm should be on every level of the home and ideally, one in the kitchen and each bedroom and one outside each sleeping area. Interconnected alarms enable wireless communication with each other and provide better full-home protection. Regularly scheduled battery replacement is recommended (e.g., daylight saving time change). For patients with hearing impairments, the alarm can also be attached to a signaling system that activates a high-volume audible and a strobe light response, to visually warn of danger. (These signaling systems also can be used to activate flashing lights in response to a doorbell, knock on the door, telephone ring, or burglar alarm.)

Clinical Note: A frequent gap in accomplishing home access is that the patient and family are provided recommendations with no community contacts to actually install the recommendations. To provide effective guidance, the therapist should be knowledgeable about community contractors experienced in home modifications for individuals with disability. The identified contractor should be available for consultation and communication with the patient, family, and rehabilitation team members throughout the planning and implementation process.

Interior Accessibility: Individual Room Consideration

Bedroom

1. The bed should be stationary and positioned to provide ample space for transfers. Stability may be improved by placing the bed against a wall or in the corner of the room (except when the patient plans to make the bed). Additional stability may be achieved by placing rubber cups under each leg.
2. The height of the sleeping surface must be optimal for transfers. Furniture risers can be used to raise bed height. Wooden and high-density rubber furniture risers are commercially available in a variety of heights with routed depressions to hold each leg of the bed (or other furniture such as chairs or tables). The use of an extra-thick mattress or box spring can also provide additional height to the bed. Using reduced-height box springs can lower the bed height.
3. The mattress should be carefully examined. It should provide a firm, comfortable surface. If the mattress is in relatively good condition, a firm bed board inserted between the mattress and box spring may suffice to improve the sleeping surface

adequately. If the mattress is badly worn, a new one should be suggested.

4. A bedside nightstand (or small table) should be available; it can be used to hold a lamp, telephone (preferably cordless with a memory dial for frequently used numbers or emergency phone numbers; cellular phones have the added advantage of always remaining with the patient), necessary medications, and call bell if assistance is needed from a caregiver.
5. The closet clothes bar may require lowering to provide wheelchair accessibility. The bar should be lowered to 52 in. (132 cm) from the floor. Nonslip hangers are often recommended. Wall hooks also may be a useful addition to the closet area and should be placed between 40 in. (101.6 cm) and 56 in. (142.2 cm) from the floor. *Wardrobe lifts* can increase closet storage capacity while maintaining accessibility (Fig. 9.8). They consist of a clothes bar attached by hinged supports; using an extended handle, the bar is pulled down and out to access clothing. Electrically powered and hydraulic wardrobe lifts are also commercially available. With height based on the patient's reaching capability, shelves also can be installed at various levels in the closet. Clothing and grooming articles frequently used by the patient should be placed in the most easily accessible bureau drawer. Freestanding modular closet units are also available in a variety of dimensions. These units typically provide clothes bar, shelves, and drawers that can be adjusted to meet the needs of the user. Figure 9.9 illustrates the basic components and dimensions of an accessible bedroom.

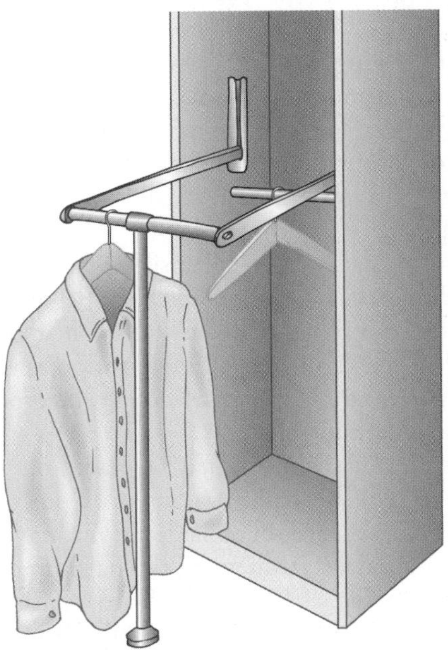

Figure 9.8 Manually operated wardrobe lift. Wardrobe lifts are available in a variety of sizes and some allow placement on either back wall or sidewalls.

Bathroom

1. If the door frame prohibits passage of a wheelchair, the patient may transfer at the door to a chair with casters attached. As mentioned, several other solutions are available to address the problem of narrow door frames (see Interior Accessibility: General Considerations, *Doors*).
2. For many patients, an elevated toilet will facilitate transfers. The simplest approach is use of a portable raised seat attachment. Some models allow the height to be custom adjusted, whereas others provide a fixed height elevation. They are also available with hand bars on each side. Base risers can be installed to elevate the entire toilet (Fig. 9.10). Finally, a standard height toilet (14 to 15 in. [36 to 38 cm]) can be replaced with a comfort (convenient) height (17 to 20 in. [43 to 51 cm]) model. Also available are power-lift toilet seats with grab bars designed to assist the patient to standing (elevation initiated from the posterior aspect of the seat). This is a costlier option and poses potential safety risks. As with other types of mechanized seat elevators, it may be difficult to stabilize one's feet as the seat is elevating (especially in area with potential for a wet floor surface). For new construction, a wall-mounted toilet may be recommended that can be placed at the optimum height for the user and provide more floor space for transfer positioning. Based on patient size, weight capacity of wall-mounted units need to be considered.
3. Grab bars securely fastened to a reinforced wall will assist in both toilet and tub transfers. Grab bars should have a circular cross-section diameter of 1.25 in. (32 mm) minimum and 2 in. (51 mm) maximum and be knurled. For use in toilet transfers, the bars should be mounted horizontally 33 to 36 in. (840 to 915 mm) from floor. The length of the grab bars should be between 42 and 54 in. (1,065 and 1,370 mm) on sidewall and between 24 and 36 in. (610 and 915 mm) on the back wall (Fig. 9.11). Ideally, two grab bars are secured horizontally to the back wall for use in tub transfers. One is placed 33 to 36 in. (840 to 915 mm) from tub floor and the second 9 in. (230 mm) above top rim of the bathtub. Grab bars may also be mounted horizontally at the foot-end wall of the bathtub (recommended length is 24 in. [610 mm] with placement at the front edge of the bathtub) and at the head-end wall of the bathtub (recommended length is 12 in. [305 mm] with placement at the front edge of the bathtub) (Fig. 9.12). Knurled surfaces are typically used on grab bars to improve grasp and prevent slipping.

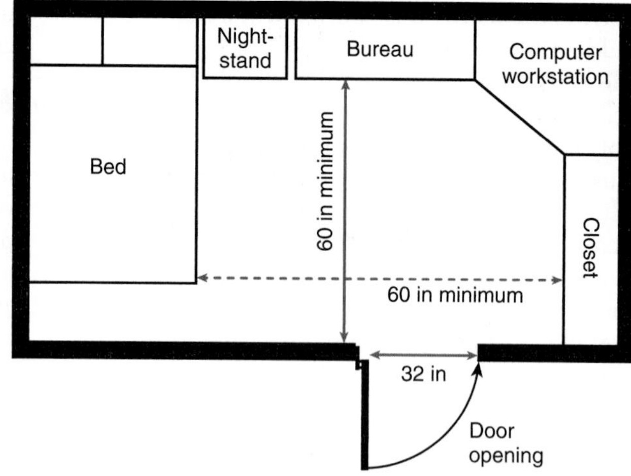

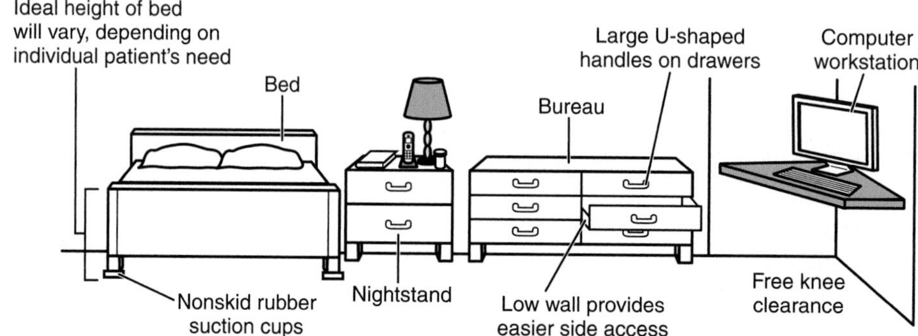

Figure 9.9 Sample dimensions and features of an accessible bedroom.

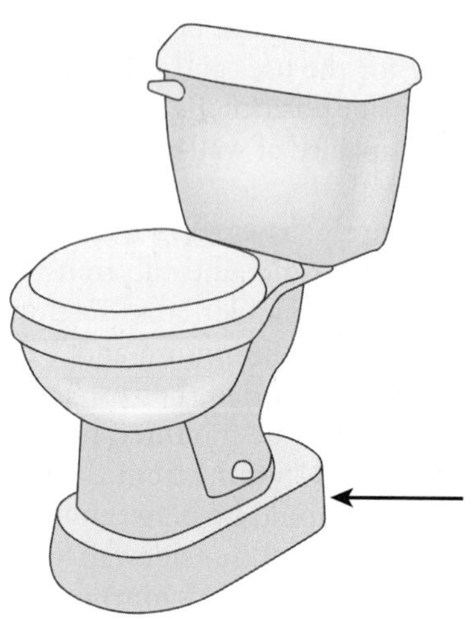

Figure 9.10 Base risers increase the height of the entire toilet to facilitate transfers.

4. A tub transfer bench (tub seat) may be recommended for bathing. Many types of commercially produced benches are available. In selecting a tub transfer bench (tub seat), function and safety are primary considerations. The bench should provide a wide base of support (some are designed with suction feet, and some provide height adjustment), a backrest, and an appropriate seating surface to facilitate transfers in and out of the tub.

Tub transfer benches with relatively long seating surfaces are typically positioned with two legs in the tub and two legs on the floor adjacent to the tub (Fig. 9.13). Smaller benches are available that require all four legs to be placed inside the bathtub.

5. A space-saving design for new construction combines a toilet and shower seat into one assembled seat (Fig. 9.14). The design has the potential benefit of allowing creation of an accessible toilet and shower area in a relatively small space. A floor drain is required.
6. In shower stall areas, a collapsible seat may be permanently attached to the wall (Fig. 9.15). When not in use, it folds flat against the wall, allowing easy shower access from a standing position as well. Many new extended shower designs incorporate a permanent, built-in seat.
7. Nonskid adhesive strips may be placed on the floor of the tub or shower area.
8. Additional bathroom considerations may include a hand-spray attachment to the bathtub or shower faucet (see Fig. 9.12 and Fig. 9.16), antiscald valves to prevent water temperature from rising above a preset limit (also called *scald-guard valves* or *high-temperature stops*), water volume–control mechanisms (to prevent a sudden surge of water with resultant change in temperature), enlarged

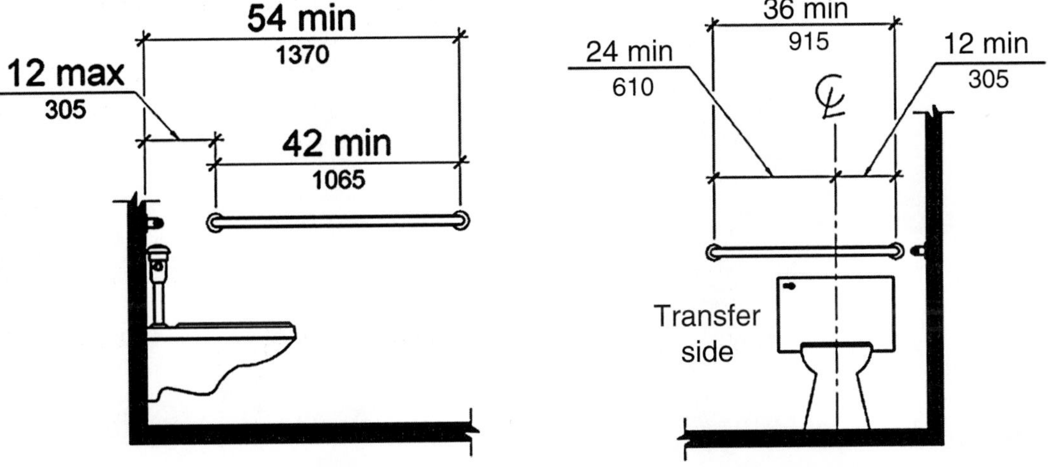

Figure 9.11 Location and dimensions of bathroom grab bars. Values denoted in inches and millimeters. The bars should be mounted horizontally 33 in. (840 mm) to 36 in. (915 mm) from the floor.[4] *(Left)* The sidewall grab bar is 42–54 in. wide and placed at a maximum of 12 in. (305 mm) from rear wall. If anchored on or near rear wall, it should extend 54 in. (1,370 mm) from the wall. *(Right)* The rear wall grab bar is 24–36 in. wide (36 in. is considered minimum if wall space allows). When 36 in. long, 24 in. of the bar (from center of toilet) is placed toward the side used for transfers. *(From 2010 ADA Standards for Accessible Design[5] [Left, p. 163; Right, p. 164].)*

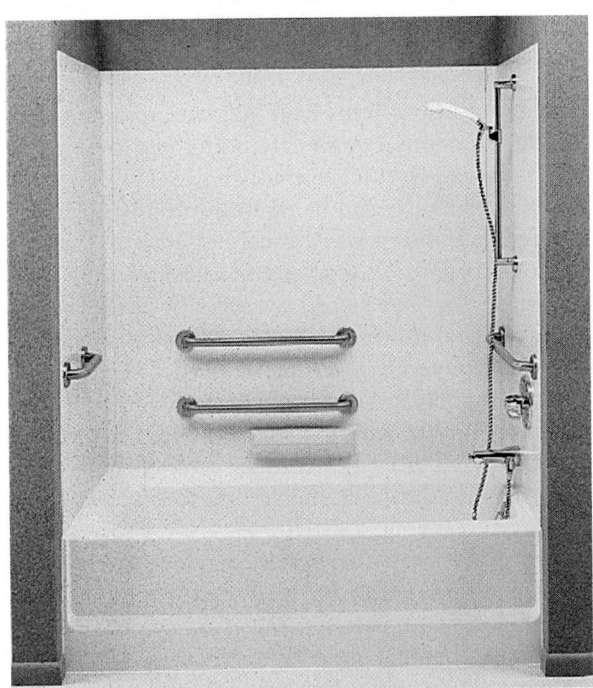

Figure 9.12 Bathtub with grab bars secured to back, foot-end, and head-end walls. The hand-spray faucet attachment facilitates control of water flow direction from a sitting position. *(Courtesy of the Swan Corporation, St. Louis, MO 63101.)*

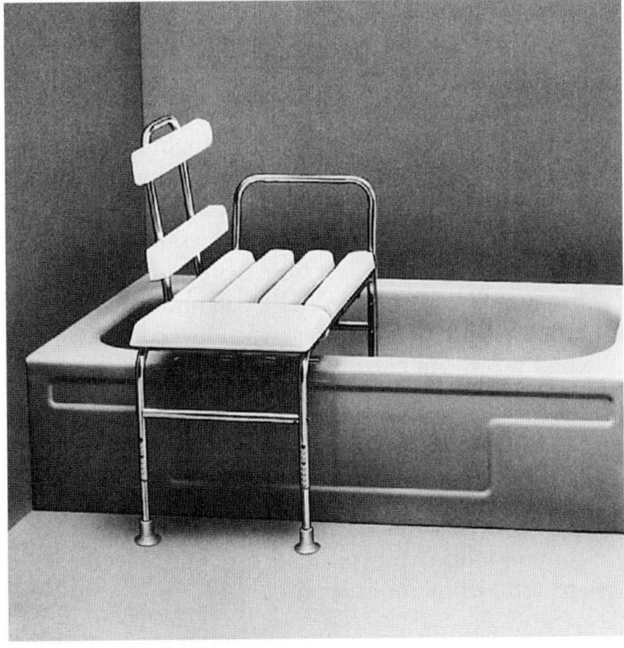

Figure 9.13 Bathtub transfer bench providing a wide base of support, a secure backrest, and a long seating surface to facilitate transfers. *(Courtesy of Lumex, Inc., Bay Shore, NY 11706.)*

faucet handles on the tub or sink (single-lever system faucets are optimal owing to their ease of use), motion-sensor faucets, a spray attachment at the sink (allows washing hair without entering the bathtub or shower), a towel rack and small shelf for toiletry articles, and a call bell within easy reach of the patient.

Clinical Note: To prevent injury in the presence of sensory impairments, patient, family, and caregiver education should include testing water temperature before bathing.

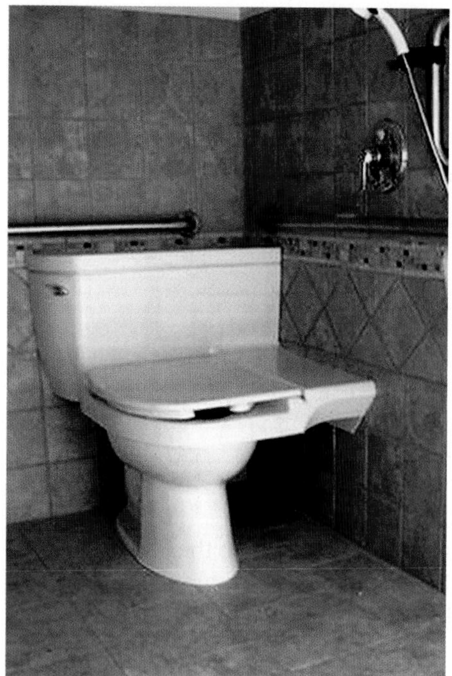

Figure 9.14 Combined toilet and shower seat into a single assembled seat. *(Courtesy of WYNG" Products, Woodlands, TX 77380).*

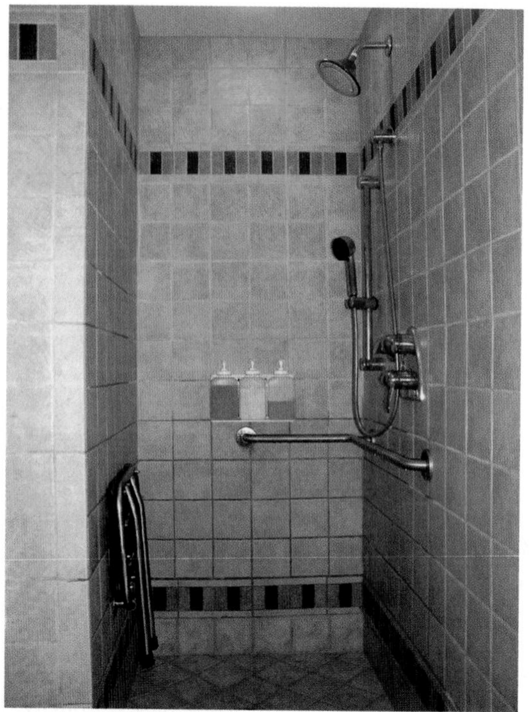

Figure 9.15 Shower stall with collapsible shower seat, grab bars, and hand-spray attachment.

9. Ideally, sinks should provide clear knee space below and any exposed hot water pipes should be insulated to prevent burns (see Fig. 9.16). In new construction, shallow sinks may be installed to increase knee clearance with faucets placed on the side for easier access. Storage space lost from beneath the sink can be partially compensated for by an under-the-sink rollout cabinet that can be easily moved for wheelchair access. An enlarged mirror over the sink with the top tilted away from the wall facilitates use from a sitting position in a wheelchair (Fig. 9.17). Forward-tilting mirrors are also available with adjustable hinges for alternating placement against and away from the wall. Hinged-wall, gooseneck, or accordion fold-up mirrors (with one side magnified) are also helpful for close work.

Figure 9.18 illustrates the minimum space requirements of a wheelchair-accessible bathroom.

Kitchen

1. The height of countertops (work space) should be appropriate for the individual. When using a wheelchair, the armrests should be able to fit under the working surface. In new construction, the ideal height of counter surfaces should be no greater than 31 in. (79 cm) from the floor with a knee clearance of 27.5 to 30 in. (70 to 76 cm). Counter space should provide a depth of at least 24 in. (61 cm). All surfaces should be smooth to facilitate sliding of heavy items from one area to another. Slide-out counter spaces are useful in providing an over-the-lap working surface (Fig. 9.19). A section of base cabinetry can be removed to provide a seated countertop workspace. For patients who are ambulatory, stools (preferably with back and footrests) may be placed strategically at the main work area(s). For patients with visual impairments, placing colored tape along the border of the countertop that contrasts sharply with the color of the counter surface will help identify boundaries of the workspace. Under-the-counter cabinets with glide-out height-adjustable shelves improve access to storage areas (Fig. 9.20).
2. Improved function and safety may be provided by a sink equipped with large blade-type handles or a single-lever style faucet, scald-guard valves, or electronic sensors that allow hands-free operation by automatically turning water off and on. A spray-hose fixture allows filling heavy pots without needing to lift them from a sink. Pressure-balanced valves can be used to equalize hot and cold water; other faucets allow preprogramming desired water temperature. Hot water dispensers are helpful for preparing coffee or tea and instant soups or cereals, minimizing the need for using the stove. Shallow sinks 5 to 6 in (12 to 15 cm) deep will improve knee clearance below. Providing sink access to an individual using a wheelchair may require removal of under-the-sink cabinets. As in the bathroom, hot water pipes under

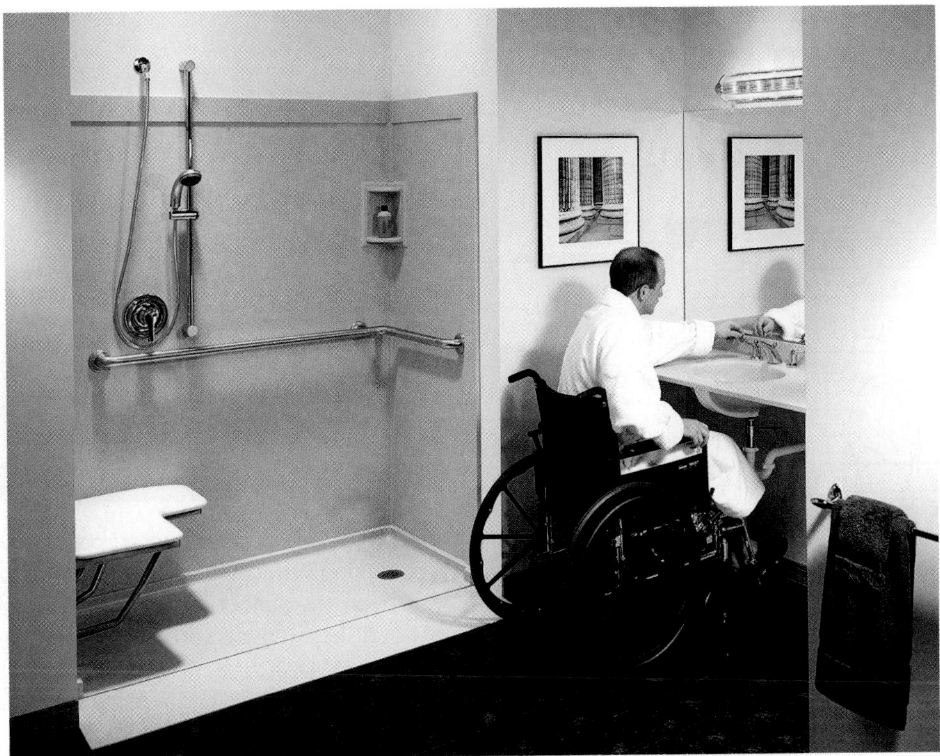

Figure 9.16 Accessible bathroom with knee clearance below sink and insulated piping. The shower entrance includes a small ramp to accommodate a difference in floor surface heights. Note that the shower hand-spray is held by a vertical slide-bar (to change height), allowing for a seated shower. Alternately, the hand-spray can be handheld to direct water flow to specific areas. *(Courtesy of the Swan Corporation, St. Louis, MO 63101.)*

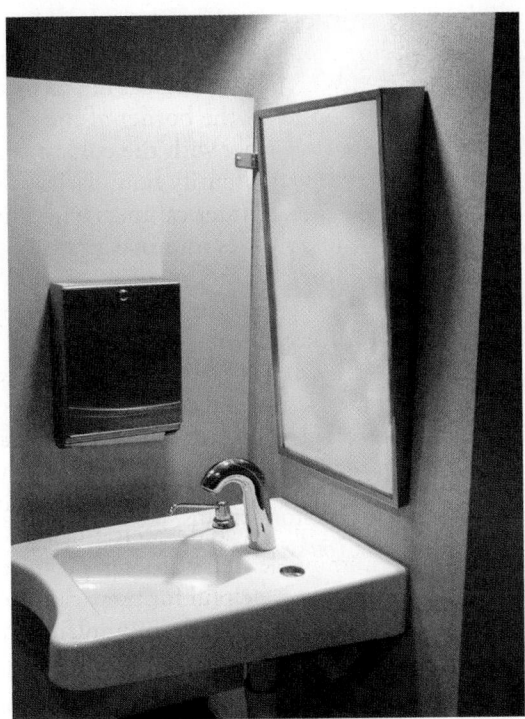

Figure 9.17 Over-sink mirror with top tilted away from wall to allow use from a seated position.

the kitchen sink should be insulated to prevent burns. In new construction, motorized adjustable sinks can be mounted against a wall between two stationary cabinets with free space beneath. By activating the control switch, the sink height can be adjusted for the individual user whether seated in a wheelchair or standing.

3. A small cart with casters may be helpful to improve ease of moving articles from refrigerator to counter or table.
4. The height of tables also should be checked and the tables may have to be raised or lowered.
5. Equipment and food storage areas should be selected with optimum energy conservation in mind. All frequently used articles should be within easy reach, and unnecessary items should be eliminated. Additional storage space may be achieved by installation of open shelving or use of pegboards for pots and pans. If shelving is added above the countertop, adjustable shelves are preferable, allowing optimal height placement for the individual patient.
6. Electric stoves are generally preferable to open-flame gas burners. For optimum safety, controls should be located on the front or side border of the stove to eliminate the need for reaching across the burners.

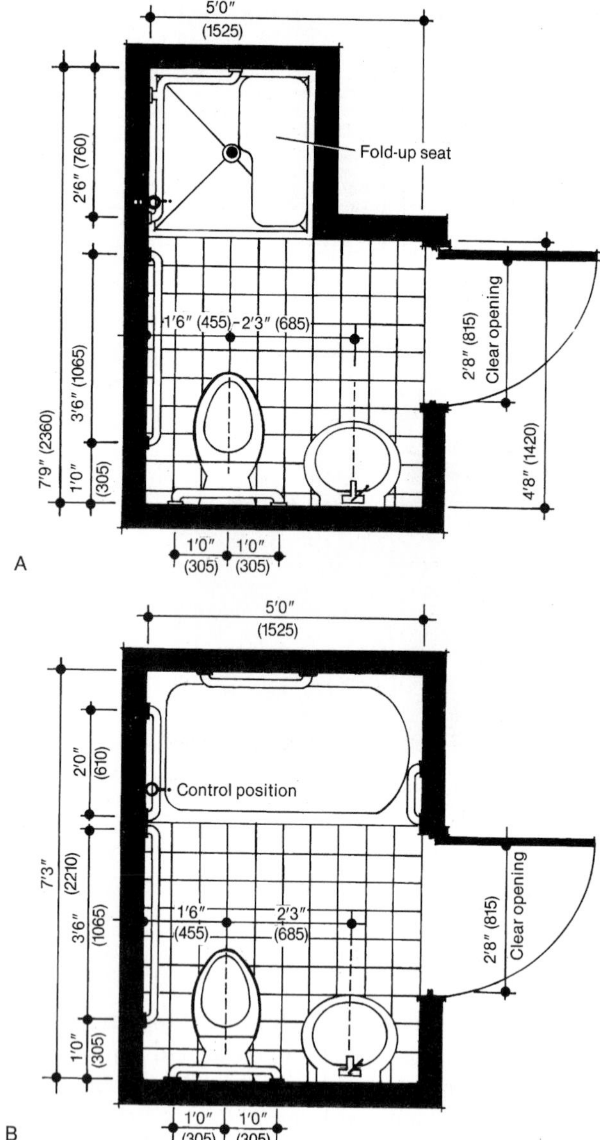

Figure 9.18 Minimum space requirements of a residential bathroom with (A) a shower stall and (B) a bathtub. The dotted line indicates lengths of wall that require reinforcement to receive grab bars or supports. *(From Nixon, V: Spinal Cord Injury: A Guide to Functional Outcomes in Physical Therapy Management. Aspen Systems Corporation, Rockville, MD, 1985, p. 186, with permission.)*

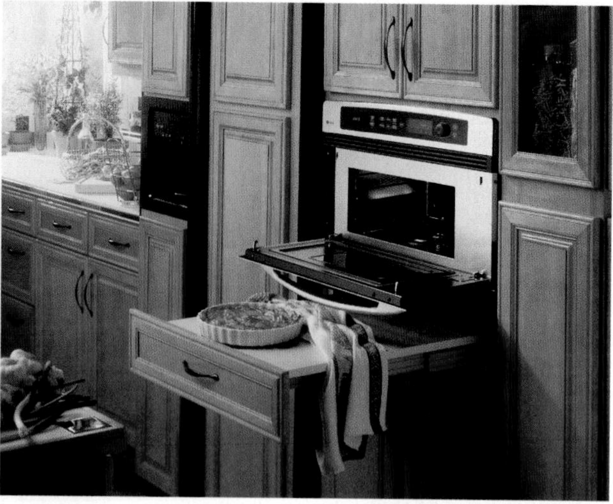

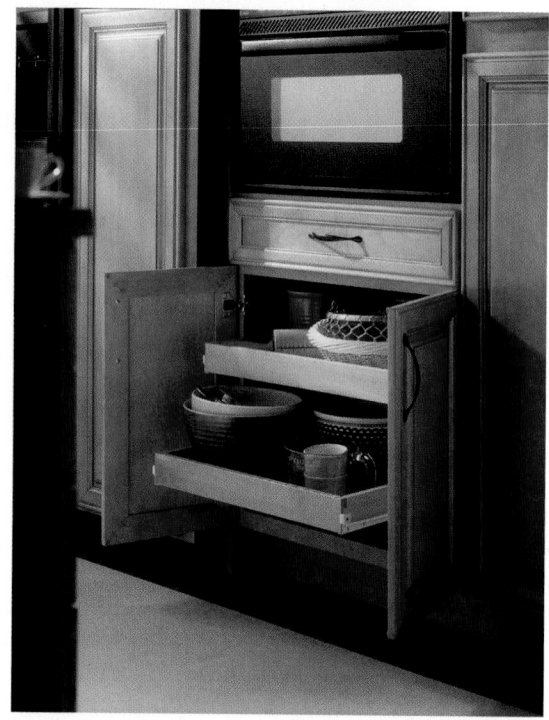

Figure 9.19 Slide-out counter spaces provide over-the-lap working surfaces. Positioned here below a built-in wall oven, the pullout surface allows for ease of transfer of hot dishes. *(Courtesy of General Electric, Appliance Park, Louisville, KY 40225.)*

Figure 9.20 Glide-out under-cabinet shelves improve ability to see and access stored items. *(Courtesy of General Electric, Appliance Park, Louisville, KY, 40225.)*

Burners that are placed beside each other provide a safer arrangement than those placed one behind the other. A heat-resistant burn-proof counter surface adjacent to the burners will facilitate movement of hot items once cooking is completed. Smooth, ceramic cooktop surfaces also reduce the amount of lifting required while cooking (Fig. 9.21). If cooktops provide knee clearance beneath, exposed or potential contact surfaces must be insulated. Induction (electromagnetic) stoves are also available that heat food without flames or heating elements.

7. For patients with visual impairments, large-print label-making devices and large-print stencil overlays can be used to enlarge appliance control indicators and dials (e.g., on/off or temperature indicators on thermostats, microwaves, stoves, and ovens). Timers, wall clocks, and telephones with large-print numbers are also available.

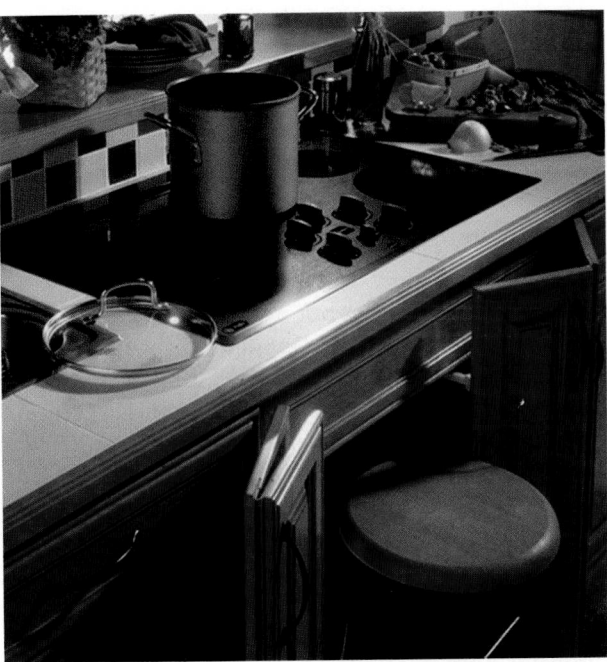

Figure 9.21 Cooktop with front-mounted controls and smooth surface that allows sliding (rather than lifting) from burner to heat-resistant countertop. Knee clearance beneath is accessed by folding doors. *(Courtesy of General Electric, Appliance Park, Louisville, KY 40225.)*

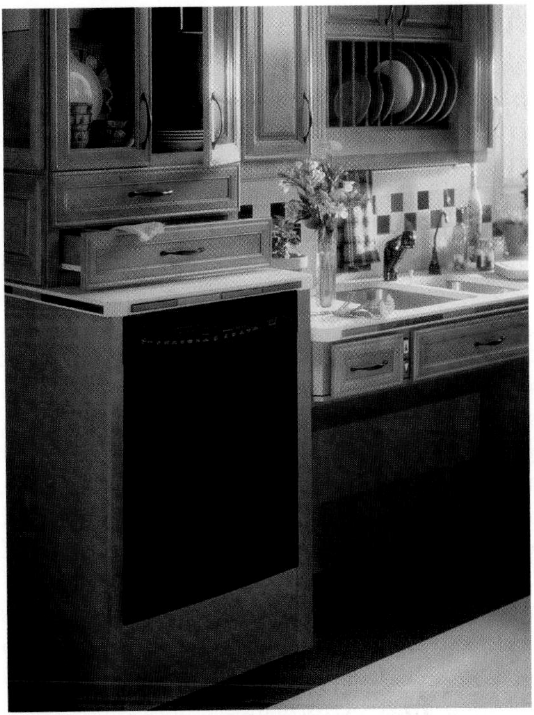

Figure 9.22 Front-loading dishwasher elevated 9 in. (23 cm) with front-mounted controls. *(Courtesy of General Electric, Appliance Park, Louisville, KY 40225.)*

8. Wall-mounted ovens (separate from the stove) should be placed 30 to 34 in. (76 to 102 cm) from the floor with a side-opening door. These cooking units are generally more easily accessible than a single, low-level combined oven and burner unit. Oven units should be self-cleaning.
9. For many individuals, a countertop microwave oven is essential for food preparation.
10. Dishwashers should be elevated 9 in. (23 cm) and be front-loading, with pullout shelves and front-mounted controls (Fig. 9.22). Elevated (9 in. [23 cm]) side-by-side clothes washers and dryers should also be front-loading with front-mounted controls (Fig. 9.23).
11. Access to the refrigerator will be enhanced by use of a side-by-side (refrigerator-freezer) model.
12. One or more, easily accessible, portable fire extinguishers should be available. It is generally recommended that fire extinguishers be mounted in open view near an exit and away from cooking appliances.

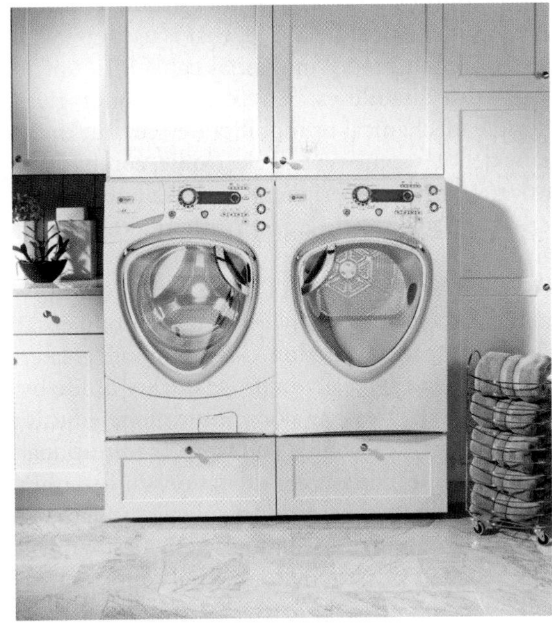

Figure 9.23 Front-loading clothes washer and dryer elevated 9 in. (23 cm) with front-mounted controls. *(Courtesy of General Electric, Appliance Park, Louisville, KY 40225.)*

Clinical Note: For older adults, specific areas of the home have been found to present greater hazards than others. Gitlin et al[60] addressed the types of difficulties older adults experience in their home. Data were collected from 296 participants (mean age 73.24 years) using interviews, self-reports, clinical assessment, and direct observation of the home environment. The researchers focused on nine areas of the home: bathroom, kitchen, bedrooms, entry to home, dining/living/family room, outdoor spaces, common rooms, stairs, and the area from street to house. The areas where subjects encountered the greatest difficulties were bathrooms (88%), kitchens (76%), bedrooms (61%), and entryways (58%).

ADAPTIVE EQUIPMENT

Recommendations for *adaptive equipment* and training in their use is an area of expertise of the occupational therapist. A large variety of adaptive equipment is commercially available to increase independence, speed, skill, and efficiency in performing activities of daily living (ADL). Adaptive equipment is available to assist performance in such areas as bathing, personal care, dressing, meal preparation, and general household tasks (e.g., built-up handles on eating utensils and personal care items, suction devices to stabilize bowls and dishes, long-handled reacher, sponge, duster, dustpan and brush, rocker knife, adapted cutting board). Use of adaptive equipment is typically considered a component of a *compensatory training approach* that focuses on achieving the highest level of function possible by using remaining abilities. This approach involves considering alternative ways to accomplish a task, use of intact segments to compensate for those lost, use of energy conservation and joint preservation techniques, and adapting the environment to optimize performance.

ASSISTIVE TECHNOLOGY

In the Assistive Technology Act of 1998, an *assistive technology device* is defined as "any item, piece of equipment, or product system, whether acquired commercially, modified, or customized, that is used to increase, maintain, or improve functional capabilities of individuals with disabilities."[61] Assistive technologies can be simple mechanical or mobility devices but the term usually denotes some type of electronic, computer (e.g., hardware, software, peripherals), tablet application, or microprocessor-based (e.g., prosthetic knee control) device.

Assistive technologies (ATs) enable individuals with disabilities to perform daily activities by compensating for lost or impaired function. They promote greater independence and typically improve quality of life by assisting in such areas as communication, education, environmental accessibility, and work or recreational activities. Three important considerations in determining the need for ATs are (1) the individual's available function, (2) the nature of the tasks or activities that will be performed, and (3) the environmental context in which it will be used.

A large variety of ATs are commercially available. Ideally, an interdisciplinary rehabilitation team is responsible for examination, evaluation, and prescription recommendation for specific items. Although influenced by the care setting and type of AT required, participating individuals typically include the patient and family, physical and occupational therapists, a speech-language pathologist, and an assistive technology professional (see below). Depending on the needs of the patient, other contributors may include a special education teacher, seating specialist, rehabilitation technology supplier, augmentative communication specialist, and social worker or funding specialist. Box 9.2 provides an overview of the general categories of AT.

An *assistive technology professional* (ATP) or *rehabilitation technology specialist* is responsible for analyzing the AT needs of the patient. Through the systematic application of technology and engineering principles, this individual addresses the patient's needs in multiple contexts, including, but not limited to, education, employment, independent living, transportation, and recreation/leisure activities. The ATP recommends and guides selection of appropriate assistive technology and educates the patient, family, and caregivers in use of the technology. The ATP or rehabilitation technology specialist may hold a degree in areas such as assistive technology engineering, assistive technology and human services, physical or occupational therapy, engineering, human factors and ergonomics, or another related field. In addition, they typically hold a certificate in assistive technology. Many such certification programs have developed across the country. An example of such a certification program is the Rehabilitation Engineering and Assistive Technology Society of North America's (RESNA's) assistive technology professional (ATP) certification program.

Environmental control units (ECUs) are an important example of how ATs can enhance function and improve independence. ECUs are electronic interfaces that allow the user to control a variety of appliances and devices (e.g., telephones, bed controls, various components of an entertainment unit, room temperature and lighting, open and close curtains, open doors). These devices combine operation of all appliances into a central control panel, providing increased independence for individuals with severe disability.

The three main components of an ECU are (1) the input device, (2) the control unit, and (3) the appliance. The *input device* controls the ECU using whatever voluntary movement the individual has available (e.g., joystick, control panel, keypad, keyboard [ECU computer software programs are available], a series of switches, touch pads and screens, light pen, optical pointers, brain implants [e.g., patients with high-level spinal cord injuries] and voice, mouth-stick, and eye control). The *control unit* is the central processor that translates the input signal to an output signal to regulate the target appliance. The *appliance* can be virtually any device that can be controlled electronically.

EXAMINATION OF THE WORKPLACE

An investigation of the workplace is an important component of a comprehensive examination of the environment. It is used to explore the *worker–job–environment relationship* and to determine the feasibility of returning

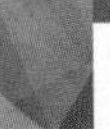

Box 9.2 Categories of Assistive Technology

Aids for Daily Living

Aids or devices that enhance performance of ADL and level of independence in such activities as eating, meal preparation, dressing, personal hygiene, bathing, or household management. *Examples*: Grab bars, ramps, stairlifts, lowered counters, bathtub seats, adapted doorknobs, eating utensils, personal hygiene items, nonslip surface to stabilize dishes or other objects, and alternative doorbells.

Augmentative Communication

Devices used to enhance personal expressive and receptive communication. *Examples*: Communication enhancement devices (electronic), book holders, communication boards, eye gaze boards, electric page turners, head wands, mouth sticks, light pointers, reading machines, personal voice amplification, signal systems, and telephone adaptations.

Computer Applications

Hardware, software, and devices to enhance computer access. *Examples*: Modified, chording, expanded or alternate keyboards; voice recognition software; alternate workstations (electrically powered height and tilt adjustments); Braille translation software (conversion from print and Braille); Braille printers; access aids (head-control sticks, light pointers, eye gaze input); alternative switches (minimal pressure, voice activated) and cursor (mouse) control; voice synthesizers, large-print software that allows user to alter background and text colors (e.g., electronic books, magazines, and newspapers); magnification screens, touch screens, onscreen keyboard, screen reader; keyguards, forearm supports; text-to-speech software; speech-to-text software; optical character recognition (OCR) system that scans written text to a computer and is read by a speech synthesis/screen review system; and robotic wheelchair mounting to support a laptop computer.

Environmental Control Systems

Electronic systems that enhance ability to control various devices. *Examples*: Electronic control of appliances, lights, doors, and security systems in the home.

Hearing Technology

Devices designed to enhance receptive communication (assistive listening devices). *Examples*: Closed captioning, FM amplification systems (isolate and amplify a sound source), hearing aids, infrared amplification systems, personal amplification systems, TDDs/TTYs, television amplifiers, telephone adaptations, and visual and tactile alerting systems.

Mobility Technology

Devices designed to provide an alternative means for walking or moving within the environment. *Examples*: Manual or powered wheelchairs; powered scooters; vehicle modification (driving adaptations, hand controls, wheelchair lifts); stairlifts; bus lifts; kneeling buses; and ambulatory assistive devices.

Seating and Positioning

Wheelchair (or other seating system) interventions to improve postural alignment, stability, and head control and reduce skin pressure. *Examples*: Custom-fitted wheelchair (reclining back, elevating leg rests), tilt-in-space wheelchair, custom-molded seating surface, control blocks, pressure-relieving seat cushions, head and neck supports, adductor cushions, abductor pommel, lumbar supports, torso supports, and pelvic and foot positioners.

Vision Technology

Devices designed to enhance interaction with the environment for individuals with visual impairments. *Examples*: Talking devices (clocks, watches, calculators, thermometers, scales, handheld spell checkers, dictionaries, and thesauruses), magnifiers, speech output devices, large-print screens, mini pocket tape recorders, voice-activated daily planners, large-button phone, large-print books, magazines, and newspapers, audio books, and books on disc (can be loaded onto a computer and read to user with a voice synthesizer).

to a former job or if reasonable accommodations will provide the needed support to resume work. The tests and measures used by physical therapists to examine work life address patient capabilities in three key areas, the ability to (1) return to work activities with or without AT, (2) obtain access to the work environment, and (3) safely perform required work activities.[3] Table 9.4 presents the tests and measures used by physical therapists to examine the patient's work life together with the tools for data-gathering and the data used in documentation.

Job Requirements

Determining the patient's ability to safely return to previous employment requires detailed information about the functional requirements of the job. If available, this information can be obtained from an existing job analysis

Table 9.4 Work Life: Examples of Tests and Measures, Data-Gathering Tools, and Data Used in Documentation.

Work life integration or reintegration is the process of assuming or resuming activities and roles in work settings. It requires abilities such as negotiating environmental terrain, gaining access to appropriate work settings, and participating in essential activities for work.

The physical therapist uses tests and measures to make judgments as to whether an individual is prepared to assume or resume work-related roles, including activities of daily living (ADL) and instrumental activities of daily living (IADL), or to assess the need for assistive technology or environmental adaptations.

Tests and Measures	Data-Gathering Tools	Documentation
Ability to assume or resume work-related activities with or without assistive technology (e.g., developmental capacity tests, activity profiles, disability indexes, functional status questionnaires, IADL scales, observations, physical capacity tests) Ability to gain access to work environments (e.g., needs assessment, barrier identification, interviews, observations, physical capacity tests, transportation assessments) Safety in performing work-related activities (e.g., ergonomic assessments, diaries, falls risk assessments, interviews, logs, observations, videographic assessments)	Cameras and photographs Equipment needed to perform developmental and physical capacity test Video cameras and video recordings	Ability to participate in a variety of work environments Clinical rationale to justify need and appropriate assistive technology Developmental level of motor ability Functional capacity for work Level of safety in work-related activities Physiological responses to work-related activities Results of ergonomic assessment

From *Guide to Physical Therapist Practice 3.0*,[3] with permission. APTA is not responsible for the translation from English.

developed by the employer when the position was first created. If a job analysis for the patient's position is not available, one will need to be created. A job analysis is a detailed description that identifies and describes the specific requirements of a job. It typically includes (1) the essential functions (fundamental duties) of a job and relative time spent on each; (2) the physical environment in which the essential functions are performed (e.g., indoors, outdoors, temperature fluctuations, noise levels); (3) the physical requirements (e.g., lifting, push/pull activities, bending, reaching); (4) the skills needed (cognitive processes, language, writing, or computer skills); and (5) the social context of the job (level of supervision, independent, contact with the public). Together with knowledge of the patient's functional capabilities, the job analysis provides an important basis for determining ability to return to work and for making recommendations for reasonable accommodations.

If a job analysis is not already available, the data can be gathered using a structured interview with the employer and patient. The interview should be designed to gather information about job requirements and tasks performed while on duty (e.g., duration of performance, weight and distance of items lifted, carried, or pulled, body positions used, repetitive exertions required on a regular basis, and so forth), as well as the characteristics of the physical space in which the individual is required to work. Interview questions are developed based on the type of employment (e.g., assembly work, food service tasks, clerical work, motor vehicle operation, manual material handling, factory work, and so forth). Table 9.5 presents an abbreviated example of questions that might be posed during development of a job analysis document for a clerical position.[62]

Functional Capacity Evaluation (FCE)

Typically, the most effective means of examining the worker–job–environment interface is an on-site visit. However, a variety of standardized functional capacity evaluation (FCE) instruments are commercially available that can be used to gather preliminary data before an on-site visit. The APTA defines FCE as "a comprehensive battery of performance-based tests that are commonly used to determine ability for work, activities of daily living, or leisure activities."[63] Depending on the job task requirements, the FCE may be all that is needed to determine ability to return to a previous job or to assume alternative job placement. The FCE provides a series of objective tests and measures designed to identify both work-related capabilities and activity limitations. Measurement parameters typically include endurance, ROM, flexibility, strength, force generation, posture, coordination, manual dexterity, and consistency of performance.[64-66]

The FCE is used to measure performance in specific components of work-related tasks. The specificity of the job will dictate the functional movements required. FCE instrument capabilities are then selected based on these requirements in order to examine the specific group of skills that comprise the employment tasks (e.g., lifting, stooping, trunk rotation, reaching). Computer-integrated FCE systems (Fig. 9.24) allow replication of physical task

Table 9.5 Suggested Interview Questions Appropriate for a Clerical Position

Interview questions are used to gather general data about functional requirements of the job and the physical space in which the individual is required to work.

1. Y	N	Do you frequently lift more than 35 pounds?
2. Y	N	Are you required to lift objects from below knee level or above shoulder level on an occasional or frequent basis?
3. Y	N	When you lift, do you reach across other objects or at arm's length in order to accomplish the lift?
4. Y	N	Do you frequently reach for objects above shoulder level during the day?
5. Y	N	Do you sit for more than 4 hours per day?
6. Y	N	Does your job require you to maintain one position or posture for 30 to 60 minutes or longer at one time? If yes, what posture is it?________
7. Y	N	Are repetitive exertions required on a regular basis (e.g., typing)?
8. Y	N	Does your job require frequent motions of the fingers, wrists, elbows, or shoulders? (If yes, circle all that apply.)
9. Y	N	Do you feel that your desk height is at a comfortable level?
10. Y	N	(a) Is your chair comfortable for you?
Y	N	(b) Do you feel that it fits you properly?
Y	N	(c) Do you know how to adjust your chair?
11. Y	N	Is there ample space for you to perform your job?
12. Y	N	Does your job involve frequent bending, twisting, or jerking movements?

From Hunter,[62, p. 68] with permission.

demands required of an individual's work environment using either standardized testing protocols or customized physical tests. A variety of tasks can be simulated, including, but not limited to, lifting, pushing, pulling, carrying capacity, turning a valve, and using a variety of tools (e.g., swinging a hammer, using a paint roller, using a manual saw). The systems may also be used for strengthening and retraining using task-specific strategies that simulate requirements of the client's real environment.

Software programs allow comparison of FCE data with normative values such as strength and ROM. Data from the FCE assist the physical therapist with the following tasks:

- Predicting the individual's work capacity and ability to safely return to work
- Identifying parameters of the physical environment needed to optimize function and prevent further injury (reasonable accommodations)
- Identifying extent of activity limitations
- Matching abilities to appropriate job placement

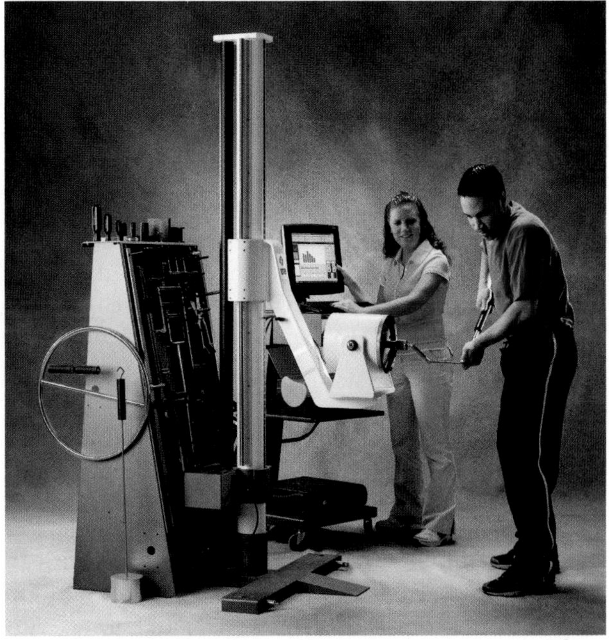

Figure 9.24 Simulator II Functional Capacity Evaluation System. *(Courtesy of BTE Technologies, Inc., Hanover, MD 21076.)*

An additional resource is the *Occupational Information Network* (O*NET) available from the U.S. Department of Labor.[67] It provides a database of occupational job requirements (e.g., required skills and knowledge, how and where the work is performed) and worker attributes. The O*NET system includes the O*NET database (files available as free downloads for application development), O*NET OnLine (access to O*NET information), and the O*NET Career Exploration Tools (career investigation and assessment tools).

On-Site Visit

The on-site visit to the workplace typically includes (1) analysis of the physical space, (2) observation of the patient/client performing work tasks within the environment in which they must be accomplished, (3) identification of safety issues, and (4) determination of the immediate or predicted risks of musculoskeletal injury for an individual worker. Data gathered during the on-site visit, information from the job analysis, and knowledge of functional abilities allow the therapist to determine if job requirements can be met and whether the patient can safely return to his or her previous employment. If return to work is feasible with modifications, these data also inform the therapist about establishing a *plan for risk reduction* with recommendations to eliminate the potential for injury, and to develop a *plan to optimize function* that includes suggestions for better fitting the job to the individual's anatomical and physiological characteristics in a way that enhances efficiency and performance. The principles of energy conservation, ergonomics, applied biomechanics, and anthropometrics provide the foundation for both prevention of injury and maximizing efficiency.

Many of the areas examined, recommendations made, and adaptive strategies employed in the home may be used in the work environment as well. Several considerations specific to the work setting are described below.

External Accessibility

A parking space should be available within a short distance of the building if the individual plans to drive to and from work. For wheelchair users, parking spaces should be a minimum of 96 in. (244 cm) wide, with an adjacent access aisle 60 in. (152 cm) wide. The location should be clearly marked as a reserved parking area. Additional aspects of external accessibility of the building should be addressed using the same guidelines as those presented for home exteriors.

Internal Accessibility

The immediate work area should be carefully examined. This includes lighting; temperature; seating surface (if other than a wheelchair); the height and size of the workstation (some patients may benefit from a variable height or tilting work surface); and exposure to noise, vibration, or fumes. Access to supplies, materials, or equipment should be considered with respect to the patient's vertical and horizontal reaching capabilities. Access to drinking fountains, dining areas, and bathrooms should also be addressed.

Given the prevalence of computer workstations in many employment settings, recommendations may likely be required to optimize efficiency and reduce the potential for trauma or repetitive stress injury from poorly designed work areas. A fully adjustable chair is an integral component of an ergonomic workstation.[68] The foundational requirements for workstation chairs are depicted in Figure 9.25. Although parameters vary for each individual, the general principles for positioning at a computer workstation include screen slightly below eye level, body centered directly in front of monitor and keyboard, forearms level or tilted slightly upward, wrists free while typing, lower back well supported, thighs horizontal on seating surface, and feet resting flat on the floor (Fig. 9.26).[68]

During examination of workstations for individuals using a wheelchair, functional sitting reach is an important consideration. From an upright wheelchair sitting position, the unobstructed high forward reach is a maximum of 48 in. (1,220 mm) from the floor and the low forward reach is a minimum of 15 in. (380 mm) from the floor (Fig. 9.27A). When the high forward reach is over a work surface of not greater than 20 in. (510 mm), the maximum reach distance is 48 in. (1,220 mm) from the floor

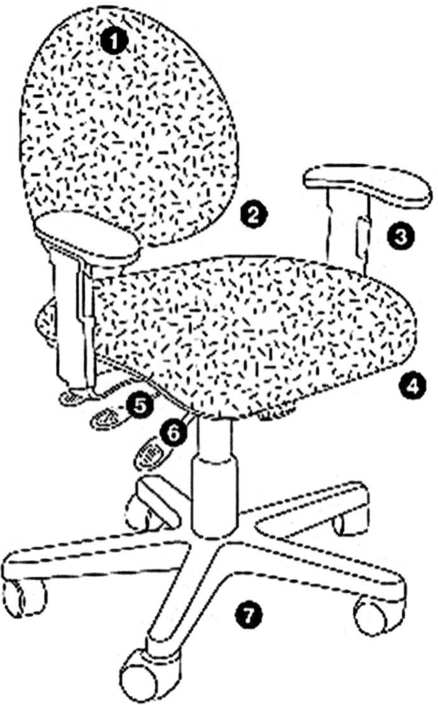

Figure 9.25 Overview of recommended features of workstation chair: (1) breathable, medium-texture upholstery; (2) adjustable lumbar support that moves up/down; (3) adjustable armrests; (4) seat with rounded front border (waterfall design); (5) adjustable seat that moves up and down and tilts forward and backward; (6) a tilt mechanism that tilts forward and backward; and (7) five-caster base with a full 360-degree swivel. *(From Workplace Ergonomics Reference Guide.[68, p. 4])*

(Fig. 9.27B). Progressively deeper work surfaces will alter the forward reach accordingly. For example, a work surface depth between 20 and 25 in. allows a maximum forward reach of not greater than 44 in. (1,120 mm) (Fig. 9.27C). With a floor obstruction of 10 in. (255 mm), the high side reach is a maximum of 48 in. (1,220 mm) and a low side reach of 15 in. (380 mm) minimum (Fig. 9. 27D). With an obstruction of a maximum of 24 in. (610 mm), the high side reach is a maximum of 46 in. (1,170 mm).[5] For individuals with good trunk control, reaching capacity will be increased.

Detailed resources are available to guide examination of the workplace. These include the *Americans with Disabilities Act (ADA) Regulations and Technical Assistance Materials*,[69] the *ADA Accessibility Guidelines* (ADAAG),[70] and the *2010 ADA Standard for Accessible Design*.[5] These documents are freely available and include the technical requirements for accessibility to buildings and facilities by individuals with disabilities under the Americans with Disabilities Act of 1990. A comprehensive source of information about the ADA is provided at the U.S. Department of Justice's ADA home page.[71]

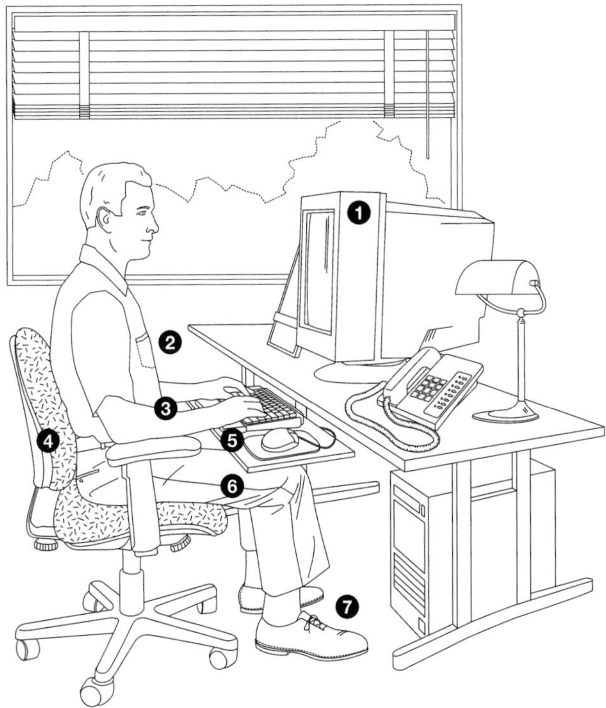

Figure 9.26 Overview of positioning recommendations for computer workstations: (1) monitor screen top slightly below eye level; (2) body centered in front of the monitor and keyboard; (3) forearms level or tilted up slightly; (4) lower back supported by chair; (5) wrists free while typing; (6) thighs horizontal; and (7) feet resting flat on the floor. *(From Workplace Ergonomics Reference Guide.[68, p. 2])*

COMMUNITY ACCESS

To attain the goal of full accessibility, community resources, services, and facilities must be investigated. When direct involvement by the therapist is not possible, this may best be accomplished by providing the patient and family with guidelines for exploring access to local facilities.

An important consideration is to refer the patient and family to community organizations such as the Arthritis Foundation, National Easter Seal Society, Multiple Sclerosis Society, the Mayor's Office, Chamber of Commerce, or the Veterans Administration. These groups can provide information on services available to individuals with a disability who reside in the community. Individuals returning to school should be encouraged to contact the campus Office for Students with Disabilities or the Student Services Office, which function to ensure appropriate and reasonable accommodations are available to facilitate an optimal learning environment for students with disabilities. Information is typically available on accessible housing and transportation, and general campus resources.

Transportation

The availability of accessible public transportation varies considerably among geographical areas. As such, careful exploration by the patient and family will be needed to determine what resources are obtainable in specific locales. Many communities provide at least part-time service of partially or completely accessible buses. These include the so-called "kneeling buses" equipped with a hydraulic unit that lowers the entrance to curb level for easier boarding (Fig. 9.28) and those designed with hydraulic lifts at the center of the bus to allow direct entry by an individual using a wheelchair (Fig. 9.29). A more recent design features a flip-out ramp for wheelchair access positioned at the front entrance to the bus.

Not all public transportation systems in the United States allow use by individuals who are nonambulatory or by those with limited ambulatory capacity. However,

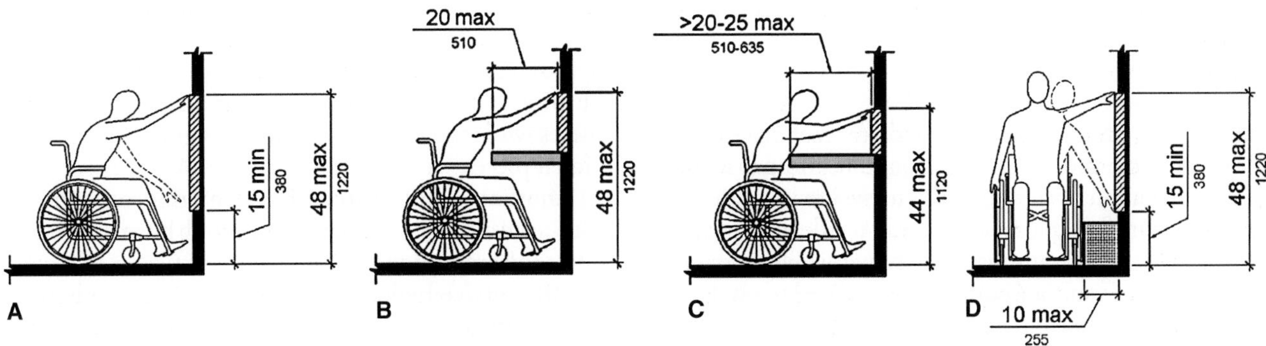

Figure 9.27 (A) Unobstructed high forward reach is a maximum of 48 in. (1,220 mm) from the floor and the low forward reach is a minimum of 15 in. (380 mm) from the floor. (B) High forward reach over a 20-in.-deep (510-mm-deep) work surface is a maximum of 48 in. (1,220 mm) from the floor. (C) A work surface depth of 20 to 25 in. (510 to 635 mm) allows a maximum forward reach of not greater than 44 in. (1,120 mm) from the floor. (D) For a reach depth of 10 in. (255 mm), the high side reach is a maximum of 48 in. (1,220 mm). With a floor obstruction of 10 in. (225 mm), the high side reach is a maximum of 48 in. (1,220 mm) and a low reach of 15 in. (380 mm) minimum. Values denoted in inches and millimeters. *(From 2010 ADA Standards for Accessible Design.[5, p.114–115])*

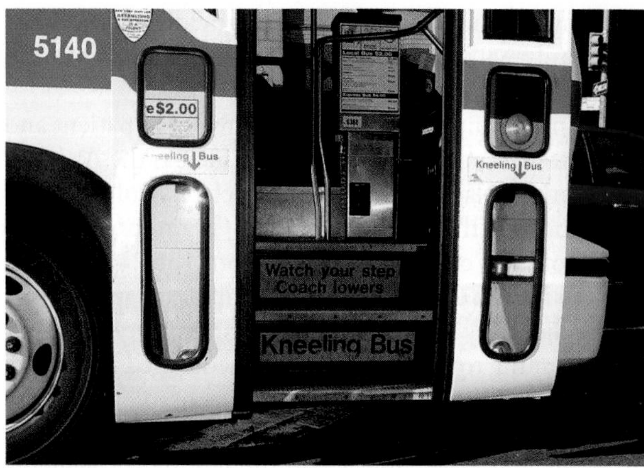

Figure 9.28 A kneeling bus lowers the steps to within 3 to 6 in. of the curb. Buses designed to kneel typically display a sign (Kneeling ↓ Bus) either on or next to the door.

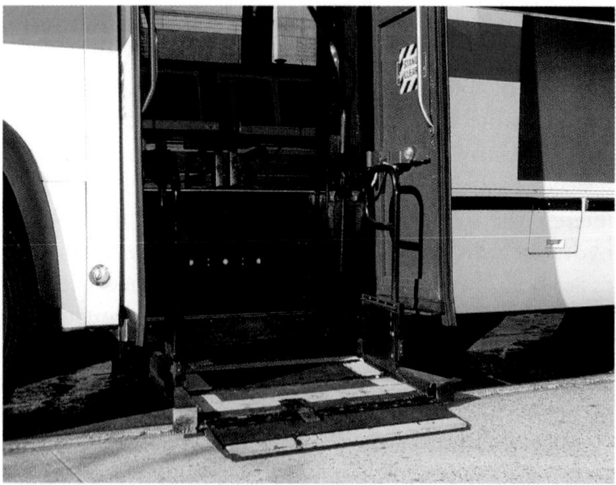

Figure 9.29 Bus lifts can accommodate wheelchairs and motorized scooters. The international wheelchair symbol for accessibility is typically displayed on the doors of the bus.

many urban transit systems are gradually making accommodations for individuals with mobility impairments (e.g., installation of elevators, alternatives to turnstile entrances, identified space for wheelchair riders). In many areas where public transportation is unavailable, door-to-door accessible van transportation is provided to residents with disabilities. Again, availability of such services may be limited in some rural locations.

Some patients will want to master driving an adapted automobile or van. This, of course, will significantly improve opportunities for community travel. Motor vehicle adaptations are selected based on the physical capabilities of the individual. Common adaptive equipment includes hand controls to operate the brakes and the accelerator; control panels mounted directly on steering wheel to control windshield wipers, turn indicators, and high/low beams; steering wheel attachments, such as knobs or universal cuffs, for individuals with limited grip strength; lifting units to assist with placement of the wheelchair into the vehicle; and, for patients with tetraplegia or high-level paraplegia, self-contained lifting platforms for entry to a van while remaining seated in a wheelchair. Driver training programs are often taught by occupational therapists and offered in most large rehabilitation centers.

For patients whose capacity for long-distance ambulation is limited and/or whose endurance is low, community-going battery-powered scooters (Fig. 9.30) may be a practical alternative for travel within a reasonable proximity of the home.

Access to Community Facilities

Area facilities used by the patient should be explored for the availability of appropriate parking areas; beveled curbs; external and internal structural accessibility of buildings; and availability of accessible drinking fountains, bathrooms, and restaurants. Theaters, auditoriums, and lecture halls must be considered with respect to accessible seating areas. Many such public presentation spaces are designed with accessible isles leading to open floor space (sufficiently wide to accommodate two wheelchairs side by side) interspersed within rows of standard seats. This allows the individual using a wheelchair the option of either sitting next to a person who is ambulatory or someone using a wheelchair. In addition to these general considerations, stores and shopping areas should also be inspected for access to merchandise (especially for individuals using a wheelchair), appropriate aisle widths, and adequate space at checkout counters.

Some theater companies offer "touch tours" for individuals who are blind or have impaired vision, allowing them to learn about the visual elements of the production. These multisensory experiences supplement for the lack of detail provided by a live performance and are led by cast, crew, and/or management. They provide an opportunity for participants to touch and handle theater pieces while tour guides explain the significance of individual pieces.[72]

Another useful source of information on community access is the guidebook offered by many larger cities (often funded by the mayor's office or as a community service by local businesses). These guides provide information on accessibility of local cultural, civic, and religious institutions; government offices; theaters; hotels; restaurants; shopping areas; transportation; and social and recreational facilities. These publications usually can be obtained from the city's chamber of commerce, the mayor's office, or the office of tourism. Many of these guides are available online. Combined use of such guides and phoning ahead for details of accessibility will facilitate travel both within and outside the local community.

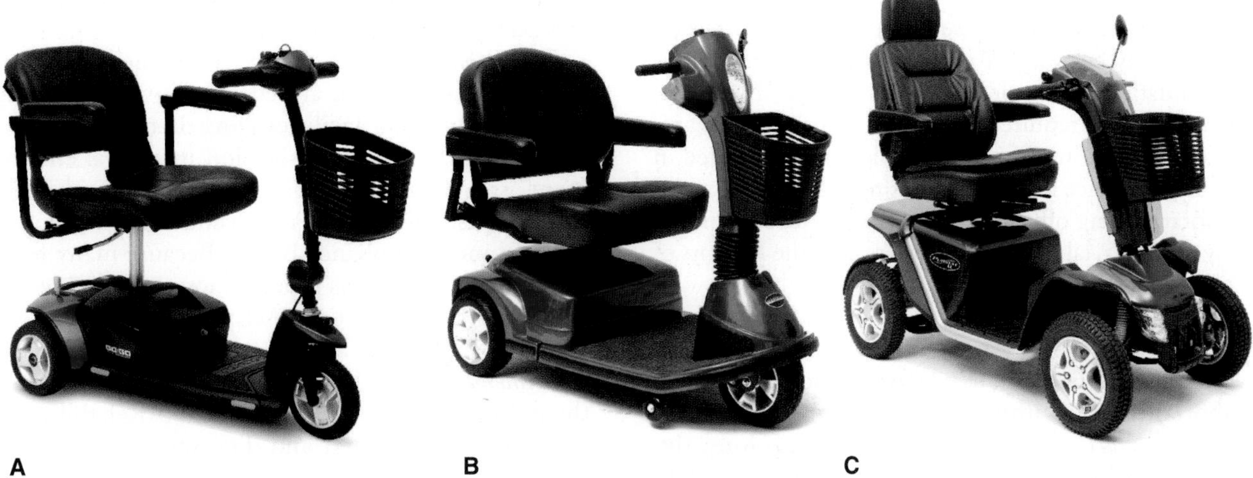

Figure 9.30 Examples of motorized scooters suitable for outdoor travel. (A) This lightweight scooter has a weight capacity of 275 lb (124.74 kg), a maximum speed of 4.25 miles per hour (mph), and a turning radius of 35.5 in. (90.17 cm). (B) This model includes a heavy-duty drivetrain with a weight capacity of 500 lb (226.8 kg), a maximum speed of 5.25 mph, with a turning radius of 50.38 in. (127.96 cm). (C) This unit features a reclining back with headrest, large pneumatic tires, a weight capacity of 400 lb (181.44 kg), a maximum speed of 8.25 mph, with a turning radius of 82.5 in. (209.55 cm). *(Courtesy of Pride Mobility Products, Exeter, PA 18643.)*

DOCUMENTATION

Once examination of the environment is complete, a final report is prepared that includes information from each participating team member. This report consists of information obtained from the home and, if applicable, the workplace or school setting. Information should also be included about the measures taken to explore general community accessibility. Data used in documentation are included in Tables 9.1 and 9.4.

Additional information should include (1) a description of the methods used to assist the patient in functional mobility (ambulation or wheelchair), (2) identification of the type and quantity of adaptive equipment required (including source and cost), and (3) explanation of recommended modifications with precise specifications for needed changes. AT recommendations, if utilized, should also be included. If an examination form, survey, or checklist was used during the on-site visit, it should be included with documentation or the data summarized in narrative form.

Documentation related to community access should include verification of the patient's knowledge of available community resources. The sources of this information, as well as whether team members were directly or indirectly involved in the community investigation, should be reported.

The completed report is then included in the patient's health record. Copies of the report are typically submitted to the patient and family, the physician, third-party payer(s) or other potential funding sources, and any community-based health care or social service agencies that will be providing care.

FUNDING SOURCES

Modifications to the physical environment and obtaining needed AT or adaptive equipment is typically very costly. Funding is not abundant and securing finances often presents a considerable challenge. The patient and family will require guidance in this area to achieve optimal accessibility and function. The social worker is an important source of information about state and local resources. The Internet also provides a rich source of funding information. Many states maintain individual websites devoted to funding sources for accessible housing and provide information about loan and grant programs.

Other potential sources of funding include home equity or other types of bank loans, the Veterans Administration, the Division of Vocational Rehabilitation, and the Workers' Compensation Commission. Local chapters of national civic groups (e.g., Kiwanis International, Veterans of Foreign Wars, Masons/Shriners Lodges, Lions International) or diagnosis-specific organizations (e.g., National Muscular Dystrophy Association, National Stroke Association, National Multiple Sclerosis Society, National Parkinson Foundation) can also be a valuable source of funding.

An important consideration is that not all patients will have current housing that is amenable to modification (e.g., an individual who previously lived in a third-floor walk-up apartment and now uses a wheelchair). In such instances, the local Housing and Urban Development Office will be an important resource. This office can provide a listing of accessible housing within the community.

Finally, creative funding for specific items (such as specialized adaptive equipment not covered by other resources) may be available through private organizations or foundations. Considerable time, research, and perseverance may be required in locating a receptive organization. General suggestions that might be considered in seeking assistance include contacting local businesses or corporate giving offices, civic or service clubs, churches or synagogues, labor unions, Jaycees, and the Knights of Columbus.

LEGISLATION

Much federal attention has been focused on the importance of environmental accessibility. Through legislation and a variety of private organizations, significant strides have been made in this area. In 1990, the *Americans with Disabilities Act* was signed into law. This legislation is among the most comprehensive of the civil rights laws enacted for individuals with disabilities. It guarantees civil rights protection and equal opportunity in the areas of government services, employment, public transportation, privately owned transportation available to the public, telephone service, and public accommodations.[73] This law requires that all "public places of accommodation" be made accessible to people with a disability unless it imposes "undue hardship" to the establishment. This law specifies that restaurants, movie theaters, hotels, professional offices, retail stores, and so forth, make reasonable accommodations.

With respect to an individual, disability is defined in the ADA as "a physical or mental impairment that substantially limits one or more major life activities of such an individual; a record of such impairment; or being regarded as having such impairment."[73, p. 4] Undue hardship includes excessive direct cost of adapting the environment, limited resources of the establishment, or situations where these changes would fundamentally alter the nature or daily operation of a business. The ADA also provides a federal tax credit incentive for measures taken by businesses to comply with this law.

The *Fair Housing Amendment Act of 1988* prohibits discrimination in housing on the basis of race, color, religion, gender, disability, familial status, and national origin. The Act includes private housing, state and local government housing, and any housing that receives federal financial support. The Act requires that accessible units be included in all new multiple-dwelling buildings with four or more units. It requires landlords to allow individuals with disabilities to make reasonable, access-related modifications to their living space, as well as common areas of the building. However, the landlord is not required to pay for these modifications. To promote adherence, the Fair Housing Amendment Act also provides accessible construction standards for multifamily housing units built for first occupancy after March 1991.

The *Rehabilitation Act of 1973* provided that access must be established in all federally funded buildings and transportation facilities constructed after 1968. The law prohibits discrimination in federal employment, stipulates accessibility within federal buildings, and established the Architectural Transportation Barriers and Compliance Board. Because many federally funded institutions provided low compliance with the 1973 Rehabilitation Act, an amendment was passed in 1978. The *Comprehensive Rehabilitation Services Amendments* (P.L. 95-602) of 1978 strengthened the enforcement of the original 1973 Rehabilitation Act. The Architectural and Transportation Barriers Compliance Board is the governing body responsible for enforcing this legislation.

The *Architectural Barrier Act of 1968* (P.L. 90-480) provided that certain buildings that were financed by federal funds be designed and constructed "to insure that physically handicapped persons will have ready access to, and use of, such buildings."[74, p. 719] Another important item of legislation related to environmental accessibility is the *Public Buildings Act of 1983,* which functioned to establish public building policies for the federal government. This Act (section 307) provided several amendments to the Architectural Barrier Act of 1968 to further strengthen and delineate the importance of accessibility. The term *fully accessible* in this Act was defined as "the absence or elimination of physical and communications barriers to the ingress, egress, movement within, and use of a building by handicapped persons and the incorporation of such equipment as is necessary to provide such ingress, egress, movement, and use and, in a building of historic, architectural, or cultural significance, the elimination of such barriers and the incorporation of such equipment in such a manner as to be compatible with the significant architectural features of the building to the maximum extent possible."[75, p. 373]

The *Telecommunications Act of 1996* applies to all telecommunication equipment and services. It stipulates that manufacturers of "telecommunications equipment or customer premises equipment shall ensure that the equipment is designed, developed, and fabricated to be accessible to and usable by individuals with disabilities, if readily achievable."[76 p. S.652-20] The Act also provides a similar accessibility directive to providers of telecommunications services.

Despite the gains made in environmental accessibility, barriers continue to exist. Inasmuch as most public transportation systems were built before 1968, accessibility is not required by law. However, the ADA indicates that all concerns that offer public transit along a fixed route must also provide buses that are accessible to individuals with disabilities, including access by wheelchairs. Other areas that continue to be problematic include revolving doors, the design of many supermarkets and shopping areas (barriers imposed by checkout areas and items displayed on high shelves), lack of available parking spaces, multiple levels of stairs at the entrance to some buildings, and the design of some theaters and auditoriums that do not have specifically designated areas for individuals using a wheelchair.

The ADA homepage[71] provides an extensive listing of links to available ADA publications, as well as links to federal resources. Appendix 9.D provides Web-based resources for clinicians, patients, and families.

SUMMARY

Examination of the environment is an important factor in facilitating the patient's transition to the home, work, and community. The rehabilitation team uses the data to determine the level of patient access, safety, and function within the environment. The information is also used to determine the need for ATs, environmental modifications, outpatient services, and adaptive equipment. In addition, the examination assists in preparing the patient, family, and/or work colleagues and employer for the individual's return to a given setting.

This chapter has presented a sample approach to examination and modification of the environment. Common features of the physical environmental that typically warrant consideration have been highlighted. Inasmuch as a return to a former environment is often a primary goal of rehabilitation, early consideration of these issues is warranted. Collaboration among team members, the patient, family, and caregivers will ensure an optimum and highly individualized patient–environment interface.

Although increasing numbers of residential spaces and public buildings are designed to provide accessibility, this area warrants further involvement from therapists. Physical therapists are particularly effective advocates for individuals with disability. They are also well prepared to assume leadership roles in assuring compliance with existing and new laws as well as providing valuable input to planning barrier-free environments and modification of existing structures.

Questions for Review

1. Differentiate among the terms barriers, accessibility, accessible design, and universal design.
2. What are the purposes for performing an examination of the environment?
3. What types of tests and measures are used for examination of environmental factors?
4. Identify an inherent shortcoming of self-report instruments designed to gather information about functional performance within the respondent's environment. How can accuracy of reporting be improved?
5. Assume you are preparing for an on-site visit to examine a patient's home environment. What preliminary information is needed that may influence the type and extent of recommendations?
6. During a home visit, you find that a wheelchair user's bathroom door width measures 31 in. wide (77.74 cm). The patient owns the 50-year-old home and plans to remain in the dwelling. What options are available to modify the environment by increasing the bathroom door width?
7. An initial aspect of examining a patient's ability to return to previous employment involves determining the functional job requirements. Describe the information required.
8. What is a functional capacity evaluation (FCE)? How are data from the FCE used (i.e., what decisions are informed by the data?)

CASE STUDY

A 78-year-old woman with a diagnosis of osteoarthritis was admitted for a right total hip replacement. The patient reported a long-standing history of discomfort. She described the hip pain as radiating posteriorly to the buttock and low back and was exacerbated by weight-bearing and stair climbing. Over the past 12 months she has experienced a very marked increase in pain and stiffness. Radiographic findings demonstrated degenerative changes of both the acetabulum and femoral head consistent with osteoarthritis. The surgical intervention replaced the right femoral head and neck with a metallic prosthesis and polyethylene (plastic) lined acetabular cup. Past medical history is unremarkable.

SOCIAL HISTORY

The patient is a retired manager of a small accounting firm that she and her husband established. Her husband is deceased. She has three grown children who all live in neighboring communities. Before the activity limitations imposed by the hip pain, the patient had been independent in all BADL and IADL. She also volunteered her accounting services one day per week to a local charity that provides meals to homebound individuals. She was a regular participant in family outings; enjoyed going to the theater, concerts, and special museum events; and was an active member of the community's historical preservation society. Recently, these activities had to be curtailed owing to the increased hip discomfort.

She essentially had no activities outside the home for 3 months before admission and used a walker to minimize weight-bearing and reduce pain. She also required the assistance of a home aide 4 hours a day, two times per week (primarily for shopping, errands, and some household management tasks). She expressed considerable distress at being unable to take a bath and having to rely on the assistance of another person for some basic care activities. She had been using aspirin for its analgesic and anti-inflammatory effects. However, the pain experienced in recent months was not alleviated by the aspirin and other conservative measures she has been instructed to use (e.g., local applications of heat, periodic rest intervals, and gentle ROM exercises). The patient has medical insurance coverage and is without financial concerns.

REVIEW OF SYSTEMS

Cognitive function: Intact.

Vision: Wears corrective lens; experiences night blindness, which she describes as seeing poorly in dim light and her eyes take several seconds longer than normal to adjust from brightness to dimness.

Hearing: Intact.

Strength—upper extremities:

- Generally, within functional limits; patient reports some sporadic episodes of wrist and finger stiffness on awakening in the morning and after periods of immobility.
- Grip strength is reduced bilaterally (manual muscle testing [MMT] of finger flexors = G–).
- Heberden's nodes noted at the distal interphalangeal (DIP) and proximal interphalangeal (PIP) joints of the left index finger. Patient denies pain in wrist or fingers.

Strength—lower extremities:

- Left: within functional limits.
- Right: within functional limits (hip motions not tested owing to surgical intervention); crepitus noted in right knee.
- Weight-bearing status on right lower extremity: partial weight-bearing.

Range of motion: Within functional limits (with the exception of the right hip, which was not tested).

Postsurgical right hip precautions: No hip flexion beyond 90°. Avoid crossing one leg or ankle over the other. Avoid internal rotation of right lower extremity.

Coordination: Within normal limits.

Sensation: Intact.

Gait: The patient is ambulating functional distances on level surfaces with supervision using bilateral standard aluminum axillary crutches with partial weight-bearing on the right lower extremity. Stair-climbing requires minimal assistance. It is anticipated the patient will be independent with household ambulation on level surfaces at time of discharge from the hospital.

PATIENT GOALS

The patient is extremely motivated to be independent in personal care and household management. The prosthetic replacement has successfully relieved much of the pain experienced in the hip before surgery (most of her current discomfort is described as "minor" and associated with the surgical incision). She would also like to return to her family, volunteer, social, and leisure activities. She is very determined to discontinue the home aide as soon as possible.

HOME ENVIRONMENT

The patient lives alone in a fifth-floor apartment in a building with an elevator. The living space is a one-bedroom apartment on a single level. At your request, one of the patient's children has provided dimensions of door frames and height of sleeping and seating surfaces together with several photographs of each room of the patient's home. The physical dimensions and photographs provide the following information:

- Bedroom: two small area rugs, a nightstand with an alarm clock, a bureau, a wooden four-poster bed in the middle of room with a sleeping surface 1.5 ft (46 cm) from the floor, and a ceiling lamp fixture controlled by a switch adjacent to the door.
- Bathroom: an area rug, standard toilet and sink, bathtub does not include a shower, a doorway entrance 30 in. (76 cm) wide.
- Kitchen: polished linoleum floors, adequate counter space, and a dining table in the center of the room with standard kitchen chairs.
- Living room: overstuffed upholstered furniture with low seating surfaces, a favorite rocking chair, a large carpet that appears to ripple in several areas, a centered coffee table, a telephone with an extra-long extension wire placed on the coffee table, a remote-controlled television, two end tables, and a bookcase.
- Hallway (between rooms): poorly lit with a long, narrow area rug.

GUIDING QUESTIONS

With general knowledge of the patient's living space, what environmental modifications, adaptive equipment, or additional instruction would you suggest or provide to optimize safety and function in each of the following areas of the home?

1. Bedroom
2. Bathroom
3. Kitchen
4. Living room
5. Hallway

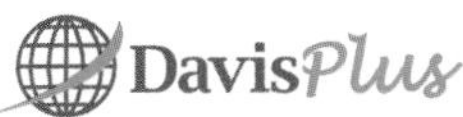

For additional resources, including answers to the questions for review and case study guiding questions, please visit **http://davisplus.fadavis.com.**

References

1. Corcoran, M, and Gitlin, L: The role of the physical environment in occupational performance. In Christiansen, CH, and Baum, CM (eds): Occupational Therapy Enabling Function and Well-Being, ed 2. Slack, Thorofare, NJ, 1997, p. 336.
2. Lawton, MP, et al: Assessing environments for older people with chronic illness. J Ment Health Aging 3:83, 1997.
3. *Guide to Physical Therapist Practice 3.0.* Alexandria, VA: American Physical Therapy Association; 2014. Available at: http://guidetoptpractice.apta.org/.
4. American National Standard Institute: Accessible and Usable Buildings and Facilities. International Code Council, Washington, DC, 2010. Retrieved September 8, 2018 from https://www.cds.hawaii.edu/projects/hvc/wp-content/uploads/sites/25/2017/08/Accessible-and-Usable-Buildings-and-Facilities-ICC-A111.1-2009-Chapter-10-Dwelling-Units-and-Sleeping-Units-2011.pdf
5. Department of Justice (DOJ): 2010 ADA Standards for Accessible Design. US DOJ, Washington, DC, 20301. Retrieved February 25, 2017, from www.ada.gov/regs2010/2010ADAStandards/2010ADAStandards.pdf.
6. World Health Organization (WHO): International Classification of Functioning, Disability and Health: ICF. WHO, Geneva, Switzerland, 2001. Retrieved February 24, 2017, from www.who.int/classifications/icf/en/.
7. Steinfeld, E, and Maisel, J: Universal Design: Designing Inclusive Environments. John Wiley & Sons, Hoboken, NJ, 2012.
8. World Health Organization (WHO): World Report on Disability. WHO, Geneva, Switzerland, 2011. Retrieved February 24, 2017, from http://www.who.int/disabilities/world_report/2011/en/.
9. Sanford, JA: Design for the Ages: Universal Design as a Rehabilitation Strategy. Springer, New York, NY, 2012.
10. The Center for Health Design (CHD): An Introduction to Evidence-Based Design: Exploring Healthcare and Design, ed 2. CHD, Concord, CA, 2010.
11. Whitemyer, D: The Future of Evidence-Based Design. Perspective (International Interior Design Association [IIDA]), Spring 2010. Retrieved February 25, 2017, from www.iida.org/resources/category/1/1/1/6/documents/sp10-ebd.pdf.
12. Connell, BR, et al: The Principles of Universal Design. The Center for Universal Design, North Carolina State University College of Design, Raleigh, NC, 1997 (updated 2011). Retrieved February 25, 2017, from www.ncsu.edu/ncsu/design/cud/about_ud/udprinciples.htm.
13. Martich, D: Telehealth Nursing: Tools and Strategies for Optimal Patient Care. Springer, New York, 2017.
14. Dewar, A, et al: Developing a measure of engagement with telehealth systems: The mHealth Technology Engagement. J Telemed Telecare 23(2):248, 2017.
15. Rajiv, J, et al: Monitoring of chronic disease in the community: Australian telehealth study on organizational challenges and economic impact. IJIC 16(6):1 (Suppl), 2016.
16. Center for Connected Health Policy (CCHPCA): What Is Telehealth? CCHPCA, Sacramento, CA. Retrieved February 27, 2017, from www.cchpca.org/what-is-telehealth.
17. Edirippulige, S, and Armfield, NR: Education and training to support the use of clinical telehealth: A review of the literature. J Telemed Telecare 23(2):273, 2017.
18. Doorenbos, AZ, et al: Enhancing access to cancer education for rural healthcare providers via telehealth. J Cancer Educ 26(4):682, 2011.
19. Mori, DL, et al: Promoting physical activity in individuals with diabetes: Telehealth approaches. Diabetes Spectr 24(3):127, 2011.
20. Young, JD, and Badowski, ME: Telehealth: Increasing access to high quality care by expanding the role of technology in correctional medicine. J Clin Med 6(2), 2017.
21. Radhakrishnan, K, and Jacelon, C: Impact of telehealth on patient self-management of heart failure: A review of literature. J Cardiovasc Nurs 27(1):33, 2012.

22. Suter, P, Suter, WN, and Johnston, D: Theory-based telehealth and patient empowerment. Popul Health Manage 14(2):87, 2011.
23. Albert, N, et al: Factors associated with telemonitoring use among patients with chronic heart failure. J Telemed Telecare 23(2):228, 2017.
24. Huijbregts, MPJ, McEwen, S, and Taylor, D: Exploring the feasibility and efficacy of a telehealth stroke self-management programme: A pilot study. Physiother Can 61(4):210, 2009.
25. Lee, ACW, and Billings, M: Telehealth implementation in a skilled nursing facility: Case report for physical therapist practice in Washington. Phys Ther 96(2):252, 2016.
26. Hwang, R, et al: Assessing functional exercise capacity using telehealth: Is it valid and reliable inpatient with chronic heart failure? J Telemed Telecare 23(2):225, 2017.
27. Lee, ACW: The VISYTER telerehabilitation system for globalizing physical therapy consultation: Issues and challenges for telehealth implementation (Case Report). J Phys Ther Educ 26(1):90, 2012.
28. Lee, ACW, and Harada, N: Telehealth as a means of health care delivery for physical therapist practice. Phys Ther 92(3):463, 2012.
29. Shaw, DK: Overview of telehealth and its application to cardiopulmonary physical therapy. Cardiopulm Phys Ther J 20(2):13, 2009.
30. American Physical Therapy Association (APTA): Telehealth—Definitions and Guidelines BOD G03-06-09-19 (Retitled: Telehealth; Amended BOD G03-03-07-12; Initial BOD 11-01-28-70) (Guideline). APTA, Alexandria, VA (document updated December 14, 2009). Retrieved February 27, 2017, from www.apta.org/uploadedFiles/APTAorg/About_Us/Policies/BOD/Practice/TelehealthDefinitionsGuidelines.pdf#search=%22Telehealth%20–%20Definitions%20Guidelines%22.
31. Sanford, JA, et al: Using telerehabilitation to identify home modification needs. Assist Technol 16(1):43, 2004.
32. Duncan, P, et al: Functional reach: A new clinical measure of balance. J Gerontol 45:M192, 1990.
33. Duncan, P, et al: Functional reach: Predictive validity in a sample of elderly male veterans. J Gerontol 47:M93, 1992.
34. Weiner, D, et al: Functional reach: A marker of physical frailty. J Am Geriatr Soc 40:203, 1992.
35. Newton, R: Balance screening of an inner city older adult population. Arch Phys Med Rehabil 78:587, 1997.
36. Newton, R: Validity of the multi-directional reach test: A practical measure for limits of stability in older adults. J Gerontol Med Sci 56A:M248, 2001.
37. Podsiadlo, D, and Richardson, S: The timed "Up and Go": A test of basic mobility for frail elderly persons. J Am Geriatr Soc 39:142, 1991.
38. Tinetti, M, et al: A fall risk index for elderly patients based on number of chronic disabilities. Am J Med 80:429, 1986.
39. Tinetti, M, and Ginter, S: Identifying mobility dysfunctions in elderly patients: Standard neuromuscular examination or direct assessment? JAMA 259:1190, 1988.
40. Faber, MJ, Bosscher, RJ, and van Wieringen, PC: Clinimetric properties of the Performance-Oriented Mobility Assessment. Phys Ther 86(7):944, 2006.
41. Berg, K, et al: Measuring balance in the elderly: Preliminary development of an instrument. Physiother Can 41:304, 1989.
42. Berg, K, et al: A comparison of clinical and laboratory measures of postural balance in an elderly population. Arch Phys Med Rehabil 73:1073, 1992.
43. Berg, K, et al: Measuring balance in the elderly: Validation of an instrument. Can J Public Health 83(Suppl 2):S7, 1992.
44. Berg, K, et al: The Balance Scale: Reliability assessment for elderly residents and patients with an acute stroke. Scand J Rehabil Med 27:27, 1995.
45. Keysor, J, Jette, A, and Haley, S: Development of the Home and Community Environment (HACE) instrument. J Rehabil Med 37(1):37, 2005.
46. Keysor, JJ, et al: Association of environmental factors with levels of home and community participation in an adult rehabilitation cohort. Arch Phys Med Rehabil 87(12):1566, 2006.
47. Home and Community Environment (HACE) Survey: Instrument and Scoring Manual, 2008. Retrieved February 28, 2017, from www.bu.edu/enact/files/2011/05/HACE-Survey-and-Manual-v1_7-30-2008.pdf.
48. Whiteneck, GG, et al: Quantifying handicap: A new measure of long-term rehabilitation outcomes. Arch Phys Med Rehabil 73(6):519, 1992.
49. Whiteneck, G, et al: Environmental factors and their role in participation and life satisfaction after spinal cord injury. Arch Phys Med Rehabil 85(11):1793, 2004.
50. Gontkovsky, ST, Russum, P, and Stokic, DS: Comparison of the CIQ and CHART Short Form in assessing community integration in individuals with chronic spinal cord injury: A pilot study. NeuroRehabilitation 24(2):185, 2009.
51. Whiteneck, GG, et al: Craig Handicap Assessment and Reporting Technique. Craig Hospital, Englewood, CO, 1992. Retrieved February 28, 2017, from https://craighospital.org/uploads/CraigHospital.CHARTManual.pdf.
52. Whiteneck, GG, Gerhart, KA, and Cusick, CP: Identifying environmental factors that influence the outcomes of people with traumatic brain injury. J Head Trauma Rehabil 19(3):191, 2004.
53. Whiteneck, GG, et al: Quantifying environmental factors: A measure of physical, attitudinal, service, productivity, and policy barriers. Arch Phys Med Rehabil 85(8):1324, 2004.
54. Ephraim, PL, et al: Environmental barriers experienced by amputees: The Craig Hospital Inventory of Environmental Factors—Short Form. Arch Phys Med Rehabil 87(3):328, 2006.
55. Craig Hospital Inventory of Environmental Factors (Version 3.0). Craig Hospital, Englewood, CO, 2001. Retrieved March 1, 2017, from www.rehabmeasures.org/Lists/RehabMeasures/Attachments/979/CHIEF%20Manual.pdf.
56. Gray, DB, et al: A subjective measure of environmental facilitators and barriers to participation for people with mobility limitations. Disabil Rehabil 30(6):434, 2008.
57. National Institutes of Health: Classification of Overweight and Obesity by BMI, Waist Circumference, and Associated Disease Risks. US Department of Health and Human Services, Washington, DC. Retrieved March 2, 2017, from www.nhlbi.nih.gov/health/educational/lose_wt/BMI/bmi_dis.htm.
58. Centers for Disease Control and Prevention (CDC): Prevalence of Obesity in the United States, 2009–2010. CDC, Atlanta, GA. Retrieved March 2, 2017, from www.cdc.gov/nchs/data/databriefs/db82.htm.
59. Schwab, C: A home that makes house calls (part 2). PN 65(2):23, 2011.
60. Gitlin, LN, et al: Factors associated with home environmental problems among community-living older people. Disabil Rehabil 23(17):777, 2001.
61. Assistive Technology Act of 1998. Retrieved March 3, 2017, from https://section508.gov/assistive-technology-act-1998.
62. Hunter, S: Using CQI to improve worker's health. PT Magazine of Physical Therapy 3(11):64, 1995.
63. American Physical Therapy Association (APTA): Glossary of Workers' Compensation Terms. APTA, Alexandria, VA, 22314, 2011. Retrieved March 4, 2017, from www.apta.org/Payment/WorkersCompensation/Glossary.
64. Talmage, JB, Melhorn, JM, and Hyman, MH (eds): AMA Guides to the Evaluation of Work Ability and Return to Work, ed 2. American Medical Association, Chicago, 2011.
65. Genovese, E, and Galper, JS (eds): Guide to the Evaluation of Functional Ability: How to Request, Interpret, and Apply Functional Capacity Evaluations. American Medical Association, Chicago, 2009.
66. Gibson, L, and Strong, J: A conceptual framework of functional capacity evaluation for occupational therapy in work rehabilitation. Austral Occup Ther J 50(2):64, 2003.
67. United States Department of Labor (DOL): O*NET—beyond information—intelligence. DOL, Washington, DC 20210. Retrieved March 4, 2017, from www.doleta.gov/programs/onet.
68. United States Department of Defense (DOD): Workplace Ergonomics Reference Guide: A Publication of the Computer/Electronic Accommodations Program, US DOD, Washington, DC 20301. Retrieved September 18, 2018, from http://cap.mil/Documents/CAP_Ergo_Guide.pdf.
69. Department of Justice (DOJ): ADA Regulations and Technical Assistance Materials. US DOJ, Washington, DC 20301. Retrieved March 4, 2017, from www.dinf.ne.jp/doc/english/Us_Eu/ada_e/ada/crt/ada/publicat.html.
70. ADA Accessibility Guidelines (ADAAG). Retrieved March 4, 2017, from www.access-board.gov/guidelines-and-standards/buildings-and-sites/about-the-ada-standards/background/adaag.
71. Department of Justice (DOJ): ADA Home Page. US DOJ, Washington, DC 20301. Retrieved March 6, 2017, from www.ada.gov.

72. Udo, JP, and Fels, DI: Enhancing the entertainment experience of blind and low-vision theatregoers through touch tours. Disabil Soc (2):231, 2010.
73. The Americans with Disabilities Act of 1990 (As Amended): Public Law 101-336. Retrieved March 4, 2017, from www.ada.gov/pubs/adastatute08.htm.
74. Architectural Barriers Act, Public Law 90-480, 1968.
75. Public Buildings Act, 98th Congress, 1st session, 1983.
76. Telecommunications Act of 1996. Retrieved March 4, 2017, from www.gpo.gov/fdsys/pkg/BILLS-104s652enr/pdf/BILLS-104s652enr.pdf.

Supplemental Readings

Aplin, T, Jonge, D, and Gustafsson, L: Understanding home modifications impact on clients and their family's experience of home: A Qualitative study. Aust Occup Ther J 62(2):123, 2015.

Bishop, M, et al: The prevalence and nature of modified housing and assistive devises use among Americans with multiple sclerosis. J Vocat Rehabil 42(2):153, 2015.

Chiatti, C, and Iwarsson, S: Evaluation of housing adaptation interventions: Integrating the economic perspective into occupational therapy practice. Scand J Occup Ther 21(5):323, 2014.

Cleland, V, et al: Environmental barriers and enablers to physical activity participation among rural adults: A qualitative study. Health Promot J Austr 26(2):99, 2015.

Heinemann, AW, et al: Measuring environmental factors: Unique and overlapping international classification of functioning, disability and health coverage of 5 instruments. Arch Phys Med Rehabil 97(12):2113, 2016.

Null, R: Universal Design: Principles and Models. Taylor and Francis Group, Boca Raton, FL, 2014.

Steinfeld, E, and Maisel, JL: Universal Design: Creating Inclusive Environments. Wiley, Hoboken, NJ, 2012.

Tepper, D: Making a house an accessible home: The role of PTs. PT in Motion 8(8):22, 2016.

Vasudevan, V, Rimmer, JH, and Kviz, F: Development of the Barriers to Physical Activity Questionnaire for people with mobility Impairments. Disabil Health J 8(4):547, 2015.

appendix 9.A

The Principles of Universal Design

The Principles of Universal Design

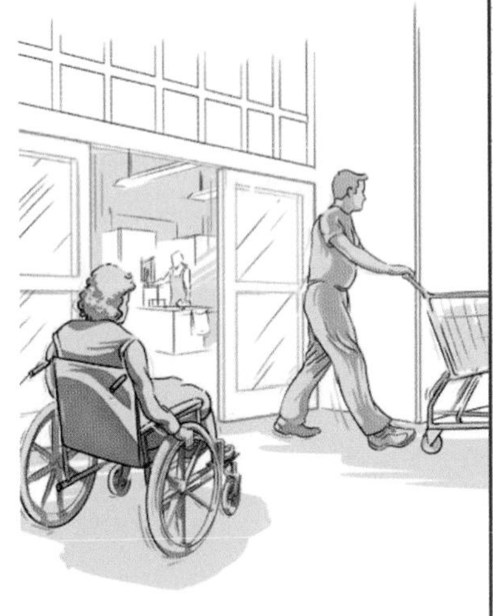

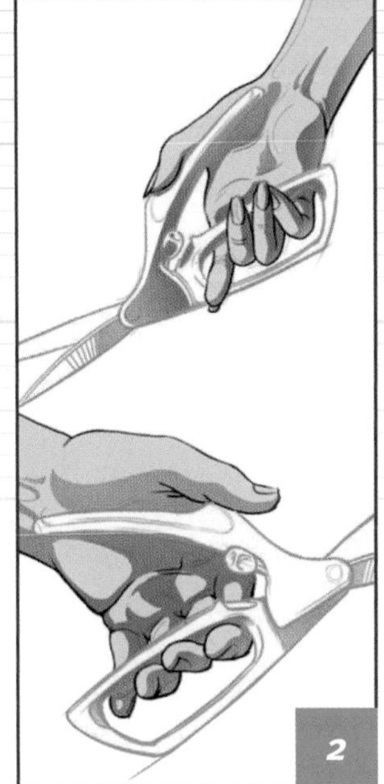

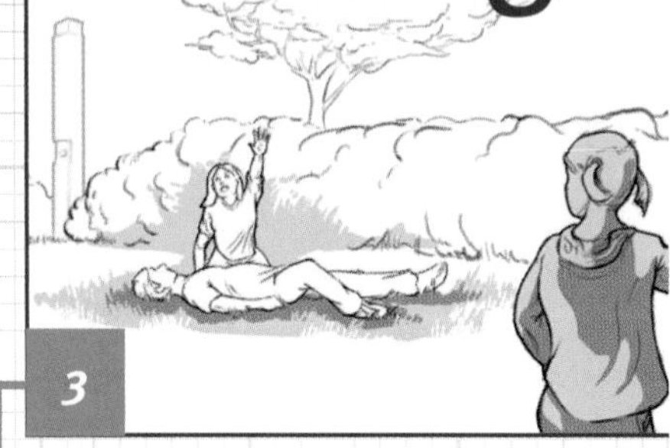

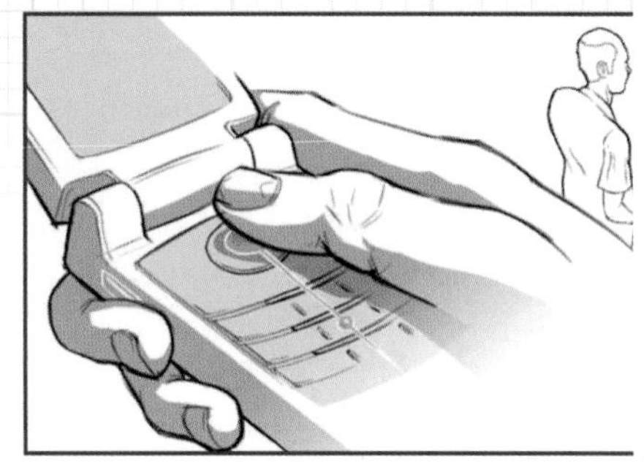

	1	2	3
PRINCIPLE	**Equitable Use** The design is useful and marketable to people with diverse abilities.	**Flexibility in Use** The design accommodates a wide range of individual preferences and abilities.	**Simple and Intuitive Use** Use of the design is easy to understand, regardless of the user's experience, knowledge, language skills, or education level.
GUIDELINES	1a. Provide the same means of use for all users: identical whenever possible; equivalent when not. 1b. Avoid segregating or stigmatizing any users. 1c. Provisions for privacy, security, and safety should be equally available to all users. 1d. Make the design appealing to all users.	2a. Provide choice in methods of use. 2b. Accommodate right- or left-handed access and use. 2c. Facilitate the user's accuracy and precision. 2d. Provide adaptability to the user's pace.	3a. Eliminate unnecessary complexity. 3b. Be consistent with user expectations and intuition. 3c. Accommodate a wide range of literacy and language skills. 3d. Arrange information consistent with its importance. 3e. Provide effective prompting and feedback during and after task completion.
EXAMPLES	• Power doors make visiting public spaces easier for all users. • E-mail makes communication easier for everyone, including people who have trouble communicating via phone.	Large grip scissors accommodates use with either hand and allows alternation between the two in repetitive tasks.	• Public emergency stations utilize recognized emergency colors and a simple design to quickly convey function to passers-by. • Intuitive ATM interfaces allow use without instruction or training.

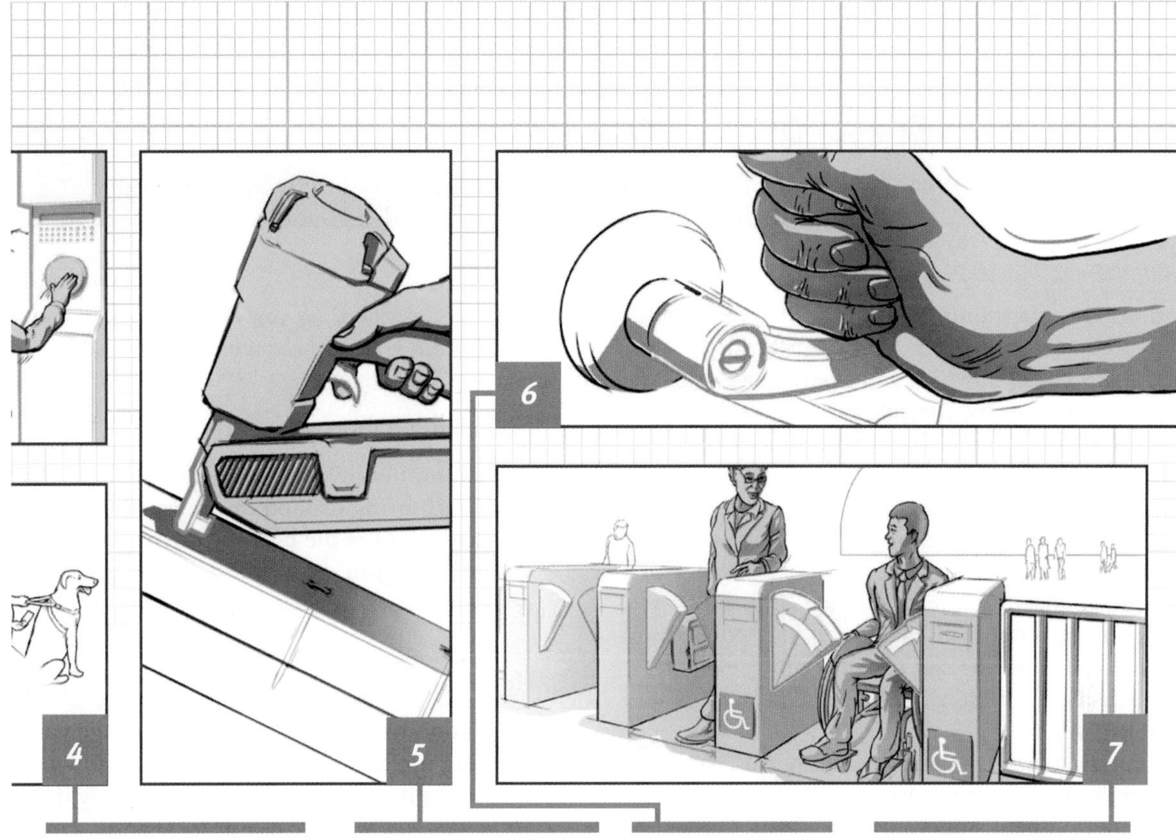

Perceptible Information

The design communicates necessary information effectively to the user, regardless of ambient conditions or the user's sensory abilities.

4a. Use different modes (pictorial, verbal, tactile) for redundant presentation of essential information.
4b. Provide adequate contrast between essential information and its surroundings.
4c. Maximize "legibility" of essential information.
4d. Differentiate elements in ways that can be described (i.e., make it easy to give instructions or directions).
4e. Provide compatibility with a variety of techniques or devices used by people with sensory limitations.

Small bumps on a cell phone keypad tell the user where important keys are without requiring the user to look at the keys.

Tolerance for Error

The design minimizes hazards and the adverse consequences of accidental or unintended actions.

5a. Arrange elements to minimize hazards and errors: most used elements, most accessible; hazardous elements eliminated, isolated, or shielded.
5b. Provide warnings of hazards and errors.
5c. Provide fail safe features.
5d. Discourage unconscious action in tasks that require vigilance.

The "sequential trip" mechanism on a nail gun prevents accidental firing when the tool is not pressed against an object.

Low Physical Effort

The design can be used efficiently and comfortably and with a minimum of fatigue.

6a. Allow user to maintain a neutral body position.
6b. Use reasonable operating forces.
6c. Minimize repetitive actions.
6d. Minimize sustained physical effort.

Door lever does not require grip strength to operate, and can even be operated by a closed fist or elbow.

Size and Space for Approach and Use

Appropriate size and space is provided for approach, reach, manipulation, and use regardless of user's body size, posture, or mobility.

7a. Provide a clear line of sight to important elements for any seated or standing user.
7b. Make reach to all components comfortable for any seated or standing user.
7c. Accommodate variations in hand and grip size.
7d. Provide adequate space for the use of assistive devices or personal assistance.

Wide gates at subway stations accommodate wheelchair users as well as commuters with packages or luggage.

appendix 9.B

Usability in My Home—A Self-Report Instrument

Directions: The questionnaire consists of two parts, with a number of questions about the design of the *physical housing environment* in which you live. You are asked to answer the questions by assessing how you feel that the design and form of the physical housing environment suits you, your needs, and your wishes.

By physical housing environment is meant here your home, the car park, garage, or parking space that you use if you have a car, your own letterbox, the dustbin/refuse storage place, the storage space, and the shared laundry, if there is one. This includes all the routes along which you move on the site to and from these places. It also includes a balcony, patio, and garden where applicable.

The questions are very general, and the aim is to capture your immediate perception of how the physical housing environment suits you.

For each question, there are seven response alternatives in the form of the numbers 1 to 7. The number 1 stands for what is the worst and lowest alternative for you, and 7 stands for the best and highest alternative. The numbers 2 to 6 describe the positions that lie between the best and the worst alternatives. The number 4 is the neutral point on the scale, neither good nor bad. Put a circle round the alternative that agrees best with your perception.

Example: If you are so dissatisfied with your physical housing environment that it could not, in your opinion, be worse for you, then circle the number 1. If you are so satisfied with the design of your physical housing environment that it could not, in your opinion, be better, then circle the number 7. You use the numbers 2 to 7 to describe how close to the best or worst alternative you find the features of your housing environment.

There now follow a number of questions about how well you feel that the design of your physical housing environment suits your needs and wishes. Some questions concern security, social interaction, and so forth, while others concern how the design of the housing environment makes it easy or difficult to do the everyday tasks you wish and need to perform.

Draw a circle round the number that you think agrees best with your own perception.

1. **In relation to how you normally manage your personal hygiene, dressing, visiting the toilet, or how you eat; to what extent is the housing environment suitably designed?** ***(If you do not manage any of these at all, cross out the whole question.)***

   1 2 3 4 5 6 7
   Not at all suitable — Very suitable

2. **In relation to how you normally manage your cooking/heating of food or preparation of snacks; to what extent is the housing environment suitably designed?** ***(If you do not manage any of these at all, cross out the whole question.)***

   1 2 3 4 5 6 7
   Not at all suitable — Very suitable

3. **In relation to how you normally manage your washing up, cleaning, care of flowers; to what extent is the housing environment suitably designed?** (***If you do not manage any of these at all, cross out the whole question.***)

   1 2 3 4 5 6 7
   Not at all suitable — Very suitable

4. **In relation to how you normally manage your washing, ironing, or repair of clothes; to what extent is the housing environment suitably designed?** (***If you do not manage any of these at all, cross out the whole question.***)

   1 2 3 4 5 6 7
   Not at all suitable — Very suitable

5. **How secure do you feel in your housing environment?**

   1 2 3 4 5 6 7
   Not at all suitable — Very suitable

6. **To what extent does the design of the housing environment allow you to be by yourself when you so wish?**

   1 2 3 4 5 6 7
   Not at all — As much as I want to

7. **To what extent does the design of the housing environment allow you to socialize with the friends and acquaintances you want to meet?**

   1 2 3 4 5 6 7
   Not at all — As much as I want to

8. To what extent does the design of the housing environment allow you to do hobbies/leisure pursuits and relax?

1 2 3 4 5 6 7
Not at all As much as I want to

9. If your health should change, to what extent would it be possible for you to make simple changes to your housing environment (e.g., to use a different parking place, to use a different toilet, to rearrange the furniture, to use a different room as a bedroom, and so forth)?

1 2 3 4 5 6 7
Not at all As much as I want to

There now follow a number of questions about how usable you feel your housing environment is. First you make an overall assessment (question 10). This is followed by a number of more detailed questions about usability in different parts of the housing environment. State the problems you perceive and make an assessment of how accessible each part of the housing environment is, with regard to the problems you have stated (questions 11 to 22). If you do not feel that there are any special problems, please say so. Do not forget to assess each part of the physical housing environment, even if you have not stated any specific problem.

10. How usable do you feel that your housing environment is in general?

1 2 3 4 5 6 7
Not at all usable Fully usable

11. What problems do you perceive in the physical environment just outside your home (e.g., paths and pavements, car park/garage/carport, the design of the refuse storage place, the placing of your letterbox, and so forth)?

____

____

12. In view of the above problems in question 11, how usable do you feel that the environment outside your home is?

1 2 3 4 5 6 7
Not at all usable Fully usable

13. What problems do you find in the design of the entrance to your home (e.g., heavy doors, narrow stairs, ramps, cramped lift, poor lighting, and so forth)?

____

____

14. In view of the above problems in question 13, how usable do you feel that the entrance to your home is?

1 2 3 4 5 6 7
Not at all usable Fully usable

15. What problems do you find in the design of the secondary spaces in your home (e.g., storerooms, attic/basement, refuse storage place, laundry [if any], and the routes you have to follow indoors to reach these places)?

____

____

16. In view of the above problems in question 15, how usable do you feel that the secondary spaces in your home are?

1 2 3 4 5 6 7
Not at all usable Fully usable

17. What problems do you have in reading and understanding markings and signs outside the building or at the entrance? (For example, are lift buttons fully visible and easy to use? Are the signs at the waste sorting station clear and easy to understand? Are the markings in staircases easy to see?) (*The questions should only be answered by people living in apartments. If you live in your own house, omit this question and question 18.*)

____

____

18. In view of the above problems in question 17, to what extent would you say that the markings and signs outside the building and at the entrance can be read and understood?

1 2 3 4 5 6 7
Not at all Perfectly easily

19. What problems do you find in the design of your balcony, patio, or garden? (*If you do not have any balcony, patio, or garden, please say so. You may then omit question 20.*)

____

____

20. In view of the above problems in question 19, how usable do you feel that the balcony, patio, or garden are?

1 2 3 4 5 6 7
Not at all usable Fully usable

21. What problems do you find in the design of the interior of your home?

____

____

22. In view of the above problems in question 21, how usable do you feel that the interior of your home is?

1 2 3 4 5 6 7
Not at all usable Fully usable

To conclude, there is a general question that allows you to express your wishes and needs.

23. If you were able to wish for anything at all concerning your home and your housing environment, what would you wish for?

____

____

____

____

____

____

____

____

Home Examination Form

appendix **9.C**

Type of Home

(Indicate apartment or single-family home)

☐ *Apartment*

Own ______________ Rent ______________

Is elevator available? ______________

What floor does patient live on? ______________

☐ *Single-family home*

Two or more floors ______________

Does patient live on only one floor, or use all floors of home? ______________

Basement. Does patient have or use basement area? ______________

Entrances to Building or Home

Location

Front Back Side (Circle one)

Which entrance is used most frequently or easily? ______________

Can patient get to entrance? ______________

Stairs

Does patient manage outside stairs? ______________

Width of stairway______________

Number of steps ________ Height of steps ________

Railing present as you go up? R ________ L ________ Both ________

Is ramp available for wheelchair? ______________

Door

Can patient unlock, open, close, lock door? (Circle for yes)

If doorsill is present, give height ________ and material ______________

Width of doorway ______________

Can patient enter ________ leave ________ via door?

Hallway

Width of hallway ______________

Are any objects obstructing the way? ______________

Approach to Apartment or Living Area

(Omit if not applicable)

Obstructions? ______________

____

Steps

Width of stairway ______________

Number of steps ________ Height of steps ________

Railing present as you go up? R ________ L ________ Both ________

Is ramp available? ______________

Door

Can patient unlock, open, close, lock door? (Circle one)

Doorsill? Give height ________ material ________

Width of doorway ______________

Can patient enter ________ leave ________ via door?

Elevator

Is elevator present? ________ Does it land flush with floor? ______________

Width of door opening ______________

Height of control buttons ______________

Can patient use elevator alone? ______________

Inside Home

Note width of hallways and of door entrances.

Note presence of doorsills and height.

Note if patient must climb stairs to reach room.

Can patient move from one part of the house to another?

Hallways ______________

Bedroom ______________

Bathroom ______________

Kitchen ______________

Living room ______________

Others ______________

Can patient move safely?

Loose rugs ______________

Electrical cords ______________

Faulty floors ______________

Highly waxed floors ______________

Sharp-edged furniture ______________

Note areas of particular danger for patient.

Hot water pipes ______________

Radiators ______________

Bedroom

Is light switch accessible? ______________

Can patient open and close windows? ______________

Bed

Height ______________ Width ______________
Both sides of bed accessible? __________ headboard present? ___________ footboard? ___________
Is bed on wheels? _________ Is it stable? _________
Can patient transfer from wheelchair-to-bed? _____
And bed-to-wheelchair? _____
Is night table within patient's reach from bed _____
Is telephone on it? _____

Clothing

Is patient's clothing located in bedroom? _________
Can patient get clothes from dresser? ___________
Closet? ____________ Elsewhere? ___________

Bathroom

Does patient use wheelchair ___________________ walker __________ in bathroom?
Does wheelchair _____ walker _____ fit into bathroom?
Light switch accessible? ________ Can patient open and close window? ________
What material are bathroom walls made of? _________
If tile, how many inches does tile extend from the floor beside the toilet? _________
How many inches does tile extend from the top of the rim of the bathtub? _________
Does patient use toilet? ______________________
Can patient transfer independently to and from toilet? ________________________
Does wheelchair wheel directly to toilet for transfers? ________________________
What is height of toilet seat from floor? __________
Are there bars or sturdy supports near toilet? _______
Is there room for grab bars? ________________
Can patient use sink? ______________ What is height of sink? ____________
Is patient able to reach and turn off faucets? _______
Is there knee space beneath sink? ______________
Is patient able to reach necessary articles? ________
Mirror? _________ Electrical outlet? __________

Bathing

Does patient take tub bath? ______ Shower? ______
Sponge bath? _______
If using tub, can patient safely transfer without assistance? ___________________
Bars or sturdy supports present beside tub? _______
Is equipment necessary? (tub seat, hand-spray attachment, tub rail, no-skid strips, grab rails, other: ___________________________)
Can patient manage faucets and drain plug? _______
Height of tub from floor to rim _____________
Is tub built-in __________ or on legs? __________
Width of tub from the inside _______________
If uses separate shower stall, can patient transfer independently and manage faucets? ___________
If patient takes sponge bath, describe method. _____
____
____

Living Room Area

Light switch accessible? ________ Can patient open and close window? __________
Can furniture be rearranged to allow manipulation of wheelchair? __________
Can patient transfer from wheelchair to and from sturdy chair? ____________
Height of chair _____________
Can patient transfer from wheelchair to and from sofa? ______________
Height of sofa ___________
Can ambulatory patient transfer to and from chair or sofa? ____________
Can patient manage television and radio? ___________

Dining Room

Light switch accessible? ____________
Is patient able to use table? ______________ Height of table ______________

Kitchen

What is the table height? ___________ Can wheelchair fit under? ____________
Can patient open refrigerator door and take food? ______________
Can patient open freezer door and take food? ________

Sink

Can patient be seated at sink? _______________
Can patient reach faucets? ______________ Turn them on and off? _______________
Can patient reach bottom of basin? _____________

Shelves and cabinets

Can patient open and close? _______________
Can patient reach dishes, pots, eating utensils, and food? ________________________
Comments: ______________________________
____
____

Transport

Can patient carry items from one part of kitchen to another? _________________________

Stove

Can patient reach and manipulate controls? _______
Manage oven door? __________________
Place food in oven and remove? ______________
Manage broiler door? __________________
Put food in and remove? _________________

Other Appliances

Can patient reach and turn on appliances? ________
Can patient use outlets? ________

Counter space

Is there enough for storage and work area? ________
Diagram (include stove, refrigerator, microwave, sink, table, counters, others if applicable)

Laundry

If patient has no facilities, how will laundry be managed?
____
____

Location of facilities in home or apartment and description of facilities present:
Can patient reach laundry area? ________
Can patient use washing machine and dryer? ________
Load and empty? ________
Manage doors and controls? ________
Can patient use sink? ________
What is height of sink? ________
Able to reach and turn on faucets? ________
Knee space beneath sink? ________
Able to reach necessary articles? ________
Is laundry cart available? ________
Can patient hang clothing on line? ________
Ironing board ________
Location: ________
Is it kept open? ________
If not kept open, can patient set up and take down ironing board? ________
Can patient reach outlet? ________

Cleaning

Can patient remove mop, broom, vacuum, pail from storage? ________
Use equipment? (mop, broom, vacuum, and so forth)
____

Emergency

Location of telephone in house: ________
Could patient use fire escape or back door in a hurry if alone? ________
Does patient have numbers for neighbors, police, fire, and physician? ________

Other

Will patient be responsible for child care? ________
If so, give number of children ________ and ages: ________
Will patient do own shopping? ________
Is family member or friend available? ________
Is delivery service available? ________
Does family have automobile? ________
Is family member or friend available to help with lawn care, changing high light bulbs, and so forth?
____
____
____

appendix 9.D

Web-Based Resources for Clinicians, Patients, and Families

Accessible Design/Universal Design Resources: www.makoa.org/accessable-design.htm

Americans with Disabilities Act of 1990, as amended: www.ada.gov/pubs/adastatute08.htm

Disability Rights in Housing: https://portal.hud.gov/hudportal/HUD?src=/program_offices/fair_housing_equal_opp/disabilities/inhousing

Home and Community Environment (HACE) Survey: Instrument and Scoring Manual: www.bu.edu/enact/files/2011/05/HACE-Survey-and-Manual-v1_7-30-2008.pdf

Information and Technical Assistance on the Americans with Disabilities Act: www.ada.gov

Occupational Information Network (O*NET): www.doleta.gov/programs/onet

Office of Disability Employment Policy: www.dol.gov/odep/

Rehabilitation Engineering and Assistive Technology Society of America: www.resna.org/

The Center for Universal Design (North Carolina State University): www.ncsu.edu/ncsu/design/cud/index.htm

2010 ADA Standards for Accessible Design. U.S. Department of Justice, Washington, DC: www.ada.gov/regs2010/2010ADAStandards/2010ADAStandards.pdf

United States Access Board: www.access-board.gov

Universal Design Institute: www.udinstitute.org/whatisud.php

Workplace Ergonomics Reference Guide: A Publication of the Computer/Electronic Accommodations Program, U.S. Department of Defense, Washington, DC: http://cap.mil/Documents/CAP_Ergo_Guide.pdf

Intervention Strategies for Rehabilitation

Strategies to Improve Motor Function

Susan B. O'Sullivan, PT, EdD

Chapter 10

LEARNING OBJECTIVES

1. Describe a model for clinical decision making that incorporates components of normal motor control and motor learning.
2. Identify factors critical to motor control and describe intervention strategies designed to optimize the acquisition of motor control.
3. Identify factors critical to motor learning and describe intervention strategies designed to optimize motor learning.
4. Differentiate between recovery and compensation at the body function/structure and activity levels.
5. Identify key factors in recovery of function and describe intervention strategies designed to optimize recovery.
6. Analyze and interpret patient data, formulate goals and expected outcomes, and develop a plan of care that presents an integrated approach to treatment when presented with a clinical case study.

CHAPTER OUTLINE

Developing strategies to improve motor function (motor control and motor learning) requires a thorough understanding of the neural processes involved in learning and producing movement and the pathologies that may affect the central nervous system (CNS). In addition, knowledge of the processes of neural plasticity and recovery following CNS insult is essential. This information allows the therapist to approach clinical decision making in an organized and informed manner. Patients with disorders of the CNS frequently demonstrate altered motor function with a wide variety of impairments, activity limitations, and restrictions in the ability to participate in normal roles. Careful examination of cognitive, sensoriperceptual, motor, and learning behaviors, along with the environmental contexts in which they occur, provides an appropriate base for planning (see Chapter 5, Examination of Motor Function: Motor Control and Motor Learning). An optimal plan of care (POC) must address the individual needs of the patient. This includes minimizing or eliminating impairments, reducing activity limitations and physical disabilities, and promoting full participation in life roles to the maximum extent possible. An effective POC also enhances overall quality of life.

■ MOTOR CONTROL

Motor control has been defined as "an area of study dealing with the understanding of the neural, physical, and behavioral aspects of biological (e.g., human) movement."[1, p. 497] Information processing of human motor behavior occurs in stages (Fig. 10.1). In the initial stage, *stimulus identification,* relevant stimuli about current body state, movement, and environment, are identified and selected. This includes somatosensory, visual, and vestibular inputs. Meaning is attached based on past sensorimotor experiences. Perceptual and cognitive processes, including memory, attention, motivation, and emotional control, all play an integral role in ensuring the ease and accuracy of information processing during this stage. Selection of relevant sensory input is sensitive to the clarity and intensity of the stimuli received. Thus, precise and stronger stimuli result in enhanced attentional mechanisms and information processing. Processing is also influenced by stimulus pattern complexity. Complicated and novel patterns of stimuli prolong stimulus identification. An intrinsic knowledge of movement (e.g., position of limb, length of limb, distance to goal, and so forth) is a critical characteristic of motor behavior.

In the *response selection stage,* the plan for movement is developed. A *motor plan* is defined as an idea or plan for purposeful movement and is made up of component motor programs. A general rather than detailed response is selected; that is, a prototype of the final movement. Decision making during this stage is sensitive to the number of different movement alternatives possible and the overall compatibility between the stimulus and response. A natural or firmly linked association between stimulus and response enhances the ease of the decision

	Within the CNS			
Stimulus ➤	Stimulus Identification	Response Selection	Response Programming	➤ Movement Output
	Sensing Perceiving Memory contact	Interpreting Planning Deciding	Translating Structuring Initiating R	
	Sensitive to: S clarity S intensity S pattern complexity	Sensitive to: Number of alternatives S-R compatibility	Sensitive to: R complexity R duration R-R compatibility	

CNS = central nervous system, S = stimulus, R = response

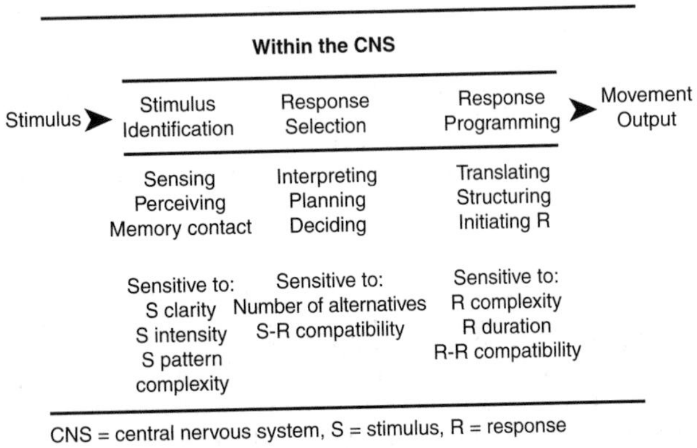

Figure 10.1 Model of information-processing stages of movement control.

making. For example, in a well-learned movement such as crossing at a streetlight, an individual easily responds to the green light by moving forward. If a crossing guard signals the individual to move forward even though the light is red, the individual is likely to be more hesitant in responding.

The final stage is termed *response programming.* Neural control centers translate and change the idea for movement into muscular actions defined by a motor program. A *motor program* is defined as "an abstract representation that, when initiated, results in the production of a coordinated movement sequence."[1, p. 497] The structuring of motor programs includes attention to specific parameters such as synergistic component parts, force, direction, timing, duration, and extent of movement. Parametric specification is based on the constraints of the individual, the task, and the environment. Information processing during this stage is sensitive to the complexity of the desired movement and duration. Thus, complex and lengthier movement sequences increase the duration of processing during this stage. Programming can also be affected by *response–response compatibility.* This is the compatibility for dual movement tasks that either occur simultaneously (e.g., bouncing a ball while walking) or when choices are required (e.g., one paired movement response must occur before another). During *response execution* (movement output), patterns of movement are selected against an appropriate background of postural control. *Feedforward control* is the sending of signals in advance of movement to ready a part of the system for incoming sensory feedback or for a future motor command.[1] It allows for anticipatory adjustments in postural activity. *Feedback* is response-produced sensory information received during or after the movement and is used to monitor movement output for corrective actions.[1] Although this simplified model gives the appearance that the information flow is linear, actual processing by the CNS is both serial and parallel. Thus, information flows in a specific pathway (serial order) and in multiple pathways (parallel order) in order to process information to more than one center. Many times, processing occurs using both serial and parallel order depending on the complexity of the movement.

The association areas of the cortex decide that a movement is called for. The premotor area (PMA) and supplementary motor areas (SMA) (collectively known as Area 6) devise a plan for the movement. The primary motor cortex (Area 4) is located just anterior to the precentral sulcus and issues the motor commands to the descending motor neurons either directly or indirectly by way of nuclei and interneurons in the brainstem and spinal cord. A major source of subcortical input arises from the loop from the cortex through the basal ganglia (BG) and back to the cortex, primarily to the SMA via the ventral lateral nucleus (VL) of the dorsal thalamus. This loop functions in assisting in the selection and initiation of voluntary movements. A second motor loop arises from the cortex through the lateral cerebellum and back to the cortex via the VL. This loop also functions in the production of voluntary movement and is concerned with execution of planned, coordinated multijoint movements (i.e., direction, timing, and force). Neurons that give rise to descending pathways are termed *upper motor neurons* (UMNs). Lateral UMN pathways are involved in the control of voluntary movements through corticospinal tracts. UMN pathways are also involved in indirect control by way of neural subsystems in the brain stem. The reticulospinal tracts and to a lesser extent rubrospinal tracts also influence voluntary movements. The tectospinal tract descends from the superior colliculus to the cervical levels and is important for reflex turning of the head. The vestibulospinal tracts are involved in control of postural adjustments and head movements. The ventral horn of the spinal cord gives rise to the peripheral nerve (*lower motor neuron* [LMN]). Activation of muscle fibers is from the motor unit.

Systems Underlying Motor Control

Contemporary theory of motor control has evolved over time and reflects current understanding and interpretation of nervous system function. The reader is referred to the work of Schmidt and Lee[1] and Shumway-Cook and Woollacott[2] for excellent reviews of this topic. The term *systems theory* is used to describe the process by which various brain and spinal centers work cooperatively to accommodate the demands of intended movements. Both internal factors (joint stiffness, inertia, movement-dependent forces) and external factors (gravity) must be taken into consideration in the planning of movements. Systems theory assumes a shifting locus of neural control, referred to as a *distributed model of control.* Thus, large areas of the CNS may be engaged for complex motor tasks, whereas relatively few centers are engaged for more automatic movements. This type of multilevel control allows for the control of a number of separate independent dimensions of movement, termed *degrees of freedom.*[3] The executive level (cortex) can be freed from the responsibility of control of some movements or the demands of having to control many degrees of freedom at one time.[4] For example, the use of central pattern generators (CPGs) in the spinal cord to initiate multijoint and intralimb coordination (coupling) for locomotion is well documented.[5,6] This is in contrast to an older theory of motor control, *hierarchical theory,* in which control was viewed as proceeding only in a descending, top-down direction from higher to lower centers, with the cortex always in control. Multiple ascending and descending systems are engaged for control of movement and posture. These include corticospinal/corticobulbar, medial (e.g., medial vestibulospinal), and lateral (e.g., reticulospinal, lateral vestibulospinal) descending pathways. Thus, both voluntary (conscious) and involuntary (automatic) pathways regulate posture and movement.

Motor programs allow for movements to occur in the absence of sensation (deafferentation) or in situations in which limitations in speed of processing feedback negate control. Motor programs also free the nervous system from conscious decisions about movement, reducing the problem of multiple degrees of freedom. Preprogrammed instructions (motor program) to a set of effectors run virtually without the influence of peripheral feedback or error detection processes, termed an *open-loop system.*[7] For example, rapid and skilled movements during piano playing occur too rapidly to benefit from feedback and function in an open-loop control system. This is in contrast to a *closed-loop control system,* which employs feedback and a reference for correctness to compute error and initiate subsequent corrections.[1] Feedback and closed-loop processes play a critical role in the learning of new motor skills (response selection) and in the shaping and correction of ongoing movements (response execution). Feedback is also essential for the ongoing maintenance of body posture and balance.[8]

The complexity of human movement negates any simplistic model of movement control. An *intermittent control hypothesis* described by Schmidt and Lee[1] proposes a blending of both open-loop and closed-loop control processes, in which both operate in concert as part of the larger system. Motor programs provide the generalized code for motor events (*schema*) rather than having every specific motor act stored in the brain. Feedback is used to refine and perfect movements.[8] Either may assume a dominant role, depending on the task at hand. Both may operate within a given movement but at different times and with different functions. Generalized motor programs include both invariant characteristics and parameters. *Invariant characteristics* are the unique features of the stored code: relative force, relative timing, and order of components. *Parameters* are the changeable features that ensure flexibility of motor programs and variations in movements from one performance to the next. These include overall force and overall duration of the movement. For example, speeding up or slowing down can change walking performance (changes in speed) while the basic order of stepping cycle and relative timing of the components (invariant characteristics) are maintained.[1]

Muscle *synergies* are used to simplify control, to reduce or constrain the degrees of freedom, and to initiate coordinated patterns of movement. Synergies are functionally linked muscles that are constrained by the CNS to act cooperatively to produce an intended motor action. Control is flexible with the cerebellum acting to generate the appropriate sequence of precise force, timing, and direction. A synergy can act in isolation for discrete movements. More frequently, synergies are combined to produce an appropriate sequence of muscle actions required for a functional task (e.g., the sequence of actions required during a transfer). Synergies are learned through motor skill practice, are flexible, and can be adapted to changes in the task or environment. For example, basic movement strategies (synergies) are well defined for postural control and balance, and include ankle, hip, and stepping strategies.[9-11] The organization and utilization of these strategies varies from quiet to perturbed stance and to positions of instability.

■ MOTOR LEARNING

Motor learning has been defined as "a set of internal processes associated with practice or experience leading to relatively permanent changes in the capability for motor skill."[1, p. 497] Learning a motor skill is a complex process that requires spatial, temporal, and hierarchical organization of the CNS. Changes in the CNS are not directly observable but rather are inferred from changes in motor behavior. See discussion in Chapter 5, Examination of Motor Function, section titled "Measures of Motor Learning."

Theories of Motor Learning

Adams's[7] theory of motor learning is based on closed-loop control (closed-loop theory). He postulated that sensory feedback from ongoing movement is compared with stored memory of the intended movement (perceptual trace) to provide the CNS with a *reference of correctness* and error detection. Memory traces are then used to produce an appropriate action and to evaluate outcomes. The stronger the perceptual trace developed through practice, the greater the capability of the learner to use closed-loop processes for learning movements. This theory helps to explain learning that occurs during slow, linear-positioning responses. It does not, however, adequately explain learning under conditions of rapid movements (open-loop control processes) or learning that occurs in the absence of sensory feedback (deafferentation studies).

Schema theory, proposed by Schmidt,[8] is an essential concept in motor learning theory. *Schema* is defined as "a rule, concept, or relationship formed based on experience."[1, p. 499] It can be viewed as a generalized motor program. Schema allows storage into short-term memory of such factors as initial conditions (body position, weight of objects, and so forth), relationships between movement elements, movement outcomes, and sensory consequences of movement. This information is then abstracted into *procedural* (motor) *memory,* defined as "the memory for movement or motor information."[1, p. 497] This type of memory is classified as nondeclarative or implicit. Movements once learned and stored into memory can be performed automatically, without attention or conscious thought. In contrast, memory for facts and events is classified as declarative or explicit memory.

Schema theory includes two types of schemas, recall and recognition. *Recall schema* are used to select and define the relationship among past parameters, past initial conditions, and past movement outcomes produced by these combinations. *Recognition schema* are used to evaluate movement responses and are based on information about the relationships among past initial conditions, past movement outcomes, and the sensory consequences produced by these combinations. Clinically, schema theory supports the concept that "we learn skills by learning rules about the functioning of our bodies—forming relationships between how our muscles are activated, what they actually do, and how these actions feel."[1, p. 448] Practicing a variety of movement tasks and outcomes would improve learning through the development of expanded rules or schema. It also enhances our understanding of how novel and open skills performed in a variable and changing environment are learned.

Stages of Motor Learning

The process of motor learning has been described as occurring in relatively distinct stages, thus providing a temporal perspective of learning. Fitts and Posner[12] developed a three-stage model, using the terms *cognitive, associated,* and *autonomous* to describe these stages. Their model is described in Chapter 5, Examination of Motor Function and is summarized in Table 10.1. It provides a useful framework for organizing a discussion of training strategies to improve motor learning.

■ MOTOR SKILLS

Motor skills are defined as a highly coordinated movement sequences for the purposes of attaining an action goal. Skilled behaviors allow for purposeful investigation and interaction with the physical and social environment (e.g., manipulation skills or walking). Skills require voluntary control, so reflexes or involuntary movements are not skilled movements. Skills are learned and are the direct result of practice and experience with actions organized in advance of movement. Skilled movements can be adapted and organized by the action goal and the environment. Thus, skilled behavior allows one to adapt movements easily to changes in task demands and the environment.

Motor development is the evolution of changes in motor behavior occurring as a result of growth, maturation, and experience. Foundational motor skills are learned in infancy and childhood with the emergence of specific markers of developmental maturation.[13-15] These skills are often referred to as *developmental motor skills,* although they are best viewed as *functional motor skills* because they remain a permanent part of movement experience throughout life. Examples include movements such as rolling, sitting up, and transitioning to standing.

Changes in motor skills are evident throughout the life span. During infancy (birth to 1 year) and childhood (1 to 10 years), changes are rapid and linked to cognitive/perceptual development and experience. During adolescence (11 to 19 years), motor skills become more complex and responsive to increasing cognitive/perceptual development and complex task and environmental demands. In adults, motor skills continue to be refined and are influenced by numerous factors, including age-related

Table 10.1 Characteristics of Motor Learning Stages and Training Strategies

Cognitive Stage Characteristics	Training Strategies
The learner develops an understanding of task; *cognitive mapping* assesses abilities, task demands; identifies stimuli, contacts memory; selects response; performs initial approximations of task; structures motor program; modifies initial responses *"What to do"* decision	Highlight purpose of task in functionally relevant terms. Demonstrate ideal performance of task to establish a *reference of correctness.* Have patient verbalize task components and requirements. Point out similarities to other learned tasks. Direct attention to critical task elements. Select appropriate feedback. • Emphasize intact sensory systems, intrinsic feedback systems. • Carefully pair extrinsic feedback with intrinsic feedback. • High dependence on vision: have patient watch movement. • *Knowledge of performance* (KP): focus on errors as they become consistent; do not cue on large number of random errors. • *Knowledge of results* (KR): focus on success of movement outcome. Ask learner to evaluate performance, outcomes; identify problems, solutions. Use reinforcements (praise) for correct performance, continuing motivation. Organize feedback schedule. • Feedback after every trial improves performance during early learning. • Variable feedback (summed, fading, bandwidth designs) increases depth of cognitive processing, improves retention; may decrease performance initially. Organize initial practice. • Stress controlled movement to minimize errors. • Provide adequate rest periods (distributed practice) if task is complex, long, or energy costly or if learner fatigues easily, has short attention, or poor concentration. • Use manual guidance to assist as appropriate. • Break complex tasks down into component parts, teach both parts and integrated whole. • Utilize bilateral transfer as appropriate. • Use blocked (repeated) practice of same task to improve performance. • Use variable practice (serial or random practice order) of related skills to increase depth of cognitive processing and retention; may decrease performance initially. • Use mental practice to improve performance and learning, reduce anxiety. Assess, modify arousal levels as appropriate. • High or low arousal impairs performance and learning. • Avoid stressors, mental fatigue. Structure environment. • Reduce extraneous environmental stimuli, distractors to ensure attention, concentration. • Emphasize closed skills initially gradually progressing to open skills.
Associated Stage Characteristics	**Training Strategies**
The learner practices movements, refines motor program: spatial and temporal organization; decreases errors, extraneous movements Dependence on visual feedback decreases, increases for use of proprioceptive feedback; cognitive monitoring decreases *"How to do"* decision	Select appropriate feedback. • Continue to provide KP; intervene when errors become consistent. • Emphasize proprioceptive feedback, "feel of movement" to assist in establishing an internal reference of correctness. • Continue to provide KR; stress relevance of functional outcomes. • Assist learner to improve self-evaluation, decision making skills. • Facilitation techniques, guided movements may be counterproductive during this stage of learning. Organize feedback schedule. • Continue to provide feedback for continuing motivation; encourage patient to self-assess achievements.

Continued

Table 10.1 Characteristics of Motor Learning Stages and Training Strategies—cont'd

Associated Stage Characteristics	Training Strategies
	• Avoid excessive augmented feedback. • Focus on use of variable feedback (summed, fading, bandwidth) designs to improve retention. Organize practice. • Encourage consistency of performance. • Focus on variable practice order (serial or random) of related skills to improve retention. Structure environment. • Progress toward open, changing environment. • Prepare the learner for home, community, work environments.
Autonomous Stage Characteristics	**Training Strategies**
The learner practices movements, continues to refine motor responses, spatial and temporal highly organized, movements are largely error-free, minimal level of cognitive monitoring *"How to succeed"* decision	Assess need for conscious attention, automaticity of movements. Select appropriate feedback. • Learner demonstrates appropriate self-evaluation, decision making skills. • Provide occasional feedback (KP, KR) when errors evident. Organize practice. • Stress consistency of performance in variable environments, variations of tasks (open skills). • High levels of practice (massed practice) are appropriate. Structure environment. • Vary environments to challenge learner. • Ready the learner for home, community, work environments. Focus on competitive aspects of skills as appropriate (e.g., wheelchair sports).

changes, overall health and nutrition, activity levels, and emerging pathology.[16-19] In middle adulthood (40 to 59 years), changes associated with aging are moderate in most systems. In older adults (60 years and older), changes are more apparent, though there is marked heterogeneity in the aging process. Spirduso et al[19] have identified a continuum of physical function among older adults varying from the high ranges of the physically elite and physically fit to a middle range of physically independent to the lower ranges of physically frail, physically dependent, and disabled. In the older adult, all stages of information processing are affected.[20] Sensory losses (decline in receptor sensitivity, recognition, and sensory encoding) affect stimulus identification. Response selection and programming are also affected by CNS changes with slowing of reaction time, especially for increasingly complex tasks. An age-related slowing of movement time is well documented.[21] Changes in motor units with a decrease in the overall number and increase in the size of motor units result in impaired coordination, especially for fine motor skills. There is a decreased ability to generate force and an increased tendency to coactivate agonist-antagonist muscles. This coactivation is most likely the result of attempts to modulate movement variability and maintain accuracy.[22] Older adults are also more sensitive to complexity of movement.[23] The principle of *speed–accuracy trade-off* typically applies as adults age—that is, the accuracy of a movement decreases as speed increases. To accommodate for this change, older adults typically move slower, especially when accuracy is required.[1] Overall movements become less efficient and more variable with age.

Secondary lifestyle factors (nutrition, body weight, exercise) have a significant impact on assisting individuals in maintaining health and in delaying dependency. Decreasing levels of cardiovascular fitness, strength, and endurance and obesity commonly associated with a sedentary lifestyle adversely affect the performance of motor skills. In addition, older adults often experience multiple disease pathologies that affect their ability to move and learn. For example, an older adult may alter the method used to roll over and sit up secondary to an increase in body weight, a decrease in overall strength and fitness, or an emerging pathology such as Parkinson's disease (PD).

Categories of Motor Skills

Motor skills can be categorized by different classification schemes. One widely used classification scheme categorizes tasks as either mobility or stability functions. *Mobility* tasks require the individual to move the body from one posture to another in a controlled manner. Both the base of support (BOS) and center of mass (COM) are moving. *Stability* tasks can be further divided into static postural control (stability) and dynamic postural control (dynamic stability). In *static postural control,* the individual is required to maintain posture in a stable, unchanging position with the COM over the BOS. During *dynamic postural control,* stability is adjusted and maintained while parts of the body (upper extremity [UE] or lower extremity [LE]) are moving. See Chapter 5, Examination of Motor Function, and Table 5.11 for a summary of characteristics and examples of movement tasks.

Additional categories of motor tasks include the following:

- Gross motor skills versus vs. fine motor skills (a major component of developmental tests and measures)
- Discrete skills vs. serial vs. continuous motor skills
- Closed vs. open motor skills
- Simple vs. complex motor skills and dual-task motor skills

Table 10.2 presents a summary of the characteristics of these skills. Terms serve as anchor points along a continuum (e.g., closed vs. open skills). It is important to remember that skills can fall anywhere along that continuum, and not just at either end. Thus, the movement may be performed in a semi-predictable environment and not just in a closed or open environment.

CONSTRAINTS ON MOTOR FUNCTION

Constraints on motor function arise from individual systems and neurological impairments, the task or movement, and the environment.

Table 10.2 Categories of Motor Skills

Categories of Tasks	Characteristics	Examples
Gross motor skills	Motor skills that involve large muscles of the body and larger movements; typically acquired during infancy and early childhood	Rolling, crawling, kneeling, standing, running
Fine motor skills	Motor skills that require control of small muscles of the body and smaller movements where precision of movement is important; typically acquired during early childhood	ADL skills: eating, buttoning clothing, writing; skills typically require a high level of hand–eye coordination.
Discrete motor skills	Skills that have a recognizable beginning and end point defined by the task	Moving from sit-to-stand, lying down, kicking or throwing a ball, locking the brake on a wheelchair
Serial motor skills	Skills that combine a series of discrete skills with a specific order of actions	Transfers from bed-to-wheelchair, Tai Chi routine
Continuous motor skills	Skills that have no recognizable beginning and end point; behavior continues until arbitrarily stopped by the performer or some external agent	Walking, running, or swimming
Closed motor skills	Skills performed in a stable, predictable environment	Walking in a quiet hall; practicing transfers in a quiet room; brushing teeth in bathroom
Open motor skills	Skills performed in a constantly changing and unpredictable environment	Walking across a busy PT gym, reception area or shopping mall; driving on a busy highway
Simple motor skills	Skills that involve a simple motor program that produces an individual movement response	Kicking a ball one time while sitting
Complex motor skills	Skills that involve multiple actions and motor programs combined to produce a coordinated movement response	Running and kicking a soccer ball during a game; gymnastics routine
Dual-task motor skills	Motor skills that involve a secondary cognitive or physical task	*Cognitive task:* walks while talking, spelling, word recall, serial subtractions, virtual gaming *Motor task:* walks while holding a tray or glass of water, stands or walks while bouncing or catching a ball

Individual Systems and Neurological Impairments

Patients with neurological lesions may demonstrate numerous impairments in voluntary movements. These include impaired motor planning or programming, impaired corrective actions (feedback adjustments), and impaired coordination. Movements can be disorganized with evidence of difficulty initiating or scaling the velocity of movements and controlling force, timing, or direction. Functionally linked synergies may be disorganized or fail to emerge and may show evidence of scaling issues. Reciprocal actions of agonists–antagonists, which normally are fine-tuned, become asynchronous. Instead of movements that are well matched to the intended movement and the environment, movements become highly stereotyped and limited. Abnormal obligatory or stereotypical synergies may emerge as is seen in the patient recovering from stroke, making it difficult to perform everyday functional tasks. Postural control and balance, a largely automatic function, becomes impaired with evidence of abnormal activation of motor strategies, increased conscious control, and difficulty in maintaining balance. Overall, the efficiency and flexibility of motor patterns is significantly reduced.

Additional constraints are imposed by specific impairments in the musculoskeletal system (e.g., weakness, contracture, postural deformity). Patients may exhibit complete loss (paralysis or plegia) or partial loss of muscle strength (paresis). Impairments can be localized to one side (hemiplegia), both LEs (paraplegia), or all four extremities (tetraplegia). Voluntary movements may become limited or absent, resulting in significant functional loss. Debilitating fatigue may be the result of centralized causes (e.g., multiple sclerosis [MS]) or peripheral causes (e.g. weak, overworked muscles in post-polio syndrome [PPS]). Abnormal tone (spasticity) impacts motor control and results in movements that are characteristically stiff and limited. Spasticity is a velocity-dependent constraint. Movements that might be possible at slow speeds become disordered or impossible at faster speeds. Alterations in the stretch-reflex response result in hyperexcitable muscles and abnormal coactivation of agonist–antagonist muscles. Overall, the number, range, and speed of movements are greatly reduced. There is altered recruitment of motor neurons, abnormal reciprocal inhibition between agonist and antagonist, impaired selective muscle activation and abnormal synergies, and increased difficulty activating and controlling movements.[2]

Constraints also emerge with impairments in sensory/perceptual and/or cognitive/behavioral systems. These include changes in sensation (absent or impaired) as well as alterations in sensory integration. Patients may demonstrate errors in stimulus identification or response selection, resulting in delayed, disorganized, or absent motor learning. Response programming may be impaired in the absence of accurate feedback to monitor and correct movement and posture. The central representation of the movement, termed *reference of correctness,* becomes inaccurate or fails to develop as a result of lack of or inaccurate feedback. Impairments in cognitive processes (attention, planning, problem solving, emotional stability) may significantly affect learning and motor control. The patient with profound cognitive deficits (e.g., the patient with traumatic brain injury [TBI]) may be unable to process feedback and develop the idea of the movement. This inability to form a *cognitive map* creates severe limitations during the initial stage of learning and is particularly evident with complex or novel movements. Cognitive interference is also readily evident during complex movements such as dual tasking and performing in novel or open environments. Patients with cognitive deficits may also demonstrate a complete lack of awareness of their deficits.

Secondary impairments associated with prolonged immobilization and decreased activity levels also constrain the patient's ability to move. These include additional changes (secondary impairments) in muscle such as weakness, decreased joint mobility, and contracture. Impairments in the cardiovascular system (e.g., limitations in endurance) can significantly affect the ability to practice and participate in rehabilitation programs.

The patient who exhibits profound impairments in motor control and learning can become poorly motivated. Every attempt at movement becomes a frustrating challenge, and activities previously done with ease become labored. The challenges of learning new motor behaviors can be overwhelming. In addition to the individual system limitations and impairments discussed above, patients with CNS dysfunction may demonstrate failure of the whole movement system to function as an integrated whole. The design of a successful POC requires careful examination of component parts, as well as the integrated whole.

Task and Environmental Constraints

The healthy individual performs a large variety of movement tasks related to daily function and activity, work, and social interests. These tasks occur in different environments under conditions of changing task and environmental demands. The patient with neurological insult and deficits in motor control typically demonstrates restrictions in the number and quality of movements resulting in significant limitations in functional performance. Movement difficulty also increases in open, variable environments in which movements must constantly be modified to match environmental demands. In planning treatment, the clinician must determine what movements are available to the patient (*where to start*) and how to structure those movements (*how to progress*). Some complex tasks will need to be broken down into component parts (*subroutines*), which are practiced first, with progression to task practice as an integrated whole. Equally important is the ability of the clinician to determine the constraints of the environment and the best possible situation for learning (*where to start*) and how to progress training (*when and how to modify the environment*).

NEURAL PLASTICITY AND RECOVERY OF FUNCTION

Recovery of motor function is defined as the reappearance of motor patterns that were present before CNS injury. *Compensation* is defined as the appearance of new motor patterns resulting from the adaptation of remaining motor elements or substitution of alternative motor strategies and body segments. Substitution occurs when functions are assumed, replaced, or substituted by different areas of the brain capable of becoming reprogrammed and engaging different effectors or body segments.[24] Thus, the preexisting movement is performed in a new manner. Recovery and compensation can be further distinguished across the different levels of the International Classification of Functioning, Disability, and Health (ICF) classification.[24]

Changes at the Body Functions/Structure Level

At the *body functions/structure level,* neuronal recovery of function is restored in the tissues that were initially lost after injury. Immediately after a brain insult, a cascade of events occurs, producing early transient depression of brain activity (*diaschisis*). Changes at a cellular level occur in the immediate area of damaged brain tissue. Disruption in blood flow and metabolism results in cerebral edema, with an accumulation of intracellular fluid and leakage of blood cells, proteins, and other toxic substances that disrupt nerve function. Initial spontaneous recovery typically occurs over a relatively short time frame (weeks) and is evidence of return to function of damaged parts of the brain with the resolution of temporary blocking factors (i.e., shock, edema, decreased blood flow, decreased glucose utilization).[25-27]

During compensation, function is assumed by neural tissue that did not demonstrate that function before injury (i.e., activation of alternative brain areas).[24] *Neural plasticity* is the primary factor allowing for the ability of brain to modify its structure and repair itself.[25] Mechanisms of neural plasticity include neuroanatomical, neurochemical, and neuroreceptive changes. Anatomical changes include nerve growth (*neural regeneration*) and activation of brain areas previously not active. Trophic molecules (*nerve growth factors*) have been shown to play a key role in growth and repair processes. Nerve cells also change their interactions with each other, with physiological changes occurring at the level of the synapses. *Regenerative synaptogenesis* refers to *sprouting* of the injured axons to innervate (reclaim) previously innervated synapses. *Reactive synaptogenesis* (*collateral sprouting*) refers to the reclaiming of synaptic sites of the injured axon by dendritic fibers from neighboring axons. Neurotransmitter release and receptor sensitivity are improved (*synaptic plasticity*). Changes in synaptic strength, known as *long-term potentiation* (LTP), firm up neuronal connections and serve as a basis for all memory and learning.[26-30]

It is important to remember that the brain is organized with parallel and distributed circuits that provide multiple inputs to many areas with overlapping functions. Different and underutilized areas of the brain (e.g., cortical supplementary and association areas) can take over the functions of damaged tissue, a process known as *cortical remapping.* Another possibility is that the CNS has backup or fail-safe systems (*parallel cortical maps*) that become operational when the primary system breaks down. The unmasking of new, redundant neuron pathways permits cortical map reorganization and restoration of function. An example of this is the increased sensitivity of the hands as a sensory information system for the person who becomes blind. In this example, the changes in sensory strategy lead to structural reorganization within the brain. Techniques in brain mapping have led to increased understanding about neuronal plasticity. These include (1) positron emission tomography (PET) scanning used to measure regional cerebral blood flow (rCBF), (2) focal transcranial magnetic stimulation (TMS) used to measure responses in motor cortical regions to focal magnetic field stimulation, and (3) functional magnetic resonance imaging (fMRI) used to measure small changes in blood flow during brain activation.[28-31] In summary, this is a complex and dynamic process, with plasticity occurring at many levels driven by changes in behavioral, sensory, and cognitive experiences and involving multiple cellular, network, and biochemical processes. It is also important to remember that these neuroplastic changes may be *adaptive,* resulting in improved function, or *maladaptive,* resulting in nonfunctional motor behaviors.

Changes at the Activity/Functional Level

Function-induced recovery (*use-dependent cortical reorganization)* refers to the ability of the nervous system to modify itself in response to changes in activity and new experiences. Task-oriented training using repetitive task practice has been shown to prevent brain degradation and atrophy and promote neural plastic changes. Improvements in individual systems and motor function have been demonstrated, including improvements in fine and gross motor coordination, sensory discrimination, postural control and balance, gait, procedural memory, functional status, and so forth.[30-38] Two examples of task-oriented training—*constraint-induced movement therapy* (CIMT) and *body weight support treadmill training* (BWSTT)—will be discussed later in this chapter.

An understanding of optimal timing and dose (intensity) of training is critical. Research on animal models suggests that there is a critical or sensitive period in which the brain is most responsive to improvements from motor training.[39] An early sensitive or critical period is also likely for humans.[40] Studies on early mobilization and patients recovering from stroke have received the most attention in the literature. In the phase 2 AVERT (A Very Early Rehabilitation Trial) protocol, researchers demonstrated preliminary evidence that early mobilization (within 24 hours of stroke onset) was safe and resulted in improvements in walking recovery.[41,42] Bernhardt and associates presented data from a larger, multinational study (AVERT: a RCT) that randomized groups of patients recovering from stroke into a higher dose, early mobilization group (92% mobilized in the first 24 hours) versus usual care group (59% mobilized in the first 24 hours). Data indicated that outcomes were less favorable for the higher dose, early mobilization group at 3 months when compared to the usual care group in terms of level of disability and accelerated walking recovery.[43] Recommendations about the critical window and appropriate dose to improve neural recovery and repair are as yet unknown and clinical trials are currently in progress.[40]

INTERVENTIONS TO IMPROVE MOTOR FUNCTION

Neurorehabilitation for the management of patients with disorders of motor function has evolved over time. Our understanding of motor function and its theoretical base is constantly changing and being updated. Clinicians need to keep abreast on *evidence-based research* that validates therapeutic interventions.

The therapist's roles include accurately examining the patient, evaluating the data, determining appropriate goals and expected outcomes, and formulating a POC that matches the patient's unique needs. Box 10.1 provides examples of general goals and outcomes for patients with disorders of motor function. The therapist must

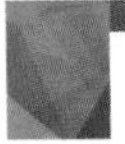

Box 10.1 Examples of General Goals and Outcomes for Patients With Disorders of Motor Function

Impact on risk reduction and prevention

- Risk factors are reduced.
- Risk of recurrence of condition is reduced.
- Risk of secondary impairment is reduced.
- Safety is improved.
- Self-management of symptoms is improved.

Impact on health, wellness, and fitness

- Fitness is improved.
- Health status is improved.
- Physical capacity is increased.
- Physical function is improved.

Impact of pathology/health condition

- Recovery of function is enhanced.
- Patient/client, family, and caregiver knowledge and awareness of the diagnosis, prognosis, goals/expected outcomes, and interventions are increased.
- Intensity of care is decreased.

Impact on impairments in body functions and structures

- Alertness, attention, and memory are improved.
- Joint integrity and mobility are improved.
- Sensory awareness and discrimination are improved.
- Motor function (motor control and motor learning) is improved.
- Coordination is improved.
- Muscle performance (strength, power, and endurance) is improved.
- Postural alignment and control are improved.
- Balance is improved.
- Aerobic capacity is increased.
- Endurance is increased.

Impact on activity limitations and participation restrictions

- Performance of and independence in activities of daily living (ADL) and instrumental activities of daily living (IADL) with or without devices and equipment are increased.
- Gait and locomotion are improved.
- Level of supervision for task performance is decreased.
- Tolerance of positions and activities is increased.
- Flexibility for varied tasks and environments is improved.
- Ability to assume or resume self-care and roles in domestic, education, work, community, social, and civic life with or without devices and equipment is improved.
- Ability to perform physical actions, tasks, or activities related to self-care and domestic, education, work, community, social, and civic life with or without devices and equipment is improved.
- Decision making is improved.

Impact on patient or client satisfaction

- Sense of well-being is improved.
- Stressors are decreased.
- Insight, self-confidence, and self-image are improved.
- Access, availability, and services provided are acceptable to the patient or client.
- Interpersonal skills of the physical therapist are acceptable to the patient or client, family, significant others, and caregivers.

Adapted from *Guide to Physical Therapist Practice 3.0*.[109]

determine an appropriate level of frequency, intensity, time (duration), and type of intervention (*FITT principle*). An important framework for practice is based on current understanding that movement arises from the interaction of three basic elements: the task, the individual, and the environment (Fig. 10.2). All three components must be considered when developing a successful POC.

Box 10.2 presents a summary of interventions to improve motor function and provides an overview of the discussion in this section. The interventions are organized from top to bottom, starting with *restorative interventions,* and are designed to promote recovery and compensation. These include motor learning strategies and task-specific training. The middle section includes interventions focusing on specific functions/body structures (impairment interventions and neuromuscular reeducation). The bottom section focuses on substitution training.

Motor Learning Strategies

Motor learning involves a significant amount of practice and feedback, with a high level of information processing related to control, error detection, and correction. Motor learning can be facilitated through effective training strategies, summarized by stages in Table 10.1.

Strategy Development

The overall goal during the early cognitive stage of learning is to facilitate task understanding and organize early practice. The learner's knowledge of the skill and any existing problems must be ascertained. The therapist

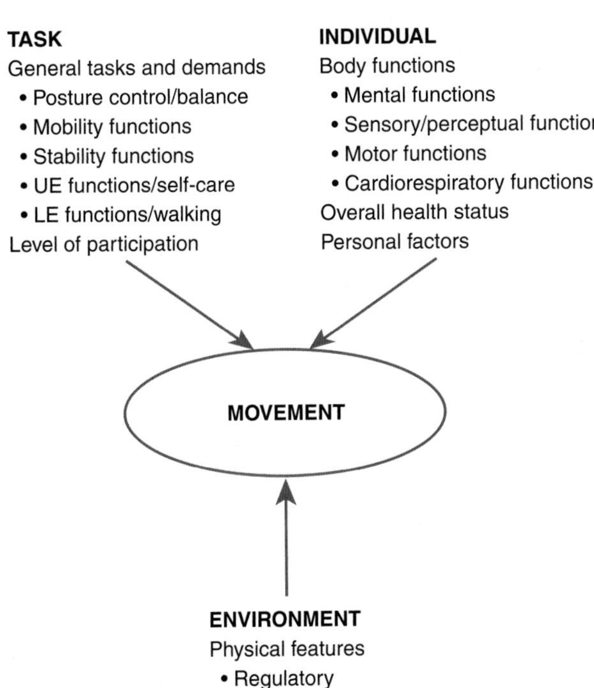

Figure 10.2 Movement emerges from interaction between the task, the individual, and the environment.

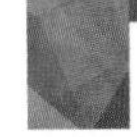

Box 10.2 Interventions to Improve Motor Function and Functional Independence

Restorative Interventions Designed to Promote Recovery and Compensation	
Task-Oriented Training	*Motor Learning Strategies*
Functional mobility skills	Strategy development
UE skills and activities of daily living	Practice
Environmental context	Feedback
Behavioral shaping	Transfer training
Safety awareness training	Active decision making and error detection
Interventions Focusing on Specific Body Functions/Structures	
Impairment Interventions	*Neuromuscular Reeducation*
Strength, power, endurance	Sensory stimulation
Flexibility	Biofeedback
Postural control and balance	Neuromuscular electrical stimulation
Coordination and agility	
Aerobic capacity/ endurance	
Substitution training	
Assistive/supportive devices	
Environmental modification	

UE = upper extremity

should highlight the purpose of the skill in a functionally relevant context. The task should seem important, desirable, and realistic to learn. The therapist should demonstrate the task (*modeling*) exactly as it should be performed (i.e., coordinated action with smooth timing and ideal performance speed). This helps the learner develop an internal cognitive map or *reference of correctness.* Attention should be directed to the desired outcome and critical task elements. The therapist should point out similarities to other learned tasks so that schema that are part of other motor programs can be retrieved from memory. Features of the environment critical to performance should also be highlighted.

Highly skilled individuals who have been successfully discharged from rehabilitation can be expert models. Their success in returning to the "real world" will also have a positive effect in motivating patients new to rehabilitation. For example, it is very difficult for a therapist with full use of muscles to accurately demonstrate appropriate transfer skills to an individual with C6 complete tetraplegia. A successful former patient with a similar level injury can accurately demonstrate how the skill should be performed. Modeling has been shown to be effective in producing learning even with unskilled patient models. In this situation, the learner/patient benefits from the cognitive processing and problem solving used while watching the unskilled model attempt to correct errors and arrive at the desired movement.[44] Demonstrations can be live or videotaped. Developing a video library of demonstrations of skilled former patients is a useful strategy to ensure availability of effective models.

Guided movement involves physically assisting the learner through the task to be learned. It can have considerable positive effects during the early period of skill acquisition.[45-47] The therapist's hands can effectively substitute for missing elements, hold a part of the body stable while constraining unwanted movements, reduce errors, and guide the patient toward correct performance. It also allows the learner to preview the kinesthetic inputs inherent in the task—that is, to learn the *sensations of movement.* The supportive use of hands also allays fears and instills confidence while ensuring safety. Verbal guidance, "talking someone through the task," is also a form of guidance that can be used to improve performance. As discussed previously, improved performance does not represent true learning or retention of a skill. Without *active trial and error discovery learning,* the changes in performance may be only temporary. The key to success in using guided movements is to limit guidance to only the amount needed and to intersperse practice with active movements as soon and as much as possible. Overuse of guided movements is likely to result in overdependence on the therapist for assistance, thus becoming a "crutch." The patient who tells you that he or she can only perform the skill if "my therapist" helps or the way "my therapist does it" is demonstrating an overreliance on guided movement. Guidance is most effective for slow postural responses (positioning tasks) and less effective during rapid or ballistic tasks.

During initial practice, the therapist should provide precise feedback, highlighting information critical for movement efficiency. The patient should not be overloaded with excessive feedback or wordy instructions. It is important to reinforce correct performance and intervene when movement errors become consistent or when safety is an issue. The therapist should *not* attempt to correct all the numerous errors that characterize early learning but rather allow for trial-and-error learning. Feedback, particularly visual feedback, is important during the early acquisition phase. The learner should be directed to watch the movements closely. The learner's initial performance trials can also be filmed for later viewing. Cued or directed viewing of the task improves learning.

During the associated and autonomous phases of learning, the patient continues to refine movement strategies with high levels of practice. Random errors decrease. As consistent errors are identified, feedback may be given and solutions generated. The focus is on refinement of skills and movement consistency in varied environments. This will ensure an overall range of movement patterns that are adaptable and match the changing demands of open environments. The patient's attention should be now focused on proprioceptive feedback, the "feel of the movement." Thus, the patient is directed to attend to the sensations intrinsic to the movement itself and to associate those sensations with the motor actions. Guided movements are counterproductive at this stage because they limit active practice. During late-stage learning, the use of distracters such as ongoing conversation or dual task training (e.g., ball skills during standing and walking) can yield important evidence of a developing level of autonomous control. It is important to remember that many patients undergoing active rehabilitation do not reach this final stage of learning. For example, in some patients with severe TBI, performance may reach consistent levels only within structured environments, whereas safe, consistent performance in open, community environments is not possible.

Practice

Practice is a major influence on motor learning. *General principles of practice* are (1) increased practice results in increased learning and (2) large and rapid improvements in performance are typically observed initially, with smaller improvements noted over time. The therapist's role is to prepare the patient for practice and to ensure that the patient practices the desired movements and has enough practice time to effect change. Practice of incorrect movement patterns can lead to a *negative learning* situation (interference) in which "faulty habits and postures" must be unlearned before the correct movements can be mastered. The organization of practice will depend on several factors, including the patient's motivation, attention span, concentration, endurance, and the type of task.

Therapists must consider the cognitive and physical resources of patients and the complexity of the tasks to be learned in determining the type of practice possible. Clinical decisions about practice include the following:

- How should practice periods and rest periods be spaced (*distribution of practice*)?
- What tasks and task variations should be practiced (*variability of practice*)?
- How should the tasks be sequenced (*practice order*)?
- How should the environment be structured (*closed vs. open*)?
- What tasks should be practiced in a parts-to-whole sequence?

Distribution: Massed Versus Distributed Practice

Massed practice refers to "a sequence of practice and rest times in which the rest time is much less than the practice time."[1, p. 497] Fatigue, decreased performance, and risk of injury are factors that must be considered when using massed practice. *Distributed practice* refers to "a sequence of practice and rest periods in which the practice time is often equal to or less than the time at rest."[1, p. 494] Although learning occurs with both, distributed practice results in the most learning per training time, although the total training time is increased. It is the preferred mode for many patients undergoing active rehabilitation who demonstrate limited performance capabilities and endurance. With adequate rest periods, performance can be improved without the interfering effects of fatigue or increasing safety issues. Distributed practice is of benefit if motivation is low or if the learner has a short attention span, poor concentration, or motor planning deficits (e.g., dyspraxia). Distributed practice should also be considered if the task itself is complex, is long, or has a high-energy cost. Massed practice can be considered when motivation and skill levels are high and when the patient has adequate endurance, attention, and concentration. For example, the patient with spinal cord injury (SCI) in the final stages of rehabilitation may spend long practice sessions acquiring the wheelchair skills needed for community access.

Blocked Versus Random Practice

Blocked practice refers to "a practice sequence in which all of the trials on one task are done together, uninterrupted by practice on any of the other tasks."[1, p. 493] *Random practice* refers to "a practice sequence in which the tasks being practiced are ordered randomly across trials."[1, p. 498] Although both allow for motor skill acquisition, random practice has been shown to have superior long-term retention effects.[48-50] For example, a variety of different types of transfers (e.g., bed-to-wheelchair, wheelchair-to-toilet, wheelchair-to-bathtub transfer seat) can be practiced all within the same training session. Although skilled performance of individual tasks may be initially delayed, improved retention of transfer skills can be expected. The constant challenge of varying the task demands provides high *contextual interference* and increases the depth of cognitive processing through retrieval practice from memory stores. The acquired skills can then be applied more easily to other task variations or environments. Constant practice will result in superior initial performance because of low contextual interference and is required in certain situations (e.g., the patient with TBI and profound cognitive and behavioral deficits who requires a high degree of structure and consistency for learning; the patient with advanced PD).

Practice Order

Practice order refers to the sequence in which tasks are practiced. *Blocked order* refers to the repeated practice of a task or group of tasks in order (three trials of task 1, three trials of task 2, three trials of task 3: 111222333). *Serial order* refers to a predictable and repeating order (practice of multiple tasks in the following order: 123123123). *Random order* refers to a nonrepeating and nonpredictable order (123321312).[1] Although skill acquisition can be achieved with all three, differences have been found. Blocked order produces improved early acquisition of skills (performance), whereas serial and random order produce better retention and generalizability of skills. This is again due to contextual interference and increased depth of cognitive processing.[48,49] The key element here is the degree to which the learner is actively involved in memory retrieval. For example, a treatment session can be organized to include practice of a number of different tasks (e.g., forward-, backward-, and side-stepping and stair climbing). Random ordering of the tasks may initially delay acquisition of the desired stepping movements but over the long-term will result in improved retention and generalizability.

Mental Practice

Mental practice is "a practice method in which performance on the task is imagined or visualized without overt physical practice."[1, p. 497] Beneficial effects result from the cognitive rehearsal of task elements. It is theorized that underlying motor programs for movement are activated but with subthreshold motor activity. Brain mapping techniques have also revealed activation of similar brain areas during imagined movements as those activated during actual movement.[50,51] Mental practice has consistently been found to facilitate the acquisition of motor skills.[52-55] It should be considered for patients who fatigue easily and are unable to sustain physical practice. Mental practice is also effective in alleviating anxiety associated with initial practice by previewing the upcoming movement experience. Mental practice when combined with physical practice has been shown to increase the accuracy and efficiency of movements at significantly faster rates than physical practice alone.[56] When using mental practice, it is important to make sure the patient understands the task and is cognitively rehearsing the correct movement. Having the patient verbalize aloud the steps being rehearsed can ensure that this occurs. It is generally contraindicated in patients with profound cognitive, communication, and/or perceptual deficits.

Part–Whole Practice

Complex motor skills can be broken down into component parts for practice. The component parts are practiced first before practice of the whole task is attempted. For example, during initial wheelchair transfer training, the individual steps are practiced in isolation (e.g., locking the brakes, lifting the foot pedals, moving forward in the chair, standing up, pivoting, and sitting down) before practicing the whole transfer. It is important to identify the key steps through accurate task analysis and to sequence them in the required order. It is also important to practice the integrated whole in conjunction with the parts practice so that the learner develops the whole idea for the required task (i.e., cognitive mapping). Delaying practice of the integrated whole can interfere with transfer effects and learning.[1] Part–whole practice is most effective with discrete or serial motor tasks that have highly independent parts. Part–whole practice is not as effective for continuous movement tasks (e.g., walking) or for complex tasks with highly integrated parts. Both require a high degree of coordination with spatial and temporal sequencing of elements. For these tasks, practice of the integrated whole will result in superior learning. Table 10.3 summarizes the types of practice and practice parameters.

Feedback

The vast body of motor learning literature affirms the critical role of feedback in promoting motor learning. Feedback can be *intrinsic* (*inherent*), occurring as a natural result of the movement, or *extrinsic* (*augmented*), incorporating sensory cues provided that are not normally received during the movement. Proprioceptive, visual, vestibular, and cutaneous signals are examples of types of intrinsic feedback; visual, auditory, and tactile cues are forms of extrinsic feedback (e.g., verbal cues, manual cues, biofeedback devices such as the electromyogram [EMG], pressure-sensing devices [force plates, foot pad]). During therapy feedback and verbal cues can be manipulated to enhance motor learning.

The use of augmented feedback serves as an important source of information and helps the learner link associations between the movement parameters and resulting action.[1] *Concurrent feedback* is given during task performance, while *terminal feedback* is given at the end of task performance. Augmented feedback about the nature of the end result produced in relation to the goal is termed *knowledge of results* (KR). Augmented feedback about the nature or quality of the movement pattern produced is termed *knowledge of performance* (KP).[1] Although both are important, the relative usefulness of KP

Table 10.3 Types of Practice and Practice Schedules[1]

	Types of Practice
Massed practice	A sequence of practice and rest times in which the rest time is much less than the practice time
Distributed practice	Spaced practice intervals in which the practice time is equal to or less than the rest time
	Practice Sequence
Blocked practice	A practice sequence organized around one task performed repeatedly, uninterrupted by practice of any other task
Random practice	A practice sequence in which a variety of tasks are ordered randomly across trials
	Practice Order
Blocked order	The repeated practice of a task or group of tasks in order; three trials of task 1, three trials of task 2, three trials of task 3 (e.g., 111222333)
Serial order	A predictable and repeating order; practice of multiple tasks in the following order (e.g., 123123123)
Random order	A nonrepeating and unpredictable order of multiple tasks (e.g., 123321312)
	Practice Strategies
Mental practice	A practice strategy in which performance of the motor task is imagined or visualized without overt physical practice
Part/whole practice	Component parts of a task are practiced before practice of the whole task
Transfer training	The gain (or loss) in the capability of task performance as a result of practice or experience on some other task • Acquisition of motor skills in one training experience enhances acquisition of similar or related skills (*positive learning*) • Acquisition of motor skills in one training experience interferes with acquisition of other skills (*negative learning*)
Practice of lead-up activities	Simpler task versions of the required complex task are practiced

and KR can vary according to the skill being learned and the availability of feedback from intrinsic sources.[57-61] For example, tracking tasks are highly dependent on intrinsic visual and kinesthetic feedback (KP), whereas KR has less influence on the accuracy of the movements. In other tasks (e.g., transfers), KR provides key information about how to shape the overall movements for the next attempt, whereas KP may not be as useful. Performance cues (KP) should focus on key task elements that lead to a successful final outcome.

Therapists must consider the cognitive and physical resources of patients and the complexity of the tasks to be learned in determining the type of feedback possible. Clinical decisions about feedback include the following issues:

- What type of feedback should be employed (*mode*)?
- How much feedback should be used (*intensity*)?
- When should feedback be given (*scheduling*)?

Choices about type of feedback involve the selection of which intrinsic sensory systems to highlight, what type of augmented feedback to use, and how to pair extrinsic feedback to intrinsic feedback. The selection of sensory systems depends on specific sensory integrity examination findings. The sensory systems selected must provide accurate and usable information. If an intrinsic sensory system is impaired and provides distorted or incomplete information (e.g., impaired proprioception with diabetic neuropathy), use of alternative sensory systems (e.g., vision) should be emphasized. Supplemental augmented feedback can be used to enhance learning. Decisions are also based on stage of learning. Early in learning, visual feedback is easily brought to conscious attention and therefore is important. Less consciously accessible sensory information such as proprioception should be emphasized during the middle and end stages of learning. Decisions about frequency and scheduling of feedback (when and how much) must be reached. Frequent augmented feedback (e.g., given after every trial) quickly guides the learner to the improved performance but slows retention and overall learning.

Conversely, feedback that is varied (not given after every trial) slows initial performance of the skill while improving performance on a retention test.[62-66] This is most likely due to the increased depth of cognitive processing that accompanies the variable presentation of feedback. In contrast, the therapist who bombards the patient immediately after task completion with excessive augmented verbal feedback may preclude active information processing by the learner.[67,68] The patient's own decision making skills are minimized, while the therapist's verbal skills dominate. Winstein[69] points out that this may well explain why many studies on the effectiveness of therapeutic approaches cite minimal carryover and limited retention of newly acquired motor skills. Finally, the withdrawal of augmented feedback should be gradual and carefully paired with the patient's efforts to correctly utilize intrinsic feedback systems. Table 10.4 summarizes the types and uses of augmented feedback.

Attentional focus and motor learning can be improved by using appropriate verbal instructions (*instructional set*). Instructions provide important information about the movement (initial positions, idea of the movement, expected outcome). Internal cues focus on specific body movements. For example, during sitting practice cues such as "Tighten your stomach and back muscles, lift your head up, straighten your back" focus on internal actions. Wulf[70] demonstrated greater movement efficiency and retention when the focus of external cues emphasized the overall outcome of the movement. For example, "Sit tall, keep your head directly over your hips with your trunk straight and pelvis neutral."[70,71]

Transfer Training

Transfer of learning refers to the gain (or loss) in the capability of task performance as a result of practice or experience on some other task. Learning can be promoted through practice using contralateral extremities, termed *bilateral transfer*. For example, a patient with stroke first practices the desired movement pattern using the less affected extremity. This initial practice enhances formation or recall of the necessary motor program, which can then be applied to the opposite, involved extremity. This method cannot, however, substitute for lack of movement potential of the affected extremities (e.g., a flaccid limb on the hemiplegic side). Transfer effects are optimal with similarity of the tasks (e.g., identical components and actions) and environments. For example, optimal transfer can be expected with practice of a UE flexion pattern first on one side, then with an identical pattern on the other side.[72]

Practice of *lead-up tasks* is commonly used in physical therapy. Lead-ups are tasks or activities presented to prepare learners for a more important or complex task or activity.[1, p. 496] The subtasks are practiced, typically in easier postures with significantly reduced degrees of freedom. Anxiety is also reduced and safety is ensured. Thus, initial upright postural control can be practiced with activities in kneeling, half kneeling, or plantigrade before standing. The patient develops the required trunk and hip extension/abduction stabilization control required for upright stance but without the demands of the full standing position or fear of falling. The more closely the lead-ups (subskills) resemble the final task, the better the transfer. For example, bridging, which involves hip extension to neutral in a supine hook-lying position, can be a lead-up to successful sit-to-stand transitions.

Motivation and Behavioral Self-Management Strategies

Fundamental psychological needs of the patient include autonomy, competence, and social-relatedness. For effective planning, the therapist needs to have a clear understanding of the patient's values (beliefs and attitudes),

Table 10.4 Types of Feedback and Feedback Schedules[1]

Concurrent feedback	Feedback is presented during the movement; KP information is provided (e.g., information about joint position; importance of forward weight shift to position the COM over the BOS during sit-to-stand training or biofeedback); best used to highlight information not readily available from intrinsic feedback and if linked to active problem-solving.
Terminal feedback	Feedback is given after the movement.
Immediate feedback	Feedback is presented immediately after the movement.
Delayed feedback	Feedback given after a brief time delay allows the learner a brief time for introspection and self-assessment (e.g., a 3-second delay). Feedback given after long delays is contraindicated, especially if other movements not related to the task occur in between, degrading learning.
Summary feedback	Feedback given after a set number of trials (e.g., after every 2nd trial or every 5th or every 20th trial).
Faded feedback	Feedback given first after every trial, then less frequently on subsequent blocks of trials (e.g., after every 1st trial progressing to every 3rd trial, then to every 5th trial).
Bandwidth-KR feedback	Feedback given only when performance deviates outside the boundaries of correct performance; error range is predetermined (e.g., top and bottom range of errors is determined).
Blocked feedback	One source of feedback is provided; KR is presented about the same segment on consecutive trials; learner processes a limited information about the task (e.g., during gait training, KR is presented about knee segment only on successive trials). Blocked KR improves performance of the identified segment but may not improve performance and learning of the whole task (multiple segments); performance deteriorates once KR is withdrawn.
Variable (random) feedback	Multiple sources of feedback are provided; KR is presented about different segments on successive trials (e.g., during gait training, KR is presented about various different body segments [trunk, hips, knees] on successive trials). Random KR is superior in improving both performance and learning of a task; encourages learner to process a wider range of information about the task.

self-perceptions (sense of confidence, self-efficacy), preferences, and outcome expectations. Motivational factors influence long-term engagement of the learner. Making the task seem important to learn and involving the patient in goal setting and collaborative planning are key motivational techniques.[1] This includes education about the task (purpose, effects of practice and exercise, expected outcomes) and identification of possible barriers. Providing feedback and encouragement is also critical to ensure motivation. Supportive statements such as, "Do the best job you can" or "You are doing very well" can go a long way toward enhancing motivation and self-confidence. Patients need to experience feelings of self-efficacy, self-control, and competence. For example, researchers found improved performance on a novel balance task when older women were provided a single statement before practice: "Active people like you, with your experience, usually do very well on this task."[73] In another study, individuals recovering from stroke were given feedback and encouragement during daily, timed walking trials. Researchers found these individuals walked significantly faster at discharge and at 3 months than the control group.[74] In a study of motor learning benefits of self-controlled practice in patients with PD, researchers found that those who demonstrated self-control in determining practice (i.e., whether to use a balance pole or not while standing on a stabilometer) were more motivated to learn the task, were less nervous, and were less concerned about their body movements than the control group.[75]

The therapist has an important role as a motivational coach, "We will work together as a team." This includes reinforcing the patient's capabilities rather than failures and pointing out successes in improving function and obstacles that have been overcome on a regular basis. "This is what you have achieved this week and how far you have come." Progress can be demonstrated through easily understood measurements (e.g., changes in timed performance, number of repetitions, weight training). Beginning and ending the therapy session with a positive and successful movement experience is also a useful strategy to improve self-efficacy.

Focus on the development of decision making skills is critical in ensuring perceived confidence, autonomy, and problem-solving success in the patient's real-world environment. Having the patient actively involved in self-monitoring, problem identification, and generating solutions encourages self-determined behavior. Trial-and-error learning can only be successful if the patient is challenged to think about the movement, to consider the feedback information received about movement performance, and to evaluate the movement outcome.[76] The therapist should allow adequate time for reflection and confirm the accuracy of the patient's responses. If the efforts do not achieve the expected outcome, the patient can be challenged to consider why. For example, the individual who consistently falls to the right while standing can be challenged with questions such as, "In what direction did you fall?" and "What do you need to do to correct this problem?" Key questions to promote active decision making and autonomy are presented in Box 10.3.

Task-Oriented Training

A task-oriented training approach is based on careful examination of motor function and activity performance (see Chapter 5, Examination of Motor Function, and Chapter 8, Examination of Function). Tasks targeted during early rehabilitation include basic activities of daily living (BADL) (e.g., feeding, dressing, hygiene, and so forth) and functional mobility skills (FMS) (e.g., bed mobility, transfers, locomotion). Later in rehabilitation, instrumental activities of daily living (IADL) (e.g., home chores, shopping), community mobility, and work activities are targeted, depending on the patient's level of recovery and discharge placement. Task analysis yields an understanding of the task, the essential elements within the task, and the context or environment in which the task occurs (see Chapter 5, Box 5.2).

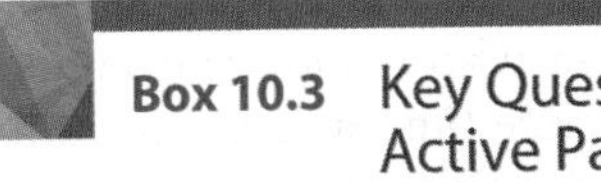

Box 10.3 Key Questions to Promote Active Patient Decision Making and Autonomy

- What is the goal of the intended movement?
- Did you accomplish the goal? If no, does the goal need to be modified?
- Did you move as planned? If no, what problems were encountered during the movement?
- What do you need to do to correct the problems in order to achieve movement success?
- For complex movements, what are the component parts or steps of the task? How should the component parts be sequenced?
- What aspects of the environment led to the success (or failure) of reaching the goal of the intended movement?
- What motivates you to keep trying?
- How confident are you in your abilities to move on your own? To be safe in your home and community environments?

Task-oriented training utilizes challenging and meaningful practice with appropriate feedback in a supportive environment that enhances the effects of interventions. Involved segments (areas of weakness) are targeted for training. For example, the patient recovering from stroke practices tasks using the more involved UE while use of the less involved UE is minimized. Tasks are selected that allow for recovery of specific functions, such as grasp and release of a cup for feeding, forward reach, UE dressing (i.e., specificity principle). Tasks are modified to permit successful early practice. For example, training using partial body weight support (BWS) and motorized treadmill training (TT) provides a means of early locomotor training for patients with stroke or incomplete SCI who are unable to walk unaided. Practice is intense with the number of repetitions reaching the physical limits of the patient (i.e., overload principle). Tasks are modified to allow for a progressive increase in the level of difficulty and adaptation and transference of skills. For example, sit-to-stand training can begin with practice standing up from a raised seat. Progressively lowering the seat height during training increases the difficulty of the task until the patient is able to stand up from a normal seat height. In a Cochrane Database of Systematic Review, researchers investigated the evidence of repetitive task training for improving functional ability after stroke (33 trials, 36 intervention-control pairs, 1,853 participants). Improvements in arm function, hand function, walking distances, and other measures of walking ability were found. The researchers concluded that additional research was needed to determine the best type and amount (intensity) of practice.[77]

Principles of promoting function-induced recovery are described by Kleim and Jones[37] and Winstein et al[78] and are summarized in Table 10.5. Examples of task-oriented training include CIMT and BWSTT, both discussed later in this section.

Intense task-oriented training is not appropriate for every patient. Its selection is dependent on the degree of recovery and severity of motor deficits (Box 10.4). There is evidence to suggest that very early intense training may actually increase the vulnerability of the brain to additional damage in animals[79,80] and in humans.[81-83] Patients who are not able to participate in task-oriented training include those who lack voluntary control or cognitive function. For example, a patient with severe TBI and profound cognitive deficits has limited potential to participate with this type of intensive training. Similarly, patients with stroke who experience profound UE paralysis and perceptual deficits would not be candidates for intense UE training. One of the consistent exclusion criteria for CIMT has been inability to perform voluntary wrist and finger extension of the more involved hand. Thus, threshold abilities to perform the basic components of the task need to be identified. Careful analysis of underlying impairments with a focus on intervention (e.g., improved strength, range of motion

Table 10.5 Principles of Experience-Dependent Neural Plasticity and Neurorehabilitation

Focus on active practice of motor skills "Use it or lose it"	Engage the patient in active practice of specific goal-directed activities that are functionally relevant and important to the individual; failure to drive specific brain functions can lead to functional degradation.
Specificity matters	The nature of the training experience dictates the nature of the plasticity.
Repetition matters	Focus on sufficient repetition to stimulate brain reorganization.
Intensity matters	Focus on sufficient intensity of training to stimulate brain reorganization, carefully matching the dynamic and changing needs of the patient.
Timing matters	Different forms of plasticity occur at different times during training; very early training may be detrimental in some cases of neural injury; delayed or absent training can limit recovery and can result in neural degradation and "learned non-use."
Age matters	Training-induced plasticity occurs more readily in younger brains; plasticity and experience-dependent brain changes in older adults may be slower and less demonstrable.
Transference "Use it and shape it to the patient's ability"	Continually challenge the patient's movement capability with acquisition of new skills to ensure continued learning; progressively modify skills to ensure transference and achieve functional outcomes.
Reinforce selection of important stimuli	Reinforce behaviorally important stimuli to enhance skill learning; create the best possible environment for learning.
Enhance attention and feedback	Actively engage the patient in evaluating goal-achievement and in making accurate adjustments of motor skills based on appropriate use of feedback.
Interference	Plasticity in response to one experience can interfere with acquisition of other behaviors.

Adapted from Kleim and Jones.[37]

[ROM]) complements task-oriented training. For example, during locomotor training using BWS and a treadmill system, stepping and pelvic motions are guided into an efficient motor pattern. To participate in this type of training, essential prerequisites include postural and head stability during upright positioning.

Environmental Context

Managing the environment is an important consideration in structuring practice sessions. During early learning, many patients benefit from practice in a stable, or predictable, *closed environment.* As learning progresses, the environment should be varied and incorporate more variable features consistent with real-world, *open environments.* Practicing walking only within the physical therapy clinic might lead to successful performance in that setting (*context-specific learning*) but does little to prepare the patient for ambulation at home or in the community. The therapist should begin to gradually modify the environment as soon as performance becomes consistent. Consideration must be given to practice in a safe environment where the patient can learn without the risk of injury or outright failure. Simulated environments (e.g., Easy Street Environments) are found in many rehabilitation centers. They can serve as an intermediate practice environment before the patient moves to the home or community setting. It is important to remember that some patients (e.g., the patient with severe TBI and limited cognitive recovery) may never be able to function in anything but a highly structured environment.

An unfamiliar and unpredictable hospital or rehabilitation environment may contribute to depression, disorientation, and decline of function. This same environment may be overly structured and protective to the point that it contributes to learned helplessness and disuse. Poor recovery after stroke may be partially explained by the impoverished and non-challenging environments that many individuals recovering from stroke are exposed to.[84] Although there are few environmental studies with humans, there is evidence that patients recovering from stroke who were treated on an acute stroke unit demonstrated better recovery and functional outcomes than patients who received a comparable amount of physical therapy while on a general medical unit.[85] This difference could also be due to the better coordination of care and expertise in specialized rehabilitation units. An important consideration is the amount of "downtime" patients typically experience while in rehabilitation. As much as 30% to 40% of the day can be spent in passive pursuits while time in therapy is limited.[86] During non-therapy time, there is often little attention to self-directed practice, thereby further limiting the potential for optimal recovery of function.[87-90]

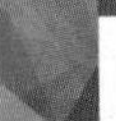

Box 10.4 Strategies for Motor Learning and Task-Oriented Training

Promote challenging and meaningful practice.

- Involve the patient in goal setting and decision making, thereby enhancing motivation and active commitment to recovery.
- Consider the patient's past and current history, health status, age, interests, and experience.

Determine the activities to be practiced.

- Select tasks that are important to the patient and enhance function.
- Determine a set of tasks to be practiced for each training goal.
- Promote transference, practice of similar behaviors.
- Target active movements of involved body segments.

Determine the parameters of practice.

- Practice at a sufficiently intense level, hours per day, days per week.
- Practice a sufficiently high number of repetitions.
- Determine optimal time for training.
- Determine practice schedule of tasks (blocked or variable).
- Determine practice order of tasks (constant, serial, random); progress to random order as soon as possible to enhance retention.
- Break down task into component parts (subroutines) as necessary; combine with practice the integrated whole.
- Control use of instructions and augmented feedback to promote active learning.
- Control use of assisted or guided movements to promote initial learning; ensure that the patient successfully transitions to active movements as soon as possible.

Enhance motivation using behavioral strategies.

- Promote self-determination (choice, control, collaboration)
- Promote self-efficacy (self-confidence in abilities)
- Provide reinforcement, emphasize positive aspects of performance and acknowledge improvements.
- Determine rest versus practice time as excessive effort and fatigue degrades performance and dampens motivation.

Promote problem-solving.

- Have the patient evaluate performance, identify obstacles, generate potential solutions, choose a solution, and evaluate outcome.
- Relate successes to overall goals.

Structure the environment.

- Promote initial practice in a supportive environment, free of distractors.
- Progress to variable practice in real-world environments (open environments).

Establish parameters for practice outside of therapy.

- Identify specific goals and strategies for unsupervised practice; maximize opportunities.
- Utilize a written behavioral contract, and have the patient agree to targeted behaviors to be carried out during the day.
- Provide home exercise program with adequate training for patient/family/caregivers.
- Have patient document unsupervised practice using an activity log or home exercise diary.

Maintain focus on active learning.

- Minimize hands-on therapy.
- Maximize role as *training coach.*

Monitor recovery closely and document progress.

- Use sensitive, valid, and reliable functional outcome measures.

Be cautious about timetables and predictions; recovery may take longer than expected.

Adapted from Kleim and Jones[37] and Winstein et al.[78]

During outpatient therapy time for post-stroke patients with hemiparesis, Lang et al[91] found time was limited to an average of 36 minutes with the number of repetitions of purposeful movements less than the number for active- and passive-exercise movements. The principles of sufficient intensity and repetition to promote recovery are clearly at issue here.

It is critical for the therapist to establish parameters for practice outside of therapy. Specific goals and strategies for unsupervised practice should be established with opportunities for meaningful practice maximized. Use of a written behavioral contract of targeted behaviors and number of repetitions per day has been successfully used in CIMT. A home exercise program should include targeted tasks with sufficient intensity and repetition. An activity log or home exercise diary can be used to document unsupervised practice.

Behavioral Shaping

Behavioral shaping refers to the use of techniques designed to systematically progress the level of difficulty of the tasks practiced. The therapist provides immediate and explicit feedback to shape and improve performance. Attention is directed toward the successful aspects of performance. Thus, the therapist serves to direct and motivate the patient toward optimal performance. The tasks chosen should be within the capabilities of the patient. Excessive effort, which can degrade performance and motivation, is avoided. The patient is kept focused on the training activity, fully informed of progress, and continually challenged.[92]

Task-Specific Training to Improve UE and ADL Function

Extensive research on CIMT in patients following stroke has demonstrated improvements in UE function with task training.[93-99] One important study is the EXCITE Randomized Clinical Trial, a large multisite trial. It consisted of a 2-week constraint-induced movement (CI) therapy intervention program with training of the more affected UE up to 6 hr/day and use of the mitt on the less affected hand for up to 90% of waking hours. Participants were also encouraged to practice two to three tasks daily at home. Measurements were taken before and after intervention and at 4-, 8- and 12-months' follow-up. Patients in the intervention group showed greater improvement than the control group in all measures of hand function (the Wolf Motor Function Test Performance Time, the Motor Activity Log Amount of Use and Quality of Movement, self-perceived hand difficulty—Stroke Impact Scale).[93,94] In a Cochrane Database Systematic Review, researchers investigated the evidence of CIMT for UEs in people with stroke (42 trials, 1,453 participants). Limited improvements were found in motor impairment and motor function, but the benefits did not convincingly reduce disability. The researchers concluded that additional research was needed on the long-term effects of CIMT and on the relationship between participant characteristics and improved outcomes.[100] Treatment-induced cortical reorganization has also been demonstrated with CIMT.[101,102]

Factors critical to successful outcomes using CI training programs include the following:

- Concentrated and repetitive task-specific practice used the more involved UE (Fig. 10.3).
- Training was intense, averaging 6 hr/day. Page et al[97] demonstrated improved function with less intensive, longer duration modified CIMT (mCIMT). All subjects started with some voluntary movement (wrist and finger extension) in their affected limb.
- Movement was constrained in the less affected UE through the use of a mitt worn up to 90% of waking hours.
- Behavioral techniques were used to enhance adherence and increased use of the affected UE in everyday life. Patients signed a behavioral contract indicating how often and with which activities they will use their affected limb. Daily administration of the Motor Activity Log also increased awareness of using the affected limb. Shaping techniques (operant conditioning) and functional training were used to develop challenging intervention tasks. Tasks were selected and tailored to address the specific motor deficits of the patient and shaped to allow for improving movement control and appropriate rest intervals. Feedback, coaching, modeling, and encouragement were provided to provide motivation. Patients were rewarded for improvement and correct movement patterns. Incorrect or poor performance was ignored in an attempt to break the cycle of learned nonuse.[92] See additional discussion in Chapter 15, Stroke.

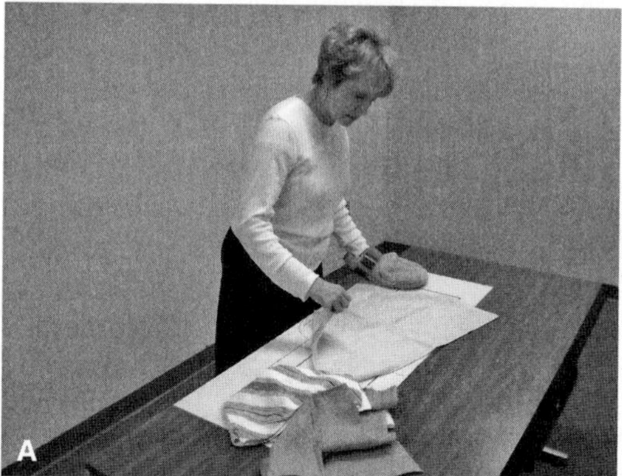

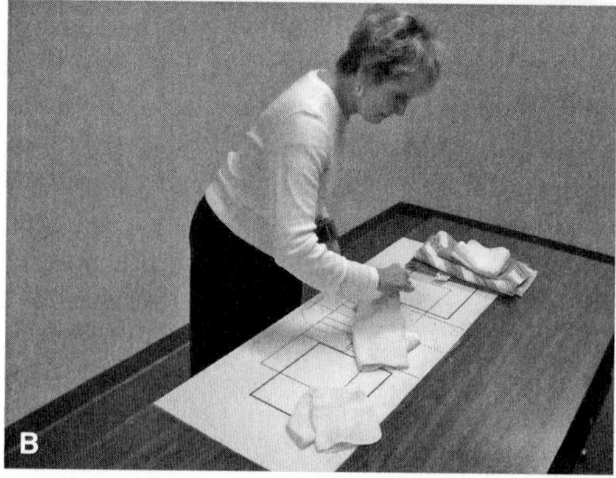

Figure 10.3 Patient is executing a task practice activity involving folding towels and stacking them during (A) early and (B) later stages of execution. *(From O'Sullivan and Schmitz,[92] with permission.)*

Task-Specific Training to Improve Gait and Locomotion

Task-specific locomotor training using treadmill training (TT) and partial body weight support (BWS) has been shown to be effective in promoting function-induced recovery.[103-106] In a Cochrane Database Systematic Review, researchers investigated BWSTT for walking after stroke (44 trials, 2,658 participants). They concluded that BWSTT improved walking velocity and walking endurance but did not significantly increase the chances of walking independently compared to other physical therapy interventions. People who demonstrated some walking ability benefited most from this intervention.[107]

Training includes intense practice (e.g., 30- to 60-minute sessions, 5 days per week for 6 to 12 weeks). The limbs are loaded to tolerance (e.g., starting at 40% BWS with progressions to 30%, 20%, 10%, and finally no BWS). Active upright posture and balance are maintained. The treadmill allows control and progression of gait speed (e.g., starting with slow speeds and progressing to faster speeds) and provides rhythmic timing of the stepping movements. Manual assistance is given to the patient's hips, pelvis, and LEs as needed to provide sensory input or to guide or adjust locomotor rhythm, limb placement, weight shifts, and symmetry (Fig 10.4). Training is progressed to no manual assistance or BWS to overground and community ambulation.[108] See additional discussion in Chapter 11, Locomotor Training, and Chapter 20, Traumatic Spinal Cord Injury.

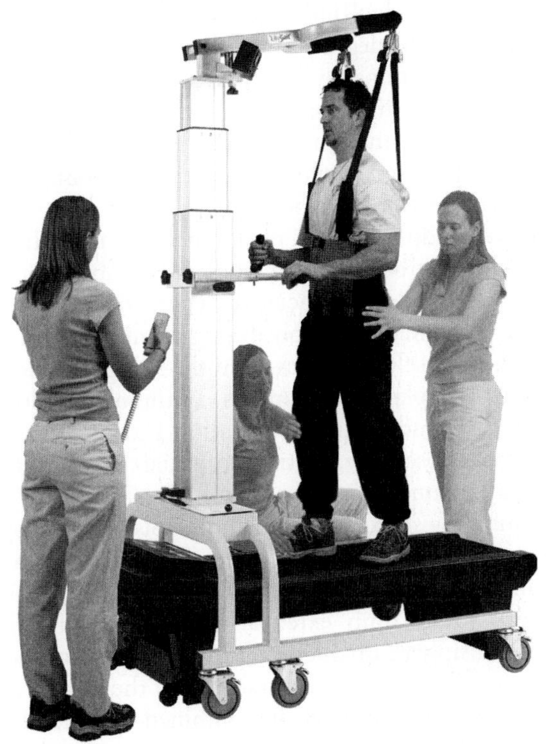

Figure 10.4 Patient in body weight support system positioned over a motorized treadmill.

Interventions to Improve Body Functions/Structure

The examination of motor function can reveal if a specific impairment or group of impairments (body functions and structure) are present. Using task analysis and evaluation, the therapist determines the links between impairments and limitations in functional performance. The therapist then needs to focus on specific interventions to improve these impairments. For example, a patient with MS demonstrates inability to stand up or transfer without moderate assistance of one. Lower extremity weakness in hip and knee extension is identified. Strength training of these muscles needs to be a targeted intervention. It is important to remember that resolution of the impairment may not yield the desired improvement in functional performance as practice is still needed within the context of the specific task. It is entirely possible that other impairments, previously masked by an inability to perform the task, were also contributing to the patient's inability to stand up independently (e.g., balance impairments). For example, early gait training in the parallel bars in which the patient with stroke requires an LE splint and maximal assistance of the therapist to move the limb forward does very little if anything to promote active locomotor control of that limb. Impairment-specific interventions must be linked to functional task training. The following section provides a brief overview of impairment-specific interventions.

Interventions to Improve Strength, Power, and Endurance

Muscle performance is defined as "the capacity of a muscle or group of muscles to generate forces." *Muscle strength* is the "muscle force exerted by a muscle or a group of muscles to overcome a resistance under a specific set of circumstances." *Muscle power* is "the work produced per unit of time or the product of strength and speed." *Muscle endurance* is "the ability to sustain forces repeatedly or to generate forces over a period of time."[109] Muscle performance is regulated by a number of factors. Neural factors include motor unit recruitment (number, type), motor neuron firing patterns, and efficiency of cooperative synergistic patterns. Muscle and biomechanical factors include initial muscle length and tension, muscle fiber composition, fuel storage and delivery, speed and type of contraction, and movement arm. Techniques that optimize these factors while addressing specific impairments and the demands of the task will yield maximum functional outcomes.

Strength Training

The benefits of strength training for patients with disorders of motor function include the following:

- Increased maximal force production due to changes in neural drive (increased motor unit recruitment, increased rate, and synchronization of firing pattern of motor units, improved reaction time).

- Changes in muscle (hypertrophy of muscle fibers, improved metabolic/enzymatic adaptations, increased size and number of myofibrils, muscle fiber type adaptation).
- Increased connective tissue tensile strength and bone mineral density.
- Improved body composition relative to body mass ratio of fat to lean.
- Improved functional performance and activity levels.
- Improved sense of well-being and self-confidence.

Basic principles of strengthening exercise include overload, specificity, cross training, and reversibility. The loads placed on muscle must be greater than those normally incurred (*overload principle*). Training effects are specific to the mode of exercise stress imposed on the exercising muscles (*specificity principle*). Thus, the training effects from an isometric protocol are specific to the exercising muscle and the point in the range that the muscle is holding. Effects do not carry over to improved dynamic performance (concentric or eccentric contractions). Nor will exercise training of the UEs transfer to improved LE performance. *Cross training* refers to a training program that includes a variety of training elements (e.g., isometric, concentric, eccentric, and endurance exercise). Cross training is used to place the broadest possible demands on the neuromuscular system and overcome the effects of specificity. *Reversibility principle* refers to the failure to sustain the benefits of strength training if muscles are not regularly engaged in exercise. Detraining effects include a reduction in muscle performance, decreased neural recruitment, and muscle fiber atrophy. The effectiveness of strength training is dependent on achieving an adequate training stimulus. Table 10.6 provides exercise guidelines for strength training.[110-113]

Open-chain exercises involve an isolated segment of the limb moving in space without simultaneous motions at adjacent joints. Muscle activation occurs predominantly in the prime mover(s) crossing the moving joint. Resistance is applied to the distal moving segment, typically in non-weight-bearing positions. *Closed-chain exercises* involve motions in which the distal part is fixed (foot or hand) while proximal segments are moving (e.g., weight shifting in standing, bilateral short-arc squats). They are performed in weight-bearing postures and involve simultaneous actions of synergistic muscles at multiple joints. The added joint approximation and stimulation of joint and muscle proprioceptors enhances neuromuscular control and joint stabilization (co-contraction). A limitation of closed-chain exercise is the substitution of other agonist muscles for specific muscle weakness. In comparison, open-chain exercises can be used to isolate contraction of a muscle or muscle group. However, the muscles trained and movements used are not well matched to normal functional movements that utilize complex movements and multisegment linkage.

Gains in strength can be obtained through progressive resistive exercises (PRE) using free weights or fixed mechanical resistance machines. A major disadvantage of PRE is that the weight selected is determined by the amount that can be lifted by the muscle at the weakest point of the range. Isokinetic training devices offer the advantage of providing accommodating resistance throughout the range. Muscle performance is therefore not limited to the weakest part of the range. The amount of force generated is recorded, providing an important objective measure of performance. Different isokinetic protocols using concentric and eccentric contractions have been developed. The speed of movement can be predetermined. This is an important consideration for training the patient who demonstrates neuromuscular impairments in timing and velocity control. For example, the patient recovering from stroke may be unable to generate the acceleration and deceleration forces needed during the different phases of gait. This results in delayed sequencing of muscle components and a general slowing of gait. Isokinetic training that focuses on the timing of these various components can improve gait function.

Strength gains can be achieved through functional training that uses task practice (e.g., repetitive practice of sit-to-stand or lunges). Resistance is provided by gravity and body weight and is applied simultaneously to multiple moving segments. It can be supplemented with manual resistance of the therapist, weights, elastic resistance bands, or resistance of water during pool therapy. Activities are selected that initially focus on specific body segments and progress to involve increasingly larger segments of the body. This serves to increase the level of difficulty and the degrees of freedom that must be controlled during the movement. Benefits of functional training include improved coordination of muscles, improved postural control and balance, and improved muscle extensibility and flexibility. Functional training helps the patient develop control of synergistic muscle groups acting in multiple axes and planes of movements. It also fosters the control of varying types and combinations of muscle contractions (concentric, eccentric, isometric) that are used interchangeably during normal movement. This is a very different focus from the straight planes of motion and isolated movements commonly employed during PRE and isokinetic training. Intrinsic sensory input (somatosensory, vestibular, visual) is maximized during functional training.

Combining strength training protocols with task-specific practice is an important strategy to maximize transfer gains to functional skills. For example, strengthening of weak lower limb extensor muscles can be first achieved using an isokinetic machine that targets both eccentric and concentric contractions of the quadriceps. This training can effectively be combined with repetitive practice of functional activities also demanding similar extensor control (e.g., partial squats, sit-to-stand transfers, and stair climbing). The important consideration

Table 10.6 Guidelines for Strength Training

Determine	Parameters of Exercise
Type of muscle contraction	Isometric, eccentric, concentric exercise
Mode of exercise training	Resistance training using weights Open chain (isolating one segment): isotonic and isokinetic exercises Closed chain: kinetic chain weight-bearing exercises (e.g., step-ups, modified squats) Circuit training: combination of varied methods Aquatic exercise Functional task training
Type of resistance/equipment	Free weights, pulleys, elastic bands, mechanical resistance machine, isokinetic resistance (dynamometry), manual resistance, body weight, water resistance (aquatics)
Recommended intensity: exercise load that best challenges the patient (*overload principle*)	Use submaximal loads • With weights, load is typically 60%–80% 1-RM with a goal. • Very weak individuals can start at 50% 1-RM and fewer than 10 repetitions (reps). Exercise progression: increase repetitions, number of sets, or load as tolerated; adjust the exercise load on the basis of exercise responses, strength measures, perceived exertion, and fatigue threshold.
Number of repetitions and sets; number of exercises per set	Initial frequency is typically 3 sets of 10–15 reps or as tolerated.
Duration	Total time of resistance training: typically, 15–30 minutes per session or as tolerated.
Frequency	Typically, 2–3 days/week, depending on intensity and level of impairment/disease.
Warm-up and cool-down periods	Include 5–10 min of warm-ups (calisthenics, stretching, ROM exercises) and 5–10 min of cool-down (muscle relaxation, stretching).
Additional considerations	Movements should be slow and controlled. Progression should occur in small increments. Reduce intensity with sudden onset of fatigue and exhaustion. Reduce intensity with prolonged and severe delayed onset muscle soreness. Regular breathing pattern should be maintained, while avoiding straining/Valsalva. Consider the interactions of exercise and medications. Exercise is contraindicated in some patients (e.g., with severe atrophic polio and recent weakness or ALS with muscle grades less than 3/5).
Outcomes	Relate strength training to functional task training. Focus the patient on improvements in functional performance in terms that are understandable and meaningful.

ALS = amyotrophic lateral sclerosis; RM = repetition max.

here is to match the strength training protocol to the requirements of the functional task in terms of ROM achieved and type, magnitude, and speed of contraction. Use of varied strength training activities and conditions also promotes development of flexibility of performance, an important goal for independence in daily life. In stroke survivors, muscle strengthening interventions have been shown to increase strength and improve function.[113-121]

Neuromuscular Reeducation

Patients with impaired motor function and weak muscles may demonstrate deficits in muscle activation. Early training should focus on isometric and eccentric contractions because muscle tension is better maintained than with concentric contractions. With isometric contractions, there is improved peripheral reflex support of contraction as opposed to the spindle unloading that occurs as the muscle moves into the shortened range of a concentric contraction. Eccentric contractions also produce greater muscle force with lower rates of motor unit discharge than concentric contractions. During training, the patient is initially asked to actively hold at midrange where the greatest tension can be generated. The patient is then asked to slowly lower the limb (an eccentric contraction) and hold (an isometric contraction). Once control is achieved in both these types of contractions, concentric contractions can be attempted.

For weak muscles, prestretching the muscle by starting the contraction in the lengthened range optimizes tension development through increased use of viscoelastic forces (*length–tension relationship*) and peripheral reflex support. Weak muscles can also be initially lightly resisted to facilitate contraction through *proprioceptive loading* (recruitment) of the muscle spindle. As the contraction proceeds through the range, weak muscles may fade out, typically by midrange. Maintaining contraction into the fully shortened range becomes difficult or impossible. A quick stretch or series of quick stretches can be applied to the agonist muscle to facilitate the contraction. Or tapping over the agonist muscle can have a similar effect of enhancing contraction through effects of proprioceptive loading. Control of velocity is also important to ensure efficiency of initial movement attempts. During concentric contractions, total tension decreases as velocity increases. Thus, patients may be able to generate a contraction at slow speeds but not at high speeds. For example, the patient with stroke who demonstrates limited control should be instructed to begin with slow and controlled movement. As movements become more efficient, they can be progressed to faster speeds. Techniques to stimulate or "jump-start" weak muscles should be reduced or eliminated as soon as active movement control becomes evident.

Muscular Endurance and Fatigue

Patients with deficits in motor function may demonstrate poor muscular endurance and fatigue. *Fatigue* is defined as the inability to contract muscle repeatedly over time. Thus, exercise cannot be sustained and exercise tolerance is reduced. The onset of fatigue is variable from patient to patient. Although many different factors may play a role, among the most important are the type and intensity of exercise. With the onset of fatigue, patients will demonstrate a decrement in force production progressing to total *exhaustion* (a ceiling effect). Fatigue can arise from neuromuscular disease affecting three primary sites: (1) the CNS (central fatigue), (2) the peripheral nerves or neuromuscular junction, or (3) the muscle itself. Examples of CNS conditions that can produce debilitating fatigue include MS, Guillain-Barré syndrome, chronic fatigue syndrome, and postpolio syndrome (PPS). The real danger of exercise training with these patients is the risk of *acute exercise overdose* producing exhaustion and possibly injury. *Overtraining,* defined as chronic overdose of exercise, is associated with both psychological and physiological decompensation, as well as musculoskeletal injury. *Overuse weakness* is manifested as aching on exertion and a prolonged decrease in absolute strength and endurance as a result of excessive activity. This is often seen in patients with PPS. For example, following an exercise session the patient with PPS demonstrates prolonged weakness and fatigue that does not recover with rest. If exercise is exhaustive, the patient may be unable to get out of bed the next day or perform normal activities of daily living (ADL). Even a simple conditioning program should be carefully monitored and progressed slowly to avoid overexertion and injury.[112]

Interventions to Improve Flexibility

Joint ROM and muscle flexibility must be adequate to allow for normal functional excursions of muscle and biomechanical alignment. Prolonged periods of disuse and immobility and motor dysfunction associated with neurological insult can lead to changes in muscle and joint function, postural alignment, and a host of indirect impairments. These include muscle tightness, atrophy, fibrosis, contracture, joint ankylosis, and postural deformity. Older adults demonstrate age-related changes affecting joint flexibility. These include increased viscosity of synovial fluid, stiffening of the joint capsule and ligaments, and calcification of articular cartilage. Proactive preventive intervention following neurological insult (e.g., stroke, TBI, SCI) is an important component of treatment. Patients with chronic and irreversible diseases (e.g., PD, MS, amyotrophic lateral sclerosis [ALS]) also need targeted intervention (tertiary prevention) to limit sequelae and degree of disability. Benefits include maintaining joint flexibility, tissue extensibility, ADL skills, and functional mobility. Additional benefits include improved circulation and tissue nutrition to the limbs and pain inhibition.

Techniques include:

- ROM exercises: active [AROM]; active assistive [AAROM]; passive.[110]
- Stretching techniques: static, dynamic, (proprioceptive neuromuscular facilitation [PNF], techniques of hold-relax [HR], contract-relax [CR]; contract-relax-agonist contract [CRAC]).[122,123]
- Low-load mechanical stretching with weights or specialized devices (serial casts, adjustable orthoses).[124,125]

The use of a warm-up period of exercise or preliminary therapeutic heat modality increases muscle temperature and elasticity and collagen extensibility. For example, calisthenics or low-resistance cycling will gradually increase tissue temperatures and elasticity, thereby enhancing the safety of stretching. Cold modalities can be used to cool muscles and decrease muscle spasm and pain.

Interventions to Improve Postural Control and Balance

Balance training focuses on improving postural control and both motor and sensory balance strategies. Targeted activities to improve balance function include biomechanical factors, static postural control (stability), dynamic postural control, anticipatory movements (proactive balance control), reactive balance control, sensory strategies, dynamic gait, dual task training, and safety training (Table 10.7).

Increased understanding of the overall coordination and strategies for balance (ankle, hip, change-in-support, sensory) negates any simplistic view of balance control. Overall, the organization of postural control and balance

Table 10.7 Postural Control and Balance Training

Parameters	Targeted Activities
Biomechanical Constraints	BOS, COM, vertical alignment ROM and strength training: trunk, LE
Static postural control/stability	Steady state static balance control: sitting or standing, without support, EO to EC Standing with reduced BOS (feet together, tandem stance)
Dynamic postural control	Weight shifts all directions to LOS, sitting or standing Reaching, all directions, sitting or standing Standing, stepping, all directions Picking up an object from the floor
Anticipatory movements (proactive balance control)	Sit-to-stand Floor-to-stand Stand on one leg, R and L Up on toes, back on heels Standing, catching a weighted ball
Reactive balance control	Responses to external perturbations, nudges: sitting and standing, all directions Stepping responses
Sensory strategies	Standing on firm surface, EO to EC Standing on foam surface, EO to EC
Dynamic gait	Walking: forward, changing BOS, changing speeds Walking: head turns, pivot turns, obstacles Walking: backward, side stepping Timed walking
Dual-task training	A secondary task is imposed during static or dynamic activities in sitting, standing, or walking; can be either motor or cognitive. Motor: batting a balloon, tossing or bouncing a ball, pouring a glass of water from a pitcher, walking while carrying a tray Cognitive: spelling forward and backward, counting backward by 2, reciting the alphabet every other letter
Safety training	Fall risk and safety awareness training Safe use of assistive/mobility devices Supportive footwear

BOS = base of support; COM = center of mass; EC = eyes closed; EO = eyes open; L = left; LOS = limits of stability; R = right

must be viewed as flexible, not rigid, involving multiple body segments and postural strategies.[126-128] In that context, patterns will vary according to a number of different factors, including initial conditions, balance requirements and challenges, movement characteristics, learning, and intention.[129] The patient needs to practice steady state, anticipatory, and reactive balance control using activities that focus on both static and dynamic postural control. The activities selected should include those required for ADL and functional mobility, as well as those required for social participation, recreation, and work, if appropriate. Sensory selection and organization should also be a part of a balance training program. The reader is referred to the work of Shumway-Cook and Woollacott[2] for a complete discussion of normal postural control.

It is important to note that some balance training activities may cause the patient distress initially. The patient will feel threatened when placed in situations where he or she is in jeopardy of falling. The therapist should ensure patient confidence by providing a clear explanation of the nature of the task, what the challenges to balance are, and the steps the therapist will take to prevent falls in terms that are easy to understand. The patient with instability can wear a gait belt or practice standing activities wearing an overhead safety harness. The therapist needs to stand close enough to the patient to guard safely but not so close as to interfere with the activity. For the very unstable patient, two spotters may be necessary. Aspects of the environment can be used to assist in ensuring safety and preventing the patient from falling. For example, standing exercises can be performed in the parallel bars, between two tables, near a wall or two walls (corner standing), or in a pool with the patient standing in waist-high or chest-high water. Support given early in training should be withdrawn as soon as possible to allow focus on active control.

An understanding of the foundational requirements of upright postures will direct the therapist in improving postural alignment and body mechanics. Sitting is a relatively stable posture with a BOS that includes contact of the buttocks, thighs, and feet with the support surface. During normal sitting, weight is equally distributed over both buttocks with the pelvis in neutral position or tilted slightly anterior. The head and trunk are vertical, maintained in midline orientation. The line of gravity passes close to the joint axes of the spine. Muscles of the cervical, thoracic, and lumbar spine are active in maintaining upright postural control and core stability. BOS can be increased by using one or both hands for additional support and reduced by sitting on a high table with the feet off the floor.

Standing is a less stable posture with a high COM and a small BOS that includes contact of the feet with the support surface. During normal quiet standing, there is minimal body sway with ankle muscle activity (primarily dorsiflexors/plantarflexors, invertors/evertors) activated to counteract body sway. Weight is equally distributed over both feet with feet positioned parallel and slightly apart; knees should be extended or in slight flexion, not hyperextended. The line of gravity falls close to most joint axes: slightly anterior to the ankle and knee joints; slightly posterior to the hip joint; posterior to the cervical and lumbar vertebrae; and anterior to the thoracic vertebrae and atlanto-occipital joint. Natural spinal curves are present but somewhat flattened in upright stance, depending on the level of postural tone (e.g., lumbar and cervical lordosis, thoracic kyphosis). The pelvis is in neutral position, with no anterior or posterior tilt. Normal alignment minimizes the need for muscle activity during erect stance.

Changes in normal alignment are common in patients with deficits in motor function. They may represent as a primary impairment or can result in corresponding changes in other body segments. For example, a slumped sitting posture (dorsal kyphosis and forward head) is typically the result of sacral sitting with the pelvis tilted posteriorly. In standing, faulty postures such as forward head and kyphosis, excessive hip and knee flexion, or pelvic asymmetries are common.

Initial physical therapy interventions should focus first on improving specific musculoskeletal impairments (e.g., limited ROM, weakness). Postural reeducation begins with demonstration of the correct posture. Verbal cues should focus on control of essential postural elements—that is, stable (neutral) pelvis, axial extension (e.g., "sit tall," "stand tall"), and normal alignment (e.g., head erect, shoulders back, weight evenly distributed over both hips [sitting] or both feet [standing]). Patients can benefit from tactile cues during initial practice (manual or surface related). For example, patients can stand (or sit) with the back positioned against a wall or patients with a lateral lean (e.g., patients with pusher syndrome following a stroke) can sit with their sound side positioned against a wall. Corner standing (against two walls) can be effective in helping patients with pronounced deficits (e.g., the patient with ataxia) maintain vertical alignment. Mirrors can provide important visual cues regarding vertical position. For example, the patient wears a shirt with a taped vertical line on it and is asked to match it to a taped vertical line on a mirror.[2] The taped lines provide useful visual feedback for achieving vertical. Mirrors are generally contraindicated for the patient with visuospatial perceptual deficits. Application of correct postures to real-life functional situations is important to ensure carryover and lasting change.

Interventions to Improve Static Postural Control

Patients who demonstrate impairments in static postural control (stability) are unable to maintain or hold a steady position for many reasons, including decreased strength, tonal imbalances (hypotonia, spasticity, dystonia), impaired voluntary control and hypermobility (ataxia, athetosis), sensory hypersensitivity (tactile-avoidance reactions), or increased anxiety or arousal (high sympathetic "fight or flight" state). Instability is associated with excessive postural sway, wide BOS, low- or high-guard hand position, holding on to an object in the environment (handhold), and loss of balance (falls).

The therapist can select any of a number of weight-bearing (antigravity) postures to develop stability control. Typical training postures include sitting and standing. Postures are selected based on (1) patient safety and level of control and (2) importance in terms of functional tasks. The patient practices active holding or resisted holding. The therapist should focus on obtaining symmetrical weight-bearing. Patients may present with specific directional instabilities, such as weight-bearing more on one side than the other. For example, after a stroke the patient typically keeps weight centered toward the less affected side. Practice should focus on redirecting the patient into a centered position by moving toward the more affected side, both in sitting and standing positions. The patient is instructed to "hold steady" while sitting or standing tall and maintaining a visual focus on a forward target. Progression is to holding for longer and longer durations. Techniques that can be used to enhance stabilizing muscle contractions include quick stretch, tapping, resistance, approximation, manual contacts, and verbal cues. For the patient unable to actively stabilize the body, the therapist can begin with resisted isometric contractions of antagonist postural muscle. For example, the patient with severe instability following TBI who is unable to sit independently may need to begin practice holding a neutral trunk position first in a supported sitting position. The therapist can then progress the patient to active sitting and to postures that demand increasing amounts of upright (antigravity) postural control (standing). If an imbalance exists, the stabilizing activity can be coupled with a strengthening activity for the weak muscles. As the trunk becomes more stable, the patient is expected to assume active control in stabilizing in the posture.

Additional strategies to improve stability include the use of elastic resistance bands to enhance *proprioceptive loading* and contraction of stabilizing muscles. For example, in standing an elastic band can be placed around both thighs. The patient is instructed to maintain the LEs apart against the resistance. This selectively loads and facilitates contraction of the hip stabilizers (abductors and extensor muscles), improving stability control at the hips.

As static postural control improves, the therapist can progress the patient to stabilizing on a moveable surface (e.g., sitting on a therapy ball). In sitting, gentle bouncing on the therapy ball provides joint approximation through the vertebral joints, facilitating extensors and an upright posture. For an additional challenge, sitting stability control can be practiced on other compliant surfaces (e.g., sitting on wobble board, or Dynadisc™). Static control in standing can be practiced while standing on foam. The therapist can also increase task difficulty by reducing the BOS (feet apart to feet together).[130,131]

Aquatic therapy can also be used to enhance proprioceptive loading. The water provides a degree of unweighting and resistance to movement. This can be quite effective in reducing hyperkinetic movements and enhancing postural stability. For example, a patient recovering from TBI who demonstrates significant ataxia may be able to sit or stand in the pool with minimal assistance whereas these same activities outside the pool are not possible.

Interventions to Improve Dynamic Postural Control

Patients who demonstrate impairments in dynamic postural control are unable to control postural stability and orientation while moving segments of the body. A number of impairments may be contributing factors, including tonal imbalances (spasticity, rigidity, hypotonia), ROM restrictions, impaired voluntary control and hypermobility (ataxia, athetosis), impaired reciprocal "actions of the antagonists (cerebellar dysfunction), or impaired proximal stabilization. Clinically, the patient demonstrates difficulty weight shifting from side to side or forward–backward. Difficulties are also apparent in maintaining balance control while moving one or more limbs. For example, one limb is moving (UE reaching or LE stepping) while the patient maintains a stable posture. These added movements increase the demands for stabilization control because the *limits of stability* (LOS, the outer point at which the COM is still maintained within the BOS) are challenged and/or the overall BOS is reduced.

Dynamic postural control is usually practiced in sitting and standing though a number of different postures can be used (e.g., quadruped, kneeling, plantigrade). Practice begins with weight shifts emphasizing smooth directional changes that engage antagonist actions. LOS should be explored. For example, in sitting or standing, the patient is instructed to slowly move in all directions (forward–backward, side to side) as far as possible while still maintaining a stable position. Loss of balance occurs when the LOS has been exceeded, for example, when the COM extends beyond the BOS. Weight shifting practice is important to assist the patient in developing an accurate perceptual awareness of stability limits, an important component of an overall CNS internal model of postural control. Because LOS changes with different tasks, a variety of functional activities should be practiced. As control improves, the movements are gradually expanded through an increasing range (*increments of range*). For the patient who has difficulty initiating or controlling movements, initial movements can be facilitated using manual contacts and verbal cues.[130,131]

Improving motor strategies is an important goal of balance training. In standing, *ankle strategies* can be promoted by having the patient practice small-range, slow-velocity anterior/posterior shifts. Attention is directed to the action of ankle muscles to move the body (COM) over the fixed feet (BOS). Standing on a rocker board (moveable surface) or foam roller with the flat side down progressing to flat side up are effective activities to increase the challenge in recruiting ankle strategies. The patient is also directed to practice weight shifts that normally recruit *hip strategies.* These include larger shifts in the COM that approach the LOS and/or faster body sway motions that are characterized by early activation of proximal hip and trunk muscles. Hip flexion and extension responses are generated during anterior–posterior shifts. Hip abductor responses are generated during lateral shifts. Patients are instructed to move their upper body forward and backward or to the side while standing.[131]

Training is progressed to include both reaching and stepping activities. Functionally important and motivating activities should be selected. For example, the patient practices reaching for a cup while maintaining a stable sitting or standing position. Items can be placed forward, backward, out to the side, overhead (e.g., on a shelf), or below the waist (e.g. emptying a dishwasher). Or a bilateral UE task (e.g., folding and stacking towels) can be used while maintaining a stable standing position (see Fig 10.3). During practice of stepping movements, the patient shifts weight over the support limb and takes a step (forward or backward, or out to the side) with the dynamic limb. Forward or lateral step-ups (placing the foot on a low stair or stool) can also be practiced.[131]

Therapy ball activities are effective in developing dynamic stability control in sitting. For example, the patient sits on a ball and gently moves the ball side to side, forward–backward, or in a combination (pelvic clock motions). Or the patient sits on the ball while performing voluntary movements of the arms or legs (e.g., alternate leg or arm raises). Progression is from unilateral to bilateral and finally to reciprocal limb movements (e.g., Mexican hat dance). Voluntary trunk motions can also be practiced while sitting on the ball (e.g., head and trunk rotation with arms held out to the side).[130]

Difficulty can be increased during static and dynamic training by adding a secondary task (*dual task training*). These can include a second motor task such as catching and throwing a ball, batting a balloon, or kicking a ball. A secondary cognitive task can also be added (e.g., spelling a word forward or backward, counting backward by 3s). By varying the cognitive demands during a balance task, the patient is forced to concentrate on the second task with less conscious control of the balance task. In real life, many falls incurred by patients with neurological insult and the elderly are experienced when distracted by secondary tasks (e.g., talking on the phone).[2]

Anticipatory Balance Control

Anticipatory postural adjustments should also be practiced, because predictive control must be operational for functional balance. Practice can include a variety of transitional functional tasks (e.g., sit-to-stand, floor-to-stand, stand on one leg, up on toes). The patient is provided with advance information (preparatory cues) about the upcoming demands of the task. For example, during catching a weighted ball while standing, verbal cues would include "I want you to catch this 5-pound weighted ball while holding a steady position." The prior knowledge serves as an important source of information for adjusting posture and performing the correct movement. Tai chi training has also been shown to improve balance control and stepping.[132-134]

Reactive Balance Control

Patients with deficits in motor function and balance are also typically unable to respond effectively to external perturbations. The therapist can utilize gentle manual pulls or pushes applied to the shoulders or hips, or use moving platforms, to provide perturbations. Small perturbations can be used to activate strategies designed to maintain a stable position (e.g., ankle or hip), whereas larger perturbations can be used activate stepping. The therapist should vary inputs so as to not be predicable in terms of the response activated (i.e., direction, type, and speed of response). An elastic band around the hips can also be used to promote stepping (forward, backward, sideward). The therapist maintains resistance of band against the hips and then suddenly releases the resistance, requiring the patient to take a step. With lateral displacements, researchers found that the typical pattern is a cross-stepping pattern, seen in 87% of lateral stepping responses, as opposed to straight sidestepping. They also found that stepping may actually be the preferred strategy to using a hip strategy for many adults.[135] Lateral destabilization is particularly problematic for a large portion of older adults who experience falls. Arm reactions in response to whole body instability were also found to be prevalent with activation of shoulder muscles occurring in 85% of destabilizing trials.[136] Patient safety and protection against falls should be maintained during all perturbation training.

Research evidence demonstrates the effectiveness of training in improving balance control.[137-143] In a Cochrane Database Review (94 studies, 9,821 participants), researchers found positive effects of exercise on balance outcome measures. Different categories of exercise were included: gait, balance and functional task training, strengthening exercise, tai chi, physical activity programs (walking, cycling), computerized balance training using visual feedback, vibration platform, and multiple exercise types (combinations of programs). Programs typically ran three times a week for three months and involved dynamic exercise in standing with few adverse effects reported. They concluded that more high quality research is needed to identify best types and intensity of training.[138]

Interventions to Improve Sensory Control of Balance

An important focus of balance training is utilization and integration of appropriate sensory systems. Normally three sources of inputs are utilized to maintain balance: somatosensory inputs (proprioceptive and tactile inputs from the feet and ankles), visual inputs, and vestibular inputs. Careful examination can identify the patient's use of inputs to maintain balance (e.g., *Clinical Test for Sensory Interaction and Balance* [CTSIB]; see Chapter 5, Examination of Motor Function, for a discussion of this test). Training is directed toward varying sensory conditions to challenge the patient. Patients who demonstrate a high degree of dependence on vision can practice balance tasks that improve utilization of surface information (somatosensory cues). The patient stands on a firm surface while vision is altered or imprecise. For example, the patient stands with eyes open (EO) to eyes closed (EC), in full lighting to reduced lighting, dark lenses to petroleum-coated lenses. Dual tasking can also be used (e.g., eyes engaged in a reading activity, reading a card held against a busy checkerboard pattern). Tasks can be practiced that improve utilization of vision (eyes remain open) while simultaneously reducing reliance on somatosensory information. For example, the patient stands on a compliant surface, progressing from carpet (low pile to high pile) to foam cushion. Standing on a moving platform (wobble board) can also be used. Tasks can be practiced that improve utilization of vestibular inputs. Examples of tasks include standing on foam EC, standing on foam with eyes engaged in a reading task, tandem standing with EC. These situations are sometimes referred to as a *sensory conflict situation,* requiring resolution of the conflict (misinformation) by the vestibular system.[131] Patients should also practice varying environmental influences such as walking outside, progressing from relatively smooth terrain (sidewalks) to uneven terrain to moving surfaces (escalator, elevator). Research evidence demonstrates the effectiveness of altering sensory contexts in improving sensory selection and organization for balance.[144-148]

Safety Training

Patients with significant sensory loss will require assistance in shifting toward the intact systems to monitor and adjust balance using alternate sensory inputs. For example, the patient with LE somatosensory losses (e.g., diabetic neuropathy, bilateral amputation) will need to learn to focus on using visual information for control in standing and walking. If deficits exist in more than one of the major sensory systems, shifts are generally inadequate and balance deficits will be pronounced. Thus, the patient with diabetic neuropathy and retinopathy will be at high risk for loss of balance and falls. Training in using an assistive device is indicated. Other patients must be encouraged to ignore distorted information (e.g., impaired proprioception and perception accompanying stroke) in favor of more accurate sensory information. Patients with low vision should practice balance activities while wearing their eyeglasses. The exception to this is when patients wear glasses with progressive or bifocal lens, which should not be worn during stair climbing training. The lower portion of the lens (designed for reading) can distort vision when looking down and interfere with depth perception.

When significant postural and balance limitations exist, patient education should focus on fall risk and balance strategies to prevent falls. Assistive devices may be indicated to ensure patient safety and to prevent a fall. Footwear designed to improve maximum support and safety is warranted (e.g., athletic shoes). Modification of the home environment is necessary to promote safety. See Chapter 9, Examination and Modification of the Environment, and Box 10.5 for strategies to promote safe balance.

Interventions to Improve Coordination and Agility

Coordination is the ability to execute smooth, accurate, and controlled movements. *Agility* is the ability to perform coordinated movements combined with upright balance. *Ataxia* is defined as uncoordinated movement that manifests when voluntary movements are attempted, influencing gait, posture, and patterns of movement. The principal causes of ataxia are cerebellar disease or lesions (e.g., cerebellar atrophy, tumor, MS, TBI, stroke, Friedreich's ataxia, chronic alcoholism). Patients with ataxia typically demonstrate impaired synergistic actions with decomposition of movement (dyssynergia), impaired ability to judge the distance or range of movement (dysmetria), and impaired ability to perform rapid alternating movements (dysdiadochokinesia), along with intention tremor and disturbances of posture and gait. Typical standing postural abnormalities include an exaggerated lumbar lordosis, anterior pelvic tilt, flexion at the hips, hyperextension at the knees, and weight placed more on the heels. Patients with ataxia also typically demonstrate mild decreases in

Box 10.5 Strategies to Promote Safe Balance

The patient is taught to do the following:

- Rely on intact senses, heightening patient awareness of available senses.
- Focus vision on a stationary visual target rather than a moving target.
- Minimize head movements during more difficult balance tasks requiring vestibular inputs (sensory conflict situations).
- Widen the BOS when turning or sitting down.
- Widen the BOS in the direction of an expected force (e.g., step position).
- Lower the COM when greater stability is needed (e.g., crouching when a threat to balance is imminent).
- Wear comfortable, well-fitting shoes with rubber soles for better friction and gripping (e.g., athletic shoes).
- Use light touch-down support as needed to increase somatosensory inputs and stability.
- Use an assistive device as needed (e.g., a cane or walker) to provide support for standing.
- Use a vertical or slant cane to increase somatosensory inputs from the hand.
- Use an augmented feedback device (e.g., auditory signals from a limb-load monitor or biofeedback cane) to provide additional sensory feedback information.
- Recognize potentially dangerous environmental situations (e.g., low light or high glare for the patient who relies heavily on vision).
- Modify the home environment (e.g., focus on adequate lighting, supportive furniture, arrangement of furniture, removal of small scatter rugs, use of handrails and grab bars).

BOS = Base of support; COM = Center of mass.

strength (asthenia) and tone (hypotonia) and hypermobility. Postural instability in the patient with ataxia is associated with excessive postural sway, wide BOS, high guard hand position, handhold, and frequent loss of balance (falls). Motor learning is also typically slowed, given the inability of the cerebellum to timely and correctly utilize feedback to modulate movement. The reader is referred to Chapter 6, Examination of Coordination and Balance, for additional information.

The benefits of training activities include the following:

- Improve postural stability and balance
- Improve accuracy of limb movements
- Improve function
- Improve safety awareness and compensatory strategies for effective movement control and fall prevention

Patients with ataxia generally benefit from the use of light resistance to slow limb and trunk movements, temporarily reducing dysmetria and tremor. This can include use of light weight cuffs (ankle, wrist), elastic bands, weighted trunk vest, weighted walkers and canes, and water resistance (pool activities). The key issue for the therapist is to provide enough resistance to enhance proprioceptive loading and movement without producing debilitating fatigue. During training, movements should be kept slow and controlled; fast movements are considerably more problematic in terms of learning and performance. Complex *gross motor skills* that engage and move large segments of the body (e.g., sit-to-stand, transfers, locomotion) are difficult for patients with ataxia. *Fine motor skills* that engage the small muscles of the hand (e.g., feeding, writing, ADL) are also difficult and can lead to functional dependence (e.g., inability to feed or dress). Augmented feedback in the form of biofeedback, rhythmic auditory stimulation (metronome, music) can be used to help modulate speed and focus attention. Devices that promote reciprocal movements and timing (e.g., cycle ergonometer, motorized treadmill with an overhead harness) can also be effective. To enhance motor learning, the patient should practice in a low-stimuli environment. Variable practice should only be attempted as skill development becomes apparent and at a much more gradual rate of progression. A distributed practice schedule is important because patients with ataxia can demonstrate low endurance and increased fatigue. For the patient with significant ataxia and postural instability, hands-on support and guidance may be necessary. Aids for mobility (assistive devices) may be necessary to ensure safety and prevent falls. Research evidence supports the effectiveness of physical therapy in improving ataxia.[149-154]

Aerobic Conditioning

The benefits of aerobic training for patients with disorders of motor function include the following:

- Enhanced brain function and neural plastic changes
- Improved cognitive function (executive function, attention/concentration, memory)
- Improved motor learning
- Improved cardiovascular and peripheral (muscular) endurance
- Decreased anxiety and depression, increased social interaction
- Enhanced physical function
- Enhanced sense of well-being

Recovery of motor function and motor learning is aided by aerobic training. Mang[155] summarized evidence of exercise-induced release of brain-derived neurotrophic factors involved in neuroprotection, neurogenesis, and angiogenesis. To capitalize on these effects the researchers suggest aerobic bouts may need to be performed in close temporal proximity to motor skill practice of experience. Aerobic training also produces positive changes in maximal oxygen uptake (Vo_{2max}) and metabolic changes.[156,157] In a Cochrane Database Systematic Review (58 trials, 2,797 patients), researchers found that cardiorespiratory training reduced disability during or after usual stroke care. Improvements in speed and walking capacity and balance were noted. They concluded that further trials were needed to investigate cognitive changes, optimal exercise prescription, and long-term benefits.[158]

An aerobic training program is determined based on the patient's level of deconditioning and specific health condition and symptoms. Aerobic training can include ergometry (two-limb or four-limb), recumbent stepper, and walking. In general, moderate intensities of exercises are appropriate for most patients undergoing active rehabilitation or with a chronic disease and disabilities (e.g., 40% to 70% of maximal oxygen consumption), whereas high intensities are contraindicated. For many patients, a frequency of 3 to 5 days per week with 20- to 60-minute sessions is often recommended. Sessions can be broken down into multiple 10-minute sessions. Most patients will require a discontinuous protocol that carefully balances exercise with rest. Clinical practice guidelines, including exercise recommendations, are available to assist the therapist in treating patients with chronic disabilities. *ACSM's Exercise Management for Persons with Chronic Diseases and Disabilities,* 4th edition, is particularly helpful for the therapist as it discusses exercise guidelines for a number of different disabilities (e.g., stroke, TBI, SCI, MS, PD).[112]

Effective management of patients with low endurance and fatigue includes the use of energy conservation techniques, activity pacing, lifestyle changes, regular rest periods during the day, and improved sleep through the use of relaxation techniques and medications. An activity log can be used to help the patient identify activities that are particularly exhausting and to document the effectiveness of rest. Unnecessary energy-consuming activities should be discontinued and essential activities restructured and paced to include regular rest periods throughout the day. Patients can monitor their level of general fatigue using the Borg

Rating of Perceived Exertion (RPE) scale[159] and should aim to keep their activities at an RPE level of "somewhat hard" (14 or lower using the 6–20 RPE scale). Ergonomic changes (e.g., seating and workstations) should be implemented to reduce energy cost of activities. Finally, stress management should be included in the educational program.

Augmented Interventions

Postural Biofeedback

Augmented feedback can be used to during training (e.g., posturography feedback, EMG-biofeedback). In posturography, a force-platform device is used to measure forces and provide *center of pressure (COP) biofeedback.* The weight on each foot is computed and converted into visual feedback regarding the locus and movement of the COP. COP displacement is associated with movement of the COM or postural sway. Although COP excursion always exceeds COM sway, this relationship is close during ankle motions (ankle strategies) when the body moves like a pendulum over the feet. However, when a hip strategy is used (upper body motion focused at the hips), the COP:COM relationship becomes distorted and does not accurately reflect sway. A computer analyzes the data and provides relevant biofeedback concerning sway path and COP position on a visual monitor. Some units also provide auditory feedback.

Posturography training can be used to shape sway movements to enhance symmetry and steadiness. The patient can be instructed to increase or decrease sway movements (weight shifts) or move the COP cursor on the computer screen to achieve a designated range or to match a designated target. It is an effective training mode for patients who demonstrate problems in force generation. For example, the patient with decreased force generation (hypometria) as typically demonstrated by individuals with PD is directed toward achieving larger and faster sway movements during posturography training. The patient with too much force (hypermetria), as typically demonstrated by the individual with cerebellar ataxia, is directed toward decreasing sway movements progressing to holding a stable, centered posture. It is also effective in improving symmetrical alignment (e.g., the patient with stroke who stands with most of the weight on the less affected limb).

Research evidence demonstrates the effectiveness of platform training in improving standing balance.[160-165] In a Cochrane Database Systematic Review (7 trials, 246 participants), researchers found that force platform feedback improved standing balance but did not improve balance during active functional activities, or overall independence.[166] Given the specificity of training principle, this is not a surprising finding that platform training did not automatically transfer to other functional activities as these require specific task practice to generate improvement.

Electromyographic Biofeedback

For patients with severe motor weakness, electromyographic biofeedback (EMG-BFB) can be used to assist the patient in regaining control of muscle actions and in neuromuscular reeducation. With careful electrode placement, it provides an accurate indication of electrical activity associated with muscular effort. It does not, however, provide an accurate indication of force of contraction. Surface electromyography (SEMG) electrodes are commonly used for recording. The signal is amplified and converted in audio and/or visual form, providing useful information about muscular performance to the patient.[167] Gaming using a virtual reality environment can also be used to provide feedback.[168]

Most neuromuscular biofeedback research focuses on the effects of biofeedback to treat UE and LE motor deficits in patients with neurological disorders. In patients recovering from stroke, EMG-BFB has been shown to improve UE function (hand and shoulder)[168-170] and LE function.[171-173] Patients who exhibit weak (trace, poor, or fair) muscle grades or deficient sensory feedback systems will benefit the most. In a Cochrane Database Systematic Review of the effects of EMG-BFB for motor function recovery following stroke (13 trials, 269 participants), Woodford et al[174] found evidence to suggest that EMG-BFB plus standard physical therapy produced improvements in motor power, functional recovery, and gait quality when compared to standard physical therapy alone. The researchers concluded that the results are limited because the trials were small, generally poorly designed, and utilized varying outcome measures.[174] The therapist must carefully structure the use of biofeedback with active task practice. External feedback must be gradually reduced to foster use of intrinsic feedback mechanisms and active movements as recovery progresses.

Neuromuscular Electrical Stimulation

Neuromuscular electrical stimulation (NMES) stimulates contraction in very weak muscles. Electrodes are placed directly over the muscle to be stimulated. Contraction is elicited by depolarizing motor neurons, with larger motor units and a greater number of Type II fibers firing first. The motor units will continue to fire until the stimulus stops. NMES has been used to reeducate muscles, improve motor function, reduce disuse atrophy and edema, and reduce spasticity with stimulation of the weak antagonist. It has also been shown to improve wrist and hand function, shoulder function and reduce subluxation, and improve gait.[175-181] In a Cochrane Database Systematic Review on the use of electrostimulation for promoting recovery of movement or functional ability after stroke (24 trials, 2,077 participants), researchers found improvement of functional motor ability when compared to no treatment. When compared to conventional physical therapy, the researchers found only improvement in motor impairment but no difference in functional improvement. They concluded there was insufficient robust data.[182]

Functional electrical stimulation (FES) uses a microprocessor to recruit muscles in a programmed synergistic sequence for the purposes of improving functional movements. Following stroke, FES of the peroneal nerve has been shown to be effective in assisting dorsiflexion (drop foot) and improving walking.[183-185] It has been effectively combined with BWS and a treadmill.[186,187] FES has been used to assist patients with incomplete SCI to exercise on bicycle ergometers (FES ergometry) and walk.[188,189]

Substitution Training

Adaptive compensation is the development of alternative or new movement patterns using involved segments. *Substitutive compensation* involves using different parts of the body, effectors, to accomplish a task.[37] For example, the patient with hemiplegia learns to dress using the less-affected UE; the patient with paraplegia regains functional rolling, transfers, and wheelchair locomotion using the UEs. During training, the patient is made aware of movement deficiencies and the changes required to complete the functional task. Alternate ways to accomplish the task are suggested, simplified, and adopted. The patient practices and relearns the task using the new movement pattern and body segments. The patient then practices the new pattern in the environment in which the function is expected to occur. Adaptation of the environment is also used to facilitate relearning of skills and optimal performance. For example, the patient with unilateral neglect is assisted in dressing by color-coding the shoes (red tape on the left shoe, yellow tape on the right shoe). The wheelchair brake toggle is extended and color-coded to allow easy identification.

One of the major criticisms of the early use of this approach is that the focus on less-involved segments may suppress recovery and contribute to *learned nonuse* of impaired segments. For example, the patient with stroke fails to learn to use the more involved extremities. Substitution training should not become the focus of treatment in patients with potential for recovery. It is important to remember that given appropriate training, motor improvements can continue well into recovery (e.g., patients with chronic stroke, greater than 1 year poststroke). Substitution training can also lead to development of *splinter skills,* which are skills acquired in a manner inconsistent with skills the individual already possesses. Splinter skills cannot be easily generalized to other task variations or to other environments.

Substitution training may be the only realistic approach possible when recovery potential is limited or the patient presents with significant comorbidities, impairments, and functional limitations with little or no expectation for additional recovery. Examples include the patient with complete SCI or the patient recovering from stroke with severe sensorimotor deficits and extensive comorbidities (e.g., severe cardiac and respiratory compromise or memory deficits associated with Alzheimer's disease). The patient in the latter example is severely limited in the ability to actively participate in rehabilitation and to relearn motor skills.

■ PATIENT/CLIENT-RELATED EDUCATION

Patient/client-related instruction is an important component of any rehabilitation POC. Components include instruction and training of patients/clients about the following:

- Current condition (pathology/pathophysiology, impairments, activity limitations, and participation restrictions)
- Accommodations to deficits in communication, cognitive, behavioral, or emotional impairments
- Goals and expected outcomes
- Strategies and preferred interventions to enhance motor function
- Risk factors for pathology/pathophysiology and prevention of additional impairments, functional limitations, and participation restrictions
- Strategies and preferred interventions to enhance health, wellness, fitness, and functional recovery

Patients with deficits in motor function need to recognize the importance of repetitive practice both in therapy and out of therapy to bring about meaningful recovery. Relevant tools to ensure high levels of practice include a behavioral contract, a caregiver contract, a daily schedule, an activity log or home diary, and a home skill assignment. These tools serve to focus the patient on the POC and ensure full, active participation in reaching successful outcomes. Patient skills in self-evaluation, problem solving, and decision making are promoted to foster independence. This empowerment serves to improve quality of life and prepare the patient for the lifelong adjustments needed when living with a disability. If patient independence is not possible because of the complexity of deficits and limitations in recovery (e.g., the patient with severe TBI), education of family, friends, and caregivers assumes paramount importance.

SUMMARY

This chapter has presented a conceptual framework for rehabilitation of the patient with deficits in motor function based on an understanding of the normal processes of motor control, motor learning, and recovery. Clinical decision making is based on a thorough examination of the patient's deficits in terms of impairments, activity limitations, and participation restrictions. The unique problems of each patient require that the therapist also recognize a number of interrelated factors, including individual needs and changing status, motivation, goals, concerns, and potential for independent function. The diversity of problems experienced by patients with disordered motor function negates the idea that any one intervention or group of interventions could be successful for all patients. Broad categories of interventions have been presented, with a major emphasis on motor learning strategies and task-oriented training. Interventions also need to promote adaptability of skills for function in real-world environments and remediation of specific impairments in structure or function. In selecting interventions, the therapist must consider those that have the greatest chance of success. The choice of interventions must also take into consideration other factors, including ability to deliver care, cost-effectiveness in terms of length of stay and number of allotted physical therapy visits, age of the patient, comorbidities, social support, and potential discharge placement. Carefully planned and structured education empowers the patient and ensures skills for lifelong learning and adjustment.

Questions for Review

1. Differentiate between the terms *motor control* and *motor learning*. How can impairments in motor control be distinguished from those of motor learning?
2. Differentiate between the three stages of motor learning. How do training strategies differ during each stage?
3. Define *neural plasticity*. What are some of the mechanisms (changes in brain function) seen during recovery of function?
4. Discuss feedback strategies designed to improve *retention and transfer of learning*. How do they differ from strategies that optimize initial learning and performance?
5. Define *recovery*. Give an example of an intervention that could be used to promote recovery for the patient with incomplete paraplegia.
6. What are the basic principles of *task-oriented training*?
7. Identify two training activities that can be used to improve *static postural control* and two to improve *dynamic postural control*.
8. Distinguish between the terms *adaptive compensation* and *substitutive compensation*. How would training strategies differ in promoting both?

CASE STUDY

HISTORY

The patient is a 36-year-old man who sustained a traumatic brain injury following a motorcycle accident. On admission to a local hospital, the patient was found to have a left frontal laceration with an underlying linear skull fracture. Computed tomography scan revealed edema, a right basal ganglia contusion, and a left frontal contusion. The patient was comatose on admission. His acute hospital course was complicated by increased intracranial pressure and severe spasticity. A gastric tube was inserted.

The patient's neurological status did not substantially improve at the acute hospital. He was transferred to a rehabilitation hospital 4 weeks after injury for intensive rehabilitation. He had a brief readmission to the acute hospital during his sixth week after injury for stabilization of acute hypothermia and hypothyroidism. He was then returned to the rehabilitation facility for continued intensive rehabilitation. His medications consisted of Tegretol (200 mg po qid), multivitamins, and Colace.

PART I: PHYSICAL THERAPY EXAMINATION FINDINGS (INITIAL ADMISSION TO REHAB, 4 WEEKS AFTER INJURY)

Behavior/cognition: He is functioning at Rancho Levels of Cognitive Functioning (RLOCF) Level V Confused–Inappropriate. The patient is able to respond to simple commands fairly consistently. With increased complexity of commands or lack of any external structure, responses are nonpurposeful, random, or fragmented. Highly distractible and lacks ability to focus on a specific task. Memory is severely impaired; often shows inappropriate use of objects. May perform previously learned tasks with structure but is unable to learn new information. Easily frustrated and responds with disinhibited behaviors (name calling and swearing).

Language–communication: Unable to examine.

Social: Married with no children. Wife is a registered nurse and very supportive of her husband.

Vital signs: Heart rate 60 beats per minute; blood pressure 122/70 mm Hg; respiratory rate 14 breaths per minute; O_2 saturation level is 92.

Sensation: Localizes to pinprick with withdrawal.

Passive range of motion:

- Right upper extremity (RUE) is limited in elbow ROM (0° to 70°); left upper extremity (LUE) elbow ROM is 10° to 100°.
- Both lower extremities (BLEs) are within normal limits except for ankle dorsiflexion 0° to 5° on R and 0° to 10° on L.

Motor Function

Tone (Modified Ashworth Scale [M-AS] grades): Severe flexor tone and spasms of the trunk that result in the patient moving in bed from a supine to a left-side-lying, curled-up (fetal) position, M-AS = 4.

- RUE extensor tone, M-AS = 3
- Right lower extremity (RLE) extensor tone, M-AS = 3
- LUE flexor tone, M-AS = 3
- Left lower extremity (LLE) extensor tone, M-AS = 2

Reflexes:

- Frequent asymmetrical tonic neck reflex posturing with head rotated to the right.
- Flexor withdrawal reflexes bilaterally in response to pain (delayed on the left with decreased intensity of response).
- Positive support reflex on the left.
- Hyperactive deep tendon reflexes throughout.
- At times, the lower extremities scissor (extend and adduct), especially when upper body flexor tone increases.

Voluntary movements:

- The patient is agitated with restless movements and is frequently diaphoretic.
- Limited head or trunk control, dependent sitting.
- Movement of RUE is spontaneous, purposeful at times, and out-of-synergy.
- Movement of the RLE is spontaneous, nonpurposeful, and out-of-synergy.
- LUE: no active movement.
- LLE movement: demonstrates abnormal obligatory extensor synergy pattern.

Coordination: Unable to assess.

Balance—sitting:

- **Static:** Poor; requires handhold support and moderate assistance; demonstrates sacral sitting with posterior tilt of the pelvis.
- **Dynamic:** Poor; unable to accept challenge or move without loss of balance.

Balance—standing:

- Static: Poor; requires maximal assist of two persons to stand in the parallel bars with splint on LLE.

Dynamic: Unable to weight shift or step.

- **Gait and locomotion** (wheelchair [w/c]): Unable.

Skin: Multiple healed lacerations on the knees and calves and pressure sores bilaterally on the lateral malleoli and calcanei from bivalve positioning splints.

Bladder and bowel: Incontinent of bowel and bladder and has external catheter in place.

Functional activities: Maximum assistance (Max A) in all ADL, FIM level 2.

PART I: (QUESTIONS 1–3)

1. Identify and prioritize the problems in motor function presented in this case in terms of impairments and activity limitations based on initial admission data (4 weeks after injury).
2. Identify the goals of physical therapy intervention for this patient at this point in his recovery (initial admission).
3. Identify the motor learning strategies and two treatment interventions appropriate for this patient at this point in his recovery (initial admission).

PART II: REEXAMINATION 12 WEEKS AFTER INJURY

Behavior/cognition: He is functioning at Rancho Levels of Cognitive Functioning (RLOCF) Level VII Automatic–Appropriate. He appears appropriate and oriented within the hospital setting; goes through daily routine automatically but frequently robot-like. Shows minimal to no confusion and has shallow recall of activities. Shows carryover for new learning but at a decreased rate. With structure is able to initiate social and recreational activities. Judgment remains impaired.

Language–communication: The patient is dysarthric; speech is usually intelligible but difficult to understand and delayed in onset. Auditory comprehension is good.

Vital signs: Within normal limits (WNL).

Skin: Lacerations are healed.

Sensation:

- **Vision and hearing** are WNL.
- **LUE:** Absent sensation.
- **LLE:** Impaired sensation, decreased proprioception.
- **RUE and RLE:** Intact.

Range of motion:

- **RUE:** elbow ROM 0° to 90°; LUE: elbow ROM 5° to 110°
- **BLEs:** WNL except for ankle dorsiflexion bilaterally of 0° to 15°

Motor function

Tone (modified Ashworth Scale grades, M-AS):

Trunk: Tone in the trunk is WNL except for occasional flexor spasms

- **RUE and RLE:** Extensor tone, M-AS = 1
- **LUE:** Flexor tone, M-AS = 2
- **LLE:** Extensor tone, M-AS = 1

Reflexes:

- Exhibits strong associated reactions in the LUE and increased flexor posturing with stressful activities.

Voluntary movements:

- **RUE and RLE:** Demonstrates purposeful, full, isolated motions through available ROM against gravity. Strength is grossly F+ in the RUE and RLE.
- **LUE:** Limited voluntary movement; extensor synergy predominates.
- **LLE:** Movement is purposeful; strength is grossly F.
- **Head and trunk:** Movement is functional and strength is grossly F.

Coordination:

- Exhibits moderate ataxia in trunk.
- Demonstrates moderate impairment in finger-to-nose and toe-tapping test in RUE; LUE not tested.

Balance—sitting:

- **Static:** Good, able to maintain balance without handhold support, limited postural sway.
- **Dynamic:** Good, able to accept moderate challenge and move without loss of balance.

Balance—standing:

- **Static:** Fair, requires handhold support to stand in the parallel bars, occasional minimal assistance.
- **Dynamic:** Fair, accepts minimal challenge; able to balance while turning head/trunk.

Functional Activities:

- **Bed mobility:** Rolls to right and left with supervision (S).
- **Supine-to-sit and sit-to-stand:** Moderate assistance (Mod A) × 1, FIM level 3.
- **Transfers:** Mod A × 1 in stand-pivot transfers, FIM level 3.
- **Wheelchair locomotion:** Maneuvers manual wheelchair with close S for safety, FIM level 5.
- **Gait:** Walks in parallel bars 10 ft with Mod A × 1, FIM level 3
- **Dressing and grooming:** Minimal assistance (Min A) × 1, FIM level 4

PART II: (QUESTIONS 4–6)

4. Identify and prioritize this patient's motor function problems in terms of impairments and activity limitations (12 weeks after injury).
5. Identify the goals and outcomes of physical therapy intervention for this patient at this point in his recovery.
6. Identify the motor learning strategies and two treatment interventions appropriate for this patient at this point in his recovery.

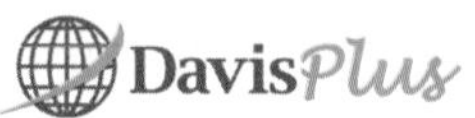

For additional resources, including answers to the questions for review and case study guiding questions, please visit **http://davisplus.fadavis.com.**

References

1. Schmidt, R, and Lee, T: Motor Control and Learning: A Behavioral Emphasis, ed 5. Human Kinetics, Champaign, IL, 2011.
2. Shumway-Cook, A, and Woollacott, M: Motor Control Theory and Practical Applications, ed 5. Lippincott Williams & Wilkins, Baltimore, 2017.
3. Bernstein, N: The Coordination and Regulation of Movements. Pergamon Press, Oxford, 1967.
4. Kelso, J: Dynamic Patterns: The Self-Organization of Brain and Behavior. MIT Press, Cambridge, MA, 1995.
5. Calancie, B, et al: Involuntary stepping after chronic spinal cord injury: Evidence for a central rhythm generator for locomotion in man. Brain 117:1143, 1994.
6. Griller S: Neurobiological bases of rhythmic motor acts in vertebrates. Science 228:143, 1989.
7. Adams, J: A closed-loop theory of motor learning. J Motor Behav 3:111, 1971.
8. Schmidt, R: A schema theory of discrete motor skill learning. Psychol Rev 82:225, 1975.
9. Nashner, L: Adapting reflexes controlling human posture. Exp Brain Res 26:59, 1976.
10. Nashner, L: Fixed patterns of rapid postural responses among leg muscles during stance. Exp Brain Res 30:13, 1977.
11. Nashner, L, and Woollacott, M: The organization of rapid postural adjustments of standing humans: An experimental-conceptual model. In Tablott, RE, and Humphrey, DR (eds): Posture and Movement. Raven, New York, 1979, pp. 243–257.
12. Fitts, P, and Posner, M: Human Performance. Brooks/Cole, Belmont, CA, 1967.
13. Bayley, N: The development of motor abilities during the first three years. Monogr Soc Res Child Dev 1(1, serial no. 1), 1935.
14. Gesell, A: The First Five Years of Life. Harper & Brothers, New York, 1940.
15. McGraw, M: The Neuromuscular Maturation of the Human Infant. Hafner, New York, 1945.
16. VanSant, A: Life span development in functional tasks. Phys Ther 70:788, 1990.
17. Woollacott, M, and Shumway-Cook, A: Changes in posture control across the life span: A systems approach. Phys Ther 70:799, 1990.
18. Woollacott, M, and Shumway-Cook, A (eds): Development of Posture and Gait Across the Life Span. University of South Carolina Press, Columbia, 1989.
19. Spirduso, W, Francis, K, and MacRai, P: Physical Dimensions of Aging. Human Kinetics, Champaign, IL, 2005.
20. Light, K: Information processing for motor performance in aging adults. Phys Ther 70:821, 1990.
21. Salthouse, T, and Somberg, B: Isolating the age deficit in speeded performance. J Gerontol 37:59, 1982.
22. Benjuva, N, Melzer, I, and Kaplanski, J: Aging-induced shifts from a reliance on sensory input to muscle cocontraction during balanced standing. J Gerontol A Biol Sci Med Sci 59A:166, 2004.
23. Light, K, and Spirduso, W: Effects of adult aging on the movement complexity factor of response programming. J Gerontol 45:107, 1990.
24. Levin, M, Kleim, J, and Wolf, S: What do motor "recovery" and "compensation" mean in patients following stroke? Neurorehabil Neural Repair 23:313, 2009.
25. Stein, D, Failowsky, B, and Will, B: Brain Repair. Oxford University Press, New York, 1995.
26. Pascual-Leone, A, et al: The plastic human brain cortex. Annu Rev Neurosci 28:377, 2005.
27. Chen, R, Cohen, LG, and Hallett, M: Nervous system reorganization following injury. Neuroscience 111(4):761, 2002.
28. Kleim, J, et al: Cortical synaptogenesis and motor map reorganization occur during late, but not early, phase of motor skill learning. J Neurosci 24:628, 2004.
29. Luscher, C, et al: Synaptic plasticity and dynamic modulation of the post synaptic membrane. Nat Neurosci 3(6):545, 2000.
30. Nudo, R: Functional and structural plasticity in motor cortex: Implications for stroke recovery. Phys Med Rehabil Clin North Am 14(1, Suppl):s5, 2003.
31. Nudo, R: Adaptive plasticity in motor cortex: Implications for rehabilitation after brain injury. J Rehabil Med 41(Suppl):7, 2003.
32. Fraser, C, et al: Driving plasticity in human adult motor cortex is associated with improved motor function after brain injury. Neuron 34:831, 2002.
33. Kleim, J, Jones, T, and Schallert, T: Motor enrichment and the induction of plasticity before and after brain injury. Neurochem Res 28:1757, 2003.
34. Shepherd, R: Exercise and training to optimize functional motor performance in stroke: Driving neural reorganization. Neural Plast 8:121, 2001.
35. Borstad, A, et al: Sensorimotor training and neural reorganization after stroke: A case series. JNPT 37:27, 2013.
36. Ward, N: Neural plasticity and recovery of function. Prog Brain Res 150:527, 2005.
37. Kleim, J, and Jones, T: Principles of experience-dependent neural plasticity: Implications for rehabilitation after brain damage. J Speech Lang Hear Res 51:S225, 2008.
38. Murphy, TH, and Corbett, D: Plasticity during stroke recovery; from synapse to behaviour. Nat Rev Neurosci 10:861, 2009.

39. Krakauer, JW, et al: Getting neurorehabilitation right: What can be learned from animal models? Neurorehagil Neural Repair 26:923, 2012.
40. Bernhardt, J, et al: Early rehabilitation after stroke. www.co-neurology.com, Current Opinion in Neurology 30(1):48, 2017.
41. Bernhardt, J, et: Very early rehabilitation trial for stroke (AVERT): Phase II safety and feasibility. Stroke 39:390, 2008.
42. Bernhardt, J, et al: Very early versus delayed mobilization after stroke. Cochrane Database Sys Rev 2009; 1:CD006187.
43. Bernhardt, J, et al: Efficacy and safety of very early mobilization within 24 h of stroke onset (AVERT): A randomized controlled trial. Lancet 386:46, 2015.
44. Lee, T, and Swanson, L: What is repeated in a repetition? Effects of practice conditions on motor skill acquisition. Phys Ther 71:150, 1991.
45. Winstein, C, Pohl, P, and Lewthwaite, R: Effects of physical guidance and knowledge of results on motor learning: Support for the guidance hypothesis. Res Quart Exer Sport 65:316–323, 1994.
46. Singer, R, and Pease, D: A comparison of discovery learning and guided instructional strategies on motor skill learning, retention, and transfer. Res Q 47:788, 1976.
47. Wulf, G, Shea, C, and Whitacre, C: Physical-guidance benefits in learning a complex motor skill. J Mot Behav 30:367–380, 1998.
48. Lee, T, Wulf, G, and Schmidt, R: Contextual interference in motor learning: Dissociated effects due to the nature of task variations. Q J Exp Psychol 44A:627, 1992.
49. Lee, T, and Magill, R: The locus of contextual interference in motor skill acquisition. J Exp Psychol Learn Mem Cogn 9:730, 1983.
50. Jeannerod, M: Neural simulation of action: A unifying mechanism for motor cognition. Neuroimage 14:103, 2001.
51. Jeannerod, M, and Frak, V: Mental imaging of motor activity in humans. Curr Opin Neurobiol 9:735, 1999.
52. Feltz, D, and Landers, D: The effects of mental practice on motor skill learning and performance: A meta-analysis. J Sports Psychol 5:25, 1983.
53. Braun, S, et al: Using mental practice in stroke rehabilitation: A framework. Clin Rehabil 22:579–591, 2008.
54. Richardson, A: Mental practice: A review and discussion (part 1). Res Q 38:95, 1967.
55. Warner, L, and McNeill, M: Mental imagery and its potential for physical therapy. Phys Ther 68:516, 1988.
56. Maring, J: Effects of mental practice on rate of skill acquisition. Phys Ther 70:165, 1990.
57. Salmoni, A, et al: Knowledge of results and motor learning: A review and critical appraisal. Psychol Bull 95:355, 1984.
58. Lee, T, et al: On the role of knowledge of results in motor learning: Exploring the guidance hypothesis. J Mot Behav 22:191, 1990.
59. Bilodeau, E, et al: Some effects of introducing and withdrawing knowledge of results early and late in practice. J Exp Psychol 58:142, 1959.
60. Magill, R: Augmented feedback in motor skill acquisition. In Singer, RN, Hausenblas, HA, and Janell, CM (eds): Handbook of Sport Psychology, ed 2. Wiley, New York, 2001, p. 86.
61. Winstein, C, et al: Learning a partial-weight-bearing skill: Effectiveness of two forms of feedback. Phys Ther 76:985, 1996.
62. Bilodeau, E, and Bilodeau, I: Variable frequency knowledge of results and the learning of a simple skill. J Exp Psychol 55:379, 1958.
63. Ho, L, and Shea, J: Effects of relative frequency of knowledge of results on retention of a motor skill. Percept Mot Skills 46:859, 1978.
64. Sherwood, D: Effect of bandwidth knowledge of results on movement consistency. Percept Mot Skills 66:535, 1988.
65. Winstein, C, and Schmidt, R: Reduced frequency of knowledge of results enhances motor skill learning. J Exp Psychol Learn Mem Cogn 16:677, 1990.
66. Lavery, J: Retention of simple motor skills as a function of type of knowledge of results. Can J Psych 16:300, 1962.
67. Boyd, L, and Winstein, C: Explicit information interferes with implicit motor learning of both continuous and discrete movement tasks after stroke. J Neur Phys Ther 30:46–57, 2006.
68. Swinnen, S, et al: Information feedback for skill acquisition: Instantaneous knowledge of results degrades learning. J Exp Psychol Learn Mem Cogn 16:706, 1990.
69. Winstein, C: Knowledge of results and motor learning: Implications for physical therapy. Phys Ther 71:140, 1991.
70. Wulf, G: Attentional focus and motor learning: A review of 15 years. Int Rev Sport Exer Psychol 6:77, 2013
71. Sturmberg, C, et al: Attentional focus of feedback and instructions in treatment of musculoskeletal dysfunction: A systematic review. Manual Ther 18:458, 2013.
72. Lee, T: Transfer-appropriate processing: A framework for conceptualizing practice effects in motor learning. In Meijer, O, and Roth, K (eds): Complex Movement Behavior: The Motor-Action Controversy. North Holland, Amsterdam, 1988, p. 201.
73. Wulf, G, Chiviacowsky, S, and Lewthwaite, R: Altering mindset can enhance motor learning in older adults. Psychol Aging 27(1):14, 2012.
74. Dobkin, B: International randomized clinical trial: Stroke inpatient rehabilitation with reinforcement of walking speed (SIRROWS), improves outcomes. Neurorehab Neural Repair 24(3):235, 2010.
75. Chiviacowsky, S, et al: Motor learning benefits of self-controlled practice in persons with Parkinson's disease. Gait Posture 35:601, 2012.
76. Gentile, A: Skill acquisition: Action, movement, and neuromotor processes. In Carr, J, and Shephard, R (eds): Movement Science. Foundations for Physical Therapy in Rehabilitation, ed 2. Aspen, Rockville, MD, 2000, p. 147.
77. French B, et al: Repetitive task training for improving functional ability after stroke. Cochrane Database of Systematic Reviews, 2016, Issue 11. Art. No.: CD006073.DOI: 10.1002/14651858.CD006073.pub3.
78. Winstein, C, et al: Infusing motor learning research into neurorehabilitation practice: A historical perspective with case exemplar from the accelerated skill acquisition program. JNPT 38:190, 2014.
79. Humm, J, et al: Use-dependent exaggeration of brain damage occurs during an early post-lesion vulnerable period. Brain Res 783:286, 1988.
80. Humm, J, et al: Use-dependent exaggeration of brain injury: Is glutamate involved? Exp Neurol 157:349, 1999.
81. Dromerick, A, et al: Very early constraint-induced movement during stroke rehabilitation. Neurology 73:195, 2009.
82. Griesbach, G, Gomez-Pinilla, F, and Hovda, D: The upregulation of plasticity-related proteins following TBI is disrupted with acute voluntary exercise. Brain Res 1016:154, 2004.
83. Biernaskie, J, Chernenko, G, and Corbett, D: Efficacy of rehabilitative experience declines with time after focal ischemic brain injury. J Neurosci 24:1245, 2004.
84. Carr, J, and Shepherd, R: Stroke Rehabilitation. Butterworth-Heinemann, London, 2003.
85. Mackey, F, et al: Stroke rehabilitation: Are highly structured units more conducive to physical activity than less structured units? Arch Phys Med Rehabil 77:1066, 1996.
86. Carr, J, and Shepherd, R: Neurological Rehabilitation: Optimizing Motor Performance, ed 2. Churchill Livingstone/Elsevier, St Louis, 2010.
87. Kwakkel, G: Impact of intensity of practice after stroke: Issues for consideration. Disabil Rehabil 28:823, 2006
88. Esmonde, T, et al: Stroke rehabilitation: Patient activity during non-therapy time. Aust J Physiother 43:43, 1997.
89. Bode, R, et al: Patterns of therapy activities across length of stay and impairment levels: peering inside the "black box" of inpatient stroke rehabilitation. Arch Phys Med Rehabil 85(12):1901, 2004.
90. Lang, C et al: Observation of amounts of movement practice provided during stroke rehabilitation. Arch Phys Med Rehabil 90(10):1692, 2009.
91. Lang, C, MacDonald, J, and Gnip, C: Counting repetitions: An observational study of outpatient therapy for people with hemiparesis post-stroke. JNPT 31:3, 2007.
92. Morris, D, and Taub, E: Constraint-induced movement therapy. In O'Sullivan, S, and Schmitz, T (eds): Improving Functional Outcomes in Physical Rehabilitation, ed 2. FA Davis, Philadelphia, 2016, p. 282.
93. Wolf, S, et al: Effect of constraint-induced movement therapy on upper extremity function 3 to 9 months after stroke: The EXCITE randomized trial. JAMA 296:2095, 2006.

94. Wolf, S, et al: The EXCITE trial: Retention of improved upper extremity function among stroke survivors receiving CI movement therapy. Lancet Neurol 7:33, 2008.
95. Hakkennes, S, and Keating, J: Constraint-induced movement therapy following stroke: A systematic review of randomized controlled trials. Aus J Physiother 51:221, 2005.
96. Dahl, A, et al: Short-and long-term outcome of constraint-induced movement therapy after stroke: A randomized controlled feasibility trial. Clinical Rehab 22:436, 2008.
97. Page, S, et al: Efficacy of modified constraint-induced movement therapy in chronic stroke: A single-blinded randomized controlled trial. Arch Phys Med Rehabil 85:14, 2004.
98. Taub, E, et al: A placebo-controlled trial of constraint-induced movement therapy for upper extremity after stroke. Stroke 37:1045, 2006.
99. Taub, E, et al: Technique to improve chronic motor deficit after stroke. Arch Phys Med Rehabil 74:347, 1993.
100. Corbetta, D, et al: Constraint-induced movement therapy for upper extremities in people with stroke. Cochrane Database of Systematic Reviews 2015, Issue 10. Art. No.: CD004433. DOI: 10.1002/14651858.CD004433.pub3.
101. Sawaki, L, et al: Constraint-induced movement therapy results in increased motor map area in subjects 3 to 9 months after stroke. Neurorehabil Neural Repair 33:505, 2008.
102. Liepert, J: Motor cortex excitability in stroke before and after constraint-induced movement therapy. Cog Behav Neurol 19:41, 2006.
103. Duncan, P, et al: Body-weight-supported treadmill rehabilitation after stroke. N Engl J Med 364:2026, 2011.
104. Ada, L: Randomized trial of treadmill walking with body weight support to establish walking in subacute stroke—the MOBILISE Trial. Stroke 41:1247, 2010.
105. Sullivan, K, et al: Effects of task-specific locomotor and strength training in adults who were ambulatory after stroke: Results of the STEPS randomized clinical trial. Phys Ther 87:1580, 2007.
106. Franceschini, M, et al: Walking after stroke: What does treadmill training with body weight support add to overground gait training in patients early after stroke? A single-blind, randomized controlled trial. Stroke 40:3079, 2009.
107. Mehrholz, J, Pohl, M, and Elsner, B: Treadmill training and body weight support for walking after stroke. *Cochrane Database of Systematic Reviews* 2014, Issue 1. Art. No.: CD002840. DOI: 10.1002/14651858.CD002840.pub3.
108. Collins, CK, and Schmitz, TJ: Interventions to improve locomotor skills. In O'Sullivan, SB, and Schmitz, TJ (eds): Improving Functional Outcomes in Physical Rehabilitation, ed 2. Philadelphia, FA Davis, 2016, p. 226.
109. *Guide to Physical Therapist Practice 3.0.* Alexandria, VA: American Physical Therapy Association; 2014. Available at: www.guidetoptpractice.apta.org. Accessed April 10, 2016.
110. Kisner, C, and Colby, L: Therapeutic Exercise Foundations and Techniques, ed 6. FA Davis, Philadelphia, 2012.
111. American College of Sports Medicine: ACSM's Guidelines for Exercise Testing and Prescription, ed 10. Lippincott Williams & Wilkins, Philadelphia, 2017.
112. American College of Sports Medicine: ACSM's Exercise Management for Persons with Chronic Diseases and Disabilities, ed 4. Lippincott Williams & Wilkins, Philadelphia, 2016.
113. Teixeira-Salmela, L, et al: Muscle strengthening and physical conditioning to reduce impairment and disability in chronic stroke survivors. Arch Phys Med Rehabil 80:1211, 1999.
114. Riolo, L, and Fisher, K: Is there evidence that strength training could help improve muscle function and other outcomes without reinforcing abnormal movement patterns or increasing reflex activity in a man who has had a stroke? Phys Ther 83:844, 2003.
115. Engardt, M et al: Dynamic muscle strength training in stroke patients: Effects on knee extension torque, electromyographic activity, and motor function. Arch Phys Med Rehabil 76(5):419, 1995.
116. Ada, L, Dorsch, D, and Canning, C: Strengthening interventions increase strength and improve activity after stroke: A systematic review. Aust J Physiother 52(4):241, 2006.
117. Yang, Y, et al: Task-oriented progressive resistance strength training improves muscle strength and functional performance in individuals with stroke. Clin Rehabil 20:860, 2006.
118. Eng, J: Strength training in individuals with stroke. Physiother Can 56:189, 2004.
119. Signal, N: Strength training after stroke: Rationale, evidence and potential implementation barriers for physiotherapists N Z J Physiother 42(2): 101, 2014.
120. Cooke, EV, et al: Efficacy of functional strength training on restoration of lower-limb motor function early after stroke: Phase I randomized controlled trial. Neurorehabil Neural Repair 24: 88, 2010.
121. Flansbjer, U, Lexell, J, and Brogårdh, C: Long-term benefits of progressive resistance training in chronic stroke: a 4-year follow-up. J Rehabil Med 44:218, 2012.
122. Page, P: Current concepts in muscle stretching for exercise and rehabilitation. Int J Sports Phys Ther 7(1):109, 2012.
123. Voss, D, et al: Proprioceptive Neuromuscular Facilitation, ed 3. Harper & Row, Philadelphia, 1985.
124. Moseley, A: The effect of casting combined with stretching on passive ankle dorsiflexion in adults with traumatic head injuries. Phys Ther 77:240, 1997.
125. Singer, B, et al: Evaluation of serial casting to correct equinovarus deformity of the ankle after acquired brain injury in adults. Arch Phys Med Rehabil 84:483, 2003.
126. Nashner, L: Adapting reflexes controlling the human posture. Exp Brain Res 26:59, 1976.
127. Nashner, L, and Woollacott, M: The organization of rapid postural adjustments of standing humans: An experimental-conceptual model. In Talbott, RE, and Humphrey, DR (eds): Posture and Movement. Raven, New York, 1979, pp. 243–257.
128. Nashner, L, Woollacott, M, and Tuma, G: Organization of rapid responses to postural and locomotor-like perturbations of standing man. Exp Brain Res 36:463, 1979.
129. Horak, F, and Nashner, L: Central programming of postural movements: Adaptation to altered support surface configurations. J Neurophysiol 55:1369, 1986.
130. O'Sullivan, SB, and Bezkor, EW: Interventions to improve sitting and sitting balance skills. In O'Sullivan, SB, and Schmitz, TJ (eds): Improving Functional Outcomes in Physical Rehabilitation, ed 2. FA Davis, Philadelphia, 2016, p. 95.
131. Moriarty-Baron, J, and O'Sullivan, S: Interventions to improve standing and standing balance skills. In O'Sullivan, SB, and Schmitz, TJ (eds): Improving Functional Outcomes in Physical Rehabilitation, ed 2. FA Davis, Philadelphia, 2016, p. 186.
132. Taggart, H: Effects of tai chi exercise on balance, functional mobility, and fear of falling among older women. Appl Nurs Res 15:235, 2002.
133. Li, F, et al: Tai chi and fall reductions in older adults: A randomized controlled trial. J Gerontol A Biol Sci Med Sci 60:187–194, 2005.
134. Gatts, S, and Woollacott, M: Neural mechanisms underlying balance improvement with short term tai chi training. Aging Clin Exp Res 18:7–19, 2006.
135. McIlroy, W, and Maki, B: Adaptive changes to compensatory stepping responses. Gait Posture 3:43, 1995.
136. Maki, B, and McIlroy, W: The role of limb movements in maintaining upright stance: The "change-in-support" strategy. Phys Ther 77:488, 1997.
137. Gillespie, L, et al: Interventions for preventing falls in elderly people. Cochrane Database of Systematic Reviews, 2011, Issue 11. Art. No.: CD004963. DOI: 10.1002/14651858.CD004963.pub3.
138. Howe, TE, et al: Exercise for improving balance in older people. Cochrane Database of Systematic Reviews, 2009, Issue 2. Art. No.: CD000340. DOI: 10.1002/14651858.CD000340.pub2.
139. Means, K, Rodell, D, and O'Sullivan, P: Balance, mobility, and falls among community-dwelling elderly persons: Effects of a rehabilitation exercise program. Am J Phys Med Rehabil 84:238–250, 2005.
140. Marigold, D, et al: Exercise leads to faster postural reflexes, improved balance and mobility, and fewer falls in older persons with chronic stroke. J Am Geriatr Soc 53:416–423, 2005.

141. Shumway-Cook, A, et al: The effect of multidimensional exercises on balance, mobility, and fall risk in community dwelling older adults. Phys Ther 77:46, 1997.
142. Nitz, J, and Choy, N: The efficacy of a specific balance-strategy training programme for preventing falls among older people: A pilot randomized controlled trial. Age Ageing 33:52–58, 2004.
143. Lubetzky-Vilnai, L, and Kartin, D: Effect of balance training on balance performance in individuals post stroke: A systematic review. J Neurol Phys Ther 34:127, 2010.
144. Hu, M, and Woollacott, M: Multisensory training of standing balance in older adults. 1. Postural stability and one-leg stance balance. J Gerontol 49:M52–M61, 1994.
145. Hu, M, and Woollacott, M: Multisensory training of standing balance in older adults. 2. Kinetic and electromyographic postural responses. J Gerontol 49:M62–M71, 1994.
146. Cass, S, Borello-France, D, and Furman, J: Functional outcome of vestibular rehabilitation in patients with abnormal sensory organization testing. Am J Otol 17:581–594, 1996.
147. Bayouk, J, Boucher, J, and Leroux, A: Balance training following stroke: Effects of task-oriented training with and without altered sensory input. Int J Rehabil Res 29:51–59, 2006.
148. Smania, N, et al: Rehabilitation of sensorimotor integration deficits in balance impairment of patients with stroke hemiparesis: A before/after pilot study. Neurol Sci 29:313–319, 2008.
149. Armutlu, K, Karabudk, R, and Nurlu, G: Physiotherapy approaches in the treatment of ataxic multiple sclerosis; a pilot study. Neurorehab Neural Repair 15:203, 2001.
150. Trujillo-Martin, M, et al: Effectiveness and safety of treatments for degenerative ataxias: A systematic review. Mov Disord 24(8):1111, 2009.
151. Miyai, I, et al. Cerebellar ataxia rehabilitation trial in degenerative cerebellar diseases. Neurorehabil Neural Repair 26(5):515, 2012.
152. Ilg, W, et al: Long-term effects of coordinative training in degenerative cerebellar disease. Mov Disord 25(13):2239, 2010.
153. Bastian, A: Moving, sensing and learning with cerebellar damage. Curr Opin Neurobiol 21(4):596, 2011.
154. Bastian, A, and Keller, J: A home balance exercise program improves walking in people with cerebellar ataxia. Neurorehabil Neural Repair 28(8):770, 2014.
155. Mang, C: Promoting neuroplasticity for motor rehabilitation after stroke: Considering the effects of aerobic exercise and genetic variation on brain-deprived neuotrophic factor. Phys Ther 93(12):1707, 2013.
156. Rimmer, J, and Wang, E: Aerobic exercise training in stroke survivors. Top Stroke Rehabil 12(1):17, 2015.
157. Carr, M, and Jones, J: Physiological effects of exercise on stroke survivors. Top Stroke Rehabil 9(4):57, 2003.
158. Saunders, DH, et al: Physical fitness training for stroke patients. *Cochrane Database of Systematic Reviews* 2016, Issue 3. Art. No.: CD003316. DOI: 10.1002/14651858.CD003316.pub6.
159. Borg, G: Borg's Perceived Exertion and Pain Scales. Human Kinetics, Champaign, IL, 1998.
160. Nichols, D: Balance retraining after stroke using force platform biofeedback. Phys Ther 77:553, 1997.
161. Winstein, C, et al: Standing balance training: Effect on balance and locomotion in hemiparetic adults. Arch Phys Med Rehabil 70:755, 1989.
162. Shumway-Cook, A, Anson, D, and Haller, S: Postural sway biofeedback: Its effect on reestablishing stance stability in hemiplegic patients after stroke. Arch Phys Med Rehabil 69:395, 1988.
163. Januario, F, Campos, I, and Amaral, C: Rehabilitation of postural stability in ataxic/hemiplegic patients. Disabil Rehabil 32(2):1775, 2010.
164. DeNunzio, A, et al: Biofeedback rehabilitation of posture and weight-bearing distribution in stroke: A center of foot pressure analysis. Funct Neurol 29(2):127, 2014.
165. van Peppen, R, et al: Effects of visual feedback therapy on postural control in bilateral standing after stroke: A systematic review. J Rehabil Med 38:3–9, 2006.
166. Barclay-Goddard, R, et al: Force platform feedback for standing balance training after stroke. Cochrane Database Syst Rev 4:D004129, 2004.
167. Giggins, O, Persson, U, and Caulfield, B: Biofeedback in rehabilitation. J Neuroeng Rehabil 10:60, 2013.
168. Merians, AS, et al: Virtual reality–augmented rehabilitation for patients following stroke. Phys Ther 82(9):898, 2002.
169. Armagan, O, Tascioglu, F, and Oner, C: Electromyographic biofeedback in the treatment of the hemiplegic hand: A placebo-controlled study. Am J Phys Med Rehabil 82:856, 2003.
170. Dogan-Aslan, M, et al: The effect of electromyographic biofeedback treatment in improving upper extremity functioning of patients with hemiplegic stroke. J Stroke Cerebrovasc Dis 21(3):187, 2010.
171. Moreland, J, Thompson, M, and Fuoco, A: Electromyographic biofeedback to improve lower extremity function after stroke: A meta-analysis. Arch Phys Med Rehabil 79:134, 1998.
172. Bradley, L, et al: Electromyographic biofeedback for gait training after stroke. Clin Rehabil 12(1):11, 1998.
173. Huang, H, Wolf, SL, and He, J: Recent developments in biofeedback for neuromotor rehabilitation. J Neuroeng Rehabil 3:11, 2006.
174. Woodford, H, and Price, C: EMG biofeedback for the recovery of motor function after stroke. Cochrane Database of Systematic Reviews 2007, Issue 2. Art. No.: CD004585. DOI: 10.1002/14651858.CD004585.pub2.
175. Kesar, T, et al: Novel patterns of functional electrical stimulation have an immediate effect on dorsiflexor muscle function during gait for people poststroke. Phys Ther 90:55, 2010.
176. Cauraugh, J, et al: Chronic motor dysfunction after stroke: Recovering wrist and finger extension by electromyography-triggered neuromuscular stimulation. Stroke 31:1360, 2000.
177. Powell, J, et al: Electrical stimulation of wrist extensors in poststroke hemiplegia. Stroke 30:1384, 1999.
178. Kowalczewski, J, et al: Upper-extremity functional electric stimulation-assisted exercises on a workstation in the sub-acute phase of stroke recovery. Arch Phys Med Rehabil 88:833, 2007.
179. Meilink, A, Hemmen, B, and Ham, S: Impact of EMG-triggered neuromuscular stimulation of the wrist and finger extensors of the paretic hand after stroke: A systematic review of the literature. Clinical Rehabil 22:291, 2008.
180. Wang, R, Chan, R, and Tsai, M: Functional electrical stimulation on chronic and acute hemiplegic shoulder subluxation. Am J Phys Med Rehabil 79:385, 2000.
181. Bogataj, U, Gros, H, and Kljajic, M: The rehabilitation of gait in patients with hemiplegia: A comparison between conventional therapy and multichannel functional electrical stimulation therapy. Phys Ther 75:490, 1995.
182. Pomeroy, V, et al: Electrostimulation for promoting recovery of movement or functional ability after stroke. Cochrane Database of Systematic Reviews 2006, Issue 2. Art. No.: CD003241. DOI: 10.1002/14651858.CD003241.pub2.
183. Yan, T, Hui-Chan, C, and Li, L: Functional electrical stimulation improves motor recovery of the lower extremity and walking ability of subjects with first acute stroke: A randomized placebo-controlled trial. Stroke 36:80, 2005.
184. Embrey, D, et al: Functional electrical stimulation to dorsiflexors and plantar flexors during gait to improve walking in adults with chronic hemiplegia. Arch Phys Med Rehabil 91:687, 2010.
185. Roche, A, Laighin, G, and Coote, S: Surface-applied functional electrical stimulation for orthotic and therapeutic treatment of drop-foot after stroke—a systematic review. Phys Ther Rev 14:63, 2009.
186. Ana, R, et al: Gait training combining partial body-weight support, a treadmill, and functional electrical stimulation on poststroke gait. Phys Ther 87:1144, 2007.
187. Daly, J, and Ruff, R: Feasibility of combining multi-channel functional neuromuscular stimulation with weight-supported treadmill training. J Neurol Sci 255:105, 2004.
188. Triolo, R, and Bogie, K: Lower extremity applications of functional neuromuscular stimulation after spinal cord injury. Top Spinal Cord Inj Rehabil 5:44, 1999.
189. Ferrante, F, et al: Cycling induced by FES improves the muscular strength and motor control of individuals with post-acute stroke. Eur J Phys Rehabil Med 44:159, 2008.

Chapter 11

Strategies to Improve Locomotor Function

George D. Fulk, PT, PhD
Lee Dibble, PT, PhD, ATC
Thomas J. Schmitz, PT, PhD

LEARNING OBJECTIVES

1. Select appropriate outcome measures to use with a client whose primary goal is to improve locomotion function.
2. Interpret change in walking ability using gait speed as an outcome measure.
3. Develop a practice schedule for locomotor interventions that enhances motor learning.
4. Utilize feedback during locomotor interventions to facilitate motor learning.
5. Explain how feedback can be used to enhance patient motivation.
6. Organize interventions to promote the recovery of locomotor function based on principles of neuroplasticity.
7. Identify benefits of using a body weight support and treadmill system to improve locomotor function.
8. Describe how to provide variable practice when utilizing a treadmill to improve locomotor function.
9. Develop a task-specific strengthening and balance exercise program that incorporates exercise guidelines and principles of neuroplasticity to improve locomotor function.
10. Design a circuit training locomotor intervention that incorporates motor learning and neuroplasticity principles.
11. Describe how to implement motor imagery to improve locomotor function.

CHAPTER OUTLINE

The recovery or improvement of walking ability is a primary goal for people with many different health conditions who seek the services of a physical therapist.[1-4] Initially, approximately two-thirds of people who experience a stroke cannot ambulate or require assistance to walk.[5] Three months later, one-third of those with a stroke still require some level of assistance to walk. People with Parkinson's disease (PD) often have impaired postural control and limited walking ability.[6] Approximately 50% of people with multiple sclerosis (MS) require assistance to walk within 15 years of their diagnosis.[7,8] Individuals with low back pain, lower extremity (LE) amputations, and a host of other health conditions often present with limited walking ability. Improving walking ability is such an important goal because people who can walk independently are likely to have a lower burden of care, be able to participate in expected social roles and desired recreational activities, have a higher quality of life, be more physically active, and have improved health status.[2,3,6,9-12]

EXAMINATION OF LOCOMOTION

Physical therapists use a variety of tests and measures to assess locomotor function. Evaluation of gait and functional walking ability assists the physical therapist in selecting appropriate interventions, measuring change, and setting goals. The major requirements for successful walking include (1) support of body mass by the LEs, (2) production of locomotor rhythm, (3) dynamic postural control of the moving body, (4) propulsion of the body in the intended direction, and (5) adaptability of the locomotor response to changing environmental and task demands. Physical therapists use observational gait analysis (OGA) as a preferred method to examine gait kinematics. One instrument used clinically is the Rancho Los Amigos (RLA) OGA System. The RLA OGA instrument gathers data on the cyclical movements of walking that occur from one stride cycle to the next. The gait cycle is divided into *stance* and *swing* phases. The physical therapist visually analyzes a patient's walking pattern, looking for asymmetries and deviations from normal. Based on these observations, the physical therapist gains insight into which body structure/function impairments may be causing the deviations.

Performance-based outcome measures that physical therapists commonly use to assess walking ability include gait speed measured over a short distance (5-meter or 10-meter walk),[13] the 6-minute walk test,[14] Functional Gait Assessment,[15] Dynamic Gait Index,[16] Community Balance and Mobility Scale,[17] Walking Index for Spinal Cord Injury,[18] Amputee Mobility Predictor,[19] mini Balance Evaluation Systems Test,[20,21] and a variety of other ordinal scales that are components of other outcome measures such as the Functional Independence Measure and the Unified Parkinson Disease Rating Scale. See Chapter 7, Examination of Gait, for additional information on outcome measures and greater detail on examination of gait.

Gait speed is likely the most widely used parameter to measure and assess walking capacity across many different patient populations, including those with stroke, PD, MS, incomplete spinal cord injury, total joint replacement, vestibular dysfunction, traumatic brain injury, LE amputation, as well as older adults and many others. Gait speed should be used with all patients for whom recovery of walking ability is a goal. It is valid, reliable, and responsive, and there are established cutoff values to assist with prediction and other clinical decisions.[22] The minimal clinically important difference (MCID) of gait speed has been established for a variety of patient populations and is useful for goal setting and interpreting change during rehabilitation. For people with stroke, the MCID ranges from 0.13 to 0.17 m/s;[23-25] for older adults, it is estimated to be 0.13 m/s;[26] for individuals who have sustained a hip fracture, it is estimated to be 0.10 m/s;[27,28] for people with chronic obstructive pulmonary disease, it is estimated to be 0.11 m/s;[29] and for patients receiving inpatient rehabilitation with a variety of health conditions (e.g., total knee arthroplasty, fracture, stroke, congestive heart failure, infection, total hip arthroplasty), it ranges from 0.12 to 0.18 m/s[30] (Table 11.1). These values differ slightly likely due to differences in the patient populations, acuity of the health condition, and differences in the anchor of importance across studies.

Table 11.1 Estimates of Minimal Clinically Important Difference of Comfortable Gait Speed

Patient Population	MCID	Anchor of Importance
Stroke	0.17 m/s[21]	Patient perception of important change in walking ability.
Stroke	0.16 m/s[22]	1-point improvement on modified Rankin Scale.
Stroke	0.13 m/s[23]	Decrease in physical assistance required to walk.
Older adults	0.13 m/s[24]	Change in SF-36 mobility questions; walk 1 block and climb 1 flight of stairs. Patient perception of important change in general mobility.
Women with hip fracture	0.10–0.17 m/s[25]	Change in SF-36 mobility questions; walk 1 block and climb 1 flight of stairs.
Older adults with hip fracture	0.10 m/s[26]	Change in Timed Up and Go. Expert opinion.
Patients with chronic obstructive pulmonary disease	0.08–0.11 m/s[27]	Change on the incremental shuttle walk. Patient self-report of feeling of improvement.
Patients undergoing inpatient rehabilitation (e.g., total knee arthroplasty, stroke, congestive heart failure, total hip arthroplasty)	0.10–0.18 m/s[28]	Patient perception of walking ability. Decrease in physical assistance required to walk. Change to less supportive assistive device. Change in gait speed categories.

Self-report measures are important, as they provide information related to the patient's perceptions of the impact of their health condition. An example of such a measure is the Multiple Sclerosis Walking Scale,[31] which is a self-report measure that was originally designed for people with MS that has been used with other patient populations.[32,33] Newly available wearable sensors that track ambulatory activity such as the StepWatch Activity Monitor (SAM) are highly accurate and provide insight into the amount of walking people do in their homes and communities as they go about their everyday lives.[34-36] Findings from these various tests and measures (OGA, performance based, self-report, and activity monitors), as well as findings from other components of the initial examination, can be used to identify what aspects of locomotion are challenging for the patient and possible causes and to develop a specific plan of care for the patient.

REHABILITATION INTERVENTIONS TO PROMOTE RECOVERY OF LOCOMOTOR FUNCTION

General Principles

There are many different interventions that physical therapists use to promote recovery of walking ability. These include locomotor training utilizing a body weight support (BWS) and treadmill (TM) system, robotic-assisted stepping, TM training, dance, virtual reality and exergaming, strengthening exercises, balance exercises, task-oriented circuit training, and motor imagery. Research into these various interventions has not found one type of intervention to be superior to another.[37-44] However, there are some general principles related to motor learning and neuroplasticity that should be incorporated as a part of any specific intervention designed to improve walking ability. *Motor learning* is a set of processes associated with practice and experience that leads to relatively permanent changes in the ability to perform movement.[45] Within the context of motor function interventions, neuroplasticity refers to changes that occur within the central nervous system (CNS) as a result of behavioral and environmental stimuli.[46]

Two key contributors to motor learning are *practice* and *feedback*. For learning to occur, a sufficient amount of practice of the task must be done. In animal models examining neuroplastic changes and in human motor learning studies, upward of 500 to 600 repetitions of the task are performed per session to demonstrate improvement in motor behavior.[47-50] Unfortunately, observational studies of physical therapy practice reveal that patients likely do not typically receive a sufficient amount of practice to optimally promote motor learning. Lang and colleagues[51] found that patients receiving outpatient physical therapy on average performed 33 active LE movements, 6 passive LE movements, and 8 purposeful movements, and took 292 steps.

The structure and conditions of practice have an impact on motor learning. *Variable* practice leads to improved retention and motor learning compared to *constant* practice. In relation to locomotor interventions, an example of variable practice would be walking on a TM at different speeds (instead of at a constant speed) or ambulating on varying surfaces. Constant practice would encompass walking on the treadmill at the same speed throughout the intervention session. Variable practice may lead to improved motor learning compared to constant practice because functionally the task of walking requires people to vary their walking speed or gait pattern depending on the environment and goal. *Random* practice, where several different tasks are practiced in a random order, instead of *blocked* practice, where all trials on one task are practiced together in a block, can also lead to improved motor learning of movement tasks.

Feedback related to performance and task completion can also be used to promote motor learning. Feedback can be *intrinsic* (feedback that comes to the performer through his or her sensory systems, such as proprioceptive, visual) or *extrinsic* (feedback that is provided, usually by the physical therapist) to augment intrinsic feedback. *Knowledge of results* (KR) is terminal, extrinsic feedback about the results of the movement's outcome. KR feedback can be delivered in a variety of ways: immediately following every trial, have a period of delay between completion of the trial and provision of KR, fading the amount of KR over successive trials, or providing summary KR after a certain number of trials. Reducing the amount of KR feedback through faded or summary feedback is more effective for motor learning than providing feedback after every trial. Observational research on how much feedback is provided during treatment sessions suggests that physical therapists may provide too much feedback, which may inhibit motor learning.[52]

Dobkin and colleagues[53] provided daily KR feedback on gait speed in people with stroke undergoing inpatient rehabilitation. Participants performed a daily timed 10-m walk. Participants in the experimental group were told that they had done well and what the specific time was. If it was faster than the day before, they were told by how much; if the time was the same, they were told they were holding their own; and if it was slower, they were encouraged and told that they would soon walk faster. Both the experimental and comparison groups received the same type and amount of physical therapy. The only difference was that the comparison group did not receive KR feedback on their gait speed. The group that received KR feedback demonstrated a significant difference in gait speed at discharge compared to the comparison group, 0.91 m/s vs. 0.72 m/s. These results illustrate the impact of feedback and its motivational potential.

Wulf and Lewthwaite[54] summarized the importance of focus of attention, motivation, and autonomy on motor learning. In a series of studies, they report that an external focus of attention (concentrating on the intended effect of the movement) rather than an internal focus of attention (concentrating on how the body is moving) was more beneficial for motor learning. For example, when balancing on a platform, subjects that were instructed to minimize the movement of the platform demonstrated better motor learning than subjects who were instructed to minimize the movement of their feet.[55] In addition to providing information related to task goal completion, feedback can be an effective motivator as well. Positive feedback after successful trials and ignoring unsuccessful trials can enhance motor learning.[56] Providing pre-task feedback to increase a patient's confidence can positively impact motor learning.[57] Enhancing patient autonomy by providing increased choice and control over the intervention can also be beneficial for motor learning. For example, participants who were allowed to decide if they wished to use an assistive device during a balance task demonstrated greater motor learning on the balance task than participants who were not given a choice.[58] Increasing motivation, self-confidence, and autonomy promote greater engagement in the task and enhance motor learning. Chapter 10, Strategies to Improve Motor Function, provides more detail on strategies to promote motor learning.

Neuroplastic changes can occur at the cellular level and synapse all the way up to cortical maps and networks. Kleim and Jones[46] suggest that neuroplasticity is the means through which the brain learns new behaviors and the damaged brain relearns motor behaviors. Intensive, task-oriented practice drives neuroplastic changes within the CNS, which in turn promotes improved movement and functional recovery.[46,59-62] Task specificity, repetition, intensity, and salience are a few of the critical principles of experience-dependent neuroplasticity.[46]

Task-specific locomotor intervention utilizing a BWS and TM system can induce neuroplastic changes as seen by increased cortical activation and improved motor function and walking capability.[61] Hornby and colleagues[63] incorporated principles of neuroplasticity with an emphasis on intensity, repetition, and variable practice to improve walking ability in people with stroke. A variety of locomotor interventions were used, including speed and skill-dependent TM walking, overground walking, and stair climbing. Participants trained at an intensity of 70% to 80% of heart rate reserve. A variety of methods were used to increase the intensity and skill, such as walking with leg weights and a weighted vest, providing perturbations while walking, stepping over obstacles, and walking in different directions. They found improvements in walking speed and endurance compared to a control group. Treatment interventions that are valued by the patient, specific to the task being (re)learned, provided at a high dosage, and challenging are likely to be associated with beneficial neuroplastic changes and improvements in function. Box 11.1 summarizes some of the important principles of motor learning and neuroplasticity that may be incorporated into locomotor interventions.

Locomotor Training With Body Weight Support and Treadmill

Locomotor training using a BWS and TM system involves suspending a patient over a TM and using the BWS system to partially unweight the patient. The ability to partially unweight the patient allows those with LE/trunk weakness or postural instability to stand and take steps in a more symmetrical, natural manner without the need for excessive upper extremity (UE) weight-bearing or compensatory movement patterns. Using this system also allows physical therapists and other rehabilitation professionals to manually assist the patient while stepping on the TM (see Fig. 20.37 in Chapter 20, Traumatic Spinal Cord Injury).

Locomotor training (LT) using a BWS and TM system was first used in patients with incomplete spinal cord injury (SCI). The rationale for its use is supported by animal studies of cats with thoracic spinal cord lesions that regained hind limb stepping patterns when supported by a harness over a moving treadmill.[64-66] These findings suggest that the spinal cord is capable of reciprocal locomotor patterns produced by central pattern generators (CPGs) at the spinal cord level in the absence of supraspinal input. Central pattern generators are also influenced by sensory input, allowing motor output modification based on environmental demands.

Behrman and colleagues[67-69] have proposed the following guiding principles for locomotor training:

- Maximally load the LEs for weight-bearing, while minimizing weight-bearing on the UEs (e.g., the

Box 11.1 Key Motor Learning and Neuroplasticity Principles for Locomotor Rehabilitation

- Task-specific practice with a high number of repetitions is critical.
- Variable and random practice promotes motor learning.
- Summary and faded knowledge of results feedback promotes motor learning.
- Feedback is beneficial for motivational purposes.
- External focus of attention.
- Provide control and autonomy to the patient.
- High intensity.
- Challenging and engaging to the patient.
- Goal directed and meaningful to the patient.

BWS system sustains sufficient body weight so that the patient can stand and step with minimal or no UE support).
- Provide sensory cues that are consistent with normal walking (e.g., manual facilitation to the extensors and flexors during stance and swing, respectively).
- Promote trunk, limb, and pelvic kinematics associated with normal walking.
- Promote balance and upright control consistent with normal walking.
- Maximize the recovery and use of normal movement patterns and minimize compensatory movement patterns.

The overarching principle is to train like the individual walks. A key element of LT using BWS and a TM is facilitation of automatic walking movements within the context of intensive, task-specific training (whole-task practice). With body weight supported, the TM speed provides a rhythmic input. Manually guided movements are used to enhance the rhythmicity of the gait pattern. The BWS and TM system provides an environment in which these LT strategies can be accomplished.

Within a task-specific and safe patient environment, LT using BWS and a TM allows the therapist access to trunk, pelvis, and LEs to manually assist, guide, or adjust locomotor rhythm, limb placement, weight shifts, and stepping symmetry. Sensory input such as appropriately timed manually assisted limb movements may promote locomotor recovery. Movements are coordinated to simulate normal gait; upright posture and balance are maintained, and speed of walking is controlled. Some of the potential advantages of LT using BWS and a TM are summarized in Box 11.2.[68]

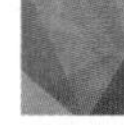

Box 11.2 Benefits of a Body Weight Support and Treadmill System

- Stepping and loading the lower extremities can be practiced before limbs are capable of fully supporting body weight.
- Gait training can be initiated earlier within an episode of care.
- Specific elements of the gait cycle (e.g., midstance limb loading; swing phase unweighting and stepping) can be promoted within a dynamic task-specific strategy.
- Owing to forced stepping movements, "learned nonuse" may be prevented by focusing attention on both involved and less involved lower extremities.
- Opportunity to practice walking is provided without undue fear of falling.
- Dynamic balance can be enhanced by decreasing BWS and increasing TM speed.
- Compensatory strategies (e.g., UE support) to compensate for LE impairment are reduced.
- Constant speed of the TM provides rhythmic input that may reinforce a coordinated reciprocal gait pattern.
- Hip extension is facilitated.

Locomotor training using a BWS and TM system can be progressed by increasing TM speed, decreasing the amount of BWS and manual guidance, and increasing the time of stepping on the TM. For example, training may be initiated at very low speeds (e.g., 0.3 m/sec) with limited LE weight-bearing (30% to 40% of BWS), constant manual guidance at both LEs and the trunk/pelvis, and a stepping trial of only 1 to 3 minutes. With continued training and patient improvement, this can be progressed to normal, age-appropriate walking speeds of 1.2 to 1.4 m/sec (4 to 4.5 ft/sec), full weight-bearing through the LEs, no manual guidance for stepping, and a stepping bout of 30 minutes without rest.

It is important to carry over the training from the BWS and TM environment to overground and community walking activities. Upon completion of walking trials on the TM with BWS, locomotor training should continue overground and in the community with activities such as walking at varying speeds, walking with vertical and horizontal head turns, walking on different surfaces, ascending/descending stairs and curbs, walking while performing a dual task, and increasing distance to improve endurance. See the "Balance and Dynamic Postural Control During Overground Walking" section for more detail on overground walking interventions.

Motor learning and neuroplasticity principles should be incorporated to enhance recovery. The BWS and TM environment provide the opportunity to practice a large number of repetitions of stepping at a high intensity. The speed can be varied during a stepping trial or across trials. Feedback in a summary or faded manner about results in terms of speed, distance, and amount of BWS can be provided. Motivational feedback can also be provided.

Locomotor training using a BWS and TM system has also been successfully combined with robotic interventions, where a robotic device moves the LEs.[70-72] Although the effectiveness of LT using a BWS and TM system has been examined in a variety of patient populations, including those with SCI,[71,73-75] stroke,[76,77] PD,[78-80] and MS,[81,82] it has not been demonstrated that it is more effective than other intervention approaches, nor is it clear what specific patients it is best suited for.[37-39,82] A BWS and TM system may be most beneficial for patients who require physical assistance to walk since these systems provide a safe environment to repetitively practice stepping at a high intensity. As patients improve and require less physical assistance to walk, progression to other task-oriented locomotor activities, at the proper dosage and skill level, may be more appropriate.

Treadmill Training

There are several concepts that may contribute to explaining the benefits observed during TM training in a variety of patient populations. Neurologically, TM walking may provide a sensorimotor environment that facilitates the recruitment of spinal cord and brain stem circuits that comprise CPGs. The recruitment of these circuits helps to produce the rhythmic, reciprocal muscle activity necessary for a coordinated gait pattern. Motor learning research strongly supports the benefits of task-specific training for the acquisition of skill. As a strategy to improve locomotor function, using a TM provides such task-specific training while allowing the clinician to closely monitor and supervise the patient in a controlled, stable environment. From a metabolic/cardiorespiratory physiological perspective, TM training provides a controllable submaximal exercise stimulus that when performed chronically contributes to increased bioenergetic efficiency required during ambulation in everyday life.

Many of the guiding principles discussed above can be incorporated into TM training to further promote walking ability. For example, variable practice can be introduced by varying the speed of the TM. Feedback on speed, distance, and time can be provided in summary form and for motivational purposes. The biomechanical characteristics of TM training make it a convenient and useful clinical tool. During overground walking, gait speed, and other spatial and temporal features may vary from step to step. In contrast, successful TM walking requires that the participant's gait speed matches that of the TM belt.

The TM imposes external spatial temporal constraints on the gait pattern, acting as an external pacemaker. Treadmill walking as an external pacemaker has been used in people with PD to improve gait rhythm and stability and may improve the symmetry of stride length as well as the consistency of cadence.[83]

There is a considerable body of research that supports the use of TM training in a variety of clinical populations. These include individuals with LE amputations, joint arthroplasty, and neurological diagnoses such as cerebrovascular accident (CVA), SCI, PD, and MS.[84-87] Outcomes from these studies suggest that TM training may result in improvements in aerobic fitness, gait speed, gait endurance, and gait symmetry. A synthesis of this literature suggests that the following parameters may be varied to manipulate the intensity of the exercise stimulus: TM speed, belt incline, and overall training time. While overground self-selected gait speed may be used as an initial guide for a starting TM speed, the speed will likely be lower for an individual unfamiliar with walking on a TM and for those during the early stages of rehabilitation. For safety and balance purposes, individuals should progress from holding on to support bars to walking without UE support. Challenge for the participant can be increased by increasing the TM speed, increasing the incline, or changing walking direction (walking sideways or backward). In all cases, individuals should be supervised and provided with the emergency stop trigger in case they lose their balance or fall. Additional adjuncts that may be utilized to improve the quality of the TM training include metronomes (to provide a model for stride to stride timing), LE manual assistance, or LE bracing (to improve gait symmetry).

While TM training can be utilized as motor skill practice with the objective of improving coordination of the limbs and trunk, it may also be used to improve cardiorespiratory endurance. When using TM training as a means of aerobic conditioning, the American College of Sports Medicine (ACSM) recommends that individuals with comorbid conditions be evaluated through the use of a submaximal or maximal exercise test, potentially with electrocardiogram monitoring. The ACSM has established dosage guidelines for moderate and vigorous exercise. These recommendations are for moderate-intensity exercise (40% to 60% of predicted maximal heart rate or a rating of perceived exertion [RPE] of 10 to 12) for at least 30 minutes on 5 or more days a week, for a total of 150 minutes per week. Vigorous-intensity exercise (60% to 85% of predicted max heart rate or a RPE of 13 to 15) for at least 20 to 25 minutes on 3 or more days a week for a total of 75 minutes per week. It should be noted that intermittent activities performed in 5- to 10-minute increments may convey some of the same health benefits as continuous activities.[88]

Virtual Reality and Exergaming

A critical factor that promotes motor learning and generalization of acquired skills to untrained tasks is the variability of practice. Although strategies to improve locomotor function such as training using a TM or walking overground in the clinic are effective, they are limited in their ability to provide varied practice environments and task challenges. In addition, adherence to basic TM training programs may pose a clinical challenge due to participants' lack of interest or boredom with the undistracted task of just walking on a TM.

Recent technological advances make virtual reality (VR) a viable option that may hold potential for addressing the barriers created by environmental restrictions, time demands, and participant lack of interest.[89,90] For the purposes of this chapter, VR is defined broadly to include the use of video or other gaming systems that allow the participant to partially or fully immerse themselves in a computer environment that mimics real-world activities. Examples of partially immersive systems include Microsoft Kinect or Nintendo Wii together with a standard television.[91] Fully immersive systems include head-worn goggles or virtual environments where video projectors provide images of between 3 and 6 sides of a room-sized environment[92,93] (Fig. 11.1).

Regardless of the patient's health condition, systematic reviews and meta-analyses of the effects of VR on gait outcomes such as gait speed, stride and step length, and composite mobility (e.g., Timed Up and Go) suggest that there may be a small but significant benefit over standard gait interventions.[89-91] The small sample sizes,

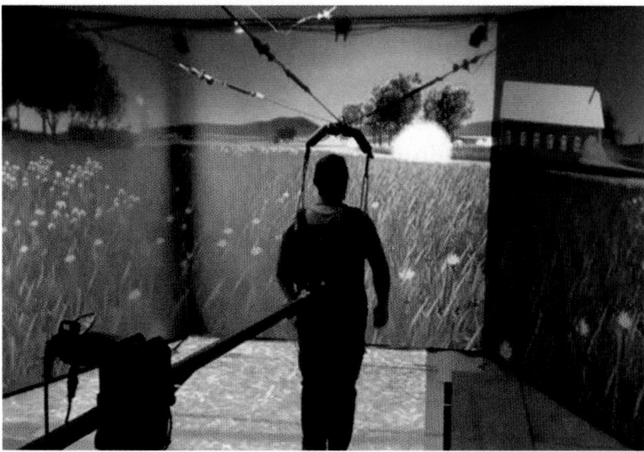

Figure 11.1 An example of an immersive virtual reality (VR) environment for gait training. In this VR environment, the participant walks on a treadmill and is provided visual input on four sides (anterior, both sides, and on the ground) that is synchronized with gait speed on the treadmill.

the variety of diagnoses studied, and the variety of intervention specifics (i.e., virtual reality systems utilized, practice dosage delivered) complicate the interpretation of a consistent effect of the intervention.

Examples of commercially available VR systems that have been utilized and shown benefit include games involving weight shifting in static stance on a Nintendo Wii balance board or dance video games on the Microsoft Kinect. Interventions ranging from 15 to 45 minutes in duration delivered 1 to 2 times per week appear to provide benefit. VR interventions provide the opportunity to incorporate many of the guiding principles discussed earlier in the chapter. For example, the games are engaging and challenging. Random practice of different gait-related tasks can easily be set up through the gaming system. The system can also provide feedback for motivational purposes that can be tracked and provided over time. Interaction with the VR environment provides an external focus of attention as well. However, there is certainly more research needed to fully understand and optimize the use of VR interventions for locomotor rehabilitation. The potential benefits of this technology that allows task-specific training that cognitively engages the participant while remaining in the clinical setting, or increasing practice time as part of a home program, warrant consideration for use in locomotor rehabilitation programs. There is also potential to use these VR systems as part of a telerehabilitation intervention.

Augmenting Muscle Force Production

A key strategy for improving muscle force production is to combine resistance training with task-specific practice. This requires repetitive practice of tasks that are *specific to the outcome* (i.e., locomotion) and *meaningful to the patient* in terms of function. Although muscle-specific resistance training (e.g., progressive resistance, isokinetic equipment) may also be indicated and complementary to locomotor rehabilitation, training of muscles involved in locomotion within the context of tasks that are specific to the positions and modes of contraction utilized during gait will optimize transfer of strength gains to locomotor skills.

Inherent to task-specific strength training is resistance provided by body weight or limb segment weight; this weight may be augmented by the addition of external resistance (e.g., resistive bands, aquatic activities, cuff weights). Task selection is based on elements of the whole task, including the body segments involved; the required mode, speed, and magnitude of contractions; and the degrees of freedom needed for the desired outcome. The goal is progression to whole task training. Activities typically begin with individual joints or body segments with progression to whole body movements.

Given that the portions of the stance phase prior to midstance require eccentric contractions of the LE to decelerate the body's momentum and the portions of stance phase subsequent to midstance require concentric contractions to accelerate the body forward, strengthening exercises must include task-specific functional activities. For example, those that focus on concentric and eccentric LE extensor muscle control might include partial wall squats, step-ups and step-downs, sit-to/from-stand transfers, and first bilateral, then single-limb heel rises to strengthen ankle plantarflexors. While a focus on extensors and flexors is appropriate for sagittal plane progression during gait, a focus on frontal plane stability requires attention to the musculature on the medial and lateral portions of the LE. Examples include strengthening of hip abductors and adductors using side-stepping, cross-stepping, and braiding (manual contact or resistive bands can be used for resistance). See Box 11.3 and Figures 11.2 to 11.4.

The goals of locomotor rehabilitation may also dictate the intensity of the resistance. For example, increases in locomotor speed or the ability to tolerate and improve walking on inclined surfaces or ascending stairs may require increases in muscle power (high muscle force delivered in a short period of time). Resistance training for this purpose should be delivered at a high intensity relative to an individual's one repetition maximum (RM) or performed in an explosive manner.[94] In contrast, sustained coordinated production of ambulation on level surfaces requires a reduced intensity of muscle contractions, but these contractions may be required over minutes to hours. Resistance training for this purpose should be delivered at intensities lower than 60% 1-RM but performed for durations of time rather than counting repetitions. The overall objective is to improve the oxidative capacity of the muscle. Owing to the varied demands of ambulation in the home and community, individuals should be trained for both muscular power and endurance.

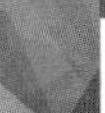

Box 11.3 Task-Specific Muscle Force Production Interventions

- Exercises for swing phase musculature
  - Standing hip flexion
  - Standing or seated knee extension
  - Standing or seated knee flexion
  - Standing or seated toe raises
- Exercises for stance phase musculature
  - Standing hip extension
  - Shallow squats with focus on concentric and eccentric control
  - Standing heel raises with focus on concentric and eccentric control
  - Step ups and step downs onto/off of 4 in step with focus on concentric and eccentric control
  - Sit to stand/stand to sit
- Exercises for frontal plane musculature
  - Standing/sidelying hip abduction
  - Standing/sidelying hip adduction

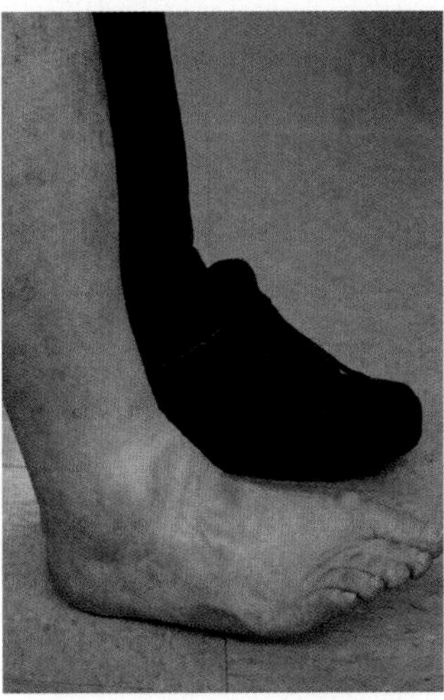

Figure 11.2 Seated ankle dorsiflexion.

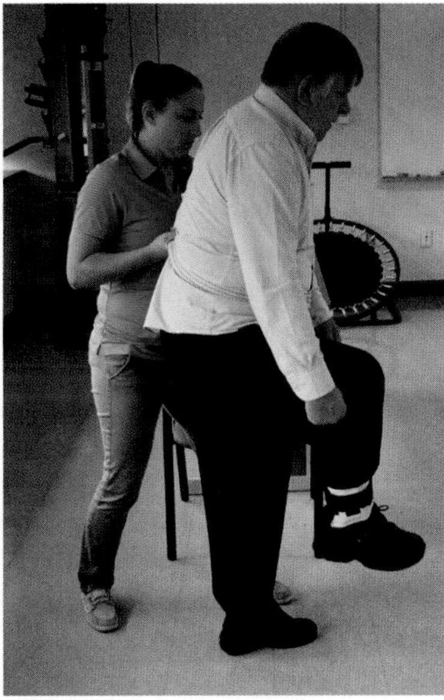

Figure 11.3 Standing hip flexion with ankle weight.

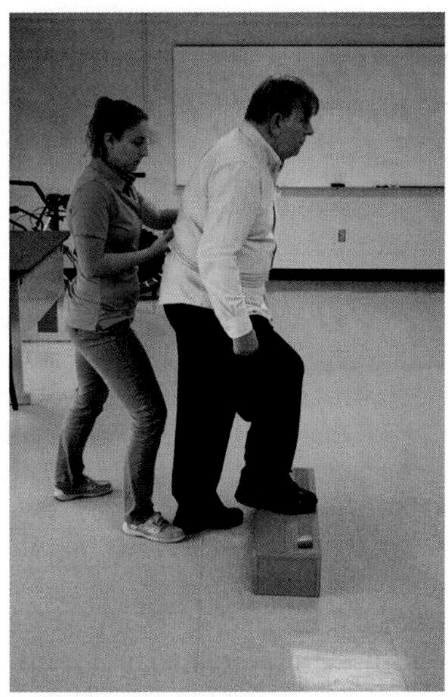

Figure 11.4 Step up onto a 4 in step.

Balance and Dynamic Postural Control During Overground Walking

Adequate standing balance and control of the center of mass (COM) are integral components of locomotion. As continuous postural adjustments are needed during locomotion, intervention strategies to improve balance should be selected that impose similar demands. Locomotion requires the ability to maintain upright stance (stability) and dynamic postural control (controlled mobility) to control movements while standing (e.g., weight shifting, LE stepping). The following provide examples of interventions to improve standing balance and dynamic postural control; balance interventions are also discussed in Chapter 10, Strategies to Improve Motor Function.

Initial standing activities may require a widening of the base of support (BOS) through the touch-down support of the hands and can be performed in the parallel bars, between two treatment tables, or next to a wall or corner of a room (corner standing). The patient is first directed to stand tall and hold steady in the posture. Enhanced postural awareness and practice of COM control can be achieved with limits of stability (LOS) training during weight shifting and in response to anticipated and unanticipated perturbations (anticipatory and reactive postural control). Active exercise to improve standing balance may include activities that require COM control while reducing the BOS (e.g., heel-rises, toe-offs), transitions to and from single-limb stance (back-kicks and sidekicks, hip and knee flexion, hip flexion with knee extension, marching in place), and tasks that change the height of the COM (partial squats). These exercises can also be performed in a pool. Adding ankle cuff weights, further alteration of the BOS (e.g., feet apart, together, tandem stance), UE position (e.g., arms overhead, reaching), and support surface (e.g., inflated disc, wobble board) can all impose greater challenge.

Engagement of ankle and hip strategies to control the COM can be promoted using incremental shifts in COM alignment and postural sway movements. Challenges can be enhanced using unstable surfaces or alterations in sensory inputs. Examples include the use of a foam cushion to degrade somatosensory input, modifying visual input by progressing from eyes open to closed, modifying the stability of the support surface (using split foam rollers [flat side down progressing to flat side up] and wobble boards), or changing the static position of the head position to alter vestibular inputs. Self-imposed or externally provided large COM shifts in all directions beyond the LOS will promote stepping strategies. Balance control can be further enhanced using manual perturbations, resistive band around pelvis during stepping (forward, backward, sideward), and mobile and compliant surfaces with alterations in BOS (feet together, tandem standing, and single-limb stance). See Box 11.4 and Figures 11.5 and 11.6.

Previous research suggests that there is a limited transfer of static standing balance activities to dynamic stability during gait.[95] For this reason, if improvements in stability during gait are desired, overground walking must be trained with the incorporation of dynamic postural control activities during gait. Examples of overground walking activities with dynamic postural control demands include modifying sensory inputs (walking on compliant surfaces, compromising vision, or asking for vertical or horizontal head movements to alter vestibular input); practicing rapid accelerations and decelerations of the COM to perform rapid starts, stops, and turns during gait; and practicing the avoidance of apparent and suddenly appearing obstacles in the gait path. Observational research suggests that the repetition of balance tasks during rehabilitation may be inadequate; therefore, consideration of increasing the practice dosage of these tasks is warranted.[96]

Although TM walking and overground walking practice may provide benefits in terms of dynamic balance, adherence to such programs over the long term may limit the overall effects. For this reason, alternative forms of exercise that provide similar benefits to gait and balance training that are more engaging are worthy of consideration. Dance is one such form of exercise. From a dynamic balance standpoint, many dance forms require repetitions of backward walking, turning, and changing speeds, all of which require the individual to control the COM (and provide variable task practice). If performed to music with a nonbalance impaired partner, additional benefits include auditory cueing, safety, working memory, and cognitive sequencing practice, as well as the social connection that occurs with the partner. Recent studies document improvements in measures of dynamic balance and gait as a result of dance interventions.[97-99] Tango and ballroom dance have been studied most often, although other forms have research support also. Studies have examined the effects of dance interventions performed between 1 to 7 days per week, 30 to 75 minutes per session, and between 2 and 18 months in overall duration.[97,100]

Box 11.4 Balance and Dynamic Postural Control During Overground Walking

- Stationary base of support/static center of mass activities
  - Static standing in wide stance, progressed to narrow or tandem stance
    - Eyes open/eyes closed, stationary head/looking up/head turns
  - Stabilization against expected and unexpected perturbations
- Stationary base of support/dynamic center of mass activities
  - Tai chi forms with feet stationary
  - Anterior/posterior/lateral/rotational upper extremity reaching
  - Picking objects up off the floor (progress from light to heavy objects)
  - Throwing and catching objects (progress from light to heavy objects)
- Moving base of support/dynamic center of mass activities
  - Stepping in different directions: backward, forward, side stepping, braiding
  - Sit to/from stand from various surfaces
  - Standing heel and toe lifts
  - Transitions to single limb stance
  - Forward, lateral, and backward step ups/downs
  - Walking on different surfaces/ascend and descend curbs, ramps, stairs
  - Walking with horizontal or vertical head turns
  - Walking while performing cognitive or motor secondary tasks
  - Obstacle course: different surfaces (carpet, mat, grass, gravel, ramp), stepping over/around objects, curbs, carrying object, varying speed, heel/toe walking, tandem walking

Circuit Training

Task-oriented locomotor circuit training involves setting up a variety of different task- oriented intervention stations, some of which are discussed in the preceding

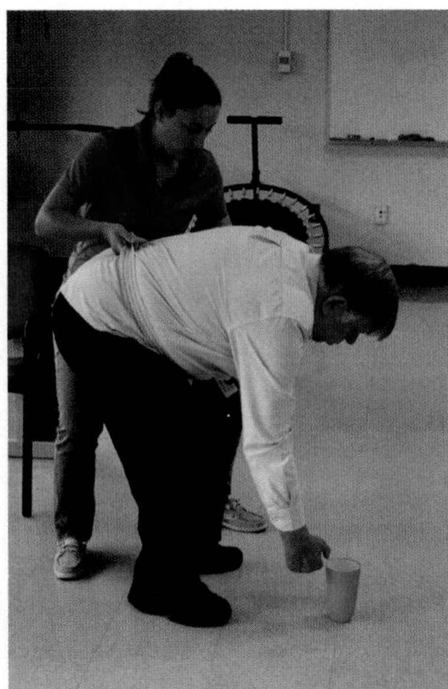

Figure 11.5 Picking up an object from the floor.

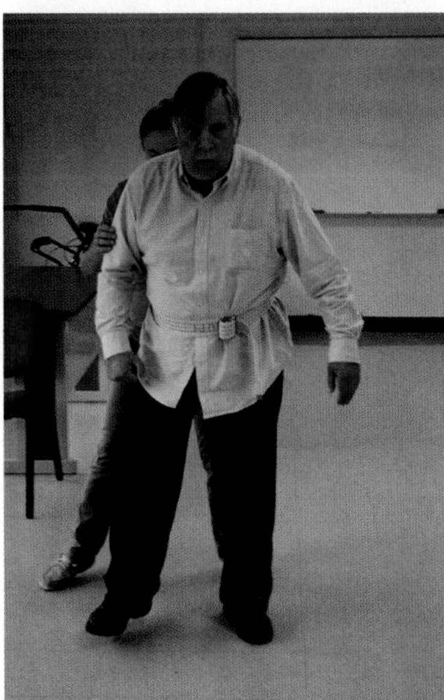

Figure 11.6 Sidestepping.

sections (e.g., augmenting force production, TM training, dynamic postural control during overground walking). At each station, the patient performs the indicated number of task repetitions (at a certain intensity) and then moves on to the next station.[101-103] For example, specific training stations may include tasks or activities such as standing and reaching, standing on different surfaces, walking through an obstacle course, transitioning from supine to sitting to standing, walking and carrying objects, walking and picking up objects from the floor, walking in different directions, walking with head turns, stepping up and down off a step, walking at varying speeds and over varying surfaces, and standing and kicking a ball. Adding ankle weights or a weighted vest, or having the patient walk against the resistance of a resistance band can vary the intensity of the task. Strength and balance exercises (described earlier) can also be incorporated into the circuit. As patient performance improves, the specific tasks are progressed by increasing the complexity and difficulty. For example, strategies to progress performance in an obstacle course might include increasing speed, carrying an object while walking through it, or stepping over higher/wider objects. A dual cognitive task can be added to the activity to increase the difficulty as well. See Box 11.5 and Figures 11.7 to 11.9.

Motor learning and neuroplasticity principles can effectively be incorporated to enhance motor learning and promote recovery. Variable and random practice is inherent to the circuit setup and different walking-related tasks at the various stations. KR feedback can be provided, for example, by informing the patient how long it took to complete the obstacle course and motivating the patient to improve on that time. An external focus of attention can be provided by instructing patients to step to or over objects instead of providing

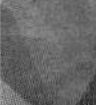

Box 11.5 Circuit Training Activities

- Obstacle course: different surfaces (carpet, mat, grass, gravel, ramp), stepping over/around objects, curbs, carrying object, varying speed, heel/toe walking, tandem walking
- Walking and picking up objects
- Stepping in different directions: backward, forward, side stepping, braiding
- Sit to/from stand from various surfaces
- Walking on different surfaces
- Stair, curbs
- Forward, lateral, and backward step ups/downs
- Standing and reaching
- Standing on different surfaces (firm, foam, carpet, grass, gravel, incline) with varying base of support (wide/narrow base of support, tandem, one foot on step and one foot on ground) and visual (eyes open/eyes closed) input
- Walking with horizontal and vertical head turns
- Walking on balance beam
- Walking on heels/toes, tandem walking
- Standing/walking and kicking ball
- Dual task: walking and carrying and/or walking with cognitive task (subtract serial 7s)
- Standing heel and toe lifts
- Walking against resistance of resistance band or with ankle weights or weighted vest
- Provide unexpected perturbations while walking
- Strength and balance exercises (see Boxes 11.3 and 11.4)

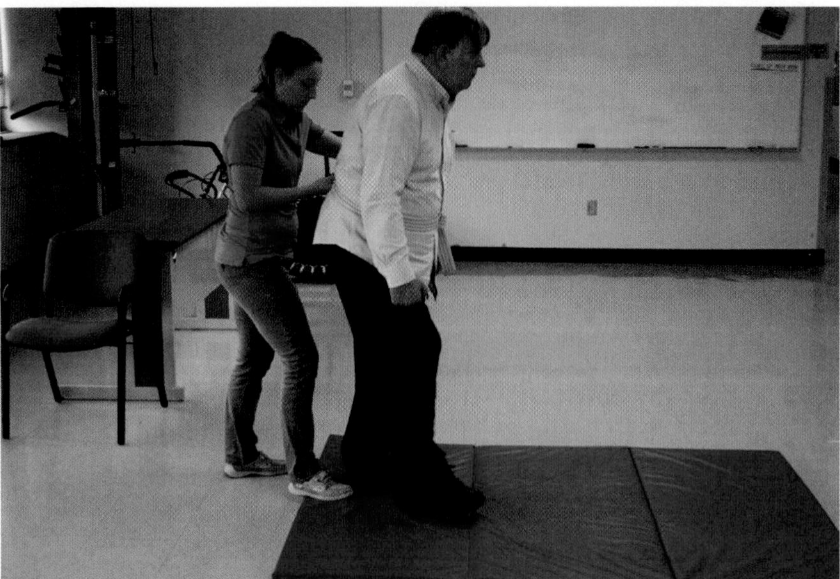

Figure 11.7 Walking on foam/uneven surface.

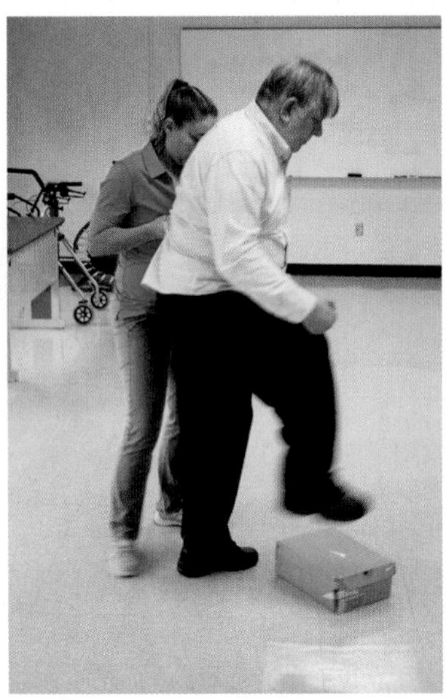

Figure 11.8 Stepping over an object while walking.

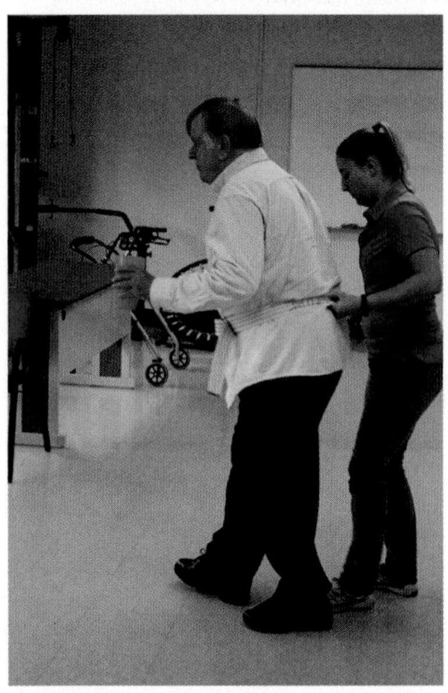

Figure 11.9 Walking while performing a motor dual task, carrying an object.

verbal instructions to lift the foot up higher when stepping (these instructions promote an internal focus of attention). Some autonomy can be provided by allowing the patient to select different objects to walk around/over in the obstacle course, to determine the height of a step up/down surface, and what objects to carry while walking. A meta-analysis by Wevers and colleagues[102] concluded that in people with chronic stroke, task-oriented circuit training is an effective intervention for improving gait speed and other gait-related activities.

Motor Imagery

Motor imagery (MI) is the mental rehearsal of a movement without the movement actually occurring.[104] Motor imagery activates some of the same cortical structures that are activated during actual movement, which may be the mechanism for improving behavioral performance.[105] Using MI as an intervention may involve either *visual imagery,* where the individual visualizes performing the activity from the third-person perspective, or *kinesthetic imagery,* where the individual imagines the sensory experience of the activity as it might normally occur from a first-person perspective.[104]

In the context of locomotion, MI is the mental practice of walking. Mental imagery practice should be relatively short (10 to 20 minutes).[104] An MI session is performed in a comfortable position (often sitting) with a short period of guided relaxation prior to initiation. The therapist guides the individual through a detailed, specific visual or kinesthetic mental rehearsal of the walking task. The tasks that are mentally rehearsed can be very specific (e.g., "See how your left foot pushes down and backward, then lifts up off the ground"). Dunsky and colleagues[106] and Dickstein and colleagues[107] provide examples of specific motor imagery sessions that incorporate both visual and kinesthetic imagery. A metronome can be added to provide auditory cues for the cadence of the imagined steps.[106] Motor imagery is often done in combination with physical practice of the task,[108,109] can be done as part of a group intervention,[110] and can be done through telerehabilitation.[111] Research supports the use of MI to improve walking ability in people with stroke,[106-108,110] PD,[104,112] and lower limb amputations.[113]

Gait Training With Assistive Devices

Appendix 11.A contains detailed information on different types of assistive devices, gait patterns with assistive devices, and gait training with assistive devices techniques.

SUMMARY

Recovery of independent walking ability is an extremely important goal for many patients who require the services of a physical therapist. It is a functional skill that directly affects performance of expected roles within the patient's social, cultural, and physical environment. A variety of interventions are available, including locomotor training with BWS and TM system, TM training, VR, strengthening, balance and overground walking training, circuit training, and MI. Although research has not found one particular intervention strategy to be more effective than another, principles of motor learning and neuroplasticity and exercise prescription guidelines should inform the development of the plan of care to improve locomotor function.

Questions for Review

1. When interpreting change in a patient's gait speed over the course of your intervention, how much should the patient's gait speed change in order for you to be confident that the patient exhibits clinically meaningful improvement in locomotor function?
2. Describe key motor learning and neuroplasticity principles that should be incorporated into any specific locomotor rehabilitation intervention.
3. Describe the guiding principles for LT using body weight support (BWS) and a treadmill (TM).
4. What variables can be manipulated to increase the intensity of locomotor training when using a treadmill?
5. Describe two task-specific interventions to increase muscle force production that would improve stance and swing phase of gait in the coronal plane.
6. List overground walking activities that promote dynamic postural control demands.
7. Describe four stations you could use in a circuit training intervention designed to promote recovery of locomotor function.

CASE STUDY

CASE STUDY PART A

You are working with a 58-year-old woman who had a left CVA 4 weeks ago in an outpatient facility. She was recently discharged home after spending 2 weeks in an inpatient rehabilitation facility. She lives alone on the fourth floor of an apartment building. She returned to work this week as an administrative assistant at a bank and takes public transportation to work. She can walk independently in her home and short distances in the community, she uses an off-the-shelf ankle-foot orthosis and straight cane. She reports her primary goal is to improve her walking ability. She has difficulty crossing the street in the city, making it on time to work because she cannot walk quickly enough to catch the bus, and has fallen once at home while walking at night to the bathroom.

CASE STUDY PART B

You find the following during your initial examination:

1. Motor Function: Fugl Meyer lower extremity motor function section: 29/34: full score on all items except:
   a. Movement combining synergies: knee flexion and ankle dorsiflexion both 1/2
   b. Movement out of synergy: knee flexion and ankle dorsiflexion both 1/2
   c. Normal reflexes: 0/2
   d. Coordination/Dysmetria: speed: 1/2
2. Sensory integrity: proprioception of right ankle is normal.
3. Muscle Performance: right ankle dorsiflexion: 22 lb of force (normative values for women aged 50–59, dominant side: 43.7 lb).
4. Balance: mini Balance Evaluation Systems Test: 19/28; test findings indicate difficulty with anticipatory postural control, postural responses to perturbation, and dynamic balance during gait both with and without cognitive task.
5. Self-Care/Domestic Life and Work Life: Stroke Impact Scale-16: 68%.
6. Specific locomotor function tests:
   a. Gait speed: 0.80 m/s (normative values for women aged 50–59: 1.31 m/s)
   b. 6-minute walk test: 318 meters (normative values for women aged 20–59: 674 m)
   c. Community Balance and Mobility Scale: 34/96; test findings indicate difficulty with support of body mass by the right lower extremity, dynamic postural control of the moving body, propulsion of the body in the intended direction, adaptability of the locomotion to changing environmental and task demands, and with stairs.
   d. Multiple Sclerosis Walking Scale: 75%; self-report outcome measure indicates that patient has difficulty with stairs, running, walking endurance, speed of walking, and need to concentrate more while walking.

CASE STUDY GUIDING QUESTIONS PART A

1. What tests and measures would you use with this patient?
2. What locomotion related tests and measures would you perform to gain more specific insight into this patient's locomotor function?

CASE STUDY GUIDING QUESTIONS PART B

1. Based on the findings from the initial examination, outline an intervention session that addresses the major locomotor impairments and limitations the patient presents with.

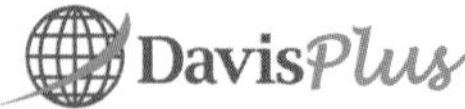

For additional resources, including answers to the questions for review and case study guiding questions, please visit **http://davisplus.fadavis.com.**

References

1. Bohannon, RA, AW, and Smith, M: Rehabilitation goals of patients with hemiplegia. Int J Rehabil Res 11:181–183, 1988.
2. Lord, SE, et al: Community ambulation after stroke: How important and obtainable is it and what measures appear predictive? *Arch Phys Med Rehabil* 85(2):234–239, 2004.
3. Jain, NB, et al: Factors associated with health-related quality of life in chronic spinal cord injury. Am J Phys Med Rehabil 86(5):387–396, 2007.
4. Williams, V, et al: What really matters to patients living with chronic obstructive pulmonary disease? An exploratory study. *Chron Respir Dis* 4(2):77–85, 2007.
5. Jorgensen, HS, et al: Recovery of walking function in stroke patients: The Copenhagen Stroke Study. Arch Phys Med Rehabil 76(1):27–32, 1995.
6. Duncan, RP, and Earhart GM. Measuring participation in individuals with Parkinson disease: Relationships with disease severity, quality of life, and mobility. Disabil Rehabil 33(15–16):1440-1446, 2011.
7. Weinshenker, BG: Natural history of multiple sclerosis. Ann Neuro 36 Suppl:S6–11, 1994.
8. Myhr, KM, et al: Disability and prognosis in multiple sclerosis: Demographic and clinical variables important for the ability to walk and awarding of disability pension. Mult Scler 7(1):59–65, 2001.
9. Ertekin, O, Ozakbas, S, and Idiman, E: Caregiver burden, quality of life and walking ability in different disability levels of multiple sclerosis. NeuroRehabilitation 34(2):313–321, 2014.
10. Kohn, CG, et al: Mobility, walking and physical activity in persons with multiple sclerosis. Curr Med Res Opin 30(9):1857–1862, 2014.
11. Schmid, A, et al: Improvements in speed-based gait classifications are meaningful. Stroke 38(7):2096–2100, 2007.
12. Kierkegaard, M, et al: The relationship between walking, manual dexterity, cognition and activity/participation in persons with multiple sclerosis. Mult Scler 18(5):639–646, 2012.
13. Fritz, S, and Lusardi, M: White paper: "walking speed: the sixth vital sign." J Geriatr Phys Ther 32(2):2–5, 2009.

14. Fulk, GD, et al: Clinometric properties of the six-minute walk test in individuals undergoing rehabilitation poststroke. Physiother Theory Pract 24(3):195–204, 2008.
15. Wrisley, DM, et al: Reliability, internal consistency, and validity of data obtained with the functional gait assessment. Phys Ther 84(10):906–918, 2004.
16. Whitney, S, Wrisley, D, and Furman, J: Concurrent validity of the Berg Balance Scale and the Dynamic Gait Index in people with vestibular dysfunction. Physiother Res Int 8(4):178–186, 2003.
17. Howe, JA, et al: The Community Balance and Mobility Scale—a balance measure for individuals with traumatic brain injury. Clin Rehabil 20(10):885–895, 2006.
18. Ditunno, JF, Jr., et al: Walking index for spinal cord injury (WISCI): An international multicenter validity and reliability study. Spinal Cord 38(4):234–243, 2000.
19. Gailey, RS, et al: The amputee mobility predictor: An instrument to assess determinants of the lower-limb amputee's ability to ambulate. Arch Phys Med Rehabil 83(5):613–627, 2002.
20. Horak, FB, Wrisley, DM, and Frank, J: The Balance Evaluation Systems Test (BESTest) to differentiate balance deficits. Phys Ther 89(5):484–498, 2009.
21. Franchignoni, F, et al: Using psychometric techniques to improve the Balance Evaluation Systems Test: The mini-BESTest. J Rehabil Med 42(4):323–331, 2010.
22. Middleton, A, Fritz, SL, and Lusardi, M: Walking speed: The functional vital sign. J Aging Phys Act 23(2):314–322, 2015.
23. Fulk, GD, et al: Estimating clinically important change in gait speed in people with stroke undergoing outpatient rehabilitation. J Neurol Phys Ther 35(2):82–89, 2011.
24. Tilson, JK, et al: Meaningful gait speed improvement during the first 60 days poststroke: Minimal clinically important difference. Phys Ther 90(2):196–208, 2010.
25. Bohannon, RW, Andrews, AW, and Glenney, SS. Minimal clinically important difference for comfortable speed as a measure of gait performance in patients undergoing inpatient rehabilitation after stroke. J Phys Ther Sci 25(10):1223–1225, 2013.
26. Perera, S, et al: Meaningful change and responsiveness in common physical performance measures in older adults. J Am Geriatr Soc 54(5):743–749, 2006.
27. Alley, DE, et al: Meaningful improvement in gait speed in hip fracture recovery. J Am Geriatr Soc 59(9):1650–1657, 2011.
28. Palombaro, KM, et al: Determining meaningful changes in gait speed after hip fracture. Phys Ther 86(6):809–816, 2006.
29. Kon, SS, et al: The 4-metre gait speed in COPD: Responsiveness and minimal clinically important difference. Eur Respir J 43(5):1298–1305, 2014.
30. Barthuly, AM, Bohannon, RW, and Gorack, W: Gait speed is a responsive measure of physical performance for patients undergoing short-term rehabilitation. Gait Posture 36(1):61–64, 2012.
31. Hobart, JC, et al: Measuring the impact of MS on walking ability: The 12-Item MS Walking Scale (MSWS-12). Neurology 60(1):31–36, 2003.
32. Danks, KA, et al: Relationship between walking capacity, biopsychosocial factors, self-efficacy, and walking activity in individuals poststroke. J Neurol Phys Ther 40:1–7, 2016.
33. Bladh, S, et al: Psychometric performance of a generic walking scale (Walk-12G) in multiple sclerosis and Parkinson's disease. J Neurol 259(4):729–738, 2012.
34. Shaughnessy, M, et al: Steps after stroke: Capturing ambulatory recovery. Stroke 36(6):1305–1307, 2005.
35. Skidmore, FM, et al: Daily ambulatory activity levels in idiopathic Parkinson disease. J Rehabil Res Dev 45(9):1343–1348, 2008.
36. Cavanaugh, JT, et al: Ambulatory activity in individuals with multiple sclerosis. J Neurol Phys Ther 35(1):26–33, 2011.
37. Mehrholz, J, Kugler, J, and Pohl, M: Locomotor training for walking after spinal cord injury. Cochrane Database Syst Rev 11:CD006676, 2012.
38. Mehrholz, J, Pohl, M, and Elsner, B: Treadmill training and body weight support for walking after stroke. Cochrane Database Syst Rev 1:CD002840, 2014.
39. States, RA, Salem, Y, and Pappas, E: Overground gait training for individuals with chronic stroke: a Cochrane systematic review. J Neurol Phys Ther 33(4):179–186, 2009.
40. Dockx, K, et al: Virtual reality for rehabilitation in Parkinson's disease. Cochrane Database Syst Rev 12:CD010760, 2016.
41. Barclay, RE, et al: Interventions for improving community ambulation in individuals with stroke. Cochrane Database Syst Rev 3:CD010200, 2015.
42. Pollock, A, et al: Physical rehabilitation approaches for the recovery of function and mobility following stroke. Cochrane Database Syst Rev 4:CD001920, 2014.
43. Tomlinson, CL, et al: Physiotherapy for Parkinson's disease: A comparison of techniques. Cochrane Database Syst Rev 6:CD002815, 2014.
44. Handoll, HH, Sherrington, C, and Mak, JC: Interventions for improving mobility after hip fracture surgery in adults. Cochrane Database Syst Rev 3:CD001704, 2011.
45. Schmidt, RA, and Lee, TD: Motor Control and Learning, ed 4. Human Kinetics, Champaign, IL, 2005.
46. Kleim, JA, and Jones, TA: Principles of experience-dependent neural plasticity: Implications for rehabilitation after brain damage. J Speech Lang Hear Res 51(1):S225–239, 2008.
47. Kleim, JA, Barbay, S, and Nudo, RJ: Functional reorganization of the rat motor cortex following motor skill learning. J Neurophysiol 80(6):3321–3325, 1998.
48. Nudo, RJ, and Milliken, GW: Reorganization of movement representations in primary motor cortex following focal ischemic infarcts in adult squirrel monkeys. J Neurophysiol 75(5):2144–2149, 1996.
49. Fine, MS, and Thoroughman, KA: Motor adaptation to single force pulses: Sensitive to direction but insensitive to within-movement pulse placement and magnitude. J Neurophysiol 96(2):710–720, 2006.
50. Boyd, L, and Winstein, C: Explicit information interferes with implicit motor learning of both continuous and discrete movement tasks after stroke. J Neurol Phys Ther 30(2):46–57; discussion 58-49, 2006.
51. Lang, CE, MacDonald, JR, and Gnip, C: Counting repetitions: An observational study of outpatient therapy for people with hemiparesis post-stroke. J Neurol Phys Ther 31(1):3–10, 2007.
52. Stanton, R, et al: Feedback received while practicing everyday activities during rehabilitation after stroke: An observational study. Physiother Res Int 20(3):166–173, 2015.
53. Dobkin, BH, et al: International randomized clinical trial, stroke inpatient rehabilitation with reinforcement of walking speed (SIRROWS), improves outcomes. Neurorehabil Neural Rep 24(3):235–242, 2010.
54. Wulf, G, and Lewthwaite, R: Optimizing performance through intrinsic motivation and attention for learning: The OPTIMAL theory of motor learning. Psychon Bull Rev 23(5):1382–1414, 2016.
55. Chiviacowsky, S, Wulf, G, and Wally, R: An external focus of attention enhances balance learning in older adults. Gait Posture 32(4):572–575, 2010.
56. Badami, R, et al: Feedback after good versus poor trials affects intrinsic motivation. Res Q Exerc Sport 82(2):360–364, 2011.
57. Wulf, G, Chiviacowsky, S, and Lewthwaite, R: Altering mindset can enhance motor learning in older adults. Psychol Aging 27(1):14–21, 2012.
58. Wulf, G, and Toole, T: Physical assistance devices in complex motor skill learning: Benefits of a self-controlled practice schedule. Res Q Exerc Sport 70(3):265–-272, 1999.
59. Nudo, RJ: Functional and structural plasticity in motor cortex: Implications for stroke recovery. Phys Med Rehabil Clin N Am 14(1 Suppl):S57–76, 2003.
60. Kolb, B: Overview of cortical plasticity and recovery from brain injury. Phys Med Rehabil Clin N Am 14(1 Suppl):S7–25, viii, 2003.
61. Dobkin, BH, et al: Ankle dorsiflexion as an fMRI paradigm to assay motor control for walking during rehabilitation. NeuroImage 23(1):370–381, 2004.
62. Taub, E, et al: The learned nonuse phenomenon: Implications for rehabilitation. Europa Medicophysica 42(3):241–255, 2006.
63. Hornby, TG, et al: Variable Intensive Early Walking Poststroke (VIEWS): A randomized controlled trial. Neurorehabil Neural Repair 30(5):440–450, 2016.
64. Barbeau, H, and Rossignol, S: Recovery of locomotion after chronic spinalization in the adult cat. Brain Res 412(1):84–95, 1987.
65. Edgerton, VR, et al: Use-dependent plasticity in spinal stepping and standing. Adv Neurol 72:233–247, 1997.

66. Lovely, RG, et al: Effects of training on the recovery of full-weight-bearing stepping in the adult spinal cat. Exp Neurol 92(2):421–435, 1986.
67. Behrman, AL, Bowden, MG, and Nair, PM: Neuroplasticity after spinal cord injury and training: An emerging paradigm shift in rehabilitation and walking recovery. Phys Ther 86(10):1406–1425, 2006.
68. Behrman, AL, and Harkema, SJ: Locomotor training after human spinal cord injury: A series of case studies. Phys Ther 80(7):688–700, 2000.
69. Harkema, S, Behrman, A, and Barbeau, H: Evidence-based therapy for recovery of function after spinal cord injury. Handb Clin Neurol 109:259–274, 2012.
70. Hidler, J, et al: Multicenter randomized clinical trial evaluating the effectiveness of the Lokomat in subacute stroke. Neurorehabil Neural Rep 23(1):5–13, 2009.
71. Field-Fote, EC, and Roach, KE: Influence of a locomotor training approach on walking speed and distance in people with chronic spinal cord injury: A randomized clinical trial. Phys Ther 91(1): 48–60, 2011.
72. Schwartz, I, et al: Robot-assisted gait training in multiple sclerosis patients: A randomized trial. Mult Scler 18(6):881–890, 2012.
73. Dobkin, B, et al: Weight-supported treadmill vs over-ground training for walking after acute incomplete SCI. Neurology 66(4):484–493, 2006.
74. Harkema, SJ, et al: Balance and ambulation improvements in individuals with chronic incomplete spinal cord injury using locomotor training-based rehabilitation. Arch Phys Med Rehabil 93(9):1508–1517, 2012.
75. Jayaraman, A, et al: Locomotor training and muscle function after incomplete spinal cord injury: case series. J Spinal Cord Med 31(2):185–193, 2008.
76. Duncan, PW, et al: Body-weight-supported treadmill rehabilitation after stroke. NEJM 364(21):2026–2036, 2011.
77. Plummer, P, et al: Effects of stroke severity and training duration on locomotor recovery after stroke: A pilot study. Neurorehabil Neural Repair 21(2):137–151, 2007.
78. Fisher, BE, et al: The effect of exercise training in improving motor performance and corticomotor excitability in people with early Parkinson's disease. Arch Phys Med Rehabil 89(7):1221–1229, 2008.
79. Toole, T, et al: The effects of loading and unloading treadmill walking on balance, gait, fall risk, and daily function in Parkinsonism. NeuroRehabilitation 20(4):307–322, 2005.
80. Miyai, I, et al: Treadmill training with body weight support: Its effect on Parkinson's disease. Arch Phys Med Rehabil 81(7):849–852, 2000.
81. Giesser, B, et al: Locomotor training using body weight support on a treadmill improves mobility in persons with multiple sclerosis: A pilot study. Mult Scler 13(2):224–231, 2007.
82. Swinnen, E, et al: Treadmill training in multiple sclerosis: Can body weight support or robot assistance provide added value? A systematic review. Mult Scler Int 2012:240–274, 2012.
83. Frenkel-Toledo, S, et al: Treadmill walking as an external pacemaker to improve gait rhythm and stability in Parkinson's disease. Mov Disord 20(9):1109–1114, 2005.
84. Nadeau, A, Pourcher, E, and Corbeil, P: Effects of 24 wk of treadmill training on gait performance in Parkinson's disease. Med Sci Sports Exerc 46(4):645–655, 2014.
85. Highsmith, MJ, et al: Gait training interventions for lower extremity amputees: A systematic literature review. Technol Innov 18(2-3):99–113, 2016.
86. Macko, RF, et al: Treadmill exercise rehabilitation improves ambulatory function and cardiovascular fitness in patients with chronic stroke: a randomized, controlled trial. Stroke 36(10):2206–2211, 2005.
87. Mehrholz, J, et al: Is body-weight-supported treadmill training or robotic-assisted gait training superior to overground gait training and other forms of physiotherapy in people with spinal cord injury? A systematic review. Spinal Cord 2017.
88. Garber, CE, et al: American College of Sports Medicine position stand. Quantity and quality of exercise for developing and maintaining cardiorespiratory, musculoskeletal, and neuromotor fitness in apparently healthy adults: Guidance for prescribing exercise. Med Sci Sports Exerc 43(7):1334–1359, 2011.
89. Laver, KE, et al: Virtual reality for stroke rehabilitation. Cochrane Database Syst Rev 2:CD008349, 2015.
90. de Rooij, IJ, van de Port, IG, and Meijer JG: Effect of virtual reality training on balance and gait ability in patients with stroke: Systematic review and meta-analysis. Phys Ther 96(12):1905–1918, 2016.
91. Ravenek, KE, Wolfe, DL, and Hitzig, SL: A scoping review of video gaming in rehabilitation. Disabil Rehabil Assist Technol 11(6):445–453, 2016.
92. van der Meer, R: Recent developments in computer assisted rehabilitation environments. Mil Med Res 1:22, 2014.
93. Kim, A, Darakjian, N, and Finley, JM: Walking in fully immersive virtual environments: An evaluation of potential adverse effects in older adults and individuals with Parkinson's disease. J Neuroeng Rehabil 14(1):16, 2017.
94. Swain DP, American College of Sports Medicine. *Acsm's Resource Manual of Guidelines for Exercise Testing and Prescription.* 7th ed. Philadelphia: Wolters Kluwer Health/Lippincott Williams and Wilkins, 2014.
95. Winstein, CJ, et al: Standing balance training: Effect on balance and locomotion in hemiparetic adults. Arch Phys Med Rehabil 70(10):755–762, 1989.
96. Lang, CE, et al: Observation of amounts of movement practice provided during stroke rehabilitation. Arch Phys Med Rehabil 90(10):1692–1698, 2009.
97. McNeely, ME, Duncan, RP, and Earhart, GM: A comparison of dance interventions in people with Parkinson disease and older adults. Maturitas 81(1):10–16, 2015.
98. Sharp, K, and Hewitt, J: Dance as an intervention for people with Parkinson's disease: A systematic review and meta-analysis. Neurosci Biobehav Rev 47:445–456, 2014.
99. Keogh, JW, et al: Physical benefits of dancing for healthy older adults: A review. J Aging Phys Act 17(4):479–500, 2009.
100. McNeely, ME, Duncan, RP, and Earhart, GM: Impacts of dance on non-motor symptoms, participation, and quality of life in Parkinson disease and healthy older adults. Maturitas 82(4):336–341, 2015.
101. Dean, CM, Richards, CL, and Malouin, F: Task-related circuit training improves performance of locomotor tasks in chronic stroke: A randomized, controlled pilot trial. Arch Phys Med Rehabil 81(4):409–417, 2000.
102. Wevers, L, et al: Effects of task-oriented circuit class training on walking competency after stroke: A systematic review. Stroke 40(7):2450–2459, 2009.
103. Fritz, S, et al: Feasibility of intensive mobility training to improve gait, balance, and mobility in persons with chronic neurological conditions: A case series. J Neurol Phys Ther 35(3):141–147, 2011.
104. Dickstein, R, and Deutsch, JE: Motor imagery in physical therapist practice. Phys Ther 87(7):942–953, 2007.
105. Ridderinkhof, KR, and Brass, M: How kinesthetic motor imagery works: A predictive-processing theory of visualization in sports and motor expertise. J Physiol Paris 109(1–3):53–63, 2015.
106. Dunsky, A, et al: Home-based motor imagery training for gait rehabilitation of people with chronic poststroke hemiparesis. Arch Phys Med Rehabil 89(8):1580–1588, 2008.
107. Dickstein, R, et al: Effects of integrated motor imagery practice on gait of individuals with chronic stroke: A half-crossover randomized study. Arch Phys Med Rehabil 94(11):2119–2125, 2013.
108. Kumar, VK, Chakrapani, M, and Kedambadi, R: Motor imagery training on muscle strength and gait performance in ambulant stroke subjects-a randomized clinical trial. J Clin Diagn Res 10(3):YC01-04, 2016.
109. Bae, YH, et al: An efficacy study on improving balance and gait in subacute stroke patients by balance training with additional motor imagery: A pilot study. J Phys Ther Sci 27(10):3245–3248, 2015.
110. Dickstein, R, et al: Motor imagery group practice for gait rehabilitation in individuals with post-stroke hemiparesis: A pilot study. NeuroRehabilitation 34(2):267–276, 2014.
111. Deutsch, JE, Maidan, I, and Dickstein, R: Patient-centered integrated motor imagery delivered in the home with telerehabilitation to improve walking after stroke. Phys Ther 92(8): 1065–1077, 2012.
112. Mirelman, A, Maidan, I, and Deutsch, JE: Virtual reality and motor imagery: Promising tools for assessment and therapy in Parkinson's disease. Mov Disord 28(11):1597–1608, 2013.
113. Cunha, RG, et al: Influence of functional task-oriented mental practice on the gait of transtibial amputees: A randomized, clinical trial. J Neuroeng Rehabil 14(1):28, 2017.

Ambulatory Assistive Devices: Types, Gait Patterns, and Gait Training

appendix **11.A**

TYPES AND GAIT PATTERNS

There are three major categories of ambulatory assistive devices: *canes, crutches,* and *walkers.* Each has several modifications to the basic design, many of which were developed to meet the needs of a specific patient problem or diagnostic group. Assistive devices are prescribed for a variety of reasons, including problems of balance, pain, fatigue, weakness, joint instability, excessive skeletal loading, and cosmesis. Another primary function of assistive devices is to eliminate weight-bearing fully or partially from a lower extremity (LE). This unloading occurs by transmission of force from the upper extremities (UEs) to the floor by downward pressure on the assistive device. Prescribing an appropriate assistive device requires knowledge of the patient's weight-bearing status. Common clinical descriptors used to identify weight-bearing status are presented in Box 11A.1. Considerations specific to the bariatric population are presented in Box 11A.2.

Canes

Most canes used in clinical practice are constructed of lightweight aluminum. Evidence supports the effectiveness of canes to improve balance[1-3] and postural stability.[1,4-6] Although canes reduce biomechanical load on LE joints,[2,7] they are not intended for use with a restricted weight-bearing status (such as non–weight-bearing [NWB] or partial weight-bearing [PWB]). Patients are typically instructed to hold a cane in the hand *opposite the affected extremity.* This positioning of the cane most closely approximates a normal reciprocal gait pattern with the opposite arm and leg moving together. It also widens the base of support (BOS) with less lateral shifting of the center of mass (COM) than when the cane is held on the ipsilateral side.

Several investigations have confirmed that contralateral positioning of the cane reduces hip abductor activity on the side opposite the cane.[4,8-10] During normal gait, the hip abductors of the stance extremity contract to counteract the gravitational moment at the pelvis on the contralateral side during swing. This prevents tilting of the pelvis on the contralateral side but results in compressive forces acting at the stance hip. Use of a cane in the UE opposite the affected hip will reduce these forces. The floor (ground) reaction force created by the downward pressure of body weight on the cane counterbalances the gravitational movement at the affected hip.[3] Thus, the need for tension in the abductor muscles is reduced, with a subsequent decrease in joint compressive forces.

Several components of floor reaction forces that create joint compression at the hip can be reduced by use of a cane. In an early study by Ely and Smidt,[11] contralateral use of a cane was found to decrease the vertical and posterior components of the floor reaction force produced by the affected foot. They noted that the reductions in vertical floor reaction peaks were probably due to a shifting of body weight toward the cane, which was a contributing factor in reducing contact force at the affected hip. In a study of patients with total hip arthroplasty (THA), Neumann[8] found that contralateral use of a cane reduced average hip abductor electromyography (EMG) activity to 31% below that generated when not using a cane. Cane use contralateral to a THA, with the addition of carrying an ipsilateral load, decreased hip abductor activity by 40% compared to walking without carrying a load or using a cane.[9]

Research supports use of a cane as an effective method for reducing forces acting at the hip.[4,6,8,9] This reduction is particularly important for activities such as stair climbing, when the forces generated at the hip are significantly increased. Contralateral cane use has also been found to reduce knee pain in patients with osteoarthritis.[7,12] Clearly, use of a cane has important implications for hip and knee involvement such as joint replacements or degenerative joint disease.

Box 11A.1 Clinical Descriptors of Weight-Bearing Status

- *Full weight-bearing*: There are no restrictions on weight-bearing; 100% of body weight can be borne on the LE.
- *Non–weight-bearing*: No weight is borne on the involved limb; foot/toes make no contact with floor/ground surface.
- *Partial weight-bearing*: Only a portion of weight can be borne on the extremity; sometimes expressed as a percentage of body weight (e.g., 20% or 50%).
- *Toe-touch weight-bearing* or *touch-down weight-bearing*: Only the toes of the affected extremity contact the floor to improve balance (not to support body weight).
- *Weight-bearing as tolerated*: Weight-bearing is limited to the amount comfortably tolerated by the patient.

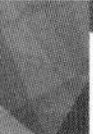

Box 11A.2 Bariatric Ambulatory Assistive Devices

As with all patients, safety and function are paramount concerns in selection of assistive devices (canes, crutches, and walkers) for patients who are morbidly obese. Important considerations include the following:

- Selecting devices with the appropriate *weight capacity*. Manufacturers of bariatric equipment typically include the maximum weight designation for each product. Standard devices have a weight capacity of 250 to 350 pounds; bariatric equipment carry weight capacities in the range of 400 to 1,000 pounds.
- Identification of the needed dimensions (height and width) of the equipment; this requires knowledge of the anthropometric characteristics (measurements and proportions) of the patient's body.
- Large patients often walk with a wide-based gait owing to lower extremity limb girth and the need to increase the base of support to carry body weight and maintain balance. If a disproportionate amount of weight falls anterior (e.g., abdominal region), upright postures will be further challenged by the need to counteract the anterior effects of gravity.

Following are general characteristics and features of commercially available walkers, crutches, and canes designed for the bariatric population. The information presents a range of available options and is not representative of any individual assistive device. As new products are continually introduced to the market, consultation with a durable medical equipment supplier will help ensure prescription of the optimal device for an individual patient.

Note: For labeling or identifying bariatric equipment in patient care settings, the term *expanded capability* is recommended over less desirable terms such as *oversized, extra-large*, or *heavy duty*.

Walkers

- Bariatric walkers typically include deeper and wider frames.
- May accommodate user heights from 5 feet 3 inches to 6 feet 10 inches.
- Overall walker height adjustments range from 31 to 41.25 inches.
- Available widths: 23.5 to 30 inches.
- May include double anterior cross bracing to increase stability.
- Weight capacity range: 500 to 700 pounds (without seat); 400 to 500 pounds (with seat).
- Walker weight: 7 to 12 pounds (without seat); 19 to 26 pounds (with seat).
- Seat dimensions: height, 22 inches; width, 17.5 to 18 inches; depth, 13 to 14 inches.
- Some models are constructed using a reinforced steel frame; for rolling walkers, large casters are typically used.

Axillary Crutches

- Bariatric axillary crutches are generally constructed of heavy-duty steel.
- May accommodate user heights from 5 feet 2 inches to 7 feet 4 inches (youth sizes available).
- Overall crutch height adjustments range from 44 to 60 inches.
- Weight capacity range: 550 to 1,000 pounds.
- Crutch tips: 2-inch diameter.
- Crutch weight: 4 pounds, 6 ounces to 5 pounds each.

Forearm Crutches

- Bariatric forearm crutches are generally constructed of heavy-duty steel.
- May accommodate user heights from 5 feet to 6 feet 7 inches (youth sizes available).
- Crutch height adjustments (handle to floor) range from 28 to 42 inches and forearm piece adjustments (handle to center of cuff) range from 8 to 9.5 inches; as with standard forearm crutches, the leg and forearm sections adjust independently.
- Weight capacity range: 500 to 700 pounds.
- Crutch tips: 2-inch diameter.
- Crutch weight: 2 pounds 6 ounces to 5 pounds 7 ounces.

Canes

- Bariatric canes are generally constructed of stainless steel or heavy-duty steel tubing; most incorporate an offset handle and a reinforcing cuff tightened by a rotation sleeve.
- May accommodate user heights from 4 feet 10 inches to 6 feet 4 inches.
- Overall height adjustments range from approximately 25 to 46 inches.
- Weight capacity range: 500 to 700 pounds.
- Cane weight: 1.8 to 2 pounds.

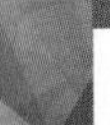

Box 11A.2 Bariatric Ambulatory Assistive Devices—cont'd

Quadruped Canes

- Bariatric quadruped canes are generally constructed of steel and often incorporate a double-plated base; most incorporate an offset handle and a reinforcing cuff tightened by a rotation sleeve.
- May accommodate user heights from 4 feet 11 inches to 6 feet 5 inches.
- Overall height adjustments range from approximately 29 to 39 inches.
- Weight capacity range: 500 to 700 pounds.
- Weight: 4 to 5 pounds.
- Footprint size: small base, 6 × 8 inches; large base, 8 × 12 inches.

Maguire et al[4] found that contralateral cane use reduced gluteus medius activity by 21.86% and tensor fascia lata activity by 19.14% in patients with subacute stroke. This finding has important implications for patients with stroke, who often use canes, because strategies to improve postural control and balance reactions may be adversely affected by reduced hip abductor activity.

In addition to altering the forces on the affected extremity, canes are selected on the basis of their ability to improve gait by providing increased dynamic stability and improving balance. This is achieved by the increased BOS provided by the additional point(s) of floor contact. The level of stability provided by canes is on a continuum. Broad-based (four-point) canes provide the greatest stability and standard (single-point) canes provide the least. The following section presents several of the more common types of canes in clinical use and identifies their advantages and disadvantages.

Types of Canes

Standard Canes

This assistive device is also referred to as a *single-point* or *straight cane* (Fig. 11A.1A). It is made of wood or acrylic and has a half-circle ("crook") or T-shaped handle.

- *Advantages.* This cane is inexpensive and fits easily on stairs or other surfaces where space is limited.
- *Disadvantages.* The standard cane is not adjustable and must be cut to fit the patient. With a half-circle handle, the point of support (shaft of cane) is anterior to the hand, not directly beneath it. The T-shaped handle shifts the point of support only slightly closer to hand.

Standard Adjustable Aluminum Cane

This assistive device (Fig. 11A.1B) has the same basic design as the standard cane. It is made of aluminum and has a half-circle handle with a molded plastic covering. The telescoping design of this cane enables the height to be adjusted using a push-button mechanism. Variations in available height range differ slightly with manufacturers. However, they are generally adjustable within the range of approximately 27 to 38.5 in. (68 to 98 cm). (*Note:* Most adjustable aluminum assistive devices [e.g., canes, crutches, walkers] use a push-button mechanism to alter height; many include a reinforcing cuff tightened by a thumbscrew or rotation sleeve.)

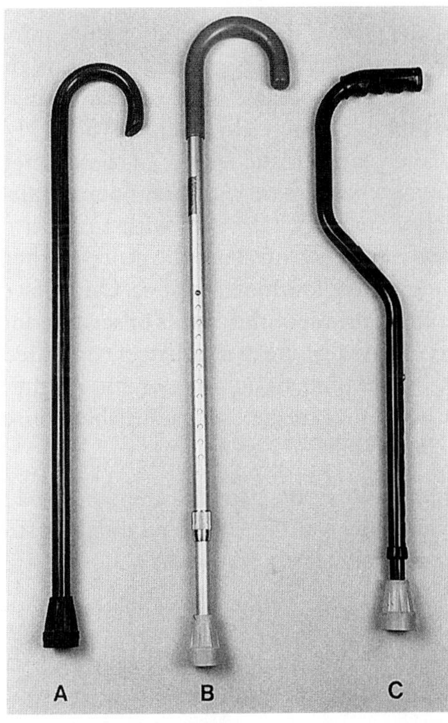

Figure 11A.1 (A) Standard wooden cane, (B) Standard adjustable aluminum cane, and (C) Adjustable offset cane.

- *Advantages.* This cane is quickly adjustable, facilitating ease of determining appropriate height. It is lightweight and fits easily on stairs.
- *Disadvantages.* The point of support is anterior to the hand, not directly beneath it. This cane is costlier than a standard wooden cane.

Adjustable Aluminum Offset Cane

The proximal component of the shaft of this cane is offset anteriorly, creating a straight *offset* handle. It is made of aluminum with a plastic or rubber molded grip-shaped handle (Fig. 11A.1C). Using a push-button mechanism, the telescoping design allows the height to be adjusted from approximately 27 to 38.5 in. (68 to 98 cm).

- *Advantages.* The design of this cane allows pressure to be borne over the center of the cane for greater stability. This cane also is quickly adjusted, is lightweight, and fits easily on stairs.
- *Disadvantages.* This cane is more costly than standard or adjustable aluminum canes.

Note: For standard and offset canes, the diameter of both the distal rubber tips and shaft of the cane is generally at least 1 in. (2.54 cm).

Quadruped (Quad) Cane

This assistive device is constructed of aluminum and is available in a variety of designs depending on the manufacturer. Both large-based quad canes and small-based quad canes are commercially available (Figs. 11A.2 and 11A.3). The characteristic feature of these canes is that they provide a broad base with four points of floor contact. Each point (leg) is covered with a rubber tip. The legs closest to the patient's body are generally shorter and may be angled to allow foot clearance. On many designs, the proximal portion of the cane is offset anteriorly. The hand piece is usually one of a variety of contoured plastic grips. A telescoping design allows for height adjustments. Quad canes are generally adjustable from approximately 28 to 38 in. (71 to 91 cm).

- *Advantages.* This cane provides a broad-based support. Bases are available in several different sizes. This cane is also easily adjustable.

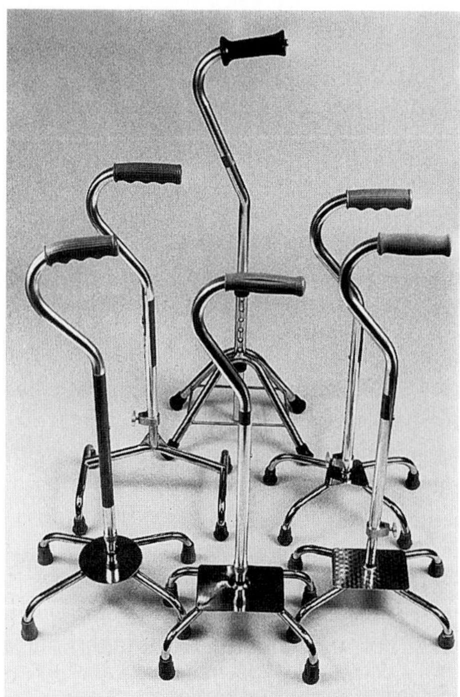

Figure 11A.2 A variety of large-based quadruped canes.

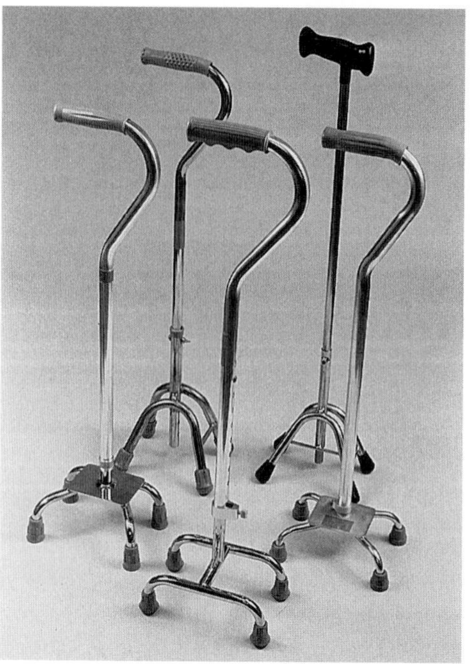

Figure 11A.3 A variety of small-based quadruped canes.

- *Disadvantages.* Depending on the specific design of the cane, the pressure exerted by the patient's hand may not be centered over the cane and may result in patient complaints of instability. As a result of the broad BOS, some quad canes may not be practical for use on stairs. Another disadvantage of broad-based canes is that they warrant use of a slower gait pattern. If a faster forward progression is used, the cane often "rocks" from rear legs to front legs, which decreases its effectiveness. Patients should be instructed to place all four legs of the cane on the floor simultaneously to obtain maximum stability.

Hemi Cane

The hemi cane also is constructed of aluminum (Fig. 11A.4). It provides a very broad base with four points of floor contact. Each point (leg) is covered with a rubber tip. The legs farther from the patient's body are angled to maintain floor contact and to improve stability. The handgrip is molded plastic around the uppermost segment of aluminum tubing. Hemi canes fold flat and are adjustable in height from approximately 29 to 37 in. (73 to 94 cm).

- *Advantages.* Hemi canes provide very broad-based support and are more stable than a quad cane. These canes also fold flat for travel or storage.
- *Disadvantages.* As with the quad canes, the specific design of a hemi cane or handgrip placement may not allow pressure to be centered over the cane. Hemi canes cannot be used on most stairs. They require use of a slow forward progression and are generally more costly than quad canes.

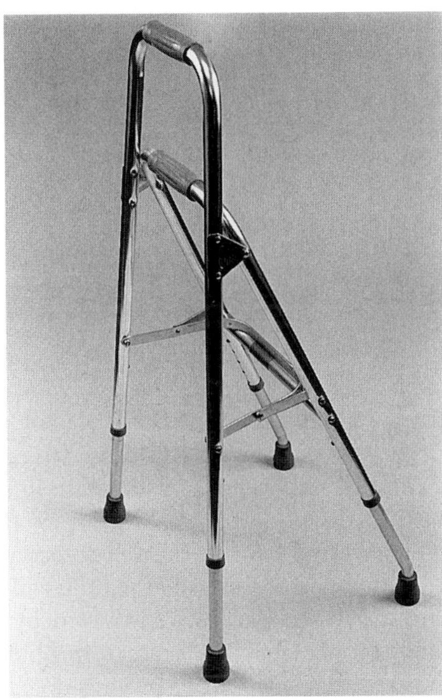

Figure 11A.4 Hemi cane.

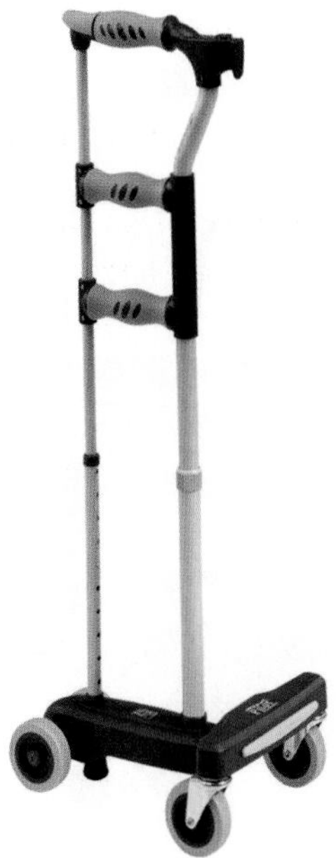

Figure 11A.5 Rolling cane. *(Courtesy of Full Life Products, LLC, Moorestown, NJ 08057.)*

Rolling Cane

Constructed of aluminum and aluminum tubing (Fig. 11A.5), this cane provides a wide, wheeled base, allowing uninterrupted forward progression. It includes a contoured handgrip, height adjustment from 28 to 37 in. (71 to 94 cm), and a pressure-sensitive brake built into the handle that is engaged using pressure from the base of the hand.

- *Advantages.* The wheeled base allows weight to be continuously applied as the need to lift and place the cane forward is eliminated. This also provides for a faster forward progression. The second and third handles placed between the uprights can assist in rising to standing (brake engaged).
- *Disadvantages.* This cane is more costly than standard quadruped canes and requires sufficient UE and grip strength to engage the braking mechanism. This cane is not suitable for patients displaying a propulsive gait pattern (e.g., Parkinson's disease).

Laser Cane

This cane incorporates a bright red laser line projected across the floor, designed to assist with overcoming freezing episodes while walking (Fig 11A.6). A walker with a laser is also available (Fig 11A.7). Donovan and colleagues[13] examined 26 patients with Parkinson's disease using either a laser cane or walker (selection based on type of device habitually used). Subjects were instructed not to look at the visual cue (laser beam) unless experiencing a freezing of gait (FOG) episode, at which time they were instructed to "step over" the light. Findings indicated a small but significant mean reduction in FOG episodes scores, and a mean reduction in fall frequency was 39.5% (±9.3%; $p = 0.002$). No significant changes in gait speed were noted. Although additional research is warranted, these initial findings suggest that assistive devices incorporating a laser beam may hold potential for addressing FOG episodes common in patients with Parkinson's disease.

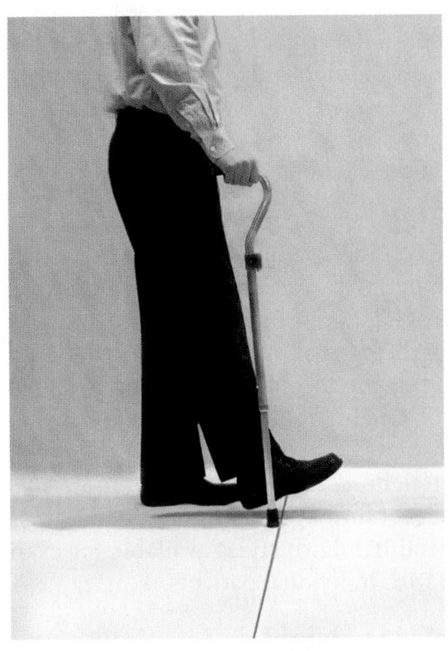

Figure 11A.6 The Laser Cane projects a bright red laser beam across the floor in front of the patient. During a freezing-of-gait episode, the beam provides a visual cue for the patient to step over. *(Courtesy of In-Step Mobility Products Corp, Skokie, IL 60076.)*

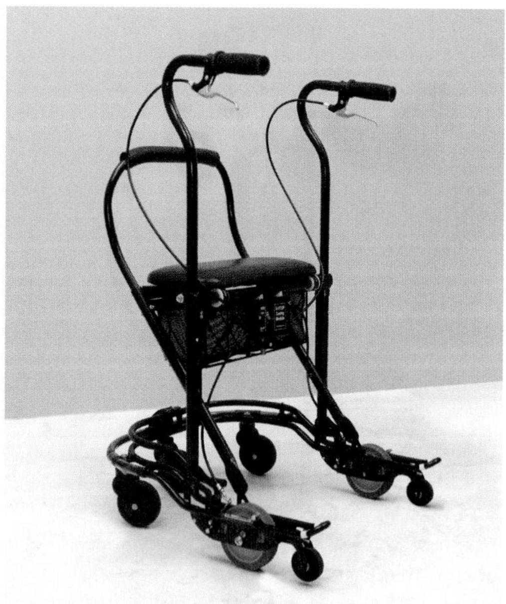

Figure 11A.7 The U-Step II walking stabilizer includes both visual (laser) and auditory (beat pattern for gait speed) cues. U-shaped base surrounds the individual for increased stability. It also includes a seat, a small projection over posterior casters to assist moving onto a curb, and a control to set rolling resistance. *(Courtesy of In-Step Mobility Products Corp, Skokie, IL 60076.)*

Handgrips

A general consideration relevant to all canes is the nature of the handgrip. A variety of styles and sizes are available. The type of handgrip should be judged and selected primarily on the basis of patient comfort and on the grip's ability to provide adequate surface area to allow effective transfer of weight from the UE to the floor. The more common types of handgrips are (1) the *crook* handle, (2) the straight *offset* handle, and (3) the *T-shaped* handle, which conforms to the patient's hand. It is useful to have several handgrip styles available for examination and trial with individual patients.

Setting Cane Height

When setting cane height, the cane (or center of a broad-based cane) is placed approximately 6 in. (15.24 cm) from the lateral border of the toes. Two landmarks typically are used during measurement: the *greater trochanter* and the *angle at the elbow*. When holding the cane, the top of the cane should come to approximately the level of the greater trochanter with the elbow flexed to about 20 to 30 degrees. Because of individual variations in body proportion and limb lengths, the degree of flexion at the elbow is generally considered the more important indicator of correct cane height.

The 20 to 30 degrees of elbow flexion serves two important functions: It allows the arm to shorten or to lengthen during different phases of gait, and it provides a shock-absorption mechanism. Finally, as with all assistive devices, the height of the cane should be considered with regard to patient comfort and the cane's effectiveness in accomplishing its intended purpose.

Gait Pattern for Use of Canes

As discussed, the cane should be held in the UE opposite the affected limb. For ambulation overground on level surfaces, the cane and the involved (or more involved) LE are advanced simultaneously (Fig. 11A.8). The cane should remain relatively close to the body and should not be placed ahead of the toe of the involved LE. These are important considerations, because placing the cane too far forward or to the side will cause lateral and/or forward bending, with a resultant decrease in dynamic stability.

When bilateral involvement exists, a decision must be made as to which side of the body the cane will be held. This question is most effectively resolved by using a problem-solving strategy with input from both the patient and therapist. Questions to be considered include the following:

- On which side is the cane most comfortable?
- Is one placement superior in terms of improving balance and/or ambulatory endurance?

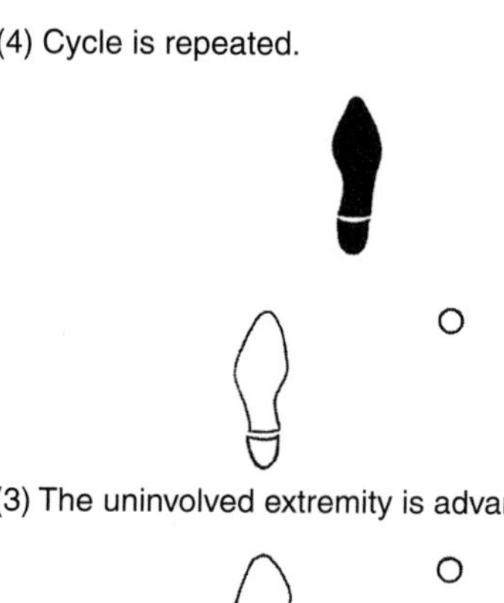

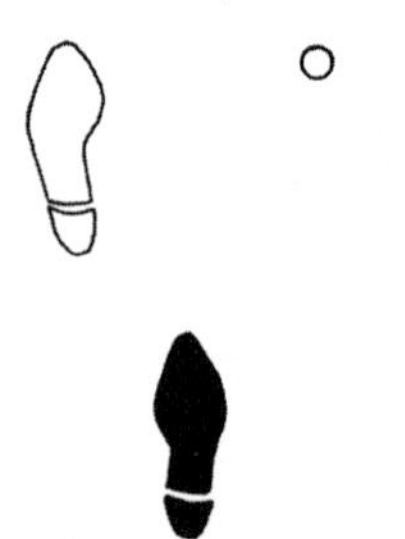

(2) The cane and involved extremity are moved forward simultaneously.

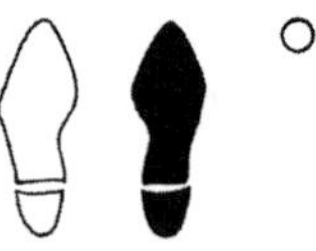

(1) Starting position. In this example, the left lower extremity is the involved limb.

Figure 11A.8 Gait pattern for use of cane.

- If gait deviations exist, is one position more effective in improving the overall gait pattern?
- Is safety influenced by cane placement (e.g., during transfers, stair climbing, or overground in community)?
- Is there a difference in strength and coordination between upper extremities (UEs)?
- Are two canes needed for stability?

Consideration of these questions will generally provide sufficient information to determine the most effective cane placement and use when bilateral involvement exists.

For some patients, optimal function is achieved using canes bilaterally (Fig 11A.9). In these situations, a two- or four-point gait pattern is used. For example, with a four-point pattern, the contralateral cane is moved forward and then the ipsilateral LE steps forward. Using a two-point pattern, the contralateral cane and ipsilateral LE are moved forward simultaneously. These gait patterns are described in the following section on crutches.

Crutches

Crutches are used most frequently to improve balance and to relieve weight-bearing, either fully or partially, on a LE. They are typically used bilaterally and function to increase the BOS, to improve lateral stability, and to allow the UEs to transfer body weight to the floor. This transfer of weight through the UEs permits functional ambulation while maintaining a restricted weight-bearing status. There are two basic designs of crutches in frequent clinical use: *axillary* and *forearm* crutches.

Types of Crutches and Attachments

Axillary Crutches

These assistive devices are also referred to as *standard crutches* (Fig. 11A.10, *left*). They are made of lightweight wood or aluminum. Their design includes an axillary bar, a hand piece, and double uprights joined distally by a single leg covered with a rubber suction tip (which should have a diameter of 1.5 to 3 in. [1.5 to 3 cm]). The single leg allows for height variations. Height adjustments for wooden crutches are made by altering the placement of screws and wing bolts in predrilled holes. The design of most aluminum crutches incorporates a push-button pin mechanism for height adjustments similar to those found on aluminum canes. Some aluminum crutches also have patient height markers adjacent to the notches to assist in adjustment. The height of the handgrips for wooden and some aluminum crutches is adjusted by placement of screws and wing bolts in predrilled holes. The handgrip height on some aluminum crutches is adjusted using a push-button mechanism with a reinforcing clip-lock (Fig. 11A.11). Both the overall height of the crutch and the height of the handgrip typically adjust in 1-in. (2.54-cm) increments.

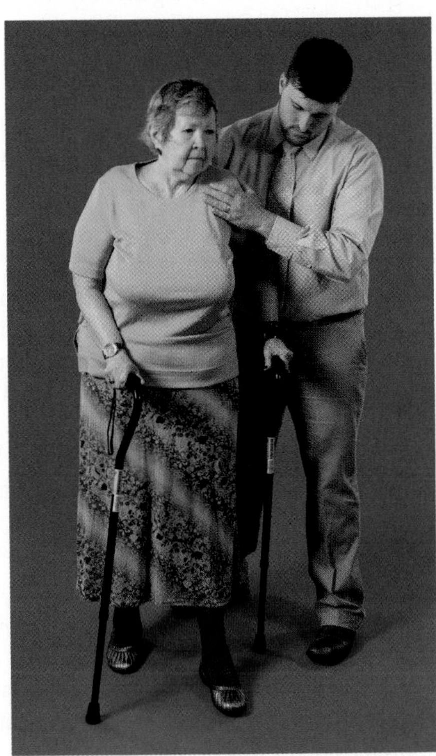

Figure 11A.9 The client is ambulating using bilateral offset canes with a four-point gait. One cane is advanced and then the opposite LE is advanced. For example, the right cane is moved forward, then the left LE, followed by the left cane and then the right LE.

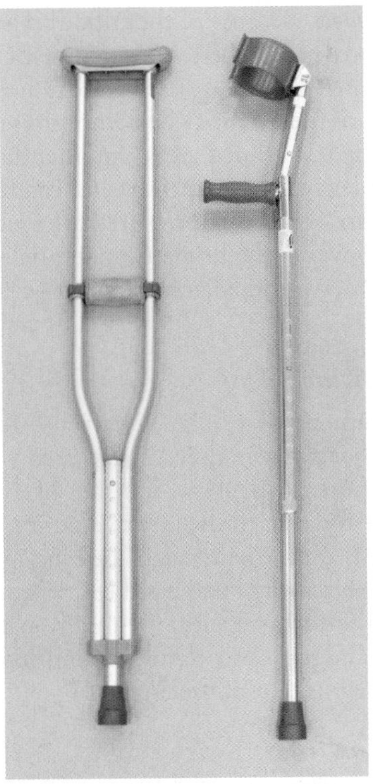

Figure 11A.10 Axillary crutch (left) and forearm crutch (right).

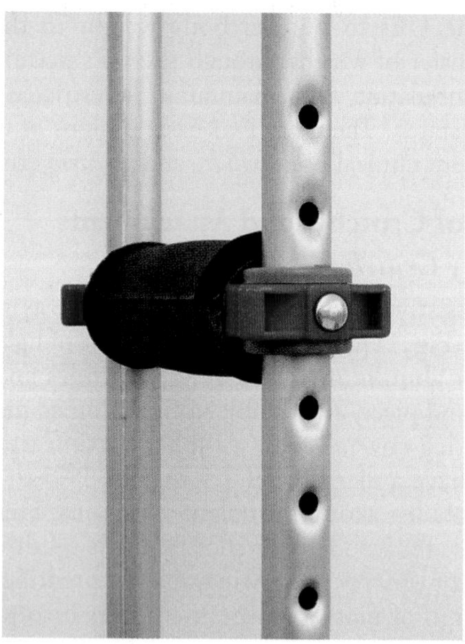

Figure 11A.11 Push-button handgrip adjustment with reinforcing clip-lock.

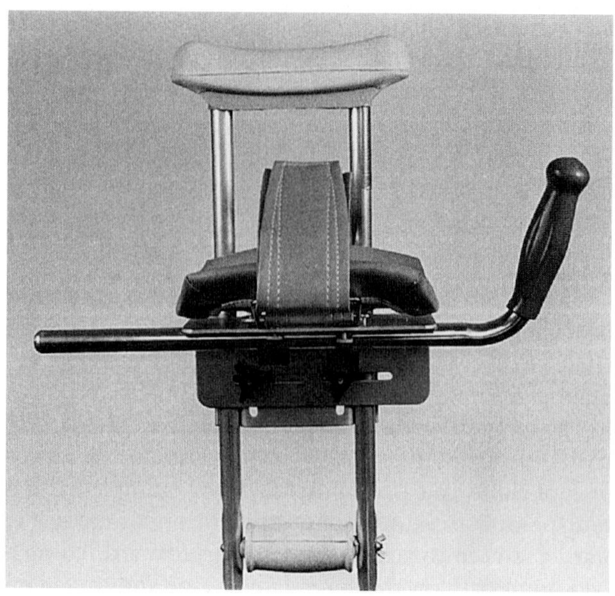

Figure 11A.12 Platform attachment to axillary crutch. These attachments can also be used on walkers.

Axillary crutches are generally adjustable in adult sizes, from approximately 48 to 60 in. (122 to 153 cm), with children's and extra-long sizes available.

- *Advantages.* Axillary crutches improve balance and lateral stability and provide for functional ambulation with restricted weight-bearing. They are easily adjusted, inexpensive when made of wood, and can be used for stair climbing.
- *Disadvantages.* Because of the tripod stance required to use crutches and the resultant large BOS, crutches are awkward in small areas. For the same reason, the safety of the user may be compromised when ambulating in crowded areas. Another disadvantage is the tendency of some patients to lean on the axillary bar. This causes pressure at the radial groove (spiral groove) of the humerus, potentially damaging the radial nerve and adjacent vascular structures in the axilla.

Platform Attachments

These attachments (Fig. 11A.12) are also referred to as *forearm rests* or *troughs*. They also are used with walkers. Their function is to allow transfer of body weight through the forearm to the assistive device. A platform attachment is used when weight-bearing is contraindicated through the wrist and hand (e.g., arthritis, Colles' fracture). The forearm piece is usually padded, has a dowel or handgrip, and has hook-and-loop straps to maintain the position of the forearm.

Forearm Crutches

These assistive devices are also known as *Lofstrand* and *Canadian* crutches (Fig. 11A.10, *right*). They are constructed of aluminum. Their design includes a single upright, a forearm cuff, and a handgrip. This crutch adjusts both proximally to alter position of the forearm cuff and distally to alter the height of the crutch. Adjustments are made using a push-button mechanism. The available heights of forearm crutches are indicated from handgrip to floor and are generally adjustable in adult sizes from 29 to 35 in. (74 to 89 cm), with children's and extra-long sizes available. The distal end of the crutch is covered with a rubber suction tip. The forearm cuffs are available with either a medial or anterior opening. The cuffs are made of metal and can be obtained with a plastic coating.

- *Advantages.* The forearm cuff allows use of hands without the crutches becoming disengaged. They are easily adjusted and allow functional stair-climbing activities, especially for individuals wearing bilateral knee-ankle-foot orthoses. Many patients feel they are more aesthetic, and they fit more easily into an automobile owing to the overall decreased height.
- *Disadvantages.* Forearm crutches provide less lateral support owing to the absence of an axillary bar. The cuffs may be difficult to remove.

Setting Crutches Height

Axillary Crutches

Several methods are available for measuring axillary crutches. The most common use a standing or a supine position. Measurement from standing is most accurate and is the preferred approach.

- *Standing.* From a supported standing position, crutches should be measured from a point approximately 2 in. (5.08 cm) below the axilla. The width of two fingers is often used to approximate this distance. During measurement, the distal end of the crutch should be resting at a point 2 in. (5.08 cm) lateral and 6 in. (15.24 cm) anterior to the foot. A general estimate of crutch height can be obtained before standing by subtracting 16 in. (40.64 cm) from the patient's height. With the shoulders relaxed, the hand piece should be adjusted to provide 20 to 30 degrees of elbow flexion.

- *Supine.* From this position, the measurement is taken from the anterior axillary fold to a surface point (mat or treatment table) 6 to 8 in. (5.08 to 7.5 cm) from the lateral border of the heel.

Forearm Crutches

Standing is the position of choice for measuring forearm crutches. From a supported standing position, the distal end of the crutch should be positioned at a point 2 in. (5.08 cm) lateral and 6 in. (15.24 cm) anterior to the foot. With the shoulders relaxed, the height should then be adjusted to provide 20 to 30 degrees of elbow flexion. The forearm cuff is adjusted separately. Cuff placement should be on the proximal third of the forearm, approximately 1 to 1.5 in. (2.5 to 3.8 cm) below the elbow.

Crutch Gait Patterns

Gait patterns are selected on the basis of the patient's balance, coordination, muscle function (strength, power, endurance), and weight-bearing status. The gait patterns differ significantly in their energy requirements, BOS, and the speed with which they can be executed.

Before initiating instruction in gait patterns, several important points should be emphasized to the patient:

- During axillary crutch use, body weight should always be borne on the hands and not on the axillary bar. This will prevent pressure on both the vascular and nervous structures located in the axillary region.
- Balance will be optimal by always maintaining a wide (tripod) BOS. Even when in a resting stance, the patient should be instructed to keep the crutches at least 4 in. (10 cm) to the front and to the side of each foot. The foot should not be allowed to achieve parallel alignment with the crutches. This will jeopardize anterior–posterior stability by decreasing the BOS.
- When using standard crutches, the axillary bars should be held close to the chest wall to provide improved lateral stability.
- The patient should also be cautioned about the importance of holding the head up and maintaining good postural alignment during ambulation.
- Stepping in a small circle rather than pivoting should be used when turning.

Three-Point

In this type of gait, three points of support contact the floor (two crutch points and a single LE). It is used when a non–weight-bearing status is required on one LE. Body weight is borne on the hands through the crutches instead of on the affected LE. The sequence of this gait pattern is illustrated in Figure 11A.13.

Partial Weight-Bearing

This gait is a modification of the three-point pattern. During forward progression of the involved extremity, weight is borne partially on both crutches and on the affected extremity (Fig. 11A.14). During instruction in the partial weight-bearing gait, emphasis should be placed on use of a normal heel-toe progression on the affected extremity. Patients may interpret "partial weight-bearing" as meaning that only the toes or ball of the foot should contact the floor. Use of this positioning over a period of days or weeks will lead to heel cord tightness. Limb load monitors are often a useful adjunct

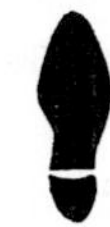
(5) Cycle is repeated.
(4) Both crutches are advanced.
(3) Weight is shifted through the upper extremities onto the crutches, and the uninvolved limb advances beyond the crutches. If this presents difficulty, the unaffected limb may initially be brought to the crutches and later progress beyond.
(2) Weight is shifted onto the uninvolved right lower extremity, and the crutches are advanced.
(1) Starting position. In this example, the left lower extremity is non–weight-bearing.

Figure 11A.13 Three-point gait pattern.

(4) Cycle is repeated.

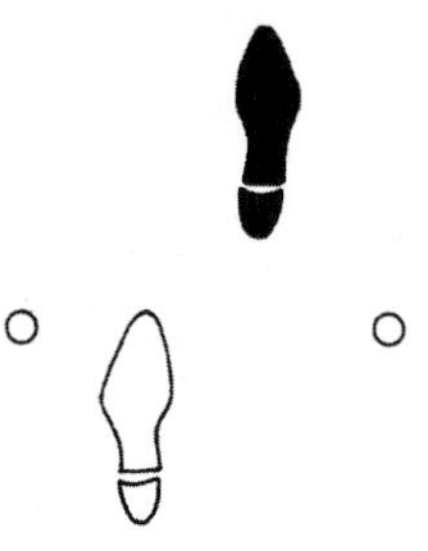

(3) Weight is shifted into the crutches and partially to the affected extremity, and the unaffected limb advances.

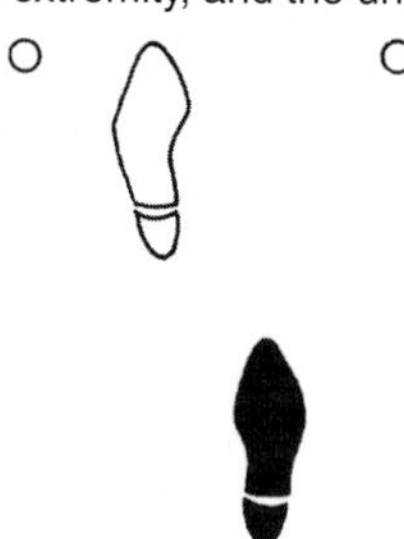

(2) Weight is shifted onto the uninvolved limb. The crutches and the affected extremity are advanced simultaneously as shown or can be broken into two components: (a) advance crutches, (b) advance affected extremity.

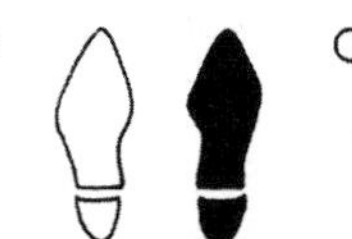

(1) Starting position. In this example, the left lower extremity is partial-weight-bearing.

Figure 11A.14 Partial weight-bearing gait; modification of the three-point gait pattern.

to partial weight-bearing gait training and are described in the "Adjunct Training Devices" section. These devices provide auditory feedback to the patient regarding the amount of weight borne on an extremity.

Four-Point

This pattern provides a slow, stable gait as three points of floor contact are maintained. Weight is borne on both LEs and typically is used with bilateral involvement due to poor balance, incoordination, or muscle weakness. In this gait pattern,1q1q one crutch is advanced and then the opposite LE is advanced. For example, the left crutch is moved forward, then the right LE, followed by the right crutch and then the left LE (Fig. 11A.15).

Two-Point

This gait pattern is similar to the four-point gait. However, it is less stable because only two points of floor contact are maintained. Thus, use of this gait requires better balance. The two-point pattern more closely simulates normal gait, inasmuch as the opposite LE and UE move together (Fig. 11A.16).

(6) Cycle is repeated.

(5) The left lower extremity is advanced.

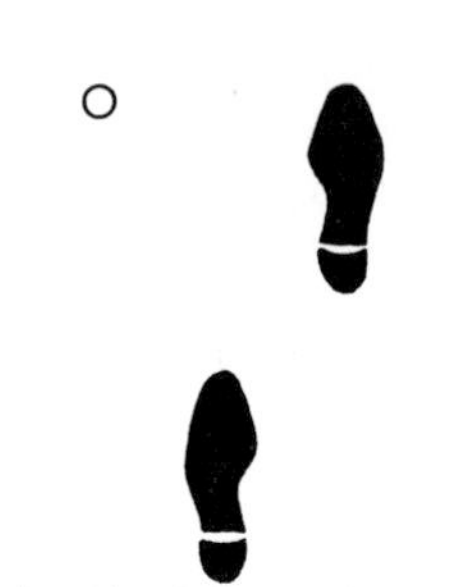

(4) The right crutch is advanced.

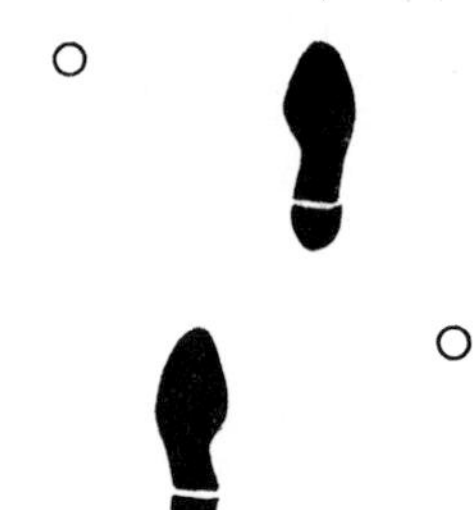

(3) The right lower extremity is advanced.

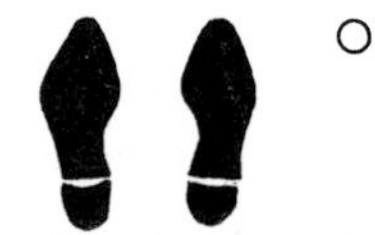

(2) The left crutch is advanced.

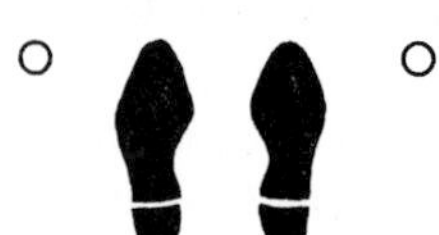

(1) Starting position. Weight is borne on both lower extremities and both crutches.

Figure 11A.15 Four-point gait pattern.

(4) Cycle is repeated.

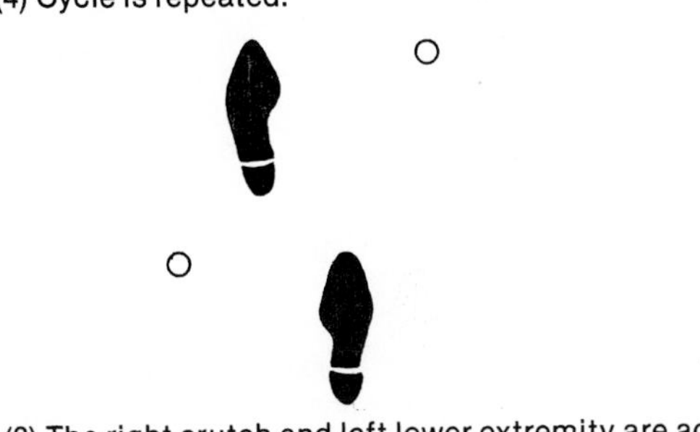

(3) The right crutch and left lower extremity are advanced together.

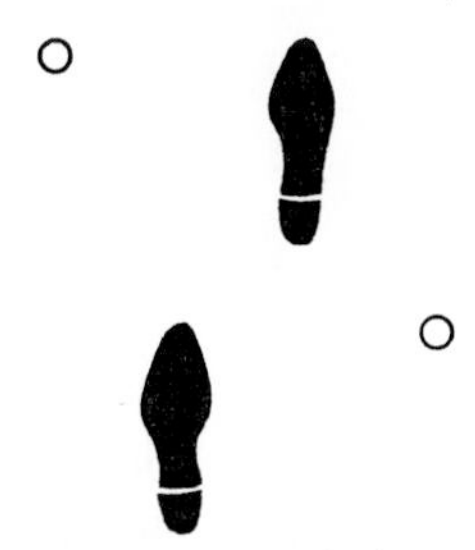

(2) The left crutch and right lower extremity are advanced together.

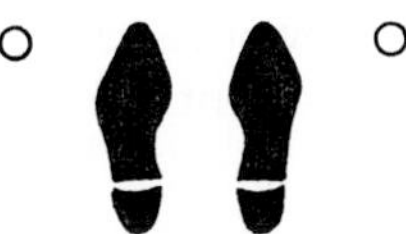

(1) Starting position. Weight is borne on both lower extremities and both crutches.

Figure 11A.16 Two-point gait pattern.

Two additional crutch gaits are the *swing-to* and *swing-through* patterns. These gaits are often used when there is bilateral LE involvement, such as in spinal cord injury (SCI). The swing-to gait involves forward movement of both crutches simultaneously, weight is shifted onto the hands, and the LEs "swing to" the crutches. In the swing-through gait, the crutches are moved forward together, weight is shifted onto the hands, and the LEs are swung beyond the crutches.

Walkers

Walkers are used to improve balance and relieve weight-bearing either fully or partially on an LE. Of the three categories of ambulatory assistive devices, walkers afford the greatest stability. They provide a wide BOS, improve anterior and lateral stability, and allow the UEs to transfer body weight to the floor.

Walkers are typically made of aluminum with molded vinyl handgrips and rubber tips. They are adjustable in adult sizes from approximately 32 to 37 in. (81 to 92 cm), with children's, youth, and tall sizes available. Several design variations and modifications to the standard design are available and are described below.

Types of Walkers and Features

Glides

Glides are small, plastic attachments placed on the posterior legs of walkers typically in combination with wheels on the front legs (Fig. 11A.17A). They promote a smooth forward progression without having to lift and place the walker with each step. They are typically made of high-density plastic in an inverted-mushroom shape. Other common glide designs include a 1-inch-diameter (2.54 cm) "disk" with a central stem that slides into the tubular leg and is tightened into place with a screwdriver and a fitted cap that is placed directly onto the walker leg (in the same manner the rubber tip is attached). Another style of glide incorporates a tennis ball within a fixed housing (Fig. 11A.18).

Folding Mechanism

Folding walkers are particularly useful for patients who travel. These walkers can be easily collapsed to fit in an automobile or other storage space (see Fig. 11A.17B).

Handgrips (Handles)

Enlarged and molded handgrips are available and may be useful for some patients with arthritis. Some walkers offer a second set of handles to assist with sit-to-stand transitions (see Fig 11A.17A).

Platform Attachments

This adaptation is used when weight-bearing is contraindicated through the wrist and hand (described in crutch section; see Figure 11A.12).

Wheel Attachments

This adaptation to walkers (often called *rolling* walkers) includes the addition of wheels (either to the two front wheels only or to all four wheels). The addition of wheels frequently allows functional ambulation for patients who are unable to lift and to move a conventional walker (e.g., frail elderly). *Swivel wheels* turn freely in a complete circle (Fig. 11A.19). *Fixed wheels* rotate around a central axis (Fig. 11A.20A). Wheels are generally available in 3-, 5-, and 6-in. (7.62-, 12.7-, 15.24-cm) diameters. Eight-inch-diameter (20.32 cm) wheels are also available and can be used to add height for tall users.

Braking Mechanism

A braking system is an essential feature of walkers designed with wheels. Walkers with four wheels frequently include hand brakes that lock the rear wheels (see Fig. 11A.19). *Spring-loaded locks* can be placed on the rear walker wheels (see Fig. 11A.20A). These locks engage when weight is placed on the posterior walker legs through the handgrips. Posterior pressure brakes are effective when wheels are placed only on the front walker legs.

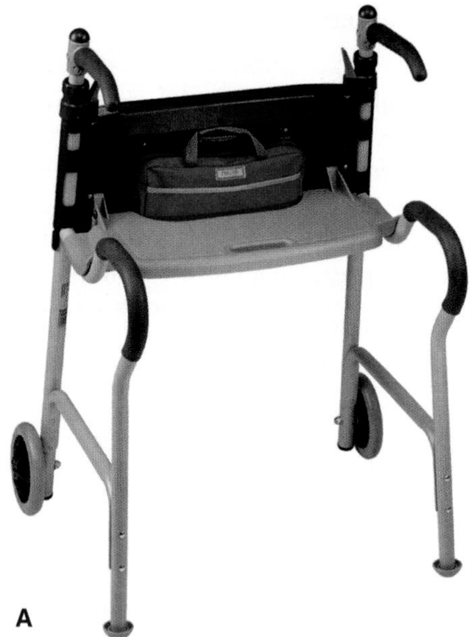

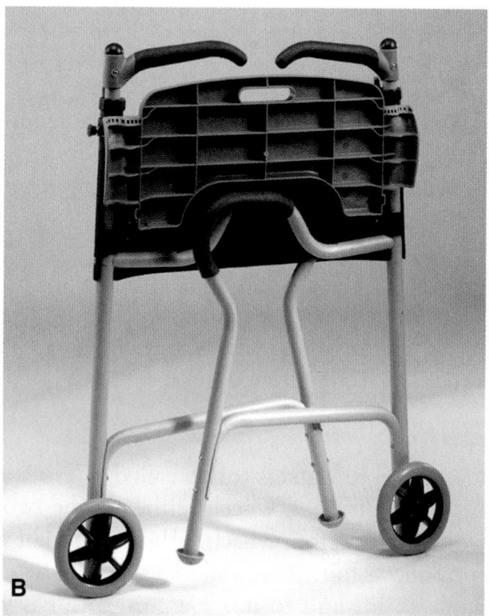

Figure 11A.17 Walker in (A) open and (B) folded position. The features on this walker include plastic posterior glides, a built-in seat with a molded back bar to support the user during rest intervals (the seat flips up for folding), large front wheels (6 in.) to improve ease of use on multiple terrains, a second set of handles set at approximately the seat level to assist sit-to-stand transitions in the absence of chair armrests or for movement on and off a toilet, and a removable walker pouch for storing personal items. Handle height adjusts using a collar and pin mechanism that eliminates having to turn the walker over to change the height. *(Courtesy of Full Life Products, LLC, Moorestown, NJ 08057.)*

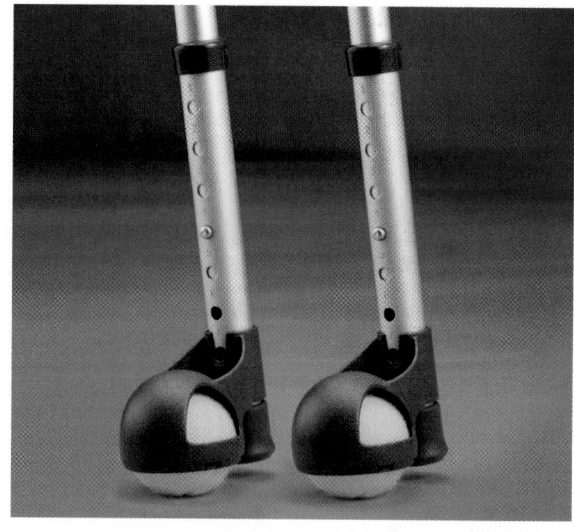

Figure 11A.18 The design of these walker glides incorporates a tennis ball within a fixed housing, a spring-loaded brake for intermittent braking during walking, and brake lock-out clips used to deactivate the braking feature for uninterrupted forward motion. The tennis ball can be manually rotated to unworn areas or completely removed to "snap in" a replacement. *(Courtesy of Invacare Corp, Elyria, OH 44036.)*

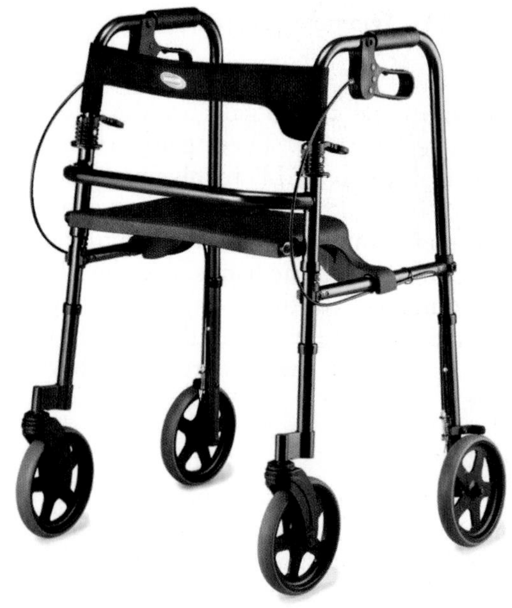

Figure 11A.19 The front wheels of this walker swivel freely in all directions. The back wheels rotate around a single axis. Handbrakes allow locking the rear wheels. A seat surface accommodates rest intervals. *(Courtesy of Invacare Corp, Elyria, OH 44036.)*

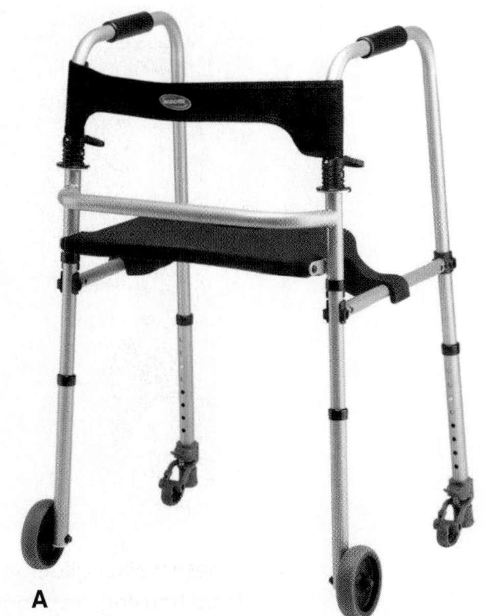

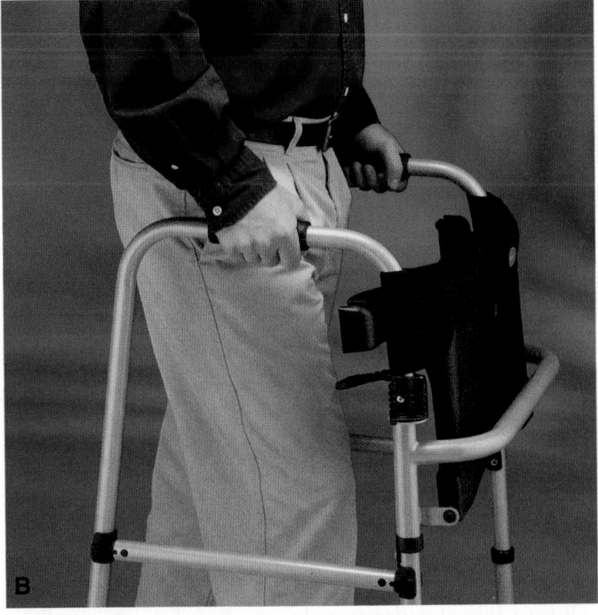

Figure 11A.20 Walker seat (A) positioned for use and (B) flipped up for ambulation. The 5-in. fixed front wheels of this walker rotate around a single axis. Features of this walker include rear spring-loaded brakes, a flexible backrest for sitting, a dual-paddle folding mechanism, and adjustable seat-to-floor height. *(Courtesy of Invacare Corp, Elyria, OH 44036.)*

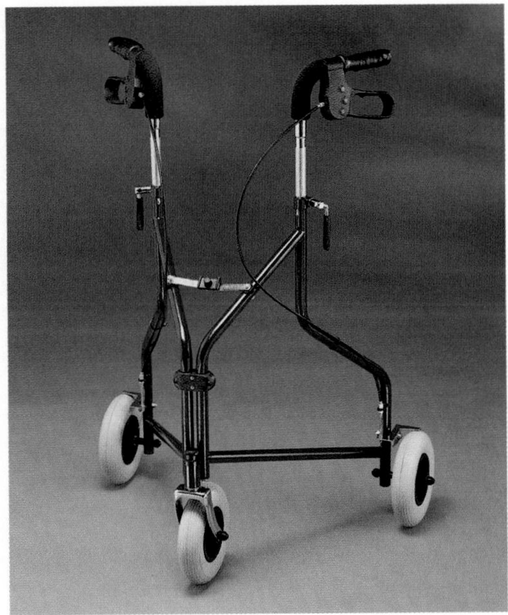

Figure 11A.21 Three-wheel walker with hand brakes and polyurethane tires to improve performance on a variety of terrains. *(Courtesy of Invacare Corp, Elyria, OH 44036.)*

Tripod Rolling Walkers

Three-wheel walkers incorporate a tripod design (Fig 11A.21); some manufacturers refer to these as *rollators.* A major advantage of this device is ease of maneuverability and turning. Height adjustments are made at the handles; the unit folds for storage and travel.

Storage Attachments

The ability to transport items is an important consideration for many patients and is often essential for those needing frequent access to medications, a cordless or cellular phone, or remote-control device. A variety of sizes and styles of attachable baskets and pouches are available (Fig. 11A.22). These storage attachments should be used judiciously and only for essential items. Overuse of the attachment creates an excessive anterior load that may pose a safety hazard and/or alter the patient's gait or ability to effectively use the walker.

Seating Surface

A variety of walker seat designs are available that fold out of the way when not in use. The structural design of many walkers also includes a contoured back support (see Figs. 11A.19 and Fig 11A.20A). Seats are an important consideration for individuals with limited endurance (e.g., postpolio syndrome), as well as for community ambulators who require periodic rest intervals. Walker seats should be carefully examined for stability and safety with respect to individual patient needs. Patient practice in use of the walker seat should be provided.

Reciprocal Walkers

These walkers are designed to allow unilateral forward progression of one side of the walker (Fig. 11A.23). A disadvantage of this design is that some inherent stability

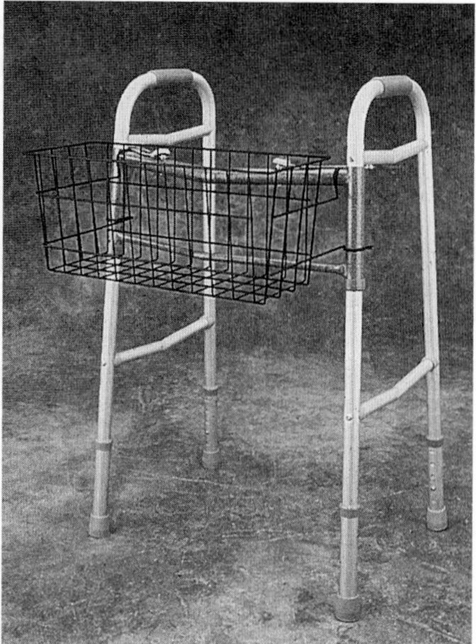

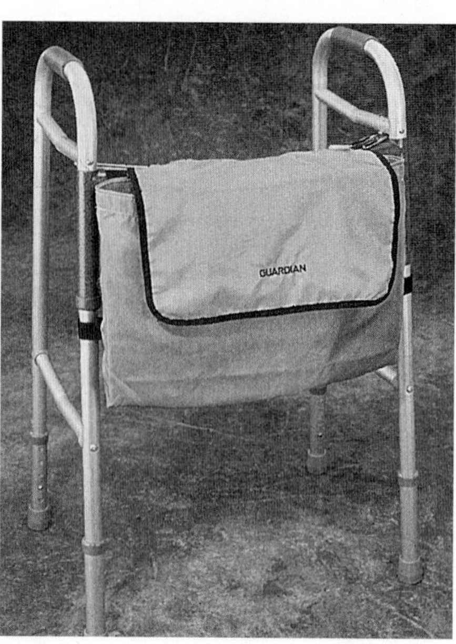

Figure 11A.22 Walker basket (left) and walker pouch (right). *(Courtesy of Sunrise Medical, Longmont, CO 80503.)*

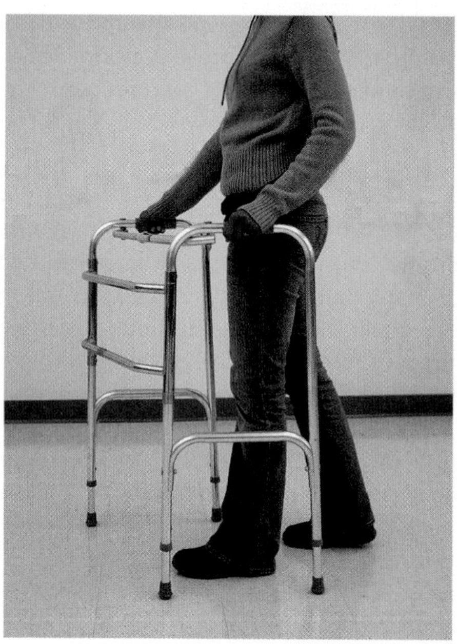

Figure 11A.23 Reciprocal walkers allow unilateral movement of one side of the walker while the opposite side remains stationary.

of the walker is lost. However, they are useful for patients incapable of lifting the walker with both hands and moving it forward (in situations in which a rolling walker might be contraindicated).

- *Advantages.* Conventional walkers provide four points of floor contact with a wide BOS. They provide a high level of stability. They also provide a sense of security for patients fearful of ambulation. They are relatively lightweight and easily adjusted.
- *Disadvantages.* Walkers tend to be cumbersome, are awkward in confined areas, and are difficult to maneuver through doorways and into cars. They eliminate normal arm swing and generally cannot be used safely on stairs.

Setting Walkers Height

The height of a walker is measured in the same way as that of a cane. The handgrip or handle of the walker should come to approximately the greater trochanter and allow for 20 to 30 degrees of elbow flexion.

Gait Patterns: Conventional Walkers

Before initiating instruction in gait patterns using a conventional walker (four points of floor contact without wheel attachments), several points related to the use of the walker should be emphasized with the patient:

- The walker should be picked up and placed down on all four legs simultaneously to achieve maximum stability. Rocking from the back to front legs should be avoided because it decreases the effectiveness and safety of using the assistive device.
- The patient should be encouraged to hold the head up and to maintain good postural alignment; forward flexion of the trunk, neck, and head should be avoided.
- The patient should be cautioned not to step too close to the front crossbar. This will decrease the overall BOS and may result in a fall.

Three types of weight-bearing gait patterns can be accomplished with conventional walkers: full weight-bearing (FWB), partial weight-bearing (PWB), and non-weight-bearing (NWB) gait (rolling devices are generally not recommended for patients with altered weight-bearing status). The sequence for each pattern with a walker follows.

Full Weight-Bearing

- The walker is picked up and moved forward about an arm's length.
- The first LE is moved forward.
- The second LE is moved forward past the first.
- The cycle is repeated.

Partial Weight-Bearing

- The walker is picked up and moved forward about an arm's length.
- The involved PWB limb is moved forward, and body weight is transferred partially onto this limb and partially through the UEs to the walker.
- The uninvolved LE is moved forward past the involved limb.
- The cycle is repeated.

Non–Weight-Bearing

- The walker is picked up and moved forward about an arm's length.
- Weight is then transferred through the UEs to the walker. The involved NWB limb is held anterior to the patient's body but does not make contact with the floor.
- The uninvolved limb is moved forward.
- The cycle is repeated.

Note: Rolling walkers generally allow use of a reciprocal step through gait pattern of the lower extremities because the walker can be rolled forward while walking. As the need to lift the walker forward following each step is eliminated, a smoother forward progression can be achieved.

GAIT TRAINING USING ASSISTIVE DEVICES

Over-ground Indoors

Several important preparatory activities should precede gait training (GT) on level surfaces with the assistive device. These activities may be completed in the parallel bars for added security. However, if the width of the bars is not adjustable, the BOS of the assistive device may make movement within the bars difficult and unsafe. An alternative is to move the patient outside but next to the parallel bars (or oval bar) or near a treatment table or wall. These preparatory activities include the following:

- Instruction in assuming the standing and seated positions with use of the assistive device. These techniques are outlined in Box 11A.3 for each category of assistive device.
- Standing balance activities with the assistive device (similar to those using the parallel bars, described earlier).
- Instruction in use of assistive device (with selected gait pattern) for forward progression and turning.

Box 11A.3 Assuming Standing and Seated Positions With Assistive Devices

I. Cane

A. *Coming to standing*

- Patient moves forward in chair.
- Cane is positioned on uninvolved side (broad-based cane) or leaned against armrest (standard cane).
- Patient leans forward and pushes down with both hands on armrests, comes to a standing position, and then grasps cane. With use of a standard cane, the cane may be grasped loosely with fingers before standing and the base of the hand is used for pushing down on armrests.

B. *Return to sitting*

- As the patient approaches the chair, the patient turns in a small circle toward the uninvolved side.
- The patient backs up until the chair can be felt against the legs.
- The patient then reaches for the armrest with the free hand, releases the cane (broad-based), and reaches for the opposite armrest. A standard cane is leaned against the chair as the patient grasps the armrest.

II. Crutches

A. *Coming to standing*

- The patient moves forward in the chair.
- Crutches are placed together in a vertical position on the affected side.
- One hand is placed on the hand pieces of the crutches; one on the armrest of the chair.
- The patient leans forward and pushes to a standing position.
- Once balance is gained, one crutch is cautiously placed under the axilla on the unaffected side.
- The second crutch is then carefully placed under the axilla on the affected side.
- A tripod stance is assumed.

B. *Return to sitting*

- As the patient approaches the chair, the patient turns in a small circle toward the uninvolved side.
- The patient backs up until the chair can be felt against the legs.

Continued

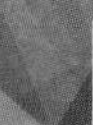

Box 11A.3 Assuming Standing and Seated Positions With Assistive Devices—cont'd

- Both crutches are placed in a vertical position (out from under axilla) on the *affected* side.
- One hand is placed on the hand pieces of the crutches, one on the armrest of the chair.
- The patient lowers to the chair in a controlled manner.

III. Walker

A. *Coming to standing*

- The patient moves forward in the chair.
- The walker is positioned directly in front of the chair.
- The patient leans forward and pushes down on armrests to come to standing.
- Once in a standing position, the patient reaches for the walker, one hand at a time.

B. *Return to sitting*

- As the patient approaches the chair, the patient turns in a small circle toward the stronger side.
- The patient backs up until the chair can be felt against the legs.
- The patient then reaches for one armrest at a time.
- The patient lowers to the chair in a controlled manner.

As mentioned, demonstrating these activities by assuming the role of the patient during verbal explanations is an effective teaching approach. Following the demonstration, manual contacts, verbal cueing, and explanations can be used again to guide performance of the activity. Following these preliminary instructions, gait training using the assistive device can be begun overground on level surfaces. The following guarding technique (Fig. 11A.24) should be used:

- The therapist stands posterior and lateral to the patient's weaker side.
- A wide BOS should be maintained with the therapist's leading LE following the assistive device. The

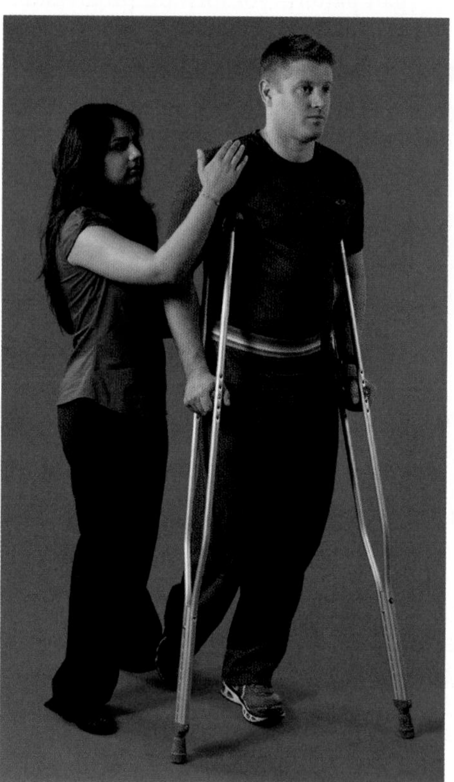

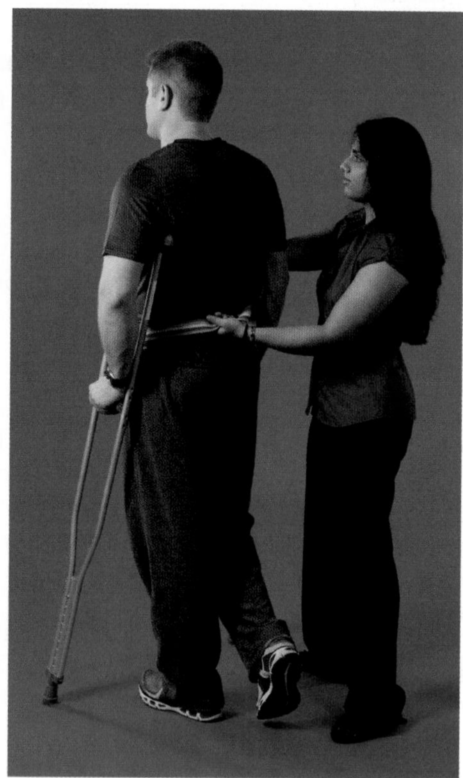

Figure 11A.24 Anterior (left) and posterior (right) views of guarding technique for level surfaces, demonstrated with use of crutches. The same positioning is used with canes and walkers.

therapist's opposite LE should be externally rotated and follow the patient's weaker LE.

- One of the therapist's hands is placed posteriorly on the guarding belt and the other anterior to, but *not touching,* the patient's shoulder on the weaker side.

Should the patient's balance be lost during training, the hand guarding at the shoulder should make contact. Frequently, the support provided by the therapist's hands at the shoulder and on the guarding belt would be enough to allow the patient to regain balance. If the balance loss is severe, the therapist should move in toward the patient so that the therapist's body and guarding hands can provide stabilization. The patient should be allowed to regain balance while "leaning" against the therapist. If balance is not recovered and it is apparent the patient must be moved to the floor, further attempts should not be made to hold the patient up because this is likely to result in injury to the patient and/or the therapist. In this situation, the therapist should continue to brace the patient against his or her body to break the fall and to protect the head and move with the patient to a sitting position on the floor. It is also important to talk to the patient (*"Help me lower you to the floor"*) so that the patient does not continue to struggle to regain balance.

Overground indoor activities on level surfaces should include instruction and practice in passage through doorways, into and out of elevators, and over thresholds. When using crutches, doorways are most easily approached from a diagonal. A hand must be freed to open the door and one crutch must be placed in a position to hold it open. The patient then gradually proceeds through the doorway, using the crutch to open the door wider if necessary.

Because many patients using a walker or cane may have balance problems, careful examination will determine the safest methods for passage through doorways. A patient using a conventional walker with sufficient balance may be able to use a technique similar to that described above.

Stair Climbing

Several general guidelines should be relayed to the patient during instruction in stair climbing. First, if a railing is available, it should always be used. This is true even if it requires placing an assistive device in the hand in which it is not normally used. For stair climbing with axillary crutches using a railing, both crutches are placed together under one arm. Second, the patient should be cautioned that the stronger LE always leads going up the stairs, and the weaker or involved limb always leads coming down (*"up with the good and down with the bad"*).

Stair-climbing techniques are presented in Box 11A.4. The therapist should use the following guarding technique during stair climbing.

Box 11A.4 Stair-Climbing Techniques*

I. Cane

A. *Ascending*

- The unaffected lower extremity leads up.
- The cane and affected lower extremity follow.

B. *Descending*

- The affected lower extremity and cane lead down.
- The unaffected lower extremity follows.

II. Crutches: Three-Point Gait (non–weight-bearing gait)

A. *Ascending*

- The patient is positioned close to the foot of the stairs. The involved lower extremity is held back to prevent "catching" on the lip of the stairs.
- The patient pushes down firmly on both hand pieces of the crutches and leads up with the unaffected lower extremity.
- The crutches are brought up to the stair that the unaffected lower extremity is now on.

B. *Descending*

- The patient stands close to the edge of the stair so that the toes of the unaffected lower extremity protrude slightly over the top. The involved lower extremity is held forward over the lower stair.
- Both crutches are moved down *together* to the *front* half of the next step.
- The patient pushes down firmly on both hand pieces and lowers the unaffected lower extremity to the step that the crutches are now on.

Continued

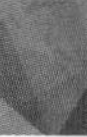

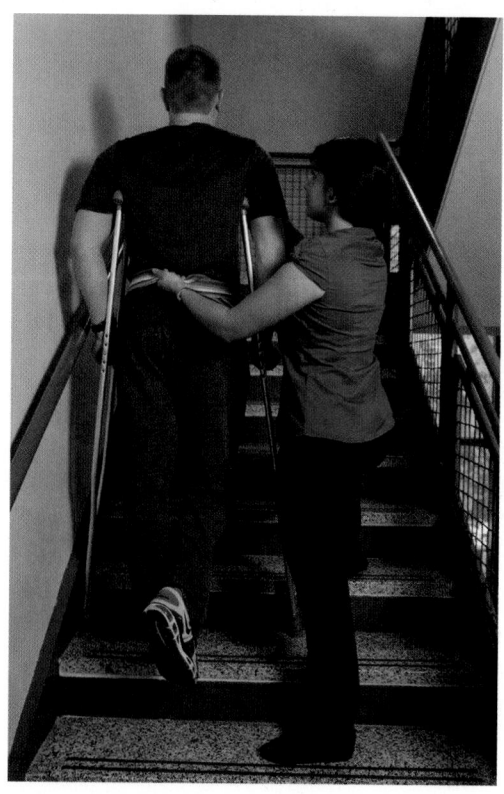

Box 11A.4 Stair-Climbing Techniques—cont'd

III. Crutches: Partial Weight-Bearing Gait

A. *Ascending*

- The patient is positioned close to the foot of the stairs.
- The patient pushes down on both hand pieces of the crutches and distributes weight partially on the crutches and partially on the affected lower extremity while the unaffected lower extremity leads up.
- The involved lower extremity and crutches are then brought up together.

B. *Descending*

- The patient stands close to the edge of the stair so that the toes protrude slightly over top of the stair.
- Both crutches are moved down *together* to the *front* half of the next step. The affected lower extremity is then lowered (depending on patient skill, these may be combined). *Note:* When crutches are not in floor contact, greater weight must be shifted to the uninvolved lower extremity to maintain a partial weight-bearing status.
- The uninvolved lower extremity is lowered to the step the crutches are now on.

IV. Crutches: Two- and Four-Point Gait

A. *Ascending*

- The patient is positioned close to the foot of the stairs.
- The right lower extremity is moved up and then the left lower extremity.
- The right crutch is moved up and then the left crutch is moved up (patients with adequate balance may find it easier to move the crutches up together).

B. *Descending*

- The patient stands close to the edge of the stair.
- Both crutches are moved down together. Alternatively, the right crutch is moved down and then the left. This pattern must be used with caution, as crutch placement on two different steps can introduce excessive and unwanted trunk rotation.
- The right lower extremity is moved down and then the left.

*The sequences presented here describe stair-climbing techniques without the use of a railing. When a secure railing is available, the patient should be instructed to use it always.

Ascending Stairs (Fig. 11A.25)

- The therapist is positioned posterior and lateral on the affected side behind the patient.
- A wide BOS should be maintained with each foot on a different stair.
- A step should be taken only when the patient is not moving.
- One hand is placed posteriorly on the guarding belt and one is anterior to, but not touching, the shoulder on the weaker side.

Descending Stairs (Fig. 11A.26)

- The therapist is positioned anterior and lateral on the affected side in front of the patient.
- A wide BOS should be maintained with each foot on a different stair.
- A step should be taken only when the patient is not moving.
- One hand is placed anteriorly on the guarding belt and one is anterior to, but not touching, the shoulder on the weaker side.

Should the patient's balance be lost during stair climbing, follow this procedure: First, contact should be made with the hand guarding at the shoulder. Next, the therapist should move toward the patient to help brace

Figure 11A.25 Guarding technique for ascending stairs.

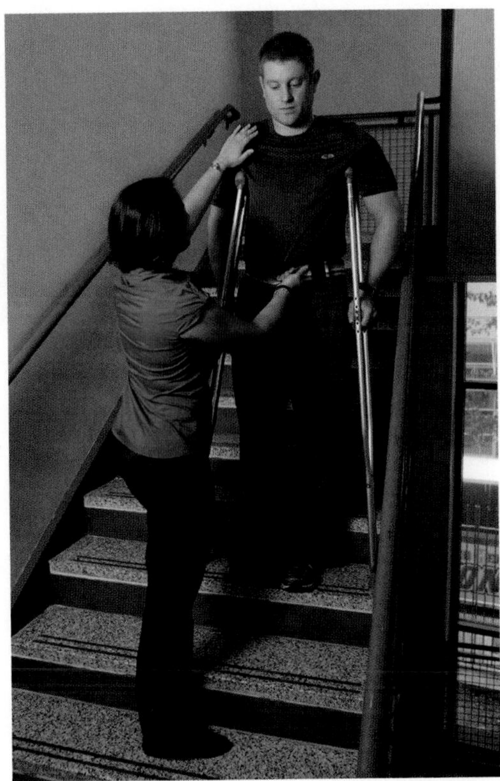

Figure 11A.26 Guarding technique for descending stairs.

him or her (the patient should never be pulled toward the therapist on stairs) or leaned toward the wall of the stairwell (if available). Finally, if needed, the therapist can move with the patient to sit the patient down on the stairs. Remember to inform the patient of your intentions (*"I'm going to sit you down"*).

Gait training using assistive devices should also include outdoor training and practice with curb climbing and negotiating ramps and sloped surfaces; even and uneven terrains; walking with imposed time requirements (e.g., crossing street at a stoplight); walking for long distances, dual-task training while walking, walking at various speeds, and negotiating open community environments with distractors, as well as outside doors and thresholds; and transportation vehicles.

Adjunct Training Devices

Limb Load Monitors

A limb load monitor is a form of biofeedback used clinically as an adjunct intervention during gait training. The limb load monitor incorporates a strain gauge attached to the sole or heel of the shoe. When a force or pressure is applied, the strain gauge is deformed and an auditory signal provides feedback to the wearer. As pressure increases, the signal becomes louder or more rapid. This feedback provides information about the amount of weight-bearing on a limb. Limb load monitors can also be used to reinforce the correctness or timing of a movement. For example, an audible noise or buzzer sounding when the heel makes contact with the floor can provide immediate feedback on foot placement. Similar devices can also be attached to a cane (often referred to as a *biofeedback cane*). The principle of operation is the same and incorporates a strain gauge. Auditory signals provide the patient with information on placement, as well as pressure applied to the cane.

Appendix 11A References

1. Bohannon, RW: Use of a standard cane increases unipedal stance time during static testing. Percept Mot Skills 112(3):726–728, 2011.
2. Hsue, BJ, and Su, FC: The effect of cane use method on center of mass displacement during stair ascent. Gait Posture 32(4): 530–535, 2010.
3. Milczarek, JJ, et al: Standard and four-footed canes: Their effect on the standing balance of patients with hemiparesis. Arch Phys Med Rehabil 74(3):281–285, 1993.
4. Maguire, C, et al: Hip abductor control in walking following stroke—the immediate effect of canes, taping and TheraTogs on gait. Clin Rehabil 24(1):37–45, 2010.
5. Laufer, Y: Effects of one-point and four-point canes on balance and weight distribution in patients with hemiparesis. Clin Rehabil 16(2):141–148, 2002.
6. Laufer, Y. The effect of walking aids on balance and weight-bearing patterns of patients with hemiparesis in various stance positions. Phys Ther 83(2):112—122, 2003.
7. Jones, A, et al: Impact of cane use on pain, function, general health and energy expenditure during gait in patients with knee osteoarthritis: a randomised controlled trial. Ann Rheum Dis 71(2):172–179, 2012.
8. Neumann, DA: Hip abductor muscle activity as subjects with hip prostheses walk with different methods of using a cane. Phys Ther 78(5):490–501, 1998.
9. Neumann, DA: An electromyographic study of the hip abductor muscles as subjects with a hip prosthesis walked with different methods of using a cane and carrying a load. Phys Ther 79(12):1163-1173; discussion 1174–1166, 1999.
10. Buurke, JH, et al: The effect of walking aids on muscle activation patterns during walking in stroke patients. Gait Posture 22(2): 164–170, 2005.
11. Ely, DD, and Smidt, GL: Effect of cane on variables of gait for patients with hip disorders. Phys Ther 57(5):507–512, 1977.
12. Jones, A, et al: Evaluation of immediate impact of cane use on energy expenditure during gait in patients with knee osteoarthritis. Gait Posture 35(3):435–439, 2012.
13. Donovan, S, et al: Laserlight cues for gait freezing in Parkinson's disease: An open-label study. Parkinsonism Relat Disord 17(4): 240–245, 2011.

Chapter 12 Chronic Pulmonary Dysfunction

Julie Ann Starr, PT, DPT, CCS

LEARNING OBJECTIVES

1. Define the disease processes (including definition, etiology, pathophysiology, clinical presentation, and clinical course) of chronic obstructive pulmonary disease, asthma, cystic fibrosis, and restrictive lung disease.
2. Describe examination procedures (including patient interview, vital signs, observation, inspection, palpation, auscultation, and laboratory tests) for a patient with pulmonary disease.
3. Identify the anticipated goals and expected outcomes of pulmonary rehabilitation.
4. Describe the rehabilitative management of a patient with chronic pulmonary dysfunction.
5. Value the therapist's role in the management of a patient with chronic pulmonary dysfunction.
6. Analyze and interpret patient data, formulate realistic goals and outcomes, and develop a plan of care when presented with a clinical case study.

CHAPTER OUTLINE

Years ago, patients with chronic pulmonary disease were given a standard prescription for rest and avoidance of exercise.[1] The stress imposed by exercise was considered deleterious to people with pulmonary disorders. A pivotal study by Pierce et al[2] provided the impetus to change direction in the treatment of pulmonary dysfunction. Exercise training effects of decreased heart rate (HR), respiratory rate (RR), minute ventilation, oxygen consumption, and carbon dioxide production at submaximal exercise levels were documented in their subjects with chronic obstructive pulmonary disease (COPD). Increased maximal aerobic capacity was also documented.[2] Reconditioning of patients with pulmonary disease was found to be possible. Pulmonary rehabilitation has emerged since that time as a multidisciplinary comprehensive program of care for patients with chronic pulmonary disease to optimize physical functioning and social participation, minimize disease symptoms, and reduce health care costs.[3]

COPD, asthma, and cystic fibrosis (CF) are the most common chronic obstructive lung diseases for which pulmonary rehabilitation is rendered. Patients with chronic restrictive lung diseases have also demonstrated improvement in functional abilities following pulmonary rehabilitation.[4] It is clear that pulmonary rehabilitation is of value for all patients in whom respiratory symptoms have resulted in a decreased functional capacity or a decreased quality of life.[3]

In this chapter, the most common chronic pulmonary diseases that present to pulmonary rehabilitation programs will be discussed, as well as the physical therapy examination and treatment of patients with chronic pulmonary disease. A brief review of ventilation and respiration is warranted for a better understanding of the disease pathologies and for understanding the rationale of the physical therapy procedures.

RESPIRATORY PHYSIOLOGY

Air is inspired through the nose or mouth, through all of the conducting airways until it reaches the distal respiratory unit, which contains the respiratory bronchiole, alveolar ducts, alveolar sacs, and alveoli (Fig. 12.1). The movement of air through the conducting airways is termed *ventilation.* At full inspiration, the lungs contain their maximum amount of air. This volume of air is called *total lung capacity* (TLC), which can be divided into four separate volumes of air: (1) tidal volume, (2) inspiratory reserve volume, (3) expiratory reserve volume, and (4) residual volume. Combinations of two or more of these lung volumes are termed *capacities.* Figure 12.2 illustrates the relationship of lung volumes and capacities.

The amount of air inspired or expired during normal resting ventilation is termed *tidal volume* (TV or V_t). As this tidal volume of air enters the pulmonary system, it travels through the conducting airways to reach the respiratory units. Tidal volume is about 500 mL/breath for a young, healthy, white male. The amount of inspired air that actually reaches the distal respiratory unit and takes part in gas exchange is about 350 mL of that 500 mL total of the tidal breath. The remaining 150 mL of the inhaled tidal breath remains in the conducting airways and does not take part in gas exchange. When only a tidal breath occupies the lungs, there is "room" for

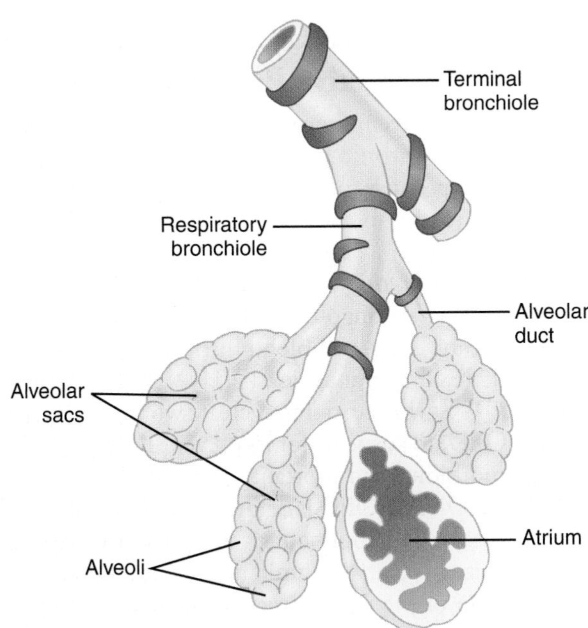

Figure 12.1 Anatomy of the distal conducting airway, the terminal bronchiole and the respiratory unit, the respiratory bronchiole, alveolar ducts, alveolar sacs, and alveoli.

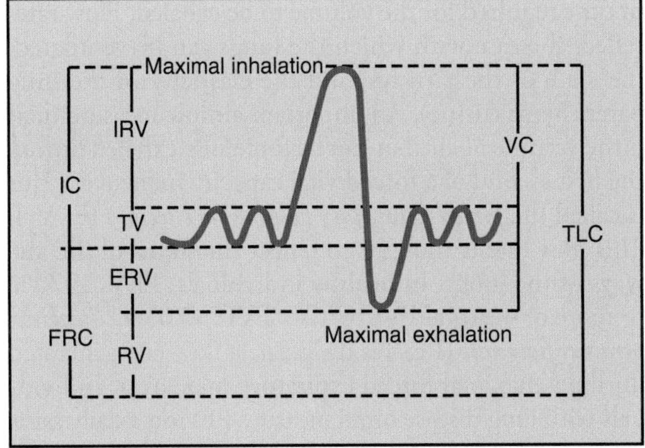

Figure 12.2 Lung volumes and capacities. ERV = expiratory reserve volume; FRC = functional residual capacity; IC = inspiratory capacity; IRV = inspiratory reserve volume; RV = residual volume; TLC = total lung capacity; TV = tidal volume; VC = vital capacity.

additional air that can be further inhaled. This inspiratory volume in excess of that used in tidal breathing is the inspiratory reserve volume (IRV). Aptly named, it is the volume of air that can be inspired when needed but is usually kept in reserve. There is a quantity of air that can potentially be exhaled beyond the end of a tidal exhalation. Although it is usually kept in reserve, the volume of air that can be exhaled in excess of tidal breathing is called the *expiratory reserve volume* (ERV). The lungs are never completely emptied of air even after maximally exhaling the expiratory reserve volume. The volume of air remaining within the lungs when ERV has been exhaled is called the residual volume (RV).

The sum of two or more volumes is referred to as a *capacity.* Tidal volume plus the inspiratory reserve volume is known as the *inspiratory capacity.* This refers to the volume of air that can be inspired beginning from a tidal exhalation. The combination of residual volume and expiratory reserve volume is the functional residual capacity (FRC). Functional residual capacity is the volume of air that remains in the lungs at the end of a tidal exhalation. The sum of inspiratory reserve volume, tidal volume, and expiratory reserve volume is called the *vital capacity* (VC). It is all of the possible volume of air within the lungs that is under volitional control. The common method of measuring VC is to achieve maximal inspiration, then forcibly exhale as hard and fast as possible into a measuring device until ERV has been exhausted. Because this is a forced expiratory maneuver, it is termed the *forced vital capacity* (FVC). As stated earlier, all volumes together equal total lung capacity: TV + IRV + ERV + RV = TLC.

Flow rates measure the volume of air moved in a period of time. Expiratory flow rates, therefore, are measurements of exhaled gas volume divided by the amount of time required for the volume to be exhaled. Flow rates reflect the ease with which the lungs can be ventilated, the state of the airways, and the elasticity of the lung parenchyma (tissue). An important airflow measurement is the volume of air that can be forcefully exhaled during the first second of a forced vital capacity maneuver. This is called the *forced expiratory volume in 1 second* (FEV_1). This flow rate is thought to reflect the status of the airways of the lungs. In healthy individuals, FEV_1 is 70% or more of the total FVC ($FEV_1/FVC > 70\%$).[5] *Peak expiratory flow rate* (PEF) is the greatest flow rate generated during a maximal forced expiratory maneuver. Individuals with lung disease often measure PEF on a daily basis with a handheld peak flow meter to track their pulmonary status. Daily peak flow rates are compared to the patient's own "best" test value.[6] A drop in a patient's peak flow rate indicates airway narrowing and may indicate the need for a physician visit and/or change in medication regimen.

Inspiratory mechanics can also be helpful in understanding a patient's pulmonary disease. *Maximum inspiratory pressure* (PI_{max}) reflects the greatest static inspiratory effort that can be generated from residual volume. It is measured as a pressure in millimeters of mercury or centimeters of water and reflects the strength of the muscles of inspiration. The maximal pressure is defined as the highest negative pressure that the patient can sustain for 1 second during the testing procedure.[7]

Lung volumes, capacities, flow rates, and mechanics depend on the size and configuration of the thorax. Therefore, height, gender, and race influence static and dynamic lung measurements. Any alteration in the properties of the lungs or chest wall due to the aging process or a disease process will also change the lung volumes, capacities, flow rates, and/or mechanics.

Respiration is a term used to describe the gas exchange within the body. This should not be confused with *ventilation,* which describes only the movement of air. External respiration is the exchange of gas that occurs at the alveolar capillary membrane between atmospheric air and the pulmonary capillaries. Internal respiration takes place at the tissue capillary level between the tissues and the surrounding capillaries. The following discussion traces the course of gas exchange, specifically that of oxygen and carbon dioxide, during both external and internal respiration (Fig. 12.3).

For external respiration to take place, there must first be an inhalation of air from the environment through the conducting airways and into the respiratory bronchioles and alveoli. Oxygen diffuses through the walls of the respiratory unit, through the interstitial space, and through the pulmonary capillary wall. Most of the oxygen (98.5%) then travels through the blood plasma into red blood cells where it occupies one of the gas-carrying sites of hemoglobin. A small portion of dissolved oxygen (1.5%) is carried in the plasma.

The now-oxygenated blood in the pulmonary capillaries travels to the left side of the heart via the pulmonary veins. From there it is pumped into the aorta, then through a network of connecting arteries, arterioles, and capillaries, until its destination, the tissue, is reached. Internal respiration begins when the arterial blood reaches the tissue level. Oxygen diffuses from the gas-carrying sites of hemoglobin, out of the red blood cell, out of the capillary, through the cell membranes, and into the mitochondria of the working cells.

Carbon dioxide (CO_2), which is produced at the tissue level as a by-product of metabolism, diffuses out of the working cells into the blood in the capillaries. Carbon dioxide is then transported to the venous system and into the right side of the heart. Once the carbon dioxide–laden blood makes its way through the right atrium, the right ventricle, the pulmonary artery, and the pulmonary capillaries, it diffuses out through the capillary membrane, through the interstitial space, and into the alveoli, where, during external respiration, it is finally exhaled into the atmosphere.

When the cycle of external and internal respiration has occurred, oxygen has been extracted from the environment and provided to the body tissues. Meanwhile, carbon dioxide has been removed from the body tissues and released into the external environment. Of course, this system is dependent on an intact cardiovascular system to pump the blood through the lungs and deliver it to the working cells, and then return it back from the working cells to the lungs, all in a timely fashion.

CHRONIC LUNG DISEASES

Chronic Obstructive Pulmonary Disease

Chronic obstructive pulmonary disease (COPD) is the most common chronic pulmonary disorder. It is the fourth-leading cause of mortality in the world.[5] It is projected to rise to the third highest cause of death by 2020.[5]

The *Global Initiative for Chronic Obstructive Lung Disease (GOLD)* is an ongoing collaborative work of the National Heart, Lung, and Blood Institute (NHLBI) and the World Health Organization (WHO). In its initial report of 2001, GOLD set out to increase worldwide awareness of COPD, to advocate for its prevention as well as to decrease morbidity and mortality from the disease. According to GOLD, COPD is defined as a preventable and treatable disease. The pulmonary component of COPD is characterized by airflow limitation caused by chronic inflammation of the small airways and air spaces in response to significant exposure to noxious particles or gases. Mucociliary dysfunction is also a characteristic of the disease. COPD is usually progressive. Additional significant extra pulmonary effects, such as a decrease in body mass index (BMI), decreased muscle strength, and exercise intolerance, contribute to the symptomology of COPD

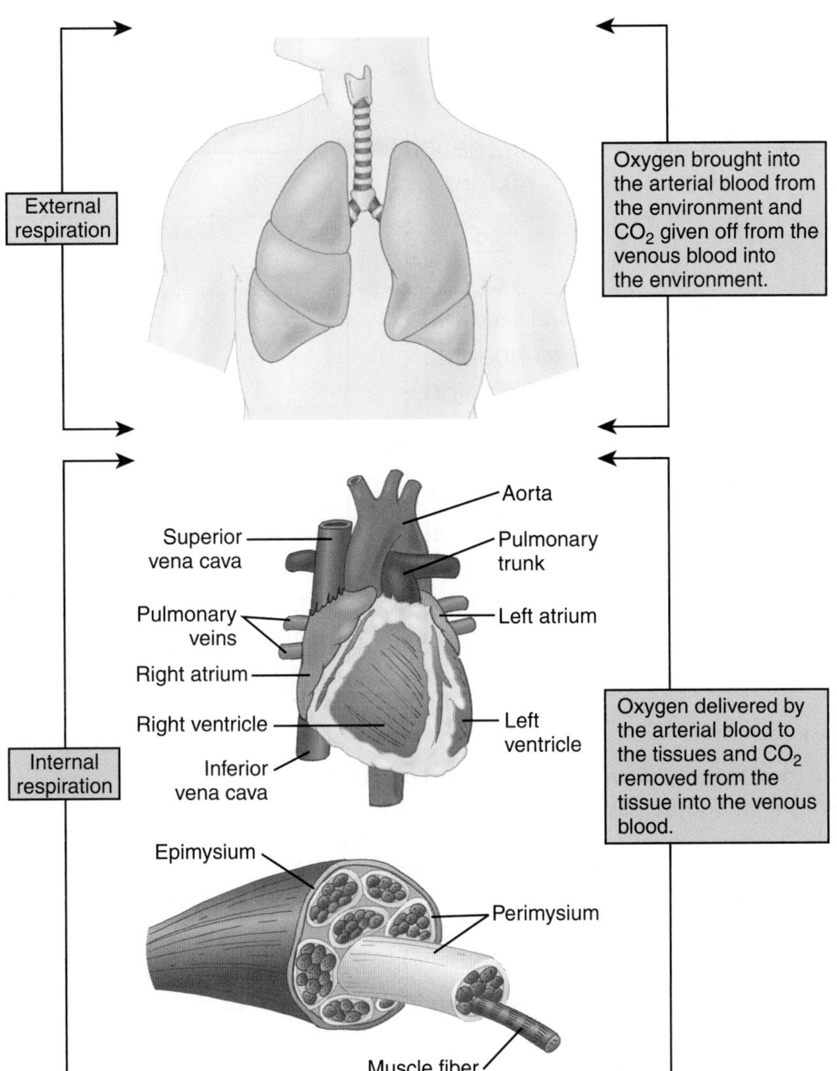

Figure 12.3 The process of external and internal respiration.

in individual patients.[5] Figure12.4 shows the ABCD assessment tool to classify disease severity based on a measurement of a patient's altered pulmonary function tests, presenting symptoms and history of exacerbations. Refer to the case study at the end of this chapter for use of this classification system.

Risk Factors

Risk factors for the development of COPD include both environmental factors and host factors. Cigarette smoking is the major environmental causal agent in the development of COPD.[5] Smoking history is quantified in units of *pack/years,* the number of packs per day times the number of years smoked. Other environmental factors that contribute to the development of COPD include occupational exposures (e.g., organic and inorganic dusts), indoor pollutants (e.g., secondhand smoke), and outdoor pollutants (e.g., urban pollution).[5]

Host factors that would make a person more susceptible to the development of COPD include hyperreactivity of the airways, overall lung growth (the amount of lung tissue developed during childhood, which is partially determined by nutritional status, health status, height, and exposure to pollutants), and genetics. It is perplexing that less than 50% of smokers go on to develop COPD in their lifetime.[8] There are a number of ongoing studies investigating the potential for a genetic influence in the development of COPD.[9]

Pathophysiology

COPD is characterized by pathological changes that can be found throughout the pulmonary system—in the airways, airspaces, and the pulmonary capillaries. Chronic inflammation, including an increase in neutrophils, macrophages, and T lymphocytes, damages the endothelial lining of the airways. Airway inflammation causes airway narrowing, which is worsened by an imbalance of proteases/antiproteases and oxidants/antioxidants in patients with COPD.[5] Disruption in the normal tissue repair process also leads to airway remodelling, and destruction

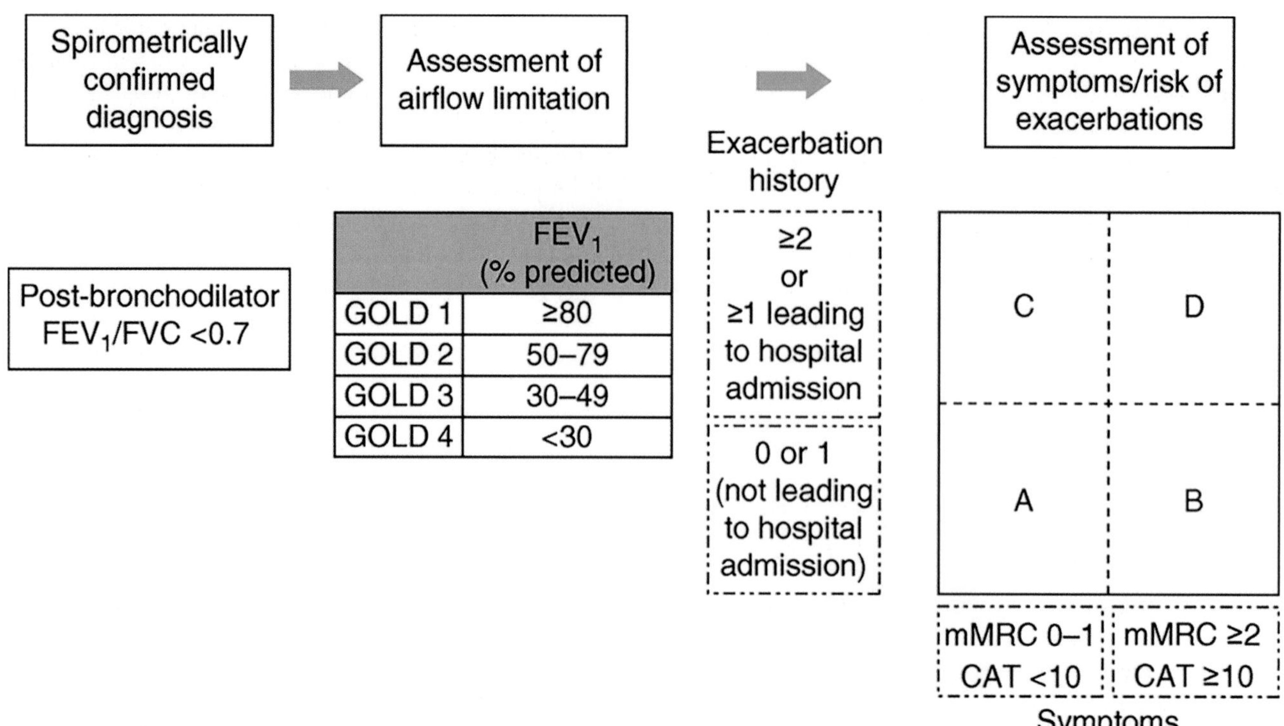

Figure 12.4 The ABCD assessment tool from the Global Initiative for Obstructive Lung Disease (GOLD). The results of spirometric assessment will categorize patients into a grade of 1 through 4. The results of the exacerbation history and the assessment of symptoms further categorizes patients into a group of A through D. *(Global Initiative for Obstructive Lung Disease [GOLD], with permission.)*

of fragile lung parenchyma. These airway changes appear to be most pronounced in the smaller peripheral airways (bronchioles).[5] These changes result in the loss of the normal elastic recoil properties of the lung tissue. Endothelial changes in the pulmonary vasculature are altered early in the development of COPD and result in thickening of the vessel walls. In advanced stages of the disease, there is destruction of the pulmonary capillary bed. In about 30% of cases of COPD (GOLD), mucus hypersecretion is present due to an increase in size of submucosal glands and the number of goblet cells within the bronchial walls. Decreases in ciliary function and alterations in physiochemical characteristics of bronchial secretions impair airway clearance and contribute to airway obstruction. Damaged and inflamed mucosa shows an increased sensitivity of irritant receptors within the bronchial walls, which in turn cause bronchial hyperreactivity.[5]

During normal inspiration, the lungs and the airways are pulled open, increasing the diameter of the airway lumen. During normal exhalation, as the thorax returns to its resting position, the airways decrease in size. In patients with COPD, during inspiration, the airways are pulled open by thoracic expansion, allowing air to enter. During exhalation, the airways, already narrowed by inflammation, remodeling, and in some cases excessive secretions, close prematurely, trapping air in the distal airways and airspaces. This air trapping causes hyperinflation, which is defined as an abnormal increase in the amount of air within the lung tissue at the end of a tidal exhalation (increased FRC).

Ventilation in the alveoli and *perfusion* in the capillary membrane are no longer well matched, resulting in *hypoxemia,* a condition of decreased amount of oxygen in the arterial blood to the tissues. As the disease progresses and more areas of the lungs become involved, hypoxemia will worsen and *hypercapnea,* a condition of increased amount of carbon dioxide within the arterial blood, will develop. Increased pulmonary vascular resistance secondary to capillary wall damage and reflex vasoconstriction in the presence of hypoxemia results in pulmonary hypertension and right ventricular hypertrophy, termed *cor pulmonale.*[10] *Polycythemia,* an increase in the number of circulating red blood cells, occurs in order to potentially increase the oxygen carrying capacity of the blood.

Clinical Presentation

Patients with COPD will usually present with a history of cigarette smoking. The most characteristic symptom of COPD is dyspnea. Dyspnea may be first evidenced during exertion. As the disease progresses, dyspnea worsens so that it occurs at progressively lower levels of activity. Severely involved patients may feel dyspneic even at rest. In a portion of patients with COPD, there is also a slow and insidious development of chronic cough and expectoration. On physical examination, the thorax appears enlarged owing to hyperinflation and the loss of lung elastic recoil properties. The anterior-posterior diameter of the chest increases and a dorsal kyphosis results. These anatomical changes give the patient a barrel-chest appearance (Fig. 12.5).

As the resting position of the thorax is now held in a more inspiratory mode, the available range of thoracic motion is limited—that is, there is decreased thoracic excursion. There are morphological changes to the ventilatory muscles due to a greater demand, both in frequency of contraction and in the power needed to move this altered thorax. The muscles of ventilation hypertrophy as a result. Figure 12.6 shows many of the accessory muscles of ventilation that may be recruited for breathing. In severe disease, these muscles are recruited even at rest to aid in the work of breathing. The length–tension relationship of muscles of ventilation is altered as the thorax increases in size with chronic hyperinflation. There are also changes in the alignment of muscle fibers, especially the fibers of the diaphragm. With hyperinflation, the diaphragm cannot return to its domed shape on exhalation. In severe disease, the diaphragm fiber alignment may become more horizontal than vertical (i.e., flatter, potentially resulting in an inward motion of the lower ribs during a diaphragm muscle contraction of inhalation) (Fig. 12.7).

Auscultation of the chest may demonstrate decreased intensity of both breath sounds and heart sounds. Partially obstructed bronchi and bronchioles may result in an expiratory *wheeze,* described as a musical, whistling sound. *Crackles* are an intermittent bubbling or popping sound that may also be present from secretions in the airways. Pursed-lip breathing, cyanosis, and digital clubbing may all be present in the advanced stages of COPD. (See "Examination" in the "Physical Therapy Management" section for clarification of terms.)

Significant and progressive airway limitation is reflected in altered pulmonary function tests. Lung volumes and capacities, especially RV and FRC, are increased from normal values due to air trapping. Figure 12.8 shows the changes in lung volumes and capacities that typically occur in obstructive pulmonary disease.

Expiratory flow rates, especially FEV_1, are decreased. The ratio of FEV_1 to FVC is decreased to less than 70%.[5] These changes in pulmonary function do not show a major reversibility in response to pharmacological agents.

Arterial blood gas analyses may reflect hypoxemia in the early stages of COPD and hypercapnea a bit later as the disease progresses. With disease progression, chest radiographs show several characteristic findings, including flattened, less domed, hemidiaphragms, alterations in pulmonary vascular markings, hyperinflation of the thorax, hyperlucency reflecting a decreased tissue density, elongation of the heart, and right ventricular hypertrophy.

The inflammatory reaction in the airways of patients with COPD can also affect other organ systems.[10] Therefore, COPD is not only a pulmonary disorder, but also

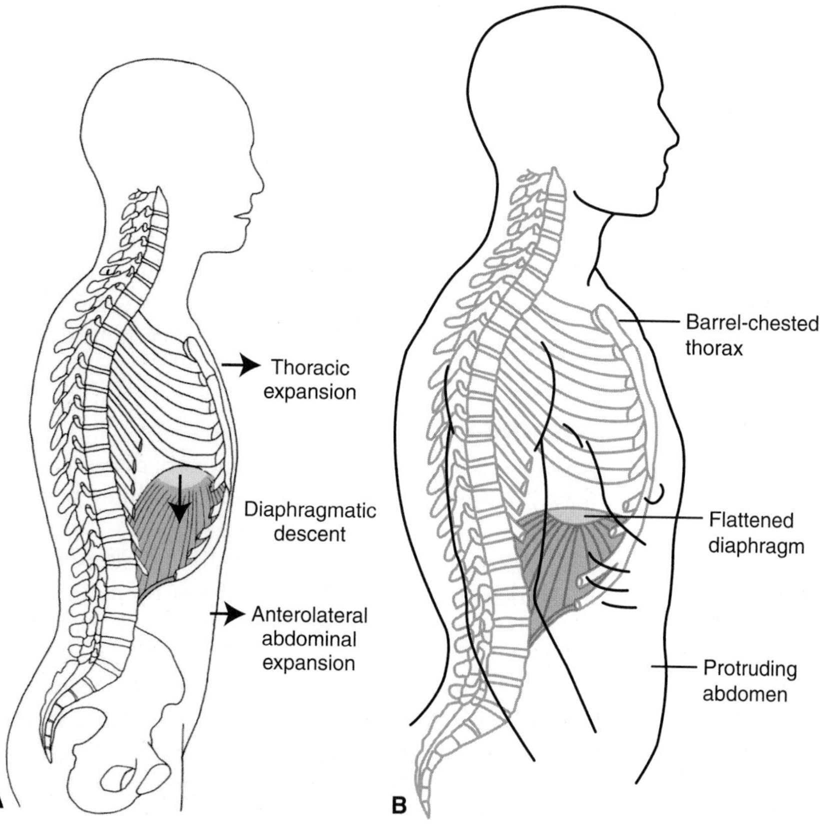

Figure 12.5 (A) normal thoracic configuration. (B) Changes in the configuration of the thorax with chronic obstructive pulmonary disease. *(Adapted from Levangie, P, and Norkin, C: Joint Structure and Function: A Comprehensive Analysis, ed 5. FA Davis, Philadelphia, 2011, p. 202, with permission.)*

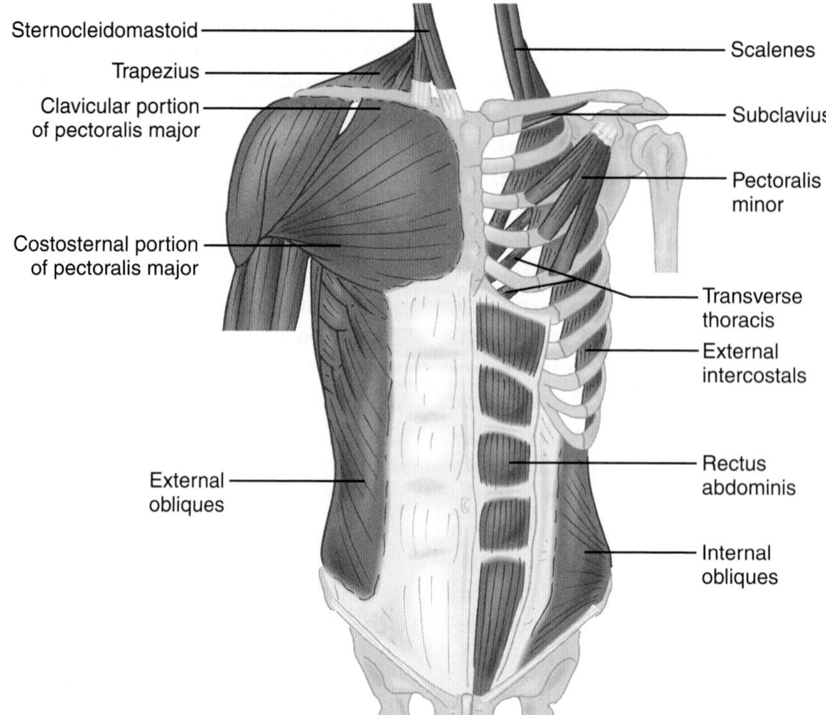

Figure 12.6 Accessory muscles of ventilation are those used during times of increased ventilatory demand. The right side of the figure shows some of the anterior superficial muscles of the thorax that can be accessory muscles of ventilation, and the left side of the thorax shows the deeper accessory muscles of ventilation.

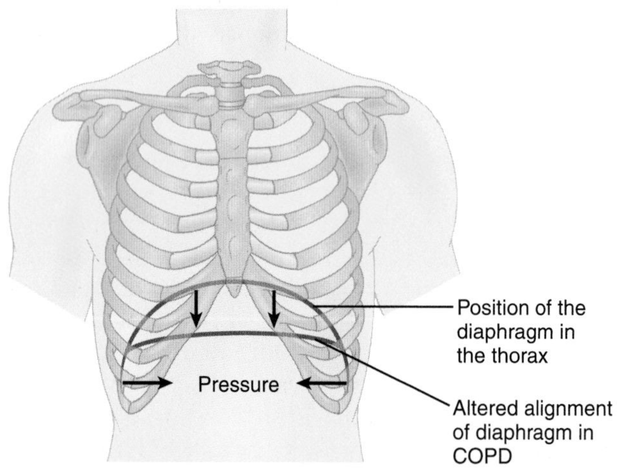

Figure 12.7 Alteration in alignment of fibers of the diaphragm due to hyperinflation. *(From Levangie, P, and Norkin, C: Joint Structure and Function, ed 5. FA Davis, Philadelphia, 2011, p. 202, with permission.)*

has extrapulmonary (i.e., systemic) effects, including changes to skeletal muscle mass and function, cardiovascular disease, osteoporosis, and depression.[11]

Course and Prognosis

The clinical course of COPD has an insidious onset with a disease progression that can develop over many years. Early identification of individuals at risk for the development of COPD has been elusive. Although smoking is the most prevalent risk factor for the development of disease, not all smokers develop clinically significant lung disease. Therefore, a smoking history in and of itself is not predictive for the development of COPD. The *BODE* index has been developed as a prognostic indicator for mortality risk in patients COPD. The index uses four domains to calculate mortality risk: body mass index (B), pulmonary obstruction (O), dyspnea (D), and exercise capacity (E).[12] This index can be found at http://reference.medscape.com/calculator/bode-index-copd. The higher the score on the BODE, the greater the mortality risk. Leading causes of death in patients with COPD are respiratory failure, lung cancer, and cardiovascular disease.

Asthma

Asthma is a common chronic pulmonary disease, affecting 17.7 million adults and 6.3 million children in the United States.[13] The *Global Initiative for Asthma* (GINA) is a collaborative work of the NHLBI and WHO. Since its launch in 1993, GINA's goal has been to reduce asthma prevalence, morbidity, and mortality. According to GINA, asthma is a disease of variable expiratory airflow limitation with symptoms of wheezing, shortness of breath, chest tightness and cough.[14] The disease is characterized by chronic airway inflammation associated with airway hyperresponsiveness (bronchospasm) to direct or indirect stimuli. Asthma exacerbations may improve

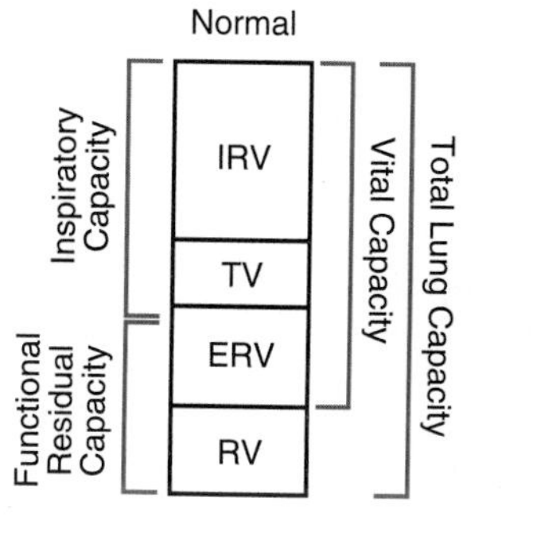

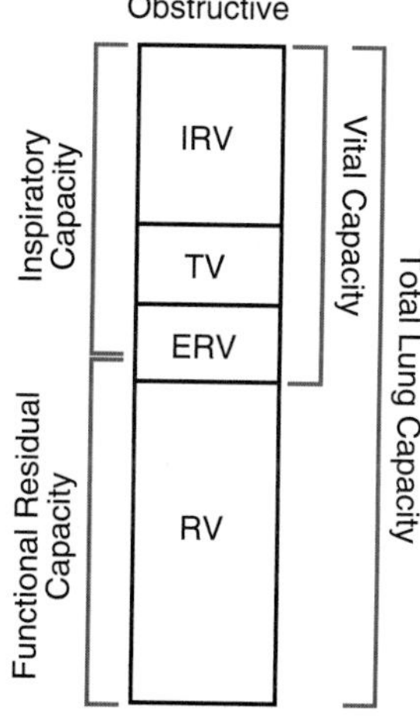

ERV: Expiratory reserve volume
IRV: Inspiratory reserve volume
RV: Residual volume
TV: Tidal volume

Figure 12.8 Lung volumes of a healthy pulmonary system compared with the lung volumes found in obstructive disease. *(Adapted from Roy, S, Wolf, S, and Scalzitti D: The Rehabilitation Specialist's Handbook, ed 4. FA Davis, Philadelphia, 2013, with permission.)*

spontaneously or with medical intervention and are interspersed with symptom-free intervals.

Diagnosis

The diagnosis of asthma is clinically based on a history of episodic wheezing, shortness of breath (SOB), tightness in the chest, and/or coughing, which may be worse at night and early morning in the absence of any other obvious cause. The FEV_1 during exacerbations will be less than 80% of the predicted value. After inhalation of a rescue drug used to quickly relieve acute symptoms (e.g., inhaled short-acting beta-2 agonist), an improvement of at least 12% (or 200 mL) in FEV_1 indicates reversibility of the airway limitation consistent with a diagnosis of asthma.[6,14]

Etiology

A number of different phenotypes of asthma have been identified. Historically, the two types of asthma that have been described are *allergic asthma* and *nonallergic asthma*. The most common phenotype of asthma is allergic (or extrinsic) asthma. Allergic asthma has an immunologic (immunoglobulin E [IgE]–mediated) response to certain environmental triggers (dust mites, pollen, mold, animal dander). Induced sputum from this group of individuals shows eosinophilic inflammation, which causes the common symptoms and pathophysiological findings of asthma. *Atopy,* or allergic sensitivity, is the strongest feature of the phenotype of allergic asthma.

Nonallergic (or intrinsic) asthma is a less common form of asthma. There are no clinical findings of atopy in nonallergic asthma; however, an inflammatory response, which is eosinophilic and/or neutrophilic does result from exposure to an irritant such as smoke, fumes, infections, or cold air.[14] Viral infections have been suggested to play a role in both the development and exacerbation of asthma.[15] Symptoms of asthma may begin at any age.

Pathophysiology

The major physiological manifestation of asthma is inflammation of the bronchial mucosa, leading to narrowing of the airways, bronchospasm, and increased bronchial secretions, all in response to a trigger (Fig. 12.9). The narrowed airways increase the resistance to airflow and cause air trapping on exhalation, leading to hyperinflation. These narrowed airways also provide an abnormal distribution of ventilation to the alveoli. Even during periods of remission, some degree of airway inflammation is present.

Clinical Presentation

The clinical symptoms of asthma *during an exacerbation* may include cough, dyspnea on exertion or at rest, and wheezing. The chest is usually held in an expanded position, indicating that hyperinflation of the lungs has occurred. Accessory muscles of ventilation may be required for breathing, even at rest. Intercostal, supraclavicular, and substernal retractions (visible inward motion of the soft tissue) may be present during inspiration. While expiratory wheezing is characteristic of asthma, crackles may also be present. With severe airway obstruction, breath sounds may be markedly decreased owing to poor air movement and wheezing may be present not only during exhalation, but may also be heard on inspiration.

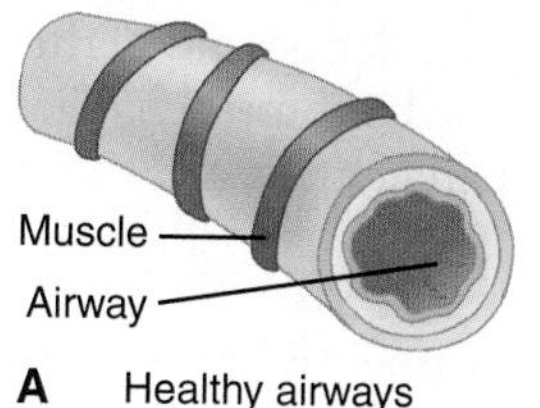

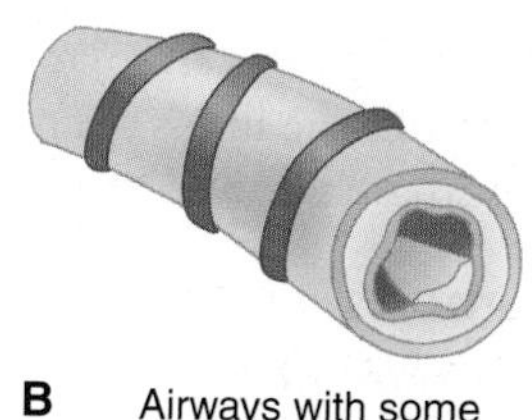

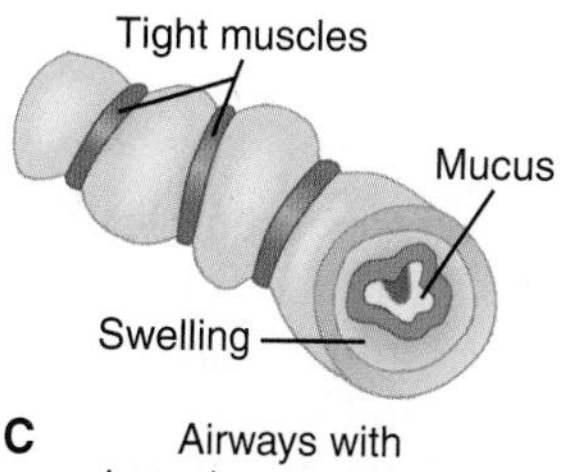

Figure 12.9 Small airways of a healthy pulmonary system, of a person showing the chronic inflammation of asthma, and of a person in an exacerbation of their asthma.

Chest radiographs taken during an asthmatic exacerbation usually demonstrate hyperinflation, as evidenced by an increase in the anterior–posterior diameter of the chest and hyperlucency of the lung fields. Less commonly, chest radiographs may reveal areas of infiltrate or *atelectasis* from the bronchial obstruction. Chest radiographs may be read as normal between asthmatic exacerbations.

The most dramatic clinical presentation during an exacerbation of asthma is a decreased forced expiratory flow rate in 1 second, FEV_1. Residual volume and FRC are increased because of air trapping at the expense of VC and IRV, which are reduced. The reversibility of these pulmonary function test abnormalities is characteristic of asthma. During remission, the patient with asthma may have normal or near-normal pulmonary function tests.

The most common arterial blood gas finding during an asthmatic exacerbation is mild to moderate hypoxemia. Usually some degree of hypocapnia is present secondary to an increased minute ventilation. With severe asthma exacerbations, hypoxemia will be more pronounced and hypercapnea may occur, indicating that the patient is experiencing decreased alveolar ventilation. Ventilator muscle fatigue and respiratory failure may follow.

Clinical Course

By the time adulthood is reached, many children with asthma no longer have symptoms of the disease. When the onset of asthma symptoms begins later in life, the clinical course is usually more progressive, showing changes in pulmonary function tests even during periods of remission. Airway remodeling in response to the chronic airway inflammation is thought to be responsible for the progressive nature of the disease.

Cystic Fibrosis

Cystic fibrosis (CF) is a chronic disease that affects the excretory glands of the body. Secretions made by these glands are thicker, more viscous than usual, and can affect a number of systems of the body, including the pulmonary, pancreatic, hepatic, sinus, and reproductive systems. Dysfunction of the pulmonary system is the most common cause of morbidity and mortality in patients with CF. Other presentations may occur due to the effect of this disease on other organ systems such as failure to thrive, diabetes, sinusitis, biliary disorders, and infertility.

Etiology

Cystic fibrosis is an autosomal recessive genetically transmitted disorder (Fig. 12.10). There are currently 30,000 people living with CF in the United States.[16]

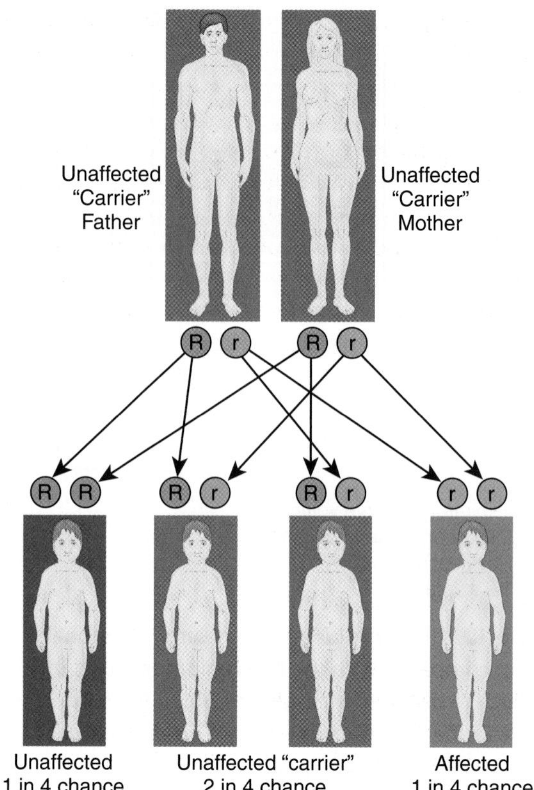

Figure 12.10 Autosomal recessive trait (Mendellian) requires that both parents be carriers of the disease or have the disease in order for their child to have the disease.

The CF gene (cystic fibrosis transmembrane conductance regulator [*CFTR*]) has been identified on the long arm of chromosome 7. The CFTR functions to transport electrolytes and water in and out of the epithelial cells of many organs in the body, including lungs, pancreas, and digestive and reproductive tracts. Defective transport of sodium, potassium, and water leaves the mucus made by excretory glands thickened and difficult to move and can often obstruct the lumen of its excretory gland. Over 1,700 mutations of this gene have been described thus far.[17]

Pathophysiology

The chronic pulmonary component of CF is related to the abnormally viscous mucus secreted in the tracheobronchial tree, which impairs the function of the mucociliary transport system. The altered secretions result in airway obstruction and hyperinflation. Exaggerated and sustained neutrophilic airway inflammation in response to infection is also a feature of this disease.[18] Partial or complete obstruction of the airways reduces ventilation to the alveolar units. Ventilation and perfusion within the lungs are not matched. Fibrotic changes are ultimately found in the lung parenchyma.

Diagnosis

Infant screening for CF was instituted in all 50 U.S. states by 2010. The diagnosis of CF may be suspected in patients who were not screened as an infant, who present with a positive family history of the disease, who present with recurrent pulmonary infections from *Staphylococcus aureus* and/or *Pseudomonas aeruginosa*, or who have a diagnosis of malnutrition and/or failure to thrive. A simple sweat test can be performed to rule out or confirm the diagnosis. A chloride ion concentration of greater than or equal to 60 mEq/L found in the sweat of children is a positive test for the diagnosis of CF. Genotyping for the most common *CFTR* mutations can also be done.

Clinical Presentation

The clinical presentation of CF can be related to any number of involved systems. Failure to thrive due to gastrointestinal dysfunction, diabetes due to pancreatic dysfunction, or frequent pulmonary infections and chronic cough due to pulmonary dysfunction are all possible presentations of the disease.

With pulmonary involvement, a patient presents with thick bronchial secretions that may be difficult to clear. With advancing disease, the chest wall will become barrel-shaped with an increased anterior–posterior (AP) diameter and an increased dorsal kyphosis due to loss of the elastic recoil properties of the underlying lungs and chronic hyperinflation. There is a resultant decrease in thoracic excursion. Breath sounds may be decreased with adventitious sounds of crackles and wheezes. Hypertrophy of accessory muscles of ventilation, pursed-lip breathing, cyanosis, and digital clubbing may all be present.

Pulmonary function studies show obstructive impairments, including decreased FEV_1, decreased PEF, decreased FVC, increased RV, and increased FRC. The abnormal ventilation–perfusion relationship within the lungs results in hypoxemia and hypercapnea, demonstrated by arterial blood gas analysis. As the disease progresses, destruction of the alveolar capillary network causes pulmonary hypertension and cor pulmonale. In advanced disease, chest radiographs show diffuse hyperinflation, increased lung marking, and atelectasis.

Course and Prognosis

Sixty-two percent of new cases of CF in 2013 in the United States were diagnosed by mandatory infant testing.[19] The course of the disease, while quite variable, has been linked to *CFTR* genotype, modifier genes, and environmental factors.[20,21] Life expectancy continues to improve owing to early diagnosis and improved medical management. Although some patients unfortunately die in early childhood, 49.7% of all patients diagnosed with CF are currently older than 18 years of age.[ED19] The predicted mean survival age of patients with CF was 40.7 years in 2013, a remarkable improvement from a mean survival age of 16 years 50 years ago.[19] Respiratory failure is the most frequent cause of death in patients with CF. Therefore, treatment of the pulmonary dysfunction, including removal of the abnormally thick secretions and prompt treatment of pulmonary infections, is important to the management of CF. Gastrointestinal dysfunction from CF can be aided by proper diet, vitamin supplements, and replacement of pancreatic enzymes. Habitual exercise has been linked to higher aerobic capacity, increased quality of life, and improved survival.[22] Nutritional status is also a powerful predictor of prognosis.[23]

Restrictive Lung Disease

Restrictive lung diseases are a group of diseases referred to collectively as *interstitial lung diseases,* with differing etiologies that result in difficulty expanding the lungs and a reduction in lung volumes. These disorders are grouped together as they have similar clinical presentations.

Etiology

This group of disorders is often divided into two groups: those with a known cause and those that are idiopathic. Rheumatic diseases, oxygen or drug-induced toxicity, inhalation of organic and inorganic dust, inhalation of noxious gases, radiation exposure, and asbestos exposure can cause damage to the pulmonary parenchyma and pleura and result in restrictive pulmonary disease. The most common restrictive lung disease is idiopathic pulmonary fibrosis (IPF), also termed *usual interstitial pneumonia*.

Pathophysiology

The particular changes occurring within the lung parenchyma and pleura depend on the etiological factors of restrictive disease. Many of the disorders begin with parenchymal changes due to chronic inflammation and a thickening of the alveoli and interstitium. As these diseases progress, distal airspaces become fibrosed, making them more resistant to expansion (i.e., less distensible). Consequently, lung volumes are reduced. A reduced pulmonary vascular bed eventually leads to hypoxemia and cor pulmonale. Asbestosis (asbestos-induced pulmonary fibrosis) is a type of restrictive lung disease that shows both parenchymal and pleural fibrosis.

Clinical Presentation

Dyspnea with activity and a persistent nonproductive cough are the classic symptoms of interstitial lung diseases. Signs of restrictive lung disease include rapid, shallow breathing, limited chest expansion, inspiratory crackles, especially over the lower lung fields, digital clubbing, and cyanosis.[24]

The plain chest radiograph reveals fine interstitial markings in a reticular, or netlike, pattern. Reduction in overall lung volume and radiographic evidence of pleural involvement, when present, can also be seen on plain chest radiographs, although their diagnostic and prognostic abilities are limited. High-resolution computed tomography is a radiological test for the diagnosis of IPF that typically shows basilar subpleural changes in a reticular pattern along with traction bronchiectasis (misshapen airways due to a pulling by fibrotic tissue on the airway wall) and honeycombing.[24,25]

Pulmonary function tests reveal a reduction in VC, FRC, RV, and TLC. Expiratory flow rates may be somewhat normal. The ratio between FVC and FEV_1 may be normal or even increased. Figure 12.11 shows the changes in lung volumes and capacities that occur in restrictive pulmonary parenchymal disease.

Arterial blood gas studies show varying degrees of hypoxemia and hypocapnia. Exercise may significantly lower oxygenation, even for patients with normal oxygenation at rest.

Course and Prognosis

Restrictive pulmonary diseases may have a slow onset but they are relentlessly progressive. Survival depends on the type of restrictive disease, the etiological factor, and the available treatments. Predictors of mortality include age, smoking history, BMI, radiological findings, pulmonary function tests, level of oxygenation, and distance walked on a 6-minute walk test.[25-27]

MEDICAL AND SURGICAL MANAGEMENT

Medical management of chronic pulmonary disease includes smoking cessation, pharmacological agents, and use of supplemental oxygen. Surgical and interventional management is a consideration for select patients with severe lung involvement. The following discussion provides an overview of these interventions.

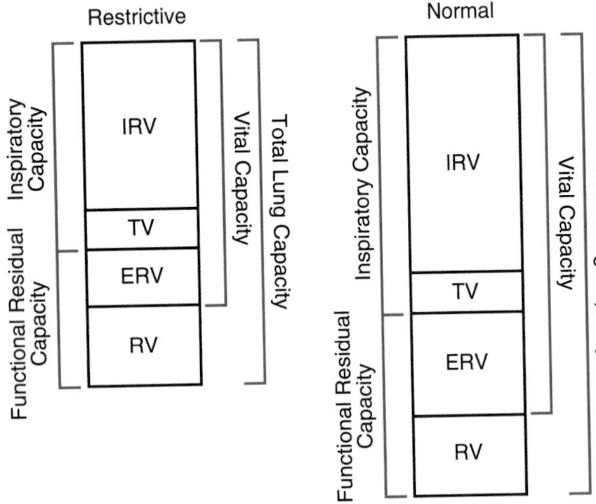

Figure 12.11 Lung volumes of a healthy pulmonary system compared with the lung volumes found in restrictive disease. *(Adapted from Roy, S, Wolf, S, and Scalzitti, D: The Rehabilitation Specialist's Handbook, ed 4. FA Davis, Philadelphia, 2013, with permission.)*

Smoking Cessation

Smoking is the major causal agent in the development of COPD, as well as a contributing cause to many other disease processes. The Global Initiative for Chronic Obstructive Pulmonary Disease states that "smoking cessation has the greatest capacity to influence the natural history of COPD."[5] The addictive properties of smoking and the withdrawal symptoms of smoking cessation make it difficult for smokers to quit. A majority of smokers who try to quit do so on their own. Unfortunately, 80% of smokers who try to quit on their own return to smoking within 1 month. Smokers report an average of six to nine attempts at smoking cessation before they are successful.[28] Using a structured smoking cessation program can increase the success of a person attempting to quit smoking.

There are two general types of smoking cessation programs: behavioral therapy and pharmacological therapy. *Behavioral therapy* includes education on the benefits of being a nonsmoker, counseling, and support through the arduous process of withdrawing from smoking. Acupuncture and hypnosis are considered part of a behavioral therapy approach because the purpose is to change smoking behavior. *Pharmacological therapy* includes the use of nicotine replacement therapy such as nicotine gum, lozenges, patches, sprays, or inhalers, and non-nicotine replacement medications such as bupropion (Zyban) and varenicline (Chantix) to assist in the cessation of smoking. Nicotine replacement therapy decreases the withdrawal symptoms linked to nicotine, such as craving for tobacco products, anger, irritability, anxiety, depression, and concentration problems.[29] Bupropion and varenicline counter the withdrawal symptoms of smoking cessation and increase the likelihood of quitting without the use of systemic nicotine.

Smoking cessation without any support has a long-term success rate of approximately 6%. Intense behavioral therapy has an improved smoking cessation rate compared to no behavioral therapy. A Cochrane Review in 2016 found that the use of intense behavioral therapy along with pharmacological therapy was the most effective method for smoking cessation, with a success rate of up to 25%.[30] Recommendations for smoking cessation need to be tailored to the individual patient as access to counseling may be difficult to obtain and adverse medication reactions may be encountered. For example, nicotine replacement therapy can be beneficial in a comprehensive smoking cessation program; however, it is not recommended following a cardiovascular event. The regional offices of the American Lung Association and the American Cancer Society are good resources for local smoking cessation programs.

Pharmacological Management

Pharmacological agents provide relief from the symptoms of chronic lung disease and improve the health and functional status of individuals with lung disease.

Each patient with a chronic pulmonary diagnosis will require a tailored plan of care. It is not unusual for patients to be on a combination of drugs for the management of their pulmonary disease. This discussion will provide information on both maintenance drugs and rescue drugs used in the care of patients with pulmonary disease. Table 12.1 provides foundational information on the pharmacological management of lung disease. Table 12.2 includes recommendations from GINA for pharmacological control of asthma symptoms.[14]

Table 12.1 Common Drugs Used in the Medical Management of Patients With Chronic Pulmonary Disease

Use	Drug Category	Example Name	Action	Adverse Reactions
Maintenance	Anticholinergic Long-acting muscarinic antagonists (LAMA)	Tiotropium (Spiriva)	Bronchodilation	Throat irritation Drying of tracheal secretions Tachycardia Palpitations
Maintenance	Long-acting Beta2 agonist (LABA)	Salmeterol (Serevent)	Bronchodilation	Tachycardia Palpitations GI distress Nervousness Tremor Headache Dizziness
Maintenance	Corticosteroids	Fluticasone (Flovent)	Anti-inflammatory effects	Increase BP Sodium retention (edema) Muscle wasting Osteoporosis GI Irritation Atherosclerosis Hypercholesterolemia Increased susceptibility to infection
Maintenance	Phosphodiesterase 4 inhibitor	Roflumilast (Daxas)	Anti-inflammatory effects	GI distress Depression Headache Insomnia Rhinitis/sinusitis Urinary tract infection
Maintenance	Leukotriene receptor antagonist	Montelukast (Singulair)	Blocks allergic reaction	GI distress Sore throat Upper respiratory tract infection Dizziness Headache Nasal congestion
Maintenance	Mucolytics	Dornase alfa (Pulmozyme)	Thins secretions	Voice changes Sore throat Runny nose or eyes Rash
Rescue	Short-acting Beta$_2$ agonist	Albuterol (Ventolin)	Bronchodilation	Tachycardia Palpitations GI distress Nervousness Tremor Headache Dizziness

Table 12.2 Suggested Pharmacological Management of Patients With Asthma

Step 1	Step 2	Step 3	Step 4	Step 5
Asthma education Risk factor modifications Environmental controls Rapid-acting B_2 agonist, as needed Consider lose dose inhaled corticosteroid				
	Low-dose inhaled corticosteroid	Low-dose inhaled corticosteroid plus long-acting beta$_2$ agonist	Medium- to high-dose corticosteroid plus long-acting beta$_2$ agonist	Refer for add-on treatment such as LAMA, anti-igE, anti-IL5
	Or leukotriene receptor agonist	Or medium- to high-dose inhaled steroid	Add tiotropium, high-dose ICS plus leukotriene receptor agonist	Add oral corticosteroids
	Or low-dose theophylline	Or low-dose inhaled steroid plus leukotriene receptor agonist	Or sustained-release theophylline	
		Or low-dose inhaled steroid plus theophylline		

Step 1 is for everyone with a diagnosis to gain and maintain control of their asthma symptoms. If Step 1 is insufficient in keeping asthma symptoms at bay, the patient needs to move to the next step(s) in order to control his or her asthma. Shaded cells are the preferred pharmacological options. Adapted from Global strategy for asthma management and prevention; Update 2016, with permission.[16]

Maintenance Drugs

Maintenance drugs are used to reduce or minimize pulmonary symptoms throughout the day. These drugs are taken on a regular schedule to keep respiratory symptoms at bay. Maintenance drugs for patients with chronic pulmonary disorders include corticosteroids, long- and short-acting muscarinic antagonists (anticholinergics), long-acting beta-2 agonists, phosphodiesterase 4 inhibitors, and leukotriene antagonists. Methylxanthines, nonselective phosphodiesterase inhibitors, are bronchodilators that are less frequently prescribed as a maintenance drug as safer medications are available. While all the above maintenance drugs are available for use, each disorder uses these drugs in a different order or combination. For example, inhaled anti-inflammatories are the mainstay of medical management of the chronic inflammation of asthma. Inhaled bronchodilators, like anticholinergics or long-acting beta agonists, are commonly prescribed for patients with COPD. And antibiotics and inhaled mucolytics may be the first line drugs to treat the respiratory symptoms that accompany cystic fibrosis.

Routes of administration of maintenance drugs are usually inhalation or ingestion. Inhalation is the advisable route of administration, when possible, as it limits systemic side effects of the drug. However, improper use of the inhalation device is a barrier to disease control. Pothirat and colleagues reported that 74.8% of patients did not use their inhalation device correctly.[31] And that even with specific training and learned correct use, Melani et al[32] reported increased errors in the use of the inhalation device over time that reduced control over the symptoms of lung disease.

Rescue Drugs

Rescue drugs are used for immediate relief of *breakthrough* symptoms of bronchoconstriction (symptoms that "break through" and become apparent even with careful management). Inhaled short-acting beta-2 agonists are used for this purpose. Patients are advised to use their prescribed inhaled short-acting beta-2 agonist on an as-needed basis. If a patient reports an increased frequency in the use of a rescue drug, it is indicative of a flaw in the maintenance drug regimen or a change in the patient's pulmonary status.

Antibiotics

Pulmonary infections are frequent in patients with chronic pulmonary diseases. They can be devastating to the patient and cause major setbacks in pulmonary rehabilitation efforts. The early signs of an infection are often noted by changes in the patient's baseline status (i.e., a change in exercise ability, peak flow rates, dyspnea, color or amount of sputum, or an increase in the use of rescue inhalers). Antibiotics are used to either kill the bacteria outright (bacteriocidal) or interfere with the growth and/or proliferation of bacteria (bacteriostatic). There are many categories of antibiotics (e.g., penicillins, cephalosporins, tetracyclines) that are effective on different infecting organisms. It is important to identify the infecting organism in order to prescribe the appropriate antibiotic. Prophylactic use of antibiotics has not demonstrated a significant decrease in hospital admissions, changes in lung function, clinically significant quality of life or mortality.[33]

Supplemental Oxygen

The long-term use of supplemental oxygen (greater than 15 hours/day) has been shown to prolong the survival of patients with COPD whose resting arterial partial pressure of oxygen ($Pa{O_2}$) is 55 mm Hg or less, which correlates with an $Sa{O_2}$ of 88% or less.[5,34] In patients with right heart failure or erythrocytosis, the cut off is less than 60 mm Hg.[5] In patients whose resting $Sa{O_2}$ is greater than 88% but their exercise abilities are limited by exertional dyspnea, supplemental oxygen during exercise may be helpful in reducing this symptom.[35] The amount of oxygen used should be titrated individually to maintain an $Sa{O_2}$ of at least 90%, if possible. The long-term use of oxygen in patients with moderate oxygen desaturation (SaO^2 >88%) at rest or with exercise did not result in quality of life or distance walked on the 6-minute walk test.[36] Various supplemental oxygen delivery methods are available; continuous flow, pulsed flow, and reservoir are among the most common.

Surgical and Interventional Management of Chronic Pulmonary Disease

There are few surgical options for the patient with pulmonary disease. Criteria used to determine the appropriateness of an intervention include the distribution of emphysema throughout the lungs, the presence of large bullae, the presence or absence of interlobar collateral ventilation, and the severity of the lung disease.

Lung volume reduction surgery (LVRS) is a surgical technique that removes nonfunctional, overdistended lung tissue, in order to restore more normal biomechanics to the thorax. LVRS may be indicated in patients with heterogeneous areas of hyperinflated, relatively nonfunctional lung tissue (with or without collateral ventilation) alongside of relatively functional lung tissue. The surgical procedure removes approximately 20% to 35% of the most diseased lung tissue, relieving the more normal lung tissue of its burden. This surgical procedure reduces RV and FRC (i.e., decreases hyperinflation), allowing for a more normal resting position of the diaphragm, an increased diaphragmatic excursion, and a more normal chest wall motion.[5] Research has shown postoperative results of increased exercise capacity, lung function, quality of life, and gas exchange in patients with moderate *upper lobe* lung disease.[5,37,38] Patients with severe pulmonary disease whose distribution is in non-upper lobe areas of the lung show only slight improvement in functional abilities and quality of life scores along with a high mortality rate.[5,37-39]

Minimally invasive, endobronchial lung volume reduction interventions are becoming available to treat the hyperinflation of emphysematous lung tissue without surgery. The placement of an endobronchial one-way valve in an airway reduces airflow into that designated area of the lung while allowing air and secretions to be expelled. The valve decreasing hyperinflation of that area of the lung, allowing improved function to the healthier adjacent lung tissue. A second means of minimally invasive lung volume reduction is by deploying lung coils into an airway in order to occlude the airway and collapse the lung tissue distal to the obstruction. A third approach is to inject a substance into overdistended areas of the lungs that causes localized inflammation leading to atelectasis, scarring and remodelling of that area. The result of all of these bronchoscopic interventions is to reduce areas of hyperinflation, allowing the more normal lung tissue room to function.[40,41]

Lung transplantation for end-stage pulmonary disease has an overall survival rate of 96.85% at 1 month, 87.5% at 1 year, and 68% at 3 years.[42] The goals of lung transplantation are to restore normal lung function, restore normal exercise capacity, and prolong life.[5] People awaiting a lung transplant include patients with COPD, CF, idiopathic pulmonary fibrosis, and pulmonary hypertension. The number of patients awaiting lung transplantation continues to grow, far exceeding the number of organs available for transplantation, making transplantation a reality for only a small number of individuals.[43]

PHYSICAL THERAPY MANAGEMENT

Chronic pulmonary diseases and their associated dysfunction have a slow yet progressive course. The person with pulmonary dysfunction often avoids activities that result in the uncomfortable sensation of dyspnea. A slow but steady decrease in these patients' functional activities follows, resulting in progressive aerobic deconditioning. It is not uncommon for someone with pulmonary disease to have lost many functional abilities before ever seeking medical help. The intended outcome of pulmonary rehabilitation is to interrupt this downward spiral of physical inability, improve exercise performance, decrease the symptom of dyspnea, and improve quality of life.[44,45]

Goals and Outcomes

The *Guide for Physical Therapist Practice 3.0*, available through the American Physical Therapy Association, provides a general framework for physical therapy intervention for patients with chronic pulmonary diseases. Tests and measures for patients with chronic pulmonary disorders include, but are not limited to, categories of aerobic capacity/endurance, circulation, ventilation and respiration, and community, social and civic life.[46] Examples of goals and outcomes for the individual patient with pulmonary dysfunction are presented in Box 12.1.

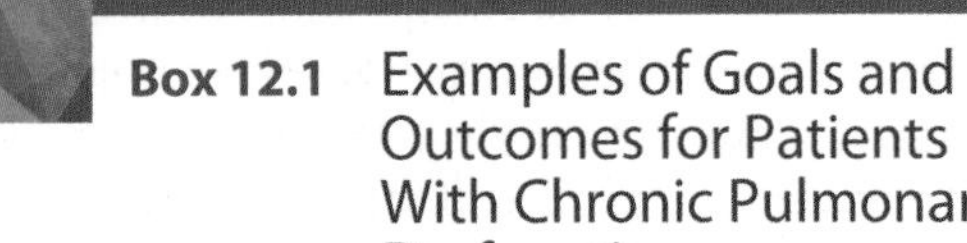

Box 12.1 Examples of Goals and Outcomes for Patients With Chronic Pulmonary Dysfunction

- Patient/client, family and caregiver understanding of disease process, expectations, goals, and outcomes is enhanced.
- Cardiovascular endurance is increased.
- Strength, power and endurance of peripheral muscles are increased.
- Performance of physical tasks, both basic activities of daily living and instrumental activities of daily living is improved.
- Strength, power and endurance of ventilator muscles are increased.
- Independence in airway clearance is improved.
- Patient/client decision making ability regarding the use of health care resources is improved.
- Patient/client self-management of symptoms and self-management of pulmonary disease are enhanced.

Examination

The examination of a patient's pulmonary status has several purposes: (1) to evaluate the appropriateness of the patient's participation in a pulmonary rehabilitation program; (2) to determine the therapeutic interventions most appropriate for the participant's plan of care (POC); (3) to monitor the participant's physiological response to exercise; and (4) to appropriately progress the participant's POC over time.

Patient History

A patient interview should begin with the chief complaint and the patient's perception of why pulmonary rehabilitation is being sought. The chief complaint is often shortness of breath and/or loss of function. A medical history contains pertinent pulmonary symptoms specific to that patient: cough, sputum production, wheezing, and SOB severity. Occupational, social, medication, smoking and family histories should also be obtained and documented.

Laboratory Tests

Various laboratory studies to examine patients with pulmonary disease may be performed and interpreted. These include radiology, pulmonary function tests (PFTs) including flow rates, arterial blood gas analysis, SaO_2 measurements, and electrocardiograms (ECGs).

Tests and Measures

Vital Signs

HR, BP, RR, oxygen saturation (SaO_2), temperature, and presence of pain (usually associated with shortness of breath) should be examined and documented (see Chapter 2, Examination of Vital Signs). An individual's height should be measured, as there is a direct relationship between height and lung volumes. Weight, for its use as a prognostic indicator, should be measured on a standard scale and each subsequent measurement should be performed on the same scale.

Observation, Inspection, and Palpation

By observing the neck and shoulders of a patient with pulmonary disease, the use of accessory muscles of ventilation can be observed (see Fig. 12.6). A normal configuration of the thorax reveals a ratio of AP to lateral diameter of 1:2. Destruction of the lung parenchyma results in an increase in the AP diameter and a reduction of this ratio (up to 1:1) (see Fig. 12.5). During inhalation and exhalation, both sides of the thorax should move symmetrically; any asymmetries should be noted and documented.

Cyanosis is a bluish discoloration of the skin that can be observed periorally, periorbitally, and in nail beds; it indicates acute tissue hypoxia. An indicator of more chronic tissue hypoxia is digital clubbing of the fingers and toes. In digital clubbing, there is an increase in the angle created by the distal phalanx and the point where the nail exits from the digit. The tip of the distal phalanx becomes bulbous (Fig. 12.12).

Auscultation of the Lungs

Auscultation involves listening over the chest wall as air enters and exits the lungs. To perform auscultation of the lungs, a stethoscope is placed firmly on the patient's thorax anteriorly, laterally, and posteriorly (Fig. 12.13). The patient is asked to inspire fully through an open mouth, then to exhale quietly. Inhalation and

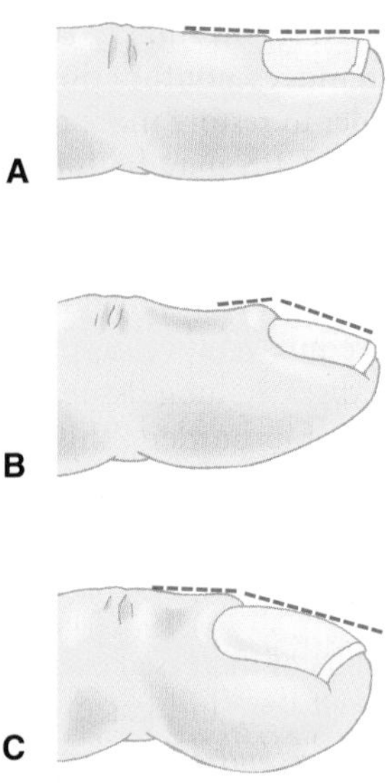

Figure 12.12 Digital clubbing is a sign of chronic tissue hypoxia. (A) Normal. (B) Early clubbing with angle present between nail and proximal skin. (C) Advanced clubbing.

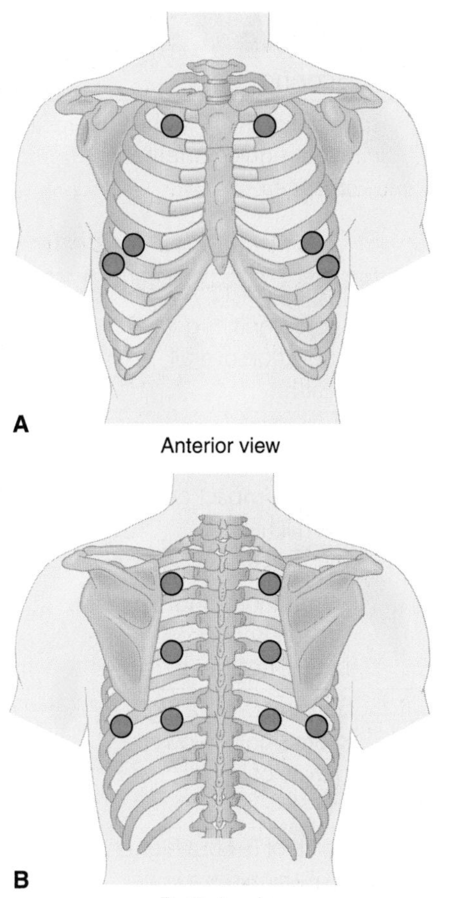

Figure 12.13 Auscultation of the lungs. A global assessment of lung sounds requires that the therapist listens through a stethoscope, which is placed anteriorly, posteriorly, and laterally on the upper, middle, and lower thorax.

the beginning of exhalation normally produce a soft rustling sound. The end of exhalation is normally silent. This characteristic of a normal breath sound is termed *vesicular.* When a louder, more hollow, and echoing sound occupies a larger portion of the ventilatory cycle, the breath sounds are referred to as *bronchial.* When the breath sounds are very quiet and barely audible, they are termed *decreased.* These three terms—*vesicular, bronchial,* and *decreased*—allow the listener to describe the intensity of the breath sound.

In addition to the description of the intensity, there may be additional sounds and vibrations heard during auscultation. These are called *adventitious* breath sounds. These sounds are superimposed on the already-described intensity of the breath sound. According to the American College of Chest Physicians and the American Thoracic Society, there are two types of adventitious sounds: crackles and wheezes.[47] *Crackles,* previously termed *rales* and *rhonchi,* sound like the rustling of cellophane and have a multitude of potential causes (tissue fibrosis, secretions in the airways, pulmonary edema, and so forth). *Wheezes* have been described as high-pitched, coarse, whistling sounds. A decrease in the size of the lumen of the airway will create a wheezing sound, much like stretching the neck of an inflated balloon narrows the passageway through which air must escape, producing a whistling sound.

Measurement of Dyspnea and Quality of Life

There are many scales that can be used to quantify dyspnea. Measured at the beginning and the end of a rehabilitation program and during periods of exacerbation can be accomplished using the clinically practical *Modified British Medical Council (mMRC) Dyspnea Scale.*[48] The *Baseline Dyspnea Index* (BDI) is another dyspnea scale that is encountered more in the research literature than in clinical practice.[49] While both these scores are reliable and valid, they are not interchangeable.[50] Quality-of-life (QOL) measures that are specific to chronic pulmonary dysfunction include the *Chronic Respiratory Questionnaire* and the *St. George's Respiratory Questionnaire.*[51,52] Shorter disease specific QOL measures such as the *COPD assessment test* (CAT) and the *COPD Control Questionnaire* (CCQ) may be more clinically useful in determining the patient's baseline health-related quality of life.[53-55] These outcome measures may be helpful in demonstrating improvement made with physical therapy intervention. Table 12.3 presents information regarding these dyspnea and QOL outcomes measures.

Measurement of Strength and Endurance

Patients with pulmonary disease may show peripheral and ventilatory muscle weakness due to deconditioning, malnutrition, steroid use, and the systemic inflammation of the disease process.[11,56-58] Muscle weakness can contribute to exercise limitations and an inability to perform activities of daily living (ADL). Therefore, measurement of peripheral muscle strength and inspiratory muscle strength will determine the need for strength training during rehabilitation. The use of *manual muscle testing* (MMT) may not be the best choice for strength assessment. The maximal effort that is required during MMT makes it likely that patients will produce a *Valsalva maneuver* while performing the test. In patients with pulmonary disease, the increased intrathoracic pressure from a Valsalva maneuver closes off the small airways, causing shortness of breath and therefore limits full participation in the test. A *Five Times Sit to Stand Test* might be a better choice to assess functional lower extremity strength in patients with pulmonary disease.[59,60] The *6-Minute Pegboard and Ring Test* is a measurement of upper extremity function that has been shown to be a reliable and valid measurement tool.[61]

Inspiratory muscle strength is determined by measuring the patient's ability to create a *negative inspiratory pressure* (PI_{max}). The standard starting patient position for the test is seated with nose clips in place. The person is asked to let out all their air before beginning the test

Table 12.3 Outcome Measures: Dyspnea and Quality of Life

Outcome Measure	Description	Scoring	MCID
Modified Medical Research Council Dyspnea Scale (mMRC dyspnea scale)[48] ICF: Body structure and function	A simple self-assessment tool that measures dyspnea ranging from 0: I only get breathless with strenuous exercise to a 4: I am too breathless to leave the house.	Score of 0–4; a higher score signifies greater dyspnea.	N/A
Baseline Dyspnea Index (BDI)[49] ICF: Participation	A self-administered 24-item questionnaire covering 3 domains of functional impairment, magnitude of task, and magnitude of effort.	Score of 0–12. A lower score signifies greater impact on overall health.	N/A
Chronic Respiratory Questionnaire (CRQ)[51] ICF: Participation	A self-administered 20 items over 4 domains of dyspnea, fatigue, emotional function, and mastery.	Score of 20–140; a higher score signifying greater impact on overall health.	0.5 points
St. George's Respiratory Questionnaire (SGRQ)[52] ICF: Participation	A self-administered questionnaire of 50 items regarding 3 domains, symptomatology, activity and impact	Score of 0–100; higher scores indicating greater impact on overall health.	4 units
COPD assessment test (CAT)[53] ICF: Participation	A self-administered tool that measures health-related quality of life and physical limitations using 8 questions to identify the impact of pulmonary disease	Score of 0–40; a higher score signifies lower quality of life.	2 points
Clinical COPD Questionnaire (CCQ)[54,55] ICF: Participation	A self-administered tool that measures health-related quality of life using 10 questions divided into three domains: symptoms, functional state, and mental state	Score of 0–60; a higher score signifies a lower quality of life.	0.4 points

(i.e., start the test at residual volume). The person is then asked to "breath in" against an occluded mouthpiece. The negative pressure is recorded using an aneroid manometer.[62] The result of this test is the negative pressure, reported in millimeters of mercury or centimeters of water, that was generated and sustained after one second of effort.[7] Normative values for inspiratory pressure are related to a person's characteristics of age and sex.[63] This ability to generate a negative inspiratory pressure reflects the strength of the muscles of inspiration.

Exercise Testing in Patients With Pulmonary Disease

An *exercise tolerance test* (ETT) can provide objective information to (1) document a patient's functional abilities, (2) document a patient's symptomatology, (3) prescribe safe exercise, (4) document changes in oxygenation during exercise and determine the need for supplemental oxygen, and (5) identify any changes in pulmonary function during exercise performance.

An ETT protocol gradually increases exercise intensity in order to stress the patient with pulmonary dysfunction to their point of limitation. Incremental cycle ergometry testing is widely used in clinical practice for patients with chronic pulmonary disorders. The *American Thoracic Society* and *American College of Chest Physicians* recommend a protocol that begins with 3 minutes of rest, 3 minutes of unloaded pedaling, and then an increase of 5 to 25 watts every minute until the patient reaches exhaustion.[64]

Heart rate, blood pressure, ECG, respiratory rate, rate of perceived exertion (RPE), rate of perceived dyspnea (RPD), and oxygen saturation (SaO_2) are monitored during the test. Documentation of peak HR, peak RPD, peak RPE, and peak workload can be used to appropriately prescribe exercise. Peak VO_2 is also a measurement that can be collected during an ETT but requires equipment not always found in the clinical setting. PFTs performed before and after an exercise test document the effects of exercise on lung function. A reduction of greater than or equal to 20% in FEV_1 is an indication that exercise provoked airway hyperresponsiveness.[65] Criteria for stopping a pulmonary ETT are presented in Box 12.2.

The *6-Minute Walk Test* (6MWT) is a functional performance measure that asks a patient to walk as far as

Box 12.2 Graded Exercise Test Termination Criteria

1. Maximal shortness of breath
2. A fall in Pa_{O_2} of greater than 20 mm Hg or a Pa_{O_2} less than 55 mm Hg
3. A rise in Pa_{CO_2} of greater than 10 mm Hg or greater than 65 mm Hg
4. Cardiac ischemia or arrhythmias
5. Symptoms of fatigue
6. Increase in diastolic blood pressure readings of 20 mm Hg, systolic hypertension greater than 250 mm Hg, decrease in blood pressure with increasing workloads
7. Leg pain
8. Total fatigue
9. Signs of insufficient cardiac output
10. Reaching a ventilatory maximum

From Brannon, F, et al: Cardiopulmonary Rehabilitation: Basic Theory and Application. FA Davis, Philadelphia, 1998, p. 300, with permission.

possible in 6 minutes. The patient is allowed to stop and rest during the administration of the test. Total distance walked is the recorded result of the test. The 6MWT has been shown to have a good correlation with a patient's functional abilities.[66]

The *Incremental Shuttle Walk Test* (ISWT) is another functional performance measure that uses a recorded audio signal to dictate incrementally increasing walking speeds over level ground. Two destination points are placed 9 meters apart, so that the walking path is 10 meters. The person is asked to reach each destination point by the time the increasingly frequent audio signal sounds. The test is terminated when the person can no longer keep up with the increasing tempo of the signals, meaning that the person is more than 0.5 meters from the cone at the time of the audio signal and cannot catch up during the next shuttle. Recording of Sa_{O_2}, HR, and RPD occurs at the beginning and end of the test. The results of the ISWT are the number of shuttles that the person completes.[67] These results have a positive correlation with maximal oxygen consumption ($V_{O_{2max}}$).[66]

Gait speed is an easy to perform outcome measure, needing only a stop watch and a length of corridor.[68] Performing the test requires a 20-meter course. The acceleration leg of the course is the first 5 meters, the deceleration leg of the course is the last 5 meters, and the timed section of the course is the middle 10 meters. The person is asked to begin at the start of the 20-meter course and walk at a comfortable pace for the length of the course. The therapist measures the time it takes to traverse the middle 10 meters. The result of this outcome measure is gait velocity reported in either meters/sec or feet/sec.

Data from these functional tests can be used to determine disability, predict hospital discharge disposition and mortality, assess the ability to perform ADL, quantify health-related quality of life, determine home and community walking abilities and the need for oxygen therapy, demonstrate the effectiveness of medication changes, and determine the prescription of exercise.[12,65,66,68]

Examining a patient's functional capabilities should be used as an outcome measure to document functional improvements following physical therapy intervention, even if an ETT has been performed. The 6MWT is easy to administer and requires minimal equipment, making it the most commonly used outcome measurements to demonstrate changes in a patient's abilities following pulmonary rehabilitation.[69] The clinically significant change from a 6MWT is between 25 and 35 meters.[70] The clinically significant change for the ISWT is 47.5 meters.[71] The clinically significant change in gait speed is 0.05 meters/second.[68] Table 12.4 presents information regarding these functional mobility outcomes measures.

Exercise Prescription

Exercise prescription for aerobic training incorporates four variables that together allow the therapist to develop a patient-specific exercise prescription designed to produce an increase in functional capacity. These variables are *mode, intensity, duration,* and *frequency*.

Mode

Any type of sustained *aerobic exercise* can be used for pulmonary rehabilitation. Lower extremity (LE) activities, including walking and cycling, are often used to improve exercise tolerance. Specificity of training remains an important factor in the choice of exercise modes so that training translates into functional abilities.[72] Upper extremity (UE) aerobic exercise (e.g., arm ergometry) can also be included. Many programs utilize a circuit approach (combining a variety of resistive and aerobic exercises) to train different muscle groups, in different ways, with interspersed rest periods.

Intensity

There are several ways to prescribe exercise intensity: oxygen consumption, HR, RPE, RPD, and a percent of peak workload. Below is a discussion of each means of prescribing exercise intensity.

Exercise Intensity as a Percent of $V_{O_{2peak}}$

Moderate intensity exercise can be prescribed using approximately 40% to 60% of the peak V_{O_2} achieved on an ETT. Vigorous intensity exercise would be approximately 60% or greater of the peak V_{O_2} achieved on an ETT.[73] Patients with mild to moderate pulmonary disease may be able to exercise for a period of time at these intensities in order to produce a training effect. While using a percentage of V_{O_2} may be the most accurate method of prescribing exercise from a graded exercise test, assuming that peak V_{O_2} was measured, it does not

Table 12.4 Outcome Measures: Functional Mobility

Outcome Measure	Description	Scoring	MCID
6-minute walk test (6MWT)[66,70] ICF: participation	The participant is asked to cover as much distance as possible in 6 minutes. Assistive devices can be used. Individuals can rest as needed, although the timer does not stop. This is a self-selected walking speed that has a good correlation to performance of ADL.	Distance walked in 6 minutes	25–35 meters
Incremental Shuttle walk test (ISWT)[67,71] ICF: Participation	Two cones are set to identify a 10-meter walking course. The participant is told to walk between cones to a walking speed dictated by an audio signal. The starting gait speed is 0.5 m/sec and increases each minute by 0.17 m/sec. The test is finished when the subject is unable to maintain the required speed and fails to complete two consecutive shuttles in the time imposed.	Distance covered from the completed number of shuttles traversed.	48 meters
Gait speed[68] ICF: Participation	Walking speed is measured by a walking course that has a 5-meter acceleration leg, a 10-meter timed leg, and a 5-meter deceleration leg.	Gait speed is calculated in m/sec.	0.05 m/sec

give the clinician a means to monitor exercise intensity during the actual performance during an exercise session.

Exercise Intensity as a Percent of Heart Rate

There is a relationship between increasing workloads, increasing VO_2, and increasing HR, making exercise HR a more practical choice for prescribing and monitoring exercise intensity in the clinical setting.[73]

Patients with mild to moderate pulmonary disease may not have a pulmonary limitation to their ability to perform exercise; therefore, their exercise test may have the expected cardiovascular end point. If these patients have no other concomitant diseases, have no musculoskeletal or neurological constraints, and are committed to exercise, 70% to 85% of their highest HR achieved on the ETT could be used to prescribe exercise intensity.[73] It should be emphasized that when prescribing exercise intensity by HR, a heart rate range should be given, rather than a single number.

Exercise Intensity by Rating of Perceived Exertion or Rating of Perceived Dyspnea

In patients with severe pulmonary impairments, dyspnea may be the limiting factor to exercise performance. Patients with severe pulmonary impairment will likely approach their ventilatory maximum on an ETT before their cardiovascular maximum is reached; that is, their peak exercise HR may be lower than their maximum HR owing to pulmonary constraints. For these patients, prescribing exercise intensity using a percentage of the peak HR may underestimate their exercise abilities. The rating of perceived dyspnea obtained from an exercise test can be used to prescribe exercise intensity for patients with COPD (Table 12.5).[74-77] A perceived dyspnea rating of up to 3 (moderate SOB) corresponds approximately to 50% of VO_{2max}. A rating of about 5 to 6 corresponds to approximately 80% of VO_{2max}. The use of RPD, especially when levels of exercise are in the vigorous intensity range (>80% peak VO_2) have been shown to be a valid and reliable means of prescribing exercise.[74]

The RPE is often used as a means of prescribing exercise intensity for patients with cardiovascular and pulmonary diseases.[73,78] Using the RPE scale allows the patient to self-regulate exercise intensity based on the perception of exertion. RPE has been correlated with VO_2, making it a useful means of prescribing and monitoring exercise intensity. Perceived exertion ratings of 12 to 13 and 14 to 17 on the 6 to 20 RPE scale were correlated with 40% to 60% and 60% to 90% of VO_{2max}, respectively[73] (see additional discussion in Chapter 13, Heart Disease and Table 13.14).

Exercise Intensity as a Percent of Peak Workload

Clinicians often prescribe exercise intensity by utilizing a combination of physiological parameters (e.g., HR, RPE, and RPD), as these measures allow for the day-to-day variations in a participant's physiological state. Using a percentage of peak workload, while not a physiological parameter, may be helpful when prescribing exercise intensity for patients with severe pulmonary disease. In this population, the exercise intensity needed to allow for a usual exercise session duration may be so low

Table 12.5 Rating of Perceived Exertion: The Borg CR10 Scale

The Borg CR10 Scale		
0	Nothing at all	"No P"
0.3		
0.5	Extremely weak	Just noticeable
1	Very weak	
1.5		
2	Weak	Light
2.5		
3	Moderate	
4		
5	Strong	Heavy
6		
7	Very strong	
8		
9		
10	Extremely strong	"Max P"
11		
12	Absolute maximum	Highest possible

Note: For correct usage of the scale, the exact design and instructions given in Borg's folders must be followed. The scale with correct instructions can be obtained from Borg Perception (see the Borg Perception website at www.borgperception.se). Also see Borg, G: Borg's Perceived Exertion and Pain Scales. Human Kinetics, Champaign, IL, 1998. Reprinted with permission.

as to produce little or no training effect.[79,80] Rather, exercise using short bursts of high-intensity activity, interspersed with low-intensity exercise or rest periods (i.e., high-intensity interval training [HIIT]) has been suggested.[81-89] According to the *Guidelines for Pulmonary Rehabilitation* from the *American College of Chest Physicians* and the *American Association of Cardiovascular and Pulmonary Rehabilitation*, an exercise intensity that uses a high percentage of the patient's peak exercise capacity is well tolerated and physiological training effects have been documented.[90] There is a dose relationship between exercise intensity and training outcomes, meaning the higher the exercise intensity, the greater the training.[73] They do caution, however, that lower-intensity exercise may be associated with better adherence.[90] Current research on interval training versus continuous exercise training is presented in Table 12.6.

It may be the case that a 6MWT is the only functional measurement available for a given patient. The 6MWT has been determined to be a moderate to vigorous intensity for patients with pulmonary dysfunction and the results can be used to predict Peak $\dot{V}O_2$.[91,92] Therefore the results of the 6MWT can be used to prescribe exercise intensity. The common workload intensity associated with a 6MWT is 80% of the average walking speed performed on the test.[93]

Duration

Exercising within prescribed exercise intensity for at least 20 to 30 minutes is recommended.[73] The duration of the training session varies according to patient tolerance, with some participants not being able to

Evidence Summary Table 12.6 Exercise Training Intensity: Interval Versus Continuous Exercise

Reference	Design	Subjects	Interventions	Results	Comments
Louvaris, Z, et al[82]	Randomized controlled study	128 patients with COPD, 85 in the interval training group, 43 in the usual care group who did not participate in pulmonary rehabilitation	12-week high-intensity exercise training exercise cycle 3x/week at 130% of baseline peak work for 30 sec of exercise and 30 sec of rest for 45 minutes, resistance training, breathing retraining, diet and education.	Training group increased their number of steps per day, 27% over baseline, increased the time spent in non-sedentary activities while the control group declined in the number of steps per day. These effects persisted 12 weeks after the cessation of the program.	High-intensity interval training not only increased the exercise potential of patients with COPD, but also there was a carryover to ADL that persisted after the cessation of the rehab program.

Continued

Evidence Summary Table 12.6 Exercise Training Intensity: Interval Versus Continuous Exercise—cont'd

Reference	Design	Subjects	Interventions	Results	Comments
Nasis, et al[83]	Non-randomized controlled parallel group study	36 participants with stable COPD, Stages II–IV, mean age 69. Participants were divided into two groups. Group 1: those who demonstrated dynamic hyperinflation during exercise testing, and Group 2: those who did not.	Group 1 was trained with 3 sessions/week for 12 weeks using 30 sec of 100% workload peak and 30 sec rest for 45 minutes. Total work load increased 5% weekly.	After training Group 1 showed an increase in peak workload, increase in Vo_2 peak, decrease in SBP, HR, and VE at submaximal levels and a decrease in dynamic hyperinflation during exercise. Group 2 showed increase in peak workload, Vo_2 peak and an increase in cardiac output.	Pulmonary rehabilitation induces cardiovascular training effects in both groups. The study used a non-invasive device to measure cardiac output in participants with COPD.
Santos C, et al[85]	Randomized controlled trial	34 subjects with stable mild to very severe COPD were divided into two treatment groups. Mean age 67.	Group 1: 30 minutes 3x/wk of treadmill training at 60% of workload max for 20 sessions. Group 2: 30 minutes, 3x/week at 80% of workload max for 20 sessions. Both groups also performed strength training and flexibility training and attended education sessions.	Both groups improved in quality of life, dyspnea, endurance, and strength greater than the known MCID for each outcome measure. There was not a statistical significant difference between the two groups.	The high-intensity workload was continuous, not interval, treadmill training at 80% of workload max found on a CPET. Other studies used discontinuous 100% to 120% of work load on a CPET. This study found that both moderate (60%) and high-intensity (80%) exercise improved quality of life, symptom control, and exercise tolerance.
Gruber, W, et al[86]	Non-randomized parallel group study	43 patients with cystic fibrosis. Interval training group included participants with Sao_2 values <90% at rest or at low levels of exercise. Standard exercise group included participants with Sao_2 values >90%	Interval training was 10 intervals of 30 sec of exercise and 60 sec of rest, totaling 16-min sessions, 5x/week for 6 weeks. Intensity was a comfortable walking pace of 3–4 km/hr at an incline of 50%	Absolute and relative Vo_{2peak}, and VE_{peak} significantly increased in both groups. Standard exercise program had a longer exercise time per session and had a superior improvement in Vo_{2peak}	The participants assigned to the IT group had more severe lung disease and were deemed inappropriate for the usual pulmonary rehabilitation program. In this more compromised group,

Evidence Summary Table 12.6 Exercise Training Intensity: Interval Versus Continuous Exercise—cont'd

Reference	Design	Subjects	Interventions	Results	Comments
		Mean age 26; mean BMI 17	max grade on steep ramped exercise test. Standard exercise program was 45 min of treadmill and sports participation at approximately 60%–70% of Vo_2 from a cycle exercise test 5x/week for 6 weeks.	and peak work.	interval training was shown to be effective in improving their functional abilities.
Butcher, S, et al[87]	Randomized cross-over design	14 subjects with moderate to severe COPD, 49–78 years, BMI 23–33, FEV1 46%–75% predicted	Steep ramp anaerobic test (SRAT) vs cardiopulmonary exercise test (CPET) for prescription of exercise intensity	Exercise intensities that used SRAT results found peak work rates to be 204% of the work rates using the results of the CPET. Participants in using the HIIT protocol had an increase of 170% of time and 95% of work over the constant workload protocol.	Usual cardiopulmonary exercise testing using an increase of 5–15 watts per minute underestimates the peak work possible in patients with mod to severe COPD.
Klijn P, et al[88]	Randomized controlled study	110 subjects with severe and very severe COPD, mean ages 61, mean FEV1 % predicted 32, mean BMI 25 were divided into two groups	Exercise program 3x/wk for 10 weeks. Group 1: nonlinear periodized exercise (NLPE), including high-volume, low-intensity exercise at 50%–60% work max and low-volume, high-intensity exercise at 100%–120% of work max. Group 2 began with 10 minutes of 30% work max and progressed to 24 minutes at 75% work max.	Improved cycle time, improved dyspnea, decreased fatigue and increased CRQ scores in both groups, significantly greater improvement in the NLPE group. Fat free mass increased minimally but significantly in the NLPE group.	Participants with severe and very severe COPD and low fat free body mass benefit from a tailored training program to improve muscle efficiency and preserve muscle mass, improve endurance, decrease dyspnea and increase quality of life scores.

BMI = Body mass index; COPD = Chronic obstructive pulmonary disease; CRQ = Chronic Respiratory Questionnaire; FEV1 = Forced expiratory volume in 1 second; IT = interval training; Vo_2 = volume of oxygen consumed.

maintain continuous exercise for 20 to 30 minutes. Oscillating between high-intensity exercise and low-intensity or rest periods can be used to accomplish a total of 20 to 30 minutes of discontinuous exercise.

Frequency

The frequency of exercise refers to the number of sessions performed on a weekly basis during the exercise-training period. The frequency of exercise is often dependent on the intensity that can be achieved and the duration that can be maintained. If 20 to 30 minutes of continuous aerobic exercise can be accomplished using a moderate intensity, three to five evenly spaced workouts per week are recommended. More frequent exercise sessions are recommended for patients with lower functional abilities. One to two daily sessions are advisable for patients with very low functional work capacities.

Pulmonary Rehabilitation

Exercise Training

A pulmonary rehabilitation exercise session includes the following components: check-in, warm-up, exercise at the prescribed intensity, and cool-down. The check-in period is a time to obtain baseline data, including resting HR, RR, BP, oxygen saturation, auscultation of the lungs, and weight. It is also the time to discuss medication schedules, any problems the patient may have encountered since last visit, and any changes that need to be addressed by a member of the pulmonary rehabilitation team, such as a change in expiratory flow rates, cough, or sputum production. Pulmonary function tests assessed with a handheld device may be performed pre- and post-exercise during a pulmonary rehabilitation session to assess the impact of the maintenance medication. Patients who use a rescue inhaler should carry this with them during the exercise session. If a patient was found to have a significant decrease in oxygenation on their exercise test, supplemental oxygen should be readied before initiation of physical activity.

The warm-up component is a time to slowly increase the HR and BP to ready the cardiovascular, pulmonary, and musculoskeletal systems for aerobic exercise. For those patients with mild to moderate lung disease who had a cardiovascular end point to their exercise test, the warm-up is usually accomplished by performing the same mode of exercise that will be used in the aerobic portion of the program but at a lower intensity, with an emphasis on controlled breathing. For example, cycling with no resistance could be used as a warm-up activity for a biking program. The warm-up for patients performing continuous exercise lasts approximately 5 minutes. For patients with severe lung disease who are prescribed short bursts of high-intensity exercise, there is little opportunity for a warm-up.

The exercise portion of the pulmonary rehabilitation session consists of a mode or modes of activity at the appropriate intensity for the advised duration. This portion of the program lasts for at least 20 minutes of either continuous or discontinuous activity. Participant monitoring can be accomplished using RPE and RPD scales, and measures of HR, RR, and Sa_{O_2} (oximetry).

The training period should be followed immediately by a cool-down period consisting of a slow decline in exercise intensity after the patient completes the exercise duration prescribed. This may consist of 5 to 10 minutes of low-level activities that slowly return the cardiovascular system to near pre-exercise levels or ramping down of the intensity of short bouts of exercise.

Finally, stretching exercises are performed to maintain joint and muscle integrity and to help prevent injury. Stretching exercises should be performed during exhalation to prevent a Valsalva maneuver, which would worsen a participant's pulmonary capabilities and put undue stress on the cardiac system. Patients often use accessory muscles of ventilation during the exercise program; therefore, the muscles of the neck and UEs should be incorporated into the stretching program.

Strength Training

Extremity Strength Training

While cardiopulmonary endurance training through continuous or discontinuous exercise is the mainstay of pulmonary rehabilitation, generalized strength training has been found to counter the systemic effects of COPD that result in peripheral and ventilatory muscle weakness. Strength of both UEs and LEs has been shown to increase with appropriate training. Weight training of the targeted muscle groups has been prescribed in a variety of ways. Vonbank et al[94] improved work capacity by using a training load that allowed for 8 to 15 repetitions before fatigue. A number of strengthening methods have been used, including free weights, isokinetic devices, stair climbing, high resistance on a cycle ergometer, and Theraband.[95,96] Regardless of the mode used for strengthening, patients should be encouraged to perform these exercises during the exhalation phase of ventilation, thus refraining from a Valsalva maneuver that may impair ventilation and affect exercise performance.

Inspiratory Muscle Training

Patients with COPD may have weak inspiratory muscles that translate into breathlessness and exercise limitations.[90] In the presence of inspiratory muscle weakness, defined as a PI_{max} of less than 60 mm Hg, many research studies have demonstrated the ability to increase inspiratory muscle strength using threshold loading devices.[97-105] Inspiratory muscle training devices provide resistance to the inspiratory phase of ventilation in order to increase the strength of these muscles. Figure 12.14 shows one type of inspiratory muscle training device (Philips Healthcare, Andover, MA). Inspiratory muscle training has also been studied for its ability to alter the perception of dyspnea. A number of researchers have demonstrated a decrease in the severity of dyspnea during the

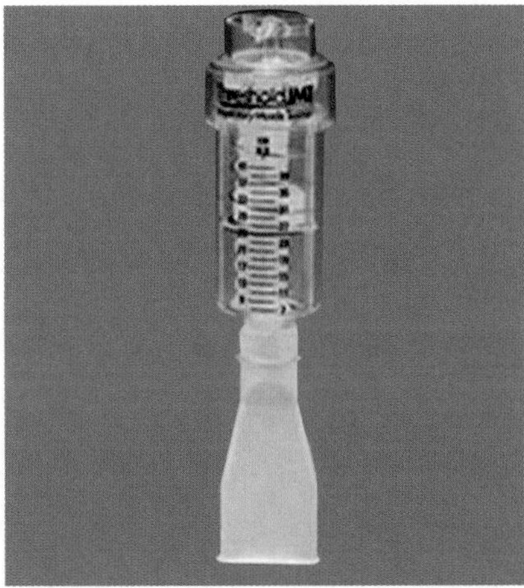

Figure 12.14 A threshold inspiratory muscle trainer for the use in improving strength and endurance of the muscles of inspiration. *(Courtesy of Philips Healthcare, Andover, MA 01810.)*

performance of ADL and exercise with inspiratory muscle training.[99,102,104,105] The use of inspiratory muscle training should be made based on the patient's type of disease, severity of disease, presence of inspiratory muscle weakness, level of dyspnea, and motivation to participate.[90] Just as there are continuous versus interval training for the general exercise portion of pulmonary rehabilitation, these two options have also been reported for inspiratory muscle training. Continuous inspiratory muscle training uses a submaximal training load, as low as 10% of the patient's PI_{max} for a prolonged duration of up to 20 to 30 minutes. Progression of this exercise prescription is to slowly increase the training load over time, upward to 60% of the initial IP_{max}.[97] Interval training uses a higher load, up to maximum load tolerable, for short bursts of 2 to 3 minutes of exercise interspersed rests of 1 to 2 minutes.[105] Both types of protocols have shown that improvements in respiratory muscle function and decreases in dyspnea. There is also literature that shows an increase in functional mobility with training of the inspiratory muscles.[105]

Exercise Progression

Exercise progression is appropriate when the individual perceives the exercise session to be easier (lower RPE or RPD) or when the same exercise workload is performed with a lower HR—that is, when physiological adaptation to exercise has occurred.

Exercise progression should first be directed toward increasing the number of continuous minutes of exercise and decreasing the amount of time spent in low-intensity exercise or rest periods. When 20 minutes of continuous activity can be accomplished, an increase in exercise duration or intensity can be proposed. Frequency should be adjusted as necessary, based on duration and intensity.

Program Duration

Improved exercise tolerance can occur in multiple settings: an inpatient rehabilitation hospital program, an outpatient pulmonary rehabilitation program, or a home-based program.[3] Because of the limited length of stay for many inpatient rehabilitation hospital admissions, most increases in functional capacity occur in an outpatient or home pulmonary rehabilitation program. Generally, conditioning exercises are conducted up to three times per week over a course of 6 to 12 weeks.[90] At the end of the rehabilitation program, QOL measurements, dyspnea measurements, and functional assessments (6MWT or ISWT) should be readministered to assess the benefits of pulmonary rehabilitation for each participant. Exercise abilities gained in a pulmonary rehabilitation program have been found to gradually decline over 12 to 18 months following completion of the program. Pulmonary rehabilitation programs that last longer than 12 weeks have shown greater sustained benefits than shorter programs.[90]

An unfortunate reality is that patients with pulmonary dysfunction often have decreased exercise ability following an exacerbation of their disease. There is evidence to support a reduction in dyspnea in patients who repeat pulmonary rehabilitation after an acute exacerbation of their COPD.[106]

Home Exercise Programs

A home exercise program (HEP) should begin while the participant is enrolled in a pulmonary rehabilitation program. When deemed appropriate (based on exercise response and laboratory data), the participant can be assigned home exercise activities. The patient uses an exercise log to record parameters such as exercise HRs, RPEs, RPD, exercise workloads, and any questions that may arise about the HEP (Fig. 12.15). At regular intervals, the therapist analyzes the data and adjusts the HEP as necessary. Progression to an independent HEP is an important rehabilitation goal to promote a participant's lifelong commitment to exercise.

Multispecialty Team

Although exercise training is integral to pulmonary rehabilitation, participants may require additional services and information to optimize their exercise capability and to improve quality of life. The pulmonary rehabilitation team may consist of a number of health care providers. While professional roles may overlap, each team member brings their own level of expertise to the participants in a pulmonary rehabilitation program. Team members may include nurses, for their expertise with medication regimens; respiratory therapists, for their knowledge of oxygen delivery systems and independent secretion removal devices; occupational therapists to teach energy conservation during the performance of activities of daily living; dieticians for nutritional support; social workers for

Activity Log

Week of: ____________

Aerobic exercise

	Monday	Tuesday	Wednesday	Thursday	Friday	Saturday	Sunday
Mode							
Average HR							
Average RPE							
Average dyspnea							
Start time							
End time							
Comments:							

Strengthening exercise:

	Monday	Tuesday	Wednesday	Thursday	Friday	Saturday	Sunday
Type							
Weight							
# of reps							
Comments:							

Figure 12.15 An exercise log that can be used to follow a patient's ability to exercise both during and independent of the pulmonary rehabilitation program.

community resources and counseling; exercise physiologists for exercise prescription and implementation; and physicians for overall care management. All of these professionals may not be present at each session of a pulmonary rehabilitation program, but the ability to refer participants to these professionals will improve overall care. The following sections address other elements of a pulmonary rehabilitation program: patient education, secretion removal techniques, and *activity pacing*. Smoking cessation should also be considered as a component of pulmonary rehabilitation. (See the section on smoking cessation in the medical management section of this chapter.)

Patient Education

The concept of self-management is promoted in the individual and group educational sessions of a pulmonary rehabilitation program.[90] Participants are given individual, one-on-one time to identify their own needs and address issues that are particular to themselves. Benefits from group discussions include support from peers regarding the patient's feelings or needs, learning from others' experiences and questions, and the socialization that only a group can provide. Key components of a patient's education program are presented in Box 12.3.

Education makes it possible for patients to assume the responsibility for their own wellness. A patient will carry out the required activities to produce the desired outcome only if the patient knows what to do, knows how to do it, and also wants to do it. This theory of self-efficacy for the patient with pulmonary disease begins with a daily routine that includes self-assessment, adherence to a medication schedule, performance of airway clearance techniques, ADL with pacing, and an appropriate HEP.

Self-assessment is used to recognize the first signs of an exacerbation of the disease: increased dyspnea, decreased exercise tolerance, change in pulmonary flow rates, sputum color or consistency, pedal edema, or any other significant change from baseline. An *exacerbation protocol* is an individually devised set of instructions

Box 12.3 Education Topics

Anatomy and physiology of respiratory disease
Airway clearance techniques
Nutritional guidelines
Energy-saving techniques
Stress management and relaxation
Benefits of being smoke free
Impact of environmental factors on COPD
Pharmacology/use of MDIs
Oxygen delivery systems
Psychosocial aspects of COPD
Diagnostic techniques
Management of COPD
Community resources
Exercise: Effects, contraindications, adherence

COPD = Chronic obstructive pulmonary disease; MDIs = Metered dose inhalers.

consistent with the participant's disease and abilities. These instructions may include the use of airway clearance techniques, pacing techniques, or a change in the exercise prescription, as well as contact with the primary care physician for a review of symptoms and pharmacological management.

Once the patient has completed a pulmonary rehabilitation program, continued support through community exercise groups is essential to maintaining the new level of physical activity obtained with pulmonary rehabilitation.[3] Access to new information and continued support is possible through groups such as the *Better Breathing Club*, sponsored by the American Lung Association. See Appendix 12.A, Web-Based Resources for Clinicians, Families, and Patients With Chronic Pulmonary Dysfunction.

Secretion Removal Techniques

Secretion retention can interfere with ventilation and the diffusion of oxygen and carbon dioxide in some patients with pulmonary disease. Patients with secretion retention may improve their exercise performance if proper secretion removal techniques have been performed before the physical activity. An individualized program for secretion removal directed to the areas of involvement can optimize ventilation and therefore gas exchange capabilities. Secretion removal techniques include programs that rely on a caregiver (postural drainage, percussion, and shaking) or independent programs, such as the active cycle of breathing technique (ACBT); positive expiratory pressure (PEP) devices, such as the TheraPEP® PEP Therapy System (Smiths Medical, Dublin, OH); airway oscillation devices, such as the Flutter® (Cardinal Health, Dublin, OH), or the Acapella® (Smiths Medical, Dublin, OH); or high-frequency chest compression (HFCC) devices, such as the Vest® System (Hill-Rom, St. Paul, MN).

Manual Secretion Removal Techniques

Postural Drainage

Positioning a patient so that the bronchus of the involved lung segment is perpendicular to the ground is the basis for *postural drainage*. Using gravity, these positions assist the mucociliary transport system in removing excessive secretions from the tracheobronchial tree. Standard postural drainage positions are presented in Figure 12.16. Although these postural drainage positions are optimal for gravity drainage of specific lung segments, such positioning may not be realistic for some patients. Modification of these standard positions may prevent any untoward effects yet still enhance secretion removal. Box 12.4 lists precautions that should be considered before instituting postural drainage with patients with signs and symptoms of increased daily pulmonary secretions. These are not absolute contraindications, but relative precautions. The list is not meant to be inclusive; however, it does provide a range of considerations that should be addressed before instituting postural drainage.

Percussion

Percussion is a force rhythmically applied with the therapist's cupped hands to the patient's chest wall. The percussion technique is applied to specific areas on the thorax that corresponds to an underlying involved lung segments. The technique is typically administered for 3 to 5 minutes over each involved lung segment. Percussion is thought to release the pulmonary secretions from the wall of the airways and into the lumen of the airway. By coupling percussion with the appropriate postural drainage position for a specific lung segment, the probability of secretion removal is enhanced. Because percussion is a force directed to the thorax, there are conditions that would necessitate caution with this technique, such as a fractured rib, a flail chest, osteoporosis, elevated coagulation studies, or a decreased platelet count. These examples are by no means inclusive, but they provide some patient presentations that might require modification (a gentler force applied to the thorax) or elimination of the percussion technique.

Shaking

Following a deep inhalation, a bouncing maneuver is applied with the therapist's open hands to the rib cage throughout the expiratory phase of breathing. This *shaking* is applied to a specific area on the thorax that corresponds to the underlying involved lung segment. Five to seven deep breaths with shaking on exhalation are appropriate to hasten the removal of secretions via the mucociliary transport system. Shaking is commonly used following percussion in the appropriate postural drainage position. Because this technique consists of a force applied to the thorax, the same circulatory and musculoskeletal considerations are needed as in the application of percussion.

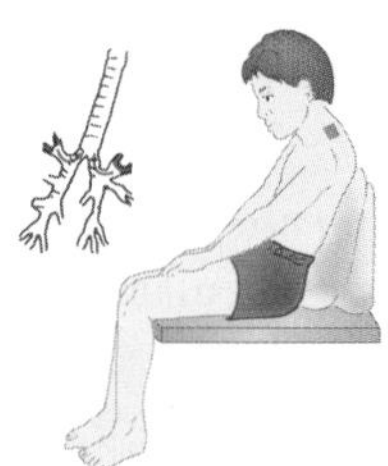

UPPER LOBES Apical Segments

Bed or drainage table flat.

Patient leans back on pillow at 30° angle against therapist.

Therapist claps with markedly cupped hand over area between clavicle and top of scapula on each side.

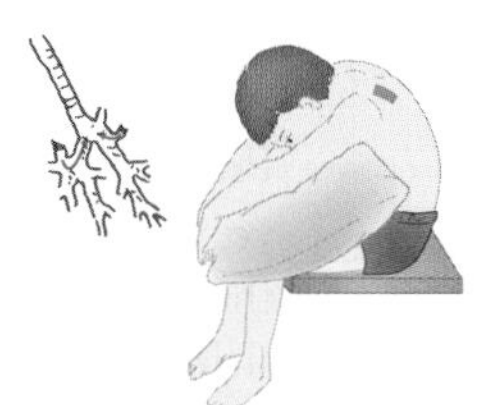

UPPER LOBES Posterior Segments

Bed or drainage table flat.

Patient leans over folded pillow at 30° angle.

Therapist stands behind and claps over upper back on both sides.

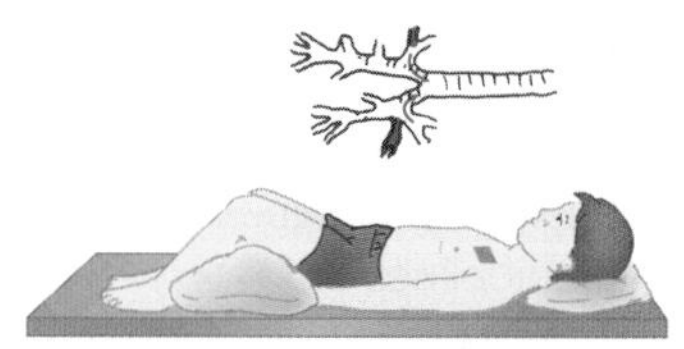

UPPER LOBES Anterior Segments

Bed or drainage table flat.

Patient lies on back with pillow under knees.

Therapist claps between clavicle and nipple on each side.

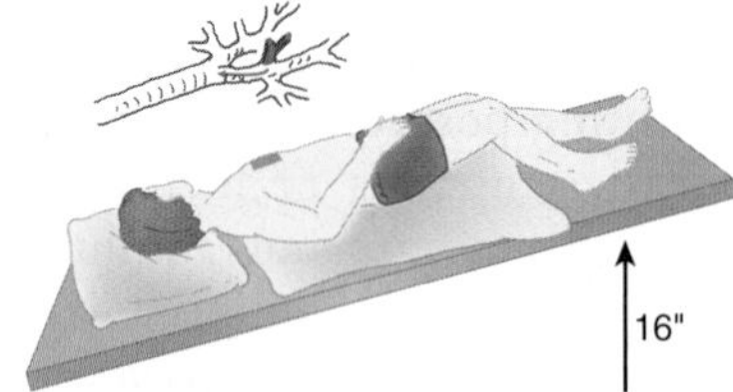

RIGHT MIDDLE LOBE

Foot of table or bed elevated 16 inches.

Patient lies head down on left side and rotates 1/4 turn backward. Pillow may be placed behind from shoulder to hip. Knees should be flexed.

Therapist claps over right nipple area. In females with breast development or tenderness use cupped hand with heel of hand under armpit and fingers extending forward beneath the breast.

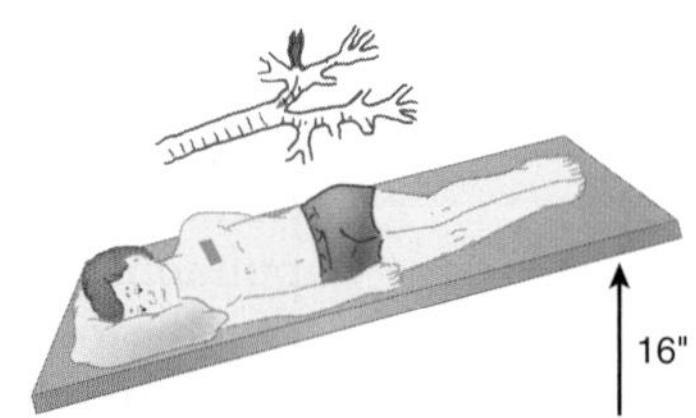

LEFT UPPER LOBE Singular Segments

Foot of table or bed elevated 16 inches.

Patient lies head down on right side and rotates 1/4 turn backward. Pillow may be placed behind from shoulder to hip. Knees should be flexed.

Therapist claps with moderately cupped hand over left nipple area. In females with breast development or tenderness use cupped hand with heel of hand under armpit and fingers extending forward beneath the breast.

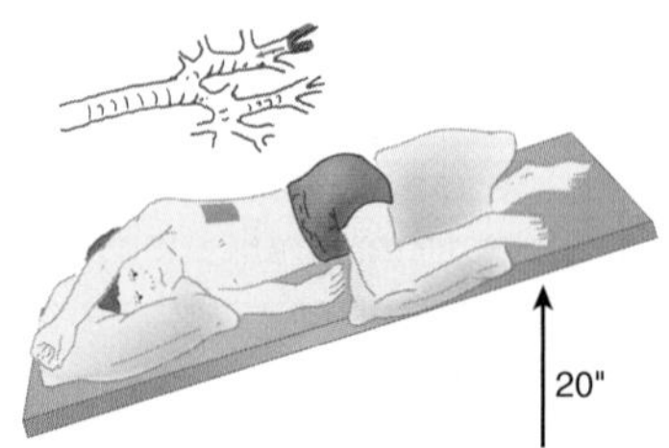

LOWER LOBES Anterior Basal Segments

Foot of table or bed elevated 20 inches.

Patient lies on side, head down, pillow under knees.

Therapist claps with slightly cupped hand over lower ribs. (Position shown is for drainage of left anterior basal segment. To drain the right anterior basal segment, patient should be on the left side in same posture).

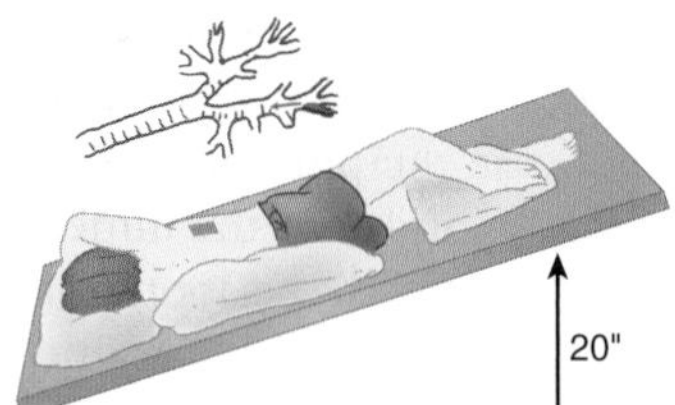

LOWER LOBES Lateral Basal Segments

Foot of table or bed elevated 20 inches.

Patient lies on abdomen, head down, then rotates 1/4 turn upward. Upper leg is flexed over pillow for support.

Therapist claps over uppermost portion of lower ribs. (Position shown is for drainage of right lateral basal segment. To drain the left lateral basal segment, patient should lie on the right side in the same posture).

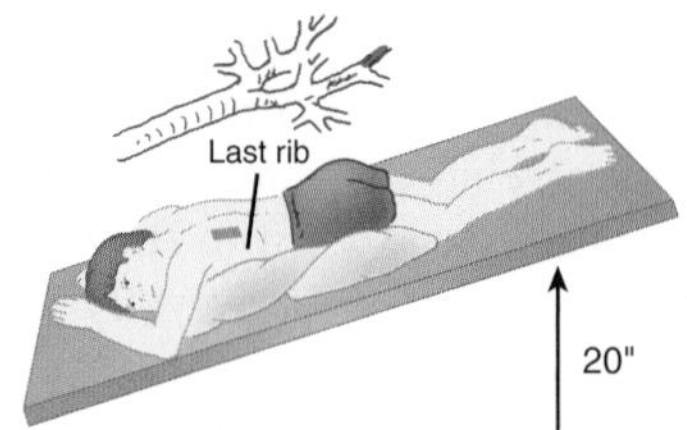

LOWER LOBES Posterior Basal Segments

Foot of table or bed elevated 20 inches.

Patient lies on abdomen, head down, with pillow under hips.

Therapist claps over lower ribs close to spine on each side.

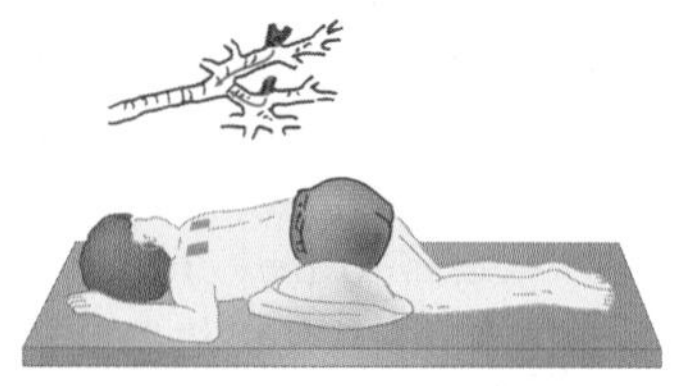

LOWER LOBES Superior Segments

Bed of table flat.

Patient lies on abdomen with two pillows under hips.

Therapist claps over middle of back at tip of scapula on either side of spine.

Figure 12.16 Positions used for postural drainage. *(From Roy, S, Wolf, S, and Scalzitti, D: The Rehabilitation Specialist's Handbook, ed 4. FA Davis, Philadelphia, 2013, with permission.)*

Airway Clearance

Once the secretions have been mobilized with postural drainage, percussion, and shaking, the task of removing the secretions from the airways is undertaken using an airway clearance technique. *Coughing* is the most common and easiest means of clearing the airway. However, it should be noted that high intrathoracic pressures, such as those generated during coughing, could force the closing of small airways in some patients with obstructive pulmonary diseases. By trapping air behind the closed airway, the forced expulsion of air during a cough becomes ineffective in clearing secretions. *Huffing* is an alternative method of airway clearance that is useful for patients with obstructive pulmonary disease. A huff uses many of the same steps of coughing, without creating the high intrathoracic pressures. The patient is asked to take a deep breath and then rapidly contract the abdominal muscles while forcefully saying "HA HA HA." This allows a forced expiration through a stabilized open airway and makes secretion removal more effective.[107]

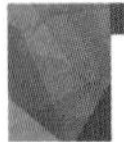

Box 12.4 Precautions for Postural Drainage

Precautions for the use of the Trendelenburg position

Circulatory: congestive heart failure, hypertension
Pulmonary: pulmonary edema, shortness of breath made worse with Trendelenberg position (head of bed lower than foot)
Abdominal: obesity, abdominal distention, hiatal hernia, nausea, recent food consumption

Precautions for the use of the side-lying position

Vascular: axillofemoral bypass graft
Musculoskeletal: arthritis, recent rib fracture, shoulder bursitis, or tendonitis, any conditioning that would make appropriate postural drainage positioning uncomfortable

Active Cycle of Breathing Techniques

ACBT is an independent breathing exercise program the patient can perform to clear secretions from the airways. This technique includes three phases: (1) a breathing control phase, (2) a thoracic expansion phase, and (3) a forced expiratory technique. ACBT begins with a few minutes at the breathing control phase, defined as relaxed, diaphragmatic, tidal volume breathing. From this breathing control phase, the patient determines what to do next. If secretions need to be loosened, the patient will perform three to four thoracic expansion exercises, defined as three to five deep inhalations with a 3-second hold followed by a passive exhalation. A return to the breathing control phase follows, which can last for a few seconds to a few minutes, while the patient assesses themselves and makes a decision of what is next needed. If the patient feels that there are secretions ready to be moved more proximally, then the forced expiratory technique completes the cycle. The forced expiratory technique, defined as one or two huffs from tidal volume down to low lung volumes, is used to move secretions into the larger, more proximal airways. The forced expiratory technique is followed by a period of breathing control for rest and reassessment. If secretions are not ready to be expelled, the patient may return to thoracic expansion exercises. Using ACBT, secretions are "milked" from smaller to larger airways. Once the secretions have moved into the larger airways, huffs from mid or high lung volumes remove the secretions from the airways. This independent technique has been demonstrated to be as effective as postural drainage, percussion, and shaking.[108] Figure 12.17 emphasizes that the patient begins at breathing control and always returns to breathing control for rest and the patient's own assessment of his or her status before moving to either thoracic expansion with breath hold or the forced expiratory technique.

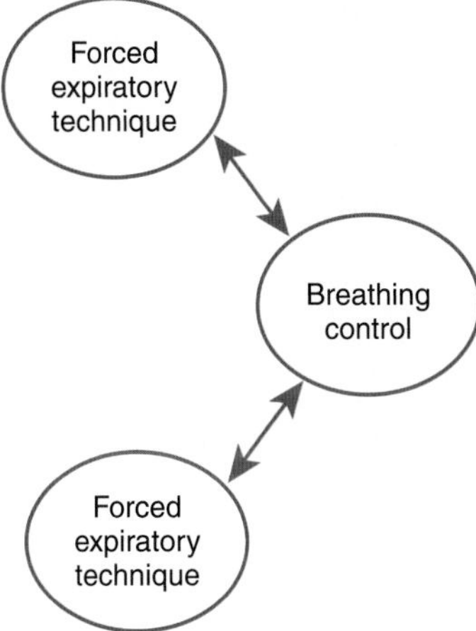

Figure 12.17 Active cycle of breathing begins with breathing control. All choices are made from the breathing control phase. After each choice is made, thoracic expansion or forced expiratory technique, the patient returns to breathing control to rest and make the next choice.

Oral Airway Oscillation Devices

Airway oscillation devices, such as the Flutter® or the Acapella® (Fig. 12.18), alter the exhaled airflow throughout the airways. The patient first inhales a normal size breath. During active exhalation through the device, the exhaled air causes an intermittent backward air pressure that oscillates the airways. The usual procedure is to exhale 10 or so breaths through the device, followed by 2 large exhaled volumes through the device and finally a huff or cough to clear mobilized secretions. This routine is repeated until secretions are cleared from the lungs. An airway oscillation device has been shown to help in the removal of secretions from airways.[109,110]

Positive Expiratory Pressure

PEP devices have a valve to regulate expiratory resistance (Fig. 12.19). Inhalation of a normal size breath through the mask or mouthpiece is unresisted. Active exhalation is against a positive expiratory pressure, measuring 10 to

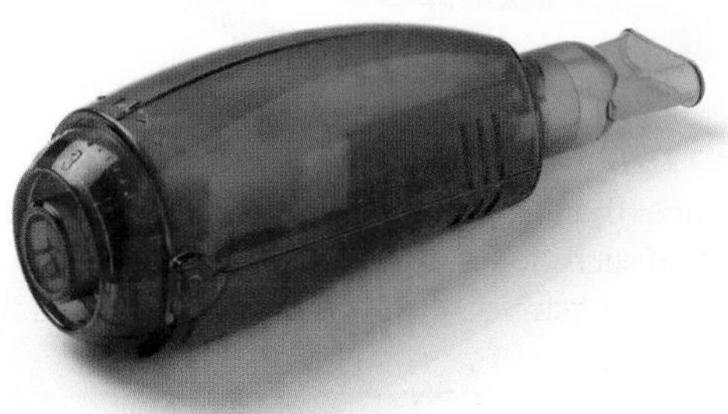

Figure 12.18 The acapella device used for an independent program of secretion removal. *(Courtesy of Smith Medical, Dublin, OH 43017.)*

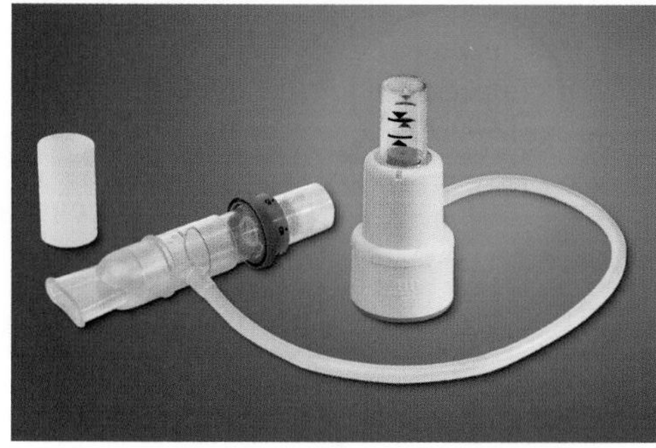

Figure 12.19 The PEP system for an independent program of secretion removal. *(Courtesy of Smith Medical, Dublin OH, 43017.)*

20 cm H_2O. A treatment session lasts approximately 10 to 20 minutes with frequent pauses to remove the mask or mouthpiece so that the patient can cough or huff to clear secretions. The session is completed when all secretions have been cleared from the airways. PEP has been shown to be as effective as postural drainage, percussion, and shaking.[111,112]

High-Frequency Chest Compression Devices

The high-frequency chest compression (HFCC) device uses an inflatable vest with air channels that is worn over the patient's thorax (Fig. 12.20). The vest is attached to an air compressor that rapidly delivers small air volumes in and out of the vest. The inflation of the vest causes compression to the chest wall and the deflation allows the chest wall to recoil back to its resting position. The patient assumes a comfortable seated position for treatments lasting between 20 and 30 minutes. Secretions may be cleared at any time throughout the treatment. HFCC has been shown to be as effective as other secretion removal techniques.[113]

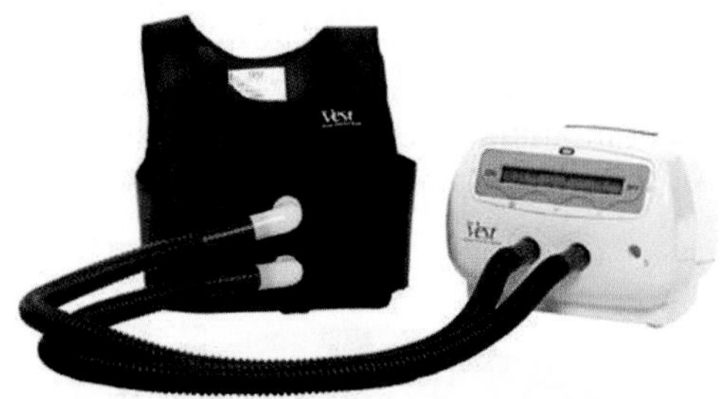

Figure 12.20 The high-frequency chest wall compression device (the Vest) can be used for an independent program of secretion removal. *(Courtesy of Hill-Rom, St. Paul, MN 55126.)*

Breathing Exercises

Pursed-lip breathing involves an unresisted inspiration followed by an active oral exhalation through a narrowed (or pursed) mouth opening. When pursed-lip breathing is used by patients with COPD, it may delay or prevent airway collapse, allowing for better gas exchange.[114,115] Most patients demonstrate this strategy during periods of dyspnea and rarely need to be taught the technique.

Although diaphragmatic breathing has been taught to patients with chronic pulmonary dysfunction for years, there is little evidence to support its use to improve pulmonary mechanics.[115] Some patients require the use of accessory muscles with exercise, with exacerbation of their disease, or with periods of dyspnea. Strengthening accessory muscles of ventilation may be a more effective treatment program than encouraging the use of an ineffective diaphragm with little ability to generate muscle force and/or limited muscle excursion. In patients with very flattened diaphragms, focusing on diaphragmatic breathing may even be detrimental.

Activity Pacing

Activity pacing refers to the performance of any activity within the limits or boundaries of that patient's breathing capacity. For example, an activity that usually causes dyspnea needs to be broken down into component parts such that each component can be performed at a rate that does not exceed breathing abilities. By breaking activities down into component parts and interspersing rest periods between each component, the total activity can be completed without dyspnea or undo fatigue. For example, patients often find that climbing stairs causes a great deal of dyspnea and discomfort. Rather than climbing the entire flight of stairs (usually done too fast and with a breath hold), the patient might be instructed as follows: "Take a deep breath. Now, on exhalation, walk up one (or two or three) stair(s). Now recover. Take in another good breath and walk up the next one (or two or three) stair(s) and recover. Repeat this technique until the flight of stairs is completed." The patient is able to reach the top of the stairs without becoming dyspneic and without undue fatigue. Pacing can and should be part of every activity that would otherwise cause dyspnea. Pacing should be used when performing ADL, ambulation, stair climbing, and other daily tasks. Pacing is not a technique to be used during the aerobic portion of a pulmonary rehabilitation program. During exercise, some shortness of breath is expected to occur.

SUMMARY

Pulmonary rehabilitation is a well-established treatment for patients with chronic pulmonary disease. Components of these programs typically include exercise training, strength training, education, secretion removal instruction, and psychosocial support. Outcomes of pulmonary rehabilitation may include increased aerobic capacity, increased skeletal muscle strength, reduced dyspnea both during exercise and ADL, and an increase in the perception of health-related quality of life. Gains made in pulmonary rehabilitation programs can make the difference between a lifestyle of dependence and one of independence. Physical therapists have the important role of evaluating patients, determining their potential, and, through exercise prescription and exercise programs, ensuring that rehabilitation goals and outcomes are realized.

Questions for Review

1. How does the clinical presentation of obstructive lung disease differ from the clinical presentation of restrictive lung disease?
2. Explain how altered airway structure leads to airflow limitation.
3. (a) What would be the expected breath sounds of a patient with COPD? Describe intensity and adventitious sounds. (b) What would be the expected breath sounds of a patient with asthma during an exacerbation? Describe intensity and adventitious sounds.
4. Identify the tests and measures required to determine the extent of pulmonary disease.
5. What are the pulmonary end points to a symptom-limited graded exercise test?
6. How does exercise prescription differ for a patient with mild pulmonary disease as compared to the patient with severe pulmonary disease?
7. (a) How do you know when to progress a patient's exercise program? (b) What is the nature of that progression? (c) Do you need a new ETT to progress a patient's exercise workload?
8. How would you respond to a patient's comment that it would take longer to climb stairs with pacing than without?
9. Design a secretion removal treatment plan for a patient with CF that can be carried out independently before coming to pulmonary rehabilitation.
10. What evidence is presented in the current literature regarding the benefits of pulmonary rehabilitation?

CASE STUDY

PATIENT WITH COPD

A 67-year-old white female was admitted to the hospital with a COPD exacerbation. She was treated with noninvasive ventilation for 2 days, inhaled bronchodilators, and intravenous antibiotics and corticosteroids. After the acute care hospital stay of 7 days, the patient was transferred to an inpatient rehabilitation facility for 7 days. She is now referred to outpatient pulmonary rehabilitation.

PAST MEDICAL HISTORY

COPD with exacerbations numbering 2 per year for the past 3 years, s/p lumpectomy of right breast 8 years ago, smoking history of 45 pack/years; quit on the day of this admission to hospital for acute bacterial pneumonia.

MEDICATIONS

2 L/min of oxygen by nasal cannula. Maintenance: Spiriva ([Tiatroprium, a long-acting muscarinic antagonist [anticholinergic] [LAMA]), Serevent (Salmeterol, a long-acting beta agonist [LABA]), Flovent (fluticasone, an inhaled corticosteroid). Rescue: Albuterol (short-acting beta-2 adrenergic [SABA]).

OCCUPATION

Secretary, works 32 hours/week. Presently on medical leave.

SOCIAL AND ENVIRONMENTAL

Lives with husband in own home. Three steps to enter home, 12 stairs within the home.

OBJECTIVE FINDINGS

Interview

Mental status: awake, alert, talks in three- to four-word sentences. Adequate historian. Chief complaint: shortness of breath limiting function. Patient is able to walk 120 ft before needing to rest to catch her breath. No complaints of increased secretions. Patient is dependent in shopping, house cleaning, and laundry.

Dyspnea and Quality of Life Measures

mMRC grade 3

COPD assessment test (CAT) score of 28

Patient Goal:

Patient's desired functional outcome is to be oxygen free and able to care for grandchildren without shortness of breath.

Resting Vital Signs

HR 72, BP 96/74, Sao_2 at rest 86% on room air, 93% on 2 L/min pulsed O_2 on 1 pulse/breath, respiratory rate 32, temperature 98.5°F.

Observation, Inspection, Palpation

Thin, frail-looking female wearing nasal cannula; kyphosis noted. Patient uses posture of forward sitting with arms supported on chair arms to enhance ventilatory accessory muscle use. Increased AP diameter of thorax, accessory muscle use at rest; labored, symmetrical breathing pattern with pursed-lip breathing. No venous distention, no edema, no cyanosis, minimal clubbing evident.

Auscultation

Decreased breath sounds throughout both lung fields, especially at bases. End expiratory wheezes at left lateral base.

Strength

The 5 times sit to stand test resulted in 24.3 seconds.

Bilateral shoulder elevation, abduction, and extension, elbow flexion and extension area are all graded as greater than or equal to a 3/5, tested in the upright sitting position. Patient unable to lie prone or supine for further testing secondary to orthopnea. Maximal resistance was not applied in order to avoid Valsalva.

Maximal inspiratory effort (PI_{max}) – 42 mm Hg.

Exercise Test Data

Patient performed a 5-minute, staged exercise test using a cycle ergometer. The test began with 3 minutes of rest sitting on the cycle. The exercise began with stage 1: 3 minutes of unresisted pedaling. Each subsequent stage was 1 minute with an increase of 15 watts. Max workload was 30 watts. ECG was within normal limits.

	Rest	Peak
HR beats/min	84	121
BP mm Hg	128/76	156/80
RR breaths/min	24	36
Tidal volume in liters	.32	.99
Sao_2 on 2 L nasal cannula	98%	93%
RPE on 0 to 10 scale	1	7
RPD on 0–10 scale	3	8
FEV_1 in l/sec	1.107 (45% predicted)	1.074
FVC in L	1.76 (64% predicted)	1.68
FEV_1/FVC	62%	
Predicted maximal minute ventilation (V_E) 35 × FEV_1	38.7 L/min	
Actual V_E in L/min	7.68	35.64

Breaths/min × L/breath

6-Minute Walk Test: 200 m on 2 L O_2 by nasal cannula.

GUIDING QUESTIONS

1. In what stage of GOLD does this patient present?
2. Did the pulmonary system or cardiovascular system stop her exercise test?
3. (a) Identify this patient's impairments, functional limitations, and disability restrictions. (b) Identify general anticipated treatment goals and expected outcomes for a 3-month (12-week) pulmonary rehabilitation program. (c) Identify outcome measures that will be used to assess the effectiveness of a pulmonary rehabilitation program.
4. (a) Formulate a physical therapy plan of care for week 1. Patient will be seen 3 times/week for this first week of therapy. (b) Briefly describe exercise progression for the first month of the program.

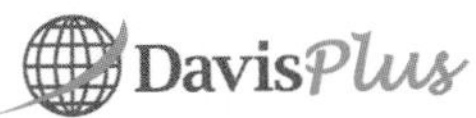

For additional resources, including answers to the questions for review and case study guiding questions, please visit **http://davisplus.fadavis.com.**

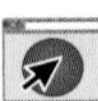

The reader is referred to video **Case Study 1 Critical Care Patient with COPD and Acute Respiratory Distress Syndrome** for additional review and study. The full written case study, including all tables, figures, charts, and three video segments (examination, intervention, and outcome) appears online at Davis*Plus*. The case study poses questions for the reader's consideration with suggested answers to the case study questions, also posted online at Davis*Plus*.

References

1. Hughes, R, and Davison, R: Limitation of exercise reconditioning in COLD. Chest 83:241,1983.
2. Pierce, A, et al: Responses to exercise training in patients with emphysema. Arch Intern Med 114:28, 1964.
3. Spruit, MA, et al: An official American Thoracic Society/European Respiratory Society Statement: Key concepts and advances in pulmonary rehabilitation. Am J Respir Crit Care Med 188(8):1011, 2013.
4. Dowman, L, et al: Pulmonary rehabilitation for interstitial lung disease. Cochrane Database of Systematic Reviews, 2014, Art. No.:CD006322.DOI:10.1002/14651858. CD006322.pub3
5. Global strategy for the diagnosis, management and prevention of COPD, global initiative for chronic obstructive lung disease (GOLD), 2016. Retrieved March, 2017, from www.goldcopd.org.
6. National asthma education and prevention program. Expert panel report 3: Guidelines for the diagnosis and management of asthma, 2007. Retrieved March 2017 from www.epa.gov/asthma/expert-panel-report-3-guidelines-diagnosis-and-management-asthma.
7. Brunetto, AF, and Alves, LA: Comparing peak and sustained values of maximal respiratory pressures in healthy subjects and chronic pulmonary disease patients. J Pneumol 29:208, 2003.
8. Rennard, SI, and Vestbo, J: COPD: The dangerous underestimate of 15%. Lancet 367(9478):2225, 2007.
9. Boueiz, A, et al: Genome-wide association study of the genetic determinants of emphysema distribution. Am J Respir Crit Care Med 195(6), 2017.
10. Chaouat, A, et al: Pulmonary hypertension in COPD. Eur Respir J 32:1371, 2008.
11. Angusti, A: Systemic effects of chronic obstructive pulmonary disease. What we know and what we don't know (but should). Proc Am Thorac Soc 4:522, 2007.
12. Celli, B, et al: The body-mass index, airflow obstruction, dyspnea, and exercise capacity index in chronic obstructive pulmonary disease. N Engl J Med 350:1005, 2004.
13. Centers for Disease Control and Prevention, National Center for Health Statistics. Asthma. Retrieved March 2017 from www.cdc.gov/nchs/fastats/asthma.htm.
14. Global Initiative for Asthma (GINA): Global strategy for asthma management and prevention. 2016. Retrieved March 2017 from http://ginasthma.org.
15. Busse, WW, et al: The role of viral respiratory infections in asthma and asthma exacerbations. Lancet 376(9743):826, 2010.
16. Cystic Fibrosis Foundation. Role of Genetics in CF. Retrieved March 2017 from https://www.cff.org.
17. Cystic Fibrosis Foundation. What is CF/Genetics/Genetic mutations. Retrieved March 2017 from https://www.cff.org.
18. Ratjen, F, and Doring, G: Cystic fibrosis. Lancet 361:681, 2003.
19. Cystic Fibrosis Foundation Patient Registry 2013. Retrieved March 2017 from https://www.cff.org/2013_CFF_Patient_Registry_Annual_Data_Report.pdf.
20. Schram, C: Atypical cystic fibrosis. Can Fam Physician 58(12):1341, 2012.
21. CFTR Science: Phenotypic factors: CFTR activity is an important influence on cystic fibrosis phenotype. Retrieved March 2017 from http://www.cftrscience.com/phenotypic-factors.
22. William, C, et al: Exercise training in children and adolescents with cystic fibrosis: Theory into practice. Int J Pediatr 2010. Retrieved March 2017 from https://www.ncbi.nlm.nih.gov/pmc/articles/PMC2945676 doi: 10.1155/2010/670640.
23. Collins, MS, et al: Improved pulmonary and growth outcomes in cystic fibrosis by newborn screening. Pediatr Pulmonal 43:648, 2008.
24. King, T: Approach to the adult with interstitial lung disease: Clinical evaluation. Retrieved March 2017 from www.uptodate.com.
25. Caminati, A, and Harari, S: IPF: New insight in diagnosis and prognosis. Respir Med 104:S2, 2010.
26. King, T: Treatment of idiopathic pulmonary fibrosis. Retrieved March 2017 from www.uptodate.com/contents/treatment-of-idiopathic-pulmonary-fibrosis.
27. King, T: Idiopathic interstitial pneumonias: Progress in classification, diagnosis, pathogenesis and management. Trans Am Clin Climatolo Assoc 115:43, 2004.
28. Benowitz, NL: Nicotine Addiction. N Engl J Med 362:2295, 2010.
29. Stead, L, et al: Nicotine replacement therapy for smoking cessation. Cochrane Database Systematic Reviews, 2012, Art. No.:CD000146. doi: 10.1002/14651858.CD000146.pub4.
30. Van Eerd, E, et al: Smoking cessation for people with chronic obstructive pulmonary disease. Cochrane Database of Systematic Reviews, 8, 2016. doi: 10.1002/14651858.CD010744.pub2.
31. Pothirat, C, et al: Evaluating inhaler use technique in COPD patients. Int J Chron Obstruct Pulmon Dis10:1291, 2015.
32. Melani, AS, et al: Inhaler mishandling remains common in real life and is associated with reduced disease control. Respir Med 105(6):9930, 2011.
33. Herath, SC, and Poole, P: Prophylactic antibiotic therapy for chronic obstructive pulmonary disease (COPD). Cochrane Database of Systematic Reviews, 2013 DOI:10.1002/14651858.CD009764.pub2.

34. Ekstrom, M: Clinical usefulness of long-term oxygen therapy in adults. NEJM 375:1683, 2016.
35. Uronis, HE, et al: Oxygen for relief of dyspnoea in people with chronic obstructive pulmonary disease who would not qualify for home oxygen: A systematic review and meta-analysis. Thorax 70:492, 2015.
36. The long-term oxygen treatment trial research group. A randomized trial of long-term oxygen for COPD with moderate desaturation: N Engl J Med 375:1617, 2016.
37. Fishman, A, et al: A randomized trial comparing lung volume reduction surgery with medical therapy for severe emphysema. N Engl J Med 348(21):2057, 2003.
38. Naunheim, K, et al: Long-term follow-up of patients receiving lung-volume-reduction surgery versus medical therapy for severe emphysema by the National Emphysema Treatment Trial research group. Ann Thorac Surg 82:431, 2006.
39. Washko, G, et al: The effect of lung volume reduction surgery on chronic obstructive pulmonary disease exacerbations. Am J Respir Crit Care Med 177:164, 2008.
40. Lee, HJ, et al: Endoscopic lung volume reduction: An American perspective. Ann Am Thorac Soc 10(6):667, 2013.
41. Klooster, K, et al: Endobronchial valves for emphysema without interlobar collateral ventilation. N Engl J Med 373:2325, 2015.
42. The Lung Institute. Lung transplant survival rates: Retrieved March 2017 from https://lunginstitute.com/blog/lung-transplant-survival-rates-for-one-month-one-year-and-three-years.
43. American Transplant Foundation: Transplantation Facts and Myths. Retrieved March 2017 from http://www.americantransplantfoundation.org/about-transplant/facts-and-myths.
44. McCarthy, B, et al: Pulmonary rehabilitation for chronic obstructive pulmonary disease. Review. Cochrane Database of Systemic Reviews 2, 2015. Art. No: CD003793. doi: 10.1002/14651858.CD003793.pub3.
45. Ries A: Pulmonary rehabilitation: Summary of an evidence-based guideline. Respir Care 53(9):1203, 2008.
46. *Guide to Physical Therapist Practice 3.0.* Alexandria, VA: American Physical Therapy Association; 2014. Available at: http://guidetoptpractice.apta.org/. Accessed March 2015.
47. American College of Chest Physicians and American Thoracic Society: ACCP-ATS joint committee on pulmonary nomenclature: Pulmonary terms and symbols: A report of the ACCP-ATS Joint Committee on Pulmonary Nomenclature. Chest 67:583, 1975.
48. Fletcher, CM, et al: The significance of respiratory symptoms and the diagnosis of chronic bronchitis in a working population. Br Med J 2(5147):257, 1959.
49. Mahler, DA, et al: The measurement of dyspnea. Contents, inter-observer agreement, and physiologic correlates of two new clinical indexes. Chest 85:751, 1984.
50. Perez, T, et al: Modified Medical Research Council scale vs Baseline Dyspnea Index to evaluate dyspnea in chronic obstructive pulmonary disease. Int J Chron Obstruct Pulmon Dis 10:1663, 2015.
51. Guyatt, GH, et al: A measure of quality of life for clinical trials in chronic lung disease. Thorax 42:73, 1987.
52. Jones, PW, et al: A self-complete measure of health status for chronic airflow limitation. The St. George's Respiratory Questionnaire. Am Rev Respir Dis 145(6):1321, 1992.
53. Jones, PW, et al: Development and first validation of the COPD assessment Test. Eur Respir J 34(3):648, 2009.
54. van der Molen, T, et al: Development, validity and responsiveness of the Clinical COPD Questionnaire. Health Qual Life Outcomes 1:13, 2003.
55. Kocks, JW, et al: Health status measurement in COPD: The minimal clinically important difference of the clinical COPD questionnaire. Respir Res 7:62, 2006.
56. Gan, W, et al: Association between chronic obstructive pulmonary disease and systemic inflammation: A systematic review and a meta-analysis. Thorax 59:574, 2004.
57. Casaburi, R: Skeletal muscle function in COPD. Chest 117:267S, 2000.
58. Gosker, HR, et al: Extrapulmonary manifestations of chronic obstructive pulmonary disease in a mouse model of chronic cigarette smoke exposure. Am J Respir Cell Mol Biol 40:710, 2009.
59. Jones, SE, et al: The five repetition sit to stand test as a functional outcome measure in COPD. Thorax 68(11):1015, 2013.
60. Ozalevli, S, et al: Comparison of the sit to stand test with 6 minute walk test in patients with chronic obstructive pulmonary disease Respir Med 101:286, 2007.
61. Zhan, S, et al: Development of an unsupported arm exercise test in patients with chronic obstructive pulmonary disease. J Cardiopulm Rehabil 26:180, 2006.
62. Black, LF, and Hyatt, RE: Maximal respiratory pressures: Normal values and relationship to age and sex. Am Rev Respir Dis 99:696, 1969.
63. Sclauser, IMB, et al: Reference values for maximal inspiratory pressure: A systematic review. Can Respir J 21(1):43, 2014.
64. Weisman, I, et al: American Thoracic Society/American College of Chest Physicians statement on cardiopulmonary exercise testing. Am J Respir Crit Care Med 167(2): 211, 2003.
65. Palange, P, et al: Recommendations on the use of exercise testing in clinical practice. Eur Respir J 29:185, 2007.
66. Singh, SJ, et al: An official systematic review of the European Respiratory Society/American Thoracic Society: Measurement properties of field walking tests in chronic respiratory disease. Eur Respir J 44:1447, 2014.
67. Singh, SJ, et al: Development of a shuttle walking test of disability in patients with chronic airways obstruction. Thorax 47(12):1019, 1992.
68. Fritz, S, and Lucardi, M: White paper: Walking speed: the sixth vital sign. J Geriatric Phys Ther 32:2, 2009.
69. American Thoracic Society: Guidelines for the 6-minute walk test. Am J Respir Crit Care Med 166:111, 2002.
70. Puhan, MA, et al: Interpretation of treatment changes in 6-minute walk distance in patients with COPD. Eur Respir J 32(3):637, 2008.
71. Singh, SJ, et al: Minimum clinically important improvement for the incremental shuttle walking test. Thorax 63:775, 2008.
72. Leung, RWM, et al: Ground walk training improves functional exercise capacity more than cycle training in people with chronic obstructive pulmonary disease (COPD): A randomized trial. J Physiother 56(2):105, 2010.
73. Garber CE, et al: American College of Sports Medicine position stand: Quantity and quality of exercise for developing and maintaining cardiorespiratory, musculoskeletal and neuromotor fitness in apparently healthy adults: guidance for prescribing exercise. Med Sci Sports Exerc 43(7):1334, 2011.
74. Horowitz, MB, et al: Dyspnea ratings for prescribing exercise intensity in patients with COPD. Chest 109(5):1169, 1996.
75. Horowitz, MB, et al: Dyspnea ratings for prescription of cross-modal exercise in patients with COPD. Chest 113(1):60, 1998.
76. Mahler, D: Hit the dyspnea target. J Cardiopulm Rehabil 23:226, 2003.
77. Mejia, R, et al: Target dyspnea ratings predict expected oxygen consumption as well as target heart rate values. Am J Respir Crit Care Med 159:1485, 1999.
78. Borg, G: Psychophysical basis of perceived exertion. Med Sci Sports Exerc 14:377, 1982.
79. Dattal, D, and ZuWallack, R: High versus low intensity exercise training in pulmonary rehabilitation: Is more better? Chronic Respir Dis 1:143, 2004.
80. Normandin, E, et al: An evaluation of two approaches to exercise conditioning in pulmonary rehabilitation. Chest 121:1085, 2002.
81. Arnardottir, R, et al: Interval training compared with continuous training in patients with COPD. Respir Med 101:1196, 2007.
82. Louvaris, Z, et al: 12 weeks of interval training induces clinically meaningful effects in amount and intensity of daily activities in COPD. Eur Respir J 48: 567, 2016.
83. Nasis, I, et al: Hemodynamic effects of high intensity interval training in COPD patients exhibiting exercise-induced dynamic hyperinflation. Respir Physiol Neurobiol 217:8, 2015.
84. Mador, M, et al: Interval training versus continuous training in patients with chronic obstructive pulmonary disease. J Cardiopul Rehab Prev 29:126, 2009.
85. Santos, C, et al: Pulmonary Rehabilitation in COPD: Effect of 2 aerobic exercise intensities on subject-centered outcomes—A randomized control trial. Respir Care 60: 1603, 2015.
86. Gruber, W, et al: Interval exercise training in cystic fibrosis-Effects on exercise capacity in severely affected adults. J Cystic Fibrosis 13:86, 2014.

87. Butcher, S, et al: The physiologic effects of an acute bout of supramaximal high-intensity interval training compared with a continuous exercise bout in patients with COPD. J Respir Med 2013. Article ID 879695, 2013.
88. Klijn, P, et al: Nonlinear Exercise Training in Advanced Chronic Obstructive Pulmonary Disease is superior to traditional exercise training. Am J Respir Crit Care Med 188:193, 2013.
89. Vogiatzis, I, et al: Dynamic hyperinflation and tolerance to interval exercise in patients with advanced COPD. Eur Respir J 24:385, 2004.
90. Ries, A, et al: Pulmonary rehabilitation joint ACCP/AACVPR evidence-based clinical practice guidelines. Chest 131:4S, 2007.
91. Ross, LM, et al: High-intensity interval training for patients with chronic diseases. J Sport Health Sci 5:139, 2016.
92. Burr, JF, et al: The 6-minute walk test as a predictor of objectively measured aerobic fitness in healthy working aged adults. Phys Sportsmed 39(2):133, 2011.
93. Zainuldin, R, et al: Prescription of walking exercise intensity from the 6-minute walk test in people with chronic obstructive pulmonary disease. J Cardiopulm Rehabil Prev 35(1):65, 2015.
94. Vonbank, K, et al: Strength training increases maximum working capacity in patients with COPD—randomized clinical trial comparing three training modalities. Respir Med 106(4):557, 2012.
95. O'Shea, SD, et al: Peripheral muscle strength training in COPD: A systematic review. Chest 126:903, 2004.
96. Spruit, MA, et al: New modalities of pulmonary rehabilitation in patients with chronic obstructive pulmonary disease. Sports Med 37:501, 2007.
97. O'Brien, K, et al: Inspiratory muscle training compared with other rehabilitation interventions in chronic obstructive pulmonary disease: A systematic review update. J Cardiopulm Rehabil Prev 28:128, 2008.
98. Scherer, TA, et al: Respiratory muscle endurance training in chronic obstructive pulmonary disease: Impact on exercise capacity, dyspnea, and quality of life. Am J Respir Crit Care Med 162:1709, 2000.
99. Riera, HS, et al: Inspiratory muscle training in patients with COPD: Effect on dyspnea, exercise performance and quality of life. Chest 120:748, 2001.
100. Weiner, P, et al: Comparison of specific expiratory, inspiratory, and combined muscle training programs in COPD. Chest 124:1357, 2003.
101. Wild, M, et al: The outcome of inspiratory muscle training in COPD patients depends on stage of the disease. Chest 120S:181S, 2001.
102. Beckerman, M, et al: The effects of 1 year of specific inspiratory muscle training in patients with COPD. Chest 128:3177, 2005.
103. Weiner, P, and Weiner, M: Inspiratory muscle training may increase peak inspiratory flow in chronic obstructive pulmonary disease. Respiration 73:151, 2006.
104. Magadle, R, et al: Inspiratory muscle training in pulmonary rehabilitation program in COPD patients. Respir Med 101: 1500, 2007.
105. Hill, K, et al: High-intensity inspiratory muscle training in COPD. Eur Respir J 27:1119, 2006.
106. Carr, RJ, et al: Pulmonary rehabilitation after acute exacerbation of chronic obstructive pulmonary disease in patients who previously completed a pulmonary rehabilitation program. J Cardiopulm Rehabil Prev 29(5):318–324, 2009.
107. Hietpas, B, et al: Huff coughing and airway patency. Resp Care 24:710, 1979.
108. Wilson, G, et al: A comparison of traditional chest physiotherapy with the active cycle of breathing in patients with chronic suppurative lung disease. Eur Respir J 8(suppl 19):171S, 1995.
109. Konstan, M, et al: Efficacy of the flutter device for airway mucus clearance in patients with cystic fibrosis. J Pediatr 124:689, 1994.
110. Gondor, M, et al: Comparison of flutter device and chest physical therapy in the treatment of cystic fibrosis during pulmonary exacerbation. Pediatr Pulmonol 28:255, 1999.
111. Van Asperen, P, et al: Comparison of a positive expiratory pressure (PEP) mask with postural drainage in patients with cystic fibrosis. Aust Paediatr J 23:283, 1987.
112. Steen, H, et al: Evaluation of the PEP mask in cystic fibrosis. Acta Paediatr Scand 80(1):51, 1991.
113. Braggion, C, et al: Short term effects of three chest physiotherapy regimens in patients hospitalized for pulmonary exacerbations of CF: A cross-over randomized study. Pediatr Pulmonol 19:16, 1995.
114. Morgan, M, and Britton, J: Chronic obstructive pulmonary disease: Non-pharmacological management of COPD. Thorax 58:453, 2003.
115. Dechman, G, and Wilson, C: Evidence underlying breathing retraining in people with stable chronic obstructive pulmonary disease. Phys Ther 84:1189, 2004.

appendix 12.A

Web-Based Resources for Clinicians, Families, and Patients With Chronic Pulmonary Dysfunction

National Heart, Lung, and Blood Institute: www.nhlbi.nih.gov

Global Initiative for Chronic Obstructive Lung Disease: www.goldcopd.org

Global Initiative for Asthma: www.ginasthma.org

American Lung Association: www.lung.org

American Thoracic Society Guidelines: www.thoracic.org

European Respiratory Society: www.ersnet.org

American Association for Respiratory Care: www.aarc.org

Cystic Fibrosis Foundation: www.cff.org

Bode calculator: http://reference.medscape.com/calculator/bode-index-copd

Better Breathing Club: www.breathingassociation.org/better-breathing-club/

Breathe Better Network: www.nhlbi.nih.gov/health/educational/copd/our-partners/

Allergies and Asthma Resources: http://acaai.org/resources

Asthma Resources: www.asthma.com; www.asthmacommunitynetwork.org/resources

Learning Lung Sounds:

1. www.easyauscultation.com
2. http://solutions.3mae.ae/wps/portal/3M/en_AE/3M-Littmann-EMEA/stethoscope/littmann-learning-institute/heart-lung-sounds/lung-sounds/
3. www.practicalclinicalskills.com

Heart Disease

Konrad J. Dias, PT, DPT, PhD, CCS

Chapter 13

LEARNING OBJECTIVES

1. Describe the etiology, pathophysiology, symptomatology, and sequelae of coronary heart disease.
2. Describe the etiology, pathophysiology, symptomatology, and sequelae of congestive heart failure.
3. Identify and describe the examination procedures used to evaluate patients with heart disease and establish a diagnosis and plan of care.
4. Describe the role of the physical therapist in assisting the patient in recovery from heart disease in terms of interventions, patient-related instruction, coordination, communication, and documentation.
5. Identify and describe strategies of intervention during various phases of cardiac rehabilitation.
6. Analyze and interpret patient data, formulate realistic anticipated goals and expected outcomes, and develop a plan of care when presented with a clinical case study.

CHAPTER OUTLINE

INTRODUCTION AND EPIDEMIOLOGY OF HEART DISEASE

Cardiovascular disease (CVD) is a term referring to the pathological process of atherosclerosis affecting the entire arterial circulation. Coronary artery disease (CAD), also called coronary heart disease (CHD), refers to the pathological process of atherosclerosis, specifically affecting the coronary arteries. CAD includes the diagnoses of angina pectoris, myocardial infarction (MI), silent myocardial ischemia, and sudden cardiac death.

The pathophysiological conditions that underlie CVD are atherosclerosis, altered myocardial muscle mechanics, valvular dysfunction, arrhythmias, and hypertension (HTN). Atherosclerosis is a disease in which lipid-laden plaque (lesions) is formed within the intimal layer of the blood vessel wall of moderate and large size arteries; over time the plaque may extend into the lumen causing a decreased lumenal diameter. Atherosclerosis is also a primary contributor to cerebrovascular disease (cerebrovascular accident [CVA]) and peripheral vascular disease (PVD).

Alteration in myocardial muscle mechanics involving the systolic and/or diastolic properties of the myocardium results in an impairment of left ventricular (LV) function.

Heart failure is a clinical diagnosis caused by impaired LV functioning and is referred to as congestive heart failure (CHF) when it is accompanied by signs and symptoms of edema (i.e., congestion). There are many causes of heart failure, including myocardial scarring and remodeling as a result of an MI, cardiomyopathy involving an enlarged, thickened, and/or hardened heart muscle from various causes, or impaired valvular function, especially within the mitral and aortic valves.

Arrhythmias are caused by a disturbance in the electrical activity of the heart, resulting in impaired electrical impulse formation or conduction. Arrhythmias may present as benign or malignant (i.e., life-threatening). Examples of malignant arrhythmias are sustained ventricular tachycardia (V-tach) and ventricular fibrillation (V-fib). An example of a common benign arrhythmia in the elderly is atrial fibrillation (A-fib) with a controlled ventricular response involving a ventricular rate between 60 and 100 beats per minute (bpm).

HTN is the most prevalent CVD in the United States and one of the most powerful contributors to cardiovascular morbidity and mortality. HTN occurs when the systolic blood pressure is consistently greater than 140 mm Hg or the DBP is equal to or greater than 90 mm Hg.

CVD remains the leading cause of death and disability in the United States. According to the American Heart Association's Heart Disease and Stroke Statistics 2016 Update, an estimated 85.6 million Americans have one or more types of CVD. Further, CVD is the leading global cause of death, accounting for more than 17.3 million deaths per year. This number is expected to grow to more than 26.3 million by the year 2030. Coronary heart disease is the most common type of heart disease, killing nearly 380,000 people annually. Heart disease is also the number one killer of women, taking more lives than all forms of cancer combined. On average, heart disease strikes an individual every 39 seconds. The direct and indirect costs of CVD and stroke including health expenditure and lost productivity total more than $316.6 billion.[1]

This chapter provides a review of normal anatomy and physiology of the cardiovascular system and its relevance to physical therapist practice followed by a discussion of various pathologies and pertinent physical therapy implications.

CARDIAC ANATOMY AND PHYSIOLOGY

The heart lies within the left thoracic cavity. The base of the heart is located superiorly, approximately between the second and third rib; the apex is located inferiorly, approximately at the level of the fifth rib (Fig.13.1). In this position, the heart is rotated in the sagittal plane so that the right ventricle (RV) is positioned anterior to the left ventricle (LV) and tipped anteriorly, bringing the apex closer to the chest wall. In the posterior–anterior view of a chest x-ray, the RV occupies a significant portion of the frontal plane. The right atrium (RA) is generally located in the area of the second intercostal space and the *angle of Louis.* When one palpates the sternum, the angle of Louis is the "bump" that demarcates the manubrium from the body of the sternum. The second intercostal spaces are lateral and slightly below the angle of Louis. The second intercostal spaces are an important auscultatory landmark; the right space is known as the *aortic area,* the left as the *pulmonic area.* The apex of the normal heart is in the fifth intercostal space at the midclavicular line. In a healthy heart, this area, known as the *point of maximal impulse (PMI),* is where the contraction of the LV is most pronounced.

Heart Tissue

The heart wall is made up of three tissue layers (Fig. 13.2). The outermost layer of the heart is a double-walled sac called the *pericardium.* The two layers of the pericardium include an outer tough, fibrous layer of dense, irregular connective tissue called the *parietal pericardium* and an

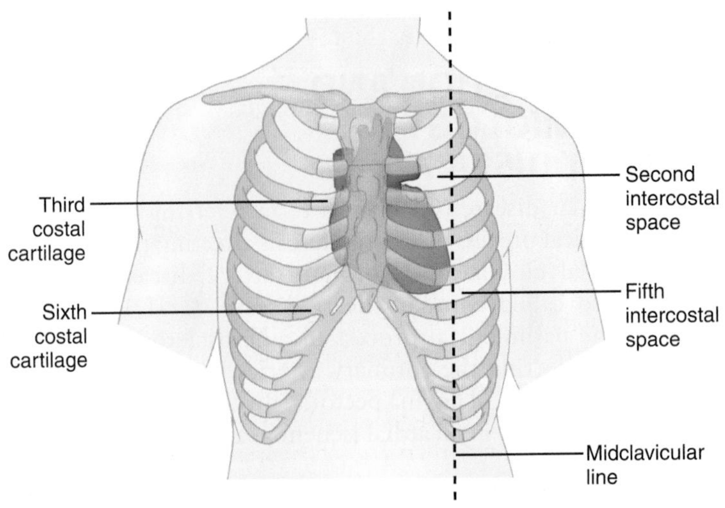

Figure 13.1 Surface anatomy of the heart.

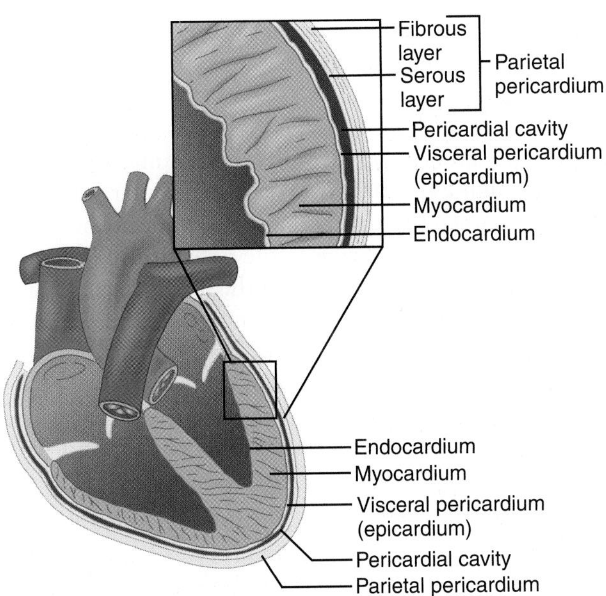

Figure 13.2 Layers of the heart.

inner thin *visceral pericardium.*[2] The visceral pericardium is also called the *epicardium.* Between the two pericardial layers is a closed space filled with 10 to 20 mL of clear pericardial fluid.[2] This fluid serves as a lubricant allowing the two surfaces to slide over each other.

Clinically, patients may develop an infection with resultant inflammation of the pericardium called *pericarditis.* The clinical signs that accompany this pathology and used to differentially diagnose pericarditis include a *pericardial friction rub* (an audible grating sound suggesting irritation of the pericardium) that can be auscultated with each heartbeat, sharp constant chest pain, possible fever and shortness of breath.[3] The presence of a pericardial friction rub in acute pericarditis has 100% specificity and 9% sensitivity.[4] In the same study, investigators found the presence of chest pain to have a 70% specificity and 70% sensitivity in determining the presence of an acute pericarditis.[4] In some patients with pericarditis, the excessive fluid accumulation within the closed pericardial space may lead to a secondary condition known as *cardiac tamponade.* Tamponade involves compression of the heart caused by fluid build-up in the space between the myocardium and pericardium. In this state, patients will demonstrate compromised cardiac function and contractility due to the excess fluid within the closed space pushing against the heart.[3]

The muscular middle layer of the heart is called the *myocardium.* It is the layer that facilitates the pumping action of the heart to move blood to the entire body. Myocardial cells may be categorized into two groups based on their function—mechanical cells contributing to mechanical contraction and conductive cells contributing to electrical conduction.

Alterations in the muscular wall of the heart are called cardiomyopathies. There are three common classifications of cardiomyopathies: *dilated, hypertrophic,* and *restrictive.*[5] Dilated cardiomyopathy is evidenced by ventricular dilation and altered cardiac muscle contractile function. CAD is the prime cause of *dilated cardiomyopathy,* causing mitochondrial dysfunction and resultant myocardial damage. Myocarditis (inflammation of the heart muscle) and alcohol abuse are additional causes of dilated cardiomyopathy. *Hypertrophic cardiomyopathy* presents as diastolic dysfunction or altered ventricular filling ability with concomitant increases in ventricular mass. Chronic HTN and aortic stenosis are conditions that lead to the development of hypertrophic cardiomyopathy. *Restrictive cardiomyopathy* also presents as diastolic dysfunction with limited filling ability owing to the presence of excessively rigid ventricular walls. The connective tissue changes of the heart associated with diabetes are an example of a restrictive cardiomyopathy. Damage to myocardial cells from cardiomyopathies and various other etiologies lead to cardiac muscle dysfunction and resultant heart failure, which will be comprehensively discussed later in this chapter.

The innermost layer of the heart is called the *endocardium.* The tissue of the endocardium forms the inner lining of the chambers of the heart and is continuous with the tissue of the valves and the endothelium of the blood vessel. Because the endocardium and valves share similar tissue, patients with infections of the endocardium are at risk for developing valvular dysfunction.[6] Endocardial infections can spread into valvular tissue developing vegetations (a mixture of bacteria and blood clots) on the valve.[6] In patients with newly developed vegetations, bronchopulmonary hygiene procedures including percussions and vibrations must be used in precaution as these procedures may cause the vegetation to dislodge, move as emboli resulting in an embolic stroke.

Coronary Arteries

The coronary arteries originate in the sinus of Valsalva located in the wall of the aorta near the aortic valve. There are three major vessels that supply the heart with oxygenated blood. These three vessels include the right coronary artery, the left anterior descending artery, and the left circumflex artery.

The right coronary originates from the area near the right aortic leaflet while the left main coronary artery arises from the area near the left aortic leaflet. When the aortic valve is open during systole, the origins of the coronary arteries are located behind the aortic leaflets within the wall; when the aortic valve is closed during diastole, the openings of the coronaries are clearly exposed, allowing them to be easily perfused.[5] The coronary arteries therefore receive the majority of their blood flow during diastole, unlike the other arteries of the body that are perfused during systole.

The left main coronary artery branches into the left anterior descending (LAD) and the circumflex (CX)

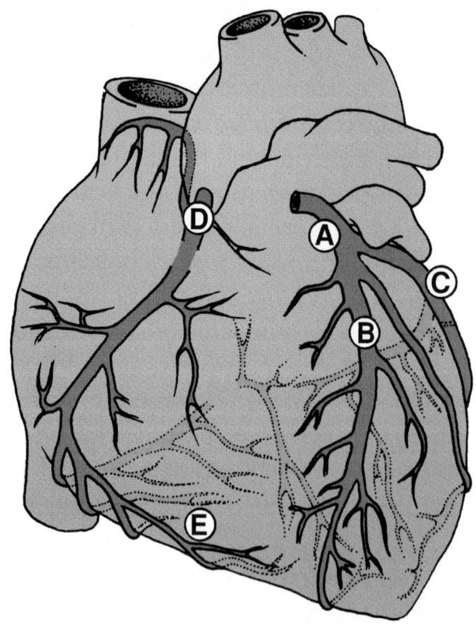

Figure 13.3 Coronary circulation. (A) left main (LM); (B) left anterior descending (LAD); (C) left circumflex (CX); (D) right coronary (RCA); (E) posterior descending (PDA). The branches of the LAD are known as diagonals; the branches of the CX are known as marginals.

(Fig. 13.3). The LAD may have further divisions, known as diagonal branches that come off the primary LAD. The LAD and its diagonal branches primarily supply the anterior and apical surfaces of the LV, as well as portions of the interventricular septum. The circumflex may also have branches, known as marginal branches. The circumflex and its marginal branches supply the lateral and part of the inferior surfaces of the LV and portions of the left atrium (LA). The right coronary artery (RCA) supplies the RA, most of the RV, part of the inferior wall of the LV, portions of the interventricular septum, and the conduction system. The posterior descending artery (PDA) is most commonly a branch of the RCA and perfuses the posterior heart. If the RCA does not perfuse the posterior heart, the CX will supply this area. When the PDA comes from the RCA, the anatomy is referred to as being right dominant; if the PDA comes from the circumflex, the anatomy is referred to as being left dominant. For physical therapists, there is no clinical importance to whether the anatomy of the myocardium is either left or right dominant.

Reduced blood flow within any of the coronary arteries will result in ischemia and possible infarction of cardiac tissue. In addition, coronary arteries may present in spasm. In this condition, the smooth muscle contraction within the walls of the artery suddenly spasm results in a profound narrowing of the coronary artery. Cigarette smoking is a major risk factor for vasospastic angina.[7] Further, there exists evidence of changes in autonomic activity detected by heart rate variability shortly before an episode of coronary spasm.[8] Finally, guide wire or balloon dilatation at the time of a percutaneous coronary intervention are risk factors of coronary spasms.[8]

Heart Valves

There exist four heart valves that ensure one-way blood flow through the heart. Two atrioventricular valves are located between the atria and ventricle. The atrioventricular valve, positioned between the right atrium (RA) and RV, is called the *tricuspid valve*; the left atrioventricular valve is the *mitral valve* (also known as the bicuspid valve). This valve is located between the left atrium (LA) and LV. The *semilunar valves* lie between the ventricles and arteries that emerge from the ventricles. These valves are named based on the vessels they correspond with (i.e., *pulmonic valve* on the right in association with the pulmonary artery, and aortic valve on the left relating to the aorta).

Flaps of tissue called *leaflets or cusps* guard the heart valve openings. The right atrioventricular valve has three cusps and is therefore called *tricuspid,* whereas the left atrioventricular valve has only two cusps and hence is called *bicuspid.* These leaflets are attached to the papillary muscles of the myocardium by chordae tendineae. The primary function of the atrioventricular valves is to prevent backflow of blood into the atria during ventricular contraction or systole, while the semilunar valves prevent backflow of blood from the aorta and pulmonary artery into the ventricles during diastole. Opening and closing of each valve depends on pressure gradient changes within the heart created during each cardiac cycle.

Patients with cardiopulmonary disease commonly present with non-specific signs and symptoms of dyspnea and fatigue. The etiology of these vague signs and symptoms can potentiate from various sources one of which is valvular dysfunction. Therefore, auscultation of the four heart valves is useful first step in determining valvular dysfunction that leads to atypical symptomology of shortness of breath and fatigue.

Cardiac Output and Cardiac Index

The goal of the heart is to provide adequate cardiac output (CO) to generate aerobic energy to meet the metabolic demands of the body. Because the energy demands of the body are constantly changing, the heart's CO must also be able to adapt to the changing systemic energy demands, as well as to its own myocardial oxygen needs. CO is defined as the amount of blood leaving the ventricles per minute, expressed in L/min. Normal CO at rest is approximately 4 to 6 L/min. It is influenced by HR (expressed as beats per minute [bpm]) and stroke volume (expressed as milliliters per minute [mL/min]).

Clinically, especially in critical care settings, the concept of cardiac index (CI) is often preferred to CO. CI expresses the CO in relationship to the body surface area (BSA) expressed in meters such that CI = CO/BSA.[9] Normal CO range at rest is 4 to 5 L/min; normal CI range is 2.5 to 3.5 L/min/m^2.[9] CI provides a more complete determination of the adequacy of an individual's CO than CO alone. For example, in comparing a 6 ft tall individual and a 5 ft tall individual each with a CO of 3 L/min, the 5-ft tall person will have a higher CI and therefore better tissue perfusion because there is less BSA requiring the 3 L of CO. Determination of BSA and CI is often done using nomograms (two-dimensional diagrams) based on the Geigy scientific tables.[9]

Stroke volume (SV) is the volume of blood ejected with each myocardial contraction and is influenced by three factors: (1) *preload,* the amount of blood filled in the ventricle at the end of diastole (also known as *left ventricular-end diastolic volume [LVEDV]*); (2) *contractility,* the ability of the ventricle to contract; and (3) *afterload,* the force the LV must generate during systole to overcome aortic pressure and open the aortic valve.[10] Afterload may also be described as the load against which the LV contracts during left ventricular ejection.

Throughout the cardiac cycle, diastole and systole place different demands on the ventricles. During diastole, the ventricles must be compliant, able to stretch to accommodate the blood entering the ventricles (preload). During systole, the ventricles must be able to contract adequately to eject the SV. The principle of Starling's length–tension relationship is applicable to the myocardium and the relationship between the properties of diastole and systole.[11] During diastole as muscle length increases (e.g., the ventricular chamber size increases) the ability of the myocardium to develop force is increased, up to a point. Beyond a certain length, however, force development is impaired owing to the inadequate alignment of the actin and myosin filaments[11] (Fig. 13.4).

In general, SV will increase with an increase in preload or contractility and will decrease with an increase in afterload. Normally about 55% to 75% of the preload is ejected as the SV. The *ejection fraction* (EF) demonstrates this relationship between SV and LVEDV such that EF = SV ÷ LVEDV. This value represents the ratio of the volume of blood ejected by the LV per contraction relative to the volume of blood received by the LV following diastole.[11] Normal EF is approximately 55% to 75% (67% ± 8%) and is widely used clinically as an index of contractility.[11]

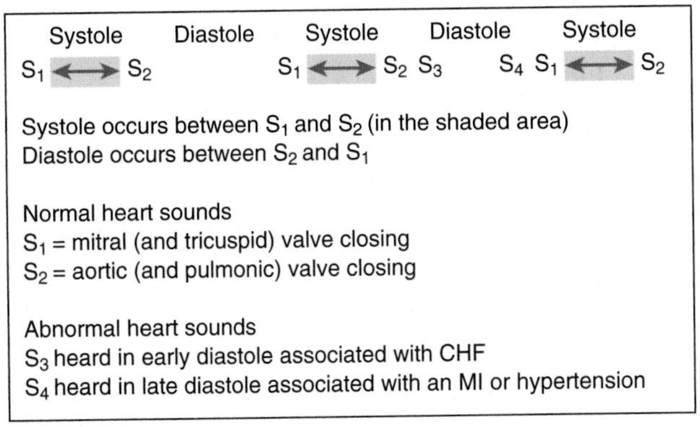

Systole Diastole Systole Diastole Systole

S_1 ⟷ S_2 S_1 ⟷ S_2 S_3 S_4 S_1 ⟷ S_2

Systole occurs between S_1 and S_2 (in the shaded area)
Diastole occurs between S_2 and S_1

Normal heart sounds
S_1 = mitral (and tricuspid) valve closing
S_2 = aortic (and pulmonic) valve closing

Abnormal heart sounds
S_3 heard in early diastole associated with CHF
S_4 heard in late diastole associated with an MI or hypertension

Figure 13.4 Heart sounds of the cardiac cycle.

Cardiac Cycle

The cardiac cycle consists of two interrelated phases: *systole,* the contraction phase, and *diastole,* the filling phase. During diastole, the ventricles fill with blood from the atria via opening of the atrioventricular valves. The atrioventricular valves lie between the atria and the ventricles and include the tricuspid valve on the right and mitral valve on the left. The first two-thirds of ventricular filling is passive; during the last one-third the atria contract and push the blood into the ventricles. This contraction is known as the *atrial kick.* After the atrial kick, diastole ends and the atrioventricular valves close. Systole begins with both the atrioventricular and semilunar valves closed. An initial *isovolumetric contraction,* like an isometric contraction of striated muscle, increases the pressure within the ventricles, and the semilunar valve opens. The LV then undergoes a concentric contraction, causing a volume to be ejected, called the *stroke volume* (SV). After the SV is ejected, the aortic valve closes and systole is complete. The cardiac cycle is defined by the presence of normal heart sounds, S_1 and S_2. Heart sounds are associated with valvular closings; S_1 is associated with atrioventricular valve closure, and S_2 is associated with semilunar valve closure. Systole occurs between S_1 and S_2, and diastole occurs between S_2 and S_1 (Fig. 13.5).

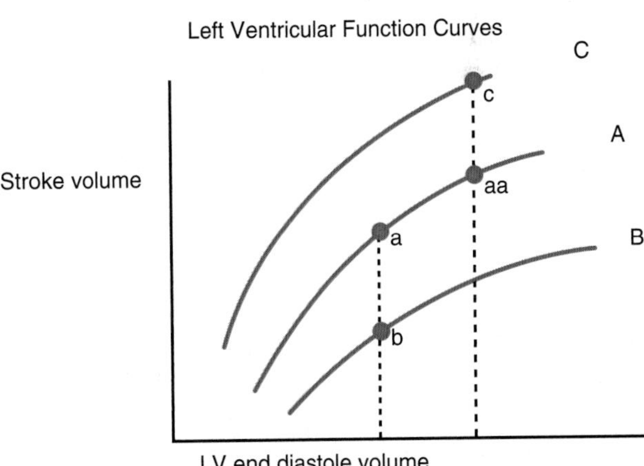

Figure 13.5 Left ventricular (LV) function curves. (A) With normal LV function, as the left ventricular volume increases, stroke volume will also increase. (B) With LV function impairment, the curve will shift to the right, and for any given length, stroke volume is decreased compared with normal (point *b* has a deceased SV compared with point *a*). (C) When normal LV function experiences an increase in sympathetic activity, the curve will shift to the left and SV will increase (note that point *c* is greater than point *aa*).

Blood Flow and Hemodynamic Values

Blood enters the heart via the superior and inferior vena cava into the RA. Blood moves forward from the RA through the tricuspid valve to the RV, and through the pulmonic valve to the pulmonary artery (PA) and pulmonary capillaries. The capillaries perfuse the alveoli, and the alveolar capillary membrane is the site of gas exchange. Newly oxygenated blood within the pulmonary veins (PVs) travels to the left atrium (LA) and passes through the mitral valve into the LV. Blood within the LV travels down to the apex, where it is squeezed in a wringing motion during systole and moved from the apex to the LV outflow tract and finally out through the aortic valve to the aorta.

Blood volume in any chamber or vessel generates a pressure. The normal pressure recordings for the cardiovascular system are presented in Table 13.1. Owing to the relationship between blood volumes and pressures, a direct measure of blood volumes within the heart is accomplished by invasive monitoring of the intravascular or chamber pressures. In a *right-sided heart catheterization,* an invasive catheter known as a Swan-Ganz catheter or Pulmonary Artery (PA) catheter, with pressure-sensitive recording ability, is inserted into the internal jugular or subclavian vein and progressed antegrade through the right side of the heart.[9] Common measurements taken with a right-sided heart catheterization are RA pressure, PA pressure, and *pulmonary capillary wedge pressure (PCWP).* The PCWP is an indirect measure of the *left ventricular end-diastolic pressure (LVEDP),* one of the most sensitive measures of LV function.[9] An advantage of right-sided heart catheterization is the ability to monitor filling pressures not only on the right side, but also left-side heart pressures, by estimation, without the need for the more difficult and risky LV catheterization.[9] The procedure of left-sided heart catheterization involves placing a catheter into the femoral or radial artery and advancing it retrograde to the flow of blood through the aorta, across the aortic valve, and into the LV where LVEDP can be directly monitored. The LV catheter lies within a high-pressure system (the left side of the heart and the aorta), and therefore can stay in place for only a short period of time (e.g., 1 hour) because of the difficulties associated with cannulation (catheter insertion) within a high-pressure system. In contrast, the right-sided heart catheter, which lies within a relatively low-pressure system (the right side of the heart), provides continuous monitoring of pressures and can be kept in place for several days.

Table 13.1 Hemodynamic Variables

Right-Sided Heart Catheterization	Normal Ranges
Central venous pressure (CVP)	0–8 mm Hg
Right atrial (mean)	0–8 mm Hg
Pulmonary artery (PA)	Systolic 20–25 mm Hg Diastolic 6–12 mm Hg Mean 9–19 mm Hg
Pulmonary capillary wedge pressure (PCWP)	6–12 mm Hg
Left-Sided Heart Catheterization	**Normal Ranges**
Left ventricular end-diastolic pressure	5–12 mm Hg
Left ventricular peak systolic pressure	90–140 mm Hg
Systemic arterial pressure	Systolic 110–120 mm Hg Diastolic 70–80 mm Hg Mean 82–102 mm Hg
Cardiac output (CO)	4–5 L/min
Cardiac index (CO ÷ body surface area)	2.5–3.5 L/min
Stroke volume	55–100 mL/beat
Systemic vascular resistance	800–1200 dynes/sec/cm^{-5}

Adapted from Braunwald, E, Zipes, D, and Libby, R (eds): Heart Disease: A Textbook of Cardiovascular Medicine, ed 6. Saunders, Philadelphia 1997, p 188; and Parrillo, JE: Current Therapy in Critical Care Medicine. BC Decker Inc., 1987, p 36.

Electrical Conduction of the Heart

It is important to note that mechanical contraction of the ventricles only occurs with appropriate electrical conduction through the heart. Effective contraction depends on an intact electrical conduction system that results in depolarization of the myocardium and timely repolarization. In *normal sinus rhythm (NSR)* the impulse begins in the sinus node and travels through the atria, the A–V node, bundle of His, Purkinje fibers, septum, and ventricles.

Electrical conduction can be viewed via the electrocardiogram (ECG) complex (Fig. 13.6). Each component of the complex reflects a certain phase of conduction pathway.

- The P wave depicts sinus node and atrial depolarization.
- The PR segment demonstrates conduction through AV node.
- The QRS complex denotes electrical flow through the ventricles causing ventricular depolarization.
- The ST segment describes the initiation of ventricular repolarization.
- The T wave illustrates the completion of ventricular repolarization.

Each ECG complex represents one cardiac cycle or one heartbeat. In a series of ECG complexes representing sinus rhythm, each QRS complex should be preceded

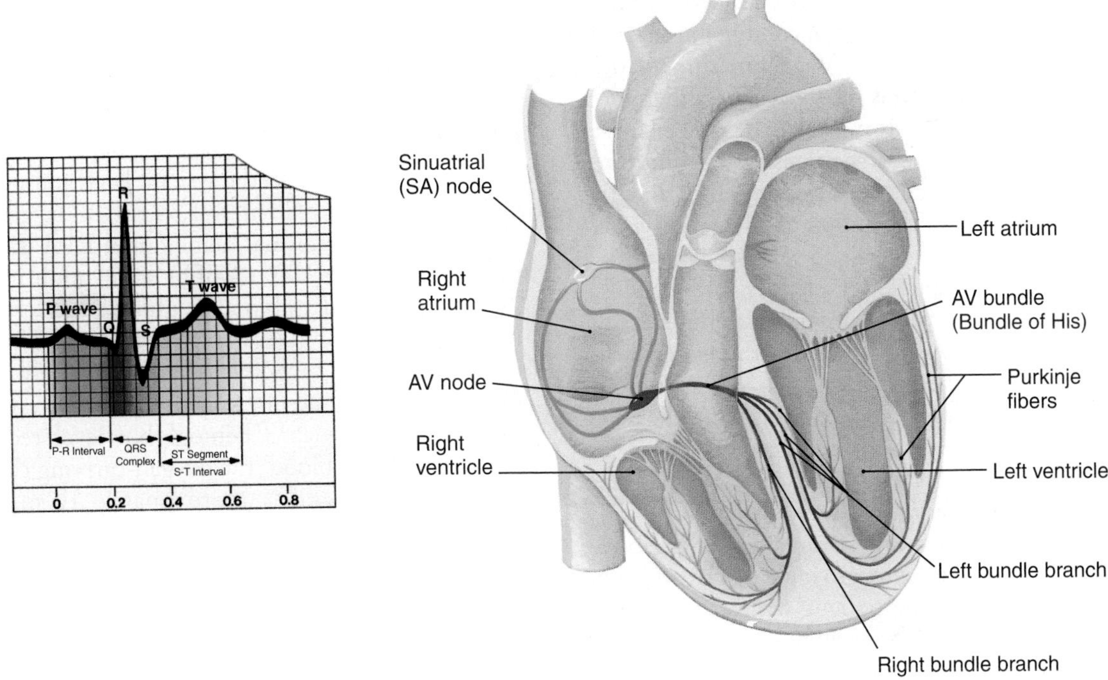

Figure 13.6 Schematic representation of the heart and normal cardiac electrical activity. The ECG is the body surface manifestation of the depolarization and repolarization waves of the heart. The P wave is generated by atrial depolarization, the QRS by ventricular muscle depolarization, and the T wave by ventricular repolarization. The PR interval is a measure of conduction time from atrium to ventricle, and the QRS duration indicates the time required for all of the ventricular cells to be activated. The QT interval reflects the duration of the ventricular action potential. *(Adapted from Taber's Cyclopedic Medical Dictionary, ed 21. FA Davis, Philadelphia, PA, 2005, p 1022, with permission.)*

by a P wave and the QRS complexes should be equally spaced apart, indicating a regular rhythm. ECG interpretation enables the clinician to differentially diagnose the cause of reduced CO that may occur from a true mechanical problem versus that occurring from an electrical problem disrupting mechanical activity of the heart.

Neurohormonal Influences on the Cardiovascular System

The autonomic nervous system (ANS) influences the heart and blood vessels through direct neural and indirect neurohormonal mechanisms. The heart has dual direct innervation from the sympathetic and parasympathetic nervous systems. The sympathetic receptors of the heart are primarily beta-adrenergic receptors and are located on the sinus node and within the myocardium. Stimulation of the receptors by the neurotransmitter norepinephrine (noradrenaline) increases the overall activity of the heart by increasing the heart rate (HR) (*chronotropy*) and force of contraction (*inotropy*), and results in coronary artery dilation. Sympathetic stimulation of the alpha-adrenergic receptors on peripheral blood vessels causes vasoconstriction and an increase in *peripheral vascular resistance (PVR).*

The sympathetic nervous system may also stimulate the adrenal cortex to secrete the catecholamine epinephrine. This blood-borne hormone has sympathetic effects that at times may be even more long lasting and potent than direct sympathetic activation. Epinephrine is released as part of the normal exercise response, especially when exercise is continued beyond a few minutes. The increase in HR and contractility noted with exercise is in part due to this hormonal influence. Many cardiovascular drugs either enhance or suppress sympathetic functioning. Those that mimic the action of the sympathetic nervous system are known as *sympathomimetics;* those that suppress sympathetic functioning are known as *sympatholytics.* Frequently used sympathomimetics are dopamine, epinephrine, and atropine, which are commonly used in the critical care setting. Dopamine and epinephrine increase cardiac output (CO), and atropine increases HR in the presence of critical *bradycardia.* Frequently used sympatholytics are the category of drugs known as beta blockers (beta-adrenergic antagonists) that suppress beta-adrenergic activity. They are commonly used as part of an anti-ischemic drug regimen and for the medical management of hypertension.

The normal parasympathetic influence via the vagus nerve has a primary impact on the resting heart, influencing resting HR substantially more than the sympathetic nervous system. Parasympathetic stimulation results in a depression of HR, decreased force of atrial contraction, and decreased speed of conduction through the atrioventricular (AV) node. Vagal fiber innervation to ventricular myocardium is relatively small; therefore, the effect on LV function is minimal. During exercise, the effects of the sympathetic nervous system and catecholamine release significantly override any effect from the parasympathetic system. The impact of direct parasympathetic influence on peripheral blood vessels is limited to a vasodilatory effect on the bowel, bladder, and genitals.

The catecholamine role in myocardial functioning during exercise is especially crucial for the patient who has lost direct sympathetic activation to the heart. For a patient who has undergone a heart transplant, the heart is essentially denervated; the sympathetic and parasympathetic fibers to the heart are excised.[12] Sympathetic influence on the denervated heart is therefore solely dependent on catecholamine stimulation of the beta-adrenergic myocardial receptors to increase HR and contractility.[12] Clinically, the patient with a denervated heart following transplantation will present with elevated resting HRs to achieve normal cardiac output, delayed elevation in HRs with exercise due to circulating catecholamines, decreased maximum HR responses, and slower decreases in HR values during the recovery phase of exercise.[12]

Myocardial Oxygen Supply and Demand

Myocardial oxygen supply and myocardial oxygen demand must be in balance. *Myocardial oxygen supply* depends on the delivery of oxygenated blood through the coronary arteries, the oxygen-carrying capacity of arterial blood, and the ability of the myocardial cells to extract oxygen from the arterial blood. *Myocardial oxygen demand* (MVO_2), the energy cost to the myocardium, is dependent on many factors. Clinically, MVO_2 is calculated as the product of HR and systolic blood pressure (SBP), known as the *rate pressure product (RPP)* or double product. Any activity that increases HR and/or BP will increase MVO_2. Therefore, any increase in systemic oxygen demand (e.g., exercise) will increase the energy cost of the heart and increase MVO_2.

The myocardium is routinely very efficient at extracting oxygen from its blood supply. Therefore, during times of increased energy demand, very little increase in extraction can occur. The primary mechanism for increasing myocardial oxygen supply during times of increased demand is by increased *coronary blood flow (CBF)*. In general, there is a linear relationship between CBF and MVO_2. During exercise, CBF may increase five times above resting level in response to the increased demand. Unlike skeletal muscle, which has the capability of both aerobic and anaerobic metabolism, the heart muscle (myocardium) is essentially dependent on aerobic metabolism and has very limited anaerobic capacity.

Laboratory Values

When managing patients with heart disease, certain laboratory values are particularly important. Table 13.2 provides reference values for various laboratory tests. The hemoglobin and hematocrit levels depict the oxygen-carrying capacity within the system. Each gram of hemoglobin carries approximately 1.34 mL of oxygen within arterial blood. A normal hemoglobin level is approximately 12 to 14 g/100 mL of blood in adult males and 14 to 16 g/100 mL of blood in adult women. For example, for a hemoglobin level of 15 g/100 mL of blood, the oxygen-carrying capacity is approximately 20 mL O_2/100 mL of blood (15 x 1.34 = 20). Now, if we consider a patient with a hemoglobin level reduced to 7.5 g/100 mL of blood, the oxygen-carrying capacity is reduced by half and is approximately 10 mL of O_2/100 mL of blood. With reduced oxygen-carrying capacity, the heart must work harder to compensate for low oxygen levels to provide sufficient oxygen to the peripheral tissue. During heart failure, increased workload placed on a failing heart will exacerbate the failure. A general rule of thumb is to use caution and lower the intensity when exercising patients with cardiovascular disease and hemoglobin levels less than 8 g/100 mL of blood.

Electrolyte levels are also important to consider before treating patients with heart disease. Appropriate levels of potassium, calcium, and magnesium allow for normal electrical conduction through the heart. *Hypokalemia*, low potassium (usually less than 3.5 mEq/L), produces arrhythmias with flattened T waves and depressed ST segments, as well as bilateral lower extremity muscle cramping. An inverted U-wave may also be noticed on the electrocardiogram. *Hypocalcemia* (low blood serum

Table 13.2 Laboratory Tests and Reference Values

Test	Reference Value
Sodium	135–145 mEq/L
Potassium	3.5–5.0 mEq/L
Chloride	95–105 mEq/L
Calcium	9–11 mg/dL
BUN	10–20
Creatinine	0.5–1.2 mg/dL
Glucose	70–110 mg/dL
Carbon dioxide	20–29 mEq/L
Magnesium	1.5–2.5 mEq/L
Hgb (g/dL)	Adult female: 12–16 Adult male: 13–18
HCT (%)	Adult female: 36-46 Adult male: 37–49

calcium levels) and *hypomagnesemia* (low magnesium in blood) have the potential of increasing ventricular ectopy within the heart. In addition, calcium enhances contractile function of muscle cells. Patients with hypocalcemia have reduced cardiac contractility whereas those with hypercalcemia present with erratic heart beats.

Renal function tests are done to determine kidney function and examine *blood urea nitrogen* (BUN) and *creatinine* levels. These levels are especially important to review in patients with heart failure and patients prescribed with diuretics. Finally, many patients with heart disease also have diabetes and therefore it is important to review blood glucose levels before exercise.

CARDIOVASCULAR RESPONSES TO AEROBIC EXERCISE

Measures of Energy Expenditure

An individual's cardiorespiratory fitness is best defined by measurement of the *maximal oxygen consumption* ($\dot{V}O_{2max}$). Oxygen consumption is measured when performing aerobic activity with increasing intensity using large muscle groups until maximum capacity. The $\dot{V}O_{2max}$ reflects the maximum amount of oxygen consumed per minute when the individual has reached maximum effort. Routinely, it is expressed relative to the body weight as milliliters or oxygen consumed, per kilogram body weight, per minute (mL/kg/min). Fick's equation defines two major factors that influence the oxygen uptake. These two factors include the cardiac output and the arterial-venous oxygen difference. Increases in cardiac output during activity reflect appropriate functioning of the central cardiovascular system in increasing exercise capacity. The arterial venous oxygen difference is the difference between oxygen content of arterial and venous blood and provides the clinician with the oxygen extraction capabilities at the level of the peripheral muscle. The arterial venous oxygen difference reflects the involvement of the peripheral muscle in increasing exercise capacity.

Energy expenditure at rest and during activity is also important to consider in the management of patients with cardiovascular disease. Energy expenditure is commonly computed from the amount of oxygen consumed at rest or while performing any given activity. Units that best quantify energy expenditure include kcal, L/O_2, mL of O_2 per kg of body weight per minute, and METs.

A single MET is defined as the amount of oxygen consumed at rest per unit of body weight for one minute. The quantity of oxygen consumed in a minute per unit body weight at rest, provides a measure of the energy expenditure to run bodily functions while the individual is at rest. Approximately 3.5 milliliters of oxygen per kilogram body weight is consumed to run bodily functions at rest and is often quantified as 1 MET.[13] During participation in an activity, the amount of oxygen consumed in a minute per unit body weight reflects the energy expenditure required to participate in that activity. Activity intensity, based on the corresponding MET level, can range from light intensity to vigorous intensity. The MET levels for a variety of activities have been determined in past research investigations and complied together in one place within the Compendium of Physical Activities.[14] This compendium is a useful resource for clinicians in determining the energy expenditure of any given activity. Activities are usually categorized as being light intensity when MET levels are less than 3 METs, moderate intensity if MET levels are between 3 and 6 METs, and vigorous intensity activities if the activity is over 6 METs.[14]

Knowledge of systemic energy requirements is important in prescribing exercise and activity guidelines, as well as in exercise testing for patients with cardiac impairments. Many charts are available that express systemic energy requirements using a variety of oxygen equivalents (Table 13.3).

Normal Responses

Heart rate and oxygen uptake increase with increasing workload. There is a direct, almost linear relationship between HR and external workload (Fig. 13.7). Therefore, if the physical therapy intervention requires an increase in systemic oxygen consumption, then HR should also increase. It is worthy to note that some cardiac medications, particularly the beta blockers, suppress the sympathetic nervous system's effect on the heart and limits the linear increase in HR. Failure of the HR to increase with increasing workloads (chronotropic incompetence) must be evaluated. Other physiological parameters may be useful to examine, including blood pressure, respiratory rate, skin color, and temperature, as well as the patient's level of cognition and perceived exertion. An adverse response in any of these parameters is an indication of the patient's inability to hemodynamically respond to the given intensity of work.

Blood pressure (BP) should be taken before and immediately after exercise with the patient in the same position (i.e., supine, sitting, standing) and from the same arm each time. Ideally, BP should be taken during exercise to determine the actual hemodynamic response to the increased workload. However, depending on the type of exercise modality, this may be technically difficult. In these cases, HR and BP must be taken immediately after exercise. As with HR, a linear increase in systolic pressure is expected with increasing levels of work (Fig. 13.7).

Abnormal Responses

Signs and symptoms of exercise intolerance are presented in Box 13.1. If a patient experiences any of these symptoms, the activity should be stopped and the patient stabilized. It is also important to inform patients that some responses may be delayed for as long as several hours after exercise (e.g. prolonged fatigue, insomnia, sudden weight gain due to fluid retention). Observation of the

Table 13.3 Metabolic Equivalent (MET) Chart

Intensity (70 kg person)	Endurance Promoting	Occupational	Recreational
1½–2 METs 4–7 mL/kg/min 2–2½ kcal/min	Too low in energy level	Desk work, driving auto, electric calculating machine operation, light housework, polishing furniture, washing clothes	Standing, strolling (1 mph), flying, motorcycling, playing cards, sewing, knitting
2–3 METs 7–11 mL/kg/min 2½–4 kcal/min	Too low in energy level unless capacity is very low	Auto repair, radio and television repair, janitorial work, bartending, riding lawn mower, light woodworking	Level walking (2 mph), level bicycling (5 mph), billiards, bowling, skeet shooting, shuffleboard, powerboat driving, golfing with power cart, canoeing, horseback riding at a walk
3–4 METs 11–14 mL/kg/min 4–5 kcal/min	Yes, if continuous and if target heart rate is reached	Brick laying, plastering, wheelbarrow (100 lb load), machine assembly, welding (moderate load), cleaning windows, mopping floors, vacuuming, pushing light power mower	Walking (3 mph), bicycling (6 mph), horseshoe pitching, volleyball (6-person, noncompetitive), golfing (pulling bag cart), archery, sailing (handling small boat), fly fishing (standing in waders), horseback riding (trotting), badminton (social doubles)
4–5 METs 14–18 mL/kg/min	Recreational activities promote endurance; occupational activities must be continuous, lasting longer than 2 min	Painting, masonry, paperhanging, light carpentry, scrubbing floors, raking leaves, hoeing	Walking (3½ mph), bicycling (8 mph), table tennis, golfing (carrying clubs), dancing (foxtrot), badminton (singles), tennis (doubles), many calisthenics, ballet
5–6 METs 18–21 mL/kg/min	Yes	Digging garden, shoveling light earth	Walking (4 mph), bicycling (10 mph), canoeing (4 mph), horseback riding (posting to trotting), stream fishing (walking in light current in waders), ice or roller skating (9 mph)
6–7 METs 21–25 mL/kg/min 7–8 kcal/min	Yes	Shoveling 10 times/min (4½ kg or 10 lb), splitting wood, snow shoveling, hand lawn mowing	Walking (5 mph), bicycling (11 mph), com-petitive badminton, tennis (singles), folk and square dancing, light downhill skiing, ski touring (2½ mph), water skiing, swimming (20 yards/min)
7–8 METs 25–28 mL/kg/min 8–10 kcal/min	Yes	Digging ditches, carrying 36 kg or 80 lb, sawing hardwood	Jogging (5 mph), bicycling (12 mph), horseback riding (gallop), vigorous downhill skiing, basketball, mountain climbing, ice hockey, canoeing (5 mph), touch football, paddleball
8–9 METs 28–32 mL/kg/min 10–11 kcal/min	Yes	Shoveling 10 times/min (5½ kg or 14 lb)	Running (5½ mph), bicycling (13 mph), ski touring (4 mph), squash (social), handball (social), fencing, basketball (vigorous), swimming (30 yards/min), rope skipping
10+ METs 32+ mL/kg/min 11+ kcal/min	Yes	Shoveling 10 times/min (7½ kg or 16 lb)	Running (6 mph = 10 METs, 7 mph = 11½ METs, 8 mph = 13½ METs, 9 mph = 15 METs, 10 mph = 17 METs), ski touring (5+ mph), handball (competitive), squash (competitive), swimming (greater than 40 yards/min)

From Fox, SM, et al: Physical activity and cardiovascular health: 3. The exercise prescription: Frequency and type of activity. Mod Con Cardiovasc Dis 41:26, 1972, with permission.

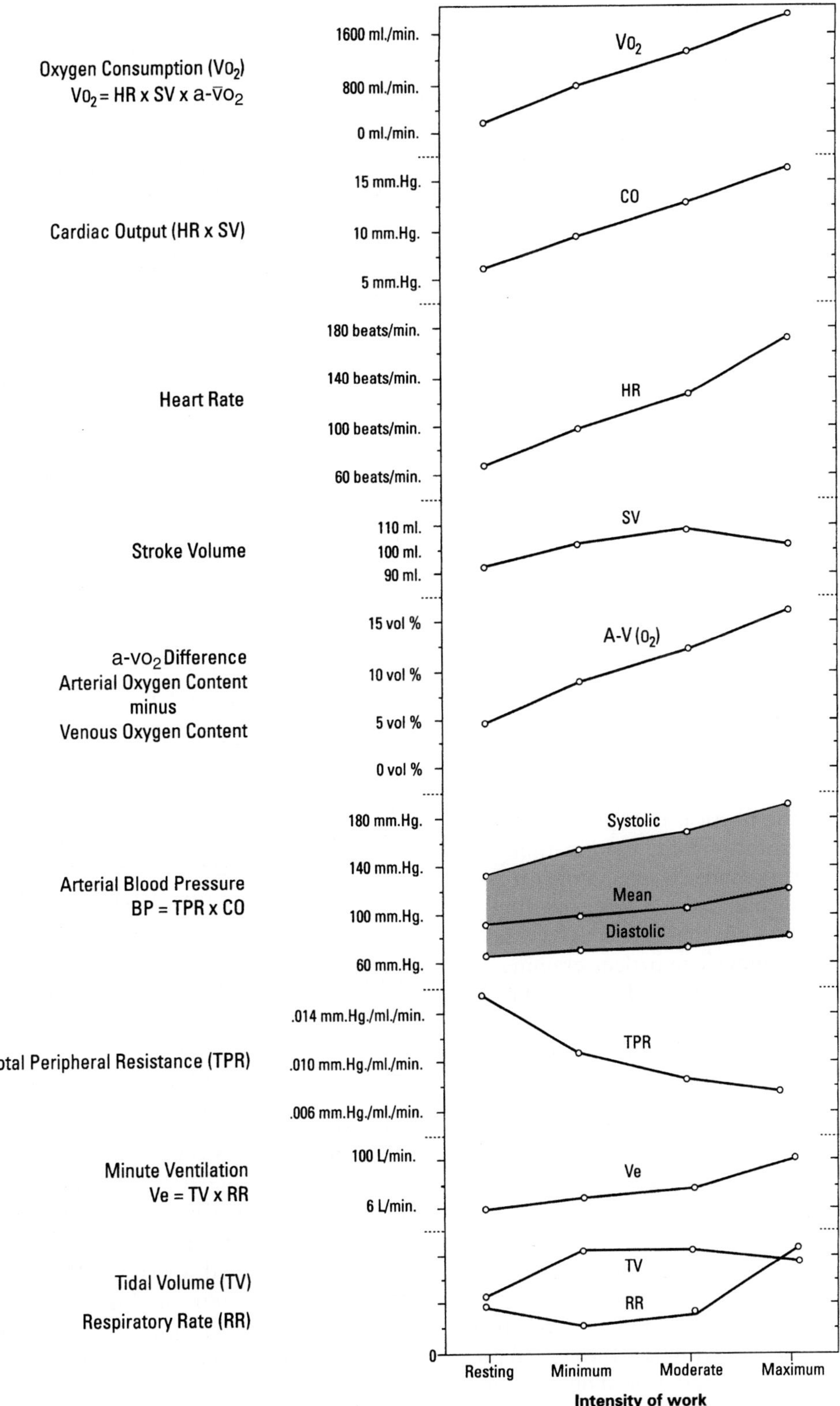

Figure 13.7 Cardiopulmonary response to acute aerobic exercise. *(Adapted from Berne, RM, and Levy, MN: Cardiovascular Physiology, ed 5. CV Mosby, St. Louis, 1986, p 237; Zadai, CC: Clinics in Physical Therapy, Pulmonary Management in Physical Therapy. Churchill Livingstone, New York, 1992, p 27; and McArdle, WD, et al: Essentials of Exercise Physiology. Lea & Febiger, Philadelphia, 1994, p 230.)*

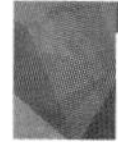

Box 13.1 Indications of Exercise Intolerance That Warrant Modification or Termination of an Exercise Session

Signs and Symptoms

- Moderately severe or increasing angina
- Marked dyspnea
- Dizziness, light-headedness, or ataxia
- Cyanosis or pallor
- Excessive fatigue
- Leg cramps or claudication

Other Abnormal Responses

- Failure of the systolic pressure to rise as exercise continues
- A hypertensive BP response, including a systolic pressure of greater than 200 mm Hg and/or a diastolic pressure greater than 110 mm Hg
- A progressive fall in systolic pressure of 10–15 mm Hg
- A significant change in cardiac rhythm detected either by palpation or by ECG monitoring (e.g., arrhythmias, ST-T wave changes).

Adapted from ACSM's Guidelines for Exercise Testing and Prescription, ed 8. Lippincott Williams & Wilkins, Philadelphia, 2010.

patient throughout the physical therapy intervention provides a mechanism for ongoing examination. The therapist must be alert to subtle changes in the patient's facial expression, skin color, tone of voice, or thought processing because these may indicate activity intolerance and may require immediate patient examination and modification of the intervention. In addition to the patient's subjective complaint of fatigue or discomfort, there are other responses that warrant termination of an exercise session. These abnormal responses are included in Box 13.1.

CARDIAC PATHOLOGIES AND PHYSICAL THERAPY IMPLICATIONS

The pathophysiological conditions that underlie heart disease include HTN, atherosclerosis within the coronary arteries, altered myocardial muscle mechanics, valvular dysfunction, and arrhythmias. The clinical presentations of CVD are diverse and depend on the source of the alterations in structure and function within the cardiovascular system including altered perfusion of coronary arteries, reduced contractility of the LV, or alterations in electrical activity. Common signs and symptoms associated with heart disease are chest pressure, dyspnea, fatigue, syncope, and palpitations. However, although these clinical manifestations are strongly associated with heart disease, they are not exclusive for heart disease. Therefore, taking a thorough patient history and performing an appropriate examination and evaluation are crucial to establishing the physical therapy movement diagnosis, goals, outcomes, and plan of care (POC).

An important consideration is that the extent of an individual's activity limitations cannot solely be based on the cardiac diagnosis and pathology. Individuals with similar cardiac pathologies may experience different degrees of activity limitations. Activity limitations are influenced by multiple factors beyond cardiac dysfunction. These factors include the degree of peripheral muscle strength, the extent of compensatory mechanism activated within the body that allow cardiac functioning to continue for a length of time before the patient becomes symptomatic and overly decompensated, and the pharmacological management provided to the patient. The following section will delineate the major pathologies affecting heart function, medical management of these conditions, and pertinent implications for physical therapist practice.

Hypertension

Hypertension (HTN) is currently the most prevalent cardiovascular disease in the United States. It has also routinely referred to as one of the most powerful contributors to cardiovascular morbidity and mortality. The National Health and Nutrition Examination Survey (NHAHES), conducted from 2005 to 2208, estimated that 29% to 31% of adults in the United States have HTN.[15] These results were extrapolated to estimate that approximately 76 million Americans above the age of 20 have HTN.[15] Further, data from the same survey indicate that only 50.1% of persons with hypertension have their blood pressure under control.[15]

In 2017 the American College of Cardiology and the American Heart Association published revised guidelines that aimed to incorporate new information from studies regarding blood pressure (BP)-related risk of cardiovascular disease (CVD), research on ambulatory BP monitoring, home BP monitoring, and appropriate threshold values to initiate antihypertensive drug treatment.[16] The new guidelines reference BP as normal, elevated, or stages 1 or 2. Normal BP is defined as <120/<80 mm Hg; elevated BP 120–129/<80 mm Hg; hypertension stage 1 is 130 to 139 or 80 to 89 mm Hg, and hypertension stage 2 is ≥140 or ≥90 mm Hg.[16] It is important to ensure that the average BP to deem an individual hypertensive be based on ≥2 readings obtained on ≥2 occasions of measurement. The guidelines additionally state that it is appropriate for clinicians to advocate for out-of-office and self-monitoring of BP measurements to confirm the diagnosis of hypertension. In some patients, the blood pressure is not consistently elevated and fluctuates between hypertensive and normal values. This is called *labile HTN* and is diagnosed following the evaluation of elevated blood pressure values over a more prolonged length of time.

Hypertensive individuals may have elevations in both systolic and diastolic values; however, in the elderly, isolated systolic hypertension (ISH) is commonly noted with elevations in the systolic blood pressure above 140 mm Hg with diastolic blood pressures in the normal range.[17]

It is also worthy to note that although somewhat controversial, home readings correlate more closely with the results of daytime ambulatory measurements of blood pressure than with blood pressure taken in the clinician's office. This is especially true in individuals with *White Coat Hypertension* defined as blood pressure that is consistently elevated at medical practitioner office readings but does not meet diagnostic criteria for hypertension based upon out-of-office home readings. The 2017 guidelines recommended that clinicians screen for white coat syndrome in adults with an untreated systolic BP (SBP) >130 but <160 mm Hg or diastolic BP (DBP) >80 but <100 mm Hg, using either ambulatory or home monitoring devices.[16]

Broadly, HTN may be divided into two major categories: *primary (or essential)* HTN and *secondary (or nonessential)* HTN. *Primary or essential HTN* is diagnosed when there is no known cause for the elevation in BP values and exists in approximately 90% to 95% of all patients with HTN. Genetic factors, environmental influences (including dietary sodium intake), stress, obesity, excessive alcohol consumption, and other risk factors (including age, lack of exercise, and glucose intolerance) have implications on the occurrence of essential HTN.[18] Regardless of the underlying cause, the pathophysiology of essential hypertension depends on the primary or secondary inability of the kidney to excrete sodium at a normal blood pressure with overall reductions in control mechanisms responsible for lowering BP.[18] *Secondary or nonessential HTN* occurs in approximately 5% to 10% of the hypertensive population and is caused by an identifiable medical problem such as primary renal disease, illicit drug use, renovascular disease, obstructive sleep apnea, Cushing's syndrome, endocrine disorders, coarctation of the aorta and more.

Uncontrolled elevated BP levels produce a variety of additional complications, including heart failure, renal failure, dissecting aneurysms, PVD, retinopathy, and stroke. These negative consequences are directly related to the level of BP. Because of this, the 2015 U.S. Preventive Services Task Force (USPSTF) guidelines indicate that all individuals 18 years or older should be screened for elevated blood pressure.[19] The document delineates that at a minimum blood pressure must be monitored with the following frequency:

- Adults 40 years or older assessed at least once annually
- Adults between 18 and 39 years screened at least once annually if they have risk factors for hypertension
- Adults between 18 and 39 years with readings <130/80 mm Hg that have no risk factors for hypertension to be screened at least every three years.

Management of Hypertension and Physical Therapy Implications

Treatment for individuals with hypertension involve a combination of nonpharmacologic therapies involving lifestyle changes coupled with antihypertensive drug therapy. Physical therapists can play an integral role in assisting patients with necessary lifestyle changes including weight loss, adopting the *Dietary Approaches to Stop Hypertension* (DASH) eating plan, reducing sodium intake, increasing physical activity, and moderating alcohol consumption.[20] The benefits of these lifestyle changes include lowering the dosage of medications and reduced occurrence of adverse side effects.

Empirical evidence has documented approximate reductions in systolic BP values with each of the lifestyle changes mentioned above. Maintenance of a normal body weight evaluated by a BMI between 18.5 to 24.9 kg/m^2 is important for all individuals. Research has documented a 5 to 20 mm Hg reduction in systolic blood pressure with a 10 kg drop in body weight.[20] Further, it is important to recommend patients follow the recommendations of the DASH diet, eating foods that are rich in fruits, vegetables, low-fat dairy products and a reduced content of saturated fat and total fat. Adopting a dietary plan based on DASH guidelines has been shown to reduce systolic BP readings by 8 to 14 mm Hg.[20] In addition, it is important to recommend a reduction of dietary sodium intake to no more than 100 meq/day.[21] A *Cochrane Database* systematic review in 2013 indicates a 2 to 8 mm Hg drop in systolic BP with the utilization of this dietary sodium restriction guideline.[21] Finally, alcohol consumption must be limited to no more than 2 drinks per day in most men and no more than 1 drink per day in women and lighter-weight individuals.

Pharmacological intervention is the most common form of medical management of HTN. Six classes of medications currently exist: beta-adrenergic blockers, alpha-adrenergic blockers, angiotensin-converting enzyme (ACE) inhibitors, diuretics, vasodilators, and calcium channel blockers.[9] In addition to pharmacology, it is important for clinicians to recommend lifestyle modifications, including weight reduction, sodium restriction, moderation of alcohol intake, and regular aerobic exercise, for patients diagnosed with HTN. The benefits of these lifestyle changes include lowering the dosage of medications and reduced occurrence of adverse side effects.[20]

Research has also shown that a combination of aerobic and resistance training exercise has the potential to decrease systolic and diastolic BP values by 4 to 6 mm Hg and 3 mm Hg, respectively, independent of weight loss.[22] In general, studies have demonstrated a reduction in blood pressure when prescribed at a frequency of three to four sessions per week of moderate-intensity with a duration of approximately 40 minutes for a period of 12 weeks. Further, a meta-analysis of 28 trials that enrolled 1,012 participants found that resting BP significantly decreased by 4/4 mm Hg with moderate-intensity resistance training.[23] The physiological factors responsible for the potential drop in BP values with aerobic exercise are incompletely understood. Most research theorizes the antihypertensive effects of exercise to be related to a reduction in sympathetic activity and an overall improvement in endothelial function.[22]

Dance therapy may also be utilized as an alternate modality of physical activity in managing patients with hypertension. A 2016 systematic review and meta-analysis investigated the effects of dance therapy in hypertensive patients. The review included four studies that met the inclusion criteria. Dance therapy resulted in a significant reduction in BP values of 12/3 mm Hg compared with the control group.[24] The authors additional document significant improvements in overall exercise capacity with the use of dance therapy.[24]

Pharmacological intervention is the most common form of medical management for patients with HTN. Six classes of medications currently exist: beta-adrenergic blockers, alpha-adrenergic blockers, angiotensin-converting enzyme (ACE) inhibitors, diuretics, vasodilators, and calcium channel blockers. It is ideally recommended that patients be evaluated two to four weeks after initial antihypertensive therapy is initiated and re-evaluated every 3 to 6 months thereafter to ensure the achievement of adequate BP control.

Acute Coronary Syndrome

Acute coronary syndrome (ACS) is the new terminology for ischemic heart disease or CAD. It involves a spectrum of entities ranging from the least involved condition on the spectrum (unstable angina) to the worst involved condition (sudden cardiac death). Additional entities on the spectrum include non-Q myocardial infarction (NQMI), non–ST-elevation myocardial infarction (NSTEMI), and Q myocardial infarction (QMI), also referred to as ST-segment elevation myocardial infarction (STEMI). The hallmark sign for any patient presenting with any condition on the spectrum is ischemic chest pain because of a dyssynchrony between the myocardial oxygen supply and demand. A discussion of physical therapy interventions for managing patients with ACS is delineated later in this chapter.

Pathophysiology of ACS

The primary impairment in acute coronary syndrome is an imbalance of myocardial oxygen supply to meet the myocardial oxygen demand ($M\dot{V}O_2$). The decrease in supply results from a narrowing of the lumen of the coronary artery, usually due to a fixed atherosclerotic lesion. Atherosclerosis is a disease in which lipid-laden plaque (lesions) is formed within the intimal layer of the blood vessel wall of moderate and large size arteries; over time the plaque may extend into the lumen causing a decreased luminal diameter. The lesion results from an initial endothelial injury that causes changes within the intima of the blood vessel and progresses to luminal narrowing.

Several risk factors have been identified that are associated with an increased risk for the formation of an atherosclerotic lesion. Cigarette smoking is an important risk factor for patients with ACS. The incidence of a myocardial infarction (MI) is increased sixfold in women and threefold in men who smoke at least 20 cigarettes per day compared with subjects who never smoked.[25] Further, the risk of acute myocardial infarction has been found to be proportional to tobacco consumption in both men and women with higher risk in inhalers compared with non-inhalers.[25] Diet is another major risk factor to be considered in patients with ACS. Dietary considerations need to include foods with a low glycemic index, low glycemic load, an increase in the consumption of fruits and vegetables, a high fiber diet, reduction in the consumption of red meat, high-fat dairy products, caffeine, and coffee.[26,27]

Clinical Manifestations

Occlusions may occur in coronary arteries and not produce symptoms. In general, symptoms of CAD are not experienced until the lumen is at least 70% occluded. There are, therefore, many patients who are unaware of their sub-acute occlusions. It is important that an individual's risk factors are known, and interventions and monitoring are adjusted according to the individual needs of the patient.

The clinical conditions resulting from atherosclerosis of the coronary arteries are due to inadequate myocardial oxygen supply to meet the myocardial oxygen demand ($M\dot{V}O_2$).[28] The three common clinical presentations of ACS include angina, injury, and infarction and are discussed in the section below.

Angina

Angina, or cardiac-related chest pain, is due to ischemia. Ischemia is characterized by reduced blood flow to the myocardium. Ischemia is a temporary condition due to the imbalance between the myocardial oxygen supply and demand. On restoring the balance between oxygen supply and demand, ischemia will be reversed and the angina will disappear.

There are three major types of angina: unstable, stable, and variant angina. *Unstable angina,* sometimes referred to as pre-infarction angina or crescendo angina. In patients with unstable angina, chest pain typically occurs at rest without any obvious precipitating factors or with minimal exertion.[28] In addition, chest pain increases in severity, frequency, and duration and therefore called crescendo angina. Chest pain in the unstable state is refractory to treatment. Unstable angina usually warrants immediate medical intervention, because the patient is at impending risk for further complications such as an MI or a lethal arrhythmia such as ventricular tachycardia or ventricular fibrillation.

The term *stable angina* is used when angina occurs during exercise or activity. Chest pain is experienced at a certain intensity of exercise when the myocardial oxygen demand exceeds the blood supply to the myocardium and is alleviated by decreasing the MVO_2.[28] As mentioned earlier, the MVO_2 is calculated as the product of HR and SBP, known as the rate pressure product (RPP). When patients experience episodes of stable angina, exercise must be terminated and HR and BP need to be taken to determine the RPP (RPP = HR x SBP). In addition to terminating exercise and resting, MVO_2 can also be reduced with nitroglycerin (NTG). In stable angina, the patient often describes the sensation as an intensity less than 5/10, which improves to 0/10 when the oxygen supply is able to balance the demand. It is important to remember that any report of angina requires intervention; the clinician cannot ignore the symptoms even when the patient describes the sensation as light (1 to 2/10). Finally, some patients may experience dyspnea as their anginal equivalent; that is, they do not have the typical chest discomfort often associated with ischemia but instead experience SOB. For these patients, treatment should be immediate and follow the guidelines for ischemia.

The third type of angina is *variant* or *Prinzmetal angina* and is caused by a vasospasm of coronary arteries in the absence of occlusive disease. Patients with this type of angina respond to NTG for short-term management of their chest pain. However, the preferred long-term pharmacological choice is a calcium channel blocker to reduce the influx of calcium into the smooth muscle cells of the coronary arteries and reduce vasospasm.

Injury and Infarction

Injury represents the presence of a new acute MI. The term *injury* is used because the myocardial tissue is being acutely injured during a sudden heart attack. Acute injury to the myocardial tissue then progresses to irreversible, dead infarcted tissue. Thus, the term *injury* illustrates the presence of a new MI, whereas the term *infarction* depicts an old heart attack with dead tissue that cannot be reversed.

Individual myocardial cells may differ in their tolerance for ischemia; however, irreversible changes start to appear 20 minutes to 2 hours from the onset of myocardial ischemia.[28] The actual process of injury and infarction evolves over a period of hours. Angina commonly precedes a MI, but the intensity of the symptoms is dramatically increased when the patient is moving into having a heart attack. Patients frequently describe their discomfort as 10 out of 10 on a pain scale during an acute MI. Whereas ischemia is due to a partial blockage of the coronary artery, an infarction results from complete occlusion of the vessel. This complete occlusion commonly results from a rupture of a vulnerable plaque with resultant formation of a thrombus. The type of plaque, more so than the size, will influence the risk of rupture. Lipid-rich and soft plaques are more vulnerable to rupture than collagen-rich and hard plaques. Angiographically, large plaque lesions are not necessarily more susceptible to rupture than smaller lesions. Because atherosclerosis begins within the walls of the artery, many vulnerable plaques are invisible via angiogram or appear smaller than their actual size.

The effects on the ventricle because of the infarction often extend beyond the acute infarction period. These long-term effects occur primarily in ventricles that have sustained a moderate to large MI. As the ventricle heals, a process of *remodeling* occurs because of the presence of the infarcted tissue and subsequent dilation. Over time, this reengineering process produces an alteration in ventricular size, shape, and function. Thus, the resultant ventricle often operates at an increased myocardial energy cost due to its inefficient muscle mechanics. Often pictured as three concentric circles (although not absolutely histologically correct), the area of infarction would be at the center of the circle surrounded first by an area of injury and then an outside area of ischemia (Fig. 13.8).

Although most MIs heal initially without incident, complications may occur. The major complications following a MI are recurrence of ischemia, LV failure, and ventricular arrhythmias. Therefore, when a patient is said to have had a *complicated MI,* it is indicative that ischemia, LV failure, or significant ventricular arrhythmias have developed in the acute post-MI period. Ischemia after MI is particularly important because it indicates that there may be vulnerable myocardium with a reduced oxygen

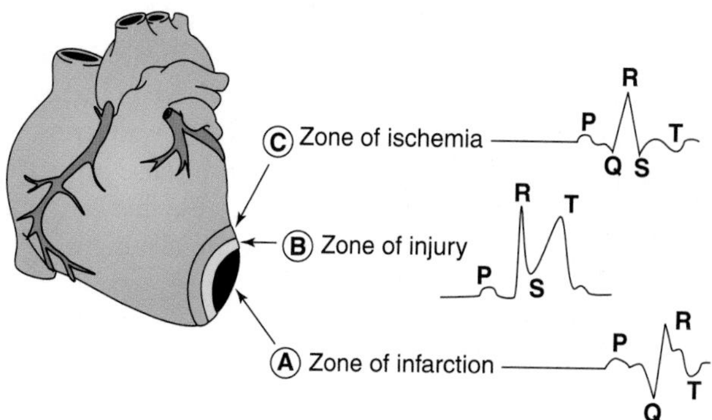

Figure 13.8 ECG following an MI. (A) *Zone of infarction*: when infarction occurs through the full thickness of the myocardium (transmural) an abnormal Q wave usually appears. (B) *Zone of injury*: ST elevation occurs in the area of injury. (C) *Zone of ischemia*: ST depression and/or T-wave inversion occurs in an area of decreased perfusion (ischemia).

supply that may go on to infarct and thereby potentially enlarge the MI.

The ultimate complication following an acute MI is cardiogenic shock characterized by inadequate CO and insufficient arterial BP to perfuse the major organs because of severe LV failure.[29] This condition necessitates extraordinary medical interventions such as the *intra-aortic balloon pump (IABP).* The IABP facilitates CO, decreases MVO_2, and increases coronary artery perfusion.[29] The IABP is a balloon catheter placed within the aorta that inflates during diastole, thereby increasing coronary artery perfusion, and deflates during systole, thereby decreasing afterload. The IABP may be used in other conditions besides post-MI cardiogenic instability. Some examples of such patients include patients with hemodynamic decompensation awaiting a heart transplantation, patients with unstable angina, patients with malignant arrhythmias such as ventricular tachycardia or ventricular fibrillation, and post–cardiac surgical patients with severe hemodynamic instability.

Evaluation of Patients With Acute Coronary Syndrome (the Evaluation Triad)

In addition to the history taking and review of systems, the evaluation of patients with ACS places emphasis on three major components: evaluating patient complaints, ECG changes, and cardiac enzyme levels (Fig. 13.9). The following reviews each component.

Patient Complaints in ACS

Most patients with myocardial ischemia will present with classic chest pain referred to as *angina pectoris.* Classic angina pectoris is diffuse and retrosternal and described as a pressure, heaviness, tightness, or constriction in the center or left of the chest. Pain is usually precipitated by exertion and relieved by rest.[30] It is important for therapists to evaluate factors that provoke chest pain. These may include activities that increase myocardial oxygen demand, including physical activity, cold, emotional stress, sexual intercourse, meals or lying down in the supine position which results in an increase in venous return and increase in myocardial wall stress.[31]

The patient usually often reports an intense pressure like “an elephant sitting on the chest.” Further, angina may present as a referred pain due to involvement of a neural reflex pathway via the thoracic and cervical nerves. This results in chest pain not being felt in a specific spot, but usually as a diffuse discomfort that may be difficult to localize. It may radiate to anywhere in the upper extremities and thorax, most specifically to the left arm and left jaw.[30] Figure 13.10 delineates common areas for referred patterns of chest pain.

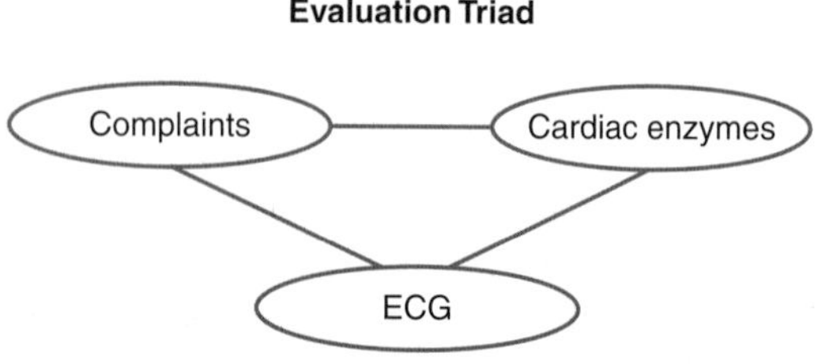

Figure 13.9 Evaluation triad for patients with acute coronary syndrome.

The hallmark approach to differentially diagnosing ischemic chest pain from non-ischemic chest pain is to observe for accompanying signs and symptoms of compromised cardiac output.[31] These signs include dizziness, light-headedness, weakness, diaphoresis (sweating), fatigue, and weakness. Thus, cardiac chest pain during ischemia or an infarction will be accompanied by signs of compromised CO, but chest pain from other etiologies including pulmonary chest pain, pleural pain, gastrointestinal related chest pain or musculoskeletal pain of the thorax will not precipitate the classic signs and symptoms of compromised cardiac output.[31]

ECG Changes in ACS

MIs are identified by 12-lead ECG findings.[32] The ECG (also referred to as EKG) is used to examine HR, rhythm, conduction delays, and coronary perfusion. Two of the most common types of ECG are the single-lead and the 12-lead ECG (Fig. 13.11). In the single-lead ECG, only one area of the heart (e.g., anterior, lateral, or inferior) may be viewed at a time. This area may be changed, however, by altering the location of the electrodes. In the 12-lead ECG, 12 areas are viewed.

The single-lead ECG is sensitive to rate and rhythm changes and is commonly used for monitoring patients during ambulation and activity. Continuous monitoring is accomplished either via telemetry (radio transmission), allowing the patient freedom to move around when wearing this portable device, or by hardwire, where the patient is attached to the monitor by a cable approximately 15 ft long, therefore limiting mobility. A variation of the single-lead ECG is the 3-lead ECG, which is usually hardwire and is used for monitoring in an inpatient setting. It can be worn continuously throughout an entire treatment session or throughout the entire hospitalization. Unlike the single-lead or 3-lead system, the 12-lead ECG does not provide continuous monitoring, except during an exercise tolerance test (ETT) completed on a treadmill or stationary bicycle ergometer. Two common uses for the 12-lead ECG are the resting ECG taken with the patient quietly supine and the ETT. Twelve-lead ECGs are invaluable in identifying perfusion impairments in the coronary arteries and in assisting with arrhythmia detection. During the ETT, the ECG is continuously monitored to determine the presence of ischemia or arrhythmias with each increase in workload. The 12-lead ECG is sensitive to changes in perfusion as well as rate, rhythm, and conduction. Each coronary artery is represented by a cluster of leads that, although not absolutely correlated with

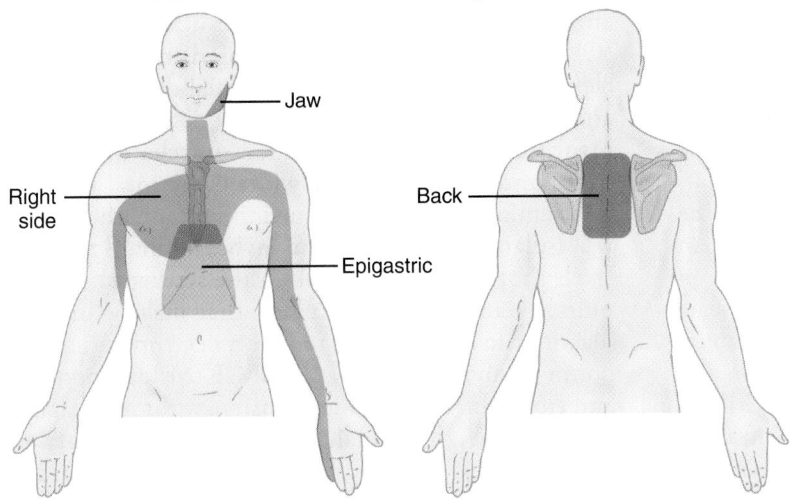

Figure 13.10 Referral pattern for chest pain.

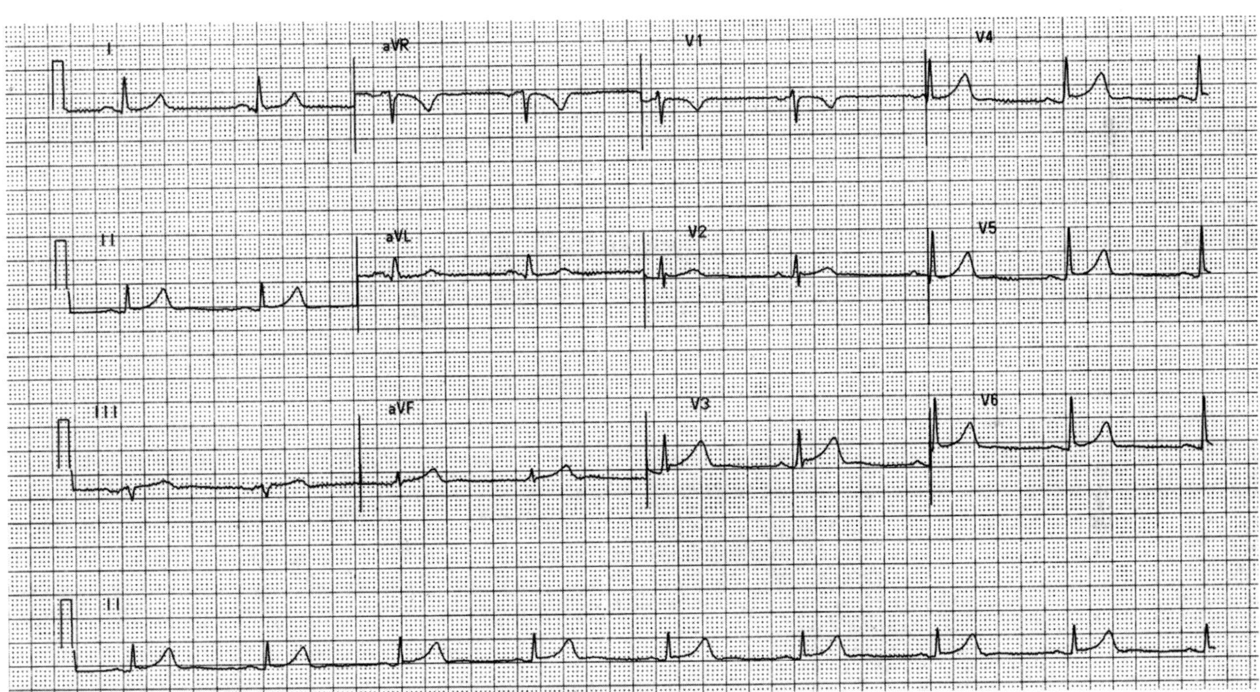

Figure 13.11 Normal 12-lead ECG from 50-year-old woman; slight ST elevation is insignificant. Twelve leads are presented; at the bottom of the page is a rhythm strip from lead II. Heart rate from the rhythm strip is approximately 52 (there are 5.8 large boxes between complex 3 and 4; therefore 300/5.8 = 52).

each individual's anatomy, gives a general schema for myocardial perfusion.

During the examination of a 12-lead ECG, the ST segment is clinically useful in identifying the presence of impaired coronary perfusion, either ischemia or injury.[32] The *J point,* the point where the S wave turns into the ST segment, is the point of reference for interpreting the ST segment.[32] If ischemia is present, the ST segment will be depressed (one or two small boxes) at two small boxes beyond the J point, and the T wave may also be inverted (flipped). Ischemic changes will be present only while the ischemia is present; when the ischemia has resolved, the ECG will return to normal.[32] Conversely, a large acute MI, with subsequent injury to the myocardial tissue, will produce ST-segment elevations on the 12-lead ECG. Large ST elevation myocardial infarction (STEMI) will produce pathological Q waves hours to days following the acute process.[32] Therefore, a QMI represents a large MI. QMIs were formerly known as a *transmural MI* because they usually involved the full thickness of the ventricular wall.

Conversely, an acute MI may be relatively smaller and not cause acute injury to the myocardial tissue. In this case, ST segments are not seen on the ECG and the MI is called an NSTEMI or an NQMI. An NQMI formerly known as a *nontransmural* or *subendocardial MI* does not involve the entire thickness of the myocardial wall, rather affects tissue primarily below the endocardium.

Anatomical classifications for MIs are based on the surfaces of the LV and not the anatomical heart. An anterior MI involves the anterior surface of the LV, an inferior MI involves the inferior surface of the LV (the diaphragmatic region), a lateral MI involves the lateral surface of the LV, a septal MI involves the septum, and a posterior MI involves the LV posterior wall.[33] MIs to different aspects of the ventricle result from compromised levels of blood flow within specific vessels. The RCA supplies blood to the inferior and posterior aspects of the LV and therefore is responsible for producing an inferior- or posterior-wall MI. The anterior and septal aspects of the LV are perfused by the LAD and therefore LAD occlusions are likely to produce anterior or septal MIs. The CX artery supplies blood to the lateral wall of the LV and thereby produces a lateral infarction when it is occluded. The involvement of occlusion within specific vessels can be determined by a 12-lead ECG.[33] RCA involvement is most likely depicted on leads II, III, and aVF (augmented unipolar limb lead). LAD pathology will be illustrated in chest leads V1, V2, V3, and V4, whereas CX pathology will most likely be demonstrated in leads I, aVL, V5, and V6 (Fig. 13.12).

Cardiac Biomarkers in ACS

Blood work also helps determine the presence of an MI. The most frequently used markers include cardiac troponins I and T as well as the MB isoenzyme of creatine kinase (CK-MB).[34] Creatine kinase MB subunit (CK-MB), an isoenzyme, is released into blood and elevates with intracellular myocardial damage.[34] Creatine kinase (CK) is found in many tissues besides the myocardium, especially striated muscle, brain, and liver. Injury to these areas will elevate total CK. To differentiate the type of tissue injured, use of CK-MB will isolate the source to the myocardium. Troponin levels should not be elevated in the setting of striated muscle trauma. Other markers that may be used to diagnose an acute MI are the proteins troponin I, troponin T, and myoglobin. Total CK-MB, troponin I, and troponin T have a high sensitivity for the diagnosis of an MI.[34] Table 13.4 provides a summary of enzyme levels that are elevated with a myocardial infarction.

I Lateral Circ	aVR	V1 Septal LAD	V4 Anterior LAD
II Inferior RCA	aVL Lateral Circ	V2 Septal LAD	V5 Lateral Circ
III Inferior RCA	aVF Inferior RCA	V3 Anterior LAD	V6 Lateral Circ

Figure 13.12 Anatomical pathology and ECG interpretation. Leads I, aVL, V5, and V6 depict problems in the lateral aspect of the left ventricle due to occlusion of blood flow within the circumflex artery. Leads II, III, and aVF depict problems in the inferior aspect of the left ventricle due to occlusion of blood flow within the right coronary artery. Leads V1 to V4 depict problems in the anterior aspect of the left ventricle due to occlusion of blood flow within the left anterior descending artery.

Medical Management of Acute Coronary Syndrome

Once the diagnosis of a MI has been reached (i.e., the patient is "ruled in" for an MI); the subsequent goal of medical management is to keep the patient hemodynamically stable and optimize the wound healing of the myocardium. Two major categories of medical interventions including revascularization procedures and pharmacological interventions are addressed in the following section.

Percutaneous Transluminal Coronary Angioplasty

Percutaneous transluminal coronary angioplasty (PTCA) uses a balloon and collapsed stent (stainless steel "cage-like" tube with multiple slots) on the tip of a catheter, inserted into the radial or femoral artery and advanced retrograde along the aorta to the openings of the coronary arteries.[35] The catheter is inserted into the coronary artery until the site of the lesion is reached. The balloon is then inflated and the stent expands, compressing the plaque against the interior artery walls, thereby increasing the lumenal area. The balloon is deflated and removed, and the stent holds the lumen open. The stent is commonly coated with a drug (e.g., paclitaxel [Abraxane]).[35] Drug-coated stents (collectively referred to as *drug-eluting stents*) are used to prevent endothelial cell proliferation, which may occur in response to endothelial trauma and the presence of a foreign object placed within the coronary artery and result in restenosis (recurrence of stenosis).[35]

The surgical and catheterization reports identify which vessels were revascularized and which vessels have less than 70% lesions and were therefore not revascularized. Because a vessel is not currently a candidate for revascularization does not guarantee that it will not be problematic later, either by rupturing or continuing to demonstrate progressive atherosclerosis. It would be short sighted to assume that a patient who

Table 13.4 Cardiac Enzymes Associated With Myocardial Injury and Infarction

Enzyme	Normal Level	Minor Cardiac Dysfunction	Major Cardiac Dysfunction	Peak Levels
Creatine kinase - myocardial band CK-MB	0%–3%	5%	10%	14–36 hours
Lactic dehydrogenase LDH	100–225 mU/mL or 127 IU	300–750 mU/mL	≥1,000 mU/mL	
Troponin	0–0.2 μg/mL	5 μg/mL	≥10 μg/mL	24–36 hours
Myoglobin	<100 ng/mL	200 ng/mL	≥500 ng/mL	

has had a revascularization procedure cannot become ischemic.

Coronary Artery Bypass Graft

Coronary artery bypass graft (CABG) uses a donor vessel to bypass the lesion (narrowed lumen) and establish an alternate improved blood supply. The donor vessel may be the radial artery of the nondominant upper extremity (UE), the saphenous vein, or the internal mammary artery. The patient's harvested saphenous vein or radial artery must be completely detached from both its proximal and distal insertions; the graph is sutured proximally into the aorta and distally into the involved artery beyond the occlusion. When the internal mammary artery is used, it maintains its native proximal attachment while the distal segment is reattached below (bypass) the area of occlusion. Bypass surgery techniques are constantly evolving; traditionally, the full sternum was cut and retracted, but newer minimally invasive techniques called *minimally invasive direct coronary artery bypass* (MIDCAB) have emerged that involve less sternal cutting, and some techniques involve no sternal cutting at all, but access the heart via the intercostal space.[36]

Most CABG procedures involve placing the patient on an artificial heart–lung machine (bypass pump), which maintains the oxygenation and circulation of the blood while the heart is stopped during the surgical procedure. Because of the bypass pump, patients may have additional fluid weight gain following surgery, may feel fatigued, and some patients may have transient A-fib and cognitive changes. Newer techniques have facilitated the use of *off-pump procedures* to limit the time on the bypass pump. Thus the surgeon operates on a beating heart for the entire or part of the procedure to limit time on the heart–lung machine and reduce the negative sequelae that result from excessive pump time.[37] Researchers who comprehensively reviewed the results from 126 experienced centers that performed off-pump procedures concluded that the off-pump CABG procedure is associated with decreased mortality and morbidity after coronary artery bypass grafting and may prove superior to conventional CABG in appropriately selected patients.[37]

Physical Therapy Clinical Implications

For patients who have had bypass surgery (e.g., CABG), recovery is somewhat slower than that for patients who have been re-vascularized through a PTCA procedure. This is because of the complexity of the surgical procedure and the incisional healing. Further, prolonged time in the crucifix position during surgery may predispose individuals to developing an ulnar nerve palsy after surgery.[38] Examination of sensation and manual muscle testing is indicated to rule out the potential for brachial plexus injuries.[38]

The number and location of incisions depend on the surgeon's technique (i.e., either a full sternal cut, partial sternal cut, or intercostal approach). The donor graph site may require additional incisions: a leg incision if saphenous vein is used, a nondominant arm incision if radial artery is used, or no additional incision if grafted with the internal mammary artery. Physical therapy intervention should address any soft tissue impairments associated with the incision to maintain appropriate tissue extensibility and range of motion (ROM), with awareness that patients often indicate soreness and/or discomfort around the donor site. Further, radial pulses cannot be obtained on the extremity where a radial graft artery was grafted for the bypass procedure.

If a sternal wound is present, appropriate posture, scapula retraction, and functional shoulder movements should be encouraged. Proprioceptive neuromuscular facilitation (PNF) UE diagonal patterns often work well, as do the traditional cardinal plane ROM exercises. Patients should be reminded that only a few repetitions at a time throughout the day are better tolerated than more intensive repetitions 1 to 2 times per day; the latter regimen often results in incisional soreness.

Sternal precautions are commonly applied to reduce dehiscence of the incision. Cited risk factors for dehiscence include diabetes, pendulous breasts, obesity, and

COPD.[39] Interestingly, there is no direct evidence that links the use of arm movements or activity to an increased risk of sternal complications after surgery. Prior research has indicated that patients with chronic sternal instability demonstrate greatest sternal separation when pushing up from a chair with sit-to-stand transfers and least sternal separation when elevating both arm overhead.[40] In addition, in normal health individuals, the greatest amount of sternal skin movement was seen with sit-to-stand and supine-to-long sitting transfers and the least movement was noted when raising a unilateral weighted UE (less than 8 lb) above shoulder height. Patients with chronic sternal instability tend to experience pain that is greater when raising a unilateral loaded UE compared with raising bilateral loaded UEs.[41]

Sternal precautions vary greatly by physician, institution, and type of surgery performed. It is important to develop a professional collegial relationship with the surgical team to discuss surgical techniques and mobility concerns to ensure the best outcome for the patient. Cahalin, LaPier, and Shaw developed an algorithm delineating sternal precaution guidelines include for patients with high, moderate, or low risk for sternal complications.[42] They present guidelines based on the risk of the patient. General considerations in sternal precaution guidelines include the following:

- Lifting, pushing, pulling objects >10 lb
- Performing shoulder and or flex >90 when upper extremity is weighted
- Encouraging shoulder AROM in pain-free range
- Avoiding scapular retraction past neutral
- Avoiding trunk flex and rotation with supine to sit transfers
- Minimizing or avoiding upper extremity use with sit to stand
- Appling sternal counter pressure (splinting) with cough
- Limiting driving

Adams and colleagues proposed an approach that applies standard kinesiological principles in the management of patients with a sternotomy.[43] The paper presents pictures and guidelines on teaching patients how to perform load-bearing movements in a way that avoids excessive stress to the sternum by keeping movement constrained within an imaginary tube around the thorax.

To avoid sternal discomfort, all patients will benefit from splinting the incision with a hand or pillow when laughing, coughing, or sneezing.[44]

Early ambulation and mobility beginning the first day after surgery will assist in the patient's physical and emotional recovery. Even though the heart function is perhaps the best it has been in quite some time, the effects of major surgery on energy level and mobility must be emphasized. The impact of fatigue on the patient's sense of well-being may be profound, and it is important that patients understand the need for rest as well as ambulation. Patients will benefit from information regarding energy conservation and rest periods.

Pharmacological Management

Cardiovascular pharmacological agents are critical in the medical management of patients with CAD. There are a variety of drugs designed to re-establish the balance of myocardial supply and demand, with new drugs being added all the time. The major anti-ischemic categories are beta blockers, calcium channel blockers, and nitrates. *Beta blockers* decrease beta-sympathetic activity on the heart, resulting in a decrease in HR and contractility and therefore reduced energy demand. *Calcium channel blockers* reduce BP and therefore decrease the work of the heart. Calcium channel blockers are also somewhat unique in preventing coronary smooth muscle spasm and thereby may increase myocardial blood supply. *Nitrates,* one of the oldest categories of drugs, are potent vasodilators that decrease preload and afterload, and therefore decrease myocardial work, as well as dilate coronary arteries. *Afterload reducers,* particularly those that affect the renin–angiotensin–aldosterone system such as *angiotensin-converting enzyme (ACE) inhibitors* and *angiotensin receptor blockers (ARBs),* are frequently used to normalize BP and reduce workload on the heart. The effect of some of the more widely used cardiac drugs on HR, BP, and ECG findings are presented in Table 13.5.

Heart Failure

Heart failure is a high prevalence syndrome characterized by impaired cardiac pump function, resulting in inadequate systemic perfusion and an inability to meet the body's metabolic demands.[45] Being a syndrome, patients in heart failure present with an array of signs and symptoms. This section presents the epidemiology, causes and types of heart failure, the pathophysiological and clinical presentation of heart failure, medical management, and evaluation for this patient population. A discussion of physical therapy interventions for managing patients with heart failure is delineated later in this chapter.

Epidemiology of Heart Failure

With the marked improvement in anti-ischemic medications, increased knowledge and management of CAD risk factors, availability of sophisticated monitoring, and revascularization techniques, more patients are living longer with coronary disease than similar patients 20 or 30 years ago. New technology and medications continually improve the understanding and management of CAD; however, an undesired effect of long-term CAD may be the increased prevalence of heart failure, also known as congestive heart failure (CHF). Technology and other advances in medicine are reducing mortality with a concomitant increase in morbidity. Therefore, patients with heart failure are less likely to die and more likely to live longer with the worldwide prevalence and incidence of heart failure approaching epidemic proportions.

Table 13.5 Effects of Medications on Heart Rate, Blood Pressure, ECG, and Exercise Capacity

Medications	Heart Rate	Blood Pressure	ECG	Exercise Capacity
I. Beta blockers (including carvedilol and labetalol)	↓ (R and E)	↓ (R and E)	↓ HR* (R) ↓ ischemia† (E)	↑(in patients with angina; ↓ or ↔ in patients without angina
II. Nitrates	↑ (R) ↑ or ↔(E)	↓ (R) ↓ or ↔ (E)	↑ HR (R) ↑ or ↔ HR (E) ↓ ischemia† (E)	↑ in patients with angina; ↔ in patients without angina; or ↔ in patients with congestive heart failure (CHF)
III. Calcium channel blockers			↓ or ↔ HR (R and E) ↓ ischemia (E)	↑ in patients with angina; ↔ in patients without angina
Amlodipine Isradipine Nicardipine Nifedipine Nimodipine	↓ or ↔ (R and E)	↓ (R and E)		
Diltiazem Verapamil	↓ (R and E)		↓ HR (R and E) ↓ ischemia† (E)	
IV. Digitalis	↓ in patients w/atrial fibrillation and possibly CHF Not significantly altered in patients w/sinus rhythm	↔(R and E)	May produce nonspecific ST-T wave changes (R) May produce ST segment depression (E)	Improved only in patients with atrial fibrillation or in patients with CHF
V. Diuretics	↔ (R and E)	↔ or ↓ (R and E)	↔ or PVCs (R) May cause PVCs and "false-positive" test results if hypokalemia occurs May cause PVCs if hypomagnesemia occurs (E)	↔ except possibly in patients with CHF
VI. Vasodilators,	↑ or ↔ (R and E)	↓ (R and E)	↑ or ↔ HR (R and E)	↔ except ↑ or ↔ in patients with CHF
ACE inhibitors and angiotensin II blockers	↔(R and E)	↓ (R and E)	↔ (R and E)	↔ except ↑ or ↔ in patients with CHF
Alpha-adrenergic blockers	↔(R and E)	↓ (R and E)	↔ (R and E)	↔
Antiadrenegic agents without selective blockade	↓ or ↔(R and E)	↓ (R and E)	↓ or ↔ HR (R and E)	↔
VII. Nicotine	↑ or ↔ (R and E)	↑ (R and E)	↑ or ↔ HR May provoke ischemia, arrhythmias (R and E)	↔ except ↓ or ↔ in patients with angina

Adapted from American College of Sports Medicine: Guidelines for Exercise Testing and Prescription, ed 8. Lippincott, Williams & Wilkins, Baltimore, 2010, pp 286, 287, and 289, with permission.

Key: ↑ = increase; ↔ = no effect; ↓ = decrease; E = exercise; R = rest.

*Beta blockers with intrinsic sympathomimetic action (ISA) lower resting HR only slightly.

†May prevent or delay myocardial ischemia.

Recent statistics show that the prevalence of HF increased nearly 20% from 5.7 million (2009–2012) to 6.5 million (2011–2014).[46]

In North America the lifetime risk of developing heart failure in both sexes at age 40 is approximately one in five. In addition, there exists an exponential rise in the prevalence of heart failure with increasing age. Heart failure has surpassed MI as the leading cause of cardiac deaths in the United States and is the most frequent cardiac diagnosis for hospital admissions and readmissions.

Causes of Heart Failure

The most common cause of heart failure is cardiac muscle dysfunction. *Cardiac muscle dysfunction* is a general term describing altered systolic and/or diastolic activity of the myocardium that usually develops because of an underlying abnormality within the cardiac structure or function. Heart failure may be caused by diseases of the myocardium, pericardium, endocardium, heart valves, coronary vessels, or by metabolic disorders.[47] Several reasons exist for the development of cardiac muscle dysfunction. Box 13.2 presents potential precursors and risk factors for the development of cardiac muscle dysfunction.

Types of Heart Failure

Heart failure is categorized from a structural and functional perspective. From a structural perspective, heart failure is described as *left-sided heart failure* or *right-sided heart failure*. Left-sided heart failure occurs with LV insult. Pathology of the LV reduces the CO leading to a backup of fluid into the LA and lungs. The increased fluid in the lungs produces the two hallmark pulmonary signs of left-sided heart failure: shortness of breath (SOB) and cough.[48] Primary right-sided heart failure occurs from direct insult to the RV caused by conditions that increase PA pressure. Increased pressure within the PA subsequently increases the afterload, thereby placing greater demands on the RV and causing it to go into failure.[49] With RV failure, blood is not effectively ejected from the RV and backs up into the RA and venous vasculature, producing two hallmark peripheral signs: jugular venous distention and peripheral edema. Often, left-sided heart failure may be severe as seen in patients experiencing a heart failure exacerbation. With severe LV pathology, fluid from the LV backs up into the lungs, increasing PA pressure and causing fluid to back up into the right side of the heart and the systemic venous vasculature. This is called *biventricular failure*. Therefore, patients with biventricular failure will present with both pulmonary and systemic signs of heart failure. Table 13.6 provides hemodynamic pressures noted with left, right, and biventricular failure.

From a functional perspective, heart failure is described as systolic or diastolic dysfunction. *Systolic dysfunction* also known as *heart failure with reduced EF (HFrEF)* is characterized by compromised contractile function of the ventricles causing reductions in the SV, CO, and EF.[47] Patients with systolic dysfunction will usually present with compromised ejection fractions (EFs) less than 40%.[47] *Diastolic dysfunction* also known as *heart failure with preserved ejection fraction (HFpEF)* is characterized by compromised diastolic function of the ventricles.[48] With this condition, the ventricles cannot relax and fill appropriately during the relaxation (diastolic) phase of the cardiac cycle. The impaired ability to fill the ventricles with blood reduces the volume of blood ejected with each contraction (the SV) and the overall volume of blood ejected per minute (the CO).[48]

Box 13.2 Causes of Cardiac Muscle Dysfunction

Precursors	Description
Hypertension	Increased peripheral arterial pressure contributes to increased afterload and pathological hypertrophy of the left ventricle.
Coronary artery disease	Acute injury to myocardial tissue damages ventricular contractility causing systolic dysfunction. Scar formation seen in infracted tissue alters relaxation and may lead to diastolic dysfunction.
Cardiac dysrhythmias	Normal electrical conduction through the heart allows for normal mechanical contraction of the ventricles. Altered electrical conduction alters the mechanical activity of the ventricles exacerbating heart failure.
Valve abnormalities	Cardiac valve pathology (stenosis or regurgitation) causes structural changes to the chamber behind the valve resulting in cardiac muscle dysfunction and failure.
Pericardial pathology	Pericarditis (fluid in the pericardial space) with resultant cardiac tamponade compresses the ventricles leading to cardiac muscle dysfunction and heart failure.
Cardiomyopathies	Damage to the myocardial cells from various pathological processes alters the systolic and/or diastolic function of the ventricles.

Table 13.6 Example of Hemodynamic Pressures Associated With Heart Failure

An increase in PAP and/or PCWP is associated with LV failure; an increase in CVP is associated with RV failure; and an increase in CVP, PAP, and PCWP is associated with biventricular failure.

Pressure (Norms)	LV Failure	RV Failure	Biventricular Failure
CVP (0–8 mm Hg)	6 mm Hg	12 mm Hg	12 mm Hg
PAP (9–19) mm Hg	22 mm Hg	16 mm Hg	22 mm Hg
PCWP (6–12) mm Hg	18 mm Hg	10 mm Hg	18 mm Hg

CVP = central venous pressure; LV = left ventricle; PAP = pulmonary artery pressure; PCWP = pulmonary capillary wedge pressure; RV = right ventricle

EF is unaltered and remains normal between 55% and 75%.[48] No reduction in the ratio is noted because there is no change in the contractile ability of the ventricles. However, there is a low volume of blood being ejected with each contraction as less blood entered the ventricle before the contraction phase.

Pathophysiology of Heart Failure

Heart failure involves a complex series of events involving pathophysiological and compensatory factors in response to cardiac muscle dysfunction.[47] When the myocardium is dysfunctional, compensatory mechanisms are activated with the goal of maintaining adequate cardiac output. Neurohormonal mechanisms including activation of the sympathetic nervous system are triggered to increase HR and maintain CO at rest. Thus, patients experiencing an acute bout of heart failure are very likely to be tachycardia at rest. Clinically, it is important to evaluate resting heart rate relative to the patient's baseline resting heart rate values. In other words, a patient with a resting heart rate that is usually 60 beats/minute and presents on a given day with a resting heart rate that is 80 beats/minute would need further assessment of other signs and symptoms that indicate the possibility of the patient moving into a state of decompensated heart failure.

When patients are in heart failure and the ventricle is ejecting low blood volumes, blood begins to accumulate within the ventricles, causing congestion. This congestion increases the LVEDV and contributes to an elevation in LV pressure. The increased pressure is transmitted retrograde toward the LA and the pulmonary veins. This increase in hydrostatic pressure in the pulmonary veins causes fluid to move from the veins into the interstitial space of the lung, resulting in pulmonary edema.[50]

It is also important to consider kidney function for patients with heart failure. Low blood volume pumped out of the heart causes less blood to perfuse the kidney and is likely to put the kidney in failure.[50] Patients experiencing an acute heart failure exacerbation often go into renal failure. It is therefore crucial for therapists to monitor BUN and plasma creatinine levels. An increase in urea production, elevated BUN and creatinine levels, and decreased urine output indicate renal dysfunction.[50]

From a musculoskeletal standpoint, patients with heart failure often present with skeletal muscle wasting and weakness, myopathies, and osteoporosis. These negative sequelae are associated with inactivity and prolonged bedrest.[51] Several studies have investigated the effects of heart failure on skeletal muscle abnormalities and found reductions in the size and number of type I and type II muscle fibers.[51] It is therefore imperative that the physical therapy POC place emphasis on interventions to improve overall muscle function and functional mobility in this patient population.

Clinical Manifestations of Heart Failure

The clinical presentation of the patient with CHF depends not only on the amount of LV failure, but also on the status of compensatory mechanisms and the impact of drug therapy. Over time, the energy cost of the compensatory mechanisms proves to be too much for the impaired myocardium. The patient then begins to present with signs and symptoms of CHF, and now moves from being asymptomatic to symptomatic. Although the terminology may be somewhat confusing, it is important to note that when a patient is referred to as being in *compensated heart failure,* the patient's congestive symptoms can be relieved by medical intervention. A patient who is *decompensated* is showing signs and symptoms of congestion and requires medical and pharmacological readjustment. Felker and colleagues define decompensated heart failure as the presence of new or worsening signs/symptoms of dyspnea, fatigue or edema that lead to hospitalization or unscheduled medical care (doctor visits or emergency department visits).[52]

The hallmark signs of decompensation are related to increased congestion and increased ventricular filling pressures.[52] Common signs and symptoms of CHF include fatigue, dyspnea, edema (pulmonary and peripheral), weight gain, presence of an S_3 heart sound, and renal dysfunction.[52] Pulmonary edema may be evident by chest x-ray and auscultation of adventitious sounds. Peripheral edema may be evident in gravity-dependent LEs by the presence of indentations in the skin when pressure is applied, that is, pitting edema. Pitting edema associated with CHF is usually bilateral and may extend from the foot to the pretibial area. Documentation should include a numerical grade based on the duration of indentation after fingertip pressure. See Chapter 14, Vascular, Lymphatic, and Integumentary Disorders, for Palpation/Pitting Scale. Weight gain and peripheral edema are among the signs of systemic volume overload.

On auscultation of the heart and lungs characteristic sounds are heard with CHF. The usual abnormal heart sound associated with CHF is the presence of an S_3 heart sound. This is a low-frequency heart sound heard in early diastole and occurs due to poor ventricular compliance and subsequent turbulence of blood within the ventricle. S_3 heart sound is correlated with increased left ventricular end diastolic pressures (LVEDP) and pulmonary capillary wedge pressures (PCWP) with sensitivity of 30% to 50% and a specificity of 80% to 90%.[53] Heart murmurs (extra heart sounds), especially those of mitral regurgitation, may also be present owing to the effect of the enlarged LV pulling on the mitral valve. Lung auscultation for patients with heart failure reveals the presence of crackles or rales.[54] These are crackling/bubbling sounds suggesting fluid in the lung. The sounds are usually heard during inspiration and represent the movement of fluid in the alveoli and subsequent opening of the alveoli that were previously closed because of the excess fluid. Negi in colleagues in 2014 discovered that patients with pulmonary crackles and an S_3 heart sound were present in more than 50% of all patients admitted to the emergency department for heart failure decompensation.[54] Further, the authors report that patients with crackles and S_3 heart sound had higher readmission rates than those without these signs, odds ratio for pulmonary crackles was 2.8; odds ratio for S_3 heart sound was 2.6.[54]

Dyspnea is one of the most common symptoms experienced with left-sided CHF. The SOB is associated with pulmonary edema.[52] When fluid accumulates in the lungs, gas exchange is altered at the alveolar capillary interface. Gas exchange (respiration) will occur at the alveolar capillary interface only when ventilation within the alveoli is matched with perfusion within the pulmonary capillary (V/Q matching). Excessive amounts of fluid within the pulmonary parenchyma cause a ventilation/perfusion mismatch, thereby reducing the amount of oxygen delivered to blood and causing dyspnea.[52]

Two other symptoms reported by patients in CHF are paroxysmal nocturnal dyspnea, orthopnea and bendopnea.[55] Paroxysmal nocturnal dyspnea (PND) is characterized by sudden episodes of SOB occurring in the night.[55] Orthopnea is increased SOB in the recumbent position.[55] The severity of orthopnea is often crudely documented by observing the number of pillows a patient needs to keep the upper body in an upright or semirecumbent position. Therefore, a patient with three- or four-pillow orthopnea suggests a greater severity of heart failure when compared with a patient with one-pillow orthopnea. Physiologically, as patients assume a recumbent position from an upright position, with their legs elevated to the same horizontal level as their trunk, fluid moves back to the heart causing an increase in preload. A failing heart cannot keep up with the additional preload and excess fluid returning to the heart and therefore causes a backup into the lungs producing increased symptoms of SOB.

Bendopnea, a relatively new sign was discovered in 2014 by Thibodeau and colleagues. This sign involves the presence of increased shortness of breath when the patient bends forward.[56] In a prospective study of 102 patients with systolic heart failure, the authors measured the time to onset of bendopnea. The researchers found that bendopnea occurred in 28% of subjects with a median time to onset of 8 seconds. Further, patients with bendopnea had higher supine right atrial pressures, PCWP, PND, orthopnea, and dyspnea on exertion compared with patients without bendopnea.[56]

One of the common complaints of patients with CHF is early onset of muscle fatigue. The cause of the muscle fatigue may be multifactorial, including a decrease in peripheral blood flow, changes within the peripheral vascular beds, peripheral vasoconstriction, atrophy of muscle fibers, and increased utilization of anaerobic metabolism for energy production.

Patients with heart failure will present with decreased exercise tolerance owing to a culmination of the pathophysiological and compensatory events associated with heart failure.[20] It is difficult for patients to exercise when they have gained weight, have SOB, and have a rapid HR. There are a variety of methods to measure exercise tolerance in patients with heart failure. Physicians utilize the New York Heart Association (NYHA) and Functional Classification Scale (Table 13.7). Classification is based on the development of symptoms and the amount of energy required to provoke them. Patients in Class I have mild heart failure and relatively better exercise tolerance compared with patients in Class IV with severe CHF and poor exercise tolerance.

Medical Examination and Evaluation of Heart Failure

Medical interventions include a variety of tests to identify the etiology and evaluate the severity of heart failure. Following an examination of signs and symptoms of heart failure in a patient, several key tests are typically performed. These include the chest x-ray, electrocardiogram analysis, laboratory tests, echocardiography, and nuclear imaging studies.

Radiological Findings in Heart Failure

Three hallmark characteristics of the chest x-ray help confirm the diagnosis of CHF (Fig. 13.13):

1. An enlarged cardiac silhouette: The enlargement of the heart in patients with CHF occurs secondary to congestion of fluid in the lungs and possible pathological hypertrophy of the ventricles.

Table 13.7 Functional Classifications of Patients With Diseases of the Heart

Functional	Continuous–Intermittent Permissible Workloads	Maximum
Class I	4.0–6.0 cal/min Patients with cardiac disease but without resulting limitations of physical activity. Ordinary physical activity does not cause undue fatigue, palpitation, dyspnea, or anginal pain.	6.5 METs
Class II	3.0–4.0 cal/min Patients with cardiac disease resulting in slight limitation of physical activity. They are comfortable at rest. Ordinary physical activity results in fatigue, palpitation, dyspnea, or anginal pain.	4.5 METs
Class III	2.0–3.0 cal/min Patients with cardiac disease resulting in marked limitation of physical activity. They are comfortable at rest. Less than ordinary physical activity causes fatigue, palpitation, dyspnea, or anginal pain.	3.0 METs
Class IV	1.0–2.0 cal/min Patients with cardiac disease resulting in inability to carry on any physical activity without discomfort. Symptoms of cardiac insufficiency or of the anginal syndrome may be present even at rest. If any physical activity is undertaken, discomfort is increased.	1.5 METs

Four-level classification system based on functional limitations.
MET = metabolic equivalent
Reprinted by permission of the American Heart Association, New York.

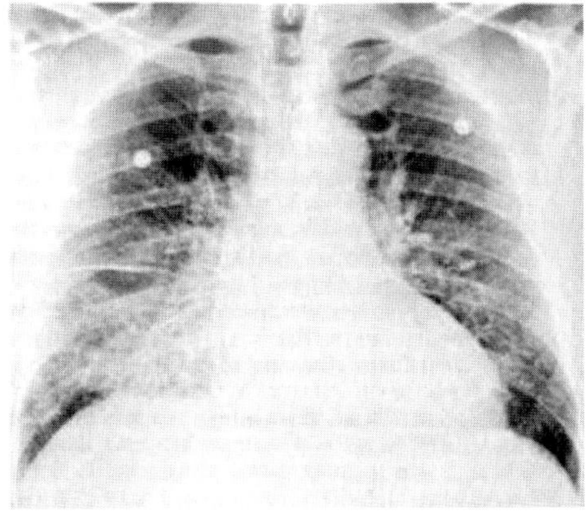

Figure 13.13 Radiographic examination to confirm CHF.

2. Opacities (white areas) in the lung field with interstitial and parenchymal edema. This occurs when excessive fluid collects in the lung when LV end-diastolic pressures exceed 25 mm Hg.[44]
3. Blunting of the costophrenic angle. The lower ribs meeting the diaphragm creates this sharp image observed on the chest x-ray. In patients with CHF, fluid settles to the lower, dependent aspect of the lung, producing an opaque appearance, and blunts the costophrenic angle.

Electrocardiogram Changes

Electrocardiogram changes in patients with acute decompensated heart failure may identify underlying predisposing or precipitating conditions for heart failure. These changes may include left ventricular hypertrophy, left atrial abnormalities, myocardial ischemia or infarction, or the presence of atrial fibrillation.

Laboratory Findings in Heart Failure

Significant laboratory data include blood counts, markers of renal function, cardiac enzymes, and B-type natriuretic peptide (BNP) and N-terminal pro-BNP (NT-proBNP) assays. Analysis of blood counts assist the clinician in identifying the presence of infection or anemia that may have precipitated the event. An assessment of cardiac enzymes is important to consider in an effort to evaluate potential myocardial injury. Finally, *natriuretic peptide assays* supplement clinical judgment when the cause of a patient's dyspnea is uncertain. Natriuretic peptides including B-type natriuretic peptide (BNP) and N-terminal pro-BNP (NT-proBNP) are released from ventricular myocytes in response to volume overload within the respective chambers.[57] These chemicals are cardiac neurohormones that target the kidney when released, to increase diuresis and decrease the overall volume of fluid within the vasculature and chambers of the heart. Circulating levels of BNP are elevated in plasma in patients with heart failure.

Markers of renal function including *blood urea nitrogen (BUN)* and serum creatinine concentrations can may be used as a marker of reduced cardiac output or elevated right sided pressures that potentiate renal venous congestion.[57] There is no level of BNP that perfectly separates patients with and without heart failure. Normal levels of BNP are less than 100 pg/mL.[57] Values above 500 are generally considered to be positive for heart failure. In some patients, the BNP level provides an indication of the extent of heart failure where higher BNP levels without renal failure indicate worsening failure of the ventricles. Therefore, a patient with a BNP of 1,000 pg/mL has more significant heart failure than a patient with a BNP of 500 pg/mL when there is no renal dysfunction present. However, in a patient with renal dysfunction, extremely high BNP levels may be noted due to an inability to respond to the BNP released from the heart. For these patients, the levels of BNP are not indicative of the extent of heart failure exacerbation. Therefore, results of B-type natriuretic peptide (BNP) and N-terminal pro-BNP (NT-proBNP) should be interpreted in the context of all available clinical data. Finally, BNP has been found to be a statistically significant ($p < 0.05$) prognostic indicator of heart failure, and studies have discovered moderate to strong (from r = 20.38 to 20.64) correlations between BNP and peak oxygen uptake (Vo_{2max}).[58]

Echocardiogram and Nuclear imaging

With ultrasound technology, the echocardiogram is used to examine wall motion integrity, valvular status, wall thickness, chamber size, and LV function.[57,59] The EF is also be calculated using the data obtained from the echocardiogram.[57] An echocardiogram may accompany a stress test and is known as a *stress echo*. The purpose of a stress echo is to compare LV function and wall motion between rest and exercise when an increased Vo_2 results in an increased MVo_2. A positive stress echo indicates a worsening of LV function as activity increases; a negative stress echo indicates that the LV has adequately adapted to the increase in energy demand. Nuclear imaging (e.g., thallium sestamibi) compares coronary perfusion between rest and exercise.[57] If there is no decrease in perfusion with increasing workloads, the test is negative; if there is a decrease, the test is considered positive. Nuclear imaging (e.g., thallium sestamibi) compares coronary perfusion between rest and exercise. If there is no decrease in perfusion with increasing workloads, the test is negative; if there is a decrease, the test is considered positive.

When a patient is unable to perform an exercise test because of limitations such as musculoskeletal or neurological impairments, a pharmacological stress test such as a *persantine thallium* test is often recommended.[59] Persantine, when given intravenously, decreases coronary vascular resistance by causing arterioles to vasodilate, and therefore increases the blood flow through the capillary beds. If an artery is atherosclerotic, its arteriole may have gradually dilated over time to increase capillary blood flow by means of pressure autoregulation. Therefore, when persantine is given, the diseased arteries may have a limitation in the amount of further arteriolar dilation that can occur. In comparison to the nondiseased arteries, there will be a relative decrease in blood flow through the capillary beds of the diseased arteries. Imaging studies will thus detect a relative decrease in blood flow to the area of the myocardium that is perfused by the diseased artery compared with that perfused by a nondiseased artery. Adenosine, which is a coronary and peripheral vasodilator (as well as an antiarrhythmic), has similar effects as persantine and may be used instead.[59]

Pharmacological Management of HF

With the advent of new medications such as combined alpha and beta blockers, ACE inhibitors, and vasodilators, the symptoms of volume overload are more effectively managed. The principles of drug management for patients with heart failure are twofold: (1) to increase the contractility or pumping ability of the heart to relieve congestion and (2) to decrease the workload on the heart by reducing either the total volume of fluid in the system (the preload) or the vascular resistance (the afterload).[47,57] Drugs that increase contractility are known as *positive inotropes;* the common drug in this category is digoxin. Diuretics decrease preload, thereby decreasing LVEDV. Patients are often on a sliding scale dosage of diuretics depending on the amount of fluid weight gain; they are instructed to weigh themselves daily and adjust diuretics accordingly. Afterload reducers, particularly those that block the effects of the renin–angiotensin system (e.g., ACE inhibitors or angiotensin receptor blockers), are often a critical component of drug management in this population. By blocking salt and water retention through aldosterone suppression, preload is decreased; by blocking vasoconstriction through angiotensin II suppression, afterload is reduced. The increase in sympathetic activity that accompanies heart failure causes an increase in MVo_2 (from beta-receptor stimulation), peripheral vasoconstriction, and resultant reduction in peripheral blood flow (from alpha-receptor stimulation). Drugs that combine both beta-receptor blockade and alpha-receptor blockade minimize these affects. Beta blockade will result in a decrease in MVo_2 and alpha blockade will result in decreased afterload due to suppression of peripheral vasoconstriction.

Mechanical and Surgical Support

For the symptomatic patient in NYHA Class III/IV, there are dramatic surgical options that may improve function, such as heart transplant, left ventricular assist devices (LVADs), myoplasty, and biventricular pacing. It is beyond the scope of this chapter to discuss in detail the complexity of each of these procedures. Heart transplantation involves replacing the patient's heart with a donor heart. The donor heart will be denervated; therefore, it will not have any direct sympathetic or parasympathetic connection and will be dependent on the intrinsic pacemaker of the SA node and hormonal stimulation to increase HR. The patient with a heart transplant requires careful pharmacological management. Immune-suppressing drugs are used to prevent the body from rejecting the organ, as well as for careful control of infection.

The LVAD is a temporary pump inserted into the patient to perform the work of the LV or to augment the function of the failing heart. The patient is connected to an external energy source but also has the option of wearing a battery pack that allows freedom of movement for hours, in which the patient can go shopping, go to the movies, and so forth. It is important for the therapist to consider the effects of a 6 lb mass (created by the external energy source) resting below the diaphragm that is likely to alter ventilator performance. Finally, gentle progression of exercise intensity must be utilized. Therapists must be vigilant to check for flow limitations (10 to 12 L/min) or changes in cardiovascular function that may occur secondary to use of a mechanically driven pump.

Myoplasty is a surgical procedure in which an enlarged LV undergoes a size reduction by removing dilated, scarred myocardium that is ineffective in contributing to contractility.

A new class of pacemaker, the biventricular pacer, includes an intraventricular conduction delay (e.g., left bundle branch block on the ECG) for patients with severe CHF.[60] This pacer coordinates the contraction of the right and left ventricles and in doing so provides a more effective LV contraction and increased CO.[60]

Valvular Heart Disease

The prevalence of valvular heart disease is rapidly increasing in the United States and worldwide. Valvular heart disease increases with age with more than one in eight people aged 75 and older presenting with moderate or severe valve disease.[61] Broadly, three major disorders encompass valvular dysfunction of one or more of the four heart valves. These include stenosis, prolapse, and regurgitation.

1. *Stenosis* involves narrowing of a heart valve limiting the flow of blood through the valve. As the pathological condition progresses, the chamber behind the valve pathologically hypertrophies to pump against the obstruction.
2. *Prolapse* involves enlarged valve cusps that become floppy and bulge backward. When the cusps and support mechanisms of the valve are destroyed, the valve droops down. As the disease progresses, prolapse may progress to regurgitation.
3. *Regurgitation* refers to the forward and backward movement of blood resulting from incomplete valve closure. During certain phases of the cardiac cycle valves must close appropriately to prevent blood from flowing in a retrograde fashion. In a regurgitant valve, the valve does not close properly leading to regurgitation of blood into the chamber behind the pathological valve.

Valve replacements are often used for treating valvular disease. Patients with stenosis or regurgitation of the aortic or mitral valves are prime candidates for valve replacement surgeries. A median sternotomy is the route to access the heart. Two major types of valves are used for valve replacement procedures: (1) mechanical valves and (2) biological valves derived from cadavers, porcine tissue, or bovine tissue.[62] Mechanical valves are preferred in patients younger than 65 because of their durability and long life.[62] However, the major disadvantage is that they tend to be thrombogenic. Patients who receive a mechanical valve must be on lifelong anticoagulation therapy. For this reason, patients who have a history of a prior bleed, wish to become pregnant, or have poor medication adherence may not be candidates for a mechanical valve.[62] For these patients, biological valves may be more appropriate. The postoperative care for patients with a valve replacement is similar to that for patients who have had a CABG. In addition, neurological monitoring must be continuous postoperatively owing to the potential for an embolic stroke that may occur during or after the procedure. Finally, recent developments in minimally invasive procedures have advanced therapeutic choices for elderly adults. Currently a transcatheter aortic valve implantation (TAVI) can be performed for patients with severe symptomatic aortic stenosis who are considered inoperable for open surgical aortic valve replacement.[63] This procedure involves the replacement of the aortic valve via a transfemoral access, subclavian access or direct aortic transapical access. Transfemoral access is the most commonly used access route performed in 95% of patients who have this procedure.[63]

Electrical Conduction Abnormalities

Arrhythmias are any alteration in the electric conduction of the heart from the normal beat. They are caused by a disturbance in the electrical activity of the heart, resulting in impaired electrical impulse formation or conduction.[64] Arrhythmias may present as benign or malignant (i.e., life-threatening). Examples of *malignant arrhythmias* are sustained ventricular tachycardia (V-tach) and ventricular fibrillation (V-fib). An example of a common *benign arrhythmia* in the elderly population would be atrial fibrillation (A-fib) with a controlled ventricular response. This section will review a few conduction abnormalities and relevant implications for the physical therapist.

Ectopic Beats

A beat that originates from a site other than the sinus node is known as an *ectopic beat*. The common ectopic beats are atrial *(premature atrial contractions [PACs])* and ventricular *(premature ventricular contractions [PVCs])*. PVCs may occur either by themselves or in groups such as couplets (two PVCs) or triplets (three PVCs), or alternating with sinus beats such as bigeminy (every other beat a PVC) or trigeminy (every third beat a PVC).[64]

A PAC is an ectopic beat that originates in the atria and may present as an irregular rhythm (Fig. 13.14B). It may be difficult to distinguish a PAC from a premature junctional contraction (PJC), an ectopic beat that originates within the area around the A-V node. Usually, PACs or PJCs will not compromise CO, and physical therapy intervention may be appropriate if accompanied by adequate hemodynamic responses.

The presence of ectopic beats results in an irregular rhythm. Usually, ectopic beats are transient, and their severity depends on their impact on CO. It is certainly common to have a few PVCs even in a normal heart. Many people may have ectopic beats during times of stress or with stimulants such as nicotine and caffeine. Even though this may be a common response in a normal heart, it is important to educate patients with myocardial impairments who may have ectopic beats or irregular rhythms to avoid these aggravators. An increase in ectopy is undesired. It is unwise for any patient with cardiac disease to engage in exercise following recent cigarette smoking. Although the specific time frame a patient may be at risk for increased ectopy is not clearly known, a good rule of thumb may be abstinence of smoking for at least 2 hours either before or after exercise. Patient education on wellness strategies and smoking cessation is always useful for any patient identified as a smoker.

Supraventricular Ectopy

Supraventricular ectopy involves the rapid firing of an ectopic focus that originates in any location above the ventricles (atrial or junctional area). Examples of supraventricular ectopy include (1) paroxysmal atrial tachycardia and (2) supraventricular tachycardia. A sudden run of PACs occurring at a fast rate (100 to 200 bpm) is known as *paroxysmal atrial tachycardia (PAT).* A run of either PACs or PJCs at a rate of 150 to 250 bpm is known as supraventricular tachycardia (SV-tach) (Fig. 13.14C). Patients with SV-tach usually respond to a carotid massage where stimulation of the baroreceptors within the carotid bodies of the carotid artery produce a parasympathetic response. Other treatment interventions to reduce heart rate for patients with SV-tach include coughing and breath-holding techniques achieved through the Valsalva maneuver or carotid sinus massage.[64] Each of these techniques are geared to increase parasympathetic drive in different ways to reduce heart rate.

Ventricular Ectopy

PVCs are ectopic beats that originate in the ventricle and may present as irregular rhythms. Two hallmark characteristics identify PVCs on the ECG: (1) A P wave is absent as the impulse originates in the ventricle and (2) a wide and bizarre QRS complex signifying abnormal electrical conduction through the ventricle (Fig. 13.14D). Single PVCs will not compromise CO if less than 7 per minute. Therefore, physical activity may be appropriate if accompanied by an adequate hemodynamic response. If the PVCs increase with activity, the activity should be stopped and the patient examined for possible signs of compromised cardiac output. PVCs may come from the same irritable site and are called *unifocal PVCs*. If they originate from different ectopic sites within the ventricle they are known as *multifocal PVCs* (Fig. 13.15A). Multifocal PVCs suggest a more irritable ventricle and are therefore more serious than unifocal PVCs. It is appropriate for the therapist to have the patient medically evaluated before beginning or continuing an activity. Finally, a rare type of PVC known as an *R-on-T PVC* occurs when PVC fires *very prematurely*, on the T wave of the preceding cardiac cycle (Fig. 13.15B). These patients must be monitored closely because they are at an increased risk for developing a life-threatening dysrhythmia such as ventricular tachycardia or ventricular fibrillation.[64]

In ventricular bigeminy (Fig. 13.14E), every other beat is a PVC; in trigeminy, every third beat is a PVC (Fig. 13.14F). These rhythms occur transiently or episodically, and many patients have frequent bursts of these rhythms. If ectopy increases with activity, the activity should be immediately stopped. When two PVCs occur together, it is known as a couplet (Fig. 13.14G); when three PVCs occur together, it is known as a triplet. Couplets and triplets are important in that they suggest a high level of ventricular irritability. Altered LV function and ischemia are two of the more common causes for ventricular ectopy; therefore, medical management is directed toward improved LV function and perfusion whenever possible, as well as arrhythmia control. Physical therapy intervention is conservative at best and depends on the hemodynamic stability of the patient.

Ventricular Tachycardia

A run of four or more PVCs in a row is known as V-tach (Fig. 13.14H). V-tach may be either sustained or nonsustained. *Sustained V-tach,* by definition, occurs at an HR of at least 100 bpm and lasts for at least 30 seconds. The patient may or may not have a palpable pulse and, if present, the pulse will be weak. Because of the severe decrease in CO and rapid hemodynamic deterioration associated with this rhythm, the presence of sustained V-tach is considered an emergency. Medical intervention must be initiated as soon as possible. No physical therapy intervention is appropriate, except assisting the patient in stabilization, initiating cardiopulmonary resuscitation (CPR) when indicated, and activating the advanced cardiac life support (ACLS) system. V-tach may deteriorate quickly into V-fib.

Nonsustained V-tach occurs either in groups of three to five PVCs known as *salvos,* or a run of six or more PVCs lasting for up to 30 seconds. Nonsustained V-tach is considered a high-risk indicator for potentially lethal arrhythmias. Because the rhythm is nonsustained, the decrease in CO may not be sufficient to cause symptoms. However, until the etiology of the arrhythmia is identified and the rhythm controlled, physical therapy intervention is generally inappropriate.

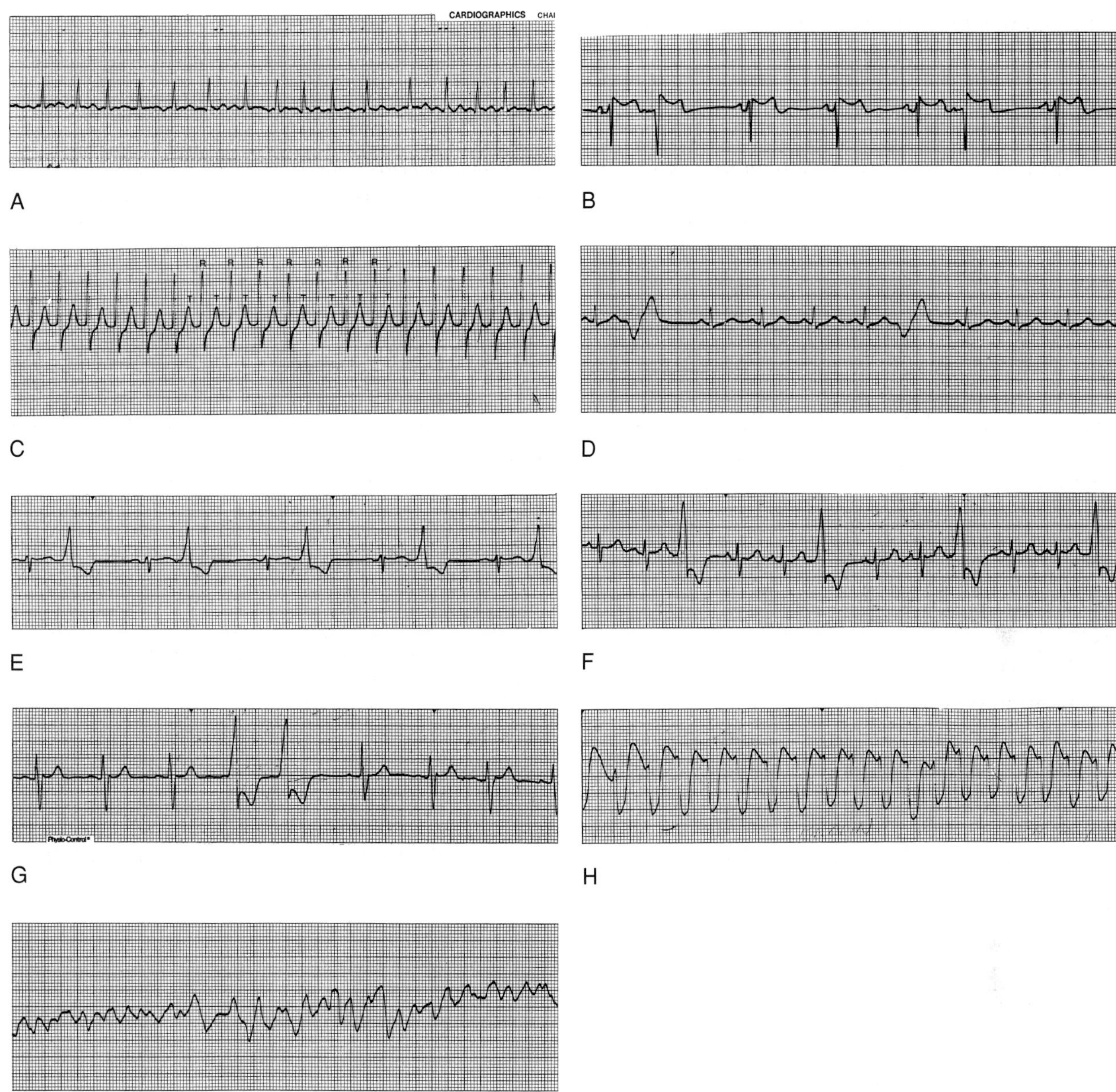

Figure 13.14 Examples of ectopy and arrhythmias. (A) Atrial fibrillation. (B) Atrial premature beat, also known as premature atrial contraction (PAC) (note third complex). (C) Supraventricular tachycardia (SVT). (D) Premature ventricular contraction (PVC) (note third complex). (E) Bigeminy (note second, fourth, and sixth complexes are PVCs). (F) Trigeminy (note second, fifth, and eighth complexes are PVCs). (G) Couplets (note fourth and fifth complexes are PVCs). (H) Ventricular tachycardia (V-tach). (I) Ventricular fibrillation (V-fib) (V-tach deteriorates into V-fib). *(From Brown, K, and Jacobson, S: Mastering Dysrhythmias: A Problem-Solving Guide. FA Davis, Philadelphia, 1988, p 30, with permission.)*

Ventricular Fibrillation

V-fib is characterized by quivering of the ventricles resulting from inadequate electrical stimulation. The ECG demonstrates a sustained run of different-looking PVCs coming from different ectopic foci (Fig. 13.14I). When the ventricles do not contract but rather quiver, there is ineffective CO. The patient will arrest and expire if this rhythm is not altered immediately. The treatment of choice is activation of ACLS, including electrical defibrillation and medication. Patients who survive ventricular fibrillation through defibrillation become candidates for an indwelling defibrillator placement known as an *automatic implantable cardiac defibrillator* (AICD).

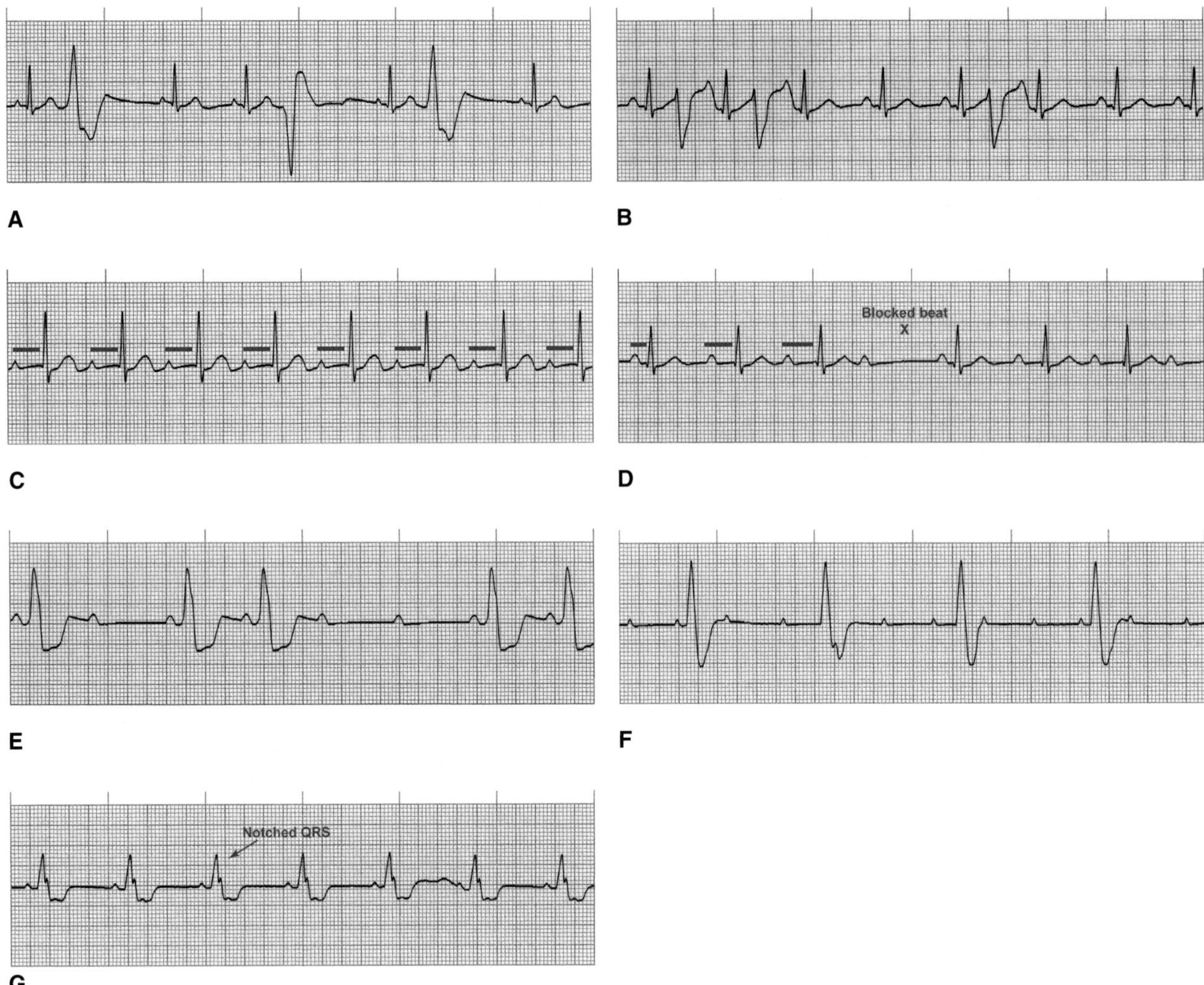

Figure 13.15 (A) Multifocal or multiform PVCs; (B) R-on-T PVC; (C) first-degree AV block; (D) Wenckebach rhythm; (E) second-degree type II; (F) third-degree AV block; (G) bundle branch block. *(From Jones, S: ECG Success: Exercises in ECG Interpretation. FA Davis, Philadelphia, 2008.)*

Automatic Implantable Cardiac Defibrillator

The *Automatic Implantable Cardiac Defibrillator* (AICD) is implanted in patients who have life-threatening ventricular arrhythmias (V-tach, V-fib).[65] The AICD is programmed to deliver an electrical shock if it detects a HR higher than its programmed HR limit.[65] Therefore, it is important for the physical therapist to know this limit and avoid an exercise intensity that may inadvertently activate the device. In addition to knowing the HR settings for the patient with an AICD, there are other considerations. ST-segment changes on the ECG may be common and are not specific for ischemia; therefore, other diagnostic studies must be done. In addition, UE aerobic or strengthening exercises should be avoided initially after placement of the pacer to avoid inadvertently dislodging the device or the lead wires. Checking with the physician when these exercises may be included is prudent. There may be a danger for patients with AICDs or pacemakers from electromagnetic signals such as anti-theft devices, either causing the AICD to discharge or causing pacers to slow down or speed up. It may be no problem for patients to walk through these devices but lingering within a few feet could be dangerous.

Atrial Fibrillation

Atrial fibrillation (A-fib) is characterized by quivering of the atria due to inadequate electrical stimulation. A varied number of non–sinus originating P waves (known as fibrillatory waves) exist for each QRS complex (Fig. 13.14A). The ventricular rhythm is said to be "irregularly irregular" because there is no regularity to the irregularity of the ventricular rhythm. It is important to note that effective contraction of the atria accounts for approximately 15% to 20% of CO—the *atrial kick*.[66] In patients with abnormal electrical conduction causing a quivering of the atria (A-fib), the mechanical contractile ability of the atria is reduced, resulting in a low atrial kick and compromised CO.[66]

Patients may exhibit A-fib continuously as their baseline rhythm or go in and out of this rhythm at rest or with activity. Physical therapy intervention may be appropriate for patients in A-fib who have a good ventricular rate at rest, with appropriate hemodynamic and HR increase with exercise. In patients with A-fib and rapid ventricular rates (greater than 120 bpm) at rest, exercise intensity must be lowered, and hemodynamic responses monitored carefully. This is because a rapid ventricular rate in addition to the loss of atrial kick further compromises the CO and results in altered hemodynamic responses. A good rule of thumb is to avoid physical activity and seek medical consultation if the patient's resting HR is greater than 115 bpm, if the patient appears uncomfortable, or if there is an inadequate hemodynamic response. Because this rhythm is irregular, it is important to monitor the HR for a full minute rather than 15 to 30 seconds to obtain an accurate pulse rate.

Conduction Delays and Blocks

Changes in the length of the PR interval, the width of the QRS complex, and the length of the QT interval are some of the ECG measurements indicative of conduction abnormalities.[67]

Conduction delays through the A-V node are classified as first-, second-, or third-degree heart blocks. *First-degree heart block* occurs when the conduction time through the A-V node is prolonged; therefore, the ECG will have an increased length of the PR interval (Fig. 13.15C).[67] There are two categories of *second-degree heart block:* Mobitz type I and Mobitz type II; each is hallmarked by the presence of dropped beats. Mobitz I, also known as *Wenckebach,* presents with a gradual increase in PR interval length in the preceding beats and then an eventual dropped beat (Fig. 13.15D); Mobitz II has normal PR intervals in all the beats preceding the dropped beat (Fig. 13.15E).[67] In *third-degree heart block,* a mismatch of atrial and ventricular conduction exists, so there is no consistency between the atrial contraction and the ventricular contraction (i.e., no relationship between P waves and QRS complex on the ECG) (Fig. 13.15F).[67] Patients in first-degree block have no limitations to exercise. Whether or not exercise is permitted with second- and third-degree blocks depends on the etiology and subsequent hemodynamic responses. Medical clearance is warranted before beginning any exercise.

Conduction delays through the bundle of His are known as either right bundle branch block (RBBB) or left bundle branch block (LBBB).[67] Bundle branch blocks are not true arrhythmias because there is no change in the actual rhythm, just in the timing of conduction through the bundle of His. The heart is still depolarized from the same pacemaker; only the route of activation is changed. Bundle branch blocks present on the ECG as a distortion of the QRS complex with an increased duration (i.e., widening) (Fig. 13.15G). The presence of an LBBB on the ECG is usually permanent and indicates a pathological condition. RBBB may occur from a variety of reasons; it may be a permanent change due to underlying disease, or it may be benign. RBBB can also occur transiently. LBBB usually indicates the presence of more significant disease than RBBB.

The presence of a new bundle branch block should be medically evaluated before beginning or progressing an exercise program. Following medical clearance, there is usually no contraindication to exercise in either the RBBB or LBBB population. Because of the alteration of the QRS complex and as a result the ST segment, the sensitivity of the ECG in detecting ischemia via ST depression is lost in the patient with LBBB. Further, during exercise a fast left bundle branch cannot be distinguished from ventricular tachycardia.[64] In such cases, patients with a left bundle branch block do not undergo exercise stress tests, rather undergo chemical stress tests to stress the heart.[64]

Pacemakers

The use of pacemakers has increased considerably, with the most common indications for placement of a permanent pacemaker being (1) an HR that is too slow (symptomatic bradycardia); (2) an HR that fails to increase appropriately with exercise (chronotropic incompetence); or (3) an electric pathway that it blocked resulting in atrioventricular delays or bundle branch blocks.[68]

A pacemaker is a device that is placed subdermally near the heart and consists of an implantable pulse generator and lead wires that connect the pacemaker to the myocardium. The pulse generator contains a long-life battery and circuitry for timing, sensing, and output functions. The life of the battery usually dictates the life of the pacemaker and varies depending on the type of battery and the extent to which the pacemaker is being used. In some cases, the patient is dependent on the pacemaker for every cardiac contraction and is likely to utilize the life of the battery in a shorter period. The average pacemaker battery life is between 5 and 10 years. Replacement of pacemaker batteries is done after serial assessments have confirmed a reduction in battery life. Battery life may be consumed more rapidly when the patient is more reliant on the pacemaker for maintaining an appropriate HR. In 2016, the U.S. Food and Drug Administration approved the newest miniature pacemaker. Empirical research has identified certain complications associated with conventional transvenous pacing systems related to the pacing lead and pocket. In light of these complications, a novel self-contained miniaturized pacemaker named Micra has been developed.[69] This pacemaker primarily does single chamber pacing and may be beneficial for some patients.

Patients are reliant on pacemakers at different levels. Some patients usually have normal electric conduction and so do not need to be reliant on the pacemaker at all times. Other patients have altered electrical conduction through the heart and may be very reliant on the pacemaker to keep them alive. Therefore, it is important for therapists to determine how reliant the patient may be on his or her pacemaker. When pacemakers trigger a pace due to altered electrical conduction through the heart, the ECG reveals a pacer spike. Thus, if the patient has a pacemaker and no pacer spikes are evident on the ECG, the therapist can infer that the heart is conducting normally, and the pacemaker is there for emergency needs only. Conversely, if the ECG demonstrates a pacer spike in every cardiac cycle, the therapist must understand that this patient is 100% reliant on the pacemaker and thus ensure that the pacemaker is adequately rate responsive during activity.

The basic functions of the pacemaker lead wires are to provide the pacemaker with information on intrinsic myocardial activity and pace the myocardium when intrinsic activity fails.[68] There are four primary functions of pacemakers: (1) the ability to sense intrinsic cardiac function, (2) the ability to stimulate cardiac depolarization in response to failed intrinsic activity, (3) the ability to respond to increased metabolic demand by providing rate-responsive pacing, and (4) the ability provide diagnostic information stored within the pacemaker.

Pacemakers have rate and rhythm sensitivity as well as the ability to override certain arrhythmias. Pacemakers may also be combined with AICD capabilities. Pacemakers are coded by either a three- or five-category system according to which chamber (atria or ventricle) is sensed, what chamber is paced (atria or ventricle), and whether the electrical stimulus will trigger a response or be inhibited (Table 13.8). Because pacemakers may fail to work properly, ECG monitoring is helpful to determine whether the pacer is working properly.

As stated previously, patients with Class III Heart Failure and LBBB may be candidates for a specialized pacemaker known as a biventricular pacemaker, the purpose of which is to synchronize LV contractility to provide a more effective CO. The biventricular pacer does not influence HR or heart rhythm.[68]

Calculating Heart Rate From Electrocardiography

HR can be determined from an ECG strip. The ECG graph paper consists of a series of small boxes (represented by light black lines) and large boxes (represented by heavy black lines). Each large box is made up of five small boxes. The horizontal axis represents time; when the ECG paper is moving at the usual speed of 25 mm/sec, five large boxes constitutes one second. Knowing that time is on the x-axis, there are many ways to calculate HR from the ECG graph paper. An easy way to calculate a minute rate is to count the number of complexes in 6 seconds (i.e., 30 large boxes) and multiply by 10. Often the ECG paper will have 3-second intervals premarked. An alternative approach is to identify an R wave from one ECG complex that is close to or on a heavy black line (i.e., a large box), and then assign each of the following heavy black lines (large boxes) a number in the following order: 300, 150, 100, 75, 60, 50, 40. The heavy line closest to the next R wave will provide an approximation of HR (Fig. 13.16). Finally, dividing 300 by the number of large boxes between two R waves will also indicate the HR. If the rate is regular, any of the preceding strategies will work. If the rate is irregular, however, the complexes will need to be counted over a long time, and a minimum of a 6-second strip should be used.

Heart Transplant

Patients who have undergone a heart transplant may present with the following: (1) calf cramps owing to the immunosuppressive drug cyclosporine; (2) decreased LE strength; (3) obesity owing to long-term corticosteroid use; (4) increased risk of fracture owing to osteoporosis associated with long-term, high-dose corticosteroids; and (5) an increased probability of developing atherosclerosis in the coronary arteries of the donor heart after the first postsurgical year. Because the heart is denervated, HR alone provides a limited measure of exercise intensity. Therefore, BP and perceived exertion should be included in the routine data collection.

Table 13.8 Pacemaker Classification System

Chamber Paced	Chamber Sensed	Response	Rate Responsive Pacing
O = none	O = none	O = none	R = rate responsive
A = atria	A = atria	I = inhibit	
V = ventricle	V = ventricle	T = trigger	
D = dual chamber	D = dual chamber	D = capacity to both inhibit and trigger	

Pacemakers are commonly identified by a three-letter code as displayed in the first three columns. Pacemakers may also have the capacity to respond to physiological stimuli to increase rate (column 4) and to override atrial tachycardia. A fifth column, for antitachycardiac function, is rarely used because of the increased sophistication of the newer implantable defibrillators/pacemakers, which renders this function unnecessary. Example: VVI pacer will provide an electrical impulse to the ventricle if it senses that there is no ventricular activity within an appropriate time frame. If there is intrinsic ventricular electrical activity, the pacemaker will be inhibited.

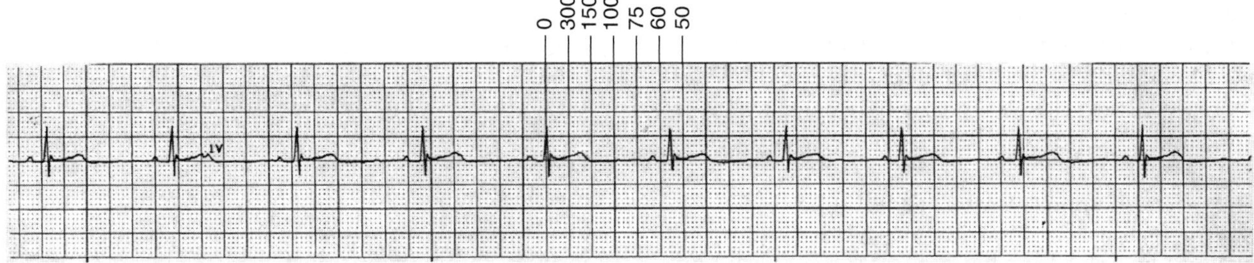

Figure 13.16 Calculation of a heart rate from a rhythm strip. Begin with the fifth complex (which falls on a large black line) and count each large black line to the right of this complex in the order of 300, 150, 100, 75, 60, 50. The sixth complex falls between two large lines (i.e., 50 and 60). There are five small lines between each large line. Between 50 and 60 there are 10 beats, therefore each small line in this case would be two beats. The heart rate would be 60 – 4 = 56. An alternate method would be to count the number of complexes in a 6-second strip and multiply by 10.

EXAMINATION OF THE PATIENT WITH HEART DISEASE

Owing to the increasing incidence and prevalence of heart disease on our society, many patients referred to physical therapy will have cardiovascular dysfunction or may be at risk for developing CVD. The history taking, review of systems, and data from specific tests and measures will guide and inform development of the physical therapy diagnosis, goals and outcomes, prognosis, and POC. This section addresses elements of the examination and tests and measures specific to the cardiovascular system.

Medical Record Review

The medical record of a patient with a history of cardiovascular impairments may at times be overwhelming. The patient interview is typically helpful if clarification of the medical record is needed. Depending on the type of setting (inpatient, outpatient, acute rehabilitation, home care), the specific contents of the medical record may vary. Important items to note within the medical record include the following:

1. Medical problems, past medical history, physician's examination
2. Medications, including type, dosage, and schedule
3. Laboratory tests
   - Blood tests for specific cardiac enzymes that may indicate an MI has occurred, such as a positive CK-MB or troponin level
   - Electrolytes, including potassium, and magnesium and calcium if ventricular arrhythmias are present
   - Complete blood count (CBC), which may indicate the presence of anemia via the hemoglobin and hematocrit values
   - Status of the kidney (BUN and creatinine) and liver function (liver function tests)
   - Presence of CAD risk factors, such as elevated lipid values (e.g., total cholesterol, low-density lipoproteins [LDLs], triglyceride), and elevated blood sugars (glucose)
   - Arterial blood gases (ABGs)
4. Results of any diagnostic studies or interventions: chest x-ray, ECGs, ETT, cardiac catheterization, surgical reports, hemodynamic monitors (e.g., pressure readings from central line and/or arterial line)
5. Nursing and other health care provider notes

The medical record contains information regarding what has happened to the patient, as well as the status of the patient within the last 24 hours or since the last health care provider intervention. Flow charts, which record vital signs, temperature, oxygenation requirements, and volume status over time, provide up-to-date patient data, especially when working with the more medically challenged patient.

Patient Interview

The formal patient interview should follow the medical record review. A determination of overall cognition (e.g., orientation, memory, learning needs, comprehension) should be made. Information regarding the patient's lifestyle, previous level of functioning, recreational interests, work requirements, and goals is important in establishing the intervention. The International Classification of Functioning Health and Disability recommends the clinician evaluate environmental and personal factors that affect a patient's overall ability for activity and participation.[70] Based on this model, it is important for therapists to assess the patient's prior level of participation in addition to the prior level of activity. An assessment of both baseline activity and participation is useful in generating goals and the appropriate functional prognosis of the patient. Further, an assessment of an individual's prior level of function should not only be limited to the level of function before the most recent hospital admission. Often times when a patient is asked their level of function before the most recent hospital admission, the therapist assumes that this level of function before the most recent admission is the patient's optimal level of function. This may not be true for a patient who had a higher level of function a few months earlier who now presents with a relatively lower level of function at this admission due to multiple recent readmissions. Clinically, it is useful to interview patients on their level of function over a prolonged length of time prior to their current state.

Data should also be obtained about the patient's response to health and illness, coping status, support systems, and knowledge of heart disease. It is important to note that not all the information from the interview needs to be obtained on the first session. During subsequent sessions, the patient may begin to feel better and less anxious and may therefore be able to communicate more easily. Patient education can often be woven into the interview process, either subtly or overtly. The patient should describe, in his or her own words, the quality and location of the symptom for which medical attention is being sought. It is common for physical therapists to ask a patient about pain; for patients with cardiac disease, one should be cautious about assuming that the patient's symptom is pain. Many patients will not use pain as their qualifier, but instead describe their symptoms as pressure, heaviness, SOB (dyspnea), aching, heartburn, or general malaise, to identify a few. Knowing the symptom presentation for each individual will make patient education and activity progression easier. It is also important to identify any consistent precipitating factors and alleviators, as well as duration and frequency of symptoms.

The interview also helps to establish rapport and trust between therapist and patient, creating an environment for mutual goal setting. This in turn facilitates patient adherence to the rehabilitation program. Patients who are recovering from an MI or from surgery need to understand the time frames for healing and convalescence. Education for family members and significant others is also crucial for patient adherence and understanding.

Tests and Measures

Following the International Classification of Functioning Health and Disability, specific examination tests and measures are presented to identify impairments in body structure and function (Table 13.9) and in functional activity limitations and participation restrictions (Table 13.10).

■ PHYSICAL THERAPY INTERVENTION FOR PATIENTS WITH HEART DISEASE

The goal of physical therapist interventions and education are to improve the individual's exercise capacity (being able to do more work), exercise efficiency (being able to do the same work with less cost), exercise tolerance (being able to do the same work with less signs and symptoms),

Table 13.9 Outcome Measures: Patients With Cardiovascular Disease

Body Structure and Function Impairment	Key Test/Measure
Baseline Hemodynamic Stability	***Resting Heart Rate and Rhythm:*** These must be assessed at rest and with activity. Normal resting heart rate is 60–100 beats/minute. Alterations in heart rate values from this range at rest must be evaluated to determine the stability of the patient at rest. Beyond an assessment of the absolute heart rate value at rest, it is also important to consider relative changes in resting heart rate values on a day-to-day basis to determine the relative stability of the patient. In other words, a patient with a routine resting heart rate of 60 beats/minute who presents on any given day with a heart rate of 80 beats/minute may be demonstrating relative instability due to an exacerbation of their pathology. Finally, if peripheral pulse is difficult to obtain, an apical pulse may be obtained by auscultating the heart at the fifth intercostal space, mid-clavicular line.
Baseline Hemodynamic Stability	***Heart Rhythm:*** The regularity of the pulse is important to assess to determine the presence of an arrhythmia. Pulses may be felt as regular, irregular, regularly irregular, or irregularly irregular. A patient who presents with any form of irregularity in their pulses will need a follow-up EKG to confirm the dysrhythmia.
Hemodynamic Stability With Exercise	***Exercise Heart Rate and Rhythm:*** An assessment of heart rate and rhythm during exercise is important to help determine the appropriateness of the cardiovascular system in meeting the metabolic needs of the body during exercise. Heart rate traditionally increases 10 beats/minute per metabolic equivalent (MET) level increase in activity. The inability to increase heart rate sufficiently or a profound increase in heart rate with activity needs further evaluation. Further, it is important to evaluate heart rate responses with activity each day to determine the relative stability of the patient on a day-to-day basis. In other words, an assessment of the patient's relative changes in heart rate to the same absolute work is useful in identifying stability on a day-to-day basis.

Table 13.9 Outcome Measures: Patients With Cardiovascular Disease—cont'd

Body Structure and Function Impairment	Key Test/Measure
Hemodynamic Stability With Exercise	***Respiratory Rate:*** Normal respiratory rate at rest in an adult is 12–20 breaths/minute. Respiratory rates greater than 30 breaths/minute at rest signify instability and will need further assessment. Further, it is important for the clinician to assess respiratory rate changes during activity at each visit to assess relative changes in stability on a day-to-day basis.
Hemodynamic Stability With Exercise	***Blood Pressure With Activity:*** Arterial BP is a product of CO and total peripheral resistance (TPR) where BP = CO × TPR. An increase in either of these factors will increase BP, and a decrease in either may decrease BP. The primary factor that changes during activity is the CO and not the TPR. Therefore, clinically, a change in blood pressure during activity is primarily due to a change in CO. Aerobic exercise of increasing intensity increases CO and concomitantly increases BP. Conversely, a drop in BP during aerobic exercise indicates a drop in CO or signifies the inability of the heart to meet the metabolic needs of the peripheral tissue. Signs of compromised CO, including fatigue, weakness, tiredness, dizziness, usually accompany this drop in BP. Therefore, BP is essential to assess in the patient who demonstrates signs of compromised CO during activity to determine whether CO is being maintained.
Hypoxemia	***Pulse Oxymetry:*** Pulse oxymetry is used to assess pulmonary respiration or gas exchange at the level of the alveolar capillary interface. Pulse oxymetry readings less than 90% indicate hypoxemia and warrant further evaluation.
Dyspnea	***Dyspnea:*** Dyspnea may be assessed by asking patients their *Perceived Level of Dyspnea* on a scale of 1–10 (0 = nothing at all; 10 = maximal). High reliability and validity have been reported.[71] Further, the Minimal Clinical Important Difference has not been established in heart disease but has been established as 1 point in patients with chronic lung disease.[72] An alternate method for measurement is the *Dyspnea Scale*, a 5-point ordinal scale (0 = no dyspnea; 4 = severe difficulty, cannot continue) (Box 13.3).
Altered Breathing Patterns	***Paroxysmal Nocturnal Dyspnea:*** An assessment of a patient's report of experiencing a sudden episode of shortness of breath at night is an important sign of an exacerbation of heart failure. It has a sensitivity and specificity of 39% to 41% and from 80% to 84%, respectively.[73]
Altered Breathing Patterns	***Orthopnea:*** Orthopnea is shortness of breath that increases in the recumbent position. This sign has a reported sensitivity of 22% to 50% and a specificity of 74% to 77% for heart failure exacerbation.[73] Patients with heart failure require increased numbers of pillows to sleep at night to avoid symptoms of orthopnea. Therefore, clinically the number of pillows required can be used to gauge the severity of heart failure.
Dyspnea on Exertion	***Dyspnea on Exertion:*** Dyspnea, especially with exertion, is one of the most common symptoms of heart failure, and it frequently appears early in the disease. Dyspnea on exertion has a sensitivity of 84% to 100% in the diagnosis of heart failure, but the specificity is much lower, ranging from 17% to 34%.[73]
Baseline Instability in Heart Failure	***Displacement of the Point of Maximum Impulse (PMI):*** The apical impulse is traditionally auscultated at the mid-clavicular line. An apical impulse recorded greater than 3 cm from the mid-clavicular line may be an accurate indicator of left ventricular enlargement with a sensitivity of 92% and a specificity of 91%.[74]
Angina	***Angina:*** The classical presentation of angina is substernal chest pressure accompanied by the *Levine sign* (the patient clenching his or her fist over the sternum). The Levine sign has a high diagnostic accuracy for ischemia.[75] For some patients, angina does not present in the classic way but rather may present as a pain or heaviness in the shoulder, jaw, arm, elbow, or upper back between scapulae. Angina may radiate from the chest to the arm or up to the throat, or it may present as indigestion or even SOB. The patient is often asked to rank his or her discomfort on the *Angina Scale* (Box 13.4).

Continued

Table 13.9 Outcome Measures: Patients With Cardiovascular Disease—cont'd

Body Structure and Function Impairment	Key Test/Measure
Abnormal Heart Sounds	***Heart Auscultation:*** Normal heart sounds are identified as S_1 (lub), which occurs at the time of the closure of the mitral (and tricuspid) valve and marks the beginning of systole and S_2 (dub), which occurs at the time of aortic (and pulmonic) valve closure and marks the end of systole. Figure 13.17 depicts locations on the chest for appropriate auscultation of each valve. The aortic valve is best auscultated at the second intercostal space, right sternal border. The pulmonic valve is heard at the second intercostal space, left sternal border. The tricuspid valve is auscultated at the fourth intercostal space, left sternal border, and the mitral valve is best heard at the fifth intercostal space, along the midclavicular line. Murmurs are abnormal heart sounds commonly the result of valvular disorders due to the changes in blood flow around and through the altered valve. A *systolic murmur* will present as audible turbulence between S_1 and S_2, and a *diastolic murmur* as turbulence between S_2 and S_1. Other abnormal sounds include are S_3 and S_4. S_3, also known as a *ventricular gallop,* occurs after S_2 and is clinically associated with acute heart failure decompensation with a specificity of 99%.[73] S_4, also known as an *atrial gallop,* occurs before S_1 and is clinically associated with an MI or chronic HTN. Finally, a *pericardial friction rub* in acute pericarditis has 100% specificity and 9% sensitivity.[4]
Abnormal Lung Sounds	***Lung Auscultation:*** Normal lung tissue produces vesicular (soft, low-pitched) sounds in the peripheral aspect of the lungs and bronchial breath (loud, high-pitched) sounds centrally along the manubrium of the sternum. Patients with LV failure often have the adventitious sounds of *crackles.* The auscultated crackles are coarse and best appreciated over the lung bases. The crackles typically occur late in inspiration.[76] Figure 13.18 demonstrates appropriate sites for the auscultation of lung fields.
Baseline instability due to increased Cardiac Filling Pressures	***Jugular Venous Distention:*** Patients with heart failure presenting with backup of fluid into the venous vasculature should be examined for the presence of jugular venous distention. To examine for this sign, the patient is placed at a 45-degree semirecumbent position.[77] The patient's head is turned away from the side to be evaluated and the clinician observes for a distention or pulsations of the jugular vein 3 to 5 cm above the sternum. The highest point of visible pulsation is determined and the vertical distance between this level and the level of the sternal angle of Louis is recorded (Fig. 13.19). Jugular venous distention has 94% specificity and 39% sensitivity in determining increased cardiac filling pressures.[77]
Peripheral Edema	***Pitting Edema and Weight Gain:*** In patients with congestive heart failure, low SV causes a reduced blood volume perfused to the periphery. This stimulates the pressoreceptors as they sense a decrease in volume. These pressoreceptors subsequently relay a message to the kidney to retain fluid. This retention of fluid increases the hydrostatic pressure within the peripheral vasculature, thereby pushing fluid into the interstitial space resulting in peripheral edema and weight gain. Edema can be assessed through girth measurements or by using the Palpation/Pitting Scale (Chapter 14). The severity of peripheral edema is categorized into four stages based on the time taken for the skin to rebound to its original contour after pitting. It is also important to note that edema can accumulate in the abdominal area (ascites) or sacral areas of the body.
Peripheral Muscle Weakness	***Muscle Strength:*** Standard manual muscle testing of major muscle groups in the upper and lower extremities is effective if weakness is suspected below functional limits. If strength of peripheral muscles is above functional limits, assessment of functional strength can be performed with a standardized sit-to-stand test called the *5 Times Sit to Stand Test* or a timed chair rise test called a *30 Second Chair Rise Test.*
Inspiratory Muscle Weakness	***Maximal Inspiratory Pressure:*** Strength of the inspiratory muscles is important in patients with heart failure. Empirical evidence suggests that patients with chronic heart failure have weak inspiratory muscles.[78] An inspiratory muscle strength of less than 60 cm H_2O traditionally depicts the presence of weak inspiratory muscles.

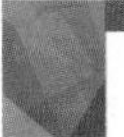

Box 13.3 Dyspnea Scale

0 = No dyspnea
1 = Mild, noticeable
2 = Mild, some difficulty
3 = Moderate difficulty, but can continue
4 = Severe difficulty, cannot continue

Box 13.4 Angina Scale

0 = No angina
1 = Light, barely noticeable
2 = Moderate, bothersome
3 = Severe, very uncomfortable: preinfarction pain
4 = Most pain ever experienced: infarction pain

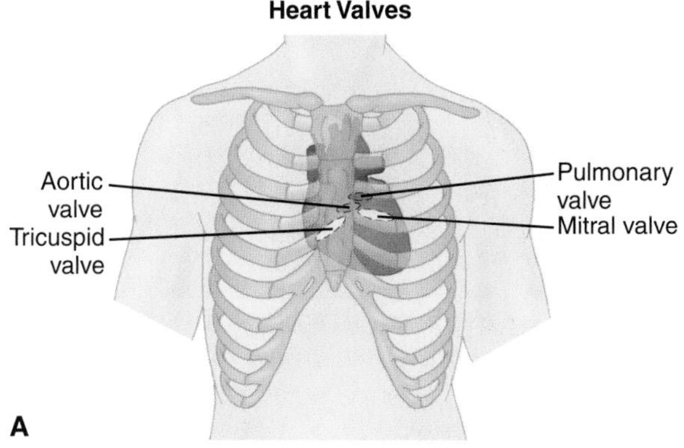

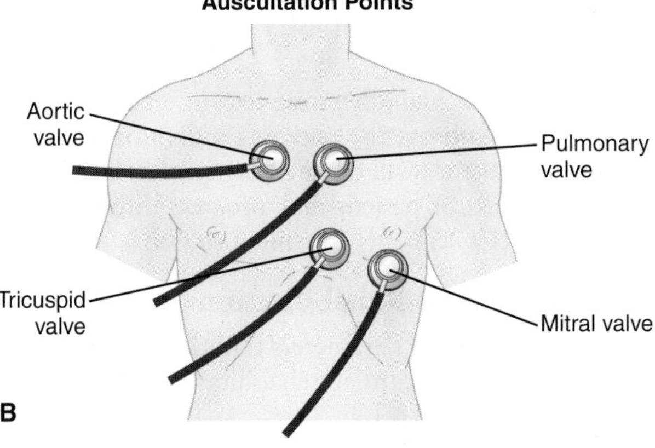

Figure 13.17 Anterior view of the chest wall of a man showing skeletal structures, heart, location of the heart valves, and auscultation points.

self-management of their cardiac pathology, and finally improve quality of life.

Therapeutic Exercise

A patient's responsiveness to functional improvement with therapeutic exercise is influenced by both central cardiovascular function and peripheral muscle weakness. Patients with greater degrees of peripheral weakness will be more responsive to exercise treatment compared with patients with greater degrees of central cardiovascular dysfunction. Additionally, the degree of improvement is variable from one individual to another and is directly dependent on the degree of purposeful exercise training that directly targets muscle weakness. Finally, a patient's presentation may differ throughout the course of treatment. For this reason, assessment of patient signs, symptoms, and hemodynamic stability must be completed at each treatment session so that interventions may be modified accordingly. For example, if a patient with heart failure has a relatively higher resting heart rate, increased weight gain, worsening lungs sounds, and increased shortness of breath, treatment will need to be modified in light of worsening stability.

Cardiac Rehabilitation

Cardiac rehabilitation is a comprehensive exercise, education, and lifestyle modification program designed to enable participants to achieve optimal physical, psychological, social, and vocational functioning. Treatment is geared to control symptoms, improve exercise capacity and tolerance, and improve overall quality of life.

Patients, especially the elderly that have been hospitalized for an acute coronary syndrome event such as a myocardial infarction or coronary artery bypass graft, or who have had a heart failure exacerbation or valve replacement surgery are at an increased risk of disability due to inactivity and bedrest. For these patients, a formal exercise prescription program is useful in improving overall activity and participation. Table 13.11 delineates current empirical evidence on the benefits of cardiac rehabilitation.

Phase I Cardiac Rehabilitation

Cardiac rehabilitation is traditionally begun in the acute hospital setting. In Phase I cardiac rehabilitation, physical therapy interventions focus on assessing the patient's hemodynamic responses to activity as well as focusing on increasing independence in functional mobility activities including bed mobility, transfers, ambulation, stair climbing, and activities of daily living. With a shortening of the length of stay in hospital settings, physical therapists are challenged to promote early ambulation, introduce patients to the goals of cardiac rehabilitation, and enroll patients in post-acute Phase II programs. In a large observational study involving 1,241 patients hospitalized for a cardiac event or cardiac surgery, researchers noted that a delay in the commencement of outpatient cardiac rehabilitation by more than 30 days was an independent predictor of a decreased improvement in exercise performance.[97]

There are a variety of inpatient cardiac rehab programs, frequently progressive based on levels of increasing energy costs (e.g., MET levels). Each facility will establish its own levels and criteria for activity progression and

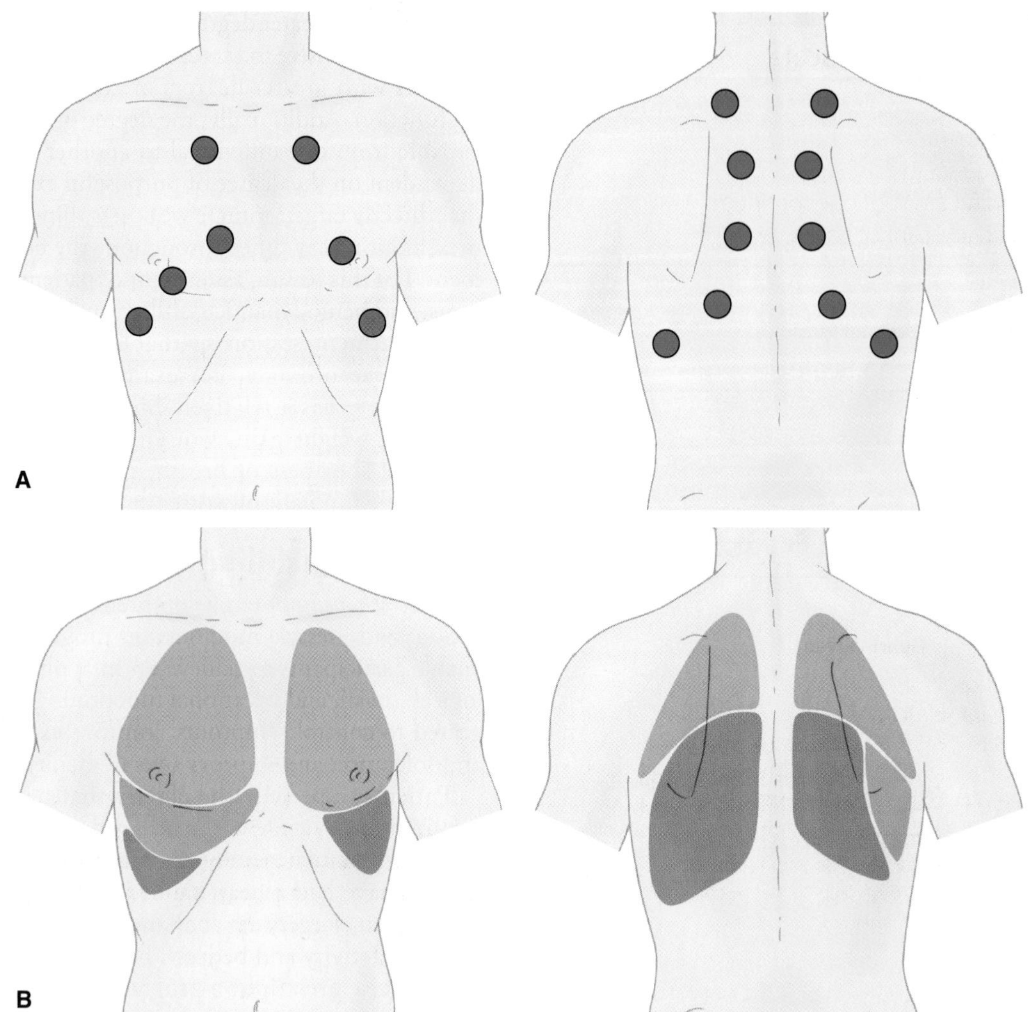

Figure 13.18 Auscultation of lungs.

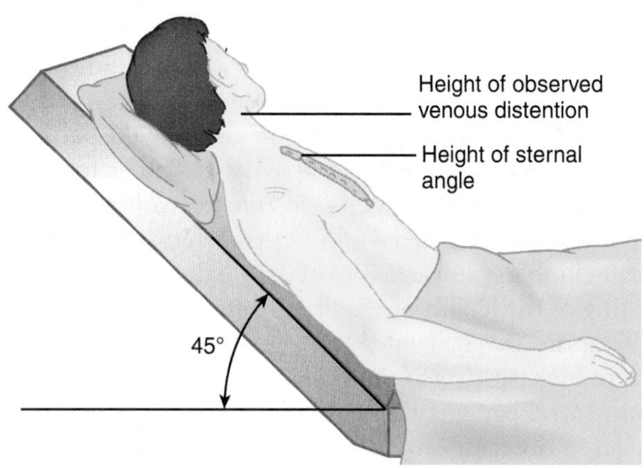

Figure 13.19 Examination of jugular venous distention.

education; an example of an inpatient program is shown in Table 13.12. Following are some general comments and recommendations about the various levels. It is important to note that activity progression occurs along a continuum and is not done in a rigid format. Although a patient must demonstrate the ability to sit at the bedside with appropriate hemodynamic response before ambulating in the hallway, the patient's individual response and medical history will dictate how quickly he or she is able to progress. A patient may progress through more than one level within any treatment session.

Phase II Cardiac Rehabilitation

Exercise prescription parameters traditionally utilized in Phase II outpatient cardiac rehabilitation programs are presented in Table 13.13.

Interventions for Patients With Heart Failure

Exercise training can be initiated when the patient is in compensated CHF. Box 13.5 provides the relative criteria for initiation and relative criteria for modification and termination of exercise in patients with heart failure. This section also outlines categories of interventions, relevant parameters, and the evidence of the benefits of exercise and other interventions in patients with heart failure. Table 13.15 provides a variety of exercise interventions utilized for patients with heart failure.

Table 13.10 Outcome Measures: Activity Limitations, and Participation Restrictions in Patients With Cardiovascular Disease	
Activity and Participation Limitation	**Key Test/ Measure**
Activity – Cardiovascular Deconditioning	***Walk Tests:*** A variety of walk tests are used to assess endurance in the patients with cardiopulmonary compromise. Two such tests include the *6 minute walk test (6MWT)* and the *2 Minute Walk Test (2MWT)*, where a participant is asked to ambulate back and forth continuously on a premeasured walkway for 6 minutes or 2 minutes, respectively. **6MWT:** The American Thoracic Society (ATS) has published guidelines for administering the 6MWT.[79] Shoemaker and colleagues report a minimal clinically important difference (MCID) for the 6MWT in patient with heart failure to be 45 m.[80] The researchers found that this change of 40 m to 45 m is a change that is greater than the measurement error and correlated with improvements in aerobic capacity and heath related quality of life.[80] Further, in a large study, Kommuri and colleagues found 6MW distances of less than 400 meters on the day of hospital discharge revealed significantly greater 30 day readmission rates compared with patients with HF and higher 6MWD scores.[81] Patients requiring readmission within 30 days had a median 6MW distance of 30 m, whereas patients not requiring readmission at 30 days walked significantly more with median score of 338 m.[81] **2MWT:** In this test the subject was asked to walk for 2 minutes. The total distance covered in 2 minutes is measured. The subject was allowed to use assistive devices when performing the test. Subject is asked to walk at a safe and comfortable pace. No verbal cues are provided during the test.
Activity – Cardiovascular Deconditioning	***2 Minute Step Test***: The 2 MST was initially developed by Rickli and Jones when space limitation or weather prohibited the subject form performing a 6MWT or 2MWT.[82] Subjects are asked to attain a standing position near a wall, doorway, next to a high back chair or countertop. Because this is not a test of balance, the subject is allowed to hold on to a high countertop or chair for support. In this test, the subject is asked to step in place for 2 minutes. Stepping involved flexing the hip and the knee to a height that is midway between the iliac crest and the knee on the opposite side. Stepping on both sides, right and left, counts as a single step. The score recorded is the total number of correct height steps taken by the one of legs within 2 minutes. If the knee height can no longer be maintained, the participant is asked to stop, or to stop and rest until proper form can be regained. During rest intervals the clock continues to run.
Activity – Cardiovascular Deconditioning	***Exercise Tolerance Tests (ETT):*** To examine the ability of the cardiovascular system to accommodate to increasing metabolic demand, an ETT, stress test, or graded exercise test is performed. The patient exercises through stages of increasing workloads, expressed in units of oxygen. Oxygen cost may be expressed in L/min, mL O_2/kg/min, kcal, or metabolic equivalents (METs)**;** the MET represents a factor of the basic systemic oxygen requirement at rest, roughly 3.5 mL O_2/kg/min. The most common modalities used in exercise testing of patients with cardiac impairments are the treadmill, bicycle, and arm ergometer (Fig. 13.20). The best indicator of an individual's aerobic capacity is through examination of the peak oxygen uptake or Vo_{2max} and anaerobic threshold measured through use of a metabolic cart. When expensive equipment like a metabolic cart is not available, field tests such as the step test, bicycle tests and walk tests can be useful in predicting the maximal oxygen consumption from the submaximal steady state heart rate. A multitude of tests are available to quantify exercise capacity. An excellent resource for these tests is the *American College of Sports Medicine's Guidelines for Exercise Testing and Prescription.*
Activity – Decrease Balance	***Tests of Balance and Fall Risk:*** A variety of functional tests including the *Timed Up and Go Test,*[83] *Berg Balance Test,*[84] and 10 meter Walk Test measuring gait speed[85] can be utilized in assessing a patient's balance and fall risk.

Continued

Table 13.10 Outcome Measures: Activity Limitations, and Participation Restrictions in Patients With Cardiovascular Disease—cont'd

Activity and Participation Limitation	Key Test/ Measure
Activity – Decrease Mobility	***Activity Measure for Post-Acute Care (AM-PAC):*** The AM-PAC is an outcome measure that assesses function in three major domains: basic mobility, daily activities and applied cognitive.[86,87] The primary goal for the development of this measure was to create a single measure to effectively measure function across all care settings within the continuum of care following an acute care stay. The AM-PAC is a patient reported outcome measure and therefore captures the patient's perspective. The measure is available in two basic formats: a computer-based version and a short-form version.
Activity – Decrease Mobility	***Mobility Measures in Post-Acute Care:*** Depending on the care setting, a variety of measures exists to document a patient's activity and functional status including the *Functional Independence Measure (FIM)* commonly used in inpatient rehabilitation facilities, the *Minimum Data Set (MDS)* used in skilled nursing facilities, and the *Outcome and Assessment Information Set (OASIS)* that is primarily used in home care (see Chapter 7).
Participation – Quality of Life	***Minnesota Living With Heart Failure Questionnaire (MLHFQ):*** The MLHFQ is a patient self-assessment of how heart failure affects a patient's daily life. It was developed by Thomas Rector in 1992 and since then has been used in multiple research investigations as a measure of quality of life in patients with heart failure. The approximate time to complete the questionnaire is 5 to 10 minutes. The content reflects most frequent and important ways heart failure affects patients' lives. All items are assessed on a 1–5 Likert scale. Sum of item responses allows for total and individual dimension scores. The test-retest/reproducibility assessed by Rector and colleagues is a Pearson correlation of 0.87.[88] Internal consistency measured by Cronbach's alpha for all items is 0.92[88] The minimally important difference is 5 points on the total score.[89] In addition, the estimated standard error of the measure is 6–7 points.[89]
Participation – Quality of Life	***Seattle Angina Questionnaire (SAQ):*** The SAQ is an outcome measure that is utilized to assess the impact of angina in a patient's quality of life within the previous four weeks of the assessment date.[90] The survey uses 19 items to assess the severity of limitations in everyday life. There are two distinct sections of the survey—the impact of angina on the patient's ability for completing ADLs and a second section involving several questions that assess the patient's health conditions. The measure has been a validated disease-specific health status instrument for coronary artery disease (CAD) with high test-retest reliability, predictive power, and responsiveness, its use in routine clinical practice.[91] However, its use has been limited by its length (19 items). Therefore, in 2014 a short version (7 items) was developed, tested, and validated to increase the feasibility of measuring patient-reported outcomes in patients with CAD.[91]

Research on Exercise Training in Heart Failure

It is worthy to note that existing research has primarily investigated the benefits of exercise training in patients who are chronically ill with HF. A paucity of research exists that investigates the benefits of exercise training in patients who are in decompensated heart failure in the acute care setting or in a state immediately after acute decompensation within the skilled nursing care, inpatient rehabilitation, or home care setting.

Davies and colleagues published a *Cochrane Database* systematic review, that investigated the effectiveness of exercise-based interventions on the mortality, hospitalization admissions, morbidity, and health-related quality of life (HRQOL) for patients with systolic heart failure.[107] Nineteen trials with 3,647 patients with HF were included within the systematic review. The findings of this review article provide substantial evidence that exercise is safe as it does not increase all-cause mortality, reduces heart failure related hospitalizations, and provides improvement in patient's Health Related Quality of Life (HRQOL). Further, the authors of this review indicate that "the effects of exercise training on total mortality, hospitalization and HRQOL were independent of the degree of left ventricular dysfunction, type of cardiac rehabilitation, dose of exercise intervention, length of follow-up, trial quality, and trial publication date."[107]

Belardinelli and colleagues took on the challenge of investigating the effects of a very long-term (10 year) exercise training program in patients with chronic HF.[108]

FUNCTIONAL CLASS	CLINICAL STATUS	O2 COST ml/kg/min	METS	STEP TEST	BICYCLE ERGOMETER	TREADMILL PROTOCOLS													
				Nagle Balke Naughton	1 watt= 6kpds	Bruce		Cornell		Balke-Ware	ACIP		mACIP		Naughton			Ware	
				2 min stages 30 steps min Step height increased 4 cm q 2 min	For 70 kg body weight	3-min stages		2-min stages		% grad at 3.3 mph 1-min stages	2-min stages First 2 stages 1 min				2-min stages			2-min stages	
				Height (cm)	KPDS	MPH	%GR	MPH	%GR		MPH	%GR	MPH	%GR	%GR 2 MPH	%GR 3 MPH	%GR 3.4 MPH	MPH	%GR
						5.5	20												
						5.0	18	5.0	18	26									
Normal and I	Healthy dependent on age, activity	56.0	16							25 24						32.5	26		
		52.5	15					4.6	17	23	3.4	24	3.4	24		30	24		
		49.0	14							22 21						27.5	22		
		45.5	13		1500	4.2	16	4.2	16	20 19	3.1	24	3.1	24		25	20		
		42.0	12	40	1350					18 17	3	21	2.7	24		22.5	18		
		38.5	11	36	1200			3.8	15	16 15						20	16		
	Sedentary healthy	35.0	10	32	1050					14 13	3	17.5	2.3	24		17.5	14	3.4	14.0
		31.5	9	28		3.4	14			12 11						15	12	3.0	15.0
	Limited	28.0	8	24	900			3.0	13	10 9	3	14	2	24		12.5	10	3.0	12.5
		24.5	7	20	750	2.5	12	2.5	12	8 7					17.5	10	8	3.0	10.0
II	Symptomatic	21.0	6	16	600			2.1	11	6 5	3	10.5	2	18.9	14	7.5	6	3.0	7.5
		17.5	5	12	450	1.7	10	1.7	10	4	3.0	7.0	2	13.5	10.5	5	4	2.0	10.5
III		14.0	4	8	300					3 2	3.0	3.0	2	7	7	2.5	2	2.0	7.0
		10.5	3	4		1.7	5	1.7	5	1	2.5	2.0	2	3.5	3.5	0		2.0	3.5
		7.0	2		150	1.7	0	1.7	0		2.0	0	2	0	0			1.5	0
IV		3.5	1															1.0	0

Figure 13.20 Estimated oxygen requirements for step, bicycle, and treadmill. The standard Bruce protocol begins at 1.7 mph and 10% grade (roughly 5 METs). Oxygen requirements increase with progressive increases in workload for all modalities. *(Adapted from Fletcher et al., p 156.)*

Table 13.11 Research on Effectiveness of Cardiac Rehabilitation Programs

Researcher	Outcomes
Suaya and colleagues	21%–34% reduction in all-cause mortality rate with the utilization of cardiac rehabilitation.[92]
Hammill and colleagues	Patients who attended 36 supervised cardiac rehabilitation sessions had lower risk for death and myocardial infraction after adjustment for demographic characteristics, comorbid conditions, and subsequent hospitalization.[93] The patients who received 36 visits showed lower death risk and lower risk for myocardial infraction than those who completed 24 sessions (hazard ratio [HR], 0.86; 95% confidence interval [CI], 0.77 to 0.97) and a 12% lower risk of MI (HR, 0.88; 95% CI, 0.83 to 0.93). In the same report, the authors indicate a 22% lower death risk and 23% lower risk of heart attack in those who completed 36 visits compared with similar patients who received 12 sessions.[93]
Taylor and colleagues	A systematic review and meta-analysis of randomized controlled trials indicated reduced all-cause mortality, greater reductions in total cholesterol level, triglyceride level, systolic blood pressure, and lower rates of self-reported smoking.[94]
Lawler and colleagues	Systematic review revealed that exercise-based cardiac rehabilitation has favorable effects on cardiovascular risk factors, including smoking, blood pressure, body weight, and lipid profile.[95]
Anderson and colleagues	Cochrane Review and Meta-analysis of 63 studies with 14,486 participants with median follow-up of 12 months delineated that cardiac rehabilitation led to reduction in cardiovascular mortality, improved quality of life, increased exercise performance, and improved adherence with medications.[96]

Table 13.12 Inpatient Cardiac Rehabilitation Program

CCU—Essentially Bedrest

Level 1

1–1.5 METs

- Evaluation and patient education
- Arms supported for meals and activities of daily living (ADL)
- Bed exercises and dangle with feet supported (if CK levels have peaked and patient has no complications)

Education

- Introduction to inpatient cardiac rehab and role of physical therapy
  - Education
  - Monitored progression of activity
  - Home exercise/activity guidelines/outpatient cardiac rehab

Sitting—Limited Room Ambulation

Level 2

1.5–2 METs

- Sitting 15–30 min, 2–4 times/day
- Leg exercises
- Commode privileges
- Reclining upright chair
- Limited ADL
- Electric razor
- Limited supervised room ambulation for small uncomplicated MI

Education

- Identification of CAD risk factors
- Concept of "healing interval" and need to pace activities

Room—Limited Hall Ambulation

Level 3

2–2.5 METs

- Room or hall ambulation up to 5 min as tolerated 3–4 times/day
- Standing leg exercises optional*
- Sit on side of bed or in bathroom to wash (per discretion nurse/physical therapist [PT])
- Manual shave
- Bathroom privileges
- Independent or assisted ambulation in room or hall as advised by PT

Education

- Size of infarct and how it relates to the need for gradual resumption of activities
- Impact of exercise on reducing the patient's risk factors
- Teach use of Borg's Scale for Rating of Perceived Exertion and appropriate parameters with activity

Progressive Hall Ambulation

Level 4

2.5–3 METs

- Hall ambulation 5–7 min as tolerated 3–4 times/day
- Standing trunk exercises optional*
- Independent or assisted ambulation in hall as advised by PT

Education

- Teach pulse taking and appropriate parameters with activity
- Reinforce benefits of outpatient cardiac rehabilitation

Table 13.12 Inpatient Cardiac Rehabilitation Program—cont'd

Progressive Hall Ambulation	Patient Outcome—No Evidence of Hemodynamic Compromise With Activity Progression (All Levels)
Level 5 3–4 METs • Hall ambulation 8–10 min as tolerated • Arm exercises optional* • Standing shower • Independent hall ambulation as advised by PT Education • Written home exercise/activity guidelines reviewed • Patient given written information on outpatient cardiac rehab Stair Climbing	No systolic drop in BP >10 mm Hg or increase >30 mm Hg No HR increase >12 if beta blocked, or no HR increase >20 if not beta blocked No complaints of dizziness, light-headedness, or angina Perceived exertion <13/20
Level 6 4–5 METs • Progressive hall ambulation as tolerated • Full flight of stairs (or as required at home) up and down one step at a time† Education • Answer patient's questions • Check for understanding of activity guidelines	**Hemodynamic Monitoring** **Level 1** • HR and BP before and after supine bed exercises • Orthostatic signs supine and dangling at bedside **Level 2** • Orthostatic signs (supine, sit, and stand) before exercises and transfer • HR and BP after leg exercises/transfer to chair • HR and BP after return to bed **Levels 3–6** • HR and BP in sitting and standing prior to activity • HR and BP immediately following activity • HR and BP 5 min after activity

From Rehabilitation Services Department, Newton Wellesley Hospital, Newton, MA, with permission.

*Optional exercises are at the discretion of the PT and may be used to establish the patient's CV response in the room, prior to moving on to more challenging hallway ambulation; or in those patients who require general strengthening exercises.

†Stair climbing activities should take place after the ETT if the scheduling of the ETT permits. Otherwise patients may, at the discretion and supervision of the PT, climb stairs on the day prior to the ETT.

Table 13.13 Exercise Prescription Parameters Utilized in Outpatient Cardiac Rehabilitation Programs

Condition	Parameters
Mode	Utilize large muscle groups, aerobic forms of exercise including walking, jogging, cycling, rowing, stepping, arm ergometry and other endurance activities. Must be enjoyable to maximize compliance.
Frequency	A minimum of three times a week but preferably must be carried out most days of the week.
Duration	Variable, but most research utilizes a duration of 12 weeks of exercise training.
Components	• 5- to 10-minute warm-up that involve stretching, flexibility movements, and aerobic activity is beneficial in allowing for an incremental increase in heart rate. • Conditioning phase of 30–45 minutes of aerobic exercise with a minimum 20 minutes of exercise. • 5- to 10-minute cool-down phase to promote venous return and avoid adverse consequences post activity including post exercise hypotension, angina, ischemic ST-T changes, and ventricular arrhythmias.[98]
Intensity	• 40%–85% of functional capacity (Vo_{2max}), corresponding to 55%–90% of maximal heart rate. • Target Heart Rate (THR) usually determined by the Karvonen method. THR = Resting Heart Rate + % intensity (symptom limited heart rate maximum – resting heart rate). • Prescribed based on the rating of perceived exertion (RPE) based on the Borg RPE scale. The Borg's RPE is a measure scale where the patient rates his or her level of exertion during the activity on a scale of 6–20 (Table 13.14). This scale is validated method that most patients can learn and apply easily and is extremely valuable during bouts of unsupervised exercise.
Progression	Progression of intensity is individualized based on several factors including patient tolerance, symptoms, motivation, and goals.

Continued

Table 13.13 Exercise Prescription Parameters Utilized in Outpatient Cardiac Rehabilitation Programs—cont'd

Condition	Parameters
Resistance Training	Resistance exercises is traditionally prescribed based on the individual's measured or estimated maximal strength or the "one-repetition maximum." General strength prescription in cardiac patients involves 30%–40% of the one-repetition maximum for upper body exercises and 40%–50% of the one-repetition maximum for lower body exercises. Exercises are performed for 12 to 15 repetitions per set, performed two to three times each week.[99]

Table 13.14 Rating of Perceived Exertion: The Borg RPE Scale*

6	No exertion at all
7	
8	Extremely light
9	Very light
10	
11	Light
12	
13	Somewhat hard
14	
15	Hard (heavy)
16	
17	Very hard
18	
19	Extremely hard
20	Maximal exertion

*Copyright Gunnar Borg. Reproduced with permission.

For correct usage of the scale(s), the exact design and instructions given in Borg's folders must be followed. See Borg, G: Borg's Perceived Exertion and Pain Scales. Human Kinetics, Champaign, IL, 1998, or www.borgproducts.com.

Box 13.5 Criteria for Modification or Termination of Exercise in Patients With Heart Failure

- Marked dyspnea or fatigue
- RR >40 breaths/min
- Development of S_3 heart sound
- Increase in pulmonary crackles
- Decrease in HR or BP of >10 bpm or mm Hg, respectively, during steady state or progressive exercise
- Increase in the CVP by 10 mm Hg
- Diaphoresis, pallor, or confusion

Criteria for Initiation of Exercise

- Compensated CHF
- Able to speak comfortably without signs of dyspnea with RR <30 breaths/min
- Less than moderate fatigue
- CI >2.0 L/min
- CVP <10 mm Hg
- Crackles in less than one half of the lungs
- Resting heart rate <120 bpm

*1 RM = 1 repetition maximum.

The primary goal of the investigation was to determine whether a 10-year supervised moderate exercise training program produces sustained improvement in functional capacity and New York Heart Association classification scores. In a randomized controlled design of 123 patients with stable HF, and ejection fraction less than 40%, subjects were assigned to either an intervention group involving 2 exercise sessions at 60% of peak oxygen consumption per week for 10 years or a control group did not participate in any regular and supervised exercise training. The authors found significant improvements in peak oxygen uptake in the exercising subjects compared with those in the control group. More specifically, peak oxygen uptake was more than 60% of age- and gender-predicted maximum each year during the 10-year study.[108] Subjects that did not exercise progressively decreased their peak oxygen uptake. In addition, there were significant improvement in quality of life, hospital readmission and cardiac mortality (hazard ratio = 0.68; 95% CI: 0.30 to 0.82, $p < 0.001$).[108] The findings of this study reveal that moderate intensity supervised exercise training performed twice weekly for 10 years maintains functional capacity greater than 60% of maximum oxygen uptake, improved quality of life, reduced hospital admissions and overall mortality in patients with HF.

The importance of exercise training in patients with HF is also depicted in a systematic review published by Smart and Marwick.[109] The researchers reviewed 81 studies including 2,387 exercising subjects with 1,197 patients enrolled in controlled studies. The studies cumulatively totaled 60,000 patient hours of exercise training.[109] Mean number of subjects was 30 ± 25; mean age of 59 years ± 7 and mean ejection fraction 27% ± 7. The investigators reported that studies utilizing aerobic exercise training ($n = 40$) demonstrated Vo_{2max} increase of 16.5%.[109] In addition, studies utilizing strength training alone ($n = 3$) demonstrated Vo_{2max} increase of 9.3% and

Table 13.15 Exercise Interventions Utilized for Patients With Heart Failure

Intervention	Parameters/ Dosage
Aerobic Exercise	• Low-impact exercise with gradual progression of intensity, frequency, and duration. • Progression of aerobic activity is appropriate if cardiac output is maintained measured by blood pressure assessment during exercise. • Intensity should be monitored using the dyspnea or perceived exertion scales and should be kept to a rating of fairly light. HR cannot be relied on for evaluating intensity because of the effects of various medications, including beta blockers.[100]
Resistance Training	Clinical guidelines for prescription of resistance exercise by NYHA class.[101] • NYHA Class I: 2–3 days/ weeks, 15–30 min., 50%–60% 1 RM,* 2–3 sets, 6–15 repetitions • NYHA Class II–III: 2 days/week, 12–15 min., 40%–50% 1 RM, 1–2 sets, 4–10 repetitions
Ventilatory Muscle Training	Guidelines for use of a threshold inspiratory muscle trainer:[102] • frequency of 6–7 days/week • 40%–60% Maximal Inspiratory Pressure (MIP) • duration of 6–12 weeks, 30 min/session or a variable session time to respiratory muscle fatigue Significant improvements with use of a threshold inspiratory muscle trainer:[103] • 20%–60% of MIP once daily or twice a day for 30 minutes for 8–12 weeks
High Intensity Interval Training	Significant improvement in patients with stable heart failure utilizing: • High-intensity interval exercise program for 10 weeks. Subjects performed 4 sets of 4 min high-intensity exercise intervals at 80%–90% of their Vo_{2max} accompanied with low-intensity exercise intervals at 50%–60% Vo_{2max} for a total time of 33 min.[104] No adverse events noted. • Four work intervals (each 4 min in length) completed at 90%–95% heart rate peak (HRpeak) accompanied by 3 min of low-intensity exercise at 50%–70% HRpeak. Total training time for the HIIT group was 38 minutes.[105]
Breathing Exercises	Diaphragmatic breathing may help reduce excessive accessory muscle use and reduce the work of breathing. Pursed-lip breathing has been shown to promote the positive end-expiratory pressure not only in patients with COPD but also in patients with CHF.[106] Pursed-lip breathing is also beneficial in helping slow down the respiratory rate in patients with heart failure.[106]
Positioning	Upright positioning is beneficial to decrease the preload and workload on the heart.
Activity Pacing/ Energy Conservation Techniques	• Frequent rest intervals before they symptoms of fatigue. • Participate in activities that require greater energy costs at times of the day when they have the most energy. • Plan and delegate as necessary. • Alternate tasks that vary in difficulty and intensity. • Adjust the environment as necessary.

*1 RM = 1 repetition maximum.

studies that combined aerobic and strength programs (n = 30) demonstrated Vo_{2max} increase of 15%.[109]

A meta-analysis conducted by van Tol et al. in 2006 investigated 35 original randomized crossover trials of patients with systolic HF.[110] The average exercise within these studies included aerobic exercise 3x/week, for 60 minutes/session for 12 weeks. The investigators found an increase in 6-minute walk distance with an effect size of 46.2 m, within 15 studies including 599 patients. In 31 studies with approximately 1,240 patients, maximum oxygen uptake was found to increase after exercise with an effect size of 2.06 mL/kg/min. In summary the researchers found significant improvement in maximum heart rate (2.5%), maximum cardiac output (21.3%), peak oxygen uptake (13%), anaerobic threshold (17.4%), 6-minute walk distance (11.6%) and health related quality of life as marked by reduced Minnesota Living With Heart Failure scores (–28%) following the 12 weeks of exercise training.[110] Interestingly, in this robust meta-analysis involving moderate intensity exercise, no significant improvements were noted in ejection fraction following exercise training. This finding clearly indicates that moderate intensity exercise training has less of an influence on central cardiovascular function and more of an influence on peripheral muscle function.

Research on Strength Training in Heart Failure

Peripheral muscle is abnormal in patients with HF. Elderly individuals with HF are at a particular risk of developing muscle wasting and resultant muscle weakness.[111]

Studies have demonstrated muscle fiber atrophy of skeletal muscle as well as alterations in arterial vasodilation capacity.[111] Research has also documented atrophy of both type I and type II muscle fibers in individuals with chronic HF.[112] In addition, in persons with HF, there exists an apparent switch in fiber-type proportion to the less fatigue resistant fast twitch type IIB fibers.[113] Further, Drexler and colleagues have reported a reduction in the quantity of aerobic enzymes and mitochondrial density in muscle tissue in patient with chronic HF.[114] Both of these factors decrease the capacity for aerobic metabolism in patients with HF. As such, it is known that the peripheral muscles in patients with HF are weaker, with a decreased mass, reduced aerobic capacity and increased fatigability. Physical therapists have the unique ability to reverse these peripheral muscle limitations through formal strength training to improve overall activity and participation in patients with HF.

Research has shown that in patients with HF, resistance exercise training coupled with aerobic exercise increases peak oxygen consumption and exercise capacity, improves New York Heart Association (NYHA) functional class, reduces mortality and improves the quality of life.[115] Gasiorowski reports that "exercise training improves skeletal muscle metabolism, increases blood flow within the active skeletal muscles, increase capillary density, promote the synthesis and release of nitric oxide, improves angiogenesis, and decrease oxidative stress."[115] The evidence is clear in indicating that the treatment for patients with HF must not only involve aerobic conditioning, but also peripheral resistance training.[101,115,116]

In such, strength training is a crucial component of the exercise plan for patients with heart failure to help improve peripheral muscle strength and endurance. Inclusion of light resistance work has been shown to be safe in this population.[142] Modalities for resistance training may include elastic bands for mild UE and LE resistance work or light weights. Closed chain or open chain exercises can be incorporated into the treatment plan. S sit-to-stand progression is extremely beneficial in increasing lower extremity muscle strength. The therapist is encouraged to evaluate the point of at which the patient begins to demonstrate compensations as a means of deciding the appropriate progression of the resistive load.

Research on Inspiratory Muscle Training in Heart Failure

Patients with heart failure are known to have poor ventilatory muscle strength.[148] Strength of the ventilator muscles can be enhanced through use of a device known as a threshold inspiratory muscle trainer. Improvements in the maximal inspiratory pressure are achieved by having the patient breathe with this device, which resists inspiration, thereby strengthening the inspiratory muscles.

Respiratory, or inspiratory, muscle training (IMT) has been empirically found to be beneficial in patients with HF. The utilization of an inspiratory muscle trainer has been found to improve peak oxygen consumption,[117] improve patient performance in functional tests,[118] and improved quality of life.[119] IMT therapy may be an alternative treatment for patients who cannot engage in conventional exercise training programs. Several recent meta-analysis and systematic reviews have document significant improvements in the overall maximum inspiratory capacity, maximum oxygen uptake, 6-minute walk tests scores and quality of life scores.[102,120,121]

Research on High Intensity Interval Training in Heart Failure

Is it beneficial and safe to work patients with heart failure harder at higher intensities? Historically, moderate continuous training) has been considered preferential as often the risk of serious medical events from moderate intensity exercise has been considered acceptable, while high intensity interval training is intuitively considered by many to carry higher risk. In addition, clinicians often believe that patients are more likely to be tolerant to moderate intensity exercise relative to high intensity work leading to greater exercise adherence. A landmark study of high intensity interval training by Wisloff and colleagues in patients with heart failure produced unsurpassed clinical improvements in peak Vo_2 (46%).[105] The underlying success of high intensity interval exercise is attributable to interval exercise which allows for rest periods. The rest intervals make it possible for patients with heart failure to perform exercise at higher intensities for shorter bouts, thereby allowing for greater degrees of adaptation. Ismail and colleagues published a systematic review and meta-analysis that aimed to investigate whether aerobic exercise training intensity produces different effect sizes for fitness, adherence, event rates, mortality rates, and hospitalization rates in patients with heart failure.[122] Seventy-four studies were included in the analysis including 76 intervention groups. Groups included 9 (11.8%) high-intensity, 38 (50%) vigorous-intensity, 24 (31.6%) moderate-intensity, and 5 (6.6%) low-intensity groups. A total of 3,265 exercising subjects and 2,612 control subjects were evaluated in these 74 studies. The authors conclude that as exercise training intensity rises, so does the magnitude of improvement in cardiorespiratory fitness, accompanied by lower study withdrawal in exercising patients. Peak Vo_{2max} for high-intensity training increased a mean of 3.33 (0.53–6.13) mL/kg/min, whereas for moderate intensity training increased by 2.19 (1.39–2.99) mL/kg/min.[122]

Research on Dance Therapy in Heart Failure

A systematic review of three studies reviewed dance therapy in patients with chronic heart failure.[123] The results indicated results indicated significant improvements in Vo_{2max} as well as QOL. The pooled homogenous effect size (CI) for quality of life was 2.09 (1.65–2.54) indicating that patients were extremely happy after dance therapy![123] In the same year, a Cochrane review evaluated the benefits of exercise based therapy on exercise capacity and quality of life.[124] Interestingly, the pooled effect size (CI) in QOL was only 0.56 (0.30–0.82).[124] The findings of these two studies indicate relatively lower improvement in quality of life with exercise based therapy compared with dance therapy which must be considered in the overall plan of care.

EDUCATION FOR PATIENTS WITH HEART DISEASE

For patients with heart disease, patient and family education develops along a continuum, depending on the patient's baseline status and readiness to attend to the information. The physical therapist, along with other members of the health care team, must determine the patient's and family's ability to understand and adhere to the information. Appropriate discharge or ongoing outpatient topics to be addressed include the following:

1. *Activity Guidelines.* Patients (and family) need to be able to understand specific activity guidelines, which include planned exercise sessions as well as leisure time and rests.
2. *Self-Monitoring.* Patients may monitor the intensity of their activity in a variety of ways; two of the more common ways are palpating a pulse and RPE. Because many older patients have decreased sensitivity in their palpation skills, the use of RPE may be easier and more reliable. Those patients who can take a pulse or choose to invest in an HR monitor may prefer to use these methods. Self-monitoring not only involves HR or the Borg RPE Scale, but awareness of other symptoms or signs that may suggest exercise intolerance, such as light-headedness, mental confusion, dyspnea, and inability to carry on a brief conversation while performing an activity. Patients with CHF commonly use the dyspnea scale and the Borg RPE Scale.
3. *Symptom Recognition and Response.* Being able to recognize their specific cardiac symptoms and to know how to respond is a key component in patient education. Patients should have written information regarding the action they should take when symptoms occur, for example, when to call their physician or go to the hospital. Angina is the most common symptom associated with coronary heart disease, whereas weight gain (2 lb over 1 to 2 days), dyspnea, LE edema, and increased pillows for sleep are common signs and symptoms for CHF.
4. *Nutrition.* Patients commonly meet with a nutritionist to discuss their usual dietary habits and to make recommendations when needed for a more heart-healthy diet. Most commonly, patients with heart disease are instructed to reduce fat intake; patients with CHF are instructed to monitor salt and fluid intake.
5. *Medications.* Patients receive written information regarding the desired action of their medications, potential side effects, dosage, and timing of medications. Patients should also know which nonprescription drugs such as cold, sinus, allergy, or anti-inflammatory medications they should avoid because of possible interactions with prescription drugs. Patients should also be encouraged to disclose all herbal remedies and supplements that they may be taking.
6. *Lifestyle Issues.* Many factors influence whether a patient will return to work after a cardiac event. Many patients with CAD return to work if they were employed before their event; patients with CHF are, in general, an older population when compared with patients with CAD and therefore may have already retired.
7. *Sexual Activity.* Resumption of sexual activity may be an uncomfortable discussion for some patients. There may be many issues of concern for the patient (e.g., fear, anxiety, performance concerns, lack of libido). Patients and their partners are encouraged to verbalize their concerns to each other and to seek appropriate information from their health care team. Some medications (e.g., beta blockers) may blunt the sexual response, and it is important that patients communicate this with their physician. Often, another medication or category of medication may be better tolerated. When patients feel ready for sex, their energy level throughout the day is satisfying for them, and they can walk outdoors and climb stairs comfortably, they are probably ready for sexual activity. It may be helpful for patients to remember that sexual activity is not unlike other physical activity with respect to energy cost, and therefore planning, pacing, and warm-up are powerful contributors for a more comfortable outcome. In some cases, the physician may recommend taking prophylactic NTG before sexual activity.

See Box 13.6 *Suggested Topics for Patient, Family, and Caregiver Education and Counselling* from the U.S. Department of Health and Human Services Clinical Practice Guidelines for Patients with CHF.

PSYCHOLOGICAL/SOCIAL ISSUES

Cardiac disease may not only create new emotional issues but also enhance some that might have existed before the cardiac event. Physical therapy practitioners need to understand the psychosocial aspects of each patient, including personality styles and coping skills. They need to recognize stages of psychosocial adaptation and help patients to progress in their own adjustment. Therapists can play an important role in reassuring patients that many of these issues are normal sequelae of their event and in encouraging patients to seek guidance and counseling in whatever arena they feel appropriate (e.g., counseling, religion). In more severe cases of generalized anxiety or depression, referral to

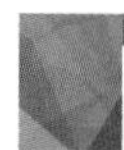

Box 13.6 Suggested Topics for Patient, Family, and Caregiver Education and Counseling

General Counseling

- Explanation of heart failure and the reason for symptoms
- Cause or probable cause of heart failure
- Expected symptoms
- Symptoms of worsening heart failure
- What to do if symptoms worsen
- Self-monitoring with daily weights
- Explanation of treatment/care plan
- Clarification of patient's responsibilities
- Importance of cessation of tobacco use
- Role of family members or other caregivers in the treatment/care plan
- Availability and value of qualified local support group
- Importance of obtaining vaccinations against influenza and pneumococcal disease

Prognosis

- Life expectancy
- Advance directives
- Advice for family members in the event of sudden death

Activity Recommendations

- Recreation, leisure, and work activity
- Exercise
- Sex, sexual difficulties, and coping strategies

Dietary Recommendations

- Sodium restriction
- Avoidance of excessive fluid intake
- Fluid restriction (if required)
- Alcohol restriction

Medications

- Effects of medications on quality of life and survival
- Dosing
- Likely side effects and what to do if they occur
- Coping mechanisms for complicated medical regimens
- Availability of lower-cost medications or financial assistance

Importance of Compliance With the Treatment Care Plan

From Clinical Practice Guidelines, Number 11, Heart Failure: Evaluation and Care of Patients With Left-Ventricular Systolic Dysfunction, AHCPR Publication No. 94-0612, p 42, with permission.

a mental health practitioner is warranted (i.e., psychiatrist, psychologist). The therapist should utilize an integrated patient/client centered approach, working together with patients to develop goals, outcomes and a POC that is congruent with their needs, values, and level of functioning. See additional discussion in Chapter 26, Psychosocial Issues in Physical Rehabilitation.

PRIMARY PREVENTION OF CORONARY ARTERY DISEASE

Patients who do not have documented CAD but who have identifiable risk factors should be encouraged to adopt lifestyle behaviors that can modify their risk factors. Health education and primary prevention programs through individualized education and exercise guidelines attempt to modify an individual's risk factors and thereby prevent CAD.

Patients are instructed in appropriate dietary guidelines, including low fat, adequate fiber, minerals and vitamins, and decreased salt, particularly if the patient has high BP. Besides lowering total dietary fat, patients are instructed to decrease their percentage of saturated fats and avoid trans-fatty acids. Elevated levels of the amino acid homocysteine appear to increase the risk of arterial endothelial disease. Folic acid, a B vitamin, lowers homocysteine levels. If weight loss is needed, patients are encouraged to see a nutritionist to design a sensible eating plan. Patients are encouraged to gradually increase their endurance activity, such as walking toward a goal of 30 to 40 minutes (not including warm-up and cool-down) four times a week.

The *American College of Sports Medicine* and the *American Heart Association* recommend that anyone over age 40 with two or more risk factors should have an ETT before beginning an aerobic or strengthening exercise program. The purpose of the ETT is to identify the presence of any latent ischemia.

If no ischemia is present, a typical aerobic exercise prescription might be as follows:

- Intensity: 70% to 85% of HR_{max} as the aerobic training zone
- Duration: 30 to 40 minutes in the aerobic training zone; appropriate warm-up of 5 to 10 minutes, and cool-down
- Frequency: minimum of three to four times per week.

Modification of the other CAD risk factors is also key to the success of any primary prevention intervention. Patients are encouraged to identify risk factors and to seek resources to assist in modifying them. There are many community-based smoking cessation programs or medically supervised programs that a patient might explore. Stress management programs are also varied and can be adapted to the individual's needs. Proper and consistent use of any medications that might be used in controlling risk factors, such as antihypertensives, antihypercholesterolemias, blood glucose–lowering agents (hypoglycemics), and antianxiety agents or antidepressants, is crucial to the success of any program.

SUMMARY

Physical activity is important for all individuals and is especially beneficial for those individuals diagnosed with CAD and HF. Individuals with heart disease should understand that a consistent exercise program is part of the management for their disease and is as necessary as their medications. Having heart disease means that the person needs to understand the parameters in which he or she may safely participate in activity either recreationally or as a prescribed exercise. The role of the physical therapist is to provide a safe exercise prescription for all patients.

During the time of illness, the effects of decreased activity can be devastating. A paradox exists, however, in that the less activity that is done, the less activity can be done because of a decreased work capacity. Therefore, the relative energy cost of all activity increases, and the heart works harder for any given task. Not encouraging the patient to resume activity when he or she is medically stable is a disservice. As physical therapists, our role is clear: to understand the pathophysiology of the disease process, to accurately examine the patient, and to establish a safe POC. The ultimate goals and outcomes of a successful rehabilitation program are to improve the patient's physiological response to exercise, decrease the work of the cardiovascular system, improve overall level of activity and participation, and improve quality of life.

Questions for Review

1. Discuss key differences between an NSTEMI and an STEMI.
2. Discuss three different types of angina. How would you instruct your patient in symptom recognition? Delineate the physical therapy management if a patient has angina during a treatment session.
3. Discuss sternal precautions that you would instruct your patient to use following a median sternotomy procedure.
4. Discuss differences between compensated and uncompensated CHF.
5. Discuss the physical therapy implications when managing patients with pacemakers.
6. Discuss appropriate goals, education, and treatment interventions for patients with acute coronary syndrome in Phase I cardiac rehabilitation.
7. Discuss appropriate goals and treatment guidelines for patients with CHF.
8. Delineate the adaptation that may be noted following an aerobic training exercise program in patients with heart failure.

CASE STUDY

A 58-year-old man presents to the local emergency department (ER) with chief complaint of SOB and difficulty sleeping last night; patient had to sit up all night to make symptoms even a little better. Patient came to the ER because he was unable to get ready for work owing to increased SOB. Patient reports that he has felt SOB off and on for a couple of months, usually associated with physical activity; symptoms, however, usually resolved with rest. Today's episode was the first related to sleeping.

PAST MEDICAL HISTORY

- Coronary artery disease: anterior MI 4 years ago
- Hypercholesterolemia
- Peripheral vascular disease

MEDICATIONS

- Digoxin, captopril, furosemide (Lasix), diltiazem, simvastatin (Zocor)

FAMILY/SOCIAL

- Patient works full-time as an engineer; travels 3 to 4 days per month.
- Married, lives with his wife in a two-story home on a 2-acre lot; three college-aged children.
- Patient is an avid golfer; enjoys gardening and landscaping.

PHYSICAL EXAMINATION

- Heart sounds: S_1, S_2 normal; S_3 present, no S_4; 2/6 systolic murmur
- Lung sounds: crackles 1/3 way
- Rhythm/rate: irregular, 140 bpm

- Blood pressure: 100/60 mm Hg
- Respiratory rate: 26 breaths/min
- Sao_2: 90%
- Jugular venous distention: 5 cm
- Echocardiogram: akinetic apex, akinetic distal septum and anterior wall; dilated atria and LV
- Chest x-ray: unavailable

LABORATORY DATA

- Enzyme pending; CBC WNL except BUN and creatinine slightly elevated.
- BNP: 900 pg/mL.
- Patient remained in the hospital for 2 days while medications were adjusted. During this time patient underwent further testing, including an ETT.

RESULTS OF ETT

- Bruce protocol: 4 minutes; estimated Vo_{2max}; 20 mL O_2/kg/min (approximately 6 METs); max VS: 130 bpm HR; 120/60 mm Hg BP
- ECG: (–) negative for ischemia, chest pain
- Reason for stopping: absolute exhaustion
- Examination immediately post-ETT: (+) S_3
- Physical and occupational therapy were requested to assist with exercise guidelines and discharge planning

PATIENT'S GOALS

- Return to work.
- Resume hiking.
- Begin to prepare his garden for spring planting within the next 5 weeks.

PHYSICAL THERAPY INTERVENTION

- Exercise tolerance via low-level exercises sitting and standing, as well as 5-minute walk.

VITAL SIGNS

- Sitting (rest): HR 90 bpm; BP 110/60 mm Hg
- Sitting exercises: HR 108 bpm; BP 110/60 mm Hg
- Standing (rest): HR 110 bpm; BP 108/60 mm Hg
- Standing exercise: HR 116 bpm: BP 110/60 mm Hg
- 5-minute walk: 1000 ft; HR 120 bpm; BP 116/60 mm Hg

HOME INSTRUCTIONS

- Meetings planned with patient and his family to discuss discharge guidelines over the next 4 to 8 weeks.

FOLLOW-UP

- Patient returns to his primary care provider 3 months after discharge. Echocardiogram is unchanged with EF 30%. Patient states that he has been following discharge guidelines.

VITAL SIGNS

- HR 100 bpm; BP 116/70 mm Hg (resting).
- Patient states that he feels great and just wants to get on with his life.

GUIDING QUESTIONS

1. What is a reasonable presenting diagnosis? Identify each piece of information (and how you interpreted it) that you used to make this diagnosis.
2. Explain the pathophysiology of the patient's presenting symptoms. Discuss the significance of his HR and heart rhythm in relation to his symptoms.
3. If the patient's symptoms and signs worsened, and he was admitted to the coronary care unit (CCU),
   a. What do you think his Swan-Ganz reading could reasonably look like?
   b. What would you expect these signs/symptoms would be that would bring the patient to the CCU?
   c. What might be a reasonable cause of his signs/symptoms worsening?
   d. What other drugs/interventions might be given in the CCU?

4. What rhythm do you think the patient is in and why? What do you think might be a reason that he is in this rhythm?
5. What do you think the chest x-ray would look like and why?
6. What is your interpretation of the patient's vital sign response to PT intervention? What is your plan for your next session?
7. What exercise prescription would you recommend for the patient at home (modality, intensity, duration, frequency)?

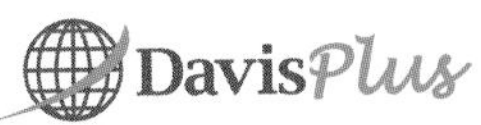

For additional resources, including answers to the questions for review and case study guiding questions, please visit **http://davisplus.fadavis.com.**

References

1. Mozaffarian D, Benjamin EJ, Go AS, et al. Heart disease and stroke statistics—2016 Update: a report from the American Heart Association. Circulation 2016;133(4):e38–360.
2. Rene Rodriguez E, Tan CD. Structure and anatomy of the human pericardium. Prog Cardiovasc Dis 2017.
3. Doctor NS, Shah AB, Coplan N, Kronzon I. Acute pericarditis: review. Prog Cardiovasc Dis 2016.
4. Hammer MM, Raptis CA, Javidan-Nejad C, Bhalla S. Accuracy of computed tomography findings in acute pericarditis. Acta radiologica (Stockholm, Sweden: 1987). 2014;55(10): 1197–1202.
5. Maron BJ, Towbin JA, Thiene G, et al. Contemporary definitions and classification of the cardiomyopathies: an American Heart Association Scientific Statement from the Council on Clinical Cardiology, Heart Failure and Transplantation Committee; Quality of Care and Outcomes Research and Functional Genomics and Translational Biology Interdisciplinary Working Groups; and Council on Epidemiology and Prevention. Circulation 2006;113(14):1807–1816.
6. Baddour LM, Wilson WR, Bayer AS, et al. Infective endocarditis in adults: diagnosis, antimicrobial therapy, and management of complications: a scientific statement for Healthcare Professionals From the American Heart Association. Circulation 2015;132(15):1435–1486.
7. Takaoka K, Yoshimura M, Ogawa H, et al. Comparison of the risk factors for coronary artery spasm with those for organic stenosis in a Japanese population: role of cigarette smoking. Int J Cardiol 2000;72(2):121–126.
8. Stern S, Bayes de Luna A. Coronary artery spasm: a 2009 update. Circulation 2009;119(18):2531–2534.
9. Nishimura RA, Carabello BA. Hemodynamics in the cardiac catheterization laboratory of the 21st century. Circulation 2012;125(17):2138–2150.
10. Badeer HS. Contractile tension in the myocardium. Am Heart J 1963;66:432–434.
11. Schwinger RH, Bohm M, Koch A, et al. The failing human heart is unable to use the Frank-Starling mechanism. Circ Res 1994;74(5):959–969.
12. Marconi C, Marzorati M. Exercise after heart transplantation. Eur J Appl Physiol 2003;90(3-4):250–259.
13. Compher C, Frankenfield D, Keim N, Roth-Yousey L. Best practice methods to apply to measurement of resting metabolic rate in adults: a systematic review. J Am Diet Assoc 2006;106(6): 881–903.
14. Ainsworth BE, Haskell WL, Herrmann SD, et al. 2011 Compendium of Physical Activities: a second update of codes and MET values. Med Sci Sports Exerc 2011;43(8):1575–1581.
15. Wright JD, Hughes JP, Ostchega Y, Yoon SS, Nwankwo T. Mean systolic and diastolic blood pressure in adults aged 18 and over in the United States, 2001-2008. National health statistics reports. 2011(35):1–22, 24.
16. Whelton PK, Carey RM, Aronow WS, et al. 2017 ACC/AHA/AAPA/ABC/ACPM/AGS/APhA/ASH/ASPC/NMA/PCNA Guideline for the Prevention, Detection, Evaluation, and Management of High Blood Pressure in Adults: A Report of the American College of Cardiology/American Heart Association Task Force on Clinical Practice Guidelines. J Am Coll Cardiol 2017.
17. Chobanian AV, Bakris GL, Black HR, et al. The Seventh Report of the Joint National Committee on Prevention, Detection, Evaluation, and Treatment of High Blood Pressure: the JNC 7 report. JAMA 2003;289(19):2560–2572.
18. Staessen JA, Wang J, Bianchi G, Birkenhager WH. Essential hypertension. Lancet *(London, England)*. 2003;361(9369): 1629-1641.
19. Siu AL. Screening for high blood pressure in adults: U.S. Preventive Services Task Force recommendation statement. Ann Intern Med 2015;163(10):778–786.
20. Eckel RH, Jakicic JM, Ard JD, et al. 2013 AHA/ACC guideline on lifestyle management to reduce cardiovascular risk: a report of the American College of Cardiology/American Heart Association Task Force on Practice Guidelines. Circulation 2014;129(25 Suppl 2):S76–99.
21. He FJ, Li J, Macgregor GA. Effect of longer-term modest salt reduction on blood pressure. The Cochrane database of systematic reviews. 2013(4):CD004937.
22. Martinez DG, Nicolau JC, Lage RL, et al. Effects of long-term exercise training on autonomic control in myocardial infarction patients. Hypertension 2011;58(6):1049–1056.
23. Cornelissen VA, Fagard RH, Coeckelberghs E, Vanhees L. Impact of resistance training on blood pressure and other cardiovascular risk factors: a meta-analysis of randomized, controlled trials. Hypertension 2011;58(5):950–958.
24. Conceicao LS, Neto MG, do Amaral MA, Martins-Filho PR, Oliveira Carvalho V. Effect of dance therapy on blood pressure and exercise capacity of individuals with hypertension: A systematic review and meta-analysis. Intl J Cardio 2016;220: 553–557.
25. Prescott E, Hippe M, Schnohr P, Hein HO, Vestbo J. Smoking and risk of myocardial infarction in women and men: longitudinal population study. BMJ (Clinical research ed.) 1998;316(7137): 1043–1047.
26. de Souza RJ, Mente A, Maroleanu A, et al. Intake of saturated and trans unsaturated fatty acids and risk of all cause mortality, cardiovascular disease, and type 2 diabetes: systematic review and meta-analysis of observational studies. BMJ (Clinical research ed.) 2015;351:h3978.
27. Chowdhury R, Warnakula S, Kunutsor S, et al. Association of dietary, circulating, and supplement fatty acids with coronary risk: a systematic review and meta-analysis. Ann Int Med 2014;160(6):398–406.
28. Ibanez B, Heusch G, Ovize M, Van de Werf F. Evolving therapies for myocardial ischemia/reperfusion injury. J Am Coll Cardiol 2015;65(14):1454–1471.
29. Reynolds HR, Hochman JS. Cardiogenic shock: current concepts and improving outcomes. *Circulation* 2008;117(5):686–697.
30. Lee TH, Cook EF, Weisberg M, Sargent RK, Wilson C, Goldman L. Acute chest pain in the emergency room. Identification and examination of low-risk patients. Arch Int Med 1985;145(1):65–69.

31. Ebell MH. Evaluation of chest pain in primary care patients. Am Fam Physician 2011;83(5):603–605.
32. Zimetbaum PJ, Josephson ME. Use of the electrocardiogram in acute myocardial infarction. N Engl J Med 2003;348(10): 933–940.
33. Thygesen K, Alpert JS, Jaffe AS, et al. Third universal definition of myocardial infarction. Circulation 2012;126(16):2020–2035.
34. Thygesen K, Alpert JS, White HD. Universal definition of myocardial infarction. Eur Heart J 2007;28(20):2525–2538.
35. Colombo A, Stankovic G, Moses JW. Selection of coronary stents. J Am Coll Cardiol 2002;40(6):1021–1033.
36. Aldea GS, Bakaeen FG, Pal J, et al.; the Society of Thoracic Surgeons Clinical Practice Guidelines on Arterial Conduits for Coronary Artery Bypass Grafting. Ann Thorac Surg 2016;101(2):801–809.
37. Cleveland JC, Jr., Shroyer AL, Chen AY, Peterson E, Grover FL. Off-pump coronary artery bypass grafting decreases risk-adjusted mortality and morbidity. Ann Thorac Surg 2001;72(4):1282–1288; discussion 1288–1289.
38. Sharma AD, Parmley CL, Sreeram G, Grocott HP. Peripheral nerve injuries during cardiac surgery: risk factors, diagnosis, prognosis, and prevention. Anesth Analg 2000;91(6):1358–1369.
39. Gualis J, Florez S, Tamayo E, Alvarez FJ, Castrodeza J, Castano M. Risk factors for mediastinitis and endocarditis after cardiac surgery. Asian cardiovascular & thoracic annals. 2009;17(6): 612–616.
40. El-Ansary D, Waddington G, Adams R. Measurement of non-physiological movement in sternal instability by ultrasound. Ann Thorac Surg 2007;83(4):1513–1516.
41. El-Ansary D, Waddington G, Adams R. Relationship between pain and upper limb movement in patients with chronic sternal instability following cardiac surgery. Physiother Theo Pract 2007;23(5):273–280.
42. Cahalin LP, Lapier TK, Shaw DK. Sternal precautions: is it time for change? precautions versus restrictions—a review of literature and recommendations for revision. Cardiopul Phys Ther J 2011;22(1):5–15.
43. Adams J, Lotshaw A, Exum E, et al. An alternative approach to prescribing sternal precautions after median sternotomy, "Keep Your Move in the Tube." Proceedings (Baylor University. Medical Center). 2016;29(1):97–100.
44. Adams J, Schmid J, Parker RD, et al. Comparison of force exerted on the sternum during a sneeze versus during low-, moderate-, and high-intensity bench press resistance exercise with and without the valsalva maneuver in healthy volunteers. Am J Cardiol 2014;113(6):1045–1048.
45. Moayedi Y, Ross HJ. Advances in heart failure: a review of biomarkers, emerging pharmacological therapies, durable mechanical support and telemonitoring. Clinical science (London, England: 1979). 2017;131(7):553–566.
46. Benjamin EJ, Blaha MJ, Chiuve SE, et al. Heart disease and stroke statistics–2017 update: a report from the American Heart Association. Circulation 2017;135(10):e146–e603.
47. Yancy CW, Jessup M, Bozkurt B, et al. 2013 ACCF/AHA guideline for the management of heart failure: executive summary: a report of the American College of Cardiology Foundation/ American Heart Association Task Force on practice guidelines. Circulation 2013;128(16):1810–1852.
48. Sharma K, Kass DA. Heart failure with preserved ejection fraction: mechanisms, clinical features, and therapies. Circulation research 2014;115(1):79–96.
49. Simonneau G, Gatzoulis MA, Adatia I, et al. Updated clinical classification of pulmonary hypertension. J Am Coll Cardiol 2013;62(25 Suppl):D34–41.
50. Borlaug BA. The pathophysiology of heart failure with preserved ejection fraction. Nature reviews. Cardiology 2014;11(9):507–515.
51. Pina IL, Apstein CS, Balady GJ, et al. Exercise and heart failure: A statement from the American Heart Association Committee on exercise, rehabilitation, and prevention. Circulation 2003;107(8):1210–1225.
52. Felker GM, Adams KF, Jr., Konstam MA, O'Connor CM, Gheorghiade M. The problem of decompensated heart failure: nomenclature, classification, and risk stratification. Am Heart J 2003;145(2 Suppl):S18–25.
53. Marcus GM, Gerber IL, McKeown BH, et al. Association between phonocardiographic third and fourth heart sounds and objective measures of left ventricular function. JAMA 2005;293(18): 2238–2244.
54. Negi S, Sawano M, Kohsaka S, et al. Prognostic implication of physical signs of congestion in acute heart failure patients and its association with steady-state biomarker levels. PloS one. 2014;9(5):e96325.
55. Martinez Ceron DM, Garcia Rosa ML, Lagoeiro Jorge AJ, et al. Association of types of dyspnea including 'bendopnea' with cardiopulmonary disease in primary care. Revista portuguesa de cardiologia: orgao oficial da Sociedade Portuguesa de Cardiologia = Portuguese journal of cardiology: an official journal of the Portuguese Society of Cardiology 2017;36(3):179–186.
56. Thibodeau JT, Turer AT, Gualano SK, et al. Characterization of a novel symptom of advanced heart failure: bendopnea. JACC. Heart failure. 2014;2(1):24–31.
57. Lindenfeld J, Albert NM, Boehmer JP, et al. HFSA 2010 Comprehensive Heart Failure Practice Guideline. J Card Fail 2010;16(6):e1–194.
58. Norman JF, Pozehl BJ, Duncan KA, Hertzog MA, Elokda AS, Krueger SK. Relationship of resting B-type natriuretic peptide level to cardiac work and total physical work capacity in heart failure patients. J Cardiopul Rehabil Prev 2009;29(5):310–313.
59. Pellikka PA, Nagueh SF, Elhendy AA, Kuehl CA, Sawada SG. American Society of Echocardiography recommendations for performance, interpretation, and application of stress echocardiography. J Am Soc Echocardiogr 2007;20(9):1021–1041.
60. Abraham WT, Hayes DL. Cardiac resynchronization therapy for heart failure. Circulation 2003;108(21):2596–2603.
61. Nkomo VT, Gardin JM, Skelton TN, Gottdiener JS, Scott CG, Enriquez-Sarano M. Burden of valvular heart diseases: a population-based study. Lancet (London, England). 2006;368(9540):1005–1011.
62. Isaacs AJ, Shuhaiber J, Salemi A, Isom OW, Sedrakyan A. National trends in utilization and in-hospital outcomes of mechanical versus bioprosthetic aortic valve replacements. J Thorac Cardiovasc Surg 2015;149(5):1262–1269.e1263.
63. Smith CR, Leon MB, Mack MJ, et al. Transcatheter versus surgical aortic-valve replacement in high-risk patients. N Engl J Med 2011;364(23):2187–2198.
64. Crawford MH, Bernstein SJ, Deedwania PC, et al. ACC/AHA guidelines for ambulatory electrocardiography: executive summary and recommendations. A report of the American College of Cardiology/American Heart Association task force on practice guidelines (committee to revise the guidelines for ambulatory electrocardiography). Circulation 1999;100(8):886–893.
65. DiMarco JP. Implantable cardioverter-defibrillators. N Engl J Med 2003;349(19):1836–1847.
66. Nicod P, Hillis LD, Winniford MD, Firth BG. Importance of the "atrial kick" in determining the effective mitral valve orifice area in mitral stenosis. Am J Cardiol 1986;57(6):403–407.
67. Lev M. Anatomic basis for atrioventricular block. Am J Med 1964;37:742–748.
68. Brignole M, Auricchio A, Baron-Esquivias G, et al. 2013 ESC Guidelines on cardiac pacing and cardiac resynchronization therapy: the Task Force on cardiac pacing and resynchronization therapy of the European Society of Cardiology (ESC). Developed in collaboration with the European Heart Rhythm Association (EHRA). Eur Heart J 2013;34(29):2281–2329.
69. Ritter P, Duray GZ, Steinwender C, et al. Early performance of a miniaturized leadless cardiac pacemaker: the Micra Transcatheter Pacing Study. Eur Heart J 2015;36(37):2510–2519.
70. Kostanjsek N. Use of The International Classification of Functioning, Disability and Health (ICF) as a conceptual framework and common language for disability statistics and health information systems. BMC public health. 2011;11 Suppl 4:S3.
71. Mador MJ, Rodis A, Magalang UJ. Reproducibility of Borg scale measurements of dyspnea during exercise in patients with COPD. Chest 1995;107(6):1590–1597.
72. Ries AL. Minimally clinically important difference for the UCSD Shortness of Breath Questionnaire, Borg Scale, and Visual Analog Scale. Copd 2005;2(1):105–110.
73. Wang CS, FitzGerald JM, Schulzer M, Mak E, Ayas NT. Does this dyspneic patient in the emergency department have congestive heart failure? JAMA 2005;294(15):1944–1956.
74. Eilen SD, Crawford MH, O'Rourke RA. Accuracy of precordial palpation for detecting increased left ventricular volume. Ann Int Med 1983;99(5):628–630.

75. Edmondstone WM. Cardiac chest pain: does body language help the diagnosis? BMJ (Clinical research ed.). 1995;311(7021): 1660–1661.
76. Marcus GM, Vessey J, Jordan MV, et al. Relationship between accurate auscultation of a clinically useful third heart sound and level of experience. Arch Intern Med 2006;166(6):617–622.
77. Drazner MH, Rame JE, Stevenson LW, Dries DL. Prognostic importance of elevated jugular venous pressure and a third heart sound in patients with heart failure. N Engl J Med 2001;345(8):574–581.
78. Cahalin LP, Arena RA. Breathing exercises and inspiratory muscle training in heart failure. Heart failure clinics. 2015;11(1):149–172.
79. ATS statement: guidelines for the six-minute walk test. Am J Resp Crit Care Med 2002;166(1):111–117.
80. Shoemaker MJ, Curtis AB, Vangsnes E, Dickinson MG. Triangulating Clinically Meaningful Change in the Six-minute Walk Test in Individuals with Chronic Heart Failure: A Systematic Review. Cardiopul Phys Ther J 2012;23(3):5–15.
81. Kommuri NV, Johnson ML, Koelling TM. Six-minute walk distance predicts 30-day readmission in hospitalized heart failure patients. Arch Med Res 2010;41(5):363–368.
82. Rikli RE, Jones CJ. Development and validation of criterion-referenced clinically relevant fitness standards for maintaining physical independence in later years. The Gerontologist. 2013;53(2):255–267.
83. Shumway-Cook A, Brauer S, Woollacott M. Predicting the probability for falls in community-dwelling older adults using the Timed Up & Go Test. Phys Ther 2000;80(9):896–903.
84. Berg KO, Wood-Dauphinee SL, Williams JI, Maki B. Measuring balance in the elderly: validation of an instrument. Can J Pub Health 1992;83 Suppl 2:S7–11.
85. Perera S, Mody SH, Woodman RC, Studenski SA. Meaningful change and responsiveness in common physical performance measures in older adults. J Am Geriatr Soc 2006;54(5):743–749.
86. Coster WJ, Haley SM, Jette AM. Measuring patient-reported outcomes after discharge from inpatient rehabilitation settings. J Rehabil Med 2006;38(4):237-242.
87. Jette DU, Stilphen M, Ranganathan VK, Passek SD, Frost FS, Jette AM. Validity of the AM-PAC "6-Clicks" inpatient daily activity and basic mobility short forms. 2014;94(3): 379–391.
88. Rector TS, Cohn JN. Assessment of patient outcome with the Minnesota Living with Heart Failure questionnaire: reliability and validity during a randomized, double-blind, placebo-controlled trial of pimobendan. Pimobendan Multicenter Research Group. Am Heart J 1992;124(4):1017–1025.
89. Rector TS, Tschumperlin LK, Kubo SH, et al. Use of the Living With Heart Failure questionnaire to ascertain patients' perspectives on improvement in quality of life versus risk of drug-induced death. J Card Fail 1995;1(3):201–206.
90. Spertus JA, Winder JA, Dewhurst TA, et al. Development and evaluation of the Seattle Angina Questionnaire: a new functional status measure for coronary artery disease. J Am Coll Cardiol 1995;25(2):333–341.
91. Chan PS, Jones PG, Arnold SA, Spertus JA. Development and validation of a short version of the Seattle angina questionnaire. Circulation 2014;7(5):640–647.
92. Suaya JA, Stason WB, Ades PA, Normand SL, Shepard DS. Cardiac rehabilitation and survival in older coronary patients. J Am Coll Cardiol 2009;54(1):25–33.
93. Hammill BG, Curtis LH, Schulman KA, Whellan DJ. Relationship between cardiac rehabilitation and long-term risks of death and myocardial infarction among elderly Medicare beneficiaries. Circulation 2010;121(1):63–70.
94. Taylor RS, Brown A, Ebrahim S, et al. Exercise-based rehabilitation for patients with coronary heart disease: systematic review and meta-analysis of randomized controlled trials. Am J Med 2004;116(10):682–692.
95. Lawler PR, Filion KB, Eisenberg MJ. Efficacy of exercise-based cardiac rehabilitation post-myocardial infarction: a systematic review and meta-analysis of randomized controlled trials. Am Heart J 2011;162(4):571–584.e572.
96. Anderson L, Oldridge N, Thompson DR, et al. Exercise-based cardiac rehabilitation for coronary heart disease: Cochrane Systematic Review and Meta-Analysis. J Am Coll Cardiol 2016;67(1):1–12.
97. Johnson DA, Sacrinty MT, Gomadam PS, et al. Effect of early enrollment on outcomes in cardiac rehabilitation. J Am Coll Cardiol2014;114(12):1908–1911.
98. Dimsdale JE, Hartley LH, Guiney T, Ruskin JN, Greenblatt D. Postexercise peril. Plasma catecholamines and exercise. JAMA 1984;251(5):630–632.
99. Thompson PD, Buchner D, Pina IL, et al. Exercise and physical activity in the prevention and treatment of atherosclerotic cardiovascular disease: a statement from the Council on Clinical Cardiology (Subcommittee on Exercise, Rehabilitation, and Prevention) and the Council on Nutrition, Physical Activity, and Metabolism (Subcommittee on Physical Activity). Circulation 2003;107(24):3109–3116.
100. Fleg JL, Cooper LS, Borlaug BA, et al. Exercise training as therapy for heart failure: current status and future directions. Circulation 2015;8(1):209–220.
101. Braith RW, Beck DT. Resistance exercise: training adaptations and developing a safe exercise prescription. Heart failure reviews 2008;13(1):69–79.
102. Smart NA, Giallauria F, Dieberg G. Efficacy of inspiratory muscle training in chronic heart failure patients: a systematic review and meta-analysis. Int J Cardiol 2013;167(4): 1502–1507.
103. Lin SJ, McElfresh J, Hall B, Bloom R, Farrell K. Inspiratory muscle training in patients with heart failure: a systematic review. Cardiopul Phys Ther J 2012;23(3):29–36.
104. Rognmo O, Hetland E, Helgerud J, Hoff J, Slordahl SA. High intensity aerobic interval exercise is superior to moderate intensity exercise for increasing aerobic capacity in patients with coronary artery disease. Eur J Cardiovasc Prev Rehabil 2004;11(3):216–222.
105. Wisloff U, Stoylen A, Loennechen JP, et al. Superior cardiovascular effect of aerobic interval training versus moderate continuous training in heart failure patients: a randomized study. Circulation 2007;115(24):3086–3094.
106. Mancini DM, La Manca J, Donchez L, Henson D, Levine S. The sensation of dyspnea during exercise is not determined by the work of breathing in patients with heart failure. J Am Coll Cardiol 1996;28(2):391–395.
107. Davies EJ, Moxham T, Rees K, et al. Exercise based rehabilitation for heart failure. The Cochrane database of systematic reviews 2010(4):CD003331.
108. Belardinelli R, Georgiou D, Cianci G, Purcaro A. 10-year exercise training in chronic heart failure: a randomized controlled trial. J Am Coll Cardiol 2012;60(16):1521–1528.
109. Smart N, Marwick TH. Exercise training for patients with heart failure: a systematic review of factors that improve mortality and morbidity. Am J Med 2004;116(10):693–706.
110. van Tol BA, Huijsmans RJ, Kroon DW, Schothorst M, Kwakkel G. Effects of exercise training on cardiac performance, exercise capacity and quality of life in patients with heart failure: a meta-analysis. Eur J Heart Fail 2006;8(8):841–850.
111. Gielen S, Adams V, Niebauer J, Schuler G, Hambrecht R. Aging and heart failure—similar syndromes of exercise intolerance? Implications for exercise-based interventions. Heart failure monitor 2005;4(4):130–136.
112. Lipkin DP, Jones DA, Round JM, Poole-Wilson PA. Abnormalities of skeletal muscle in patients with chronic heart failure. Int J Cardiol 1988;18(2):187–195.
113. Magnusson G, Gordon A, Kaijser L, et al. High intensity knee extensor training, in patients with chronic heart failure. Major skeletal muscle improvement. Eur Heart J 1996; 17(7):1048–1055.
114. Drexler H, Riede U, Munzel T, Konig H, Funke E, Just H. Alterations of skeletal muscle in chronic heart failure. Circulation 1992;85(5):1751–1759.
115. Gasiorowski A, Dutkiewicz J. Comprehensive rehabilitation in chronic heart failure. *Ann* Agric Environ Med 2013;20(3): 606–612.
116. Piepoli MF, Guazzi M, Boriani G, et al. Exercise intolerance in chronic heart failure: mechanisms and therapies. Part I. European journal of cardiovascular prevention and rehabilitation: official journal of the European Society of Cardiology, Working Groups on Epidemiology & Prevention and Cardiac Rehabilitation and Exercise Physiology 2010;17(6):637–642.

117. Winkelmann ER, Chiappa GR, Lima CO, Viecili PR, Stein R, Ribeiro JP. Addition of inspiratory muscle training to aerobic training improves cardiorespiratory responses to exercise in patients with heart failure and inspiratory muscle weakness. Am Heart J 2009;158(5):768.e761–767.
118. Dall'Ago P, Chiappa GR, Guths H, Stein R, Ribeiro JP. Inspiratory muscle training in patients with heart failure and inspiratory muscle weakness: a randomized trial. J Am Coll Cardiol 2006;47(4):757–763.
119. Padula CA, Yeaw E, Mistry S. A home-based nurse-coached inspiratory muscle training intervention in heart failure. Appl Nurs Res 2009;22(1):18–25.
120. Neto MG, Martinez BP, Conceicao CS, Silva PE, Carvalho VO. Combined Exercise and Inspiratory Muscle Training in Patients With Heart Failure: a systematic review and meta-analysis. 2016;36(6):395–401.
121. Montemezzo D, Fregonezi GA, Pereira DA, Britto RR, Reid WD. Influence of inspiratory muscle weakness on inspiratory muscle training responses in chronic heart failure patients: a systematic review and meta-analysis. Arch Phys Med Rehabil 2014;95(7):1398–1407.
122. Ismail H, McFarlane JR, Dieberg G, Smart NA. Exercise training program characteristics and magnitude of change in functional capacity of heart failure patients. Int J Cardiol 2014;171(1):62–65.
123. Gomes Neto M, Menezes MA, Oliveira Carvalho V. Dance therapy in patients with chronic heart failure: a systematic review and a meta-analysis. Clin Rehabil 2014;28(12): 1172–1179.
124. Sagar VA, Davies EJ, Briscoe S, et al. Exercise-based rehabilitation for heart failure: systematic review and meta-analysis. Open heart 2015;2(1):e000163.

Web-Based Resources for Clinicians, Families, and Patients With Heart Disease

appendix **13.A**

American Heart Association
www.americanheart.org

National Heart, Lung and Blood Institute
www.nhlbi.nih.gov/

Heart Disease
www.nlm.nih.gov/medlineplus/heartdiseases.html

Cardiac Rehabilitation
http://www.nhlbi.nih.gov/health/health-topics/topics/rehab/

American Association of Cardiovascular and Pulmonary Rehabilitation
www.aacvpr.org

World Health Organization
www.who.int/topics/cardiovascular_diseases/

Centers for Disease Control and Prevention
www.cdc.gov/heartdisease/

Clinical Practice Guidelines
www.guideline.gov/content.aspx?id=10856

American Association of Physical Medicine and Rehabilitation
www.aapmr.org

Chapter 14

Vascular, Lymphatic, and Integumentary Disorders

Deborah Graffis Kelly, PT, DPT, MSEd

LEARNING OBJECTIVES

1. Understand basic concepts about the anatomy, physiology, and pathophysiology of the vascular, lymphatic, and integumentary systems.
2. Describe wound physiology as it relates to normal and abnormal wound healing.
3. Recognize the characteristics and risk factors of common disorders of the vascular, lymphatic, and integumentary systems.
4. Identify the components of a comprehensive examination of a patient with a disorder related to the vascular, lymphatic, and/or integumentary systems.
5. Analyze and integrate wound examination data to complete the physical therapy evaluation.
6. Interpret the rationale for skin and wound care treatment with particular attention to moist wound healing, arterial wound hydration, venous wound compression, lymphedema treatment, and foot care for the patient with diabetes.
7. Design an appropriate plan of care for an individual with a vascular, lymphatic, and/or integumentary disorder.
8. Using the case study example, apply clinical decision making skills to design a plan for advanced wound care.

CHAPTER OUTLINE

Patients and clients with disorders of the vascular, lymphatic, and integumentary systems have complex and often interrelated health problems to be understood before healing can occur. In recent years, options for intervention have expanded significantly, providing the physical therapist with challenging and rewarding clinical treatments for clients. This chapter provides foundational material on which to build sound clinical decisions. Though interrelated, the systems discussed have unique characteristics and functions. This chapter facilitates understanding of the separate systems and then illustrates how the systems are intricately and essentially related. The elements of examination and the intervention strategies for all of the disorders are combined to ensure that the overlapping signs, symptoms, impairments, and activity limitations will be addressed and considered in the plan of care (POC). In this text, information about thermal injuries is complementary and supplemental to the information in this chapter (see Chapter 24, Burns).

ANATOMY AND PHYSIOLOGY OF THE VASCULAR, LYMPHATIC, AND INTEGUMENTARY SYSTEMS

In the microscopic world of circulation, blood and lymph vessels permeate most tissues, carrying oxygen and nutrients while removing carbon dioxide and wastes. Not all vessels involved are the "large tubes" so often associated with the circulatory system. Capillaries are woven throughout most of the tissues of the body, around muscle fibers, through connective tissues, and below the basement membrane of the epithelium.[1] Since arteries and veins are too large and too thick to allow diffusion between the bloodstream and surrounding tissues, a delicate network of blood and lymph capillaries controls all chemical and gaseous exchange between blood, interstitial fluid, and lymph.[1] In the normal system, homeostatic mechanisms adjust blood flow across the capillary walls to meet the needs of peripheral tissues. Every year, new information is uncovered that further elucidates the complexities of the circulatory system and how it interacts with the other systems of the body. It is important to have a clear understanding of the delicate vessels that carry blood to the peripheral tissues and the normal processes that occur there to gain insight into the disorders discussed later in the chapter.

Vascular

Arterial

Arteries carry rich, oxygenated blood away from the heart, branching off into sections with smaller diameters called *arterioles,* leading ultimately to capillaries. Arteries have three-layered walls that give them strength and elasticity. The walls of arteries are generally thicker than those of veins because they have to bear strong blood flow pressures generated by the heart. Arteries are strong and durable, able to keep their cylindrical shape when stretched. The movement of blood through arteries is dependent on heart function. Arteries have the ability to change in diameter when the volume of blood passing through them changes. They can also change in diameter when the sympathetic division of the autonomic nervous system is triggered, either contracting (*vasoconstriction*) or relaxing (*vasodilation*). Because they have contractile abilities, arteries do not need valves to effect blood flow. These terms and concepts will be important when the chapter discussion turns to topics such as peripheral vascular disease, capillary blood flow, and wound healing.

Venous

Veins return oxygen-depleted blood from tissues and organs to the heart. At the beginning of the venous system, superficial blood capillaries empty into venules that carry blood toward medium-sized veins (about the size of muscular arteries). Superficial veins run above the fascia of the muscles. Deep veins run below the fascia. Perforating veins run between the superficial and the deep, penetrating the fascia to connect the superficial and deep vessels. Veins also have three-layered walls, but they do not need to be as muscular or elastic as arteries because the blood pressure in veins is lower than in arteries. Venous walls are so thin that they do not hold their shape well under stress, collapsing or tearing when stretched. As blood moves through the outermost regions of the body (the peripheral vascular system) from the arteries to the veins, blood pressures decrease. The blood pressure in the medium-sized veins is so low that it cannot oppose the force of gravity without structural assistance.[1] In the limbs, medium-sized veins contain *valves* that project from the inner walls of the veins, pointing in the direction of blood flow. Under normal conditions, the valves allow blood to flow in one direction, preventing backflow of blood. When the valves are working normally, any movement that compresses or pulls on a vein will help to push blood toward the heart. Skeletal muscle contraction will squeeze venous blood toward the heart. The act of walking helps to empty veins and move blood out of the lower extremities (LEs). When the walls of veins weaken, or are enlarged, the valves cannot function properly and blood pools in the veins. Eventually the veins become distended, leading to varicose veins. If a valve or valves do not close properly, this leads to a condition known as *venous reflux.* These terms and concepts will be important when the chapter discussion leads to topics such as chronic venous disease and LE swelling.

Lymphatic

Although parallel, and working in concert with the venous system, the lymphatic system is separate and unique. Because of its many roles and diffuse locations throughout the body, anatomists place discussion of the lymphatic system with the immune system, the circulatory system, and the integumentary system. The two primary functions of the lymphatic system are to protect the body from infection and disease via the immune response and to facilitate movement of fluid back and forth between the bloodstream and the interstitium, removing excess fluid, blood waste, and protein molecules in the process of fluid exchange. *Lymphatics* are located in all portions of the body except the central nervous system (CNS) and cornea.[2] The lymphatic system includes lymph vessels (superficial, intermediate, and deep; also referred to as *lymphatics*), lymph fluid, and lymph tissues and organs (lymph nodes, tonsils, spleen, thymus, and the thoracic duct).

Lymph fluid, also called *lymph,* is first absorbed at the capillary level, then channeled through small vessels called *precollectors,* and finally picked up by the larger, valved vessels called *collectors.* The collectors have contractile properties, smooth muscle, and valves. Lymphatics are even thinner and more likely to collapse under pressure than veins.[2-4] Lymph moves throughout the body by a number of mechanisms. Superficially, the process of diffusion and filtration moves lymph fluid. Below the dermis, intrinsic contractions within the vessels themselves drive lymph propulsion in the deeper collectors. Drainage depends on contraction of the valved lymph vessels that create a pumping force. Classic literature reports information about lymph flow but new knowledge about the lymphatic system is continually expanding.[4-10] The human body is wonderfully equipped to provide a variety of stimuli that have an impact on lymphangion contraction:

- Parasympathetic, sympathetic, and sensory *nerve stimulation.*
- *Contraction of muscles* adjacent to a vessel.
- *Pulsation of arteries* adjacent to a lymph vessel (even pre-capillary arterioles have pulsation).
- Abdominal and thoracic cavity pressure changes that occur during *breathing.*
- *Volume changes* within each lymphangion (internal receptors respond to tension and trigger a contraction).
- *Mild mechanical stimulation* of dermal tissue such as *manual lymphatic drainage* (MLD) techniques will increase the frequency of lymphangion contractions.

Excess lymph fluid is transported through the thoracic duct and emptied into the venous angles at the left and right jugular vein trunks. Under normal conditions, lymph flow is not adversely affected by gravity. Under abnormal conditions such as morbid obesity or *chronic venous insufficiency* (CVI), the lymphatic system may exhibit excess lymph pooling related to gravity, especially in the LEs.

Integumentary

Also referred to as an *organ,* the integumentary system is the most often seen and touched by a physical therapist of all the body systems. The integumentary system has a functional relationship to many other body systems. The health of this system is dependent on the normal functions of the arterial, venous, and lymphatic capillaries (dermal circulation). A thorough review of the functions of the skin illustrates the importance of even a small area of damage to this organ. The discussion on skin anatomy, with diagrams, in this textbook will supplement the overview here (see Chapter 24, Burns). The *epidermis,* the outermost layer of skin, is avascular and water-resistant. It provides protection from infection, abrasion, and chemicals and assists with heat regulation, retention, and dissipation. Melanocytes, which are present in this layer, determine skin color and provide protection from ultraviolet radiation. The epidermis regenerates rapidly, allowing individuals to heal quickly when conditions are normal. The *dermis,* or next layer of skin, is 20 to 30 times thicker than epidermis. It contains blood vessels and lymphatics, nerves and nerve endings, and sensory neurons that all supply the epidermis. The dermis also contains hair follicles, sweat glands, sebaceous glands, and nails. All of these project through the epidermis to the surface of the skin. These appendages are a deep source of epithelial cells, needed to resurface a wound during healing. The contents of the dermis are surrounded and supported by collagen, elastin, and ground substance that provide structure, strength, flexibility, and elasticity. The *hypodermis* (also referred to as the *subcutaneous layer*) is not part of the integument but is important in stabilizing skin over skeletal muscles and organs. It consists of loose connective tissue and fat cells and provides insulation and protection to underlying structures. The hypodermis plays an important role in the prevention of *pressure injuries,* especially over the ischial tuberosities and greater trochanters.

When there is an injury to the integument, some or all of the components of the integument are impaired, resulting in many possible sequelae such as decreased lubrication, loss of elasticity, increased scar formation, loss of tensile strength, decreased ability to resist infection, and an increase or decrease in sensitivity.

■ WOUND PHYSIOLOGY

Normal Wound Healing

In the human body, an elegant sequence of events takes place to ensure that when injury occurs, wounds will heal. Within the endogenous fluids of the body, every cell and chemical mediator is programmed and ready to act when needed. When conditions are normal, the body is equipped to heal itself.

Phases of Healing

The classic model of overlapping phases of wound healing describes a process that is continuous, its phases not entirely distinct. The model is used in this chapter to draw attention to the normal process and to provide guidelines for what can be expected in normal healing. The number of days to complete each phase will vary based on factors such as age, size of wound, comorbidities, continued trauma, nutrition, blood flow, medications, stress, and infection. The process of repair is the same for all wounds but the sequence will be much quicker in more shallow wounds with less tissue loss. In all stages of healing, wounded tissues are striving to achieve homeostasis. Italicized words below stress important concepts during each phase.

Inflammation (Phase I)

- The *normal* immune system reaction to injury.
- The *central activity* in wound healing.
- Temporary repair initiated by coagulation (clotting factors, platelets) and *short-term decreased* blood flow.
- *Necrosis* occurs after cells have been injured or destroyed.
- The spread of pathogens is slowed: debris and bacteria are attacked by a host of cells. If the wound is

acute, some periwound edema, erythema, and drainage can be expected. If fluid accumulates at the injury site, it is called *pus.*
- Oxygen is delivered via *increased* blood flow to keep the phagocytic cells alive and functioning.
- Permanent repair is facilitated by creating a clean wound, *setting the stage* for the next phase of healing; signals are generated that re-epithelialization can begin.
- Time frame: day of injury to approximately day 10.
- *Rate* of inflammatory process is affected by the size of the wound, blood supply, available nutrients, and the extrinsic environment.
- If this phase is interrupted or delayed, *chronic inflammation can result,* lasting from months to years (see the "Abnormal Wound Healing and the Chronic Wound" section).

Proliferation (Phase II)

- *New tissue* fills in the wound as fibroblasts secrete collagen.
- Skin integrity is restored by re-epithelialization and/or contraction (see discussion below).
- Angiogenesis occurs: new blood vessel growth from endothelial cells and fragile capillary buds grow into the wound bed; new reddish, slightly bumpy tissue is called *granulation tissue.*
- Epithelial cells differentiate into type I collagen. *Collagen synthesis* occurs but the resulting new scar tissue is fragile and must be protected; trauma during this phase may return the wound to the inflammatory process.
- Time frame: day 3 of injury to approximately day 20.
- *Rate* of proliferation is affected by the size of the wound, blood supply, available nutrients, and the extrinsic environment.
- If this phase is interrupted or delayed, the result may be a chronic wound.

Maturation/Remodeling (Phase III)

- Maturation or remodeling of new tissue begins while granulation tissue is forming during the prior (proliferative) phase.
- Epithelial cells continue to differentiate into type I collagen.
- New skin has *tensile strength* that is 15% of normal. Scar tissue is rebuilding but at best reaches 80% of original tensile strength.
- Underlying granulation tissue is replaced by *less vascular* tissue.
- In deep wounds, dermal appendages are rarely repaired (hair follicles, sebaceous and sweat glands, nerves) but instead are replaced by *fibrous tissue.*
- Over time the scar tissue matures, changing from red to pink to white and from raised and rigid to flat and flexible.
- Time frame: approximately day 9 of injury up to 2 years.
- *Rate of maturation/remodeling* is affected by the size of the wound, blood supply, available nutrients, and the extrinsic environment.

The Role of Oxygen in Wound Healing

The need for oxygen to sustain life is apparent, not only at the systemic level, but also at the cellular level of human physiology. Oxygen reaches the wound bed through blood flow to the area. When oxygenated blood flows to the tissues of the body, it is called *perfusion.* Wound contraction, collagen deposition, angiogenesis, and granulation are examples of wound healing steps supported by oxygen perfusion. As a safeguard, most cells in the wound environment have an enzyme that converts oxygen to a form that allows the cell to support wound healing.[11] Wound tissue oxygenation or perfusion is so important that it is a sensitive indicator for the risk of post-operative infection.[12] A decrease in oxygen availability in any type of wound results in increased likelihood of infection. Wound perfusion may be limited for a variety of reasons but the two most common problems are edema and necrosis. The presence of edema and/or necrotic tissue can make it more difficult for oxygen to reach the wound. Since compression can reduce edema and débridement can reduce the presence of necrotic tissue, these procedural interventions are important components of most wound care. Unless contraindicated owing to arterial disease, compression and débridement will assist wound oxygenation. Peripheral vasoconstriction can also limit wound perfusion. Problems with vasoconstriction cannot always be improved readily. Interventions that will increase wound perfusion and are appropriate for all individuals include keeping the wound area warm, avoiding smoking, hydrating the individual, and controlling pain and anxiety. Improvement of oxygen levels in wound tissue alone may trigger wound healing. Adequate oxygen levels will also enhance the effectiveness of growth factors and a host of other cells that require oxygenation to maintain their function. The delivery of exogenous oxygen will be discussed later in the chapter in the "Hyperbaric Oxygen Therapy" section. The nutritional status of the individual, as discussed below, will also have an impact on oxygenation since hemoglobin, iron, vitamin B_{12}, and folic acid are needed to enable red blood cells to carry oxygen to healing tissues.

The Role of Moisture in Wound Healing

In the past, the goal of wound care was to create and maintain a dry wound, packed with dry dressings, dried by heat lamps, and exposed to the air. Modern wound management is based on the concept of creating and maintaining a *moist wound environment* to facilitate wound healing. More than 50 years ago, research confirmed that a dry wound creates an environment that is hostile to wound healing. A dry wound allows the formation of wound scab and *eschar,* which inhibit migration of epithelial cells, provide food for pathogens, and affect blood flow to the wound bed. A dry wound also allows cooling of the wound surface; without a protective barrier, the surface temperature of the wound is decreased and healing is slowed. Adhesion of gauze or other dry dressings to the wound bed causes trauma to the wound bed and pain to the individual upon removal. As the wound dries through evaporation or by the removal of dry dressings, the rich endogenous fluids that contain the elements necessary for wound healing are significantly decreased or lost.

Wound management experts agree that adequate wound hydration is the most important external factor responsible for optimal wound healing.[13-15] Wounds are typically covered with an occlusive or semi-occlusive dressing. This type of dressing is also called a *moisture-retentive dressing* because it retains fluids on the wound bed. There are many types and styles of dressings that will facilitate a moist environment (see the "Dressings" section for further discussion). Maintaining a moist wound with an occlusive dressing should hold an appropriate amount of endogenous fluids on the wound, preserving the cells needed for healing and keeping them in contact with the wound bed. Some chronic wound fluid may contain substances that can delay healing so a balance must be maintained between moisture and exudate removal.[16] Moisture softens wound scab and eschar; under the right conditions, the body's own enzymes will dissolve the eschar in a process called *autolytic débridement.* Occlusive dressings help to maintain the appropriate wound surface temperature to prevent delays in healing and to protect the wound surface from trauma and from bacteria and other contaminants.

Basic principles of moist wound healing include covering the wound with a barrier (occlusive dressing) that preserves adequate wound hydration; limiting fluid loss from the wound surface while the dressing is in place; allowing gaseous exchange; maintaining periwound integrity; controlling heavy *exudate;* and removing the dressing when exudate begins to leak out from edges of dressing.

It has long been believed that occlusive dressings should not be applied over infected wounds because trapped bacteria could fulminate. Studies have produced evidence that the opposite may be true in many cases.[17-19] Because in acute wounds, and some chronic wounds, endogenous fluids have bacteria-fighting chemical elements, evidence of colonized bacteria in the wound does not automatically preclude the use of occlusive dressings. Specially selected dressings such as hydrocolloids are a good choice in this situation.

With the use of a systemic antibiotic and a close watch for signs of change in the patient's symptoms, clinicians may be able to utilize occlusive or moisture-retentive dressings over some types of wounds that are infected. The use of this dressing technique may broaden if the evidence continues to build in strength. Meanwhile, there is ongoing investigation into the contents of chronic wound exudate and its power to break down growth factors and prolong the inflammatory phase of wound healing. Information on this level should guide the use of occlusive dressings in the chronic wound healing environment.[20]

Despite half a century of research to support the concepts of moist wound healing, there are still practitioners who ignore the evidence and utilize outdated methods of wound management. Clinicians must strive to educate patients, families, and all members of the wound care team about appropriate wound care concepts.

The Role of Nutrition in Wound Healing

It is well established that nutritional status can have a significant impact on wound healing. Adequate protein intake is required for collagen synthesis, as well as the formation of new blood vessels and muscle tissue.[21] Literature abounds with information about important nutritional issues such as the role of specific nutrients in wound healing, how poor nutritional status can delay wound healing, the use of special pharmacological interventions, and appropriate routes for nutritional support (enteral versus parenteral). Newer literature supports the classic understanding that the function of nutrients is crucial to wound healing.[22-30]

Issues related to wound healing and nutrition are important across the life span. Pediatric patients in long-term care, recovering from surgery, or with wounds, burns, or trauma are at risk for pressure injuries.[31] As with adults, adequate protein intake is essential for healing to occur on time. Another patient population of concern is the elderly, whose tissues are fragile and whose immune systems are easily compromised. Nutrition plays a role in the prevention and management of pressure injuries in this population as well.[32]

Nutrients that must be present for a wound to close and heal on time include iron, vitamin B_{12} and folic acid (essential so that red blood cells can deliver oxygen to tissues), vitamin C and zinc (essential for tissue repair), vitamin A (essential to stimulate collagen cross-linking), and arginine (enhances healing and immune function).[33,34] High protein intake provides the amino acids required to build new tissue. Protein and calorie needs will vary depending on the size of the wound and the medical condition of the patient. In response to the available information and the need for more research, nutrition and metabolic support of acutely and chronically ill patients is emerging as an important branch of medicine.

As a part of the wound care team, a physical therapist will make contributions to the plans for nutritional support of the patient. Clinicians will collect data through medical record review, observation, history taking, and the use of dietary examination methods. Because exercise, hydration, and improved appetite often are interrelated, a physical therapist should pay close attention to a patient's activity level, strength, conditioning, and mobility issues while encouraging fluid and nutrient intake.

Wound Characteristics

Wound characteristics describe the physical appearance of the wound but may also provide the clues to the cause of the wound, the phase of healing, and likelihood of closure. The characteristics of wounds may be defined as dry, wet, or granulating. Wounds can also be defined by their etiology, such as diabetic, vascular, or traumatic. Wound characteristics can provide valuable information needed to make sound clinical judgments about treatment. For example, the location of the wound may prompt the clinician to select a particular dressing, change patient positioning, or prescribe orthotic footwear. When wound characteristics are described in documentation, they can indicate progress (or failure to progress) toward closure and healing. Wound characteristics should be identified during the initial examination and then monitored at least weekly during the wound healing phase. Depending on the etiology and chronicity of the wound, some characteristics may not be evident on initial examination but could appear at a later date as complications of the wound healing process. The following are characteristics that should be tracked and documented throughout the phases of wound healing:

- *Location*: where on the body.
- *Size*: depth, width, and length.
- *Shape*: irregular versus distinct.
- *Edges*: condition and shape of wound edges, evidence of premature healing.
- *Tunneling, undermining, sinus tracts*: presence and depth.
- *Base*: characteristics of the wound base compared to sides and edges.
    - Necrosis, eschar, slough: amount, color, texture, adherence to wound bed
    - Exudate: amount, color, odor
    - Granulation tissue: presence or absence, amount, location
    - Epithelialization: presence or absence, premature or on schedule
    - Exposed structures: color and condition of bone, tendon, ligament
- *Periwound area*: edema, induration, maceration.
- *Pain*: although not a visible characteristic, it is measurable and significant to the intervention.
- *Quantity of bacteria*: amount present in a wound. This is referred to as the *bio-burden.*

The quantitative biopsy is the gold standard for obtaining a wound culture, but it is not used universally owing to cost, lack of laboratory facilities, and potential pain for the patient.[11] A swab culture is often used as an alternative, but it is limited to detecting surface contamination, not tissue infection. Clinical intuition is also important in determining if infection is probable.

The examination will include data about the characteristics that have been gathered using methods such as observation, palpation, measurement, photography, and tracing. A clinician who is new to the wound care team should remember that these are skills that take practice to master.

Wound Closure

Primary Intention

Healing by primary intention occurs when a health care provider closes a wound by bringing the edges together. Approximating the edges can occur through the use of sutures, staples, glue, skin grafts, or skin flaps. (For more information on skin grafting, see Chapter 24, Burns.) Wounds closed by primary intention still pass through the phases of wound healing but usually in a shorter time span. A wound closed by primary intention that later opens up again owing to maceration or infection has opened by the process of *dehiscence* (Fig. 14.1). Following dehiscence, a wound is almost always allowed to close by secondary intention.

Secondary Intention

Closure and subsequent healing by secondary intention occurs when a wound is left open to heal on its own. The mechanisms of healing by secondary intention are contraction, re-epithelialization, or a combination of both. Deeper wounds heal by replacing injured tissue with scar tissue as collagen fills the wound bed.

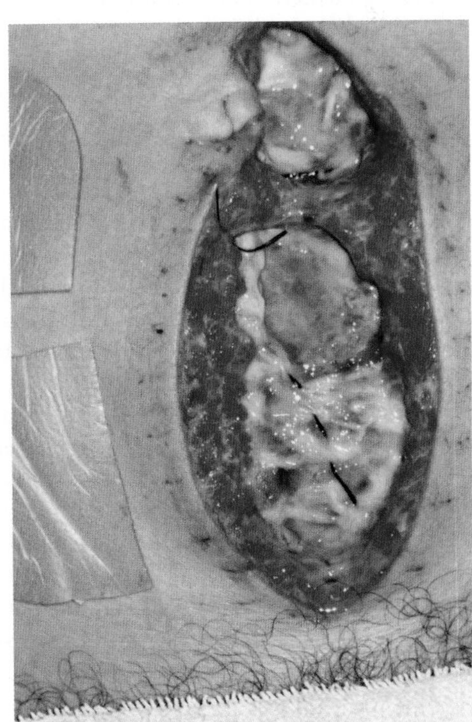

Figure 14.1 Wound dehiscence following appendectomy.

Contraction occurs when growth factors trigger myofibroblasts to pull the wound edges inward. During the process of contraction, existing tissue migrates, pulling the wound edges toward the center of the wound. This process forms no new tissue. New tissue may be forming in the wound simultaneously but not via contraction. Growth factors and myofibroblasts can be influenced positively or negatively by physiological factors such as the amount of oxygen and nutrients available, and by mechanical factors such as external compression and the shape of the wound. Even though contraction is a normal occurrence in certain types of wound healing, if it is too rapid, it can cause disfiguring scars and impaired tissue function. Since there is centripetal movement of the entire thickness of the surrounding skin, tissue elongation may not keep up with the pace of contraction, causing significant functional and cosmetic deformity. Clinicians should intervene by applying special types of pressure to the tissues to slow the deforming forces of contraction (scar management is discussed later in the chapter).

Epithelialization is another response used by the body to close a wound. As noted in the phases of normal wound healing, chemical mediators send signals for re-epithelialization to begin in phase I (the inflammatory phase). Actual repair begins in phase II when new tissue is formed to cover the wound. Growth factors stimulate specialized epithelial cells, called *keratinocytes,* to begin to migrate from the edges of the wound toward the center. In partial-thickness wounds in which the dermal appendages have not been destroyed, the cells will also migrate from the hair follicles, sebaceous glands, and sweat glands. In smaller, shallower wounds, this process may be triggered to begin as early as 12 hours after wounding. In larger wounds, it may be 10 days or longer before the cells begin to migrate. In a chronic wound, there are many reasons why this process is not triggered or is interrupted. (See discussion under "Abnormal Wound Healing and the Chronic Wound.")

When epithelial cells meet at the center of the wound, the wound is covered with new skin, migration ends, and cells will stop dividing. This is referred to as *contact inhibition.* At the time of contact inhibition or full re-epithelialization, wound *closure* has occurred. Wound *healing,* however, may continue for several years. A significant amount of intervention is still required to support the wound successfully from "closed" to "healed" status. A physical therapist will provide routine surveillance as well as specific intervention for the many possible sequelae of a wound. When a wound is closing and healing by secondary intention, the rate of closure and the physiology of closure are impacted by a number of factors that a clinician will monitor and document:

- *Wound shape*: linear wounds (surgical) contract most rapidly; circular wounds (pressure injuries) contract most slowly.
- *Wound depth*: all things equal, the shallower the wound, the quicker the closure.[35-38]
  - *Superficial* (loss of the epidermis): closes by re-epithelialization.
  - *Partial-thickness* (loss of the epidermis and dermis): closes primarily by re-epithelialization with minimal contraction.
  - *Full-thickness* (loss of all layers of the epidermis, dermis, and deeper structures): closes by contraction and scar formation; however, epithelial cells will migrate from the wound edges to assist in wound closure if the environment is homeostatic.
- *Wound location*: areas with least pressure, most perfusion (face) will close more rapidly than areas with most pressure, least perfusion (sacrum, heel).
- *Wound etiology*: least traumatic (surgery) will close more rapidly than most traumatic (pressure injury, burn).

As deeper wounds heal, the wound is filled with tissue but the repair process does not replace lost muscle, fat, or dermis with those same types of tissue. The wound is filled with scar tissue made up primarily of collagen. Because the original tissue is not replaced with more of the same, a wound that is closed, and finally healed, does not return to its prewounded state. This concept is particularly important to understanding the position on reverse staging of pressure injuries as described in the "Tests and Measurements" section. It is also important to understand this concept when planning protection, positioning, patient education, footwear, and exercise programs for individuals with all types of wounds whether they are acute, closed, healed, or chronic wounds.

Tertiary Intention

Also called *delayed primary,* this type of closure occurs when a wound is allowed to heal by secondary intention and then is closed by primary intention as the final treatment. The delay in primary closure is usually owing to the presence of infection.

Abnormal Wound Healing and the Chronic Wound

When the sequence of events that leads to normal wound closure and healing does not occur, a chronic wound results. The characteristics and causes of chronic wounds vary owing to the diverse nature of individuals with wounds, their medical histories, and the etiologies of the wounds. Even if the chronic wound moves through the classic phases of wound healing, it does so in an abnormal manner. Vital actions and reactions necessary for wound healing are interrupted, stunted, or absent in the chronic wound.

Although the characteristics of abnormal wound closure and healing may be varied, concepts can be used to illustrate the failure of a wound to pass through phases of wound healing in a timely manner. The following discussion highlights what may happen if there is an interruption to any of the classic phases of wound healing:

- Inflammation (Phase I): If there is inadequate blood flow and oxygen supply to support cellular life and activity, cells may not initiate the repair sequence. Debris and bacteria may build up, and pathogens spread more rapidly. Bio-burden, if measured, is greater than 10^5 organisms/g of tissue, the classic definition of infection.
  - Clinical signs: increase in amount of drainage, change in color or odor, lingering swelling, eschar/necrosis from ischemic conditions, periwound maceration, chronic inflammation, *tunneling, undermining,* and infection may develop if the host's immune system is unable to resist the impact of the bacterial load.
- Proliferation (Phase II): If collagen synthesis is delayed in this phase, skin integrity will be poor. If angiogenesis is delayed, there will not be enough myofibroblasts to initiate wound contraction. The need for oxygen and nutrients will be very high and without them, available cells will be unable to reproduce rapidly, resulting in delayed epithelialization.
  - Clinical signs: Keratinocytes do not migrate because the wound bed is not moist, healthy, clean, and granulating. Epithelial cells may attempt to migrate from the wound edges but without a wound bed that is ready, they will build up at the wound edge and may migrate over the edge, forming a lip that curls under. Granulation tissue is either absent, pale, or delayed; new tissue is weak and breaks down or bleeds easily; tunneling, eschar, and periwound maceration may be evident. Necrosis, if it has not been removed, will delay angiogenesis. Changes in drainage color, amount, odor, or lingering swelling may signal a return to the inflammation stage.
- Maturation/Remodeling (Phase III): If the synthesis and lysis of collagen is out of balance, weakened tissue will break down too easily or hypertrophic scarring will build up too rapidly.
  - Clinical signs: newly formed skin breaks down with little provocation, or scar tissue may build up within the outline of the original wound (hypertrophic) or beyond the margins of the original wound (keloid).

Infection in Wound Healing

Wound infection is a significant problem for any individual. Infection may turn life-threatening if the patient is elderly or critically ill. Regardless of the condition of the individual, wound infection is detrimental to wound closure and healing time. Bio-burden has a greater impact on wound healing than most underlying medical conditions.[39] True infection is identified if the presence of bacteria or microorganisms is greater than 10^5 per gram of tissue determined by a quantitative culture. This determination can only be made with a biopsy. Surface swabs that are cultured may or may not be conclusive for actual infection since there are many types of bacteria that exist on the skin all the time.

- Effects of infection
  - Inefficient cellular activity, decreased collagen metabolism, chemical mediators absent or dilute, cells absent or confused by lack of instructions from chemical mediators and presence of other cells; when the bio-burden is greater than 10^5 organisms/g of tissue, epithelialization may not occur.
  - Decreased oxygen in the wound bed; insufficient oxygen to support the regeneration of tissue and to assist in the prevention of infection
  - Increased rate of cell necrosis
  - Overall decline of body systems contributes to strain on the specialized cells
  - Risk of wound sepsis, osteomyelitis, gangrene
- Signs of potential infection
  - Change in wound drainage (amount, color, odor)
  - Swelling
  - Periwound redness or warmth (less obvious with darker skin)
  - Increase in pain or tenderness
  - Change in the quality of granulation tissue or failure to produce good quality tissue (may be pale, soft, easily broken down)
  - No measurable wound contraction within 2 to 4 weeks
  - Tissue culture/punch biopsy results of greater than 10^5 organisms/g of tissue
  - Fever, nausea, fatigue, loss of appetite

Clinicians should use a structured approach to identify clinical infection. Careful identification of infection may help to avoid the risk of overuse of antibiotics.[40] The punch biopsy is the gold standard for confirming infection, but a physical therapist should watch for the early signs of infection: *warmth, redness, swelling, fever, malaise,* and *loss of appetite.*

Factors Contributing to Abnormal Wound Healing

The factors or triggers that may contribute to abnormal wound healing are varied but can be placed into broad categories for better understanding. Most abnormal wound healing will be influenced by factors from all the categories. Treatment intervention that addresses factors from one category and not the others will be incomplete.

Intrinsic Factors

Intrinsic or internal factors are conditions within the body that may contribute to abnormal healing. These factors relate primarily to the wound and periwound areas, and include aging skin and inadequate blood flow or decreased oxygen supply from an underlying disease. As the integument ages, there is a decrease in moisture content leading to an increase in brittle quality and a delay in the renewal time affecting the stratum corneum. *Rete pegs,* undulations between contact layers of the epidermis and dermis, become less functional with increased risk of shearing.

Changes in the dermis include a decrease in elasticity, collagen, and mast cell production, along with a decrease in the vascularity and number of pain receptors. Available fat in the subcutaneous layer begins to resorb during aging, leading to a decrease in protection against pressure and shearing. Finally, underlying disease is an intrinsic factor that may affect acute and chronic wound healing. The more common conditions known to affect healing are diabetes, cancer, circulatory insufficiencies, HIV infection, and connective tissue diseases.

Extrinsic Factors

Extrinsic or environmental factors are those influences that come from outside the body. The medical professionals caring for a person with a wound may be able to moderate the impact of extrinsic factors on the wound environment. Examples of extrinsic factors include the effects of radiation therapy or chemotherapy; incontinence; medication, smoking, recreational drugs, and alcohol (all slow or eliminate cellular reactions needed for healing); dehydration and malnutrition (both slow the delivery of oxygen to wound tissues); bio-burden/infection (healing is slowed by pathogens, necrotic tissue, granulomas); and stress (negative effects of stress can lead to impaired healing).[37,41-46]

Iatrogenic Factors

Iatrogenic refers to any injury or illness that occurs as the result of medical care. Theoretically, these factors are under the control of the medical professionals who care for the patient and are therefore preventable. Factors include, but are not limited to, poor wound management, frequent disruption of the wound through inappropriate cleansing, use of inappropriate dressings and dressing techniques, use of cytotoxic topical agents that lead to inefficient cellular activity, and lack of moisture resulting in delayed or absent migration of keratinocytes. Frequent dressing changes not only disturb the fragile surface of the wound but will also slow wound healing by reducing wound temperature. It can take more than 30 minutes for a wound to return to normal temperature after a dressing change. Infection can be an iatrogenic factor when caused by cross-contamination, improper use of gloves and other protective devices, inadequate use of sterile and clean technique, lack of proper hand washing, and lack of adherence to standard precautions. Other iatrogenic factors that contribute to abnormal wound healing include shear injuries (skin tears) that occur during transfers and repositioning and ischemia from unrelieved pressure owing to inadequate turning schedules or absent or inadequate *pressure-redistributing devices* (PRDs).

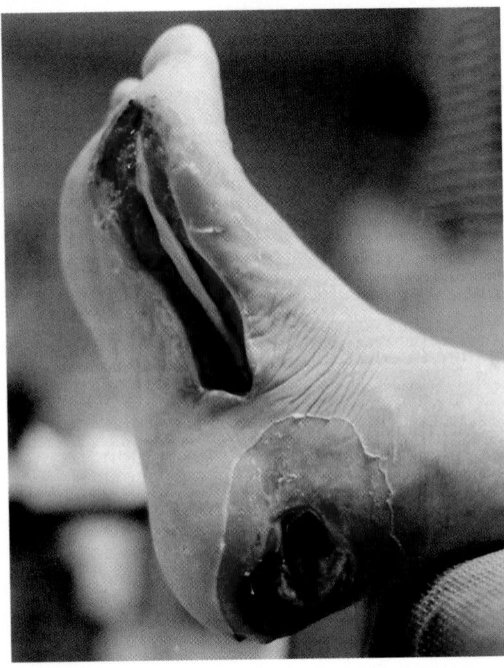

Figure 14.2 Chronic wound as a result of diabetic neuropathy.

Complications of Chronicity

A chronic wound creates a complex and serious health problem for an individual (Fig. 14.2). Chronic wounds may lead to complications, including any or all of the following: impairments of body function and structures, restrictions in activities and participation, need for assisted living or home care, decreased quality-of-life perceptions, depression, infection, malnutrition and weight loss, protein depletion, tissue fibrosis, loss of limb, and death. Every year millions of Americans are treated for chronic wounds at a cost of billions of dollars, making this type of wound one of the most costly challenges in health care. A chronic wound fails to close and heal because of an underlying pathology and will not progress readily until the cause is corrected or improved. The clinician must determine the factors contributing to abnormal wound healing and then develop an appropriate POC to overcome or address the obstacles.

■ VASCULAR, LYMPHATIC, AND INTEGUMENTARY DISORDERS

Arterial Insufficiency and Ulceration

Arterial insufficiency refers to a lack of adequate blood flow to a region or regions of the body. Many different disorders may arise from arterial insufficiency and can be classified by a variety of descriptors. For the purposes of this chapter, references will be to arterial insufficiency owing to organic disruption of blood flow to the extremities or to *peripheral vascular disease* (PVD). PVD is a general term used to describe any disorder that interferes with arterial or venous blood flow of the extremities. PVD caused by arterial insufficiency may be related to smoking, cardiac disease, diabetes, hypertension, renal disease, and/or elevated cholesterol and triglycerides. Obesity and a sedentary lifestyle are related contributors in the cycle of disease and vessel obstruction. When several of these factors are combined, as they often can be, the possibility for health problems is almost 100%. The damage caused by these factors is reflected in structural changes in the walls of the arteries, causing abnormal blood flow. The following is a brief overview of disorders that occur with abnormal arterial blood flow:

- *Arteriosclerosis*: thickening, hardening, and loss of elasticity of arterial walls.
- *Atherosclerosis*: the most common form of arteriosclerosis, associated with damage to the endothelial lining of the vessels and the formation of lipid deposits, eventually leading to plaque formation.
- *Arteriosclerosis obliterans*: a peripheral manifestation of atherosclerosis characterized by *intermittent claudication,* rest pain, and trophic changes. This is the arterial disease most likely to lead to ulceration. Known risk factors for development of the disease are smoking, diabetes mellitus, hypertension, hyperlipidemia, and hyperhomocysteinemia.
- *Thromboangiitis obliterans* (Buerger's disease): inflammation leads to arterial occlusion and tissue ischemia, especially in young men who smoke.
- *Raynaud's disease:* a vasomotor disease of small arteries and arterioles that is most often characterized by pallor and cyanosis of the fingers. In some cases, both the hands and feet may be affected. The cause of Raynaud's is unknown but attacks are usually triggered by cold or emotional upset.
- *Ulceration*: a peripheral sign of a long-standing disease process; by definition, arterial ulcers are associated with arterial insufficiency.

Between 10% and 25% of LE ulcers are caused by arterial disease.[47] The incidence of arterial disease and LE ulceration is significantly lower than that for venous disease and ulceration; however, arterial wounds more frequently lead to loss of limb and death. These important facts signal the significance of taking a thorough history, performing a systems review, and adequate skin inspection during the initial visit with any individual who might have arterial disease.

Clinical Presentation

- Wounds will most frequently be located on the LEs: lateral malleoli, dorsum of feet, toes.
- When wounds are present on an ischemic limb, atherosclerotic occlusion of the peripheral vasculature is almost always present.
- The majority of patients with arterial insufficiency also have diabetes.
- Trophic changes are present and include abnormal nail growth, decreased leg and foot hair, and dry skin.
- Skin is cool on palpation.
- Wounds are painful and patient may also describe pain in the legs and/or feet (see discussion below about intermittent claudication).
- Wound base is usually necrotic and pale, lacking granulation tissue.
- Skin around the wound may be black, mummified (dry gangrene).
- Other signs of arterial insufficiency will be evident: decreased pulses, *pallor* on leg elevation, and *rubor* when dependent.

History

Painful cramping or aching of the LEs during walking is the most common complaint of patients with chronic arterial occlusion of the LEs. The pain is caused by intermittent claudication that occurs when exercising muscles are not receiving the blood perfusion needed for normal function. Patients should be examined for other signs of arterial insufficiency if intermittent claudication is occurring. Rest pain that develops at night, awakens the patient, or requires analgesics for relief is considered more severe than claudication. The individual with vascular dysfunction may also be diabetic. Diabetes will contribute to slower healing times and difficulty fighting infection. A wound in a distal, ischemic area is not likely to close or heal on time unless the vascular supply is enhanced or restored. Individuals with arterial disease and diabetes are more likely to have hypertension and may have previous bypass grafts or amputations of the toes, pain on ambulation or rest, pain with elevation, cold hands and feet, and color changes of fingers and toes. Owing to the long latency period between injury to the arterial circulation and clinical appearance of disorders, health care providers, families, caregivers, and patients must join forces with education, prevention, and vigilance.

Tests and Measurements

One of the most important screening tests for individuals with arterial disease is performed using a handheld Doppler ultrasound unit to measure blood flow to the LEs. The readings are calculated and the end result is called the *Ankle-Brachial Index* (ABI). Results provide useful information about the potential loss of perfusion in the LEs. Refer to "Arterial Perfusion" in the "Tests and Measurements" section under "Examination and Evaluation."

Intervention

If ulceration is present, intervention should enhance chemical and gaseous homeostasis in the wound bed, facilitate superficial blood flow to target tissues, and educate patients about the importance of facilitating blood flow to the extremities. Treatment will include appropriate wound care as well as important adjuncts to wound care. Results of the ABI will guide the therapist and referring practitioner in the appropriate use of compression. In a diagnosis of mixed arterial and venous disease, the condition that is more severe should be treated first. If the arterial condition is worse, compression may be inappropriate even when edema is present. A nonhealing wound on an ischemic limb can lead to gangrene, amputation, further amputation, and/or loss of life (Fig. 14.3). In the most severe cases, conditions are inhospitable to wound closure. Conditions for closing and healing the wound are poor. In this case, necrotic tissue should not be débrided, since the dead tissue will not be replaced with new tissue. Skin grafts may not adhere to the virtually lifeless wound bed. Antibiotics cannot reach the wound systemically and topical agents are too superficial to stop infection. At this point, vascular surgery may be an option for some individuals. A bypass graft may be used to restore arterial circulation to the ischemic tissue. For others, living with a chronic nonhealing wound or coming to terms with amputation are the only options. Most experts agree that the single most important intervention in PVD is prevention of smoking. The second most important intervention is exercise for weight control. Exercise will also improve collateral circulation, lipid profiles, and management of hypertension. A physical therapist plays a crucial role in wound care for arterial wounds and should address patient education and exercise in the intervention plan.

Venous Insufficiency and Ulceration

Venous insufficiency refers to inadequate drainage of venous blood from a body part, usually resulting in edema and/or skin abnormalities and ulcerations. Chronic venous insufficiency (CVI) refers to venous insufficiency that persists over a long period of time. The majority of individuals with PVD are diagnosed with CVI. CVI is the most common cause of leg ulcers.[48] In current literature, venous insufficiency is synonymous with venous hypertension, defining the beginning of a chain of pathophysiological events that often end in ulceration. Some authors still use the term *venous stasis ulcer,* but it has been shown that blood stasis (blood pooling) is not the cause of these wounds.[49] Although it is clear that ulcerations are the result of inadequate venous circulation, the mechanism by which this happens is not well understood. Research has focused on how skin breakdown is affected by dysfunction of circulating white blood cells (WBCs), endothelial cell dysfunction, fibrin deposition, edema, and lymphatic congestion.[50,51]

The incidence of venous ulceration is much higher than that of arterial ulceration (Fig. 14.4). In fact, 80% of all leg ulcers are caused by venous disease.[47] The higher incidence is not clearly understood even though years of clinical and laboratory research have been devoted to understanding venous disease. The path from CVI to ulceration can take many turns. Aging, lack of exercise, obesity, pregnancy, long hours of standing or sitting, heredity, and history of deep vein thrombosis (DVT) will predispose an individual to venous hypertension and subsequent CVI.[52]

Clinical Presentation

- Swelling of unilateral or bilateral LEs relieved in the early stages by elevation
- Complaints of itching, fatigue, aching, heaviness in involved limb(s)
- Skin changes including *hemosiderin staining* and *lipodermatosclerosis*
- *Fibrosis* of the dermis
- Increase in skin temperature of lower legs
- Wounds:
  - Most frequently located on the LEs: proximal to the medial malleolus although can occur anywhere (arterial wounds may also occur at this location).
  - Not significantly painful; usually complaints of minor dull leg pain are relieved with elevation.

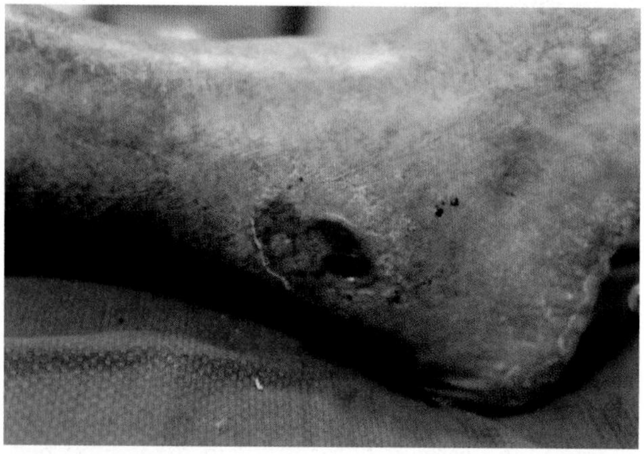

Figure 14.3 Clinical presentation of arterial insufficiency.

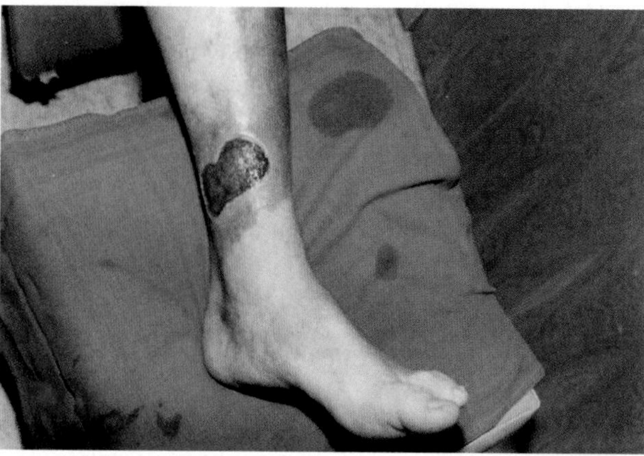

Figure 14.4 Venous insufficiency with leg ulcer.

- Granulation tissue is usually present in the wound bed.
- Tissue is *wet* from a typically large amount of draining *exudate.*
- Signs and symptoms of lymphedema may be present (it is common to see the impact of chronic inflammation and fluid overload as triggers for the onset of lymphedema).

History

Because the incidence of CVI increases with age, clinicians should be suspicious of the disease in older patients. The slow development of venous disease and ulceration usually implies a history of lingering swelling, slow healing, repeated infection, and frequent recurrence of skin breakdown. Once ulceration occurs, venous wounds can exist for years. This progression of symptoms frequently leads to a mechanical overload of the lymphatic system and subsequent development of lymphedema. If the individual is older than age 50, it is likely there are comorbidities such as diabetes, hypertension, congestive heart failure (CHF), or history of DVT. Owing to the long latency period between injury to the venous circulation and clinical manifestations, health care providers, patients, families, and caregivers must join forces using the tools of education, prevention, and vigilance.

Tests and Measurements

With the exception of mixed arterial and venous disease, the vascular examination results for venous insufficiency will show strong distal pulses and a normal ABI. On palpation, the skin temperature of the lower leg may be elevated. This sign can imply a worsening or impending complication of CVI.[53,54] The use of instrumentation to measure skin temperature can be invaluable during the examination. Measuring skin temperature will be covered later in this chapter. Existing edema may decrease with elevation unless it occurs in the advanced stages of disease or in combination with lymphedema. With venous disease, pitting edema may occur in the periwound area, the foot and ankle, or anywhere on the body. Advanced edema and lymphedema are generally unaffected by elevation and require compression as part of treatment. However, before adding compression, it will be important to address the possibility of an arterial component to the venous pathology. If there is arterial insufficiency, healing will be impaired and compression may be contraindicated.[47,53] Results from the ABI will give preliminary information about potential arterial insufficiency, but more sophisticated laboratory tests may be indicated to confirm or rule out arterial disease in the individual who also has venous insufficiency.

Intervention

The most important therapeutic measure for prevention and treatment of venous leg ulcers is *compression therapy.* Compression refers primarily to specialized bandaging and specialized garments but can also include intermittent pneumatic compression. All of these treatment interventions will be discussed later in the chapter. Even though edema is a natural characteristic of the first phase of wound healing, excessive edema can delay wound healing by slowing perfusion of tissues and facilitating the growth of bacteria.[13] Along with compression and appropriate wound care for CVI, treatment will include exercise to increase mobility and positioning to support and enhance venous blood flow.[48] Compression therapy is essential for timely healing if arterial disease has been ruled out. As mentioned earlier, in a diagnosis of mixed arterial and venous disease, the more severe pathology is treated first. Significant arterial disease will most likely preclude the use of compression. For the individual with a diagnosis of venous disease or mixed (mild) arterial/venous disease, a combination of therapeutic measures will accelerate positive outcomes.[55] These include compression bandaging and garments, gait training, manual lymphatic drainage, and exercise, including range of motion (ROM). A wound care plan should not include whirlpool owing to the risks of dependent positioning, cross-contamination, cytotoxic additives, and unnecessary costs.

Lymphedema

Lymphedema is a chronic disorder characterized by an abnormal accumulation of lymph fluid in the tissues of one or more body regions.[2,56,57] The accumulation of fluid can be caused by a number of events but is most often owing to a mechanical insufficiency of the lymphatic system. This means that some components of the lymphatic system are not functioning sufficiently to manage the lymph fluid present in the body region. Lymphedema can be classified as primary or secondary lymphedema. *Primary lymphedema* (Fig. 14.5) is caused by a condition that is congenital or hereditary. With

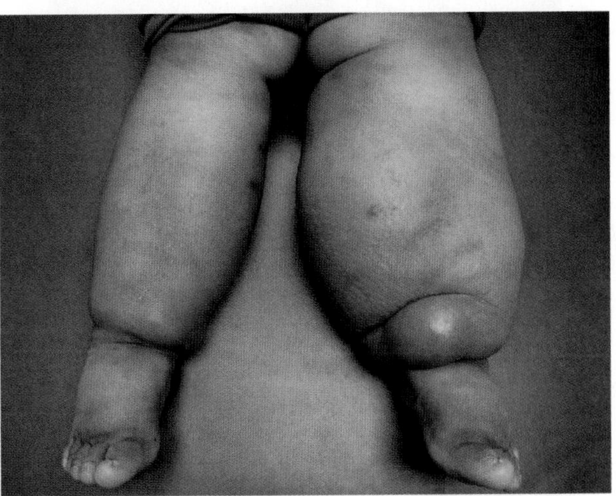

Figure 14.5 Primary lymphedema of bilateral LEs with one extremity more involved than the other.

primary lymphedema, lymph node or lymph vessel formation is abnormal. The most common abnormality is *hypoplasia,* a condition in which there are fewer lymphatic vessels and they are smaller than normal. One of the more common forms of primary lymphedema appears in *Milroy's disease. Secondary lymphedema* (Fig. 14.6) is caused by injury to one or more components of the lymphatic system: Some portion of the lymphatic system has been blocked, dissected, fibrosed, overloaded, or otherwise damaged or altered.

Secondary lymphedema is more prevalent than primary. In developed countries, the most common cause of secondary lymphedema is surgery and/or radiation therapy as part of breast cancer treatment. The rise in incidence of other types of cancer and the subsequent treatments for those cancers has led to an increase in reports of lymphedema following treatment for cancer of the prostate, bladder, uterus, ovaries, and skin. Cancer is not the only causative factor for lymphedema. It is common for an individual with CVI to develop lymphedema, triggered by long-standing fluid overload in the LEs.[58] Secondary lymphedema can also be triggered by the complications of paralysis, disuse in chronic regional pain syndrome, or trauma to regional lymph nodes following liposuction, pelvic fracture, hernia repair, and other surgical interventions where lymph nodes or lymph vessels are located.[59-61] Lymphedema is a common disease, and health care providers can expect an increase in the number of patients with this condition over the next decade.[62]

Through the efforts of experts in the field of physical therapy, there has been compelling evidence to support a *prospective surveillance model* as the standard of care in breast cancer treatment.[63,64] Surveillance includes regular follow-up visits performed by physical therapists to identify and monitor changes that might signal adverse effects of treatment. Studies have shown that this model is more cost-effective than treating the late adverse effects of treatment such as advanced-stage lymphedema.[63-65] This model should also apply to individuals undergoing treatment for other types of cancer and those at risk of developing lymphedema for other reasons. The collection of data on the incidence of non-cancer-related secondary lymphedema is limited by the lack of specific education related to lymphedema among health care professionals and by a lack of clinical suspicion when examining individuals with a history of swelling.[66] In the tropical and subtropical regions of the world, secondary lymphedema is most often caused by *filariasis.* In filariasis, nematode worm larvae live a full life cycle in the lymphatic vessels, causing inflammation and blocked lymphatic vessels.

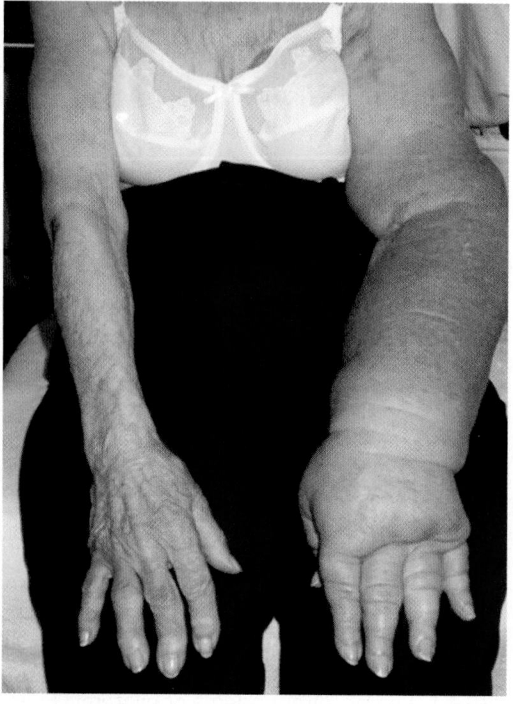

Figure 14.6 Secondary lymphedema of unilateral UE.

Clinical Presentation

- Swelling distal to or adjacent to the area where lymph system function has been impaired
- Swelling usually not relieved by elevation
- Pitting edema in the early stages of disease, nonpitting edema in later stages, as fibrotic changes occur
- Feelings of fatigue, heaviness, pressure, or tightness in the affected region
- Numbness and tingling as swelling becomes more severe
- Discomfort varying from mild to intense
- Fibrotic changes of the dermis
- Dermal abnormalities such as *cysts, fistulas, lymphorrhea, papillomas, hyperkeratosis*
- Increased susceptibility to infection, at first local to the affected region but often becoming systemic
- Loss of mobility and ROM
- Impaired wound healing

History

A patient history consistent with lymphatic system damage or deformity will be pivotal in the diagnosis of lymphedema. A patient's history might include cancer, cancer treatment, radiation therapy, lymph node disruption, CVI, trauma, surgery, or (in primary lymphedema) onset of swelling at birth or puberty. There may be a long latency period between injury to the lymphatics and clinical manifestations; thus, health care providers and patients must adhere to prevention guidelines and be suspicious of any signs and symptoms that might suggest lymphedema. The condition can develop within a few weeks of the initial insult to the system or as long as 30 years later.

Tests and Measurements

For most individuals, the diagnosis of lymphedema can be made without the use of special tests. A patient history consistent with lymph system damage or deformity, a systems review, differential diagnosis, inspection, and palpation of the integument and girth measurements are adequate for accurate diagnosis in most cases. Unique findings might include the *Stemmer's sign,* skin texture changes, skin folds, fibrosis, increase in girth, *papules,* lymph leakage, and *elephantiasis. Severity* is determined by a collection of data, including presence of fibrotic tissue changes (brawny or woody [hardened] and/or lobular [rounded projection]); number of episodes of cellulitis; condition of the superficial integument of the lymphedematous limb (papules, leakage, fungus, venous wounds); circumference or volume differences between involved and uninvolved limbs; and quality-of-life issues (sleep, mobility, activities of daily living [ADL], relationships). A noninvasive test called *lymphoscintigraphy* is a special test using radioactive tracer and a gamma camera to provide images of the lymphatic system. This test is useful for differential diagnosis and to characterize the severity of lymphedema.[62,67,68]

Intervention

A physical therapist should be cautious about the application of pressure to an edematous or lymphedematous body part. Although compression is an essential intervention, pressures that are too high will occlude superficial lymph capillaries and prevent the initial step of fluid absorption needed to control edema and lymphedema.[4]

Current intervention for the patient/client with lymphedema requires attention to detail and a level of expertise not often provided in entry-level professional educational programs. Practitioners are best served by gaining additional education to better prepare them to treat these patients. The current recommended course of care is a two-phase program of *complete decongestive therapy* (CDT).[69-72] Phase I (intensive) includes skin care, MLD, lymphedema bandaging, exercise, and compression garment at the *end* of phase I. Phase II (self-management) includes skin care, compression garment during the day, exercise, lymphedema bandaging at night, and MLD as needed. A good source of information on training programs or other information on CDT, trained therapists, and patient education related to lymphedema is the National Lymphedema Network (NLN; available at www.lymphnet.org).

As with many progressive, chronic disorders, the effectiveness of treatment is significantly improved by early intervention. Accurate and early diagnosis occurs when health care professionals are sensitized to the signs and symptoms and carefully evaluate the examination data. In the POC, the number and frequency of treatments should not be determined by lymphedema staging or by circumferential differences between limbs (the severity of the condition is not determined by these data alone). Some individuals with lymphedema may present with more involved signs and symptoms than the measurements imply. The physical therapist should pay close attention to indicators such as a history of cellulitis, brawny tissue changes, and increasing impairment in developing the POC and number of visits needed.

Pressure Injuries

A *pressure injury* is a wound caused by unrelieved pressure to the dermis and underlying vascular structures, usually between bone and support surfaces. When pressure is not relieved in time, the damage is of such magnitude that the tissues cannot repair and recover on their own. As deeper vessels are occluded, decreased blood flow leads to cell death, tissue necrosis, and finally a visible wound. The superficial dermis can tolerate *ischemia* for 2 to 8 hours before breakdown occurs. Deeper muscle, connective, and fat tissues tolerate pressures for 2 hours or less. Thus, there may be significant damage to underlying tissues while initially the epidermis and dermis remain intact. The clinical implications of this phenomenon are discussed below and in the "Tests and Measurements" section. Readers can gain greater understanding about depth of damage to the integument by referring to Chapter 24, Burns, to view cross sections of skin, illustrating which components of the skin are lost at descending levels of damage.

Pressure injuries occur most frequently among individuals who are immobilized for long periods of time. Although pressure injuries can occur at any age during prolonged periods of immobility, they are more likely to occur on individuals who are hospitalized, elderly, incontinent, and/or underweight and among individuals of all ages following spinal cord injury (SCI).[40,73-75] Up to 25% of hospital-acquired pressure injuries may originate during surgery.[76] According to Reed et al,[77] the presence of low albumin levels, confusion, and a *do not resuscitate (DNR)* order are also pressure injury risk factors.[77] Pressure injuries increase the risk of death for elderly individuals whether at home or in a hospital or long-term care setting.[78] In developed countries, the incidence of chronic wounds, including pressure injuries, is increasing as the population ages.

Clinical Presentation

The severity of pressure injury can be estimated by observing clinical signs. A progression from least tissue damage to most severe damage is presented here.[79] More details on the challenges of identifying pressure injury depth will be covered later in the chapter.

- The first clinical sign of pressure injury is *blanchable erythema* along with increased skin temperature. If pressure is relieved, tissues may recover in 24 hours. If pressure is unrelieved, nonblanchable erythema occurs.
- Progression to a superficial abrasion, blister, or shallow crater indicates involvement of the dermis.
- When full-thickness skin loss is apparent, the ulcer appears as a deep crater. Bleeding is minimal, and

tissues are *indurated* and warm. Eschar formation marks full-thickness skin loss. Tunneling or undermining is often present (the official staging classification for pressure injuries will be covered later in this chapter).

- The majority of all pressure injuries develop over six primary bony areas (Fig. 14.7): sacrum (Fig. 14.8), coccyx, greater trochanter, ischial tuberosity, calcaneus (heel), and lateral malleolus.

History

If an individual has a history of a period of immobility followed by the discovery of a warm, red spot over a bony prominence, a pressure injury can usually be confirmed.

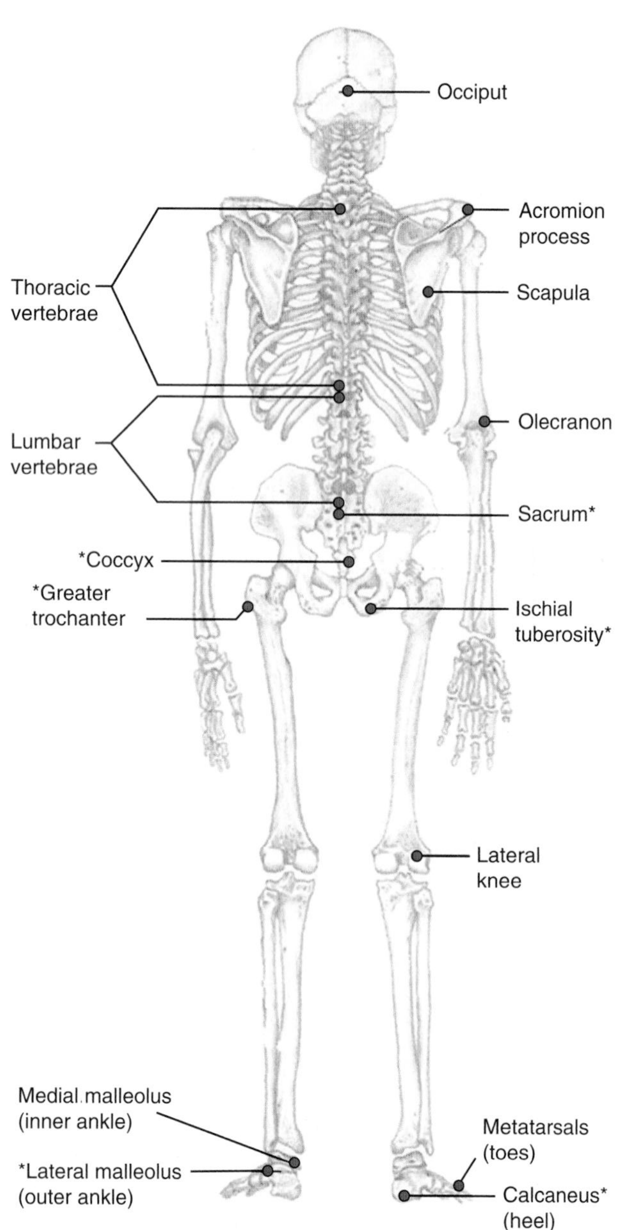

Figure 14.7 Pressure points of bony prominences.

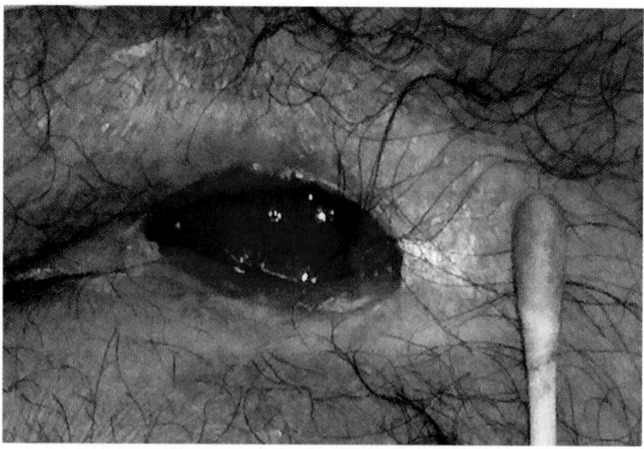

Figure 14.8 Sacral pressure injury.

If the spot is unnaturally soft to the touch, sometimes referred to as "boggy," this is enough evidence to suspect that damage is deeper than the epidermis.

Tests and Measurements

During examination, along with general wound characteristics, pressure injuries are classified by grading or staging systems that describe the degree of tissue damage observed. It can also be important to use a tool to measure an individual's risk of developing a pressure injury before a tissue injury exists. Refer to the "Integumentary Integrity" section for more information on risk assessment for pressure injuries (Fig. 14.9).

Intervention

A physical therapist treats integumentary disorders that involve the epidermis, dermis, hypodermis, or below into exposed bone, tendon, muscle, and organs. For closure and subsequent healing to occur, intervention for disorders of the integument must facilitate local and regional homeostasis of the vascular and lymphatic systems. In addition to appropriate wound care, it is imperative that

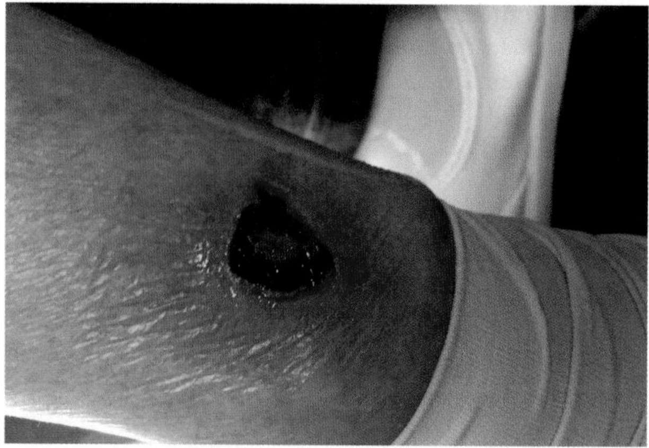

Figure 14.9 Unstageable pressure injury: obscured full-thickness skin and tissue loss.

the underlying cause of pressure be addressed. Wounds will not close and remain healed unless the reduction of pressure and prevention of future breakdown are top priorities in the intervention plan. Pressure management is accomplished with the use of PRDs, *pressure mapping* to determine pressure loads, *positioning/turning schedules,* and *education* of the patient, family, and caregivers. Other factors that contribute to ulceration or risk of ulceration should be considered and/or addressed. These factors include shear, friction, mobility, sensation, moisture, nutrition, age, and underlying medical condition. With appropriate wound care, control of pressure, and attention to risk factors, a wound should progress through the phases of wound healing, showing signs of improvement in a matter of weeks.[36]

Neuropathy

Neuropathy can be defined as any disease of nerves and can include peripheral nerves, cranial nerves, and/or autonomic nerves. Neuropathy exists in many disease processes; however, the most common disease process seen with neuropathy is diabetes. For most chronic diseases, including diabetes, the effects of neuropathy are peripheral. The etiology of diabetic neuropathy is not well understood but thought to be related to high levels of glucose in the blood over a long period of time. *Diabetic neuropathy* is a generic term for any diabetes mellitus–related disorder of the peripheral or autonomic nervous systems or the cranial nerves. The majority of symptoms from diabetic neuropathy will be located in the LE with foot insensitivity and subsequent ulceration being the most common (Fig. 14.10).

It is estimated that 15% of individuals with diabetes will develop a foot ulcer sometime in their life, making them almost 40 times more likely to undergo amputation because of a nonhealing wound than the nondiabetic population.[47] To complicate matters, many individuals with diabetes have coexisting arterial disease because the conditions are not mutually exclusive. Although the incidence is lower than for venous and arterial wounds in general, the underlying diabetic condition creates a difficult environment in which to close a wound. The incidence of neuropathic LE wounds is likely to grow as the population ages and the incidence of diabetes continues to escalate. According to the Centers for Disease Control and Prevention (CDC), almost half of all adults now are at risk for diabetes.[80] Diabetes affects more than 29 million people of all ages in the United States. This figure represents 9.3% of the population. About 60% to 70% of people with diabetes have mild to severe forms of neuropathy, and more than 60% of the nontraumatic lower-limb amputations that are performed in the United States occur among people with diabetes.[80] If current trends prevail, the impact of diabetic neuropathy on future wound care needs will continue to expand.

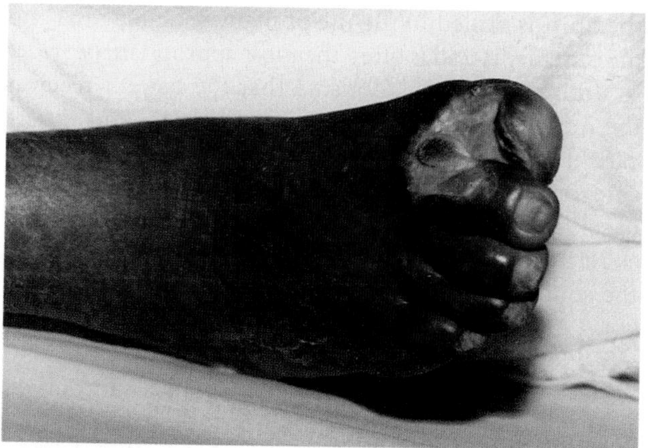

Figure 14.10 Chronic wound as a result of diabetic neuropathy.

Clinical Presentation

- Ulceration is usually located on the weight-bearing surfaces of the foot
- Usually anesthetic, round, over bony prominences but can be located anywhere
- Sensory neuropathy, if present:
  - Patient unable to sense pain and pressure
  - Risk of skin breakdown without patient awareness
  - Mechanical, repetitive stresses most common causative factors of wounds
- Motor neuropathy, if present:
  - Loss of intrinsic muscles
  - Hammer-toe, claw-toe deformities adding to risk of breakdown owing to poor weight distribution and rubbing from shoes
  - Foot drop
- Autonomic neuropathy, if present:
  - Decreased or absent sweat and oil production leading to dry, inelastic skin
  - Increased susceptibility to skin breakdown and injury
  - Propensity for heavy callus formation
- Dysvascular symptoms, if present:
  - Usually arterial disorders but can be complicated by reduced cardiac function from autonomic causes
  - Ischemia
  - Impaired healing time (also present owing to diabetes)
  - Impaired transport of oxygen, antibiotics, and nutrients needed for healing

History

A history of diabetes is sufficient to warrant investigation of diabetic neuropathy. If the individual has had diabetes for a number of years or has had trouble regulating insulin levels even for a few years, the presence of diabetic neuropathy is very likely. When ulceration is visible, the history will include specific details about the wound in addition to information about other symptoms.

Tests and Measurements

During the examination, every patient with diabetes should be checked, using monofilaments, for the presence of *protective sensation* in the LEs. This should be part of a systems review for patients with diabetes even when diabetes is not the primary diagnosis. Data on skin temperature of the LEs should also be recorded during the examination. Information about blood glucose levels should be obtained as part of the examination and must be considered for safe development of the POC.

Intervention

Physical therapists are in an ideal position to provide education and comprehensive foot care intervention for the diabetic population. In addition to appropriate wound care and maintenance of acceptable blood glucose levels, intervention must include some method of decreasing weight-bearing stresses. Options for off-loading include crutches or walker, changes in gait patterns, walking casts or splints, and specialized footwear. It would not be unusual to utilize all of the off-loading options over the course of treatment for foot ulceration. Intervention must include a comprehensive program, including elements of wound care, foot care, education, PRDs, orthotics, exercise, and modalities. Every effort should be made by clinicians and patients alike to improve or retain skin integrity of the foot. (Refer to Appendix 14.A for patient education information on foot care.) In addition to other medical complications of diabetes, altered circulation to the foot can complicate symptoms from diabetic neuropathy. Intervention should address the worst problem first but with lower expectations for healing when vascular disorders coexist with neuropathy.

The five most common disorders of the vascular, lymphatic, and integumentary systems have been discussed. Other disorders caused by surgery, trauma, malignancy, hematologic disease, connective tissue disease, and thermal injury *will* affect the systems discussed in this chapter. Owing to space restrictions, however, they will not be discussed at this time. Interested readers should seek one of the texts mentioned in the reference list to supplement information presented here.[1,2,37,49,56] Examination and treatment of other disorders would utilize the same tests and measurements and treatment interventions discussed in this chapter based on the patient's unique characteristics.

■ EXAMINATION AND EVALUATION

Examination

History

Many of the disorders discussed in this chapter have a slow or insidious onset, making history taking challenging but important. See Chapter 1, Clinical Decision Making, to review the type of data that may be generated from taking a thorough history. A thorough history will include seeking information on systems beyond the local affected area. As noted in Chapter 1, physical therapy examinations for all disorders begin with gathering data from the patient, family, and other involved individuals. For the disorders discussed in this chapter, information needed from the history will be similar which makes the inclusion of these topics in one chapter ideal.

Systems Review

It might be tempting to skip a systems review before using other tests and measurements in the examination process to save time. This step, however, is of utmost importance as physical therapists move toward greater autonomy. Results may alert the physical therapist to problems that may require referral to another practitioner. A systems review is particularly important here because the disorders discussed in this chapter are often the result of dysfunction in other systems of the body. For example, diabetes may lead to wounds of the feet, breast cancer surgery may lead to lymphedema, heart disease may lead to arterial wounds of the legs, and paralysis may lead to pressure injuries. A comprehensive approach to observing and examining the patient will set the stage for the investigation and data collection that follow.

Tests and Measurements

Owing to the close relationship among disorders of the vascular, lymphatic, and integumentary systems; the importance of differential diagnosis; and the likelihood of a patient or client presenting with more than one disorder, a physical therapist will use a wide variety of available tests and measurements during the examination. The tests and measurements discussed in this chapter are described in the order in which they are presented in the *Guide to Physical Therapist Practice 3.0*.[81] A review of the test and measurement categories themselves should serve as a reminder of the responsibility of the examining therapist to document thoroughly. A physical therapist is skilled in the use of many valuable tests and measurements and is often the most appropriate provider to utilize these tools to assure that the patient receives the most patient-centered, comprehensive, and timely care. For purposes of space, only the most essential categories have been addressed. An annotated version of selected tests and measurements has been included to assist the reader in greater understanding of the tests and the conditions under examination.

Aerobic Capacity/Endurance

Aerobic capacity during functional activities is important to measure since activity will be encouraged as part of long-term management of the disorders in this chapter. In addition to information obtained during the systems review, the gathering of additional data will depend on the individual patient. This might include the use of angina, claudication, and dyspnea scales, pulmonary function tests, and electrocardiogram (ECG). A determination of heart rhythm sounds, as well as breath and voice sounds, may also be required.

Anthropometric Characteristics

Height and Weight: Data on height and weight are necessary to address and track normal weight values, especially for the patient with a disorder that results in abnormal fluid retention such as diabetes, edema, lymphedema, venous disease, or underlying cardiopulmonary disease.

Volumetric Measurement: Volumetrics are performed utilizing special containers that hold water and a graduated cylinder for water collection (Fig. 14.11). This method is accurate for measuring changes in body dimensions with the most common measurements taken for the hand, full arm, foot, or full lower leg; however, it is time-consuming, awkward to administer, and may be inappropriate when open wounds are present owing to cross-contamination risks.

Girth Measurement: Girth is recorded using a tape measure to determine circumferential body dimensions (Fig. 14.12). Ideally, a tape measure specially designed to measure girth should be used. Although bony landmarks are sometimes used as reference points in taking girth measurements, the standard among experts who treat edema is to use consistent centimeter intervals instead. For example, in measuring the LE, circumferential measurements are taken in centimeter (cm) intervals, starting from the floor or weight-bearing surface to the groin. Clinicians choose intervals of 4, 6, 8, or 10 cm. The smaller the interval, the better the representation of body dimensions. Special measuring boards (Fig. 14.13) can be obtained for measuring the LE, or a well-placed clipboard under the foot can be used to establish the beginning "floor" measurement if the patient is in supine position. A physical therapist must remember that girth measurements by themselves should not be used to determine severity, frequency of visits, or duration of the episode of care. Advanced fibrotic changes can occur to the dermis and underlying connective tissue without a significant increase in the girth of a limb.[2,60]

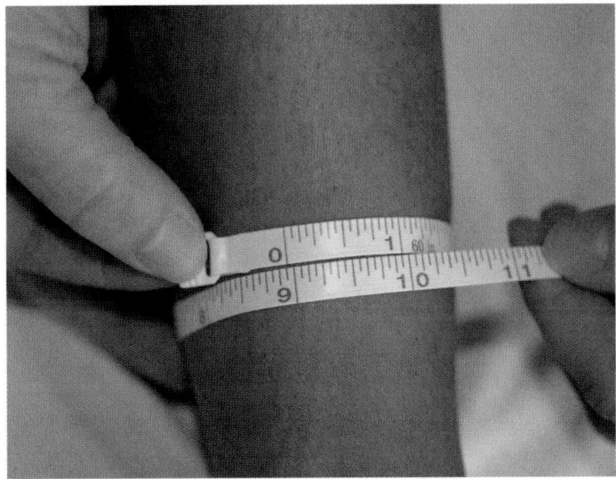

Figure 14.12 Tape measure examination for girth measurement.

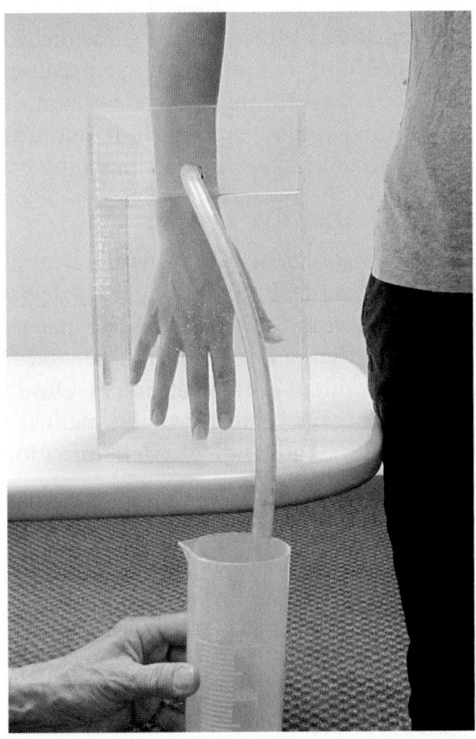

Figure 14.11 Volumetric examination for edema.

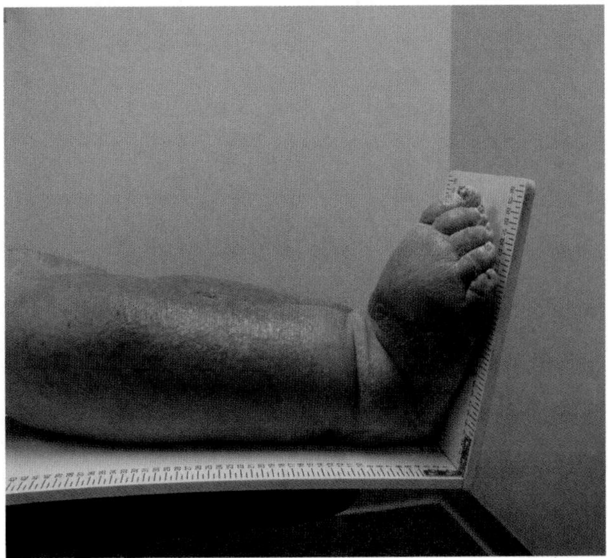

Figure 14.13 Use of footboard with ruler to establish consistent intervals for measuring lower extremity circumferences.

Additional Tools

Data on anthropometric measurements may be collected using *tonometry* or *bioelectrical impedance.* Although not a standardized procedure, soft-tissue tonometry uses a device that measures tissue tension at the surface of the skin. Less pliable skin creates a higher tension reading, suggesting the presence of fluid and/or tissue fibrosis. Data from tonometry can be useful for subclinical evidence of edema, lymphedema, and fibrotic changes before they are visible or palpable. Bioelectrical impedance analysis provides accurate measurements to help predict the onset of lymphedema, often many months before a clinical diagnosis is possible. The technique involves passing a very small amount of alternating current (AC) through the limb to be tested and measuring the impedance to its flow at various frequencies. This technique is more sensitive than limb volume measurements in detecting changes in the extracellular fluid volume. In studies thus far, the false-negative rate has been zero.[82-85]

Palpation/Pitting Scale

Palpation of soft tissues must be a regular part of vascular, lymphatic, and integumentary examinations. There is no universal pitting scale currently used by health care professionals. Some scales are based on how deep an indentation is left after applying fingertip pressure. Other scales are based on how severe the examiner believes the pitting to be. The following scale, most commonly used by physical therapists and physicians, gives a numerical grade to the pitting based on how long it remains after fingertip pressure is applied:

1+: Indentation is barely detectable.
2+: Slight indentation visible when skin is depressed, returns to normal in 15 seconds.
3+: Deeper indentation occurs when pressed and returns to normal within 30 seconds.
4+: Indentation lasts for more than 30 seconds.

If using a pitting scale during an examination, it is wise to document an explanation of the grades or scoring system used. It is common for a physical therapist to assess pedal edema because it may be attributed to chronic wounds, inflammation, infection, cellulitis, diabetes, liver disease, renal disease, CVI, lymphedema, phlebolymphedema, CHF, or trauma.

Staging or Grading of Lymphedema

In an effort to categorize levels of severity, some professionals use staging or grading systems for edema and lymphedema in addition to one or more of the measurement techniques above.[2] Grading or staging of edema and lymphedema is not universally used by health professionals and should be accompanied by objective information in the examination results. One of the most frequently used systems is the *International Society of Lymphology Staging System* as described in their most recent consensus document[57]:

- Stage 0: Subclinical state where the peripheral swelling is not visible, but lymphatic transport is impaired. Symptoms and subtle tissue changes may be noted.
- Stage I: Early onset of swelling that is visible and subsides with elevation. Pitting may be present.
- Stage II: Consistent volume change with pitting present. Elevation rarely reduces the swelling and progressive tissue fibrosis occurs.
- Stage III: Skin changes such as thickening, hyperpigmentation, increased skin folds, fat deposits and warty overgrowths occur. Tissue is very fibrotic and pitting is absent.

Stages 0 and I are considered early stage lymphedema. Another term would be *preclinical lymphedema* as the patient begins to feel "heaviness" in the limb or body part but may not be able to see it. Stage II is considered moderate/established lymphedema. Stage III is late stage lymphedema and often appears as elephantiasis due to the appearance of the skin.

Arousal, Attention, and Cognition

After evaluating screening results during the history and systems review, the physical therapist will decide whether there is a clinical indication for tests and measurements in this category. It is important for the therapist to understand the patient's level of motivation, orientation, attention, and ability to process instructions. Many of the disorders in this chapter, such as diabetic neuropathy, chronic venous insufficiency, and lymphedema, require lifelong adherence to the self-care component of the treatment in order to retain the gains made during intervention. Most of the information regarding cognition can be obtained through interviews and observations. Additional tools would include cognitive and behavior scales, safety checklists, and learning profiles.

Assistive and Adaptive Devices

It is very likely that patients with vascular, lymphatic, or integumentary disorders will need assistive devices during the intervention and self-care phases of management. Increasing mobility is a key factor in timely recovery or symptom management of these disorders. Observation, gait analysis, functional screening, and manual muscle testing are often used to guide this determination.

Circulation

Collecting data about the movement of blood and lymph through the arterial, venous, and lymphatic systems is interrelated with the tests and measurements for integumentary integrity. Tests and measurements for skin changes that may occur with impairment of the circulation are discussed under the "Integumentary Integrity" section. The presence or risk of pathology of the circulatory systems can be detected in many cases by skilled observation and palpation (e.g., temperature and pulses).

Temperature

To further examine circulation, skin temperature can be assessed by palpation. Objective data should also be collected and quantified using a *radiometer* or a *thermistor,* because superficial skin temperature changes are often indicative of pathology (Fig. 14.14). A decrease in skin temperature can indicate poor arterial perfusion. An increase can indicate infection or active disease processes such as cellulitis or a *Charcot joint.* An increase in temperature can also indicate a worsening or impending complication of CVI.[54]

Arterial Perfusion

The therapist collects data to determine whether adequate blood flow is reaching distal tissues. If blood flow is adequate, the oxygen supply will be adequate. Some noninvasive tests and measurements are designed to determine *blood flow* and *skin perfusion,* whereas others address *oxygen levels* in the tissues. Pulses should be palpated initially to provide information about possible vascular system involvement. The examination should include palpation of the following arteries: brachial and radial, femoral, popliteal, dorsalis pedis, and posterior tibialis. The following scale, commonly used by physical therapists and physicians, gives a numerical grade and a descriptive word to describe the pulse quality:

0 = *Absent,* no perceptible pulse
1+ = *Thready,* barely perceptible
2+ = *Weak,* palpable but diminished
3+ = *Normal,* easy to palpate
4+ = *Bounding,* very strong, may imply the possibility of an aneurysm or other pathological condition

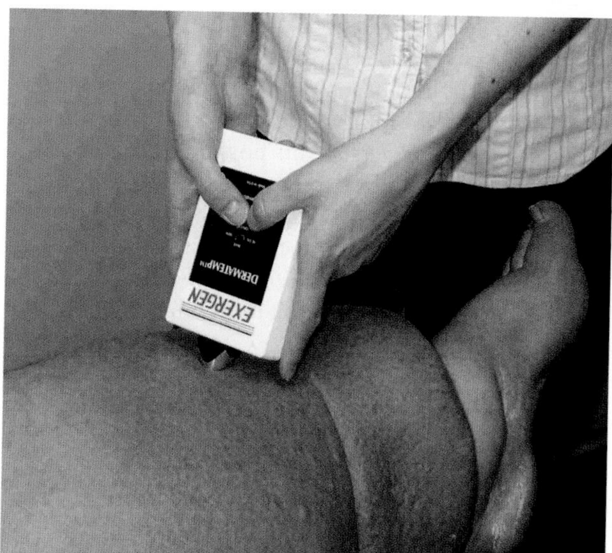

Figure 14.14 Skin temperature examination using a skin thermometer.

Auscultation by stethoscope of major pulse points may identify a *bruit.* If turbulent blood flow is heard, the patient may have partial blockage of the artery. Barriers to effective pulse taking include scar tissue, edema, fibrosis, and tissue induration.

Doppler ultrasound is considered an essential component of the vascular examination.[49,86,87] The examiner uses a handheld probe to direct a sound wave into the vessel to be tested. The sound wave is reflected by red blood cells moving in the vessel. The sound wave signal is changed into audible sound that is transmitted from a small, handheld unit. The ABI is the most frequently performed test using Doppler ultrasound. A blood pressure cuff is inflated to occlude blood flow temporarily and is then deflated as the examiner listens for the return of flow. Blood flow is observed on the upper extremity (UE) at the brachial artery and on the LE at the posterior tibial and the dorsalis pedis arteries (Fig. 14.15). The ABI is a ratio of the LE pressure divided by the UE pressure. Table 14.1 presents the ranges of ABI values and potential vascular indications. Obtaining an ABI will provide useful information about the arterial system since the ABI is an indicator of loss of perfusion in the LE. Results will guide the therapist in decisions about the use of compression and débridement, and will help predict the likelihood of wound closure. When the examiner cannot occlude blood flow with the blood pressure cuff, calculations may show a falsely elevated ABI. Arteriosclerosis or calcified vessels (from diabetes) can make it difficult for the cuff to compress enough to get an accurate ABI. The target arteries would be documented as *noncompressible vessels.* Test options when the vessels are noncompressible include taking toe pressures with a special cuff, proceeding with transcutaneous oxygen testing (see below), or recommending referral for a vascular laboratory workup.

Trophic Changes

Trophic changes occur in the soft tissue of the LEs when circulation is impaired by poor arterial blood flow and

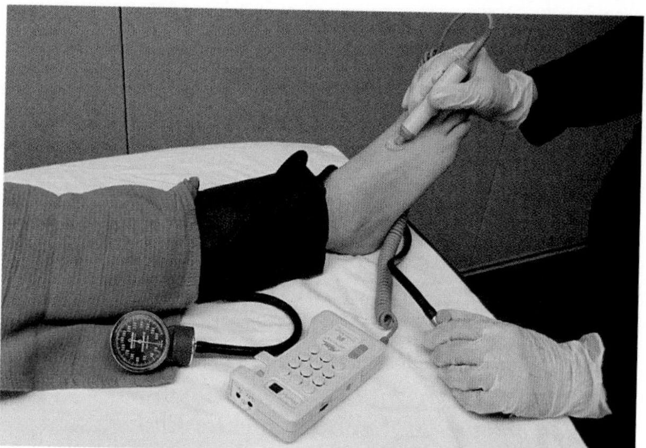

Figure 14.15 ABI test performed using a handheld Doppler ultrasound instrument.

Table 14.1 Ankle–Brachial Indices With Corresponding Indications

ABI Ranges	Possible Indication
>1.2	Falsely elevated, arterial disease, diabetes
1.19–0.95	Normal
0.94–0.75	Mild arterial disease, + intermittent claudication
0.74–0.50	Moderate arterial disease, + rest pain
<0.50	Severe arterial disease

interruptions in nerve supply. Observation is the most accurate way to note trophic changes. Changes include dry, shiny skin (pale in Caucasians), decreased or absent leg hair, and thick toenails. It should be noted that these signs are also a predictable part of aging but not to the same degree as can be seen with trophic changes. The presence of changes indicates the need for other tests of circulation.

Pain

When related to circulation, a thorough pain history may be all that is necessary to suggest the possibility of arterial disease. Reports of pain indicate the need for further tests and measurements of the vascular system. Pain as the result of intermittent claudication (IC) is described earlier in this chapter. Rest pain that develops at night, awakens the patient, or requires analgesics for relief is considered more severe than IC. Pain can be measured for severity on a Visual Analog Scale (VAS). The degree of impairment from IC is often measured in terms of how far an individual can walk before experiencing acute leg pain or fatigue. IC can be classified objectively with a rating scale to indicate severity based on distance walked before onset of pain. The *Walking Impairment Questionnaire* (WIQ) is a disease-specific questionnaire commonly used to examine claudication. It does not, however, measure the impact of claudication on quality of life (QOL).[88] The most extensively researched disease-specific QOL questionnaire for IC is the *Claudication Scale*.[88-90]

Special Tests

There are many other noninvasive and invasive tests used to detect, examine, diagnose, or confirm arterial disease and dysfunction. Appendix 14.B presents a brief description of special tests for arterial and venous function, including *rubor of dependency, air plethysmography (APG), transcutaneous oxygen ($TcPO_2$)* measurement, and *skin perfusion pressure (SPP)* measurement. Although some of the tests are useful for predicting healing of ulcers and amputation wounds, they may not be readily reimbursed when performed by a physical therapist. The APG, $TcPO_2$, and SPP are used primarily for research purposes because they are time-consuming to perform.

Venous Patency

Venous disease and dysfunction can be detected with a wide range of tests and measurements. The amount of time available for examination, as well as reimbursement issues, may influence decisions about which tests to use. Refer to Appendix 14.B for a brief description of *Venous Filling Time, Percussion Test,* and the *Trendelenburg Test.* Owing to inconsistencies in interpretation and administration, the *Homans' Test,* or Homans' sign (pain in the calf when the foot is passively dorsiflexed), should not be relied on to detect a DVT. A physician should be contacted and a Doppler study used if an individual exhibits two of the following signs: change in skin temperature, change in skin color (darker), pain in the calf (experienced by approximately half of patients), or swelling. Many clinicians utilize the Well's Criteria for DVT because it can provide objective data based on clinical findings to assist in decision making.[91,92]

Lymph Vessel Integrity

Patient history and clinical findings are used most often to make a diagnosis of lymphedema. Most invasive tests have lost popularity because of the risk of triggering the onset of lymphedema or an exacerbation of existing lymphedema owing to the irritation caused by dye and/or needle puncture. When invasive tests are indicated, the most common test procedure is *lymphoscintigraphy.* This test, using dye and a special camera and computer, can visualize many lymphatic system functions.[2,93]

Gait, Locomotion, and Balance

It is always important to utilize tests and measurements to assess and document a patient's ability to move. The importance of movement to improve blood and lymphatic flow and to facilitate the overall return to function for most individuals makes this category essential. During the initial examination, gathering data through observation, gait analysis, and postural control tests is usually adequate. The examination results may indicate the need for additional tests such as inventories, or batteries of tests to further document safety (fall risk) or equipment needs. Individuals who are morbidly obese have unique challenges with gait that should be addressed during the examination.

Integumentary Integrity

Collection of data about skin and subcutaneous tissues is interrelated with the tests and measurements for circulation and cutaneous sensation.

Observation and Palpation

Characteristics of the skin are noted almost entirely by observation and palpation. A comparison between involved and normal integument is made with careful attention to color, moisture, texture, firmness, temperature, elasticity, symmetry, and shape. In the presence of a wound, the wound tissue, the periwound area, and the wound exudate should all be observed and data recorded regarding the observations. The location of a wound, presence of edema, and presence of lymphedema can be documented using a *body diagram.*

Trophic Changes

Because they are an important part of many disorders involving the integument, trophic changes are mentioned again under this section. Readers who are making a quick reference specifically to integumentary integrity in this chapter are reminded to refer to all sections related to trophic changes. As in the section on circulation, observation is an important approach to noting changes.

Fibrosis

The best way to detect fibrotic changes of the skin is through palpation of the affected tissue. The superficial skin and underlying tissue will feel thickened, firm, and unyielding or immobile. Fibrosis is common in later stages of CVI and lymphedema. Testing for the presence or absence of the *Stemmer's sign* is an objective measurement that can be added to the examination for lymphedema. When the dorsal skin folds of the toes or fingers are resistant to lifting, or cannot be lifted at all, the Stemmer's sign is said to be "present." The clinician must be cautious, however, because a negative or "absent" skin fold test does not rule out lymphedema.

Coloration

Skin color will vary based on the underlying disease. Observation is the best way to note comparisons between normal tissues and those under examination. The most abnormal color changes include red, purple, and brown. Color changes may indicate a chronic condition such as hemosiderin staining or an acute situation such as redness associated with DVT. If color changes are intermittent, they may signal a disease such as Raynaud's.

Temperature

The temperature of the skin is most often examined by palpation, but data can be objectively collected and quantified using a radiometer or a thermistor (see Fig. 14.14). Maintenance of normal skin temperatures is essential for good wound healing. Abnormal skin temperatures can signal problems related to the dermis or other structures. A decrease in superficial skin temperature may indicate poor arterial perfusion. An increase may indicate infection or active disease processes.

Wounds

Size and Depth

A number of tools and scales are available for gathering data about wounds, edema, lymphedema, and other aspects of integumentary integrity. Wounds not classified with staging or grading can be described based on the depth of tissue damage. The descriptions used for depth of burn injury, *superficial, partial,* and *full thickness,* can also be used to describe depth in other types of wounds. Objective measures included in documentation are vital for communication about the patient. A calibrated grid, photographs, tracings, graphs, and specifically designed forms are most commonly used to document wound size and depth.

Drainage

Drainage is usually measured by observation and is often described in terms of color and thickness. In the case of heavy drainage where suction might be needed, the liquid exudate may be collected in a canister and measured. Examination of wound drainage may be very important because it may indicate a normal response to trauma (few days) or a prolonged response to necrotic tissue, a foreign substance in the wound, or infection. The most common language for describing wound drainage is described in Table 14.2.

Staging

Pressure injuries are typically classified using a *staging* or *grading* system that gives information about the severity

Table 14.2 Descriptions of Drainage by Color and Thickness

Drainage Type	Color	Thickness
Transudate	Clear	Thin, watery
Serosanguineous	Clear or tinge of red/brown	Thin, watery
Exudate	Creamy, yellowish	Moderate to very thick, expected with autolytic débridement
Pus	Yellow, brown	Moderate to very thick
Infected pus	Hues of yellow, blue, green	Thick, usually indicates infection (but may be normal as white blood cells macrophage necrotic cells and turn them into slough); drainage can be foul and yet the wound may not be infected

of the wound based on depth of tissue destruction. Both the National Pressure Ulcer Advisory Panel (NPUAP) and the Agency for Health Care Research and Quality (AHRQ) support the use of the universal classification system described in Table 14.3.[94-96]

Staging can be challenging because tissue damage may be deeper than what appears on the surface, wounds cannot be staged when necrotic tissue is present, and darker skin does not always show the reddened alterations indicating Stage 1. To respond to these challenges, the NPUAP has redefined the definition of a pressure injury and the stages of pressure injuries. The new terminology includes the use of Arabic numbers instead of Roman numerals for the stages. The revised stages and the change in terminology from *pressure ulcer* to *pressure injury* more accurately describes pressure injuries. These improvements describe injuries to both intact and ulcerated skin. The staging descriptions are intended for use with pressure injuries and not to describe the severity of other wound types.

Wound Healing Tools

A variety of tools can be utilized to document wound status and wound healing. Since there is no single wound characteristic that can be used alone to monitor healing or predict outcomes, it is best to use a tool that includes multiple characteristics as measures of wound healing. The three tools with the most well-established reliability and validity are the *Sussman Wound Healing Tool*,[38] the *Pressure Ulcer Scale for Healing*,[38,97] and the *Pressure Sore Status Tool*.[38] The *Wagner Ulcer Grade Classification* system is a tool designed for examination of the diabetic foot when neuropathy and ischemia are present.[98]

Risk Factor Assessment

Although all individuals may be subjected to the same intensities of pressure for similar amounts of time, they all will not develop pressure injuries. As a result, factors related to individual risk, susceptibility, or tolerance capacity should be determined. A physical therapist will find that data from a risk assessment can be helpful in planning cost-effective intervention strategies. As discussed earlier in the chapter, there are many factors that put individuals at risk for developing pressure injuries, such as poor peripheral circulation, diabetes, nutritional status, mobility, and continence issues, to name a few. To objectify and standardize risk assessment, a number of reliable tools have been validated by research:

- *Norton Risk Assessment Scale*: original risk assessment instrument scores individuals on physical condition, mental condition, activity, mobility, and incontinence.[99]
- *Gosnell Scale–Pressure Sore Risk Assessment*: refinement of Norton's scale includes changes to the following scoring categories: nutrition, mental condition, activity, mobility, continence, skin appearance, medication, diet, and fluid balance.[100]
- *Braden Scale for Predicting Pressure Sore Risk*: the six scoring categories of this instrument include sensory perception, moisture, activity, mobility, nutrition, and friction/shear.[101]

Muscle Performance

Muscle strength screening during the systems review and specific manual muscle testing during the examination should be included for the individual with a disorder of the vascular, lymphatic, or integumentary system. Functional muscle strength identified during an examination of functional mobility skills and ADL is also important. Lack of strength and immobility go hand in hand, often leading to problems such as pressure injuries, CVI, increased LE edema and lymphedema, varicosities, and poor control of diabetic sequelae.

Orthotic, Protective, and Supportive Devices

There are many situations in which an individual who has disorders mentioned in this chapter would need to be assessed for an orthotic, protective, or supportive device. Those individuals already using a device may need a modification. For the individual with impaired sensation of the feet, *extra-depth* shoes may be indicated. Existing shoes should be checked periodically for fit and wear. A referral to another professional for protective footwear may be needed. Supportive devices may allow an individual to increase his or her activity level, offsetting the risks of a sedentary lifestyle. Compression garments and bandaging, considered *supportive devices,* must be checked periodically for fit and function to ensure that they retain their effectiveness. Garments and bandages will be essential intervention choices for most individuals with edema and lymphedema. In the later stages, a patient's need for devices may provide a way to quantify the remediation of impairments or activity limitations imposed by the symptoms of the disorder. A physical therapist is skilled in selecting, fitting, and monitoring the best devices in this category. A poorly fitted device will do more harm than good.

Pain

Pain is often a cause of psychological distress for individuals with chronic wounds. The presence or absence of pain, its location and intensity, its effect on sleep, and other QOL factors should be measured (see Chapter 25, Chronic Pain). Pain scales, drawings, and maps are effective for documentation. Owing to the high incidence of comorbidity in patients with disorders of the vascular, lymphatic, and integumentary systems, the measurement of pain may also assist in making a differential diagnosis.

Posture

Indications for examination of posture include pain, heavy or large limbs, scar tissue, poor body image (e.g., following cancer treatment), obesity, and decreased

Table 14.3 Pressure Injury Staging Criteria Revised by NPUAP

Pressure injuries are staged to indicate the extent of tissue damage. The stages were revised based on questions received by NPUAP from clinicians attempting to diagnose and identify the stage of pressure injuries. Schematic artwork for each of the stages of pressure injury was also revised and is available for use at no cost through the NPUAP website (http://www.npuap.org/resources/educational-and-clinical-resources/pressure-injury-staging-illustrations/).

Stage 1 Pressure Injury: Non-blanchable erythema of intact skin
Intact skin with a localized area of non-blanchable erythema, which may appear differently in darkly pigmented skin. Presence of blanchable erythema or changes in sensation, temperature, or firmness may precede visual changes. Color changes do not include purple or maroon discoloration; these may indicate deep tissue pressure injury.

Stage 2 Pressure Injury: Partial-thickness skin loss with exposed dermis
Partial-thickness loss of skin with exposed dermis. The wound bed is viable, pink or red, moist, and may also present as an intact or ruptured serum-filled blister. Adipose (fat) is not visible and deeper tissues are not visible. Granulation tissue, slough, and eschar are not present. These injuries commonly result from adverse microclimate and shear in the skin over the pelvis and shear in the heel. This stage should not be used to describe moisture associated skin damage (MASD) including incontinence associated dermatitis (IAD), intertriginous dermatitis (ITD), medical adhesive related skin injury (MARSI), or traumatic wounds (skin tears, burns, abrasions).

Stage 3 Pressure Injury: Full-thickness skin loss
Full-thickness loss of skin, in which adipose (fat) is visible in the ulcer and granulation tissue and epibole (rolled wound edges) are often present. Slough and/or eschar may be visible. The depth of tissue damage varies by anatomical location; areas of significant adiposity can develop deep wounds. Undermining and tunneling may occur. Fascia, muscle, tendon, ligament, cartilage and/or bone are not exposed. If slough or eschar obscures the extent of tissue loss this is an Unstageable Pressure Injury.

Stage 4 Pressure Injury: Full-thickness skin and tissue loss
Full-thickness skin and tissue loss with exposed or directly palpable fascia, muscle, tendon, ligament, cartilage, or bone in the ulcer. Slough and/or eschar may be visible. Epibole (rolled edges), undermining and/or tunneling often occur. Depth varies by anatomical location. If slough or eschar obscures the extent of tissue loss this is an Unstageable Pressure Injury.

Unstageable Pressure Injury: Obscured full-thickness skin and tissue loss
Full-thickness skin and tissue loss in which the extent of tissue damage within the ulcer cannot be confirmed because it is obscured by slough or eschar. If slough or eschar is removed, a Stage 3 or Stage 4 pressure injury will be revealed. Stable eschar (i.e. dry, adherent, intact without erythema or fluctuance) on the heel or ischemic limb should not be softened or removed.

Deep Tissue Pressure Injury (DTPI): Persistent non-blanchable deep red, maroon or purple discoloration
Intact or non-intact skin with localized area of persistent non-blanchable deep red, maroon, purple discoloration, or epidermal separation revealing a dark wound bed or blood filled blister. Pain and temperature change often precede skin color changes. Discoloration may appear differently in darkly pigmented skin. This injury results from intense and/or prolonged pressure and shear forces at the bone–muscle interface. The wound may evolve rapidly to reveal the actual extent of tissue injury or may resolve without tissue loss. If necrotic tissue, subcutaneous tissue, granulation tissue, fascia, muscle, or other underlying structures are visible, this indicates a full thickness pressure injury (unstageable, Stage 3, or Stage 4). Do not use DTPI to describe vascular, traumatic, neuropathic, or dermatologic conditions.

Additional pressure injury definitions.

Medical Device–Related Pressure Injury: This describes an etiology. Medical device–related pressure injuries result from the use of devices designed and applied for diagnostic or therapeutic purposes. The resultant pressure injury generally conforms to the pattern or shape of the device. The injury should be staged using the staging system.

Mucosal Membrane Pressure Injury: Mucosal membrane pressure injury is found on mucous membranes with a history of a medical device in use at the location of the injury. Due to the anatomy of the tissue these injuries cannot be staged.

Source: http://www.npuap.org/resources/educational-and-clinical-resources/npuap-pressure-injury-stages/

sensation. Data can be obtained with the combined use of a posture grid, tape measure, observation, and palpation. A physical therapist will begin a posture assessment initially by observation the moment the client enters the room and will continue to assess and observe posture formally and informally during the examination and intervention.

Range of Motion

The need for adequate ROM and the impact of decreased ROM cannot be underestimated. Following ROM screening during the systems review, specific ROM measurements are often indicated, especially with persons for whom movement is an essential part of symptom management. Examples are numerous but include ankle ROM for the person with CVI, shoulder ROM following breast cancer surgery, or knee ROM in the individual with lymphedema of the LE. A universal goniometer and a tape measure are required to obtain objective ROM data.

Self-Care and Home Management

Activity limitations and disability are common with disorders of the vascular, lymphatic, and integumentary systems. Examination, education, and training that allow the patient to safely perform self-care and home management activities are of great importance in planning and implementing the self-management phase. Descriptions and quantifications are needed for documentation and goal setting. Examination tools should include functional measures of both basic activities of daily living (BADL) and instrumental activities of daily living (IADL), as well as fall risk scales (see Chapter 8, Examination of Function).

Sensation

Information from the history and systems review may indicate the need for a detailed examination of sensory function. Therapists should not rely on history alone as an indication for sensory testing, however, because many individuals are unaware of their deficits until tested. Sensory tests are particularly important when symptoms are long-standing or include complaints of numbness, tingling, or burning. Patients who should routinely be tested are those who may receive LE compression treatments, and all individuals who have a diagnosis of peripheral neuropathy, diabetes, and/or arterial disease. In addition to observation and palpation, initial tests should include testing for protective sensation using filaments such as the *Semmes-Weinstein monofilaments*. The filaments are supplied in varying sizes and are each mounted on a handle. The filament is applied to the skin until it bends. The patient is asked to report, with eyes closed, whether the filament is touching the body part. Each monofilament supplies a specific amount of force when it is placed on the test area and gently bent. The monofilaments are available in a large set but most testing can be accomplished using a few filaments. An individual has *normal sensation* when the 4.17 monofilament (1 *g* of force) can be felt. An individual has *protective sensation* intact when the 5.07 filament (10 *g* of force) can be felt (Fig. 14.16). With loss of protective sensation, the individual cannot sense trauma to the foot, often leading to foot ulceration. For the individual who has lost protective sensation, the use of special protective footwear is indicated. Lack of sensation, especially protective sensation, can be a characteristic of long-standing diabetes. Decreased sensation may signal a disorder such as *scleroderma*. To test for sharp/dull sensation, vibratory sensation, pressure, and other sensations, tools for gathering data include a pressure scale, tuning fork, and/or aesthesiometer. Additional information can be obtained in this textbook (see Chapter 3, Examination of Sensory Function).

Ventilation and Respiration

Tests and measures should be used to determine if the patient has adequate ventilation and respiration to meet normal oxygen demands. The presence of pathology might be indicated from a predictable source such as breath sounds or the color of nail beds. A less predictable sign, such as swelling around the ankles, could also indicate pathology. Initial data may be gathered by examining arterial blood gases, observing the work of breathing, or utilizing a spirometer. Additional appropriate tests include the airway clearance test and use of a pulse oximeter (see Chapter 12, Chronic Pulmonary Dysfunction).

Evaluation

Diagnosis, Prognosis, and Plan of Care

Once the examination is complete, the physical therapist evaluates the data and determines the diagnosis and prognosis. The physical therapist needs to consider a number of factors, including clinical findings, overall

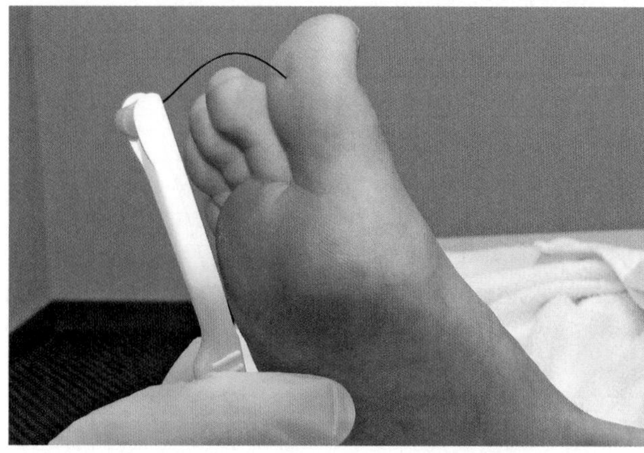

Figure 14.16 A monofilament used to assess presence of protective sensation. Bowing of the filament indicates that appropriate pressure has been applied.

physical function and health status, social support, multisystem involvement and comorbid conditions, and chronicity, severity, and stability of the condition. This information is outlined in the *Guide to Physical Therapist Practice 3.0*[81] and presented in this textbook (see Chapter 1, Clinical Decision Making). The next step is the design and implementation of the POC, including procedural interventions.

INTERVENTION

Physical therapist intervention for disorders of the vascular, lymphatic, and/or integumentary systems should include a variety of techniques to address the problems identified during the examination. It is common for patients with disorders in these systems to present with multiple factors contributing to the primary diagnosis. The intervention plan should reflect a holistic view of the patient. For example, an individual with signs and symptoms of venous disease may also present with poor ankle ROM, an LE wound, and lymphedema. The wound must be cleansed and dressed but the limb should also receive compression for optimum healing. Ankle ROM must be improved because ambulation will enhance calf pump function. Another example of the need to view patients holistically would be an individual with signs and symptoms of arterial disease who also presents with decreased LE strength, diabetes, and peripheral neuropathy. Exercise is important for this person, but it must be carefully coordinated to address arterial health, diabetes management, and skin protection.

A natural component of viewing patients holistically is to be able to identify the need for interdisciplinary care. This concept may be more important for individuals with disorders of the vascular, lymphatic, or integumentary systems for the very reasons listed in the previous paragraph: These populations present with complicated, multisystem problems that are often best addressed using a team approach. Integrated care facilitates an exchange of information among all the health professionals that are involved in the care of the patient. This model of care might be delivered by a team of individuals who work together every day or it might be coordinated by a physical therapist who pulls together certain professionals for a particular patient's needs.

Coordination, Communication, and Documentation

In keeping with practice standards, the physical therapist coordinates intervention efforts to ensure the patient receives the highest quality of care. Critical to this goal is open communication among the health care team, patient, family, and caregivers. The team will most likely include a physician, nurse, physical therapist, occupational therapist, dietitian, and social worker. Referrals to other health care professionals (e.g., podiatrist) who can support the patient can also be made. Meticulous documentation will have a significant impact on issues such as continuity of care, receiving adequate number of visits for procedures, and a stronger working relationship with referring practitioners. Photographs, special forms for data collection, and body graphs are very effective tools to enhance communication and documentation. Appendix 14.C provides an example of an examination form that might be used to document data collected for a patient with a disorder of the vascular, lymphatic, or integumentary system.

Patient/Client-Related Instruction

Disorders of the vascular, lymphatic, and integumentary systems represent major health events for patients and their families and require lifelong management strategies. Patients and families often react with anger, despair, or at least confusion when learning about a condition that may be permanent. The value of patient and family education cannot be underestimated. Patient education will be the key to preparing individuals to manage their symptoms, prevent recurrence, and remain vigilant about their condition. Information should be provided that is appropriate to the patient/family/caregiver's educational level with provisions for follow-up and repetition. Motivational strategies are important to ensure adherence to self-management. For many chronic disorders, high-quality patient education has been shown to result in positive changes in health behaviors, QOL perceptions, and adherence to home programs. Instruction for the patient should include resources, education materials, and a home program.

- Resources
  - Community services and support groups related to the patient's diagnosis
  - Counseling services, as needed, especially for assistance with QOL issues
  - Internet sites (Appendix 14.D lists Web-based resources for clinicians, families, and patients with vascular, lymphatic, and integumentary disorders)
  - Family member participation in care
- Education materials
  - Instructional materials, multimedia tools
  - Self-management strategies
  - Available resources include materials found on the Internet (see Appendix 14.D)
- Home program
  - Skin and/or wound care; prevention practices; scar management
  - Compression garment or bandage wear and care
  - Exercise
  - Edema control
  - Pressure-redistributing devices
  - Foot care for patients with diabetes (see Appendix 14.A for a foot care guide)

Outpatient or home therapy may be required for some patients. Follow-up visits at regularly scheduled intervals may be the best way to facilitate adherence to the home program and to prevent recurrence or exacerbation of symptoms.

Procedural Interventions

This section has been organized in the order in which a physical therapist would provide patient care. Within each section, information has been organized from most invasive/least selective (nonspecific) to least invasive/most selective (highly specific). In developing the POC, a physical therapist should select interventions that are least invasive/most selective, always trying to create an environment that is conducive to healing. The ultimate goal should be to optimize the body's opportunity to heal. Despite tremendous gains in the management of vascular, lymphatic, and integumentary disorders, there are still an alarming number of practitioners using outdated and often harmful methods to treat these disorders. Overused agents such as povidone-iodine, wet-to-dry dressings, whirlpool, and compression pumps have been replaced for at least two decades with more advanced, biocompatible, and cost-effective methods of treatment. The use of inappropriate agents can delay healing and may cause harm. Supporting literature abounds for the clinician seeking evidence-based practice. Elements of skin and wound care that are often overlooked or underestimated for their impact include PRDs, positioning, exercise, patient education, compression, and orthotics.

The therapist treating a patient with a wound should strive to establish an ideal wound environment. The choices made about intervention should be guided by the goal of achieving this ideal environment, described as moist, free from necrotic tissue, free from exudate, warm, protected from trauma, and protected from infection. Physical therapists may manage wound care in a primary care role, or in consultation with a physician and/or other providers. Interventions involving pharmaceuticals will always require physician consultation for a prescription. "Although practice may change based on new evidence, the search for healing in the most humane way and fastest time possible persists as the goal."[102, p. S1]

Cleansing

Wound cleansing is differentiated from wound débridement, which follows in the next section. The wound cleansing method should be selected based on its ability to support or return a wound bed to homeostasis. Chemical and mechanical trauma should be minimized even in the presence of infection. A decision to cleanse should be made carefully, because many wounds do not need to be cleansed at every dressing change. Often the negative effects to the wound from cleansing outweigh the positives. Not only is there a potential loss of endogenous fluids from the wound surface but also there is significant slowing of cellular activity for up to 3 hours after wound cleansing.[103]

Whirlpool

Since whirlpool can be classified as a means of cleansing and mechanical débridement, it is discussed in both categories of intervention. Despite at least a decade of investigation, with little evidence to support its use, whirlpool is still used for both nonselective mechanical débridement and for wound cleansing. However, many clinicians involved in wound care have decreased their use of whirlpool significantly in response to the evolution of wound care and subsequent publication of the AHRQ guidelines. Standards have changed with the increased knowledge of the microenvironment in the wound bed and a greater understanding of the chemical mediators necessary for homeostasis.

The historical rationale for use of whirlpool was based on its use in deodorization, skin and wound cleansing, mechanical nonselective débridement, wound decontamination and infection control, and softening adherent necrotic tissue in preparation for débridement. There is little evidence to support whirlpool as the *optimal* method for achieving these. If using whirlpool for an infected wound, the AHRQ recommends that whirlpool be discontinued when the ulcer is clean. First issued in 1994, the guidelines are considered to still be current.[95] The guidelines include more than 300 references, bibliographic sources, and updates that can be easily obtained.

Evidence-based rationale for a decrease in the use of whirlpool is based on a number of factors. There is risk of contamination from waterborne pathogens and from patient cross-contamination. The dependent position can initiate or increase venous congestion and extremity edema. With whirlpool, there is loss of endogenous fluids from the wound bed and heat loss affecting core body temperature and the local wound area. Even mild changes in core body temperature (hypothermia) have negative effects on the cells that are important to wound healing. In addition, mechanical disruption of granulation tissue, epithelial cells, and new skin grafts occurs, primarily from the use of water agitation. Immersion in a whirlpool saturates wound tissue and surrounding skin, creating the potential for maceration, skin breakdown, and temporary inactivation of normal skin defenses. Thus, there is the potential to prolong inflammation and delay wound healing. Whirlpool can also increase heart and respiratory rates. Finally, the use of whirlpool is labor intensive and costly in terms of use of water, utilities, linen, and staff.[3,104-109]

Based on current standards of care and guidance from the literature, it may be possible to justify the use of whirlpool in some situations. Wounds that need intensive cleansing that cannot be accomplished with other methods might benefit from whirlpool. Minimal agitation of water is recommended with only small body areas treated for short amounts of time (5 to 10 minutes) to limit the negative effects of temperature and pressure changes. Unless infection is confirmed with tissue culture, cytotoxic agents in the water should be avoided (e.g., povidone-iodine, chlorine). Wounds that need softening of loosely adherent tissue before sharp, enzymatic, or autolytic débridement might benefit from whirlpool when other tissue-softening methods are not appropriate. (*Note*: There is little to no reimbursement for the use of whirlpool to soften tissue before débridement.) Wounds that would benefit from stimulation of peripheral circulation might benefit from whirlpool. Neutral warmth or normothermia (normal body temperature, 98.6°F [37°C]) is recommended.

Pulsatile Lavage With Suction

Pulsatile lavage with suction (*PLWS,* also referred to as *forceful irrigation*) is a method of wound irrigation combined with suction (Fig. 14.17).[110] Pulsed irrigation and simultaneous suction removes the irrigation fluid, wound exudate, and loose debris. In use for over 25 years, this wound cleansing and débridement method has several advantages over whirlpool cleansing. PLWS uses less water, less staff support, and less treatment time and requires less cleanup time. PLWS can be performed bedside and in the home. (*Note*: Family or visitors should not be allowed in the room during the procedure owing to aerosolization of microorganisms.[111,112]) This type of cleansing collects wound exudate and debris efficiently and delivers topical antibiotics, antiseptics, and antibacterial solutions efficiently. PLWS speeds healing by rapid removal of contaminants and treats tunneling wounds and undermining wounds using special cannula tips (Fig. 14.18). Risk of periwound maceration and cross-contamination is eliminated with use of disposable equipment.

Although the advantages are clear, there are disadvantages to using PLWS. These include risk of overuse, especially with clean, granulating wounds, and risk of trauma to newly formed tissue from plastic tips, pulsed irrigant, and/or suction. Treatment may be painful to the patient. PLWS use should be limited to experienced therapists who are well versed in anatomy, especially when irrigating tracts, areas of undermining, or exposed bone, tendon, blood vessels, cavity linings, grafts, or flaps. All staff involved in treatment must wear disposable personal protective equipment (PPE). Compared to other irrigation options, disposable, single-use equipment contributes to landfill burden. There is considerable cost when labor, PPE, and equipment are calculated.

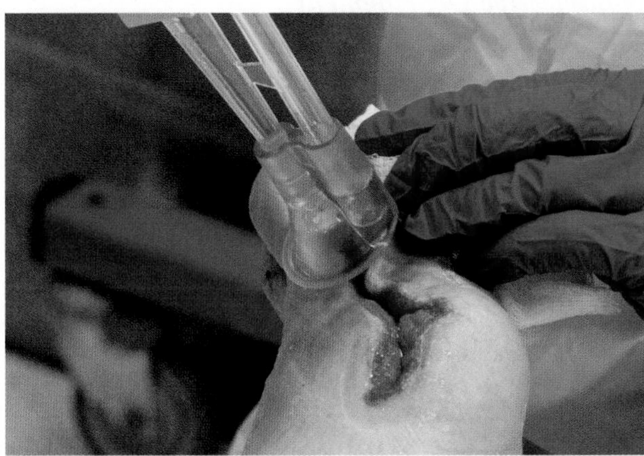

Figure 14.17 Physical therapist guides the PLWS shield close to the wound surface.

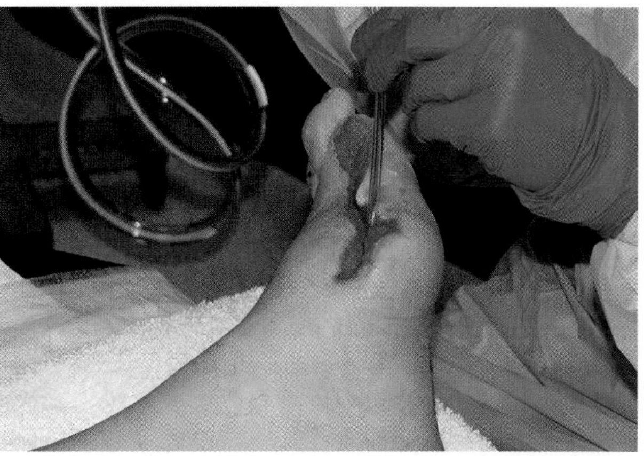

Figure 14.18 A special tip may be used to gently cleanse a deeper wound with PLWS.

Nonforceful Irrigation

As soon as possible, wound cleansing should be accomplished with minimal pressure or force on the wound bed by nonforceful irrigation. This can be accomplished by pouring a solution over a wound or using a bulb syringe or other device designed to deliver an irrigant to the wound (Fig. 14.19). There are several products that

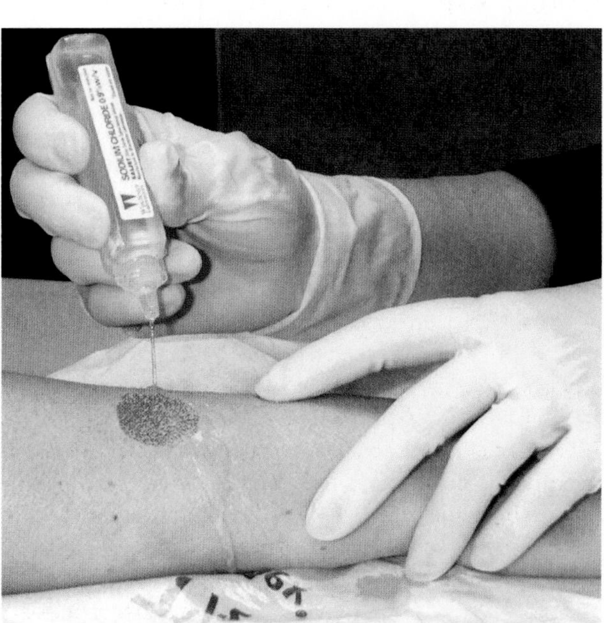

Figure 14.19 Wound cleansing with nonforceful irrigation.

package saline specifically for wound cleansing: Blairex™ Wound Wash Saline, manufactured by Blairex Laboratories, Columbus, IN 47202; and Saljet™, single-dose sterile saline manufactured by Winchester Laboratories, LLC, St. Charles, IL 60174. Several manufacturers produce a spray container that delivers saline or a surfactant at very gentle pressures (Fig. 14.20). Infected wounds can also be effectively cleaned with nonforceful irrigation. Wounds with necrotic tissue or debris, however, may respond best to a few sessions of a more forceful type of cleansing. For wounds that are clean, with new tissue growth, cleansing should be done only to remove excess endogenous fluids or residue left by dressing products.

Commercial Skin and Wound Cleansers

There are many skin and wound cleansers designed as topical solutions and marketed to treat acute and chronic wounds. For many years solutions have been used indiscriminately without consideration or measurement of the potential side effects on the new cells trying to proliferate in the wound bed. These topical cleansers may have some antimicrobial effects but most have significant antimitotic (inhibiting mitosis) effects as well.[113] This means that cleansers may adversely affect important cells such as fibroblasts and epidermal keratinocytes during tissue repair. The cells most affected are the all-important cells that fill and cover a wound. Information on the toxicity of the most common cleansers has been created to assist health care providers in selecting or rejecting the use of cleansers.[113] It is no surprise that acetic acid is extremely cytotoxic to the cells in a wound but of greater concern is the fact that ordinary bath soaps, even moisturizing body washes, are very cytotoxic. A physical therapist utilizing commercial cleansers or ordinary soap must consider the rationale behind the use of each topical agent applied to the wound and weigh the cost to the wound: some contribute to wound healing whereas others contribute to aspects other than wound healing.

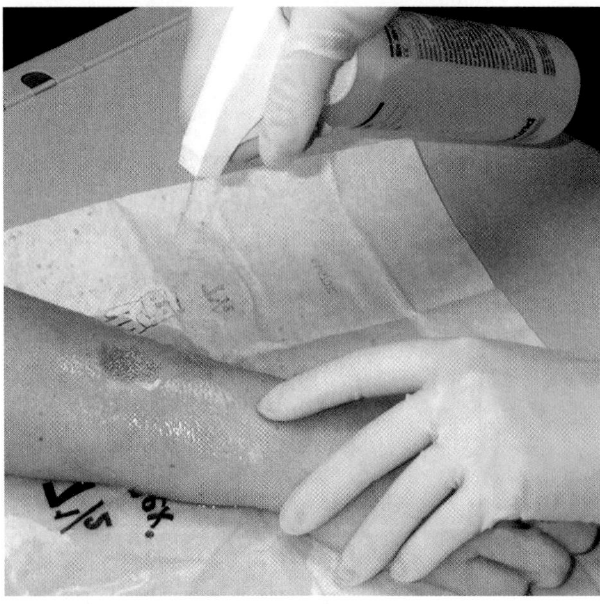

Figure 14.20 Wound cleansing with a spray cleanser.

Débridement

Débridement is defined as the removal of foreign material and dead or damaged tissue. Removal of devitalized or infected tissue is an important intervention to prevent or control bacterial growth, encourage normal cellular activity in the wound bed, and enhance the rate of tissue repair. For clarity in this chapter, *nonselective débridement* refers to techniques that remove all tissue both necrotic and living. Methods in this category may be quick but are often painful and frequently cause damage to nearby healthy tissue. *Selective débridement* refers to techniques that remove necrotic tissue in a controlled method. Selective methods are more comfortable and gentle to the wound bed but may remove tissue more slowly.

The importance of physical therapist proficiency in sharp débridement is reflected in the Physical Therapist Licensure Examination Content Outline (the content outline can be accessed at www.fsbpt.org/FreeResources/NPTECandidateHandbook.aspx), the Commission on Accreditation in Physical Therapy Education (CAPTE) evaluative criteria (the Accreditation Handbook can be accessed at www.capteonline.org/Accreditation Handbook) and the *Guide to Physical Therapist Practice 3.0*.[81] In response, most professional-level programs include instruction in sharp débridement within the curriculum. In the majority of states, débridement is included in the scope of practice for physical therapists. Physical therapists should consult their state's practice act to ensure that débridement is within their scope of practice in that state before providing this intervention.

When choosing a method of débridement, clinicians must consider not only the wound status but also the physiological, emotional, and financial status of the patient. Modern wound management experts avoid débridement techniques that cause the wound to bleed owing to the highly damaging effects to the wound tissues.

Nonselective Débridement

Wet-to-Dry Dressings A wet-to-dry (WTD) dressing consists of wet gauze applied to the wound bed and allowed to dry on the wound. Removal of the dry dressing débrides the wound, pulling away any cellular material that has adhered to the gauze. This method of débridement removes necrotic tissue, as well as rich endogenous fluids, fibrin, and other cells critical to wound healing. It is frequently uncomfortable for the patient, often causing bleeding and trauma to the wound bed. There is literature to describe the use of WTD dressings for débridement, but the efficacy of the procedure has not been demonstrated.[114,115] Wound management experts have agreed for over two decades with a multidisciplinary panel: "One of the most routinely and inappropriately used forms of non-selective mechanical débridement is the wet-to-dry dressing."[116, p. 28] Once believed to be less costly than other dressing options, it has been shown that WTD gauze dressings are actually more costly than advanced dressings. Evidence in the literature clearly highlights the many negative aspects of WTD dressings.[117-127]

Since WTD dressings can be classified as a tool for mechanical débridement and/or a primary wound dressing, the procedure has been discussed here and in the section on dressings.

Surgical Débridement Surgical débridement provides rapid results when treating life-threatening necrosis, large wounds, tunneling wounds, and necrotic or infected bone. Wide excision, removing viable and nonviable tissue, is usually done in the operating room with anesthesia. Laser débridement, another form of surgical débridement, may be appropriate when an individual is not a candidate for operating room procedures. Surgical débridement is not within the scope of practice of a physical therapist.

Pulsatile Lavage with Suction PLWS will provide nonselective débridement while cleansing a wound. Refer to the detailed discussion of PLWS in the "Cleansing" section earlier.

Whirlpool Whirlpool can be used for mechanical débridement through its feature of water agitation. It can also be used to soften necrotic tissue in preparation for sharp, enzymatic, or autolytic débridement. There are, however, often better methods of preparing tissue for débridement than whirlpool. See discussion in the "Cleansing" section earlier.

Selective Débridement

Sharp Sharp débridement is defined as the removal of dead or necrotic tissue or foreign material from and around a wound using sterile instruments such as a scalpel (Fig. 14.21), scissors, and/or forceps (Fig. 14.22). Considered the *gold standard* of methods for removal of necrotic tissue, sharp débridement is a minor, tissue-sparing procedure that is performed bedside or in a procedure room. In the vast majority of U.S. states, it is within the scope of practice for a physical therapist to perform sharp débridement. It is incumbent on the therapist to be aware of his or her state practice act regarding regulations. The American Physical Therapy Association (APTA) position statement indicates that sharp débridement should be performed exclusively by physical therapists, not other personnel. For a full copy of this statement, go to www.apta.org/uploadedFiles/APTAorg/About_Us/Policies/HOD/Practice/ProceduralInterventions.pdf. Additional information can be found in the *Guide to Physical Therapist Practice 3.0*.[81] To maintain current standards, a physical therapist should not débride except in the presence of necrotic tissue.

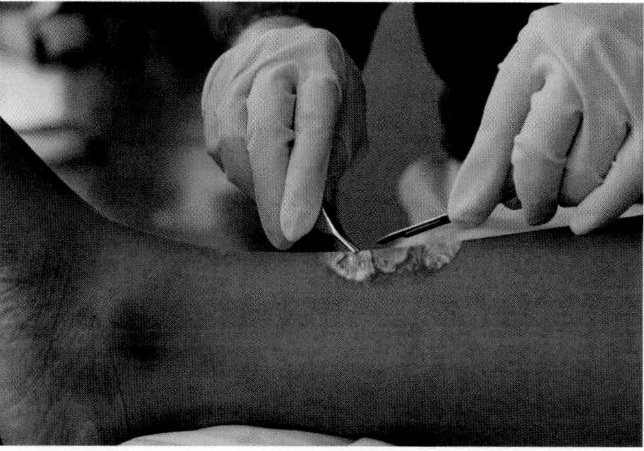

Figure 14.21 Use of scalpel and forceps for sharp débridement.

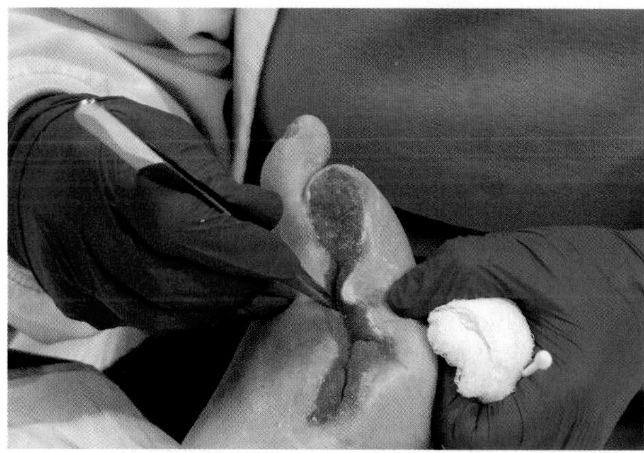

Figure 14.22 Selective débridement of necrotic tissue can be accomplished using forceps.

Even though sharp débridement is effective for all types of necrotic tissue, there are situations where this form of débridement is not appropriate. It is contraindicated for vascular wounds with limited blood flow where eschar may be serving as a cap or cover for a chronic open wound. Without adequate perfusion in this scenario, there is little hope of wound closure. Sharp débridement is not appropriate for wounds with tunneling (when the wound bed cannot be seen) or areas affected by dry gangrene. Patients with low platelet counts, on anticoagulants, or with other conditions that inhibit clotting are not suitable candidates. It may be contraindicated for pressure injuries on the heels covered with dry eschar. (*Note:* Some experts maintain that in this scenario, eschar provides protection as long as there is no infection present; others maintain that eschar must be removed because it inhibits epithelial cell growth.)

Chemical or Enzymatic Enzymatic débridement is a type of selective débridement that includes the application of a topical agent containing enzymes that act by dissolving necrotic tissue. There are several types and brands of enzymatic agents, each designed to affect a certain type of necrotic tissue. Advantages for this type of treatment are that débridement is selective, patient discomfort is minimal, and application procedures are simple. Disadvantages include the potential development of dermatitis of the intact periwound skin, frequent dressing changes disrupting the wound bed, and the need to crosshatch existing eschar with a scalpel so that the enzyme can penetrate the wound. Enzymatic débridement agents do not have an impact on pathogen levels in the wound bed and should not be considered antimicrobial. Some enzymatic débridement preparations contain the protein papain. Topical drug products containing papain were taken off the market in the United States in November 2008 because they have not been approved by the Food and Drug Administration (FDA). When utilizing other types of enzymatic agents still on the market, a referral for treatment and a prescription for the enzymatic agent are currently required in most regions of North America.

Biosurgery Biosurgery as a form of selective débridement is also referred to as *maggot débridement therapy* (MDT), or maggot or larval therapy (Fig. 14.23). Although it has been in use in the Western world for over 150 years, its popularity declined with the advent of antibiotics. Biosurgery is now generating new interest owing to the rise of multidrug-resistant bacteria such as methicillin-resistant *Staphylococcus aureus* (MRSA). Sterile, newly hatched larvae are placed on chronic wounds and held in place with dressings or a *biobag* for 2 to 5 days before removal. Biosurgery has been shown to remove devitalized tissue, decrease the risk of infection, and improve wound healing without side effects in a wide variety of wound types. Biosurgery is recommended for osteomyelitis and deep wound infections that remain unresponsive to more conventional antibiotic and surgical therapy. Although moist wound healing is compatible with biosurgery, a very wet wound environment has an adverse effect on larval survival. Certain types of moisture-retentive wound dressings are more compatible with larval survival than others.[128-135]

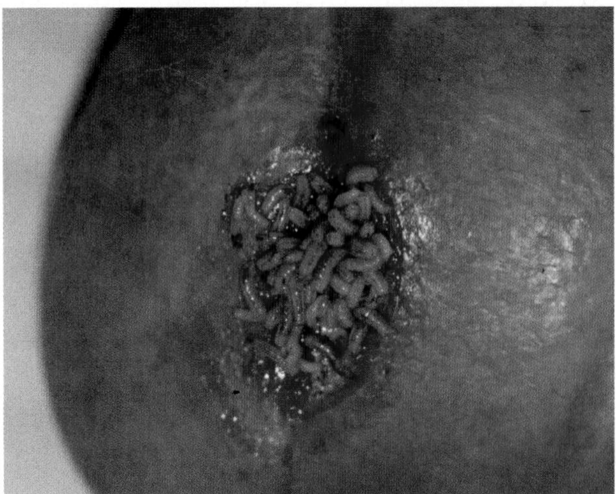

Figure 14.23 Maggot therapy for a cavity wound. *(Courtesy of the Biosurgical Research Unit, Surgical Materials Testing Laboratory, Bridgend, UK.)*

Medical-Grade Honey

The use of medical-grade honey as a wound dressing has been shown to enhance débridement and healing. Honey dressings are available in hydrocolloid, alginate, and liquid categories. They have been shown to facilitate autolytic débridement, decrease or eliminate wound odor, prevent biofilm (thin layer of bacteria) formation, and soften necrotic tissue.[136-139]

Autolytic

Autolytic débridement uses the endogenous enzymes on the wound bed to digest devitalized tissue and promote granulation tissue formation. In practice, the body's natural fluids are held in contact with the wound base with a moisture-retentive dressing for 3 to 7 days. By increasing the moisture content of slough and necrotic tissue with enzyme-rich body fluids, autolytic activity is facilitated. Although this method is the least invasive/most selective, as well as inexpensive, painless, and biocompatible, each patient is examined to determine if this type of débridement is best for the existing wound. The type of moisture-retentive dressing selected to promote autolytic débridement will be based on the health of the periwound tissues and the level of fungal or bacterial loads. The presence of infection does not rule out the use of occlusive dressings, as described earlier in the discussion on moist wound healing.

Topical Agents

Current standards for chronic wound care have decreased the use of topical agents even in the presence of infection. In the literature, these agents may be referred to as *antiseptics, disinfectants,* and/or *antimicrobials.* Other topical agent categories include *antibiotics* and *analgesics.* Guidelines reveal that almost all human-made products are cytotoxic to WBCs even when diluted.[95] Many agents once thought to be safe are now known to be unsafe to healing tissue, causing adverse reactions at any concentration. Many agents once thought to be effective as antibacterial or decontaminating agents are now known to be ineffective. When striving for wound bed homeostasis, preserving cellular life in endogenous fluids is almost always more desirable than destroying it with additives. Many physicians and wound management experts use the following adage to guide in the decision making process: "It is desirable never to put anything in the wound that cannot be tolerated comfortably in the conjunctival sac."[13, p. 179] In plain terms, "If you can't put it in your eyes don't put it in the wound." Even under Direct Access, in most states physical therapists are not permitted to prescribe medications, even over-the-counter products, for wound care. If, during the examination or intervention, a physical therapist determines that a topical agent may be indicated, the patient's physician should be contacted and the findings discussed. Consideration of topical agents should always include the risks and benefits of the topical agent in relation to potential cytotoxicity, biocompatibility, safety, and efficacy.

Antiseptics

Povidone-Iodine Povidone-iodine (PVI) is a combination of iodine plus a polymer that provides bactericidal effects. One commonly known product name is Betadine® (Purdue Products LP, Stamford, CT 06901). Used indiscriminately for many years on acute and chronic wounds, it is now recommended mainly for wounds infected with *Staphylococcus aureus.* The AHRQ guidelines published in 1994 state: "Do not clean ulcer wounds with skin cleansers or antiseptic agents (e.g., povidone-iodine, iodophor, sodium hypochlorite solution [Dakin's solution], hydrogen peroxide, acetic acid)."[95, p. 15] Although the guidelines address pressure injuries, the wound-healing evidence is applicable to all wound treatments. This evidence implies that the use of PVI, as well as other antiseptics, is inconsistent with practice standards. In rare instances when such agents are recommended by a physician and are indeed appropriate, clinicians should document sound reasoning behind the use of these products because they will be held accountable to these published and respected guidelines. An example of a situation such as this would be when other, less cytotoxic treatments have failed to reduce the bacterial load in an infected wound. The literature does not provide adequate clinical or legal reasons to use PVI for managing wounds. In addition, the FDA has not approved the use of PVI solution or PVI surgical scrub solution for wounds. PVI has been shown to reduce bacterial counts in infected wounds, and currently there is no antimicrobial resistance to PVI.[140] Its use is contraindicated for the noninfected wound.[95]

Sodium Hypochlorite Solutions: Dakin's Solution (Bleach and Boric Acid), Sodium Hypochlorite (Household Bleach) Sodium hypochlorite is cytotoxic even at very dilute concentrations. It damages fibroblasts and endothelial cells and causes cellular damage to granulation tissue. It is irritating to the skin and can initiate severe reactions in some individuals. It is used in the management of wounds with purulent exudate. Treatment should be discontinued when the wound is clean. Its use is contraindicated for the noninfected wound.[95]

Acetic Acid Solution Acetic acid is traditionally used to inhibit bacterial infections; however, the solution has been found to be more damaging to fibroblasts than to bacteria. A common form of acetic acid is found in vinegar. It is corrosive and cytotoxic at any dilution. Most recently, it has been used to manage contamination by ***Pseudomonas aeruginosa.*** Its use is contraindicated for the noninfected wound.[95]

Oxidizing Agents: Hydrogen Peroxide Solution When this solution comes in contact with tissue, there is a release of oxygen and temporary antimicrobial activity. Its bubbling action is used for nonselective débridement to loosen small debris. It is cytotoxic unless diluted to a very weak concentration. Its use is contraindicated for wounds that are noninfected, tunneling, or granulating.[95]

Antibacterials

This section includes a sample of commonly used topical antimicrobials, antibiotics, and antibacterials. Each of these topical agents is effective against a variety of bacteria and is selected by the physician based on the species cultured for an individual patient. All share a risk of similar side effects such as burning, itching, contact dermatitis, and/or allergic sensitivity. There is little evidence in the literature to show levels of cytotoxicity in these topical agents. Examples include the following:

- Bacitracin/Baciguent: associated with allergic reactions.
- Neosporin/neomycin sulfate: causes greatest incidence of allergic reactions.
- Silvadene/silver sulfadiazine: primarily for thermal injuries, silver is selectively toxic to bacteria but may inactivate topical proteolytic enzymes.[141]
- Furacin/nitrofurazone: cytotoxic in animal studies.[142]
- Sulfamylon/mafenide acetate: diffuses easily through eschar, primarily for thermal injuries.
- Bactroban/mupirocin ointment: currently effective against all species of staphylococcus.
- Gentamicin/Garamycin: currently effective against all species of staphylococcus and streptococcus.

Owing to the paucity of information on cytotoxicity, the risk of side effects, and the growing incidence of antibiotic-resistant bacteria, use of these products for chronic wounds should be considered carefully and is usually contraindicated for the noninfected wound.

Creams and Ointments (Over-the-Counter) Some antibacterial ointments and creams such as Bacitracin and Neosporin® can be purchased without a prescription. These are minimally bacteriostatic owing to their dilution. Once they lose their antibacterial strength, the ointments may trap bacteria and encourage bacterial growth from surface contamination. If ointments or creams are used, the wound should be cleansed regularly to remove potential contamination; however, frequent cleansing may disrupt the healing process. These preparations can be used to provide moisture to a dry wound, but they may create a greasy wound bed, making early epithelial cell migration difficult. A more biocompatible ointment that will provide moisture to a healing wound is Aquaphor® (Beiersdorf Inc., Wilton, CT 06897).

Analgesics

The use of topical anesthetics to control wound pain is controversial in the literature. Conflicting reports and the lack of substantial research have led to concerns about the impact of anesthetics on the wound bed. This issue is further complicated by the broad profile of patients with wounds, their etiologies, and comorbidities. The more common agents used topically are lidocaine or a mixture of lidocaine and prilocaine. Amitriptyline, a tricyclic antidepressant, has local anesthetic properties and has shown promise as an option for treating wound pain when applied topically.[143] While topical anesthetics may be under scrutiny for their effects, vasoconstriction in particular, there is a need for more investigation since pain is a major issue for most patients with wounds.[144]

Growth Factors

Growth factors are substances that stimulate cell growth and proliferation. These substances serve as the messaging center to signal other cells in the area to act. They usually consist of a group of proteins but can also include hormones. Growth factors normally abound in the fluids of a wound. In most chronic wounds the normal timetable for healing has been delayed or stopped due in part to a decrease in the amount of growth factors in the wound. Growth factors that are decreased or absent can be added topically to the wound bed. Increasing strength of evidence supports the practice of adding growth factors to a wound to facilitate healing. The practice of applying exogenous growth factors in conjunction with good wound care has been accepted for over 20 years.[16,145-148] Growth factors can be isolated from an individual's own tissue, added to a liquid formula in a laboratory, and then applied to the wound. Growth factors can also be cultivated in a laboratory from human platelets and packaged in a gel form. An example of an autologous growth factor product with a name familiar to many clinicians is Aurix System™ (Cytomedix Inc., Gaithersburg, MD 20877).[149] Recombinant DNA technology has resulted in other products such as Becaplermin gel (Regranex® Gel; Smith & Nephew Inc, Andover, MA 01810).[150] Reimbursement for application of growth factors varies and should be checked before use. For example, Becaplermin gel is FDA approved for the treatment of LE diabetic neuropathic ulcers that extend into the subcutaneous tissue or beyond but currently may not be approved for the treatment of pressure, venous, or other nondiabetic-related wounds.

Topical Agents and Acute Wounds

The use of antiseptics and antibiotics to reduce bacterial levels in acute, traumatic wounds follows a different rationale from that of chronic wounds. For wounds resulting from trauma or thermal injury, the risk for contamination is high. It is accepted practice to use cytotoxic products such as povidone-iodine or Silvadene (silver sulfadiazine) in the *early* management of acute traumatic wounds. The goal is to discontinue use of cytotoxic agents as soon as the wounds are clean and able to produce and support endogenous fluids.

Mechanical Modalities

Procedures for use of modalities vary based on unique patient characteristics and individual patient response. A useful place to begin is with protocols recommended in comprehensive wound management texts such as *Wound Healing: Evidence-Based Management* by McCulloch and Kloth[151] and *Wound Care: A Collaborative Practice Manual for Health Professionals* by Sussman and Bates-Jensen.[152] Owing to the ever-changing rules of reimbursement, it is prudent to check current reimbursement and documentation guidelines when billing for these services. The decision to use mechanical modalities rests in the hands of the physical therapist unless physician authorization is required in order to receive reimbursement. The reimbursement requirement may vary from state to state and sometimes between payers in the same state. In some cases, individual physicians may develop their own protocols that require physical therapists to contact them before changing a POC.

Ultrasound

Therapeutic ultrasound (US) application for wound management differs from its use as a modality to treat pain. Ultrasound stimulates cell activity, accelerating processes such as inflammation. Once thought to target only the sluggish wound in the inflammatory stage, evidence now demonstrates that the effects can be seen throughout all wound-healing phases. Basic science evidence and clinical research have established that skin repair and wound contraction can be accelerated, collagen secretion can be stimulated, and elastin properties can be affected to strengthen scar tissue. One option for the treatment is to cover the wound with a sheet of hydrogel or an application of amorphous hydrogel. US is then delivered with a handheld applicator. Another option for treatment is to apply US transmission gel to the periwound area and treat from this region in addition to or instead of the wound bed.[153-155] The newest option for delivery of US is to use a system that provides noncontact, nonthermal, low-frequency ultrasound (Fig. 14.24).

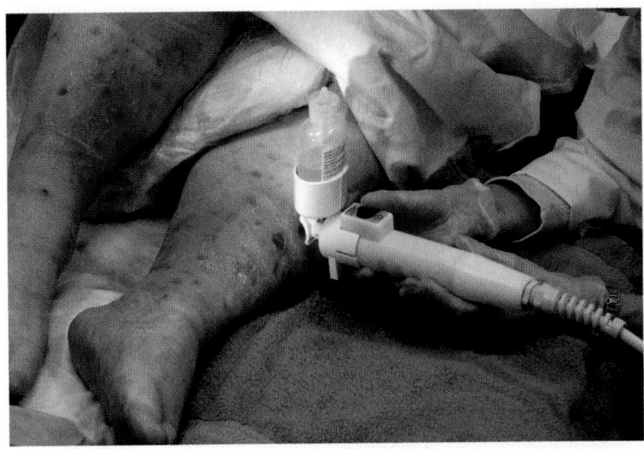

Figure 14.24 Application of noncontact, nonthermal, low-frequency ultrasound treatment to leg wounds. *(Courtesy of Alliqua Biomedical, Yardley, PA 19067.)*

A mist of sterile saline is propelled toward the wound and the ultrasound is transferred from the device to the patient without contact or pain. Studies have provided evidence (Table 14.4) that this type of US treatment reduces bacterial quantity in a wound and promotes healing, especially in wounds that have been slow to heal.[156-162]

Electrical Stimulation

The use of electrical stimulation (ES) to treat chronic and, more recently, acute wounds is well documented. Electrical stimulation is recommended to eliminate bacterial load, promote granulation, decrease inflammation, reduce edema, reduce wound-related pain, and augment blood flow. Human skin, wounds, and the cells that facilitate wound healing all have measurable electrical currents. Electrical stimulation affects various types of

Table 14.4 Evidence Summary Does Non-Contact Low-Frequency Ultrasound (MIST) Decrease the Healing Time of Chronic Wounds?

White, J, et al. Non-contact low-frequency ultrasound therapy compared with UK standard of care for venous leg ulcers: A single-centre, assessor-blinded, randomized controlled trial. Int Wound J. 13(5):833, 2015.

Design	Randomized controlled trial (RCT)
Level of Evidence	1
Subjects	Inclusion: Adults with chronic venous leg ulcers (≥6 weeks and ≤ 5 year durations, between 5 and 100 cm^2 area) and an ankle brachial pressure index of >0.8 Exclusion: Uncontrolled DM (HbA1c >12% in last 3 months), active infection of wound on day of inclusion, renal failure, exposed tendon/ligament/muscle/bone in the ulcer, osteomyelitis/cellulitis/gangrene in the limb, arterial ulcer, pregnant or breastfeeding women, women of child-bearing age not willing to use highly effective contraception, planned surgical procedure during study period for the wound, prior skin replacement/negative-pressure therapy/or ultrasound therapy to the wound 2 weeks prior, radio or chemotherapy currently or within last 3 months, ultrasound required near or on electronic implant or prosthesis, not capable of providing informed consent, enrolled in another trial currently or last 30 days.
Intervention	MIST US was applied to a clean wound bed for 3–12 minutes, dependent upon wound size, three times per week. This was followed by application of a non-adherent dressing and strong compression therapy (3x/wk).
Results	Both control and NLFU groups saw significant improvement in wound size; however, there was no significant difference between the two groups.
Comments	Limitations: difference of frequency between two treatment groups (Standard of Care: At least 1x/wk vs NLFU: 3x/wk).

Beheshti, A, et al. Comparison of high-frequency and MIST ultrasound therapy for the healing of venous leg ulcers. Adv Clin Exp Med 23(6):969, 2014.

Design	Comparative
Level of Evidence	2
Subjects	Inclusion: Wound duration longer than 4 weeks and no clinical improvement after using the clinic's standard of care for healing during a 2-week period. Exclusion: Allergy to ultrasound contact gel, pregnancy, known contraindications to US, ankle or knee prosthesis, metal in lower leg, suspected or confirmed local cancers or metastatic disease and neuropathy, no evidence of infections including active cellulites, suspicious thrombophlebitis and no history of antibiotic therapy at time of enrollment, PAD, DM, or RA.

Continued

Table 14.4 Evidence Summary Does Non-Contact Low-Frequency Ultrasound (MIST) Decrease the Healing Time of Chronic Wounds?—cont'd

Design	Comparative
Intervention	HFU therapy was applied for 5–10 min around edge of the ulcer. Mist therapy delivered low-intensity (0.1–0.8 W/cm^2), low-frequency (40 kHz) ultrasound energy to wound bed for 4–12 min.
Results	No significant difference between groups for complete wound healing duration. No significant difference in edema between groups at 2 months. Significant difference noted in edema in ultrasound groups compared to standard of care at 4 months. Significant reduction in pain in HFU and MIST groups compared to standard of care at 2 months, no significant difference between HFU and MIST.

Ennis, W, et al: Ultrasound therapy for recalcitrant diabetic foot ulcers: Results of a randomized, double-blind, controlled, multicenter study [corrected] [published erratum appears in OSTOMY WOUND MANAGE 2005;51(9):14]. Ostomy Wound Manage. 51(8):24, 2005.

Design	RCT
Level of Evidence	2
Subjects	Inclusion: Subjects over 18 y/o with type 1 or 2 diabetes and a chronic diabetic foot ulcer (>30 days) of Wagner grade 1 or 2 on plantar surface of foot, glycosylated hemoglobin level <12, no exposure of bone/ligament/tendons in the wound, no clinical signs of infection, not currently taking antibiotics.
Intervention	Intervention and control group both received standard of care treatment. Intervention group received US treatment for 4 minutes, device was held 5–15 mm away from the wound bed. Control group received a sham treatment that was designed to simulate the US treatment by providing same parameters of pressure and time to the wound bed. Both interventions were performed 3x/week.
Results	Significant reduction in exudate at 5 weeks in US group compared to control. No significant difference in granulation tissue between groups; 40.7% of US group healed compared to 14.3% of control. Significantly shorter healing time frames found in US group compared to control.
Comments	Despite no clinical evidence of infection in the tissue when evaluated, 86% of US group and 93% of control group showed presence of aerobic bacteria on biopsy. This information was not made available to the investigators during the study and may have had influence on the results.

Kavros, S, et al: Expedited wound healing with noncontact, low-frequency ultrasound therapy in chronic wounds: A retrospective analysis. Adv Skin Wound Care. 21(9):416, 2008.

Design	Retrospective
Level of Evidence	2
Subjects	Inclusion: Below the knee wounds that received MIST therapy 3x/wk for 90 days or until wound healed. Inclusion for compare group: Met criteria for MIST therapy but were not able to accommodate for required 3x/wk treatment visits. Exclusion: Patients who did not meet criteria for US therapy 3x/wk, had significant discontinuity of treatments, did not complete the treatment regimen at the wound center, or had participated in a previous study of MIST therapy in the critical limb ischemia at the wound center.
Intervention	MIST therapy system utilizing noncontact US delivering low-intensity (0/1–0.8 W/cm^2) and low-frequency (40 kHz) ultrasound energy through atomized sterile saline mist to the wound bed. Treatment times ranged from 3–20 minutes based on size of wound.
Results	A faster rate of healing was noted for the patients who received MIST therapy compared to standard of care ($P = 0.002$) and a greater percentage of wounds treated with MIST therapy healed compared to standard of care ($P = 0.009$).

Kavros SJ, Miller JL, and Hanna SW: Treatment of ischemic wounds with noncontact, low-frequency ultrasound: The Mayo clinic experience, 2004-2006. Adv Skin Wound Care. 20(4):221, 2007.

Table 14.4 Evidence Summary Does Non-Contact Low-Frequency Ultrasound (MIST) Decrease the Healing Time of Chronic Wounds?—cont'd

Design	Prospective, parallel, RCT
Level of Evidence	2
Subjects	Inclusion: Non-healing foot/ankle/leg wound with documented critical ischemia present for a minimum of 8 weeks. Exclusion: patients undergoing chemotherapy and patients unable or unwilling to attend 3 treatment sessions per week.
Intervention	MIST therapy was delivered with low-intensity (0.1 W–0.8 W/cm^2), low-frequency (40 kHz) US energy via saline mist to wound bed without directly contacting the body or wound. This was performed three times a week in conjunction with standard care.
Results	Significant improvement in wound healing noted at 12 weeks in intervention group compared to standard care alone.

Olyaie, M, et al: High-frequency and noncontact low-frequency ultrasound therapy for venous leg ulcer treatment: A randomized, controlled study. Ostomy Wound Manage. 59(8):14, 2013.

Design	RCT
Level of Evidence	2
Subjects	Inclusion: Patient with a venous leg ulcer >4 weeks that did not respond to standard of care treatment for 2 weeks. Exclusion: Patients who were pregnant or who had a known allergy to US gel, known US contraindications, history of antibiotic therapy at time of enrollment, RA, DM, or peripheral artery disease (ABI < 0.8 or signs of artery disease).
Intervention	HFU: High-intensity (0.5–1 W/cm^2), high-frequency (1–3 MHz) ultrasound was applied for 5–10 minutes to skin surrounding ulcer. NCLFU: Low-intensity (0.1–0.8 W/cm^2), low-frequency (40 kHz) ultrasound was delivered to wound bed using atomized sterile saline mist without direct contact to the body or wound. Treatment time was based on total wound area ranging from 3–20 minutes.
Results	At 4-month follow-up, the HFU and NCLFU showed significant improvement in wound size ($P = 0.04$) compared to standard of care alone. Significant difference was also noted in edema and pain rating at 4-month follow-up in HFU and NCLFU compared to standard of care ($P < 0.05$).
Comments	Limitations: Small sample size and use of perpendicular axis for measurement of wound bed. Researchers note use of more precise imaging and histopathological assessment methods may have enhanced study accuracy.

Yao, M, et al: A pilot study evaluating non-contact low-frequency ultrasound and underlying molecular mechanism on diabetic foot ulcers. Int Wound J 11(6):586, 2014.

Design	Prospective RCT pilot study
Level of Evidence	2
Subjects	Inclusion: age 18–90 yo, DM I/II, presence of chronic diabetic foot wound (0.5–15 cm^2 area) of Wagner grade 1 or 2, $TcPO_2$ >30 mm Hg or ABI >0.6. Exclusion: Treatment with non-contact US during the 4 weeks prior to study, LE malignancy (either limb), critical limb ischemia, local infection of limb with the target ulcer, systemic infection, pregnancy, end stage renal disease, severe liver disease, venous leg ulcer with or without DM, or known/suspected lidocaine allergy.
Intervention	NCLFU therapy was utilized with a frequency of 40 kHZ and an intensity ranging from 0.2–0.6 W/cm^2. The transducer was held 0.5–1.5 cm away from wound bed and US waves were delivered in a continuous mode through a sterile saline mist. Treatment duration varied with wound area with a single session lasting approximately 5 min.

Continued

Table 14.4 Evidence Summary Does Non-Contact Low-Frequency Ultrasound (MIST) Decrease the Healing Time of Chronic Wounds?—cont'd

Design	Prospective RCT pilot study
Results	Subjects who received NCLFU three times per week showed significant wound area reduction at weeks 3, 4, and 5 compared to control and those who received NCLFU one time per week (*P* <0.05). Biochemical and histological analyses showed trend toward reduction of pro-inflammatory cytokines, matrix metalloproteinase-9, vascular endothelial growth factor, and macrophages in both NCLFU groups.
Comments	Researchers of this pilot study note the need for more research in the area to determine possible effects of NCLFU on pro-inflammatory cytokines.

ABI = Ankle–Brachial Index; DM = Diabetes mellitus; HFU = High-frequency ultrasound; LE = Lower extremity; NCLFU = Noncontact low-frequency ultrasound; PAD = Peripheral artery disease; RA = Rheumatoid arthritis; US = Ultrasound.

cells and their activities by supporting, altering, or providing electrical currents to accelerate wound healing. A clear understanding of medical electricity will assist the clinician in applying an appropriate ES treatment. The available literature is diverse and instructive.[163-170] There are a variety of options for treatment setup, depending on the goals of treatment, the type of wound, and the condition of the patient. Standard equipment for the direct method of application will include an ES unit, treatment and nontreatment electrodes, and a substance such as saline-soaked gauze or a hydrogel dressing applied to the wound bed or cavity to enhance electrical conductivity under the treatment electrode (Fig. 14.25). For the indirect method, gel electrodes straddle the wound and interface with the periwound skin. Clinical decisions related to voltage, electrode placement, dosage, and other variables must be made on a case-by-case basis. Information about treatment protocols, strength of evidence, and guidelines for treatment can be found in detailed wound care texts.[171,172]

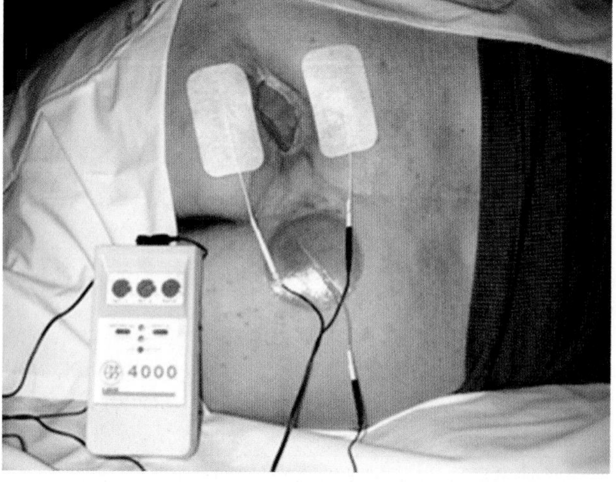

Figure 14.25 Conductively coupled bipolar treatment electrodes of opposite polarity positioned on opposite sides of a wound. *(From McCulloch and Kloth: Wound Healing: Evidence-Based Management, ed 4. FA Davis, Philadelphia, Figure 26–28, with permission.)*

Thermal and Nonthermal Diathermy

Pulsed shortwave diathermy (PSWD), continuous shortwave diathermy (CSWD), and nonthermal pulsed radiofrequency stimulation (PRFS) have been used successfully to treat chronic open wounds, facilitating progress from one phase of wound healing to the next. These diathermy treatments utilize radio waves to provide thermal and nonthermal effects, respectively. All models transmit radiation from an applicator head to the target tissues. PSWD heats superficial and deep tissues. CSWD heats deep muscle and joint tissues. PRFS is nonthermal and can influence tissue at the cellular level. Individuals with arterial insufficiency are not good candidates for PSWD or CSWD because their tissues are not able to dissipate heat well enough to avoid burns. Wound sites treated with diathermy have demonstrated increased fibroblast proliferation, collagen formation, tissue perfusion, and metabolic rate. The number of clinical studies is smaller than that of other modalities, and there are only a few well-controlled clinical studies. The evidence for the role diathermy plays in wound healing will need to be stronger for this modality to be readily utilized in clinical settings. Physical therapists have used diathermy for wound care since the publication of a number of studies regarding the nonthermal effects of pulsed diathermy and the production of smaller, more portable, user-friendly diathermy units.[173,174] Equipment needed for treatment includes a diathermy unit/electronic console and one or two applicator heads. Treatment is usually delivered without touching the skin. Wounds should be carefully prepared before treatment according to guidelines provided by the distributor.

Ultraviolet Radiation

Ultraviolet (UV) radiation energy is a form of radiation between x-ray and visible light on the electromagnetic spectrum.[175] UV wavelengths have been divided into wavelengths and bands. The three bands most useful for their effects on human skin are UVA, UVB, and UVC. UV has cutaneous and bactericidal effects that include increased blood flow, enhanced granulation tissue formation, destruction of bacteria, stimulation of vitamin D production, and thickening of the stratum corneum. The varied physiological effects make this treatment appropriate for a variety of skin diseases, as well as acute and chronic wounds.[153] The effects of UV radiation on antibiotic-resistant bacteria make it a potentially effective tool in wound care; however, there are only a few up-to-date, well-controlled clinical studies emerging at this time.[176,177] Early supporting literature is now quite dated, leaving room for new clinical studies to provide evidence of the efficacy of the intervention. UVC in particular has been found to be effective in the treatment of *methicillin-resistant Staphylococcus aureus* (MRSA), *vancomycin-resistant Enterococcus* (VRE), and some strains of *Pseudomonas aeruginosa*.[178,179] The treatment is typically delivered to a clean wound with dressings removed, using a UVB or UVC lamp. Treatment distance, dosage, frequency, and subsequent clinical outcomes will vary based on the goals of the treatment and the status of the wound.[180] Handheld UV units to treat wounds can be obtained through Biomation at www.biomation.com/wound. Physical therapists planning to utilize UV for wound care might partner with a wound care team, a resourceful vendor, and the latest evidence to devise a treatment plan.

Hyperbaric Oxygen Therapy

Hyperbaric oxygen therapy (HBOT) delivers 100% oxygen to an individual resting inside a sealed chamber. The oxygen is delivered at a pressure greater than the atmosphere. This *systemic* treatment increases the amount of oxygen available for cell metabolism, improving oxygen delivery to hypoxic tissue. Systemic HBOT is, however, associated with risks related to oxygen toxicity. The literature demonstrates positive responses to this treatment when used as an adjunct to other forms of wound care but few controlled, randomized trials have been completed.[153,181-183] Chambers to deliver *topical* oxygen have been available for at least a decade. These smaller chambers enclose a limb or a segment of the body instead of requiring coverage of the entire body.

Following physician referral, a physical therapist may assist or coordinate a systemic or topical treatment. Often, a trained technician will manage the equipment controls and the delivery chamber. Wound care may occur before or after the HBOT or the topical HBOT, depending on the preferences of the physician and the protocol of the facility. Discussion among investigators comparing the effects of systemic versus topical oxygen is ongoing. In some studies, topical oxygen is also referred to as *topical hyperbaric oxygen* (THBO) and *O_2 therapy*.[12,184] Instead of the full-body chamber used for HBOT, THBO is portable and is delivered in a localized limb chamber.[12,184,185] THBO has been combined with electrical stimulation and also with cold laser for the treatment of pressure injuries and neuropathic foot wounds.[186] Investigations have examined whether topical O_2 therapy will enhance the effects of growth factors but there is a lack of high-level evidence at this time. Renewed interest by investigators should lead to more refined protocols and improved strength of evidence in the field.[187] If investigations continue to provide positive results, the use of topical O_2 in wound care could result in more cost-effective and efficient care, fewer risks, and applicability to a wider population as compared to systemic O_2.

Negative Pressure Wound Therapy

Negative pressure wound therapy (NPWT) is used as an adjunct to wound healing to facilitate wound closure in acute surgical wounds, as well as with more challenging, slow-to-heal wounds. The procedure is known by several terms but the most well-known is *vacuum-assisted closure* or *VAC*® (Kinetic Concepts, Inc., San Antonio, TX 78265). An open cell foam dressing is placed in the wound and a suction tube is connected from the foam to a portable pump. An airtight seal is created over the foam and the suction tube with a clear, occlusive film (Figs. 14.26, 14.27, and 14.28). A controlled amount of negative (subatmospheric) pressure is applied through the foam to the entire wound bed. Typically, for the first few days (48 hours) the negative pressure is applied continuously via the portable pump system. After a significant amount of excess wound fluid has been withdrawn, the pump is programmed to apply pressure intermittently. The foam dressing is changed every 12 hours (infected wounds) to 48 hours or longer (clean wounds). A recent addition to the features of the wound VAC is an automated system that will rinse a wound regularly with either saline or an antiseptic or antibiotic solution and then remove the fluids with the regular suction treatment. This feature is most often recommended for the severely infected orthopedic and trauma wounds.[188] The strength of evidence is mounting as basic research explores the effects of this treatment.

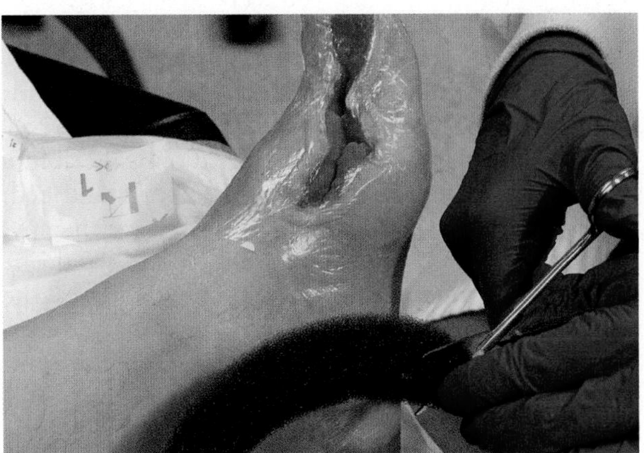

Figure 14.26 Reticulated foam dressing is cut to the shape of the wound outline in preparation for applying NPWT.

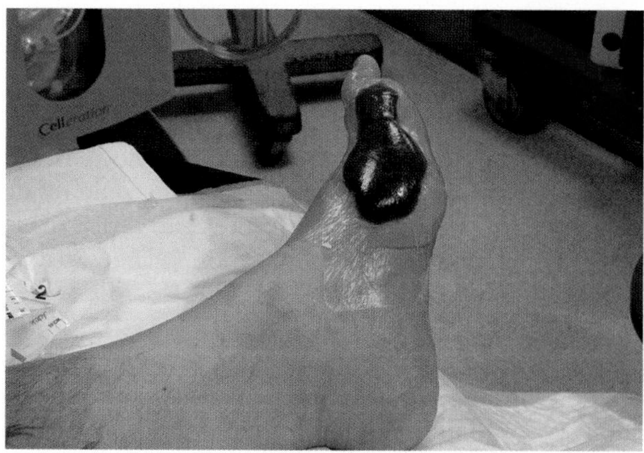

Figure 14.27 Reticulated foam dressing covered with a polyurethane sheet before tubing and suction are applied.

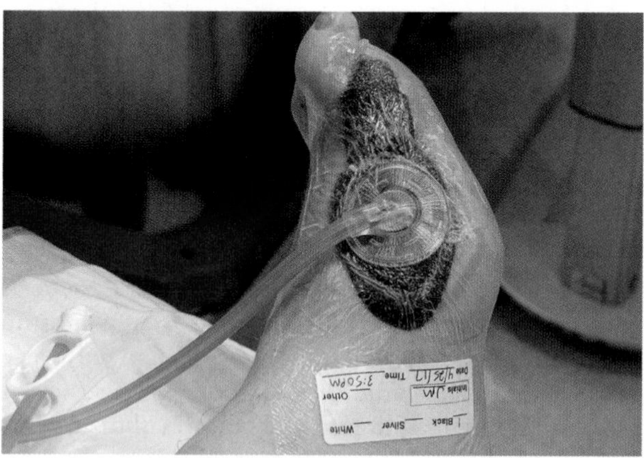

Figure 14.28 A wound treated with a NPWT with reticulated foam dressing, tubing, and polyurethane sheet covering the entire wound to maintain the vacuum during treatment with vacuum-assisted closure.

NPWT has been shown to enhance granulation tissue formation, promote wound edge approximation, remove edema from wounds, and improve oxygen levels in the wound.[189-194] Studies have also shown that with the use of NPWT, the healing time for selected wounds decreased in comparison to standard wound care.[195,196] One claim that is still under investigation is the ability of the VAC to remove bacteria from the wound bed. Although a physician must order this type of therapy, many are unaware of this intervention and would be responsive to an appropriate recommendation by the therapist. In different environments, physical therapists, nurses, or other clinical staff may perform administration of the technique.

Cold Laser Therapy

Cold laser is also referred to in the literature as *low-level cold laser, low-level infrared laser,* or *monochromatic infrared photo energy* (MIRE). Low-energy laser treatment uses light in the infrared spectrum. This therapy has been promoted for augmenting wound healing[197] and reversing the symptoms of peripheral neuropathy in individuals with diabetes.[198] It is thought that the effects of laser may increase circulation and reduce pain by increasing the release of nitric oxide into the microcirculation. Supportive, peer-reviewed literature is modest, published studies citing success with this treatment are inconclusive as investigative debates continue.[199-201] Despite the term *cold laser,* light in the infrared spectrum can also be used to deliver heat as a treatment modality. Owing to the perceived lack of adequate evidence, some third-party payers do not cover cold laser treatment except when used as a heat modality.

Dressings

The type of wound dressings selected for a wound may have a profound effect on healing time. There are hundreds of choices for the discerning clinician. Information on indications, contraindications, and expected outcomes can be obtained from individual vendors listed in Appendix 14.E, as well as from texts devoted entirely to wound care.[151,152] Physical therapists who are monitoring a wound on a regular basis and are knowledgeable about dressing alternatives are often the most appropriate clinicians to make the decision about dressing selections. This chapter includes introductory information necessary to make clinical decisions about dressings: the characteristics of the dressing categories and the effects of the dressings on the wound bed.

The dressing that is applied directly to the wound is referred to as the *primary* dressing. The dressing that is applied over the primary dressing is referred to as the *secondary* dressing. Some advanced dressings serve as the primary and secondary, including adhesive and absorptive qualities in the same dressing. Choosing or recommending appropriate dressings should be directed by the characteristics of the wound and periwound tissues, not by what is available in the supply closet. A product that preserves wound hydration by limiting or controlling fluid loss is usually ideal. To understand the wide range of options and to assist in selecting the appropriate dressing, refer to Appendix 14.F for a listing of dressings categorized by treatment goal (purpose) and also by type of wound (indication).

Gauze/Fiber

Gauze dressings (Fig. 14.29) are considered by many wound management experts to be outside the description of modern wound dressings.[114] Used and misused for decades, there are more reasons not to use gauze than there are indications for use. As a primary dressing, gauze leaves contaminating fibers in the wound, contributes to desiccation, is permeable to bacteria, can be adherent to the wound, releases excessive amounts of bacteria into the air on removal, causes a loss of normothermia, and is painful on removal if it adheres to the wound surface.

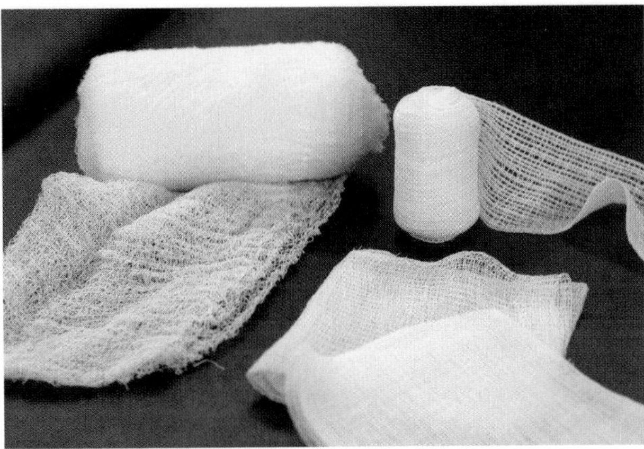

Figure 14.29 Samples of gauze dressings.

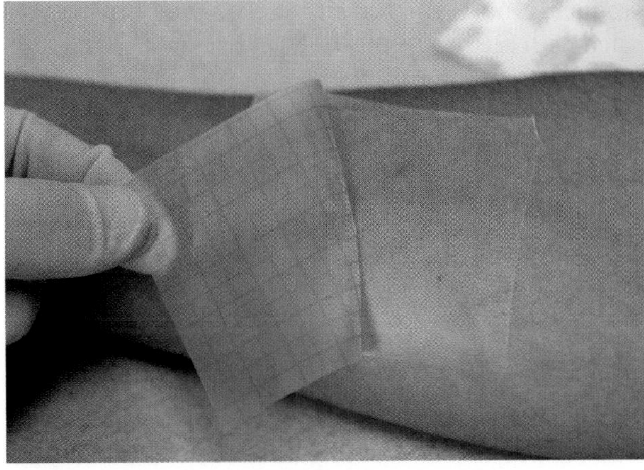

Figure 14.30 Application of a film dressing.

Once thought to be cost-effective, it has been shown in more than one study to be more costly than other dressing choices. Gauze ribbon can be used to maintain an opening for drainage in a tunneling wound. It can also be used successfully to gently support a cavity wound but should not be used to aggressively pack any shape of wound. It was once thought that cavity wounds should be packed very full but it has since been established that granulation tissue and epithelial cells do not flourish with aggressive gauze packing. The additional pressure from a tightly packed wound will impede the flow of oxygen and nutrients to the granulating wound bed. Gauze can be an effective secondary dressing, especially if the dressings will be changed frequently or if exudate is heavy. Gauze 4 × 4s and a roll of gauze are typically used to create a WTD dressing. WTD dressings were previously discussed under the section on débridement because of their nonselective removal of tissue during dressing changes. Because WTD dressings can be classified as a tool for mechanical débridement or as a primary wound dressing, they are discussed in both categories. Refer to that section of the chapter for more details.

Impregnated Gauze

Designed to be less adherent, this category includes products made of tightly meshed synthetic fibers or woven products such as cellulose acetate. Fiber materials are impregnated with a petroleum emulsion such as Vaseline®, intended to prevent the gauze from sticking to the wound surface. Used as a primary dressing this choice is minimally absorptive, provides minimal protection, does not enhance a moist environment, and may create a greasy wound bed. One of its more appropriate uses is as a primary dressing over new sutures to prevent them from catching or sticking in a gauze secondary dressing.

Transparent Films

Films are made of a transparent membrane with an acrylic adhesive layer (Fig.. 14.30). Transparent films do not allow bacteria or moisture into the wound. They facilitate a moist wound environment, trapping endogenous fluids in the wound bed to assist with autolytic débridement, wound bed homeostasis, and *angiogenesis.* Films assist in protecting skin from the effects of shearing, friction, and the contaminating effects of incontinence. Removal of a film dressing must be done with great caution because this can cause skin tears, especially with fragile or aging skin. Currently, few films have absorptive qualities and cannot be used on highly exuding wounds.

Foam

Foams are highly absorbent pads, sheets, or ropes of polyurethane or polyvinyl alcohol available in many sizes with many features (Fig. 14.31). They are available with or without adhesive backing so that they can be used as a primary and/or a secondary dressing. Foam dressings are highly absorptive but also help to create an occlusive environment for moist wound healing. They should not be used alone on a dry wound but could serve as a secondary dressing if the primary dressing was a gel

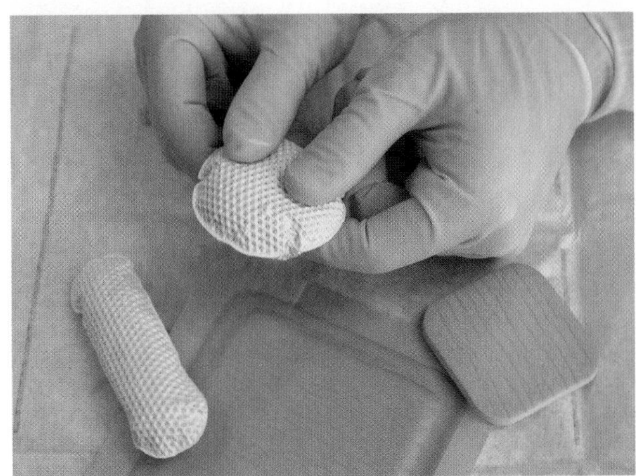

Figure 14.31 Samples of foam dressings.

product. One of the newest foam dressings is impregnated with methylene blue and gentian violet to provide broad-spectrum antibacterial protection (Fig. 14.32). Methylene blue and gentian violet are nontoxic organic pigments that assist in controlling bioburden without the risk of being cytotoxic to living tissue. Since the blue pigments do not absorb into the skin, the dressings can be used for long periods of time as the wound closes and heals.[202,203]

Hydrogels

Hydrogels are categorized as *amorphous,* referring to a liquid-like gel, or as *sheets,* consisting of a thin, flexible sheet of polymer containing at least 90% water (Fig. 14.33). Both types are used to increase moisture in a dry wound bed, soften necrotic tissue, and support autolytic débridement. Both have some absorptive qualities and will swell slightly until they are saturated. The amorphous gel (Fig. 14.34) must be contained in the wound with a secondary dressing. The flexible sheets usually require a secondary dressing but are available through some vendors with tape attached to the borders. Patient response is usually very positive to the soothing sensation of the hydrogel application.

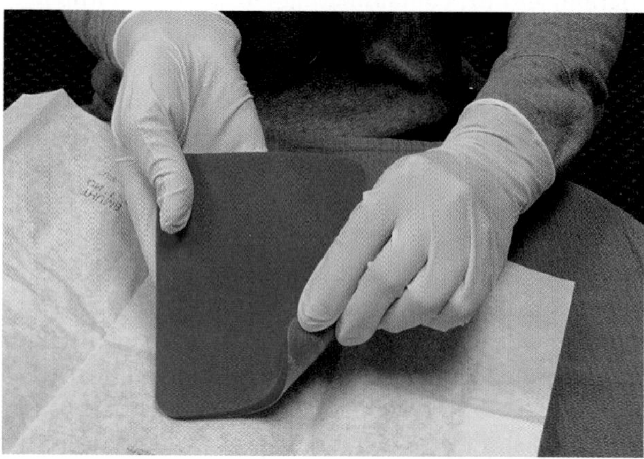

Figure 14.32 Sample of a gentian violet and methylene blue antibacterial foam dressing.

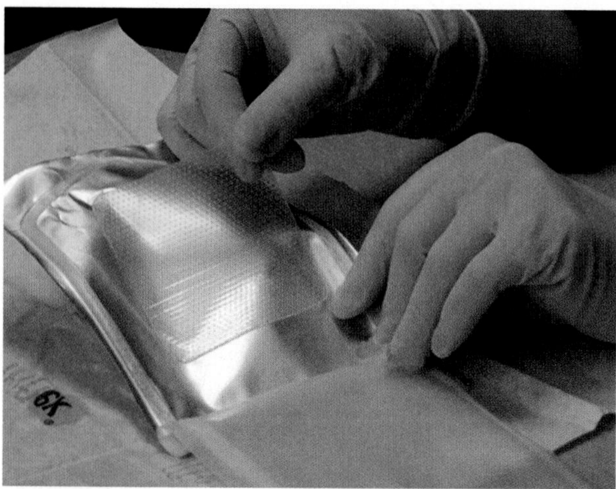

Figure 14.33 Sample of a hydrogel sheet dressing.

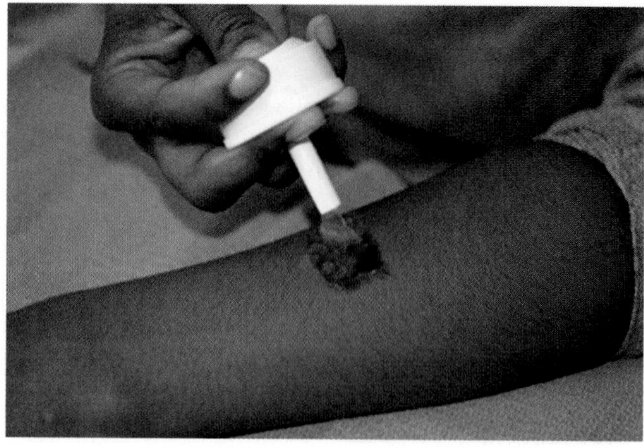

Figure 14.34 Application of an amorphous gel dressing.

Hydrocolloids

Considered the most occlusive of the moisture-retentive dressings, hydrocolloids are also available in less occlusive or semipermeable styles as well. As with foams, these dressings come in a variety of styles and shapes, including pastes, granules, powder, and sheets. They typically consist of an absorbent colloidal material combined with a film or foam backing (Fig. 14.35). Hydrocolloid dressings work best on mild to moderate exudating wounds. When wound exudate combines with the colloidal polymer, a soft, gelatinous, often yellow, and malodorous mass is formed. Patients, families, caregivers, and other health care providers must be informed about this harmless reaction so that infection is not assumed. Hydrocolloids have been used successfully as occlusive dressings over infected wounds without fulmination of existing bacteria. They are also the dressing of choice to cover and protect larvae during maggot débridement therapy.

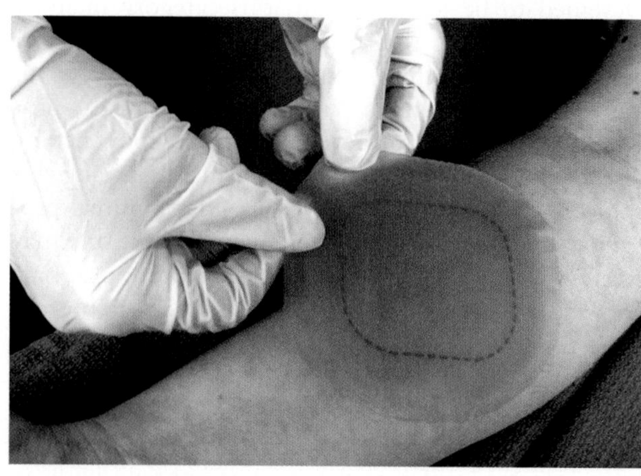

Figure 14.35 Sample of a hydrocolloid dressing.

Alginates

This dressing category is also known as *calcium alginate* because the dressings are manufactured using the calcium salts of alginic acid derived from marine algae and kelp (seaweed). The raw material is woven and then converted into flat sheets, ropes, or ribbon shapes (Fig. 14.36). Alginates absorb 20 to 30 times their own weight, are gentle to apply and remove, and are biocompatible with the wound bed. A chemical reaction between the dressing and wound exudate creates a gel substance that helps to maintain a moist wound environment while absorbing excess exudate. Because they are permeable, alginates do not provide a barrier against bacteria. This characteristic makes them an effective choice when an infected wound cannot be covered with an occlusive dressing. Most alginates currently require a secondary dressing to hold them in place. Several manufacturers are combining alginates with other products, such as hydrocolloids, to maximize their effectiveness. There is growing interest in the use of silver in advanced dressings to combine the antimicrobial action of silver with the absorptive qualities of alginates. Long-term effects remain unclear. There is a need for more clinical trials and longer follow-up times to look at the long-term effects on healing.[204]

Hydrofibers

Hydrofiber or hydroactive dressings are designed to have a selective absorptive capacity. They have the combined positive characteristics of alginate, foam, and gel dressings. When in contact with the wound, the synthetic fibers absorb exudate and align themselves perpendicular to the wound surface. This vertical wicking process keeps debris and wound fluid contained within the dressing.[205] There is considerably less pain on removal of a hydrofiber dressing because the fibers do not stick to the wound or dry out.[205,206] The dressing properties allow growth factors and other peptides to survive on the wound bed. Aquacel® is a spun Hydrofiber™ dressing that readily absorbs moisture (Fig. 14.37). Aquacel® Ag adds ionic silver to the absorbent dressing (ConvaTec, Skillman, NJ 08558).

Composite Dressings

Composite dressings represent a general category of wound dressings that combine different types of dressings into a single dressing. They usually have three layers that each have their own functions. The layer closest to the wound will allow moisture to pass through and will be non-stick. The next layer will be absorbent, pulling drainage away from the wound. The outer layer will usually be waterproof so that the wound is protected but drainage can't leak out as easily. A composite dressing could be a primary or secondary dressing.

Biological Dressings/Skin Substitutes

Considered by some to be topical applications and by others to be dressings, human skin equivalents and bioengineered tissues are finding their place in the wound care arena. Skin substitutes are created using a variety of techniques and substances. Cells are derived from sources such as neonatal male foreskin and porcine (pig) dermal collagen. The products are produced in laboratories, shipped either frozen or cooled, and then applied to the patient's wound by a member of the wound care team. Although a physician would prescribe the use of a skin substitute, other health care professionals can apply the product to the wound based on individual facility protocol. Skin substitutes consist of living skin applications that resemble skin structure and function and may include epidermal and dermal layers. They are useful as temporary coverage, providing skin protection for the wound bed. Some have been shown to stimulate endogenous cell activity. Most are marketed to use on wounds that have not responded to conventional therapy such as chronic diabetic foot ulcers, venous leg ulcers, and deep burn wounds.[207] Examples to look for when

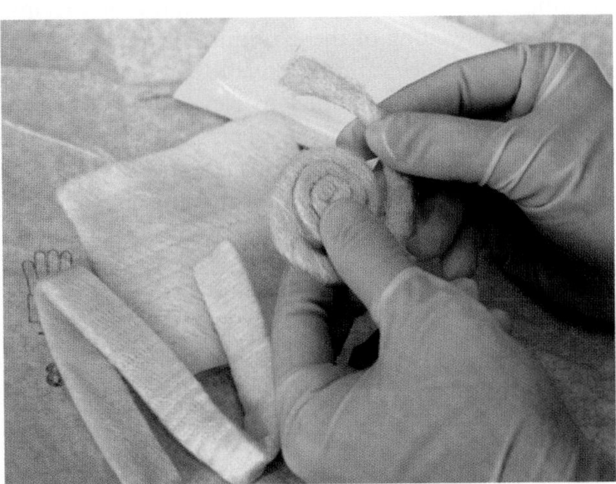

Figure 14.36 Samples of alginate dressings.

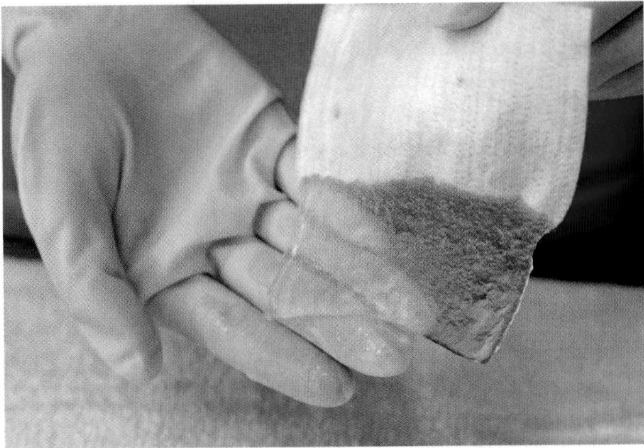

Figure 14.37 Sample of a synthetic fiber dressing simulating the change in consistency from dry to gel as wound drainage is absorbed.

investigating skin substitutes are Apligraf® (Novartis, East Hanover, NJ 07936), Dermagraft® (Organogenesis, Canton, MA 02021) and Biobrane™ (Smith & Nephew, Auckland, New Zealand 1140).[208]

Innovative Dressings

New products are entering the market yearly as research and development continue to grow and expand in the area of wound care. One of the driving forces in the creation of new products is the ever-growing list of resistant bacterial strains. Cost is another factor that drives development as clinicians search for the most economical dressing that will establish the ideal wound environment, facilitate débridement, maintain moisture, absorb bacteria and decrease the number of dressing changes. New products are too numerous to mention all but include options such as polysaccharide dressings, absorptive fillers, hydrophilic fiber, dressings that contain collagen, new skin substitutes, and dressings made with a hyaluronic acid derivative applied directly to the wound.

Manual Lymphatic Drainage

MLD is a specialized manual therapy technique that affects primarily superficial lymphatic circulation. It is considered to be one of the five elements of an effective treatment intervention for lymphedema and many types of edema. This manual therapy provides a gentle stretch to the skin that enhances lymph capillary activity. MLD will increase the frequency of lymphangion contractions; improve lymph transport capacity; redirect lymph flow toward collateral vessels, anastomoses, and uninvolved lymph regions; and mobilize excess lymph fluid that has overwhelmed a body segment or region.[72,209] The techniques of MLD are gentle and specific, requiring specialized education to be performed accurately (Fig. 14.38). To obtain contact information for training facilities that provide specialized education in MLD as a part of CDT, refer to the special section in Appendix 14.D for contact information. The benefits of this treatment are not limited to the population with lymphedema. MLD is used successfully for edema from CVI, sports injury, neurological injury, and post-operative swelling, but there is a need for more well-designed randomized controlled trials to provide high-ranking evidence.[210,211] The use of MLD is contraindicated for treating cardiac-, pulmonary-, or renal-related edema because the amount of fluid that will be mobilized may overwhelm one or all of those systems when disease is present.[212]

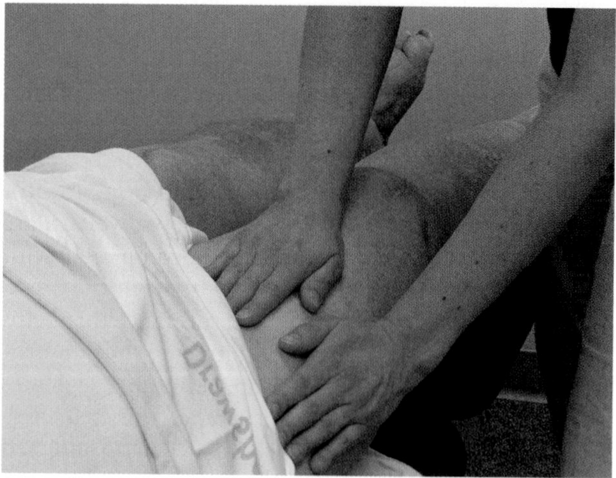

Figure 14.38 Manual lymphatic drainage on the LE.

Compression Therapy

Controlling edema or lymphedema is critical to all stages of healing. Edema inhibits wound healing primarily by affecting perfusion of tissues. Unless there are red flags, compression should be part of every treatment for individuals with lymphedema, edema, and CVI. Compression therapy should be introduced as soon as clinical signs of swelling or fibrosis appear. A physical therapist may find indications for compression therapy during the examination or later, during the intervention. In most situations, the therapist will decide what type and/or style of compression should be applied. Physician authorization, however, may be necessary for reimbursement. When leg wounds are present, compression is essential for timely wound healing. For the individual with mixed arterial and venous disease, an ABI test is indicated to provide information about the safety of using compression on the LE. A greater understanding of how the lymphatic system functions has created a paradigm shift in the way intervention for all types of swelling is planned and delivered. Aggressive compression techniques were once used to "milk" the fluid out of a limb. It is now understood that deep pressure and mechanical "milking" techniques are counterproductive and harmful to the superficial capillary network that filters lymph and interstitial fluids.[4]

Elevation

Elevation is used as a means of controlling some types of swelling and is often a precursor to compression therapy. Mild, acute swelling of the extremities may be relieved temporarily with elevation. Active ROM exercises (e.g., ankle pumps) can be added to elevation to facilitate blood flow in the extremities. Patients should be educated about how to elevate safely, paying attention to positioning so that optimal venous and lymphatic circulation is facilitated. Elevation should be viewed as a temporary or complementary measure while other means of controlling swelling are employed.

Unna's Boot

Compression for the LE with a venous wound can be applied using zinc paste–impregnated gauze or Unna's boot. The moist gauze roll is wrapped over the wound, around the foot and ankle, and then covered with compression bandaging. It is an inexpensive means of covering a wound, providing compression, and supporting the calf pump to empty venous blood from the LE. For the appropriate patient, an Unna's boot can be left in place for up to 1 week. Examples of conveniently packaged products are Medicopaste® (Graham-Field, Atlanta, GA 30360), Unna-FLEX® (ConvaTec, Skillman, NJ 08558), and Gelo-Cast® (BSN-JOBST, Charlotte, NC 28209). Despite the abundance of materials available for applying the boot, there is little information in the literature to support the topical application of zinc for wound healing. The success of this treatment application is most likely owing to the compression. Unna's boot is not appropriate for arterial or mixed arterial/venous ulcers due to the potentially negative effects of compression when arterial disease is present. Although the treatment is used frequently, there are other methods for combining compression with wound care to treat venous wounds.[213,214]

Four-Layer Bandage System

Similar to the Unna boot, yet distinctive, four-layer compression bandaging systems have been designed for the management of venous leg ulcers. The systems include a wound covering with modest absorptive qualities and several layers of different types of compression bandaging. The bandage system has been shown to be comfortable and cost-effective, but new literature compares the four-layer systems to other types of compression and finds that there are other options that may be even more cost effective.[215,216] An example of a well-known system is Profore® (Smith & Nephew, Largo, FL 33773). For the appropriate patient, a four-layer bandage system can be left in place for up to 1 week. As with all compression, watch for signs of ischemia, don't use with an ABI below .8, and rule out arterial disease before using.

Long-Stretch and Short-Stretch Bandages

Both long-stretch and short-stretch bandages are used to control edema and to supply therapeutic levels of compression to support the venous and lymphatic systems. Long-stretch bandages such as Ace™ (3M, St. Paul, MN 55144) bandages provide a *high resting pressure,* which means that they continue to constrict when the wearer is resting. Owing to their extensibility or stretchiness, they do not provide significant *working pressure,* the ability to resist muscle contraction during activity. Long-stretch bandages are readily available and require minimal training to apply. Short-stretch bandages such as Comprilan® (BSN Medical, Charlotte, NC 28209) and Rosidal (Lohmann & Rauscher, Topeka, KS 66619) provide *low resting pressure* and *high working pressure* (Fig. 14.39). They are less extensible or stretchy, providing a more rigid shell when applied to a limb. This feature makes short-stretch bandages more appropriate for treating edema and lymphedema. Higher working pressures increase the efficiency of the muscle pump during activity, whereas lower resting pressures make the bandages more tolerable to wear. The appropriate application

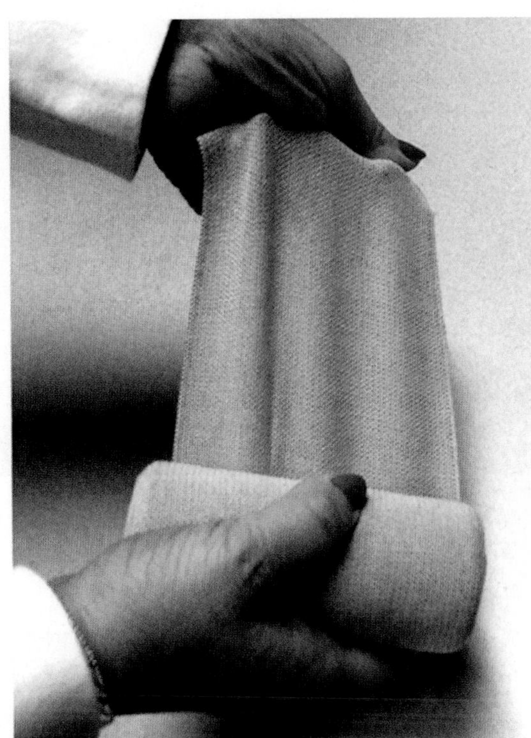

Figure 14.39 Sample of short-stretch bandage.

of short-stretch bandages is a complex skill that requires special training to utilize safely. For a successful outcome as an intervention to reduce, support or retain limb size, a physical therapist will need training, experience, knowledge and clinical intuition. The amount of working and resting pressure delivered to a limb that is bandaged will depend on several important factors: the number of layers of bandage, the age and condition of the bandages, the tension on the bandage when it is applied, and the skill of the clinician.[217]

Lymphedema Bandaging

This highly specialized form of bandaging utilizes multiple layers of unique padding materials and short-stretch bandages to create a supportive structure for edematous and lymphedematous body segments. Lymphedema bandaging provides support for tissues that have lost elasticity; facilitates a mild increase in tissue pressure, assisting lymph vessels to empty; prevents refilling of the interstitium between MLD treatments; improves the efficiency of the muscle pump during activity; and provides localized pressure where indicated to soften fibrotic tissue.

Bandaging protocols include techniques for applying compression to the head and neck, fingers, and hands (Figs. 14.40 and 14.41), the UE (Fig. 14.42), and the LE (Fig. 14.43). The chest, abdomen, genital area, and back can also receive specialized support from compression products.[217]

As with MLD, the benefits of this treatment are not limited to the population with lymphedema. When

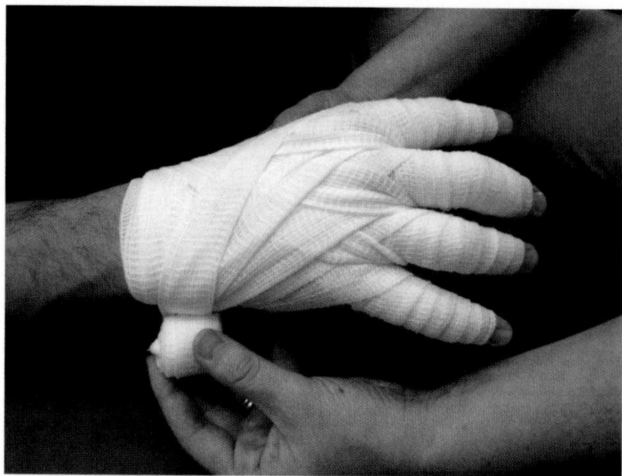

Figure 14.40 Application of lymphedema bandaging to fingers and hand.

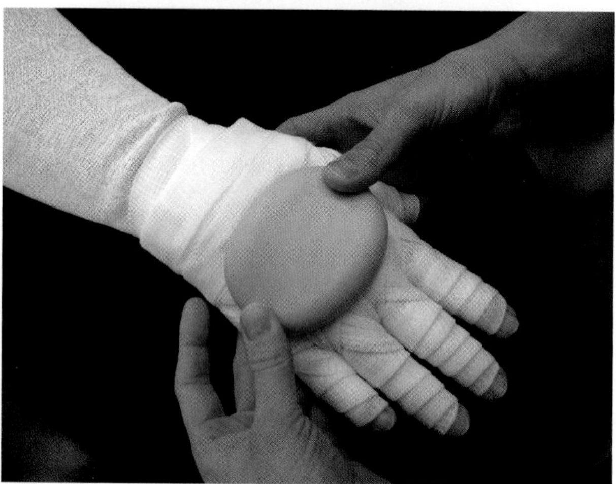

Figure 14.41 Use of foam padding to enhance the effects of lymphedema bandaging.

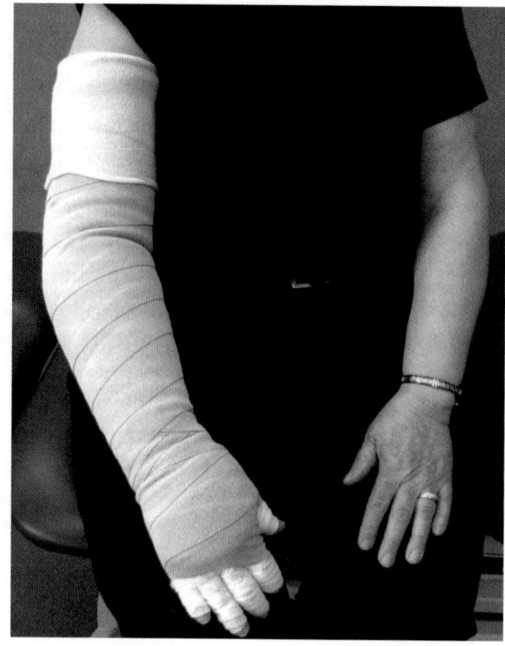

Figure 14.42 Lymphedema bandaging of the UE.

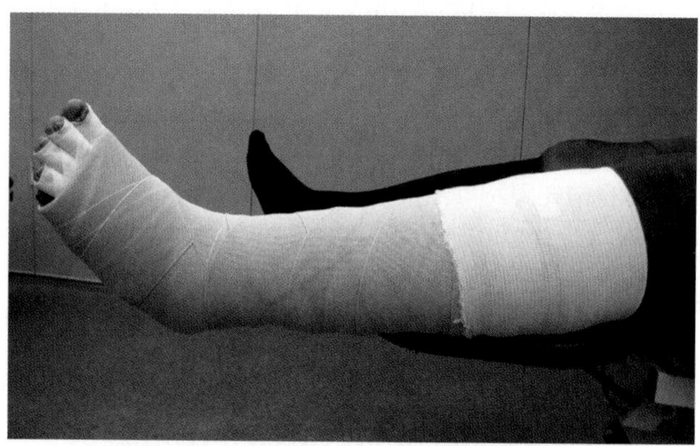

Figure 14.43 Lymphedema bandaging of the foot, ankle, and calf.

compression is indicated, standard or modified lymphedema bandaging can be beneficial to the population with edema (e.g., postoperative, CVI, venous ulcers, orthopedic injury).[218-223] To obtain contact information for training facilities that provide specialized education in bandaging as a part of CDT, refer to Appendix 14.D.

Compression Garments

Many patient/client populations use compression garments (Fig. 14.44). Originally designed to assist venous blood flow in the LEs, they are now specifically designed to manage burn and surgical scars, provide support to venous circulation, and prevent re-accumulation of fluid in the lymphedematous limb. There are a variety of garment styles and fabrics, custom and off-the-shelf, to meet the unique needs of different populations. Varying amounts of pressure are woven into the fabric during manufacturing. The amounts of pressure are conveyed as millimeters of mercury (mm Hg). Low pressure would start at 12 to 25 mm Hg and higher pressures go up to 30 to 40 mm Hg. It is important to understand that garments must be appropriately selected and fitted by a trained professional. When worn correctly by a patient who has been prepared for garment wear and educated about compression, the garments serve an essential role in managing chronic, lifelong conditions such as CVI and lymphedema.[217,223]

Garments should not be used as a treatment to remove excess fluids from an extremity. If applied to an extremity that has not been adequately evacuated, the garments will be uncomfortable and may worsen the patient's symptoms.[224-226] Currently, manufacturers are participating in clinical research supporting the use of silver in compression garments. Juzo® (Juzo, Cuyahoga Falls, OH 44223) adds permanently bonded silver to the textile

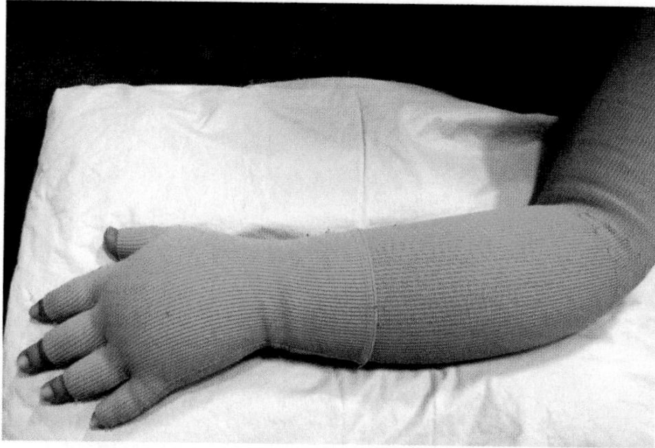

Figure 14.44 Patient wearing custom-fitted UE compression sleeve and separate glove with open fingertips.

fiber of LE garments such as stockings to inhibit bacterial growth and reduce odor.

Limb Containment Systems

Another option for some individuals is a quilted compression device or limb containment system. These unique compression options may be easier to don and doff, can be worn under short stretch wraps or alone, and can be custom made to any part of the body (Figs. 14.45 and 14.46). This option may be useful for a person who is unable to apply a more fitted support garment independently or whose skin is compromised or fragile. The garments are often chosen by patients to wear at night instead of bandaging. There are many styles of therapeutic nightwear to add to a home program to help retain limb reductions achieved in physical therapy. These specialized garments can be made to support venous circulation or lymphatic drainage through altering the style and the stitching channels to complement the diagnosis. A physical therapist can consult with the leading manufacturers to get information on garment options to integrate this type of compression into the POC or the after-care by contacting www.lohmann-rauscher.us and/or www.bsnmedical.us.

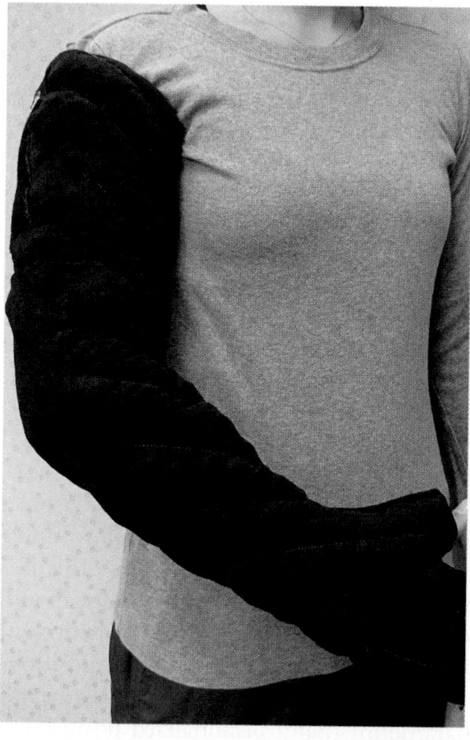

Figure 14.45 Individual wearing a quilted, custom limb containment system as part of a lymphedema management plan.

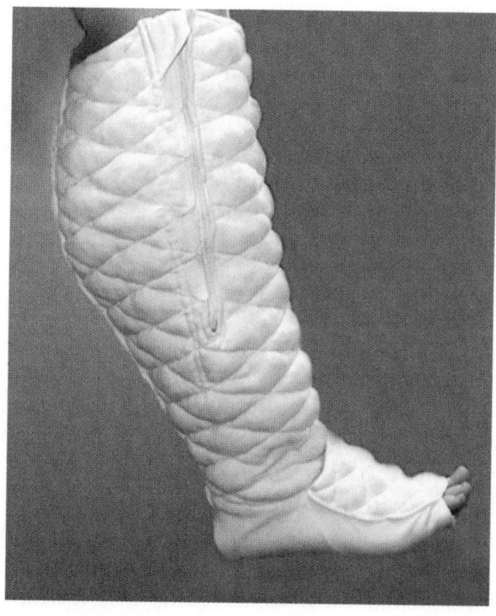

Figure 14.46 Quilted channel compression garment for venous insufficiency.

Compression Guidelines

Compression treatment should be customized to the characteristics of each individual. Since there is inherent risk in the application of compression, relative contraindications for compression should be evaluated, including history of DVT, acute local infection, CHF, cor pulmonale, and acute dermatitis. To assist in clinical decision making, the following is a summary of general guidelines for compression bandaging and garments for edema and lymphedema:

- Arterial wounds: No compression or very light compression with close involvement of the referring practitioner. Long-stretch bandaging or off-the-shelf low compression garment (12 to 25 mm Hg) can be used. Edema will not be significant and will evacuate quickly.
- Venous wounds: Compression is an essential component of treatment for wound healing and support

of the venous system.[227-229] Short-stretch bandaging with high working pressure and low resting pressure will facilitate the effects of the calf pump during activity. High pressure of 40 mm Hg at the ankle has been suggested.[229] Compression garments at pressures of 20 to 30 mm Hg to 30 to 40 mm Hg are used depending on location and severity of swelling, as well as ability of the patient to don and doff garments.

- Neuropathic wounds: Compression is contingent on blood flow. Fifteen percent of patients with a neuropathic condition also have an arterial component to their disease and must have an ABI calculated before compression is applied. If no arterial involvement, compress with short-stretch wrap. Follow up with compression garments for long-term use at lower compression of 12 to 25 mm Hg up to 20 to 30 mm Hg.
- Lymphedema: Short-stretch compression wrap worn 23 hours a day until limb reduction goal reached, then moderate to high compression garments at 20 to 30 mm Hg to 30 to 40 mm Hg, depending on location and severity of swelling, as well as ability of the patient to don and doff garments.[225]
- Edema: Case studies and reports from the field establish that the compression treatment for lymphedema also works well for edema.[230] Short-stretch compression bandages are worn 23 hours/day, graduating to daytime only, decreasing as edema resolves. Off-the-shelf garments at lower levels of compression provide support for skin and help to retain reductions that therapy has achieved.

Intermittent Pneumatic Compression

Until the 1990s, intermittent pneumatic compression (IPC) was one of the few clinical interventions used to treat swelling (Fig. 14.47). Since then, new information about the physiology of edema and lymphedema, as well as lymphatic system function, has limited its value in treating some edema and most lymphedema. Intermittent compression pumps can facilitate venous return and may be an important adjunct to other forms of compression for the individual with a venous disorder.[3,227] A review of the evidence provided only modest support for the use of IPC for the treatment of venous leg ulcers.[228,229] Many individuals with long-standing venous insufficiency also have lymphedema. There is even less evidence and more controversy related to the use of IPC for lymphedema.[230-233] If a trial of IPC is indicated, MLD should be delivered before and after each treatment to offset the negative effects of fluid pooling that occurs adjacent to the edge of the limb sleeves. If indicated for treatment, IPC pressure settings must be kept very low to avoid collapse of the superficial lymph capillaries. Each client should be carefully examined by an experienced health care professional before IPC is applied. Blood pressure readings should be taken before each treatment to confirm that IPC will be safe to use. Increasing total peripheral resistance with pneumatic compression will increase the work of the heart, increasing blood pressure. Pneumatic compression treatment is contraindicated for individuals with hypertension or a blood pressure reading greater than 140/90 mm Hg. Other contraindications to intermittent compression include acute inflammation or trauma, local infection, presence of thrombus, cardiac or kidney dysfunction, obstructed lymphatic channels, and impaired cognitive function.

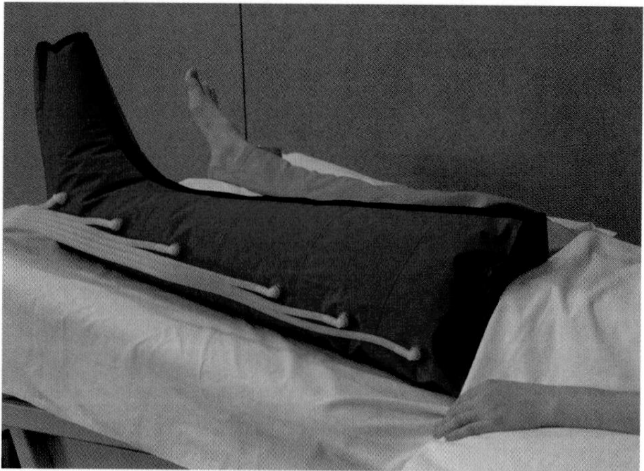

Figure 14.47 Intermittent pneumatic compression pump.

Sequential Pneumatic Compression With Truncal Component

Advances in compression systems include more pneumatic chambers that inflate and deflate in a sequential pattern at very low pressures. The newest home use models include truncal decongestion and clearance in preparation for receiving lymph from affected areas. This appliance style mimics the benefits of MLD in the clinic setting (Fig. 14.48). Manual treatments clear the trunk proximally before treating more distal segments of the body. Stretch fabric is incorporated into the appliance design to further mimic the light stretch to the skin that is applied with MLD.[72,234-236]

Positioning

Positioning techniques are used to prevent or protect pressure injuries, as well as other types of wounds, edema, lymphedema, and vascular disorders. This important aspect of intervention, as well as PRDs, should not be overlooked or underestimated during treatment planning. Devices and techniques selected for positioning should be compatible with the individual's health status. It is paramount that a personalized positioning and repositioning schedule be developed and prominently displayed for any patient who cannot position or reposition independently. The standard time intervals

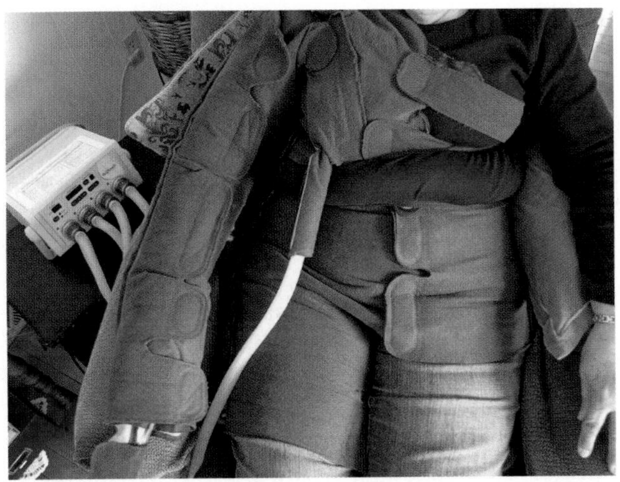

Figure 14.48 Sequential pneumatic compression with truncal component designed to retain and support the benefits of in-clinic lymphedema therapy at home.

used for turning schedules (i.e., every 2 hours) are often too long for individuals who are frail, have fragile skin, or have existing wounds. A turning schedule could be as frequent as every 30 minutes in some cases, whereas for other individuals, every 4 hours may be enough. Suggestions for patient positioning programs include the following[237-239]:

- The patient's heels should be protected and elevated off the surface of the bed.
- The head of bed should not be elevated past 30° unless medically necessary.
- An individualized turning schedule should be provided.
- PRDs should be used in conjunction with a turning schedule.
- Positioning with weight-bearing directly over the greater trochanter should be avoided.
- Positioning with full weight-bearing over an existing wound should be avoided.
- Donut-shaped devices for seating solutions should not be used.
- Pillows and wedges should be used to separate bony prominences from bed and other body parts.

Pressure-Redistributing Devices

Pressure has a direct influence on perfusion or vascularity of a wound site. PRDs should be used to prevent skin breakdown, during the wound healing phase, and during the self-management phase, for lifelong protection and prevention. One of the most often used PRD has adjustable air-filled cushions that mimic the pressure relieving properties of water, and aim to remove friction while sitting (Fig. 14.49). Along with positioning, patients and their caregivers must be educated about pressure redistribution and prevention of pressure-related trauma.[240] Advances in support surfaces that redistribute

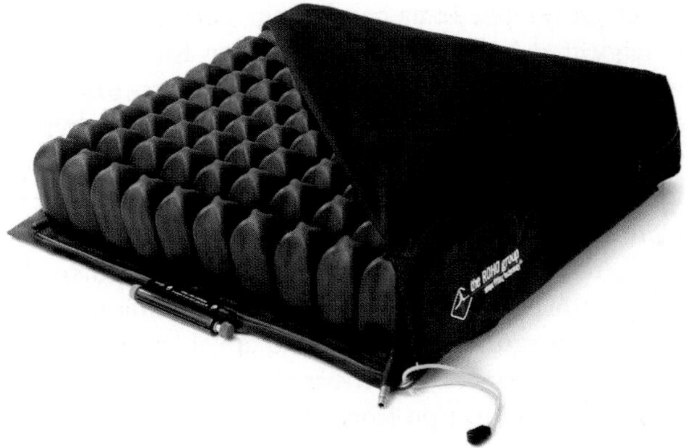

Figure 14.49 ROHO® QUADTRO SELECT® HIGH PROFILE® Cushion for pressure redistribution and skin protection. *(Courtesy of Permobil ROHO Seating and Positioning, Inc., Belleville, IL 62221.)*

weight have made them more sophisticated and effective (Fig. 14.50). Experts in positioning systems are readily available to advise and instruct clinicians working with special populations.[241] Groups such as the Consortium for Spinal Cord Medicine, NPUAP, and the Department of Health and Human Services have made recommendations and algorithms for positioning and pressure redistributing devices that can be used for intervention planning.[74,95,242]

Exercise

The powerful impact of exercise to the rate of recovery should be appreciated for a variety of reasons, including, but not limited to, increased strength and joint ROM, improved quality of movement, increased ADL, improved QOL perceptions, increased blood flow to the extremities, improved calf pump activity, prevention of pressure injuries, prevention of falls, and enhanced

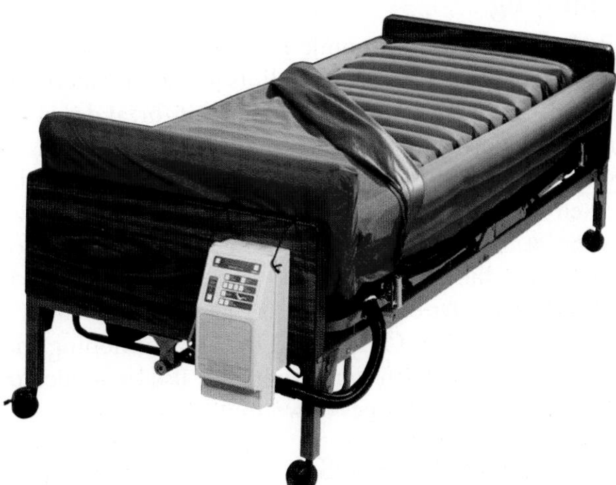

Figure 14.50 *Select*Air® MAX, a low-air-loss support system for pressure relief. *(Courtesy of Permobil ROHO Seating and Positioning, Belleville, IL 62221.)*

effects of lymphedema bandaging. Too often, exercise is neglected in the intervention plan for individuals with vascular, lymphatic, and integumentary disorders, especially those with wounds or edema. The physical therapist is viewed as the movement expert and should intentionally promote activities in the POC related to increasing activity levels as appropriate.

Exercise prescription should be customized to the patient's needs and medical status. A walking program can benefit most individuals who are able to ambulate even short distances. Water-based exercise programs can facilitate the transition from bed or chair to land-based exercise. Individuals with wounds can participate in water-based exercise if it is appropriate to cover the wounds with occlusive dressings. The hydrostatic pressure of water contributes to support of edematous and lymphedematous body segments and creates an ideal setting for exercise for most individuals with swelling. The implementation of active exercise for individuals with lymphedema or who are at risk of developing lymphedema is under investigation. Early literature appears to prove that specific, active exercise may help and not hurt those individuals.[243,244]

Patients should be educated about the concept that movement, activity, and formal exercise are all important for long-term management of the conditions listed in this chapter. Physical therapists introduce these concepts, provide expert instruction, and develop appropriate home exercise programs. Patients are guided to accept responsibility for following the exercise prescriptions at home and for making them a part of their everyday lives. Exercise might be contraindicated or planned with caution when medical issues arise such as the need to be non-weight-bearing on a foot wound, unstable cardiopulmonary conditions, or related orthopedic problems that would limit activity.

Orthotics

Splinting

Patients who are immobile may benefit from resting splints to retain, or dynamic splints to regain, functional ROM. Splinting can also prevent skin breakdown by retaining normal positioning of joints during periods of immobility. Extra precautions (i.e., padding) must be taken to protect aging or fragile skin from breakdown when semi-rigid thermoplastic materials are used for splinting. The use of splinting to manage burn scar is an essential part of the POC for an individual with a thermal injury (see Chapter 24, Burns). Positioning and splinting information found there can also be applied to patients with other types of wounds.

Total Contact Casting

One method for reduction of weight-bearing stresses on the foot is the application of a *total contact cast* (TCC). This method can be useful for the individual with a neuropathic ulcer on the plantar surface of the foot. After infection and swelling have been controlled, a plaster cast is applied from the toes to below the knee. A specially trained individual uses plaster, padding techniques, and the placement of a rubber insert on the weight-bearing part of the cast to complete the application. A TCC is usually worn for 7 to 10 days at a time, removed for skin care, and then reapplied.[245,246]

Neuropathic Walker

A removable ankle-foot orthosis (AFO) can be custom fabricated or ordered prefabricated to provide weight distribution and cushioning for the individual with an insensate foot, a chronic foot ulcer, or Charcot joint (Fig. 14.51). This option is versatile in fit and allows skin checks, dressing changes, and pressure alterations as needed.

Cast Shoes

Cast shoes or post-operative shoes can be utilized as an inexpensive, temporary alternative for wound off-loading. These shoes, however, do not provide any means of controlling foot motion and little cushioning protection for the chronic wound. This option should be considered temporary. Patients wearing cast shoes for pressure distribution should be monitored closely for signs of complications.

Extra-Depth Shoes

Extra-depth shoes have a roomy toe box and a deep sole to provide shock absorption and cushion. The shoes should redirect foot pressure away from bony prominences and wounds (Fig. 14.52).[247] Available in many styles, they can be purchased from an orthotist or at a specialty shoe store. Individuals with insensate feet, with or without wounds, should strongly consider wearing this type of shoe to support skin protection and ulcer prevention.

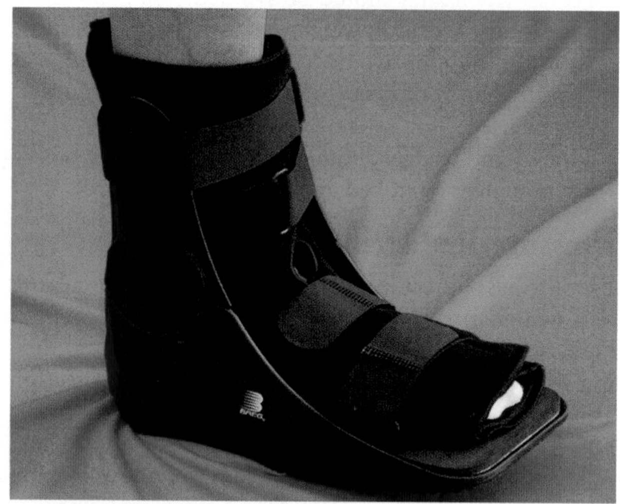

Figure 14.51 An ankle-foot orthosis specifically designed to allow distributed weight-bearing for individuals with neuropathy.

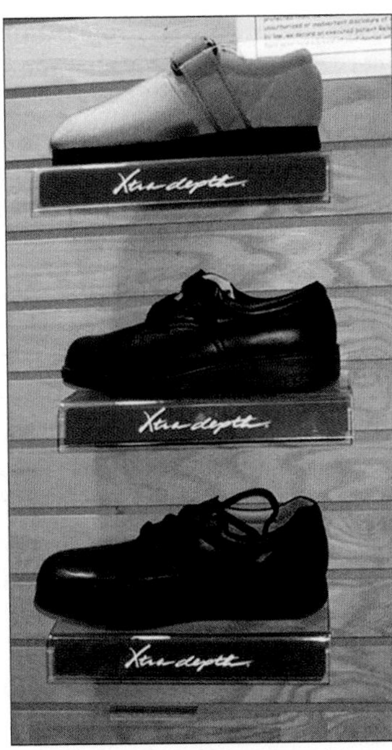

Figure 14.52 Extra-depth shoes that redirect foot pressures away from problem areas.

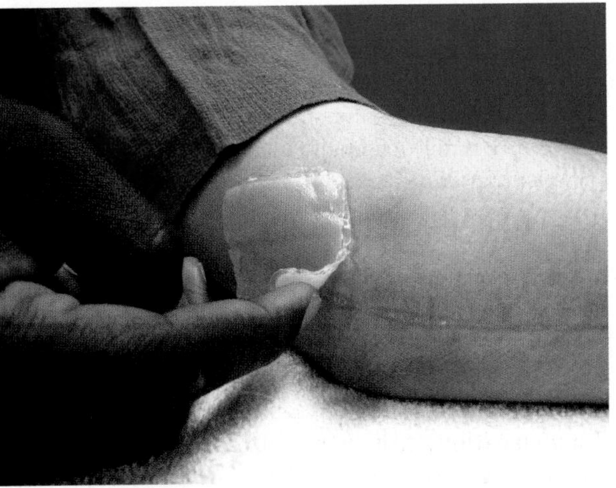

Figure 14.53 Application of a silicone gel sheet to scar tissue during the maturation phase of wound healing.

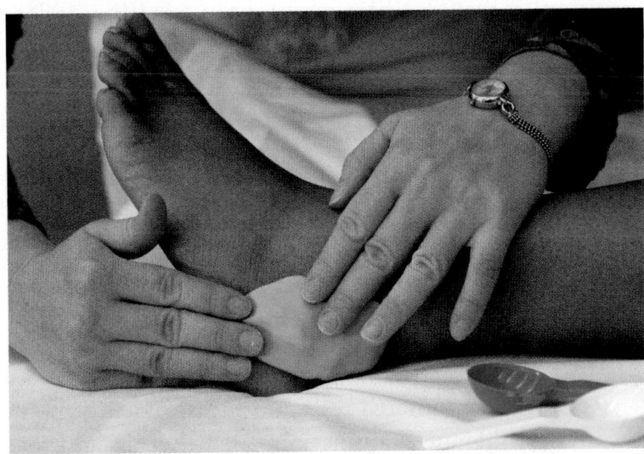

Figure 14.54 Application of elastomer putty to scar tissue during the maturation phase of wound healing.

Scar Management

As described earlier in this chapter, scar formation is a component of wound healing.[248] After the wound is filled with collagen, the tissue must be remodeled and shaped into the finely structured end product. Contraction of scar tissue can lead to disfigurement and loss of function, especially if the scar tissue is located over a joint surface. Issues of disfigurement and dysfunction are greatest following thermal injury (see Chapter 24, Burns). Currently, the mechanisms by which scar can be controlled are not completely understood. Although some interventions do seem to help, there is room for further investigation into how to achieve optimal control of scar formation. Most scar tissue is managed by a physical therapist using compression garments, stretching exercises, orthotics, positioning, specific types of massage, and the use of topical adjuncts such as silicone gel sheets (Fig. 14.53) and elastomer putty (Fig. 14.54). Topical creams, oils, and ointments have some positive effects on scar but it is not known if the massaging actions used to apply the agents or the agents themselves provide the therapeutic effects. Early and adequate intervention can prevent most of the complications of scarring. Since the process of scar formation usually continues for 6 to 24 months, follow-up care should be part of the intervention plan. Individuals with scar tissue must learn how to safely massage the skin at home because frequent pressure applications have the greatest influence on new connective tissue orientation. When conservative measures of scar management have not controlled scarring, surgical intervention may be indicated. Following surgery, the individual will have a new wound and subsequent new scar to manage.

SUMMARY

These are exciting times for clinicians interested in the care of patients with vascular, lymphatic, and integumentary disorders. Skin and wound care practices continue to advance with clinical trials, randomized controlled studies, and empirical data all contributing to the pool of knowledge. New information about the microcirculation of blood and lymph has changed intervention strategies. The role of the skin as an organ has gained new respect. It is not surprising that there is an explosion of research, literature, and products to serve the needs of individuals with disorders affecting these systems. Current and future generations are facing health care challenges of a magnitude never before seen in our society, including an increase in the number of individuals with conditions related to the disorders discussed in this chapter. The incidence of diabetes, obesity, vascular and lymphatic disease, chronic wounds, and antibiotic-resistant pathogens is on the rise. Issues compounding the challenges include a growing population of older individuals, health care reimbursement challenges, and numerous ethical dilemmas in daily practice.

This chapter provides support for clinicians in their efforts to provide excellent patient care. Topics of particular importance include current strategies for wound management, the importance of adequate and appropriate patient education, pressure injury prevention and precautions, advanced foot care for individuals with diabetic neuropathy, optimal compression for lymphedema, the essential role of moisture in wound healing, and the importance of exercise as part of the POC.

There is great need for ongoing research to establish the level of strength of evidence for a variety of topics that may or may not be important in the world of vascular, lymphatic, and integumentary disorders. Some of the concepts that deserve a second look are the impact of bio-burden on the wound infection continuum, the preparation of the wound bed, the use of exogenous oxygen applications, noncontact US, nonthermal radiofrequency stimulation, cold laser, biosurgery/maggot therapy, bioengineered tissue, exogenous growth factors, medical-grade honey, and topical silver preparations. In addition to expanding the evidence, improvements in the standardizing of wound care education are needed. The interdisciplinary nature of wound care calls for more communication among health care professionals. Wise clinicians must keep abreast of new information and current standards of care, approaching new entries to the field with a strong sense of clinical intuition, as well as a firm grasp of the scientific evidence.

Questions for Review

1. Discuss the differences, similarities, and relationships among the arterial, venous, and lymphatic systems. Compare anatomy, method of fluid movement, and function.
2. Outline some of the unique characteristics that can be identified clinically for disorders of the vascular, lymphatic, and integumentary systems.
3. Prepare a list of factors that contribute to abnormal wound healing. Divide the list into intrinsic, extrinsic, and iatrogenic factors.
4. Review the annotated tests and measurements included in this chapter that should be used during a physical therapy examination. Identify tests and measurements routinely performed for patients with vascular, lymphatic, or integumentary disorders.
5. Design a checklist of examination categories for examining a patient with a disorder of the vascular, lymphatic, and/or integumentary systems.
6. Create a general list of the primary components of a POC for a patient with a wound.
7. Explain how a physical therapist should respond to the knowledge that many vascular, lymphatic, and integumentary disorders have a long latency period and require a heightened level of vigilance and proactivity in order to identify symptoms and begin treatment as early as possible.
8. Explain the rationale for each of the following treatments in skin and wound care: moist wound healing, arterial wound hydration, venous wound compression, lymphedema treatment, and foot care for the individual with diabetes.

CASE STUDY

REFERRAL

A 78-year-old woman with a primary diagnosis of Alzheimer's disease has been living in a residential facility for 10 months. The physician at the facility refers her to physical therapy. Referral is for advanced wound care.

PAST MEDICAL HISTORY

Unremarkable until onset of symptoms of Alzheimer's 3 years ago.

CURRENT MEDICAL HISTORY

Health conditions include mild hypertension controlled by medication and a Stage 3 pressure injury over the right ischial tuberosity.

MEDICAL INTERVENTION PREVIOUS TO CURRENT REFERRAL

Pressure injury treated for 4 weeks (30 days) with bid hydrogen peroxide flushes followed by dry gauze 4 × 4s covered with gauze pad and adhesive tape. No changes in wound bed for 4 weeks. No other intervention in place.

PSYCHOSOCIAL

The patient's husband also resides at the same facility and lives in the same room. He is frail but mobile and contributes to care for wife. There are no children. The patient enjoys music and trips by wheelchair to the facility's activity center.

COGNITIVE

Patient disoriented to place and time. Becomes agitated during wound care. She is unable to follow weight shift and turning schedules independently and has difficulty following instructions.

PHYSICAL THERAPY EXAMINATION DATA

Body Structure/Function

- *Wound:* Stage 3 pressure injury over right ischial tuberosity. Measures 2.36 × 1.57 in. (6 × 4 cm) with depth of 1.57 in. (4 cm). The wound bed is 50% necrotic yellow tissue and 50% red granulation tissue. Periwound tissue is intact. Drainage is moderate, yellow-brown, and thin with minimal odor. The wound is currently contaminated but not infected (i.e., colonized bacteria are present but not to the level of clinical infection).
- *Strength and ROM:* Patient unable to follow commands consistently for examination of strength but appears to have functional strength and ROM of bilateral upper extremities (BUEs). Gross bilateral lower extremity (BLE) strength is impaired perhaps owing to declining activity levels. Active ROM appears functional in BUEs. Bilateral hip flexion contractures of 30° can be reduced to 15° with passive ROM.

Activity Limitations—Mobility

Patient is either in wheelchair or bed 24 hours/day. Patient is unable to roll independently but can often assist using BUEs when instructed. Requires maximum assist of two to pivot transfer. The patient is unable to ambulate at this time.

Participation Restrictions

Requires close supervision during social engagement due to propensity to become agitated.

GUIDING QUESTIONS

1. What are the contributing factors that have most likely led to the chronicity of this wound?
2. What other factors might contribute to the slow healing time of this wound?
3. What combination of interventions to clean and débride would allow removal of necrotic tissue while protecting granulation tissue?
4. Clinically, which electromodalities are biocompatible for the treatment of this wound (irrespective of payment) and how will they contribute to wound healing?
5. Other than local wound care, what intervention will be essential for wound closure?
6. Once progress has been made in wound healing, if the wound were to become dry, what dressing types could be used to create a moist wound environment?
7. If using an occlusive dressing, why should this patient be closely monitored?
8. Assuming this patient's wound will close, what are the expectations for the condition of her skin over the wound site?

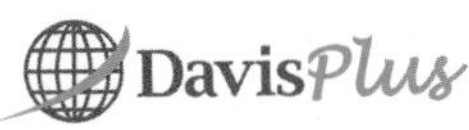

For additional resources, including answers to the questions for review and case study guiding questions, please visit **http://davisplus.fadavis.com.**

References

1. Martini, FH: Fundamentals of Anatomy and Physiology, ed 4. Prentice-Hall, Upper Saddle River, NJ, 2008.
2. Lawenda, B, Mondry, T, and Johnstone, P: Lymphedema: A primer on the identification and management of a chronic condition in oncologic treatment. CA Cancer J Clin 59(1):8, 2009. doi:10.3322/caac.20001.
3. McCulloch, JM: Therapeutic modalities stimulate wound management. Biomechanics 67, April 2004.
4. Eliska, O, and Eliskova, M: Are peripheral lymphatics damaged by high pressure manual massage? Lymphology 28:21, 1995.
5. Casley-Smith, JR: Varying total tissue pressures and the concentration of initial lymphatic lymph. Microvasc Res 25:369, 1983.
6. Mortimer, PS, et al: The measurement of skin lymph flow by isotope clearance—reliability, reproducibility, injection dynamics and the effect of massage. J Invest Dermatol 95(6):677, 1990.
7. Olszewski W: Physiology, biology, and lymph biochemistry. In Lee, B-B, Bergan J, Rockson, SG (eds): Lymphedema, Springer, London, 2011, p. 65. doi: 10.1007/978-0-85729-567-5_8.
8. Bertram, CD, Macaskill, C, and Moore, JE, Jr: Simulation of a chain of collapsible contracting lymphangions with progressive valve closure. J Biomech Eng 133(1):011008, 2011.
9. Gashev, AA: Lymphatic vessels: Pressure-and flow-dependent regulatory reactions. Ann NY Acad Sci 1131:100, 2008.
10. Belgrado, JP et al: Near-infrared fluorescence lymphatic imaging to reconsider occlusion pressure of superficial lymphatic collectors in upper extremities of healthy volunteers. Lymphat Res and Biol 14(2): 70, 2016. doi.org/10.1089/lrb.2015.0040.
11. Sen, CK: The general case of redox control of wound repair. Wound Repair Regen 11(6):431, 2003.
12. Gordillo, GM, and Sen, CK: Revisiting the essential role of oxygen in wound healing. Am J Surg 186:259, 2003.
13. Atiyeh, BS, et al: Management of acute and chronic open wounds: The importance of moist environment to optimal wound healing. Curr Pharm Biotechnol 3:179, 2002.
14. Bolton, L: Operational definition of moist wound healing. J Wound Ostomy Continence Nurs 34(1):23, 2007.
15. Okan, D, et al: The role of moisture balance in wound healing. Adv Skin Wound Care 20:39, 2007.
16. Schultz, GS, et al: Wound bed preparation: A systematic approach to wound management. Wound Rep Reg 11:1, 2003.
17. Lee, JE, et al: An infection-preventing bilayered collagen membrane containing antibiotic-loaded hyaluronan microparticles: Physical and biological properties. Artif Organs 26(7): 636, 2002.
18. Thomas, DW, et al: Randomized clinical trial of the effect of semi-occlusive dressings on the microflora and clinical outcome of acute facial wounds. Wound Repair Regen 8(4):258, 2000.
19. Koupil, J, et al: The influence of moisture wound healing on the incidence of bacterial infection and histological changes in healthy human skin after treatment of interactive dressings. Acta Chir Plast 45(3):89, 2003.
20. Ratliff, CR: Wound exudate: An influential factor in healing. Adv Nurs Pract 16(7):32, 2008.
21. Sherman, A, and Barkley M: Nutrition and wound healing. J Wound Care 20(8):357, 2011. doi.org/10.12968/jowc.2011.20.8.357.
22. Mechanick, JI: Practical aspects of nutritional support for wound-healing patients. Am J Surg 188(1, Suppl 1):52, 2004.
23. Shepherd, AA: Nutrition for optimum wound healing. Nurs Stand 18(6):55, 2003.
24. Gray, M: Does oral supplementation with vitamins A or E promote healing of chronic wounds? J Wound Ostom Continen Nurs 30(6): 290, 2003.
25. Gray, M: Does vitamin C supplementation promote pressure ulcer healing? J Wound Osteom Continen Nurs 30(5):245, 2003.
26. Collins, N: The right mix: Using nutritional interventions and an anabolic agent to manage a Stage IV ulcer. Adv Skin Wound Care 17(1):36, 2004.
27. Collins, N: Diabetes, nutrition and wound healing. Adv Skin Wound Care 16(6):292, 2003.
28. Williams, JZ, and Barbul, A: Nutrition and wound healing. Surg Clin North Am 83:571, 2003.
29. Zulkowski, K, and Albrecht, D: How nutrition and aging affect wound healing. Nursing 33(8):70, 2003.
30. Barnes, P, Sauter, T, and Azheri, S: Subnormal prealbumin levels and wound healing. Tex Med 103(8):65, 2007.
31. Rodriguez-Key, M, and Alonzi, A: Nutrition, skin integrity, and pressure ulcer healing in chronically ill children: An overview. Ostomy Wound Manage 53(6):56, 2007.
32. Stechmiller, JK: Understanding the role of nutrition and wound healing. Nutr Clin Pract 25(1):61, 2010.
33. Zhang, XJ, et al: Enternal [corrected] arginine supplementation stimulates DNA synthesis in skin donor wound. Clin Nutr 30(3): 391, 2011.
34. McMahon, L, et al: A randomized phase II trial of arginine butyrate with standard local therapy in refractory sickle cell leg ulcers. Br J Haematol 151(5):516, 2010.
35. Goldberg, SR, and Diegelmann, RF: Wound healing primer. Surg Clin North Am 90:1133, 2010.
36. Dunn, SL: The wound healing process. In Kloth, LC, and McCulloch, JM (eds): Wound Healing: Evidence-Based Management, ed 4. FA Davis, Philadelphia, 2010.
37. Sussman, C, and Bates-Jensen, BM: Wound healing physiology and chronic wound healing. In Sussman, C, and Bates, BM (eds): Wound Care: A Collaborative Practice Manual for Physical Therapists and Nurses, ed 3. Lippincott Williams & Wilkins, Baltimore, MD, 2007, p. 21.
38. Bates-Jensen, BM, and Sussman, C: Tools to measure wound healing. In Sussman, C, and Bates, BM (eds): Wound Care: A Collaborative Practice Manual for Physical Therapists and Nurses, ed 3. Lippincott Williams & Wilkins, Baltimore, MD, 2007, p. 144.
39. Weed, T, Ratliff C, and Drake DB: Quantifying bacterial bioburden during negative pressure wound therapy. Ann Plast Surg 52(3): 276, 2004.
40. Lindholm, C: Pressure ulcers and infection—understanding clinical features. Ostomy Wound Manage 49(5A):4, 2003.
41. Beitz, JM, and Goldberg, E: The lived experience of having a chronic wound: A phenomenologic study. Medsurg Nurs 14(1):51, 2005.
42. Glasper, ER, and Devries, AC: Social structure influences effects of pair-housing on wound healing. Brain Behav Immun 19(1): 61, 2005.
43. Detillion, CE, et al: Social facilitation of wound healing. Psychoneuroendocrinology 29(8):1004, 2005.
44. Ebrecht, M, et al: Perceived stress and cortisol levels predict speed of wound healing in healthy male adults. Psychoneuroendocrinology 29(6):798, 2004.
45. Christian, L, et al: Stress and wound healing. Neuroimmunomodulation 13(5-6):337, 2006..
46. Vileikyte, L: Stress and wound healing. Clin Dermatol 25(1):49, 2007. doi.org/10.1016/j.clindermatol.2006.09.005.
47. Valencia, IC, et al: Chronic venous insufficiency and venous leg ulceration. J Am Acad Dermatol 44(3):401, 2001.
48. Kunimoto, B, et al: Best practices for the prevention and treatment of venous leg ulcers. Ostomy Wound Manage 47(2):34, 2001.
49. Seiggreen, MY, and Kline, RA: Vascular ulcers. In Baranoski, S, and Ayello, EA (eds): Wound Care Essentials: Practice Principles. Lippincott Williams & Wilkins, Springhouse, PA, 2004, p. 271.
50. Word, R: Medical and surgical therapy for advanced chronic venous insufficiency. Surg Clin North Am 90(6):1195, 2010.
51. Kolbach, DN, et al: Severity of venous insufficiency is related to the density of microvascular deposition of PAI-1, uPA and von Willebrand factor. J Vasc Dis 33(1):19, 2004.
52. Berard, A, et al: Risk factors for the first-time development of venous ulcers of the lower limbs: The influence of heredity and physical activity. Angiology 53(6):647, 2002.
53. Gloviczki, P, et al: The care of patients with varicose veins and associated chronic venous diseases: Clinical practice guidelines of the Society for Vascular Surgery and the American Venous Forum. J Vasc Surg 53(5 Suppl):2S, 2011.
54. Kelechi, TJ, et al: Skin temperature and chronic venous insufficiency. J Wound Ostomy Continence Nurs 30(1):17, 2003.
55. Strossenreuther, RHK, et al: Guidelines for the application of MLD/CDT for primary and secondary lymphedema and other selected pathologies. In Foldi, M, Foldi, E, and Kubik, S (eds): Textbook of Lymphology for Physicians and Lymphedema Therapists, ed 5. Elsevier, Munich, Germany, 2003, p. 590.
56. Foldi, E, et al: Lymphostatic diseases. In Foldi, M, Foldi, E, and Kubik, S (eds): Textbook of Lymphology for Physicians and

Lymphedema Therapists, ed 5. Elsevier, Munich, Germany, 2003, p. 232.
57. International Society of Lymphology. The diagnosis and treatment of peripheral lymphedema: 2013 Consensus Document of the International Society of Lymphology. Lymphology 46(1):1, 2013.
58. Bunke, N, Brown, K, and Bergan, J: Phlebolymphedema, usually unrecognized, often poorly treated. Perspect Vasc Surg Endovasc Ther 21(2):65, 2009.
59. Gaber, Y: Secondary lymphoedema of the lower leg as an unusual side-effect of a liquid silicone injection in the hips and buttocks. Dermatology 208:342, 2004.
60. Halaska, MJ, et al: A prospective study of postoperative lymphedema after surgery for cervical cancer. Int J Gynecol Cancer 20(5):900, 2010.
61. Kasper, DA, and Meller, MM: Lymphedema of the hand and forearm following fracture of the distal radius. Orthopedics 31(2): 172, 2008.
62. Szuba, A, et al: The third circulation: Radionuclide lymphoscintigraphy in the evaluation of lymphedema. J Nucl Med 44:43, 2003.
63. Stout, N, et al: Breast cancer-related lymphedema: comparing direct costs of a prospective surveillance model and a traditional model of care. Phys Ther; 92(1):152, 2012.
64. Armer, J, et al: Best-practice guidelines in assessment, risk reduction, management, and surveillance for post-breast cancer lymphedema. Curr Breast Cancer Rep 5:134, 2013. doi:10.1007/s12609-013-0105-0.
65. Stout, N, et al: Preoperative assessment enables the early diagnosis and successful treatment of lymphedema. Cancer 112(12):2809, 2008.
66. Leard, T, and Barrett, C: Successful management of severe unilateral lower extremity lymphedema in an outpatient setting. Phys Ther 95(9):1295, 2015.
67. Tartaglione, G, et al: Intradermal lymphoscintigraphy at rest and after exercise: A new technique for the functional assessment of the lymphatic system in patients with lymphoedema. Nucl Med Commun 31(6):547, 2010.
68. Yuan, Z, et al: The role of radionuclide lymphoscintigraphy in extremity lymphedema. Ann Nucl Med 20(5):341, 2006.
69. Hamner, JB, and Fleming, MD: Lymphedema therapy reduces the volume of edema and pain in patients with breast cancer. Ann Surg Onc 14(6):1904, 2007.
70. Mondry, TF, Riffengurgh, RH, and Johnstone, PA: Prospective trial of complete decongestive therapy for upper extremity lymphedema after breast cancer therapy. Cancer J 10:42, 2004.
71. Koul, R, et al: Efficacy of complete decongestive therapy and manual lymphatic drainage on treatment-related lymphedema in breast cancer. Int J Radiat Oncol Biol Phys 67(3):841, 2007.
72. Mayrovitz, HN: The standard of care for lymphedema: Current concepts and physiological considerations. Lymphat Res Biol 7(2):101, 2009.
73. Baumgarten, M, et al: Pressure ulcers and the transition to long-term care. Adv Skin Wound Care 16(6):299, 2003.
74. Consortium for Spinal Cord Medicine: Pressure Ulcer Prevention and Treatment Following Spinal Cord Injury: A Clinical Practice Guideline for Health-Care Professionals. Paralyzed Veterans of American, Washington, DC, 2000. Retrieved July 4, 2011, from www.pva.org.
75. Langemo, DK, Anderson, J, and Volden, C: Uncovering pressure ulcer incidence. Nurs Manage 34(10):64, 2003.
76. Scott, EM, et al: Effects of warming therapy on pressure ulcers—a randomized trial. J Periop Nurs, May 2001.
77. Reed, RL, et al: Low serum albumin levels, confusion, and fecal incontinence: Are these risk factors for pressure ulcers in mobility-impaired hospitalized adults? Gerontology 49(4):255, 2003.
78. de Souza, DM, and de Gouveia Santos, VL: Incidence of pressure ulcers in the institutionalized elderly. J Wound Ostomy 37(3):272, 2010.
79. Institute for Clinical Systems Improvement (ICSI): Pressure Ulcer Prevention and Treatment. Health Care Protocol. ICSI, Bloomington, MN, 2010.
80. Centers for Disease Control and Prevention: National Diabetes Fact Sheet: National Estimates and General Information on Diabetes and Prediabetes in the United States, 2014. US Department of Health and Human Services, Centers for Disease Control and Prevention, Atlanta, 2014.
81. *Guide to Physical Therapist Practice 3.0.* Alexandria, VA: American Physical Therapy Association; 2014. Available at http://guidetoptpractice.apta.org/. Accessed March 28, 2017.
82. Ridner, SH, et al: Comparison of upper limb volume measurement techniques and arm symptoms between healthy volunteers and individuals with known lymphedema. Lymphology 40(1): 35, 2007.
83. Warren, AG, et al: The use of bioimpedance analysis to evaluate lymphedema. Ann Plast Surg 58(5):541, 2007.
84. Cornish, BH, et al: Early diagnosis of lymphedema using multiple frequency bioimpedance. Lymphology 34(1):2, 2001.
85. Czerniec, SA, et al: Assessment of breast cancer–related arm lymphedema—comparison of physical measurement methods and self-report. Cancer Invest 28(1):54, 2010.
86. McCulloch, JM: Assessing the circulatory and neurological systems. In Kloth, LC, and McCulloch, JM (eds): Wound Healing: Evidence-Based Management, ed 4. FA Davis, Philadelphia, 2010, p. 94.
87. Patterson, GK: Vascular evaluation. In Sussman, C, and Bates, BM: Wound Care: A Collaborative Practice Manual for Physical Therapists and Nurses, ed 3. Lippincott Williams & Wilkins, Baltimore, 2007, p. 180.
88. Mehta, T, et al: Disease-specific quality of life assessment in intermittent claudication: Review. Eur J Endovasc Surg 25:202, 2003.
89. Lehert, P: Quality-of-life assessment in comparative therapeutic trials and causal structure considerations in peripheral occlusive arterial disease. Pharmacoeconomics 19(2):121, 2001.
90. Marquis, P, Comte, S, and Lehert, P: International validation of the CLAUS-S Quality-of-Life Questionnaire for Use in Patients with Intermittent Claudication. Pharmacoeconomics 19(6):667, 2001.
91. Wells, PS, Anderson DR, Bormanis, J, et al: Value of assessment of pretest probability of deep-vein thrombosis in clinical management. Lancet 350(9094):1795–1798, 1997.
92. Silveira, PC, et al: Performance of Wells Score for deep vein thrombosis in the inpatient setting. JAMA Intern Med. 175(7): 1112–1117, 2015.
93. Tiedjen, KU, et al: Radiological diagnostic procedures in edema of the extremities. In Foldi, M, Foldi, E, and Kubik, S (eds): Textbook of Lymphology for Physicians and Lymphedema Therapists, ed 5. Elsevier, Munich, Germany, 2003, p. 434.
94. Black, J: National Pressure Ulcer Advisory Panel's updated pressure ulcer staging system. Adv Skin Wound Care 20(5):269, 2007.
95. Bergstrom, N, et al: Pressure Ulcer Treatment, Clinical Practice Guideline, Quick Reference Guide for Clinicians, No. 15. AHRQ Pub. No. 95-0653. U.S. Department of Health and Human Services, Public Health Service Agency, Agency for Health Care Research and Quality, Rockville, MD, December 1994.
96. National Pressure Ulcer Advisory Panel, European Pressure Ulcer Advisory Panel and Pan Pacific Pressure Injury Alliance. Prevention and Treatment of Pressure Ulcers: Quick Reference Guide. Emily Haesler (ed.). Cambridge Media: Osborne park, Western Australia; 2014.
97. Hon, J, et al: A prospective, multicenter study to validate use of the PUSH in patients with diabetic, venous, and pressure ulcers. Ostomy Wound Manage 56(2):26, 2010.
98. Gul, A: Role of wound classification in predicting the outcome of diabetic foot ulcer. J Pak Med Assoc 56(10):444, 2006.
99. Schoonhoven, L, et al: Prospective cohort study of routine use of risk assessment scales for prediction of pressure ulcers. BMJ 12:325, 2002.
100. Mortenson, WB, et al: A review of scales for assessing the risk of developing a pressure ulcer in individuals with SCI. Spinal Cord 46(3):168, 2008.
101. Beeson, T, et al: Thinking about the Braden Scale. Clin Nurse Spec 24(2):49, 2010.
102. Ayello, EA: New evidence for an enduring wound-healing concept: Moisture control. J Wound Ostomy Continence Nurs 33(65):S1, 2006.
103. Sarsam, SE, Elliott, JP, and Lam, GK: Management of wound complications from cesarean delivery. Obstet Gynecol Surv 60(7):462, 2005.
104. McCulloch, JM, and Boyd, V: The effects of whirlpool and the dependent position on LE volume. J Orthop Sports Phys Ther 16:169, 1992.

105. Sussman, C: Whirlpool. In Sussman, C, and Bates, BM (eds): Wound Care: A Collaborative Practice Manual for Physical Therapists and Nurses, ed 3. Lippincott Williams & Wilkins, Baltimore, 2007, p. 644.
106. Burke, DT, et al: Effects of hydrotherapy on pressure ulcer healing. Am J Phys Med Rehabil 77(5):394, 1998.
107. Hess, CL, Howard, MA, and Attinger, CE: A review of mechanical adjuncts in wound healing: Hydrotherapy, ultrasound, negative pressure therapy, hyperbaric oxygen, and electrostimulation. Ann Plast Surg 51(2):210, 2003.
108. Ho, CH, and Bogie, K: The prevention and treatment of pressure ulcers. Phys Med Rehabil Clin North Am 18:235, 2007.
109. Tao, H, et al: The role of whirlpool in wound care. J Am Coll Clin Wound Spec. 4: 7, 2013. doi.org/10.1016/j.jccw.2013.01.002.
110. Luedtke-Hoffmann, KA, and Schafer, DS: Pulsed lavage in wound cleansing. Phys Ther 80:292, 2000.
111. Loehne, HB, et al: Aerosolization of microorganisms during pulsatile lavage with suction. Presented at Combined Sections Meeting/American Physical Therapy Association, February 2000, New Orleans, LA.
112. Sonnergren, H, et al: Aerosolized spread of bacteria and reduction of bacterial wound contamination with three different methods of surgical wound débridement: A pilot study. J Hosp Infect 85(2):112, 2013. doi.org/10.1016/j.jhin.2013.05.011.
113. Wilson, JR, et al: A toxicity index of skin and wound cleansers used on in vitro fibroblasts and keratinocytes. Adv Skin Wound Care 18(7):373, 2005.
114. Spear, M: Wet-to-dry dressings—evaluating the evidence. Plast Surg Nurs 28(2):92, 2008.
115. Cowan, LJ, and Stechmiller, J: Prevalence of wet-to-dry dressings in wound care. Adv Skin Wound Care 22(12):567, 2009.
116. Rodeheaver, G, et al: Wound healing and wound management: Focus on débridement. Adv Wound Care 7(1):22, 1994.
117. Ovington, LG: Hanging wet-to-dry dressings out to dry. Home Health Nurse 19(8):477, 2001.
118. Shinohara, T, et al: Prospective evaluation of occlusive hydrocolloid dressing versus conventional gauze dressing regarding the healing effect after abdominal operations: Randomized controlled trial. Asian J Surg 31(1):1, 2008.
119. Singh, A, et al: Meta-analysis of randomized controlled trials on hydrocolloid occlusive dressing versus conventional gauze dressing in the healing of chronic wounds. Asian J Surg 27(4):326, 2004.
120. Vermeulen, H, et al: Dressings and topical agents for surgical wounds healing by secondary intention (review). Cochrane Database Syst Rev 1; CD003554, 2004.
121. Bergstrom, N, et al: The national pressure ulcer long-term care study: Outcomes of pressure ulcer treatments in long-term care. J Am Geriatr Soc 53:1721, 2005.
122. Jones, KR, and Fennie, K: Factors influencing pressure ulcer healing in adults over 50: An exploratory study. J Am Med Dir Assoc 8:378, 2007.
123. Lawrence, JC: Dressings and wound infection. Am J Surg 167(1A):21S, 1994.
124. Lawrence, JC, Lilly, HA, and Kidson, A: Wound dressings and airborne dispersal of bacteria. Lancet 339:807, 1992.
125. Kohr, R: Moist healing versus wet to dry. Can Nurse 97(1):17, 2001.
126. Payne, WG, et al: A prospective, randomized clinical trial to assess the cost-effectiveness of a modern foam dressing versus a traditional saline gauze dressing in the treatment of Stage II pressure ulcers. Ostomy Wound Manage 55(2):50, 2009.
127. Capasso, VA, and Munro, BH: The cost and efficacy of two wound treatments. J Perioper Nurs 77(5):984, 2003.
128. Hall, S: A review of maggot débridement therapy to treat chronic wounds. Br J Nurs 19(15):S26, 2010.
129. Sherman, RA: Maggot therapy takes us back to the future of wound care: New and improved maggot therapy for the 21st century. J Diabetes Sci Technol 3(2):336, 2009.
130. Mumcuoglu, KY: Clinical applications for maggots in wound care. Am J Clin Dermatol 2(4):219, 2001.
131. Jones, M: An overview of maggot therapy used on chronic wounds in the community. Br J Community Nurs 14(3):S16, 2009.
132. Allen, CS: Merit in maggots. Physical Therapy Products, p. 44, May/June 2003.
133. Paul, AG, et al: Maggot débridement therapy with Lucilia cuprina: A comparison with conventional débridement in diabetic foot ulcers. Int Wound J 6(1):39, 2009.
134. Hunter, S, et al: Maggot therapy for wound management. Adv Skin Wound Care 22(1):25, 2009.
135. Durnville JC, et al: VenUS II: a randomized controlled trial of larval therapy in the management of leg ulcers. Health Technol Asses 13(55):1–182, 2009.
136. Gethin, G, and Cowman, S: Manuka honey vs hydrogel—a prospective, open label, mulitcentre, randomized controlled trial to compare desloughing efficacy and healing outcomes in venous ulcers. J Clin Nurs 18:466, 2009.
137. Robson, V: Leptospermum honey used as a debriding agent. Nurse 2(11):66, 2002.
138. Cutting, KF: Honey and contemporary wound care: An overview. Ostomy Wound Manage 53(11):49, 2008.
139. Molan, PC: Re-introducing honey in the management of wounds and ulcers—theory and practice. 48(11):28, 2002.
140. Landis, SJ: Chronic wound infection and antimicrobial use. Adv Skin Wound Care 21:531, 2008.
141. Bates-Jensen, BM, and Ovington, LG: Management of exudate and infection. In Sussman, C, and Bates, BM (eds): Wound Care: A Collaborative Practice Manual for Physical Therapists and Nurses, ed 3. Lippincott Williams & Wilkins, Baltimore, 2007, p. 215.
142. Takahashi, M, et al: Possible mechanisms underlying mammary carcinogenesis in female Wistar rats by nitrofurazone. Cancer Lett 156(2):177, 2000.
143. Popescu, A, and Salcido, R: Wound pain: A challenge for the patient and the wound care specialist. Adv Skin Wound Care 17(1):14, 2004.
144. White, R: Pain assessment and management in patients with chronic wounds. Nursing Standard 22(32):62, 2008.
145. Nagai, MK, and Embil, JM: Becaplermin: Recombinant platelet derived growth factor, a new treatment for healing diabetic foot ulcers. Expert Opin Biol Ther 2(2):211, 2002.
146. Barrientos, S, et al: PERSPECTIVE ARTICLE: Growth factors and cytokines in wound healing. Wound Repair Regen 16(5):585, 2008. doi: 10.1111/j.1524-475X.2008.00410.x
147. Edmonds, M, et al: New treatments in ulcer healing and wound infection. Diabetes/Metab Res Rev Suppl 1:S51, September–October 2000.
148. Goldman, R: Growth factors and chronic wound healing: Past, present, and future. Adv Skin Wound Care 17(1):24, 2004.
149. Rappl, LM: Effect of platelet rich plasma gel in a physiologically relevant platelet concentration on wounds in persons with spinal cord injury. Int Wound J 8:187, 2011.
150. Gilligan, AM, Waycaster, CR, and Motley, TA: Cost-effectiveness of becaplermin gel on wound healing of diabetic foot ulcers. Wound Rep Regen 23(3):353–360, 2015.
151. McCulloch, JM, and Kloth, LC: Wound Healing: Evidence-Based Management, ed 4. FA Davis, Philadelphia, 2010.
152. Sussman, C, and Bates-Jensen, BM: Wound Care: A Collaborative Practice Manual for Health Professionals, ed 4. Lippincott Williams & Wilkins, Philadelphia, 2012.
153. Kloth, LC, and Niezgoda, JA: Ultrasound for wound débridement and healing. In Kloth, LC, and McCulloch, JM (eds): Wound Healing: Evidence-Based Management, ed 4. FA Davis, Philadelphia, 2010, p. 545.
154. Sussman, C, and Dyson, M: Therapeutic and diagnostic ultrasound. In Sussman, C, and Bates, BM (eds): Wound Care: A Collaborative Practice Manual for Physical Therapists and Nurses, ed 3. Lippincott Williams & Wilkins, Baltimore, 2007, p. 612.
155. Baba-Akbari, SA, et al: Therapeutic ultrasound for pressure ulcers. Cochrane Database Syst Rev CD001275, 2006.
156. White, J, et al: Non-contact low-frequency ultrasound therapy compared with UK standard of care for venous leg ulcers: A single-centre, assessor-blinded, randomized controlled trial. Int Wound J 13(5):833, 2015.
157. Beheshti, A, et al. Comparison of high-frequency and MIST ultrasound therapy for the healing of venous leg ulcers. Adv Clin Exp Med 23(6):969, 2014.
158. Ennis, W, et al: Ultrasound therapy for recalcitrant diabetic foot ulcers: Results of a randomized, double-blind, controlled, multicenter study [corrected] [published erratum appears in OSTOMY WOUND MANAGE 2005;51(9):14]. Ostomy Wound Manage. 51(8):24, 2005.

159. Kavros, S, et al: Expedited wound healing with noncontact, low-frequency ultrasound therapy in chronic wounds: A retrospective analysis. Adv Skin Wound Care 21(9):416, 2008.
160. Kavros, SJ, Miller, JL, and Hanna, SW: Treatment of ischemic wounds with noncontact, low-frequency ultrasound: The Mayo Clinic experience, 2004–2006. Adv Skin Wound Care 20(4): 221, 2007.
161. Olyaie, M, et al: High-frequency and noncontact low-frequency ultrasound therapy for venous leg ulcer treatment: A randomized, controlled study. Ostomy Wound Manage. 59(8):14, 2013.
162. Yao, M, et al: A pilot study evaluating non-contact low-frequency ultrasound and underlying molecular mechanism on diabetic foot ulcers. Int Wound J 11(6):586, 2014.
163. Kloth, LC: Electrical stimulation for wound healing: A review of evidence from in vitro studies, animal experiments, and clinical trials. Int J Low Extrem Wounds 4(1):23, 2005.
164. Demir, H, Balay, H, and Kirnap, M: A comparative study of the effects of electrical stimulation and laser treatment on experimental wound healing in rats. J Rehabil Res Dev 41(2):147, 2004.
165. Ojingwa, JC, and Isseroff, RR: Electrical stimulation of wound healing. J Invest Dermatol 121(1):1, 2003.
166. Houghton, PE, et al: Effect of electrical stimulation on chronic leg ulcer size and appearance. Phys Ther 83(1):17, 2003.
167. Edsberg, LE, et al: Topical hyperbaric oxygen and electrical stimulation: Exploring potential synergy. Ostomy Wound Manage 48(1):42, 2003.
168. Houghton PE: Clinical trials involving biphasic pulsed current, microcurrent, and/or low-intensity direct current. Adv wound Care (New Rochelle) 3(2):166–183, 2014.
169. Isseroff, RR, and Dahle, SE: Electrical stimulation therapy and wound healing: Where are we now? Adv Wound Care (New Rochelle) 1(6):238–243, 2012.
170. Ashrafi, M, et al: The efficacy of electrical stimulation in experimentally induced cutaneous wounds in animals. Vet Dermatol 27(4):235-e57. doi: 10.1111/vde.12328. Epub 2016 May 18, 2016.
171. Kloth, LC, and Pilla, AA: Electromagnetic stimulation for wound repair. In Kloth, LC, and McCulloch, JM (eds): Wound Healing: Evidence-Based Management, ed 4. FA Davis, Philadelphia, 2010, p. 514.
172. Sussman, C: Electrical stimulation for wound healing. In Sussman, C, and Bates, BM (eds): Wound Care: A Collaborative Practice Manual for Physical Therapists and Nurses, ed 3. Lippincott Williams & Wilkins, Baltimore, 2007, p. 505.
173. Johnson, W, and Draper, DO: Increased range of motion and function in an individual with breast cancer and necrotizing fasciitis—manual therapy and pulsed short-wave diathermy treatment. Case Report Med 2010. Volume 2010, Article ID 179581. doi: 10.1155/2010/179581. [Epub July 14, 2010.] https://www.hindawi.com/journals/crim/2010/179581/ref/
174. Al-Mandeel, MM, and Watson, T: The thermal and nonthermal effects of high and low doses of pulsed short wave therapy (PSWT). Physiother Res Int 15(4):199, 2010.
175. Conner-Kerr, T et al: Phototherapy in wound management. In Sussman, C, and Bates, BM (eds): Wound Care: A Collaborative Practice Manual for Physical Therapists and Nurses, ed 3. Lippincott Williams & Wilkins, Baltimore, 2007, p. 591.
176. Rennekampff, HO: Is UV radiation beneficial in postburn wound healing? Med Hypotheses 75(5):436, 2010.
177. Ennis, WJ, Lee, C, and Meneses, P: A biochemical approach to wound healing through the use of modalities. Clin Dermatol 25(1):63, 2007.
178. Thai, T, et al: Ultraviolet light C in the treatment of chronic wounds with MRSA: A case study. Ostomy Wound Manage 48(11):52, 2002.
179. Murugan, S, et al: Prevalence and antimicrobial susceptibility patter of metallo lactamase producing *Pseudomonas aeruginosa* in diabetic foot infection. Int J Microbiol Res 1(3):123, 2010.
180. Gupta A, et al: Ultraviolet radiation in wound care: Sterilization and Stimulation. Adv Wound Care 2(8):422–437, 2013.
181. Londahl, M, et al: Hyperbaric oxygen therapy facilitates healing of chronic foot ulcers in patients with diabetes. Diabetes Care 33(5):998, 2010.
182. Duzgun, AP, et al: Effect of hyperbaric oxygen therapy on healing of diabetic foot ulcers. J Foot Ankle Surg 47(6):515, 2008.
183. Boykin, JV, and Baylis, C: Hyperbaric oxygen therapy mediates increased nitric oxide production associated with wound healing: A preliminary study. Adv Skin Wound Care 20(7):382, 2007.
184. Kalliainen, L, et al: Topical oxygen as an adjunct to wound healing: A clinical case series. Pathophysiology 9:81, 2003.
185. Rodriguez, P, et al: The Role of Oxygen in Wound Healing: A Review of the Literature. Dermatol Surg 34(9):1159, 2008. doi: 10.1111/j.1524-4725.2008.34254.x.
186. Landau, Z, et al: Topical hyperbaric oxygen and low-energy laser for the treatment of chronic ulcers. Eur J Intern Med 17(4): 272, 2006.
187. Braun, L, et al: Diabetic foot ulcer: An evidence-based treatment update. Am J Clin Dermatol 15(3):267, 2014.
188. Gabriel, A, Kahn, KM: New advances in instillation therapy in wounds at risk for compromised healing. Surg Technol Int 24: 75, 2014.
189. Gupta, S, Gabriel, A, and Shores, J: The perioperative use of negative pressure wound therapy in skin grafting. Ostomy Wound Manage 50(4A Suppl):32, 2004.
190. Armstrong, DG, et al: Plantar pressure changes using a novel negative pressure wound therapy technique. J Am Podiatr Med Assoc 94(5):456, 2004.
191. Mendez-Eastman, S: Determining the appropriateness of negative pressure wound therapy for pressure ulcers. Ostomy Wound Manage 50(4A Suppl):13, 2004.
192. Wanner, MB, et al: Vacuum-assisted wound closure for cheaper and more comfortable healing of pressure sores: A prospective study. Scand J Plast Reconstr Surg 37(1):28, 2003.
193. Zannis, J, et al: Comparison of fasciotomy wound closures using traditional dressing changes and the vacuum-assisted closure device. Ann Plast Surg 62(4):407, 2009.
194. Borgquist, O, Ingemansson, R, and Malmsjo, M: Individualizing the use of negative pressure wound therapy for optimal wound healing: A focused review of the literature. Ostomy Wound Manage 57(4):44, 2011.
195. Vuerstaek, JD, et al: State-of-the-art treatment of chronic leg ulcers: A randomized controlled trial comparing vacuum-assisted closure (VAC) with modern wound dressings. J Vasc Surg 44(5):1029, 2006.
196. Eginton, MT, et al: A prospective randomized evaluation of negative-pressure wound dressings for diabetic foot wounds. Ann Vasc Surg 17(6):645, 2003.
197. Hunter, S, et al: The use of monochromatic infrared energy in wound management. Adv Skin Wound Care 20(5):265, 2007.
198. Leonard, DR, Farooqi, MH, and Myers, S: Restoration of sensation, reduced pain, and improved balance in subjects with diabetic peripheral neuropathy: A double-blind, randomized, placebo-controlled study with monochromatic near-infrared treatment. Diabetes Care 27(1):168, 2004.
199. Lavery, L, et al: Does anodyne light therapy improve peripheral neuropath in diabetes? A double-blind, sham-controlled, randomize trial to evaluate monochromatic infrared photoenergy. Diabetes Care 31(2):316, 2008.
200. Powell, MW, Carnegie, DE, and Burke, TJ: Reversal of diabetic peripheral neuropathy and new wound incidence: The role of MIRE. Adv Skin Wound Care 17(6):295, 2004.
201. Harkless, LB, et al: Improved foot sensitivity and pain reduction in patients with peripheral neuropathy after treatment with monochromatic infrared photo energy—MIRE. J Diabetes Complications 20(2):81, 2006.
202. Edwards, K: New twist on an old favorite: Gentian violet and methylene blue antibacterial foams. Adv Wound Care 5(1): 11, 2016.
203. Applewhite, A, et al: Gentian violet and methylene blue polyvinyl alcohol foam antibacterial dressing as a viable form of autolytic débridement in the wound bed. Surg Technol Int 26:65, 2015.
204. Carter, MJ, Tingley-Kelley, K, and Warriner, RA: Silver treatments and silver-impregnated dressings for the healing of leg wounds and ulcers: A systematic review and meta-analysis. J Am Acad Dermatol 63(4):668, 2010.
205. Cohn, S, et al: Open surgical wounds: How does Aquacel compare with wet-to-dry gauze? J Wound Care 13(1):10, 2004.
206. Bethell, E: Why gauze dressings should not be the first choice to manage most acute surgical cavity wounds. J Wound Care 12(6): 237, 2003.

207. Allie, DE, et al: Novel treatment strategy for leg and sternal wound complications after coronary artery bypass graft surgery: Bioengineered Apligraf. Ann Thorac Surg 78(2):673, 2004.
208. Greenwood, JE, Clausen, J, and Kavanagh, S: Experience with Biobrane: Uses and Caveats for Success. Eplasty 9:e25, 2009.
209. Williams, A: Manual lymphatic drainage: Exploring the history and the evidence base. Br J Community Nurs 15(4):S18, 2010.
210. Molski, P, et al: Patients with venous disease benefit from manual lymphatic drainage. Int Angiol 28(2):151, 2008.
211. Vairo, GI, et al: Systematic review of efficacy for manual lymphatic drainage techniques in sports medicine and rehabilitation: An evidence-based practice approach. J Man Manip Ther 17(3): 80, 2009.
212. Strossenreuther, RHK, et al: Practical instructions for therapists—manual lymph drainage according to Dr. E. Vodder. In Foldi, M, Foldi, E, and Kubik, S (eds): Textbook of Lymphology for Physicians and Lymphedema Therapists, ed 2. Elsevier, Munich, Germany, 2006, p. 526.
213. Koksal, C, and Bozkurt, AK: Combination of hydrocolloid dressing and medical compression stockings versus Unna's boot for the treatment of venous leg ulcers. Swiss Med Wkly 133(25-26): 364, 2003.
214. Polignano, R, et al: A randomized controlled study of four-layer compression versus Unna's boot for venous ulcers. J Wound Care 13(1):21–24, 2004.
215. Iglesias, C, et al: VenUS I: a randomized controlled trial of two types of bandage for treating venous leg ulcers. Health Technol Assess 8(29):1–105, 2004.
216. Ashby RL, et al: VenUS IV (Venous leg Ulcer study IV)—compression hosiery compared with compression bandaging in the treatment of venous leg ulcers: A randomized controlled trial, mixed-treatment comparison and decision-analytic model. Health Technol Assess 18(57):1–293, 2014.
217. Weissleder, H, and Schuchhardt, C: Lymphedema: Diagnosis and therapy. In Weissleder, H, and Schuchhardt, C (eds): Therapy Concepts, ed 4. Viavital Verlag, Essen, Germany, 2008, p. 403.
218. Leduc, O, Peeters, A, and Borgeois, P: Bandages: Scintigraphic demonstration of its efficacy on colloidal protein reabsorption during muscle activity. Progress in Lymphology—XII. Elsevier, Philadelphia, 1990.
219. Johansson, K, et al: Effects of compression bandaging with or without manual lymph drainage treatment in patients with postoperative arm lymphedema. Lymphology 32:103, 1999.
220. Schmid-Schonbein, GW: Microlymphatics and lymph flow. Physiol Rev 70(4):987, 1990.
221. Simon, DA, Dix, FP, and McCollum, CN: Management of venous leg ulcers. Br Med J 328:1358, 2004.
222. Weiss, J: Treatment of leg edema and wounds in a patient with severe musculoskeletal injuries. Phys Ther 78(10):1104, 1998.
223. Asmussen, PD, and Strossenreuther, RHK: Compression therapy. In Foldi, M, Foldi, E, and Kubik, S (eds): Textbook of Lymphology for Physicians and Lymphedema Therapists, ed 5. Elsevier, Munich, Germany, 2003, p. 528.
224. Yasuhara, H, Shigematsu, H, and Muto, T: A study of the advantages of elastic stocking for leg lymphedema. Int Angiology 15(3):272, 1996.
225. Harris, SR, et al: Clinical practice guidelines for the care and treatment of breast cancer: 11. Lymphedema. Can Med Assoc J 164(2):191, 2001.
226. Badger, CM, Peacock, JL, and Mortimer, PS: A randomized, controlled, parallel-group clinical trial comparing multiplayer bandaging followed by hosiery versus hosiery alone in the treatment of patients with lymphedema of the limb. Cancer 88(12): 2832, 2000.
227. Apaqut, U, and Dayioglu, E: Importance and advantages of intermittent external pneumatic compression therapy in venous stasis ulceration. Angiology 56(1):19, 2005.
228. Nelson E, Hillman A, and Thomas K: Intermittent pneumatic compression for treating venous leg ulcers. Cochrane Database of Systematic Reviews 2014 (5) Art. No.: CD001899. doi: 10.1002/14651858. CD001899.pub4.
229. Comerota, AJ: Intermittent pneumatic compression: Physiologic and clinical basis to improve management of venous leg ulcers. J Vasc Surg 53(4):1121, 2011.
230. Haghighat, S, et al: Comparing two treatment methods for post mastectomy lymphedema: Complex decongestive therapy alone and in combination with intermittent pneumatic compression. Lymphology 43(1):25, 2010.
231. Partsch, H, et al: Clinical trials needed to evaluate compression therapy in breast cancer related lymphedema (BCRL). Proposals from an expert group. Int Angiol 25(5):442, 2010.
232. Devoogdt, N, et al: Different physical treatment modalities for lymphoedema developing after axillary lymph node dissection for breast cancer: A review. Eur J Obstet Gynecol Reprod Biol 149(1):3, 2010.
233. Rockson, SG: Current concepts and future directions in the diagnosis and management of lymphatic vascular disease. Vasc Med 15(3):223, 2010.
234. Adams, KE, et al: Direct evidence of lymphatic function improvement after advanced pneumatic compression device treatment of lymphedema. Biomed Opt Express 1(1):114, 2010.
235. Ridner, SH, et al: Home-based lymphedema treatment in patients with cancer-related lymphedema or noncancer-related lymphedema. Oncol Nurs Forum 35(4):671, 2008.
236. Wilburn, O, Wilburn, P, and Rockson, SG. A pilot, prospective evaluation of a novel alternative for maintenance therapy of breast cancer–associated lymphedema. BMC Cancer 6:84, 2006.
237. Van Rijswijk, L: Pressure ulcer prevention updates. Am J Nurs 109(8):S6, 2009.
238. Brienza, DM, Geyer MJ, Sprigle, S, et al: Seating, positioning, and support surfaces. In Baranoski, S, and Ayello, EA (eds): Wound Care Essentials: Practice Principles, ed 4. Lippincott Williams & Wilkins, Philadelphia, 2012.
239. National Pressure Ulcer Advisory Panel, European Pressure Ulcer Advisory Panel: Pressure ulcer treatment recommendations. In Prevention and Treatment of Pressure Ulcers: Clinical Practice Guideline. National Pressure Ulcer Advisory Panel, Washington, DC, 2009.
240. Brienza, D, et al: A randomized clinical trial on preventing pressure ulcers with wheelchair seat cushions. J Am Geriatr Soc 58(12):2308, 2010.
241. Stockton, L, Gebhardt, KS, and Clark, M: Seating and pressure ulcers: Clinical practice guidelines. J Tissue Viability 18(4):98, 2009.
242. McInnes, E, et al: Support surfaces for pressure ulcer prevention. Cochrane Database of Systematic Reviews 2015 Sept 3;(9) CD001735. doi: 10:1002/14651858.
243. Zhang, L, et al: Combining manual lymph drainage with physical exercise after modified radical mastectomy effectively prevents upper limb lymphedema. Lymphat Res Biol 14(2):104, 2016.
244. Schmitz, K et al: Weight lifting in women with breast-cancer-related lymphedema. N Engl J Med 361:664, 2009.
245. Armstrong, DG, et al: Evaluation of removable and irremovable cast walkers in the healing of diabetic foot wounds. Diabetes Care 28.3:551, 2005.
246. Vaseenon, T, et al: Off-loading total contact cast in combination with hydrogel and foam dressing for management of diabetic plantar ulcer of the foot. J Med Assoc Thai 97(12):1319, 2014.
247. Cavanagh, PR, and Bus, SA: Off-loading the diabetic foot for ulcer prevention and healing. Plast Reconstr Surg 127:248S, 2011.
248. Shaw, TJ, Kishi, K, and Mori, R: Wound associated skin fibrosis: Mechanisms and treatments based on modulating the inflammatory response. Endocr Metab Immune Disord Drug Targets 10(4):320, 2010.

Patient Education: Skin Care and Footwear Instructions

appendix **14.A**

INSPECT YOUR SKIN

1. Look at your feet every day. Use a mirror, a magnifying glass, or the assistance of a family member to help you see all over your feet including between your toes and the bottoms of your feet.
2. Look for these things on your feet: blisters, sores, corns, calluses, red spots, swelling, pain, drainage from a sore, broken toenails, cracked skin, odor. Notify your health care provider if you see any of these things on your feet or if you injure either of your feet.

TAKE CARE OF YOUR SKIN

1. Wash your feet gently every day using lukewarm water and mild soap. Test the water temperature with your hand before you wash your feet. If your hand is not sensitive to temperature, use a thermometer. The temperature should be about 85°F (29.44°C).
2. Dry your feet well, especially between your toes.
3. You may want to use a lanolin-based lotion or petroleum jelly to soften dry skin. Do not apply any lotion between your toes. You may use powder or cornstarch between your toes.
4. Never try to treat corns, calluses, or toenails with sharp instruments, home remedies, or store-bought foot care products. These items can all hurt your skin.
5. Cut toenails straight across; do not cut into corners. Use an emery board for sharp edges. A pumice stone can be used to treat small corns and calluses. Alert your health care provider about your foot care practices.
6. For padding and air circulation, use small bits of lamb's wool between the toes. Change the lamb's wool every day. Be sure to use new pieces after you wash your feet. Do not use cotton or cotton balls because the fibers may irritate your skin.
7. Put on a clean pair of white socks after your skin care routine.
8. Do not walk barefoot.
9. If your feet are cold at bedtime, wear cotton socks; do not use a hot water bottle or heating pad to warm your feet.

CHECK YOUR SHOES

1. Check your shoes every day before you put them on. Look inside for small things that could cause a sore on your foot. Alternate shoes each day to allow them to breathe and dry completely.
2. Be sure that your shoes are the right size and width.
3. Do not wear old worn-out shoes or socks.
4. Shop for shoes in the afternoon when your feet are the largest.
5. Break in your new shoes gradually.

SEE YOUR HEALTH CARE PROVIDER

1. Get help in controlling your diabetes.
2. Have regular appointments with your doctor.
3. Call your health care provider immediately if you find a wound on your foot.

appendix

14.B Special Tests for Arterial and Venous Function

Special Tests	Description
Rubor of dependency	A noninvasive test to examine the lower extremity (LE) for the presence of ischemia. Following elevation of the limb, lowering of the limb should return the skin of the limb to a pink color. If the color is dark red and takes more than 30 seconds to appear, the test is positive for arterial insufficiency.
Air plethysmography (APG)	A noninvasive test of both the arterial and venous circulation. Changes in LE volume are measured using a pressure cuff that quantifies volume changes during rest, standing, and light walking. Venous obstruction and arterial inflow can be observed with this test.
Transcutaneous oxygen ($TcPO_2$)	A noninvasive examination tool for arterial circulation. A special probe and a heating element measure profusion. Measurement of oxygen at the skin level gives information about what is happening at the cellular level. Also found in the literature as *transcutaneous partial pressure of oxygen* and *transcutaneous oxygen tension measurement.* The results are predictive for healing of ulcers and amputation wounds.
Skin perfusion pressure (SPP) measurement	A noninvasive test that measures blood flow in the skin. To take the measurements, a modified laser Doppler probe is secured in the bladder of a specialized blood pressure cuff. Results are predictive for healing of ulcers and amputation wounds.
Venous filling time	The extremity is elevated and then lowered into a dependent position. The time it takes for the veins on top of the foot to refill is recorded. Normal filling time is 15 seconds. Greater than 15 seconds indicates arterial disease whereas less than 15 indicates venous disease.
Percussion test	With LE in a dependent position, the greater saphenous vein is palpated distal to the knee with one hand while it is tapped 6 in. (15.2 cm) proximal to the knee with the other hand. If a wave of fluid is detected under the distal palpation site, this indicates the possibility of valvular incompetency.
Trendelenburg test	Test measures the time required to refill the veins in the dorsum of the foot. The LE is elevated to allow venous blood to empty. A tourniquet on the thigh prevents backflow. After 1 minute, the individual stands. If veins fully distend within 5 seconds before the tourniquet is released, valvular incompetence in the deep veins is suspected. If distention occurs within 5 seconds after the tourniquet is released, incompetence of superficial veins is suspected.

Sample Wound Examination Form

appendix **14.C**

Name ______________________________

B/P __________ Resp __________ HR __________ Temp __________ Weight __________

Date: Orientation to time/place/person? ( ) Yes ( ) No

Arrived: ( ) Ambulatory ( ) Cane ( ) Crutches ( ) Walker ( ) Wheelchair ( ) Stretcher ( ) N/A

( ) Initial Examination Reviewed: Changes in medicine, allergies, or health history since last visit? ( ) Yes ( ) No (If yes, indicate changes)

Wound Number				
Wound Location				
Wound Type	Ulcer: ☐ Pressure ☐ Venous ☐ Arterial ☐ Diabetic ☐ SDTI ☐ Burn ☐ Donor site ☐ Other: ______ ☐ Infected ☐ Contaminated ☐ Unknown ☐ Biopsy: ☐ Yes, Date: ______ ☐ No ☐ Other: ______	Ulcer: ☐ Pressure ☐ Venous ☐ Arterial ☐ Diabetic ☐ SDTI ☐ Burn ☐ Donor site ☐ Other: ______ ☐ Infected ☐ Contaminated ☐ Unknown ☐ Biopsy: ☐ Yes, Date: ______ ☐ No ☐ Other: ______	Ulcer: ☐ Pressure ☐ Venous ☐ Arterial ☐ Diabetic ☐ SDTI ☐ Burn ☐ Donor site ☐ Other: ______ ☐ Infected ☐ Contaminated ☐ Unknown ☐ Biopsy: ☐ Yes, Date: ______ ☐ No ☐ Other: ______	Ulcer: ☐ Pressure ☐ Venous ☐ Arterial ☐ Diabetic ☐ SDTI ☐ Burn ☐ Donor site ☐ Other: ______ ☐ Infected ☐ Contaminated ☐ Unknown ☐ Biopsy: ☐ Yes, Date: ______ ☐ No ☐ Other: ______
Wound Stage (Circle)	I II III IV U/S	I II III IV U/S	I II III IV U/S	I II III IV U/S
Length				
Width				
Depth				
Tunnels/ Undermining	( ) Yes ( ) No	( ) Yes ( ) No	( ) Yes ( ) No	( ) Yes ( ) No
Granulation				
Slough				

Eschar	( ) Yes ( ) No	( ) Yes ( ) No	( ) Yes ( ) No	( ) Yes ( ) No
Odor	( ) Yes ( ) No	( ) Yes ( ) No	( ) Yes ( ) No	( ) Yes ( ) No
Drainage Amount	( ) None ( ) Minimal ( ) Moderate ( ) Heavy	( ) None ( ) Minimal ( ) Moderate ( ) Heavy	( ) None ( ) Minimal ( ) Moderate ( ) Heavy	( ) None ( ) Minimal ( ) Moderate ( ) Heavy
Drainage Color	( ) Serous ( ) Serosanguineous ( ) Sanguineous ( ) Purulent ( ) Yellow/Green ( ) NA	( ) Serous ( ) Serosanguineous ( ) Sanguineous ( ) Purulent ( ) Yellow/Green ( ) NA	( ) Serous ( ) Serosanguineous ( ) Sanguineous ( ) Purulent ( ) Yellow/Green ( ) NA	( ) Serous ( ) Serosanguineous ( ) Sanguineous ( ) Purulent ( ) Yellow/Green ( ) NA
Wound Margin ( ) Yes ( ) No	( ) Well Defined ( ) Poorly Defined	( ) Well Defined ( ) Poorly Defined	( ) Well Defined ( ) Poorly Defined	( ) Well Defined ( ) Poorly Defined
Exposed Bone	( ) Yes ( ) No	( ) Yes ( ) No	( ) Yes ( ) No	( ) Yes ( ) No
Exposed Muscle/ Tendon/Ligament	( ) Yes ( ) No	( ) Yes ( ) No	( ) Yes ( ) No	( ) Yes ( ) No
Periwound	( ) Maceration ( ) Intact	( ) Maceration ( ) Intact	( ) Maceration ( ) Intact	( ) Maceration ( ) Intact
Appearance	( ) Callus ( ) Necrotic ( ) Erythema	( ) Callus ( ) Necrotic ( ) Erythema	( ) Callus ( ) Necrotic ( ) Erythema	( ) Callus ( ) Necrotic ( ) Erythema

■ PAIN MANAGEMENT

Pain Scale: None 0 1 2 3 4 5 6 7 8 9 10 Severe

Locations(s):

Described as: ( ) Sharp ( ) Dull ( ) Burning
( ) Throbbing ( ) Radiating ( ) Constant
( ) Intermittent ( ) AM ( ) PM
( ) Only with dressing change

Relieved by: ( ) Elevation of Legs/offloading/rest
( ) Medication
( ) Standing/walking ( ) Other ______
Comments: ______________________

Pain Management Measures: ( ) LAT ( ) Lidocaine ( ) NA ( ) Refused ( ) Other:

Strength/ROM/ADL/Gait/Transfers/Mobility: ( ) Impaired ( ) Not Impaired
Comments:

Other Test Results: ABI: Monofilaments:

■ PLAN OF CARE

Cleansing:

Dressing:

Modalities:

Débridement:

Exercise:
Education:
Pressure Relief:
Compression:

Other:
ABI: Ankle–Brachial Index
LAT: Lidocaine, Adrenaline, and Tetracaine
ROM: Range of motion
Stage Descriptions:

SDTI:	Suspected deep tissue injury (purple or maroon localized area of discolored intact skin)
Stage I:	Skin intact, light skin: nonblanchable red area; dark skin: warm, indurated, hard edema
Stage II:	Partial-thickness skin loss
Stage III:	Full-thickness skin loss
Stage IV:	Muscle/bone/joint(s) involved
U/S:	Unstageable (full thickness tissue loss/base covered by slough and/or eschar)

Signature: ___________________________

Date/Time: ___________________________

appendix 14.D

Web-Based Resources for Clinicians, Families, and Patients With Vascular, Lymphatic, and Integumentary Disorders

FOR CLINICIANS

American Academy of Wound Management (AAWM)	www.abwmcertified.org
American College of Certified Wound Specialists (ACCWS)	www.accws.org
World Wide Wounds	www.worldwidewounds.com
The Wound Care Institute	www.wcei.net
National Lymphedema Network	www.lymphnet.org
Consortium for Spinal Cord Medicine/Paralyzed Veterans of America	www.pva.org
Wound Care Consultants	www.woundcarecenters.org
Association for the Advancement of Wound Care	https://aawconline.memberclicks.net
American Podiatric Medical Association (APMA)	www.apma.org
Wound Care Associates	www.woundcareresources.com
Wound, Ostomy and Continence Nurses Society (WOCN)	www.wocn.org
Centers for Disease Control and Prevention (CDC)	www.cdc.gov

SELECTED LIST OF PROGRAMS FOR SPECIALIZED EDUCATION IN CDT AND MLD

National Lymphedema Network	www.lymphnet.org
Academy of Lymphatic Studies	www.acols.com
Dr. Vodder School International	www.vodderschool.com
Klose Training & Consulting	www.klosetraining.com
Norton School of Lymphatic Therapy	www.nortonschool.com
Complex Lymphatic Therapy	www.casleysmithinternational.org

FOR PATIENTS AND FAMILY MEMBERS

National Lymphedema Network	www.lymphnet.org
American Cancer Society	www.cancer.org
Lymph Notes	http://www.lymphnotes.com

appendix 14.E

Selected Wound Dressing Manufacturer Web Sites

Coloplast	www.coloplast.com
ConvaTec	www.convatec.com
DeRoyal	www.deroyal.com
Hollister	www.hollister.com
Jobst	www.jobst-usa.com
Johnson & Johnson	www.jnj.com
Smith & Nephew	www.smith-nephew.com

appendix 14.F

Dressings by Treatment Goal (Purpose) and Wound Type (Indication)

I. Dressings by Treatment Goal

Purpose	Dressing
Space filling (cavities, undermining, tunnels, or sinuses)	Gauze ribbons Foams (some) Hydrogels (amorphous or sheet) Alginates Impregnated gauze Absorptive dressings (beads, powders, and pastes) Composite dressings (some)
Mechanical débridement	Gauze
Exudate absorption	Gauze Foams Absorptive dressings (beads, powders, and pastes) Alginates Hydrocolloids Collagen
Hydration	Hydrogels (amorphous or sheets) Saline-moistened gauze (do not allow to dry)
Autolytic débridement	Transparent films Hydrocolloids Hydrogels (amorphous or sheet) Foams Alginates Impregnated gauze Absorptive dressings (beads, powders, and pastes) Composites
Protection for newly formed tissue	Transparent films Hydrocolloids Hydrogel sheets (some) Composites (some) Foams (some)
Hemostasis	Alginates Collagen
Friction reduction	Transparent films Hydrocolloids Hydrogel sheets (some)
Insulation to promote warmth	Transparent films Hydrocolloids Hydrogels (amorphous or sheet) Foams Composites (some)

Continued

Pain reduction	Transparent films Hydrocolloids Hydrogels (amorphous or sheet) Foams Alginates Composites
Odor reduction	Hydrocolloids Hydrogel sheet (some) Alginates (some) Foams (charcoal) Absorptive dressings (beads, powders, and pastes) (some)
Cushioning	Hydrocolloids Hydrogel sheet (some) Foams Composites (some) Gauze (some)
Antibacterial	Silver-based dressings Iodine-based dressings Methylene blue and gentian violet-based dressings

II. Dressings by Wound Type and Dressing Goals

Indication	Dressing
Infected wounds: prevent or treat bacterial growth	Gauze (some) Alginates Hydrogels Hydrogel sheets Impregnated gauze Foams (with or without added antibacterial protection)
Burns	Alginates Hydrocolloids Hydrogels Transparent films Impregnated gauze Foams Biological dressings Collagen
Stage 1 pressure injuries	Transparent films Foams
Stage 2 pressure injuries	Alginate Hydrocolloids Hydrogel sheets Transparent films Impregnated gauze Foams Collagen
Stage 3 and 4 pressure injuries	Alginates Hydrocolloids Hydrogel sheets Impregnated gauze Foams Collagen

Venous ulcers	Alginates Hydrocolloids Hydrogels Foams
Arterial ulcers	Alginates (do not allow to dry) Hydrogel sheets Foams
Diabetic ulcers	Alginates Hydrocolloids Transparent films Foams
Donor sites	Alginates Hydrocolloids Hydrogel sheets Transparent films Impregnated gauze Collagen

Chapter 15 Stroke

Judith E. Deutsch, PT, PhD
Susan B. O'Sullivan, PT, EdD

LEARNING OBJECTIVES

1. Describe the epidemiology, etiology, pathophysiology, symptomatology, and sequelae of stroke.
2. Identify and describe the procedures used to examine and evaluate patients with stroke to establish a diagnosis, prognosis, and plan of care.
3. Describe the role of the physical therapist in assisting the patient in recovery from stroke in terms of interventions, patient/client-related instruction, coordination, communication, and documentation.
4. Describe and practice clinical reasoning used to examine and evaluate client care, formulate realistic goals, and develop a plan of care for a clinical case study.

CHAPTER OUTLINE

Stroke (cerebrovascular accident [CVA]) is the sudden loss of neurological function caused by an interruption of blood flow to the brain. *Ischemic stroke* is the most common type, affecting about 80% of individuals with stroke, and can be the result of a thrombosis, embolism, or hypoperfusion. A thrombus is a local occlusion of a blood vessel, and an embolus is material from a distant site that either blocks or impairs blood flow, depriving the brain of essential oxygen and nutrients. Lack of oxygen and nutrients results in tissue necrosis and penumbral area where the cells may be damaged but preserved.[1]

Hemorrhagic stroke occurs when blood vessels rupture, causing leakage of blood in or around the brain. Clinically, a variety of focal deficits are possible, including changes in the level of consciousness and impairments of sensory, motor, cognitive, perceptual, and language functions. To be classified as stroke, neurological deficits must persist for at least 24 hours. Motor deficits are characterized by paralysis *(hemiplegia)* or weakness *(hemiparesis),* typically on the side of the body opposite the side of the lesion. The term *hemiplegia* is often used generically to refer to the wide variety of motor problems that result from stroke. The location and extent of brain injury, the amount of collateral blood flow, and early acute care management determine the severity of neurological deficits in an individual patient. Impairments may resolve spontaneously as brain swelling subsides (reversible ischemic neurological deficit), generally within 3 weeks. Residual neurological impairments are those that persist longer than 3 weeks and may lead to lasting disability. Strokes are classified by etiological categories (thrombosis, embolus, or hemorrhage), specific vascular territory (anterior cerebral artery syndrome, middle cerebral artery syndrome, and so forth), and management categories (transient ischemic attack, minor stroke, major stroke, deteriorating stroke, young stroke).

■ EPIDEMIOLOGY AND ETIOLOGY

Stroke is the fifth leading cause of death and the leading cause of long-term disability among adults in the United States. An estimated 7.2 million Americans older than 20 years of age have experienced a stroke. Each year, approximately 795,000 individuals experience a stroke; approximately 610,000 are first attacks and 185,000 are recurrent strokes. Women have a lower age-adjusted stroke prevalence than men. However, this prevalence is reversed in older ages; women over 85 years of age have an elevated prevalence compared to men. Compared to whites, African Americans have twice the risk of first-ever stroke; rates are also higher in Mexican Americans, American Indians, and Alaskan Natives. The incidence of stroke increases dramatically with age, effectively doubling in the decade after 65 years of age. Approximately 10% of all strokes occur in individuals 18 to 50 years of age. Between 5% and 8% of persons who survive an initial stroke will experience another one within 1 year; within 5 years, stroke will recur in 16%. Current data reveal that stroke incidence has been declining in recent years in a largely white adult cohort.[2]

The incidence of stroke deaths is greater than 133,000 annually, and strokes account for 1 of every 20 deaths in the United States. Death rates due to stroke have been declining since 2007. The type of stroke is significant in determining survival. Of patients with stroke, hemorrhagic stroke accounts for the largest number of deaths, with mortality rates of 37% to 38% at 1 month, whereas ischemic strokes have a mortality rate of only 14.7% at 1 month. Survival rates are dramatically lessened by increased age, hypertension, heart disease, and diabetes. Loss of consciousness at stroke onset, lesion size, persistent severe hemiplegia, multiple neurological deficits, and history of previous stroke are also important predictors of mortality.[2,3]

Stroke is the leading cause of *serious* long-term disability in the United States. Of ischemic stroke survivors 65 or older, incidences of disabilities observed at 6 months include hemiparesis (50%), inability to walk without assistance (30%), dependence in activities of daily living (ADL) (26%), aphasia (19%), and depression (35%). Stroke survivors represent the largest group admitted to rehabilitation hospitals, and about a third of patients receive outpatient rehabilitation services. Another indicator of disability is the fact that approximately 26% of patients with stroke are institutionalized in a long-term care facility. Direct and indirect costs of stroke are in the tens of billions.[2]

Atherosclerosis is a major contributory factor in cerebrovascular disease. It is characterized by plaque formation with an accumulation of lipids, fibrin, complex carbohydrates, and calcium deposits on arterial walls that leads to progressive narrowing of blood vessels. Interruption of blood flow by atherosclerotic plaques occurs at certain sites of predilection. These generally include bifurcations, constrictions, dilations, or angulations of arteries. The most common sites for lesions to occur are at the origin of the common carotid artery or at its transition into the middle cerebral artery, at the main bifurcation of the middle cerebral artery, and at the junction of the vertebral arteries with the basilar artery.

Ischemic strokes are the result of thrombus, embolism, or conditions that produce low systemic perfusion pressures. The resulting lack of cerebral blood flow (CBF) deprives the brain of needed oxygen and glucose, disrupts cellular metabolism, and leads to injury and death of tissues. A thrombus results from platelet adhesion and aggregation on plaques. *Cerebral thrombosis* refers to the formation or development of a blood clot within the cerebral arteries or their branches. It should be noted that lesions of extracranial vessels (carotid or vertebral arteries) can also produce symptoms of stroke. Thrombi lead to ischemia, or occlusion of an artery with resulting *cerebral infarction* or tissue death *(atherothrombotic brain infarction [ABI]).* Thrombi can also become dislodged and travel to a more distal site in the form of an intra-artery embolus. *Cerebral embolus (CE)* is composed of bits of matter (blood clot, plaque) formed elsewhere and released into the bloodstream, traveling to the cerebral arteries where they lodge in a vessel, producing occlusion and infarction. The most common source of CE is disease of the cardiovascular system. Occasionally, systemic disorders may produce septic, fat, or air emboli that affect the cerebral circulation. Ischemic strokes may also result from low systemic perfusion, the result of cardiac failure or significant blood loss with resulting systemic hypotension. The neurological deficits produced with systemic failure are global in nature with bilateral neurological deficits.

Hemorrhagic strokes, with abnormal bleeding into the extravascular areas of the brain, are the result of rupture of a cerebral vessel or trauma. Hemorrhage results in increased intracranial pressures with injury to brain tissues and restriction of distal blood flow. *Intracerebral hemorrhage (IH)* is caused by rupture of a cerebral vessel with subsequent bleeding into the brain. Primary *cerebral hemorrhage* (nontraumatic spontaneous hemorrhage) typically occurs in small blood vessels weakened by atherosclerosis producing an *aneurysm. Subarachnoid hemorrhage (SH)* occurs from bleeding into the subarachnoid space typically from a saccular or berry aneurysm affecting primarily large blood vessels. Congenital defects that produce weakness in the blood vessel wall are major contributing factors to the formation of an aneurysm. Hemorrhage is closely linked to chronic hypertension. *Arteriovenous malformation (AVM)* is another congenital defect that can result in stroke. AVM is characterized by a tortuous tangle of arteries and veins with agenesis of an interposing capillary system. The abnormal vessels undergo progressive dilation with age and eventually bleed in about 50% of cases. Sudden and severe cerebral bleeding can result in death within hours, because intracranial pressures rise rapidly and adjacent cortical tissues are compressed or displaced as in brainstem herniation.

■ RISK FACTORS AND STROKE PREVENTION

Cardiovascular diseases affecting the brain and heart share a number of common risk factors important to the development of atherosclerosis. Major risk factors for stroke are hypertension, diabetes mellitus (DM), disorders of heart rhythm, high blood cholesterol and other lipids, smoking/tobacco use, and heart disease (HD). In patients with ABI, approximately 70% have hypertension, 30% HD, 15% congestive heart failure (CHF), 30% peripheral arterial disease (PAD), and 15% DM.[3] Blood pressure (BP) is a powerful determinant of risk for both ischemic stroke and intracranial hemorrhage. Individuals with BP less than 120/80 mm Hg have approximately half the lifetime risk of stroke of those with hypertension.[2, p. e380] Patients with marked elevations of hematocrit are also at an increased risk of occlusive stroke owing to a generalized reduction of CBF. Cardiac disorders (e.g., rheumatic heart valvular disease, endocarditis) and cardiac surgery (e.g., coronary artery bypass graft [CABG]) increase the risk of embolic stroke. Atrial fibrillation is a powerful risk factor for ischemic stroke with a three- to fivefold increased risk. End-stage renal disease and chronic kidney disease also increase the risk of stroke. Sleep apnea is an independent risk factor for stroke, almost doubling the risk of stroke or death. Control of these chronic diseases and conditions is essential in reducing stroke risk.[2,3]

A number of stroke risk factors are specific to women. Women with early menopause (before 42 years of age) have twice the risk of ischemic stroke as women with later menopause. The use of estrogen alone or estrogen plus progestin increases the risk of ischemic stroke (up to 44% to 55% or higher). Pregnancy, birth, and the first 6 weeks postpartum can also increase risk of stroke, especially in older women and African Americans. Preeclampsia is an independent risk factor for stroke.[2]

Modifiable risk factors include cigarette smoking, physical inactivity, obesity, and diet. Risk of stroke is two to four times higher in current smokers than in nonsmokers or those who have quit for more than 10 years. Exposure to secondhand smoke increases the risk of stroke by 20% to 30%. Physical activity (moderate to vigorous exercise) is associated with an overall 35% reduction in stroke risk, whereas light exercise (walking) does not appear to have the same benefit. As with a cardiac risk profile, the more risk factors present or the greater the degree of abnormality of any one factor, the greater the risk of stroke. Stroke risk factors considered nonmodifiable include family history, age, gender, and race (African American).

Lifestyle changes can greatly reduce the risk of stroke. Achieving the greatest ideal cardiovascular health metrics, including avoiding smoking and tobacco products; engaging in daily physical activity; eating a healthy diet; maintaining a healthy weight; and keeping cholesterol, BP, and glucose at healthy levels, is associated with a lower risk of stroke. Table 15.1 indicates the definitions of cardiovascular health, take from the AHA 2020 Goals.[2,4]

Effective stroke prevention depends on improving public awareness concerning the *early warning signs of stroke.* Only about 60% of Americans can recognize even one warning sign, and only 55% can identify one stroke symptom.[2] Early warning signs identified by the American Heart Association and National Stroke Association, known as FAST, are presented in Box 15.1.[5] The significance of recognizing early warning signs rests with prompt initiation of emergency care under the rule that "time is brain." *FAST* is used as a mnemonic to help improve responsiveness to stroke victims by calling out the most common warning signs. Patients and families are encouraged to call 911 immediately, even if these symptoms go away quickly or are not painful.

Early computed tomography (CT) is used to differentiate between atherothrombotic stroke and hemorrhagic stroke. If the stroke is atherothrombotic, clot-dissolving enzymes (e.g., tissue plasminogen activator [tPA]) can be used for thrombolysis. To be effective, thrombolytic therapy such as tPA must be given within 3 to 4.5 hours of symptom onset. It cannot be given to patients with hemorrhagic stroke or patients with active intracranial bleeding (e.g., serious head trauma) because the drug may

Table 15.1 Definitions of Cardiovascular Health[2,4]

	Level of Cardiovascular Health for Each Metric for Adults 20 Years of Age and Older		
	Poor	*Intermediate*	*Ideal*
Current Smoking	Yes	Never or quit >12 mo	Former ≥23 mo
BMI	≥30 kg/m^2	25–29.9 kg/m^2	<25 kg/m^2
Physical Activity	None	1–149 min/wk moderate or 1–74 min/wk vigorous or 1–149 min/wk moderate + 2× vigorous	>150 min/wk moderate or ≥75 min/wk vigorous or ≥150 min/wk moderate + 2× vigorous
Healthy Diet Pattern, Number of Components (AHA Diet Score) ‡	<2 (0–39)	2–3(40–79)	4–5 (80–100)
Total Cholesterol, mg/dL	≥240	200–239 or treated to goal	<200
Blood Pressure	SBP ≥140 mm Hg or DBP ≥90 mm Hg	SBP 120–139 mm Hg or DBP 80–89 mm Hg or treated to goal	<120 mm Hg/80 mm Hg
Fasting Plasma Glucose, mg/dL	≥126	100–125 or treated to goal	<100

‡In the context of a healthy dietary pattern that is consistent with a Dietary Approaches to Stop Hypertension [DASH]–type eating pattern, to consume ≥4.5 cups/d of fruits and vegetables, ≥2 servings/wk of fish, and ≥3 servings/d of whole grains and no more than 36 oz/wk of sugar-sweetened beverages and 1,500 mg/d of sodium. The consistency of one's diet with these dietary targets can be described using a continuous AHA diet score, scaled from 0 to 100. Modified from Lloyd-Jones et al[4] with permission. Copyright © 2010, American Heart Association, Inc.

worsen bleeding. It is also contraindicated in patients with severe uncontrolled hypertension. Within this window of opportunity, the patient must recognize the situation as a medical emergency, be transported to an appropriate hospital, be evaluated by emergency department (ED) staff (including a CT scan of the brain), and be treated.[6,7] Although this treatment has been available since the mid-1990s and has been shown to be safe and to dramatically reduce death and disability, fewer than half of individuals experiencing stroke arrive at the ED within 2 hours of symptoms.[8] Women are less likely than men to arrive in time. Of those arriving at the ED within 2 hours of symptoms, only 65% received imaging within 1 hour of ED arrival.[9]

In the United States, there is a Stroke Center Network dedicated to providing the highest quality of acute stroke care. Direct access to a *comprehensive stroke center (CSC)* is associated with a shorter onset-to-treatment time and better outcomes for ischemic stroke treated with thrombolysis.[10] Even with policy changes that allow emergency first responders to transmit individuals directly to a CSC, only about half of patients have timely access.[11] A significant predictor in successfully accessing emergency care is the "executive" spouse or significant other who is able to make the decision to seek treatment immediately. Patients who do receive tPA are at least 33% more likely to recover from their stroke with little or no disability after 3 months as compared to those who do not receive the treatment.[12] Major heart and stroke organizations currently promote the use of the term *brain attack,* comparable to heart attack, to help individuals recognize the importance of seeking immediate emergency care.

PATHOPHYSIOLOGY

Sudden cessation of CBF and oxygen-glucose deprivation sets in motion a series of pathological events. Within minutes, neurons die in the ischemic core tissue, while the majority of neurons in the surrounding penumbra survive for a slightly longer time. Cell survival depends largely on the severity and the duration of the ischemic episode. For cells to survive, 20% to 25% of regular blood flow is required. Without timely reperfusion, cells in the penumbra die, neuronal activity ceases, and the infarct expands. Ischemia triggers a number of damaging cellular events, termed *ischemic cascade.* The release of excess neurotransmitters (e.g., glutamate and aspartate) produces a progressive disturbance of energy metabolism and anoxic depolarization, which results in an inability of brain cells to produce energy, particularly adenosine triphosphate (ATP). This is followed by excess influx of calcium ions and pump failure of the neuronal membrane. Excess calcium reacts with intracellular phospholipids to form free radicals. Calcium influx also stimulates the release of nitric oxide and cytokines. Both mechanisms further damage brain cells. Research efforts

Box 15.1 Stroke Early Warning Signs

SPOT A STROKE F.A.S.T.

F.A.S.T. is an easy way to remember the sudden signs of a stroke.

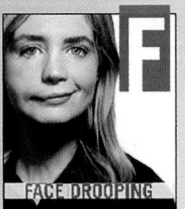

Face Drooping
Does one side of the face droop or is it numb? Ask the person to smile.

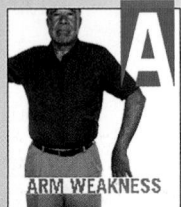

Arm Weakness
Is one arm weak or numb? Ask the person to raise both arms. Does one arm drift downward?

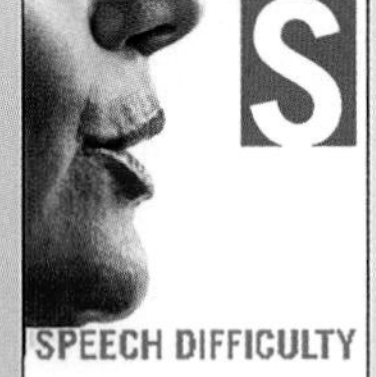

Speech Difficulty
Is speech slurred, are they unable to speak, or are they hard to understand? Ask the person to repeat a simple sentence, like "the sky is blue." Is the sentence repeated correctly?

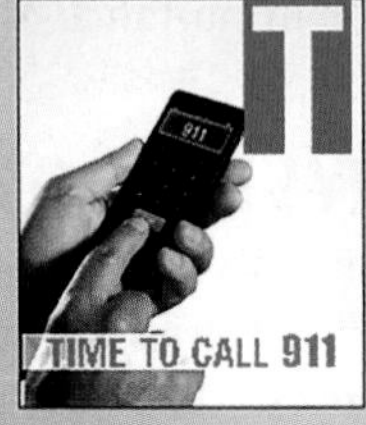

Time to call 9-1-1
If the person shows any of these symptoms, even if the symptoms go away, call 9-1-1 and get them to the hospital immediately.

Beyond F.A.S.T. – Other Symptoms you should know

- Sudden numbness or weakness of the leg
- Sudden confusion or trouble understanding
- Sudden trouble seeing in one or both eyes
- Sudden trouble walking, dizziness, loss of balance or coordination
- Sudden severe headache with no known cause

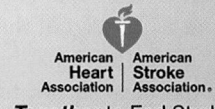

Together to End Stroke™

StrokeAssociation.org/warningsigns

are ongoing toward development of drugs that might promote angiogenesis, restore blood supply, stimulate neuroprotective genes, and reverse the metabolic changes of the ischemic penumbra area.[13]

Ischemic strokes produce *cerebral edema,* an accumulation of fluids within the brain that begins within minutes of the insult and reaches a maximum by 3 to 4 days. It is the result of tissue necrosis and widespread rupture of cell membranes with movement of fluid from the blood into brain tissues. The swelling gradually subsides and generally disappears by 2 to 3 weeks. Significant edema can elevate intracranial pressures, leading to intracranial hypertension and neurological deterioration associated with contralateral and caudal shifts of brain structures *(brainstem herniation).* Clinical signs of *elevating intracranial pressure (ICP)* include decreasing level of consciousness (stupor and coma), widened pulse pressure, increased heart rate, irregular respirations *(Cheyne-Stokes respirations),* vomiting, unreactive pupils (cranial nerve [CN] III signs), and papilledema. Cerebral edema is the most frequent cause of death in acute stroke and is characteristic of large infarcts involving the middle cerebral artery and the internal carotid artery.

Management Categories

Transient ischemic attack (TIA) refers to the temporary interruption of blood supply to the brain. Symptoms of focal neurological deficit may last for only a few minutes or for several hours but by definition do not last longer than 24 hours. After the attack, there may be evidence of residual brain damage or permanent neurological dysfunction. It is therefore recommended that they be considered like acute strokes.[1] TIAs may result from a number of different etiological factors, including occlusive episodes, emboli, reduced cerebral perfusion (arrhythmias, decreased cardiac output, hypotension, overmedication with antihypertensive medications, subclavian steal syndrome), or cerebrovascular spasm. The major clinical significance of TIA is as a precursor to susceptibility for both cerebral infarction and myocardial infarction. The risk for recurrent stroke is 3.5%, 8%, and 9.2% at 2, 30, and 90 days post-TIA respectively.[14]

Patients are classified as having a *major stroke* in the presence of stable, usually severe, impairments. The term *deteriorating stroke* refers to the patient whose neurological status deteriorates after admission to the hospital. This change in status may be due to cerebral or systemic causes (e.g., cerebral edema, progressing thrombosis). The category of *young stroke* describes a stroke affecting persons younger than age 45. Causes of stroke in children include perinatal arterial ischemic stroke, sickle cell disease, congenital HD, thrombophlebitis, and trauma.[2]

Vascular Syndromes

CBF varies with the patency of the vessels. Progressive narrowing secondary to atherosclerosis decreases blood flow. As in coronary heart disease, symptomatic changes generally result from a restriction of flow greater than 80%. The severity and symptoms of stroke are dependent on a number of factors, including (1) the location of the ischemic process, (2) the size of the ischemic area, (3) the nature and functions of the structures involved, and (4) the availability of collateral blood flow. Presenting symptoms may also depend on the rapidity of the occlusion of a blood vessel because slow occlusions may allow collateral vessels to take over, whereas sudden events do not.

CBF is controlled by numerous *autoregulatory mechanisms* (cerebral) that modulate a constant rate of blood flow through the brain. These mechanisms provide homeostatic balance, counteracting fluctuations in systolic BP (SBP) while maintaining a normal flow of 50 to 60 mL per 100g of brain tissue per minute. The brain has high energy requirements and very little metabolic reserves. Thus, it requires a continuous, rich perfusion of blood to deliver oxygen and glucose to the tissues. Cerebral flow represents approximately 17% of available cardiac output. Chemical regulation of CBF occurs in response to changes in blood concentrations of carbon dioxide or oxygen. Vasodilation and increased CBF are produced in response to an increase in $Paco_2$ or a decrease in Pao_2, whereas vasoconstriction and decreased CBF are produced by the opposite stimuli. Blood flow is also altered by changes in the blood pH. A fall in pH (increased acidity) produces vasodilation, and a rise in pH (increased alkalinity) produces a decrease in blood flow. Neurogenic regulation alters blood flow by vasodilating vessels in direct proportion to local function of brain tissue. Released metabolites probably act directly on the smooth muscle in local vessel walls. Changes in blood viscosity or ICP may also influence CBF. Changes in BP produce minor alterations of CBF. As pressure rises, the artery is stretched, resulting in contraction of smooth muscle in the vessel wall. Thus, the patency of the vessel is decreased, with a consequent decrease in CBF. As pressure falls, contraction lessens and CBF increases. Following stroke, autoregulatory mechanisms may be impaired.[15]

Knowledge of cerebral vascular anatomy is essential to understand the symptoms, diagnosis, and management of stroke. Extracranial blood supply to the brain is provided by the right and left internal carotid arteries and by the right and left vertebral arteries. The *internal carotid artery* begins at the bifurcation of the common carotid artery and ascends in the deep portions of the neck to the carotid canal. It turns rostromedially and ascends into the cranial cavity. It then pierces the dura mater and gives off the ophthalmic and anterior choroidal arteries before bifurcating into the middle and anterior cerebral arteries. The anterior communicating artery communicates with the anterior cerebral arteries of either side, giving rise to the rostral portion of the circle of Willis (Fig. 15.1). The *vertebral artery* arises as a branch off the subclavian artery. It enters the vertebral foramen of the sixth cervical vertebra and travels through the foramina of the transverse processes of the upper six cervical vertebrae to the foramen magnum and into the brain. There it travels in the posterior cranial fossa ventrally and medially and unites with the vertebral artery from the other side to form the basilar artery at the upper border of the medulla. At the upper border of the pons, the basilar artery bifurcates to form the posterior cerebral arteries and the posterior portion of the circle of Willis. Posterior communicating arteries connect the posterior cerebral arteries with the internal carotid arteries and complete the circle of Willis.

Anterior Cerebral Artery Syndrome

The *anterior cerebral artery (ACA)* is the first and smaller of two terminal branches of the internal carotid artery. It supplies the medial aspect of the cerebral hemisphere (frontal and parietal lobes) and subcortical structures, including the basal ganglia (anterior internal capsule, inferior caudate nucleus), anterior fornix, and anterior four-fifths of the corpus callosum (Fig. 15.2). Because

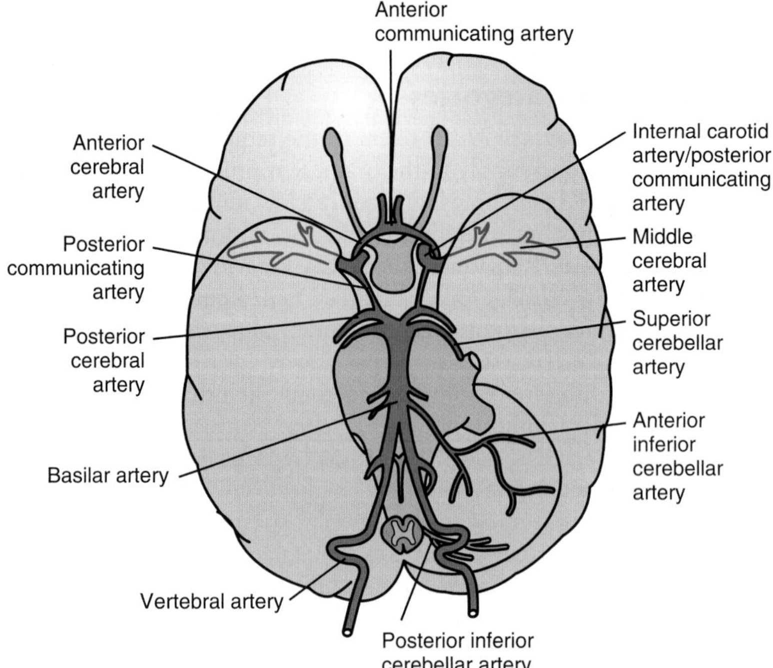

Figure 15.1 Cerebral circulation: circle of Willis.

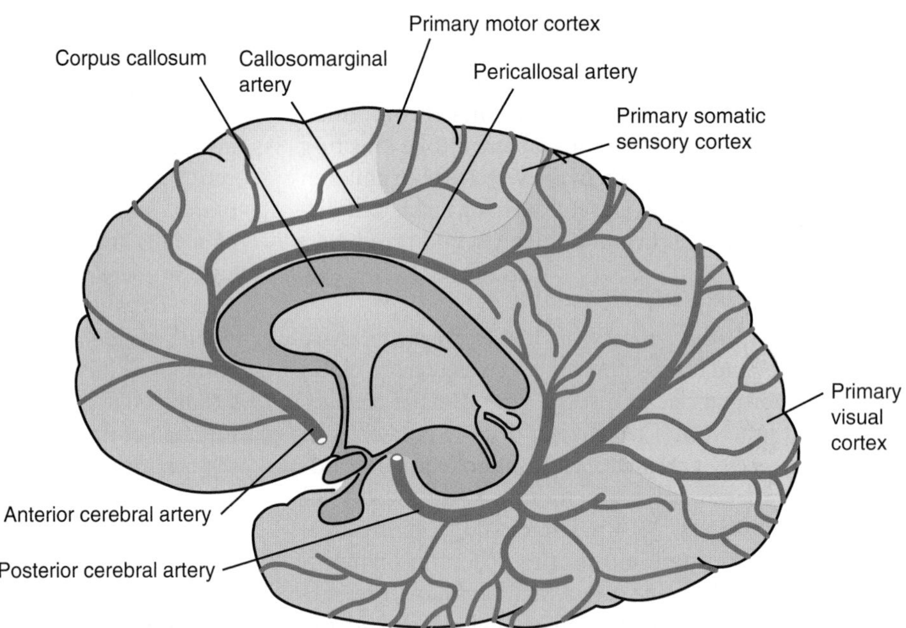

Figure 15.2 Cerebral circulation: Diagram of a midsagittal view of the brain illustrates the distribution of the anterior and posterior cerebral arteries.

the anterior communicating artery allows perfusion of the proximal ACA from either side, occlusion proximal to this point results in minimal deficit.

More distal lesions produce more significant deficits. Table 15.2 presents the clinical manifestations of *anterior cerebral artery (ACA) syndrome.* The most common characteristics of ACA syndrome include contralateral hemiparesis and sensory loss with greater involvement of the lower extremity (LE) than the upper extremity (UE) because the somatotopic organization of the medial aspect of the cortex includes the functional area for the LE.

Middle Cerebral Artery Syndrome

The *middle cerebral artery (MCA)* is the second of the two main branches of the internal carotid artery and supplies the entire lateral aspect of the cerebral hemisphere (frontal, temporal, and parietal lobes) and subcortical structures, including the internal capsule (posterior portion), corona radiata, globus pallidus (outer part), most of the caudate nucleus, and the putamen (Fig. 15.3). Occlusion of the proximal MCA produces extensive neurological damage with significant cerebral edema. Increased ICP typically leads to loss of consciousness, brain herniation, and possibly

Table 15.2 Clinical Manifestations of Anterior Cerebral Artery Syndrome

Signs and Symptoms	Structures Involved
Contralateral hemiparesis involving mainly the LE (UE is more spared)	Primary motor area, medial aspect of cortex, internal capsule
Contralateral hemisensory loss involving mainly the LE (UE is more spared)	Primary sensory area, medial aspect of cortex
Urinary incontinence	Posteromedial aspect of superior frontal gyrus
Problems with imitation and bimanual tasks, apraxia	Corpus callosum
Abulia (akinetic mutism), slowness, delay, lack of spontaneity, motor inaction	Uncertain localization
Contralateral grasp reflex, sucking reflex Can be asymptomatic if circle of Willis is competent.	Uncertain localization

LE = lower extremity; UE = upper extremity.

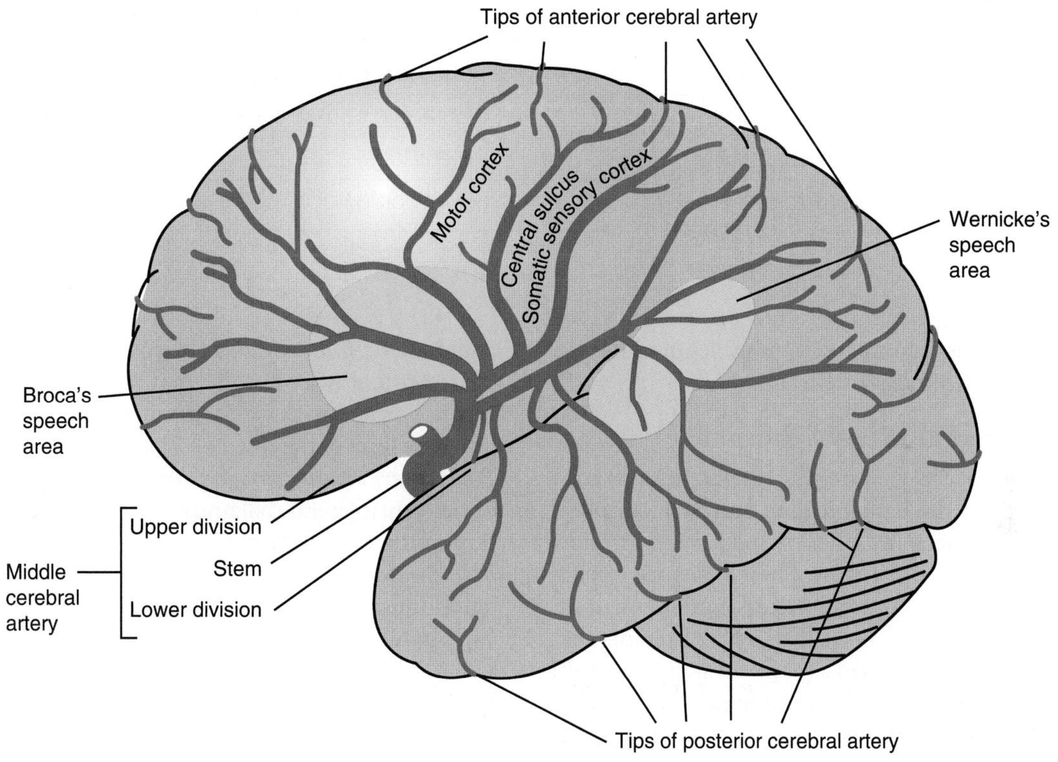

Figure 15. 3 Cerebral circulation: Diagram of a lateral view of the brain illustrates the distribution of the middle cerebral artery.

death. Table 15.3 presents the clinical manifestations of *MCA syndrome.* The most common characteristics of MCA syndrome are contralateral spastic hemiparesis and sensory loss of the face, UE, and LE, with the face and UE more involved than the LE. Lesions of the parieto-occipital cortex of the dominant hemisphere (usually the left hemisphere) typically produce aphasia. Lesions of the right parietal lobe of the nondominant hemisphere (usually the right hemisphere) typically produce perceptual deficits (e.g., *unilateral neglect, anosognosia, apraxia,* and *spatial disorganization*). *Homonymous hemianopsia* (a visual field defect) is also a common finding. The MCA is the most common site of occlusion in stroke.

Internal Carotid Artery Syndrome

Occlusion of the *internal carotid artery (ICA)* typically produces massive infarction in the region of the brain supplied by the MCA. The ICA supplies both the MCA and the ACA. If collateral circulation to the ACA from the circle of Willis is absent, extensive cerebral infarction in the areas of both the ACA and MCA can occur.

Table 15.3 Clinical Manifestations of Middle Cerebral Artery Syndrome

Signs and Symptoms	Structures Involved
Contralateral hemiparesis involving mainly the UE and face (LE is more spared)	Primary motor cortex and internal capsule
Contralateral hemisensory loss involving mainly the UE and face (LE is more spared)	Primary sensory cortex and internal capsule
Motor speech impairment: Broca's or nonfluent aphasia with limited vocabulary and slow, hesitant speech	Broca's cortical area (third frontal convolution) in the dominant hemisphere, typically the left hemisphere
Receptive speech impairment: Wernicke's or fluent aphasia with impaired auditory comprehension and fluent speech with normal rate and melody	Wernicke's cortical area (posterior portion of the temporal gyrus) in the dominant hemisphere, typically the left
Global aphasia: nonfluent speech with poor comprehension	Both third frontal convolution and posterior portion of the superior temporal gyrus
Perceptual deficits: unilateral neglect, depth perception, spatial relations, agnosia	Parietal sensory association cortex in the nondominant hemisphere, typically the right
Limb-kinetic apraxia	Premotor or parietal cortex
Contralateral homonymous hemianopsia	Optic radiation in internal capsule
Loss of conjugate gaze to the opposite side	Frontal eye fields or their descending tracts
Ataxia of contralateral limb(s) (sensory ataxia)	Parietal lobe
Pure motor hemiplegia (lacunar stroke)	Upper portion of posterior limb of internal capsule

LE = lower extremity; UE = upper extremity.

Significant edema is common with possible uncal herniation, coma, and death (mass effect).

Posterior Cerebral Artery Syndrome

The two posterior cerebral arteries (PCAs) arise as terminal branches of the basilar artery, and each supplies the corresponding occipital lobe and medial and inferior temporal lobe (see Fig. 15.2). They also supply the upper brainstem, midbrain, and posterior diencephalon, including most of the thalamus. Table 15.4 presents the clinical manifestations of *(PCA) syndrome.* Occlusion proximal to the posterior communicating artery typically results in minimal deficits owing to the collateral blood supply from the PCA (similar to ACA syndrome). Occlusion of thalamic branches may produce hemianesthesia (contralateral sensory loss) or *central poststroke (thalamic) pain.* Occipital infarction produces homonymous hemianopsia, *visual agnosia, prosopagnosia,* or, if bilateral, cortical blindness. Temporal lobe ischemia results in amnesia (memory loss). Involvement of subthalamic branches may involve the subthalamic nucleus or its pallidal connections, producing a wide variety of deficits. Contralateral hemiplegia occurs with involvement of the cerebral peduncle.

Lacunar Strokes

Lacunar strokes are caused by small vessel disease deep in the cerebral white matter (penetrating artery disease). They are strongly associated with hypertensive hemorrhage and diabetic microvascular disease. Lacunar syndromes are consistent with specific anatomical sites. *Pure motor lacunar stroke* is associated with involvement of the posterior limb of the internal capsule, pons, and pyramids. *Pure sensory lacunar stroke* is associated with involvement of the ventrolateral thalamus or thalamocortical projections. Other lacunar syndromes include *dysarthria/clumsy hand syndrome* (involving the base of the pons, genu of anterior limb, or the internal capsule), *ataxic hemiparesis* (involving the pons, genu of internal capsule, corona radiata, or cerebellum), *sensory/motor stroke* (involving the junction of the internal capsule and thalamus), and *dystonia/involuntary movements* (choreoathetosis with lacunar infarction of the putamen or globus pallidus; hemiballismus with involvement of the subthalamic nucleus). Deficits in consciousness, language, or visual fields are not seen in lacunar strokes because the higher cortical areas are preserved. A hypertensive hemorrhage affecting the thalamus can also produce central poststroke pain.[15]

Vertebrobasilar Artery Syndrome

The *vertebral arteries* arise from the subclavian arteries and travel into the brain along the medulla where they merge at the inferior border of the pons to form the basilar artery. The vertebral arteries supply the cerebellum (via posterior inferior cerebellar arteries) and the medulla (via the medullary arteries). The basilar artery supplies the pons (via pontine arteries), the internal ear (via

Table 15.4 Clinical Manifestations of Posterior Cerebral Artery Syndrome

Signs and Symptoms	Structures Involved
Peripheral Territory	
Contralateral homonymous hemianopsia	Primary visual cortex or optic radiation
Bilateral homonymous hemianopsia with some degree of macular sparing	Calcarine cortex (macular sparing is due to occipital pole receiving collateral blood supply from MCA)
Visual agnosia	Left occipital lobe
Prosopagnosia (difficulty naming people on sight)	Visual association cortex
Dyslexia (difficulty reading) without agraphia (difficulty writing), color naming (anomia), and color discrimination problems	Dominant calcarine lesion and posterior part of corpus callosum
Memory defect	Lesion of inferomedial portions of temporal lobe bilaterally or on the dominant side only
Topographic disorientation	Nondominant primary visual area, usually bilaterally
Central Territory	
Central poststroke (thalamic) pain Spontaneous pain and dysesthesias; sensory impairments (all modalities)	Ventral posterolateral nucleus of thalamus
Involuntary movements; choreoathetosis, intention tremor, hemiballismus	Subthalamic nucleus or its pallidal connections
Contralateral hemiplegia	Cerebral peduncle of midbrain
Weber's syndrome Oculomotor nerve palsy and contralateral hemiplegia	Third nerve and cerebral peduncle of midbrain
Paresis of vertical eye movements, slight miosis and ptosis, and sluggish pupillary light response	Supranuclear fibers to third cranial nerve

LE = lower extremity; MCA = middle cerebral artery; UE = upper extremity.

labyrinthine arteries), and the cerebellum (via the anterior inferior and superior cerebellar arteries). The basilar artery then terminates at the upper border of the pons, giving rise to the two posterior arteries (see Fig. 15.1). Occlusions of the vertebrobasilar system can produce a wide variety of symptoms with both ipsilateral and contralateral signs because some of the tracts in the brainstem will have crossed and others will not. Numerous cerebellar and cranial nerve abnormalities also are present. Table 15.5 presents the clinical manifestations of *vertebrobasilar artery syndromes.*

Locked-in syndrome (LIS) occurs with basilar artery thrombosis and bilateral infarction of the ventral pons. LIS is a catastrophic event with sudden onset. Patients develop acute hemiparesis rapidly progressing to tetraplegia and lower bulbar paralysis (CNs V through XII are involved). Initially the patient is dysarthric and dysphonic but rapidly progresses to mutism (anarthria). There is preserved consciousness and sensation. Thus the patient cannot move or speak but remains alert and oriented. Horizontal eye movements are impaired but vertical eye movements and blinking remain intact. Communication can be established via these eye movements. Mortality rates are high (59%), and those patients who do survive are left with severe impairments associated with brainstem injury.[15]

Extracranial injuries to the vertebral arteries as they travel through the cervical spine can also produce vertebrobasilar signs and symptoms. Forceful neck motions (e.g., whiplash or aggressive neck manipulations) are among the more common types of injuries.

■ NEUROLOGICAL SEQUELAE AND ASSOCIATED CONDITIONS

Altered Consciousness

Altered level of consciousness (coma, decreased arousal levels) may occur with extensive brain damage (e.g., large proximal MCA occlusion). The *Glasgow Coma Scale* developed by Teasdale and Jennett[16] is used to document level of coma (see Chapter 19, Traumatic Brain Injury). Three areas of function are examined: eye opening, best motor response, and verbal responses. The therapist may document levels of consciousness using standard descriptive terms: *normal, lethargy, obtundation, stupor,* and *coma* (see Chapter 5, Examination of Motor Function: Motor

Table 15.5 Clinical Manifestations of Vertebrobasilar Artery Syndrome

Signs and Symptoms	Structures Involved
Medial medullary syndrome	Occlusion vertebral artery, medullary branch
Ipsilateral to lesion Paralysis with atrophy of half the tongue with deviation to the paralyzed side when tongue is protruded	CN XII, hypoglossal, or nucleus
Contralateral to lesion Paralysis of UE and LE	Corticospinal tract
Impaired tactile and proprioceptive sense	Medial lemniscus
Lateral medullary (Wallenburg's) syndrome	Occlusion of posterior inferior cerebellar artery or vertebral artery
Ipsilateral to lesion Decreased pain and temperature sensation in face	Descending tract and nucleus of CN V, trigeminal
Cerebellum or inferior cerebellar peduncle	Cerebellar ataxia: gait and limbs ataxia
Vertigo, nausea, vomiting	Vestibular nuclei and connections
Nystagmus	Vestibular nuclei and connections
Horner's syndrome*:* miosis, ptosis, decreased sweating	Descending sympathetic tract
Dysphagia and dysphonia: paralysis of palatal and laryngeal muscles, diminished gag reflex	CN IX, glossopharyngeal, and CN X, vagus, or nuclei
Sensory impairment of ipsilateral UE, trunk, or LE	Cuneate and gracile nuclei
Contralateral to lesion Impaired pain and thermal sense over 50% of body, sometimes face	Spinal lemniscus—spinothalamic tract
Complete basilar artery syndrome (locked-in syndrome)	Basilar artery, ventral pons
Tetraplegia (quadriplegia)	Corticospinal tracts bilaterally
Bilateral cranial nerve palsy: upward gaze is spared	Long tracts to cranial nerve nuclei bilaterally
Coma	Reticular activating system
Cognition is spared	
Medial inferior pontine syndrome	Occlusion of paramedian branch of basilar artery
Ipsilateral to lesion Paralysis of conjugate gaze to side of lesion (preservation of convergence)	Pontine center for lateral gaze PPRF
Nystagmus	Vestibular nuclei and connections
Ataxia of limbs and gait	Middle cerebellar peduncle
Diplopia on lateral gaze	CN VI, abducens, or nucleus
Contralateral to lesion Paresis of face, UE, and LE	Corticobulbar and corticospinal tract in lower pons
Impaired tactile and proprioceptive sense over 50% of the body	Medial lemniscus
Lateral inferior pontine syndrome	Occlusion of anterior inferior cerebellar artery, a branch of the basilar artery
Ipsilateral to lesion Horizontal and vertical nystagmus, vertigo, nausea, vomiting	CN VIII, vestibular, or nucleus

Table 15.5 Clinical Manifestations of Vertebrobasilar Artery Syndrome—cont'd

Signs and Symptoms	Structures Involved
Facial paralysis	CN VII, facial, or nucleus
Paralysis of conjugate gaze to side of lesion	Pontine center for lateral gaze (PPRF)
Deafness, tinnitus	CN VIII, cochlear, or nucleus
Ataxia	Middle cerebellar peduncle and cerebellar hemisphere
Impaired sensation over face	Main sensory nucleus and descending tract of fifth nerve
Contralateral to lesion Impaired pain and thermal sense over half the body (may include face)	Spinothalamic tract
Medial midpontine syndrome	Occlusion of paramedian branch of the mid-basilar artery
Ipsilateral to lesion Ataxia of limbs and gait (more prominent in bilateral involvement)	Middle cerebellar peduncle
Contralateral to lesion Paralysis of face, UE, and LE	Corticobulbar and corticospinal tract
Deviation of eyes	Abducent nerve nucleus, medial longitudinal fasciculus
Lateral midpontine syndrome	Occlusion of short circumferential artery
Ipsilateral to lesion Ataxia of limbs	Middle cerebellar peduncle
Paralysis of muscles of mastication	Motor fibers or nucleus of CN V, trigeminal
Impaired sensation over side of face	Sensory fibers or nucleus of CN V, trigeminal
Medial superior pontine syndrome	Occlusion of paramedian branches of upper basilar artery
Cerebellar ataxia	Superior or middle cerebellar peduncle
Internuclear ophthalmoplegia	Medial longitudinal fasciculus
Contralateral to lesion **Paralysis of face, UE, and LE**	Corticobulbar and corticospinal tract
Lateral superior pontine syndrome	Occlusion of superior cerebellar artery, a branch of the basilar artery
Ipsilateral to lesion Cerebellar ataxia of limbs and gait, falling to side of lesion	Middle and superior cerebellar peduncles, superior surface of cerebellum, dentate nucleus
Dizziness, nausea, vomiting	Vestibular nuclei
Horizontal nystagmus	Vestibular nuclei
Paresis of conjugate gaze (ipsilateral)	Uncertain
Loss of optokinetic nystagmus	Uncertain
Horner's syndrome: miosis, ptosis, decreased sweating on opposite side face	Descending sympathetic fibers
Contralateral to lesion Impaired pain and thermal sense of face, limbs, and trunk	Spinothalamic tract
Impaired touch, vibration, and position sense, more in LE than UE (tendency to incongruity of pain and touch deficits)	Medial lemniscus (lateral portion)

CN = cranial nerve; LE = lower extremity; PPRF = paramedian pontine reticular formation; UE = upper extremity.

Control and Motor Learning). Since the patient's behaviors can be expected to fluctuate, frequent repeat observations are necessary.

Speech and Language Deficits

Patients with lesions involving the cortex of the dominant hemisphere (typically the left hemisphere) demonstrate speech and language impairments. *Aphasia* is the general term used to describe an acquired communication disorder caused by brain damage and is characterized by an impairment of language comprehension, formulation, and use. Aphasia has been estimated to occur in 30% to 36% of all patients with stroke.[3] There are many different types of aphasias; major classification categories are fluent, nonfluent, and global. In *fluent aphasia (Wernicke's/sensory/receptive aphasia),* speech flows smoothly with a variety of grammatical constructions and preserved melody of speech. Auditory comprehension is impaired. Thus, the patient demonstrates difficulty in comprehending spoken language and in following commands. The lesion is located in the auditory association cortex in the left lateral temporal lobe. In *nonfluent aphasia (Broca's/expressive aphasia),* the flow of speech is slow and hesitant, vocabulary is limited, and syntax is impaired. Speech production is labored or lost completely whereas comprehension is good. The lesion is located in the premotor area of the left frontal lobe. *Global aphasia* is a severe aphasia characterized by marked impairments of both production and comprehension of language. It is often an indication of extensive brain damage. Severe problems in communication may limit the patient's ability to learn and often impede successful outcomes in rehabilitation. See Chapter 28, Neurogenic Disorders of Speech and Language, for a complete discussion of these impairments and their management.

Patients with stroke commonly present with *dysarthria* with a reported incidence ranging from 48% to 57%.[3] This term refers to a category of motor speech disorders caused by lesions in parts of the central or peripheral nervous system that mediate speech production. Respiration, articulation, phonation, resonance, and/or sensory feedback may be affected. The lesion can be located in the primary motor cortex, the primary sensory cortex, or the cerebellum. Volitional and automatic actions such as chewing and swallowing and movement of the jaw and tongue are impaired, resulting in slurred speech. In patients with stroke, dysarthria can accompany aphasia, complicating the course of rehabilitation (see Chapter 28).

It is important to establish a reliable mode of communication before proceeding with the examination. Close collaboration with the speech-language pathologist will aid in making an accurate determination of the patient's communication abilities. It is important to distinguish between a motor disorder (dysarthria) and a language disorder (aphasia). Preservation of receptive language functions (auditory comprehension, reading comprehension) and expressive language function (word finding, fluency, writing) abilities will guide the communication strategy. Gestures, demonstration, communication boards, and simple language are strategies to enhance communication.

Dysphagia

Dysphagia, an inability to swallow or difficulty in swallowing, occurs in about 51% of patients with stroke. It can be seen in hemispheric stroke, brainstem stroke, or pseudobulbar and suprabulbar palsy. In brainstem stroke, the reported incidence is as high as 81%. Cranial nerve involvement results in swallowing dysfunction of the oral stage (CN V [trigeminal], CN VII [facial]), the pharyngeal stage (CN IX [glossopharyngeal], CN X [vagus], and CN XI [accessory]), or oral and pharyngeal (CN XII [hypoglossal]). Dysphagia is also common in patients with multiple strokes. The most common problems seen in patients with dysphagia include delayed triggering of the swallowing reflex, reduced pharyngeal peristalsis, and reduced lingual control. Altered mental status, altered sensation, poor jaw and lip closure, impaired head control, and poor sitting posture also contribute to the patient's swallowing difficulties. Most patients demonstrate multiple problems that can include drooling, difficulty ingesting food, compromised nutritional status, and dehydration. *Aspiration,* the penetration of food, liquid, saliva, or gastric reflux into the airway, occurs in about one-third of patients with dysphagia. Aspiration can lead to acute respiratory distress within hours, aspiration pneumonia, and, if left untreated, death.[17,18]

A referral to a dysphagia specialist or multidisciplinary dysphagia team is indicated. Team members typically include the physician, nurse, occupational therapist, speech-language pathologist, and dietitian. Clinical evaluation of dysphagia includes an examination of oral-motor function, pharyngeal function, functional status (e.g., upright sitting position, use of adaptive feeding equipment), examination of abnormal reflexes, and a feeding trial. Instrumental testing can include a *modified barium swallow (MBS), videofluoroscopic evaluation of swallowing,* and a *fiberoptic endoscopic evaluation of swallowing* (FEES).[19] If dysphagia is severe enough, patients may be placed on nothing-by-mouth (NPO) precautions. The use of tube feeding, either a nasogastric (NG) tube for short periods of time or an invasive gastrostomy (G) tube for more long-term care, is required. Nutrition can also be provided through an intravenous route (total parenteral nutrition [TPN]).

Cognitive Deficits

Cognitive deficits may include impairments in alertness, attention, orientation, memory, or executive functions. Premorbid changes associated with aging may also account for some of the limitations noted and may be determined from interviews with family, significant others, or caregivers. Difficulty with *alertness* results from lesions in the prefrontal cortex and reticular formation with the person appearing lethargic. *Disorientation* presents as the person being unable to provide information about self, time of day, physical or geographical location, or disability and is the result of lesions affecting the prefrontal cortex, limbic system, and limbic cortex. *Attention* is the ability to select and attend to a specific stimulus while simultaneously suppressing extraneous stimuli. Attention disorders include impairments in sustained attention, selective attention, divided attention, or alternating attention. Altered attention results from lesions in the prefrontal cortex and reticular formation. *Memory* is defined as the ability to store experiences and perceptions for later recall. Immediate and short-term memory impairments are common, occurring in about 36% of patients with stroke, whereas long-term memory typically remains intact.[2] Thus, the person cannot remember the instructions for a new task given only minutes or hours ago but can easily remember events from 30 years ago. Short-term memory loss is associated with lesions of the limbic system, limbic association cortex (orbitofrontal areas), or temporal lobes. Long-term memory loss is associated with lesions of the hippocampus of the limbic system. Memory gaps may be filled with inappropriate words or fabricated stories, an impairment termed *confabulation* that also results from lesions in the prefrontal cortex. The patient may be confused, demonstrating disorientation and an inability to understand the specific context of a conversation. *Confusion* is the result of disruption of the prefrontal cortex. *Perseveration* is the continued repetition of words, thoughts, or acts not related to current context. Thus, the patient gets "stuck" and repeats words or acts without much success at stopping. Preservation results from lesions in the premotor and/or prefrontal cortex.

Executive functions, defined as those abilities that enable a person to engage in purposeful behaviors, include volition, planning, purposeful action, and effective performance. Patients with lesions of the prefrontal cortex typically demonstrate impairments in executive function including some or all of the following: impulsiveness, inflexible thinking, lack of abstract thinking, impaired organization and sequencing, decreased insight, impaired planning ability, and impaired judgment. Patients are unable to realistically appraise their environment and the people and events in it. They also demonstrate difficulty in self-monitoring and self-correcting behaviors, thereby posing safety risks.[20,21] (See Chapter 27, Cognitive and Perceptual Dysfunction, for a complete discussion of these impairments and their management.)

Multi-infarct dementia (vascular dementia) results from multiple small infarcts of the brain and is seen in 6% to 32% of patients. It is more common in individuals over age 60 and is associated with episodes of cerebral ischemia (microvascular or small vessel disease) and hypertension. Other contributing factors include arrhythmias, myocardial infarct, TIAs, diabetes, obesity, and smoking. Scattered areas of the brain are involved, evidenced by focal neurological deficits. Onset is frequently abrupt. The person exhibits impairments in memory and cognition and may fluctuate between periods of impaired function and periods of improved function. This stepwise and paroxysmal deterioration of intellectual function is in contrast to the gradual onset and steadier, widespread decline seen in Alzheimer's dementia.[20]

Delirium, also known as *acute confusional state,* is seen more commonly in the acute care setting and results from a number of factors following acute stroke. Deprivation of oxygen to the brain, metabolic imbalance, or adverse drug reactions can all induce confusion. Additional contributory factors can include sensory and perceptual losses coupled with an unfamiliar hospital environment and inactivity. Delirium is characterized by a clouding of consciousness or dulling of cognitive processes and impaired alertness. Thus, the patient is inattentive, incoherent, and disorganized with fluctuating levels of consciousness. Hallucinations and agitation are also common. Nighttime may be particularly problematic. Patients with significant sensory loss following stroke may experience sensory deprivation problems evidenced by irritability, confusion, psychosis, delusions, and even hallucinations. These problems are more frequently seen in the acute phase, especially with patients who have been confined to a bed or whose bed is positioned to limit social interaction (e.g., with the more involved side toward the door). Some patients are equally unable to deal with a sensory overload, produced by too much stimulation. Altered arousal levels are implicated.

It is important to examine cognitive abilities early because they may affect the validity of other tests and measures. An examination of orientation (to person, place, time, and circumstance [e.g., awareness of event causing need for medical care]), attention (selective, sustained, alternating, divided), memory (immediate, short- and long-term), and ability to follow instructions (one-, two-, and three-level commands) can be made from observations of the patient's interactions and responses to specific questions. Higher cortical functions can be examined using tests of simple arithmetic and abstract reasoning (grasp of information, abstract thinking and problem-solving, calculating ability, constructional ability). The *Mini-Mental Status Examination (MMSE)* provides a valid and reliable quick screen of cognitive function.[22] A determination of learning impairments (retention and generalization) usually requires repeat sessions with the patient before a complete picture can be ascertained. Difficulties arise in reaching an accurate determination of cognition when the person presents with impairments in communication or perception. Close collaboration with the occupational therapist, speech-language pathologist, and the rest of team is essential.

Affective Status

Lesions of the brain affecting the frontal lobe, hypothalamus, and limbic system can produce a number of emotional changes. The patient with stroke may demonstrate *pseudobulbar affect* (PBA), also known as *emotional lability* or *emotional dysregulation syndrome*. PBA occurs in about 18% of cases and is characterized by emotional outbursts of uncontrolled or exaggerated laughing or crying that are inconsistent with mood. The patient quickly changes from laughing to crying with only slight provocation. The patient is typically unable to control these episodes or to inhibit the expression of spontaneous emotions. Frequent crying may also accompany depression. *Apathy* occurs in about 22% of cases and is characterized by a shallow affect and blunted emotional responses. In such patients, apathy is frequently misconstrued as depression or poor motivation. Patients can also demonstrate *euphoria* (exaggerated feelings of well-being), increased levels of irritability or frustration, and social inappropriateness. Changes in the ability to sense, move, communicate, think, or act as before are enormously frustrating by themselves and create high stress levels for the patient with stroke. Increased levels of anxiety, irritability, and frustration are the natural outcomes of high stress levels. These behaviors along with a poor perception of one's self and environment may lead to increasing isolation and social withdrawal.[21]

Depression occurs in approximately 31% of persons poststroke. It decreases to 25% and 23% at 1 and 5 years poststroke respectively.[23] It is characterized by persistent feelings of sadness accompanied by feelings of hopelessness, worthlessness, and/or helplessness. Depressed patients may also experience a loss of energy or persistent fatigue, an inability to concentrate, and decreased interest in daily life along with changes in weight and sleep patterns, generalized anxiety, and recurrent thoughts of death or suicide. Depression is seen with lesions in the left frontal lobe (acute stage) and with lesions in the right parietal lobes (subacute stage).[24] Most patients remain significantly depressed for many months, with an average time of 7 to 8 months. The period from 6 months to 2 years after a CVA is the most likely time for depression to occur.[25] Depression occurs in both mildly and severely involved patients and thus is not significantly related to the degree of motor impairment. Patients with lesions of the left hemisphere may experience more frequent and more severe depression than patients with right hemisphere or brainstem strokes. These findings suggest that poststroke depression is not simply a result of psychological reaction to disability but rather a direct impairment of the CVA.[26] Anxiety can coexist with depression during any phase of recovery.[24] Prolonged poststroke depression can interfere with the success of rehabilitation and result in poorer long-term functional outcomes. Refer to Chapter 26, Psychosocial Issues in Physical Rehabilitation, for a more complete discussion of psychosocial impairments and their management.

Hemispheric Behavioral Differences

Individuals with stroke differ widely in their approach to processing information and in their behaviors. Those with *left hemisphere lesions* (right hemiplegia) demonstrate difficulties in communication and in processing information in a sequential, linear manner. They are frequently described as cautious, anxious, and disorganized. This makes them more hesitant when trying new tasks and increases the need for feedback and support. They tend, however, to be realistic in their appraisal of their existing problems. Individuals with *right hemisphere lesions* (left hemiplegia), on the other hand, demonstrate difficulty in spatial–perceptual tasks and in grasping the whole idea of a task or activity. They are frequently described as quick and impulsive. They tend to overestimate their abilities while acting unaware of their deficits. This lack of insight and concreteness impairs the patient's ability to participate in rehabilitation. Safety is a far greater issue for patients with left hemiplegia, where poor judgment is common. These patients also require a great deal of feedback when learning a new task. The feedback should be focused on slowing down the activity, checking sequential steps, and relating them to the whole task. Patients also need help recognizing the consequences and risks of their actions. The patient with left hemiplegia frequently cannot attend to visuospatial cues effectively, especially in a cluttered or crowded environment. Table 15.6 summarizes the behavioral differences attributed to damage of the left and right hemispheres.

Emotional states and behavioral styles can best be examined through observation of the patient in a variety of situations over a number of sessions. It is important to correlate findings with those reported by other team members and by the family regarding premorbid behaviors and emotional characteristics. Families who report a "personality change" after stroke are likely responding to presenting emotional impairments and disinhibition. Episodes of euphoria and crying should be carefully documented and links to situational or environmental circumstances explored. Duration and frequency of these episodes should also be documented along with strategies that are successful in bringing about an end to the episode (redirecting strategies). The patient's response to new or stressful situations should also be carefully observed for evidence of anxiety (e.g., excessive worrying, restlessness, irritability). The therapist should examine for evidence of depression. Depressed patients can also be irritable, angry, or hostile and wish to be left alone.[21] The *Beck Depression Inventory*[27] is a useful instrument for depression screening. It consists of 21 statements that are

Table 15.6 Hemispheric Differences Commonly Seen Following Stroke

Right Hemisphere Lesion	Left Hemisphere Lesion
Left-side hemiplegia/paresis	Right-side hemiplegia/paresis
Left-side sensory loss	Right-side sensory loss
Visual–perceptual impairments: Left-side unilateral neglect Agnosias Visuospatial disorders Disturbances of body image and body scheme Difficulty processing visual cues	***Speech and language impairments:*** Dominant hemisphere: • Nonfluent (Broca's) aphasia • Fluent (Wernicke's) aphasia • Global aphasia Difficulty processing verbal cues, verbal commands
Behavioral deficits: Quick, impulsive behavioral style Poor judgment, unrealistic Inability to self-correct Poor insight, awareness of impairments, denial of disability Increased safety risk	***Behavioral deficits:*** Slow, cautious behavioral style Disorganized Often very aware of impairments, extent of disability
Intellectual deficits: Difficulty with abstract reasoning, problem solving Difficulty synthesizing information and grasping whole idea of task Rigidity of thought Memory impairments, typically related to spatial-perceptual information	***Intellectual deficits:*** Disorganized problem solving Difficulty initiating tasks, processing delays Highly distractible Memory impairments, typically related to language Perseveration
Emotional deficits: Difficulty with ability to perceive emotions	***Emotional deficits:*** Difficulty with expression of positive emotions
Difficulty with expression of negative emotions	
Task performance: Fluctuations in performance	***Task performance:*** Apraxia common: difficulty planning and sequencing movements • Ideational • Ideomotor
Deficits of either hemisphere depending on lesion location: Visual field defects: Homonymous hemianopsia Emotional abnormalities: Lability, apathy, irritability, low frustration levels, anxiety, depression Cognitive deficits: Confusion, short attention span, loss of memory, executive functions	

scored on a scale from 0 to 3 (the short version has 13 questions and takes 5 minutes to complete).

Perceptual Deficits

Stroke can produce visual–perceptual deficits, with a reported incidence ranging from 32% to 41%.[3] They are frequently the result of lesions in the right parietal cortex and are seen more with left hemiplegia than right. These may include disorders of *body scheme/body image, spatial relations,* and *agnosias.* Body scheme refers to a postural model of the body, including the relationship of the body parts to each other and the relationship of the body to the environment. Body image is the visual and mental image of one's body that includes feelings about one's body. Both may be distorted following stroke. Specific impairments of body scheme/body image include *unilateral neglect, anosognosia, somatagnosia, right–left discrimination,* and *finger agnosia.* Spatial relations syndrome refers to a constellation of impairments that have in common a difficulty in perceiving the relationship between the self and two or more objects in the environment. It includes specific impairments in *figure–ground discrimination, form discrimination, spatial relations, position in space,* and *topographical disorientation.* Agnosia is the inability to recognize incoming information despite intact sensory capacities. Agnosias can include visual object agnosia, auditory agnosia, or tactile agnosia (astereognosis). Significant information on sensory and perceptual deficits will be gained by close collaboration with the occupational therapist. Refer to Chapter 27 for a more complete discussion of these deficits and their management.

Because the patient with left hemiplegia may behave in ways that tend to minimize his or her disabilities, it is easy for staff to overestimate the patient's perceptual abilities. For the patient with visuospatial deficits, the use of gestures or visual cues may decrease this patient's ability to perform tasks, whereas verbal cues may increase chances for success. Equally important strategies include carefully structuring the environment to minimize clutter and activity, providing adequate lighting, and providing clear boundaries and reference points.

Problems in *unilateral neglect* (lack of awareness of part of the body or the external environment) will limit movement and use of the more involved extremities (usually the nondominant left side). The patient typically does not react to sensory stimuli (visual, auditory, or somatosensory) presented on the more involved side. Careful observation of spontaneous use of affected limbs, as well as specific responses to inquiries for movement on or toward the hemiplegic side, will provide important information about neglect. Persistent neglect may result in bruising or trauma to the hemiplegic limbs during activity and negatively affect rehabilitation outcomes.

Seizures

Seizures occur in a small percentage of patients with stroke and are slightly more common in occlusive carotid disease (17%) than in MCA disease (11%). Seizures are common right after stroke during the acute phase (e.g., in about 15% of cases with cerebral hemorrhage); late-onset seizures can also occur several months after stroke. They tend to be of the partial motor type. Seizures are potentially life threatening if not controlled. Anticonvulsant medications may be indicated (e.g., phenytoin [Dilantin], carbamazepine [Tegretol], phenobarbital [Solfoton]).[3]

Bladder and Bowel Dysfunction

Disturbances of bladder function are common during the acute phase, occurring in about 29% of cases.[3] Urinary incontinence can result from bladder hyperreflexia or hyporeflexia, disturbances of sphincter control, and/or sensory loss. A toileting schedule for prompted voiding is often implemented to reduce the incidence of incontinence and to accommodate for factors that cause functional incontinence, such as inattention, mental status changes, or immobility. Generally, this problem improves quickly. Persistent incontinence is often due to a treatable medical condition (e.g., urinary tract infection). Absorbent pads and special undergarments or external collection devices may be used if incontinence proves refractory. Urinary retention can be controlled pharmacologically and with intermittent or indwelling catheterization. Early treatment is desirable to prevent further complications such as chronic urinary tract infection and skin breakdown. Patients who are incontinent often suffer embarrassment, isolation, and depression. Persistent incontinence is associated with a poor long-term prognosis for functional recovery.

Disturbances of bowel function can include incontinence and diarrhea or constipation and impaction. Patients who are constipated may require stool softeners and dietary/fluid modifications and medications to resolve this problem. Physical activity is also helpful.

Cardiovascular and Pulmonary Dysfunction

The majority of strokes are caused by vascular disease. Persons who had a stroke as a result of underlying coronary artery disease (CAD) may demonstrate impaired cardiac output, cardiac decompensation, and serious rhythm disorders. If these problems persist, they can directly alter cerebral perfusion and produce additional focal signs (e.g., mental confusion). Patients with stroke typically exhibit low peak VO_2 levels during exercise (about half of that achieved by age-matched healthy individuals).[28] These vary according to age, level of disability, number and severity of comorbidities, secondary complications, and medications. Cardiac limitations in exercise tolerance may restrict rehabilitation potential and requires diligent monitoring and careful exercise prescription by the physical therapist.

Many persons with stroke are deconditioned and exhibit low work capacities, the result of acute illness, bedrest, and limited activity levels. Some individuals may have been inactive before the stroke. Changes in the cardiovascular system associated with deconditioning include reduced cardiac output, decreased maximal heart rate, increased resting and exercise BPs, decreased maximal oxygen uptake, and decreased vital capacity. Changes in the musculoskeletal system (e.g., decreased muscle mass and strength, decreased bone mass, decreased flexibility) and decreased glucose tolerance also affect exercise tolerance and endurance levels. Decreased activity levels may also be related to depression, a common finding in stroke.

Pulmonary function is often impaired in individuals with stroke. Decreased lung volume, decreased pulmonary perfusion and vital capacity, and altered chest wall excursion are all common findings. The decreased respiratory output is accompanied by increased oxygen demands required during activity using altered and unfamiliar movement patterns. For example, walking using an orthosis and assistive device dramatically increases the energy demands of the activity. The end result for the patient with stroke is increased fatigue and decreased endurance.

Deep Vein Thrombosis and Pulmonary Embolus

Deep vein thrombosis (DVT) and *pulmonary embolus* (PE) are potential complications for all immobilized patients. The incidence of DVT in patients with stroke is as high as 47% with an estimated 10% of deaths attributed to PE.[3] The dangers are particularly high during the acute phase when venous stasis from immobility and prolonged bedrest, limb paralysis, hemineglect, and reduced cognitive status significantly elevate the risk. About 50% of cases do not present with clinically detectable symptoms and can be identified only by Doppler duplex ultrasonography (the gold standard for rapid screening), radiocontrast venography, or impedance plethysmography. Patients with symptoms may report calf pain and tenderness, or a tight feeling in the calf. Swelling can vary from minimal to high and typically affects the foot and ankle. Prompt diagnosis and treatment of acute DVT are necessary to reduce the risk of fatal PE. About half of patients at time of diagnosis of DVT have already had a PE. Signs and symptoms of PE include chest pain, tachypnea, tachycardia, anxiety, restlessness, and apprehension together with persistent cough. About 10% to 15% of patients with PE will die. Symptomatic treatment of DVT consists of continuous infusion or subcutaneous injections of low-molecular-weight heparin (LMWH) followed by long-term oral anticoagulants (warfarin [Coumadin]). Bedrest is instituted (up to 24 hours) until anticoagulation from medications takes effect. The patient is then mobilized out of bed and will wear compression stockings. In select cases, surgical removal of the thrombus or placement of intracaval filters is undertaken. Treatment of PE involves supplemental oxygen or intubation in severe cases, anticoagulants, and thrombolytic drugs and, in some cases, surgical intervention. Primary prevention of DVT and PE involves prophylactic administration of anticoagulants, exercising the legs to improve blood flow, early mobilization, and use of elastic support stockings.[29]

Osteoporosis and Fracture Risk

Osteoporosis, a bone disease characterized by a loss of bone mass per unit volume, is common in the elderly and results from decreased physical activity, changes in protein nutrition, hormonal deficiency, and calcium deficiency. Patients with stroke who are immobilized and restricted in weight-bearing demonstrate increased risk of osteoporosis and disuse muscle atrophy. Fall risk is also increased with incidence rates ranging between 23% and 50% for individuals with chronic stroke.[30] Risk of falls in patients with stroke is multifactorial, arising from sensorimotor deficits, impaired balance, confusion, attention deficits, perceptual deficits, visual impairments, behavioral impulsivity, depression, and communication problems.[31-33] Increased risk of fracture, especially vertebral and hip fracture, is the natural outcome of osteoporosis and falls. In patients with stroke, osteoporosis and hip fracture are more likely on the more involved side.[34] Paradoxically, persons who receive rehabilitation are more likely to experience a fall.

■ MEDICAL DIAGNOSIS OF THE STROKE HEALTH CONDITION

History and Examination

An accurate history profiling the timing of neurological events is obtained from the patient or from family members in the case of the unconscious or noncommunicative patient. Of particular importance are the exact time and pattern of symptom onset. An abrupt onset with worsening symptoms and decreasing level of consciousness is suggestive of cerebral hemorrhage. Severe headache described as "the worst headache of my life" is suggestive of subarachnoid hemorrhage. An embolus also occurs rapidly, with no warning, and is frequently associated with heart disease and/or heart complications. A more variable and uneven onset is typical with thrombosis. The patient's past history, including episodes of TIAs or head trauma, presence of major or minor risk factors, and medications; pertinent family history; and any recent alterations in patient function (either transient or permanent) are thoroughly investigated.[35] Stroke can mimic a number of other conditions that must be ruled out, including seizures, space-occupying lesions (e.g., subdural hematoma, cerebral abscess/infection, tumor), syncope, somatization, and delirium secondary to sepsis.[36]

The physical examination includes measuring vital signs (heart rate [HR], respiratory rate [RR], BP); signs of cardiac decompensation; and function of the cerebral hemispheres, cerebellum, cranial nerves, eyes, and sensorimotor system. The presenting symptoms will help to determine the location of the lesion, and comparison of both sides of the body will reveal the side of the lesion. Bilateral signs are suggestive of brainstem lesions or massive cerebral involvement.[35]

Tests and Measures

The *National Institutes of Health Stroke Scale (NIHSS)* is a valuable screening tool that focuses on initial and serial examination of impairments following acute stroke. The scale includes 11 items and uses a variable ordinal scale. Some items are scored 0–2 or 0–3 (level of consciousness, best gaze, visual fields, facial palsy, limb ataxia, sensory, best language, dysarthria, extinction, and inattention); other items are scored 0–4 (motor arm and motor leg). Specific descriptors are attached to each score. It was designed to be completed in 5 to 8 minutes. (The NIHSS is available at https://stroke.nih.gov/documents/NIH_Stroke_Scale.pdf.).[37] An examination scoring service for the NIHSS is maintained by the National Stroke Association. The NIHSS has been used to discriminate between stroke subtypes.[38-40] It has also been recommended as the measure for stroke severity, from acute to chronic patients, in stroke recovery research trials.[41]

A number of biomarkers can be used to help identify acute cerebral ischemia. These include inflammatory mediators such as interleukin-6, matrix metalloproteinase (MMP-9), markers of glial activation, and so forth. Biomarker assays may play an increasing role in the diagnosis of acute stroke as more research becomes available.[36] Biomarkers using neuroimaging techniques will serve as measures to predict structural and functional stroke recovery.[42]

A standardized set of blood analyses is performed, including hematological studies, serum electrolyte levels, and renal and hepatic tests. These tests are used to rule out metabolic abnormalities as well as blood, kidney, or liver conditions.

Cerebrovascular Imaging

Cerebrovascular imaging is the main tool to establish the diagnosis of suspected ischemic stroke and to rule out hemorrhagic stroke and other types of central nervous system (CNS) lesions (e.g., tumor or abscess). Advanced neuroimaging can rapidly identify the occluded artery and estimate the size of the core and the penumbra. It is also used to guide ischemic stroke therapy. Lack of imaging use is high in acute stroke primarily because many patients arrive beyond the strict 3-hour time window.[43]

Computed Tomography

Computed tomography (CT) scan is the most commonly used and readily available neuroimaging technique. CT resolution allows identification of large arteries and veins and venous sinuses. It demonstrates poor sensitivity for detecting small infarcts and infarction in the posterior fossa. Many times, CT scans during the acute phase are negative with no clear evidence of abnormalities. However, acute bleeding and hemorrhagic transformation are visible on CT scanning (Fig. 15.4). In the subacute phase, CT scans can delineate the development of cerebral edema (within 3 days), which then fades over the next 2 to 3 weeks. Cerebral infarction (within 3 to 5 days) is visible with the addition of contrast material by showing areas of decreased density. Long-term parenchymal changes consistent with scar formation are also visible on CT. It is important to remember that the extent of CT lesion does not necessarily correlate with clinical signs or changes in function.

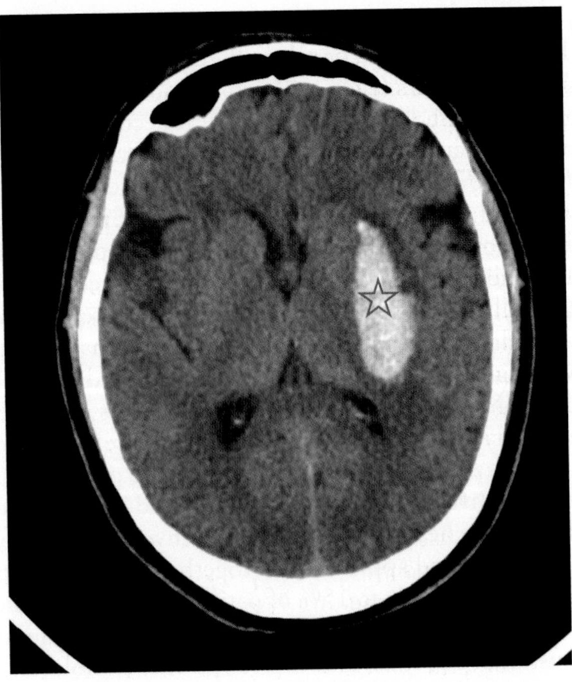

Figure 15.4 CT demonstrating an acute intracerebral hemorrhage (star). *(From Weber, E, Vilensky, J, and Fog, A: Practical Radiology: A Symptom-Based Approach. FA Davis, Philadelphia, PA, 2013, with permission.)*

Magnetic Resonance Imaging

Magnetic resonance imaging (MRI) has evolved to become the first-line imaging in some stroke centers, whereas in other facilities it is used when CT has not provided clear evidence of lesion location. MRI measures nuclear particles as they interact with a powerful magnetic field. MRI, especially diffusion/perfusion MRI, shows greater resolution of the brain and its structural detail than does a CT scan (Fig. 15.5). MRI is more sensitive in the diagnosis of acute strokes, allowing detection of cerebral ischemia as early as 30 minutes after vascular occlusion and infarction within 2 to 6 hours. It is also able to detail the extent of infarction or hemorrhage and can detect smaller lesions than a CT scan. Use of contrast enhancement allows documentation of changes

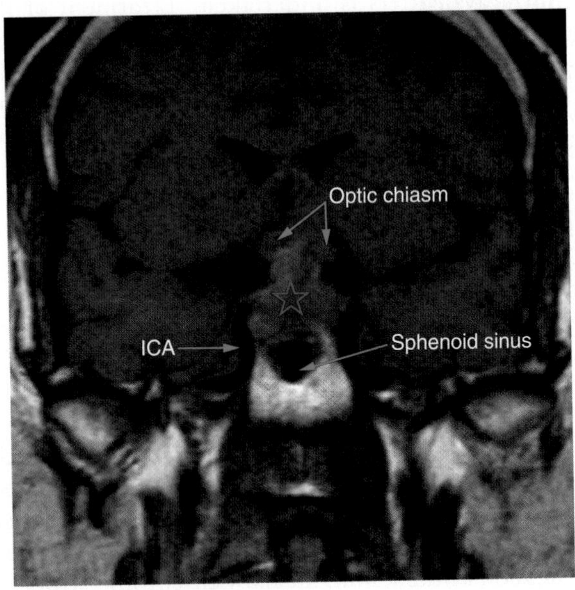

Figure 15.5 Coronal MRI without contrast enhancement on a pregnant patient with headache and visual field defect. The T1 hyperintensity of the greatly enlarged pituitary (star) indicates subacute hemorrhage. ICA = internal carotid artery. *(From Weber, E, Vilensky, J, and Fog, A: Practical Radiology: A Symptom-Based Approach. FA Davis, Philadelphia, PA, 2013, with permission.)*

in an infarct over the first 2 to 3 weeks. MRI scans cannot be performed on individuals with certain implantable devices (e.g., pacemakers) or on patients who are claustrophobic.[43]

Magnetic Resonance Angiography

Magnetic resonance angiography (MRA) is a type of magnetic resonance image that uses special software to create an image of the arteries in the brain. It is used to identify vascular abnormalities (e.g., stenosis) and alterations in blood flow as a result of embolus or thrombosis. It provides similar information as classical angiography (x-ray of blood vessels following dye injection) with increased sensitivity of detection and with lowered risks.[43]

Doppler Ultrasound

Doppler ultrasound imaging is a noninvasive technique that sends sound waves into the body. Echoes bounce off the moving blood and artery and are formed into an image. Diagnostically, transcranial Doppler is used to examine the posterior circulation of the brain (the vertebrobasilar system). Carotid Doppler is used to examine the carotid arteries and typically precedes carotid endarterectomy. It is also used to examine the peripheral arteries in the diagnosis of PAD.

Arteriography and Digital Subtraction Angiography

Arteriography is an x-ray of the carotid artery with a special dye injected into an artery in the leg or arm. Digital subtraction angiography (DSA) is also an x-ray of the carotid artery with less dye used. These procedures are considered invasive and carry a small risk of causing a stroke.

MEDICAL, PHARMACOLOGICAL, AND NEUROSURGICAL MANAGEMENT OF STROKE

Medical Management

Medical management of completed stroke includes strategies to achieve the following:

- Improve cerebral perfusion by reestablishing circulation and oxygenation and assist in stopping progression of the lesion to limit deficits. Oxygen is delivered via mask or nasal cannula. Patients in a coma may require intubation or assisted ventilation and suctioning.
- Maintain adequate BP. Hypotension or extreme hypertension is treated; antihypertension agents have the added risk of inducing hypotension and decreasing cerebral perfusion.
- Maintain sufficient cardiac output. If the causes of stroke are cardiac in origin, medical management focuses on control of arrhythmias and cardiac decompensation.
- Restore/maintain fluid and electrolyte balance.
- Maintain blood glucose levels within the normal range.
- Control seizures and infections.
- Control edema, intracranial pressure, and herniation using antiedema agents. Ventriculostomy may be indicated to monitor and drain cerebrospinal fluid.
- Maintain bowel and bladder function, which may include urinary catheter. Catheterization is typically short-term but may be long-term with the patient in coma.
- Maintain integrity of skin and joints by instituting protective positioning, a turning schedule every 2 hours, and early physical and occupational therapy.
- Decrease the risk of complications such as DVT, aspiration, decubitus ulcers, and so forth.

Pharmacological Management

Pharmacological interventions for completed stroke and its comorbidities are summarized in Box 15.2.[44,45]

Neurosurgical Management[46]

Neurosurgical interventions may include the following:

- In hemorrhagic stroke, surgery may be indicated to repair a superficial ruptured aneurysm or AVM, prevent rebleeding, and evacuate a clot (hematoma). Larger, deeper intracranial or brainstem vascular lesions are generally not amenable to surgery. Surgery may also be indicated for resection of a superficial unruptured AVM when there is high risk of rupture and stroke.
- Mechanical thrombectomy is the removal of a large blood clot by sending a stent retriever to the site of the blocked blood vessel in the brain. To remove the brain clot, a catheter is threaded through an artery in the groin up to the blocked artery in the brain where the clot is removed. The procedure should be done within 6 hours of acute stroke symptoms, and only after a patient receives tPA.
- Carotid endarterectomy is a surgical procedure used to remove fatty deposits from the carotid artery. It is a useful procedure to prevent recurrent strokes or the development of stroke in individuals with TIAs. Stenosis of 60% to 99% is the typical guideline used when surgery is considered and can reduce stroke risk by as much as 55%. It cannot be performed with acute stroke because altered pressures could subject ischemic areas to further damage.

FRAMEWORK FOR REHABILITATION

Integrated Framework for Clinical Decision Making

Rehabilitation has an important role in increasing participation in societal roles by promoting activity and reducing body function structure deficits. Prevention of

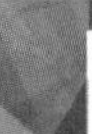

Box 15.2 Medications Commonly Used to Treat Patients With Stroke[44,45]

- ***Thrombolytics*** (alteplase [Activase or tPA]): Converts plasminogen to plasmin, degrades fibrin present in clots, dissolves clots and reestablishes blood flow (e.g., lysis of thrombi causing ischemic stroke; also used to dissolve clots in coronary arteries, pulmonary emboli, deep vein thrombosis).
  Possible adverse effects: The most common complication is brain hemorrhage.
- ***Anticoagulants*** (e.g., warfarin [Coumadin], heparin, dabigatran etexilate [Pradaxa]): Used to reduce the risk of blood clots and prevent existing clots from getting bigger by thinning the blood; indications include DVT prophylaxis, stroke prevention, peripheral vascular disease. With Coumadin, clotting times are closely monitored. Heparin is given intravenously and is faster acting.
  Possible adverse effects: Increased risk of bleeding and hemorrhage, hematomas.
- ***Antiplatelet therapy*** (e.g., acetylsalicylic acid [aspirin]; clopidogrel bisulfate [Plavix]; dabigatran etexilate [Pradaxa]; ticlopidine hydrochloride [Ticlid, Aggrenox, Persantine]): Prevent platelets (blood cells) from sticking together; long-term, low-dose is used to decrease the risk of thrombosis and recurrent stroke; higher doses may be used in place of anticoagulants and may be recommended for patients with atrial fibrillation.
  Possible adverse effects: Increased risk of gastric ulcers and bleeding.
- ***Antihypertensive agents*** (e.g., ACE inhibitors, alpha-blockers [Minipress], beta-blockers, calcium channel blockers, direct vasodilators, diuretics, postganglionic neuron inhibitors): Used to control hypertension.
  Possible adverse effects: Dizziness, hypotension, among other symptoms.
- ***Angiotensin II receptor antagonists*** (telmisartan [Micardis], losartan potassium [Cozaar, Hyzaar]): Block angiotensin II, a chemical that triggers muscle contraction around blood vessels, narrowing them; enlarges blood vessels and reduces blood pressure.
  Possible adverse effects: Dizziness, hypotension, among other symptoms.
- ***Anticholesterol agents/statins*** (atorvastatin calcium [Lipitor], rosuvastatin calcium [Crestor], simvastatin [Zocor], lovastatin [Mevacor], fluvastatin [Lescol]): Lower cholesterol by inhibiting the enzyme in the blood that produces cholesterol in the liver; for management of hypercholesterolemia and mixed dyslipidemias.
  Possible adverse effects: Dizziness, headache, insomnia, weakness.
- ***Antispasmodics/spasmolytics*** (e.g., carisoprodol [Soma], chlorzoxazone [Parafon Forte], cyclobenzaprine [Flexeril], diazepam [Valium], methocarbamol [Robaxin], orphenadrine [Norflex/Norgesic]): Used to relax skeletal muscle and decrease muscle spasm.
  Possible adverse effects: May cause drowsiness, dizziness, dry mouth, among other symptoms.
- ***Antispastics*** (e.g., baclofen [Lioresal], dantrolene sodium [Dantrium], diazepam [Valium], tizanidine [Zanaflex]): Used to relax skeletal muscle and decrease muscle spasm.
  Possible adverse effects: May cause drowsiness, dizziness, confusion, weakness, among other symptoms.
- ***Anticonvulsants*** (e.g., carbamazepine [Tegretol], clonazepam [Klonopin], diazepam [Valium], phenobarbital [Luminal], phenytoin [Dilantin]): Used to control seizures; act as a generalized CNS depressant.
  Possible adverse effects: May cause drowsiness, ataxia, sedation, among other symptoms.
- **Antidepressants** (e.g., fluoxetine [Prozac], monoamine oxidase inhibitors, sertraline [Zoloft], tricyclics [Amitriptyline]): Used to control depression.
  Possible adverse effects: May cause anxiety, tremor, insomnia, nausea.
- ***GABA (gamma-amino butyric acid) receptor antagonists*** (e.g., baclofen [Kemstro, Lioresal]): Inhibit the action of GABA, which inhibits neurotransmitters and regulates the nervous system. May be used to manage spasticity.
  Possible side effects: Drowsiness, dizziness, or headache.
- ***Neurotoxins*** (e.g., botulinum toxin [Botox]): Interact with proteins in nerves to relax muscles.
  Possible side effects: Pain or swelling at site of injection, drowsiness.

secondary complications is an important component of rehabilitation. Patient-centered care and shared clinical decision making facilitate goal setting to develop a *comprehensive plan of care* (POC).[47] The team of rehabilitation specialists includes the physician, nurse, physical therapist, occupational therapist, speech-language pathologist, and social worker. Additional disciplines may include a neuropsychologist, nutritionist, and recreational therapist or vocational counselor. The patient/client, family, and caregivers, as important members of the team, should be involved in all decision making regarding the POC. Interdisciplinary communication is critical for effective team function and occurs through case conferences, informal interactions, patient care rounds, and patient/client family meetings. Effective case management also includes a coordinated education plan and accurate and effective documentation. It is critical for the team to provide a supportive environment to assist patients and their family members in their adjustment to this life-altering event.

The National Stroke Association has instituted a process to certify stroke rehabilitation specialists. The designation of *clinical stroke rehabilitation specialist (CSRS)* ensures that therapists are expert stroke clinicians through a rigorous set of courses and written examination and a nationally recognized credential, the CSRS certification. Additional information can be found at www.stroke.org.

In this chapter, the examination and intervention for the person poststroke is guided by the integrated framework for clinical reasoning.[47] *Guide to Physical Therapist Practice 3.0*[48] forms the structure of the model. It incorporates the International Classification of Functioning Disability and Health (ICF), which provides enablement language and a structure for organizing information.[49] The hypothesis-oriented algorithm for clinicians (HOAC) II represents the iterative process of generating and testing hypotheses at each step of the patient client management.[50] Both enablement (ICF) and disablement (Nagi) models guide the interview and screening of the patient. Standardized assessments and task analysis guide examination. The formulation of the POC, inclusive of prognosis, is informed by the individual's goals and the clinician's assessment of his or her ability to achieve them based on the body function structure limitations that restrict activity and participation coupled with evidence from the literature. Factored into the decision making are the patient's abilities (assets), priorities, and resources, including family, home, and community resources. Interventions are *restorative* (aimed at improving impairments, activity limitations, and participation restrictions), *preventive* (aimed at minimizing potential complications and indirect impairments), and *compensatory* (aimed at modifying the task, activity, or environment to improve function). See discussion in Chapter 1, Clinical Decision Making and Examination.

The overall focus for patients with moderate to severe stroke is on long-range planning, with consideration of anticipated episodes of care that typically include hospital-based care (acute care, inpatient rehabilitation, or subacute rehabilitation), outpatient rehabilitation, and home/community-based care.

Resources to guide evidence-based practice for persons poststroke include clinical practice guidelines, recommendations for examination tools for persons poststroke from the StrokEDGE task force,[51] and synthesized evidence found at https://www.PTNow.org. These evidence-based resources coupled with patient preferences and clinician expertise form the evidence-based triad for practice.

Stage of recovery and severity of the stroke will influence the setting and therapy for a person poststroke. Stages of recovery have recently been defined on the basis of links to biology.[52] These time periods are helpful in understanding the therapeutic approach one might take considering events such as cell death (in the hyperacute phase, 0 to 24 hours), period of inflammation and scarring 1 to 7 days poststroke (acute phase) and the endogenous plasticity (the nervous system's ability to repair itself) that starts in the acute phase, peaks in the early subacute phase (7 days to 3 months) and plateaus in the late subacute (3 to 6 months) through the chronic phase (more than 6 months).[52] Episodes of care may include hospital-based care (acute care, inpatient rehabilitation or subacute rehabilitation), outpatient rehabilitation, and home/community-based care.

Acute Phase

The patient may be first seen in a neurological intensive care unit (ICU) or specialized stroke care unit in a facility that also provides comprehensive rehabilitation services. Evidence supports the benefits of specialized stroke units in improving functional outcomes when compared to patients not receiving specialized care. Individuals who received this care were more likely to be alive, independent, and living at home 1 year after stroke.[53,54] The therapist needs to be aware of the patient's current status by reviewing the medical record and communicating with the medical team. During acute care, the therapist assists in ongoing monitoring of the patient's recovery and is alert for changes in the patient's status (e.g., changes in vital signs [HR, BP, RR], drop in O_2 saturation levels, skin changes, alterations in mental status and consciousness). Early mobilization prevents or minimizes the harmful effects of bedrest and deconditioning. Early, frequent, short bouts of mobilization have been shown to produce better outcomes at 3 months than do long bouts.[55] Early mobilization may also increase the patient's level of consciousness and foster return to independence. Functional reorganization is promoted through early stimulation and use of the hemiparetic side. *Learned nonuse* of the hemiparetic extremities and maladaptive patterns of movement are minimized. Mental deterioration, depression, and apathy can be reduced through the fostering of a positive outlook toward the rehabilitation process. Interventions include but are not limited to functional mobility training (e.g., bed mobility, sitting, transfers, locomotion), ADL training, range of motion (ROM), splinting, and positioning.

Instruction, education, and training of patients and their families/caregivers is initiated early regarding current condition (pathophysiology, impairments, activity limitations) and risk factors for disability. It includes an overview of the recovery process, the rehabilitation POC, and expected transitions across care settings. It is important to remember that this is a highly stressful time for patients and families, and information needs to be graded in appropriate amounts and repeated and reinforced throughout the course of treatment. The therapist should establish effective communication. This includes speaking to the patient in a normal tone and volume, speaking slowly and giving the patient enough time to respond, using simple yes/no questions, and using gesture and tactile cues whenever appropriate.

Controlling the environment and reducing distractions will also help to ensure the patient's attention and promote good communication. Awareness of the presence of visual field defect (homonymous hemianopsia) and perceptual changes (unilateral neglect) will influence choice of the therapist's position when interacting with the patient.

Current trends are toward shorter acute care hospital stays (average stay is about 5 days).[2] However, early discharge has resulted in an increase in the number of serious medical complications seen during subacute rehabilitation or at home. These complications may result in delays during active rehabilitation and, for some, temporary cessation of therapy or transfer back to the acute hospital until medical complications are resolved. It is important to monitor patients for potential risk of complications and medical emergencies (e.g., cardiac arrhythmias, DVT, uncontrolled BP, and recurrent stroke).

Subacute Phase

Persons poststroke with moderate or severe residual body function structure or activity limitations may benefit from intensive inpatient rehabilitation provided in a freestanding rehabilitation facility or in a rehabilitation unit within the acute care hospital. Rehabilitation programs certified by the Commission on Accreditation of Rehabilitation Facilities (CARF) and the Joint Commission on Accreditation of Healthcare Organizations (JCAHO) can be expected to adhere to uniform standards and provide high-quality care.[3] Evidence supports the value of physical therapy in producing improved functional outcomes for persons with stroke.[56-70] They are referred to inpatient rehabilitation if they can tolerate an intensity of services consisting of two or more rehabilitation disciplines, 6 days a week for a minimum of 3 hours of active rehabilitation per day. If the patient requires less intensive services, transfer to a transitional care unit (TCU) within a skilled nursing facility is instituted. Here rehabilitation services are less intense, ranging from 60 to 90 minutes of therapy services 5 days per week.[3]

The timing of rehabilitation services is an important factor in predicting outcome. In general, a shorter onset-to-admission interval, within the first 20 days, has been shown to significantly improve functional outcomes when compared to longer intervals.[65] Additional factors that influence the timing of rehabilitation efforts include medical stability, severity of cognitive–perceptual deficits, motivation, patient endurance, and recovery. In an era of time-limited payment for comprehensive rehabilitation services, selecting the optimal time for rehabilitation services may prevent unnecessary patient failures and improve long-term functional outcomes.

Chronic Phase

Rehabilitation services during the chronic phase, generally defined to be more than 6 months poststroke, are typically delivered in an outpatient rehabilitation facility, in a community setting, or at home. Outpatient services are prescribed for the patient who is discharged from inpatient rehabilitation, is in need of continuing rehabilitation, and can enter and exit the home with ease. Many of the interventions begun during inpatient rehabilitation are continued and progressed in order to sustain the gains made and improve functional performance.[56,58,60-64] Other interventions, including constraint-induced movement therapy (CIMT),[57] bilateral training,[59] virtual reality (VR) training,[65] and electromechanical-assisted walking,[66] may be implemented. Some patients with mild involvement who did not require intense inpatient rehabilitation also benefit from outpatient rehabilitation services. A complete record of past medical and rehabilitation services should be made available to these agencies. The intensity of services provided varies but is generally less than that of inpatient rehabilitation (e.g., 60 to 90 minutes per visit, two to three times per week). Outpatient intervention programs that target progressive improvements in flexibility, strength, balance, locomotion, endurance, and UE function have been shown to be effective in producing meaningful outcomes.[69] The patient and family are instructed in a home exercise program (HEP) and educated about the importance of maintaining exercise levels, health promotion, fall prevention, and safety.

The patient may receive home care rehabilitation services, typically for the patient who is unable to exit the home independently. The challenges of being home can impose additional daily stresses for the patient and family. Difficulties should be addressed promptly as they arise. The therapist needs to emphasize the development of problem-solving skills to ensure successful adaptation to variable home and community environments. Fall risk factors should be eliminated or minimized as appropriate or possible. Examination of the environment and recommendations for modification of the environment are important parts of the preparation for return to home (see Chapter 9, Examination and Modification of the Environment).

Finally, the patient should be assisted in resuming participation in community and recreational activities. With increasing activity levels, it is important to monitor the patient's endurance levels carefully and provide instruction in activity pacing and energy conservation techniques as needed. Community fitness programs[63] and water-based activities[70] have been shown to improve function after stroke. A small number of stroke survivors can be evaluated and assisted in return to work. As the patient becomes successful in the home and community environments, services should be gradually phased out, but a wellness program should be in place (see Chapter 29, Promoting Health and Wellness). Follow-up visits at periodic intervals are recommended to identify problems as they develop and to ensure long-term maintenance of function.

Note: Although there is a large body of research on the efficacy of stroke rehabilitation and more than

15 Cochrane Systematic Reviews,[56-70] the Cochrane researchers often conclude that further high-quality research is needed to determine the most effective interventions. Additional research is also needed to investigate the effect of rehabilitation interventions on quality of life, participation, overall cost–benefit ratios, and the differential effects of stroke severity, latency, and age.

EXAMINATION

The three basic components of a comprehensive physical therapy examination include patient/client history, systems review, and tests and measures. The selection of examination procedures will vary depending on a number of factors, including patient's goals, age, location and severity of stroke, stage of recovery, phase of rehabilitation, and home/community/work situation, as well as other factors.

The purposes of the examination are to

- Screen for likely benefit from rehabilitation services and the most appropriate choice of a care setting.
- Develop a specific POC, including patient and clinician goals, expected outcomes, prognosis, and interventions.
- Measure progress toward projected goals and outcomes.
- Determine if referral to another practitioner is indicated.
- Plan for discharge.

The interview that preceded the formal examination allows the clinician and the person poststroke to identify the relevant goals for this episode of care. This shared decision-making process guides the system review, screening, selection of tests and measures that inform the prognosis, diagnosis, and development of the POC. Examination findings are coordinated with other members of the rehabilitation team in order to arrive at an integrated POC. Box 15.3 presents Elements of the Examination of the Patient with Stroke[48] highlighting possible body function structure limitations observed in persons poststroke. Many of these examination procedures, tests, and measures are discussed in earlier chapters (see Chapters 2 through 9).

The order of the examination may vary. In this chapter, we propose that examination of participation and activities is done first, followed by determination of underlying body function structure limitations. The examination can be performed using standardized tests as well as task analysis and movement observation and analysis.

There are many standardized tests used to assess persons poststroke. The ones presented in this chapter (see Table 15.7) are a synthesis of those recommended by the Academy of Neurologic Physical Therapy's (ANPT) StrokEDGE workgroup (www.neuropt.org/docs/stroke-sig/strokeedge_taskforce_summary_document.pdf?sfvrsn=2)[51] and the interdisciplinary task force on stroke recovery research.[41] The ANPT StrokEDGE workgroup reviewed 54 outcomes measures for persons poststroke. They then rated them on the basis of their psychometric properties and clinical utility for persons poststroke. Further, they recommended, on the basis of a Delphi study, a core set of measures that entry-level PT students should learn (www.neuropt.org/docs/edge-documents/strokedge_entrylevel_recs.pdf?sfvrsn=2) and measures that should be used in different settings. Table 15.7 is organized on the basis of the ICF model and by practice setting.

Participation

Examination of participation begins by understanding the patient's participation goals during the interview. The *Goal Attainment Scale (GAS)* allows for customization of goals and a specific way of measuring them. The GAS requires an interview and a follow-up assessment if goals were achieved or not.[71] Information on test administration can be found at www.rehabmeasures@sralab.org. Alternatively, participation can be examined with a stroke-specific standardized test.

Stroke Impact Scale

The *Stroke Impact Scale (SIS)* is a self-report measure developed to assess function and quality of life after stroke. It is therefore both an activity and a participation measure. It includes 59 items organized into 8 subgroups: strength, memory and thinking, emotions, communication, ADL, mobility, hand function, and participation. The participation domain has 8 questions covering work, social activities, quiet recreation, active recreation, role as a family member or friend, participation in spiritual or religious activities, feeling emotionally connected, and ability to help others. The final item of the SIS asks the person to rate perceived recovery on a scale of 0 to 100 with 100 representing full recovery and 0 representing no recovery. It takes about 30 minutes to complete. The SIS is a valid, reliable, and sensitive measure of change in this population.[72,73] A unique score can be calculated for the participation domain, and responses may be accurately provided by proxy.[74] The form and user agreement are available at www.rehabmeasures@sralab.org.

Activity

Examination of activity may be done using a task analysis supported by observation of movement as well as standardized tests. Activities can be grouped according to their different motor control requirements, posture and balance, gait, and upper limb use. There are also tests of function, which combine the motor control requirements into whole body ADL.

Postural Control and Balance

Postural control and balance (when measured at the activity level with the standardized tests described in this

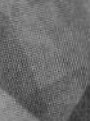

Box 15.3 Elements of the Examination of the Patient With Stroke

Patient/Client History

- Goals (emphasis on participation and activity)
- Quick communication and cognition screen (see details below)
- Age, sex, race/ethnicity, primary language, education
- Social history: cultural beliefs and behaviors, family and caregiver resources, social support systems
- Occupation/employment/work
- Living environment: home/work barriers
- Hand dominance
- General health status: physical, psychological, social, and role function, health habits
- Family history
- Medical/surgical history
- Medications
- Medical/laboratory test results
- Functional activity level: premorbid

Systems Review

- Neuromuscular
- Musculoskeletal
- Cardiovascular/pulmonary
- Integumentary

Tests and Measures

Tests and measures are selected based on their ability to quantify or describe each of the following:
Participation: Work, community, and leisure activities: ability to assume/resume activities, safety; use of the GAS or the SIS

Activities:

- ***Postural control and balance*:** sensorimotor integration, balance strategies (static and dynamic); safety PASS
  Primary impairments: altered balance, increased fall risk
- ***Gait and locomotion***: speed, distance, steps, temporal-spatial description, use of assistive devices/orthotic devices, safety. 10MWT, 6MWT
- ***Upper limb use*:** active isolated movement against gravity, ARAT, MAL
- ***Functional status and activity level:*** performance-based examination of functional skills (FIM level), basic and instrumental ADL; functional mobility skills; home management skills; assistive or adaptive devices: fit, alignment, function, use; safety

Body Function Structure:

- ***Level of consciousness, arousal, attention, and cognition*: mental status, *insight, motivation***
  Primary impairments: impaired alertness and attention, perseveration, confabulation, confusion, disorientation, distractibility, memory deficits, impaired judgment
- ***Emotional status***
  Primary impairments: depression, pseudobulbar affect, apathy, euphoria
  Secondary impairments: depression
- ***Behavioral style***
  Primary impairments: impulsive or cautious behavioral styles; frustration, irritability
- ***Communication and language:*** coordinate efforts with the speech-language pathologist
  Primary impairments: fluent, nonfluent, or global aphasia, dysarthria
- ***Circulation;*** cardiovascular signs and symptoms
  Common comorbidities: hypertension, CAD, CHF, diabetes, DVT
- ***Ventilation and respiration/gas exchange***: pulmonary signs and symptoms
  Common comorbidities: chronic pulmonary disease
- ***Anthropometric characteristics***: body mass index, girth, length
  Secondary impairments: edema, common in hand and foot
- ***Integumentary integrity***: skin condition, pressure-sensitive areas; effectiveness of protective pressure-relieving devices
  Secondary impairments: altered skin integrity, decubitus ulcers
- ***Pain:*** intensity and location
  Primary impairments: central poststroke pain
  Secondary impairments: hemiplegic shoulder and/or hand pain
- ***Cranial and peripheral nerve integrity***
  Primary impairments: visual field defects (CN II); impaired facial sensation (CN V) and facial movements (CNs V and VII); vestibular/auditory dysfunction (CN VII), dysphagia and dysarthria (CNs IX, X, XII)
- ***Sensory integrity and integration***
  Primary impairments: homonymous hemianopsia, tactile/proprioceptive/kinesthetic losses, astereognosis
- ***Perceptual function***: collaborate with an occupational therapist on assessment as needed
  Primary impairments: spatial relations syndrome, body scheme/body image disorders, unilateral neglect, agnosia, topographical disorientation
- ***Joint integrity, alignment, and mobility:*** ROM (active and passive); muscle length and soft tissue extensibility
  Secondary impairments: altered biomechanical alignment; loss of joint ROM, muscle and soft tissue length
- ***Posture:*** alignment and position, symmetry (static and dynamic, sitting and standing); ergonomics and body mechanics
  Secondary impairment: altered biomechanical alignment
- ***Motor function: motor control and motor learning***
  Primary impairments:
  Abnormal (obligatory) synergies: flexion and extension synergy patterns

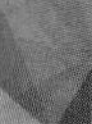

Box 15.3 Elements of the Examination of the Patient With Stroke—cont'd

Altered voluntary movement patterns: altered initiation, sequencing, timing of muscle contractions; altered force production
Altered reflex integrity: hyperreflexia, tonic reflexes, associated reactions
Abnormal tone: flaccidity initially; spasticity: spastic posturing
Coordination, dexterity, agility: coordination deficits
Motor planning: ideomotor or ideational apraxia

- ***Muscle performance: strength, power, and endurance***
Primary impairments: paralysis or weakness; fatigue
Secondary impairments: disuse atrophy
Primary impairments: altered sequencing, timing, balance, endurance
- ***Aerobic capacity and endurance***: functional activity testing, graded exercise testing
Secondary impairments: decreased endurance
- ***Wheelchair management and mobility***: safety and endurance
- ***Orthotic, protective and supportive devices***: fit, alignment, function, use, safety

Adapted from the Guide to PT Practice[48]

Table 15.7 Standardized Assessments Organized by the ICF and Setting

ICF Domain	Test	Acute Care	In-patient	Out-patient	Stroke Research	Entry-Level Education
Participation	Goal Attainment Scale		X	X		
	Stroke Impact Scale			X		X
Activity						
Posture and Balance	Postural Assessment Scale	X	X	X		X
	Functional Reach	X	X	X		X
	Berg Balance Scale		X	X		X
	Timed Up and Go	X	X	X		
Gait	6-Minute Walk Test	X	X	X		X
	10-Meter Walk Test	X	X	X	X	X
	Dynamic Gait Index					X
Upper Limb Use	Action Research Arm Test				X	X
	Motor Activity Log		X	X		
Function	Functional Independence Measure		X			
Body Function Structure	Ashworth					X
	Fugl Meyer-Motor Performance				X	X
	Orpington Prognostic Scale	X			X	X

chapter) may be categorized as an activity at the body function structure level when looking at basic features of the postural control (such as using anticipatory control, balance strategies, and sensory integration). In this chapter, they are kept together because the examination and intervention begin at the task level, then go to the body function structure level to interpret deficits. Postural control and balance are disturbed following stroke and are characterized by asymmetries in alignment and movement. Common postural alignment deviations following stroke are presented in Table 15.8. Control of balance may be impaired when reacting to a destabilizing external force *(reactive postural control)* and/or during self-initiated movements *(proactive or anticipatory postural control)*. Thus, the patient may be unable to maintain stable balance in sitting or standing or to move in the posture without loss of balance. Disruptions of central sensorimotor processing contribute to an inability to recruit effective postural strategies and adapt postural movements to changing task and environmental demands. Persons with stroke typically demonstrate uneven weight distribution and increased postural sway in standing. Patients with stroke often experience delays in the onset of motor activity, abnormal timing and sequencing of muscle activity, and abnormal co-contraction, resulting in disorganization of normal postural synergies. For example, proximal muscles are typically activated in advance of distal muscles or, in some patients, very late. Compensatory responses typically include excessive hip and knee movements. Corrective responses to perturbations or destabilizing forces are inadequate and result in loss of balance and frequent falls. Patients with hemiplegia typically fall in the direction of weakness.[75-79] Examination should include both the static and dynamic balance control in both sitting and standing.

The patient's ability to maintain a stable position (steadiness) and position (symmetry) within the base of support (BOS) is determined. Dynamic stability control can be examined by having the patient move within a given posture (weight shift) or reach within his or her limits of stability (LOS). The patient is directed to shift weight in all directions, especially to the more involved side where greater impairments are expected. Functional tasks that utilize moving from one posture to another (e.g., supine-to-sit, sit-to-stand) can also be used to examine dynamic postural control.[80]

Performance-based postural control and balance scales highly recommended by the Strokedge group are either stroke specific, such as the *Postural Assessment Scale for Stroke Patients (PASS),* or have been validated for persons poststroke, such as the *Functional Reach, Berg Balance Scale,* and *Timed Up and Go* (the latter three can be found in Chapter 6, Examination of Coordination and Balance).

- The *PASS* examines the postural abilities in lying, sitting, and standing, and changing posture (supine-to-affected side, supine-to-unaffected side, supine-to-sitting, sitting-to-standing, and standing picking up a pencil off the floor). The 12 items are scored using an ordinal scale with descriptors ranging from "cannot perform" to "perform with little help" to "perform without help." It demonstrates good

Table 15.8 Common Postural Alignment Deviations Associated With Stroke

Body Segment	Postural Alignment Deviations
Pelvis	• Asymmetrical weight-bearing with majority of weight borne on the stronger side • In sitting, posterior pelvic tilt (sacral sitting) • In standing, unilateral retraction and elevation on the more affected side
Trunk	• With sacral sitting, a flattened lumbar curve with exaggerated thoracic curve and forward head • Lateral flexion with trunk shortening on more affected side
Shoulders	• Unequal height with more affected shoulder depressed • Humeral subluxation with scapular downward rotation and lateral flexion of trunk • Scapular instability (winging) may be present
Head/Neck	• Protraction with lateral trunk flexion • Lateral flexion of the head with rotation away from the more affected side
Upper Extremities	• More affected UE typically held in a flexed, adducted position, with internal rotation and elbow flexion, forearm pronation, wrist and finger flexion; limb is non–weight-bearing • Stronger UE used for postural support
Lower Extremities	• In sitting: More affected LE typically held in hip abduction and external rotation with hip and knee flexion (flexion synergy pattern) • In standing: More affected LE typically held in hip and knee extension with adduction and internal rotation (scissoring pattern); ankle plantar flexion • Unequal weight bearing on feet, similar to pelvis in sitting

construct validity and high interrater and intrarater reliability.[81] It has been shown to be highly responsive to change in acute patients (14 to 30 days poststroke), moderately responsive to change in subacute patients (30 to 90 days poststroke), and least responsive in chronic patients (180 days poststroke) except when the latter are severe, in which case the responsiveness is high.[82] The minimal detectable change for acute patients is 2.2 points.[83] A minimal clinically important difference (MCID) is not established, but extensive predictive and criterion validity can be viewed at www.rehabmeasures@sralab.org.

Ipsilateral Pushing

Ipsilateral pushing (also known as *pusher syndrome* or *contraversive pushing*) is motor behavior characterized by active pushing with the stronger extremities toward the hemiparetic side with a lateral postural imbalance.[84] The end result is a tendency to fall toward the hemiparetic side. Ipsilateral pushing occurs in about 10% of patients with acute stroke and results from stroke affecting the posterolateral thalamus.[85,86] The result is an altered perception of the body's orientation in relation to gravity. Karnath et al[84] found that patients experienced a misperception of subjective postural vertical position, perceiving their body as vertical when it was actually tilted about 20° toward the hemiparetic side. They also found that the visual and vestibular input for orientation perception to vertical remained intact as patients were able to align their bodies with the help of visual cues and conscious strategies. No significant association between ipsilateral pushing and hemineglect, anosognosia, aphasia, or apraxia has been found.[85]

Functional skills are significantly impaired for patients with ipsilateral pushing. During sitting, the push results in a strong lateral lean toward the weaker side; when sitting in a wheelchair, ipsilateral push often thrusts the patient over onto the wheelchair arm. In standing, a strong push creates an unstable situation with a high risk of falls because the hemiparetic LE typically cannot support the body weight. The patient shows no fear even when active pushing leads to instability and strongly resists any attempts to passively correct posture to midline, symmetrical weight-bearing. This pattern is totally opposite the expected postural deficiency seen in most patients after stroke, that is, increased weight-bearing to the stronger side to compensate for deficits on the hemiparetic side. Patients also typically demonstrate severe problems in transfers and gait. During transfers to the less involved side, the patient demonstrates increased pushback away from that side.

During walking, the patient typically exhibits inadequate extension of the hemiparetic LE with inability to transfer weight toward the less involved LE. During swing, strong scissoring (adduction) of the more involved LE is typically evident. The use of a cane during ambulation is problematic because patients use the cane to increase push to the hemiplegic side. Pedersen et al[85] demonstrated that patients with ipsilateral pushing behavior have poorer rehabilitation outcomes with longer hospital stays and prolonged recovery times. They also had significantly lower functional scores on admission and discharge with increased levels of dependence at discharge. However, with training, the brain can compensate well. The syndrome is rarely still evident at 6 months.[87]

Examination of the patient with ipsilateral pushing should include a focus on several criteria of behavior, including the following: (1) spontaneous body posture with tilting toward the more paretic side, (2) an increase of pushing force by the less involved extremities evidenced by increased abduction and extension, and (3) resistance to passive correction of the posture. Broetz and Karnath[88] developed the *Clinical Assessment Scale for Contraversive Pushing (SCP),* which scores each of these three criteria in both sitting and standing. A subjective rating scale is used. The scores for each criteria range from 0 to 1. Because the criteria are examined in both sitting and standing, the maximum for each is 2 with a maximum possible overall score of 6. Patients are diagnosed with pushing behaviors if all three criteria are present and a score of 1 or more exists in each of the three criteria. Functional examination will reveal consistent difficulties with transfers to the less affected side and difficulties with independent sitting, standing, and walking.[89]

Gait and Locomotion

Gait is altered following stroke owing to a number of factors such as lack of selective capacity (ability to isolate movement), weakness, sensory loss, impaired balance, and loss of balance confidence. An examination of gait typically includes an *observational gait analysis (OGA).* The therapist examines the movements occurring at the ankle, foot, knee, hip, pelvis, and trunk during walking (kinematic gait analysis). Gait is observed from the different planes of motion, and deviations are identified. Digital video recording of a patient's gait for subsequent OGA can improve identification of gait deviations, provides a visual record of performance, and offers a useful teaching tool (patient feedback) to assist with remediation of gait problems. Quantitative measures of distance and time, cadence, velocity, and stride times should also be obtained using measured walkways and a stop watch. Kinetic gait analysis examines the forces involved in the production of movement during walking and requires sophisticated instrumentation (force plates). See Chapter 7, Examination of Gait.

Persons poststroke often present with slow gait that is asymmetrical. Typically, stance time on the stroke-affected side is reduced and step length is increased relative to the less affected side. There is a decreased push-off on the stroke affected leg, which further compromises step length on the stroke-affected side. There may be a lack of dissociation between the right and left sides of the body, with the stroke-affected side moving as a unit rather than with a dissociating arm swing from the lower extremity on forward progression.

StrokEDGE recommends both a measure of gait speed, the 10-meter walk test (10MWT), and a measure of endurance, the 6-minute walk test (6MWT), as well as a more global measure of gait performance, the Dynamic Gait Index (see Chapter 7). Ambulation profiles and scales can be used to determine locomotor function following stroke. These tests have been examined for reliability and/or validity and are reviewed in Chapter 7.

Gait speed has been found to be particularly useful in classifying a patient's ability to ambulate in different environments. Perry et al[90] constructed a walking ability questionnaire and surveyed a group of 147 patients with chronic stroke about the effects of their limited walking ability. They then developed the *Classification of Walking Handicap After Stroke.* The use of functional categories (physiological walker, household walker, and community walker) provides a useful method of identifying customary level of walking at home and in the community. For example, a *physiological walker* walks for exercise only either at home or in parallel bars during physical therapy. A *limited household walker* relies on walking to some extent for home activities and requires assistance for some walking activities, uses a wheelchair, or is unable to perform others. A *community walker* can walk unlimited distances outside.

Factors that differentiated household from community ambulators included strength, proprioception, isolated knee control (flexion and extension), and velocity. This classification system can be used to improve communication among clinicians, treatment planning, and documentation. It also forms the basis for the *Functional Ambulation Classification Scale.*[91]

More recently, Fulk et al[92] were able to classify walking ability based on population studies[93-95] that quantified the numbers of steps walked, walking speed, and walking endurance. This newer classification offers concrete measures to differentiate between walking categories. For example, a person poststroke who walks more than 7,500 steps/day, or 287 meters on the 6MWT, can be classified as an unlimited community walker. The new scale offers the clinician the choice to examine step frequency or use the 6MWT to identify walking category. Table 15.9 compares the two classifications.

Upper Limb Use

Upper limb use poststroke is compromised and can present with no active movement to limited movement and, when resolved, as isolated selective movement. Measurement of upper limb is recommended by the StrokEDGE group using the combination of the performance-based *Action Research Arm Test (ARAT)* and the self-report *Motor Activity Log (MAL).*

The ARAT has 19 UE functional tasks/movements with four subscales: grasping, gripping, pinching, and gross movement. Ordinal scoring is used for the 19 items, where 0 indicates no movement and 3 indicates normal movement. Items in each subscale are totaled for grasping (18 point maximum), gripping (12 point maximum), pinching (18 point maximum), and gross movement (9 point maximum), with a total scale score of 57, indicating normal UE use. It takes between 5 and 20 minutes to administer the ARAT. The test is valid and reliable.[96-99] However, it does have significant floor effects at 14 days post-stroke (greater than 21% of participants) and notable ceiling effects (greater than 21% of participants) at 30, 90, and 180 days poststroke.[100] The

Table 15.9 Classification of Ambulation

	Household Walker	Limited Community Walker	Community Walker
Perry et al[90] description and criteria	• Able to walk throughout home • Does not use wheelchair in the home • Difficulty on stairs • Gait speed: <0.40 m/s	• Can enter and leave home independently • Ascends/descends curbs independently • Manages stairs • Independent walking in some (1–2) moderate community settings (i.e., visit friend in local restaurants) • Gait speed: 0.40–0.80 m/s	• Independent walking in home and all community activities • Can walk in crowded areas and on uneven terrain • Gait speed: >0.80 m/s
Fulk et al[91] description and criteria	• 100–2,499 steps/day • Gait speed: <0.49 m/s • 6MWT distance: <205 meters	• 2,500–7,499 steps/day • Gait speed: 0.49–0.92 m/s • 6MWT distance: 205–287 meters	• ≥7,500 steps/day • Gait speed: >0.92 m/s • 6MWT distance: >287 meters

Adapted from Perry et al,[90, p. 985] with permission, and Fulk.[92]
6MWT = six-minute walk test; m/s = meters per second.

MCID of the ARAT if the dominant hand is affected is 12 points, and if the nondominant hand is affected, it is 17 points.[101]

The MAL is a self-report measure, which uses a semi-structured interview to assess arm function. Individuals are asked to rate quality of movement (QOM) and amount of movement (AOM) during 30 daily functional tasks (original MAL), 28 functional tasks (MAL 28), or 14 tasks (MAL 14).[102-104] Target tasks include object manipulation (e.g., pen, fork, comb, and cup) as well as the use of the arm during gross motor activities (e.g., transferring to a car, steadying oneself during standing, pulling a chair into a table while sitting). The AOM as well as QOM of the weaker arm are scored for each item on a 5-point scale ranging from no movement (0) to movement and quality comparable to before the stroke (5).[102,103] The MAL is recommended for use with people who are already in the community, and it may be scored by a caregiver.[102,103]

Functional Status

Functional measures are used to quantify activity limitations, inform the POC, monitor progress, ascertain efficacy of stroke rehabilitation efforts, and make recommendations for long-term care or placement. Instruments can include items to examine *functional mobility skills* (bed mobility, movement transitions, transfers, locomotion, stairs), *basic ADL (BADL) skills* (feeding, hygiene, dressing), and *instrumental ADL (IADL) skills* (communication, home chores). Information on functional disability following stroke is typically gained through performance-based measures. The *Barthel Index*[105] and the *Functional Independence Measure (FIM)*[106] have been extensively tested and demonstrate excellent reliability, validity, and sensitivity. The FIM is now in widespread use in rehabilitation facilities across the United States. Higher FIM scores have been correlated to successful outcomes, discharge home, and return to the community for patients with stroke.[107] See Chapter 8, Examination of Function, for a more detailed discussion of the FIM.

Body Function Structure

Limitations of body function structure may explain difficulty with activities required for participation. It is important to determine the person's cognitive and communication abilities, as this information will further influence the therapist's examination and intervention strategies. Specific body function structures may be examined completely or selectively based on the clinician's hypothesis of which may be limiting activity. For example, if during gait observation the clinician observes difficulty clearing of the affected LE, the clinician may hypothesize weakness of the affected lower extremity and perform strength testing. In the event of a comprehensive examination, the clinician may want to clear passive body functions and structures such as flexibility, tone, integumentary system, and sensation before looking at active structures such as motor performance.

Flexibility and Joint Integrity

An examination of joint flexibility may be performed as a gross active screen and include passive ROM using a goniometer for limited ROM areas that will be targeted for therapy as well as examination for joint hypermobility/hypomobility and soft-tissue changes (swelling, inflammation, or restriction) that could affect ROM. The shoulder and wrist should be examined closely because joint malalignment problems are common. Flaccidity will result in a shoulder subluxation, which should be carefully evaluated and monitored. The UE is placed in a non-supported position and the gap in the glenohumeral joint is measured with a tape measure. Edema of the wrist often produces malaligned carpal bones with resulting impingement during wrist extension. Measurement may be affected by tonal changes or spasticity, so the clinician should attend to those fluctuations and standardize position for measurement. Active ROM (AROM) may be limited or impossible for the patient in early or middle recovery in the presence of paresis, spasticity, or obligatory synergies that can preclude isolated voluntary movements. ROM limitations and developing contractures should be carefully documented.

Contractures can develop anywhere but are particularly apparent in the paretic limbs. As contractures progress, edema and pain may develop and further restrict mobility. In the UE, limitations in the shoulder motions of flexion, abduction, and external rotation are common. Contractures are likely in the elbow flexors, wrist and finger flexors, and forearm pronators. In the LE, plantarflexion contractures are common.

Muscle Tone and Spasticity

Flaccidity (hypotonicity) is present immediately after stroke and is due primarily to the effects of cerebral shock. It is generally short-lived, lasting a few days or weeks. Flaccidity may persist in a small number of patients with lesions restricted to the primary motor cortex or cerebellum. Spasticity (hypertonicity) emerges early in about 90% of cases and occurs on the side of the body opposite the lesion. Spasticity in upper motor neuron syndrome occurs predominantly in antigravity muscles (see Chapter 5, Table 5.3). In the patient with stroke, UE spasticity is frequently strong in scapular retractors; shoulder adductors, depressors, and internal rotators; elbow flexors and forearm pronators; and wrist and finger flexors. In the neck and trunk, spasticity may cause increased lateral flexion to the hemiplegic side. In the LE, spasticity is often strong in the pelvic retractors, hip adductors and internal rotators, hip and knee extensors, plantar flexors and supinators, and toe flexors. Spasticity results in tight (stiff) muscles. Posturing of the limbs (e.g., a tightly fisted hand with the elbow flexed and held tightly against the chest or a stiff extended knee with a plantarflexed foot) is common with moderate to severe spasticity. Spastic posturing can lead to development of painful spasms (similar to muscle cramping), degenerative changes, and fixed contractures. The automatic adjustment of postural muscles that occurs normally in preparation for and during a movement task is also impaired. Thus, patients with stroke may lack the ability to adjust and stabilize proximal limbs and trunk appropriately during movement, with resulting postural abnormalities, balance impairments, and increased risk for falls.

Passive motion testing can be used to determine the presence of hypotonicity or spasticity. Severity of spasticity can be graded on the basis of speed dependent resistance to passive stretch using the *Modified Ashworth Scale (MAS)* (see Chapter 5, Table 5.4). The position of the affected limbs at rest (resting postures) and during voluntary movements should be observed for tonal influences.

Sensation and Vision

Deficits in somatic sensations (touch, temperature, pain, and proprioception) are common after stroke. The type and extent of impairment are related to the location and size of the vascular lesion. Specific localized areas of dysfunction are common with cortical lesions, whereas diffuse involvement throughout one side of the body suggests deeper lesions involving the thalamus and adjacent structures. Impairment in touch sensation (64% to 94%), proprioception (17% to 52%), vibration (44%), and loss of pinprick sensation (35% to 71%) have been reported.[108-110] Sensory loss has also been reported in the ipsilateral, less affected limbs, though to a lesser extent (12% to 25%). Symptoms of crossed anesthesia (ipsilateral facial impairments with contralateral trunk and limb involvement) typify brainstem lesions. Disturbances in cortical sensory modalities (two-point discrimination, stereognosis, kinesthesia, graphesthesia) are also found.)[111,112] Profound sensory impairments will negatively affect motor performance, motor learning, and rehabilitation outcomes and contribute to unilateral neglect and *learned nonuse* of limbs. Sensory impairment is also associated with pressure sores, abrasions, and shoulder pain and subluxation.

The visual system should be carefully investigated, including tests for visual field defects (CN II, optic radiation, visual cortex), acuity (CN II), pupillary reflexes (CNs II and III), and extraocular movements (CNs III, IV, and VI). Ocular motility disturbances, such as diplopia, oscillopsia, visual distortions, or paralysis of conjugate gaze, may be present with brainstem strokes. Visual field defects (homonymous hemianopsia) need to be differentiated from visual neglect, a perceptual deficit characterized by an inattention to or neglect of visual stimuli presented on the involved side. The patient with pure hemianopsia is typically aware of the deficit and may spontaneously compensate by moving the eyes or head toward the side of deficit; the patient with visual neglect will be unaware (inattentive) of the deficit (see Chapter 27). The use of prescriptive eyeglasses should be determined before any testing; the therapist should ensure that eyeglasses are worn and clean.

Central poststroke pain (CPSP) is defined as pain arising as a direct consequence of a lesion or disease affecting the central somatosensory system and occurs in about 10% of strokes.[113] It can result from lesions at any level of the somatosensory pathways including the medulla, thalamus, and cortex. The thalamus is thought to play an important part in the underlying pathophysiology of central pain. CPSP can be severe and persistent (described as "burning," "aching"), spontaneous and intermittent (described as "lacerating" or "shooting" pain), or evoked by mechanical (stroking the skin, pressure) or thermal (heat or cold) stimuli. Symptoms may be focal, affecting the hand/arm or foot/leg, or in severe cases affect half the body. Development of pain is typically within the first few months after stroke, though onset may be delayed for many months. Spontaneous recovery is rare and chronic suffering common. The debilitating nature of CPSP frequently limits participation in rehabilitation programs and outcomes.[114]

A sensory examination should include testing of superficial sensations (e.g., touch, pressure, sharp or dull discrimination, temperature) and deep sensations (proprioception, kinesthesia, vibration). Combined (cortical) sensations such as stereognosis, tactile localization, two-point discrimination, and texture recognition should also be examined once the integrity of the superficial sensations of touch and pressure is established. Sensory testing procedures are described in detail in Chapter 3, Examination of Sensory Function. The quality of sensory impairments experienced can range from mild altered perception to marked changes in sensory thresholds, delayed perceptions, uncertainty of responses, altered time for sensory adaptation, and sensory persistence.[108] Impairments may be evident in one sensory modality and not in others. Differences can also be expected between upper and lower hemiplegic extremities, depending on lesion location. Comparisons with the intact side should be viewed with caution because impairments may exist in the supposedly "normal" extremities due to aging and comorbidities. Sensory testing may be difficult or need to be deferred owing to cognitive or communication deficits.

Integumentary Integrity

Ischemic damage and subsequent necrosis of the skin results in skin breakdown and pressure ulcers (decubitus ulcers). The skin breaks down typically over bony prominences from pressure, friction, shearing, and/or maceration. Intense pressure for a short time or low pressure for a long time results in pressure ulcers. Friction occurs as the skin rubs or is dragged against the supporting surface, for example, when the patient slides down in bed or is pulled up. Spasticity and contractures also contribute to increased friction. Shearing occurs from sliding of adjacent structures in opposite directions (skin vs. underlying bone), for example, during transfers from bed to wheelchair. Maceration is caused by excess moisture, for example, with urinary incontinence. Additional risk factors include reduced activity (bedfast or chairfast), immobility, decreased sensation, abnormal patterns of movement, poor nutrition, and decreased level of consciousness. The incidence of pressure sores is increased with comorbid medical conditions such as infections, peripheral vascular disease, edema, and diabetes.

Daily systematic inspection of the skin is indicated for high-risk patients, particularly over areas prone to breakdown. The skin must be kept clean, dry, and protected from injury. Adherence to proper techniques for positioning, turning, and transferring is essential. The therapist collaborates with nursing to develop and monitor a positioning schedule and time in each position. Pressure-relieving devices (PRDs) are used to minimize high concentrations of pressure (e.g., foam pads, alternating pressure mattress, water mattress, air-fluidized bed, sheepskin, heel and elbow protectors, multipodus boots, and seating cushions). Proper use of PRDs and positioning (seating) in the wheelchair should be closely examined.

Motor Control

Stages of Motor Recovery

Initially, flaccid paralysis is present *(stage 1)*. This is replaced by the development of spasticity, hyperreflexia, and mass patterns of movement, termed ***obligatory synergies***, all characteristics of upper motor neuron syndrome. Muscles involved in obligatory synergy patterns are strongly linked in a highly stereotyped, abnormal pattern; isolated joint movements outside the obligatory pattern are not possible. During *stage 2* (early synergy), facilitatory stimuli will elicit partial range synergies. As recovery progresses, spasticity is marked with full ROM and obligatory synergies *(stage 3)*. Synergy influence begins to decline in *stage 4* as some isolated out-of-synergy joint movements emerge. During *stage 5*, relative independence of synergy, spasticity continues to decreased and isolated joint movements become more apparent, and during *stage 6*, patterns of movement are near normal. This general pattern of recovery was initially described by Twitchell[115] and Brunnstrom[116,117] and confirmed by additional investigators[118,119] (Box 15.4). Several important points merit consideration. Progression through these stages exists, though individual recovery is highly variable. Some patients experience mild involvement with early full recovery, whereas other patients demonstrate severe involvement with incomplete recovery. The degree of recovery depends on a number of factors, including lesion location and severity and capacity for adaptation through training. Finally, recovery differs within patients. For example, the UE may be more involved and demonstrate less complete recovery than the LE, as is seen in MCA syndrome.

Abnormal and highly stereotyped obligatory synergies emerge with spasticity following stroke. Thus, the patient is unable to perform an isolated movement of a single limb segment without producing movements in the remainder of the limb. For example, efforts to flex the elbow also result in shoulder flexion, abduction, and external rotation. Two distinct abnormal synergy patterns have been described for each extremity: a flexion synergy and an extension synergy (Table 15.10). An inspection of the synergy components reveals that certain muscles are not usually involved in either the flexion or extension synergy. These muscles include the (1) latissimus dorsi, (2) teres major, (3) serratus anterior, (4) finger extensors, and (5) ankle evertors. These muscles, therefore, are generally difficult to activate while the patient is exhibiting

Box 15.4 Sequential Motor Recovery Stages Following Stroke

STAGE 1	Recovery from hemiplegia occurs in a stereotyped sequence of events that begins with a period of *flaccidity* immediately following the acute episode. *No movement of the limbs* can be elicited.
STAGE 2	As recovery begins, the basic limb synergies or some of their components may appear as associated reactions, or *minimal voluntary movement* responses may be present. At this time, spasticity begins to develop.
STAGE 3	Thereafter, the patient gains *voluntary control of the movement synergies,* although full range of all synergy components does not necessarily develop. Spasticity has further increased and may become severe.
STAGE 4	Some *movement combinations that do not follow the paths of either synergy are mastered,* first with difficulty, then with more ease, and *spasticity begins to decline.*
STAGE 5	If progress continues, more *difficult movement combinations are learned* as the basic limb synergies lose their dominance over motor acts.
STAGE 6	With the *disappearance of spasticity, individual joint movements become possible and coordination* approaches normal. From here on, as the last recovery step, normal motor function is restored, but this last stage is not achieved by all, for the recovery process can plateau at any stage.

From Brunnstrom, S: Movement Therapy in Hemiplegia. Harper & Row, New York, NY, 1970, with permission.

Table 15.10 Obligatory Synergy Patterns Following Stroke

	Flexion Synergy Components	Extension Synergy Components
Upper extremity	Scapular retraction/elevation or hyperextension Shoulder abduction, external rotation Elbow flexion* Forearm supination Wrist and finger Flexion	Scapular protraction Shoulder adduction,* internal rotation Elbow extension Forearm pronation* Wrist and finger flexion
Lower extremity	Hip flexion,* abduction, external rotation Knee flexion Ankle dorsiflexion, inversion Toe dorsiflexion	Hip extension, adduction,* internal rotation Knee extension* Ankle plantarflexion,* inversion Toe plantarflexion

*Generally the strongest component.

these patterns. Obligatory synergies are often incompatible with normal ADL and functional mobility skills. For example, the patient with a strong LE extensor synergy will have difficulty walking owing to foot plantarflexion and inversion with hip and knee extension and adduction (scissoring gait pattern). As recovery progresses, spasticity and obligatory synergies begin to disappear and more normal synergies with isolated joint control become possible.

Fugl-Meyer Assessment of Physical Performance

The *Fugl-Meyer Assessment of Physical Performance (FMA)* is a standardized way to test for motor recovery.[120] It is based on the work of Twitchell[115] and Brunnstrom.[116,117] This is an impairment-based test with items organized by sequential recovery stages. A three-point ordinal scale is used to measure impairments of volitional movement with grades ranging from 0 (item cannot be performed) to 2 (item can be fully performed). Specific descriptions for performance accompany individual test items. Subtests exist for UE function, LE function, balance, sensation, ROM, and pain. The cumulative test score for all components is 226 with availability of specific subtest scores (e.g., UE maximum score is 66, LE score 34; balance score 14). This instrument has good construct validity and high reliability ($r = 0.99$) for determining motor function following stroke.[121, 122] The instrument requires an estimated 30 to 45 minutes to administer. A shortened version consists of combining the UE and LE sections to form the *Fugl-Meyer Motor Scale*. This version has also been shown to be a useful measure of stagewise recovery and outcomes with a shortened administration time.[123] The motor section is recommended for stroke research recovery.[41] For the LE motor score, a change of greater than 5 points is required to be outside of measurement error,[124] and 5.4 is the MDC for the UE score.[73] This test is used in many of the studies of stroke recovery and rehabilitation.

Selective Capacity

Clinicians may use the synergies to describe movement, but examination should focus on the person's selective capacity or ability to isolate movement. Voluntary movement patterns should be examined to determine if the person has movement that is *active, isolated,* and *against gravity*. In early stages of recovery, movement can be partially active, partially isolated, and also gravity eliminated. The assessment consists of asking the person to voluntarily move a limb in one direction at a specific joint (e.g., shoulder or hip flexion) and then observing the extent to which the person can move through the full available ROM without moving the other joints in that limb. For example, the person poststroke may be able to actively flex his or her shoulder 50% against gravity while maintaining the elbow extended and wrist/hand relaxed; after this point, the elbow and wrist may flex and the shoulder may abduct.

While testing for active isolated movement, the clinician may observe *associated reactions,* which also typically present in patients with stroke who exhibit strong spasticity and obligatory synergies. These consist of unintentional movements of the hemiparetic limb caused by voluntary action of another limb or by other stimuli such as yawning, sneezing, or coughing. For example, when the patient vigorously contracts the elbow flexors of the stronger UE, the hemiparetic elbow also flexes; or when the patient flexes the hip to lift the hemiparetic LE in sitting, the hemiparetic UE also flexes.

Muscle Performance

If the patient demonstrates some degree of selective capacity, then testing of muscle strength is indicated. Paresis is found in 80% to 90% of all patients after stroke and is a major factor in impaired motor function, activity limitation, and disability. Patients are unable to generate the force necessary for initiating and controlling movement. The degree of primary weakness is related to the location and size of the brain injury and varies from a complete inability to achieve any contraction (hemiplegia) to hemiparesis with measurable impairments in force production.[125] Deficits on the contralateral side typically include hemiparesis (opposite UE and LE). Owing to the high incidence of MCA strokes, the UE is frequently more affected than the LE. About 20% of individuals with MCA strokes fail to regain any functional use of the affected UE. Typically, distal muscles exhibit greater strength deficits than proximal. This can be explained by the greater facilitation of distal muscles than proximal by the corticospinal system. Mild weakness also occurs on the ipsilateral, "supposedly normal" side.[126,127] This can be explained by the fact that only 75% to 90% of the corticospinal fibers cross in the medulla to the contralateral side. The remainder are transmitted to the spinal cord ipsilaterally in the anterior or ventral corticospinal tract. Once in the spinal cord, some of these fibers cross while the rest remain uncrossed, thereby explaining bilateral weakness.[128] The amount of weakness experienced by the patient may also vary according to the extent and level of inactivity (disuse atrophy) and the specific functional tasks attempted. Thus, a patient may appear stronger in some tasks than others.[129]

Poststroke weakness is associated with a number of changes in both the muscle and the motor unit. Changes occur in muscle composition, including atrophy of muscle fibers. There is a selective loss of type II fast-twitch fibers with subsequent increase in the percentage of type I fibers (a finding also reported in the elderly). This selective loss of type II fibers results in slowed force production; difficulty with initiation and production of rapid, high-force movements; and rapid onset of fatigue.[111,129-131] The number of functioning motor units and discharge firing rates also decrease. This is explained by the presence of transsynaptic degeneration of alpha motor neurons that occurs with loss of corticospinal innervation. Abnormal recruitment of motor units with altered timing occurs.[132-134] Thus, patients demonstrate inefficient patterns of muscle activation and higher levels of co-contraction. This opposing muscle activation can contribute to muscle weakness and incoordination. These impairments in force production and coordination have been reported in both paretic and less affected UEs after stroke.[135,136] Patients demonstrate increased effort and fatigability with frequent complaints of feelings of weakness. Denervation potentials on electromyography (EMG) are common, also the result of denervation changes in the corticospinal tracts. Overall reaction times are increased, a finding also reported in the less affected extremities and for the elderly in general. Movement times are prolonged, a timing abnormality that contributes to impairment of coordinated motor sequences.

Although an examination of strength is necessary, the traditional manual muscle test (MMT) poses problems of validity in the presence of strong spasticity, reflex, and synergy dominance. The patient who is not able to isolate specific movements should not be examined using MMT. In this situation, an estimation of strength can be made from observation of active movements during functional activities (functional strength testing). The patient's self-report can also yield important indicators of weakness and fatigue. The patient in later recovery with improving motor control and isolated movement can be examined using traditional MMT or handheld dynamometry. Use of a computerized isokinetic dynamometer can reveal important objective data regarding forces generated, peak torque, time to peak torque, and total work normalized to body weight. See Chapter 4, Musculoskeletal Examination.

Coordination

Proprioceptive losses can result in sensory ataxia. Strokes affecting the cerebellum typically produce cerebellar ataxia (e.g., lateral medullary syndrome, basilar artery syndrome, pontine syndromes) and motor weakness. The resulting problems with timing and sequencing of muscles can significantly impair function and limit adaptability to changing task and environmental demands. Basal ganglia involvement (posterior cerebral artery syndrome) may lead to slowed movements (bradykinesia) or involuntary movements (choreoathetosis, hemiballismus).

Coordination tests can be used to examine movement control. The therapist focuses on elements of speed/rate control, steadiness, response orientation, and reaction and movement times. Fine motor control and dexterity should be examined using writing, dressing, and feeding tasks (see Chapter 6). Although more significant impairments can be expected on the hemiparetic side, it is important to remember that subtle deficits can occur on the less involved side. Thus, it is important to examine both unilateral and bilateral movements, including symmetrical, asymmetrical, and unrelated movements. Performance may vary as the patient moves from supine to sitting to standing positions with the resultant increased postural demands and greater degrees of freedom.

Motor Planning

Motor praxis is the ability to plan and execute coordinated movement. Lesions of the premotor frontal cortex of either hemisphere, left inferior parietal lobe, and corpus callosum can produce *apraxia.* Apraxia is more evident with left hemisphere damage than right and is commonly seen with aphasia. The patient demonstrates difficulty planning and executing purposeful movements that cannot be accounted for by any other reason (i.e., impaired strength, coordination, sensation, tone, cognitive function, communication, or uncooperativeness). There are two main types of apraxia. *Ideational apraxia* is an inability of the patient to produce movement either on command or automatically and represents a complete breakdown in the conceptualization of the task. The patient has no idea how to do the movement and thus cannot formulate the required motor programs. With *ideomotor apraxia,* the patient is unable to produce a movement on command but is able to move automatically. Thus, the patient can perform habitual tasks when not commanded to do so and often perseverates, repeating the activity over and over. Significant information on apraxia will be gained by close collaboration with the occupational therapist. Refer to Chapter 27 for a more complete discussion of these deficits and their management.

Cranial Nerves

The therapist should examine for facial sensation (CN V), facial movements (CNs V and VII), and labyrinthine/auditory function (CN VIII). The presence of swallowing difficulties and drooling necessitates an examination of the motor nuclei of the lower brainstem cranial nerves (CNs IX, X, and XII) affecting the muscles of the face, tongue, larynx, and pharynx. This includes determination of motor function of the lips, mouth, tongue, palate, pharynx, and larynx. The gag reflex should be examined because hypoactivity may lead to aspiration into the airway. Adequacy of cough mechanisms should also be carefully examined. The therapist needs to be able to recognize the presence of swallowing difficulties and initiate prompt referral.

Aerobic Capacity and Endurance

A supervised exercise test with electrocardiogram (ECG) monitoring may be indicated for survivors of stroke with cardiovascular disease in the subacute phase. Performance measures include significant ECG changes, HR, BP, *rating of perceived exertion (RPE)*, and other signs of ischemic intolerance. The mode of testing will depend on the individual patient and can include leg cycle ergometry, semirecumbent cycle ergometry, a combination arm-leg ergometer, treadmill (TM) walking, or a seated stepper. If balance is impaired, recumbent equipment or an overhead safety harness on a TM should be used. Test protocols are individualized and are generally submaximal with a gradual progression in intensity. An intermittent protocol with rest periods may be required for some patients. Clinical endpoints of testing are similar as for other patients with cardiovascular disease (serious dysrhythmias, greater than 2 mm ST-segment depression or elevation, SBP greater than 250 mm Hg or diastolic BP [DBP] greater than 115 mm Hg, volitional fatigue).[28]

For ambulatory patients, walking endurance can be measured using a *6- or 12-minute walk test* (see discussion in Chapter 7). The time, total distance, number of rest stops, and symptoms at rest stops are recorded. Shorter distances (e.g., a 2-minute walk test) have been used for patients with acute stroke.[137] Table 15.9 shows the usefulness of the information gleaned from the 6MWT.

PROGNOSIS AND DIAGNOSIS

Formulating a POC involves weighing the person's resources and limitations, interpreting the results of the examination tests that are predictive, and consulting the literature on the health condition. For example, administering the *Orpington Prognostic Scale (OPS)* is recommended by Strokedge to assess the person in the first two weeks poststroke because it is valid and reliable and the scores predict discharge setting.[138,139] It has four domains, balance, cognition, motor, and proprioception, which are often measured anyway. Using the OPS, the clinician could in the prognosis predict the discharge setting as follows: a score of less than 3.2 indicates discharge to home within 3 weeks of stroke, a score of greater than 5.2 requires long-term care, and a score between 3.2 and 5.2 requires intensive rehabilitation (see Table 15.7).[139]

Evidence from basic science is accumulating to support motor recovery poststroke and the findings of specific tests are being recommended for inclusion in stroke recovery clinical trials. A consensus panel recommended assessing the integrity of the *corticospinal track (CST)* using diffusion tensor imaging across the continuum of recovery. The integrity of the CST has demonstrated a moderate to strong relationship with sensorimotor recovery. Similarly, the panel recommended, for inclusion in stroke recovery trials of the upper limb, the use of motor evoked potentials (MEPs), which are measured using transcranial magnetic stimulation. They propose that we classify participants based on the presence of MEP (+) or absence of MEP (–) to understand how they respond to treatments. The presence of a MEP indicates a better prognosis. Once this type of information is available, the clinician will be able to select therapies based on the likelihood of motor recovery.[42]

Clinical tests may also be predictive. Strong evidence has been reported supporting the clinical measurement of the upper limb impairment as predictive of recovery, demonstrating that the lesser the degree of UE impairment early on, the greater the recovery. This finding had only moderate evidence for recovery of the lower limb.[140] It has also been suggested that the NIH Stroke Scale (NIHSS) be used as a measure of stroke severity with the goal of having severity guide prognosis.[41] Additional factors known to moderate prognosis are discussed under Recovery and Outcomes later in this chapter.

GOALS AND OUTCOMES

Examples of long-term participation and activity goals with short-term body function structure goals for patients with stroke are presented in Box 15.5. These examples illustrate the logic of having short-term goals reflect the underlying body function structure or activity limitation that interfere with participation. They refer to person who had an MCA stroke 3 weeks prior and is currently receiving physical therapy in a subacute rehabilitation facility.

PHYSICAL THERAPY INTERVENTIONS

Therapists select interventions based on an accurate examination and evaluation of the existing body function

Box 15.5 Example of Participation, Activity and Related Body Function Structure Goals*

Participation Goal

Patient will participate with close supervision in his daughter's wedding ceremony and reception in 2 months.

Related Activity Goals

1. Patient will sit in a folding chair with no arm rests for 30 minutes in 1 month.
2. Patient will independently transition from sit-stand-sit on a folding chair with no arm rests 5 times in 20 seconds in 1 month.
3. Patient will walk escorting (arm in arm) the PT 300 meters on a level surface using a single point cane in 2 months.
4. Patient will increase walking speed (10MWT) from 0.50 m/s to 0.75 m/s in 2 months.
5. Patient will increase his Berg Balance Scale from 48 to 54 in 2 months.
6. Patient will safely and independently transfer in and out of his car in 1 month.

Related Body Function Structure Goals

1. Patient will increase the affected ankle dorsiflexion, eversion, and plantarflexion by half a grade in 1 month.
2. Patient will increase PROM of the affected hip extension by 5° in 2 weeks.
3. Patient will respond to external perturbations in the anterior posterior direction using an ankle or hip strategy five out of five times in 6 weeks.

*Goals refer to person who had an MCA stroke 4 weeks prior and is currently receiving physical therapy in a subacute rehabilitation facility.

structure and activity limitations that interfere with activity and participation goals. The intervention is modified on the basis of the patient's resources, capabilities, and affective state. Physical therapy can take the form of remediation, compensation, or prevention.[48] Remediation is indicated whenever there is the potential for structural and behavioral plasticity. In more severe cases with limited recovery potential, compensation strategies may be employed. Repetitive task-specific training based on motor learning coupled with exercise and physical activity are the core principles that organize the approach to intervention. PT interventions are centered around a meaningful salient goal with consideration of how to (1) structure the environment, (2) schedule practice, (3) provide feedback, (4) dose the intervention, (5) progress the program, and (6) encourage problem-solving, reflection, and self-management. If available, an algorithm may guide intervention selection based on specific criteria (see later section in this chapter, Interventions to Improve Upper Limb Use).

Evidence-based practice (EBP) promotes the use of current best research evidence along with individual clinical expertise in order to reach informed decisions about patient care. EBP allows therapists to identify the best (most effective) techniques and to take responsibility for evaluating their practice on an ongoing basis. For example, in the 2014 Cochrane review of interventions to improve mobility and function, there was no difference between neurophysiological (neurodevelopmental treatment [NDT], proprioceptive neuromuscular facilitation [PNF]) and other forms of active exercise, such as task-based training. Therefore, to improve mobility and function, based on this evidence, one approach was not superior to another, and the authors recommended that clinicians select the intervention on the basis of their skill and the needs of the patient.[56] In contrast, a 2014 Cochrane review on interventions for improving upper limb use for persons poststroke did not find any quality evidence for the use of NDT.[141] The clinician who practices EBP will regularly consult the literature to select interventions based on best available evidence. Using a combination of synthesis evidence, such as clinical practice guidelines (CPGs) and systematic reviews (SR) with meta-analyses, is recommended as the starting point for reviewing the evidence because SRs may find limited evidence in an area where the CPG can fill the gap. This may be followed by high-quality randomized controlled trials (RCTs) that will have specific protocols for practice. It is important to note that in some instances the available evidence may be a single small study or even a case study, particularly when an area of study is new and not well developed. Then the clinician may draw upon his or her prior knowledge and patient preferences to make a decision about the intervention that is selected.

There is not one optimal intervention for all persons poststroke. As they are a diverse group with variable levels of function, interventions must be carefully selected on the basis of individual abilities and needs. The choice of interventions must also take into consideration a number of other factors, including phase of poststroke recovery (acute, postacute, chronic), severity of the stroke, age of the patient, number of comorbidities, cognitive abilities, communication status, affective status, social and financial resources, and potential discharge placement.

Structure of the Intervention

Motor skill learning is based on the brain's capacity for recovery through mechanisms of reorganization and adaptation. An effective rehabilitation plan capitalizes on this potential and encourages active participation with the goal of acquiring skills. Activities are selected that are meaningful and important to the patient. Optimal motor learning can be promoted through attention to a number of factors, most important, (1) task and learner, (2) structuring the environment, (3) practice schedules, (4) feedback, (5) dose, (6) progression, and (7) self-monitoring. Carr and Shepherd[142] describe many of these strategies in their book *A Motor Relearning Programme for Stroke*. See also Chapter 10, Strategies to Improve Motor Function

Task, Goal, and Learner

The patient's goals influence task selection. The type of task (serial, continuous) and the stage of the learner (cognitive, associative, and autonomous) also guide the intervention. (See Table 10.1 in Chapter 10.) The therapist first assists the patient in learning the desired task (cognitive stage). Explicit verbal instructions are used to direct the patient's attention to the task. More specifically, critical task elements and successful outcomes are identified. The desired task is demonstrated at the ideal performance speeds. The patient then begins to practice. Ideally, there should be whole task practice. If the task has a number of interrelated steps, practice of component parts may also be part of therapy (see later section Practice Schedule). The therapist should give clear, simple, and precise verbal instructions and not overload the patient with excessive or wordy instructions. There is some evidence to suggest that providing excessive information about the task can be disruptive to learning, especially for patients with MCA stroke involving the sensorimotor cortex. This interference may block formation of the implicit motor plan.[143,144] Correct performance should be reinforced and intervention provided when movement errors become consistent (see later section Feedback). The learner is an active participant in the therapy process, reflecting on his or her performance while developing task analysis and problem-solving.

Structuring the Environment

The environment can be structured using Gentile's taxonomy.[145] Gentile's taxonomy has three organizing categories: (1) the environment conditions (open or closed environment) which also includes the environmental context (stationary or in motion: with or without intertrial variability), (2) the desired outcome of the action (body stability or body transport) and (3) manipulation (use or no use of the limbs).[145] It is a useful tool for structuring the environment relative to the task. For example, a patient practicing sitting on a plinth in a quiet room would be in a closed environment that is stationary and has no trial variability working on stability without manipulations. The addition of another support surface such as a chair or a bed would add some intertrial variability but keep the rest of the conditions the same. Giving the person an upper limb task in addition to the sitting would add a manipulation component.

A simplified version of the taxonomy has four categories that emphasize the environmental context and the movement goal:

1. Stationary individual in stationary environment
2. Moving individual in a stationary environment
3. Stationary individual in a moving environment
4. Moving individual in a moving environment.

This hierarchy represents a guideline for progression. In the first context, a patient may be practicing sitting on a mat table in a closed treatment space; in the second, the patient may practicing sitting on a therapeutic ball or the hospital bed; in the third, the patient may be sitting in a wheelchair in the PT gym; and in the fourth, the patient may be navigating the wheelchair in the PT gym. Each level increases is complexity. The first level is a stationary individual in a stationary environment with no manipulation, and in the fourth level there is a moving individual in a moving environment with manipulation.[145]

Other considerations in the environment are sounds, lighting, and interaction with other people. Persons with stroke and cognitive/perceptual deficits may initially benefit from training in a *closed environment* with limited distractions. Later, the environment can be varied, providing an appropriate level of *contextual interference*. Thus, the patient is progressed toward performing the same skill in a more *open environment*, with variable and real-life challenges. Ultimately, the closer the environmental demands of the practice setting, the greater the likelihood of transfer of skill.

Practice Schedule

Practice is essential for motor skill learning and recovery. The therapist needs to organize the patient's therapy session to ensure optimal practice. *Blocked practice* (constant repetition of a single task) is used to improve *initial* performance and motivation, especially for patients with disorganized movements. It also provides a mechanism for strengthening when you need repetition of a movement. Most hospitalized patients also initially require a *distributed practice schedule* with adequate rest periods owing to limited endurance, as both physical and cognitive fatigue can result in decreased performance. The patient should be encouraged to self-monitor practice sessions and recognize when fatigue may be setting in and rest is required. *Variable practice* (practice of more than one task within a session) using a serial or random order should begin as soon as possible. Variable practice improves performance and results in better retention of learned skills and improved ability to adapt to changing task demands. Patient, staff, and family efforts should be coordinated to ensure continued and consistent practice during off-therapy times. Practice schedules are reviewed in Chapter 10.

Feedback

Feedback can be intrinsic (naturally occurring as part of the movement response) or extrinsic (provided by the therapist). During early motor learning, the therapist provides extrinsic feedback (e.g., verbal cueing, manual cueing) and manual guidance to shape performance. It is important to monitor performance carefully and provide accurate feedback. The patient's attention should be directed to naturally occurring intrinsic feedback. Feedback can be provided verbally using *knowledge of performance* (KP) to address the kinematic features of the movement and *knowledge of results* (KR) to emphasize achievement of task goals. Augmented feedback can also be provided manually, using sensory input as well as manual contacts to maintain normal alignment or guide movement when the patient lacks active control or has reduced sensation. Manual techniques can be drawn from some of the neurofacilitation approaches with a clear understanding of the intent of the feedback. Great care must be taken to avoid dependence on the therapist (i.e., the patient is only able to move with the therapist's manual or verbal assistance) by providing decreasing amounts of physical guidance and augmented feedback systematically. This requires careful consideration during each treatment session. Therapists should allow the patient adequate time for introspection about the movements and available intrinsic feedback (see Table 10.5 in Chapter 10).

Dose and Progression

Therapy, for persons poststroke has to be dosed with high enough intensity, be it frequency, duration, or repetitions, to achieve neuroplastic and behavioral changes.[146] The frequency, intensity, time, type (FITT) principle can guide dose considerations (see Chapter 10). Although it is challenging to achieve similar doses to those reported in the literature, the therapist has to approximate them as best as possible. Therapy needs to be challenging enough but not too difficult to discourage active participation in therapy.[147]

Increased challenge can be achieved by using the Gentile taxonomy to progress the difficulty of the (1) environment, going from a closed to an open environment; (2) environmental context, introducing variability in the environment; (3) movement goal, from stability to mobility; and (4) manipulation, adding a manipulation component to the task. Progression can also be achieved by modifying the dose parameters of frequency, intensity, and duration. In reviewing the literature, it is important to note, where available, the dose and progression used in research studies.

Motivation and Self-Management

Motivation and self-efficacy (confidence) are key to successful learning. Self-management has been shown to aid in the transfer of skill from the therapeutic to the real-world setting for persons poststroke.[148] Motivational factors influence long-term engagement of the learner. This includes education about the task (purpose, effects of practice and exercise, expected outcomes) and identification of possible barriers. Providing feedback (both KP and KR, but also positive feedback) and encouragement is important to ensure motivation. Patients need to experience feelings of self-efficacy, self-control, and competence. The patient should be fully involved in collaborative goal setting from the beginning and be reminded of the goal, the task, what progress has been made, and the expected outcomes. Task salience, goal setting, and collaborative planning are key motivational techniques.[149] Treatment sessions should include positive experiences, ensuring the patient experiences success in therapy and instilling self-confidence. Beginning and ending the therapy session on a positive note (a successful activity) is a helpful strategy. Self-efficacy ratings and summary comments can be used to monitor progress (e.g., "What successes did you achieve in therapy today?"). Supportive strategies should be discussed with family and caregivers.

Interventions to Improve Participation

Participation is best trained at the task level in the environmental context where the goals are to be achieved. Often, this is not feasible, so the therapist uses the results of the task analysis to reproduce the activities in the therapeutic setting to be as close as possible to the environmental and contextual conditions required for participation.

Participation goals may be addressed with interventions that target both cognitive and motor operations. These interventions include mental practice through motor and motivational (focusing on feelings of accomplishment) imagery, virtual environments, and dual tasking to promote cognitive motor interference. They are discussed in more detail under specific categories.

Interventions to Improve Activities

Most of the interventions presented in this chapter are in this section on improving activities. This arrangement is consistent with a task-based training approach. The tasks are organized as postural control and balance, locomotion and gait, upper limb use, functional and aerobic capacity, and physical activity. Included in this section are also relevant body function structure interventions that support the tasks, such as increasing range of motion, selective capacity of the limbs, and muscle strength. The clinician will address the task and then move into body function structure interventions as needed.

Postural Control and Balance

Postural control and balance can be viewed at both the body function structure or the activity level. For persons poststroke, balance training in the context of the task produces better outcomes.[146] Therefore, in this intervention section, training balance in the context of the task is illustrated along with stimulating specific postural responses that aim directly at eliciting a specific balance strategy or target a specific body function structure limitation, such as decreased vision or proprioception.

Training at the task level begins by having the person poststroke either hold a position or move in and out of the position. Observation of the deficits will guide the intervention starting point. For example, for the person poststroke seen in an outpatient setting who is a librarian returning to work, the intervention may start with the person in standing placing books on a shelf. If that person had difficulty with the task, one intervention option is an environmental modification, lowering the height of the shelf as a way of reducing the force generation requirement for the UE and the balance demand on the LEs. The person may need additional KP cues to modify the kinematics of the movement or force generation through the LEs to modify the way the person shifts the weight. Another option would be promoting a stepping response to adjust for a loss of balance while placing the book. As a second example, for a person with a recent acute stroke, the intervention may start at the bedside observing the person's ability to hold a sitting position at the edge of the bed. The therapist focuses on identifying the patient's ability to hold the position and alignment. Often, the person poststroke may not be able to symmetrically hold or move into a position. Instruction for alignment would precede using some form of manual guidance. KP or KR is provided to guide the attainment of a safe position with the best biomechanics.

Stroke results in significant changes in postural control and balance. Patients typically exhibit delayed, varied, or absent balance responses with deficits in latency, amplitude, and timing of muscle activity. Falls and fracture can occur and lead to a loss of confidence in balance and locomotor skills.[150] It is therefore important to challenge the patient's balance while maintaining safety. The goals of training are to progressively increase the level of difficulty (e.g., range and speed of self-initiated movements) while encouraging consistency, symmetry, and maximum use of the more affected side. Supportive devices such as a posterior leg splint, gait belt, or body-weight-support harness can be used to assist in early standing to promote confidence and prevent falls.

Progression for balance training can be viewed broadly as first attaining postural alignment and static stability in upright postures followed by center-of-mass (COM) control training. In sitting and standing, the patient is instructed to explore his or her limits of stability (LOS) through low-frequency weight shifting. The patient learns how far in any one direction he or she can safely move and how to align the COM within the base of support (BOS) to maintain upright stability. KP about symmetrical weight-bearing as well as activities that promote use of more affected side are encouraged. Weight-bearing on the more affected hip (sitting) and lower limb (standing) is encouraged ,while unnecessary activity of the less affected limbs (grabbing for support) is discouraged. The therapist increases the difficulty of the balance activity by manipulating the following:

- *BOS:* Sitting, LEs uncrossed to crossed; standing, wide to narrow to tandem position; standing on one LE (beginning with less affected, progressing to more affected LE)
- *Support surface:* Sitting on a mat to sitting on a therapy ball; standing on the floor to standing on dense foam, standing on woodchips, standing on a moving surface[151]
- *Sensory inputs:* Eyes open (EO) to eyes closed (EC); feet on firm surface or foam[152]
- *UE position/support:* Light touchdown support; UEs extended out to the side to UEs folded across the chest
- *UE movements:* Single UE raises to bilateral UE raises (symmetrical, asymmetrical); reaching movements with emphasis to the more affected side; picking objects off table, stool, floor
- *LE movements:* Single LE support, stepping (forward-backward, side; step-ups); marching in place; foot on ball, moving ball
- *Trunk movements:* Head and trunk rotations; looking up at ceiling or down to floor
- *Destabilizing functional activities:* Sit-to-stand, sit-down, turning, floor-to-standing, lunges[146]
- *Walking activities:* Forward, backward, sideward, crossed step[146,153]
- *Dual-task training (combined motor-cognitive dual tasks):* Standing while catching or kicking a ball; standing while talking; standing while holding a tray with a glass of water;[154,155] combined motor-cognitive dual tasks[156]
- *Modifying environmental conditions:* Closed to open environments

Postural strategy training is an important component of intervention. Ankle strategies can be promoted through small-range anterior-posterior shifts or by applying a small perturbation at the hips (forward-backward). Standing on a half-foam roller or wobble board also promotes ankle strategies but may be too advanced for some patients during early rehabilitation. Hip strategies can be promoted through larger anterior-posterior shifts or stronger perturbations. Medial-lateral hip strategies are promoted by tandem stance (on floor or half foam roller). Stepping strategies are promoted by increased displacements of the COM (e.g., forward, backward, or sideward leans that move the COM outside of the BOS). The therapist can apply an elastic band around the hips, offering resistance to the forward lean. Resistance that is quickly released once the patient achieves the desired lean will necessitate a step to control balance. Step-ups (small step to large; foam surface) should also be practiced.

The therapist provides well-timed feedback to help the patient correct alignment and adjust postural control. During balance training, the patient should be encouraged to actively problem solve. The patient is presented with challenges, identifies potential problems, and recruits safe strategies to maintain balance. Adaptability of skills needed for successful community reentry is promoted. Safety education about fall prevention and fall recovery is a critical factor in ensuring maintenance of the patient's hard-won functional independence.[157]

Research supports the effectiveness of balance training programs in improving balance ability for patients with stroke. Review of balance training for persons in the chronic phase poststroke showed that balance can be improved after treatment measured by the Berg Balance Scale (BBS), Functional Reach (FR), and Sensory Organization Test (SOT). Those gains were retained for the BBS but not for the SOT, suggesting that the participants may have compensated rather than changed their underlying strategy or acquiring a new skill.[153] There was too much variability in the type of training to propose a dose. However, training performed in the context of the task is more efficient that balance training in isolation. Both one-on-one training and group programs have produced positive results. Finally, there is limited evidence that balance performance may deteriorate once the intervention is stopped.[158,159]

Training With Visual Feedback

The use of visual feedback has been shown to improve balance in persons poststroke. The patient's balance is detected either with a force platform represented as his or her center of pressure or with motion sensing equipment represented as an avatar in a virtual environment.

Force platform biofeedback (center-of-pressure biofeedback) promotes practice of voluntary movement shifts in response to computer-generated visual feedback. Patients can also practice responding to unexpected platform tilts (perturbations) in order to improve reactive balance control. A safety harness may be required during early training; holding on with one or both hands is discouraged. Improvements with biofeedback/forceplate training have been found in steadiness (reduced sway),[160,161] postural symmetry,[160,161] and dynamic stability.[161-163] Evidence is stronger and more consistent for the latter two parameters than for changes in steadiness.[164] There is very limited evidence of carryover of improved balance during functional skills, specifically transfer skills and endurance,[163] functional reach,[165] and measures of ADL and mobility.[161] Carryover to improved locomotor performance has not been demonstrated.[160,163] Failure to find significant correlations to gait is most likely related to specificity of training, specifically a dissimilarity between training mode and outcome measure. A Cochrane review (that included 254 participants) summarizing the study of platform force feedback for balance concluded that it was suitable to improve static balance but did not transfer balance as measured by the BBS or locomotion. It may therefore have limited benefit for persons poststroke.[166]

VR, such as commercial and customized virtual environments coupled with TMs, and video games played on a Nintendo Wii console, have been recently tested for rehabilitation of postural control and activity level balance.[167] There is a small but consistent benefit for VR and video games compared to an active control when measuring balance with the BBS and the Timed Up and Go (TUG) test. The improvement, however, did not reach the MCID.[168-171] In a review that compared the efficacy between off-the-shelf games and customized systems for persons in the chronic phase poststroke, it was found that customized systems are superior.[170] VR and video games may be an appropriate tool to engage a subset of persons poststroke for balance training.

The Patient With Ipsilateral Pushing (Pusher Syndrome)

The patient with ipsilateral pushing presents with an entirely different set of postural control and balance problems. The patient sits or stands asymmetrically, but with most of the weight shifted toward the weaker side. The patient uses the stronger UE or LE to push over to the weaker side, often resulting in instability and falls. Efforts by the therapist to passively correct the patient's tilted posture often result in the patient pushing more forcefully. Training needs to emphasize upright positions with *active* movement shifts toward the stronger side. Use of visual stimuli is effective, as patients retain the ability to correct posture with such stimuli but may not be able to do so spontaneously. Patients should be asked to look at their posture and see if they are upright. Environmental prompts can be used to assist orientation. These can include use of a mirror if visuospatial deficits are not present or vertical structures in the environment. For example, the therapist can sit on the patient's less involved side and instruct the patient to "lean over to me." Or the patient can be positioned with the stronger side next to a wall and instructed to "lean toward the wall."[89] Therapists can provide verbal and tactile cues for postural orientation. To improve sitting posture, training activities can include sitting on a therapy ball to promote symmetry and sitting. In early standing, the weaker LE is often flexed and has difficulty supporting the body on that side. Extension can be assisted by the use of an air splint or a posterior leg splint or by direct tapping over the quadriceps muscle. The modified plantigrade position is effective for early supported standing; however, the therapist should focus on unilateral support using the weaker UE. Again, an air splint can be used to assist extension of the weaker arm. If a cane is used, it can be shortened to encourage weight shift to the stronger side. An environmental boundary can be used to achieve symmetrical standing (e.g., standing in a doorway or corner standing). It is important to limit pushing with the sound extremities. For example, in sitting or standing, the therapist should block the stronger limb from drifting laterally into abduction and extension and pushing.[172,173] During wheelchair sitting, the patient should be assisted to maintain upright posture and midline orientation. Motor learning strategies are very effective in reducing the effects of this disorder and enhancing recovery. In particular, the therapist should demonstrate correct orientation to vertical, provide consistent feedback about body orientation, and practice correct orientation and weight shifts. The patient should be fully involved in problem-solving. For example, the therapist should ask questions such as "What direction are you tilted?" and "What direction do you have to move in order to achieve vertical?" Karnath et al[87] indicate that the prognosis for recovery is good with effective training.

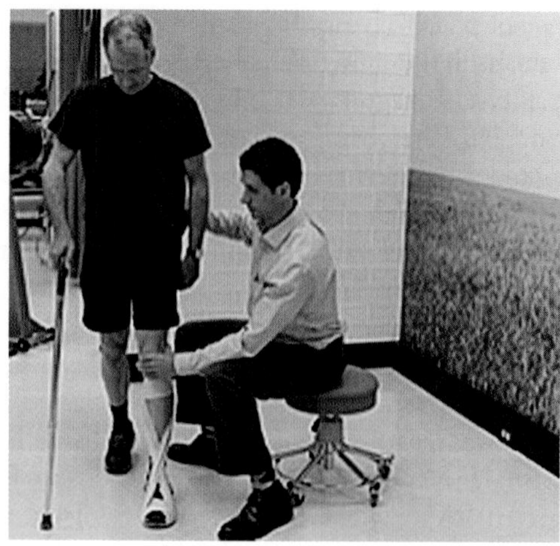

Figure 15.6 Gait practice where the clinician aids the patient with maintaining proper alignment during walking.

Interventions to Improve Gait and Locomotion

Improving gait for persons poststroke can be addressed in several ways: task-specific overground locomotor training (LT), LT using a motorized treadmill (TM), TM training aided by a harness (body-weight-supported treadmill training [BWSTT]), robotic-assisted LT, high intensity-stepping, functional electrical stimulation, and motor imagery and virtual reality. Additional strategies include rhythmic auditory cueing, community-based training, circuit training, LE strengthening, management of LE spasticity, improving LE range of motion, and standing balance practice. Varying levels of evidence support each approach. In this section, the approaches and supporting evidence (and wherever possible differentiating based on level of acuity) are provided.

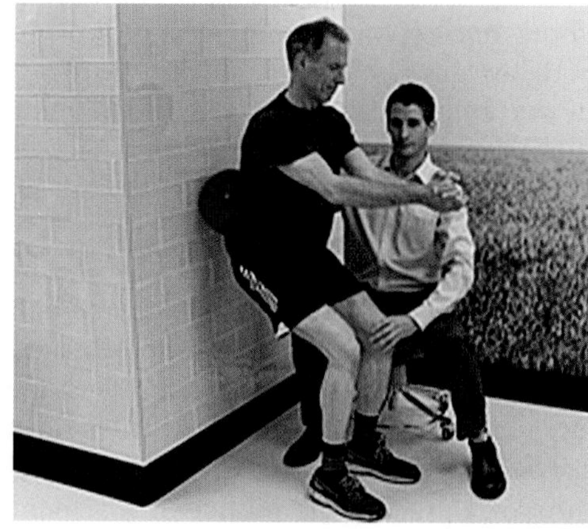

Figure 15.7 The clinician breaks from task-based training to address lower extremity strengthening in a weight-bearing position.

Task-Specific Overground Locomotor Training

Task-specific overground LT focuses on practicing walking to improve speed and endurance. Whole practice is emphasized, but when deficits (such as strength, selective capacity, balance and endurance) are encountered, then specific aspects of gait may be repeated (blocked, part task training) to improve performance. Figure 15.6 illustrates gait practice where the clinician aids the patient with maintaining proper alignment during walking, and Figure 15.7 illustrates how the clinician breaks from task-based training to address LE strengthening in a weight-bearing position.

The patient practices functional, task-specific skills, including the following:

- Walking in all directions.
- Walking on different surfaces.
- Stair climbing, step-over-step.
- Walking in a simulated home environment: Through doorways, over and around obstacles, stairs in/out of the home.
- Walking in a community environment: Walking on ramps, curbs, uneven terrain, over and around obstacles.
- Activities that involve coincident timing: Crossing at a streetlight, stepping on and off elevators or escalators, walking through automatic doors.
- Dual-task activities: Walking while holding a ball, bouncing a ball, carrying a tray, carrying on a conversation.

In a Cochrane review published in 2009, task-based training was shown to have a small positive effect for persons in the chronic phase poststroke for walking distance (26.6 m increase on the 6MWT) and walking speed (0.07 m/s).[174] More recently, in a systematic review of 19 RCTs that included 1,008 persons poststroke, task-based training decreased anxiety for persons poststroke who are walking independently.[146] Outcomes for walking distance, walking ability, and balance differed depending on level of recovery. Persons in the chronic phase poststroke were able to improve walking distance and walking ability but not balance. Persons in the late phase (subacute) were able to improve balance and walking ability not walking distance. Persons in the acute phase did not improve at all.[146] This finding highlights the relevance of phase of recovery when selecting an intervention. Persons in the earlier recovery phases may have lacked the capacity to engage in overground walking activities. In addition, given the open-loop nature of these tasks, it may be difficult to achieve a high intensity of training. The greatest challenge with this task-based approach is to provide a high enough training intensity protocol, particularly to persons in the early recovery poststroke.

Locomotor Training Using a Treadmill Without a Harness

LT on a TM without using a harness for support has been shown (in 16 RCTS with a total of 610 participants) to improve maximum gait speed and temporal spatial parameters of gait for persons in all phases of recovery.[146] The ability to increase walking speed on the TM resulted in the gait speed improvement as well as an increase in step width.

Locomotor Training Using Body Weight Support and Motorized Treadmill Training

Body weight support (BWS) and motorized treadmill training (TT) allows the clinician to use a closed-loop training environment to improve recovery of walking ability after stroke using intensive task-oriented training. Normal kinematics and phase relationships of the full gait cycle are promoted, including limb loading in midstance and unweighting and stepping during swing. Initially, manual assistance can be provided by trainers to normalize gait in the presence of muscle weakness and impaired balance. For example, one therapist provides manual assistance to foot placement during stepping movements of the weaker LE while a second therapist stands behind the patient and provides manual assistance to pelvic rotation movements (Fig. 15.8). An overhead harness is used to support a portion of the patient's weight (e.g., 30% progressing down to 20%, then 10%). The harness controls the upright position of the patient in the absence of good postural stability and reduces fear of falling. The use of a harness also eliminates the need for adaptive UE support to compensate for LE weakness (e.g., as seen with the use of a walker). As improvements in walking occur, the harness is removed and full weight-bearing is allowed. At this point, the patient is practicing supervised walking on a TM. Initially the TM speeds are slow (e.g., 0.52 mph [0.23 m/sec]) and are gradually increased as the patient's walking ability is improved (e.g., 0.95 mph [0.42 m/sec]). Progression is to task-specific practice and overground walking. See Chapter 11, Locomotor Training, for additional discussion.

TT and BWS is a relatively safe task-oriented LT activity that has been extensively studied in patients recovering from stroke.[175-190] In a Cochrane Systematic Review,[61] the researchers identified 44 trials with 2,648 poststroke participants. They concluded TT with BWS was not superior to other forms of PT in gaining independence. It did, however, have a positive effect on walking velocity (0.07 m/s) and walking distance (26.35 m/s). These gains

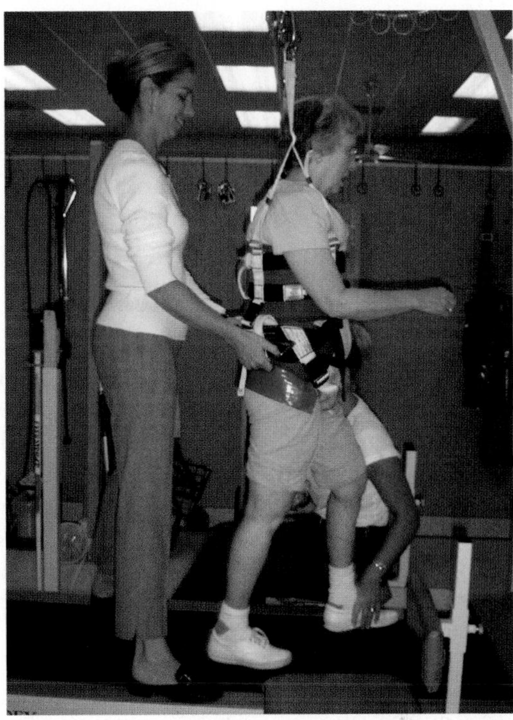

Figure 15.8 Locomotor training using body-weight support and a motorized treadmill. One therapist manually assists pelvic motions while a second therapist assists stepping of the hemiparetic left LE.

were mostly not retained at follow-up except for people who were already ambulating, who retained their walking distance.[61] Serious adverse events were uncommon. TT appears to be a safe intervention for patients with acute and subacute stroke[175,176,183-185,188] as well as for chronic stroke.[177-179,186]

The *Locomotor Experience Applied Poststroke (LEAPS)* was the largest multicenter RCT conducted on BWSTT.[190] Four hundred eight participants were recruited from six inpatient rehabilitation centers and stratified according to walking impairment. Those with moderate impairment were able to walk 0.4 to less than 0.8 m per second, and those in the severe group were able to walk less than 0.4 m per second. Participants were randomly assigned to one of three treatment groups: (1) early LT using BWSTT 2 months after stroke, (2) late LT using BWSTT 6 months after stroke, and (3) home exercise using therapist-directed exercise training 2 months after stroke. The latter group received exercises designed to improve flexibility, strength, coordination, and balance along with encouragement for daily walking. Each intervention had similar intensity and duration (36 sessions of 90 minutes each for 12 to 16 weeks). The researchers found that all participants increased their functional walking ability. No significant differences were found between the groups in terms of improvements in walking speed, motor recovery, balance, functional status, and quality of life. Outcomes of participants in the early and late LT groups also revealed no significant differences at 1 year. The researchers concluded that early intervention may accelerate gains in walking ability after stroke. The research reviewed supports the benefits of physical therapy in improving walking outcomes. There is no clear evidence of the superiority of one type of intervention over another. What appears to be critical is training intensity.

Robotic-Assisted Locomotor Training

Electromechanical, robotic-assisted LT is used in rehabilitation to improve walking after stroke. In a Cochrane Systematic Database review, Mehrholz et al[66] reviewed 23 trials involving 999 participants. When combined with conventional physiotherapy, these devices were found to increase the odds of patients becoming independent walkers. Increases in gait speed or walking capacity were not found. Study differences were noted in variations of (1) initial level of patient independence in walking, (2) duration and frequency of treatment, and (3) use of electrical stimulation used in some devices. This made it difficult to interpret their results. A systematic review of studies recruiting nonambulatory patients early after stroke (six studies involving 549 participants) found that mechanically assisted LT with BWS resulted in more people walking independently at 4 weeks and at 6 months.[191]

Electromechanical-assisted gait training may be coupled with using functional electrical stimulation (FES) to activate selected muscles. A review assessed both modes. The researchers found that electromechanical-assisted gait training without FES resulted in improved gait speed, walking distance, peak heart rate, and basic ADL. Only persons in the early phase of rehabilitation who were dependent for walking improved their comfortable gait speed, walking ability, and balance.[192,193] Findings were similar when electromagnetic-assisted TT was coupled with FES. Balance and walking improved only for the persons in the early phase poststroke who were dependent.[193]

Assistance for advancing the LEs can also be provided manually. It is interesting to note that there were no differences in functional ambulatory capacity in a systematic review (16 studies that included a total of 558 patients) comparing conventional LT or TT with BWS and manual assistance versus TT with BWS and robotic assistance.[193] In contrast, Lewek et al[194] found that therapist-assisted LT when compared to robotic-assisted LT resulted in significant improvements in coordination of intralimb kinematics, lending support to the value of variable practice versus constant practice. As with other interventions, phase of recovery and severity affect the decision to use the intervention. Electromechanical-assisted gait training appears to be most beneficial for persons early in their recovery who are dependent in walking.

High-Intensity Stepping

High-intensity stepping is an intervention that combines task-based training; oveground, speed-dependent TT; and a high-intensity (based on frequency of steps, cardiovascular parameters, and perceived effort). It addresses walking recovery as a multidimensional problem. In a pilot study, researchers determined the feasibility of the stepping intervention,[194] and then in cross-over study with persons more than 6 months poststroke, the researchers confirmed that intensity was relevant.[195] A third study, an RCT, was conducted with persons between 1 and 6 months poststroke. A high-intensity group was compared to a usual-care group where each received 40 sessions over 10 weeks. The first week consisted of walking on a BWS treadmill with assist for the swing phase of gait. Nylon straps were used to stabilize the pelvis as necessary to ensure successful stepping. Successful stepping was defined as positive step lengths, lack of stance-phase limb collapse, and sagittal/frontal plane stability. After the second week, variability was the focus, alternating approximately every 10 minutes between speed-dependent TT (at 70% to 80% HR reserve and RPE ≥14), skill-dependent (e.g., perturbations, obstacles, weights) TT, overground training (high speeds or variable tasks), and stair climbing. Walking speed and distance as well as steps in community were greater for the high intensity group.[196] This type of therapy is promising. However, it is a challenge to implement that dose and intensity in the clinic.

Functional Electrical Stimulation

FES can be used to stimulate dorsiflexor function and improve the gait pattern of patients with drop foot. Sufficient strength in the quadriceps muscle is needed to prevent the knee from buckling. This requirement limits the number of patients who can successfully use the device. The patient wears a small, lightweight cuff that fits just below the knee. Electrodes are positioned to stimulate the anterior tibialis and the peroneus longus muscles. A gait sensor attaches to the patient's shoe and transmits a wireless signal to the stimulator. The level of stimulation can be adjusted by a handheld remote control, which also allows the patient to turn the device off and on. The device can be used as a bridge to the recovery of normal motor function or, in the absence of recovery, can be used indefinitely. FES training should be paired with a comprehensive physical therapy POC. In a systematic review of the literature (30 studies), Roche et al[197] reported that FES had a significant positive effect on gait with improvements noted in gait speed and physiological cost index (PCI) in patients with chronic stroke. FES is theorized to have a positive effect on brain plasticity with its provision of high-level sensory-motor input into the CNS.[198] This may explain research findings of improved gait function with FES when compared to orthotic intervention.[199]

Motor Imagery and Virtual Reality

Motor imagery (MI) and *VR* using video games allow simulation of real-world environments for walking training. Imagining walking has been studied at the strategy level and the task level.[200-202] At the strategy level, individuals poststroke imagined walking and changing the kinematics and kinetics of their movement, for example, loading the affected lower extremity and taking a larger step with the less affected extremity. This type of training improved gait speed.[200] In a second study, the training was done at the task level. Persons poststroke had to imagine themselves walking in different environments with an emphasis on the task. This intervention resulted in an increased gait speed but no significant increase on falls self-efficacy when compared to the active control group that engaged in an upper limb intervention.[201]

In a final study from the same group, the therapy was delivered in the home combining physical practice plus motor imagery. The therapy was customized to the participant and included walking in and outside the home. The clinician first observed the task performed and then adjusted the cues for the intervention. There were cues for movement as well as increasing self-efficacy. For example, the participant was observed walking in his or her home environment that required stair climbing to get from the basement to the kitchen. On the stairs, the participant tripped and was helped by the caregiver to maintain balance. During the imagery practice, the participant imagined tripping and then successfully catching himself or herself without assistance. Then the participant imagined feeling good about having overcome the "tripping." This type of motivational imagery aids with increasing confidence. The therapy that was delivered using a combination of in-person and telerehabilitation sessions was found to be feasible.[202] The appeal of motor imagery is that is portable and low cost. To use this intervention, it is important to determine that the person poststroke is able to imagine. This can be assessed by administering the Kinesthetic and Visual Imagery Questionnaire (KVIQ), which has been validated for persons poststroke.[203,204]

As with balance training, gait training with VR has been implemented with a TM coupled to a virtual environment, off-the-shelf video games, and specialized systems.[167] There has been a small but consistent effect favoring VR for improving gait speed.[169-171,205] This finding applies to persons in the subacute and chronic phases poststroke. The challenge with this technology currently is that some of the systems are not available in the clinic. However, this is an area of rapid development, and transfer of the technology to the clinic is accelerating.

Orthotics and Assistive Devices for the Lower Extremity

Orthotics and assistive devices are compensations for lack of active control and balance. An orthosis may be required when persistent problems prevent safe ambulation (e.g., inadequate ankle dorsiflexion during swing, mediolateral ankle instability, and insufficient push-off during late stance). Orthotic prescription will depend on the unique problems each patient presents. The pattern of instability and weakness at the ankle and knee and the extent and severity of spasticity and sensory deficits of the limb are major considerations when prescribing an orthosis. Temporary devices (e.g., dorsiflexor assists) may be used during the early stages while recovery is proceeding to allow the patient to practice standing and walking. Use of a temporary orthosis also provides insight into the type of components that will most effectively address the patient's needs. Permanent devices are prescribed once the patient's status stabilizes. Consultation with a certified orthotist and clinic team is initiated if a permanent orthosis is needed.

- *Foot–ankle controls:* An *ankle–foot orthosis* (AFO) is commonly prescribed to control impaired ankle–foot function. Examples include a custom-molded polypropylene AFO *(posterior leaf spring [PLS], modified AFO, or solid ankle AFO)* or *conventional double upright/dual channel AFO.* The least restrictive AFO is the PLS used to control drop foot. An AFO of higher-density plastic that covers more surface area can provide additional control of calcaneal and forefoot inversion and eversion. A solid ankle molded AFO provides maximum stabilization through its lateral trim lines that project more anteriorly. Movement in all planes (dorsiflexion, plantarflexion, inversion, and eversion) is limited. The conventional double upright metal AFO may be indicated for patients who cannot tolerate plastic AFOs owing to sensory impairments, girth fluctuations, or diabetic neuropathy or who require additional controls. A posterior stop can be added to limit plantarflexion, while a spring assist can be added to assist dorsiflexion (Klenzak joint). Advantages of a conventional AFO include better stabilization of the ankle, allowing improved heel-strike and push-off. Disadvantages include heavier weight, less cosmetic appearance, and increased difficulty donning and doffing.
- *Knee controls:* Knee instability following stroke can be controlled with an AFO by adjusting the position of the ankle. An ankle set in 5° dorsiflexion limits knee hyperextension, whereas an ankle set in 5° plantarflexion decreases the flexor moment and stabilizes the knee during midstance. A patient with knee hyperextension without foot and/or ankle instability may benefit from the application of a *Swedish Knee Cage* or strapping to protect the knee. Extensive bracing using a knee-ankle-foot orthosis (KAFO) is rarely indicated or successful. The added weight and restrictions in normal knee joint motion significantly increase energy costs and limit independent function.

The need for an orthosis or a particular type of orthosis may change with continuing recovery. The therapist may need to recommend a change in prescription or discontinuing the use of a device. With limited reimbursements, ordering a new orthosis may prove problematic and speaks to the need to anticipate changes when ordering the initial device. For example, a good option for the patient who needs a custom-molded solid AFO is to order a hinged AFO with a plantarflexion stop. As the patient regains sufficient knee and dorsiflexor control, the device can be adjusted to remove the stop and allow the hinges to work. Orthotic training includes donning and doffing, skin inspections, and education in safe use of the device during gait. See Chapter 30, Orthotics, for a more complete description of orthotic devices, examination, and training.

Wheelchairs

Many persons poststroke require the use of a wheelchair for mobility at some point during their recovery. Persons with stroke exhibit postural asymmetries, which need to be carefully evaluated. These include the following:

- Trunk laterally flexed to the weaker side; head may also be flexed to the weaker side.
- Pelvic posterior tilt with some obliquity (lower on the unaffected side).
- LE rolled out into abduction and external rotation; if spasticity is present, increased hip extension, adduction, and internal rotation with knee extension may occur; foot is typically plantarflexed and inverted.
- UE held flexed and adducted to the trunk with increased elbow, wrist, and finger flexion. With flaccidity, the shoulder is subluxed with the hand dangling in a dependent position.

Positioning in a wheelchair needs to correct for these postural asymmetries and ensure correct sitting posture. Refer to Chapter 32, The Prescriptive Wheelchair, for a more complete discussion of general principles of prescription and wheelchair adaptations.

A patient with stroke can learn to propel a wheelchair using the stronger UE and LE. The seat-to-floor height is critical in ensuring successful use of the foot for steering and propulsion. A *hemi-height wheelchair* with a lower seat-to-floor height (17.5 in [44.45 cm]) may be required. A standard wheelchair has a seat-to-floor height of 19.5 in (49.53 cm). One-arm drive chairs in which both handrims are placed on one wheel were designed for individuals with only one functional UE. The patient with stroke is rarely successful in using this type of chair because it takes a great deal of strength and coordination to propel the wheelchair in a forward direction. It is contraindicated in patients with significant perceptual and cognitive impairments. A power wheelchair may be required for some individuals who cannot successfully use a manual wheelchair and will depend on a wheelchair as their primary means of locomotion. The therapist needs to consider individual needs and reimbursement policies when ordering a wheelchair. It is important to balance both present and future needs, as providers restrict frequent reordering of a new wheelchair. It is also important to remember that prolonged used of a wheelchair contributes to learned nonuse and may limit recovery, especially if walking is a primary goal of therapy. Wheelchair training activities include patient and caregiver instruction in the use, maintenance, and safety of all parts of the wheelchair (e.g., brakes, leg rests, removable armrests). The patient needs to be instructed in methods of propulsion and given the opportunity to practice on level and varied surfaces (e.g., ramps, outdoor terrain). Transfers (to and from bed, toilet, tub, car) should also be practiced once the patient receives the prescriptive wheelchair.

Interventions to Improve Upper Limb Use

Restitution of skilled upper limb use includes management of musculoskeletal impairments, sensory retraining, strengthening, and improvement of selective capacity. This intervention is typically done in close collaboration with the occupational therapist. Patients with MCA syndrome may exhibit severe sensory, motor, and functional impairments of the UE with limited recovery. These patients benefit from early mobilization, ROM, and positioning strategies. Compensatory training strategies and environmental adaptations should be considered to maximize function. For patients who achieve some recovery of voluntary movement, training strategies should focus on repetitive, task-specific practice. The tasks selected should be relevant and important to the patient (e.g., reaching and manipulation, walking with devices, stair climbing). UE training activities should be closely coordinated with the occupational therapist.

Algorithm for Selecting Upper Limb Interventions

An international group has developed an algorithm to guide upper limb rehabilitation[206] (see Box 15.6). The algorithm is based on the shoulder abduction finger extension (SAFE) model.[207,208] This model has shown that in those persons poststroke demonstrating some voluntary finger extension and some visible shoulder abduction on day 2 after stroke had a 98% probability of achieving upper limb function. A number of patients do not develop the finger extension in the first 2 days but do so in the first 12 weeks poststroke. For this reason, the 12-week period poststroke is used as the first question in the algorithm (dividing interventions based on this time frame). The ViaTherapy app can be downloaded for free in the app store or found online at www.viatherapy.org. It guides management of the upper limb with task-specific training as well as management of body function structure deficits.

Several questions guide the user on how to select interventions:

1. Is the person with the first 12 weeks of stroke onset? (If the answer is YES, the interventions are found in boxes 1 to 4; if the answer is NOT YET, the interventions are found in boxes 5 to 8.)

Box 15.6 Algorithm for Selecting Upper Limb Interventions[206]

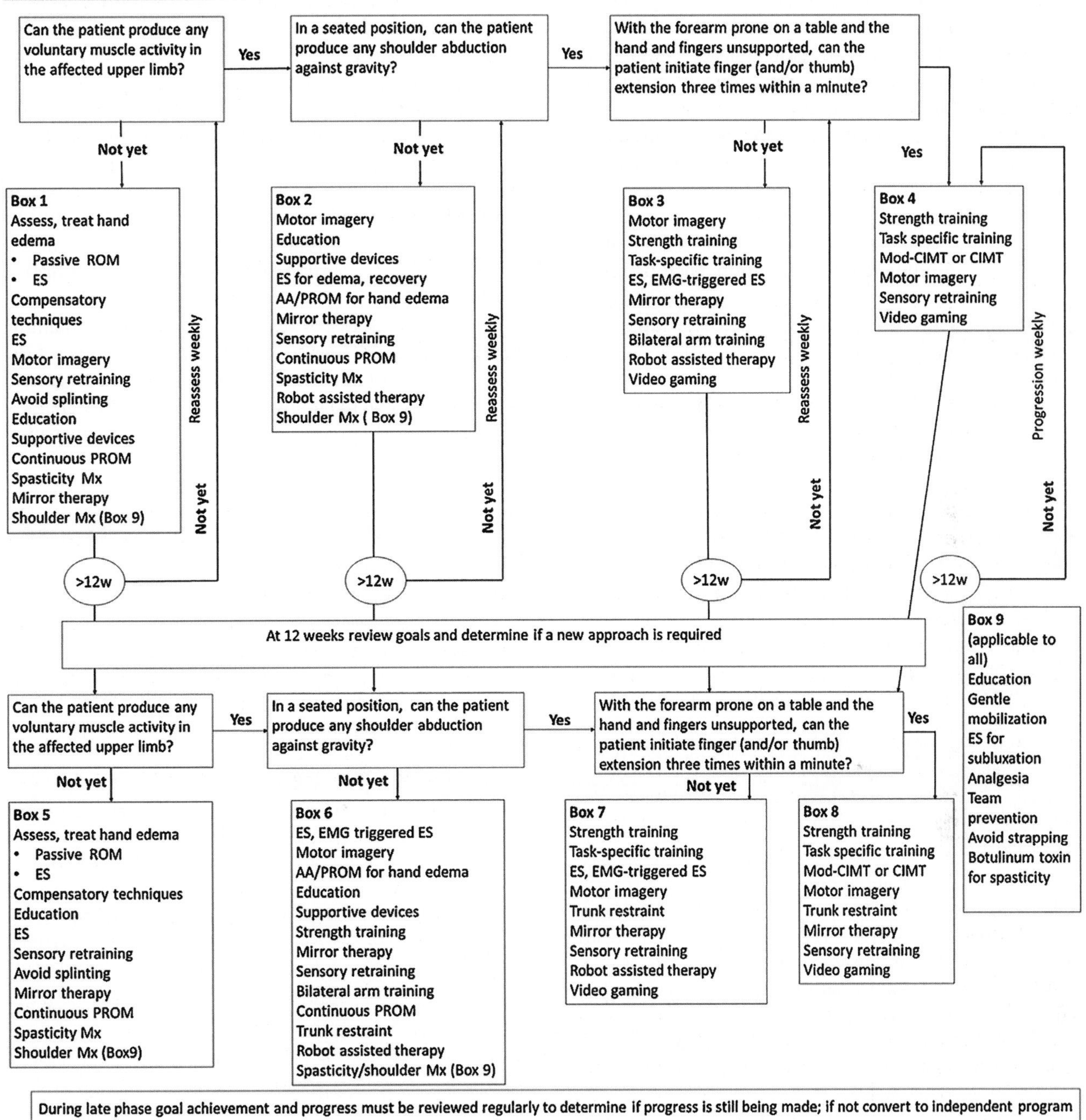

From Wolf, SL, et al: Group upper extremity stroke algorithm working. Best practice for arm recovery post stroke: An international application. Physiotherapy 102(1):1, 2016, with permission.

2. The following three questions refine the search:
   a. Is there voluntary muscle activity?
   b. Is there shoulder abduction?
   c. Is there finger extension?

Responses to these questions will take the user to the appropriate box containing a list of interventions that have been rated with an A if there is at least one RCT. There is also a star rating (with four being the highest rating) based on expert opinion that takes into account time, equipment required, and ease of use. Treatment dose is offered and is based on the references reviewed. The references supporting the recommendations are available in the app. Outcome measures are also suggested. To guide the clinician in deciding if the intervention is suitable for the patient, the app reports both on who has not been studied and on the exclusion criteria for specific interventions. Finally, because shoulder pain can occur with persons poststroke at many phases of recovery, management is presented in a separate box (Box 9), which can apply to any patient.

In the absence of voluntary movement, most of the interventions are the same for the first 12 weeks after the stroke (Box 1) and beyond 12 weeks (Box 5). These interventions involve maintaining ROM, preventing or managing edema, sensory retraining, managing spasticity, positioning, patient education, eliciting movement by using imagery, mirror therapy and electrical stimulation, patient education, providing supportive devices, and teaching compensatory techniques. As the person poststroke acquires movement, some of the interventions are discontinued and others are added. For example, task-specific training is proposed when there is some active shoulder movement starting in boxes 3 and 7, and constraint-induced movement therapy applies only once people have some active finger movement applying only to boxes 4 and 8. Any patient who presents with shoulder pain can be managed with the recommended interventions in Box 9.

Interventions to Improve Range of Motion

Soft tissue/joint mobilization and ROM exercises are initiated early to maintain joint integrity and mobility and prevent contractures. Passive ROM (PROM), and AROM when possible, with terminal stretch should be performed daily in all motions. If a contracture is developing, more frequent ROM (twice daily or more) is necessary.

Positioning strategies are also important in maintaining soft tissue length (Box 15.7). Effective positioning of the hemiparetic extremities encourages proper joint alignment while positioning the limbs out of the good biomechanical alignment. ROM and positioning should be viewed as

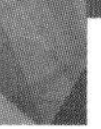

Box 15.7 Positioning Strategies to Reduce Common Malalignments

Supine Position

- Head/neck: Neutral and symmetrical; supported on pillow.
- Trunk: Aligned in midline.
- More affected UE: Scapular protracted, shoulder forward and slightly abducted; arm supported on a pillow; elbow extended with hand resting on a pillow; wrist neutral, fingers extended, and thumb abducted.
- More affected LE: Hip forward (pelvis protracted); knee on a small pillow or towel roll to prevent hyperextension; nothing against the soles of feet. For persistent plantarflexion, a splint can be used to position the foot and ankle in neutral position.

Side-Lying on Less Affected Side

- Head/neck: Neutral and symmetrical.
- Trunk: Aligned in midline; small pillow or towel can be placed under the rib cage to elongate the hemiplegic side.
- More affected UE: Scapular protracted, shoulder forward; arm on a supporting pillow with elbow extended, wrist neutral, fingers extended, and thumb abducted.
- More affected LE: Hip forward and flexed, knee flexed and supported on a pillow.

Side-Lying on More Affected Side

- Head/neck: Neutral and symmetrical.
- Trunk: Aligned in midline.
- More affected UE: Scapular protracted; shoulder forward; arm placed in slight abduction and external rotation; elbow extended, forearm supinated, wrist neutral, fingers extended, and thumb abducted.
- More affected LE: Hip extended and knee flexed and supported by pillows. An alternative position is slight hip and knee flexion with pelvic protraction.

Sitting in an Armchair or Wheelchair

- Head/neck: Neutral and symmetrical; head directly above pelvis.
- Trunk: Spine extension.
- Pelvis: Aligned in neutral with weight-bearing on both buttocks.
- More affected UE: Shoulder protracted and forward; elbow supported on an arm trough or lapboard; forearm, wrist neutral, fingers extended, and thumb abducted (resting splint as needed).
- Both LEs: Hips flexed to 90°, positioned in neutral with respect to rotation.

a whole-body intervention because the malalignment of the LEs and the trunk could then influence the position of the upper limbs. Coordination with team members, staff, family, and caregivers is essential for long-term management.[209]

In the UE, correct PROM techniques require careful attention to external rotation and distraction of the humerus, especially as ranges approach 90° of flexion or more. The scapula should be mobilized on the thoracic wall with an emphasis on upward rotation and protraction to prevent soft tissue impingement in the subacromial space during overhead movements of the arm (Figure 15.9) and to prepare for forward reach patterns. The use of overhead pulleys for self-ROM is *contraindicated* because of failure to achieve the above requirements for scapulohumeral movement. Full extension of the elbow is important because the majority of patients with stroke develop tightness in elbow flexors as a result of excess flexor spasticity. Normal length of wrist and finger extensors should also be maintained, as tightness is typical in flexion. This can be achieved functionally through sitting, weight-bearing on the extended paretic UE with the wrist extended and fingers open and extended (Figure 15.10). Edema and tonal changes may produce impingement with wrist extension. In this situation, grade 1 and grade 2 mobilization to the carpal bones before stretching at the wrist is indicated. The edema can also be managed with gentle retrograde massage.[209]

Strategies to teach patients safe self-ROM activities should be instituted early. Suggested activities include the following:

- In *arm cradling,* the stronger UE cradles and lifts the more affected UE to 90° humeral flexion; the arm is moved into positions of horizontal abduction and adduction. Active trunk rotation is combined with the arm movements.
- In *tabletop polishing,* the more affected UE is positioned in humeral flexion with scapular protraction and elbow extension; both hands are positioned on a towel. The less affected hand moves the paretic hand by pulling on the towel (forward and side-to-side). Trunk movements and ROM are optimized by placing the chair slightly back from the table.
- Sitting, the patient leans forward and reaches both hands down to the floor. This position encourages forward flexion of the humerus with scapular protraction, and extension of the elbow, wrist, and fingers.
- Supine, hands are clasped together and placed behind the head, the elbows fall flat to the mat. This activity should be considered only if scapula upward mobility is present. Hands clasped, self-overhead movements are contraindicated if scapulohumeral rhythm is lacking.

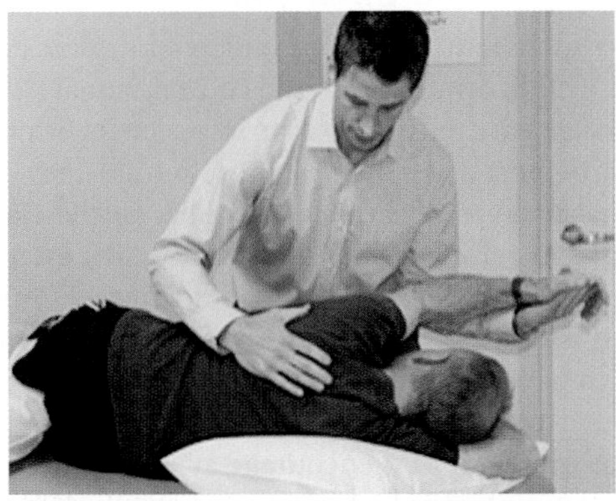

Figure 15.9 Range-of-motion exercises for the hemiparetic UE. The therapist carefully mobilizes the scapula during arm elevation.

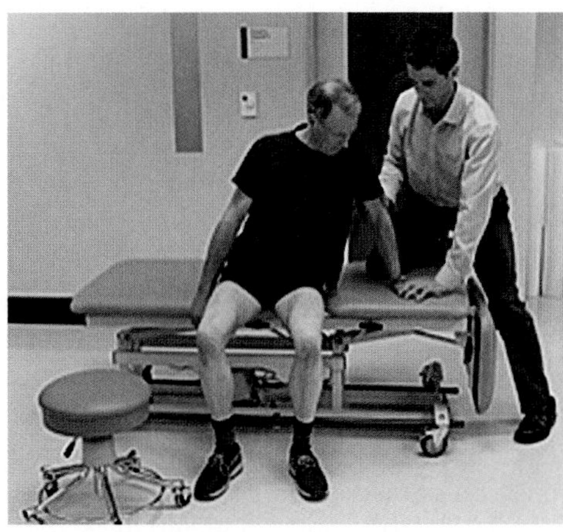

Figure 15.10 Sitting, with extended arm support. The therapist assists in stabilizing the elbow and fingers in extension.

When sitting in a wheelchair, the patient's paretic UE can be positioned on an arm trough (shallow elbow/forearm support) attached to the armrest. The shoulder is positioned in 5° of abduction and flexion and neutral rotation; elbow in 90° flexion and slightly forward; forearm pronated; and hand in a functional resting position. Routine use of splinting is not recommended in the literature; however, it may still be evaluated on a case-by-case basis.[209]

Interventions to Manage Spasticity

Patients who demonstrate spasticity (resistance to rapid stretch) can benefit from interventions designed to manage the secondary effects of spasticity (immobility, soft-tissue contracture, and deformity). These include early mobilization and daily stretching to maintain the length of spastic muscles and soft tissues and promote optimal positioning.[210] It is important to note that the methodological quality of research studies in this area is diverse and not well controlled, and available evidence about the effectiveness of stretching is inconclusive.[211,212] Once full range is achieved, the limb is positioned in the lengthened position. For example, the shoulder is extended, abducted, and externally rotated with the elbow, wrist, and fingers extended. The hand is positioned in weight-bearing to the patient's side (see Fig. 15.10) and maintained for several minutes. The benefits of *sustained stretching* include relaxation through mechanisms of autogenic inhibition. In sitting, slow rocking movements can be added to increase relaxation effects from influences of slow vestibular stimulation. Side sitting on the hemiparetic side provides sustained stretch to the spastic side flexors. The patient, family members, and caregivers should be taught safe ROM and stretching techniques.

Modalities can be used to treat spasticity. These include the application of cold, massage, and electrical stimulation. Cold slows nerve conduction and decreases muscle spindle activity. These factors can lead to a temporary reduction of tone. Cold can be applied with ice packs or ice massage (duration 10 to 20 minutes) or using vapocoolants. The effects of cold are short-lived, generally lasting for about 20 to 30 minutes. FES can be used to target the weak antagonist muscles (e.g., peroneal nerve stimulators) and works to decrease tone through the effects of reciprocal inhibition. FES has been used with some success to decrease tone during the treatment time.[212] There is no evidence to support the use of airsplints around the paretic arm to reduce tone. Use of botulinum toxin injections are supported by the Canadian Stroke Guidelines for spasticity management of both upper and lower limb for persons poststroke.[209]

Interventions to Improve Sensory Function

Patients who have significant sensory impairments may demonstrate impaired or absent spontaneous movement. The more the patient can be encouraged to use the affected side, the greater the chance of increased awareness and function. Conversely, the patient who refuses to use the hemiplegic side contributes to the problems imposed by lack of sensorimotor experience. Without attention during treatment, this *learned nonuse* phenomenon can contribute to further deterioration.[213]

Multiple interventions for UE sensory impairment after stroke have been described. These can be categorized into sensory retraining and sensory stimulation approaches. *Sensory retraining programs* include use of mirror therapy (described below), repetitive sensory discrimination activities, bilateral simultaneous movements, and repetitive task practice. *Sensorimotor integrative treatment* focuses on normalizing tone, practice of functional activity, and use of augmented sensory cues. *Sensory stimulation intervention* includes compression techniques (weight-bearing, manual compression, inflatable pressure splints, intermittent pneumatic compression), mobilizations, electrical stimulation, thermal stimulation, or magnetic stimulation. In a review of 13 studies, Cochrane reviewers[60] found significant clinical and methodological diversity, limited RCTs, generally small sample sizes with inadequate data, variability in outcome measures, and limited used of functional performance and participation outcome measures. They concluded there was insufficient evidence to support or refute the effectiveness of many of these interventions in improving sensory function. Limited evidence was found in support of the following:

- Mirror therapy for improving detection of light touch, pressure, and temperature pain.
- Thermal stimulation intervention for improving rate of recovery of sensation.
- Intermittent pneumatic compression for improving tactile and kinesthetic sensation.

The results of a systematic review of sensory retraining by Schabrun and Hillier[214] were similar with additional support found for electrical stimulation interventions. More recently, two RCTs provided evidence of sensory retraining by matching the sensation between the hands and vision. They reported improved sensory discrimination, motor control, actual use, perceived performance, and satisfaction with upper limb tasks.[215,216] This intervention required 45 minutes a day for at least 10 sessions.

Sensory retraining may be incorporated into functional training. The therapist may maximize weight-bearing and compression of the sensory-deficient limbs. Approximation can be applied with the sensory-deficient UE by weight-bearing in sitting or standing/modified plantigrade position and to the pelvis during standing activities. While sitting on a ball, the patient can practice bouncing. The compression and approximation that occur through the spine enhance activity in the postural extensors. During the application of sensory stimulation to the more involved limbs, the therapist directs the patient's attention and assists in shaping the patient's responses.[217,218]

A safety education program should be instituted early for patients, family, and caregivers to improve awareness of sensory impairments and ensure protection of anesthetic limbs. This is particularly important for preventing UE trauma during transfer and wheelchair activities.

Hemianopsia and Unilateral Neglect

Patients with hemianopsia or unilateral neglect demonstrate a lack of awareness of the contralesional side. The impairments are more pervasive in patients with neglect and in its most severe form (anosognosia) may extend to a total unawareness of the disability or the extent of the problems. The interventions that follow are recommended in the Canadian Stroke Guidelines,[209] but were not consistently supported in the Cochrane review.[219] This is in part because many of these interventions have not been extensively studied. These patients benefit from training strategies that encourage awareness and use of the environment on the hemiparetic side and use of the hemiparetic extremities. It is important to teach active visual scanning movements through turning of the head and axial trunk rotation to the more involved side.

Cueing (e.g., visual, verbal, or motor cues) is used to direct the patient's attention. For example, a red anchor line can be taped on the floor and the patient directed to visually follow the line from one side to the other. Or a red ribbon can be attached to the patient's hemiparetic wrist and the patient directed to keep the red ribbon in sight. Scanning movements can also be stimulated using visual tracking tasks using a computer. Imagery has also been shown to help (e.g., "Imagine you are a lighthouse beam; use your beam to sweep and scan the floor from one side to the other"). During therapy, the therapist stimulates and encourages active voluntary movements of the neglected limbs while encouraging the patient to look at his or her limbs while moving. UE exercises that involve crossing the midline toward the hemiparetic side are important (e.g., PNF chop or lift patterns). Functional activities that encourage bilateral interaction are also valuable (e.g., pouring a drink and drinking from a cup; picking up an object with the more involved hand and placing it in the other; "dusting a tabletop" with a cloth held by both hands). The therapist needs to maximize the patient's attention by optimizing visual, tactile, and proprioceptive stimuli on the more affected side. These can include stroking, brushing, tapping, or vibrating the hemiparetic limbs. The therapist also needs to consistently reorient the patient as inattention develops. Patients with very low levels of arousal are likely to be less responsive to therapy efforts.[220-222]

Supportive Devices for the Upper Extremity

The use of supportive devices is controversial. Recent There is no evidence that support slings prevent glenohumeral subluxation or glenohumeral pain.[146] However, the practice guidelines acknowledge the need to protect the shoulder joint, especially when the upper limb is flaccid, during movement transitions and when the arm is in a dependent position.[209] This is because a patient with hypotonia is at increased risk of shoulder *traction injury*. Slings may be used to prevent soft-tissue stretching (e.g., supraspinatus, capsular stretching) and relieve pressure on the neurovascular bundle (e.g., brachial plexus/brachial artery). They support the weight of the arm and protect the patient. They also free up the therapist to attend to postural/trunk control during functional activities. However, slings have a number of negative features. They do little to reduce subluxation or improve shoulder function, especially if scapular and trunk malalignment are not adequately addressed. Most slings have the additional negative feature of positioning the arm close to the body in adduction, internal rotation, and elbow flexion. With prolonged use, contractures and increased flexor tone may develop. Slings also contribute to body scheme disorders and body neglect. Prolonged use of slings blocks spontaneous use of the UE and contributes to learned nonuse. Slings may also block balance reactions involving the UE. They are recommended for use when patients do not acquire active movement.

Close collaboration with the occupational therapist is important in the appropriate selection and use of slings. Gillen[223] suggests the following guidelines:

- Therapists should minimize sling use during rehabilitation.
- Slings may be useful for initial transfer and gait training.
- Slings that position the UE in flexion are less desirable and should be used only for select upright activities and only for short time periods.
- No one sling is appropriate for all patients; selection and use should be carefully evaluated and sling effectiveness carefully reevaluated.
- Effective alternatives to use of a sling should be considered: humeral taping (strapping) to facilitate or inhibit musculature surrounding the scapula and neuromuscular electrical stimulation (NMES), which has been shown to reduce shoulder subluxation.[146] The hand can also be positioned in a garment pocket.

The patient, family members, and caregivers should be instructed in and allowed to practice proper use of the support. As recovery progresses and voluntary movement emerge, spontaneous reduction of shoulder subluxation may occur eliminating the need for a sling.

For patients using a wheelchair, an arm board or lap tray can provide support for the flaccid arm. A lateral elbow guard and/or straps may be necessary if the patient's arm slips off the side. Patients with decreased sensation are at risk for hand injury if the hand becomes stuck in the spokes of the wheelchair; elbow trauma can occur if the elbow slips off the side (e.g., the elbow hits as the patient is going through a doorway).

Motor Imagery

Motor imagery (MI) is the systematic application of imagery techniques for improving motor performance and learning. It can be practiced in a visual or kinesthetic mode. The patient is instructed to either see or feel the movement as he or she imagines executing it. Mental practice can be facilitated through the use of audiotapes and has been successfully combined with physical practice to enhance UE recovery.[224,225] There is strong evidence that it can be used to improve arm-hand activities from the earliest stages of recovery as long as the patient is cognitively able to engage in the practice.[146,209] It is best when combined with physical practice. As noted in the gait section, it is important to determine that the patient has the ability to imagine by using the KVIQ or a quick mental chronometry screen. For this screen, the clinician compares the executed to imagined times for specific task for congruence. For example, if the person executes a sequential finger movement task in 10 seconds but needs only 3 seconds to imagine the same task, there is no congruence and perhaps the person is not able to effectively imagine.

Mirror Therapy

The use of a mirror can be an effective adjunct for some patients to improve motor function using visual feedback. *Mirror therapy (MT)* is a therapeutic intervention that focuses on moving the less impaired limb while watching its mirror reflection. A mirror is placed in the patient's midsagittal plane, presenting the patient with the mirror image of his or her less affected limb as if it were the hemiparetic limb. It is believed that mirror neurons help create the illusion that the affected hand is moving. It can be practiced in a unimanual or bimanual mode. It was first introduced by Ramachandran et al[226] for individuals with arm amputation. For patients with stroke, MT has been shown to improve LE recovery and ankle dorsiflexion,[227] UE recovery and distal motor function, as well as recovery from hemineglect.[228,229] These findings were reported in studies to which MT was added to conventional therapy.

A Cochrane review by Thieme et al[230] included 14 studies with patients in the subacute and chronic phases poststroke with a wide range of abilities. Therapy was either unimanual (five studies) or bimanual (six studies) with 10 to 60 minutes provided 1, 2, 5, and 7 days/week for 2 to 4 weeks in inpatient setting or the home. They found that MT improved motor function, which was retained after 5 months. There were also improvements in ADLs and decreased shoulder pain.

MT is being combined with task-specific training, MI, as well as NMES.[231-233] It has been shown that the combination of task-specific training plus MT is better at improving upper limb use than either in isolation.[232] The recommended dose on the ViaTherapy app is 30 minutes a day 1 to 3 days a week at least for 4 weeks. This, however, is only a guideline, and studies are underway to determine the dose. It is important to note that use of mirrors is contraindicated in patients with marked visuospatial perceptual impairments. A video of MT with a stroke patient can be viewed online (https://www.youtube.com/watch?v=1BnsQO7a4Og).

Electrical Stimulation

Electrical stimulation of the peripheral nerves and muscles with external electrodes has been applied to the UEs of persons poststroke while performing selected movements as well as task-based movements.[234] It can take the form of NMES or EMG-triggered NMES, both of which have been used with persons recovering from stroke to reduce spasticity, improve sensory awareness, prevent or reduce shoulder subluxation, and stimulate volitional movements.[235-238] NMES has been shown to increase the ability of muscle to exert force by preferentially activating the fast-contracting motor units. Effective treatment results have been reported for improving function of the deltoid and supraspinatus muscles whereby the glenohumeral alignment was improved and subluxation reduced. Optimal results have been obtained when combined with task-specific training.[238]

EMG-NMES to the affected wrist and finger extensors has been shown to improve motor function of the paretic arm, arm-hand activities, and active ROM.[146] The electrical stimulation findings do not appear to differ between persons in the early or late stages poststroke. For this reason, it is included boxes 1, 2, 3 and 5, 6, 7 of the UL algorithm of the ViaTherapy app. Once the person has selective capacity of the upper limb, electrical stimulation is not used.

Simultaneous Bilateral Training

Simultaneous bilateral training involves using both arms simultaneously alone or in combination with augmented sensory feedback. Bilateral arm training with rhythmic auditory cueing (BATRAC) is an example of this intervention.[239] It is theorized that similar movement in the less affected extremity facilitates movement in the more affected extremity. Positive results have been reported in improving motor recovery after stroke.[239-241] When compared to usual or conventional care, simultaneous bilateral training was not shown to be significantly better than other UE interventions in terms of improvements in ADL, arm or hand movements, or scores on motor impairment measures. The Cochrane reviewers cited lack of high-quality evidence in these findings.[59]

Robotic-Assisted Training

Robotic devices have been developed to assist the patient with moderate to severe motor impairments in improving UE function and recovery. They are used in conjunction with task-oriented training and motor learning principles. Robots work to restore lost motor function and can include pneumatic actuators (acting as muscles) to power the device or passive robotic systems using elastic bands or springs. Reach and grasp/release movements are typically targeted. They can be unilateral or bilateral. These devices are used to augment therapist–patient interventions and enable high levels of intensive practice.[242] They can target proximal, distal, and proximal plus distal UL muscles. Unilateral proximal (shoulder elbow) robots have been found to improve motor function of the shoulder, muscle strength, and pain.[146] Bilateral elbow wrists robots were shown to improve motor function of the paretic arm and strength.[146] Limited evidence exists of treatment efficacy that can be generalized to arm and hand use during ADL.[243] In a large randomized trial of persons with moderate to severe stroke, robotic devices were not found to be any better in improving motor function on the FMA than standards of care delivered at high intensity.[244] High cost of equipment currently limits widespread use in the clinical setting.

Strengthening

Muscle weakness is a major impairment after stroke and contributes to significant activity limitations (e.g., walking, sit-to-stand transfers, stair climbing, UE activities).

It is discussed in the upper limb section because it is found in boxes 3, 4, 6, 7 and 8 of the upper limb algorithm (Box 15.6). It is also discussed here because of its importance to postural control and function and is relevant for gait and locomotion. Progressive resistive strength training has been shown to improve muscle strength in individuals with stroke,[245-257] with no evidence of a detrimental increase in spasticity or reduction in ROM.[245,246] Most studies have indicated improvements in function,[246,250,251,253,257] although some have failed to demonstrate carryover to improved function.[245] Specificity of training as well as variable intensities of training may explain this inconsistency.

Exercise modalities for strengthening include free weights, elastic bands or tubing, and machines (progressive resistive exercise [PRE], isokinetics). For patients who are very weak (less than 3/5), gravity-minimized exercises using powder boards, sling suspension, or aquatic exercise is indicated. Gravity-resisted active movements are indicated for patients who demonstrate 3/5 strength (e.g., arm lifts, leg lifts). Patients who demonstrate adequate strength in independent gravity-resisted movement (e.g., 8 to 12 repetitions) can be progressed to exercise using added resistance (e.g., free weights, bands, or machines). Ideally, resistance training should occur 2 to 3 times a week; three sets of 8 to 12 repetitions per exercise should be used.[28]

Combining resistance training with task-oriented functional activities enhances carryover in terms of improving function (e.g., sit-to-stand transfers [Fig. 15.11], partial wall squats [Fig. 15.7], step-ups, stair climbing while the patient is wearing weighted cuffs). Circuit training workstations can be used to maximize muscle training.[253] Lifting free weights or using elastic bands places added demands for postural stability in sitting and standing and is an important element of training to improve postural control.

Exercise Precautions for Strengthening

Many patients with stroke demonstrate poor hand function with no effective grasp. Specially designed gloves may be necessary to ensure maintained contact with exercise equipment (e.g., leather mitts with Velcro, wrist cuffs). Patients with impaired sensation are at increased risk for injury and should be monitored closely. Patients with postural deficits should be safely positioned to prevent falls (e.g., stable seat, corner standing while lifting free weights).

In determining a safe exercise prescription, it is important to remember the high incidence of hypertension and cardiac disease in patients with stroke. High-intensity strengthening exercises (sustained maximal effort) is generally contraindicated in patients with recent stroke and unstable BP. Isometric exercise that is accompanied by the Valsalva maneuver and dangerous elevations in BP is also contraindicated. Dynamic exercises performed in an upright position (sitting) produce less elevations in BP than recumbent/supine exercises. For patients at risk, submaximal protocols using low-intensity exercises (e.g., 30% to 50% of maximal voluntary contraction) are appropriate for initial exercise. Varying the exercises is also an effective strategy to reduce cardiovascular risk. The therapist needs to ensure that warm-ups and cool-downs are adequate and the overall exercise progression is gradual.

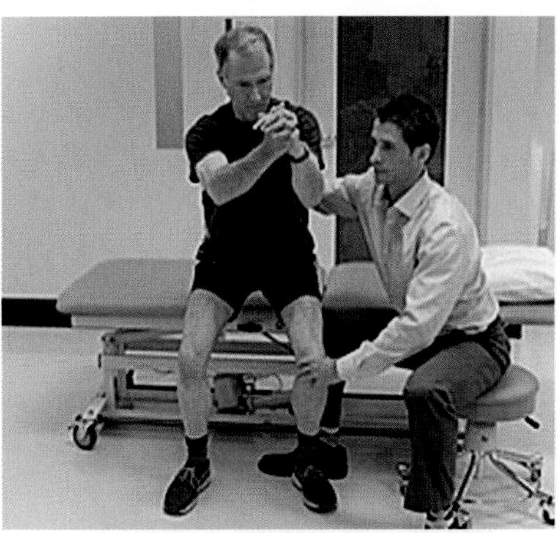

Figure 15.11 Sit-to-stand transitions. The therapist assists the patient in straightening the hemiparetic knee while bringing the center of mass forward. Hands are clasped together.

Task-Specific Training for the Upper Limb

Task-specific training is included in boxes 3, 4, 7, and 8 of the ViaTherapy app's upper limb algorithm (Box 15.6). This suggests that some active control is required for task-specific training of the upper limb. The upper limb can be used as a stabilizer, an assist, and a manipulator. During a reaching movement, the hand is transported by the arm. During that trajectory, the hand, as the distal effector, begins to assume the shape it needs in order to grasp an objective. Van Vliet's work has shown that functional task modifies the kinematics of the reach and grasp in persons poststroke.[258] This suggests that reaching tasks should be done with meaningful objects.

Task-specific training can be done in concert with reducing the obligatory synergistic postures. This can be done by promoting a postural shift toward the more affected side using the arm as a stabilizer by weight-bearing on the extended arm and stabilized hand on a support surface. This early activity promotes proximal stabilization and counteracts the effects of excess flexor hypertonus and a dominant flexion synergy. Approximation can be used to increase activity of shoulder/scapular stabilizers, and tapping can facilitate the elbow extensors. Weight-bearing activities are performed in sitting (Fig. 15.9), modified plantigrade (Fig. 15.12), and standing positions. Control may progress from holding to dynamic stabilization activities. For example, the

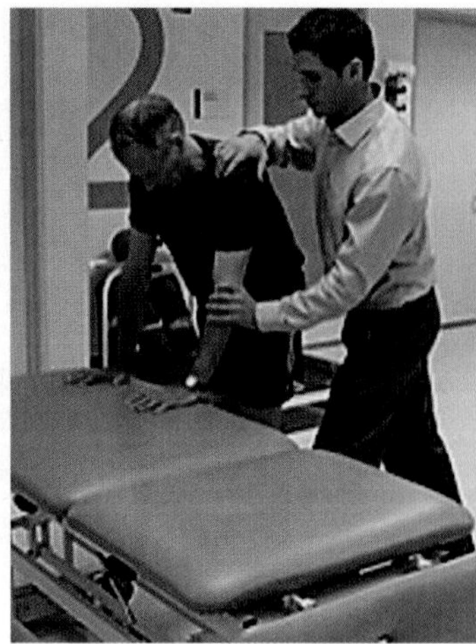

Figure 15.12 Standing in modified plantigrade, both UEs extended and weight-bearing. The therapist assists elbow extension of the hemiparetic UE while providing approximation through the shoulder.

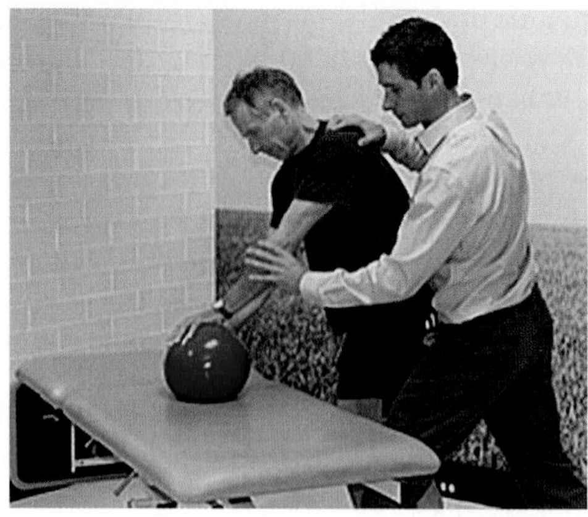

Figure 15.13 Standing in modified plantigrade with hemiparetic hand positioned on small ball. The patient practices rolling the ball from side-to-side; the therapist stabilizes the elbow and shoulder.

patient stabilizes with the more affected UE while performing weight shifts and functional tasks with the stronger UE (e.g., reaching). As previously mentioned, the more affected UE should also be recruited for postural assistance during functional training activities (e.g., pushing up from side-lying into sitting).[223]

Patients with stroke have difficulty regaining control of scapular upward rotation and protraction, elbow extension, and wrist and finger extension necessary for forward reach and manipulation. Reaching and manipulation also requires accurate processing and use of visual–perceptual information. Patients with limited voluntary control can practice initial reaching in a supported position (e.g., side-lying with arm supported by therapist or on a powder board, sitting with the UE resting on a tabletop). The patient is encouraged to slide the hand forward over the tabletop, recruiting shoulder flexors, scapular protractors, and elbow extensors. A cloth can be used to decrease friction effects as the patient practices wiping or polishing a table. The patient can also practice reaching forward and downward touching the floor. More advanced reaching activities include independent lifting and reaching forward (e.g., UE placed into a shirt sleeve). Combining reaching with increased balance challenges in modified plantigrade or standing should also be incorporated. For example, the patient can practice pushing a ball side-to-side or forward-backward while standing in modified plantigrade (Fig. 15.13). Or in standing, the patient can practice reaching to pick an object up off a shelf, a low stool, or the floor. Varying the height and distance reached, increasing the weight of objects held in the hand, or increasing the speed and accuracy requirements can increase difficulty. Substitution movements (e.g., trunk or head lateral movements) or excessive shoulder elevation should, be discouraged.[223]

Meaningful task-oriented practice involving grasp and manipulation is important for stimulating recovery. Initial hand movements typically include gross grasp and release while advanced hand patterns (fine motor control) may not be present unless there is more advanced recovery. Voluntary release is generally much more difficult to achieve than voluntary grasp, and stretching/positioning and inhibitory techniques may be necessary to facilitate extension movements. Initial hand tasks can include using the more affected hand to stabilize (e.g., hand stabilizes paper while the stronger hand writes, hand stabilizes food while the stronger hand cuts) or holding a book with both hands for reading. The patient should be encouraged to use the weaker hand to assist in ADL (e.g., washing the upper body with a washcloth, bringing food to mouth). Forks, toothbrushes, and pens may need to have built-up handles for grasp. Task training should combine reach patterns with hand activity (e.g., picking sock up off floor, reaching for an object off a shelf). Advanced hand activities include practice of wrist and finger extension, opposition, and manipulation of objects (e.g., using utensils to eat; drinking from a cup; writing; picking up and reorienting coins, paperclips, or other objects). Pronation often predominates, whereas active supination without elbow and shoulder flexion is difficult to achieve. The therapist must observe movements carefully and assist in eliminating those aspects of movement patterns that interfere with effective and efficient control. Graded physical assist and use of mental practice/imagery techniques can be helpful to improve learning and performance.[223,259]

Virtual Reality and Video Games

Video games are recommended in the ViaTherapy app for boxes 3, 4, 7, and 8. Therefore, participants need some active isolated movement of the upper limb to play these games. This is especially true if they are not interfaced with a robotic device. The most recent Cochrane review by Laver et al[65] provided support for VR-augmented therapy enhancing the use of the UL for persons post-stroke. In subgroup analyses, they reported greater gains for persons in the early phase poststroke compared to persons in the chronic phase. A second analysis showed that persons who received more than 15 hours of therapy did better than those who received less than 15. It should be noted that most of the studies included in the review were performed with VR systems and not off-the-shelf video games. A recent trial using the Wii during recreational therapy, compared to standard recreational therapy, did not show any differences for persons within 3 months poststroke with moderate deficits.[260] If a video game is incorporated into clinical practice a clear understanding of the game and its application may enhance its efficacy. There are two games analyses that may be useful in applying video games in practice.[261,262]

Constraint-Induced Movement Therapy

CIMT is a multifaceted intervention designed to promote increased use of the more affected UE. The patient is engaged in intense task-oriented practice of the more affected UE for up to 6 hours a day, performed on consecutive weekdays for 10 to 15 days (Fig. 15.14). The less affected UE is restrained from use by having the patient wear a safety mitt for up to 90% of waking hours.[263] The therapist uses shaping techniques to modify and progress performance (e.g., an object is lifted and placed at increasing distances away from the patient). Feedback, coaching, modeling, and encouragement are provided during practice. Behavioral methods designed to ensure adherence to exercise and developing task-oriented behaviors include engaging the patient in the following:

- Self-monitoring of target behaviors (e.g., mode of activity, duration, frequency, perceived exertion, and overall response to activity).
- Problem-solving to identify obstacles and generate potential solutions.
- Behavioral contracting to engage the patient in carrying out behaviors throughout the day.
- Social support strategies to educate and enlist caregivers in providing optimal support.

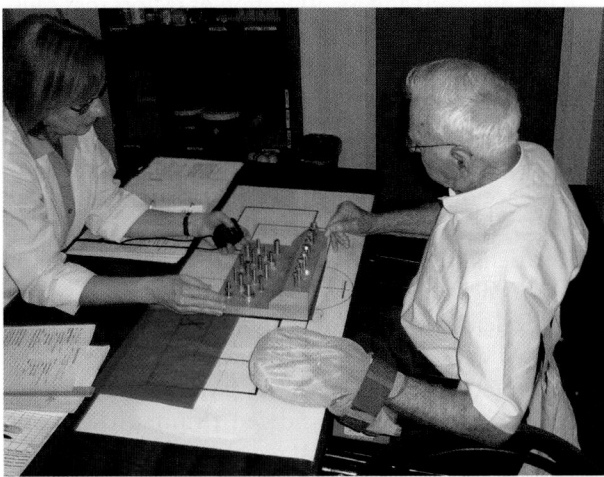

Figure 15.14 Constraint-induced movement therapy (CIMT). The patient practices a pegboard task using the hemiparetic hand while the less affected hand wears a mitt. The therapist times the activity while encouraging the patient.

Refer to the work of Morris and Taub[264,265] for a more complete description of these techniques. *Modified CIMT* (mCIMT) has also been used for patients with stroke. For example, Page et al[266,267] used 30 minutes of functional task practice and shaping techniques 3 days per week and restraint of the less affected UE for up to 5 hours per day. Training occurred over an extended 10-week period. This outpatient protocol increased the use and function of the more affected arm.[266,267]

Significant gains in motor function and a moderate reduction in disability following CIMT have been demonstrated in patients with stroke.[57,268,269] The *EXCITE trial* was a large prospective, single-blind, randomized, multisite study that included 222 patients after stroke. CIMT was compared to customary care and found to significantly improve outcomes as measured by the Wolf Motor Function test and the Motor Activity Log.[270] Associated changes in brain organization with CIMT have also been demonstrated on functional magnetic resonance imaging (fMRI), including an apparent shift in motor cortical activation toward other ipsilateral areas and the contralesional hemisphere.[271] Significant gains have also been reported in the patients receiving mCIMT.[265,266,272] It is important to note that patients were included in the studies if they had potential for recovery and some residual upper arm and hand movement (active wrist and finger extension) but tended not to use the arm. Limited pain or spasticity and absence of cognitive impairment were also inclusion criteria. Many early studies involved patients with chronic stroke (greater than 1 year). Evidence also exists for positive results with subacute stroke patients (less than 1 year)[270] and acute patients (less than 2 weeks after stroke).[273] The Cochrane researchers in their most recent review of the literature concluded that the evidence supported limited improvements after CIMT in motor function and motor impairment, but these benefits did not reduce disability. Studies showing long-term benefits are also limited.[57]

In contrast, another review, which separated CIMT into three categories—(1) original CIMT, (2) high-intensity mCIMT, and (3) low-intensity mCIMT—reported gains. Specifically, the original CIMT (based on 41 RCTs and 1,342 participants) showed positive effects for arm-hand activities, self-reported a significant increase in amount of arm-hand use in daily life, and self-reported quality of arm-hand movements in daily life.[149, p.11] The high-intensity mCMIT (based on 17 RCTs and 512 subjects) found a significant increase in the amount of arm-hand use in daily life and self-reported arm-hand quality and quantity. These effects were found for participants early after stroke but not for those in the chronic phase.[149] For the low-intensity mCIMT (23 RCTs with 627 participants), there were positive effects for motor function of the paretic arm, arm-hand activities, self-reported amount of use, and quality in daily life and basic ADLs. These findings applied to those who were early in rehabilitation and chronic but not to those in between.[146] CIMT is a therapy that has been extensively studied and has several variations. It is becoming easier to know what changes occur and where in the recovery patients benefit from the different types of CIMT therapy. Refer to additional discussion in Chapter 10.

Management of Shoulder Pain

Shoulder pain is Box 9 in the ViaTherapy app's UL algorithm and can apply at any point in the recovery poststroke. Several causes of hemiplegic shoulder pain have been identified that can be broadly divided into flaccid and spastic presentations. In the flaccid stage, proprioceptive loss, lack of muscle tone, and muscle paralysis reduce the support and normal seating action of the rotator cuff muscles, particularly the supraspinatus. The ligaments and capsule thus become the shoulder's sole support. The normal orientation of the glenoid fossa is upward, outward, and forward, so that it keeps the superior capsule taut and stabilizes the humerus mechanically. In the absence of supporting musculature, any abduction or forward flexion of the humerus, or scapular depression and downward rotation, reduces this stabilization and causes the humerus to sublux. Initially, the subluxation is not painful, but mechanical stresses resulting from traction and gravitational forces produce persistent malalignment and pain. Glenohumeral friction–compression stresses also occur between the humeral head and superior soft tissues during flexion or abduction movements in the absence of normal scapulohumeral rhythm *(shoulder impingement syndrome).* During the spastic stage, abnormal muscle tone may contribute to poor scapular position (depression, retraction, and downward rotation) leading to subluxation and restricted movement. Secondary tightness in ligaments, tendons, and joint capsule can develop quickly. *Adhesive capsulitis* (intracapsular inflammation and "frozen shoulder") can occur. Poor handling and positioning of the more affected UE have been implicated in producing joint microtrauma and pain. Activities that traumatize the shoulder include PROM without adequate mobilization of the scapula (promoting normal scapulohumeral rhythm), traction or pulling on the UE during a transfer, or using reciprocal pulleys.[274-276] An incorrectly aligned joint can significantly impair the patient's ability to move. Additional interventions aimed at reducing subluxation can include NMES therapy, EMG biofeedback, taping, and slings (previously discussed).

Complex regional pain syndrome type 1 (CRPS-1), also known as shoulder-hand syndrome (SHS) or reflex sympathetic dystrophy, is caused by proximal trauma to the shoulder or neck or can occur with stroke and may be the result of autonomic nervous system (ANS) changes. Clinical factors associated with its development include motor deficits, spasticity, sensory deficits, and initial coma.[277] Early on, pain is intermittent and limited to the shoulder. During later stages, pain is intense and involves the whole extremity. CRPS-1 is associated with a range of other symptoms. Stiffness and limitations in ROM occur. The wrist tends to assume a flexed position with intense pain likely during wrist extension movements. The elbow is not typically involved. Early *stage 1* vasomotor changes include discoloration (pale pink or cool) and alterations in temperature. The skin may be hypersensitive to touch, pressure, or temperature variations. The patient typically guards against movement attempts. *Stage 2* is characterized by subsiding pain and early dystrophic changes: muscle and skin atrophy, vasospasm, hyperhidrosis (increased sweating), and coarse hair and nails. There is radiographic evidence of early osteoporosis. In *stage 3,* the atrophic phase, pain and vasomotor changes are rare. There is progressive atrophy of the skin, muscles, and bones (severe osteoporosis is evident). Pericapsular fibrosis and articular changes become pronounced. The hand typically becomes contracted in a clawed position with MP extension and IP flexion (similar to the intrinsic minus hand). There is marked atrophy of the thenar and hypothenar muscles with flattening of the hand. Chances of reversal of signs and symptoms are high for stage 1 and variable for stage 2, whereas stage 3 changes are largely irreversible.[277]

Early diagnosis and identification of factors that cause CRPS is essential. Interventions are selected on the basis of examination findings. Because of close daily contact with the patient, the physical therapist is frequently one of the first to recognize and report early signs and symptoms. A prevention protocol should be implemented.[278] In the flaccid stage, the arm should be supported at all times. Proper positioning and handling are essential. In bed, patients should be positioned so they cannot roll onto the more affected UE, compressing it. In supine and wheelchair sitting, the scapula/shoulder should be supported with the arm forward in slight abduction and neutral rotation. During transfers and standing supportive devices should be considered to prevent traction injury. Interventions aimed at reducing pain and stiffness include appropriate PROM and mobilization techniques (gentle grade 1 to 2 mobilizations). PROM to the UE without scapular mobilization is *not* permitted. PROM of the shoulder should be limited to 90° during flexion and abduction or to the point of pain, not beyond the pain position. The therapist needs to ensure that everyone involved in assisting the patient (e.g., family member, caregiver, nurses, and aides) has been instructed in proper handling/mobilization of the UE and recognizes the importance of avoiding trauma and traction injuries during PROM, transfers, and wheelchair activities. Active movements of the UE are encouraged to promote shoulder ROM (e.g., pushing away a tabletop therapy ball while standing). Interventions to manage edema are also a consideration. Additional considerations include no infusions into the veins of the hemiplegic hand. Persistent pain may be managed with oral analgesics or local injection techniques (corticosteroids). Repeat steroid injections are not recommended due to likely weakening of the rotator cuff. With intractable pain, surgical nerve blocks may be considered.[276]

Interventions to Improve Functional Status

Intervention to restore functional status most often takes place in acute care, inpatient acute rehabilitation, or a subacute facility. The loss of sensory and motor function on one side will present a tremendous challenge for the patient struggling to relearn postural control and functional mobility. Observation of the movement will identify body function structure limitations that may be incorporated into the intervention. For example, when a person rolls to the less affected side the stroke, the affected arm is left behind. This could be due to weakness, incoordination, sensory loss. The clinician needs to identify which one and work on remediating the problem in the context of the task. If it is weakness or incoordination, the task may be set up so that the movements at first are gravity assisted. If it is sensory, the patient may have to look at the limb or use a mirror. Or, at first the patient may compensate and use the other limb to assist with movement of the affected limb. If the person is unable to do the movement, he or she may require guided movements progressing to active assisted movement and then finally to active movement.

Persons poststroke present with asymmetrical posture and movement. Whenever possible, that should be reduced to provide better biomechanics for movement, but it cannot be the sole focus of the therapy. If they are able to change their initial conditions (posture) or the therapist can change the environment, then they may have success with the movement.

Normal function implies variability of movements. Muscles need to be activated in varied activities using varied types of contractions. All three types—eccentric, isometric, and concentric—are important to include in an exercise program. For the patient with stroke who demonstrates very weak movements, isometric and eccentric contractions should be practiced before concentric contractions because they utilize elastic elements and muscle spindle support more efficiently. For the same amount of tension, fewer motor units are required. Practice of functional tasks that utilize variations of contractions should also be implemented.

Bed Mobility

Rolling to both sides should be practiced; rolling onto the less affected side will prove more difficult. Extremity movement patterns (e.g., PNF D1 flexion of the LE) can be used to enhance the movement. Care must be taken to ensure the patient does not leave the more affected UE behind but rather brings it forward. This can be accomplished by having the patient clasp the hands together first. The more affected LE can be used to assist in rolling by pushing off from a flexed and neutral, hook-lying position (Fig. 15.15). Rolling onto the more affected side and into a side-lying-on-elbow position is important to promote early weight-bearing. This position has the added benefit of elongating the lateral trunk flexors, which may be shortened.

The patient practices moving from supine-to-sit leading from both sides, with an emphasis on rising with the more involved side leading (closest to the edge of bed or mat). The therapist can provide assistance from side-lying on the more affected side by shifting the LEs over the edge of the bed or mat while the patient pushes up into sitting using both UEs for support. Controlled lowering should also be practiced.

Bridging activities help develop trunk and hip extensor control important for use of a bedpan, pressure relief on the buttocks, initial bed mobility (scooting), and sit-to-stand transfers. It also develops advanced LE out-of-synergy control (hip extension with knee flexion) and stimulates early weight-bearing through the foot (see Fig. 15.16). Bridging activities include independent assumption of the posture, holding in the posture, and moving in the posture (lateral weight shifts, bridge-and-placing hips to one side). If the more affected LE is unable to hold in a hook-lying position, the therapist will need to assist by stabilizing the foot. Lifting the less affected foot off the surface (placing it on a small ball) while maintaining the pelvis level significantly increases the difficulty and can be used to increase

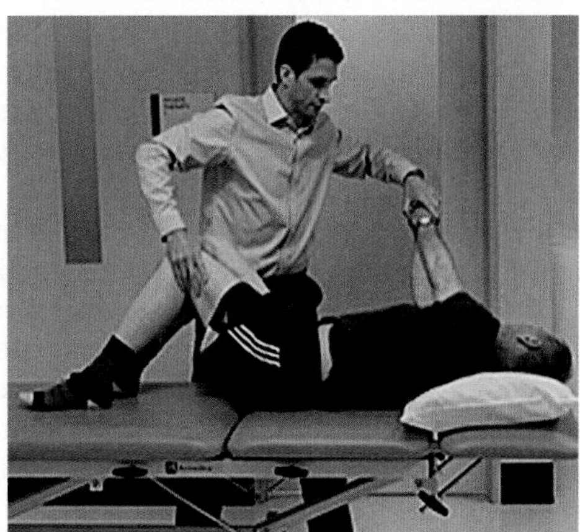

Figure 15.15 Early mobility activities: Rolling onto the unaffected side. The therapist assists the movement through contacts on the knees and clasped hands.

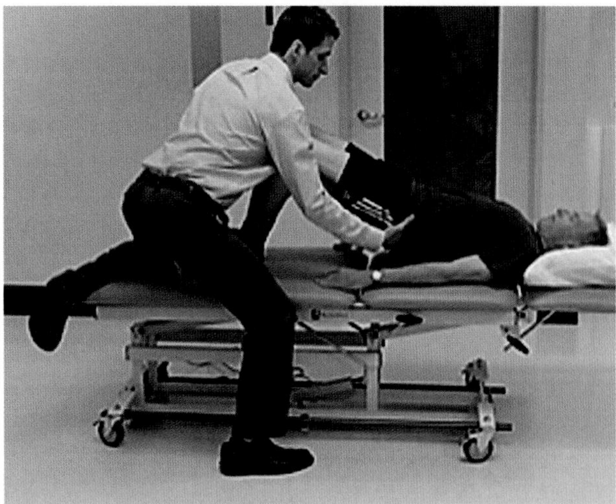

Figure 15.16 The patient practices bridging, combining hip extension with knee flexion. The therapist cues the patient to activate the hip extensors on the hemiparetic LE.

demands on the more affected side. Difficulty can also be increased by varying the position of the UEs, from extended and abducted at the sides to arms folded across the chest or hands clasped together overhead in a prayer position.

Sitting

Early training in sitting should focus on achieving a symmetrical posture with proper spine and pelvic alignment. The pelvis should be neutral, spine straight. Feet should be flat on the support surface. A good initial posture will make it easier for the person to transition to other positions. Typically, patients with stroke will sit asymmetrically with weight borne more on the less affected side, pelvis in a posterior tilt, and upper trunk flexed (kyphotic). Lateral flexion to the affected side is also common. The therapist models correct sitting position and provides verbal instruction for correction and, if needed, manual cues. Early sitting can be assisted by having the patient use the UEs for bilateral support at sides or in front on tabletop, a large ball, or the therapist's shoulders with the therapist sitting directly in front of the patient. Sitting on a therapy ball may also be used to promote pelvic alignment and mobility and trunk upright alignment (gentle bouncing). Sitting control can start with reaching beyond the base of support and then, if that is not possible, work to move in smaller ranges or practice holding the position. The patient should also practice scooting in sitting ("butt walking") to ensure mobility for dressing (putting pants on) and practice initial positioning for sit-to-stand transitions (coming to the edge of the seat to place the feet back and under the body).

Summarized data from studies training sitting balance (six RCTs, 150 participants) showed no gain in symmetry while sitting and standing. However, when data were pooled from studies that used a strategy of reaching beyond arm's length, the researcher found positive effects for sitting balance.[146]

Sit-to-Stand and Sit-Down Transfers

Sit-to-stand transfers should be practiced with a focus on symmetrical weight-bearing, coordinated muscular responses, and adequate timing. To perform the sit-to-stand task, the patient must first actively flex the trunk and use momentum to shift the body mass forward *(flexion-momentum phase),* then extend the hips and knees to move vertically into the upright position *(extension phase),* and finally, stabilize in erect standing *(stabilization phase).* Patients with stroke can demonstrate difficulty with each of these phases. To assist the patient in relearning this task, the patient's feet can be placed evenly side by side in mild ankle dorsiflexion to allow forward movement of the body. Placement of the UEs forward with hands clasped together also assists with the *flexion-momentum stage.* To assist with the *extension phase,* the height of the seat can be initially elevated to decrease the extensor force required; the therapist can also provide tactile and proprioceptive cues to assist hip and knee extension (Fig. 15.11) and to guide the direction of the weight shift. Increased weight-bearing on the stronger LE can be achieved by varying the initial foot position, placing the stronger foot slightly behind the weaker foot. Performance during the stabilization stage can be initially practiced with a wider BOS and support of the hemiplegic arm to maximize trunk alignment and balance. The patient with stroke typically accomplishes sit-to-stand very slowly. With repetitive practice, the patient should be encouraged to focus on increasing the speed of the movement to retrain timing of limb movements, alignment, and balance during this task. The task of stand-to-sit requires eccentric control throughout the trunk and LEs and must also be retrained. Eccentric movements (small-range movements) can be practiced with the patient positioned back against a wall doing partial wall squats as part of a mat exercise program (e.g., bridging, low trunk rotation) or by performing scooting to the right and left while sitting at the edge of a mat.

Standing

Modified plantigrade is an option for an early standing posture to develop postural and extremity control if the person is unable to attain standing without upper limb support. The more affected UE is extended and weight-bearing (an out-of-synergy posture), while the more affected LE is holding in extension (also an out-of-synergy pattern of hip flexion with knee extension). The forward trunk position creates an extension moment at the knee, thus assisting weak knee extensors. In addition, the posture has a wide (four-limb) BOS and is very stable (see Fig. 15.12). Progression may be from holding in the posture to moving in the posture (weight shifts) to reaching tasks.

Initial upright standing can be enhanced using fingertip light touchdown support on a high table or wall. As soon as possible, the patient should be encouraged to practice standing with unilateral UE support (more affected side) and then freestanding (no UE support). If standing with dynamic reaching is not possible, then the person may start by first holding in the posture, then moving in the posture (weight shifts), and finally withstanding challenges to dynamic balance (e.g., reaching in all directions, stepping). The patient is instructed in proper symmetry and alignment. Gentle resistance can be applied to assist in holding, using the PNF technique of rhythmic stabilization. Weight shifts should incorporate moving forward-backward, side-to-side, and diagonally (incorporating upper trunk rotation). Lateral weight shifts to the more affected side are the most difficult. Manual contacts in the direction of the movement combined with gentle resistance can provide cues for movement direction.

Transfers

During early transfers, the patient may require maximal assistance. Adjusting the hospital bed to the height of the chair or wheelchair will help to decrease the difficulty of the transfer. Staff often emphasize the sound side by placing the chair to that side and having the patient stand and pivot a quarter turn on the stronger LE before sitting down. Although this compensatory strategy promotes early transfers, it neglects the weaker side and may make subsequent training more difficult. The patient should be taught to transfer to both sides, with emphasis on moving toward the more affected side. Practice to both sides has functional significance, because most bathrooms are not large enough to allow positioning of the wheelchair on both sides of a tub or toilet. Also, the patient is not likely to be able to reposition the wheelchair once he or she transfers into bed so that a transfer toward the same direction can be achieved when getting out of bed. When transferring, the patient's affected arm can be stabilized in elbow extension and shoulder external rotation against the therapist's body. Alternatively, the patient's UEs (hands in prayer position) can be placed in front or to one side on the therapist's shoulders. The therapist can then assist by using manual contacts, either at the upper trunk or pelvis. The more affected LE may be stabilized by the therapist's knee exerting a counterforce on the patient's knee as needed. Transfer training should include practice in transferring to various different surfaces and heights (e.g., wheelchair, toilet, tub seat, car).

Functional training is begun early and continued throughout the course of rehabilitation. Training activities and postures are varied according to individual needs. Advanced functional training should include practice in getting down to and up from the floor in the event of a fall. Incorporating ROM or strength training while practicing function will make the session more efficient.

Interventions to Improve Body Function Structure

The management of body function structure (BFS) deficits is integrated with task-level training. There is strong evidence that strength training is important to address BFS deficits in stroke rehabilitation (see Strengthening earlier in this section). Evidence to support strengthening of the lower extremity exists for water-based exercises, neuromuscular stimulation (NMES) of the paretic leg, transcutaneous electrical nerve stimulation (TENS), strength training, mixed cardiorespiratory and strength exercises, and high-intensity practice.[149] Therefore, the clinician can work at the BFS or the task level to achieve strengthening. Other BFS may need to be addressed in preparation for task-based training, such as increasing and maintaining ankle ROM through passive stretching, administration of pharmacological agents to reduce spasticity, and positioning in the wheelchair or bed[209] (see Table 15.7).

A sequence for the intervention would start with joint mobilization and retrograde massage of the affected ankle in advance of sit-stand training. Increasing joint ROM and reducing edema are preparatory interventions to practice sit-stand-walk tasks that require a specific amount of ankle ROM to be performed in a biomechanically correct way. This is an example where the clinician uses BFS interventions to create initial conditions for the tasks practice that will increase likelihood of success.

Aerobic Capacity and Physical Activity

Persons poststroke are deconditioned, predisposed to a sedentary lifestyle, and at increased risks for falls and recurrence of cardiovascular disease. They require greater energy expenditure than prior to the stroke, so they are prone to fatigue. The inactive lifestyle leads to secondary complications such as reduced cardiorespiratory fitness, increased fatigability, muscle atrophy/weakness, osteoporosis, and impaired circulation to the lower extremities in stroke survivors. In addition, diminished self-efficacy, greater dependence on others for ADL, and reduced ability for normal societal interactions can have a profound negative psychological impact.[279] Therefore, physical activity (PA) and exercise are important for both rehabilitation and prevention of secondary conditions.

Individuals recovering from stroke can benefit from PA and endurance (aerobic) training to improve cardiovascular function. It is important to promote PA across the continuum of recovery. During the early acute stages, it is essential to minimize bedrest by having early mobilization (within 24 hours after stroke),[280] and functional activity training is appropriate. During the post-acute stage, patients/clients may be able to engage in more traditional exercise training modes such as TM walking, cycle ergometry (upper and lower body ergometer), or seated stepper. Patients with balance impairments will benefit from TT or overground walking with a safety harness or from a recumbent cycle ergometer. The therapist should assess barriers and facilitators to PA.[209] To ensure safety, patients should receive a thorough examination and supervised exercise test. Stroke guidelines (2014) recommend a graded exercise test with ECG monitoring.[279] The 6MWT, although used with many diagnoses to measure cardiorespiratory fitness, should be interpreted with caution when used with persons with stroke because the correlation between distance walked and peak VO_2 test is low to moderate.[279]

Exercise prescription elements include mode (type of exercise), frequency, intensity, and duration[281] (see Chapter 13, Heart Disease). Choice of training mode depends on the individual's abilities and interests. Intensity guidelines for acute persons poststroke suggest using an RPE of 11 or less (6–20 category scale) and heart rate of 10 to 20 beats above resting.[279] For post-acute persons who have greater motor ability and are more medically stable, intensity can be increased. The moderate-intensity continuous exercise (MICE) guidelines are (1) 40% to 70% of $\dot{V}O_{2Max}$ or heart rate reserve, (2) 55% to 80% of HR maximum, (3) 11 to 14 RPE, (4) 20 to 60 minutes, (5) 5 to 10 minutes of warm up and cool down, (6) 3 to 5 days a week.[279] Greater intensity may be achieved with high-intensity interval training (HIIT). It consists of short bursts of activity followed by recovery (standing, walking, stepping in place or sitting). A HIIT protocol was studied with persons in the chronic phase poststroke who could walk at 0.75 m/s. It was found that after a 5-minute warm-up, 30-second bursts followed by combination of 30- and 60-second recovery provided the highest aerobic intensity based on TM speed and step count.[282] The same investigators have determined that HIIT is safe for future study among persons with stroke who have been prescreened with an ECG, have had a graded exercise test, and use a harness.[283]

The use of a training log or exercise diary is an excellent way to help the patient keep track of prescriptive elements, objective measurements (heart rate, BP), and subjective reactions (RPE, perceived enjoyment). Wearing a pedometer may serve as feedback and incentive for activity. Adequate supervision, monitoring, and safety education about warning signs for impending stroke and heart attack are critical components.[28,279]

Exercise Precautions

Careful monitoring of exercise is essential. For patients at risk, BP, HR, and RPE should be taken initially, during, and after each exercise. As exercise progresses, less frequent monitoring can be implemented. The therapist also needs to monitor breathing rate and pattern, ensuring that breath holding and Valsalva do not occur. Patients should be instructed in how to measure their own HR and RPE. They should also be taught the warning signs for when to stop exercising. These include the following:

- Lightheadedness or dizziness
- Chest heaviness, pain, or tightness; angina
- Palpitations or irregular heart beat
- Sudden shortness of breath not due to increased activity
- Volitional fatigue and exhaustion

Patients who are on medications that limit cardiac output (e.g., beta blockers) will demonstrate reduced HR responses and lower peak HRs. Patients taking diuretics to reduce fluid volume may demonstrate altered electrolyte balance with resulting dysrhythmias. Patients taking vasodilators may require a longer cool-down period after exercise to prevent postexercise hypotension.[28]

Patients undergoing an aerobic conditioning program demonstrate improvements in physical fitness, functional status, psychological outlook, and self-esteem. Regular exercise may have the additional benefit of reducing risk of recurrent stroke or heart attack. Patients who participate in a regular conditioning program may be more successful in adopting continuing, life-long exercise habits and in moving beyond the disability associated with stroke.

Physical fitness for persons poststroke was assessed in a Cochrane Database Systematic Review by Saunders et al.[63] They reviewed 28 trials with 1,408 participants and found that cardiorespiratory fitness training after stroke improved maximal walking speed and preferred gait speed. Their review also included mixed training (cardiorespiratory plus strengthening) and found that preferred walking speed and walking capacity as well as balance improved. Some mobility benefits persisted after training. A separate review reported that combining cardiovascular and strengthening activities has been shown to have beneficial effects for physical activity, walking distance, maximum gait speed, and aerobic capacity.[149] Boyne et al. confirmed these findings and added that intensity of training yielded better results, and specificity of training was relevant when training walking.[284] Clinicians may wish to combine therapies to increase their efficiency in delivering care unless their primary aerobic fitness goal is walking, in which case they should train walking.

One strategy to combine interventions of aerobic training and functional training is *circuit class training (CCT).* When used to improve mobility of persons poststroke who were either inpatients or dwelling in the community, CCT has been found, in a Cochrane review, to be safe and effective.[64] It may also reduce inpatient length of stay. Rose et al[285] reported on the effectiveness of a circuit training physical therapy (CTPT) program in the acute rehabilitation setting. Patients received a 60-minute training session, 5 days a week, using four task-specific stations. Activities were stratified and tailored to patients' specific mobility levels (nonambulatory, severe, moderate, and mild groups). In addition, a 30-minute daily session was dedicated to critical inpatient rehabilitation issues (family and home program education, wheelchair and orthotic prescription). When compared to standard physical therapy (SPT) of the same intensity, the CTPT groups showed significantly greater improvements in gait speed, primarily in ambulatory patients.

PATIENT/CLIENT-RELATED INSTRUCTION

Stroke represents a major health crisis for patients and their families. Ignorance about the cause of the illness or the recovery process and misconceptions concerning the rehabilitation program and potential outcomes can negatively influence coping responses and progress in rehabilitation. Frequently, the problems seem unmanageable and overwhelming for the family, especially when faced with alterations in the patient's behavior, cognition, and emotion. Patients may feel depressed, isolated, irritable, or demanding. Families often demonstrate reactions that include initial relief and hope for full recovery, followed by feelings of entrapment, depression, anger, or guilt when complete recovery does not occur. These changes and feelings can strain even the best of relationships. Therapists can often have a dramatic influence on this situation because of the high frequency of contact and the often close relationships that develop with patients and their families. There are many important guidelines to follow when planning educational interventions:

- Give accurate, factual information; counsel family members about the patient's capabilities and limitations; *avoid* predictions that categorically define expected function or future recovery.
- Structure interventions carefully, giving only as much information as the patient or family need or can assimilate; provide reinforcement and repetition.
- Adapt interventions to ensure they are appropriate to the educational and cultural background of the patient and family.
- Offer a variety of educational interventions: didactic sessions, books, brochures, and videotapes, and family participation in therapy (see Appendix 15.A).
- Provide a forum for open discussion and communication.
- Be supportive and sensitive and maintain a positive, hopeful manner.
- Assist patients and families in confronting alternatives and developing problem-solving abilities.
- Motivate and provide positive reinforcement in therapy; enhance patient satisfaction and self-esteem.
- Refer patients and families to support and self-help groups such as the following national associations (see Appendix 15.A, American Stroke Association).

Psychotherapy and counseling (e.g., sexual, leisure, vocational) can assist in improving overall quality of life and should be recommended as needed.

DISCHARGE PLANNING

Planning for discharge begins early in rehabilitation and involves the patient and family. Potential placement (safe place of residence), level of family and community support, and need for continued medical and rehabilitation services should be explored. Family members should regularly participate in therapy sessions to learn exercises and activities designed to support the patient's independence. Discharge should be considered when reasonable treatment goals/outcomes are attained. Indication of the attainment of a functional ceiling can be considered when there is lack of evidence of progress at two successive evaluations. Home visits should be made before discharge to determine the home's physical structure and accessibility. Potential problems can be identified, and corrective measures initiated. See Chapter 9 for additional discussion. Home adaptations, assistive devices, and supportive services should be in place before the patient is discharged to home. A home exercise program coupled with patient and caregiver training should be instituted. Caregiver training of gait and mobility related function and activities has been reported to have a positive impact on improving basic ADL and reducing caregiver strain.[149] Patients with residual impairments or activity limitations who will be receiving outpatient or home therapy should be given all the necessary information concerning these services. Community services should be identified and information provided to the patient and family. Long-term follow-up at regularly scheduled intervals should be initiated in order to maintain patients at their highest possible functional level.

RECOVERY AND OUTCOMES

Recovery from stroke is generally fastest in the first weeks and months after onset. Patients can continue to make measurable functional gains generally at a reduced rate for months or years after insult. Late recovery of function has been consistently demonstrated for patients with chronic stroke (defined as greater than 1 year post-stroke) who undergo extensive task-specific functional training that emphasizes use of the more involved extremities. Prolonged recovery with improvements occurring over a period of years is especially apparent in the areas of language and visuospatial function. Rates of motor recovery vary across management categories: patients suffering minor stroke recover rapidly with few or no residual deficits, whereas severely impaired individuals demonstrate more limited and prolonged recovery. The initial grade of paresis, measured on initial hospital admission, is an important predictor of motor recovery. In the case of complete paralysis on admission, complete motor recovery occurs in less than 15% of patients. In an extensive review of the literature, Hendricks et al[286] found no significant difference in potential for motor recovery between type of stroke (hemorrhage vs. infarction) and location (brainstem vs. hemispheric infarction).

Functional mobility skills are impaired following stroke and vary considerably from individual to individual. The ability to recover functional tasks is influenced by a number of factors. Motor and perceptual impairments have the greatest impact on functional performance, but other limiting factors include sensory loss, disorientation, communication disorders, and decreased cardiorespiratory endurance. Enablement factors include high motivation, stable supportive family, financial resources, and intensive training with repetitive practice.[287-289]

Patients who receive inpatient stroke rehabilitation (skilled occupational, physical, and speech therapy) demonstrate improved motor recovery, functional status, and quality of life at discharge.[286-293] In a systematic review of the literature (151 studies), Van Peppen et al[292] found strong evidence in support of task-oriented exercise and intensive training. Inpatient rehabilitation admission averaged a little over 2 weeks. Approximately 80% of patients were discharged home.[292] Post-discharge outpatient treatment or home care for stroke survivors is often indicated because functional status typically is not stabilized at discharge from a rehabilitation hospital, and effects diminish over time with no treatment. Patients who demonstrate less successful rehabilitation outcomes tended to include those with (1) advanced age, (2) severe motor impairments (e.g., prolonged paralysis, apraxia), (3) persistent medical problems (e.g., incontinence), (4) impaired cognitive function (e.g., decreased alertness, poor attention span, judgment, memory, learning difficulty), (5) severe language disturbances, (6) severe visuospatial hemineglect, and (7) other less well-defined social and economic problems.[290-293] Researchers who studied long-term follow-up at 2 years poststroke (148 patients) found that only 12% demonstrated a decline in mobility. Depression was cited as the single major risk factor for mobility decline.[294]

SUMMARY

Stroke results from many different vascular events that interrupt cerebral circulation and impair brain function, including cerebral thrombosis, emboli, and hemorrhage. The location and size of the ischemic process, the nature and functions of the structures involved, the availability of collateral blood flow, and effectiveness of early emergency medical management all influence the symptomatology that evolves. For many patients, stroke represents a major cause of disability, with diffuse problems affecting widespread areas of function. Examination using standardized assessments of participation, activity, and body function and structure are complemented with task analysis and movement observation. Effective rehabilitation should take advantage of the brain's capacity for repair and recovery. A patient-centered approach to rehabilitation interventions promotes recovery and independence through restitution, compensation, and prevention. Task-oriented training using motor learning constructs, coupled with exercise science, form the basis of the intervention. Ultimately, management should be customized to address the individual as well as factors such as stroke location, stroke severity, and phase of recovery.

The author wishes to acknowledge the following individuals who reviewed parts of the manuscript and offered advice or content: Phyllis Bowlby, Kathy Gill Body, Kari Dunning, George Fulk, and my students who helped with research and writing: Lisa Ricker, Aurora James Palmer, and Brittany Hoehlein.

Questions for Review

1. Differentiate between anterior cerebral artery syndrome and middle cerebral artery syndrome in terms of expected deficits.
2. Differentiate between lesions of the right and left hemispheres in terms of expected behavioral deficits.
3. What are the major types of aphasia that can result from stroke? Where are the lesions located?
4. Differentiate between the following stroke-specific instruments: the Fugl-Meyer Assessment of Physical Performance (FMA) and the Stroke Impact Scale.
5. Describe the behaviors of the patient with stroke who demonstrates ipsilateral pushing. What is the primary focus of rehabilitation intervention?
6. Describe the steps for structuring a therapeutic session to promote motor skill acquisition.
7. What are the essential elements of constraint-induced movement therapy to improve UE function poststroke?
8. Describe high intensity stepping and how it relates to locomotor training and aerobic training.
9. Describe how the Orpington scale and information from the transcranial magnetic stimulation can guide prognosis.
10. What important guidelines should be followed when planning an educational program for the patient with stroke and for family members?

CASE STUDY

HISTORY

The patient/client is a 41-year-old man admitted to an acute care hospital with a diagnosis of CVA with R hemiparesis (L MCA). He was admitted to a rehabilitation facility 7 days later. His goal is to walk independently and resume his responsibilities as a spouse and provider.

PAST MEDICAL HISTORY

- History of mild hypertension well controlled with medication.
- Smokes 1 pack/day; 20-year history.

MEDICATIONS

- Persantine 50 mg po tid
- Tenormin 25 mg po qd
- Aspirin 10 grains po bid

SOCIAL HISTORY

Patient lives with his wife and three teenage children and was independent and active before CVA. He has a college education and has worked for 18 years as a computer programmer. There is a two-step access to a rented, single-family house.

COGNITION

- Mild disorientation to time and place.
- Attention span for up to 5 minutes on task.
- Difficult to examine further owing to language impairment; cognitive deficits likely.

LANGUAGE/COMMUNICATION

- Auditory comprehension: Reliable yes/no.
- Verbal expression: Limited to only occasional automatic words.
- Reading comprehension: Can read sentences.
- Written expression: To be determined.
- Gestures: Spontaneous use of gestures not evident.

PHYSICAL THERAPY EXAMINATION

(Not assessed in this order, documented according to facility standards)

Passive Range of Motion

- BUEs WNL; R shoulder pain at end ranges
- BLEs WNL except R dorsiflexion 0° to 5°

Sensation

- RUE and RLE unable to test due to communication deficits.
- Patient reports pain in RUE, end ranges of shoulder motions.

Motor Control

- RUE: Active movement (1/2 range) (shoulder and elbow flexion); unable to isolate against gravity but can isolate into flexion and extension in a gravity-eliminated position. Unable to isolate movement of the hand, which is in flexion.
- RLE: Full motion in both extensor and flexor synergy patterns with extensor pattern dominating; able to isolate hip flexion and extension and knee extension in the full range in a gravity-eliminated position

Strength

- LUE and LLE: Full isolated movement with G+ to N strength.
- RUE: Poor strength in the shoulder and elbow flexors
- RLE: Fair strength in the hip flexors and extensors and knee extensors, poor strength in the ankle dorsiflexors

Coordination

- LUE and LLE intact.
- RUE and RLE: Limited movements; unable to test.

Postural Control/Balance

- Sitting control: Maintains balance without support and proper alignment for 10 minutes. Able to displace COM over BOS independently and to both sides.

- Standing control: Able to maintain independent standing in parallel bars for up to 1 minute with LUE handhold. Able to displace COM over BOS with supervision to both sides.
- Berg Balance Scale: 46.

Functional Status

- Rolls to R: Independent with bed rail
- Rolls to L: min assist with upper limb
- Scoots up in bed: Supervision
- Supine-to-sit: min assist
- Sit-to-supine: min assist
- Transfers bed-to-chair: Stand pivot transfer, min assist (FIM 4)
- Eating: Supervision (FIM 5)
- Bathing: mod assist RUE and RLE (FIM 3)
- Dressing: mod assist RUE and RLE (FIM 3)

Gait and Locomotion

- W/C mobility: Propels 150 ft with supervision (FIM 5); uses LUE and L foot for propulsion.
- Locomotion: Ambulates 0.4 m/s using a hemi cane and a temporary dorsiflexor assist and close supervision to contact guard. Presents step asymmetry, decreased clearance of the stroke-affected leg, decreased stance time on the stroke-affected leg. Lacks a loading response and push off
- Stairs: Unable to test.

Upper Limb Control

- Using extremity as a stabilizer when positioned in sitting.

Endurance

- Tolerates 3/4-hour treatment session with frequent rests.

Other Tests

Orpington Score: 3.4.

PSYCHOSOCIAL

Patient is motivated and cooperative. He appears anxious about his future and exhibited a brief episode of crying during the initial therapy session. His main goal is to walk again. Family is supportive and anxious to have him home again.

GUIDING QUESTIONS

1. Identify/categorize this patient's problems in terms of
   a. participation limitations.
   b. activity limitations.
   c. body function structure limitations.
2. Identify three activity-based long-term goals (3 weeks) and three body function structure goals (2 to 3 weeks) for this patient.
3. For each of the following, formulate a treatment intervention that could be used during the first 2 weeks of therapy. Provide a brief rationale that justifies your choices.
   a. To address an upper limb deficit
   b. To address function
   c. To address gait and locomotion
4. Describe how you would structure the intervention for the initial physical therapy sessions with this patient.

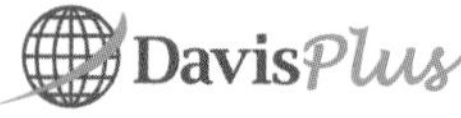

For additional resources, including answers to the questions for review and case study guiding questions, please visit **http://davisplus.fadavis.com.**

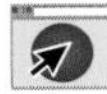

The reader is referred to the following video case studies for additional review and study:

- Case Study 9: Patient With Right Hemorrhagic CVA
- Case Study 10: Patient With Left Ischemic CVA
- Case Study 11: Patient With Right Thalamic Ischemic Infarct and Left Lateral Medullary Ischemia
- Case 12: Patient With Right Basal Ganglia Intraparenchymal Hemorrhage

These case studies including full written summaries, all tables, figures, charts, and three video segments (examination, intervention, and outcome), appear online at Davis*Plus*. The case studies pose questions for the reader's consideration with suggested answers to the case study questions, also posted online at Davis*Plus*.

References

1. Gonzalez-Castellon, M, and Kitago, T: Pathophysiology and management of acute stroke. In Stein, J, et al (eds), Stroke Recovery and Rehabilitation, ed 2. Demos Medical, New York, NY, 2015, pp. 42–55, 2015.
2. Benjamin, EJ, et al: AHA heart disease and stroke statistical—2017 update: A report from the American Heart Association. 2017. Circulation 135(10):e146.
3. Gresham, GE, and Post-Stroke Rehabilitation Guideline Panel: Post-Stroke Rehabilitation Guideline Panel: Post-Stroke Rehabilitation Clinical Practice Guideline. Aspen, Gaithersburg, MD, 1996 (formerly published as AHCPR Publication No. 95-0662, May 1995).
4. Lloyd-Jones, DM, et al: Defining and setting national goals for cardiovascular health promotion and disease reduction: The American Heart Association's strategic Impact Goal through 2020 and beyond. Circulation 121(4):586, 2010.
5. American Heart Association/American Stroke Association: Stroke Warning Signs and Symptoms. American Heart Association, Dallas, TX, 2011. Retrieved May 6, 2017, from http://www.strokeassociation.org/STROKEORG/WarningSigns/Stroke-Warning-Signs-and-Symptoms_UCM_308528_SubHomePage.jsp.
6. NINDS Group: Tissue plasminogen activator for acute ischemic stroke. N Engl J Med 333(24):1581, 1995.
7. NINDS t-PA Stroke Study Group: Generalized efficacy of t-PA for acute stroke: Subgroup analysis of the NINDS t-PA stroke trial. Stroke 28(11):2119, 1997.
8. Hertzberg, V, et al: Methods and processes for the reanalysis of the NINDS tissue plasminogen activator for acute ischemic stroke. Clin Trials 5:308, 2008.
9. Kwan, J, et al: A systematic review of barriers to delivery of thrombolysis for acute stroke. Age Ageing 33(2):116, 2004.
10. De la Ossa, N, et al: Influence of direct admission to comprehensive stroke centers on the outcome of acute stroke patients treated with intravenous thrombolysis. J Neurol 256(8):1270, 2009.
11. Barclay, L: ACCESS: Acute cerebrovascular care in emergency stroke systems. Arch Neurol 67(10):1210, 2010.
12. Kwiatkowski, T, et al: Effects of tissue plasminogen activator or acute ischemic stroke at one year. N Engl J Med 340(23):1781, 1999.
13. Mitsios, N, et al: Pathophysiology of acute ischaemic stroke: An analysis of common signaling mechanisms and identification of new molecular targets. Pathobiology 73(4):159, 2006.
14. Wu, CM, et al: Early risk of stroke after transient ischemic attack: a systematic review and meta-analysis. Arch Intern Med 167(22): 2417, 2007.
15. Kaplan, P, Cailliet, R, and Kaplan, C: Rehabilitation of Stroke. Butterworth-Heinemann, Woburn, MA, 2003.
16. Teasdale, G, and Jennett, B: Assessment of coma and impaired consciousness: A practical scale. Lancet 2(7872):81, 1974.
17. Smithard, DG, et al: The natural history of dysphagia following stroke. Dysphagia 12(4):188, 1997.
18. Meng, N, Wang, T, and Lien, I: Dysphagia in patients with brainstem stroke: Incidence and outcome. Am J Phys Med Rehabil 79(2):170, 2000.
19. Avery, W: Dysphagia management. In Gillen, G (ed): Stroke Rehabilitation: A Function-Based Approach. Elsevier/Mosby, St. Louis, MO, 2011, pp 629–647.
20. Sachdev, P, et al: Clinical determinants of dementia and mild cognitive impairment following ischaemic stroke: The Sydney Stroke Study. Dement Geriatr Cogn Disord 21(5–6):275, 2006.
21. Chemerinski, E, and Robinson, R: The neuropsychiatry of stroke. Psychosomatics 41(1): 5, 2000.
22. Folstein, MF, et al: Mini Mental State: A practical method for grading the cognitive state of patients for the clinician. J Psychiatr Res 12(3):189, 1975.
23. Hackett, ML, and Pickels, K: Part I: Frequency of depression after stroke: An updated systematic review and meta-analysis of observational studies. Int J of Stroke 9(8):1017, 2014.
24. Barker-Collo, S: Depression and anxiety 3 months post stroke: Prevalence and correlates. Arch Clin Neuropsychol 22(4):519, 2007.
25. Berg, A, et al: Post stroke depression: An 18-month follow-up. Stroke 34(1):138, 2003.
26. Robinson, RG: Vascular depression and post-stroke depression: Where do we go from here? Am J Geriatr Psychiatry 13(2):85, 2005.
27. Beck, A, and Beck, R: Screening depressed patients in family practice: A rapid technique. Postgrad Med 52(6):81, 1972.
28. Palmer-McLean, K, and Harbst, K: Stroke and brain injury. In American College of Sports Medicine: ACSM's Exercise Management for Persons with Chronic Diseases and Disabilities, ed 3. Human Kinetics, Champaign, IL, 2009, p 287.
29. Porth, C: Pathophysiology, ed 7. Lippincott Williams & Wilkins, Philadelphia, 2005.
30. Harris, J, et al: Relationship of balance and mobility to fall incidence in people with chronic stroke. Phys Ther 85(2):150, 2005.
31. Teasall, R, et al: The incidence and consequences of falls in stroke patients during inpatient rehabilitation: Factors associated with high risk. Arch Phys Med Rehabil 83(3):329, 2002.
32. Tutuarima, J, et al: Risk factors for falls of hospitalized stroke patients. Stroke 28(2):297, 1997.
33. Forster, A, and Young, J: Incidence and consequences of falls due to stroke: A systematic inquiry. Br Med J 311(6997):83, 1995.
34. Ramnemark, A, et al: Fractures after stroke. Osteoporos Int 8(1):92, 1998.
35. Yew, K, and Cheng, E: Acute stroke diagnosis. Am Fam Physician 80(1):33, 2009.
36. Nor, A, and Ford, G: Misdiagnosis of stroke. Expert Rev Neurotherapeutics 7(8):989, 2007.
37. National Institute of Neurological Disorders and Stroke: NIH Stroke Scale. 2003. Retrieved March 7, 2012, from www.ninds.nih.gov/doctors/NIH_Stroke_Scale.pdf.
38. Leira, E, et al: Baseline NIH Stroke Scale responses estimate the probability of each particular stroke subtype. Cerebrovasc Dis 26(6):573, 2008.
39. Wityk, RJ, Pessin, MS, and Kaplan, RF: Serial assessment of acute stroke using the NIH Stroke Scale. Stroke 25(2):362, 1994.
40. Goldstein, LB, and Samsa, GP: Reliability of the National Institutes of Health Stroke Scale. Stroke 28(2):307, 1997.
41. Kwakkel G, et al: Standardized measurement of sensorimotor recovery in stroke trials: Consensus-based core recommendations for the Stroke Recovery and Rehabilitation Roundtable. Int J of Stroke 12(5):451, 2017.
42. Boyd LA, et al Biomarkers of stroke recovery: Consensus-based core recommendations from the Stroke Recovery and Rehabilitation roundtable. Int J of Stroke 12(5): 480, 2017.
43. Hakimelahi, R, and Gonzalez, R: Neuroimaging of ischemic stroke with CT and MRI: Advancing towards physiological based diagnosis and therapy. Expert Rev Cardiovasc Ther 7(1): 29, 2009.

44. National Stroke Association: Explaining Stroke-Related Medications. Retrieved May 8, 2017, from www.stroke.org/we-can-help/survivors/stroke-recovery/first-steps-recovery/preventing-another-stroke/medications?pagename=med_adherence#explain.
45. Deglin, JH, Vallerand, AH, and Sanoski CA: Davis's Drug Guide for Nurses, ed 14. FA Davis, Philadelphia, 2015.
46. National Stroke Association: Stroke Treatment. Retrieved May 1, 2017, from www.strokeassociation.org/STROKEORG/AboutStroke/Treatment/Stroke-Treatment_UCM_492017_SubHomePage.jsp.
47. Schenkman, M, Deutsch, JE, and Gill-Body, K: An integrated framework for decision making in neurologic physical therapy practice. Phys Ther 86(12):1681, 2006.
48. American Physical Therapy Association: Guide to Physical Therapist Practice 3.0. 2014. Retrieved April 10, 2016, from http://guidetoptpractice.apta.org.
49. World Health Organization (WHO): International Classification of Functioning, Disability and Health: ICF. WHO, Geneva, Switzerland, 2001. Retrieved September 10, 2016, from www.who.int/classifications/icf/en
50. Rothstein, JM, Echternach, JL, and Riddle, DL: The hypothesis-oriented algorithm for clinicians II (HOAC II): A guide for patient management. Phys Ther 83(5):455, 2003.
51. Strokedge: The Academy of Neurology Outcome Measures Recommendations. Retrieved March 15, 2017, from www.neuropt.org/special-interest-groups/stroke/strokedge.
52. Bernhardt, J, et al: Agreed definitions and a shared vision for new standards in stroke recovery research: The Stroke Recovery and Rehabilitation Roundtable Taskforce. Int J Stroke 12(5):444, 2017.
53. Langhorne, P, et al: Do stroke units save lives? Lancet 342(8868): 395, 1993.
54. Stroke Unit Trialists Collaboration: Organised inpatient (stroke unit) care after stroke (review). Cochrane Database of Systematic Reviews 2007, Issue 4. Art. No.: CD000197. DOI: 10.1002/14651858.CD000197.pub2.
55. Bernhardt, J, et al: Prespecified dose-response analysis for a very early rehabilitation trial (AVERT). Neurology 86(23): 2138, 2016.
56. Pollock, A, et al: Physical rehabilitation approaches for the recovery of function and mobility following stroke. Cochrane Database of Systematic Reviews 2014, Issue 4. Art. No.: CD001920. DOI: 10.1002/14651858.CD001920.pub3.
57. Corbetta, D, et al: Constraint-induced movement therapy for upper extremities in people with stroke. Cochrane Database of Systematic Reviews 2015, Issue 10. Art. No.: CD004433. DOI: 10.1002/14651858.CD004433.pub3.
58. Winter, J, et al: Hands-on therapy interventions for upper limb motor dysfunction following stroke (review). Cochrane Database of Systematic Reviews 2011, Issue 6. Art. No.: CD006609. DOI: 10.1002/14651858.CD006609.pub2.
59. Coupar, F, et al: Simultaneous bilateral training for improving arm function after stroke (review). Cochrane Database of Systematic Reviews 2010, Issue 4. Art. No.: CD006432. DOI: 10.1002/14651858.CD006432.pub2.
60. Doyle, S, et al: Interventions for sensory impairment in the upper limb after stroke (review). Cochrane Database of Systematic Reviews 2010, Issue 6. Art. No.: CD006331. DOI: 10.1002/14651858.CD006331.pub2.
61. Mehrholz, J, Pohl, M, and Elsner, B: Treadmill training and body weight support for walking after stroke. Cochrane Database of Systematic Reviews 2014, Issue 1. Art. No.: CD002840. DOI: 10.1002/14651858.CD002840.pub3.
62. French, B, et al: Repetitive task training for improving functional ability after stroke. Cochrane Database of Systematic Reviews 2016, Issue 11. Art. No.: CD006073. DOI: 10.1002/14651858.CD006073.pub3.
63. Saunders, DH, et al: Physical fitness training for stroke patients. Cochrane Database of Systematic Reviews 2016, Issue 3. Art. No.: CD003316. DOI: 10.1002/14651858.CD003316.pub6.
64. English, C, Hillier, SL, and Lynch EA: Circuit class therapy for improving mobility after stroke (review). Cochrane Database of Systematic Reviews 2017, Issue 6. Art. No.: CD007513. DOI: 10.1002/14651858.CD007513.pub3.
65. Laver, KE, et al: Virtual reality for stroke rehabilitation. Cochrane Database of Systematic Reviews 2015, Issue 2. Art. No.: CD008349. DOI: 10.1002/14651858.CD008349.pub3.
66. Mehrholz, J, et al: Electromechanical-assisted training for walking after stroke. Cochrane Database of Systematic Reviews 2013, Issue 7. Art. No.: CD006185. DOI: 10.1002/14651858.CD006185.pub3.
67. Coupar, F, et al: Home-based therapy programmes for upper limb functional recovery following stroke. Cochrane Database of Systematic Reviews 2012, Issue 5. Art. No.: CD006755. DOI: 10.1002/14651858.CD006755.pub2.
68. Laver, KE, et al: Telerehabilitation services for stroke. Cochrane Database of Systematic Reviews 2013, Issue 12. Art. No.: CD010255. DOI: 10.1002/14651858.CD010255.pub2.
69. Outpatient Service Trialists: Therapy-based rehabilitation services for stroke patients at home (review). Cochrane Database of Systematic Reviews 2009, Issue 1. Art. No.: CD002925. DOI: 10.1002/14651858.CD002925.
70. Mehrholz, J, Kugler, J, and Pohl, M: Water-based exercises for improving activities of daily living after stroke (review). Cochrane Database of Systematic Reviews 2011, Issue 1. Art. No.: CD008186. DOI: 10.1002/14651858.CD008186.pub2.
71. Turner-Stokes, L: Goal attainment scaling (GAS) in rehabilitation: a practical guide. Clinical Rehabilitation 23(4): 362, 2009.
72. Duncan, PW, et al: The Stroke Impact Scale version 2.0: Evaluation of reliability, validity, and sensitivity to change. Stroke 30(10): 2131, 1999.
73. Lin, K, et al: Psychometric comparisons of the Stroke Impact Scale 3.0 and the Stroke-Specific Quality of Life Scale. Qual Life Res 19(3):435, 2010.
74. Duncan, PW, et al: Evaluation of proxy responses to the Stroke Impact Scale. Stroke 33(11):2593, 2002.
75. Sackley, CM: The relationships between weight-bearing asymmetry after stroke and function and activities of daily living. Physiother Theory Pract 6(4):179, 1990.
76. Badke, MB, and Duncan, P: Patterns of rapid motor responses during postural adjustments when standing in healthy subjects and hemiplegic patients. Phys Ther 63(1):13, 1983.
77. Dickstein, R, and Ablaffio, N: Postural sway of the affected and nonaffected pelvis and leg in stance of hemiparetic patients. Arch Phys Med Rehabil 81(3):364, 2000.
78. DiFabio, R, and Badke, M: Relationship of sensory organization to balance function in patients with hemiplegia. Phys Ther 70(9): 543, 1990.
79. Shumway-Cook, A, Anson, D, and Haller, S: Postural sway biofeedback: Its effect on reestablishing stance stability in hemiplegic patients. Arch Phys Med Rehabil 69(6):395, 1988.
80. Gustavsen, M, Aamodt, G, and Mengshoel, A: Measuring balance in subacute stroke rehabilitation. Adv Physiother 8(1):15, 2006.
81. Benaim, C, et al: Validation of a standardized assessment of postural control in stroke patients: The Postural Assessment Scale for Stroke Patients (PASS). Stroke 30(9):1862, 1999.
82. Mao, HF, et al: Analysis and comparison of the psychometric properties of three balance measures for stroke patients. Stroke 33(4):1022, 2002.
83. Chien, CW, et al: A comparison of psychometric properties of the smart balance master system and the postural assessment scale for stroke in people who have had mild stroke. Arch Phys Med Rehabil 88(3):374, 2007.
84. Karnath, H, Ferber, S, and Dichgans, J: The origin of contraversive pushing: Evidence for a second graviceptive system in humans. Neurology 55(9):1298, 2000.
85. Pedersen, P, et al: Ipsilateral pushing in stroke: Incidence, relation to neuropsychological symptoms, and impact on rehabilitation. The Copenhagen stroke study. Arch Phys Med 77(1): 25, 1996.
86. Karnath, H, Ferber, S, and Dichgans, J: The neural representation of postural control in humans. PNAS 97:13931, 2000.
87. Karnath, H, et al: Prognosis of contraversive pushing. J Neurol 249(9):1250, 2002.
88. Broetz, D, and Karnath, H: New aspects for the physiotherapy of pushing behavior. Neurorehabil 20:133, 2005.
89. Karnath, H, and Broetz, D: Understanding and treating "pusher syndrome." Phys Ther 83(12):1119, 2003.
90. Perry, J, et al: Classification of walking handicap in the stroke population. Stroke 26(6):982, 1995.
91. Viosca, E, et al: Proposal and validation of a new functional ambulation classification scale for clinical use. Arch Phys Med Rehabil 86(6):1234, 2005.
92. Fulk, GD, et al: Predicting home and community walking activity poststroke. Stroke 48(2):406, 2017.

93. Tudor-Locke, C, and Bassett, DR Jr. How many steps/day are enough? Preliminary pedometer indices for public health. Sports Med 34(1):1, 2004.
94. Tudor-Locke, C, Johnson, WD, and Katzmarzyk, PT. Accelerometer-determined steps per day in US adults. Med Sci Sports Exerc 41(7):1384, 2009.
95. Tudor-Locke, C, et al: Revisiting how many steps are enough?. Med Sci Sports Exerc 40(suppl 7):S537, 2008.
96. Van der Lee, JH, et al: The intra- and interrater reliability of the Action Research Arm Test: A practical test of upper extremity function in patients with stroke. Arch Phys Med Rehabil 82(1):14, 2001.
97. Hsieh, C, et al: Inter-rater reliability and validity of the Action Research Arm Test in stroke patients. Age Ageing 27(2):107, 1998
98. Platz, T, et al: Reliability and validity of arm function assessment with standardized guidelines for the Fugl-Meyer Test, Action Research Arm Test and Box and Block Test: A multicentre study. Clin Rehabil 19(4):404, 2005.
99. Lang, CE, et al: Measurement of upper-extremity function early after stroke: Properties of the Action Research Arm Test. Arch Phys Med Rehabil 87(12):1605, 2006.
100. Lin, J, et al: Psychometric comparisons of 4 measures for assessing upper-extremity function in people with stroke. Phys Ther 89(8): 840, 2009.
101. Lang, CE, et al: Estimating minimally clinically important differences of upper-extremity measures early after stroke. Arch Phys Med Rehabil 89(9):1693, 2008.
102. Uswatte, G, et al: The Motor Activity Log-28: Assessing daily use of the hemiparetic arm after stroke. Neurology 67(7): 1189, 2006.
103. Uswatte, G, et al: Reliability and validity of the upper extremity Motor Activity Log-14 for measuring real-world arm use. Stroke 36(11):2493, 2005.
104. Van der Lee, JH, et al: Clinimetric properties of the motor activity log for the assessment of arm use in hemiparetic patients. Stroke 35(6):1410, 2004.
105. Mahoney, F, and Barthel, D: Functional evaluation: Barthel Index. Md State Med J 14:61, 1965.
106. Keith, RA, et al: The Functional Independence Measure. Adv Clin Rehabil 1:6, 1987.
107. Uniform Data Service, Data Management Service: UDS Update. State University of New York at Buffalo, 1993.
108. Hunter, SM, and Crome, P: Hand function and stroke. Rev Clin Gerontol 12(1):66, 2002.
109. Tyson, SF, et al: Sensory loss of in-hospital admitted people with stroke: Characteristics, associated factors, and relationship with function. Neurorehab Neural Re 22(2):166, 2008.
110. Carey, L: Somatosensory loss after stroke. Crit Rev Phys Med Rehabil 7(1):51, 1995.
111. Rand, D, Gottlieb, D, and Weiss, P: Recovery of patients with a combined motor and proprioception deficit during the first six weeks of post stroke rehabilitation. Phys Occup Ther Geriatr 18(3):69, 2001.
112. Connell, LA, Lincoln, NB, and Radford, KA: Somatosensory impairment after stroke: Frequency of different deficits and their recovery. Clin Rehabil 22(8):758, 2008.
113. Canavero, S, and Bonicalzi, V: Central pain syndrome: Elucidation of genesis and treatment. Expert Rev Neurotherapeutics 7(11):1485, 2007.
114. Klit, H, Finnerup, N, and Jensen, T: Central post-stroke pain: Clinical characteristics, pathophysiology, and management. Lancet Neurol 8(9):857, 2009.
115. Twitchell, T: The restoration of motor function following hemiplegia in man. Brain 47:443, 1951.
116. Brunnstrom, S: Motor testing procedures in hemiplegia based on recovery stages. J Am Phys Ther Assoc 46(4):357, 1966.
117. Brunnstrom, S: Movement Therapy in Hemiplegia. Harper & Row, New York, NY, 1970.
118. Gray, C, et al: Motor recovery following acute stroke. Age Ageing 19(3):179, 1990.
119. Wade, D, et al: Recovery after stroke: The first 3 months. J Neurol Neurosurg Psychiatry 48(1):7, 1985.
120. Fugl-Meyer, A, et al: The post stroke hemiplegic patient, 1. A method for evaluation of physical performance. Scand J Rehabil Med 7(1):13, 1976.
121. Duncan, P, et al: Reliability of the Fugl-Meyer Assessment of Sensorimotor Recovery following cerebrovascular accident. Phys Ther 63(10):1606, 1983.
122. Gladstone, DJ, Danells, CJ, and Black, SE: The Fugl-Meyer assessment of motor recovery after stroke: A critical review of its measurement properties. Neurorehabil NeuralRepair 16(3):232, 2002.
123. Crowe, J, and Harmeling-vander Wel, B: Hierarchical properties of the motor function sections of the Fugl-Meyer Assessment Scale for people after stroke: A retrospective study. PhysTher 88(12):1555, 2008.
124. Beckerman, H, et al: A criterion for stability of the function of the lower extremity in stroke patients using the Fugl-Meyer Assessment Scale. Scand J. Rehabil Med 28:3, 1996.
125. Patten, C, Lexell, J, and Brown, H: Weakness and strength training in persons with post-stroke hemiplegia: Rationale, method and efficacy. J Rehabil Res Dev 41(3A):293, 2004.
126. Carin-Levy, G, et al: Longitudinal changes in muscle strength and mass after acute stroke. Cerebrovasc Dis 21(3):201, 2006.
127. Adams, R, Gandevia, S, and Skuse, N: The distribution of muscle weakness in upper motoneuron lesions affecting the lower limb. Brain 113(5):1459, 1990.
128. Davidoff, R: The pyramidal tract. Neurology 40(2):332, 1990.
129. Andrews A, and Bohannon, R: Distribution of muscle strength impairments following stroke. Clin Rehabil 14(1):79, 2000.
130. Canning, C, Ada, L, and O'Dwyer, N: Slowness to develop force contributes to weakness after stroke. Arch Phys Med Rehabil 80(1):66, 1999.
131. Eng, J: Strength training in individuals with stroke. Physiother Can 56(4):189, 2004.
132. Dattola, R, et al: Muscle rearrangement in patients with hemiparesis after stroke: An electrophysiological and morphological study. Eur Neurol 33(2):109, 1993.
133. Stoeckmann, T, Sullivan, K, and Scheidt, R: Elastic, viscous, and mass load effects on poststroke muscle recruitment and co-contraction during reaching: A pilot study. Phys Ther 89(7): 665, 2008.
134. Chae, J, et al: Delay in initiation and termination of muscle contraction, motor impairment, and physical disability in upper limb hemiparesis. Muscle Nerve 2(25):568, 2002.
135. McCrea, PH, Eng JJ, and Hodgson, A: Time and magnitude of torque generation is impaired in both arms following stroke. Muscle Nerve 28(1):46, 2003.
136. Desrosiers, J, et al: Performance of the "unaffected" upper extremity of elderly stroke patients. Stroke 27(9):1564, 1996.
137. Miller, P, Moreland, J, and Stevenson, T: Measurement properties of a standardized version of the two-minute walk test for individuals with neurological dysfunction. Physiother Can 54(4): 241, 2002.
138. Rieck, M, Moreland, J: The Orpington Prognostic Scale for patients with stroke: Reliability and pilot predictive data for discharge destination and therapeutic services. Disabil and Rehabil 27(23):1425, 2005.
139. Kalra, L, Crome, P: The role of prognostic scores in targeting stroke rehabilitation in elderly patients. J Am Geriat Soc 41(4):396, 1993.
140. Coupar, FA, et al: Predictors of upper limb recovery after stroke: A systematic review and meta-analysis. Clin Rehabil 26(4):291, 2012.
141. Pollock, A, et al: Interventions for improving upper limb function after stroke. Cochrane Database of Systematic Review 2014, Issue 11 Art No.: Cd010820. DOI: 10.1002/14651858. CD010820.pub2.
142. Carr, J, and Shepherd, R: A Motor Relearning Programme for Stroke, ed 2. Aspen, Gaithersville, MD, 1987.
143. Boyd, L, and Winstein, C: Impact of explicit information on implicit motor-sequence learning following middle cerebral artery stroke. Phys Ther 83(11):976, 2003.
144. Orrell, A, Eves, F, and Masters, R: Motor learning of a dynamic balancing task after stroke: Implicit implications for stroke rehabilitation. Phys Ther 86(3):369, 2006.
145. Gentile, A: Skill acquisition: Action, movement, and neuromotor processes. In Carr, J, and Shephard, R (eds): Movement Science: Foundations for Physical Therapy in Rehabilitation, ed 2. Aspen, Rockville, MD, 2000, p. 147.
146. Veerbeek, JM, et al: What is the evidence for physical therapy poststroke? A Systematic Review and Meta-Analysis. PLoS One 9(2):e87987, 2014.

147. Platuz, EJ, et al: Effects of repetitive motor training on movement representations in adult squirrel monkeys role of use versus learning. Neurbiol Learn Mem, 74(1):27, 2000.
148. Hellstrom, K, et al: Self-efficacy in relation to impairments and activities of daily living disability in elderly patients with stroke: A prospective investigation. J Rehabil Med 35(5):202, 2003.
149. Schmidt, R, and Lee, T: Motor Control and Learning: A Behavioral Emphasis, ed 5. Human Kinetics, Champaign, IL, 2011.
150. Eng, J, Pang, M, and Ashe, M: Balance, falls, and bone health: Role of exercise in reducing fracture risk after stroke. J Rehabil Res Dev 45(2):297, 2008.
151. Bayouk, JF, Boucher, JP, and Leroux, A: Balance training following stroke: Effects of task-oriented exercises with and without altered sensory input. Int J Rehabil Res 29(1):51, 2006.
152. Bonan, IV, et al: Reliance on visual information after stroke. Part II: Effectiveness of a balance rehabilitation program with visual cue deprivation after stroke: A randomized controlled trial. Arch Phys Med Rehabil 85(2):274, 2004.
153. van Duijnhoven, HJ, et al: Effects of exercise therapy on balance capacity in chronic stroke: Systematic review and meta-analysis. Stroke 47(10):2603, 2016.
154. Wang, XQ, et al: Cognitive motor interference for gait and balance in stroke: a systematic review and meta-analysis. Eur J Neurol 22(3):555, 2015.
155. Ghai, S, Ghai, I, and Effenberg, AO: Effects of dual tasks and dual-task training on postural stability: A systematic review and meta-analysis. Clin Interv Aging 12:557, 2017.
156. An, HJ, et al: The effect of various dual task training methods with gait on the balance and gait of patients with chronic stroke. J Phys Ther Sci 26(8):1287, 2014.
157. Rose, D: Fall Proof: A Comprehensive Balance and Mobility Training Program, ed 2. Human Kinetics, Champaign, IL, 2010.
158. Lubetzky-Vilnai, A, and Kartin, D: The effect of balance training on balance performance in individuals poststroke: A systematic review. J Neurol Phys Ther 34(3):127, 2010.
159. Hammer, A, Nilsagarad, Y, and Wallquist, M: Balance training in stroke patients—a systematic review of randomized, controlled trials. Adv Physiother 10(4):163, 2008.
160. Winstein, C, et al: Standing balance training: Effect on balance and locomotion in hemiparetic adults. Arch Phys Med Rehabil 70(10):755, 1989.
161. Sackley, C, and Lincoln, N: Single blind randomized controlled trial of visual feedback after stroke: Effects on stance symmetry and function. Disabil Rehabil 19(12):536, 1997.
162. Hamman, R, et al: Training effects during repeated therapy sessions of balance training using visual feedback. Arch Phys Med Rehabil 73(8):738, 1992.
163. McRae, J, et al: Rehabilitation of hemiplegia: Functional outcomes and treatment of postural control. Phys Ther 74(Suppl):S119, 1994.
164. Nichols, D: Balance retraining after stroke using force platform biofeedback. Phys Ther 77(5):553, 1997.
165. Fishman, M, et al: Comparison of functional upper extremity tasks and dynamic standing. Phys Ther 76(Suppl):79, 1996.
166. Barclay-Goddard, R, et al: Force platform feedback for standing balance training after stroke. Cochrane Database of Systematic Reviews 2004, Issue 3. Art. No.: CD004129. DOI: 10.1002/14651858.CD004129.pub2.
167. Deutsch, JE, and Westcott McCoy, S: Virtual reality and serious games in neurorehabilitation of children and adults: Prevention, plasticity, and participation. Pediatr Phys Ther 29(Suppl 3): S23, 2017.
168. Li, Z, et al: Virtual reality for improving balance in patients after stroke: A systematic review and meta-analysis. Clinical Rehabil 30(5):432, 2016.
169. Gibbons EM, et al: Are virtual reality technologies effective improving lower limb outcomes for patients following stroke—A systematic review with meta-analysis. Top Stroke Rehabil: 23(6):440, 2016.
170. Iruthayarajah, J, et al: The use of virtual reality for balance among individuals with chronic stroke: A systematic review and meta-analysis. Top Stroke Rehabil 24(1):65, 2017.
171. de Rooij, IJ, et al: Effect of virtual reality training on balance and gait ability in patients with stroke: Systematic review and meta-analysis. Phys Ther 96(12):1905, 2016.
172. Davies, P: Steps to Follow: The Comprehensive Treatment of Patients with Hemiplegia, ed 2. Springer-Verlag, New York, 2000.
173. Paci, M, and Nannetti, L: Physiotherapy for pusher behavior in a patient with post-stroke hemiplegia. J Rehabil Med 36(4):183, 2004.
174. States, R, Salem, Y, and Pappas, E: Overground gait training for individuals with chronic stroke: A Cochrane systematic review. J Neurol Phys Ther 33(4):179, 2009.
175. Malouin, F, et al: Use of an intensive task-oriented gait training program in a series of patients with acute cerebrovascular accidents. Phys Ther 72(11):781, 1992.
176. Richards, C, et al: Task-specific physical therapy for optimization of gait recovery in acute stroke patients. Arch Phys Med Rehabil 74(6):612, 1993.
177. Hesse, S, et al: Restoration of gait in nonambulatory hemiparetic patients by treadmill training with partial body-weight support. Arch Phys Med Rehabil 75(10):1087, 1994.
178. Visintin, M, et al: A new approach to retrain gait in stroke patients through body weight support and treadmill stimulation. Stroke 29(6):1122, 1998.
179. Barbeau, H, and Visintin, M: Optimal outcomes obtained with body-weight support combined with treadmill training in stroke subjects. Arch Phys Med Rehabil 84(10):1458, 2003.
180. Nilsson, L, et al: Walking training of patients with hemiparesis at an early stage after stroke: A comparison of walking training on a treadmill with body weight support and walking training on the ground. Clin Rehabil 15(5):515, 2001.
181. Pohl, M, et al: Speed-dependent treadmill training in ambulatory hemiparetic stroke patients: A randomized controlled trial. Stroke 33(2):553, 2002.
182. Sullivan, K, Knowlton, B, and Dobkin, BH: Step training with body weight support: effect of treadmill speed and practice paradigms on poststroke locomotor recovery. Arch Phys Med Rehabil 83(5):683, 2002.
183. Ada, L, et al: Randomized trial of treadmill walking with body weight support to establish walking in subacute stroke: The MOBILISE trial. Stroke 41(6):1247, 2010.
184. Eich, HJ, et al: Aerobic treadmill plus Bobath walking training improves walking in subacute stroke: A randomized controlled trial. Clin Rehabil 18(6):640, 2004.
185. Dean, C, et al: Treadmill walking with body weight support in subacute non-ambulatory stroke improves walking capacity more than overground walking: A randomized trial. J Physiother 56(2):97, 2010.
186. Macko, RG, Ivey, FM, and Forrester, LW: Treadmill exercise rehabilitation improves ambulatory function and cardiovascular fitness in patients with chronic stroke: A randomized controlled trial. Stroke 36(10):2206, 2005.
187. Hesse, S: Treadmill training with partial body weight support after stroke: A review. NeuroRehabil 23(1):55, 2008.
188. Franceschini, M, et al: Walking after stroke: What does treadmill training with body weight support add to overground training in patients with very early stroke? A single-blind randomized controlled trial. Stroke 40(9):3079, 2009.
189. Sullivan, K, et al: Effects of task-specific locomotor and strength training in adults who were ambulatory after stroke: Results of the STEPS randomized clinical trial. Phys Ther 87(12):1580, 2007.
190. Duncan, PW, et al: Body-weight-supported treadmill rehabilitation after stroke. N Engl J Med 364(21):2026, 2011.
191. Tefertiller, C, et al: Efficacy of rehabilitation robotics for walking training in neurological disorders: A review. J Rehabil Res Dev 48(4):387, 2011.
192. Ada, L, et al: Mechanically assisted walking with body weight support results in more independent walking than assisted overground walking in non-ambulatory patients early after stroke: A systematic review. J Physiother 56(3):153, 2010.
193. Lewek, M, et al: Allowing intralimb kinematic variability during locomotor training poststroke improves kinematic consistency: A subgroup analysis from a randomized clinical trial. Phys Ther 89(8):829, 2009.
194. Holleran, CL., et al: Feasibility and potential efficacy of high-intensity stepping training in variable contexts in subacute and chronic stroke. Neurorehab Neural Re, 28(7):643, 2014.
195. Holleran, CL, et al: Potential contributions of training intensity on locomotor performance in individuals with chronic stroke. JNPT, 39(2):95, 2015.
196. Hornby, TG, et al: Variable intensive early walking poststroke (VIEWS). Neurorehab Neural Re, 30(5):440, 2016.

197. Roche, A, Laighin, G, and Coote, S: Surface-applied functional electrical stimulation for orthotic and therapeutic treatment of drop-foot after stroke—A systematic review. Phys Ther Rev 14(2):63, 2009.
198. Weingarden, H, and Ring, H: Functional electrical stimulation–induced neural changes and recovery after stroke. Eur J Phys Rehabil Med 42(2):87, 2006.
199. Swigchem, R, et al: Effect of peroneal electrical stimulation versus an ankle-foot orthosis on obstacle avoidance ability in people with stroke-related drop foot. Phys Ther 92(3):398, 2012.
200. Dunsky, AR, et al: Home-based motor imagery training for gait rehabilitation of people with chronic poststroke Hemiparesis. Arch Phys Med Rehabil 89(8):1580, 2008.
201. Dickstein, R, et al: Effects of integrated motor imagery practice on gait of individuals with chronic stroke: A half-crossover randomized study. Arch Phys Med Rehabil 94(11):2119, 2013.
202. Deutsch, JE, Maidan I, and Dickstein, R. Patient-centered integrated motor imagery delivered in the home with telerehabilitation to improve walking after stroke. Phys Ther 92(8):1065, 2012.
203. Malouin, F, et al: The Kinesthetic and Visual Imagery Questionnaire (KVIQ) for assessing motor imagery in persons with physical disabilities: A reliability and construct validity study. J Neurol Phys Ther 31(1):20, 2007.
204. Malouin, F, et al: Clinical assessment of motor imagery after stroke. Neurorehab Neural Re 22(4):330, 2008.
205. Corbetta D, Imeri, F, and Gatti R. Rehabilitation that incorporates virtual reality is more effective than standard rehabilitation for improving walking speed, balance and mobility after stroke: A systematic review. J Physiother 61(3):117, 2015.
206. Wolf, SL, et al: Group upper extremity stroke algorithm working. Best practice for arm recovery post stroke: An international application. Physiotherapy 102(1):1, 2016.
207. Nijland, RH, et al: Presence of finger extension and shoulder abduction within 72 hours after stroke predicts functional recovery: early prediction of functional outcome after stroke: The Epos cohort study. Stroke 41(4):745, 2010.
208. Stinear, C: Prediction of recovery of motor function after stroke. Lancet Neurol 9 (12):1228, 2010.
209. Hebert, D, et al: Canadian stroke best practice recommendations: Stroke rehabilitation practice guidelines, update 2015. Int J Stroke 11(4): 459, 2016.
210. Gracies, JM, et al: Pathophysiology of impairment in patients with spasticity and use of stretch as a treatment of spastic hypertonia. Phys Med Rehabil Clin North Am 12(4):747, 2001.
211. Bovend'Eerdt, TJ, et al: The effects of stretching in spasticity: A systematic review. Arch Phys Med Rehabil 89(7):1395, 2008.
212. Watanabe, T: The role of therapy in spasticity management. Am J Phys Med Rehabil 83(10):S45, 2004.
213. Taub, E: Somatosensory deafferentation research with monkeys. In Ince, L (ed): Behavioral Psychology in Rehabilitation Medicine: Clinical Applications. Williams & Wilkins, Baltimore, MD, 1980, p. 371.
214. Schabrun, SM, and Hillier, S: Evidence for the retraining of sensation after stroke: A systematic review. Clin Rehabil 23(1): 27, 2009.
215. Carey, L, Macdonell L, and Matyas, TA: SENSe: Study of the effectiveness of neurorehabilitation on sensation: A randomized controlled trial. Neurorehab Neural Re 25(4):304, 2011.
216. Hunter, SM, et al: Dose-response study of mobilisation and tactile stimulation therapy for the upper extremity early after stroke: A phase I trial. Neurorehab Neural Re 25(4):314, 2011.
217. Dannenbaum, R, and Dykes, R: Sensory loss in the hand after sensory stroke: Therapeutic rationale. Arch Phys Med Rehabil 69(10):833, 1988.
218. Weinberg, J, et al: Training sensory awareness and spatial organization in people with right brain damage. Arch Phys Med Rehabil 60(11):491, 1979.
219. Pollock, A, et al: Interventions for visual field defects in patients with stroke. Cochrane Database of Systematic Reviews, 2011, Issue 10. Art. No.: CD008388. DOI:10.1002/14651858.CD008388.pub2.
220. Bailey, M, Riddoch, M, and Crome, P: Treatment of visual neglect in elderly patients with stroke: A single-subject series using either a scanning and cueing strategy or a left-limb activation strategy. Phys Ther 82(8):782, 2002.
221. Bailey, M, and Riddoch, M: Hemineglect in stroke patients. Part 2. Rehabilitation techniques and strategies: A summary of recent studies. Phys Ther Rev 4(2):77, 1999.
222. Wiart, L, et al: Unilateral neglect syndrome rehabilitation by trunk rotation and scanning training. Arch Phys Med Rehabil 78(4):424, 1997.
223. Gillen, G: Upper extremity function and management. In Gillen, G, and Burkhardt, A (eds): Stroke Rehabilitation: A Function-Based Approach, ed 3. Mosby, St. Louis, MO, 2011, p. 218.
224. Page, S, et al: Mental practice combined with physical practice for upper-limb motor deficit in subacute stroke. Phys Ther 81(8): 1455, 2001.
225. Barclay-Goddard, R. E., et al: Mental practice for treating upper extremity deficits in individuals with hemiparesis after stroke. Cochrane Database of Systematic Reviews, 2011, Issue 5. Art No.: CD005950. DOI: 10.1002/14651858.CD005950.pub4.
226. Ramachandran, VS, and Roger-Remachandran, D: Synaesthesia in phantom limbs induced with mirrors. Proc R Soc Lond B Biol Sci 263(1369):431, 1996.
227. Sübeyaz, S, et al: Mirror therapy enhances lower-extremity motor recovery and motor functioning after stroke: A randomized controlled trial. Arch Phys Med Rehabil 88(5):555, 2007.
228. Dohle, C, et al: Mirror therapy promotes recovery from severe hemiparesis: A randomized controlled trial. Neurorehab Neural Re 20(3):1, 2008.
229. Yavuzer, G, et al: Mirror therapy improves hand function in subacute stroke: A randomized controlled trial. Arch Phys Med Rehabil 89(3):393, 2008.
230. Thieme, H, et al: Mirror therapy for improving motor function after stroke. Cochrane Database of Systematic Reviews, 2012, Issue 3. Art. No.: CD008449. DOI: 10.1002/14651858.CD008449.pub2.
231. Yun, JG, et al: The synergistic effects of mirror therapy and neuromuscular electrical stimulation for hand function in stroke. Ann Rehabil Med 35(3): 316, 2011.
232. Khandare, S, et al: Comparison of task specific exercises and mirror therapy to improve upper limb function in subacute stroke patients. IOSR-JDMS 7(1):5, 2013.
233. Arya, KN, et al: Task-based mirror therapy augmenting motor recovery in poststroke hemiparesis: a randomized controlled trial. J Stroke Cerebrovasc Dis 24(8):1738, 2015.
234. Pomeroy, VM., et al: Electrostimulation for promoting recovery of movement or functional ability after stroke. Cochrane Database of Systematic Reviews, Issue 2, 2006. Art. No.: CD003241. DOI:10.1002/14651858.CD003241.pub2.
235. Chae, J, et al: Neuromuscular stimulation for upper extremity motor and functional recovery in acute hemiplegia. Stroke 29(5): 975, 1998.
236. Hardy, J, et al: Meta-analysis examining the effectiveness of electrical stimulation in improving the functional use of the upper limb in stroke patients. Phys Occup Ther Geriatr 21(4):67, 2003.
237. Ada, L, and Foongchomcheay, A: Efficacy of electrical stimulation in preventing and treating subluxation of the shoulder after stroke: A meta-analysis. Aust J Physiother 48(4):257, 2002.
238. Price, C, and Pandyan, A: Electrical stimulation for preventing and treating post-stroke shoulder pain. Cochrane Database of Systematic Reviews, 2000, Issue 4. Art. No.: CD001698. DOI: 10.1002/14651858.CD00169.
239. Whitall, J, et al: Repetitive bilateral arm training with rhythmic auditory cueing improves motor function in chronic hemiparetic stroke. Stroke 31(10):2390, 2000.
240. Richards, LG, et al: Bilateral arm training with rhythmic auditory cueing in chronic stroke: Not always efficacious. Neurorehab Neural Re 22(2):180, 2008.
241. Stewart, KC, Cauraugh, J, and Summers, J: Bilateral movement training and stroke rehabilitation: A systematic review and meta-analysis. J Neurol Sci 244(1–2):89, 2006.
242. Fasoli, S: Rehabilitation technologies to promote upper limb recovery after stroke. In Gillen, G, and Burkhardt, A (eds): Stroke Rehabilitation: A Function-Based Approach, ed 3. Mosby, St. Louis, MO, 2011, p. 280.
243. Brewer, B, McDowell, S, and Worthen-Chaudhari, L: Poststroke upper extremity rehabilitation: A review of robotic systems and clinical results. Top Stroke Rehabil 14(6):1562, 2003.
244. Lo, Albert C., et al: Robot-assisted therapy for long-term upper-limb impairment after stroke. New Engl J Med 362(19):1772, 2010.

245. Morris, S, Dodd, K, and Morris, M: Outcomes of progressive resistance strength training following stroke: A systematic review. Clin Rehabil 18(1):27, 2004.
246. Ada, L, Dorsch, S, and Canning, C: Strengthening interventions increase stroke and improve activity after stroke: A systematic review. Aust J Physiother 52(4):241, 2006.
247. Flansbjer, U, et al: Progressive resistance training after stroke: Effects on muscle strength, muscle tone, gait performance, and perceived participation. J Rehabil Med 40(1):42, 2008.
248. Carr, M, and Jones, J: Physiologic effects of exercise on stroke survivors. Top Stroke Rehabil 9(4):57, 2003.
249. Moreland, JD, et al: Progressive resistance strengthening exercises after stroke: A single-blind randomized controlled trial. Arch Phys Med Rehabil 84(10):1433, 2003.
250. Ouellette, M, et al: High-intensity resistance training improves muscle strength, self-reported function, and disability in long-term stroke survivors. Stroke 35(6):1404, 2004.
251. Weiss, A, et al: High intensity strength training improves strength and functional performance after stroke. Am J Phys Med Rehabil 79(4):369, 2000.
252. Badics, E, et al: Systematic muscle building exercises in the rehabilitation of stroke patients. Neuro Rehab 17(3):211, 2002.
253. Yang, YR, et al: Task-oriented progressive resistance strength training improves muscle strength and functional performance after stroke. Clin Rehabil 20(10):860, 2006.
254. Patten, C, et al: Combined functional task practice and dynamic high intensity resistance training promotes recovery of upper-extremity motor function in post-stroke hemiparesis: A case study. J Neurol Phys Ther 30(3):99, 2006.
255. Kim, CM, et al: Effects of isokinetic strength training on walking in persons with stroke: A double-blind controlled pilot study. J Stroke Cerebrovasc Dis 10(6):265, 2001.
256. Sharp, SA, and Brouwer, BJ: Isokinetic strength training of the hemiparetic knee: Effects on function and spasticity. Arch Phys Med Rehabil 78(11):1231, 1997.
257. Butefisch, C, et al: Repetitive training of isolated movements improves the outcome of motor rehabilitation of the centrally paretic hand. J Neurol Sci 130(1):59, 1995.
258. van Vliet, P, et al: The influence of functional goals on the kinematics of reaching following stroke. J of Neurol Phys Ther 19(1):11, 1995.
259. Carr, J, and Shepherd, R: Stroke Rehabilitation—Guidelines for Exercise and Training to Optimize Motor Skill. Butterworth Heinemann, Elsevier, Philadelphia, PA, 2003.
260. Saposnik, GL, et al: Efficacy and safety of non-immersive virtual reality exercising in stroke rehabilitation (EVREST): A randomised, multicentre, single-blind, controlled trial. Lancet Neurol 15(10): 1019, 2016.
261. Deutsch, JE, et al: Nintendo Wii sports and Wii fit game analysis, validation, and application to stroke rehabilitation. Top Stroke Rehabil 18(6):701, 2011.
262. Levac, D, et al: "Kinect-ing" with clinicians: A knowledge translation resource to support decision making about video game use in rehabilitation. Phys Ther 95(3):426, 2015.
263. Mark, V, and Taub, E: Constraint-induced movement therapy for chronic stroke hemiparesis and other disabilities. Restorative Neurol Neurosci 22(3–5):317, 2002.
264. Morris, D, and Taub, E: Constraint-induced movement therapy. In O'Sullivan, S, and Schmitz, T (eds): Improving Functional Outcomes in Physical Rehabilitation, ed 2. FA Davis, Philadelphia, PA, 2016, p 282.
265. Morris, D, Taub, E, and Mark, V: Constraint-induced movement therapy: Characterizing the intervention protocol. Eura Medicophy 42(3):257, 2006.
266. Page, S, et al: Efficacy of modified constraint-induced movement therapy in chronic stroke: A single-blinded randomized controlled trial. Arch Phys Med Rehabil 85(1):14, 2004.
267. Page, S, and Levine, P: Modified constraint-induced therapy in patients with chronic stroke exhibiting minimal movement ability in the affected arm. Phys Ther 87(7):872, 2007.
268. Bjorklund, A, and Fecht, A: The effectiveness of constraint-induced therapy as a stroke intervention: A meta-analysis. Occup Ther Health Care 20(2):31, 2006.
269. Hakkennes, S, and Keating, JL: Constraint-induced movement therapy following stroke: A systematic review of randomized controlled trials. Aus J Physiother 51(4):221, 2005.
270. Wolf, SL, et al: Effect of constraint-induced movement therapy on upper extremity function 3 to 6 months after stroke: The EXCITE randomized clinical trial. JAMA 296(17):2095, 2006.
271. Schaechter, JD, et al: Motor recovery and cortical reorganization after constraint-induced movement therapy in stroke patients: A preliminary study. Neurorehab Neural Re 16(4): 326, 2002.
272. Richards, L, et al: Limited dose response to constraint-induced movement therapy in patients with chronic stroke. Clin Rehabil 20(12):1066, 2006.
273. Dromerick, A, Edwards, DF, and Hahn, M: Does the applications of constraint-induced movement therapy during acute rehabilitation reduce arm impairment after ischemic stroke? Stroke 31(12):2984, 2000.
274. Jespersen, HF, et al: Shoulder pain after a stroke. Int J Rehabil Res 18(3):273, 1995.
275. Turner-Stokes, L, and Jackson, D: Shoulder pain after stroke: A review of the evidence base to inform the development of an integrated care pathway. Clin Rehabil 16(3):276, 2002.
276. Snels, I, et al: Treating patients with hemiplegic shoulder pain. Am J Phys Med Rehabil 81(2):150, 2002.
277. Daviet, JC, et al: Clinical factors in the prognosis of complex regional pain syndrome type 1 after stroke. Am J Phys Med Rehabil 81(1):34, 2002.
278. Davis, J: The role of the occupational therapist in the treatment of shoulder-hand syndrome. Occup Ther Pract 1(3):30, 1990.
279. Billinger, SA, et al: Physical activity and exercise recommendations for stroke survivors. A statement for healthcare professionals from the American Heart Association/American Stroke Association. Stroke 45(8); 2532, 2014.
280. Cumming, TB, et al: Very early mobilization after stroke fast-tracks return to walking: Further results from the phase II AVERT randomized controlled trial 42(1):153, 2011.
281. Billinger, SA, et al: Does aerobic exercise and the FITT principle fit into stroke recovery? Curr Neurol Neurosci Rep 15(2): 519. 201.
282. Carl, DL, et al: Preliminary safety analysis of high-intensity interval training (HIIT) in persons with chronic stroke. Appl Physiol Nutr Metab 42(3):331, 2017.
283. Boyne, PK, et al: Within-session responses to high-intensity interval training in chronic stroke. Med Sci Sports Exerc 47(3):476, 2015.
284. Boyne, PJ, et al: Factors influencing the efficacy of aerobic exercise for improving fitness and walking capacity after stroke: A meta-analysis with meta-regression. Arch Phys Med Rehabil 98(3):581, 2017.
285. Rose, D, et al: Feasibility and effectiveness of circuit training in acute stroke rehabilitation. Neurorehab Neural Re 25(2):140, 2011.
286. Hendricks, H, et al: Motor recovery after stroke: A systematic review of the literature. Arch Phys Med Rehabil 83(11):1629, 2002.
287. Meijer, R, et al: Prognostic factors for ambulation and activities of daily living in the subacute phase after stroke. A systematic review of the literature. Clin Rehabil 17(2):119, 2003.
288. Studenski, S, et al: Daily functioning and quality of life in a randomized controlled trial of therapeutic exercise for subacute stroke survivors. Stroke 36(8):1764, 2005.
289. Chen, M: Effects of exercise on quality of life in stroke survivors. Stroke 42(3):832, 2011.
290. Ottenbacher, KJ, et al: Trends in length of stay, living setting, functional outcome, and mortality following medical rehabilitation. JAMA 292(14):1687, 2004.
291. Karges, J, and Smallfield, S: A description of outcomes, frequency, duration and intensity of occupational, physical, and speech therapy in inpatient stroke rehabilitation. J Allied Health 38(1):e1, 2009.
292. Van Peppen, RPS, et al: The impact of physical therapy on functional outcomes after stroke: What's the evidence? Clin Rehabil 18(8):833, 2004.
293. Dobkin, V: Rehabilitation after stroke. N Engl J Med 352(16): 1677, 2005.
294. vanWijk, I, et al: Change in mobility activity in the second year after stroke in a rehabilitation population: Who is at risk for decline? Arch Phys Med Rehabil 87(1):45, 2006.

Web-Based Resources for Clinicians, Families, and Patients With Stroke

appendix **15.A**

Resource	Website
American Heart Association	https://www.americanheart.org
American Stroke Association—a division of the American Heart Association	www.strokeassociation.org
National Stroke Association	www.stroke.org
American Stroke Foundation	https://americanstroke.org
World Stroke Organization	https://www.world-stroke.org
Stroke Association—UK	https://www.stroke.org.uk
Heart and Stroke Foundation of Canada	www.heartandstroke.ca
Veterans Affairs—search stroke	https://www.va.gov
Americans with Disabilities Act: ADA home page	https://www.ada.gov
Medicare information	https://www.cms.hhs.gov
Social Security Online	https://www.ssa.gov
National Institute of Neurological Disorders and Stroke	https://www.ninds.nih.gov
National Library of Medicine	https://www.nlm.nih.gov
American Association of Physical Medicine and Rehabilitation	https://www.aapmr.org/about-physiatry/conditions-treatments/rehabilitation-of-central-nervous-system-disorders/stroke
American Academy of Neurology (AAN) home page	https://www.aan.com
AAN's neurology journals	http://www.neurology.org
National Rehabilitation Information Center (NARIC)	https://www.naric.com
Stroke rehab forum at Med Help	https://www.medhelp.org/forums/Stroke/show/62
Rehabilitation Research & Training Center on Stroke Rehabilitation	https://www.sralab.org/research/labs/rehabilitation-research-and-training-center-rrtc
National Aphasia Association	https://www.aphasia.org
National Easter Seals Society	www.easter-seals.org
Disease prevention	https://www.heart.org/en/healthy-living
Agency for Healthcare Research & Quality	https://www.ahrq.gov
Stroke Information Directory	http://www.stroke-info.com
Clinical trials—National Institutes of Health (NIH)—stroke	https://www.clinicaltrials.gov/search/term=stroke
Stroke survivors	www.stroke.org/we-can-help/survivors
Resource center for clinicians and families	https://www.icelearningcenter.com
The Stroke Network, Inc	www.strokenetwork.org
Caregiver Action Network	http://caregiveraction.org
Well Spouse Foundation	https://wellspouse.org
Ability Hub—assistive technology solutions	www.abilityhub.com
ABLEDATA—assistive technology information	https://abledata.acl.gov

Chapter 16

Multiple Sclerosis

Tara L. McIsaac, PT, PhD
Nora E. Fritz, PhD, PT, DPT, NCS
Susan B. O'Sullivan, PT, EdD

LEARNING OBJECTIVES

1. Describe the etiology, epidemiology, pathophysiology, signs and symptoms, diagnosis, and course of multiple sclerosis (MS).
2. Describe elements of the medical management of patients with MS.
3. Identify and describe the examination procedures used to inform the evaluation of patients with MS to establish the physical therapy diagnosis, prognosis, and plan of care.
4. Describe the role of the physical therapist in the management of patients with MS in terms of direct interventions and patient/client-related instruction to maximize function and quality of life.
5. Describe appropriate elements of the exercise prescription for patients with MS.
6. Review current research findings concerning the rehabilitation of patients with MS.
7. Identify the psychosocial impact of MS and describe appropriate interventions.
8. Analyze and interpret patient data, formulate realistic goals and outcomes, and develop a plan of care when presented with a clinical case study.

CHAPTER OUTLINE

Multiple sclerosis (MS) is a progressive autoimmune disease characterized by inflammation, selective demyelination, and gliosis. It causes both acute and chronic symptoms and can result in significant disability and impaired quality of life. MS affects approximately 400,000 persons in the United States; worldwide, MS affects approximately 2.1 million people.[1] It was first defined by Dr. Jean Charcot in 1868 by its clinical and pathological characteristics: paralysis and the cardinal symptoms of intention tremor, scanning speech, and nystagmus, later termed *Charcot's triad*. Using autopsy studies, he identified areas of hardened plaques and termed the disease *sclerosis in plaques*.[2]

The onset of MS typically occurs between ages 20 and 50 years and is uncommon in children. Only 3% to 5% of all individuals with MS have symptoms begin before the age of 16, although cases as young as 2 years have been reported.[3] The onset of symptoms after the age of 50 occurs in approximately 9% of individuals with MS.[4] The disease is more common in women than in men by a ratio of 2:1 to 3:1, but men display a more progressive disease course and more rapid disability.[5] Interestingly, when symptoms occur after age 50, the prevalence is approximately equal for men and women, and approximately half of all individuals experience the progressive form of the disease.[5] Although the incidence and prevalence of MS overall have increased over the past five decades, this increase appears to be mostly related to an increased prevalence in women.[6] There are also ethnic differences. MS affects predominantly white populations. African Americans demonstrate approximately half the risk of acquiring the disease. However,

African Americans tend to experience a more progressive disease course, have more frequent relapses with less recovery, are more likely to have optic nerve and spinal cord involvement, and are more likely to develop greater disability over the same time period than their Caucasian counterparts.[7,8] Low rates of MS are also reported in Asians and Native Americans.[8]

Epidemiological studies have established a geographical pattern of MS prevalence with areas of high, medium, and low frequency. High-frequency areas include the temperate zones of the northern United States, the Scandinavian countries, northern Europe, southern Canada, New Zealand, and southern Australia. Areas of medium frequency closer to the equator include the southern United States and Europe and the rest of Australia, and low-frequency tropical areas include Asia, Africa, and South America. Migration studies indicate that the geographical risk associated with an individual's birthplace is retained if emigration occurs after age 15 years. Individuals migrating before this age assume the risk of their new location.[9,10]

ETIOLOGY

The risk of developing MS in the general population is 0.1%, while the risk of MS is increased in persons with an affected family member. The risk is 2% for a child of a person with MS, 5% for a sibling, or a fraternal co-twin of a person with MS, rising to 25% for an identical co-twin.[3] Genetic studies have revealed more than 100 interacting alleles that may contribute to MS susceptibility with mutations in the human leukocyte antigen major histocompatibility complex (MHC) gene most strongly correlated. It appears that although individuals do not inherit the disease, they may inherit a genetic susceptibility to immune system dysfunction.[11]

When persons with a genetic susceptibility are exposed to a viral agent, the immune system responds with activated myelin-reactive lymphocytes, a concept known as *molecular mimicry*. Implicated viruses in this process under investigation include the Epstein-Barr virus, measles, canine distemper, human herpesvirus-6, and *Chlamydia pneumoniae,* though none have been definitely proven to trigger MS. The viruses may be retained in the body, resulting in a self-perpetuating autoimmune process. Risk of MS may also be increased with vitamin D deficiency and smoking.[11]

PATHOPHYSIOLOGY

In patients with MS, an abnormal immune-mediated response attacks the *myelin* nerve coating, the *oligodendrocytes* (myelin producing cells), and the nerve fibers themselves in the central nervous system (CNS). The response triggers activation of immune cells (e.g., selective activation of helper T cells and killer T cells, with a corresponding decrease in regulatory T cells, and B cell activation) that cross the blood-brain barrier, entering the CNS and initiating a damaging inflammatory cascade of events (the *outside-in model*).[12] Recently the *inside-out model* has been proposed in which oligodendrocyte damage and loss occur first, which then triggers immune attacks and inflammation.[13] Along with inflammation and phagocytic activity of macrophages, mitochondrial damage is thought to contribute to demyelination, oligodendrocyte loss and axonal damage.[1,12] Myelin serves as an insulator, speeding up the conduction along nerve fibers from one node of Ranvier to another (termed *saltatory conduction*). It also serves to conserve energy for the nerve because depolarization occurs only at the nodes. Disruption of the myelin sheath and active demyelination slows neural transmission and causes nerves to fatigue rapidly. With severe disruption, conduction block occurs with resulting disruption of function.

The acute inflammatory attack on myelin gradually subsides, contributing to the pattern of fluctuations in function that characterize this disease (*relapses,* defined as periods of acute worsening of neurological function, and *remissions,* defined as periods without disease progression and partial or complete abatement of signs and symptoms). With repeat attacks, the anti-inflammatory processes become less effective and are unable to keep up. During the early stages of MS, oligodendrocytes survive the initial insult and can produce remyelination. This process is often incomplete and, as the disease becomes more chronic, stalls altogether. When the oligodendrocytes become damaged myelin repair cannot occur. One form of MS, primary-progressive MS in which relapses and remissions do not occur, appears to be closely associated with oligodendrocyte damage and neurodegeneration.[14] Demyelinated areas eventually become filled with fibrous astrocytes and undergo a process called gliosis. Gliosis refers to the proliferation of neuroglial tissue within the CNS and results in glial scars (*plaques*). The axon itself becomes interrupted, undergoes neurodegeneration, and is believed to be the main cause of permanent neurological disability. It has long been thought that MS progresses in a two-stage process: inflammatory damage with associated demyelination and some axonal damage as the first stage; and degenerative changes including axonal and oligodendrocyte destruction as the second stage. Recent studies suggest that rather than two distinct sequential stages, both neuroinflammation and neurodegeneration may occur simultaneously.[15]

In advanced cases of relapsing-remitting MS and earlier in progressive forms of MS, there are both acute and degenerative lesions of varying size scattered throughout the CNS (brain, brainstem, cerebellum, and spinal cord). Lesions primarily affect white matter early, with lesions of gray matter evident in more advanced disease. Lesions may also include small perivascular areas of demyelination and pial surface lesions. Brain atrophy, the loss of axons and myelin throughout the brain, is evident even in early stages of the disease and is progressive.[1] There are certain areas of predilection, such as the optic nerves, periventricular white matter, spinal cord (corticospinal tracts, posterior white columns), and cerebellar peduncles.[1]

DISEASE COURSE

MS is highly variable and unpredictable from person-to-person and within a given individual over time. In 1996, the U.S. National Multiple Sclerosis Society (NMSS) Advisory Council on Clinical Trials in Multiple Sclerosis defined the clinical course descriptions (phenotypes) of multiple sclerosis.[16] The NMSS gave standardized definitions for four MS clinical courses: relapsing-remitting (RR), secondary progressive (SP), primary progressive (PP), and progressive relapsing (PR). These phenotype descriptions were intended to represent the spectrum of MS subtypes, but were based on subjective views of the time and lacked objective biological supports that are now available. These descriptions of MS phenotypes were revised in 2013, maintaining the basic features of the original descriptions, with clarifications and modifications, eliminating the PRMS subtype.[17]

A new disease course was added in the 2013 revisions; *Clinically Isolated Syndrome (CIS)*, not included in the 1996 clinical descriptors, refers to a first episode of inflammatory demyelination in the central nervous system that could become MS if additional activity occurs. CIS can be further characterized as *not active* (no clinical relapses or new MRI activity) or *active* (with relapses and/or evidence of new MRI activity) in which case it becomes relapsing-remitting MS. *Relapsing-remitting MS (RRMS)* is the most common course, affecting approximately 85% of patients with MS. It is characterized by discrete attacks or relapses followed by remissions and can also be further characterized as *active* or *not active*. Most people diagnosed with RRMS will eventually transition to *secondary-progressive MS (SPMS)*. SPMS begins with a relapsing-remitting course followed by progression to steady and irreversible worsening of neurologic function and accumulation of disability. As with CIS and RRMS, SPMS can be further characterized as either *active* or *not active* but is also characterized as *with progression* (evidence of disease worsening on an objective measure of change over time, with or without relapses) or *without progression*, referring to progressive accumulation of disability. *Primary-progressive MS (PPMS)* is a less common form occurring in about 15% of cases. It is characterized by a nearly continuous worsening of the disease from the onset without distinct attacks and is further characterized as *active* or *not active* and as *with progression* or *without progression*. Because the course of the disease may alter (RRMS to SPMS), clinicians need to be alert to changes in signs or symptoms in terms of severity, frequency, and impact on function.[1,17] The 1996 category of progressive-relapsing MS is eliminated since these patients are now classified as PPMS with disease activity. Box 16.1 summarizes the 1996 disease-course definitions and the 2013 revisions of disease-course (or clinical subtype) of multiple sclerosis.

Box 16.1 Four Major Clinical Subtypes of MS[17]

1996 MS Clinical Description Subtypes	2013 MS Disease Modifiers Phenotypes
	Clinically Isolated Syndrome (CIS) • Not Active • Active
• **Relapsing-Remitting Disease (RRMS)** • With full recovery from relapses • With sequelae/residual deficit after incomplete recovery	• **Relapsing-Remitting Disease (RRMS)** • Not Active • Active
Progressive Disease • **Primary-Progressive (PPMS)** • Progressive accumulation of disability from onset with or without temporary plateaus, minor remissions and improvements	*Progressive Disease* • **Primary-Progressive (PPMS)** • Progressive accumulation of disability from onset • Active and with progression • Active but without progression • Not active but with progression • Not active and without progression (stable disease)
• **Secondary-Progressive (SPMS)** • Progressive accumulation of disability after initial relapsing course, with or without occasional relapses and minor remissions	• **Secondary-Progressive (SPMS)** • Progressive accumulation of disability after initial relapsing course • Active and with progression • Active but without progression • Not active but with progression • Not active and without progression (stable disease)
• **Progressive-Relapsing (PRMS)** • Progressive accumulation of disability from onset, but clear acute clinical attacks, with or without full recovery.	

Exacerbating Factors

MS relapses (*exacerbations*) are defined by new and recurrent MS symptoms lasting more than 24 hours but generally of longer duration that are unrelated to another etiology. Several exacerbating factors have been identified. Avoiding these factors is important in ensuring the patient's optimal function. An individual whose overall health deteriorates is more likely to have a relapse than one who remains healthy. Viral or bacterial infections (e.g., common cold, influenza, urinary tract infection, sinus infection) and diseases of major organ systems (e.g., hepatitis, pancreatitis, asthma attacks) are associated with relapses of disease. There is also a modest link between stress and acute attacks. Both major stresses (divorce, death, job loss, trauma) and minor stresses (exhaustion, dehydration, malnutrition, and sleep deprivation) can affect the immune system and an already compromised nervous system.

Pseudoexacerbation refers to the temporary worsening of MS symptoms. The episode typically comes and goes quickly, usually within 24 hours. The overwhelming majority of individuals with MS demonstrate an adverse reaction to heat, known as *Uthoff's symptom*. Anything that raises the body temperature can bring on a pseudoattack. External heat stressors include sun exposure, hot muggy environmental temperatures, or a hot bath. Internal elevations in temperature can be produced by fever or prolonged exercise; however, studies indicate exercise is a safe and essential component of health for individuals with MS.[18] The effects are usually immediate and dramatic in terms of reduced function and increased fatigue. Most pseudoattacks resolve within 24 hours of cooling off and/or the end of a fever.

■ SYMPTOMS

Symptoms of MS vary considerably, depending on the location of specific lesions within the central nervous system. Early symptoms typically include minor visual disturbances (e.g., episodes of double vision) and paresthesias progressing to numbness, weakness, and fatigability. In more advanced stages, patients demonstrate multiple symptoms with varying involvement. Common MS symptoms are presented in Box 16.2.[19,20] The onset of symptoms can develop rapidly over a course of minutes or hours; less frequently, onset is insidious, occurring over a period of weeks or months. An early remission may lead the individual to postpone initial neurological workup for months or longer.

Sensory

Complete loss of any single sensation (anesthesia) is rare. Focal deficits can produce limited areas of diminished sensation. Altered sensations are far more common and can include *paresthesias* (pins-and-needles sensation) or numbness of the face, body, or extremities. Disturbances in position sense are also common, as are lower extremity (LE) impairments of vibratory sense.[20]

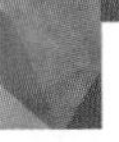

Box 16.2 Common Symptoms in Multiple Sclerosis

Sensory Symptoms
- Hypoesthesia, numbness
- Paresthesias

Pain
- Paroxysmal limb pain, dysesthesias
- Headache
- Optic or trigeminal neuritis
- Lhermitte's sign
- Hyperpathia
- Chronic neuropathic pain

Visual Symptoms
- Blurred or double vision (diplopia)
- Diminished acuity/loss of vision
- Scotoma
- Nystagmus
- Lateral gaze palsy

Cognitive Symptoms
- Short-term memory deficits
- Difficulty performing multiple tasks simultaneously
- Diminished attention, concentration
- Diminished executive functions
- Diminished information processing
- Diminished visual–spatial abilities

Affective Symptoms
- Depression
- Anxiety
- Pseudobulbar affect

Motor Symptoms
- Paresis or paralysis
- Fatigue
- Spasticity, spasms
- Ataxia: incoordination, intention tremor
- postural tremor
- Impaired balance and gait

Speech and Swallowing
- Dysarthria
- Diminished verbal fluency
- Dysphonia
- Dysphagia

Bladder and Bowel Symptoms
- Spastic bladder
- Flaccid bladder
- Dyssynergic bladder
- Constipation
- Diarrhea and incontinence

Sexual Symptoms
- Impotence
- Decreased libido
- Impaired ability to achieve orgasm

Pattern of Symptoms
- Varies greatly from person to person
- Varies over time in each individual affected
- First symptoms usually transient; typically sensory and/or visual
- Diagnosis involves evidence of damage occurring in at least two separate areas of CNS and at two separate points in time at least one month apart (*dissemination of lesions in space and time*)

CNS = central nervous system.

Pain

Approximately 80% of patients with MS experience pain, with clinically significant pain occurring in about 55% of individuals and almost half experience chronic pain.[21] Patients often experience acute, paroxysmal pain characterized by sudden and spontaneous onset. The pains are described as intense, sharp, shooting, electric shock–like, and burning. The most common types are trigeminal neuralgia, paroxysmal limb pain, and headache. *Trigeminal neuralgia* (tic douloureux) results from demyelination of the sensory division of the trigeminal nerve innervating the face, cheek, and jaw. Eating, shaving, or simply touching the face may trigger painful episodes. A common sign of posterior column damage in the spinal cord is Lhermitte's sign in which flexion of the neck produces an electric shock–like sensation running down the spine and into the LEs. Paroxysmal limb pain presents as abnormal burning, aching pain (*dysesthesias*) that can affect any part of the body but is more common in the LEs. It is the most common type of pain in MS and is often worse at night and after exercise. It can be aggravated by temperature elevations. *Hyperpathia,* a hypersensitivity to minor sensory stimuli, can occur. For example, a light touch or light pressure stimulus elicits a severe pain reaction. Headache is more frequent in MS than in the general population and can be migraine or tension type. Chronic *neuropathic pain* can result from demyelinating lesions in spinothalamic tracts or in the sensory roots. It is more common in patients with minimum disability and is described as a burning, aching, "pins and needles" pain similar to pain described by individuals with disk herniation. Musculoskeletal pain associated with muscle and ligament strain can develop from mechanical stress, abnormal postures, and immobility, often the result of weak muscles, powerful spasticity, and tonic spasms. Anxiety and fear can worsen pain symptoms.[21]

Visual

Visual symptoms are common with MS and are found in approximately 80% of patients. Involvement of the optic nerve produces altered visual acuity; blindness is rare. *Optic neuritis,* inflammation of the optic nerve, is a common problem, and produces an icepick-like pain behind the eye with blurring or graying of vision or blindness in one eye. A *scotoma* or dark spot may occur in the center of the visual field. Neuritis rarely affects both eyes and is usually self-limiting. Vision generally improves within 4 to 12 weeks. Damage to the optic nerve will also affect light reflexes. Relative afferent pupillary defect (RAPD) (*Marcus Gunn pupil*) often develops in individuals with MS who have had an episode of optic neuritis. Shining a bright light into the healthy eye will produce reflex contraction in both eyes (consensual light reflex). If the light is then shone in the affected eye only, a paradoxical widening (dilation) of both pupils occurs.

Eye movements can be disturbed in a variety of ways. *Nystagmus* is common in patients with MS and results from lesions affecting the cerebellum or central vestibular pathways. This involves involuntary and rapid cyclical movements of the eyeball (horizontal or vertical) that develop when the patient looks to the sides or vertically (gaze-induced nystagmus) or when the patient moves the head. *Internuclear ophthalmoplegia* (INO) produces incomplete eye adduction (lateral gaze palsy) on the affected side and nystagmus of the opposite abducting eye with gaze to one side. It is caused by demyelination of the pontine medial longitudinal fasciculus (MLF). Additional impairments in conjugate gaze and control of eye movements may also be present with brainstem lesions affecting cranial nerves III, IV, and VI or the MLF. *Diplopia,* double vision, occurs when the muscles that control the eyes are not well coordinated. Visual disturbances frequently remit and are seldom the primary cause of disability. The effects of impaired vision on balance and movement should be carefully examined.[22]

Motor

Patients with corticospinal lesions demonstrate signs and symptoms of upper motor neuron (UMN) syndrome. Paresis, spasticity, brisk tendon reflexes, involuntary flexor and extensor spasms, clonus, Babinski's sign, exaggerated cutaneous reflexes, and loss of precise autonomic control all characterize UMN involvement. (See discussion in Chapter 5, Examination of Motor Function: Motor Control and Motor Learning.)

Weakness

Patients with UMN syndrome demonstrate movements that are slow, stiff, and weak, the result of loss of orderly recruitment and reduced firing rate modulation of motor neurons. Reduced muscle strength, power, and endurance, along with impaired synergistic relationships, are evident. Patients with cerebellar lesions demonstrate asthenia or generalized muscle weakness along with ataxia. Patients can also experience muscle weakness secondary to inactivity. Muscle weakness can vary from a mild paresis, often transient at first, to total paralysis of the involved extremities.[20]

Spasticity

Spasticity is an extremely common problem in patients with MS; spasticity can range from mild to severe, depending on the duration of the disease, number of relapses, and worsening symptoms in recent months. It occurs in the muscles of the upper extremities (UEs) and particularly the LEs. Clinical indications of spasticity include impaired voluntary control of movement (abnormal co-contraction); increased deep tendon reflexes (DTRs); clonus; and decreased range of motion (ROM). Spasticity also results in increased fatigue, impaired functional mobility, and impaired activities of daily living (ADL). Spasticity can cause pain, disabling contractures, abnormal posturing, problems in maintaining skin integrity, and falls. For some patients, spasticity can be beneficial to sitting and standing,[23] acting to support weak musculature. Spasticity fluctuates on a daily basis and can be exacerbated by certain factors, such as fatigue, stress, overheating (fever, environmental), cold temperatures, infections, or noxious stimuli (e.g., pain, bladder, renal, bowel, skin lesions/injury).[23] Certain antidepressant agents (serotonin-reuptake inhibitors such as fluoxetine, sertraline, and paroxetine) can exacerbate spasticity. Spasticity does not typically abate during spontaneous remissions. In patients with advanced disease, spasticity can be quite disabling and difficult to manage.[23]

Fatigue

Fatigue is a frequent and often disabling symptom of MS. The definition of fatigue differs widely among patients, physicians, and researchers; typically reported by patients as feelings of overwhelming tiredness, exhaustion, and weakness together with difficulty concentrating and mental dullness.[24] Fatigue in MS may onset abruptly without warning and typically worsens throughout the day. A large majority of patients report that fatigue is one of their most troubling symptoms and consistently report that fatigue interferes with physical functioning, overall role performance, social participation, and perceived health status.[24] Despite its prevalence, the pathophysiology of fatigue in MS is still not completely understood. A recently proposed definition and model of fatigue is "the decrease in physical and/or mental performance that results from changes in central, psychological, and/or peripheral factors."[25] These changes depend on the task being performed, the environment, and the individual's mental and physical capacity.[25] Central factors contributing to fatigue in MS include inflammation, axonal conduction velocity, imbalance of neurotransmitter levels, and decreased cerebral glucose metabolism. Psychological factors include perceived effort, self-efficacy, motivation, and cognitive impairment. Peripheral factors of fatigue in MS involve slowed contractile properties and decreased metabolic response of muscles.[25] A patient's level of fatigue can be influenced by physical exertion, exposure to heat and humidity, disturbed or reduced sleep, depression, anxiety, cognitive impairment, and medical conditions (e.g., respiratory infection). Side effects of medications also affect fatigue, including analgesics, anticonvulsants, antidepressants, antihistamines, antihypertensive agents, and anti-inflammatory agents.[26]

Coordination and Balance

Demyelinating lesions in the cerebellum and cerebellar tracts are common in MS, producing cerebellar symptoms. Clinical manifestations include ataxia, postural and intention tremors, hypotonia, and truncal weakness. Ataxia is a general term used to describe uncoordinated movements characterized by dysmetria, dyssynergia, and dysdiadochokinesia. Progressive ataxia of the trunk and LEs is often apparent. During sitting or standing, when a limb or the body must be supported against gravity, the patient typically presents with *postural tremor* (shaking, back-and-forth oscillatory movements). *Intention (action) tremors* are involuntary, rhythmic, shaking movements that occur when purposeful movement is attempted and results from the inability of the cerebellum to dampen motor movements (see Chapter 6, Examination of Coordination and Balance). Tremors vary in severity from slight, barely perceptible quivering (fine tremor) to wide oscillations (gross tremors). Severe tremors impose significant limitations in performance of functional activities, particularly in such areas as eating, speaking clearly, writing, personal hygiene, and walking. Tremor can be exacerbated by stress, excitement, and anxiety, all adrenalin-releasing conditions producing a temporary aroused condition.[20] Severe numbness of the feet can contribute to difficulty with standing balance or walking (sensory ataxia).

Lesions affecting the cerebellum or central vestibular pathways can produce vestibular dysfunction. Patients may experience symptoms of dizziness, disequilibrium, vertigo, and nausea. Symptoms are precipitated or made worse by movements of the head or eyes (see Chapter 21, Vestibular Disorders).

Gait and Mobility

Individuals with MS experience difficulty walking as a result of muscle weakness, fatigue, spasticity, impaired balance, impaired sensation, visual problems, and ataxia. Approximately half of patients with RRMS will require some form of assistance during walking within 15 years of their diagnosis. Weakness in one or both LEs may result in asymmetric step lengths and increased variability of gait, while severe LE extensor spasticity may produce a scissoring gait pattern. Staggering, uneven steps, poor foot placement, uncoordinated limb movements, and frequent loss of balance characterize ataxic gait. It is often mistaken for drunkenness, a finding that frequently results in the patient revealing the disease for the first time. Gait and balance impairments increase the risk of falls and fall injury. Approximately half of patients with MS report recent falls. Fear of falling is associated with self-imposed restrictions in mobility and contributes to disability and social isolation.[19] Safe and goal-oriented walking requires higher-level cognitive processing, highlighting the strong relationship between cognitive function and gait.[27] Deficits in both walking and cognitive function are common in MS. These impairments are compounded when performing walking and cognitive tasks simultaneously (dual-tasking), referred to as *cognitive-motor interference* (CMI). While walking performance declines in people with MS as a result of CMI, a recent systematic review and meta-analysis of 13 studies found only minimal difference in the CMI between individuals with and without MS.[28]

Speech and Swallowing

Speech problems are the result of muscle weakness, spasticity, tremor, or ataxia. As many as 44% of individuals with MS experience impairment of speech or voice after disease onset.[29] Dysarthria is characterized by slurred or poorly articulated speech with low volume, unnatural emphasis, and slow rate. Dysphonia is characterized by changes in vocal quality including harshness, hoarseness, breathiness, or hypernasal sounds. Poor coordination of the tongue, oral, and pharyngeal muscles can also result in dysphagia, difficulty in swallowing. Signs of swallowing dysfunction include difficulty chewing and maintaining a lip seal, inability to swallow (ingest food), and spitting or coughing or throat clearing during or after meals. Aspiration pneumonia is a serious complication that can develop if foods or liquids are inhaled into the trachea. Signs of aspiration include coughing or throat clearing after intake, a wet voice quality with gurgling or sounds of congestion, and fever. The patient is also at risk for poor nutritional intake and dehydration and may experience weight loss. Poor coordination of breath control and posture contributes to speech and feeding difficulties.[30]

Cognitive

Cognitive impairment is common in MS and may appear in either early or later stages of the disease, with prevalence rates of up to 70%.[31] Multiple aspects of cognition are impacted by MS, most commonly in decreased information processing speed.[32] Other deficits in selective cognitive domains include impaired attention and concentration, executive functioning (concept formation, abstract reasoning, problem solving, planning, and sequencing), visuospatial functions, verbal fluency, and working memory.[31-34] Overall intellectual functioning, long-term memory, conversational skills, and reading comprehension are typically intact. Cognitive impairments are related to the specific locations and total volume of the lesions, cerebral atrophy, third ventricle width, and corpus callosum size.[31,33] With increasing lesion load over time, neuroplastic changes occur to compensate and maintain cognitive function, but eventually are ineffective.[31] Cognitive function is not associated with overall severity of the disease, its course, or the patient's disability status. Focal frontal lobe lesions can produce cognitive inflexibility and poor impulse control. Secondary factors that can influence cognition include depression, anxiety, fatigue, medications, and comorbid conditions (e.g., cardiovascular or cerebrovascular disease).[34,35] Level of cognitive dysfunction is a major factor in determining quality of life, social functioning, employment status, and function.[1,34]

Depression

Depression is a common symptom of MS; indeed major depressive disorder, the most severe form, occurs in up to 50% of individuals.[35] The age-standardized incidence of depression is 71% higher and prevalence is roughly 10% higher than in the matched population.[36,37] Inflammation may be a contributing factor to depression in MS, as individuals with other neuroinflammatory diseases, such as inflammatory bowel disease and rheumatoid arthritis also experience depression at similar rates to individuals with MS.[38] Depressive symptoms can include feelings of hopelessness or despair, diminished interest or pleasure in activities, changes in appetite and significant weight loss or gain, insomnia or hypersomnia (daytime sleepiness), feelings of lethargy or worthlessness, fatigue or loss of energy, decreased concentration, and recurrent thoughts of death and suicide.[35] Depression can occur from a complex interaction of pathological processes in MS, a pre-existing or predisposition to a mood disorder as a side effect of some drugs (e.g., corticosteroids, interferon), as a psychological reaction to the stresses of this far-reaching and unpredictable disease, and normal grieving of the losses associated with MS.[35] Other mood disorders also occur more frequently in MS; the prevalence of anxiety disorders is up to 36%, adjustment disorder is up to 22%, and bipolar disorder (alternating periods of depression and mania) is up to 13%.[35,37] Denial, anger, aggression, and substance abuse can also occur. Patients with MS face enormous issues related to the ambiguity of their health status, the unpredictable course of disease activity, unpredictable future status, and the loss of effective functioning during the prime of their lives.

Emotional

Affective disorders in MS occur as a direct result from effects of the disease on the brain and can include changes in mood, feelings, emotional expression, and control. Pseudobulbar affect (PBA), also known as *involuntary emotional expression disorder* or *emotional incontinence,* occurs in about 10% of people with MS and is characterized by sudden and unpredictable episodes of crying, laughing, or other emotional displays.[35,39] PBA may occur when the disease damages the area of the brain that controls normal expression of emotion, including the limbic system and paralimbic networks.[39] Euphoria is an exaggerated feeling of well-being, a sense of optimism incongruent with the patient's incapacitating disability, which is less common and can occur in more advanced MS or with significant cognitive changes.[40,41] Apathy is the lack of motivation affecting cognitive, emotional and behavioral domains, which occurs in MS with a prevalence of up to 40% and is correlated to more severe cognitive dysfunction.[41,42]

Bladder

Urinary bladder dysfunction occurs in about 80% of patients. Demyelinating lesions affecting the lateral and posterior spinal tracts unmask the sacral reflex arc producing loss in volitional and synergistic control of the micturition reflex. Types of bladder dysfunction in MS can include a small, spastic bladder (a failure to store problem), a flaccid or big bladder (a failure to empty problem), or a dyssynergic bladder. The dyssynergic bladder represents a problem with coordination between the bladder contraction and sphincter relaxation. Common symptoms include urinary urgency, urinary frequency, hesitancy in starting urination, nocturia (frequency at night), dribbling, and incontinence. The severity of bladder symptoms is associated with severity of other neurological symptoms, particularly pyramidal tract involvement. Progressive loss of functional mobility (e.g., hand skills, sitting balance and transfer skills, ambulation) contributes to personal hygiene problems, emotional distress, and functional incontinence (inability to toilet or manage dysfunction). Emptying dysfunction with large residual urine volume increases the risk of recurrent urinary tract infections (UTIs) and kidney damage from frequent UTIs.[43]

Bowel

Constipation is the most common bowel complaint in MS and results from lesions affecting control of the gastrocolic reflex. It is associated with the presence of spasticity of the pelvic floor muscles and is also a frequent consequence of inactivity, lack of fluid intake, poor diet and bowel habits, depression, and medication side effects. Bowel impaction is a serious complication that requires immediate attention. Diarrhea and incontinence are less problematic but can also occur as a result of loss of rectal control, sphincter abnormalities, or other, secondary problems (e.g., gastroenteritis, inflammatory bowel disease, medication side effect).[44]

Sexual

Sexual dysfunction is common, affecting as many as 91% of men and 72% of women. In women, symptoms can include changes in sensation, vaginal dryness, trouble reaching orgasm, and loss of libido. In men, symptoms can include erectile dysfunction, decreased sensation, difficulty or inability to ejaculate, and loss of libido. Sexual activity is also affected by the appearance of other symptoms such as spasticity, uncontrollable spasms, pain, weakness and fatigue, bladder or bowel incontinence, losses in functional mobility, and changes in self-image. Psychological factors have a large impact on function. Sexual dysfunction has tremendous functional and psychosocial implications for both patient and partner.[45]

■ DIAGNOSIS

The early and accurate diagnosis of MS is important to take advantage of the recent advances in effective medication treatments for relapsing-remitting MS. Misdiagnosis or delayed diagnosis is not uncommon because the initial presentation of MS is highly variable and patients can present to a wide range of health care professionals.[46] There is no definitive diagnostic test for MS, rather a diagnosis of exclusion that is made by a neurologist based on a careful medical history, a complete neurological examination, and supportive laboratory tests. Diagnosis of MS relies on two key features determined from evidence of lesions seen on MRI: dissemination in space (*DIS*) and dissemination in time (*DIT*). Dissemination in space can be satisfied by at least one T2-weighted MRI lesion seen in two of the four MS typical areas of the CNS: periventricular, juxtacortical, infratentorial, or spinal cord. Dissemination in time can be satisfied by a single scan in a patient with a clinically silent contrast-enhancing (gadolinium) lesion and another clinically silent T2-weighted (non-enhancing) lesion at any time. Alternatively, any new T2 lesion seen after the original scan can fulfil dissemination in time.[47] The revised 2010 *McDonald Criteria of the International Panel on Diagnosis of MS* has resulted in earlier diagnosis of MS with improved specificity and sensitivity (TipSheet is available at www.nationalmssociety.org/).[47,48] In addition, other possible diagnoses that mimic MS must be ruled out. The mnemonic VITAMINS is helpful in ruling out the many diseases/disorders of Vascular, Infectious, Traumatic, Autoimmune, Metabolic/toxic, Ideopathic/genetic, Neoplastic, and Psychiatric origin that can mimic MS.[1,49] Among the common differential diagnoses are *acute disseminating encephalomyelitis* (*ADEM*), acute and subacute *transverse myelitis*, and *neuromyelitis optica* spectrum disorders (*NMO*).[50]

Laboratory tests used to help confirm the diagnosis include magnetic resonance imaging (MRI), evoked potentials (EP), and lumbar puncture (LP) with cerebrospinal fluid (CSF) analysis. MRI is highly sensitive for detecting MS plaques/lesions in the white matter of the brain and spinal cord (Fig. 16.1). The Consortium of Multiple Sclerosis Centers recently revised their guidelines for diagnostic and follow-up standardized MRI protocol.[51] A brain MRI with gadolinium (GAD) is recommended for the diagnosis of MS, because it is specifically used to see vascular structures and breakdown in the blood-brain barrier. Most new lesions are characterized by an area of GAD enhancement seen as areas of signal hyperintensity, "bright spots," often ovoid and arranged at right angles to the corpus callosum as if radiating from this area. When seen in sagittal view, they are referred to as *Dawson's Fingers*, which are relatively specific to MS and may help differentiate from other conditions, such as NMO (Fig. 16.1).[52] A spinal cord MRI is additionally recommended if the brain MRI is nondiagnostic or if the presenting symptoms are at the level of the spinal cord. Follow-up MRIs with GAD are recommended to demonstrate dissemination in time and ongoing disease activity that is "clinically silent" (active lesion without correlated clinical signs) while on medication treatment. In addition, follow-up MRIs should be done to evaluate unexpected clinical worsening and as a new baseline prior to starting or modifying medications, with routine brain MRIs every 6 months to 2 years for all patients with relapsing MS.[51] MS lesions that appear as hypointense areas on T1-weighted MRIs, "black holes," are thought to indicate axonal loss, tissue destruction, and neurodegeneration.[53,54] Most patients with

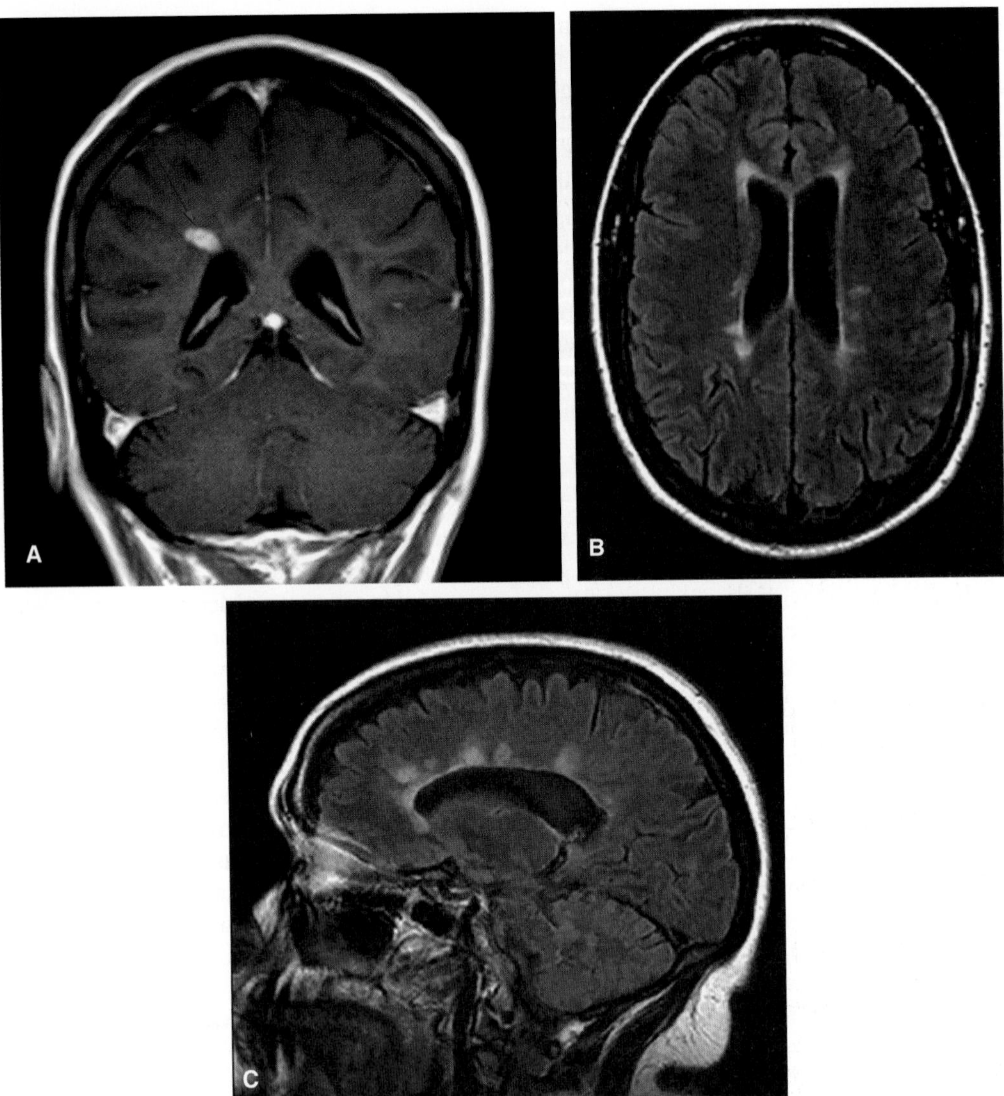

Figure 16.1 (A) Coronal contrast-enhanced T1 MRI. The contrast enhancement of a periventricular white matter lesion (arrow) indicates that this is an active MS plaque. Other (older) plaques in this case that were T2 hyperintense showed no enhancement. *(From Weber et al[54] with permission.)* (B) Axial and (C) Sagittal T2-weighted MRI demonstrating common periventricular lesional pattern in persons with MS *(From Raz et al[52] with permission).* The pattern seen in (C) is known as Dawson's Fingers, and indicates demyelinating plaques through the corpus callosum; this pattern of T2 hyperintensities is relatively specific to MS and may help in the differentiation between MS and other demyelinating conditions, such as NMO.[52]

clinically defined MS have well-defined MRI changes; however 5% of individuals with clinically defined MS do not exhibit MRI changes. Lesions seen on MRI in "silent" areas of the brain that don't cause symptoms make it difficult to correlate the MRI findings of lesion load and the individual's clinical signs and symptoms, called the clinical-radiological paradox.[55] Additionally, some healthy individuals can exhibit bright spots on MRI.[1,56]

Up to 90% of individuals with MS demonstrate abnormal EP. The presence of demyelinating lesions on visual, auditory, and somatosensory pathways produces slowed central conduction. Of the three, visual evoked potentials (VEPs) have been found to be the most helpful in the diagnostic process.[50]

Patients with MS show elevated total immunoglobulin (IgG) in CSF and the presence of oligoclonal IgG bands in response to inflammatory demyelinating lesions. Patients with PPMS have higher levels of immunoglobulins in spinal fluid than patients with RRMS.[50]

MEDICAL MANAGEMENT

A number of medications are used to help treat and prevent relapses and slow the progression of neurological disability. Medications are also given to provide symptom relief.

Management of Acute Relapses

Corticosteroid therapy (methylprednisolone) is used to treat acute disease relapses (exacerbations), shortening the duration of the episode. These drugs exert powerful anti-inflammatory and immunosuppressive effects, including diminished swelling within the CNS, decreased T-cell activation, limited immune cell penetration of the CNS, and enhanced apoptosis of activated immune cells. The drugs do not modify the disease course or degree of recovery. Typically, corticosteroids are given in high doses (500 to 1,000 mg/day), administered intravenously for a brief course (e.g., 3 to 5 days), followed by tapered dosage of oral medication over a period of 1 to 3 weeks. There are a number of potential adverse side effects, including mood changes, increased blood pressure, fluid retention, hyperglycemia, acne, and insomnia. Chronic use is associated with hypertension, diabetes, aseptic femoral necrosis, osteopenia, and peptic ulcer.[15]

Plasmapheresis (plasma exchange) may be used to enhance recovery from an acute relapse in patients who fail to respond to steroids. It is used for an exacerbation of RRMS and is not recommended for PPMS or SPMS.

Disease-Modifying Therapeutic Agents

Since 1993 the U.S. Food and Drug Administration (FDA) has approved drugs to reduce disease activity in people with MS. The goal of these drugs is to prevent future disease activity, rather than to return function that has been lost. The Multiple Sclerosis Coalition developed a consensus paper in 2014 and updated in 2016, summarizing current evidence about disease modification in MS and providing support for access to disease-modifying therapies (DMT) for people with MS in the United States.[15] The consensus paper identified four important themes from the evidence in DMTs in MS: (1) early and successful control of disease activity is important for reducing the accumulation of disability, helping individuals with MS to stay active, and protecting quality of life; (2) early disease activity and progression result in physical impairments as only one aspect of disability; (3) prognosis is variable and unpredictable among individuals; and (4) treatment adherence is important to efficacy and barriers to adherence should be identified and addressed early. The 14 DMTs that have been approved by the U.S. Food and Drug Administration (FDA) through July 2016 are listed in Table 16.1. Synthetic interferon drugs (interferon beta 1a [Avonex® and Rebif®]) interferon beta-1b [Betaseron®, Extavia®], and peginterferon beta 1a [Plegridy®]) are first-line injectable drugs that have substantial immunomodulating properties. These are close copies of a naturally occurring human chemical, interferon beta. Interferons slow down the immune system response by reducing inflammation, swelling, and rapid proliferation of T and B cells. They also block activated T cells from crossing the blood-brain barrier. Other disease-modifying drugs include daclizumab (Zinbryta™), glatiramer acetate (Copaxone®, Glatopa™), dimethyl fumarate (Tecfidera®), fingolimod (Gilenya®), teriflunomide (Aubagio®), alemtuzumab (Lemtrada®), mitoxantrone (Novantrone®), and natalizumab (Tysabri®). A promising agent for treating primary progressive MS is ocrelizumab (Ocrevus®), a monoclonal antibody that binds to a molecule on the surface of B cells and depletes them from circulation.[57] Patients may show reduced relapses, reduced number of new lesions on MRI, and reduced severity of attack as evidenced by acquired neurological deficits. For patients with new and suspected MS (clinical isolated syndrome [CIS]), the medications may delay time to a second clinical episode and a confirmed diagnosis of MS. Continued, frequent relapses or excessive MRI activity may indicate the need to switch drug therapy to higher doses or combination therapies. These agents cannot, however, reverse existing deficits. All of these medications are contraindicated for women who are pregnant or trying to become pregnant, or who are breastfeeding.[15]

Common adverse effects of the injectable interferon drugs include injection-site skin reactions (soreness, redness, pain, bruising, or swelling) and flu-like symptoms following injection that lessen over time (fever, chills, sweating, muscle aches, and fatigue). Injection sites are varied to reduce adverse effects. Rare and more severe adverse reactions include depression, allergic reactions, and liver reactions. Copaxone® can produce similar injection-site reactions and an initial flushing reaction immediately after injection (anxiety, chest pain, palpitations, shortness of breath). It has the advantage of not causing flu-like symptoms or depression.

Patients receive Novantrone® by intravenous (IV) infusion in a medical facility and must be closely monitored for serious heart and liver damage. Tysabri® poses serious risks for a rare brain infection (progressive multifocal leukoencephalopathy [PML]). Following the first dose of Gilenya®, patients must be monitored for changes in heart and pulmonary function. An additional disadvantage is the significant annual cost of these drugs (in the thousands or tens of thousands of dollars) that may not be covered fully by private insurance plans.[15]

Problems with adherence using immunomodulating agents are well documented, especially for the injectable medications.[15] Health professionals can have a significant impact on promoting acceptance and maintenance of immunomodulating therapy. In discussions with the patient, the therapist needs to determine the patient's understanding of the treatment benefits and risks, perception of his or her illness, general mood and level of self-esteem, lifestyle and daily living situation, and level of family and community support. Professionals need to support the patient's hope for a positive outcome from drug therapy and emphasize the benefits of early treatment and the importance of consistency in management.[15]

Table 16.1 Disease-Modifying Therapeutic Agents for MS[15]

Agent	FDA-Approved Indications	Select Side Effects	Contraindications/ Boxed Warning	Delivery System and Frequency
daclizumab (Zinbryta™)	Relapsing forms of MS, generally for patients who have had an inadequate response to two or more MS therapies	• nasopharyngitis • upper respiratory tract infection • rash • depression • increased liver enzymes • influenza • dermatitis	• hepatic injury and other immune-mediated disorders • depression and suicide	Injection, monthly
glatiramer acetate (Copaxone®) (and therapeutic equivalent Glatopa™)	Relapsing forms of MS	• injection site reactions • lipoatrophy • vasodilation, rash, dyspnea • chest pain	• immediate post-injection reactions • lipoatrophy & skin necrosis • potential effects on immune response	SC injection, every day or 3 times weekly
interferon beta-1a (Avonex®)	Relapsing forms of MS	• flu-like symptoms • depression • increased liver enzymes	• depression, suicide • hepatic injury • anaphylaxis • CHF • seizures	IM injection, weekly
interferon beta-1a (Rebif®)	Relapsing forms of MS	• flu-like symptoms • depression • increased liver enzymes • abdominal pain • hematologic abnormalities	• depression, suicide • hepatic injury • anaphylaxis • seizures • injection site necrosis	SC injection, 3 times weekly
interferon beta-1b (Betaseron®), (Extavia®)	Relapsing forms of MS	• flu-like symptoms • injection site reactions • depression • increased liver enzymes • decreased white blood cells	• depression, suicide • hepatic injury • anaphylaxis • seizures • injection site necrosis • CHF	SC injections, every other day
peginterferon beta-1a (Plegridy®)	Relapsing forms of MS	• flu-like symptoms • injection site reactions • depression • increased liver enzymes • decreased white blood cells	• depression, suicide • hepatic injury • anaphylaxis • seizures • injection site necrosis • CHF	SC injections, every 2 weeks
dimethyl fumarate (Tecfidera®)	Relapsing forms of MS	• flushing • GI symptoms • rash	• PML • anaphylaxis • flushing • lymphopenia	Oral, twice daily capsule
fingolimod (Gilenya®)	Relapsing forms of MS	• bradycardia on first dose • headache • influenza • diarrhea • back pain • increased liver enzymes	• bradyarrhythmia • infection risk • PML and other encephalopathies • decreased pulmonary function tests	Oral, once daily capsule

Table 16.1 Disease-Modifying Therapeutic Agents for MS[15]—cont'd

Agent	FDA-Approved Indications	Select Side Effects	Contraindications/ Boxed Warning	Delivery System and Frequency
		• macular edema • lymphopenia • bronchitis	• hepatic injury • contraindicated for recent MI, unstable angina, stroke, TIA	
teriflunomide (Aubagio®)	Relapsing forms of MS	• increased liver enzymes • alopecia • diarrhea • influenza • nausea • paresthesia	• hepatotoxicity and risk of teratogenicity	Oral, once daily capsule
alemtuzumab (Lemtrada®)	Relapsing forms of MS, generally for patients who have had an inadequate response to two or more MS therapies	• infusion reactions: • rash • fever • headache • anaphylaxis • cardiac arrhythmias • urinary tract infection • upper respiratory infection • diarrhea • paresthesia • dizziness • nausea	• Because of the risk of autoimmunity, life threatening infusion reactions, and malignancies, alemtuzumab is available only through restricted distribution under a Risk Evaluation Mitigation Strategy (REMS) program.	IV infusion in a medical center on 5 consecutive days followed 12 months later by IV infusion on 3 consecutive days
mitoxantrone (Novatrone®)	worsening relapsing forms and SPMS	• discolored urine & sclera • nausea • alopecia • amenorrhea & infertility • infections • cardiac toxicity	• cardiotoxicity and secondary leukemia (monitoring required long term)	IV infusion in a medical center every 3 months, (max cumulative dose of 140 mg/m^2)
natalizumab (Tysabri®)	Relapsing forms of MS	• headache • fatigue • urinary tract infection • lower respiratory infection • arthralgia • gastroenteritis • vaginitis • depression • diarrhea	• Because of the risk of progressive multifocal leukoencephalopathy, natalizumab is available only through a restricted distribution program called the TOUCH® Prescribing Program.	IV infusion in a medical center monthly
Ocrelizumab (Ocrevus®)	Primary-progressive MS and relapsing forms			IV infusion in a medical center every 6 months

CHF = congestive heart failure; FDA = Food and Drug Administration; IM = intramuscular; IV = intravenous; MI = myocardial infarct; PML = progressive multifocal leukoencephalopathy; SC = subcutaneous; SPMS = secondary-progressive MS; TIA = trans-ischemic attack

MS Coalition Consensus paper on DMTs available at: http://ms-coalition.org/cms/images/stories//dmt_consensus_ms_coalition092016.pdf. Information on ocrelizumab available at: https://www.mstrust.org.uk/a-z/ocrelizumab.

Management of Symptoms

Pharmacological agents are used for symptomatic relief of a wide range of symptoms in MS. The clinician should have a thorough understanding of the medications the patient is taking, the expected benefit, and potential adverse reactions.

Spasticity

Management of spasticity and spasms includes the use of muscle relaxants. Oral baclofen (Lioresal®) is commonly used and is highly effective in reducing muscle tone and decreasing the frequency of spasms and clonus. Dosage is progressed gradually to obtain optimal effects. Other examples of oral agents include tizanidine (Zanaflex®), dantrolene sodium (Dantrium®), and diazepam (Valium®). The reduction in spasticity must be balanced with the possibility of adverse effects from overdosing that may include sedation (drowsiness), weakness, and fatigue. The therapist must be alert to these changes and communicate with the physician to achieve optimal dosing for rehabilitation. The therapist must also recognize that at times spasticity can be used to enhance function, substituting for lack of strength. For example, extensor spasticity can be used to assist standing during a stand-pivot transfer. Significant reduction of spasticity with medications might serve to produce loss of function. Carbamazepine (Tegretol®) can be effective in reducing paroxysmal (sudden, sharp-onset) spasms. Patients who do not adequately respond to standard drug treatment (e.g., those with intractable spasticity or spasms) may benefit from intrathecal administration of baclofen directly into the CSF of the lumbar spine via a catheter. A programmable implanted pump controls the dosage. Significant reduction in spasticity and spasms has been reported in the LEs and trunk with less improvement reported in the UEs. Adverse effects can include sedation, dizziness, impaired vision, and impaired speech. Pump failure, infection, programming error and lead displacement can also occur.[58]

Botulinum toxin (BT) injections are used as the most common chemodenervation agent (neurolytic) to provide localized relief of muscle tone and spasms. Efficacy is short term and generally lasts up to 3 months. Excessive use of BT can overly weaken muscles, so it is typically reserved for patients with significant problems. Physical therapy stretching of the limb for at least 4 weeks after injection is an important adjunct. Phenol injections have also been used but are more unpredictable in degree and duration of response and are associated with sensory side effects.[58]

Surgical intervention may be considered for patients with intractable spasticity. The typical surgical candidate presents with spastic paralysis for many years resulting in a nonfunctional limb and serious complications (e.g., contractures and skin breakdown). Interventions include severing tendons (*tendonotomy*), nerves (*neurectomy*), or nerve roots (*rhizotomy*).[1,58]

Pain

A variety of drugs are available to manage pain and clinical decisions are based on type of pain. Tricyclic antidepressants, selective serotonin and norepinephrine reuptake inhibitors (SSNRIs) (e.g., duloxetine hydrochloride [Cymbalta®]) and pregabalin (Lyrica®) are used to treat burning, central neuropathic pain similar to the use with peripheral neuropathic pain. Paroxysmal pain responds to carbamazepine (Tegretol®), amitriptyline (Elavil®), phenytoin (Dilantin®), diazepam (Valium®), or gabapentin (Neurontin®). Dysesthesias are managed with low doses of amitriptyline (Elavil®), imipramine (Tofranil®), or desipramine (Norpramin®). Antiepileptic drugs (carbamazepine) are used with trigeminal neuralgia. The discomfort and pain associated with spasticity and spasms may be managed with over-the-counter or prescription anti-inflammatory drugs. Sometimes pain can be managed with mild painkillers (acetaminophen or ibuprofen). Strong opioids (oxycodone, methadone, morphine) have limited effectiveness and are not typically prescribed.[19,21]

Fatigue

Amantadine (Symmetrel®) and modafinil (Provigil®) have demonstrated moderate benefit in managing MS-related fatigue in some patients. In patients receiving disease-modifying agents, glatiramer acetate is associated with less fatigue than interferon beta-1b.[15] A recent meta-analysis of MS fatigue management with exercise, education and medication found that rehabilitation interventions had stronger and more significant effects on reducing the impact or severity of self-reported fatigue than did medication.[59]

Tremor

Agents to decrease tremor have been used with varying degrees of success. Some patients respond well to a single drug, some to combinations of drugs, and some find no benefit. Medications used to decrease tremor include anti-tuberculosis agent isoniazid (INH), antihistamines (Atarax®, Vistaril®), the beta blocker propranolol (Inderal®), anti-anxiety medications clonazepam (Klonopin®) and buspirone (Buspar®), antidiuretic acetazolamide (Diamox®), and anticonvulsive primidone (Mysoline®). Dizziness and vertigo can be managed with antinausea drugs (meclizine [Antivert®] and ondansetron [Zofran®]) or with scopolamine patches. Severe tremor can also be treated with deep brain stimulation, which involves implanting electrodes into the thalamus.[60]

Cognitive and Emotional Impairments

Cognitive rehabilitation training has been used to improve function in patients with MS.[31,61] Compensatory training strategies (e.g., memory aids, organizational tools) can improve function in everyday activities together with modifying the home environment to limit distractions. Acetylcholinesterase inhibitors used for the treatment of Alzheimer's disease (donepezil [Aricept®], memantine [Namenda®]) have been shown to provide only modest benefits in memory deficits and verbal learning in some patients.[34]

Depression can be managed effectively with psychotherapy and psychopharmcology. Commonly used antidepressant medications are fluoxetine (Prozac®), paroxetine (Paxil®), sertraline (Zoloft®), duloxetine hydrochloride (Cymbalta®), venlafaxine (Effexor®), and bupropion (Wellbutrin®). Some antidepressants can also decrease fatigue. Patients with pseudobulbar affect can be effectively treated with the antidepressant medication amitriptyline (Elavil®). Complementary therapies such as mindfulness meditation, yoga, journaling, and support groups often help the patient cope with the stresses of this unpredictable disease. Exercise and an active lifestyle are important components to reduce depression and anxiety.[34]

Bladder and Bowel Impairments

Urinary problems require a complete urodynamic workup to identify the specific cause of the problem and to arrive at the appropriate course of treatment. Treatment for an overactive, spastic bladder (storage dysfunction) typically involves pharmacological management with anticholinergic medications (tolterodine [Detrol®], oxybutynin [Ditropan®], imipramine [Tofranil®]) to regulate bladder emptying. Adverse effects can include dry mouth, constipation, blurred vision, dry eyes, and less commonly tachycardia. Dietary recommendations include drinking 8 glasses of fluid per day (water) while limiting intake of caffeine or alcohol. A flaccid bladder (emptying dysfunction) is managed with alternate techniques for emptying, including instruction in the *Crede maneuver* (the application of manual downward pressure over the lower abdomen) or intermittent self-catheterization (ISC) performed four to five times per day. Pharmacological agents may include cholinergic stimulation with urecholine. Dietary recommendations include limiting intake of citrus and tomato products (ketchup, salsa, pizza sauce). The acidity in cranberry juice, which is often recommended for urinary tract infections, is a bladder irritant and can worsen urgency of an already spastic bladder. A dyssynergic bladder (combined dysfunction) is managed with alpha-adrenergic blocking agents (e.g., terazosin [Hytrin®], prazosin [Minipress®], tamsulosin [Flomax®]) and antispasticity agents (e.g., baclofen [Lioresal®], tizanidine hydrochloride [Zanaflex®]). On rare occasions when bladder symptoms cannot be controlled with medication and/or ISC, continuous catheterization (indwelling or Foley catheter; condom, or Texas catheter) or surgical urinary diversion (suprapubic catheter) may be necessary. For example, the patient with advanced disease and significant ataxia of the UEs may be unable to manually perform self-catheterization. Urinary tract infections result from retention of urine in the bladder and from catheterization procedures. Antibiotic therapy is the mainstay of treatment.[1,43]

Constipation is a common problem and may be associated with medications that can exacerbate constipation (e.g., antihypertensives, analgesics/narcotics, tricyclic antidepressants, anticholinergics, diuretics, sedatives/tranquilizers, antacids). It is typically managed with dietary changes including increased fluid intake (six to eight glasses daily) and fiber in the diet. Bulk-forming supplements (Metamucil®, FiberCon®, Citrucel®, Benefiber®) or stool softeners (docusate [Colace®], polyethylene glycol [miraLax®]) can also be used. Regular or continuous use of stimulant laxatives and enemas is not recommended. Bowel training may also include manual disimpaction. Incontinence management includes dietary changes such as avoidance of irritants (caffeine, alcohol); adjustment of medications used to reduce spasticity, which can contribute to the problem; or addition of medications to control bowel spasms (tolterodine [Detrol®], propantheline [Pro-Banthine®]).[44]

■ FRAMEWORK FOR REHABILITATION

The chronicity of this disease, along with its variable and unpredictable course, may lead some to view individuals with MS as poor rehabilitation candidates. Although the disease or its direct impairments cannot be altered, there is strong evidence to support physical therapy rehabilitation in producing significant gains in enhancing levels of activity and participation.[62] Multidisciplinary rehabilitation, including cognitive-behavior therapy for depression and information-provision interventions for patient knowledge, shows moderate evidence for gains over a longer period at the level of activity and participation.[62] A systematic review (SR) of 39 SR studies between 2001 and 2016 evaluated the range of rehabilitation interventions in MS.[62] The most common interventions focused on improving strength, mobility, aerobic capacity, and quality of life.. There was also strong evidence for comprehensive fatigue management interventions for patient-reported fatigue, followed by cognitive/psychological intervention for depression.

Rehabilitation referral should be initiated early in the disease when behavioral and lifestyle changes may be easier to implement. Referral is recommended at diagnosis for baseline assessments, education on exercise, health and wellness concerns, and early support for cognitive and work-related difficulties.[62-67] Periodic reassessment should be done to establish and revise goals and to measure outcomes[67] Focusing on patient engagement strategies, the consensus statement of the Multiple Sclerosis in the 21st Century Steering Group recommends education and encouragement for patients from credible sources of accurate information.[68] The physical therapist is a crucial member of the health care team in educating the newly diagnosed individual with MS and discussing healthy lifestyle, fitness and wellness programs.

Individuals with neurodegenerative diseases such as MS benefit from *restorative intervention,* aimed at remediating or improving impairments, activity limitations, and participation restrictions.[69] Direct CNS impairments are not responsive to intervention whereas indirect impairments caused by evolving multisystem dysfunction from inactivity and disuse can be modified (Fig. 16.2). For example, strength training can result in meaningful improvements in balance and gait. Goals and outcome statements reflective of restorative intervention focus on remediating impairments and regaining functional independence while promoting self-management skills. As the disease progresses, important goals and outcomes also include assisting the patient in effective coping skills by promoting acceptance and adjustment to limitations and disabilities and enhancing quality of life. The enhancement of quality of life at every stage of the disease may in fact be the most meaningful outcome for patients in the face of chronic neurodegenerative disease.

Preventive intervention is aimed at minimizing potential complications, impairments, activity limitations, or disabilities at every stage of the disease. Preventive interventions for the patient with MS are geared toward decreasing the duration and severity of symptoms, reducing effects of inactivity, or delaying the emergence of disease sequelae through early detection and intervention, termed *secondary prevention*. Prevention is also aimed at minimizing the degree of disability, termed *tertiary prevention*. Goal and outcome statements reflective of preventive intervention focus on promotion of health, wellness, and fitness, and preservation of optimal function.[69]

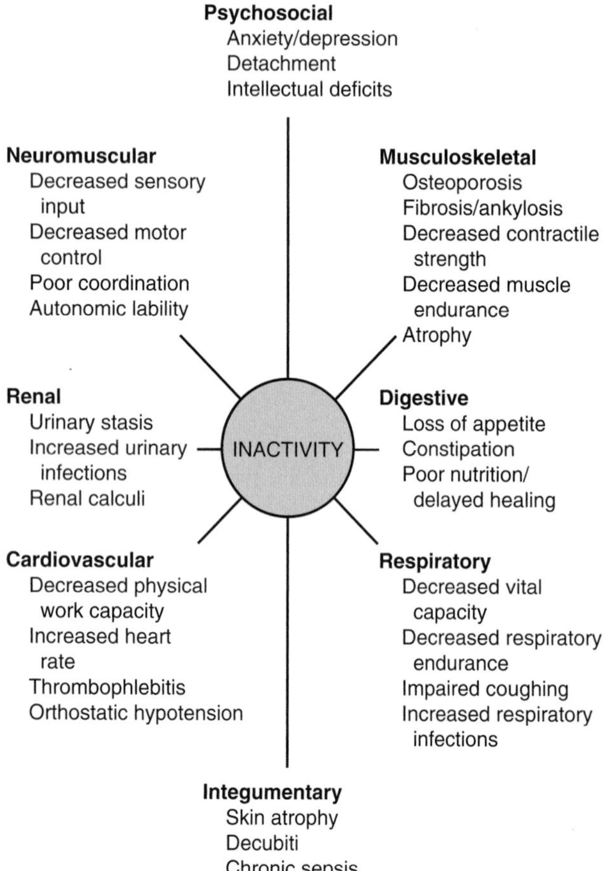

Figure 16.2 Clinical manifestations of inactivity.

Compensatory intervention is aimed at modifying the task, activity, or environment to maintain optimal function within the scope of existing impairments and limitations. Goal and outcome statements reflective of compensatory intervention focus on regaining/maintaining function.[69]

Maintenance therapy is defined as a series of occasional clinical, educational, and administrative services designed to maintain the patient's current level of function. Individuals with MS who benefit from maintenance therapy typically are in the late stages of the disease (Expanded Disability Status Scale [EDSS] stages 7.0 to 9.5; the EDSS is discussed later in the section titled Tests and Measures). Maintenance programs have historically not been well funded by insurance and require careful documentation. The Centers for Medicare & Medicaid Services (CMS), which covers services for the elderly and the disabled, covers maintenance therapy if the *professional skills of a therapist* (one having specialized knowledge and judgment) are needed to prevent or slow deterioration of a person's condition and maintain the maximal predictable level of function. As the result of a legal settlement agreement on January 24, 2013, in the case of *Jimmo v. Sibelius,* CMS issued a clarification that the coverage of skilled services does not turn on the presence or absence of a beneficiary's potential for improvement, but rather on the beneficiary's need for skilled care.[70] For example, risk of secondary impairment and loss of functional capabilities is reduced, or safety of caregivers is enhanced. A variety of interventions are used to achieve goals and outcomes, including limited direct interventions, patient/client-related instruction, and supportive counseling. The therapist tapers the frequency of the visits as the patient or family/caregivers are able to assume independent self-management of the care plan. Indeed, recent models of rehabilitation delivery that promote routine 6- to 12-month reassessments of function to optimize management of care in Parkinson's disease may also show benefit for management of MS.[1,72]

A coordinated interdisciplinary team is necessary to oversee the comprehensive examination and management needed to address the patient's complex and multifaceted problems.[63] The team typically includes the physician, nurse, physical therapist, occupational therapist, speech-language pathologist, nutritionist, psychologist, and social worker. As with any team, the patient is the central figure, with family and caregivers being key members. The ideal rehabilitation program considers the patient's disease history, course, and symptoms, including impairments, activity limitations, and disability. Of equal importance are the patient's abilities (assets), priorities, and resources (e.g., family, home, community). The focus is on long-range planning with anticipated episodes of care, including hospital-based, outpatient, and home/community-based care. Dal Bello-Haas[73] discusses a continuum of care based on disease stage (early, middle, and late) for individuals with neurodegenerative diseases. Considerations for the patient with MS are presented in Table 16.2.

PHYSICAL THERAPY EXAMINATION

MS may impact many different areas of the CNS; thus, it is imperative that a careful examination is performed to determine the extent of neurological and functional

Table 16.2 Stages of MS: Common Impairments, Activity Limitations, and Intervention Strategies

Stage of MS	Common Impairments and Activity Limitations	Intervention Strategies
Early/Mild	• Few/minimal impairments and activity limitations with independence maintained • Motor symptoms present but do not interfere with daily activities • Symptoms for RRMS are more variable and do not progress at the same rate as PPMS • SPMS initially presents with relapsing-remitting course followed by a more progressive course	*Preventive and Restorative* • Regular exercise to improve/maintain motor performance, strength, mobility, flexibility, ROM, balance, locomotion, endurance, and perceived quality of life • Community classes to improve/maintain socialization, camaraderie, positive outlook, and life purpose *Compensatory* • Patient/family/caregiver education about disease process, rehabilitation, energy conservation • Determine need for adaptive or assistive devices • Determine need for environmental modification of home/workplace • Provide psychological support with early referral to support groups for patient and family/caregiver • Referral to other health care professionals as needed
Middle/ Moderate	• Progressive course with increasing number and severity of impairments • Minimal to moderate activity limitations, participation restrictions • ADL with modified dependence (assistance) • Difficulty with balance and gait, postural instability	*Preventive and Restorative* • Regular exercise to maintain/improve motor performance, strength, mobility, flexibility, ROM, balance, locomotion, endurance, and perceived quality of life • Community classes to improve/maintain socialization, camaraderie, positive outlook and life purpose *Compensatory* • Assistive devices to maintain function • Motorized wheelchair or scooter for community mobility • Environmental modifications to home • Patient/family/caregiver education and training • Psychological support for patient and family/caregiver • Referral to other health care professionals as needed
Late/ Advanced	• Progressive course with numerous impairments with increasing severity • Severe activity limitations with dependence in most activities • Great difficulty walking; typically in wheelchair or bed most of the day • Assistance needed with all ADL • Severe participation restrictions: • Not able to live alone • Typically requires full-time assistance or placement in chronic care facility • Social interactions restricted • Cognitive problems may be prominent, including dementia, hallucinations, and delusions	*Preventive* • Maximize upright posture, out-of-bed time • Maximize participation in ADL • Prevention of contractures, pressure wounds, pneumonia, and so forth *Compensatory* • Family/caregiver education and training: safety education, transfers, positioning, turning, skin care • Pressure-relieving devices • Hospital bed, wheelchair, mechanical lift • Psychological support for patient and family/caregiver • Referral to other health care professionals as needed

Adapted from Dal Bello-Haas.[73]

ADL = activities of daily living; PPMS = primary-progressive multiple sclerosis; ROM = range of motion; RRMS = relapsing-remitting multiple sclerosis; SPMS = secondary-progressive multiple sclerosis involvement. Subsequent re-examinations at specified intervals are used to distinguish change in status as well as effects of treatment. It may not always be possible to differentiate change in status associated with remission of symptoms from treatment outcomes. Considering the variability of symptoms of any individual patient, it is often beneficial to observe performance over a period of a few days to obtain a representative sample of baseline functioning. Fatigue and exacerbating factors should be considered when scheduling the examination.

Physical therapy examination data can be obtained through the patient's history and systems review and relevant tests and measures. The selection of examination procedures and level of inquiry are determined by the patient's unique status. The severity of problems, stage of disease (early/mild, middle/moderate, and late/advanced), age, setting of rehabilitation, and other factors must all be considered in structuring the examination.

Patient/Client History

Data obtained through interview with the patient/family and review of the medical record will provide information on general demographics, medical/surgical history, social and employment history, family history, living environment, general health status, social and health habits, and disease duration. The patient's current/primary complaints and current functional status and activity level should be ascertained. Coexisting health problems and medications should also be identified.

Systems Review

Data obtained from the history and medical record will inform the systems review and help focus selection of appropriate tests and measures (Box 16.3). Review of the following systems is included: (1) cardiovascular/pulmonary, (2) cognitive, affective, and communication, (3) genitourinary, (4) integumentary, (5) musculoskeletal, and (6) neuromuscular.

Tests and Measures

The following are specific areas and relevant tests and measures that can be used to examine function in patients with MS (for more detailed descriptions, see earlier chapters in this text focusing on examination).

Cognition

Memory function, attention, concentration, conceptual reasoning, problem solving, and speed of information processing should be examined, as well as the effects of fatigue on cognitive performance. An expert panel convened by the Consortium of MS Centers in 2001 developed the *Minimal Examination of Cognitive Function in MS (MACFIMS).* This 90-minute battery of seven neuropsychological tests examines processing speed/working memory, learning and memory, executive function, visual–spatial processing, and word retrieval.[74] In 2012, the *Brief International Cognitive Assessment for MS (BICAMS)* was introduced.[75] The BICAMS includes a 15-minute battery of three neuropsychological tests and is sensitive and specific to cognitive impairment defined by the MACFIMS.[76] A brief screen of cognitive function can be achieved using the *Mini-Mental Status Examination (MMSE),*[77] though many individuals with MS may experience ceiling effects. The Symbol Digit Modalities Test (SDMT) may be the most appropriate cognitive test if >5 minutes are available to the examiner;[75] the SDMT has been shown to have excellent validity for predicting diagnosis, course and work disability and is easy to administer.[78]

Affective and Psychosocial Function

Emotional stability should be examined. The presence of emotional lability, euphoria, emotional dysregulation, or depression (symptoms, severity, length, effect on functional performance); the level of stress and anxiety; coping strategies; and presence of sleep disorders should be documented. A useful instrument is the Beck Depression Inventory.[79] Many of these domains may also be assessed with Quality of Life scales, which are discussed later in this chapter under General Health Measures. As previously mentioned, it is imperative that the physical therapist be familiar with the patient's medications, because numerous medications will have effects on the affective and psychosocial domain.

Sensation

Given the extent of variability in sensory deficits in individuals with MS, a detailed examination of superficial and deep sensations should be completed (see Chapter 3, Examination of Sensory Function). Additionally, sensory deficits and their effects on quality of life (QOL) in individuals with MS can be quantified by using quantitative measures such as the *Nottingham Sensory Assessment,*[80] neurothesiometer, Semmes-Weinstein monofilaments,[81] or Vibratron.[82] Sensory function may also be assessed with the *Visual Analog Scale*[81] or *Guy's Neurological Disability Scale,*[83] a comprehensive multidimensional scale designed to assess the wide range of disability in patients with MS. Caution should be used when selecting measures, as only the neurothesiometer, visual analog scale and Vibratron have established reliability in persons with MS.[81,82] Vibration sensation is assessed in the neurologic examination with a tuning fork; quantitative assessment of vibration with the Vibratron demonstrates strong correlations with balance performance and integrity of the spinal cord white matter in persons with MS.[82,84]

Pain

The presence of acute, paroxysmal pain (Lhermitte's sign, dysesthesias) and chronic pain including pain behaviors and reactions during specific movements and provoking stimuli should be documented. The *McGill Pain Questionnaire*[85] or the *Neuropathic Pain Scale,*[86]

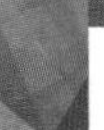

Box 16.3 Elements of the Examination of the Patient With Multiple Sclerosis[69]

History

- Demographic information: age, sex, race/ethnicity, primary language, education
- Social history: cultural beliefs and behaviors, family and caregiver resources, social support systems
- Occupation/employment/work information
- Living environment: home/work barriers
- Hand dominance
- General health status: physical, psychological, social, and role function, health habits
- Social and health habits (current and past)
- Family history
- Medical/surgical history
- Current conditions/chief complaints
- Medications
- Medical/laboratory/clinical test results
- Functional status and activity level: premorbid and current

Systems Review

- Cardiovascular/pulmonary
- Cognitive/affective
- Genitourinary
- Integumentary
- Musculoskeletal
- Neuromuscular

Tests and Measures

- Aerobic capacity and endurance: during functional activities and standardized exercise protocols; cardiovascular signs and symptoms in response to exercise and activity; pulmonary signs and symptoms in response to exercise and activity
- Anthropometric characteristics: body mass index, girth, length
- Assistive or adaptive devices: fit, alignment, function, use; safety
- Assistive technology
- Balance: degree of postural instability, balance strategies; safety
- Circulation: response to position change/degree of orthostatic hypotension
- Communication
- Cranial and peripheral nerve integrity
- Environment, home, and work barriers
- Functional status and activity level: performance-based examination of functional skills (FIM level), basic and instrumental ADL; functional mobility skills; home management skills
- Gait and locomotion: gait pattern and speed, safety
- Integumentary integrity: skin condition, pressure sensitive areas; activities, positioning, and postures to relieve pressure
- Joint integrity, alignment, and mobility: range of motion (active and passive); muscle length and soft tissue extensibility
- Mental functions: cognition, memory
- Motor function: motor control and motor learning
- Muscle performance: strength, power, and endurance
- Neuromotor development and sensory processing
- Pain: intensity and location
- Perceptual function: visuospatial skills
- Posture: alignment and position, symmetry (static and dynamic, sitting and standing); ergonomics, and body mechanics
- Psychosocial function: motivation
- Range of motion
- Reflex integrity
- Self-care and domestic life
- Sensory integrity and integration
- Skeletal integrity
- Ventilation and gas exchange
- Work, community, and leisure activities: ability to participate in activities, safety

developed to assess distinct pain qualities associated with neuropathic pain, can be used. (See discussion in Chapter 25, Chronic Pain.) The *Brief Pain Inventory*[87] assesses pain severity and pain interference and has established reliability and validity in persons with MS.

Visual Acuity

Acuity, tracking, and accommodation should be examined; the presence of visual deficits (blurred vision, field defects [scotoma], diplopia) should be documented.

Cranial Nerve Integrity

Motor and sensory cranial nerve function should be examined; the presence of deficits (optic pain [optic neuritis], oculomotor dyscontrol, dysphagia, impaired gag reflex, trigeminal neuralgia) should be documented.

Range of Motion

Passive range of motion (PROM) and active range of motion (AROM) should be examined; the presence of specific range of motion (ROM) impairments should be documented.

Muscle Performance

Functional strength using manual muscle testing (MMT) and dynamometers (isokinetic, grasp and pinch dynamometers) should be examined; strong spasticity may be a contraindication to standard MMT positions.

Fatigue

The frequency, duration, and severity of fatigue should be examined; precipitating factors, activity levels, and efficacy of rest attempts should be documented.[88] The *Modified Fatigue Impact Scale (MFIS)* developed by Fisk et al[89,90] is a structured, self-report, 21-item questionnaire addressing the effects of fatigue on cognitive, physical, and psychosocial function using a 5-point ordinal scale with 0 equal to never and 4 equal to almost always. Each area (subscale) can be scored separately; the total MFIS score range is from 0 to 84 (http://www.nationalmssociety.org/For-Professionals/Researchers/Resources-for-Researchers/Clinical-Study-Measures/Modified-Fatigue-Impact-Scale-(MFIS)). An abbreviated version of the MFIS has five items (the *MFIS-5*). Additionally, the *Fatigue Scale for Motor and Cognitive Functions (FSMC)* is a 20-item scale developed as a measure of cognitive and motor fatigue for people with MS.[91] To measure fatigue during the examination and treatment process, the Visual Analog Scale—Fatigue can be used as a single-item self-report of fatigue (Table 16.3).

Temperature Sensitivity

The degree of temperature sensitivity and its effect on fatigue and weakness should be examined. A tympanic membrane thermometer (ear thermometer) can be used before, during, and after moderate-intensity exercise.

Table 16.3 Selected Outcome Measures for Persons With Multiple Sclerosis by ICF Domain

Outcome Measure and *ICF Category*	Description	Scoring	MDC/MDIC
Fatigue Scale for Motor and Cognitive Functions[91] *Body Function and Structure*	20-item self-report measure evaluating motor and cognitive fatigue in persons with MS	Cognitive (10 items) and motor (10 items) subscales are scored for a total score (max 20 points)	MDC: not established MDIC: not established
Trunk Impairment Scale[221] *Body Function and Structure* *Activity*	A measure examining motor function of the trunk in sitting	Items are scored out of a possible 23 points with static sitting (0–7), dynamic sitting (0–10) and coordination (0–6) subscales.	MDC: not established MDIC: not established
Visual Analog Scale – Fatigue[88,222] *Body Function and Structure*	Single-item self-report measure for fatigue	(various versions) 2 examples: 0–10 scale: 10 indicates major fatigue problem 100 mm line: right end of scale indicates extremely tired	MDC: 3.47 points on 0–10 scale (rheumatoid arthritis)[223] MDIC: -0.82 to -1.12 for meaningful improvement and 1.13 to 1.26 for meaningful worsening on a 0–10 scale (rheumatoid arthritis)[223]

Table 16.3 Selected Outcome Measures for Persons With Multiple Sclerosis by ICF Domain—cont'd

Outcome Measure and *ICF Category*	Description	Scoring	MDC/MDIC
12-item MS Walking Scale[105] *Activity*	12-item self-report measure evaluating the impact of MS on walking ability.	Items are scored 1-5 and the sum of the scores is then: [(Sum of scores -12)/48] * 100	MDC: 22% (MS) (224) MDIC: not established
6 Minute Walk Test[225] *Activity*	Measure of distance walked in 6 minutes	Utilize a marked course and measuring wheel to obtain distance traveled in 6 minutes	MDC: +/– 88–92.16 m (MS)[224,226] MDIC: decline of 53–55m detects individuals with MS who are deteriorating vs. individuals who are stable[226]
9-Hole Peg Test[227] *Activity*	Timed performance test; the individual removes 9 pegs from a peg board to a well, one at a time and then returns the pegs to the pegboard, one at a time.	Time to complete this task is measured in seconds for both the dominant and non-dominant hands.	MDC: not established MDIC: 20% change (MS)[228]
MS Quality of Life –54[111] *Activity* *Participation*	54-item self-report measure of health-related quality of life; contains the SF-36 and 18 additional MS-specific items.	There is no overall summary score, rather there are 2 combined summary scores (mental health composite and physical health composite)	MDC: not established MDIC: not established
Rivermead Mobility Index[229] *Activity*	15-item (14 self-report items and 1 performance item) measure examining mobility	Items are scored on a 2-point scale (0 = no; 1 = yes) for a maximal score of 15 points	MDC: 3 points (stroke,[230] CIDP[231]) MDIC: 2 points (MS)[229,232]
Timed 25-Foot Walk[23] *Activity*	A measure of fast walking speed	Time to walk 25 feet at the individual's quickest safe speed is recorded	MDC: 2.7 seconds (MS)[224] MDIC: not established
Outcome Measures Balance: **Berg Balance Scale** **Functional Reach** **Dynamic Gait Index** **Timed Up and Go (TUG); TUG Cognitive & Manual** **Dynamic Gait Index** **Activities-Specific Balance Confidence Scale**	***See discussion in Chapter 6, Examination of Coordination and Balance and Table 6.7***		
Functional Independence Measure (FIM)	***See discussion in Chapter 8, Examination of Function***		

All measures "highly recommended" or "recommended" by the MS EDGE Task Force for use across settings (acute, inpatient rehabilitation, home health, skilled nursing facility and outpatient) *and* required at entry-level education (http://www.neuropt.org/docs/ms-edge-documents/final-ms-edge-document.pdf?sfvrsn=4) and (http://www.neuropt.org/docs/ms-edge-documents/ms-edge-summary-recommendations.pdf?sfvrsn=4).

A determination of the correlation between temperature changes and worsening of neurological symptoms can be made. This transient increase in symptoms following a raise in core temperature, which may be seen with exercise, has been more accurately termed a *pseudoexacerbation,* and occurs due to transient increased blockade of nerve conduction in demyelinated fibers.[92,93]

Motor Function

The therapist should examine for the presence of corticospinal signs (paresis, spasticity, hyperactive DTRs, positive Babinski's sign, and involuntary spasms [flexor or extensor]).

Spasticity can be examined using a subjective rating scale. The *Ashworth Spasticity Scale*[94] led to the more widely used *Modified Ashworth Scale.*[95] These are ordinal scales designed to measure tone intensity; the modified Ashworth has an additional grade at the lower end allowing for more discrete rating. A determination should be made of the differences between lower limbs versus upper limbs; right and left sides; and factors that influence tone.

The therapist should examine for the presence of cerebellar signs (ataxia, intention tremor, nystagmus, dysarthria). The effects of position change (e.g., sitting-to-standing) may produce an increase in ataxic movements with increased demands for postural stability and should be documented.

The therapist should examine for the presence of vestibular dysfunction (dizziness, vertigo, nystagmus, blurred vision with head and body movements, and postural imbalance; see Chapter 21, Vestibular Disorders).

Posture

Static and dynamic postural control in various different positions (e.g., sitting, standing) should be examined. The presence of postural abnormalities and postural tremor should be documented. Instruments can include posture grids, plumb lines, and still photography with light-emitting diodes.

Balance, Gait, and Locomotion

The therapist should examine static and dynamic balance, reactive and anticipatory control, sensory interaction, and synergistic strategies. Useful instruments include the *Clinical Test for Sensory Interaction in Balance,*[96] dynamic posturography,[97,98] the *Berg Balance Scale,*[99,100] the *Tinetti Performance Oriented Mobility Examination (POMA),*[101] and the *Balance Evaluation Systems Test (BESTest).*[102] Balance tests are noted in Table 16.3; additional information on the *Timed Up and Go, Activities Balance Confidence Scale,* and *Functional Reach* can be found in Chapter 6: Examination of Coordination and Balance and Table 6.7 Outcome Measures: Examination of Balance.

Gait parameters and characteristics should be examined including gait speed, kinematics, stability, safety, and endurance. Examination of patients with significant ataxia can be enhanced by use of videotaped performance. Useful tests include timed walk tests (10-Meter Walk Test, 6-Minute Walk Test, 2-minute walk test, the Timed 25 Foot Walk, which is a component of the MSFC and the standard walking test included in MS Clinical Trials), the *Dynamic Gait Index;*[103] and the *Ambulation Index (AI).*[104] Self-reported walking function can be assessed with the *Multiple Sclerosis Walking Scale-12 (MSWS-12),*[105] and lower extremity coordination may be assessed with the *Six Spot Step Test (SSST).*[106,107] Additional walking tests recommended by the APTA's MSEDGE are located at http://www.neuropt.org/docs/ms-edge-documents/final-ms-edge-document.pdf.

Alignment and fit, safety, practicality, and ease of use of orthotic and assistive devices should be examined along with energy conservation and expenditure. Wheelchair skills, including functional mobility, management, safety, transfers, and energy conservation and expenditure, should be examined.

Aerobic Capacity and Endurance

Vital signs (heart rate, blood pressure, respiratory rate) and breathing patterns should be examined at rest, during and after exercise. Exertional symptoms (dyspnea; elevated blood pressure) and perceived exertion during and after activity should be documented. Useful scales include the *Rating of Perceived Exertion Scale (the Borg RPE Scale)*[108] and the *Dyspnea Scale.*[109]

Skin Integrity and Condition

Skin integrity and condition should be examined. Areas of insensitivity, bruising, moisture buildup, and skin breakdown should be examined and documented, along with level of urinary continence; bed and wheelchair positioning; effectiveness of pressure-relieving compensatory strategies and pressure-relieving devices (PRDs); and cognitive status and safety awareness.

Functional Status

An examination of functional mobility skills, basic activities of daily living (BADL), and instrumental activities of daily living (IADL) is indicated, together with social functioning and community and work adaptive skills. A commonly used instrument for patients undergoing active rehabilitation is the *Functional Independence Measure (FIM)*[110] (see Chapter 8, Examination of Function).

Environment (Home, Community, and Work)

Physical space for barriers, access, and safety should be examined; a specific task-analysis (patient performance-based examination) in relevant environments (home, work) may be included (see Chapter 9, Examination and Modification of the Environment).

General Health Measures

General health measures are used to examine outcomes across a broad spectrum of global or long-term health outcomes. Instruments involve self-report of the patient's perceptions of limitations and quality of life (e.g., physical and social function, general health and vitality, emotional well-being, bodily pain, and so forth). The *Health Status Questionnaire (SF-36)*[111] is widely acknowledged as the gold standard of generic measures of health status. The properties of this instrument have been investigated in patients with MS. Freeman et al[112] found limitations in evaluating change in moderate to severely disabled patients participating in inpatient rehabilitation with significant floor and ceiling effects in four of eight SF-36 dimensions.

Disease-Specific Measures

Disease-specific measures are designed to examine attributes common in a specific disease entity. Items are included to provide information about the disease process and outcomes, and ideally document clinically meaningful change over time. Thus, the instruments have greater responsiveness or sensitivity to change than general health measures.

Expanded Disability Status Scale (EDSS) for Patients With Multiple Sclerosis

In 1955, Kurtzke developed a 10-point scale for rating overall disability in MS (the *Disability Status Scale or DSS*).[113] This scale was expanded in 1983 to increase its clinical sensitivity by including half-point increments, becoming the EDSS (https://www.nationalmssociety.org/NationalMSSociety/media/MSNationalFiles/Brochures/10-2-3-29-EDSS_Form.pdf).[114] This scale has been widely adopted by clinicians and has been used as a standard in MS research. Based on a standard neurological examination, patients are first graded on presenting symptoms in seven specific functional systems (pyramidal, cerebellar, brainstem, sensory, bowel and bladder, visual, mental), plus other functions. Functional system scores (FSS) are obtained using an ordinal clinical rating scale ranging from 0 to 5 or 6. The EDSS is based on the grades obtained from the FSS and uses a 0 to 10 ordinal scale graded in half-point increments, with 0 equal to normal neurological function and 10.0 equal to death owing to MS. For example, patients classified in EDSS step 2.5 demonstrate minimal disability in two FSS (two FSS grade 2, others 0 or 1). The EDSS focuses on ambulation as the primary indicator of disability (see scores 3.0 through 6.5 for levels of ambulation; patients with scores 7.0 or greater are unable to walk). Criticisms of the EDSS include its lack of sensitivity to changes that do not include functional mobility (ambulation), problems in interrater reliability with patients whose performance is less impaired (scores in the lower ranges, ambulation less impaired)[115,116] and because high variability and nonlinearity of the scale make determination of change over time challenging.[117,118]

MS Functional Composite (MSFC)

The *MS Functional Composite (MSFC)* is a 21-item test that includes 3 different functional subtests: the Timed 25-Foot Walk (T25FW), the 9-Hole Peg Test (9HPT), and the Paced Auditory Serial Addition Test (PASAT). The *MSFC Administration and Scoring Manual* can be obtained from the National Multiple Sclerosis Society at http://www.nationalmssociety.org/NationalMSSociety/media/MSNationalFiles/Brochures/10-2-3-31-MSFC_Manual_and_Forms.pdf.

Multiple Sclerosis Quality Of Life—54 (MSQOL-54)

The *Multiple Sclerosis Quality of Life—54 (MSQOL-54)* is a multidimensional health-related quality-of-life measure that combines both generic and MS-specific items into a single instrument.[111] The generic items are from the SF-36 to which 18 items were added to provide more information regarding MS-specific issues.[119] No overall summary score is used: the MSQOL-54 consists of 12 subscales, 2 combined summary scores, and 2 single-item measures. The subscales are physical function, role limitations—physical, role limitations—emotional, pain, emotional well-being, energy, health perceptions, social function, cognitive function, health distress, overall quality of life, and sexual function. The summary scores are the physical health composite summary and the mental health composite summary. The single-item measures are satisfaction with sexual function and change in health.

MS Quality of Life Inventory (MSQLI)

The *MS Quality of Life Inventory (MSQLI)* is a comprehensive outcomes examination that includes a battery of 10 self-report scales (138 items) that provide information about health-related quality of life in MS, including the Health Status Questionnaire (SF-36), Modified Fatigue Impact Scale (MFIS), MOS Pain Effects Scale (PES), Sexual Satisfaction Scale (SSS), Bladder Control Scale (BLCS), Bowel Control Scale (BWCS), Impact of Visual Impairment Scale (IVIS), Perceived Deficits Questionnaire (PDQ), Mental Health Inventory (MHI), and MOS Modified Social Support Survey (MSSS). The battery can be administered in approximately 45 minutes in most cases. Abbreviated versions of some of the scales can reduce the set to 81 items requiring approximately 30 minutes to administer. A *User's Manual* can be obtained from http://www.nationalmssociety.org/NationalMSSociety/media/MSNationalFiles/Brochures/MSQLI_-A-User-s-Manual.pdf.

Functional Examination of Multiple Sclerosis (FAMS)

The *Functional Examination of MS (FAMS)* is a 59-item index of health-related quality-of-life measures with six subscales (mobility, symptoms, emotional well-being [depression], general contentment, thinking/fatigue, and family/social well-being). The mobility subscale strongly correlates with the EDSS.[120]

Multiple Sclerosis Impact Scale (MSIS-29)

The *MS Impact Scale (MSIS-29)* measures the physical and psychological impact of MS.[121] The scale was primarily developed for community-based populations though testing with hospital-based populations (patients admitted for inpatient rehabilitation, IV corticosteroid treatment for MS relapses, and patients admitted with PPMS) revealed consistency of psychometric properties.[122]

The *Neurology Section Multiple Sclerosis Outcome Measures Taskforce* of the American Physical Therapy Association (APTA) has compiled a list of measures for each relevant International Classification of Functioning, Disability, and Health (ICF) category together with instrument analysis, recommendations for use, and relevant references. The document can be found at http://www.neuropt.org/docs/ms-edge-documents/final-ms-edge-document.pdf. Selected outcome measures are listed in Table 16.3.

Goals and Outcomes

The general goals and outcomes for patients with progressive disorders of the CNS, adapted from the *Guide to Physical Therapist Practice,*[69] are presented in Box 16.4. These general goals will provide the basis for development of specific anticipated goals and expected outcomes for an individual patient.

In this document the reader will find relevant information on patient/client diagnostic classification; examination components; considerations for evaluation, diagnosis, and prognosis; and suggested interventions. Thus, the *Guide to Physical Therapist Practice* serves as a primary resource to help physical therapists design an appropriate plan of care (POC) and document the services provided and outcomes achieved.

PHYSICAL THERAPY INTERVENTIONS

Management of Sensory Deficits and Skin Care

In patients with MS, inflammation causes a disruption in neuronal signaling, causing a variety of sensory symptoms. Strategies should be instituted to increase awareness of sensory deficits, compensate for sensory loss, and promote safety. It is important to remember that sensory deficits may remit, so ongoing examination is necessary. The success of compensatory training strategies depends on the availability of other intact sensory systems. For example, visual compensation techniques can be instituted when deficits in proprioception produce imbalance and place the patient at risk for falls. If multiple sensory systems are involved (e.g., vision is also impaired), sensory compensatory strategies are not likely to be successful.

Patients with proprioceptive losses demonstrate impairments in movement control and motor learning. They require increased use of other sensory systems, especially vision. Tapping, verbal cueing, and/or biofeedback can

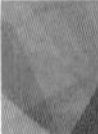

Box 16.4 Examples of General Goals and Outcomes for Patients With Progressive Disorders of the Central Nervous System[69]

1. **Impact of pathology/pathophysiology is reduced.**
   - *Decrease:* risk of secondary impairment; intensity of care
   - *Improve:* patient/client, family, and caregiver knowledge of disease, prognosis and plan of care; symptom management
2. **Impact of impairments is reduced.**
   - *Decrease:* pain
   - *Improve:* cognitive function; joint integrity; mobility; sensory awareness; skin integrity; motor function; muscle performance; postural control and balance; gait and locomotion; management of fatigue; aerobic capacity
3. **Ability to perform physical actions, tasks, or activities is improved.**
   - *Improve:* independence with ADL; tolerance of positions and activities; activity pacing and energy conservation; problem solving and decision making skills; safety of patient, family and caregivers
4. **Disability associated with chronic illness is reduced.**
   - *Improve:* ability to assume/resume self-care and home management; ability to assume work (job/school/play), community and leisure roles; patient/client and family knowledge and awareness of personal and environmental factors associated with condition worsening; awareness and use of community resources
5. **Health status and quality of life are improved.**
   - *Decrease:* stressors
   - *Improve:* sense of well-being; insight, self-confidence and self-management skills; health, wellness and fitness
6. **Patient/client satisfaction is enhanced.**
   - *Improve:* acceptability of access and availability of services and quality of rehabilitation services to patient/client and family; coordination of care with patient/client, family, caregivers, and other professionals.

Adapted from the *Guide to Physical Therapist Practice.*[69]

all be effective forms of augmented feedback. Proprioceptive loading through exercise, light tracking resistance, resistance bands or weights, and the use of a pool may heighten residual proprioceptive function and improve movement awareness.

Visual loss will interfere with movement and postural control. Blurred vision, especially at night or in low light situations, can occur after episodes of optic neuritis. When individuals with MS have to stand in an upright position in the dark, the likelihood of falls increases.[123] It is therefore important to instruct the patient to maintain adequate lighting at all times (e.g., use of a bright light at night) and reducing clutter to improve safety. Adding color contrast between items in the environment (e.g., stair markings) can also improve safety. Double vision is frequently the result of impaired coordination and weak eye muscles. It can be controlled by placing a patch over one eye and is an important strategy for improving reading, driving, or watching television. However, eye patching should not be used all the time, because it will prevent possible adaptation of the CNS. Eye patching also interferes with depth perception. The symptoms of visual blurring and double vision also fluctuate and can be heightened with fatigue, an increase in temperature, stress, and infection. If low vision persists, the patient should be referred to a low-vision specialist or one of the national service organizations that provide help to individuals with vision impairments (*National Association for Visually Handicapped, National Federation of the Blind, American Foundation for the Blind*).

One of the most common early sensory symptoms of MS is decreased sensitivity to touch and vibration.[124,125] This may result in reduced sensitivity on the soles of the feet and difficulty with proprioception and kinesthetic awareness. This sensory ataxia may result in difficulty with foot placement and an increased risk of falls in individuals with MS. Persons with MS are also at an increased risk of developing pressure ulcers owing to the symptoms of MS, including loss of sensation, immobility, loss of bowel and bladder control, and nutritional state. Changes in skin turgor, static posturing, and prolonged pressure over bony prominences increase the likelihood of skin breakdown. Patients may not feel the discomfort of a prolonged position or may be unable to shift position because of weakness or spasticity. In addition, spasticity and/or spasms may cause friction effects between the skin and supporting surfaces. Awareness, protection, and care of desensitized parts should be taught early in the rehabilitation process and consistently reinforced by all members of the team. It has been demonstrated that patient education programs result in 50% reductions in pressure sore incidence.[126] The patient/family/caregiver should be educated in the following principles of skin care:

- The skin should be kept clean and dry. Soiled skin should be cleansed and dried promptly.
- The skin should be inspected regularly (at least once a day) and carefully, with particular attention to persistent areas of redness and over bony prominences.
- Clothing should be breathable and comfortable (soft, not too loose or wrinkled, or too tight). Seams, buttons, and pockets should not press on the skin, particularly in weight-bearing areas.
- Regular pressure relief is essential. Patients should be instructed to change their position or be changed frequently, typically every 2 hours in bed and every 15 to 30 minutes when sitting in a wheelchair.[127]

Pressure-relieving devices (PRDs) may be necessary to protect insensitive areas and should be implemented as appropriate. These can include mattresses (water, gel, air, or alternating pressure) to distribute body weight and reduce shear and friction in bed. Sheepskins, air or foam cushions, cuffs, and/or boots may be necessary to protect body areas prone to breakdown (shoulder blades, elbows, ischial tuberosities, sacrum, trochanters, knees, malleoli, or heels). Cushions (foam; fluid or air pressure–relieving cushions) are necessary for patients who spend prolonged periods of time sitting in their wheelchair. When evaluating a PRD, it is imperative that a pressure mapping system be used to determine its effectiveness and to ensure that the areas of high pressure are adequately protected.[127]

Prevention is the best strategy. Important measures for maintaining skin integrity and function include maintaining good nutrition and drinking plenty of fluids. Studies suggest that for patients with MS with pressure sores, there are increased requirements for specific nutrients; particularly zinc and iron supplementation should be considered.[128] The patient must be cautioned against activities that might traumatize the skin. Dragging, bumping, or scraping body parts during a transfer or bed mobility activities can injure the skin. Thermal injury can result from contact with hot water or hot objects. If nonblanchable skin redness develops (lasting longer than 30 minutes), patients should be instructed to stay off the area until the redness disappears. If the redness does not disappear within 24 hours, the individual should seek medical attention. Blisters, blue areas, or open sores indicate more serious injury and require immediate attention. This may include systemic antibiotic therapy for infection and wound management techniques (cleansing and débridement, topical antibiotic agents, and protective dressings).

Management of Pain

Pain can be classified into four categories: pain directly from MS, pain secondary to other symptoms of MS, pain as a result of drug treatment for MS, and pain independent of MS. The management of pain depends on an accurate determination of its causes. Musculoskeletal strain or joint malalignment from chronically weakened muscles are important considerations and are responsive to physical therapy intervention. Patients may experience relief of pain with regular stretching or exercise, massage, and ultrasound. Postural retraining and correction of faulty movement patterns along with orthotic and/or adaptive seating devices can reduce malalignment and pain. Stabbing pain from Lhermitte's sign may be relieved with a soft cervical collar to limit neck flexion. Hydrotherapy or pool therapy using *lukewarm* water may have a beneficial effect on painful dysesthesias. Pressure stockings or gloves can also be used to relieve pain, converting the sensation of pain to one of pressure. Neutral warmth may be an additional factor in the pain relief experienced with stockings or gloves. Patients with chronic pain may benefit from referral to a total management approach for chronic pain, for example, the *multidisciplinary pain clinic* (see Chapter 25, Chronic Pain). Stress management techniques, relaxation training, biofeedback, and meditation are often helpful in reducing both anxiety and pain. The use of transcutaneous electrical nerve stimulation (TENS) to modulate pain in patients with MS has had conflicting results, with some patients experiencing improvement and some a worsening of symptoms.[20,21] Pain is linked to depression, fatigue, anxiety, and sleep in persons with MS,[129] so management of pain requires examination of other contributing factors. Behavioral approaches such as self-management,[130] self-hypnosis,[131] and positive psychology[132] have demonstrated success in improving pain outcomes in persons with MS and warrant further examination.

Exercise Training

Exercise training is safe for individuals with MS; it is not associated with an increased risk of either relapses or adverse events.[133] Muscle weakness and decreased endurance are common findings in patients with MS. As a result, persons with MS may adopt a sedentary lifestyle and limit their physical activity. Thus, early education on the importance of exercise is crucial. The benefits of exercise have been firmly established in terms of producing meaningful physiological and psychological changes, improving function while lessening disability, and enhancing quality of life. In a systematic review of systematic reviews investigating rehabilitation in MS, researchers identified 53 systematic reviews.[134] The researchers found strong evidence to support physical therapy to improve activity and participation domains in persons with MS as well as strong evidence to support the reduction of patient-reported fatigue. Individuals with minimal to moderate impairments (i.e., EDSS scores between 1 and 6) demonstrate the best exercise tolerance. This speaks to the need to institute exercises early in the course of the disease. Additional systematic reviews and meta-analyses demonstrate the positive effect of exercise therapy on depression,[135,136] fatigue,[137] cognition,[138,139] gait and gait endurance,[140,141] balance,[140] arm/hand function,[142] strength,[143-145] cardiorespiratory fitness,[145] respiratory function,[146] and disability in both relapsing[134] and progressive MS[147], as well as strength, activity and respiratory function in nonambulatory persons with MS.[148]

The use of technology may augment rehabilitation for persons with MS. Virtual reality and gaming[149-151] may be useful and motivational alternatives or additions to traditional exercise therapy to improve arm movement and control, walking and anticipatory postural control in persons with MS. Virtual reality is also an effective interface for wheelchair users.[152] Training programs focusing on whole body vibration may improve muscle strength, walking endurance and reduce fall risk in persons with MS.[141,153,154]

Exercise responses of the patient with MS are influenced by a host of factors that require careful attention during exercise, including fatigue, spasticity, incoordination, impaired balance, sensory loss (numbness), tremor, and heat intolerance. As a result of exercise-induced increases in core body temperature, individuals with heat intolerance may be more tolerant to resistance exercise than endurance or aerobic exercise.[155] Additionally, depression may affect adherence to an exercise program. Therapists therefore need to provide constant reinforcement and a positive environment.

Individuals with MS will vary greatly in their responses to exercise. The focus and pace of therapy must be readjusted according to the patient's specific abilities and needs at that time. Patients with RRMS who are experiencing an exacerbation should not exercise until remission is evident. Exercise therapy can be reinstituted when the deterioration has stabilized, and no new symptoms are appearing. Patients with PPMS can exercise within the limits of their capabilities as exercise may slow further deterioration and optimize remaining function.[109] Table 16.4 presents a summary of selected systematic reviews and meta analyses related to exercise and MS.

Strength and Conditioning

Maximal muscle force during sustained isometric or isokinetic exercise is lower for persons with MS secondary to reduced ability to activate muscles (reduced force/unit muscle mass), reduced muscle metabolic responses, and muscle weakness secondary to muscle fiber atrophy, spasticity, and disuse. Determining an appropriate exercise prescription to improve strength and endurance is challenging and needs to be carefully individualized for each patient. Prescription is based on four interrelated elements: frequency of exercise, intensity of exercise, type of exercise, and time or duration (the *FITT equation*). The following guidelines can be used:[156]

- Exercise sessions should be scheduled on alternate (non-endurance) days and during optimal times, such as in the morning, when body core temperatures tend to be lowest and before fatigue sets in. Patients with greater neurological involvement may require more frequent exercise (e.g., daily exercise time).

Table 16.4 Evidence Summary Exercise and Multiple Sclerosis

Reference	Study Design/Intervention/Results
Campbell et al (2016)[147]	*Subjects:* 13 studies identified *Design/Intervention:* Systematic review examining the effect of physical therapy rehabilitation for persons with progressive MS *Results:* Studies were underpowered or power analyses were not performed. Multidisciplinary rehabilitation results in improvements in disability on the FIM as well as fatigue and quality of life. Inspiratory muscle training had a positive impact on maximal inspiratory and expiratory pressure in persons with progressive MS. Therapeutic standing significantly improved hip and ankle passive range of motion and reduced leg spasms. Results were inconclusive for exercise therapy, BOTOX injections, acupuncture, and BWSTT. *Comments:* There was a large variety of interventions considered (8 different types across 13 studies) ranging from exercise training to inspiratory muscle training to treadmill training to BOTOX injections.
Cruickshank et al (2015)[143]	*Subjects:* 7 of 20 identified studies included individuals with MS *Design/Intervention:* Systematic review and meta-analysis of strength training in individuals with MS or Parkinson's disease. *Results:* Strength training has a positive impact on muscle strength (effect size of 0.31), fatigue, functional capacity, quality of life, power and EMG activity in persons with MS with EDSS ≤6.5. *Comments:* The majority of studies examined muscle strength as the primary outcome with secondary outcomes of fatigue, quality of life or muscle power. Improvements in muscle power, fatigue and strength may underlie improvements in functional capacity.
Dalgas et al (2015)[136]	*Subjects:* 15 studies identified *Design/Intervention:* Systematic review and meta-analysis of RCTs examining the effect of exercise on depressive symptoms in persons with MS *Results:* The overall effect size of −0.37 indicated a small, yet beneficial effect of exercise on depressive symptoms. *Comments:* Baseline depression score, disability level, outcomes used, and intensity of exercise can influence the observed results of exercise training.
Gunn et al (2015)[140]	*Subjects:* 15 studies identified *Design/Intervention:* Systematic review and meta-analysis of randomized and quasi-randomized studies examining interventions targeting fall reduction and balance improvement in persons with MS *Results:* General exercise programs and gait, balance and functional training demonstrated significant improvements in balance outcomes, which may not significantly impact fall risk. *Comments:* Providing intensive practice and challenging balance activities is critical for maximizing effectiveness of balance interventions
Heine et al (2015)[137]	*Subjects:* 45 studies identified; 36 studies had sufficient data for meta-analysis *Design/Intervention:* Systematic review and meta-analysis examining the impact of exercise on fatigue in MS *Results:* 26 of 45 studies utilized a non-exercise control: exercise therapy produced a significant effect of fatigue (SMD −0.53; $p < 0.01$), particularly endurance training, mixed training, and "other" training. *Comments:* The majority of studies did not include individuals with progressive MS or an EDSS greater than 6.0.

Continued

Table 16.4 Evidence Summary Exercise and Multiple Sclerosis—cont'd

Reference	Study Design/Intervention/Results
Kantele et al (2015)[141]	*Subjects:* 7 studies identified *Design/Intervention:* Meta-analysis of RCTs examining effects of long-term whole-body vibration on mobility in MS *Results:* Improved 2–6 minute walking endurance following long-term whole body vibration (effect size 0.25). *Comments:* There was no improvement on walking speed (effect size 0.17) or balance (effect size -0.10) with whole body vibration. All studies targeted individuals with low disability levels.
Khan et al (2017)[134]	*Subjects:* 39 studies identified; 15 of 39 were *Cochrane Reviews* *Design/Intervention:* Systematic review of systematic reviews investigating rehabilitation in MS *Results:* There is "strong" evidence for physical therapy to improve: activity (disability), participation, depression (with cognitive behavioral therapy), patient knowledge (with information-provision interventions) There is "limited" evidence for improved patient outcomes (i.e., fatigue, spasticity) using psychological and symptom management programs *Comments:* High-quality evidence is needed to support many rehabilitation approaches. The cost-effectiveness, optimal dosage, or economic benefit of various interventions is not discussed.
Kjølhede et al (2012)[144]	*Subjects:* 16 studies identified *Design/Intervention:* Systematic review of studies utilizing progressive resistance training in persons with MS at EDSS <6.5. *Results:* Progressive resistance training improves muscle strength in persons with MS. The results are less consistent for improvements in muscle hypertrophy and neural changes, functional capacity, balance, and self-reported fatigue, mood and quality of life. *Comments:* Heterogeneity of the results may be a result of varied training protocols, sample sizes, outcome measures, and type and severity of MS.
Martín-Valero et al (2014)[146]	*Subjects:* 15 studies identified *Design/Intervention:* Systematic review and meta-analysis examining respiratory training interventions in MS *Results:* Respiratory muscle training resulted in improvements in maximum inspiratory pressure and maximum expiratory pressure. *Comments:* Training protocols were heterogeneous with regards to intensity, frequency and duration.
Platta et al (2016)[145]	*Subjects:* 20 studies included *Design/Intervention:* Systematic review examining the effects of exercise, physical activity and physical fitness on cognition in MS *Results:* Exercise training results in significant changes in muscular (effect size 0.27) and cardiorespiratory (effect size 0.47) fitness outcomes. *Comments:* Studies that did not include a measure of physical fitness were not included in this analysis.
Sandroff et al (2016)[139]	*Subjects:* 26 studies identified *Design/Intervention:* Systematic review examining the effects of exercise, physical activity and physical fitness on cognition in MS *Results:* Exercise: Class U (inadequate or conflicting data) with 4 of 9 studies supporting improvements in cognition with chronic exercise Physical activity: Class C (possibly effective) with 4 of 6 studies supporting improvements in cognition with physical activity

Table 16.4 Evidence Summary Exercise and Multiple Sclerosis—cont'd

Reference	Study Design/Intervention/Results
	Physical fitness: Class C (possibly effective) with 7 of 8 studies supporting improvements in cognitive performance with physical fitness *Comments:* Many studies included cognition as a secondary outcome and may be underpowered to detect changes.
Spooren et al (2012)[142]	*Subjects:* 11 studies identified *Design/Intervention:* Systematic review examining upper extremity training in MS *Results:* Motor training programs can improve arm and hand performance in MS. Effect sizes were not calculated. *Comments:* 10 of 11 studies included upper extremity training in conjunction with lower extremity training.
Toomey et al (2012)[148]	*Subjects:* 16 studies identified *Design/Intervention:* Systematic review examining rehabilitation interventions for non-ambulatory individuals with MS *Results:* 5 of 16 studies targeted exercise (i.e., aerobic exercise, strength training, respiratory muscle training) and suggest improvements in the target muscle trained, without carryover to other activities. 4 of 16 studies examined multidisciplinary rehabilitation interventions and noted improvements at impairment and activity levels. 5 of 16 studies examined cooling suits and found inconclusive results on fatigue. 1 of 16 studies examined therapeutic standing, resulting in significant improvements in hip and ankle range of motion that did not carryover to other activities. *Comments:* All studies identified were low-grade; high-grade evidence is needed to improve recommendations for non-ambulatory persons with MS.

BWSTT = body weight support treadmill training; EDSS = expanded disability status scale; EMG = electromyography; RCT = randomized controlled trial; SMD = standardized mean difference

- Resistance training modes can include weight machines, free or pulley weights, latex resistance bands, or isokinetic machines.
- Circuit training, in which improved work capacity is developed through the use of various different stations that alternate work between UEs and LEs, distributes the load among muscles and may prove beneficial for reducing the likelihood of fatigue.
- Sessions should involve discontinuous work, carefully balancing exercise with adequate rest periods.
- Progression is generally slower than with healthy individuals.
- Precautions should be taken to prevent the deleterious effects of overwork. Exercising to the point of fatigue is contraindicated and can result in worsening of symptoms, most notably temporary increased weakness. This may have additional adverse effects on the continuing motivation of the patient.
- Precautions should be taken to monitor the effects of fatigue. *Time to fatigue* varies greatly among individuals with MS and is *not* correlated with the level of physical impairment or disability.
- Precautions should be taken to manage core body temperature and prevent overheating.[157,158] Environmental temperatures should be carefully controlled. Air-conditioning is a medical necessity in many climates. Additional cooling can be achieved through the use of fans, wet neck wraps, spray bottles for misting the skin with cool water, and immersion in cool water with aquatic exercises. Surface cooling devices have emerged as effective tools in managing body temperatures, controlling fatigue, and improving function. These include cooling suits or vests.[159-161]
- Precautions should be taken with certain impairments. Tactile and proprioceptive losses or incoordination and tremors may make the use of some equipment (e.g., free weights) unsafe. Visual feedback, when intact, should be used to monitor exercise performance. An alternative suggestion would be to use synchronized arm/leg ergometers to control limb movements.
- Precautions should be taken with cognitive and memory impairments. Individuals may require written or posted exercise instructions/diagrams including reminders of the number of repetitions, proper form, and correct use of equipment.
- Functional training activities (e.g., closed chain exercises) can be used to promote strength and functional endurance. Individuals with ataxia and

balance problems may require the use of more stable postures (e.g., modified plantigrade, quadruped, or supported sitting).
- Group exercise classes can provide valuable motivation and social support. The therapist's primary role is one of educator and group leader. Successful management of group classes requires careful, individualized examination of group members to determine specific goals and exercises.
- Outcome measures can include isokinetic dynamometry, MMT (may be unreliable if spasticity is present), functional tests (e.g., sit-to-stand), fatigue (MFIS), and quality-of-life measures (HRQoL).

Recent work suggests that 8 weeks of individualized progressive resistance training in a group setting is sufficient to improve hip strength in persons with MS.[162]

Aerobic Conditioning

Individuals with MS demonstrate expected physiological responses to submaximal aerobic exercise; that is, heart rate (HR), blood pressure (BP), and oxygen uptake (V_{O_2}) all increase in a linear fashion in response to increasing workloads. Respiratory responses (respiratory rate [RR] and minute ventilation) also increase. However, HR and BP responses may be blunted if cardiovascular dysautonomia is present. A direct relationship exists between the duration and extent of disease[163] and the likelihood of autonomic cardiovascular dysfunction. Patients with MS can also demonstrate respiratory muscle dysfunction (weakness, dyssynergia), contributing to reduced exercise tolerance.

Exercise tolerance and maximal aerobic power ($V_{O_{2max}}$) are reduced in individuals with reduced cardiorespiratory fitness secondary to physical inactivity. Decreased physical work capacity, decreased vital capacity, increased HR at rest and in response to exercise, decreased muscular strength, increased fatigue, increased anxiety, and depression are common findings.

Determining an appropriate exercise prescription to improve cardiovascular conditioning needs to be carefully individualized for each patient. While predicting exercise capacity and cardiorespiratory fitness is challenging for individuals with MS, peak V_{O_2} and exercise capacity can be predicted through submaximal testing.[164-165] The following guidelines for *clinical exercise testing* can be used.[156]

- The preferred mode is either an upright or recumbent leg cycle ergometer. A recumbent device is indicated if sitting balance is impaired. Combination leg and arm ergometry or UE ergometry alone may be necessary in the presence of significant LE involvement. Toe clips and heel straps are recommended to control foot placement especially in patients with spasticity, tremor, or weakness.
- Performance measures include HR, ratings of perceived exertion (RPE), BP, and expired gas analysis (V_{O_2}). Using the RPE scale, peripheral (muscles, joints) exertion is consistently rated as more stressful (higher) than central (cardiopulmonary) exertion.
- A continuous or discontinuous protocol (3- to 5-minute stages) can be used; the discontinuous protocol is indicated with symptomatic disease, especially fatigue.
- A submaximal test should be used. Most individuals with MS can achieve 70% to 85% of their age-predicted maximal heart rate (HR_{max}).
- Recommendations for increasing workloads for each stage are 12 to 25 watts for LE work and 8 to 12 watts for combined UE and LE work.
- Termination criteria include achievement of peak HR, peak V_{O_2}, volitional fatigue, significant BP changes (systolic blood pressure [SBP] greater than 250 mm Hg or diastolic blood pressure [DPB] greater than 115 mm Hg or a hypotensive response), or a decrease in oxygen uptake with increasing work rate.
- Precautions should be taken to monitor for attenuated HR or BP responses during exercise. A category-ratio RPE scale can be used to estimate central and peripheral exertion.[108]
- Precautions should be taken to manage core body temperature and prevent overheating (e.g., use of a fan for cooling).
- Precautions should be taken to monitor the effects of fatigue.
- Precautions should be taken to prevent the deleterious effects of overwork.
- Precautions should be taken with certain medications that can affect results: amantadine hydrochloride (HCl) may temporarily reduce fatigue; baclofen and amitriptyline HCl may cause muscle weakness; prednisone can also cause muscle weakness along with reduced sweating and hypertension.
- Morning is the optimal time for testing.

Prescription is again based on the four interrelated elements of the FITT equation. Recommendations for exercise programming to improve aerobic conditioning include the following:[156]

- Recommended training frequency is 3 to 5 days/week, on alternate days. Daily exercise at lower levels of intensity is recommended for individuals with more limited exercise capacities (e.g., 3 to 5 metabolic equivalents [METs]).
- Training intensity should be limited to 60% to 85% HR_{peak} or 50% to 70% peak V_{O_2}.
- Recommended duration is 30 minutes per session or, for more involved individuals, three 10-minute sessions per day.
- Type of exercise can include cycling, walking, swimming, or water aerobics.
- Circuit training may prove best for optimizing training.
- Individuals with balance problems or sensory loss will require non–weight-bearing activities.

- Exercise precautions: discussed in previous section.
- Outcome measures include graded exercise test results, HR (which may be difficult to monitor with dysautonomia; sensory loss in the fingers may make self-monitoring difficult), tests of lung function (forced vital capacity [FVC]), body composition, RPE, fatigue (FI, MFIS), functional status, and quality-of-life measures (HRQoL).

Patient education is particularly important because the overall success of a fitness program is influenced by the individual's level of understanding of the basic principles of training, independence in self-monitoring, and skill in decision making relative to level of impairment and exercise modifications required, as well as lifestyle and general health and safety considerations.

Flexibility Exercises

Stretching and ROM exercises are necessary to ensure adequate joint motion and to counteract the effects of spasticity (Fig. 16.3). Sedentary or inactive persons who are dependent on wheelchairs often develop tightness in hip flexors, adductors, hamstrings, and plantarflexors. Limited overhead ROM is seen with tightness in the pectoralis major/minor, and latissimus dorsi and is associated with a slumped, forward posture. Patients confined to bed typically present with tightness in hip/knee extensors, adductors, and plantarflexors. Stretching and ROM exercises should be performed daily. For adequate stretching, holding at end range should be a minimum of 30 to 60 seconds repeated for a minimum of two repetitions. The use of orthoses or dynamic splinting is an appropriate option for prevention and in some cases reversal of contractures.[166,167] Considering the gait deviations and difficulty with transfers/bed mobility that arise from limited ROM and spasticity, it is important to also include aggressive trunk ROM to allow for full function of the core musculature, most notably the quadratus lumborum (Fig. 16.4). More active patients may benefit from Tai Chi, which provides additional important benefits of relaxation and balance training. ROM measurement using goniometry is an appropriate outcome measure.

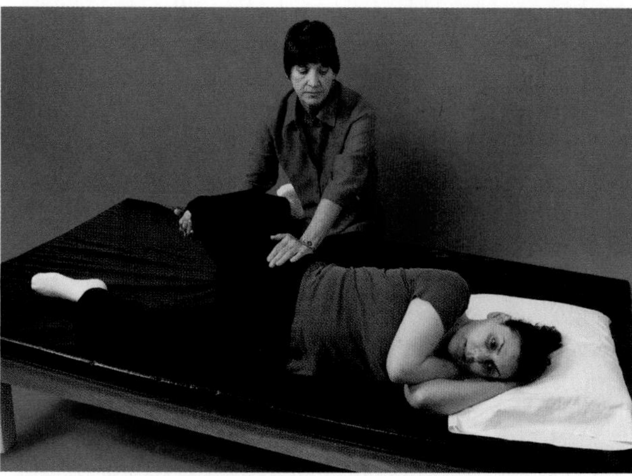

Figure 16.3 Side-lying hip flexor/rectus femoris stretch. This position allows the therapists to control the hip and ensure that excessive lumber lordosis is prevented while also modulating the amount of stretch between the iliopsoas and the rectus femoris.

Management of Bladder Control

The prevalence of urinary incontinence among individuals with MS is greater than 50%. Many individuals benefit from physical therapy intervention to address bladder control in conjunction with care from a urologist. Timed voiding on a schedule is useful when individuals have impaired bladder sensation, whereas fluid restriction at certain times of the day may minimize incontinence events (e.g., restrict evening fluid intake to avoid nocturia).[168] Biofeedback and physical therapy targeting the strength of the pelvic floor muscles are successful at combating urgency, improving incontinence, and improving quality of life.[169,170] Functional training may also assist patients who may be unsteady when hurrying to the restroom, which has been linked to increased fall risks among persons with MS.[171]

Management of Fatigue

With approximately 75% of individuals with MS describing persistent or sporadic symptoms, fatigue is among the most debilitating. Fatigue is characterized

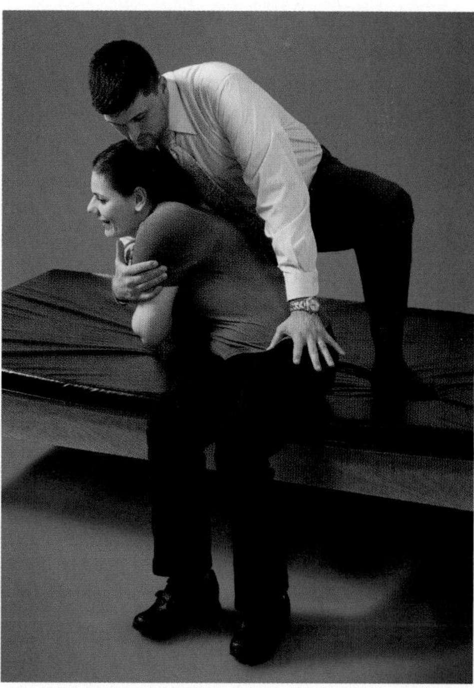

Figure 16.4 Seated trunk stretch. The pictured position allows the therapist to control the pelvis to ensure trunk stretching while maintaining control of the individual's trunk to apply the correct emphasis to the desired muscle groups.

by overwhelming sleepiness, excessive tiredness, and sense of weakness that comes on suddenly and severely. Aversion to activity for fear of bringing on fatigue is also common. The resultant lowered activity levels have important implications for diminished health status and deconditioning. Therapists are faced with a balancing act, on one hand prescribing exercise, while on the other hand avoiding overwork and the development of fatigue. Aerobic exercise training (previously discussed) and *energy effectiveness strategies (EES)* are central to any intervention plan to lessen fatigue.[26] During exercise prescription and physical therapy sessions, it is imperative that a skilled therapist recognize the difference between MS-related fatigue and the expected exercise-related fatigue. MS-related fatigue during exercise is often associated with thermal stress, which can be offset with adequate rest and the use of cooling and precooling treatments during exercise.[159-161]

Patients are instructed to keep an *activity diary* in which they record how they slept the night before, daily activities by hour, and how costly those activities were. For each activity, they can be asked to rate their level of fatigue (*F*), the value or importance of the activity (*V*), and satisfaction perceived with performance of the activity (*S*) by assigning a number between 1 and 10 with 1 being very low and 10 being very high. For example, the activity might be fixing lunch. Scores reported for this activity might be $F = 7$, $V = 3$, and $S = 2$. Aggravating factors associated with increasing fatigue (e.g., heat stress) and MS symptoms that appear or worsen during the day are also recorded. An *MS Daily Activity Diary* is available online at: http://www.hail.ku.edu.

Based on this information, therapists can initiate training sessions, teaching energy effectiveness strategies. *Energy conservation* refers to the adoption of strategies that reduce overall energy requirements of the task and overall level of fatigue. These can include modifying the task or modifying the environment to ensure successful completion of daily activities. For example, a motorized scooter or powered wheelchair can be considered for community or home mobility to help conserve energy and maintain independence. Other mobility equipment such as walkers, crutches, or orthotics can also be considered. Activities that are difficult or have high energy needs can be broken down into component parts, requiring accurate activity analysis. *Activity pacing* refers to the balancing of activity with rest periods interspersed throughout the day. For the patient with chronic fatigue, *rest–activity ratios* are developed, with periodic rest periods planned in advance. Time-outs with complete rest should be instituted if an activity becomes exhaustive. Overall levels of energy can be improved if patients learn to set priorities and limit their activities, saving their energy for those activities that are truly important to them (e.g., activities that are enjoyable and meaningful in terms of the individual's lifestyle). The occupational therapist addresses EES and can provide valuable suggestions in terms of planning, work simplification, and developing energy-efficient activities for self-care and home management. The vocational rehabilitation counselor can provide useful strategies for behavioral modification and vocational rehabilitation. Team efforts with the physical therapist and others are important for consistency and reinforcement. Weekly review of activities and recommended modifications is used to evaluate progress. The MFIS should be administered on a regular basis to monitor ongoing fatigue status. Finally, stress management techniques are important components of symptom management.

The occupational and physical therapist should complete a direct environmental examination of the home and/or job site (see Chapter 9, Examination and Modification of the Environment). A number of adaptations may be considered to improve efficiency and safety, including air-conditioning, home, or work modifications, or ergonomic equipment. The patient/family/caregivers should be educated as to the importance of these recommendations for improved function. Periodic review of equipment and environmental modifications is also recommended. Additional referrals or collaboration with neuropsychology may also be useful to combat fatigue. Recent work suggests that behavioral interventions may also improve fatigue in persons with MS.[130,172]

Proper communication between the occupational and physical therapist and the patient's physician can ensure that the correct doses of the pharmacological treatments are in place, as the therapist has the unique opportunity of observing the patient in various circumstances and activity levels.

Management of Spasticity

Although spasticity varies greatly from person to person, muscles that typically demonstrate strong tone include the antigravity muscles. For example, in the LEs, the quadriceps, hip adductors, and plantarflexors are often spastic while in the UEs the elbow, wrist, and finger flexors together with shoulder adductors are spastic. Individuals with MS typically demonstrate stronger spasticity in the LEs than the UEs. Spasticity is functionally limiting and contributes to the development of a number of secondary impairments such as contractures, postural deformity, and decubitus ulcers.

A variety of physical therapy interventions can be used, including cryotherapy, hydrotherapy, therapeutic exercise, stretching, positioning, or any combination thereof. The responses to these interventions must be monitored closely and carefully balanced with pharmacological interventions. The therapist must closely monitor the effects of the antispasticity medications prescribed and optimize physical therapy interventions with the dosing cycle. For example, patients on baclofen will respond better to stretching techniques if they are applied in the middle of the dosing cycle rather than at the end or beginning. Physical therapists must also recognize contributing factors that affect tone and respond appropriately. For example, infection or fever that increases tone may require a referral to the physician. It is important to reduce or eliminate all factors that can aggravate spasticity (e.g., heat, humidity, stress).

Topical cold (ice packs or wraps) or hydrotherapy (cool bath) can temporarily reduce spasticity by decreasing tendon reflex excitability and clonus and by slowing conduction of impulses in nerves and muscles. The effects of cryotherapy are relatively short-lived, although some patients may experience enhanced ability to move that lasts for minutes or hours. It is important to remember that some patients, particularly those with intact sensation, may react to the unpleasant sensation of cold with *fight or flight* (autonomic nervous system) responses, such as increased HR, increased RR, or nausea. Cryotherapy is contraindicated in these patients.

Stretching and ROM exercises begun early in the course of the disease and continued daily can help patients maintain joint integrity and mobility in the presence of spasticity. Combining stretching with movements using rhythmic rotation (gentle rotation of the limb) or proprioceptive neuromuscular facilitation (PNF) stretching techniques (hold–relax active contraction [HRAC], contract–relax active contraction [CRAC]) is effective in gaining ROM.[173] See Chapter 10, Strategies to Improve Motor Function, for a discussion of these techniques. Maintained stretch, held for 30 minutes to 3 hours, also can be used to decrease stretch reflex activity. Maintained stretch can be achieved with prolonged positioning (e.g., tilt table standing with toe wedges), low-load weights applied using skin traction, or serial casts. Air splints also provide an effective mechanism to maintain limbs in lengthened, out of spasticity positions. Patients/family members/clients should be taught stretching exercises as part of a home exercise program (HEP). Fast, ballistic stretching movements are contraindicated, because spasticity is velocity sensitive. Stretching movements need to proceed slowly to gradually achieve the desired range.

Active exercises at slow or self-selected speeds should focus on expanding the available ROM. Emphasis on contracting the antagonist muscles can assist through mechanisms of reciprocal inhibition. Electrical stimulation of muscles antagonist to the spastic muscles can also be used to decrease spasticity. Movements that encourage abnormal postures should be discouraged. Patients with abnormal co-contraction may benefit from exercises focused on improving motor control (timing exercises) or biofeedback. Tai Chi, yoga, and aquatic exercises combined with cool water temperatures (less than 85°F [29.44°C]) can also be helpful in producing desired relaxation.[12]

Functional activities aimed at reducing tone should concentrate on trunk and proximal segments, because many patterns of hypertonus seem to be fixed from the action of the stronger proximal muscles. Extensor tone seems to predominate, so activities that stress LE flexion with trunk rotation are generally the most effective. For example, lower trunk rotation (LTR) in hook-lying can be effective in reducing proximal extensor tone. One very effective strategy is to position the patient in hook-lying with a therapy ball under the flexed legs and gently rock the ball back and forth. Moving from quadruped position to side-sitting can also be effective in reducing extensor tone in some patients as the activity combines LTR with prolonged inhibitory pressure on the quadriceps.[174]

For the patient with limited functional mobility (EDSS levels of 7.0 or above) positioning out of abnormal spastic postures is an important component of the management program. In general, prolonged or static positioning in any fixed posture can be deleterious to the patient with strong spasticity and should be avoided. For example, the patient who remains in bed all day with the LEs positioned in extension, adduction, and plantarflexion may be unable to flex enough at the hips and knees to sit in a wheelchair. Similarly, the feet will remain fixed in plantarflexion and cannot be positioned on the footrests. A positioning schedule using varied positions (in bed, chair, or wheelchair) will help keep the patient from getting stuck in any one posture. Mechanical positioning devices (e.g., resting splints, toe spreader, finger spreader, ankle splint) are helpful in maintaining position and preserving joint structures.

Management of Coordination and Balance Deficits

Cerebellar deficits (ataxia, postural instability) are common in MS. Impairments in somatosensory, visual, vestibular systems are also common and can significantly impair coordination and balance. Spasms and muscle weakness can affect balance by changing the force and sequence of muscle contraction.[175] These combined effects result in difficulty in sustaining upright postures, walking, and other functional activities, leading to an increased risk of falls.

Interventions directed at promoting postural control should first focus on static control (holding) in weight-bearing, antigravity postures (e.g., sitting, quadruped, kneeling, modified plantigrade, and standing). Progression through a series of postures is used to gradually increase postural demands by varying the base of support (BOS), raising the center of mass (COM), and increasing the number of body segments (degrees of freedom) that must be controlled. Specific exercise techniques that can be used to promote stability include joint approximation applied through proximal joints (shoulders or hips) or spine and rhythmic stabilization (PNF). Patients with significant ataxia will not be able to hold steady and may benefit from the application of the technique of PNF dynamic reversals (slow reversals), progressing through decrements of range.[173] Dynamic postural control can be challenged by incorporating activities such as weight shifting and UE reaching (Fig. 16.5) or LE stepping. In

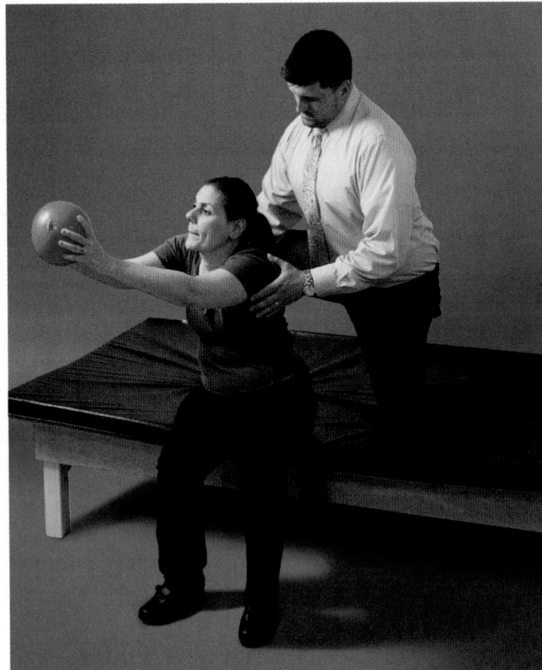

Figure 16.5 Dynamic postural control is promoted through weight shifting and upper trunk rotation to the right.

sitting, combining UE movements with trunk movements (flexion with rotation and extension with rotation) is an excellent activity. This can be progressed to more advanced dynamic activities with the patient sitting on a therapy (Swiss) ball as opposed to sitting on a hard, flat surface (Fig. 16.6). Core musculature is engaged while the demands on ankle and knee musculature are minimized. This allows for a more focused core balance program that can progress to standing.[176]

An important goal of therapy is to promote safe and functional balance. Effective training should involve a variety of everyday functional tasks that challenge balance. Figure 16.7 demonstrates a dynamic postural control activity of combined stepping and reaching. Figure 16.8 demonstrates sit-to-stand movement transitions. As training progresses, tasks are modified (e.g., wide base to narrow base to tandem stance, stable surface to moveable surface) to promote adaptation of skills. Sensory contexts are also varied to promote adaptive control in various different perceptual contexts (e.g., eyes open to eyes closed, firm surface to thick foam surface).[174] Patients with MS and central vestibular dysfunction may benefit from vestibular rehabilitation to improve impaired balance and disability due to dizziness or disequilibrium[177] (Fig. 16.9). See Chapter 21, Vestibular Disorders, for additional discussion.

The pool is an important therapeutic medium to practice static and dynamic postural control in both sitting and standing, as well as walking. Water provides graded resistance that slows down the patient's ataxic movements, while the buoyancy aids in upright balance. Water aerobics have been shown to be effective in improving strength, decreasing muscular fatigability, increasing endurance, and improving overall fatigue and quality of life in patients with MS.[178-180] When recommending aquatic exercise programs, it is imperative to assess the individual's tolerance to heat. It is commonly recommended that persons with MS exercise in a pool that is 80° to 85°F (26.66° to 29.44°C).

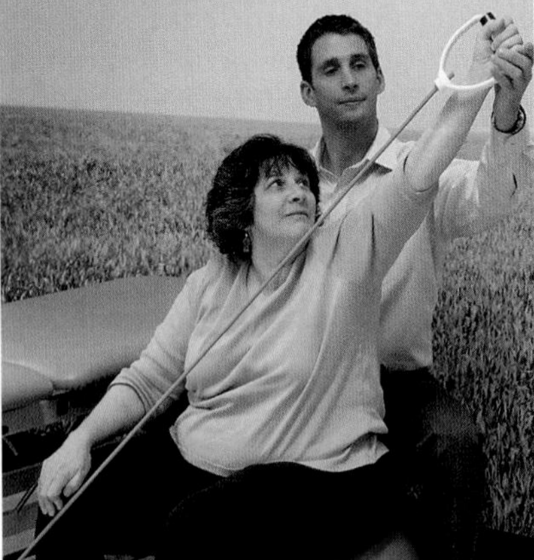

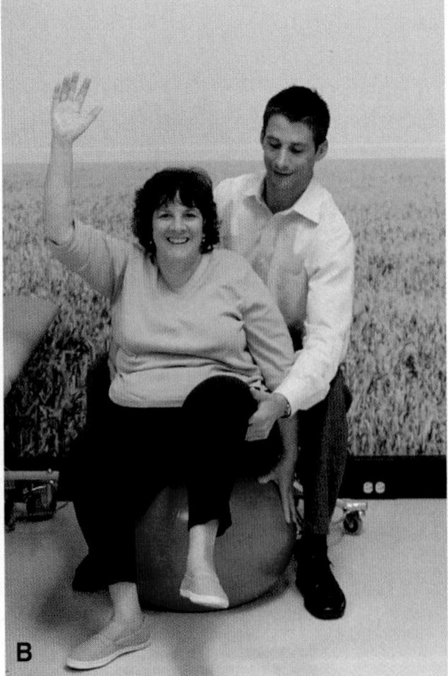

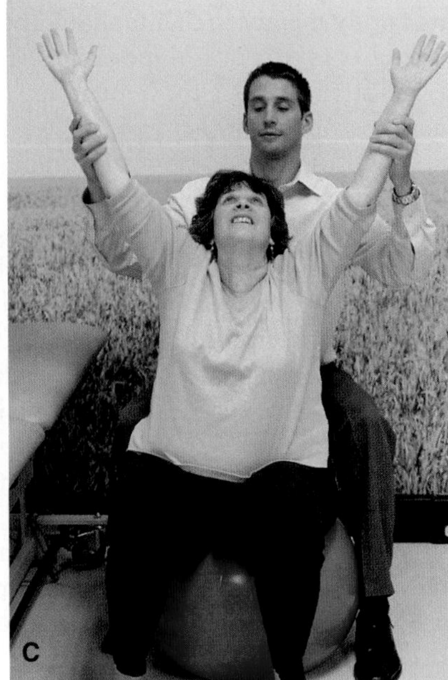

Figure 16.6 Sitting on the ball, the patient practices dynamic postural control activities: (A) unilateral resisted overhead reach, (B) reciprocal stepping and overhead arm swing, and (C) resisted overhead reaching.

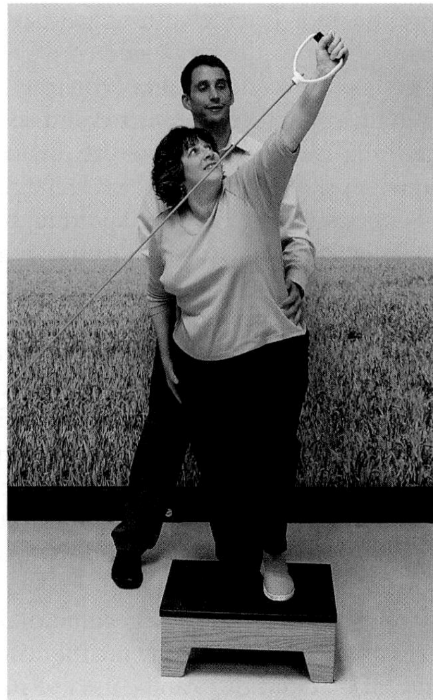

Figure 16.7 Dynamic postural control activities. This position demonstrates an advanced stepping and reaching activity with the added challenge of a resistance tube.

Biofeedback training using augmented feedback can be used to improve balance function. Augmented visual feedback[181] and augmented proprioceptive feedback (e.g., whole body vibration platform training)[182] have been used to improve function in patients with MS. Training on a moveable force platform (e.g., SMART Balance Master® [NeuroCom International, Inc., Clackamas, OR 97015]) can also improve balance. The added biofeedback from visual and/or auditory feedback displays on force platform training machines is especially useful for patients with somatosensory deficits. The patient with ataxia needs to learn how to reduce excess postural sway (frequency and amplitude) and to control center of alignment position. Prolonged latencies (onset of responses) should be expected.

Control of ataxic limb movements (tremor and dysmetria) can be achieved through proprioceptive loading and light resistance. For example, the therapist can use dynamic reversals with light tracking resistance to modulate force output and reciprocal actions of muscles. Ataxic movements have sometimes been helped by the application of latex resistance bands or light weights to stabilize movements. Velcro® weight cuffs (wrist or ankle), weighted boots, or a weighted jacket or belt can reduce tremors of the limbs or trunk. The extra weight will also increase energy expenditure and must therefore be carefully balanced against the increased fatigue they might cause. Weighted canes or walkers can be used to reduce ataxic UE movements that interfere with the use of an assistive device during ambulation. Weighted spoons or forks can be used to enhance eating. For patients with significant tremor, these devices may mean the difference between dependent and independent function. External devices (braces or splints) can be used to stabilize ataxic limbs but also have the undesirable effect of adding weight to limb movements. Air splints can also stabilize limb movements and should be considered, because they are lighter and less energy costly. A soft cervical collar can be used to stabilize head and neck tremors. All these strategies, however, should be viewed as temporary and compensatory. Once the devices are removed, ataxic movements will return or in some cases may actually temporarily worsen.

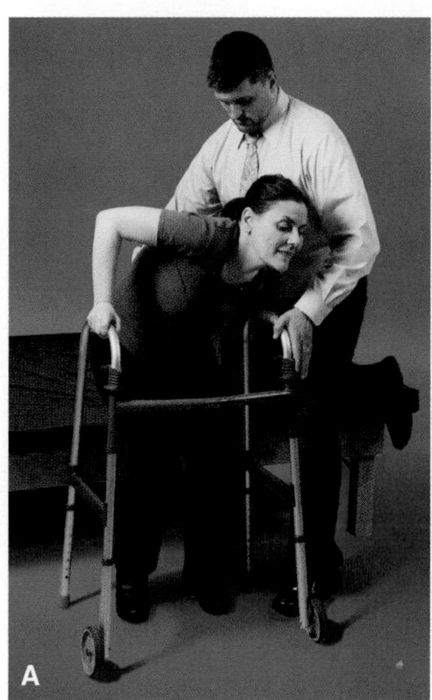

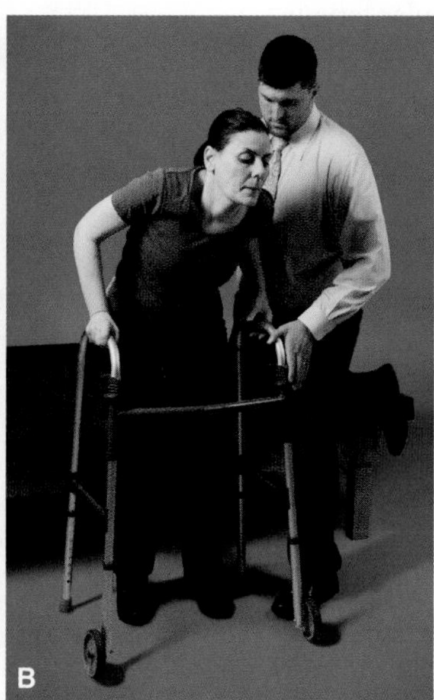

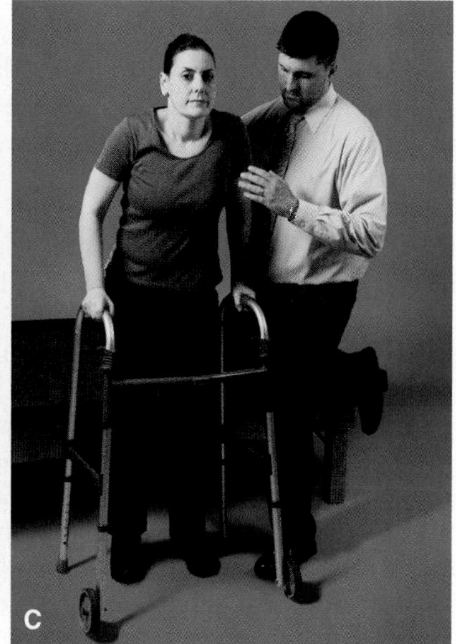

Figure 16.8 Sit-to-stand movement transition. The sit-to-stand transition is an important component of pre-gait/gait training, transfer training, and balance training.

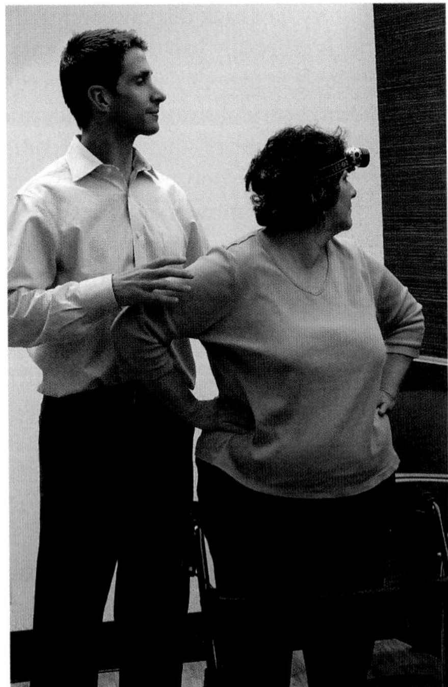

Figure 16.9 Head turns for vestibular training.

Unwanted movements are worse under conditions of stress, anxiety, and excitement. The increased arousal, the result of adrenalin pumping through the system, increases existing tremors while decreasing function. Stress management techniques are therefore an important component of the POC. In general, patients do better in a low-stimulus environment that allows full concentration on control of movements. They benefit from augmented feedback (verbal cueing of knowledge of results and knowledge of performance; biofeedback) and repetition to improve motor learning. The patient with MS is often restricted in practice by neuromuscular fatigue and neurological deficits that impair sensory feedback, attention, memory, and concentration. The successful therapist will need to carefully identify the patient's resources and abilities and capitalize on them to maximize motor learning.

Locomotor Training

Walking ability is frequently impaired. However, at least 65% of patients with MS are still walking after 20 years.[20] Early gait problems often include poor balance and heaviness of one or more limbs. Patients frequently report difficulty lifting their legs (hip flexor weakness). Weak dorsiflexors are also common, resulting in foot drop. Problems with foot clearance may result in a circumducted gait pattern, among other gait deviations. Later problems evolve owing to clonus, spasticity, sensory loss, and/or ataxia. Weakness generally extends to include the quadriceps and hip abductors. Quadriceps weakness typically results in hyperextension of the knee and forward flexion of the trunk with increased lumbar lordosis. Hip abductor weakness results in a Trendelenburg gait pattern with a strong lateral lean to the weak side.

A well-designed exercise program of tone management, stretching, strengthening exercises and task-specific walking training can improve walking. Standing and walking activities should stress safety and maintaining a stable BOS; maximum weight-bearing through the LEs; and adequate weight transfer and forward progression with trunk, limb, and pelvic kinematics consistent with safe walking. Verbal and manual cueing can assist the patient in the correct mechanics of gait. A variety of functional activities should be practiced. These include walking forward and backward, side-stepping, and cross-stepping (Fig. 16.10). Braiding, which combines side-stepping and cross-stepping is a complex, higher-level walking activity. Stair climbing, negotiating curbs and ramps, navigation around obstacles, and walking on varied surfaces should also be practiced for safety in community mobility. See Chapter 11, Locomotor Training, for further discussion. As previously mentioned, the pool is an important medium that can be used to assist training of the more involved patient with ataxia while reducing tone and fatigue.

Locomotor training (LT) using an antigravity treadmill or a treadmill training (TT) with body weight support (BWS) results in improvements in muscle strength, spasticity, endurance, balance, walking speed, and quality of life. Level of effort was reduced while detrimental effects on fatigue are not evident.[183,184] BWSTT is also safe and beneficial for individuals with progressive disease and

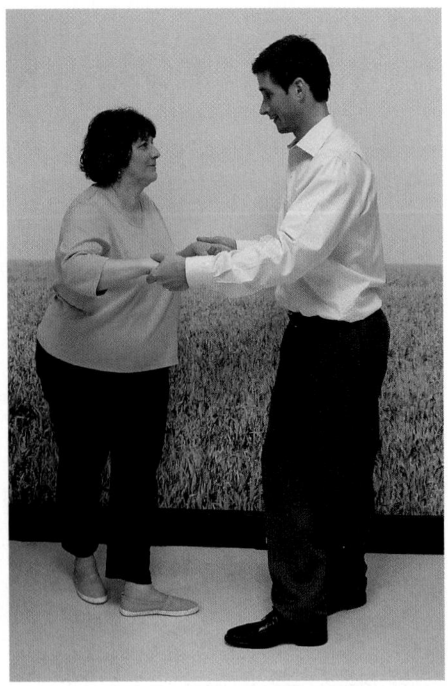

Figure 16.10 Patient practices cross-stepping. Dynamic standing activities are an integral component of an exercise program geared toward improving gait/locomotion.

results in improvements in fatigue and quality of life.[185] Robot-assisted treadmill training (RATT) with BWS has also been used and when compared with conventional BWSTT, patients in both groups experienced similar improvements in outcome measures.[186,187] When RATT was compared with conventional gait training, no difference in outcomes was found between the groups.[188] Recent work suggests that eccentric training may be particularly useful for persons with MS; downhill treadmill walking resulted in significant improvements in fatigue, mobility, balance, and strength when compared with uphill walking.[189] Other forms of stepping, as in recumbent stepping may be promising rehabilitation tools, particularly for individuals with progressive disease.[185] In summary, LT with BWS is an activity-dependent intervention that is feasible and safe and has the potential to result in significant improvements in function for patients with MS.

Balance and LT may also be paired with secondary cognitive or motor demands during training to target dual-task deficits. The ability to perform tasks simultaneously is frequently impaired in persons with MS due to motor and cognitive impairments. A systematic review of dual-task training studies in neurodegenerative disorders concluded that virtual reality training may improve dual-task performance.[190]

Orthotics and Assistive Devices

Patients with MS often require orthotic devices as ambulation skills decline. Improvements in energy efficiency and safety are also important outcomes. Ankle–foot stability can be achieved by the addition of an ankle–foot orthosis (AFO). AFOs are prescribed for foot drop, poor knee control (especially hyperextension), minimal to moderate spasticity, and poor somatosensation. The most common types used are the standard polypropylene AFO (Fig. 16.11) and the carbon fiber AFO, which are lightweight and have the added benefit of cosmesis. An AFO with an articulated joint can be prescribed to provide more rigid control for the ankle with the addition of a plantarflexion stop. Functional electrical stimulation (FES) devices have become prevalent in treatment and compensation for foot drop with improvements in walking performance and satisfaction reported. Patients also experienced fewer falls and reduced fatigue.[191-193] In order to effectively use any orthotic or FES device for foot drop, an individual must have adequate hip flexion strength. Relative contraindications to the prescription of these devices include severe spasticity, foot edema, and weakness (nonfunctional grades of LE muscles, especially hip flexors). Although knee–ankle–foot orthoses (KAFOs) can provide additional stabilization control of the knee, they are rarely used because of the increased energy expenditure required.

Canes, forearm crutches, or a walker may be necessary to compensate for deficits in fatigue, strength, sensory loss (numbness), or balance (Fig. 16.12). For many patients, acceptance of an assistive device involves full recognition of their disability, so early discussion and introduction of these devices may smooth the transition when these devices are required. They need to be convinced that use of these devices is far

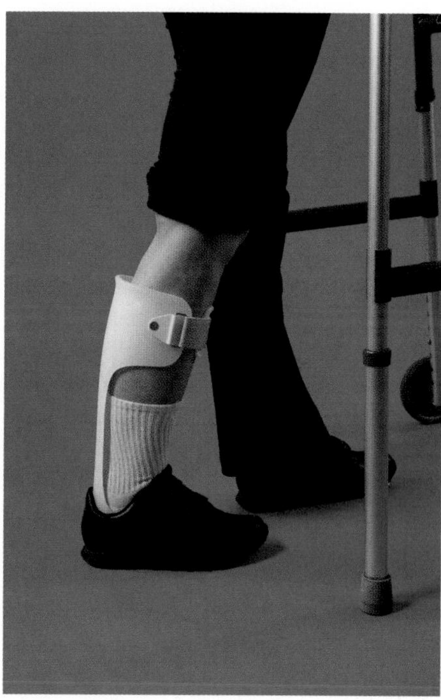

Figure 16.11 Patient is wearing an ankle–foot orthosis (AFO) to stabilize the ankle and prevent foot drop.

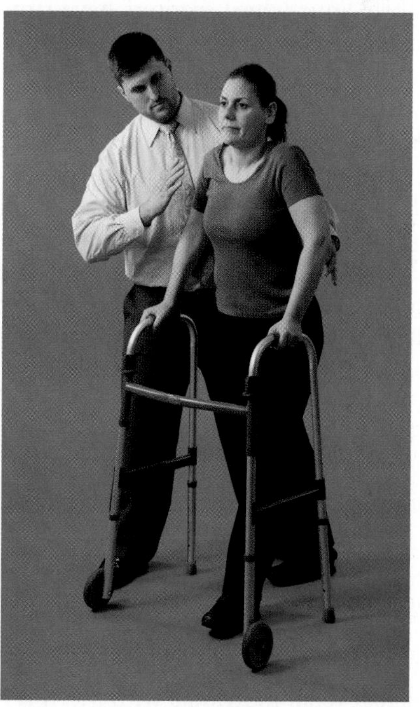

Figure 16.12 Locomotor training with a front-wheeled rolling walker.

safer than "wall walking" or "furniture walking." Devices also provide recognition to the community at large that patients are not staggering or losing their balance because they are "drunk," a frequent occurrence with many patients. The devices may be the difference between community participation or remaining homebound because of fear of falling. Patients should be encouraged to try out different devices to determine which works best for them. For example, the patient with significant fatigue levels may benefit from a large-wheeled walker with locking hand brakes and a seat that allows for frequent rests. Recent technological advancements have brought a new breed of mechanical upright walking devices that have integrated computer chips, sensors, and motors to aid an individual in ambulation. Cosmesis is an important factor in promoting acceptance. There are many innovations in assistive technology that make the choices easier. For example, designer canes now come in many different colors and styles, including clear Lucite. ABLEDATA (www.abledata.com) is a federally funded project that offers product information, resources, and links to manufacturers.

As the disease progresses, many patients benefit from a wheeled mobility device (powered scooter or wheelchair). The course and progression of the disease and presenting symptoms should be taken into consideration when deciding on a device. For patients with adequate trunk stability, UE function, and appropriate visual, perceptual, and cognitive skills, a scooter provides needed mobility while conserving energy. Scooters also do not carry the same negative stigma as that of a wheelchair. Both three- and four-wheel scooters are available. Four-wheel scooters have superior outdoor and uneven terrain performance but are not as easily transported. Features that should be recommended include a seat that rotates for easy mounting and dismounting, easy dismantling for loading into the car, and steering mechanisms that minimize the work of the UEs. One disadvantage of scooters is that seating cannot always be customized. They are often not designed for prolonged sitting or for patients with moderate to severe postural instability. Some new three-wheeled scooters are designed to turn in very small areas while others have a wide turning radius and may not be suitable for in-home use. The individual with MS must be adequately educated on the safety precautions of a scooter, because the trunk strength and stability requirements are significantly higher than those of a power wheelchair.

A wheelchair should be considered when postural demands necessitate increased support. A standard wheelchair requires additional energy expenditure and coordination for propulsion. When prescribing a manual wheelchair to an individual with MS it is important to include education on proper wheelchair propulsion for both preservation of shoulder strength and energy conservation. A power wheelchair should be considered when impairments prevent or limit manual propulsion or when fatigue is a major limiting factor in mobility (Fig. 16.13). However, they are costlier and require specialized transportation by a wheelchair-accessible van or bus. Most patients will navigate using a joystick. For patients with impaired hand strength and sensation, the joystick can be adjusted to increase sensitivity. Wheelchair seating should ensure proper alignment of the pelvis, trunk and head, and limbs while enhancing function. Common malalignments include posterior tilting of the pelvis (sacral sitting) with kyphosis, typically the result of spasticity in the hamstring muscles. This can be improved with the addition of a seat cushion. Postural alignment can also be assisted by the addition of contoured seating (custom built). A solid back support and adjustable lateral trunk supports may be needed to enhance postural alignment and upright sitting. Footrests should be positioned to ensure that the thighs are parallel to the floor. If extensor spasms are strong, they can actually propel the patient out of the chair. A strong lap belt that secures firmly around the pelvis is necessary for safety. For patients with strong adductor spasticity, a medial knee block (pommel) may be necessary. Heel loops and straps may be required to maintain foot position on the footrests. Patients who no longer demonstrate adequate trunk and head stability require an alternate seating design. A tilt-in-space wheelchair with head/neck support is a better option than a reclining

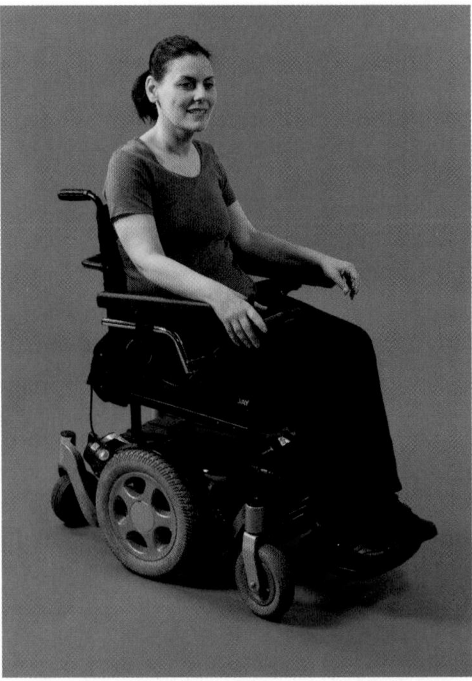

Figure 16.13 An individual with MS using a power wheelchair with joystick control for mobility. The correct power wheelchair prescription can encourage proper alignment of the pelvis, trunk, head, and limbs.

wheelchair with high back and elevating legrests. The former maintains the normal hip sitting angle; the latter produces extension of the hips and may feed into strong extensor spasticity. Elevating legrests tend to stretch hamstring muscles and may cause posterior pelvic tilting when spasticity is present. The reclining wheelchair with elevating legrests also creates greater environmental access problems. Motorized control of the seat back available in tilt-in-space wheelchairs will allow the patient to make easy adjustments in position, thus preventing skin breakdown. See Chapter 32, The Prescriptive Wheelchair, for additional discussion.

Patients should be instructed in transfer and wheelchair mobility/management skills. A transfer board or hydraulic lift may be necessary as UE function deteriorates. Attention to good sitting posture and pressure-relief techniques is essential to maintain alignment and prevent skin breakdown. Patients should be encouraged to balance time in the wheelchair with other activities, such as walking or exercising, and should be extra diligent in stretching muscles that tend to contract as a result of prolonged sitting (e.g., hip and knee flexors).

One of the constraints the therapist will have to deal with is financial reimbursement for the changing mobility needs of the patient with chronic MS. Private or public insurance organizations require a statement of medical necessity for payment. Because symptoms are not static in MS but rather typically exacerbate or remit, the therapist needs to provide clear and convincing documentation of need, stressing improved function and safety. Many third-party payers will not reimburse for new wheelchairs prescribed within specified time intervals or may be hesitant to finance expensive specialty wheelchairs such as the tilt-in-space chair or a second lightweight chair for traveling. The therapist will need to provide careful documentation of potential adverse outcomes to justify the cost of the new chair. For example, a likely deleterious outcome for a patient who is denied reimbursement for a tilt-in-space chair may be skin breakdown. The costs of nursing and surgical care for decubitus ulcers can then be compared with the cost of the new wheelchair, which can be justified as a preventive measure. It is equally important to anticipate future needs as they relate to rate of disease progression when ordering equipment.

Functional Training

Functional training should focus on problem solving and the development of appropriate decision making skills required to meet the challenges of being disabled. Skills should be adapted and practiced to ensure safe performance in both the home and community environments. Training in functional mobility skills (e.g., bed mobility, transfers, locomotion) is typically directed by the physical therapist whereas ADL (e.g., dressing, personal hygiene, bathing, toileting, grooming, and feeding) and IADL (e.g., cooking, laundry, and bed making) training is directed by the occupational therapist and training in communication skills by the speech-language pathologist. Close communication and coordination among team members is necessary to ensure that training methods are applied consistently and successfully. Full participation of the patient in all phases of planning and training will increase personal involvement while decreasing dependency and passivity.

Many individuals with MS will use multiple adaptive devices. This requires careful attention to appropriate prescription of devices and environmental modifications to assist the patient in conserving energy and maintaining function. Assistive devices are discussed earlier in this chapter in *Orthotics and Assistive Devices*. Adaptive equipment can include bed or bathroom grab bars, overhead trapeze, raised seats, transfer board, or hydraulic lift. Appropriate positional and functional splints to facilitate writing or typing and plates and cups with lips to minimize spills are often helpful in assisting with hand function. Long-handled shoehorns, reachers, button hooks, sock aids, or Velcro® closures can assist in dressing. Effective communication may require built-up writing utensils or a universal cuff for written communication or more sophisticated computerized devices. Patients with severe speech problems may require voice amplification devices, electronic aids, or computer-assisted alternative communication systems. The team must recognize when a device is indicated and assist the patient in acceptance and in learning how to use the device *before* significant deterioration of function occurs.

Management of Speech and Swallowing

Impairments in communication and swallowing have been identified in individuals with MS.[194] Approximately 44% of MS patients experience impairments of speech and voice early in the disease course, while 35% to 43% of MS patients can acquire voice, chewing, and swallowing disorders.[195] Respiratory deconditioning, characterized by reduced diaphragmatic support and shortening of the intercostal muscles, contributes to speech disorders and increases the likelihood of respiratory infections. Thus, collaborating with a speech-language pathologist to develop a *resistive breathing training* (RBT) program paired with activities to improve trunk stability, head control, and sitting balance is an important component of the POC for patients with MS. Improved respiration can be facilitated through the implementation of prolonged phonation exercises, resistive breathing exercises, and incentive spirometry. The therapist should focus on diaphragmatic and segmental chest expansion, expiratory training, and volitional and effortful coughing.[196] NMES is more effective for the treatment of adult dysphagia patients of variable aetiologies than traditional treatment.[197]

When dysphagia or difficulty in swallowing occurs, physical therapists should work closely with speech-language pathologists to preserve safety of swallowing.

Often a detailed examination is needed to investigate the deceptively complex swallowing mechanism. Diagnostic methods include *Videofluoroscopic Swallowing Studies (VFSS)* and *Flexible Endoscopic Evaluation of Swallowing (FEES)*.[198] The role of the physical therapist is important in assisting with improving sitting position, body posture, and head control. An upright body posture with a slightly forward and downward-pointing chin position can be helpful in achieving a safe swallow and preventing aspiration.[199] Application of transcutaneous neuromuscular electric stimulation (NMES) to the submental muscles (suprahyoid triangle) to facilitate muscle reeducation was cleared by the FDA in late 2002, after the submission of data from over 800 patients (adults and children). NMES of the submental muscles paired with selected oral–motor exercises and swallowing maneuvers (e.g., Mendelsohn maneuver, effortful swallow, super-supraglottic swallow) can improve the strength, ROM, and coordination of the swallowing musculature.[196]

Thermal-tactile stimulation (TTS) is a sensory technique whereby stimulation is provided to the anterior faucial pillars to improve swallowing reflexes and the pharyngeal phase of swallowing. Anecdotally, the use of cold and icy beverages such as a shakes, fruit slushes, and ice chips provide heightened sensory input, which can improve the initiation of swallowing for many patients. Some patients also benefit from alternating small (teaspoon sized) sips of liquids with their food during mealtime. Most patients should be discouraged to engage in consecutive swallowing because it increases demand on the respiratory system and decreases airway protection. Resistive sucking through a straw can also be helpful, though therapists should use caution as use of straws can result in a larger amount of liquid compared with single sips. Thick liquids such as honey-thick and nectar-thick liquids can provide some resistance to facilitate muscle strengthening,[200] and provide an alternate means of hydration when patients are unable to drink thin liquids due aspiration risk. Moist foods (with sauces, broth, water, or milk) are easier to manage than dry ones. Semisolid and pureed foods are easier than regular solids. Foods that irritate the throat (e.g., vinegar) and crumbly or stringy foods (e.g., cake, cookies, potato chips, celery, cheeses) should be avoided. Patients also benefit when instructed to focus their effort on eating and never attempting to talk during active eating (mastication). Maintaining a quiet and peaceful environment during meals is helpful in improving attention and focus. Fatigue can also affect food intake. Many patients with MS benefit from reducing the size of their meals and eating smaller, more frequent meals or smaller, more nutrient-dense meals throughout the day. Percutaneous endoscopic gastrostomy (PEG) feeding tubes and/or nasogastric tubes may become medically necessary for individuals with severe dysphagia.[201] For overall safety, it is important that family members, caregivers, and health care providers alike are educated in the use of the Heimlich maneuver in the event of an emergency.[202]

Cognitive Training

Cognitive impairments can present major difficulties for the patient and for the rehabilitation team in general. Referral to a neuropsychologist may be indicated to determine the patient's strengths and weaknesses and to assist in the adaptive process. Compensatory strategies for memory deficits can be helpful. These include the use of memory aids, timing devices, and environmental strategies. Memory can be assisted by using a memory notebook to log daily events and reminders. With the increasing availability of mobile technologies, mobile devices, such as smartphones, have proven helpful for individuals with cognitive impairment related to memory and attention. A pill dispenser can assist the patient in maintaining a correct medication schedule. Cueing devices such as an alarm clock, bell timer, or watch alarm can help patients remember when to do certain tasks (e.g., taking medications, performing pressure relief). Structuring and labeling the environment are also effective strategies to assist memory (e.g., labeled drawers, cabinets). Directions for functional tasks (e.g., transfers, self-stretching techniques) should be carefully written down for both patients and caregivers. Complex tasks can be broken down with clear written directions provided for each step. Directions can be posted in different areas of the home (e.g., steps to follow for toilet or tub transfer posted in the bathroom). Additional cognitive strategies that may be helpful include mental rehearsal, requesting assistance, maximizing alertness, avoidance of difficult situations, and mental exercises. Poor follow-through should be expected among patients with severe cognitive deficits, because often there is very little insight. In this situation, the efforts of family and caregivers must be fully maximized.[34] As with healthy individuals, regular physical activity may have a positive effect on cognitive function, self-efficacy, and quality of life.[139,203,204]

Cognitive-behavioral therapy (CBT) for patients with MS can yield significant improvement in the ability to deal with distress, debilitating symptoms such as pain, fatigue and depression, impairment and disease exacerbation, and progression.[205] The goal of CBT is to change the way the individual thinks or feels about a particular impairment or problem. Significant improvements in quality of life[206] and depressive symptoms result when CBT was applied in those with newly diagnosed MS.[207]

Cognitive Rehabilitation conducted in both individual and group settings and through both in-person and computer-based methods is also useful for individuals with cognitive impairment[208-213] and has been shown to improve multiple domains of cognition including memory, attention, and information processing speed. Cognitive training may be more effective if the patient with

MS is referred to a neuropsychologist for neuropsychological test assessment prior to treatment. This battery of tests can guide the focus of cognitive rehabilitation by identifying cognitive domains that are particularly impaired in the individual.

PSYCHOSOCIAL ISSUES

Individuals with MS and their families experience a variety of losses such as loss of social functioning, interpersonal relationships, employment status, independence, and functional skills. In contrast, these individuals are typically young adults who are normally engaged in establishing independence, careers, and social relationships. Disabilities emerge as the disease progresses over time. Various different psychosocial adaptations can be seen, including anger, denial, and depression. The unique feature of a relapsing-remitting disease course is that it requires continual readjustment every time a new set of symptoms appears. Patients who appear well adjusted at one stage may regress as the disease worsens. The uncertainty of MS produces significant cognitive and emotional stress. Patients often feel out of control and unsure of themselves. Living with MS requires not only initial acceptance, but also a tremendous flexibility to deal with this lack of closure. Patients also experience the cumulative effects of smaller, everyday stresses that are associated with fluctuating symptoms, inability to perform ADL, dependency on others, and architectural barriers. Many factors play a role in determining how an individual reacts to MS. These include the overall effect of the disease on daily life functioning, previous coping skills, perceived self-efficacy, extent of social support, and spiritual well-being. They may experience attitudes of "wait and see" or "nothing can be done." This may explain why many individuals with MS do not take medications to help control their MS despite medical guidelines recommending disease-modifying drugs. The longer they are influenced by these attitudes, the less likely they are to seek help. Learned helplessness, low self-efficacy, and lack of environmental mastery have been identified as major factors contributing to depression and fatigue.[214]

As mentioned, depression does not necessarily correlate to the severity of the disease. For example, a person with mild disease can be severely depressed, whereas the person with severe disability is not. The therapist must be alert to the signs of depression and intervene as appropriate. Chapter 26, Psychosocial Disorders, presents a complete discussion of this topic.

Despite the negative psychosocial effects of the disease, studies indicate that while initial diagnosis was met with negative reactions, over time positive changes in terms of values and outlook often occur. Interventions that target re-examination of the individual's role and identity result in an increased appreciation for life and can assist individuals with MS in better managing the disease and enjoying their lives. [215] *Self-efficacy* is the belief that an individual will be able to deal with particular situations that may contain novel, unpredictable, and stressful elements. Strategies that enhance self-efficacy and self-management (elements of CBT) empower the patient with MS.[216] Additional interventions include education, involvement in goal-setting and treatment planning, wellness forums, and support or psychotherapy groups. The use of stress reduction techniques (e.g., relaxation techniques, meditation, and exercise) can also be helpful in promoting effective coping. Family and multidisciplinary support are key elements in effective psychosocial management.[217-218] Finally, referral for counseling or psychological services may be useful.

PATIENT AND FAMILY/ CAREGIVER EDUCATION

The primary roles of the clinician can be categorized as caring professional, expert teacher, and competent practitioner. A positive, affirming attitude can effectively influence patients' attitudes and assist them to view rehabilitation from a more positive perspective. The development of a strong collaborative relationship with the patient and family/caregivers in which there is respect, compassion, and effective communication is key to successful rehabilitation outcomes.[216] The overall focus should be on the maintenance of *hope* and *encouragement* tempered with *realism.*

As an educator, the therapist has an important role in assisting the patient and family/caregivers in providing information on the following:

- The disease process, clinical manifestations, and their significance in terms of management
- Prevention of secondary complications, indirect impairments, and activity limitations
- The rehabilitation process, the POC, and its specific interventions
- The HEP, including interventions that can be carried out independently
- Monitoring the effects and possible adverse reactions of medications
- Use of assistive devices and adaptive equipment
- General health and stress management techniques
- Community resources
- Ongoing monitoring that includes wellness visits every 6 to 12 months to progress HEP and prevent decline as a result of deconditioning
- Referral to appropriate services including other health providers and community fitness and support services

Prompt referral to community resources including a support group can provide a necessary stabilizing base for patients and their families/caregivers. Within this environment individuals can gain accurate and useful information about the disease, discuss common problems and methods of coping, and share anxieties and resources.

Thus, it provides a valuable forum to assist in the continual adjustment process. The National Multiple Sclerosis Society (www.nationalmssociety.org) provides education, emotional support, and a variety of programs and services to individuals with MS and their families through their local chapters. Web-based resources are provided in Appendix 16.A.

A significant number of patients with MS (one out of every two patients) will require the assistance of another person at some point in the course of their disease. This places an extra burden on family members and on the financial resources of the patient if outside caregivers must be utilized. The majority of caregivers experience moderate levels of stress associated with their caregiving duties. As the level and duration of physical care increases, caregivers can experience a variety of signs and symptoms, including physical (e.g., fatigue, headache, sleep disturbances, appetite changes), psychological (e.g., anxiety, depression, frustration), social (e.g., family conflicts, decreasing social experiences or "lack of life"), and spiritual changes (e.g., hopeless and meaningless life and work).[219] This can also put stress on relationships, as the caregiver is often a spouse and the dependency and the degree of support needed to perform certain tasks can be a source of tension.[215] The therapist will need to be sensitive to these changes and to conflicts, problems, and tensions as they develop. Considerable time and energy will be devoted to counseling and educating caregivers and coordinating home management. Attention should also be paid to the children of patients with MS, because studies have indicated that parental MS has a negative impact on children's psychological well-being. This is due, in part, to lack of understanding about the disease, and education may help ameliorate some of the negative effects.[220]

SUMMARY

Timely referral to neurorehabilitation services is the key to successful management of activity limitations, disability, and quality-of-life issues in patients with MS. Neurorehabilitation should be initiated early in the disease process, even at diagnosis, to discuss the importance of exercise, initiate a wellness HEP, and establish the therapist-patient relationship. Too often services are not begun until the individual becomes severely disabled. A comprehensive POC that addresses the needs of the whole patient and emphasizes meaningful functional activities, patient education, and self-management is ideal for such a complex neurodegenerative disorder. Activities that prove attainable and safe ensure patient success and build self-efficacy. Many patients with MS report that they lack the knowledge and skills needed to exercise safely. Promoting self-efficacy, self-management, and mastery can be achieved through supervised programs that focus on regular exercise, activity pacing, energy conservation, and overall healthy behaviors. Comprehensive efforts of the interdisciplinary team are needed to provide the coordinated and continuing care required with anticipated inpatient, outpatient, and home/community episodes of care.

Acknowledgments

The authors wish to thank Maja Abdinovic, MA, CCC-SLP, Evan Cohen, PT, MA, PhD, NCS, and Tamara Roehling, PT, DPT, for their contributions to this chapter.

Questions for Review

1. What are the pathophysiological processes involved in MS? What are the primary areas of CNS involvement?
2. Differentiate among the various disease courses (clinical subtypes) of MS.
3. How is the diagnosis of MS established? What tests and measures are used to confirm the diagnosis?
4. What is the role of disease-modifying drugs used in the medical management of MS? What are their indications and potential adverse effects?
5. Discuss the Expanded Disability Status Scale (EDSS) for patients with MS and indications for use.
6. Discuss the guidelines for an effective exercise prescription for the patient with MS to improve strength and conditioning.
7. Discuss the guidelines for an effective exercise prescription for the patient with MS to improve aerobic performance.
8. Discuss the problem of fatigue in MS and how it influences the design of an exercise program.
9. What strategies can be used to assist in the psychosocial adjustment of the patient with relapsing-remitting MS?

CASE STUDY

HISTORY

The patient is a 27-year-old graduate student who was admitted to an acute care facility with a chief complaint of double vision for 2 weeks. She reported that both lower extremities (LEs) seemed weaker recently. Four months earlier, she had noticed persistent tingling of her fingers on the left hand and some numbness on the left side of her face.

Neurological examination showed a scotoma in the upper field of the left eye, weakness of the left medial rectus muscle, horizontal nystagmus on left lateral gaze, and mild weakness of the left central facial muscles. All other muscles had normal strength. The deep tendon reflexes were normal on the right and brisk on the left, and there was a left extensor plantar response. The sensory system was unremarkable. A diagnosis of suspected MS was made. The patient was discharged a few days later, seemingly improved after corticosteroid treatment.

The patient was readmitted to a neurological service 10 months later because she noticed increased difficulty in walking and her speech had become thickened.

NEUROLOGIST REPORT

Patient presents with wide-based ataxic gait, minor slurring of speech, bilateral tremor in the finger-to-nose test, and dysdiadochokinesia. CT scan is within normal limits. MRI scan reveals numerous white areas indicative of lesions. Lumbar puncture shows 56 mg of protein with increased level of gamma-globulin. All other CSF findings are normal. Treatment with high doses of intravenous corticosteroids seemed to improve the neurological symptoms. Patient was discharged home with a referral for outpatient rehabilitation.

Two months later, the patient's symptoms worsened, and she is now admitted for intensive rehabilitation.

MEDICATIONS

Prednisone 20 mg po qid
Maalox 30 mL po qid
Valium 10 mg po qid
Copaxone 20mg subcutaneously qid

SOCIAL HISTORY

Patient has been living on her own for several years until her recent illness. She has taken a medical leave from graduate school and had returned home to live with her parents. They are both supportive and would like some advice as to how to modify their two-story home. There are five entry stairs with a handrail on both sides. There is a first-floor bathroom, and they plan to convert the first-floor study into a bedroom. The patient was driving but is currently relying on her parents for transportation. Patient does not have easy access to health care, having to travel close to an hour to therapy. Her parents are both in their early 60s and in good health. Both the patient and her parents are very anxious about their daughter's rapidly deteriorating condition. The patient is highly motivated to participate in therapy and to return to her prior level of function.

PHYSICAL THERAPY EXAMINATION FINDINGS

Mental Status

Alert, oriented
Memory: minimal impairment
At times lacks insight, seems unaware of the seriousness of her condition
Euphoric at times; other times she is depressed and cries easily

Communication

Speech is dysarthric, difficult to understand at times

Vision

Transient double vision
Gaze-evoked nystagmus to both left and right
Ocular dysmetria
Upper field defect of left eye

Endurance/Fatigue

Moderate impairment
Tolerance to activity is approximately 10 minutes before rest is required

Skin

WNL except for small bruise on right lateral malleolus

ROM

WNL except for 0° right dorsiflexion; 0° to 5° left dorsiflexion

Tone

Moderate extensor spasticity (2 on the modified Ashworth Scale) in both lower extremities (BLEs), left greater than right

Occasional BLE extensor spasms, which are a major safety risk when they occur during transfers

Sensation

Paresthesias in BLEs with moderate proprioceptive losses, ankle joints greater than proximal joints

Both upper extremities (BUEs): mild decrease in light touch, left greater than right

Strength

Moderate weakness in BLEs; generally functional muscle grades (able to move against gravity), with the greatest weakness noted at the hips

Standard MMT positions not used owing to spasticity

BUEs 3+/5 (fair+) to 4/5 (good) strength

Coordination

BUEs: Intention tremors with mild limb ataxia; voluntary movements are hypermetric; rapid alternating movements are moderately impaired

BLEs: Movements restricted by spasticity and spasms; unable to test

Gait

Ataxic

Wide BOS

Increased double support time

Decreased weight shift

Decreased gait speed

Increased pressure through UE's on walker

Forward flexion of trunk

Decreased hip extension

Decreased (B) heel strike

Decreased hip and knee flexion (B)

Balance

Berg Balance Scale: 10

Sitting balance:

- *Static:* With eyes open (EO), able to maintain position independently up to 5 minutes with minimal postural tremor; with eyes closed (EC), truncal ataxia is pronounced
- *Dynamic:* With EO, able to weight shift to left and right to about 40% of limits of stability (LOS); with EC, experiences loss of balance (LOB) with minimal weight shifts

Standing balance:

- *Static:* Able to maintain standing position in parallel bars with min assist × 1 for up to 3 minutes; during standing, patient is unable to maintain centered alignment; demonstrates moderate postural tremor; with EC, sway is increased dramatically, and patient quickly loses her balance
- Tends to keep her hips and knees stiff in extension/hyperextension
- *Dynamic:* Unable to weight shift or step without bilateral handhold

Functional

Functional Independence Measure (FIM):

- Eating: FIM 6; requires adaptive equipment
- Grooming: FIM 6; requires adaptive equipment
- Bathing: FIM 5; requires setup and adaptive equipment
- Dressing—upper and lower: FIM 4; minimal assist
- Toileting: FIM 4; minimal assist for balance
- Sphincter control—bladder FIM 6; bowel FIM 6
- Transfers—bed, chair, wheelchair: FIM 4, minimal contact assist for stand pivot transfers
- Transfers—toilet and tub: FIM 4; minimal contact assist
- Locomotion—walk: FIM 4; minimal contact assist, uses walker for up to 100 ft.

- Locomotion—stairs: FIM 2; less than 4 to 6 stairs, maximal assist
- Locomotion—wheelchair: FIM 5; supervision, uses manual wheelchair for distances up to 150 ft; posture in wheelchair: sacral sitting
- Requires a lap belt due to extensor spasms, which can cause her to fling out of the chair
- Communication—expression: FIM 6; requires extra time, mild dysarthria
- Communication—comprehension: FIM 6; complete understanding, requires extra time for processing
- Social interaction: FIM 7
- Problem solving: FIM 6; requires extra time, slight difficulty initiating decisions
- Memory: FIM 6; slight difficulty remembering daily routines and executing requests without need for repetition

Expanded Disability Status Scale (EDSS) score: 6.5

PATIENT'S GOALS

She would like to regain ambulation skills and independent living status. She recognizes the need to live with her parents for the time being but sees this as only temporary.

GUIDING QUESTIONS

1. Using the ICF WHO model, identify/categorize body function and structure impairments, activity limitations, participation restrictions, and environmental and personal limiting factors.
2. Identify two outcome measures that will best address the patient's current functional level that represent the activity section of the ICF model. Provide a brief rationale for each.
3. Formulate four treatment interventions that could be used at the start of therapy to achieve the stated outcomes and goals. Provide a brief rationale for each.
4. What strategies can be used to develop self-management skills and promote self-efficacy and quality of life?

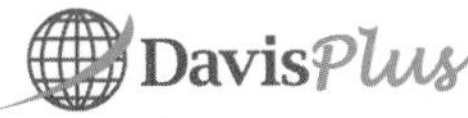

For additional resources, including answers to the questions for review and case study guiding questions, please visit **http://davisplus.fadavis.com.**

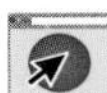

The reader is referred to Video Case Study 14: Patient with Multiple Sclerosis. This case study including full written summary, tables, figures, charts, and three video segments (examination, intervention, and outcome), appear online at Davis*Plus*. The case study poses questions for the reader's consideration with suggested answers to the case study questions, also posted online at Davis*Plus*.

References

1. Cohen, JA, and Rae-Grant, A: Handbook of Multiple Sclerosis, ed 2. [electronic resource]. Springer Healthcare Ltd., London, 2012. Retrieved January 19, 2017, from http://dx.doi.org.p.atsu.edu/10.1007/978-1-907673-50-4.
2. Rolak, LA: History of Multiple Sclerosis. National Multiple Sclerosis Society, New York, 2015. Retrieved January 19, 2017, from www.nationalmssociety.org/Programs-and-Services/Resources/History-of-Multiple-Sclerosis?page=1&orderby=3&order=asc.
3. National Multiple Sclerosis Society: What is MS? Who gets MS? Retrieved January 19, 2017, from www.nationalmssociety.org/What-is-MS/Who-Gets-MS.
4. Bove, RM, et al: Effect of gender on late-onset multiple sclerosis. Multiple sclerosis 18(10):1472, 2012.
5. Bove, R, et al: No sex-specific difference in disease trajectory in multiple sclerosis patients before and after age 50. BMC Neurology 13(1):73, 2013.
6. Celine, J, Coyle, P, and Duquette, P: Gender issues in multiple sclerosis: An update. Women's Health 6(6):797, 2010.
7. Cree, BAC, et al: Clinical characteristics of African Americans vs Caucasian Americans with multiple sclerosis. Neurology 63(11):2039, 2004.
8. National Multiple Sclerosis Society: Resources for specific populations. Retrieved January 19, 2017 from www.nationalmssociety.org/Resources-Support/Resources-for-Specific-Populations/African-American-Resources.
9. Alter, M, et al: Migration and risk of multiple sclerosis. Neurology 28:1089, 1978.
10. Koch, MW, et al: Environmental factors and their regulation of immunity in multiple sclerosis. J Neurol Sci 324(1-2):10, 2013.
11. Sawcer, S, Franklin, RJM, and Ban, M: Review: Multiple sclerosis genetics. Lancet Neurology 13:700, 2014.
12. Witte, ME, et al: Mitochondrial dysfunction contributes to neurodegeneration in multiple sclerosis. Trends Mol Med 20(3):179, 2014.
13. Traka, M, et al: Oligodendrocyte death results in immune-mediated CNS demyelination. Nat Neurosci 19(1):65, 2016.
14. Ellwardt, E, and Zipp, F: Molecular mechanisms linking neuroinflammation and neurodegeneration in MS. Exp Neurol 262 Pt A:8, 2014.
15. Costello, K, et al: The Use of Disease-Modifying Therapies in Multiple Sclerosis: Principles and Current Evidence—A Consensus Paper, Multiple Sclerosis Coalition, New York, 2014. Retrieved January 22, 2017, from http://ms-coalition.org/cms/images/stories//dmt_consensus_ms_coalition092016.pdf.
16. Lublin, F, and Reingold, S: Defining the clinical course of multiple sclerosis: Results of an international survey. Neurology 46:907, 1996.
17. Lublin, FD, et al: Defining the clinical course of multiple sclerosis: the 2013 revisions. Neurology 83(3):278, 2014.
18. Opara, JA, et al: Uhthoff's phenomenon 125 years later—what do we know today? J Med Life 9(1):101, 2016.

19. Cohen, B (ed): Managing symptoms in multiple sclerosis. In Neurology: Multiple Sclerosis 2013 Edition. Living Medical eTextbook. Retrieved January 22, 2017, from http://lmt.project_sinknowledge.com/Activity/index.cfm?jn=2023&sj=2023.01&i=8.
20. Shapiro, R: Managing the Symptoms of Multiple Sclerosis, ed 6. Demos Medical Publishers, New York, 2014.
21. Maloni, H: Pain in multiple sclerosis. Clinical Bulletin for Health Professionals, National Multiple Sclerosis Society, New York, 2016. Retrieved January 22, 2017, from www.nationalmssociety.org/.
22. Frohman, E: Vision problems in multiple sclerosis. Clinical Bulletin for Health Professionals, 2015, National Multiple Sclerosis Society, New York, 2015. Retrieved January 22, 2017, from www.nationalmssociety.org/.
23. Kushner, S, and Brandfass, K: Spasticity. Clinical Bulletin for Health Professionals. National Multiple Sclerosis Society, New York, 2012. Retrieved January 22, 2017, from www.nationalmssociety.org/.
24. Krupp, LB, Serafin, DJ, and Christodoulou, C: Multiple sclerosis-associated fatigue. Expert Rev Neurother 10(9):1437, 2010.
25. Rudroff, T, Kindred, JH, and Ketelhut, NB: Fatigue in Multiple Sclerosis: Misconceptions and Future Research Directions. Front Neurol 7:122, 2016.
26. National Clinical Advisory Board of the National Multiple Sclerosis Society: Fatigue: What you should know. National Multiple Sclerosis Society, New York, 2016. Retrieved January 22 2017, from www.nationalmssociety.org/.
27. Al-Yahya, E, et al: Cognitive motor interference while walking: A systematic review and meta-analysis. Neurosci Biobehav Rev 35(3):715, 2011.
28. Learmonth, YC, Ensari, I, and Motl, RW: Cognitive motor interference in multiple sclerosis: Insights from a systematic, quantitative review. Arch Phys Med Rehabil, 2016.
29. Hartelius, L, and Svensson, P: Speech and swallowing symptoms associated with Parkinson's disease and multiple sclerosis: A survey. Folia Phoniatr Logop 46(1):9, 1994.
30. Logemann, J: Swallowing disorders and their management in patients with multiple sclerosis. Clinical Bulletin for Health Professionals. National Multiple Sclerosis Society, New York, NY, 2011. Retrieved January 22, 2017, from www.nationalmssociety.org/.
31. Chiaravalloti, ND, Genova, HM, and DeLuca, J: Cognitive rehabilitation in multiple sclerosis: the role of plasticity. Front Neurol 6:67, 2015.
32. Bergendal, G, Fredrikson, S, and Almkvist, O: Selective decline in information processing in subgroups of multiple sclerosis: an 8-year longitudinal study. Eur Neurol 57(4):193, 2007.
33. Rocca, MA, et al: Clinical and imaging assessment of cognitive dysfunction in multiple sclerosis. Lancet Neurol 14(3):302, 2015.
34. Benedict, R: Cognitive dysfunction in multiple sclerosis. Clinical Bulletin for Health Professionals. National Multiple Sclerosis Society, New York, 2011. Retrieved January 22, 2017, from www.nationalmssociety.org/.
35. Minden, S, et al: Emotional disorders in multiple sclerosis. Clinical Bulletin for Health Professionals. National Multiple Sclerosis Society, New York, 2014. Retrieved January 22, 2017, from www.nationalmssociety.org/.
36. Marrie, RA, et al: Differences in the burden of psychiatric comorbidity in MS vs the general population. Neurology 85(22):1972, 2015.
37. Marrie, RA, et al: The incidence and prevalence of psychiatric disorders in multiple sclerosis: a systematic review. Mult Scler 21(3):305, 2015.
38. Miller, AH, Raison, CL: The role of inflammation in depression: from evolutionary imperative to modern treatment target. Nat Rev Immunol 16(1):22, 2016.
39. Minden, S: Pseudobulbar affect. Clinical Bulletin for Health Professionals. National Multiple Sclerosis Society, New York, 2012. Retrieved January 22, 2017, from www.nationalmssociety.org/.
40. Duncan, A, et al: The Incidence of Euphoria in Multiple Sclerosis: Artefact of Measure. Mult Scler Int 2016:5738425, 2016.
41. Rosti-Otajarvi, E and Hamalainen, P: Behavioural symptoms and impairments in multiple sclerosis: a systematic review and meta-analysis. Mult Scler 19(1):31, 2013.
42. Raimo, S, et al: Apathy in multiple sclerosis: A validation study of the apathy evaluation scale. J Neurol Sci 347(1-2):295, 2014.
43. Holland, N: Urinary dysfunction and multiple sclerosis. Brochure. National Multiple Sclerosis Society, New York, 2016. Retrieved January 22, 2017, from www.nationalmssociety.org/.
44. Holland, N and Kennedy, P: Bowel management in multiple sclerosis. Clinical Bulletin for Health Professionals. National Multiple Sclerosis Society, New York, 2017. Retrieved January 22, 2017, from www.nationalmssociety.org/.
45. Foley, F: Assessment and treatment of sexual dysfunction in multiple sclerosis. Clinical Bulletin for Health Professionals. National Multiple Sclerosis Society, New York, 2017. Retrieved January 22, 2017, from www.nationalmssociety.org/.
46. Brownlee, WJ, et al: Diagnosis of multiple sclerosis: progress and challenges. Lancet, 2016. DOI: http://dx.doi.org/10.1016/S0140-6736(16)30959-X.
47. Polman, C, et al: Diagnostic criteria for multiple sclerosis: 2010 revisions to the McDonald criteria. Ann Neurol 69(2):292, 2011.
48. McDonald, W, et al: Recommended diagnostic criteria for multiple sclerosis: Guidelines from the International Panel on the Diagnosis of Multiple Sclerosis. Ann Neurol 50(1):121, 2001.
49. National Multiple Sclerosis Society, Professional Resource Center. Differential Diagnosis, 2016. Retrieved January 22, 2017, from www.nationalmssociety.org/For-Professionals/Clinical-Care/Diagnosing-MS/Differential-Diagnosis.
50. Olek, MJ: Diagnosis of multiple sclerosis in adults. In: UpToDate, Gonzalez-Scarano F (ed): UpToDate, Waltham, MA. Retrieved on February 3, 2017, from www.uptodate.com/contents/diagnosis-of-multiple-sclerosis-in-adults.
51. Traboulsee, A, et al: Revised Recommendations of the Consortium of MS Centers Task Force for a Standardized MRI Protocol and Clinical Guidelines for the Diagnosis and Follow-Up of Multiple Sclerosis. Am J Neuroradiol 37(3):394, 2016.
52. Raz, E, et al: Periventricular lesions help differentiate neuromyelitis optica spectrum disorders from multiple sclerosis. Mult Scler Int 2014:986923, 2014.
53. Sahraian, MA, et al: Black holes in multiple sclerosis: definition, evolution, and clinical correlations. Acta Neurologica Scand 122(1):1, 2010.
54. Weber, E, Vilensky, J, and Fog, A: Practical Radiology: A Symptom-Based Approach. FA Davis, Philadelphia, 2013.
55. Rocca, MA, Messina, R, and Filippi, M: Multiple sclerosis imaging: recent advances. J Neurol 260(3):929, 2013.
56. National Multiple Sclerosis Society: Diagnosing Tools – MRI. Retrieved on February 3, 2017, from www.nationalmssociety.org/Symptoms-Diagnosis/Diagnosing-Tools/MRI.
57. National Multiple Sclerosis Society: News on ocrelizumab. Retrieved on February 3, 2017, from www.nationalmssociety.org/About-the-Society/News/Ocrelizumab-Granted-Breakthrough-Therapy-Designat.
58. Hughes, C and Howard, IM: Spasticity Management in Multiple Sclerosis. Phys Med Rehabil Clin 24(4):593, 2013.
59. Asano, M and Finlayson, ML: Meta-analysis of three different types of fatigue management interventions for people with multiple sclerosis: exercise, education, and medication. Mult Scler Int 2014:798285, 2014.
60. National Multiple Sclerosis Society, New York, 2017. Tremor. Retrieved February 5, 2017 from www.nationalmssociety.org/Symptoms-Diagnosis/MS-Symptoms/Tremor.
61. Mitolo, M, et al: Cognitive rehabilitation in multiple sclerosis: A systematic review. J Neurol Sci 354(1-2):1, 2015.
62. Khan, F and Amatya, B: Rehabilitation in Multiple Sclerosis: A Systematic Review of Systematic Reviews. Arch Phys Med Rehabil 98(2):353, 2017.
63. Newsome, SD, et al: A Framework of Care in Multiple Sclerosis, Part 1. Internat J MS Care 18(6):314, 2016.
64. Sandroff, BM, et al: Systematic, Evidence-Based Review of Exercise, Physical Activity, and Physical Fitness Effects on Cognition in Persons with Multiple Sclerosis. Neuropsychol Rev 26(3):271, 2016.
65. Sweetland, J, Playford, DE and Radford, KA: What is early intervention for work related difficulties for people with multiple sclerosis? A case study report. J Neurol Neurophysiol 5:252, 2014.
66. Sandroff, BM, et al: Association between physical fitness and cognitive function in multiple sclerosis: does disability status matter? Neurorehabil Neural Repair 29(3):214, 2015.
67. National Clinical Care Committee, National Multiple Sclerosis Society, Rehabilitation Recommendations for Persons with

Multiple Sclerosis (abridged). Retrieved January 22, 2017, from www. nationalmssociety.org/For-Professionals/Clinical-Care/Managing-MS/Rehabilitation.

68. Rieckmann, P, et al: Achieving patient engagement in multiple sclerosis: A perspective from the multiple sclerosis in the 21st Century Steering Group. Mult Scler Relat Disord 4(3):202, 2015.
69. *Guide to Physical Therapist Practice 3.0*. Alexandria, VA: American Physical Therapy Association; 2014. Retrieved January 22, 2017, from http://guidetoptpractice.apta.org/.
70. Medicare Benefit Policy Manual, Covered Medical and Other Health Services, Transmittal 179, Change Request (CR) 8458 dated January 2014. Retrieved January 16, 2017, from https://www.cms.gov/Regulations-and-Guidance/Guidance/Transmittals/Downloads/R179BP.pdf.
71. Frazzitta, G, et al: Intensive rehabilitation treatment in early Parkinson's disease: a randomized pilot study with a 2-year follow-up. Neurorehabil Neural Repair 29(2):123, 2015.
72. Ellis, T and Motl, RW: Physical activity behavior change in persons with neurologic disorders: overview and examples from Parkinson disease and multiple sclerosis. J Neurol Phys Ther 37(2):85, 2013.
73. Dal Bello-Haas, V: A framework for rehabilitation of neurodegenerative diseases: Planning care and maximizing quality of life. Neurology Report (now JNPT) 26(2):115, 2002.
74. Benedict, R, et al: Minimal neuropsychological examination of MS patients: A consensus approach. Clin Neuropsychol 16(3):381, 2002.
75. Langdon, DW, et al: Recommendations for a brief international cognitive assessment for multiple sclerosis (BICAMS). Mult Scler 18(6):891. 2012.
76. Dusankova, JB, et al: Cross cultural validation of the minimal assessment of cognitive function in multiple sclerosis (MACFIMS) and the brief international cognitive assessment for multiple sclerosis (BICAMS). Clin Neuropsychol 26(7):1186, 2012.
77. Folstein, M: Mini-Mental State: A practical method for grading the cognitive state of patients for the clinician. J Psychiatr Res 12:189, 1975.
78. Drake, AS, et al: Psychometrics and normative data for the multiple sclerosis functional composite: replacing the PASAT with the symbol digit modalities test. Mult Scler 16(2):228, 2010.
79. Beck, A, and Beck, R: Screening depressed patients in family practice: A rapid technique. Postgrad Med 52:81, 1972.
80. Lincoln, NB, Jackson, JM, and Adams, SA: Reliability and revision of the Nottingham Sensory Assessment for stroke patients. Physiother 84(8):358, 1998.
81. Uszynksi, M, Purthill, H, and Coote, S: Interrater reliability of four sensory measures in people with multiples sclerosis. Int J MS Care 18(2):86, 2016.
82. Newsome, SD, et al: Quantitative measures detect sensory and motor impairments in multiple sclerosis. J Neurol Sci 305(1):103, 2011.
83. Sharrack, B, and Hughes, R: The Guy's Neurological Disability Scale (GNDS): A new disability measure for multiple sclerosis. Mult Scler 5(4):223, 1999.
84. Zackowski, KM, et al: Sensorimotor dysfunction in multiple sclerosis and column-specific magnetization transfer-imaging abnormalities in the spinal cord. Brain 132 (pt 5):1200, 2009.
85. Melzack, R: The McGill Pain Questionnaire: Major properties and scoring methods. Pain 1:227, 1975.
86. Rog, DJ, et al: Validation and reliability of the Neuropathic Pain Scale (NPS) in multiple sclerosis. Clin J Pain 23(6):473, 2007.
87. Osborne, TL, et al: The reliability and validity of pain interference measures in persons with multiple sclerosis. J Pain Symptom Manag 32(2):217, 2006.
88. Flachenecker, P, et al: Fatigue in multiple sclerosis: A comparison of different rating scales and correlation to clinical parameters. Mult Scler 8(6):523, 2002.
89. Fisk, JD, et al: The impact of fatigue on patients with multiple sclerosis. Can J Neurol Sci 21(1):9, 1994.
90. Fisk, JD, et al: Measuring the functional impact of fatigue: Initial validation of the fatigue impact scale. Clin Infect Dis Suppl 1:S79, 1994.
91. Penner, IK, et al: The Fatigue Scale for Motor and Cognitive Functions (FSMC): Validation of a new instrument to assess multiple sclerosis related fatigue. Mult Scler 15(12):1509, 2009.
92. Karpatkin, HI: Multiple sclerosis and exercise: A review of the evidence. Int J MS Care 7(2):36, 2005.
93. Vukusic, S, and Confavreux, C: The natural history of multiple sclerosis. In Cook, SD (ed): Handbook of Multiple Sclerosis. Marcel Dekker, New York, 2001, p 443.
94. Lee, K, et al: The Ashworth Scale: A reliable and reproducible method of measuring spasticity. J Neuro Rehab 3:205, 1989.
95. Bohannon, R, and Smith, M: Interrater reliability of a modified Ashworth scale of muscle spasticity. Phys Ther 67:206, 1987.
96. Shumway-Cook, A, and Horak, F: Assessing the influence of sensory interaction on balance. Phys Ther 66:1548, 1986.
97. Fritz, NE, et al: The impact of dynamic balance measures on walking performance in multiple sclerosis. Neurorehabil Neural Repair 29(1):62, 2015.
98. Fritz, NE, et al: Longitudinal relationships among posturography and gait measures in multiple sclerosis. Neurology 84(20):2048, 2015.
99. Berg, K, et al: Measuring balance in the elderly: Preliminary development of an instrument. Physiother Can 41:304, 1989.
100. Berg, K, et al: Measuring balance in the elderly: Validation of an instrument. Can J Public Health Suppl 2(Jul-Aug):S7–11, 1992.
101. Tinetti, M: Performance-oriented examination of mobility problems in elderly patients. J Am Geriatr Soc 34:119, 1986.
102. Horak, FB, Wrisley, DM, and Frank, J: The Balance Evaluation Systems Test (BESTest) to differentiate balance deficits. Phys Ther 89(5):484, 2009.
103. Shumway-Cook, A, et al: Predicting the probability of falls in community dwelling older adults. Phys Ther 77:812, 1997.
104. Schwid, S, et al: The measurement of ambulatory impairment in multiple sclerosis. Neurology 49:1419, 1997.
105. Hobart, JC, et al: Measuring the impact of MS on walking ability: the 12-item MS walking scale (MSWS-12). Neurology 60(1):31, 2003.
106. Nieuwenhuis, MM, et al: The six spot step test: a new measurement for walking ability in multiple sclerosis. Mult Scler 12(4):495, 2006.
107. Fritz, NE, et al: Utility of the six-spot step test as a measure of walking performance in ambulatory individuals with multiple sclerosis. Arch Phys Med Rehabil 97(4):507, 2016.
108. Borg, G: Psychophysical bases of perceived exertion. Med Sci Sports Exerc 14:377, 1982.
109. American College of Sports Medicine: ACSM's Guidelines for Exercise Testing and Prescription, ed 8. Lippincott Williams & Wilkins, Philadelphia, 2010.
110. Sharrack B, et al: The psychometric properties of clinical rating scales used in multiple sclerosis. Brain 122 (Pt 1):141-159, 1999.
111. Vickrey, BG, et al: A health-related quality of life measure for multiple sclerosis. Qual Life Res 4:187, 1995.
112. Freeman, JA, et al: Clinical appropriateness: A key factor in outcome measure selection: The 36 item short form health survey in multiple sclerosis. J Neurol 68(2):150, 2000.
113. Kurtzke, J: On the evaluation of disability in multiple sclerosis. Neurology 11:686, 1961.
114. Kurtzke, J: Rating neurological impairment in multiple sclerosis: An expanded disability status scale (EDSS). Neurology 33:1444, 1983.
115. Noseworthy, J, et al, and Canadian Cooperative MS Study Group: Interrater variability with the Expanded Disability Status Scale (EDSS) and Functional Systems (FS) in a multiple sclerosis clinical trial. Neurology 40:971, 1990.
116. Meyer-Moock, S, et al: Systematic literature review and validity evaluation of the Expanded Disability Status Scale (EDSS) and the Multiple Sclerosis Functional Composite (MSFC) in patients with multiple sclerosis. BMC Neurol 14:58, 2014.
117. Amato, MP, and Ponziani, G: Quantification of impairment in MS: a discussion of the scales in use. Mult Scler 5: 216-219, 1999.
118. Hyland, M, and Rudick, RA: Challenges to clinical trials in multiple sclerosis: outcome measures in the era of disease-modifying drugs. Curr Opin Neurol 24:255–226, 2011.
119. Vickrey, BG, et al: Comparison of a generic to disease-targeted health-related quality of life measure for multiple sclerosis. J Clin Epidemiol 50:557, 1997.
120. Cella, DF, et al: Validation of the Functional Assessment of Multiple Sclerosis quality of life instrument. Neurology 47(1):129, 1996.

121. Hobart, JC, et al: The Multiple Sclerosis Impact Scale (MSIS-29): A new patient-based outcome measure. Brain 124:962, 2001.
122. Riazi, A, et al: Multiple Sclerosis Impact Scale (MSIS-29): Reliability and validity in hospital based samples. J Neurol Neurosurg Psychiatry 73(6):701, 2002.
123. Cattaneo, D, and Jonsdottir, J: Sensory impairments in quiet standing in subjects with MS. Mult Scler 15(1):59, 2009.
124. Fox, RJ, et al: Prevalence of multiple sclerosis symptoms across lifespan: data from the NARCOMS Registry. Neurodegener Dis Manag 5(6 Suppl):3, 2015.
125. Xia, Z, et al: Assessment of early evidence of multiple sclerosis in a prospective study of asymptomatic high-risk family members. JAMA Neurol. DOI: 10.1001/jamaneurol.2016.5056, 2017.
126. Cramp, A, et al: The incidence of pressure ulcers in people with MS and persons responsible for their management. Int J M S Care 6(2):52, 2004.
127. Shelley, A, et al: Impact of sitting time on seat-interface pressure and on pressure mapping with MS patients. Arch Phys Med Rehabil 86:1221, 2005.
128. Williams, C, et al: Iron and zinc status in MS patients with pressure sores. Eur J Clin Nutr 42(4):321, 1988.
129. Amtmann, D, et al: Pain affects depression through anxiety, fatigue, and sleep in multiple sclerosis. Rehabil Psychol 60(1):81, 2015.
130. Ehde, DM, et al: Efficacy of a telephone- delivered self-management intervention for persons with multiple sclerosis: a randomized controlled trial with a one-year follow-up. Arch Phys Med Rehabil 96(11):1945, 2015.
131. Jenson, MP, et al: Effects of self-hypnosis training and cognitive restructuring on daily pain intensity and catastrophizing in individuals with multiple sclerosis and chronic pain. Int J Clin Exp Hypn 59(1):45, 2011.
132. Müller, R, et al: Effects of a tailored positive psychology intervention on well-being and pain in individuals with chronic pain and a physical disability: a feasibility trail. Clin J Pain 32(1):32, 2016.
133. Pilutti, LA, et al: The safety of exercise training in multiple sclerosis: a systematic review. J Neurol Sci 343(1-2):3, 2014.
134. Khan. F, and Amatya, B: Rehabilitation in multiple sclerosis: a systematic review of systematic reviews. Arch Phys Med Rehabil 98(2):353, 2017.
135. Adamson, BC, et al: Effect of exercise on depressive symptoms in adults with neurologic disorders: a systematic review and meta-analysis. Arch Phys Med Rehabil 96:1329, 2015.
136. Dalgas, U, et al: The effect of exercise on depressive symptoms in multiple sclerosis based on meta-analysis and critical review of the literature. Eur J Neurol 22:443, 2015.
137. Heine, M, et al: Exercise therapy for fatigue in multiple sclerosis (review). Cochrane Library (9), 2015.
138. Kalron, A, et al: Efficacy of exercise intervention programs on cognition in people suffering from multiple sclerosis, stroke and Parkinson's disease: a systematic review and meta-analysis of current evidence. NeuroRehabilitation 37:273, 2015.
139. Sandroff, BM, et al: Systematic, evidence-based review of exercise, physical activity, and physical fitness effects on cognition in persons with multiple sclerosis. Neuropsychol Rev. 26(3):271, 2016.
140. Gunn, H, et al: Systematic review: the effectiveness of interventions to reduce falls and improve balance in adults with multiple sclerosis. Arch Phys Med Rehabil 96:898, 2015.
141. Kantele, S, Karinkanta, S, and Sievänen, H: Effects of long-term whole-body vibration training on mobility on patients with multiple sclerosis: a meta-analysis of randomized controlled trials. J Neurol Sci 358(1):31, 2015.
142. Spooren, A, Timmermans, A, and Seelen, H: Motor training programs of arm and hand in patients with MS according to different levels of the ICF: a systematic review. BMC Neurology 1(49):1, 2014.
143. Cuickshank, TM, et al: A systematic review and meta-analysis of strength training in individuals with multiple sclerosis or Parkinson disease. Medicine 94(4):1, 2015.
144. Kjølhede, T, Vissing, K, and Dalgas, U: Multiple sclerosis and progressive resistance training: a systematic review. Mult Scler J 18(9):1215, 2015.
145. Platta, M, et al: Effect of exercise training on fitness in multiple sclerosis: a meta-analysis. Arch Phys Med Rehabil 98(2):1565, 2016.
146. Martin-Valero, R, Zamora-Pascual, N, and Armenta-Peinado, JA: Training of respiratory muscles in patients with multiple sclerosis: a systematic review. Respir Care 59(11):1764, 2014.
147. Campbell, E, et al: Physiotherapy rehabilitation for people with progressive multiple sclerosis: a systematic review. Arch Phys Med Rehabil 97:141, 2016.
148. Toomey, E, and Coote, SB: Physical rehabilitation interventions in nonambulatory people with multiple sclerosis: a systematic review. Int J Rehabil Res 35(40):281, 2012.
149. Kalron, A, et al: The effect of balance training on postural control in people with multiple sclerosis using the CAREN virtual reality system: a pilot randomized controlled trial. J Neuroeng Rehabil 13:13, 2016.
150. Massetti, T, et al: Virtual reality in multiple sclerosis—a systematic review. Mult Scler Relat Disord 8:107, 2016.
151. Peruzzi, A, et al: An innovative training program based on virtual reality and treadmill: effects on gait of persons with multiple sclerosis. Disabil Rehabil 1, 2016.
152. Mahajan, H, et al: Preliminary evaluation of variable compliance joystick for people with multiple sclerosis. J Rehabil Res Dev 51(6):951, 2014.
153. Kang, H, Lu, J, and Xu, G: The effects of whole body vibration on muscle strength and functional mobility in persons with multiple sclerosis: a systematic review and meta-analysis. Mult Scler Relat Disord 7:1, 2016.
154. Yang, F, et al: Effects of controlled whole-body vibration training in improving fall risk factors among individuals with multiple sclerosis: a pilot study. Disabil Rehabil 15:1, 2016.
155. Skjerbæk, AG, et al: Heat sensitive persons with multiple sclerosis are more tolerant to resistance exercise than to endurance exercise. Mult Scler 19(7):932, 2013.
156. Jackson, K, and Mulcare, J: Multiple sclerosis. In American College of Sports Medicine: ACSM's Exercise Management for Persons with Chronic Diseases and Disabilities, ed 3. Human Kinetics, Champaign, IL, 2009.
157. Ku, YE, et al: Physiologic and functional responses of MS patients to body cooling. Am J Phys Med Rehabil 79:427, 2000.
158. Davis, SL, et al: Thermoregulation in multiple sclerosis. J Appl Physiol 109(5):1531, 2010.
159. Meyer-Heim, A, et al: Advanced lightweight cooling-garment technology: Functional improvements in thermosensitive patients with multiple sclerosis. Mult Scler 13(2):232, 2007.
160. Nilsagård, Y, Denison, E, and Gunnarsson, LG: Evaluation of a single session with cooling garment for persons with multiple sclerosis—a randomized trial. Disabil Rehabil Assist Technol 1(4):225, 2006.
161. White, AT, et al: Effect of precooling on physical performance in multiple sclerosis. Mult Scler 6:176, 2000.
162. Keller, JL, et al: Adapted resistance training improves strength in weight weeks in individuals with multiple sclerosis. J Vis Exp (107):53449, 2016.
163. Gunal, D, et al: Autonomic dysfunction in multiple sclerosis: correlation with disease-related parameters. Eur Neurol 48(1):1, 2002.
164. Langeskov-Christensen, M, et al: Aerobic capacity in persons with multiple sclerosis: a systematic review and meta-analysis. Sports Med 45(6):905, 2015.
165. van den Akker, LE, et al: Feasibility and safety of cardiopulmonary exercise testing on multiple sclerosis: a systematic review. Arch Phys Med Rehabil 96(11):2055, 2015.
166. Curran, SA, and Willis, FB: Chronic ankle contracture reduced: A case series. Foot Ankle Online J 4(7):2, July 2011.
167. Harvey, L, Herbert, R, and Crosbie, J: Does stretching induce lasting increases in joint ROM? A systematic review. Physiother Res Int 7(1):1, 2002.
168. Yang, CC, et al: Bladder management in multiple sclerosis. Phys Med Rehabil Clin N Am 24(4):673, 2013.
169. Block, V, et al: Do physical therapy interventions affect urinary incontinence and quality of life in people with multiple sclerosis?: An evidence-based review. Int J MS Care 17(4):172, 2015.
170. Ferreira, AP, et al: Impact of a pelvic floor training program among women with multiple sclerosis: a controlled clinical trial. Am J Phys Med Rehabil 95(1):1, 2016.

171. Coote S, Hogan N, and Franklin S. Falls in people with multiple sclerosis who use a walking aid: prevalence, factors, and effect of strength and balance interventions. Arch Phys Med Rehabil 94:616, 2013.
172. van den Akker, LE, et al: Effectiveness of cognitive behavioural therapy for the treatment of fatigue in patients with multiple sclerosis: a systematic review and meta-analysis. J Psychosom Res. 90:33, 2016.
173. Adler, S, Beckers, D, and Buck, M: PNF in Practice, ed 3. Springer, New York, 2008.
174. O'Sullivan, S, and Schmitz, T: Improving Functional Outcomes in Physical Rehabilitation, ed 2. FA Davis, Philadelphia, 2016.
175. Kelleher, K, et al: Ambulatory rehabilitation in multiple sclerosis. Disabil Rehabil 31(20):1625, 2009.
176. Freeman, JA, et al: The effect of core stability training on balance and mobility in ambulant individuals with multiple sclerosis: A multi-center series of single case studies. Mult Scler 16(11):1377, 2010.
177. Hebert, J, et al: Effects of vestibular rehabilitation on multiple sclerosis–related fatigue, upright postural control: A randomized controlled trial. Phys Ther 91(8):1166, 2011.
178. Kargarfard, M, et al: Effect of aquatic exercise training on fatigue and health-related quality of life in patients with multiple sclerosis. Arch Phys Med Rehabil 93(10):1701, 2012.
179. Marinho-Buzelli, AR, et al: The effects of aquatic therapy on mobility of individuals with neurological diseases: a systematic review. Clin Rehabil 29(8):741, 2015.
180. Roehrs, T, and Karst, G: Effects of an aquatics exercise program on quality of life measures for individuals with progressive multiple sclerosis. JNPT 28(2):63, 2004.
181. Cattaneo, D, et al: Effects of balance exercises on people with multiple sclerosis: A pilot study. Clin Rehabil 21:771, 2007.
182. Prosperini, L, et al: Visuo-proprioceptive training reduces risk of falls in patients with multiple sclerosis. Mult Scler 16(4):491, 2010.
183. Giesser, B, et al: Locomotor training using body weight support on a treadmill improves mobility in persons with multiple sclerosis: A pilot study. Mult Scler 13:224, 2007.
184. Newman, MA: Can aerobic treadmill training reduce the effort of walking and fatigue in people with multiple sclerosis? A pilot study. Mult Scler 13:113, 2007.
185. Pilutti, L, et al: Exercise training in progressive multiple sclerosis: a comparison of recumbent stepping and body weight-supported treadmill training Int J MS Care 18:221, 2016.
186. Wier, LM, et al: Effect of robot-assisted versus conventional body-weight-supported treadmill training on quality of life for people with multiple sclerosis. J Rehabil Res Dev 48(4):483, 2011.
187. Lo, AC, and Triche, EW: Improving gait in multiple sclerosis using robot-assisted, body weight supported treadmill training. Neurorehabil Neural Repair 22(6):661, 2008.
188. Schwartz, I, et al: Robot-assisted gait training in multiple sclerosis: A randomized trial. Mult Scler 18(6):881, 2012.
189. Samaei, A, et al: Uphill and downhill walking in multiple sclerosis: a randomized controlled trial. Int J MS Care 18(1):34, 2016.
190. Wajda, DA, et al: Intervention modalities for targeting cognitive-motor interference in individuals with neurodegenerative disease: a systematic review. Expert Rev Neurother 12:1, 2016.
191. Chag, Y, et al: Decreased central fatigue in multiple sclerosis patients after 8 weeks of surface functional electrical stimulation. J Rehabil Res Dev 48(5):555, 2011.
192. Esnouf, JE, et al: Impact on activities of daily living using a functional electrical stimulation device to improve dropped foot in people with multiple sclerosis, measured by the Canadian Occupational Performance Measure. Mult Scler 16(9):1141, 2010.
193. Paul, L, et al: The effect of functional electrical stimulation on the physiological cost of gait in people with multiple sclerosis. Mult Scler 14:954, 2008.
194. Achiron, A, et al: Aphasia in multiple sclerosis: clinical and radiologic correlations. Neurol 42:2195, 1992.
195. Beukelman, DR, Kraft, GH, and Freal, J: Expressive communication disorders in persons with multiple sclerosis. Arch Phys Med Rehabil 66:675, 1985.
196. Blumenfeld, L, et al: Transcutaneous electrical stimulation versus traditional dysphagia therapy: A nonconcurrent cohort study. Otolaryngol Head Neck Surg 135:754, 2006.
197. Tan, C, et al: Transcutaneous neuromuscular electrical stimulation can improve swallowing function in patients with dysphagia caused by non-stroke diseases: a meta-analysis. J Oral Rehabil 40(6):2013.
198. Mari, F, et al: Predictive value of clinical indices in detecting aspiration in patients with neurological disorders. J Neurol Neurosurg Psychiatry 63(4):456, 1997.
199. Calcagno, P, et al: Dysphagia in multiple sclerosis—prevalence and prognostic factors. Acta Neurol Scand 105(1):40, 2002.
200. Regan, J, Walshe, M, and Tobin, WO: Immediate effects of thermal-tactile stimulation on timing of swallow in idiopathic Parkinson's disease. Dysphagia 25(3):207, 2010.
201. Thomas, FJ, et al: Dysphagia and nutritional status in multiple sclerosis. J Neurol 246(8):677, 1999.
202. Duffy, JR: Motor Speech Disorders: Substrates, Differential Diagnosis, and Management, ed 2. Mosby, St Louis, 2005.
203. Motl, R: Physical activity and cognitive function in multiple sclerosis. J Sport Exerc Psychol 33(5):734, 2011.
204. Motl, R, and Snook, E: Physical activity, self-efficacy, and quality of life. Ann Behav Med 35:111, 2008.
205. Dennison, L, and Moss-Morris, R: Cognitive-behavioral therapy: What benefits can it offer people with multiple sclerosis? Expert Rev Neurother 10(9):1383, 2010.
206. Genty, M, et al: Effect of cognitive behavioral therapy on MS patients' quality of life. A multi-centre controlled trial. Ann Phys Rehabil Med 59:41, 2016.
207. Kiropoulos, LA, et al: A pilot randomized controlled trial of a tailored cognitive behavioral therapy based intervention for depressive symptoms in those newly diagnosed with multiple sclerosis. BMC Psychiatry 16(1):435, 2016.
208. Chiaravalloti, ND, et al: An RCT to treat learning impairment in multiple sclerosis: The MEMREHAB trial. Neurology 81(24):2066, 2013.
209. das Nair, R, Martin, KJ, and Lincoln NB: Memory rehabilitation for people with multiple sclerosis. Cochrane Database Syst Rev 23:3, 2016.
210. Pedullà L, et al: Adaptive vs. non-adaptive cognitive training by means of a personalized app: a randomized trial in people with multiple sclerosis. J Neuroeng Rehabil 13(1):88, 2016.
211. Rilo, O, et al: Integrative group-based cognitive rehabilitation efficiency in multiple sclerosis: a randomized clinical trial. Disabil Rehabil 7:1, 2016.
212. Rosti-Otajärvi EM, and Hämäläinen PI: Neuropsychological rehabilitation for multiple sclerosis. Cochrane Database Syst Rev 11(2):9131, 2014.
213. Shatil, E, et al: Home-based personalized cognitive training in MS patients: A study of adherence and cognitive performance. Neurorehabil 26(2):143, 2010.
214. Shnek, Z, et al: Helplessness, self-efficacy, cognitive distortions and depression in multiple sclerosis and spinal cord injury. Ann Behav Med 19:287, 1997.
215. Irvine, H, et al: Psychosocial adjustment to multiple sclerosis: Exploration of identity redefinition. Disabil Rehabil 31(8): 599, 2009.
216. Leino-Kilpi, H, et al: Elements of empowerment and MS patients. J Neurosci Nurs 30:116, 1998.
217. Malcomson, KS, Dunwoody, L, and Lowe-Strong, AS: Psychosocial interventions in people with multiple sclerosis—a review. J Neurol 254:1, 2007.
218. Plow, M, Mathiowetz, V, and Resnik, L: Multiple sclerosis: Impact of physical activity on psychosocial constructs. Am J Health Behav 32(6):614, 2008.
219. Bello-Hass, V, Bene, M, and Mitsumoto, H: End of life: Challenges and strategies for the rehabilitation professional. Neurology Report (now J Neurol Phys Ther) 26(4):174, 2002.
220. Bogosian, A, Moss-Morris, R, and Hadwin, J: Psychosocial adjustment in children and adolescents with a parent with multiple sclerosis: A systematic review. Clin Rehabil 24(9):789, 2010.
221. Verheyden, G, et al. The Trunk Impairment Scale: a new tool to measure motor impairment of the trunk after stroke. Clin Rehabil 18(3):326, 2004.
222. Kos, D, et al. Origin of fatigue in multiple sclerosis: review of the literature. Neurorehabil Neural Repair 22(1):91, 2008.
223. Khanna, D, et al. The minimally important difference for the fatigue visual analog scale in patients with rheumatoid

arthritis followed in an academic clinical practice. J Rheumatol 35(12):2339, 2008.
224. Learmonth, YC, et al. The reliability, precision and clinically meaningful change of walking assessments in multiple sclerosis. Mult Scler 19(13):1784, 2013.
225. Goldman, MD, et al. Evaluation of the six_ minute walk in multiple sclerosis subjects and healthy controls. Mult Scler 14(3):383, 2008.
226. Paltamaa, J, et al. Measuring deterioration in international classification of functioning domains of people with multiple sclerosis who are ambulatory. Phys Ther 88(2):176, 2008.
227. Solari, A, et al. The multiple sclerosis functional composite: different practice effects in the three test components. J Neurol Sci 228(1):71, 2005.
228. Schwid, SR, et al. Quantitative functional measures in MS: what is a reliable change? Neurology 58(8):1294, 2002.
229. Collen, FM, et al. The Rivermead Mobility Index: a further development of the Rivermead Motor Assessment. Int Disabil Stud 13(2):50, 1991.
230. Hsieh, CL, Hsueh, IP, and Mao, HF. Validity and responsiveness of the rivermead mobility index in stroke patients. Scand J Rehabil Med 32(3):140, 2000.
231. Molenaar, DS, van Doorn, PA, and Vermeulen, M. Pulsed high dose dexamethasone treatment in chronic inflammatory demyelinating polyneuropathy: a pilot study. J Neurol Neurosurg Psychiatry 62(4):388, 1997.
232. Lord, SE, Wade, DT, and Halligan, PW. A comparison of two physiotherapy treatment approaches to improve walking in multiple sclerosis: a pilot randomized controlled study. Clin Rehabil 12(6):477, 1998.
233. Cutter, GR, et al. Development of a multiple sclerosis functional composite as a clinical trial outcome measure. Brain 122:101, 1999.

Web-Based Resources for Clinicians and Patients/Families Living With Multiple Sclerosis

appendix 16.A

Resource	Website
National Multiple Sclerosis Society	www.nationalmssociety.org
Americans with Disabilities Act	www.ada.gov www.dol.gov/general/topic/disability/ada
Medicare information	http://cms.hhs.gov
Social Security Online	www.ssa.gov
National Institute of Neurological Disorders and Stroke	www.ninds.nih.gov
National Library of Medicine	www.nlm.nih.gov
JAMA Neurology	http://jamanetwork.com/journals/jamaneurology/issue
Neurology	www.neurology.org
CenterWatch Clinical Trials Listing Service	www.centerwatch.com
Veterans Affairs MS Centers of Excellence	www.va.gov/ms
CLAMS: Computer Literate Advocates for Multiple Sclerosis	www.clams.org
Consortium of Multiple Sclerosis Centers	www.mscare.org
The Heuga Center—MS Can Do program	www.mscando.org
Multiple Sclerosis International Federation	www.msif.org
The Multiple Sclerosis Society of America	www.mymsaa.org
The Consortium of Multiple Sclerosis Centers	www.mscare.org
MSWorld	www.msworld.org
The Myelin Project—MS research	www.myelin.org
Rocky Mountain MS Center	www.mscenter.org
National Family Caregivers Association (NFCA)	http://caregiveraction.org
Well Spouse Foundation	www.wellspouse.org
American Academy of Neurology (AAN)	www.aan.com
National Rehabilitation Information Center (NARIC)	www.naric.com
Paralyzed Veterans of America (PVA)	www.pva.org
Ability Hub—assistive technology	www.abilityhub.com
ABLEDATA—assistive technology	www.abledata.com
Apple Computer Accessibility	www.apple.com/accessibility
IBM Accessibility	www.ibm.com/able
Microsoft Accessibility Technology for Everyone	www.microsoft.com/enable

Chapter 17

Amyotrophic Lateral Sclerosis

Vanina Dal Bello-Haas, PT, PhD

LEARNING OBJECTIVES

1. Describe the epidemiology, risk factors, etiology, pathogenesis, diagnosis, and general prognosis of amyotrophic lateral sclerosis (ALS).
2. Compare and contrast the El Escorial and Awaji-Shima diagnostic criteria for ALS.
3. Differentiate among impairments related to lower motor neuron, upper motor neuron, and bulbar pathology.
4. Discuss the medical and health care management of individuals with ALS.
5. Outline a framework for rehabilitation for individuals with ALS.
6. Describe the components of the physical therapy examination for ALS.
7. Describe the role of the physical therapist in the management ALS and the factors that influence intervention options.
8. Compare and contrast overwork damage and disuse atrophy as it relates to ALS.
9. Describe considerations that must be taken into account when designing an exercise program for an individual with ALS.
10. Describe common impairments associated with ALS and the physical therapy interventions to address these impairments.
11. Determine the goals and expected outcomes for an individual with ALS based on physical therapist examination findings.
12. Design a physical therapy plan of care for the individual with ALS.

CHAPTER OUTLINE

Motor neuron diseases (MNDs) include a heterogeneous spectrum of inherited and sporadic (no family history) clinical disorders of the upper motor neurons (UMNs), lower motor neurons (LMNs), or a combination of both[1] (Table 17.1). Amyotrophic lateral sclerosis (ALS),* commonly known as Lou Gehrig's disease, is the most common and devastatingly fatal MND among adults. "Pure" ALS is typically characterized by the degeneration and loss of motor neurons in the spinal cord, brainstem, and brain, resulting in a variety of UMN and LMN clinical signs and symptoms.[2] It is important to note that ALS is increasingly being considered a multisystem disorder or syndrome, with variable pathological involvement of extra-motor networks and connections, in addition to the LMNs and UMNs.

Table 17.1 Motor Neuron Disorders

Subtype	Nervous System Pathology
Amyotrophic lateral sclerosis	Degeneration of the corticospinal tracts, neurons in the motor cortex and brainstem, and anterior horn cells in the spinal cord
Primary lateral sclerosis	Degeneration of upper motor neurons
Progressive bulbar palsy	Degeneration of motor neurons of cranial nerves IX to XII
Progressive muscular atrophy	Loss or chromatolysis of motor neurons of the spinal cord and brainstem

Adapted in part from Rowland.[1]

EPIDEMIOLOGY

It is estimated that 30,000 individuals in the United States have ALS at any one time and 15 cases are diagnosed every day. Except in a very few high-incidence areas, such as Guam, Western New Guinea, and the Kii Peninsula of Japan (geographical foci, Western Pacific form of ALS), the overall incidence of ALS has been reported to be in the range of 0.4 to 2.4 cases per 100,000, with the incidence increasing with each decade of life, until at least the seventh decade. The prevalence of ALS has been reported to be 4 to 10 cases per 100,000.[3-7]

ALS can occur at any age; however, the average age at onset is the mid-to-late 50s.[4,5,7,8] Most studies have found that the disease affects men slightly more than women, with an approximate ratio of 1.7:1;[3,5,6] after age 65, this gender-related incidence is less pronounced.[3] About 5% to 10% of individuals have a family history of ALS (*familial ALS*, [FALS]).[3,9,10] Familial ALS is phenotypically and genetically heterogeneous. Although most familial cases of ALS are autosomal dominant, recessive and X-linked forms have been described. Rare cases of juvenile-onset ALS have been reported and are inherited in an autosomal recessive pattern.[11]

FALS is categorized by mode of inheritance and subcategorized by specific gene or chromosomal locus (Appendix 17.A).[9] More than 20 chromosomal regions and a number of identified genes have been linked to ALS. Of the hereditary adult ALS cases, approximately 20% are a result of one of more than 100 mutations in superoxide dismutase 1 (SOD1),[12,13] a gene that encodes the copper-zinc superoxide dismutase enzyme. About 50% of individuals with an *SOD1* ALS variant are symptomatic by 46 years of age, and 90% are symptomatic by 70 years of age.[9] The very large majority of adult individuals with ALS have no family history of the disease *(sporadic ALS),* although a very small percentage of individuals with sporadic ALS do have a mutation in *SOD1*.[14,15]

Approximately 70% to 80% of individuals develop *limb-onset ALS,* with initial involvement in the extremities; 20% to 30% develop *bulbar-onset ALS,* with initial involvement in the bulbar muscles.[6,16,17] Bulbar-onset ALS is more common in middle-aged women, and initial symptoms may include difficulty speaking, chewing, or swallowing.[2,6]

ETIOLOGY

Epidemiologic evidence has identified several known and possible risk factors for ALS (Fig. 17.1). However, other than the small percentage of hereditary cases, etiology for the most part is unknown. It is thought that no one single mechanism but rather multiple or cumulative mechanisms including oxidative stress, aberrant RNA processing, exogenous neurotoxicity, excitotoxicity, impaired axonal transportation, axonal dysfunction, mitochondrial disruption, protein misfolding, protein aggregation, apoptosis (programmed cell death), and lifestyle factors may be responsible for neuron degeneration in ALS:[13]

1. *Superoxide dismutases* are a group of enzymes that eliminate oxygen free radicals that, although products of normal cell metabolism, have been implicated in neurodegeneration. There are three isoforms of SOD in humans: *cytosolic copper-zinc superoxide dismutase (CuZnSOD), mitochondrial manganese superoxide dismutase (MnSOD),* and *extracellular superoxide dismutase (ECSOD).* SOD1, a gene on chromosome 21, encodes CuZnSOD. Genetic studies of individuals with adult-onset FALS have determined that about 20% of these individuals have mutations in SOD1; however, the primary gene defect is unknown. When the SOD enzyme activity is decreased, as has been observed in individuals with FALS with SOD1 mutations, free radicals may accumulate causing damage.[13,18,19]

*The term MND is used to describe the disease in the United Kingdom, whereas the term ALS is used in North America and Europe. In Europe, ALS is also called Charcot's disease.

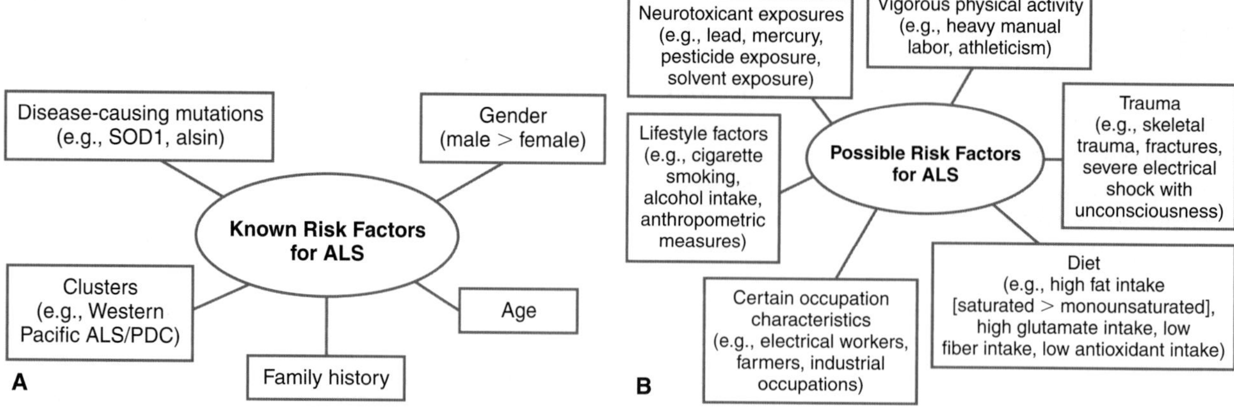

Figure 17.1 (A) Known risk factors for ALS. (B) Possible risk factors for ALS. ALS/PDC = amyotrophic lateral sclerosis and parkinsonism dementia complex.

Most mutations identified in FALS show modest loss in enzyme activity,[20] suggesting the mutant SOD-1 protein may have toxic properties that cause motor neurons to die. However, the mechanism has yet to be determined.[13]

2. *Glutamate,* an excitatory neurotransmitter, has also been implicated in neurodegeneration. Excess glutamate triggers a cascade of events leading to cell death.[13] Increased levels of glutamate in the cerebrospinal fluid (CSF), plasma, and in postmortem tissue of individuals with ALS have been reported.[21,22] A deficiency in excitatory amino acid transporter 2 (EAAT2), a specific glutamate transporter protein, in the motor cortex and spinal cord of postmortem ALS tissue was reported and lends support to the theory of excitotoxicity causing neurodegeneration.[23,24]
3. Clumping of neurofilament proteins into spheroids in the cell body and proximal axon is one of the histopathological characteristics of ALS.[13,25,26] Whether abnormal accumulation is secondary to the pathology or contributes to motor neuron degeneration has yet to be determined.[13]
4. Several studies have implicated an autoimmune reaction in the etiology of ALS.[7,27-29] For example, serum factors toxic to anterior horn motor neurons in individuals with ALS have been reported,[27] and antibodies to calcium channels have been identified in individuals with ALS.[29]
5. It has been hypothesized that a lack of neurotrophic factors could contribute to the development of ALS and other neurodegenerative disorders.[30] In vivo experiments and experiments with isolated motor neurons in cell culture have shown that neurotrophic factors are important in motor neuron survival.[31,32] However, factor deficits in ALS have not been conclusive. For example, a postmortem study found decreased amounts of ciliary neurotrophic factor (CNTF) in the ventral horn of the spinal cord, but not in the motor cortex; nerve growth factors were decreased in the motor cortex, but increased in the lateral column of the spinal cord.[33]
6. Other potential theories thought to contribute to neurodegeneration in ALS, which have anecdotal, limited, or indirect evidence, include exogenous or environmental factors,[34] apoptosis,[35] and viral infections.[36]

■ PATHOPHYSIOLOGY

Amyotrophic lateral sclerosis is typically characterized by a progressive degeneration and loss of motor neurons in the spinal cord, brainstem, and motor cortex (Fig. 17.2). However, as noted previously, there is increasing evidence

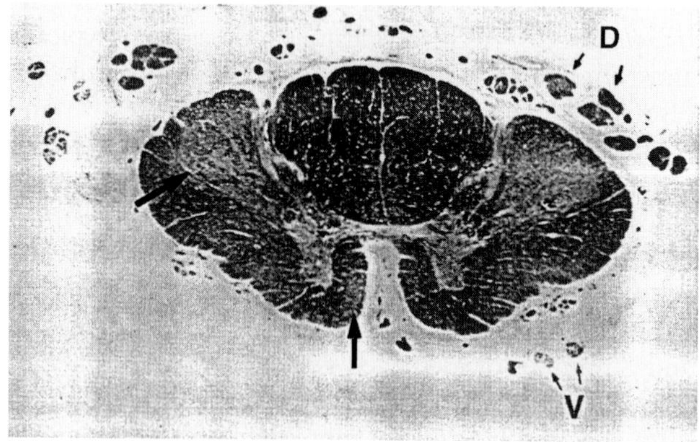

Figure 17.2 Luxol Fast B stained cross-section of spinal cord at the high cervical level from a patient with classical ALS. Marked pallor, secondary to degeneration of the lateral and anterior corticospinal tracts, can be seen (large arrows). The ventral roots (V, small arrows) are atrophied, especially compared to the dorsal roots (D, small arrows). *(From King, PH, and Mitsumoto, H: Neuropathology of amyotrophic lateral sclerosis. In Belsh, JM, and Schiffman, PL [eds]: Amyotrophic Lateral Sclerosis: Diagnosis and Management for the Clinician. Blackwell Publishing, Oxford, UK, 1996, p 205, with permission.)*

that ALS should be regarded as a multisystem health condition. Neuropathological and imaging findings have confirmed that ALS includes various non-motor areas,[37-39] and the discovery of the C9orf72 gene, which is linked to ALS-*frontotemporal dementia (FTD)*, reinforces the concept that ALS is comprised of multiple, complex pathophysiological mechanisms.[40] Regions beyond the motor system affected by ALS include the autonomic nervous system, the basal ganglia, and the cerebellar, frontotemporal, oculomotor and sensory systems.[41,42]

UMNs in the cortex are affected, as are the corticospinal tracts. Brainstem nuclei for cranial nerves V (trigeminal), VII (facial), IX (glossopharyngeal), X (vagus), and XII (hypoglossal) and anterior horn cells in the spinal cord are also involved.[2] Brainstem nuclei for cranial nerves controlling external ocular muscles (III: oculomotor, IV: trochlear, and VI: abducens) are usually spared; if degeneration occurs, it does so late in the course of the disease.[43] Motor neurons of the *Onufrowicz nucleus (Onuf's nucleus),* located in the ventral margin of the anterior horn in the second sacral spinal level, are also generally spared; if they are affected, it is to a very limited extent.[44,45] These neurons control striated muscles in the pelvic floor, including anal and external urethral sphincters.[46]

The sensory system is generally spared in ALS. Some studies suggest that sensory neurons may be involved in ALS, but to a much lesser extent than the motor neurons. Morphologic studies have found that peripheral sensory nerves exhibit axonal atrophy, demyelination, and degeneration,[47,48] and dorsal root ganglia cells at autopsy reveal loss of large ganglion cells.[49] Degeneration of Clarke's neurons and of the spinocerebellar tracts has also been reported.[50-52] Degeneration of the spinocerebellar tracts is a well-recognized pathological feature of FALS and has been described in sporadic ALS, although it is rare.[50] Posterior column degeneration is more common in FALS, but is rare in sporadic ALS.[53]

As motor neurons degenerate, they can no longer control the muscle fibers they innervate. Healthy, intact surrounding axons can sprout and reinnervate the partially denervated muscle[54] (Fig. 17.3), in essence assuming the role of the degenerated motor neuron and preserving strength and function early in the disease; however, the surviving motor units undergo enlargement.[55,56] Reinnervation can compensate for the progressive degeneration until motor unit loss is about 50%,[55,56] and electromyography (EMG) studies have found evidence of motor unit reinnervation in individuals with ALS.[57,58] As the disease progresses, reinnervation cannot compensate for the rate of degeneration,[57] and a variety of impairments develop (Table 17.2).

The progression of ALS is thought to spread in a *contiguous* manner, e.g., within spinal cord segments (cervical segments to cervical segments), before developing rostral or caudal symptoms.[17,59] Thus, signs and symptoms spread locally within a region (e.g., bulbar, cervical, thoracic, lumbosacral) before moving to other regions. Caudal-to-rostral spread within the spinal cord and spread from the cervical to bulbar region appears to occur faster than rostral-to-caudal spread within the spinal cord.[17,59]

CLINICAL MANIFESTATIONS

The phenotypic expression of ALS is highly variable. Clinical manifestations of ALS vary depending on the localization and extent of motor neuron loss, the degree and combination of LMN and UMN loss, extrapyramidal areas affected and associated signs and symptoms, pattern of onset and progression, body region(s) affected, and stage of the disease. At onset, signs or symptoms are usually asymmetrical and focal.[2] Progression of the disease leads to increasing numbers and severity of impairments.

Impairments Related to LMN Pathology

The most frequent presenting impairment, occurring in the majority of people with ALS, is focal, asymmetrical muscle weakness beginning in the lower extremity (LE) or upper extremity (UE), or weakness of the bulbar muscles.[3,7] Onset in the LE is more common for individuals with FALS.[9]

Muscle weakness is considered the cardinal sign of ALS and may be caused by LMN or UMN loss. The weakness associated with LMN loss causes more significant dysfunction than the weakness from UMN loss.[60] Initial muscle weakness usually occurs in isolated muscles, most often distally, and is followed by progressive

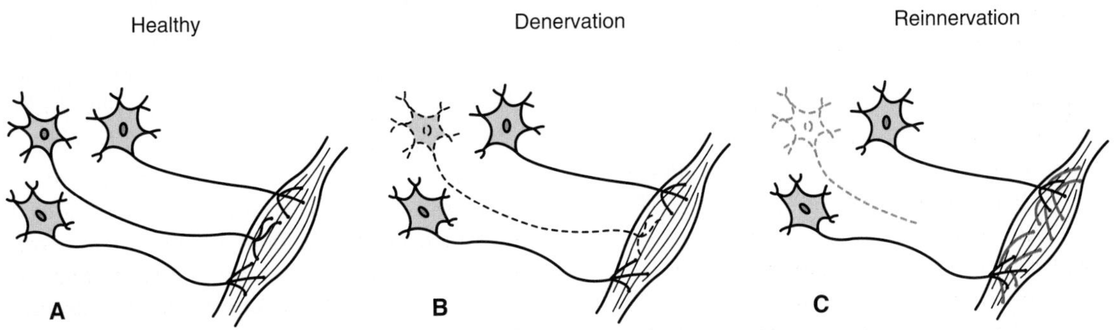

Figure 17.3 Sprouting: (A) normal motor neurons; (B) denervation; (C) reinnervation.

Table 17.2 Common Impairments Associated with Amyotrophic Lateral Sclerosis

Pathology/System Affected	Clinical Manifestations/Impairments
LMN pathology	Muscle weakness, hyporeflexia, hypotonicity, atrophy, muscle cramps, fasciculations
UMN pathology	Spasticity, pathologic reflexes, hyperreflexia, muscle weakness
Bulbar	Bulbar muscle weakness, dysphagia, dysarthria, sialorrhea, pseudobulbar affect
Respiratory	Respiratory muscle weakness (inspiratory and expiratory), dyspnea, exertional dyspnea, nocturnal respiratory difficulty, orthopnea, hypoventilation, secretion retention, ineffective cough
ALS-FTD, ALSci, ALSbi	Frontotemporal dementia-related impairments (e.g., loss of insight, emotional blunting), cognitive impairments (e.g., attention deficits, deficits in cognitive flexibility), behavioral impairments (e.g., irritability, social disinhibition)
Other	*Rare impairments:* sensory impairments, bowel and bladder dysfunction, ocular palsy *Indirect and composite impairments:* Fatigue, weight loss, cachexia, decreased range of motion, tendon shortening, joint contracture, joint subluxation, adhesive capsulitis, pain, balance and postural control impairments, gait disturbances, deconditioning, depression, anxiety

Adapted in part from Swash.[2]
ALS = amyotrophic lateral sclerosis; ALSbi = ALS with behavioral impairment; ALSci = ALS with cognitive impairment; ALS-FTD = ALS with frontotemporal dementia; LMN = lower motor neuron; UMN = upper motor neuron.

weakness[2,60] and activity limitations. For example, at onset an individual may notice difficulty with fine motor movements, such as buttoning, pinching, or writing, or may notice foot "slapping" or increased frequency of tripping while walking. Individuals with bulbar onset may notice changes in their voice, difficulty moving the tongue, or decreased ability to move the lips or open or close the mouth.

In people with ALS, cervical extensor weakness is typical.[2,60] Individuals may initially notice neck stiffness, feel "heavy-headed" after reading or writing, or may have difficulty stabilizing the head with unanticipated movements, such as in an accelerating car. As weakness progresses, the head may begin to fall forward, and in more advanced stages the neck becomes completely flexed with the head dropped forward, causing cervical pain and impairments in ambulation and feeding (Fig. 17.4).

Muscle weakness leads to secondary impairments, including decreased range of motion (ROM), predisposing the patient to joint subluxation (e.g., shoulder), tendon shortening (e.g., Achilles), joint contractures (commonly claw-hand deformity), and adhesive capsulitis. Weakness also results in ambulation difficulties, deconditioning, and impaired postural control and balance. Foot drop, secondary to distal weakness, and instability, secondary to proximal weakness, are common. The pattern and progression of LE weakness are characterized by greater losses of muscle force in distal muscles compared to proximal muscles.[61,62] A retrospective study found that decreases in walking ability from independent walking, to walking in the community with assistance, to walking only at home, to being unable to walk were precipitated by relatively small changes in muscle force.[62] Falls are also common, reported to occur in 46% of individuals with ALS.[63]

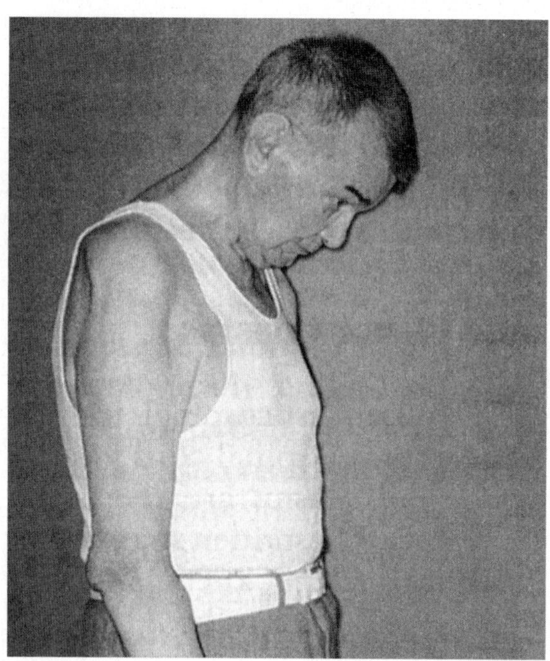

Figure 17.4 Marked head droop in a 65-year-old man with ALS who first developed progressive weakness in both upper extremities. *(From Mitsumoto, H, Chad, DA, and Pioro, EK: Clinical features: Signs and symptoms. In Mitsumoto, H, Chad, DA, and Pioro, EK (eds): Amyotrophic Lateral Sclerosis. F.A. Davis, Philadelphia, 1998, p 47, with permission.)*

As muscle fibers progressively denervate, their volume decreases resulting in atrophy. *Fasciculations*, random spontaneous twitching of muscle fibers often seen through the skin, are common in individuals with ALS, although they are rarely an initial symptom. The etiology of fasciculations remains unclear and is thought to be related to hyperexcitability of motor axons.[60]

Other LMN signs include hyporeflexia, decreased or absent reflexes, decreased muscle tone or flaccidity, and muscle cramping.[2,60] The etiology of muscle cramping is not well understood and is also thought to be related to hyperexcitability of motor axons. In individuals with ALS, muscle cramps can occur in uncommon sites such as the tongue, jaw, neck, or abdomen, as well as in the UEs, hands, and calf or thigh.[2]

Impairments Related to UMN Pathology

UMN loss is characterized by spasticity, hyperflexia, clonus, and pathological reflexes, such as a Babinski or Hoffmann sign, and may also cause muscle weakness. As the disease progresses, UMN signs may decrease.[2,60]

Spasticity can eventually lead to contractures and deformities, as well as cause dyssynergic movement patterns, abnormal timing, loss of dexterity, and fatigue, all of which affect motor control and function.[64,65] For example, difficulties with the swing phase of gait secondary to distal spasticity and decreased balance owing to generalized spasticity are often seen in individuals with ALS.

Impairments Related to Bulbar Pathology

As bulbar UMNs and LMNs degenerate, *spastic bulbar palsy* or *flaccid bulbar palsy* (respectively) develops. In individuals with ALS a mixed palsy, which includes both flaccid and spastic components, is common.[60]

Dysarthria, impaired speech, can occur with either spastic or flaccid palsy, owing to weakness of the tongue and muscles of the lip, jaw, larynx, and pharynx. Initial symptoms include the inability to project the voice (e.g., shouting, singing) and problems with enunciation. With spastic dysarthria, the voice sounds forced, as more effort is needed to move air through the upper airway; whereas in flaccid dysarthria, the voice sounds hoarse or breathy. With pharyngeal weakness, air in the mouth leaks into the nose during enunciation, resulting in a nasal tone. As the disease progresses, speech becomes more difficult and unintelligible, and eventually the individual becomes *anarthric*.[2,60]

Dysphagia, impaired chewing or swallowing, can also occur with either spastic or flaccid palsy. Manipulating food inside the mouth or moving food into the esophagus is difficult, and swallowing is impaired. With flaccid bulbar palsy, liquids may regurgitate into the nose because of pharyngeal weakness and the cough reflex may be weak or absent, greatly increasing the risk of aspiration. Individuals with spastic bulbar palsy will have uncoordinated closure of the epiglottis, which may allow liquids or solids to pass to the larynx.[2,60] Choking and slowed eating patterns are associated with dysphagia, placing the patient at risk for less than optimal fluid and caloric intake that results in weight loss and potentially cachexia.[60]

Individuals with ALS frequently experience *sialorrhea*, excessive saliva and drooling, owing to absence of automatic, spontaneous swallowing to clear excessive saliva, or because the lower facial muscles are too weak to close the lips tightly to prevent leakage.[60] Individuals with bulbar onset will experience this symptom relatively early. Initially, the individual may begin to notice drooling at night (e.g., the pillow is wet in the morning); this eventually leads to needing to use a tissue repeatedly to wipe away the saliva.

Respiratory Impairments

Respiratory impairments in people with ALS are related to loss of respiratory muscle strength and a decrease in vital capacity (VC). A VC reduced to 50% of predicted is often associated with respiratory symptoms.[66] Early signs and symptoms of respiratory muscle weakness may include fatigue, dyspnea on exertion, difficulty sleeping in supine, frequent awakening at night, recurrent sighing, excessive daytime sleepiness, and morning headaches due to hypoxia.[67,68] Patients experiencing a gradual increase in respiratory muscle weakness will not complain of respiratory symptoms because they tend to decrease their overall level of physical activity owing to muscle weakness in the extremities.[69] Although the decline of respiratory muscle strength differs among individuals, for the most part it tends to progress at a linear rate.[70] As weakness progresses, truncated speech, orthopnea, dyspnea at rest, paradoxical breathing, accessory muscle use, and a weak cough are typically evident. A VC of less than 25% to 30% of predicted indicates significant risk of impending respiratory failure or death.[66] If an individual does not receive ventilatory support, eventual CO_2 retention will lead to acidosis, coma, and respiratory failure.[69]

Cognitive Impairments

Neuropathological findings suggest that ALS affects the frontotemporal pathway and may be part of a wide clinicopathological spectrum of brain disorders known as TAR DNA-binding protein 43 (TDP-43) proteinopathies.[71] Although once considered rare outside the western Pacific region, cognitive impairments ranging from mild deficits[72] to severe FTD[73] are now considered part of the ALS disease spectrum.[74] A large prospective study found that 35.6% of patients with ALS showed clinically significant cognitive impairment.[75] ALS-associated FTD has been characterized by cognitive decline; executive functioning impairments; difficulties with planning, organization, and concept abstraction; and personality and behavior changes.[73,76-78] Individuals with ALS, without FTD, have been reported to have a variety of cognitive impairments, including difficulties with verbal fluency, language comprehension, memory, abstract reasoning, and generalized impairments in intellectual function.[75,78-80] Studies have found that patients with bulbar-onset ALS are more likely to have cognitive impairments than patients with limb-onset disease.[78,79] Cognitive and behavioral impairments have important clinical implications, including increased caregiver burden and stress, as well implications related to effective communication, legal issues, and end-of-life decision making.[81] As well, cognitive and behavioral impairments have been linked with less adherence with management recommendations and decreased survival.[82,83]

Other Impairments

Pseudobulbar affect is a term used to describe poor or pathological emotional control.[84] Spontaneous crying or laughter occurs in the absence of emotional triggers or emotional responses are exaggerated and not related to the context.[84] This symptom is commonly seen in individuals with spastic bulbar palsy,[2,60] and can occur in as many as 50% of individuals.[85]

Several factors affect fatigue levels in patients with ALS, thus fatigue is considered a composite impairment. As motor neurons die, the remaining neurons or sprouted neurons are overburdened. Weak muscles must work at a higher percentage of their maximal strength to perform the same activity. This hastens muscle fatigue.[86] Fatigue may also be related to sleep disturbances, respiratory impairments, hypoxia, and depression. Sanjak et al[87] demonstrated that individuals with ALS have abnormal physiologic and metabolic responses to single bouts of exercise. Sharma et al[88] found that in individuals with ALS, tetanic and maximal voluntary force during sustained contraction were decreased compared to controls. No impairment was found in the muscular membrane or neuromuscular transmission, suggesting that muscle fatigue in ALS, in part, is due to impaired contraction activation.[88]

Many individuals with ALS report pain, even though the disease does not typically affect pain pathways. Pain is typically a secondary impairment: musculoskeletal impairments, immobility, loss of ROM, decreased support from weakened muscles, positioning difficulty, dependent edema, and acute injuries (sprains, strains, and falls) can all cause pain. Spasticity and cramps, especially if severe, and pre-existing conditions can also cause pain. Pain is associated with decreased quality of life,[89] and may exacerbate depression and fatigue, both of which have been associated with decreased quality of life in individuals with ALS.[90] The reader is referred to the 2016 clinical guidelines on motor neurone disease[91] and the review article by Chiò et al[92] for summaries of possible causes of pain in individuals with ALS.

Rare Impairments

Sensory pathways are spared, for the most part, with ALS. Some individuals may complain of vague, ill-defined sensory symptoms of paresthesia or focal pain in the limbs.[60] External ocular muscles are usually spared in people with ALS; if degeneration occurs, it does so late in the course of the disease.[43] Patients who have been maintained on ventilators for long periods of time may develop the inability to voluntarily close the eyes or *ophthalmoplegia,* complete ocular paralysis.[43]

Motor neurons controlling the anal and vesicourethral sphincter muscles and muscles of the pelvic floor are generally spared. Urinary symptoms, such as urgency, obstructive micturition, or both, have been reported, suggesting that supranuclear control over sympathetic, parasympathetic, and somatic neurons may be abnormal in ALS.[60]

■ DIAGNOSIS

No definitive diagnostic test or diagnostic biologic marker exists for ALS. For individuals with a clinical presentation of ALS, laboratory studies, EMG, nerve conduction velocity (NCV) studies, muscle and nerve biopsies, and neuroimaging studies are used to support the diagnosis and to exclude other diagnoses. Studies have found that the time interval from symptom onset to diagnosis confirmation ranges from 8 to 15 months,[93,94] which may represent a significant proportion of disease duration.

The diagnosis of ALS requires the *presence* of (1) LMN signs by clinical, electrophysiologic, or neuropathological examination; (2) UMN signs by clinical examination; and (3) progression of the disease within a region or to other regions by clinical examination or via the medical history. The *absence* of (1) electrophysiological and pathological evidence of other diseases that may explain the UMN and LMN signs; and (2) neuroimaging evidence of other disease processes that may explain the observed clinical and electrophysiologic signs are also evaluated.[95]

Because of the variability in clinical findings in the early stages of ALS and the lack of absolute biological diagnostic markers, the *World Federation of Neurology Research Group on Motor Neuron Diseases* established the *El Escorial criteria* in 1994, and these were revised in 1998.[95] These widely accepted criteria are considered standard for the diagnosis of ALS for clinical practice, therapeutic trials, and other research purposes. In the absence of pathological evidence, the diagnosis of ALS is classified into *clinically definite, clinically probable, clinically probable with laboratory support,* and *clinically possible* categories (Fig. 17.5).[95] A diagnosis of *clinically definite ALS* is defined as both UMN and LMN findings in at least three of four regions (bulbar, cervical, thoracic, or lumbosacral) or UMN and LMN signs in the bulbar region and at least two spinal regions. *Clinically probable* ALS is defined as UMN and LMN signs in two regions, with at least one UMN finding rostral to the LMN findings. *Clinically probable, laboratory-supported* ALS is defined as UMN and LMN clinical signs in one region only, or UMN signs alone present in one region and LMN signs defined by EMG criteria present in at least

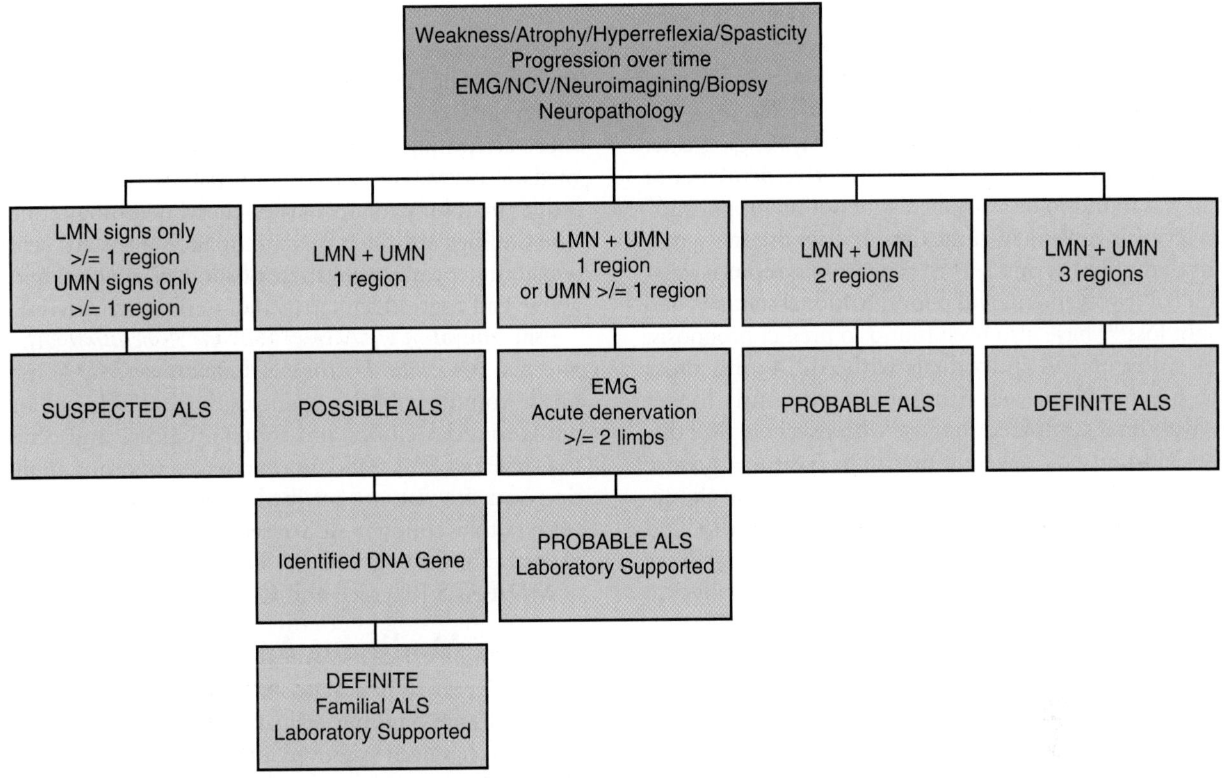

Figure 17.5 El Escorial Criteria for the Diagnosis of ALS. *(Note: The Suspected ALS category was removed when the El Escorial criteria were revised.)*

two regions. The EMG criteria include signs of active denervation, such as fibrillation potentials and positive sharp waves; and signs of chronic denervation, such as large motor unit potentials (increased duration, increased proportion of polyphasic potentials, increased amplitude) and unstable motor unit potentials. *Clinically possible* ALS is defined as UMN and LMN signs found together in only one region, or UMN signs found alone in two or more regions, or LMN signs found rostral to UMN signs and the inability to establish a diagnosis of clinically probable, laboratory-supported ALS.[95]

Awaji-Shima criteria were developed to address the criticism that the El Escorial criteria favor clinical signs over electrodiagnostic findings, thereby reducing sensitivity.[96] The Awaji-Shima criteria are as follows: (i) *Clinically definite ALS*—clinical or electrophysiologic evidence of LMN and UMN signs in the bulbar region and at least two spinal regions, or the presence of LMN and UMN in three spinal regions. (ii) *Clinically probable ALS*—clinical or electrophysiologic evidence of LMN and UMN in at least two regions, with some UMN signs necessarily rostral to the LMN signs. (iii) *Clinically possible ALS*—clinical or electrophysiologic signs of LMN and UMN signs in one region; or UMN signs are found alone in two or more regions; or LMN signs are found rostral to UMN signs.[96]

Despite these new criteria, there have been recent calls to revise currently available criteria, which are considered inconsistent and do not enable inclusion of the highly variable nature of ALS and clinical phenotypes, to improve both patient care and ALS research.[97]

■ DISEASE COURSE

ALS has a progressive and deteriorating disease trajectory, and the progression from pathology to impairments to activity limitations to participation restrictions is inevitable. Although the disease course varies among individuals, with time from onset to death ranging from several months to 20 years, studies have found the average duration of ALS to be between 27 and 43 months, and the median duration to be between 23 and 52 months.[3,5,7,98,99] Five-year and 10-year survival rates range from 9% to 40% and 8% to 16%, respectively.[7,98,100,101] A 50% survival probability after the first symptom of ALS appears is slightly greater than 3 years, unless mechanical ventilation is used to sustain breathing.[6] In most patients, death occurs within 3 to 5 years after symptom onset and usually results from respiratory failure.[5] However, about 10% of patients have a much slower disease progression, living 10 years or longer.[102]

■ PROGNOSIS

Age at time of onset has the strongest relationship to prognosis. Studies have found that patients less than 35 to 40 years of age at onset had better 5-year survival rates than older individuals.[5,6,99,103,104] Individuals with limb-onset ALS have a better prognosis than those with bulbar-onset ALS with 5-year survival rates reported to be 37% and 44%, compared to survival rates of 9% and 16% for patients with bulbar-onset ALS.[103,104] Delay between symptom onset and diagnosis has also been found to predict prognosis. Individuals with ALS who had a delay of less than 6 months had a mortality rate of 45% compared to 6% mortality in those with longer delays (e.g., greater than 25 months).[105] Presence of executive dementia or FTD was found to be associated with poorer prognosis.[83] Less severe involvement at the time of diagnosis, no symptoms of dyspnea at onset,[5,6,106] time from symptom onset to bulbar involvement, and poor nutritional status[107] and weight loss[108] have also been found to predict prognosis.

A study of 144 individuals with ALS found those with psychological well-being had significantly longer survival times compared to those with psychological distress. Mortality rates were found to be 6.8 times greater in those experiencing psychological distress, and the relationship was independent of age, disease severity, and length of time from diagnosis.[109] These findings were confirmed in a later study that found degree of physical disability, disease progression, and survival could be predicted by the patient's psychological status.[110]

■ MANAGEMENT

Patients with ALS may receive care in a variety of health care settings. Care via specialized centers or clinics that provide a comprehensive and multidisciplinary approach is considered the most advantageous owing to the progressive nature of the disease and continually changing patient status (Fig. 17.6). A study comparing a cohort of patients attending a multidisciplinary clinic versus those attending a general neurology practice found the median survival of the ALS clinic cohort was 7.5 months longer than for patients in the general neurology cohort. The findings indicated that attendance at the ALS clinic was an independent covariate of survival, suggesting that active and aggressive management enhances survival.[111]

The *Amyotrophic Lateral Sclerosis Association (ALSA)* and the *Muscular Dystrophy Association (MDA)*, nonprofit voluntary health agencies, have developed standards for ALS clinics and centers. Clinics and centers that meet ALSA's standards and pass a rigorous application and site visit are certified as ALSA Centers. MDA centers that conduct ALS research and have staff with expertise in dealing with ALS earn special designations as MDA ALS Research and Clinical Centers.

Disease-Modifying Agents

Currently, there is no cure for ALS, although clinical drug trials are ongoing. Riluzole (Rilutek), a glutamate inhibitor, has been approved by the U.S. Food and Drug Administration (FDA) for the treatment of ALS. The standard dose of riluzole is one 50 mg tablet two times

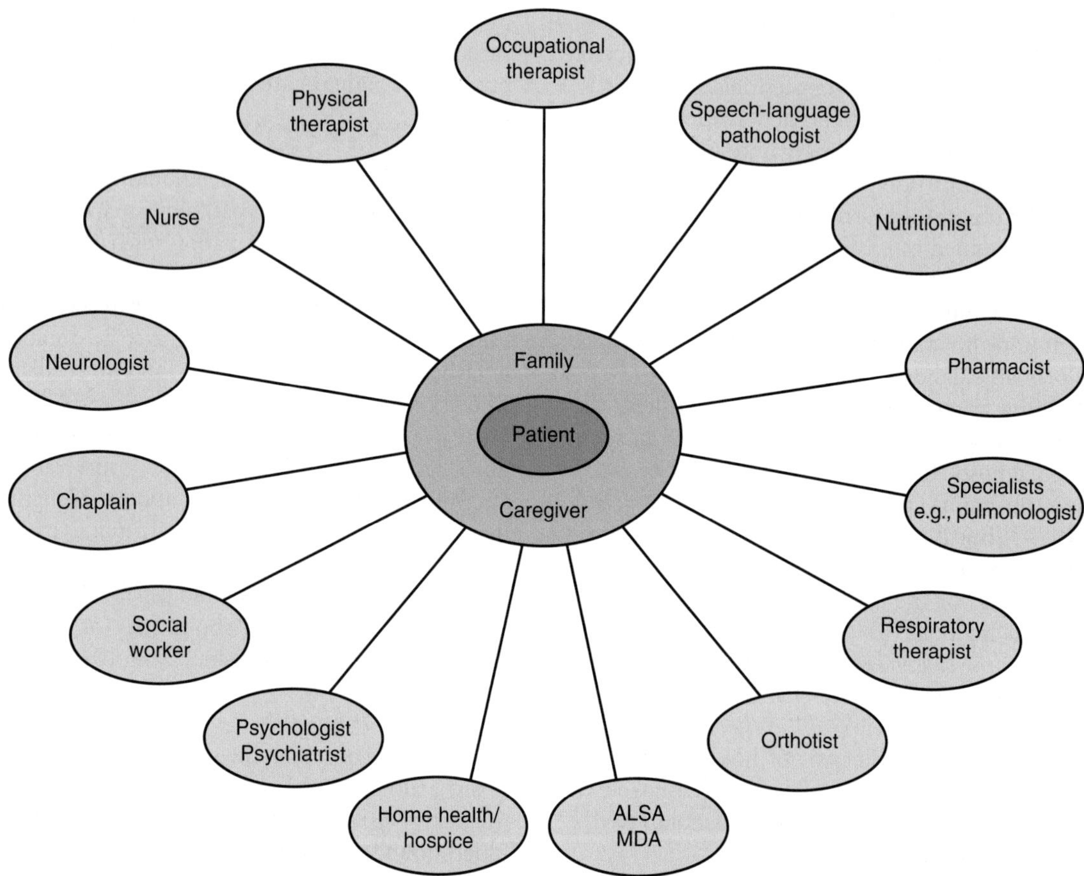

Figure 17.6 Multidisciplinary approach to the care of the individual with ALS. ALSA = Amyotrophic Lateral Sclerosis Foundation; MDA = Muscular Dystrophy Association.

a day, and side effects include liver toxicity (which requires discontinuation), asthenia, nausea, vomiting, and dizziness. Evidence suggests the effects of riluzole to be modest, extending survival for 2 to 3 months.[112,113]

After more than 20 years since the approval of riluzole, the FDA recently approved a second drug, Radicava/Radicut® (edaravone), for the treatment of ALS. Radicava, a free radical scavenger, seems to be more effective in the earlier stages of the disease, with less severe signs and symptoms and a greater forced vital capacity (FVC).[114] Radicava is delivered intravenously daily for 14 days, followed by no drug for the next 14 days. This initial course of treatment is then followed by another intravenous administration over 10 of the next 14 days, followed by another 14-day period without the drug. This cycle continues for as long as the treatment is to be administered.[114] The clinical trial conducted in Japan that led to the FDA approval found that those who received Radicava had less decline compared to the placebo group, as measured by the ALSFRS-R.[115] Side effects of Radicava reported in the clinical trial included: contusion, gait disturbance, headache, dermatitis, eczema, respiratory issues (failure, disorder, hypoxia), glycosuria, and tinea infection.[115]

Symptomatic Management

Disease-modifying agents currently available are not curative and may extend survival for a very short time. Because the pathological process cannot be reversed and is progressive in nature, the context of medical management for individuals with ALS may be considered "palliative" by definition. As defined by the World Health Organization, palliative care is "an approach that improves the quality of life of patients and their families facing the problem associated with life-threatening illness, through the prevention and relief of suffering by means of early identification and impeccable assessment and treatment of pain and other problems, physical, psychosocial and spiritual."[116, p. 1]

Although there is no cure for ALS, it is still considered a "treatable disease," and rehabilitation plays an integral role in the overall comprehensive care of the patient. Medical management is symptomatic and individualized and involves supportive care to address impairments as they arise.

Consensus-based recommendations are available[117,118] for ALS management related to: (1) informing the patient and family about the diagnosis and prognosis; (2) management of communication problems, insomnia, anxiety, depression, spasticity, fatigue, cramps, *sialorrhea,* and *pseudobulbar affect;* (3) nutrition management and percutaneous endoscopic gastrostomy (PEG) decisions; (4) management of respiratory insufficiency and ventilation decisions; (5) diagnosis and management of cognitive and behavioral impairments; (6) drug therapies; and (7) multidisciplinary management and palliative care. Clinical decision making algorithms (practice parameters) for the management of nutrition and respiratory signs and symptoms are presented in Figures 17.7 and 17.8. Full guidelines for other recommendations and information regarding definitions of the levels of recommendations and classifications of evidence can be found at the *American Academy of Neurology* (AAN) website (www.aan.com).

More recently, the AAN *Quality Measurement and Reporting Subcommittee* undertook a literature review and evidence search of 378 recommendation statements from 20 guidelines and consensus papers.[119] Following extensive consultation, 11 final recommendation statements measures (Table 17.3) that were rated highest on: clinical importance, linked to desired outcomes, the evidence base, the level of evidence, gaps in care associated with the recommendation, and validity and feasibility related to the implementation of the recommendation in practice were approved by the subcommittee and other AAN committees.[119] The full reports reported as data supplements is available at: https://www.ncbi.nlm.nih.gov/pmc/articles/PMC3863352/bin/supp_81_24_2136__index.html.

Nicholson et al describe the types of symptoms reported by individuals with ALS. In order of decreasing prevalence, the following symptoms were reported: fatigue (90%), muscle stiffness (84%), muscle cramps (74%), shortness of breath (66%), sleep difficulty (60%), pain (59%), anxiety (55%), depression (52%), increased saliva (52%), constipation (51%), pseudobulbar affect (38%), loss of appetite (37%), and weight loss (29%).[120]

The recommendations related to symptom management, per the AAN Subcommittee, are summarized in Table 17.3, and may include the prescription of anticramping and antispasticity agents, drying agents for sialorrhea, and antidepressants; recommendations and referrals for *percutaneous endoscopic gastrostomy* tubes and ventilatory support (non-invasive ventilation, tracheostomy); and discussion of advanced care directives.[2,60,117-119,121] Unfortunately, it has been reported that there is low treatment prevalence of many ALS-related symptoms,[120] highlighting that more can and should be offered to individuals with ALS.

Sialorrhea and Pseudobulbar Affect

Management of *sialorrhea* in people with ALS and other diseases is often directed toward prescription of anticholinergic medications that decrease saliva production. Examples include glycopyrrolate (Robinul), benztropine (Cogentin), transdermal hyoscine (scopolamine), atropine, and trihexyphenidyl hydrochloride (Artane).[121] Side effects include constipation, difficulty urinating, dry eyes, and confusion. For patients with associated thick mucus production, mucolytics or beta-blockers such as propranolol (Inderal) or metoprolol (Toprol) may be prescribed. Botulinum type injections into the parotid and submandibular glands and low-dose radiation have

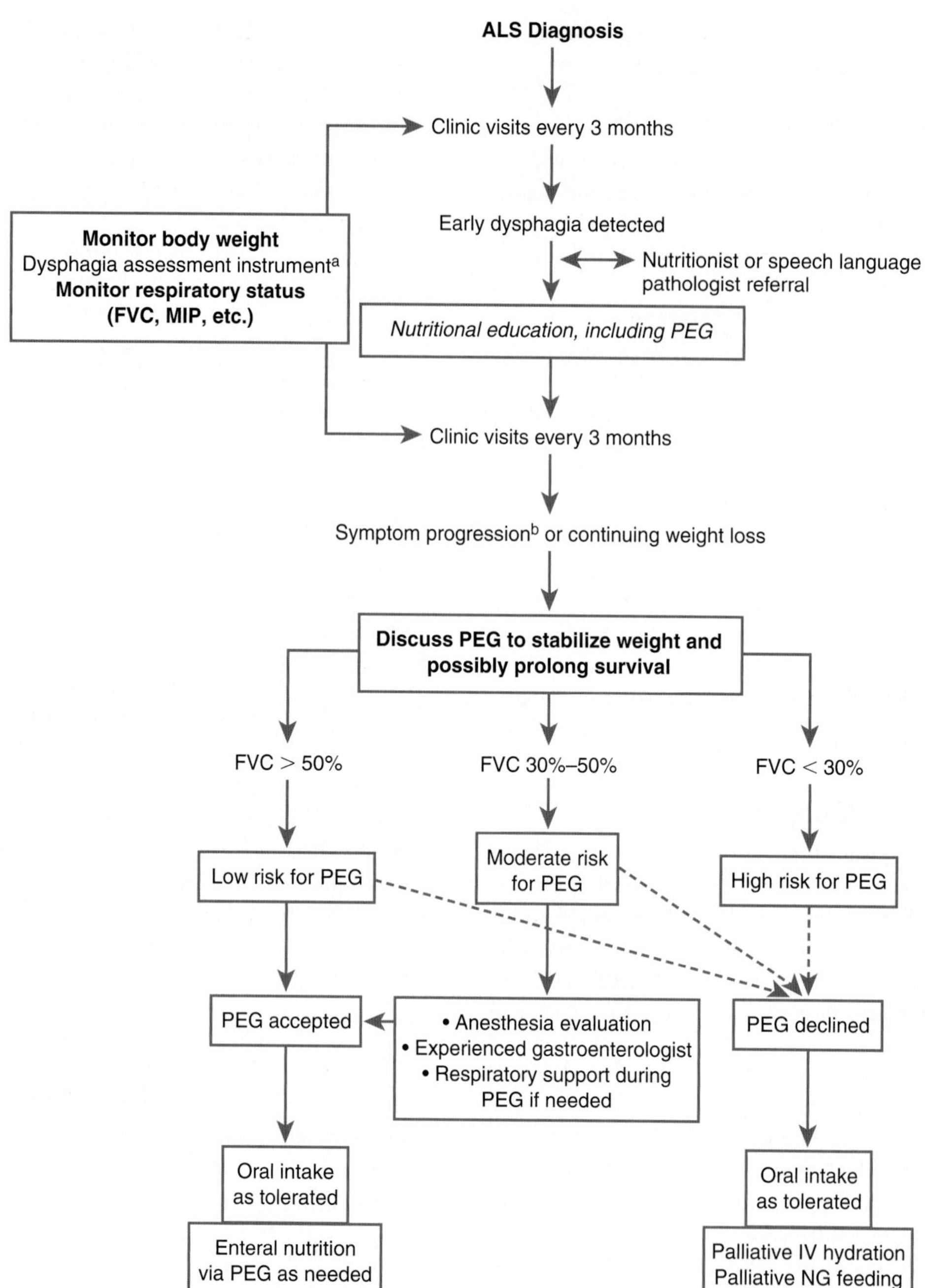

Figure 17.7 Algorithm for nutrition management. Note that **bolded text represents evidence-based information;** *text in italics denotes consensus-based information.*[a]
For example, Questions #1 to 3 (bulbar questions) from the Amyotrophic Lateral Sclerosis Functional Rating Scale—Revised (ALSFRS-R), or other instrument.[b]
For example, prolonged mealtime, ending meal prematurely because of fatigue, accelerated weight loss due to poor caloric intake, family concern about feeding difficulties.
FVC = forced vital capacity (supine or erect); IV = intravenous; MIP = maximum inspiratory pressure; NG = nasogastric; PEG = percutaneous endoscopic gastrostomy. *(From Miller, RG, et al (ALS Practice Parameters Task Force): The care of the patient with amyotrophic lateral sclerosis (an evidence-based review). Report of the quality Standards Subcommittee of the American Academy of Neurology. Neurology 52(7):1311, 1999, p 1316, with permission.)*

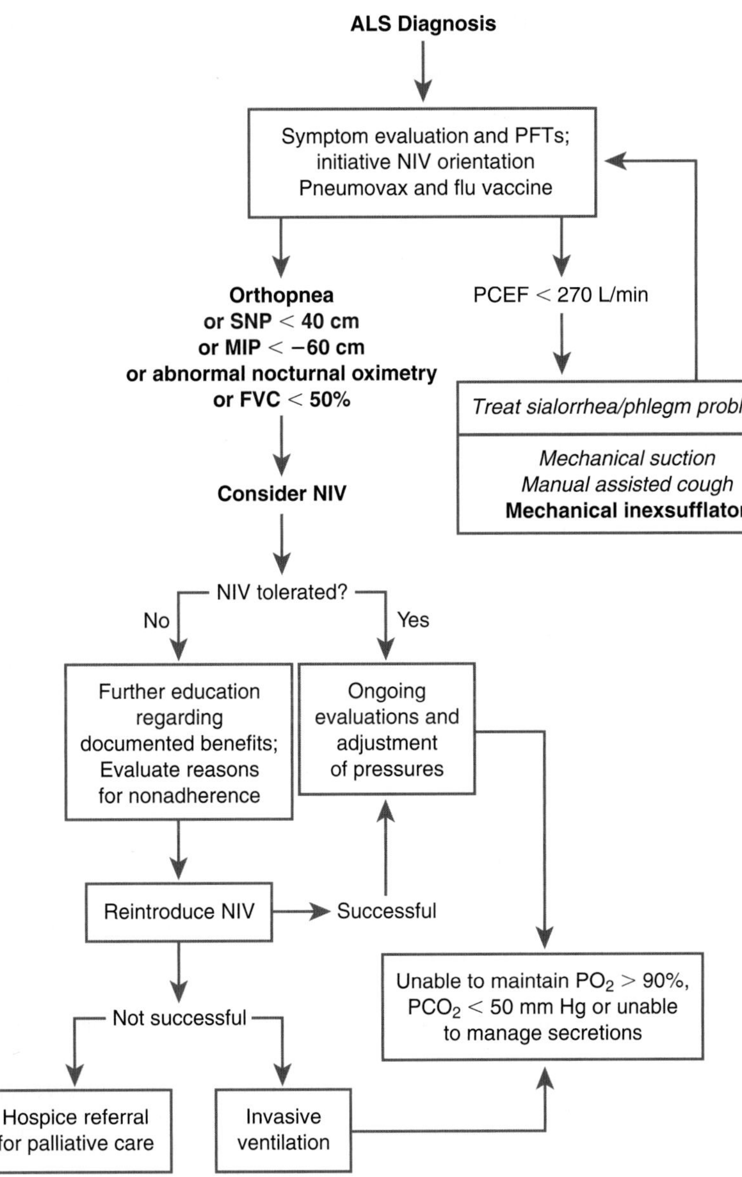

Figure 17.8 Algorithm for respiratory management. Note that **bolded text represents evidence-based information;** *text in italics denotes consensus-based information.* FVC = forced vital capacity (supine or erect); MIP = maximal inspiratory pressure; NIV = non-invasive ventilation; PCEF = peak cough expiratory flow; PFT = pulmonary function tests; SNP = sniff nasal pressure. *(From Miller, RG, et al (ALS Practice Parameters Task Force): The care of the patient with amyotrophic lateral sclerosis (an evidence-based review). Report of the quality Standards Subcommittee of the American Academy of Neurology. Neurology 52(7):1311, 1999, p 1317, with permission.)*

Table 17.3 Amyotrophic Lateral Sclerosis Performance Measurement Set. Data adapted from Miller 2013[119]

Measure	Description
1. Multidisciplinary Care Plan Development/Updating	Multidisciplinary care plan should include a neurologist and at least four of the following: dentist, dietician, gastroenterologist, genetic counselor, occupational therapist, palliative care specialist, physiatrist, physical therapist, psychiatrist, psychologist, pulmonologist, respiratory therapist, social worker, specialized nurse, speech-language pathologist. Plan should be updated at least once annually.
2. Disease-Modifying Pharmacotherapy for ALS Discussion	Riluzole should be offered.
3. Cognitive and Behavioral Impairment Screening	Screen for cognitive impairment at least once annually.

Continued

Table 17.3 Amyotrophic Lateral Sclerosis Performance Measurement Set. Data adapted from Miller 2013[119]—cont'd

Measure	Description
4. Symptomatic Therapy Treatment Offering	Symptomatic treatment should be offered for pseudobulbar affect, sialorrhea, and other ALS-related symptoms, if present.
5. Respiratory Insufficiency Querying and Referral for Pulmonary Function Testing	Query about symptoms of respiratory insufficiency (at each clinical visit). Vital capacity, maximum inspiratory pressure, sniff nasal pressure, or peak cough expiratory flow testing at least every three months.
6. Non-invasive Ventilation Treatment for Respiratory Insufficiency Discussion	Discuss treatment options of non-invasive respiratory support (e.g., non-invasive ventilation, assisted cough) at least once annually.
7. Screening for Dysphagia, Weight Loss, and Impaired Nutrition	Screen for dysphagia, weight loss, or impaired nutrition at least every three months.
8. Nutritional Support Offering	Dietary or enteral nutritional support via percutaneous endoscopy gastrostomy or radiographic-inserted gastrostomy at least once annually for those with dysphagia, weight loss, or impaired nutrition.
9. Communication Support Referral	Refer to a speech-language pathologist for augmentative/alternative communication evaluation at least once annually for those with dysarthria.
10. End of Life Planning Assistance	Assistance in planning for end-of-life issues, e.g., advanced directives, invasive ventilation, and hospice at least once annually.
11. Falls Querying	Query about falls within the past 12 months (at each clinical visit).

been found to be effective for individuals with ALS with medically refractory sialorrhea.[122] Use of mechanical suction to remove oropharyngeal secretions and nonpharmacologic treatments that are used for clearing respiratory secretions (see section that follows titled, Management of Respiratory Impairments) may also be useful.

For patients with pseudobulbar affect, tricyclic antidepressants, such as amitriptyline (Elavil), or selective serotonin reuptake inhibitors (SSRIs), such as fluvoxamine (Luvox), are often prescribed.[121] Research has found that a fixed-dose combination of dextromethorphan/quinidine reduced the severity and frequency of crying and laughing behaviors. However, side effects, including somnolence, dizziness, and nausea, were common.[122]

Dysphagia

It is recommended that screening for dysphagia, weight loss or impaired nutrition should take place at least every 3 months; and dietary or enteral nutritional support via percutaneous endoscopy gastrostomy or radiographic inserted gastrostomy at least once annually for those with dysphagia, weight loss, or impaired nutrition.[119]

Early, mild dysphagia is addressed by a nutritionist or registered dietitian together with a speech-language pathologist (SLP). Speech-language pathologists conduct swallowing examinations such as video fluoroscopy to determine the degree and nature of the swallowing impairment and to assist in formulating a plan of care (POC). Nutritionists provide counseling and diet management throughout the course of the disease.

Nutrition status has been identified as a prognostic factor for survival and disease complications.[107,122] A study of 1,600 hospitalized patients with ALS found the most common concurrent diagnosis was dehydration and malnutrition, present in 36% of patients.[123] Regardless of whether poor nutritional status results from dysphagia, hypermetabolism, or inability to eat due to UE muscle weakness, research findings emphasize the need for careful attention to nutritional and hydration status, in particular with individuals with impaired oral intake or arm or hand weakness limiting self-feeding.

Initial treatment of dysphagia is directed toward (1) dietary modifications, such as adapting foods and fluid consistencies for easier and safer swallowing; (2) patient education regarding dietary strategies for maximizing calories and nutrients and maintaining adequate hydration; and (3) adaptations to promote swallowing such as tucking the chin down during swallowing or performing a clearing cough after each swallow.[124]

As dysphagia progresses, the time required to consume a meal gradually increases owing to fatigue, increased difficulty chewing, and frequent choking. It is not uncommon for these eating difficulties to cause an accelerated weight loss. In these circumstances a percutaneous endoscopic gastrostomy (PEG) may be recommended. A PEG is a type of gastrostomy tube inserted via endoscopic surgery that creates a permanent opening into the stomach for the introduction of food. A PEG is useful for stabilizing body weight/mass.[117] Although there is no firm evidence, for optimal safety and efficacy the PEG procedure should be offered to the patient and completed before the individual's VC falls below 50% of predicted at the time of the procedure.[125] Studies have found that PEG insertion may prolong survival. Patients with PEG were found to live 1 to 4 months longer than those individuals who refused PEG or were deemed ineligible for the procedure. Survival was greatest for patients with a VC greater than 50% predicted at the time of the procedure.[126,127] It is important for physical therapists to be aware that a PEG does not prevent the risk of aspiration.[128,129]

Respiratory Impairments

Respiratory impairments place the patient at risk for respiratory tract infections. Important management considerations include (1) pneumococcal and yearly influenza vaccinations;[69] (2) prevention of aspiration; and (3) effective oral and pulmonary secretion management. Supplemental oxygen must be used with caution because it can suppress respiratory drive, exacerbate hypoventilation, and ultimately lead to hypercarbia and respiratory arrest. Typically, supplemental oxygen is recommended only for individuals with concomitant pulmonary disease or as a comfort measure for patients who decline ventilatory support.[69]

Symptoms of respiratory insufficiency should be queried at each clinical visit, and VC, maximum inspiratory pressure (MIP), sniff nasal pressure (SNiF), or peak cough expiratory flow (PCEF) testing should be conducted at least every 3 months.[119]

When VC decreases to 50% of predicted, positive-pressure non-invasive ventilation (NIV) is recommended.[69,125] Non-invasive ventilation has been shown to decrease symptoms of hypoventilation and increase survival time by several months.[130-133] In addition, improvement in cognition has been noted after NIV initiation.[111] When NIV can no longer be tolerated or it is no longer effective, a decision must be made between invasion ventilation (IV) with tracheostomy via surgical intervention or hospice care to address late-stage respiratory symptoms. Owing to the emotional, social, and financial burden of IV, patients and families must be carefully informed of the multiple costs and benefits of the intervention. No controlled studies of specific strategies for ventilation withdrawal have been published, although case studies provide practical advice.[117] Conditions for withdrawal of ventilation are discussed before, or at the time of, instituting IV because the patient may become unable to communicate his or her wishes as the disease progresses.[69,125]

Communication

Communication impairments are managed primarily by a SLP. Initial speech changes are usually managed with intelligibility strategies, such as having the individual exaggerate articulation or decrease the rate of speech; and environmental modifications, such as decreasing background noise. It is recommended that a referral to a SLP for augmentative/alternative communication evaluation should be offered at least once annually for those with dysarthria.[119]

As the severity of dysarthria progresses, management will focus on decreasing the patient's dependence on speech as the primary method of communication. Interventions first include "low-tech" devices, such as using a writing board or pad and pen for patients with adequate hand function or using an alphabet board. A progression is then made to more "high-tech" devices, such as computers with voice synthesizers or single-switch, scanning computerized communication systems.[134,135]

A *palatal lift prosthesis* may be prescribed for individuals with good articulation but who have a breathy voice quality or decreased loudness because of excessive air loss through the nose. The device, a dental appliance designed to attach to the existing teeth and to elevate the soft palate, is custom-made by a prosthodontist. It allows the soft palate to close around the surrounding structures such as the pharynx, making verbal communication more understandable by reducing or eliminating hypernasal speech. The device also lowers the hard palate, which reduces tongue movement allowing speech to be less fatiguing.[134] Findings from a retrospective study of 25 patients with ALS treated with a palatal lift indicated 21 patients showed improvement in their dysarthria, specifically in reduction of hypernasality, with 19 patients benefiting at least moderately for 6 months.[136]

Muscle Cramps, Spasticity, Fasciculations, and Pain

Anticonvulsant medication such as phenytoin (Dilantin) and carbamazepine (Atretol, Tegretol) may be prescribed for muscle cramps, if they are not relieved with a program of muscle stretching and adequate hydration and nutrition. Both of these medications can cause gastrointestinal upset and rash, and carbamazepine can cause sedation. Benzodiazepines, such as diazepam (Valium), clonazepam (Klonopin), or lorazepam (Ativan) can also be prescribed for muscle cramps, and side effects may include sedation, dizziness, respiratory depression, and increased weakness. Benzodiazepines, especially diazepam, may be prescribed for spasticity, although baclofen (Lioresal) and tizanidine (Zanaflex) are more commonly used. Side effects include weakness, fatigue, sedation, and hypotension.[60,120,137]

Patients with brisk, widespread fasciculations are generally instructed to avoid or minimize caffeine and nicotine. Lorazepam (Ativan) may be prescribed to decrease the intensity of the fasciculations.[60] Depending on the etiology of pain, a variety of management strategies may be utilized, as there are no pain medication trials that have been conducted in individuals with ALS. Mild pain or pain associated with joint discomfort is usually addressed with analgesics, such as acetaminophen or non-steroidal anti-inflammatory drugs (NSAIDs). For more severe refractory pain, opiates or opioids such as codeine, hydrocodone, or methadone may be prescribed. In the terminal stages of ALS, morphine may be administered to provide analgesia, sedation, and relief from respiratory distress.[60,120,137]

Anxiety and Depression

Anxiety and depression can greatly affect a patient's and his or her family's quality of life, as well as the ability to cope with and adapt to the progressive changes and losses of the disease. Thus, pharmacotherapy and psychological counseling are important management strategies for addressing the anxiety and depression that can develop. Individuals with depression may be prescribed a selective serotonin reuptake inhibitor (SSRI), such as fluoxetine (Prozac) or sertraline (Zoloft), or serotonin and norepinephrine reuptake inhibitor (SNRI). It is important to note that antidepressant effects may not occur for several weeks after initiation of the medications, and side effects may include agitation and insomnia. If the patient presents with depression and insomnia or agitation, a tricyclic antidepressant, such as amitriptyline (Elavil) or imipramine (Tofranil), is preferred.[60,120,137]

Benzodiazepines, such as chlordiazepoxide (Librium), clorazepate, diazepam, and flurazepam (Dalmane), may be prescribed for anxiety or for patients with depression and insomnia. For patients whose respiratory status is affected, a non-benzodiazepine anxiolytic, such as buspirone (BuSpar), is preferred.[60,120,137]

FRAMEWORK FOR REHABILITATION

As previously described, the course of ALS cannot be altered and eventually the individual will become dependent in essentially all aspects of mobility and self-care. However, appropriate rehabilitation programs should be designed and implemented to allow the individual to maintain independence and function for as long as possible, within the context of his or her goals and resources, throughout the disease and across health care settings. Examples of general goals and outcomes for individuals with ALS can be found Box 17.1. Consideration of the rehabilitation framework[138] elements will help guide the physical therapist in developing patient-specific goals.

Because of the progressive nature of ALS, it is imperative that the physical therapist not only addresses an individual's current problems, but also plans ahead for future problems.[138] A large body of evidence to help guide physical therapy decision making is currently unavailable. As identified earlier, ALS has a progressive and deteriorating disease trajectory, with inevitable progression to disability. However, there is great variability among individuals across the disease trajectory. Staging ALS into *early, middle* (early-middle and late-middle), and *late* stages based on impairments, activity limitations, and participation restrictions may assist the therapist in designing appropriate and realistic interventions throughout the disease process, as well as anticipate the evolving needs of individual patients[138] (Fig. 17.9).

In the *early* stage of the disease, ALS will manifest as a variety of signs and symptoms recognized by the

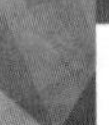

Box 17.1 Examples of General Goals and Outcomes for Individuals with ALS

Impact of Pathology/Pathophysiology is Addressed

- Patient/client, family, and caregiver awareness and knowledge of the disease, prognosis, and plan of care are enhanced.
- Symptom management is addressed and enhanced.
- Changes associated with disease progression are monitored and addressed.
- Risk of secondary impairments is reduced.
- Composite impairments are addressed.
- Intensity of care is optimized.

Impact of Impairments is Reduced

- Cognitive and psychosocial function are considered and addressed where possible.
- Pain is prevented, and if present decreased.
- Respiratory impairments are addressed and decreased to the extent possible.
- Dysarthria, dysphagia, and sialorrhea are considered and addressed.
- Joint integrity issues are prevented, and if present addressed.
- Motor function is addressed and enhanced to the extent possible.
- Muscle performance (strength, power, and endurance) issues are addressed and enhanced to the extent possible.
- Postural control and balance issues are addressed and enhanced to the extent possible.
- Mobility, gait, and locomotion are addressed and enhanced to the extent possible.
- Aerobic capacity is addressed and enhanced to the extent possible.

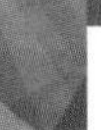

Box 17.1 Examples of General Goals and Outcomes for Individuals with ALS—cont'd

Ability to Perform Physical Actions, Tasks, or Activities is Optimized, and, Where Possible, Enhanced

- ADLs are addressed and optimized.
- Activity tolerance is optimized.
- Problem-solving and decision making skills are enhanced.
- Safety of patient/client, family, and caregivers is increased.

Effects of Disability are Addressed and Where Possible Reduced to the Extent Possible

- Ability to engage in self-care and home management is optimized.
- Ability to engage in work (job/school), community, and leisure roles is optimized.
- Awareness and use of community resources are improved.

Health Status is Optimized and Quality of Life of Patient/Client, Family, and Caregivers is Enhanced

- Sense of well-being is enhanced.
- Stressors are reduced.
- Self-confidence and self-management skills are optimized and enhanced.
- Health, wellness, and fitness are optimized.

Patient/Client Satisfaction is Enhanced

- Access and availability of services are acceptable to patient/client and family.
- Quality of rehabilitation services is acceptable to patient/client and family.
- Care is optimized.
- Care is coordinated with patient/client, family, caregivers, and other health care professionals.
- Living arrangements are optimized.

Adapted from Guide to Physical Therapist Practice 3.0, with permission of the American Physical Therapy Association.® 2014 American Physical Therapy Association. APTA is not responsible for the translation from English.

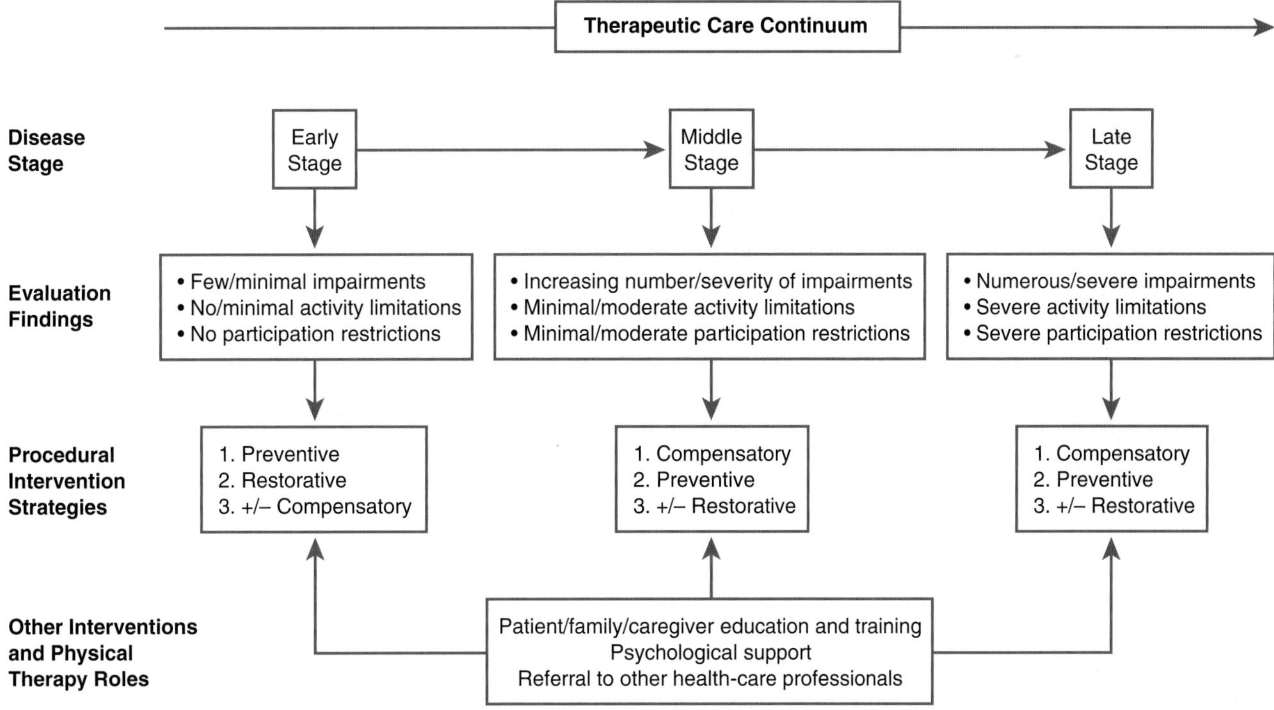

Figure 17.9 Framework for rehabilitation for individuals with ALS. *(From Dal Bello-Haas, V p 116[138] with permission.)*

patient as abnormal. The resultant impairments may or may not cause minor activity limitations and no participation restrictions are present. In the *middle* stage of ALS, the patient experiences increasing signs and symptoms, and develops an increase in the number of impairments and the severity of impairments. Minimal to moderate activity limitations will be noted and participation restrictions will develop. In the *late* stage of ALS, disease progression leads to numerous and increasingly more severe impairments. The patient becomes increasingly limited functionally owing to lack of voluntary motor control and numerous participation restrictions ensue. The patient becomes dependent in essentially all aspects of mobility and self-care, and may require mechanical ventilation to address respiratory compromise, if not already ventilated.[138]

Within this framework, impairments, activity limitations, and participation restrictions are managed through restorative, compensatory, or preventative physical therapy interventions.[138] These interventions should be tailored to the stage of the disease, keeping in mind individual variability throughout disease course (e.g., presence of cognitive impairments or respiratory signs and symptoms) and disease progression (e.g., slowly progressing versus fast progressing), and grounded in evidence-based research whenever possible. The patient's goals are paramount, and psychosocial factors that may influence the patient's decision making, such as acceptance of the diagnosis, and social and financial resources must be considered.[138]

PHYSICAL THERAPY EXAMINATION

At any one time, a variety of body regions can be affected by ALS and in various combinations. Impairments may occur as a direct result of the pathology (*direct impairment*), as sequelae to the pathology (*indirect impairment*), or as the result of multiple underlying origins (*composite impairments*). Therefore, a careful and comprehensive examination is required to determine the extent of involvement as well as the impact of involvement on activity limitations and participation restrictions. Elements of the examination for the individual with ALS are summarized in Box 17.2. Reexamination at regular intervals is necessary to determine the extent and rate of progression of the disease. However, at times it may be difficult to differentiate between the progressive course of the disease and the lack of impact of the interventions. In considering the tests and measures to include in a reexamination, the benefits should be carefully weighted against the psychological impact of repeating tests and measures when the patient is progressively deteriorating. This is especially true in the late-middle and late stage of the disease. It is important for the physical therapist to re-examine, monitor, and evaluate changes, because some medical decisions may be based on the physical

Box 17.2 Elements of the Examination for the Individual with Amyotrophic Lateral Sclerosis

Patient/Client History

- Age, sex, race/ethnicity/cultural heritage, primary language, education level
- Social history: cultural beliefs and behaviors, family, caregiver and other resources, social support systems
- Occupation/employment/work, volunteer activities
- Leisure, hobbies
- Living environment: home/work barriers
- Hand dominance
- General health status: physical, psychological, social and role function, health and wellness habits
- Family history
- Medical/surgical history
- Current conditions/chief complaints
- Medications
- Medical/laboratory test results
- Premorbid functional activity level

Systems Review

- Neuromuscular
- Musculoskeletal
- Cardiovascular/pulmonary
- Integumentary
- Cognitive and Psychological

Tests and Measures (see narrative) for:

- Cognition and behavior
- Psychosocial function
- Pain
- Muscle performance, strength, power and endurance
- Motor function
- Tone and reflexes
- Cranial nerve integrity
- Sensation
- Postural alignment and position symmetry
- Postural control and balance
- Gait and mobility
- Respiratory function
- Anthropometrics
- Integument
- Functional status
- Environmental barriers
- Fatigue

therapist's findings, for example, the patient's percent predicted VC and the timing of PEG placement.

The patient's goals and individual psychosocial factors, rate of disease progression, extent and area of involvement, stage of the disease, and respiratory and bulbar involvement that may affect the patient's ability to participate all need to be considered when structuring the initial examination. The types of data generated from the patient history and interview are presented in Chapter 1, Clinical Decision Making. When collecting these data, determining what is important, relevant, and valued by the individual patient is key. By understanding what is most meaningful to a patient, the physical therapist can narrow the gap between a patient's expectations and hopes and actual experiences through realistic and appropriate interventions. For example, a young mother with ALS may inform the physical therapist her priority is caring for her children rather than maintaining employment. Thus, the initial examination would be structured around abilities and activities related to home, rather than work.

Many of the tests and measures described in this text are generally appropriate components of a comprehensive examination for an individual with ALS. However, selection is always based on specific patient need. The tests and measures frequently applicable to patients with ALS include examination of sensory function, muscle performance, motor function, coordination and balance, gait, functional status, the environment, respiratory function, and cognitive function (see Chapters 3, 4, 5, 6, 7, 8, 9, 12, and 27). The following section presents areas that typically warrant emphasis during the examination.

Cognition

The ALS Cognitive Behavioral Screen (ALS-CBS) assesses executive function via two components: (i) *cognitive*, which evaluates attention, concentration, working memory, fluency, and tracking[139] using four subscales with a total score of 20; and (ii) *behavioral*, which evaluates changes in empathy, personality, judgment, language, and insight using 15 questions completed by the caregiver with scores ranging from 0 to 45.[139] Studies have found that the cognitive section differentiated patients with cognitive impairments with 71% specificity and 85% sensitivity, and that the behavioral section predicted ALS-frontotemporal dementia (ALS-FTD) with 80% sensitivity and 88% specificity.[139] The utility of incorporating screening instruments into a busy ALS clinic has been documented,[140] and it is recommended that patients with ALS be screened at least once annually for cognitive impairment, e.g., FTD screening, cognitive and behavioral impairment screening.[119] As cognitive impairment is often best identified through neuropsychological evaluation comprised of standardized measures and normative data, referral to a neuropsychologist may be warranted to identify specific cognitive impairments.

The Edinburgh Cognitive and Behavioural ALS Screen (ECAS) is an additional tool that incorporates short cognitive tests that have been shown to be sensitive to cognitive impairment in ALS.[141] Executive functions, memory, language, visuospatial skills, and social cognition are assessed. It also includes a short series behavioral and psychosis interview questions for family or caregivers. The ECAS takes about 15 minutes to administer (score range from 0 to 136).[141]

Psychosocial Function

As depression and anxiety are common in individuals with ALS, screening is important and referral to a psychologist or psychiatrist for further evaluation may be indicated. The *Beck's Depression Inventory,*[142] the *Center of Epidemiologic Study Depression Scale,*[143] the *Hospital Anxiety and Depression Scale* (HADS),[144] and the *State-Trait Anxiety Inventory*[145] have been used in clinical studies. The 12-item Amyotrophic Lateral Sclerosis Depression Inventory (ADI-12) is a short self-report screening questionnaire comprised of 12 items, rated on a 4-point scale, none of which refer to somatic or motor-related symptoms.[146] The ADI-12 has not undergone extensive or rigorous cross-cultural methodology or psychometric testing.

Pain

Pain is common in individuals with ALS and should be examined subjectively and objectively, using a *Visual Analogue Scale* (VAS) for example. Pain is not necessarily a direct impairment of ALS, but rather an indirect (decreased ROM, adhesive capsulitis) or a composite impairment (joint malalignment secondary to spasticity and faulty posture). Further examination of underlying causes of pain is often required.

Joint Integrity, Range of Motion, and Muscle Length

Functional ROM, active, active-assisted, and passive range ROM, muscle length, and soft tissue flexibility and extensibility should be examined using standard methods.

Muscle Performance

Specific deficits of muscle strength, power and endurance, and muscle performance during functional activities should be determined. Specific deficits can be measured with manual muscle testing (MMT), isokinetic muscle strength testing, or handheld dynamometry.

In clinical trials, muscle strength has been examined as *maximum voluntary isometric contraction* (MVIC) using a strain gauge tensiometer system.[147] This method eliminates muscle length and velocity as factors in testing and produces reliable, valid, interval data.[147-150] MVIC is considered the most direct technique for investigating motor unit loss, and has been used extensively for examining muscle strength in individuals with ALS for the past 10 years. Its range and sensitivity have been validated by several natural history studies.[5,17,151] However, MVIC testing requires specialized equipment and training in its use. Test reliability of MMT and MVIC scores among uniformly trained physical therapists at several institutions has been examined. Reproducibility between MMT and MVIC was found to be equivalent. Sensitivity to detect progressive muscle strength changes in individuals with ALS favored MMT. However, six muscles were tested with MVIC and 34 muscles were tested with MMT; thus, the difference in detecting change was largely accounted for by the number of muscles sampled by MMT versus MVIC.[152]

Motor Function

Impairments in dexterity, coordination of large movement patterns, as well as gross and fine motor control, may be evident owing to spasticity and muscle weakness. Hand function and initiation, modification, and control of movement patterns should be examined.

Tone and Reflexes

Muscle tone may be examined using the *Modified Ashworth Scale.*[153] Deep tendon and pathological reflexes should be tested to distinguish between UMN and LMN involvement. See Chapter 5: Examination of Motor Function: Motor Control and Motor Learning.

Cranial Nerve Integrity

The cranial nerves commonly affected by ALS include V, VII, IX, X, and XII. Cranial nerves should be tested to determine the extent of bulbar involvement (see Chapter 5). Screening for oral motor function, phonation, and speech production can be accomplished through the interview and observation. Referral to a SLP is recommended.

Sensation

If the patient complains of sensory symptoms or if sensory involvement is suspected, sensory testing should be completed, as described in Chapter 3, Examination of Sensory Function.

Postural Alignment, Control, and Balance

Static and dynamic postural alignment and body mechanics during self-care, functional mobility skills, functional activities, and work conditions and activities should be examined. Postural stability, reactive control, anticipatory control, and adaptive postural control should also be determined. See Chapter 6, Examination of Coordination and Balance for more information.

Falls in people with ALS lead to morbidity and mortality,[154] with fall-related deaths occurring in 1.7% of all patients with ALS.[154] Similar to other patient populations, those with ALS should be queried about falls since the last visit, and should be evaluated for known fall risk factors. Sanjak et al reported 37% of ambulatory individuals with ALS had decreased ability to use vestibular input and increased reliance on visual input for postural orientation to sustain equilibrium, despite relatively normal clinical balance and mobility test findings.[155] The authors suggest these findings may be reflective of peripheral and central pathological abnormalities or ALS-related cerebellum pathology.[155]

No ALS-specific balance test or measure exists. A variety of balance status measures, originally designed for use with other patient populations, including the *Tinetti Performance Oriented Mobility Assessment* (POMA),[156] the *Berg Balance Scale*,[157] the *Timed Up and Go Test* (TUG),[158] and the *Functional Reach Test*,[159] can be used. Low total *Tinetti Balance Test* scores, indicating impaired balance, were found to be moderately to strongly related to LE muscle weakness and disability in individuals with ALS.[160,161] Kloos et al[160] suggest that the POMA is a reliable measure for individuals in the early or early-middle stages of ALS. A study of 31 individuals with ALS who underwent monthly TUG, Amyotrophic Lateral Sclerosis Functional Rating Scale—Revised (ALSFRS-R), FVC, MMT, and quality-of-life assessments for 6 months found that the TUG was significantly associated with the chance of falling.[162]

Gait

No ALS-specific gait test or measure exists. Documentation of gait within a particular time period (e.g., within 15 seconds) or over a certain distance (e.g., 10 feet [3 meters]) has been measured in clinical trials. Gait stability, safety, and endurance should be examined. Energy expenditure, alignment, fit, practicality, safety, and ease of use of orthotic and assistive devices should also be examined at regular intervals.

Respiratory Function

Determination of respiratory status and function includes regular (at each clinical visit) querying about symptoms of respiratory insufficiency (dyspnea, orthopnea, excessive daytime sleepiness, insomnia, fatigue, morning headache),[119] examination of respiratory symptoms and muscle function, breathing pattern, chest expansion, respiratory sounds, cough effectiveness, and regular (at least every 3 months) pulmonary function testing.[119] VC or FVC may be assessed using a handheld spirometer. Supine FVC may be a better indicator of diaphragm weakness than erect FVC, and if possible VC should be measured in standing, sitting, and lying.[163] Maximal inspiratory pressure may be useful in respiratory function monitoring because it can detect early respiratory insufficiency.[94] Sniff nasal pressure (SNP) may be effective in detecting hypercapnia and nocturnal hypoxemia and may be used for monitoring of inspiratory muscle strength, especially for those with bulbar involvement who cannot perform VC effectively.[163] Peak cough expiratory flow is the most widely used measure of cough effectiveness.[117,119]

Aerobic capacity and cardiovascular–pulmonary endurance may be tested in the early stages of ALS using standardized, modified protocols to evaluate and monitor responses to aerobic conditioning.

Integument

In general, even in the late stage of ALS skin integrity is rarely a problem. Skin inspection should be used to examine contact points between the body and assistive, adaptive, orthotic, protective, and supportive devices, mobility devices, and the sleeping surface. Such inspection is especially important when the patient's mobility becomes increasingly more dependent. If present, swelling should also be examined and monitored. Swelling of the distal limb may develop owing to lack of muscle-pumping action in a weakened extremity.

Functional Status

Functional mobility skills, safety, and energy expenditure are important considerations. Basic and instrumental activities of daily living and the need for adaptive equipment should be examined. The *Functional Independence Measure* (FIM)[164] has been used to document functional status in clinical trials.

The *Schwab and England Activities of Daily Living Scale*[165] is an 11-point global measure of functioning that asks the rater to report activities of daily living (ADL) function from 100% (normal) to 0% (vegetative functions only), and has been used to examine function in individuals with ALS (Appendix 17.A). The ALS CNTF Treatment Study Group found the scale to have excellent test-retest reliability, to correlate well with qualitative and quantitative changes in function, and to be sensitive to changes over time.[166]

Environmental Barriers

The patient's home, work, and leisure environments should be examined for current and potential barriers, access, and safety.

Fatigue

Fatigue is very common in individuals with ALS. No ALS-specific measures exist; the *Fatigue Severity Scale*[167] has been used in clinical trials.

DISEASE-SPECIFIC AND QUALITY-OF-LIFE MEASURES

Disease-Specific Measures

The *ALS Functional Rating Scale* (ALSFRS)[166] and the revised version, ALSFRS-R[167] (Appendix 17.C) examine the functional status of patients with ALS. The patient is asked to rate his or her function using a scale from 4 (normal function) to 0 (unable to attempt the task). The original scale, the ALSFRS, correlated positively with objective measures of UE and LE strength and was found to be valid and reliable for measuring the decline in function that results from loss of muscular strength.[166] The ALSFRS-R was expanded to include additional respiratory items, and was found to have internal consistency and construct validity, and to have retained the properties of the original scale.[167,168] Telephone administration of the ALSFRS-R has also been found to be reliable.[169] Other disease-specific scales include the *Appel ALS Scale* (AALS),[170] the *ALS Severity Scale* (ALSSS),[171] and the *Norris Scale.*[172]

Quality-of-Life Measures

Quality of life in individuals with ALS has been examined with generic measures, such as the SF-36,[173] the *Schedule for Evaluation of Individual Quality of Life—Direct Weighting* (SEIQoL-DW),[174] and the *Sickness Impact Profile* (SIP).[175]

The *Amyotrophic Lateral Sclerosis Assessment Questionnaire* (ALSAQ-40),[176] an ALS-specific quality of life measure, contains 40 items that represent five distinct areas of health: mobility (10 items), ADL (10 items), eating and drinking (3 items), communication (7 items), and emotional functioning (10 items). The questions refer to the patient's condition during the past 2 weeks and responses are given on a five-point Likert scale. The ALSAQ-40 measures health status in each domain using a summary score from 0 (best health status) to 100 (worst health status). The validity and reliability of this instrument have been examined and reported.[176,177] The *ALSAQ-40* has been shortened to 11 items and also appears to be valid and reliable.[178]

PHYSICAL THERAPY INTERVENTIONS

The role of the physical therapist in management of individuals with ALS and the extent of interventions provided vary depending on whether the therapist is working as a member of a team specialized in ALS care or as an independent or clinic-based therapist. Additional variables include the availability of other health care professionals in the practice setting and the reason the individual is seeking physical therapy (e.g., specific ALS-related issue versus a co-morbidity condition such as arthritis).

Restorative intervention is directed toward remediating or improving impairments and activity limitations. In the early and middle stages of ALS, restorative interventions are temporary at best because disease progression is expected and permanent loss of function and disability is likely. Restorative interventions in the late stage of ALS are for the most part directed solely toward remediation of impairments that result from other systems pathology (e.g., pressure sores, edema, pneumonia, atelectasis, adhesive capsulitis).

Compensatory intervention is directed toward modifying activities, tasks, or the environment to minimize activity limitations and participation restrictions. In the early and middle stages of ALS, tasks or activities may be adapted to achieve function. As the disease progresses, increasing environmental adaptations will be necessary to maintain and promote function.[138]

In the early and early-middle stages of ALS, *preventative intervention* is directed toward minimizing potential impairments such as loss of ROM, aerobic capacity, or strength, preventing pneumonia or atelectasis, and activity limitations. Beginning an early prevention program may alter impairments and maintain physical function temporarily, and may also improve well-being and decrease fatigue, as well as the secondary effects of immobility. In the late-middle and late stages, the pathology is more advanced and mobility becomes progressively restricted. In these stages, it may be extremely difficult or impossible to prevent impairments and activity limitations that are directly related to the nervous system pathology. Thus, the role of prevention is *tertiary,* to mitigate the effects of the pathology that lead to impairments in other systems (e.g., educating caregivers about a passive ROM exercise program to prevent adhesive capsulitis in the shoulder).[138] In general, the role of the physical therapist includes the following:

- Promoting independence and maximizing function throughout the stages of the disease, through restorative and compensatory interventions that address impairments, activity limitations, and participation restrictions
- Promoting health and wellness in the early and early-middle stages of the disease through restorative and preventive interventions
- Providing alternative means of carrying out functional activities with adaptive equipment and alternate methods for performing tasks and activities through compensatory interventions as the disease progresses
- Minimizing or preventing complications through preventive interventions throughout the course of the disease
- Providing education, psychological support, and recommendations for equipment and community resources to assist in adapting to the disease progression[138]

Owing to the individual variability of the disease presentation, onset, course, and progression, patients with ALS will present with unique and different sets of problems; thus, interventions will vary. As described earlier, interventions are directed mainly toward addressing activity limitations and participation restrictions, because often the impairments causing the limitations and restrictions cannot be altered. However, in the early and early-middle stages of ALS, it may be possible to direct treatment toward the underlying central nervous system (CNS) impairments, and perhaps postpone the onset of particular activity limitations. For example, a study of patients in the early stages of ALS (FVC ≥90% predicted and ALSFRS ≥30) who engaged in moderate load, moderate resistance exercises were found to have higher ALSFRS scores and SF-36 Physical Function scores compared to a matched control group who performed stretching exercises.[179] Patients and therapists must understand that any beneficial effects of an early prevention program will be short term and will not have an impact on the overall course of the disease. Much more research into the effectiveness of specific physical therapy and other interventions for individuals with ALS is needed.

In developing a POC, in addition to the patient's goals, the therapist must also consider the rate of disease progression, the extent and area of involvement, stage of the disease, respiratory and bulbar factors that may affect participation, timing of the intervention, patient acceptance and motivation, life support choices, availability of psychosocial support, and resources.

Some patients may view the need to use adaptive equipment, such as an ambulatory assistive device or wheelchair, as a definitive marker for disease progression and impending death. This may cause the patient to be hesitant to accept the recommended aid or device as a means of maintaining some aspect of control over the disease. The physical therapist will be required to maintain a balance between being realistic about what can be achieved and providing a sense of hope, not helplessness, when discussing intervention options. An overview of ALS disease stages and general intervention strategies is presented in Table 17.4. Common impairments and activity limitations associated with ALS and their respective interventions are described as follows.

Cervical Muscle Weakness

Progressive cervical extensor weakness will cause the head to fall forward, resulting in overstretching of the posterior musculature and soft tissues. This may cause bouts of acute pain or develop into anterior muscle tightness or a chronic cervical syndrome. Some patients will compensate for the forward head position by increasing lordosis, as they attempt to maintain their posture during ambulation.

For mild to moderate cervical weakness, a soft foam collar may be worn during specific activities. Soft collars are comfortable and usually well tolerated. However, wear-induced compressibility requires that they be replaced frequently. For moderate to severe weakness, a semi-rigid or rigid collar is prescribed. These are usually made of padded rigid plastic or leather and provide very firm support. Patients may find the collars very warm; may experience discomfort at points of body contact, such as the chin, mandible, sternum, or over clavicles; may feel pressure on the trachea; and may feel confined. Several types of collars are presented in Figures 17.10 and 17.11, and the advantages and disadvantages of individual collar types are summarized in Table 17.5.

Some patients with combined cervical and upper thoracic weakness may benefit from a cervical-thoracic

Table 17.4 Amyotrophic Lateral Sclerosis Disease Stages and Common Intervention Strategies: Framework for Rehabilitation for Individuals with ALS

Stage	Common Impairments and Activity Limitations	Interventions
Early	Mild to moderate weakness in specific muscle groups Difficulty with ADL and mobility toward the end of this stage	**Restorative/Preventative** • Strengthening exercises* • Endurance exercises • Active ROM, active-assisted ROM, stretching exercises **Compensatory** • Determine potential need for adaptive or assistive devices. • Determine potential need for ergonomic modifications of home/workplace • Energy conservation • Educate the patient about the disease process, energy conservation, and support groups
Middle	Progressive decrease in mobility throughout stage Wheelchair needed for long distances; increased wheelchair use toward end of stage Severe muscle weakness in some groups; mild to moderate weakness in other groups Progressive decrease in ADL skills throughout stage Pain	**Compensatory** • Support weak muscles (assistive and supportive devices, adaptive equipment, slings, and orthoses) • Modifications to workplace/home (e.g., install ramp, move bedroom to first floor) • Wheelchair prescription • Education of caregivers regarding functional training **Preventative** • Active, active-assistive, and passive ROM, stretching exercises • Strengthening exercises (early middle) • Endurance exercises (early middle) • Determine need for pressure-relieving devices (e.g., pressure-distributing mattress)
Late	Wheelchair dependent or restricted to bed Complete dependence with ADL Severe weakness of UE, LE, neck and trunk muscles Dysarthria, dysphagia Respiratory compromise Pain	**Preventative** • Passive ROM • Pulmonary care* • Hospital bed and pressure-relieving devices • Skin care, hygiene* **Compensatory** • Caregiver education regarding transfers, positioning, turning, skin care • Mechanical lift

Adapted from Dal Bello-Haas,[138, p. 123] with permission.
*May be restorative
ADL = activities of daily living; LE = lower extremity; ROM = range of motion; UE = upper extremity.

orthosis, or a Sternal Occipital Mandibular Immobilizer (SOMI). These devices provide greater support, but are more expensive and heavy and may be difficult to don and doff. For severe or intractable neck weakness, referral to an orthotist for a custom-made device may be necessary.

In addition to wearing collars, individuals with cervical weakness may also benefit from taking frequent rest periods; supportive seating, such as high-back chairs or recliners; tilt-in-space or reclining wheelchairs; elevating reading material; and education about good arm support for prolonged sitting, proper use of head rest when riding in a car, and ergonomic changes for workstations. It is important to note that when trunk weakness accompanies neck weakness, positioning for head support becomes more challenging.

Dysarthria and Dysphagia

In collaboration with the SLP and nutritionist, the physical therapist can play a role in managing dysarthria and dysphagia by addressing the patient's head and trunk control and sitting position. In addition, the physical therapist can reinforce the use of strategies for eating and swallowing (e.g., chin tuck), the use of prescribed communication devices, and the need for food consistency modifications. Because patients are at risk for aspiration, education of the patient, family, and caregiver is imperative (see section that follows, titled Respiratory Muscle Weakness).

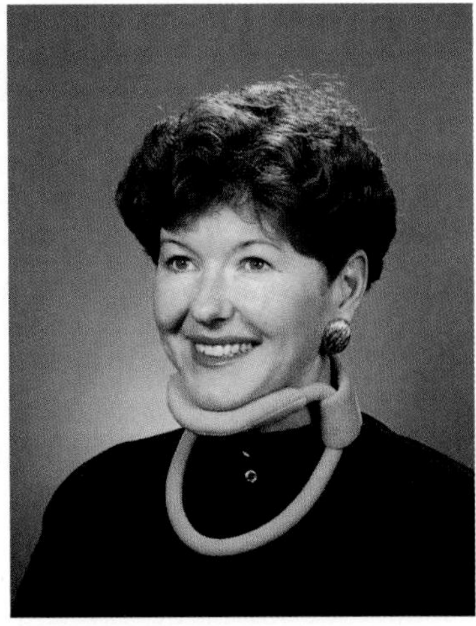

Figure 17.10 The Headmaster Collar. *(Courtesy of Symmetric Designs, Salt Spring Island, BC, Canada, V8K 1C9.)*

Pain

Pain has been poorly studied in people with ALS and is often poorly managed.[180] As noted earlier, pain is typically a secondary impairment resulting from decreased ROM, decreased mobility, and positioning issues. Shoulder, neck, and back pain are common.[181] It is imperative that pain be addressed, as pain has been found to be associated with decreased quality of life.[90] Pain intervention is dependent on what is causing the pain. Although the "best treatment" for pain is prevention, interventions may include modalities, ROM exercises, passive stretching, joint mobilizations, and education about proper positioning and joint support and protection. As well, simple interventions such as asking individuals about comfort (pain) levels while seated or lying and making adjustments to the chair, wheelchair or bed to provide adequate support may be all that is required.

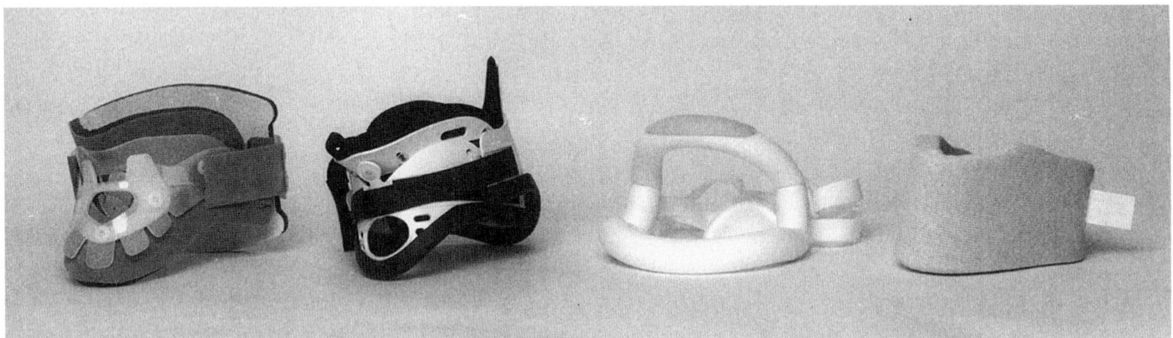

Figure 17.11 Types of collars. From left to right: Aspen Collar, Miami-J Collar, Executive Collar, and Soft Collar.

Table 17.5 Types of Semi-rigid and Rigid Cervical Collars

Type	Examples	Advantages	Disadvantages
Collars without anterior neck access	Philadelphia Collar[a]	Offers good support	Patient may feel confined. May cause pressure on trachea Patient may experience difficulty breathing or swallowing. Can be uncomfortably warm
Collars with anterior neck access (for tracheostomy)	Miami-J Collar[b] Aspen Collar[c] Malibu Collar[d]	Padding absorbs and wicks moisture away from skin Suitable for individuals with cervical weakness in all three planes	Patient may feel confined. May be uncomfortably warm More expensive
	Canadian Collar[e] Headmaster Collar[e]	Open design allows for circulation of air Lightweight No pressure on trachea Some patients consider collar more cosmetically appealing	May put pressure on chin and sternum Some models more expensive Some models require custom cutting. Not adequate if rotation and lateral flexion weakness is also present

[a]Philadelphia® Cervical Collar Co, Thorofare, NJ.
[b]Jerome Medical, Moorestown, NJ.
[c]Aspen Medical Products Inc, Irvine, CA.
[d]Seattle Systems, Poulsbo, WA.
[e]Symmetric Designs Ltd., Salt Spring Island, BC, Canada.

For example, severe muscle weakness in the LE may result in distal edema (and subsequent pain) due to lack of active muscle pump, and concomitant pain, when sitting in a wheelchair.

Shoulder Pain

Individuals with ALS may develop shoulder pain and present with capsular patterns of restriction. Pain may be caused by several factors: abnormal scapulohumeral rhythm secondary to spasticity or weakness causing imbalance that may lead to impingement; overuse of strong muscles; muscle strain; faulty resting position; glenohumeral subluxation secondary to weakness; or a fall.

A 20% incidence of adhesive capsulitis in individuals with ALS has been found. Recommendations for managing the pain and decreased ROM include a protocol of an intra-articular analgesic and anti-inflammatory cocktail injection, followed by a course of aggressive ROM exercises. Some patients reported an acute resolution of pain, whereas others reported improvements over 2 to 3 weeks.[182]

UE Muscle Weakness

Weakness of the UEs greatly affects the patient's ability to carry out ADL. There is a large variety of adaptive equipment available that may help the patient prolong function for as long as possible (see section that follows titled, Activities of Daily Living).

Patients with a painful shoulder due to subluxation may benefit from a sling, similar to those used with patients following stroke with decreased tone, although subluxation cannot be corrected completely. Splinting of the wrist or hand may be indicated to prevent contractures or to improve the patient's function, such as the ability to grasp.

Respiratory Muscle Weakness

Education is extremely important. Patients and caregivers must be taught how to balance activity and rest, and educated about energy conservation techniques. Patients and caregivers should also be educated about signs and symptoms of aspiration; positioning to avoid aspiration, such as upper cervical spine flexion during eating; causes and signs of respiratory infection; and strategies for managing oral secretions (use of oral suction device) or choking episodes (Heimlich maneuver). Specific breathing exercises and positioning to optimize ventilation/perfusion matching may also be incorporated, although their effectiveness in ALS has not been determined.

A small sample size double-blind study randomly assigned nine people with ALS to an inspiratory muscle training (IMT) group. Subjects completed daily IMT training sessions (10 minutes per session) three times per day. After 12 weeks of training, subjects in the IMT group demonstrated trends toward improvement in FVC, VC, MIP, and SNP, compared to a control group who completed sham training (n = 10), and gains in inspiratory muscle strength that were partially reversed after an 8-week period of training cessation.[183]

Clinical and research interest in cough augmentation techniques for individuals with ALS has been increasing. Airway clearance techniques may be necessary when conditions that cause secretion retention, such as pneumonia or atelectasis, arise. To compensate for a weakened cough, the patient and caregiver may be instructed in the use of manually assisted coughing techniques or the use of a mechanical insufflation–exsufflation (MI-E) device to facilitate clearance of respiratory and oral secretions (Fig. 17.12).

The MI-E device is designed to inflate the lung with positive pressure and assist cough with negative pressure through the flip of a switch. A positive-pressure breath of 30 to 50 cm H_2O over a 1- to 3-second period via an oral–nasal mask or tracheal airway is provided. The airway pressure is then reversed abruptly to –30 to –50 cm H_2O and maintained for 2 to 3 seconds. A peak expiratory cough flow (PECF) within normal range is achieved, thereby assisting with the clearance of secretions.[184] A systematic review of the effects of MI-E and the breath-stacking technique for reducing morbidity and mortality and enhancing quality of life in people with ALS/ MND is currently underway.[185]

Studies of cough flows and pressures during cough augmentation have found that manual assistance increased flow 11% in those with bulbar ALS and 13% in those with non-bulbar ALS. MI-E increased flow by 26% in those with bulbar ALS and 28% in those with non-bulbar ALS. The greatest improvements were in patients with the weakest coughs.[186]

The effectiveness of MI-E has not been definitely demonstrated in people ALS, but case reports have described the benefits from regular use of a mechanical insufflation device.[187,188] A comparison study of MI-E versus breath-stacking found no statistically significant differences. The authors attribute this lack of

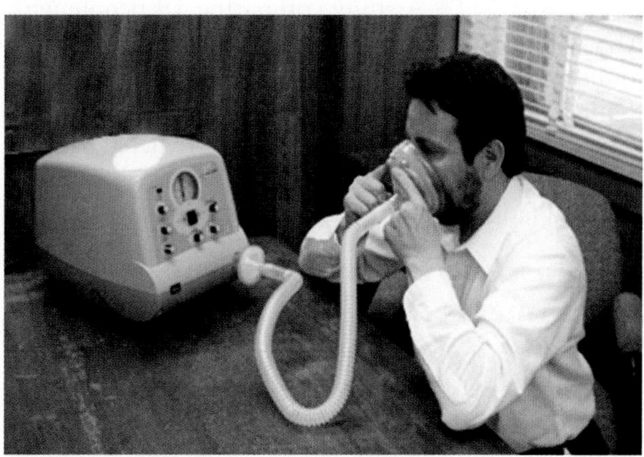

Figure 17.12 Mechanical insufflation–exsufflation (MI-E) device. *(Courtesy of JH Emerson Co., Cambridge, MA 02140.)*

significance to under-powering and multiple confounders, and suggest the need for larger sample size trials.[189]

The lung volume recruitment (LVR) technique (breath stacking, deep lung insufflation) may also be used to facilitate secretion clearance. LVR involves the administration of a series of stacked breaths using a resuscitator bag, which expands the lungs to a volume greater than spontaneous inspiratory capacity. LVR allows for the initiation of a cough from a higher lung volume. Thus, the greater respiratory system elastic recoil pressure generates a greater cough flow. LVR has been shown to increase peak cough flow in people with various neuromuscular diseases (NMDs) and ALS.[186, 190, 191]

In people with NMD with respiratory muscle weakness, reduced tidal volumes, and decreased sighing and cough effectiveness leads to reduced compliance ("stiffening") of the lungs and chest wall over time, further contributing to respiratory insufficiency.[192] It has been proposed that in this context, the regular use of LVR can be viewed as a "range-of-motion" exercise for the respiratory system to maintain normal compliance of the system and possibly delay the onset of ventilatory failure.[193]

Kaminsky et al examined LVR in people with NMD, including eight individuals with ALS.[194] The authors reported that after 3 months of regular LVR use, there was high acceptability and willingness to use LVR, and that there was a significant increase in lung inspiratory capacity-FVC difference, even though FVC declined (total subject analysis). Interestingly, adherence to LVR was highest in the participants with ALS.[194]

High-frequency chest wall oscillation (HF-CWO) has garnered some interest in its applicability to the ALS population. HF-CWO is an external non-invasive modality that transmits high-frequency oscillatory pressures through the chest wall, thereby mobilizing secretions from the small peripheral airways and enhancing secretion clearance and gas exchange. HF-CWO has been effectively used in patient populations in which secretion retention and hypersecretion are issues (e.g., cystic fibrosis).[195,196] A study comparing 19 people with ALS who used HF-CWO to 16 who were not treated found that after 6 months, those using the device had significantly less breathlessness. In addition, those users with an FVC between 40% and 70% predicted had significantly less mean decrease in FVC and less breathlessness and fatigue.[197]

LE Muscle Weakness and Gait Impairments

Orthoses may be recommended to improve function by offering support to weakened muscles and the joints they surround, decrease the stress on remaining functioning or compensatory muscles, conserve energy, or minimize local or general muscle fatigue. Controlling knee impairments can often be achieved through an ankle–foot orthosis (AFO); as such, addressing the ankle should be considered first. It is also important to consider the weight of the orthosis, as individuals with ALS will have energy expenditure issues, and it may be more fatiguing for the patient to ambulate with a heavy orthosis than to ambulate without the impairment being corrected. For this reason, a knee-ankle-foot orthosis (KAFO) is not recommended.

Deciding between a commercially manufactured versus a custom-made orthosis is certainly dependent on the patient's resources, but the rate of disease progression should also be considered. For an individual with rapidly progressive ALS and who is likely to use the orthosis for a limited time, a commercially manufactured orthosis may suffice. Solid AFOs are a good choice for patients who have medial/lateral instability of the ankle with quadriceps weakness. The fixed-ankle position, combined with the quadriceps weakness, may make it difficult for sit-to-stand transfers, climbing stairs, and negotiating inclines. Hinged AFOs allow dorsiflexion and may be appropriate for the patient with adequate knee extensor strength and mild ankle strength loss.

The type of ambulatory assistive device prescribed is dependent on the degree of proximal muscle strength or instability; function of the UEs; the pattern, extent, and rate of disease progression; acceptance by the patient; and financial constraints. Again, weight of the device is an important factor to consider in decision making, while also considering which device will ensure optimal function and safety. Wheeled walkers, which do not require the patient to lift the device, are usually recommended. In general, individuals with ALS are rarely prescribed crutches. If crutches are warranted, Loftstrand (Canadian) crutches are preferred.

Activities of Daily Living

A large variety of adaptive equipment is available to assist individuals with muscle weakness perform everyday tasks. However, the benefits and effectiveness of adaptive equipment for people with ALS have not been evaluated systematically. No one type of device is suitable for every patient or for every stage of the disease. Reimbursement for the equipment is variable and although a piece of adaptive equipment can help the patient maintain independence, limited financial resources may prevent recommending or purchasing the item. For example, in the early stages of ALS a universal cuff with a pocket for writing or feeding utensils may be beneficial. As the disease progresses and proximal shoulder weakness increases, a mobile arm support may be incorporated to allow the patient to maintain independence in eating. In the late stage of ALS when the patient is dependent on the caregiver for eating, a long straw and straw holder may be recommended to assist the caregiver with the activity. Examples of common adaptive equipment that may be beneficial for performing ADL are presented in Table 17.6.

Table 17.6 Common Types of Adaptive Equipment

Feeding and eating	Foam tubing to increase the size of utensil handles; utensils and cups with modified handles or holders; long-levered jar opener; plate guard; serrated or rocker knife; wrist splint/adapted cuff (for holding tools and instruments); mobile arm support; Dycem
Self-care and bathing	Bathing benches; bath tub seats; shower commode; handheld shower head; grab bars; raised toilet seat; long-handled sponge; electric toothbrush or shaver; strap-fitted hairbrushes
Dressing	Zipper pulls or hooks; button hooks; long-handled shoehorn; hook and loop clothing closures; elastic shoelaces
Writing and reading	Foam tubing to increase the size of the pen or pencil; triangular pencil grip; pen holders; book holders; automatic page turner; adjustable angle table
Other	Key holders; doorknob adapters; lamp extension switch; personal alarm system; switch-operated environmental controls; speaker phone with automatic dialing; telephone holder; use of telecommunication devices for the deaf

Decreased Mobility

Patients with LE weakness may have difficulty with sit-to-stand or car transfers. Simple interventions include placing a firm cushion 2 to 3 in (5 to 7.6 cm) thick under the buttocks in the chair or elevating the chair by placing the legs in prefabricated blocks (Fig. 17.13). Self-powered lifting cushions are relatively inexpensive and portable, but the individual needs adequate trunk control and balance to use the device safely (Fig. 17.14). Upholstered reclining chairs with powered seat lifts may also be recommended, but are more expensive. All these interventions increase the biomechanical advantage and make it easier for the patient to rise from a sitting position.

Caregivers will need to be educated regarding assisting the patient with transitional movements. Transfer boards may be used for transfers once the individual is unable to stand, either alone if the person has adequate arm strength and good sitting balance, or the caregiver can be instructed in how to assist the patient. Other useful devices to assist the patient's mobility are transfer belts and swivel cushions or seats. Transfer belts ease the burden of the transfer for the caregiver and prevent potential pulling on the patient's UEs. Swivel cushions are lightweight, cushioned seats that swivel in both directions and make getting in and out of a car easier (Fig. 17.15).

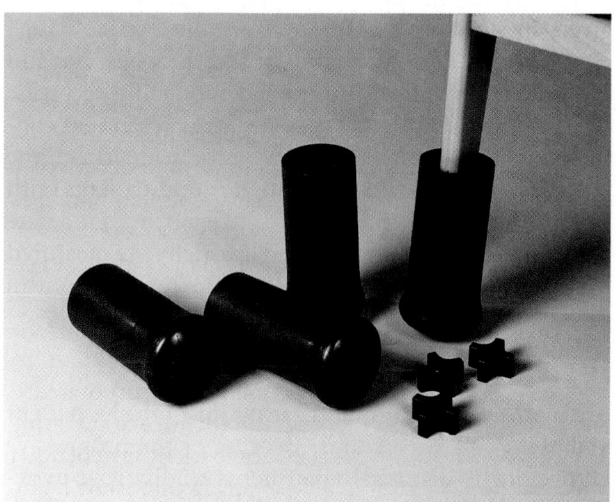

Figure 17.13 Prefabricated blocks. *(Courtesy of Homecraft AbilityOne, Kirkby-in-Ashfield, Nottinghamshire, England NG17 7ET.)*

Once an individual cannot perform transfers, even with the assistance of a caregiver, a hydraulic or mechanical lift is required. Commonly recommended lifts devices include the Easy Pivot™ (Rand-Scot Inc., Fort Collins, CO), and the Hoyer Lift® (Sunrise Medical, Longmont, CO). Use of an electric hospital bed may facilitate bed mobility and transfers both for the patient and caregiver, and, depending on resources, home modifications and automobile adaptations may also be considered.

Chair glides or stairway lifts can be suggested for those individuals who live in multilevel homes, but who cannot or should not climb stairs (see Chapter 9, Examination and Modification of the Environment). These lifts are measured and custom-made for individual staircases and are very expensive. Insurance companies usually do not reimburse for stairway lifts, but some medical supply companies offer "rent-to-own" options. In addition, local ALSA or MDA chapters may have lifts that have been recycled.

At some time point as the disease progresses, the extent of muscle weakness or the energy requirements for ambulation will necessitate wheelchair use for mobility. In the early or early-middle stage of ALS a manual wheelchair, preferably lightweight, may be used for traveling long distances as an energy conservation technique. This wheelchair should be rented on a short-term basis or loaned from a local ALSA or MDA chapter or other source, because most insurance companies will reimburse for only one wheelchair purchase. As the disease progresses, a power wheelchair system tailored to the patient's

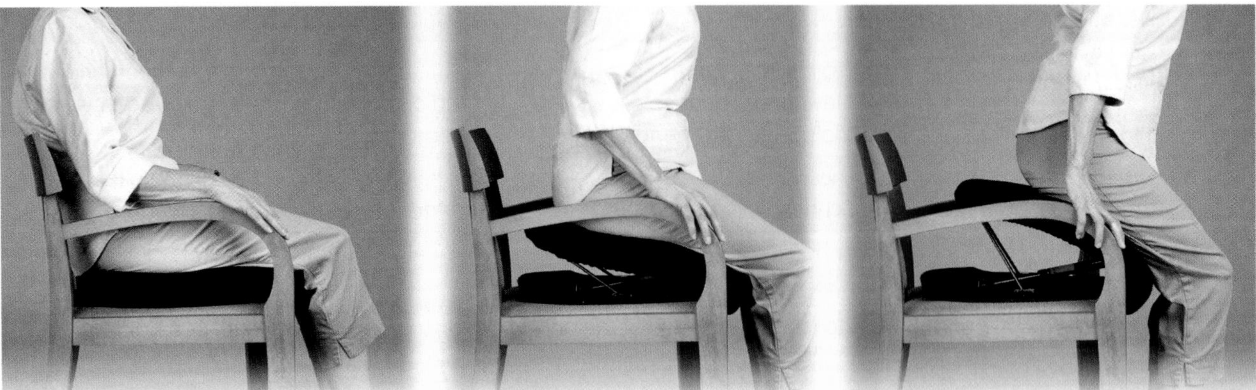

Figure 17.14 UpLift Seat. *(Courtesy of Uplift Technologies Inc., Dartmouth, NS, Canada, B3B 1M2.)*

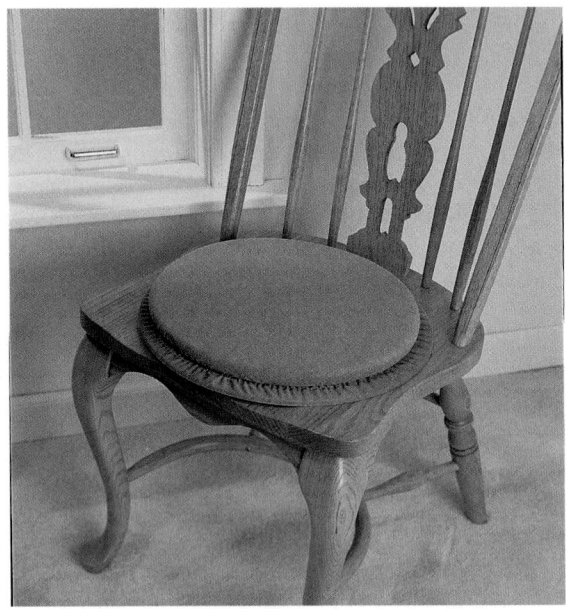

Figure 17.15 Swivel cushion. *(Courtesy of Sammons Preston Rolyan Canada, Mississauga, Ontario, Canada, L4Y 4C5.)*

current needs and potential future needs will be necessary. Numerous customized wheelchair features and options are available that can assist the individual in maintaining a maximum level of independence and comfort (see Chapter 32: Seating and Wheeled Mobility). A referral to a wheelchair and seating clinic may be the best option owing to the numerous, specialized, and evolving needs of the individual with ALS.

Trail et al[198] surveyed 42 patients with ALS and moderate disability, as documented on the AALS, about the wheelchair features they found most beneficial. Sixty-one percent of patients reported that their wheelchairs allowed them to maintain their previous activity levels. In order of priority, manual wheelchair users cited a lightweight frame, small turning radius, high reclining back and supports for the head, trunk, and extremities as most desirable; undesirable features included low, sling, non-reclining back; non-motorized; static, non-adjustable leg rests; heaviness or large size; and non-removable armrests. Desirable features for patients who used powered wheelchairs included independent mobility, maneuverability, overall comfort and tilt-in-space/recline features; undesirable features included low, non-reclining back, heaviness, or large size, uncomfortable seat, non-adjustable leg rests, and general discomfort.[198]

Although power scooters may be suitable for a patient with adequate UE and trunk strength in the earlier stages of ALS, the vehicle becomes limiting as the disease progresses and should not be prescribed. If the patient has already been reimbursed for a scooter, most insurance companies will not pay for a power wheelchair, because the scooter is considered a power mobility device. If a scooter is to be recommended at all, the patient should rent or borrow the device for short-term use.

Muscle Cramps and Spasticity

Muscle cramps may be alleviated with massage and a stretching program. Cold can temporarily decrease spasticity. Physical therapists can perform and instruct caregivers in slow prolonged stretches and passive ROM exercises to address spasticity. In addition, postural and positioning techniques can be incorporated to decrease spasticity and splinting may be necessary to prevent contractures. A published Cochrane review identified one randomized, controlled study that found patients with ALS who engaged in a 15-min, twice-daily, moderate intensity exercise had decreased spasticity, as measured by the *Modified Ashworth Scale,* compared to a control group who engaged in usual daily activities.[199]

Psychosocial Issues

A diagnosis of ALS is devastating for both the patient and family–caregiver unit. Because of the progressive nature of the disease, impairments readily lead to activity limitations and participation restrictions, which may affect quality of life. The emotional responses of the person experiencing the disease, family members, and individuals caring for the patient are multifaceted and may fluctuate throughout the stages of the disease. Much is lost when living with a terminal, progressive disease: physical health and abilities, body image, work and family roles, identity, family and social networks, lifestyle, independence, control, hope, meaning, and the anticipated future.[200,201] The physical therapist must be able to recognize the patient's ability to cope and adapt, and his or her psychological reactions, level of acceptance, and willingness and ability to integrate therapeutic recommendations. It is also imperative that the physical therapist be able to differentiate between normal reactionary grief to losses or a change in physical function and the presence of clinical anxiety and depression, and refer the patient to the appropriate health care team member, when necessary.[202]

When pervasive, anxiety and depressive symptoms need to be treated aggressively with pyschopharmacologic medications, because left untreated these psychosocial impairments can adversely affect an individual's ability to adapt, cope, and participate in the POC. Depression may also lead to suicide. In addition, anxiety and depression may also be prevalent among family members or caregivers.[202]

EXERCISE AND ALS

Despite the high incidence of muscle weakness in individuals with ALS, the effects of exercise programs have not been extensively studied and, thus, are not well understood. Often physical therapy programs involve ROM and stretching exercises only. Despite the lack of research evidence, some discourage exercise programs because of fear of overuse weakness and believe that no exercise other than everyday activities is indicated.

Studies of individuals with other neuromuscular diseases such as poliomyelitis; Duchenne's muscular dystrophy; myotonic dystrophy; hereditary motor and sensory neuropathy; spinal muscular atrophy; and limb-girdle, Becker, and fascioscapulohumeral dystrophy have found that exercise programs are beneficial and do not produce overuse weakness.[203-210] The research evidence[203-210] from these patient populations suggests the following:

- Overuse weakness does not occur in muscles with an MMT grade of 3 (fair) or greater out of 5 (normal).
- Moderate resistance exercises can increase strength in muscles with an MMT grade of 3 or greater out of 5.
- Strength gains are proportional to initial muscle strength.
- Heavy eccentric exercise should be avoided.
- Exercise may produce functional benefits.
- Psychological benefits have yet to be determined.

When prescribed appropriately, exercise may be beneficial, especially in the early stages of the disease. Exercise may not improve the strength of muscles already weakened by ALS, certainly not those below grade 3. However, general active ROM and stretching of affected joints, resistive strengthening exercises of unaffected muscles with low to moderate weights, and aerobic activities, such as swimming, walking, and bicycling, at submaximal levels, may be prescribed.

When designing a strengthening exercise program for a patient with ALS, the physical therapist must consider the balance between overuse fatigue and disuse atrophy. Evidence from patients with other neuromuscular diseases suggests that highly repetitive or heavy resistance exercise can cause prolonged loss of muscle strength in weakened, denervated muscle.[211,212]

Some animal studies have found that neuromuscular activity has inhibitory effects on sprouting in partially denervated muscle,[213-215] whereas other studies have reported no effect[216,217] or that activity can promote sprouting or reinnervation.[218,219] ALS animal model studies found that endurance exercise training at moderate intensities slowed disease progression;[220-222] while high-endurance exercise training had detrimental effects on male mice only.[223] As well, swimming-induced benefits sustained motor function, increased the lifespan of ALS mice and induced relative maintenance of the fast phenotype in fast-twitch muscles in the animals.[224]

On the other hand, a marked reduction in activity level secondary to ALS can lead to cardiovascular deconditioning and disuse weakness beyond the amount caused by the disease itself. Therefore, the type and intensity of the exercise program should be carefully monitored and adjusted by the physical therapist to prevent excessive fatigue, while at the same time promoting optimal use of intact muscle groups. Patients should be advised not to carry out any activities to the point of extreme fatigue, and should keep track of *symptoms of overuse*, such as the inability to perform daily activities following exercise due to exhaustion or pain, increased fasciculations, or increased muscle cramping. They may also be advised to exercise for several brief periods throughout the day, with sufficient rest in between.

Disuse Atrophy

Reduced physical activity, particularly if prolonged, reduces function of the neuromuscular system, in addition to the skeletal and other organ systems. With insufficient activity, disuse atrophy develops when muscle contractions are less than 20% of the total tension a muscle is capable of producing. As contractile proteins are lost, the muscle weakness progresses at a rate of 3% per day.[225] Strength loss through inactivity and disuse can significantly debilitate individuals with ALS, making them highly susceptible to deconditioning, and muscle and joint tightness leading to contractures and pain.

Overuse Fatigue

The potential for inducing overwork damage in individuals with ALS through excessive exercise is a common concern. Sanjak et al[87] found that individuals with ALS demonstrate abnormal physiologic and metabolic responses to single bouts of exercise. Oxygen consumption during submaximal exercise was increased in individuals with ALS compared to controls, and Vo_{2max} and work capacity were decreased. In addition, it was found that several metabolic substrates of plasma and muscle compartments did not increase to the same level as untrained control subjects, indicating that the availability of substrate for energy production is affected.[87]

In individuals with ALS, the safe range for therapeutic exercise narrows, and the degree to which the range narrows is dependent on the extent of disease involvement and the rate of disease progression[225] (Fig 17.16). A weak or denervated muscle is more susceptible to overwork damage because it is already functioning close to its maximal limits. ADL alone may cause impaired muscles to act as though in training and exercise that would improve normal muscles may actually cause overwork damage in impaired muscles. The remaining motor units will respond to training, and these motor units must work harder to handle a given amount of exercise stress.[225] Thus, special attention must be paid to developing an exercise program for patients with ALS, and

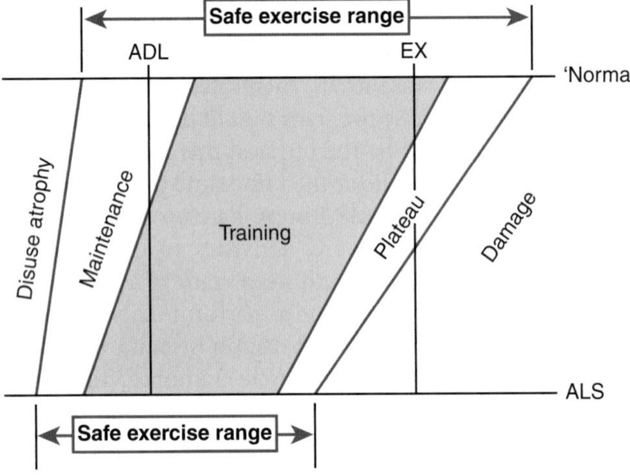

Figure 17.16 Exercise should be considered along a continuum from disuse, to maintenance and upper limit plateau, and if extreme, overwork (damage). With destroyed or lost motor units, the safe training range is decreased or narrowed depending on the extent of disease, the rate of progression, and individual variability. The range continues to narrow as the disease progresses. Exercise is safe when the activity is sufficient to prevent disuse atrophy and less than the amount causing overwork damage. Within this window, effective training can occur. *Note*: As impaired muscles are already functioning close to maximal limits, activities of daily living alone may cause them to act as though in "training." As such, exercise that would improve normal muscles may actually cause overwork damage in impaired muscles.
Adapted from Coble, NO, and Mahoney, FP.[225]

physical therapists should prescribe exercise training at moderate to low intensities.

The literature related to exercise in individuals with ALS is limited. Two early case studies demonstrated positive effects of specific strengthening and endurance exercises.[226,227] The effects of exercise in individuals with ALS have been evaluated with "larger samples." These studies found significantly less decline in function scores and other outcome measures[179,228-230] in the exercise group. A 2013 update to a Cochrane Review[231] found no new trials, and this review is in the process of being updated. The results are pending for two recently completed exercise trials: *Muscle Training of Patients with Amyotrophic Lateral Sclerosis* (NCT01504009, Sweden) and *Trial of Resistance and Endurance Exercise in Amyotrophic Lateral Sclerosis* (NCT01521728 United States).

The physical therapist needs to be prepared for two common questions: *Can I exercise*? and *What exercises can I do*? The reader is referred to Dal Bello-Haas and Krivickas[232] for recommendations that consider physical therapy assessment findings, the rehabilitation framework,[138] the nature and course of ALS, and the evidence. Evidence related to exercise for people with ALS is presented in Table 17.7.

PATIENT/CLIENT-RELATED INSTRUCTION

A diagnosis of ALS is devastating for individuals and their families. They are faced with continual, multiple changes and losses, and eventual death. Assisting the individual and his or her family and caregivers to accept the impact of the disease is an important role for the physical therapist, and providing psychological support and opportunities for expression of feelings, frustrations, and concerns is imperative. Collaborating with and educating the patient, family, and caregivers in an open and encouraging environment may empower patients in their efforts to cope with their disease, foster a sense of purpose and self-efficacy, and enhance the overall effectiveness of the intervention by increasing adherence with recommendations.[138]

Patient and family/caregiver education is integral throughout all stages of the disease. In addition to education topics discussed throughout this chapter, the broad scope of education topics can include, but is not limited to, the following:

- Providing accurate, factual information about the disease process and clinical manifestations, and their significance in overall medical and physical therapy management
  - Give only as much information as the patient, family, and caregivers need; information should be provided in a manner appropriate to their understanding.
- Instructing patients, family members, and caregivers regarding interventions that can be carried

Table 17.7 Evidence Summary Exercise and ALS

Dal Bello-Haas, V, and Florence J: Therapeutic exercise for people with amyotrophic lateral sclerosis/motor neuron disease. Cochrane Database Syst Rev:5, 2013; CD005229.

Design	Systematic review of randomized and quasi-randomized trials examining effects of exercise on people with amyotrophic lateral sclerosis (ALS) or motor neuron disease (MND). Databases used to identify relevant studies: CENTRAL, Cochrane Neuromuscular Disease Group Specialized Register, MEDLINE, EMBASE, AMED, CINAHL Plus, LILACS, and Ovid HealthSTAR.
Level of Evidence	1a—systematic review of randomized controlled trials
Subjects	Participants with a diagnosis of definite, probable, probable with laboratory support, or possible ALS were included.
Intervention	Exercise interventions included: • Progressive resistance or strengthening exercises • Endurance or aerobic exercise Control group: no exercise or standard care (e.g., range of motion or stretching exercises)
Results	The review identified two randomized controlled trials, with 43 participants, who met the inclusion criteria: • Strengthening exercise group—significant improvement in Amyotrophic Lateral Sclerosis Functional Rating Scale (ALSFRS) scores.
Comments	Only two randomized controlled trials were included. It is difficult to determine the extent of beneficial outcomes resulting from strengthening exercises in patients with ALS. A thorough literature search was conducted that included: • Dissertations and theses • Reference lists of included studies Author(s) of included studies were contacted to obtain additional unpublished data. Quality of studies was assessed independently by two reviewers.

Radunovic, A, et al: Mechanical ventilation for amyotrophic lateral sclerosis/motor neuron disease. Cochrane Database Syst Rev:3, 2013. CD004427.

Design	Systematic review of randomized and quasi-randomized trials examining efficacy of noninvasive or tracheostomy assisted ventilation in people with a clinical diagnosis of ALS. Databases used to identify relevant studies: Cochrane Neuromuscular Disease Group Specialized Register, CENTRAL, EMBASE, CINAHL Plus, AMED, and MEDLINE.
Level of Evidence	1a—systematic review of randomized controlled trials
Subjects	Participants with clinical diagnosis of ALS or MND were included.
Intervention	Interventions included: • Noninvasive ventilation • Tracheostomy assisted ventilation Control group: no intervention or standard care.
Results	Two randomized controlled trials were identified involving 54 participants. The results were only based on one of the studies (41 participants) as the other trial published incomplete data. • Significant difference in median survival for noninvasive ventilation group. • Significant difference in survival and quality of life in sub-group with normal to moderate bulbar impairments. • Participants with poor bulbar function showed significant improvement in the Sleep Apnea Quality of Life Index, but not in the Short Form-36 Mental Component Summary score.
Comments	A thorough literature search was conducted which included: • Identification of unpublished theses • Inspection of reference lists of included studies Author(s) of included studies were contacted to obtain additional unpublished data. Quality of studies was assessed independently by four reviewers.

Continued

Table 17.7 Evidence Summary Exercise and ALS—cont'd

Sanjak, M, et al: Vestibular deficits leading to disequilibrium and falls in ambulatory amyotrophic lateral sclerosis. Arch Phys Med Rehabil 95(10), 2014.

Design	Cohort study. This study investigated the use of sensory information to maintain equilibrium in ambulatory in patients with ALS. The Sensory Organization Test (SOT) was used to provide information regarding vestibular input.
Level of Evidence	2b—cohort study
Subjects	Participants included 19 ambulatory patients with ALS and 15 healthy controls. Inclusion criteria for those with ALS included: • Confirmed ALS diagnosis • Ambulatory without the use of assistive devices • No falls during the Clinical Test of Sensory Interaction on Balance • Berg Balance Scale (BBS) score of ≥45, Dynamic Gait Index score ≥18, Timed-Up-and-Go Test ≤11 seconds
Intervention	Not applicable
Results	• Ambulatory participants with ALS had no signs of motor deficits or risk of falling; however, their equilibrium scores on the SOT were significantly lower compared to healthy controls. • Ambulatory participants with ALS with normal clinical balance testing scores had impaired vestibular function and required reliance on visual input to maintain equilibrium.
Comments	• Generalizability is limited as the participants were recruited from a specialized ALS clinic using convenience sampling. • Previous research has found that the SOT alone is not a useful indicator of balance and functional changes in people with vestibular deficits.

Andersen T: Laryngeal response patterns influence the efficacy of mechanical assisted cough in amyotrophic lateral sclerosis. Thorax 72(3): 221, 2016.

Design	Cross sectional study. To better understand treatment to improve cough effectiveness in people with ALS, this study examined the mechanical insufflation-exsufflation (MI-E) procedure using laryngoscopy.
Level of Evidence	2b—cross sectional study
Subjects	Included 20 participants with ALS and 20 healthy age-matched and sex-matched control participants.
Intervention	Not applicable
Results	This study found: • All ALS participants with bulbar symptoms adducted their laryngeal structures during insufflation at the supraglottic level, compromising airflow. • Healthy controls and those with ALS without bulbar symptoms were able to coordinate their cough during MI-E. • It is important to provide an individualized approach such as adjusting settings of MI-E for people with ALS to achieve desired outcomes.
Comments	• Effects of confounding factors were adjusted by recruiting healthy age-matched and sex-matched control participants. • Small cohort size may lead to risk of failure in detecting significant difference that may have been present.

Table 17.7 Evidence Summary Exercise and ALS—cont'd

Pupillo, E: Physical activity and amyotrophic lateral sclerosis: A European population-based case-control study. Ann Neurol 75(5):708, 2014.

Design	This population based, case-control study examined whether physical activity is a risk factor for ALS. Participants were interviewed to gain a better understanding of their history of physical activity, occupation, sport, leisure activities, and accidental injuries.
Level of Evidence	3b—case control study
Subjects	Case eligibility criteria included newly diagnosed patients with ALS who were 18 years or older. The study consisted of 652 individuals with ALS from European population-based registries and 1,166 age-matched, sex-matched, and residency matched population controls.
Intervention	Not applicable
Results	• Physical activity, including work-related physical activity, was associated with decreased odds of having ALS. • An inverse correlation was found between ALS and sports in women, but not in men, and in participants with repeated traumatic events.
Comments	Some of the study limitations include: • Recall bias as the participants were required to provide information regarding their history of physical activity, sports, occupation, and leisure activities. • Several questionnaires were completed by proxy for some case and control participants.

Jones, U, Enright, S, and Busse, M. Management of respiratory problems in people with neurodegenerative conditions: A narrative review. Physiother 98:1, 2012.

Design	This review was conducted to assess the efficacy of current physiotherapy interventions used to manage respiratory problems in patients with neurodegenerative conditions. Databases searched: HUGEnet, SIGLE, British Library Direct, CINAHL, MEDLINE, EMBASE, and AMED.
Level of Evidence	Narrative review
Subjects	Participants included people with neurodegenerative conditions.
Intervention	Not applicable. Studies included in this review examined interventions such as manually assisted cough, MI-E, high frequency chest wall oscillation (HFCWO), use of mechanical glottis, noninvasive ventilation, and respiratory muscle training to address ineffective cough.
Results	Thirty-five relevant articles were identified. Overall, there was weak evidence for positive effects of respiratory interventions in people with ALS.
Comments	Some of the limitations of this review include: • Studies included in the review had heterogeneous populations and were often nonrandomized. • Review process was conducted by one reviewer instead of two. • Number and quality of studies.

Rafiq, MK: A preliminary randomized trial of the mechanical insufflator-exsufflator versus breath-stacking technique in patients with amyotrophic lateral sclerosis. Amyotroph Lateral Scler Frontotemporal Degener 16(7–8):448, 2015.

Design	Randomized controlled trial. Patients were randomized to two intervention groups: breath stacking technique or a MI-E intervention. Participants were asked to document symptoms of respiratory tract infection, use of antibiotics, and hospital admissions due to respiratory complications. Outcome measures included chest infections, hospitalizations, and quality of life.
Level of Evidence	2b—randomized controlled trial
Subjects	• Diagnosis of clinically definite or probable ALS • Inclusion criteria included evidence of respiratory failure. • Individuals with ALS who were able to tolerate noninvasive ventilation

Continued

Table 17.7 Evidence Summary Exercise and ALS—cont'd

Intervention	Breath stacking technique versus MI-E
Results	Main study findings: • 33% of the participants with ALS assigned to breath-stacking intervention group and 32% in the MI-E group reported antibiotic use. • 46% of participants with ALS in the breath-stacking group and 32% in the MI-E group were hospitalized. • The quality of life measure was maintained above 75% of baseline for a median of 329 days in breath-stacking group and 205 days in MI-E group. • Overall, there were no statistically significant difference found between the two groups.
Comments	Participants were assigned to treatment and control groups using minimization algorithm to balance the groups' variables such as age, body mass index, bulbar function, and "relaxed" vital capacity. Limitations: • Variable adherence to the planned intervention and deaths unrelated to ALS • Small sample size from a single site

out independently such as monitoring the effects and side effects of medications, use of assistive devices and adaptive equipment, and preventing secondary impairments and complications

- Advising the patient about methods to promote general health
  - Instruction regarding energy conservation, balancing rest and activity, and relaxation techniques may be beneficial in assisting the patient to cope with the daily constraints of the disease.
- Counseling regarding care and life decisions, if the patient asks about these issues
- Referring patients to support groups or psychological counseling
- Providing information on health and available social and support services[138]

The ALSA and the MDA are two national voluntary organizations that provide many functions and programs for individuals with ALS and their families and caregivers, including the provision of written and video educational materials, local education programs, patient and caregiver support groups, equipment loan programs, respite programs, transportation programs, advocacy programs, and ALS Awareness Programs. Patients and families can contact the ALSA and MDA for information and can explore available resources on the websites:

Amyotrophic Lateral Sclerosis Association (national headquarters)
1275 K Street NW, Suite 250
Washington, DC 20005
202-407-8580
www.alsa.org

Muscular Dystrophy Association—USA (national office)
161 N. Clark
Suite 3550
Chicago, Illinois 60601
800-572-1717
https://www.mda.org/office/chicago

In addition, there are numerous international organizations whose websites provide various resources, including information about ALS, information about clinical trials, evidence-based reviews and practice guidelines, and publications about living with ALS. Appendix 17.D includes web-based resources for clinicians, families, and patients with ALS.

SUMMARY

ALS, the most common and devastatingly fatal motor neuron disease among adults, causes a progressive increase in the number and severity of impairments, activity limitations, and participation restrictions. Other than a small percentage of cases, etiology for the most part is unknown, and it is hypothesized that multiple mechanisms may be responsible for the disease. Although there is no cure for ALS and its course cannot be altered, it should be considered a "treatable disease." Medical management is primarily symptomatic, and a team approach to care is considered optimal. Rehabilitation management is focused on maximizing function and promoting independence to the highest level possible, and ensuring optimal quality of life throughout the course of the disease and across health care settings.

The physical therapist plays an integral role in designing and implementing therapeutic interventions for individuals with ALS that will allow them to maintain independence and function for as long as possible. The selection of interventions, grounded in evidence-based research whenever possible, is based on the stage and progression of the disease and may be restorative, compensatory, or preventive. These interventions should take into consideration the individual's goals and psychosocial factors that may affect decision making, such as the individual's acceptance of the diagnosis and the individual's social and financial resources. Because of the progressive nature of ALS, the physical therapist must not only address the patient's current problems, but also plan for future needs.

Acknowledgments

Special thanks to Humna Malik for her for assistance with the editorial and administrative aspects of the manuscript; and to Ashley Chapman, Tasha Kravchenko, and Gabi Watson for their assistance with previous versions. Sincerest thanks to Peggy Ingels-Allred for her thoughtful and critical review of earlier editions of this chapter.

Questions for Review

1. Describe the clinical manifestations of ALS. Differentiate among impairments associated with upper and lower motor neuron pathology, bulbar pathology, and respiratory system pathology. What cognitive, rare, indirect, composite, and other impairments might you see in an individual with ALS?
2. What medical examination procedures are used to help support the diagnosis of ALS?
3. Identify and define the major classifications of ALS included in the El Escorial criteria and the Awaji-Shima criteria.
4. Describe the disease course of ALS. What factors have indicated a relationship to improved prognosis and poorer prognosis?
5. Considering the variety of impairments associated with ALS, what factors does a physical therapist need to consider when deciding on which tests and measures should be included in a comprehensive examination?
6. Differentiate among *restorative, compensatory,* and *preventive* interventions.
7. When designing an exercise program for a patient with ALS, what factors need to be considered?
8. What information should be considered and included when developing a plan for patient and family education following the diagnosis of ALS?

CASE STUDY

The patient is a right-handed 36-year-old male recently diagnosed with ALS. Seven months ago, the patient experienced cramping in his left calf and a few months later noted that his left foot slapped and that he "caught his toes" and tripped while playing basketball or walking on the golf course. He also noticed painless twitching of the muscles in his right hand, forearm, and upper arm and reported difficulty fastening the snaps on his youngest son's pajamas.

PAST MEDICAL HISTORY

No significant past medical history.

SOCIAL HISTORY

The patient has been married for 10 years. He has a 3-year-old and a 9-month-old son, and his wife is pregnant with their third child. He lives in a two-story house with four steps up to the front door (no railing), 12 stairs between levels (bilateral railing), and 10 stairs to the basement with a railing on the right.

He stopped playing basketball and baseball because he is embarrassed about the frequent tripping, but continues to play golf on the weekend. He uses a golf cart because he is unable to keep up with his friends on the golf course. He would like to be more active.

OCCUPATION

He is a manager at a computer graphics business and reports his voice becomes hoarse on occasion after long presentations. He reports significant fatigue if he works on the computer for long periods of time or if he has to stand for long periods for presentations. He attributes this to "getting older."

DIAGNOSTIC TESTS

Electromyographic studies showed (1) low compound motor action potentials in all extremities; (2) normal sensory nerve conduction; (3) fibrillations and fasciculations in all extremities; and (4) widespread neurogenic changes in motor unit action potentials, abnormal recruitment patterns in the distal leg musculature, and mild to moderate changes in the upper extremities.

PHYSICAL EXAMINATION FINDINGS

- Observation: Marked wasting of the interossei regions bilaterally.
- Speech: No abnormalities noted.
- ROM: Within normal limits (WNL) for all joints, except the thumbs and the L ankle. Patient was only able to oppose thumbs to the third digits. He lacks 5° of L dorsiflexion.
- Strength: Bilateral LE strength graded as 5/5, except for the hip flexor group (R = 4/5; L = 4+/5) and the L ankle dorsiflexors (3–/5). Shoulder muscle strength graded as 4+/5 (R) and 4/5 (L); elbow muscle strength graded as 4/4 (R) and 4+/5 (L).
- Hand strength: R = 12 lb; L = 24 lb (handheld dynamometer).
- Pinch strength: R-tripod = 2 lb; lateral = 3 lb; L-tripod = 5 lb; lateral = 3 lb (see following for normative data on grip and pinch strength). *Note:* Tripod pinch is a component of manual dexterity that involves opposition of the thumb and the first two fingers as a "tripod." Pinch strength measures are obtained using a pinch gauge.
- Manual coordination: Purdue Pegboard Testing, R—6 peg holes in 30 sec; L—3 peg holes in 30 sec.
- Tone: 1 for both UEs and 1+ for both LEs (Modified Ashworth spasticity scores).
- Reflexes: A clonic jaw reflex is evident; hyperreflexia in both UEs; hyporeflexia in both LEs; positive Babinski reflex bilaterally.
- Gait: Independent of assistive devices; positive for L foot drop and hip hiking; 15-ft walk test = 3.6 sec.
- Balance (standing): Unilateral stance/eyes open, R = 25 sec; L = 6 sec.
- Respiratory: FVC and MIP are within normal limits.
- Functional status: The patient rated himself at 90% on the Schwab and England Rating Scale (see Appendix 17.B). ALSFRS-R scores (see Appendix 17.C):

ALSFRS-R Scores

Item	Score
Speech	4
Salivation	3
Swallowing	3
Handwriting (pre-ALS dominant hand)	3
Cutting food and handling utensils (patients without gastrostomy)	3
Dressing and hygiene	3
Turning in bed; adjusting bed clothes	4
Walking	3
Climbing stairs	3
Dyspnea	3
Orthopnea	4
Respiratory insufficiency	4

Grip and Pinch Strength Values (Pounds) for Men 35 to 39 (n = 25)

	Hand	Mean	SD	SE	Low	High
Grip	R	119.7	24.0	4.8	76	176
	L	112.9	21.7	4.4	73	157
Tip	R	18.0	3.6	.73	12	27
	L	17.7	3.8	.76	10	24
Palmar	R	26.1	3.2	.65	21	32
	L	25.6	3.9	.77	18	32
Lateral (Key)	R	26.2	4.1	.83	19	36
	L	25.9	5.4	1.17	14	40

From Mathiowetz, V, et al: Grip and pinch strength: Normative data for adults. Arch Phys Med Rehabil 66:69, 1984.

GUIDING QUESTIONS

1. What El Escorial diagnostic criteria would you anticipate to be documented in the patient's medical record?
2. Identify the patient's problems as direct, indirect, or composite impairments.
3. What impact do the impairments have on the patient's ability to function (i.e., activity limitations)?
4. What additional tests and measurements should be conducted? What consultations should be recommended?
5. At present, what are the initial key areas of patient education that should be addressed?
6. Identify the general elements of a physical therapy POC for the patient.

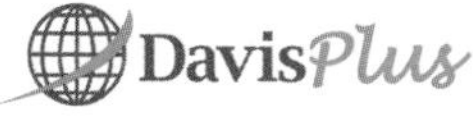

For additional resources, including answers to the questions for review and case study guiding questions, please visit **http://davisplus.fadavis.com.**

References

1. Rowland, LP: Diverse forms of motor neuron diseases. Adv Neurol 36:1, 1982.
2. Swash, M: Clinical features and diagnosis of amyotrophic lateral sclerosis. In Brown, R, Jr, Meininger, V, and Swash, M (eds): Amyotrophic Lateral Sclerosis. Martin Dunitz Ltd, London, 2000, p 3.
3. Norris, F, et al: Onset, natural history and outcome in idiopathic adult motor neuron disease. J Neurol Sci 118(1):48, 1993.
4. Pradas, J, et al: The natural history of amyotrophic lateral sclerosis and the use of natural history controls in therapeutic trials. Neurology 43(4):751, 1993.
5. Ringel, SP, et al: The natural history of amyotrophic lateral sclerosis. Neurology 43(7):1316, 1993.
6. Haverkamp, LJ, Appel, V, and Appel, SH: Natural history of amyotrophic lateral sclerosis in a database population: Validation of a scoring system and a model for survival prediction. Brain 118:707, 1995.
7. Gubbay, SS, et al: Amyotrophic lateral sclerosis. A study of its presentation and prognosis. J Neurol 232(5):295, 1985.
8. Appel, SH, et al: Amyotrophic lateral sclerosis. Associated clinical disorders and immunological evaluations. Arch Neurol 43(3): 234, 1986.
9. Siddique T: Molecular genetics of familial amyotrophic lateral sclerosis. Adv Neurol 56:227, 1991.
10. Strong, MJ, Hudson, AJ, and Alvord, WG: Familial amyotrophic lateral sclerosis, 1850–1989: A statistical analysis of the world literature. Can J Neurol Sci 18:45, 1991.
11. Hamida, MB, and Hentati, F: Juvenile amyotrophic lateral sclerosis. In Brown, R, Jr, Meininger, V, and Swash, M (eds): Amyotrophic Lateral Sclerosis. Martin Dunitz Ltd, London, 2000, p 59.
12. Rosen, DR: Mutations in Cu/Zn superoxide dismutase gene are associated with familial amyotrophic lateral sclerosis. Nature 362:59, 1993.
13. Jackson, M, and Rothstein, JD: Amyotrophic lateral sclerosis. In Marcoux, FW, and Choi, DW (eds): Central Nervous System Neuroprotection. Springer, New York, 2002, p 423.
14. Jackson, M, et al: Analysis of chromosome 5q13 genes in amyotrophic lateral sclerosis: Homozygous NAIP deletion in a sporadic case. Ann Neurol 39(6):796, 1996.
15. Robberecht, W, et al: D90A heterozygosity in the SOD1 gene is associated with familial and apparently sporadic amyotrophic lateral sclerosis. Neurology 47(5):1336, 1996.
16. Caroscio, JT, Calhoun, WF, and Yahr, MD: Prognostic factors in motor neuron disease: A prospective study of longevity. In Rose, FC (ed): Research Progress in Motor Neuron Disease. Pitman, London, 1984, p 34.
17. Brooks, BR: The natural history of amyotrophic lateral sclerosis. In Williams, AC (ed): Motor Neurone Disease. Chapman & Hall, London, 1994, p 121.
18. Hosler, BA, and Brown, RH, Jr: Copper/zinc superoxide dismutase mutations and free radical damage in amyotrophic lateral sclerosis. Adv Neurol 68:41, 1995.
19. Rothstein, JD, et al: Chronic inhibition of superoxide dismutase produces apoptotic death of spinal neurons. Proc Natl Acad Sci USA 91(10):4155, 1994.
20. Borchelt, DR, et al: Superoxide dismutase 1 with mutations linked to familial amyotrophic lateral sclerosis possesses significant activity. Proc Natl Acad Sci USA 91(17):8292, 1994.
21. Plaitakis, A, and Caroscio, JT: Abnormal glutamate metabolism in amyotrophic lateral sclerosis. Ann Neurol 22(5):575, 1987.
22. Rothstein, JD, et al: Abnormal excitatory amino acid metabolism in amyotrophic lateral sclerosis. Ann Neurol 28(1):18, 1990.
23. Rothstein, JD, Martin, LJ, and Kuncl, RW: Decreased glutamate transport by the brain and spinal cord in amyotrophic lateral sclerosis. N Engl J Med 326(22):1464, 1992.

24. Rothstein, JD, et al: Selective loss of glial glutamate transporter GLT-1 in amyotrophic lateral sclerosis. Ann Neurol 38(1): 73, 1995.
25. Carpenter, S: Proximal axonal enlargement in motor neuron disease. Neurology 18:841, 1968.
26. Hirano, A, et al: Fine structural study of neurofibrillary changes in a family with amyotrophic lateral sclerosis. J Neuropathol Exp Neurol 43(5):471, 1984.
27. Wolfgang, F, and Myers, L: Amyotrophic lateral sclerosis: Effect of serum on anterior horn cells in tissue culture. Science 179:579, 1973.
28. Troost, D, Van den Oord, JJ, and Vianney de Jong, JM: Immunohistochemical characterization of the inflammatory infiltrate in amyotrophic lateral sclerosis. Neuropathol Appl Neurobiol 16(5):401, 1990.
29. Smith, RG, et al: Serum antibodies to L-type calcium channels in patients with amyotrophic lateral sclerosis. N Engl J Med 24(327):1721, 1992.
30. Appel, SH: A unifying hypothesis for the cause of amyotrophic lateral sclerosis, parkinsonism, and Alzheimer disease. Ann Neurol 10(6):499, 1981.
31. Lindsay, RM: Brain-derived neurotrophic factor: an NGF-related neurotrophin. In Loughlin, SE, and Fallon, JH (eds): Neurotrophic Factors. Academic Press, San Diego, 1993, p 257.
32. Thoenen, H, Hughes, RA, and Sendtner, M: Trophic support of motoneurons: Physiological, pathophysiological, and therapeutic implications. Exp Neurol 124(1):47, 1993.
33. Anand, P, et al: Regional changes of ciliary neurotrophic factor and nerve growth factor levels in post mortem spinal cord and cerebral cortex from patients with motor disease. Nat Med 1(2):168, 1995.
34. Strong, MJ: Exogenous neurotoxins. In Brown, R, Jr, Meininger, V, and Swash, M (eds): Amyotrophic Lateral Sclerosis. Martin Dunitz Ltd, London, 2000, p 279.
35. Brown, R, Jr: Apoptosis in amyotrophic lateral sclerosis: A review. In Brown, R, Jr, Meininger, V, and Swash, M (eds): Amyotrophic Lateral Sclerosis. Martin Dunitz Ltd, London, 2000, p 363.
36. Mitsumoto, H, Chad, DA, and Pioro, EK: Hypotheses for viral and other transmissible agents in amyotrophic lateral sclerosis. In Mitsumoto, H, Chad, DA, and Pioro, EK (eds): Amyotrophic Lateral Sclerosis. FA Davis, Philadelphia, 1998, p 239.
37. Brettschneider, J, et al: Microglial activation and TDP-43 pathology correlate with executive dysfunction in amyotrophic lateral sclerosis. Acta Neuropathol 123:395, 2012.
38. Cistaro, A, et al: Brain hypermetabolism in amyotrophic lateral sclerosis: A FDG PET study in ALS of spinal and bulbar onset. Eur J Nucl Med Mol Imaging 39:251, 2012.
39. Prell, T, et al: Diffusion tensor imaging patterns differ in bulbar and limb onset amyotrophic lateral sclerosis. Clin Neurol Neurosurg 115:1281, 2013.
40. Sabatelli, M, et al: New ALS-related genes expand the spectrum paradigm of amyotrophic lateral sclerosis. Brain Pathol 26(2):266, 2016.
41. McCluskey, L, et al: ALS-Plus syndrome: Non-pyramidal features in a large ALS cohort. J Neurol Sci 345:118, 2014.
42. Brooks, BR: ALS-Plus – where does it begin, where does it end? J Neurol Sci 345:1, 2014.
43. Mizutani, T, et al: Amyotrophic lateral sclerosis with ophthalmoplegia and multisystem degeneration in patients on long-term use of respirators. Acta Neuropathol 84(4):372, 1992.
44. Iwata, M, and Hirano, A: Sparing of the Onufrowicz nucleus in sacral anterior horn lesions. Ann Neurol 4(3):245, 1978.
45. Mannen, T, and et al: Preservation of certain motor neurone group of the sacral cord in amyotrophic lateral sclerosis: Its clinical significance. J Neuropathol Exp Neurol 47:642, 1988.
46. Barr, ML, and Kiernan, JA: The Human Nervous System: An Anatomical Viewpoint, ed 6. JB Lippincott, Philadelphia, 1993.
47. Bradley, WG, et al: Morphometric and biochemical studies of peripheral nerves in amyotrophic lateral sclerosis. Ann Neurol 14(3):267, 1983.
48. Heads, T, et al: Sensory nerve pathology in amyotrophic lateral sclerosis. Acta Neuropathol 82(4):316, 1991.
49. Kawamura, Y, et al: Morphometric comparison in the vulnerability of peripheral motor and sensory neurons in amyotrophic lateral sclerosis. J Neuropathol Exp Neurol 40(6):667, 1988.
50. Swash, M, et al: Selective and asymmetric vulnerability of corticospinal and spinocerebellar tracts in motor neuron disease. J Neurol Neurosurg Psychiatry 51(6):785, 1988.
51. Averback, P, and Crocker, P: Regular involvement of Clarke's nucleus in sporadic amyotrophic lateral sclerosis. Arch Neurol 39(3):155, 1982.
52. Takahaski, H, et al: Clarke's column in sporadic amyotrophic lateral sclerosis. Acta Neuropathol 84(5):465, 1992.
53. Hudson, AJ: Amyotrophic lateral sclerosis and its association with dementia, parkinsonism and other neurological disorders: A review. Brain 104(2):217, 1981.
54. Wohlfart, G: Collateral regeneration in partially denervated muscles. Neurology 8(3):175, 1958.
55. Hansen, S, and Ballantyne, JP: A quantitative electrophysiological study of motor neurone disease. J Neurol Neurosurg Psychiatry 41(9):773, 1978.
56. McComas, AJ, et al: Functional compensation in partially denervated muscles. J Neurol Neurosurg Psychiatry 34(4):453, 1971.
57. Swash, M, and Schwartz, MS: A longitudinal study of changes in motor units in motor neuron disease. J Neurol Sci 56(2–3):185, 1982.
58. Swash, M, and Schwartz, MS: Staging motor neurone disease: Single fibre EMG studies of asymmetry, progression and compensatory reinnervation. In Rose, FC (ed): Research Progress in Motor Neuron Disease. Pitman, London, 1984, p 123.
59. Brooks, BR, et al: Natural history of amyotrophic lateral sclerosis: Quantification of symptoms, signs, strength and function. In Serratrice, G, and Munsat, TL (eds): Advances in Neurology: Pathogenesis and Therapy of Amyotrophic Lateral Sclerosis. Lippincott-Raven, Philadelphia, 1995, p 163.
60. Mitsumoto, H, Chad, DA, and Pioro, EK: Clinical features: Signs and symptoms. In Mitsumoto, H, Chad, DA, and Pioro, EK (eds): Amyotrophic Lateral Sclerosis. FA Davis, Philadelphia, 1998, p 47.
61. Brooks, BR: Natural history of ALS: Symptoms, strength, pulmonary function, and disability. Neurology 47(Suppl):S71, 1996.
62. Jette, DU, et al: The relationship of lower-limb muscle force to walking ability in patients with amyotrophic lateral sclerosis. Phys Ther 79(7):672, 1999.
63. Dal Bello-Haas, V, et al: Development, analysis, refinement, and utility of an interdisciplinary amyotrophic lateral sclerosis database. Amyotroph Lateral Scler Other Motor Neuron Disord 2(1):39, 2001.
64. Sahrmann, SA, and Norton, BJ: The relationship of voluntary movement to spasticity in the upper motor neuron syndrome. Ann Neurol 2(6):460, 1977.
65. Mayer, NH: Clinicophysiologic concepts of spasticity and motor dysfunction in adults with an upper motoneuron lesion. Muscle Nerve Suppl 6:S1, 1997.
66. Fallat, RJ, et al: Spirometry in amyotrophic lateral sclerosis. Arch Neurol 36(2):74, 1979.
67. Rochester, DF, and Esau, SA: Assessment of ventilatory function in patients with neuromuscular disease. Clin Chest Med 15(4):751, 1994.
68. Vitacca, M, et al: Breathing pattern and respiratory mechanics in patients with amyotrophic lateral sclerosis. Eur Respir J 10(7):1614, 1997.
69. Krivickas, L: Pulmonary function and respiratory failure. In Mitsumoto, H, Chad, DA, and Pioro, EK (eds): Amyotrophic Lateral Sclerosis. FA Davis, Philadelphia, 1998, p 382.
70. Schiffman, PL, and Belsh, JM: Pulmonary function at diagnosis of amyotrophic lateral sclerosis. Rate of deterioration. Chest 103(2):508, 1993.
71. Trojsi, F, et al: Widespread structural and functional connectivity changes in amyotrophic lateral sclerosis: Insights from advanced neuroimaging research. Neural Plast 2012:473, 2012.
72. Abe, K, et al: Cognitive function in amyotrophic lateral sclerosis. J Neurol Sci 148(1):95, 1997.
73. Kew, JJM, et al: The relationship between abnormalities of cognitive function and cerebral activation in amyotrophic lateral sclerosis. A neuropsychological and positron emission tomography study. Brain 116:1399, 1993.
74. Wilson, CM, et al: Cognitive impairment in sporadic ALS: A pathologic continuum underlying a multisystem disorder. Neurology 57(4):651, 2001.

75. Massman, PJ, et al: Prevalence and correlates of neuropsychological deficits in amyotrophic lateral sclerosis. J Neurol Neurosurg Psychiatry 61(5):450, 1996.
76. Lomen-Hoerth, C, et al: Are amyotrophic lateral sclerosis patients cognitively normal? Neurology 60(7):1094, 2003.
77. Neary, D, et al: Frontal lobe dementia and motor neuron disease. J Neurol Neurosurg Psychiatry 53(1):23, 1990.
78. Strong, MJ, et al: A prospective study of cognitive impairment in ALS. Neurology 53(8):1665, 1999.
79. Abrahams, S, et al: Verbal fluency and executive dysfunction in amyotrophic lateral sclerosis (ALS). Neuropsychologia 38(6): 734, 2000.
80. Abrahams, S, et al: Relation between cognitive dysfunction and pseudobulbar palsy in amyotrophic lateral sclerosis. J Neurol Neurosurg Psychiatry 62(5):464, 1997.
81. EFNS Task Force on Diagnosis and Management of Amyotrophic Lateral Sclerosis, et al: EFNS guidelines on the clinical management of amyotrophic lateral sclerosis (MALS)—Revised report of an EFNS task force. Eur J Neurol 19(3):360, 2012.
82. Olney, RK, et al: The effects of executive and behavioral dysfunction on the course of ALS. Neurology 65:1774, 2005.
83. Elamin, M, et al: Executive dysfunction is a negative prognostic indicator in patients with ALS without dementia. Neurology 76(14): 1263, 2011.
84. Schiffer, RB, Cash, J, and Herndon, RM: Treatment of emotional lability with low-dosage tricyclic antidepressants. Psychosomatics 24(12):1094, 1983.
85. Gallagher, JP: Pathologic laughter and crying in ALS: A search for their origin. Acta Neurol Scand 80(2):114, 1989.
86. Kilmer, DD: The role of exercise in neuromuscular disease. Phys Med Rehabil Clin North Am 9(1):115, 1998.
87. Sanjak, M, et al: Physiologic and metabolic response to progressive and prolonged exercise in amyotrophic lateral sclerosis. Neurology 37(7):1217, 1987.
88. Sharma, KR, et al: Physiology of fatigue in amyotrophic lateral sclerosis. Neurology 45(4):733, 1995.
89. Rivera, I, et al: Prevalence and characteristics of pain in early and late stages of ALS. Amyotroph Lateral Scler Frontotemporal Degener 14:369, 2013.
90. Pizzimenti, A, et al: Depression, pain and quality of life in patients with amyotrophic lateral sclerosis: A cross-sectional study. Funct Neurol 28:115, 2013.
91. National Institute for Health and Care Excellence (NICE). Motor neurone disease: Assessment and management. Clinical Guideline NG42. NICE, London, 2016. Retrieved August 15, 2017, from www.nice.org.uk/guidance/ng42.
92. Chiò, A, Mora, G, and Lauria, G: Pain in amyotrophic lateral sclerosis. Lancet Neurol 16(2):144, 2017.
93. Cellura, E, et al: Factors affecting the diagnostic delay in amyotrophic lateral sclerosis. Clin Neurol Neurosurg 114(6):550, 2012.
94. Pagnoni S, et al: Diagnostic timelines and delays in diagnosing amyotrophic lateral sclerosis (ALS). Amyotroph Lateral Scler Other Motor Neuron Disord 15(0):453, 2014.
95. Brooks, BR, et al: El Escorial revisited: Revised criteria for the diagnosis of amyotrophic lateral sclerosis. Amyotroph Lateral Scler Other Motor Neuron Disord 1(5):293, 2000.
96. de Carvalho, M, et al: Electrodiagnosis criteria for diagnosis of ALS. Clin Neurophysiol 119(3):497, 2008.
97. Al-Chalabi, A, et al: Amyotrophic lateral sclerosis: Moving towards a new classification system. Lancet Neurol 15(11):1182, 2016.
98. Juergens, SM, et al: ALS in Rochester, Minnesota. Neurology 30(5):463, 1980.
99. Caroscio, JT, et al: Amyotrophic lateral sclerosis: Its natural history. Neurol Clin 5(1):1, 1987.
100. Kristensen, O, and Melgaard, B: Motor neuron disease: Prognosis and epidemiology. Acta Neurol Scand 56(4):299, 1977.
101. Granieri, E, et al: Motor neuron disease in the province of Ferrara, Italy, in 1964–1982. Neurology 38(10):1604, 1988.
102. Chiò, A, et al: Prognostic factors in ALS: A critical review. Amyotroph Lateral Scler 10(5-6):310, 2009.
103. Tysnes, OB, Vollset, SE, and Aarli, JA: Epidemiology of amyotrophic lateral sclerosis in Hordaland county, western Norway. Acta Neurol Scand 83(5):280, 1991.
104. Rosen, AD: Amyotrophic lateral sclerosis. Clinical features and prognosis. Arch Neurol 35(10):638, 1978.
105. Wolf, J, et al: Factors predicting one-year mortality in amyotrophic lateral sclerosis patients—data from a population-based registry. BMC Neurol 14:197, 2014.
106. Tysnes, OB, et al: Prognostic factors and survival in amyotrophic lateral sclerosis. Neuroepidemiology 13(5):226, 1994.
107. Marin, B, et al: Alteration of nutritional status at diagnosis is a prognostic factor for survival of amyotrophic lateral sclerosis patients. J Neurol Neurosurg Psychiatry 82:628, 2011.
108. Shimizu, T, et al. Reduction rate of body mass index predicts prognosis for survival in amyotrophic lateral sclerosis: a multicenter study in Japan. Amyotroph Lateral Scler. 13:363, 2012.
109. McDonald, ER, et al: Survival in amyotrophic lateral sclerosis: The role of psychological factors. Arch Neurol 51(1):17, 1994.
110. Johnston, M, et al: Mood as a predictor of disability and survival in patients diagnosed with ALS/MND. Br J Health Psych 4(2):1999, 1999.
111. Traynor, BJ, et al: Effect of a multidisciplinary amyotrophic lateral sclerosis (ALS) clinic on ALS survival: A population based study, 1996–2000. J Neurol Neurosurg Psychiatry 74(9):1258, 2003.
112. Bensimon, G, Lacomblez, L, and Meininger, V: A controlled trial of riluzole in amyotrophic lateral sclerosis. ALS/Riluzole Study Group. N Engl J Med 330(9):585, 1994.
113. Lacomblez, L, et al: Dose-ranging study of riluzole in amyotrophic lateral sclerosis. Amyotrophic Lateral Sclerosis/Riluzole Study Group II. Lancet 347(9013):1425, 1996.
114. US Food and Drug Administration (FDA): FDA Approves Drug to Treat ALS. Retrieved August 15, 2017, from https://www.fda.gov/NewsEvents/Newsroom/PressAnnouncements/ucm557102.htm.
115. Abe, KA, et al: Safety and efficacy of edaravone in well defined patients with amyotrophic lateral sclerosis: A randomised, double-blind, placebo-controlled trial. Lancet Neurol 16(7):505, 2017.
116. World Health Organization (WHO): WHO Definition of Palliative Care. WHO, Geneva, Switzerland. Retrieved August 15, 2017, from www.who.int/cancer/palliative/definition/en/.
117. Miller, RG, et al: Practice parameter update: The care of the patient with amyotrophic lateral sclerosis: Drug, nutritional, and respiratory therapies (an evidence-based review): Report of the Quality Standards Subcommittee of the American Academy of Neurology. Neurology 73(15):1218, 2009.
118. Miller, RG, et al: Practice parameter update: The care of the patient with amyotrophic lateral sclerosis: Multidisciplinary care, symptom management, and cognitive/behavioral impairment (an evidence-based review): Report of the Quality Standards Subcommittee of the American Academy of Neurology. Neurology 73(15):1227, 2009.
119. Miller, RG, et al. Quality improvement in neurology: Amyotrophic lateral sclerosis quality measures: Report of the quality measurement and reporting subcommittee of the American Academy of Neurology. Neurology 81(24):2136, 2013.
120. Nicholson, K, et al: Improving symptom management for people with amyotrophic lateral sclerosis. Muscle Nerve. 2017; May 31. doi: 10.1002/mus.25712. [Epub ahead of print]
121. Gordon, PH: Amyotrophic lateral sclerosis: Pathophysiology, diagnosis and management. CNS Drugs 25(1):1, 2011.
122. Desport, JC, et al: Nutritional status is a prognostic factor for survival in ALS patients. Neurology 53(5):1059, 1999.
123. Lechtzin, N, et al: Hospitalization in amyotrophic lateral sclerosis: Causes, costs, and outcomes. Neurology 56(6):753, 2001.
124. Hillel, AD, and Miller, R: Bulbar amyotrophic lateral sclerosis: Patterns of progression and clinical management. Head Neck 11(1):51, 1989.
125. Miller, RG, et al (ALS Practice Parameters Task Force): The care of the patient with amyotrophic lateral sclerosis (an evidence-based review): Report of the Quality Standards Subcommittee of the American Academy of Neurology. Neurology 52(7):1311, 1999.
126. Mathus-Vliegen, LMH, et al: Percutaneous endoscopic gastrostomy in patients with amyotrophic lateral sclerosis and impaired pulmonary function. Gastrointest Endosc 40(4):463, 1994.
127. Mazzini, L, et al: Percutaneous endoscopic gastrostomy and enteral nutrition in amyotrophic lateral sclerosis. Neurology 242(10):695, 1995.
128. Jarnagin, WR, et al: The efficacy and limitations of percutaneous endoscopic gastrostomy. Arch Surg 127(3):261, 1992.

129. Kadakia, SC, Sullivan, HO, and Starnes, E: Percutaneous endoscopic gastrostomy or jejunostomy and the incidence of aspiration in 79 patients. Am J Surg 164(2):114, 1992.
130. Piper, AJ, and Sullivan, CE: Effects of long-term nocturnal nasal ventilation on spontaneous breathing during sleep in neuromuscular and chest wall disorders. Eur Respir J 9(7):1515, 1996.
131. Cazzolli, PA, and Oppenheimer, EA: Home mechanical ventilation for amyotrophic lateral sclerosis: Nasal compared to tracheostomy-intermittent positive pressure ventilation. J Neurol Sci 139(Suppl):123, 1996.
132. Pinto, AC, et al: Respiratory assistance with a non-invasive ventilator (BiPAP) in MND/ALS patients: Survival rates in a controlled trial. J Neurol Sci 129(Suppl):19, 1995.
133. Aboussouan, LS, et al: Effect of noninvasive positive-pressure ventilation on survival in amyotrophic lateral sclerosis. Ann Intern Med 127(6):450, 1997.
134. Yorkston, KM, et al: Speech deterioration in amyotrophic lateral sclerosis: Implications for the timing of intervention. J Med Speech-Language Pathol 1:35, 1993.
135. Adams, L, and Kazandijan, M: Managing communication and swallowing difficulties. In Mitsumoto, M, and Munsat, T (eds): Amyotrophic Lateral Sclerosis: A Guide for Patients and Families. Demos Medical Publishing, New York, 2001, p 133.
136. Esposito, SJ, Mitsumoto, H, and Shanks, M: Use of palatal lift and palatal augmentation prostheses to improve dysarthria in patients with amyotrophic lateral sclerosis: A case series. J Prosthet Dent 83(1):90, 2000.
137. Gelinas, DF, and Miller, RG: A treatable disease: A guide to management of amyotrophic lateral sclerosis. In Brown, R, Jr, Meininger, V, and Swash, M (eds): Amyotrophic Lateral Sclerosis. Martin Dunitz Ltd, London, 2000, p 405.
138. Dal Bello-Haas, V: A framework for rehabilitation in degenerative diseases: Planning care and maximizing quality of life. Neurology Report 26(3):115, 2002.
139. Woolley, SC: Utility of the ALS Cognitive Behavioral Screen. Neurodegen Dis Manage 1:473, 2011.
140. Gordon, PH, et al: A screening assessment of cognitive impairment in patients with ALS. Amyotroph Lateral Scler 8:362, 2007.
141. Edinburgh Cognitive and Behavioural ALS Screen (ECAS) English version 2013. Retrieved August 16, 2017, from https://www.era.lib.ed.ac.uk/handle/1842/6592.
142. Beck, AT, et al: An inventory for measuring depression. Arch Gen Psychiatry 4:561, 1961.
143. Radloff, LS: CES-D scale: A self-report depression scale for research in the general population. Appl Psychol Meas 1(3):385, 1977.
144. Zigmond, AS, and Snaith, RP: The hospital anxiety and depression scale. Acta Psychiatr Scand 67(6):361, 1983.
145. Spielberger, CS, Gorsuch, RL, and Lushene, RE: Manual for the State Trait Anxiety Inventory. Consulting Psychologists Press, Palo Alto, CA, 1970.
146. Kübler, A, et al: Das ALS-Depressionsinventar (ADI). Z Klin Psychol Psychother (Gott) 34(1):19, 2005.
147. Andres, PL, et al: Quantitative motor assessment in amyotrophic lateral sclerosis. Neurology 36(7):937, 1986.
148. deBoer, A, Boukes, RJ, and Sterk, JC: Reliability of dynamometry in patients with neuromuscular disorders. N Engl J Med 11(11): 169, 1982.
149. Scott, OM, et al: Quantification of muscle function in children: A prospective study in Duchenne muscular dystrophy. Muscle Nerve 5(4):291, 1982.
150. Munsat, TL, Andres, P, and Skerry, L: Therapeutic trials in amyotrophic lateral sclerosis: Measurement of clinical deficit. In Rose, C (ed): Amyotrophic Lateral Sclerosis. Demos, New York, 1990, p 65.
151. Brooks, BR, et al: Design of clinical therapeutic trials in amyotrophic lateral sclerosis. Adv Neurol 56:521, 1991.
152. Great Lakes ALS Study Group: A comparison of muscle strength testing techniques in amyotrophic lateral sclerosis. Neurology 61(11):1503, 2003.
153. Bohannon, RW, and Smith, MB: Interrater reliability of a modified Ashworth scale of muscle spasticity. Phys Ther 67(2):206, 1987.
154. Gil, J, et al: Causes of death amongst French patients with amyotrophic lateral sclerosis. A prospective study. Eur J Neurol 15(11):1245, 2008.
155. Sanjak, M, et al: Vestibular deficits leading to disequilibrium and falls in ambulatory amyotrophic lateral sclerosis. Arch Phys Med Rehabil 95(10):1933, 2014.
156. Tinetti, ME: Performance-oriented assessment of mobility problems in elderly patients. J Am Geriatr Soc 34(2):119, 1986.
157. Berg, KO, et al: Measuring balance in the elderly: Validation of an instrument. Can J Public Health 83(2 Suppl):S7, 1992.
158. Podsiadlo, D, and Richardson, S: The timed "Up and Go": A test of basic functional mobility for frail elderly persons. J Am Geriatr Soc 39(2):142, 1991.
159. Duncan, PW, et al: Functional reach: A new clinical measure of balance. J Gerontol 45(6):M192, 1990.
160. Kloos, A, et al: Interrater and intrarater reliability of the Tinetti Balance Test for individuals with amyotrophic lateral sclerosis. JNPT 28(1):12, 2004.
161. Kloos, A, et al: Validity of the Tinetti Balance Assessment in individuals with amyotrophic lateral sclerosis. Proceedings of the 9th International Symposium on ALS/MND, Munich, Germany.
162. Montes, J, et al: The Timed Up and Go test: Predicting falls in ALS. Amyotroph Lateral Scler 8(5):292, 2007.
163. Heffernan, C, et al: Management of respiration in MND/ALS patients: An evidence based review. Amytroph Lateral Scler 7(1): 5, 2006.
164. Guide for the Uniform Data Set for Medical Rehabilitation (including the FIM instrument), Version 5.0. State University of New York, Buffalo, 1996.
165. Schwab, R, and England, A: Projection technique for evaluating surgery in Parkinson's disease. In Gillingham, J, and Donaldson, I (eds): Third Symposium on Parkinson's Disease. Livingstone, Edinburgh, Scotland, 1969.
166. The ALS CNTF Treatment Study (ACTS) Phase I–II Study Group: The amyotrophic sclerosis functional rating scale: Assessment of daily living in patients with amyotrophic lateral sclerosis. Arch Neurol 53:141, 1996.
167. Krupp, LB, et al: The fatigue severity scale. Application to patients with multiple sclerosis and systemic lupus erythematosus. Arch Neurol 46(10):1121, 1989.
168. Cedarbaum, JM, et al: The ALSFRS-R: A revised ALS functional rating scale that incorporates assessments of respiratory function. J Neurol Sci 169:13, 1999.
169. Kaufmann, P, et al: Excellent inter-rater, intra-rater, and telephone-administered reliability of the ALSFRS-R in a multicenter clinical trial. Amyotroph Lateral Scler 8(1):42, 2007.
170. Appel, V, et al: A rating scale for amyotrophic lateral sclerosis: Description and preliminary experience. Ann Neurol 22(3):328, 1987.
171. Hillel, AD, et al: Amyotrophic Lateral Sclerosis Severity Scale. Neuroepidemiology 8(3):142, 1989.
172. Norris, F, et al: The administration of guanidine in amyotrophic lateral sclerosis. Neurology 24(8):721, 1974.
173. Ware, JE, et al: SF-36 Health Survey: Manual and Interpretation Guide. Health Institute, New England Medical Center, Boston, 1993.
174. Hickey, AM, et al: A new short form individual quality of life measure (SEIQoL-DW): Application in a cohort of individuals with HIV/AIDS. Br Med J 313(7048):29, 1996.
175. Bergner, M, et al: The Sickness Impact Profile: Development and final revision of a health status measure. Med Care 19(8):787, 1981.
176. Jenkinson, C, et al: Development and validation of a short measure of health status for individuals with amyotrophic lateral sclerosis/motor neuron disease: The ALSAQ-40. J Neurol 246:16, 1999.
177. Jenkinson, C, et al: Evidence for the validity and reliability of the ALS assessment questionnaire: the ALSAQ-40. Amyotroph Lateral Scler Other Motor Neuron Disord 1(1):33, 1999.
178. Jenkinson, C, and Fitzpatrick, R: Reduced item set for the amyotrophic lateral sclerosis assessment questionnaire: Development and validation of the ALSAQ-5. J Neurol Neurosurg Psychiatry 70(1):70, 2001.
179. Dal Bello-Haas, V, et al: A randomized controlled trial of resistance exercise in individuals with ALS. Neurology 68(23):2003, 2007.
180. Wallace, VC, et al: The evaluation of pain in amyotrophic lateral sclerosis: A case controlled observational study. Amyotroph Lateral Scler Frontotemporal Degener 15:520, 2014.
181. Ho, DT, Ruthazer, R, and Russell, JA. Shoulder pain in amyotrophic lateral sclerosis. J Clin Neuromuscul Dis 13:53, 2011.

182. Ingels, PL, et al: Adhesive capsulitis: A common occurrence in patients with ALS. Amyotroph Lateral Scler Other Motor Neuron Disord 2(S2):60, 2001.
183. Cheah, BC, et al: INSPIRATIonAL—INSPIRAtory muscle training in amyotrophic lateral sclerosis. Amyotroph Lateral Scler 10(5-6):384, 2009.
184. Bach, JR: Respiratory muscle aids for the prevention of pulmonary morbidity and mortality. Semin Neurol 15(1):72, 1995.
185. Rafiq, MK, et al: Mechanical cough augmentation techniques in amyotrophic lateral sclerosis/motor neuron disease (Protocol). Cochrane Database Syst Rev 12, 2016; CD012482.
186. Mustfa, N, et al: Cough augmentation in amyotrophic lateral sclerosis. Neurology 61(9):1285, 2003.
187. Lahrmann, H, et al: Expiratory muscle weakness and assisted cough in ALS. Amyotroph Lateral Scler Other Motor Neuron Disord 4(1):49, 2003.
188. Hanayama, K, Ishikawa, Y, and Bach, JR: Amyotrophic lateral sclerosis: Successful treatment of mucous plugging by mechanical insufflation-exsufflation. Am J Phys Med Rehabil 76(4):338, 1997.
189. Rafiq, MK, et al: A preliminary randomized trial of the mechanical insufflator-exsufflator versus breath-stacking technique in patients with amyotrophic lateral sclerosis. Amyotroph Lateral Scler Frontotemporal Degener. 16(7-8):448, 215.
190. Kang, SW, and Bach, JR: Maximum insufflation capacity: Vital capacity and cough flows in neuromuscular disease. Am J Phys Med Rehabil 79:222, 2000.
191. Sancho, J, et al: Efficacy of mechanical insufflation-exsufflation in medically stable patients with amyotrophic lateral sclerosis. Chest 125:1400, 2004.
192. Estenne, M, et al: Lung volume restriction in patients with chronic respiratory muscle weakness: The role of microatelectasis. Thorax 48:698, 1993.
193. Kang, SW, and Bach, JR. Maximum insufflation capacity. Chest 118:61, 2000.
194. Kaminska, M, et al: Feasibility of lung volume recruitment in early neuromuscular weakness: A comparison between amyotrophic lateral sclerosis, myotonic dystrophy, and postpolio syndrome. Phys Med Rehabil 7:677, 2015.
195. Scherer, TA, et al: Effect of high-frequency oral airway and chest wall oscillation and conventional chest physical therapy on expectoration in patients with stable cystic fibrosis. Chest 113(4):1019, 1998.
196. Arens, R, et al: Comparison of high frequency chest compression and conventional chest physiotherapy in hospitalized patients with cystic fibrosis. Am J Respir Crit Care Med 150(4):1154, 1994.
197. Lange, DJ, et al: High-frequency chest wall oscillation in ALS: An exploratory randomized, controlled trial. Neurology 67(6):991, 2006.
198. Trail, M, et al: Wheelchair use by patients with amyotrophic lateral sclerosis: A survey of user characteristics and selection preferences. Arch Phys Med Rehabil 82(1):98, 2001.
199. Ashworth, NL, Satkunam, LE, and Deforge, D: Treatment for spasticity in amyotrophic lateral sclerosis/motor neuron disease (Cochrane review). The Cochrane Library, Issue 4. Jon Wiley & Sons, Chichester, UK, 2004.
200. Kemp, C: Psychosocial needs, problems, and interventions: The individual. In Terminal Illness: A Guide to Nursing Care. Lippincott, Philadelphia, 1999, p 17.
201. Doka, KJ: Mourning psychosocial loss: Anticipatory mourning in Alzheimer's, ALS, and irreversible coma. In Rando, TA (ed): Clinical Dimensions of Anticipatory Mourning: Theory and Practice in Working with the Dying, Their Loved Ones, and Their Caregivers. Research Press, Champaign, IL, 2000, p 477.
202. Dal Bello-Haas, V, Delbene, M, and Mitsumoto, H: End of life: Challenges and strategies for the rehabilitation professional. Neurological Report 26(4):174, 2002.
203. Kilmer, DD, et al: The effect of a high resistance exercise program in slowly progressive neuromuscular disease. Arch Phys Med Rehabil 75(5):560, 1994.
204. Lindeman, E, et al: Strength training in patients with myotonic dystrophy and hereditary motor and sensory neuropathy: A randomized clinical trial. Arch Phys Med Rehabil 76(7):612, 1995.
205. Aitkens, SG, et al: Moderate resistance exercise program: Its effect in slowly progressive neuromuscular disease. Arch Phys Med Rehabil 74(7):711, 1993.
206. Milner-Brown, HS, and Miller, RG: Muscle strengthening through high-resistance weight training in patients with neuromuscular disorders. Arch Phys Med Rehabil 69(1):14, 1988.
207. Florence, JM, and Hagberg, JM: Effect of training on the exercise responses of neuromuscular disease patients. Med Sci Sports Exerc 16(5):460, 1984.
208. Vignos, PJJ: Physical models of rehabilitation in neuromuscular disease. Muscle Nerve 6(5):323, 1983.
209. Einarsson, G: Muscle conditioning in late poliomyelitis. Arch Phys Med Rehabil 72(1):11, 1991.
210. McCartney, N, et al: The effects of strength training in patients with selected neuromuscular disorders. Med Sci Sports Exerc 20(4):362, 1988.
211. Bennett, RL, and Knowlton, GC: Overwork weakness in partially denervated skeletal muscle. Clin Orthop 12:22, 1958.
212. Johnson, EW, and Braddom, R: Over-work weakness in facioscapulohumeral muscular dystrophy. Arch Phys Med Rehabil 52(7):333, 1971.
213. Tam, SL, et al: Increased neuromuscular activity reduces sprouting in partially denervated muscles. J Neurosci 21(2):654, 2001.
214. Gardiner, PF, Michel, R, and Iadeluca, G: Previous exercise training influences functional sprouting of rat hind limb motoneurons in response to partial denervation. Neurosci Lett 45(2):123, 1984.
215. Rafuse, VF, Gordon, T, and Orozco, R: Proportional enlargement of motor units after partial denervation of cat triceps surae muscles. J Neurophysiol 68(4):1261, 1992.
216. Michel, RN, and Gardiner, PF: Influence of overload on recovery of rat plantaris from partial denervation. J Appl Physiol 66(2):732, 1989.
217. Seburn, KL, and Gardiner, PF: Properties of sprouted rat motor units: Effects of period of enlargement and activity level. Muscle Nerve 19(9):1100, 1996.
218. Ribchester, RR: Activity-dependent and independent synaptic interactions during reinnervation of partially denervated rat muscle. J Physiol (Lond) 401:53, 1988.
219. Einsiedel, LJ, and Luff, AR: Activity and motor unit size in partially denervated rat medial gastrocnemius. J Appl Physiol 76(6):2663, 1994.
220. Kirkinezos, IG, et al: Regular exercise is beneficial to a mouse model of amyotrophic lateral sclerosis. Ann Neurol 53(6):804, 2003.
221. Veldink, JH, et al: Sexual differences in onset of disease and response to exercise in a transgenic model of ALS. Neuromusc Disord 13(9):737, 2003.
222. Carreras, I, et al: Moderate exercise delays the motor performance decline in a transgenic model of ALS. Brain Res 1313:192, 2010.
223. Mahoney, DJ, et al: Effects of high-intensity endurance exercise training in the G93A mouse model of amyotrophic lateral sclerosis. Muscle Nerve 29(5):656, 2004.
224. Deforges, S, et al: Motoneuron survival is promoted by specific exercise in a mouse model of amyotrophic lateral sclerosis. J Physiol (Lond) 587(14):3561, 2009.
225. Coble, NO, and Maloney, FP: Effects of exercise in neuromuscular disease. In Maloney, FP, Burks, JS, and Ringel, SP (eds): Interdisciplinary Rehabilitation of Multiple Sclerosis and Neuromuscular Disorders. Lippincott, New York, 1985, p 228.
226. Bohanon, RW: Results of resistance exercise on a patient with amyotrophic lateral sclerosis. Phys Ther 63(6):965, 1983.
227. Sanjak, M, Reddan, W, and Brooks, BR: Role of muscular exercise in amyotrophic lateral sclerosis. Neurol Clin 5(2):251, 1987.
228. Pinto, AC, et al: Can amyotrophic lateral sclerosis patients with respiratory insufficiency exercise? J Neurol Sci 169:69, 1999.
229. Drory, VE, et al: The value of muscle exercise in patients with amyotrophic lateral sclerosis. J Neurol Sci 191(1-2):133, 2001.
230. Lunetta, C, et al: Strictly monitored exercise programs reduce motor deterioration in ALS: preliminary results of a randomized controlled trial. J Neurol 263(1):52, 2016.
231. Dal Bello-Haas V, Florence JM. Therapeutic exercise for people with amyotrophic lateral sclerosis or motor neuron disease. Cochrane Database Syst Rev 5, 2013; CD005229.
232. Dal Bello-Haas, V, and Krivickas, L: Amyotrophic lateral sclerosis. In Durstine, JL, Moore, GE, and Painter, PL (eds): ACSM's Exercise Management for Persons with Chronic Diseases and Disabilities, ed 3. Human Kinetics, Champaign, IL, 2008, p 336.

Supplemental Readings

Andersen, PM, et al: EFNS guidelines on the clinical management of amyotrophic lateral sclerosis (MALS)—revised report of an EFNS task force. Eur J Neurol 19(3):360, 2012.

Blackhall, LJ: Amyotrophic lateral sclerosis and palliative care: Where we are, and the road ahead. Muscle Nerve 45(3):311, 2012.

Dal Bello-Haas, V, Kloos, A, and Mitsumoto, H: Physical therapy for the stages of amyotrophic lateral sclerosis: A case report. Phys Ther 78(12):1312, 1998.

Lancioni, GE, et al: Technology-aided programs for assisting communication and leisure engagement of persons with amyotrophic lateral sclerosis: Two single-case studies. Res Dev Disabil 33(5):1605, 2012.

Majumdar S, Wu J, and Paganoni S: Rehabilitation in amyotrophic lateral sclerosis: Why it matters. Muscle Nerve 50(1):4, 2014.

MND Guideline Development Group: Guidelines for the Physiotherapy Management of Motor Neuron Disease (MND). The Irish Hospice Foundation, 2012. Retrieved August 17, 2017, from http://imnda.ie/wp-content/uploads/2014/09/MND-guidelines-on-Physiotherapy.pdf.

Paganoni S, et al: Comprehensive rehabilitative care across the spectrum of amyotrophic lateral sclerosis. NeuroRehabilitation 37(1):53, 2015.

Paganoni, S, et al: Functional decline is associated with hopelessness in amyotrophic lateral sclerosis (ALS). J Neurol Neurophysiol 8(2):423, 2017.

Pagnini, F, et al: Respiratory function of people with amyotrophic lateral sclerosis and caregiver distress level: A correlational study. Biopsychosoc Med 6(1):14, 2012.

Rodrigues, MC, et al: Neurovascular aspects of amyotrophic lateral sclerosis. Int Rev Neurobiol 102:91, 2012.

Amyotrophic Lateral Sclerosis Genetics. Data summarized from Alsultan et al.,[a] Chen et al.,[b] Yamashita and Ando,[c] and Renton, Chiò, and Traynor[d]

appendix **17.A**

Percentage of Individuals with FALS	Locus (*Gene*) Chromosome	Inheritance	Clinical Phenotype	Protein Functional Change
~20% (range: 12%-23.5%)	ALS1 (*SOD1*) 21q22.11	AD, AR	ALS, LL>UL>bulbar onset Primary lateral sclerosis Progressive muscular atrophy	Superoxide dismutase 1 (Cu-Zn) Oxidative stress
Rare	ALS2 (*ALS2*) 2q33.2	AR	Juvenile ALS (slowly progressive, predominantly UMN) Primary lateral sclerosis Infantile ascending hereditary spastic paraplegia	ALSin/Rho Guanine nucleotide exchange factors
Rare	ALS3 18q21	AD	ALS, typically lower limb onset	Alsin
Rare	ALS4 (*SETX*) 9q34.13	AD	Juvenile ALS, LL>UL onset Ataxia-ocular apraxia 2	Senataxin DNA/RNA processing
Rare	ALS5 (*SPG11*) 15q21.1	AR	ALS (slowly progressive), bulbar onset, limb onset Hereditary spastic paraplegia	Spatacsin Transmembrane protein
<5%	ALS6 (*FUS*) 16p11.2	AD	ALS, UL, bulbar>LL onset FTD FTSD	RNA-binding protein FUS
Rare	ALS7 (*unknown*) 20p13	AD	ALS	Unknown
Rare	ALS8 (*VAPB*) 20q13.33	AD	ALS, limb onset Finkel-type spinal muscular atrophy Spinal muscular atrophy IV	Vesicle-associated membrane, protein-associated protein B and C Altered axonal transport
Rare	ALS9 (*ANG*) 14qq11.2	AD	ALS, limb onset, bulbar onset	Angiogenin
<5%	ALS10 (*TARDBP*) 1p36.22	AD	ALS, limb onset, bulbar onset FTD FTDS	TAR DNA-binding protein (TDP-43) RNA/DNA processing
Rare	ALS11 (*FIG4*) 6q21	AD	ALS (rapidly progressive), bulbar>limb onset	Polyphosphoinositide phosphatase

Continued

Percentage of Individuals with FALS	Locus (*Gene*) Chromosome	Inheritance	Clinical Phenotype	Protein Functional Change
Rare	ALS12 (OPTN) 10p13	AD, AR	ALS (slowly progressive, limb onset, predominant UMN) Primary open-angle glaucoma Parkisonism	Optineurin
~5%	ALS13 (*ATXN2*) 12q24.12	AD	ALS, limb onset, bulbar onset Cerebellar ataxia Corticobasal syndrome Parkisonism	RNA processing
Unknown	ALS14 (*VCP*) 9q13.3	AD	ALS, limb>bulbar onset FTD FTDS Multisystem proteinopathy	Valocin-containing protein
<2%	ALS15 (*UBQLN2*) X11p.21	x-linked AD	ALS, limb onset, bulbar onset FTD FTDS ALS, limb onset, bulbar onset Primary lateral sclerosis Multisystem proteinopathy	Ubiquilin 2 Ubiquitination, protein degradation Profilin 1 Actin binding protein, actin polymerization Heterogeneous nuclear ribonucleoprotein mRNA processing
Rare	ALS16 (SIGMAR1) 9p13.2-21.3	AR	Juvenile ALS, LL>UL onset FTD	Sigma non-opioid intracellular receptor
1%	ALS17 (*CHMP2B*) 3p11.2	AD	ALS, bulbar onset, limb onset FTD Progressive muscular atrophy Parkinsonism	Endosomal trafficking, autophagy
2.5%	ALS18 (*PFN1*) 17p13.2	AD	Limb-onset ALS	Cytoskeleton, axonal growth
Rare	ALS19 (*ERBB4*) 2q34	AD	UL onset, bulbar onset ALS	Neuronal development
Rare	ALS20 (*hnPRNPA1*) 12q13.13	AD	FTD	RNA processing
<2%	ALS21 (*MATR3*) 5q31.2	AD	FTD ALS, bulbar onset, limb onset	RNA processing
<2%	ALS22 (*TUBA4A*) 2q35	AD	ALS	Cytoskeleton

Percentage of Individuals with FALS	Locus (*Gene*) Chromosome	Inheritance	Clinical Phenotype	Protein Functional Change
23%-30%	ALS-FTD (*C9orf72*) 9p21.2	AD	ALS FTD FTDS	Chromosome 9 open reading frame 72 Unknown
	ALS-FTD (*TBKI*) 12q154.2	AD, sporadic	ALS FTD	TANK-binding kinase 1 Multifunctional kinase active in autophagosome-mediated degradation of ubiquinated proteins Neuroinflammation
~3.5%	ALS-FTD (*CHCHD10*) 22q11.23	AD	*CHCHD10*-related ALS/FTD *(ALS-related MND, with both UMN and LMN involvement)*	Coiled-coil-helix-coiled-coil-helix domain-containing protein 10, mitochondrial function

AD = Autosomal dominant; ALS = Amyotrophic lateral sclerosis;
AR = Autosomal recessive; FALS = Familial amyotrophic lateral sclerosis;
FTD = Frontotemporal dementia; FTSD = Frontotemporal spectrum disorder;
LL = Lower limb; LMN = Lower motor neuron; MND = Motor neuron disease;
UL = Upper limb; UMN = Upper motor neuron

a. Alsultan, AA, et al: The genetics of amyotrophic lateral sclerosis: Current insights. Degener Neurol Neuromuscul Dis 6:49, 2016.
b. Chen, S, et al: Genetics of amyotrophic lateral sclerosis: An update. Mol Neurodegener 8:28, 2013.
c. Yamashita, S, and Ando, Y: Genotype-phenotype relationship in hereditary amyotrophic lateral sclerosis. Transl Neurodegener 4:13, 2015.
d. Renton, AE, Chiò, A, and Traynor, BJ: State of play in amyotrophic lateral sclerosis genetics. Nat Neurosci 17:17, 2014.

appendix

17.B Schwab and England Activities of Daily Living Scale

100% =	Completely independent; able to do all chores without slowness, difficulty, or impairment; essentially normal; unaware of any difficulty
90% =	Completely independent; able to do all chores with some degree of slowness, difficulty, and impairment; may take twice as long as usual; beginning to be aware of difficulty
80% =	Completely independent in most chores; takes twice as long as normal; conscious of difficulty and slowness
70% =	Not completely independent; more difficulty with some chores; takes three to four times as long as normal in some instances; must spend a large part of the day with some chores
60% =	Some dependency; can do most chores, but exceedingly slowly and with considerable effort and errors; some chores impossible
50% =	More dependent; needs help with half the chores, slower, and so forth; difficulty with everything
40% =	Very dependent; can assist with all chores but does few alone
30% =	With effort, now and then does a few chores alone or begins alone; much help needed
20% =	Does nothing alone; can be a slight help with some chores; severe invalid
10% =	Totally dependent and helpless; complete invalid
0% =	Vegetative functions such as swallowing, bladder, and bowels are not functioning; bedridden

From Schwab, R, and England, A[165] with permission.

Amyotrophic Lateral Sclerosis Functional Rating Scale—Revised*

appendix **17.C**

1. Speech

4 Normal speech processes.
3 Detectable speech disturbance.
2 Intelligible with repeating.
1 Speech combined with non-vocal communication.
0 Loss of useful speech.

2. Salivation

4 Normal.
3 Slight but definite excess of saliva in mouth; may have nighttime drooling.
2 Moderately excessive saliva; may have minimal drooling.
1 Marked excess of saliva with some drooling.
0 Marked drooling; requires constant tissue or handkerchief.

3. Swallowing

4 Normal eating habits.
3 Early eating problems—occasional choking.
2 Dietary consistency changes.
1 Needs supplemental tube feeding.
0 NPO (exclusively parenteral or enteral feeding).

4. Handwriting

4 Normal.
3 Slow or sloppy; all words are legible.
2 Not all words are legible.
1 Able to grip pen but unable to write.
0 Unable to grip pen.

5a. Cutting Food and Handling Utensils (Patients without Gastrostomy)

4 Normal.
3 Somewhat slow and clumsy, but no help needed.
2 Can cut most foods, although clumsy and slow; some help needed.
1 Food must be cut by someone, but can still feed slowly.
0 Needs to be fed.

OR

5b. Cutting Food and Handling Utensils (Alternate Scale for Patients with Gastrostomy)

4 Normal.
3 Clumsy but able to perform all manipulations independently.
2 Some help needed with closures and fasteners.
1 Provides minimal assistance to caregiver.
0 Unable to perform any aspect of task.

6. Dressing and Hygiene

4 Normal function.
3 Independent and complete self-care with effort or decreased efficiency.
2 Intermittent assistance or substitute methods.
1 Needs attendant for self.
0 Total dependence.

7. Turning in Bed and Adjusting Bed Clothes

4 Normal.
3 Somewhat slow and clumsy, but no help needed.
2 Can turn alone or adjust sheets, but with great difficulty.
1 Can initiate, but not turn or adjust sheets alone.
0 Helpless.

8. Walking

4 Normal.
3 Early ambulation difficulties.
2 Walks with assistance.
1 Non-ambulatory functional movement only.
0 No purposeful leg movement.

9. Climbing Stairs

4 Normal.
3 Slow.
2 Mild unsteadiness or fatigue.
1 Needs assistance.
0 Cannot do.

10. Dyspnea

4 None.
3 Occurs when walking.
2 Occurs with one or more of the following: eating, bathing, dressing (ADL).
1 Occurs at rest, difficulty breathing when either sitting or lying.
0 Significant difficulty, considering using mechanical respiratory support.

11. Orthopnea

4 None.
3 Some difficulty sleeping at night due to shortness of breath, does not routinely use more than two pillows.
2 Needs extra pillows to sleep (more than two).
1 Can only sleep sitting up.
0 Unable to sleep.

12. Respiratory Insufficiency

4 None.
3 Intermittent use of BiPAP.
2 Continuous use of BiPAP during the night.
1 Continuous use of BiPAP during the night and day.
0 Invasive mechanical ventilation by intubation or tracheostomy.

*The original ALSFRS consists of items 1 through 9 and the original item 10 below:

10. Breathing

4 Normal.
3 Shortness of breath with minimal exertion (e.g., walking, talking).
2 Shortness of breath at rest.
1 Intermittent (e.g., nocturnal) ventilatory assistance.
0 Ventilator dependent.

BiPAP = bidirectional positive airway pressure; NPO = *non per os*, nothing by mouth.

From Cedarbaum, JM, et al,[168] with permission.

Web-Based Resources for Clinicians, Families, and Patients with Amyotrophic Lateral Sclerosis

appendix **17.D**

Organization/Resource	Website
American Academy of Neurology	www.aan.com*
Amyotrophic Lateral Sclerosis Association • Section titled, For People with ALS and Caregivers	www.alsa.org http://www.alsa.org/als-care/
Amyotrophic Lateral Sclerosis Society of Canada • Resources, e.g., A Manual for People Living with ALS; Coping with Grief	www.als.ca https://www.als.ca/about-als/resources/
European Academy of Neurology	www.ean.org*
International Alliance of ALS/MND Associations • Position Statements • Useful Links	www.alsmndalliance.org https://www.alsmndalliance.org/about-us/policies/ https://www.alsmndalliance.org/useful-links/
Motor Neuron Disease Association • Information Resources	https://www.mndassociation.org https://www.mndassociation.org/about-mnd/information-resources/
Muscular Dystrophy Association	www.mda.org*
National Institute of Neurological Disorders and Stroke	www.ninds.nih.gov*†
National Institute for Health and Care Excellence • Motor Neuron Disease: Assessment and management, NICE guideline [NG42]	www.nice.org.uk*† https://www.nice.org.uk/guidance/ng42
World Federation of Neurology Research Group on Motor Neuron Diseases/Amyotrophic Lateral Sclerosis (WFN-ALS)	www.wfnals.org

*Search term: Amyotrophic lateral sclerosis or ALS.
†Search term: Motor neuron(e) disease(s).
ALS = amyotrophic lateral sclerosis; ALS/MND = amyotrophic lateral sclerosis and motor neuron disease.

Chapter 18

Parkinson's Disease

Edward W. Bezkor, PT, DPT, OCS, MTC
Tara L. McIsaac, PT, PhD
Susan B. O'Sullivan, PT, EdD

LEARNING OBJECTIVES

1. Describe the etiology, pathophysiology, clinical manifestations, and sequelae of Parkinson's disease.
2. Identify and describe the examination procedures used to evaluate people with Parkinson's disease to establish a diagnosis, prognosis, and plan of care.
3. Describe the role of the physical therapist in assisting a person with Parkinson's disease in terms of direct interventions to maximize function, and in education to client, family/caregiver, community program instructors, and health care team to optimize outcomes and participation.
4. Describe appropriate elements of the exercise prescription for individuals with Parkinson's disease.
5. Identify the neuropsychological effects and social impact of Parkinson's disease and describe appropriate interventions to maximize function, participation and quality of life.
6. Analyze and interpret patient data, formulate realistic goals and outcomes, and develop a plan of care when presented with a clinical case study.

CHAPTER OUTLINE

Parkinson's disease (PD) is a progressive disorder of the central nervous system (CNS) with both motor and nonmotor symptoms. Motor symptoms include the *cardinal features* of *rigidity, bradykinesia, tremor, and postural instability.* Nonmotor symptoms (NMSs) may precede the onset of motor symptoms by several years. These early premotor symptoms can include loss of sense of smell (anosmia), constipation, rapid eye movement (REM) sleep behavior disorder, depression, anxiety and orthostatic hypotension. Other nonmotor symptoms include excessive daytime sleepiness, fatigue (a sense of exhaustion rather than sleepiness), pain (often unilateral and in affected limb), altered bladder function, erectile dysfunction, excessive saliva, integumentary changes, difficulty speaking and swallowing, apathy, and cognitive problems (reduced concentration and attention, slowed thinking, confusion, and in some cases dementia). Onset is insidious with a slow rate of progression. Disruptions in daily functions, roles, and activities are common in individuals with PD.[1,2]

■ INCIDENCE

PD is the second most common neurodegenerative disorder and affects an estimated 1 million Americans and an estimated 7 to 10 million people worldwide. More than 2% of people older than 65 years of age have PD, second only to Alzheimer's disease among neurodegenerative disorders. The prevalence of the disease is expected to increase substantially in the coming years due to the aging of the population. The average age of onset is 50 to 60 years. Only 4% to 10% of patients are diagnosed with early-onset PD (less than 50 years of age). Young-onset PD is classified as beginning between 21 and 50 years of age, and juvenile-onset PD affects individuals less than 21 years of age. Men are affected 1.2 to 1.5 times more frequently than women, but this varies across the globe.[3,4]

ETIOLOGY

The term *parkinsonism* is a generic term used to describe a group of bradykinetic syndromes with primary disturbances in the dopamine systems of basal ganglia (BG). Both genetic and environmental influences have been identified. Parkinson's disease, or idiopathic parkinsonism, is the most common form, affecting approximately 78% of patients. *Secondary parkinsonism* results from a number of different identifiable causes, including viruses, toxins, drugs, and tumors (Box 18.1). The term *atypical parkinsonism* (Parkinson Plus Syndrome) refers to those conditions that mimic PD in some respects, but the symptoms are caused by other neurodegenerative disorders.[1,4]

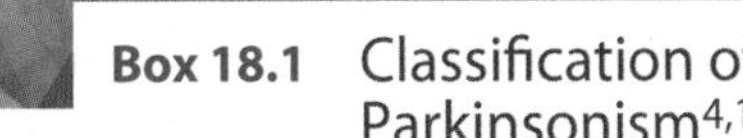

Box 18.1 Classification of Parkinsonism[4,14]

Idiopathic Parkinson's Disease

Late-onset (>50 years; generally sporadic)
Early-onset (<50 years; often familial)
- Young-onset (>21 years)
- Juvenile (<21 years)

Parkinsonism due to Identifiable Causes

Drug-induced (e.g., phenothiazines, reserpine, butyrophenones, metoclopramide)
Hemiparkinsonism, hemiatrophy
Hydrocephalus (e.g., normal pressure hydrocephalus [NPH])
Hypoxia
Infectious (e.g., postencephalitic)
Metabolic
- Wilson's disease
- Hepatocerebral degeneration
- Hallervorden-Spatz disease
- Hypoparathyroidism

Toxins (e.g., carbon monoxide, manganese, methyl-phenyl-tetrahydropyridine [MPTP])
Trauma
Tumors of basal ganglia
Vascular disease (multi-infarct)

Parkinsonism in Other Neurodegenerative Disorders

Cortical–basal ganglionic degeneration (CBD)
Disorders with prominent and often early dementia:
- Diffuse cortical Lewy body disease (DLBD)
- Alzheimer's disease with parkinsonism (AD)
- Frontotemporal dementia (FTD)

Disorders with cerebellar/autonomic/pyramidal manifestation:
- Multiple-system atrophy (MSA)
- Sporadic Olivopontocerebellar atrophy (OPCA)
- Shy-Drager syndrome
- Striatonigral degeneration
- Machado-Joseph disease

Parkinsonism–dementia–ALS complex of Guam
Progressive pallidal atrophy
Progressive supranuclear palsy (PSP)

Parkinson's Disease

Parkinson's disease was first described as "the shaking palsy" by James Parkinson[5] in 1817 and refers to those cases where the etiology is idiopathic (unknown) or genetically determined. Two clinical subgroups (motor phenotypes) have been identified. One group includes individuals whose dominant symptoms include postural instability and gait disturbances (*postural instability gait disorder [PIGD] phenotype*). Another group includes individuals with tremor as the main feature (*tremor-dominant [TD] phenotype*). Patients who are tremor-dominant typically demonstrate fewer problems with bradykinesia or postural instability, have lower prevalence of non-motor symptoms, including lower risk of developing dementia, and are less likely to have the known genetic mutations associated with PD.[4,6,7]

Genetic forms of PD represent less than 10% of cases overall. In a small number of families, several gene mutations have been identified (e.g., SNCA, PARK1, PINK1, LRRK2, DJ-1, and glucocerebrosidase, among others).[1] Genes have been grouped into two categories: (1) causal genes, which actually produce the disease; and (2) associated genes that do not cause PD but increase the risk of developing it.[8]

Secondary Parkinsonism

Postencephalitic Parkinsonism

The influenza epidemics of encephalitis lethargica that occurred from 1917 to 1926 affected large numbers of individuals. The onset of parkinsonian symptoms typically occurred after many years, giving rise to the theory that a slow virus infected the brain. In the absence of a recent outbreak, this type of parkinsonism is no longer seen. Moving case histories are portrayed in the book *Awakenings* by Oliver Sacks.[9]

Toxic Parkinsonism

Parkinsonian symptoms occur in individuals exposed to certain environmental toxins, including pesticides (e.g., permethrin, beta-HCH, paraquat, maneb, Agent Orange) and industrial chemicals (e.g., manganese, carbon disulfide, carbon monoxide, cyanide, methanol).

The most common of these toxins is manganese, which represents a serious occupational hazard to many miners from prolonged exposure.[10,11] Severe and permanent parkinsonism has been inadvertently produced in individuals who injected a synthetic heroin containing the chemical MPTP (1-methyl-4-phenyl-1,2,3,6- tetra/hydropyridine).[12] It is important to note that simple exposure is never enough to cause the disease.

Drug-Induced Parkinsonism (DIP)

A variety of drugs can produce extrapyramidal dysfunction that mimics the signs of PD. These drugs are thought to interfere with dopaminergic mechanisms either presynaptically or postsynaptically. They include (1) *neuroleptic drugs* such as chlorpromazine (Thorazine®), haloperidol (Haldol®), thioridazine (Mellaril®), and thiothixene (Navane®); (2) *antidepressant drugs* such as amitriptyline (Triavil®), amoxapine (Asendin®), and trazodone (Desyrel®); and (3) *antihypertensive drugs* such as methyldopa (Aldomet®) and reserpine. High doses of these medications are particularly problematic in the elderly. Withdrawal of these agents usually reverses the symptoms within a few weeks, although in some cases the effects can persist and may be related to subclinical PD.[13]

Parkinsonism can be caused in rare cases by metabolic conditions, including disorders of calcium metabolism that result in BG calcification. These include hypothyroidism, hyperparathyroidism, hypoparathyroidism, and Wilson's disease.[4]

Parkinson-Plus Syndromes

A group of neurodegenerative diseases can affect the substantia nigra and produce parkinsonian symptoms along with other neurological signs. These diseases include cortical–basal ganglionic degeneration (CBGD); progressive supranuclear palsy (PSP); multiple system atrophy (MSA) syndromes (striatonigral degeneration [SND], Shy-Drager syndrome, sporadic olivopontocerebellar atrophy [OPCA], and motor neuron disease-parkinsonism]). In addition, parkinsonian symptoms can be exhibited in patients with multi-infarct vascular disease; dementia syndromes (Alzheimer's disease, diffuse Lewy body disease [DLBD], and frontotemporal dementia [FTD]); normal pressure hydrocephalus (NPH); Creutzfeldt-Jakob disease (CJD), Wilson's disease (WD); and juvenile Huntington's disease. Many of these conditions are rare and affect relatively small numbers of individuals. Early in their course, these diseases may present with rigidity and bradykinesia indistinguishable from PD. However, other diagnostic symptoms eventually appear (e.g., cognitive impairment in Alzheimer's disease). Another diagnostic feature is that Parkinson-plus syndromes typically do not show measurable improvement from the administration of anti-Parkinson medications such as levodopa therapy (termed the *apomorphine test*).[14]

■ PATHOPHYSIOLOGY

The BG is a network of subcortical nuclei consisting of the *caudate nucleus*, the *putamen*, the *globus pallidus*, and the *subthalamic nucleus* along with the *substantia nigra*. The caudate and the putamen together are called the *striatum* (Fig. 18.1). The BG engages in a number of parallel circuits or loops, only a few of which are motor. The *direct motor loop* through the BG consists of signals transmitted from the cortex to putamen to globus pallidus, to ventrolateral (VL) nucleus of the thalamus, and back to cortex (supplementary motor area [SMA]) (Fig. 18.2). This VL-SMA connection is excitatory and facilitates discharge of cells in the SMA. The BG thus serves to activate the cortex via a positive-feedback loop

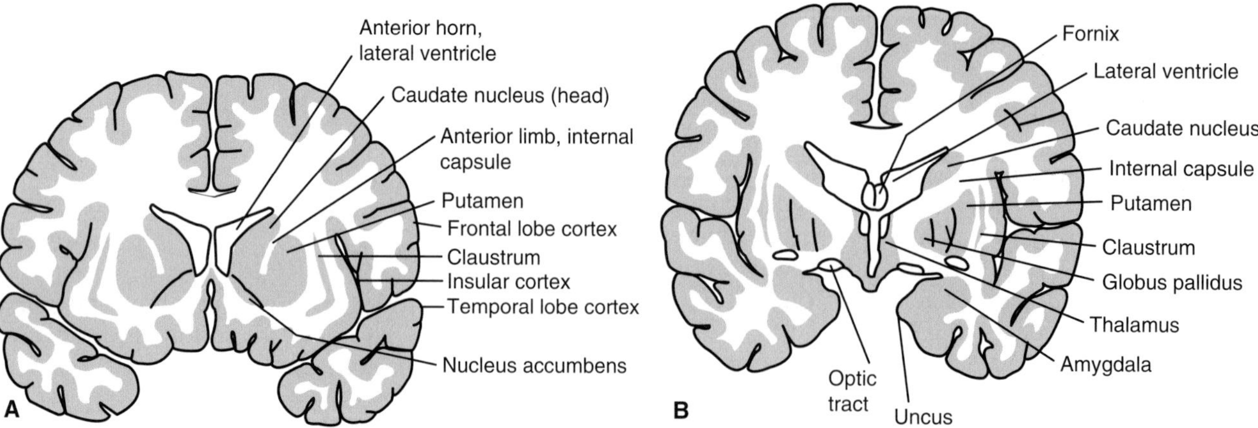

Figure 18.1 The major structures of the basal ganglia. (A) Coronal section through the rostral part of the frontal lobe showing the relation of the caudate nucleus, putamen, and nucleus accumbens to the surrounding telencephalic structures. (B) Coronal section through the caudal part of the front lobe showing the location of the lentiform nucleus later to, and the body of the caudate nucleus dorsal to, the diencephalon.

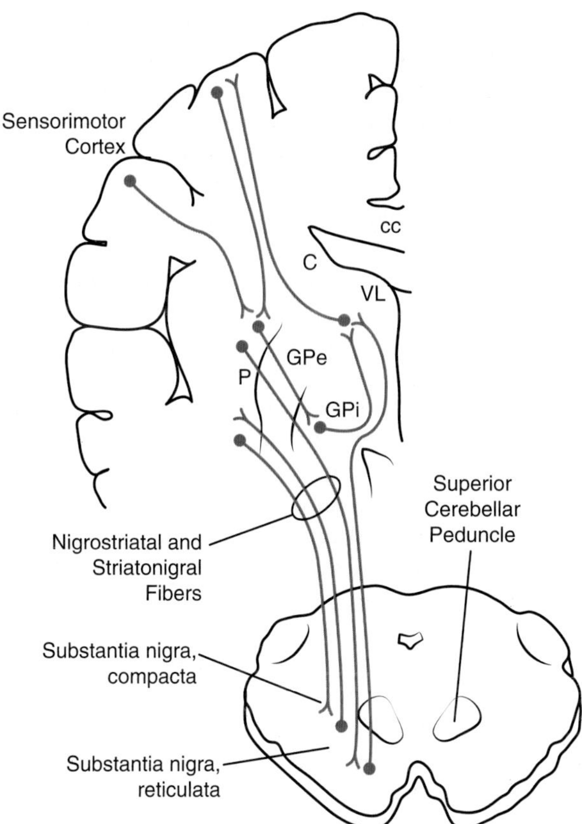

Figure 18.2 The direct loop through the putamen and the connections of the striatum with the substantia nigra pars compacta. The striatonigral fibers represented in this diagram arise in the putamen. However, most striatonigral fibers arise from the caudate. C = caudate nucleus; cc = corpus callosum; GPe = globus pallidus pars externa; GPi = glogus pallidus pars interna; P = putamen; VL = ventral lateral nucleus of the thalamus.

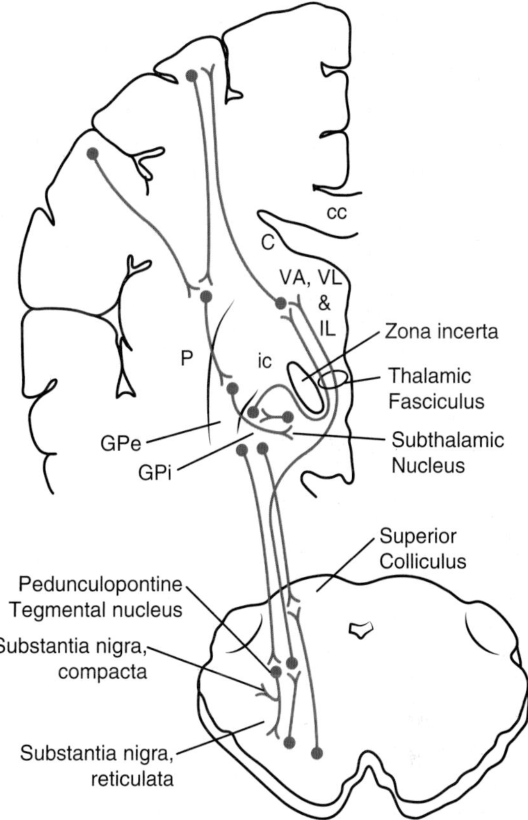

Figure 18.3 The indirect loop through the subthalamic nucleus; also represented are the efferents from the globus pallidus interna and substantia nigra pars reticulata to the superior colliculus and midbrain tegmentum. C = caudate nucleus; GPe = globus pallidus pars externa; GPi = globus pallidus pars interna; ic = internal capsule; IL = intralaminar nuclei of the thalamus; P = putamen; VA = ventral anterior nucleus of the thalamus; VL = ventral lateral nucleus of the thalamus.

and assists in the initiation of voluntary movement. Inhibition of the thalamus by the BG is thought to underlie the hypokinesia seen in PD. An *indirect loop* through the BG involves the subthalamic nucleus, the globus pallidus interna, and substantia nigra pars reticulata to the superior colliculus and midbrain tegmentum (Fig. 18.3). This indirect loop serves to decrease thalamocortical activation. The BG projection to the superior colliculus assists in regulation of saccadic eye movements. The BG projection to the reticular formation assists in the regulation of trunk and limb musculature (via extrapyramidal pathways), sleep and wakefulness, and arousal. Other circuits in the BG are involved with memory and cognitive functions.[15]

Parkinson's disease is characterized by (1) degeneration of dopaminergic neurons in the BG in the pars compacta of the substantia nigra that produce *dopamine* and (2) as the disease progresses and neurons degenerate, the presence of *alpha-synuclein* cytoplasmic inclusions (misfolded proteins that clump), called *Lewy bodies.* Substantial neurodegeneration occurs in PD before the onset of motor symptoms with clinical signs emerging at approximately 60% degeneration of neurons. Loss of the melanin-containing neurons produces characteristic changes in depigmentation in the substantia nigra with a characteristic pallor.[14] Numerous other brain regions of people with PD show structural and functional changes, including impaired modulation of other neurotransmitters (acetylcholine, serotonin, noradrenaline, glutamate, and GABA).[6] Changes are seen in the *pedunculopontine nucleus* (PPN) and *nucleus basalis of Meynert* (nbM) that release acetylcholine (ACh), and the *locus coeruleus* that releases noradrenaline, also show alpha-synuclein deposition very early in the disease.[17-19]

STAGES OF BRAIN PATHOLOGY

Postmortem studies by Braak and colleagues have yielded evidence supporting the view that PD is a widely dispersed neurodegenerative disease that demonstrates a progression through different stages of brain pathology. Early on (*stage 1*) lesions are found in the olfactory bulb, olfactory nucleus, and/or the dorsal IX/X nuclei in the brainstem. In *stage 2,* pathology is expanded to involve lesions in the pontine tegmentum (locus coeruleus, magnocellular nucleus of the reticular formation, and raphe nuclei). In *stage 3,* involvement of the nigrostriatal system is apparent (pars compacta of the substantia nigra). In *stage 4,* lesions are also found in the hypothalamus, parts of the thalamus, and cortex (temporal mesocortex and allocortex). In *stage 5,* pathology is extended to involve the sensory association areas of the neocortex and prefrontal neocortex. In *stage 6,* pathology is extended to involve the first-order association areas and primary areas of the neocortex.[17-20]

CLINICAL PRESENTATION

Cardinal Motor Symptoms

Rigidity

Rigidity is one of the clinical hallmarks of PD and is defined as increased resistance to passive motion regardless of movement velocity. Patients frequently complain of "heaviness" and "stiffness" of their limbs. It is felt uniformly in both agonist and antagonist muscles and in movements in both directions. Spinal stretch reflexes are normal. Rigidity is fairly constant regardless of the task, amplitude, or speed of movement. Two descriptive terms are sometimes used: cogwheel and lead pipe. Cogwheel rigidity is a jerky, ratchet-like resistance to passive movement as muscles alternately tense and relax. It occurs when tremor is superimposed on a background increased tone. Lead pipe rigidity is a sustained resistance to passive movement in all directions, with no fluctuations. Rigidity is often asymmetrical, especially in the early stages of PD. It typically affects proximal muscles first, especially the shoulders and neck, and it progresses to involve muscles of the face and extremities. Rigidity may initially affect the left or right side, eventually spreading to involve the whole body. As the disease progresses, rigidity becomes more severe. Rigidity decreases the ability to move easily. For example, loss of bed mobility or lack of reciprocal arm swing during gait, seen even early in the disease, is often related to the degree of truncal rigidity. Active movement, mental concentration, or emotional stress may all increase rigidity. Prolonged rigidity results in decreased range of motion (ROM) and serious secondary complications of contracture and postural deformity. Rigidity also has a direct impact on increasing resting energy expenditure and fatigue levels.[21,22]

Bradykinesia

Bradykinesia refers to slowness of movement and is the one cardinal feature common to all parkinsonian disorders, including PD. Weakness, tremor, and rigidity may contribute to bradykinesia but do not fully explain it. The principle deficit is the result of insufficient recruitment of muscle force during initiation of movement. Patients underscale movement commands in internally generated movements. The introduction of external cues (e.g., vision, sound) can partially ameliorate this and is used in treatment to guide movement. It is one of the most disabling symptoms of PD, with prolonged movement and reaction times resulting in increased time on task and dependence in daily activities. Slowness of thought, *bradyphrenia,* can contribute to bradykinesia.[23]

Akinesia refers to a poverty of spontaneous movement. For example, the patient with PD demonstrates *hypomimia* or masked facial expression, with significant social consequences. Other examples of akinesia include the absence of associated movements (e.g., arm swing during walking) or freezing (sudden, short, and transient inhibitions of movements while walking [*freezing of gait; FOG*], or during other movements such as while writing, talking, or driving). Akinesia can be influenced by the degree of rigidity, as well as stage of disease, fluctuations in drug action, and disturbances in attention and depression.[24-26]

Hypokinesia refers to slowed and reduced movements and can also be seen in PD. For example, patients with moderate or severe PD typically present with handwriting that may start out strong but becomes smaller and smaller as writing proceeds (micrographia). During walking, rotational movements of the trunk with arm swing may also start out strong and decrease over time.

Tremor

Tremor, a third cardinal feature of PD, involves involuntary shaking or oscillating movement of a part or parts of the body resulting from contractions of opposing muscles. In the early stages of the disease, about 70% of patients experience a slight tremor of the hand or foot on one side of the body, or less commonly in the jaw or tongue. It tends to be mild and occurs for only short periods. Tremor in PD tends to be of low frequency (4–6 Hz). The tremor is known as a *resting tremor* because it is present at rest, suppressed briefly by voluntary movement, and disappears with sleep. Tremor in the lower limbs is most apparent while the patient is supine. Tremor of the head, trunk, and limbs (postural tremor) can be seen when muscles are used to maintain sustained postures against gravity. Tremor that continues with movement (action tremor/kinetic tremor) can occur in patients and is seen more often as the disease progresses. Tremor tends to be less severe when the patient is relaxed and unoccupied. It is aggravated by emotional stress or excitement. With disease progression, tremor can become severe, spread to the other side, and interfere with activities of daily living (ADL).[27,28]

Postural Instability

The ability to achieve, maintain and regain balance during posture and movement are all components of postural control that are impaired in individuals with PD, resulting in postural instability. Throughout the disease, several problems become evident across a broad spectrum of movement control. Patients demonstrate abnormal and inflexible postural responses controlling their center of mass (COM) within their base of support (BOS). They have smaller functional limits of stability (LOS) compared with healthy adults of the same age, reduced more anteriorly with forward lean than posteriorly with backward lean.[29] Narrowing of the BOS (tandem stance or single-limb stance) or competing attentional demands (alternating and divided attention situations) increases postural instability. Individuals with PD experience difficulty during dynamic destabilizing activities such as self-initiated movements (e.g., functional reach, walking, turning) and perform poorly under conditions of perturbed balance.[30] The response to instability is an abnormal pattern of coactivation, resulting in a rigid body and an inability to utilize normal postural synergies to recover balance.[30] Patients also demonstrate difficulty in regulating feed-forward, anticipatory adjustments of postural muscles during voluntary movements. These anticipatory postural adjustments (APAs) are abnormally slow in people with PD (see section on Gait). Sensorimotor integration is impaired as evidenced by difficulty in adapting movement strategies to changing sensory conditions.[31] Visuospatial impairment has been identified in people with PD and correlates with lower scores in mobility, freezing episodes and self-reported cognitive impairment.[26,32] Some patients are unable to perceive the upright or vertical position, which may indicate an abnormality in processing of vestibular, visual, and proprioceptive information contributing to balance. Contributing factors to postural instability include rigidity, decreased muscle torque production and weakness, loss of available ROM particularly of trunk motions, axial rigidity, and freezing. Medication side effects (e.g., postural hypotension and dyskinesias) also contribute.

Progressive development of postural deformity occurs. Weakness of antigravity muscles contributes to the adoption of a flexed, stooped posture with increased flexion of the neck, trunk, hips, and knees.[33] This results in a significant change in the center-of-alignment position, placing the individual at the forward limits of stability. In the lower extremities (LEs), *contractures* develop in hip and knee flexors, hip rotators and adductors, and plantarflexors. In the spine, dorsal spine and neck flexors are involved, and in the upper extremities (UEs), shoulder adductors and internal rotators and elbow flexors are involved. Function becomes progressively more limited by these musculoskeletal constraints. Older individuals with reduced activity levels and poor diet are likely to develop *osteoporosis.*

Frequent falls and fall injury are twice as likely to occur for individuals with PD as those without PD and recurrent falls are 9 times more likely in PD.[34] Falls can occur early in the disease, become increasingly prevalent during the middle portion of disease progression, and as the patient becomes progressively immobile, disappear during late disease. About 70% of patients with PD report experiencing falls within the past year and 50% report recurrent falls. The rate of fall injury is about 40%. Although most injuries are not severe, some lead to hospitalization. Within 10 years of diagnosis, approximately 25% of patients will have developed a hip fracture. In a long-term study of over 3 million people in Sweden that explored fall-risk *prior to* clinical diagnosis of PD (*prodromal/preclinical*), researchers found the risk of falls with injury was increased 10 years before diagnosis.[35] Disease severity, postural instability, and gait impairment including freezing are clearly linked to increased risk for falls.[26,30,36,37] Other risk factors include dementia, depression, postural hypotension, and involuntary movements associated with long-term use of anti-parkinsonian medication (dyskinesias).[34,38] Falls can lead to "fear of falling" with increasing levels of immobility and dependency with a deteriorating quality of life.

Other Motor Symptoms

Muscle Performance

A reduction in strength is evident in patients with PD. Torque production is decreased at all speeds resulting in activity limitations and muscle weakness.[39-41] Changes in strength may be dopamine related as patients on dopamine replacement ("on" state) demonstrate increases in strength when compared with testing the same muscles during an "off" state.[42] Electromyography (EMG) studies reveal that motor unit recruitment is delayed with under-recruitment of muscles and breakdown in the agonist-antagonist-agonist (triphasic) pattern of muscle activity. Once initiated, contraction is characterized by multiple bursts and *asynchronization,* that is, pauses and an inability to smoothly increase firing rate as contraction continues.[43-47] These difficulties are compounded during the production of complex movements. As the disease progresses, disuse weakness evolves from inactivity and increases movement difficulties.

In patients with PD, *fatigue* is among the most common symptoms reported. The patient has difficulty in sustaining activity and experiences increasing weakness and lethargy as the day progresses. Repetitive motor acts may start out strong but decrease in strength and amplitude as the activity progresses. Performance decreases dramatically with great physical effort or stress. Rest or sleep may restore mobility. When levodopa therapy is initiated, the patient may notice a dramatic improvement initially and feel significantly less fatigued. In long-standing disease and drug therapy, fatigue typically reappears. A common perception among patients is an increased sense of effort associated with movement that is manifested by difficulty activating and sustaining responses.[48]

Motor Function

The striatum of the BG (caudate nucleus, putamen, and nucleus accumbens) receive input from all cortical areas and project throughout the thalamus to frontal lobe areas (prefrontal, premotor, and supplementary motor areas) concerned with motor planning. In PD, motor planning deficits are evident, involving a loss of regulatory control of both automatic and voluntary movement responses directed through the pyramidal system.[49] Paucity of movement occurs with less accurate movements overall. This deficit in accuracy becomes more pronounced as the patient attempts to increase the speed of movement (*speed-accuracy trade-off*). This is a commonly observed problem in the elderly in general. Patients have trouble performing complex, sequential, or simultaneous movements. The difficulties combining tasks or shifting attentional sets from one to another can also be seen with cognitive tasks or when combining cognitive and motor tasks (*dual-task control*). Movement preparation (i.e., the when, where, and how to initiate movement) is significantly prolonged (a finding also seen with advancing age). This *start hesitation* is especially evident as the disease progresses.[50] For example, the patient is delayed and slow in initiating movement during a transfer sequence.

Motor learning deficits are seen in patients with PD but are not universal. Deficits in learning new motor skills, fine-tuning skills, and learning complex and sequential tasks have been demonstrated in all stages of disease.[51-53] Healthy adults achieve better learning (determined by retention and transfer testing) with random order practice conditions and high levels of *contextual interference* (see Chapter 10, Strategies to Improve Motor Function). In contrast, for individuals with PD learning is improved with lower levels of contextual interference through blocked practice conditions and with slower learning-rates than healthy adults.[54] Learning deficits can be expected to be severe if multiple motor programs are required either simultaneously or sequentially (i.e., switching among tasks). For example, the patient may freeze when asked to carry out a second task while walking, when performing any two tasks that have separate task goals (*dual-tasking*),[55] or when performing a complex task that requires increased cognitive processing.[56,57] Compounding variables that degrade learning include the severity of disease, dementia, and visual–perceptual deficits. Differences in learning can also be expected based on medication levels as motor learning is degraded when patients are in the "off" state of medication.[51-57]

Gait

More than 25% of patients present with gait disturbances and postural instability as their initial motor symptom and comprise a PIGD group.[58] The patient with PD demonstrates a number of significant gait changes that can generally be divided into continuous and episodic disturbances.[59] Continuous gait control problems have been characterized as three primary gait impairments that are relatively independent: (1) slowness (pace and rhythm), (2) increased variability and asymmetry, and (3) poor postural control.[30] Slowed walking is a hallmark characteristic of PD observed throughout the disease and primarily caused by bradykinesia (slower steps), hypokinesia (shorter steps), and rigidity (increased tone). Reduction in arm swing and trunk rotation, also due to bradykinesia/hypokinesia, are seen throughout the disease. Axial rigidity (neck, trunk, and hips) contributes to an abnormal stooped posture, slowed gait, and an *en bloc* turning style with reduced speed and more steps to complete the turn. Variability of gait, seen as step width (medio-lateral) and step length (anterior-posterior) fluctuations from stride to stride, is increased in people with PD and seen even early in the disease before the onset of shortened step length.[60,61] Asymmetry of arm swing (an early sign of abnormal gait in PD), step length and time are increased in people with PD and may partially relate to the asymmetric onset of bradykinesia and rigidity.[62] All three components of postural control, achieving, maintaining, and restoring balance, are impaired in people with PD.[30] Postural sway is increased, particularly in the medio-lateral direction, and limits of stability (peak displacement of center of mass [COM] without changing base of support) are decreased in standing especially in the backward direction, which is seen even in very early disease.[63,64] In addition, people with PD have slow and small preparatory balance adjustments for an upcoming voluntary movement (anticipatory postural adjustment; APA). These reduced APAs contribute to the delayed step initiation and narrowed stance/step commonly seen in those with PD.[65] For example, in order to step with the right foot one must first shift COM laterally toward that side in order to subsequently shift COM toward the stance side and allow right swing. The PD-related narrowed stance and slowed and small lateral-shifting APAs contribute to poorer gait initiation and balance during gait. Balance while walking is a complex temporal coupling of trunk control and stepping (posture and gait).[66]

Episodic gait disturbances refer to the intermittent, unpredictable and context-specific characteristics of *festination* (unintentionally rapid short steps) and *freezing of gait* (FOG) (trembling of the legs and transient inability to effectively step, or absence of leg movement/akinesia, described as being "stuck to the ground").[59] Gait can be *anteropulsive* (a forward festinating gait) or *retropulsive* (a backward festinating gait), typically seen when the individual is attempting to regain balance lost backward and is often unsuccessful. Freezing episodes affect 26% of people with mild PD and 80% of those with severe PD.[67,68] FOG can be triggered by confrontation of competing stimuli. For example, the patient slows and stops walking when exposed to a narrowed space, an obstacle or even a visual barrier such as a hallway, doorway, or change in flooring pattern. These freezing behaviors are consistent with findings from brain imaging studies in people with PD that indicate those with FOG have disruptions in the "executive-attention" and visual neural networks, compared with those who do not freeze.[26,69] The cognitive aspects that contribute to freezing are inhibition, attention, and visuospatial functions.[70] Stress and increased cognitive load, such as when dual-tasking, can exacerbate freezing episodes. Turning or changing direction is particularly difficult and typically accomplished by taking multiple small steps, which itself can elicit festination and freezing episodes.[71] In early disease stage, FOG is generally short in duration and rarely leads to falls. With disease progression FOG becomes more frequent and disabling, often leading to falls.[36,58,72] Patients who are in the "off" medication state experience increased FOG and deterioration in gait performance whereas gait patterns often improve with "on" medication levels. Most patients with mild gait deficits can compensate at least partially using external cues and attentional and self-cueing strategies.[72] Problems with controlling posture and balance limit independence, community ambulation, and safety.

Nonmotor Symptoms

Typically a person with PD will experience from 8 to 13 nonmotor symptoms (NMSs), regardless of the motor stage or duration of disease.[1,73] Seventeen NMSs are more common in early nonmedicated PD patients than adults of the same age without PD. Fifteen of these NMSs are associated in 4 clusters: (1) rapid eye movement sleep behavior disorder (RBD) symptoms (frequent nightmares, dream-enacting behaviors) and constipation, (2) cognition-related (memory complaints, fatigue, inattention, excessive daytime sleepiness), (3) mood-related (anhedonia, apathy, mood disturbance), and (4) sensory and disautonomia (taste loss, chest pain, unexplained pain, excessive sweating, postprandial fullness) clusters. The most commonly reported early onset NMSs (from 2 to >10 years before motor symptoms) are smell loss, constipation, RBD symptoms and mood disorders.[74]

Sensory Symptoms

Patients with PD do not suffer from primary sensory loss. However, 60% to 80% experience paresthesias and pain as early symptoms PD, including sensations of numbness, tingling, cold, aching pain, and burning.[75,76] Pain related to PD presents in five classifications: musculoskeletal, dystonic, neuropathic/radicular, central or primary, *akathisia* (a feeling of inner restlessness and an inability to remain still).[75] The pathophysiology of PD-related pain is not clear, but likely is complex and multifaceted. Central or primary pain may be due to abnormal modulation of pain cause by dopamine deficiency in the basal ganglia.[75] Pain is most commonly reported in the lower back and legs, and shoulders, but can also affect the face, head, mouth, pharynx, and internal/visceral regions.[75] Symptoms are typically intermittent, and vary in intensity and location, often starting or being more severe on the side of the appearance of the first motor symptoms. Hypersensitivity to pain (*hyperalgesia*) is common and is linked to the motor fluctuations experienced during levodopa therapy (e.g., pain is more intense in an "off" state).[77] Pain may also be increased in patients experiencing depression.[1]

Proprioceptive regulation of voluntary movement and integration of somatosensory inputs may also be impaired. Patients with PD perform significantly worse than do control subjects on tests of kinesthesia and proprioceptive position sense for the limbs and the trunk. Without visual guidance, patients demonstrate increased difficulty in accurately perceiving the extent of movement, consistently underscaling their movements.[78,79] Combined with the deficits in visuospatial skills that are common in PD, kinesthetic and proprioceptive impairments can contribute to balance and motor control problems. Patients demonstrate significantly more errors than normal on visual perception tasks involving spatial organization.

Olfactory dysfunction is common, with some studies showing up to 100% of patients affected. Most patients with PD report a decline or loss of sense of smell (*anosmia*), often years before motor symptoms develop. Loss of smell therefore has important implications for diagnosis of early disease. It also increases the difficulty individuals have in maintaining a healthy diet and adequate nutrition.[1]

Visual perception disturbances are reported in over 70% of people with PD. These include visual hallucinations; misjudging objects and distances; impaired contrast sensitivity; abnormal color discrimination; peripheral visual disturbance; impaired face and emotion recognition; altered detection of visual motion, line orientation, pattern and depth perception; and oculomotor changes, particularly with voluntary saccades.[80] Smooth pursuit movements may have a jerky quality. Decreased blinking can produce bloodshot, irritated eyes that burn and itch. Conventional drugs (e.g., anticholinergic drugs) used in PD can also cause visual disturbances (e.g., blurred vision and sensitivity to light [photophobia]). These drugs can worsen the normal visual changes associated with aging (presbyopia).

Dysphagia

Dysphagia, impaired swallowing, is present in as many as 95% of patients and is the result of rigidity, reduced mobility, and restricted range of movement.[81] It is often an early symptom of the disease though it is present in all stages.[82] Individuals with PD experience problems in all four phases of swallowing: oral preparatory, oral, pharyngeal, and esophageal. Thus, the patient demonstrates abnormal tongue control and problems with chewing, bolus formation, delayed swallow response, and peristalsis. Dysphagia can lead to choking or aspiration pneumonia and impaired nutrition with significant weight loss. Nutritional inadequacy can contribute to the fatigue and exhaustion typically experienced by patients with PD. Patients also typically experience excessive drooling (*sialorrhea*) because of increased saliva production and decreased spontaneous swallowing. Drooling is particularly problematic while sleeping or initiating speech and in advanced cases increases the risk of aspiration. Excessive drooling has important negative social implications.[82]

Speech Disorders

Speech is impaired in 90% of people with PD and is the result of primary symptoms of PD (rigidity, bradykinesia, hypokinesia, and tremor).[83] People with PD experience *hypokinetic dysarthria,* which is characterized by decreased voice volume, monotone/monopitch speech, imprecise or distorted articulation, and uncontrolled speech rate. Vocal quality is degraded with speech described as hoarse, breathy, and harsh. In addition, patients experience timing difficulty of vocal onsets and offsets. Reduced mobility, restricted range, and uncontrolled rate of movement of muscles controlling respiration, phonation, resonation, and articulation are present. Reduced vital capacity results in reduced air expended during phonation. In advanced cases, the patient may speak in whispers or not at all, demonstrating *mutism.* Sensory problems may also contribute to speech difficulties. Patients who are instructed to upscale their speech sounds to produce increased volume consistently describe their speech as "too loud." Speech difficulties contribute to social isolation and impaired activity participation.[82,83]

Cognitive Dysfunction

Impairment in cognitive function is subtly present from the earliest stages of PD and prior to beginning medication (*de novo*).[84,85] Compared with similarly-aged healthy controls, most people with early stage PD demonstrate executive dysfunction (deficits in cognitive processing speed, attention and set-shifting, verbal fluency, planning and abstract reasoning), and almost half have visuospatial and verbal and visual memory deficits.[85-87] *Mild cognitive impairment* (*MCI*) is a state between normal cognition and early dementia. The frequency of MCI due to PD (*PD-MCI*) in newly diagnosed is between 15% and 40% and predicts an increased risk of dementia within 5 years.[88] Although many people with PD-MCI during the first year after diagnosis went on to develop *PD dementia* (*PDD*), about 25% of patients with PD-MCI actually reverted to normal cognition by the fifth year.[88] The reasons for this are unclear but appear to be related to early diagnosis and treatment. The incidence of PD-MCI is 7% per year and increases to >10% per year in patients diagnosed at 65 years and older. Older patients appear to be at greatest risk for progressing to dementia, with reported rates 4.4 times higher for individuals 80 years of age or older.[86,87] The conversion from PD-MCI to PDD is characterized by deterioration of previous impairments and the development of language deficits (aphasia symptoms and confrontation naming/word-retrieval difficulties).[86] Dementia is associated with increased mortality rates. Coexisting Alzheimer's disease and multi-infarct dementia secondary to atherosclerotic disease are also common in the elderly and may be contributory factors in some patients. Dementia associated with PD is characterized by progression of impairments seen in PD-MCI. *Bradyphrenia,* slowed thinking, is seen in patients with PD and may be one of the early nonspecific features of the disease. Cognitive performance is degraded in the "off" state. Hallucinations, delusions, and psychosis are common complications owing to levodopa toxicity.

Depression, Anxiety, and Apathy

Depression is one of the first NMSs to appear in people with PD. Major depression is reported to occur in approximately 40% of patients and subclinical depression in nearly 55% of those in early stage PD.[89] A significant number of patients develop depression before or just after onset of motor symptoms, suggesting an endogenous cause that may be related to genetic mutations associated with PD, underlying deficiencies of dopamine, serotonin, and norepinephrine.[89] Patients demonstrate a variety of symptoms, including feelings of guilt, hopelessness, and worthlessness; loss of energy; poor concentration; deficits in short-term memory; loss of ambition or enthusiasm; and disturbances in appetite and sleep. Suicidal thoughts may also be present. Hypomimia, a reduction in facial expressiveness, can give the appearance of depression. Patients can also demonstrate *dysthymic disorder* characterized by chronic depression and dysphoric mood, resulting in poor appetite or overeating, insomnia or hypersomnia, low energy, low self-esteem, and poor concentration.

Anxiety is a common symptom in PD with a prevalence of 31%. Clinically patients may present with symptoms of a panic attack (e.g., palpitations, sweating, trembling, shortness of breath, and so forth) as well as social phobia (social withdrawal), agoraphobia, obsessive-compulsive disorder, or panic disorder. Anxiety symptoms may not be simply related to the psychological or social difficulties patients experience, but due to specific neurobiological processes associated with the disease. Patients who are in the "off" medication state experience significant worsening of depression and anxiety.[90]

Apathy is characterized by decreased motivation, a reduction in goal-directed behavior, and includes affective, cognitive, and behavioral aspects. Apathy is found in 20% to 36% of people newly diagnosed with PD who have not begun medication treatment. The frequency appears to decrease with the onset of dopaminergic therapy and increases again after 5 to 10 years of disease to 40% in patients without dementia and to 60% in PDD.[91]

Autonomic Dysfunction

Autonomic dysfunction occurs early in PD and is a direct manifestation of the disease, as evidenced by the presence of Lewy bodies found in the autonomic nervous system and relationship to disease progression. Thermoregulatory dysfunction includes *hyperhidrosis* (excessive sweating) and abnormal or uncomfortable sensations of warmth and coldness. Patients in the "off" state experience impaired peripheral vasodilation with difficulty dissipating body heat. *Seborrhea* (increased oil secretion of the sebaceous glands of the skin) and *seborrheic dermatitis* (oily, chafing, and reddened skin) are also common. Patients with PD exhibit abnormally slow pupillary responses to light and pain and reduced overall response to changes in light.[92-94]

Gastrointestinal disorders include poor motility (impaired gastric emptying occurs in up to 70% to 100%), changes in appetite, inadequate hydration, sialorrhea, and weight loss.[95] *Constipation* is a common problem for most patients and typically occurs early in PD. *Urinary incontinence* occurs with associated symptoms of urinary frequency, urgency, and nocturia. Most individuals with PD report changes in libido, *erectile dysfunction* in males and *anorgasmia* in females, including impotence and reduced rates of sexual activity.[92-94]

Early and progressive sympathetic denervation of the heart occurs in most people with PD. This results in diminished heart function, which may be a contributory factor to the fatigue that most patients experience. People with mild to moderate PD exhibit blunted cardiovascular and metabolic responses to peak exercise (lower heart rate [HR], oxygen uptake [VO_2] and systolic blood pressure [SBP]) compared with their healthy peers. The motor limitations of PD may create a higher energy demand at the same absolute workload than for people without PD. Taking this into account, studies of submaximal exercise using ventilator thresholds as indicators of *relative* levels of intensity show that HR is lower and Vo_2 and SBP are similar to healthy adults at this similar intensity. Thus, the blunted response to exercise in people with PD is present even at submaximal levels of exercise and worsens with increased intensity of exercise.[96,97]

Orthostatic hypotension (OH) is common in middle and late PD and is caused by a sharp drop in BP (20 mm Hg systolic and 10 mm Hg diastolic within 3 min) that occurs with position changes (e.g., supine-to-sit or sit-to-stand). Typical symptoms include light-headedness or dizziness. Patients can also experience pallor, diaphoresis, weakness, trembling, nausea, difficulty thinking, or syncope. The condition puts individuals at risk for loss of balance, falls, and fall injury. Medications (e.g., levodopa/carbidopa, bromocriptine) can contribute to orthostatic hypotension.[93]

Patients with PD demonstrate respiratory impairments, reported in as many as 84% of patients. *Airway obstruction* (e.g., air trapping, lung insufflation) is the most frequently reported pulmonary problem and has been linked to episodes of pulmonary failure. The etiology remains unknown but may be linked to bradykinetic disorganization of respiratory movements. *Restrictive lung dysfunction* is common and is linked to the decreased chest expansion that occurs because of rigidity of the trunk muscles, loss of musculoskeletal flexibility, and kyphotic posture. Patients with PD demonstrate lower forced vital capacity (FVC), lower forced expiratory volume in 1 second (FEV_1), and higher residual volume (RV) and residual airway resistance (RAW) values when compared with age-matched controls. Daily function and activity participation are reduced in patients with pulmonary dysfunction.[98-100] A sedentary lifestyle with decreased activity levels contributes to cardiopulmonary deconditioning.

Sleep Disorders

Individuals with PD can experience *excessive daytime somnolence* (sleepiness). At night, *insomnia* (disturbed sleep pattern) may occur. This includes problems in falling asleep, staying asleep, and good quality of sleep. REM sleep behavior disorder (RBD) occurs early in the prodromal phase of PD (prior to motor signs appearing), affects as many as 50% to 60% of patients and is the biomarker with the highest diagnostic strength potential.[101] In a person with RBD, the paralysis that normally occurs during REM sleep is incomplete or absent, allowing the person to "act out" his or her dreams that are vivid, intense, and violent. Dream-enacting behaviors include agitation and physical activity during sleep (e.g., talking, yelling, punching, kicking, arm flailing, and grabbing).[1] Box 18.2 provides a summary of the cardinal features and clinical manifestations of PD.

MEDICAL DIAGNOSIS

Diagnosis at onset of PD is difficult with accurate diagnosis possible only with continued observation of evolving clinical motor and nonmotor signs and symptoms. There is no single definitive test or group of tests used to diagnose the disease. The diagnosis is made based on history and clinical examination. The most widely accepted clinical criteria for diagnosis of PD, introduced in 1992 by the Parkinson's Disease Society UK Brain Bank criteria, focus on motor symptoms and exclude NMSs which are now know to be central to PD.[102] To address this issue, in 2015 the Movement Disorder Society (MDS) proposed a revised set of criteria for PD diagnosis that retains the original motor criteria and now includes NMS in determining the likelihood that the motor syndrome is specific to PD. The MDS Clinical Diagnostic Criteria for Parkinson's Disease identifies parkinsonism (bradykinesia plus rest tremor or rigidity) as the core feature of the disease.[103] Then, determining PD as the cause of parkinsonism relies on three categories of diagnostic features: (1) absolute exclusion criteria ruling out PD, (2) red flags that are potential signs that

Box 18.2 Cardinal Features and Clinical Manifestations of Parkinson's Disease

Cardinal Features

- Rigidity
- Bradykinesia/Akinesia
- Tremor
- Postural instability

Clinical Manifestations

Motor Performance

- Decreased torque production
- Fatigue
- Contractures and deformity common
- Masked face
- Micrographia
- Hypometria / undershooting target with limbs and with gaze

Motor Planning

- Start hesitation
- Freezing episodes
- Poverty of movement
- Visuomotor transformation difficulties

Motor Learning

- Slower learning rates, reduced efficiency
- Increased context-specificity of learning; impaired contextual flexibility
- Procedural learning deficits for complex and sequential tasks

Gait

- Reduced stride length; increased step-to-step variability
- Reduced step width
- Reduced speed of walking
- Cadence (steps per minute) typically intact; may be reduced in advanced PD
- Increased time: double-limb support
- Insufficient hip, knee, and ankle flexion: shuffling steps
- Insufficient heel strike with increased forefoot loading
- Reduced trunk rotation: decreased or absent arm swing
- Festinating gait: anteropulsion common
- Freezing of gait (FOG)
- Difficulty turning: increased steps per turn
- Difficulty stepping backward: retropulsion or decreased step initiation
- Difficulty sidestepping: decreased step initiation and narrowed steps
- Difficulty with dual-tasking: simultaneous motor and/or cognitive tasks
- Difficulty with attentional demands of complex environments

Posture

- Kyphosis with forward head and scapular protraction
- Leaning to one side with tonal asymmetries
- Increased fall risk

Sensation

- Paresthesias
- Pain
- Akathisia
- Proprioceptive and kinesthetic deficits

Speech, Voice, and Swallowing Disorders

- Hypokinetic dysarthria
- Dysphagia

Cognition and Behavior

- Dementia
- Bradyphrenia
- Visuospatial deficits
- Depression
- Dysphoric mood
- Apathy
- Anxiety

Autonomic Nervous System

- Excessive sweating
- Abnormal sensations of heat and cold
- Seborrhea
- Sialorrhea
- Constipation
- Urinary bladder dysfunction
- Orthostatic hypotension

Cardiopulmonary Function

- Low resting blood pressure (BP)
- Compromised cardiovascular response to exercise
- Impaired respiratory function

may rule out PD, and (3) supportive criteria that lend support to the diagnosis of PD, such as clear and dramatic benefit from dopaminergic therapy. Using these criteria, diagnosis can be made of either *clinically probable PD* or *clinically established PD*.[103] Exclusion of Parkinson-plus syndromes is necessary. The presence of extrapyramidal signs that are bilaterally symmetrical and do not respond to levodopa and dopamine agonists (apomorphine test) is suggestive of these syndromes, not PD. Imaging can be used to rule out other pathologies. In vivo functional imaging (magnetic resonance imaging [MRI]) using chemical markers to identify dopaminergic deficits in PD and related disorders identifies dopamine deficiency but does not discriminate between PD and other causes of parkinsonism. Handwriting samples, speech analysis, interview questions that focus on developing symptoms, and physical examination are used. In the prodromal stage, nonmotor symptoms predominate. There is an increasing focus on use of questionnaires and tests (e.g., olfactory testing, imaging of cardiac sympathetic innervation) that focus on nonmotor symptoms. Often symptoms of loss of smell, sleep disturbances, vivid dreams with REM alterations, foot dystonia and foot cramping, restless legs syndrome, orthostatic hypotension, and constipation are symptoms that are present many years before a clinical diagnosis of PD is made.[73,104-106]

■ CLINICAL COURSE

The disease is progressive, with a long preclinical period (without apparent clinical manifestations) estimated to be 5 to 25 years.[101] Mean PD duration is approximately 10 to 20 years with a life expectancy nearly that of the general population. There is variability of the rate of progression. Patients with a young age at onset or who are tremor predominant typically demonstrate a slower progression. Patients with PD who present with postural instability and gait disturbances (the PIGD group) tend to have more pronounced deterioration with a more rapid disease progression. Neurobehavioral disturbances and dementia are also more common in this group.[107] With dopaminergic therapy, progression is generally slower with an overall improvement in mortality rates. The most common causes of death are cardiovascular disease and pneumonia.[108]

Hoehn and Yahr Classification of Disability Scale

An estimate of the stage and severity of the disease can be made using a staging scale. The most widely used in clinical practice and research trials is the *Hoehn and Yahr Classification of Disability Scale* (H & Y) (Table 18.1).[109] It provides a broad measure for charting the progression of the disease using motor signs and elements of functional status. H & Y Stage I is used to indicate minimal disease involvement, whereas H & Y Stage V is indicative of severe deterioration in which the patient is confined to bed or a wheelchair.

Table 18.1 Hoehn and Yahr Classification of Disability[109]

Stage	Character of Disability
I	Minimal or absent; unilateral if present.
II	Minimal bilateral or midline involvement. Balance not impaired.
III	Impaired righting reflexes. Unsteadiness when turning or rising from chair. Some activities are restricted, but patient can live independently and continue some forms of employment.
IV	All symptoms present and severe. Standing and walking possible only with assistance.
V	Confined to bed or wheelchair.

Movement Disorders Society Unified Parkinson's Disease Rating Scale

The *Unified Parkinson's Disease Rating Scale (UPDRS)* has been the "gold standard" for measuring the progression of PD since 1987.[110] Goetz and colleagues reported on a modification of this scale renamed the Movement Disorder Society–sponsored revision of the Unified Parkinson's Disease Rating Scale (MDS-UPDRS).[28,111] The goals of the revision were to improve ability to detect slower and smaller changes in mildly disabled patients and increase focus on nonmotor symptoms. Descriptors are added for each question. Parts I and II have been renamed: Part I is now *Non-motor Aspects of Experiences of Daily Living* and Part II is now *Motor Experiences of Daily Living*. Part III is *Motor Examination* (same title) and Part IV is renamed *Motor Complications*.[28] The total time to administer the test is an estimated 30 minutes, with Parts I and II designed to be self-administered by the patient. This instrument can be found at: http://www.movementdisorders.org/MDS-Files1/PDFs/Rating-Scales/MDS-UPDRS_Vol23_Issue15_2008.pdf.

■ MEDICAL MANAGEMENT

Medical management is directed at slowing disease progression using neuroprotective strategies, and symptomatic treatment of motor and nonmotor symptoms. Management becomes increasingly more challenging over time for patients with moderate and advanced disease (i.e., H & Y Stage III or higher).

Pharmacological Management

Several agents are available as first-line neuroprotective and symptomatic therapy. Table 18.2 outlines the current pharmacological agents for treatment of PD, organized by type, mechanism of action, and potential side effects. Selection is individualized according to the patient's characteristics with the benefits and risks of adverse side effects carefully weighed. Starting medication early has been shown to be beneficial in slowing the progression of the disease.[112,113] Drug delivery should be as close to constant as possible to avoid large peaks and valleys. The importance of taking the medication on a fixed schedule should be stressed to patients, family members, and caregivers. When patients with PD are hospitalized it is important that they continue to receive their medication on schedule.[114-116] The *Aware in Care kit* from the National Parkinson Foundation can be helpful for these issues during hospital stays (www.awareincare.org).

Carbidopa/Levodopa

Carbidopa/levodopa (Sinemet®) is the gold standard drug therapy for PD. Levodopa was first introduced in 1961 as an experimental drug and came into widespread clinical use in the late 1960s. It is a dopamine precursor that is

Table 18.2 Pharmacological Agents for Treatment of PD[119,123]

Class / Type and Medication (available in U.S.)	Mechanism of Action	Potential Side Effects
Levodopa **(carbidopa/levodopa in 1:4 ratio)**		
• carbidopa/levodopa (Sinemet®) • controlled-release (Sinemet CR®) • orally disintegrating tablet (Parcopa®) • with entacapone (Stalevo®) • extended-release capsules (Rytary®) • enteral suspension (Duopa®)	Replaces dopamine lost in PD. Carbidopa prevents levodopa from being converted to dopamine until after it crosses blood-brain barrier.	• Low BP • Nausea • Dry mouth • Dizziness • Fluctuations & "wearing-off" of benefit between doses • Dyskinesias
Dopamine Agonists		
• apomorphine (Apokyn®) • bromocriptine (Parlodel®) • pramipexole (Mirapex®) • ropinirole (Requip®) • rotigotine transdermal patch (Neupro®)	Stimulates dopamine receptors in the basal ganglia.	• Low BP • Nausea • Leg swelling • Hallucinations • Sleepiness • Impulse control disorders • Dyskinesias
COMT Inhibitors **(Catechol-O-Methyl Tranferase)**		
• entacapone (Comtan®) • tolcapone (Tasmar®)	Prolongs effects of levodopa by blocking its breakdown in the body. Used to alleviate "wearing-off," the return of PD symptoms between doses.	• Low BP • Nausea • Indigestion • Abdominal pain • Constipation • Back pain • Insomnia • Aggravation of dopaminergic side effects
MAO-B Inhibitors		
• rasagiline (Azilect®) • selegiline or deprenyl (Eldepryl®)	Boosts the effects of levodopa by blocking enzyme in brain that breaks it down. Used early in PD as alternatives to levodopa, and to control mild wearing-off phenomena. Low risk of inducing dyskinesias.[122]	• Low BP • Nausea • Agitation • Insomnia • Dizziness • Headache • Back pain • Mouth sores • Indigestion • Dyskinesias • Hallucinations
Anticholinergics		
• benztropine mesylate (Cogentin®) • trihexyphenidyl (formerly Artane®)	Reduces excessive acetylcholine influence caused by depleted dopamine. May reduce tremor and dystonias. Less commonly used due to many side effects. Central toxicity indicated by impaired memory, confusion, hallucinations, and delusions.	• Blurred vision • Dry mouth • Constipation • Urinary retention • Memory problems

Table 18.2 Pharmacological Agents for Treatment of PD[119,123]—cont'd

Class / Type and Medication (available in U.S.)	Mechanism of Action	Potential Side Effects
Amantadine		
• (Symmetrel®) • (Symadine®)	An antiviral (influenza A) with unknown mechanism for PD, recently found to block effects of glutamate (excitatory amino acid). May reduce dyskinesias.[121]	• Dry mouth • Constipation • Urinary retention • Ankle swelling • Mottled skin rash • Aggravate hallucinations
Norepinephrine Precursors		
• droxidopa (Northera®)	Targets neurogenic orthostatic hypotension by increasing norepinephrine levels.	• Nausea • Headache • Confusion • High BP when lying down
Cholinesterase Inhibitors		
• rivastigmine tartrate (Exelon®)	Inhibits enzymes that breakdown acetylcholine. Used to improve memory function and gait stability.[123]	• Diarrhea • Dizziness • Weakness • Drowsiness • Insomnia • Increased sweating • Loss of appetite • Nausea
Atypical Antipsychotics		
• pimavanserin (Nuplazid®)	Blocks some effects from serotonin. Used to reduce hallucinations and psychosis from side effects of other PD medications.[124]	• Leg swelling • Nausea • Confusion • Constipation • Difficulty walking

BP = blood pressure

metabolized to dopamine in the brain. Thus, administration of the drug represents an attempt to correct the essential neurochemical imbalance. Most of levodopa (almost 99%) is metabolized before reaching the brain, requiring administration of high doses that can produce numerous side effects. Today, levodopa is commonly administered with carbidopa, a decarboxylase inhibitor that allows a higher percentage of levodopa to enter the brain. Thus, lower doses of levodopa can be used with fewer adverse side effects. Sinemet® is available in immediate-release (IR) and controlled-release (CR) formulations. The IR form has a short half-life requiring multiple oral dosing throughout the day. The CR form is a long-acting, sustained-release preparation. Both are equally effective.[117-119]

The primary benefits of dopamine replacement include controlling the PD motor symptoms of bradykinesia and rigidity. Increased movement velocity, initial burst of motor activity, and increased strength are all positive outcomes.[119] The effects on reduction of tremor are varied. Some individuals demonstrate little or no response to levodopa whereas others demonstrate a positive reduction in tremor amplitude. The "on" state refers to the motor state when tremor, akinesia or rigidity symptoms have improved with the medication, typically 20 to 60 minutes after dosing. The "off" state applies to the motor state when the patient experiences tremor, akinesia, or rigidity because no medication or not enough was taken, or because the medication taken is not effective.

Symptoms that are less or non-responsive to dopaminergic therapy include postural instability, freezing, speech abnormalities, cognitive changes, dementia, depression, sensory abnormalities, and many autonomic dysfunctions.[117] However, these variations in responsiveness of different symptoms to levodopa may in fact be due to *relative* under- or over-dosing.[87,117] Different regions of the basal ganglia-thalamocortical circuitry (the motor, cognitive, affective, and behavioral "loops" discussed in the Pathophysiology section) are thought to be affected by dopaminergic loss along a gradient of depletion. This *gradient of dopaminergic depletion* is thought to be greatest in the dorsal striatum involving the "motor loop" and weakest in the ventral striatum involving the "affective loop." [87] For example, freezing is a symptom that abates at a higher dosage of levodopa than is typically given to alleviate bradykinesia or rigidity.[72] At the other end of the dopamine-depletion gradient for which there is not as much loss of dopamine are circuits for mood and behavioral symptoms (e.g., gambling, reversal learning). These symptoms are effectively "overdosed" at the therapeutic level for cardinal motor symptoms.[87] The decision about when to start levodopa/carbidopa is determined by the neurologist and is different for every person. Initial dosing improves low levels of levodopa often with dramatic improvements in functional status.

Complications of chronic dopamine replacement therapy include motor fluctuations, dyskinesias and dystonias. As the disease progresses the window becomes smaller between therapeutic benefit (4 to 6 years) and motor complications when the optimal benefit wears off (termed *wearing-off state*). Motor fluctuations include both the "on–off" phenomenon and wearing-off. The term *"on–off" phenomenon* refers to abrupt, random fluctuations in motor performance and responses. Production of movement errors is common. *Wearing-off* refers to *end-of-dose deterioration*, a worsening of symptoms toward the end of the expected timeframe of medication effectiveness. The levodopa-related motor fluctuations are further complicated by disease severity and duration.[117,120,121] Early in the disease, remaining dopaminergic neurons act to store the dopamine converted from the therapeutically administered levodopa. The neurons buffer the pulsatile aspect of taking levodopa medication and allow for gradual release of dopamine and a more stable motor response. As the disease progresses and more dopaminergic neurons have disappeared there is less buffer storage capacity for the administered medication. As this happens, the effects of dopamine more directly follow the fluctuating (pulsatile) blood levels of levodopa medication, and more frequent dosing is needed to keep an adequate and constant level of dopamine. These unbuffered peaks of dopamine concentration in the basal ganglia lead to drug-induced hyperkinetic movements (levodopa-induced dyskinesia).[120]

Levodopa-Induced Dyskinesias (LID) are dynamic uncontrolled or involuntary movements that include choreic, athetotic, dystonic, and ballistic qualities. They are described based on their pattern of appearance within the "on–off" cycle of medication state. *Peak dose* or *"on"* state dyskinesia occurs with high plasma levels of levodopa when the patient has the maximum benefit of reducing akinesia and rigidity. These are often choreic in quality and are seen in the neck, face, trunk, and upper limbs. *Diphasic dyskinesia* appears when the patient is transitioning between "on" and "off" states when the plasma levels of levodopa are rising or falling. These dyskinetic movements are more repetitive, slow, and stereotyped, or resemble ballisms and can affect walking and balance. Risk factors for developing dyskinesias within 5 years of treatment include duration of levodopa therapy and younger age of onset of PD. LID occurs in 50% of those with age of onset of 40 to 59 years, 25% with age of onset of 60 to 69 years, and 16% after the age of 70 years.[121,122]

Dystonia, a prolonged involuntary contraction that causes twisting or torsion of body segments, can also occur. The patient typically complains of clawing of the toes or fingers, or cramping of the calf, neck, face, or paraspinal muscles. Dystonia is associated with pain and occurs typically during "off" periods. Patients may experience akathisia and significant disruptions in sleep and relaxation. This affects as many as 25% of patients and is relieved with movement (e.g., walking). *Akathisia* is associated with advanced PD and is more commonly seen in the "off" state.

Unsupervised reduction or sudden discontinuation of levodopa/carbidopa is contraindicated and may produce dangerous, life-threatening adverse effects. Adverse interactions can occur with several medications, including antacids, antiseizure drugs, antihypertensives, and antidepressants.[119]

Patients may also experience other changes that are dose related and may indicate the need for drug modification. These include (1) disabling psychiatric toxicity (visual hallucinations, delusions, and paranoia); (2) depression; (3) gastrointestinal changes (nausea, dry mouth); (4) cardiovascular changes (hypotension, dizziness, arrhythmias); (5) genitourinary changes (dysuria); and (6) sleep disturbances (insomnia, sleep fragmentation).[119]

Dopamine Agonists

Dopamine agonists (DAs) are a class of drugs designed to directly stimulate postsynaptic dopamine receptors. They are administered alone as a first-line monotherapy or along with levodopa/carbidopa, allowing lower doses to be administered with prolonged effectiveness. The greatest benefit of these drugs is reducing rigidity, bradykinesia, and motor fluctuations. Adverse effects are similar to those of levodopa with nausea, sedation, dizziness, constipation, and hallucinations being the most common. These medications have also been linked to an increased risk of impulse control disorders (see above for discussion of *relative overdosing*; e.g., pathological gambling, compulsive shopping, hypersexuality, overeating).[119]

Other Agents

The other categories of pharmacological agents that are used in the treatment of PD include catechol-o-methyltransferase (COMT) inhibitors, monoamine oxidase B (MAO-B) inhibitors, anticholinergic agents, and amantadine. Norepinephrine precursors target orthostatic hypotension, cholinesterase inhibitors target memory function and gait stability, and atypical antipsychotics are used to treat hallucinations and psychosis.[119] Refer to Table 18.2 for details.

Implications for the Physical Therapist

The therapist needs to be fully aware of each of the medications the patient is taking and potential adverse effects. It is important to remember that patients on dopamine replacement will develop motor complications at some point. Optimal performance can be expected at peak dosage whereas worsening performance is associated with end-of-dose cycle and medication depletion.[117,120] Timing of physical therapy examination and intervention should be consistent and occur whenever possible during optimal dosing cycle. Therapists are involved in monitoring drug effectiveness on motor performance, function, and activity participation. As the disease progresses, patients may develop an intolerance for a medication, necessitating a change in prescription. Often, it is the therapist who first notices a change in functional status as the patient's system adapts to either the amount or type of drug prescribed. Accurate observation, examination, and reporting of these changes greatly assists the physician in modifying a drug prescription. Therapists may also be involved with clinical drug trials as new medications or combinations are developed.

Nutritional Management

A high-protein diet can block the effectiveness of levodopa. The dietary amino acids in protein compete with levodopa absorption. This is particularly problematic in patients with chronic disease who exhibit fluctuations in motor performance. Thus, patients are generally advised to follow a high-calorie, low-protein diet. Generally, no more than 15% of calories should come from protein. Dietary recommendations may also include shifting the intake of daily protein to the evening meal when patients are less active. These modifications minimize motor fluctuations and maximize responsiveness to levodopa therapy. Patients are also advised to increase their daily intake of water and dietary fiber to help control problems of constipation.

Rigidity and bradykinesia can limit upright posture and UE feeding movements. Learned motor plans, for example, using a cup or eating utensils, may also be difficult. Occupational therapy intervention to improve feeding and recommend adaptive eating devices is of considerable importance in helping to maintain nutrition and general health status. The speech-language pathologist also has an important role in the evaluation of dysphagia and the recommendation of strategies to assist with swallowing dysfunction. Patient, family, and caregiver education should focus on the importance of maintaining good nutritional intake. Percutaneous endoscopic gastrostomy (PEG) is reserved for advanced disease when all other strategies for dysphagia fail.

Deep Brain Stimulation

Deep brain stimulation (DBS) involves the implantation of electrodes into the brain where stimulation of a relatively small area can result in network-wide changes that can improve symptoms of PD.[125] While the exact mechanisms of symptom improvement by DBS are unknown, it is believed that cell bodies close to the electrodes are inhibited, axons are excited, neurochemical changes are triggered, neurovascular and neurogenic changes are induced, and changes in the oscillatory behavior of certain groups of neurons of the basal ganglia appear to play important roles.[125,126] Brain electrodes are most often placed in the subthalamic nucleus (STN) or the globus pallidus internus (GPi) with the location being chosen according to individual patient needs. The GPi is considered if there are dyskinesias, cognitive or behavioral concerns; whereas the STN might be considered if medication reduction is the goal.[125] More recently the pedunculopontine nucleus (PPN) and substantia nigra have been explored as targets for DBS to specifically improve gait and balance difficulties that are unresponsive to medication and DBS in the STN or GPi.[125] An impulse generator (IPG), similar to a pacemaker, is implanted in the subclavicular area and a thin wire goes under the skin to connect to the brain electrodes. High-frequency stimulation is provided. The patient can control the pacemaker's "on–off" switch using a controller while the physician determines the amount of stimulation it delivers, tailoring it to the individual's needs.

DBS in either the STN or GPi have shown overall improvements in tremor and motor symptoms particularly in the off-periods. Advantages of the STN target for DBS are greater medication reduction early after implantation and less frequent IPG battery changes. DBS of the GPi has the advantage of a more robust suppression of dyskinesias, greater flexibility of medication adjustments long-term, and easier programming DBS parameters to optimize effects. Other motor symptoms of akinesia, rigidity, weakness, and reduced walking speed may improve with DBS though the responses are more variable across individuals. Adverse effects can include confusion, depression, headache, speech problems, gait disturbances, and falling. Surgical risks (intracerebral hemorrhage, infection) and mechanical problems with the device (lead breakage, generator malfunction) are also possible.[125-129]

The most critical factor for successful DBS outcomes is selection of appropriate patients. DBS is effective for the treatment of PD in 10% to 20% of patients that are screened as good candidates. Levodopa responsiveness is considered the single best predictor of DBS outcome. Symptoms that are under- or unresponsive to levodopa (gait, postural instability, speech, and posture) will likely not improve with DBS and may in fact worsen. A multidisciplinary evaluation is important for uncovering potential risks and benefits and to individualize alternative approaches. These teams include the neurologist, neurosurgeon, psychologist, psychiatrist, speech-language pathologists, and physical and occupational therapists. After separate evaluations by each team member the decision to reject or to recommend DBS surgery is made.[125-129]

FRAMEWORK FOR REHABILITATION

Rehabilitation has an important role in reducing activity limitations while promoting activity participation and independence. In addition, known complications of PD can be reduced or prevented while quality of life is promoted. Optimal management involves a coordinated interdisciplinary team to oversee a comprehensive plan of care to address the patient's individual clinical problems, concerns, and needs. The team typically includes the physician, nurse, physical therapist, occupational therapist, speech-language pathologist, and social worker. Referral to other specialists may also be necessary, for example, psychologist, nutritionist, gastroenterologist, urologist, or pulmonologist. As with any team, the patient is the central figure with family and caregivers being key members.

The ideal rehabilitation program considers the patient's age of onset, disease history, course, and symptoms, together with impairments, activity limitations, and participation restrictions. Of equal importance are the patient's abilities (assets), priorities, and resources, including family, home, work, and community resources. Eventual medication-induced fluctuations in performance and deterioration of condition should be expected, but early intervention with moderate to high physical activity can slow this deterioration. Depression and anxiety are common and should be carefully monitored. The overall focus is on improving level of physical activity and associated health behavior changes throughout all stages of the disease, followed by long-range planning, with anticipated episodes of care including hospital-based, outpatient, and home/community-based care.

Therapeutic Care Continuum

A therapeutic care continuum based on disease stage (early, middle, late) is an effective way to organize care.[130] Interventions are restorative (aimed at improving impairments, activity limitations, and participation restrictions), preventive (aimed at minimizing potential complications and indirect impairments), and compensatory (aimed at modifying the task, activity, or environment to improve function) (see discussion in Chapter 1). It is critical for the whole team to provide a supportive environment to assist patients and their family members in the difficult adjustment to living with a chronic and progressive disease. This approach and focus on the relief of symptoms, pain, and stress of a serious illness, called *palliative care*, is misunderstood as end-of-life care. However, palliative care is appropriate throughout *all* stages of the disease and can be provided in parallel with curative treatments with the goal of improved quality of life for patients and families.[131,132]

In the *early* stage of the disease, patients are functional and independent with minimal impairments. Traditionally, referral for physical therapy has been delayed at this stage, although benefits could clearly be obtained in improving fitness levels and delaying or preventing indirect impairments. Recently results of multidisciplinary intensive rehabilitation in newly diagnosed individuals with PD have suggested that early and intensive exercise might slow the progression of motor decline, delay the need for increasing drug treatment, and therefore have a neuroprotective effect.[133,134] Patients in early stage are typically seen on an outpatient basis.

During the *middle* stage of the disease, symptoms are more apparent and activity limitations emerge. The patient may still be independent in gait and ADL, although performance is slowed and less efficient. Some assistance may be required. The patient may be seen as an outpatient, during home care, or during a brief inpatient admission. There are numerous benefits to rehabilitation services. Exercise training programs have been shown to be effective for patients with mild to moderate PD in improving motor performance.[133-138] Perceived quality of life and subjective well-being are also improved.[139] Family and caregiver instruction is intensified to assist the patient in remaining as functionally independent as possible.

In the *late* stage, disease progression leads to increased and more severe impairments and complications. Patients are dependent in many or most of their daily functional mobility skills and ADL and are typically wheelchair bound or bedridden. Family and community resources are vital in maintaining the patient in the home. Some patients may require placement in a chronic care facility. These changes can be a source of great anxiety and frustration to the patient and family. Goals need to be restructured. The therapist needs to focus on preventive care to avoid secondary complications that may be life-threatening (e.g., pneumonia, pressure ulcers). Compensatory training focuses on maintaining function, including being upright and out of bed as much as possible. Safety for both the caregiver and the patient becomes a primary concern as maximal assist dependent transfers become the norm. Often, environmental adaptations may mean the difference between total dependence and modified dependence. The rehabilitation team should be supportive of the patient's efforts no matter how small they may be. Patients in late-stage PD demonstrate extremely limited skills to interact with their environment, with increasing social isolation and withdrawal. Families also suffer from the increasing demands of care, burnout, and social isolation. Therapists need to maximize psychosocial support and be readily available for consultation.

Maintenance therapy is defined as a series of occasional clinical, educational, and administrative services designed to maintain the patient's current level of function. Individuals with PD who benefit from maintenance therapy typically are in the late stages of the disease. Maintenance programs have historically not been well funded by insurance and require careful documentation. The Centers for Medicare & Medicaid Services (CMS), which covers services for the elderly and the disabled, covers maintenance therapy if the *professional skills of a therapist* (specialized knowledge and judgment) are needed to prevent or slow deterioration of a person's condition and maintain the maximal predictable level of function. As the result of a legal settlement agreement on January 24, 2013, in the case of *Jimmo v. Sibelius*, CMS issued a clarification that the coverage of skilled services "does not turn on the presence or absence of a beneficiary's potential for improvement, but rather on the beneficiary's need for skilled care."[140] For example, risk of secondary impairment and loss of functional capabilities is reduced or safety of caregivers is enhanced. A variety of interventions are used to achieve goals and outcomes, including limited direct interventions, patient-related instruction, and supportive counseling. The therapist tapers the frequency of the visits as the patient or family/caregivers can assume independent self-management of the care plan. Recent models of rehabilitation delivery have been proposed which promote routine 6- to 12-month reassessment of function to optimize management of care.[134,135,138] More information on the *Jimmo* settlements and implementation resources can be found on the Academy of Neurologic Physical Therapy (ANPT) website (http://neuropt.org/professional-resources/advocacy/jimmo-implementation-information). Table 18.3 presents an overview of Parkinson's disease stages and intervention strategies.[130]

Table 18.3 Parkinson's Disease Stages, Common Impairments and Activity Limitations, and Intervention Strategies[130]

Stage	Common Impairments and Activity Limitations	Intervention Strategies
Early/Mild PD	• Few/minimal cognitive and motor impairments and activity limitations with independence maintained • Movement symptoms present but do not interfere with daily activities • Movement symptoms, often tremor, occur on one side of the body • Changes noted in posture, walking ability, or facial expression • Parkinson's medications effectively suppress movement symptoms • Nonmotor symptoms present, but usually do not interfere with daily activity	*Preventive and Restorative* • Regular exercise to improve/maintain cognition, motor performance, strength, mobility, flexibility, range of motion (ROM), balance, locomotion, endurance, and perceived quality of life • Community classes to improve/maintain socialization, camaraderie, positive outlook and life purpose *Compensatory* • Patient/family/caregiver education about disease process, rehabilitation, energy conservation • Determine need for adaptive or assistive devices • Determine need for environmental modification of home/workplace • Provide psychological support with early referral to support groups for patient and family/caregiver • Referral to other health care professionals as needed
Middle/ Moderate PD	• Increasing number and severity of cognitive and motor impairments • Minimal to moderate activity limitations, participation restrictions • Nonmotor symptoms increasing in number and severity • Movement symptoms occur on both sides of the body • The body moves more slowly against increasing stiffness • ADL with modified dependence (assistance) • Difficulty with balance, postural instability; stooped posture; increasing number of falls • Gait impairments evident; freezing episodes may occur	*Preventive and Restorative* • Regular exercise to maintain/improve cognition, motor performance, strength, mobility, flexibility, ROM, balance, locomotion, endurance, and perceived quality of life • Community classes to improve/maintain socialization, camaraderie, positive outlook, and life purpose *Compensatory* • Assistive devices to maintain function • Wheelchair for community mobility • Environmental modifications to home • Patient/family/caregiver education and training

Continued

Table 18.3 Parkinson's Disease Stages, Common Impairments and Activity Limitations, and Intervention Strategies[130]—cont'd

Stage	Common Impairments and Activity Limitations	Intervention Strategies
	• Locomotion with modified dependence (assistance) • Parkinson's medications may "wear off" between doses • Parkinson's medications may cause side effects, including dyskinesias	• Psychological support for patient and family/caregiver • Referral to other health care professionals as needed; occupational therapy may provide strategies for maintaining independence

Late/ Advanced PD	• Numerous cognitive and motor impairments with increasing severity
	• Severe activity limitations with dependence in most activities:
	  • Great difficulty walking; typically in wheelchair or bed most of the day
	  • Assistance needed with all ADL
	• Severe participation restrictions:
	  • Not able to live alone
	  • Typically requires full time assistance or placement in chronic care facility
	• Social interactions restricted
	• Cognitive problems may be prominent, including dementia, hallucinations, and delusions
	• Increasing medication intolerance with dyskinesias
	• Balancing the benefits of medications with their side effects becomes more challenging
		Preventive
		• Maximize upright posture, out-of-bed time
		• Maximize participation in activities of daily living
		• Prevention of contractures, pressure wounds, pneumonia, and so forth
		Compensatory
		• Family/caregiver education and training: safety education, transfers, positioning, turning, skin care
		• Pressure relieving devices
		• Hospital bed, wheelchair, mechanical lift
		• Psychological support for patient and family/caregiver
		• Referral to other health care professionals as needed

PHYSICAL THERAPY EXAMINATION AND EVALUATION

A comprehensive examination is required to determine the level of impairments and degree of function. Subsequent re-examination at specified intervals is used to distinguish change in status as well as effects of treatment. Data are obtained from the history, systems review, and relevant tests and measures (Box 18.3).[139] The selection of examination procedures and instruments is determined by the patient's unique status. The severity of problems, stage of disease, age, phase and setting of rehabilitation, and other factors must all be considered in structuring the examination and evaluating data. During the early stages of PD, measures of impairment and physical performance are relatively stable. During middle and late stages of the disease and under conditions of fluctuating symptoms with pharmacological instability, measures can be expected to be less stable. [141]

This section presents strategies for examination as well as relevant tests and measures. Complete descriptions of many of the tests and measures identified are provided in earlier chapters focusing on examination.

Cognitive Function

Learning and memory, visuospatial processing, orientation, conceptual reasoning, problem solving, and judgment should be examined. Speed of information processing, attention, and concentration are particularly important to determine if bradyphrenia is suspected. A brief screen of cognitive function across multiple cognitive domains (visuospatial and executive function, attention, orientation, naming, memory, language, abstraction) can be obtained using the *Montreal Cognitive Assessment (MoCA)*.[142]

Psychosocial Function

The therapist should determine overall levels of depression, stress and anxiety, and available coping strategies. It is important to ask the patient about the presence of symptoms such as sadness, apathy, passivity, insomnia, anorexia, weight loss, inactivity and dependency, inability to concentrate and impaired memory, or suicidal ideation. Instruments recommended for screening and measuring severity of depression in PD include the *Geriatric Depression Scales* (GDS-15 and GDS-30) and the *Hamilton Depression Rating Scale* (HAMD-17).[143-145] Anxiety is prevalent and disabling in this patient

Box 18.3 Elements of the Examination for a Patient With Parkinson's Disease[139]

History

- Demographic information: age, sex, race/ethnicity, primary language, education
- Social history: cultural beliefs and behaviors, family and caregiver resources, social support systems
- Occupation/employment/work information
- Living environment: home/work barriers
- Hand dominance
- General health status: physical, psychological, social, and role function, health habits
- Social and health habits (current and past)
- Family history
- Medical/surgical history
- Current conditions/chief complaints
- Medications
- Medical/laboratory/clinical test results
- Functional status and activity level: premorbid and current

Systems Review

- Cardiovascular/pulmonary
- Cognitive/affective
- Genitourinary
- Integumentary
- Musculoskeletal
- Neuromuscular

Tests and Measures/Impairments

- Aerobic capacity and endurance: during functional activities and standardized exercise protocols including cardiovascular signs and symptoms in response to exercise and activity (see Autonomic); pulmonary signs and symptoms in response to exercise and activity
- Anthropometric characteristics: body mass index, girth, length; edema
- Assistive or adaptive devices: fit, alignment, function, use; safety
- Autonomic nervous system integrity: thermal responses, sweating; gastrointestinal signs and symptoms, constipation/bowel incontinence, urinary urgency/incontinence; salivation/drooling; orthostatic hypotension; cardiac sympathetic denervation
- Circulation: response to position change, degree of orthostatic hypotension (see Autonomic)
- Cognition: mental status, learning, memory, hesitation, slowness of thought processes, attention, visuospatial processing
- Communication
- Cranial and peripheral nerve integrity
- Environment, home, and work barriers
- Functional status and activity level: performance-based examination of functional skills (FIM level), basic and instrumental ADL; functional mobility skills; home management skills
- Gait and locomotion: gait pattern and speed, safety
- Integumentary integrity: skin condition, pressure-sensitive areas; activities, positioning, and postures to relieve pressure
- Joint integrity, alignment, and mobility: range of motion (active and passive); muscle length, and soft tissue extensibility
- Motor function: motor control and motor learning: tone, voluntary movement patterns; involuntary movements; hesitation, slowness, arrests of movements; poverty of movements
- Muscle performance: strength, power, and endurance
- Neuromotor control and sensory processing
- Oromotor function: communication (fluctuations, reduced volume), swallowing
- Pain: intensity, quality, behavior, and location
- Perceptual function: visuospatial skills
- Postural control and balance: degree of postural instability, balance strategies, safety
- Posture: alignment and position, symmetry (static and dynamic); ergonomics, and body mechanics
- Procedural learning for complex and sequential tasks
- Psychosocial function: motivation, apathy, anxiety, depression
- Range of motion (see Joint integrity)
- Reflex integrity
- Self-care and domestic life
- Sensory integrity and integration
- Skeletal integrity
- Ventilation and gas exchange
- Work, community, and leisure activities: ability to participate in activities, safety

population. The *Geriatric Anxiety Inventory* (GAI) and the *Parkinson's Anxiety Scale* (PAS) are recommended for use in detecting and grading the severity of anxiety in PD without dementia.[146-148]

Sensory Function

A screening examination of sensation is indicated (superficial and deep sensations, combined cortical sensations). Sensory changes can be expected with aging, such as blunting of touch sensations and proprioception with greater losses in LEs than UEs, and distal more than proximal. Specific areas of sensory loss may be indicative of comorbid pathology, for example, stroke and diabetic neuropathy. The patient with PD should be asked about the presence of paresthesias (sensations of numbness or tingling) and pain. Mild aching and cramp-like sensations are common and are often poorly localized. It is important to examine for musculoskeletal aches and pains linked to lack of movement, faulty movements or posture, and ligamentous strain.

An examination of vision should include a determination of acuity, peripheral vision, color discrimination, contrast sensitivity, tracking, accommodation, light and dark adaptation, and depth perception. Visual changes in PD include loss of visual acuity (both distance and near acuity), blurring of vision and difficulty reading not improved by corrective lenses, loss of color discrimination, difficulty detecting low contrast (shades of gray), problems with eye pursuit (cogwheeling), and age-related decreased adaptation to light, and sensitivity to light and glare.[149] Medications may also produce impaired or fuzzy vision, for example, antidepressants and anticholinergics.

Musculoskeletal Function

Joint Flexibility and Posture

An examination of musculoskeletal ROM and flexibility is important. The therapist can document specific active range of motion (AROM) and passive range of motion (PROM) impairments using goniometric measurement. Patients with PD are likely to present with losses in hip and knee extension, dorsiflexion, shoulder flexion, elbow extension, dorsal spine and neck extension, and axial rotation.

It is particularly important to examine spinal ROM (ability to rotate, flex, and extend the spine) because patients with PD have been shown to exhibit impairments in this area.[150] All segments of the spine should be examined, including cervical, thoracic, and lumbar segments. Spinal inclinometers such as the Back Range of Motion II™ (BROM II) and Cervical Range of Motion™ (CROM) instruments have been shown to be valid and reliable in measuring spinal ROM and forward head posture (www.spineproducts.com).[151] The use of a head-mounted laser and wall measurements is a novel way to assess transverse plane spine ROM. Standing with feet stationary, the patient rotates as far as possible to one side. An objective measurement of full body (trunk) rotation is obtained by measuring the distance that the laser moves along the wall. This multisegmental measurement may be a better predictor of functional trunk mobility than isolated measurements of cervical and lumbar ROM. The mobility of the spine can also be examined using a series of functional movements, such as axial rotation (looking behind) in sitting and standing and walking. Hamstring length can be determined using a straight leg test.

An examination of resting posture and changes in posture that occur with movement is indicated. The therapist can use posture grids, plumb lines, still photography, or videotape to document changes. A flexible ruler contoured to the patient's spine in standing and then traced onto graph paper can be used to record static sagittal plane posture. This technique is affordable, with good intratester and intertester reliability, and was shown to have a high correlation to radiographic measurements of the lumbar and thoracic spine.[152-154] In standing, patients with PD typically assume a flexed, stooped posture (kyphosis with forward head) with the COM placed forward within the reduced LOS (Fig. 18.4). In supine, the flexed posture with forward head is still evident (shadow pillow posture) (Fig. 18.5).

Muscle Performance

An examination of strength and endurance is indicated. The therapist can measure strength using manual muscle

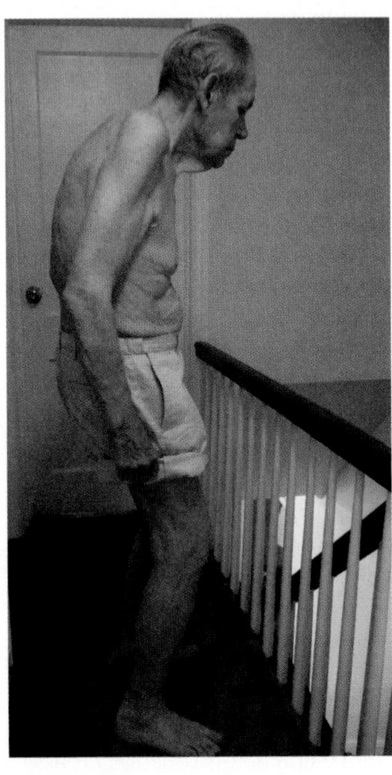

Figure 18.4 In standing, patient with PD demonstrates the typical flexed, stooped posture with kyphosis, forward head, and hip and knee flexion.

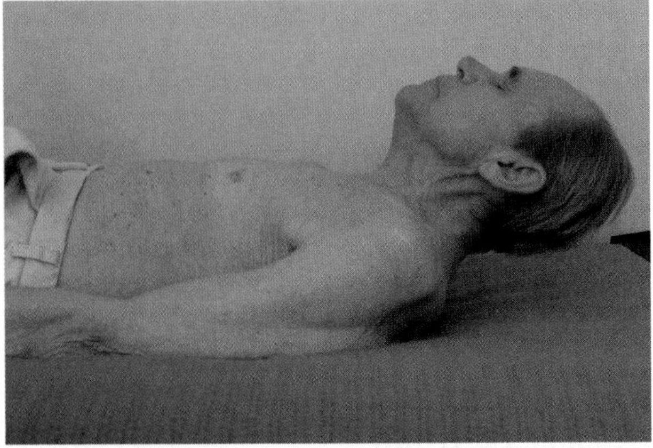

Figure 18.5 In supine, the patient with PD demonstrates the typical flexed posture (shadow pillow posture).

testing (MMT). Handheld and isokinetic dynamometry can be used to quantify peak force (torque output). Patients with PD have been shown to exhibit impairments in the rate of force development and in maximum torque production capability. Isokinetic dynamometry can also be used to document muscle endurance and has been suggested for documenting tremor, using slow speeds of movement (25 mm/sec) and low torques.[41]

Motor Function

Rigidity

Rigidity is usually equal in both agonist and antagonist muscle groups. As mentioned earlier, it can be sustained (lead pipe) or intermittent (cogwheel). Distribution of rigidity is often asymmetrical especially in the early stages of the disease and can vary during the day, at some point in the medication cycle, and with stress. It is therefore important to determine which body segments are affected and the severity of involvement. The patient should be seated or supine in a relaxed position. The therapist moves each extremity through full PROM. For head and neck and spinal PROM the patient can be seated on a mat or at the edge of a chair, perch sitting, to allow for excursion of spinal motions (flexion, extension, rotation). A determination of severity of rigidity can be made based on the level of resistance to passive movement and availability of ROM. See item 3.3 in Part III of the MDS-UPDRS for test examples.[28] Deficits in functional mobility and postural reactions should be suspected in the presence of significant trunk rigidity. The patient should also be examined for facial mobility (e.g., hypomimia or masked face) including ability to produce spontaneous expressions and part the lips; the ability to smile or use the muscles of facial expression should also be examined. An inspection of voluntary repetitive movements should be performed to determine active limitations imposed by rigidity.

Bradykinesia

Initially movements are slowed, then movements decrease in amplitude (hypokinesia); in later stages, movements become arrhythmic with frequent start hesitations and arrests (akinesia). A stopwatch can be used to quantify detectable slowing of movement (*movement time*) and start hesitancy or *reaction time* (elapsed time between the patient's desire to move and the actual movement response). The therapist should examine overall amplitude of movement and fluctuations in amplitude. For example, impaired coordination and asymmetry of arm swing during walking is a common finding in early PD. As the disease progresses, movements are characterized by marked slowness, poverty, and reduced amplitude. Timed tests for rapid alternating movements (RAM) can be used to determine the effects of bradykinesia. Examples of RAM include repeated opposition of the forefinger and thumb, alternating between pronation and supination, opening and closing of hands, and tapping (finger or foot tapping). Dexterity in complex motor tasks (e.g., writing, dressing, skilled object manipulation) can be expected to be impaired and should be examined. This is also true for motor tasks involving simultaneous use of both sides (e.g., bilateral RAM between pronation and supination). See items 3.4 to 3.8 and 3.14 in Part III of the MDS-UPDRS[28], and Chapter 6, Examination of Coordination and Balance, for additional test examples.

More sophisticated methods have been used to study movement in patients with PD, largely in the research setting. EMG has been used to quantify the effects of rigidity and bradykinesia on motor performance. Long-latency EMG responses (50 to 120 msec) have been observed when muscles are subjected to sudden stretch. Abnormal patterns of motor unit recruitment have also been observed.[45]

Tremor

The location, persistence, and severity (amplitude) of tremor should be recorded. The therapist should determine if tremor is present at rest (initial typical pattern) or present with action and interferes with function. This latter pattern may occur in severe, long-standing disease. UE functional skills such as drinking from a cup, feeding, dressing, and writing can be used to test for the effects of tremor during movement. With severe tremor, the patient will be unable to complete the functional task. Stress can increase tremor. See items 3.15 to 3.18 in Part III of the MDS-UPDRS for test examples.[28]

Postural Control and Balance

A thorough examination of postural control and balance is indicated. The therapist should first observe the patient's resting posture in sitting and standing. The patient's perception of trunk rotation and of vertical may be impaired; some patients with advanced disease will perceive themselves as fully upright when they are actually leaning forward.[79]

Clinical measures of balance performance have been shown to be reliable and sensitive in the examination of functional performance and balance in patients with Parkinson's disease.[155] These include the *Berg Balance Scale* (BBS),[156] the *Functional Reach Test* (FRT),[157] the *Timed Up and Go test* (TUG),[158] the *Cognitive Timed Up and Go* (CTUG),[159] and the *Dynamic Gait Index* (DGI).[160] These tests are discussed in Chapter 6, Examination of Coordination and Balance and Table 6.7 Outcome Measures: Examination of Balance. The BBS correlates well with the UPDRS and has been found to be a good overall measure of function in this population.[161,162] Dibble and Lange[163] demonstrated that each of these tests can be used to discriminate among people with PD who had a history of falls from those without a history of falls and suggested cutoff scores to maximize sensitivity and minimize false negatives. False negatives can also be reduced when interpretation is based on the collective interpretation of multiple balance tests. A clinical decision making algorithm that involves the serial use of clinical balance tests has been proposed.[164] Studies evaluating the BBS, the *Fullerton Advanced Balance Scale (FAB)*,[165] the Functional Gait Assessment (FGA),[166] the *Balance Evaluation Systems Test (BESTest)*,[167] and the *Mini Balance Evaluation Systems Test (Mini-BESTest)*[168] have shown that all tests demonstrated high reliability scores.[169,170] The FAB, Mini-BESTest and BBS showed similar accuracy in predicting falls and the BESTest was most sensitive for identifying fallers.[169-171] The BBS, FGA and DGI all have ceiling effects in early stage PD.[155,171] Steffen and Seney[172] found high reliability scores for the BBS, the 6-Minute Walk Test (6-MWT), and gait speed. In contrast, the *Tinetti Gait Assessment (TGA)* was not sensitive for detecting change in gait impairments in people with moderately disabling PD.[155,173] Strong stability of measurements on balance tests occurs during the "on" phase of the medication cycle while stability of measurements is not maintained during the "off" period.[174] See Table 18.4, Selected Outcome Measures for Persons With PD, for descriptions, scoring, and minimal detectible change values.

Reduced postural control is evident during quiet standing (static control), with increased oscillations in both medial-lateral and anterior-posterior planes.[175] During dynamic posturographic tests, postural restabilization strategies are often inadequate to maintain balance. Available postural strategies and reactions should be carefully

Table 18.4 Selected Outcome Measures for Persons With Parkinson disease by ICF Domain

Outcome Measure and ICF Category	Description	Scoring	MDC/MCID
Montreal Cognitive Assessment [MoCA][142] *Body Function and Structure*	16-item screen of multiple cognitive domains to detect mild cognitive impairment	Criteria are given for scoring each item for a total score (max 30 points). Cutoff scores: <26/30 mild cognitive impairment (PD-MCI); <22/30 dementia (PDD)	MDC: not established MCID: not established
Mini Balance Evaluation Systems Test [Mini-BESTest][168] *Body Function and Structure* *Activity*	14-item clinical balance assessment in 4 domains, shortened version of the BESTest*	Items are scored on a 3-point scale (0–2) for a total score (max 28)	MDC: 17.1% or 5.52 points (PD) MCID: 4 points (balance disorders)
Parkinson Fatigue Scale [PFS-16][195] *Body Function and Structure* *Activity*	16-item self-report measure for physical fatigue and its impact on daily function	Items are scored from 1–5 and summed for a total score (16–80)	MDC: not established MCID: not established
Movement Disorders Society sponsored Unified Parkinson Disease Rating Scale [MDS-UPDRS][111] *Body Function and Structure* *Activity* *Participation*	4-part comprehensive clinical rating scale for assessment of the extent and burden of PD	Items are scored from 0–4 and summed for each part Parts I and II (13 questions each) rate non-motor and motor experiences of daily living. Part III motor exam has 33 scores on 18 items. Part IV has 6 questions on motor complications.	MDC: not established MCID: not established
Nonmotor Symptoms Questionnaire [NMSQuest][73] *Activity* *Participation*	30-item self-report questionnaire covering 10 domains based on the previous month to screen the presence of NMS in PD and their impact of quality of life	Items scored as "yes," "no," or "don't know"	MDC: not established MCID: not established

Table 18.4 Selected Outcome Measures for Persons With Parkinson disease by ICF Domain—cont'd

Outcome Measure and ICF Category	Description	Scoring	MDC/MCID
Nonmotor Symptoms Scale [NMSS][199] *Body Function and Structure* *Activity* *Participation*	30-item scale covering 9 dimensions based on the previous month for the assessment of frequency and severity of NMS in PD	Items scored on Severity (0–3) and on Frequency (1–4). Each item Severity and Frequency scores are multiplied, then summed within each domain. Total score is sum of domain scores	MDC: not established MCID: not established
Parkinson's Disease Questionnaire-39 [PDQ-39][221] or **Parkinson's Disease Questionnaire-8 [PDQ-8]** *Participation*	39-item self-report questionnaire based on previous month for assessment of PD-related health quality in 8 dimensions 8-item version of the PDQ-39	Items scored from 0-4 on previous month's experience. Scores are summed for each dimension, divided by max possible dimension score, and multiplied by 100. Overall summary index is sum of dimension total scores divided by 8	MDC: 12 to 24 points across dimensions MCID: −11.4 to 1.3 points across dimensions
New Freezing of Gait Questionnaire [NFOG-Q][185] *Activity* *Participation*	9-item questionnaire in 3 parts based on previous month: Part I Distinction of freezer or non-freezer; Part II Severity; Part III Impact on daily life	Criteria are given for scoring each item for a total score (max 29 points). High score indicates more severe freezing	MDC: not established MCID: not established
6 Minute Walk Test[172] *Activity*	A measure of walking endurance	Utilize a marked course (33 meters) and measuring wheel to obtain distance travelled in 6 minutes	MDC: 82 meters or 269 feet (PD) MCID: 54–80 meters (COPD, geriatrics, stroke)
10 Meter Walk Test[179] *Activity*	A measure of comfortable and fast walking speeds	Times are recorded to walk 10 meters at the individual's (1) comfortable and (2) fastest safe speed	MDC: 0.02–0.18 m/s comfortable speed; 0.09–0.25 m/s fastest speed (PD) MCID: 0.10–0.16 m/s (geriatrics, stroke)
9-Hole Peg Test [211] *Activity*	A measure of manual dexterity; the individual removes 9 pegs from a peg board to a well, one at a time and then returns the pegs to the pegboard, one at a time.	Time to complete this task is measured in seconds for both the dominant and non-dominant hands.	MDC: 2.6 s dominant, 1.3 s non-dominant hand (PD) MCID: not established
***Activities-Specific Balance Confidence Scale** *Activity* *Participation*	16-item self-report measure evaluating confidence performing home and community functional activities on a 0% to 100% scale	Sum of the scores divided by 16 gives the final average score. Higher scores indicate better balance confidence	MDC: not established MCID: not established
***Berg Balance Scale** *Activity*	14-item balance performance test	Items are scored 0-4 for a maximal score of 56. Scores ≤45 are associated with greater fall risk	MDC: 5 points (PD) MCID: not established

Continued

Table 18.4 Selected Outcome Measures for Persons With Parkinson disease by ICF Domain—cont'd

Outcome Measure and ICF Category	Description	Scoring	MDC/MCID
***Dynamic Gait Index** *Activity*	8-item walking test examining changing task demands when walking (i.e., head turns, change in speed, obstacles, turns, stops, stairs)	Items are scored 0–3 for a maximal score of 24.	MDC: 2.9 points and 13.3% (PD)[179] MCID: 4 points (migraine and vestibular disorders)
***Functional Reach** *Activity*	A measure of the maximal forward reach of an individual	A yardstick is secured to the walk at shoulder height; the individual flexes their arm forward 90 degrees with the hand in a fist. After reaching as far forward as possible, the distance is recorded at the third metacarpal head	MDC: 9 cm (PD) MCID: not established
Functional Gait Assessment[166] *Activity*	10-item assessment of dynamic gait	Items scored from 0–3 for a maximum score of 30	MDC: 5 points (stroke) MCID: not established
Five Times Sit to Stand Test[215-217] *Activity*	A measure of functional leg strength	Time to stand up from and return to sitting in a chair 5 times consecutively is recorded Cutoff score of 16 seconds discriminates PD fallers from non-fallers	MDC: 10 seconds MCID: not established
***Timed Up and Go** *Activity*	A measure of dynamic balance	Time to stand from a chair, walk 3 m, turn, and return to sitting in the chair is recorded	MDC: 3.5–11 seconds (PD) MCID: not established
Timed Up and Go Cognitive[159] *Activity*	A measure of dynamic balance with the addition of a secondary challenge	Time to perform the TUG with a cognitive task (subtract by 3's)	MDC: not established MCID: not established

*Please reference Chapter 6: Examination of Coordination and Balance, for additional information on these balance measures.
All measures but the NMSQ and NMSS are "highly recommended" or "recommended" by the *PD EDGE Task Force* for use across settings (acute, inpatient rehabilitation, home health, skilled nursing facility, and outpatient) AND required at entry-level education (http://www.neuropt.org/docs/default-source/parkinson-edge/pdedge-all-documents-combined.pdf?sfvrsn=2).

documented (e.g., use of ankle, hip, and stepping strategies). Healthy individuals typically respond initially using an ankle strategy with small shifts in their COM, followed by hip and stepping strategies with larger shifts in the COM. Persons with PD and the elderly population in general typically respond to destabilizing forces with postural strategies involving more the hip joints than ankle joints. Start hesitation, abnormal coactivation patterns (rigid body) with an inability to recover a stable posture, is common. An absence of postural strategies (i.e., patient would fall if not for overhead body support harness) is also seen in advanced disease. During complex postural situations involving sensory conflict (e.g., the Sensory Organization Test), persons with advanced PD typically demonstrate reduced postural performance, suggesting inadequate sensory organization.[176] Balance control can also be expected to degrade under conditions of reduced cognitive monitoring. Patients with PD especially in the early stages of the disease may not demonstrate balance impairments in response to steady standing with normal BOS or self-initiated movements as along as their attention is fully directed to the task at hand. However, if competing attentional demands are instituted (i.e., *dual-task interference* such as talking while balancing), instability can be seen.[177] Balance confidence is also related to functional mobility and falls in people with PD.[178]

Gait

Parameters and characteristics of gait that should be examined during unobstructed walking on level surfaces include start time or gait initiation, speed of walking, stride length, cadence, stability, variability, and safety. The *10-Meter Walk Test* can be used to determine speed, average stride, and cadence or more sophisticated kinetic analysis can be obtained from embedded force plates, body markers, and computerized equipment (motion analysis systems typically seen in the laboratory setting). Persons with PD frequently demonstrate decreased step length and trunk rotation, difficulty initiating gait, and difficulty attaining increased walking speed. When instructed to walk as fast as possible, the movements produced are smaller and more variable when compared with healthy elders.[30,179]

Gait should be examined for kinematic or qualitative changes, including reductions in hip, knee, and ankle motions that result in a short-stepped, shuffling (festinating) gait pattern with reduced trunk rotation and arm swing. Postural abnormalities that contribute to the development of a festinating gait pattern should be documented (i.e., flexed, stooped posture). Gait should be examined in all movement directions: forward, backward, and sideward. A complex gait pattern such as cross-stepping or braiding can be used to examine deficits in motor planning. Patients with advanced PD typically have trouble with adaptability and cannot easily vary walking or walk in complex confined areas such as narrow doorways or open environments. Walking should be examined in varied environments (e.g., community environment) or negotiating an obstacle course. Increased difficulty in walking is also experienced in response to varying attentional demands and dual-task interference. Changes in gait speed, stride length, and cadence can be observed while simultaneously performing a secondary cognitive task (e.g., talking while walking) or walking while simultaneously performing a secondary motor task (e.g., buttoning a coat). The degree of change was similar to type of dual-task interference.[180] Clinical measures of locomotor performance shown to be reliable and sensitive for people with PD include the DGI, the FGA, and the TUG (all previously discussed). Huang et al[181] identified the minimal detectable change values for both the TUG and the DGI.

Freezing of Gait

Freezing of gait, an episodic inability to generate effective stepping in the absence of any known cause, has a dramatic effect on quality of life and risk of falls for patients with PD.[36,59,70,182,183] Assessment is often difficult due to the unpredictable nature of the episodes. The therapist needs to document triggers or provoking factors. Common triggers for FOG include initiating gait, walking through narrow passages (e.g., doorway) or turning in tight spaces, a change in the environment or attentional demands, and walking under time pressure, anxiety, or stress. In the early stages of the disease, episodes are levodopa sensitive and more common in the "off" time. In advanced stages, FOG can occur during the "on" time.[184] The *New Freezing of Gait Questionnaire (NFOG-Q)* is a reliable three-part questionnaire and short video to detect and rate FOG severity and impact.[185]

Fall Risk

A determination of fall history and fall injuries is an important component of the examination of balance and gait function. There is a strong association between duration and severity of PD with increased risk of falls. Of significance are balance and walking impairments including FOG, anterior displacement of COM, decreased postural righting reactions, and the presence of dyskinesias. Other linked factors include postural hypotension, dementia, depression, and prior history of falls.[186-188] A *fall risk diary* can be used to assist the patient and family/caregivers in accurately recording a fall event and the context of daily life in which the fall occurred. For example, activity at the time of the fall, relation to timing of medication and food intake, type of footwear, degree of fatigue and injury, and other risk factors all should be documented. The need for assisted gait and frequency of contact guarding from family members or caregivers during walking should also be documented.

Fatigue

Fatigue is a common impairment associated with PD. As the disease process progresses so does the prevalence of fatigue and its impact on quality of life.[189-191] The Movement Disorders Society (www.movementdisorders.org) created a task force to evaluate and make recommendations on available fatigue rating scales.[191,192] Following the systematic review, the task force recommended the *Multidimensional Fatigue Inventory (MFI)*, the *Fatigue Severity Scale (FSS)*, and the *Parkinson Fatigue Scale (PFS-16)* for assessment of fatigue in patients with PD. The MFI is a 20-item self-report scale that measures general fatigue, physical fatigue, mental fatigue, reduced motivation, and reduced activity.[193] The FSS is a self-administered 9-item rating scale that emphasizes the functional impact of fatigue.[194] The PFS-16 is a 16-item self-reported measure of physical fatigue and its impact on daily function,[195] described in Table 18.4.

Dyskinesias

Drug-induced dyskinesias have a profound effect on physical and social functioning. Risk factors include high total dosage of dopaminergic drugs, young age at onset of PD, and extended duration of the disease process.[121,122] The *Rush Dyskinesia Scale* assesses functional disability by grading the subject walking, drinking from a cup, and putting on and buttoning a coat.[196] This scale has been used extensively in clinical trials and patient care, and has undergone extensive clinimetric testing.[197] The *Unified*

Dyskinesia Rating Scale (UDysRS) is a four-part comprehensive rating tool recently developed by the Movement Disorders Society (MDS) to assess dyskinesias using the patient perspective, objective impairment, and objective disability approaches.[198] The therapist can explore the impact of motor fluctuations using questions that address changes in performance during the day.

Nonmotor Symptoms (NMS)

The Nonmotor Symptoms Questionnaire (NMSQuest) was the first comprehensive self-report measure to assess the presence nonmotor symptoms of PD and their impact on activities and quality of life.[73] The Nonmotor Symptom Scale (NMSS) was developed in conjunction with the NMSQuest to assess the frequency and severity of NMS in PD patients across all stages.[199]

Swallowing and Speech

An examination of swallowing function, feeding, and speech is important. Referral to a speech-language pathologist may be indicated if the patient demonstrates significant limitations in any of these areas.

Autonomic Function

The therapist should examine for problems with autonomic dysfunction. Excessive drooling (salivation) or sweating, greasy skin, and abnormalities in thermoregulation should be noted. Excessive sweating and flushing during the "on" state are linked to the presence of dyskinesias.

Cardiorespiratory Function

Endurance may be reduced because of impaired cardiorespiratory function and long-standing inactivity, both common problems in PD. An examination of respiratory function should include inspection of rib cage compliance, chest wall mobility, and thoracic expansion. Visual inspection of breathing patterns and an examination of the influence of posture and activity on breathing should be performed. Objective measurements include respiratory rate (RR) and circumferential measurements of the chest. Specific ventilation parameters may be determined in patients with significant respiratory compromise. These can include FVC, FEV_1, maximal expiratory flow (MEF), maximal inspiratory flow (MIF), total lung capacity (TLC), residual volume (RV), and RAW.

Individuals with mild PD (H & Y Stages I and II) can demonstrate aerobic exercise capacities similar to healthy adults. Individuals with more advanced disease (H & Y Stages III and IV) demonstrate greater variability and lower aerobic capacities compared with healthy adults. It is important to remember that many older adults are at high risk for latent cardiovascular disease. Exercise testing can be used to determine the patient's level of fitness before commencing an exercise program. Patients who have balance deficits or freezing episodes should not be tested on a treadmill without the use of a safety harness. Cycle ergometry (arm or leg) may be an acceptable alternative. A *6- or 12-Minute Walk Test* can be used to determine endurance capacity and walking velocity. The therapist should document vital signs (HR, RR, BP), exertional symptoms (dyspnea, dizziness or confusion, excessive fatigue, pallor, and so forth), time, distance, and number of rest stops.[200] For patients with advanced PD (H & Y Stages III and IV), Light et al (201) used a *2-Minute Walk Test* to evaluate walking endurance and found it to be a sensitive and feasible test. Perceived exertion can be documented using Borg's Rating of Perceived Exertion Scale (RPE Scale).[202]

Orthostatic Hypotension

Orthostatic hypotension (OH) with positional change should be examined. Subjective signs and symptoms of OH on sitting up and standing up are documented (e.g., dizziness, light-headedness, pallor, diaphoresis, or syncope). A drop in systolic blood pressure (SBP) of 20 mm Hg, or a drop of 10 mm Hg in diastolic blood pressure (DBP), *and* a 10% to 20% increase in pulse rate is diagnostic of the condition. The examination begins with the patient resting in supine for 2 to 3 minutes. Resting BP and HR are taken. The patient is then asked to move from supine-to-sitting. After at least 1 minute, BP and HR are taken. If the patient is stable after at least 3 minutes (no symptoms), testing can be performed in the standing position. The patient is asked to move from sitting-to-standing with BP and HR again taken after at least 1 minute and repeated between 3 and 5 minutes. BP that continues to drop after at least 1 minute of standing is problematic and is evident in advanced PD.[203]

Integumentary Integrity

Sympathetic skin responses may be abnormal. For example, the skin may become oily (e.g., on face). Seborrhea or seborrheic dermatitis occurs frequently in patients with PD. The therapist should examine the patient closely for areas of bruising and skin breakdown. Patients who are severely disabled (H & Y Stage V) are restricted to bed, wheelchair, or both. Incontinence may occur during late-stage disease. The effect of these problems on skin integrity should be carefully documented. Use and effectiveness of pressure-relieving strategies and devices should also be documented.

Functional Status

An examination of functional status is indicated, including performance of functional mobility skills, basic activities of daily living (BADL), and instrumental activities of daily living (IADL). For patients undergoing inpatient rehabilitation, the *Functional Independence Measure (FIM)* is commonly administered[204] (see Chapter 8, Examination of Function). Need for and appropriate use of protective and supportive devices is an important component of the functional status examination. Close collaboration with the occupational therapist is essential.

Hand function is impacted by PD with dexterity problems being reported as one of the top contributors to disease burden.[205] For example, problems are common with ADL such as fastening clothes, tying shoes, using eating utensils, handling coins, turning pages, handwriting, dialing a cell phone, and typing on a touch screen tablet. Contributing factors include bradykinesia, tremor, dyskinesias, reduced coordination of the wrist and fingers, difficulty making sequential movements, impaired planning, and abnormal grip force adjustments.[206-209] There are few recommendations for outcome measures to assess hand function and its impact on quality of life in people with PD.[210] The *9-Hole Peg Test* is commonly used, has shown high test-retest reliability, and its performance has been related to scores of bradykinesia and freezing of gait.[211] The *Dexterity Questionnaire 24 (DextQ-24)* is a recently developed, valid and reliable tool for evaluating dexterity in patients with PD.[212]

During functional performance tests, each skill should be analyzed to determine the impact of direct and indirect impairments on performance. For example, sit-to-stand transfers typically present a significant challenge for patients with moderate to severe PD as evidenced by increased time and increased falls. These changes have been attributed to hypokinesia, decreased rates of force production, and changes in distal muscle timing.[213,214] The *Five Times Sit-to-Stand Test (FTSS)* is a timed test that has been used to determine performance in patients with PD at different disease stages and to discriminate between fallers and nonfallers with PD.[215,216] The average time for FTSS performance for community-dwelling individuals with PD was 20 seconds with a cutoff time of 16 seconds discriminating between fallers and nonfallers. Peterson et al[217] reported the minimal detectible change for the FTSS at 10 seconds. Timed performance can also be used for other functional tasks such as rolling over in bed or moving from supine-to-sitting that are likely to prove difficult. These activities have a large rotational component of the trunk, typically lacking in many patients with PD.

Functional testing should be balanced with adequate rest to ensure that fatigue does not degrade performance with resultant fluctuations. Repeat testing should be undertaken at the same time of day and importantly at the same time in the medication cycle. Filming task activities can provide an objective record of functional performance. This is particularly useful to document motor fluctuations and dyskinesias. An examination of functional performance in the home (or work) environment is also indicated. The patient's physical environment is examined for barriers, access, and safety.

Profile of Function and Impairment Level Experience With Parkinson's Disease

The *Profile of Function and Impairment Level Experience with Parkinson's Disease* (*PROFILE PD*) was developed to assist the physical therapist's examination and evaluation of individuals with PD in the early and middle stages of disease. Half the test relates to deficits in body systems and cognitive/emotional factors. These include questions on tremor (with activity and at rest), rigidity, posture, postural stability, dyskinesia, dystonia, clinical fluctuations, falling, FOG, bradykinesia, speech, depression, memory, and involvement (routine daily/leisure/social activities). The other half of the test focuses on functional activities that are typically difficult for individuals with PD (e.g., dressing, hygiene, mealtime activities, transfers, bed mobility, chair rise, gait, fine and gross motor performance). Initial testing revealed it to be a reliable and valid scale and an estimated administration time of 15 minutes.[218]

Global Health Measures

Global health measures can be used to determine individual outcomes across a broad spectrum of populations. Instruments typically include items that examine ability to perform routine daily activities and quality of life (e.g., physical and social function, general health and vitality, emotional well-being, bodily pain). General health measures have been used to study large populations and are most useful in determining long-term health outcomes. They lack the sensitivity needed to document short-term outcomes of treatment. Commonly used measures of general health status include the *Rand 36-Item Health Survey SF-36*[219] and the *Sickness Impact Profile.*[220]

Disease-Specific Measures

Disease-specific measures are designed to determine attributes unique to a specific disease entity. Items are included that provide information about the disease process and outcomes, and ideally document clinically meaningful change over time. Thus, these instruments have greater responsiveness or sensitivity to change than general health measures. The *Parkinson's Disease Questionnaire (PDQ-39)* is a 39-item questionnaire developed from in-depth interviews with patients with PD.[221] It focuses on the subjective report of the impact of PD on daily life and addresses eight health-related quality-of-life dimensions (mobility, ADL, emotional well-being, stigma, social support, cognition, communication, and bodily discomfort). The PDQ-39 produces a profile of scores on the eight individual dimensions, and a summary score using the *Parkinson's Disease Summary Index* (PDSI) can also be determined. It provides a useful indication of the global impact of PD on health status. Internal and test–retest reliability was moderate to high. Construct validity was good with significant and high correlations were found between the PDQ-39 and the SF-36 and the H & Yahr staging score.[221]

The *Neurology Section Parkinson Disease Outcome Measures Taskforce* of the American Physical Therapy Association (APTA) has compiled a list of measures for each relevant International Classification of Functioning, Disability, and Health (ICF) category together with instrument analysis, recommendations for use, and relevant references. The document can be found at http://www.neuropt.org/docs/default-source/parkinson-edge/pdedge-all-documents-combined.pdf?sfvrsn=2. Selected outcome measures are listed in Table 18.4.

Goals and Outcomes

The general goals and outcomes for patients with progressive disorders of the CNS, adapted from the *Guide to Physical Therapist Practice*,[139] are presented in Box 18.4.

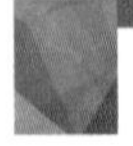

Box 18.4 Examples of General Goals and Outcomes for Patients with Progressive Disorders of the Central Nervous System[139]

Impact of pathology/pathophysiology is reduced.

- *Decrease:* risk of secondary impairment; intensity of care
- *Improve:* patient/client, family and caregiver knowledge of disease, prognosis, and plan of care; symptom management

Impact of impairments is reduced.

- *Decrease:* pain
- *Improve:* cognitive function; joint integrity; mobility; sensory awareness; skin integrity; motor function; muscle performance; postural control and balance; gait and locomotion; management of fatigue; aerobic capacity

Ability to perform physical actions, tasks, or activities is improved.

- *Improve:* independence with ADL; tolerance of positions and activities; activity pacing and energy conservation; problem solving and decision making skills; safety of patient, family, and caregivers

Disability associated with chronic illness is reduced.

- *Improve:* ability to assume/resume self-care and home management; ability to assume work (job/school/play), community and leisure roles; patient/client and family knowledge and awareness of personal and environmental factors associated with condition worsening; awareness and use of community resources

Health status and quality of life are improved.

- *Decrease:* stressors
- *Improve:* sense of well-being; insight, self-confidence, and self-management skills; health, wellness, and fitness

Patient/client satisfaction is enhanced.

- *Improve:* acceptability of access and availability of services and quality of rehabilitation services to patient/client and family; coordination of care with patient/client, family, caregivers, and other professionals

These general goals will provide the basis for development of specific anticipated goals and expected outcomes for an individual patient.

In this document the reader will find relevant information on patient/client diagnostic classification; examination components; considerations for evaluation, diagnosis, and prognosis; and suggested interventions. Thus, the *Guide to Physical Therapist Practice* serves as a primary resource to help physical therapists design an appropriate plan of care (POC) and document the services provided and outcomes achieved.

PHYSICAL THERAPY INTERVENTION

A combined approach of physical therapy and pharmacological intervention plays a key role in the management of the patient with PD. Despite best efforts, progressive disability develops and affects the patient's quality of life. A variety of interventions to maximize functional ability and minimize secondary complications are used to achieve goals and outcomes, including direct interventions, supervision of assistive personnel, patient/family/caregiver instruction, environmental modification, and supportive counseling. Early intervention is critical in preventing the devastating musculoskeletal impairments these patients are so prone to develop. Interventions also focus on improvement of motor function, exercise capacity, functional performance, and activity participation. Education and support of patients, family members, and caregivers at each stage of the disease is critical to attaining optimal outcomes. The research team for the *Cochrane Database of Systematic Reviews* found that there was insufficient evidence to support or refute the efficacy of any given form of physical therapy over another in PD. The researchers stressed the need for improved research in this area, including large well-designed placebo-controlled randomized controlled trials (RCTs) to demonstrate the efficacy and effectiveness of "best practice" physical therapy in PD.[222,223]

Motor Learning Strategies

Patients with PD typically demonstrate motor learning deficits, including slower learning rates, reduced efficiency, and increased context-specificity of learning. Learning complex movement sequences and movements dependent on internally generated cues are more difficult than those dependent on external cues. In the early and middle stages of the disease, patients can improve their performance through practice and by using additional sensory information. The amount and persistence of learning are variable and can be expected to be lower than in healthy age-matched people. In more advanced stages and in the presence of pronounced cognitive deficits, training will likely be less successful.[54,224-227] The therapist needs to structure treatment sessions to optimize motor learning.

Critical elements of practice include many repetitions to develop procedural skills. The therapist should instruct the patient to deliberately focus his or her full attention on the desired movement, emphasizing self-awareness of the amplitude of movements. The environment should also be modified to reduce clutter and competing attentional demands that may trigger freezing episodes. The task should be modified to minimize competing cognitive demands (e.g., dual-tasking). Long and complex movement sequences should be limited initially, or broken down into component parts, then progressed in complexity as the patient gains success. Initially, *random practice order* (i.e., practice in which the patient switches back and forth between tasks) should be avoided in favor of a *blocked practice order,* thereby reducing the effects of contextual interference. Use of *structured instructional sets* has been shown to improve movement speed and consistency.[228] For example, walking patterns can be improved with focused instructions of "swing your arms," "walk fast," or "take large steps." For the patient with advanced disease and cognitive deficits, repetitive drill-like practice should be used together with an increased focus on caregiver training to ensure safety.

Cueing Strategies

External cues have been shown to be effective in triggering sequential movements and improving movement characteristics in individuals with mild to moderate PD.[229] *Visual cues* include stationary floor markings (e.g., brightly colored lines on the floor placed perpendicular to the gait path and spaced about one step length apart) and dynamic transportable cues (e.g., laser light signals). A laser light that projects a line onto the floor in front of the patient can be mounted on an assistive device (cane or walker) or on a subject's chest harness. Visual cues have been shown to improve stride length and velocity while cadence was relatively unchanged.[230] Freezing episodes are also reduced. *Rhythmic auditory stimulation (RAS)* includes use of a metronome beat or a steady beat from a musical listening device. RAS has been shown to improve gait speed, cadence, and stride length, but for freezers a slight increase in frequency (10%) of the beat resulted in *reduced* step length compared with the *increased* step length for non-freezers.[231-233] The beat is typically set 25% faster than the patient's preferred pace. Auditory cues such as "Big step" have also been shown to improve gait. Cues should be consistent, not rushed and have a rhythmical quality to them. Auditory cues appear to have a greater influence on the temporal components of movement (e.g., gait cadence, stride synchronization) rather than on spatial components. *Multisensory cueing* (use of both visual and auditory cueing) has been used for patients with PD. When sensory enhanced therapy using multisensory cueing was compared with conventional therapy, significant improvements were found in the sensory training group.[234-238] However, the possible gait benefits of auditory cueing came at a cost in energy and poorer walking economy for patients walking on the treadmill at self-selected and slightly faster walking speed.[239]

External cues appear to facilitate movement by utilizing different brain areas. For example, the premotor cortex is active in the generation of movement in response to visual or auditory stimuli. Normally the supplementary motor area (SMA) with inputs from the BG is involved in the initiation of self-generated movements and the performance of well-learned, repetitive movement sequences. External cues heighten patient attention through a common mode of action, that is, to bypass the diminished internal cueing of the BG. Thus, focus is shifted to less automatic movement using alternative, more conscious motor control pathways. This is supported by the finding that when patients were requested to carry out a secondary task while walking (dual-tasking), the beneficial effects of visual and attentional cues was reduced.[240]

Selection of the type of cue and successful use will depend on the individual patient with predicted long-term benefit of a cue linked to its initial success. External cues are clearly not effective for all patients with PD. For patients with advanced disease and severe reductions in stride length, cueing is not effective. When cueing is withheld, performance can be expected to deteriorate. Focused attention with cueing requires constant vigilance and is cognitively demanding. Thus, cueing is not suitable for patients with dementia.

Exercise Training

Amplitude-based behavioral intervention is a concept that can be applied in different contexts in the treatment of PD.[241] These approaches are based on the concept that repetitive high-amplitude movements with high effort yield greater improvements in motor performance, following principles of neuroplasticity.[242-246] Patients are guided by a physical therapist to exercise at a high intensity (8/10 Borg's RPE Scale) with large amplitude, multiple repetitions, and whole body movements that increase in complexity. These vigorous large movements of the trunk and extremities are counter to the paucity of movement normally associated with PD. Improvements in UPDRS motor scores, TUG, and timed 10 m walking have been reported after 4 weeks of high-amplitude, high-effort training 4 times per week.[247] Hirsch et al[248] reviewed studies of exercise-induced neuroplasticity in people with PD (N = 144), suggesting exercise elicits plasticity-related events including corticomotor excitation, changes in gray matter volume, and changes in brain-derived neurotrophic factor (BDNF).

Relaxation Exercises

Gentle rocking can be used to produce generalized relaxation of excessive muscle tension owing to rigidity. Professor Charcot, who noted dramatic improvement in patients with PD following rides in bumpy, horse-drawn carriages, first described this effect almost 100 years ago in Paris. Following this observation, he constructed a vibrating chair to use with his patients.[249]

Another strategy to promote relaxation is emphasis on diaphragmatic breathing during exercise. For example, yoga and Pilates movements and coordinated breathing with large amplitude trunk and arm movements overhead can be used to expand the restricted chest and promote shoulder ROM (Fig. 18.6). The patient's attention can be focused on deep inspiration during arm elevation ("breathe in deeply") and on expiration ("breathe out deeply") while lowering the arms. Patients may also benefit from cognitive imaging, motor imagery or meditation techniques.[250-253] Relaxation audiotapes can be used at home as part of the home exercise program (HEP). Stress management techniques are an important adjunct to relaxation training. A daily schedule needs to be planned to accommodate the restrictions of the disease and the functional needs of the patient. Lifestyle modifications and time management strategies reduce anxiety associated with movement difficulties and prolonged times required to complete basic functional tasks.

Flexibility Exercise

The purpose of flexibility exercise (stretching) is to improve ROM and physical function. A combination of static (PROM) and dynamic (AROM) exercises is used to achieve maximum ROM. Flexibility exercises should be performed a minimum 2 to 3 days per week and ideally 5 to 7 days per week. A minimum of 4 repetitions per stretch held for 15 to 60 seconds is recommended.[200] Special consideration should be given to stretching common areas of limitation (Table 18.5). Stretching can be combined with joint mobilization techniques to reduce tightness of the joint capsule or of ligaments around a joint (Fig. 18.7). By using selected grades of accessory movement, both improved ROM and decreased pain can be achieved. The stretching will be more effective if the muscles have been warmed with active exercise or with an external heating modality. Stretching exercises are an important component of the HEP. The patient and caregiver should be instructed in the appropriate stretching exercises. A yoga sequence can be used effectively to focus attention on developmental postures, core stability, and stretching of structures that are traditionally restricted with PD, as well as to promote relaxation (Appendix 18.A).[25]

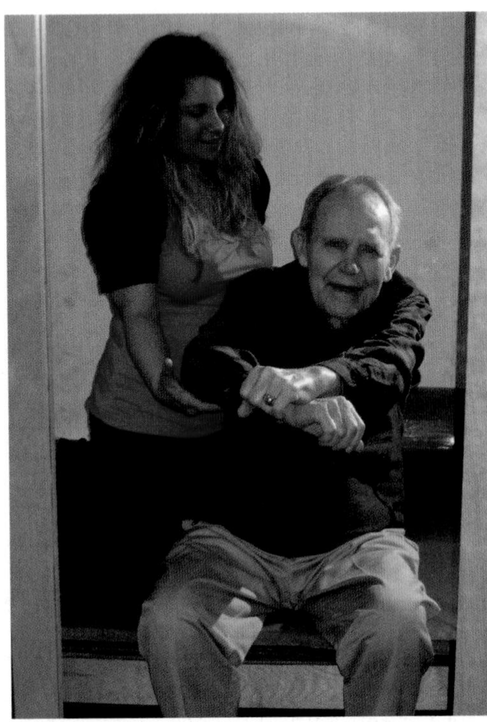

Figure 18.6 The patient with PD performs bilateral arm raises in diagonal patterns while sitting (note the difficulty in achieving full shoulder flexion).

Patients with PD benefit from additional attention and cueing strategies during active stretching exercises. Patients are instructed to think of the end (goal) of the movement, and to "move BIG, with purpose and power" through the whole range with full focus and attention on the ending position for each repetition. Additional tactile or visual cueing can assist in maximizing range during active motions. For example, during active trunk rotation and reaching movements in sitting, the patient can be cued to touch an object or target. Ballistic stretches (high-intensity bouncing stretches) should be avoided because they are linked to increased injury. Muscle tears or ruptures of weakened tissues are especially prevalent in elderly, sedentary individuals. Vigorous stretching can stimulate pain receptors and cause rebound muscle contraction. Patients with PD who are elderly and have long-standing disease must be considered at risk for osteoporosis and therefore must be stretched accordingly.

Positioning can also be used to stretch tight muscles and soft tissues. Patients in late-stage PD are likely to demonstrate severe flexion contractures of the trunk and limbs. Early on, the patient may benefit from daily positioning in prone-lying. As the disease progresses and significant postural deformity and cardiorespiratory impairments develop, the patient may not tolerate this position. The patient with a developing lateral curvature can be positioned in side-lying with a small pillow under the lateral trunk. Positional stretching is prolonged, with times typically ranging from 20 to 30 minutes. Additional mechanical stretching can be achieved using a tilt table, for example, the patient is positioned with fixed leg straps to reduce hip and knee flexion contractures and toe wedges to reduce plantarflexion contractures.

Resistance Training

Resistance training is indicated for patients with PD who demonstrate primary muscle weakness with impaired motor unit recruitment and rate of force development

Table 18.5 Common Areas of Limitation and Suggested Stretching Exercises

Areas of Limitation	Suggested Stretching Exercises
Cervical retraction	• Sitting, back against wall (or supine), head retractions (chin tuck position)
Cervical rotation	• Sit (or supine), with head retracted, head turns side to side
Shoulder flexion with trunk extension	• Sitting, hands clasped together, overhead arm lifts with thoracic extension • Supine, pillow under thoracic spine, hands clasp together, overhead arm lifts with thoracic extension
Elbow extension	• Sitting (or standing, modified plantigrade) weight-bearing with both upper extremities (UEs), elbows extended
Wrist and fingers extension	• Sitting or standing, palms together with fingers spread and pointing upward • Sitting or standing, roll tennis ball between fingers
Trunk extension	• Sitting, thoracic extension over the back of a chair with elbows bent and shoulders retracted • Prone lying, prone push-ups (press-ups) • Standing trunk extension, hands positioned on hips
Trunk rotation	• Supine, upper trunk rotation, hands clasped together (or holding a small ball), arms move with trunk rotation side to side • Hook-lying, lower trunk rotation, knees move with trunk rotation side-to-side • Sitting or standing, both arms out to one side (clasped together or holding a small ball), arms move with trunk rotation side-to-side
Hip extension	• Supine with one lower extremity (LE) over edge of mat (hip extended, knee flexed), other knee held to chest • Supine, hips and knees extended • Hook-lying bridging • Standing, active hip extension or forward lunge • High-kneeling with hips extended
Hip abduction	• Supine, one LE extended and abducted, other LE in hook-lying
Knee extension	• Standing, forward lean with wall push-ups
Ankle dorsiflexion	• Standing, both forefeet on edge of step or block, heels off step, lower heels down with light touch-down support of both hands • Standing, forward lean with wall push-ups
Toe dorsiflexion / Foot intrinsics	• Sitting, place foot on tennis ball, roll arch of foot back and forth over ball

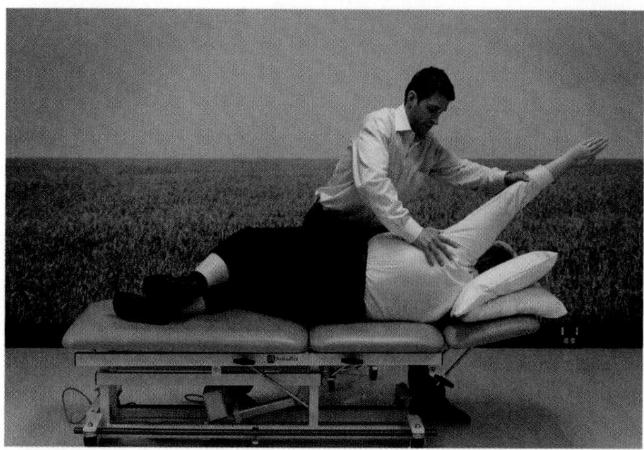

Figure 18.7 Shoulder ROM with scapular mobilization performed in the side-lying position.

and disuse weakness associated with prolonged inactivity. Specific areas of weakness are targeted, such as the antigravity extensor muscles. Weakness of these muscles is associated with poor posture (e.g., a flexed, stooped posture) and functional deficits (e.g., inability to get out of a chair, limitations in gait function). Weakness also contributes to postural instability, falls, and fall injury, as well as increased sense of effort. Strength training has been shown to improve muscle force, bradykinesia, functional mobility, balance, gait, fall risk, and quality of life in patients with PD. Toole et al[255] compared two different exercise training programs for patients with PD. They found significantly greater improvements in balance and strength using a combined program of balance training and high-intensity resistance training for knee extensors and flexors and ankle plantarflexors as compared with balance training alone.[256-263]

Resistance training is based on the *progressive overload principle*. The amount of resistance is increased during training. Load can be applied using resistance machines, free weights, elastic resistance bands, or manually. With older adults the recommendation is to begin at a lower intensity (e.g., using an RPE Scale of somewhat hard, 5 to 6 on a 10-point scale), ensuring that 10 to 12 repetitions per set can be completed.[200] Progression is as tolerated. Each repetition should be held for 10 seconds. Strength training can be performed 2 days per week on nonconsecutive days. Exercise machines may be safer than free weights for patients with more advanced disease because the movements are more controlled, especially for the patient who demonstrates dyskinesias at peak dose or cognitive changes.[200] Because patients with PD already demonstrate too much stiffness and coactivation, isometric training is generally contraindicated. Functional training activities (see next section) can also be effective interventions to improve strength.

Corcos et al[264] found a significant interaction between medication and strength. Withdrawal of levodopa during an "off" state period caused a decrease in strength and rate of force development. Exercise training should therefore optimally be timed for "on" periods when the patient is at his or her best (i.e., 45 minutes to 1 hour after medication has been taken). Exercising during an "off" period may not be possible or pose great difficulty for the patient. The patient should consistently exercise at the same time during a medication cycle.

Functional Training

An exercise program should be based on focused practice of functional skills. The overall emphasis is on improving functional mobility with specific emphasis on improving mobility of axial structures, the head, trunk, hips, and shoulders. Progression to more difficult motor activities should be gradual. The more severely involved patient may benefit initially from assisted movements progressing to active movements to improve initial motor performance.

Bed mobility skills (i.e., rolling, bridging, supine-to-sit transitions) are essential skills that are often very difficult owing to truncal rigidity and bradykinesia. Side-lying rolling activities that emphasize segmental rotation patterns (i.e., isolated upper and lower trunk rotations) should be practiced rather than a log-rolling pattern. Patients with very stiff trunks may benefit from compensatory rolling strategies using the UE or LE to reach over and initiate the movement. Utilizing large amplitude and high effort movements is particularly helpful for patients working on bed mobility and managing the bedsheets. For example, an overhead and diagonal reach with high and explosive effort can facilitate trunk rotation and a momentum strategy of rolling. Rolling should be practiced on different surfaces progressing from firm to soft and finally simulating the patient's bed surface at home. Bridging is an important activity that improves scooting in bed as well as sit-to-stand transfers. Practicing large amplitude, purposeful, and effortful steps with each leg then trunk and shoulders facilitates bridging and scooting (Fig. 18.8).

Sitting can be enhanced through exercises designed to improve pelvic and hip mobility as the patient with PD typically sits with a stiff and posteriorly tilted pelvis (i.e., sacral sitting position) along with a flexed upper trunk and legs close together with little hip abduction or rotation. Anterior and posterior tilts, side-to-side tilts, and pelvic clock exercises with legs apart (hips in full abduction) can be practiced while sitting on a therapy ball, which enhances ease of movement (Fig. 18.9). These

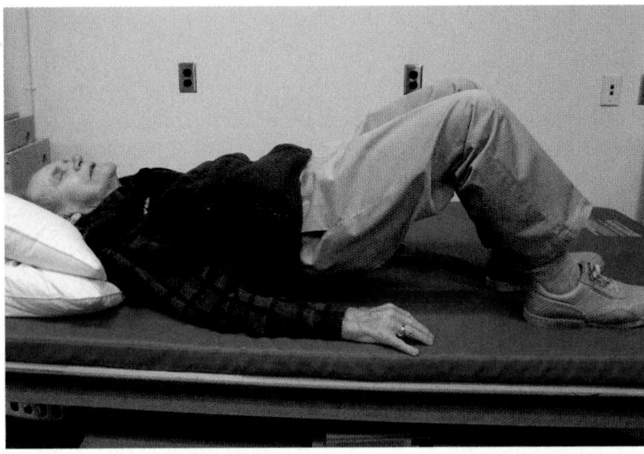

Figure 18.8 The patient with PD practices bridging (note the difficulty in achieving full hip extension).

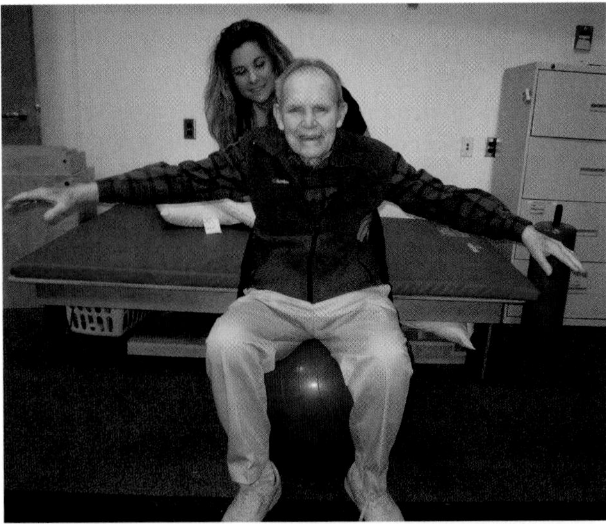

Figure 18.9 The patient with PD practices sitting on ball with UEs abducted to the sides, hands open.

activities can then be progressed to sitting on a stationary surface such as a mat table using an inflatable disc to finally no apparatus. Sitting activities should include weight shifting emphasizing upper trunk rotations and reaching. Diagonal movement patterns with the arms in sitting can be used to enhance trunk mobility, especially rotation.

Sit-to-stand (STS) is a difficult activity for many patients with PD, especially with moderate or advanced disease or when in the "off" state. Issues in poor dynamic stability and inadequate limb support contribute to falls. Patients demonstrate poor timing in controlling their COM forward velocity, which tends to be slower. Insufficient upward momentum (LE extension torques) in standing up is also problematic.[265] Other factors include level of agonist-antagonist coactivation and rigidity. STS training begins with the patient scooting to the edge of the mat and placing both feet under the knees and apart. Forward trunk and hip flexion can be enhanced through reaching forward and toward the floor between widespread knees. Cueing strategies (e.g., counting, placing one hand between the patient's shoulder blades) can be used to assist the forward lean. Sitting on an inflated disc can also assist in the forward weight shift and seat-off. Strengthening of the hip and knee extensors can be achieved through repeated sit-to-stand and partial squats while standing at the sink or counter. Practice standing up from a firm *raised* seat decreases the total excursion and work of extensor muscles and promotes ease of rise. Once control is achieved, progression is then to lower, standard height seats. Standing directly in front of the patient should be avoided, because this may block initial standing attempts. Instead, the therapist or caregiver should stand to the patient's side. If safety issues are apparent, a safety gait belt should be used. The more involved patient can practice STS from a chair with both hands on armrests.[266]

Standing activities can model the progression used in sitting. The patient needs to first gain the fully upright position with symmetrical weight-bearing over the BOS. Tactile cueing or light resistance can be used on the anterior pelvis to encourage movement of the hips forward into full extension. Once standing, weight shifts and rotational movements of the trunk should be practiced (e.g., reciprocal arm swings or reaching movements). Step-ups using a low platform step (forward, lateral) should be practiced. Backward stepping can be used to strengthen hip and spinal extensors and promote upright posturing. To increase the challenge during stepping, elastic resistive bands can be used (Fig. 18.10). The patient can also practice standing with UEs extended and hands weight-bearing on a wall to promote upper trunk extension.

Patients with PD typically experience a high number of falls and should be taught how to get up after a fall. To that end, skills in quadruped creeping should be practiced with the same large amplitude movements mentioned previously, so the patient is able to move to a nearby stable chair or couch at home. The patient should also practice transitions moving from quadruped to kneeling to half-kneeling and finally to standing using UE support. Blocked, repetitive practice of powerful, rapid, and purposeful movements should be practiced. For example, during the transition from floor on hands-knees to one hip flexed, the patient steps that foot forward beside the hand, then pushes up and extends hips and trunk to upright with arms opened up and out to half-kneeling, then pushing up with UEs to standing.

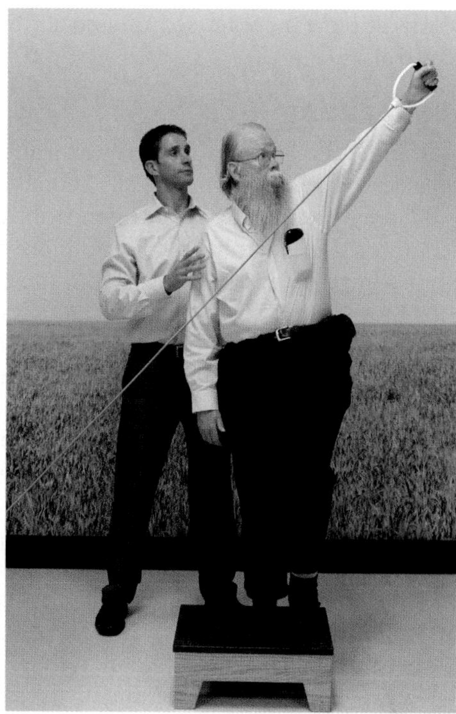

Figure 18.10 The patient with PD practices maintaining a step-up position while performing resisted UE shoulder abduction and flexion using elastic band resistance. The patient is encouraged to turn and look at the hand.

Mobilizing facial muscles is another important component of the exercise program because the patient will have limited social interaction and poor feeding skills in the presence of marked facial rigidity and bradykinesia. These factors can greatly influence the patient's overall psychological state, motivation, and social participation. Massage, stretch, manual contacts, and verbal cueing can be used to enhance facial movements. The patient can be instructed to practice lip pursing, movements of the tongue, swallowing, and facial movements such as smiling, frowning, and so forth. A mirror can be used to provide visual feedback. In cases where eating is impaired by immobility, the movements of opening and closing the mouth and chewing should be combined with neck stabilization in a neutral position.

Verbal skills should be practiced in association with breath control.

Balance Training

It is important to recall that learning is task and context specific. Thus, a balance training program should include a variety of activities that alter task demands and expose the patient to varying environmental conditions. Whenever possible the therapist should try to duplicate the conditions the patient will encounter in everyday life. The level of challenge is important. A therapist should know the limitations of the patient and the specific demands of the task and environment to select and progress tasks accordingly and ensure patient safety. See Chapter 10, Strategies to Improve Motor Function, for a more complete discussion of balance training.

An important focus of balance training for the patient with PD is COM and LOS control training. Patients should be instructed in how COM influences balance and how to improve posture in sitting, in standing, and during dynamic movement tasks. Patients should also explore their LOS and practice working toward expanding them in both sitting and standing. In standing, patients with PD typically demonstrate restricted LOS with forward displacement of center of foot pressure. Patients should be instructed in how to improve postural alignment and in ways to avoid postural disturbances and falls. The therapist can assist with postural and safety awareness by using appropriate verbal, visual, tactile, or proprioceptive cues to facilitate the desired responses. A standing platform training device (i.e., posturography system) can be valuable in providing COM position and LOS biofeedback. The patient is instructed in weight shifting that expands the LOS. The Nintendo Wii Balance Board is a widely available and economical force platform and biofeedback system. When compared with a laboratory-grade force platform the Nintendo Wii Balance Board was valid in quantifying center of pressure, an important component of standing balance.[267,268] Subjects with poor positional awareness who trained on the Wii Balance Board with real-time visual biofeedback demonstrated significant improvements in weight-bearing symmetry.[269] Subjects with PD who trained with this device for 30 minutes 3 times a week over a 4-week period improved on average 3.3 points on the BBS, 2.8 points of the DGI and decreased their variability of postural sway by 31%.[270]

Balance training should emphasize practice of dynamic stability tasks (e.g., weight shifts, alternating unilateral weight-bearing, reaching, axial rotation of the head and trunk, axial rotation combined with reaching, stepping to reach in all directions). Seated activities can include sitting on a compliant surface (inflatable disc) or a therapy ball. Challenges to balance can also be introduced in quadruped (Fig. 18.11), kneeling (Fig. 18.12), half-kneeling (Fig. 18.13), and standing on a disc (Figs. 18.14 and 18.15). Altering arm positions (e.g., arms out to side, arms folded across chest, reaching); altering foot/leg positions (e.g., feet apart, feet together); or adding voluntary movements (e.g., overhead arm clapping, head and trunk rotations, single leg raises, stepping or marching in place) can all be used to increase difficulty of the activity. Training should focus on achieving faster initiation and execution movement times (i.e., large, fast and powerful) supported by the use of appropriate cueing strategies.[228] Strategies for varying environmental demands include altering the support surface (e.g., standing on foam), visual inputs (e.g., reduced lighting,

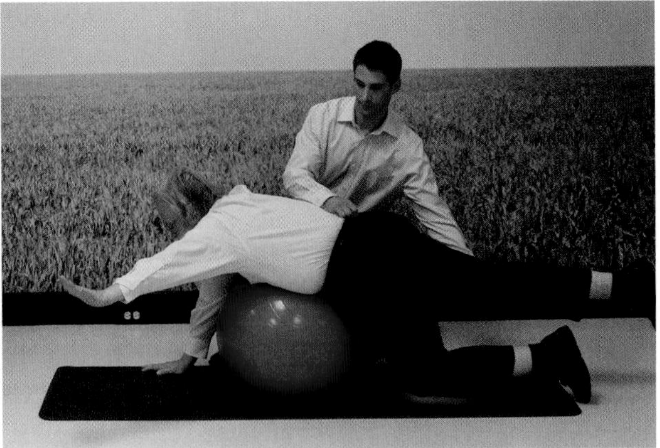

Figure 18.11 The patient with PD practices contralateral UE/LE lifts in quadruped over a ball.

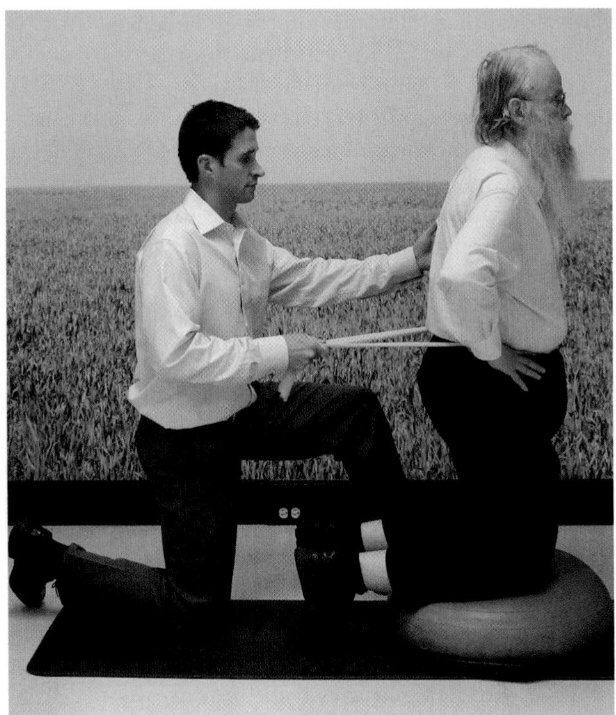

Figure 18.12 The patient with PD practices kneeling on a BOSU™ disc. The therapist provides resistance using an elastic band to promote full hip extension.

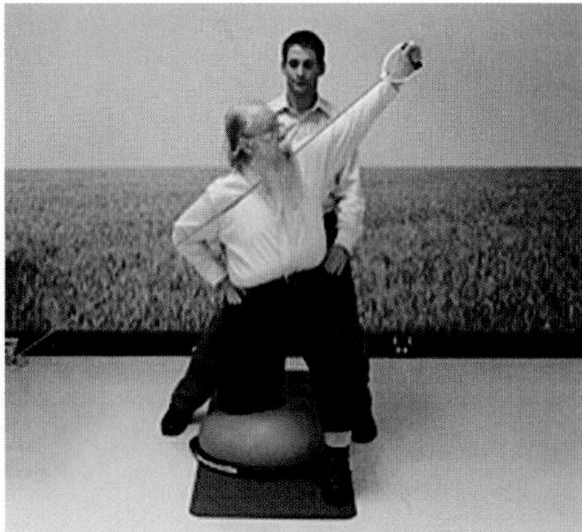

Figure 18.13 The patient with PD practices half-kneeling on a BOSU™ disc while performing resisted UE shoulder abduction and flexion using elastic band resistance.

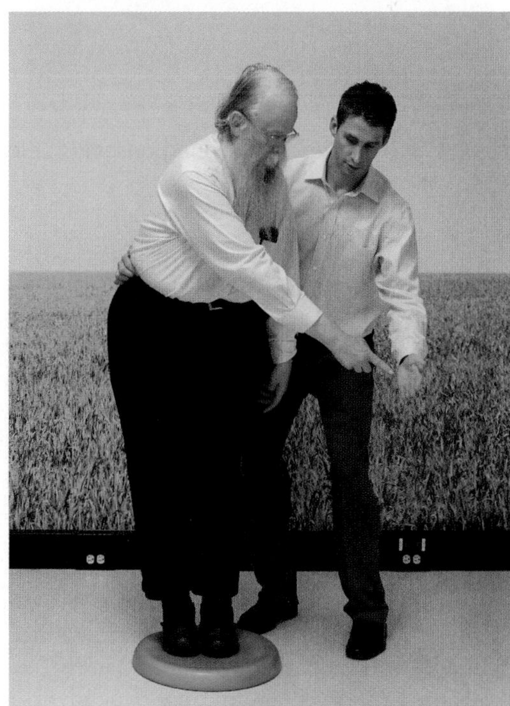

Figure 18.14 The patient with PD practices standing on an inflated disc while reaching across, promoting upper trunk rotation.

eyes closed), or challenging the patient with a variable open environment (e.g., busy clinic setting).

Adequate strength and ROM are important components needed to withstand the challenges of balance. The patient can be instructed in standing exercises to enhance balance, including heel-rises and toe-offs, partial squats and chair rises, single-limb stance with side-kicks or back-kicks, and marching in place. Collectively these exercises are sometimes referred to as the *kitchen sink exercises* and are important components of the HEP for

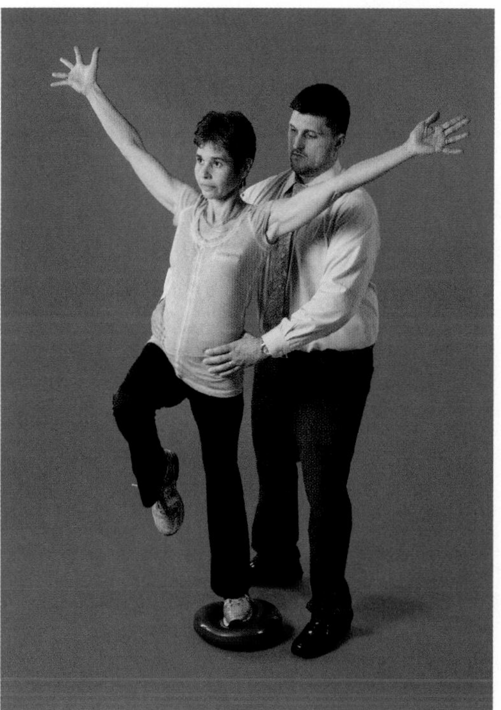

Figure 18.15 The patient with young-onset PD practices standing with one foot on an inflated disc with bilateral "Big arms" and hands open, palms up.

patients with balance deficiencies. The patient may require light touch-down support of the hands to start to stabilize yet keep the center of mass over the feet; the goal is to progress to no support as soon as possible.

Locomotor Training

Locomotor training goals focus on reducing primary gait impairments, which typically include slowed speed, decreased stride length, lack of a heel-toe sequence with forward progression characterized by a shuffling (festinating) gait pattern, diminished contralateral trunk movement and arm swing, and an overall attitude of flexion while walking. Goals also focus on increasing the patient's ability to safely perform functional mobility activities and prevent falls.[271] Effective strategies for improving upright alignment and safety include having the patient walk with vertical poles (pole walking) (Fig. 18.16). Strategies to enhance posture, step length, velocity, and arm swing include the use of *verbal instructional sets* (e.g., "Walk tall," "Walk fast," "Take large steps," "Swing both arms"). Behrman et al[272] found that commands for large step and arm swing were more effective instructional strategies than the command to walk fast. As previously discussed, visual (transverse more than parallel) and auditory cues are also effective in improving gait speed and step length.[273] Strategies to improve foot placement can include use of floor markers or footprints on the floor. Strategies to improve step height include practice marching in place progressing to walking using

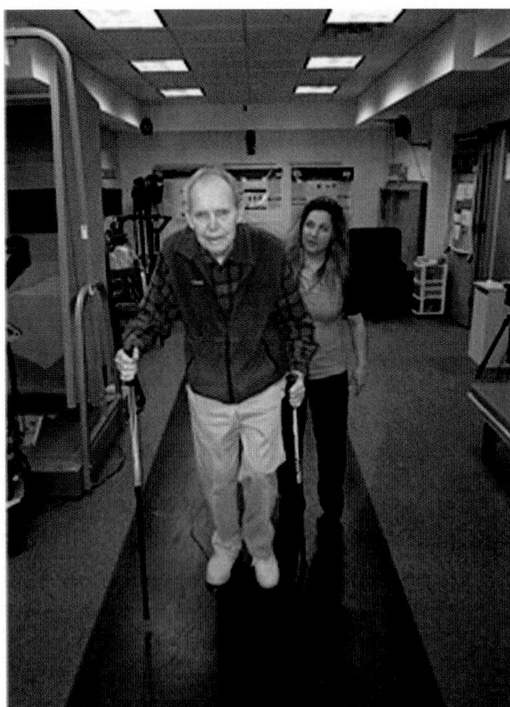

Figure 18.16 The patient with PD practices walking using two vertical poles.

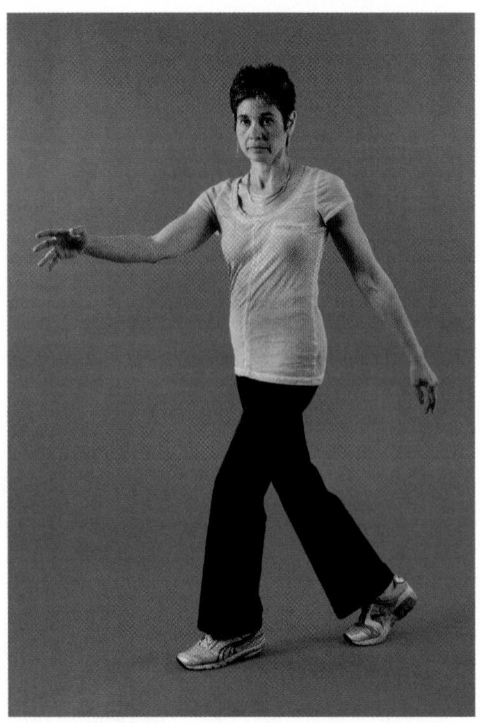

Figure 18.17 The patient with young-onset PD practices cross-step walking.

an exaggerated high stepping pattern. Brisk marching music can be used to enhance pace. Sidestepping and crossed-step walking can be practiced. The activity of braiding, which combines side-stepping with alternate crossed-stepping, is a good activity for the patient with early PD because it emphasizes lower trunk rotation with stepping and side-stepping movements. It can be practiced with the patient holding on lightly to a dowel held jointly with therapist or as a free walking pattern. However, braiding fails to encourage large steps, hip abduction, and external rotation, and instead can elicit festination and freezing. Advanced stepping and balancing that includes large hip and pelvic movements can be achieved by having the patient practice juggling scarves (Fig. 18.17) or move through an agility course. Agility courses can include turns, multidirectional stepping, crossing obstacles of different heights, changing surfaces, reaching, boxing, creeping through tunnels or under bars, crawling, floor-to-stand transitions, and more.[70] Reciprocal arm swing during gait can be enhanced by having the patient and therapist hold onto a set of two dowels (one in each hand). The therapist walks behind the patient and uses his or her arm swing to assist the patient's. Alternatively, from behind the therapist can lightly facilitate trunk rotation at the shoulders/upper trunk, thereby arm swing occurs passively because of the "natural" trunk rotation.

Patients with PD who practiced locomotor training on a motorized treadmill with an overhead harness demonstrated improvements in postural stability, gait (e.g., walking speed, step and stride length), motor function, and quality of life.[274-278] Both body weight support (e.g., up to 20%)[279] and no body support have been used.[280] In a long-term study, Miyai et al[281] found that gains in walking speed and number of steps following this type of training were maintained at 4 months. The researchers stated that attentional strategies were not used and speculate that the enhancement of gait might be due to activation of central pattern generators as is thought the case in stroke and spinal cord injury (SCI) studies. The treadmill may be acting as an external cue to enhance gait rhythmicity and reduce gait variability.[282] The benefits of treadmill training, as with exercise training in general, are dose dependent. More pronounced improvements are noted with high-intensity practice and incremental increases in treadmill speed.[283] High-intensity treadmill training has been shown to normalize corticomotor excitability in early PD and to increase neuroplasticity of dopaminergic signalling in the basal ganglia.[274,284] The motorized treadmill can also be used for step training in people with PD. While supported in a safety harness, patients practice stepping in all four directions in response to suddenly turning the treadmill on and off[285] or by turning 90 or 180 degrees to change direction of walking without pausing the treadmill, for patients in earlier stages of PD.

Locomotor training should also include task-specific training designed to promote full participation in social roles pertaining to family life, leisure, and community participation. This includes varying the walking task (e.g., walking on a tile floor, on carpet, outdoors on sidewalks and grassy terrain). Additional challenges include walking in the community (e.g., variable open environments), stair climbing, up and down curbs and ramps, over obstacles, and while also carrying out another task (e.g., buttoning a coat/shirt, talking on the phone, getting coins from a purse or pocket). Patients with PD often demonstrate difficulties in obstacle stepping due to deficits in cognitive and sensory-motor processing[286] and to reduced foot clearance. Foot clearance can be improved with repeated practice of stepping over horizontal floor markers or laser light signals.

Patients in the advanced stage of the disease will be limited in terms of walking and variations that can be utilized. The overall goal at this stage is to promote regular walking while maintaining safety and preventing falls. Compensatory training strategies are indicated. Caregiver instruction regarding assisted walking and safety is imperative.

Freezing of Gait

Freezing episodes are common and are often resistant to drug therapy. The therapist and patient should identify and practice strategies for unfreezing gait.[72] For example, some compensatory strategies include cueing or "trick" movements such as dropping a tissue that the patient must step over. Having the patient focus extra attention to gait, making wide turns, walking and turning with wide and rocking steps, high-knees marching, and modifying the environment to reduce exposure to closed, tight spaces can also be successful strategies in reducing freezing.

Action observation training (AOT) is a recent approach that is based on the concept of the mirror neuron system in the frontal and parietal lobes.[287,288] Patients with freezing episodes watched video clips of strategies and movements that were helpful in reducing freezing, 3 times a week for 4 weeks. Each 60-minute session consisted of 24 minutes of observation and 36 minutes of imitation performed separately. The control group watched the same number and length of video clips of static landscapes followed by performance of the same movements/actions of the AOT group. After treatment, both groups showed reduced severity of freezing, but only the AOT group showed improved motor impairment (MDS-UPDRS scores), walking speed, balance, and quality of life at 1 month post training. These motor improvements were associated with functional MRI (fMRI) findings of increased recruitment of motor regions and areas of the brain involved in attention, goal-directed processing, and the mirror neuron system.

Freezing of gait is associated with cognitive dysfunction, specifically in the areas of response inhibition, conflict resolution, visuospatial function, and switching or divided attention.[26,289-292] Cognitive training for people with PD has shown to be successful.[293-295] Considering the evidence that indicates an overlap of cognition and mobility, combining cognitive and physical exercise training for people with PD may reduce freezing from a restorative versus compensatory perspective.[70] Peterson et al[70] suggest example activities that could be done with patients to specifically challenge the deficits in cognitive domains associated with freezing. For example, an agility course (divided attention) as described previously, a Trail Making Test walking task in which one walks from a letter to a number alternating in ascending order (attention shifting),[296] a Stroop walking task (inhibition),[297] and a Go-No-Go boxing task with congruent and incongruent visual and verbal cues (inhibition, selection), among others.

Motor-Cognitive Dual-Task Training

Many activities of daily living require doing two or more tasks at once such as driving, having a phone conversation while walking, and conversing while preparing dinner. Dual-tasking is the simultaneous execution of two tasks that can be performed independently, can be measured separately, and that have distinct task goals.[298] *Dual-task interference* is a measure often used to represent the degree of performance deterioration from single task (ST) to dual-task (DT) conditions.[299] Successful dual-task performance relies on the cognitive ability to process and integrate the requirements of both tasks and to perform tasks automatically to some degree.[300,301] Individuals with PD have deficits in cognitive/executive functions, automaticity and movement control, as discussed earlier in the chapter. These deficits influence dual-tasking which can lead to problems including imbalance and falls,[188,302-304] and impaired driving and car accidents.[305-307] Most commonly, dual-task interference during walking is seen as decreased gait speed and stride length, and increased variability and asymmetry.[308] Drivers with PD and dual-task interference show decreased steering accuracy and speed adaptation, and increased braking reaction time.[309]

Dual-task training (DTT) has been traditionally considered to be hazardous for people with PD and that underlying cognitive / executive function and automaticity deficits were not likely to change with intervention.[310,311] Therefore, clinical guidelines have recommended people with PD avoid or limit dual-task situations in their daily lives.[312,313] However, recent evidence of the benefits from dual-task training has contributed to the discussion of whether it is advisable to "train hazardous behavior."[310,314] Table 18.6, Evidence Summary, presents a review of selected research in the area of motor-cognitive dual-task training for people with PD.

In a systematic review to assess the effectiveness of motor-cognitive DTT compared with usual care in individuals with neurologic disorders, Fritz et al[315] found that, regardless of the method used, motor-cognitive DTT interventions improved single and dual-task walking (stride length and velocity). Furthermore, DTT resulted in more moderate improvements in balance and cognition. See Table 18.6 for details.

Table 18.6 Evidence Summary Motor-Cognitive Dual-Task Training (DTT) for Patients With Parkinson's Disease

Fritz, NE, Cheek, FM, and Nichols-Larsen, DS: Motor-cognitive dual-task training in persons with neurologic disorders: A systematic review.[315]

Design	SR to determine the effectiveness of motor-cognitive dual-task training compared with usual care on mobility and cognition in individuals with neurologic disorders.
Level of Evidence	Level I
Subjects	Subjects with PD and Alzheimer's disease (AD)
Intervention	Cued walking, cognitive tasks paired with gait, balance, and strength training and virtual reality or gaming.
Results	DTT improves single-task gait velocity and stride length in subjects with PD and AD, dual-task gait velocity and stride length in subjects with PD, AD, and brain injury, and may improve balance and cognition in those with PD and AD.
Comments	Improvement of dual-task ability in individuals with neurologic disorders holds potential for improving gait, balance, and cognition.

Killane, I, et al: Dual motor-cognitive virtual reality training impacts dual-task performance in freezing of gait.[316]

Design	RCT to examine the effect of dual motor-cognitive virtual reality training on dual-task performance in freezing of gait (FOG) in individuals with PD.
Level of Evidence	Level II
Subjects	Twenty community dwelling participants with PD (13 with FOG, 7 without FOG).
Intervention	Eight 20-minute intervention sessions consisting of a virtual reality maze through which participants navigated by stepping in place on a balance board combined with a cognitive task (Stroop test).
Results	Significant improvement in dual-task cognitive and motor parameters (stepping time and rhythmicity), dual-task effect for those with FOG and a noteworthy improvement in FOG episodes. Improvements were less significant for those without FOG.
Comments	A dual motor-cognitive approach to treatment improves dual-task performance and decreases FOG in subjects with PD.

Conradsson, D, et al: The effects of highly challenging balance training in elderly with Parkinson's disease: A randomized controlled trial.[136]

Design	RCT to evaluate the short-term effects of the HiBalance program, a highly challenging balance-training regimen that incorporates both dual-tasking and PD-specific balance components.
Level of Evidence	Level II
Subjects	Ninety-one elderly participants with mild to moderate PD
Intervention	Participants randomized either into a 10-week program of highly challenging balance-training incorporating DTT or usual care for elderly with mild to moderate PD.
Results	Training group demonstrated significantly improved balance and gait performance. In addition, the training group improved their performance of the cognitive task while walking.
Comments	The HiBalance program showed promising transfer effects to everyday living.

Yitayeh, A, and Teshome, A: The effectiveness of physiotherapy treatment on balance dysfunction and postural instability in persons with Parkinson's disease: A systematic review and meta-analysis.[318]

Design	SR to determine the effectiveness of conventional physiotherapy interventions in the management of balance dysfunction and postural instability in persons with idiopathic PD.
Level of Evidence	Level I
Subjects	248 participants with idiopathic PD
Intervention	Highly challenging balance training that incorporates both dual-taking and PD-specific balance components in the form of stance and gait tasks which require feedforward and feedback postural control and in the form of technology-assisted balance training.

Table 18.6 Evidence Summary Motor-Cognitive Dual-Task Training (DTT) for Patients With Parkinson's Disease—cont'd

Results	Training that incorporates both dual-tasking and PD-specific balance components significantly benefited balance and gait abilities when compared with usual care. Repetitive exercises, highly challenging balance training, and incremental speed-dependent treadmill training improved range of motion, endurance, gait parameters, functional reaching activities and postural stability. In addition, it was demonstrated that these exercises help to decrease fall rate and fear of falling.
Comments	Results of study on high balance training can only be generalized to elderly, community dwelling individuals with mild to moderate-stage PD without cognitive impairments.
Ford, M, et al: The effect of dual task activities on the walking gait of individuals with Parkinson's disease.[319]	
Design	SR to determine the effectiveness of dual-task gait training (DTGT) on individuals with PD
Level of Evidence	Level I
Subjects	Subjects with PD
Intervention	Dual-task gait training
Results	DTGT improved gait speed, stride length, cadence and balance. The addition of gait patterns and rhythmic music produced positive effects on dual-task walking.
Comments	DTGT can offset the negative effects of PD on patient's ability to dual-task while ambulating.
Strouwen, C, et al: Training dual tasks together or apart in Parkinson's disease: Results from the DUALITY trial.[300]	
Design	RCT to evaluate and compare the efficacy and possible fall risk of two dual-task training (DTT) interventions for improving gait delivered in the home for 6 weeks.
Level of Evidence	Level II
Subjects	One hundred twenty-one patients with PD, H & Y II-III
Intervention	Participants randomized into either (1) a consecutive task training (CTT) group which trained on gait and cognitive tasks separately, or (2) an integrated dual-task training (IDT) group which trained gait and cognitive tasks simultaneously. Posttests occurred immediately after training and at 12-week follow-up.
Results	Both groups improved in dual-task gait velocity which was retained after 12 weeks. Fall risk was unchanged for both groups.
Comments	Gains in dual-task walking are likely due to *both* improved task automaticity from the CTT *and* more efficient integration of task-related neural networks from the IDT. Dual-task training can be safe, even when delivered in the home.

SR: systematic review; RCTs: randomized controlled trials

Specifically exploring the effects of DTT intervention for FOG using virtual reality, Killane et al[316] found that the participants with FOG improved in dual-task cognitive and gait measures (reaction time, stepping time, and rhythmicity), whereas the non-FOG group only improved in stepping time. In addition, for the FOG group the number of FOG episodes per trial was reduced after DTT intervention compared with before. The authors suggest that virtual reality DTT interventions such as these, that integrate cognitive and motor tasks together in training, could be used in the home and improve the quality of life for patients who experience FOG.

FOG is a risk factor for falls, as discussed earlier in the chapter. Therefore, an intervention that uses cognitive functions known to contribute to falls in people with PD, and with FOG in particular, may pose a safety risk.[310] Strouwen et al[300,317] addressed this issue and the efficacy of two different DTT programs for improving dual-task gait delivered in the home, consecutive task training (CTT) and integrated dual-task training (IDT). In CTT, gait training and cognitive exercises (verbal fluency, reciting switching and working memory tasks) were delivered separately to improve task *automaticity*. IDT consisted of gait practice and cognitive training done simultaneously to improve dual-task *integration*. Results showed that dual-task gait improved after training, regardless of which method was used, and benefits were retained 12 weeks later. Importantly, the risk of falls did not increase with either of the two community-delivered interventions. The authors note that the improved dual-task performance gains are likely due to improved task automaticity after CTT *and* to better integration of task-related neural networks after IDT.

Spinal Orthotics

Spinal bracing may be an appropriate adjunct to therapy for patients with postural deformities common to PD (e.g., increased thoracic kyphosis, decreased costal expansion, and forward head posture). The Spinomed thoracolumbar orthosis is unique in that it not only corrects faulty posture but also has been shown to increase trunk stability, increase respiratory vital capacity, and improve a patient's self-report of well-being.[321,322] When the brace was worn for 6 months the subjects had a 73% increase in back extensor strength and a 58% increase in abdominal flexor strength. These strength gains are attributed to increased muscular activity in response to the proprioceptive biofeedback of the brace.[323] A study investigating gait stability and physical functioning in women with postmenopausal osteoporosis demonstrated decreased double limb stance time associated with a beneficial impact on gait stability.[324] Further research is warranted to determine if this type of orthotic intervention holds potential for patients with PD.

Pulmonary Rehabilitation

The four main classifications of respiratory disorders in patients with PD are medication complications, upper airway obstructions, restrictive disorders, and aspiration pneumonia.[98,325] Since respiratory dysfunction in the neurological movement disorders population is linked to a high rate of disability and mortality, it is critical that the prevention and treatment of these dysfunctions take priority. Components include diaphragmatic breathing exercises, air-shifting techniques, and exercises that recruit neck, shoulder, and trunk muscles. Manual techniques such as vibration and shaking can be used to ensure complete exhalation, distal alveoli opening, and to assist with secretion clearance. The patient should be instructed in deep-breathing exercises to improve chest wall mobility and vital capacity. Air shifts are promoted to lesser-ventilated areas of the lung. For example, basal expansion can be promoted using side-lying recumbent positioning, manual stretch, and resistance to those segments. Upper body resistance training exercises are indicated. These can include raising and lowering a dowel with light weights added to increase resistance. Weights are increased as function improves. As previously mentioned, chest wall mobility can be improved by arm raises in multiple and diagonal directions. Light weights (wrist cuffs) can also be added to these exercises. Patients are encouraged to coordinate breathing with UE movement. Exercises are performed in unsupported sitting to promote trunk stabilization. A focus on improving trunk extension is especially important in improving breathing patterns in patients with postural kyphosis. Pulmonary rehabilitation programs have been shown to be safe and effective for patients with PD in improving pulmonary function[326,327] and perception of dyspnea.[328]

Speech Therapy

The quality of speech in patients with PD is often a breathy monotone, soft voice that is perceived by the patient to be of normal loudness. Hypophonia is caused by a bradykinetic bellows mechanism (chest wall and diaphragm) and patients' inaccurate perception of their own speech effort. Speech deficits are seen in 80% of patients with PD and have a dramatic effect on function with 30% reporting it as the most disabling part of the disease.[329] The Lee Silverman Voice Treatment (LSVT) was designed specifically for patients with PD.[330] It focuses on intensive high-effort exercise with a single functionally relevant target (loudness) and a recalibration of self-perception of vocal loudness. This technique effectively increases vocal loudness and improves facial expressions in patients with PD.[331,332]

Aerobic Exercise

An individualized exercise prescription is developed based on the ACSM guidelines for frequency, intensity, time (duration), and type of intervention (the FITT equation).[200] Intensities will be less than normal training intensities or submaximal (i.e., 60% to 80% of maximum HR), based on the patient's level of disease, fitness, and lifestyle. When lower intensities are used, longer-duration or more frequent exercise sessions are necessary to improve fitness. Careful monitoring is indicated, because autonomic dysfunction is common. Long-term levodopa use can produce arrhythmias and OH along with dyskinesias. The therapist should monitor vital signs (HR, RR, BP), RPE, fatigue levels, and symptoms of exertional intolerance (e.g., significant dyspnea, and hypotensive response). Endurance exercise training at a relatively high level improves cardiorespiratory capacity and endurance through increased Vo_{2max} in mild and moderate PD.[333] Aerobic capacity and cognitive function improved in people with PD after a high-intensity aerobic exercise training program on a stationary recumbent bike, 3 times/week for 12 weeks, starting at 5 minutes/week up to 40 min/week.[334] These changes were correlated with functional changes measured with fMRI in brain areas involved in motor learning (increased activity in the hippocampus, striatum, and cerebellum).[335]

Training modes can include leg and arm ergometry and walking. Selection will depend on the specific abilities of the patient; for example, postural instability and increased risk of falls may rule out use of a treadmill without an overhead harness. Recumbent or seated LE ergometry is a suitable alternative. A community-based indoor tandem cycling program, 3 times per week for 10 weeks, was designed to promote a high-cadence, consistency and intensity of practice.[336] The authors found that the vast majority of participants with PD achieved their training goals for target HR of 60% to 75% max and cadence of 80 to 90 revolutions per minute, and had 100% attendance. For most patients, a program of regular walking is recommended. The duration, speed, and terrain covered can be modified, based on individual ability. Accessibility to a supervised walking program using an indoor walking track is important for some to ensure safety. A shopping mall can provide an acceptable environment for community walkers in case of inclement or extremes of weather. A supervised aerobic pool program can also provide an acceptable mode of exercise for some patients. The warmth of the water may be relaxing, and the buoyancy may enhance stepping movements. The minimum recommended aerobic exercise frequency is 3 sessions per week. Daily walking with short multiple bouts (20 to 30 minutes) spaced throughout the day is recommended for individuals with lower functional capacity. Intermittent exercise with adequate rest intervals is indicated for those patients who are elderly and deconditioned, and who present with restrictive pulmonary dysfunction. Aerobic training programs have been shown to be safe and effective for patients with PD in improving aerobic capacity.[333-336]

Group and Home Exercises

Community-based group exercise classes can be valuable for patients with PD. Patients benefit from the positive support, camaraderie, and communication the group situation offers.[337,338] Exercise classes directed by a physical therapist can provide an integrated focus on PD-related issues. Careful evaluation of each patient before admission into a group or class is essential to ensure appropriate matching of the patient's fitness level with the class demands. Patients should be able to perform the therapeutic core of the class. Selecting patients with similar levels of disability is often advisable because the sense of competition can frequently be a key factor in motivating groups. The ratio of staff to patients should be kept small (ideally, 1:8 or 1:10), and extra staff should be added if patients are unable to work on their own. A variety of activities can be used to stimulate and motivate patients. The patients can begin in the seated position and progress to standing, using light, touch-down support of the back of the chair. Stretching exercises or calisthenics involving large muscle groups and multijoint compound movements can be used as an initial warm-up activity. Progression is to combination movements (UEs and LEs with axial trunk rotation) and to chained, sequential movements. Well-structured, low-impact aerobics are an appropriate focus for a group class. For example, patients can march in place, first in sitting, then in standing. The group can then practice walking with an emphasis on taking large, high steps. Music is used to provide necessary stimulation to movement and movement pacing. Exercise stations set up as a circuit class (e.g., stationary bicycle, mats, pulleys, and agility course) can also be used. Exercises done by the whole group together should focus on important exercise goals (e.g., improving ROM, and mobility). Recreational activities can follow the aerobic portion, such as line dancing, partnered tango, ball activities, beanbag toss, partnered boxing, and drumming. The activities selected should be interesting and varied. A relaxation segment should be incorporated into each class. Polestriding groups (walking with trekking poles) are gaining in popularity and is another effective way to exercise at moderate to high intensity.[137,339] Yoga, Pilates, Alexander Technique, and Tai Chi group classes effectively address multiple components of PD by improving posture, flexibility, core stability, functional mobility, balance, relaxation, and socialization.[253,254,340-344] King and Horak[345] recommend incorporating Tai Chi with other agility exercises (e.g., kayaking, boxing, lunges, agility training, and Pilates exercises) to delay loss of mobility in people with PD.

The home exercise program (HEP) includes exercises designed to improve relaxation, flexibility, strength, and cardiopulmonary function (all previously discussed). A key element is stressing the importance of regular daily exercise and avoidance of prolonged periods of inactivity. The HEP should be realistic and of moderate duration and intensity. Early morning warm-up exercises and stretches are often helpful in reducing the increased stiffness patients may experience on arising. Stretching and strengthening exercises are performed in supine, sitting, and standing positions. Home ROM exercises can often be assisted by use of adaptive equipment. For example, to reduce the effects of forward head and kyphotic posture, the patient can be instructed to hang by the hands using an overhead bar. Standing, corner wall stretches can also be used to provide a maintained stretch on the upper trunk flexors. Use of a wand or cane can be effective in promoting overhead motions. In standing, a countertop or back of a sturdy chair can be used to assist in stabilization during standing calisthenics and balance activities. Home-based exercise programs have been found to be effective in improving postural control, mobility, functional status, and motor complications in people with PD.[346-350]

ADAPTIVE AND SUPPORTIVE DEVICES

Attention should be directed toward needs for adaptive and supportive devices that can improve function. To promote bed mobility, the patient can be helped to assume a sitting position by elevating the head of an electronic hospital bed or with commercially available blocks approximately 4 in (10 cm) high (furniture legs fit into a recess in the block). A simpler solution might include attaching a knotted rope or canvas "ladder" to the end of the bed to pull on. The bed should be stable and the mattress firm to facilitate mobility. Satin sheets and pajamas have sometimes been helpful to enhance bed mobility. Patients should be instructed to select firm chairs with armrests and avoid soft, low seats such as a low sofa. The chair can be raised (i.e., 4 in [10 cm] and secured with blocks or tilted forward by elevating only the back legs about 2 in [5 cm]). Some patients benefit from the use of a rocking chair to facilitate independent sit-to-stand transfers. Chairs that have spring-loaded seats that push the patient into standing are heavily marketed to the geriatric population but should be used with caution. The patient is propelled into standing but may have difficulty stopping the movement and/or getting his or her balance within an appropriate time frame when first reaching the standing position. A raised toilet seat and toilet rails are also essential devices to facilitate ease of sit-to-stand transitions in the bathroom.

Loose-fitting clothing and sneakers with hook and loop closures can be used to facilitate dressing. If the patient demonstrates a shuffling gait, shoes should have leather or hard composition soles, because shoes with crepe or rubber soles will not slide easily and can result in falls. A festinating gait can sometimes be alleviated by the addition of modified heel or shoe wedges. A flat heel or toe wedge may slow down a propulsive gait. The use of assistive devices can be problematic owing to movement difficulties. A cane can be helpful for patients with mild to moderate disease to assist in balance or cue stepping (inverted walking stick). It is important that the height of the device not promote increased flexion of the trunk. Vertical poles (previously mentioned) can also be helpful to improve upright posture, trunk rotation, and arm swing during walking. Patients with more pronounced movement difficulties and poor balance are not likely to benefit from assistive devices. Walkers with wheels are particularly hazardous and are likely to increase a festinating gait; hand brakes are an essential requirement.

Most patients use adaptive devices to assist in ADL. Reachers can be used to assist in dressing as well as for other activities. Eating can be facilitated in several ways. The patient should be seated properly, close to the table, with good posture. Specially adapted utensils, plate guards, and enlarged handles can aid the patient's efforts. Because eating time will be prolonged, heated plates or pads may help keep food warm and palatable. Drooling and/or spills should be anticipated and clothing protected. Extra time should be planned, and the patient should not feel rushed.

PSYCHOSOCIAL ISSUES

The progressive nature of PD necessitates frequent personal and social adjustments and affects all aspects of life for both the patient and family. Disruptions in daily functions, roles, and activities are experienced. Some of the changes associated with PD are socially isolating (masked face, progressive immobility, and unintelligible speech) whereas other changes (increased salivation, perspiration, decreased sexual function) are distressing and can be socially embarrassing. The patient may feel increasingly isolated and family relationships may suffer. The principal goal for team members is to assist the patient and family in their understanding of the disease and in developing insights and adjustments that lead to more effective self-management. Some individuals can successfully deal with the changes associated with the disease; others are not. Coping skills can be facilitated. First and foremost, education is the key to assisting patients and family members assume responsibility. Feelings of hopelessness and dependency are reduced as the patient develops a sense of control over his or her own life. Self-management skills that should be promoted include advanced planning of activities, effective time management strategies, and stress management techniques. It is equally important to ensure that patients do not become isolated and that appropriate services are available. Team members must be vigilant regarding their assumptions and expectations. A condescending or pessimistic and limiting attitude can become a self-fulfilling prophecy. Patients and family members need reassurances and encouragement. An overall emphasis on what patients *can do* rather than what they cannot do helps to empower patients. Therapists need to provide a message of *hope tempered with realism.*

PATIENT, FAMILY, AND CAREGIVER EDUCATION

The interdisciplinary team provides information about a variety of topics related to living with PD. These are presented in Box 18.5. Interventions can take the form of direct one-on-one instruction, group sessions, printed materials, and video or computer presentations. The therapist's overall approach needs to be positive and supportive.

Community support groups are available for patients and their families. They disseminate information and offer a chance to discuss common issues, problems, and management tips. They also can provide a stabilizing influence, assisting patients and families to focus on healthy behaviors, coping skills, and effective self-management. For some patients in the early stages of the disease, participation in a support group may increase levels of anxiety as they observe more disabled patients. Groups particularly targeted to patients with early-stage disease and similar ages may be more helpful.

Educational pamphlets, newsletters, and location of support groups can be obtained through national PD associations.

National Parkinson Foundation (NPF)
200 SE 1st Street, Suite 800
Miami, FL 33131
Website: www.parkinson.org
Phone: 800-473-4636
E-mail: contact@parkinson.org

Parkinson's Disease Foundation (PDF)
1359 Broadway, Suite 1509
New York, NY 10018
Website: www.pdf.org
Phone: 800-457-6676
E-mail: info@pdf.org

Web-based resources for clinicians and patients/families living with PD are presented in Appendix 18.B.

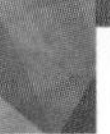

Box 18.5 Elements of a Patient, Family, and Caregiver Education Program

- Parkinson's disease: clinical presentation, strategies to manage symptoms
- Medications: purpose, dosage, possible adverse side effects, signs of either overmedication or undermedication
- Preventive measures to minimize the secondary complications and impairments
- Impact of PD on movement and effective strategies to manage movement problems
- Barriers to exercise and effective solutions to regular exercise participation
- Impact of PD on function and effective strategies to maintain independent function in home, community, or work environments
- Strategies for energy conservation and activity pacing
- Strategies for ensuring activity participation in valued leisure and family activities
- Community resources for patients: support groups, in-home interventions, community training programs, day programs
- Community resources for caregivers: counseling, support groups, exercise programs, respite care

SUMMARY

PD is a chronic, progressive disorder of the BG characterized by the cardinal features of rigidity, bradykinesia, tremor, and postural instability. Additional impairments include the development of abnormal fixed postures, poverty of movement, fatigue, masked face, contractures, a festinating gait pattern, swallowing and communication difficulties, visual and sensorimotor disturbances, cognitive and behavioral dysfunction, autonomic dysfunction, and cardiopulmonary changes. Pharmacological interventions have become the mainstay of treatment and provide protective and symptomatic treatment. Effective rehabilitation focuses on the patient's stage of disease and symptoms, activity limitations and participation restriction, and residual abilities and assets. Interventions are restorative; that is, rehabilitation is focused on the improvement of strength, ROM, mobility, balance, functional skills, and endurance. Individuals with PD also benefit from functional maintenance programs designed to manage the effects of progressive disease. Strategies are developed to prevent or reduce indirect impairments and promote regular exercise, good health, and self-management skills. A comprehensive team approach including active involvement of patient and family provides optimal benefits. Team members need to be active during all stages of the disease, assisting the patient and family in maintenance of function and providing psychosocial support as needed.

Questions for Review

1. What are the major CNS structures involved in Parkinson's disease and what are the pathophysiological changes associated with the disease?
2. Differentiate between cogwheel rigidity and lead pipe rigidity.
3. What impairments in postural stability are typically seen in patients with PD?
4. What are the nonmotor impairments in cognition associated with PD?
5. What are the major adverse effects associated with long-term use of levodopa/carbidopa?
6. How might the goals/outcomes and interventions vary by stage of disease?
7. Orthostatic hypotension is a common problem in patients with PD. How should it be examined?
8. Identify appropriate motor learning strategies for the patient with PD in terms of practice and feedback.
9. Describe the gait impairments common in patients with PD. What interventions can be used to improve locomotor function?
10. What guidelines for aerobic training are appropriate for the patient with early- to middle-stage PD?

CASE STUDY

Patient presented for physical therapy evaluation with his wife. The patient is a 63-year-old male with an 8-year history of PD. Patient reports a recent progression of decreased function, feelings of heaviness throughout his body. Wife reports that he has been moving more slowly with increased episodes of freezing and a new onset of hopelessness and depression. Patient referred to physical therapy to improve safety with ambulation and ability to perform activities of daily living with improved independence.

HISTORY

The patient is a retired construction foreman/supervisor and a martial arts teacher/boxing trainer. He lives in a private house with his wife. The patient's initial onset of Parkinson's disease manifested with slight bilateral hand and lower extremity tremors right greater than left. He lived a very active life until recently when symptoms progressed to include freezing, shuffling gait pattern, decreased coordination of upper and lower body, rigidity, and decreased balance. Bed mobility has deteriorated, including difficulty getting in and out of bed and freezing in bed. Speech volume has also deteriorated over time. Patient has a history of a fall out of a window and cervical trauma sustained during a martial arts practice that has left him with chronic cervical and bilateral shoulder pain.

CURRENT STATUS

The patient is currently taking trihexyphenidyl, ropinirole, and rasagiline. His chief complaints include the following:

- Difficulty walking, especially on uneven terrain, when getting up from office chair, and when moving in tight confined spaces
- Episodes of gait blocks (freezing of gait) that are worse with dual-tasking, stopping and starting movement, and changing positions and directions with turns
- Increased bouts of uncontrolled or unsteady balance and 3 falls in the past year
- Decreased endurance with ambulation; currently able to walk only 200 feet before requiring a break
- Increased difficulty rolling and getting into and out of bed
- Inability to dress independently
- Increased trunk rigidity
- Decreased speech volume
- Due to decreased hand coordination and respiratory tidal volume, patient frustrated that he is no longer able to play the harmonica
- Bilateral shoulder pain left greater than right aggravated with movement and sleep postures

EXAMINATION FINDINGS

Cognition

Alert, oriented × 3

Psychosocial

Patient is showing signs of depression and frustration with progression of disease. He has always prided himself on how active he was with martial arts and activities of daily living. Patient presents with a fear of falling in unfamiliar places.

Speech

Mild dysarthria, hypophonia

Sensation

Slightly decreased proprioception bilaterally in both ankles; otherwise intact

Tone

Rigidity (cogwheel type) moderate in all extremities R > L

Marked rigidity throughout neck and trunk

Mask-like face

Range of Motion

Decreased due to moderate rigidity; with limitations in the following:

- Bilateral cervical rotation (0° to 30°)
- Bilateral shoulder abduction (0° to 130°)
- Bilateral elbow extension (10° to 140°)
- Bilateral hip extension (0° to 10°)
- Bilateral knee extension (10° to 115°)
- Bilateral ankle dorsiflexion (0° to 10°).

Strength
Generally fair (3/5) to good minus (4–/5)
Poor (2/5) bilateral shoulder abduction, bilateral ankle dorsiflexion

Motor Function
Moderate to severe resting tremors, R hand > L hand.
Bradykinesia: marked slowness, poverty of movement.
Hesitation on initiation of movement

Posture
Forward head position; flexed; kyphotic spine
Stands with flexion of elbows and hips

Balance
Decreased limits of stability
The Lower Extremity Functional Scale (LEFS) score: 40/80, LOB negotiating steps, freezing, and hesitation of movement ambulating through doorways and elevators.
Single Leg Stance: Right and Left 0 seconds. Ankle strategies used to maintain static standing on even surfaces
Berg Balance Measure: 43/56 requires increased time for turning 360° (10 sec), turns clockwise 10 steps and counter clockwise 9 steps, shuffling/freezing throughout, loss of balance with tandem stance.
Sitting static control: good (able to maintain balance without handhold).
Sitting dynamic control: fair (accepts minimal challenge; able to lift both arms).
Standing static control: good (able to maintain balance without handhold).
Standing dynamic control: poor (unable to accept minimal challenge without handhold).
He has slowed reactions to loss of balance with decreased rotational movements of head/trunk and ineffective use of stepping strategies.
Timed Up and Go score is 38 seconds.

Functional Mobility
Generally decreased.
Requires moderate assist: rolling in bed and supine-to-sit and sit-to-stand transfers. Retropulsion during sit to stand transfer, poor eccentric control with transfer to sofa with a low soft surface, poor posture and body mechanics, and slowness of movement with car transfers.

Locomotion
Patient ambulates independently with a narrow base of support with narrow-based gait pattern evident with changes of directions and when negotiating around obstacles. Poor hip/trunk dissociation with minimal trunk rotation with no arm swing worse on the left. Poverty and slowness of movement with shuffling gait pattern more pronounced when negotiating small/confined spaces and through doorways. Difficulty negotiating busy environments, dual-task challenge gait deviations worsen with talking/carrying object.

Self-Care
Requires minimal assistance to supervision for feeding.
Requires minimal to moderate assist for dressing/bathing.

Cardiopulmonary Function/Endurance
Shallow (upper respiratory) breathing pattern
Generally decreased functional capacity (estimated functional work capacity [FWC] is 6 metabolic equivalents [METs])
Fatigues easily and requires frequent rest periods

Skin
Intact, no areas of breakdown

GUIDING QUESTIONS

1. Identify/categorize this patient's problems in terms of:
   a. Direct impairments
   b. Indirect impairments
   c. Activity limitations
   d. Participation restrictions/disability
2. Identify two outcomes (the remediation of activity limitations and disability) and two goals (remediation of impairments) for this patient.

3. Determine four interventions that could be used at the start of therapy to achieve the outcomes and goals provided for question 2. Provide a brief rationale for each.
4. What motor learning strategies will assist in improving his motor function?

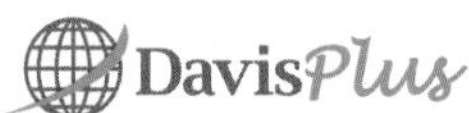

For additional resources, including answers to the questions for review and case study guiding questions, please visit **http://davisplus.fadavis.com.**

The reader is referred to video Case Study 6: Patient with Parkinson's Disease for additional review and study. The full written case study, including tables, figures, charts, and three video segments (examination, intervention, and outcome), appears online at Davis*Plus*. The case study poses questions for the reader's consideration with suggested answers to the case study questions, also posted online at Davis*Plus*.

References

1. Sauerbier, A, Chaudhuri, KR: Nonmotor symptoms of Parkinson's disease. In: Tolosa, E, Jankovic, J (Eds.): Parkinson's disease & movement disorders, 6 ed., Philadelphia : Wolters Kluwer, [electronic book], 2015, p. 42.
2. Todorova, A, Jenner, P, Ray Chaudhuri, K: Non-motor Parkinson's: Integral to motor Parkinson's, yet often neglected. Pract Neurol 14(5):310, 2014.
3. de Lau, LM, Breteler, MM: Epidemiology of Parkinson's disease. Lancet Neurol 5(6):525, 2006.
4. Goldman, SM, Tanner, CM: Epidemiology of Parkinson's disease. In: Tolosa, E, Jankovic, J (Eds.): Parkinson's disease & movement disorders, 6 ed., Philadelphia : Wolters Kluwer, [electronic book], 2015, p. 28.
5. Parkinson, J: An essay on the Shaking Palsy. Originally published by Sherwood, Neely, and Jones, London, 1817. [Available from Classic Pieces Series (Parkinson's Disease)]. J Neuropsychiatry Clin Neurosci 14(2):223, 2002.
6. Wu, Y, et al: Non-motor symptoms and quality of life in tremor dominant vs postural instability gait disorder Parkinson's disease patients. Acta Neurol Scand 133(5):330, 2016.
7. Ba, F, et al: Parkinson Disease: The relationship between non-motor symptoms and motor phenotype. Can J Neurol Sci 43(2):261, 2016.
8. Brockmann, K, Gasser, T: Genetics of Parkinson's disease. In: Tolosa, E, Jankovic, J (Eds.): Parkinson's disease & movement disorders, 6 ed., Philadelphia : Wolters Kluwer, [electronic book], 2015, p. 65.
9. Sacks, O: Awakenings, New York : Harper Collins, 1990.
10. Wright, J, Keller-Byme, J: Environmental determinants of Parkinson's disease. Arch Environ Occup Health 60:32, 2005.
11. Dauer, W, Przedborski, S: Parkinson's disease: Mechanisms and models. Neuron 39(6):889, 2003.
12. Langston, JW, et al: Chronic Parkinsonism in humans due to a product of meperidine-analog synthesis. Science 219(4587):979, 1983.
13. Mehta, SH, Sethi, KD, Morgan, JC: Drug-induced movement disorders. In: Tolosa, E, Jankovic, J (Eds.): Parkinson's disease & movement disorders, 6 ed., Philadelphia : Wolters Kluwer, [electronic book], 2015, p. 357.
14. Przedborski, S: Etiology and pathogenesis of Parkinson's disease. In: Tolosa, E, Jankovic, J (Eds.): Parkinson's disease & movement disorders, 6 ed., Philadelphia : Wolters Kluwer, [electronic book], 2015, p. 51.
15. Obeso, JA, et al: Functional organization of the basal ganglia: Therapeutic implications for Parkinson's disease. Mov Disord 23(S3):S548, 2008.
16. Barone, P: Neurotransmission in Parkinson's disease: beyond dopamine. Eur J Neurol 17(3):364, 2010.
17. Braak, H, et al: Stages in the development of Parkinson's disease-related pathology. Cell Tissue Res 318(1):121, 2004.
18. Braak, H, et al: Staging of brain pathology related to sporadic Parkinson's disease. Neurobiol Aging 24(2):197, 2003.
19. Del Tredici, K, Braak, H: Lewy pathology and neurodegeneration in premotor Parkinson's disease. Mov Disord 27(5):597, 2012.
20. Goedert, M, et al: 100 years of Lewy pathology. Nat Rev Neurol 9(1):13, 2013.
21. Fung, VS, Burne, JA, Morris, JG: Objective quantification of resting and activated parkinsonian rigidity: A comparison of angular impulse and work scores. Mov Disord 15(1):48, 2000.
22. Fung, VSC, Thompson, PD: Rigidity and spasticity. In: Tolosa, E, Jankovic, J (Eds.): Parkinson's disease & movement disorders, 6 ed., Philadelphia : Wolters Kluwer, [electronic book], 2015, p. 420.
23. Berardelli, A, et al: Pathophysiology of bradykinesia in Parkinson's disease. Brain 124(Pt 11):2131, 2001.
24. Rosin, B, et al: Physiology and pathophysiology of the basal ganglia—thalamo—cortical networks. Parkinsonism Relat Disord 13(Suppl 3):S437, 2007.
25. Cohen, RG, et al: Freezing of gait is associated with a mismatch between motor imagery and motor execution in narrow doorways, not with failure to judge doorway passability. Neuropsychologia 49(14):3981, 2011.
26. Peterson, DS, et al: Dual-task interference and brain structural connectivity in people with Parkinson's disease who freeze. J Neurol Neurosurg Psychiatry 86(7):786, 2015.
27. Lee, HJ, et al: Tremor frequency characteristics in Parkinson's disease under resting-state and stress-state conditions. J Neurol Sci 362:272, 2016.
28. Goetz, CG, et al: Movement Disorder Society-sponsored revision of the Unified Parkinson's Disease Rating Scale (MDS-UPDRS): scale presentation and clinimetric testing results. Mov Disord 23(15):2129, 2008.
29. Mancini, M, et al: Effects of Parkinson's disease and levodopa on functional limits of stability. Clin Biomech 23(4):450, 2008.
30. Peterson, DS, Horak, FB: Neural control of walking in people with parkinsonism. Physiology 31(2):95, 2016.
31. Müller, MLTM, et al: Thalamic cholinergic innervation and postural sensory integration function in Parkinson's disease. Brain 136(Pt 11):3282, 2013.
32. Maeshima, S, et al: Visuospatial impairment and activities of daily living in patients with Parkinson's disease: a quantitative assessment of the cube-copying task. Am J Phys Med Rehabil 76(5): 383, 1997.
33. Ashour, R, Jankovic, J: Joint and skeletal deformities in Parkinson's disease, multiple system atrophy, and progressive supranuclear palsy. Mov Disord 21(11):1856, 2006.
34. Weaver, TB, et al: Falls and Parkinson's disease: Evidence from video recordings of actual fall events. J Am Geriatr Soc 64(1):96, 2016.
35. Nystrom, H, Nordstrom, A, Nordstrom, P: Risk of injurious fall and hip fracture up to 26 y before the diagnosis of Parkinson disease: Nested case-control studies in a nationwide cohort. PLoS Med 13(2):e1001954, 2016.
36. Okuma, Y: Freezing of gait and falls in Parkinson's disease. J Parkinsons Dis 4(2):255, 2014.
37. Bloem, BR, et al: Falls and freezing of Gait in Parkinson's disease: A review of two interconnected, episodic phenomena. Mov Disord 19(8):871, 2004.

38. Robinson, K, et al: Falling risk factors in Parkinson's disease. Neuro Rehabilitation 20(3):169, 2005.
39. Corcos, DM, et al: Strength in Parkinson's disease: Relationship to rate of force generation and clinical status. Ann Neurol 39(1): 79, 1996.
40. Pedersen, SW, Oberg, B: Dynamic strength in Parkinson's disease. Quantitative measurements following withdrawal of medication. Eur Neurol 33(2):97, 1993.
41. Stelmach, GE, et al: Force production characteristics in Parkinson's disease. Ex Brain Res 76(1):165, 1989.
42. Yanagawa, S, Shindo, M, Yanagisawa, N: Muscular weakness in Parkinson's disease. Adv Neurol 53:259, 1990.
43. Berardelli, A, et al: Scaling of the size of the first agonist EMG burst during rapid wrist movements in patients with Parkinson's disease. J Neurol Neurosurg Psychiatry 49:1273, 1986.
44. Pfann, KD, et al: Muscle activation patterns in point-to-point and reversal movements in healthy, older subjects and in subjects with Parkinson's disease. Ex Brain Res 157(1):67, 2004.
45. Dengler, R, et al: Behavior of motor units in parkinsonism. Adv Neurol 53:167, 1990.
46. Vaillancourt, DE, et al: Effects of deep brain stimulation and medication on strength, bradykinesia, and electromyographic patterns of the ankle joint in Parkinson's disease. Mov Disord 21(1):50, 2006.
47. Allen, NE, et al: Bradykinesia, muscle weakness and reduced muscle power in Parkinson's disease. Mov Disord 24(9):1344, 2009.
48. Berardelli, A, et al: Pathophysiology of pain and fatigue in Parkinson's disease. Parkinsonism Relat Disord 18(Suppl 1): S226, 2012.
49. Herrero, MT, Barcia, C, Navarro, JM: Functional anatomy of thalamus and basal ganglia. Childs Nerv Syst 18(8):386, 2002.
50. Pendt, LK, Reuter, I, Muller, H: Motor skill learning, retention, and control deficits in Parkinson's disease. PLoS One 6(7): e21669, 2011.
51. Mentis, MJ, et al: Enhancement of brain activation during trial-and-error sequence learning in early PD. Neurology 60(4):612, 2003.
52. Hayes, HA, Hunsaker, N, Dibble, LE: Implicit motor sequence learning in individuals with Parkinson disease: A meta-analysis. J Parkinsons Dis 5(3):549, 2015.
53. Ruitenberg, MF, et al: Sequential movement skill in Parkinson's disease: A state-of-the-art. Cortex 65:102, 2015.
54. Nieuwboer, A, et al: Motor learning in Parkinson's disease: Limitations and potential for rehabilitation. Parkinsonism Relat Disord 15(Suppl 3):S53, 2009.
55. McIsaac, TL, Benjapalakorn, B: Allocation of attention and dual-task effects on upper and lower limb task performance in healthy young adults. Ex Brain Res 233(9):2607, 2015.
56. Heremans, E, et al: Cognitive aspects of freezing of gait in Parkinson's disease: A challenge for rehabilitation. J Neural Transm (Vienna, Austria: 1996) 120(4):543, 2013.
57. Nieuwboer, A, Giladi, N: Characterizing freezing of gait in Parkinson's disease: Models of an episodic phenomenon. Mov Disord 28(11):1509, 2013.
58. Shulman, LM, et al: The evolution of disability in Parkinson disease. Mov Disord 23(6):790, 2008.
59. Giladi, N, Horak, FB, Hausdorff, JM: Classification of gait disturbances: Distinguishing between continuous and episodic changes. Mov Disord 28(11):1469, 2013.
60. Hausdorff, JM: Gait dynamics in Parkinson's disease: Common and distinct behavior among stride length, gait variability, and fractal-like scaling. Chaos 19(2):026113, 2009.
61. Baltadjieva, R, et al: Marked alterations in the gait timing and rhythmicity of patients with de novo Parkinson's disease. Eur J Neurosci 24(6):1815, 2006.
62. Zampieri, C, et al: The instrumented timed up and go test: potential outcome measure for disease modifying therapies in Parkinson's disease. J NeurolNeurosurg Psychiatry 81(2):171, 2010.
63. Horak, FB, Dimitrova, D, Nutt, JG: Direction-specific postural instability in subjects with Parkinson's disease. Exp Neurol 193(2): 504, 2005.
64. Mancini, M, et al: Postural sway as a marker of progression in Parkinson's disease: A pilot longitudinal study. Gait Posture 36(3): 471, 2012.
65. Mancini, M, et al: Anticipatory postural adjustments prior to step initiation are hypometric in untreated Parkinson's disease: An accelerometer-based approach. Eur J Neurol 16(9):1028, 2009.
66. Mille, ML, et al: Posture and locomotion coupling: a target for rehabilitation interventions in persons with Parkinson's disease. Parkinson Dis 2012:754186, 2012.
67. Giladi, N, Kao, R, Fahn, S: Freezing phenomenon in patients with parkinsonian syndromes. Mov Disord 12(3):302, 1997.
68. Macht, M, et al: Predictors of freezing in Parkinson's disease: A survey of 6,620 patients. Mov Disord 22(7):953, 2007.
69. Herman, T, Giladi, N, Hausdorff, JM: Neuroimaging as a window into gait disturbances and freezing of gait in patients with Parkinson's disease. Curr Neurol Neurosci Rep 13(12):411, 2013.
70. Peterson, DS, et al: Cognitive contributions to freezing of gait in Parkinson disease: Implications for physical rehabilitation. Phys Ther 95(5):659, 2016.
71. Nonnekes, J, et al: Short rapid steps to provoke freezing of gait in Parkinson's disease. J Neurol 261(9):1763, 2014.
72. Nonnekes, J, et al: Freezing of gait: A practical approach to management. Lancet Neurol 14(7):768, 2015.
73. Chaudhuri, KR, et al: International multicenter pilot study of the first comprehensive self-completed nonmotor symptoms questionnaire for Parkinson's disease: The NMSQuest study. Mov Disord 21(7):916, 2006.
74. Pont-Sunyer, C, et al: The onset of nonmotor symptoms in Parkinson's disease (the ONSET PD study). Mov Disord 30(2): 229, 2015.
75. Young Blood, MR, et al: Classification and characteristics of pain associated with Parkinson's disease. Parkinson Dis (20420080): 1, 2016.
76. Beiske, AG, et al: Pain in Parkinson's disease: Prevalence and characteristics. Pain 141(1-2):173, 2009.
77. Thompson, T, et al: Pain perception in Parkinson's disease: A systematic review and meta-analysis of experimental studies. Ageing Res Rev 35:74, 2017.
78. Konczak, J, et al: Proprioception and motor control in Parkinson's disease. J Mot Behav 41(6):543, 2009.
79. Wright, WG, et al: Axial kinesthesia is impaired in Parkinson's disease: Effects of levodopa. Exp Neurol 225(1):202, 2010.
80. Weil, RS, et al: Visual dysfunction in Parkinson's disease. Brain 139(11):2827, 2016.
81. Kalf, JG, et al: Review: Prevalence of oropharyngeal dysphagia in Parkinson's disease: A meta-analysis. Parkinsonism Relat Disord 18:311, 2012.
82. Ciucci, MR, et al: Early identification and treatment of communication and swallowing deficits in Parkinson disease. Semin Speech Lang 34(3):185, 2013.
83. Theodoros, DG: Speech disorder in Parkinson disease. In: Ramig, LO, Theodoros, DG (Eds.): Communication and swallowing in Parkinson disease, San Diego : Plural Publishing, 2011, p. 51.
84. Aarsland, D, et al: Cognitive impairment in incident, untreated Parkinson disease: The Norwegian ParkWest study. Neurology 72(13):1121, 2009.
85. Muslimovic, D, et al: Cognitive profile of patients with newly diagnosed Parkinson disease. Neurology 65(8):1239, 2005.
86. Pagonabarraga, J, Kulisevsky, J: Cognitive impairment and dementia in Parkinson's disease. Neurobiol Dis 46(3):590, 2012.
87. Kehagia, AA, Barker, RA, Robbins, TW: Cognitive impairment in Parkinson's disease: The dual syndrome hypothesis. Neurodegener Dis 11(2):79, 2013.
88. Pedersen, KF, et al: Natural course of mild cognitive impairment in Parkinson disease: A 5-year population-based study. Neurology 88(8):767, 2017.
89. Borgonovo, J, et al: Changes in neural circuitry associated with depression at pre-clinical, pre-motor and early motor phases of Parkinson's disease. Parkinsonism Relat Disord 35:17, 2017.
90. Broen, MP, et al: Prevalence of anxiety in Parkinson's disease: A systematic review and meta-analysis. Mov Disord 31(8):1125, 2016.
91. Pagonabarraga, J, et al: Apathy in Parkinson's disease: Clinical features, neural substrates, diagnosis, and treatment. Lancet Neurol 14(5):518, 2015.
92. Kim, JB, et al: Autonomic dysfunction according to disease progression in Parkinson's disease. Parkinsonism Relat Disord 20: 303, 2014.
93. Cersosimo, MG, Benarroch, EE: Autonomic involvement in Parkinson's disease: Pathology, pathophysiology, clinical features and possible peripheral biomarkers. J Neurol Sci 313(1-2):57, 2012.

94. Malek, N, et al: Autonomic dysfunction in early Parkinson's disease: Results from the United Kingdom Tracking Parkinson's Study. Mov Disord Clin Pract, 2016.
95. Heetun, ZS, Quigley, EM: Gastroparesis and Parkinson's disease: A systematic review. Parkinsonism Relat Disord 18(5):433, 2012.
96. Kanegusuku, H, et al: Blunted maximal and submaximal responses to cardiopulmonary exercise tests in patients with Parkinson disease. Arch Phys Med Rehabil 97(5):720, 2016.
97. Speelman, AD, et al: Cardiovascular responses during a submaximal exercise test in patients with Parkinson's disease. J Parkinsons Dis 2(3):241, 2012.
98. Hampson, NB, et al: Prospective evaluation of pulmonary function in Parkinson's disease patients with motor fluctuations. Int J Neurosci 127(3):276, 2017.
99. Hovestadt, A, et al: Pulmonary function in Parkinson's disease. J Neurol Neurosurg Psychiatry 52(3):329, 1989.
100. Sabate, M, et al: Obstructive and restrictive pulmonary dysfunction increases disability in Parkinson disease. Arch Phys Med Rehabil 77(1):29, 1996.
101. Postuma, RB, Berg, D: Advances in markers of prodromal Parkinson disease. Nat Rev Neurol 12(11):622, 2016.
102. Hughes, AJ, et al: Accuracy of clinical diagnosis of idiopathic Parkinson's disease: A clinico-pathological study of 100 cases. J Neurol Neurosurg Psychiatry 55(3):181, 1992.
103. Postuma, RB, et al: MDS clinical diagnostic criteria for Parkinson's disease. Mov Disord 30(12):1591, 2015.
104. Berg, D, et al: MDS research criteria for prodromal Parkinson's disease. Mov Disord 30(12):1600, 2015.
105. Martinez-Martin, P, et al: The impact of non-motor symptoms on health-related quality of life of patients with Parkinson's disease. Mov Disord 26(3):399, 2011.
106. Chaudhuri, KR, et al: The burden of non-motor symptoms in Parkinson's disease using a self-completed non-motor questionnaire: A simple grading system. Parkinsonism Relat Disord 21(3):287, 2015.
107. Herman, T, et al: Cognitive function and other non-motor features in non-demented Parkinson's disease motor subtypes. J Neural Transm 122(8):1115, 2015.
108. Pinter, B, et al: Mortality in Parkinson's disease: A 38-year follow-up study. Mov Disord 30(2):266, 2015.
109. Hoehn, MM, Yahr, MD: Parkinsonism: Onset, progression and mortality. Neurology 17(5):427, 1967.
110. Fahn, S, Elton, R: Unified Parkinson's disease rating scale. In: Fahn, S, Marsden, C, Calne, D, Goldstein, M (Eds.): Recent developments in Parkinson's disease, Florham Park, NJ : MacMillan Healthcare Information, 1987, p. 153.
111. Goetz, CG, et al: Movement Disorder Society-sponsored revision of the Unified Parkinson's Disease Rating Scale (MDS-UPDRS): Process, format, and clinimetric testing plan. Mov Disord 22(1):41, 2007.
112. Lotia, M, Jankovic, J: New and emerging medical therapies in Parkinson's disease. Expert Opin Pharmacother 17(7):895, 2016.
113. Ahlskog, JE: Cheaper, simpler, and better: Tips for treating seniors with Parkinson disease. Mayo Clin Proc 86(12):1211, 2011.
114. Ahlskog, JE: Parkinson disease treatment in hospitals and nursing facilities: Avoiding pitfalls. Mayo Clin Proc 89(7):997, 2014.
115. Aminoff, MJ, et al: Management of the hospitalized patient with Parkinson's disease: Current state of the field and need for guidelines. Parkinsonism Relat Disord 17(3):139, 2011.
116. Magdalinou, KN, Martin, A, Kessel, B: Prescribing medications in Parkinson's disease (PD) patients during acute admissions to a district general hospital. Parkinsonism Relat Disord 13(8):539, 2007.
117. Nonnekes, J, et al: Unmasking levodopa resistance in Parkinson's disease. Mov Disord 31(11):1602, 2016.
118. Fahn, S, et al: Levodopa and the progression of Parkinson's disease. N Engl J Med 351(24):2498, 2004.
119. PDF: Treatments. Parkinson's Disease Foundation 2017. Retrieved March 27, 2017, from www.parkinson.org.
120. Vlaar, A, et al: The treatment of early Parkinson's disease: Levodopa rehabilitated. Pract Neurol 11(3):145, 2011.
121. Coelho, M, Ferreira, JJ: Epidemiology of levodopa-induced dyskinesia. In: Fox, SH, Brotchie, JM (Eds.): Levodopa-induced dyskinesia in Parkinson's disease, London : Springer-Verlag, 2014, p. 33.
122. Katzenschlager, R: Pharmacological treatments options for levodopa-induced dyskinesia. In: Fox, SH, Brotchie, JM (Eds.): Levodopa-induced dyskinesia in Parkinson's disease, London: Springer-Verlag, 2014, p. 69.
123. Henderson, EJ, et al: Rivastigmine for gait stability in patients with Parkinson's disease (ReSPonD): A randomised, double-blind, placebo-controlled, phase 2 trial. Lancet Neurol 15(3):249, 2016.
124. Sarva, H, Henchcliffe, C: Evidence for the use of pimavanserin in the treatment of Parkinson's disease psychosis. Ther Adv Neurol Disord 9(6):462, 2016.
125. Martinez-Ramirez, D, Peng-Chen, Z, Okun, MS: Surgery for Parkinson's disease. In: Tolosa, E, Jankovic, J (Eds.): Parkinson's disease & movement disorders, 6 ed., Philadelphia: Wolters Kluwer, [electronic book], 2015, p. 496.
126. Okun, MS: Deep-brain stimulation for Parkinson's disease. N Engl J Med 367(16):1529, 2012.
127. Okun, MS, Foote, KD: Parkinson's disease DBS: What, when, who and why? The time has come to tailor DBS targets. Expert Rev Neurother 10(12):1847, 2010.
128. Williams, NR, Foote, KD, Okun, MS: Subthalamic nucleus versus globus pallidus internus deep brain stimulation: Translating the rematch into clinical practice. Mov Disord Clin Pract 1(1):24, 2014.
129. Combs, HL, et al: Cognition and depression following deep brain stimulation of the subthalamic nucleus and globus pallidus pars internus in Parkinson's disease: A meta-analysis. Neuropsychol Rev 25(4):439, 2015.
130. Dal Bello-Haas, V: A framework for rehabilitation of neurodegenerative diseases: Planning care and maximizing quality of life. J Neurol Phys Ther 26(3):115, 2002.
131. Boersma, I, et al: Palliative care and neurology: Time for a paradigm shift. Neurology 83(6):561, 2014.
132. Kluger, BM, et al: Palliative care and Parkinson's disease: Meeting summary and recommendations for clinical research. Parkinsonism Relat Disord 37:19, 2017.
133. Frazzitta, G, et al: The beneficial role of intensive exercise on Parkinson disease progression. Am J Phys Med Rehabil 92(6):523, 2013.
134. Frazzitta, G, et al: Intensive rehabilitation treatment in early Parkinson's disease: A randomized pilot study with a 2-year follow-up. Neurorehabil Neural Repair 29(2):123, 2015.
135. Ellis, T, et al: Effectiveness of an inpatient multidisciplinary rehabilitation program for people with Parkinson disease. Phys Ther 88(7):812, 2008.
136. Conradsson, D, et al: The effects of highly challenging balance training in elderly with Parkinson's disease: A randomized controlled trial. Neurorehabil Neural Repair 29(9):827, 2015.
137. Bombieri, F, et al: Walking on four limbs: A systematic review of Nordic Walking in Parkinson disease. Parkinsonism Relat Disord, 2017.
138. Kaseda, Y, et al: Therapeutic effects of intensive inpatient rehabilitation in advanced Parkinson's disease. Neurol Clin Neurosci 5(1):18, 2017.
139. APTA: Guide to Physical Therapist Practice 3.0, Alexandria, VA: APTA, 2014.
140. CMS: Transmittal 179, Change Request 8458, in: Department of Health and Human Services (Ed.) 2014.
141. Tanji, H, et al: A comparative study of physical performance measures in Parkinson's disease. Mov Disord 23(13):1897, 2008.
142. Zadikoff, C, et al: A comparison of the mini mental state exam to the Montreal cognitive assessment in identifying cognitive deficits in Parkinson's disease. Mov Disord 23(2):297, 2008.
143. Yesavage, JA, et al: Development and validation of a geriatric depression screening scale: A preliminary report. J Psychiatr Res 17(1):37, 1982.
144. Hamilton, M: A rating scale for depression. J Neurol Neurosurg Psychiatry 23:56, 1960.
145. Torbey, E, Pachana, NA, Dissanayaka, NN: Depression rating scales in Parkinson's disease: A critical review updating recent literature. J Affect Disord 184:216, 2015.
146. Dissanayaka, NN, Torbey, E, Pachana, NA: Anxiety rating scales in Parkinson's disease: A critical review updating recent literature. Int Psychogeriatr 27(11):1777, 2015.
147. Pachana, NA, et al: Development and validation of the Geriatric Anxiety Inventory. Int Psychogeriatr 19(1):103, 2007.
148. Leentjens, AF, et al: The Parkinson Anxiety Scale (PAS): Development and validation of a new anxiety scale. Mov Disord 29(8):1035, 2014.

149. Nowacka, B, et al: Ophthalmological features of Parkinson disease. Med Sci Monit 20:2243, 2014.
150. Wright, WG, et al: Axial hypertonicity in Parkinson's disease: Direct measurements of trunk and hip torque. Exp Neurol 208(1):38, 2007.
151. Breum, J, Wiberg, J, Bolton, JE: Reliability and concurrent validity of the BROM II for measuring lumbar mobility. J Manipulative Physiol Ther 18(8):497, 1995.
152. Youdas, JW, Suman, VJ, Garrett, TR: Reliability of measurements of lumbar spine sagittal mobility obtained with the flexible curve. J Orthop Sports Phys Ther 21(1):13, 1995.
153. Dunleavy, K, et al: Reliability and minimal detectable change of spinal length and width measurements using the Flexicurve for usual standing posture in healthy young adults. J Back Musculoskelet Rehabil 23(4):209, 2010.
154. Lundon, KM, Li, AM, Bibershtein, S: Interrater and intrarater reliability in the measurement of kyphosis in postmenopausal women with osteoporosis. Spine (Phila Pa 1976) 23(18):1978, 1998.
155. Bloem, BR, et al: Measurement instruments to assess posture, gait, and balance in Parkinson's disease: Critique and recommendations. Mov Disord 31(9):1342, 2016.
156. Berg, KO, et al: Measuring balance in the elderly: validation of an instrument. Can J Public Health 83(Suppl 2):S7, 1992.
157. Duncan, PW, et al: Functional reach: a new clinical measure of balance. J Gerontol 45(6):M192, 1990.
158. Podsiadlo, D, Richardson, S: The timed "Up & Go": A test of basic functional mobility for frail elderly persons. J Am Geriatr Soc 39(2):142, 1991.
159. Campbell, CM, et al: The effect of cognitive demand on timed up and go performance in older adults with and without Parkinson disease. Neurology Report 27(1):2, 2003.
160. Shumway-Cook, A, et al: Predicting the probability for falls in community-dwelling older adults. Phys Ther 77(8):812, 1997.
161. Brusse, KJ, et al: Testing functional performance in people with Parkinson disease. Phys Ther 85(2):134, 2005.
162. Landers, MR, et al: Postural instability in idiopathic Parkinson's disease: Discriminating fallers from nonfallers based on standardized clinical measures. J Neurol Phys Ther 32(2):56, 2008.
163. Dibble, LE, Lange, M: Predicting falls in individuals with Parkinson disease: A reconsideration of clinical balance measures. J Neurol Phys Ther 30(2):60, 2006.
164. Dibble, LE, et al: Diagnosis of fall risk in Parkinson disease: An analysis of individual and collective clinical balance test interpretation. Phys Ther 88(3):323, 2008.
165. Rose, DJ, Lucchese, N, Wiersma, LD: Development of a multidimensional balance scale for use with functionally independent older adults. Arch Phys Med Rehabil 87(11):1478, 2006.
166. Wrisley, DM, et al: Reliability, internal consistency, and validity of data obtained with the functional gait assessment. Phy Ther 84(10):906, 2004.
167. Horak, FB, Wrisley, DM, Frank, J: The Balance Evaluation Systems Test (BESTest) to differentiate balance deficits. Phys Ther 89(5):484, 2009.
168. Franchignoni, F, et al: Using psychometric techniques to improve the Balance Evaluation Systems Test: The mini-BESTest. J Rehabil Med 42(4):323, 2010.
169. Schlenstedt, C, et al: Comparison of the Fullerton Advanced Balance Scale, Mini-BESTest, and Berg Balance Scale to predict falls in Parkinson disease. Phys Ther 96(4):494, 2016.
170. Leddy, AL, Crowner, BE, Earhart, GM: Functional Gait Assessment and Balance Evaluation System Test: Reliability, validity, sensitivity, and specificity for identifying individuals with Parkinson disease who fall. Phys Ther 91(1):102, 2011.
171. King, LA, et al: Comparing the Mini-BESTest with the Berg Balance Scale to evaluate balance disorders in Parkinson's disease. Parkinson Dis 2012:7, 2012.
172. Steffen, T, Seney, M: Test-retest reliability and minimal detectable change on balance and ambulation tests, the 36-Item Short-Form Health Survey, and the Unified Parkinson Disease Rating Scale in people with parkinsonism [corrected] [published erratum appears in Phys Ther 2010 Mar;90(3):462]. Phys Ther 88(6):733, 2008.
173. Behrman, AL, Light, KE, Miller, GM: Sensitivity of the Tinetti Gait Assessment for detecting change in individuals with Parkinson's disease. Clin Rehabil 16(4):399, 2002.
174. Curtze, C, et al: Levodopa Is a double-edged sword for balance and gait in people with Parkinson's disease. Mov Disord 30(10):1361, 2015.
175. Adkin, AL, Bloem, BR, Allum, JH: Trunk sway measurements during stance and gait tasks in Parkinson's disease. Gait Posture 22(3):240, 2005.
176. Gera, G, et al: Identification of balance deficits in people with Parkinson disease: Is the Sensory Organization Test enough? Int J Phys Med Rehabil 4(1), 2016.
177. Paul, SS, et al: Motor and cognitive impairments in Parkinson disease: Relationships with specific balance and mobility tasks. Neurorehabil Neural Repair 27(1):63, 2013.
178. Mak, MK, Pang, MY: Balance confidence and functional mobility are independently associated with falls in people with Parkinson's disease. J Neurol 256(5):742, 2009.
179. Dibble, LE, et al: Maximal speed gait initiation of healthy elderly individuals and persons with Parkinson disease. J Neurol Phys Ther 28(1):2, 2004.
180. Strouwen, C, et al: Are factors related to dual-task performance in people with Parkinson's disease dependent on the type of dual task? Parkinsonism Relat Disord 23:23, 2016.
181. Huang, SL, et al: Minimal detectable change of the timed "up & go" test and the dynamic gait index in people with Parkinson disease. Phys Ther 91(1):114, 2011.
182. Schlenstedt, C, et al: Postural control and freezing of gait in Parkinson's disease. Parkinsonism Relat Disord 24:107, 2016.
183. Beck, EN, Ehgoetz Martens, KA, Almeida, QJ: Freezing of gait in Parkinson's disease: An overload problem? PLoS One 10(12):e0144986, 2015.
184. Browner, N, Giladi, N: What can we learn from freezing of gait in Parkinson's disease? Curr Neurol Neurosci Rep 10(5):345, 2010.
185. Nieuwboer, A, et al: Reliability of the new freezing of gait questionnaire: agreement between patients with Parkinson's disease and their carers. Gait Posture 30(4):459, 2009.
186. Paul, SS, et al: Two-year trajectory of fall risk in people with Parkinson disease: A latent class analysis. Arch Phys Med Rehabil 97(3):372, 2016.
187. Canning, CG, Paul, SS, Nieuwboer, A: Prevention of falls in Parkinson's disease: A review of fall risk factors and the role of physical interventions. Neurodegener Dis Manag 4(3): 203, 2014.
188. Plotnik, M, et al: Postural instability and fall risk in Parkinson's disease: Impaired dual tasking, pacing, and bilateral coordination of gait during the "ON" medication state. Exp Brain Res 210 (3-4):529, 2011.
189. Kostić, VS, Tomić, A, Ječmenica-Lukić, M: The pathophysiology of fatigue in Parkinson's disease and its pragmatic management. Mov Disord Clin Pract 3(4):323, 2016.
190. Friedman, JH: Is fatigue in early Parkinson's disease a minor inconvenience or major distress? The answer is "Yes!". Eur J Neurol 19(7):931, 2012.
191. Friedman, JH, et al: Fatigue in Parkinson's disease: Report from a mutidisciplinary symposium. NPJ Parkinsons Dis 2, 2016.
192. Friedman, JH, et al: Fatigue rating scales critique and recommendations by the Movement Disorders Society task force on rating scales for Parkinson's disease. Mov Disord 25(7):805, 2010.
193. Smets, EM, et al: The Multidimensional Fatigue Inventory (MFI) psychometric qualities of an instrument to assess fatigue. J Psychosom Res 39(3):315, 1995.
194. Krupp, LB, et al: The fatigue severity scale. Application to patients with multiple sclerosis and systemic lupus erythematosus. Arch Neurol 46(10):1121, 1989.
195. Brown, RG, et al: The Parkinson fatigue scale. Parkinsonism Relat Disord 11(1):49, 2005.
196. Goetz, CG, et al: Utility of an objective dyskinesia rating scale for Parkinson's disease: Inter- and intrarater reliability assessment. Mov Disord 9(4):390, 1994.
197. Colosimo, C, et al: Task force report on scales to assess dyskinesia in Parkinson's disease: Critique and recommendations. Mov Disord 25(9):1131, 2010.
198. Goetz, CG, Nutt, JG, Stebbins, GT: The Unified Dyskinesia Rating Scale: Presentation and clinimetric profile. Mov Disord 23(16):2398, 2008.
199. Chaudhuri, KR, et al: The metric properties of a novel non-motor symptoms scale for Parkinson's disease: Results from an international pilot study. Mov Disord 22(13):1901, 2007.

200. ACSM: ACSM's guidelines for exercise testing and prescription, 9 ed., Philadelphia : Wolters Kluwer Health/Lippincott Williams & Wilkins, 2014.
201. Light, KE, et al: The 2-minute walk test: A tool for evaluating walking endurance in clients with Parkinson's disease. Neurol Rep 21(4):136, 1997.
202. Borg, GA: Psychophysical bases of perceived exertion. Med Sci Sports Exerc 14(5):377, 1982.
203. PDF: Understanding Parkinson's neurogenic orthostatic hypotension, New York : Parkinson's Disease Foundation, 2015.
204. Guide for the Uniform Data Set for Medical Rehabilitation including the FIM Instrument, Buffalo: State University of New York at Buffalo, 1996.
205. Pohar, SL, Allyson Jones, C: The burden of Parkinson disease (PD) and concomitant comorbidities. Arch Gerontol Geriatr 49(2):317, 2009.
206. Rand, MK, et al: Control of aperture closure initiation during reach-to-grasp movements under manipulations of visual feedback and trunk involvement in Parkinson's disease. Exp Brain Res 201(3):509, 2010.
207. Lukos, JR, et al: Parkinson's disease patients show impaired corrective grasp control and eye–hand coupling when reaching to grasp virtual objects. Neuroscience 254(0):205, 2013.
208. Muratori, LM, et al: Impaired anticipatory control of force sharing patterns during whole-hand grasping in Parkinson's disease. Exp Brain Res 185(1):41, 2008.
209. Lukos, J, Poizner, H, Sage, J: Hand function in Parkinson's disease. In: Duruöz, MT (Ed.): Hand function, New York: Springer, 2014, p. 133.
210. Proud, EL, et al: Evaluation of measures of upper limb functioning and disability in people with Parkinson disease: A systematic review. Arch Phys Med Rehabil 96(3):540, 2015.
211. Earhart, GM, et al: The 9-hole peg test of upper extremity function: Average values, test-retest reliability, and factors contributing to performance in people with Parkinson disease. J Neurol Phys Ther 35(4):157, 2011.
212. Vanbellingen, T, et al: Reliability and validity of a new dexterity questionnaire (DextQ-24) in Parkinson's disease. Parkinsonism Relat Disord 33:78, 2016.
213. Bishop, M, et al: Changes in distal muscle timing may contribute to slowness during sit to stand in Parkinson's disease. Clin Biomech (Bristol, Avon) 20(1):112, 2005.
214. Ramsey, VK, Miszko, TA, Horvat, M: Muscle activation and force production in Parkinson's patients during sit to stand transfers. Clin Biomech (Bristol, Avon) 19(4):377, 2004.
215. Guralnik, JM, et al: Lower-extremity function in persons over the age of 70 years as a predictor of subsequent disability. New Engl J Med 332(9):556, 1995.
216. Duncan, RP, Leddy, AL, Earhart, GM: Five times sit-to-stand test performance in Parkinson's disease. Arch Phys Med Rehabil 92(9):1431, 2011.
217. Petersen, C, et al: Reliability and Minimal Detectable Change for Sit-to-Stand Tests and the Functional Gait Assessment for individuals with Parkinson disease. J Geriatr Phys Ther, 2016.
218. Schenkman, M, McFann, K, Baron, AE: PROFILE PD: Profile of function and impairment level experience with Parkinson disease—clinimetric properties of a rating scale for physical therapist practice. J Neurol Phys Ther 34(4):182, 2010.
219. McHorney, CA, Ware, JE, Jr., Raczek, AE: The MOS 36-Item Short-Form Health Survey (SF-36): II. Psychometric and clinical tests of validity in measuring physical and mental health constructs. Med Care 31(3):247, 1993.
220. Gilson, BS, et al: The Sickness Impact Profile: Development of an outcome measure of health care. Am J Pub Health 65(12):1304, 1975.
221. Jenkinson, C, et al: Self-reported functioning and well-being in patients with Parkinson's disease: Comparison of the short-form health survey (SF-36) and the Parkinson's Disease Questionnaire (PDQ-39). Age Ageing 24(6):505, 1995.
222. Tomlinson Claire, L, et al: Physiotherapy for Parkinson's disease: A comparison of techniques. Cochrane Database Syst Rev, 2014(6):CD002815, 2014.
223. Tomlinson Claire, L, et al: Physiotherapy versus placebo or no intervention in Parkinson's disease. Cochrane Database Syst Rev, 2012(7):CD002817, 2012.
224. Rochester, L, et al: Evidence for motor learning in Parkinson's disease: Acquisition, automaticity and retention of cued gait performance after training with external rhythmical cues. Brain Res 1319:103, 2010.
225. van Tilborg, I, Hulstijn, W: Implicit motor learning in patients with Parkinson's and Alzheimer's disease: Differences in learning abilities? Motor Control 14(3):344, 2010.
226. Chiviacowsky, S, et al: Motor learning benefits of self-controlled practice in persons with Parkinson's disease. Gait Posture 35(4):601, 2012.
227. Peterson, DS, Dijkstra, BW, Horak, FB: Postural motor learning in people with Parkinson's disease. J Neurol, 2016.
228. Behrman, AL, Cauraugh, JH, Light, KE: Practice as an intervention to improve speeded motor performance and motor learning in Parkinson's disease. J Neurol Sci 174(2):127, 2000.
229. Lim, I, et al: Effects of external rhythmical cueing on gait in patients with Parkinson's disease: A systematic review. Clin Rehab 19(7):695, 2005.
230. Azulay, J-P, Mesure, S, Blin, O: Influence of visual cues on gait in Parkinson's disease: Contribution to attention or sensory dependence? J Neurol Sci 248(1-2):192, 2006.
231. Brodie, MA, et al: Symmetry matched auditory cues improve gait steadiness in most people with Parkinson's disease but not in healthy older people. J Parkinsons Dis 5(1):105, 2015.
232. Willems, AM, et al: The use of rhythmic auditory cues to influence gait in patients with Parkinson's disease, the differential effect for freezers and non-freezers, an explorative study. Disabil Rehabil 28(11):721, 2006.
233. Willems, AM, et al: Turning in Parkinson's disease patients and controls: The effect of auditory cues. Mov Disord 22(13):1871, 2007.
234. Arias, P, Cudeiro, J: Effects of rhythmic sensory stimulation (auditory, visual) on gait in Parkinson's disease patients. Expl Brain Res 186(4):589, 2008.
235. Mak, MK, Yu, L, Hui-Chan, CW: The immediate effect of a novel audio-visual cueing strategy (simulated traffic lights) on dual-task walking in people with Parkinson's disease. Eur J Phys Rehabil Med 49(2):153, 2013.
236. Nieuwboer, A, et al: The short-term effects of different cueing modalities on turn speed in people with Parkinson's disease. Neurorehabil Neural Repair 23(8):831, 2009.
237. van Wegen, E, et al: The effect of rhythmic somatosensory cueing on gait in patients with Parkinson's disease. J Neurol Sci 248 (1-2):210, 2006.
238. Rochester, L, et al: The effect of external rhythmic cues (auditory and visual) on walking during a functional task in homes of people with Parkinson's disease. Arch Phys Med Rehabil 86(5):999, 2005.
239. Gallo, PM, McIsaac, TL, Garber, CE: Walking economy during cued versus non-cued self-selected treadmill walking in persons with Parkinson's disease. J Parkinsons Dis 4(4):705, 2014.
240. Lewis, GN, Byblow, WD, Walt, SE: Stride length regulation in Parkinson's disease: The use of extrinsic, visual cues. Brain 123 (10):2077, 2000.
241. Farley, BG, et al: Intensive amplitude-specific therapeutic approaches for Parkinson's disease: Toward a neuroplasticity-principled rehabilitation model. Top Geriatr Rehabil 24(2): 99, 2008.
242. Hirsch, MA, Farley, BG: Exercise and neuroplasticity in persons living with Parkinson's disease. Eur J Phys Rehabil Med 45(2): 215, 2009.
243. Farley, BG, Koshland, GF: Training BIG to move faster: the application of the speed-amplitude relation as a rehabilitation strategy for people with Parkinson's disease. Exp Brain Res 167(3): 462, 2005.
244. Kleim, JA, Jones, TA: Principles of experience-dependent neural plasticity: Implications for rehabilitation after brain damage. J Speech Lang Hear Res 51(1):S225, 2008.
245. Petzinger, GM, et al: The effects of exercise on dopamine neurotransmission in Parkinson's disease: Targeting neuroplasticity to modulate basal ganglia circuitry. Brain Plast 1(1):29, 2015.
246. Petzinger, GM, et al: Exercise-enhanced neuroplasticity targeting motor and cognitive circuitry in Parkinson's disease. Lancet Neurol 12(7):716, 2013.
247. Ebersbach, G, et al: Comparing exercise in Parkinson's disease—the Berlin BIG Study. Mov Disord 25(12):1902, 2010.

248. Hirsch, MA, Iyer, SS, Sanjak, M: Exercise-induced neuroplasticity in human Parkinson's disease: What is the evidence telling us? Parkinsonism Relat Disord 22(Suppl 1):S78, 2016.
249. Kapur, AS, Stebbins, GT, Goetz, CG: Vibration therapy for Parkinson's disease: Charcot's stuides revisited. J Parkinsons Dis 2(2012):23, 2012.
250. Smart, K, et al: A potential case of remission of Parkinson's disease. J Complement Integ Med, 13(3):311, 2016.
251. Tang, Y-Y, Holzel, BK, Posner, MI: The neuroscience of mindfulness meditation. Nat Rev Neurosci 16(4):213, 2015.
252. Caligiore, D, et al: Action observation and motor imagery for rehabilitation in Parkinson's disease: A systematic review and an integrative hypothesis. Neurosci Biobehav Rev 72:210, 2017.
253. Kwok, JY, Choi, KC, Chan, HY: Effects of mind-body exercises on the physiological and psychosocial well-being of individuals with Parkinson's disease: A systematic review and meta-analysis. Complement Ther Med 29:121, 2016.
254. Kakde, N, et al: Development and validation of a yoga module for Parkinson disease. J Complement Integ Med 14(3), 2017.
255. Toole, T, et al: The effects of a balance and strength training program on equilibrium in parkinsonism: A preliminary study. NeuroRehabilitation 14(3):165, 2000.
256. Falvo, MJ, Schilling, BK, Earhart, GM: Parkinson's disease and resistive exercise: Rationale, review, and recommendations. Mov Disord 23(1):1, 2008.
257. Dibble, LE, et al: High intensity eccentric resistance training decreases bradykinesia and improves quality of life in persons with Parkinson's disease: A preliminary study. Parkinsonism Relat Disord 15(10):752, 2009.
258. Lima, LO, Scianni, A, Rodrigues-de-Paula, F: Progressive resistance exercise improves strength and physical performance in people with mild to moderate Parkinson's disease: A systematic review. J Physiother 59(1):7, 2013.
259. Roeder, L, et al: Effects of resistance training on measures of muscular strength in people with Parkinson's disease: A systematic review and meta-analysis. PLoS One 10(7):e0132135, 2015.
260. Schlenstedt, C, et al: Resistance versus balance training to improve postural control in Parkinson's disease: A randomized rater blinded controlled study. PLoS One 10(10):e0140584, 2015.
261. Chung, CL, Thilarajah, S, Tan, D: Effectiveness of resistance training on muscle strength and physical function in people with Parkinson's disease: A systematic review and meta-analysis. Clin Rehabil 30(1):11, 2016.
262. Ni, M, et al: Power training induced change in bradykinesia and muscle power in Parkinson's disease. Parkinsonism Relat Disord 23:37, 2016.
263. Saltychev, M, et al: Progressive resistance training in Parkinson's disease: A systematic review and meta-analysis. BMJ 6(1): e008756, 2016.
264. Corcos, DM, et al: A two-year randomized controlled trial of progressive resistance exercise for Parkinson's disease. Mov Disord 28(9):1230, 2013.
265. Mak, MK, Yang, F, Pai, YC: Limb collapse, rather than instability, causes failure in sit-to-stand performance among patients with Parkinson disease. Phys Ther 91(3):381, 2011.
266. Bolen, M: Health professionals guide to physical management of Parkinson's disease, Champaign, IL : Human Kinetics, 2009.
267. Park, DS, Lee, G: Validity and reliability of balance assessment software using the Nintendo Wii balance board: Usability and validation. J Neuroeng Rehabil 11:99, 2014.
268. Clark, RA, et al: Validity and reliability of the Nintendo Wii Balance Board for assessment of standing balance. Gait Posture 31(3):307, 2010.
269. McGough, R, et al: Improving lower limb weight distribution asymmetry during the squat using Nintendo Wii Balance Boards and real-time feedback. J Strength Cond Res 26(1):47, 2012.
270. Mhatre, PV, et al: Wii Fit balance board playing improves balance and gait in Parkinson disease. PM R 5(9):769, 2013.
271. Morris, ME: Locomotor training in people with Parkinson disease. Phys Ther 86(10):1426, 2006.
272. Behrman, AL, Teitelbaum, P, Cauraugh, JH: Verbal instructional sets to normalise the temporal and spatial gait variables in Parkinson's disease. J Neurol Neurosurg Psychiatry 65(4):580, 1998.
273. de Melo Roiz, R, et al: Analysis of parallel and transverse visual cues on the gait of individuals with idiopathic Parkinson's disease. Int J Rehabil Res 34(4):343, 2011.
274. Fisher, BE, et al: Treadmill exercise elevates striatal dopamine D2 receptor binding potential in patients with early Parkinson's disease. Neuroreport 24(10):509, 2013.
275. Ganesan, M, et al: Effect of partial weight-supported treadmill gait training on balance in patients with Parkinson disease. PM&R 6(1):22, 2014.
276. Nadeau, A, Pourcher, E, Corbeil, P: Effects of 24 wk of treadmill training on gait performance in Parkinson's disease. Med Sci Sports Exerc 46(4):645, 2014.
277. Tseng, IJ, Yuan, RY, Jeng, C: Treadmill training improves forward and backward gait in early Parkinson disease. Am J Phys Med Rehabil, 2015.
278. Picelli, A, et al: Effects of treadmill training on cognitive and motor features of patients with mild to moderate Parkinson's disease: A pilot, single-blind, randomized controlled trial. Funct Neurol 31(1):25, 2016.
279. Miyai, I, et al: Long-term effect of body weight-supported treadmill training in Parkinson's disease: A randomized controlled trial. Arch Phys Med Rehabil 83(10):1370, 2002.
280. Pohl, M, et al: Immediate effects of speed-dependent treadmill training on gait parameters in early Parkinson's disease. Arch Phys Med Rehabil 84(12):1760, 2003.
281. Miyai, I, et al: Treadmill training with body weight support: Its effect on Parkinson's disease. Arch Phys Med Rehabil 81(7):849, 2000.
282. Frenkel-Toledo, S, et al: Treadmill walking as an external pacemaker to improve gait rhythm and stability in Parkinson's disease. Mov Disord 20(9):1109, 2005.
283. Cakit, BD, et al: The effects of incremental speed-dependent treadmill training on postural instability and fear of falling in Parkinson's disease. Clin Rehabil 21(8):698, 2007.
284. Fisher, BE, et al: The effect of exercise training in improving motor performance and corticomotor excitability in people with early Parkinson's disease. Arch Phys Med Rehabil 89(7):1221, 2008.
285. Protas, EJ, et al: Gait and step training to reduce falls in Parkinson's disease. NeuroRehabilitation 20(3):183, 2005.
286. Maidan, I, et al: Altered brain activation in complex walking conditions in patients with Parkinson's disease. Parkinsonism Relat Disord 25:91, 2016.
287. Agosta, F, et al: Brain plasticity in Parkinson's disease with freezing of gait induced by action observation training. J Neurol 264(1): 88, 2017.
288. Pelosin, E, et al: Action observation improves freezing of gait in patients with Parkinson's disease. Neurorehabil Neural Repair 24(8):746, 2010.
289. Shine, JM, et al: Attentional set-shifting deficits correlate with the severity of freezing of gait in Parkinson's disease. Parkinsonism Relat Disord 19(3):388, 2013.
290. Cohen, RG, et al: Inhibition, executive function, and freezing of gait. J Parkinsons Dis 4(1):111, 2014.
291. Vandenbossche, J, et al: Conflict and freezing of gait in Parkinson's disease: Support for a response control deficit. Neuroscience 206:144, 2012.
292. Nantel, J, et al: Deficits in visuospatial processing contribute to quantitative measures of freezing of gait in Parkinson's disease. Neuroscience 221:151, 2012.
293. Leung, IHK, et al: Cognitive training in Parkinson disease: A systematic review and meta-analysis. Neurology, 2015.
294. París, AP, et al: Blind randomized controlled study of the efficacy of cognitive training in Parkinson's disease. Mov Disord 26(17): 1251, 2011.
295. Sammer, G, et al: Training of executive functions in Parkinson's disease. J Neurol Sci 248(1-2):115, 2006.
296. Perrochon, A, Kemoun, G: The Walking Trail-Making Test is an early detection tool for mild cognitive impairment. Clin Interv Aging 9:111, 2014.
297. Perrochon, A, et al: Walking Stroop carpet: An innovative dual-task concept for detecting cognitive impairment. Clin Interv Aging 8: 317, 2013.
298. McIsaac, TL, Lamberg, EM, Muratori, LM: Building a framework for a dual task taxonomy. Biomed Res Int 2015:591475, 2015.
299. O'Shea, S, Morris, ME, Iansek, R: Dual task interference during gait in people with Parkinson disease: Effects of motor versus cognitive secondary tasks. Phys Ther 82(9):888, 2002.

300. Strouwen, C, et al: Training dual tasks together or apart in Parkinson's disease: Results from the DUALITY trial. Mov Disord, 2017.
301. Wu, T, Hallett, M: A functional MRI study of automatic movements in patients with Parkinson's disease. Brain 128 (Pt 10):2250, 2005.
302. Pelosin, E, et al: Attentional control of gait and falls: Is cholinergic dysfunction a common substrate in the elderly and Parkinson's disease? Front Aging Neurosci 8, 2016.
303. Jacobs, JV, et al: Dual tasking during postural stepping responses increases falls but not freezing in people with Parkinson's disease. Parkinsonism Relat Disord 20(7):779, 2014.
304. Lapointe, LL, Stierwalt, JAG, Maitland, CG: Talking while walking: Cognitive loading and injurious falls in Parkinson's disease. Int J Speech Lang Pathol 12(5):455, 2010.
305. Stolwyk, RJ, et al: Self-regulation of driving behavior in people with Parkinson disease. Cogn Behav Neurol 28(2):80, 2015.
306. Crizzle, AM, Classen, S, Uc, EY: Parkinson disease and driving: An evidence-based review. Neurology 79(20):2067, 2012.
307. Rizzo, M, et al: Driving difficulties in Parkinson's disease. Mov Disord 25(Suppl 1):S136, 2010.
308. Kelly, VE, Eusterbrock, AJ, Shumway-Cook, A: A review of dual-task walking deficits in people with Parkinson's disease: Motor and cognitive contributions, mechanisms, and clinical implications. Parkinson Dis 2012:918719, 2012.
309. Stolwyk, RJ, et al: Effect of a concurrent task on driving performance in people with Parkinson's disease. Mov Disord 21(12):2096, 2006.
310. Strouwen, C, et al: Dual tasking in Parkinson's disease: Should we train hazardous behavior? Expert Rev Neurother 15(9):1031, 2015.
311. Uc, EY, Rizzo, M: Driving and neurodegenerative diseases. Curr Neurol Neurosci Rep 8(5):377, 2008.
312. Keus, SH, et al: Evidence-based analysis of physical therapy in Parkinson's disease with recommendations for practice and research. Mov Disord 22(4):451, 2007.
313. Keus, SHJ, et al: European Physiotherapy Guideline for Parkinson's disease, The Netherlands: KNGF/ParkinsonNet, 2014.
314. Yogev-Seligmann, G, Hausdorff, JM, Giladi, N: Do we always prioritize balance when walking? Towards an integrated model of task prioritization. Mov Disord 27(6):765, 2012.
315. Fritz, NE, Cheek, FM, Nichols-Larsen, DS: Motor-cognitive dual-task training in persons with neurologic disorders: A systematic review. J Neurol Phys Ther 39(3):142, 2015.
316. Killane, I, et al: Dual motor-cognitive virtual reality training impacts dual-task performance in freezing of gait. IEEE J Biomed Health Inform 19(6):1855, 2015.
317. Strouwen, C, et al: Protocol for a randomized comparison of integrated versus consecutive dual task practice in Parkinson's disease: The DUALITY trial. BMC Neurology 14(1):61, 2014.
318. Yitayeh, A, and Teshome, A: The effectiveness of physiotherapy treatment on balance dysfunction and postural instability in persons with Parkinson's disease: A systematic review and meta-analysis. BMC Sports Sci Med Rehabil 8(1): 2016.
319. Ford, M, et al: The effect of dual task activities on the walking gait of individuals with Parkinson's disease. Clin Kinesiol 69(1): 2015.
320. Pfeifer, M, et al: Effects of two newly developed spinal orthoses on trunk muscle strength, posture, and quality-of-life in women with postmenopausal osteoporosis: A randomized trial. Am J Phys Med Rehabil 90(10):805, 2011.
321. Pfeifer, M, Begerow, B, Minne, HW: Effects of a new spinal orthosis on posture, trunk strength, and quality of life in women with postmenopausal osteoporosis: A randomized trial. Am J Phys Med Rehabil 83(3):177, 2004.
322. Lantz, SA, Schultz, AB: Lumbar spine orthosis wearing. II. Effect on trunk muscle myoelectric activity. Spine 11(8):838, 1986.
323. Schmidt, K, et al: [Influence of spinal orthosis on gait and physical functioning in women with postmenopausal osteoporosis]. Orthopade 41(3):200, 2012.
324. Mehanna, R, Jankovic, J: Respiratory problems in neurologic movement disorders. Parkinsonism Relat Disord 16(10):628, 2010.
325. Koseoglu, F, et al: The effects of a pulmonary rehabilitation program on pulmonary function tests and exercise tolerance in patients with Parkinson's disease. Funct Neurol 12(6):319, 1997.
326. Inzelberg, R, et al: Inspiratory muscle training and the perception of dyspnea in Parkinson's disease. Can J Neurol Sci 32(2):213, 2005.
327. Bergen, JL, et al: Aerobic exercise intervention improves aerobic capacity and movement initiation in Parkinson's disease patients. NeuroRehabilitation 17(2):161, 2002.
328. Meyer, TK: The larynx for neurologists. Neurologist 15(6):313, 2009.
329. Fox, CM, et al: The science and practice of LSVT/LOUD: Neural plasticity-principled approach to treating individuals with Parkinson disease and other neurological disorders. Semin Speech Lang 27(4):283, 2006.
330. Spielman, JL, Borod, JC, Ramig, LO: The effects of intensive voice treatment on facial expressiveness in Parkinson disease: Preliminary data. Cogn Behav Neurol 16(3):177, 2003.
331. Mahler, LA, Ramig, LO, Fox, C: Evidence-based treatment of voice and speech disorders in Parkinson disease. Curr Opin Otolaryngol Head Neck Surg 23(3):209, 2015.
332. Lamotte, G, et al: Effects of endurance exercise training on the motor and non-motor features of Parkinson's disease: A review. J Parkinsons Dis 5(1):21, 2015.
333. Duchesne, C, et al: Enhancing both motor and cognitive functioning in Parkinson's disease: Aerobic exercise as a rehabilitative intervention. Brain Cogn 99:68, 2015.
334. Duchesne, C, et al: Influence of aerobic exercise training on the neural correlates of motor learning in Parkinson's disease individuals. Neuroimage Clin 12:559, 2016.
335. McGough, EL, et al: A Tandem cycling program: Feasibility and physical performance outcomes in people with Parkinson disease. J Neurol Phys Ther 40(4):223, 2016.
336. States, RA, et al: Physical functioning after 1, 3, and 5 years of exercise among people with Parkinson's disease: A longitudinal observational study. J Geriatric Phys Ther, epub ahead of print(April), 2016.
337. Ellis, T, et al: Factors associated with exercise behavior in people with Parkinson disease. Phys Ther 91(12):1838, 2011.
338. Krishnamurthi, N, et al: Polestriding intervention improves gait and axial symptoms in mild to moderate Parkinson disease. Arch Phys Med Rehabil 98(4):613, 2017.
339. Ni, M, et al: Comparative effect of power training and high-speed yoga on motor function in older patients with Parkinson disease. Arch Phys Med Rehabil 97(3):345, 2016.
340. Cohen, RG, et al: Lighten Up: Specific postural instructions affect axial rigidity and step initiation in patients with Parkinson's disease. Neurorehabil Neural Rep 29(9):878, 2015.
341. Stallibrass, C, Sissons, P, Chalmers, C: Randomized controlled trial of the Alexander technique for idiopathic Parkinson's disease. Clin Rehabil 16(7):695, 2002.
342. Kim, HD, et al: The effects of tai chi based exercise on dynamic postural control of Parkinson's disease patients while initiating gait. J Phys Ther Sci 23(2):265, 2011.
343. Li, F, et al: Tai chi and postural stability in patients with Parkinson's disease. New Engl J Med 366(6):511, 2012.
344. King, LA, Horak, FB: Delaying mobility disability in people with Parkinson disease using a sensorimotor agility exercise program. Phys Ther 89(4):384, 2009.
345. Cubo, E, et al: Prospective study on cost-effectiveness of home-based motor assessment in Parkinson's disease. J Telemed Telecare 23(2):328, 2017.
346. Ginis, P, et al: Feasibility and effects of home-based smartphone-delivered automated feedback training for gait in people with Parkinson's disease: A pilot randomized controlled trial. Parkinsonism Relat Disord, 22:28, 2015.
347. Bhidayasiri, R, et al: What is the evidence to support home environmental adaptation in Parkinson's disease? A call for multidisciplinary interventions. Parkinsonism Relat Disord 21(10):1127, 2015.
348. King, LA, et al: Effects of group, individual, and home exercise in persons with Parkinson disease: A randomized clinical trial. J Neurol Phys Ther 39(4):204, 2015.
349. Caglar, AT, et al: Effects of home exercises on motor performance in patients with Parkinson's disease. Clin Rehabil 19(8): 870, 2005.

Yoga Sequence for Early/Mild Parkinson's Disease

appendix **18.A**

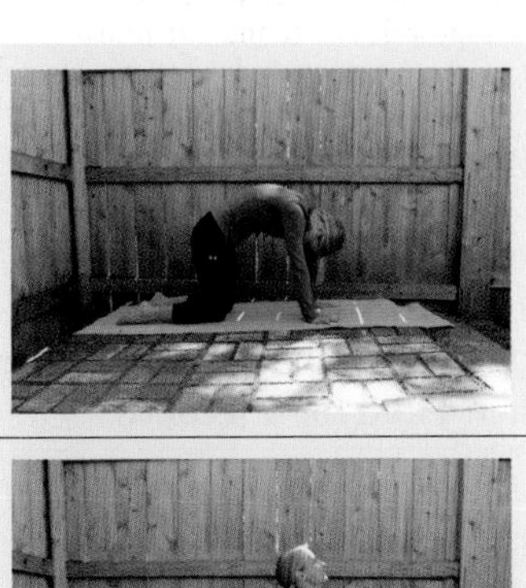

Marjaryasana (Cat Pose)

1. Start on your hands and knees. Tabletop position.
2. As you exhale round your spine toward the ceiling. Hold for 5 seconds.

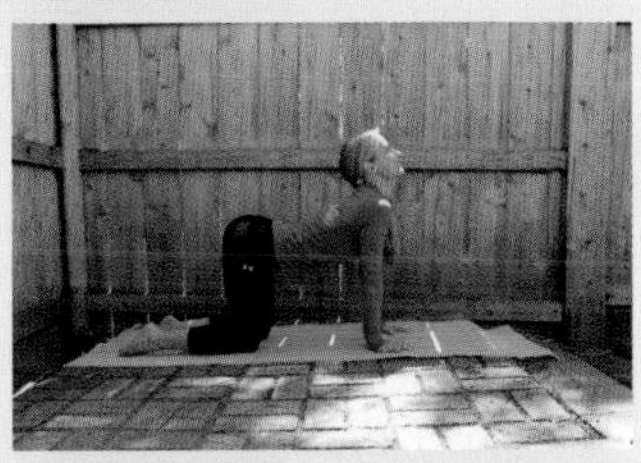

Bitilasana (Cow Pose)

1. As you inhale lift your sitting bones and chest toward the ceiling. Hold for 5 seconds.

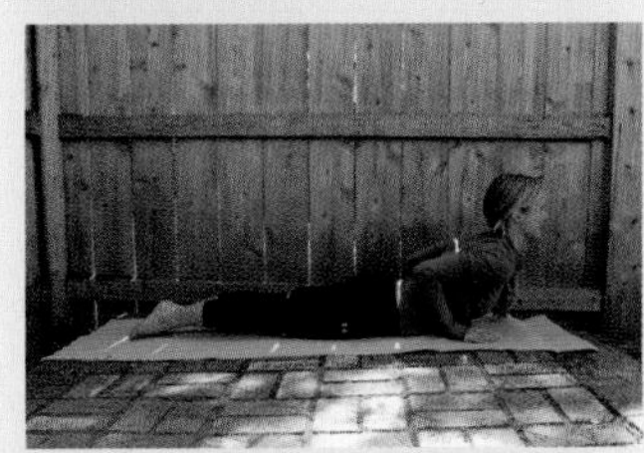

Bhujanga (Cobra Pose)

1. Lie on your stomach with your hands under your shoulders.
2. As you inhale press the shoulders and torso off the mat and look up. Hold for 5 seconds.

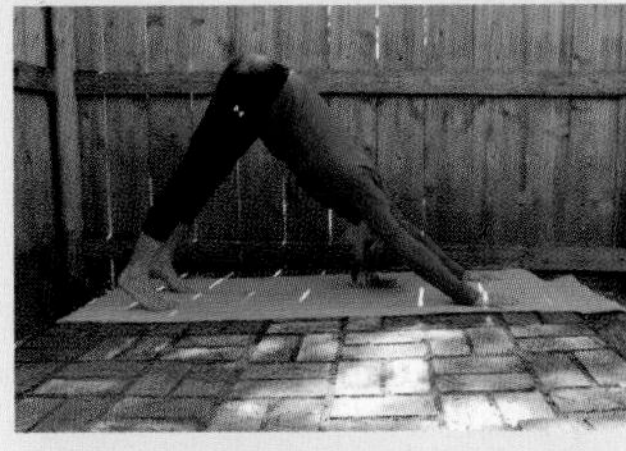

Adho Mukha Svanasana (Downward-Facing Dog)

1. Start in the tabletop position.
2. As you exhale lift your knees and torso from the ground forming an inverted "V."
3. Push your shoulder blades against your back and heels to the ground.
4. Hold for 5 seconds.

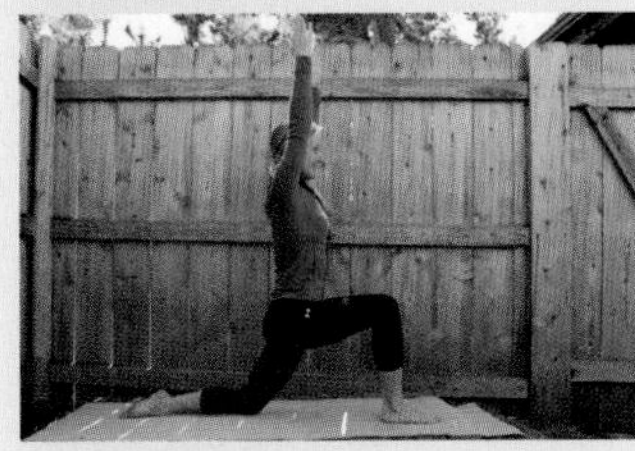

Anjaneyasana (Low Lunge)

1. Step your right foot forward and maintain your left knee on the ground.
2. As you inhale raise your arms to the sky and stretch your torso forward.

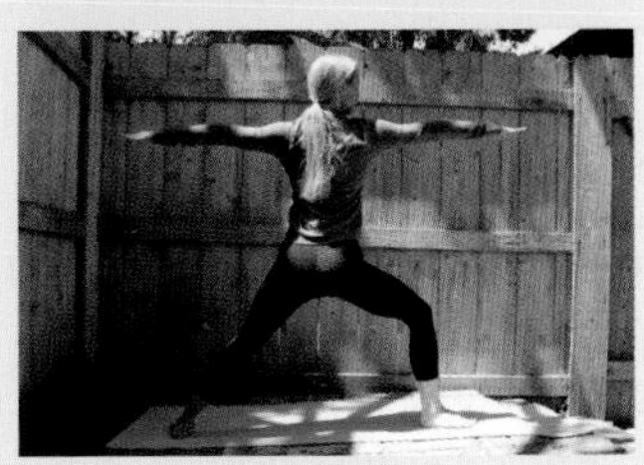

Virabhadrasana II (Warrior II Pose)

1. Rise up from low lunge maintaining the right knee bent and the left knee straight.
2. Right foot should be straight ahead, and the left foot should be turned out 90 degrees.
3. Ensure that outside border of the left foot stays on the ground.
4. With the right arm straight forward and the left arm straight back, sink into the pose looking over the fingers of your right hand.

Yoga Sequence for Late Parkinson's Disease

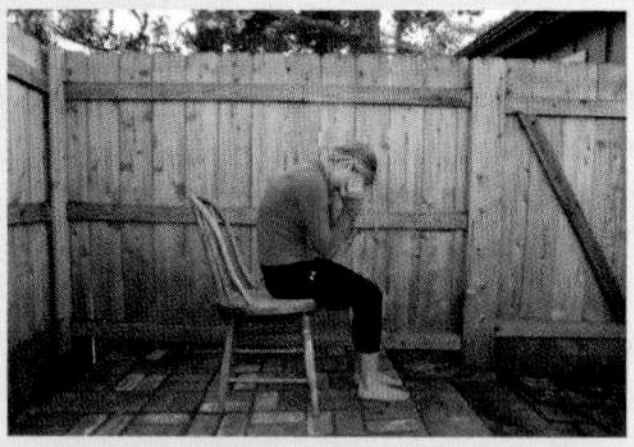

Pose	Instructions
Marjaryasana (Chair Cat Pose)	**1.** Start perch sitting (body at front of chair), sitting tall and hands on the side of your head. **2.** As you exhale, round your spine toward the back of the chair and bring your shoulders and head forward while bringing your elbows together. Hold for 5 seconds.
Bitilasana (Chair Cow Pose)	**1.** As you inhale, arch your back and look up to the sky. Open your chest and spread your elbows wide. Hold for 5 seconds.
Parighasana (Chair Gate Pose)	**1.** Start sitting tall with your right hand on the chair and left arm raised to the sky palm facing in. **2.** Inhale deeply. **3.** As you exhale, side-bend your torso to the right and look up to your left hand. Hold for 5 seconds. **4.** Repeat on the opposite side.
Ardha Matsyendrasana (Chair Spinal Twist)	**1.** Start sitting tall with your hands on the side of your head. **2.** Inhale deeply. **3.** As you exhale, rotate to one side. Hold for 5 seconds. **4.** Repeat on the opposite side.
Eka Pada Rajakapotasana (Chair Pigeon Pose)	**1.** Start sitting tall with your legs crossed, right ankle on top of left knee. **2.** As you exhale, lean forward from the hips keeping your spine long. Hold for 5 seconds. **3.** Repeat on the opposite side.
Anjaneyasana (Modified Low Lunge) Variation A (Advanced) Variation B (Beginner)	Variation A: **1.** Stand holding on to a stable surface for stability. **2.** Left foot is supported on chair behind you. **3.** With a tall upright spine, exhale and bend the right knee while moving the pelvis forward. Hold for 5 seconds. **4.** Repeat on the opposite side.

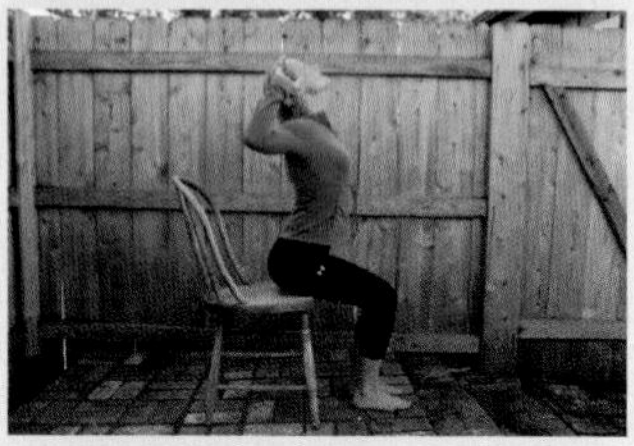

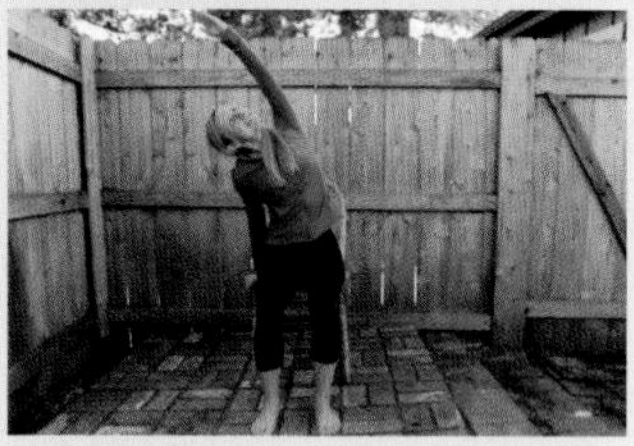

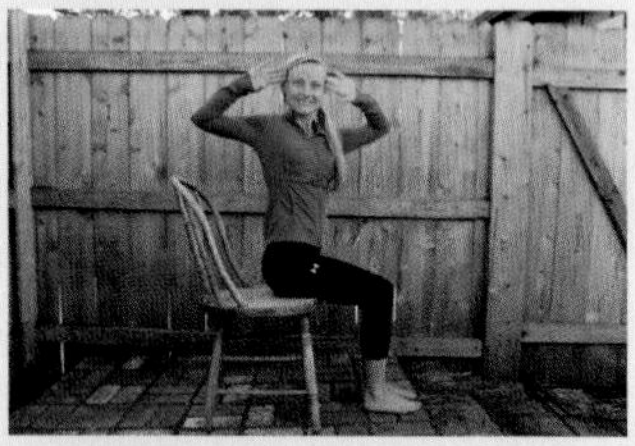

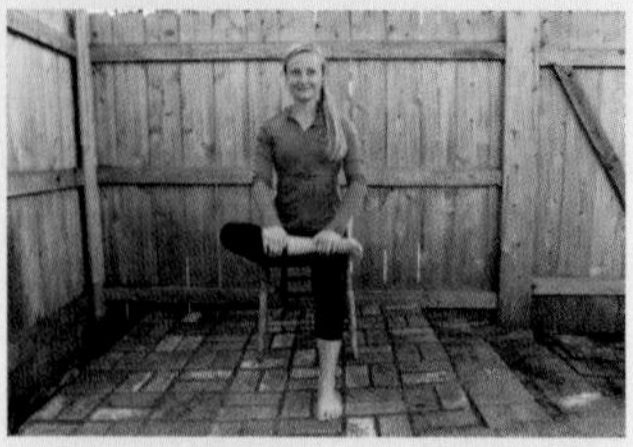

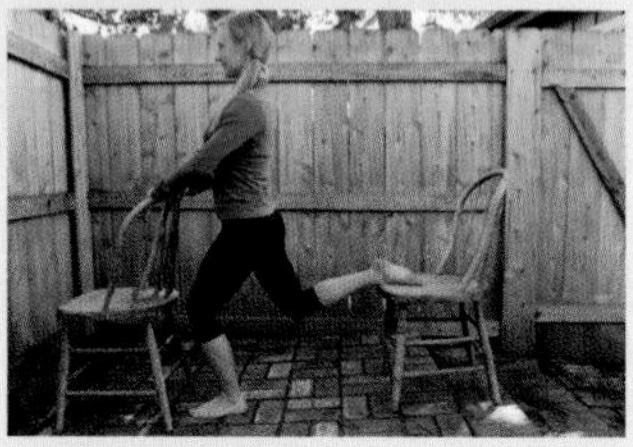

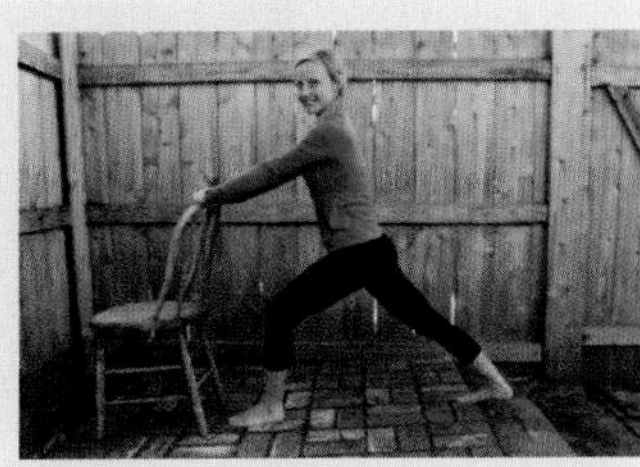		Variation B: **1.** Stand holding on to a stable surface for stability. Left is foot forward and right foot back. **2.** With a tall upright spine, exhale while bending the left knee and maintaining the right leg straight. Hold for 5 seconds. **3.** Repeat on the opposite side.
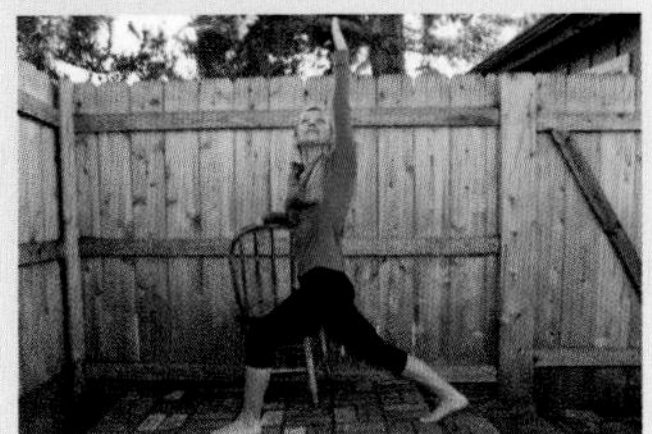	Utthita Parsvakonasana (Modified Extended Side Angle Pose)	**1.** Hold on to a stable surface with your right hand. Left foot is forward and right foot back. **2.** While maintaining a long spine, bend the left knee moving the pelvis forward and keeping the right knee straight. **3.** As you exhale, raise the left arm to the sky and turn your head to the left looking up to your left hand. Hold for 5 seconds. **4.** Repeat on the opposite side.

appendix 18.B

Web-Based Resources for Clinicians and Patients/Families Living With Parkinson's Disease

Resource	Web Address
National Parkinson Foundation (NPF)	www.parkinson.org www.parkinson.org/books (free publications available for download) www.parkinson.org/pd-library (broader library resources for professionals) www.parkinson.org/find-help/resources-in-your-community (registry of health professionals or support groups by local area) helpline@parkinson.org: provides dialogue for outreach and education www.toolkit.parkinson.org (Aware in Care kit for patients to bring with them for hospital stays)
Parkinson's Disease Foundation (PDF)	www.pdf.org
American Parkinson Disease Association (APDA)	www.apdaparkinson.org
World Parkinson Coalition (WPC)	www.worldpdcoalition.org
Parkinson Society Canada	www.parkinson.ca
Michael J. Fox Foundation for Parkinson's Research	www.michaeljfox.org
The Parkinson Alliance	www.parkinsonalliance.net
Americans With Disabilities Act: ADA home page	www.ada.gov
Medicare information	http://cms.hhs.gov
Social Security Online	www.ssa.gov
National Institute of Neurologic Disorders and Stroke (Parkinson's Disease Information Page)	https://www.ninds.nih.gov/Disorders/All-Disorders/Parkinsons-Disease-Information-Page
National Library of Medicine	www.nlm.nih.gov
Journal of the American Medical Association (JAMA) – Neurology	http://jamanetwork.com/journals/jamaneurology/newonline
Neurology	www.neurology.org
Veterans Affairs	www.va.gov
Caregiver Action Network (CAN)	www.caregiveraction.org
Parkinson's Disease Caregiver Information	www.myparkinsons.org
Well Spouse Foundation	www.wellspouse.org
American Academy of Neurology (AAN)	www.aan.com (AAN members, professionals) www.aan.com/public (public education)
National Rehabilitation Information Center (NARIC)	www.naric.com
ABLEDATA—assistive technology	www.abledata.com

Traumatic Brain Injury

George D. Fulk, PT, PhD
Coby Nirider, PT, DPT

Chapter 19

LEARNING OBJECTIVES

1. Describe the pathophysiology of traumatic brain injury.
2. Analyze the impact of cognitive, neurobehavioral, and neuromuscular impairments, activity limitations, and participation restrictions on outcomes of people with traumatic brain injury.
3. Identify the different team members and settings in the management of the patient with traumatic brain injury.
4. Compare and contrast persistent vegetative state and minimally conscious state.
5. Identify key components of the physical therapy examination during the acute stage of recovery in patients with severe to moderate traumatic brain injury.
6. Create a plan of care for a patient with a severe to moderate traumatic brain injury that presents with disorder of consciousness in the acute stage of recovery.
7. Select evidence-based outcome measures to use during the physical therapy examination of a patient with moderate to severe traumatic brain injury during the active rehabilitation stage of recovery.
8. Explain the impact of cognitive and neurobehavioral impairments on the physical therapy plan of care in the active rehabilitation stage of recovery.
9. Create a plan of care for a patient with a severe to moderate traumatic brain injury in the active rehabilitation stage of recovery.
10. Select evidence-based outcome measures to use during the physical therapy examination of a patient with a mild traumatic brain injury.
11. Outline a return to play/activity timeline for a patient with a mild traumatic brain injury.
12. Create a plan of care for a patient with a mild traumatic brain injury.

CHAPTER OUTLINE

A traumatic brain injury (TBI) is defined as "an alteration in brain function, or other evidence of brain pathology, caused by an external force."[1] The TBI population is one of the most challenging and rewarding that a physical therapist (PT) is likely to encounter. Because of the multiple body systems affected by a brain injury and the strong likelihood of secondary impairments, a PT must be proficient in a wide variety of examination procedures and intervention techniques. Owing to behavioral difficulties encountered during recovery, a PT working with this population must also possess strong communication and interpersonal skills, be able to react quickly and effectively to suddenly changing situations, and have keen observation skills. These factors and others can make working with this population challenging and exhausting—cognitively, emotionally, and physically. However, the rewards of assisting a patient with a severe brain injury to return to home, work, or school vastly outweigh the challenges of rehabilitation.

The patient with a brain injury is treated across a wide continuum of care, which includes the intensive care unit (ICU), acute hospital, inpatient rehabilitation center, skilled nursing facility (subacute rehabilitation), and long-term care facility. Additional services may include outpatient services, community reintegration programs, comprehensive day treatment, and residential programs for assisted living and neurobehavioral services. Because of the wide variety of presenting impairments, activity limitations, and participation restrictions, rehabilitation for the patient with TBI requires a strong interdisciplinary team. A PT is an important member of this team. It is crucial that there be open communication between and among all team members to ensure safe, timely, and consistent treatment. Regardless of the setting, it is important to remember that the patient is the central member of the team.

PREVALENCE AND IMPACT

Traumatic brain injury is the leading cause of injury-related death and disability in the United States. In 2013, approximately 2.8 million people are admitted to emergency departments, are hospitalized, or die as a result of a TBI. Of these, approximately 56,000 people die as a result of the injury and 280,000 require hospitalization.[2] In all likelihood, these numbers underrepresent the true incidence of TBI. They do not take into account military personnel, people who seek medical attention in settings other than emergency departments, and many sports-related brain injuries that often go unrecognized.[3]

Falls are the leading cause of TBI, followed by struck by/against events and motor vehicle/traffic accidents. Older adults (>75 years) are at greatest risk of TBI, followed by infants (0–4 months) and older adolescents/young adults (14–24 years).[2] Hospitalization and death as a result of TBI is most common in older adults (>65 years).[4,5] Motor vehicle accidents are the most common cause of moderate to severe TBI in younger adults, which decreases with age. Falls are the most common cause in older adults.[6]

The long-term consequences of TBI on the health care system, society, and the individual are high. There are approximately 3.2 to 5.3 million people in the United States who are disabled as a result of TBI.[7-9] The annual economic burden is estimated to be $37.8 billion, including direct medical costs, injury-related disability and work loss, and lost income due to premature death.[10] One in five individuals who receive inpatient rehabilitation services post-TBI die within 5 years and of those who survive, 50% are readmitted to the hospital at least once.[11] Approximately 60% of people with moderate to severe TBI are unemployed, and of those who are employed, one-third of them work part-time.[12] One-quarter to one-third of people with severe to moderate TBI require assistance with activities of daily living (ADL), and approximately 30% to 40% report poor mental and physical health.[11,13]

MECHANISM OF INJURY AND PATHOPHYSIOLOGY

Traumatic brain injury is a heterogenous injury, with a wide variety of pathophysiological mechanisms.[14] The brain damage results from external forces that cause brain tissue to make direct contact with an object (bony skull or penetrating object), rapid acceleration or deceleration forces, or blast waves from an explosion.[15] Generally speaking, brain tissue damage can be categorized as either primary injury that is due to direct trauma to the parenchyma or secondary injury that results from a cascade of biochemical, cellular, and molecular events that evolve over time due to the initial injury and injury-related hypoxia, edema, and elevated intracranial pressure (ICP).[14,16]

Primary Injury

Primary TBI results from either brain tissue coming into contact with an object (e.g., bony skull or external object such as a bullet or sharp instrument creating a penetrating injury) or rapid acceleration/deceleration of the brain creating cortical disruption. Contact injuries often result in contusions, lacerations, and intracerebral hematomas. This damage is generally focal in nature as the brain comes into contact with bony protuberances on the inside surface of the skull or damage from the penetrating object. Common areas of focal injury are the anterior temporal poles, frontal poles, lateral and inferior temporal cortices, and orbital frontal cortices.

Acceleration and deceleration cause shear, tensile, and compression forces within the brain, which causes diffuse axonal injury (DAI), tissue tearing, and intracerebral hemorrhages.[16] DAI is the predominant mechanism of injury in most individuals with severe to moderate TBI.[17] It is common in high-speed motor vehicle accidents and can be seen in some sports-related TBIs.[18,19]

The term *diffuse* is somewhat misleading because DAI most often occurs in discrete areas: the parasagittal white matter of the cerebral cortex, the corpus callosum, and the pontine-mesencephalic junction adjacent to the superior cerebellar peduncles.[20] The mechanism of DAI is microscopic, so there may be minimal initial findings on computed tomography (CT) and magnetic resonance imaging (MRI). The acceleration/deceleration forces disrupt neurofilaments within the axon, leading to Wallerian-type axonal degeneration.[20]

Blast Injury

Blast injury is considered a signature injury of the U.S. military conflicts in the Middle East.[21,22] When an explosive device detonates, a transient shock wave is produced, which can cause brain damage.[21,23] Primary blast injury results from the direct effect of blast overpressure on organs (in this case the brain), secondary injury results from shrapnel and other objects being hurled at the individual, and tertiary injury occurs when the victim is flung backward and strikes an object. Although the exact mechanisms are not fully understood, there appear to be three mechanisms by which primary blast brain injury may occur: (1) direct transcranial blast wave propagation; (2) the transfer of kinetic energy from the blast wave through the vasculature, which triggers pressure oscillations in the blood vessels leading to the brain; and (3) elevations in cerebrospinal fluid (CSF) or venous pressure caused by compression of the thorax and abdomen and by propagation of a shock wave through the blood vessels or CSF.[21,23] Blast-related brain injury can result in edema, contusion, DAI, hematomas, and hemorrhage.[24,25] A wide spectrum of injury severities, ranging from mild (blast concussion) to severe to fatal, can result from blast TBI.

Secondary Injury

Secondary cell death occurs as a result of a chain of cellular events that follow tissue damage in addition to the secondary effects of hypoxemia, hypotension, ischemia, edema, and elevated ICP. Secondary processes develop over hours and days, and include glutamate neurotoxicity, influx of calcium and other ions, free radical release, cytokines, and inflammatory responses that can lead to cell death.[15,16] The release of glutamate and other excitatory neurotransmitters exacerbates ion-channel leakage and contributes to brain swelling and raised ICP.[15] Hypoxic-ischemic injury results from a lack of oxygenated blood flow to the brain tissue. It can be caused by systemic hypotension, anoxia, or damage to specific vascular territories of the brain. Because the rigid skull surrounds the brain, swelling, abnormal brain fluid dynamics, or hematoma can result in elevated ICP. Hematomas are usually classified according to their site (epidural, subdural, or intracerebral). Normal ICP is 5 to 20 mmHg.[26] Severely increased ICP typically results in herniation of the brain, requiring prompt emergency treatment. Common types of herniations are uncal, central, and tonsillar.

It is important to keep in mind that both primary and secondary mechanisms of injury are not mutually exclusive and often do not occur in isolation. This is one reason that the impact of TBI is so widespread across the International Classification of Functioning, Disability, and Health (ICF) spectrum.

SEQUELAE OF TRAUMATIC BRAIN INJURY

Traumatic brain injury is associated with a wide spectrum of body structure/function impairments, activity limitations, and participation restrictions that can lead to diminished quality of life.[11,27-30] Box 19.1 identifies some of the prevalent body structure/function impairments,

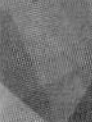

Box 19.1 Impairments, Limitations, and Restrictions Commonly Associated With Traumatic Brain Injury

Neuromuscular
- Paresis
- Abnormal tone
- Motor function
- Postural control

Cognitive
- Arousal level
- Attention
- Concentration
- Memory
- Learning
- Executive functions

Neurobehavioral
- Agitation/aggression
- Disinhibition
- Apathy
- Emotional lability
- Mental inflexibility
- Impulsivity
- Irritability

Communication

Swallowing

Activity limitations
- Walking
- Basic mobility
- Dressing
- Bathing
- Grooming
- Eating

Participation restrictions
- Return to employment
- Family role
- Community/social role

activity limitations, and participation restrictions associated with TBI. Although physical therapy interventions primarily address physical limitations related to mobility, the cognitive and behavioral changes associated with TBI are often more disabling.

Body Structure/Function Impairments

Neuromuscular Impairments

Individuals with TBI commonly exhibit impaired motor function.[31] Upper extremity (UE) and lower extremity (LE) paresis,[31,32] impaired coordination,[31-33] impaired postural control,[34-38] abnormal tone,[32] and abnormal gait[37,39,40] may be present as lifelong impairments. Abnormal, involuntary movements such as tremor and chorea form and dystonic movements are less common.[31] Patients may also present with impaired somatosensory function, depending on the location of the lesion.

Cognitive Impairments

Cognition is the mental process of knowing and applying information. Owing to the complex nature of many cognitive processes, it is difficult to localize the exact neuroanatomical structures responsible for many different cognitive functions. However, many cognitive functions are controlled in the frontal lobes. This makes people with TBI particularly susceptible to cognitive impairments. Cognition includes many complex neural processes, including arousal, attention, concentration, memory, learning, and executive functions.[41-43] Executive functions can be categorized into the following main areas: planning, cognitive flexibility, initiation and self-generation, response inhibition, and serial ordering and sequencing.[42] Chapter 27, Cognitive and Perceptual Dysfunction, provides an in-depth discussion.

Soon after injury, patients often present with disorders of consciousness.[44,45] Between 10% and 15% of patients with severe TBI are discharged from the acute hospital in a *vegetative state,*[46] and the prevalence of a *minimally conscious state* is greater than that of vegetative state.[47] Coma, vegetative state, and minimally conscious state are disordered arousal states seen after severe brain injury.[47,48] The term *unresponsive wakefulness* has been proposed for use in place of *vegetative state*; however, it has not yet gained wide acceptance.[49] It can be difficult to distinguish among the disordered arousal states. Many severe injuries begin with coma, where the arousal system is not functioning. The patient's eyes are closed, there are no sleep/wake cycles, and the patient is ventilator dependent. There is no auditory or visual function and no cognitive or communicative function.[45,47] Abnormal motor and postural reflexes may be present. A coma is usually not permanent. Patients may become brain dead, enter a vegetative or minimally conscious state, or go onto full recovery.

In a vegetative state, there is disassociation between wakefulness and awareness.[50] The higher central nervous system (CNS) centers are not integrated with the brain stem. The brain stem manages the basic cardiac, respiratory, and other vegetative functions, and the patient can be weaned off the ventilator. Sleep/wake cycles are present. The eyes may be open, though awareness of surroundings is absent. Patients may startle to visual or auditory stimuli and briefly orient to sound or visual stimuli. Meaningful cognitive and communication function is absent. Reflexive smiling/crying may be present.[44,47] A withdrawal response to noxious stimuli is present. Although patients in a vegetative state may appear to have purposeful movements, they are merely reflexive in response to external stimuli. Movement will also not be reproducible. Patients in a permanent vegetative state may have no meaningful motor or cognitive function and a complete absence of awareness of self or the environment for a period greater than 1 year after TBI and greater than 3 months after anoxic brain injury.[33,44,51]

In a minimally conscious state, there is some evidence of self or environmental awareness. Cognitively mediated behaviors occur inconsistently and are reproducible or sustained such that they can be differentiated from reflexive behaviors.[44,47] Similar to a vegetative state, sleep/wake cycles are present. However, instead of withdrawing or posturing to stimuli, patients in a minimally conscious state will localize to stimuli and may inconsistently reach for objects. Patients may localize to sound location and demonstrate sustained visual fixation and visual pursuit.[44,47]

Commonly used terms to describe other altered levels of consciousness are *stupor* and *obtunded.* Stupor is an unresponsive state from which the patient can be aroused only briefly with vigorous, repeated sensory stimulation. The patient in an obtunded state sleeps often and when aroused exhibits decreased alertness and interest in the environment and delayed reactions.

Neurobehavioral Impairments

Patients can exhibit profound behavioral changes as they progress through recovery. These changes can be closely linked to cognitive impairments and are often more debilitating in the long run than physical disability. Common behavioral sequelae include low frustration tolerance, agitation, disinhibition, apathy, emotional lability, mental inflexibility, physical and verbal aggression, impulsivity, and irritability.[42]

Communication

Language and communication deficits after brain injury are generally nonaphasic in nature[52] and are related to cognitive impairment. Common language and communication deficits include disorganized and tangential oral or written communication, imprecise language, word-retrieval difficulties, and disinhibited and socially inappropriate language. Patients may also exhibit difficulties communicating in distracting environments, reading social cues, and adjusting communication to meet the demands of the situation.[53] These communication deficits can affect employability, social integration, and quality of life.[54,55] Chapter 28, Neurogenic Disorders of Speech and Language, provides more detail on communication deficits and intervention strategies.

Dysautonomia

Elevated sympathetic nervous system activity occurs as a normal response to trauma; following TBI, this response may become overactive. Increased sympathetic activity results in increased heart rate, respiratory rate, and blood pressure; diaphoresis; and hyperthermia.[56,57] Other symptoms of dysautonomia include decerebrate and decorticate posturing, hypertonia, and teeth grinding.[56] The term *paroxysmal sympathetic hyperactivity* (also known as *sympathetic storming*) accurately describes this phenomenon.[57] The incidence of paroxysmal sympathetic hyperactivity ranges from 8% to 33% in patients with TBI in the ICU.[56]

Post-Traumatic Seizures

Between 12% and 50% of people with severe TBI develop post-traumatic seizures.[58-60] Antiepileptic/anticonvulsant medications such as phenytoin and fosphenytoin are used for seizure prophalixis.[61-63]

Secondary Impairments and Medical Complications

Due to the high potential of prolonged immobility and concomitant injury, patients with TBI are at risk of developing a number of secondary impairments and other medical issues. Up to 50% of patients with severe brain injury develop gastrointestinal difficulties, 45% develop genitourinary problems, 34% develop respiratory problems, 32% develop cardiovascular problems, and 21% develop dermatological complications.[64] Box 19.2 lists some of the more common secondary impairments and concomitant injuries associated with TBI,[60,65-67] including urinary and bowel incontinence, deep vein thrombosis (DVT), heterotopic ossification, pressure ulcer, pneumonia, and chronic pain.

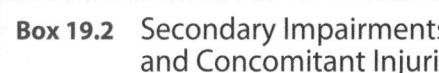

Box 19.2 Secondary Impairments and Concomitant Injuries

- Deep vein thrombosis
- Heterotopic ossification
- Pressure ulcer
- Pneumonia
- Chronic pain
- Contractures
- Decreased endurance
- Muscle atrophy
- Fracture
- Peripheral nerve damage

Activity Limitations

The activity domain of functioning in the ICF is related to the execution of a task or action by an individual. Activity limitations involve difficulties with walking, carrying/handling objects, changing and maintaining body position, washing/bathing, dressing, eating, drinking, and other ADLs.[68] People with TBI are likely to have limitations in walking ability;[69,70] high-level mobility;[71] and eating, dressing, bathing, grooming, and other ADLs.[72,73] Individuals with TBI are more likely to experience long-lasting limitations in cognitive-related activities such as problem-solving, memory, and cognitive comprehension rather than experience motor-related activity limitations such as ADLs and basic mobility.[13]

Participation Restrictions

According to the ICF, the participation domain of functioning is related to one's life situations, including but not limited to his or her role in the home, vocation, leisure, and recreational involvement.[68] Participation restrictions involve the difficulties one may experience while attempting to engage in typical life situations due to the presence of disability related to their health condition. Although many people with TBI are able to return to some level of independence in relation to basic ADLs,[13,28] given that TBI can vary in severity and implicate all brain functions, persons with TBI may experience significant, long-term participation restrictions.[11,12,28-30] Survivors may not be able to return to their prior roles in workforce, family, or community. Although the evidence is not yet conclusive, there appears to be a significant relationship between age of onset, overall brain injury severity, severity of cognitive impairments, preinjury employment, and length of ICU stay and return to gainful employment post-TBI.[74,75] A TBI Model System study found that within the first 5 years post-injury for those who were employed prior to the injury, the rate of unemployment was 55%.[11] Additionally, one study found that higher levels of mobility were associated with higher quality of life and greater social participation.[76]

Long-Term Sequalae

In addition to the immediate and near-term effects of TBI, there is also a correlation between TBI and the development of certain neurodegenerative and psychiatric diseases. In a review of the topic, Young and colleagues suggest that for those with traumatic brain injury, as the brain ages, there is a long-term risk of developing Alzheimer's disease, Parkinson's disease, frontotemporal dementia, and chronic traumatic encephalopathy.[77] There also appears to be a relationship between the presence of a TBI and the development of depressive and anxiety disorders.[77]

DIAGNOSIS AND PROGNOSIS

Traumatic brain injury is generally categorized as severe, moderate, or mild using the *Glasgow Coma Scale* (GCS) (Fig. 19.1).[78] The GCS, developed by Teasdale and Jennett, is the most widely used clinical scale that helps define and classify the severity of injury. The GCS is comprised of three response scores: motor response, verbal response, and eye opening. The scores from the separate responses are summed to provide a score between 3 and 15. Scores of 8 or less are classified as severe, scores between 9 and 12 are defined as moderate, and scores of 13 to 15 are classified as mild. Table 19.1 provides an overview of some of the characteristics that distinguish mild, moderate, and severe brain injury. However, these terms can be somewhat misleading in that a mild TBI can have a profound impact across the ICF spectrum.

Glasgow Coma Scale

Activity	Score
Eye Opening	
Spontaneous	4
To speech	3
To pain	2
No response	1
Best Motor Response	
Follows motor commands	6
Localizes	5
Withdraws	4
Abnormal flexion	3
Extensor response	2
No response	1
Verbal Response	
Oriented	5
Confused conversation	4
Inappropriate words	3
Incomprehensible sounds	2
No response	1

Figure 19.1 Glasgow Coma Scale. *(From Teasdale and Jennett,[78] with permission.)*

Table 19.1 Characteristics of Mild, Moderate, and Severe Traumatic Brain Injury

Mild TBI	Moderate TBI	Severe TBI
LOC: 0–30 min	>30 min and <24 hr	>24 hr
AOC: brief >24 hr	>24 hr	>24 hr
PTA: 0–1 day	>1 and <7 days	>7 days
GCS: 13–15	9–12	<9
Neuroimaging: normal	Normal or abnormal	Normal or abnormal

AOC = alteration of consciousness; GCS = Glasgow Coma Scale; LOC = loss of consciousness; PTA = post-traumatic amnesia; TBI = traumatic brain injury

Owing to the wide range of cognitive, motor, and neurobehavioral impairments that accompany brain injury, it can be difficult to establish and predict long-term outcomes and set goals for these patients, even for an experienced clinician. However, researchers have identified some factors that are useful in estimating future outcomes. Low initial scores on the GCS, particularly motor score and pupillary reactivity, have been identified by a number of studies as a predictor of poor recovery in patients with moderate to severe TBI.[79-83] Other factors associated with poor outcomes are age, race, and lower education level.[79,80,82,84] Petechial hemorrhages, subarachnoid bleed, obliteration of third ventricle or basal cisterns, midline shift, and subdural hematoma findings on initial CT scan are also predictive of poor outcomes.[79,82,83]

The *Medical Research Council* CRASH (corticosteroid randomization after significant head injury) study provides a Web-based calculator (www.crash2.lshtm.ac.uk/Risk%20calculator/index.html) that allows clinicians to enter demographic and prognostic information (i.e., country, age, GCS score, pupil reactivity to light, presence of major extra cranial injury, and CT findings if available); it calculates the 14-day mortality risk and unfavorable outcome at 6 months, along with the 95% confidence interval.[79] Unfavorable outcome is defined as dead, vegetative state, or severe disability as measured by the *Glasgow Outcome Scale* (GOS).

Duration of post-traumatic amnesia (PTA), the length of time between the injury and the time at which the patient is able to consistently remember ongoing events, is also an important factor in predicting recovery. Brown et al[85] found that duration of PTA as measured by the *Galveston Orientation and Amnesia Test* (GOAT), the revised GOAT, or the *Orientation Log* (O-Log) during inpatient rehabilitation can predict functional independence, employment, good overall recovery, and independent living 1 year after injury. Patients with PTA less than 48.5 days are likely to have higher *Functional Independence Measure* (FIM) scores at discharge from inpatient rehabilitation; patients with PTA less than 27 days are likely to be employed; patients with PTA less than 34 days are likely to have a good overall recovery (as measured by the GOS); and those with PTA less than 53 days are likely to be living without assistance.[85] Perrin and colleagues[86] found that PTA was a stronger predictor of discharge FIM scores than either GCS scores or time to follow commands.

CONTINUUM OF CARE AND INTERDISCIPLINARY TEAM

The rehabilitation of patients with TBI occurs across a continuum of care in a variety of settings (Fig. 19.2). Patients who are in a persistent vegetative state may receive ongoing therapy in a nursing home or other long-term

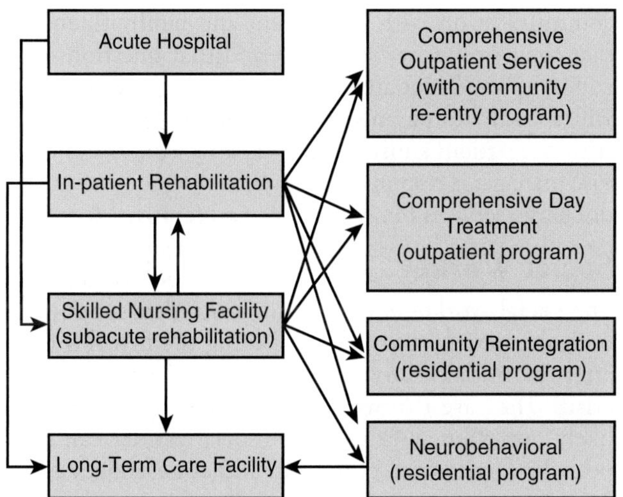

Figure 19.2 Rehabilitation settings for individuals with TBI across the continuum of care.

care facility once they are medically stable. Patients who are beginning to recover from coma with moderate to severe cognitive, behavioral, and physical impairments often continue rehabilitation in either an acute or subacute inpatient rehabilitation facility. As patients progress in recovery, they will be discharged to other community-based settings depending on the needs of the individual patient.

The foundation for successful rehabilitation following TBI is an *interdisciplinary team*. An interdisciplinary team approach is essential to providing the most comprehensive care that will lead to maximizing functional recovery. An interdisciplinary approach to rehabilitation for this population has been shown to be effective for improving activity levels and participation in society.[87-89]

Within the context of the team, individual members collaborate, contributing their expertise in a specific area, thereby enhancing the team's overall effectiveness. Communication and open-mindedness are key to any team. The different members must share their skills and findings with the whole team and be willing to learn from other team members to promote optimal recovery. The PT must be willing to share a unique knowledge of movement and motor control, but be open to learning from other team members. Each team member should develop an approach to treatment that considers information obtained from all other participating disciplines. This will lead to a consistent and comprehensive approach to care.

Some members may play more prominent roles depending on the setting and stage of recovery. For example, a recreational therapist will not likely be involved with a patient in the acute hospital but would play a vital role in a community-reentry setting. The following sections identify some of the team members involved in the care of individuals with brain injury and their roles in an acute rehabilitation hospital.

Patient and Family

The patient and his/her family are at the center of the team. The lives of both the patient and family members are likely to be dramatically changed as a result of the injury. Familial roles often change. The patient who previously took care of the children may now be on the receiving end of care. The team must garner information regarding the patient's work, school, financial status, and social history. Family members should be interviewed to obtain information about the patient's lifestyle (work/school/leisure), favorite social and recreational activities, and so forth. Information about the family dynamics should be ascertained. What is the patient's role in the family (e.g., head of the household, primary wage earner)? Is the patient responsible for taking care of children? Is the patient in school? What level? Is the patient working? All of these and many other similar questions should be answered to develop a comprehensive plan of care (POC).

Physician

In the acute rehabilitation hospital, the physician overseeing the care of the patient with a brain injury is usually a physiatrist or neurologist. The physiatrist has expertise and training in physical medicine and rehabilitation. A neurologist's skills lie in the realm of the brain and nervous system. A neurologist will have particular knowledge related to how the brain may recover and what impairments and activity limitations are likely to be seen given the location and the extent of the injury. Both a physiatrist and neurologist have vast knowledge in neuropharmacology, an extremely important part of management with this patient population. Certain medications may have harmful side effects that may not be readily apparent. For example, the physician may be able to prescribe a less-sedating drug than would normally be used to treat a certain clinical problem in other patient populations.

Speech-Language Pathologist

Owing to the nature of a brain injury, the speech-language pathologist (SLP) plays an important and diverse role in rehabilitation. The SLP examines, evaluates, and treats communication, swallowing, and cognitive impairments. As can be seen from the cognitive and communication impairments described above, this can be a challenging task. It is important for the PT to be in close communication with the SLP to provide consistency of care in relation to cognitive, swallowing, and communication impairments. With the guidance of the SLP, the team will be able to devise the most effective and consistent way to communicate with the patient. He or she will also be able to instruct the team in how the patient's cognitive impairments may impede new learning, which in turn will affect everyone's interactions with the patient and their approach to treatment.

Occupational Therapist

The occupational therapist (OT) examines, evaluates, and treats the patient's diminished ability to perform ADLs, visual/perceptual impairments, UE functional loss, and sensory integration problems, and will often work with the SLP in treating cognitive impairments. Basic ADL includes dressing, self-feeding, bathing, and grooming. Instrumental ADL includes home management, housekeeping, grocery shopping, driving, and telephone use. In the rehabilitation hospital, the occupational and physical therapists often work very closely together. A useful treatment approach is co-treatments with the OT. Having two trained professionals working at the same time with the patient can be very productive. This is especially true with patients who have severe motor control and cognitive deficits. One example would be a scavenger hunt in the community with a higher functioning patient. The patient is given a list of tasks to do or items to find in a community setting such as a grocery store. During the scavenger hunt, the PT might address specific mobility barriers or dual-task deficits in balance, whereas the OT might work toward improving problem-solving and social skills. The OT will also educate the nursing staff on the best ways to assist the patient with ADL.

Rehabilitation Nurse

In a rehabilitation hospital, the nurse is responsible for continually assessing the patient's medical status and the level of emotional and behavioral stability. Additional responsibilities include dispensing medications and closely monitoring their effects, initiating and managing programs for bowel and bladder retraining to assist the patient in learning to become continent again. Bowel and bladder control is extremely important for self-esteem and is related to discharge placement. The nurse performs daily monitoring of vital signs to make sure the patient remains medically stable. He or she will inspect the patient's skin daily to ensure there are no signs of skin breakdown. The nurse also has the difficult task of consistently following through with the team's treatment plan throughout the day. For example, each shift of nursing staff must follow splinting schedules established by the physical and occupational therapists. The nurse often has the most interaction on a regular basis with the patient and family.

Case Manager/Team Coordinator

The case manager acts as the coordinator for the team. The case manager is often a nurse, social worker, or other health professional. The case manager will direct team meetings, schedule family conferences, and act as a liaison with third-party payers. He or she must promote good communication among all team members to ensure that the rehabilitation care being provided is truly team oriented. The case manager will also be in constant communication with the patient and family to ensure that their needs are being met and that questions and concerns are adequately addressed. The case manager will coordinate payment and insurance benefit issues with the patient's insurance company. In addition, the case manager is responsible for scheduling follow-up and discharge services for the patient and family.

Social Worker

The social worker provides much needed support to both the patient and family. During the first few days after the initial injury, the family is often in a state of crisis. They are thrown into a world that they, most likely, never knew existed. The social worker can support the family with education and counseling. As the patient progresses with recovery, the social worker will also provide counseling for the patient. This is particularly important as the patient begins to develop greater awareness and insight into his or her deficits. If the patient has behavioral impairments, the social worker can provide counseling to both the patient and family and can help develop coping strategies for what may be a lifelong disability.

Neuropsychologist

The neuropsychologist plays an important role on the team. He or she will often perform neuropsychological testing when appropriate to determine the patient's baseline cognitive functioning. He or she will also assist the team in developing a cognitive and behavioral management program. When the patient with a brain injury has severe behavioral impairments, the neuropsychologist may assume the role of the team leader.

Other Team Members

Many patients with severe brain injury may require ventilatory support. The respiratory care practitioner is a vital participant in the evaluation and treatment of respiratory impairments. In the rehabilitation hospital, the respiratory therapist helps monitor the patient's pulmonary status and provides appropriate treatment.

A recreational therapist assists the patient's return to activities enjoyed before the accident, or helps identify new activities that the patient will find rewarding. Therapeutic recreation is an extremely important part of rehabilitation. Being able to participate in some type of leisure or recreational activities is a significant step in returning to a fulfilling lifestyle.

EARLY MEDICAL MANAGEMENT

Medical treatment following brain injury starts at the scene of the accident. Early resuscitation with the goal of stabilizing the cardiovascular and respiratory systems is important to maintain sufficient blood flow and oxygen to the brain.[90,91] Once the patient arrives at the medical center, the primary goals are to minimize secondary brain injury by optimizing cerebral blood flow and oxygenation, stabilize vital signs, perform a complete examination, identify and treat any non-neurological injuries, and continuously monitor the patient.[90-92] Systolic blood pressure should be kept above 90 mm Hg and oxygen saturation above 90%.[90] Patients with severe injury and some with moderate injury will need to be intubated. The patient's neck should be stabilized with a collar and the head elevated 30 degrees.[90] This is done to protect the spine in case of instability, as well as avoid an increase in ICP. The GCS is used to determine the severity of the brain injury. A complete neurological examination is also done. Additional information about the extent of the injury is obtained through x-ray films and neuroimaging studies such as CT and MRI. This is done to determine if neurosurgery is warranted. Intracranial hematomas or other mass lesions may need to be addressed surgically.

Cerebral perfusion pressure (CPP) and ICP is monitored.[93] For patients with a GCS of 8 or less, any acute abnormality on CT, a systolic pressure of less than 90 mm Hg, or age greater than 40 years, ICP monitoring is recommended.[90] However, some patients may not require continuous ICP monitoring.[94] External ventricular drains, a subdural bolt, and a fiber-optic catheter provide methods of monitoring ICP. Elevated ICP can be treated with the use of sedating medications, moderate head-up positioning (head elevated to 30°), osmotherapy, hypothermia, surgical decompression, and barbiturates.[90,91] Intracranial pressure should be less than 20 mm Hg and CPP greater than 60 mm Hg.[90] If ICP cannot be treated successfully, inducing a pharmacological coma or surgical decompression may be necessary.

The CNS neurotransmitter dopamine is thought to increase arousal and attention through the reticular activating system. Medications that act as dopamine and norepinephrine agonists may increase arousal in patients with disorders of consciousness.[95,96] Amantadine is used to increase levels of arousal and the rate of recovery.[97,98] Other medications that can be used to increase levels of arousal are methylphenidate and bromocriptine.[95] Methylphenidate has been shown to decrease ICU and hospital length of stay in patients with severe TBI.[99] Conversely, dopamine antagonists such as haloperidol should be avoided, as they may delay or slow recovery.[100,101] Transcranial magnetic stimulation and deep brain stimulation are other promising interventions that may help improve levels of arousal and outcomes in patients with disordered levels of consciousness; however, the efficacy of these treatments has not yet been demonstrated.[95]

The remainder of this chapter is divided into three main sections: (1) physical therapy management of patients with severe to moderate TBI during the early stages of recovery, (2) physical therapy management of patients with severe to moderate TBI during active rehabilitation, and (3) physical therapy management of patients with mild TBI. Patients in the early stage of recovery after severe to moderate TBI often demonstrate an altered level of consciousness (see above for detailed discussion). The primary goals of physical therapy in this early stage of recovery are early mobilization, preventing secondary complications due to the TBI and associated prolonged bedrest/immobilization, and initiating family education. The examination and intervention procedures described in the section on physical therapy management during active rehabilitation are likely to be used with patients early after injury and who have higher levels of consciousness.

Examination

The first step in beginning an examination at this early stage of recovery is to conduct a complete medical record review. Because the patient may not be medically stable and will likely have various contraindications, precautions, and complications that may impact physical therapy interventions, it is important to obtain all critical information from the medical record, nursing staff, and physician before actually seeing the patient. The patient may be on a ventilator with ongoing monitoring. He or she may have weight-bearing restrictions owing to musculoskeletal injuries or open wounds. A thorough medical record review provides a comprehensive perspective about the patient's condition, as well as a complete understanding of the precautions and contraindications that must be observed during the examination and subsequent treatment. Because the patient's medical status may be dynamic at these stages, it is important to check with the patient's primary nurse before beginning any session. Team members should always observe universal precautions and may need to wear gowns, gloves, and/or masks or other personal protective equipment when treating the patient.

It is vital to perform a comprehensive and standardized examination to determine level of consciousness (coma vs. vegetative state vs. minimally conscious state).[45,102] There are a variety of challenges associated with accurately determining the patient's level of consciousness. Limited motor function, communication impairments, sedating medications, impaired sensation, and impaired executive function can impact the patient's ability to respond to sensory stimuli and commands. The examination should be performed in a closed environment, in a structured manner at multiple times in order to capture the patient's response over a period of time as he or she may not be consistent. The entire team should do the exam with all members carefully documenting the patient's response. The Coma Recovery Scale–Revised (CRS-R, see below for details on this test) is strongly recommended for this purpose.[48,103] An appropriate determination of level of consciousness is critical, as patients with disordered levels of consciousness are easily misdiagnosed. A misdiagnosis at this early stage of recovery can lead to a lack of appropriate rehabilitation services and poorer outcomes.

In addition to examining arousal, attention, and cognition, other key areas to examine include the following:

- Integument integrity
- Sensory integrity
- Motor function
- Range of motion
- Reflex integrity
- Ventilation and respiration/gas exchange

Patients with severe TBI who are in a low arousal state may present with abnormal tone and posturing. Primitive postures may include those associated with decorticate or decerebrate rigidity. In decorticate rigidity, the upper extremities are in a flexed posture and the lower extremities are extended. With decerebrate rigidity, both the upper and lower extremities are positioned in extension. Abnormal tone may take the form of spastic hypertonia. This may range from spasticity that severely affects the entire body and greatly inhibits normal, functional movement, to lesser levels of tone that affect individual muscle groups.

If not medically contraindicated, the examination should include early mobilization such as assisted bed mobility and sitting, and if possible supported upright posture/standing. The therapist should monitor vital signs and observe for changes in arousal and motor function during assisted mobilization. A more upright posture may change the patient's level of arousal compared to when he/she is supine in bed. When appropriate, the patient should be transferred into a wheelchair. The patient may require the assistance of two to three people to transfer at this stage. In most cases, a reclining or tilt-in-space wheelchair is the best option for positioning, with a specialized pressure-reducing cushion. Often it may require several treatment sessions to complete the entire examination. Because early patient status is often dynamic, any signs of progress or regression should be carefully monitored and documented.

Outcome Measures

Arousal, Attention, and Cognition

The *Coma Recovery Scale–Revised* (CRS-R) is recommended to assess patients with disordered consciousness.[104] The CRS-R is a valid and reliable 23-item measure with six subscales: auditory, visual, motor, oromotor, communication, and arousal.[105] Scores range from 0 to 23. Data are useful in distinguishing between different states of consciousness (vegetative state, minimally conscious state, and emerging), determining the prognosis, and informing treatment planning.[105]

The *Disorders of Consciousness Scale* (DOCS) is a valid and reliable scale also designed to measure arousal and neurobehavioral recovery in patients with disorders of consciousness.[106,107] It consists of 23 items, which assess social knowledge, taste/swallowing, olfactory function, proprioception, tactile sensation, auditory function, and visual function. Scoring is based on patient response and includes no response, generalized response, or localized response. The DOCS can be used to differentiate states of consciousness (i.e., vegetative state and minimally conscious state) and assist in determining prognosis for recovery. A manual and video training are available for the DOCS at www.queri.research.va.gov/tools/docs_training/.

The *Rancho Los Amigos Levels of Cognitive Functioning* (LOCF) scale is a descriptive scale used to examine cognitive and behavioral recovery in individuals with TBI (Box 19.3) as they emerge from coma.[108] This scale does not address specific cognitive deficits but is useful for communicating general cognitive and/or behavioral status and for treatment planning. The eight categories describe typical cognitive and behavioral progress after a brain injury. Patients may plateau at any level. The LOCF has been shown to be a reliable and valid measure of cognitive and behavioral function for individuals with brain injury.[109]

Plan of Care

Outcomes/Goals

A list of general goals and outcomes anticipated for patients in Levels I, II, and III (LOCF) are presented in Box 19.4. These can be used to guide the development of specific anticipated goals and expected outcomes for an individual patient.

Interventions

Early Mobilization

There is a developing body of evidence that early, assisted mobilization is an important intervention for individuals with disorders of consciousness and that patients with disordered consciousness can benefit from early rehabilitation.[72,102,110,111] Studies of patients in the ICU have found that early, assisted mobilization is safe and results in shorter length of stays, greater likelihood of home discharge, lower incidence of secondary complications such as infections and pressure ulcers, and improved outcomes.[112-115] Contraindications to early mobilization include unstable spine and increased ICP. Precautions include weight-bearing restrictions, skin and joint integrity, autonomic instability, and cardiovascular status.

Early mobilization should be undertaken in a systematic manner. The physical therapist should closely monitor vital signs and observe for changes in level of arousal during the intervention session. A hard cervical collar may be useful to assist with head control. A tilt table, or specialized tilt table with a stepping system built in, can be used to safely assist the patient into a standing position and has been shown to improve level of consciousness.[116] A body weight support (BWS) system used either overground or over a treadmill can be used to safely assist the patient to a standing position and take assisted steps.[111] Other interventions that can promote early mobilization include passive seated bikes that use a powered system to pedal, functional electrical

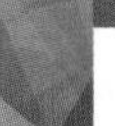

Box 19.3 Rancho Los Amigos Levels of Cognitive Functioning (LOCF)[a]

I. No Response

Patient appears to be in a deep sleep and is completely unresponsive to any stimuli.

II. Generalized Response

Patient reacts inconsistently and nonpurposefully to stimuli in a nonspecific manner. Responses are limited and often the same regardless of stimulus presented. Responses may be physiological changes, gross body movements, and/or vocalization.

III. Localized Response

Patient reacts specifically but inconsistently to stimuli. Responses are directly related to the type of stimulus presented. May follow simple commands such as closing eyes or squeezing hand in an inconsistent, delayed manner.

IV. Confused-Agitated

Patient is in a heightened state of activity. Behavior is bizarre and nonpurposeful relative to immediate environment. Does not discriminate among persons or objects; is unable to cooperate directly with treatment efforts. Verbalizations frequently are incoherent and/or inappropriate to the environment; confabulation may be present. Gross attention to environment is very brief; selective attention is often nonexistent. Patient lacks short- and long-term recall.

V. Confused-Inappropriate

Patient is able to respond to simple commands fairly consistently. However, with increased complexity of commands or lack of any external structure, responses are nonpurposeful, random, or fragmented. Demonstrates gross attention to the environment but is highly distractible and lacks ability to focus attention on a specific task. With structure, may be able to converse on a social automatic level for short periods of time. Verbalization is often inappropriate and confabulatory. Memory is severely impaired; often shows inappropriate use of objects; may perform previously learned tasks with structure but is unable to learn new information.

VI. Confused-Appropriate

Patient shows goal-directed behavior but is dependent on external input or direction. Follows simple directions consistently and shows carryover for relearned tasks such as self-care. Responses may be incorrect due to memory problems, but they are appropriate to the situation. Past memories show more depth and detail than recent memory.

VII. Automatic-Appropriate

Patient appears appropriate and oriented within the hospital and home settings; goes through daily routine automatically but frequently robot-like. Patient shows minimal to no confusion and has shallow recall of activities. Shows carryover for new learning but at a decreased rate. With structure is able to initiate social or recreational activities; judgment remains impaired.

VIII. Purposeful-Appropriate

Patient is able to recall and integrate past and recent events and is aware of and responsive to environment. Shows carryover for new learning and needs no supervision once activities are learned. May continue to show a decreased ability relative to premorbid abilities, abstract reasoning, tolerance for stress, and judgment in emergencies or unusual circumstances.

[a]Condensed form.

From Professional Staff Association, Ranchos Los Amigos Hospital, with permission.[108]

stimulation (FES) bikes, and assisted sitting. Importantly, physical therapists should not automatically assume that patients with low levels of arousal cannot be mobilized. Early mobilization may be an important active ingredient to promote beneficial neuroplastic changes to improve outcomes.

Preventing Secondary Impairments

Because of the patient's inability to move at these levels, he or she is susceptible to secondary impairments such as contractures, decubiti, pneumonia, and DVT.[64] If prevention is not addressed early, these impairments are likely to impede future progress and can be life-threatening. Proper positioning both in bed and in a wheelchair is essential. Appropriate positioning will assist in preventing skin breakdown and contractures, improve pulmonary hygiene and circulation, and may modify muscle tone. When the patient is in bed, the head should be kept in neutral. The hips and knees should be slightly flexed, but range of motion (ROM) should be monitored to ensure that contractures do not develop. Splints may be used to assist in positioning. Special boots can be used to position the foot to prevent foot drop and skin breakdown on the heel (Fig. 19.3). Turning will help prevent skin breakdown and pneumonia. Patients should be repositioned every 2 hours when in bed. Specialized air mattresses are

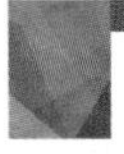

Box 19.4 General Goals and Outcomes Anticipated for Patients With Severe to Moderate Traumatic Brain Injury in the Acute Stage

- Impact of impairment is reduced
  - Risk of secondary impairments is reduced.
  - Motor function is improved.
  - Joint integrity and mobility are improved or remain functional.
  - Level of arousal and alertness is increased.
- Ability to improve physical actions, tasks, or activities is improved.
  - Tolerance of upright postures and activities is improved.
  - Functional mobility is improved.
  - Safety of patient, family, and caregivers is improved.
- Patient satisfaction is enhanced
  - Family and caregivers are educated on patient's diagnosis, physical therapy interventions, goals, and outcomes.
  - Care is coordinated among all team members.

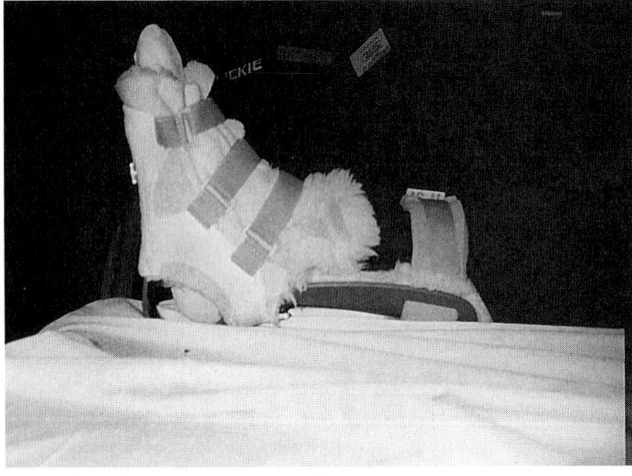

Figure 19.3 Multi-podus boot used for ankle and foot positioning and to prevent skin breakdown on the heel. This type of positioning device may not be beneficial for the patient with moderate to severe tone at the ankle; it is not strong enough to prevent the ankle from plantarflexing.

another effective way to assist with the prevention of pressure sores.

Serial casting may be used to maintain or improve ROM.[117-119] Serial casting is often used for plantarflexor or biceps contractures. With a plantarflexion contracture, the ankle is stretched into as much dorsiflexion as possible and then a short leg cast is applied (Fig. 19.4). In approximately 2 to 5 days, the cast is removed. The muscle is stretched again and another cast is applied. This procedure is repeated until satisfactory gains in ROM have been achieved or until no further progress is made. Because the individual with brain injury is likely to have impaired sensation and communication, as well as behavioral deficits, there is a risk of skin breakdown or the patient hurting himself or herself or others with the cast. The decision to use casts should be made carefully. The benefits and possible side effects should be thoroughly discussed with input from appropriate team members. It is also important to monitor the patient after the cast is applied. Hands-on experience under the supervision of a skilled clinician is recommended before attempting cast applications.

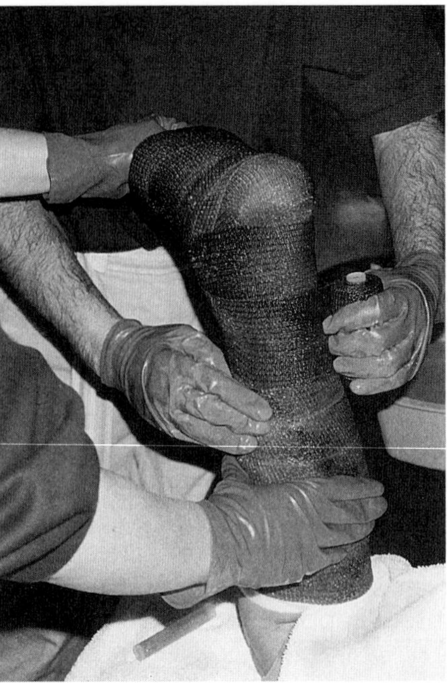

Figure 19.4 Serial casting: Fiberglass casting material is wrapped around the lower leg and foot. One clinician does the wrapping while another holds the leg and foot in the proper position.

Proper wheelchair positioning is important.[120] Because of reduced postural control at these levels, a reclining wheelchair or a tilt-in-space wheelchair is typically required. Proper pelvic positioning and head positioning are key elements in promoting good posture in a wheelchair. Refer to Chapter 32, Seating and Wheeled Mobility, for further discussion of this topic. Respiratory care practitioners, physical therapists, and nurses often use postural drainage, percussion, vibration, and positioning to prevent pulmonary complications and improve pulmonary function.[121]

Sensory Stimulation

Sensory stimulation is an intervention used to increase the level of arousal and elicit movement in individuals with low levels of arousal. The theory is that by providing stimulation in a controlled, multisensory manner, with a balance of stimulation and rest, the reticular activating system may be stimulated, causing a general increase in arousal.[122] In general, multisensory stimulation involves the presentation of sensory stimulation in a highly structured and consistent manner while the patient is closely monitored to determine his or her behavioral response to the sensory stimulation. The following sensory systems are systematically stimulated: auditory, olfactory, gustatory, visual, tactile, kinesthetic, and vestibular.

The value of sensory stimulation for patients who are slow to recover remains in debate. A systematic review published by the Cochrane Library suggests that there is no reliable evidence to support or rule out the effectiveness of sensory stimulation programs for this patient population.[123] A different result was found in a more recent systematic review that suggested strong evidence for multimodal stimulation to increase arousal and alertness of persons in coma and persistent vegetative state.[124] The different findings by these two systematic reviews may be due to when the reviews were conducted, the limited number of studies in both reviews, small sample sizes in most of the studies, difficulties with accuracy and consistency related to measuring level of consciousness, and limited number of studies with strong research designs.

Family Education

Family education at this early stage after injury is critical. It is important to provide a realistic and consistent message to family members regarding prognosis. Family members should be included in decision making when determining the plan of care and goals of physical therapy. Families should be educated on how patients with disorders of consciousness present and the differences between reflexive and purposeful movements. Since family members may be with the patient often, they can be taught how to perform ROM exercises and learn how to position the patient to help prevent secondary complications. Family members can also assist with early mobilization interventions described above. Because some patients with TBI may not achieve full independence, family members should also be instructed in how to provide assistance with basic ADLs. Although family members value physical therapy, they may also view it negatively if they perceive it causes the patient pain or distress, so it is important to promote open communication with them.

PHYSICAL THERAPY MANAGEMENT OF MODERATE TO SEVERE TRAUMATIC BRAIN INJURY DURING ACTIVE REHABILITATION

As patients with severe to moderate TBI recover, they require extensive and protracted rehabilitation across a variety of settings throughout the continuum of care. This may include acute and subacute inpatient rehabilitation, postacute rehabilitation, day treatment program, and outpatient or home care. The many cognitive, physical, and/or behavioral impairments that affect activity levels and social participation often necessitate multiple episodes of physical therapy care over the patient's lifetime. Goals and interventions should be focused on the patient's abilities and personal goals regardless of setting and episode of care.

Examination

Regardless of injury chronicity, some patients with TBI will have cognitive and behavioral impairments that pose barriers to the examination process. These barriers may include disorientation, confusion, physical aggression, memory deficits, and limited attention span. It may be difficult to gather data using standardized tests and measures, such as goniometry or manual muscle testing, because the patient may be unable to cooperate. In these cases, the therapist must utilize observational skills as the patient moves to gain insight to the extent of the body structure/function impairments and activity restrictions. The physical therapist should determine the patient's cognitive abilities, because these will affect the capacity to relearn motor skills, including orientation, attention span, memory, insight, safety awareness, and alertness. Key initial questions that warrant consideration include the following:

- Is the patient able to follow commands: one-step, two-step, or multistep commands?
- Is the patient oriented to person, place, and/or time?
- Does the patient recognize family members?
- Does the patient demonstrate any insight into what has happened?

It is beneficial to consult with other team members, especially the SLP and OT, to obtain additional information about the patient's cognitive status. As the patient's cognitive and behavioral impairments become less obtrusive to the process, the physical therapy examination should include the elements and outcome measures found in Box 19.5.

Depending on the status of the individual patient, some of these areas may be screened whereas others require more in-depth examination. Determination of the patient's functional abilities should be done in a variety of environments, because some patients may perform well in the closed environment of a private room, but performance may deteriorate in an open environment with multiple distractions. Section One of this book (Chapters 1 through 9 on clinical decision making and examination) provides a detailed description of procedures, tests and measures, and specific outcome measures for examining the above-mentioned areas. A brief description of some of the more clinically useful outcome measures for individuals with TBI follows.

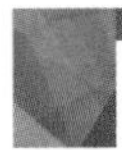

Box 19.5 Elements of the Examination and Outcome Measures

- Aerobic capacity/endurance
- Balance
  - *Berg Balance Scale, Community Balance and Mobility Scale, High-Level Mobility Assessment Tool*
- Behavioral status
  - *Supervision Rating Scale, Neurobehavioral Rating Scale–Revised, Agitated Behavior Scale*
- Community, Social, and Civic Life
  - *Mayo-Portland Adaptability Inventory, Community Integration Questionnaire, Quality of Life After Brain Injury*
- Cranial nerve integrity
- Gait
  - *Rancho Los Amigos (RLA) OGA System, 10-Meter Walk Test, 6-Minute Walk Test, Modified Walking and Remembering Test*
- Integumentary integrity
- Joint integrity and mobility
- Mental functions
  - *Coma Recovery Scale–Revised, Disorders of Consciousness Scale, Rancho Los Amigos Levels of Cognitive Functioning, Moss Attention Rating Scale, Test of Everyday Attention, Trail Making Test Part B, Galveston Orientation and Amnesia Test, Orientation Log*
- Mobility
  - *Functional Independence Measure, Functional Assessment Measure*
- Motor function
- Muscle performance, including strength, power, and endurance
- Neuromotor development and sensory processing
- Pain
- Posture
- Range of motion
- Reflex integrity
- Self-care and domestic life
  - *Functional Independence Measure, Functional Assessment Measure*
- Sensory integrity
- Ventilation and respiration
- Work life
  - *Mayo-Portland Adaptability Inventory, Community Integration Questionnaire, Quality of Life After Brain Injury*

Outcome Measures: Body Structure/Function

Balance

The Berg Balance Scale is a valid and clinically useful measure of balance in individuals with TBI.[125-127] The Berg Balance Scale, together with functional status measured using the FIM, may assist predicting inpatient rehabilitation length of stay, falls during rehabilitation stay, and functional gains during rehabilitation.[125,126] However, as patients improve the Berg Balance Scale may exhibit a ceiling effect.[128]

The *Community Balance and Mobility Scale* (CB&M) by Howe et al[129] is an instrument developed specifically for patients with persistent balance deficits following TBI. The CB&M is a reliable and valid tool that assesses higher-level balance abilities typically associated with community mobility. This tool shares similarities to the *High-Level Mobility Assessment Tool* (HiMAT) developed by Williams et al.[130,131] The HiMAT is a unidimensional measure of higher-level motor performance for individuals with TBI. The test items in both are more difficult than general measures of balance and functional mobility and are intended to quantify abilities required of physically demanding vocational and social roles, as well as sporting activities. A revised version of the HiMAT has a minimal detectable change score of 2 points.[132]

Attention and Cognition

The *Moss Attention Rating Scale* (MARS) is an observational rating scale that provides a reliable and valid measure of attention-related behavior after TBI. The scale allows the therapist to rate a patient's behavior on a 5-point scale across 22 items that capture the effects of impaired attention on cognitive and motor performance.[133] Other measures of attention most often employed by neuropsychologists include the *Test of Everyday Attention*[134] and the *Trail Making Test Part B.*[135] Though all three of these measures capture attentional deficits and may serve as useful global outcome measures, they will be less helpful in measuring changes in attention behavior attributable to physical therapy interventions.

The *Galveston Orientation and Amnesia Test* is a measure of PTA.[136] The GOAT is administered by asking a series of standardized questions related to orientation and the ability to recall events before and after the injury. Scores between 100 and 76 are considered normal and patients with scores below are considered to have PTA. The GOAT has high interrater reliability and is a valid measure of PTA.[136,137] The O-Log measures orientation to time, place, and circumstance.[138] It can be used for serial assessment of orientation to document improvements during rehabilitation.[139] It is reliable and valid, and can be used to predict outcome.[138,140] Measures of dual-task performance (see later discussion) are more specific to physical therapy practice.

Behavior and Safety

Rehabilitation teams often use an outcome measure that captures the impact of behavior and safety on overall independence. The *Agitated Behavior Scale* measures the type and degree of agitation after TBI.[141] The *Supervision Rating Scale*[142] provides a one-step method for rating a patient's current level of supervision, ranging from independent to full-time direct supervision. The *Neurobehavioral Rating Scale–Revised* is a 29-item multidimensional, clinician-based assessment instrument designed to measure neurobehavioral disturbances.[143] The items cover numerous cognitive and behavioral constructs such as memory, attention, communication, mood, and agitation.

Outcome Measures: Activity and Participation

Global Functioning

The FIM[144,145] is a commonly used measure of functional mobility, ADL function, cognition, and communication. It was designed to measure level of disability and burden of care in individuals undergoing inpatient rehabilitation and is useful for monitoring patient progress and evaluating outcomes. The *Functional Assessment Measure* (FAM)[146,147] was developed as an adjunct to the FIM. It includes functional areas not addressed in the FIM that are important for individuals with TBI and stroke. The other items include community access, reading, writing, safety, employability, and adjustment to limitations. The FIM, in combination with the FAM, is a valid and reliable measure of disability after TBI.[148] In addition to measuring the amount of physical assistance required to perform a functional task, the therapist should also analyze how the patient performs the task. A thorough movement analysis[149] of how functional tasks (sit to/from stand, rolling, etc.) are performed will aid the therapist in identifying the motor function and other impairments that underlie specific activity limitations.

Community Reintegration and Quality of Life

Rehabilitation teams commonly employ the use of a participation-level measure that quantifies the extent of reintegrate into social, familial, and vocational roles. One such measure is the *Mayo-Portland Adaptability Inventory,*[150,151] which is frequently used in postacute TBI rehabilitation. Another, similar measure is the *Community Integration Questionnaire* (CIQ).[152] The CIQ consists of 15 items relevant to home integration, social integration, and productive activities. Whiteneck and colleagues[153] developed the *Participation Assessment With Recombined Tools-Objective* (PART-O), which combines aspects of other participation level measures. The PART-O is a 24-item participation measure that is currently being used by the Traumatic Brain Injury Model System for use in clinical trials and outcome measure validation studies.[154] Another useful measure is the *Quality of Life After Brain Injury* tool.[155,156] This is a health-related quality-of-life measure with 37 items and 8 subscales addressing issues of thinking, feelings and emotion, autonomy in daily life, negative feelings and perceived restrictions. Given that subjective reports of dizziness are common following head trauma, the *Dizziness Handicap Inventory* may be helpful.[157] This 25-item inventory is designed to evaluate the patient's perception of the effects of dizziness on their daily functioning as measured across functional, emotional, and physical domains. The measure specifically addresses the perceived impact of dizziness on daily life in the home and community, making it most appropriate for use in later stages of recovery (e.g., outpatient setting).

Locomotion

Gait deficits are common following TBI.[69] Classification systems of gait disorders can assist in clinical decision making, selecting interventions, and determining a prognosis. Williams and colleagues[40] developed a gait classification system for people with TBI that includes six categories: spastic hemiparesis, nonspastic hemiparesis, ataxia/dyspraxia unilateral, spastic bilateral paresis, nonspastic bilateral paresis, and ataxia/dyspraxia bilateral. These descriptors provide a common, clinically useful method when describing gait limitations and communicating findings.

Physical therapists use *observational gait analysis* (OGA) as a preferred method in the clinic to evaluate gait.[158] One instrument used clinically is the *Rancho Los Amigos (RLA) OGA System.* Refer to Chapter 7, Examination of Gait, for further discussion of this instrument. The RLA OGA instrument gathers data on the cyclical movements of walking that occur from one stride cycle to the next. The gait cycle is divided into stance and swing phases. The PT visually analyzes a patient's walking pattern, looking for asymmetries and deviations from normal. Based on these observations, the PT gains insight into which impairments may be causing the deviations. Specific interventions are then designed to address the possible causes of the gait deviations. However, caution should be used when interpreting OGA findings. Some gait abnormalities identified by quantitative gait analysis may not be detected by OGA.[69] Chapter 7 also reviews instrumented walkways and other methods of more precisely and accurately measuring specific kinematics and kinetics associated with gait.

Gait speed is also an important measure of walking ability. The *10-Meter Walk Test* (10MWT) is a reliable measure of both fast-paced and self-paced gait speed in patients with TBI.[159-161] Caution should be used when interpreting gait speed measured with the 10MWT, because there is evidence suggesting that the 10MWT may not fully reflect the many different demands of walking in the community (e.g., crossing a busy street, walking in a crowded mall, walking on uneven surfaces, etc.).[161]

Fatigue and deconditioning are common following TBI.[162,163] As such, measuring walking endurance is clinically useful. The *6-Minute Walk Test* (6MWT) is a common, reliable, and valid way to measure this aspect of walking ability.[164,165] Normative values from healthy adults are available for this test.[166] Other methods of assessing cardiorespiratory fitness have also been validated for patients with TBI, including the *graded exercise test*[167] and a *modified shuttle test.*[168]

Several tests of dynamic balance (see above) and walking ability are appropriate for this population; however, they do not offer insight into how walking and balance are affected by the addition of a cognitive load. Measures of *dual-task performance* allow the therapist to examine the extent to which deficits in attention and memory affect gait speed and safety. These two cognitive abilities (attention and memory) are strongly associated with dual-task performance and also commonly impaired in persons with TBI.[169,170] There are a variety of clinical tests of dual-task performance that can be used for clients with acquired brain injury. A review of several dual-task performance measures is available.[171] One such measure is the *Modified Walking and Remembering Test* (WART) developed by McCulloch et al.[169] The WART involves a single-task condition (simple walking task) and a dual-task condition (walking task and cognitive task).

Further information on these and other outcome measures specifically used in TBI rehabilitation can be found at the *Center for Outcome Measurement in Brain Injury* website (www.tbims.org/combi/index.html), at the Shirley Ryan AbilityLab Rehabilitation Measures Database (www.sralab.org/rehabilitation-measures), and at the Academy of Neurologic Physical Therapy Outcome Measures Recommendations webpage (www.neuropt.org/professional-resources/neurology-section-outcome-measures-recommendations/traumatic-brain-injury). Table 19.2 contains more detail on selected, highly recommended tests.

Plan of Care

Goals/Outcomes

People with moderate to severe TBI present with a wide variety of physical, cognitive, and behavioral impairments that may greatly impact the patient's ability to fully participate in his/her desired social roles. As the

Table 19.2 Outcome Measures

OUTCOME MEASURE and ICF Category	DESCRIPTION	SCORING	MDC and MCID
6-Minute Walk Test ICF = 2	Performance-based test: assesses functional walking endurance.	Distance walked in 6 minutes when walking as fast as possible.	MDC = 61 meters, (estimated data based on data from Mossberg[164]) MCID: NA
10-Meter Walk Test ICF = 2	Performance-based test: assesses walking capacity.	Time to walk 10 m, usually performed with a 2-meter acceleration and deceleration phase.	MDC: 0.10 m/s (estimated based on data from Van Loo et al[159]) MCID: NA
Berg Balance Scale ICF = 2	Performance-based test: assess balance during 14 functional tasks.	14 items scored on a 5-point ordinal scale of 0 to 4, where 0 is unable to perform/needs assistance and 4 is able to perform safely and independently.	MDC = 4 (estimated based on data from Newstead et al[127]) MCID: NA
Community Balance and Mobility Scale ICF = 1, 2	Performance-based test: assess balance and mobility in ambulatory patients with TBI who have balance impairments that impact their ability to fully participate in normal social activities. Less of a ceiling effect than the Berg Balance Scale.	13 items scored on a 6-point ordinal scale of 0 to 5, where 0 is unable to perform or requires assistance and 5 is completes task independently, safely, in a coordinated manner and in allotted time frame.	MDC: 8-10 points (Howe et al[129]) MCID: NA
Functional Assessment Measure ICF = 1, 2, 3	Performance-based test with 12 items that are added to the Functional Independence Measure (FIM) that address functional areas that are not addressed in the FIM, such as community functioning and behavior.	12 items added to 18 items of the FIM for a total of 30 items scored on a 7-point ordinal scale 1 to 7, where 1 is complete dependence and 7 is independent without assistive device.	MDC: NA MCID: NA

Table 19.2 Outcome Measures—cont'd

OUTCOME MEASURE and ICF Category	DESCRIPTION	SCORING	MDC and MCID
Quality of Life After Brain Injury ICF = 3	Self-report measure that assesses health-related quality of life. Contains 6 subscales: cognition, self, daily life and autonomy, social relationships, emotions, and physical problems.	Items scored on a 5-point ordinal scale, 1 to 5. Scale means are converted to a 0–100 scale, with a lowest possible value of 0 (worst possible quality of life) and a maximum value of 100 (best possible quality of life).	MDC: NA MCID: NA
Coma Recovery Scale Revised ICF = 1	Observational measure used to assist with differential diagnosis, prognostic assessment, and treatment planning in patients with disorders of consciousness. It has 6 subscales: auditory, visual, motor, oromotor, communication, and arousal functions.	Scores are based on the presence or absence of operationally defined behavioral responses to specific sensory stimuli.	MDC: NA MCID: NA
Agitated Behavior Scale ICF = 1, 2	Observation-based test: measures behavioral aspects of agitation during the early stages of recovery. In addition to total score, subscores for disinhibition, aggression, and lability can be calculated.	14 items, each item scored on an ordinal scale of 1 to 4, where 1 is behavior not present and 4 is behavior is present to an extreme degree.	MDC: NA MCID: NA

ICF CATEGORY: 1 = Body Structure/Function, 2 = Activity, 3 = Participation; MCID = minimal clinically important difference; MDC = minimal detectable change; NA = not available

patient progresses, goals and outcomes will move from basic mobility and self-care toward skills that facilitate community inclusion and social participation. Examples include the following:

- Impact of impairment is reduced.
  - Risk of secondary impairments is reduced.
  - Joint integrity and mobility are improved.
  - Motor function is improved.
  - Muscle performance is improved.
  - Cognition is improved.
  - Postural control is improved.
- Ability to improve physical actions, tasks, or activities is improved.
  - Walking ability is improved.
  - Independence in ADLs is increased.
  - Tolerance of upright postures and activities is increased.
  - Safety of patient, family, and caregivers is improved.
- Ability to participate in social roles is enhanced.
  - Ability to assume/resume home management is improved.
  - Ability to assume/resume work, community, and leisure roles is improved.
  - Awareness and use of community resources are improved.

These can be used to guide the development of specific anticipated goals and expected outcomes tailored to each individual patient.

Interventions

Motor (Re)Learning Strategies

Treatment sessions should be thoughtfully planned to maximize the patient's motor learning capabilities. Practice should be *distributed,* with frequent rest periods. Owing to cognitive impairments, patients may experience mental as well as physical fatigue during treatment sessions. Signs of mental fatigue may include increased irritability, decreased attention and concentration, deterioration in performance of physical skills, and delayed initiation. Treatment sessions should include sufficient rest periods to minimize both physical and mental fatigue and maximize motor relearning.

The impact of manipulating motor learning variables on motor skill acquisition and generalizability has not been thoroughly studied in patients with TBI. Refer to Chapter 10 , Strategies to Improve Motor Function, for an in-depth discussion of motor learning principles. There are a few studies with a limited number of subjects, however, that suggest the use of *video self-modeling*[172] and the *concept of self-generation*[173] may be beneficial to the relearning of functional tasks. With video self-modeling, the patient watches himself or herself engaging in skillful behavior on edited videotapes. The self-generation concept is a phenomenon whereby items that are self-generated are better learned and remembered compared to information that is provided. As the cognitive and behavioral barriers to treatment become less intrusive, sessions can be progressively more challenging both mentally and physically. A *random practice schedule* may be more beneficial to learning,[174] although this schedule can be employed only after the patient has demonstrated some initial learning of the task's dynamics.[175] Feedback is also very important. Owing to cognitive, sensory, and perceptual impairments, *explicit or augmented feedback* may be more beneficial in the early stages of motor learning as opposed to intrinsic feedback. However, care should be taken not to overwhelm the patient with feedback.

Restorative Versus Compensatory-Based Interventions

As discussed earlier, an early, interdisciplinary approach to rehabilitation after TBI has been shown to be beneficial. There are many intervention approaches available to the PT that can promote functional recovery following brain injury. Two basic treatment strategies are a *compensatory* and a *restorative* (recovery) approach. The compensatory approach seeks to improve functional skills by compensating for the lost ability. A simple example of this would be teaching one-handed dressing techniques to a patient with UE hemiparesis resulting from a TBI. A restorative approach seeks to restore the "normal" use of the affected UE. Both approaches seek to reinstitute functional independence.

Compensation is commonly defined as the resumption of the ability to complete a task using alternative motor patterns and strategies. The definition of recovery varies. Some feel that it refers to the resumption of the ability to complete a task using the same motor patterns and strategies as before. Another, more liberal, definition is completing a task using similar strategies despite inferior efficiency, speed, and/or accuracy. Levin et al[176] addressed this topic and proposed explicit definitions for recovery and compensation. The authors argue that the definitions of recovery and compensation will change based on whether performance or function is measured. To make this point clearer, the authors used the framework of the *World Health Organization's ICF Model.* Refer to Table 19.3 for more details.

In most cases involving moderate to severe TBI, clinical management will likely require a balance between both restorative and compensatory approaches. As an example, a therapist may determine that a restorative approach to gait training is indicated but may also choose to ensure that the client and caregiver have adequate training in the use of an assistive device for safety during the earlier stages of recovery should it be needed. Current literature offers little guidance for the practitioner attempting to choose between approaches. Table 19.4 offers questions that can guide this aspect of clinical

Table 19.3 Motor Recovery and Compensation Across Three Levels of the ICF

Level	Recovery	Compensation
ICF: Health Condition (neuronal)	*Restoring function in neural tissue that was initially lost after injury.* May be seen as reactivation in brain areas previously inactivated by the circulatory event. Although this is not expected to occur in the area of the primary brain lesion, it may occur in areas surrounding the lesion (penumbra) and in the diaschisis.	*Neural tissue acquires a function that it did not have prior to injury.* May be seen as activation in alternative brain areas not normally observed in nondisabled individuals.
ICF: Body Functions/ Structure (performance)	*Restoring the ability to perform a movement in the same manner as it was performed before injury.* This may occur through the reappearance of premorbid movement patterns during task accomplishment (voluntary joint range of motion, temporal and spatial interjoint coordination, etc.).	*Performing an old movement in a new manner.* May be seen as the appearance of alternative movement patterns (i.e., recruitment of additional or different degrees of freedom, changes in muscle-activation patterns such as increased agonist/antagonist coactivation, delays in timing between movements of adjacent joints, etc.) during the accomplishment of a task.
ICF: Activity (functional)	*Successful task accomplishment using limbs or end effectors typically used by nondisabled individuals.*[a]	*Successful task accomplishment using alternate limbs or end effectors.* For example, opening a package of chips using one hand and the mouth instead of two hands.

ICF = World Health Organization International Classification of Functioning.
[a]Note that task performance may be successful using compensatory motor strategies and movement patterns.
Levin, MF, Kleim, JA, and Wolf, SL: What do motor "recovery" and "compensation" mean in patients following stroke? Neurorehabilitation and Neural Repair 23(4):313–319, 2009.[176] Reprinted by permission of SAGE Publications.

Table 19.4 Compensation Versus Restoration: Guiding Questions to Consider

Injury Severity	• Are sensorimotor deficits so severe that restorative approaches are not possible or appropriate? • Do secondary complications or comorbidities exist that pose barriers to recovery (e.g., contractures, fractures)? • Is an appropriate motor recovery program (specificity, intensity, frequency, duration, difficulty) feasible? • How chronic is the injury?
Motor Learning	• What strengths and weaknesses does the patient have relative to his or her ability to learn motor tasks? • Are there significant cognitive, behavioral, or medical barriers? • Does the patient have any financial or support barriers?
Resources	• Will funding lapse before functional recovery occurs? • Do financial resources suggest that a more rapid approach be used? • What impact will discharge destination have on the prescribed treatment approach?

decision making. After a thorough examination and consideration of the patient's unique personal and environment barriers and facilitators, these questions can help lead the clinician and patient to a shared agreement about which approach will be used.

The last decade of translational and applied research in the areas of neural plasticity, motor learning, and neurological rehabilitation has heightened awareness that relearning is directly related to the rehabilitative experiences patients are exposed to. Using the example above, interventions that seek compensation will result in learning how to use the less-affected UE as well as learning not to use the more affected UE. Alternatively, a restorative rehabilitative experience that allows the patient to practice using the affected arm for everyday tasks will result in greater functional independence and affected UE use. This knowledge is useful in clinical decision making when developing the POC.

Restorative Interventions and Neural Plasticity

No studies to date have identified what types of restorative interventions are the most beneficial for persons with TBI. Current research has demonstrated that task-specific interventions with large amounts of practice can induce beneficial neuroplastic changes in the CNS and restore function.[177-179] Studies involving monkey and rat models of brain injury have demonstrated the importance of intensive, task-oriented training on neuroplastic changes in the motor cortex and functional recovery.[180,181] This line of research was extended to include human models with neurological deficits and later the sum of these findings was translated into tangible principles of experience-dependent neural plasticity.[177,182] Table 19.5 provides examples of several of these principles. Current evidence suggests that treatment interventions that are most beneficial will be specific to the function/task being retrained, meaningful to the client, and challenging to the cortical systems involved in the activity.

Table 19.5 Principles of Experience-Dependent Neuroplasticity

Principle	Description
Use It or Lose It	Failure to drive specific brain functions can lead to functional degradation.
Use It and Improve It	Training that drives a specific brain function can lead to an enhancement of that function.
Specificity	The nature of the training experience dictates the nature of the plasticity.
Repetition Matters	Induction of plasticity requires sufficient repetition.
Intensity Matters	Induction of plasticity requires sufficient training intensity.
Time Matters	Different forms of plasticity occur at different times during training.
Salience Matters	The training experience must be sufficiently salient to induce plasticity.
Age Matters	Training-induced plasticity occurs more readily in younger brains.
Transference	Plasticity in response to one training experience can enhance the acquisition of similar behaviors.
Interference	Plasticity in response to one experience can interfere with the acquisition of other behaviors.

From Kleim, JA, and Jones, TA: Principles of experience-dependent neural plasticity: Implications for rehabilitation after brain damage. J Speech Lang Hear Res 51(1):S225–239, 2008, with permission.[182]

Task-Oriented Approach

Also in line with these principles, current theories of motor control and motor learning advocate for a task-oriented approach to interventions for individuals with neurological deficits.[175] The majority of research on the principles that underpin effective, task-oriented interventions for clients with neurological disorders has been done with persons with stroke. Despite this, these same principles will serve the PT well in selecting and applying appropriate interventions for persons with TBI.[183] Locomotor training, utilizing BWS with and without a treadmill,[184-186] and constraint-induced movement therapy (CIMT) for improving UE function[187,188] are two interventions that have shown potential. See additional discussion in Chapters 15, Stroke, and 20, Traumatic Spinal Cord Injury.

Another task-oriented approach for improving mobility skills such as walking and running was developed by Williams and Schache.[262] They used a conceptual framework based on the hierarchical ordering of high-level mobility tasks based on the HiMAT (see above) and biomechanical parameters associated with normal walking and running as the basis for the specific interventions. Easier items on the HiMAT are set as goals and mastered before moving on to more difficult tasks. For example, once a patient can walk backward, the next, more difficult tasks—walking on toes and walking over obstacles—are set as goals. Important biomechanical aspects of walking and running, such as the generation of ankle and hip flexion power at push-off and initial swing, are targeted through the specific interventions.

Similarly, Peters and colleagues[189] utilized an intensive, task-oriented, mobility training intervention to improve walking ability. Participants received BWS gait training on a treadmill, overground gait training, sit to/from stand transfer training, standing balance activities, resistance training, coordination training, and ROM exercises for a total of 150 minutes per session for 20 sessions.

An important consideration for these and other task-oriented strategies is treatment dosing. Dosage entails more than just the number of PT sessions/week and length of the individual session. When critically examining the treatment dosage, the following factors should be considered: sessions/week (or day), amount of practice time per task within a session, number of repetitions of the task performed within a session, and the intensity at which the task is being performed. Although not well researched for persons with TBI, literature on UE rehabilitation and locomotor training after stroke suggest that these interventions are commonly underdosed[190,191] and that there is a dose–response relationship.[192]

Locomotor Training With Body Weight Support

Locomotor training with BWS and a treadmill involves suspending the client in a parachute-like overhead harness that allows for a percentage of body weight to be relieved. Therapists assist the patient by providing trunk/pelvic stabilization, assistance with weight shifting, and advancing the LEs. Locomotor training with BWS is commonly combined with treadmill ambulation (Fig. 19.5) but can be done overground as well. Locomotor training with BWS and a treadmill allows for repetitive training throughout a complete gait cycle. Progressively decreasing the amount of BWS and increasing the treadmill speed allows the physical therapist to gradually increase the difficulty of the task as walking ability improves. Locomotor training with BWS and a treadmill has a solid theoretical basis. However, it is not clear what the optimal parameters for treatment should be for patients with TBI, and it has not been demonstrated that it is more effective than conventional gait training (see Chapter 20, Traumatic Spinal Cord Injury).

Constraint-Induced Therapy

Constraint-induced movement therapy involves promoting the use of the more affected UE for up to 90% of waking hours and reducing the use of the least affected UE. Intensive, task-oriented training is provided for the affected UE for up to 6 hours per day over a 2- to 3-week period.[193] Most of the research published on CIMT has been done in people with stroke. However, this same intervention may also be useful for people with TBI.[187,188] Given the frequency of behavioral and cognitive impairments after TBI, patients undergoing CIMT may require greater structure and caregiver support outside of therapy to maximize their adherence to the protocol.

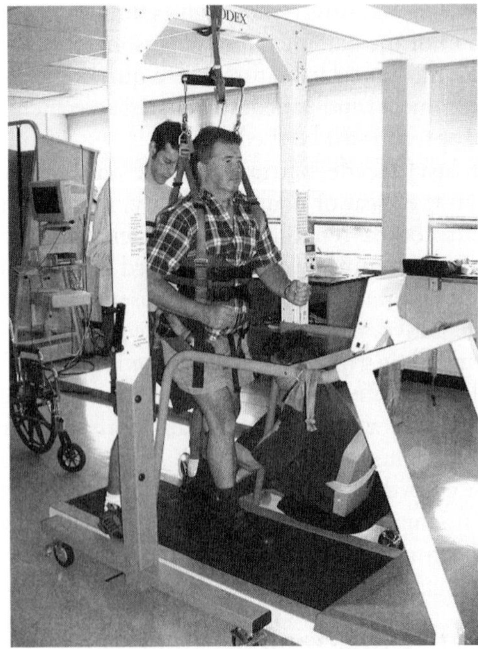

Figure 19.5 Locomotor training utilizing a body weight support system and treadmill. One trainer is assisting with the trunk and pelvic stability and weight shifting, while another trainer is facilitating stepping at the left LE.

Aerobic and Endurance Conditioning

Fatigue and cardiopulmonary pathology are common after TBI.[162] The severity of deconditioning found in persons with TBI is significantly greater than that found in sedentary persons without disabilities.[163] Aerobic training is effective for persons with TBI.[183,194] Appropriately dosed aerobic exercise has the potential to reduce long-term cardiovascular risks, improve sleep hygiene, and reduce both depression and reports of fatigue.[194]

There are many options when developing an endurance-training program. The mode of training can vary, from traditional exercises (e.g., walking, jogging, treadmill, elliptical machines, and ergometers) to circuit training.[195] Intensity should be at 60% to 90% of age predicted maximal heart rate, for 20 to 40 minutes per session, three to four times a week.[194] Hassett et al[196] studied a program that combined both aerobic and strengthening exercises for 62 participants with severe TBI. They found that the program, whether performed in a fitness center or at home, had a positive impact on cardiorespiratory fitness. The PT will need to carefully consider both cognitive and physical abilities when developing an aerobic conditioning program for an individual patient.

There is a growing line of research investigating the relationship between aerobic exercise and improved cognitive performance. The majority of this research to date has involved persons with stroke[197] but recently has been investigated in a small sample of persons with TBI. In a small group of persons with TBI, Chin and colleagues[198,199] found that an aerobic exercise program led to improvements in cognitive function in addition to aerobic function and fatigue.

Resistance Training

Interventions aimed at improving force-production capacity may be beneficial supplements to the physical therapist's POC.[200,201] There is currently a dearth of literature investigating the role of strength training in TBI rehabilitation. There is, however, evidence of a positive effect in other progressive and nonprogressive neurological disorders. A review by Pak and Patten[202] suggest that for persons with stroke, resistance training is associated with improved force production, functional abilities, and quality of life. Similar findings have been demonstrated for persons with Parkinson's disease,[203] and it is plausible that patients with TBI might also achieve similar benefits. Strength training should be done 2 to 3 days a week at an intensity of 3 sets of 8 to 12 repetitions at 10 repetition max.[204] Postural and balance impairments may require modification of positions used.

Electrical Stimulation

Functional electrical stimulation (FES) is a useful tool to combine with other motor rehabilitation interventions. Several manufacturers have developed various types of FES foot-drop stimulators. All rely on peroneal nerve stimulation to increase active dorsiflexion during the swing phase of gait. The devices range from traditional electrical stimulation with manual stimulation triggers to cuff-type units that employ inclinometers or pressure sensors. Similar units can be used to augment active wrist extension during UE reaching tasks. Little research exists on use of this modality with patients with TBI,[205] and there is limited evidence as to their long-term efficacy in other populations.[206] These devices, however, can be used to increase both the quality and number of repetitions of a desired task (e.g., steps or reaching) and can be an effective addition to early, task-oriented training sessions.

Dual-Task Performance

As mentioned above, many patients make significant improvements in physical function at this stage of rehabilitation. Many will demonstrate independence with basic ambulation as measured by gait speed and dynamic balance tests. Most will also have persisting cognitive deficits. Beyond basic locomotor recovery, another important consideration is how these ongoing cognitive deficits affect mobility and community reentry. As discussed in the examination section, a dual-task paradigm can give valuable insight into how safely and efficiently patients will ambulate when also performing secondary, cognitive tasks. Research suggests that dual-task decrements, such as reduced walking speed and postural stability, are common after brain injury.[171]

Like many other interventions, improvements in dual-task performance are training specific. This should be taken into consideration when designing and progressing a dual-task training regimen. The tasks and environments used in training should match those that the patient is anticipated to return to. Progressing this type of training can involve manipulation of the training environment, motor task (type and difficulty), and the cognitive demands of the secondary task. A training program to improve dual-task performance can coincide with the achievement of independence in walking across different terrains. For example, once independent with walking down a corridor, progressively more challenging cognitive tasks such as serial subtraction or visual scanning tasks can be added. Furthering this example, the client might be asked to ambulate in a parking lot and scan for vehicles with certain characters in their license plate or walk the aisle of a busy grocery store and find specific items. Training speed can also be varied to add challenge. Walking on a treadmill while reading is one example of a dual-task intervention.

Patient/Family/Caregiver Education

Patient/family/caregiver education and training are important goals across each level of rehabilitation. The goals of this education and training will vary based on the cognitive and behavioral abilities of the patient.

Clients in the early phase of recovery may go through a period where they are significantly confused and agitated. It is difficult to provide education for the patient at this level; the patient has very little, if any, ability for new learning. However, it is extremely important to provide education for the patient's family. Above all, the family should understand that the patient does not have control of his or her behavior. The patient is not striking out or cursing because of intent to hurt others, but because of agitation and confusion. Many times families do not understand why a patient is acting a certain way. They should be educated that these behaviors are a symptom of the brain injury, just as the patient's inability to walk or eat is. It is important to educate the family that these behaviors are actually a good sign because it indicates the patient is moving toward the next level of recovery. Aggressive behaviors are usually short-lived, typically lasting only a few weeks at most. Family members should also be taught to use specific behavioral strategies (see below) when interacting with their loved one. Consistency is important for everyone. If a behavioral plan is being implemented, the family should be part of devising it and carrying it out.

It is important to emphasize safety awareness education with the patient and caregivers. The individual is beginning to exhibit improved mobility skills at these levels but may lack the insight to recognize that he or she may not yet be safe to ambulate or transfer alone. Family members and caregivers should learn how to safely assist the patient with functional mobility. This typically includes training in bed mobility, transfers, ambulation, and wheelchair mobility skills. They should be instructed in proper body mechanics when assisting with functional mobility, so as to avoid risking injury to the patient or themselves. Family members/caregivers should be educated about how to assist the patient with strengthening exercises, passive ROM, and other elements of the exercise program. They should also be made aware of methods to enhance the patient's decision making skills and safety awareness. Family members typically become the primary caregiver for the patient upon discharge to home.

Behavioral Factors

Therapists may encounter a variety of behavioral barriers to examining and treating patients with moderate to severe TBI. As the patient begins to emerge from coma, he or she often experiences a period of acute post-traumatic agitation.[42,207,208] The confusion, amnesia, and disorientation during this phase of recovery often result in agitation, aggression, noncompliance, and combative behavior.[42,208] The therapist should incorporate creativity and flexibility when designing and providing interventions. This is particularly true with individuals who are in the confused and agitated stage of recovery. At this stage, the therapist should work near the patient's physical level of function using familiar activities, rather than progress to more challenging skills that require new learning, because the patient does not have the capacity for new learning at this stage. Interventions should be done in a closed environment so as not to overstimulate or distract the patient.

The neuropsychologist can assist the team by providing insight into different ways to manage the patient's agitated behavior and may set up a behavioral modification program. Behavioral modification techniques such as positive reinforcement using a point or reward system, redirection, and compliance training are useful in managing these inappropriate behaviors and improving participation in therapy.[207] Different medications may be effective in helping the patient manage behavior as well.[208] These include propranolol, trazadone, SSRIs, Tegretol, and Seroquel. Ativan should only be used with severe agitation. Table 19.6 summarizes special considerations for managing patients who display significant cognitive and/or neurobehavioral impairments.

Professionals who frequently encounter aggressive and disruptive behaviors from patients with TBI may benefit from further training in managing these events. *Nonviolent Crisis Intervention Training* and *Brain Injury Specialist Training* through the Brain Injury Association of America are two such training programs.

Community Reentry

Many clients will make significant progress in the early phase of rehabilitation. Before discharge from physical therapy, it is crucial to begin weaning the patient from the external structure provided by the hospital setting that was so important in the early and middle stages of recovery. As the patient becomes better able to control himself or herself, external control provided by the environment should be lessened. Doing so will prepare the patient for the challenges of the next level of rehabilitation—postacute community-reentry programming.

This level of therapy is often delivered in a comprehensive day treatment setting, with an interdisciplinary emphasis on community reentry, return to work or school, and cognitive, behavioral, and psychosocial issues.[209,210] In this setting, the patient goes to therapy throughout the day for 4 to 5 days a week and returns home in the late afternoon. Individuals with more severe physical impairments may continue their rehabilitation in a residential-based community reentry program, whereas those with continued, severe behavioral issues may require a residential neurobehavioral program.

The major goal of treatment at this level is to assist the patient in integrating the cognitive, physical, and emotional skills necessary to function in the community. Skills in judgment, problem-solving, planning, self-awareness, health and wellness, and social interaction are emphasized. For the demands of treatment to approximate the demands of the real world, treatment focuses on advanced activities such as community skills, social skills, and daily living skills. Examples of these skills are presented in Table 19.7. The interdisciplinary

Table 19.6 Special Considerations for Confused and Agitated Patients

Strategy	Rationale and Clinical Application
Consistency	• Consistency is important. All team members, including family members, should interact and address inappropriate behaviors in a consistent manner. • Remember that the patient is confused. To help decrease confusion, the patient should be seen by the same person at the same time and in the same location every day. • Establishing a daily routine is very important. It is calming and reassuring to have a sense of familiarity. Additionally, orientation (i.e., person, place, and time) should be provided frequently and in a nonthreatening manner. At this level, it is often better to provide orientation information than to challenge the patient to provide it, particularly if the patient is not expected to succeed.
Expect No Carryover	• Teaching new skills at this level is unrealistic. The patient may begin to perform a functional task, such as brushing teeth or ambulating. However, this does not indicate a general learning ability, because brushing one's teeth and especially walking are automatic skills with an ingrained neural network. • The use of charts or graphs may be useful to help the patient progress each day. Without the use of such aids, the patient is likely to have no recall of the previous day's performance.
Model Calm Behavior	• The patient is likely to perceive, and may reflect, the demeanor of the caregiver. Therefore, it is important for the therapist to assume a calm and focused affect. • The patient may not be able to control his or her behavior and may not feel safe. To help the patient feel safe, it is important for the therapist to be perceived as in control of his or her emotions and behavior.
Expect Egocentricity	• At this level of recovery, the patient cannot be expected to see another's point of view. He or she will tend to think only of himself or herself, and at this point, it is unwise to stress the patient with attempts to do otherwise.
Flexibility/Options	• The patient will have a limited attention span and may not be able to concentrate on any given activity for a very long time. It is important to be prepared with numerous activities. If the patient cannot be redirected to the selected task, it is appropriate to attempt to engage him or her in another. For example, it may be difficult for a client to tolerate a full constraint-induced therapy protocol. You might, however, be able to engage the client in a variety of UE reaching tasks in various environments, allowing the patient's level of attention and tolerance to dictate the duration of each. • Treat the patient at an appropriate age level. • Give control to the patient when it is safe and appropriate. Control can be given while maintaining focus on therapeutic goals by phrasing questions as, "Would you rather play ball or go for a walk?" This prevents situations where the patient chooses an undesirable or unrealistic activity if asked, "What would you like to do?" or the case where the patient simply answers "No" when asked, "Would you like to . . . ?" • Provide safe choices for the patient. This allows the patient to feel that he or she has some control over the situation. This is important, because the patient typically feels considerable loss of control during prolonged hospitalization.
Safety	• Owing to the patient's often unpredictable and inappropriate behaviors, it is important to keep the patient and those interacting with him or her safe. • In addition to utilizing some of the previously mentioned behavioral strategies, patients in this level of recovery may be kept on a locked unit of the hospital. Patients may require one-to-one staff supervision and assistance throughout the day.
Environment	• Initially interventions should be performed in a closed environment with limited distractions. Open environments such as a busy rehab gym will likely have too many distractions and can lead to increased agitation and limited ability to participate in the intervention. • Progress to more open environment to challenge the patient as he/she improves.

Table 19.7 Components of Community Skills, Social Skills, and Daily Living Skills Programs

Daily Living	Social Skills	Community Skills
Food preparation	Introductions	Shopping
Housekeeping	Nonverbal communication	Public transport
Money management	Assertiveness	Map reading
Meal planning	Listening skills	Leisure planning
Telephone use	Giving/receiving feedback	Community resources
Time management		

team emphasizes patient assumption of self-responsibility. Because the patient now has some insight into his or her own strengths and weaknesses, it is important to involve the individual in decision making.

Independent and cooperative work with others is encouraged. Group treatment sessions are often the basis of interventions. Honest feedback from the therapist and support group is crucial for the patient to learn how to function in society with his or her present abilities and limitations. Trial periods of independent living and supported work are important. The success and failures of these trials should be communicated to the interdisciplinary team so that clinical decisions regarding intervention modification or progression can be made. Adaptations are often required by the family, work, and school to accommodate the needs of the individual.

Living with a TBI is a lifelong proposition, and, like neurologically healthy individuals, persons with TBI benefit from lifelong exercise. The physical therapist should prescribe exercises that form the basis of a well-rounded health and wellness program to positively impact general health and mobility. There is a high prevalence of fatigue and cardiovascular deconditioning found in the TBI population. This, combined with the possibility that cardiovascular training may have positive cognitive benefits and be neuroprotective against chronic neurodegenerative changes, emphasizes the need for patients to engage in regular bouts of cardiovascular training.[197] The program should also include general strengthening and flexibility exercises that may sustain the levels of balance and mobility attained during the course of physical therapy.

■ MILD TRAUMATIC BRAIN INJURY

The military conflicts in the Middle East and increased media attention to sports-related concussion have highlighted the impact of mild TBI (mTBI) or post-concussion injury and the need for appropriate assessment and management. Between 1.6 and 3.8 million sports-related mTBIs occur annually in the United States,[3] and approximately 12% of military personnel report symptoms consistent with blast-related mTBI.[211] A mTBI is a type of TBI induced by biomechanical forces that disrupt physiological brain function.[212] It results from forces transmitted to the brain as a result of a direct blow to the head, neck, or elsewhere on the body. Mild TBI is primarily a functional injury of the CNS, which is thought to be due to metabolic dysfunction, neurotransmitter disturbances, and microstructural changes.[213,214] The impact of an mTBI is typically short. Most individuals with mTBI fully recover in approximately 7 to 10 days.[212] However, up to 10% to 20% of people with mTBI experience *post-concussion syndrome* and have deficits months to years after the initial injury.[215-217]

The GCS defines mTBI as a score between 13 and 15. Generally speaking, mTBI is characterized by varying degrees of loss of consciousness (0 to 30 minutes; it is important to recognize that no loss of consciousness may occur) and PTA and altered mental state for up to 24 hours. Individuals with mTBI often experience a combination of neurocognitive deficits and postural control and balance impairments, and they self-report symptoms such as blurred vision, nausea, light sensitivity, sleep disturbance, and ringing in the ears. It is also important to keep in mind that the appearance of symptoms may be delayed several hours.

A clinical diagnosis of mTBI is made by assessing the mechanism of injury and symptoms. These can include cognitive impairments (i.e., disturbances in memory, attention; intellectual dullness; mental rigidity), personality changes, rapid mood swings, postural control and balance impairments, visual disturbances, behavioral impairment, and possible sleep disturbance.[212,218] If any of these elements are present, an mTBI should be suspected. Commonly reported symptoms of an mTBI are listed in Box 19.6. Because an mTBI results in functional changes, neuroimaging is usually not indicated.[212] Recent research suggests that certain biomarkers (e.g. S-100) may be useful to assist with the diagnosis, but there is insufficient evidence at this time for their use.[212,219,220]

Physical Therapy Management

The Proponency Office for Rehabilitation and Reintegration, Office of the Surgeon General, and the United States Army developed physical therapy guidelines for assessment and intervention of working service members with mTBI.[221] The main areas recommended to assess and provide intervention for are patient education, activity intolerance, vestibular dysfunction, high-level balance dysfunction, post-traumatic headache, temporomandibular disorder, attention and dual-task performance, and participation in exercise (Box 19.7). The 2016 full mTBI

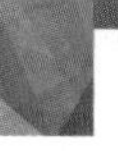

Box 19.6 Commonly Reported Symptoms in Patients With Mild Traumatic Brain Injury

- Headache
- Nausea
- Dizziness
- Poor balance
- Fatigue
- Difficulty sleeping
- Eyestrain
- Visual difficulties
- Feeling confused or foggy
- Frustration
- Light sensitivity
- Noise sensitivity
- Difficulty hearing
- Irritable
- More emotional
- Difficult concentrating and remembering

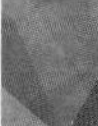

Box 19.7 Areas for Physical Therapist to Examine and Intervene in Patients With Mild Traumatic Brain Injury

- Patient education
- Activity intolerance
- Vestibular dysfunction
- High-level balance dysfunction
- Post-traumatic headache
- Temporomandibular disorder
- Cervical dysfunction
- Attention and dual-task performance
- Participation in exercise

guidelines developed by the Department of Defense and Veterans Affairs is available online at www.healthquality.va.gov/guidelines/Rehab/mtbi/mTBICPGFullCPG50821816.pdf.

Collins and colleagues[218] describe six clinical trajectories of mTBI that may emerge in people with persistent (>7 days post-injury) sports-related post-mTBI symptoms: cognitive/fatigue, vestibular, ocular motor, post-traumatic migraine, affective, and cervical. They argue that sports-related mTBI are heterogeneous and as such require interventions that are individualized for the patient depending on their presentation. Although physical therapists may play a role in the treatment of patients across all of these clinical trajectories, the physical therapist is most likely to play a prominent role in patients with vestibular (vestibular/balance rehabilitation), oculomotor (gaze stabilization exercises), and cervical trajectories (musculoskeletal interventions).

Return to Play/Activity

Return to play or activity after an mTBI should follow a graduated, stepwise progression of increasing activity levels with an initial 24-hour rest period (Table 19.8).[212,222] It is important to recognize that in addition to physical activity, activities that require attention and concentration (e.g., school work, playing video games) may exacerbate symptoms and prolong recovery. Each step should take 24 hours, so that it will take approximately 1 week to return to full activities or full-contact sports. If any symptoms return during the progressive increase in activity, the patient should step back to the previous stage and attempt to progress again after a 24-hour period of rest.

Although rest is commonly prescribed after mTBI, too much rest may actually be detrimental to recovery.[223,224] However, the duration and type of rest is not well defined. Recent guidelines and research suggest that graded exercise and return to activity at levels that do not exacerbate mTBI symptoms may be beneficial for patients with persistent symptoms.[224-228] The Progressive Return to Activity Following Mild TBI Working Group (PAWG) developed return-to-activity clinical recommendations for service members with mild post-mTBI symptoms that persist longer than 24 hours or preinjury symptoms.[224] The PAWG recommendations utilize symptom severity as measured by the Neurobehavioral Symptom Inventory (NSI)[229] to guide progression of activity through six stages—rest, light routine activity, light occupational activity, moderate activity, intense activity, and unrestricted activity. After an initial 24-hour rest period, individuals can progress to the next activity level as long as symptom severity on the NSI does not exceed mild and there are no symptoms such as altered consciousness, pupillary asymmetry, vomiting, diplopia, and confusion that may indicate an acute neurological event. For each activity stage, there are specific cardiovascular responses to exercise/activity guidelines and restrictions. For example, video games and driving are restricted in stages 1 through 3. These guidelines also provide more specific guidance related to amount and type of physical and cognitive rest/activity.

A similar individualized, balanced approach between rest and cognitive activity and graded increase in cognitive activity should be taken when students with concussion return to the classroom (Return to Learn).[230,231] If the student's ability to concentrate or tolerate stimulation is less than 30 minutes, then he or she should likely stay at home. Light neurocognitive tasks such as light reading or interaction may be done. Computer, video games, and texting should be avoided. Once the student is able to tolerate 30 to 45 minutes of neurocognitive activity without provoking symptoms, a return to school should be considered. Adjustments in the school such as taking frequent breaks, resting in a quiet area, reducing brightness levels on computer screens, wearing sunglasses, eating lunch in a quiet area, being dismissed

Table 19.8 Graduated Return-to-Play Protocol

Rehabilitation Stage	Functional Exercise at Each Stage of Rehabilitation	Objective of Each Stage
1. No activity	Complete physical and cognitive rest.	Recovery.
2. Light aerobic exercise	Walking, swimming, or stationary cycling, keeping intensity at 70% of maximum predicted heart rate. No resistance training.	Increase heart rate.
3. Sport-specific exercise	Skating drills in ice hockey, running drills in soccer. No head-impact activities.	Add movement.
4. Noncontact training drills	Progression to more complex training drills (e.g., passing drills in football and ice hockey). May start progressive resistance.	Exercise, coordination, and cognitive load.
5. Full-contact practice	Following medical clearance, participate in normal training activities.	Restore confidence and assess functional skills by coaching staff.
6. Return to play	Normal game play.	

From McCrory, P, et al: Consensus Statement on Concussion in Sport: The 3rd International Conference on Concussion in Sport held in Zurich, November 2008. British Journal of Sports Medicine 43(Suppl 1):i76–90, 2009, with permission.[222]

early from class to avoid noisy hallways during transitions, and requesting extra time on tests may be helpful during the initial period of return to school/learning.

Physical Therapy Examination

The PT examination should be conducted in a closed, quiet environment (quiet, dimly lit area, without distractions such as a television) that is not likely to exacerbate symptoms and thus confound the test results. This allows for better isolation of symptom causation. The physical exam should begin with the tests least likely to provoke symptoms and progress to tests that are more likely to provoke symptoms. Because the exam is likely to provoke symptoms, it may not be possible to perform all the desired tests during one session. Further testing is likely to be necessary to fully understand the patient's presentation.

Symptoms

There are many self-report symptom scales.[232] These scales ask patients to rate the severity of postconcussion symptoms such as headache, dizziness, vision difficulties, difficulty concentrating, fatigue, depression, sleep disturbance, and sensitivity to light and noise. The NSI asks the patient to rate 22 symptoms using a 5-point Likert scale (ranging from none to very severe). The NSI appears to measure four different factors: somatosensory, affective, cognitive, and vestibular.[229] The Post-Concussion Scale (revised)[233,234] is a 22-item symptom list that the patient uses to rate the severity of symptoms using a 7-point Likert scale (ranging from no symptoms to severe). Self-report measures specific to the impact of dizziness and impaired balance include the Dizziness Handicap Inventory and the Activities-Specific Balance Confidence scale.[235]

Cognition

Computerized tests have been developed to assess cognition after mTBI. One such test is the Immediate Post-Concussion Assessment and Cognitive Testing (ImPACT). The ImPACT assesses attention span, working memory, sustained and selective attention time, response variability, nonverbal problem-solving, and reaction time. The ImPACT can be used to track recovery and assist in the return-to-play decision after mTBI.[236-238]

Vestibular and Balance

The incidence of vestibular-related symptoms (e.g., dizziness, vertigo, imbalance) after blast mTBI ranges from 24% to 83% and is seen in the acute (1 to 3 days), subacute (3 to 30 days), and chronic (30 to 360 days) stage.[239] Vestibular and postural control deficits are also seen in sports-related mTBI.[240,241] Vestibular dysfunction after blast-related mTBI includes benign paroxysmal positional vertigo of the posterior or lateral canals and unilateral vestibular hypofunction of central origin.[242] Positional tests, such as the Dix-Hallpike test and supine roll test, and dynamic visual acuity testing should be performed.[221] Chapter 21, Vestibular Disorders, provides detailed information on these and other tests of vestibular function.

The NeuroCom Sensory Organization Test (SOT) is a computerized, force plate–based, dynamic posturography test that assesses the ability to use and integrate sensory information from the visual, somatosensory, and vestibular systems to maintain balance.[240] The Balance Error Scoring System (BESS) is a clinical analog to the SOT. Both of these measures (SOT and BESS) have been used to demonstrate impaired postural control in people with sports-related mTBI.[241,243]

Other measures of high-level balance activity such as the HiMAT,[130,131] Dynamic Gait Index,[244,245] Functional Gait Assessment,[246] and Balance Evaluation Systems Test[247]can also be used to assess balance. However, they may not be appropriate in the early stages of recovery. Sensor-based systems that utilize accelerometers and magnetometers to measure balance/postural control may be more sensitive than clinical measures but less expensive and more portable than force-plate measures.[248-250]

Oculomotor

Oculomotor dysfunction is present in approximately 65% of patients with mTBI as a result of blast injury,[251] which may result in impairments in vergence, accommodation, version, and alignment and cause headaches, blurred vision, and difficulty reading. Mucha and colleagues[252] developed the Vestibular/Ocular Motor Screening (VOMS) tool, which examines five aspects of vestibular oculomotor function: smooth pursuit, horizontal and vertical saccades, near point convergence distance, horizontal vestibular ocular reflex, and visual motion sensitivity. Patients rate symptom provocation and severity while they undergo the vestibular/oculomotor tests. The VOMS was able to accurately distinguish between subjects who had a concussion and healthy controls.[252]

Other

The Sport Concussion Assessment Tool 3 (SCAT3) is a short test that can be completed on the sideline of a sports event within minutes of injury to assess mental status, symptom severity, balance, coordination, and cervical involvement.[212] The SCAT3 incorporates the Standardized Assessment of Concussion and the Maddocks questions and is designed for on the field/sideline assessment of acute concussion and should not replace more a comprehensive evaluation.

The Buffalo Concussion Treadmill Test (BCTT) is a standardized, progressive exercise test that can diagnose physiological dysfunction after concussion and differentiate between factors other than exercise tolerance that may be impacting post-concussion symptoms.[227,228]

Post-traumatic headache, temporomandibular disorder, and cervical dysfunction can be assessed using a standard musculoskeletal examination of the neck, shoulders, and jaw along with standardized pain questionnaires. Dual-task performance should be assessed as described above. Box 19.8 lists some of the more commonly used outcome measures and tests and measures.

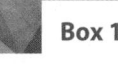

Box 19.8 Tests and Measures/Outcome Measures Commonly Used in Patients With Mild Traumatic Brain Injury

- Sport Concussion Assessment Tool 3
- Vestibular positional tests
- Vestibular Ocular Motor Screening
- Sensory Organization Test
- Balance Error Scoring System
- Dynamic Gait Index
- Functional Gait Assessment
- Buffalo Concussion Treadmill Test
- Post-Concussion Scale–Revised
- Neurobehavioral Symptom Inventory
- Dizziness Handicap Inventory
- Activities-Specific Balance Confidence Scale

Interventions

As described above, recovery from mTBI should include a graded progression of increasing physical activity/exercise that does not exacerbate symptoms and balances rest. However, that does not mean that patients should avoid all activity. Limiting all activities can prolong the course of recovery. A graded approach to increasing exercise and other activities along with properly managing sleep is appropriate. Patients should be carefully monitored during treatment sessions to determine if the intervention exacerbates any symptoms. If so, the intensity, duration, and frequency should be reduced. Systematic reviews[253-255] suggest that exercise and vestibular rehabilitation are beneficial. Interventions should be targeted to the findings of the examination and patient's presentation.[218]

Vestibular, Balance, and Dual Task

Although the overall level of evidence is relatively low, a recent systematic review by Murray and colleagues[253] concluded that vestibular therapy and balance interventions are indicated for patients with mTBI who present with persistent vestibular/balance impairment. Repositioning techniques (canalith repositioning maneuvers), habituation exercise, gaze stability exercises (e.g. VORx1), substitution exercises, and balance exercises can be prescribed to improve dizziness and vertigo, visual impairment, balance, and gait. Schneider and colleagues[256] found that a combination of vestibular rehabilitation and physical therapy directed at the cervical spine decreased the time for return to play. See Chapter 21, Vestibular Disorders, for specifics on these interventions.

High-level, task-oriented balance and gait training as described above in the section on interventions for persons with moderate to severe TBI can be performed. Activities that are challenging to the vestibular system such as walking with head turns and on uneven, varied surfaces are recommended, as well as sport-specific skill training.[221] Balance training that incorporates the use of different sensory modalities such as standing on dense foam with eyes open and eyes closed can be performed. Balance training using computerized dynamic posturography can also be done. Dual-task training as described above is another important intervention. See additional discussion in Chapter 10, Strategies to Improve Motor Function. Table 19.9 contains more detail and specific findings on selected studies that incorporated vestibular therapy interventions with patients with mTBI.[235,256-258]

Exercise

Aerobic exercise has wide-ranging beneficial effects, including improving neuronal function.[259] While deconditioning with prolonged rest that may occur follow mTBI may have detrimental effects, progressive aerobic exercise on a treadmill at levels that do not provoke symptoms in athletes with persistent post-concussion symptoms has been shown to be safe and results in a decrease in symptoms.[227] Leddy and colleagues[227,228] recommend 20 minutes of aerobic training on the treadmill at 80% of heart rate threshold (established by the BCTT, level of exercise at which symptoms are exacerbated) five times a week and progressively increasing the intensity by 5 to 10 beats per minute every 2 weeks as long as symptoms are not exaggerated.

Other

Musculoskeletal-based interventions such as stretching, strengthening, and manual therapy and modalities can be used when appropriate for patients with cervical involvement, post-traumatic headache, or temporomandibular disorder.[218,221]

Patient Education

Patients should be provided with educational material about the symptoms of mTBI and told that in most cases symptoms will resolve in days to a few months. They should also be informed about the dangers of *second impact syndrome*. This is rare but can occur if the

Table 19.9 Evidence Summary Selected Studies Examining the Effectiveness of Vestibular Therapy for Patients With Mild Traumatic Brain Injury

	Schneider et al, 2014[256]
Design	Randomized controlled trial
Level of Evidence	Level II
Subjects	31 patients with sports-related concussion with persistent symptoms (>10 days). Mixed adults and children, 12–30 years old, median age of 15.
Intervention	x1/week (or until medically cleared to participate in sport) Control group: Non-provocative ROM, stretching, and postural reeducation as indicated. Rest until symptom-free, followed by graded exercise/exertion. Intervention group: Cervical spine physical therapy: joint mobilization, therapeutic exercise, and sensorimotor retraining exercises. Vestibular therapy: habituation, gaze stabilization, adaptation exercises, balance exercises, and canalith repositioning. Graded exercise/exertion.
Results	Odds ratio of 10.27 (p<0.001) for return to sport in 8 weeks for the intervention group compared to control group.
Comments	Low risk of bias
	Alsalaheen et al, 2010[235]
Design	Retrospective chart review
Level of Evidence	Level III
Subjects	114 patients with concussion, both adults (aged 19–73) and children (aged 8–18)
Intervention	1–13 sessions of vestibular rehabilitation consisting of gaze-stabilization exercises (VOR × 1 in sitting and standing), standing balance on foam surface with EO and EC, walking with balance challenges, and canalith repositioning maneuvers when indicated.
Results	Significant improvement in all self-report measures and performance measures: ABC, DHI, DGI, FGA, gait speed, TUG, FTST, and SOT.
Comments	Retrospective review.

Table 19.9 Evidence Summary Selected Studies Examining the Effectiveness of Vestibular Therapy for Patients With Mild Traumatic Brain Injury—cont'd

	Hoffer et al, 2004[257]
Design	Prospective cohort
Level of Evidence	Level III
Subjects	58 active duty or retired military personnel within 1–3 days post-mTBI; subjects subdivided into three groups: post-traumatic positional vertigo, PTMAD, and post-traumatic spatial disorientation
Intervention	6–8 weeks of vestibular rehabilitation for the PTMAD and post-traumatic spatial disorientation groups consisting of VOR exercises, COR exercises, somatosensory exercises, and aerobic activity.
Results	84% of PTMAD group and 27% of post-traumatic spatial disorientation group demonstrated improvement in VOR tests. Significantly shorter time to return to work and resolution of symptoms in the PTMAD group compared to post-traumatic spatial disorientation group.
Comments	Low-quality study.
	Gottshall and Hoffer, 2010[258]
Design	Prospective cohort
Level of Evidence	Level III
Subjects	82 soldiers with mild traumatic brain injury due to blast injury (aged 19–34)
Intervention	Vestibular therapy x2/week with home exercise program over 8–12 weeks. Vestibular therapy targeted VOR, COR, depth perception, somatosensory training, dynamic gait, and aerobic exercise.
Results	Improvement in perception time, target acquisition, target following, dynamic visual acuity, gaze stabilization tests, SOT, and DGI.
Comments	Low level of evidence

ABC = Activities-Specific Balance Confidence scale; COR = cervico-ocular reflex; DGI = Dynamic Gait Index; DHI = Dizziness Handicap Inventory; EC = eyes closed; EO = eyes open; FGA = Functional Gait Assessment; FTST = Five Time Sit to Stand; PTMAD = post-traumatic migraine-associated dizziness; SOT = Sensory Organization Test; TUG = Timed Up and Go; VOR = vestibular-ocular reflex

patient experiences a second mTBI after an initial mTBI. The brain swells rapidly and can result in death. If appropriate, depending on the patient's symptoms and status, patients can be taught how to perform neck ROM and isometric strengthening exercises, appropriate sleep posture, vestibular positional techniques, gaze stabilization exercises, and balance exercises. Patients can also be instructed to begin an aerobic and strengthening exercise program.

Mild TBI Summary

Mild TBI is an area of rapid research, and clinical guidelines are evolving quickly. For example, in an update to clinical practice guidelines (CPGs), Marshall and colleagues[260] found ten different CPGs published between 2008 and 2012. Most of the recommendations of these different CPGs are based on lower levels of evidence and expert, consensus opinion. Because of the rapidly evolving evidence related to the assessment and treatment of mTBI, it is important for the reader to employ evidence-based practice skills to remain up to date.

Although the term *mild* is used, an mTBI can lead to debilitating impairments, limitations, and restrictions. In most cases the symptoms subside relatively quickly and patients are able to return to prior level of activity. However, with some patients symptoms can persist for long periods of time post-injury.[261] Patients with mTBI can be challenging to work with because it can be difficult to develop a targeted plan of care with the appropriate balance of rest and activity. Just as with patients with severe to moderate TBI, because of the wide spectrum of signs and symptoms it is important to consult and work with other health care professionals to support the patient with mTBI to maximize their recovery.

SUMMARY

A TBI is a devastating and life-changing event for the individual and his or her family. The resulting complexity of impairments, activity limitations, and participation restrictions make working with the patient with brain injury extremely rewarding and challenging. There are a multitude of issues to consider. The physical therapist must adapt traditional PT examination procedures and interventions to the unique motor function, cognitive, and behavioral challenges presented. The interdisciplinary team offers a unique opportunity for the physical therapist to learn and collaborate with experienced professionals. By working together with a team, the physical therapist is able to provide appropriate care that will help the individual with a TBI to maximize performance of activities and enhance social participation.

Questions for Review

1. List primary and secondary mechanisms of TBI.
2. Identify common neuromuscular, cognitive, and neurobehavioral impairments that result from TBI.
3. Contrast persistent vegetative state and minimally conscious state.
4. Identify key prognostic factors for individuals with TBI.
5. Identify and describe the roles of the interdisciplinary team members working with a patient with TBI.
6. Discuss the primary goals of physical therapy during the early stage of recovery in patients with severe to moderate TBI.
7. Select key outcome measures to use during the active rehabilitation stage in patients with severe to moderate TBI.
8. Describe strategies that should be taken into account when designing a plan of care for a patient with a severe to moderate TBI with cognitive and neurobehavioral deficits.
9. Contrast restorative-versus compensation-based interventions. Give an example of each.
10. Develop a physical therapy plan of care for a patient with a severe to moderate TBI, which incorporates principles of experience-dependent neuroplasticity.
11. Outline a graduated return to play for a patient who has experienced a mild TBI.
12. Develop a physical therapy plan of care for a patient with a mild TBI.

CASE STUDY

The patient is a 22-year-old male who was involved in a motor vehicle accident. He was struck by another car as he exited his car. The patient suffered a severe closed brain injury, GCS score of 7 at the emergency department, and both pupils were reactive to light. He was taken to a local hospital. CT scan revealed a left parietal subarachnoid hemorrhage. He also experienced a fracture of his right scapula. Two weeks after his injury, the patient is now transferred to an acute rehabilitation hospital.

MEDICATIONS

Ritalin, Tegretol, Zanaflex, and Ativan prn.

SOCIAL HISTORY

Patient is a graduate student in a computer science program at a local college. His parents live approximately 2 hours away. They are very supportive, and his mother has taken a leave of absence from her job in order to be with him and assist in his rehabilitation. He has private insurance through his parents, which covers inpatient and outpatient rehabilitation.

PHYSICAL THERAPY EXAMINATION

I. Screening: cardiopulmonary: HR 78, BP 110/76; integumentary: intact; musculoskeletal: see below; neuromuscular: see below.

II. Arousal, attention, and cognition: Rancho Los Amigos Levels of Cognitive Functioning: Level V. Easily distracted.

  A. Agitated behavior scale: 26/56

  B. Galveston Orientation and Amnesia Test: 66

  C. Moss Attention Rating Scale:

    1. Total Raw Score: 84

    2. Average MARS Item Score: 3.82

    3. Factor 1 (Restlessness/Distractibility) Score: 4.60

    4. Factor 2 (Initiation) Score: 4.00

    5. Factor 3 (Consistent/Sustained Attention) Score: 3.67

III. Assistive and adaptive devices: currently uses a standard wheelchair in the hospital environment with gel cushion and solid back.

IV. Balance

  A. Sitting balance: able to sit on edge of bed or mat with supervision

  B. Standing balance: able to stand with close supervision × 30 seconds, decreased WB on right LE, Berg Balance Scale score: 36/56

V. Locomotion

  A. Able to ambulate with small-based quad cane with minimal assistance for 150 feet using 3-point step to/through pattern

  B. Gait speed: 0.44 m/s

  C. Observational gait assessment: difficulty clearing right foot in swing, right knee in extension throughout swing phase, circumducts and hip hikes right hip to clear foot, initial contact with mid foot on right

VI. Joint mobility: decreased posterior and inferior glide R glenohumeral joint

VII. Motor function: tone: increased extensor tone in right hip and knee and ankle, 2 on Modified Ashworth Scale (MAS), increased flexor tone in right UE, 2 on MAS. Able to fractionate movement in left UE and LE, not able to fractionate movement in right UE or LE. However, he does exhibit active right dorsiflexion, wrist, and finger extension.

VIII. Orthotic, protective, and supportive devices:

  A. Has a bivalve cast at ankle and elbow from the acute care hospital for positioning ankle into dorsiflexion and elbow into extension.

IX. Range of motion: passive WNL except:

  A. Right LE

    1. Dorsiflexion: has 5-degree plantar flexion contracture

    2. Knee extension: has 5-degree flexion contracture

  B. Right UE

    1. Shoulder flexion: 95; abduction: 90; external rotation: 65; internal rotation: 80; extension: 45

    2. Elbow extension: has a 10-degree flexion contracture

    3. Wrist extension: 0 degrees

X. Self-care and home management:

A. FIM score:

Self-Care	Score	Self-Care	Score	Self-Care	Score
Eating	4	Bowel	4	Cognition	4
Grooming	4	Transfers	4	Comprehension	4
Bathing	3	Toilet	3	Expression	4
Dressing UE	3	Tub/shower	3	Problem-solving	3
Dressing LE	2	Bed/wheelchair	4	Memory	2
Toileting	3	Locomotion	4	Social interaction	3
Sphincter control	4	Walk/wheelchair	4	Total	75
Bladder	4	Stairs	2		

XI. Sensory integrity:

A. Proprioception, light touch, and sharp/dull discrimination intact right and left extremities

CASE STUDY GUIDING QUESTIONS

1. List factors that support a good prognosis for this patient, as well as factors that support a poor prognosis.
2. What factors make a restorative intervention approach appropriate for this patient? What factors make a compensatory approach appropriate for this patient?
3. List three long-term goals for this patient related to balance, walking ability, and transfer ability that are appropriate for discharge from the acute rehabilitation hospital.
4. Describe interventions to improve his walking ability.

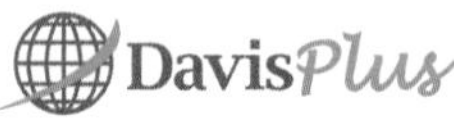

For additional resources, including answers to the questions for review and case study guiding questions, please visit **http://davisplus.fadavis.com.**

References

1. Menon, DK, et al: Position statement: definition of traumatic brain injury. Arch Phys Med Rehabil 91(11):1637–1640, 2010.
2. Taylor, CA, et al: Traumatic brain injury-related emergency department visits, hospitalizations, and deaths—United States, 2007 and 2013. MMWR Surveill Summ 66(9):1–16, 2017.
3. Langlois, JA, Rutland-Brown, W, and Wald, MM: The epidemiology and impact of traumatic brain injury: A brief overview. J Head Trauma Rehabil 21(5):375–378, 2006.
4. Rutland-Brown, W, et al: Incidence of traumatic brain injury in the United States, 2003. J Head Trauma Rehabil 21(6):544–548, 2006.
5. Faul, M, et al: Traumatic brain injury in the United States: Emergency department visits, hospitalizations and deaths 2002–2006. Atlanta (GA): Centers for Disease Control and Prevention, National Center for Injury Prevention and Control; 2010.
6. Cuthbert, JP, et al: Epidemiology of adults receiving acute inpatient rehabilitation for a primary diagnosis of traumatic brain injury in the United States. J Head Trauma Rehabil 30(2):122–135, 2015.
7. Selassie, AW, et al: Incidence of long-term disability following traumatic brain injury hospitalization, United States, 2003. J Head Trauma Rehabil 23(2):123–131, 2008.
8. Thurman, DJ, et al: Traumatic brain injury in the United States: A public health perspective. J Head Trauma Rehabil 14(6):602–615, 1999.
9. Zaloshnja, E, et al: Prevalence of long-term disability from traumatic brain injury in the civilian population of the United States, 2005. J Head Trauma Rehabil 23(6):394–400, 2008.
10. Max, W, Mackenzie, EJ, and Rice, DP: Head injuries: Costs and consequences. J Head Trauma Rehabil 6(2):76–91, 1991.
11. Corrigan, JD, et al: US population estimates of health and social outcomes 5 years after rehabilitation for traumatic brain injury. J Head Trauma Rehabil 29(6):E1-9, 2014.
12. Cuthbert, JP, et al: Unemployment in the United States after traumatic brain injury for working-age individuals: Prevalence and associated factors 2 years postinjury. J Head Trauma Rehabil 30(3):160–174, 2015.
13. Andelic, N, et al: Disability, physical health and mental health 1 year after traumatic brain injury. Disabil Rehabil 32(13): 1122–1131, 2010.
14. Povlishock, JT, and Katz, DI: Update of neuropathology and neurological recovery after traumatic brain injury. J Head Trauma Rehabil 20(1):76–94, 2005.
15. Maas, AI, Stocchetti, N, and Bullock, R: Moderate and severe traumatic brain injury in adults. Lancet Neurol 7(8):728–741, 2008.
16. Kochanek, PM, Clark, RSB, and Jenkins, LW: TBI: Pathobiology. In: Zasler, ND, Katz, DI, and Zafonte, RD (eds): Brain Injury Medicine: Principles and Practice. Demos Medical Publishing, New York, 2007.
17. Bennett, M, et al: Clinicopathologic observations in 100 consecutive patients with fatal head injury admitted to a neurosurgical unit. Ir Med J 88(2):60–62, 59, 1995.
18. Powell, JW, and Barber-Foss, KD: Traumatic brain injury in high school athletes. JAMA 282(10):958–963, 1999.
19. Tegner, Y, and Lorentzon, R: Concussion among Swedish elite ice hockey players. Br J Sports Med 30(3):251–255, 1996.

20. Meythaler, JM, et al: Current concepts: Diffuse axonal injury-associated traumatic brain injury. Arch Phys Med Rehabil 82(10):1461–1471, 2001.
21. Hicks, RR, et al: Neurological effects of blast injury. J Trauma 68(5):1257-1263, 2010.
22. Warden, D: Military TBI during the Iraq and Afghanistan wars. J Head Trauma Rehabil 21(5):398–402, 2006.
23. Kocsis, JD, and Tessler, A: Pathology of blast-related brain injury. J Rehabil Res Dev 46(6):667–672, 2009.
24. Levi, L, et al: Wartime neurosurgical experience in Lebanon, 1982–85. II: Closed craniocerebral injuries. Isr J Med Sci 26(10):555–558, 1990.
25. Schwartz, I, et al: Cognitive and functional outcomes of terror victims who suffered from traumatic brain injury. Brain Inj 22(3):255–263, 2008.
26. Pleasure, SJ, and Fishman, RA: Ventricular volume and transmural pressure gradient in normal pressure hydrocephalus. Arch Neurol 56(10):1199–1200, 1999.
27. Lippert-Gruner, M, et al: Health-related quality of life during the first year after severe brain trauma with and without polytrauma. Brain Inj 21(5):451–455, 2007.
28. Jacobsson, LJ, et al: Functioning and disability 6-15 years after traumatic brain injuries in northern Sweden. Acta Neurol Scand 120(6):389–395, 2009.
29. Ponsford, JL, et al: Longitudinal follow-up of patients with traumatic brain injury: Outcome at two, five, and ten years post-injury. J Neurotrauma 31(1):64–77, 2014.
30. Sandhaug, M, et al: Community integration 2 years after moderate and severe traumatic brain injury. Brain Inj 29(7-8):915–920, 2015.
31. Walker, WC, and Pickett, TC: Motor impairment after severe traumatic brain injury: A longitudinal multicenter study. J Rehabil Res Dev 44(7):975–982, 2007.
32. Brown, AW, et al: Impairment at rehabilitation admission and 1 year after moderate-to-severe traumatic brain injury: A prospective multi-centre analysis. Brain Inj 21(7):673–680, 2007.
33. Haaland, KY, et al: Recovery of simple motor skills after head injury. J Clin Exp Neuropsychol 16(3):448–456, 1994.
34. Lehmann, JF, et al: Quantitative evaluation of sway as an indicator of functional balance in post-traumatic brain injury. Arch Phys Med Rehabil 71(12):955–962, 1990.
35. Newton, RA: Balance abilities in individuals with moderate and severe traumatic brain injury. Brain Inj 9(5):445–451, 1995.
36. Wober, C, et al: Posturographic measurement of body sway in survivors of severe closed head injury. Arch Phys Med Rehabil 74(11):1151–1156, 1993.
37. Basford, JR, et al: An assessment of gait and balance deficits after traumatic brain injury. Arch Phys Med Rehabil 84(3):343–349, 2003.
38. Campbell, M, and Parry, A: Balance disorder and traumatic brain injury: Preliminary findings of a multi-factorial observational study. Brain Inj 19(13):1095–1104, 2005.
39. Williams, G, et al: Spatiotemporal deficits and kinematic classification of gait following a traumatic brain injury: A systematic review. J Head Trauma Rehabil 25(5):366–374, 2010.
40. Williams, G, et al: Classification of gait disorders following traumatic brain injury. J Head Trauma Rehabil 30(2):E13–23, 2015.
41. Anderson, CA, and Arciniegas, DB: Cognitive sequelae of hypoxic-ischemic brain injury: A review. NeuroRehabilitation 26(1):47–2010.
42. Riggio, S, and Wong, M: Neurobehavioral sequelae of traumatic brain injury. Mt Sinai J Med 76(2):163–172, 2009.
43. Marsh, NV, Ludbrook, MR, and Gaffaney, LC: Cognitive functioning following traumatic brain injury: A five-year follow-up. NeuroRehabilitation 38(1):71–78, 2016.
44. Giacino, JT: The vegetative and minimally conscious states: Consensus-based criteria for establishing diagnosis and prognosis. NeuroRehabilitation 19(4):293–298, 2004.
45. Giacino, JT, Katz, DI, and Whyte, J: Neurorehabilitation in disorders of consciousness. Semin Neurol 33(2):142–156, 2013.
46. Levin, HS, et al: Vegetative state after closed-head injury. A Traumatic Coma Data Bank Report. Arch Neurol 48(6):580–585, 1991.
47. Giacino, JT, et al: The minimally conscious state: Definition and diagnostic criteria. Neurology 58(3):349–353, 2002.
48. American Congress of Rehabilitation Medicine BI-ISIGDoCTF, Seel, RT, et al: Assessment scales for disorders of consciousness: Evidence-based recommendations for clinical practice and research. Arch Phys Med Rehabil 91(12):1795–1813, 2010.
49. van Erp, WS, et al: The vegetative state/unresponsive wakefulness syndrome: A systematic review of prevalence studies. Eur J Neurol 21(11):1361–1368, 2014.
50. Fine, RL: From Quinlan to Schiavo: Medical, ethical, and legal issues in severe brain injury. Proceedings 18(4):303–310, 2005.
51. The Multi-Society Task Force on PVS: Medical aspects of the persistent vegetative state (1). N Engl J Med 330(21):1499–1508, 1994.
52. Ylvisaker, M: Communication outcomes following traumatic brain injury. Semin Speech Lang 13:239–250, 1992.
53. Leblanc, J, et al: Early prediction of language impairment following traumatic brain injury. Brain Inj 20(13-14):1391–1401, 2006.
54. Galski, T, Tompkins, C, and Johnston, MV: Competence in discourse as a measure of social integration and quality of life in persons with traumatic brain injury. Brain Inj 12(9):769–782, 1998.
55. Wehman, P, et al: Critical factors associated with the successful supported employment placement of patients with severe traumatic brain injury. Brain Inj 7(1):31–44, 1993.
56. Bower, RS, et al: Paroxysmal sympathetic hyperactivity after traumatic brain injury. Neurocrit Care 13(2):233–234, 2010.
57. Rabinstein, AA: Paroxysmal sympathetic hyperactivity in the neurological intensive care unit. Neurol Res 29(7):680–682, 2007.
58. Annegers, JF, et al: A population-based study of seizures after traumatic brain injuries. N Engl J Med 338(1):20–24, 1998.
59. Salazar, AM, et al: Epilepsy after penetrating head injury. I. Clinical correlates: A report of the Vietnam Head Injury Study. Neurology 35(10):1406–1414, 1985.
60. Safaz, I, et al: Medical complications, physical function and communication skills in patients with traumatic brain injury: A single centre 5-year experience. Brain Inj 22(10):733–739, 2008.
61. Chang, BS, and Lowenstein, DH: Practice parameter: Antiepileptic drug prophylaxis in severe traumatic brain injury: Report of the Quality Standards Subcommittee of the American Academy of Neurology. Neurology 60(1):10–16, 2003.
62. Ostahowski, PJ, et al: Variation in seizure prophylaxis in severe pediatric traumatic brain injury. J Neurosurg Pediatr 18(4): 499–506, 2016.
63. Thompson, K, et al: Pharmacological treatments for preventing epilepsy following traumatic head injury. Cochrane Database Syst Rev 8:CD009900, 2015.
64. Kalisky, Z, et al: Medical problems encountered during rehabilitation of patients with head injury. Arch Phys Med Rehabil 66(1):25–29, 1985.
65. Vitaz, TW, et al: Outcome following moderate traumatic brain injury. Surg Neurol 60(4):285–291, 2003.
66. Hammond, FM, and Meighen, MJ: Venous thromboembolism in the patient with acute traumatic brain injury: Screening, diagnosis, prophylaxis, and treatment issues. J Head Trauma Rehabil 13(1):36–50, 1998.
67. Nampiaparampil, DE: Prevalence of chronic pain after traumatic brain injury: A systematic review. J Am Med Assoc 300(6): 711–719, 2008.
68. Organization, WH: International Classification of Functioning, Disability and Health (ICF). 2017; Retrieved February 24, 2017, from www.who.int/classifications/icf/en/.
69. Williams, G, et al: Incidence of gait abnormalities after traumatic brain injury. Arch Phys Med Rehabil 90(4):587–593, 2009.
70. Katz, DI, et al: Recovery of ambulation after traumatic brain injury. Arch Phys Med Rehabil 85(6):865–869, 2004.
71. Moen, KT, et al: High-level mobility in chronic traumatic brain injury and its relationship with clinical variables and magnetic resonance imaging findings in the acute phase. Arch Phys Med Rehabil 95(10):1838–1845, 2014.
72. Whyte, J, et al: Functional outcomes in traumatic disorders of consciousness: 5-year outcomes from the National Institute on Disability and Rehabilitation Research Traumatic Brain Injury Model Systems. Arch Phys Med Rehabil 94(10):1855–1860, 2013.
73. Jourdan, C, et al: A comprehensive picture of 4-year outcome of severe brain injuries. Results from the PariS-TBI study. Ann Phys Rehabil Med 59(2):100–106, 2016.

74. Andelic, N, et al: Associations between disability and employment 1 year after traumatic brain injury in a working age population. Brain Inj 26(3):261–269, 2012.
75. Jourdan, C, et al: Predictive factors for 1-year outcome of a cohort of patients with severe traumatic brain injury (TBI): Results from the PariS-TBI study. Brain Inj 27(9):1000–1007, 2013.
76. Williams, G, and Willmott, C: Higher levels of mobility are associated with greater societal participation and better quality-of-life. Brain Inj 26(9):1065–1071, 2012.
77. Young, JS, Hobbs, JG, and Bailes, JE: The impact of traumatic brain injury on the aging brain. Curr Psychiatry Rep 18(9):81, 2016.
78. Teasdale, G, and Jennett, B: Assessment of coma and impaired consciousness. A practical scale. Lancet 2(7872):81–84, 1974.
79. Perel, P, et al: Predicting outcome after traumatic brain injury: Practical prognostic models based on large cohort of international patients. BMJ 336(7641):425–429, 2008.
80. Steyerberg, EW, et al: Predicting outcome after traumatic brain injury: Development and international validation of prognostic scores based on admission characteristics. PLoS Med 5(8):e165; discussion e165, 2008.
81. Marmarou, A, et al: Prognostic value of the Glasgow Coma Scale and pupil reactivity in traumatic brain injury assessed pre-hospital and on enrollment: an IMPACT analysis. J Neurotrauma 24(2):270–280, 2007.
82. Murray, GD, et al: Multivariable prognostic analysis in traumatic brain injury: Results from the IMPACT study. J Neurotrauma 24(2):329-337, 2007.
83. Husson, EC, et al: Prognosis of six-month functioning after moderate to severe traumatic brain injury: A systematic review of prospective cohort studies. J Rehabil Med 42(5):425–436, 2010.
84. Mushkudiani, NA, et al: Prognostic value of demographic characteristics in traumatic brain injury: Results from the IMPACT study. J Neurotrauma 24(2):259–269, 2007.
85. Brown, AW, et al: Predictive utility of weekly post-traumatic amnesia assessments after brain injury: A multicentre analysis. Brain Inj 24(3):472–478, 2010.
86. Perrin, PB, et al: Measures of injury severity and prediction of acute traumatic brain injury outcomes. J Head Trauma Rehabil 30(2):136–142, 2015.
87. Semlyen, JK, Summers, SJ, and Barnes, MP: Traumatic brain injury: Efficacy of multidisciplinary rehabilitation. Arch Phys Med Rehabil 79(6):678–683, 1998.
88. Malec, JF: Impact of comprehensive day treatment on societal participation for persons with acquired brain injury. Arch Phys Med Rehabil 82(7):885–895, 2001.
89. Braverman, SE, et al: A multidisciplinary TBI inpatient rehabilitation programme for active duty service members as part of a randomized clinical trial. Brain Inj 13(6):405–415, 1999.
90. Ling, GS, and Marshall, SA: Management of traumatic brain injury in the intensive care unit. Neurol Clin 26(2):409–426, 2008.
91. Clausen, T, and Bullock, R: Medical treatment and neuroprotection in traumatic brain injury. Curr Pharm Des 7(15):1517–1532, 2001.
92. Donnelly, J, et al: Regulation of the cerebral circulation: Bedside assessment and clinical implications. Crit Care 20(1):129, 2016.
93. Thomas, E, et al: Calculation of cerebral perfusion pressure in the management of traumatic brain injury: Joint position statement by the councils of the Neuroanaesthesia and Critical Care Society of Great Britain and Ireland (NACCS) and the Society of British Neurological Surgeons (SBNS). Br J Anaesth 115(4):487–488, 2015.
94. Tang, A, et al: Intracranial pressure monitor in patients with traumatic brain injury. J Surg Res 194(2):565–570, 2015.
95. Cossu, G: Therapeutic options to enhance coma arousal after traumatic brain injury: State of the art of current treatments to improve coma recovery. Br J Neurosurg 28(2):187–198, 2014.
96. Patrick, PD, et al: The use of dopamine enhancing medications with children in low response states following brain injury. Brain Inj 17(6):497–506, 2003.
97. Giacino, JT, et al: Placebo-controlled trial of amantadine for severe traumatic brain injury. N Engl J Med 366(9):819–826, 2012.
98. Hughes, S, et al: Amantadine to enhance readiness for rehabilitation following severe traumatic brain injury. Brain Inj 19(14):1197–1206, 2005.
99. Moein, H, Khalili, HA, and Keramatian, K: Effect of methylphenidate on ICU and hospital length of stay in patients with severe and moderate traumatic brain injury. Clin Neurol Neurosurg 108(6): 539–542, 2006.
100. Hoffman, AN, et al: Administration of haloperidol and risperidone after neurobehavioral testing hinders the recovery of traumatic brain injury-induced deficits. Life Sci 83(17-18): 602–607, 2008.
101. Kline, AE, et al: Chronic administration of antipsychotics impede behavioral recovery after experimental traumatic brain injury. Neurosci Lett 448(3):263–267, 2008.
102. Whyte, J, and Nakase-Richardson, R: Disorders of consciousness: outcomes, comorbidities, and care needs. Arch Phys Med Rehabil 94(10):1851–1854, 2013.
103. McCulloch, KL, et al: Outcome measures for persons with moderate to severe traumatic brain injury: Recommendations from the American Physical Therapy Association Academy of Neurologic Physical Therapy TBI EDGE Task Force. J Neurol Phys Ther 40(4):269–280, 2016.
104. Seel, RT, et al: Assessment scales for disorders of consciousness: evidence-based recommendations for clinical practice and research. Arch Phys Med Rehabil 91(12):1795–1813, 2010.
105. Giacino, JT, Kalmar, K, and Whyte, J: The JFK Coma Recovery Scale-Revised: Measurement characteristics and diagnostic utility. Arch Phys Med Rehabil 85(12):2020–2029, 2004.
106. Pape, TL, et al: A measure of neurobehavioral functioning after coma. Part I: Theory, reliability, and validity of Disorders of Consciousness Scale. J Rehabil Res Dev 42(1):1–17, 2005.
107. Pape, TL, et al: A measure of neurobehavioral functioning after coma. Part II: Clinical and scientific implementation. J Rehabil Res Dev 42(1):19–27, 2005.
108. Hagen, C, Malkmus, D, and Durham, P: Levels of Cognitive Functioning. Ranchos Los Amigos Hospital, Downey, CA, 1972.
109. Gouvier, WD, et al: Reliability and validity of the Disability Rating Scale and the Levels of Cognitive Functioning Scale in monitoring recovery from severe head injury. Arch Phys Med Rehabil 68(2):94–97, 1987.
110. Seel, RT, et al: Specialized early treatment for persons with disorders of consciousness: program components and outcomes. Arch Phys Med Rehabil 94(10):1908–1923, 2013.
111. Eifert, B, Maurer-Karattup, P, and Schorl, M: Integration of intensive care treatment and neurorehabilitation in patients with disorders of consciousness: a program description and case report. Arch Phys Med Rehabil 94(10):1924–1933, 2013.
112. Klein, K, et al: Clinical and psychological effects of early mobilization in patients treated in a neurologic ICU: A comparative study. Crit Care Med 43(4):865–873, 2015.
113. Engels, PT, et al: Physical rehabilitation of the critically ill trauma patient in the ICU. Crit Care Med 41(7):1790–1801, 2013.
114. Bernhardt, J, et al: Early rehabilitation after stroke. Curr Opin Neurol 30(1):48–54, 2017.
115. AVERT Trial Collaboration group, Bernhardt J, Langhorne P, et al. Efficacy and safety of very early mobilisation within 24 h of stroke onset (AVERT): A randomised controlled trial. Lancet 386(9988):46–55, 2015.
116. Krewer, C, et al: Tilt table therapies for patients with severe disorders of consciousness: A randomized, controlled trial. PLoS One 10(12):e0143180, 2015.
117. Lannin, NA, et al: Splinting the hand in the functional position after brain impairment: A randomized, controlled trial. Arch Phys Med Rehabil 84(2):297–302, 2003.
118. Moseley, AM: The effect of casting combined with stretching on passive ankle dorsiflexion in adults with traumatic head injuries. Phys Ther 77(3):240–247; discussion 248-259, 1997.
119. Mortenson, PA, and Eng, JJ: The use of casts in the management of joint mobility and hypertonia following brain injury in adults: A systematic review. Phys Ther 83(7):648–658, 2003.
120. Kanyer, B: Meeting the seating and mobiity needs of the client with traumatic brain injury. J Head Trauma Rehabil 7(3):81–93, 1992.
121. Ciesla, ND: Chest physical therapy for patients in the intensive care unit. Phys Ther 76(6):609–625, 1996.
122. Ansell, BJ: Slow-to-recover brain-injured patients: Rationale for treatment. J Speech Hear Res 34(5):1017–1022, 1991.
123. Lombardi, F, et al: Sensory stimulation for brain injured individuals in coma or vegetative state. Cochrane Database Syst Rev 2:CD001427, 2002.

124. Padilla, R, and Domina, A: Effectiveness of sensory stimulation to improve arousal and alertness of people in a coma or persistent vegetative state after traumatic brain injury: A systematic review. Am J Occup Ther 70(3):7003180030p7003180031-7003180038, 2016.
125. Feld, JA, et al: Berg balance scale and outcome measures in acquired brain injury. Neurorehabil Neural Repair 15(3): 239–244, 2001.
126. Juneja, G, Czyrny, JJ, and Linn, RT: Admission balance and outcomes of patients admitted for acute inpatient rehabilitation. Am J Phys Med Rehabil 77(5):388–393, 1998.
127. Newstead, AH, Hinman, MR, and Tomberlin, JA: Reliability of the Berg Balance Scale and balance master limits of stability tests for individuals with brain injury. J Neurol Phys Ther 29(1): 18–23, 2005.
128. Inness, EL, et al: Measuring balance and mobility after traumatic brain injury: Validation of the Community Balance and Mobility Scale (CB&M). Physiother Can 63(2):199–208, 2011.
129. Howe, JA, et al: The Community Balance and Mobility Scale—a balance measure for individuals with traumatic brain injury. Clin Rehabil 20(10):885–895, 2006.
130. Williams, G, et al: The high-level mobility assessment tool (HiMAT) for traumatic brain injury. Part 1: Item generation. Brain Inj 19(11):925–932, 2005.
131. Williams, GP, et al: The high-level mobility assessment tool (HiMAT) for traumatic brain injury. Part 2: content validity and discriminability. Brain Inj 19(10):833–843, 2005.
132. Williams, G, Pallant, J, and Greenwood, K: Further development of the High-level Mobility Assessment Tool (HiMAT). Brain Inj 24(7-8):1027–1031, 2010.
133. Whyte, J, et al: The Moss Attention Rating Scale for traumatic brain injury: Initial psychometric assessment. Arch Phys Med Rehabil 84(2):268–276, 2003.
134. Robertson, IH, et al: The structure of normal human attention: The Test of Everyday Attention. J Int Neuropsychol Soc 2(6): 525–534, 1996.
135. Gaudino, EA, Geisler, MW, and Squires, NK: Construct validity in the Trail Making Test: What makes Part B harder? J Clin Exp Neuropsychol 17(4):529–535, 1995.
136. Levin, HS, O'Donnell, VM, and Grossman, RG: The Galveston Orientation and Amnesia Test. A practical scale to assess cognition after head injury. J Nerv Ment Dis 167(11):675–684, 1979.
137. Bode, RK, Heinemann, AW, and Semik, P: Measurement properties of the Galveston Orientation and Amnesia Test (GOAT) and improvement patterns during inpatient rehabilitation. J Head Trauma Rehabil 15(1):637–655, 2000.
138. Novack, TA, et al: Validity of the Orientation Log, relative to the Galveston Orientation and Amnesia Test. J Head Trauma Rehabil 15(3):957–961, 2000.
139. Alderso, AL, and Novack, TA: Measuring recovery of orientation during acute rehabilitation for traumatic brain injury: Value and expectations of recovery. J Head Trauma Rehabil 17(3):210–219, 2002.
140. Jackson, WT, Novack, TA, and Dowler, RN: Effective serial measurement of cognitive orientation in rehabilitation: The Orientation Log. Arch Phys Med Rehabil 79(6):718–720, 1998.
141. Corrigan, JD: Development of a scale for assessment of agitation following traumatic brain injury. J Clin Exp Neuropsychol 11(2):261–277, 1989.
142. Boake, C: Supervision rating scale: a measure of functional outcome from brain injury. Arch Phys Med Rehabil 77(8): 765–772, 1996.
143. McCauley, SR, et al: The neurobehavioural rating scale-revised: Sensitivity and validity in closed head injury assessment. J Neurol Neurosurg Psychiatry 71(5):643–651, 2001.
144. Dodds, TA, et al: A validation of the functional independence measurement and its performance among rehabilitation inpatients. Arch Phys Med Rehabil 74(5):531–536, 1993.
145. Stineman, MG, et al: The Functional Independence Measure: Tests of scaling assumptions, structure, and reliability across 20 diverse impairment categories. Arch Phys Med Rehabil 77(11):1101–1108, 1996.
146. Gurka, JA, et al: Utility of the functional assessment measure after discharge from inpatient rehabilitation. J Head Trauma Rehabil 14(3):247–256, 1999.
147. Hall, KM: The Functional Assessment Measure (FAM). J Rehab Outcomes 1(3):63–65, 1997.
148. Hawley, CA, et al: Use of the functional assessment measure (FIM+FAM) in head injury rehabilitation: A psychometric analysis. J Neurol Neurosurg Psychiatry 67(6):749–754, 1999.
149. Hedman, LD, Rogers, MW, and Hanke, TA: Neurologic professional education: Linking the foundation science of motor control with physical therapy interventions for movement dysfunction. J Neurol Phys Ther 20(1):9–13, 1996.
150. Malec, JF: The Mayo-Portland Participation Index: A brief and psychometrically sound measure of brain injury outcome. Arch Phys Med Rehabil 85(12):1989–1996, 2004.
151. Kean, J, et al: Rasch measurement analysis of the Mayo-Portland Adaptability Inventory (MPAI-4) in a community-based rehabilitation sample. J Neurotrauma 28(5):745–753, 2011.
152. Willer, B, Ottenbacher, KJ, and Coad, ML: The community integration questionnaire. A comparative examination. Am J Phys Med Rehabil 73(2):103–111, 1994.
153. Whiteneck, GG, et al: Development of the participation assessment with recombined tools-objective for use after traumatic brain injury. Arch Phys Med Rehabil 92(4): 542–551, 2011.
154. Malec, JF, Whiteneck, GG, and Bogner, JA: Another look at the PART-O using the Traumatic Brain Injury Model Systems National Database: Scoring to optimize psychometrics. Arch Phys Med Rehabil 97(2):211–217, 2016.
155. von Steinbuchel, N, et al: Quality of Life after Brain Injury (QOLIBRI): Scale validity and correlates of quality of life. J Neurotrauma 27(7):1157–1165, 2010.
156. von Steinbuchel, N, et al: Quality of Life after Brain Injury (QOLIBRI): Scale development and metric properties. J Neurotrauma 27(7):1167–1185, 2010.
157. Jacobson, GP, and Newman, CW: The development of the Dizziness Handicap Inventory. Arch Otolaryngol Head Neck Surg 116(4):424–427, 1990.
158. Krebs, DE, Edelstein, JE, and Fishman, S: Reliability of observational kinematic gait analysis. Phys Ther 65(7):1027–1033, 1985.
159. van Loo, MA, et al: Test-re-test reliability of walking speed, step length and step width measurement after traumatic brain injury: A pilot study. Brain Inj 18(10):1041–1048, 2004.
160. van Loo, MA, et al: Inter-rater reliability and concurrent validity of walking speed measurement after traumatic brain injury. Clin Rehabil 17(7):775–779, 2003.
161. Moseley, AM, et al: Ecological validity of walking speed assessment after traumatic brain injury: A pilot study. J Head Trauma Rehabil 19(4):341–348, 2004.
162. Englander, J, et al: Fatigue after traumatic brain injury: Association with neuroendocrine, sleep, depression and other factors. Brain Inj 24(12):1379–1388, 2010.
163. Mossberg, KA, et al: Aerobic capacity after traumatic brain injury: Comparison with a nondisabled cohort. Arch Phys Med Rehabil 88(3):315–320, 2007.
164. Mossberg, KA: Reliability of a timed walk test in persons with acquired brain injury. Am J Phys Med Rehabil 82(5):385–390; quiz 391–382, 2003.
165. Mossberg, KA, and Fortini, E: Responsiveness and validity of the six-minute walk test in individuals with traumatic brain injury. Phys Ther 92(5):726–733, 2012.
166. Gibbons, WJ, et al: Reference values for a multiple repetition 6-minute walk test in healthy adults older than 20 years. J Cardiopulm Rehabil 21(2):87–93, 2001.
167. Mossberg, KA, and Greene, BP: Reliability of graded exercise testing after traumatic brain injury: Submaximal and peak responses. Am J Phys Med Rehabil 84(7):492–500, 2005.
168. Hassett, LM, et al: Validity of the modified 20-metre shuttle test: Assessment of cardiorespiratory fitness in people who have sustained a traumatic brain injury. Brain Inj 21(10):1069–1077, 2007.
169. McCulloch, KL, et al: Balance, attention, and dual-task performance during walking after brain injury: Associations with falls history. J Head Trauma Rehabil 25(3):155–163, 2010.
170. McFadyen, BJ, et al: Modality-specific, multitask locomotor deficits persist despite good recovery after a traumatic brain injury. Arch Phys Med Rehabil 90(9):1596–1606, 2009.
171. McCulloch, K: Attention and dual-task conditions: Physical therapy implications for individuals with acquired brain injury. J Neurol Phys Ther 31(3):104–118, 2007.

172. McGraw-Hunter, M, Faw, GD, and Davis, PK: The use of video self-modelling and feedback to teach cooking skills to individuals with traumatic brain injury: A pilot study. Brain Inj 20(10):1061–1068, 2006.
173. Goverover, Y, Chiaravalloti, N, and DeLuca, J: Pilot study to examine the use of self-generation to improve learning and memory in people with traumatic brain injury. Am J Occup Ther 64(4):540–546, 2010.
174. Giuffrida, CG, et al: Functional skill learning in men with traumatic brain injury. Am J Occup Ther 63(4):398–407, 2009.
175. Shumway-Cook, A, and Woollacott, MH: Motor Control: Translating Research into Clinical Practice, ed 5. Lippincott Williams and Wilkins, Philadelphia, 2016.
176. Levin, MF, Kleim, JA, and Wolf, SL: What do motor "recovery" and "compensation" mean in patients following stroke? Neurorehabil Neural Repair 23(4):313–319, 2009.
177. Nudo, RJ: Neural bases of recovery after brain injury. J Commun Disord 44(5):515–520, 2011.
178. Birkenmeier, RL, Prager, EM, and Lang, CE: Translating animal doses of task-specific training to people with chronic stroke in 1-hour therapy sessions: A proof-of-concept study. Neurorehabil Neural Repair 24(7):620–635, 2010.
179. Wolf, SL, et al: Effect of constraint-induced movement therapy on upper extremity function 3 to 9 months after stroke: The EXCITE randomized clinical trial. J Am Med Assoc 296(17): 2095–2104, 2006.
180. Nudo, RJ: Functional and structural plasticity in motor cortex: Implications for stroke recovery. Phys Med Rehabil Clin N Am 14(1 Suppl):S57–76, 2003.
181. Kolb, B: Overview of cortical plasticity and recovery from brain injury. Phys Med Rehabil Clin N Am 14(1 Suppl):S7–25, viii, 2003.
182. Kleim, JA, and Jones, TA: Principles of experience-dependent neural plasticity: Implications for rehabilitation after brain damage. J Speech Lang Hear Res 51(1):S225–239, 2008.
183. Hellweg, S, and Johannes, S: Physiotherapy after traumatic brain injury: A systematic review of the literature. Brain Inj 22(5): 365–373, 2008.
184. Brown, TH, et al: Body weight-supported treadmill training versus conventional gait training for people with chronic traumatic brain injury. J Head Trauma Rehabil 20(5): 402–415, 2005.
185. Mossberg, KA, Orlander, EE, and Norcross, JL: Cardiorespiratory capacity after weight-supported treadmill training in patients with traumatic brain injury. Phys Ther 88(1):77–87, 2008.
186. Wilson, DJ, and Swaboda, JL: Partial weight-bearing gait retraining for persons following traumatic brain injury: Preliminary report and proposed assessment scale. Brain Inj 16(3):259–268, 2002.
187. Shaw, SE, et al: Constraint-induced movement therapy for recovery of upper-limb function following traumatic brain injury. J Rehabil Res Dev 42(6):769–778, 2005.
188. Karman, N, et al: Constraint-induced movement therapy for hemiplegic children with acquired brain injuries. J Head Trauma Rehabil 18(3):259–267, 2003.
189. Peters, DM, et al: Individuals with chronic traumatic brain injury improve walking speed and mobility with intensive mobility training. Arch Phys Med Rehabil 95(8):1454–1460, 2014.
190. Lang, CE, et al: Estimating minimal clinically important differences of upper-extremity measures early after stroke. Arch Phys Med Rehabil 89(9):1693–1700, 2008.
191. Lang, CE, MacDonald, JR, and Gnip, C: Counting repetitions: An observational study of outpatient therapy for people with hemiparesis post-stroke. J Neurol Phys Ther 31(1):3–10, 2007.
192. Moore, JL, et al: Locomotor training improves daily stepping activity and gait efficiency in individuals poststroke who have reached a "plateau" in recovery. Stroke 41(1):129–135, 2010.
193. Morris, DM, Taub, E, and Mark, VW: Constraint-induced movement therapy: Characterizing the intervention protocol. Eura Medicophys 42(3):257–268, 2006.
194. Mossberg, KA, Amonette,WE, and Masel, BE: Endurance training and cardiorespiratory conditioning after traumatic brain injury. J Head Trauma Rehabil 25(3):173–183, 2010.
195. Bhambhani, Y, Rowland, G, and Farag, M: Effects of circuit training on body composition and peak cardiorespiratory responses in patients with moderate to severe traumatic brain injury. Arch Phys Med Rehabil 86(2):268–276, 2005.
196. Hassett, LM, et al: Efficacy of a fitness centre-based exercise programme compared with a home-based exercise programme in traumatic brain injury: A randomized controlled trial. J Rehabil Med 41(4):247–255, 2009.
197. Zheng, G, et al: Aerobic exercise ameliorates cognitive function in older adults with mild cognitive impairment: A systematic review and meta-analysis of randomised controlled trials. Br J Sports Med 2016.
198. Chin, LM, et al: Improved cardiorespiratory fitness with aerobic exercise training in individuals with traumatic brain injury. J Head Trauma Rehabil 30(6):382–390, 2015.
199. Chin, LM, et al: Improved cognitive performance following aerobic exercise training in people with traumatic brain injury. Arch Phys Med Rehabil 96(4):754–759, 2015.
200. Killington, MJ, Mackintosh, SF, and Ayres, M: An isokinetic muscle strengthening program for adults with an acquired brain injury leads to meaningful improvements in physical function. Brain Inj 24(7-8):970–977, 2010.
201. Killington, MJ, Mackintosh, SF, and Ayres, MB: Isokinetic strength training of lower limb muscles following acquired brain injury. Brain Inj 24(12):1399–1407, 2010.
202. Pak, S, and Patten, C: Strengthening to promote functional recovery poststroke: An evidence-based review. Top Stroke Rehabil 15(3):177–199, 2008.
203. Scandalis, TA, et al: Resistance training and gait function in patients with Parkinson's disease. Am J Phys Med Rehabil 80(1):38–43; quiz 44–36, 2001.
204. Palmer-McLean, K, and Harbst, KB: Stroke and brain injury. In: Durstine, JL, and Moore, GE (eds): ACSM's Exercise Management for Persons wiht Chronic Diseases and Disabilities. American College of Sports Medicine, Champaign, IL, 2003.
205. Everaert, DG, et al: Does functional electrical stimulation for foot drop strengthen corticospinal connections? Neurorehabil Neural Repair 24(2):168–177, 2010.
206. Kluding, PM, et al: Foot drop stimulation versus ankle foot orthosis after stroke: 30-week outcomes. Stroke 44(6): 1660–1669, 2013.
207. Slifer, KJ, et al: Antecedent management and compliance training improve adolescents' participation in early brain injury rehabilitation. Brain Inj 11(12):877–889, 1997.
208. Kim, E: Agitation, aggression, and disinhibition syndromes after traumatic brain injury. NeuroRehabilitation 17(4):297–310, 2002.
209. Cicerone, KD, et al: A randomized controlled trial of holistic neuropsychologic rehabilitation after traumatic brain injury. Arch Phys Med Rehabil 89(12):2239–2249, 2008.
210. Klonoff, PS, Lamb, DG, and Henderson, SW: Outcomes from milieu-based neurorehabilitation at up to 11 years post-discharge. Brain Inj 15(5):413–428, 2001.
211. Schneiderman, AI, Braver, ER, and Kang, HK: Understanding sequelae of injury mechanisms and mild traumatic brain injury incurred during the conflicts in Iraq and Afghanistan: Persistent postconcussive symptoms and posttraumatic stress disorder. Am J Epidemiol 167(12):1446–1452, 2008.
212. McCrory, P, et al: Consensus statement on concussion in sport: The 4th International Conference on Concussion in Sport, Zurich, November 2012. J Athl Train 48(4): 554–575, 2013.
213. Inverson, GL, Zasler, N, and Lange, RT: Post concussive disorder. In Zasler, N, Katz, DI, and Zafonte, R (eds): Brain Injury Medicine: Principles and Practice. Demos Medical Publishing, New York, 2007.
214. Barkhoudarian, G, Hovda, DA, and Giza, CC: The molecular pathophysiology of concussive brain injury—an update. Phys Med Rehabil Clin N Am 27(2):373–393, 2016.
215. Hartlage, LC, Durant-Wilson, D, and Patch, PC: Persistent neurobehavioral problems following mild traumatic brain injury. Arch Clin Neuropsychol 16(6):561–570, 2001.
216. Vanderploeg, RD, et al: Long-term morbidities following self-reported mild traumatic brain injury. J Clin Exp Neuropsychol 29(6):585–598, 2007.
217. Sosnoff, JJ, et al: Previous mild traumatic brain injury and postural-control dynamics. J Athl Train 46(1):85–91, 2011.
218. Collins, MW, et al: A comprehensive, targeted approach to the clinical care of athletes following sport-related concussion. Knee Surg Sports Traumatol Arthrosc 22(2):235–246, 2014.

219. Calcagnile, O, Anell, A, and Unden, J: The addition of S100B to guidelines for management of mild head injury is potentially cost saving. BMC Neurol 16(1):200, 2016.
220. Manzano, S, et al: Diagnostic performance of S100B protein serum measurement in detecting intracranial injury in children with mild head trauma. Emerg Med J 33(1):42–46, 2016.
221. Weightman, MM, et al: Physical therapy recommendations for service members with mild traumatic brain injury. J Head Trauma Rehabil 25(3):206–218, 2010.
222. McCrory, P, et al: Consensus statement on concussion in sport: The 3rd International Conference on Concussion in Sport held in Zurich, November 2008. Br J Sports Med 43 Suppl 1:i76–90, 2009.
223. Howell, DR, et al: Physical activity level and symptom duration are not associated after concussion. Am J Sports Med 44(4):1040–1046, 2016.
224. McCulloch, KL, et al: Development of clinical recommendations for progressive return to activity after military mild traumatic brain injury: Guidance for rehabilitation providers. J Head Trauma Rehabil 30(1):56–67, 2015.
225. Silverberg, ND, and Iverson, GL: Is rest after concussion "the best medicine"? Recommendations for activity resumption following concussion in athletes, civilians, and military service members. J Head Trauma Rehabil 28(4):250–259, 2013.
226. Baker, JG, et al: Return to full functioning after graded exercise assessment and progressive exercise treatment of postconcussion syndrome. Rehabil Res Pract 2012:705309, 2012.
227. Leddy, JJ, et al: A preliminary study of subsymptom threshold exercise training for refractory post-concussion syndrome. Clin J Sport Med 20(1):21–27, 2010.
228. Leddy, JJ, and Willer, B: Use of graded exercise testing in concussion and return-to-activity management. Curr Sports Med Rep 12(6):370–376, 2013.
229. Meterko, M, et al: Psychometric assessment of the Neurobehavioral Symptom Inventory-22: The structure of persistent postconcussive symptoms following deployment-related mild traumatic brain injury among veterans. J Head Trauma Rehabil 27(1): 55–62, 2012.
230. Halstead, ME, et al: Returning to learning following a concussion. Pediatrics 132(5):948–957, 2013.
231. Santiago, S: Adolescent concussion and return-to-learn. Pediatr Ann 45(3):e73–75, 2016.
232. Alla, S, et al: Self-report scales/checklists for the measurement of concussion symptoms: a systematic review. Br J Sports Med 43 Suppl 1:i3–12, 2009.
233. Lovell, MR, and Collins, MW: Neuropsychological assessment of the college football player. J Head Trauma Rehabil 13(2):9–26, 1998.
234. Lovell, MR, et al: Measurement of symptoms following sports-related concussion: Reliability and normative data for the post-concussion scale. Appl Neuropsychol 13(3):166–174, 2006.
235. Alsalaheen, BA, et al: Vestibular rehabilitation for dizziness and balance disorders after concussion. J Neurol Phys Ther 34(2): 87–93, 2010.
236. Iverson, GL, et al: Tracking neuropsychological recovery following concussion in sport. Brain Inj 20(3):245–252, 2006.
237. Iverson, GL, Lovell, MR, and Collins, MW: Interpreting change on ImPACT following sport concussion. Clin Neuropsychol 17(4):460–467, 2003.
238. Schatz, P, et al: Sensitivity and specificity of the ImPACT Test Battery for concussion in athletes. Arch Clin Neuropsychol 21(1):91–99, 2006.
239. Hoffer, ME, et al: Blast exposure: Vestibular consequences and associated characteristics. Otol Neurotol 31(2):232–236, 2010.
240. Guskiewicz, KM: Balance assessment in the management of sport-related concussion. Clin Sports Med 30(1):89–102, ix, 2011.
241. Guskiewicz, KM, et al: Alternative approaches to the assessment of mild head injury in athletes. Med Sci Sports Exerc 29(7 Suppl): S213–221, 1997.
242. Scherer, MR, et al: Evidence of central and peripheral vestibular pathology in blast-related traumatic brain injury. Otol Neurotol 2011.
243. Riemann, BL, and Guskiewicz, KM: Effects of mild head injury on postural stability as measured through clinical balance testing. J Athl Train 35(1):19–25, 2000.
244. Whitney, S, Wrisley, D, and Furman, J: Concurrent validity of the Berg Balance Scale and the Dynamic Gait Index in people with vestibular dysfunction. Physiother Res Int 8(4):178–186, 2003.
245. Kleffelgaard, I, et al: Associations among self-reported balance problems, post-concussion symptoms and performance-based tests: A longitudinal follow-up study. Disabil Rehabil 34(9): 788–794, 2012.
246. Moore, BM, Adams, JT, and Barakatt, E: Outcomes following a vestibular rehabilitation and aerobic training program to address persistent post-concussion symptoms. J Allied Health 45(4): e59–e68, 2016.
247. Horak, FB, Wrisley, DM, and Frank, J: The Balance Evaluation Systems Test (BESTest) to differentiate balance deficits. Phys Ther 89(5):484–498, 2009.
248. Mancini, M, et al: Mobility lab to assess balance and gait with synchronized body-worn sensors. J Bioeng Biomed Sci Suppl 1:007, 2011.
249. Mancini, M, et al: ISway: A sensitive, valid and reliable measure of postural control. J Neuroeng Rehabil 9:59, 2012.
250. King, LA, et al: Instrumenting the balance error scoring system for use with patients reporting persistent balance problems after mild traumatic brain injury. Arch Phys Med Rehabil 95(2): 353–359, 2014.
251. Capo-Aponte, JE, et al: Visual dysfunctions and symptoms during the subacute stage of blast-induced mild traumatic brain injury. Mil Med 177(7):804–813, 2012.
252. Mucha, A, et al: A brief Vestibular/Ocular Motor Screening (VOMS) assessment to evaluate concussions: Preliminary findings. Am J Sports Med 42(10):2479–2486, 2014.
253. Murray, DA, Meldrum, D, and Lennon, O: Can vestibular rehabilitation exercises help patients with concussion? A systematic review of efficacy, prescription and progression patterns. Br J Sports Med 51(5):442–451, 2017.
254. Schneider, KJ, et al: The effects of rest and treatment following sport-related concussion: A systematic review of the literature. Br J Sports Med 47(5):304–307, 2013.
255. Sawyer, Q, Vesci, B, and McLeod, TC: Physical activity and intermittent postconcussion symptoms after a period of symptom-limited physical and cognitive rest. J Athl Train 51(9): 739–742, 2016.
256. Schneider, KJ, et al: Cervicovestibular rehabilitation in sport-related concussion: A randomised controlled trial. Br J Sports Med 48(17):1294–1298, 2014.
257. Hoffer, ME, et al: Characterizing and treating dizziness after mild head trauma. Otol Neurotol 25(2):135–138, 2004.
258. Gottshall, KR, and Hoffer, ME: Tracking recovery of vestibular function in individuals with blast-induced head trauma using vestibular-visual-cognitive interaction tests. J Neurol Phys Ther 34(2):94–97, 2010.
259. Ahlskog, JE, et al: Physical exercise as a preventive or disease-modifying treatment of dementia and brain aging. Mayo Clin Proc 86(9):876–884, 2011.
260. Marshall, S, et al: Updated clinical practice guidelines for concussion/mild traumatic brain injury and persistent symptoms. Brain Inj 29(6):688–700, 2015.
261. Laker, SR, et al: Retirement and activity restrictions following concussion. Phys Med Rehabil Clin N Am 27(2):487–501, 2016.
262. Williams, G, and Schache, A. Evaluation of a conceptual framework for retraining high-level mobility following traumatic brain injury: two case reports. J Head Trauma Rehabil 25(3):164–172, 2010.

appendix

19.A Internet Resources

- Brain Injury Association of America: www.biausa.org/
- Traumatic Brain Injury Model Systems Knowledge Translation Center: www.msktc.org/tbi/model-system-centers
- National Resource Center for Traumatic Brain Injury: www.tbinrc.com
- Centers for Disease Control and Prevention: Heads Up: www.cdc.gov/headsup/basics/index.html
- mTBI Guidelines: Department of Defense and Veterans Affairs: www.healthquality.va.gov/guidelines/Rehab/mtbi/mTBICPGFullCPG50821816.pdf
- Brainline: www.brainline.org/index.html
- Center for Outcome Measurement in Brain Injury: www.tbims.org
- Academy of Neurologic Physical Therapy PT Outcome Measures Recommendations: Traumatic Brain Injury: www.neuropt.org/professional-resources/neurology-section-outcome-measures-recommendations/traumatic-brain-injury
- Shirley Ryan AbilityLab Rehabilitation Measures Database: www.sralab.org/rehabilitation-measures

Traumatic Spinal Cord Injury

George D. Fulk, PT, PhD
Mark Bowden, PT, PhD
Andrea L. Behrman, PT, PhD, FAPTA

Chapter 20

LEARNING OBJECTIVES

1. Identify the major etiological factors associated with traumatic spinal cord injury.
2. Describe the clinical presentation following damage to the spinal cord.
3. Given a patient with a spinal cord injury, identify the motor and sensory level of injury and the American Spinal Injury Association Impairment Scale classification.
4. Analyze the impact of complications associated with spinal cord injury on the physical therapy plan of care and outcomes.
5. Identify the expected functional outcomes for patients with spinal cord injury at various lesion levels.
6. Explain how common precautions will affect physical therapy interventions.
7. Evaluate different outcome measures commonly used in people with spinal cord injury.
8. Analyze and interpret patient data, formulate goals and expected outcomes, and develop a plan of care when presented with a clinical case study.
9. Justify the selection of different interventions for the acute and active rehabilitation stages of recovery.
10. Discuss the use of neurotechnologies for people with spinal cord injury.

CHAPTER OUTLINE

Spinal cord injury (SCI) is a relatively low-incidence, high-cost injury that results in tremendous change in an individual's life. Paralysis of the muscles below the level of the injury can lead to limited and altered mobility, self-care, and ability to participate in valued social activities. In addition to the musculoskeletal system, many other body systems are impaired after an SCI, including the cardiopulmonary, integumentary, gastrointestinal, genitourinary, and sensory systems. The psychosocial impact of SCI can be just as great as the physical impact. Changes in body image and sexual function, incontinence, and having to rely on others to complete everyday tasks that were previously done without thought or effort can profoundly influence a person's identity. Rehabilitation is an important element toward achieving a fulfilling and active life after SCI. Physical therapists play a key role in the rehabilitation process.

DEMOGRAPHICS AND ETIOLOGY

It is estimated that approximately 17,000 new cases of SCI occur in the United States annually. Between 243,000 and 347,000 individuals with SCI are currently living in the United States. The average age at injury is 42.[1] However, there is a bimodal distribution of age at injury. The first peak occurs in young adults between the ages of 15 and 29, and a second peak occurs in older adults (65 or older).[2] This may be due to the aging of the U.S. population and an increase in falls as a cause of injury.[1] The majority of persons with SCI are male (80% male vs. 20% female).[1]

Spinal cord injuries can be grossly divided into two broad etiological categories: *traumatic* and *nontraumatic*. Trauma is the most frequent cause of injury in adult rehabilitation populations. Traumatic injury results from damage caused by events such as motor vehicle accidents (38%), falls (30.5%), violence (13.5%), and sports-related injuries (9%).[1] Falls are the most common cause of SCI in older adults.[3] Nontraumatic damage in adult populations generally results from disease or pathological influence. Conditions that may damage the spinal cord are vascular dysfunction (arteriovenous malformation, thrombosis, embolus, or hemorrhage); spinal stenosis; spinal neoplasms; syringomyelia; infection; and neurological diseases, such as multiple sclerosis and amyotrophic lateral sclerosis.[4,5] Nontraumatic etiologies account for approximately 38% of all SCIs.[4] Outcomes after rehabilitation tend not to differ between people with traumatic and nontraumatic SCI.[6]

Incomplete tetraplegia (45%) is the most common neurological category, followed by incomplete paraplegia (21.3%), complete paraplegia (20%), and complete tetraplegia (13.3%).[1] The length of hospital stay, both in acute care and inpatient rehabilitation, has decreased considerably since the 1970s.[1,7] The median length of stay in the acute care hospital has decreased from 24 days in the 1970s to 11 days in 2016. This trend is true for length of stay of inpatient rehabilitation as well—98 days in the 1970s compared to 35 days in 2016.[1]

Life expectancy for people with SCI has not significantly improved since the 1980s[8] and is lower than people without SCI. Factors that influence life expectancy are age at onset and level and extent of neurological injury. Individuals with an incomplete neurological SCI have a longer life expectancy than those with a complete injury, and individuals with more caudal injuries also have a greater life expectancy. A 20-year-old healthy individual without an SCI has a life expectancy of an additional 59.5 years (total life expectancy of 79.5 years). A person who experiences an SCI at age 20 with a neurologically incomplete injury has a life expectancy of an additional 52.9 years, a person with complete paraplegia an additional 45.5 years, low tetraplegia (C5–C8) an additional 40.7 years, and a person with high tetraplegia (C1–C4) an additional 36.9 years. Mortality rate is also higher during the first year after injury.[1]

The financial impact of SCI is extremely high. Spinal cord injury is characterized by lengthy hospitalization, medical complications, extensive follow-up care, attendant care, and recurrent hospitalizations. Expenses during the first year post-injury vary based on level and type of injury and range from $423,152 for high tetraplegia (C1–C4), $293,529 for low tetraplegia (C5–C8), and $191,431 for paraplegia.[9] Average lifetime costs for an individual injured at 25 years of age are $3.5 million for high tetraplegia (C1–C4), $2.5 million for low tetraplegia (C5–C8), and $1.6 million for paraplegia.[10] These numbers do not take into account lost wages, fringe benefits, and productivity.

This brief presentation of demographic information provides some important general perspectives on characteristics of SCI. It is a relatively low-incidence disability affecting predominantly younger males and is associated with lengthy and costly care as well as a shorter life expectancy.

CLASSIFICATION OF SPINAL CORD INJURIES

Spinal cord injuries typically are divided into two broad functional categories: tetraplegia and paraplegia. *Tetraplegia* refers to motor and/or sensory impairment of all four extremities and trunk, including the respiratory muscles, and results from lesions of the cervical cord. *Paraplegia* refers to motor and/or sensory impairment of all or part of the trunk and both lower extremities (LEs), resulting from lesions of the thoracic or lumbar spinal cord or cauda equina.[11]

Neuroanatomical Organization and Structure

Before considering designation of spinal cord lesions, it is useful to briefly review the anatomy of the spinal cord and its relationship with nerve roots to the vertebral bodies. The spinal cord exits the foramen magnum and extends to approximately the L1 vertebral level. It contains white matter, which consists mainly of ascending sensory tracts, descending motor tracts, and an H-shaped central area of gray matter. The primary ascending tracts are the dorsal column (conveys proprioception, vibratory sensation, deep touch, and discriminative touch); anterolateral system, consisting of the spinothalamic, spinoreticular, and spinotectal tracts (conveys pain, temperature, and crude touch); and the dorsal and ventral spinocerebellar tracts (conveys unconscious proprioception) (Fig. 20.1). The primary descending tracts are the lateral corticospinal (voluntary movement); anterior corticospinal (voluntary movement of axial muscles, minimal functional significance due to small size); medial vestibulospinal (positioning of head and neck); lateral and medial vestibulospinal (posture and balance); lateral and

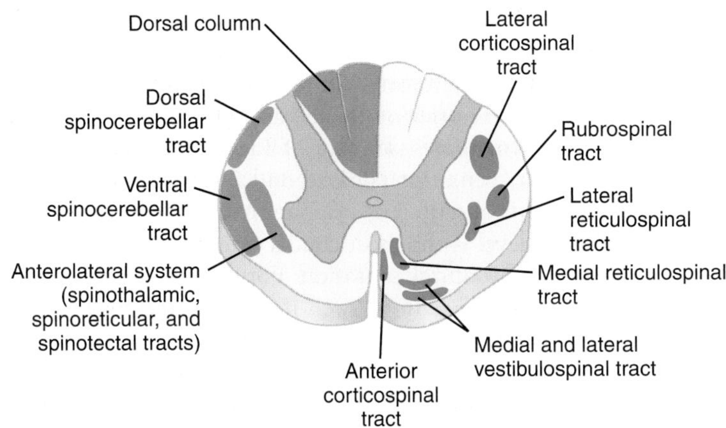

Figure 20.1 Main ascending sensor tracts: dorsal column, spinothalamic, spinoreticular, spinotectal, dorsal, and ventral spinocerebellar tracts. Main descending motor tracts: lateral corticospinal, anterior corticospinal, lateral and medial vestibulospinal, lateral and medial reticulospinal, and rubrospinal tracts.

medial reticulospinal (posture, balance, automatic gait-related movements); and rubrospinal (movement of limbs) (see Fig. 20.1). In addition to these long tracts, the white matter contains axons of interneurons, which convey information between spinal cord segments. The H-shaped gray matter is arranged such that the dorsal section in each half contains neurons involved in sensory function, the middle portion contains interneurons, and the ventral section contains neurons involved in motor function (anterior horn cells) that project to the peripheral muscles.[11,12]

There are 31 pairs of spinal nerves: 8 cervical, 12 thoracic, 5 lumbar, 5 sacral, and 1 coccygeal (Fig. 20.2). The cervical nerves are relatively horizontal as they exit the intervertebral foramina. The nerve roots for C1–C7 exit above the corresponding vertebrae. C8 exits below the C7 vertebrae. The remaining nerves exit in a downward direction and do not emerge at the corresponding vertebral level. During fetal development, the cord fills the entire length of the vertebral canal and the spinal nerves run in a horizontal direction. As the vertebral column elongates with growth, the spinal cord, which does not elongate at the same rate or as much, is drawn upward. In adults the spinal cord ends in the conus medullaris at the L1 vertebral level. The nerve roots assume an increasingly oblique and downward direction, running in an almost vertical direction in the lumbar area, giving the appearance of a "horse's tail" (cauda equina) (see Fig. 20.2). Because of this, in more caudal injuries the vertebral level of injury does not correspond directly to the spinal cord segment level of injury.

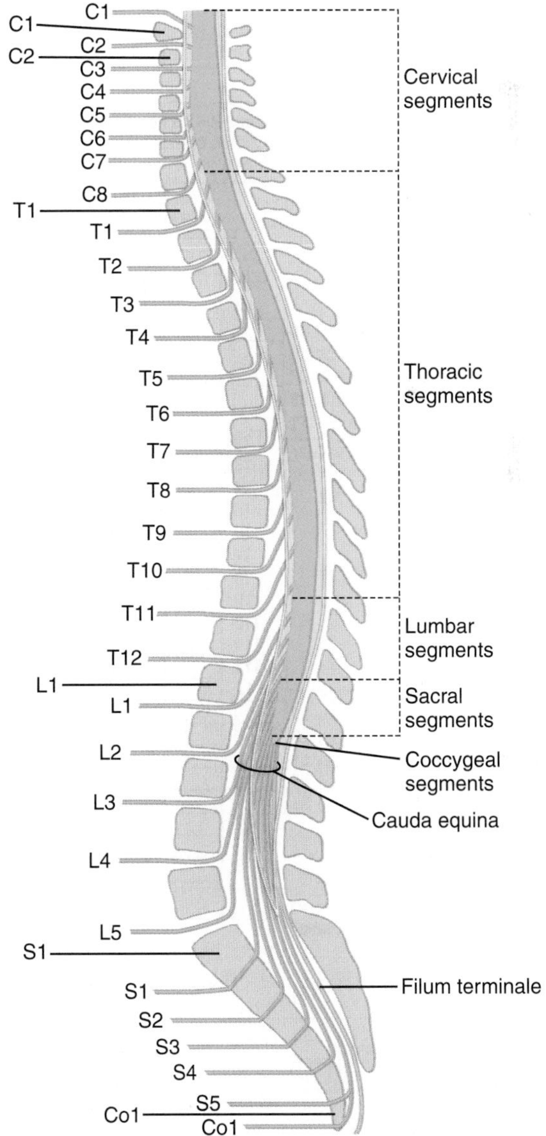

Figure 20.2 Relationship between spinal cord and nerve roots to vertebral bodies.

Designation of Lesion Level

It is extremely important for clinicians and researchers to be able to accurately determine the extent of neurological impairment in terms of motor and sensory loss when working with individuals with SCI. The extent of motor and sensory function after injury has a large impact on the medical and rehabilitation needs of the individual. In an effort to standardize the way in which severity of injury is determined and documented, the American Spinal Injury Association (ASIA) created the *International Standards for Neurological Classification of Spinal Cord Injury* (ISNCSCI)[11,13] (Fig. 20.3). The ISNCSCI provides a standardized examination method to determine the extent of motor and sensory function loss after a SCI. It promotes better communication between and among professionals, provides guidance for establishing the prognosis, and is an important tool for clinical research trials.

The *neurological level of injury* is defined as the most caudal level of the spinal cord with normal motor and sensory function on both the left and right sides of the body. *Motor level* is determined testing the strength of 10 key muscles on the right and left side of the body (see Fig. 20.3 for key muscles). Key muscle strength is scored using the 6-point ordinal scale commonly used for manual muscle testing (MMT). The motor level is the lowest myotome with a key muscle that has a grade of at least 3, provided that the muscle function in the key muscles above this level are normal (MMT = 5). *Sensory level* is determined by testing the patient's sensitivity to light touch and pinprick on the left and right side of the body at key dermatomes (see Fig. 20.3 for key sensory points). Scoring of sensation is based on a 3-point ordinal scale, where 0 is absent, 1 is impaired, and 2 is normal. The sensory level is the most caudal level with normal light touch and pinprick sensation. For an individual patient, the motor and sensory levels may differ and may be different between the left and right sides of the body.[11,13]

Assigning a single muscle to represent one myotome is a generalization. Most muscles are innervated by more than one segmental nerve root; usually two nerve roots innervate each muscle. For example, the extensor carpi radialis longus receives innervation from the C6 and C7 spinal nerve roots. The ISNCSCI key muscles have two levels of innervation, adding to the validity of the scoring. For the purpose of determining motor and neurological

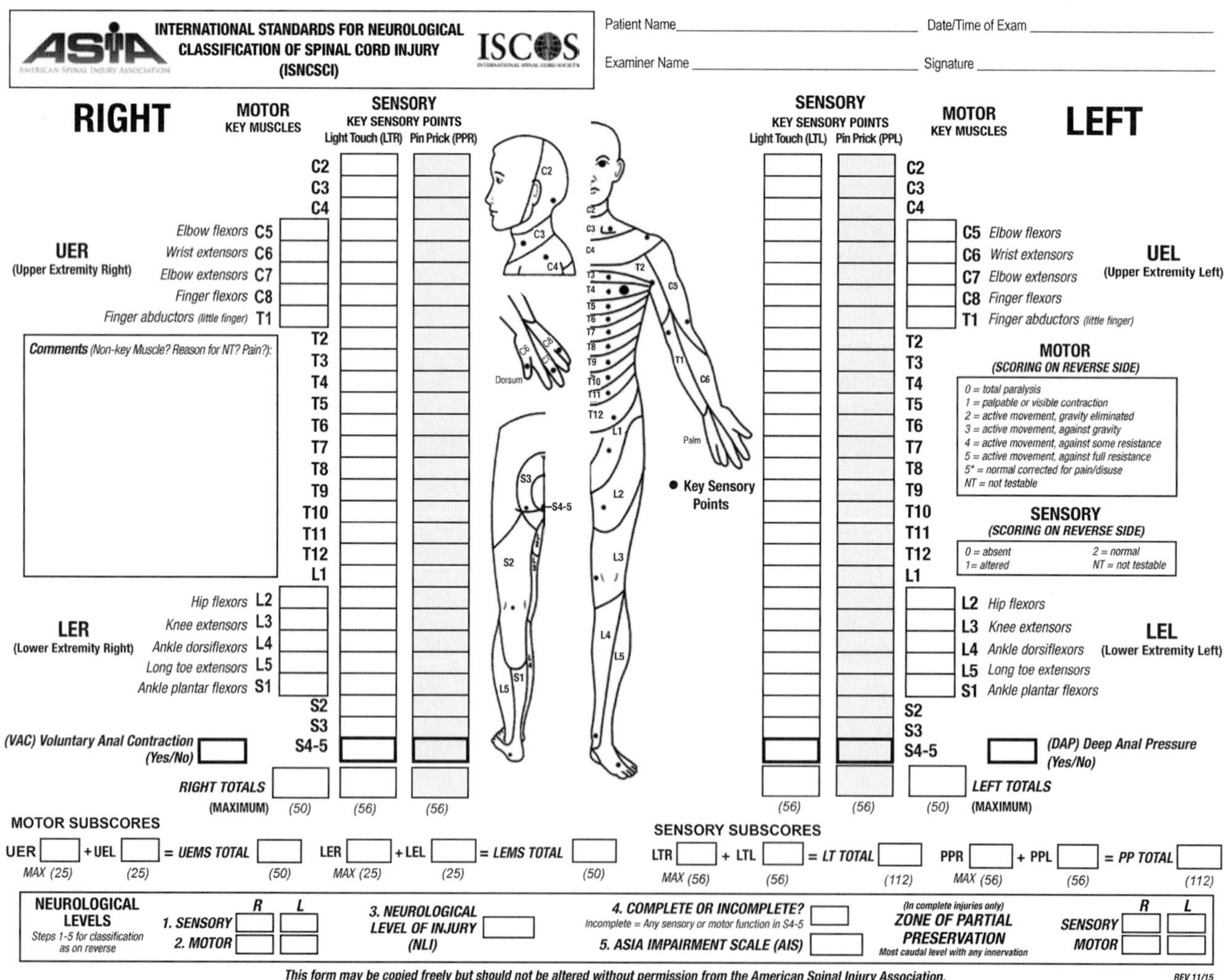
ASIA (American Spinal Injury Association) INTERNATIONAL STANDARDS FOR NEUROLOGICAL CLASSIFICATION OF SPINAL CORD INJURY (ISNCSCI) ISCoS

Patient Name ____ Date/Time of Exam ____

Examiner Name ____ Signature ____

RIGHT — MOTOR KEY MUSCLES — SENSORY KEY SENSORY POINTS Light Touch (LTR) Pin Prick (PPR)

C2 C3 C4

UER (Upper Extremity Right): Elbow flexors C5; Wrist extensors C6; Elbow extensors C7; Finger flexors C8; Finger abductors (little finger) T1

Comments (Non-key Muscle? Reason for NT? Pain?):

T2 T3 T4 T5 T6 T7 T8 T9 T10 T11 T12 L1

LER (Lower Extremity Right): Hip flexors L2; Knee extensors L3; Ankle dorsiflexors L4; Long toe extensors L5; Ankle plantar flexors S1

S2 S3 S4-5

(VAC) Voluntary Anal Contraction (Yes/No)

RIGHT TOTALS (MAXIMUM) (50) (56) (56)

SENSORY KEY SENSORY POINTS Light Touch (LTL) Pin Prick (PPL) — MOTOR KEY MUSCLES — LEFT

C2 C3 C4

UEL (Upper Extremity Left): C5 Elbow flexors; C6 Wrist extensors; C7 Elbow extensors; C8 Finger flexors; T1 Finger abductors (little finger)

T2 T3 T4 T5 T6 T7 T8 T9 T10 T11 T12 L1

MOTOR (SCORING ON REVERSE SIDE)
0 = total paralysis
1 = palpable or visible contraction
2 = active movement, gravity eliminated
3 = active movement, against gravity
4 = active movement, against some resistance
5 = active movement, against full resistance
5* = normal corrected for pain/disuse
NT = not testable

SENSORY (SCORING ON REVERSE SIDE)
0 = absent 2 = normal
1 = altered NT = not testable

LEL (Lower Extremity Left): L2 Hip flexors; L3 Knee extensors; L4 Ankle dorsiflexors; L5 Long toe extensors; S1 Ankle plantar flexors

S2 S3 S4-5

(DAP) Deep Anal Pressure (Yes/No)

LEFT TOTALS (MAXIMUM) (56) (56) (50)

MOTOR SUBSCORES
UER ☐ + UEL ☐ = UEMS TOTAL ☐ — MAX (25) (25) (50)
LER ☐ + LEL ☐ = LEMS TOTAL ☐ — MAX (25) (25) (50)

SENSORY SUBSCORES
LTR ☐ + LTL ☐ = LT TOTAL ☐ — MAX (56) (56) (112)
PPR ☐ + PPL ☐ = PP TOTAL ☐ — MAX (56) (56) (112)

NEUROLOGICAL LEVELS (Steps 1-5 for classification as on reverse): 1. SENSORY R L; 2. MOTOR R L
3. NEUROLOGICAL LEVEL OF INJURY (NLI)
4. COMPLETE OR INCOMPLETE? Incomplete = Any sensory or motor function in S4-5
5. ASIA IMPAIRMENT SCALE (AIS)
ZONE OF PARTIAL PRESERVATION (In complete injuries only) Most caudal level with any innervation: SENSORY R L; MOTOR R L

This form may be copied freely but should not be altered without permission from the American Spinal Injury Association. REV 11/15

Figure 20.3 International Standards for Classification of Spinal Cord Injury. *(With permission from American Spinal Injury Association: International Standards for Neurological Classification of Spinal Cord Injury, revised 2011; Atlanta, GA, Revised 2011, Updated 2015.)*

level, the key muscle is defined as having intact innervation if it has an MMT score of at least 3/5 (fair) and the rostral key muscles exhibit 5/5 (normal) strength. If the rostral key muscle does not demonstrate 5/5 strength but the therapist feels that the muscle would test normally except for factors that would impede normal testing (e.g., pain with testing or difficulty with positioning), then this information should be carefully documented. For myotomes that are not clinically testable (i.e., C1–C4, T2–L1, and S2–S5), the motor level is defined as the same as the sensory level.

As mentioned, when determining neurological level, there may be differences in the level of sensory and motor function and between the left and right sides of the body. For example, a patient's sensory level may be at C5 on the left and C8 on the right, and the motor level may be C5 on the left and T1 on the right. In these cases, it is still necessary to assign a neurological level so that ASIA Impairment Scale (AIS) classification can be assigned by determining the number of key muscles intact below the neurological level (see AIS Impairment section below). However, it should be noted that in some cases the neurological level assignment can be misleading in that the patient may have a mixed presentation of intact motor and/or sensory function below that level.

Complete Injuries, Incomplete Injuries, and Zone of Partial Preservation

A complete anatomical transection of the spinal cord is rare. However, even if the injury is not anatomically complete, it may present as neurologically complete. The ISNCSCI defines a *complete injury* as having no sensory or motor function in the lowest sacral segments (S4 and S5), with no sacral sparing. Sacral sparing is determined by sensory function at S4–5 dermatome, ability to feel deep anal pressure, or voluntary anal sphincter contraction. An *incomplete injury* is classified as having motor and/or sensory function below the neurological level that includes sensory and/or motor function at S4 and S5, with presence of sacral sparing. If an individual has motor and/or sensory function below the neurological level but does not have sacral sparing, then the areas of intact motor and/or sensory function below the neurological level are termed *zones of partial preservation.*[11,14]

ASIA Impairment Scale

Individuals with incomplete injuries may have variable clinical presentations in terms of motor and/or sensory function below the neurological level. For example, one patient may have close to normal sensory and motor function below the level of the lesion, whereas another with the same lesion level may have impaired sensation and no motor function below the neurological level. The AIS (Box 20.1) was created to distinguish among different types of SCI—complete, sensory incomplete, and motor incomplete.

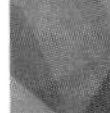

Box 20.1 ASIA Impairment Scale (AIS)

A = Complete: No motor or sensory function is preserved in the sacral segments S4–S5.

B = Sensory Incomplete: Sensory but not motor function is preserved below the neurological level and includes the sacral segments S4–S5 (light touch or pin prick at S4–5 or deep anal pressure) and no motor function is preserved more than three levels below the motor level on either side of the body.

C = Motor Incomplete: Motor function is preserved at the most caudal sacral segments for voluntary anal contraction OR the patient meets the criteria for sensor incomplete status (sensory function preserved at the most caudal sacral segments (S4-5) by LT, PP, or DAP), and has some sparing of motor function more than three levels below the ipsilateral motor level on either side of the body.
(This includes key or non-key muscle functions to determine motor incomplete status) For AIS C less than half of key muscle functions below the single NLI have a muscle grade ≥3.

D = Motor Incomplete: Motor incomplete status as defined above, with at least half (half or more) of key muscle functions below the single NLI having a muscle grade ≥3.

E = Normal: If sensation and motor function as tested with the ISNCSCI are graded as normal in all segments, and the patient had prior deficits, then the AIS grade is E. Someone without an initial SCI does not receive an AIS grade.

Using ND: To document the sensory, motor, and NLI levels, the ASIA Impairment Scale grade, and/or the zone of partial preservation (ZPP) when they are unable to be determined based on the examination results.

From American Spinal Injury Association, with permission. American Spinal Injury Association: International Standards for Neurological Classification of Spinal Cord Injury, revised 2011; Atlanta, GA., Revised 2011, Updated 2015.

Clinical Syndromes

Despite the disparity associated with incomplete lesions, several syndromes have emerged with consistent clinical features. Approximately one-fifth of all SCIs result in an injury pattern similar to clinical SCI syndromes.[15] Information related to the anticipated sensory and motor functions of these syndromes is useful in establishing anticipated goals, expected outcomes, and plan of care (POC). The approximate area of cord damage of each syndrome is presented in Figure 20.4. The corresponding clinical features of the different syndromes are explained by the anatomical organization of the motor and sensory pathways described earlier. Patients who are identified as having one of these syndromes should still

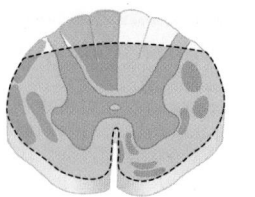

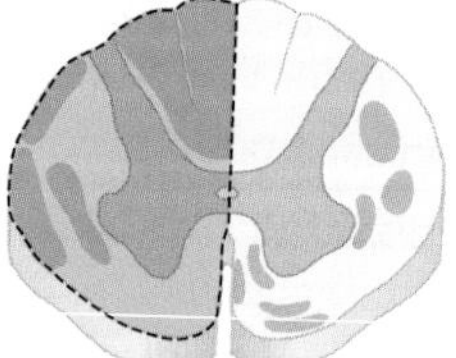

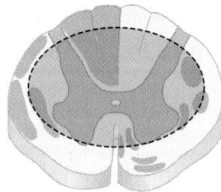

Figure 20.4 Areas of spinal cord damage in clinical syndromes.

receive a neurological, motor, and sensory-level designation and be assigned an AIS classification.

Brown-Sequard Syndrome

Brown-Sequard syndrome occurs from hemisection of the spinal cord (damage to one side) and is typically caused by penetration wounds—that is, gunshot or stab. Partial lesions (termed *Brown-Sequard plus syndrome*) occur more frequently; true hemisections are rare. The clinical features of this syndrome are asymmetrical. On the *ipsilateral* (same) side as the lesion, there is paralysis and sensory loss. The ipsilateral loss of proprioception, light touch, and vibratory sense is due to damage to the dorsal column; paralysis results from damage to the lateral corticospinal tract. Damage to the spinothalamic tracts results in loss of sense of pain and temperature on the side *contralateral* (opposite) to the lesion.[8] This loss begins several dermatome segments below the level of injury.[9] This discrepancy in levels and impairment on sides of the body occurs because the lateral spinothalamic tracts ascend two to four segments on the same side before crossing and the descending motor tract decussating in the medulla.[11,12] Individuals with Brown-Sequard syndrome typically achieve good functional gains during inpatient rehabilitation.[15]

Anterior Cord Syndrome

Anterior cord syndrome is frequently related to flexion injuries of the cervical region with resultant damage to the anterior portion of the cord and/or its vascular supply from the anterior spinal artery. There is typically compression of the anterior cord from fracture, dislocation, or cervical disk protrusion. This syndrome is characterized by loss of motor function (corticospinal tract damage) and loss of the sense of pain and temperature (spinothalamic tract damage) below the level of the lesion. Proprioception, light touch, and vibratory sense are generally preserved, because they are mediated by the dorsal columns with a separate vascular supply from the posterior spinal arteries.[12,15] Individuals with anterior cord syndrome often require a longer length of stay during inpatient rehabilitation compared to people with other types of SCI clinical syndromes.[15]

Central Cord Syndrome

Central cord syndrome is the most common SCI syndrome.[15] It generally occurs from hyperextension injuries to the cervical region.[16] It also has been associated with congenital or degenerative narrowing of the spinal canal. The resultant compressive forces give rise to hemorrhage and edema, producing damage to the most central aspects of the cord. There is characteristically more severe neurological involvement of the upper extremities (UEs) (cervical tracts are more centrally located) than of the LEs (lumbar and sacral tracts are located more peripherally).[15] Varying degrees of sensory impairment occur but tend to be less severe than motor deficits. With complete preservation of sacral tracts, normal sexual, bowel, and bladder function may be retained. Patients with central cord syndrome typically recover the ability to ambulate. Some distal UE weakness and loss of fine motor control remain, which can result in moderate to severe limitations in the ability to perform functional tasks.

Cauda Equina Injuries

The spinal cord tapers distally to form the conus medullaris at the lower border of the first lumbar vertebra. Although some anatomical variations exist, this is the typical termination point of the spinal cord. Below this level is the collection of long nerve roots known as the *cauda equina.* Complete transections in this area are rare. Cauda equina lesions are frequently anatomically incomplete owing to the great number of nerve roots involved and the comparatively large surface area they encompass (i.e., it would be unlikely that an injury to this region would involve the entire surface area and all the nerve roots).

Individuals with cauda equina injuries exhibit areflexic bowel and bladder and saddle anesthesia. Lower extremity paralysis and paresis is variable, depending on the extent of the injury to the cauda equina.[15] Cauda equina lesions are peripheral nerve (*lower motor neuron* [LMN]) injuries. As such, they have the same potential to regenerate as peripheral nerves elsewhere in the body. However, full return of innervation is not common because (1) there is a large distance between the lesion and the point of innervation; (2) axonal regeneration may not occur along the original distribution of the nerve; (3) axonal regeneration may be blocked by glial-collagen scarring; (4) the end organ may no longer be functioning once reinnervation occurs; and (5) the rate of regeneration slows and finally stops after about 1 year.

Conus medullaris syndrome occurs when the very distal portion of the spinal cord is damaged. This type of injury often results in a mixture of LMN and *upper motor neuron* (UMN) damage. ASIA has an excellent website with educational materials that provide more detail on the ISNCSCI (http://asia-spinalinjury.org).

IMPACT OF SPINAL CORD INJURY ACROSS THE ICF

Spinal cord injury results in a disruption of communication from higher centers in the central nervous system (CNS) to the periphery. This disruption results in many different body structure/function impairments, activity limitations, and participation restrictions.

Body Structure/Function Impairments

Spinal Shock

Immediately following SCI, there is a period of areflexia that is part of *spinal shock*. This period of transient reflex depression is not clearly understood.[17] It is believed to result from the very abrupt withdrawal of connections between higher centers and the spinal cord. It is characterized initially by an absence of all reflex activity and impairment of autonomic regulation, resulting in hypotension and loss of control of sweating and piloerection (goose bumps). In addition to the loss of deep tendon reflexes, there is a loss of the bulbocavernosus reflex, cremasteric reflex, Babinski response, and a delayed plantar response.

Spinal shock evolves over time. The initial period of total areflexia lasts approximately 24 hours. This is followed by a gradual return of reflexes 1 to 3 days after injury and a period of increasing hyperreflexia lasting 1 to 4 weeks.[17]

Motor and Sensory Impairments

Following SCI, there will be either complete (paralysis) or partial (paresis) loss of muscle function below the level of the lesion. Disruption of the ascending sensory fibers following SCI results in impaired or absent sensation below the level of the lesion.

The clinical presentation of motor and sensory impairments depends on the specific features of the lesion. These include the neurological level and the completeness of the lesion.

Autonomic Dysreflexia

Autonomic dysreflexia (AD), also referred to as autonomic hyperreflexia, is a pathological autonomic reflex that can be life-threatening. Typically, AD occurs in lesions above T6 (above the sympathetic splanchnic outflow).[18] However, it has been reported in patients with lower injuries. The incidence of AD is approximately 45%.[19,20] Although AD is more common in the chronic stage of recovery (more than 3 to 6 months after injury), it may also occur in the early stages after SCI.[21,22] It is more common with complete injury, but it may also occur with an incomplete SCI.[23]

This clinical syndrome produces an acute onset of autonomic activity from noxious stimuli below the level of the lesion. Afferent input from these stimuli reach the lower spinal cord (lower thoracic and sacral areas) and initiate a mass reflex response resulting in elevation of blood pressure. Normally, the impulses stimulate the receptors in the carotid sinus and aorta, which signal the vasomotor center to readjust peripheral resistance. Following SCI, however, impulses from the vasomotor center cannot pass the site of the lesion to counteract the hypertension by vasodilation.[24] This is a critical, emergency situation. Owing to the lack of inhibition from higher centers, hypertension will persist if not treated promptly. Hypertension triggered by AD can result in seizures, cardiac arrest, subarachnoid hemorrhage, stroke, or even death.[25]

Initiating Stimuli

The most common cause of this pathological reflex is bladder and bowel distention/irritation.[24] Common bladder issues that may trigger AD are distended bladder, blocked catheter, urinary tract infection, kidney stones, and irritation of bladder or urethra during catheterization or other procedures. Other precipitating stimuli include pressure injuries, noxious cutaneous stimuli below the level of the lesion, kidney malfunction, electrical stimulation below the level of the lesion, sexual activity, labor, and skeletal fracture below the level of the lesion.[24] Table 20.1 summarizes stimuli that may trigger an onset of AD, as well as common associated signs and symptoms.

Symptoms

The symptoms of AD include hypertension, bradycardia, headache (often severe and pounding), profuse sweating, increased spasticity, restlessness, vasoconstriction below the level of the lesion, vasodilation (flushing) above the level of the lesion, constricted pupils, nasal congestion, piloerection, and blurred vision.[24] Less commonly, AD may also present as asymptomatic. A rise in systolic blood pressure of 20 to 30 mm Hg is diagnostic of an episode of AD.[18] People with SCI typically have lower than normal resting blood pressure; systolic may be in the range of 90 to 110 mm Hg for those with neurological level above T6. During an episode of AD, systolic blood pressure may rise to 250 to 300 mm Hg and diastolic to 200 to 220 mm Hg.

Intervention

The onset of symptoms should be treated as a medical emergency. If lying flat, the patient should be brought to an upright position, inasmuch as blood pressure will be lowered in this position, and loosen any tight clothing or restrictive devices. Blood pressure and pulse should be monitored. The individual should be questioned as to possible triggers, starting with urinary system. Because bladder distention is a primary cause of AD, the drainage system should be examined first. If the patient is using an indwelling catheter, it should be checked to make sure it is not blocked. If any type of blockage is found, it should be removed immediately. If the patient

Table 20.1 Initiating Stimuli and Signs and Symptoms of Autonomic Dysreflexia

Initiating Stimuli	Signs and Symptoms
Bladder distention/irritation*	Hypertension (rise in systolic BP 20–30 mm Hg)
Bowel distention/irritation*	Bradycardia
Stimuli that would normally be painful below level of lesion	Severe headache
Gastrointestinal irritation	Feeling of anxiety
Sexual activity	Constricted pupils
Labor	Blurred vision
Skeletal fracture below level of injury	Flushing and piloerection above level of lesion
Electrical stimulation below level of lesion	Dry, pale skin below level of lesion (due to vasoconstriction)
	Nasal congestion
	Increased spasticity
	May be asymptomatic

*Most common triggers of AD.

catheterizes intermittently, a catheter should be placed and the bladder drained. The patient should then be questioned about when the last bowel movement occurred and checked for an impaction. The patient's body should be examined for triggering stimuli such as tight clothing, restricting catheter straps, abdominal binders, or anything that may be a noxious stimulus.[26]

If hypertension and other symptoms do not subside with the identification and elimination of specific triggers, medical and/or nursing assistance should be sought emergently. Antihypertensive medications are commonly prescribed to lower blood pressure acutely,[21,27] and clonidine is used in recurrent cases of AD.[27]

Education related to triggers, signs and symptoms, and management of AD is critical. One study found that 41% of people with SCI above T6 reported never having heard about AD, and 22% of those who did know about it did not know how to respond to an episode.[28] Because, in most cases, AD is not manifested until the patient is discharged from the hospital and in rehabilitation, people with SCI may no longer be in a health care setting when they first experience an episode. Those who are at risk of experiencing AD should be educated on initiating stimuli, symptoms, and management. The Consortium for Spinal Cord Medicine has developed clinical practice guidelines for acute management of AD that are available at the Paralyzed Veterans Association website (www.pva.org/CMSPages/GetFile.aspx?guid=2e9169c3-d2d9-4b4c-b3f1-c06f50aeba65).[26]

Spastic Hypertonia

Individuals with SCI and other CNS disorders such as traumatic brain injury, multiple sclerosis, and stroke often present with spastic hypertonia. Approximately 65% of people with SCI have spasticity, and it is more common in people with cervical-level injuries.[29] Spastic hypertonia is part of UMN syndrome, which encompasses a range of conditions, including spasticity, muscle spasms, abnormally high muscle tone, hyperactive stretch reflexes, and clonus.[30] These terms are sometimes used interchangeably in the literature. The classic definition of spasticity is a velocity-dependent increase in resistance to passive stretch.[31] Spastic hypertonia is thought to be a result of altered input at the spinal segmental level, which causes an imbalance between excitation and inhibition of the spinal motor neurons. Descending, suprasegmental signals are altered or eliminated following SCI, the anterior horn cell may become hyperexcitable, and there are changes in afferent input.[30]

Spastic hypertonia typically emerges below the level of the lesion after spinal shock evolves. There is a gradual increase in spastic hypertonia during the first 6 months, and a plateau is usually reached 1 year after injury. Various stimuli, including positional changes, cutaneous stimuli, environmental temperatures, tight clothing, bladder or kidney stones, fecal impactions, catheter blockage, urinary tract infections, decubitus ulcers, and emotional stress, may trigger or increase spasticity and muscle spasms.

Spasticity varies in the degree of severity. Approximately 50% of people with SCI report that their spasticity is problematic and negatively impacts their function.[29,32,33] Spasticity is also associated with poorer health.[34] Patients with minimal to moderate involvement may learn to trigger the spasticity or muscle spasm at appropriate times to assist in functional activities. However, strong spasticity can be a deterrent to independent function. For example, severe spasms during transfers may cause loss of balance and a fall. The management of spasticity must balance the potential benefits against the negative effects.

Spasticity is generally managed through a variety of methods, including stretch, modalities, and medications.[35-37] Although stretch is commonly used in the clinic, a systematic review found that stretch had no clinically important impact on spasticity in people with neurological conditions.[38] This may be due to the differences in how spasticity was measured and length of time and force used while providing the stretch between studies.

Medications typically used include muscle relaxants and spasmolytic agents such as baclofen,[30,32] tizanidine,[33] diazepam,[34] and dantrolene sodium.[34] Intrathecal baclofen (where an implanted pump delivers small amounts of baclofen directly at the spinal cord level to minimize side effects) can be used in cases of severe spasticity when individuals do not respond well to oral administration.[35] Intramuscular injection of botulinum neurotoxin can be used to manage focal spasticity.[36] Pharmacological management is often not successful in alleviating spasticity,[39] and its limited benefits must be weighed against potentially adverse side effects (e.g., weakness, dizziness, drowsiness). There is also some evidence that the use of antispasmodic medications may actually be associated with reduced recovery during inpatient rehabilitation.[40]

Cardiovascular Impairment

In healthy individuals with an intact spinal cord, cardiovascular function is regulated by the brain stem and hypothalamus via the sympathetic and parasympathetic nervous systems of the autonomic nervous system. Parasympathetic signals to the heart arise from the vagus nerve, decreasing heart rate and contractility. Sympathetic outflow comes from spinal segments T1 to L2 through the sympathetic trunk, increasing heart rate and heart contractility and peripheral vasoconstriction.[41] More specifically, sympathetic outflow to the heart and blood vessels of the upper body comes from the cervical and upper thoracic region (above T6), while sympathetic outflow to blood vessels of the lower body come from below T5 (T6–L2). Thus, a higher SCI (above T6) will result in loss of sympathetic control to the heart and blood vessels below the level of the injury and intact parasympathetic input to the heart. An SCI at T6 and below has intact sympathetic and parasympathetic control to the heart but loss of sympathetic control to the blood vessels below the level of the injury. The resulting imbalance between sympathetic and parasympathetic control of the cardiovascular system can result in a variety of cardiovascular impairments.[41,42] These include AD (discussed above), neurogenic shock, bradyarrhythmias, hypotension, orthostatic hypotension, and impaired cardiovascular reflexes.[42]

A rostral SCI (above T6) may result in neurogenic shock because sympathetic output to the heart is lacking and vagal (parasympathetic) input is unopposed. Neurogenic shock is defined as systolic blood pressure below 100 mm Hg and heart rate below 80 beats per minute. Neurogenic shock results in bradyarrhythmias, atrioventricular conduction block, and hypotension. Neurogenic shock may resolve in weeks post-injury.[41] Acutely, patients may experience bradycardia (heart rate below 50). This is more likely in individuals with cervical and upper thoracic–level injuries.[41,42]

Because of the disrupted balance between sympathetic and parasympathetic input (bradycardia, hypotension, heart rate response, and dilation of the peripheral vasculature below the level of the lesion), as well as a lack of or decrease in active muscle contraction and prolonged time in bed, orthostatic hypotension is often experienced early after injury. Symptoms of orthostatic hypotension include blurred vision, ringing in the ears, light-headedness, and fainting. Orthostatic hypotension is usually only significant in people with SCI above T6. Although the exact mechanism is not clearly understood, the cardiovascular system, over time, gradually reestablishes sufficient vasomotor tone to allow assumption of the vertical position.[43,39]

To minimize these effects when mobilizing patients early after SCI, the cardiovascular system should be allowed to adapt gradually by a slow progression to the vertical position. This frequently begins with elevation of the head of the bed and progresses to a reclining wheelchair with elevating legrests and use of a standing frame or tilt table. Vital signs should be monitored carefully. Use of compressive stockings, ace wraps on the LEs, and an abdominal binder may further minimize these effects.[44] Pharmacological therapy may be indicated (e.g., ephedrine to increase blood pressure or low-dose diuretics to relieve persistent edema of legs, ankles, or feet). As vasomotor stability returns, tolerance to the vertical position will gradually improve.

Past the acute stage of injury, people with SCI below or within the thoracolumbar sympathetic output will exhibit a reduced exercise tolerance, lower stroke volume, and reduced cardiac output.[45,46] Individuals with cervical SCI are likely to demonstrate a lower peak heart rate, post-exercise hypotension, and other abnormal cardiovascular responses to exercise.[47,48] Deconditioning often occurs due to physical inactivity and an impaired cardiovascular system. A regular cardiovascular fitness exercise program is an important component of rehabilitation. Programs should be designed based on the level of injury and include careful patient monitoring.[46]

Impaired Temperature Control

After damage to the spinal cord, the hypothalamus can no longer control cutaneous blood flow or level of sweating. This autonomic (sympathetic) dysfunction results in loss of internal thermoregulatory responses. The ability to shiver below the level of the injury is also lost. The degree of impaired thermoregulation will vary depending on the level of the injury and whether the injury is complete or incomplete. Individuals with cervical-level injuries and complete injuries demonstrate more impairment. Initially after injury, hypothermia may occur due to peripheral vasodilation. Later, hyperthermia is more likely due to the lack of sympathetic control of sweat glands. Although some improvement in thermoregulatory responses occurs over time, patients with tetraplegia typically experience long-term impairment of body temperature regulation, especially in response to extreme environmental changes.

Pulmonary Impairment

Ventilatory and respiratory function varies considerably, depending on the level of lesion. As with other impairments following SCI, the more rostral the injury, the greater impact on function. Pulmonary complications are a leading cause of death both in the early and late stages of recovery.[1,49]

The primary muscle of inspiration is the diaphragm. The scalenes and intercostals also play important roles by stabilizing and elevating the ribs. Other important accessory and stabilizing muscles of inspiration are the sternocleidomastoid, serratus anterior, pectoralis major and minor, serratus posterior superior, trapezius, levator scapulae, and abdominals. The primary muscles of expiration are the abdominals and internal intercostals. Normally, relaxed expiration is essentially a passive process that occurs through elastic recoil of the lungs and thorax. However, the abdominals and internal intercostals contribute several important functions related to movement of air out of the lungs. Loss of these muscles significantly decreases expiratory efficiency. Control of the abdominal muscles originates from T6–T12. When fully innervated, they play an important role in maintaining intrathoracic pressure for effective respiration. They support the abdominal viscera and assist in maintaining the position of the diaphragm. They also function to push the diaphragm upward during forced expiration. With paralysis of the abdominal musculature, this support is lost, causing the diaphragm to assume an unusually low position. This lowered position and lack of abdominal pressure to move the diaphragm upward during forced expiration results in a decreased expiratory reserve volume. This subsequently decreases cough effectiveness and the ability to expel secretions. Table 20.2 presents the level of innervation of inspiratory and expiratory muscles in relation to level of SCI.[12,50-53]

With high spinal cord lesions at C1 and C2, phrenic nerve innervation and spontaneous respiration are lost. The only muscles of respiration that are intact are accessory muscles of inspiration: sternocleidomastoid and upper trapezius. An artificial ventilator or phrenic nerve stimulator is required to sustain life. Expiration is passive; as a result, individuals with SCI at these levels require assistance for airway clearance. C3- and C4-level injuries have partial diaphragm innervation, as well as scalenes and levator scapulae function. In the acute stage of recovery, individuals with an injury at these levels will require mechanical ventilation. With recovery and training, they will likely be able to breathe on their own.[54] However, they may need part-time ventilatory support, especially individuals with C3-level injury. These individuals do not have innervation to muscles of expiration (abdominals or intercostals), so they will need assistance for airway clearance.

Patients with mid to lower cervical-level injuries have better pulmonary function than those with higher cervical-level injuries. Injuries at C5–C8 have a fully innervated diaphragm, as well as many accessory muscles of inspiration. They are not likely to require ventilator support. However, forced expiration is severely impaired. Although some cough ability is preserved, it is usually weak.

Although individuals with paraplegia have better respiratory function than people with tetraplegia, they still have impaired respiratory function compared to healthy

Table 20.2 Innervation of Muscles of Inspiration and Expiration

Level of Spinal Cord Injury	Inspiratory Muscles* (Innervation)	Forced Expiratory Muscles* (Innervation)
C1–2	Sternocleidomastoid and upper trapezius (accessory cranial nerve)	
C3–C4	Partial diaphragm (C3–C5), levator scapulae (C3–C5), scalenes (C3–C8)	
C5	Diaphragm (C3–C5)	Pectoralis major—clavicular (C5–6)
C6–8	Pectoralis major—sternal (C7–T1), pectoralis minor (C6–T1), serratus anterior (C5–C7)	
T1–T5	Intercostals (T1–T11), serratus posterior superior (T1–T3)	Intercostals (T1–T11)
T6–T10	Abdominals (T6–L1)	Abdominals (T6–L1), serratus posterior inferior (T9–T12)
T11 and below	All of the above	All of the above, quadratus lumborum (T12–L4)

*Lower-level SCI have intact innervation to muscles above level of SCI. There are slight differences among sources in regards to muscle innervation levels.

individuals without an SCI.[55] Individuals with weak or absent abdominal and intercostal musculature will have impaired airway clearance ability and be at a greater risk for developing pneumonia and atelectasis.

Other factors may further impair respiratory status. Additional trauma sustained at the time of injury, premorbid respiratory problems, age, weight, and smoking history can all further compromise respiratory function.[55,56]

Bladder and Bowel Impairment

Bladder Dysfunction

The effects of bladder dysfunction following SCI pose a serious medical complication requiring consistent and long-term management. Urinary tract infections (UTIs) are a major cause of mortality and morbidity in people with SCI. Forty percent of people with SCI report having a UTI 1 year after injury.[20] Spinal cord injury alters the complex reflexive and voluntary control of *micturition*. As a result, people with SCI often require a catheter to drain the bladder.

Spinal control for micturition originates from the sacral segments of S2, S3, and S4.[12] The level of the SCI dictates the type of bladder dysfunction. Patients with lesions that occur above the conus medullaris and sacral segments develop a *spastic* or *hyperreflexic bladder*.[12] This is also termed a *UMN bladder*. Following a lesion of the sacral segments or conus medullaris, a *flaccid* or *areflexic bladder* develops.[12] This is also termed an *LMN bladder*.

A spastic or hyperreflexic bladder (UMN lesion) contracts and reflexively empties in response to a certain level of filling pressure.[57] The reflex arc is intact with this type of injury. The detrusor muscle is generally hyperreflexive. There can be increased tone of the sphincter, contraction of the detrusor with small urine volumes, and lack of coordination between detrusor and sphincters (dyssynergia). A flaccid or areflexive bladder (LMN lesion) is essentially flaccid because there is no reflex action of the detrusor muscle.

There are generally two types of bladder dysfunction: failure to store urine and failure to empty urine.[57] These can be due to detrusor muscle or sphincter impairment. Inability to store urine may be due to an areflexive sphincter or spastic detrusor muscle. Inability to empty the bladder sufficiently may be due to an areflexive bladder or a sphincter that is unable to relax. Dyssynergia between the detrusor and sphincter can also cause incomplete drainage of the bladder.[57]

Bladder Management

The primary goal of bladder management is to prevent or minimize urinary tract complications. These include UTIs, *hydronephrosis* (swelling of kidney due to backup of urine), renal calculi, bladder calculi, and *vesicoureteral reflux* (backward flow of urine up the ureter).[57] Because urinary incontinence has very strong psychosocial implications for the patient, a coordinated approach to this problem is particularly important. Knowledge of and participation in the bladder management program is an important consideration for the physical therapist.

In the early stage of recovery, while the patient is still in spinal shock, the bladder is flaccid and an indwelling catheter is inserted. After the patient is stable during rehabilitation, the most frequently used method of bladder management is *intermittent catheterization*.[57,58] Briefly stated, the program involves establishing a fluid intake pattern of approximately 2,000 mL/day. Intake is stopped late in the day to reduce the need for catheterization during the night. Initially, the patient is catheterized every 4 hours. A record is maintained of voided and residual urine. While in the hospital, sterile intermittent catheterization should be done; after discharge, a clean technique is often used.

Although intermittent catheterization is the most common method of bladder management after discharge from the rehabilitation hospital, many males switch to the use of an external condom catheter.[58] Other methods of bladder management include suprapubic tapping and the Valsalva maneuver. *Suprapubic tapping* involves tapping directly over the bladder with fingertips, causing a reflexive emptying of the bladder. This technique only works for individuals with an UMN bladder without dyssynergia between the detrusor and sphincter, because the sphincter must open for the bladder to reflexively drain.[57,58] Individuals with an areflexive bladder can use the *Valsalva maneuver*, which is done by straining.[57,58] Some individuals may elect to use an indwelling, suprapubic catheter.[59]

The exact method or combination of methods used for bladder management will depend on a variety factors: type of bladder dysfunction, level of injury, functional ability, and personal preference. Whichever method(s) is used, the goal is for the patient to be catheter free, have low postvoid residual volume of urine in the bladder, and be without high bladder pressure during voiding.[60] Urodynamic testing is done after spinal shock resolves, approximately 3 months after injury, to help diagnose the specific type of bladder dysfunction and guide the selection of management strategies.

Because of impaired bladder function, over 60% of people with SCI will develop UTIs in the first year postinjury.[20] Further urinary system complications linked to chronic UTIs are development of bladder and kidney stones and kidney dysfunction.

Bowel Dysfunction

As with bladder dysfunction, bowel dysfunction is a major concern after SCI. Over 98% of people with SCI report problems with bowel care and 34% require some level of assistance with bowel care.[61] People with SCI report that bowel function has a greater impact on daily life than many other impairments after SCI, including sexual function, bladder function, pain, spasticity, and skin integrity.[61-63] Bowel function also has a large impact on social activities and quality of life.[62] Neurogenic bowel conditions that develop after spinal shock subsides are of two main types. In spinal cord lesions above S2, there is a *spastic* or *reflex bowel* (UMN lesion). Because the parasympathetic and internal sphincter connections from S2–S4 are intact, reflex defecation can occur when the rectum fills with stool. In S2–S4 or cauda equina (peripheral nerves) lesions, a *flaccid* or *areflexive bowel* (LMN lesion) develops. With an areflexive bowel, the parasympathetic connections from S2–S4 are not intact, so the bowel will not reflexively empty. This can cause feces to become impacted and, because the external sphincter is flaccid, incontinence can occur.[57]

Bowel Management

Safety and an appropriate, well-timed bowel care routine are common goals for bowel management. Safety includes continence in order to maintain intact and healthy skin, prevent damage to colorectal structures, and prevent AD due to bowel dysfunction.[60] In addition to type of neurogenic bowel (UMN or LMN), the bowel care program will also depend on presence of other health conditions that may affect gastrointestinal function, medications, dietary habits, fluid intake, and functional ability.[57] A typical bowel program involves establishing a daily (or every other day) pattern of eliciting a bowel movement. The exact time of day is chosen by the patient based on lifestyle needs and should be done consistently at the same time of day. This is usually in the morning or late evening. People with a reflex bowel require the use of suppositories and digital stimulation techniques to cause a reflex defecation. Digital stimulation involves manual stretch of the anal sphincter, either with a lubricated gloved finger or an orthotic digital stimulator. This stretch stimulates peristalsis of the colon and evacuation of the rectum (mediated by S2, S3, and S4).[57] Valsalva maneuver and abdominal massage may also be performed. Nonreflex bowel management relies on manual evacuation techniques and gentle Valsalva.[57] Other factors that can play a role in maintaining a consistent, safe bowel program include eating a diet with appropriate amount of fiber, fluid intake, physical activity, stool softeners, laxatives, and bulking agents.

Sexual Dysfunction

Sexuality encompasses much more than just the physical ability to have sexual intercourse. It is an important part of an individual's makeup and sense of self-esteem. Spinal cord injury not only affects the physiological ability to have intercourse but also the psychosocial aspect of sexuality. People with paraplegia report that improved sexual function is the primary factor that would improve their quality of life. For people with tetraplegia, it is the second most important after regaining hand function.[63] Education so that the patient can fully understand the impact of SCI on sexual function and psychosocial support so the patient can become confident in his or her new sexuality are an important part of rehabilitation.

Male Response

Sexual response is directly related to level and completeness of injury. As with bowel and bladder function, sexual capabilities are broadly divided between UMN (damage to the cord above S2–S4) and LMN lesions. Generally speaking, erectile capacity is greater in UMN lesions than in LMN lesions and greater in incomplete lesions than in complete lesions. There are two types of erections: reflexogenic and psychogenic. *Reflexogenic erections* occur in response to external physical stimulation of the genitals or perineum. An intact reflex arc is required (mediated through S2, S3, and S4). *Psychogenic erections* occur through cognitive activity such as erotic fantasy. They are mediated from the cerebral cortex either through the thoracolumbar or sacral cord centers.[12,57] Medications such as Viagra, Levitra, and Cialis; injectable medications that relax penile smooth muscle; topical agents; and mechanical devices can also be used to improve erectile function.[57,64,65]

There is a higher incidence of ability to ejaculate with LMN lesions than with UMN lesions and incomplete as compared with complete lesions.[57] Historically, relatively few patients with SCI were able to sire children. This low level of fertility was associated with impaired spermatogenesis and an inability to ejaculate. However, vibratory stimulation and electroejaculation may improve ejaculatory response and promote higher semen quality for fertility purposes.[65]

Female Response

Female sexual responses also follow a pattern related to location of lesion. In patients with UMN lesions, the reflex arc remains intact. Therefore, components of sexual arousal (vaginal lubrication, engorgement of the labia, and clitoral erection) will likely occur through reflexogenic stimulation, but psychogenic response will be lost. Conversely, with LMN lesions, psychogenic responses will most likely be preserved and reflex responses lost.[57]

Fertility is not affected as severely in women as men with SCI. The menstrual cycle typically is interrupted for a period of 4 to 5 months following injury. After this time, normal menses return and the potential for conception remains unimpaired.[57] Women with SCI who want to bear children should be closely supervised during pregnancy. They are more likely to encounter complications during pregnancy and childbirth than woman without SCI. Problems include UTIs, anemia, and venous thrombosis.[66] Labor and delivery must be monitored. Depending on the neurological level of injury, the woman may not feel labor. There is a risk of AD during labor. See review by Smeltzer and Wetzel-Effinger[67] for an in-depth review of pregnancy in women with SCI.

As with men with SCI, there is little information available on the impact of SCI on orgasm in women.

Women with SCI appear to be less likely to achieve orgasm than women without SCI and those with LMN are less likely to achieve orgasm than those with UMN.[57]

A major consideration for the physical therapist regarding sexual dysfunction is that a patient will often direct questions to the individuals with whom he or she feels most comfortable. It is not uncommon for such a discussion to arise during a physical therapy session. These questions or issues should be addressed openly and honestly. In addition, the therapist must anticipate and be prepared for these situations by (1) obtaining accurate information about the patient's physiological state and anticipated sexual function and (2) having knowledge of referral options and support services available to the patient for appropriate examination and counseling.

Pain

Pain is a common occurrence following SCI both in the acute and chronic stages of recovery.[68-70] Between 26% and 96% of people with SCI report having chronic pain.[71] Pain can limit the performance of activities of daily living (ADL), affect sleep, and contribute to a lower quality of life.[72,73] Pain can be grossly divided into two broad categories: *nociceptive pain* and *neuropathic pain.* Nociceptive pain can be musculoskeletal or visceral in origin. Neuropathic pain can be below, at, or above the level of injury.[74]

Nociceptive Pain

Shoulder pain and pain in other UE joints and soft tissue is common in people with SCI.[75,76] Musculoskeletal injuries are often due to overuse or poor posture and commonly occur in the shoulder, wrist, or elbow joints involving capsule, tendon, ligament, and muscle tissue.[77] A variety of factors can cause musculoskeletal pain: mechanical injury to soft and bony tissue structures, inflammation, and muscle spasm. Muscular imbalances in the shoulder girdle, poor seated posture in a wheelchair, decreased flexibility, incorrect positioning in bed, older age, and higher body mass index (BMI) can all contribute to shoulder pain.[76] Overuse musculoskeletal injuries can be due to repetitive stress from propelling a wheelchair while in a biomechanically poor position, increased weight-bearing on the UEs while transferring or using pressure-relief techniques, and using assistive device(s) during ambulation or to improve function. Specific musculoskeletal injuries that may occur are biceps tendinitis, lateral epicondylitis, shoulder impingement, rotator cuff tears, carpal tunnel syndrome, and wrist tendonitis.[77]

Neuropathic Pain

Neuropathic pain is caused by injury to the central or peripheral nervous system. It can occur below, at, or above the level of the spinal cord lesion. Neuropathic pain below the level of the lesion is due to spinal cord damage and may take the form of *allodynia* (central pain in response to a normal non-painful stimulation) or *hyperalgesia* (increased sensitivity to pain caused by damage to nociceptors). Damage to nerve roots or the spinal cord may be the cause of neuropathic pain at the level of the lesion. Neuropathic pain at the level of the lesion may also take the form of allodynia or hyperalgesia. Neuropathic pain above the level of the lesion is likely due to peripheral nerve damage associated with nerve impingement or compression. Neuropathic pain may be burning, shooting, or sharp. This type of pain below the level of the lesion is diffuse.[74]

Neuropathic pain is particularly challenging to treat and no single intervention option has established efficacy.[78,79] Nonpharmacological options include transcutaneous electrical nerve stimulation, massage, acupuncture, and mental imagery.[80] Pharmacological interventions commonly used are anticonvulsants such as gabapentin (Neurontin), pregabalin (Lyrica), and valproic acid (Depakote, Valparin); the antidepressant amitriptyline (Elavil, Vanatrip); and analgesics such as tramadol (Rybix, Ultram).[78,81] Chapter 25, Chronic Pain, provides an in-depth discussion of different types of pain, as well as interventions for pain management.

Secondary and Other Impairments

Individuals with SCI are at great risk for secondary impairments throughout their life because of prolonged immobilization and the wide-ranging effects of the SCI on multiple body systems. One year after injury, common secondary complications include pressure injuries, heterotopic ossification, deep vein thrombosis, and musculoskeletal injuries.[20]

Contractures

Contractures develop secondary to prolonged shortening of structures across and around a joint, resulting in limitation in motion. Contractures initially produce alterations in muscle tissue but progress to involve capsular and pericapsular changes. Lack of active muscle function eliminates the normal reciprocal stretching of a muscle group and surrounding structures as the opposing muscle contracts. In addition, spasticity, positioning in wheelchair or bed for prolonged periods of time, and abnormal muscle tone are all factors that place people with SCI at a high risk for developing contractures. All joints are at risk for contractures. Contractures of the ankle, knee, hip, elbow, and shoulder joints may have significant negative impact on a person's ability to perform important activities and participate in valued social roles. Contractures may also be painful, make positioning and hygiene difficult, and lead to skin breakdown. The most important management consideration related to the potential development of contractures is prevention. Once contractures have developed, it is extremely difficult to reverse the process.[38] A consistent and concurrent program of range of motion (ROM) exercises, positioning, and splinting is important to maintain joint motion and prevent contracture.

Heterotopic (Ectopic) Ossification

Heterotopic ossification (HO) is osteogenesis in soft tissues, usually near joints, below the level of the lesion. The etiology of this abnormal bone growth is unknown. The incidence of HO ranges from 10% to 53%.[82] Factors associated with HO include complete injury, trauma, severe spasticity, UTI, and pressure injuries.[83,84] Care should be taken while performing passive range of motion (PROM). If it is too vigorous, it may cause trauma, which may be a causative factor for HO. It most often occurs in the hip and knee joints. Early symptoms of HO include swelling, joint and muscle pain, decreased ROM, erythema, and local warmth near a joint.[85] Heterotopic ossification can lead to contractures, pressure injuries, impaired mobility, and compromised ability to perform ADLs.

Management of ectopic bone formation utilizes several approaches, including pharmacological management, physical therapy (maintaining ROM), and, with severe activity limitations, surgery. NSAIDs are effective in preventing the formation of HO. Bisphosphonates are an effective pharmacological intervention but are most effective when used early when radiographs may still be normal.[85] Pulsed low-intensity electromagnetic field may also be an effective method to prevent HO formation. Finally, surgical excision is used when HO causes extreme limitations in activities and social participation.

Osteoporosis and Skeletal Fracture

Individuals with SCI may experience significant loss of bone both early after injury and long-term. There is a rapid bone mineral loss in the first 4 to 6 months after injury. Bone mineral density (BMD) continues to decrease up to 3 years after injury; however, this may continue longer.[86,87] Although the exact etiology is not clear, the reduction in bone mineral density is thought to be due primarily to a combination of no (or limited) muscle action and limited (or no) weight-bearing.[86,87] It is most common in the LEs, although osteoporosis may also occur in the UEs in people with cervical SCIs.

The reduction in BMD places people with SCI at a significant risk for fracture. Fracture incidence may be as high as 46%.[86] Risk factors for fracture include being female, having a lower BMI, complete injury, paraplegia versus tetraplegia, and longer time since injury.[86,87] Falls or a forced maneuver during a transfer, ADL such as dressing, and stretching are common activities that precipitate a fracture. The onset of a fracture can also be nontraumatic.[88] Intervention strategies focus on prevention in the early stage after injury or limiting/reversing BMD loss once osteoporosis has begun. Bisphosphonate is used in the early and later stages to prevent and reduce BMD loss.[86] Rehabilitation strategies used to prevent or reduce BMD loss are functional electrical stimulation and weight-bearing activities with either a standing frame or orthotics and assistive devices. The effectiveness of these rehabilitation interventions is not fully established.[86,87] This may be associated with study designs that did not have subjects standing for long enough and/or standing without sufficient loading on the LEs.

Activity Limitations, Participation Restrictions, and Quality of Life

As discussed below in the section on outcomes and goals, the neurological level of injury and whether the injury is complete or incomplete plays a major role in determining an individual's independence with functional mobility tasks and ADL. Spinal cord injury has a large impact on employability. At 1 year post-SCI, 2% of people were employed. By 20 years post-injury, this increased to 34%.[1] Individuals who had a college degree prior to injury or who were injured at a younger age are more likely to be employed after their injury.[89,90] Reported barriers to employment are transportation; health and physical limitations; lack of experience, education, or training; environmental barriers, discrimination, and loss of benefits.[90] Generally, people with SCI report a lower quality of life (QOL) compared to nondisabled individuals. However, QOL is not consistently related to severity of injury and activity limitations.[91] Individuals with cervical and lower levels of SCI report similar levels of health-related QOL as measured by the SF-36.[92]

PROGNOSIS FOR RECOVERY OF WALKING AND MOTOR FUNCTION

One of the most common questions that patients and families have after an SCI is how much recovery of motor function will occur and will the individual be able to walk again. The potential for recovery from SCI is directly related to the neurological level of the lesion and completeness of the injury.[93] An incomplete lesion (AIS B, C, or D) is a good prognostic indicator of recovery of motor function (see Box 20.1).[94,95] Patients with an AIS impairment A are unlikely to regain the ability to walk, approximately 33% of patients with AIS B, 65% of patients with AIS C, and almost 100% of patients with AIS D regain some ability to walk.[93,96] However, even with complete lesions (AIS A), 70% of patients with cervical-level injuries are likely to experience one level of motor recovery below the original neurological level.[97]

Preservation of pinprick sensation after injury in the LEs or sacral region is associated with a good prognosis for motor recovery and walking ability at 1 year after injury.[98,99] Lower-extremity ASIA motor score, quadriceps and gastrocnemius strength in particular, can be a useful predictor of functional walking ability in people with motor incomplete injuries. The *European Multicenter*

Study on Human Spinal Cord Injury has published a clinical prediction rule for predicting ambulation after SCI.[100] In a cohort study of almost 500 patients, findings indicated that age, motor scores of quadriceps and gastrocnemius, and light touch sensory scores at L3 and S1 were able to accurately distinguish between independent home ambulators and those who require assistance or cannot ambulate. The clinical prediction rule was 96% accurate. As with any clinical prediction guide, it is important to keep in mind that these factors should only be used as a *guide* to assist in the development of goals and the POC. Other factors such as psychosocial support, insurance coverage, and patient psychological status and motivation can affect outcomes. Additionally, new therapies may be developed that improve neurological recovery. Recovery of motor function generally plateaus around 12 to 18 months after injury.[95,101]

EARLY MEDICAL MANAGEMENT

Emergency Care

Management of SCI begins at the location of the accident. Techniques used in stabilizing, moving, and managing the patient immediately following the trauma can influence prognosis and recovery of motor function. Rescue personnel must be adept at questioning and examining for signs of SCI before moving the individual. Signs of SCI after a traumatic event include paresthesias, lack of or impaired movement or sensation in the extremities, spinal pain, and altered cognitive status or level of alertness. When an SCI is suspected, efforts should be made to avoid both active and passive movements of the spine. If the injury caused a displaced fracture, further damage to the spinal cord can occur. Movement of the spine is minimized by strapping the patient to a spinal backboard or a full-body adjustable backboard, using a supporting cervical collar, immobilizing the head, and obtaining assistance from multiple personnel in moving the patient to safety.[102] These measures assist in maintaining the spine in a neutral, anatomical position and may prevent further neurological damage.

On arrival at the emergency department, initial attention is focused on stabilizing the patient medically with a primary emphasis on ventilation and circulation. Cardiac, hemodynamic, and respiratory status are closely monitored.[102,103] Diagnosis of SCI is based on the physical examination, neurological assessment, and imaging.[103] A complete neurological examination is performed once the patient is stabilized. Imaging studies assist in determining the extent of damage and plans for medical management. Attention is directed toward preventing progression of neurological impairment by restoration of vertebral alignment and early immobilization of the fracture site. A urinary catheter typically is inserted, and secondary injuries are addressed.

High doses of methylprednisolone had previously been used early after injury with the intention of reducing edema and improving motor recovery.[104-107] However, its use has been called into question. More recent studies find that the use of steroids early after injury does not lead to improved motor or functional outcomes.[108,109] Also, there may be serious complications associated with taking high doses of steroids over a prolonged time.[110,111] Current guidelines do not advocate for routine use of steroids.[108,109,112,113] Local and systemic hypothermia have also been studied as an intervention to reduce secondary damage and provide neuroprotection to the spinal cord early after injury and improve outcomes.[114,115] The evidence suggests that local and systemic hypothermia is safe, but further research is needed to establish the effectiveness and optimal dosage.

Fracture Stabilization

The goal of fracture/spinal injury site management is to stabilize the spinal column to prevent further damage to the cord. Reduction and immobilization of spinal injuries can be achieved via conservative or operative methods. Indications for surgical stabilization are unstable fracture site, gross malalignment, cord compression, and deteriorating neurological status. In people with acute, traumatic SCI, early (within 24 hours) surgical decompression and stabilization is recommended. Approximately 60% of patients with SCI admitted to model SCI system centers underwent surgical stabilization.[116] Closed reduction is indicated for patients with cervical subluxation or fracture dislocation injuries. It is achieved with the use of traction devices. Patients with thoracic or lumbar injuries that are managed conservatively without surgery require immobilization by positioning in a regular or rotating bed.

Immobilization

Following reduction of the fracture site, through either conservative or surgical means, the spine is immobilized for a period of time through the use of spinal orthoses and recumbent positioning. *Halos* are used commonly to immobilize cervical fractures after both open and closed reduction. This spinal orthosis (Fig. 20.5) consists of a halo ring with four steel screws that attach directly to the outer skull. The halo is attached to a body jacket or vest by four vertical steel posts. A halo is extremely effective at limiting cervical motion in all planes. The most common complication of a halo orthosis is loosening of the pin site. This can create instability at the injury site in the vertebral column and/or be a sign of infection. Skin breakdown may also occur under the vest portion of the halo.

Although a halo is an effective means of immobilizing and protecting the injury site, it can make learning mobility skills even more challenging. The orthosis limits shoulder motion and changes the user's center of gravity. This may cause patients to feel unstable. It can also make bed and wheelchair positioning difficult.

The *Minerva* is another type of cervical orthosis (CO) that also effectively limits motion in all planes. Like the

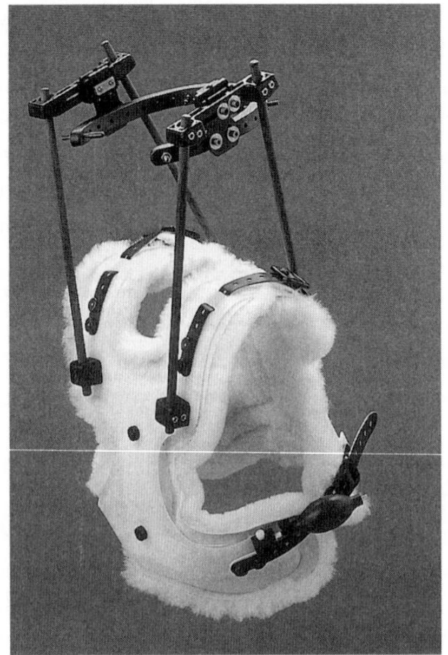

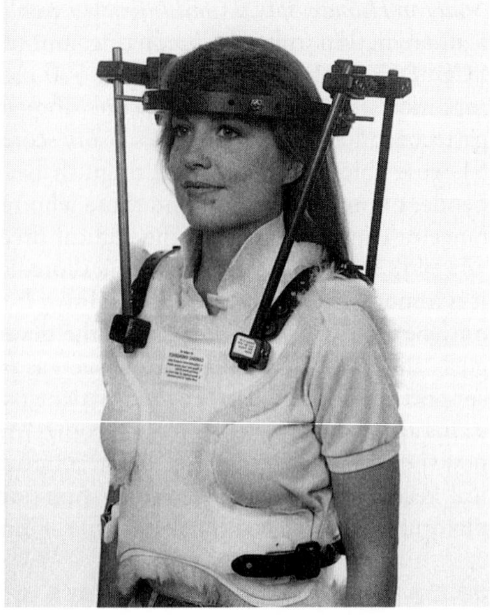

Figure 20.5 Halo orthosis.
(Courtesy of PMT Corp., Chanhassen, MN 55317.)

halo, because it provides excellent cervical stability, the Minerva allows for early mobility and rehabilitation after SCI. The sterno–occipital–mandibular immobilizer is another type of CO. It is less effective in limiting cervical ROM than either the halo or Minerva. There are also a variety of cervical collars that can be used. Generally, these are constructed of semi-rigid foam and plastic and consist of two halves, which are held together with hook-and-loop closures. They do not effectively immobilize the spine. However, they may be used as transitional support following removal of a more rigid device (e.g., halo). Common types of collars include Philadelphia collar, Miami J collar, Aspen collar, and foam soft collar.

A thoracolumbosacral orthosis (TLSO) is commonly used to immobilize the spine in patients with thoracic or lumbar injuries. A TLSO is made by an orthotist who takes a cast of the patient's trunk and makes the molded body jacket from the impression. Body jackets are typically bivalved and connected by hook-and-loop closures, which allows for removal during bathing and skin inspection. An extension is necessary with high thoracic injuries and low lumbar injuries in order to provide effective immobilization of the spine in these areas. A Jewett orthosis is a prefabricated device made of a metal frame and pads. The Jewett orthosis is not as effective for immobilizing the spine as a body jacket. See Chapter 30, Orthotics, for a more in-depth discussion.

PHYSICAL THERAPY MANAGEMENT EARLY AFTER INJURY

While hospitalized during the acute stage of recovery, the patient may be on a period of bed rest and immobilization. However, physical therapy and early mobility should begin once the surgeon has cleared the patient for activity. The primary goals of physical therapy during this early stage of recovery are to begin early mobilization, prevent secondary complications, and provide patient education.

Physical Therapy Examination

Before beginning the initial examination, the patient and fracture site must be sufficiently stable to undergo the examination and the therapist must be aware of any precautions. Spinal instability, orthotic devices, concomitant injuries, and need for medical support (e.g., ventilator) may preclude certain movements or positions. During this early stage of recovery, the examination focuses on sensory and motor function, respiratory function, skin integrity, PROM, and performance of early mobility skills.

Motor and Sensory Function

Motor and sensory function should be assessed using the ISNCSCI to determine the level of neurological injury (see Fig. 20.3). Care should be taken when performing MMT, particularly if the spine is not yet stabilized or fully healed after surgery. Forceful contraction of muscles that originate from the spine may cause instability at the fracture site. Discretion should be used in applying resistance around the shoulders in tetraplegia and around the lower trunk and hips in paraplegia. However, if the surgeon has indicated that the fracture site is stable after surgery, then these precautions are not likely needed. In addition to testing the key muscles identified in the ISNCSCI, other muscle groups should be tested throughout the myotomes that have intact innervation. For example, if the C5 myotome is intact as indicated by normal strength in the biceps, then the strength of other muscles such as the deltoids and supraspinatus that are innervated by the C5 nerve root should also be determined. Standard techniques should be used for the manual muscle testing and examination of sensation (see Chapter 3, Examination of Sensory Function). Any alteration in testing position or procedure should be recorded. Reflexes should also be tested (see Reflex Integrity section below).

Respiratory

The physical therapist should assess the strength of the diaphragm and intercostal muscles through observation while the patient is breathing. Normally, the epigastric region should rise and the chest wall expands during inhalation while in supine. Contractions of the sternocleidomastoids and scalenes or paradoxical breathing patterns indicate weakness or lack of innervation of the diaphragm or intercostal muscles. Respiratory rate should be assessed while the patient is unaware that it is being done. Normal respiratory rate is between 12 and 20 breathes per minute. To compensate for a weak diaphragm, the respiratory rate will typically increase.

Maximal chest excursion can be assessed using a tape measure with the patient supine. At both the level of the axilla and xiphoid process, the physical therapist should measure the chest's diameter at maximal exhalation and inhalation. Chest expansion measurements are the difference between chest measurements at maximal exhalation and at maximal inhalation. Normal chest expansion ranges from 2.5 to 3 in. (6.35 to 7.62 cm), and negative values are an indication of paradoxical chest motions.

Vital capacity (VC) should be measured during the early stages of recovery. Vital capacity can be measured with a handheld spirometer and is strongly related to other measures of pulmonary function.[117] Forced vital capacity and volume of pulmonary secretion and gas exchange are predictive of airway management.[118] Typically, VC is approximately less than 25% of normal in individuals with high cervical lesions (above C3), 25% to 50% in mid cervical lesions, 50% to 75% in lower cervical and upper thoracic lesions, and 70% to 80% in mid to lower thoracic lesions.[56,119,120]

Owing to lack of full abdominal musculature innervation in many people with SCI, respiratory capability changes when the patient is sitting compared to supine. In sitting, the lack of abdominal muscle innervation causes abdominal contents to fall forward and pull down on the central tendon. This changes the motion of the diaphragm when it contracts during inspiration, resulting in an inefficient breathing pattern.[121]

The lack of full abdominal muscle function also impairs the ability to cough and clear the airway. The ability to effectively cough is vital for the removal of secretions. The abdominal muscles are the major contributors to generating enough force to expel secretions or foreign objects. Cough function can be categorized into three types: functional, weak functional, and nonfunctional.[122,123] A *functional cough* is loud and forceful, and the patient is able to generate two or more coughs with one exhalation. In this case the patient is able to clear all respiratory secretions. A *weak functional cough* is soft, and the patient is only able to generate one per exhalation. The patient can clear small amounts of secretions and clear the throat. A *nonfunctional cough* is not a true cough; it is a clearing of the throat and has no expulsive force. In this case, assistance is needed to clear secretions from the airway.

Integument

During the acute phase, meticulous and regular skin inspection is a shared responsibility of the patient and the entire medical/rehabilitative team. As management progresses into the active rehabilitation phase and throughout his or her life, the patient will gradually assume greater responsibility for this activity. Patient education related to skin care is crucial and should be initiated early. The patient may view frequent position changes and skin inspection as bothersome or distracting from sleep if there is not adequate awareness of the importance and purpose of these activities.

Assessment for pressure injuries should combine both direct skin inspection, which combines both visual observation and palpation, with assessment of risk factors. The patient's entire body should be observed regularly with particular attention to areas most susceptible to pressure (Table 20.3). Palpation is useful for identifying skin temperature changes that may be indicative of a hyperemic reaction. This is particularly important in examining individuals with dark pigmented skin, because early skin responses to pressure may not be readily apparent. Skin reactions to excess pressure include redness, local warmth, local edema, and small open or cracked skin areas. If the patient is wearing a halo, vest, or other orthotic device, contact points between the body and the orthosis must also be inspected.

In addition to skin inspection, factors that increase the risk for pressure injuries should be considered. Spasticity, bladder or bowel incontinence, and nutritional deficiencies can increase the risk of developing pressure injuries. A number of specific scales can be used to assess the risk of developing a pressure injury in people with SCI.[124] The Braden Scale is commonly used for a variety of patient groups who are at risk for developing pressure injuries, including those with SCI.[124,125] The Braden Scale is more sensitive (75%) than specific (57%) and is easy to administer and has adequate validity.[124] The Spinal Cord Injury Pressure Ulcer Scale (SCIPUS) and SCIPUS-Acute were designed specifically for people with SCI in acute care and in active rehabilitation.[124-126] The SCIPUS is more specific (84%) than sensitive (37%), whereas the SCIPUS-Acute is more sensitive (88%) than specific (59%).[124] Both of these scales have adequate validity and are easy to administer.

If a patient develops a pressure injury, there are a variety of tools that can be used to examine the wound. The location, shape, size, and stage of the wound should be documented. A photograph of the wound on a grid

Table 20.3 Areas Most Susceptible to Pressure in Recumbent Positions

Supine	Prone	Side-Lying
• Occiput • Scapulae • Vertebrae • Elbows • Sacrum • Coccyx • Heels	• Ears (head rotated) • Shoulders (anterior aspect) • Iliac crest • Male genital region • Patella • Dorsum of feet	• Ears • Shoulders (lateral aspect) • Greater trochanter • Head of fibula • Knees (medial aspect from contact between knees) • Lateral malleolus • Medial malleolus (contact between malleoli)

is also an effective method of documenting the wound. Chapter 14, Vascular, Lymphatic, and Integumentary Disorders, provides more detailed information on wound examination.

Range of Motion

Goniometry can be used to assess joint ROM. Shoulder ROM is particularly important for patients with tetraplegia. Depending on the motor level of injury, people with tetraplegia may require more than normal ROM to perform certain mobility skills,[123] and decreased shoulder ROM is associated with shoulder pain.[127] Hamstring length, hip extension, and ankle dorsiflexion are important to measure as well, owing to the potential for contractures in these joints.

Mobility Skills

During this early phase of recovery, patients may have restrictions on certain motions and positions, as well as limited ability to tolerate an upright posture for extended periods of time (sitting or standing). Before a detailed, accurate, and specific determination of functional skills is done, the therapist should again be sure the surgeon has provided clearance for these activities and indicates that the fracture sites are stable. Basic mobility skills that should be examined are rolling in bed, transitioning supine to and from sitting, management of LEs, long and short sitting balance, and transfers. The section on active rehabilitation below has specific outcome measures that may be used to assess these and other mobility skills.

Physical Therapy Interventions

The extent to which the following interventions are implemented is dependent on the medical stability of the patient, stability of healing fracture and surgical sites, status of other injuries that may have occurred during the initial event that caused the SCI, and clearance from the surgeon. The physician/surgeon should be consulted regarding any rehabilitation activities that may place stress on the spine while the spine is still unstable. Although the interventions described below are usually initiated in the early stages of recovery, they should be continued throughout the rehabilitation process and be incorporated into the patient's lifestyle to manage the long-term consequences of the SCI.

Respiratory Management

Respiratory care will vary according to the level of injury and individual respiratory status. Primary goals of management include improved ventilation, increased effectiveness of cough, and prevention of chest tightness and ineffective substitute breathing patterns.

Individuals with cervical injuries at and above C5 often require ventilatory support using an intermittent positive pressure ventilator. Invasive mechanical ventilation is often done through a tracheostomy and can be provided through a stationary or portable ventilator. Noninvasive positive pressure ventilation provides an alternative to invasive mechanical ventilation.[53] Intubation may impair the function of the airway cilia, leading to chronic bacterial colonization and chronic inflammatory changes of the airway. Patients may also prefer noninvasive ventilation.

Respiratory Muscle Training

Similar to other muscles, strength training can improve respiratory muscle strength and endurance. Two systematic reviews concluded that respiratory muscle training is effective for improving respiratory muscle strength, vital capacity, maximal inspiratory pressure, maximal expiratory pressure, and residual volume.[128,129] Diaphragmatic breathing should be encouraged. To facilitate diaphragmatic movement and increase VC, the therapist can apply light pressure during both inspiration and expiration. Manual contacts can be made just below the sternum. This will assist the patient to concentrate on deep-breathing patterns even in the absence of thoracic and abdominal sensation.

Inspiratory muscles can be trained using relatively inexpensive handheld devices, which increase the resistive or threshold inspiratory load on muscles of inspiration (Fig. 20.6). There are two general categories of handheld inspiratory muscle training devices: resistive or threshold trainers. Breathing through these devices increases the resistive or threshold inspiratory load on the muscles. The load can be progressively increased as the patient progresses. Inspiratory muscle training can improve pulmonary function, reduce dyspnea, and improve cough

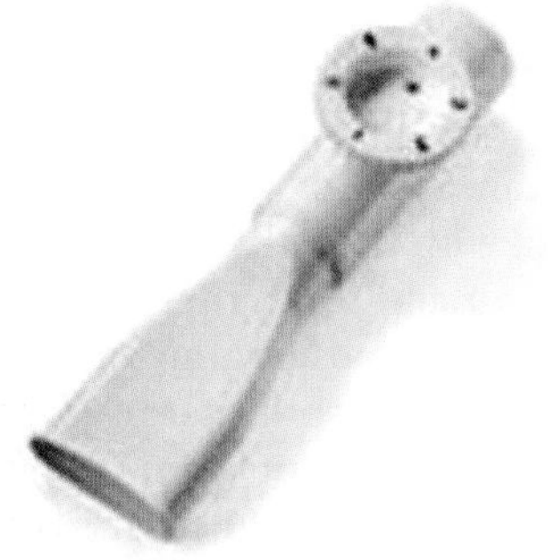

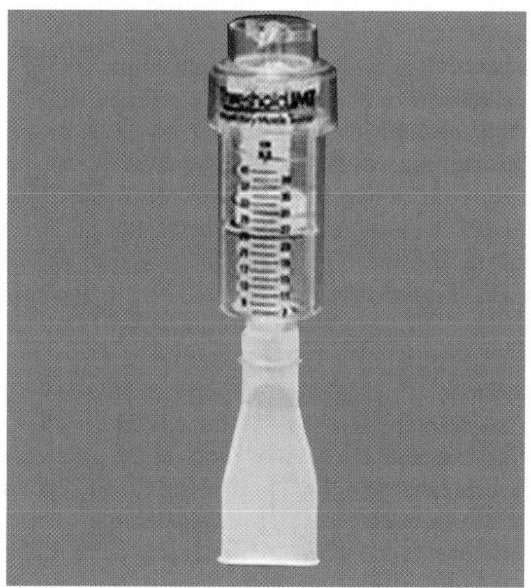

Figure 20.6 Inspiratory muscle trainers. *(Courtesy of Respironics, Inc., Murrysville, PA 15668-8525.)*

function.[130] Another method of strengthening inspiratory muscles is to provide manual resistance (and progress to weighted resistance) to the epigastric area as the patient breathes.

Expiratory muscle training can assist in improving pulmonary function.[128,131] Similar to inspiratory muscle training, expiratory muscle training is done by breathing through a device with a small diameter that limits the airflow, increasing the resistance to expiration (resistive training), or breathing with enough force to overcome a valve and allow airflow (threshold training). The impact of respiratory muscle strengthening on functional outcomes and quality of life are not clear. Also, the most effective dosage of strength training has not been established.

Patients who are not able to produce a functional cough should be taught to perform a self-assisted cough. Those who cannot perform a self-assisted cough may benefit from a manually assisted cough to help remove secretions (Fig. 20.7).[132] To assist with coughing and movement of secretions, manual contacts are placed over the epigastric area. The therapist pushes quickly in an inward and upward direction as the patient attempts to cough.

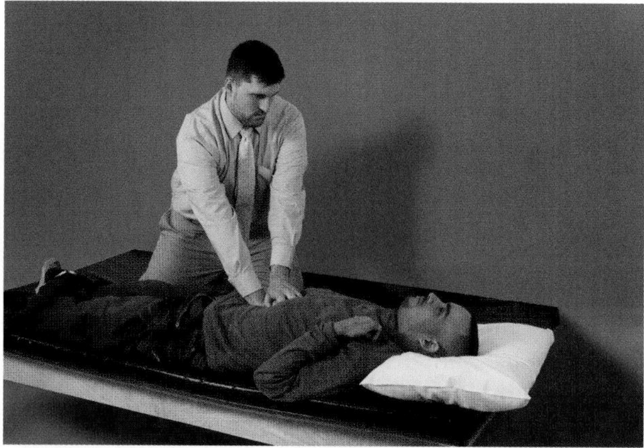

Figure 20.7 Assisted cough using abdominal thrust maneuver to clear secretions.

Glossopharyngeal Breathing

Glossopharyngeal breathing may be appropriate for patients with high-level cervical lesions who are dependent on a mechanical ventilator for ventilation, as well as for patients with mid to high cervical–level injuries who are not dependent on mechanical ventilation. Glossopharyngeal breathing utilizes the lips, pharyngeal muscles, and the tongue to inhale air.[133,134] The patient is instructed to take in small amounts of air, using a "gulping" pattern, thus utilizing available facial and pharyngeal muscles. The patient repeats this 6 to 10 times. By using this technique, enough air is gradually inspired. Exhalation occurs owing to the elastic recoil of the lungs. Glossopharyngeal breathing provides a method for individuals with high cervical lesions who are dependent on mechanical ventilation to breathe independently for a period of time in emergency situations[133] and as a way to increase vital capacity in people with cervical lesions who are not dependent on a mechanical ventilator. Teaching a patient to perform glossopharyngeal breathing requires specialized skills and experience beyond entry level.[123]

Abdominal Binder

An abdominal binder may improve respiratory function,[44,135] cough ability,[136] and speech[135] in patients with high thoracic and cervical lesions. An abdominal binder may improve respiratory mechanics by compensating for nonfunctioning abdominal muscles. The binder compresses abdominal contents to increase intra-abdominal pressure and elevate the diaphragm into a more optimal position for breathing. In addition, abdominal binders may provide the secondary benefits of maintaining intrathoracic pressure and decreasing postural hypotension.

Manual Stretching

Mobility and compliance of the thoracic wall can be facilitated by manual stretching chest wall muscles in supine. This is done by placing one hand around the side of the chest wall with the fingertips on the transverse processes and the other on top of the chest with the base of the hand on the edge of the sternum. The hands are moved in a wringing motion. Pressure should be distributed across the surface of the hands. Wetzel[134] provides an in-depth discussion of interventions to enhance respiratory function.

Skin Care

Prevention is the most effective intervention for skin care; this entails positioning, consistent and effective pressure relief, skin inspection, and education. Areas that are susceptible to skin pressure injury (see Table 20.3) should be adequately protected when the patient is in bed by using pillows, foam, and positioning devices (Fig. 20.8). Positioning should also be used to prevent development of joint contractures and secondary pulmonary complications. Specific positioning of the extremities to prevent contractures will depend on the level of the SCI. Certain joints may be more prone to contracture, depending on which muscles surrounding the joint are innervated. For example, a patient with a C5-level injury may tend to position the shoulder in adduction and the elbow in flexion. When positioning this patient, the shoulders should be abducted and elbows extended when possible.

When in bed, patients should be repositioned at least every 2 hours.[137] Increased and consistent pressure over bony prominences, shear forces, heat, and moisture should be minimized. A variety of beds and rotating beds with foam, air, low air loss, and air fluidized mattresses and overlays can assist in the prevention of pressure injuries and aid with healing (Fig. 20.9).

The wheelchair and seating system should also assist in promoting optimal positioning for reducing pressure and shear forces on susceptible areas. The pelvis should be positioned in a neutral position or slightly tilted anteriorly and be symmetrical (i.e., left anterior-superior iliac spine [ASIS] even with the right ASIS). A variety of wheelchair cushion types are designed to assist with positioning and redistribution of pressure. Positioning should optimize weight-bearing on the ischial tuberosities while minimizing pressure on the greater trochanters and sacrum/coccyx, which are able to accommodate much less pressure without the breakdown of skin tissue. The main types of cushions are foam, gel, air, and flexible matrix and differ in the balance between support and pressure compensation. Cushions are often contoured to further assist in the redistribution of pressure and to reduce shear. No one type of cushion is the most effective. The exact type of cushion selected should be based on the individual patient. Chapter 32, Seating and Wheeled Mobility, provides more detail about wheelchairs and seating systems, as well as their advantages and indications for use.

Patients should perform a pressure-relief maneuver every 15 minutes when in the wheelchair, either with assistance or independently.[138] From the seated position, this can be done by using a push-up maneuver, leaning to the side, or leaning forward (Fig. 20.10). If using a forward lean, the lean should be greater than 45 degrees.[139]

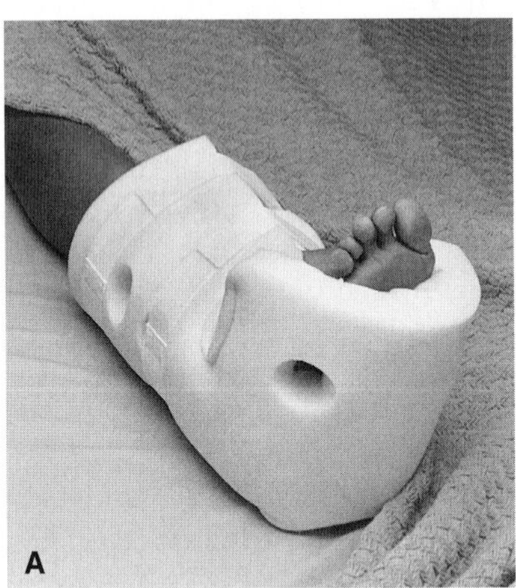

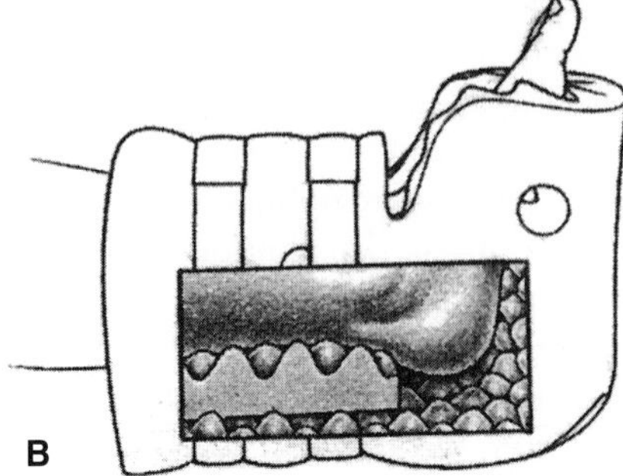

Figure 20.8 Ankle/foot positioning to prevent skin breakdown and contracture. *(Courtesy of DM Systems, Inc., Evanston, IL 60201.)*

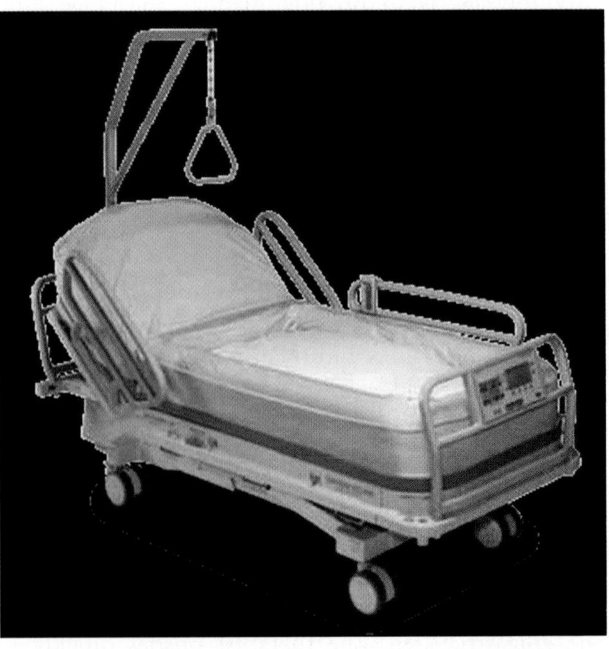

Figure 20.9 Air fluidized bed. *(Courtesy of Hill-Rom, Inc., Batesville, IN 47006.)*

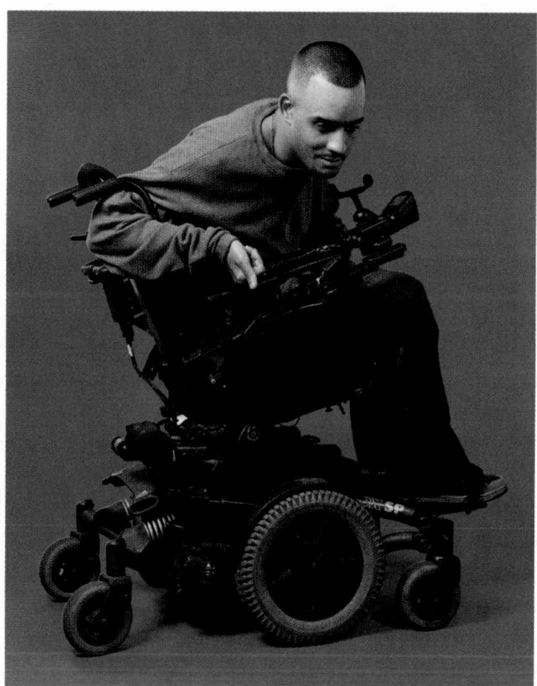

Figure 20.10 Lateral lean in wheelchair for pressure relief.

Patients who are not able to perform these maneuvers initially can be assisted or their wheelchair can be tilted back. If tilting the entire wheelchair back, it should be tilted to at least 65 degrees in order to adequately shift the pressure off the ischial tuberosities. All pressure-relief maneuvers should be maintained for at least 2 minutes to be effective.[140] A tilt-in-space or reclining wheelchair can also be used to redistribute pressure.

The patient's skin should be routinely inspected to ensure there are no developing pressure injuries. Enhanced education on prevention and management with consistent follow-up can reduce the development and recurrence of pressure injuries.[141] As the rehabilitation program progresses, the patient gradually assumes responsibility for skin care. Preparation for assumption of this responsibility will include patient education about the potential risks of pressure sores, the importance of hygiene, instruction in skin inspection techniques, the use of pressure-relief equipment and procedures, and what to do if a pressure injury develops.

If the patient develops a skin pressure injury, the preventive measures described above should continue to be employed. Various therapies directed at wound healing should be initiated. Chapter 14, Vascular, Lymphatic, and Integumentary Disorders, provides a comprehensive perspective on these and other specific wound healing interventions.

Strength and Range of Motion

Range of motion exercises should be completed daily. If the site of the vertebral fracture was surgically stabilized and the surgeon has placed no restrictions on movement, then ROM and strengthening exercises can be initiated. However, if the fracture site is designated as unstable, then ROM or strengthening exercises that place increased stress on the fracture site are contraindicated. For example, to avoid stress on an unstable surgical site in the lumbar region while performing ROM exercises, straight leg raises may be restricted to no more than approximately 60 degrees and hip flexion (during combined hip and knee flexion) limited to no greater than 90 degrees. With an unstable cervical spine, motion of the head and neck may be contraindicated and shoulder flexion and abduction limited to no more than 90 degrees.

Patients with SCIs do not require full ROM in all joints. Some joints benefit from allowing tightness to develop in certain muscles to enhance function. For example, with tetraplegia, tightness of the lower trunk musculature may improve sitting posture and prevent vertebral telescoping (where the trunk elongates but the pelvis does not lift off the seating surface) during transfers by increasing trunk stability; tightness in the long finger flexors will provide an improved tenodesis grasp. Conversely, some muscles require a fully lengthened range. The hamstrings may require stretching to achieve a straight leg raise of approximately 100 degrees. This ROM is required for many functional activities such as long sitting and LE dressing. However, care should be taken not to overstretch the hamstring muscles because some tightness in this muscle group provides passive pelvic stabilization in sitting. This process of understretching some muscles and full stretching of others to improve function is referred to as *selective stretching*.

Positioning of the wrist, hands, and fingers is an important early consideration. Alignment of the fingers, thumb, and wrist must be maintained for functional activities or possible future splinting. Individuals with functional, active wrist extension can learn to use a tenodesis grasp to perform ADLs, manipulate objects, and hold objects without active finger control. The tenodesis grasp occurs through the biomechanics of the wrist and finger joints. When the wrist is actively extended, the finger flexor tendons are shortened, causing the fingers to passively flex and assume a grasp position. When the wrist is flexed, the tension on the tendons is released and the hand opens providing release (Fig. 20.11) An *intrinsic-plus splint* can be used to position the wrist (20 degrees of extension), metacarpal phalangeal joints (80 to 90 degrees of flexion), interphalangeal joints (full extension or slight flexion), and the thumb (natural opposition) to maintain the joints in optimal intrinsic-plus position[142] (Fig. 20.12). This position helps reduce edema, preserve tenodesis function, and prevent contractures. As with any splint, the user's skin should be inspected for redness, irritation, or open areas and a progressive schedule should be used to slowly build up the wearing time to prevent skin irritation.

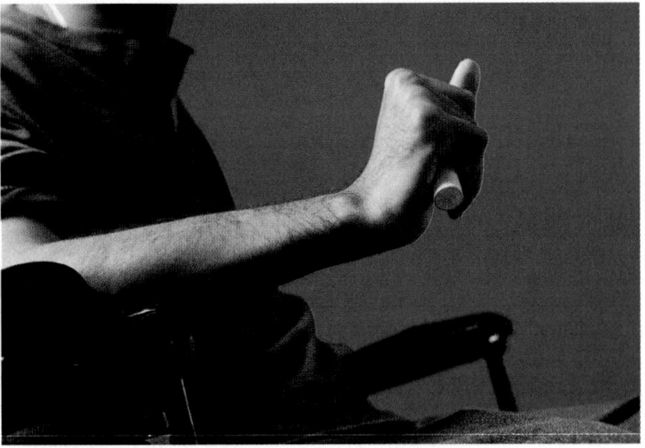

Figure 20.11 Patient extends the wrist, which causes the shortened long finger flexors to passively flex, allowing a grasp.

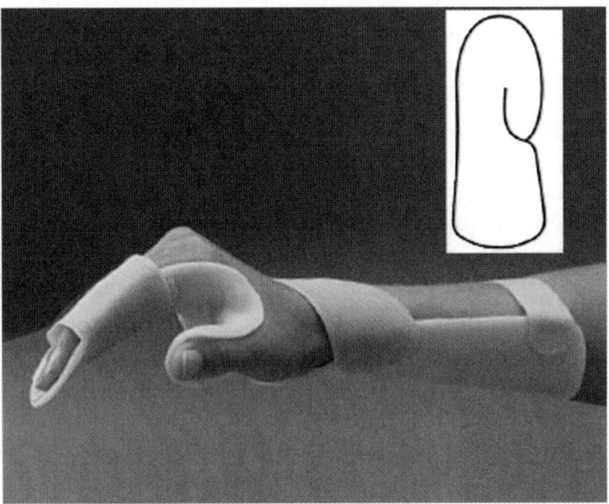

Figure 20.12 Intrinsic-plus splint. *(Courtesy 3Tailer, Charlotte, NC.)*

During the course of rehabilitation, all innervated musculature is strengthened maximally. However, as noted above, resistive exercises may be contraindicated if the fracture site is unstable. Key muscles and strengthening techniques are discussed below.

Mobility Interventions

Once the patient is physician-cleared to assume an upright posture, functional mobility skills can be initiated. The patient typically will experience symptoms of orthostatic hypotension (e.g., dizziness, nausea, ringing in ears, loss of vision, or loss of consciousness) when first assuming sitting and/or standing (if able). A gradual acclimation to upright postures is necessary. The use of an abdominal binder and elastic stockings may reduce venous pooling and prevent orthostatic hypotension. During early upright positioning, elastic wraps may also be used in combination with (placed over) the elastic stockings.

Initially, upright activities can be initiated by slowly elevating the head of the bed and progressing to a reclining or tilt-in-space wheelchair with elevating legrests. Use of a standing frame provides another option for orienting the patient to a vertical position. A tilt table can also be used. Vital signs should be monitored carefully and documented during this acclimation period to ensure that systolic and diastolic blood pressure values do not fall below a safe range. If the patient experiences any of the signs or symptoms of orthostatic hypotension during sitting or standing activities, the patient should be brought safely to a supine position (or trunk reclined) with the legs elevated.

When the patient is acclimated to upright postures (sitting and standing), specific training can begin on basic mobility skills. Interventions designed to teach bed mobility skills such as rolling and transitioning supine to/from long and short sitting and transfer skills can be initiated. These and other functional mobility skills become the focus of rehabilitation once the patient is stable. Specific intervention techniques on these and other functional mobility skills are discussed below.

Education

Living with an SCI requires significant adaptations and changes on the part of the patient and his or her family. In order to meet the challenges presented by an SCI, patients must fully understand all the consequences of the injury. Patient and family/caregiver education should begin early after injury and address the impact of SCI on various body systems, secondary complications, and prognosis. Later in the recovery process, it may be particularly helpful to introduce the patient to individuals with long-standing SCI who have successfully completed rehabilitation and are functioning in the community. Such contacts will provide the patient with further understanding and insight into the impact of SCI on day-to-day life.

■ ACTIVE REHABILITATION

The overarching goal of rehabilitation is for the patient to become as independent as possible and to achieve the functional mobility necessary for everyday life, work, and recreation. Independent mobility can be achieved in a way that (1) uses new movement strategies to compensate for neuromuscular impairments or (2) uses the neuromuscular system to accomplish the task with a movement pattern similar to that before the injury.[143,144] *Compensation* refers to use of an alternative or new movement strategy, or technology to compensate for neuromuscular deficits to accomplish a daily task.[145] *Recovery of function* refers to the restoration of the neuromuscular system so that the motor task is performed in a similar manner as it was before the SCI.[144,145]

For instance, if a patient cannot actively flex the fingers to grasp a bottle owing to weakness or paralysis of finger flexor muscles, use of wrist "tenodesis" is often taught as a compensatory strategy (Fig. 20.11). Active wrist extension simultaneously produces passive finger flexion and can be used to achieve a functional grasp. Knee-ankle-foot orthoses (KAFOs) may help a patient achieve the goal of standing but do not have a therapeutic effect on retraining the neuromuscular system in the once familiar task of standing. Once the KAFOs are removed, the LEs cannot perform the task of standing. The braces compensate for the inability to activate antigravity LE muscles due to weakness or paralysis. The task of moving from sitting to standing with KAFOs entails the use of assistive devices and weight-bearing through the arms, further altering the preinjury movement pattern to accomplish the task. Transfers from a wheelchair to a bed that also incorporate weight-bearing through the arms and a *head-hips* movement strategy (the head moves in one direction to move the hips in the opposite direction; see below) is another example of a compensatory behavior using a biomechanical advantage to achieve a functional goal in a new way. Focusing on recovery of the once-familiar task of sit-to-stand would require a movement pattern that included a weight shift from the buttocks forward over the feet, a powerful activation of antigravity muscles to lift the body off the chair, the head moving up and forward, and then full extension of the limbs and trunk to achieve standing without the arms weight-bearing.

How a goal is achieved (or expected to be achieved) is thus important in treatment planning and goal-setting. Historically, rehabilitation for persons after SCI has employed compensation strategies using muscles spared above the level of the lesion, substitution, novel movement patterns, and assistive devices/braces as the primary means for achieving independent functional mobility skills. Recent advances in our understanding of the neurobiological control of walking and in activity-dependent plasticity have provided the basis for new, alternative therapies that generate activity below the level of the lesion with the goal of recovery.[144] Our assumption that the spinal cord was simply a conduit for neural signals from the brain was incorrect. In fact, the spinal cord is quite responsive to the ensemble of sensorimotor information provided during task execution to generate a motor output. Activity elicited through such therapies (e.g., locomotor training, task-specific practice) is used to retrain the neuromuscular control required for function, then used in everyday activities, and finally integrated into daily use.[146-148]

Although both compensation and recovery-based approaches (activity-based therapies) are used in rehabilitation for SCI, compensation dominates current clinical practice. However, a large and expanding body of literature is providing new insights about integration of activity-based therapies into the POC,[149,150] their potential for improving outcomes with combinatorial approaches,[149,151,152] and the impact of these therapies on functional outcomes to advance recovery and quality of life.

If independence cannot be achieved, whether using compensation or recovery-based strategies, then the patient may be interdependent on others for assistance in accomplishing certain tasks of daily life (e.g., the patient with a complete high cervical lesion). The patient, family, friends, and caregivers receive thorough instructions and training in the knowledge and skills required to address the individual's daily needs.

Physical Therapy Examination

All the examination procedures completed during the acute phase are continued during the active rehabilitation phase. In as much as greater patient mobility is now allowed, more complete testing of muscle strength, ROM, and functional skills can be performed. A variety of standardized outcome measures and tests are available to the physical therapist (Table 20.4). Using a modified Delphi process, the Spinal Cord Injury Special Interest Group of the Academy of Neurologic Physical Therapy developed recommendations for use of outcome measures in clinical practice, research, and entry-level physical therapy education. These recommendations and psychometric properties of the recommended outcome measures are available at: www.neuropt.org/professional-resources/neurology-section-outcome-measures-recommendations/spinal-cord-injury. The Shirley Ryan AbilityLab Rehabilitation Measures Database (www.sralab.org/rehabilitation-measures) and the Spinal Cord Injury Research Evidence (https://scireproject.com) websites are also useful resources for information on outcome measures. Some of the more frequently used and recommended tests and measures are discussed here.

Body Structure/Function

Aerobic Capacity/Endurance

The *6-minute arm test (6MAT)* can be used to assess aerobic capacity and cardiovascular endurance.[153] The 6MAT requires the patient to perform 6 minutes of submaximal cycling on an arm ergometer at a single, steady-state power output. It is a valid and reliable measure for people with either tetraplegia or paraplegia. Steady-state power output for clients with tetraplegia should be set between 10 and 30 watts based on use of a manual versus power wheelchair and activity level. For clients with paraplegia, the power output should be set between 30 and 60 watts, depending on gender, AIS motor score, and activity level. Heart rate is continuously recorded and the final steady state heart rate averaged over the last 30 seconds. Ratings of perceived exertion should also be documented.[153]

Integumentary Integrity

See discussion in the "Physical Therapy Management Early After Injury" section. Also see Chapter 14, Vascular, Lymphatic, and Integumentary Disorders for additional information on examination and treatment of pressure injuries.

Table 20.4 Outcome Measures

Outcome Measure and ICF Category	Description	Scoring	MDC and MCID
International Standards for Neurological Classification of Spinal Injury, ASIA Impairment Scale (AIS) ICF: 1	Observation-based measure: assesses and classifies the current level of motor and sensory deficits.	Ability to sense and differentiate sharp and dull sensation as well as ability to resist the examiner at varying muscles. Classified between AIS A = complete to AIS E = no deficits.	MDC[210]: 3.87 (total sensory), 1.87 (total motor) (all AIS classifications) MCID[210]: 5.19 (total sensory), 4.48 (total motor) (all AIS classifications)
Handheld dynamometry ICF: 1	Performance-based test: assesses muscular strength during grip task.	Force production (kg, N, or lb) during maximal isometric contraction for 3–5 seconds ("make") or examiner applies force to overcome patient ("break")	MDC[164]: 5.1–8.2 lb (biceps), 6–6.7 lb (triceps), 0.7–4.8 lb (wrist extensors) (estimated based on data from Aufsesser et al[164]) (both paraplegia and tetraplegia) MCID: NA
Wheelchair User's Shoulder Pain Index (WUSPI) ICF: 1	Self-reported measure: assesses shoulder pain in wheelchair users during functional activities and tasks that include transfers, wheelchair mobility, self-care, and general activities.	15 items across the 4 domains; each have a 10-cm visual analog scale (VAS) that is anchored from "no pain" at 0 cm to "worst pain ever experienced" at 10 cm.	MDC: NA MCID: NA
6-Minute Walk Test (6MWT) ICF: 2	Performance-based test: assesses functional walking endurance.	Distance walked in 6 minutes when walking as fast as possible.	MDC[164,194]: 45.8m (150 ft) (incomplete SCI) (estimated based on data from van Hedel et al[193]) MCID: NA
10-Meter Walk Test (10MWT) ICF: 2	Performance-based test: assesses walking speed over a short time period.	Time to walk 10 m, usually performed with a 2-m acceleration and deceleration phase.	MDC[194]: 0.13 m/s (incomplete SCI) MCID: NA
Berg Balance Scale (BBS) ICF: 2	Performance-based test: assesses both static and dynamic balance during 14 functional tasks.	14 items scored on a 5-point ordinal scale of 0 to 4, where 0 is unable to perform/needs assistance and 4 is able to perform safely and independently.	MDC: NA MCID: NA
Walking Index for Spinal Cord Injury (WISCI) ICF: 2	Performance-based test: assesses the need for physical assistance and/or assistive devices for ambulation.	Amount of assistance needed over 10-m walk ranked on 20-point ordinal scale, where 0 is unable to stand or participate and 20 is ambulates with no assistance.	MDC[190]: 0.78 (self-selected level), 0.16 (maximum level); estimated based on data from Burns et al[190] (both paraplegia and tetraplegia) MCID: NA
Capabilities of UE Functioning Instrument (CUE) ICF: 2	Self-reported measure: assesses impact of tetraplegia on upper extremity motor function.	32 items scored on a 7-point ordinal scale of 1 to 7, where 1 is totally limited and cannot do at all and 7 is not at all limited.	MDC[198]: 33.8 (estimated based on data from Marino et al[211]) (tetraplegia, mostly AIS A) MCID: NA

Table 20.4 Outcome Measures—cont'd

Outcome Measure and ICF Category	Description	Scoring	MDC and MCID
World Health Organization Quality of Life—BREF ICF: 3	Self-reported measure: assesses impact of injury on domains in physical health, psychological health, social relationships, and one's environment in the past 4 weeks.	25 items across 4 domains scored on a 5-point Likert scale from 1–5, with scores indicating various meanings. Greater scores in total indicate greater quality of life.	MDC: 6.6–21.5 (estimated based on data from Lin et al[185]) MCID: NA
Spinal Cord Independence Measure (SCIM) ICF: 2	Observation-based test with interview component: assesses ability to self-care, bladder/bowel management, and general mobility.	19 items are scored over 3 domains that together in total range from 0–100, with greater scores indicating increased independence.	MDC: NA MCID: NA
Graded and Redefined Assessment of Sensibility Strength and Prehension (GRASSP) ICF: 2	Performance-based test: assesses hand (L/R) function, neurological recovery, and sensation in those with tetraplegia from cervical spinal cord injuries.	5 total subtests over 3 domains that measure sensory function (6 locations), from 0–4; strength (10 locations), from 0–5; prehension (3 grasps), from 0–4, and prehension performance (6 tasks), from 0–5.	MDC: 5.1 (R), 5.3 (L; strength), 1.8 (R), 1.7 (L; prehension ability), 7 (R), 4.9 (L; prehension performance; estimated based on data from Kalsi-Ryan, et al[213] (tetraplegia) MCID: NA
Wheelchair Skills Test ICF: 2	Performance-based test: assesses ability to navigate and utilize wheelchair for necessary tasks and activities.	32 items of increasing difficulty from indoor, outdoor, and community environment. Scored as "pass, safe" to "fail, unsafe" or "no part" for indicated skills.	MDC: NA MCID: NA
Needs Assessment Checklist (NAC) ICF: 3	Self-reported measure: assesses independence in ADLs, mobility, and reintegration.	199 items across 9 domains with scores achieved by summing sub-scale items and deriving a percentage from 0% to 100% for each subscale, with greater scores indicating increased independence.	MDC: NA MCID: NA
Life Satisfaction Questionnaire (LISAT-9) ICF: 3	Self-reported measure: assesses self-care ability and relationships.	9 domains that score a single item for life satisfaction and 8 additional items for each domain using a 6-point Likert scale, with 1 being very dissatisfied to 6 bring very satisfied.	MDC: 0.14–0.19 (estimated based on data from Geyh et al[181]) MCID: NA
Craig Handicap Assessment and Reporting Technique (CHART) ICF: 3	Self-reported measure: assesses degree of handicap within physical, social, and cognitive aspects in the community.	6 domains with 32 total items with each subscale, ranging from 0–100 for a total score of 0–600, with greater scores indicating lesser handicap.	MDC[178]: 53.3 (total score) MCID: NA

ICF category: 1 = body structure/function, 2 = activity, 3 = participation
MDC = minimal detectable change
MCID = minimal clinically important difference
NA = not available
Table created by John LaRue, Doctor of Physical Therapy student at Clarkson University

Mental Functions

It is particularly important to screen patients for cognitive impairment, because up to 60% of people who experience a traumatic SCI may also have a concomitant traumatic brain injury (TBI).[154,155] Motor vehicle accidents and falls are common causes of SCI that may also result in a TBI. In some cases, the impact of the TBI may be subtle and not easily recognized. A concomitant TBI, whether mild or severe, can have a profound impact on recovery and the rehabilitation POC. Although they have not been validated in people with SCI, the *Mini Mental State Exam* and the *Montreal Cognitive Assessment* are useful tools to screen for cognitive impairment.[156,157] If it is suspected that a patient has a TBI, a referral should be made to a neuropsychologist or psychiatrist.

Motor Function/Muscle Performance/Sensory Integrity

As described earlier, the ASIA ISNCSCI[158] standards should be used to determine the level of lesion and intact motor and sensory function. The presence of spastic hypertonia should be assessed as part of the motor function examination. The *modified Ashworth Scale* (MAS) is a commonly used 6-point ordinal scale that rates a joint's resistance to passive movement.[159] (See Chapter 5 , Examination of Motor Function: Motor Control and Motor Learning, for a description of the MAS.) The *Penn Spasm Frequency Scale* is a valid and reliable two-part self-report measure that assesses the frequency and severity of spasms.[160,161]

Further MMT should be performed for all muscle groups that are innervated based on findings from the ASIA ISNCSCI. For example, if the biceps are intact, then other muscles innervated by C5 such as the deltoids and rotator cuff muscles should also be tested. Although not included as key muscles in the ISNCSCI, examination of other functionally important muscles such as deltoids, pronators/supinators, gluteals, and hamstrings will assist in establishing goals and expected outcomes. Handheld dynamometry can also be used to examine muscle strength, including trunk strength.[162-164] There are several unique considerations when performing MMT for people with SCI. Patients often learn to functionally move joints by substituting intact muscle contraction for weak or paralyzed muscles. For example, supination of the forearm allows gravity to extend the wrist, and lower abdominal muscles can substitute for hip flexion by causing the pelvis to tilt posteriorly. The physical therapist should carefully stabilize proximal areas to reduce substitution and palpate to ensure that the test muscle is contracting. Abnormal muscle tone and spasms can cause involuntary muscle contractions or a weak muscle to appear stronger. Orthoses and spinal precautions may preclude the patient from assuming a recommended test position or forcefully contract certain muscles. The use of alternate (nonstandard) test positions should be documented.

A complete sensory examination should be performed (see Chapter 3, Examination of Sensory Function).

Pain

Pain should be examined continually. A *numeric pain rating scale* can be used to identify the intensity of pain. The patient rates pain on a scale from 0 to 10, where 0 is no pain and 10 is severe, disabling pain. There are also self-report measures of pain designed specifically for people with SCI. The *Wheelchair User's Shoulder Pain Index* measures the impact of shoulder pain on transfers, self-care, wheelchair mobility, and general activities.[165,166] Wheelchair users rate the amount of pain experienced while performing various activities on a scale from 0 to 10. Total score ranges from 0 to 150, with higher scores indicating a greater impact of pain.

Range of Motion

Joint ROM should be assessed using standard goniometry techniques.

Reflex Integrity

Deep tendon reflexes, graded on a 0 to 4+ scale, with 2+ being normal, should be tested. Reflex testing assists in determining the resolution of spinal shock and distinguishing between UMN and LMN injuries. See Chapter 5, Examination of Motor Function: Motor Control and Motor Learning.

Ventilation and Respiration

See the "Physical Therapy Management Early After Injury" section.

Activity/Participation

Assistive Technology

Individuals with SCI benefit from a variety of assistive technologies to increase independence with mobility and ADL and to enhance participation in desired social roles and activities. These range from high-tech devices such as exoskeletons, power wheelchairs, environmental control units, and speech recognition software to lower-tech devices such as adaptive writing devices, a trapeze over the bed, and reaching devices. The Psychosocial Impact of Assistive Devices is a self-report tool that can be used to assess the impact of assistive technology on independence, well-being, and quality of life.[167,168]

Balance

Sitting balance can be examined using the modified Functional Reach Test.[169,170] For patients with some capability to stand and walk, balance can be assessed using the Berg Balance Scale (BBS). See Chapter 6, Examination of Coordination and Balance, for a description of this instrument. Although originally developed for patients with stroke and older adults, the BBS has been validated for people with incomplete spinal cord injury (iSCI).[171,172]

Community, Social, and Civic Life

The ultimate goal of rehabilitation is to allow the individual to return to his or her normal roles and fully participate in society. Measures of participation provide insight into how the individual is functioning in the home and community. Some commonly used outcome measures are the *Craig Handicap Assessment and Reporting Technique*,[173-178] *Life Satisfaction Questionnaire*,[179-181] *Short Form 36*,[182,183] *Satisfaction with Life Scale*,[174] *Reintegration to Normal Living Index*,[184] and *World Health Organization Quality of Life*.[185]

Gait

Gait and walking ability should also be examined in patients who maintain some ability to stand and walk. An observational gait analysis tool such as the *Rancho Los Amigos Observational Gait Analysis*[186] can be used to identify gait deviations. See Chapter 7, Examination of Gait, for a description of this instrument. Identifying abnormal gait patterns will inform selection of additional tests and measures needed to determine the underlying impairments that may be causing the abnormal movements as well as guide development of the POC.

The *Walking Index for Spinal Cord Injury* examines level of physical assistance, type of assistive device, and amount of bracing required to ambulate 10 meters.[187-190] Scores range from 0 (unable to stand or walk with assistance) to 20 (ambulates with no assistance, no braces, and no assistive device). The *Spinal Cord Injury Functional Ambulation Inventory* is another outcome measure used to assess walking ability in people with iSCI.[191] It involves a 2-minute observational gait analysis performed using the patient's usual assistive device. Documentation includes the frequency and distances the patient typically walks in the home and community.

The *10-Meter Walk Test*[189,192-194] and *6-Minute Walk Test*[189,193,194] are reliable, valid, and responsive to change in people with iSCI. A change of 0.13 m/sec in gait speed is an indication that significant clinical change has occurred.[194] Gait speed can also be used as a predictor of functional walking ability. People with iSCI who walk at 0.09 m/sec are likely to be supervised ambulators. Walking speed of 0.15 m/sec is an indication that the person can likely walk indoor but use a wheelchair outside the home. Walking speed of 0.44 m/sec is an indication that the person will likely use an assistive device or orthosis to walk in and outside the home. Finally, a walking speed of 0.70 m/sec indicates the person can walk in and outside the home without an assistive device or orthotic.[192] The minimal detectable change of the 6-Minute Walk Test is 46 meters.[194]

Mobility

Most individuals with SCI will rely on a wheelchair as their primary means of mobility in the home and community. As such, it is important to examine the patient's ability to perform wheelchair skills. This includes setting and releasing the wheel locks, removing footrests and armrests, propelling the wheelchair on level surfaces, performing wheelies, ascending and descending curbs, and various other wheelchair skills necessary for independent mobility in the community. The *Wheelchair Skills Test* examines a wheelchair user's skills in performing 32 representative wheelchair skills.[195-197] The skills are categorized according to three levels that reflect difficulty and the setting in which they will be performed: indoor, community, and advanced. There are separate tests for manual and power wheelchair users. The Wheelchair Skills Test can be used as a diagnostic measure to determine which wheelchair skills need to be addressed in therapy and to document improvement during rehabilitation. (For in-depth information about the test and wheelchair skills training, see www.wheelchairskills program.ca/eng/index.php). The *Wheelchair Circuit* is another outcome measure that is designed to assess three aspects of manual wheelchair mobility: tempo, technical skill, and physical capacity.[198,199]

Other basic mobility skills such as transfers, rolling, and transitioning to/from supine should also be examined. Outcome measures that address these skills are highlighted in the "Self-Care and Domestic Life" section.

The *Neuromuscular Recovery Scale (NRS)* is an outcome measure used to examine the ability to perform a functional movement in the manner used by the intact neuromuscular system before injury and without compensation.[200-203] In comparison, the Functional Independence Measure (FIM; see below) examines performance of functional tasks based on the level of assistance required (i.e., burden of care). Some measures include time as an element of task performance (e.g., 10-Meter Walk Test for walking speed). The FIM and 10-Meter Walk Test allow compensation as a movement strategy and address only whether a goal is achieved, not how it is accomplished. The NRS uniquely examines how a goal is attempted (or achieved) and does not allow the use of compensation strategies during task performance. Thus, the gold standard for recovery is not only whether a goal is achieved, but also whether it is accomplished in the manner (i.e., behavioral pattern) used before injury. This scale is particularly relevant because newer interventions for rehabilitation after SCI are now beginning to target recovery to preinjury status as opposed to compensation for injury-related impairments. The NRS consists of 11 items ranging from sitting to sit-to-stand to walking.

Self-Care and Domestic Life

Among the main goals of rehabilitation is to promote independence in functional mobility skills and self-care. In addition to wheelchair propulsion skills and gait (if appropriate), it is important to carefully examine the patient's ability to perform other mobility skills such as transfers, bed mobility, and ability to perform pressure relief. The amount of physical assistance, method of performing the task, verbal cues required, use of adaptive/assistive devices, characteristics of environment, and degree of safety should all be carefully documented. To be truly independent, the patient must be able to complete the task safely, without assistance, in a timely manner, without undue effort, in an open environment, in different environments, and consistently. It may be tempting to provide a small amount of assistance such as stabilizing the wheelchair while the patient transfers (to prevent sliding) and still document that the patient was independent with the bed-to-wheelchair transfer. However, in this case the patient was not truly independent with the task. The patient must be able to complete the task without assistance but with the physical therapist present. The physical therapist must actually observe the patient performing the task because patients may overestimate their own ability (e.g., self-report).

The *Functional Independence Measure* (FIM®)[204-206] scores task completion based on the amount of assistance required based on the percentage of active patient participation. The amount of assistance is scored on a 7-point ordinal scale that ranges from 1 (total assistance; patient performs less than 25% of the effort) to 7 (independent). The FIM assesses burden of care across 18 basic ADLs; 13 motor tasks, such as dressing, bathing, and transfers; and 5 cognitive tasks, such as comprehension, problem-solving, and memory. Additional information on the FIM is provided in Chapter 8, Examination of Function.

Several SCI-specific outcome measures are available to examine self-care and domestic life. The *Spinal Cord Injury Independence Measure (SCIM)* was specifically created to assess function in people with SCI. It includes 19 items divided into 3 subcategories: self-care, respiration and sphincter management, and mobility. Total scores range from 0 to 100, where higher scores indicate greater independence. The SCIM is valid and reliable and may be more responsive in people with SCI than the FIM.[207-210]

The *Capabilities of Upper Extremity Instrument (CUEI)* is a self-report measure that assesses the ability to unilaterally and bilaterally grasp, release, and lift; it assesses wrist and finger actions as well.[211] Each item is scored on a 7-point ordinal scale, where 1 is totally limited (cannot do at all) and 7 is not at all limited. Total scores range from 32 to 224, where higher scores indicate better UE function. The CUEI is reliable, valid, and responsive.[211,212] The MDC is estimated to be 34 points.[211] The *Graded and Redefined Assessment of Sensibility, Strength, and Prehension* is a performance-based measure that assesses hand function, neurological recovery, and sensation in people with tetraplegia.[213]

Contextual Factors

Environment

It is also essential that the physical therapist examine the patient's home, community, and work environments to determine accessibility. Because structural modifications and/or additions to the home may be required to ensure patient safety and access, the rehabilitation team should perform an examination of the home environment early in the rehabilitation process (see Chapter 9, Examination and Modification of the Environment).

Outcomes and Goals

Functional outcome after SCI is dependent on many factors; primary among these, especially for individuals with complete injuries, is level of motor function. With complete lower-level lesions (i.e., more musculature intact), there is greater potential for independence in mobility tasks and ADL. With incomplete lesions (AIS A, B, C, or D), there is greater functional potential as compared to AIS A injuries; AIS D injuries represent greater functional independence than that of AIS B or C injuries. Other factors that may affect functional outcomes include age, concomitant injury, preexisting health conditions, secondary complications, body type, and psychosocial support.[214-217] Table 20.5 provides a guide to expected functional outcomes for people with complete SCI based on level of injury. The physical therapist, rehabilitation team, and patient can use these expected outcomes to establish goals and outcomes. However, as mentioned earlier, factors other than motor level may affect functional recovery.

Goals should reflect what is important and meaningful to the patient. This will increase motivation, promote achievement of goals, and enhance patient autonomy. Early after injury, patients are not likely to fully understand the consequences of an SCI and are still in the process of adjusting to the injury. It is important to educate them on the impact of SCI and review the findings of the initial examination and all reexaminations. Potential functional goals should be discussed and the patient encouraged to suggest his or her own goals as well. Long-term goals should focus on activity and social participation, not body structure and function impairments. Goals should be specific by stating what the patient will achieve. The level of assistance, the environment/conditions, and the length of time to achieve the goal should all be documented.

Table 20.5 Functional Expectations for Patients With Spinal Cord Injury*

Motor Level and Key Muscles	Available Movements	Functional Capabilities	Equipment and Assistance Required
C1, C2, C3, C4			
Face and neck muscles, cranial nerve innervation, diaphragm (partial innervation at C3 and C4)	Talking Mastication Sipping Blowing Scapular elevation	Activities of daily living (ADL) Dependence in basic ADL (BADL) Activation of computer, light switches, page turners, call buttons, electrical appliances, and speaker phones	Dependent Environmental control units (ECU) Brain-computer interface (BCI) Adaptive equipment such as head or mouth stick *Full-time attendant required, directs care provided by attendants*
		Bowel and bladder	Dependent, directs care provided by attendants
		Wheelchair mobility and pressure relief in wheelchair	Independent with power wheelchair Typical components include adaptive controls such as head, chin, tongue, or sip-and-puff control Electronically controlled seating system (tilt and/or recline) Wheelchair cushion and head/trunk support Portable ventilator (depending on innervation of diaphragm) Dependent with positioning in wheelchair
		Bed mobility	Dependent Adjustable bed with pressure-reducing mattress Directs care provided by attendants
		Transfers	Dependent, attendants use mechanical lift Directs care provided by attendants
		Ambulation	Unable
		Driving	Unable
C5			
Biceps Brachialis Brachioradialis Deltoid Infraspinatus Rhomboid (major and minor) Supinator	Elbow flexion and supination Shoulder external rotation Shoulder abduction and flexion to ~90°	ADL Feeding Grooming, washing face, and oral hygiene Bathing and dressing (dependent) Activation of computer, light switches, page turners, call buttons, electrical appliances, and speakerphones	Some assistance and/or setup required, depending on the activity Mobile arm supports, deltoid aid Adapted utensils and splinting Adapted equipment (wash mitt, adapted toothbrush, etc.) Dependent Adapted computer keyboard Hand splints Adapted typing sticks ECU *Part-time attendant required, directs care provided by attendants*
		Bowel and bladder	Dependent, directs care provided by attendants
		Wheelchair mobility and pressure relief in wheelchair	Independent to some assist with manual wheelchair on level surfaces Requires plastic-coated hand rims/extensions

Continued

Table 20.5 Functional Expectations for Patients With Spinal Cord Injury—cont'd

Motor Level and Key Muscles	Available Movements	Functional Capabilities	Equipment and Assistance Required
			Benefit from power-assist wheelchair Independent with power wheelchair using handheld joystick An electronically controlled seating system (tilt and/or recline) Wheelchair cushion and trunk support, dependent with positioning in wheelchair Manual wheelchair: independent to some assistance indoors on level surfaces, some/total assistance outdoors
		Bed mobility	Assistance to dependent Adjustable bed with pressure-reducing mattress Bed rails and loops Directs care provided by attendants
		Transfers	Dependent, attendants use mechanical lift Directs care provided by attendants May be able to perform with assistance and transfer board
		Ambulation	Unable
		Driving	Independent with van with adaptive controls
C6			
Extensor carpi radialis Infraspinatus Latissimus dorsi Pectoralis major (clavicular portion) Pronator teres Serratus anterior Teres minor	Shoulder flexion, extension, internal rotation, and adduction Scapular abduction, protraction, and upward rotation Forearm pronation Wrist extension (tenodesis grasp)	ADL	Assistance to independent with setup and/or equipment
		Feeding	Universal cuff, adaptive utensils
		Grooming, washing face, and oral hygiene	Adaptive equipment, universal cuff
		Dressing	Upper body: independent with adaptive equipment Lower body: assistance with adaptive equipment
		Bathing	Assistance with adaptive equipment
		Home management	Assistance, may be independent with certain tasks with adaptive equipment (e.g., light meal prep) *Part-time attendant required*
		Bowel and bladder care	May be able to be independent with adaptive equipment, likely to require assistance/dependent
		Wheelchair mobility and pressure relief in wheelchair	Independent with manual wheelchair on level surfaces and independent/some assistance in community May require power wheelchair in community Requires plastic-coated hand rims/extensions

Table 20.5 Functional Expectations for Patients With Spinal Cord Injury—cont'd

Motor Level and Key Muscles	Available Movements	Functional Capabilities	Equipment and Assistance Required
			May benefit from power-assist wheelchair Independent with pressure relief in wheelchair
		Bed mobility	Independent to some assistance with adaptive equipment and/or electric bed (e.g., bed rails, loops, etc.)
		Transfers	Independent to some assistance level surfaces Some assistance to total assistance with uneven transfers
		Ambulation	Unable
		Driving	Independent with car/van with adaptive controls
C7			
Extensor pollicis longus and brevis Extrinsic finger extensors Flexor carpi radialis Triceps	Elbow extension Wrist flexion Finger extension	ADL	Independent
		Feeding Grooming, washing face, and oral hygiene Dressing Bathing	Independent with most ADL with adaptive equipment (e.g. shower chair, hand rails, button hook, adaptive utensils) and wheelchair-accessible environment
		Home management	Likely to require assistance with heavy household tasks
		Bowel and bladder care	Independent with adaptive equipment
		Wheelchair mobility and pressure relief in wheelchair	Independent with manual wheelchair in home and community with plastic-coated hand rims May need some assist with ramps, curbs, and uneven terrain May benefit from power assist Independent with pressure relief
		Bed mobility	Independent, may require adaptive equipment (i.e., bed rails, leg loops)
		Transfers	Independent, may require assistance between uneven surfaces
		Ambulation	Unable
		Driving	Independent with car with adaptive controls
C8			
Extrinsic finger flexors Flexor carpi ulnaris Flexor pollicis longus and brevis Intrinsic finger flexor	Finger flexion	ADL	Independent
		Feeding Grooming, washing face, and oral hygiene Dressing Bathing	Independent in all ADLs, may require adaptive equipment (e.g., shower chair, hand rails, reacher, adaptive utensils) for some tasks and wheelchair-accessible environment
		Home management	Better able to perform with less need for adaptive equipment due to improved hand function compared to higher cervical-level injuries

Continued

Table 20.5 Functional Expectations for Patients With Spinal Cord Injury—cont'd

Motor Level and Key Muscles	Available Movements	Functional Capabilities	Equipment and Assistance Required
		Bowel and bladder care	Independent with adaptive equipment
		Wheelchair mobility and pressure relief in wheelchair	Independent with manual wheelchair in home and community Better able to propel on ramps, curbs, and uneven terrain due to improved hand function compared to higher cervical level injuries, may need assistance on uneven surfaces May benefit from power assist Independent with pressure relief
		Bed mobility	Independent to some assistance, may require adaptive equipment (i.e., bed rails, leg loops)
		Transfers	Independent, may require assistance between uneven surfaces May be able to transfer from floor into wheelchair
		Ambulation	Unable
		Driving	Independent with car with adaptive controls
T1 to T12			
Intercostals Long muscles of back (sacrospinalis and semispinalis) Abdominal musculature (~T7 and below)	Improved trunk control with more caudal SCI Increased respiratory reserve Pectoral girdle stabilized for lifting objects	ADL	Independent Independent in all areas Generally tasks become easier and require less adaptive equipment to perform with improved trunk control with more caudal SCI
		Bowel and bladder care	Independent with adaptive equipment
		Wheelchair mobility and pressure relief in wheelchair	Independent with manual wheelchair in home and community Independent on ramps, curbs, and uneven terrain Independent with pressure relief Wheelchair mobility becomes easier and more efficient with improved trunk control with more caudal SCI
		Bed mobility	Bed mobility independent, skills become easier and more efficient with improved trunk control with more caudal SCI
		Transfers	Independent Able to transfer from floor into wheelchair Transfers become easier and more efficient with improved trunk control with more caudal SCI

Table 20.5 Functional Expectations for Patients With Spinal Cord Injury—cont'd

Motor Level and Key Muscles	Available Movements	Functional Capabilities	Equipment and Assistance Required
		Ambulation	Independent with physiological standing and ambulation for exercise over short distances in the home Assistive devices (e.g., forearm crutches) Orthoses: hip-knee-ankle-foot-orthosis (HKAFO), knee-ankle-foot orthosis (KAFO)
		Driving	Independent with car with adaptive controls
L1, L2, L3			
Gracilis Iliopsoas Quadratus lumborum Rectus femoris Sartorius	Hip flexion Hip adduction Knee extension	Ambulation	Independent with short distances in home and possibly community Many choose to use wheelchair in the community due to high energy demands of community ambulation Assistive devices (e.g., forearm crutches) Orthoses: HKAFO, KAFO, AFO (depending on which muscles are innervated)
L4, L5, SI			
Quadriceps (L4) Anterior tibialis (L5) Hamstrings (L5–S1) Gastrocnemius (S1) Gluteus medius and maximus (L5–S1) Extensor digitorum, posterior tibialis, peroneals, flexor digitorum (L5, S1)	Strong hip flexion Strong knee extension Knee flexion Ankle dorsiflexion Ankle plantarflexion Ankle eversion Toe extension	Ambulation	Independent ambulation in home and community (L4-level injury may elect to use wheelchair for long distances) Assistive devices (e.g., forearm crutches, canes) Orthoses: AFO Less supportive assistive device and orthoses the more caudal the SCI

*This table presents general functional expectations at various lesion levels. Each progressively lower motor includes the muscles from the previous levels. Although the key muscles listed frequently receive innervation from several spinal levels, they are listed here at the key neurological levels where they add to functional outcomes. Although intact musculature plays a main role in determining functional capability, many other factors influence function, including concomitant injuries, premorbid health status, age, body type, and psychosocial factors. Individuals with an incomplete injury will likely have greater functional abilities.

Table updated by John LaRue, Doctor of Physical Therapy student, Clarkson University.

Examples of general goals and outcomes for patients with SCI as adapted from the *Guide to Physical Therapist Practice 3.0* are presented in Box 20.2.

For patients with high cervical SCI who may not be able to physically perform certain functional mobility tasks, goals should be directed toward patient ability to independently direct an attendant caregiver to perform the task appropriately.

Physical Therapy Interventions

Improvements in body structure/function impairments, the ability to perform activities that are important to the individual, and a return to participating in normal, desired social roles can be achieved through interventions that are based on compensatory strategies, restorative strategies, or a combination of the two. The intervention

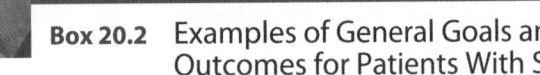

Box 20.2 Examples of General Goals and Outcomes for Patients With SCI

- Impact of pathology/pathophysiology is reduced.
  - Decrease risk of secondary impairment (i.e., pressure injury).
  - Educate patient family/caregiver regarding health condition, prognosis, and plan of care.
- Impact of body structure/function impairments is reduced.
  - Airway clearance is improved.
  - Muscle performance is increased.
  - Aerobic capacity is increased.
  - Joint mobility and integrity are improved or remain functional.
- Ability to perform physical actions, tasks, or activities is improved.
  - Tolerates upright sitting posture.
  - Independence with bed mobility tasks.
  - Independence with wheelchair mobility.
  - Independence with transfers.
  - Independence with self-directing care.
  - Independence with pressure relief.
- Disability associated with chronic health condition is reduced.
  - Independence with self-care and home management.
  - Resume work, community, and leisure roles.
  - Education on community resources.

Box 20.3 Common Precautions to Consider When Performing Interventions With People With Spinal Cord Injury

- Orthopedic/stress at the fracture site
- Skin integrity
- Blood pressure
- Fall risk
- Overstretching
- Overuse/stress

strategy selected is largely based on the amount of preserved motor function. Independence in functional skills in patients with complete motor SCI (AIS A and B [see Box 20.1]) is largely achieved through compensatory mechanisms, and interventions are developed accordingly. For example, a person with a C6 injury (AIS A) is taught to transfer from bed-to-wheelchair using a sit pivot method. Patients with AIS C or D, depending on the degree of motor return, may relearn how to perform functional tasks using more normal movement strategies. For example, a person with an AIS C or D may relearn to walk through locomotor training using a body-weight support (BWS) and treadmill (TM) system, an intervention that promotes normal movement patterns during gait training. This restorative approach attempts to minimize compensatory movement strategies and promote normal movement patterns to drive beneficial neuroplastic changes within the CNS.[216]

Because SCI affects many different body systems, certain precautions (Box 20.3) and general principles must be considered when performing interventions. Common principles used across compensatory intervention strategies to promote functional independence in mobility tasks are momentum, head–hips relationship, and muscle substitution. These compensatory strategies allow performance of functional mobility by substituting for lost motor function and strength below the lesion level. For example, a patient with a T1 AIS A will use momentum by swinging the arms across the body multiple times to roll from supine to side-lying as a compensation for lost trunk or LE muscles that would normally assist in performing the task.

For compensatory training, the overarching goal is to teach techniques to move the body using available musculature and motor control. These techniques will vary from individual to individual based on multiple factors, among them preexisting health conditions, body type, and ability to incorporate motor learning. Even individuals with the same level of injury may adapt seemingly very different techniques to maximize independence with function. There are, however, several principles that can be applied to all compensatory strategies, and examples of how these may be incorporated are covered in later sections:

- **Head-hips relationship:** This compensatory strategy is applicable to a variety of functional tasks. It involves moving the head in one direction in order to cause the movement of the hips in the opposite direction. For example, a compensatory strategy for sit-pivot transfers or wheelchair positioning is to lead with the hips while the head leans in the opposite direction.
- **Momentum:** Body segments with available motor function can be used to generate momentum (force × velocity) to facilitate movement of denervated body segments.
- **Muscle substitution:** To improve function, individuals with SCI typically become very adept at using intact muscles to substitute for those that are lost. If deemed safe and effective, these substitutions should be incorporated into movement training.
- **Task modification:** Modifying the task to make it easier allows for a progression and builds patient confidence and self-efficacy. Examples include placing a wedge behind the back to assist with early rolling activities, modifying the height for uneven transfers, or using adaptive equipment (e.g., trapeze

system over the bed to promote independence with bed mobility).
- **Working in and out of the task:** Failure to complete a functional task might be due to a lack of skill or a lack of required components (flexibility, strength, stability). Patients benefit from both task-specific skill training and out-of-task impairment-focused training (e.g., muscle strengthening and stretching).

Motor learning concepts should be incorporated into the POC. In the early stages of motor learning, when the patient is not skillful and cannot perform the task independently, extrinsic feedback regarding task performance may be useful. For example, the physical therapist may provide tactile and verbal cues on correct hand placement on the hand rim when the patient is practicing and learning how to perform wheelies. Extrinsic feedback provided on a faded schedule promotes motor learning. In later stages of motor learning, it is beneficial to have the patient use intrinsic feedback and rely less on extrinsic feedback. The practice schedule and environment can also be set up to promote motor learning. A random practice schedule is more beneficial to learning than a blocked practice schedule. The environment should be varied as the patient develops more skill in performing the task. For example, the patient should practice transferring to and from a variety of different surfaces (e.g., wheelchair to/from mat, bed, chair, car, sofa, etc.) once basic competence in the skill has been achieved.

For mobility tasks, it is often beneficial to break down the task into component parts for practice followed closely by practice of the integrated whole (parts-to-whole practice). For example, when learning to move from supine to long sitting, practice first focuses on a component part such as transitioning to supine on elbows. See Chapter 10, Strategies to Improve Motor Function, for a discussion of motor learning strategies.

Strengthening

As described earlier, strengthening all remaining innervated musculature is an important component of the POC. Key UE muscles to strengthen include serratus anterior, latissimus dorsi, pectoralis major, rotator cuff muscles, and triceps brachii.[218,219] These muscles are particularly important for independent transfers. Initially, strengthening exercises may be done daily during early rehabilitation. A variety of methods can be used to implement strengthening exercises such as pulley systems, free weights, manual resistance, elastic bands, and weight cuffs. With very weak muscles (grade ≤2) strengthening can be performed in gravity-reduced positions on a powder board or with active assistive ROM. Strengthening can be done in functional postures as well. For example, push-ups can be performed in prone-on-elbows and supine-on-elbows. Regardless of the strengthening modality or baseline level of strength, it is important to dose on the basis of 60% to 80% of the 1Repetition Max (RM) (or 100% of the 10RM, the intensity required to complete 10 repetitions before fatigue).[220,221]

Cardiovascular/Endurance Training

As with able-bodied people, cardiovascular training has important health benefits for people with SCI. A number of studies have shown that endurance training can improve aerobic fitness.[222-224] Upper extremity–based exercises such as arm ergometry, wheelchair propulsion, and swimming are the most common method of aerobic training. In people with iSCI who have sufficient walking capacity, locomotor training on a TM with or without BWS is another method of endurance training.[225] The American College of Sports Medicine recommends endurance training 3 to 5 days a week, with a total duration per day of 20 to 60 minutes at 50% to 80% of peak heart rate (HR).[220] If individuals are not capable of increasing HR secondary to sympathetic nervous system damage, a rating of perceived exertion (RPE) of 13 to 17 may be substituted for maximum HR percentage.[226] The duration and intensity of the training should be gradually increased for those not able to initially tolerate these training levels. Surface functional electrical stimulation (FES)–induced cycling or walking is also an effective means of improving cardiovascular fitness.[227] Surface electrodes are attached bilaterally to the hamstrings, quadriceps, and gluteal muscles; a computer controls the intensity of the muscle stimulation and cadence based on the position of the pedals (Fig. 20.13). Any activity, including functional training and strength training, that keeps the HR or RPE in the target zone for 20 to 60 minutes constitutes cardiovascular training and may be an appropriate substitution for those who are not capable of utilizing traditional endurance training techniques or equipment.

Bed Mobility Skills

Bed mobility skills are necessary to promote independence in functional mobility. These skills include rolling, transitioning supine to/from sitting on the edge of the bed, and LE management. Independence in these skills is also necessary for dressing, positioning in bed, and skin inspection. The degree to which these skills can be performed independently depends on the individual's level of injury and other factors. The exact method of performing the task will vary with the individual. The skills and intervention techniques described below provide a general guide; however, these may need to be adapted depending on the unique presentation of the patient. Again, certain precautions need to be observed when teaching patients these techniques. For example, excessive friction on the elbows while weight shifting in prone-on-elbows may result in skin breakdown. Patients may begin training wearing protective elbow pads.

At first, bed mobility skills are learned and practiced on an exercise mat, which is firmer and larger than a typical bed. However, as skill improves, they should be

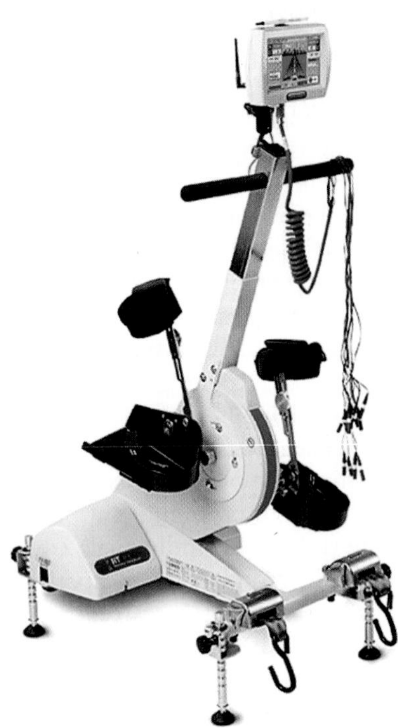

Figure 20.13 FES-powered lower extremity ergometer. *(Courtesy of Restorative Therapies, Baltimore, MD 21224.)*

practiced on a bed similar to that used at home. A patient may be independent performing these skills on a mat but still require more practice to become independent performing the same task on a bed due to the softer and smaller surface.

Individuals with complete SCI will need to use compensatory movement strategies (e.g., momentum, muscle substitution, and head-hips principle) to move the entire body. For example, a patient with a T1 AIS A injury will swing the arms up and across the body to generate momentum that will cause the trunk and legs to roll to the side-lying position from supine. A patient with a T10 AIS A injury will use muscle substitution by using the UEs to lift the legs up onto the mat from a short sitting position when transitioning to supine from sitting. Individuals with iSCI may be able to use more normal movement strategies to perform these tasks, depending on the extent of motor recovery. Regardless of whether the injury is complete or incomplete, the recovery of normal movement patterns should be attempted and assessed.

Rolling

Rolling is a frequent focal point of mat programs, and it is a prerequisite skill for other bed mobility tasks and provides an early lesson in developing functional patterns of movement. It requires the patient to learn to use the head, neck, and UEs, as well as momentum, to move the trunk and/or LEs. It is usually easiest to begin rolling activities from the supine position, working toward the prone position. If asymmetric involvement exists, rolling should be initiated with movement toward the weaker side. While rolling is a prerequisite skill for many other functional tasks, it is also very difficult and may require an extended period of time to master.

To develop maximum independence, adaptive devices such as bed rails, ropes, canvas "ladders," or overhead devices such as trapezes should be avoided, if possible. However, if these adaptive devices allow more efficient or independent task performance or when the task cannot be otherwise accomplished, they should be incorporated into the overall POC. In addition, the patient should work toward achieving independent rolling when covered by sheets and blankets. To begin training and facilitate rolling, several strategies can be used:

- Flexion of the head and neck with rotation may be used to assist movement from supine to prone positions.
- Extension of the head and neck with rotation may be used to assist movement from prone to supine positions.
- Bilateral, symmetrical UE rocking with outstretched arms produces a pendular motion when moving from supine to prone positions. The patient rhythmically rocks the outstretched arms and head from side to side and then forcefully "tosses" them to the side to which the patient is rolling. The trunk and hips will follow (Fig. 20.14). The head and arms should be synchronized. Use of wrist cuff weights (2 to 3 lb) may be used initially to increase kinesthetic awareness and momentum. The number of rocking motions necessary will depend on the patient's skill, level of SCI, and body type.
- Crossing the ankles will also facilitate rolling initially (see Fig. 20.14). The therapist crosses the patient's ankles so that the upper limb is toward the direction of the roll (e.g., the right ankle would be crossed over the left when rolling toward the left). When first learning, flexing the hip and knee of the top LE and placing it over the opposite limb (e.g., the hip and knee of the right LE would be flexed and placed over the left when rolling toward the left) can assist.
- In moving from the supine position to the prone position, pillows may be placed under one side of the pelvis (or scapula, if needed) to create initial rotation in the direction of the roll. The activity can be started with two pillows, progress to one, and then to rolling without the use of pillows. If difficulty is encountered in initiating the roll, the activity can be started from a side-lying position. To facilitate movement from prone to supine positions, pillows may be placed under one side of the chest and/or pelvis. Again, the number and height of pillows should be reduced gradually and eventually eliminated.
- Several *proprioceptive neuromuscular facilitation* (PNF) patterns are useful during early rolling

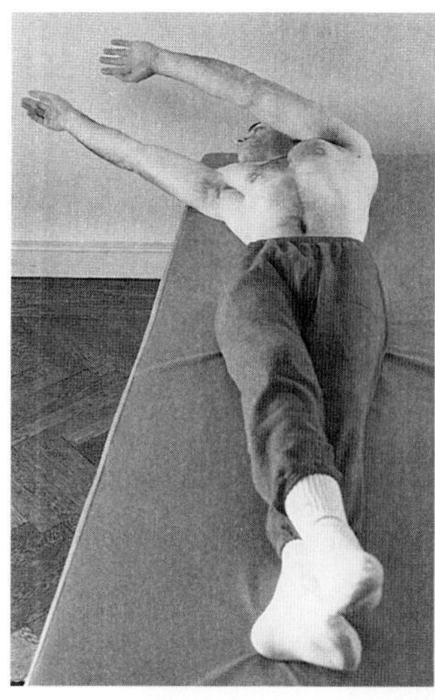
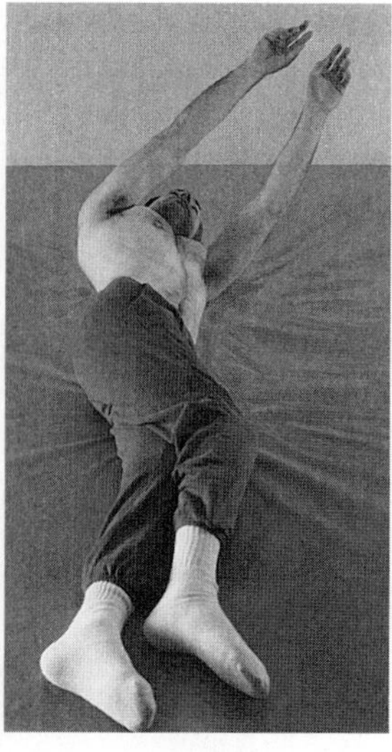
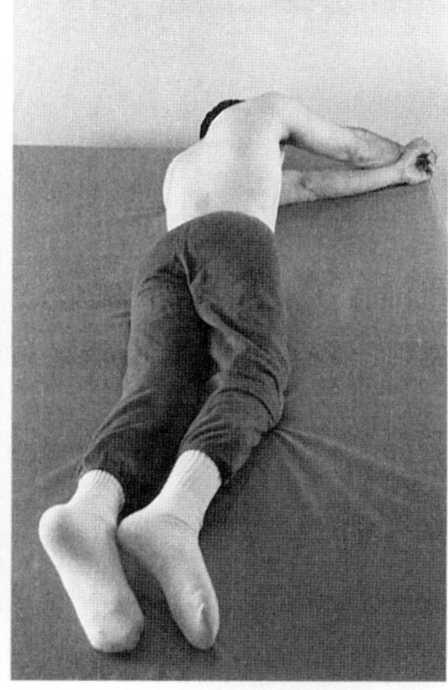

Figure 20.14 Rolling from supine to prone using UE momentum and crossing the ankles.

activities. The UE flexion-adduction-external rotation and extension-adduction-internal rotation patterns, and reverse chop will facilitate rolling toward the prone position. The UE lift pattern will facilitate rolling toward the supine position from side-lying.

Transitioning Supine to/From Sitting

The ability to transition from supine in bed to sitting on the edge of the bed is a critical skill necessary for independent mobility. Before a person can transfer out of bed to a wheelchair, the ability to sit up on the edge of the bed must be first achieved. There are two basic methods (with variations) to transition from supine to sitting: (1) "walking" onto elbows from prone or side-lying and (2) coming straight up from supine. Both of these methods transition the patient from supine to long sitting. The patient then must learn to manage the LEs to move into short sitting on the edge of the bed. In addition to rolling, two important prerequisite skills/postures that are necessary to come to long sitting from supine are the ability to assume and move within prone-on-elbows and supine-on-elbows. Long-sitting requires at least 90 degrees of hamstring length bilaterally and may be substituted by having the patient long-sit with external rotation of the hips with the knees slightly flexed.

Prone on Elbows

Prone-on-elbows can be assumed from either prone or side-lying. In prone, the shoulders can be either abducted (elbows out away from the body) or adducted (elbows at the side of the trunk) and the patient weight shifts from side to side while moving the unweighted arm to eventually position both elbows directly underneath the shoulder joints (Fig. 20.15A and B). From side-lying, the patient pushes the elbow that is on the mat down into the mat by extending the shoulder, then swings the top arm forward while rolling to prone so the elbow comes onto mat in the prone-on-elbows position.

Transitioning into prone-on-elbows is a challenging skill, particularly for individuals without functioning triceps. The patient can be assisted into the position and practice stability and controlled mobility interventions initially.

- Weight-bearing in the prone-on-elbows position will improve stability and strength at the upper trunk, neck, and shoulders.
- The PNF technique of rhythmic stabilization may be used to increase stability and strength at the head, neck, shoulders, and scapula.
- Weight shifting assists with development of controlled mobility and is usually easiest in a lateral direction with a progression to anterior or posterior movements.
- Unilateral weight-bearing on one elbow can be achieved in the prone-on-elbows position by having the patient lift one arm. This further facilitates co-contraction in the weight-bearing limb.
- Movement within this posture can be achieved by walking on elbows to both sides, up toward the head of the mat, and backward toward the foot of the mat.
- Strengthening of the serratus anterior and other scapular muscles can be achieved with prone-on-elbows push-ups. This is accomplished by having the patient push the elbows down into the mat and tuck in the chin while lifting and rounding out the shoulders and upper thorax. This is similar to the "cat/camel" maneuver used in the quadruped position. The patient lowers the upper chest to the mat again by allowing the scapula to adduct.

Supine-on-Elbows

There are several approaches to assuming the supine-on-elbows position. If control of abdominal muscles is present, the patient may have sufficient strength to achieve the position by pushing the elbows into the mat and lifting into the position. A common technique is for

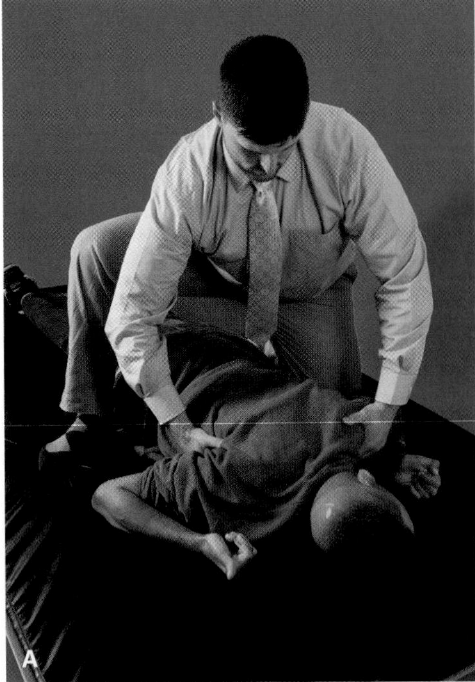

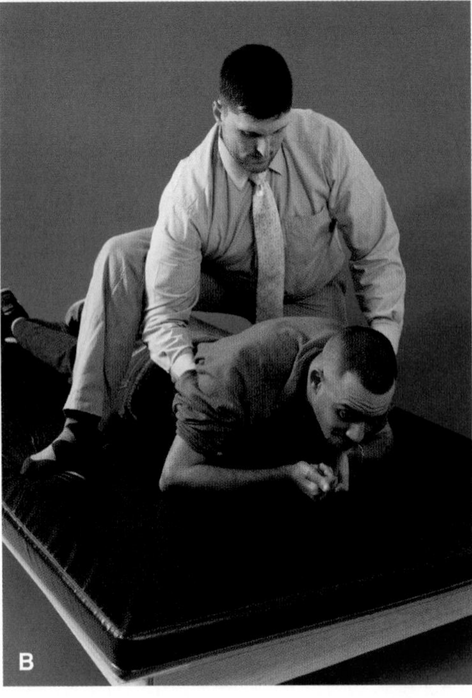

Figure 20.15 Transitioning from prone (A) to prone on elbows (B) with shoulders initially abducted and weight shifting.

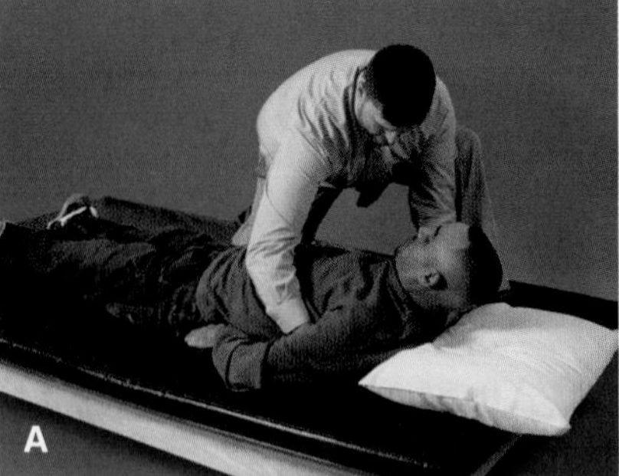

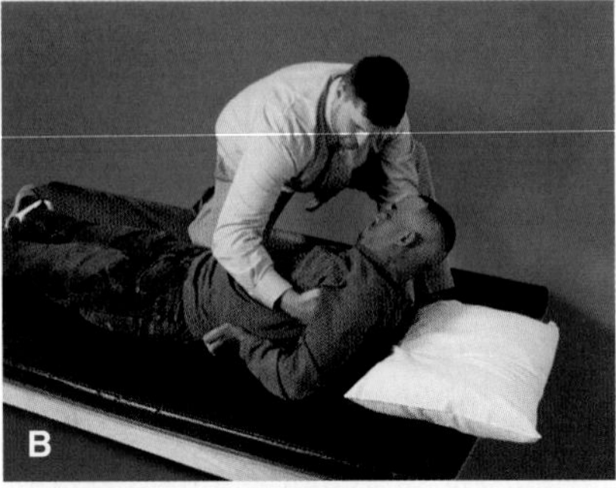

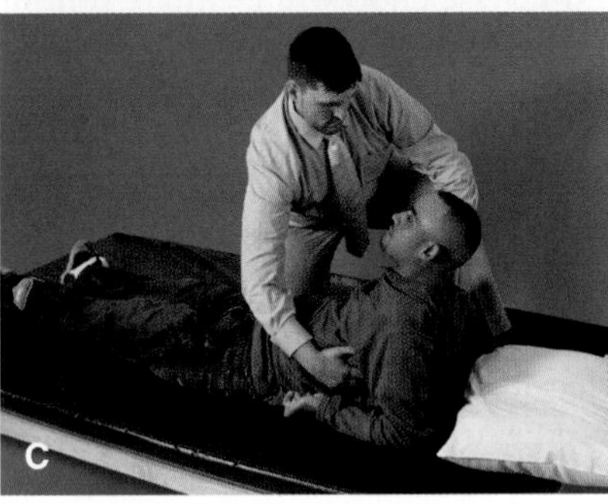

Figure 20.16 Patient transitioning from supine (A) to supine-on-elbows (B) by stabilizing hands under pelvis, forcefully pulling up by contracting the biceps, weight shifting side to side, and placing elbows farther underneath the shoulder joints (C).

the patient to "wedge" the hands under the hips or to hook the thumbs into pants pockets or belt loops. By contracting the biceps and/or wrist extensors, the patient can pull up partially into the posture. By shifting weight from side to side, the elbows can then be positioned under the shoulders (Fig. 20.16A, B, and C).

Some patients may find it easiest to assume this position from side-lying. The lower elbow is first positioned and pushed into the mat. The patient then rolls toward the supine position and quickly extends the upper arm, landing on the elbow as close to the shoulder as possible. By weight shifting, placement of the elbows can then be adjusted.

Much of the inherent benefit of this activity is achieved in learning to assume the posture and then move into long sitting. In addition to its direct functional significance, this activity is also an important strengthening exercise for shoulder extensors and scapular adductors.

- Rhythmic stabilization may be used to increase stability and strength at the head, neck, shoulder, and scapula.
- Lateral weight shifting can be practiced in this position.
- Side-to-side movement in this posture will enhance the patient's ability to align the trunk with the

LEs when in bed or in preparation for positional changes.

- Precautions should be taken with this posture because it may cause increased shoulder pain due to the pressure exerted on the anterior shoulder joint capsule.

Walking on Elbows to Assume Long Sitting

From prone the patient walks on elbows toward one side into a "C" position. The patient then unweights the elbow closest to the legs and hooks it around the knees and pulls the trunk toward the legs. At a certain point, the patient can then shift weight off the weight-bearing elbow to the palm and push with one arm while pulling with the other up to a long sitting position (Fig. 20.17A, B, C, and D).

This method of coming to long sitting does not require as much ROM in the shoulders as coming to sitting straight up from supine (see below). Practicing component parts of the task (e.g., walking on elbows or pulling up with one arm once in the "C" position), followed closely by practicing the whole task can be used to facilitate learning.

Coming Straight to Long Sitting From Supine

To come to long sitting from supine requires a more than normal amount of shoulder extension and strong elbow flexors and wrist extensors. From supine, the patient should assume the supine-on-elbows position as described above. From this position, the patient unweights one elbow by shifting onto the opposite elbow. For the patient with a midlevel cervical SCI, the unweighted UE is thrown back into hyperextension and external rotation with the elbow extended so that the palm is on the mat. The patient then rotates the upper trunk onto the UE that was just thrown back in order to unweight the other UE. The unweighted UE is now thrown back in a similar manner so that the patient is now weight-bearing on both hands, then weight shifts side to side and walks the hands up to assume a long sitting position (Fig. 20.18A, B, and C). Again, it is useful to practice parts of the task to assist in learning how to perform the entire skill.

Patients without sufficient strength or ROM, or due to other factors, may use adaptive equipment such as bed rails, loop ladder, suspended trapeze, or suspended loops to assist in coming to long sitting.

Once in long sitting, patients must learn to move the LEs off the edge of the bed to come to short sitting, back onto the bed when moving from short sitting to supine, and to position themselves in bed using their UEs. Patients without full finger and hand musculature innervation can slide the wrist under a leg so that the palm of the hand is facing the mat and extend the wrist to help move the legs. Alternatively, leg loops can be placed around the thighs to slide the hand in and extend the wrist to lift the leg.

Sitting Balance

Independent sitting balance, both in short sitting and long sitting, is an important skill for many different functional tasks such as transfers, dressing, and wheelchair mobility. Sitting posture will vary considerably with lesion level. Patients with low thoracic lesions can be expected to sit with a relatively erect trunk. Individuals with low cervical and high thoracic lesions maintain sitting balance by forward head displacement and trunk flexion (Figs. 20.19 and 20.20).

Owing to sensory and motor impairments, patients need to relearn their center of balance and limits of stability

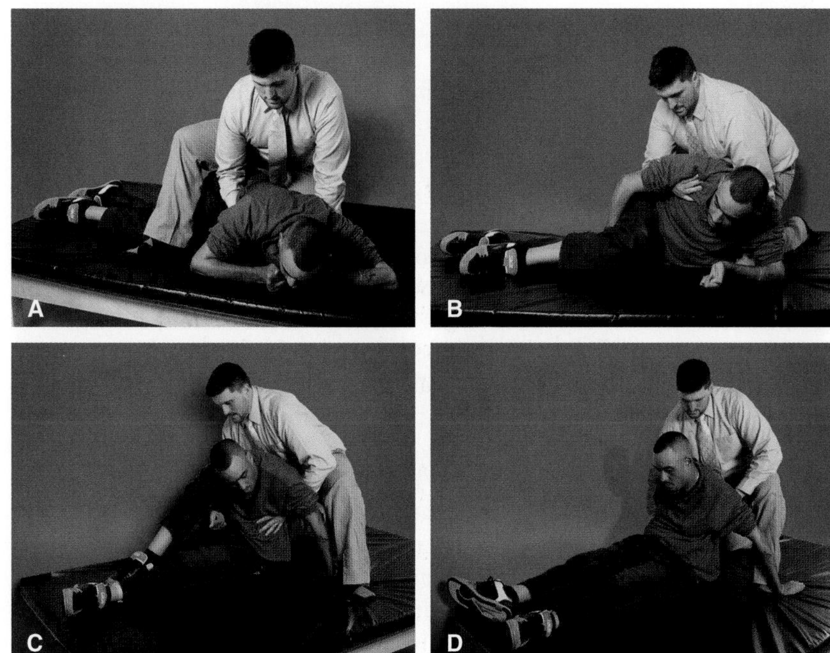

Figure 20.17 Patient transitioning from prone-on-elbows (A) to long sitting (B), walks into a "C" position (C), pulls trunk up to long sitting position (D).

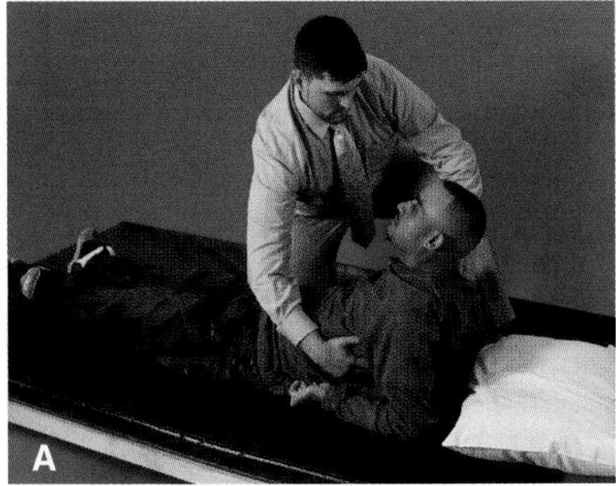

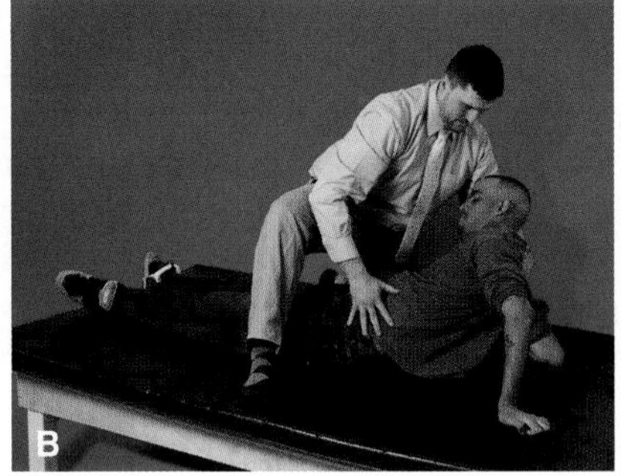

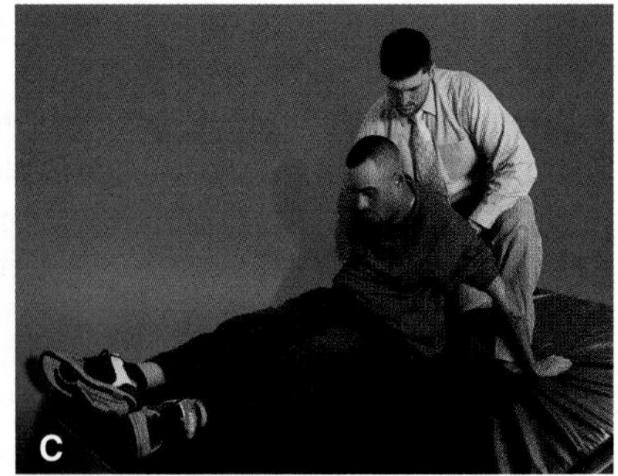

Figure 20.18 Patient transitioning to long sitting from supine-on-elbows (A). Bears weight on one elbow while the other UE is thrown back into shoulder extension with the elbow extended to bear weight on the other UE (B); then weight shifts onto the other UE and throws other UE back into shoulder extension with elbow extended to come into long sitting (C).

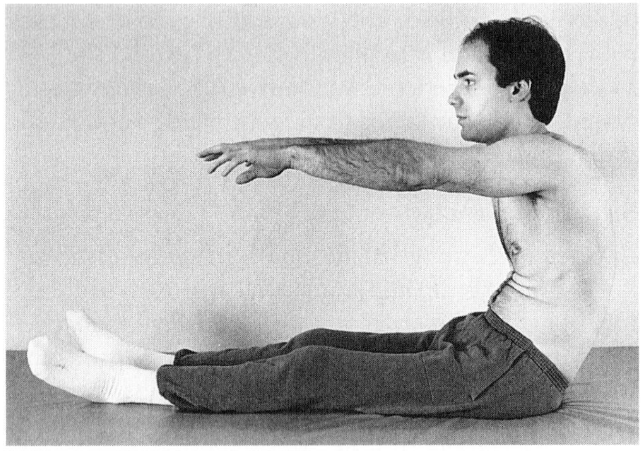

Figure 20.19 Individual with a T4 AIS A injury in long sitting.

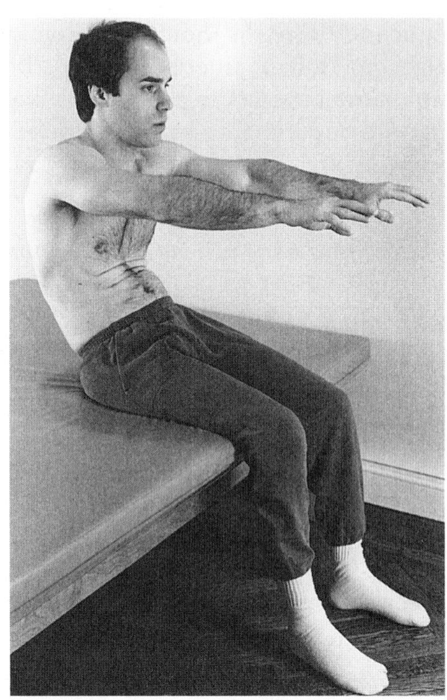

Figure 20.20 Individual with a T4 AIS A injury in short sitting.

as well as how to maintain postural control. The following are some suggestions that can be incorporated to improve sitting balance, both in long and short sitting.

- Sitting balance training is initially done by assisting the patient into a balanced short or long sitting position. In short sitting, the patient should initially be positioned with the feet firmly supported on the floor and the hips and knees flexed to 90 degrees. In long sitting, patients should have approximately 90 to 100 degrees of straight leg raise ROM to avoid overstretching the low back muscles. Initially, it is easier to maintain balance in long sitting due to the larger BOS. The LEs can be placed with the hips in external rotation and slight abduction to allow knee flexion to avoid overstretching the low back muscles if there is insufficient hamstring flexibility.
- Patients may initially need to bear weight through the UEs to maintain the sitting position. For patients with cervical-level lesions who utilize a tenodesis grasp to hold and manipulate objects, the fingers should be flexed at the proximal and distal interphalangeal joints when the wrist is in full extension to prevent overstretching the finger flexor tendons. Patients who do not have triceps innervation need to learn to keep the elbows extended through muscle substitution. In a closed-chain position, extended elbows combined with shoulder external rotation will assist in maintaining the tripod position. The patient throws back the shoulder into full extension while externally rotating the shoulder and supinating the forearm. When the UE is weight-bearing in this position, the patient can contract the anterior deltoids to flex the shoulder in a closed chain, which will extend the elbow.
- Stability in sitting can be enhanced by providing manual resistance to the upper trunk using PNF

techniques of stabilizing reversals and rhythmic stabilization.
- Sitting practice should include altering UE support (bilateral, unilateral, with progression to no support). Reaching for objects with one and both UEs can improve anticipatory balance reactions. Patients should also practice maintaining postural control while manipulating objects and performing ADL in sitting.
- Patients should safely learn their new limits of stability. This can be accomplished by weight shifting until the point is reached where balance can no longer be maintained; close supervision/assistance is warranted.
- Providing unexpected perturbations in a safe manner can be used to practice reactive postural control.
- Balance interventions should be practiced on a variety of surfaces: firm mat, bed, dense foam, sofa cushion, and so forth. Balance interventions should also be practiced while sitting in the patient's wheelchair.

Transfers

There are three components to the sit-pivot transfer (e.g., bed to/from wheelchair in a seated position): preparatory phase, lift phase, and descent phase.[228] During the *preparatory phase,* the trunk flexes forward, leans laterally, and rotates toward the trailing arm in order to lead with the hips (see description of head-hips relationship below) (Fig. 20.21A). The *lift phase* starts when the buttocks lift off the sitting surface and continues while the trunk is lifted halfway between the two surfaces (Fig. 20.21B). The *descent phase* denotes the period when the trunk is lowered to the other seating surface, from the halfway point until the buttocks are on the other surface (Fig. 20.21C).

The following are key components and intervention strategies that can be used to improve transfer ability:

- Provide support and assistance so the patient feels safe and comfortable while learning transfers.
- Confidence and skill in maintaining sitting balance is critical (see above strategies).
- The head–hips relationship is important. Moving the head and upper trunk in one direction causes the lower trunk and buttocks to move in the opposite direction. For example, if the patient wants to transfer from bed to the wheelchair, which is positioned to the patient's right, the patient rocks the head and upper trunk forward/downward and to the left. In combination with protracting the scapulae to lift the buttocks, this will cause the lower trunk and buttocks to lift upward and swing to the right into the wheelchair.
- For patients without innervated triceps, the strategies described above can be used to place and maintain the elbows in extension. For patients without full finger function, overstretching the finger flexors as described above should be avoided.

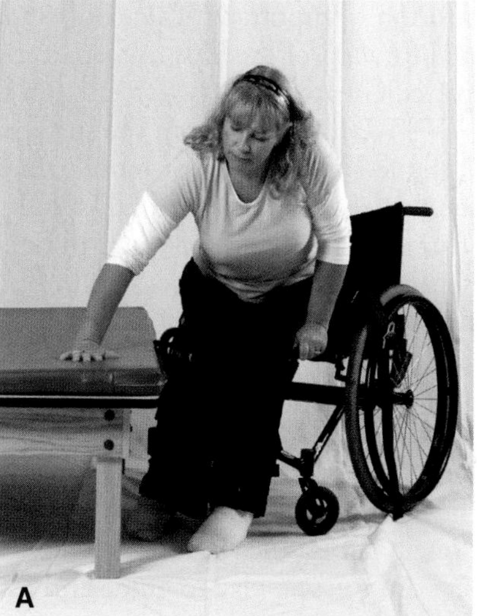

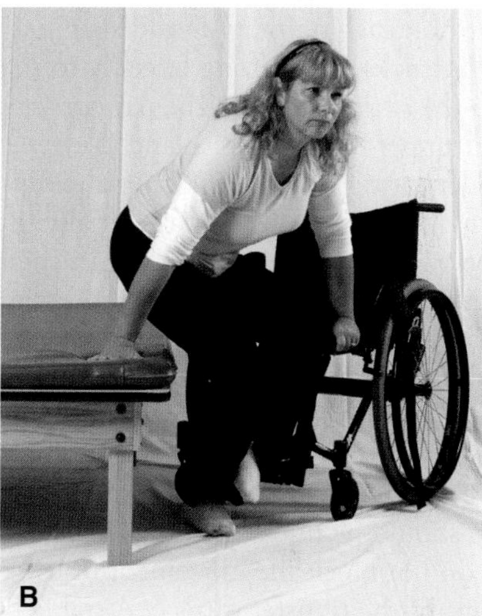

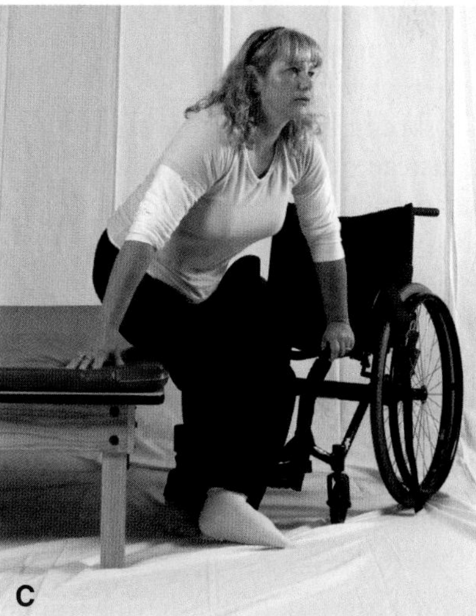

Figure 20.21 (A) Preparatory phase of the transfer; trunk is flexed forward and laterally away from surface transferring to. (B) Lift phase; buttocks are lifted off the seating surface as the trunk rotates. (C) End of the descent phase when the buttocks are on the other sitting surface. *(From O'Sullivan, S, and Schmitz, T: Improving Functional Outcomes in Physical Rehabilitation. FA Davis, Philadelphia, 2010, with permission.)*

- Hand position is important. The hands should be positioned forward of the hips to form a tripod with the buttocks. Greater force is generated in the trailing UE[228,229] (UE farthest from the surface transferring to); if one UE is weaker or more painful, it should be the lead UE. The lead UE should be farther from the trunk/buttocks and the trailing UE closer to the trunk/buttocks.
- Part to whole task training protracting the scapulae while leaning head and upper trunk forward and down (head–hips relationship) should be practiced to lift the buttocks off the sitting surface. The physical therapist can assist by placing his or her hands under the patient's hips and assisting the lift or by placing one hand on the front of the chest and the other between the scapulae to guide and assist the forward/downward lean and lift.
- Part to whole task training should also include lifting the buttocks and shifting laterally to the left and right on the sitting surface. The patient should lean the head/upper trunk forward and downward, then twist to left or right to lift and shift the hips in the opposite direction. Patients may initially lift the hips and then twist the upper trunk to shift the lower trunk and buttocks in the opposite direction in two motions. As the patient improves, these two movements should be performed as a single motion.
- Lower extremities should be positioned with the feet supported and the hips and knees at approximately 90 degrees of flexion or slightly more at the hips. The legs should be midway between the two surfaces so they do not block the movement of the trunk and body toward the transfer surface. A stable position of the feet, even in those without LE motor control, will provide a pivot point and increase stability during the transfer.
- Emphasis should be placed on lifting and shifting laterally instead of sliding/scooting to the side to avoid shearing of the skin. Control of movement should be promoted during the descent phase to avoid trauma to the skin. A transfer board may be used initially until the patient gains more skill with the task. Some patients with mid-cervical SCI may always require a transfer board.
- Transfer training should include a variety of surfaces from the wheelchair (bed, sofa, toilet, car, etc.) and to varying heights (higher and lower than the wheelchair surface).

In addition to the task of transferring from one surface to another, there are important complementary skills that patients must be able to perform to be fully independent with transfers. These include positioning the wheelchair, setting wheel locks, removing and replacing armrests on the wheelchair, removing and replacing legrests on the wheelchair, managing LEs, and managing body position in the wheelchair.

Floor-to-Wheelchair Transfers

There are several basic floor-to-wheelchair techniques, including forward (Fig. 20.22A–D) and sideways (Fig. 20.23A–C) approaches. *Improving Functional Outcomes in Physical Rehabilitation*[230] and *Spinal Cord Injury: Functional Rehabilitation*[123] provide more detail on how to perform these transfers and other interventions to improve transfer ability.

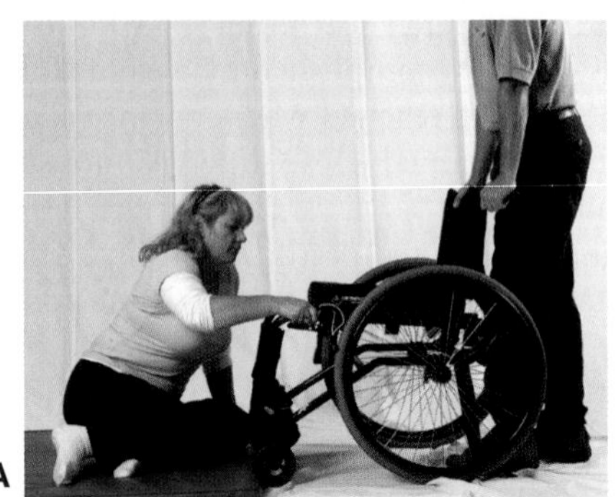

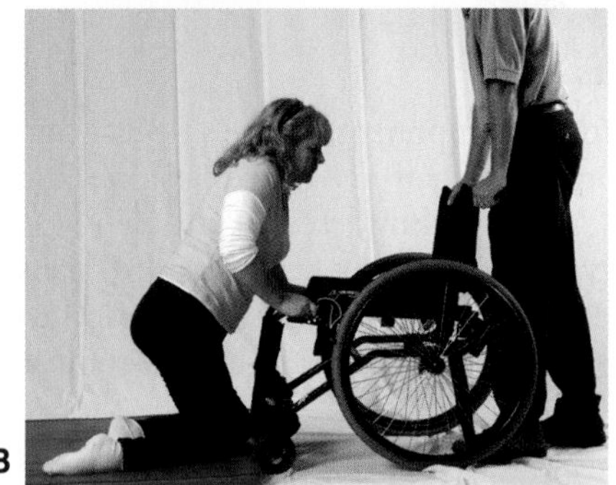

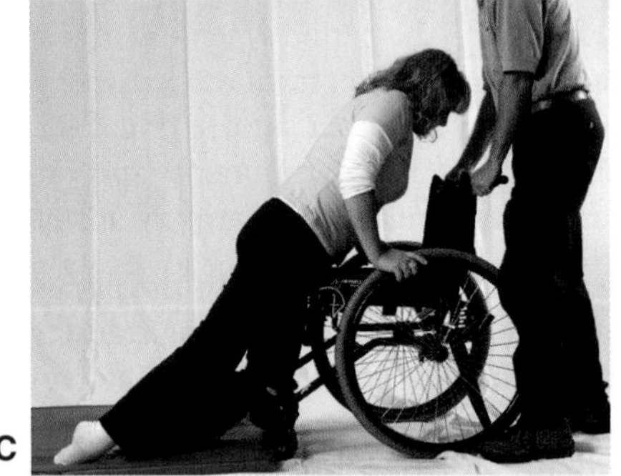

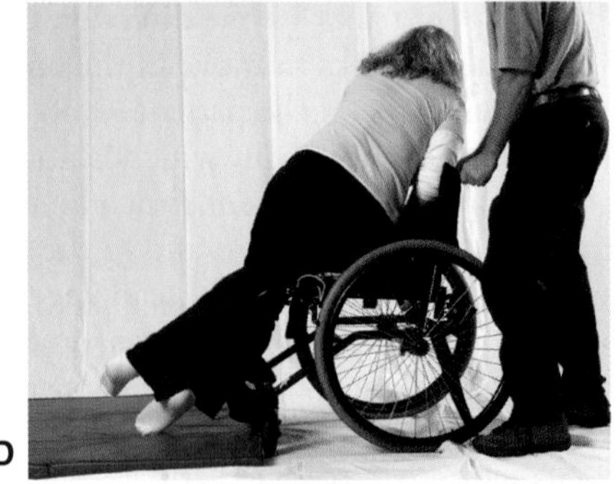

Figure 20.22 (A–D) Floor to wheelchair transfer using a frontward approach. *(From O'Sullivan, S, and Schmitz, T: Improving Functional Outcomes in Physical Rehabilitation. FA Davis, Philadelphia, 2016, with permission.)*

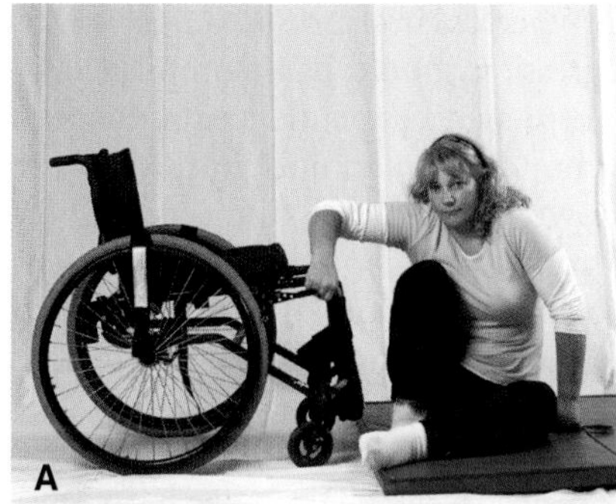

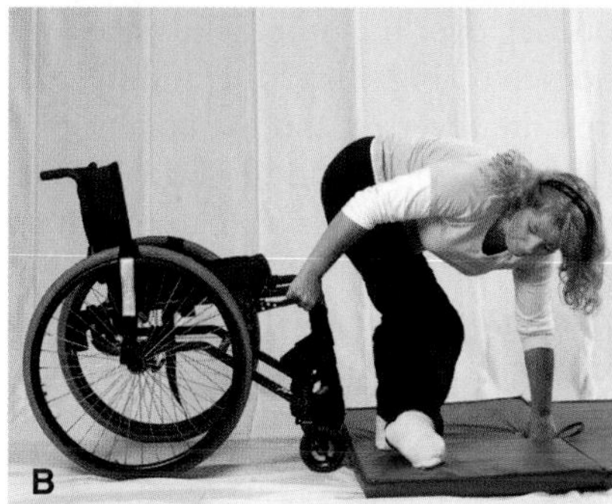

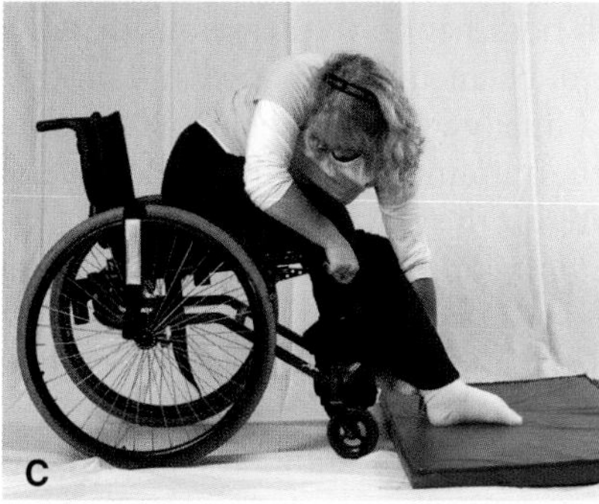

Figure 20.23 (A–C) Floor to wheelchair transfer using a sideways approach. *(From O'Sullivan, S, and Schmitz, T: Improving Functional Outcomes in Physical Rehabilitation. FA Davis, Philadelphia, 2016, with permission.)*

Locomotor Rehabilitation

Regaining the ability to walk is a common goal for most individuals following SCI. A number of factors will influence the success or failure in attaining this goal. Patients must possess adequate muscle strength, postural alignment, ROM, and sufficient cardiovascular endurance to become functional ambulators. Becoming a functional ambulator following a complete SCI is very difficult. Walking with orthoses and assistive devices is slower and requires considerably more energy than walking before the injury. Many individuals with motor complete SCI who learn to walk with these devices may not continue walking once they stop rehabilitation. Patients with motor iSCI (AIS C and D) are more likely to regain functional ambulation skills than those with complete or sensory incomplete injuries.[209,211,212]

This section on strategies to improve locomotor function is divided into two parts. The first deals with gait retraining using a compensatory-based approach for people with motor complete SCI. The second part highlights a recovery and activity-based approach for people with motor iSCI.

Compensatory-Based Approach

When initiating a program to improve locomotor function for individuals with complete SCI, therapists should be realistic and provide a clear picture of the costs and potential benefits. Patients who wish to relearn to ambulate following SCI should be given this option even if their potential for functional ambulation is limited. Although some patients may not become functional ambulators, standing alone may provide other important benefits such as improved circulation, skin integrity, bowel and bladder function, sleep, and a sense of well-being.[231-233]

Individuals with complete SCI rely on orthotic and assistive devices, adequate ROM, and maximizing strength of neurologically intact musculature for standing and walking. Full ROM in hip extension is essential in attaining balance in the upright position. The patient learns to lean into the anterior ligaments of the hip with the trunk extended to stabilize the trunk and pelvis (often referred to as the "parastance" position). The absence of knee flexion and plantarflexion contractures is also important in attaining upright standing balance.

Adequate cardiovascular endurance also is a criterion for functional ambulation. Because the energy cost of ambulation for a patient with complete paraplegia is higher than it is for people without SCI, endurance becomes an important factor in determining success or failure and continued ambulation once rehabilitation is complete. In addition, the energetic cost (oxygen utilization per unit distance) of walking with braces and compensatory strategies is very high compared to normal ambulation.[231]

Other factors that may restrict ambulation include severe spasticity, loss of proprioception (particularly at the hips and knees), pain, obesity, and the presence of secondary complications such as pressure injuries, heterotopic bone formation at the hips, or deformity. In addition, the patient's motivation plays a key role in determining success or failure in ambulation. A highly motivated patient can learn to walk using KAFOs and assistive devices. However, these patients may eventually find that the energy cost of ambulation is too great.

Follow-up studies of long-term continuation of ambulation have not been extensive. Mikelberg and Reid[232] surveyed 60 individuals with SCI for whom orthotics had been prescribed. From this group, 60% used their wheelchairs as the primary means of mobility. Thirty-one percent completely discarded their orthoses. Those who did use their orthoses reserved them primarily for standing and exercise activities. It was reported as early as 1973 that functional ambulation required knee control in at least one leg,[233] and there is little data to suggest that individuals with SCI become long-term functional ambulators using bilateral KAFOs.

For patients with complete SCI, training emphasis is on strengthening available musculature; using assistive devices and orthoses to support weak or denervated muscles; and learning new, compensatory methods of walking. Forearm crutches are most often selected for patients with paraplegia. These crutches provide several advantages. They are lightweight; they allow use of the hand without the crutch becoming disengaged; they fit more easily into an automobile; and, most importantly, they improve function in ambulation and stair climbing by allowing full hip extension and unrestricted movement at the shoulders. See Chapter 30, Orthotics, that provides a detailed discussion of different types of orthoses.

Swing-through (Fig. 20.24) and four-point gait patterns are two common walking patterns learned by patients with complete SCI using KAFOs. Initial standing balance and gait training should be done in the parallel bars and then progressed to the appropriate assistive device when the patient is ready. Relevant training activities include those described below.

Performed in Sitting or Supine

- *Putting on and removing orthoses.* The patient is first taught the correct way to don and doff the orthoses. The patient must be cautioned to continuously monitor skin for pressure areas, particularly after brace removal.

Performed in Parallel Bars

- *Sit-to-stand activities.* These activities should be practiced using a wheelchair, then progressed to using the forearm crutches. The patient must learn to slide to the edge of the chair and unlock and lock the orthoses. Initially the patient is taught to pull to standing, using the parallel bars (a progression is made to using the wheelchair armrests to push to standing). This progression should be accomplished as quickly as possible to avoid dependence on the pulling mechanism. Once in an upright position, the patient pushes down on the hands and tilts the pelvis forward in front of the shoulders. Return to sitting is a reversal of this procedure. To begin this activity with crutches, the patient first places the crutches behind the chair, leaning against the push handle(s). To assume a standing position with crutches, the patient moves forward in the chair, locks both knee joints, crosses one leg over the other, and then rotates the trunk and pelvis (Fig. 20.25). Hand placements on the armrest are reversed and the patient pushes to standing by pivoting around to face the chair. The reverse of this technique is used to return to the chair.
- *Static standing balance.* The patient learns to balance in standing with the hips in hyperextension and the upper trunk, head, feet, and arms behind the pelvis. The feet are 3 to 5 in. (7.6 to 12.7 cm) apart. The patient should first practice maintaining this position with both hands on the parallel bars, then progress to balancing with one hand off the parallel bars, and finally with both hands off the bars. The greater the amount of dorsiflexion at the ankle, the more anterior the pelvis can be.
- *Weight shifting in standing.* This entails controlling the pelvic position using UE support and positioning the head and shoulders forward ahead of the pelvis. The head–hips relationship applied in transfers also applies in standing. The patient must be taught recovery to overcome and/or to prevent jackknifing from happening during ambulation. Jackknifing occurs when the patient's center of mass (COM) falls anterior to the hips, causing the patient to flex forward suddenly.

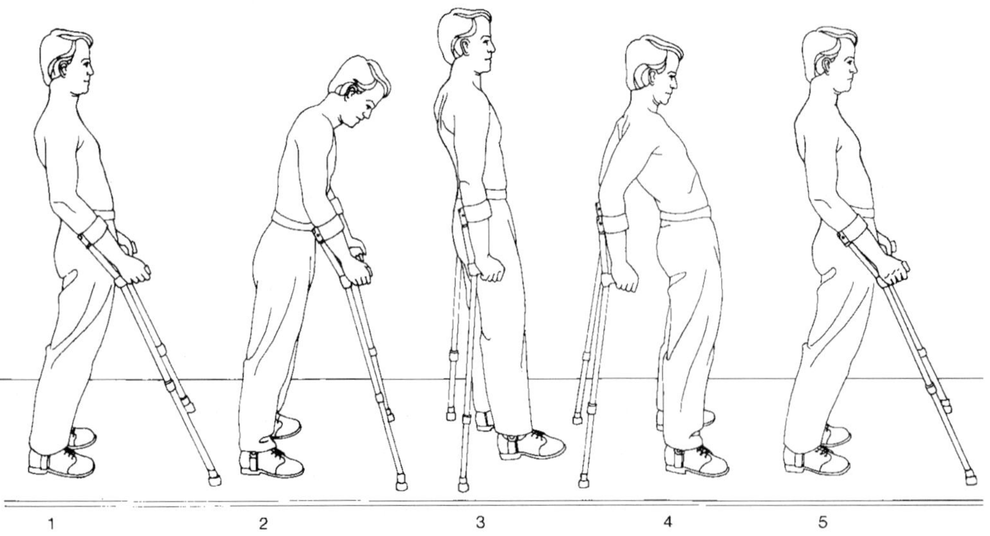

Figure 20.24 Swing-through gait pattern.

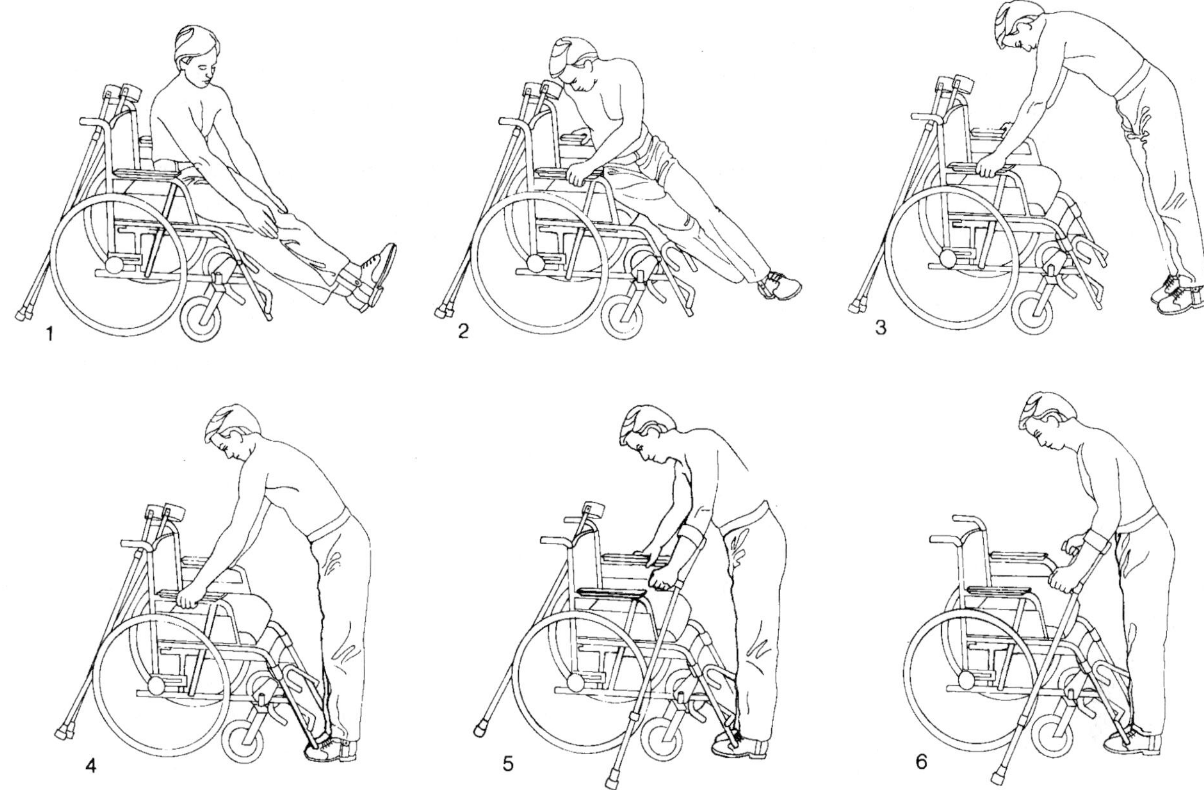

Figure 20.25 Standing from wheelchair using forearm crutches and KAFOs. The reverse sequence is used to return to sitting in the wheelchair.

- *Push-ups.* This includes lifting the body off the floor using elbow extension and scapulae depression and protraction, tucking the head to gain added height, and controlled lowering of the body.

Performed in Parallel Bars Progressed to Overground

- *Swing-through pattern.* From a balanced standing position with the hands posterior to the pelvis, the patient moves the hands forward, causing the trunk to flex. Then the patient lifts up by extending the elbows and protracting/depressing the scapulae and tucking the head. Gravity will cause the trunk and legs to swing forward. When the heels strike the ground, the patient quickly extends the upper trunk and head and pushes the pelvis forward to come back to the starting position (Fig. 20.24).
- *Four-point pattern.* This gait pattern is slower but safer than a swing-through pattern; three points are always in contact with the ground, as opposed to a swing-through pattern, in which there are times when only two points are in contact with the ground. From a standing position with the pelvis forward, both feet on the ground, and hands posterior to the pelvis, one hand/crutch is lifted up and placed forward. Weight is shifted away from the contralateral LE so it can swing forward as the hip is hiked and the head is moved down and away from the swing leg. This unweighting and hip hiking allows gravity to assist the forward swing. This process is repeated on the opposite side.

Recovery and Activity-Based Approach

Locomotor training (LT) for patients with iSCI using partial BWS, a TM, and manual assistance by trainers is an important therapeutic intervention to retrain walking after iSCI. Terms to describe this training include *body weight supported treadmill training, partial body weight supported treadmill training,* or *weight supported treadmill training.* These terms emphasize the exercise or training equipment currently advocated for retraining walking by medical equipment manufacturers and by some clinicians and researchers; however, the terms fail to describe the critical elements of the training[234] and the specific rehabilitation goal. What does a therapist actually do with a patient to retrain walking using this equipment? This section provides (1) a global perspective on LT and how it differs from LT for persons with complete SCI; (2) the clinical guidelines for selection and use of LT strategies; and (3) evidence regarding use of LT following SCI.

Locomotor training is a product of translational research that emerged from animal models of the neural control of locomotion. Knowledge gained by basic science researchers concerning the neurobiological control of walking laid the foundation for developing a therapeutic intervention with application to human clinical populations. Scientists discovered that when mid-thoracic spinalized cats (i.e., cats that had a complete transaction of the spinal cord) were placed on a TM, suspended by a sling, and repetitively trained for hind-limb stepping with assistance of trainers for loading and limb placement, the animals learned to hind-limb step (on the TM) independent of supraspinal input. With continued training, the cats were ultimately able to step on the TM independent of manual assistance.[235,236] Furthermore, this intense training was task-specific in that the spinalized cats could be trained to stand, or to step, but that training to perform one task did not transfer to performance of the other task.[237] Seminal research in this arena provided the impetus for Hugues Barbeau, Anton Wernig, Volker Dietz, Susan Harkema, and other translational scientists to translate this knowledge into human clinical populations.

Barbeau and coworkers published the first studies in which humans were partially suspended with a BWS apparatus over a TM to examine its impact on gait[238,239] and then provided training similar to that experienced by the cats for persons with SCI.[240] Though a suspension system and TM appear to be strong common denominators of the training, the equipment is likely not the dominant, critical component. The equipment provides an effective and controlled environment for consistent and intense practice of walking that can closely approximate the sensory experience of walking. The successes of the spinalized cats and improvements in walking by humans after iSCI were attributed to activity-dependent plasticity of the neural axis.[241] Activity-dependent plasticity, or the responsiveness of the neural circuitry of the spinal cord to task-specific practice and its capacity to learn, was a new concept and revolutionary for the rehabilitation of persons after SCI.[242] The spinal cord and neural axis were responsive to the ensemble of sensory information specific to walking and generated a motor response for stepping below the level of the lesion. Many researchers and clinicians continue to translate knowledge from basic science into developing a rehabilitation intervention to retrain walking after neurological injury or disease.[149,243-246] In parallel, other researchers have focused on testing the efficacy of this intervention and effectiveness for the recovery of walking after SCI.[150,247,248]

Locomotor training occurs across three environments: (1) on the TM with use of BWS and manual facilitation (Fig 20.26), (2) assessment of the patient's ability to apply new skills overground, and (3) community integration. Retraining the neuromuscular system may occur most effectively in the TM environment where BWS and speed can be controlled, and manual facilitation can be provided by trainers to optimize afferent input. Transfer of skills learned in the TM environment is assessed off the TM. Overground locomotion allows level of independence and community integration (home and community-based activities) to be assessed. LT encourages incorporation of movement patterns consistent with movement strategies

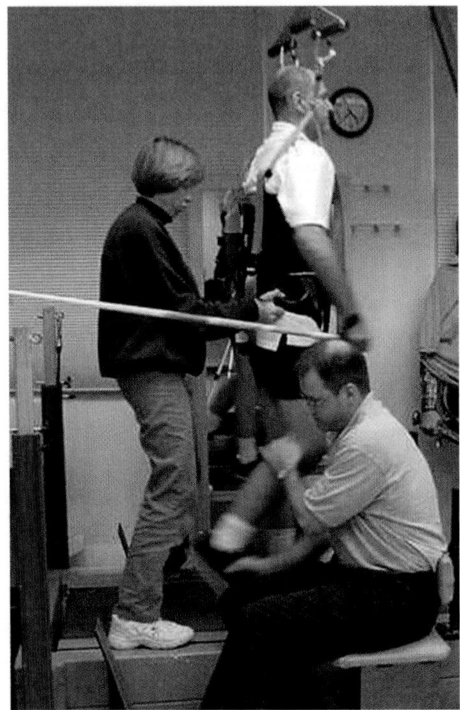

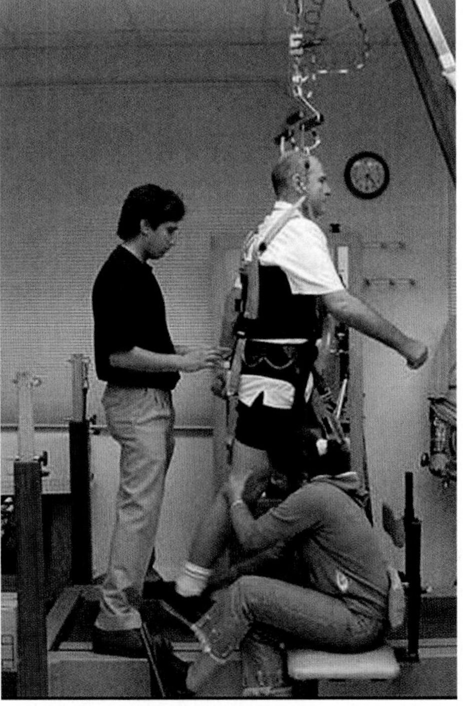

Figure 20.26 Locomotor training for a person with an incomplete spinal cord injury using body weight support, treadmill, and manual assistance by trainers. *(From Behrman et al, 2005,[249] with permission.)*

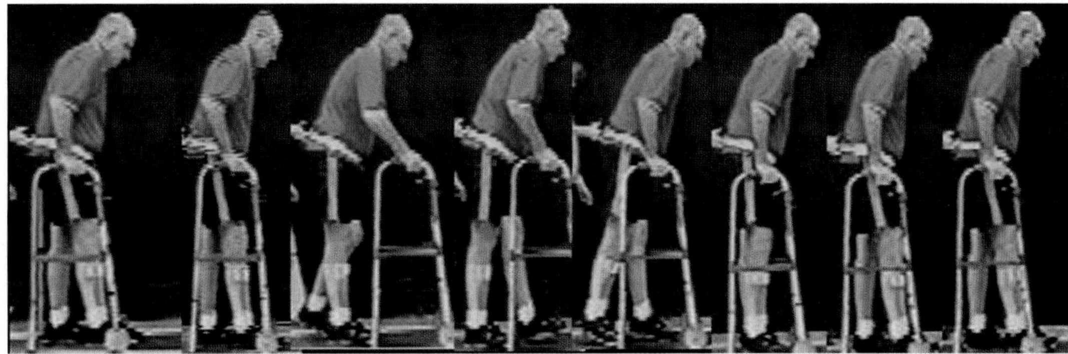

Figure 20.27 Gait pattern of a person with an incomplete spinal cord injury using a rolling walker and a right ankle-foot orthosis. *(From Behrman et al, 2005,[249] with permission.)*

present before the injury, encouraging individuals after SCI to "train like you walk." This approach translates into the following practical LT guidelines:

- The LEs are maximally loaded for weight-bearing, minimizing or eliminating loading of the arms.
- Sensory cues provided are consistent with the task of walking (e.g., TM speed, manual cues to facilitate flexor or extensor muscle activation).
- The posture, trunk, pelvis, and limb kinematics are coordinated and specific to the task of walking.
- Compensatory strategies for movement (i.e., hip hiking) are minimized or eliminated, with recovery of preinjury movement patterns as the goal.[147,249]

The same training principles should be applied outside of the BWS-TM system overground in the clinic, home, and community. Adaptations can be made for advancing skills for walking when off the TM and should be consistent with LT principles. In the example from Fig. 20.27, the rolling walker may permit a faster walking speed; however, this individual's posture and inability to flex the right knee preclude any faster speed. The lack of upright posture also limits hip extension range and loading, likely necessary precursors to initiating swing. Several suggestions for treatment are to have this individual practice upright standing with his back to a wall using the walker to load the LEs as opposed to his arms (Fig. 20.28), to practice weight-bearing solely on the left LE with the right leg flexed on a stool or chair (Fig. 20.29A and B), and to elevate the height of the walker to encourage upright posture. A posterior walker may also encourage a more upright posture. Certainly, use of the BWS system and TM has advantages and may be the optimal environment for consistent practice and retraining the neuromuscular system. The transition and application to community ambulation is critical (Fig. 20.30).

Locomotor training principles can thus be applied while on the TM with a BWS system and continued overground for community ambulation (see Fig. 20.29). Transferring skills acquired in one environment to another is an important element for learning and can be reinforced by a daily examination of the walking abilities overground and on the TM with BWS. Modifying the parameters of training in both environments will challenge the use of new skills, reinforce new patterns and independence, and inform goal setting across environments.

Engaging the client in each aspect of goal setting and understanding of the LT principles empowers the client to extend "training" beyond the time in the clinic to the rest of the day. The choices that the therapist and client make daily may significantly affect the rate and magnitude of the client's recovery and achievement of goals. For instance, a client's choice to walk using a grocery

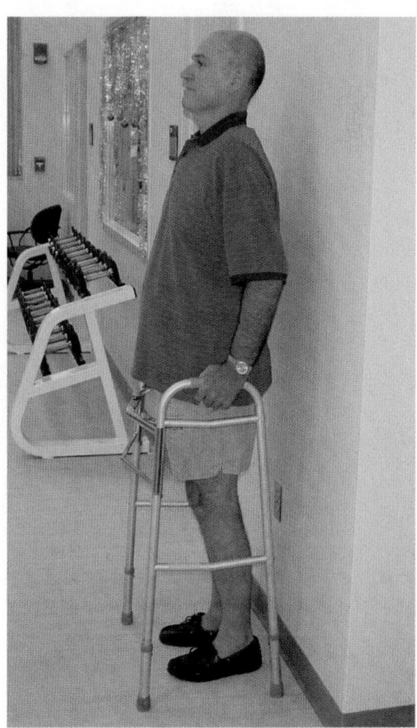

Figure 20.28 Locomotor training principles applied to the task of standing with upright posture for a person with an incomplete spinal cord injury. *(From Behrman et al, 2005,[249] with permission.)*

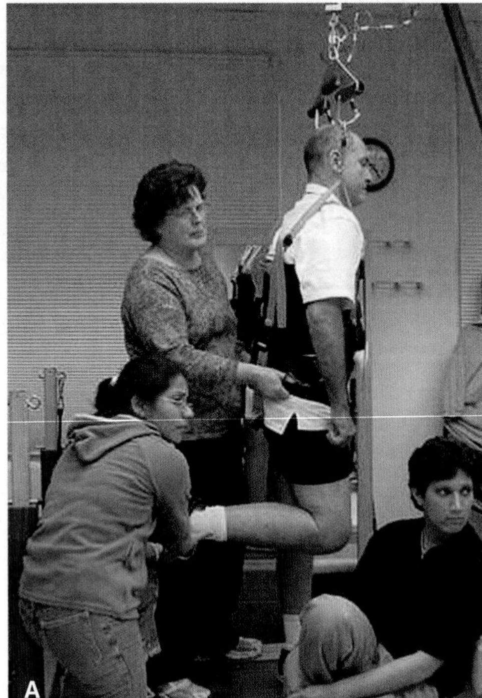

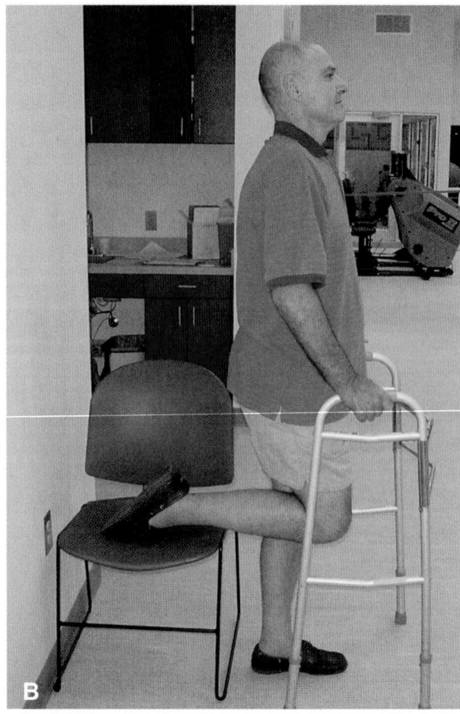

Figure 20.29 Locomotor training principles applied to standing upright while practicing loading and extension on the left lower limb while the right lower limb is unloaded and flexed on the treadmill with body weight support (A) and overground with a walker (B). *(From Behrman et al, 2005,[249] with permission.)*

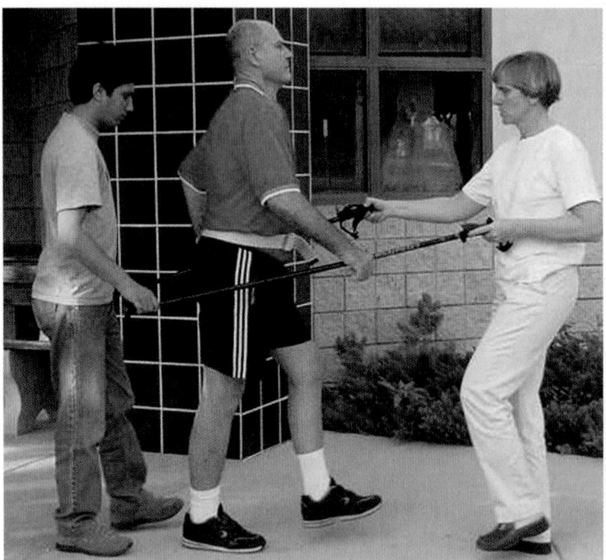

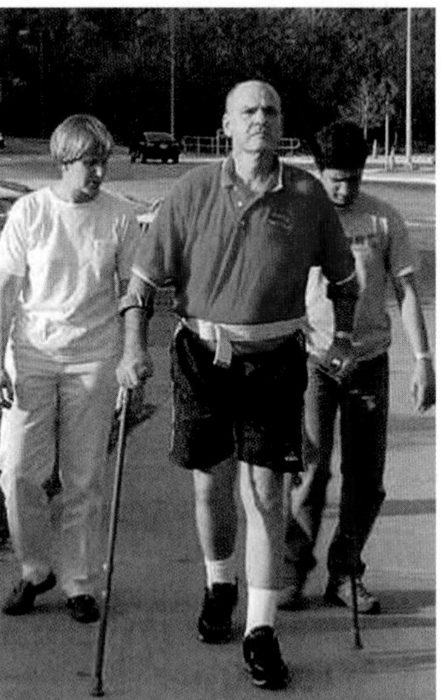

Figure 20.30 Translation of skills acquired on the treadmill to walking overground and community ambulation. *(From Behrman et al, 2005,[249] with permission.)*

cart instead of shopping from a wheelchair reinforces the principle of maximizing weight-bearing through the LE. Similarly, setting the assistive device higher than normally prescribed will decrease the ability to bear excessive weight through the UEs and promote a more upright posture. If the individual walks with an upright posture, the goal is further enhanced with increased load-bearing on the LE versus the arms and achievement of hip extension during loading. This simple choice will advance the individual's recovery. Many more choices can be made by the client to support recovery regardless of where one is on a continuum of recovery.

Clinical guidelines for LT and for safe and effective use of therapeutic equipment are essential to the practice of evidence-based physical therapy following SCI. As research findings are published, clinicians should seek information to guide their decision-making and practice. Such future research may identify the following:

- Who will benefit from LT with the aim of improving the ability to walk? Persons classified according to AIS A, B, C, or D impairments or persons classified according to the NRS; persons who already walk but not well; persons who have a particular clinical motor or sensory presentation; or persons at a particular neurological level of injury (i.e., severity of injury)?
- When is the best time after injury to provide an intervention for optimal recovery of walking? In the acute stage of rehabilitation, after discharge from rehabilitation, or at some other point after SCI (and if so, what is the appropriate time after injury)?
- Will early engagement of recovery-based walking limit the onset of maladaptive plasticity observed in the chronic phases of other neurological conditions?[250]
- What is the optimal dose of therapy (i.e., intensity, frequency, and duration of the training)?
- How to train and progress a patient, how to use the BWS system and TM equipment, how to examine new training equipment as it reaches the market (e.g., suspension systems, robotic devices, etc.), and how to monitor the trainers' body ergonomics during training?
- Any medical precautions and safety issues for persons with SCI and their effect on LT locomotor training (e.g., AD, skin, bowel and bladder, falling, osteoporosis, spasticity, cardiovascular health, etc.)?
- What therapies may augment LT or what combined therapies enhance the recovery of walking (e.g., strengthening, FES)?[150]
- What is the cost–benefit ratio (i.e., cost to provide this intervention in the clinic, including equipment and personnel; reimbursement policies; and outcomes and value to the patient and community)?

An important area for research is the benefits of LT to a person's health after SCI, whether an incomplete or a complete injury. Additional questions that need to be answered include the following: Does LT decrease the risk of pressure injuries or bladder infections; reduce bone loss or muscle atrophy? Do benefits for health warrant increased access to LT? Can robotic devices provide an avenue to cost-effectively provide this service? What is the impact of LT outcomes on the quality of life of the person with SCI and the impact on the family or caregiver(s)?

The advent of recovery and activity-based approaches represents a new era in management of patients with SCI. This era, brought forth by partnership among basic scientists, rehabilitation scientists, physicians, and clinicians, encompasses knowledge of the neurobiological control of walking and the physiological promise of activity-dependent plasticity as bases for developing new interventions and advancing the potential for recovery after SCI. Whereas LT alone may provide a means for recovery of preinjury abilities and fostering neuromuscular activity below the level of the lesion, the next generation of interventions may employ combinatorial approaches. Such approaches may include advancing technology, epidural stimulation, stem cell transplants, and pharmacological approaches to bolster the neuroplasticity of the neural environment. Locomotor training in combination with these approaches or others may be an essential component and catalyst to achieve an effective therapeutic outcome.[152,251] For additional information on LT and other interventions to improve locomotor function, refer to Chapter 11, Strategies to Improve Locomotor Function.

Activity-Based Upper Extremity Training

For people with a cervical SCI, the recovery of UE function is a primary goal.[252] Interventions aimed at improving functional use of the UE have primarily been compensatory in nature. For example, patients with active wrist extension are taught how to manipulate and pick up objects using a tenodesis grasp, use the hand as a hook, and use different types of orthoses to feed themselves. More recently, researchers have begun to explore the use of massed practice interventions to promote functional recovery and corticomotor and spinal reorganization.[253-255]

Based on massed practice principles used in constraint-induced movement therapy, Field-Fote and colleagues[253-255] applied similar training techniques by having patients practice unimanual or bimanual UE activities 2 hours per day, 5 days a week for 3 weeks. Patients did not have a UE constrained. Applying sensory electrical stimulation to the volar surface of the wrist over the median nerve while the patients performed the different tasks augmented the massed practice. Patients with cervical iSCI practiced five main types of unimanual or bimanual UE activities: finger isolation, grasp, grasps with rotation, pinch, and pinch with rotation. The researchers found significant improvements in hand and arm function after the intervention.

Health and Wellness

Just as with people without SCI, regular exercise is an important part of a healthy lifestyle. Patients should be provided a comprehensive home exercise program that incorporates stretching, balance, aerobic, and strengthening exercises. Aerobic exercises such as UE ergometer should be done 3 to 5 days a week for a total of 20 to 60 minutes per session at an intensity of 50% to 80% of maximum HR. Strengthening exercises should be done 2 to 4 days a week at an intensity of 8 to 10 repetitions at 60% to 80% of one repetition maximum.[220] When developing the exercise program, attention should be directed to the unique precautions associated with SCI such as the possibility of overuse injuries (particularly in the shoulders), AD, thermal dysregulation, and exaggerated HR response to exercise.[46]

Patient-Related Education

Because SCI can affect many different body systems and drastically change an individual's life, ongoing education about the consequences of SCI is critical. Education should begin early after injury and continue throughout rehabilitation and cover the extensive impact of SCI discussed above (e.g., skin care, AD, self-directing care, wheelchair mobility and maintenance, sexuality, etc.). Without education, patients will not be able to make informed decisions regarding their care or informed choices regarding community reintegration.

Peer mentoring with others who have experienced an SCI and are living in the community can be an effective method of providing education, support, and assistance with the rehabilitation process.[256] For example, a person with an AIS A T2 SCI will be able to realistically demonstrate how to transfer from the bed to a wheelchair to a person recently injured who is undergoing rehabilitation. This person may also be able to discuss the impact of SCI on everyday life in a way a physical therapist could not.

An important aspect of rehabilitation involves planning for discharge and community reintegration. Consideration must be given to multiple issues, including accessible housing, nutrition, transportation, finances, maintaining functional skills and level of physical fitness, employment or further education, and methods for involvement in desired social or recreational activities. Each of these issues must be addressed early and continued throughout the course of rehabilitation in consultation with the patient, family, and appropriate team members. Educating the patient will allow him or her to make informed decisions regarding medical care and lifestyle choices throughout the life span. A plethora of Internet resources are available, which patients should be encouraged to explore. Appendix 20.A lists some of the many resources available for patients, families, and clinicians.

■ PRESCRIPTIVE WHEELCHAIR/SEATING SYSTEM AND WHEELCHAIR SKILLS TRAINING

Many people with SCI will use a wheelchair as their primary means of mobility. A wheelchair acts as a mobility base and serves to provide postural support. Because patients with SCI will have varying degrees of trunk, hip, and shoulder girdle paralysis, the wheelchair and accompanying seating system provides postural support to keep the pelvis, spine, and extremities in optimal alignment. Postural alignment affects a variety of areas, including respiration, bowel and bladder function, skin integrity, and mobility. Poor posture in the wheelchair can negatively affect all of these areas. Because most patients will be using a wheelchair exclusively, it should be custom-ordered (prescribed) for each individual. When prescribing a wheelchair, consideration should be given to the patient's goals and characteristics, as well as the activities and environment in which it will be used.

The first choice is between a power and manual wheelchair. Generally, individuals with intact triceps function can independently propel a manual wheelchair. Individuals with a C6- or C5-level injury may also be able to independently propel a manual wheelchair but may not have the endurance or strength for community wheelchair mobility. The selection of a manual or power wheelchair in these cases should be done on an individual basis. Individuals with higher cervical injuries generally rely on a power wheelchair for their mobility needs (see Table 20.5). Before prescribing a wheelchair, a series of trials with different types of chairs with different components will assist with making an informed decision on what specific type of wheelchair to obtain.

There are two basic frames for manual wheelchairs—a *folding* or a *rigid* frame—and three weights (standard, lightweight, and ultralight). Folding chairs are an important consideration for patients who plan to transfer into a car because they can be folded compactly for storage without having to remove as many parts. Folding frames typically incorporate a below-seat crossbar and generally provide a smoother ride on uneven surfaces. Potential drawbacks include heavier and more moveable parts, causing it to be less energy efficient during propulsion than rigid frames.

A rigid frame is generally lighter, is more energy efficient, and often has an adjustable seat-to-back angle. This type of frame may be more difficult to store in a car. Both wheels must be removed for storage. A rigid frame is often more durable than a folding frame.

A variety of different components and options can be selected for a manual wheelchair. There are benefits and drawbacks to the different options. For example, the wheel locks can be mounted high or low on some wheelchair frames. High-mounted wheel locks are easier to access but can be an obstacle to transfers. Conversely, low-mounted wheel locks are more difficult to access but are not in the way of transfers or during propulsion.

Power wheelchairs are indicated for all patients with C4 lesions and above. Patients with C5-level lesions may also elect to use power wheelchairs, particularly for community mobility. A tilt-in-space or reclining seating system provides improved postural control and allows the user to independently perform pressure relief. There are various types of controls, ranging from a hand-operated joystick to a sip-and-puff control.

Some patients may require more than one wheelchair. Many lightweight "everyday" chairs are not suitable for sport and recreational activities. Depending on the interests of the patient, a second chair specifically designed for a particular sport such as tennis or racing may be desired.

Chapter 32, Seating and Wheeled Mobility, provides detail on the wheelchair and seating evaluation, drawbacks, and benefits of different wheelchair components, seating systems, and a variety of other issues associated with selecting a wheelchair and seating system.

Wheelchair Skills

For individuals who use a manual wheelchair, the ability to propel and maneuver over and around various obstacles and terrains in their home and community is essential for functional independence. In order to propel a manual wheelchair independently in the home and community environments, patients must be able to perform certain basic wheelchair mobility skills: propelling forward and backward, turning, ascending and descending inclines, assuming and maintaining a wheelie, and propelling on uneven terrain.

Propulsion on Even Surfaces

To propel the wheelchair forward, the patient reaches back and grasps the wheelchair hand rims (Fig. 20.31), then pushes forward, releasing the hand rims after the hands have passed in front of the hips. Patients should practice reaching far back on the hand rims to initiate the stroke and pushing far forward before releasing the hand rims. A longer pushing stroke is more efficient. Patients who do not have the ability to grasp the hand rims propel the wheelchair by pressing their palms against the lateral aspect of the hand rims and then pushing forward. These patients will often use hand rim projections or have plastic-coated hand rims.

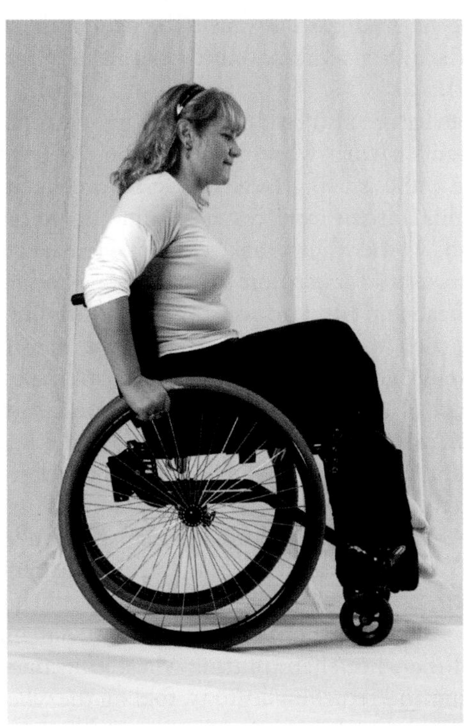

Figure 20.31 Propelling wheelchair forward. *(From O'Sullivan, S, and Schmitz, T: Improving Functional Outcomes in Physical Rehabilitation. FA Davis, Philadelphia, 2016, with permission.)*

The technique used to turn depends on how quickly the patient needs to turn, as well as the size of the turning radius. To make a large radius or slow turn, the patient just pushes harder with one arm (e.g., if turning to the right, the patient pushes harder with the left arm). To make a tight and/or quick turn, the patient pushes forward with one hand while pulling back with the other (e.g., if turning to the right quickly, the patient pushes forward with the left arm while pulling back with the right arm).

Inclines

There are a variety of surfaces with inclines that wheelchair users need to negotiate to be independent in their home and community. These include ramps, curb cutouts, slopes, and hills. The basic techniques used to ascend and descend these inclines are the same. To ascend an incline, the patient takes shorter and quicker strokes and pushes on the hand rims more forcefully. If possible, the patient should lean forward with the head and trunk while pushing forward to prevent the chair from tipping backward.

To control or slow the descent of the wheelchair, grip the hand rim and slowly release the grip in a controlled manner. Patients without full hand function control the descent of the wheelchair by applying pressure to the hand rims with the palms and slowly releasing the pressure.

Wheelies

The ability to perform a wheelie (Fig. 20.32) is an essential skill in order to negotiate curbs, steep declines, uneven terrain, and other areas of the community. To attain a wheelie, the patient reaches back on the hand rim and forcefully pushes forward to lift the front casters off the ground (as if attempting to tip the wheelchair over backward). When first learning any skill that involves a wheelie or if there is a risk of the wheelchair tipping over, the patient should always be closely supervised and guarded. To ensure safety while practicing wheelies, a gait belt is looped through the frame of the wheelchair. The therapist is positioned behind the wheelchair, holding the gait belt in one hand with the other hand placed on the patient's shoulder or push handle of the wheelchair (Fig. 20.33).

The type of wheelchair and its configuration impact how easy or difficult it is to attain a wheelie. Achieving a wheelie in a heavier wheelchair and one with a posterior axle plate is more difficult. An axle that is more forward, so that the user's COM is behind the axle, causes the wheelchair to be less stable and more "tippy." This makes it easier to assume a wheelie.

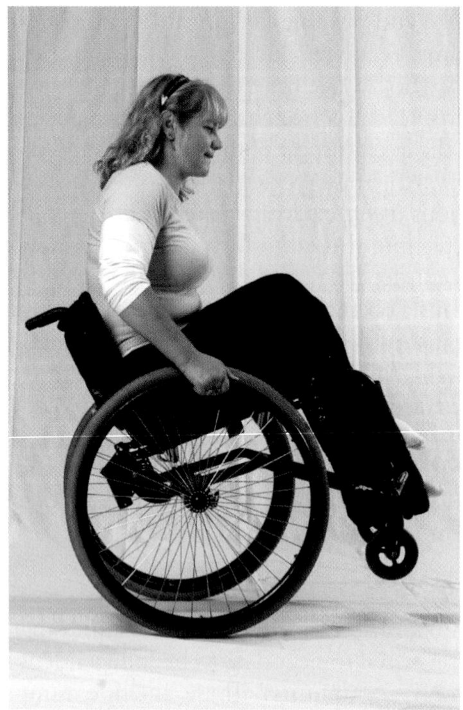

Figure 20.32 Performing a wheelie. *(From O'Sullivan, S, and Schmitz, T: Improving Functional Outcomes in Physical Rehabilitation. FA Davis, Philadelphia, 2016, with permission.)*

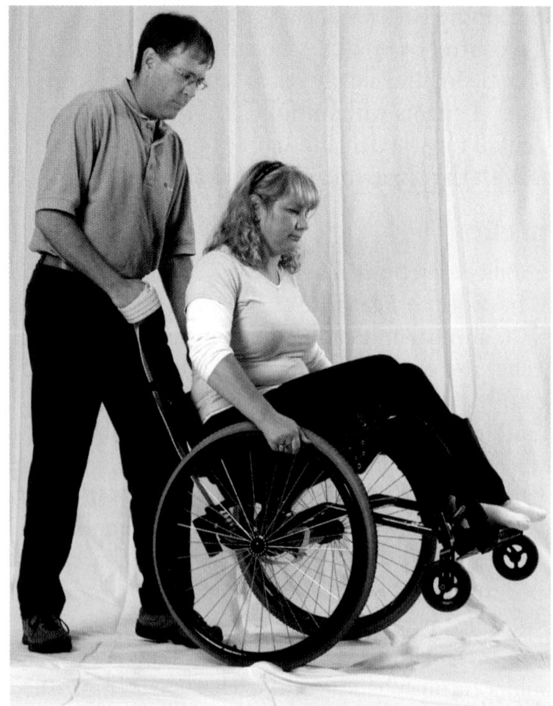

Figure 20.33 Technique to safely spot a patient while she practices performing wheelies. *(From O'Sullivan, S, and Schmitz, T: Improving Functional Outcomes in Physical Rehabilitation. FA Davis, Philadelphia, 2016, with permission.)*

The ability to maintain a wheelie should be learned in conjunction with attaining a wheelie. Both of these skills are important lead-up activities to more advanced wheelie skills such as ascending and descending curbs and propelling over uneven terrain. The therapist should assist the patient into the *balance point* in which the front casters are off the ground with the wheelchair in equilibrium. The patient's hands should lightly grip the hand rim in a position near the hips. Pushing forward on the hand rims causes the chair to tip backward, and pulling backward causes the wheelchair to tip forward onto the casters and back into a stable position. The patient should practice lightly pushing and pulling on the hand rim to learn the balance point; the hand rim should slide through the patient's grip as he or she does this. The patient should not keep the hand firmly grasped at the same point on the hand rim.

When propelling a wheelchair on uneven surfaces (e.g., gravel, grass), there is a possibility of the front casters catching, causing the wheelchair to tip over in a forward direction. Being able to propel the wheelchair forward while maintaining a wheelie can minimize this risk and allow the patient to propel the wheelchair independently over a variety of terrains. When learning to propel the wheelchair forward and backward and while turning in a wheelie position, the patient should be instructed again not to use a firm grip but to allow the hand rims to slide within his or her grip.

On some uneven surfaces, it may be easier to "pop up" into a wheelie for only a brief time (not maintain the wheelie) and push forward. The patient then crosses the surface in a series of short wheelies while pushing forward.

Wheelies are also used to ascend and descend curbs. To ascend a curb while moving, the patient pops a wheelie while moving forward just before reaching the curb. This lifts the front casters so they are up on top of the curb. As the wheels make contact with the curb, the patient pushes forward on the hand rims and leans his or her head and trunk forward (Fig. 20.34A–C). To descend a curb, the patient pushes the wheelchair forward, and just as the casters approach the edge of the curb, the patient pops a wheelie. The wheelie is maintained as momentum carries the back wheels off the curb. The patient maintains the wheelie so the back wheels land first; then the casters land (Fig. 20.35A–C).

Other wheelchair skills that patients should learn include falling from a wheelchair, picking up objects off the floor, opening and closing doors, and negotiating obstacles. Patients should also learn how to manage the parts of the wheelchair: putting wheel locks on and off, removing and returning legrests, folding the wheelchair, removing the cushion, moving armrests, and removing and putting the wheels back on.

In addition to developing the Wheelchair Skills Test described earlier, Kirby and colleagues also developed the *Wheelchair Skills Training Program*. Based on the

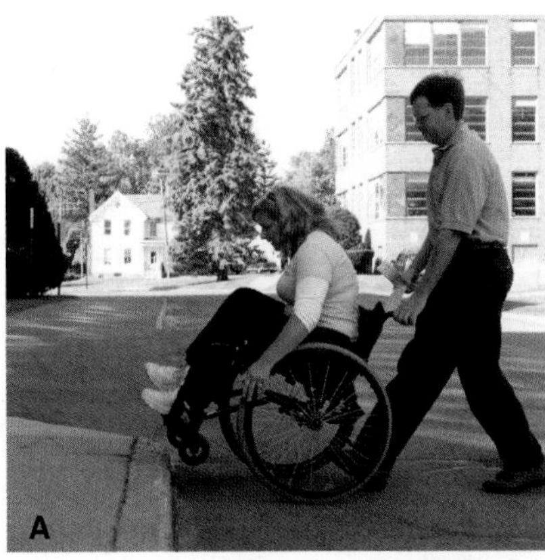

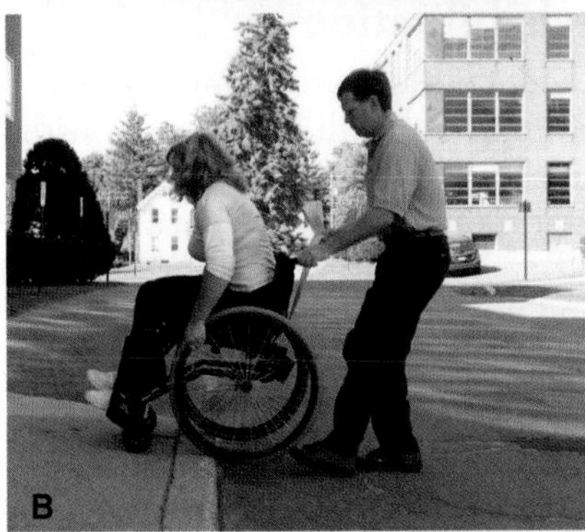

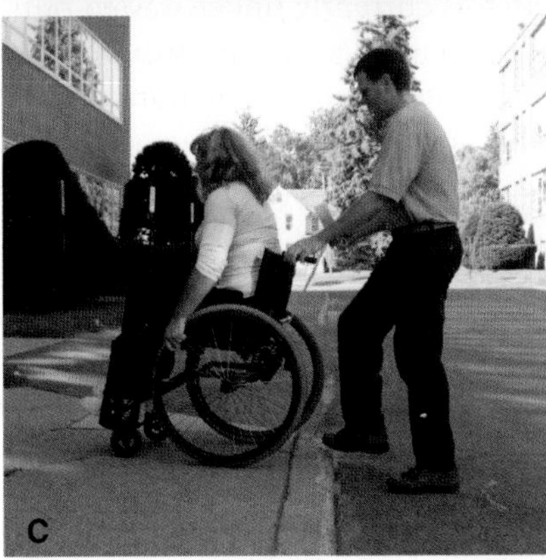

Figure 20.34 (A–C) Ascending a curb in a wheelie. *(From O'Sullivan, S, and Schmitz, T: Improving Functional Outcomes in Physical Rehabilitation. FA Davis, Philadelphia, 2016, with permission.)*

skills of the Wheelchair Skills Test and principles of motor learning, the Wheelchair Skills Training Program was designed to improve manual wheelchair user performance and safety. Research has shown it to be a safe and effective training method for new wheelchair users, community-based wheelchair users, and caregivers.[257-259] Detailed information on both the Wheelchair Skills Test and Wheelchair Skills Training Program is available at www.wheelchairskillsprogram.ca/. *Spinal Cord Injury: Functional Rehabilitation*[123] and *Improving Functional Outcomes in Physical Rehabilitation*[260] are other resources that provide more detail on interventions to improve the above-mentioned and other wheelchair skills.

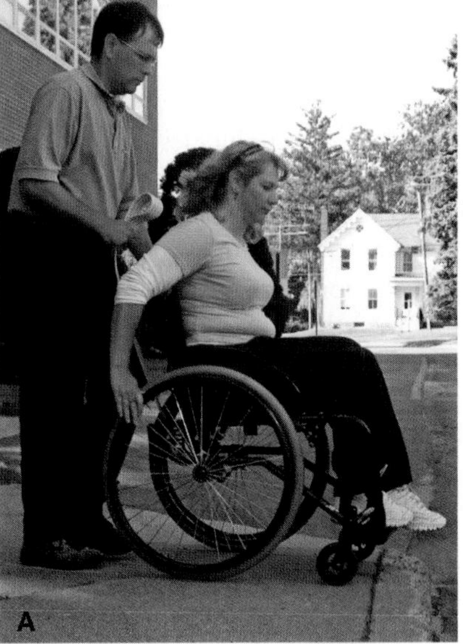

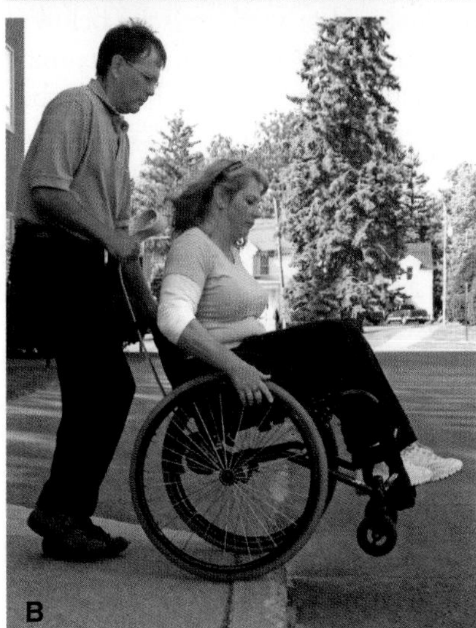

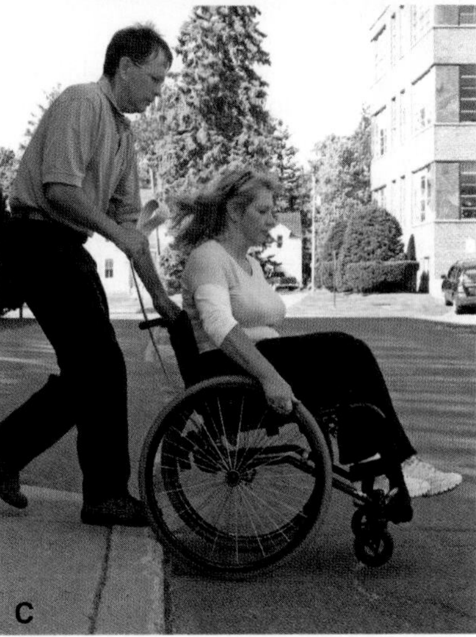

Figure 20.35 (A–C) Descending a curb in a wheelie. *(From O'Sullivan, S, and Schmitz, T: Improving Functional Outcomes in Physical Rehabilitation. FA Davis, Philadelphia, 2010, with permission.)*

NEUROTECHNOLOGIES

People with SCI also benefit from recent advances in neurotechnologies designed to improve function and quality of life. Neurotechnologies can fall into four main areas: (1) neuromodulation, which is use of electrical stimulation to improve control of an intact portion of the nervous system; (2) neural prosthesis, which is use of electrical stimulation to replace or improve function of a paralyzed or weak limb; (3) neurorehabilitation, which is applying technologies to promote normal recovery of impaired body functions; and (4) neuro-sensing and diagnostics, which encompasses technologies to monitor the nervous system or diagnose a condition.

Neuromodulation

Electrical stimulation can be used in a variety of ways. One of the most common is to use FES to cause the contraction of paralyzed or weak muscles below the level of the lesion for exercise, walking, and functional use of the UEs. As discussed above, surface FES can be used with an LE ergometer as a method of cardiovascular training.[227,261] Surface FES can also be applied to LEs to allow standing and walking in people with SCI.[262] Surface electromyography has been paired with FES to provide patients with a method of triggering the FES to produce a more normal walking pattern than FES alone.[263] Implanted FES systems allow people with SCI to stand and walk,[264] as well as those with high cervical SCI to use their hand to grasp and manipulate objects.[265] Implanted FES systems can also be used for phrenic nerve stimulation to allow patients with high cervical SCI to breathe without a ventilator[266] and to provide patients with bladder control.[267,268]

Neuroprostheses

Brain-computer interface devices (BCIs) acquire brain signals (electroencephalogram) and translate them into commands that are relayed to output devices that perform an action such as controlling a mouse on the computer screen.[269] People with high cervical SCI with little motor function are able to use BCIs to use a computer, play video games, drive a power wheelchair, and control a robot.[270-273]

Robotic devices can be used during LT to move the LEs in a stepping pattern to promote recovery of walking ability.[274] Exoskeleton robots assist people with complete SCI in walking overground.[275] In 2014, the U.S. Food and Drug Administration approved the use of robotic exoskeletons for use in the home and community. These devices range from those which provide full movement support at the hip and knee (e.g., ReWalk™, Berkley Bionics eLEGS™, and Indego®) to those that require at least some movement to engage locking and unlocking mechanisms at the knee (OttoBock E-MAG). The devices range in weight from approximately 20 pounds to over 200 pounds and may be used by individuals up to 6'4" in height. While the devices are expensive and are currently not covered by most third-party payers, the technology is progressing rapidly and may provide more full-time walking assistance for some individuals with SCI.

Neurorehabilitation

Harkema and colleagues[149] combined epidural spinal electrical stimulation with LT on a TM with BWS and stand training in an individual with a chronic AIS B C7 injury. After training, the individual was able to stand with full LE weight-bearing requiring assistance only for balance and was able to voluntarily activate some LE muscles when the stimulator was on. The authors speculate that this combination therapy (epidural electrical stimulation with task-specific locomotor and stand training) may be a viable method to improve function after SCI. Research is currently under way to translate these invasive stimulation techniques to noninvasive direct current stimulation, both at the level of the brain and directly at the spinal cord.[276,277]

Neurodiagnostics

Tools such as transcranial magnetic stimulation can be used to assess the connection between motor cortex and peripheral muscles and demonstrates potential to quantify changes to the neuromotor system as a result of rehabilitation efforts.[278] As the primary motor effect of SCI is to block conduction of signals in the descending corticospinal tract (CST), this technology allows for investigation of improved CST function. Early research demonstrated improvements in the amplitude of the muscle motor evoked potential, as well as the rate of recruitment of LE muscles after engaging in locomotor training.[279] These neurodiagnostic tools demonstrate great potential to understand the effects not only of neuromodulation and neurorehabilitation, but also of activity-based therapies on the corticospinal reorganization.[280]

These examples offer some insight into how technology is being used and glimpses of the future of rehabilitation that provide exciting opportunities to increase activity levels, improve social participation, and enhance the quality of life for people with SCI.

SUMMARY

Spinal cord injury has a profound impact on many different body systems, which can greatly affect a person's ability to move, perform everyday tasks, and participate in expected social roles. This chapter has reviewed the impact of SCI on different body systems, common impairments that result from SCI, classification of different types of SCI, and secondary complications associated with SCI. Physical therapists play a role across the continuum of care from the acute care hospital through rehabilitation to community reintegration. Use of standardized outcome measures are an important element of the examination process. The POC should be individually tailored to the patient's presentation, concerns, and goals. Interventions may be compensatory or recovery based, depending on the presentation of the patient. Patient education is a critical component of the POC. Patients unable to perform certain activities should be educated to direct others about their care. People with SCI, no matter at what level, can lead a productive, healthy, and high-quality life.

Questions for Review

1. Identify the clinical features of Brown-Sequard, anterior, central, and posterior cord syndromes.
2. Define *spinal shock.*
3. Describe complications associated with spinal cord injury.
4. What is autonomic dysreflexia? Describe the initiating stimuli and symptoms of this syndrome. What action would you take if a patient experienced an onset of symptoms during a physical therapy treatment?
5. Identify two primary factors affecting prognosis following spinal cord injury.
6. What is included in a physical therapy examination during the acute phase of recovery? How might some of the standard examination techniques need to be modified?
7. What is meant by the term *selective stretching*?
8. Describe potential goals and interventions to improve respiratory function during the acute phase of management.
9. Identify tests and measures and outcome measures used during the active rehabilitation phase of management.
10. List factors that will have an impact on the prognosis for recovery of walking ability.
11. Outline interventions to improve transfers for a patient with C6 and AIS A tetraplegia. Describe the specific activities you would include. What type of progressive strengthening and endurance training activities would you suggest for each patient as an adjunct to the mat program?
12. Describe how you would modify training parameters when performing LT using a BWS and TM system for an individual with an incomplete SCI.

CASE STUDY

HISTORY

The patient is a 21-year-old white man who was transferred to a rehabilitation hospital yesterday. He suffered a traumatic cervical spinal cord injury 8 days ago. He was given methylprednisolone in the emergency department. He had surgery to stabilize the fracture site, internal fixation and decompression using a right iliac bone graft. He was discharged to your facility yesterday and is currently wearing a Philadelphia collar. He is able to extend his elbows but cannot flex his fingers in either hand. He is a senior in college, majoring in computer science. He lives in an on-campus apartment, which is not wheelchair accessible. His parents live in the next state.

MEDICATIONS

Lovenox, midodrine, amitriptyline, Oxycontin, and Dulcolax.

PHYSICAL THERAPY EXAMINATION

Cardiopulmonary

HR: 75

BP: supine, 110/72; sitting, 100/66 (only able to tolerate sitting for about 10 minutes, then blood pressure drops due to orthostatic hypotension)

Forced vital capacity: 2.2 liters

Weak functional cough

Communication/Cognition

Alert, oriented ×3, able to follow multistep commands; MMSE: 30/30

Muscle Performance

Bilateral: biceps, 5/5; wrist extensors, 5/5; triceps, 4/5; no active contraction below C7

Sensory Integrity

Intact pinprick and light touch bilaterally C2–T4, absent below T4

Intact anal sensation

Functional Mobility

Bed mobility: moderate assistance to roll to the left and right

Supine ↔ short sit: maximal assistance

Supine ↔ long sit: maximal assistance

Transfer wheelchair ↔ bed: FIM score 2 (requires maximal assistance with transfer board)

Transfer wheelchair ↔ toilet: FIM score 2 (requires maximal assistance with transfer board)

Locomotion

Unable to ambulate.

Able to propel wheelchair 150 ft on level surface with minimal assistance.

Wheelchair Skills

Requires assistance with locking wheel locks, removing footrests and armrests, and to perform pressure relief. Wheelchair Skills Test score: 4%.

Currently uses a lightweight, folding wheelchair with hand rim projections.

Gel cushion.

Tolerates sitting in wheelchair for 20 to 30 minutes.

Balance

Long sitting: able to maintain balance on mat for 1 minute with UEs in weight-bearing position with supervision.

Short sitting: able to maintain balance on edge of mat for 1 minute with UEs in weight-bearing position with minimal assistance, 0 inches for modified functional reach.

Motor Function

Increased spasticity in bilateral hip flexors, 1+ on modified Ashworth Scale.

Passive ROM

WNL except bilateral ankle dorsiflexion is 5° from neutral.

Skin Integrity

Stage 1 wound on right heel.

Self-Care

Dressing upper body: FIM score 2 (requires maximal assistance)

Dressing lower body: FIM score 1 (dependent)

Bathing: FIM score 1 (dependent using shower chair)

Feeding: FIM score 3 (moderate assistance with adapted utensils)

Grooming: FIM score 3 (moderate assistance with adapted utensils)

Toileting: FIM score 2 (maximal assistance)

Bowel and Bladder

Bladder: FIM score 1 (just began intermittent catheterization program and requires total assist to manage)

Bowel: FIM score 1 (just began bowel training program with nursing, has been incontinent of bowel during the past day)

CASE STUDY GUIDING QUESTIONS

1. What is the patient's neurological level of injury, motor level of injury, and sensory level of injury? What is the patient's AIS classification?

2. Identify/categorize this patient's problems in terms of:
   a. Body structure/function impairments.
   b. Activity limitations.
   c. Restrictions in social participation.
3. Identify three anticipated goals and three expected outcomes for this patient.
4. Formulate three interventions with one progression that could be used during the first 3 weeks of therapy to improve bed mobility skills.

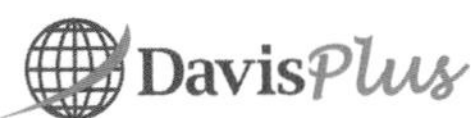

For additional resources, including answers to the questions for review and case study guiding questions, please visit **http://davisplus.fadavis.com.**

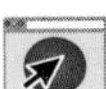

The reader is referred to the following video case studies for additional review and study:
- Case Study 4: Patient With Spinal Cord Injury, T12/L1 Complete
- Case Study 5: Patient With Spinal Cord Injury, C5/6 Incomplete

The full written case study, including all tables, figures, charts, and three video segments (examination, intervention, and outcome), appears online at Davis*Plus*. The case studies pose questions for the reader's consideration with suggested answers to the case study questions, also posted online at Davis*Plus*.

References

1. National Spinal Cord Injury Statistical Center. Spinal Cord Injury: Facts and Figures at a Glance, 2016. Retrieved February 7, 2017, from www.nscisc.uab.edu/.
2. van den Berg, ME, et al: Incidence of spinal cord injury worldwide: A systematic review. Neuroepidemiology 34(3):184–192, 2010.
3. Smith, SR, Purzner, T, and Fehlings, MG: The epidemiology of geriatric spinal cord injury. Top Spinal Cord Inj Rehabil 15(3):54–64, 2010.
4. McKinley, W: Nontraumatic spinal cord injury/disease: Etiologies and outcomes. Top Spinal Cord Inj Rehabil 14(2):1–9, 2008.
5. Gupta, A, et al: Non-traumatic spinal cord lesions: Epidemiology, complications, neurological and functional outcome of rehabilitation. Spinal Cord 47(4):307–311, 2009.
6. Gupta, A, et al: Traumatic vs non-traumatic spinal cord lesions: Comparison of neurological and functional outcome after in-patient rehabilitation. Spinal Cord 46(7):482–487, 2008.
7. Ottenbacher, KJ, et al: Trends in length of stay, living setting, functional outcome, and mortality following medical rehabilitation. JAMA 292(14):1687–1695, 2004.
8. Shavelle, RM, et al: Improvements in long-term survival after spinal cord injury? Arch Phys Med Rehabil 96(4):645–651, 2015.
9. DeVivo, MJ, et al: Costs of care following spinal cord injury. Top Spinal Cord Inj Rehabil 16(4):1–9, 2011.
10. Cao, Y, Chen, Y, and DeVivo, MJ: Lifetime direct costs after spinal cord injury. Top Spinal Cord Inj Rehab 16(4):10–16, 2011.
11. Kirshblum, SC, et al: International standards for neurological classification of spinal cord injury (revised 2011). J Spinal Cord Med 34(6):535–546, 2011.
12. Blumenfeld, H: Neuroanatomy Through Clinical Cases, ed 2. Sinauer Associates, Sunderland, MA, 2010.
13. Kirshblum, SC, et al: Reference for the 2011 revision of the International Standards for Neurological Classification of Spinal Cord Injury. J Spinal Cord Med 34(6):547–554, 2011.
14. Kirshblum, S, and Waring, W, 3rd: Updates for the International Standards for Neurological Classification of Spinal Cord Injury. Phys Med Rehabil Clin N Am 25(3):505–517, 2014.
15. McKinley, W, et al: Incidence and outcomes of spinal cord injury clinical syndromes. J Spinal Cord Med 30(3):215–224, 2007.
16. Yadla, S, Klimo, P, and Harrop, JS: Traumatic central cord syndrome: Etiology, management, and outcomes. Top Spinal Cord Inj Rehabil 15(3):73–84, 2010.
17. Ditunno, JF, et al: Spinal shock revisited: A four-phase model. Spinal Cord 42(7):383–395, 2004.
18. Teasell, RW, et al: Cardiovascular consequences of loss of supraspinal control of the sympathetic nervous system after spinal cord injury. Arch Phys Med Rehabil 81(4):506–516, 2000.
19. Lindan, R, et al: Incidence and clinical features of autonomic dysreflexia in patients with spinal cord injury. Paraplegia 18(5):285-292, 1980.
20. Stillman, MD, et al: Complications of spinal cord injury over the first year after discharge from inpatient rehabilitation. Arch Phys Med Rehabil 98(9):1800–1805, 2017.
21. Krassioukov, A, et al: A systematic review of the management of autonomic dysreflexia after spinal cord injury. Arch Phys Med Rehabil 90(4):682–695, 2009.
22. Krassioukov, AV, Furlan, JC, and Fehlings, MG: Autonomic dysreflexia in acute spinal cord injury: An under-recognized clinical entity. J Neurotrauma 20(8):707–716, 2003.
23. Curt, A, et al: Assessment of autonomic dysreflexia in patients with spinal cord injury. J Neurol Neurosurg Psychiatry 62(5):473–477, 1997.
24. Karlsson, AK: Autonomic dysreflexia. Spinal Cord 37(6):383–391, 1999.
25. Wan, D, and Krassioukov, AV: Life-threatening outcomes associated with autonomic dysreflexia: A clinical review. J Spinal Cord Med 37(1):2–10, 2014.
26. Acute management of autonomic dysreflexia: Individuals with spinal cord injury presenting to health-care facilities. J Spinal Cord Med 25 Suppl 1:S67–88, 2002.
27. Caruso, D, Gater, D, and Harnish, C: Prevention of recurrent autonomic dysreflexia: A survey of current practice. Clin Auton Res 25(5):293–300, 2015.
28. McGillivray, CF, et al: Evaluating knowledge of autonomic dysreflexia among individuals with spinal cord injury and their families. J Spinal Cord Med 32(1):54–62, 2009.
29. Skold, C, Levi, R, and Seiger, A: Spasticity after traumatic spinal cord injury: Nature, severity, and location. Arch Phys Med Rehabil 80(12):1548–1557, 1999.
30. Meythaler, JM: Concept of spastic hypertonia. Phys Med Rehabil Clin N Am 12(4):725–732, 2001.
31. Young, RR, and Delwaide, PJ: Drug therapy: Spasticity (first of two parts). N Engl J Med 304(1):28–33, 1981.
32. Walter, JS, et al: A database of self-reported secondary medical problems among VA spinal cord injury patients: Its role in clinical care and management. J Rehabil Res Dev 39(1):53-61, 2002.

33. van Cooten, IP, et al: Functional hindrance due to spasticity in individuals with spinal cord injury during inpatient rehabilitation and 1 year thereafter. Spinal Cord 53(9):663–667, 2015.
34. Milinis, K, and Young, CA: Trajectories of outcome in neurological conditions. Systematic review of the influence of spasticity on quality of life in adults with chronic neurological conditions. Disabil Rehabil 1–11, 2015.
35. Gracies, JM: Physical modalities other than stretch in spastic hypertonia. Phys Med Rehabil Clin N Am 12(4):769–792, vi, 2001.
36. Gracies, JM: Pathophysiology of impairment in patients with spasticity and use of stretch as a treatment of spastic hypertonia. Phys Med Rehabil Clin N Am 12(4):747–768, vi, 2001.
37. Adams, MM, and Hicks, AL: Spasticity after spinal cord injury. Spinal Cord 43(10):577–586, 2005.
38. Katalinic, OM, Harvey, LA, and Herbert, RD: Effectiveness of stretch for the treatment and prevention of contractures in people with neurological conditions: A systematic review. Phys Ther 91(1):11–24, 2011.
39. Taricco, M, et al: Pharmacological interventions for spasticity following spinal cord injury. Cochrane Database Syst Rev 2: CD001131, 2000.
40. Theriault, ER, et al: Antispasmodic medications may be associated with reduced recovery during inpatient rehabilitation after traumatic spinal cord injury. J Spinal Cord Med 1–9, 2016.
41. Biering-Sorensen, F, et al: Alterations in cardiac autonomic control in spinal cord injury. Auton Neurosci 209:4–18, 2017.
42. Hagen, EM, et al: Cardiovascular and urological dysfunction in spinal cord injury. Acta Neurol Scand Suppl 191:71–78, 2011.
43. Naso, F: Cardiovascular problems in patients with spinal cord injury. Phys Med Rehabil Clin N Am 3(4):741–749, 1992.
44. Wadsworth, BM, et al: Abdominal binder use in people with spinal cord injuries: A systematic review and meta-analysis. Spinal Cord 47(4):274–285, 2009.
45. Gondim, FA, et al: Cardiovascular control after spinal cord injury. Curr Vasc Pharmacol 2(1):71–79, 2004.
46. Jacobs, PL, and Nash, MS: Exercise recommendations for individuals with spinal cord injury. Sports Med 34(11):727–751, 2004.
47. Machac, S, et al: Cardiovascular response to peak voluntary exercise in males with cervical spinal cord injury. J Spinal Cord Med 39(4):412–420, 2016.
48. Claydon, VE, et al: Cardiovascular responses and postexercise hypotension after arm cycling exercise in subjects with spinal cord injury. Arch Phys Med Rehabil 87(8):1106–1114, 2006.
49. Osterthun, R, et al: Causes of death following spinal cord injury during inpatient rehabilitation and the first five years after discharge. A Dutch cohort study. Spinal Cord 52(6):483–488, 2014.
50. Schilero, GJ, et al: Pulmonary function and spinal cord injury. Respir Physiol Neurobiol 166(3):129–141, 2009.
51. Warren, PM, Awad, BI, and Alilain, WJ: Drawing breath without the command of effectors: The control of respiration following spinal cord injury. Respir Physiol Neurobiol 203:98–108, 2014.
52. Neumann, DA: Kinesiology of the Musculoskeletal System: Foundations for Rehabilitation. Elsevier, St. Louis, MO, 2017.
53. Berlly, M, and Shem, K: Respiratory management during the first five days after spinal cord injury. J Spinal Cord Med 30(4):309–318, 2007.
54. Wallbom, AS, Naran, B, and Thomas, E: Acute ventilator management and weaning in individuals with high tetraplegia. Top Spinal Cord Inj Rehabil 10(3):1–7, 2005.
55. Jain, NB, et al: Determinants of forced expiratory volume in 1 second (FEV1), forced vital capacity (FVC), and FEV1/FVC in chronic spinal cord injury. Arch Phys Med Rehabil 87(10): 1327–1333, 2006.
56. Stolzmann, KL, et al: Longitudinal change in FEV1 and FVC in chronic spinal cord injury. Am J Respir Crit Care Med 177(7): 781–786, 2008.
57. Benevento, BT, and Sipski, ML: Neurogenic bladder, neurogenic bowel, and sexual dysfunction in people with spinal cord injury. Phys Ther 82(6):601-612, 2002.
58. Garcia Leoni, ME, and Esclarin De Ruz, A: Management of urinary tract infection in patients with spinal cord injuries. Clin Microbiol Infect 9(8):780–785, 2003.
59. Lane, GI, et al: A cross-sectional study of the catheter management of neurogenic bladder after traumatic spinal cord injury. Neurourol Urodyn 37(1):360–367, 2018.
60. Warms, C, et al: Bowel and bladder function and management. In Field-Fote, EC (ed): Spinal Cord Injury Rehabilitation. FA Davis, Philadelphia, PA, 2009.
61. Coggrave, M, Norton, C, and Wilson-Barnett, J: Management of neurogenic bowel dysfunction in the community after spinal cord injury: A postal survey in the United Kingdom. Spinal Cord 47(4):323–330; quiz 331–323, 2009.
62. Liu, CW, et al: Relationship between neurogenic bowel dysfunction and health-related quality of life in persons with spinal cord injury. J Rehabil Med 41(1):35–40, 2009.
63. Anderson, KD, et al: The impact of spinal cord injury on sexual function: Concerns of the general population. Spinal Cord 45(5):328–337, 2007.
64. Watanabe, T, et al: Epidemiology of current treatment for sexual dysfunction in spinal cord injured men in the USA model spinal cord injury centers. J Spinal Cord Med 19(3):186–189, 1996.
65. Elliott, S: Sexuality after spinal cord injury. In Field-Fote, EC (ed): Spinal Cord Injury Rehabilitation. FA Davis, Philadelphia, PA, 2009.
66. Baker, ER, and Cardenas, DD: Pregnancy in spinal cord injured women. Arch Phys Med Rehabil 77(5):501-507, 1996.
67. Smeltzer, SC, and Wetzel-Effinger, L: Pregnancy in women with spinal cord injury. Top Spinal Cord Inj Rehabil 15(1):29–42, 2009.
68. Demirel, G, et al: Pain following spinal cord injury. Spinal Cord 36(1):25–28, 1998.
69. Finnerup, NB, et al: Pain and dysesthesia in patients with spinal cord injury: A postal survey. Spinal Cord 39(5):256–262, 2001.
70. Widerstrom-Noga, EG, et al: Perceived difficulty in dealing with consequences of spinal cord injury. Arch Phys Med Rehabil 80(5):580–586, 1999.
71. Dijkers, M, Bryce, T, and Zanca, J: Prevalence of chronic pain after traumatic spinal cord injury: A systematic review. J Rehabil Res Dev 46(1):13–29, 2009.
72. Widerstrom-Noga, EG, Felipe-Cuervo, E, and Yezierski, RP: Chronic pain after spinal injury: Interference with sleep and daily activities. Arch Phys Med Rehabil 82(11):1571–1577, 2001.
73. Westgren, N, and Levi, R: Quality of life and traumatic spinal cord injury. Arch Phys Med Rehabil 79(11):1433–1439, 1998.
74. Widerstrom-Noga, EG: Pain after spinal cord injury: Etiology and management. In Field-Fote, EC (ed): Spinal Cord Injury Rehabilitation. FA Davis, Philadelphia, PA, 2009.
75. MacKay-Lyons, M: Shoulder pain in patients with acute quadriplegia: A retrospective study. Physiother Can 46(4):255–258, 1994.
76. Dyson-Hudson, TA, and Kirshblum, SC: Shoulder pain in chronic spinal cord injury, Part I: Epidemiology, etiology, and pathomechanics. J Spinal Cord Med 27(1):4–17, 2004.
77. Irwin, RW, Restrepo, JA, and Sherman, A: Musculoskeletal pain in persons with spinal cord injury. Top Spinal Cord Inj Rehabil 13(2):43–57, 2007.
78. Teasell, RW, et al: A systematic review of pharmacologic treatments of pain after spinal cord injury. Arch Phys Med Rehabil 91(5):816–831, 2010.
79. Cardenas, DD, and Jensen, MP: Treatments for chronic pain in persons with spinal cord injury: A survey study. J Spinal Cord Med 29(2):109–117, 2006.
80. Fattal, C, et al: What is the efficacy of physical therapeutics for treating neuropathic pain in spinal cord injury patients? Ann Phys Rehabil Med 52(2):149–166, 2009.
81. Attal, N, et al: Chronic neuropathic pain management in spinal cord injury patients. What is the efficacy of pharmacological treatments with a general mode of administration? (oral, transdermal, intravenous). Ann Phys Rehabil Med 52(2):124–141, 2009.
82. van Kuijk, AA, Geurts, AC, and van Kuppevelt, HJ: Neurogenic heterotopic ossification in spinal cord injury. Spinal Cord 40(7):313–326, 2002.
83. Lal, S, et al: Risk factors for heterotopic ossification in spinal cord injury. Arch Phys Med Rehabil 70(5):387–390, 1989.
84. Bravo-Payno, P, et al: Incidence and risk factors in the appearance of heterotopic ossification in spinal cord injury. Paraplegia; 30(10): 740–745, 1992.
85. Teasell, RW, et al: A systematic review of the therapeutic interventions for heterotopic ossification after spinal cord injury. Spinal Cord 48(7):512–521, 2010.

86. Ashe, MC, et al: Prevention and treatment of bone loss after a spinal cord injury: A systematic review. Top Spinal Cord Inj Rehabil 13(1):123–145, 2007.
87. Giangregorio, L, and McCartney, N: Bone loss and muscle atrophy in spinal cord injury: Epidemiology, fracture prediction, and rehabilitation strategies. J Spinal Cord Med 29(5):489–500, 2006.
88. Fattal, C, et al: Osteoporosis in persons with spinal cord injury: The need for a targeted therapeutic education. Arch Phys Med Rehabil 92(1):59–67, 2011.
89. Krause, JS, et al: Prediction of postinjury employment and percentage of time worked after spinal cord injury. Arch Phys Med Rehabil 93(2):373-375, 2012.
90. Lidal, IB, Huynh, TK, and Biering-Sorensen, F: Return to work following spinal cord injury: A review. Disabil Rehabil 29(17): 1341–1375, 2007.
91. Dijkers, MP: Quality of life of individuals with spinal cord injury: A review of conceptualization, measurement, and research findings. J Rehabil Res Dev 42(3 Suppl 1):87–110, 2005.
92. Tavakoli, SA, et al: Is level of injury a determinant of quality of life among individuals with spinal cord injury? A tertiary rehabilitation center report. Oman Med J 31(2):112–116, 2016.
93. Scivoletto, G, et al: Who is going to walk? A review of the factors influencing walking recovery after spinal cord injury. Front Hum Neurosci 8:141, 2014.
94. Waters, RL, et al: Motor and sensory recovery following incomplete tetraplegia. Arch Phys Med Rehabil 75(3):306–311, 1994.
95. Waters, RL, et al: Motor and sensory recovery following incomplete paraplegia. Arch Phys Med Rehabil 75(1):67–72, 1994.
96. van Middendorp, JJ, et al: Diagnosis and prognosis of traumatic spinal cord injury. Global Spine J 1(1):1–8, 2011.
97. Steeves, JD, et al: Extent of spontaneous motor recovery after traumatic cervical sensorimotor complete spinal cord injury. Spinal Cord 49(2):257–265, 2011.
98. Oleson, CV, et al: Prognostic value of pinprick preservation in motor complete, sensory incomplete spinal cord injury. Arch Phys Med Rehabil 86(5):988–992, 2005.
99. Oleson, CV, et al: Influence of age alone, and age combined with pinprick, on recovery of walking function in motor complete, sensory incomplete spinal cord injury. Arch Phys Med Rehabil 97(10):1635–1641, 2016.
100. van Middendorp, JJ, et al: A clinical prediction rule for ambulation outcomes after traumatic spinal cord injury: A longitudinal cohort study. Lancet 377(9770):1004–1010, 2011.
101. Waters, RL, et al: Motor and sensory recovery following complete tetraplegia. Arch Phys Med Rehabil 74(3):242–247, 1993.
102. Fehlings, MG, Cadotte, DW, and Fehlings, LN: A series of systematic reviews on the treatment of acute spinal cord injury: a foundation for best medical practice. J Neurotrauma 28(8): 1329–1333, 2011.
103. Sheerin, F: Spinal cord injury: acute care management. Emerg Nurse 12(10):26–34, 2005.
104. Bracken, MB: Steroids for acute spinal cord injury. Cochrane Database Syst Rev 1:CD001046, 2012.
105. Bracken, MB, et al: A randomized, controlled trial of methylprednisolone or naloxone in the treatment of acute spinal-cord injury. Results of the Second National Acute Spinal Cord Injury Study. New Eng J Med 322(20):1405–1411, 1990.
106. Bracken, MB, et al: Administration of methylprednisolone for 24 or 48 hours or tirilazad mesylate for 48 hours in the treatment of acute spinal cord injury. Results of the Third National Acute Spinal Cord Injury Randomized Controlled Trial. National Acute Spinal Cord Injury Study. JAMA 277(20):1597–1604, 1997.
107. Bracken, MB, et al: Methylprednisolone or tirilazad mesylate administration after acute spinal cord injury: 1-year follow up. Results of the third National Acute Spinal Cord Injury randomized controlled trial. J Neurosurg 89(5):699–706, 1998.
108. Walters, BC, et al: Guidelines for the management of acute cervical spine and spinal cord injuries: 2013 update. Neurosurg 60 Suppl 1:82–91, 2013.
109. Sunshine, JE, et al: Methylprednisolone therapy in acute traumatic spinal cord injury: Analysis of a Regional Spinal Cord Model Systems Database. Anesth Analg 124(4):1200–1205, 2017.
110. Qian, T, Campagnolo, D, and Kirshblum, S: High-dose methylprednisolone may do more harm for spinal cord injury. Med Hypotheses 55(5):452–453, 2000.
111. Gerndt, SJ, et al: Consequences of high-dose steroid therapy for acute spinal cord injury. J Trauma 42(2):279–284, 1997.
112. Evaniew, N, et al: Methylprednisolone for the treatment of patients with acute spinal cord injuries: a systematic review and meta-analysis. J Neurotrauma 33(5):468–481, 2016.
113. Evaniew, N, et al: Methylprednisolone for the treatment of patients with acute spinal cord injuries: A propensity score-matched cohort study from a Canadian multi-center spinal cord injury registry. J Neurotrauma 32(21):1674–1683, 2015.
114. Alkabie, S, and Boileau, AJ: The role of therapeutic hypothermia after traumatic spinal cord injury—a systematic review. World Neurosurg 86:432–449, 2016.
115. Martirosyan, NL, et al: The role of therapeutic hypothermia in the management of acute spinal cord injury. Clin Neurol Neurosurg 154:79–88, 2017.
116. Waters, RL, et al: Emergency, acute, and surgical management of spine trauma. Arch Phys Med Rehabil 80(11):1383–1390, 1999.
117. Roth, EJ, et al: Pulmonary function testing in spinal cord injury: Correlation with vital capacity. Paraplegia 33(8):454–457, 1995.
118. Berney, SC, et al: A classification and regression tree to assist clinical decision making in airway management for patients with cervical spinal cord injury. Spinal Cord 49(2):244–250, 2011.
119. Anke, A, et al: Lung volumes in tetraplegic patients according to cervical spinal cord injury level. Scan J Rehabil Med 25(2):73–77, 1993.
120. Roth, EJ, et al: Ventilatory function in cervical and high thoracic spinal cord injury. Relationship to level of injury and tone. Am J Phys Med Rehabil 76(4):262–267, 1997.
121. Manning, H, et al: Oxygen cost of resistive-loaded breathing in quadriplegia. J Applied Physiol 73(3):825–831, 1992.
122. Alvarez, SE, Peterson, M, and Lunsford, BR: Respiratory treatment of the adult patient with spinal cord injury. Phys Ther 61(12):1737-1745, 1981.
123. Somers, MF: Spinal Cord Injury: Functional Rehabilitation, ed 3. Pearson, Upper Saddle River, NJ, 2010.
124. Mortenson, WB, and Miller, WC: A review of scales for assessing the risk of developing a pressure ulcer in individuals with SCI. Spinal Cord 46(3):168–175, 2008.
125. Salzberg, CA, et al: A new pressure ulcer risk assessment scale for individuals with spinal cord injury. Am J Phys Med Rehabil 75(2):96–104, 1996.
126. Salzberg, CA, et al: Predicting pressure ulcers during initial hospitalisation for acute spinal cord injury. Wounds 11:45–57, 1999.
127. Eriks-Hoogland, IE, et al: Passive shoulder range of motion impairment in spinal cord injury during and one year after rehabilitation. J Rehabil Med 41(6):438–444, 2009.
128. Berlowitz, DJ, and Tamplin, J: Respiratory muscle training for cervical spinal cord injury. Cochrane Database Syst Rev 7: CD008507, 2013.
129. Van Houtte, S, Vanlandewijck, Y, and Gosselink, R: Respiratory muscle training in persons with spinal cord injury: A systematic review. Respir Med 100(11):1886–1895, 2006.
130. Sheel, AW, et al: Effects of exercise training and inspiratory muscle training in spinal cord injury: A systematic review. J Spinal Cord Med 31(5):500–508, 2008.
131. Roth, EJ, et al: Expiratory muscle training in spinal cord injury: A randomized controlled trial. Arch Phys Med Rehabil 91(6): 857–861, 2010.
132. Reid, WD, et al: Physiotherapy secretion removal techniques in people with spinal cord injury: A systematic review. J Spinal Cord Med 33(4):353–370, 2010.
133. Warren, VC: Glossopharyngeal and neck accessory muscle breathing in a young adult with C2 complete tetraplegia resulting in ventilator dependency. Phys Ther 82(6):590–600, 2002.
134. Wetzel, JL: Management of respiratory dysfunction. In Field-Fote, EC (ed): Spinal Cord Injury Rehabilitation. FA Davis, Philadelphia, PA, 2009.
135. Wadsworth, BM, et al: Abdominal binder improves lung volumes and voice in people with tetraplegic spinal cord injury. Arch Phys Med Rehabil 93(12):2189–2197, 2012.
136. Julia, PE, Sa'ari, MY, and Hasnan, N: Benefit of triple-strap abdominal binder on voluntary cough in patients with spinal cord injury. Spinal Cord 49(11):1138–1142, 2011.
137. Royster, RA, Barboi, C, and Peruzzi, WT: Critical care in acute cervical spinal cord injury. Top Spinal Cord Inj Rehab 9(3): 11–32, 2004.

138. Gittler, MS: Acute rehabilitation in cervical spinal cord injury. Top Spinal Cord Inj Rehabil 9(3):60–73, 2004.
139. Henderson, JL, et al: Efficacy of three measures to relieve pressure in seated persons with spinal cord injury. Arch Phys Med Rehabil 75(5):535–539, 1994.
140. Coggrave, MJ, and Rose, LS: A specialist seating assessment clinic: Changing pressure relief practice. Spinal Cord 41(12):692–695, 2003.
141. Rintala, DH, et al: Preventing recurrent pressure ulcers in veterans with spinal cord injury: Impact of a structured education and follow-up intervention. Arch Phys Med Rehabil 89(8): 1429–1441, 2008.
142. Bohn, AS, and Peljovich, AE: Upper extremity orthotic and post surgical management. In Field-Fote EC (ed): Spinal Cord Injury Rehabilitation. FA Davis, Philadelphia, PA, 2009.
143. Behrman, A, et al: Assessment of functional improvement without compensation reduces variability of outcome measures after human spinal cord injury. Arch Phys Med Rehabil 93(9): 1518–1529, 2012.
144. Behrman, AL, and Harkema, SJ: Physical rehabilitation as an agent for recovery after spinal cord injury. Phys Med Rehabil Clin N Am 18(2):183–202, v, 2007.
145. Levin, MF, Kleim, JA, and Wolf, SL: What do motor "recovery" and "compensation" mean in patients following stroke? Neurorehabil Neural Rep 23(4):313–319, 2009.
146. Dietz, V, and Harkema, SJ: Locomotor activity in spinal cord-injured persons. J App Physiol 96(5):1954–1960, 2004.
147. Harkema, S, Behrman, A, and Barbeau, H: Locomotor Training: Principles and Practice. Oxford University Press, 2011.
148. Harkema, SJ: Neural plasticity after human spinal cord injury: Application of locomotor training to the rehabilitation of walking. Neuroscientist 7(5):455–468, 2001.
149. Harkema, S, et al: Effect of epidural stimulation of the lumbosacral spinal cord on voluntary movement, standing, and assisted stepping after motor complete paraplegia: A case study. Lancet 377(9781):1938–1947, 2011.
150. Field-Fote, EC, and Roach, KE: Influence of a locomotor training approach on walking speed and distance in people with chronic spinal cord injury: A randomized clinical trial. Phys Ther 91(1):48–60, 2011.
151. Edgerton, VR, and Harkema, S: Epidural stimulation of the spinal cord in spinal cord injury: Current status and future challenges. Expert Rev Neurother 11(10):1351–1353, 2011.
152. Musienko, P, et al: Multi-system neurorehabilitative strategies to restore motor functions following severe spinal cord injury. Exp Neurol 235(1):100–109, 2012.
153. Hol, AT, et al: Reliability and validity of the six-minute arm test for the evaluation of cardiovascular fitness in people with spinal cord injury. Arch Phys Med Rehabil 88(4):489–495, 2007.
154. Macciocchi, S, et al: Spinal cord injury and co-occurring traumatic brain injury: Assessment and incidence. Arch Phys Med Rehabil 89(7):1350–1357, 2008.
155. Budisin, B, et al: Traumatic brain injury in spinal cord injury: Frequency and risk factors. J Head Trauma Rehabil 31(4): E33–42, 2016.
156. Nasreddine, ZS, et al: The Montreal Cognitive Assessment, MoCA: A brief screening tool for mild cognitive impairment. J Amer Geriatr Soc 53(4):695–699, 2005.
157. Folstein, MF, Folstein, SE, and McHugh, PR: "Mini-mental state": A practical method for grading the cognitive state of patients for the clinician. J Psychiatr Res 12(3):189–198, 1975.
158. Scivoletto, G, et al: Distribution-based estimates of clinically significant changes in the International Standards for Neurological Classification of Spinal Cord Injury motor and sensory scores. Eur J Phys Rehabil Med 49(3):373–384, 2013.
159. Haas, BM, et al: The inter rater reliability of the original and of the modified Ashworth scale for the assessment of spasticity in patients with spinal cord injury. Spinal Cord 34(9):560–564, 1996.
160. Adams, MM, Ginis, KA, and Hicks, AL: The spinal cord injury spasticity evaluation tool: Development and evaluation. Arch Phys Med Rehabil 88(9):1185–1192, 2007.
161. Hornby, TG, et al: Windup of flexion reflexes in chronic human spinal cord injury: A marker for neuronal plateau potentials? J Neurophysiol 89(1):416-426, 2003.
162. Sisto, SA, and Dyson-Hudson, T: Dynamometry testing in spinal cord injury. J Rehabil Res Dev 44(1):123–136, 2007.
163. Larson, CA, et al: Assessment of postural muscle strength in sitting: Reliability of measures obtained with hand-held dynamometry in individuals with spinal cord injury. J Neurol Phys Ther 34(1):24–31, 2010.
164. Aufsesser, PM, Horvat, M, and Austin, M: The reliability of hand held muscle testers with individuals with spinal cord injury. Clin Kinesiology 57(4):71–75, 2003.
165. Curtis, KA, et al: Development of the Wheelchair User's Shoulder Pain Index (WUSPI). Paraplegia 33(5):290–293, 1995.
166. Curtis, KA, et al: Reliability and validity of the Wheelchair User's Shoulder Pain Index (WUSPI). Paraplegia 33(10):595–601, 1995.
167. Day, H, Jutai, J, and Campbell, KA: Development of a scale to measure the psychosocial impact of assistive devices: Lessons learned and the road ahead. Disabil Rehabil 24(1–3):31–37, 2002.
168. Demers, L, et al: The Psychosocial Impact of Assistive Devices Scale (PIADS): Translation and preliminary psychometric evaluation of a Canadian-French version. Qual Life Res 11(6):583–592, 2002.
169. Lynch, SM, Leahy, P, and Barker, SP: Reliability of measurements obtained with a modified functional reach test in subjects with spinal cord injury. Phys Ther 78(2):128–133, 1998.
170. Gabison, S, et al: Trunk strength and function using the multidirectional reach distance in individuals with non-traumatic spinal cord injury. J Spinal Cord Med 37(5):537–547, 2014.
171. Lemay, JF, and Nadeau, S: Standing balance assessment in ASIA D paraplegic and tetraplegic participants: Concurrent validity of the Berg Balance Scale. Spinal Cord 48(3):245–250, 2010.
172. Wirz, M, Muller, R, and Bastiaenen, C: Falls in persons with spinal cord injury: Validity and reliability of the Berg Balance Scale. Neurorehabil Neural Rep 24(1):70–77, 2010.
173. Whiteneck, GG, et al: Quantifying handicap: A new measure of long-term rehabilitation outcomes. Arch Phys Med Rehabil 73(6):519–526, 1992.
174. Hill, MR, et al: Quality of life instruments and definitions in individuals with spinal cord injury: A systematic review. Spinal Cord 48(6):438–450, 2010.
175. Noonan, VK, et al: Comparing the content of participation instruments using the international classification of functioning, disability and health. Health Qual Life Outcomes 7:93, 2009.
176. Noonan, VK, et al: A review of participation instruments based on the International Classification of Functioning, Disability and Health. Disabil Rehabil 31(23):1883–1901, 2009.
177. Noonan, VK, et al: A review of instruments assessing participation in persons with spinal cord injury. Spinal Cord 47(6): 435–446, 2009.
178. De Wolf, A, et al: Measuring community integration after spinal cord injury: Validation of the Sydney psychosocial reintegration scale and community integration measure. Qual Life Res 19(8):1185–1193, 2010.
179. Post, MW, et al: Validity of the Life Satisfaction questions, the Life Satisfaction Questionnaire, and the Satisfaction With Life Scale in persons with spinal cord injury. Arch Phys Med Rehabil 93(10):1832–1837, 2012.
180. van Koppenhagen CF, et al: Changes and determinants of life satisfaction after spinal cord injury: A cohort study in the Netherlands. Arch Phys Med Rehabil 89(9):1733–1740, 2008.
181. Geyh, S, et al: Cross-cultural validity of four quality of life scales in persons with spinal cord injury. Health Qual Life Outcomes 8:94, 2010.
182. Forchheimer, M, McAweeney, M, and Tate, DG: Use of the SF-36 among persons with spinal cord injury. Am J Phys Med Rehabil 83(5):390–395, 2004.
183. Lee, BB, et al: The SF-36 walk-wheel: A simple modification of the SF-36 physical domain improves its responsiveness for measuring health status change in spinal cord injury. Spinal Cord 47(1):50–55, 2009.
184. May, LA, and Warren, S: Measuring quality of life of persons with spinal cord injury: External and structural validity. Spinal Cord 40(7):341–350, 2002.
185. Lin, MR, et al: Comparisons of the brief form of the World Health Organization Quality of Life and Short Form-36 for persons with spinal cord injuries. Am J Phys Med Rehabil 86(2):104–113, 2007.
186. Perry, J, and Burnfield, JM: Gait Analysis: Normal and Pathological Function, ed 2. Slack, Thorofare, NJ, 2010.

187. Ditunno, JF, et al: Validation of the walking index for spinal cord injury in a US and European clinical population. Spinal Cord 46(3):181–188, 2008.
188. Ditunno, JF, Jr., et al: Walking index for spinal cord injury (WISCI): An international multicenter validity and reliability study. Spinal Cord 38(4):234-243, 2000.
189. Jackson, AB, et al: Outcome measures for gait and ambulation in the spinal cord injury population. J Spinal Cord Med 31(5): 487–499, 2008.
190. Burns, AS, et al: The reproducibility and convergent validity of the walking index for spinal cord injury (WISCI) in chronic spinal cord injury. Neurorehabil Neural Repair 25(2):149–157, 2011.
191. Field-Fote, EC, et al: The Spinal Cord Injury Functional Ambulation Inventory (SCI-FAI). J Rehabil Med 33(4):177–181, 2001.
192. van Hedel, HJ: Gait speed in relation to categories of functional ambulation after spinal cord injury. Neurorehabil Neural Repair 23(4):343–350, 2009.
193. van Hedel, HJ, Wirz, M, and Dietz, V: Assessing walking ability in subjects with spinal cord injury: Validity and reliability of 3 walking tests. Arch Phys Med Rehabil 86(2):190–196, 2005.
194. Lam, T, Noonan, VK, and Eng, JJ: A systematic review of functional ambulation outcome measures in spinal cord injury. Spinal Cord 46(4):246–254, 2008.
195. Hosseini, SM, et al: Manual wheelchair skills capacity predicts quality of life and community integration in persons with spinal cord injury. Arch Phys Med Rehabil 93(12):2237–2243, 2012.
196. Kirby, RL, et al: The wheelchair skills test (version 2.4): Measurement properties. Arch Phys Med Rehabil 85(5):794–804, 2004.
197. Lindquist, NJ, et al: Reliability of the performance and safety scores of the wheelchair skills test version 4.1 for manual wheelchair users. Arch Phys Med Rehabil 91(11):1752–1757, 2010.
198. Kilkens, OJ, et al: The Wheelchair Circuit: Construct validity and responsiveness of a test to assess manual wheelchair mobility in persons with spinal cord injury. Arch Phys Med Rehabil 85(3):424–431, 2004.
199. Kilkens, OJ, et al: The wheelchair circuit: reliability of a test to assess mobility in persons with spinal cord injuries. Arch Phys Med Rehabil 83(12):1783–1788, 2002.
200. Basso, DM, et al: Interrater reliability of the Neuromuscular Recovery Scale for spinal cord injury. Arch Phys Med Rehabil 96(8):1397–1403, 2015.
201. Behrman, AL, et al: Test-retest reliability of the Neuromuscular Recovery Scale. Arch Phys Med Rehabil 96(8):1375–1384, 2015.
202. Tester, NJ, et al: Responsiveness of the Neuromuscular Recovery Scale during outpatient activity-dependent rehabilitation for spinal cord injury. Neurorehabil Neural Repair 30(6):528–538, 2016.
203. Velozo, C, et al: Validity of the Neuromuscular Recovery Scale: A measurement model approach. Arch Phys Med Rehabil 96(8):1385–1396, 2015.
204. Dodds, TA, et al: A validation of the functional independence measurement and its performance among rehabilitation inpatients. Arch Phys Med Rehabil 74(5):531–536, 1993.
205. Hamilton, BB, et al: Relation of disability costs to function: Spinal cord injury. Arch Phys Med Rehabil 80(4):385–391, 1999.
206. Heinemann, AW, et al: Relationships between disability measures and nursing effort during medical rehabilitation for patients with traumatic brain and spinal cord injury. Arch Phys Med Rehabil 78(2):143–149, 1997.
207. Catz, A, et al: SCIM—spinal cord independence measure: A new disability scale for patients with spinal cord lesions. Spinal Cord 35(12):850–856, 1997.
208. Rudhe, C, and van Hedel, HJ: Upper extremity function in persons with tetraplegia: Relationships between strength, capacity, and the spinal cord independence measure. Neurorehabil Neural Repair 23(5):413–421, 2009.
209. Dawson, J, Shamley, D, and Jamous, MA: A structured review of outcome measures used for the assessment of rehabilitation interventions for spinal cord injury. Spinal Cord 46(12):768–780, 2008.
210. Scivoletto, G, et al: The spinal cord independence measure: How much change is clinically significant for spinal cord injury subjects. Disabil Rehabil 35(21):1808–1813, 2013.
211. Marino, RJ, Shea, JA, and Stineman, MG: The Capabilities of Upper Extremity instrument: Reliability and validity of a measure of functional limitation in tetraplegia. Arch Phys Med Rehabil 79(12):1512–1521, 1998.
212. Mulcahey, MJ, Smith, BT, and Betz, RR: Psychometric rigor of the Grasp and Release Test for measuring functional limitation of persons with tetraplegia: A preliminary analysis. J Spinal Cord Med 27(1):41-46, 2004.
213. Kalsi-Ryan, S, et al: The Graded Redefined Assessment of Strength Sensibility and Prehension: Reliability and validity. J Neurotrauma 29(5):905–914, 2012.
214. Roth, EJ, Lawler, MH, and Yarkony, GM: Traumatic central cord syndrome: Clinical features and functional outcomes. Arch Phys Med Rehabil 71(1):18–23, 1990.
215. Consortium for Spinal Cord Injury Medicine Clinical Practice Guidelines. Outcomes following traumatic spinal cord injury: Clinical practice guidelines for health-care professionals. Paralyzed Veterans of American, 1999.
216. Al-Habib, AF, et al: Clinical predictors of recovery after blunt spinal cord trauma: Systematic review. J Neurotrauma 28(8): 1431–1443, 2011.
217. Bombardier, CH, et al: Do preinjury alcohol problems predict poorer rehabilitation progress in persons with spinal cord injury? Arch Phys Med Rehabil 85(9):1488–1492, 2004.
218. Nyland, J, et al: Preserving transfer independence among individuals with spinal cord injury. Spinal Cord 38(11):649–657, 2000.
219. Mulroy, SJ, et al: Strengthening and optimal movements for painful shoulders (STOMPS) in chronic spinal cord injury: A randomized controlled trial. Phys Ther 91(3):305–324, 2011.
220. Figoni, SF: Spinal cord disabilities: Paraplegia and tetraplegia. In Durstine, JL, and Moore, GE (eds): ACSM's Exercise Management for Persons with Chronic Diseases and Disabilities. American College of Sports Medicine, Champaign, IL, 2003.
221. Flansbjer, UB, et al: Progressive resistance training after stroke: Effects on muscle strength, muscle tone, gait performance and perceived participation. J Rehabil Med 40(1):42–48, 2008.
222. de Groot, PC, et al: Effect of training intensity on physical capacity, lipid profile and insulin sensitivity in early rehabilitation of spinal cord injured individuals. Spinal Cord 41(12):673–679, 2003.
223. Davis, G, Plyley, MJ, and Shephard, RJ: Gains of cardiorespiratory fitness with arm-crank training in spinally disabled men. Can J Sport Sci 16(1):64–72, 1991.
224. Valent, LJ, et al: Effects of hand cycle training on physical capacity in individuals with tetraplegia: A clinical trial. Phys Ther 89(10):1051–1060, 2009.
225. Soyupek, F, et al: Effects of body weight supported treadmill training on cardiac and pulmonary functions in the patients with incomplete spinal cord injury. J Back Musculoskelet Rehabil 22(4):213–218, 2009.
226. Kaufman, C, et al: Ratings of perceived exertion of ACSM exercise guidelines in individuals varying in aerobic fitness. Res Q Exerc Sport 77(1):122–130, 2006.
227. Janssen, TW, and Pringle, DD: Effects of modified electrical stimulation-induced leg cycle ergometer training for individuals with spinal cord injury. J Rehabil Res Dev 45(6):819–830, 2008.
228. Perry, J, et al: Electromyographic analysis of the shoulder muscles during depression transfers in subjects with low-level paraplegia. Arch Phys Med Rehabil 77(4):350–355, 1996.
229. Forslund, EB, et al: Transfer from table to wheelchair in men and women with spinal cord injury: Coordination of body movement and arm forces. Spinal Cord 45(1):41–48, 2007.
230. Fulk, G, and Nirider, CD: Interventions to improve transfers skills. In O'Sullivan, S, and Schmitz, T (eds): Improving Functional Outcomes in Physical Rehabilitation. FA Davis, Philadelphia, PA, 2016.
231. Hanada, E, and Kerrigan, DC: Energy consumption during level walking with arm and knee immobilized. Arch Phys Med Rehabil 82(9):1251–1254, 2001.
232. Mikelberg, R, and Reid, S: Spinal cord lesions and lower extremity bracing: An overview and follow-up study. Paraplegia 19(6): 379–385, 1981.
233. Hussey, RW, and Stauffer, ES: Spinal cord injury: Requirements for ambulation. Arch Phys Med Rehabil 54(12):544–547, 1973.
234. Behrman, AL, and Plummer-D'Amato, P: "What's in a Name?" Revisited. Phys Ther 88(1):6–9, 2008.
235. Barbeau, H, and Rossignol, S: Recovery of locomotion after chronic spinalization in the adult cat. Brain Res 412(1):84–95, 1987.
236. Lovely, RG, et al: Effects of training on the recovery of full-weight-bearing stepping in the adult spinal cat. Exp Neurol 92(2):421–435, 1986.

237. Edgerton, VR, et al: Use-dependent plasticity in spinal stepping and standing. Adv Neurol 72:233–247, 1997.
238. Barbeau, H, Wainberg, M, and Finch, L: Description and application of a system for locomotor rehabilitation. Med Biol Eng Comput 25(3):341–344, 1987.
239. Finch, L, Barbeau, H, and Arsenault, B: Influence of body weight support on normal human gait: Development of a gait retraining strategy. Phys Ther 71(11):842–855; discussion 855–846, 1991.
240. Barbeau, H, Danakas, M, and Arsenault, B: The effects of locomotor training in spinal cord injured subjects: A preliminary study. Restorative Neurol Neurosci 5(1):81–84, 1993.
241. Hodgson, JA, et al: Can the mammalian lumbar spinal cord learn a motor task? Med Sci Sport Exerc 26(12):1491–1497, 1994.
242. Edgerton, VR, et al: A physiological basis for the development of rehabilitative strategies for spinally injured patients. J Am Paraplegia Soc 14(4):150–157, 1991.
243. Visintin, M, and Barbeau, H: The effects of body weight support on the locomotor pattern of spastic paretic patients. Can J Neurol Sci 16(3):315–325, 1989.
244. Beres-Jones, JA, and Harkema, SJ: The human spinal cord interprets velocity-dependent afferent input during stepping. Brain 127(Pt 10):2232–2246, 2004.
245. Harkema, SJ, et al: Human lumbosacral spinal cord interprets loading during stepping. J Neurophysiol 77(2):797–811, 1997.
246. Ferris, DP, et al: Muscle activation during unilateral stepping occurs in the nonstepping limb of humans with clinically complete spinal cord injury. Spinal Cord 42(1):14–23, 2004.
247. Field-Fote, EC, Lindley, SD, and Sherman, AL: Locomotor training approaches for individuals with spinal cord injury: A preliminary report of walking-related outcomes. J Neurol Phys Ther 29(3):127–137, 2005.
248. Dobkin, B, et al: Weight-supported treadmill vs over-ground training for walking after acute incomplete SCI. Neurology 66(4):484–493, 2006.
249. Behrman, AL, et al: Locomotor training progression and outcomes after incomplete spinal cord injury. Phys Ther 85(12): 1356–1371, 2005.
250. Takeuchi, N, and Izumi, S: Maladaptive plasticity for motor recovery after stroke: Mechanisms and approaches. Neural Plast 2012:359728, 2012.
251. Fong, AJ, et al: Recovery of control of posture and locomotion after a spinal cord injury: Solutions staring us in the face. Prog Brain Res 175:393–418, 2009.
252. Snoek, GJ, et al: Survey of the needs of patients with spinal cord injury: Impact and priority for improvement in hand function in tetraplegics. Spinal Cord 42(9):526–532, 2004.
253. Beekhuizen, KS, and Field-Fote, EC: Sensory stimulation augments the effects of massed practice training in persons with tetraplegia. Arch Phys Med Rehabil 89(4):602–608, 2008.
254. Beekhuizen, KS, and Field-Fote, EC: Massed practice versus massed practice with stimulation: Effects on upper extremity function and cortical plasticity in individuals with incomplete cervical spinal cord injury. Neurorehabil Neural Repair 19(1): 33–45, 2005.
255. Hoffman, LR, and Field-Fote, EC: Functional and corticomotor changes in individuals with tetraplegia following unimanual or bimanual massed practice training with somatosensory stimulation: A pilot study. J Neurol Phys Ther 34(4):193–201, 2010.
256. Ljungberg, I, et al: Using peer mentoring for people with spinal cord injury to enhance self-efficacy beliefs and prevent medical complications. J Clin Nurs 20(3–4):351–358, 2011.
257. MacPhee, AH, et al: Wheelchair skills training program: A randomized clinical trial of wheelchair users undergoing initial rehabilitation. Arch Phys Med Rehabil 85(1):41–50, 2004.
258. Best, KL, et al: Wheelchair skills training for community-based manual wheelchair users: A randomized controlled trial. Arch Phys Med Rehabil 86(12):2316–2323, 2005.
259. Coolen, AL, et al: Wheelchair skills training program for clinicians: A randomized controlled trial with occupational therapy students. Arch Phys Med Rehabil 85(7):1160–1167, 2004.
260. Fulk, G, and Hastings, J: Interventions to improve wheelchair skills. In O'Sullivan, S, and Schmitz, T (eds): Improving Functional Outcomes in Physical Rehabilitation. FA Davis, Philadelphia, PA, 2016.
261. Mohr, T, et al: Long-term adaptation to electrically induced cycle training in severe spinal cord injured individuals. Spinal Cord 35(1):1–16, 1997.
262. Mushahwar, VK, et al: New functional electrical stimulation approaches to standing and walking. J Neural Eng 4(3):S181–197, 2007.
263. Dutta, A, Kobetic, R, and Triolo, RJ: Gait initiation with electromyographically triggered electrical stimulation in people with partial paralysis. J Biomech Eng 131(8):081002, 2009.
264. Johnston, TE, et al: Implanted functional electrical stimulation: An alternative for standing and walking in pediatric spinal cord injury. Spinal Cord 41(3):144–152, 2003.
265. Kilgore, KL, et al: An implanted upper-extremity neuroprosthesis using myoelectric control. J Hand Surg Am 33(4):539–550, 2008.
266. DiMarco, AF, Takaoka, Y, and Kowalski, KE: Combined intercostal and diaphragm pacing to provide artificial ventilation in patients with tetraplegia. Arch Phys Med Rehabil 86(6):1200–1207, 2005.
267. Kutzenberger, J, Domurath, B, and Sauerwein, D: Spastic bladder and spinal cord injury: Seventeen years of experience with sacral deafferentation and implantation of an anterior root stimulator. Artif Organs 29(3):239–241, 2005.
268. Jezernik, S, et al: Electrical stimulation for the treatment of bladder dysfunction: Current status and future possibilities. Neurol Res 24(5):413–430, 2002.
269. Shih, JJ, Krusienski, DJ, and Wolpaw, JR: Brain-computer interfaces in medicine. Mayo Clin Proc 87(3):268–279, 2012.
270. Machado, S, et al: EEG-based brain-computer interfaces: An overview of basic concepts and clinical applications in neurorehabilitation. Rev Neurosci 21(6):451–468, 2010.
271. Mason, SG, et al: Real-time control of a video game with a direct brain—computer interface. J Clin Neurophysiol 21(6):404–408, 2004.
272. McFarland, DJ, et al: Emulation of computer mouse control with a noninvasive brain-computer interface. J Neural Eng 5(2): 101–110, 2008.
273. Millan, JD, et al: Combining brain-computer interfaces and assistive technologies: State-of-the-art and challenges. Front Neurosci 4, 2010.
274. Tefertiller, C, et al: Efficacy of rehabilitation robotics for walking training in neurological disorders: A review. J Rehabil Res Dev 48(4):387–416, 2011.
275. Ferris, DP: The exoskeletons are here. J Neuroengin Rehabil 6:17, 2009.
276. Song, W, et al: Combined motor cortex and spinal cord neuromodulation promotes corticospinal system functional and structural plasticity and motor function after injury. Exp Neurol 277:46–57, 2016.
277. Bocci, T, et al: Cathodal transcutaneous spinal direct current stimulation (tsDCS) improves motor unit recruitment in healthy subjects. Neurosci Lett 578:75–79, 2014.
278. McKay, WB, et al: Neurophysiological examination of the corticospinal system and voluntary motor control in motor-incomplete human spinal cord injury. Exp Brain Res 163(3):379–387, 2005.
279. Thomas, SL, and Gorassini, MA: Increases in corticospinal tract function by treadmill training after incomplete spinal cord injury. J Neurophysiol 94(4):2844–2855, 2005.
280. Hajela, N, et al: Corticospinal reorganization after locomotor training in a person with motor incomplete paraplegia. Biomed Res Int 2013:516427, 2013.

Web-Based Resources for Clinicians and Patients/Families Living With Spinal Cord Injury

appendix **20.A**

WEB-BASED RESOURCES FOR PATIENTS, FAMILIES, AND CLINICIANS

Spinal Cord Injury Information Network: www.spinalcord.uab.edu
Christopher and Dana Reeve Paralysis Foundation: www.christopherreeve.org
Model Spinal Cord Injury System Dissemination Center: www.mscisdisseminationcenter.org
WheelchairNet: www.wheelchairnet.org
Wheelchair Skills Program: www.wheelchairskillsprogram.ca
National Council on Independent Living: www.ncil.org
Paralyzed Veterans Association: www.pva.org
Paralyzed Veterans Association, Clinical Practice Guidelines: www.pva.org/publications/clinical-practice-guidelines
American Spinal Injury Association: www.asia-spinalinjury.org
National Spinal Cord Injury Association: www.spinalcord.org
NeurotechNetwork: www.neurotechnetwork.org
Think First: www.thinkfirst.org
Sports'n Spokes: www.pvamagazines.com/sns
New Mobility: www.newmobility.com
Shake-A-Leg: www.shakealeg.org
The Cleveland Center: http://fescenter.case.edu
The Miami Project to Cure Paralysis: www.miamiproject.miami.edu
disABILITY Information and Resources: www.makoa.org
Spinal Cord Injury Rehabilitation Evidence: www.scireproject.com
Shirley Ryan AbilityLab Rehabilitation Measures Database: www.sralab.org/rehabilitation-measures
Physiotherapy Exercises for People With Spinal Cord Injury and Other Neurological Conditions: www.physiotherapyexercises.com
Academy of Neurologic Physical Therapy SCI EDGE: www.neuropt.org/professional-resources/neurology-section-outcome-measures-recommendations/spinal-cord-injury
PT Now SCI Clinical Summaries: www.ptnow.org/clinical-summaries
Access to Independence: www.atilange.com/Resources.html

Chapter 21 Vestibular Disorders

Michael C. Schubert, PT, PhD

LEARNING OBJECTIVES

1. Differentiate vestibular symptom pathology from other manifestations of vertigo, dizziness, and dysequilibrium.
2. Identify the examination procedures used to evaluate patients with vestibular dysfunction to establish a diagnosis, prognosis, and plan of care.
3. When presented with a clinical case study, analyze and interpret examination data and determine appropriate interventions for the clinical problems presented.
4. Determine appropriate elements of the rehabilitation program for patients with vestibular dysfunction.

CHAPTER OUTLINE

Physical therapists are likely to encounter patients with vestibular disorders in a variety of clinical settings, including the emergency department. At an incidence of 5.5%, dizziness in the United States affects more than 15 million people each year.[1] The reported prevalence of dizziness as a medical symptom in community-dwelling adults varies based on subjects' age, sex, and definition of the complaint (1% to 35%).[2-6] Dizziness is among the most common complaints adults report to their physicians and prevalence increases with age.[7,8] A cross-sectional study of emergency department visits for dizziness found that otologic/vestibular pathology was the number one cause (32%).[9] Among community-dwelling adults, it has been suggested that nearly one-third of the U.S. population has a vestibular disorder.[10,11] Patients who experience dizziness report a significant disability that reduces their quality of life.[12-14] Furthermore, it has been reported that greater than 70% of patients with initial complaints of dizziness will not have a resolution of symptoms at a 2-week follow-up. Of patients with persistent dizziness, 63% reported recurrent symptoms continuing beyond 3 months.[15]

Cawthorne[16] and Cooksey[17] were the first clinicians to advocate exercises for persons suffering from dizziness and vertigo. It has only been within the last two decades, however, that our knowledge of vestibular function and related disorders has profoundly changed rehabilitation approaches. Once an accurate diagnosis involving the vestibular pathways has been made, activity limitations are minimized and progression toward disability can be prevented. Evidence suggests that an individualized approach to vestibular rehabilitation is important for a better outcome.

The peripheral vestibular system serves as the primary focus of this chapter because it is the most common origin for patient signs and symptoms. The physical therapist, however, must recognize patterns of signs and symptoms from a central pathology as well. With an appreciation of the complexity of the vestibular system coupled with an understanding of tests to measure its function, the reader will be able to discern anomalies of the system and begin to formulate effective rehabilitation strategies.

ANATOMY

Peripheral Vestibular System

The three primary functions of the peripheral vestibular system are (1) stabilizing visual images on the fovea of the retina during head movement to allow clear vision; (2) maintaining postural stability, especially during movement of the head; and (3) providing information used for spatial orientation.

Semicircular Canals

Within the petrous portion of each temporal bone (base of the skull between the sphenoid and occipital bones) lies the membranous vestibular labyrinth. Each labyrinth contains five neural structures that detect head acceleration: three *semicircular canals* and two *otolith* organs (Fig. 21.1). The three semicircular canals (SCCs) (*horizontal, posterior* [inferior], and *superior* [anterior]) respond to angular acceleration and are orthogonal (at right angles) with respect to one another. Alignment of the SCCs in the temporal bone is such that each canal has a contralateral coplanar mate. The horizontal canals form a coplanar pair while the posterior and contralateral anterior SCCs form coplanar pairs. The anterior aspect of the horizontal SCC is inclined 30° upward from a plane connecting the external auditory canal to the lateral canthus. The posterior and anterior SCCs are inclined about 92° and 90°, respectively, from the plane of the horizontal SCC.[18] Angular head rotation stimulates each canal to varying degrees.[19]

The SCCs are filled with *endolymph* (fluid) that has a density slightly greater than water.[20] Endolymph moves freely within each canal in response to the direction of the angular head rotation. The SCCs enlarge at one end to form the *ampulla*. Within the ampulla lies the *cupula*, a gelatinous barrier that contains the sensory hair cells (Fig. 21.2). The *kinocilia* (mechanosensing cilia involved in the sense of movement) and *stereocilia* (mechanosensing organelles) of the hair cells are seated in the *crista ampullaris* (sensory organ of angular rotation). Deflection of the stereocilia caused by motion of the endolymph results in an opening (or closing) of the transduction channels of hair cells, which results in changes in the membrane potential of the hair cells. Deflection of the stereocilia toward the kinocilia in each hair cell leads to excitation (*depolarization*) and deflection of the stereocilia away from the kinocilia leads to inhibition (*hyperpolarization*).

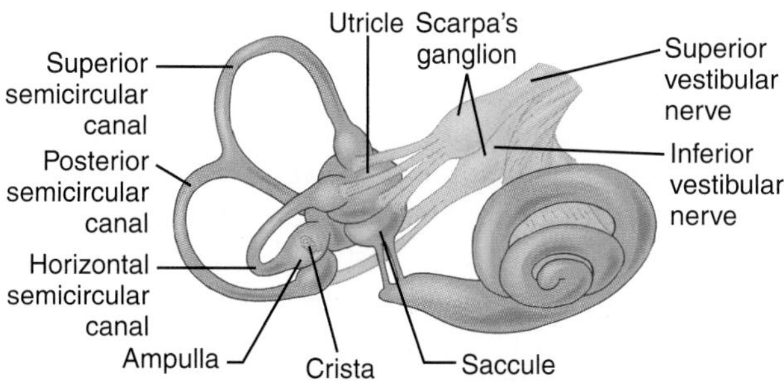

Figure 21.1 Anatomy of the vestibular labyrinth. Structures include the utricle, sacculus, superior semicircular canal, posterior semicircular canal, and the horizontal semicircular canal. The three semicircular canals (SCCs) are orthogonal with each other. Note the superior vestibular nerve innervating the superior (anterior) and horizontal semicircular canals as well as the utricle. The inferior vestibular nerve innervates the posterior semicircular canal and the saccule. The cell bodies of the vestibular nerves are located in Scarpa's ganglion (Gangl. Scarpae). Also note that the semicircular canals enlarge at one end to form the ampulla.

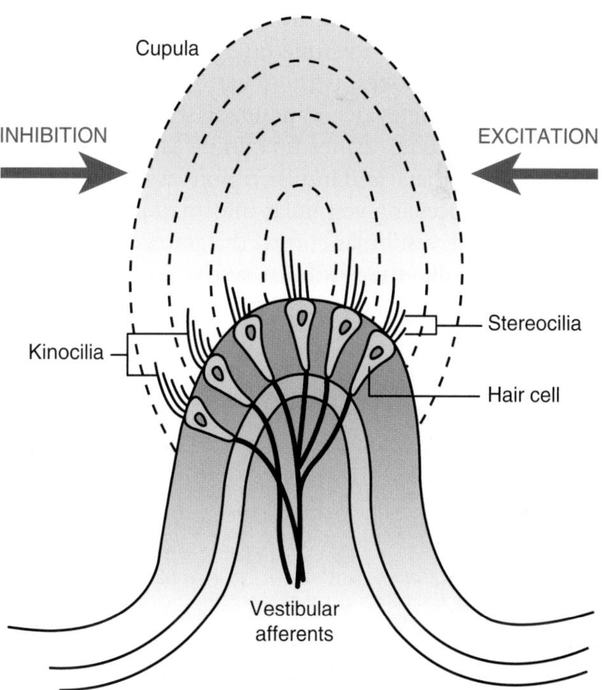

Figure 21.2 The cupula of the ampulla is a flexible, gelatinous barrier that partitions the canal. The crista ampullaris contains the kinocilia and stereocilia sensory hair cells. The hair cells generate action potentials in response to cupular deflection. Deflection of the stereocilia toward the kinocilia causes excitation; deflection in the opposite direction causes inhibition.

Each of the SCCs responds best to motion in its own plane with coplanar pairs exhibiting a *push–pull dynamic.* For example, as the head is turned to the right, the hair cells in the right horizontal SCC are excited, while hair cells in the left horizontal SCC are inhibited. The brain detects the direction of head movement by comparing input from the coplanar labyrinthine mates.

Otolith Organs

The saccule and utricle make up the otolith organs of the membranous labyrinth and respond to linear acceleration and static head tilt. Sensory hair cells project into a gelatinous material that has calcium carbonate crystalline-structure material (otoconia) embedded in it, which provides the otolith organs with an inertial mass (Fig. 21.3). Similar to the SCCs, motion toward the kinocilia causes excitation, while motion away leads to inhibition. Utricular excitation occurs during horizontal linear acceleration and/or static head tilt and saccular excitation occurs during vertical linear acceleration.

Central Vestibular System

Brain stem processes provide primary control of many vestibular reflexes. Tracing techniques, used to follow axonal projections from their source to point of termination, have identified extensive connections between the vestibular nuclei and the reticular formation, thalamus, and cerebellum[21-23] (Fig. 21.4). In addition, vestibular pathways appear to terminate in a unique cortical area. Primate studies have identified the junction of the parietal and insular lobes as the location for a vestibular cortex.[24-26] Recent evidence in human studies using functional magnetic resonance imaging (fMRI) appears to confirm the parietal and insular regions as the cortical location for processing vestibular information.[27] Connections with the vestibular cortex, thalamus, and reticular formation enable the vestibular system to contribute to the integration of arousal and conscious awareness of the body, as well as to discriminate between movement of self and the environment.[28,29] The cerebellar connections help maintain calibration of the vestibulo-ocular reflex (VOR), which stabilizes images on the retina during head movements, contributes to posture during static and dynamic activities, and influences the coordination of limb movements.

Vestibular connections with the autonomic nervous system contribute to cardiovascular function (i.e., blood pressure), validated in astronauts who upon returning to Earth's gravitational field (and the return of vestibular afference of gravity) suffer orthostatic intolerance after long-duration space exposure.[30]

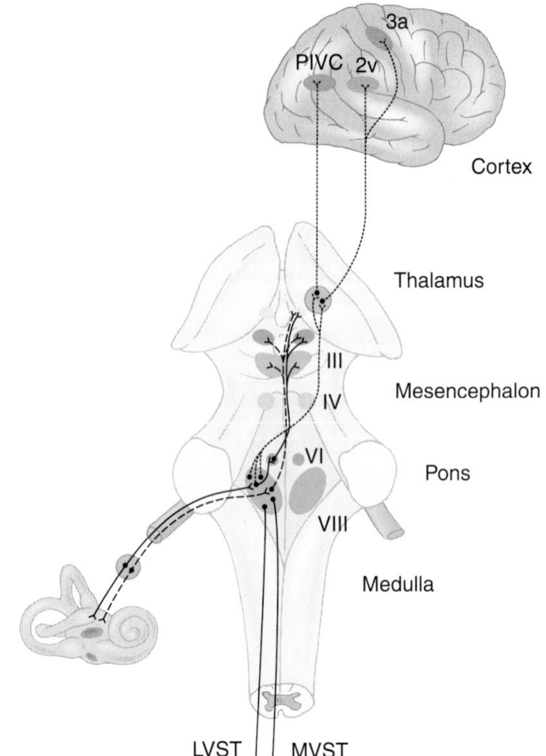

Figure 21.4 The semicircular canal (angular) and otolith (linear) input is sent to the vestibular nuclei. From the vestibular nuclei, the input travels to the ocular motor nuclei (III, IV, VI) for mediation of the vestibulo-ocular reflex. For arousal and conscious awareness of the head and body in space, information proceeds further to the thalamus and cortex. For maintenance of postural control, the peripheral vestibular input is sent distally as the medial and lateral vestibulo-spinal tracts (MVST, LVST). PIVC = Parieto-insular vestibular cortex.

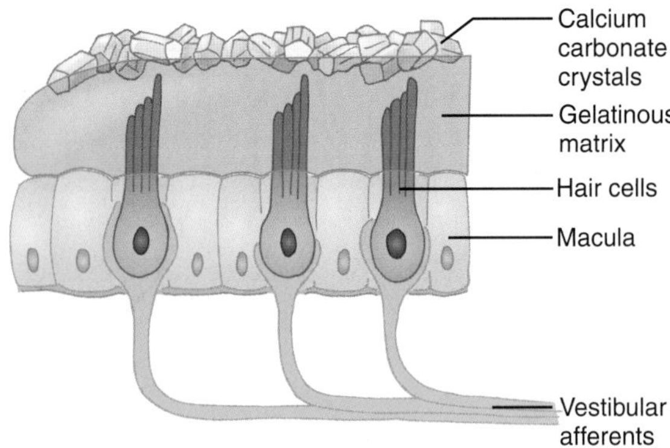

Figure 21.3 Otoconia are calcium carbonate crystals that are embedded in a gelatinous matrix that provides an inertial mass. Linear acceleration shifts the gelatinous matrix and excites or inhibits the vestibular afferents depending on the direction in which the stereocilia are deflected.

■ PHYSIOLOGY AND MOTOR CONTROL

Foundational knowledge of vestibular neurophysiology is important for understanding the signs and symptoms of vestibular dysfunction. Important principles of the vestibular system include the *tonic-firing rate, VOR, push–pull mechanism, inhibitory cutoff,* and *velocity storage system.*

Tonic Firing Rate

In primates, primary vestibular afferents of the healthy vestibular system have a resting firing rate that is typically 70 to 100 spikes/sec.[31,32] The presence of the high tonic firing rate means each vestibular system can detect head motion through excitation or inhibition. During angular head rotations, ipsilateral vestibular afferents and ipsilateral central vestibular neurons are excited.[31] Such head movements also result in inhibition of peripheral afferents and of many central vestibular neurons receiving innervation from the contralateral labyrinth.

Vestibulo-Ocular Reflex

The VOR is responsible for maintaining stability of an image on the fovea of the retina during rapid head movements. To do this, the VOR must generate rapid compensatory eye movements in the direction opposite the head rotation. The VOR achieves this with relatively simple patterns of connectivity in the central vestibular pathways. In its most basic form, the pathways controlling the VOR can be described as a three-neuron arc:

- Primary vestibular afferents from the anterior SCC synapse in the ipsilateral vestibular nuclei.
- Secondary ipsilateral vestibular neurons receiving innervation from the ipsilateral labyrinth decussate and synapse in the contralateral oculomotor nucleus.
- Motor neurons from the contralateral oculomotor nucleus then synapse at the neuromuscular junction of the ipsilateral superior rectus and the contralateral inferior oblique muscles, respectively (Fig. 21.5).

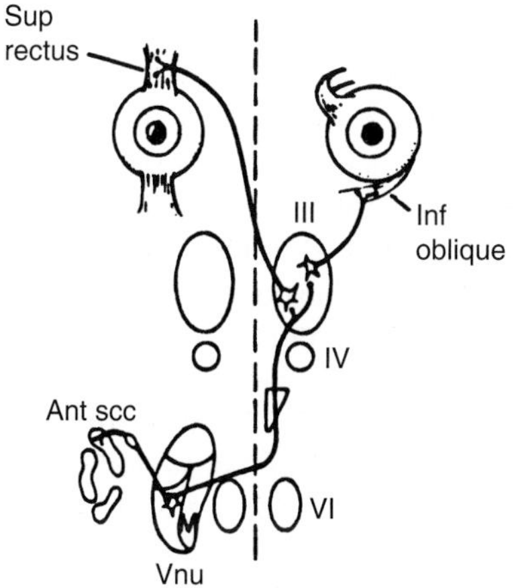

Figure 21.5 From the anterior semicircular canal (Ant Scc), afferent input travels to the vestibular nuclei (Vnu). The signal continues to the contralateral oculomotor nuclei (III). From there, motoneurons synapse with the superior rectus muscle that moves the eye upward, and the inferior oblique muscle that moves the eye upward and torsionally. Also shown are the oculomotor nuclei IV, and VI. *(Adapted from Baloh and Honrubia,[33, p. 52] with permission.)*

Similar patterns of connectivity exist for each SCC and the eye muscles that receive innervations from them (Table 21.1). See Figure 21.6 for insertions of the ocular muscles.

VOR Gain and Phase

Normally, as the head moves in one direction, the eyes move in the opposite direction with equal velocity. This relationship of eye velocity to head velocity is expressed as the gain (*VOR gain*) of the vestibular system (eye velocity/head velocity = −1). For example, when the head is moved down, the anterior SCCs are stimulated. Excitation of the anterior SCC afferents rotates both eyes in the direction opposite the angular head movement, or up (see Fig. 21.5). *VOR phase* is a second useful measure of the vestibular system and represents the amplitude relationship between the eye and head. VOR phase should represent an equal but opposite head and eye position relationship. Therefore, if the head moves 10 degrees to the right, the eyes should be positioned 10 degrees to the left. When the head and eyes are equally positioned but oppositely directed, this is described as a zero phase shift. *Note*: VOR phase is not equivalent with VOR gain, which examines the difference between head and eye velocity.

In individuals with healthy oculomotor function, for head velocities below 60°/sec, *gaze stability* can be maintained fairly well using *smooth pursuit* (the ability to move the eyes with smooth, continuous motions in order to follow the movement of a target of interest and maintain the moving image on the fovea).[33] In situations where head velocity is greater than 60°/sec, the vestibular system is primarily responsible for generating eye movement (in the direction opposite the head movement) to maintain *gaze* on the target.[34] The VOR operates at head velocities as great as 350° to 400°/sec.[35]

Push–Pull Mechanism

The brain detects head movement and direction through comparison of inputs between the two vestibular systems. The SCCs each work in coplanar fashion as mentioned earlier; as the head is turned to the right, the right horizontal SCC will have an increased firing rate while the left horizontal SCC has a decreased firing rate. This is called the *push–pull mechanism* (Fig. 21.7). The brain is then responsible for recognizing the difference and interpreting movement. A faulty interpretation will lead to difficulties with gaze stabilization, postural stability, and motion perception.

Inhibitory Cutoff

Recall that during angular head rotations (rotations about an axis) ipsilateral vestibular afferents can be excited up to 400 spikes/sec.[35] A simultaneous hyperpolarization (reduction of the spontaneous firing rate) of the opposite labyrinth also occurs. However, the inhibition of the hair cells in the opposite labyrinth can only reduce the firing rate to zero, at which point the inhibition is cut off

Table 21.1 Innervation Pattern of Excitatory Input From the Semicircular Canals

Primary Afferent	Secondary Neuron[a]	Extraocular Motor Neuron		Muscle
Horizontal (left)	Medial vestibular nucleus	Left oculomotor nucleus[b]	→	Left medial rectus
		Right abducens nucleus	→	Right lateral rectus
Posterior (left)	Medial vestibular nucleus	Right trochlear nucleus	→	Left superior oblique
		Right oculomotor nucleus	→	Right inferior rectus
Anterior/Superior (left)	Lateral vestibular nucleus	Right oculomotor nucleus	→	Left superior rectus
			→	Right inferior oblique

[a]Ascending secondary neurons travel in the medial longitudinal fasciculus.
[b]In the horizontal semicircular canal, secondary neurons also travel in the ascending tract of Dieters.

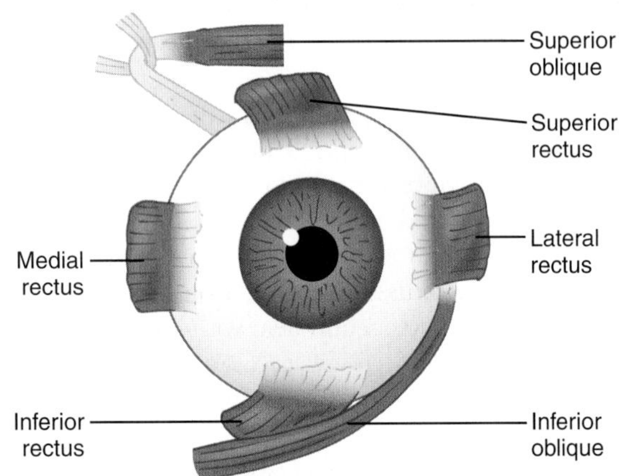

Figure 21.6 Muscle insertions of the left eye. Six extraocular muscles insert into the sclera and can be considered as complementary pairs. The medial and lateral rectus muscles rotate the eyes horizontally, the superior and inferior rectus muscles rotate the eyes vertically, and the superior and inferior oblique muscles rotate the eyes torsionally with some vertical component. By convention, the torsional rotation is noted as it relates to the superior poles of the eyes. The superior oblique muscle rotates the eye downward and toward the nose, whereas the inferior oblique muscle rotates the eye upward and away from the nose. The superior oblique muscle travels through the fibrous trochlea, which attaches to the anteromedial superior wall of the orbit.

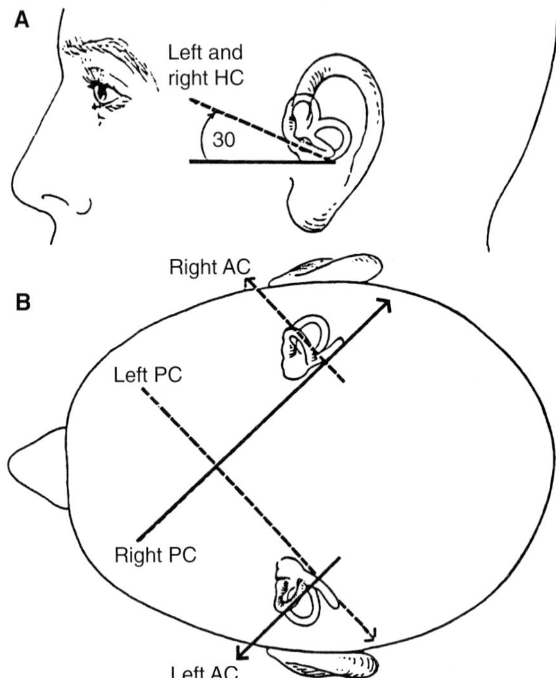

Figure 21.7 (A) Orientation of the horizontal semicircular canals (HC) in situ, with the head neutrally aligned. (B) The semicircular canals (ipsilateral anterior and contralateral posterior, and each horizontal) work in pairs. The arrows indicate the angular pitch direction of individual SCC stimulation. The dashed and continuous lines illustrate each SCC has an equally opposing SCC, sensitive to the opposite angular pitch direction of the head, for example, the left anterior canal (left AC) is paired with the right posterior canal (right PC) and collectively recognized as the left anterior right posterior (LARP) plane. *(Adapted from Baloh and Honrubia,[33, p. 52] with permission.)*

(*inhibitory cutoff*). Thus, for ipsilateral rapid head rotations, the contralateral vestibular afferents cannot detect head rotation when the ipsilateral head velocity is greater than the inhibitory cutoff of those contralateral afferents. The response to head movements that hyperpolarize the hair cells is therefore limited to a velocity range up to 70° to 100°/sec. For example, if the tonic firing rates of the vestibular afferents are 80 spikes/sec, with a rotation to the right of 120°/sec the vestibular afferents increase their firing rate from 80 to 200 spikes/sec (tonic firing rate + rotational velocity). In contrast, the left ear will decrease from 80 to 0 (zero), not to negative 40 (–40), which limits the afferents from the left ear from adequately detecting the head velocity. (It is generally accepted that a 1:1 ratio exists between head velocity and spikes per second neuronal firing rate.) Because the resting discharge rate of these afferents and central vestibular neurons averages 70 to 100 spikes/sec, inhibitory cutoff is more likely to occur than is excitation saturation.

Velocity Storage System

The signal generated by movement of the cupula is brief, lasting only as long as the cupula is deflected (~ 6 sec).[36]

The response is sustained, however, by a circuit of neurons involving the medial vestibular nucleus and the cerebellum, extending the duration of nystagmus beyond 10 seconds in people with normal vestibular function. It is generally believed that the purpose of sustaining vestibular input is to assist the brain in detecting low-frequency head rotation.

■ EXAMINATION

History and Systems Review

Physical therapists examining people who report dizziness and imbalance have the difficult task of sorting through potential causes. Capturing a thorough history and performing a systems review are critical components of the process. Key elements of taking the history are identification of symptoms, as well as their duration and the circumstances under which the symptoms occur.

Identification of Symptoms

Many patients use the imprecise term *dizziness* to describe a vague sensation of light-headedness or a feeling that they have a tendency to fall. The imprecision of the term can entangle clinical management decisions. It is essential to determine what the patient is experiencing when the term *dizziness* is used. Most complaints of being "dizzy" can be categorized as vertigo, light-headedness, dysequilibrium, or oscillopsia (targets in visual field appear to move during head motion). Generally, dizziness is vaguely defined as the sensation of whirling or feeling a tendency to fall. Ideally, patients should be directed away from using the word and to use more precise terms that will help the clinician develop more direct treatment approaches.

Vertigo is defined as an illusion of movement. Many patients use the term *vertigo* incorrectly and thus the clinician must be certain to inform patients of the true definition, as well as identify their unique experience. Patients may describe that they sense their environment is moving or that they see the environment moving (spinning). Vertigo tends to be episodic and to indicate pathology at one or more locations along the vestibular pathways. It is most common during the acute stage of unilateral vestibular hypofunction (UVH) but may also manifest itself via displaced otoconia (benign paroxysmal positional vertigo), or an acute unilateral brain stem lesion affecting the root entry zone of the peripheral vestibular neurons or the vestibular nuclei.

Light-headedness is often defined as a feeling that fainting is about to occur and can be caused by nonvestibular factors such as hypotension, hypoglycemia, or anxiety.[37] Light-headedness is vague and less localizing than vertigo.

Dysequilibrium is defined as the sensation of being off balance. Typically, acute and chronic vestibular lesions will produce dysequilibrium. Often, however, this symptom is associated with nonvestibular problems such as decreased somatosensation or weakness in the lower extremities (LEs) (Table 21.2).

Oscillopsia is the subjective experience of motion of objects in the visual environment that are known to be stationary. Oscillopsia can occur with head movements in patients with vestibular hypofunction since the vestibular system is not generating an adequate compensatory eye velocity during the head motion. Such a deficit in the VOR results in motion of images on the fovea and in a decline in visual acuity. The severity of gaze instability, however, varies across individuals with vestibular hypofunction.[38-41]

Duration and Circumstances of Symptoms

The physical therapist must determine how recently the patient has had an acute attack of vertigo, light-headedness, dysequilibruim, or oscillopsia and whether the symptom is constant or episodic. If the symptom is episodic, the clinician must attempt to determine the average duration of the episodes in seconds, minutes, or hours. For example, vertigo lasting seconds to minutes commonly suggests benign paroxysmal positional vertigo. In contrast, vertigo lasting minutes to hours suggest Ménière's disease (see below, "Diagnoses Involving the Vestibular System"), and vertigo lasting for days implies vestibular neuronitis or migraine-associated dizziness.

The physical therapist must also determine under what circumstances the patient experiences symptoms. It is important to discern whether the patient experiences symptoms with particular movements, positions, or at rest. For example, is the patient sensitive to motion as the passenger in a moving car? Or does the patient experience a vigorous vertigo when the head is moved into certain positions?

Tests and Measures

Visual Analogue Scale

Use of a *visual analogue scale* (VAS) is an effective tool to obtain subjective intensity ratings of vertigo,

Table 21.2 Symptoms and Possible Causes

Symptom	Possible Cause
Vertigo	BPPV, UVH, unilateral central lesion affecting the vestibular nuclei, migraine affecting the central vestibular pathways
Light-headedness	Orthostatic hypotension, hypoglycemia, anxiety, panic disorder
Dysequilibrium	BVH, chronic UVH, lower extremity somatosensation loss, upper brainstem/vestibular cortex lesion, cerebellar and motor pathway lesions

BPPV = benign paroxysmal positional vertigo; BVH = bilateral vestibular hypofunction; UVH = unilateral vestibular hypofunction.

light-headedness, dysequilibrium, and oscillopsia.[42,43] The patient is asked to answer a question (e.g., *How intense are your symptoms?*) and mark on a 10-cm line (on a continuum from "none" to "worst possible intensity") where the symptoms exist at that moment. The clinician then measures the line and obtains a quantified value.

Dizziness Handicap Inventory

The *Dizziness Handicap Inventory* (DHI) is a popular tool used to measure a patient's self-perceived handicap as a result of vestibular disorders (Table 21.3).[44] The DHI has excellent test–retest reliability (r = 0.97) and good internal consistency reliability (r = 0.89). Patients respond to 25 questions, subgrouped into functional, emotional, and physical components. The DHI provides quantification of the patient's perception of dysequilibrium and its impact on daily activities. It is useful to establish subjective improvement. Measures of subjective impairment and physiological improvement are often not correlated;[45,46] therefore, it is likely that factors other than organic recovery of vestibular function are responsible for subjective impairment.

Vestibular Rehabilitaiton Benefit Questionnaire

The *Vestibular Rehabilitation Benefit Questionnaire* (VRBQ) was developed to specify the benefit from vestibular physical therapy and includes questions that address avoidance behavior, which is often absent in similar measures.[47] The VRBQ is a 22-item questionnaire that uses seven unique choices (word descriptors) to answer questions from one of four subscales: Dizziness, Anxiety, Motion-Provoked Dizziness, and Quality of Life. The VRBQ has excellent test–retest reliability (r = 0.92) and is moderately correlated with the DHI (0.59).

Motion Sensitivity Quotient

The *Motion Sensitivity Quotient* (MSQ) was developed to provide a subjective score of an individual's sensitivity to motion.[48] The test involves placing patients into positions incorporating head or entire body motion to determine whether the movement reproduces dizziness (Fig. 21.8). If the patient reports an increased symptom intensity moving into a provoking position, the intensity is assigned a point, graded by the patient between 1 (mild) and 5 (severe). The duration of symptoms is also assigned points from 0 to 3 (0 to 4 seconds = 0; 5 to 10 seconds = 1; 11 to 30 seconds = 2; greater than 30 seconds = 3). The symptom intensity and duration values are then added together for a score. The MSQ is calculated by multiplying the number of positions that provoked symptoms by the score. This number is then divided by 2,048. An MSQ score of 0 indicates no symptoms, whereas a score of 100 means severe dizziness in all positions.

Table 21.3 Sample of the Types of Questions Included in the Dizziness Handicap Inventory, Based on the Three Subcomponents

Physical Domain
Does looking up increase your problem?
Does walking down the aisle of a supermarket increase your problem?
Does performing more ambitious activities like sports, dancing, or household chores (such as sweeping or putting dishes away) increase your problem?
Does bending over increase your problem?
Emotional Domain
Because of your problem, do you feel frustrated?
Because of your problem, are you afraid to leave your home without having someone accompany you?
Has your problem placed stress on your relationships with members of your family or friends?
Because of your problem, are you afraid to stay home alone?
Functional Domain
Because of your problem, do you restrict your travel for business or recreation?
Because of your problem, do you have difficulty getting into or out of bed?
Does your problem significantly restrict your participation in social activities such as going out to dinner, going to the movies, dancing, or going to parties?
Because of your problem, is it difficult for you to walk around the house in the dark?

The patient instructions are as follows: The purpose of these questions is to identify difficulties that you may be experiencing because of your dizziness. Please answer "yes," "no," or "sometimes" to each question. Answer each question as it pertains to your dizziness or balance problem only.

Name: ______________ Age: ______ Gender: ______ Date: ______

Baseline Symptoms	INTENSITY	DURATION	SCORE
1. Sitting-to-supine			
2. Supine-to-left side			
3. Supine-to-right side			
4. Supine-to-sit			
5. Left Hallpike-Dix test			
6. Return from Hallpike-Dix test			
7. Right Hallpike-Dix test			
8. Return from Hallpike-Dix test			
9. Sitting: nose toward left knee			
10. Return to sitting			
11. Sitting: nose toward right knee			
12. Return to sitting			
13. Sitting: head rotation 5×			
14. Sitting: head flexion and extension 5×			
15. Standing: turn right (180°)			
16. Standing: turn left (180°)			
Intensity: rated from 0 to 5 (0 = no symptoms; 5 = severe symptoms) Duration: rated from 0 to 3 (5-10 sec = 1 point, 11-30 sec = 2 points, ≥30 sec = 3 points)			

Motion sensitivity quotient: $\frac{\#\text{Provoking positions} \times \text{score} \times 100}{2048}$ = ________ Total

Note: An MSQ score of zero means no symptoms and 100 means severe dizziness in all positions.

Figure 21.8 Motion sensitivity quotient. *(Adapted from Smith-Wheelock et al,[48, p. 221] with permission.)*

Examination of Eye Movements

Owing to the direct relationship between vestibular receptors in the inner ear and eye movements produced by the VOR, the examination of eye movements is critical for defining and localizing vestibular pathology. The key tests include observation for nystagmus, the Head Impulse Test (examination of the VOR at high acceleration), the Head-Shaking Induced Nystagmus (HSN) test, positional testing, and the Dynamic Visual Acuity (DVA) test.

Observation for Nystagmus

Nystagmus is the primary diagnostic indicator used in identifying most peripheral and central vestibular lesions. An involuntary eye movement, nystagmus due to a *peripheral vestibular lesion* is composed of both slow and fast components. The direction of the nystagmus is named by the direction of the fast component. For individuals with a unilateral vestibular lesion, the slow component is due to relative excitation of one side of the vestibular system. The fast component is generated from the parapontine reticular formation in the brain stem and repositions the eye to the center of the orbit. For example, in left-beating nystagmus, the eyes move slowly to the right (VOR), and the resetting eye movement is to the left (fast component). Therefore, the direction opposite the quick component of the nystagmus localizes the side of the vestibular reduced firing rate (possible hypofunction).

Nystagmus due to a vestibular lesion is most commonly seen after an acute unilateral insult, *spontaneous* (at rest) *nystagmus*. This type of nystagmus occurs in the absence of motion because of the asymmetry between the healthy functioning and reduced/absent functioning vestibular systems. The brain perceives the asymmetry as active stimulation from the more neutrally active (i.e., healthy) ear. Resolution of spontaneous nystagmus in the light typically occurs within 3 to 7 days but may vary, and it can last as long as 2 months.[49,50] Spontaneous nystagmus may always be present in the dark after a unilateral loss of vestibular function. Regardless, resolution of spontaneous nystagmus in the light or dark occurs when symmetry between the resting firing rates of both vestibular systems is reestablished.[51]

Vestibular nystagmus can be suppressed in light and when a person visually fixates on a target.[52] As a result, the observation of nystagmus should be performed under conditions in which the person cannot see. This can be achieved with Frenzel lenses or an infrared camera system. Frenzel lenses look like large goggles with magnifying lenses that enable the clinician to observe for nystagmus while preventing the patient from fixating on a target. An infrared camera uses infrared light to illuminate the eyes while the patient remains in complete darkness.

Head Impulse Test (Examination of the VOR at High Acceleration)

The head impulse test (HIT) is a widely accepted clinical tool used to examine semicircular canal function.[53-57] Cervical range of motion (ROM) should be determined before performing the head impulse test and the physical therapist should explain why the head must be moved quickly. The head impulse test is performed by having the patient first fixate on a near target (e.g., the clinician's nose). Patients are asked to keep their eyes focused on a target while their head is manually rotated in an unpredictable direction using a small-amplitude (5° to 15°), moderate-velocity (approximately 200°/sec), and high-acceleration (3,000° to 4,000°/sec^2) angular impulse (Figs. 21.9 and 21.10). When the VOR is functioning normally, the eyes move in the direction opposite to the head movement and gaze will remain on the target. In a patient with a loss of vestibular function, the VOR will not move the eyes as quickly as the head rotation and the eyes move off the target. The patient will then make a corrective saccade (a rapid eye movement used to reposition the eyes to the target of interest) to reposition the eyes (fovea) on the target. The appearance of corrective saccade indicates vestibular hypofunction as determined by the HIT and occurs because inhibition of vestibular afferents and central vestibular neurons on the intact side (persons with unilateral vestibular hypofunction) are less effective in encoding the amplitude of a head movement than excitation. A patient who has a unilateral peripheral lesion or pathology of the central vestibular neurons will not be able to maintain gaze when the head is rotated quickly toward the side of the lesion. A patient with a bilateral loss of vestibular function will make corrective saccades after a head impulse to either side. The HIT provides a sensitive indication of vestibular hypofunction in patients with complete loss of function in the affected labyrinth that occurs following ablative surgical procedures, such as labyrinthectomy.[53,56-58] The test is less sensitive in detecting hypofunction in patients with incomplete loss of function.[59-62]

Head-Shaking Induced Nystagmus Test

The head-shaking induced nystagmus (HSN) test is a useful aid in the diagnosis of a unilateral peripheral vestibular defect. During this test, vision is occluded. The patient is instructed to close his or her eyes. The clinician flexes the head 30° before oscillating horizontally for 20 cycles at a frequency of two repetitions per second (2 Hz). When the oscillation stops, the patient opens the eyes and the clinician checks for nystagmus. In subjects with normal vestibular function, nystagmus will not be present. An asymmetry between the peripheral vestibular inputs to central vestibular nuclei, however, may result in HSN. Typically, a person with a UVH will manifest a horizontal HSN, with the quick phases of the nystagmus directed toward the healthy ear and the slow phases directed toward the lesioned ear.[63] Not all patients with a UVH will have HSN. Patients with a complete loss of vestibular function bilaterally will not have HSN because neither system is functioning. As a result, there is no asymmetry between the tonic firing rates. The presence of vertical nystagmus after either horizontal or vertical head shaking suggests a central lesion.

Positional Testing

Positional testing is commonly used to identify whether otoconia have been displaced into the SCC, causing a condition referred to as *benign paroxysmal positional vertigo* (BPPV). The addition of the otoconia into the endolymph makes the semicircular canals sensitive to changes in head position. The Dix-Hallpike test is the most common positional test used to examine for BPPV.[64] The patient is moved from a long-sitting position with the head rotated 45° to one side, to a supine position with the head extended 30° beyond horizontal, head still rotated 45° (Fig. 21.11). The maneuver places each of the SCCs in a gravity-dependent position and the physical therapist should observe the eyes for nystagmus. The direction of the nystagmus is unique to the involved SCC. The direction and duration of the resultant nystagmus can help determine whether the patient has BPPV or a central lesion. An alternative form of the Dix-Hallpike test asks the patient to move into a side-lying position (Fig. 21.12). In both versions illustrated, the ear toward the ground is the labyrinth being tested. If horizontal SCC BPPV is suspected, the roll test can be used instead (Fig. 21.13). In this test, the patient is positioned supine with the head flexed 20°. Rapid rotations to the sides are done separately and the clinician observes for nystagmus and vertigo. To prevent neck injury, the patient may perform his or her own head rotation.

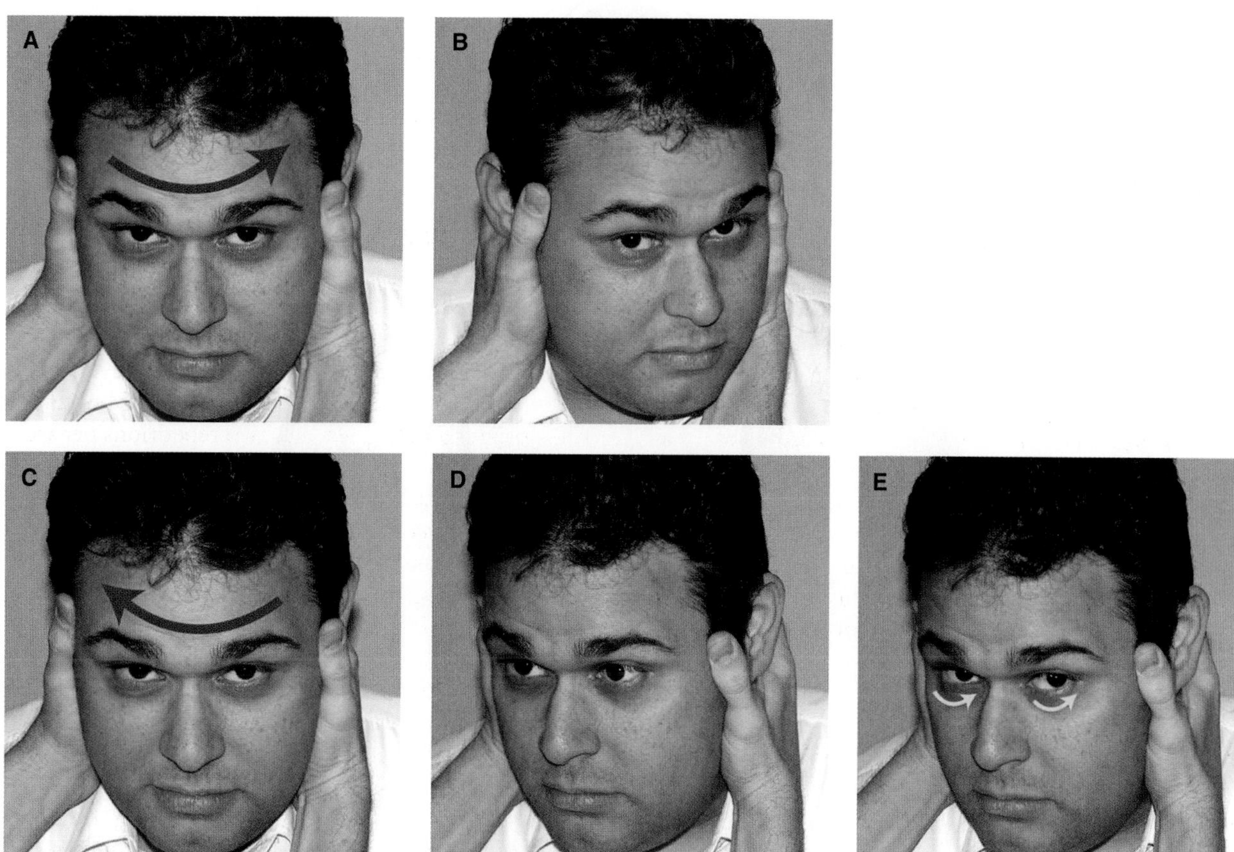

Figure 21.9 Normal horizontal canal head impulse test to the left (A, B), abnormal to the right (C–E). The examiner applies the head impulse test (HIT) to the patient. Large arrow denotes direction the head will be turned. (A) Initial starting position places subject's head into cervical flexion; eyes are focused on the target. (B) On stopping the head turn, the eyes are still on target and no corrective saccade is observed. In photographs A and B, the subject's eyes stay fixed on the examiner's nose throughout the test. (C) Initial starting position places subject's head into cervical flexion; eyes are focused on the target. (D) As the head is turned rapidly to the right, the eyes fall off the target and move with the head. (E) The subject must make a corrective saccade (small arrows) to bring the eyes back to the target of interest. For patients with cervical spine pathology, the clinician may choose to perform the horizontal canal HIT by first positioning the head in 15 degrees of rotation and then returning the head to center. *(From Schubert et al[62, p. 153] with permission of the American Physical Therapy Association.)*

Dynamic Visual Acuity Test

Dynamic visual acuity (DVA) is the measurement of visual acuity during horizontal motion of the head. A "bedside" and computerized form of the test can be used to identify the functional significance of the vestibular hypofunction.[65,66] Head velocities need to be greater than 100°/sec at the time DVA is measured to ensure that the vestibular afferents from the contralateral side are driven into inhibition and the letters (acuity chart) are not identified with a smooth pursuit eye movement. To perform the test, static visual acuity is determined first. The patient is asked to "Read the lowest line you can see" on a wall-mounted acuity chart. Lighthouse ETDRS (Early Treatment Diabetic Retinopathy Study) wall charts are recommended because they provide uniform light luminance for each of the letters. The patient then attempts to read the chart while the clinician horizontally oscillates the patient's head at a frequency of 2 Hz. A metronome can be useful to ensure correct frequency of the oscillation. For patients with loss of vestibular function, the eyes will not be stable in space during head movements. This causes a decrement in DVA compared with visual acuity when the head is still. Using the acuity chart, a three-line or more decrement in visual acuity during head movement is suggestive of vestibular hypofunction.[66] For people with normal vestibular function, head movement results in little or no change of visual acuity compared with the head still (less than one-line difference). Computerized DVA has been found to correctly identify the side of lesion in patients with unilateral hypofunction for self-generated and unpredictable head motion[66,67] and can be used to identify single SCC lesions.[68]

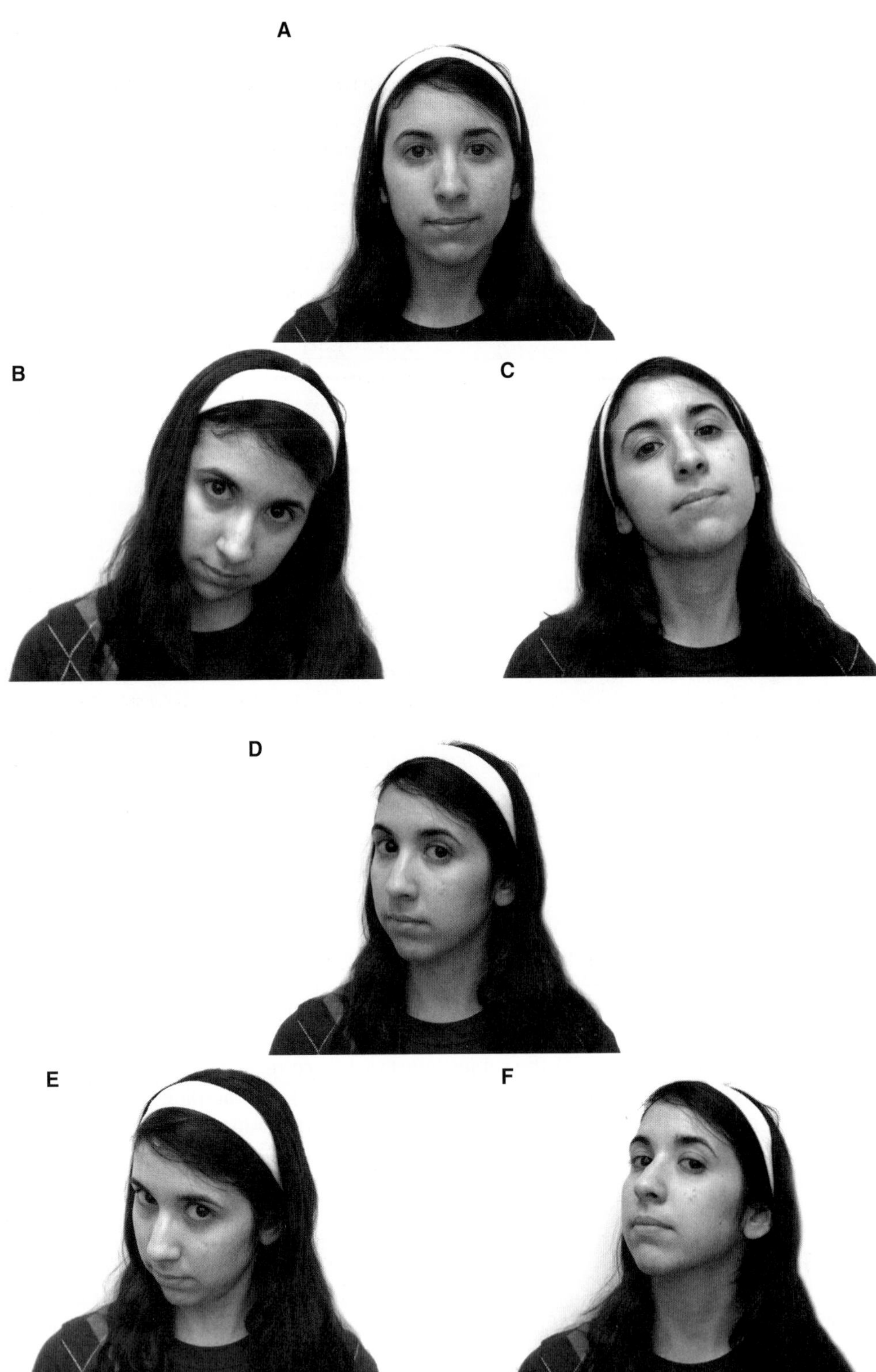

Figure 21.10 Vertical semicircular canal head impulse test (HIT), examiner's hands not shown here. There are two ways to investigate the VOR from each coplanar pair; methods A–C and D–F illustrate the two methods for the left anterior right posterior (LARP) VOR. (A) The head is placed in a neck neutral position. Next the head is rapidly moved pitch down while being rolled to the left, (B) as if the head were moving diagonally. This examines the VOR from the left anterior SCC. From here, the clinician should return to (A) before rapidly moving the head pitch up and rolled to the right (C). This examines the VOR from the right posterior canal. Alternatively, the head is rotated 45° to the right (D). From this static position, the head is rapidly pitched down (E), examining the left anterior SCC. The head should be returned to the start position (D) and then the head rapidly moved pitch up to examine the right posterior SCC (F). In this figure, the HIT is normal for the LARP plane, since the eyes remain gazing straight ahead.

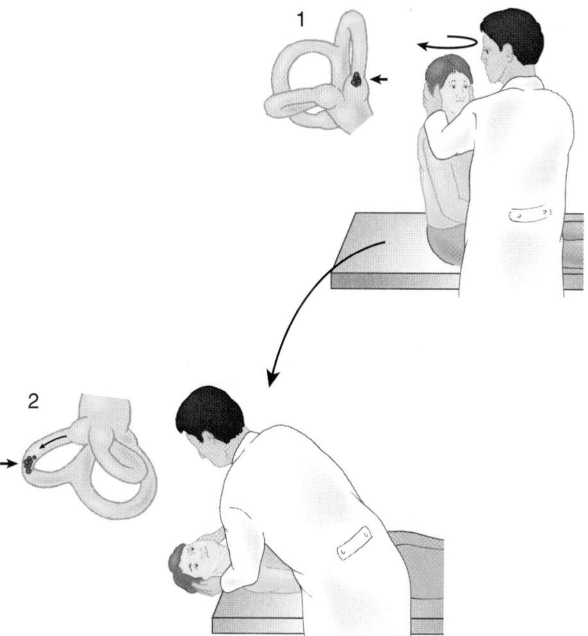

Figure 21.11 The Dix–Hallpike test. (1) The patient sits on the examination table and the clinician turns the head horizontally 45°. (2) As the examiner maintains the 45° rotation, the patient is quickly brought to a supine position with the neck extended 30° beyond the horizontal. The examiner must look for nystagmus and ask the patient if vertigo is being experienced. The patient is then slowly brought back to the starting position, and the other side is tested. The side that reproduces nystagmus and vertigo is the side that has the benign paroxysmal positional vertigo (BPPV). Shown here for testing right posterior or right anterior semicircular canal BPPV.

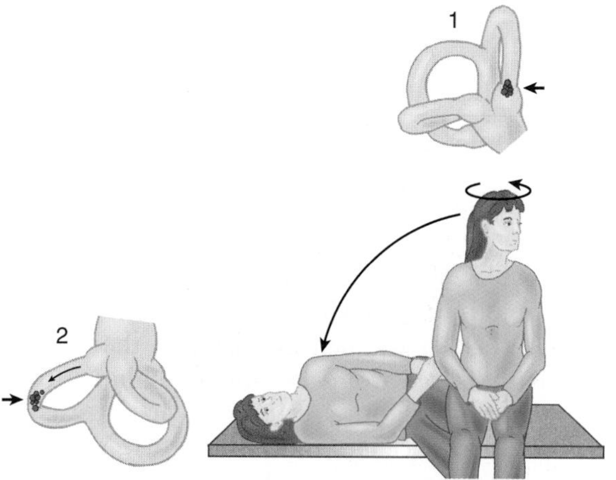

Figure 21.12 The Dix–Hallpike test (side-lying). (1) The patient sits on the edge of the examination table. The clinician turns the head horizontally 45°. (2) As the examiner maintains the 45° rotation, the patient is quickly brought down to the side opposite the head rotation (pictured here as the right side). The examiner checks for nystagmus and vertigo, and then slowly brings the patient to the starting position. The other side is then tested.

Examination of Gait and Balance

Examination of gait and balance problems is important for determination of a patient's functional status. Testing should address both static and dynamic balance (e.g., weight shifting, automatic postural responses, and ambulation). Gait and balance tests *cannot* uniquely identify pathology within the vestibular system. Table 21.4 includes common balance tests and expected results.

Vestibular Function Tests

Semicircular Canal Tests

The more common SCC tests include *electro* or *videonystagmography* (ENG, VNG) testing and *rotational chair tests* and are commonly performed in a clinical vestibular function test laboratory. ENG includes a battery of tests that measure central and vestibular *oculomotor* function. The test also examines for nystagmus in different head positions. The ENG oculomotor tests typically examine saccadic and smooth pursuit including velocity, latency, and gain. The vestibular component includes the *caloric test* and infuses the external auditory canal with separate cold and warm air or water. This stimulus introduces a temperature gradient. In the presence of gravity, this temperature gradient results in the convective flow of endolymph that deflects the cupula and generates nystagmus from the horizontal SCC. This test is particularly useful for determining the side of the deficit, because each labyrinth is stimulated separately. A variation with ice water is useful to determine whether minimal function exists in the vestibular system for patients with severe loss. However, the caloric test provides limited information since only the horizontal SCCs can be stimulated and that stimulation corresponds to a frequency (0.025 Hz) that is much lower than the natural frequencies of head movement (1 to 20 Hz).[69]

The rotational chair test stimulates each horizontal SCC by rotating subjects in the dark. In subjects with normal vestibular function, nystagmus should be generated by the rotation. In the presence of a vestibular disorder, the extent of pathology can be determined by comparing VOR gain and phase from rotations toward one ear with rotations toward the opposite ear. In addition, VOR gain and phase of people with normal vestibular function can be compared with that of people with suspected vestibular hypofunction. The rotational chair test is considered the standard test for bilateral vestibular hypofunction. Rotational chair testing is limited because only the horizontal SCCs are routinely tested to determine extent of pathology.

Otolith Tests

Advances in vestibular diagnostic testing have extended the region of identifiable pathology to include the otolith organs.[70-72] The *vestibular-evoked myogenic potential* (VEMP) test is a laboratory test that has gained broad clinical use and includes two subtypes: *cervical* and *ocular* VEMP. Both types use the threshold and

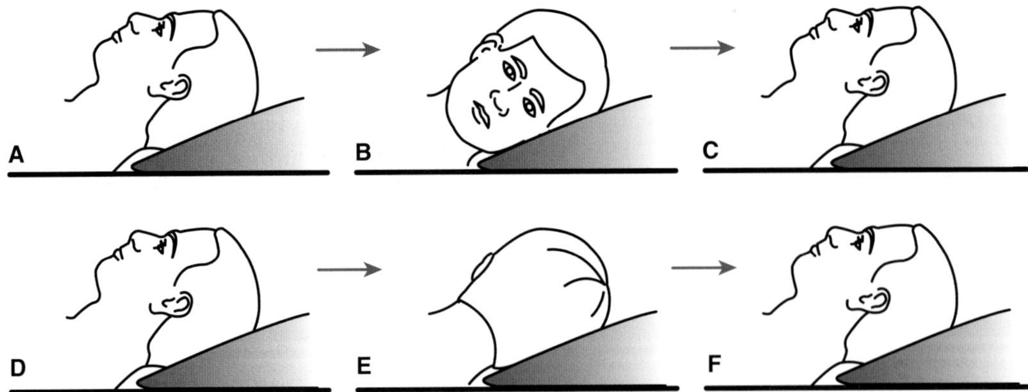

Figure 21.13 Roll test for horizontal semicircular canal BPPV. The patient is positioned in supine. (A) Initially, the patient's head should be placed in 20° cervical flexion. (B) The head is quickly turned 90° to the left side. The clinician then checks for nystagmus and vertigo. (C) The head is then gently returned to the neutral starting position. (D–F) The test is repeated to the other side (head is quickly turned 90° to the right side). The therapist again must check for nystagmus and vertigo. The head is then returned to the neutral starting position.

Table 21.4 Common Balance Tests and Expected Results Related to Specific Diagnosis

Test	BPPV	UVH	BVH	Central Lesion
Romberg	Negative	Acute: positive Chronic: negative	Acute: positive Chronic: negative	Often negative
Tandem Romberg	Negative	Positive, eyes closed	Positive	Positive
Single-legged stance	Negative	May be positive	Acute: positive Chronic: negative	May be unable to perform
Gait	Normal	Acute: wide-based, slow, decreased arm swing and trunk rotation Compensated: normal	Acute: wide-based, slow, decreased arm swing and trunk rotation Compensated: mild gait deviation	May have pronounced ataxia
Turn head while walking	May produce slight unsteadiness	Acute: may not keep balance Compensated: normal	May not keep balance or slows cadence	May not keep balance, increased ataxia

BPPV = benign paroxysmal postural vertigo; BVH = bilateral vestibular hypofunction; UVH = unilateral vestibular hypofunction.

amplitude of a muscle contraction (electromyography [EMG]) to classify pathology. The cervical VEMP test exposes patients to aural stimuli in the form of a series of ipsilateral loud (95-decibel [dB]) clicks. During the sound application, the ipsilateral sternocleidomastoid (SCM) muscle is tested for myogenic potentials. In people with healthy vestibular function, an initial inhibitory potential (occurring at a latency of 13 milliseconds [msec] after the click) is followed by an excitatory potential (occurring at a latency of 21 msec after the click). For patients with vestibular hypofunction, the VEMPs are absent on the side of the lesion. The saccule has been implicated as the site of afferent stimulation during cervical VEMP testing because saccular afferents provide ipsilateral inhibitory disynaptic input to the SCM muscle,[73] are responsive to click noise,[74-76] and are positioned close to the footplate of the stapes (inner most auditory ossicle) and therefore are subject to mechanical stimulation.[71,74]

The ocular VEMP exposes subjects to loud clicks (aural stimuli) or bone vibration applied to the central forehead (Fz), at the hairline. During the stimulus, EMG is measured from the inferior oblique muscle while subjects look upward to bring the muscle belly closer to the surface electrode. The ocular VEMP is a crossed, excitatory otolith-oculomotor response and in patients with UVH will be absent from the contralateral superior oblique.[77] The ocular VEMP is considered a test of the utricle and the superior vestibular nerve based on its absence in patients with abnormal caloric but preserved cervical VEMP.[77]

The *subjective visual vertical* (SVV) and *subjective visual horizontal* (SVH) tests are used to examine otolith function, though they cannot be used to uniquely detect saccular or utricular pathology. During the SVV test, patients are asked to align a dimly lit luminous bar (in an otherwise darkened room) with what they perceive as being vertical. The SVH test asks patients to align a bar with what they perceive as being horizontal. In the absence of vestibular problems, subjects typically align the bar within 1.5° of true horizontal. Patients with UVH generally align the bar more than 2° from true vertical or horizontal with the bar tilted toward the lesioned side.[72,78]

VESTIBULAR SYSTEM DYSFUNCTION

Peripheral Pathology

Mechanical

The most common cause of vertigo, BPPV, is a biomechanical disorder. Symptoms of BPPV include nystagmus and vertigo with change in head position, and occasionally nausea with or without vomiting, and dysequilibrium. In the most common form, latency to onset of the vertigo and nystagmus occurs within 15 seconds once the head is in the provoking position. The duration is usually less than 60 seconds. The vertigo and nystagmus are direct impairments caused by the misplaced otoconia. BPPV is believed to occur via one of two mechanisms: *cupulolithiasis* and *canalithiasis.* Both of the theories involve the otoliths becoming dislodged from the utricle and falling into the SCCs. Schuknecht[79] first theorized that fragments of otoconia break away and adhere to the cupula of one of the SCCs (cupulolithiasis). When the head is moved into certain positions, the weighted cupula is deflected by the pull of gravity. This abnormal signal results in vertigo and nystagmus, which persists as long as the patient is in the provoking position. Cupulolithiasis, therefore, does not explain the brief duration of the vertigo common in BPPV.[80] A second theory was proposed, canalithiasis, in which the otoconia are floating freely in one of the SCCs.[81] When a patient changes head position, the pull of gravity causes the freely floating otoconia to move inside the SCC, resulting in endolymph movement and deflection of the cupula. Figure 21.14 illustrates BPPV occurring from cupulolithiasis or canalithiasis.

Decreased Receptor Input

The most common causes of UVH leading to decreased or eliminated receptor input are viral insults, trauma, and vascular events.[82,83] Patients who sustain a UVH will experience direct impairments of vertigo, spontaneous nystagmus, oscillopsia during head movements, postural instability, and dysequilibrium. Initially, the patient will experience the vertigo and nystagmus impairments due to the asymmetry created when one vestibular system is no longer functioning. This resolves within 3 to 7 days, assuming the patient is exposed to common

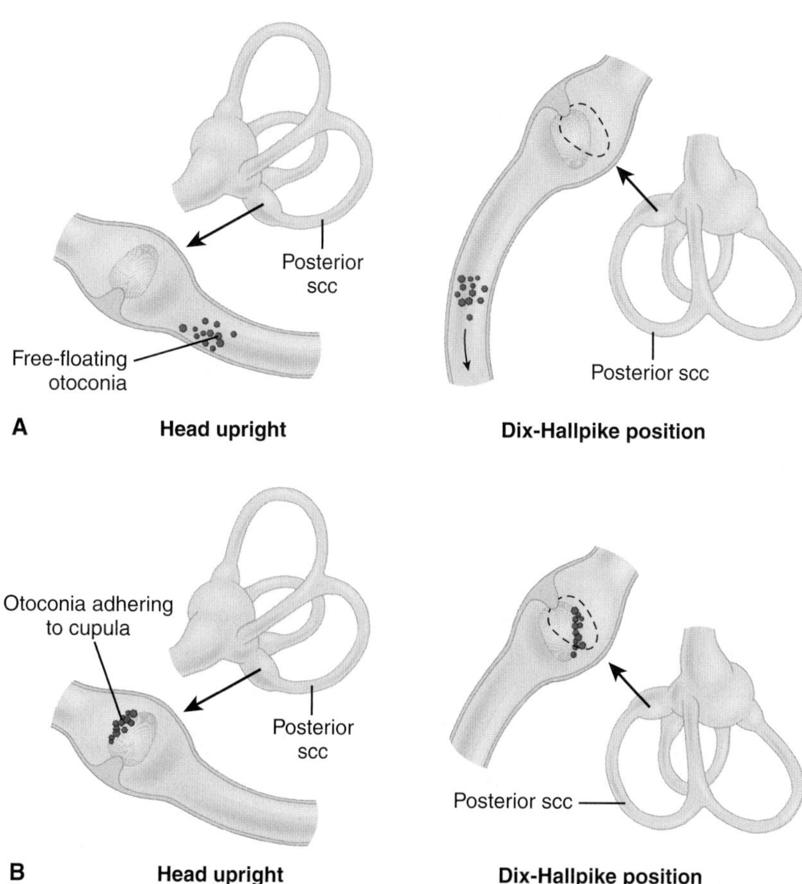

Figure 21.14 Illustrated is benign paroxysmal positional vertigo (BPPV) of the posterior SCC. (A) Canalithiasis indicates free-floating otoconia within the SCC. When the head is moved into a position that places the SCC parallel to the pull of gravity (e.g., Dix-Hallpike position), the free-floating otoconia move to the dependent position within the canal. The movement of the free-floating otoconia results in deflection of the cupula. (B) Cupulolithiasis indicates otoconia adhering to the cupula. When the head is moved to a position placing one of the SCCs parallel to the pull of gravity (e.g., Dix–Hallpike position), the cupula is continually displaced. Illustrated is BPPV of the posterior SCC; also note the cupular deflection. Note that the cupula is drawn with the superior aspect detached from the ampulla.

daylight conditions.[84] Spontaneous nystagmus in room light, beyond this time period, should alert the clinician to a possible central lesion or an unstable peripheral vestibular lesion. The direct impairments of visual blurring, postural instability, and dysequilibrium respond to physical therapy intervention. Because vertigo owing to asymmetry typically resolves within 7 days, persistent symptoms of vertigo beyond 2 weeks should be considered chronic, also necessitating vestibular rehabilitation.

The most common cause of a bilateral vestibular hypofunction (BVH) is ototoxicity. Certain classes of antibiotics such as aminoglycosides (e.g., gentamicin, streptomycin) are readily taken up by the hair cells of the vestibular apparatus and continue to build in this system even after the person has stopped using the antibiotic. Less common causes of BVH include meningitis, autoimmune disorders, head trauma, tumors on each eighth cranial nerve (including bilateral vestibular schwannoma), transient ischemic episodes of vessels supplying the vestibular system, and sequential unilateral vestibular neuronitis.[85-87] The primary complaint is dysequilibrium, though oscillopsia and gait ataxia are common clinical signs with a BVH diagnosis, all direct impairments. Unless the BVH is asymmetrical, the patient will not experience nausea, vertigo, or nystagmus because there is no asymmetry in the tonic firing rate of the vestibular neurons. Halmagyi et al[88] reported that patients with gentamicin ototoxicity have posture and gait abnormalities, decreased visual acuity with head movement, and reduced VOR gains resulting in a positive head impulse test. These impairments are likely permanent though patients with BVH can return to high levels of activity.

Central Nervous System Pathology

Various central nervous system (CNS) injuries can affect the vestibular system.[89] Cerebrovascular insults involving the *anterior-inferior cerebellar artery (AICA), posterior-inferior cerebellar artery (PICA),* and *vertebral artery* may cause vertigo, though other signs associated with these infarcts are present and help clarify the site of pathology. Signs and symptoms between an AICA and PICA infarct can be difficult to distinguish though hearing loss is usually more common with AICA infarcts. Lesions of the vertebral artery may affect the cerebellum only and can mimic a peripheral vestibular hypofunction in its clinical presentation. Most patients with cerebellar lesions, however, will have associated signs such as dysdiadochokinesia or past pointing.[90] Individuals with transient ischemic attacks may present with sudden vertigo that lasts minutes and also include complaint of hearing loss. For more thorough reading discerning types of central vestibular pathology, see Brandt and Dieterich[89] and Delaney.[90]

Signs and symptoms associated with *vertebrobasilar insufficiency* (VBI) typically do not involve the classic signs and symptoms of vestibular pathology. The most common cause of VBI is motor vehicle accident.[91] A recent study identified the most common symptoms of VBI as visual field cuts,[92] whereas an older study reported visual dysfunction, drop attacks (sudden, spontaneous falls), and unsteadiness/incoordination as the three most common symptoms.[93] Another cause of VBI is cervical spondylosis. In these patients, vertigo and decreased blood flow velocity through vertebral arteries after head rotation has been reported.[94]

Patients who have sustained a traumatic brain injury (TBI) due to labyrinthine or skull fractures may complain of vertigo.[95] As much as 78% of patients sustaining a mild head injury had acute complaints of vertigo, and 20% to 37% still experienced the vertigo 6 months to 5 years later.[96,97] Abnormal central processing as well as reduced receptor input may cause the perseveration of the vertigo reported in patients with TBI.

Demyelinating diseases such as multiple sclerosis (MS) can affect cranial nerve VIII where it enters the brain stem. In such a case, signs and symptoms may be identical to a UVH. A magnetic resonance image scan will need to be performed to ensure an accurate diagnosis of MS.

Discerning Peripheral Vestibular Pathology From Central Vestibular Pathology

Observation of nystagmus is a useful tool for assisting in determining a diagnosis of CNS pathology. Nystagmus from a cerebellar lesion may be in a pure vertical direction.[98] The nystagmus may not have a slow component and the eyes therefore oscillate at equal speeds, called *pendular nystagmus.* Pendular nystagmus is often indicative of congenital disorders, such as the absence of central vision (cortical visual processing). Another clue to discern a central versus a peripheral vestibular pathology is the recovery time. Unlike nystagmus following a peripheral vestibular lesion, nystagmus from a central vestibular lesion often never resolves.

Vertigo can be a symptom with central pathology but is rare and if present, is often much less intense than with a peripheral vestibular lesion.[99] Patients with lesions of the vestibular nuclei can present with vertigo, nystagmus, and dysequilibrium similar to the patient with a peripheral vestibular lesion. However, central lesions above the level of the vestibular nuclei will manifest lateropulsion, head tilt, and visual perceptual difficulties, as well as oculomotor signs. *Lateropulsion* refers to the person's tendency to fall to one side.

Brandt et al[100] classify central vestibular syndromes from a clinical consensus of establishing perceptual, oculomotor, and postural signs. They report that the most sensitive signs of unilateral brainstem infarct are tilt of the patient's SVV and ocular torsion. *Ocular torsion* refers to the superior pole of the eyes moving together in a role direction.

Ocular torsion combined with head tilting and skew deviation encompass a triad of signs termed a complete *ocular tilt reaction* (OTR) (Fig. 21.15).[101] Skew deviation of the eyes appears as one eye being superiorly displaced in comparison with the other eye. Kattah et al[102] examined 101 subjects with symptoms that may have been due to a central pathology (acute vertigo, nystagmus, nausea/vomiting, head-motion intolerance, unsteady gait). Each subject underwent neuroimaging and admission (generally 72 hours after symptom onset). Cerebrovascular accidents (CVAs) were diagnosed by magnetic resonance imaging (MRI) or computed tomography (CT). The initial MRI diffusion-weighted imaging was falsely negative in 12% (48 hours after symptom onset) of subjects. However, the presence of normal horizontal head impulse test, direction-changing nystagmus in eccentric gaze, or skew deviation was 100% sensitive and 96% specific for stroke. Furthermore, the presence of skew deviation correctly predicted lateral pontine stroke in two of three cases in which an abnormal horizontal head impulse test erroneously suggested peripheral localization. In conclusion, skew is an important predictor of brainstem involvement and can identify CVA when an abnormal horizontal head impulse test may falsely suggest a peripheral lesion. The study recommended a three-step bedside oculomotor examination (HINTS: Head-Impulse, Nystagmus, Test-of-Skew) as a more sensitive measure for stroke than early MRI.[102]

"Red flags" that should alert the physical therapist to a central vestibular etiology include horizontal or vertical diplopia lasting longer than 2 weeks after the onset of signs or symptoms thought to be due to UVH, persistent pure vertical *positional nystagmus* (anterior canal cupulolithiasis should be ruled out), a spontaneous upbeating nystagmus (rare), and a positive test for skew deviation. The therapist should refer a patient with these manifestations to a neurologist.

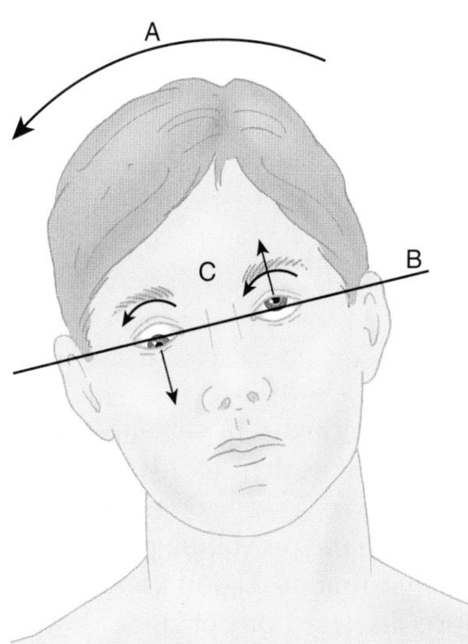

Figure 21.15 The ocular tilt reaction (OTR) consists of a triad of signs: (A) Head tilting to the right, indicated with the large arrow. (B) Skew deviation of the eyes (right eye is down, left eye is up), indicated with the bisecting line and straight arrows. (C) Torsion of the eyes to the right, indicated with the two smaller rounded arrows.

It is not within the scope of this chapter to expand on the differential diagnosis within the CNS, identifying the site of lesion. However, the physical therapist must recognize the difference between central and peripheral vestibular dysfunction because this guides the treatment strategy. The symptoms presented in Table 21.5 can be used to discern central vestibular pathology from peripheral vestibular pathology.

INTERVENTIONS

Benign Paroxysmal Positional Vertigo

The development of specific goals and outcomes for the individual patient with BPPV is based on the following general goals:

- The otoconia will be returned into the vestibule.
- The patient will demonstrate reduced vertigo associated with head motion.
- The patient will demonstrate reduced or absent nystagmus associate with head motion.
- The patient will demonstrate improved balance.
- The patient will demonstrate independence in daily activity (basic activities of daily living [BADL]; instrumental activities of daily living [IADL]) involving head motion.

Because BPPV is the most common peripheral vestibular pathology, physical therapists should be familiar with treating this disorder. The type of nystagmus generated as result of placing the SCCs in gravity-dependent positions indicates which SCC is involved (Table 21.6) and directs the clinician to choose an appropriate treatment approach. Three different treatment approaches have been developed, each based on pathophysiological theories of this disorder. The techniques include the canalith repositioning maneuver, the Liberatory (Semont) maneuver, and Brandt–Daroff exercises.

The *canalith repositioning maneuver* (CRM) is based on the canalithiasis theory of free-floating debris in the SCC.[103] The patient's head is moved into different positions in a sequence that will move the debris out of the involved SCC and into the vestibule (general term for the location of the utricle and saccule) (see Fig. 21.1). Once the debris is in the vestibule, the signs and symptoms should resolve. The positions used in the treatment of posterior and anterior SCC canalithiasis can be the same. Figure 21.16 illustrates the CRM as applied to either the left posterior or left anterior SCC. It is important to instruct the patient that horizontal movement of the head is not contraindicated and should be performed to prevent stiff neck muscles. Patients may wish to limit vertical head motion. CRM has also been adapted for application to the horizontal SCC (Fig. 21.17), although BPPV is less common in either the horizontal or anterior

Table 21.5 Common Symptoms Associated With Central Versus Peripheral Vestibular Pathology

Central Vestibular Pathology	Peripheral Vestibular Pathology
Ataxia often severe.	Ataxia mild.
Abnormal smooth pursuit and abnormal saccadic eye movement tests.	Smooth pursuit and saccades usually normal; positional testing may reproduce nystagmus.
SX usually do not include hearing loss; if so, it is often sudden and permanent.	SX may include hearing loss (insidious—may recover), fullness in ears, tinnitus.
SX might include diplopia, altered conscious, lateropulsion.	SX of acute vertigo usually suppressed by visual fixation.
SX of acute vertigo not usually suppressed by visual fixation.	SX of acute vertigo usually intense (more than central vestibular pathology).
Pendular nystagmus (eyes oscillate at equal speeds).	Nystagmus will incorporate slow and fast phases (jerk nystagmus).
Pure persistent vertical nystagmus persists regardless of positional testing (persistent downbeat nystagmus in Hallpike–Dix test may indicate anterior canal BPPV).	Spontaneous horizontal nystagmus usually resolves within 7 days in a patient with UVH.

BPPV = benign paroxysmal postural vertigo; SX = symptoms; UVH = unilateral vestibular hypofunction.

Table 21.6 Type of Nystagmus Based on SCC Location and Mechanism of BPPV

SCC[a]	Mechanism	Nystagmus[b]	Incidence[c] (%)[12]
Right posterior	Cupulolithiasis Canalithiasis	Persistent UBN and right torsion[d] Transient UBN and right torsion	62
Left posterior	Cupulolithiasis Canalithiasis	Persistent UBN and left torsion Transient UBN and left torsion	
Horizontal[e]	Cupulolithiasis Canalithiasis	Persistent ageotropic[f] Transient geotropic[g]	35
Right superior	Cupulolithiasis Canalithiasis	Persistent DBN and right torsion Persistent DBN and right torsion	3
Left superior	Cupulolithiasis Canalithiasis	Persistent DBN and left torsion Persistent DBN and left torsion	

[a]Testing for BPPV in the SCC assumes the patient is in the appropriate positional test.
[b]Nystagmus is labeled by the direction of the fast component. Up-beat nystagmus (UBN) means the fast component of the nystagmus is beating upward; DBN = down-beat nystagmus.
[c]The incidence of BPPV refers to the affected semicircular canal, not the type of BPPV.
[d]Torsional rotation is noted as it relates to the superior poles of the eyes, from the perspective of the examiner.
[e]When BPPV occurs in the horizontal SCC, nystagmus will be present when the head is positioned to either side.
[f]Ageotropic nystagmus = fast component beats away from the ground.
[g]Geotropic nystagmus = fast component beats toward the ground.

SCC.[104] The original post-CRM instructions asked patients to remain upright for one to two nights (sleep in a recliner chair) and then to avoid sleeping on the involved side for five additional nights. There is no evidence to support sleeping upright after CRM.[105] Recurrence of BPPV varies depending on the study involved.[106,107] There is no evidence that prophylactic CRM prevents recurrence.[108]

The *Liberatory (Semont) maneuver* was first offered as a treatment for posterior SCC BPPV based on the cupulolithiasis theory.[109] It involves rapidly moving the patient through positions designed to dislodge the debris from the cupula (Fig. 21.18). Data suggest it is effective as an alternative treatment for canalithiasis, though it is more difficult for the patient to tolerate.[110,111]

Brandt–Daroff exercises were originally designed to habituate the CNS to the provoking position.[109] Evidence now suggests that Brandt–Daroff exercises are not effective to remove displaced otoconia.[112] They may still be useful to treat motion-induced dizziness that is not caused by BPPV, or perhaps to habituation dizziness sensations once BPPV has been resolved. Figure 21.19 illustrates the exercises. The exercise should be performed for 5 to 10 repetitions, three times a day until the patient has no vertigo for 2 consecutive days. If the patient has severe vertigo or complaints of nausea, decreasing the number

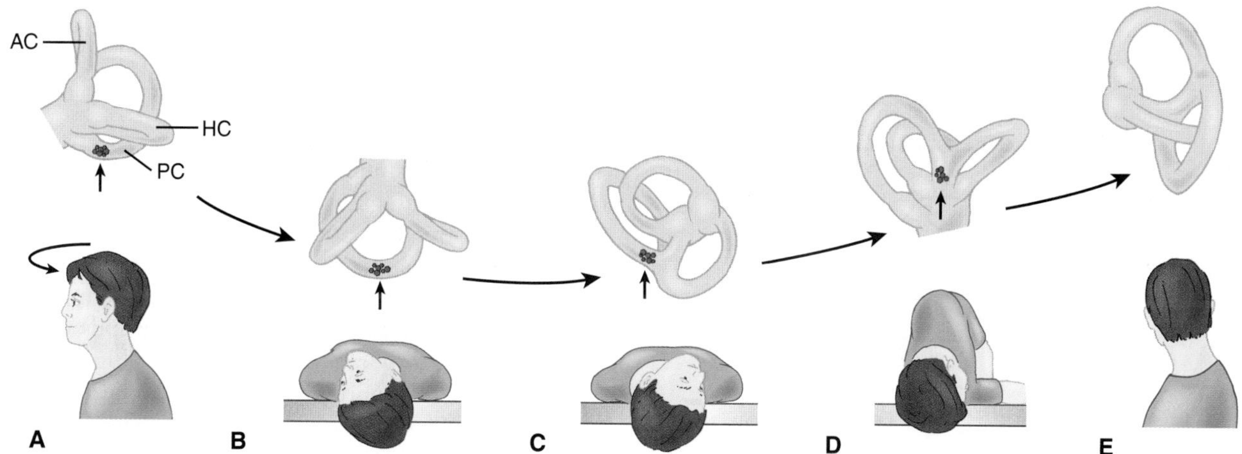

Figure 21.16 Canalith repositioning maneuver (CRM) for posterior or anterior semicircular canal BPPV. (A) The patient's head is first rotated 45° toward the involved side, pictured here at the left. (B) The patient is then moved into the Dix–Hallpike position with the affected left ear toward the ground. (C) Next, the head is rotated 90° to the right. It is important to maintain the 30° neck extension during this step. The head should now be positioned 45° to the right. (D) The patient is rolled onto the right shoulder and (E) slowly brought up to sitting position, head still rotated 45° to the right. The patient may then be fitted with a soft collar. Note the orientation of the labyrinth for each stage. The arrow points to the free-floating debris and shows its movement through the canal into the common crus (D). AC = anterior SCC; PC = posterior SCC; HC = horizontal SCC. Between each step, the clinician should wait 1 to 2 minutes or until the vertigo and nystagmus has stopped to ensure otoconia flow through the canal.

of repetitions to three, performed three times a day, may render the exercises more tolerable. It is important to explain to the patient that the movements must be performed rapidly and that this will probably provoke vertigo. Education should also include informing the patient that it is normal to have some residual symptoms of dysequilibrium and nausea on completing the exercises. The residual symptoms are usually temporary and patients need to continue the exercises.

The goal of performing CRM and liberatory procedures is to replace the otoconia into the vestibule, where the calcium crystals can be reabsorbed or perhaps dissolved. The Brandt–Daroff exercises, although originally designed to habituate the peripheral vestibular response, have also led to a complete remission of symptoms, sometimes after the first exercise session.[113] Physical therapy outcomes should also include teaching the patient how to use the appropriate techniques at home, in the case of recurrence. See Table 21.7 for suggested guidelines for use of the CRM, the Liberatory (Semont) maneuver, and Brandt–Daroff exercises.

Unilateral Vestibular Hypofunction

The development of specific goals and expected outcomes for the individual patient with UVH is based on the following general goals:

- The patient will demonstrate improved stability of gaze during head movement.
- The patient will demonstrate diminished sensitivity to motion.
- The patient will demonstrate improved static and dynamic postural stability.
- The patient will be independent in a home exercise program (HEP) that includes walking.

Patients with UVH should be informed that recovery time after initiating vestibular rehabilitation averages 6 to 8 weeks. To ensure adherence with the vestibular rehabilitation exercises, patients should be encouraged frequently and the mutually agreed on goals and outcomes regularly reinforced.

Gaze Stability Exercises

The purpose of these exercises is to improve the VOR and other systems that are used to assist gaze stability with head motion. There is some evidence suggesting VOR gain does change after performing gaze stability exercises.[114] Vestibular adaptation exercises are designed to expose patients to retinal slip. *Retinal slip* occurs when the image of an object moves off the fovea of the retina, resulting in visual blurring. Retinal slip is necessary as this is the signal used to drive vestibular adaptation within the brain. Because the brain can tolerate small amounts of retinal slip yet see a target clearly, the patient must try to keep the target in focus. Otherwise, head motion that is too rapid will result in excessive retinal slip. The two primary paradigms of vestibular adaptation are ×1 (times 1) and ×2 (times 2) exercises.[42] In the ×1 exercise, the

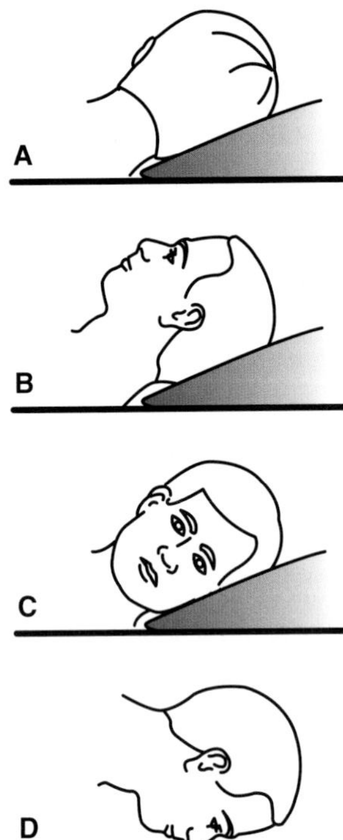

Figure 21.17 Canalith repositioning maneuver (CRM) for right horizontal semicircular canal BPPV. Initially, the patient's head should be placed in 20° cervical flexion. (A) For treating a right-sided horizontal canal BPPV, the patient's head is initially placed 90° to the right. (B) Next, the head is rotated 90° to the left. The therapist should wait in this position for 15 seconds or until the vertigo and nystagmus stops. (C) The head should then be rotated another 90° to the left; again, the therapist must wait for 15 seconds or until the vertigo and nystagmus stops. (D) The patient must then roll into prone position and await the signs or symptoms to stop. The therapist must attempt to keep the head in 20° flexion during the transition from C to D. If the CRT has been successful, nystagmus and vertigo should resolve once the patient is in the prone position. The patient may need assistance to sit up from the prone position.

patient is asked to move the head horizontally (and vertically if appropriate) as quickly as possible while maintaining focus on a stable target. The patient must learn to slow the head movement if the target becomes blurred. A good target to use is a business card, asking the patient to focus on a word or a letter within a word. The starting target distance should be an arm's length away. The ×2 paradigm requires the patient to move the head and target in opposite directions (Fig. 21.20). Both paradigms should be made increasingly more difficult as the patient improves. Examples of increasing difficulty include the use of a distracting background while the patient attempts to focus on the letter or word (checkerboard, venetian blinds), varying the distance from which the patient performs the exercises, moving the head more rapidly, and performing the exercise while standing or walking. The *computerized DVA* test is a useful measure of improved gaze stability for individuals with UVH and TBI.[66,115]

Postural Stability Exercises

The purpose of postural stability exercises is to improve balance by encouraging the development of balance strategies within the patient's limitations, be they somatosensory, visual, or vestibular. The exercises should challenge the patient and be safe enough to perform independently (Table 21.8). Exercises must be updated and progressed to incorporate more challenges (Fig. 21.21). In addition, it is important to incorporate head movement into the exercises because many patients with vestibular loss tend to decrease their head movement.

Habituation Exercises (Motion Sensitivity)

Habituation exercises are warranted when a patient with a UVH has continual complaints of dizziness. *Habituation* is defined as the reduction in response to a repeatedly performed movement. These exercises were the first successful methods used to treat persons with vestibular disorders. Various investigators[48,116] have developed versions of positional tests based on the original exercises and studies by Cawthorne,[16] Cooksey,[17] Norre and DeWeerdt,[117] and Dix.[118,119] As our knowledge of the vestibular system improves, however, we are able to provide more specific exercises than what habituation offers. Clinicians should not use habituation exercises to treat all patients with vestibular disorders.

To determine which habituation exercises to prescribe, the physical therapist must determine the provoking positions first (see Fig. 21.8). When a position elicits a mild to moderate dizziness, the patient remains in the provoking position for 30 seconds or until the symptoms abate, whichever comes first.[48] The patient is provided with an HEP based on the results of the positional test.[48,113] The provoking exercises are performed from three to five times each, two to three times a day. Figure 21.22 provides an example of an HEP using vestibular habituation training. An activity diary can be a useful method to monitor response to training. The exercises are designed to reproduce the dizziness and the patient should be encouraged that the symptoms normally decrease within 2 weeks. If after 2 weeks the symptoms are no better, the habituation exercises should first be changed. If this is not helpful, the patient should be referred to either a physical therapist with special training in vestibular rehabilitation and/or a physician for further evaluation.

Bilateral Vestibular Hypofunction

The development of specific goals and expected outcomes for the individual patient with BVH is based on the following general goals:

- The patient will demonstrate improved stability of gaze during head movement.

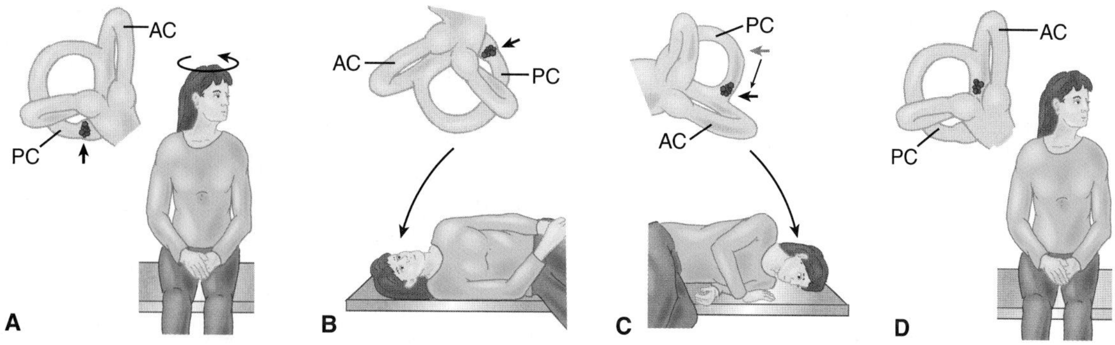

Figure 21.18 Liberatory (Semont) maneuver for right posterior SCC BPPV. The physical therapist should assist the patient through this positioning procedure. Note the otoconia adherent to the cupula in A and B. (A) The head is rotated 45° to the left side. (B) With assistance, the patient is then moved from sitting to right side-lying and stays in this position for 1 minute. (C) The patient is then rapidly moved 180°, from right side-lying to left side-lying. The head should be in the original starting position, left rotated (nose down in final position) in this example. Note that the otoconia have been dislodged from the cupula. After 1 minute in this position, (D) the patient returns to sitting. AC = anterior SCC; PC = posterior SCC.

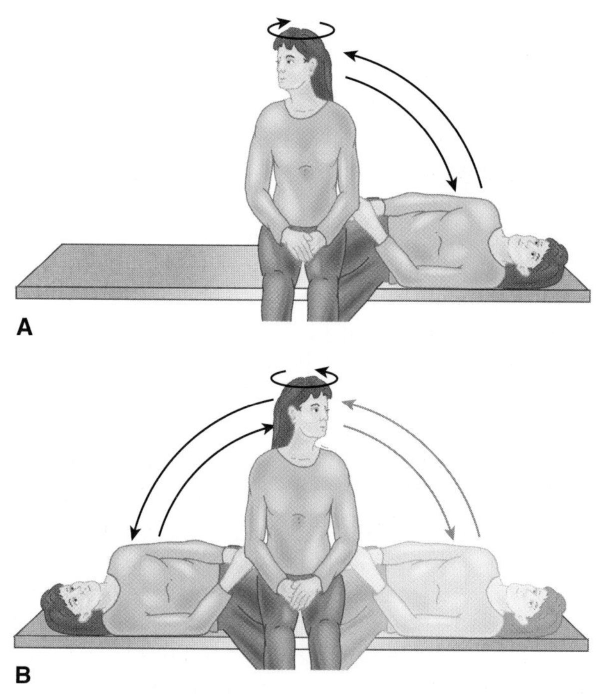

Figure 21.19 Brandt–Daroff exercises for posterior SCC BPPV. (A) The patient starts in a sitting position and turns the head 45° to one side (*right*), then quickly lies down on the opposite shoulder (*left*). The patient should be instructed to remain in this position for 30 seconds or until the vertigo stops. The patient then slowly returns to the starting position (A), maintaining the head rotation (*right*) until sitting upright. (B) Next, the patient turns the head to the opposite direction (*left*) and lies down on the other shoulder (*right*), observing the similar 30-second time guidelines. The exercise should be done 10 to 20 times, three times per day until the patient is without vertigo for 2 consecutive days.

Table 21.7 Benign Paroxysmal Positional Vertigo Treatment Techniques[a]

Treatment Procedure	Diagnosis/Symptoms
CRM	BPPV due to canalithiasis Posterior SCC canalithiasis is the most common
Liberatory maneuver	BPPV due to canalithiasis or cupulolithiasis
Brandt–Daroff exercises	Persistent/residual or mild vertigo (even after CRM) For the patient who may not tolerate CRM

BPPV = benign paroxysmal positional vertigo; CRM = canalith repositioning maneuver; SCC = semicircular canal.

[a]Note: This table presents an overview of the treatment procedures for BPPV. For more in-depth content on the many different CRM for each semicircular canal, please see Gold et al in Supplemental Reading.

- The patient will demonstrate reduced subjective complaints of gaze instability.
- The patient will demonstrate improved static and dynamic balance.
- The patient will be independent in an HEP that includes walking.
- The patient will demonstrate enhanced decision making skills during performance of basic and instrumental activities of daily living.

Treatment of patients with a BVH is designed to address the primary complaints of gaze instability during head motion, dysequilibrium, and gait ataxia. Gaze stability exercises can be similar to the ×1 paradigm described in treatment for UVH. Use of the ×2 paradigm

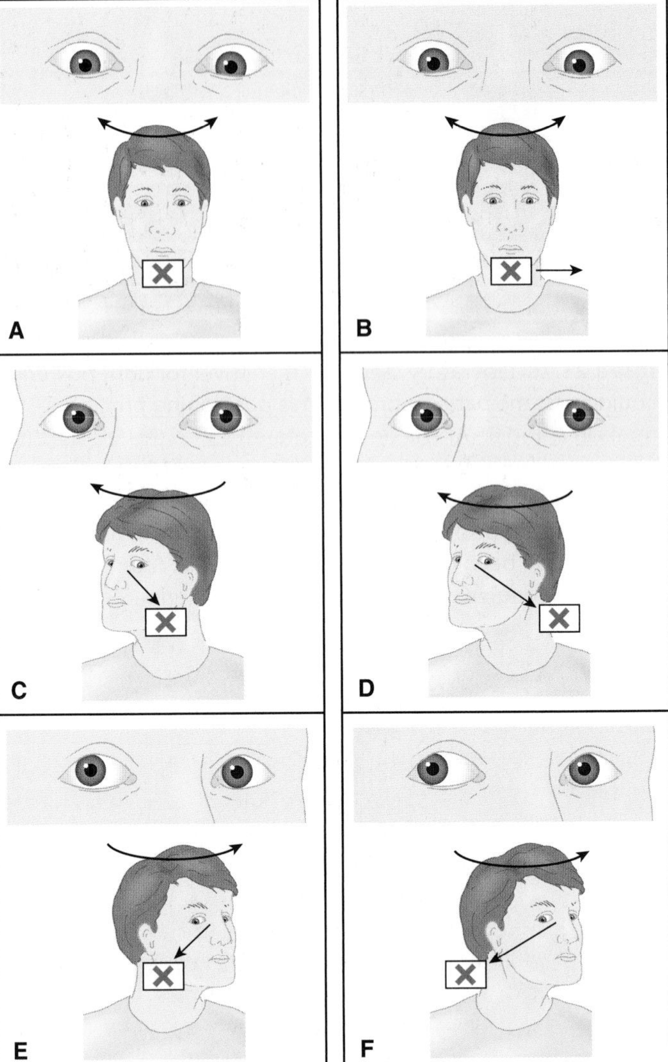

Figure 21.20 Gaze stability exercises. (A, C, E) ×1 paradigm: The patient is instructed to focus the eyes on a near target. While maintaining focus on the target, the patient horizontally rotates the head keeping the target still. (B, D, F) ×2 paradigm: The patient is instructed to focus the eyes on a near target. While the focus is maintained, the patient horizontally rotates the head and the target in *opposite* directions. Both ×1 and ×2 paradigms require vigilance of the patient to ensure clear vision during the motions. Both exercises are typically performed for 1 to 2 minutes, five times a day. It can be repeated using vertical head movements.

Table 21.8 Balance Exercises and Progressions

Begin With	Progress To	Purpose
1. Stand with feet shoulder-width apart, arms across the chest.	Bringing feet closer together. Close eyes. Stand on a sofa cushion or foam.	Enhances the use of vestibular cues for balance by decreasing base of support. Eyes closed increases reliance on vestibular cues for balance.
2. Practice ankle sways: medial-lateral and anterior-posterior.	Doing circle sways. Close eyes.	Teaches the patient to use a correct ankle strategy.
3. Attempt to walk with heel touching toe on firm surface.	Doing the same exercise on carpet.	Enhances the use of vestibular cues for balance by decreasing base of support. Doing the exercise on carpet alters proprioceptive input, increasing difficulty.
4. Practice walking five steps and turning 180° (left and right).	Making smaller turns. Close eyes.	Turning provides a greater challenge to the vestibular system.
5. Walk and move the head side to side, up and down.	Counting backward from 100 by threes.	Uses distracting cognitive or motor demands to challenge balance.

Note: This table presents a limited number of exercises that are effective at improving functional balance. Each of the balance exercises should be performed three times a day for 1–2 minutes each repetition.

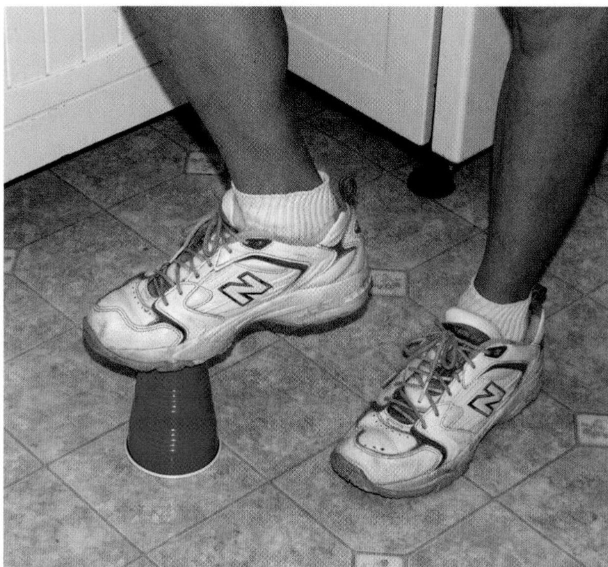

Figure 21.21 Example of a more difficult balance exercise. Instruct the patient to gently place his or her foot on a plastic cup and maintain his or her balance without crushing the cup. Initially, the patient should be advised to use a handhold. The exercise can be progressed to eyes closed, no handhold, or stepping while alternating foot placement on the cup.

is generally not recommended for a patient with a BVH because this exercise may cause excessive retinal slip. (However, many patients have an asymmetrical BVH, in which the ×2 exercise may be useful.) Instead, exercises that incorporate sequenced eye and head movements and the use of imaginary targets may improve gaze stability by enhancing central preprogramming of eye movements (Table 21.9).

Patients with BVH depend on somatosensation and/or vision to maintain postural stability. Balance exercises should enhance the use of these cues. Care must be taken that the exercises are performed safely because people with BVH are likely to fall.[120] It is imperative to begin the patient on a walking program, daily if tolerated. This can be progressed to ambulating on different surfaces (grass, gravel, sand) and in different environments (grocery store, mall). Recovery from a lesion involving both vestibular systems takes much longer than a unilateral lesion. Patients should be informed that as long as 2 years may be necessary to ensure as complete a recovery as possible. For this reason, patient education emphasizing daily activity is a high priority. Daily activity must continue beyond the course of vestibular rehabilitation. Other recommended activities include exercises in a pool and tai chi. A pool provides an environment of buoyancy, allowing the patient to move safely without the risk of falling quickly to the ground. Tai chi incorporates slow, controlled motions used to improve balance, flexibility, and increase strength. In most cases, a person with a BVH will incur an activity limitation or disability. Certain activities may always be limited, such as walking in the dark, night driving, or sports involving quick movements of the head.[121] Older patients may have to use an assistive device such as a cane for safe ambulation at night or on uneven surfaces. Habituation exercises do not work for the patient with a bilateral vestibular loss.[48]

Vestibular adaptation exercises are an excellent starting point for rehabilitation of patients with vestibular

Instructions for the Patient:

Once in the provoking position, wait for 10 seconds to determine if the dizziness will occur. If you experience symptoms of dizziness, remain in the position for an additional 20 seconds (30 seconds total) or until the dizziness abates, whichever comes first. If you do not experience any symptoms you may return to your starting position. Now that you have returned to your starting position, remain here for 10 seconds to monitor your dizziness. If you are dizzy, remain in the return position for an additional 20 seconds (30 seconds total) or until the symptoms abate, whichever comes first. Repeat five times.

Example of Exercises:

1.) Quickly move from sitting upright to bending at the trunk as if to touch your nose to your knee.
2.) Quickly move from sitting at the edge of the bed to lying flat.
3.) In supine, roll onto your left then right side.

Guidelines for the Therapist:

Often, the patient may complain of a certain movement that provokes the symptoms which the examination does not incorporate. This movement can be adapted to be a part of the patient's home exercise program.

	Mon	Tues	Wed	Thur	Fri	Sat	Sun
Duration (0–30 seconds)							
Intensity (0–5)							

Figure 21.22 Example of a home exercise program using habituation therapy. Intensity refers to symptoms (or dizziness) on a five-point scale (0 = none; 5 = most severe).

Table 21.9 Bilateral Vestibular Lesion Exercises to Improve Gaze Stability

Begin With	Progress To
1. In sitting, hold two targets at arm's length from your head (i.e., X and Y). Look with your eyes first to one of the targets (X) and make sure your nose is pointed to the "X" as well. Now look at the "Y" with your eyes only, followed by turning your head horizontally to point your nose to the "Y." Repeat this sequence of alternating between the two targets. Attempt to do this for 60 seconds. The patient should be instructed to always first make an eye rotation followed by a head rotation.	Progress to increasing the distance used to see the target. Use a busy background (checkerboard, venetian blinds). Progress to doing this standing.
2. In sitting perform exercise #1 above using vertical head turns.	Same as above.
3. In sitting, hold one target at arm's length from your head. Close your eyes and turn your head horizontally away from the target, attempting to keep your eyes focused on the target. Open your eyes only after having turned your head.	Progress to doing this standing. Progress to decreasing base of support.

hypofunction (UVH and BVH). Research supports the beneficial effects of vestibular adaptation exercises on gait, posture, and DVA.[42,114,122-130] For a thorough report on the beneficial effects of vestibular rehabilitation, see the systematic review of literature by Hall and colleagues.[131] The Evidence Summary in Table 21.10 presents outcome studies using gaze stability exercises for vestibular hypofunction.

Abnormal Central Vestibular Function

The development of specific goals and expected outcomes for the individual patient with a central vestibular lesion is based on the following general goals:

- The patient will demonstrate enhanced decision making skill regarding fall prevention strategies and necessary safety precautions to allow safe functioning within the home and community.
- The patient will demonstrate enhanced decision making skills regarding use of compensatory strategies to assist in gaze stability.
- The patient will be independent in performance of an HEP that includes walking.

Once an accurate diagnosis of central vestibular pathology is made, expectations for recovery should be described initially to the patient. Generally, the time to recover will be 6 months or more, and may be incomplete.[132] Many of the adaptive mechanisms thought responsible for recovery of the vestibular system are central processes that may have been damaged in the initial central lesion. Physical therapists treating patients with TBI

Table 21.10 Evidence Summary Outcome Studies Using Gaze Stability Exercises to Improve Gait, Balance, and Dynamic Visual Acuity in Subjects With Vestibular Hypofunction

Reference	Subjects	Design/ Intervention	Duration	Results	Comments
Herdman et al, 2003[42]	21 patients with UVH E: $N = 13$; mean age 65.1 ± 16.5 C: $N = 8$; mean age 64.9 ± 16.2. EC: normal DVA, BVH.	RCT; double blind; repeated measures with control E: VOR adaptation exercises and balance retraining C: smooth pursuit and balance exercises; DVA measured weekly for 4 weeks	E and C groups exercised 4–5x/day for 20–30 minutes in addition to 20 minutes of balance exercises	12 of 13 individuals in the E group demonstrated DVA that returned to age-matched normal values; no change in DVA for control group; only the type of exercise contributed to change in DVA	Important first study showing the beneficial effect of VOR adaptation exercises to improve gaze stability in persons with UVH as measured by the DVA

Table 21.10 Evidence Summary Outcome Studies Using Gaze Stability Exercises to Improve Gait, Balance, and Dynamic Visual Acuity in Subjects With Vestibular Hypofunction—cont'd

Reference	Subjects	Design/ Intervention	Duration	Results	Comments
Herdman et al, 2007[128]	13 patients with BVH E: $N = 8$; mean age 63.6 ± 9.4 C: $N = 8$; mean age 63.6 ± 10.8 EC: presence of nystagmus in room light, static visual acuity with the worse than logMAR 0.500, minors/people incapable of understanding the purpose.	RCT; double blind; repeated measures with control E: VOR adaptation exercises and balance retraining C: smooth pursuit and balance exercises; DVA measured weekly for 6 weeks; VAS-O measured	E and C groups exercised 4–5x/day for 20–30 minutes in addition to 20 minutes of balance exercises	7 of 8 individuals in E group only had improvement in DVA; those in C group did not. Change in VAS-O did not correlate with change in DVA	Only type of exercise was correlated with change in DVA, not age, time from onset, initial DVA, or complaints of oscillopsia and dysequilibrium
Hillier and Hollohan, 2007[129]	21 trials in the review	Cochrane review of RCT on vestibular rehabilitation in adults living in the community, diagnosed with symptomatic unilateral peripheral vestibular hypofunction	Included studies addressing the effectiveness of vestibular rehabilitation against control/sham interventions, nonvestibular rehabilitation interventions, by comparing the subjects in each group who had significant resolution of symptoms and/ or improved function	Individual and pooled data showed a statistically significant effect in favor of the vestibular rehabilitation over control or no intervention; there were no reported adverse effects	Moderate to strong evidence that vestibular rehabilitation is a safe, effective management for UVH
Schubert et al, 2008[114]	E: n = 4 UVH and 1 BVH; mean age 54.4 ± 8.9 years; C: n = 5 age matched healthy controls, mean 54 ± 12.8 years EC: patients with dizziness not confirmed as true vestibular hypofunction, BPPV	Age-matched control intervention study E: VOR adaptation and balance exercises 4–5x/day for 20–30 minutes C: No intervention	Mean 5.0 ± 1.4 visits; over 66 ± 24 days Outcome measures: a VOR gain and DVA	DVA improved (mean, 51% ± 25%, range 21%–81%) A VOR gain during the head rotation increased in each patient mean range, 0.7 ± 0.2 to 0.9 ± 0.2 (35%) For control subjects, a VOR	First study to show mechanistic effect of exercises explaining improved DVA Saccade system also modifiable with gaze stability exercises

Continued

Table 21.10 Evidence Summary Outcome Studies Using Gaze Stability Exercises to Improve Gait, Balance, and Dynamic Visual Acuity in Subjects With Vestibular Hypofunction—cont'd

Reference	Subjects	Design/ Intervention	Duration	Results	Comments
				gain during DVA was always near 1 Patients also increased use of compensatory saccades	
Morimoto et al 2011 (122)	Healthy young adults E: *N*=28; mean age 19.1 ± 0.6 C: *N*=13; mean age 19.4 ± 1.2.	Random placement E: VOR adaptation and oculomotor exercises (pursuit and saccades)	E did all exercises in sitting for 5 minutes daily for 3 weeks C did no exercises	Improved DVA, reduced postural sway velocity standing on forceplate actively rotating head at 2Hz	DVA was performed using paper and 2Hz head rotation monitored with metronome. Pursuit and Saccades have been shown to be ineffective at improving gaze stability[48,123,128]

BVH = bilateral vestibular hypofunction; C = control group; DVA = dynamic visual acuity; E = experimental group; EC = exclusion criteria; UVH = unilateral vestibular hypofunction; VAS-O = visual analogue scale oscillopsia.

must be cautious not to be too aggressive, thereby greatly exacerbating the patient's symptoms. Though vestibular rehabilitation offers promise for treating persons with TBI,[132] it may not always be the treatment of choice owing to its irritative nature.

The physical therapy intervention for a central vestibular lesion at the level of the brain stem (vestibular nuclei) likely will be similar to a UVH, with the same expectations for recovery. Vestibular cortical lesions may also recover, similar to the process in which recovery from a CVA might occur.

Because many patients with central vestibular lesions complain of dizziness, a good treatment approach is to start with habituation exercises. However, the exercises should not be too aggressive, thereby aggravating the patient's condition. In addition, gait and balance exercises designed to incorporate somatosensory, visual, and vestibular contributions are also effective with this patient population.

Patient Education

The vestibular system requires movement to recover from most lesions. This basic tenet should be thoroughly discussed when educating patients about returning to daily activity, exercising independently at home, and as a general guideline for their recovery. (Appendix 21.A includes Web-based resources for clinicians, families, and patients with vestibular disorders.) The vestibular system will not improve to its greatest extent without head motion. The challenge for both outpatient and inpatient management is determining the amount of exertion the patient can tolerate and creating an effective vestibular rehabilitation strategy without causing deleterious effects.

DIAGNOSES INVOLVING THE VESTIBULAR SYSTEM

Ménière's Disease

Ménière's disease is confirmed by a documented low-frequency hearing loss and episodic vertigo.[133] The patient may also complain of a sense of fullness in the ear and tinnitus. The symptoms gradually increase in severity and can last several hours per episode. During an episode, vestibular exercises are not recommended. Chronic Ménière's disease, however, can result in a UVH, for which rehabilitation is appropriate. The pathophysiology of Ménière's disease, in part, probably involves an increase in endolymphatic fluid causing distention of the membranous tissues.[134] Medical treatment is therefore directed toward reducing or preventing fluid buildup. Many patients can manage the symptoms well with a controlled diet. Patients with Ménière's disease are often placed on a 2 g/day or less sodium diet. This is the most important dietary restriction to follow. Other substances to be avoided are caffeine and alcohol. Sometimes medical management includes use of a diuretic to control the amount of water in the body. Surgery to either prevent the fluid buildup in the inner ear (endolymphatic shunt placement) or to stop the abnormal vestibular signal (vestibular nerve section, or chemical ablation using transtympanic gentamicin injection) may be indicated if the episodes are frequent enough to disturb daily function. Physical therapy is beneficial in treating the effects of a UVH owing to chronic Ménière's disease, although the therapy will not stop the episodes of vertigo. Gaze and postural stability exercises may be appropriate. Physical therapy is also useful in the treatment of dysequilibrium occurring after a vestibular neurectomy or chemical ablation.

Perilymphatic Fistula

Perilymphatic fistula (PLF) is most commonly caused by a rupture of the oval or round windows, membranes that separate the middle and inner ear. A rupture of these membranes results in leakage of the perilymph into the middle ear. The result is vertigo and hearing loss. Normally, perilymph bathes the SCCs and serves as a protective barrier between the bony and membranous labyrinth. PLF usually is caused from a traumatic event, such as excessive pressure changes as in deep-water diving, blunt head trauma without skull fracture, or extremely loud noise.[135] This diagnosis is much debated and the treatment for PLF is similarly ambiguous. Patients often are treated first with bedrest in hopes of allowing the membrane to heal. Surgical patches of the fistula are also performed. Physical therapy is contraindicated for most patients with PLF; however, it can be beneficial for those who experience continual dysequilibrium or develop a vestibular hypofunction postoperatively. Medical management will likely include strict limitations on activities, warranting good communication between physical therapist and physician.

A form of PLF not debated is *superior semicircular canal dehiscence.* In this condition, the region of the temporal bone normally covering the superior SCC is thin or missing, rendering the membranous SCC susceptible to stimuli that it normally should not (e.g., sound, change of cranial pressure, vibrations).[136] The patient will notice a disturbing syndrome of vestibular and auditory signs that may include eye movements induced by loud noises or effort that increase intracranial pressure (e.g., coughing), sudden or progressive hearing loss, conductive hyperacusis, conductive hearing loss that can mimic otosclerosis (abnormal bone growth near middle ear), autophony (person's own voice sounds amplified), imbalance with noise, vertigo, or motion sensitivity. Some patients even report hearing their eyeballs, "as if scratching sandpaper"!

Vestibular Schwannoma

Vestibular schwannomas (VSs), historically known as *acoustic neuromas,* are benign tumors arising from the Schwann cell of the eighth cranial nerve, often in the internal auditory canal (IAC). The IAC also contains the facial nerve (cranial nerve VII) and the internal auditory artery along with the vestibulocochlear nerve. Symptom presentation is usually related to where the tumor arises. If the tumor arises in the IAC, then tinnitus and hearing loss are often the first symptoms. However, if the growth occurs in the cerebellar-pontine angle, the tumor may become quite large before symptoms of hearing loss are revealed. Thus, although unilateral hearing loss is often the initial sign of VS, the pathogenesis of the associated structures within the space can sometimes result in vestibular (i.e., vertigo, imbalance), facial, or even vascular symptoms. Generally, VS tumors grow slowly. As a result, the extent of impaired vestibular or facial nerve function is often not appreciated until the tumor is removed. This is because the tumor gradually compresses the cranial nerves, and in the case of vestibular function, allows the brain to compensate. However, as the VS enlarges, symptoms of hearing loss, tinnitus, and vestibular hypofunction worsen, resulting in the primary deficits. Treatment usually involves surgical excision of the tumor, though gamma knife radiation is also an option. On tumor removal, most unilateral vestibular afference is lost and the brain now perceives asymmetrical vestibular input. Optimally, physical therapy is initiated during the early postoperative period to help the patient resolve symptoms of dysequilibrium and oscillopsia.[123] Outpatient treatment should be considered similar to the treatment for a UVH.

Vestibular Atelectasis

Atelectasis commonly refers to the collapse of a lung. However, previously described histologic studies suggests that the peripheral vestibular labyrinth, too, might suffer from a collapse of the endolymph-containing portions of the labyrinth.[137] In a retrospective case series, Wenzel et al[138] described four patients with bilateral vestibular hypofunction, sound and/or pressure-evoked nystagmus, and normal hearing thresholds. None of these patients presented with a history suggestive of damage to the end-organ (i.e., exposure to toxins, aminoglycosides, head trauma). The physical therapist may be one of the clinicians treating patients with vestibular atelectasis; therefore, familiarity with the clinical vestibular examination remains critical when treating patients with symptoms of dizziness.

Vestibular Paroxysmia

Vestibular paroxysmia refers to a vascular compression of the eighth cranial nerve. Compression of cranial nerves is thought to cause their demyelination, affecting firing rate and perhaps making the nerve susceptible to aberrant excitation.[139] Patients with putative vestibular paroxysmia typically report frequent, spontaneous, brief attacks of vertigo or dizziness that generally last less than 1 minute. MR imaging has revealed the neurovascular compression of the eighth nerve.[140] Treatment includes surgical decompression or anti-epileptic medication. Physical therapy would not be expected to be helpful.

Motion Sickness

Motion sickness is a normal sensation that in some people becomes debilitating. The predominant explanation for motion sickness is the *sensory conflict theory.*[141] The three sensory inputs of proprioception, vestibular, and visual information do not match stored neural patterns the brain expects to recognize. As a result, persons experience pallor, nausea, emesis, diaphoresis, and motion sensitivity. Physical therapy has been successfully used to reduce motion sensitivity.[142] Other methods reported to combat motion sickness include the use of cognitive-behavioral management, medications, biofeedback, and habituation training.[143-146]

Mal de Debarquement

Mal de debarquement (MdD) literally means feeling sick upon disembarkment, as when exiting from a water or airborne vessel. Patients with MdD report a persistent rhythmic motion (sense of rocking, swaying) while at rest that typically resolves during motion. The diagnosis should be made when the history includes a phantom self-motion perception that occurs after exposure to passive motion (e.g., boat, plane).[147] MdD is not to be confused with the commonly felt "sea legs" that occurs after return to land and resolves within 24 hours. Instead, MdD persists. Treatment options are limited and include mediation[147] and cross-axis habituation techniques.[148] There is limited evidence that physical therapy offers much benefit.[149]

Migraine-Related Dizziness

Migraine-related dizziness can be deceptively similar to a peripheral vestibular lesion, be it BPPV or UVH. Migraine-related symptoms include vertigo, dizziness, imbalance, and motion sickness. A recent study reported 100% of migraineurs had abnormal nystagmus during a migraine episode, if they were positionally tested as part of an oculomotor examination.[150] The prevalence of migraine is significant, affecting 6% of men and 15% to 18% of women between the ages of 25 and 55.[151] The clinical examination will often provide the differential diagnosis between vestibular pathology and migraine. The history is crucial, and important questions to patients in whom migraine is suspected include asking if symptoms worsen when barometric pressure changes, and whether headache or eating certain foods are associated with any of the symptoms. If the therapist suspects migraine, the patient should be referred to a neurologist, preferably one with a special interest in headache. Migraine is often well controlled with medication and diet. Migraine that is not controlled may become worse with exercises such as vestibular rehabilitation, which stimulate the peripheral vestibular end organ and central VOR pathways.[152] Vestibular rehabilitation in patients with migraine can be very helpful, but patients with both vestibular hypofunction and migraine do not respond as well.[153] Strupp et al[154] provide a thorough discussion of this topic.

Multiple Sclerosis

MS can affect cranial nerve VIII where it enters the brain stem and causes identical symptoms to a unilateral vestibular pathology. An MRI scan will ensure an accurate diagnosis of MS.

Multiple System Atrophy

Multiple system atrophy (MSA) is a progressive degenerative disease of the nervous system involving four clinical domains: *cerebellar ataxia, autonomic dysfunction, Parkinson's disease–like symptoms,* and *corticospinal dysfunction.* MSA has been found to be a cause of dizziness and imbalance.[155] The effect of physical therapy for persons with MSA has not been thoroughly investigated, though a case study has been reported.[156]

Cervicogenic Dizziness

Cervicogenic dizziness is a term meant to imply that the cause of symptoms such as dizziness or imbalance arise from pathology affecting the cervical spine or related soft tissue. Unfortunately, *cervical vertigo* is a term still often used, which implies true vertigo as a result of cervical pathology, not documented in humans. The mechanisms of involvement are believed to be from at least two sources. First, the upper cervical spine sends proprioceptive input to the contralateral vestibular nucleus.[157] Soft tissue injury and joint dysfunction might alter the afferent input contributing to spatial orientation. Vestibular rehabilitation appears to be warranted for these individuals.[158] Second, a patient might have VBI (see earlier section titled Central Nervous System Pathology). If VBI is suspected, vascular compromise must first be ruled out as a cause of the patient's symptoms. The VBI test can be performed while the subject is seated, though little evidence exists for the sensitivity and specificity of this test. The patient leans forward and extends the neck. The neck is then rotated 45° to the suspicious side. Persons suspected of having VBI should be referred to a neurologist immediately. Repeated episodes of vertigo without the associated VBI symptoms usually suggest a peripheral vestibular diagnosis.

■ CONTRAINDICATIONS TO VESTIBULAR REHABILITATION

Physical therapy is not appropriate for unstable vestibular disorders such as Ménière's disease (with the exception mentioned above), uncontrolled migraine, PLF, or an unrepaired superior semicircular canal dehiscence. Other contraindications the physical therapist should be alert to include sudden loss of hearing, increased feeling of pressure or fullness to the point of discomfort in one or both ears, and severe ringing in one or both ears. When treating patients who have had a surgical procedure, the clinician must be observant for discharge of fluid from the ears or nose, which may indicate cerebrospinal fluid leak. Patients with acute neck injuries may not be able to tolerate some components of the physical examination, the CRM, or some of the gaze stability exercises.

SUMMARY

High incidence and prevalence rates of vestibular disorders oblige the physical therapist to recognize signs and symptoms associated with inner ear disorders. It is essential to differentiate a peripheral pathology from a central one. Peripheral and central lesions have separate manifestations and may require different intervention strategies. In addition, all vestibular disorders should not be treated similarly. The most common form of vertigo, BPPV, is a biomechanical problem readily treated often with a single maneuver. This is in stark contrast to a patient with a BVH, which requires a greater rehabilitation effort. Evidence supports the use of vestibular adaptation exercises for patients with vestibular hypofunction.

Research in vestibular rehabilitation is ongoing and remains imperative to answer important questions related to dosing, recruitment of compensatory strategies to assist gaze stability, recurrence prevention for BPPV, and more. Exciting future treatments may involve instrumentation to improve the VOR, virtual reality, vibrotactors to alert patients of abnormal posture, and the inclusion of computer gaming platforms. Currently, humans are being implanted with a vestibular prosthesis as part of an early efficacy and safety trial. Within the next 5 years, we will have good evidence realizing the utility of such prosthetics to improve quality of life for those suffering from BVH. Regardless of technological advances, rehabilitation will still be important for these patients.

The *Vestibular Disorders Association* (VEDA) has a list of physical therapists in each state, interested in treating patients with vestibular disorders. VEDA can be contacted via phone (800-837-8428; 24-hour voice mail), fax (503-229-8064), or through the "contact us" link on their website (www.vestibular.org). The supplemental reading list contains other excellent literature for the reader interested in pursuing a greater depth of knowledge in vestibular rehabilitation.

Questions for Review

1. Why is it important to perform the head impulse test using a rapid velocity?
2. What is the name of the linear accelerometers within the vestibular labyrinth?
3. Why does the patient with an acute unilateral vestibular lesion experience spontaneous nystagmus?
4. How will cupulolithiasis present differently than canalithiasis of the posterior semicircular canal?
5. What are the key elements in taking a history for a patient with a suspected vestibular disorder?
6. Explain inhibitory cutoff.
7. Differentiate the ×1 exercise paradigm from the ×2 exercise paradigm.
8. In a patient with vestibular nystagmus, which part of the eye movement (slow or fast) is from the vestibular system? Why?
9. Describe how the Dix–Hallpike test would elicit nystagmus for posterior SCC BPPV.
10. Differentiate between adaptation and habituation training for patients with vestibular dysfunction.

CASE STUDIES

CASE STUDY 1

You are performing an initial examination of a patient with new onset of complaints of imbalance and dizziness. In a sitting position, at rest, the patient is observed to have a purely torsional and vertical nystagmus. You also notice that the patient's head is tilting to the left. The nystagmus is not altered with any change in head position, and the head-shaking induced nystagmus test (HSN) is negative.

GUIDING QUESTIONS

1. Do you suspect a central or peripheral pathology as a cause of the imbalance and dizziness?
2. Is physical therapy appropriate at this time?

CASE STUDY 2

On your patient's return to sitting up after you have performed the canalith-repositioning maneuver (CRM) for a left posterior canalithiasis, you notice left beating nystagmus that stops after 15 seconds. The patient is complaining of vertigo.

GUIDING QUESTIONS

1. Where do you suspect the otoconia is now located?
2. What positional test might you use to confirm where the otoconia are located?
3. How will you treat for benign paroxysmal positional vertigo (BPPV) the second time?
4. Following the second treatment for BPPV, the patient complains of dizziness and neck pain. The vertigo and nystagmus are gone. Can you prescribe any other forms of exercise for the remaining dizziness? What about the neck pain?

CASE STUDY 3

A patient with a unilateral vestibular hypofunction (UVH) complains of feeling worse after 7 days of starting a vestibular rehabilitation program. The patient has had no falls. The complaints consist of increased dizziness with head motion, nausea, and fatigue.

GUIDING QUESTIONS

1. Is your rehabilitation program making the patient worse?
2. How can you modify the program?
3. What information will you tell your patient with a UVH regarding time to recover? What will you tell patients with BPPV, BVH, or central nervous system pathology regarding times to recover?

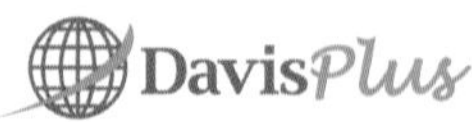

For additional resources, including answers to the questions for review and case study guiding questions, please visit **http://davisplus.fadavis.com.**

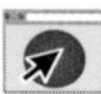

The reader is referred to video **Case Study 13: Patient With Vestibular Disorder** for additional review and study. The full written case study, including tables, figures, charts, and three video segments (examination, intervention, and outcome), appears online at Davis*Plus*. The case study poses questions for the reader's consideration with suggested answers to the case study questions, also posted online at Davis*Plus*.

References

1. Kroenke, K, and Mangelsdorff, AD: Common symptoms in ambulatory care: Incidence, evaluation, therapy, and outcome. Am J Med 86(3):262, 1989.
2. Yardley, L, et al: Prevalence and presentation of dizziness in a general practice community sample of working age people. Br J Gen Pract 48(429):1131, 1998.
3. Sloane, PD: Dizziness in primary care. Results from the National Ambulatory Medical Care Survey. J Fam Pract 29(1):33, 1989.
4. Tinetti, ME, et al: Dizziness among older adults: A possible geriatric syndrome. Ann Intern Med 132(5):337, 2000.
5. Colledge, NR, et al: The prevalence and characteristics of dizziness in an elderly community. Age Ageing 23(2):117, 1994.
6. Sloane, PD, et al: Dizziness in a community elderly population. J Am Geriatr Soc 37:101, 1989.
7. Sloane, PD, et al: Dizziness: State of the science. Ann Intern Med 134:823, 2001.
8. Kroenke, K, et al: How common are various causes of dizziness? A critical review. South Med J 93:160, 2000.
9. Newman-Toker, DE, et al: Spectrum of dizziness visits to US emergency departments: Cross-sectional analysis from a nationally representative sample. Mayo Clin Proc 83(7):765, 2008.
10. Agrawal, Y, et al: Disorders of balance and vestibular function in US adults: Data from the National Health and Nutrition Examination Survey, 2001–2004. Arch Intern Med 169(10), 2009.
11. Gopinath, B, et al: Dizziness and vertigo in an older population: The Blue Mountains prospective cross-sectional study. Clin Otolaryngol. 34(6):552, 2009.
12. Hsiao, CJ, et al: National Ambulatory Medical Care Survey: 2007 Summary Number 27, November 3, 2010. National Health Statistics Reports 2010. Retrieved March 13, 2017, from www.cdc.gov/nchs/data/nhsr/nhsr027.pdf.
13. Grimby, A, and Rosenhall, U: Health related quality of life and dizziness in old age. Gerontology 41:286, 1995.
14. National Institute on Deafness and Other Communication Disorders (NIDCD): Strategic Plan 2012–2014. National Institutes of Health, Bethesda, MD. Retrieved March 13, 2017, from https://www.nidcd.nih.gov/about/strategic-plan/2012-2016.
15. Kroenke, K, et al: Causes of persistent dizziness: A prospective study of 100 patients in ambulatory care. Ann Intern Med 117(11):898, 1992.
16. Cawthorne, T: The physiological basis for head exercises. J Charter Soc Physiother 30:106, 1944.

17. Cooksey, FS: Rehabilitation in vestibular injuries. Proc R Soc Med 39:273, 1946.
18. Della Santina, CC, et al: Orientations of human vestibular labyrinth semicircular canals. In Proceedings of the 2004 Midwinter Meeting of the Association for Research in Otolaryngology, Daytona Beach, FL (February 22–26, 2004). Association for Research in Otolaryngology, Mt Royal, NJ, 2004.
19. Cremer, PD, et al: Semicircular canal plane head impulses detect absent function of individual semicircular canals. Brain 121:699, 1998.
20. Smith, CA, et al: The electrolytes of the labyrinthine fluids. Laryngoscope 64:141, 1954.
21. Troiani, D, et al: Relations of single semicircular canals to the pontine reticular formation. Arch Ital Biol 114(4):337, 1976.
22. Buttner, U, and Henn, V: Thalamic unit activity in the alert monkey during natural vestibular stimulation. Brain Res 103(1): 127, 1976.
23. Brodal, A, and Brodal, P: Observations on the secondary vestibulocerebellar projections in the macaque monkey. Exp Brain Res 58:62, 1985.
24. Buttner, U, and Buettner, UW: Parietal cortex (2v) neuronal activity in the alert monkey during natural vestibular and optokinetic stimulation. Brain Res 153:392, 1978.
25. Grusser, OJ, et al: Localization and responses of neurones in the parieto-insular vestibular cortex of awake monkeys (Macaca fascicularis). J Physiol 430:537, 1990.
26. Their, P, and Erickson, RG: Vestibular input to visual-tracking neurons in area MST of awake rhesus monkeys. Ann N Y Acad Sci 656:960, 1992.
27. Brandt, T, et al: Visual-vestibular and visuovisual cortical interaction: New insights from fMRI and PET. Ann N Y Acad Sci 956:230, 2002.
28. Dieterich, M, et al: fMRI signal increases and decreases in cortical areas during small-field optokinetic stimulation and central fixation. Exp Brain Res 148:117, 2003.
29. Brandt, T, and Dieterich, M: Vestibular syndromes in the roll plane: Topographic diagnosis from brainstem to cortex. Ann Neurol 36:337, 1994.
30. Buckey JC, et al. Orthostatic intolerance after spaceflight. J Appl Physiol (1985) 81(1):7, 1996.
31. Goldberg, JM, and Fernandez, C: Physiology of peripheral neurons innervating semicircular canals of the squirrel monkey. I: Resting discharge and response to constant angular accelerations. J Neurophysiol 34:635, 1971.
32. Lysakowski, AM, et al: Physiological identification of morphologically distinct afferent classes innervating the cristae ampullares of the squirrel monkey. J Neurophysiol 73:1270, 1995.
33. Baloh, RW, and Honrubia, V: Clinical Neurophysiology of the Vestibular System. FA Davis, Philadelphia, 1990.
34. Meyer, CH, et al: The upper limit of human smooth pursuit velocity. Vision Res 25:561, 1985.
35. Fernandez, C, and Goldberg, JM: Physiology of peripheral neurons innervating semicircular canals of the squirrel monkey. II: Response to sinusoidal stimulation and dynamics of peripheral vestibular system. J Neurophysiol 34:661, 1971.
36. Dai, M, et al: Model-based study of the human cupular time constant. J Vestib Res 9(4):293, 1999.
37. Baloh, RW: Dizziness: Neurological emergencies. Neurol Clin 16:305, 1998.
38. Gillespie, MB, and Minor, LB: Prognosis in bilateral vestibular hypofunction. Laryngoscope 109:35, 1999.
39. Telian, SA, et al: Bilateral vestibular paresis: Diagnosis and treatment. Otolaryngol Head Neck Surg 104:67, 1991.
40. Grunfeld, EA, et al: Adaptation to oscillopsia: A psychophysical and questionnaire investigation. Brain 123(pt 2):277, 2000.
41. Bhansali, SA, et al: Oscillopsia in patients with loss of vestibular function. Otolaryngol Head Neck Surg 109:120, 1993.
42. Herdman, SJ, et al: Recovery of dynamic visual acuity in unilateral vestibular hypofunction. Arch Otolaryngol Head Neck Surg 129(8):819, 2003.
43. Dixon, JS, and Bird, HA: Reproducibility along a 10 cm vertical visual analog scale. Ann Rheum Dis 40:87, 1981.
44. Jacobson, GP, and Newman, CW: The development of the Dizziness Handicap Inventory. Arch Otolaryngol Head Neck Surg 116:424, 1990.
45. Robertson, D, and Ireland, D: Dizziness Handicap Inventory correlates of computerized dynamic posturography. J Otolaryngol 24:118, 1995.
46. Jacobson, GP, and McCaslin, DL: Agreement between functional and electrophysiologic measures in patients with unilateral peripheral vestibular system impairment. J Am Acad Audiol 14(5):231, 2003.
47. Morris, A, Lutman, ME, and Luxon, L: Measuring outcome from vestibular rehabilitation, part II: Refinement and validation of a new self-report measure. Int J Audiol 48(1):24, 2008.
48. Smith-Wheelock, M, et al: Physical therapy program for vestibular rehabilitation. Am J Otol May 12(3):218, 1991.
49. Fetter, M, and Dichgans, J: Adaptive mechanisms of VOR compensation after unilateral peripheral vestibular lesions in humans. J Vestib Res 1:9, 1990.
50. Cass, SP, et al: Patterns of vestibular function following vestibular nerve section. Laryngoscope 102:388, 1992.
51. Maioli, C, et al: Short- and long-term modifications of vestibulo-ocular response dynamics following unilateral vestibular nerve lesions in the cat. Exp Brain Res 50:259, 1983.
52. Watabe, H, Hashiba, M, and Baba, S: Voluntary suppression of caloric nystagmus under fixation of imaginary or after-image target. Acta Otolaryngol Suppl 525:155, 1996.
53. Halmagyi, GM, and Curthoys, IS: A clinical sign of canal paresis. Arch Neurol 45:737, 1998.
54. Halmagyi, GM, et al: The human horizontal vestibulo-ocular reflex in response to high-acceleration stimulation before and after unilateral vestibular neurectomy. Exp Brain Res 81:479, 1990.
55. Minor, LB, et al: Symptoms and signs in superior canal dehiscence syndrome. Ann N Y Acad Sci 942:259, 2001.
56. Aw, ST, et al: Unilateral vestibular deafferentation causes permanent impairment of the human vertical vestibulo-ocular reflex in the pitch plane. Exp Brain Res 102:121, 1994.
57. Cremer, PD, et al: Semicircular canal plane head impulses detect absent function of individual semicircular canals. Brain 121:699, 1998.
58. Foster, CA, et al: Functional loss of the horizontal doll's eye reflex following unilateral vestibular lesions. Laryngoscope 104:473, 1994.
59. Harvey, SA, and Wood, DJ: The oculocephalic response in the evaluation of the dizzy patient. Laryngoscope 106:6, 1996.
60. Harvey, SA, et al: Relationship of the head impulse test and head-shake nystagmus in reference to caloric testing. Am J Otolaryngol 18:207, 1997.
61. Beynon, GJ, et al: A clinical evaluation of head impulse testing. Clin Otolaryngol 23:117, 1998.
62. Schubert, MC, et al: Optimizing the sensitivity of the head thrust test for identifying vestibular hypofunction. Phys Ther 84:151, 2004.
63. Hain, TC, et al: Head-shaking nystagmus in patients with unilateral peripheral vestibular lesions. Am J Otolaryngol 8:36, 1987.
64. Dix, R, and Hallpike, CS: The pathology, symptomatology and diagnosis of certain common disorders of the vestibular system. Ann Otol Rhinol Laryngol 6:987, 1952.
65. Longridge, NS, and Mallinson, AI: The dynamic illegible E (DIE) test: A simple technique for assessing the ability of the vestibulo-ocular reflex to overcome vestibular pathology. J Otolaryngol 16:97, 1987.
66. Herdman, SJ, et al: Computerized dynamic visual acuity test in the assessment of vestibular deficits. Am J Otolaryngol 19:790, 1998.
67. Tian, JR, et al: Dynamic visual acuity during passive and self-generated transient head rotation in normal and unilaterally vestibulopathic humans. Exp Brain Res 142(4):486, 2002.
68. Schubert, MC, Migliaccio, AA, and Della Santina, CC: Dynamic visual acuity during passive head thrusts in canal planes. J Assoc Res Otolaryngol 7(4):329, 2006.
69. Grossman, GE, et al: Frequency and velocity of rotational head perturbations during locomotion. Exp Brain Res 70:470, 1988.
70. Colebatch, JG, and Halmagyi, GM: Vestibular evoked potentials in human neck muscles before and after unilateral vestibular deafferentation. Neurology 42:1635, 1992.
71. Halmagyi, GM, et al: Tapping the head activates the vestibular system: A new use for the clinical reflex hammer. Neurology 45:1927, 1995.

72. Curthoys, IS, et al: Human ocular torsional position before and after unilateral vestibular neurectomy. Exp Brain Res 85:218, 1991.
73. Kushiro, K, et al: Saccular and utricular inputs to sternocleidomastoid motoneurons of decerebrate cats. Exp Brain Res 126:410, 1999.
74. Young, ED, et al: Responses of squirrel monkey vestibular neurons to audio-frequency sound and head vibration. Acta Otolaryngol 84:352, 1977.
75. Murofushi, T, et al: Responses of guinea pig primary vestibular neurons to clicks. Exp Brain Res 103:174, 1995.
76. Murofushi, T, et al: Response of guinea pig vestibular nucleus neurons to clicks. Exp Brain Res 111:149, 1996.
77. Iwasaki, S, et al: The role of the superior vestibular nerve in generating ocular vestibular-evoked myogenic potentials to bone conducted vibration at Fz. Clin Neurophysiol 120(3):588, 2009.
78. Tabak, S, et al: Deviation of the subjective vertical in long-standing unilateral vestibular loss. Acta Otolaryngol 117:1, 1997.
79. Schuknecht, HF: Cupulolithiasis. Arch Otolaryngol 90:765, 1969.
80. Furuya, M, et al: Experimental study of speed-dependent positional nystagmus in benign paroxysmal positional vertigo. Acta Otolaryngol 123(6):709, 2003.
81. Hall, SF, et al: The mechanics of benign paroxysmal vertigo. J Otolaryngol 8(2):151, 1979.
82. Cooper, CW: Vestibular neuronitis: A review of a common cause of vertigo in general practice. Br J Gen Pract 43:164, 1993.
83. Jayarajan, V, and Rajenderkumar, D: A survey of dizziness management in general practice. J Laryngol Otol 117(8):599, 2003.
84. Fetter, M, and Dichgans, J: Adaptive mechanisms of VOR compensation after unilateral peripheral vestibular lesions in humans. J Vestib Res 1:9, 1990.
85. Baloh, RW: Vertebrobasilar insufficiency and stroke. Otolaryngol Head Neck Surg 112:114, 1995.
86. Schuknecht, HF, and Witt, RL: Acute bilateral sequential vestibular neuritis. Am J Otolaryngol 6:255, 1985.
87. Barber, HO, and Dionne, J: Vestibular findings in vertebro-basilar ischemia. Ann Otol Rhinol Laryngol 80:805, 1971.
88. Halmagyi, GM, et al: Gentamicin vestibulotoxicity. Otolaryngol Head Neck Surg 111:571, 1994.
89. Brandt, T, and Dieterich, M: Vestibular syndromes in the roll plane: Topographic diagnosis from brainstem to cortex. Ann Neurol 36:337, 1994.
90. Delaney, KA: Bedside diagnosis of vertigo: Value of the history and neurological examination. Acad Emerg Med 10(12):1388, 2003.
91. Beaudry, M, and Spence, JD: Motor vehicle accidents: The most common cause of traumatic vertebrobasilar ischemia. Can J Neurol Sci 30(4):320, 2003.
92. Purvin, V, Kawasaki, A, and Zeldes, S: Dolichoectatic arterial compression of the anterior visual pathways: Neuro-ophthalmic features and clinical course. J Neurol Neurosurg Psychiatry 75(1):27, 2004.
93. Grad, A, and Baloh, RW: Vertigo of vascular origin. Clinical and electronystagmographic features in 84 cases. Arch Neurol 46(3):281, 1989.
94. Olszewski, J, et al: The association between positional vertebral and basilar artery flow lesion and prevalence of vertigo in patients with cervical spondylosis. J Otolaryngol Head Neck Surg 134:680, 2006.
95. Berman, J, and Frederickson, J: Vertigo after head injury: A five year follow-up. J Otolaryngol 7:237, 1978.
96. Tuohimma, P: Vestibular disturbances after acute mild head injury. Acta Otolaryngol Suppl (Stockh) 359:7, 1978.
97. Masson, F, et al: Prevalence of impairments 5 years after a head injury, and their relationship with disabilities and outcome. Brain Inj 10(7):487, 1996.
98. Leigh, RJ, and Zee, DS: Diagnosis of central disorders of ocular motility. In Leigh, RJ and Zee, DS (eds): The Neurology of Eye Movements, ed 4. Oxford University Press, New York, 2006, p. 598.
99. Kluge, M, et al: Epileptic vertigo: Evidence for vestibular representation in human frontal cortex. Neurology 55(12):1906, 2000.
100. Brandt, T, et al: Vestibular cortex lesions affect the perception of verticality. Ann Neurol 35:403, 1994.
101. Brandt, T, et al: Plasticity of the vestibular system: Central compensation and sensory substitution for vestibular deficits. Brain Plast Adv Neurol 73:297, 1997.
102. Kattah, JC, et al: HINTS to diagnose stroke in the acute vestibular syndrome: Three-step bedside oculomotor examination more sensitive than early MRI diffusion-weighted imaging. Stroke 40(11):3504, 2009. [Epub September 17, 2009.]
103. Epley, JM: The canalith repositioning procedure: For treatment of benign paroxysmal positional vertigo. Otolaryngol Head Neck Surg 107:399, 1992.
104. Chung, KW, et al: Incidence of horizontal canal benign paroxysmal positional vertigo as a function of the duration of symptoms. Otol Neurotol 30(2):202, 2009.
105. Fyrmpas, G, et al: Are postural restrictions after an Epley maneuver unnecessary? First results of a controlled study and review of the literature. Auris Nasus Larynx 36(6):637, 2009.
106. Simhadri, S, Freyss, G, and Vitte, E: Efficacy of particle repositioning maneuver in BPPV: A prospective study. Am J Otolaryngol 24(6):355, 2003.
107. Sakaida, M, Freyss, G, and Vitte, E: Long-term outcome of benign paroxysmal positional vertigo. Neurology 60(9):1532, 2003.
108. Helminski, JO, Janssen, I, and Hain, TC: Daily exercise does not prevent recurrence of benign paroxysmal positional vertigo. Otol Neurotol 29(7):976, 2008.
109. Semont, A, Freyss, G, and Vitte, E: Curing the BPPV with a liberatory maneuver. Adv Otorhinolaryngol 42:290, 1988.
110. Campanini, A, and Vicini, C: Semont maneuver vs. particle repositioning maneuver: Comparative study. Acta Otorhinolaryngol Ital 21(6):331, 2001.
111. Campanini, A, et al: Efficacy of the Semont maneuver in benign paroxysmal positional vertigo. Arch Otolaryngol Head Neck Surg 129(6):629, 2003.
112. Amor-Dorado, JC, et al. Particle repositioning maneuver versus Brandt-Daroff exercise for treatment of unilateral idiopathic BPPV of the posterior semicircular canal: A randomized prospective clinical trial with short- and long-term outcome. Otol Neurotol 33(8):1401, 2012.
113. Brandt, T, and Daroff, RB: Physical therapy for benign paroxysmal positional vertigo. Arch Otolaryngol 106:484, 1980.
114. Schubert, MC, et al: Mechanism of dynamic visual acuity recovery with vestibular rehabilitation. Arch Phys Med Rehabil 89(3):500, 2008.
115. Gottshall, K, et al: Objective vestibular tests as outcome measures in head injury patients. Laryngoscope 113(10):1746, 2003.
116. Shumway-Cook, A, and Horak, FB: Vestibular rehabilitation: An exercise approach to managing symptoms of vestibular dysfunction. Semin Hearing 10:196, 1989.
117. Norre, ME, and DeWeerdt, W: Treatment of vertigo based on habituation. J Laryngol Otol 94:971, 1980.
118. Dix, MR: The rationale and technique of head exercises in the treatment of vertigo. Acta Otorhinolaryngol Belg 33:370, 1979.
119. Dix, MR: The physiological basis and practical value of head exercises in the treatment of vertigo. Practitioner 217:919, 1976.
120. Herdman, SJ, et al: Falls in patients with vestibular deficits. Am J Otol 21:847, 2000.
121. Cohen, HS, et al: Driving disability and dizziness. J Safety Res 34(4):361, 2003.
122. Morimoto, H, et al: Effect of oculo-motor and gaze stability exercises on postural stability and dynamic visual acuity in healthy young adults. Gait Posture 33(4):600, 2011.
123. Herdman, SJ, et al: Vestibular adaptation exercises and recovery: Acute stage after acoustic neuroma resection. Otolaryngol Head Neck Surg 113(1):77, 1995.
124. Strupp, M, et al: Vestibular exercises improve central vestibulospinal compensation after vestibular neuritis. Neurology 51(3):838, 1998.
125. Cohen, HS, and Kimball, KT: Increased independence and decreased vertigo after vestibular rehabilitation. Otolaryngol Head Neck Surg 128(1):60, 2003.
126. Krebs, DE, et al: Vestibular rehabilitation: Useful but not universally so. Otolaryngol Head Neck Surg 128(2):240, 2003.
127. Patten, C, et al: Head and body center of gravity control strategies: Adaptations following vestibular rehabilitation. Acta Otolaryngol 123(1):32, 2003.

128. Herdman, SJ, et al: Recovery of dynamic visual acuity in bilateral vestibular hypofunction. Arch Otolaryngol Head Neck Surg 133(4):383, 2007.
129. Hillier, SL, and Hollohan, V: Vestibular rehabilitation for unilateral peripheral vestibular dysfunction. Cochrane Database Syst Rev 17(4):CD005397, 2007.
130. Giray, M, et al: Short-term effects of vestibular rehabilitation in patients with chronic unilateral vestibular dysfunction: A randomized controlled study. Arch Phys Med Rehabil 90(8):1325, 2009.
131. Hall, CD, et al. Vestibular rehabilitation for peripheral vestibular hypofunction: An evidence-based clinical practice guideline: FROM THE AMERICAN PHYSICAL THERAPY ASSOCIATION NEUROLOGY SECTION. J Neurol Phys Ther 40(2):124, 2016.
132. Gurr, B, and Moffat, N: Psychological consequences of vertigo and the effectiveness of vestibular rehabilitation for brain injury patients. Brain Inj 15(5):387, 2001.
133. Sharon, JD, et al: Treatment of Menière's Disease. Curr Treat Options Neurol 17(4):341, 2015.
134. Arenberg, IK: Ménières disease: Diagnosis and management of vertigo and endolymphatic hydrops. In Arenberg, IK (ed): Dizziness and Balance Disorders. Kugler Publications, New York, 1993, p. 503.
135. Bruno, E, et al: Perilymphatic fistula following trans-tympanic trauma: A clinical case presentation and review of the literature. An Otorrinolaringol Ibero Am 29(4):359, 2002.
136. Minor, LB: Superior canal dehiscence syndrome. Am J Otol 21(1):9, 2000.
137. Merchant, SN, and Schuknecht, HF: Vestibular atelectasis. Ann Otol Rhinol Laryngol 1988; 97 (6 Pt 1):565–76.
138. Wenzel, A, et al: Patients with vestibular loss, tullio phenomenon, and pressure-induced nystagmus: Vestibular atelectasis? Otol Neurotol 35(5):866–872, 2014.
139. Love, S, and Coakham, HB: Trigeminal neuralgia: pathology and pathogenesis. Brain 124(Pt 12):2347–2360, 2001.
140. Brandt, T, et al: Vestibular paroxysmia: A treatable neurovascular cross-compression syndrome. J Neurol 263:90, 2016.
141. Dobie, TG, and May, JG: Cognitive-behavioral management of motion sickness. Aviat Space Environ Med 65(Suppl 10):C1, 1994.
142. Rine, RM, et al: Visual-vestibular habituation and balance training for motion sickness. Phys Ther 79:949, 1999.
143. Reason, JT: Motion sickness adaptation: A neural mismatch model. J R Soc Med 71:819, 1978.
144. Bagshaw, M, and Stott, JR: The desensitization of chronically motion sick aircrew in the Royal Air Force. Aviat Space Environ Med 56:1144, 1985.
145. Golding, JF, and Stott, JR: Objective and subjective time courses of recovery from motion sickness assessed by repeated motion challenges. J Vestib Res 7:421, 1997.
146. Banks, RD, et al: The Canadian Forces airsickness rehabilitation program, 1981–1991. Aviat Space Environ Med 63:1098, 1992.
147. Cha, YH: Mal de Debarquement. Semin Neurol 29(5):520, 2009.
148. Dai, M, et al: Readaptation of the vestibulo-ocular reflex relieves the mal de debarquement syndrome. Front Neurol 15(5):124, 2014.
149. Liphart, J: Use of sensory reweighting for a woman with persistent mal de debarquement: A case report. J Geriatr Phys Ther 38(2):96, 2015.
150. Polensek, SH, and Tusa, RJ: Nystagmus during attacks of vestibular migraine: An aid in diagnosis. Audiol Neurootol 15(4):241, 2010.
151. MacGregor, EA, et al: Migraine prevalence and treatment patterns: The global Migraine and Zolmitriptan Evaluation survey. Headache 43(1):19, 2003.
152. Murdin, L, Davies, RA, and Bronstein, AM: Vertigo as a migraine trigger. Neurology 73(8):638, 2009.
153. Wrisley, DM, Whitney, SL, and Furman, JM: Vestibular rehabilitation outcomes in patients with a history of migraine. Otol Neurotol 23(4):483, 2002.
154. Strupp, M, Versino, M, and Brandt, T: Vestibular migraine. Hand Clin Neurol 97:755, 2010.
155. Wang, SR, and Young, YI: Multiple system atrophy manifested as dizziness and imbalance: A report of two cases. Eur Arch Otorhinolayrngol 260:404, 2003.
156. Wedge, F: The impact of resistance training on balance and functional ability of a patient with multiple system atrophy. J Geriatr Phys Ther 31(2):79, 2008.
157. Hikosaka, O, and Maeda, M: Cervical effects on abducens motor neurons and their interaction with vestibulo-ocular reflex. Exp Brain Res 18:512, 1973.
158. Wrisley, DM, et al: Cervicogenic dizziness: A review of diagnosis and treatment. J Orthop Sports Phys Ther 30(12):755, 2000.

Supplemental Readings

Baloh, RW, Honrubia, V, and Kerber, KA: Baloh and Honrubia's Clinical Neurophysiology of the Vestibular System, ed 4. Oxford University Press, New York, 2011.

Epley, JM: The canalith repositioning procedure: For treatment of benign paroxysmal positional vertigo. Otolaryngol Head Neck Surg 107:399, 1992.

Hall, CD, et al: Efficacy of gaze stability exercises in older adults with dizziness. J Neurol Phys Ther 34(2):64, 2010.

Gold, DR, et al: Repositioning maneuvers for benign paroxysmal positional vertigo. Curr Treat Options Neurol 16(8):307, 2014.

Rine, RM, et al: New portable tool to screen vestibular and visual function—National Institutes of Health Toolbox initiative. J Rehabil Res Dev 49(2):209, 2012.

Schubert, MC, et al: Oculomotor strategies and their effect on reducing gaze position error. Otol Neurotol 31(2):228, 2010.

Strupp, M, et al: Vestibular migraine. Hand Clin Neurol 97:755, 2010.

appendix 21.A

Web-Based Resources for Clinicians, Families, and Patients With Vestibular Disorders

Organization	Website
Vestibular Disorders Association (VEDA)	www.vestibular.org
National Institute for Deafness and Other Communication Disorders (NIDCD)	www.nidcd.nih.gov
Johns Hopkins University School of Medicine	www.hopkinsmedicine.org/otolaryngology
Micromedical Technologies	www.micromedical.com
Interacoustics	http://www.interacoustics.com/vf405
Neurokinetics	www.neuro-kinetics.com
Natus EquiTest	http://www.natus.com/index.cfm?page=products_1&crid=270

Amputation

Margery A. Lockard, PT, PhD
Bella J. May, PT, EdD, FAPTA, CEEAA

Chapter 22

LEARNING OBJECTIVES

1. Discuss the role of the physical therapist in the care of any individual following lower extremity amputation.
2. Describe the major etiological factors leading to lower extremity amputation.
3. Explain the major concepts involved in lower extremity amputation surgery.
4. Develop an evaluation plan for any individual following lower extremity amputation.
   a. Prioritize data gathering for the acute postsurgical period and the preprosthetic phase.
5. Design an effective plan of care for the acute postsurgical period.
   a. Explain the rationale for, and teach patient and caregiver, proper positioning.
   b. Teach sitting and standing balance to enhance transfers and mobility.
   c. Ensure continuity of care following discharge from acute care.
6. Design an effective plan of care for the preprosthetic period.
   a. Teach proper residual limb care, including bandaging as indicated.
   b. Teach standing balance to help the patient attain the highest functional level of mobility with appropriate ancillary support.
   c. Teach residual limb strengthening exercises to facilitate eventual prosthetic fitting.
   d. Teach range of motion exercises to prevent/alleviate secondary contractures.
7. Respond appropriately to patient/family from an awareness of the psychological impact of lower extremity amputation.
8. Analyze and interpret patient data, formulate realistic goals and expected outcomes, and develop a plan of care when presented with a clinical case study.

CHAPTER OUTLINE

There are about 1.9 million people living with limb loss in the United States today with an estimated 185,000 new amputations per year.[1] This number of individuals with limb loss is expected to increase and it has been projected that by 2050 the prevalence of amputation will reach 3.6 million Americans.[2] The most common causes of amputation are peripheral vascular disease (about 54%), trauma (about 45%), malignancy (< 1%), and congenital limb deficiency (< 1%).[3]

CAUSES OF AMPUTATION

The primary cause of lower extremity (LE) amputation continues to be peripheral vascular disease (PVD), particularly with associated diabetes. The Centers for Disease Control (CDC) reports that 9.3% (29.1 million people in 2014) of the U.S. population has diabetes.[4] About 60% of non-traumatic LE amputations among individuals 20 years of age or older occur in people with diabetes.[4] Stated another way, an adult with diabetes is 10 times more likely to have an amputation than a non-diabetic individual.[5] However, among those with diabetes some are disproportionally affected by amputation. Amputation has its highest incidence in diabetics who are 75 years of age or older, male, and black.[6] It is also interesting to note that 90% of diabetics who undergo LE amputation had a preexisting foot ulcer.[7] Overall, in the U.S. Medicare population, the incidence of diabetic foot ulcers is approximately 6 per 100 individuals with diabetes per year and the incidence of LE amputation is about 4 per 1,000 persons with diabetes per year.[8] Despite these data, the rate of amputation as a complication of diabetes has been decreasing in the United States over the past two decades.[9] Much of the credit for this reduction in amputation rates has been attributed to improved foot surveillance programs, interdisciplinary foot care, and diabetes education addressing the seriousness of foot ulcers and how to prevent them.[3,10,11] However, because the prevalence of diabetes has been increasing over the same time period, the rate of amputation in the overall population has not decreased.[9]

Major amputation (level of amputation above the ankle or wrist)—considered a treatment of last resort for conditions, including infected diabetic foot ulcers and critical limb ischemia, like all major surgeries—carries mortality risk. Perioperative (30-day) mortality has been variously reported between 7% and 13%. High 30-day mortality rates for both transtibial and transfemoral amputations are predicted by older age (> 80 yr), dependent functional status before surgery, dialysis, steroid use, preoperative sepsis, impaired mental status (confusion or delirium), thrombocytopenia, and renal insufficiency or failure.[12] The overall 5-year mortality rate for amputations in diabetic dysvascular (poor vascular status) patients is very high: 40% to 80% after transtibial amputation and 40% to 90% after transfemoral amputation.[13] This is higher than the 5-year mortality rate for breast cancer, colon cancer, and prostate cancer together.[14] When planning rehabilitation programs for patients with amputation, it is also important to be aware of the status of the contralateral or remaining lower limb. Five years after a major amputation in persons with PVD, 52% had undergone a major amputation of the contralateral lower limb. An independent risk factor for contralateral limb amputation is atherosclerosis with or without diabetic neuropathy.[15] Additionally, 41% had a revision or additional amputation to the originally amputated lower limb in the same time frame.[15] Stated in a simpler but dramatic way: about 50% of patients with amputation owing to poor vascular status will die in the 5 years following surgery; of those who live, 50% will have a contralateral limb amputation! Many of the patients that therapists treat in all types of settings have diabetes and/or peripheral arterial disease (PAD). Therapists can be more effective by being knowledgeable about diabetes and PAD and by making patient education for prevention of amputation an integral part of the plan of care (POC). Several studies have indicated a positive relationship between early patient education and proper foot care and a reduction in amputations.[16-18]

The second leading cause of amputation is trauma, usually from motor vehicle accidents, accidents with machines, war, or gunshot injury. Individuals with traumatic amputations are often young adults, more frequently men, and have often been involved in an active lifestyle before amputation. The incidence of civilian trauma-related amputation has been declining over the past several decades with the majority of amputations involving the upper limb (approximately 67%).[19] Civilian trauma-related amputations of the lower limb have a high incidence of post-surgical complications, including pneumonia, acute kidney injury, deep-vein thrombosis (DVT)/thrombophlebitis, and revision amputation. Significant predictors of need for revision amputation include injury severity, crush fracture, and compartment syndrome.[20] The presence of these complications may extend hospital stays and delay prosthetic fitting. Combat-related amputations during the wars in Afghanistan and Iraq have increased the numbers of service members with amputation returning to civilian life, due to higher survival rates in the war zones.[21] During these wars, the mean amputation rate was 5.9 per 100,000 deployed troops: 41% transtibial amputation (TTA), 40% transfemoral (TFA) or through-the-knee amputation, and 14% upper limb amputation.[21] Thirty percent of service members with amputations have multiple amputations, which is significantly greater than in any other American wars. The most common combinations are TFA/TFA (27%), TTA/TTA (20%), and TFA/TTA (16%).[21]

The incidence of amputation from malignancy, primarily osteogenic sarcoma, has been reduced owing to improved imaging techniques, more effective chemotherapy, and better limb salvage procedures. Osteogenic sarcoma is most prevalent in adolescents and young adults. Amputation may be necessary if the tumor is large and cannot be resected without substantial removal of bone and tissue. However, the surgeon may choose to remove the tumor and incorporate one of several limb salvage procedures. Many factors go into this decision, including the age of the patient, the size of the tumor, and, if the patient is young, the potential for future growth.[22] Limb salvage with adjunctive chemotherapy, however, is now the treatment of choice in 90% of these patients, since studies have shown no difference in survival rates compared to those treated with amputation.[23]

Congenital limb deficiency may be caused by genetic variation, exposure to environmental teratogens or gene-environment interaction.[3,24] The incidence of congenital deficiencies is quite small (2–7 per 10,000 live births or 0.8% of all limb losses) and has been stable over 10 years.[3] However, when limb deficiencies do occur, they are most common in the upper limb.

Regardless of the cause of amputation, physical therapists have a major role in rehabilitation. Early initiation of rehabilitation influences the eventual outcome of the episode of care. It is critically important, especially for the older individual, for the therapist in the acute care center to ensure continuity of care once the patient is discharged from the hospital. Too often, the patient is sent home and is not seen again for several weeks or months. By that time, the patient may have become debilitated and developed contractures that interfere with prosthetic use and function.

■ LEVELS OF AMPUTATION

Traditionally, levels of amputation have been identified by anatomical considerations such as below knee and above knee. In 1974, the Task Force on Standardization of Prosthetic-Orthotic Terminology developed an international classification system to define amputation levels. Table 22.1 describes the major terms in common use today.

Amputations following trauma may be performed at any level. The surgeon tries to maintain the greatest bone length and save all possible joints, while providing adequate soft tissue coverage to produce a *residual limb* (RL) that will be comfortable and functional in a prosthetic socket. A variety of surgical techniques may be necessary to create a functional residual limb. Guillotine amputations (skin, muscle, and bone all transected at approximately the same level) may precede secondary closure with skin flaps; occasionally, free tissue flaps, taken from some other area of the body, may be used to cover the wound. Amputations for vascular diseases are generally performed at partial foot (transmetatarsal), transtibial, or transfemoral levels.

Patients with unilateral transtibial amputations regardless of age are quite likely to become functional prosthetic users; many individuals with bilateral transtibial

Table 22.1 Levels of Amputation

Partial toe	Excision of any part of one or more toes.
Toe disarticulation	Disarticulation at the metatarsal phalangeal joint.
Partial foot/ray resection	Resection of the 3rd, 4th, 5th metatarsals and digits (a ray is a metatarsal and its associated phalanges).
Transmetatarsal	Amputation through the midsection of all metatarsals.
Tarsometatarsal (Lisfranc)	Amputation through the tarsometatarsal joint (the distal bones in the foot are the cuneiforms and the cuboid).
Ankle disarticulation (Syme's)	Ankle disarticulation with attachment of heel pad to distal end of tibia; may include removal of malleoli and distal tibial/fibular flares.
Long transtibial (below knee)	More than 50% of tibial length.
Transtibial (below knee)	Between 20% and 50% of tibial length.
Short transtibial (below knee)	Less than 20% of tibial length.
Knee disarticulation	Amputation through the knee joint; femur intact.
Long transfemoral (above knee)	More than 60% of femoral length.
Transfemoral (above knee)	Between 35% and 60% of femoral length.
Short transfemoral (above knee)	Less than 35% of femoral length.
Hip disarticulation	Amputation through hip joint; pelvis intact.
Transpelvectomy or Hemipelvectomy	Resection of part of the pelvis.
Hemicorporectomy	Amputation both lower limbs and pelvis below L4–L5 level.

amputations also become functional ambulators with a prosthesis. Older adults with unilateral transfemoral amputations who have good balance, cognitive ability, and good pre-amputation functional status are also able to successfully use a prosthesis for functional mobility.[25] Patients with bilateral transfemoral amputations may become prosthetic users with microprocessor-controlled and externally powered prosthetic components. However, this is a difficult task and requires good balance, strength, endurance, and coordination. Hip disarticulations, transpelvectomies, and hemicorporectomies are generally performed either for tumors or for severe trauma and represent a small percentage of the population of individuals with amputations. The most important factor in determining the prosthetic potential of an individual is her or his level of activity prior to amputation.[25,26] In addition, good hip strength and balance are also predictive of the ability to ambulate functionally with a prosthesis.[27] Comorbidities and the extent of injuries from war and trauma must be considered, but the individual who led an active life before amputation—even an individual with diabetes and related comorbidities—is likely to become a functional prosthetic user if he or she can demonstrate good balance, hip strength, and coordination.[26,27]

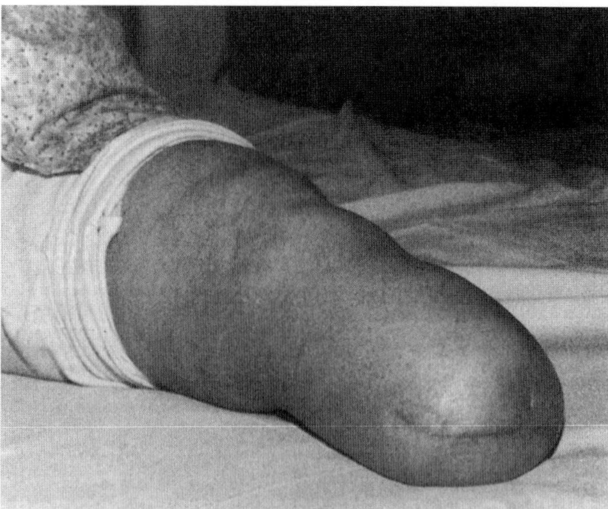

Figure 22.1 Transtibial residual limb with incision from equal-length flaps.

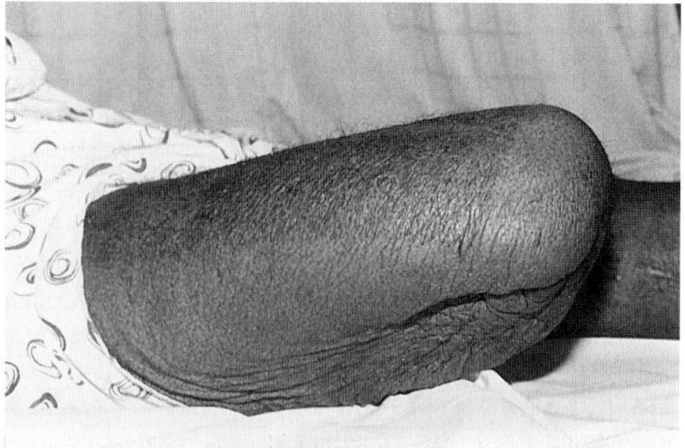

Figure 22.2 Transfemoral residual limb with incision from equal-length flaps.

■ AMPUTATION SURGERY

The specific type of surgery is determined by the surgeon, whose decision depends on the status of the extremity at the time of amputation. The surgeon must allow for primary or secondary wound healing and construct a RL for optimal prosthetic fitting and function. Numerous factors affect the selection of level of amputation. Conservation of RL length, uncomplicated wound healing, and the creation of a pain free limb that can be fitted with a prosthesis that maximizes the individual's functional mobility are all important considerations.[28] Although a description of each type of surgical procedure is beyond the scope of this chapter, an understanding of the basic principles of amputation surgery is important.[29]

Skin flaps are as broad as possible and the scar should be pliable, painless, and nonadherent. For most transfemoral and some transtibial amputations without vascular impairment, equal length anterior and posterior flaps are used, placing the scar at the distal end of the bone (Figs. 22.1 and 22.2). Long posterior flaps are often used in transtibial amputations with compromised circulation because the posterior tissues have better blood supply than the anterior skin. Additionally, the calf muscles provide better distal cushioning for the tibia and fibula. A long posterior flap places the scar anteriorly over the distal end of the tibia; care must be taken to ensure that the scar does not become adherent to the bone (Fig. 22.3). Some surgeons believe the skew flap, developed in England, is a better approach for individuals with severely compromised distal circulation. The skew flap is an angular medial–lateral incision that places the scar away from bony prominences. Research on the use of different skin flaps does not clearly delineate the most advantageous approach, and all indicate similar results in terms of rehabilitation.[30,31]

Stabilization of the major muscles that are cut during surgery allows for retention of muscle tension and maximum muscle function. Muscle stabilization may be achieved by myofascial closure, myoplasty, myodesis, or tenodesis. In most transtibial and transfemoral amputations, a combination of *myoplasty* (muscle to muscle closure) and *myofascial* (muscle to fascia) closure is used to ensure that the muscles are properly stabilized and do not slide over the end of the bone. *Myodesis* (muscle attached to periosteum or bone) may also be used to provide a very stable muscle attachment. More rarely, a *tenodesis* (tendon attached to bone) may be used for muscle stabilization, particularly in partial foot amputations where extrinsic muscle tendons are cut. Whatever the technique, muscle stabilization under some tension is

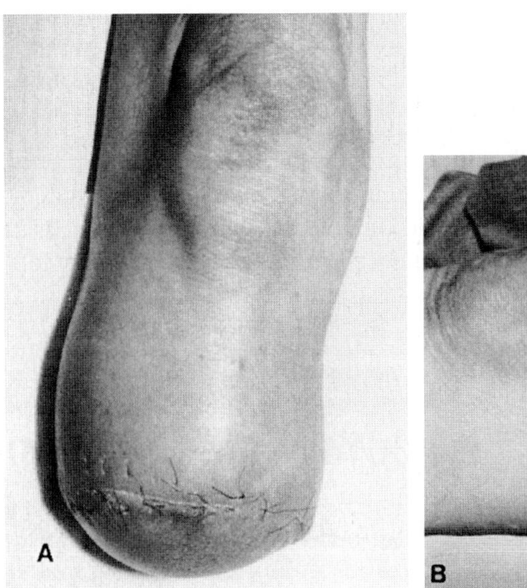

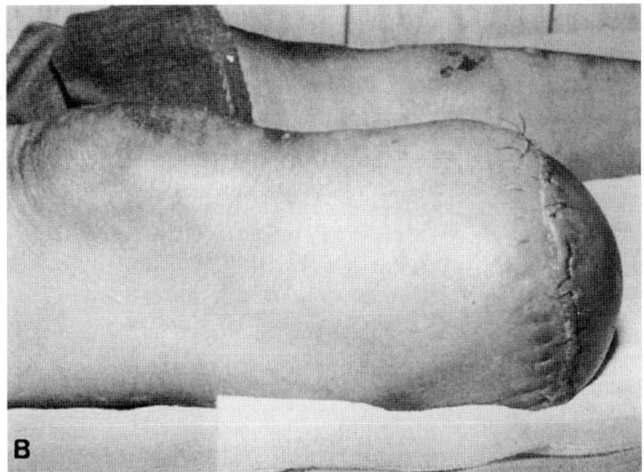

Figure 22.3 (A) Anterior view and (B) lateral view of a transtibial residual limb with anterior incision from a long posterior flap.

desirable to ensure that the transected muscles can contract to maintain muscle bulk and function.

Severed peripheral nerves form *neuromas* (a collection of nerve cell ends) in the RL. The neuroma must be well surrounded by soft tissue so as not to cause pain and interfere with prosthetic wear. Surgeons identify the major nerves, pull them down under some tension, and then cut them cleanly and sharply and allow them to retract into the soft tissue of the residual limb. Neuromas that form close to scar tissue or bone generally cause pain and may require later resection or revision. *Hemostasis* is achieved by ligating major veins and arteries; *cauterization* is used only for small bleeders. Care is taken not to compromise circulation to distal tissues, particularly the skin flaps, which are important to uncomplicated wound healing.

Bones are sectioned at a length to allow wound closure without excessive redundant tissue at the end of the RL and without placing the incision under great tension that might impair healing. Sharp bone ends are smoothed and rounded without disturbing or stripping the periosteum; disruption of the periosteum from the bone may cause development of *osteophytes* (bone spicules) and RL pain during prosthetic use. In transtibial amputations, the anterior portion of the distal tibia is *beveled* and the fibula is cut slightly shorter than the tibia (approximately 1 cm) to reduce pressure between the end of the bones and the prosthetic socket. Alternatively, an Ertle or *osteoplasty* procedure may be performed during transtibial amputation. In this procedure, an autologous piece of bone (often from the amputated fibula) is placed between the ends of the tibia and fibula, secured, and allowed to solidly fuse in place. This results in a more cylindrically shaped RL, which may permit better fitting with a prosthetic socket and increase the ability to take direct end-pressure on the RL.[32,33] Whatever procedure is used, care is taken to ensure that the bone is physiologically prepared for the pressures of prosthetic wear. Tissue layers are approximated under normal physiological tension and the incision is closed, usually with regular sutures. A drainage tube may be inserted as necessary.

In a traumatic amputation, the surgeon attempts to save as much bone length and viable skin as possible and preserve proximal joints while providing for appropriate healing of tissues without secondary complications such as infection. In potentially "dirty" (involving foreign substances) amputations, the incision may be left open with the proximal joint immobilized in a functional position for 5 to 9 days to prevent invasive infection. Secondary closure also allows the surgeon to shape the RL appropriately for prosthetic wear and function.

Osteointegration is a newer technique that has developed over the last few decades as a solution for individuals who are unable to successfully use a conventional prosthesis that attaches to the RL with a socket and suspension system. This is often the case in individuals who have very short or atypically shaped transfemoral or transhumeral RLs due to trauma or tumor resection amputations. In osteointegration, the prosthesis is surgically connected into the residual bone, similarly to dental implants or the insertion of a prosthesis in a total hip arthroplasty.[33] The basic components include a fixture that is inserted into the intramedullary canal of the bone and a percutaneous abutment that is attached to the fixture and connects the prosthesis directly to the bone. Benefits of this approach include elimination of pain due to socket-residual limb fit issues and improved sensory feedback owing to direct connection of the prosthesis into the skeleton.[34] Despite these benefits, problems can arise due to infections at the skin-implant interface or occasionally long bone fracture.[34] In the United States, this procedure only received FDA (Food and Drug Administration) approval in 2015; however, research on this technique and the rehabilitation of individuals who have had the procedure has been conducted in Sweden, Australia, and the United Kingdom.[34-36]

Amputation for vascular disease is generally considered an elective procedure; the surgeon determines the level of amputation by examining tissue viability through a variety of measures. Segmental limb blood pressures can be determined by Doppler systolic blood pressure measurement. Transcutaneous oxygen measurement and skin blood flow by radioisotope or plethysmography are also determined. Doppler systolic blood pressure measures have been reported to be quite accurate in predicting viable level of amputation. Improvements in noninvasive examination techniques have greatly reduced the use of arteriography to determine amputation level. Videos of actual amputation surgery at transtibial and transfemoral levels may be seen at the Amputation Surgery Education Center website (www.ampsurg.org).

■ HEALING PROCESS

Numerous factors influence the course of the healing process in each patient. One of the greatest postoperative concerns is infection, whether from external or internal sources. Individuals with contaminated wounds from injury, infected foot ulcers, or other causes are at greater risk of infection. Research indicates that smoking is a major deterrent to wound healing; one study reported that cigarette smokers had a 2.5% higher rate of infection and reamputation than nonsmokers.[37] Other factors affecting wound healing are the severity of the vascular problems, diabetes, renal disease, and other physiological problems such as cardiac disease.[29] The physical therapist can influence optimal wound healing by teaching proper bed mobility, avoiding pressure on the newly amputated limb, and facilitating mobilization as soon as it is medically approved.

■ POSTSURGICAL DRESSINGS

Surgeons have several options regarding the postoperative dressing, including (1) rigid dressing, (2) semirigid dressing, or (3) soft dressing. It is important for some type of edema control to be used because excessive edema in the RL can compromise healing and cause pain. Table 22.2 outlines the major postsurgical dressings in use today with their advantages and disadvantages.

Rigid Dressings

Rigid dressings, developed in the early 1960s, can be applied as a removable rigid dressing or as an *immediate*

Table 22.2 Postsurgical Dressings

Type of Dressing	Advantages	Disadvantages
Elastic roller bandage	Readily available, accessible Inexpensive Easy access to incision	Can be difficult for patients and family members to learn to apply correctly with appropriate pressure. May produce areas of high pressure that may impair healing. Minimal residual limb (RL) protection. Requires frequent rewrapping. Increased likelihood of developing knee flexion contracture with transtibial amputation.
Shrinker	Easy to apply, particularly for transfemoral level Can effectively control edema with even pressure	Not used until sutures are removed. Requires changing as RL shrinks. Can be expensive to replace. Increased likelihood of knee flexion contracture with transtibial amputation.
Semirigid dressing	Better edema control than soft dressing RL protection	Needs frequent changing. Cannot be applied by patient. No access to incision.
Removable rigid dressing	Effective edema control RL protection Access to incision	Requires skilled practitioner to fabricate or may be expensive to purchase.
IPOP	Excellent edema control Excellent RL protection Control of RL pain Decreased time to fitting with prosthesis	No access to incision. More expensive than other dressings. Requires proper training for use. Requires skilled practitioner for frequent reapplications and fittings. Patient must carefully adhere to all procedures.

IPOP = immediate postoperative prosthesis; RL = residual limb *postoperative prosthesis* (IPOP).[38,39] In either case, the socket may be custom or handmade from plaster or fiberglass casting materials or purchased as a prefabricated device made from plastic or other materials in various sizes. The IPOP socket is applied by the surgeon or a prosthetist in the operating room over wound dressings and padding to protect the wound, skin, and bony prominences. The IPOP cast, most commonly used with transtibial amputations, extends to midthigh and immobilizes the knee in extension.[40,41] A removable pylon (pipe that replaces the missing tibia) and prosthetic foot is added to the cast so that the patient is able to walk with very limited weight-bearing on the first day following surgery. In about 2 weeks the cast is removed to inspect the incision and remove sutures. The cast and pylon are reapplied and the patient continues with this process until fitted with a temporary or definitive prosthesis. Prefabricated IPOP devices that use pneumatic compression have also been used. As healing progresses the patient is able to increase the amount of weight-bearing on the device. Advantages of this system include early mobilization, decreased RL edema and pain, improved balance and safety during transfers, protection of the wound from trauma, prevention of knee flexion contracture, decreased time to fitting with a prosthesis, and the psychological benefit of early prosthetic fitting. Not all patients, however, are good candidates for this method. Patients must be free of infection, have been ambulatory prior to surgery, and able and willing to follow all directions carefully.[40] *Removable rigid dressings* (RRDs) whether handmade from plaster or fiberglass casting materials or prefabricated are applied over dressings, a RL sock, stockinette, or a silicone gel liner.[42-44] Prefabricated RRDs are adjustable as the limb shape and volume changes and may be removed as needed for wound inspection. RRDs used with transtibial amputations can extend over the knee to maintain knee extension or end below the knee to permit active knee flexion.

Use of immediate postoperative rigid dressings varies greatly and is more prevalent in some areas of the country than others. Rigid postsurgical dressings, whether used immediately after surgery or in the early postoperative period, have been found to be successful in reducing postoperative edema and pain, enhancing healing, and reducing the time to fitting with a prosthesis.[39-41]

Semirigid Dressings

There are a number of semirigid dressings that have been reported in the literature. All provide better control of edema than the soft dressing but each has some disadvantage that limits its use. *Unna's dressing* (Unna boot), gauze impregnated with a compound of zinc oxide, gelatin, glycerin, and calamine, may be applied in the operating room. Its major disadvantage is that it may loosen easily and is not as rigid as the plaster of Paris dressing. However, it has been shown to be superior to the soft dressing in enhancing healing and reducing edema.[45]

Soft Dressings

The soft dressing is the oldest method of postsurgical management of the RL and probably the one that most physical therapists in acute care hospitals will encounter. A soft postoperative dressing typically includes a nonadherent dressing over the incision, gauze pads and fluff placed over the distal and anterior aspect of the RL secured with roll-over gauze. Typically, but not always, an elastic bandage is applied over the dressing to control edema. After the fluff gauze is no longer needed, edema is managed with an elastic bandage or an elastic or silicone shrinker.[39,41]

Elastic Wraps

For most individuals with a LE amputation, an elastic bandage, 4 inches wide or more, may be applied over the postsurgical dressing with care taken to ensure proper compression. The elastic bandage must apply even pressure without areas of excessive pressure that might impair circulation and healing. The patient or a family member should learn to apply the wrap using effective technique as soon as possible after wound care is no longer necessary. Many older individuals with transfemoral amputations may not have the necessary balance and coordination to wrap effectively.

Some surgeons prefer delaying elastic wrapping until the incision has healed and the sutures have been removed. Leaving the RL without any compression allows for full development of postoperative edema, which may increase pain and interfere with circulation in the small vessels in the skin and soft tissue, thereby potentially compromising healing. The therapist can discuss the benefits of early wrapping with the surgeon if no other form of rigid dressing is used. There is strong evidence in the literature of the benefits of either the IPOP or the RRD.[39-44]

One of the major drawbacks of the elastic wrap is that it needs frequent rewrapping. Movement of the RL against the bedclothes, bending and extending the proximal joints, and general body movements cause slippage and changes in pressure. Covering the finished wrap with stockinet helps to reduce some of the slippage; however, careful and frequent rewrapping is the only effective way to prevent complications. Nursing staff, family members, and the patient, as well as the physical therapist or physical therapist assistant, need to assume responsibility for frequent inspection and rewrapping of the RL. Residual limb wrapping is described in detail later in this chapter.

Elastic Shrinkers

Shrinkers are sock-like garments manufactured from an elastic material; they are conical in shape and come in a variety of sizes (Fig. 22.4). It is difficult to use a shrinker

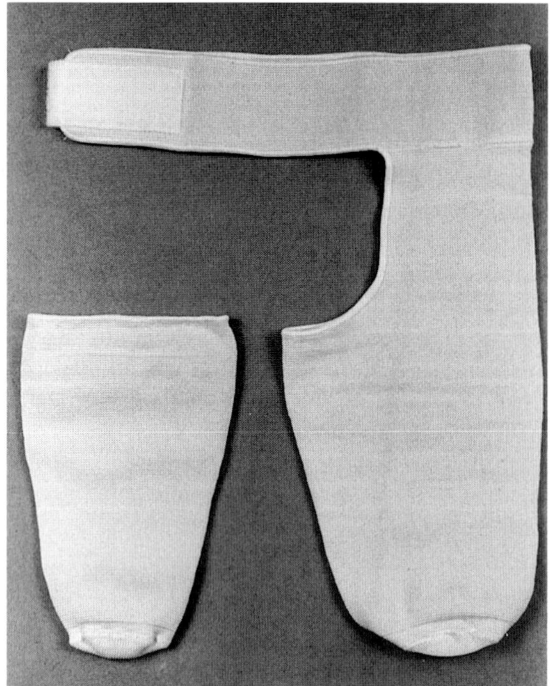

Figure 22.4 (Left) Transtibial shrinker. (Right) Transfemoral shrinker.

in the early postoperative period because the process of pulling it onto the RL during donning may put undesirable stress on the unhealed incision. Silicone liners are applied with a "roll-on" process that is less traumatic to the incision.[43] Another potential disadvantage of a shrinker is that as the RL shrinks in volume, new smaller shrinkers will need to be purchased several times before limb volume stabilizes. Shrinkers are best used after healing has taken place and the initial postoperative edema has been reduced.

PHASES OF CARE

Early onset of rehabilitation produces greater potential for success. A long delay is likely to result in the development of complications such as joint contractures, general debilitation, and depressed psychological state. The rehabilitation program can be arbitrarily divided into two phases: (1) the *postsurgical phase* is the time between surgery and discharge from the acute care hospital where surgery occurred; (2) the *preprosthetic phase* runs from acute care hospital discharge to prosthetic fitting or a decision that the patient is not a candidate for prosthetic fitting.[46] These, of course, are arbitrary periods but each has different goals and emphases within the POC. The desired expected outcome of the episode of care is to help the patient regain the presurgical level of function. For some, it will mean return to gainful employment with an active recreational life. For others, it will mean independence in the home and community. For still others, it may mean living in an assisted living environment or nursing home. If the amputation resulted from long-standing chronic disease, the rehabilitation approach may be to help the person function at a higher level than immediately before surgery.

Preoperative Phase

In the case of traumatic amputation, there is no option for a preoperative phase of rehabilitation. However, when amputation is presented as a likely intervention for patients with peripheral vascular disease (PVD) and critical limb ischemia, optimal rehabilitation care begins before the amputation with multidisciplinary medical, physical, and functional assessments, including assessment of the contralateral limb and psychosocial and cognitive factors that can affect functional prognosis.[47-51] Patient education, including discussions with the patient and family members about phantom and RL pain and realistic short- and long-term goals, is also important at this stage. Patients whose pain expectations are realistic for the postamputation year are more satisfied with their rehabilitation outcomes, regardless of their actual reported pain levels.[52] When possible, patients should also begin a cardiorespiratory conditioning program prior to surgery.[49] Learning about prosthetic rehabilitation, seeing a prosthesis, and even meeting or talking with a successful prosthesis user helps individuals be less fearful of amputation as a treatment option.

Postsurgical Phase

The postsurgical phase is the time between surgery and discharge from the acute care hospital. The primary goal of this phase of care is to prepare the patient for discharge to the appropriate placement site for continued rehabilitation. Box 22.1 presents the general goals of the postsurgical phase of care.

Box 22.2 outlines the data necessary for the therapist to develop a physical therapy POC for the hospitalized patient following amputation. This data is collected from

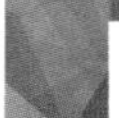

Box 22.1 Postsurgical Phase General Goals[49,50]

- Promote residual limb (RL) wound healing
- Residual limb pain management and control
- Phantom limb pain/sensation management
- Optimize range of motion of both lower and upper limbs, without impairing RL healing
- Optimize strength of both lower and upper limbs, without impairing RL healing
- Protect remaining limb (if dysvascular)
- Demonstrate functional sitting and standing balance
- Perform independent transfers and bed mobility
- Ambulate with appropriate assistive device
- Demonstrate proper sitting and bed positioning
- Begin psychological adjustment
- Understand the process of prosthetic rehabilitation

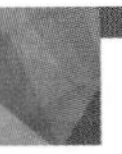

Box 22.2 Postsurgical Phase Examination[50]

- Medical Record Review
  - Onset and duration of symptoms and reason for admission
  - Height, weight, BMI
  - Tobacco use
  - Comorbid chronic conditions (e.g., diabetes, PAD, CAD, MI, COPD, CHF)
  - Medications and relevant laboratory results
  - Previous or ongoing medical or surgical treatments
  - Type and level of amputation; relevant specifics of amputation surgery
  - Status of residual limb incision healing, infection
  - Social history, including prior functional level and use of mobility aids, home environment, social support, and patient goals and expectations
  - Out-of-bed status; orders that affect mobility
- Physical Examination
  - Observation
    - Lines and tubes
    - Residual limb position and dressings; presence of devices (e.g., knee immobilizer)
    - Mental status, cognition, communication
    - Affect and psychological considerations (e.g., fear, anxiety, emotional lability)
  - Systems review
    - Vital signs, Spo_2—at rest and following activity
    - Cardiovascular (e.g., pulses, edema, pitting edema)
    - Respiratory (signs of respiratory distress; effort of breathing, dyspnea)
    - Integumentary (e.g., skin integrity, wounds, scars); remaining intact foot
    - Neuromuscular (e.g., sensation, protective sensation in intact foot)
  - Pain
    - Residual limb pain; incisional pain
    - Phantom limb pain or sensation
    - Other
  - Musculoskeletal
    - Range of motion of residual limb joints and intact UEs and LEs
    - Gross functional muscle performance, UEs and intact LE (e.g., strength, coordination)
  - Balance (sitting, standing, response to perturbation)
  - Functional status
    - Bed mobility, transfers, sitting, standing
    - Ambulation with ambulatory aid (distance, assistance required)
    - Safety awareness during functional activities

CAD = coronary artery disease; CHF = congestive heart failure; COPD = chronic obstructive pulmonary disease; MI = myocardial infarction; PAD = peripheral vascular disease

review of the medical record and patient interview and examination. Data gathering must be prioritized according to the person's physiological status and cause of amputation; however, the information obtained on initial and subsequent examinations will influence discharge planning and future care. Thus, it is important that the therapist include evidence of the patient's physical capabilities required to qualify for various post-hospitalization levels of care. For example, to qualify for some inpatient rehabilitation facilities, patients must be able to tolerate 3 hours of therapy per day. Patients may be discharged to home with home services (including physical and occupational therapy) or outpatient services. Other options include discharge to an inpatient rehabilitation facility or a subacute/skilled rehabilitation facility. Physical therapists must advocate for their patients to ensure appropriate continuation of rehabilitation services following hospital discharge. Studies show that persons with amputation who receive rehabilitation at comprehensive inpatient rehabilitation facilities achieve a higher level of mobility success with their prostheses and are more satisfied with their mobility when compared to those who went home or to subacute/skilled facilities.[53-55] For all patients, current cardiovascular status, physiological response to surgery, presence of infection, pain level, and medication will influence to what extent the patient will be able to actively participate in the therapy program. Individuals with amputations secondary to severe trauma, blast injuries in war, and similar problems will require a somewhat different approach from individuals with vascular disease. The type of postsurgical dressing will also influence both data gathering and interventions. The person with a rigid dressing may be able to move more easily in bed than someone with a soft dressing. Typically, an individual in the early postsurgical phase will have limited mobility and functional capabilities. They may also have compromised endurance, RL postoperative pain and phantom limb pain/sensation that may interfere with participation in the program. The specific POC is developed to achieve patient goals based on critical examination findings.

Intervention: Postsurgical Phase

The therapist treating a patient in the hospital has only limited time in which to achieve the goals because hospital lengths of stay are typically short. Interventions must be aimed at preparing the patient for discharge from acute care to appropriate continuing rehabilitation care. Box 22.3 outlines interventions included in the postsurgical rehabilitation POC.

Positioning

Persons with amputation are at risk for developing RL joint contractures that make it difficult to comfortably wear and use a prosthesis. The development of contractures also delays fitting with a definitive prosthesis. The most common type that develops in a transtibial

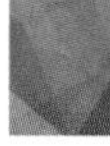

Box 22.3 Postsurgical Phase Interventions

- Interventions to prevent development of residual limb joint contractures
  - Positioning (e.g., prone lying; for transtibial amputations, devices to maintain full knee extension of residual limb)
  - Active range of motion exercise; caution to prevent unwanted stress to the incision
- Functional training
  - Bed mobility (rolling, supine to and from sitting, supine to and from prone)
  - Transfers (bed, chair, wheelchair, toilet)
- Standing and sitting balance training
- Ambulation training with crutches or a walker; stairs, if appropriate
- Exercises for intact extremities (upper limbs and remaining lower extremity)
  - Active exercise to maintain joint ROM and muscle function
  - Exercise to maintain cardiorespiratory endurance necessary for functional activities
- Residual limb care and protection; edema management (when appropriate, elastic bandage, rigid dressing, shrinker)
- Care of the remaining lower extremity (if circulation compromised)
- Patient and caregiver education
  - Education on amputation rehabilitation and prosthetics
  - Safety awareness during all functional activities

amputation is a knee flexion contracture. Frequently seen with transfemoral amputations are hip flexion and abduction contractures owing to muscle imbalance. For example, the hamstrings are cut and secured, but the iliopsoas is unaffected by the amputation; the long adductor muscles are cut and secured, but the abductor muscles are intact. Additionally, persons with lower limb amputations tend to spend much of their time sitting, which can predispose to development of flexion contractures. Persons with partial foot amputations may develop plantarflexion contractures, particularly if weight-bearing is restricted for a long period of time. When a tarsometatarsal amputation is performed, the foot may assume an inverted position because of loss of the attachment of peroneus longus, resulting in eversion weakness. Figure 22.5 illustrates the positioning strategies appropriate for either a patient with a transtibial or transfemoral amputation. Although the figure represents someone with a transtibial amputation, the general principles are the same. It is critical in both instances to prevent hip flexion contractures and the patient should be encouraged to spend at least 30 minutes in the prone position each day, if at all possible. A pillow under the RL while the patient is supine is never recommended, nor is prolonged sitting. In the early days, the patient will want to avoid side-lying on the amputated side and the RL should be kept in extension at both hip and knee. Some facilities use a knee immobilizer or a posterior splint to maintain knee extension following a transtibial amputation. If a knee immobilizer is used, care must be taken to avoid excessive pressure to the RL. It is also most likely not safe to use the knee immobilizer during ambulation. A rigid dressing usually extends to midthigh and maintains knee extension. Patients can also perform active ROM of the joints of the RL; however, prior to healing, care must be taken to avoid movements that place excessive tension on the incision.

Functional Training

The loss of part of a limb shifts the body's center of mass (COM) and alters weight distribution among the limbs and trunk. As a result, some patients may have difficulty turning in bed or moving from a supine to sitting position. Usual procedures for teaching functional mobility are typically effective in helping patients to achieve independence in bed mobility. Transfers require the patient to demonstrate good sitting and standing balance. The shift in COM owing to the amputation will require the patient to adjust his or her balance responses accordingly. Persons with intact vision, vestibular function, and proprioception accommodate quickly. Those with impairments in these functions may require more time and training. It is important to include safety awareness during transfer training, since at this point postamputation, most patients have phantom sensations (nonpainful sensations in the part of the limb that has been amputated and removed) and may default to learned motor patterns that include the now-absent limb. Patients will need to learn new motor patterns for functional activities and transfers. During transfer training in the early postsurgical period, the person should stand and transfer leading with the unamputated limb to protect the RL from possible injury against the chair or bed.

Balance Training

Sitting balance is usually not a problem with unilateral amputations; however, persons with a transfemoral amputation may have difficulty in unsupported sitting, if pushed in a posterior direction. Individuals with bilateral amputations may require more specific training in sitting balance. For persons with unilateral amputation, standing balance exercises on the remaining extremity are helpful to regain appropriate balance responses. The better the person can balance on the remaining extremity the more likely he or she will be to use crutches and lead an active life during the period before prosthetic fitting.

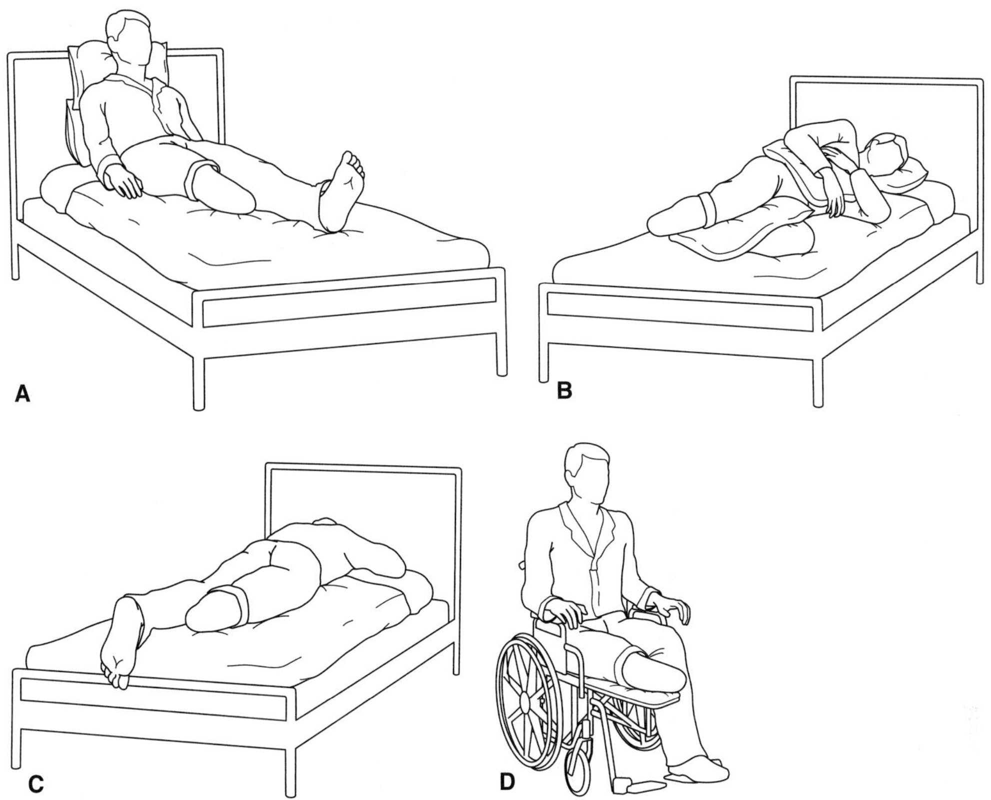

Figure 22.5 Proper transtibial position: (A) Supine. (B) Side-lying. (C) Prone. (D) Sitting. *(From May and Lockard,[46, p. 67] with permission.)*

A variety of balance exercises may be used, including balancing on a compliant surface.

Ambulation and Gait Training

Many physical therapists fit patients with a walker for ambulation. Although this is appropriate for some individuals, teaching the patient safe and independent mobility with crutches is more beneficial because the crutch gait pattern is similar to the pattern that will be used when walking with a prosthesis. While there is more stability in a walker, there is greater flexibility in accomplishing activities of daily living (ADL) with crutches, particularly when forearm (Loftstrand) crutches are used. The added balance needed for crutches will also serve the individual well when it is time for prosthetic fitting.

If the patient has been fitted with an IPOP rigid dressing and has good control of weight-bearing, a pylon and prosthetic foot may be added to the rigid dressing, making partial weight-bearing gait possible. In this instance, the patient must be fitted with crutches because the walker will inhibit the natural function of the prosthetic components.

When teaching mobility to someone with diabetes or any vascular compromise, it is important that the patient wear a shoe on the remaining foot. The remaining foot must be protected from injury, and hospital-provided slippers, or any slippers, do not provide the necessary protection. The family should bring in an appropriate shoe (low heel, cushion sole, good heel support, and laces to firmly secure the shoe to the foot). If the patient has lost protective sensation or has deformity in the intact foot, consider fitting the foot with an accommodative shoe to prevent trauma.[56]

Residual Limb Care

The physical therapist should discuss volume containment for edema management with the patient and family and provide instruction in how to properly implement the technique. If the patient has been fitted with an IPOP or RRD, the physical therapist must be alert to excessive bleeding or drainage through the cast. A primary focus at this point is to teach the patient how to protect the RL while moving in bed, coming to sitting, and transferring. Patients should not put pressure on the limb or drag it on the bed. Slightly raising the RL and moving it to the side while rolling to the unamputated side is the best way to come to sitting. Careful monitoring of RL healing status is important during postsurgical rehabilitation. The patient should be encouraged to move the limb gently within a pain-free range both at the knee (transtibial) and at the hip (both levels). Gentle hip extension performed several times a day (for transtibial amputations, with the knee straight) is an excellent exercise to teach the patient while lying prone or on the unamputated side. Resistive exercises for the RL are contraindicated at this time.

Care of the Remaining Lower Extremity

Since the majority of individuals undergoing amputation do so as a result of poor circulation, it is important to evaluate the status of the remaining extremity and teach the patient and family proper care, as presented in Chapter 14, Vascular, Lymphatic, and Integumentary Disorders. A proper shoe must be obtained before standing and mobility activities.[56] Range of motion (ROM) and strengthening exercises can be implemented as appropriate for the status of the remaining limb.

Patient Education

The more the patient and family understand about the amputation and rehabilitation process the better the outcome.[51] Throughout the examination and implementation of the POC, the physical therapist continuously involves the patient and caregivers, answering questions and providing information at a level and rate commensurate with the capabilities of the individuals. The goals are to have the patient and caregivers assume responsibility for care and safety awareness during functional activities, understand the need for continued care, and become active participants in the rehabilitation program.[57] Regardless of the specific discharge placement, the patient should be given a home program and encouraged to be as mobile as possible.

Discharge Planning

Physical therapists, as part of the multidisciplinary team caring for the patient, should actively participate in discharge planning and placement discussions. As mentioned, evidence shows that persons with amputation who receive rehabilitation at comprehensive inpatient rehabilitation facilities achieve a higher level of mobility success with their prostheses and are more satisfied with their mobility when compared to those who went home or to subacute/skilled facilities.[53-55,58] When discharge to home is planned, physical therapists must coordinate with the occupational therapist and social services to ensure that appropriate equipment, an ambulatory aid, and continued rehabilitation services are arranged for safety and continuity of care.

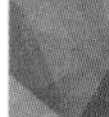

Box 22.4 Preprosthetic Phase General Goals

- Independent in residual limb care
  - Volume containment and edema management: elastic bandage, shrinker, or removable rigid dressing application; IPOP care
  - Skin care and desensitization
  - Positioning
- Independent in mobility, transfers, and functional activities
  - If fitted with IPOP, partial weight-bearing crutch walking; full weight-bearing when tolerated
  - Single-leg ambulation with crutches/walker if fitted with soft dressing or removable rigid dressing; demonstration of a gait pattern that will allow easy transition to prosthetic gait
  - Ability to ambulate safely on level surfaces, uneven surfaces, inclines and steps, as appropriate for the ability of the patient
  - Ability to perform all transfers, including in the bathroom, car transfers, and to and from the floor, as appropriate for the ability of the patient
- Perform an exercise program accurately and with good form
  - ROM and resisted exercises for all parts of residual lower extremity
  - ROM and strengthening exercises for the unamputated lower extremity and trunk
  - Muscle strengthening and endurance exercises for upper extremities, to support functional needs
- Perform appropriate care of the remaining lower extremity if amputation was for vascular reasons
- Demonstrate cardiorespiratory endurance necessary for prosthetic use and community mobility

IPOP = immediate postoperative prosthesis

Preprosthetic Phase

The preprosthetic phase is the time between discharge from the acute care hospital and fitting with a preparatory (temporary) or definitive prosthesis, or the decision not to fit the patient with an artificial limb. Regrettably, for many individuals this period lasts too long and does not include a regular program of physical therapy, resulting in poor outcomes. The general goals for the preprosthetic phase of care are presented in Box 22.4. Box 22.5 provides a guide for preprosthetic examination.

Examination

Residual Limb

Approximately 7 to 12 days after surgery, depending on the condition of the RL, the amount of healing, and the postsurgical dressing, specific data about the RL and adjacent joint(s) can be gathered. Residual limb girth and length measurements are taken after initial postsurgical edema has diminished. Circumferential measurements are then taken regularly throughout the preprosthetic phase to document RL shaping and shrinkage. Measurements are made at regular intervals over the length of the limb to reflect the specific limb shape. Circumferential measurements of the transtibial RL are started at the medial tibial plateau (medial joint line of the knee) and taken every 2 to 3 in. (5 to 8 cm), depending on the length of the limb. Length of the RL is measured from the medial tibial plateau to the end of the bone, then to the end of the skin. Circumferential measurements of the transfemoral RL are started at the ischial tuberosity, greater trochanter, or the insertion of the adductor longus tendon onto the pubic ramus, whichever is most reliably palpable, and are

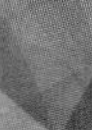

Box 22.5 Preprosthetic Phase Examination Guide

General and Social History

- Patient demographics (age, sex, body weight, BMI)
- Family and social data
  - Living arrangements, home architectural challenges or hazards
  - Social support/caregivers
- Preamputation status (work, physical activity level, avocation, independence, community mobility)
- Insurance status, relative to coverage for prosthesis, durable medical equipment and continued rehabilitation
- Psychological and emotional status (adjustment to and acceptance of amputation; body image)
- Other as relevant

History of Present Illness (HPI) and Past Medical History (PMH)

- Amputation history
  - Cause of amputation (disease, tumor, trauma, congenital)
  - Date of surgery, hospital, surgeon; any surgical/medical complications
- Associated diseases/symptoms (e.g., diabetes, neuropathy, visual disturbances, cardiopulmonary disease, cardiovascular disease, renal disease, stroke, arthritis, congenital anomalies, history of depression/anxiety)
- Other relevant surgeries (e.g., total joint replacements, fracture repairs with open reduction internal fixation [ORIF])
- Medications

Systems Review

- Cardiopulmonary
  - Vital signs and Spo_2 measured with pulse oximeter, at rest and after activity
  - Observation for signs of respiratory distress, dyspnea at rest and after activity
  - Auscultation of heart and lungs, if required
- Integumentary
  - Lesions (location, size, shape, open, scar tissue)
  - Skin condition, turgor, and texture (moist, dry, scaly, cracked, callous)
  - Trophic changes (changes due to neuropathy, such as dryness, loss of hair, nail thickening)
  - Grafts (location, type, healing)
  - Dermatological lesions (psoriasis, eczema, rashes, maceration, cysts)
- Neuromuscular
  - Mental status, cognition and communication
  - Pain (location, intensity, nature, frequency, duration)
    - Residual limb pain
    - Phantom limb sensation and phantom limb pain
    - Other locations
  - Sensation (absent, diminished, hyperesthesia; protective sensation in intact foot)
  - Balance (sitting, standing, with perturbation)
  - Coordination (quality of movements)
- Vascular (both lower limbs)
  - Pulses (femoral, popliteal, dorsalis pedis, posterior tibial)
  - Color (red, pallor, cyanosis)
  - Temperature (glove-stocking presentation)
  - Edema (location, type [pitting or nonpitting]; girth measurements)
  - Intermittent claudication in intact lower extremity
- Musculoskeletal (all four extremities and trunk)
  - Range of motion (patients are vulnerable to insidious development of joint contractures during this phase; therapists must monitor and carefully measure and remeasure)
  - Muscle strength and endurance (core trunk strength is very important to prosthetic control and should be assessed in addition to the extremities)

Continued

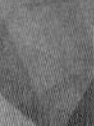

Box 22.5 Preprosthetic Phase Examination Guide—cont'd

Residual Limb

- Length
  - Bone length (transtibial limbs measured from medial tibial plateau; transfemoral limbs measured from ischial tuberosity or greater trochanter)
  - Soft tissue length (note distal redundant tissue)
- Shape
  - Cylindrical (desirable), conical, bulbous end, and so forth
  - Abnormalities ("dog ears," adductor roll)
- Incision (healed, adherent, invaginated, flat, dehiscence, signs of necrotic flap)
- Skin condition

Functional Status

- Transfers
  - Bed-to-chair, to toilet and tub/shower, to car
  - Assistance required; safety awareness
- Mobility and ambulation
  - Wheelchair or type of ambulatory aid
  - Required assistance or supervision; safety awareness, balance and recovery from balance loss
  - Distance and cardiorespiratory response to sustained mobility
- Basic activities of daily living (bathing, dressing)
- Instrumental activities of daily living (cooking, cleaning)
- Functional Outcome Measures (choose instrument to measure progress or regression)
  - Performance-based measurement
  - Quality of life measurement

taken every 3 to 4 in. (8 to 10 cm). Length is measured from the same proximal landmark to the end of the bone, then to the end of the skin. For accuracy of repeat measurements, exact landmarks are carefully noted. If the ischial tuberosity is used in transfemoral measurements, hip joint position is noted as well. Other information gathered about the RL includes a description of its shape (conical, bulbous, or cylindrical; presence of redundant tissue), skin condition, sensation, and joint proprioception.

Range of Motion

Gross ROM estimations are generally adequate for examination of the uninvolved extremity, unless there are specific limitations or contractures. Specific goniometric measurements are necessary for the amputated side, bilateral hip extension, and ankle dorsiflexion of the unamputated side. Functional balance requires good ankle motion, and many older individuals have developed limited range in ankle dorsiflexion leading to catching the toes during swing, stumbling, or falling. Hip and knee measurements are taken following transtibial amputation. Hip flexion, extension, abduction, and adduction measurements are taken following transfemoral amputation. Measurement of internal and external hip rotation is difficult to obtain and unnecessary if no gross abnormality or pathology is evident. Hip flexion contractures are particularly important to note because the patient will not be able to stand and bear weight properly using a prosthesis without adequate hip extension (Fig. 22.6). Additionally, hip extension participates in prosthetic knee control for some transfemoral prostheses.

Muscle Strength

Manual muscle testing (MMT) of functional muscle groups in the upper extremities (UEs) and uninvolved LE is performed as part of the initial examination. MMT of the involved LE must usually wait until most healing has occurred. With a transtibial amputation, good strength in the hip extensors and abductors, as well as the knee extensors and flexors, is needed for satisfactory prosthetic ambulation. For the patient with a transfemoral amputation, good strength of the hip extensors and abductors is a requirement. The POC should include monitoring and strengthening of these muscles throughout the preprosthetic phase. Hip extensor strength has been identified as a predictor of successful prosthetic use.[27,28] Strength of the muscles that stabilize the trunk must also be assessed. Trunk strength is important for successful prosthetic use but is often not included in preprosthetic examinations and subsequent exercise programs.

Status of the Uninvolved Limb

The vascular status of the uninvolved LE is determined and documented. Data gathered include condition of

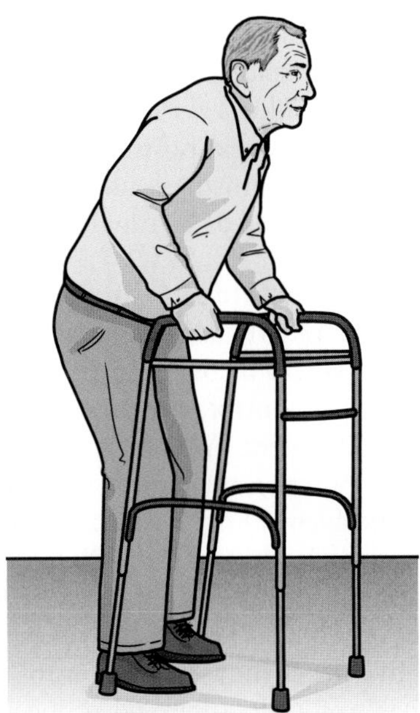

Figure 22.6 Hip flexion contractures alter upright postural alignment and lower extremity weight-bearing.

the skin, presence of pulses, sensation, temperature, edema, pain on exercise or at rest, presence of wounds, ulceration, or other abnormalities. Chapter 14, Vascular, Lymphatic, and Integumentary Disorders, presents further information on examination and evaluation of peripheral vascular status. In addition to examination of the remaining lower limb's vascular status, ROM, and strength, the presence of deformities and other orthopedic problems should also be identified. Contralateral knee pain is a common complaint after amputation that affects function.[59] The presence of preexisting conditions, such as arthritis, should be noted early so that accommodations can be made to prevent them from limiting function in the future.

Functional Status

Activities of daily living and functional mobility skills, including transfer and ambulatory status, are examined, measured, and documented. Sitting balance and standing balance on the remaining extremity are important and should be examined. Data regarding presurgical activity level and the person's own expected outcomes are obtained through interview and are often indicative of potential functional prosthetic use.[25,26] An individual who had an active lifestyle before the amputation, regardless of age, is more likely to be able to learn to use a prosthesis well. Individuals with a long history of a sedentary lifestyle may encounter more difficulty, particularly if the amputation is at the transfemoral level. A performance-based functional outcome measure should be included in the examination to be used as a baseline for subsequent assessment of function.[60] Functional outcome measures are discussed at the end of this chapter.

Phantom Limb

The majority of individuals will encounter *phantom limb sensations* following amputation.[61] Phantom sensation is the perception that the part of the limb that has been amputated is still present. The phantom, which may occur initially immediately after surgery, is variably described as feeling normal in character, feeling warmth or tingling, or feeling that part of the amputated limb is held in a particular position. Occasionally the person may feel the whole extremity. The phantom is more often described as "telescoping" in which the patient perceives the distal part of the limb without sensation from the midportion of the limb.[62] Phantom limb sensations are reported as strongest in amputations above the elbow and weakest in amputations below the knee. Most phantom sensations generally resolve after 2 to 3 years without treatment, except when phantom pain develops.[62] Phantom pain occurs when the phantom sensations are noxious, often interfering with prosthetic use and function. It is most commonly described as burning, aching, or cramping. The prevalence of phantom limb pain (PLP) is variably reported but is generally present to some extent in about 80% of persons with amputation.[63] PLP may be localized or diffuse, continuous or intermittent, or may be triggered by some external stimuli. It may diminish over time or become a permanent and disabling condition. However, despite its commonality among individuals with amputation, a specific etiology for PLP has not been determined. A leading theory suggests that phantom phenomena are due to maladaptive neuroplasticity (changes to the cerebral cortex, particularly the motor and sensory cortex) driven by the deafferentation that occurs with amputation.[61,62]

During examination, it is important to document the presence of phantom sensation and pain. Patients should be asked to describe their sensation, rate its intensity using a numerical rating scale, and describe the frequency of occurrence and the duration of the episodes. In addition, patients should be asked to qualify or quantify the effect of their phantom on activities of daily living and quality of life. The effects of phantom limb sensation/pain should be noted in functional outcome measurements. Physical exam may not be very useful in understanding a person's PLP, except in the few patients who may have trigger points on the RL that reproduce PLP.[62] Some clinicians have reported altered sensitivity or "coldness" to touch in the RLs of some patients with PLP.[62] Baseline data documenting the status of phantom limb sensations during the preprosthetic phase should be recorded as a basis for evaluating the effects of time or interventions.

Emotional and Psychological Status

Initial reaction to the traumatic loss of a limb may be grief and depression. The person may experience insomnia and restlessness and have difficulty concentrating. Some individuals may actually mourn the possible loss of a job or the ability to participate in a favorite sport or other activities rather than the lost limb per se. In the early stages, the person's grief may alternate with feelings of hopelessness, despondency, bitterness, and anger. Socially the patient may feel lonely, isolated, and the object of pity. Concerns about the future, about body image and sexual function, about the responses of family and friends, and about employment all affect the individual's reactions.[64,65] If the amputation is the result of vascular disease or other long-term problem, the amputation may actually come as a relief. The fight to save the limb, sometimes long and painful, is finally over. However, regardless of the cause of amputation, responses are variable among individuals. Despite this variation, about one-third of all individuals with an amputation, regardless of cause, report experiencing depressed mood, which is higher in adults aged 64 years or younger (about 35%) as compared to older persons (about 20%).[63] During examination, therapists should encourage patients to express personal feelings about their limb loss and address concerns with patient education or referral for counselling. Although it is difficult to predict long-range adjustment initially, there is some evidence that early counseling and the opportunity to explore the feelings associated with amputation and rehabilitation may be beneficial for individuals in all age groups.[65] Often seeing others in the treatment area with similar problems, particularly if involved in prosthetic training, may help the patient with a new amputation realize what can be achieved.

Social integration is another important factor to evaluate. Social integration refers to the contacts and interactions between the person with amputation and his or her social network. Increased social interaction is associated with both improved function and quality of life.[66] Therapists should identify and facilitate patients' participation in important social relationships.

Cognition

Cognitive impairment from vascular disease can affect memory, concentration, problem-solving, and reasoning.[67] Rehabilitation following amputation requires learning new methods of performing functional mobility and ADL, which may prove challenging for persons with a vascular amputation and impaired cognition. Although there is no evidence that those with cognitive impairment should be excluded from consideration for prosthetic fitting and rehabilitation, therapists must be aware of their patients' cognitive abilities when planning and implementing rehabilitation plans of care. Effective learning styles for each patient should be identified and alternative or supplemental methods to facilitate learning and remembering safe procedures should be included.[67] Evaluation of cognitive abilities in persons with a vascular amputation should be performed at intervals in the postamputation period. Overall, cognitive performance appears poorest before surgery, but improves after amputation. Cognitive improvement generally stabilizes between 6 and 12 weeks postsurgery.[68] Individuals with better attention and working memory at 6 weeks postsurgery are more likely to have higher levels of prosthesis use, functional mobility, and social integration at 1 year after amputation.[69]

Clinical Note (the Older Adult With Amputation): Elderly individuals are subject to considerable stress from concerns about financial limitations, loss of control over their lives, and fear of becoming dependent. An elderly individual who requires an amputation must often cope with multiple physical problems. Loss is a part of normal aging—loss of physiological capabilities, loss of a spouse or friends, loss of the self-esteem related to one's career or job, and now loss of function. It is helpful to give the client as much control over decision making as possible, to provide opportunities to be involved in goal setting and sequencing of activities. As with any client during examination, physical therapists need to learn about the stressors affecting the individual and assist with coping by being reflective listeners and enablers.

It is a myth that elderly individuals cannot learn a new skill, have difficulty remembering, and cannot achieve functional independence. Some elderly individuals may have difficulty learning a new skill, but many are able to adapt successfully to a disability such as an amputation and lead a full and normal life. Although some suffer from dementia, others who are labeled as having dementia because of confusion in the acute care setting may actually only be responding to medications, metabolic imbalances, infection toxicity, insecurity in a strange environment, or the sequelae of anesthesia. It is important to reassess cognition in postacute care rehabilitation settings because cognition typically improves postsurgery.[68] Understanding the client's cognitive capabilities is necessary to structure learning experiences appropriately. Goal-oriented statements may be clearer than step-by-step instructions. For example, asking the patient to "stand up" may be more successful than instructions involving multiple steps. We do many activities almost automatically—getting up from a chair, turning in bed, and walking. Most of us have developed particular patterns of movements over the years. The physical therapist can draw on such patterns while focusing on the movement goals.

Intervention: Preprosthetic Phase

Residual Limb Care and Edema/Volume Management

Changes in RL volume occur due to postoperative edema and overall body weight. The limb should be healed and postoperative edema minimized to be ready for prosthetic fitting. The RL is subjected to considerable and varied pressures during prosthetic walking and is generally not fully healed and prepared for these stresses for 8 to 12 weeks after surgery. Although using the IPOP method enables partial weight-bearing with a prosthesis earlier than this timeframe, it is only variably used in the United States.[40,41] Individuals not fitted with an IPOP or rigid dressing use elastic bandages or shrinkers to reduce the size of the RL. The patient, family member, or professional staff member applies the bandage, which is worn 23 hours a day (full time, except when bathing). Using an elastic wrap or a shrinker to reduce edema is a slow process. Edema may be difficult to control in individuals with diabetes, particularly if they have renal disease or congestive heart failure.

Body weight also contributes to the size of the RL. After amputation, some individuals gain weight because their appetite returns or they become less active. Others lose weight because they become more active. Body weight must be monitored by regular weighing, just as RL girth measurements must be taken to monitor edema reduction. Patients require education regarding the importance of maintaining a stable body weight because fluctuations in body weight will make prosthetic socket fit difficult.

Residual Limb Wrapping

The basic principles of wrapping are presented in Box 22.6. When the wrap is complete, all skin of the RL should be covered with a smooth (wrinkle-free), snug wrap. The shape of the RL should be cylindrical. All wraps will slip and move, regardless of how well they are applied; rewrapping should be performed about every 4 hours. Whenever possible, patients should be able to independently wrap their own RL using good technique; a family member or caregiver should also be able to apply a good wrap. This usually requires considerable practice and should be a treatment goal.

Figure 22.7 and Box 22.7 illustrate and describe the wrapping technique for the transtibial amputation. Figure 22.8 and Box 22.8 illustrate and describe the wrapping technique for the transfemoral amputation. An alternate view of the wrapping techniques from the patient's perspective is available online.[50]

Shrinkers

The transtibial elastic shrinker is rolled onto the RL to midthigh and is designed to be self-suspending. Individuals with heavy thighs may need additional suspension with a waist belt to prevent distal slippage. Transfemoral shrinkers typically incorporate a hip spica (encircles the pelvis), which provides good suspension except with obese individuals (see Fig. 22.4). Care must be taken that the patient understands the importance of proper suspension; any rolling of the edges or slipping of the shrinker can create a tourniquet around the proximal part of the RL and form an adductor roll. Shrinkers are easier to apply than elastic bandages and may be a better alternative, particularly for the transfemoral RL. Shrinkers are more expensive to use than elastic wrap; the initial cost is greater, and new shrinkers of smaller sizes must be purchased as the limb volume decreases. However, shrinkers are a viable option for individuals

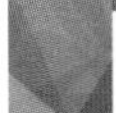

Box 22.6 General Principles of Residual Limb (RL) Elastic Bandaging

- The general direction of wrapping should be from distal to proximal.
- Use figure-of-8 wrapping pattern, with diagonal turns—NOT circular turns that can constrict or choke.
- Diagonal turns should be about 45° from horizontal and should form an X pattern as the diagonal turns cross each other.
- Each turn should partially overlap previous turns so there are no gaps in the wrap and pressure is even throughout the wrap.
- Apply the wrap diagonally over the distal "corners" of the RL to prevent "dog ears" or a bulbous shape. After the RL is wrapped, the shape should be cylindrical.
- Pressure should be even throughout the wrap, with a slight gradient from more distally to less proximally.
- The elastic in the wrap should be stretched about half of its available elasticity for a snug wrap.
- There should be about three layers of wrap evenly applied over the RL; more layers in one area will cause localized higher pressure.
- Secure with tape applied wrap to wrap. Do not apply tape to skin or secure the wrap with clips or pins.
- When the wrap is complete, the RL should be totally covered with no gaps between turns.
- There should be no wrinkles or folds in the wrap; wrinkles cause increased pressure.
- In the transtibial (TT) RL, the patella may be covered or left open; the full wrap should cover the supracondylar region of the thigh.
- Wrapping the transfemoral (TF) RL requires a hip spica (about two wraps around the waist to prevent the RL wrap from sliding down).
- While applying the TF wrap, make sure that the wrapping does not pull the RL into hip flexion or abduction by moving the RL into good position while wrapping.
- While applying the TT wrap, ensure that the wrapping does not pull the RL into knee flexion by maintaining the knee in extension during wrapping.
- Two elastic bandages are usually required, but the number is determined by the size of the RL
  - TT usually use two 4-inch wraps
  - TF usually use one 4-inch and one 6-inch wrap; a large TF may require three wraps
- Wraps should be removed and reapplied about every 4 hours or whenever slippage occurs.

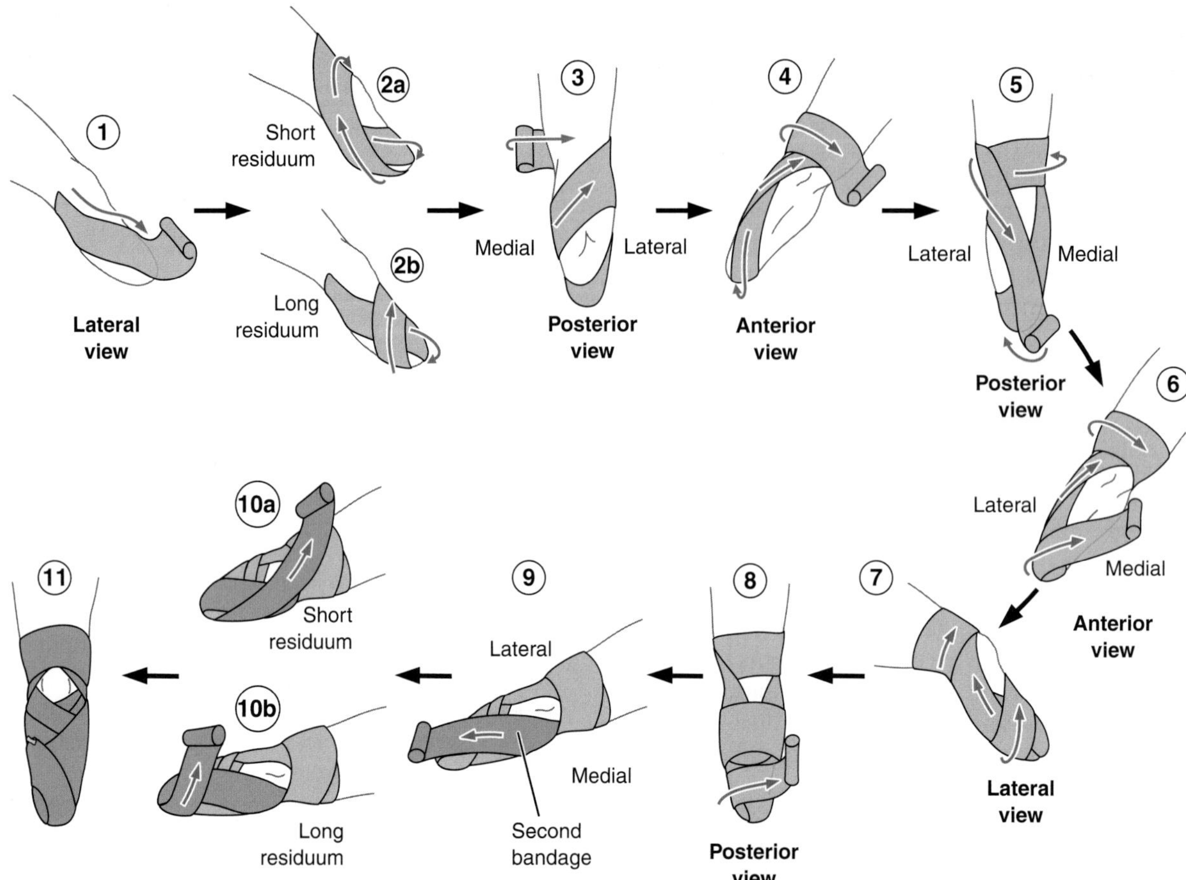

Figure 22.7 Transtibial residual limb bandaging. *(From May and Lockard,[46, p. 75] with permission.)*

Box 22.7 Transtibial Residual Limb Bandaging Technique*

- **Step 1:** Start the wrap at the medial or lateral tibial condyle and wrap diagonally over the anterior surface of the residual limb (RL) to the distal end, covering the midline of the incision. Continue diagonally over the posterior RL, to the beginning turn as an anchor. If the incision is anterior, wrap from posterior to anterior over the distal end to pull the soft tissue forward over the bone to facilitate a distal muscle cushion under the bone at the end of the RL.
- **Step 2:** The wrap may be brought directly over the beginning point (step 2a) or across the front of the residual limb in an X design (step 2b). The latter is useful with long RLs and aids in bandage suspension. Anchoring turns over the distal thigh suspend the wrap and shape the supracondylar region of the thigh for prosthetic fitting.
- **Steps 3–5:** After anchoring above the knee, the bandage is brought back around the opposite tibial condyle and down to the distal end of the RL. The bandage should overlap the midline of the incision and the other wrap by 1/2 inch to ensure adequate distal support.
- **Steps 5–8:** The figure-of-8 pattern is continued until the bandage is used up making sure to distribute the turns so the wrap is not too thick in any area from the distal end of the RL to the supracondylar region of the thigh. The patella may be covered or left open, depending on the specific needs of the individual.
- **Steps 9–11:** The second bandage is wrapped like the first, except that it is started at the opposite tibial condyle from the first wrap. Bringing the weave of each bandage in contraposition exerts a more even pressure. Effort is made to bring the angular turns across each other rather than in the same direction.
- After completing the wrap, check for and correct any gaps or wrinkles. Check to make sure that the knee has not been pulled into flexion by the wrap.

*Step numbers refer to Figure 22.7.

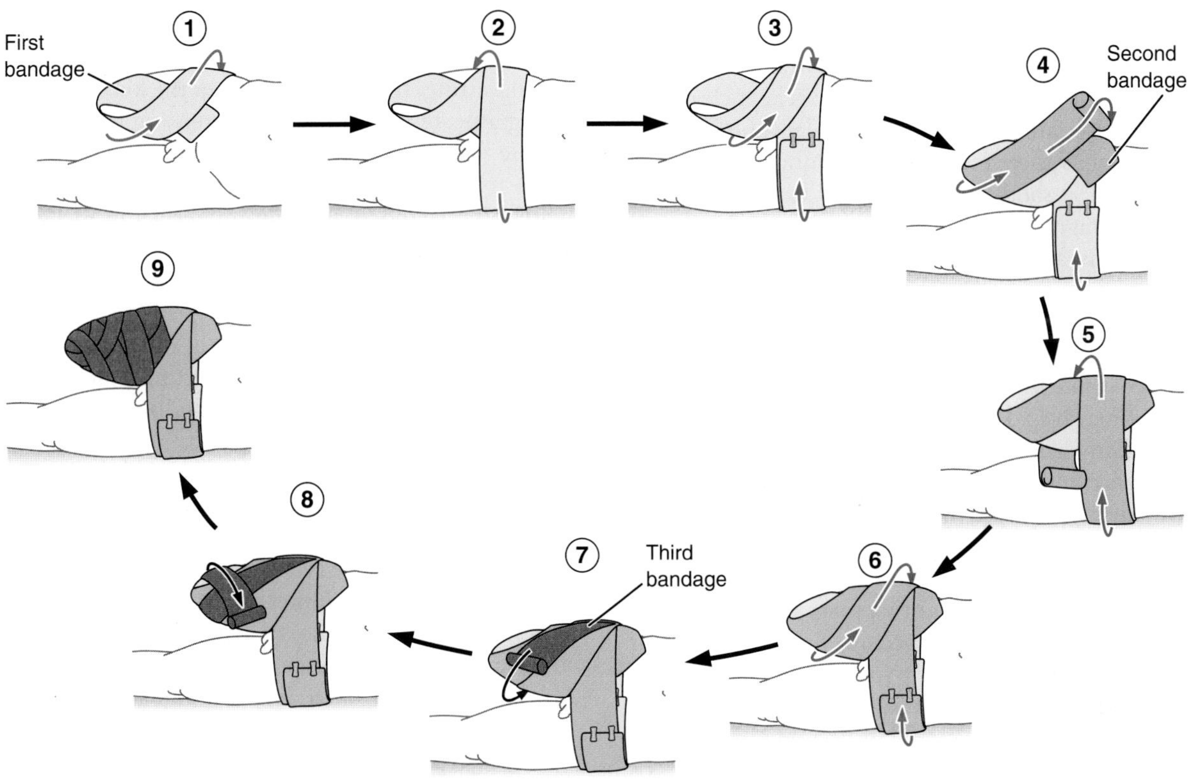

Figure 22.8 Transfemoral residual limb bandaging. *(From May and Lockard,[46, p. 76] with permission.)*

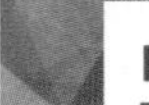

Box 22.8 Transfemoral Residual Limb Bandaging Technique*

- Positioning in side-lying or standing is preferred. Wrapping in sitting or supine can result in pulling the residual limb (RL) into flexion or abduction.
- A combination of 6- and 4-inch elastic bandages are used depending on RL size. Double length wraps can be purchased. Two or 3 wraps may be used.
- **Step 1:** Start the first bandage in the groin; wrap diagonally over the anterior surface to the distal lateral corner, covering at least half of the distal end of the RL. Continue diagonally up the posterior RL and cross and anchor the beginning of the wrap high in the groin. Continue around the iliac crest to form a hip spica. Move the hip into extension to prevent a flexion and abduction pull by the wrap.
- **Steps 2 and 3:** Continue figure-of-8 wraps with diagonal turns. The wrap must be high in the groin (to the pubic ramus) to prevent an adductor roll (proximal soft tissue that is not contained within the wrap). An adductor roll makes prosthetic socket fitting difficult and socket wear painful.
- **Steps 4–6:** The second bandage is wrapped like the first but is started more laterally; it is anchored in a hip spica after the first figure-of-8. Prevention of an adductor roll is important but be careful not to create a proximal tourniquet effect.
- **Steps 7–9:** If a third 4-in. bandage is used, it should exert greater pressure over middle and distal areas of the RL without a spica. Start laterally to bring the wrap across the previous wraps.
- After completing the wrap, check for and correct any gaps or wrinkles. Check to make sure that the hip has not been pulled into flexion or abduction by the wrap.

*Step numbers refer to Figure 22.8.

who are not able to properly wrap the limb. Shrinkers are not used until the incision is healed and the sutures removed; distraction forces that may occur during donning can cause wound dehiscence (splitting open). A small study of individuals with transtibial amputation who were taught proper bandaging techniques found that wrapping was slightly more effective in reducing edema.[70] However, a systematic review of the management of RL volume revealed limited evidence that can be used to guide clinical decision making.[71]

Skin Care

Proper hygiene and skin care are important. The RL is treated as any other part of the body; it is kept clean and dry. The application of lotions is usually not recommended, unless there is a specific reason; however, if a lotion is used, it should be non-alcohol based, hypoallergenic, and fragrance-free. Care must be taken to avoid abrasions, cuts, and other skin problems. Appropriate scar massage techniques can be used to prevent or mobilize adherent scar tissue. The massage is done gently, after the wound is healed and when no infection is present. Properly performed gentle friction massage to mobilize the scar and RL tissues may help decrease hypersensitivity to touch and pressure. Early handling of the RL by the patient is an aid to acceptance and is encouraged, particularly for individuals who may be repulsed by the limb. For individuals with hypersensitivity, desensitization techniques can be used, including gently brushing the RL with a soft material, progressing to rougher materials or tapping.[72]

The patient is taught to inspect the limb with a mirror each night to ensure there are no sores or impending problems, especially in areas not readily visible. If the person has diminished sensation, careful inspection is particularly important. Because the RL tends to become edematous after bathing, nightly bathing is recommended, particularly once a prosthesis has been fitted. The elastic bandage, shrinker, or removable rigid dressing is reapplied after bathing. If the person has been fitted with a prosthesis, the RL is wrapped at night and any time the prosthesis is not worn until it is fully mature (i.e., does not develop edema when not wearing a prosthesis).

The skin of the RL may be affected by a variety of dermatological problems such as eczema, psoriasis, contact dermatitis, or other rashes. Specific care is prescribed and coordinated among the physician, therapist, and prosthetist.

Range of Motion Exercise

An important deterrent to successful and comfortable use of a prosthesis is contractures of the hip or knee. In fact, contractures have been shown to predict poor prosthetic functional mobility.[73] The most common and functionally limiting contractures in the transfemoral RL are flexion and abduction; in the transtibial RL hip and knee flexion contractures are most common and limiting. These contractures make prosthetic fitting difficult and walking with a prosthesis painful, slow, or inefficient. Joint contractures in the intact limb also affect gait and must be identified and reduced. The best treatment for contractures is prevention. Patients should understand the importance of proper positioning and regular exercise in preparing for eventual prosthetic fit and ambulation. For all levels of amputation, full ROM in hip extension is critical in allowing the individual to assume a balanced upright posture without the need for pelvic or spinal compensations that may lead to gait asymmetries and back pain.[63,69]

With the transtibial amputation, full ROM in both hips and the knee, particularly in extension, is needed. While sitting, the patient can keep the knee extended by using a posterior splint or an extension board attached to the wheelchair; some facilities recommend using a knee immobilizer during sitting or lying. The patient with a transfemoral amputation needs full ROM in the hip, particularly in extension and adduction. Prolonged sitting should be avoided by all. At least 30 minutes each day should be spent in the prone position.

Some individuals, however, will develop hip or knee flexion contractures. Mild contractures may respond to various stretching techniques, including active and passive exercises and neurophysiological techniques, such as contract-relax and hold-relax methods. Although low load-prolonged stretching exercises are effective for improving ROM, they are often difficult to administer in the presence of amputation because the RL lever arm length may be too short to effectively position and load the shortened tissues. It is very difficult to reduce moderate to severe contractures by manual stretching, especially hip flexion contractures. An alternative method to reduce a transtibial knee flexion contracture for an individual who is ready for prosthetic fitting is to provide a prosthesis that is aligned to place the hamstrings on stretch with each step. If this "stretch during walking" technique is used, therapists must carefully instruct and monitor the patient while walking to ensure that stretching occurs without excessive abnormal socket pressure on the RL. This technique requires careful monitoring and frequent alignment adjustments to produce a good outcome. Hip flexion contractures are frequently found in persons with transfemoral amputations. It is difficult to "walk out" a hip flexion contracture with the transfemoral prosthesis because prosthetic knee instability and falls may result. Alternatively, pelvic and spinal compensation may occur that lead to low back pain. In some instances, depending on the severity of the contracture and the length of the RL, the contracture can be accommodated in the alignment of the prosthesis. A knee flexion contracture of less than 15° is not usually a problem. Prevention, however, continues to be the best treatment for contractures.

Exercises to Improve Muscle Function

Although there are few research studies that document the effectiveness of exercise programs for persons with amputation, there is evidence that physical fitness is a factor that predicts prosthetic success.[28,74,75] Thus, exercise programs to improve muscle function are included in preprosthetic rehabilitation. Exercises to improve muscle strength and endurance are prescribed for the RL as well as the intact lower limb and upper extremities. The type of postsurgical dressing, volume containment, degree of postoperative pain, and healing of the incision will determine when resistive exercises for the involved extremity can be started. The exercise program can take many forms and must include exercises that the patient performs independently when not in therapy. The hip extensors and abductors, core trunk stabilizer muscles, and knee extensors are particularly important for effective prosthetic ambulation.[27,75,76] Figures 22.9 and 22.10 depict examples of exercises to strengthen key muscles around the hip and knee. Exercises in which the patient pushes the RL against a towel roll or bolster to lift the trunk using hip extensors (Fig 22.9F) and resistive hip abduction exercises (Fig 22.10E) performed in supine and side-lying are important because they simulate activity of important muscles used during gait. These exercises also expose the RL to contact pressures, simulating the pressure imposed by the prosthetic socket while walking. Exercises to

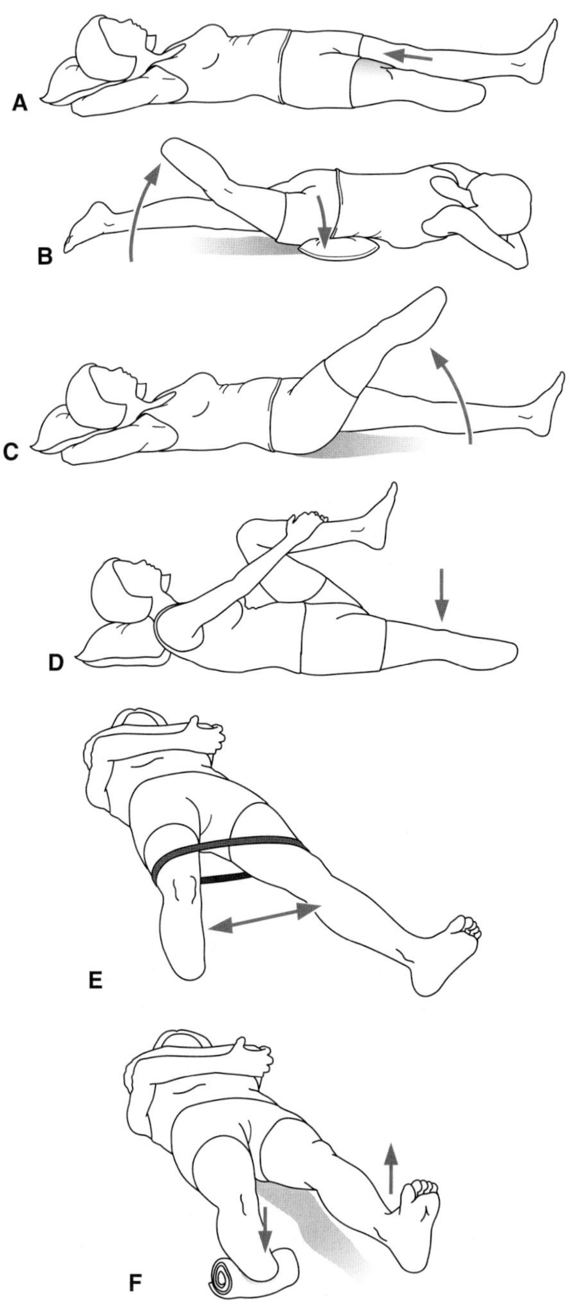

A

B

C

D

E

F

Figure 22.9 Transtibial exercises: (A) quadriceps sets. (B) Hip extension with knee straight. (C) Straight leg raise. (D) Hip and knee extension of the residual limb with opposite knee against chest. (E) Hip abduction against resistance (also performed in side-lying). (F) Hip extension against a towel roll "bridging." *(From May and Lockard,[46, p. 77] with permission.)*

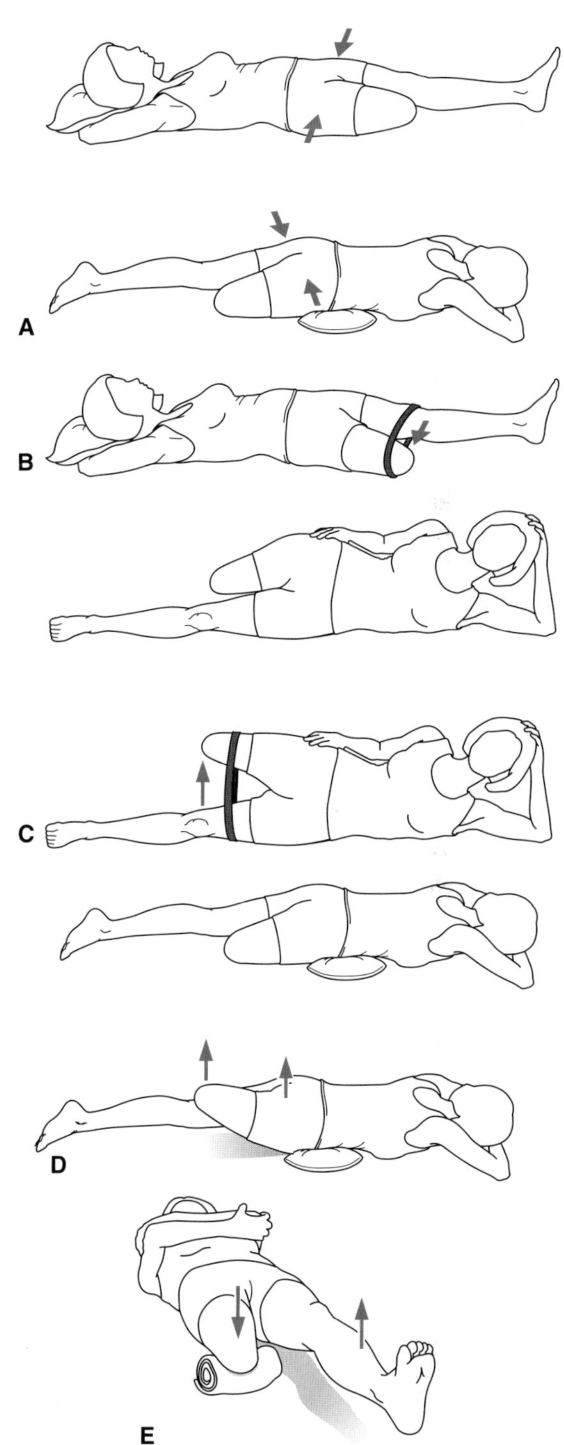

Figure 22.10 Transfemoral exercises: (A) Gluteal sets. (B) Hip abduction supine against resistance. (C) Hip abduction side-lying active and resistive. (D) Hip extension prone. (E) Hip extension against a towel roll "bridging." *(From May and Lockard,[46, p. 78] with permission.)*

strengthen trunk and spine stabilizer muscles are also important for all persons with amputation. Exercises must be progressed with increased resistance or modifications to increase the challenge when appropriate and to remain relevant.

Balance and Mobility Activities

Early mobility and independence in functional activities is important to physiological and psychological recovery following amputation. Balance is a key element to safe and effective mobility. Poor balance and fear of falling have been found to negatively affect successful prosthetic rehabilitation and social activity.[77,78] Although individuals with unilateral amputation usually do not have a problem with unperturbed sitting balance, it is important for the individual to develop good standing balance on the remaining limb. Poor balance confidence is a persistent problem after amputation.[78] Even after prosthetic fitting, many prosthesis users continue to report that they modify their participation because of the potential for falls.[79] Patients with amputation have lost some of the proprioceptive input and response strategies used for balance. In addition, research has shown that the postural responses to balance perturbation are altered and slower in the amputated and intact lower limbs in LE prosthesis users.[80] Activities to help patients develop balance skills and confidence must begin early in rehabilitation. Single leg balance exercises can be designed by progressively introducing balance challenges with compliant surfaces, upper limb movements, and distracting activities, such as throwing/catching a ball. Figure 22.11 illustrates one type of standing balance exercise on a compliant surface. Weight-bearing through the RL is also beneficial to future prosthetic training. This can only be safely achieved in patients with transtibial amputations. Figure 22.12 depicts a person kneeling on a cushion placed on a chair of appropriate height, shifting weight on and off the amputated side. Weight-bearing and shifting activities can also be performed in kneeling on a mat table with progression to "stepping" forward and backward with alternate knees.

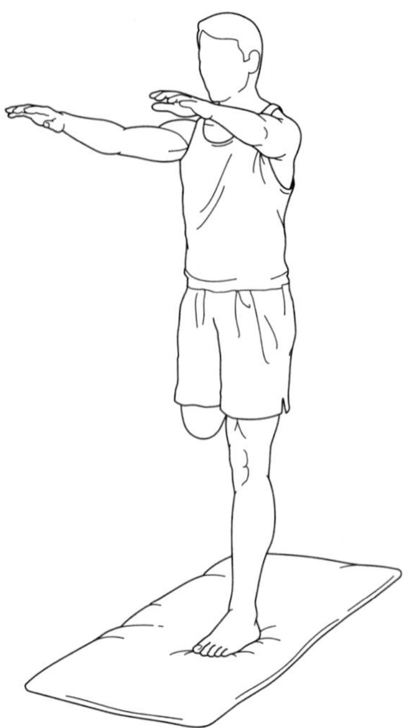

Figure 22.11 Standing balance exercise on a compliant surface. *(From May and Lockard,[46, p. 73] with permission.)*

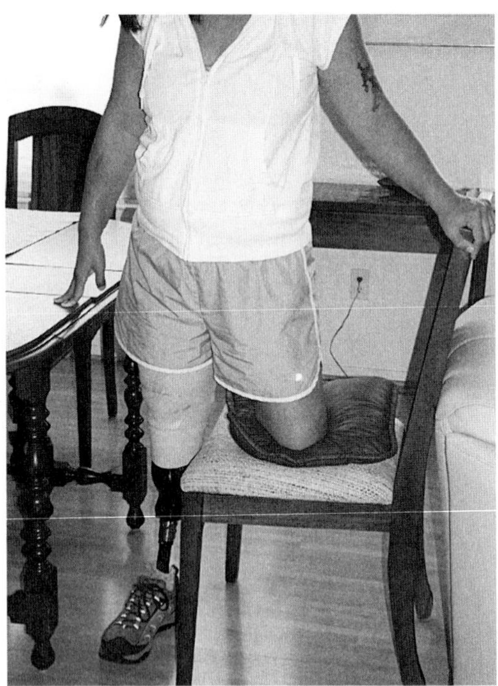

Figure 22.12 Kneeling on a pillow on a chair provides an opportunity for some weight-bearing. *(From May and Lockard,[46, p. 74] with permission.)*

Walking is an excellent exercise and necessary for independence in daily life. Gait training can start early and the person with a unilateral LE amputation can become quite independent using a three-point gait pattern on crutches. Many older individuals have difficulty learning to walk on crutches. Some are afraid, some lack the necessary balance and coordination, and others lack endurance. Walking with crutches without a prosthesis requires a greater expenditure of energy than walking with a prosthesis.

Independence in crutch walking is an outcome worthy of therapy time. The individual who can ambulate with crutches will develop a greater degree of general fitness than the person who spends most of the time in a wheelchair. Crutch walking is good preparation for prosthetic ambulation and the person who can learn to use crutches generally will not have difficulty learning to use a prosthesis. However, the individual who cannot learn to walk with crutches independently may be independent using a walker.

A walker is more stable than crutches but cannot be used safely on stairs and curbs. It is sometimes difficult for the person who has used a walker following the amputation to switch to crutches or a cane when fitted with a prosthesis. The gait pattern used with a walker is not appropriate with a prosthesis and should not be used for prosthetic training. A walker encourages a flexed posture and a step-to gait pattern, whereas efficient prosthetic use requires an erect, extended posture and a step-through gait pattern. However, all individuals with an amputation need to learn some form of safe mobility without a prosthesis for use at night or when the prosthesis cannot be worn. For some individuals, this may need to be a walker.

Exercise for Cardiopulmonary Endurance

Ambulation and functional activity require energy expenditure. At rest in healthy individuals the rate of metabolic energy expenditure (oxygen consumption or VO_2) is 3.5 mL/kg per minute. As the rate of ambulation or functional activity increases, oxygen consumption and heart rate response increase linearly, using aerobic metabolism. When the intensity of the activity requires an individual to consume oxygen ≥ 50% of his or her maximum capacity (VO_{2max}), the anaerobic threshold (AT) is reached, and a portion of the metabolism becomes anaerobic. Continued higher intensity activity will be limited by the accumulation of metabolites and muscle fatigue. The relationship between energy expenditure and ambulation speed with an amputation is also linear, but the slope is greater than in normal individuals. Thus, at any walking speed, individuals with an amputation use metabolic energy at a higher rate and will reach AT at a slower walking speed. In addition, they exhibit a greater heart rate response and increased cardiac work load compared to individuals without amputation walking at the same speed.[81] Another important variable to consider when evaluating the metabolic consequences of ambulation with an amputation is energy cost. Energy cost is oxygen consumption relative to the distance walked, rather than per unit of time. Thus, this variable defines endurance, or how long a person can continue to walk before fatigue causes him or her to stop. The energy cost of ambulation with a prosthesis has been variably reported but is increased at all levels of lower limb amputation.[81] Box 22.9 shows the impact of amputation cause and level on the energy cost of ambulation with a prosthesis. Ambulation without a prosthesis using crutches is more energy expensive than walking with a prosthesis.[82] Additionally, walking with a prosthesis and crutches shows increased energy expenditure compared to walking with a prosthesis alone.[83] Many additional factors may affect the energy cost of walking, including prosthetic componentry, gait pattern and symmetry, the level of walking skill or efficiency, and balance confidence. However, in general, prosthesis users, particularly older persons with high-level vascular amputations, have a higher energy cost of walking, walk at slower, less efficient speeds, resulting in poorer walking endurance.[84,85] Prosthesis users may be able to walk at the same speed as peers without amputation, but they are working at a higher percentage of their maximum aerobic capacity, thus they use more energy and may not be able to sustain the speed. Therefore, peak aerobic capacity is an important determinant for walking ability, and appropriately prescribed aerobic exercise training must be included in rehabilitation programs at all levels.[85] Various types of exercise can be used to increase aerobic capacity, walking distance, and speed, but it is important to define the aerobic training stimulus with a specific target heart rate and duration and frequency of the exercise. Some examples include LE ergometry using the intact leg alone, UE ergometry and treadmill training, with or without body weight support.[86-89] It is of importance to note that military personnel with traumatic amputations who were provided with a comprehensive, intensive rehabilitation program achieved metabolic energy expenditure with their prostheses that was equivalent to their able-bodied peers.[90]

Box 22.9 Metabolic Costs of Ambulation with a Prosthesis[81]

- Partial foot: increased approx. 15%
- Traumatic transtibial: increased approx. 25%
- Vascular transtibial: increased approx. 40%
- Traumatic transfemoral: increased approx. 68%
- Vascular transfemoral: increased approx. 100%

Management of Phantom Limb Pain

Postoperative RL pain usually improves as healing progresses, edema is reduced and mobility restored. However, persons with trauma-related amputations were 1.5 times more likely to report persistent RL pain.[63] This may be associated with trauma-related structural abnormalities, neuromas, bone spicules, or heterotopic ossifications in the RL, which may require surgical revision. Phantom limb pain (PLP), however, can become persistent and debilitating. In a national survey of persons with amputations of all ages and from all causes, 80% reported PLP, regardless of time since amputation; the average intensity reported was 5.5 (1 = extremely mild pain; 10 = extremely intense pain). Eighty-one percent of those with phantom pain were bothered by it, and about 33% reported they were extremely bothered.[63] Severe and constant PLP is reported most often by those with upper limb amputation. Seventy-three percent of individuals reported their PLP was intermittent.[63] Thus, PLP must be identified and addressed early. There is some evidence that preemptive epidural anesthesia and immediate postoperative regional analgesia may prevent the development of PLP, but the results of studies are equivocal and many persons develop PLP.[91]

There are many and varied treatments for PLP because its specific cause is still undetermined. Treatments are classified as pharmacological and nonpharmacological. Usual analgesics, such as acetaminophen and NSAIDs may mildly reduce pain intensity.[91] Opioids, such as morphine, and ketamine offer some short-term pain relief but have significant adverse effects, which interfere with usual functional activity.[92] Gabapentin also may offer some short-term pain relief without the adverse effects, but effectiveness is unclear. The effects of medications, such as tricyclic antidepressants and anticonvulsants, used to treat chronic neuropathic pain, are variable and unclear when used to treat PLP.[91,92] Botulinum toxin A and calcitonin did not seem effective.[92] Owing to the lack of evidence for the effectiveness of pharmacological treatments for PLP and the relatively high occurrence of adverse effects, there is a greater focus on nonpharmacological interventions.

Nonpharmacological treatments for PLP include invasive and noninvasive interventions.[91] Invasive neuromodulation interventions include deep brain stimulation and spinal cord or dorsal root ganglion stimulation.[91,93] In some small studies, dorsal root ganglion stimulation has shown some success, without significant negative side effects.[93] Noninvasive techniques that have shown some efficacy in small trials include transcranial direct current stimulation of the motor cortex, transcutaneous electric nerve stimulation (TENS), acupuncture, and hypnosis.[94-97]

A current theory for the cause of PLP that has accrued considerable supporting evidence is neuroplastic changes in the brain due to deafferentation caused by amputation. Based on this theory, treatments have been developed that target neuroplastic mechanisms to restore neural representation of the missing limb through motor imagery.[98] Therapies in this domain include the use of visual feedback via mirrors or virtual reality, whereby the patient observes movements executed by their intact limb, viewed in a mirror or a virtual environment, and then couple the observed movement with movement of the phantom limb.[99,100] In augmented virtual reality, myoelectric signals from activation of the muscles of the RL are used to create a virtual body part that executes motor tasks in a virtual environment. Using a conventional webcam and monitor, patients observe themselves with a virtual limb (replacing their phantom) that they can actively move to accomplish virtual tasks by activating their RL muscles. Because the virtual limb images are created from myoelectric signals from the RL, unlike mirror therapy, this treatment can be used by persons with bilateral amputations. Early results have been quite favorable.[101,102]

Psychological Support

The patient needs to receive reassurance and understanding from the entire rehabilitation team. Team members should create an open and receptive environment and be willing to listen to the patient's questions and concerns. The patient should know what to expect during the entire process. The physician and therapists should carefully explain the steps and expectations of rehabilitation, using methods that are compatible with the patient's preferred learning style. The Amputee Coalition of America (ACA) is a national, nonprofit consumer education and advocacy organization representing people who have experienced amputation or were born with limb differences (www.amputee-coalition.org). The ACA provides training for peer visitors, individuals with amputations who are trained to provide emotional support and motivation by visiting individuals with recent amputations. Therapists should be cognizant of local ACA chapters and make use of the organization to support and educate their patients. A peer visitation program can also be developed from previous successful patients.

Patients have various attitudes and goals regarding a prosthesis. Some are most concerned with regaining the greatest level of function possible; others are more concerned about its appearance and cosmesis. Therapists must be sensitive to the specific concerns of each patient and advocate for their individual goals in prosthetic prescription and training. Good predictors for adjustment to the prosthesis are active involvement in the rehabilitation program and consistent attempts to return to an active lifestyle and social interaction. Therapists must foster and develop active participation by the patient.

Preparatory and Definitive Prostheses

Many individuals are not fitted with a prosthetic appliance until the RL is healed and free from edema. During this 6- to 12-week period, the patient is limited to mobility using a wheelchair or ambulation with crutches or a walker. The first prosthesis may be a temporary or preparatory prosthesis, made with simple components. However, separate temporary prostheses are not used often today in the United States. A definitive prosthesis is one that is permanent. Since definitive prosthetic componentry is modular (parts can be changed out or replaced without affecting the rest of the prosthesis), if the RL continues to shrink and the socket is too large, a new socket can be manufactured to replace the original one without replacing the rest of the prosthesis. Once fitted with a first prosthesis, the RL may continue to change in size and a second socket is often required within the first 2 years. Many third-party payers (insurers) will not fund a temporary prosthesis, so early permanent fitting is advocated, even though the socket may become too big quite quickly and require replacement.

Early bipedal ambulation is a desired goal for most individuals following amputation. The longer the delay in fitting with a prosthesis, the lower the potential for effective rehabilitation. Care should be taken that the patient is fitted with optimum components for his or her expected level of function. Too often, older individuals are fitted with low-cost, low-function components when they probably could achieve a higher level of function with more functional components. Therapists must clearly and objectively document functional performance and potential and justify the prescription of an appropriate prosthesis that will maximize function and ambulation.

Patient Education

Patient education is an integral and ongoing part of the rehabilitation program. Information on the care of the RL; proper care of the uninvolved extremity, positioning, exercises, and diet (if the patient has diabetes or is overweight), is necessary for the patient to be a full participant in the rehabilitation program. Discussions should also be held regarding patient goals, projected activity levels, funding, and prosthetic components. If the patient underwent the amputation for vascular problems, the education program should include information on proper footwear.

Care must be taken not to overwhelm the patient with too much information at one time; information overload leads to forgetfulness. It is more effective to prioritize the information and ask the person to remember one new thing each session rather than try to teach a complex program at one time. Visual materials using media compatible with the client's preferred learning style are necessary to supplement the teaching and help the patient remember what is required. It is also important for the program to be tailored to the individual's way of life. Involving the patient in establishing priorities enhances adherence. Appendix 22.A includes Web-based resources for clinicians, families, and patients with amputation.

Bilateral Amputation

Intervention for the person with bilateral LE amputations is similar to the program developed for someone with a unilateral amputation. If the individual was previously fitted with a prosthesis and ambulated after unilateral amputation, the prosthesis is useful for transfer activities and limited ambulation. Some individuals may be able to use the prosthesis with external support to get around more easily, particularly for bathroom activities.

Most individuals with bilateral amputations need a wheelchair on a permanent basis, even if they use prostheses for ambulation because there will always be times when the prostheses cannot be worn. The chair should be as narrow as possible (for the size of the patient with prostheses, if worn) and lightweight to facilitate community mobility. Removable desk arms and removable leg rests are necessary. Elevating armrests are useful to assist in sit-to-stand transfers. Amputee wheelchairs with offset rear wheels and no leg rests are not recommended unless the therapist is sure that the person will never be fitted with prostheses. It is easier to add antitipping devices to the rear of the wheelchair or attach small weights to the front uprights (counterbalance) for use when the footrests are removed and no prostheses are worn.

The exercise program includes mat activities designed to help the person regain a sense of body position and balance; balance is usually more challenging for individuals with bilateral lower limb amputations. Upper extremity and RL strengthening and ROM exercises are also important. Functional mobility training should stress independence in bed mobility, transfers, and wheelchair use. With bilateral amputations, individuals spend considerable time sitting and are therefore more prone to develop flexion contractures, particularly around the hip joints. The patient should be encouraged to sleep prone if possible, or at least spend time in the prone position each day. With the variety of prosthetic componentry options available today, many persons with bilateral lower limb amputations can walk functionally with prostheses. Thus, rehabilitation for persons with bilateral amputations should be similar to, and as intensive as, rehabilitation for individuals with unilateral amputations. Energy expenditure during functional activities with or without prostheses is quite high. Thus, all programs for persons with bilateral amputations must include cardiopulmonary exercise training to maximize functional potential.

■ PREDICTING PROSTHETIC POTENTIAL

The ability to accurately predict prosthetic functional mobility from pre- and postamputation patient characteristics has been pursued for many years. Recognition of characteristics that predict prosthetic use and positive functional outcomes at different levels of amputation would help the patient with poor vascular status and critical limb ischemia and his or her surgeon to decide on the best surgical approach to disease management.[28] Evidence that certain patient characteristics are strongly associated with successful prosthetic mobility would also help therapists and physicians advocate for patients with third-party payors to provide for prostheses and prosthetic rehabilitation. To this end, researchers developed and validated the AMPREDICT, an instrument that can be used by clinicians to predict mobility outcome after LE amputation at different levels secondary to vascular compromise.[28] This instrument utilizes the presence or absence of patient characteristics that were identified as important to predict the probability of achieving independent basic or advanced functional mobility with a prosthesis.[28] A recent systematic literature review identified characteristics of all types of patients (not just those with dysvascular amputation) that predict prosthetic walking ability following lower limb amputation.[103] The most strongly supported factors for considering prosthetic candidacy were amputation level (lower), age (younger), physical fitness (cardiorespiratory endurance/aerobic capacity), and no or few comorbidities. Moderately supported factors for prosthetic candidacy included cognition/mood disturbance, etiology, ability to stand on one leg, and preamputation living status. Another research group identified clinical assessments administered to patients after amputation, but before the decision to fit with a prosthesis, that yield predictors of prosthetic use.[73] The report indicated that age (younger), level of amputation (lower), absence of contractures, ability to stand on one leg for ≥ 10 seconds (a proxy for balance and strength), and cognitive function (as measured by the Trail Making Test) were predictive of successful functional mobility with a prosthesis.[73] Another study identified balance on the remaining leg and RL hip extensor strength as predictive of successful prosthetic use.[27]

Although recognition of the factors associated with successful prosthetic use is helpful, it still leaves unanswered questions regarding the decision to fit a particular patient with a prosthesis. For example, there is evidence that being older and having a higher level of amputation makes it less likely that a patient will become an independent prosthetic user, but, in fact, some older individuals with transfemoral amputations do become independent in ambulation with a prosthesis. Thus, an instrument that predicts the likelihood that a particular individual with an amputation will be able to ambulate successfully with a prosthesis based on his or her current performance is most desirable.

Medicare developed a functional classification system for persons with amputation. It is used to classify individuals according to their potential to achieve independent functional mobility with a prosthesis at home and in the community, as well as to achieve advanced sports or work-related activities. The classification levels are described in Box 22.10. These levels are used to determine the medical necessity of a prosthesis and to determine the types of prosthetic components (e.g., types of prosthetic knees and feet) available to patients in each category. Although the classification system is promulgated by Medicare, it is used by many insurers to determine coverage for a prosthesis for an individual. Thus, it is important for therapists to be able to objectively measure individual patient functional capabilities. However, substantiating and justifying a prosthetic prescription requires an instrument that measures current physical performance without a prosthesis to predict ability to ambulate with a prosthesis. The Amputee Mobility Predictor (AMP) is a reliable instrument that has been validated to make this prediction.[104] For patients with unilateral amputation, versions are available for those with a prosthesis (AMPPRO) as well as for those without a prosthesis (AMPnoPRO). It is a 20-item assessment of a patient's ability to perform functional tasks required for successful prosthetic ambulation. It can be administered and scored in about 15 minutes.[104] To make the instrument usable for individuals with bilateral amputations (AMP-B), five items were modified and the scoring system adjusted.[105] All instruments have been shown to predict performance on the 6-Minute Walk Test.[104,105]

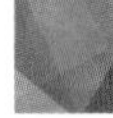

Box 22.10 Medicare Functional Classification Levels

- **Functional level 0 (K0):** The patient does not have the ability or potential to ambulate or transfer safely with or without assistance and a prosthesis does not enhance his or her quality of life or mobility.
- **Functional level 1 (K1):** The patient has the ability or potential to use a prosthesis for transfers or ambulation on level surfaces at fixed cadence. Typical of the limited and unlimited household ambulator.
- **Functional level 2 (K2):** The patient has the ability or potential for ambulation with the ability to traverse low-level environmental barriers such as curbs, stairs, or uneven surfaces. Typical of the limited community ambulator.
- **Functional level 3 (K3):** The patient has the ability or potential for ambulation with variable cadence. Typical of the community ambulator who has the ability to traverse most environmental barriers and may have vocational, therapeutic, or exercise activity that demands prosthetic utilization beyond simple locomotion.
- **Functional level 4 (K4):** The patient has the ability or potential for prosthetic ambulation that exceeds basic ambulation skills, exhibiting high-impact, stress, or energy levels. Typical of the prosthetic demands of the child, active adult, or athlete.

PROSTHETIC TRAINING

The major goal of prosthetic rehabilitation is to attain a smooth, energy-efficient gait that allows the individual to perform ADL and participate in desired social, employment, and recreational activities. Prosthetic ambulation is a skilled psychomotor activity and the person must learn to adapt well-developed patterns of movement to new situations. Box 22.11 outlines general motor skills required to achieve an effective prosthetic gait. In general, gait training must guide the individual to integrate the prosthesis into all mobility activities. Table 22.3 presents basic prosthetic training elements, starting with basic balance and progressing to ambulation.[106] Although the table depicts training with a transfemoral prosthesis, the sequence is equally appropriate for transtibial prosthetic training other than the knee control step.

Some gait or prosthetic control skills are specific for certain prosthetic components. For example, certain types of microprocessor-controlled knees and power knees require specific techniques to operative their control features.[107,108] Walking with a microprocessor knee is different from walking with a prosthesis with a

Box 22.11 Skills Required for Efficient Prosthetic Gait

- Accept and support body weight on each leg at the instant of initial contact
- Balance on one foot in single-limb support without excessive sway
- Symmetrical stance time on prosthetic and intact lower limb
- Maintain erect trunk and spine stability in stance and swing; minimize pelvic tilt and excessive frontal plane trunk compensatory movements
- Execute anterior transverse pelvic rotation (on the prosthetic side) during stance to advance pressure on the prosthetic foot all the way to the toe
- Advance each limb with symmetrical step lengths
- Adapt to environmental demands, such as uneven terrain, obstacle avoidance, inclines, and steps without stumble

conventionally controlled knee. The therapist must be knowledgeable of the requirements of each type of componentry and teach the appropriate gait skills. To use energy storing and releasing (ESAR) prosthetic feet effectively, users must shift weight onto the foot at initial contact and advance the pelvis over the foot through late stance phase to ensure deflection of the toe and optimal use of foot features. Box 22.12 provides examples of specific exercises that can be used in prosthetic gait training with an ESAR prosthetic foot.[109]

It is important to accomplish as much training as possible without the use of external support, as walking is more efficient without it. If found necessary, a cane may be added for safety once there is good control of weight shifting on and off the prosthesis and a step-through progression has been achieved. Therapists should not plan to begin prosthetic training with a walker and progress to a cane or less restrictive device because this will most likely not be successful. In addition, it is very

Table 22.3 Prosthetic Training Elements

Element	Activity	Details
Stability—both legs (TT/TF)	Secure standing without hand support; reaching for objects.	Hold an object a reachable distance; patient reaches and touches objects with either hand looking at object. Objects placed high/low/right/left encouraging goal-oriented weight shifting.
Knee control (TF)	Secure standing without hand support; slightly bend and straighten prosthetic knee to varying degrees.	Encourage patient to develop kinesthetic feel of knee position by socket pressures.

Continued

Table 22.3 Prosthetic Training Elements—cont'd

Element	Activity	Details
Stability on prosthesis (TT/TF) 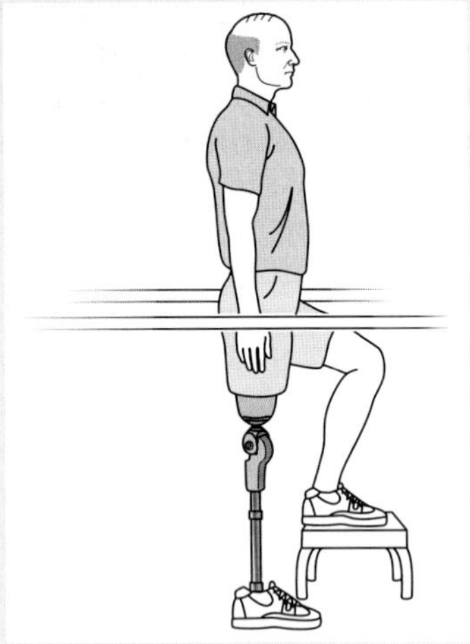	Secure standing without hand support; place 6–8 in. stool directly in front of patient.	In a controlled manner, patient places unamputated foot on stool and back on the floor.
Stability on prosthesis (TT/TF) 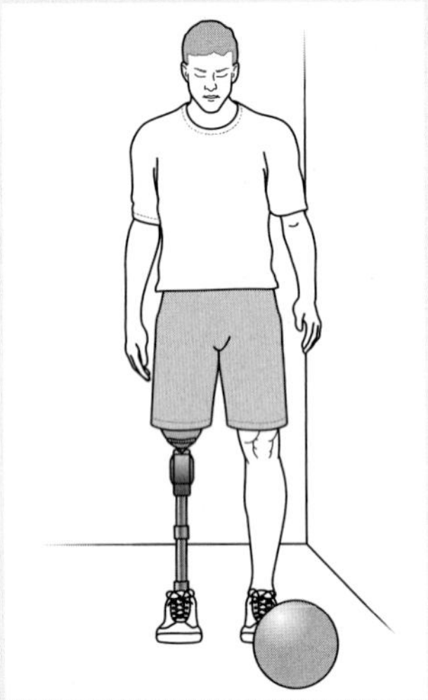	Secure standing without hand support; place soccer ball in front of unamputated leg.	In a controlled manner, patient kicks the ball with the unamputated foot.
Prosthetic control (TT/TF) 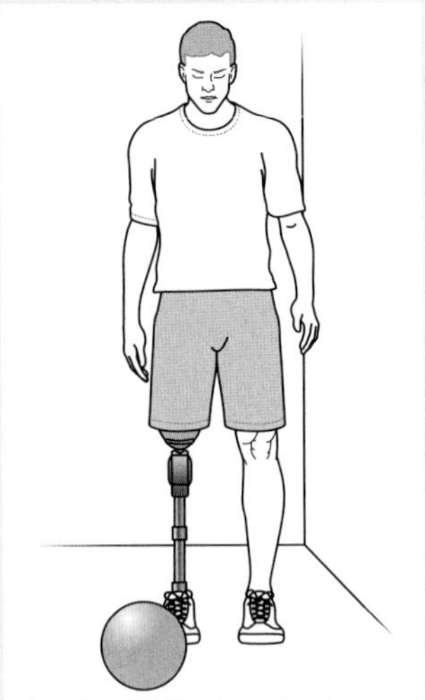	Secure standing without hand support; place soccer ball in front of prosthesis.	In a controlled manner, patient kicks the ball with the prosthetic leg.

Table 22.3 Prosthetic Training Elements—cont'd

Element	Activity	Details
Proprioception (TT/TF) 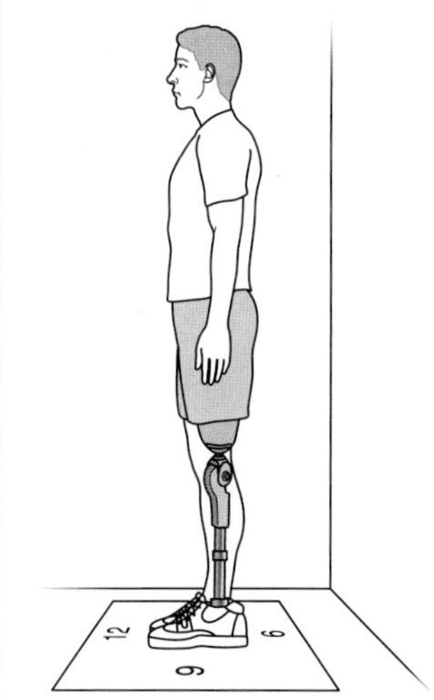	Secure standing both legs on a piece of paper with a clock face drawn and without hand support.	On command, patient shifts weight to 12, 3, 6, and 9 o'clock in random order. Learns to recognize where prosthetic foot is in relation to weight-bearing.
Pelvic control (TT/TF) 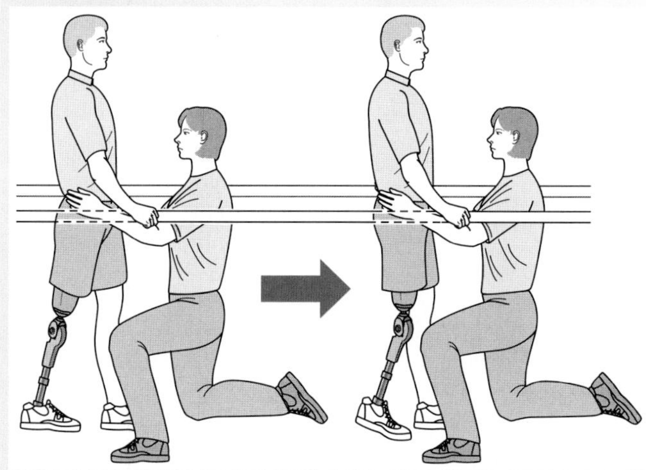	Secure standing without hand support prosthetic leg behind unamputated leg. Provide resistance to forward pelvic progression at initial contact to foot flat.	Encourage patient to transfer weight smoothly with forward and slight lateral pelvic motion by providing resistance as patient brings prosthesis forward.
Stepping with prosthesis (TT/TF) 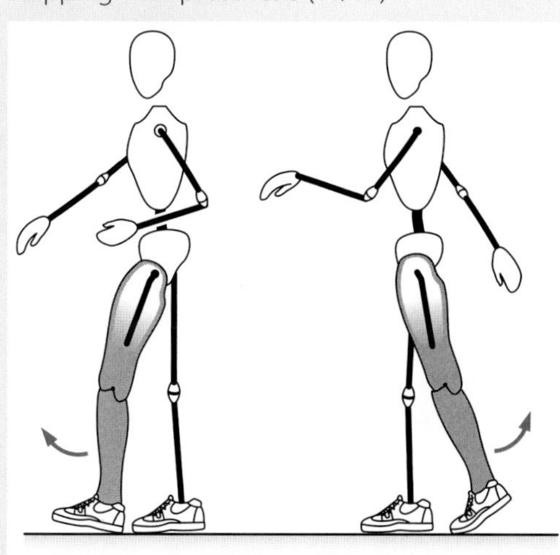	Secure standing without hand support, step forward and back with prosthesis.	Start with double leg stance, shift weight to unamputated leg and steps forward with prosthesis. Returns prosthesis to position behind sound leg. Emphasize knee control with TF.

Continued

Table 22.3 Prosthetic Training Elements—cont'd

Element	Activity	Details
Stepping with sound leg (TT/TF) 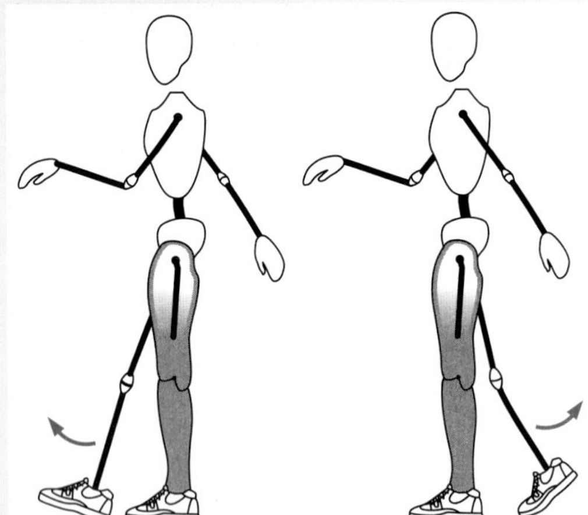	Secure standing without hand support, step forward and back with unamputated leg	As above but with unamputated leg. Make sure patient brings weight to forward part of foot before stepping on unamputated leg. Emphasize toe-off on TF to activate swing initiation.
Sidestepping; backward stepping (TT/TF) 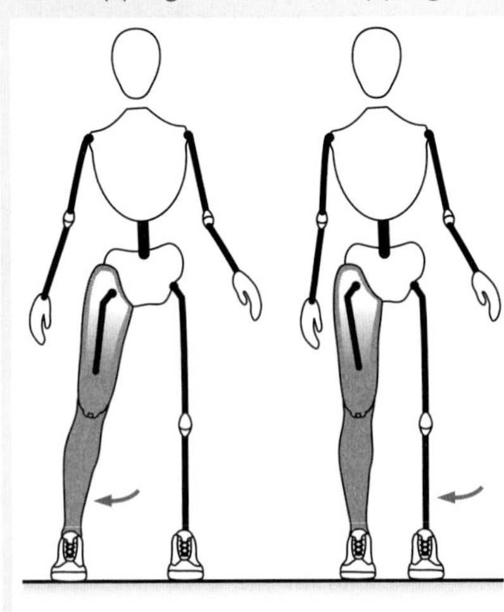	Consecutive steps to the right, then to the left without hand support. Stepping backward several steps.	Sidestepping, emphasize picking up the leg and placing it several inches to the side, then picking up the other leg to the first leg. TF backward stepping generally requires a larger prosthetic step than the unamputated for knee control.

From May and Lockard,[46, pp. 136–141] with permission.
TF = patient with transfemoral prosthesis; TT = patient with transtibial prosthesis

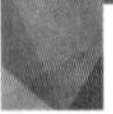

Box 22.12 Gait Training Exercises for Patients Using an Energy Storing and Releasing (ESAR) Prosthetic Foot[109]

- Stool stepping to improve single limb standing balance on the prosthetic foot
- Resistive gait training to enhance transverse pelvic rotation, pelvic advancement, and symmetry of movement during ambulation
- Resistive ambulation to promote dynamic balance and proper prosthetic toe-loading during late stance
- Ball rolls (with the intact foot) in three planes to increase the speed of hip muscle contraction to maintain prosthetic single limb balance during stance
- Trunk rotation to assist with balance and symmetry of movement
- Change of direction and turning skills; agility skills
- Addition exercises: www.amputee-coalition.org/military-instep/ten-exercises.html

difficult to use an appropriate prosthetic gait pattern with a walker. Leaning on a walker makes it almost impossible to advance the pelvis in the transverse plane to achieve proper weight-bearing through the prosthesis. A walker should be reserved for situations where the individual is so limited that it is the only safe option.

Gait Training

In addition to prosthetic training to teach patients how to correctly use the prosthesis and its components, gait training is required to improve the quality and efficiency of gait. Abnormal gait patterns, particularly gait asymmetries and over-dependence on the intact lower limb can lead to musculoskeletal overuse injuries and arthritis. Knee pain in the intact lower limb and back pain are common problems reported by prosthesis users.[59,63] People with limb loss commonly complain of back pain, which may be associated with a variety of possible causes, including poor posture, abnormal movements during gait, leg length discrepancy, poor prosthetic fit or alignment, or general deconditioning.[59] Knee pain and osteoarthritis in the intact leg is common and may be caused by increased stress and loading of the intact lower limb during walking and functional activities.[59] Physical therapy should include gait training to improve spaciotemporal and kinematic symmetry and the bioenergetics or efficiency of gait. A variety of gait training techniques are used, but few large or randomized controlled trials are published. A recent systematic literature review identified studies that reported on prosthetic gait training.[110] They classified studies as overground or treadmill training and reported with high confidence that gait training under skilled supervision is effective in improving spaciotemporal gait parameters in patients with LE amputations.[110] In addition to traditional gait training techniques, success has been reported using body-weight-supported treadmill training, virtual reality environments with moving platforms to improve balance, and gaming, such as Wii Fit. Table 22.4, the Evidence Summary Table, presents studies that investigated a variety of usual and novel interventions to improve gait and gait symmetry in persons with amputation.

Advanced Training

Changing the environment is an integral part of the gait training program. Functional ambulation takes place in complex environments. Walking around furniture, through narrow doorways, on rugs, and around obstacles

Table 22.4 Evidence Summary Prosthetic Gait Training

Highsmith, MJ, et al: Gait training interventions for lower extremity amputees: A systematic literature review. Technol Innov 18(2–3):99, 2016.

Design	Systematic review
Level of Evidence	II
Subjects	Individuals with transfemoral and transtibial amputations
Intervention	Prosthetic gait training
Results	13 studies using overground training and 5 studies using treadmill training met the inclusion criteria. Eight evidence statements were synthesized: 3 with moderate evidence, 5 with low evidence.
Comments	Therapeutic gait training under supervision with appropriate prosthetic component prescription is effective.

Agrawal, V, et al: Influence of gait training and prosthetic foot category on external work symmetry during unilateral transtibial amputee gait. Prosthet Orthot Int 37(5):396, 2013.

Design	Randomized repeated measures trial
Level of Evidence	III
Subjects	5 subjects with transtibial amputations, K-level 2; 5 subjects with transtibial amputations, K-level 3
Intervention	Each subject was tested with 4 different prosthetic feet on the same socket: SACH, SAFE, Talux, Proprio and standardized gait training
Results	The Talux (J-ankle, heel to toe footplate) provided the best symmetry of work for K-level 2 subjects.
Comments	Gait training can influence gait symmetry; K-level 2 subjects achieved greater work symmetry with K-3 feet (Talux, J-foot)

Continued

Table 22.4 Evidence Summary Prosthetic Gait Training—cont'd

Kaufman, K, et al: Task-specific fall prevention training is effective for warfighters with transtibial amputation. Clin Orthop Rel Res 472:3076, 2014.

Design	Prospective cohort study
Level of Evidence	III
Subjects	11 males with traumatic transtibial amputations, ages 18–40; all experienced prosthesis users
Intervention	Trip-specific fall prevention training program with a microprocessor controlled treadmill to provide bidirectional trip stimulus; 6 30-min training sessions over 2 weeks.
Results	Post-tests were at completion of training, 3 months, and 6 months. All subjects decreased trunk flexion angle (indicator of decreased falls risk on perturbation) and increased stepping ability on both legs and improved in balance confidence.
Comments	Results were maintained at 3 and 6 months.

Miller, CA, et al: Using Nintendo Wii Fit and body weight support to improve aerobic capacity, balance, gait ability, and fear of falling: Two case reports. J Geriatr Phys Ther 35(2):95, 2012.

Design	2 case reports
Level of Evidence	IV
Subjects	2 male subjects with transfemoral amputations; ages 58 and 62 yr.
Intervention	Wii Fit balance program and body weight supported treadmill gait training for 12 sessions over 6 weeks; 20 minutes of each intervention per session.
Results	Clinically important improvement in dynamic balance, balance confidence, spaciotemporal gait measures, and gait velocity. Decreased oxygen consumption for walking.
Comment	Neither subject reached performance equal to age matched control.

Imam, B, et al: A randomized controlled trial to evaluate the feasibility of the Wii Fit for improving walking in older adults with lower limb amputation. Clin Rehabil 31(1):82, 2015.

Design	Randomized controlled trial, with evaluator blinding
Level of Evidence	II
Subjects	Persons with lower limb amputation > 50 yr old wearing prosthesis at least 2 hours/day; 12 subjects in each study arm.
Intervention	Wii Fit training 3 times/week for 4 weeks; 40-min sessions. Controls played cognitive games.
Results	Steps per day and Walk While Talking test scores improved; effect size of walk test improvements was medium.
Comments	Improvements were retained after 3 weeks; subjects preferred supervised group training, but also liked training at home.

Darter, BJ, et al: Home-based treadmill training to improve gait performance in persons with chronic transfemoral amputation. Arch Phys Med Rehabil 94(12):2440, 2013.

Design	Repeated measures cohort
Level of Evidence	IV
Subjects	8 subjects with transfemoral amputations, who had lost their limb due to trauma or cancer at least 3 years ago.
Intervention	Home-based treadmill walking for 30 min/day, 3 days/week for 8 weeks. Each session involved walking at 3 speeds.
Results	Improvement in all outcome measures: stance phase duration and step length, energy expenditure, and energy cost; self-selected walking speed and maximum walking speed; and 2-min walk test.
Comments	Home-based treadmill walking is an effective method to improve gait in patients with transfemoral amputations, even beyond the traditional rehabilitation period.

Table 22.4 Evidence Summary Prosthetic Gait Training—cont'd

Sheehan, RC, et al: Use of perturbation based training in a virtual environment to address mediolateral instability in an individual with unilateral transfemoral amputation. Phys Ther 96(12):1896, 2016.

Design	Case Report
Level of Evidence	IV
Subjects	One 43-year-old subject, 7 years post-transfemoral amputation with frontal plane gait abnormalities.
Intervention	Perturbation-based gait training with virtual reality; 8 sessions over 4 weeks.
Results	Post-tested immediately at end of program and at 5 weeks. Significant increase in gait speed and decreased step width, indicating improved medial-lateral stability.
Comments	Positive effects retained at 5-week follow-up.

Darter, BJ, and Wilken, JM: Gait training with virtual reality-based real-time feedback: Improving gait performance following transfemoral amputation. Phys Ther 9(10):1385, 2011.

Design	Case Report
Level of Evidence	IV
Subjects	One 24-year-old male subject with a transfemoral amputation.
Intervention	Visual feedback with CAREN virtual reality and verbal feedback from physical therapist. Twelve 30-minute sessions over 3 weeks.
Results	Clinically important improvement in gait kinematics and Vo_2
Comments	Improvements were retained over 3 weeks. Improvements were 2–3 times larger than is expected with usual gait training.

is very different from walking in the clear open space of the physical therapy gym. Placing obstacles on the floor to step around or over, walking in a busy hallway or on a sidewalk, picking something up from the floor, and carrying an object while walking are all advanced activities that require balance, coordination, and the ability to shift one's weight on and off the prosthesis smoothly in different body positions. During advanced training, the client is taught to get up and down from chairs of different heights and seat resilience, including toilet seats, as well as how to get up and down from the floor. Obstacle avoidance is also important and can be practiced by creating an obstacle course using chairs, single steps, cones, and blocks to walk around, and should also be practiced using a variety of walking surfaces.

Steps and Ramps

Individuals wearing transtibial prostheses generally have little difficulty mastering steps and ramps once they have achieved good balance and prosthetic control. Going up step over step requires good quadriceps strength and is easier for individuals with medium to long RL length. Descending steps requires accommodating for lack of prosthetic ankle dorsiflexion by placing it over the edge of the step. Safety descending steps is important; those with poor balance should use a step-to pattern, placing the prosthesis down first until balance has improved. Some gait adaption may be needed for steep ramps or hills, depending on the type of prosthetic foot. The more limitation of dorsiflexion, the harder it is to go up a steep hill step over step. Going down a steep hill requires good quadriceps strength and prosthetic control but can be accomplished by most individuals.

The technique for going up and down stairs and ramps will vary for an individual wearing a transfemoral prosthesis based on the type of knee component. Generally, the person will ascend stairs one step at a time leading with the unamputated leg, unless the prosthesis has a powered knee. A power knee joint permits ascending stairs using a foot-over-foot pattern, although it is quite energy expensive. Individuals fitted with a microprocessor controlled knee with stance phase control can descend steps using a foot-over-foot pattern. The patient should be carefully instructed to operate the features of the prosthetic knee correctly. For descending stairs with many fluid/hydraulic prostheses, it is necessary to place the prosthetic heel only on the step and "sit back" to create a flexion moment at the knee, thereby allowing the knee to flex. Table 22.5 presents examples of advanced training activities for individuals with a transfemoral prosthesis. Once good balance, prosthetic control, and gait have been achieved, many individuals develop their own method of doing each of these activities.

Table 22.5 Advanced Activities (Transfemoral)

Activity	Procedure
Sitting on the floor	Place the prosthesis about half a step behind the sound foot, keeping the weight on the sound foot. Bend from the waist and flex at the knees and hips, reaching for the floor with both arms outstretched and pivoting to the sound side. Then gradually lower the body to the floor. This activity is one continuous movement.
Getting up from the floor	Get on the hands and knees; place the sound leg forward, well under the trunk, with the foot flat on the floor while balancing on the hands and the prosthetic knee. Then extend the sound knee while maintaining the weight over the sound leg. Move to an erect position by pushing strongly with the sound leg and the arms bringing the prosthesis forward when almost erect.
Kneeling	Place the sound foot ahead of the prosthetic foot keeping the weight on the sound leg. Slowly flex the trunk, hip, and knee until the prosthetic knee can be gently placed on the floor. Clients with transfemoral limbs usually kneel on the prosthetic leg. Getting up from a kneeling position is like getting up from the floor.
Picking up an object from the floor	Place the sound foot ahead of the prosthetic foot with the body weight remaining on the sound leg. Bend forward at the waist flexing the hips and knees until the object can be reached. Care must be taken to maintain the weight on the sound leg if wearing a mechanical knee. Some individuals like to bend sideways rather than forward, whereas others find it easier to keep the prosthetic knee straight and bend the sound leg until the object can be picked up.

Adapted from May and Lockard.[106, p. 147]

FUNCTIONAL OUTCOME MEASUREMENTS

Use of standardized functional outcome measures is an important strategy to monitor change in patients over time, identify effective interventions, and enhance the quality of the care provided. Since 2013, the Centers for Medicare and Medicaid Services (CMS) require therapy providers to document patients' initial function and their achieved outcomes during and after treatment by including G codes (and modifiers) on requests for reimbursement.[111] These codes are used to document functional activity limitations and participation restrictions, as defined by the International Classification of Functioning, Disability and Health (ICF). Thus, it is important for clinicians to include appropriate measurements of functional status in all patient examinations, including clients with amputation. There are many types of functional status instruments available. Some are designed to be used with individuals regardless of specific diagnostic group, while others are designed for a particular group, such as persons with amputation. Functional status measures are grouped into two general categories: self-report or performance-based assessments. Instrument selection should be based on available data addressing reliability as well as its validity for use with the patient population. Other important psychometric information about the instrument include its responsiveness to change, and how much change must occur to be real or clinically important (minimally detectable change [MDC]; minimal clinically important difference [MCID]). Additional factors considered when selecting an instrument include: ease of completion, time required to administer, and space or specialized equipment requirements. It is important to note whether it can be used with individuals with or without a prosthesis, or if the instrument is limited only to current prosthesis users. Many functional status outcome measures are used with persons with amputation.[104,105,109,112-119] Table 22.6 presents examples of commonly used outcome measures that are valid, reliable, responsive to change, and relatively easy to administer. Assessment of functional status is an important component of determining effectiveness of physical therapy treatment and justifying reimbursement. Interventions used for patients with amputation, whether an exercise or a prosthetic component, should have an effect on function that is measurable. If interventions are not effective, they should be abandoned and an alternative approach pursued.

Table 22.6 Outcome Measures: Self-Report and Performance-Based Functional Status Measures for Persons With Amputation

Outcome Measure and ICF Category	Description	Scoring	MDC and MCID
	Self-Report Functional Status Measures		
Prosthetic Evaluation Questionnaire (PEQ) **ICF: 2**	82 questions divided into 4 domains; 12- item mobility subscale (PEQ-MS) assesses prosthetic ambulation and transfers	0–4 Likert scale; score is average of all items. Available online at http://www.prs-research.org/Texts/PEQ_Evaluation_Guide.pdf	MDC: 0.8–1.4 PEQ-MS, 0.8;[112,113] 0.55[115]
Locomotor Capabilities Index (LCI-5)[113,114] **ICF: 2**	14 questions about ambulation in various circumstances and performing activities while walking	5-level ordinal scale (0–4); higher scores indicate better locomotor capabilities using prosthesis	NA
Prosthetic Limb Users Survey of Mobility (PLUS-M) **ICF: 2**	Version 1 is designed for clinical practice; includes 44 mobility items; 2 short forms (12 and 7 items)	5-point rating of difficulty in walking and performing activities; Raw score is converted to T-score and percentile. Available online at www.plus-m.org	MDC: 5.59 (7-item); 5.36 (12-item)[115]
Activities-Specific Balance Confidence Scale (ABC)[116] **ICF: 2**	16-item scale; patients rate level of balance confidence while performing functional mobility activities	5-level ordinal rating scale (no, low, moderate, high, and complete confidence). Score is average of all ratings.	MDC: 0.49[115]
Patient Reported Outcomes Measurement Information System (PROMIS-29) **ICF: 2, 3**	Measures 8 symptoms and QoL constructs: physical function, anxiety, depression, fatigue, sleep disturbance, social role satisfaction, pain interference, pain intensity.	T-score and percentiles	MDC: Physical function subscore 7.3; others range from 2.3 (pain intensity) to 9.2 (fatigue)[115]
	Performance-Based Measures		
Timed "Up & Go" (TUG) **ICF: 2**	Patient rises from a chair, walks 3 m, turns, returns to chair and sits.	Time in seconds from buttocks off chair to buttocks back on chair. Can be used with all patient populations, but has been validated for use with patients with LE amputations.	MDC: (90% confidence): 0.96 sec for lower limb amputees;[112] May have ceiling effect for more active patients.
L Test **ICF: 2**	Modification of the TUG for more active patients with amputation; arise from armless chair, walk 3 m, make right-angle turn, continue walking 7 m and turn 180° and walk back along same path and sit down (20 m total)	Time in seconds from buttocks off chair to buttocks back on chair.	MCID: 4.5 sec[117]

Continued

Table 22.6 Outcome Measures: Self-Report and Performance-Based Functional Status Measures for Persons With Amputation—cont'd

Outcome Measure and ICF Category	Description	Scoring	MDC and MCID
Six-minute Walk Test (6MWT) **ICF: 2**	Patient walks on a smooth, level surface 100-foot path; Instructions: Walk as far as possible for 6 minutes, but don't run or jog; patient may stop and rest, but clock continues.	Total distance walked in meters in 6 minutes.	MDC (90% confidence): 45 m[112]
Two-minute Walk Test (2MWT) **ICF: 2**	The same as the 6MWT, but patient only walks for 2 minutes.	Total meters walked in 2 minutes.	MDC (90% confidence): 34.3 m[112]
Amputee Mobility Predictor, with Prosthesis (AMPPRO), without prosthesis (AMPnoPRO); AMP for patients with bilateral amputations (AMP-B)[104,105,109] **ICF: 2**	Patient is asked to perform 21 tasks in 4 categories (sitting balance, simple mobility, standing balance, gait, functional activities).	Based on quality of performance; score is sum of ratings for all items; scoring adjustments made for those with unilateral amputations who do not have a prosthesis and for those with bilateral amputations, for who some tasks will be difficult, even for very able individuals.	MDC: 3.4[112]
Comprehensive High-Level Activity Mobility Predictor (CHAMP)[118,119] **ICF: 2**	Developed for military servicemembers who demonstrate proficient strength, balance, postural stability, prosthetic control and endurance; designed to test speed, power and agility.	Scores for each item are added to produce a composite score, with 40 the highest level of performance.	MDC (95% confidence): for total CHAMP score: 3.74

ICF CATEGORY: 1 = body structure/function; 2 = activity; 3 = participation
LE = lower extremity; MCID = minimal clinically important difference; MDC = minimal detectable change; NA= not available (not established); QoL = quality of life

SUMMARY

Most individuals with LE amputations can return to a full and useful life following the loss of a limb. A program of postoperative care that includes consideration of physical and emotional needs will enable most patients to become functional prosthetic users. Many prosthetic problems can be avoided by properly preparing the individual for prosthetic wear. In this chapter, concepts related to the postoperative and preprosthetic management of the individual with LE amputation have been presented. Through a process of careful evaluation and open communication, a comprehensive program designed to meet the needs of an individual patient can be achieved.

Questions for Review

1. Describe the advantages and disadvantages of the following postoperative dressings: (a) compressible soft dressing, (b) semirigid dressing, (c) removable rigid dressing, and (d) immediate postoperative prosthesis.
2. What are the general goals of the postsurgical phase of amputation care?

3. What critical information would you provide a family member about patient positioning following a transtibial amputation?
4. A 72-year-old man with a history of diabetes, cardiovascular disease, and PVD has been referred for physical therapy 24 hours post–right transtibial amputation performed due to an infected foot ulcer. What examination data are needed to plan an appropriate treatment program? Which are the most critical to obtain on the first visit?
5. Describe the patient data that you would gather to justify prescribing a prosthesis for a patient.
6. Plan three gait training activities that could be used to improve stability during weight bearing on the prosthesis.

CASE STUDY

REFERRAL

The patient is a 68-year-old female status post–right transtibial amputation yesterday secondary to an infected non-healing plantar pressure ulcer on the foot.

CURRENT MEDICAL HISTORY

Type 2 diabetes since age 48 controlled by insulin 20 units bid. Arteriosclerosis; hypertension controlled by medication; treated for a pressure ulcer on the plantar surface of right first metatarsal area for past 4 months. Ulcer did not heal leading to amputation. Body mass index (BMI) is 29.

PAST MEDICAL HISTORY

Hysterectomy at age 42; otherwise unremarkable.

SOCIAL HISTORY

Widow who lives alone. Three grown children and six grandchildren in the area.

Retired school teacher; enjoys gardening, and until her foot ulcer, she was active in volunteer activities, including teaching in an English as a second language (ESL) program.

She does not smoke; drinks wine occasionally; does not use drugs.

Physical activity was moderate: she took a yoga class twice per week. She had decreased physical activity during wound treatments and has been sedentary for the last 4 months.

PHYSICAL THERAPY EXAMINATION (INITIAL)

Chart Review

Patient alert and awake in no apparent distress. Right residual limb wrapped in soft gauze dressing covered with an elastic wrap. Drain in place. Incision clean on dressing change.

BP: 142/70, pulse 66, respiration normal.

Respiratory therapist reports patient using spirometer properly, normal cough, and no evidence of respiratory problems; Spo_2 is 97%.

Patient complains of some pain in residual limb (pain medication prescribed). Reports some uncomfortable phantom limb sensation, but denies pain.

Patient has been sitting at the side of the bed twice/day.

Examination Data

Gross muscle strength of left lower extremity (LE) and both upper extremities (UEs) grossly within functional limits (WFL). Muscle strength of right hip flexion, abduction, and adduction grossly WFL; hip extension tested side-lying and graded 3+/5. Demonstrates active motion of right knee flexion and extension with no resistance given at this time.

Residual limb measurements deferred until initial healing has taken place.

Gross range of motion of left LE and both UEs WFL. Left hip extension measurements deferred until patient can lie prone or on right side. Gross ROM of the right hip WFL except hip extension to 0° measured side-lying. Right knee flexion and extension grossly WFL. Specific measurement deferred until dressing can be removed.

Left LE is hairless below the ankle. Skin is warm to touch. Dorsalis pedis pulse not palpable. Toes are warm to touch. Proprioceptive sensation at the ankle and toes is intact. She is unable to detect the 5.07 Semmes Weinstein monofilament under metatarsal heads on the left. Diminished sensation over plantar surface of left foot and dorsum of first metatarsal. No evidence of edema in left LE. Sensation testing of right residual limb deferred owing to presence of dressing.

FUNCTIONAL STATUS

Bed Mobility

Rolling to left: independent; rolling to right and prone: not tested.

Supine-to-sit and return: modified independent using side rail of bed.

Sitting Balance

Independent

Standing Balance

Single leg balance (without hand support): 5 seconds

Transfers

Sit-to-stand with walker: moderate assistance. No orthostatic hypotension.

Stand-to-sit in chair or bed: moderate assistance.

Locomotion

Ambulation with walker: moderate assistance for 5 feet. Complains of increased residual limb pain when her right leg is dependent.

Vital signs (post-ambulation): HR, 82; BP, 150/72; residual limb pain rated: 7/10

Expected outcomes of physical therapy episode of care (achieved before discharge from hospital):

1. The patient will be independent in all transfers and bed mobility.
2. The patient will be independent in ambulation with crutches or walker for 40 feet.
3. The patient will demonstrate knowledge of proper residual limb positioning, bandaging, and care.
4. The patient will demonstrate knowledge of basic residual limb exercises.
5. The patient will demonstrate knowledge of proper care of the left lower extremity.

PREPROSTHETIC HOME CARE PHYSICAL THERAPY

The patient is discharged on day 5 to the home of one of her daughters. She is referred to home care physical therapy.

Examination Data

Examination data obtained following discharge from hospital by home care physical therapist:

Residual limb: Sutures in place, incision healing well, no drainage; length 5.4 in. (13.6 cm) from medial tibial plateau (MTP) to end of residual limb.

Circumferential measurements from MTP:

- 2 in. (5 cm) below MTP = 14 in. (35 cm)
- 4 in. (10 cm) below MTP = 15 in. (38 cm)
- 5 in. (12 cm) below MTP = 14.5 in. (37 cm)

RL Sensation intact. She continues to have phantom limb sensation (throbbing, like the wound she had before the amputation), but denies phantom limb pain. She rates her RL pain: 5/10.

Psychosocial. She is somewhat anxious because she doesn't want to be a burden to her daughter. She is able to look at and touch her residual limb and is anxious to get moving. She acknowledges that she is worried because she has never known anyone with an amputation and is not sure she can learn to use a prosthesis. She also is fearful that she will fall, so she stays in her chair unless someone is with her.

ROM right knee: WFL.

ROM right hip: extension to 0° (all other motions WFL).

The patient's daughter is present and tells you that she is worried because her mother seems more forgetful now than she was before the surgery. The daughter is concerned that her mother will forget safe procedures and fall or not be able to learn to use a prosthesis.

Expected Outcomes

Expected outcomes for physical therapy episode of care during preprosthetic home care intervention:

1. The patient will be independent in care of residual limb, including bandaging or using a shrinker.
2. The patient will be independent in crutch (or walker) ambulation in and around the home and community.
3. The patient will be independent in home exercise program (HEP).
4. The patient will be independent in self-care and functional activities in the home.

Ten weeks after surgery the patient is fitted with a transtibial prosthesis (total surface bearing socket with seal-in liner, suction suspension, and energy storing and releasing [ESAR] prosthetic foot). When she receives the prosthesis, she will be admitted to an acute rehabilitation hospital for 10 days of prosthetic training. Her goal is to return to her own home when discharged from rehabilitation.

GUIDING QUESTIONS

1. The patient's residual limb was wrapped in a soft dressing after amputation. Discuss the advantages and disadvantages of the volume containment options (rigid, semirigid, and soft dressings) for this patient.
2. Review the initial examination data given for the patient. What data would be important to obtain on the first postoperative visit and what can be deferred? What other data would you obtain and when?
3. As the home health therapist:
   a. What additional examination data do you need to develop an appropriate POC?
   b. Describe your initial plan of interventions.
   c. Describe your mobility program.
   d. How will you address your patient's anxiety regarding falling and her ability to be successful with a prosthesis?
   e. Describe possible causes for your patient's cognitive issues and how you will address her daughter's concerns.
4. When the patient receives her prosthesis and is admitted to the acute rehabilitation hospital, what will be the focus of her prosthetic training program? Outline your program.
   a. Describe your initial balance training program.
   b. How will you teach her to use her ESAR prosthetic foot effectively? What gait training techniques will you include to ensure that she develops a symmetrical gait pattern?
   c. How would you teach this person to get down to and up from the floor?

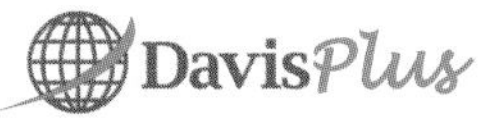

For additional resources, including answers to the questions for review and case study guiding questions, please visit **http://davisplus.fadavis.com.**

The reader is referred to video **Case Study 3: Patient With Transtibial (Below Knee) Amputation** for additional review and study. The full written case study, including tables, figures, charts, and three video segments (examination, intervention, and outcome), appears online at Davis*Plus*. The case study poses questions for the reader's consideration with suggested answers to the case study questions, also posted online at Davis*Plus*.

References

1. Amputee Coalition: Limb Loss Resource Center: Limb Loss Statistics. Amputee Coalition, Manassas, VA, 19110, 2017. Retrieved March 25, 2017, from http://www.amputee-coalition.org/limb-loss-resource-center/resources-by-topic/limb-loss-statistics/.
2. Ziegler-Graham, K, et al: Estimating the prevalence of limb loss in the United States 2005–2050. Arch Phys Med Rehabil 89(3): 422, 2008.
3. Varma, P, Stineman, MJ, and Dillingham, TR: Epidemiology of limb loss. Phys Med Rehabil Clin N Am 25:1, 2014.
4. Centers for Disease Control and Prevention National Diabetes Statistics Report: Estimates of Diabetes and Its Burden in the United States, 2014. US Department of Health and Human Services, Atlanta, GA, 2014.
5. Hoffstad, O, et al: Diabetes, lower-extremity amputation, and death. Diabetes Care 38(10):1852, 2015.
6. Li, Y, et al: Declining rates of hospitalization for non-traumatic lower-extremity amputation in the diabetic population aged 40 years or older, U.S., 1988–2008. Diabetes Care 35(2):273, 2012.
7. Markowitz, JS, et al: Risk of amputation in patients with diabetic foot ulcers: A claims-based study. Wound Repair Regen 14(1): 11, 2006.
8. Feinglass, J, et al: How "preventable" are lower extremity amputations? A qualitative study of patient perceptions of precipitating factors. Disabil Rehabil 34(25):2158, 2012.
9. Gregg, EW, et al: Changes in diabetes-related complications in the United States, 1990–2010. N Engl J Med 370(16):1514, 2014.
10. Baba, M, et al: Temporal changes in the prevalence and associates of diabetes-related lower extremity amputations in patients with type 2 diabetes: The Fremantle diabetes study. Cardiovasc Diabetol 14:152, 2015.
11. Tseng, CL, et al: Trends in initial lower extremity amputation rates among Veterans Health Administration health care systems users from 2000–2004. Diabetes Care 35(4):1157, 2011.
12. Nelson, MT, et al: Preoperative factors predict mortality after major lower-extremity amputation. Surgery 152(4):685, 2012.
13. Thorud, JC, et al: Mortality after nontraumatic major amputation among patients with diabetes and peripheral vascular disease: A systematic review. J Foot Ankle Surg 55(3):591, 2016.
14. Robbins, JM, et al: Mortality rates and diabetic foot ulcers. J Am Podiatr Med Assoc 98(6):489, 2008.
15. Glaser, JD, et al: Fate of the contralateral limb after lower extremity amputation. J Vasc Surg 58(6):1571, 2013.

16. Dorresteijn, JA, et al: Patient education for preventing diabetic foot ulceration. Cochrane Database of Syst Rev 2014, Issue 12. Art No: CD001488. doi: 10.1002/14651858.CD001488.pub5.
17. Price, P: How can we improve adherence? Diabetes Metab Res Rev 32(Suppl 1):201, 2016.
18. Bus, SA, et al: IWGDF guidance on the prevention of foot ulcers in at risk patients with diabetes. Diabetes Meab Res Rev 32(Suppl 1):16, 2016.
19. Dillingham, TR, Pezzin, LE, and MacKenzie, EJ. Limb amputation and limb deficiency: Epidemiology and recent trends in the United States. South Med J 95(8):875, 2002.
20. Low, EE, Inkellis, E, and Morshed, S: Complications and revision amputation following trauma-related lower limb loss. Injury, Int J Care Injured 48(2):364, 2017.
21 Krueger, CA, Wenke, JC, and Ficke, JR: Ten years at war: Comprehensive analysis of amputation trends. J Trauma Acute Care Surg 73(6) Supplement 5:S438, 2012.
22. Nagarajan, R, et al: Limb salvage and amputation in survivors of pediatric lower-extremity bone tumors: What are the long-term implications? J Clin Oncol 20:4493, 2002.
23. Schwartz, AJ, et al: Cemented distal femoral endoprosthesis for musculoskeletal tumor. Clin Orthop Relat Res 468:2198, 2010.
24. Rosano, A, et al: Limb defects associated with major congenital anomalies: Clinical and epidemiological study from the international clearinghouse for birth defects monitoring systems. Am J Med Genet 93(2):110, 2000.
25. van Eijk, MS, et al: Predicting prosthetic use in elderly patients after major lower limb amputation. Prosthet Orthot Int 36(1): 45, 2012.
26. Stevens, P: The balancing act: Are amputees falling for it? The O&P Edge pp 5–7, May 2010. Retrieved March 31, 2017, from www.oandp.com/articles/2010-05_03.asp.
27. Raya, MA, et al: Impairment variables predicting activity limitation in individuals with lower limb amputation. Prosthet Orthot Int 34(1):73, 2010.
28. Czerniecki, JM, el al: The development and validation of the AMPREDICT model for predicting mobility outcome after dysvascular lower extremity amputation. J Vasc Surg 65(1): 162, 2017.
29. Smith, DG: General principles of amputation surgery. In Smith, DG, Michael, JW, and Bowker, JH: Atlas of Amputations and Limb Deficiencies: Surgical, Prosthetic, and Rehabilitation Principles, ed 3. American Academy of Orthopaedic Surgeons, Rosemont, IL, 2004, p. 21.
30. Bowker, JH: Transtibial amputation: Surgical management. In Smith, DG, Michael, JW, and Bowker, JH: Atlas of Amputations and Limb Deficiencies: Surgical, Prosthetic, and Rehabilitation Principles, ed 3. American Academy of Orthopaedic Surgeons, Rosemont, IL, 2004, p. 481.
31. Tisi, PV, and Than, MM: Type of incision for below knee amputation. Cochrane Database Systematic Reviews, 8(4): 2014. Art. No. CD 003749. doi: 10.002/14651858.CD003749.pub3.
32. Schnur, D, and Meier, RH: Amputation surgery. Phys Med Rehabil Clin N Am 25:35, 2014.
33. Taylor, BC, and Poka, A: Osteomyoplastic amputation: The Ertl technique. J Am Acad Orthop Surg 24(4):259, 2016.
34. Li, Y, and Branemark, R: Osteointegration prosthesis for rehabilitation following amputation: The pioneering Swedish model. Unfallchirurg 120(4):285, 2017.
35. Muderis, MA, et al: The Osteointegration Group of Australia Accelerated Protocol (OGAAP-1) for two-stage osteointegrated reconstruction of amputated limbs. Bone Joint J 98-B(7):952, 2016.
36. Food and Drug Administration (FDA): FDA authorized use of prosthesis rehabilitation of above-the-knee amputations, Silver Springs, MD, 2015. Retrieved October 10, 2018 from https://www.meddeviceonline.com/doc/fda-authorizes-use-of-prosthesis-for-rehab-of-above-the-knee-amputations-0001.
37. Lind, J, et al: The influence of smoking on complications after primary amputations of the lower extremity. Clin Orthop 267:211, 1991.
38. Burgess, EM, and Romano, RL: the management of lower extremity amputees using immediate postsurgical prostheses. Clin Orthop Relat Res 57:137, 1968.
39. Smith, DG, et al: Postoperative dressing and management strategies for transtibial amputations: A critical review. J Rehabil Res Dev 40(3):213, 2003.
40. Ali, MM, et al: A comparative analysis of immediate postoperative prosthesis placement following below-knee amputation. Ann Vasc Surg 27(8):1146, 2013.
41. Sumpio, B, et al: Comparison of immediate postoperative rigid and soft dressings for below-knee amputations. Ann Vasc Surg 27(6):774, 2013.
42. Wu, Y: An innovative removable rigid dressing technique for below-the-knee amputation. J Bone Joint Surg Am 61(5): 724, 1979.
43. Johannesson, A, et al: Comparison of vacuum-formed removable rigid dressing with conventional rigid dressing after transtibial amputation: Similar outcome in a randomized controlled trial involving 27 patients. Acta Orthop 79(3):361, 2008.
44. Duwayri, Y, et al: Early protection and compression of residual limbs may improve and accelerate prosthetic fit: A preliminary study. Ann Vasc Surg 26(2):242, 2012.
45. Wong, CK, and Edelstein, JE: Unna and elastic post-operative dressings: Comparisons of their effect on function of adults with amputations and vascular disease. Arch Phys Med Rehabil 81:1191, 2000.
46. May, BJ, and Lockard, MA: Postsurgical management. In May, BJ, and Lockard, MA: Prosthetics and Orthotics in Clinical Practice: A Case Study Approach. FA Davis, Philadelphia, 2011, p. 59.
47. Hakimi, KN: Pre-operative rehabilitation evaluation of the dysvascular patient prior to amputation. Phys Med Rehabil Clin N Am 20:677, 2009.
48. Esquenazi, A: Amputation rehabilitation and prosthetic restoration, from surgery to community reintegration. Disabil Rehabil 26(14–15):831, 2004.
49. Esquenazi, A, and DiGiacomo, R: Rehabilitation after amputation. J Am Podiatr Med Assoc 91(1):13, 2001.
50. Brigham and Woman's Hospital, Department of Rehabilitation Services, Physical Therapy: Standard of Care: Lower Extremity Amputation. Brigham and Women's Hospital, 2011. Retrieved October 10, 2018, from http://www.brighamandwomens.org/assets/BWH/patients-and-families/rehabilitation-services/pdfs/general-le-amputation-bwh.pdf.
51. Uustal, H: Prosthetic rehabilitation issues in the diabetic and dysvascular amputee. Phys Med Rehabil Clin N Am 20(4): 689, 2009.
52. Williams, RM: The role of expectations in pain after dysvascular lower extremity amputation. Rehabil Psychol 59(4):459, 2014.
53. Czerniecki, JM, et al: The effect of rehabilitation in a comprehensive inpatient rehabilitation unit on mobility outcome after dysvascular lower extremity amputation. Arch Phys Med Rehabil 93(8):1384, 2012.
54. Sauter, CN, Pezzin, LE, and Dillingham, TR: Functional outcomes of persons who underwent dysvascular lower extremity amputations. Am J Phys Med Rehabil 92(4):287, 2013.
55. Roth, EV, et al: Prosthesis use and satisfaction among persons with dysvascular lower limb amputations across postacute care discharge settings. PMR 6(12):1128, 2014.
56. Lockard, MA: Shoes and orthoses for foot impairments. In May, BJ, and Lockard, MA: Prosthetics and Orthotics in Clinical Practice: A Case Study Approach. FA Davis, Philadelphia, 2011, p. 221.
57. May, BJ: Patient education past and present. J Phys Ther Educ 13(3):3–7, 1999.
58. Stineman, MG, et al: The effectiveness of inpatient rehabilitation in the acute postoperative phase of care after transtibial or transfemoral amputation. Study of an integrated health care delivery system. Arch Phys Med Rehabil 89(10):1863–1872, 2008.
59. Gailey, RS, et al: Review of secondary physical conditions associated with lower-limb amputation and long-term prosthesis use. J Rehabil Res Dev 45(1):15, 2008.
60. Agrawal, V: Clinical outcome measures for rehabilitation of amputees—A review. Phys Med Rehabil Int 3(2):1080, 2016.
61. Ramachandran, VS, and Hirstein, WL: The perception of phantom limbs: The D. O. Hebb Lecture. Brain 9(121): 1603–1630, 1998.
62. Manchikanti, L, and Singh, V: Managing phantom pain. Pain Physician 7(3)365, 2004.
63. Ephraim, PL, et al: Phantom pain, residual limb pain, and back pain in amputees: Results of a national survey. Arch Phys Med Rehabil 86(10):1910, 2005.

64. Racy, J: Psychological adaptation to amputation. In Smith, DG, Michael, JW, and Bowker, JH: Atlas of Amputations and Limb Deficiencies: Surgical, Prosthetic, and Rehabilitation, ed 3. American Academy of Orthopaedic Surgeons, Rosemont, IL, 2004, p. 727.
65. May, BJ: Psychosocial issues. In May, BJ, and Lockard, MA: Prosthetics and Orthotics in Clinical Practice: A Case Study Approach. FA Davis, Philadelphia, 2011, p. 39.
66. Hawkins, AT, et al: The effect of social integration on outcomes after major lower extremity amputation. J Vasc Surg (63)1: 154, 2016.
67. Frengopoulos, C, et al: Association between Montreal Cognitive Assessment scores and measures of functional mobility in lower extremity amputees after inpatient rehabilitation. Arch Phys Med Rehabil 98(3):450, 2017.
68. Williams, RM, et al: Changes in cognitive function from presurgery to 4 months post-surgery in individuals undergoing dysvascular amputation. Arch Phys Med Rehabil 95(4):663, 2014.
69. Williams, RM: Relationship between cognition and functional outcomes after dysvascular lower extremity amputation: A prospective study. Am J Phys Med Rehabil 94(9):707, 2015.
70. Louie, WS, et al: Residual limb management for person with transtibial amputation: Comparison of bandaging technique and residual limb sock. JPO 22(3):194–201, 2010.
71. Sanders, JE, and Fatone, S: Residual limb volume change: Systematic review of measurement and management. J Rehabil Res Dev 48(8):949, 2011.
72. Rossbach, P: First Step (vol 5): Care of Your Wounds After Amputation Surgery. Amputee Coalition of America, Manassus, VA, Retrieved April 6, 2017, from http://www.amputee-coalition.org/wp-content/uploads/2015/08/Care-of-Your-Wounds-After-Amputation-Surgery.x32243.pdf.
73. Sansam, K, et al: Can simple clinical tests predict walking ability after prosthetic rehabilitation? J Rehabil Med 44(11):968, 2012.
74. Wong, CK, et al: Exercise programs to improve gait performance in people with lower limb amputation: A systematic review. Prosthet Orthot Int 40(1):8, 2014.
75. Corio, F, Troiano, R, and Magel, JR: The effects of spinal stabilization exercises on the spatial and temporal parameters of gait in individuals with lower limb loss. J Prosthet Orthot 22(4):230–236, 2010.
76. Longlois, K, et al: Influence of physical capabilities of males with transtibial amputation on gait adjustments on sloped surfaces. J Rehabil Res Dev 51(12):193, 2014.
77. Miller, WC, Speechley, M, and Deathe, AB: Balance confidence among people with lower-limb amputations. Phys Ther 82: 856, 2002.
78. Miller, WC, and Deathe, AB: The influence of balance confidence on social activity after discharge from prosthetic rehabilitation for first lower limb amputation. Prosthet Orthot Int 35(4): 379, 2011.
79. Fogelberg, DJ, et al: What people want in a prosthetic foot: A focus group study. J Prosthet Orthot 28(6):145, 2016.
80. Rusaw, D, et al: Bilateral electromyogram response latency following platform perturbation in unilateral transtibial prosthesis users: Influence of weight distribution and limb position. J Rehabil Res Dev 50(4):531, 2013.
81. Czerniecki, JM: Rehabilitation in limb deficiency. 1. Gait and motion analysis. Arch Phys Med Rehabil 77(3 Suppl):S-3, 1996.
82. Mohanty, RK, et al: Comparison of energy cost in transtibial amputees using "prosthesis" and "crutches without prosthesis" for walking activities. Ann Phys Rehabil Med 55(4):252, 2012.
83. Vllasolli, TO, et al: Energy expenditure and walking speed in lower limb amputees: A cross sectional study. Orthop Traumatol Rehabil 16(4):419, 2014.
84. Wezenberg, D, et al: Peak oxygen consumption in older adults with a lower limb amputation. Arch Phys Med Rehabil 93(11): 1934, 2012.
85. Wezenbery, D, et al: Relation between aerobic capacity and walking ability in older adults with a lower-limb amputation. Arch Phys Med Rehabil 94(9):1714, 2013.
86. Chin, T, et al: Effect of endurance training programs based on anaerobic threshold (AT) for lower limb amputees. J Rehabil Res Dev 38(1):7, 2001.
87. Chin, T, et al: Physical fitness of lower limb amputees. Am J Phys Med Rehabil 81(5):321, 2002.
88. Darter, BJ, et al: Home-based treadmill training to improve gait performance in persons with a chronic transfemoral amputation. Arch Phys Med Rehabil 94(12):2440, 2013.
89. Miller, CA, et al: Using the Nintendo Wii Fit and body weight support to improve aerobic capacity, balance, gait ability, and fear of falling: Two case reports. J Geriatr Phys Ther 35(2):95, 2012.
90. Jarvis, HL, et al: Temporal, spatial and metabolic measures of walking in highly functional individuals with lower limb amputations. Arch Phys Med Rehabil 2016 Nov 16. doi: 10.1016/j.apmr.2016.09.134.
91. Luo, Y, and Anderson, TA: Phantom limb pain: A review. Int Anesthesiol Clin 54(2):121, 2016.
92. Alviar, MJ, Hale, T, and Dungca, M: Pharmacologic interventions for treating phantom limb pain. Cochrane Database Syst Rev, 2016, Issue 10. Art. No.: CD006380. doi: 10.1002/14651858.CD006380.pub3.
93. Eldabe, S. et al: Dorsal root ganglion (DRG) stimulation in the treatment of phantom limb pain (PLP). Neuromodulation 18(7):610, 2015.
94. Bolognini, N, et al: Immediate and sustained effects of 5-day transcranial direct current stimulation of the motor cortex in phantom limb pain. J Pain 16(7):657, 2015.
95. Mulvey, MR, et al: Transcutaneous electrical nerve stimulation for phantom pain and stump pain in adult amputees. Pain Pract 13(4):289, 2012.
96. Trevelyan, EG, et al: Acupuncture for the treatment of phantom limb syndrome in lower limb amputees: a randomized controlled feasibility study. Trials 17(1):519, 2016.
97. Batsford, S, Ryan, GC, and Martin, DJ: Non-pharmacolgical conservative therapy for phantom limb pain: A systematic review of randomized controlled trials. Physiother Theory Pract 33(3):173, 2017.
98. Ramachandran, VS, and Altschuler, EL: The use of visual feedback, in particular mirror visual feedback, in restoring brain function. Brain 132(Pt 7): 1693, 2009.
99. Chan, BL, et al: Mirror therapy for phantom limb pain. N Engl J Med 357(21):2206, 2007.
100. Dunn, J, et al: Virtual and augmented reality in the treatment of phantom limb pain: A literature review. NeuroRehabilitation. 2017 Feb 13. doi: 10.3233/NRE-171447.
101. Ortiz-Catalan, M, et al: Treatment of phantom limb pain (PLP) based on augmented reality and gaming controlled by myoelectric pattern recognition: A case study of a chronic PLP patient. Front Neurosci 25(8):24, 2014.
102. Ortiz-Catalan, M, et al: Phantom motor execution facilitated by machine learning and augmented reality as treatment for phantom limb pain: A single group, clinical trial in patients with chronic intractable phantom limb pain. Lancet 10(388): 2885, 2016.
103. Kahle, JT, et al: Predicting walking ability following lower limb amputation: An updated systematic literature review. Technol Innov 18(2–3):125, 2016.
104. Gailey, RS, et al: The amputee mobility predictor: An instrument to assess determinants of the lower limb amputee's ability to ambulate. Arch Phys Med Rehabil 83(5):613–627, 2002.
105. Raya, MA, et al: Amputee mobility predictor-bilateral: A performance-based measure of mobility for people with bilateral lower-limb loss. J Rehabil Res Dev 50(7):961, 2013.
106. May, BJ, and Lockard, MA: Prosthetics and Orthotics in Clinical Practice: A Case Study Approach. FA Davis, Philadelphia, 2011.
107. Highsmith, MJ, et al: A method for training step-over-step stair descent gait with stance yielding prosthetic knees. J Prosthet Orthot 24(1):10, 2012.
108. Highsmith, MJ, et al: Stair ascent and ramp gait training with the Genium knee. Technol Innov 15:349, 2014.
109. Gailey, RS, et al: Application of self-report and performance-based outcome measures to determine functional differences between four categories of prosthetic feet. J Rehabil Res Dev 49(4):597, 2012.
110. Highsmith, MJ, et al: Gait training interventions for lower extremity amputees: A systematic literature review. Technol Innov 18(2–3):99, 2016.
111. Resnik, LL: Medicare mandate for claims-based functional data collection: An opportunity to advance care, or a regulatory burden? Phys Ther 93(5):587, 2013.

112. Resnik, LL, and Borgia, M: Reliability of outcome measures for people with lower-limb amputations: Distinguishing true change from statistical error. Phys Ther 91(4):555, 2011.
113. Deathe, BA, et al: Selection of outcome measures in lower extremity amputation rehabilitation: ICF activities. Disabil Rehabil 31(18):1455, 2009.
114. Franchignoni, AG, et al: Rasch analysis of the locomotor capabilities index-5 in people with lower limb amputation. Prosthet Orthot Int 31(4):394, 2007.
115. Hafner, BJ, et al: Psychometric evaluation of self-report outcome measures for prosthetic application. J Rehabil Res Dev 53(6): 797, 2016.
116. Sakakibara, BM, Miller, WC, and Backman, CL: Basch analyses of the activities-specific balance confidence scale with individuals 50 years and older with lower-limb amputation. Arch Phys Med Rehabil 92(8):1257, 2011.
117. Rushton, PW, Miller, WC, and Deathe, BA: Minimal clinically important difference of the L test for individuals with lower limb amputation: A pilot study. Prosthet Orthot Int 39(6): 470, 2014.
118. Gailey, RS, et al: Development and reliability testing of the comprehensive high-level activity mobility predictor (CHAMP) in male servicemembers with traumatic lower limb loss. J Rehabil Res Dev 50(7):905, 2013.
119. Gailey, RS, et al: Construct validity of comprehensive high-level activity mobility predictor (CHAMP) for male servicemembers with traumatic lower-limb loss. J Rehabil Res Dev 50(7): 919, 2013.

Supplemental Readings

May, BJ, and Lockard, MA: Prosthetics and Orthotics in Clinical Practice: A Case Study Approach. FA Davis, Philadelphia, 2011.
Smith, DG, Michael, JW, and Bowker, JH (eds): Atlas of Amputations and Limb Deficiencies: Surgical, Prosthetic, and Rehabilitation Principles, ed 3. American Academy of Orthopaedic Surgeons, Rosemont, IL, 2004.

appendix 22.A

Web-Based Resources for Clinicians, Families, and Patients With Amputation

Connects to multiple websites related to prostheses and orthoses, including manufacturers.	www.oandp.com
The website of the American Academy of Orthotists and Prosthetists and the *Journal of Prosthetics and Orthotics.* This is the professional organization of prosthetists and orthotists.	https://www.oandp.org.
Amputee Coalition of America. Largest organization for amputees, families, and clinicians. Good source of high-quality patient education materials.	www.amputee-coalition.org
Disabled Sports Organization. Has regional chapters. Provides opportunities for community sports, recreation, and educational programs.	www.disabledsportsusa.org
Website of the U.S. Paralympic team.	www.teamusa.org/US-Paralympics
National Amputee Golf Association.	www.nagagolf.org
Website of the American Diabetes Association.	www.diabetes.org

Chapter 23

Arthritis

Maura Daly Iversen, PT, DPT, SD, MPH, FNAP, FAPTA
Marie D. Westby, PT, PhD

LEARNING OBJECTIVES

1. Discriminate between the epidemiology, pathophysiology, disease course, and clinical manifestations of two common rheumatic diseases: rheumatoid arthritis and osteoarthritis.
2. Identify the medical (clinical) diagnostic procedures commonly used in the examination of patients with arthritis, including laboratory tests and imaging.
3. Apply common principles of medical and rehabilitation management to the plan of care for individuals with rheumatoid arthritis and osteoarthritis.
4. Identify and understand when, why, and how to apply and interpret clinical examination and outcome measures commonly used in assessing individuals with rheumatoid arthritis or osteoarthritis.
6. Describe environmental, psychosocial, and other personal factors associated with arthritis that affect participation, adherence to treatment, achievement of anticipated goals, and expected outcomes.
7. Explain the importance of a team-based chronic disease management approach for persons with arthritis.
8. Analyze and interpret patient data, formulate realistic intervention goals and outcomes, and develop a plan of care when presented with a clinical case study.

CHAPTER OUTLINE

The terms *arthritis*, *rheumatism*, and *rheumatic disease* are generic references to an array of more than 100 diseases that are divided into 10 classification categories. Two major forms of arthritis are considered in this chapter. *Rheumatoid arthritis (RA)*, a systemic inflammatory disease, and *osteoarthritis (OA)*, a more localized process that has been known previously as *degenerative joint disease (DJD)*. Rheumatoid arthritis and osteoarthritis account for most arthritis cases treated by physical therapists.

RHEUMATOID ARTHRITIS

RA is a major subclassification within the category of diffuse inflammatory connective tissue diseases that also includes juvenile idiopathic arthritis, systemic lupus erythematosus (SLE), progressive systemic sclerosis or scleroderma, polymyositis, and dermatomyositis. RA is primarily a disease of the *synovium.* The first clinical description of RA is attributed to A. J. Landré-Beauvais in 1800, although analysis of pictorial art of the late Renaissance suggests the existence of RA in earlier times. Early descriptions of patient symptomatology were complicated by the lack of uniform agreement about the distinguishing disease characteristics, given its wide spectrum of clinical presentations. The term *rheumatoid arthritis* was first used by Sir Alfred Baring Garrod in 1858 but was not accepted by the American Rheumatism Association (ARA) as the official terminology until 1941.[1] Diagnostic criteria and terminology have been developed and, in some cases, revised based on current data.[2,3]

Epidemiology

The estimated prevalence of RA among adults in the United States is approximately 1.3 million,[4] and its prevalence increases with age. Women are affected two to four times more often than men. Differences in prevalence exist among certain subpopulations, which suggest a possible role for genetic or environmental factors in the etiology of the disease. For example, African Americans have a lower prevalence of RA than Caucasians, whereas several Native American groups demonstrate higher prevalence rates. There also is a lower prevalence of RA in native Japanese and native Chinese peoples compared to Caucasians.[4,5]

Etiology

RA is an autoimmune disease of unknown complex etiology. RA is presently believed to have a genetic basis demonstrated by the increased disease risk and clustering in families.[6] Among the genetic factors associated with RA risk, Human Leukocyte Antigen–DR isotype (*HLA–DRB1*) positivity is the strongest genetic risk factor, increasing disease risk by roughly threefold.[7,8]

Briefly, an *antigen* is a substance, usually foreign to the host, which provokes the immune system into action. The immune system may respond to the antigen directly (cellular immunity) or by the production of *antibodies* that circulate in the serum (humoral immunity). These responses involve two general types of lymphocytes: T cells, which are responsible for cellular immunity, and B cells, which produce circulating antibodies specific to the antigen. Antibodies are immunoglobulins, a type of serum protein.[1]

Given that individuals with RA produce antibodies to their own immunoglobulins, such as rheumatoid factor (RF) and anti-citrullinated protein antibody (ACPA), and these antibodies precede the clinical presentation of RA by years,[9,10] RA is considered an autoimmune disease.[10] It is not clear, however, whether this antibody production is a primary event or results as a response to a specific antigen from an external stimulus. Current theory and research on the cellular basis of autoimmunity suggest that aberrant functioning of cell-mediated immunity and defective T lymphocytes may trigger the autoimmune response that underlies RA.[10] A specific etiological agent for RA has not been identified. However, external agents may trigger disease expression through various and differing mechanisms. Behavioral risk factors, such as low fish intake, obesity, poor dental health, and smoking are associated with an increased risk of developing rheumatoid arthritis.[11-15] Bacterial organisms, including streptococcus, clostridia, diphtheroids, and mycoplasmas, have been suggested as triggers but no connections have been definitively proven. There has also been discussion of a viral etiology for RA. As with other investigations seeking to identify an etiology for RA, research remains speculative.[1]

RFs are antibodies specific to immunoglobulin G (IgG) and are found in the sera of approximately 70% of all patients with RA. Current theory suggests that RFs arise as antibodies to "altered" autologous (the patient's own) IgG. Some modification of IgG changes its configuration and renders it an autoimmunogen, stimulating the production of RF. IgM is the first class of immunoglobulins formed after contact with an antigen and most RFs are of this class, although RFs may be of any immunoglobulin class.[1] The exact biological role of RF is unknown. Although RF has been implicated in the pathogenesis of RA, the disease occurs in the absence of RF in a substantial number of individuals.[16] Research indicates that the presence of RF affects disease severity, because those who have RF, or seropositive disease, have increased frequency of subcutaneous nodules, vasculitis, and polyarticular involvement.[1]

Ollier and Worthington[6] examined the literature investigating a genetic predisposition to the development of RA.[6] HLAs found on the surface of most human cells are capable of generating *an immune response* when genetically incompatible tissues are grafted to each other, for example, during organ transplants. Genes controlling these HLAs are found on the sixth chromosome. Four loci have been described: HLA-A, HLA-B, HLA-C, and HLA-D. RA has been associated with increased HLA-D and HLA-DR (D-related) antigens, suggesting that certain genes determine whether a host is more or less at risk for an immunological response that leads to RA.[6] A "*rheumatoid epitope*" has been identified through DNA typing of HLA-DR4 as a particular sequence of amino acids common among patients with RA.[17] A national case-control study conducted in Sweden focused on citrulline-modified proteins, proteins not normally present in healthy adults but found in about two-thirds of patients with RA, to determine if smoking and the presence of shared epitope (SE) HLA genes triggered RA. The investigators concluded that the interaction of smoking and carrying two copies of the SE gene increases the risk of developing RA by 21-fold.[18,19] Further studies of genomic organization of the HLA-D region specifically implicate a short sequence on the HLA-DRB1 gene and suggest that HLA-DRB1 alleles (alternate forms of a gene) modify disease expression and progression.[1] Various studies of different ethnic groups have also shown that particular variations of the HLA-DRB1 allele are overrepresented in people with RA.[1]

Pathophysiology

In early RA, synovial inflammation leads to pain, stiffness, and restricted range of motion (ROM). As the disease progresses, the joint capsule becomes inflamed and immune cells degrade the cartilage. With longstanding RA the synovium appears grossly edematous with slender villous or hair-like projections into the joint cavity (Fig. 23.1). Distinctive vascular changes, including venous distention, capillary obstruction,

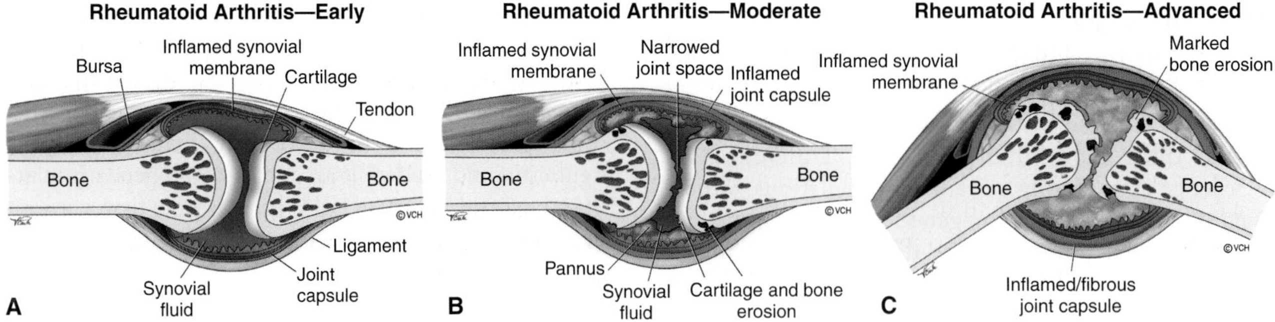

Figure 23.1 Progression of joint changes due to RA inflammation: Early to advanced disease. *(From Mary Pack Arthritis Program, Vancouver Coastal Health, with permission.)*

neutrophilic infiltration of the arterial walls, and areas of thrombosis and hemorrhage, may be evident. Synovial proliferation of vascular granulation tissue, known as *pannus,* dissolves collagen as it extends over the joint cartilage. Eventually, with disease progression, the granulation tissue leads to adhesions, fibrosis, or bony ankylosis of the joint. Chronic inflammation associated with RA weakens the joint capsule and its supporting ligamentous structures, altering joint structure and function. Tendon rupture and fraying tendon sheaths produce imbalanced muscle pull on pathologically altered joints resulting in the characteristic musculoskeletal deformities seen in advanced RA.[20]

Following alterations in blood flow, rapid changes in the cellular content and volume of the synovial fluid may result, owing to low pressure in the joint space and the lack of a limiting membrane between the joint space and synovial blood vessels. High-molecular-weight substances such as macroglobulins and fibrinogens can pass through the synovial capillaries during periods of inflammation and are not easily cleared.[1] Antigen–antibody complexes may be isolated within the joint cavity and stimulate phagocytosis and further development of pannus. Although sustained requires the proliferation of new blood vessels, the exact mechanism of capillary growth is not understood. One hypothesis suggests that activated macrophages, responding to antigen–antibody complexes, may stimulate this development. With established synovitis, polymorphonuclear (PMN) leukocytes are drawn into the joint cavity and coupled with lysosomal enzyme activity contribute to destruction of synovial tissues.[16]

Laboratory Tests

Elevated *erythrocyte sedimentation rate (ESR)* and *C-reactive protein (CRP)* are acute phase reactants that indicate the presence of active inflammation. Although patients with RA characteristically have active inflammation, up to 40% may have normal values for these tests despite clinical evidence of inflammation. Normal ESR and CRP values are nonspecific and alone cannot confirm or refute a diagnosis of RA. RF is the result of the binding of two immunoglobulins. The presence or absence of RF alone neither confirms nor rules out a diagnosis of RA. Nearly 25% of people with RA do not have a positive RF (seronegative RA), whereas a positive RF is seen in a number of other immunologic conditions (e.g., leprosy, tuberculosis, chronic hepatitis) and occasionally in individuals with no disease. A positive RF in combination with clinical criteria may help to confirm a clinical impression.[17]

A *complete blood count (CBC)* is routinely ordered because many findings are commonly associated with RA. Red blood cell counts are often decreased, indicating the anemia of chronic disease found in approximately 20% of individuals with RA. By comparison, the white blood cell count is generally normal. *Thrombocytosis,* a high platelet count, is not uncommon in active RA.

Synovial fluid analysis can greatly enhance the process of differential diagnosis. Normal synovial fluid is transparent, yellowish, viscous, and without clots. Synovial fluid from inflamed joints is cloudy, less viscous owing to a change in hyaluronate proteins, and will clot. Significant inflammation also increases the number of fluid proteins. A culture can be performed to identify potential bacterial agents as the cause of joint inflammation. If the joint is inflamed, white blood cells will be elevated in the fluid. Crystals are not common. If present they may confirm the diagnosis of **gout** (urate crystals) or *pseudogout* (calcium pyrophosphate crystals). A mucin clot test (a measure of viscosity) of the synovial fluid can be used to discriminate between acute infectious arthritis and inflammatory arthritis, such as RA. Poor clotting accompanies acute infectious arthritis whereas RA produces fair mucin clotting.[1]

Radiography/Imaging

Radiographic study is essential in a diagnostic workup for RA.[20] Physical therapists practicing in rheumatology should develop a basic proficiency in identifying abnormalities in joint structure and the surrounding soft tissues as these abnormalities influence the course and outcome of rehabilitation. To identify radiographic abnormalities, the therapist must be able to describe how a normal joint appears on a radiograph. Therapists can orient themselves to a radiograph by considering several parameters: alignment, bone density and surface, and cartilaginous spacing (Figs. 23.2 and 23.3). Normal alignment is present when the long axes of the proximal and distal bones of the joint are in their normal spatial relationships and the convex surface of one bone fits well with the concavity of the other. Bone density, in the absence of *osteoporosis,* should be somewhat opaque and milky and appear evenly distributed throughout. The cortices of each bone should be distinct, appropriately thick, and well defined. The joint soft tissues should conform to known anatomical shape. Soft tissue swelling and evidence of uneven spacing between joint surfaces on radiograph may suggest activity limitations. Uneven, reduced, or absent spacing suggests joint cartilage loss or joint surface erosion. A normal joint surface should be smooth and should conform to known anatomical shape without osteophytes. RA progression can be characterized in four sequential stages using periodic radiographic examination. Radiographic changes evident in early RA are nonspecific and usually limited to soft tissue swelling, joint effusion, and periarticular demineralization. Diagnostic confirmation is made when the disease process leads to bilateral joint space narrowing and erosions in the hands and feet.[1]

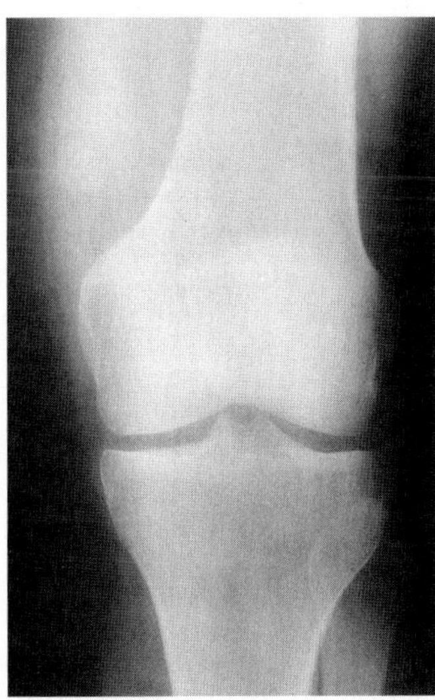

Figure 23.2 Frontal view of the normal knee. *(From the American College of Rheumatology, with permission.)*

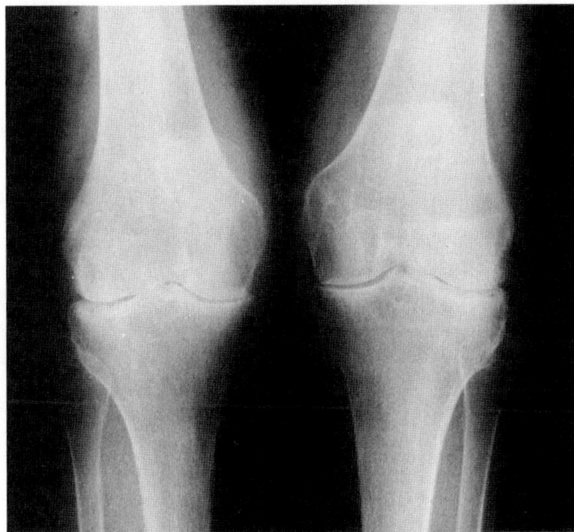

Figure 23.3 Frontal view of the knee with characteristics of rheumatoid arthritis. *(From the American College of Rheumatology, with permission.)*

Ultrasound and magnetic resonance imaging (MRI) may also be used to assess RA-associated changes and to monitor disease activity. Both are more sensitive to use than physical examination of the joints.[21] A recent systematic review comparing MRI and ultrasound to assess joint inflammation indicates that ultrasound is a valid technique for identifying synovitis in the hand and wrist joints and is easier and more practical to implement than MRI.[22]

Classification and Diagnostic Criteria

The differential diagnosis of RA is predicated on the history, clinical examination of signs and symptoms, and careful exclusion of other disorders. The *American College of Rheumatology* (ACR) classification criteria,[2] developed using data from patients in outpatient clinics, are commonly used to confirm whether an individual's clinical presentation should be confirmed as a case of RA. Originally these criteria had four classifications of RA: classical, definite, probable, and possible. Some of these classifications were judged to be problematic. The 1987 revised criteria can be found at the following link: www.rheumatology.org. In 2010 the ACR and the *European League Against Rheumatism* (EULAR) revised the 1987 classification criteria for RA[2] to help identify early RA. These criteria are based on a combination of signs, symptoms, and laboratory findings that have persisted for a specified period of time.[3] A diagnosis of definite RA is now established on the confirmed presence of synovitis in at least one joint, absence of an alternative diagnosis that better explains the synovitis, and a total score of 6 or greater (out of a possible 10) from four domains. The domains are (1) *Joint Involvement,* designating the number and site of involved joints (score range 0–5); (2) *Serology,* indicating serologic abnormalities (score range 0–3); (3) *Acute-Phase Reactants,* describing elevated acute-phase response (score range 0–1); and (4) *Duration of Symptom* (two levels; range 0–1).[3] The inclusion of criteria for early RA may help rheumatologists to target treatment at earlier stages of the disease and decrease RA progression. A full explanation of the revised classification criteria can be found at: www.rheumatology.org.

Patients with RA can also be classified based on global functional status criteria.[23] There are four functional classifications based on a person's ability to complete functional and self-care activities ranging from independence to full dependence. In addition to their clinical relevance, these functional classifications enable clinicians and researchers to classify subjects in clinical trials and inform evidence-based clinical recommendations for therapies (Table 23.1).

Disease Onset and Course

RA is commonly characterized by an exacerbating and remitting disease course. Disease onset is accompanied by complaints of generalized joint pain and stiffness, usually in multiple small joints (*polyarthritis)* though it may be localized to a single joint. Symptoms may appear spontaneously or over a prolonged period of time. Disease progression is highly variable. High titers of RF indicate a more severe disease course. Spontaneous remissions can occur. Some patients experience an intermittent course, characterized by partial to complete remissions longer than the periods of exacerbations. A third group of patients experiences the full unremitting destructive process of progressive RA.[1] Comparisons of elderly-onset RA with early-onset RA revealed that abrupt onset and large joint involvement, particularly of the shoulder girdle, were more common in the older adults. The elderly-onset group demonstrated clinical features more commonly associated with *polymyalgia rheumatica,* a separate and distinct disease affecting the shoulder and pelvic musculature leading to muscle inflammation.[24]

Clinical Presentation

Systemic

Systemic features of RA include weight loss, fever, and extreme fatigue. Fatigue greatly affects function and participation in daily life and is often underappreciated on physical examination.[25] Fatigue may result from chronic pain, and is associated with cerebral inflammation and physical inactivity.[17] A hallmark clinical feature of RA is *morning stiffness* in and around the joints lasting at least 1 hour before maximal improvement.[3] In contrast, OA-induced stiffness results from inactivity. Morning stiffness can be qualified in its severity and duration, both of which are directly related to the degree of disease activity.

Joint Impairments (Articular and Nonarticular)

RA is characterized by bilateral and symmetrical synovial joint involvement (see Figure 23.4). Clinically, patients present with limited mobility and signs of inflammation including pain, redness, swelling, and warm joints. The most common joints involved are the hands, feet, and cervical spine. The hands are generally affected early in the disease course and severity of hand involvement is indicative of severity of disease.[25] The term *arthralgia* refers to joint pain. The joint examination may reveal *crepitus,* an audible or palpable grating or crunching evident as the joint is moved through its ROM. Crepitus is the result of uneven degeneration of the joint surface.

Cervical Spine and Temporomandibular Joint

The cervical spine is often involved in RA and on examination ROM may be limited in all planes. The occipitoatlantal (occiput–C1) and atlantoaxial (C1–C2) joints are frequently affected due to their extensive synovial tissue. The midcervical region is also a common site of inflammation, leading to decreased ROM, particularly in rotation, accompanied by instability. Three patterns of cervical spine involvement are described: atlantoaxial subluxation (65%), atlantoaxial impaction (20% to 25%), and subaxial subluxation (10% to 15%).[26] Involvement of the C1 and C2 vertebrae may produce life-threatening situations if the transverse ligament of the atlas should rupture or if the odontoid process should fracture or herniate through the foramen magnum, compressing the upper cervical cord. Patients presenting with cervical radiculopathy and neurological signs should be immediately referred to a physician. MRI is the most effective tool to visualize both the spinal column and the cord.[26] *Ankylosing* (i.e., fusion) of one or more vertebrae of the spine may accompany RA and can lead to loss of ROM and function of the involved joints.

The temporomandibular joint (TMJ) is usually among the last joints involved. Inflammation of the TMJ results in pain, swelling, and limited movement and eventually to ankylosis. With juvenile RA, involvement of the TMJ can lead to destruction of the condyle and potential alterations in mandibular growth and facial deformity. With early disease, TMJ x-rays are usually negative but with time and chronic inflammation can demonstrate bone destruction. The recent use of cone-beam computed tomography (CBCT) has been helpful

Table 23.1 American College of Rheumatology Revised Criteria for Classification of Functional Status in Rheumatoid Arthritis[a]

Class I	Completely able to perform usual activities of daily living (self-care, vocational, and avocational)
Class II	Able to perform usual self-care and vocational activities, but limited in avocational activities
Class III	Able to perform usual self-care activities, but limited in vocational and avocational activities
Class IV	Limited in ability to perform usual self-care, vocational, and avocational activities

From Hochberg, MC, et al: The American College of Rheumatology 1991 revised criteria for the classification of global functional status in rheumatoid arthritis. Arthritis Rheum 35:498, 1992, with permission.

[a]Usual self-care activities include dressing, feeding, bathing, grooming, and toileting. Avocational (recreational and or leisure) and vocational (work, school, homemaking) activities are patient-desired and age- and sex-specific.

in early identification of degenerative TMJ changes, which may affect the ability to open the mouth fully (approximately 2 in [5.08 cm]) with normal side-to-side gliding and protrusion.[27] In resting position, the normal approximation of the upper and lower teeth may be altered following persistent inflammation.

Shoulders and Elbows

Shoulder involvement may be evident in the glenohumeral, sternoclavicular, or acromioclavicular joints leading to joint surface degeneration, pain, and loss of ROM. Shoulder pain is often referred to the deltoid region. The scapulothoracic articulation may secondarily exhibit a loss of ROM as well. Chronic shoulder inflammation causes the capsule and the ligaments to become distended and thinned. As joint surfaces erode, the shoulder eventually becomes unstable. In addition, **tendinitis** and **bursitis** may complicate management. Typical elbow joint findings include effusions between the lateral epicondyle and olecranon prominence, bilateral swelling of the olecranon bursa (more prevalent with severe disease), and rheumatoid nodules on the olecranon or extensor surface of the proximal ulna.[26] Inflammation, capsular and ligamentous distention, and joint erosion may lead to instability and irregular or catching movements. Flexion contractures frequently develop, due to patient posturing to reduce pain and persistent spasm.

Wrists

The ulnar styloid may be tender on examination, suggesting inflammatory synovitis. Early synovitis among the carpal bones and the ulna leads to a fairly rapid development of a flexion contracture, which ultimately diminishes the ability to grasp. Additionally, *carpal tunnel syndrome* may occur due to compression of the median nerve in the carpal tunnel. Chronic inflammation around the ulnar styloid coupled with laxity of the

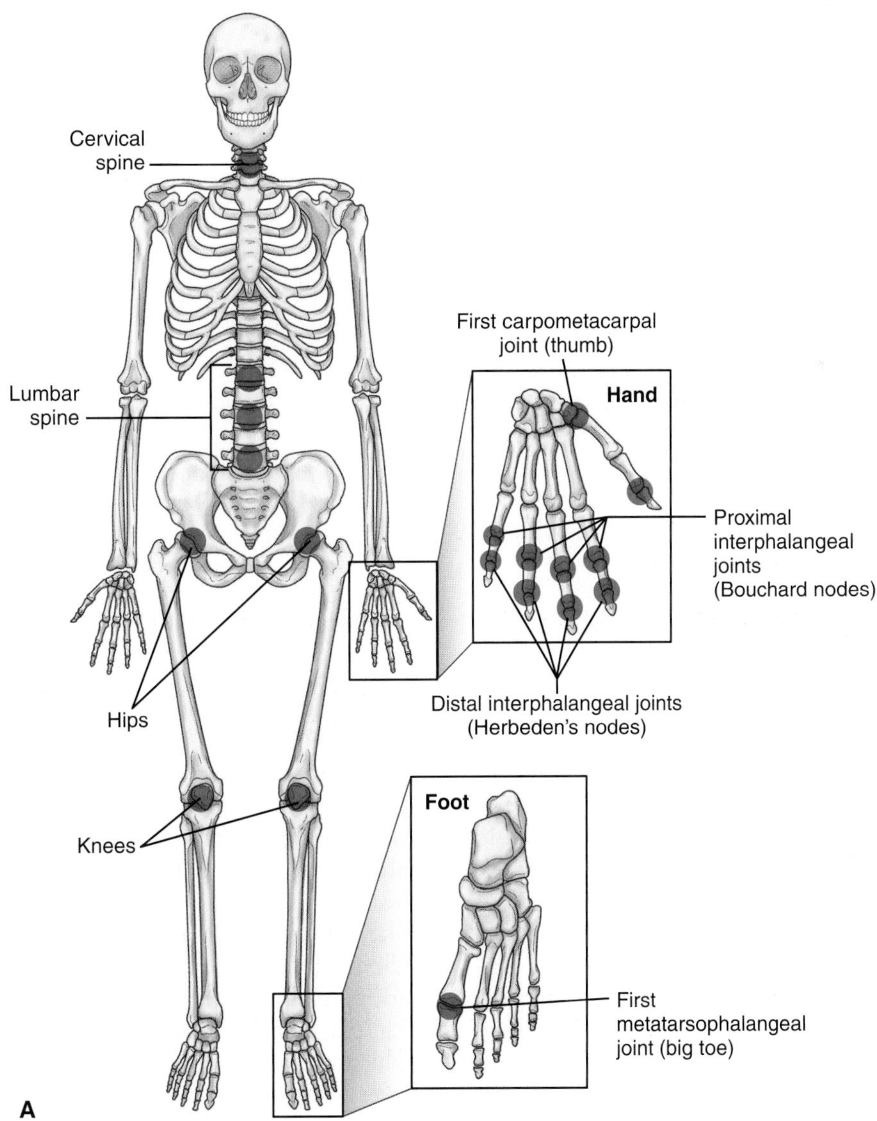

Figure 23.4 A Homunculus showing common joints affected by OA.

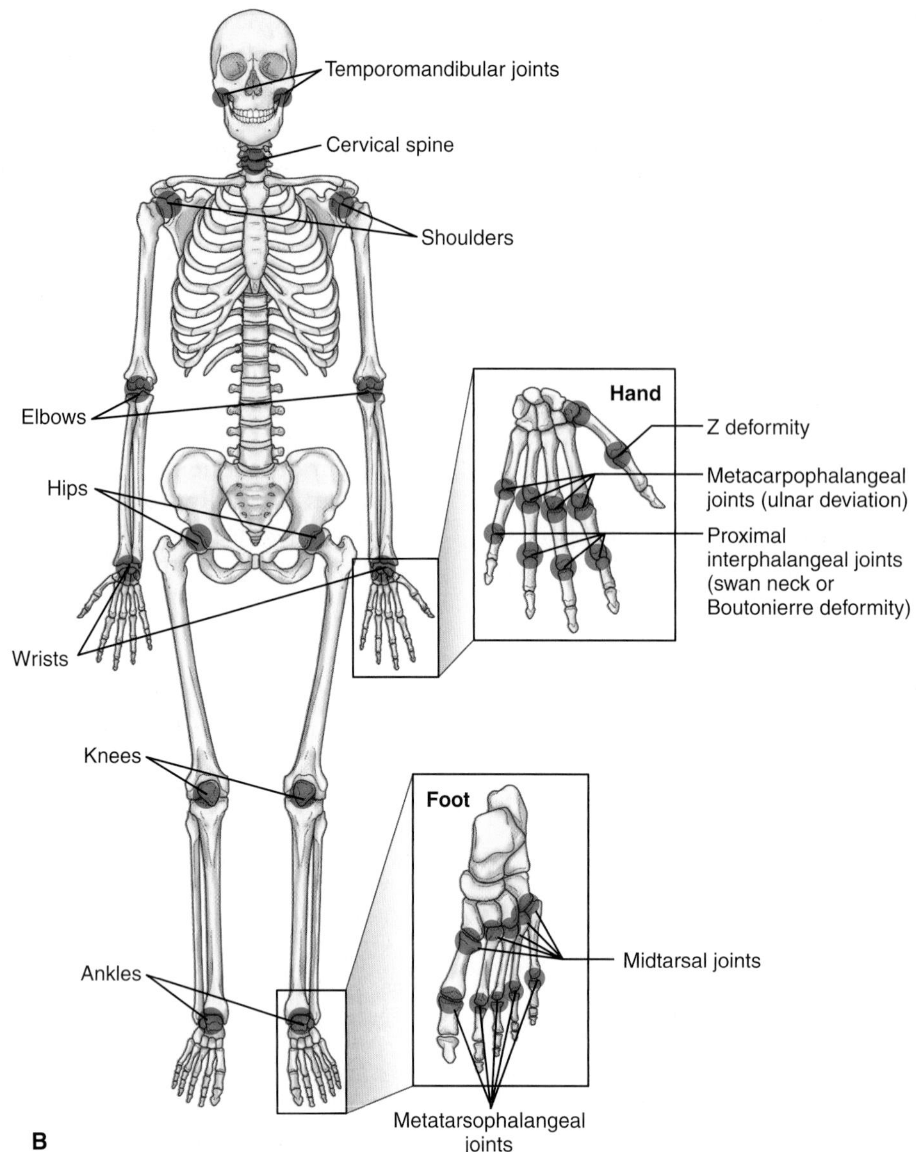

Figure 23.4 B Homunculus showing common joints affected by RA.

radioulnar ligament produces the *piano key sign* on examination. The piano key sign is defined as an up and down movement of the styloid in response to point pressure from the examiner. Over time ulnar deviation or drift may occur from chronic inflammation causing movement of the wrist toward the ulna (Fig. 23.5). Chronic inflammation of the proximal row of carpals can lead to a volar *subluxation* of the wrist and hand on the radius, accentuating the normal 10° to 15° of volar inclination of the carpus on the distal radius (Fig. 23.6). In addition, radial deviation of the distal carpals can occur due to loss of radial ligamentous support, destruction of the extensor carpi ulnaris and the fibrocartilage on the distal side of the ulna. This allows the proximal carpals to slide down the distal radius toward the ulna, contributing to radial deviation of the distal row of carpals relative to the two bones of the forearm, where normally there is 5° to 10° of ulnar deviation.[28] Stenosing tenosynovitis of the first dorsal compartment of the wrist (*de Quervain's disease*) may also occur.

Hand Joints

Metacarpophalangeal: Soft-tissue swelling around the metacarpophalangeal (MCP) joints, especially the index and long fingers, is common. The volar subluxation and **ulnar drift** of the MCPs frequently seen in RA results from exaggeration of the joints' normal structural shape that tilt the proximal phalanges in an ulnar direction. Ulnar "drift" is normal feature of gripping and repeated gripping can further lead to this deformity. The anatomical placement and length of the collateral ligaments, which are most stretched during MCP flexion, and the insertions of the intrinsics, which also pull from an ulnar direction, contribute to ulnar drift at the MCPs during hand motion. Weakened ligaments cannot resist a pull

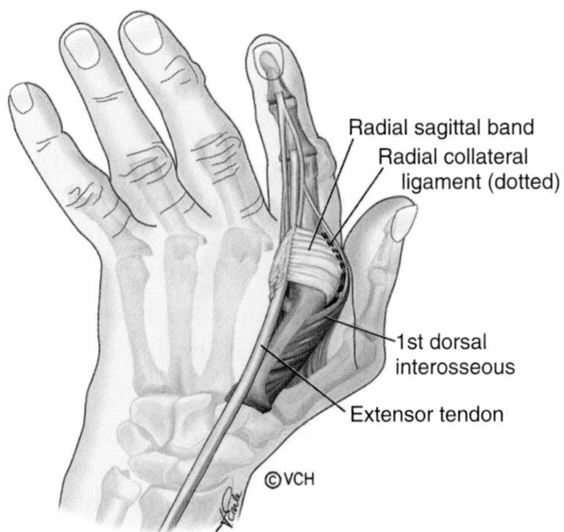

Figure 23.5 Ulnar drift (deviation) of the fingers. This drawing depicts the impact of metacarpophalangeal joint swelling, soft tissue laxity due to synovitis, which leads to ulnar deviation of the fingers in RA.

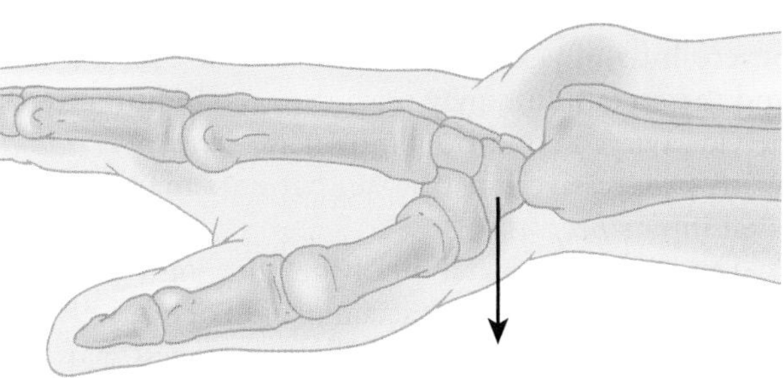

Figure 23.6 Volar subluxation of the wrist seen with rheumatoid arthritis. The chronic inflammation of the proximal carpals can eventually lead to a volar subluxation of the wrist and hand on the radius, accentuating the normal 10° to 15° of volar inclination of the carpus on the distal radius.

toward volar subluxation during power pinch or grasp when flexor tendons bowstring across MCPs through frayed tendon sheaths damaged by long-term synovitis. The *bowstring effect* results from moving the fulcrum of the flexor tendons distally, placing an ulnar and volar pull on the proximal phalanges (Fig. 23.7). Radial deviation of the carpals further enhances MCP ulnar drift as the phalanges try to compensate for the loss of normal ulnar deviation at the wrist. This is known as the *zigzag effect,* where forces in the hand try to move the index finger back into its normal functional position in line with the radius. *A trigger finger* may be evident whereby a snapping sensation is felt when flexing or extending the finger due to flexor tenosynovitis and resultant slippage of the tendon, friction with movement, or presence of tendon nodules.[26,29]

Proximal Interphalangeal: Swelling of the proximal interphalangeal (PIP) joints is common and is easily appreciated with lateral joint palpation. There are two

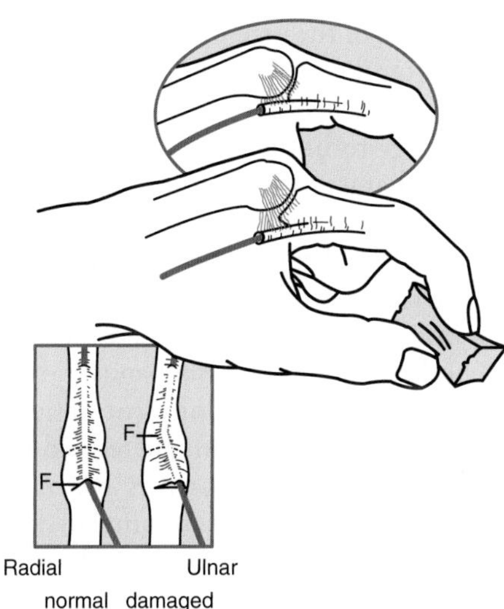

Figure 23.7 Influence of the long flexors (F) in metacarpophalangeal drift deformity. *(Adapted from Melvin,[19, p. 283] with permission.)*

characteristic irreversible deformities (if not surgically repaired early) seen at the PIPs in individuals with severe RA. The first of these is known as *swan neck deformity* and consists of PIP hyperextension and distal interphalangeal (DIP) flexion (Fig. 23.8). Swan neck deformities arise in three distinct ways, depending on the site of initial involvement. Most commonly, swan neck deformity follows from initial synovitis of the MCP, where the pain of chronic synovitis leads to reflex muscle spasm of the intrinsics. The biomechanical force of the intrinsics then combines with the hypermobility found in the chronically inflamed and structurally changed PIP, resulting in volar subluxation and PIP hyperextension. Swan neck deformity may also result when the volar capsule of the PIP is stretched, the lateral bands move dorsally, and tension is placed on the flexor digitorum profundus by the PIP flexes the DIP. In these instances, a rupture of the flexor digitorum sublimis further predisposes an individual to swan neck deformity. A third mechanism for developing swan neck deformity

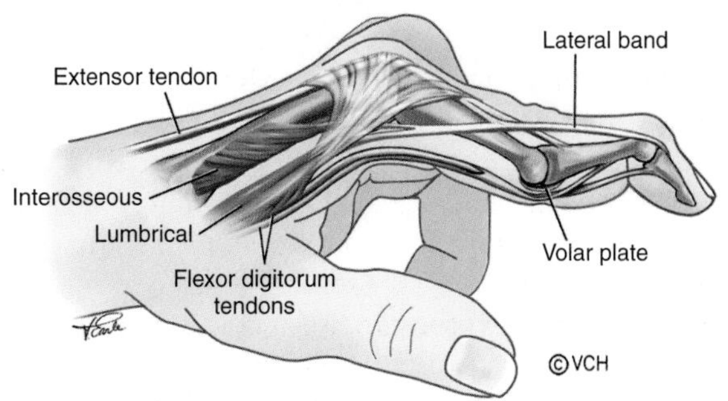

Figure 23.8 Swan neck deformity is characterized by PIP hyperextension and DIP flexion. *(From Mary Pack Arthritis Program, Vancouver Coastal Health, with permission.)*

involves a rupture of the extensor digitorum communis at its insertion on the DIP resulting in DIP flexion and PIP hyperextension owing to unrestrained pull by the flexor digitorum profundus.[26,28]

The other characteristic deformity of the PIP is known as a *boutonniere deformity* and consists of DIP extension with PIP flexion (Fig. 23.9). As a result of chronic synovitis, the insertion of extensor digitorum communis into the middle phalanx (known as the central slip) lengthens, and the lateral bands slide volarly to force the PIP into flexion. Bony formation or outgrowths around the end of a joint are termed *osteophytes.* Those found at the PIP are known as *Bouchard's nodes,* and may be seen in OA. They are unrelated to RA, although an individual may have both kinds of arthritis at the same time.[26,29]

Distal Interphalangeal: The distal interphalangeal (DIP) joints are rarely affected in RA. Osteophytes are, however, common in OA and are called *Heberden's nodes.* Occasionally, a *mallet finger* deformity will result from rupture of the tendon of the extensor digitorum communis, pulling the DIP into flexion as force from the flexor digitorum profundus is unopposed.[29]

Thumb: Many deformities can occur in the thumb due to synovitis. The most prevalent is a *flail IP* in which the patient loses the ability to flex the interphalangeal (IP) joint. The fibers of the dorsal hood mechanism over the MCP, the joint capsule and the collateral ligaments, and the tendons of extensor pollicis brevis and extensor pollicis longus are particularly affected. The exact mechanism of thumb deformities depends on the particular combination of affected structures. Similar to other hand deformities, the actual presentation depends on the site of initial synovitis, the direction of imbalanced muscle forces, and the integrity of the surrounding joint structures. A *type I deformity*, consisting of MCP flexion with IP hyperextension without involvement of the carpometacarpal (CMC) joint, is most commonly seen. *Type II deformity* is assigned when the CMC is subluxed and the IP is held in hyperextension. CMC subluxation and MCP hyperextension is classified as a *type III deformity* and is more common in RA than a type II deformity.[26-29]

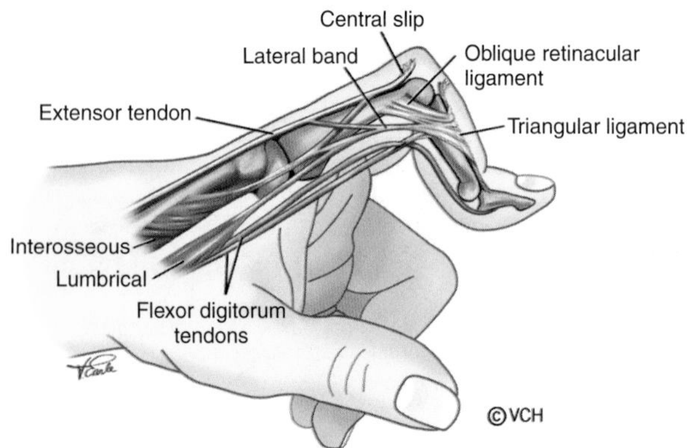

Figure 23.9 Features of a boutonniere deformity include DIP extension with PIP flexion. *(From Mary Pack Arthritis Program, Vancouver Coastal Health, with permission.)*

Mutilans Deformity (Opera-Glass Hand): Grossly unstable thumbs and severely deformed phalanges are indicative of *mutilans-type deformity.* Also known as opera-glass hand, the transverse folds of the skin of the thumb and fingers resemble a folded telescope. Radiographic study of the bones of the hand reveal severe bone resorption, erosion, and shortening of the MCP, PIP, radiocarpal, and radioulnar joints especially. The negative impact of this deformity on hand function and activities of daily living (ADL) is significant.[29]

Hips and Knees

Hip synovitis is less frequent in early RA. Hip synovitis often presents as pain in the groin or lower buttock. Pain over the greater trochanter often is secondary to trochanteric bursitis. Radiographic hip disease is evident in approximately half of all patients with RA.[29] Severe inflammatory destruction of the femoral head and the acetabulum may push the acetabulum into the pelvic cavity, a condition known as *protrusio acetabuli.* With progressive hip disease, patients may require a total hip *arthroplasty*.[26]

The clinical presentation of the knee joint frequently includes synovitis, causing accumulation of relatively large amounts of fluid. The knee ballottement test is used to examine for excess fluid. The examiner presses on the patella with the index finger, resulting in a downward motion of the patella; a sensation of bogginess indicates effusion of the knee. Posterior accumulation of fluid in the knee produces a *Baker's cyst.* If a Baker's cyst ruptures it produces pain, swelling, and heat in the posterior calf similar to symptoms of a deep vein thrombosis. The bulge test is a simple procedure to examine for anterior synovitis. With this procedure the examiner strokes the medial aspect of the knee in an upward motion, then presses on the lateral aspect of the knee. A positive sign is a *wavelike* movement of fluid medially. Chronic synovitis results in distention of the joint capsule, attenuation of the collateral and cruciate ligaments, and destruction of the joint surfaces. Painful knees may be held in slightly flexed positions, ultimately resulting in joint tightness or flexion contractures.[26]

Ankles and Feet

Early inflammation of the feet is often evident in the forefoot where patients note pain with compression of the forefoot on examination. Chronic synovitis accentuates the natural tendency of the talus to glide medially and plantarward, resulting in pressure on the calcaneus and leading to hindfoot pronation. The spring ligament is also stretched by these occurrences, flattening the medial longitudinal arch (Fig. 23.10).

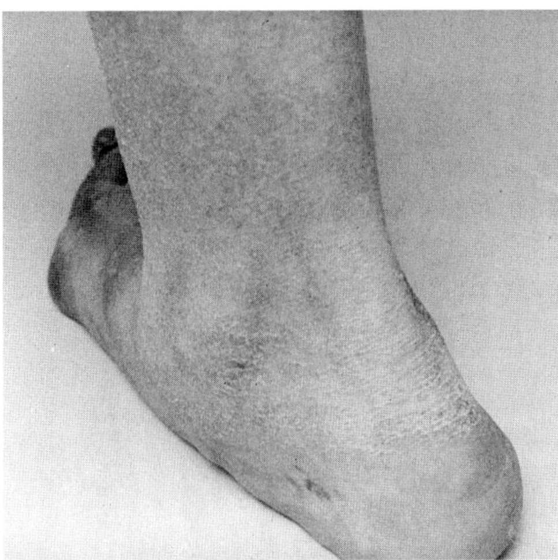

Figure 23.10 Posterior–medial view of the foot and ankle showing calcaneal valgus, pes planus (flatfoot), and hallux valgus, with major foot and ankle deformities seen in rheumatoid arthritis.

The calcaneus may erode or develop bony *exostoses* known as spurs. As synovitis weakens the transverse arch, the metatarsals spread and a splayed forefoot (*splayfoot*) may develop (Fig. 23.11). Instability of the talocalcaneal joint, if severe, can lead to the need for surgical fusion. Synovitis of the metatarsophalangeal (MTP) joints is extremely common and *metatarsalgia* (pain over the metatarsal heads) may develop. A *hallux valgus* and *bunion* (a painful bursitis over the medial aspect of the first MTP joint) may also be present. When volar subluxation of the MTP combines with flexion of the PIP and hyperextension of the DIP joints, this condition is commonly referred to as *hammer toes* (Fig. 23.12). The MTPs may also exhibit volar subluxation of the metatarsal head with flexion of the PIP and DIP joints, known as *cock-up* or ***claw toes*** (Fig. 23.13). As the capsule and intertarsal ligaments are weakened and stretched, the proximal phalanges move dorsally on the metatarsal head (Fig. 23.14). Similar to conditions observed in the hand, the long toe extensors "bowstring" over the PIP joints while the flexors are displaced into the intertarsal spaces.[26]

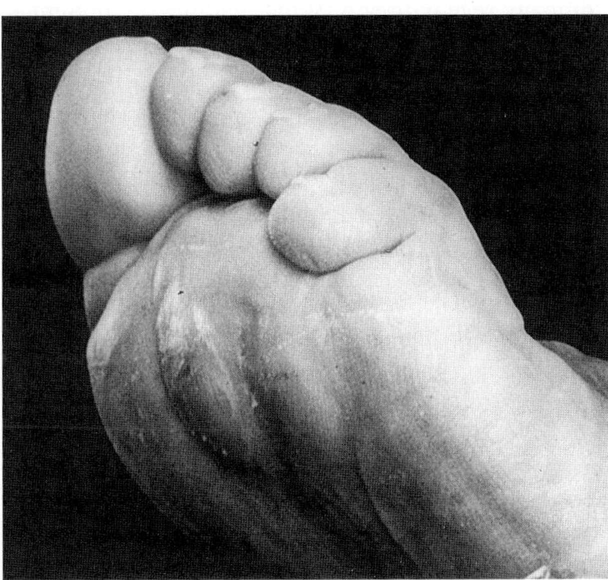

Figure 23.11 Metatarsophalangeal subluxation. *(Used by permission of the American College of Rheumatology.)*

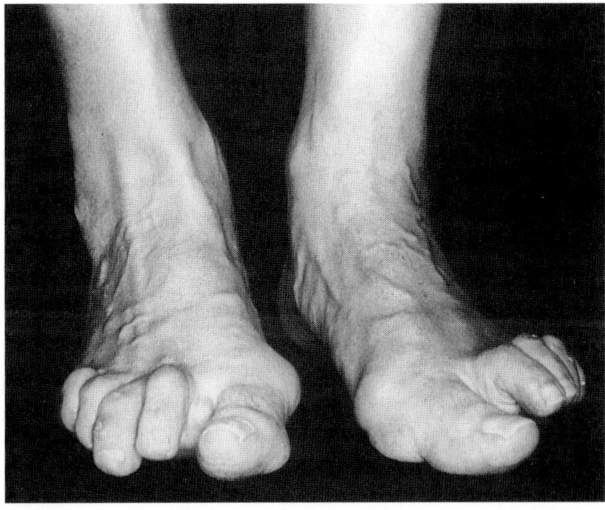

Figure 23.12 Common deformities of the rheumatoid foot. Evident in this photo are hallux valgus of the great toe, hammer toes, and cock-up toes due to metatarsophalangeal joint subluxation. *(Used by permission of the American College of Rheumatology.)*

Muscle Involvement

Muscle atrophy around affected joints may be present early. Roughly 50% of patients with RA will develop *rheumatoid cachexia*, a loss of muscle loss with concurrent increase in fat mass and increase in body mass index.[30] It is not definitively known, however, whether this atrophy results from disuse or selective attrition of muscles owing to some unknown mechanism specifically related to the disease process. It appears that individuals

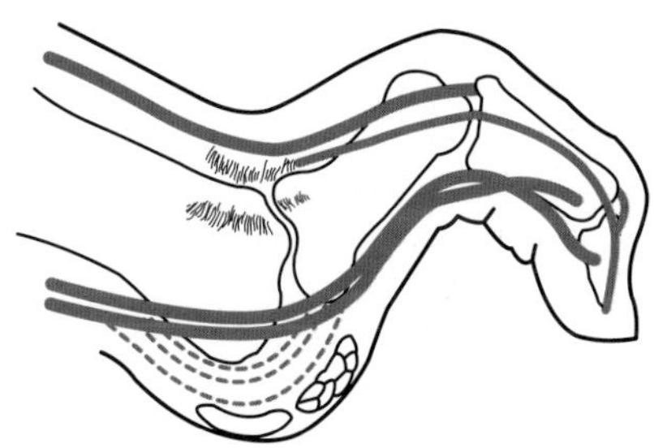

Figure 23.13 Relationship of structures to the metatarsal heads in metatarsalgia. *(From Moncur, C, and Shields, M: Clinical management of metatarsalgia in the patient with arthritis. Clin Manage Phys Ther 3:7, 1983, p 10, with permission.)*

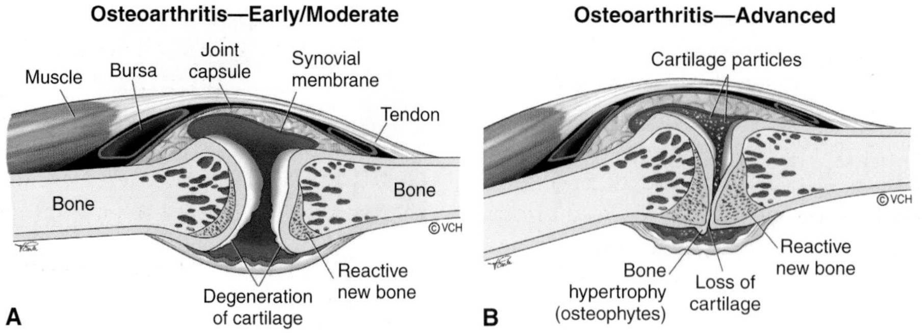

Figure 23.14 Early-advanced osteoarthritis joint changes. Early joint changes are characterized by superficial damage to articular cartilage and mild inflammation. Progression to moderate joint changes includes joint space narrowing with full-thickness damage to cartilage and thickening of the subchondral bone. Advanced joint changes are marked by bony hypertrophy (marginal osteophytes), significant joint space narrowing, and possible angulation (deformity). *(From Mary Pack Arthritis Program, Vancouver Coastal Health, with permission.)*

with RA who have rheumatoid cachexia experience selective attrition of Type II (phasic) muscle fibers through some unknown mechanism.[30,31] Evidence suggests that elevated production of *cytokines* (i.e., TNF-α and IL-1β) may contribute to rheumatoid cachexia. Specifically, the cytokines can trigger cell death by nuclear apoptosis in skeletal muscle[30] perhaps leading to muscle loss in RA.[32] There is also some evidence that Type I (tonic) muscle fibers of the quadriceps will undergo selective atrophy following anterior cruciate ligament damage.[31] Loss of muscle bulk may also be the result of a peripheral neuropathy or steroid-induced myopathy. Muscle weakness may be due to either reflex inhibition secondary to pain or atrophy.[30-32]Atrophy in the hand intrinsics and the quadriceps is particularly evident in long-standing disease, although the mechanisms for these changes may not be the same.

Tendon Involvement

Tenosynovitis, inflammation of the lining of the sheath that surrounds a tendon, may occur with active disease and interferes with the smooth gliding of the tendon through the sheath. Inflammation may directly damage the tendon, eventually leading to a tendon rupture. Common sites of tenosynovitis are wrist flexors, thumb flexors, patella, and Achilles tendons. Trigger finger and *de Quervain's tenosynovitis* may occur. A patient with tendon damage or muscle weakness may exhibit a *lag phenomenon,* which refers to a substantial difference in passive versus active ROM. This is a nonspecific finding that therapists need to examine carefully to determine its cause and design appropriate treatment.[29]

Deconditioning

Deconditioning is a significant clinical feature of RA. Research assessing physical fitness in persons with RA has demonstrated diminished cardiorespiratory status, muscular strength and endurance, flexibility, and altered body composition among these individuals when compared with healthy individuals of the same age and gender without arthritis. Deconditioning results from both direct and indirect impairments.[30-32] Direct impairments of RA include loss of Type II muscle fibers, systemic fatigue, cachexia (wasting of lean body mass),[30-32] and shortening of contractile tissues. Indirect impairments of RA include deconditioning secondary to inactivity and elevated resting energy expenditure (calories required by the body during a 24-hour period under resting conditions). Immune system activity and inflammation, even in individuals with well-controlled disease, create an increased metabolism with subsequent loss of lean body tissue.[31,33]

Rheumatoid Nodules

Rheumatoid nodules occur in approximately 20% to 25% of patients and are associated with a positive serological test for RF. Nodules are generally tender and accompany severe disease. When nodules are present in early RA they are suggestive for a greater likelihood of severe *extra-articular* manifestations. Nodules are found in the subcutaneous or deeper connective tissues in areas subjected to repeated mechanical pressure such as the olecranon bursae, the extensor surfaces of the forearms, and the Achilles tendons. The presence of nodules on tendon mechanisms may lead to mechanical breakdown and tenosynovitis.[26,29]

Vascular and Neurologic Complications

Vasculitis, or inflammation of the blood vessels, has been found in 25% to 30% of individuals with RA on autopsy.[29] Most forms of vascular lesions associated with RA are silent and difficult to diagnose due to variability in the size of blood vessels affected. Skin vasculitis is the easiest to observe and can present as discoloration of the nail beds, purpura (red or purple discoloration), and petechiae (red or purple spots). The fulminant form of *rheumatoid arteritis* (arterial inflammation associated with a rheumatoid disorder) can be life threatening, and accompanied by malnutrition, infection, congestive heart failure (CHF), and gastrointestinal bleeding. Vasculitis of the vessels supplying nerves can lead to peripheral neuropathies such as foot or wrist drop.[1] Peripheral neuropathies may also occur secondary to mechanical compression of nerves such as carpal tunnel or tarsal tunnel syndrome. Spinal cord compression may result from inflammation in the cervical spine (see section on cervical spine and TMJ), and if clinical signs of cord compression are present, this requires immediate medical attention.[1]

Cardiovascular and Pulmonary Complications

Morbidity and mortality from cardiovascular disease is elevated in persons with RA due to a greater prevalence of ischemic heart disease, secondary to accelerated atherosclerosis. In fact, patients with RA have nearly a twofold increase risk of developing coronary artery disease (CAD), a risk similar to adults with diabetes.[33] Although the exact etiology of accelerated atherosclerosis is unclear, it is hypothesized that metabolic and vascular effects of chronic inflammation may be the causative factor.[33,34] Subclinical pericarditis may be present and has been demonstrated at autopsy. Heart failure is also more prevalent among adults with RA, especially among patients who are RF positive as compared to those who are RF negative. However, patients with RA who have heart failure have an atypical presentation making it harder to detect and resulting in less aggressive management. Some evidence suggests patients with RA have heart failure related to diastolic dysfunction.[35]

Pulmonary involvement is frequent and more prevalent in men than women and among those with high rheumatoid titers. Nodes are more commonly found in the periphery of the upper and middle regions of the lung. *Pleuritis* and pulmonary nodules may be present. Pulmonary nodules are related to presence of nodules elsewhere and found among seropositive patients with profuse synovitis. Nodules may be 0.40 to 3 in (1 to 8 cm) in size and affect gas exchange.[26]

Ocular Complications

Keratoconjunctivitis, inflammation of the cornea and conjunctiva, is the most common ocular complication in RA, impacting about 10% of all patients. The severity of this condition, however, is not proportional to the severity of RA. *Uveitis,* inflammation of the uvea located between the sclera and retina may be present in RA leading to blurred vision dark, floating spots, eye pain, redness, and light sensitivity. *Episcleritis* is a benign and self-limiting process that typically correlates with RA disease activity. With episcleritis patients present with red and painful eyes and the distribution may be diffuse or nodular. *Scleritis,* inflammation of the sclera, is associated with long-standing disease. Patients with scleritis experience eye pain, redness, redness, blurred vision, tearing, and sensitivity to light. If scleritis goes untreated it may lead to *scleromalacia,* thinning of the sclera and eventual blindness. The difference between episcleritis and scleritis is difficult to detect with clinical symptoms. Therefore, patients with RA should undergo annual eye examinations, and, if symptoms of suspected eye disease are present, they should be referred to an ophthalmologist.[29]

Activity Limitation and Participation Restriction

Patients with milder forms of RA may suffer from activity limitations and decreased participation in ADL due to joint destruction. Almost 50% of individuals with RA will eventually have marked restrictions in ADL.[1] Late-onset RA is generally associated with better functional outcomes and less activity limitations and participation restrictions, though the cause of these findings is unclear. Table 23.1 presents a broad classification of functional status in RA that characterizes the progressive impact of the disease.[23] Loss of income is a major consequence of RA and is directly attributable to work disability. In a large international comparison study, work disability rates were high in persons with RA and disability was associated with disease factors as well as societal factors.[36]

Prognosis

RA causes increased morbidity and reduces life span. The question of mortality associated with RA is controversial. Previously, it was believed that RA itself was not usually a cause of death, although conditions such as systemic vasculitis and atlantoaxial subluxation could be fatal. There is presently a growing body of evidence that individuals with RA have decreased survival compared to their siblings and may not live as long as their counterparts without disease, especially if the early years of RA were marked by aggressive disease and poor functional status. Causes of death occurring more frequently in patients with RA as compared to the general population are infections; ischemic heart disease; and renal, respiratory, and gastrointestinal disease.[26,29,37]

Although numerous prognostic factors have been identified in the literature, there is no firm consensus regarding specific prognostic factors. Research demonstrates that individuals with a positive RF are more likely to progress to severe disease, as are those with high ESR and CRP at baseline. Baseline CRP is also associated with radiographic changes later in life.[38,39] Similarly, baseline radiographics are strongly associated with pattern of progression. Genetic research suggests that a shared epitope in the hypervariable region of the HLA-DR is associated with disease severity in a dose-dependent manner.[40]

Remission Criteria

In 2011, in response to the increasing ability to achieve remission with appropriate medical management, the ACR, the European League Against Rheumatism

(EULAR), and the ACR Outcomes Measures in Rheumatology Initiatives developed a rigorous set of remission criteria. *Remission*, described as little if any active disease, can be operationally confirmed based on one of two definitions: (a) when scores on the tender joint count, swollen joint count, CRP (in mg/dL), and the *Patient Global Assessment* (0–10 scale rating how patient feels overall) are all less than or equal to 1, or (b) when the score on the *Simplified Disease Activity Index* (numerical sum of all of the above plus the score on the Physician Global Assessment) is less than or equal to 3.3.[41]

OSTEOARTHRITIS

Osteoarthritis (OA) is primarily confined to one or more synovial joints and its surrounding soft tissues. Two predominant, pathological features once defined OA: the progressive destruction of articular cartilage and the formation of bone at the margins of the joint.[1] OA is now recognized as a disease involving the entire joint including the periarticular musculature[42] (Fig. 23.14). Accordingly, the impairment, activity limitations, and participation restrictions related to OA extend far beyond the boundaries of the synovial joint. Data on the personal and societal impact of OA increasingly demonstrate its importance as an individual and public health issue.

Epidemiology

Osteoarthritis is the most common form of arthritis and extremely prevalent among individuals over 40 years of age. Based on data from the *Medical Expenditure Panel Survey* (MEPS), it is estimated that 30.8 million adults in the United States (13.4% of U.S. adult population) are living with OA.[43] It is widespread in adults older than 65, and affects men more than women before age 50, but reverses after age 50.[1] Studies concerning racial predisposition to OA have yielded conflicting data, depending on the joint studied. Several longitudinal studies have revealed that the prevalence of radiographic and symptomatic knee OA was highest in non-Hispanic African Americans compared to non-Hispanic whites or Mexican Americans, which had similar prevalence rates.[44] Chinese women were found to have a higher prevalence of radiographic and symptomatic knee compared with white females of the same age. Conversely, radiographic hip OA is lower among Chinese women whereas similar rates are reported when comparing African-Americans and Caucasians.[44]

Etiology

Similar to RA, no single factor that predisposes an individual to OA has been identified. Although aging is indeed strongly associated with OA, it must be emphasized that aging in itself does not cause OA, nor should OA be considered synonymous with the "normal" aging process.[1,45] In fact, many OA-related changes seen at both a cellular and tissue level are opposite those seen with normal aging.[46] Several factors related to aging may, however, contribute to its development. Genetic factors account for between 39% and 65% of radiographic OA of the hand, hip, and knee in women and as much as 70% of OA cases of the spine.[47] Trauma before adulthood may initiate a remodeling of bone that alters joint mechanics and nutrition in a way that becomes problematic only later in life. The role of repetitive *microtrauma* in the etiology of OA has also received attention.[1] Specifically, occupational tasks involving heavy lifting are associated with the development of hip OA,[48] and those involving kneeling and heavy lifting are related to the development of knee OA.[49,50] Malalignment, including *varus* and *valgus* deformities, and leg length discrepancy are associated with greater prevalence of knee and hip OA, respectively.[50,51] The strongest predictor of disease progression in the knee is varus malalignment.[52] At the hip, there is increasing recognition of the role of *femoroacetabular impingement* (FAI) (a mechanical mismatch between the femoral head and acetabulum) in development of OA.[53] Finally, obesity has been shown to be a risk factor for the development of OA in later life; it is most evident in the knee joint and to a lesser extent in the hip and hands.[1,51] Obesity is also associated with greater functional decline in knee OA.[54] The relationship between obesity and incidence of OA is stronger in women than in men.[51] Risk factors for OA can be classified as either systemic or local (Box 23.1), and OA most likely results from the combined effect of multiple factors acting on a vulnerable joint that leads to disease.[51,55] It is imperative that physical therapists understand and are able to counsel patients on those factors that are modifiable and amenable to therapeutic interventions.

Pathophysiology

Normal Cartilage

Healthy articular cartilage is composed of an extracellular matrix and *chondrocytes*. Water makes up between 65% and 80% of the matrix by weight, mostly Type II

Box 23.1 Risk Factors for Osteoarthritis[1,50,51]

Systemic Factors	Local Factors
Age	Obesity
Gender	Major joint trauma (e.g., ACL rupture)
Race	Repetitive stress (occupation)
Genetics	Muscle weakness/imbalance
Metabolic/endocrine	Altered joint biomechanics
High bone density	Joint malalignment
Nutritional status (e.g., vitamin D deficiency)	Proprioceptive impairments
Congenital/developmental	
Obesity	

collagen contributes approximately 10%, and *proteoglycans* (molecules found in articular cartilage), noncollagenous proteins, and glycoproteins the remainder.[50,55] It is the matrix that protects the chondrocytes from damage during normal joint use. Chondrocytes, the only cells in articular cartilage, secrete the matrix yet make up only 1% of the total volume of adult human articular cartilage.[50] Chondrocytes are dispersed throughout the extracellular matrix but most concentrated in the deep layer. The superficial layer has the highest concentration of water and collagen fibers giving this zone the greatest tensile stiffness and strength and ability to resist shearing forces.[50] Proteoglycans consist of a protein core and one or more glycosaminoglycans (GAGs), including hyaluronic acid (HA) and chondroitin sulfate. Proteoglycan concentration is highest in the middle and deep zones.[50]

Articular cartilage contains no nerves, blood vessels, or lymphatic vessels. It receives its nutrition and eliminates waste via diffusion through synovial fluid and by facilitated *imbibition* (absorption of fluid by a solid body).[50] The multiple roles of articular cartilage include decreasing friction between articulating joint surfaces, distributing static and dynamic joint forces to the underlying bone and absorbing shock.[50,56] Cartilage's shock-absorbing function is minimal (1% to 3% of load forces), however, compared to that of subchondral bone (30%)[50] and periarticular muscles (which requires timely and coordinated muscle contraction). These joint structures together with ligaments, menisci, capsule, synovium, and synovial fluid serve to protect the joint from regular wear and tear and damaging forces. Regular forces acting on the articular cartilage include body weight, muscle contractions, and ground reaction forces that vary with the rate and duration of loading and the available load-bearing surface.[50,55] Extremes of joint loading in either direction can lead to detrimental morphological and metabolic changes in the cartilage whereas moderate, cyclic loading enhances proteoglycan synthesis and concentration.[42,50]

Joint Pathology

The first osteoarthritic change in articular cartilage, which has been confirmed in humans, is an increase in water content. This increase suggests that the proteoglycans have become swollen with water far beyond normal. This process, together with disruption of other components of the extracellular matrix, decreases the stiffness of the matrix and leads to further mechanical damage.[50,55]

In later stages of disease progression, proteoglycans are lost, which diminishes the water content of cartilage. As proteoglycans are lost, articular cartilage loses its compressive stiffness and elasticity, which, in turn, results in the transmission of compressive forces to underlying bone. Collagen synthesis is increased initially, although there is a shift from type II collagen fibers to a larger proportion of type I collagen, the kind found in skin and fibrous tissue. Chondrocytes attempt to respond to this early tissue damage by synthesizing new matrix molecules and proliferating and forming clusters of cells.[50,56] As the articular cartilage is destroyed, the joint space narrows.[42] In summary, the early phases of cartilage degeneration are characterized by biosynthesis and repair as the chondrocytes attempt to restore the damaged matrix while the later phase is degradative in nature as catabolic enzyme activity digests the matrix and erodes the cartilage. Age-related oxidative stress and *cell senescence* (reduced proliferation of cells) can further contribute to increased production of inflammatory *cytokines* and these catabolic matrix metalloproteinases.[45,50,56]

One of the first noticeable changes in cartilage is the mild fraying or "flaking" of superficial collagen fibers. Deeper fraying, or "fibrillation," of the upper third of the cartilage follows in areas of greater weight-bearing and may progress to full-thickness fissures (Fig. 23.15). As the cartilage degenerates, there are accompanying changes in the subchondral bone including increased bone density or subchondral sclerosis, creation of cyst-like bone cavities, and formation of marginal *osteophytes*.[1,50,57] The cartilage may degenerate to the point that the exposed subchondral bone becomes necrotic and *eburnated* (polished or ivory-like) (Fig. 23.16). The stiffer than normal subchondral bone further decreases the shock-absorbing properties of the joint and results in greater impact loading.[50] The traditional view of OA is that the disease process starts with an unrepaired injury to articular cartilage; however, there is also evidence that reduced compliance in subchondral bone and periarticular structures may initiate the degenerative processes.[50,56]

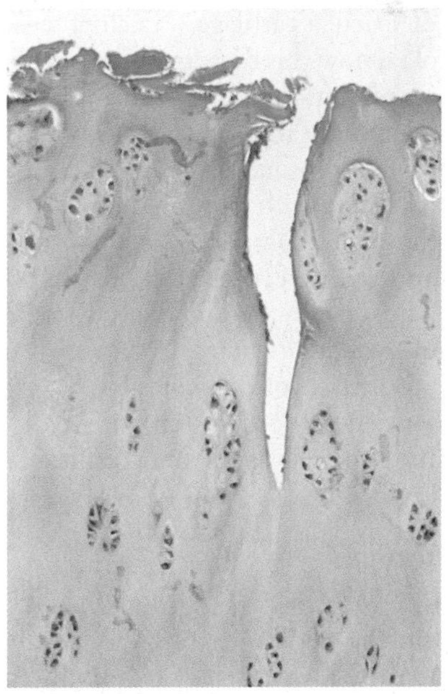

Figure 23.15 Osteoarthritis: cartilage, clefts and fibrillation (histological specimen). *(Used by permission of the American College of Rheumatology.)*

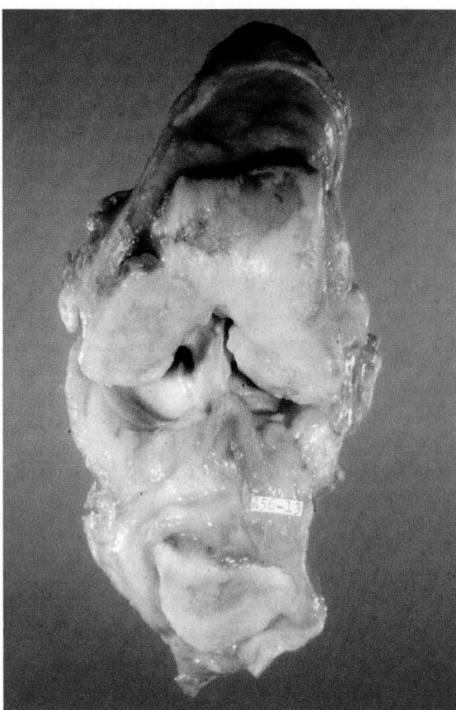

Figure 23.16 Osteoarthritis: knee, gross pathology. *(Used by permission of the American College of Rheumatology.)*

Osteophytes may be fibrous, cartilaginous, or bony in composition and marginal prominences are palpable and often tender in more superficial joints.[1,50,57] The process of osteophyte formation in OA is not well understood. Current hypotheses have implicated increased vascularity in the deepest layers of the degenerated cartilage, venous congestion from subchondral cysts and thickened subchondral trabeculae, and the continued sloughing of articular cartilage.[57] Each of these hypotheses may explain how this bony growth contributes to the pain and loss of motion that accompany OA. Subchondral cysts containing myxoid, fibrous, or cartilaginous tissue along with bone marrow lesions identified through MRI, are associated with painful knee OA.[56,59]

Although traditionally viewed as a non-inflammatory disease, improved detection methods suggest that inflammation does play a role and that inflammatory pathways are up-regulated (increased responsiveness) with increased production of cytokines.[1,45,50,56] Further inflammatory reactions occur in response to cartilage fragments in the synovial cavity and resultant low-grade synovitis.[50]

OA Phenotypes

A number of *phenotypes* (subgroups) have been identified within the heterogeneous OA population and differentiated by a number of factors including presentation of joint involvement, radiographic severity, depression, body mass index (BMI), muscle strength, and pain.[56,58] Recognizing these phenotypes of patients may help to detect OA in its early stages and distinguish patients who are at higher risk of progression. This in turn could be used to guide clinical decision making and lead to phenotype-specific therapeutic interventions.[55,58]

Disease Onset and Course

Osteoarthritis usually starts in an insidious fashion and may progress undetected in some individuals when early, aneural articular cartilage is the only involved tissue. Pain is initially episodic and triggered by specific activity. In later disease, pain becomes a chronic, dull ache accentuated with episodic severe pain.[42] It is pain that leads an individual to seek medical help. Unlike RA, there are no systemic features such as fatigue, fever, or malaise with the onset of OA.

OA is typically a slowly progressive condition; however, most people with radiographic evidence of joint damage in their hips or knees stabilize and do not require joint replacement surgery.[1] The pathological process involved in OA appears to be cyclical with active periods of increased matrix protein turnover interspersed with inactive phases.[60] The prognosis is variable and not necessarily bad. However, in combination with normal aging, comorbidities often present in older adults, and high levels of inactivity in this population, OA can contribute to increasing disability.[1]

Classification and Diagnostic Criteria

OA is typically differentiated in two ways: *primary* (*idiopathic*) and *secondary* disease.[1] When the etiology of the disease is unknown with no known prior event, it is termed primary or idiopathic OA. This category can be further divided into *localized* (one or two joints affected) or *generalized* OA (affecting three or more joints).[1] Generalized OA typically involves the hands in a more symmetrical fashion not unlike inflammatory forms of arthritis and has a stronger genetic association.[1] OA is classified as secondary when the etiology (e.g., trauma, biomechanical factors, congenital malformation, or other musculoskeletal disease) can be identified. There is increasing evidence that many cases categorized as idiopathic are more appropriately recognized as secondary disease as our ability to detect subtle and early biochemical, histological, morphological, and biomechanical factors improve.

Most researchers have used Kellgren and Lawrence's *radiographic classification system* and their grade 2 definition (the presence of definite osteophytes) as the criterion for identifying disease, although a few others have required evidence of joint space narrowing (grade 3 corresponding to clinically identified disease) to designate OA.[61] This five-point system remains the most widely used criteria for grading radiographic changes both clinically and for purposes of research.[61]

- Grade 0: normal radiograph
- Grade 1: doubtful narrowing of the joint space and possible osteophytes

- Grade 2: definite osteophytes and absent or questionable narrowing of the joint space
- Grade 3: moderate osteophytes and joint space narrowing, some sclerosis, and possible deformity
- Grade 4: large osteophytes, marked narrowing of joint space, severe sclerosis, and definite deformity

It is widely recognized, however, that radiographic findings are not strongly related to clinical symptoms and pain severity[51] and add little to the accuracy of the clinical diagnosis. In knee OA, muscle strength and pain are more explanatory of functional loss than radiographic findings.[62] Radiographs are frequently used to confirm the extent of joint damage and disease progression and continue to be a component of the ACR diagnostic criteria.[42]

The clinical criteria for hip,[63] knee,[64] and hand[65] OA are described primarily in terms of pain and limitation of motion (Box 23.2).

Radiography/Imaging

In Figure 23.17, early OA changes of the right hip are depicted. Newer imaging techniques including high-resolution MRI are able to detect early structural changes and pathology in pain-sensitive structures well before changes are observable on radiographs.[42,66] Real-time ultrasound allows visualization of both bony and soft tissue structures and is more sensitive than clinical examination in detecting effusion, synovitis, and early osteophytes in OA.[66] In Figure 23.18, an ultrasound image of a popliteal or Baker's cyst in the knee is shown. Ultrasound imaging has greater potential for routine use in clinical practice than MRI.

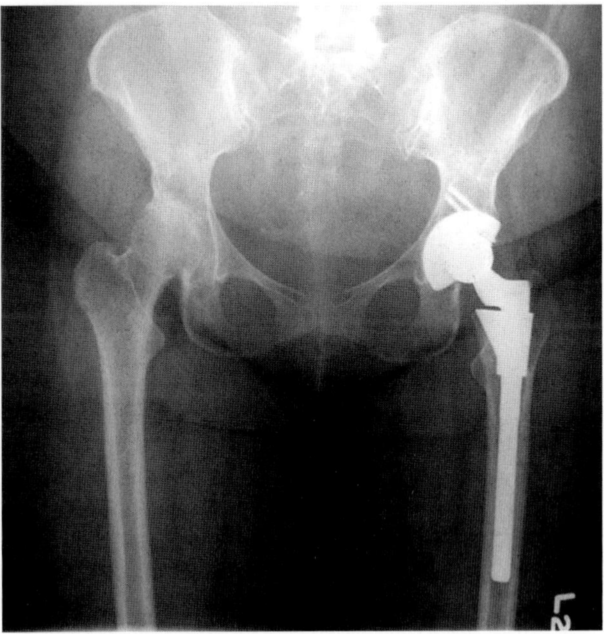

Figure 23.17 Osteoarthritis: Mild degenerative changes right hip, total hip replacement in left. *(Used by permission of the American College of Rheumatology.)*

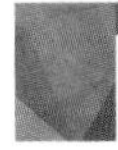

Box 23.2 Clinical Classification Criteria for Knee, Hip, and Hand Osteoarthritis

Knee Osteoarthritis[a64]

- Persistent knee pain
- Limited morning stiffness ≤30 minutes
- Reduced function
- Crepitus
- Bony enlargement
- Restricted movement

Hip Osteoarthritis[b63]

Pain present in combination with either:

- Hip internal rotation ≥15°; morning stiffness ≤60 minutes; and age >50 years, and pain on internal rotation, *or*
- Hip internal rotation <15° and hip flexion <115°

Hand Osteoarthritis[c65]

- Presence of Heberden's nodes
- Age >40 years
- Family history of nodes
- Joint space narrowing in any finger joint

[a]Correctly diagnoses 99% of knee OA when all six criteria are met.[64]
[b]86% sensitivity, 75% specificity.[63]
[c]Correctly diagnoses 88% of patients when all four criteria are met.[65]

Clinical Presentation

Signs and Symptoms (Impairments)

As noted already, the clinical diagnosis is often made on the basis of signs and symptoms (e.g., pain and swelling, loss of ROM, and bony deformity). Not all joints are equally affected by OA. In the upper extremity (UE), the finger DIP and PIP joints and CMC of the thumb are commonly involved. The cervical and lumbar spine, hips, knees, and MTP of the great toe are also sites for OA. The MCP joints, wrists, elbows, and shoulders are usually spared in primary OA.[1] Unlike RA, OA does not have a bilateral, symmetrical presentation (with the exception of generalized OA).[1] (See Figure 23.4A-OA homunculus.) A single joint or any combination of joints may be affected and of differing etiological origins. OA is not a systemic disease and is therefore not associated with systemic complaints of fatigue, generalized morning stiffness, fever, or loss of appetite. Severe fatigue, however, is reported by nearly half of patients with hip and knee OA and is associated with factors such as greater pain, less physical activity, and depression.[67] Individuals with OA may experience some stiffness in particular joints on awakening that is similar to the stiffness felt when moving the same joints after inactivity during the day, but this stiffness (articular gelling) typically does not last more than 30 minutes, nor is it generalized to

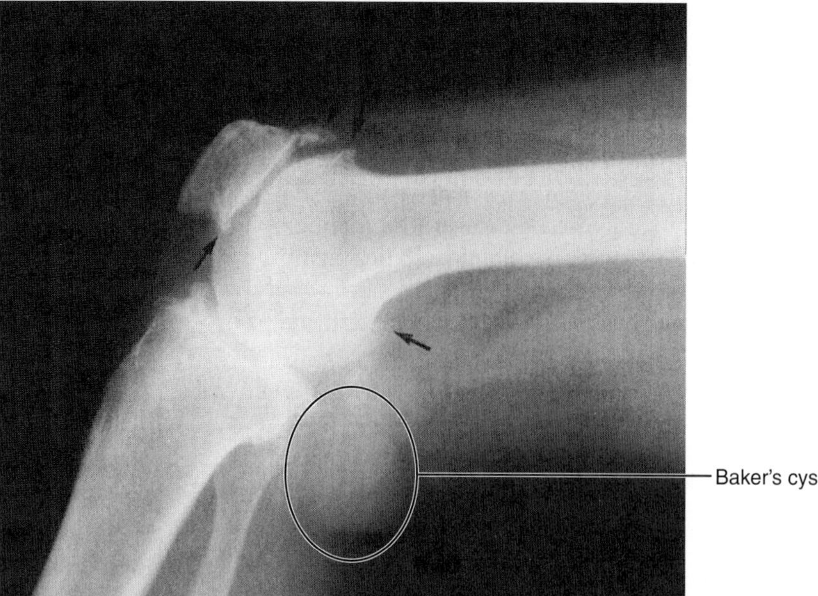

Figure 23.18 Baker's cyst via ultrasound.

the entire body.[1,42] Crepitus is a common clinical finding in OA and may progress from a painless grating sensation to an extremely painful, high-pitched sound as a result of bone-on-bone articulation.

Although cartilage degeneration is the primary manifestation of OA, cartilage is aneural, and therefore not the cause of a person's pain. Pain in OA can arise from any innervated tissue and may be attributed to incongruent articulations of joint surfaces, periosteal elevation secondary to bone proliferation at the joint margin (osteophytes), vasocongestion in subchondral bone, trabecular microfractures, distention of the joint capsule and ligaments, and muscle spasm or strain.[42,56,59] Many patients will also experience a secondary synovitis and effusion, especially when the knee is involved.[56,59]

As noted earlier, symptoms do not always match the severity of the disease on radiographs. Further, some patients with OA may have an amplified pain experience and central pain sensitization at the spinal or cortical level.[56] Unlike individuals with RA who often report more pain and stiffness at rest, the pain associated with OA is likely to occur or worsen with motion, except in the later stages of the disease when it is present at rest and with activity.[1,42]

Joints

OA may present differently and result in varied levels of impairment depending on the joints involved. The most commonly affected joints are described and noted on the homunculus (Fig 23.4).

Hands and Fingers: OA may present differently and result in varied levels of impairment depending on the joints involved. In the hand, DIP and PIP involvement may result in reduced ROM, poor grip strength, bony nodes, and joint angulation as a result of stretched collateral ligaments or bone erosion. Bouchard's nodes at the PIP joints and Heberden's nodes at the DIP joints are often tender in the early stages and can lead to marked restrictions in finger ROM and fine motor skills later in the disease (Fig 23.19). Osteoarthritic damage in the first CMC joint results in pain or aching at the base of the thumb and can lead to decreased pinch strength and squaring of the thumb (thickening and prominence of CMC due to subluxation of first metacarpal) as a result of weakness and contracture of the thenar muscles.[68] This in turn affects abduction, extension, and opposition ROM of the thumb and greatly affects grip strength and hand function.[69] In cases of generalized OA, the hands are always affected and in a more symmetrical pattern.[1] Painful inflammation with synovitis, erosive changes, cystic swellings, and osteophytes are present in this less common form of OA and may lead to ankylosis of the DIP and PIP joints.[1,68]

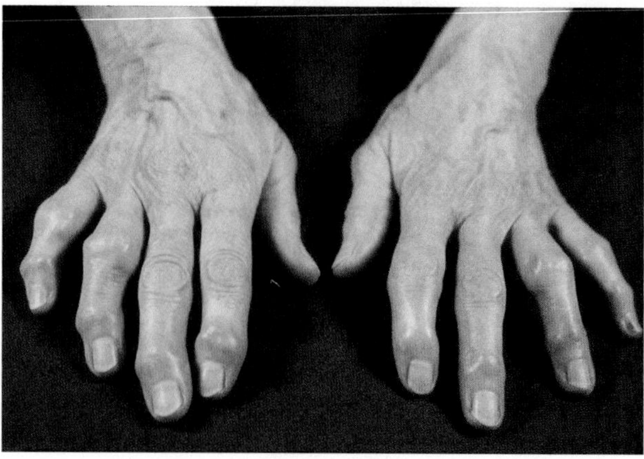

Figure 23.19 Osteoarthritis: Heberden's and Bouchard's nodes, hand. *(Used by permission of the American College of Rheumatology.)*

Hips: Symptoms of hip OA are usually insidious in onset and may include a limp and decreased ROM with a tendency for the hip to be held in a somewhat flexed, abducted, and externally rotated position. Internal rotation is usually restricted and painful.[70] Pain arising from the hip joint is commonly experienced in the groin, but can also be felt in the buttock, trochanteric, or knee region.[70,71] Lateral hip pain is most often associated with gluteus medius and minimus tendinopathy and often misdiagnosed as trochanteric bursitis.[72] Decreased hip ROM is associated with decreased walking speed, decreased stride length, poor balance, and increased energy expenditure.[71] Even early hip OA is associated with a 52% increased risk of falls.[73]

Knees: Early presentation of knee OA includes pain with weight-bearing activities such as climbing stairs and squatting. In later stages, both pain and stiffness are reported after prolonged sitting such as with watching a movie. Symptoms of joint locking and buckling (giving way) may also occur with damage to stabilizing menisci and ligaments[70] and lead to increased risk of falls.[42] Proximal hip weakness, most notably the gluteal muscles, and soft tissue shortening, especially in the rectus femoris, are also common.[74] Knee OA more commonly affects the medial joint due to the higher weight-bearing load placed on this compartment. As a result, medial joint space narrowing often results in *pseudolaxity* of the medial collateral ligament, stretching of the lateral collateral counterpart, and a genu varus deformity (Fig. 23.20). Genu valgus as a result of greater lateral compartment involvement is less common. A *flexion deformity* of several degrees can develop quickly in the painful knee and contribute to a functional leg length discrepancy, decreased step length, and quadriceps muscular fatigue or strain. Patellofemoral compartment OA, with its hallmark anterior knee pain, can occur in isolation as a result of patella malalignment, abnormal tracking and loading and direct trauma to the patella.[70]

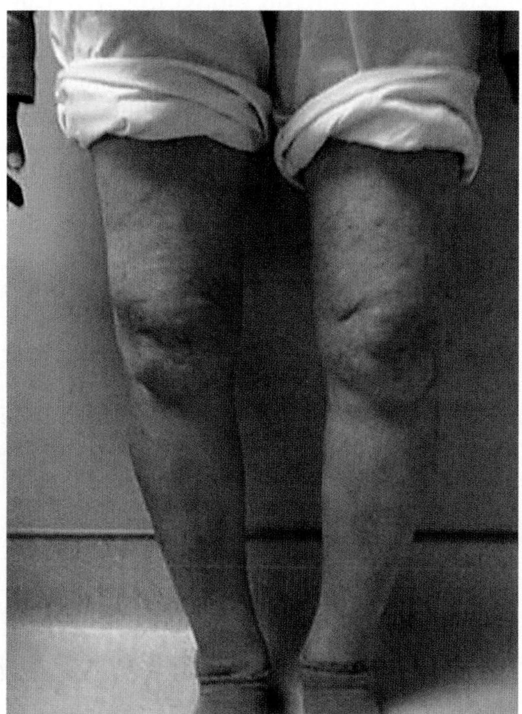

Figure 23.20 Bilateral genu varum. *(Dr. Basram Masri, with permission.)*

Feet and Toes: Two distinct phenotypes of foot OA are suggested. Isolated first MTP joint OA is the most common and may result in hallux rigidus or hallux valgus deformities, first interphalangeal joint hyperextension, and hindfoot eversion. Polyarticular foot OA with changes in the other MTP joints, toes, and medial tarsal joints can lead to shortening of the long extensors, hammer toes, reduced MTP flexion, and flattened sagittal arch.[75,76] Forefoot involvement contributes to painful and limited push-off in the terminal stance phase of gait, slower walking speed, and balance issues (Fig 23.21).[75,76]

Spine: The lower cervical and mid to lower lumbar regions of the spine are most susceptible to OA. All spinal articulations can experience degenerative changes; however, the facet (zygapophyseal) joints are the only true synovial joints in the spine.[77] Degeneration of the intervertebral disks may precede facet joint involvement by many years and lead to increased compressive loads and degenerative changes. Facet joint osteophytes can contribute to lateral and central lumbar stenosis and subsequent nerve root impingement[77] (Fig. 23.22). Pain from lumbar facet joint OA can originate from the joint itself and affected nerve roots (radicular pain) and in the lumbar area, and typically increases with spinal extension, rotary motions, and with prolonged standing or sitting.[77]

Consequences of OA

Although not a systemic illness, OA has been linked to an increased risk of cardiovascular disease (CVD) and all-cause mortality. In a large Canadian cohort of older adults with hip/knee OA followed over 10 years, greater self-reported functional disability, walking disability and use of a walking aid were associated with all-cause mortality and risk for a serious CVD event even after controlling for comorbidities such as obesity, diabetes, and hypertension.[78] Physical therapy interventions to reduce walking disability may have an important protective effect.

Activity Limitations and Participation Restrictions

Overall, OA of the knee can impose functional limitations to a degree equivalent to heart disease, CHF, and chronic obstructive pulmonary disease (COPD) and accounts for a substantial proportion of the burden of disability among community-living elders.[79]

Patients with the most severe disease may not move their joints as often or in the ways that exacerbate their symptoms. Therefore, pain, disease severity, and functional

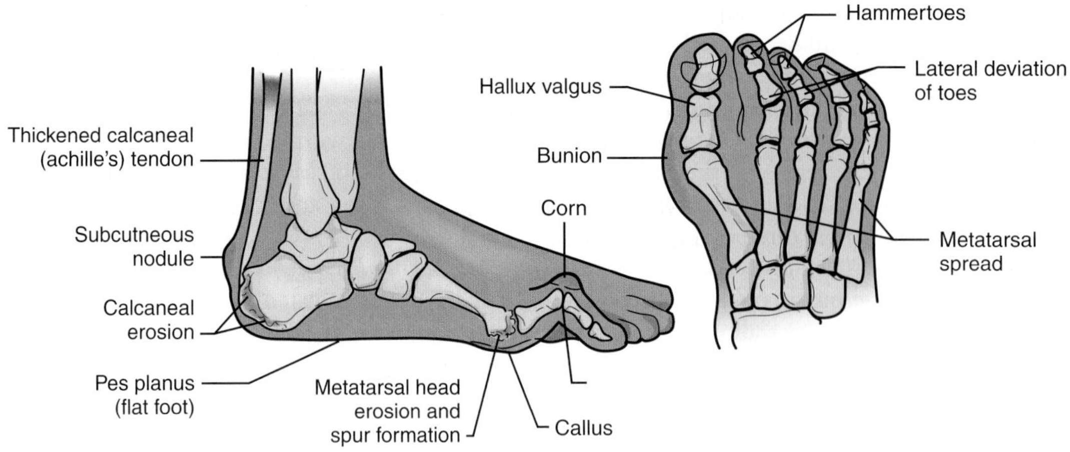

Figure 23.21 Osteoarthritic foot.

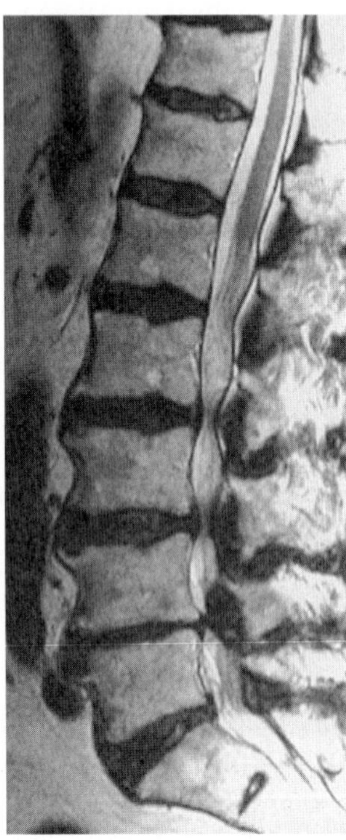

Figure 23.22 Spinal stenosis: lumbar spine, MRI image. *(Used by permission of the American College of Rheumatology.)*

disability in individuals with OA are interrelated. Among elders, it has been shown that the functional loss associated with severe radiographic OA without pain is more likely than the loss associated with symptomatic but milder disease.[80] One explanation of this finding is that individuals with OA limit their functional activities to avoid movements that are painful. In the clinical examination it is important to determine functional status even in the absence of pain. Given that individuals with OA may reduce or eliminate their symptoms by avoiding certain activities, clinicians should explore activity limitations and physical inactivity-related symptoms in patients with OA separately from the evaluation of symptoms.

Greater self-reported disability in advanced knee OA was associated with pain, joint laxity, age, and BMI among Finnish adults ages 60 to 80 years while performance-based functioning was related to the self-report *Western Ontario and McMasters Universities Arthritis Index* (WOMAC) function score, pain, and obesity.[62] Of interest, the authors found no association between radiographic severity of knee OA and self-reported and performance-based function.[62] The comprehensive *International Classification of Functioning, Disability, and Health* (ICF) *Core Set* of impairments, activity limitations, and participation restrictions has been established through an international team of researchers, clinicians, and patients to identify those areas of functioning that are affected by OA, with the shorter Brief ICF Core Set created for clinical purposes.[81,82] OA is a leading cause of disability and major contributor to work-related disability, reduced productivity, and absenteeism.[83]

Prognosis

OA is a slow-progressing disease that can be self-limiting or can progress to advanced joint and soft tissue damage leading to complete failure of that joint. In such a case, joint surgery including *arthrodesis* of some joints in the foot, or *arthroplasty* (replacement), for example, of the hip or knee is the final treatment option to help the patient regain function. However, rapidly progressive joint damage is uncommon; in most cases, patients stabilize.[1] Increasing disability may be more related to advancing years and comorbidities such as obesity and inactivity.

■ MEDICAL MANAGEMENT

Pharmacological Therapy in Rheumatoid Arthritis

Joint destruction and irreversible damage are most pronounced early in the disease course. Current medical management is based on the implementation of an early, aggressive, treat-to-target approach to disease management designed to reach remission or low disease activity and eventually to halt or decrease progression.[84] Medical therapies also focus on decreasing pain and inflammation. Early aggressive pharmacological therapy is associated with diminished joint damage and long-term maintenance of function. The major classifications of drugs used in RA management include non-steroidal anti-inflammatory drugs (NSAIDs) and disease-modifying anti-rheumatic drugs (DMARDs), which include the biological response modifiers (BRMs) and corticosteroids.[84]

Nonsteroidal Anti-Inflammatory Drugs

NSAIDs provide both *analgesic* and *anti-inflammatory* effects depending on the dose prescribed; however, they do not alter disease progression. Discontinuance of NSAIDs quickly leads to exacerbation of symptoms. Thus, NSAIDs are generally given in combination with other disease-modifying agents. At lower doses, the NSAID effect is analgesic, through the peripheral inhibition of pro-inflammatory prostaglandin synthesis. At higher doses, the effect is anti-inflammatory, probably through both prostaglandin inhibition and alterations in macrophage and neutrophil function. Due to the mechanism of action of these medications, adverse effects include gastrointestinal (GI) complaints and renal effects. Mild GI adverse effects include distress and nausea. However, approximately 2% to 4% of patients experience serious adverse effects including gastrointestinal bleeding, ulcers, and perforation. Patients are encouraged to take these medications with food, to monitor GI signs, and or are given prophylactic therapy to decrease gastrointestinal damage. Renal and other adverse effects associated with continued use and high doses of NSAIDs include dizziness, drowsiness, headache, tinnitus (ringing in the ears), kidney dysfunction, and elevation of liver enzymes. Complete blood counts (CBCs) and stool guaiac analyses for occult blood should be conducted every 3 to 4 months to monitor for potential adverse effects.[84]

There are two primary categories of NSAIDs, based on whether they inhibit COX-1 and COX-2 enzymes or COX-2 enzymes alone. These enzymes are responsible for synthesis of prostaglandins. Traditional NSAIDs block both COX-1 and COX-2 enzymes. The main function of the COX-1 enzyme is synthesis of prostaglandins in the endothelium and gastric mucosa, tissues present in the stomach lining and kidneys. Caution should be taken when prescribing NSAIDs to specific groups of patients at risk for GI complications such as the elderly, smokers, those taking corticosteroids, and those with severe arthritis, comorbidities, and history of GI symptoms. The selective COX-2 inhibitors were designed to decrease the risk of GI toxicity by inhibiting only the COX-2 enzyme, which is responsible for the pain and swelling associated with inflammation. Early studies of short duration exposure supported the reduced risk of GI side effects and increased tolerability of COX-2 inhibitors.[85] However, studies of longer selective COX-2 exposure and systematic evaluation of the data from numerous trials indicate that patients on selective COX-2 inhibitors are at greater risk of acute myocardial infarction and other cardiovascular events.[86-88]

NSAIDs are an accessible and relatively inexpensive drug to manage inflammation; however, the decision to prescribe an NSAID must be based on risk factors, known toxicities, and dosing preferences. Individual response to an NSAID is extremely variable in effectiveness and tolerance. Therefore, it often requires several month-long trials to find the best product. Taking more than one NSAID increases the risk of toxicity with no increase in benefit. NSAIDs are prescribed for patients with RA at the onset of symptoms to provide rapid pain relief and control of inflammation while waiting for the slower-acting DMARD to become effective.

Disease-Modifying Antirheumatic Drugs

DMARDs are the primary class of drugs for managing disease progression in RA. These include an array of drugs with varying chemical structures, modes of actions, clinical indications, and toxicities. Typical DMARDs used to manage RA include anti-malarials, methotrexate (MTX), sulfasalazine, and leflu*no*mide. Although DMARDs are effective in reducing disease progression, these medications do not provide an analgesic effect and are slow acting, taking from 3 weeks to 3 months to take effect. A drug that is classified as a DMARD must show evidence of affecting the course of RA for at least 1 year (improved function, reduced inflammation, and slowing or prevention of structural damage). Given its relative low cost and safety profile, oral MTX is the most widely used conventional DMARD (cDMARD).[89] DMARDs may be given alone or in combination for best effectiveness. Individuals taking DMARDs should be monitored regularly for the toxicities accompanying the specific drug. DMARDs are most often used to treat adult-onset RA; however, some are used to treat juvenile RA, ankylosing spondylitis, psoriatic arthritis, and systemic lupus erythematosus.[29] Advances in medical management and the treat-to target approach have led to a recognition of the importance of initiating conventional synthetic (csDMARD) therapy in combination with low-dose glucocorticoids. Additionally, it is well noted that methotrexate given in proper doses and in conjunction with folate, is the major player in the management of RA.[89]

Biological Response Modifiers

BRMs are a class of disease-modifying agents in use since 1998 that are biologically engineered to mimic the activities of targeted immune cells to reduce or block the inflammatory process. These drugs are approved to treat moderate to severe RA that is nonresponsive to traditional therapy. Unlike other RA medications, these drugs are engineered to target specific components of the immune system. The mechanism of action of BRMs varies and includes inhibition of cytokine activity, by blocking tumor necrosis factor–alpha (a pro-inflammatory cytokine) or interleukin-1 to their receptors. Some biologics are immunoglobulin isotypes, such as IgG1, fusion proteins that block the co-stimulatory signal required for T-cell activation (T cells or T-lymphocytes, are a subtype of white blood cells), a central component of the RA inflammatory response. Thus, the drug will work "upstream" in the inflammatory cascade compared with other biologic agents. Another form of biologic therapy is a monoclonal antibody (MAb) that binds to CD20, a cell marker expressed on mature B-cells (B-lymphocytes) and pre-B-cells, leading to selective depletion of CD20+ B-cells via several mechanisms.[90] The half-life and dosing of these drugs are important considerations as they impact the frequency, cost and mode of drug delivery (e.g., intravenous). Evidence demonstrates these drugs result in both inhibition of the progression of structural damage and improvement of physical function in RA. Biologics represent a significant advance in the treatment of RA. Patients who begin BRMs usually continue with their NSAIDs, corticosteroids, or other RA medication. These medications can be given by injection or infusion. In fewer than 30% of patients, there may be a rash and an injection site reaction. Severe allergic reaction is also a potential outcome so patients are routinely monitored during infusion of the medication. Adverse effects of these medications can be quite serious and patients must be monitored for signs of infection, including colds and flus, which can rapidly progress during immunosuppression. Those with a history of tuberculosis (TB) are at risk for reactivation of TB and may be excluded from this form of therapy. The number of diseases in which these agents are useful continues to expand as do the number and types of agents available.[90]

Corticosteroids

Corticosteroids are powerful anti-inflammatory drugs creating rapid and potent suppression of inflammation. Corticosteroids are generally not given alone and may be administered orally, intravenously, or via intra-articular or periarticular injection. Often, they are given in conjunction with a slower-acting DMARD until the DMARD has reached therapeutic levels. Unfortunately, these potent inflammatory medications also produce serious adverse effects when used long term or in high doses. Potential adverse effects include thinning of the skin, osteoporosis, muscle wasting, adrenal suppression, increased susceptibility to infections, impaired wound healing, cataracts, glaucoma, hyperlipidemia, and aseptic bone necrosis. Resistance exercise or heavy physical activity in the presence of high-dose steroids can lead to tendon rupture.[91]

Corticosteroids are generally prescribed in the presence of unremitting disease and severe extra-articular inflammation and are given in combination with other RA medications (e.g., DMARDs). Corticosteroids are often prescribed in *pulse doses* (low tapering doses over a specific time period) to reduce the risk of side effects. Patients on corticosteroids should have their blood counts, serum potassium, and glucose levels monitored and be observed for potential side effects.[29] When inflammation is confined to a specific location, steroid injections into a joint, bursa, tendon, or tendon sheath may be administered. However, use of steroid injections is commonly limited to no more than two to four per year to reduce the risk of osteonecrosis and soft tissue damage.

Pharmacological Therapy in Osteoarthritis

To date, drug therapy in OA has no effect on disease progression and is ancillary to nonpharmacological approaches to pain management including patient education and self-management, weight loss, joint protection, and exercise.[52,92-97] The goals of drug therapy in patients with OA are to relieve pain and decrease inflammation when it is present. Oral analgesics, oral and topical NSAIDs, and corticosteroid injections are the primary medications used in OA management.[1,92-97]

Acetaminophen, an oral analgesic, is usually the drug of first choice.[52,92-97] Acetaminophen-containing compounds (Tylenol, Panadol, Anacin-3) have been cited as having almost no toxicity in recommended doses (up to 4 g/day) and little or no GI side effects. However, there is no anti-inflammatory effect; acetaminophen cannot be substituted for NSAIDs in this regard. Earlier clinical studies in OA demonstrated symptom relief from acetaminophen (3 to 4 g/day) greater than that of a placebo and slightly less than that of NSAIDs.[98] However, newer evidence suggests that acetaminophen has minimal clinically important effects on pain and no significant effect on stiffness or physical function in patients with symptomatic knee OA.[96] Further, acetaminophen use can lead to liver and, less commonly, kidney toxicity, especially in individuals who drink excessive amounts of alcohol. As well, there is increasing evidence of an increased incidence of hospitalization due to GI perforation, peptic ulceration, and bleeding with acetaminophen use of >3 g/day compared to lower doses (<3g/day).[96]

NSAIDs have a place in the management of persons with OA who do not respond to acetaminophen and nonpharmacological measures.[94,95,99] NSAIDs may be used in combination with acetaminophen, and should be kept to the lowest effective dose to minimize GI toxicity. The COX-2 NSAIDs, described for RA management, had been prescribed for people who are at increased risk for GI problems until longer-term trials called their safety into question.

Intra-articular corticosteroid injections are often used for acute episodes with a moderate effect for pain relief, irrespective of the number of injections.[94] The knee is the most common site; however, soft tissue injections for subacromial, anserine, and trochanteric bursitis also may be effective.

Viscosupplementation or intra-articular injections of the knee with a form of HA is conditionally recommended in some guidelines.[92,94] A number of synthetic forms are available (Synvisc, Hyalgan, Artzal). HA is a naturally occurring polysaccharide that contributes to the thickness and viscosity of joint fluid in the healthy joint. In the OA knee, the levels of HA are lower and the joint fluid is thinner and less dense, reducing the ability of the fluid to lubricate and attenuate shock. Viscosupplementation therapy consists of a series of weekly injections. The reported effects of treatment are reduced pain and stiffness and improved function in people with mild to moderate knee OA, which may last for several months.[94] It is not clear if HA injections are more effective than corticosteroid injections, NSAIDs, or placebo injections. The injected HA does not replace normal joint fluid to achieve its effect as most is absorbed and cleared from the joint within a week. The risk of adverse effects is low. The most serious reported adverse event is an allergic reaction and less serious effects are injection site reactions and joint swelling. There is no evidence that supports increased efficacy of one product over another; however, high-molecular-weight hylan (Synvisc) may have greater efficacy.[94]

Glucosamine sulphate (GS) and glucosamine hydrochloride (GH) have been examined in placebo-controlled trials and found to be moderately effective for pain relief; however, the size of the effect diminishes when only high-quality trials are considered.[96] In one long-term follow-up study, patients who had taken GS, 1500 mg/day for at least 12 months, were half as likely to undergo total knee replacement (TKR) at 5 years.[96] The structural-modifying effects of glucosamine products in hip and knee OA remain uncertain.

Topical agents include analgesics and anti-inflammatory preparations. Topical analgesics may be rubefacients, which contain methyl salicylate, chemical compounds that produce a counterirritant effect, or capsaicin compounds, which reduce pain through depletion of the neurotransmitter substance P in peripheral nerves. To date, the only topical analgesic to show consistent efficacy in controlled clinical trials is capsaicin. Capsaicin is an alkaloid derived from red chili peppers and is available in topical analgesic creams in varying concentrations (Zostrix, Capsaicin-P, Dolorac). It has been shown to decrease pain approximately 33% when applied to specific joints four times daily.[94] The initial stinging or burning sensation disappears after several days of use; however, the need for frequent daily applications may limit the acceptability of this therapy for some patients. Topical NSAIDs (diclofenac sodium) are recommended as alternative or adjunctive therapy in symptomatic peripheral joint OA and the EULAR and Osteoarthritis Research Society International (OARSI) guidelines recommend topical NSAIDs over oral NSAIDs for patients with knee or hand OA.[94,97] Topical preparations delivered through gel, liquid, or patch formulations are absorbed through the skin with the help of an absorption enhancer and are slightly less or equally effective as oral NSAIDs with fewer adverse events.[42,94,100]

■ REHABILITATIVE MANAGEMENT

The chronic progressive nature of arthritis dictates a plan of care (POC) that includes patient education and self-management beyond the initial presentation. Although RA is systemic and OA is a more localized condition, both diseases can significantly affect health, function, participation, and quality of life. The rehabilitation of persons with arthritis requires comprehensive and coordinated efforts of a team of health professionals, including physical therapists, and ensures that the patient is first in treatment planning. The patient's ability to self-manage successfully is a major predictor of better health outcomes.[101] The physical therapist plays a pivotal role in helping the patient to minimize disability and gain confidence and experience in using self-management skills to deal with the condition. The general goals and outcomes for persons with RA and OA are similar.

The remainder of this chapter will discuss physical therapist examination and interventions for people with RA and OA of the hip and knee. Although OA also presents at other joints, these two are the most common and disabling sites for OA and are most frequently seen by a physical therapist.

Physical Therapy Examination

A comprehensive and multisystem examination and history is an essential component of physical therapy management. Whether the patient is a direct access client or seen in a system-based clinical setting, collaboration and communication with other care providers working with the patient is imperative. As with all patient-centered care, the patient is the primary stakeholder and should be actively engaged in goal setting and in the development of the POC.

Careful observation of the patient during the initial meeting and history can help inform the process. For example, observation of the patient's gait, ability to remove outerwear, and transfer into a chair for the history will provide the therapist with a quick assessment of functional ability.

History

The medical and social history will direct and inform the examination and provide insight into the development of a POC and need for potential resources. Ascertaining the patient's understanding of the disease and the implications of the disease is an important component of the interview process. In particular, the therapist should be concerned with identifying "red flag" signs and symptoms that indicate the need for immediate medical follow up (Table 23.2). Pain assessment questions should include location, duration, pattern, quality, and intensity. Specific details regarding joint inflammation such as joint heat, swelling, and erythema should be recorded and confirmed during the physical examination.[102] A determination of joint stiffness (morning versus after prolonged static posture), previous activity level, pattern and degree of fatigue, presence of comorbidities, and current medication is also essential. Use and effectiveness of previous therapeutic interventions and complementary approaches should be noted. Although many physical therapy tests and measures are used during the examination, specific adaptations may be made to tailor the examination to the person with RA or OA. Especially in RA, the tender and swollen joint count appears to be a sensitive measure of systemic disease activity and guides the exercise prescription.[24]

Observation, Joint Tenderness, and Sensory Integrity

Clinical examination of the patient begins with careful observation of posture, gait, and functional transfers during the initial meeting and interview process. A general guideline for clinical observation of any RA joint begins with a careful joint inspection. Examine the joint and surrounding tissues for swelling, muscle wasting, thinning and bruising of the skin (an indication of long-term steroid use), deformity, presence of nodules, rashes, and scars. In the hands and feet, be sure to examine the nails for pitting or nail fold vasculitis. Compare the joint on one side with the other to determine whether changes are symmetric or asymmetric. Check the skin temperature (best to use dorsal side of hand while examining).

Palpate soft tissue to determine whether there is tendon thickening or joint pain. To assess joint pain, gently compress the joint (e.g., for MCPs squeeze MCPs using a medial–lateral pressure). Check peripheral pulses. With RA, alternations in sensation may be evident with the presence of *Raynaud's disease* or with compression of nerves due to inflammation or joint derangement. Any indication of peripheral neuropathy or nerve involvement should be investigated using standard examination procedures (see Chapter 3, Examination of Sensory Function). Sensory changes resulting from other comorbidities or from the normal aging process should be considered when appropriate.

Range of Motion

Tenderness and subjective reports of pain with passive range of motion (PROM), are highly indicative of inflammation; thus, gentle pressure and appropriate hand position is paramount during examination. Goniometric measurement of PROM is indicated and necessary at all affected joints after a gross joint screening to assist in monitoring treatment effectiveness. Standardized procedures (e.g., testing positions) are essential for reliable and valid measures.[103] Otherwise, potential variations in intra-rater and inter-rater reliability will reduce the accuracy of data comparison throughout the disease course. If joint pain or poor activity tolerance prohibits measurement of PROM, the therapist may consider substituting a functional ROM test by asking the patient to touch various body parts (e.g., the top of the

Table 23.2 "Red Flags" Suggesting the Need for Urgent Evaluation and Management

Flag	Differential Diagnosis
History of significant trauma	Soft tissue injury, internal derangement, or fracture
Hot, swollen joint	Infection, systemic rheumatic disease, gout, pseudogout
Constitutional signs (e.g., fever, weight loss, malaise)	Infection, sepsis, systemic rheumatic disease
Weakness	
Focal	Focal nerve lesion (compartment syndrome, entrapment neuropathy, mononeuritis multiplex, motor neuron disease, radiculopathy[a])
Diffuse	Myositis, metabolic myopathy, paraneoplastic syndrome, degenerative neuromuscular disorder, toxin, myelopathy,[a] transverse myelitis
Neurogenic pain (burning, numbness, paresthesia)	
Asymmetrical Symmetrical	Radiculopathy,[a] reflex sympathetic dystrophy, entrapment neuropathy myelopathy,[a] peripheral neuropathy
History of significant trauma	Soft tissue injury, internal derangement, or fracture
Claudication pain pattern	Peripheral vascular disease, giant cell arteritis (jaw pain), lumbar spinal stenosis

[a]Radiculopathy and myelopathy may be due to infectious, neoplastic, or mechanical processes.

head and small of the back) to determine the available ROM for performing self-care activities. The therapist should note any tenderness, crepitus, or pain during examination of ROM.

Regardless of whether the patient has OA and monoarticular involvement or RA with polyarticular involvement, the impact of an involved joint on the kinematic chain or on the contralateral side should not be overlooked. When there is OA in a hip or knee, active motion in functional positions should be examined in all joints of both lower extremities (LEs). It is important to observe motion for symmetry and smoothness during gait, stair climbing, and rising from a chair. In RA patients, the impact of ankle and foot involvement should not be overlooked. Data have shown that elevated midfoot peak plantar pressures, self-reported foot impairment, and vascular disease are associated with falls among adults with RA.[104] Ascending stairs requires the greatest amount and velocity of knee flexion and may be one of the best activities to determine knee function. Decreased ROM at the hip and knee increases the risk for injury and falls. Approximately 50° hip flexion and 90° knee flexion are required to recover balance from a stumble during walking.[105]

Strength

Pain and joint effusions impede muscle contraction, limiting examination of strength. A patient may be able to generate force in the pain-free range but unable to completely contract in the painful range secondary to reflex inhibition. Traditional strength tests (e.g., manual muscle tests) are not appropriate in the presence of severely deformed and or deranged joints. Functional strength assessments are more appropriate and will provide sufficient data to formulate treatment goals. Individuals who demonstrate a *lag phenomenon* will have limited active range and will not be candidates for traditional grading systems, because these are not sensitive to changes in the quality and quantity of muscle contraction. When documenting strength, it is important to include information on required modifications made to standardized testing positions, grade of strength exhibited in that arc of motion, and the method of strength testing used (e.g., break test, isometric holding at the end of range, or resistance throughout the ROM). Modifying the test protocol to include an isometric break test at midrange or most comfortable joint position generally yields higher grades than would be received if full range testing were done (see Chapter 4, Musculoskeletal Examination). Any modifications to standardized test protocols must be carefully documented. It is also important to document the time of day the patient was tested, as well as the use and timing of medications that might alter performance or exercise tolerance.

The functional threshold for LE strength has yet to be determined. However, reports from studies that have examined knee strength as a percentage of body weight suggest that isokinetic strength measured at velocities between 60° and 180° per second should be 20% to 30% body weight for knee extension and 20% to 25% for knee flexion.[106] It is also important to perform strength testing of the muscle groups proximal to the affected joints to detect deficits that can affect function and contribute to abnormal biomechanics. It is important to note that the severity of knee pain, obesity, and perceived helplessness to manage OA have been identified as important determinants of disability.[107] Thus, pain experience will influence the strength assessment.

Joint Stability

Joint stability is essential for normal biomechanics, function, and independence. Inflammatory aspects of RA can lead to joint instability and eventual deformity. Intra-articular ligaments are highly susceptible to inflammatory and erosive changes in RA. Thus, ligamentous laxity of any affected joint should be fully investigated. More RA-specific tests for joint stability of the wrist and hand are well-described in the literature.[108,109] *Pseudolaxity*, often detected in unicompartmental knee OA, should be differentiated from *true ligamentous laxity*. Standard ligamentous integrity tests including those for the anterior and posterior cruciate, and collateral ligaments of the knee are appropriate for both knee OA and knee involvement from RA.

Cardiovascular Status

Fatigue is one of the systemic manifestations of RA and frequently unappreciated.[17] Individuals with OA also report fatigue.[67] To best ascertain the impact of fatigue on patient functioning and independence, assessments should be made over the course of a single day and over several days. The increased incidence of asymptomatic cardiovascular disease, elevated risk for ischemic heart disease, and decreased cardiovascular fitness of individuals with RA[33–35] demands specific attention. Heart rate, respiratory rate, blood pressure, and ratings of perceived exertion should all be measured during a functional activity that is reasonably stressful for the patient's current level of fitness. Excessive increases in perceived exertion may indicate the presence of inflammation or impairment of pulmonary and cardiac function that requires more extensive and formal evaluation. It is also important to determine cardiovascular fitness in individuals with OA, because cardiovascular deficits and increased risk for coronary artery disease are clearly associated with long-standing or severe disease, inactivity, and walking disability.[78]

Functional Examination

Functional examination measures provide a rich and patient-centered approach to assessment. Functional measures may include *patient-reported outcome measures* (PROs), physician-reported data that may merge laboratory findings with the physician's judgment of the patient's function, or performance-based measures (see Chapter 8, Examination of Function). The selection of a functional measure is based on the demographic features of the patient (e.g., age, gender), the level depth of information required, the measure's sensitivity and responsiveness in gauging the efficacy of treatment and clinical feasibility (e.g., available resources, space). As with goniometric measurement, the reliability and validity are important for individual and comparative purposes.

PROs in arthritis are be used for patients with many forms of arthritis or may be used for patients with a specific form of arthritis. The revised *Arthritis Impact Measurement Scales 2* (AIMS2) includes physical function, performance in psychological and social domains, and has been used in persons with RA, OA, psoriatic arthritis, ankylosing spondylitis, and fibromyalgia.[110,111] The AIMS2 also measures the patient's satisfaction with current functional status and individual preferences for outcome. The AIMS2 is not well suited for program evaluation or clinical purposes due to its complicated scoring algorithm and associated costs (Table 23.3).

For patients with RA, the *Health Assessment Questionnaire* (HAQ)[116] consists of the following five domains or subscales: disability, discomfort, pain, drug side effects (toxicity), and costs of care. The HAQ is a component

Table 23.3 Outcome Measures for RA and OA Organized by ICF Categories

Outcome Measure (ICF Category)	Description of Measure and Link to Measure	Scoring	Clinically Important Change Values
		General Arthritis	
Arthritis Impact Measurement Scales 2 (AIMS2)[110,111] (body structure & function, activity and participation)	This PRO measures physical, social, and emotional well-being using a series of items that ask about the level of disability the person is experiencing for each item. The AIMS2 also includes a measure of satisfaction with health. The AIMS-2 has been proven a valid and reliable measure in many forms of arthritis. See form at: http://www.aqol.com.au/documents/MIC/OSTEOARTHRITIS_MIC_qnr_180711.pdf	The response format for each item is a five-point scale. Items are scored separately without weights. Greater disability = higher score. Total health score is calculated by summing the standardized scores for mobility, physical and household activities, dexterity, pain, and depression.	SRMs for changes in AIMS2-SF scores over 3 months range from 0.36 (small) to 0.8 (high).
		Rheumatoid Arthritis	
Clinical Disease Activity Index (CDAI)[112,113] (body structure and function)	This is a provider and patient assessment measure. The CDAI includes the provider's assessment of 28 joints as either swollen (SJC-28) or tender (TJC-28) and the patient's self-assessment of overall RA disease activity (scale 1–10 where 10 is maximal activity and the provider's global disease activity (scale 1–10; 10 is maximal activity) http://www.rheumatology.org/CDAI	Total score created by summing the four components of the measure. Interpretation as follows: Disease in remission CDAI ≤2.8 Low disease activity CDAI >2.8 and ≤10 Moderately active disease CDAI >10 and ≤22 Highly active disease CDAI >22	In general MID is five points. MID cutpoints for improvement in adults with high disease activity, reduction of >11 units), (patients with moderate disease reduction of 6 units, low disease activity, reduction >2 units

Table 23.3 Outcome Measures for RA and OA Organized by ICF Categories—cont'd

Outcome Measure (ICF Category)	Description of Measure and Link to Measure	Scoring	Clinically Important Change Values
		Rheumatoid Arthritis	
Disease Activity Score (DAS)[114] (body structure and function)	This measure includes the provider assessment and laboratory data. It is a four-item tool to assess RA disease activity in patients by counting tender joints and painful joints calculated by the Ritchie Articular Index (RAI), a 44 swollen joint count (44JSC), erythrocyte sedimentation rate (ESR), and a patient global assessment of disease activity (PtGA) or General Health (GH) using a Visual Analogue Scale (VAS). Validated for patients with RA. http://www.das-score.nl/das28/en/	Scores for each item are calculated as follows: The RAI ranges from 0–78, the 44SJC ranges from 0–44, the GH/PtGA VAS ranges from 0–100, and the ESR ranges from 0–100 mm/hr. The DAS ranges from 0-10. The level of disease activity is classified as follows: in remission, low, moderate, or high if the scores are between 0–1.6, 1.6–2.4, 2.4–3.7, and 3.7–10 respectively.	A change in the DAS >1.2 is a significant change. Change is classified as good, nonresponsive, or moderate if scores and follow up scores are >1.2 and <2.4, >0.6 or improvement between 0.6 and 1.2 and a follow-up >3.7. All other responses are classified as moderate.
Disease Activity Score (28)[115] (body structure and function)	Provider assessment plus laboratory data. This four-item tool is a modified version of the DAS. It is used to assess rheumatic disease activity in patients using a 28 swollen joint count (28SJC), a 28 tender joint count (28TJC), ESR, and a PtGA or GH using a VAS. Validated for patients with RA. http://www.das-score.nl/das28/en/	Scores for each item are calculated as follows: The 28TJC and 28SJC range from 0–28, the GH/PtGA VAS ranges from 0–100, and the ESR ranges from 0–100 mm/hr. The DAS28 ranges from 0–9.4. The level of disease activity is classified as in remission, low, moderate, or high if the scores are 0–1.6, 1.6–2.4, 2.4v3.7, and 3.7–10, respectively.	A change in the DAS28 >1.2 is a significant change. Change is classified as good, nonresponsive, or moderate if scores and follow up scores are >1.2 and <2.4, >0.6, or improvement between 0.6 and 1.2 and a follow-up >3.7. All other responses are classified as moderate.
Health Assessment Disability Questionnaire (HAQ)[116] **Health Assessment Disability Questionnaire_ Disability Index (HAQ-DI)**[116,117] (body structure & function and activity)	Twenty-item patient reported tool assessing physical function in daily living and the use of aids or help from others. Validated for patients with a variety of rheumatic conditions. http://www.rheumatoid-arthritis-decisions.com/HAQ.html HAQ-DI has 41 items (20 for daily activities, 13 for assistive devices, eight items for help from others). https://integrationacademy.ahrq.gov/sites/default/files/HAQ-DI_0.pdf	HAQ scores are calculated for each subcategory on a scale from 0 (no difficulty) to 3 (unable to do) in 0.125 increments. Scores are adjusted upward by 1 for each category if aids/assistance are used and the score for that category was reported at 0 or 1. Scores process similar. The eight scores of the eight sections are summed and divided by 8.	MCID for scores is ~0.22, although the value can range from 0.07–0.87. MCID for HAQ_DI is a change of 0.22–0.25. A recent study suggests, the minimum clinically important improvement (MCII) is a decrease of 0.375.

Continued

Table 23.3 Outcome Measures for RA and OA Organized by ICF Categories—cont'd

Outcome Measure (ICF Category)	Description of Measure and Link to Measure	Scoring	Clinically Important Change Values
		Rheumatoid Arthritis	
Multidimensional Health Assessment Questionnaire (MDHAQ)[118] (body structure and function, activity, participation)	Patient reported 10-item tool assessing physical function in daily living and use of assistive devices or aid from others. Includes more difficult activities such as playing sports and walking >2 miles. Validated for patients with a variety of rheumatic diseases. A short form MDHAQ is recommended for routine clinical use. http://www.corptransinc.com/sites/mdhaq-rapid3/home	Scores calculated for each item on a scale from 0 (no difficulty) to 3 (unable to do). If at least 9/10 questions were answered, the scores are summed and then divided by the number of questions answered to reach a final score of 0–3 and rounded to the nearest 0.1.	MDHAQ scores found to be significantly associated with amount of morning stiffness as compared to pain, fatigue, joint counts, and patient global and independently predict 10-year mortality.
Patient Activity Scale (PAS), and (PAS-II)[120,121] (body structure & function)	Patient reported outcome that includes three primary components: patient pain score (pain VAS) and PtGA via health assessment questionnaire (PAS) or using the health assessment questionnaire II (PAS II). (PAS) http://www.arthritis-research.org/research/pas (PAS II) http://www.arthritis-research.org/research/pas	Take the mean of the sum the three subscales (but in the process of summing a weighting applied to the HAQ score, multiply HAQ × 0.33). Similar process for PAS-II. Scores range 0 to 10. Disease activity cutoffs (both): Remission (0–0.25) Low disease (0.26–3.7) Moderate (3.71 < 8.0) High (> = 8.0)	As this is a composite of three known measures treated with equal weighting, ability to detect change is moderate to good.
Patient-Reported Outcomes Measurement Information System (PROMIS)[122–124] (body structure and function, activity, and participation)	Patient-reported physical function and disability measure is one measure of the PROMIS set. These measures are part of a series of generic measures available for free from the national institutes of health. PROMIS also measures pain, fatigue, depression, anxiety, and social function. www.nihpromis.org	For best information on scoring see: http://www.healthmeasures.net/promis-scoring-manuals	MCID for physical function from a longitudinal cohort study in RA was 0.2 SD.
Routine Assessment of Patient Index Data 3 (RAPID-3)[125]	Patient reported Three primary components: patient pain score, pain VAS and the Multidimensional HAQ [MDHAQ). http://mdhaq.org/Public/Questionnaires.aspx	(MDHAQ × 3.33 + pain VAS + patient global assessment VAS)/3	As this is a composite of three known measures treated with equal weighting, ability to detect change is moderate to good.

Table 23.3 Outcome Measures for RA and OA Organized by ICF Categories—cont'd

Outcome Measure (ICF Category)	Description of Measure and Link to Measure	Scoring	Clinically Important Change Values
		Rheumatoid Arthritis	
Simplified Disease Activity Index (SDAI)[126,127] (body structure & function)	This measure combines physician assessment and laboratory data to determine disease activity. It includes a physician global assessment, patient global assessment, 28 total tender joint count and 28 total swollen joint count plus CRP level. http://www.rheumatology.org/SDAI	The score is calculated by taking the total of the 28 tender joint count score + 28 swollen joint count score + provider global assessment + patient global assessment + CRP.	As this is a composite of three known measures treated with equal weighting, ability to detect change is moderate to good.
		Osteoarthritis	
Disabilities of the Arm, Shoulder, and Hand (DASH)[128] (body structure and function, activity)	A 30-item self-report questionnaire designed to assess musculoskeletal disorders of the upper limbs. It has two shortened versions, the QuickDASH and the QuickDASH-9. http://www.dash.iwh.on.ca/	Each item scored 1 (no difficulty, not at all, not limited, none, strongly disagree) to 5 (unable, extremely, unable, strongly agree). Online version and scoring at: http://www.orthopaedicscore.com/scorepages/disabilities_of_arm_shoulder_hand_score_dash.html	MDC = 12.75 in adults with upper extremity musculoskeletal problems.
Hip disability and Osteoarthritis Outcome Score (HOOS)[129,130] (body structure and function, activity, and participation)	A 40-item tool that assesses pain, symptoms, function in daily living, function in sports and recreation, and quality of life over the past week. Validated for hip OA and THR patients. A short form HOOS-PS is recommended for routine clinical use (Rolfson, 2016). www.koos.nu	Scores calculated for each subscale with 0 being lowest score and 100 being highest.	MCII 1 year after THA is 24 points for pain subscale and 17 for quality of life (QOL) subscale.
Knee injury and Osteoarthritis Outcome Score (KOOS)[130,131] (body structure and function, activity, and participation)	A 42-item tool that assesses pain, symptoms, function in daily living, function in sports and recreation and quality of life over the past week. Validated for knee injury (e.g., ACL), OA, and TKR. A short form KOOS-PS is recommended for routine clinical use www.koos.nu	Scores calculated for each subscale with 0 being lowest score and 100 being highest.	MDC for knee OA ranges from 13.4 points for pain subscale to 21.1 for QOL subscale.

Continued

Table 23.3 Outcome Measures for RA and OA Organized by ICF Categories—cont'd

Outcome Measure (ICF Category)	Description of Measure and Link to Measure	Scoring	Clinically Important Change Values
		Osteoarthritis	
Lower Extremity Functional Scale (LEFS)[132] (activity)	A 20-item tool that assesses current (i.e., today) ability to undertake activities at home, work, school, recreation and sport. Validated for hip and knee OA and TJR. (Binkley, 1999) http://www.rehab.msu.edu/_files/_docs/LEFS.pdf	Scored 9 to 80 with higher score representing better function.	MDC and MCID is 9 points.
Oswestry Disability Index[133] (body structure and function, activity, participation)	A 10-item tool that assesses pain intensity, personal care, lifting, walking, sitting, standing, sleeping, sex (if applicable), social, and travel. http://www.rehab.msu.edu/_files/_docs/Oswestry_Low_Back_Disability.pdf	Each item scored 0 (least disability) to 5 (greatest disability) for total score of 0 to 50. Online version and scoring at: http://www.orthopaedicscore.com/scorepages/oswestry_low_back_pain.html	MDC = 12.72 for population with chronic back pain.
Patient Specific Functional Scale (PSFS)[134] (activity and participation)	Patients select activities important to them and rate their current ability to complete each on an 11-point scale. http://www.rehab.msu.edu/_files/_docs/Patient-specific%20functional%20scale.pdf	Each item rated 0 (unable to perform) to 10 (able to perform at prior level).	MDC = 1.4 for low back pain MCID = 1.34 for spinal stenosis

MCII: minimal clinically important improvement; MDC: minimal detectable change; MCID: minimal clinically important difference; SRMs: standardized response means SRMs.
[a]See Appendix 23.D, Web-Based Resources.

of the ACR core measures for RA and has been shown to correlate highly with measures of disease progression in RA (x-ray changes). There are numerous versions of the HAQ available.[116-119] The *Modified HAQ*, an abbreviated version of the HAQ, is an instrument that assesses the impact of disease activity on function and disability. It is quick and easy to complete and score. The *Multidimensional HAQ* includes a sports item and walking more than 2 miles to reduce floor effects found with the HAQ.[118] Online versions are available for free.

Assessment of RA disease activity is an important component of disease management. Although there are numerous (more than 60 at current count) disease activity measures in RA, the six most highly recommended include: the *Disease Activity Score* (DAS) with 28-joint counts (erythrocyte sedimentation rate or CRP),[115] the *Clinical Disease Activity Index* (CDAI),[112] the *Patient Activity Scale* (PAS), PAS-II,[120,121] the *Routine Assessment of Patient Index Data with 3 measures* (RAPID-3),[125] and *Simplified Disease Activity Index* (SDAI).[126] These measures were recommended following a systematic review of the literature and input from an expert panel of clinician researchers due to their accuracy; sensitivity to change; and ability to discriminate adults with low, moderate, and high disease activity states.[121] All measures have criteria to establish remission and are easy to use in the clinic. As an example, both the DAS28[115] and the Rheumatoid Arthritis Disease Activity Index (RADAI)[122] combine data from the physician's physical examination of the patient with clinical laboratory biomarkers of inflammation. These measures are used frequently to assess and monitor disease activity in RA and determine whether the patient has achieved either remission or low disease activity in response to medical therapy (Table 23.2).

In OA, the *Western Ontario and McMaster Universities Osteoarthritis Index* (WOMAC) is a widely used, valid, and reliable self-report instrument of 24 items in three categories specific to OA of the hip and or knee (pain, stiffness, and function).[135] The WOMAC, however, requires a licensing fee to use making it less appropriate for routine clinical use.[130] The *Knee Injury and Osteoarthritis Outcome* (KOOS)[131] was developed using the WOMAC as a base and includes sports, recreation, and quality of life items. This measure is readily accessible; is relatively easy to score; and demonstrates strong validity, reliability, and responsiveness in adults.[135] A modified version of the KOOS was developed for persons with hip osteoarthritis (HOOS)[131] and short forms of both tools are recommended for routine clinical use[130] (Table 23.2). The *Lower Extremity Functional Scale* (LEFS) is another short (20-item) tool that has been validated in the OA population, is feasible for clinical use, and enables comparison of disability across a variety of LE conditions.[132]

Based on recent evidence and expert opinion, the Osteoarthritis Research Society International (OARSI) has suggested the use of five performance tests thought to be the most valuable for patients aged >40 years with knee and hip OA or undergoing joint arthroplasty surgery.[136] The selected tests encompass different aspects of functional mobility and aerobic capacity. The *30-second Chair Stand Test* (30CST) evaluates sit-to-stand ability, the 4-by-10 meter fast-paced walk test is a test of walking activity and walking speed over short distances with changing directions, the *Timed Up and Go* (TUG) evaluates functional mobility and gait speed, the timed stair climb test assesses stair negotiation, and the 6-minute walk test (6MWT) acquires information regarding aerobic capacity and walking longer distances. These tests were chosen to be complementary to the established PROs and are considered the best available clinimetric evidence. However, OARSI acknowledges the need for further evidence.

Mobility, Gait, and Balance

A complete and detailed gait examination is one of the most important contributions of the physical therapist to the rehabilitation team's understanding of the individual's functional abilities and serves to identify additional areas for examination and intervention. (See Chapter 7, Examination of Gait, for a complete discussion.) Substantial differences in fall risks, knee ROM, and gait velocity between patients with either OA or RA and their peers without arthritis have been demonstrated. Persons with RA demonstrate alterations in joint kinematics and kinetics as a result of chronic synovitis, in some instances joint derangement, and high prevalence of significant foot and ankle involvement. Studies of 3D gait analysis indicate that persons with arthritis develop an antalgic gait pattern with reduced walking speed, stride length, and cadence. These individuals also demonstrate reduced joint motions, prolonged weight-bearing periods, and diminished joint power. At the foot, there is decreased plantarflexion, reduced and often delayed heel rise in early stance, and diminished power.[137]

During ambulation, adults with knee OA and medial compartment involvement tend to outwardly rotate their leg, and walk at a slower speed with a reduced knee extensor moment. Ligamentous instability further alters normal knee biomechanics during level ground walking and stair negotiation. Gait patterns in individuals with hip OA tend to be altered to accommodate reduced hip range of motion, hip pain, and lateral muscle weakness. Typically, these individuals demonstrate increased cadence and ankle power generation, maintenance of anterior pelvic tilt throughout the gait cycle, decreased step width, reduced hip extension, and a dropped pelvis (Trendelenburg gait) during stance. These deviations are quite different from comparisons with age and gender-matched healthy controls.[137]

Psychological Status

Individuals with chronic arthritis experience years of functional and social loss that would stress any person's ability to cope and adapt.[138] Although pain is significantly correlated with self-reports of depression, no firm association with function has been identified. The overall psychological status of the individual with RA is generally similar to those individuals with other chronic diseases that threaten a severe change in body image and disruption of social integration (see Chapter 26, Psychosocial Issues in Physical Rehabilitation). Individuals respond to these threats with various coping strategies to maintain psychological well-being. No single strategy can be deemed definitely better than another, although for individual patients some strategies will lead to better coping and more positive outcomes than others. Exploration of the patient's attitude toward rehabilitation and readiness to make health behavior changes, as well the availability of social support, can assist the therapist in shared goal setting and identifying realistic expectations of future functional ability. Persons with RA face the additional challenges of living with a chronic disease that is characterized by a fluctuating disease course and must learn to adapt their lifestyle, activity level, and medication and sleep schedule according to their disease activity. Thus, it is paramount that the therapist works with the patient to set realistic, achievable goals and educate the patient about warning signs of flares to help the patient self-manage.

Anxiety and depression are also common in patients with OA and may alter the pain experience, function, and response to treatment interventions.[139] Chronic pain, fatigue, loss of function, and reduced activity levels can all contribute to emotional distress. It is therefore important to recognize the signs of anxiety and depression and, if indicated, refer to appropriate screening services and resources to help individuals manage their psychological symptoms through improved coping skills.[140] Participation in the *Arthritis Self-Management Program* has been shown to improve coping.[140,141]

Environmental Factors

Therapists should be aware of environmental factors in the home, work, and leisure environments that might serve as facilitators or barriers to functioning and warrant specific identification, examination, and recommendations to address (see Chapter 9, Examination and Modification of the Environment). A discussion about the home and work environments may reveal conditions that threaten independence that can be addressed through ergonomic and environmental modifications and school or workplace accommodations. The cost of such changes may be a limiting factor for implementing these recommendations. The work environment affects employment and disability in more ways than the physical setting and task requirements.[142] Acceptance and understanding by supervisors and co-workers of the disease and self-management requirements of the worker with arthritis are important determinants of maintaining employment and income. Other environmental factors common to both the RA and OA ICF Core Sets include technology and assistive devices for ADL, mobility, transportation, and employment; design and access to buildings; climate; and attitudes of family, friends, and health professionals.[143-145]

Physical Therapy Intervention

The development of specific goals and expected outcomes for the individual with arthritis is based on the following general goals and expected outcomes developed in conjunction with the patient (Box 23.3).

The specific goals and outcomes identified for each patient will depend on the type of arthritis, disease activity level, clinical presentation, and patient preferences in line with patient-centered care. Mutual goal setting promotes patient participation in treatment. It is the physical therapist's responsibility to document the POC, implement that plan safely and effectively, and delegate responsibility appropriately to ensure that the patient's goals can be reached. The therapist should ensure that treatment goals and objectives are measurable, attainable (e.g., SMART or specific, measurable, attainable, relevant, and time-bound goals), and documented, with specific time frames included (e.g., increase left shoulder flexion ROM by 10° in 2 weeks, and independent ambulation with platform crutches on level surfaces for at least 250 feet without fatigue within 1 month). Failure to achieve goals within the stated time frame indicates the need for re-evaluation and reformulation of the goals. Goals and outcomes should be revised to reflect changes owing to both personal and environmental factors that may affect progress or alter the proposed time frames (see Chapter 1, Clinical Decision Making).

Modalities for Pain Relief

A variety of therapeutic modalities are available to relieve pain and prepare the patient for passive and dynamic stretching and other exercise interventions. The most common form is thermotherapy.

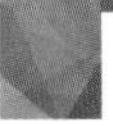

Box 23.3 Examples of General Goals and Outcomes for Patients with Arthritis

Reduce impact of impairments

- Decreased pain
- Maximized ROM of all joints sufficient for functional activities
- Maximized muscle activation and strength sufficient for functional activities
- Maximized joint stability and decreased biomechanical stress on all affected joints to prevent deformity
- Increased endurance for all functional activities and desired leisure activities
- Improved ability to perform physical actions, tasks, or activities
- Greater independence in ADL, including dressing, transfers, and self-care
- Improved efficiency and safety of gait pattern and balance with reduced fall risk
- Established adequate physical activity or exercise patterns to maintain or improve musculoskeletal and cardiovascular fitness and general health

Improve health status and quality of life

- Improved capacity for self-management, including joint protection, through education of patient, family, and caregivers

Adapted from Guide to Physical Therapist Practice, 2011.

Heat

Superficial heat, heat that penetrates only a few millimeters, produces localized analgesia and increases circulation in the vicinity where it is applied. Types of superficial heat include moist hot packs, dry heating pads, lamps, paraffin wax, and hydrotherapy. The evidence supporting the effectiveness of these modalities is weak, but patients often report that they gain comfort from moist heat. Paraffin is particularly useful in delivering superficial heat to irregularly shaped joints or to individuals who cannot tolerate the weight of a moist hot pack. Hydrotherapy allows the therapist to combine heating of tissues with exercise, and provides the patient the experience of aquatic therapy, although it is expensive. Systematic reviews of heat and cold therapy in arthritis suggest small to modest effects.[146]

Deep heating modalities, such as ultrasound, may affect the viscoelastic properties of collagen and increase the plastic stretch of ligaments, providing modest improvements in pain and function in individuals with knee OA.[147] However, their efficacy in RA is not demonstrated.[148] Their use in treating individuals with RA during the acute stage of inflammation is contraindicated because they may stimulate collagenase activity within the joint, furthering its destruction.[149]

Furthermore, modalities that do not readily translate to home use foster a dependency on clinical care and do not promote self-management.

Cold

Local applications of cold will also produce local analgesia, increase superficial circulation at the site of application following an initial period of vasoconstriction, and decrease intra-articular temperature.[149] Cold is particularly useful around joints that are inflamed and swollen, a condition that usually worsens with the application of superficial heat modalities. Therapists may use either wet or dry cold application techniques. Contrast baths, where the hand or foot is alternately immersed in hot and cold water for a specified ratio of time, have been used to decrease swelling, stiffness, and pain; however, there is no common approach or consistent findings.[150] Superficial cold is contradicted in patients with Raynaud's phenomenon or *cryoglobulinemia,* linked to an abnormal protein (cryoglobulins) in the blood that gels at low temperatures. Both may be associated with RA.

Electrotherapy Modalities

Therapists may also wish to consider using other modalities for pain relief in treating the individual with RA, including transcutaneous electrical nerve stimulation (TENS), although the value of TENS as reported in the literature is inconsistent. A meta-analysis of studies investigating TENS for knee OA pain concluded that the mode of TENS applied did affect results, repeated use was more effective than a single application, and use for at least 4 weeks was the most effective.[151] A more recent meta-analysis found high-frequency TENS provided moderate pain relief while interferential current (IFC) resulted in even greater pain reduction when compared to control or sham interventions.[152] International guidelines are uncertain or provide conditional recommendations regarding the use of TENS,[92,94] and none include IFC in their recommendations for OA.[92-97]

Orthoses, Splints, and Braces

As hand involvement occurs both early in RA and is an indication of disease severity, hand and wrist orthoses are used to immobilize specific joints and help reduce pain and swelling by providing local rest and support.[153] There are three primary types of splints: resting splints (used to maintain joint alignment and reduce pain), functional splints (used to restore or improve function), and corrective (used to improve alignment). Resting splints are worn at night or periodically during the day to reduce synovitis and tenosynovitis or in patients with end-stage disease to reduce contractures of the intrinsic and extrinsic muscles of the hand. If volar subluxation at the metacarpal phalangeal joint (MCP) is present, the splint should be designed to apply a gentle force on the volar aspect of the proximal phalange to reduce volar subluxation.[109] There is little to no evidence that resting splints are effective in reducing pain and inflammation and improving function.[154-156]

A functional metacarpal phalangeal (MCP) splint can be useful for patients who have moderate synovitis and or early-to-moderate soft tissue changes. This splint provides support to MCPJs in slight flexion and neutral deviation. It is believed that the splint can reduce pain, decrease flexion forces during grip, and help to keep joints in good alignment. To optimize hand function, splints should only be recommended for the involved joints. MCP splints are contraindicated with significant proximal phalangeal synovitis, as the splint may increase joint forces and may be too restrictive for daily function and gripping. When patients understand the use of the splint, how to properly wear the splint, and any restrictions associated with the splint, they are more adherent.[157]

There is evidence of small benefits for pain reduction and increased function with the use of functional splints. Hand splints may improve grip and pincher strength. There is evidence that wearing functional wrist splints decreases grip strength and does not affect pain, morning stiffness, pinch grip, or quality of life with regular wear.[158] A study that investigated the effects of functional wrist splint wear on task performance reported that wearing a commercially available elastic wrist orthosis resulted in some decrement in performance speed on a number of common tasks, though pain was significantly reduced for all tasks.[159] There is consistent evidence supporting the use of splints for short- and long-term pain relief in OA of the first CMC joint.[160]

Foot orthoses also may be used to alleviate pain through biomechanical support or correction for individuals with knee OA. A lateral wedge insole designed to reduce medial compartment stress compared to no insole appears to reduce pain and NSAID use in some individuals with knee OA.[161] Other methods that show promise in treating knee OA pain are patellofemoral taping,[162] and load shifting or unloader knee braces (stress shifted away from most involved area).[163] All orthotic interventions require professional evaluation, selection, education, and monitoring of use.

Rest

Complete bed rest is rarely recommended. Adequate quality and quantity of sleep at night and short rests during the day are preferred. General recommendations include 8 to 10 hours of sleep per night and brief 30-minute rest periods during the day. Inactivity is a common problem for people with arthritis and may lead to deconditioning, depression, lower pain thresholds, diminished bone and soft tissue health, and increased risk for other serious health conditions. Thus, a major goal of therapy is to assist the person to maintain or regain adequate levels of physical activity and avoid the unnecessary consequences of inactivity.[24,164]

Range of Motion and Flexibility Exercise

A major factor affecting joint mobility in individuals with RA is the level of inflammation and resting position in which specific joints are maintained. For example, intra-articular pressure is reduced when joints are in flexion. Although helpful in reducing joint pain, this flexed position may lead to capsular and musculotendinous shortening and eventual contracture. Patients should be taught proper positioning when resting and should be encouraged to perform daily, active ROM as tolerated to maintain motion. Active-assisted, passive, and proprioceptive neuromuscular facilitation (PNF) techniques may also be applied to shortened muscles. Pain should be respected at all times and should be minimal during and after exercise. Evoking a pain response during stretching may lead to a reflex contraction of the agonist muscle as opposed to creating a relaxation response. Stretching exercises to lengthen shortened muscles should be performed slowly, held for 20 to 30 seconds two to three days a week or more often if indicated. It is important to educate the patient not to do stretching exercises that involve inflamed, swollen joints because they are at risk for capsular stretching and rupture.[24,164] Common wisdom recommends that *exercise-induced pain should subside within 1 hour*. If the patient reports discomfort lasting longer than 1 hour, it may indicate that either the technique, intensity, or duration of the exercise was too great and should be reduced or modified at the next exercise session. Patients should be encouraged to exercise on their own during those times of the day when they feel best. Local pain-relieving modalities before or immediately after exercise may be useful and increase exercise adherence.

In hip and knee OA, manual therapy may offer some additional benefit within a comprehensive treatment program that includes exercise.[166] In a systematic review of manual therapy techniques including passive physiological and accessory movements, muscle stretching and soft tissue mobilization, moderate to large effects for pain and self-reported function were found when compared to alternate interventions and exercise alone.[166] Manual therapy is not generally recommended for individuals with RA who have joint inflammation or resultant laxity.

Strengthening Exercise

Decreased muscle function (strength, endurance, power) in persons with arthritis arises from both direct and indirect effects of the disease. These include intra-articular and extra-articular inflammatory disease elements, side effects of medication, disuse, reflex inhibition in response to pain and joint effusion, impaired proprioception, and loss of mechanical integrity around the joint. A variety of conditioning programs can be effective for improving strength, endurance, and function without exacerbation of pain or disease activity. Exercise has also been shown to reduce RA-related cachexia with concurrent increases in fat-free body mass.[167]

Initially, isometric exercise may be indicated to improve muscle tone, strength, and static endurance; to recruit or activate specific muscles; and to prepare joints for more vigorous activity. Although isometric exercise does avoid dynamic joint stress and mechanical irritation, it can produce other unwanted effects. Isometric exercise performed at more than 50% of maximal voluntary contraction constricts blood flow through the exercising muscle, leading to post-exercise muscle soreness, and the increased peripheral vascular resistance produces increased blood pressure.[164] In the knee and hip, high-intensity isometric contractions are associated with significant increases in intra-articular pressure and reductions in synovial circulation.[168–170] Patients with cardiovascular disease should perform these exercises with caution and be sure to breathe during the contraction because holding one's breath can increase intra-abdominal pressure (*Valsalva maneuver*). Patient instructions for isometric exercise should include the cautions to (1) maintain the contraction for no more than 6 seconds; (2) avoid maximal effort because it is neither necessary nor desirable; (3) exhale during the contraction and inhale during a similar time period of relaxation; and (4) not contract more than two muscle groups at a time.

Dynamic exercise includes both shortening (concentric) and lengthening (eccentric) contractions. Strength and endurance may be improved through resistance (physiological overload) supplied by weight of the body part or external resistance in the form of free weights, elastic bands, or a variety of resistive exercise equipment. A cautious approach to resistance training is recommended to protect unstable or inflamed joints from damage. Strengthening exercise should be performed within the pain-free range. Maximum benefit and maintenance can be achieved by incorporating functional movements and body positions in the recommended exercise routine. The use of well-controlled smooth movement toward the end part of the range is advised, and modifications to resistance, repetitions, or frequency are recommended as needed. Gradual progression of resistance and repetition over a 2- to 3-week period is recommended. Reduce exercise intensity, frequency, or motion if increased joint swelling or pain occurs (local inflammatory response).[24]

Individuals with RA benefit from maintaining or restoring muscular fitness. A number of systematic reviews and meta-analyses of the literature illustrate that there is moderate level evidence for the benefits of both short (8–12 weeks) and long-term progressive land-based and aquatic resistance exercise (a year or more) of up to 70% of one repetition of maximal contraction (1RM) for muscle strength and functional performance. Studies of higher intensity tended to yield greater improvements. Data are presented in Table 23.4 Evidence Summary.[171-179] Loads of up to 70% 1RM used in a circuit training resistance program for persons with controlled RA demonstrated no exacerbation in joint

Table 23.4 Evidence Summary Systematic Reviews and Meta-analyses of Exercise Interventions for Adults with Rheumatoid Arthritis (RA)

Author (Yr)	Subjects	Methods	Duration/Dosage	Results/Comments
Swärdh et al (2016)[171]	Adults with RA: total number not provided	17 RCTs of aerobic and strengthening exercise performed at least 2x/week, sessions a minimum of 20 minutes each, total duration ≥6 weeks, and intensity of at least 40%–50% of Vo_2max, and or ≥ 30%–50% 1 RM.	Evaluated outcomes stratified by short-term and long-term interventions. Durations ranged 8 to 104 weeks. Frequency of exercise ranged 2–7x/ week. See results for specific descriptions.	**Short-term land-based aerobic exercise**: Moderate quality evidence that exercise 3x/week for 30–75 minutes/session at ≥ 40% Vo_2max progressing to 65% Vo_2max improves cardiorespiratory fitness but not strength. **Short-term water-based aerobic exercise:** Moderate quality evidence that exercise for 8-12 weeks at 3x/week for ≥ 60 minutes/session at ≥ 40% Vo_2max progressing to 80% Vo_2max improves cardiorespiratory fitness. **Short-term land-based aerobic and strengthening exercise**: Moderate quality evidence that exercise 12–26 weeks at 2–5x/week for ≥ 30 to 75 minutes/session at ≥40% Vo_2max progressing to 85% Vo_2max and increasing resistance up to 70% 1RM improves cardiorespiratory fitness and muscle strength. **Long-term land-based aerobic and strengthening exercise**: Exercise of 52–104 weeks at 3x/week for ≥ 30 to 80 minutes/session at ≥ 40% Vo_2max progressing to 75%–80% Vo_2max and increasing resistance up to 70% 1RM improves cardiorespiratory fitness and muscle strength.
Hammond et al (2016)[172]	665 adults with mean age of 59 years (one study had adults with early RA)	Seven RCTs of supervised home hand exercise therapy: ROMS and resistance exercise (three RCTs with low risk of bias and 4 with moderate risk of bias assessed with PEDro scale)	Duration ranged from 4 weeks to 52 weeks. Frequency ranged from 1 individualized session with home exercise follow-up to daily, supervised sessions.	Data indicated significant short-term gains in hand function, pain, and grip strength. Long-term improvements for found for hand and upper extremity function and pinch strength. Data suggest high-intensity home hand exercise programs led to better short-term outcomes than low-intensity programs, and these programs are cost-effective.
Bergstra et al (2014)[173]	482 adults; mean age 48 to 59 years across studies	Eight studies (seven RCTs) on treatments for hand RA.	Interventions ranged from 10 days to 14 weeks and from 15 to 336 sessions	Exercise programs varied by study but all included resistance and or active ROM exercises. Grip strength improved and daily

Continued

Table 23.4 Evidence Summary Systematic Reviews and Meta-analyses of Exercise Interventions for Adults with Rheumatoid Arthritis (RA)—cont'd

Author (Yr)	Subjects	Methods	Duration/Dosage	Results/Comments
			during those periods.	function without adverse effects on pain or disease activity. Changes in ROM were less impacted. Longer duration of treatment and higher intensity led to greater improvements.
Baillet et al (2012)[174]	547 adults with mean age ranging from 42 to 61 years. Functional class (reported in select studies) was II-III. Only two RCTs specifically included adults with early RA	Meta-analysis of 10 RCTs comparing resistance exercise to no resistance exercise; quadriceps exercises (three studies); upper and lower extremity (five studies); shoulder strengthening (one study); hand strengthening (one study); supervised exercise (five studies).	Duration ranged from 3 weeks to 104 weeks. Frequency ranged from 2 times per week to daily.	The mean Jadad score was 2.3/ 3, suggesting moderate quality studies. Significant improvements found for isokinetic strength (WMD = 23.7%, $P < 0.001$), isometric strength (WMD = 35.8%, $P < 0.001$), grip strength (WMD = 26.4%, $P < 0.001$) and disability (HAQ scores) (WMD= 0.22, $P < 0.001$). Resistance exercise led to significant improvements in the 50-ft walk (WMD = −1.90 seconds, $P < 0.001$) and disease activity as measured by ESR (WMD = −5.17, $P = 0.005$). Adverse events (RR = 1.08, 95% CI 0.72, 1.63) were similar across groups. Trend toward higher efficacy associated with higher intensity exercise.
Hurkmans et al (2009)[175]	575 adults mean age was 52 years (except one trail mean age = 62 years), low to moderate disease activity	Eight RCTs of supervised dynamic exercise of short-term (<3 months) and long-term (>3 months) duration (aerobic, resistive exercise both on land and in water). Exercise had to be performed ≥2x/week >20 minutes; duration >6 weeks; aerobic exercise intensity >55% of the max HR and/or muscle strengthening starting at 30% to 50% of 1RM	Duration of interventions ranged from 8 weeks to 2 years. Frequency ranged from 2 x/week to 5 x/week	**Short-term, land-based aerobic**: Moderate evidence for improvements in aerobic capacity (pooled effect size 0.99) (95% CI 0.29 to 1.68). **Short-term, land-based aerobic and muscle strength:** Moderate evidence for gains in aerobic capacity and muscle strength (pooled effect size 0.47) (95% CI 0.01 to 0.93). **Short-term, water-based aerobic:** Limited evidence for benefits for functional ability and aerobic capacity. **Long-term, land-based aerobic and muscle strength training:** Moderate evidence for benefits for aerobic capacity and muscle strength. No deleterious effects found in any study.

Table 23.4 Evidence Summary Systematic Reviews and Meta-analyses of Exercise Interventions for Adults with Rheumatoid Arthritis (RA)—cont'd

Author (Yr)	Subjects	Methods	Duration/Dosage	Results/Comments
Cairns et al (2009)[176]	467 adults with early, stable, and active disease	12 RCTs of dynamic exercise alone or in combination (pool, resistance, and aerobic). Mean study quality score was 6.9/10	Duration ranged from 2 weeks to 52 weeks Frequency of exercise ranged from 2x/weeks to 6x/weeks.	Improvements found for muscle strength, physical function, and aerobic capacity. Some studies also reported benefits for disease activity, and small improvements in hip bone mineral density. One study reported significantly less progression of radiographic damage in the small feet joints. However, one study found worse radiographic damage in large joints in patients who had preexisting large joint damage.
Gaudin et al (2008)[177]	647 adults, mean age was 53 years, most had stable disease	Nine RCTs of dynamic exercise with a median quality score of 8/10	Duration ranged from 2 months to 2 years. Frequency ranged from 2x/week to 5x/week.	Improvements were found for aerobic capacity and muscle strength. There was insufficient evidence for improvements in functional capacity.
Han et al (2007)[178]	217 adults	Five studies of tai chi (two RCTs and three CCTs) with low quality	Duration ranged from 6 to 12 wk. Frequency ranged from once to twice weekly.	The evidence was not convincing to suggest tai chi as an effective treatment for RA given low study quality and low frequency of intervention.
Lee et al (2004)[179]	206 adults	Four RCTs of tai chi	Duration ranged up to 12 weeks.	There is silver evidence that tai chi provides benefits for ankle, knee, and hip ROM. No evidence regarding improvements in joint symptoms. No deleterious effects, and patients reported they felt as if they improved with exercise.

1RM = one repetition of maximum voluntary contraction; Vo_2max = maximal oxygen uptake; ROM = range of motion; CCT = non-randomized controlled clinical trials.

symptoms and significant improvements in strength and function.

Designing exercise interventions for individuals with RA requires careful consideration of the patient's disease activity, disease severity, and systemic disease features. Persons with RA in an active flare-up should limit their exercise to daily ROM exercises incorporated into ADLs to promote adherence to active joint movement and isometric exercises to promote strength. It is also important to use caution with resistance exercise in individuals on high doses on corticosteroids to reduce the risk of tendon rupture and osteoporosis-related fractures. Walking as tolerated, is encouraged together with daily periods of rest and a full night of sleep to manage fatigue. When the disease activity subsides, the exercise program can be progressed by adding dynamic strengthening exercises, with caution to avoid stress on deranged joints or cysts, and greater repetitions of isometric exercises as well as greater engagement in physical activity. When the disease is in remission, aerobic exercises and dynamic exercises with resistance should be considered to promote cardiovascular health and improve strength and conditioning. When RA affects the large weight-bearing joints, patients should be cautious with high-intensity impact exercise especially in the presence of established joint changes.[176]

In persons with knee OA, the evidence is strong and consistent that LE exercise that includes neuromuscular and functional training reduces pain and improves function. Interventions have included isometric, isotonic, functional, and aquatic exercise, as well as proprioceptive and balance training. Interventions have been tested in both clinically supervised and self-directed settings with positive results and acceptable adherence.[180] Evidence supporting the use of exercise in the management of knee and hip OA is presented in Table 23.5 Evidence Summary.[180-188] Physical therapists should routinely incorporate strategies to enhance patient motivation and adherence to the therapeutic exercise and home exercise programs (HEPs) including exercise booster sessions (periodic follow-up appointments), goal setting, and other self-efficacy enhancing practices.[164,189]

Cardiovascular Training

Individuals with RA or OA are usually deconditioned compared to their age-matched peers. A number of systematic reviews have reported significant improvements in aerobic capacity and activity levels through regular cardiovascular conditioning without aggravating joints and other disease symptoms. If weight-bearing is a barrier to exercise, low- or non-weight-bearing activities such as stationary cycling, pool-based aerobics, or deep water running may be options.[16,127,145] For most people, walking and stationary bicycles are a safe and effective means of aerobic exercise.[16,190] Furthermore, patients who have engaged in such a program often report an increase in self-esteem and improved emotional status.[16] Medical screening as appropriate for age and medical condition (e.g., *Revised Physical Activity Readiness Questionnaire* [PAR-Q]) (http://eparmedx.com) should be completed before beginning an aerobic exercise program.

Physical Activity

Patients with RA and OA are less physically active than their healthy counterparts. Recent studies indicate that patients with RA engage in suboptimal physical activity and this low level of participation in physical activity remains despite improvements in disease activity.[191] The U.S. Department of Health and Human Services has established *Physical Activity Guidelines*.[192] These guidelines recommend accumulating (minimum 10-minute bouts) 30 minutes of moderate-intensity physical activity five times per week for a total of 150 minutes each week. Recommendations for vigorous physical activity are set at 75 minutes total per week for adults with chronic illness. In a study by Lee et al, 42% of patients with RA accumulated no moderate/vigorous physical activity over

Table 23.4 Evidence Summary Mobile and Internet Applications for Tracking and Promoting Physical Activity

Application	Description and Link
Arthritis Power	Mobile application where you can enter exercise as well as data on fatigue, sleep, and medications, and you can track your disease symptoms. Available for Android phones. https://arthritispower.creakyjoints.org
Health Log	This mobile app for smartphones helps a patient record and track exercise, weight, hours of sleep, mood, and other useful functions. Available for free only with Android phones. https://play.google.com/store/apps/details?id=andrew.arproductions.healthlog&hl=en
MyRA	This RA symptom tracking app allows you to record information about your joint pain, fatigue, and other RA-related symptoms in your phone. You can also print out the information to share with your rheumatologist or rheumatology health professional. Available for iPhones and Androids. https://trackmyra.com
RheumaTrack	This mobile app allows you to track your RA symptoms as well as physical activity. It includes a personal lock system to keep health information safe. Available for both iPhones and Androids https://play.google.com/store/apps/details?id=com.rheumatrack&hl=en
Track+React	Developed by the Arthritis Foundation, this app enables people with RA to track their fitness, nutrition, sleep, and self-management activities to see what impact it has on their symptoms. http://www.arthritis.org/living-with-arthritis/tools-resources/track-and-react/track-and-react-app.php
tRAppen	This newly developed mobile internet service was designed specifically to help adults with RA self-manage their disease. A recent study of its use suggests tRAppen may support a physically active lifestyle. http://rmdopen.bmj.com/content/rmdopen/2/1/e000214.full.pdf
Walk with Ease	This internet-based and mobile app (available for smartphones including iPhone and Androids) allows you to track your steps. The application is based on the Arthritis Foundation's Walk with Ease 6-week program. http://www.arthritis.org/living-with-arthritis/tools-resources/walk-with-ease/about.php

a 1-week period.[193] In a longitudinal study of a large cohort of adults, those with knee OA spent two-thirds of their daily time in sedentary behavior.[194] With sedentary behavior (e.g., watching TV, using computer, reading) being an independent risk factor for increased morbidity and mortality, it is vital that physical therapists counsel and support their patients to "move more and sit less" throughout the day.

Fortunately, there are many technologies (mobile apps used with smartphones, wearable devices, internet tracking programs, etc.) that can help motivate patients to be physically active, enable them to track their progress and serve as a coaching tool for physical therapists.

Functional Training

Functional training for the individual with arthritis proceeds in the same fashion as for other individuals with similar deficits. Therapists may choose to reduce the functional demands of an activity either temporarily, such as under conditions of acute inflammation, or permanently by incorporating a variety of adaptive equipment into ADL that substitute for lost ROM and strength. To ensure patients with RA can engage in functional training activities, modifications can be made to handles of devices for easier grasp. There are aids for dressing and grooming, as well as personal hygiene. By breaking down functional tasks, such as rising from a chair or climbing stairs, into smaller movements and incorporating these into a therapeutic exercise program, the therapist can help the patient identify faulty movement patterns and address specific components of the movement that are causing difficulty. Functional exercises aim to replicate daily activities including house, yard, work, and leisure activities that are important to the patient. Such exercises often incorporate body weight for resistance and the use of actual tools/equipment or movements that make up that activity.

UE involvement in RA, particularly of the wrist and hands, may complicate the choice of an ambulatory assistive device by precluding any weight-bearing on these affected joints. In these instances, platform attachments can be used to transform the forearm into a weight-bearing surface. Rearranging the home or work environment also can improve a person's functional abilities. Raising beds or chairs can reduce the effort needed to stand up. Railings placed around the bed, bath, and along stairways also can help increase an individual's independence.

Gait and Balance Training

Specific deviations will be evident throughout the gait cycle in both RA and OA. These may include gait asymmetries, decreased velocity, cadence and stride length, prolonged period of double support, inadequate initial contact and push-off, and diminished joint excursion through both swing and stance. Gait deviations in the patient with RA, specifically owing to foot pain or deformities, may also be evident (Table 23.6).[137,195] Therapists should address the underlying joint and muscle impairments that contribute to these deviations in the gait training program with persons with any type of arthritis.

The degree to which the gait of an individual with arthritis should, or can, approximate normal is one of the most difficult questions in designing a therapeutic program. Some "abnormalities" such as antalgic limping may in fact reduce joint loading. Joint destruction may necessitate the introduction of assistive devices as simple as a standard cane or walking poles, or as cumbersome as platform crutches or rolling walkers with platform attachments. The gait of the individual with RA or OA should be safe, functional, and cosmetically acceptable to the patient rather than an unattainable idealized version of the norm. Use of a properly fitted, standard cane in the contralateral hand is associated with decreased joint loading and pain in individuals with both hip and knee OA.

Decreased walking speed in arthritis is common, and there is general agreement that increased speed is a meaningful measure of functional capacity and improvement.[196] For example, a person's ability to walk fast enough to cross the street with the timing of the traffic light is important for functional and safe community locomotion. However, increased walking speed without attention to joint biomechanics may be undesirable. In a clinical trial of a nonsteroidal drug for persons with knee OA, all with a varus deformity, gait variables were included as outcome measures. The researchers found that self-reported pain diminished and walking speed increased in the active therapy group. At the same time, kinetic analysis of joint forces showed the increased speed was accompanied by increased adductor moment at the knee and greater loading of the medial compartment.[197] This additional loading of the joint and increased stress on lateral supporting tissue may not be worth the gains of increased speed. Attention to biomechanical factors thus should be considered in comprehensive management, even when drug therapy decreases pain and improves gait speed.

Decreased proprioceptive input, impaired neuromuscular reflexes, altered joint biomechanics, pain, and muscle weakness contribute to static and dynamic balance problems in the individual with LE arthritis. Balance training may include progression from static postures moving from double- to single-limb support, stable to unstable surfaces, and adding perturbations where safe. Dynamic balance activities include maintaining postural alignment while shifting weight from one limb to the other in various directions and walking on different surfaces to challenge the vestibular and proprioceptive systems. A systematic review of 17 randomized controlled trials and clinical controlled trials

Table 23.6 Analysis of Gait Deviations, Physical Examination Findings, and Treatment Goals

Gait Deviations	Physical Examination Findings	Treatment Goals
Pronated Foot		
Shuffled progression Decreased step length Initial contact with medial border of foot Decreased single-limb balance Prolonged double-support phase Late heel rise Plantarflexion of ipsilateral ankle in swing Genu valgus with weight-bearing	Tenderness over subtalar midtarsal area Limited inversion range Weak and painful posterior tibialis muscle Pronated weight-bearing posture of foot Lax medial collateral ligament of knee	Relieve subtalar and midtarsal joint stresses Increase ankle inversion Strengthen posterior tibialis muscle Stabilize hypermobile joints with rigid orthosis Maintain neutral alignment in stance by foot positioning
Hallux Valgus		
Lateral and posterior weight shift Late heel rise Decreased single-limb balance	Lateral deviation of great toe Swelling of first MTP joint Shortening of flexor hallucis brevis muscle Tenderness of great toe Weakness of great toe abduction	Accommodate foot with wide toe box shoe Increase extension of great toe Relieve weight-bearing stresses
Metatarsophalangeal Joint Subluxation		
Diminished roll off Decreased single-limb stance Apropulsive progression Decreased single-limb balance	Painful MTP heads with weight bearing Callus formation over MTP heads Ulcerations over MTP heads Limited MTP flexion Prominent MTP heads	Redistribute pressure with metatarsal bar Relieve pressure with soft cutout shoe insert Increase flexion mobility of MTP joints Accommodate foot with extra-depth shoe
Hammer or Claw Toes		
Diminished roll off Decreased single-limb stance Apropulsive progression Decreased single-limb balance	Posture of MTP joint hyperextension with proximal and distal interphalangeal joint flexion Posture of MTP and distal interphalangeal joint hyperextension with proximal interphalangeal flexion Callus formation at plantar tips and dorsum of proximal interphalangeal joint Limited MTP flexion	Improve toe alignment with metatarsal bar Accommodate foot with extra-depth shoe Diminish pressure with soft insert Increase toe mobility
Painful Heel		
Toe-heel pattern No heel contact in stance Decreased stride length Decreased velocity Plantarflexion of ankle in swing Increased hip flexion in swing Decreased step length of contralateral limb	Painful active plantarflexion Painful passive and active dorsiflexion Swelling and pain at Achilles insertion Tenderness over spur Decreased ankle dorsiflexion range	Decrease inflammation with steroid injection or modalities Relieve weight-bearing stress Decrease pressure over spur with soft shoe insert Maintain ankle mobility

From Dimonte and Light[195] with permission.
MTP = metatarsal-phalangeal.

found no studies that separately evaluated balance training, rather exercise programs were comprehensive in nature including muscle strengthening, endurance and functional activities[198] (see Chapter 10, Strategies to Improve Motor Function).

Joint Protection

Joint protection is a key component of arthritis management, due to the impact of the disease on the joint and supportive structures. A randomized controlled trial for persons with hand OA compared the effects of a 3-month educational–behavioral joint protection program to standard education (each consisting of a 20-minute session and provision of a piece of Dycem [nonslip matting] to use when opening jars). This single-blinded study demonstrated that patients in the joint protection and exercise group increased grip strength by 25% and both groups reported better hand function with the joint protection information.[199] Patients should be encouraged to incorporate joint care into all ADL to minimize pain and conserve energy (see *Appendix 23.A, Joint Protection, Rest, and Energy Conservation*).

In addition to reducing pain and improving function, orthoses also may provide support and protection for vulnerable and painful joints. Foot orthotics or specially designed shoes can serve the dual purpose of relieving biomechanical stresses and enhancing function for the person with RA foot involvement.[200] The cost of special shoes may not be reimbursable under many insurance programs. A good shoe will provide support and eliminate unnecessary joint motion in the talocalcaneal joint with a firm and wide heel counter. It should also help to maintain normal bony alignment and accommodate all existing foot deformities within a toe box of adequate dimensions. Pressure should be evenly distributed along the plantar surface of the foot during weight-bearing. Commercially available gel inserts may be helpful and are inexpensive; however, with more advanced biomechanical changes in the foot, the fabrication of orthoses may be required. A *rocker sole* (shoe sole that is curved at the toe) can be used to facilitate push-off with limited ankle motion. A controlled trial was conducted of the effect of off-the-shelf extra-depth orthopedic footwear for people with RA and at least 1 year of foot pain. Outcomes were measures of pain, gait, and physical function after 2 months of wearing the extra-depth shoes. The footwear group improved significantly on self-reported disability, weight-bearing and non-weight-bearing pain, and gait. In addition to extra depth in the shoe toe box, the shoes provided greater rear foot stability, an arch support, a stiff shank, and a padded heel collar above the counter for improved fit. This study reported that walking pain accounted for 75% of the variability in physical function level of the subjects.[201] In a systematic review, the authors were unable to draw conclusions about the long-term effects of different footwear on knee and hip OA pain.[202] They did suggest, however, that there was increasing evidence that shock-absorbing insoles, subtalar taping, and avoidance of high heels and sandals early in life may prevent lower extremity joint pain later in life.

Education and Self-Management

Patient education in the rheumatic diseases has been shown to result in positive changes in knowledge, health behavior, beliefs, and attitudes that affect health status, quality of life, and health care utilization. In a review of the literature, researchers documented the well-established benefits of self-management programs on mental health.[101] As in any chronic illness, education should include information needed to deal with the condition (taking medications, exercise), self-management skills necessary to carry out important social and vocational roles, and resources needed to deal with the emotional consequences of chronic illness such as depression, fear, and frustration. The evidence is overwhelming that education designed to teach self-management skills and increase client self-efficacy for these tasks is the most effective.[101,203] The *Arthritis Foundation* (www.arthritis.org) can supply the clinician or the individual with a variety of resources and self-help courses that will increase cognitive understanding of the disease process and self-management skills. (See *Appendix 23.B for overview of their programs.*) Many local chapters of the Arthritis Foundation hold individual and family support groups to increase psychosocial adaptation, as well as conduct aquatic and land exercise programs in public facilities. The *Association of Rheumatology Health Professionals,* a division of the American College of Rheumatology (www.rheumatology.org), can provide the therapist with scientific and clinical resources for enhanced practice, as well as a network of professional colleagues who work in rheumatology. See Appendix 23.C for *Web-based Patient and Professional Resources.*

SUMMARY

Rheumatoid arthritis and osteoarthritis are the two most common forms of arthritis in adults. Both exact a high toll with respect to physical functioning and limitations in participation and quality of life. Rheumatoid arthritis, due to its exacerbating and remitting course and systemic features, also impacts mental well-being. Advances in medical therapies for both conditions combined with physical therapy and physical activity allow patients to achieve maximum functioning. Physical therapy for these patients covers a broad array of interventions from modalities and orthotics, to exercise and self-management strategies. Exercise has the strongest evidence for benefits; equivalent to the effects of non-steroidal medications whereas the evidence for other interventions is less strong. Overall, data have shown that maintaining a physically active lifestyle is important for both joint and cardiovascular health and should be a component of all counseling discussions with patients.

Questions for Review

1. What epidemiological factors are associated with a diagnosis of RA?
2. What are the major pathological changes seen in RA?
3. State two hypotheses concerning the pathogenesis of RA.
4. Describe four modifiable risk factors that may predispose an individual to OA.
5. Describe two changes in articular cartilage associated with OA that differ from normal aging.
6. Name at least two laboratory tests used in the diagnosis of RA and state their purposes.
7. Describe the parameters used in examining radiographs of arthritic joints.
8. Describe the typical joint changes seen with RA for the following joints: occipitoatlantal, atlantoaxial, temporomandibular, carpals, knees, and talocalcaneal.
9. Define the following deformities: ulnar drift, swan neck, boutonnière, hammer toes, claw toes, and hallux valgus.
10. Describe the typical radiographic joint changes seen in advanced OA.
11. Describe the overall goals of medical management for RA and OA.
12. What are the primary indications for surgery in RA?
13. Describe the key points in taking a history for the individual with arthritis.
14. What adaptations of standard tests and measures might be required in examining the individual with RA?
15. What are the general physical therapy goals for individuals with RA or OA?
16. Explain the goals, modifications, and progression of a typical strengthening program.
17. Discuss treatment strategies for increasing ROM.
18. Design a cardiovascular conditioning program for an individual with LE arthritic joint involvement.
19. Describe strategies to enhance patients' adherence to therapeutic exercise programs.
20. State at least four principles of joint protection and give a practical application of each.
21. What criteria guide the selection of shoes for the individual with RA?
22. What are the purposes of splints?
23. What changes in gait are commonly associated with RA? What impairments contribute to static and dynamic balance problems in the individual with LE arthritis?

CASE STUDIES

Two case studies are presented: Case 1 presents a patient with rheumatoid arthritis and Case 2 considers a patient with osteoarthritis.

CASE 1: RHEUMATOID ARTHRITIS

HISTORY

The patient is a 52-year-old woman who has two children in high school. She is a nurse and works about 40 hours a week. She has had symptoms of joint swelling and pain, fatigue, and increasing weakness for 2 years. During initial onset of symptoms, a primary care physician diagnosed her with carpal tunnel syndrome, knee osteoarthritis, and eventually, fibromyalgia. Her symptoms continued to worsen on NSAIDs. She was also prescribed antidepressants and she referred to a rheumatologist 3 months ago. Based on her history, physical examination, laboratory values (Disease Activity Score [DAS] = 3.2; RF= 12.30; ESR = 26), and radiographic evidence, the rheumatologist confirmed a diagnosis of seropositive RA. She began a course of methotrexate and has been referred to physical therapy.

PHYSICAL THERAPY EXAMINATION

At the initial physical therapy examination, she reports her morning stiffness is now less than 30 minutes (previous high of 3 hours). The pain and swelling in her hands, feet, and elbows is markedly decreased, and she is feeling more energetic. Systems review of the integumentary system is unremarkable except for a slight edema and redness of the distal finger joints and wrist R > L. Her blood pressure and respiratory rate are within normal limits. Her resting heart rate is 72 but increases to 96 with modest exertion.

ROM is limited at the shoulder, elbows, wrists, and MCPs. She lacks 10° of knee extension and has no ankle dorsiflexion or hip extension beyond neutral. Bilateral strength is good minus. She exhibits a forward head, rounded shoulder posture, with the beginning of a marked kyphosis. Her pain is most prominent in her wrists, elbows, and ankles (4/10 visual analogue scale [VAS]) and indicates general fatigue. She has flat feet and moderate swelling of the metatarsal heads. She is relieved that at last she has been diagnosed with a condition for which there is effective treatment and she trusts her rheumatologist. Her immediate goals are to regain comfortable motion, strength, and stamina and to avoid deformity.

GUIDING QUESTIONS

1. Identify the general anticipated goals and expected outcomes of physical therapy for this patient.
2. What self-management strategies would you recommend and or instruct the patient to use?
3. Describe the types of community resources you would recommend the patient explore.
4. What supportive devices might be used to decrease symptoms and increase function?
5. How would her physical therapist optimally schedule her return visits to clinic?

CASE 2: OSTEOARTHRITIS

HISTORY

The patient is a 58-year-old Caucasian woman whose low back and bilateral knee pain have increased over the past year. She is 5 feet 7 inches tall and weighs 195 pounds. She has hypertension and chronic renal insufficiency for which she takes prescribed medication. She works part time as a teacher's assistant in a local elementary school and lives alone in a third floor walk-up apartment. On weekends, she serves as the assistant building manager, which includes both cleaning and minimal maintenance duties. She has difficulty using stairs, getting up and down from sitting, getting on and off the bus, and walking for more than 15 minutes at a time. She has had progressively greater knee pain and stiffness for the past 3 years and has recently experienced episodes of "giving way" in the right knee. Her low back pain is worse after prolonged sitting, vacuuming, and at the end of the day. She avoids over-the-counter medications due to her underlying kidney disease but reports moderate pain relief with topical diclofenac applied to both knees three times a day. The patient recently joined an aquafit class at a local pool but admits to rarely attending classes.

On a recent visit to her primary care physician, she underwent radiographs of both knees, which revealed bilateral joint space narrowing, with the right knee more affected than left and greater lateral compartment involvement than medial. There is evidence of bony sclerosis, osteophytes, and mild malalignment (genu valgum) greater on the right. Her physician has suggested continued use of the topical NSAID, use of a cane, losing weight, and referred her to a physical therapist for evaluation and exercise advice. The patient and her doctor have agreed to discuss surgical options for the knee if she is not satisfied with her condition in 3 to 6 months.

PHYSICAL THERAPY EXAMINATION

During the initial history and systems review, the patient reports that she is finding both of her part-time jobs difficult, and in particular her cleaning responsibilities in the apartment building. She is divorced with one grown son who lives out of town. She is frequently tired and lacks the energy to go to the pool classes despite enjoying the session she last attended about 2 months ago. The patient admits to not sleeping well and having to take occasional sick days from her school-based job. She is concerned about finances and feels that she needs to continue working for at least another 3 years. Her pain is intermittent during the day but wakes her up frequently during the night. Her heart rate is 82, her blood pressure is 140/85, and her respiratory rate is 16. Her skin and circulation in the lower extremities are unremarkable and sensory integrity and reflexes are intact. Her concerns are being able to keep working and to avoid knee surgery.

Selected tests and measures reveal weakness and loss of motion in hips and knees bilaterally, and an antalgic and slow gait. Her spinal ROM is restricted in extension and rotation. Anterior–posterior knee stability is good, but there is moderate pseudolaxity of the lateral collateral ligaments bilaterally. Using a numeric pain rating scale, she rates her left knee pain as 7 out of 10 while walking and 8 out of 10 while climbing stairs, and right knee pain at 6 out of 10 for all activities. She is wearing unsupportive slip-on shoes and shows marked ankle pronation on the right and bilateral hallux valgus. Her static dynamic and balance are poor in both legs and her fast-paced walking speed is 0.94 m/second.

GUIDING QUESTIONS

1. What anticipated goals should the physical therapist discuss with the patient for the episode of care?
2. Formulate a home exercise program for this patient and determine an optimal schedule for follow-up by the physical therapist.
3. What kind of orthotic device(s) or equipment would reduce this patient's symptoms and increase her function?
4. What should be included in patient-related instruction to maximize this patient's function?
5. What strategies would maximize this patient's adherence to a home exercise program and regular physical activity?
6. What other health professional(s) and or community resources would you recommend for this patient?

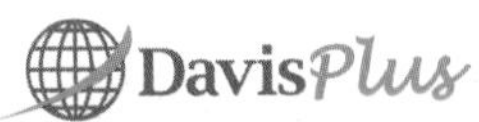

For additional resources, including answers to the questions for review and case study guiding questions, please visit **http://davisplus.fadavis.com**

References

1. Klippel, JH, Stone, JH, Crofford, JH, Le, J, and White, PH (eds). Primer on the Rheumatic Diseases, ed 13. Arthritis Foundation and Springer Publishing, Atlanta, GA, 2011.
2. Arnett FC, et al: The American Rheumatism Association 1987 revised criteria for the classification of rheumatoid arthritis. Arthritis Rheum 31(3):315–324, 1988.
3. Aletaha, D, et al: Rheumatoid arthritis classification criteria. Arthritis Rheum 62(9):2569–2581, 2010. doi: 10.1002/art.27584.
4. Hemlick, CG, et al: Estimates of the prevalence of arthritis and other rheumatic conditions in the United States. Arthritis Rheum 58(1):15–25, 2008. doi: 10.1002/art.23177.
5. Symmons, DPM: Epidemiological concepts and the classification of musculoskeletal conditions. In Hochberg M, Silman AJ, Smolen JS, Weinblatt M, eds. Rheumatology, ed 6. Mosby Elsevier, Philadelphia, PA, 2014, pp 1–8.
6. Worthington, J, and Eyre S: Principles of genetic epidemiology. In Hochberg, M, Silman, AJ, Smolen, JS, Weinblatt, M, eds. Rheumatology, ed 6. Mosby Elsevier, Philadelphia, PA, 2014, pp 80–85.
7. Raychaudhuri, S, et al: Five amino acids in three HLA proteins explain most of the association between MHC and seropositive rheumatoid arthritis. Nat Genet 44(3):291–296, 2012. doi: 10.1038/ng.1076.
8. Fernando, MM, et al: Defining the role of the MHC in autoimmunity: a review and pooled analysis. PLoS Genet 4(4):e1000024, 2008. doi: 10.1371/journal.pgen.1000024.
9. Nielsen, MM, et al: Specific autoantibodies precede the symptoms of rheumatoid arthritis: A study of serial measurements in blood donors. Arthritis Rheum 50(2):380–386, 2004.
10. Rantapaa-Dahlqvist, S, et al: Antibodies against cyclic citrullinated peptide and IgA rheumatoid factor predict the development of rheumatoid arthritis. Arthritis Rheum 48(10):2741–2749, 2003.
11. Lahiri, M, et al: Modifiable risk factors for RA: prevention, better than cure? Rheumatology (Oxford) 51(3):499–512, 2012. doi: 10.1093/rheumatology/ker299.
12. Sugiyama, D, et al: Impact of smoking as a risk factor for developing rheumatoid arthritis: a meta-analysis of observational studies. Ann Rheum Dis 69(1):70–81, 2010. doi: 10.1136/ard.2008.096487.
13. Qin, B, et al: Body mass index and the risk of rheumatoid arthritis: a systematic review and dose-response meta-analysis. Arthritis Res Ther 17:86, 2015. doi: 10.1186/s13075-015-0601-x.
14. Di Giuseppe, D, et al: Fish consumption and risk of rheumatoid arthritis: a dose-response meta-analysis. Arthritis Res Ther 16(5):446, 2014. doi: 10.1186/s13075-014-0446-8.
15. Mikuls, TR, et al: Periodontitis and Porphyromonas gingivalis in patients with rheumatoid arthritis. Arthritis Rheumatol 66(5):1090–1100, 2014. doi: 10.1002/art.38348.

16. McInnes, IB, and Schett G: The pathogenesis of rheumatoid arthritis. N Engl J Med 365(23): 2205–2219, 2011. doi: 10.1056/NEJMra1004965.
17. Klareskog, L, Catrina, AI, and Paget, S: Rheumatoid arthritis. Lancet 373:659–672, 2009.
18. Hutchinson, D, et al: Heavy cigarette smoking is strongly associated with rheumatoid arthritis (RA), particularly in patients without a family history of RA. Ann Rheum Dis 60(3):223–227, 2001.
19. Klareskog, L, Gregersen, PK, and Huizinga, TW: Prevention of autoimmune rheumatic disease: State of the art and future perspectives. Ann Rheum Dis 69(12):2062–2066, 2010. doi: 10.1136/ard.2010.142109.
20. Pravin, P, and Dasgupta, B: Role of diagnostic ultrasound in the assessment of musculoskeletal diseases. Ther Adv Musculoskelet Dis 4(5):341–355, 2012. doi:10.1177/1759720X12442112.
21. D'Agostino, MA, et al: Novel algorithms for the pragmatic use of ultrasound in the management of patients with rheumatoid arthritis: from diagnosis to remission. Ann Rheum Dis 75(11): 1902–1908, 2016. doi: 10.1136/annrheumdis-2016-209646.
22. Takase-Minegishi, K, et al: Diagnostic test accuracy of ultrasound for synovitis in rheumatoid arthritis: systematic review and meta-analysis. Rheumatology (Oxford) 2017. doi: 10.1093/rheumatology/kex036.
23. Hochberg, MC, et al: The American College of Rheumatology 1991 revised criteria for the classification of global functional status in rheumatoid arthritis. Arthritis Rheum 35(5):498–502, 1992.
24. Iversen, MD, and Kale, MK: Physical therapy management of select rheumatic conditions in older adults. In Nakasato Y, Yung RL, eds. Geriatric rheumatology: A comprehensive approach. Springer, New York, NY, 2011, pp 101–110.
25. Iversen, MD, Finckh, A, and Liang, MH: Exercise prescriptions for the major inflammatory and non-inflammatory arthritides. In Frontera WR, Dawson DM, Slovik DM, eds. Exercise in Rehabilitation Medicine. Human Kinetics, Champaign, IL, 2005, pp 157–179.
26. Brasington, RD: Clinical features of rheumatoid arthritis. In Hochberg M, Silman AJ, Smolen JS, Weinblatt M, eds. Rheumatology, ed 6. Philadelphia, PA, Mosby Elsevier, 2014, 704–711.
27. Sodhi A, et al: Rheumatoid arthritis affecting temporomandibular joint. Contemp Clin Dent 6(1):124–127, 2015. doi: 10.4103/0976-237X.149308.
28. Ilan, DI, and Rettig, ME: Rheumatoid arthritis of the wrist. Bulletin Hosp for Joint Dis 61(3):179–185, 2004.
29. Turkiewicz, AM, and Moreland, LW: Rheumatoid arthritis. In Bartlett, SJ, Bingham CO, Maricic MJ, Iversen MD, Ruffing V, (eds). *Clinical Care Text in the Rheumatic Diseases*, ed 3. Atlanta, GA: Association of Rheumatology Health Professionals, American College of Rheumatology, 2006, pp 157–166.
30. Summers, GD, et al: Rheumatoid cachexia: a clinical perspective. Rheumatol 47(8):1124–1131, 2008.
31. Fiori, MG, et al: Selective atrophy of the type IIb muscle fibers in rheumatoid arthritis and progressive systemic sclerosis (scleroderma). A biopsy histochemical study. European J Rheumatol Inflammation 6(2):168–181, 1983.
32. Always, SE, Morissette, MR, and Siu, PM: Aging and apoptosis in muscle. In Masoro EJ, Austad S (eds). ed 7. Handbook of the Biology of Aging. Academic Press, San Diego, CA, 2011, pp 64–118.
33. Solomon, DH, Goodson, NJ, and Katz, JN, et al: Patterns of cardiovascular risk in rheumatoid arthritis. Ann Rheum Dis 65(12):1608–1612, 2006.
34. Metsios, GS, et al: Rheumatoid arthritis, cardiovascular disease and physical exercise: A systematic review. Rheumatol 47:239, 2008.
35. Davis, JM, 3rd, et al: The presentation and outcome of heart failure in patients with rheumatoid arthritis differs from that in the general population. Arthritis Rheum 58(9):2603v2611, 2008. doi: 10.1002/art.23798.
36. Sokka, T, et al: Work disability remains a major problem in rheumatoid arthritis in the 2000s: Data from 32 countries in the QUEST-RA study. Arthritis Res Ther 12(2):R42, 2010. doi: 10.1186/ar2951.
37. Kumar, N, et al: Causes of death in patients with rheumatoid arthritis: Comparison with siblings and matched osteoarthritis controls. J Rheumatol 34(8):1695–1698, 2007.
38. Lindqvist, E, et al: Prognostic laboratory markers of joint damage in rheumatoid arthritis. Ann Rheum Dis 64(2):196–201, 2005.
39. Landewe, R: Predictive markers in rapidly progressing rheumatoid arthritis. J Rheum Suppl 80:8–15, 2007.
40. Gough, A, et al: Genetic typing of patients with inflammatory arthritis at presentation can be used to predict outcome. Arthritis Rheum 37(8):1166–1170, 1994.
41. Felson, DT, et al: American College of Rheumatology/ European League Against Rheumatism provisional definition of remission in rheumatoid arthritis for clinical trials. Arthritis Rheum 70(3)404–413, 2011. doi: 10.1136/ard.2011.149765.
42. Felson, DT: Developments in the clinical understanding of osteoarthritis. Arthritis Res Ther 2009;11(1):203. doi: 10.1016/j.joca.2015.02.164.
43. Cisternas, MG, et al: Alternative methods for defining osteoarthritis and the impact on estimating prevalence in a US population-based survey. Arthritis Care Res (Hoboken) 68(5):574–580, 2016.
44. Allen, KD: Racial and ethnic disparities in osteoarthritis phenotypes. Curr Opin Rheumatol 22:528–532, 2010.
45. Loeser, RF: Aging processes and the development of osteoarthritis. Curr Opin Rheumatol 25(1):108–113, 2013.
46. Bland, JH, Melvin, JL, and Hasson S. Osteoarthritis: In Melvin J, Ferrell KM (eds). Rheumatologic Rehabilitation Series: Adult Rheumatic Diseases, vol 2. Bethesda, MD: American Occupational Therapy Association; 2000:81–92.
47. Valdes, AM, and Spector, TD: The contribution of genes to osteoarthritis. Med Clin North Am 93(1):45–66, 2009.
48. Jensen, L: Hip osteoarthritis: Influence of work with heavy lifting, climbing stairs or ladders, or combining kneeling/squatting with heavy lifting. Occup Environ Med 65(1):6–19, 2009.
49. Jensen, LK: Knee osteoarthritis: Influence of work involving heavy lifting, kneeling, climbing stairs or ladders, or knee/squatting combined with heavy lifting. Occup Environ Med 65(2):72–89, 2008.
50. Garstang, SV, and Stitik, TP: Osteoarthritis: Epidemiology, risk factors, and pathophysiology. Am J Phys Med Rehabil 85(11 Suppl):S2–S11, 2006.
51. Felson, DT: Risk factors for osteoarthritis: Understanding joint vulnerability. Clin Orthop Rel Res 427 suppl:S16–S21, 2004.
52. Altman, RD: Early management of osteoarthritis. Am J Manage Care 16:S41–S47, 2010.
53. Reid, GD, et al: Femoroacetabular impingement syndrome: An underrecognized cause of hip pain and premature osteoarthritis? J Rheumatol 37(7):1395–1404, 2010.
54. White, D, et al: Trajectories of functional decline in knee osteoarthritis: the Osteoarthritis Initiative. Rheumatology (Oxford) 55:801–808, 2016.
55. Martel-Palletier, J, et al: Osteoarthritis. Nat Rev Dis Primers 2:16072, 2016. doi: 10.1038/nrdp.2016.72.
56. Dieppe, PA, and Lohmander, LS: Pathogenesis and management of pain in osteoarthritis. Lancet 365(9463):965–973, 2005.
57. van Der Kraan, PM: Osteophytes: relevance and biology. Osteoarthritis Cartilage 15(3):237–244, 2007.
58. Kittelson, AJ, Stevens-Lapsley, JE, and Schmiege, SJ: Determination of pain phenotypes in knee osteoarthritis: A latent class analysis using data from the Osteoarthritis Initiative. Arthritis Care Res (Hoboken) 68(5):612–620, 2016.
59. Witt, KL, and Vilensky JA: Anatomy of osteoarthritis joint pain. Clin Anat 27:451–454, 2014.
60. Sharif, M, et al: Suggestion of nonlinear or phasic progression of knee osteoarthritis based on measurements of serum cartilage oligomeric matrix protein levels over five years. Arthritis Rheum 50(8):2479–2488, 2004.
61. Kohn, MD, et al: Classifications in Brief: Kellgren-Lawrence classification of osteoarthritis. Clin Orthop Relat Res 474(8): 1886–1893, 2016.
62. Kauppila, AM, et al: Disability in end-stage knee osteoarthritis. Disabil Rehabil 31(5):370–380, 2009.
63. Altman, R, et al: The American College of Rheumatology criteria for the classification and reporting of osteoarthritis of the hip. Arthritis Rheum 34(5):505–514, 1991.
64. Zhang, W, et al: EULAR evidence-based recommendations for the diagnosis of knee osteoarthritis. Ann Rheum Dis 69(3):483–489, 2010.
65. Zhang, W, et al: EULAR evidence-based recommendations for the diagnosis of hand osteoarthritis: Report of a task force of ESCISIT. Ann Rheum Dis 68(1):8–17, 2009.

66. Iagnocco, A, and Naredo, E: Ultrasound of the osteoarthritis joint. Clin Exp Rheumatol 2017 Feb 10. [Epub ahead of print] PMID: 28229810.
67. Snijders, GF, et al: Fatigue in knee and hip osteoarthritis: the role of pain and physical function. Rheumatology (Oxford) 50(10):1894–1900, 2011.
68. Beasley, J: Therapist's evaluation and conservative management of arthritis of the upper extremity. In Skirven, TM, Osterman, AL, Fedorczyk, J, Amadio, PC, eds. Rehabilitation of the Hand and Upper Extremity, ed 6. Mosby, Philadelphia, PA, 2011, pp 1330–13436.
69. Haugen, IK: Hand osteoarthritis: current knowledge and new ideas. Scand J Rheumatol 45(suppl 128):58–63, 2016.
70. Ling, SM, and Rudolph, K. Osteoarthritis: In Bartlett, SJ, Bingham, CO, Maricic, MJ, Iversen, MD, and Ruffing, V (eds). Clinical Care Text in the Rheumatic Diseases, ed 3. Association of Rheumatology Health Professionals, American College of Rheumatology, Atlanta, GA, 2006, pp 127–134.
71. Cibulka, MT, et al: Hip pain and mobility deficits-hip osteoarthritis: Clinical practice guidelines linked to the International Classification of Functioning, Disability and Health from the Orthopaedic Section of the American Physical Therapy Association. J Orthop Sports Phys Ther 39(4):A1–A25, 2009.
72. Grimaldi, A, and Fearon, A: Gluteal tendinopathy: Integrating pathomechanics and clinical features in its management. J Orthop Sports Phys Ther 45(11):910–922, 2015.
73. Smith, TO, et al: Is there an increased risk of falls and fractures in people with early diagnosed hip and knee osteoarthritis? Data from the Osteoarthritis Initiative. Int J Rheum Dis 2016 May 6. doi: 10.1111/1756-185X.12871. [Epub ahead of print]
74. Iversen, MD, et al: Physical examination findings and their relationship with performance-based function in adults with knee osteoarthritis. BMC Musculoskelet Disord 17:273, 2016. doi: 10.1186/s12891-016-1151-3.
75. Kalichman, L, Hernandez-Molina, G: Midfoot and forefoot osteoarthritis. Foot 24:128–134, 2014.
76. Menz, HB, and Lord, SR: The contribution of foot problems to mobility impairment and falls in community-dwelling older people. J Am Geriatr Soc 49:1651–1656, 2001.
77. Laplante, BL, and DePalma MJ: Spine osteoarthritis. Phys Med Rehabil 4:S28–S36, 2012.
78. Hawker, GA, et al: All-cause mortality and serious cardiovascular events in people with hip and knee osteoarthritis: a population-based cohort study. PLoS One 9(3):e91286, 2014.
79. Guccione, AA, et al: The effects of specific medical conditions on the functional limitations of elders in the Framingham Study. Am J Publ Health 84:351–358, 1994.
80. Cross, M, et al: The global burden of hip and knee osteoarthritis: estimates from the global burden of disease 2010 study. Ann Rheum Dis 73(7):1323–1330, 2014.
81. Dreinhöfer, K, et al: ICF Core Sets for osteoarthritis. J Rehabil Med 44 Suppl:75–80, 2004.
82. Bossman, T, et al: Validation of the comprehensive ICF Core Set for osteoarthritis: The perspective of physical therapists. Physiotherapy 97(1):3–16, 2011.
83. Gignac, MA, et al: Examination of arthritis-related workplace activity limitations and intermittent disability over four and a half years and its relationship to job modifications and outcomes. Arthritis Care Res 63(7):953–962, 2011.
84. Singh, JA, et al: 2015 American College of Rheumatology guidelines for the treatment of rheumatoid arthritis. Arthritis Care Res 68:1–26, 2016. doi: 10.1002/acr.22783
85. Watson, DJ, et al: Gastrointestinal tolerability of the selective cyclooxygenase-2 (COX-2) inhibitor rofecoxib compared with nonselective COX-1 and COX-2 inhibitors in osteoarthritis. Arch Intern Med 160(19):2998–3003, 2000.
86. Solomon, DH, Schneeweiss, S, and Glynn, RJ: Relationship between selective cyclooxygenase inhibitors and acute myocardial infarction in older adults. Circulation 109(17):2068–2073, 2004.
87. Shaya, FT, et al: Selective cyclooxygenase inhibition and cardiovascular effects. Arch Intern Med 165(2):181–186, 2005. doi:10.1001/archinte.165.2.181.
88. Sowers, JR, et al: The effects of cyclooxygenase-2 inhibitors and nonsteroidal anti-inflammatory therapy on 24-hour blood pressure in patients with hypertension, osteoarthritis and type 2 diabetes mellitus. Arch Intern Med 2005;165(2):161–168, 2005.
89. Visser, K, and van der Heijde, D: Optimal dosage and route of administration of methotrexate in rheumatoid arthritis: a systematic review of the literature. Ann Rheum Dis 68:1094–1099, 2009.
90. Curtis, JR, and Singh, JA: The use of biologics in rheumatoid arthritis: Current and emerging paradigms of care. Clin Ther 33(6):679–707, 2011. doi: 10.1016/j.clinthera.2011.05.044.
91. Saag, KG, et al: Low dose long-term corticosteroid therapy in rheumatoid arthritis: an analysis of serious adverse events. Am J Med 96:115–123, 1994.
92. Hochberg, MC, et al: American College of Rheumatology 2012 recommendations for the use of nonpharmacologic and pharmacologic therapies in osteoarthritis of the hand, hip, and knee. Arthritis Care Res (Hoboken) 64(4):465–474, 2012.
93. American Society of Orthopaedic Surgeons: Treatment of osteoarthritis of the knee (non-arthroplasty), 2013. ed 2. Retrieved March 25, 2017, from www.aaos.org/research/guidelines/GuidelineOAKnee.asp.
94. McAlindon, TE, et al: OARSI guidelines for the non-surgical management of knee osteoarthritis. Osteoarthritis Cartilage 22:363–388, 2014.
95. Zhang, W, et al: OARSI recommendations for the management of hip and knee osteoarthritis, part II: OARSI evidence-based, expert consensus guidelines. Osteoarthritis Cartilage 16(2): 137–162, 2008.
96. Zhang, W, et al: OARSI recommendations for the management of hip and knee osteoarthritis part III: Changes in evidence following systematic cumulative update of research published through January 2009. Osteoarthr Cartil 18(4):476–499, 2010.
97. Fernandes, L, et al: EULAR recommendations for the non-pharmacological core management of hip and knee osteoarthritis. Ann Rheum Dis 72(7):1125–1135, 2013.
98. Towheed, T, et al: Acetaminophen for osteoarthritis. Cochrane Database Syst Rev 1, 2006. Art. No.: CD004257. doi: 10.1002/14651858.CD004257.pub2.
99. Da Costa, BR, et al: Effectiveness of non-steroidal anti-inflammatory drugs for the treatment of pain in knee and hip osteoarthritis: a network meta-analysis. Lancet 387(10033): 209302105, 2016.
100. Tieppo Francio, V, et al: Oral versus topical diclofenac sodium in the treatment of osteoarthritis. J Pain Palliat Care Pharmacother 1–8, 2017. doi: 10.1080/15360288.2017.1301616. [Epub ahead of print]
101. Iversen, MD, Hammond, A, and Betteridge, N: Self-management of rheumatic diseases—state of the art and future perspectives. Ann Rheum Dis 69(6):955–964, 2010. doi: 10.1136/ard.2010.129270.
102. American College of Rheumatology Ad Hoc Committee on Clinical Guidelines: Guidelines for the initial evaluation of the adult patient with acute musculoskeletal symptoms. Arthritis Rheum 39(1):1–8, 1996. doi: 10.1002/art.1780390102.
103. Norkin, CC, and White, DJ: Measurement of joint motion: A guide to goniometry. ed 5. F.A. Davis Company, Philadelphia, PA, 2016.
104. Brenton-Rule, A, et al: Foot and ankle characteristics associated with falls in adults with established rheumatoid arthritis: a cross-sectional study. BMC Musculoskelet Disord 17:22, 2016. doi: 10.1186/s12891-016-0888-z.
105. Grabiner, MD, et al: Kinematics of recovery from a stumble. J Gerontol 48(3):M97–102, 1993.
106. Jesevar, DS, et al: Knee kinematics and kinetics during locomotor activities of daily living in subjects with knee arthroplasty and in healthy controls. Phys Ther 73(4):229–239, 1993.
107. Creamer, P, Lethbridge-Cejku, M, and Hochberg, MC: Factors associated with functional impairment in symptomatic knee osteoarthritis. Rheumatology (Oxford) 39(5):490–496, 2000.
108. Bielefield, T, and Neumann, DA: The unstable metacarpophalangeal joint in rheumatoid arthritis: anatomy, pathomechanics, and physical rehabilitation considerations. Curr Opin Rheumatol 24(2):215–221, 2012. doi: 10.1097/BOR.0b013e3283503361.
109. Porter, BJ, and Brittain, A: Splinting and hand exercise for three common hand deformities in rheumatoid arthritis: a clinical perspective. Curr Opin Rheumatol 24(2):215–221, 2012. doi: 10.1097/BOR.0b013e3283503361.

110. Meenan, RF, et al. AIMS2: the content and properties of a revised and expanded Arthritis Impact Measurement Scales health status questionnaire. Arthritis Rheum 35:1–10, 1992.
111. Ren, XS, Kazis, L, and Meenan, RF: Short-form Arthritis Impact Measurement Scales 2: Tests of reliability and validity among patients with osteoarthritis. Arthritis Care Res 12(3):163–171, 1999.
112. Aletaha, D, et al: Acute phase reactants add little to composite disease activity indices for rheumatoid arthritis: validation of a clinical activity score. Arthritis Res Ther 7:R796–R806, 2005.
113. Curtis, JR, et al: Determining the minimally important difference in the clinical disease activity index for improvement and worsening in early rheumatoid arthritis. Arthritis Care Res (Hoboken) 67(10):1345–1353, 2015. doi: 10.1002/acr.22606.
114. Van der Heijde, DM, et al: Judging disease activity in clinical practice in rheumatoid arthritis: first step in the development of a disease activity score. Ann Rheum Dis 49(11):916–920, 1990.
115. Prevoo, ML, et al: Modified disease activity scores that include twenty-eight–joint counts: development and validation in a prospective longitudinal study of patients with rheumatoid arthritis. Arthritis Rheum 38(1):44–48, 1995.
116. Fries, JF, et al: Measurement of patient outcome in arthritis. Arthritis Rheum 23(2):137–145, 1980.
117. Ward, MM, Guthrie, LC, and Alba, MI: Clinically important changes in individual and composite measures of rheumatoid arthritis activity: thresholds applicable in clinical trials. Ann Rheum Dis 74(9):1691–1696, 2015. doi: 10.1136/annrheumdis-2013-205079.
118. Pincus, T, Yazici, Y, and Bergman, M: Development of a Multidimensional Health Assessment Questionnaire (MDHAQ) for the infrastructure of standard clinical care. Clin Exp Rheumatol 23(Suppl): S19–28, 2005.
119. Maksa L, Anderson J, Michaud K. Measures of functional status and quality of life in rheumatoid arthritis: Health Assessment Questionnaire Disability Index (HAQ), Modified Health Assessment Questionnaire (MHAQ), Multidimensional Health Assessment Questionnaire (MDHAQ), Health Assessment Questionnaire II (HAQ-II), Improved Health Assessment Questionnaire (Improved HAQ), and Rheumatoid Arthritis Quality of Life (RAQoL). Arthritis Care Res (Hoboken) 2011; 63(S11): S4–S13. DOI: 10.1002/acr.20620.
120. Wolfe, F, Michaud, K, and Pincus, T: A composite disease activity scale for clinical practice, observational studies, and clinical trials: The Patient Activity Scale (PAS/PAS-II). J Rheumatol 32:2410–2415, 2005. [PubMed: 16331773]
121. Anderson, J, et al: Rheumatoid Arthritis Disease Activity Measures: American College of Rheumatology Recommendations for Use in Clinical Practice. Arthritis Care Res (Hoboken) 64(5): 640–647, 2012. doi: 10.1002/acr.21649.
122. Hays, RD, et al: Responsiveness and minimally important difference for the Patient-Reported Outcomes Measurement Information System (PROMIS) 20-item physical functioning short form in a prospective observational study of rheumatoid arthritis. Ann Rheum Dis 74:104–107, 2015.
123. Oude Voshaar, MA, et al. Relative performance of commonly used physical function questionnaires in rheumatoid arthritis and a patient-reported outcomes measurement information system computerized adaptive test. Arthritis Care Res (Hoboken) 66:2900–2908, 2014.
124. Bartlett, SJ, et al: How well do generic patient reported outcomes measurement information system instruments capture health status in rheumatoid arthritis? Arthritis Rheum 65(10 Suppl): S972–S973, 2013.
125. Pincus, T, et al: RAPID3 (Routine Assessment of Patient Index Data 3), a rheumatoid arthritis index without formal joint counts for routine care: proposed severity categories compared to Disease Activity Score and Clinical Disease Activity Index categories. J Rheumatol 35:2136–2147, 2008. [PubMed: 18793006].
126. Smolen, JS, et al: A Simplified Disease Activity Index for rheumatoid arthritis for use in clinical practice. Rheumatology (Oxford) 42:244 –257, 2003.
127. Lassere, MN, et al: Reliability of measures of disease activity and disease damage in rheumatoid arthritis: implications for smallest detectable difference, minimal clinically important difference, and analysis of treatment effects in randomized controlled trials. J Rheumatol 28:892–903, 2001.
128. Hudak, P, et al: Development of an upper extremity outcome measure: The DASH (Disabilities of the Arm, Shoulder, and Hand). Am J Industrial Med 29:602–608, 1996.
129. Klassbo, M, Larsson, E, and Mannevik, E. Hip disability and osteoarthritis outcome score. An extension of the Western Ontario and McMaster Universities Osteoarthritis Index. Scand J Rheumatol 32(1):46–51, 2003.
130. Rolfson, O, et al: Defining an international standard set of outcome measures for patients with hip or knee osteoarthritis: Consensus of the International Consortium for Health Outcomes Measurement Hip and Knee Osteoarthritis Working Group. Arthritis Care Res (Hoboken) 68(11):1631–1639, 2016.
131. Roos, EM, et al: Knee Injury and Osteoarthritis Outcome Score (KOOS)—development of a self-administered outcome measure. J Orthop Sports Phys Ther 28:88–96, 1998.
132. Binkley, JM, et al: The lower extremity functional scale (LEFS): scale development, measurement properties, and clinical application. Phys Ther 79:371–383, 1999.
133. Fairbank, JCT, and Pynsent PB: The Oswestry Disability Index. Spine 25 (22):2940–2953, 2000.
134. Stratford, P, et al: Assessing disability and change on individual patients: a report of a patient specific measure. Physiotherapy Canada 47:258–263, 1995.
135. Katz, P: Patient outcomes in rheumatology, 2011. Arthritis Care Res 63(S11): S1–S490, 2011.
136. Dobson, F, et al: OARSI recommended performance-based tests to assess physical function in people diagnosed with hip or knee osteoarthritis. Osteoarthritis and Cartilage 21(8):1042–1052, 2013.
137. Brostrom, EW, et al: Gait deviations in individuals with inflammatory joint diseases and osteoarthritis and the usage of three-dimensional gait analysis. Best Practice Res Clinical Rheumatol 26(3):409–422, 2012.
138. Parker, JC, Wright, GE, and Smarr, KL: Psychological assessment. In Bartlett, SJ, Bingham, CO, Maricic, MJ, Iversen, MD, Ruffing, V (eds). Clinical Care Text in the Rheumatic Diseases, ed 3. Association of Rheumatology Health Professionals, American College of Rheumatology, Atlanta, GA, pp 67–72, 2006.
139. Marks, R: Comorbid depression and anxiety impact hip osteoarthritis disability. Disabil Health J 2(1):27–35, 2009. doi: 10.1016/j.dhjo.2008.10.001.
140. Keefe, FJ, Somers, TJ, and Martire, LM: Psychologic interventions and lifestyle modifications for arthritis pain management. Rheum Dis Clin North Am. 2008;34(2):351–368. doi: 10.1016/j.rdc.2008.03.001.
141. Brady, TJ, et al: A meta-analysis of health status, health behaviors, and healthcare utilization outcomes of the Chronic Disease Self-Management Program. Prev Chronic Dis e10, 2013. doi:10.5888/pcd10.120112.
142. Verstappen, SM: Rheumatoid arthritis and work: The impact of rheumatoid arthritis on absenteeism and presenteeism. Best Pract Res Clin Rheumatol 29(3):495–511, 2015. doi: 10.1016/j.berh.2015.06.001.
143. Stucki, G, et al: ICF Core Sets for rheumatoid arthritis. J Rehabil Med 44(Suppl):87–93, 2004. doi: 10.1080/16501960410015470.
144. Gebhardt, C, et al: Validation of the comprehensive ICF Core Set for rheumatoid arthritis: The perspective of physicians. J Rehabil Med 42(8):780–788, 2001. doi: 10.2340/16501977-0599.
145. Coenen, M, et al: Validation of the International Classification of Functioning, Disability and Health (ICF) Core Set for rheumatoid arthritis from the patient perspective using focus groups. Arthritis Res The. 8(4):R84, 2006. doi:10.1186/ar1956.
146. Ottawa Panel: Ottawa Panel evidence-based clinical practice guidelines for electrotherapy and thermotherapy interventions in the management of rheumatoid arthritis in adults. Phys Ther 84(11):1016–1043, 2004.
147. Zeng, C, et al: Effectiveness of continuous and pulsed ultrasound for the management of knee osteoarthritis: a systematic review and network meta-analysis. Osteoarthritis Cartilage 22(8), 1090–1099, 2014.
148. Casimiro, L, et al: Therapeutic ultrasound for the treatment of rheumatoid arthritis. Cochrane Database Syst Rev 3, 2002. CD003787. doi: 10.1002/14651858.CD003787.

149. Oosterveld, F, and Rasker, JJ: Effects of local heat and cold treatment on surface and articular temperature of arthritic knees. Arthitis Rheum 37(11):1578–1582, 1994.
150. Breger Stanton, DE, Lazaro, R, and MacDermid, JC: A systematic review of the effectiveness of contrast baths. J Hand Ther 22(1):57–69, 2009.
151. Rutjes, AWS, et al: Transcutaneous electrostimulation for osteoarthritis of the knee. Cochrane Database Syst Rev 7(4): CD002823, 2009. doi: 10.1002/14651858.CD002823.pub2.
152. Zeng, C, et al: Electrical stimulation for pain relief in knee osteoarthritis: systematic review and network meta-analysis. Osteoarthritis Cartilage 23(2):189–202, 2015.
153. Johnsson, PM, and Eberhardt, K: Hand deformities are important signs of disease severity in patients with early rheumatoid arthritis. Rheumatology 48:1398–1401, 2009.
154. Adams, J, et al: The clinical effectiveness of static resting splints in early rheumatoid arthritis: a randomized controlled trial. Rheumatology 47:1548–1553, 2008.
155. Fess, EE, and Philips, CA: Hand Splinting: Principles and Methods, ed 2. Mosby Inc., St Louis, MO, 1987.
156. Silva, AC, et al: Effectiveness of a night-time hand positioning splint in rheumatoid arthritis: a randomized controlled trial. J Rehabil Med 40:749–754, 2008.
157. Mary Pack Arthritis Program: Best practice recommendations for management of ulnar drift deformity in rheumatoid arthritis. 2011. Retrieved March 20, 2016, from: http://mpap.vch.ca/wp-content/uploads/sites/16/2014/08/Best-Practise-Recommendations-for-Management-of-Ulnar-Drift-Deformity-in-Rheumatoid-Arthritis.pdf
158. Egan, M, et al: Splints and orthosis for treating rheumatoid arthritis. Cochrane Database Syst Rev 1:CD004018, 2003. doi: 10.1002/14651858.CD004018.
159. Pagnotta, A, et al: The effect of a static wrist orthosis on hand function in individuals with rheumatoid arthritis. J Rheumatol 25(5):879–885, 1998.
160. Kjeken, I, et al: Systematic review of design and effects of splints and exercise programs in hand osteoarthritis. Arthritis Care Res (Hoboken) 63(6):834–848, 2011. doi: 10.1002/acr.20427.
161. Duivenvoorden, T, et al: Braces and orthoses for treating osteoarthritis of the knee. Cochrane Database Syst Rev 16(3): CD004020, 2015.
162. van Jonbergen, HPW, Poolman, RW, and van Kampen, A: Isolated patellofemoral osteoarthritis: A systematic review of treatment options using the GRADE approach. Acta Orthop 81(2):199–205, 2010.
163. Raja, K, and Dewan, N: Efficacy of knee braces and foot orthoses in conservative management of knee osteoarthritis: A systematic review. Am J Phys Med Rehabil 90(3):247–252, 2011. doi: 10.1097/PHM.0b013e318206386b.
164. Westby, M, and Minor, M: Exercise and physical activity. In Bartlett, SJ, Bingham, CO, Maricic, MJ, Iversen, MD, Ruffing, V (eds). Clinical Care Text in the Rheumatic Diseases, ed 3. Association of Rheumatology Health Professionals, American College of Rheumatology, Atlanta, GA, 2006, pp 211–220.
165. Kisner, C, and Colby LA: Therapeutic Exercise. Foundations and Techniques, ed 6. F.A. Davis, Philadelphia, PA, 2013.
166. Salamh, P, et al: Treatment effectiveness and fidelity of manual therapy to the knee: A systematic review and meta-analysis. Musculoskeletal Care 2016. doi: 10.1002/msc.1166. [Epub ahead of print]
167. Perandini, LA, et al: Exercise as a therapeutic tool to counteract inflammation and clinical symptoms in autoimmune rheumatic diseases. Autoimm Rev 12:218–224, 2012.
168. James, MJ, et al: Effect of exercise on 99mTc-DPTA clearance from knees with effusions. J Rheumatol 21(3):501–504, 1994.
169. Krebs, DE, et al: Exercise and gait effects on in vivo hip contact pressures. Phys Ther 71(4):301–309, 1991.
170. Jawed, S, Gaffney, K, and Blake, DR: Intra-articular pressure profile of the knee joint in a spectrum of inflammatory arthropathies. Ann Rheum Dis 56(11):686–689, 1997.
171. Swärdh, E, and Brodin N: Effects of aerobic and muscle strengthening exercise in adults with rheumatoid arthritis: a narrative review summarising a chapter in physical activity in the prevention and treatment of disease. Br J Sports Med 50:362–367, 2016.
172. Hammond, A, and Prior, Y: The effectiveness of home hand exercise programmes in rheumatoid arthritis: a systematic review. Br Med Bull 119(1):49–62, 2016.
173. Bergstra, SA, et al: A systematic review into the effectiveness of hand exercise therapy in the treatment of rheumatoid arthritis. Clin Rheumatol 33:1539–1548, 2014. doi:10.1007/s10067-014-2691-2.
174. Baillet, A, et al: Efficacy of resistance exercises in rheumatoid arthritis: Meta-analysis of randomized controlled trials. Rheumatology (Oxford) 51(3):519–527, 2012. doi:10.1093/rheumatology/ker330.
175. Hurkmans, E, et al: Dynamic exercise programs (aerobic capacity and/or muscle strength training) in patients with rheumatoid arthritis. Cochrane Database Syst Rev 4, 2009. Art. No.: CD006853. doi: 10.1002/14651858.CD006853.pub2.
176. Cairns, AP, and McVeigh, JG: A systematic review of the effects of dynamic exercise in rheumatoid arthritis. Rheumatol Int 30(2):147–158, 2009. doi: 10.1007/s00296-009-1090-1095.
177. Gaudin, P, et al: Is dynamic exercise beneficial in patients with rheumatoid arthritis? Joint Bone Spine 75(1):11–17, 2008.
178. Han, A, et al: Tai Chi for treating rheumatoid arthritis (Cochrane review) [with consumer summary]. Cochrane Database Syst Rev 3, 2004. doi: 10.1002/14651858.CD004849.
179. Lee, MS, Pittler, MH, and Earnest E: Tai chi for rheumatoid arthritis: systematic review. Rheumatology 46:1648–1651, 2007. doi:10.1093/rheumatology/kem151.
180. Williams, SB, et al: Feasibility and outcomes of a home-based exercise program on improving balance and gait stability in women with lower-limb osteoarthritis or rheumatoid arthritis: A pilot study. Arch Phys Med Rehabil 91(1):106–114, 2010.
181. Brosseau, L, et al: The Ottawa panel clinical practice guidelines for the management of knee osteoarthritis. Part one: Introduction, and mind-body exercise programs. Clin Rehabil 31(5): 582–595, 2017. doi: 10.1177/0269215517691083. [Epub ahead of print]
182. Brosseau, L, et al. The Ottawa panel clinical practice guidelines for the management of knee osteoarthritis. Part two: strengthening exercise programs. Clin Rehabil 31(5):596–611, 2017.
183. Brosseau, L, et al. The Ottawa panel clinical practice guidelines for the management of knee osteoarthritis. Part three: aerobic exercise programs. Clin Rehabil 31(5):612–624, 2017.
184. Fransen, M, et al: Exercise for osteoarthritis of the knee. Cochrane Database Syst Rev 1:CD004376, 2015.
185. Brosseau L, et al: Ottawa panel evidence-based clinical practice guidelines for therapeutic exercise in the management of hip osteoarthritis. Clin Rehabil 30(10):935–946, 2016.
186. Fransen, M, et al: Exercise for osteoarthritis of the hip. Cochrane Database Syst Rev (4):CD007912, 2014.
187. Pisters, MF, et al: Long-term effectiveness of exercise therapy in patients with osteoarthritis of the hip or knee: a systematic review. Arthritis Rheum 57(7):1245–1253, 2007.
188. Bartels, EM, et al: Aquatic exercise for the treatment of knee and hip osteoarthritis. Cochrane Database Syst Rev 3:CD005523, 2016.
189. Nicolson, PJ, et al: Interventions to increase adherence to therapeutic exercise in older adults with low back pain and/or hip/knee osteoarthritis: A systematic review and meta-analysis. Br J Sports Med 2017. doi: 10.1136/bjsports-2016-096458. [Epub ahead of print]
190. Westby, MD: A health professional's guide to exercise prescription for people with arthritis: A review of aerobic fitness activities. Arthritis Rheum 45(6):501–511, 2001.
191. Iversen, MD, et al: Correlates of physical activity participation over 3 years in adults with rheumatoid arthritis. Arthritis Care Res 18, 2016. doi: 10.1002/acr.23156.
192. Office of Disease Prevention and Health Promotion (ODPHP): Translating scientific evidence about total amount and intensity of physical activity into guidelines, 2008. Retrieved April 22, 2016, from: http://health.gov/paguidelines/guidelines/appendix1.aspx.
193. Lee, J, et al: Public health impact of risk factors for physical inactivity in adults with rheumatoid arthritis. Arthritis Care Res (Hoboken) 64(4):488–493, 2012.
194. Lee, J, et al: Sedentary behaviour and physical function: Objective evidence from the Osteoarthritis Initiative. Arthritis Care Res (Hoboken) 67(3):366–373, 2015.

195. Dimonte, P, and Light, H: Pathomechanics, gait deviations, and treatment of the rheumatoid foot. Phys Ther 62(8):1148–1156, 1982.
196. Middleton, A, Fritz, SL, and Lusardi, M: Walking speed: the functional vital sign. J Aging Phys Act 23(2):314–322, 2015. doi: 10.1123/japa.2013-0236.
197. Schnitzer, TJ, et al: Effect of piroxicam on gait in patients with osteoarthritis of the knee. Arthritis Rheum 36(9):1207–1213, 1993.
198. Silva, KN, et al: Balance training (proprioceptive training) for patients with rheumatoid arthritis. Cochrane Database Syst Rev (5): CD007648, 2010. doi: 10.1002/14651858.CD007648.pub2. 01.
199. Stamm, T, et al: Joint protection and home hand exercises improve hand function in patients with hand osteoarthritis: A randomized control trial. Arthritis Rheum 47(1):44–49, 2002.
200. Clark, A, et al. A critical review of foot orthoses in the rheumatoid arthritic foot. Rheumatology (Oxford) 45(2):139–145, 2006. doi: https://doi.org/10.1093/rheumatology/kei177.
201. Fransen, M, and Edmonds J: Off-the-shelf footwear for people with rheumatoid arthritis. Arthritis Care Res 10(4):250–256, 1997.
202. Wagner, A, and Luna, S: Effect of footwear on joint pain and function in older adults with lower extremity osteoarthritis. J Geriatr Phys Ther 2016. doi: 10.1519/JPT.0000000000000108.
203. Marks, R, Allegrante, JP, and Lorig, K: A review and synthesis of research evidence for self-efficacy-enhancing interventions for reducing chronic disability: Implications for health education practice (part II). Health Promot Pract 6(2):148–156, 2005.

appendix

23.A Joint Protection, Rest, and Energy Conservation

JOINT PROTECTION

Why Is Joint Protection Important?

Overuse and abuse of arthritic joints may lead to progressive deterioration of the joint and its surrounding tissues. Positive action is necessary to protect joints, conserve energy, and preserve function.

During activity, a normal joint is protected by the muscles around it that absorb the forces on the joint, preventing undue strain on the tendons, ligaments, and cartilage. A diseased joint is mechanically weak and poorly stabilized, which can contribute to the overstretching of the tendons and ligaments and damage to the cartilage. This increased stress can increase the destruction of the joint and cause increased pain.

How Can Joints Be Protected?

The main idea in joint protection is to minimize the strain on joints in daily activities. Joint protection techniques try to reduce the force on the joint, to slow down the joint damage. Good posture and positioning, changing the method of an activity, and pacing all help to protect the joint.

Which Joints Need Protection?

People with a local type of arthritis, such as osteoarthritis, need to pay close attention to the joints that are involved with the arthritis. People with a systemic or whole-body type of arthritis, such as rheumatoid arthritis, need to reduce the stress on all their joints. In addition to the joint protection principles and examples listed below, people with rheumatoid arthritis should look at the section that follows titled, "Additional Reminders for Protection of the Rheumatoid Hand."

In planning your joint protection, start by concentrating on the joints that are currently giving the most trouble. Check off the principles that apply most strongly to you and list several examples of how you can apply that principle to your problem joints.

Joint Protection Principles	Your Examples
☐ 1. Respect Pain.	
It is important to distinguish between discomfort and pain.	________
Pain that lasts for more than 1 to 2 hr after an activity indicates that the activity is too stressful and needs to be modified.	________
If there is a sharp increase in pain during activity, stop and rest, then modify the activity.	________
If there is unusual pain or stiffness the next day, look back at the previous day's activities to see if they were too strenuous.	________
☐ 2. Avoid Positions of Deformity.	
The foremost position of deformity for most joints is flexion, bending of the joint.	
Maintaining a bent position increases the possibility of deformity.	
Stand erect, with weight evenly divided on both feet.	________
Lay as flat as possible in bed; do not curl up or prop yourself up on several pillows.	________
Work with your hands flat.	________
Avoid tight grip or squeezing.	________
☐ 3. Avoid Awkward Positions.	
Use each joint in its most stable and functional position. Extra strain is placed on a joint when it is twisted or rotated.	
Rise straight up from sitting, rather than leaning to one side for support.	________
Reposition feet rather than twisting trunk or knees.	________
Stand on a stool to reach overhead.	________
Reposition yourself closer to object rather than stretch your reach.	________
Sit to clean or garden, rather than squatting or kneeling down.	________
Use good posture when you stand, sit, and lie down.	________

Joint Protection Principles	Your Examples
☐ 4. Use Strongest Joints or Distribute the Force over Several Joints.	
The stress on each individual joint is less if it is divided over several joints. The larger joints have greater muscles surrounding them to absorb the stress.	
Use two hands whenever possible.	________
Carry packages in both arms rather than in one.	________
Carry a shoulder purse or purse handle over forearm rather than in fingers.	________
Use knapsack to carry packages on back.	________
Lift objects from underneath, using wrist and elbow, rather than pinch gripping the sides.	________
Lift objects with your knees bent, and your back straight.	________
Move large objects with body weight behind it, the push coming from the legs.	________
Push with open palm or forearm rather than fingers.	________
☐ 5. Use Adapted Equipment.	
Find equipment that will reduce the stress on the joint or make the job easier.	
The Self-Help Manual for People with Arthritis is a catalog of adapted equipment available from the local Arthritis Foundation.	________
Equipment can be modified by:	
Building up the handle so it is easier to grasp.	________
Extending the handle so it is easier to reach.	________
Equipment available:	
Walking aids	
Self-care aids	
Bathroom safety	
Homemaking equipment	
Job modification equipment	
Joints that need protection:	________
Activities to be modified:_____	
________	
________	
________	

■ ADDITIONAL REMINDERS FOR THE PROTECTION OF THE RHEUMATOID HAND

1. Maintain wrist extension (ability to pick hand up off table) through exercise to ensure power grip.
2. Maintain supination (ability to turn palm up) through exercise to ensure ability to hold and to carry objects.
3. Avoid positions of deformity.
   a. Finger flexion
      1. Avoid making fist or tight grip—use built-up handles.
      2. Work with hand flat—use dust mitts, sponges.
      3. Avoid prolonged holding of objects: pen, book, pan, and needle.
      4. Avoid putting any pressure on bent knuckles.
   b. Ulnar deviation (tendency of fingers to slide to little finger side)
      1. Avoid pressure toward little finger side of hand.
      2. Any twisting of hand, open door knobs, jars, and so forth should be turned toward thumb.
      3. Grip objects parallel across palm, not diagonal; for example, hold utensil like dagger to cut food, stir with wooden spoon.
4. Avoid stress on small joints of hand.
   a. Use two hands whenever possible.
   b. Substitute larger stronger joints: for example, lift or carry with palms or forearm, not small finger joints; carry bag over elbow or shoulder, not in fingertips.
   c. Avoid activities involving pinching motions.
   d. Avoid twisting and squeezing motions with hands.

■ GETTING ADDITIONAL REST

Rest is important because it reduces the pain and fatigue that accompany arthritis. In addition, it aids the body's healing process and helps control the inflammation. Rest also may reduce the stress on joints and protect them from further damage. All of these benefits are important in managing arthritis.

Each day you need to make sure you get enough whole body rest, local joint rest, and emotional rest. There are many options: Mark off the options that may be possible for you.

☐ **1.** *Plenty of Nightly Rest*
Get the usual 8 to 10 hours of nightly rest. It is not as important that you sleep for that length of time, but make sure you stretch out with your joints supported, so that your body can rest.

☐ **2.** *Daily Rest Periods*
Ideally, several times a day you can stretch out for 15 to 60 minutes with your joints supported. Again, it is the body rest, not sleep, that is most important.

☐ **3.** *Five-Minute "Breathers"*
Partway through a task, sit back and take it easy for a few minutes. This will allow you to finish the task almost as quickly but more comfortably and with less fatigue.

☐ **4.** *Local Joint Rest*
When a joint hurts, stop and rest. If your hip or knee hurts while walking, sit down for a few minutes with your legs supported; if your hand hurts while writing, stop and lay it flat for a few minutes. Splints can be used to rest painful wrists or fingers. If your neck hurts, lay down with just a small pillow supporting the curve of your neck. Any painful joint can be given extra rest.

☐ **5.** *Take Time for Relaxing Activities*
Listening to music, reading, playing cards, or other light leisure activities all can be a pleasant change of pace and can be restful and refreshing for you. There are unlimited options for getting additional rest. It takes creativity to find ways to fit extra rest into your schedule; then it takes self-discipline to make sure you follow through, incorporating the additional rest in your activities. Making the effort to get more rest can pay off in a reduction of pain and fatigue.
Ways to get more rest: ____
Systemic, whole body rest
Local joint rest __________
Emotional rest __________

ENERGY CONSERVATION TO REDUCE FATIGUE

Why Is Energy Conservation Important?

One of the major symptoms of arthritis may be fatigue—getting tired very easily. In the inflammatory types of arthritis, fatigue may be part of the disease process. In all types of arthritis, pain and difficult movement may use up energy, so you tire more easily.

It is important to avoid getting overtired. Fatigue may increase the possibility of a flare-up in inflammatory types of arthritis such as rheumatoid arthritis. In all types of arthritis, fatigue may make the pain and stiffness seem worse, and it will make activities more difficult. We hope to reduce this fatigue by conserving energy and using it carefully.

How Can You Reduce Fatigue?

Some people try to conserve energy and reduce fatigue by staying in bed all day. Others stop doing anything that is not absolutely necessary each day. Unfortunately, the activities that are usually cut out are the leisure activities—the enjoyable things people do for themselves or for fun. These are not good ideas.

You can conserve energy and reduce fatigue by modifying and simplifying your activities, pacing yourself, getting additional rest, and using adapted equipment.

Energy Conservation

By conserving your energy, you may be able to do as much or more activity with less pain and fatigue. We are trying to avoid both overactivity and underactivity. Conserving your energy and simplifying your work is *not* being lazy. It is not sensible to overtire yourself. Overwork will not keep your joints mobile, but it may damage your joints further.

It is not so much *what* you do, but *how* you do it that can help control your fatigue. An attempt should be made to modify any activities that leave you overly tired or cause pain that continues for more than 1 to 2 hours.

You will need to identify ways that your own daily activities can be simplified. As you read through the energy conservation strategies, check off strategies that may work for you, and list several of your own examples.

☐ **1.** *Plan the Task.*
Your Examples
a. Think the task through. ____
b. Decide when and where the job is best done. ____
c. Plan out the simplest approach to the job. ____
d. Gather all supplies before you begin. ____
e. Arrange step sequence so that it moves in one direction (usually left to right). ____
f. Use fewer, more efficient movements to complete task. ____

☐ **2.** *Eliminate Extra Trips.*
a. Organize your shopping list according to how the store is laid out. ____
b. Stay in the laundry room until your laundry is finished. ____
c. Clean one area at a time. ____

☐ **3.** *Use Good Posture and Body Mechanics.*
   a. Sit to work; you will be more stable and use your strength more efficiently. ____
   b. Use large strong muscle groups, rather than straining individual muscles and joints. ____
   c. Lift with your knees bent, your back straight. ____
   d. Carry objects close to your body. ____
   e. Push objects, with body weight behind it, rather than pulling or carrying. ____
   f. Avoid awkward bending, reaching, and twisting. ____

☐ **4.** *Don't Fight Gravity.*
   a. Slide rather than lift objects. ____
   b. Use wheeled cart. ____
   c. Use lightweight equipment. ____
   d. Stabilize pitcher on surface and tilt to pour, rather than picking it up. ____

☐ **5.** *Pace Yourself.*
   a. Get plenty of nightly rest. ____
   b. Plan several rest periods during the day. ____
   c. Rest before you get tired. ____
   d. Avoid a rush. ____
   e. Work at a steady rate with rest period. ____
   f. Develop a rhythm to your movements. ____

☐ **6.** *Use Energy-Saving Devices.*
   a. Convenience foods. ____
   b. Adapted equipment. ____

Strategies to be tried:	Activities to be modified:
__________	__________
__________	__________
__________	__________

Excerpted from Brady, TJ: Home Management of Arthritis: Developing Your Own Plan. Arthritis Foundation, Minnesota Chapter, Minneapolis, 1983. Used by permission of the author.

appendix 23.B

Arthritis Foundation Patient Resources

Topic	Purpose of program and web tool	Link
Where does it hurt?	Diagram of the body with stars over common sites of pain. Patients can hover the cursor where they are hurting. A bubble pops up with a link for more information.	http://www.arthritis.org/about-arthritis/where-it-hurts/
Breaking the arthritis pain chain	This tool has links to walk a patient through arthritis pain, common causes, different types of pain, and effective treatments/professionals who can help.	http://www.arthritis.org/toolkits/arthritis-pain/
Better living toolkit	This "toolkit" provides four links that give patients access to research. Links include: learn about your disease, health tracker, set goals, and communicate with your doctor.	http://www.arthritis.org/toolkits/better-living/
Your coverage and care	This site explains the patient options for health care, their rights vis à vis Medicare/Affordable Care Act, and so forth, how to appeal denied claims, and resources to appeal those denied claims.	http://www.arthritis.org/toolkits/arthritis-coverage-claims/
Arthritis Resource Finder	The drop-down menu allows patients to choose between Arthritis Foundation events, health care professional resources, fitness programs and professionals, and community health care resources.	http://resourcefinder.arthritis.org/?_ga=1.226263582.508921375.1491376887
Ease of use	Provides information on products for persons with arthritis (health and wellness, home and hobbies, and work products)	http://www.arthritis.org/living-with-arthritis/tools-resources/ease-of-use/
Your local weather	Predict the weather's effect on joint pain by entering in your zip code.	http://www.arthritis.org/living-with-arthritis/tools-resources/weather/
Drug guide	Extensive list of medications for treating arthritis and details about side effects, adverse events, use, and dosage. Helpful for clinicians as well.	http://www.arthritis.org/living-with-arthritis/treatments/medication/drug-guide/
Arthritis support networks	Provides patient support networks	http://www.arthritis.org/arthritisintrospective/

Topic	Purpose of program and web tool	Link
Arthritis helpline	Information on how patients can set up a healthline.	http://blog.arthritis.org/news/arthritis-foundation-phone-helpline/?_ga=1.226263582.508921375.1491376887
Online community	Forum for persons with arthritis to talk about arthritis related topics	https://www.inspire.com/groups/arthritis-foundation/?ga=freshen
Your exercise solution	Exercise recommendations;also links to a mobile app	http://www.arthritis.org/living-with-arthritis/tools-resources/your-exercise-solution/
Walk with ease	Links to the Walk with Ease program	http://www.arthritis.org/living-with-arthritis/tools-resources/walk-with-ease/
Track and React	Links to a page where patients can discuss the Track and React program/app	http://www.arthritis.org/living-with-arthritis/tools-resources/track-and-react/
BMI calculator	Basic BMI calculator for patients to determine their BMI	http://www.arthritis.org/living-with-arthritis/tools-resources/bmi-calculator.php

appendix 23.C

Web-Based Resources for Clinicians, Families, and Patients with Arthritis

Association of Rheumatology Health Professionals (ARHP) (US)	www.rheumatology.org Clinical classification and response criteria: www.rheumatology.org/practice/clinical/classification/index.asp Guidelines for RA management: http://www.rheumatology.org/Practice-Quality/Clinical-Support/Clinical-Practice-Guidelines/Rheumatoid-Arthritis Guidelines for OA management: http://www.rheumatology.org/Practice-Quality/Clinical-Support/Clinical-Practice-Guidelines/Osteoarthritis Roles of Members of the Rheumatology Health Care Team http://www.rheumatology.org/I-Am-A/Patient-Caregiver/Health-Care-Team Health Professional Education (online courses) http://www.rheumatology.org/I-Am-A/Health-Professional/Health-Professional-Education
Arthritis Foundation (US)	www.arthritis.org Exercises for Arthritis: http://www.arthritis.org/living-with-arthritis/exercise/ Tools and Resources: http://www.arthritis.org/living-with-arthritis/tools-resources/ (includes a variety of exercise and fitness tools, links to online community and support networks, and daily living tools)
The Arthritis Society (Canada)	www.arthritis.ca Standardized Assessment of Joint Inflammation web tool: http://arthritis.ca/healthcare-professionals/standardized-assessment-of-joint-inflammation Living Well with Arthritis: http://arthritis.ca/manage-arthritis/living-well-with-arthritis (includes a range of tools on physical activity and exercise, nutrition, arthritis in the workplace and complementary therapies)
Arthritis Health Professions Association (AHPA) (Canada)	https://www.ahpa.ca/ (links to variety of clinical resources and online education for arthritis health professionals)
Mary Pack Arthritis Program (Canada)	www.mpap.vch.ca http://mpap.vch.ca/resources-for-professionals/assessment-tools-treatment-approaches/physical-therapy (includes best practice recommendations for common RA hand problems, assessment tools, and exercise programs)
Stanford Patient Education Resource Center (US)	http://patienteducation.stanford.edu/research/ (links to variety of self-reported measures of disease self-efficacy, self-management behaviors, and health status) Health Assessment Questionnaire-Disability Index: http://patienteducation.stanford.edu/research/haq20.html

Centers for Disease Control and Prevention (US)	CDC Arthritis Information https://www.cdc.gov/arthritis/ Physical Activity Basics https://www.cdc.gov/physicalactivity/basics/index.htm CDC-Recommended and Promising Programs https://www.cdc.gov/arthritis/interventions/index.htm
Osteoarthritis Research Society International (OARSI)	www.oarsi.org Guidelines for Managing OA: https://www.oarsi.org/education/oarsi-guidelines
The European Language Against Rheumatism (EULAR)	www.eular.org Recommendations for management of early RA http://ard.bmj.com/content/early/2017/03/31/annrheumdis-2016-210602 Non-pharmacological management of OA http://ard.bmj.com/content/72/7/1125
Orthopedic Scores	www.orthopaedicscore.com Commercial website containing orthopedic scores and scoring systems for all regions of the musculoskeletal system
Rehabilitation Measures Database	http://www.rehabmeasures.org/default.aspx A repository of outcome measures to screen and monitor patients with clinimetric information and links to the tools
RheumInfo (Canada)	http://rheuminfo.com/ Commercial website containing information and resources for patients and health professionals including screening, assessment, and counseling tools.

Chapter 24 Burns

R. Scott Ward, PT, PhD, FAPTA
Ingrid Parry, PT, MS
Reginald L. Richard, PT, MS

LEARNING OBJECTIVES

1. Describe the anatomy and physiology of the skin as an organ in the healthy state and damaged condition that occurs with a burn injury.
2. Discuss the pathology, symptoms, and sequelae of burn injuries.
3. Compare the treatment for various depths and extent of burn injury in relation to medical, surgical, and physical therapy management.
4. Identify the consequences of contracture formation after burn injury and the treatment of this condition.
5. Differentiate the options for management of hypertrophic scars.
6. Determine the type of skin care necessary after burn wound healing.
7. Design a physical therapy plan of care that appropriately incorporates positioning, splinting, and exercise.
8. Analyze and interpret patient data, formulate realistic goals and outcomes, and develop a plan of care when presented with a clinical case study.

CHAPTER OUTLINE

Burn injuries are one of the major health problems of the industrial world. In the United States, 450,000 to 500,000 burn injuries require medical treatment each year with an estimated 3,500 related deaths.[1] In addition, it has been estimated that burn injuries account for 40,000 hospitalizations per year, with about 30,000 patients being admitted to specialized burn treatment centers and the balance to other types of medical facilities.[1]

Although these data report the extent of the health care problem caused by burn injury, recent medical advances have significantly reduced the number of deaths from burn injuries and have improved the prognosis and functional abilities of surviving patients.[1-3] The survival rate has improved annually owing to improved resuscitation techniques, the acute medical and surgical care now practiced, and continued research into the management and care of the patient with burns. The American Burn Association (ABA) reported an overall survival rate of 96.8% from 2005 to 2014.[1] As a result of improvements in care, treatment, and survival of patients with burns, more physical therapists will become responsible for treating these patients for a significant portion of their rehabilitation in settings other than a hospital burn center (e.g., outpatient clinics, community hospitals).

This chapter introduces the clinical presentation of different depths of burn injury and the complications that can result from thermal destruction of the skin. Current techniques used in the medical, surgical, and rehabilitative management of the patient who has been burned will be described. For more in-depth information regarding the examination and treatment of the patient with a burn injury, the reader is referred to additional sources.[4-8]

EPIDEMIOLOGY OF BURN INJURIES

Although the morbidity and mortality rate of patients with burns has dramatically decreased in recent years, the epidemiology of burns remains basically the same.

The most common cause of burn injury in children 1 to 5 years of age is scalds from hot liquids.[9-12] Fires are the most common cause of burn injury in other age groups. Men are twice as likely as women to suffer a burn injury.[1,9] Fire and flame burns make up 43% of the admissions to burn centers, with scald injuries contributing 34% of admissions, then contact burns (9%), electrical injury (4%), chemical burns (3%), and a collection of other causes equaling 7%.[1] The majority of burn injuries occur in the home (73%), followed distantly by occupational sites (8%), motor vehicles (5%), and recreation/sport activities (5%), with 9% of injuries occurring in other settings.[1] The chances of dying of fire or smoke inhalation is about 1 in 1,442. The number of burn-related accidents has decreased, presumably because of better preventive measures, such as smoke detectors, education, and more stringent fire codes.[13]

A major reason for the improved prognosis and survival of patients with severe burn injury is the availability of specialized burn centers.[2] The advent of the burn center and the concentrated team care and focused research that has been generated by these facilities have improved the outcome of the most severely burned patient, as well as reduced the average hospital stay in most cases. The ABA[14] has established criteria for admission to a designated burn center as follows:

- Partial-thickness burns greater than 10% of total body surface area (TBSA)
- Burns that involve the face, hands, feet, genitalia, perineum, or major joints
- Third degree burns in any age group
- Electrical burns, including lightning injury
- Chemical burns
- Inhalation injury
- Burn injury in patients with preexisting illness that could complicate management, prolong recovery, or affect mortality.
- Burns and concomitant trauma (such as fractures) when the burn injury poses the greatest risk of morbidity or mortality. If the trauma poses the greater immediate risk, the patient's condition may be stabilized initially in a trauma center before transfer to a burn center. Physician judgment will be necessary in such situations and should be in concert with the regional medical control plan and triage protocols.
- Burns in children; children with burns should be transferred to a burn center verified to treat children. In the absence of a regional pediatric burn center, an adult burn center may serve as a second option for the management of pediatric burns.
- Burn injury in patients who will require special social, emotional, or rehabilitative intervention.

Thirty-five years ago, there were only 12 specialized burn centers in the United States. Today there are over 125 specialized centers for the care of patients with burn injuries and other skin disorders.[15] This accounts for approximately 1,700 beds. Burn centers can now undergo a process of verification (voluntary quality assurance review) through the ABA.[16] Currently, more than half of the burn centers in the United States are verified.

A burn center is staffed by specialists from multiple disciplines—physicians, nurses, physical therapists, occupational therapists, dietitians, psychiatrists, psychologists, social workers, child life therapists, chaplains, pharmacists, vocational rehabilitation specialists, and other support personnel—who direct their professional expertise toward the care, treatment, and rehabilitation of the patient with a burn injury. Each member is an integral part of the team, and the most effective burn centers are successful because of their team approach to the care of each patient.[2] It is historically noteworthy that burn personnel, with the founding and establishment of the ABA in 1967, initiated the interdisciplinary "team" approach to patient care.

SKIN ANATOMY AND BURN WOUND PATHOLOGY

The skin is the largest organ of the body, comprising approximately 15% of total body weight. Anatomically, the skin consists of two distinct layers of tissue: the *epidermis,* which is the outermost layer exposed to the environment, and the deeper layer, termed the *dermis* (subdivided into the *papillary* and *reticular* dermis).[17] Although not part of the skin per se, a third layer involved in the anatomical consideration of the skin is the subcutaneous fat cell layer directly under the dermis and above muscle fascial layers. These layers are illustrated in Figure 24.1.

The epidermis is avascular. Notwithstanding, it performs several vital functions. The *stratum corneum* gives the skin its waterproof characteristic and serves the role of protection from infection. The *stratum granulosum* is the layer responsible for water retention. The *stratum spinosum* adds a layer of protection to the underlying stratum basale layer. Cells in the *stratum basale* layer enable the epidermis to regenerate. This layer also contains

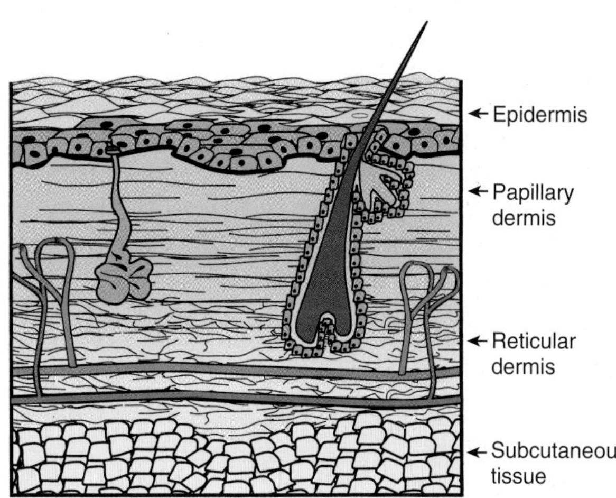

Figure 24.1 Cross section of skin.

melanocytes, the cells that determine skin pigmentation. The interface between the epidermis and the dermis is termed the *rete peg region*. This area consists of an extensive series of epidermal-dermal ridges and valleys that serve to increase the surface area between the epidermis and the dermis. These ridges act as a reservoir of skin and are needed to overcome frictional forces that skin is exposed to in daily activity. Lack of these ridges in the healed burn wound will result in blisters from abrasion and poor adherence of the new epidermal tissue when it comes in contact with clothing or other surfaces.

In earlier literature, the dermis is often referred to as the *corium* or "true skin," because it contains blood vessels, lymphatics, nerves, collagen, and elastic fibers. It also encloses the epidermal appendages (sweat ducts and sebaceous glands, and hair follicles), which provide a deep source of epidermal cells for wound healing. The dermis is 20 to 30 times thicker than the epidermis. It is composed primarily of interwoven collagen and elastic fibers, which provide the skin with its tensile strength and elasticity to resist deformation. The predominantly parallel orientation of normal collagen in the dermis is different from the whorls of collagen typically seen in scar tissue that result from burn injury.[18] The tiered location of sensory receptors in the skin is an important consideration in determining depth of burn injury (Table 24.1). The dermis is subdivided into two layers: the superficial *papillary* layer and the deep *reticular* layer.[17] The papillae of the papillary layer project upward and interlock with the epidermis. The papillae are vascular plexuses that serve, in part, to nourish the epidermis through osmosis. Morphologically, this layer is composed of a loose basket-weave network of collagen fibers. The reticular dermis lies below the papillary dermis and is composed of densely interwoven collagen fibers. The reticular dermis attaches to the subcutaneous tissue by an irregular interlacing network of fibrous connective tissue.

In addition to the functions mentioned already, the skin is important in temperature regulation through the emission of sweat and electrolytes, secretion of oils from the sebaceous glands to lubricate the skin, vitamin D synthesis, and contributes to cosmetic appearance and identity. As the result of a burn injury, some or all of these functions may be impaired and/or lost, and a patient's protective barrier defense mechanisms will be compromised.

One basic pathophysiological consideration in a burn injury is the alteration of vascular integrity, which results in the formation of edema in the interstitial spaces. Edema formation occurs in the area of burn as well as in adjacent tissues. An initial concern of the physical therapist on the burn team is a decrease in joint range of motion (ROM) due to swelling.

The amount of skin destruction is based on temperature and length of time the tissue is exposed to heat.[19] The type of insult (i.e., flame, liquid, chemical, or electrical) also will affect the amount of tissue destruction. A tremendous amount of heat is not required to cause damage. At temperatures below 111°F (44°C), local tissue damage will not occur unless the exposure is for prolonged periods. In the temperature range between 111°F and 124°F (44°C and 51°C), the rate of cellular death doubles with each degree rise in temperature, and short exposures will lead to cell destruction.[19,20] At temperatures higher than 124°F (51°C), exposure time needed to damage tissue is extremely brief.

Table 24.1 Sensory Receptors, Location by Layer of Skin, and Sensation Mediated

Sensory Receptor	Location	Sensation Mediated
Free nerve ending	Epidermis	Pain, itch
Free nerve ending	Dermis	Pain
Merkel's disks	Stratum spinosum	Touch
Meissner's corpuscle	Papillary dermis	Touch
Ruffini's corpuscle	Papillary dermis	Warmth
Krause's end bulb	Papillary dermis	Cold
Pacinian corpuscle	Reticular dermis	Pressure, vibration

CLASSIFICATIONS OF BURN INJURY

In the past, burn injury depth was categorized as *first, second,* and *third* degree. Although the lay public may use these classifications, most medical literature now classifies burn injuries by the depth of skin tissue destroyed (Table 24.2).[20] *The Guide to Physical Therapist Practice* includes classification of wounds based on etiology and depth of tissue destruction.[21] The depth to which a burn injury causes damage depends on many factors, including the duration and intensity of heat, skin thickness of area, the distance of the area from the source of heat, the extent (percentage) of body area exposed, vascularity, and age.

The different classifications of burn wounds will present different clinical pictures, and each can change dramatically during the course of treatment. In addition to the amount of direct tissue damage from a burn, a patient's metabolic, physiological, and psychological condition can greatly affect clinical status. This

Table 24.2 Burn Wound Classification: Differential Diagnosis

Depth of Burn	Color/Vascularity	Surface Appearance/Pain	Swelling/Healing/Scarring
Epidermal	Erythematous, pink or red; irritated dermis	No blisters, dry surface; delayed pain, tender	Minimal edema; spontaneous healing; no scars
Superficial partial-thickness	Bright pink or red, mottled red; inflamed dermis; erythematous with blanching and brisk capillary refill	Intact blisters, moist weeping, or glistening surface when blisters removed; very painful, sensitive to changes in temperature, exposure to air currents, light touch	Moderate edema; spontaneous healing; minimal scarring; discoloration
Deep partial-thickness	Mixed red, waxy white; blanching with slow capillary refill	Broken blisters, wet surface; sensitive to pressure but insensitive to light touch or soft pinprick	Marked edema; slow healing; excessive scarring
Full-thickness	White (ischemic), charred, tan, fawn, mahogany, black, red (hemoglobin fixation); no blanching; thrombosed vessels; poor distal circulation	Parchment-like, leathery, rigid, dry; anesthetic; body hairs pull out easily	Area depressed; heals with skin grafting; scarring
Subdermal	Charred	Subcutaneous tissue evident; anesthetic; muscle damage; neurological involvement	Tissue defects; heals with skin graft or flap; scarring

section presents general clinical signs and symptoms seen in each of the burn wound classifications (see Table 24.2).

Epidermal Burn

An epidermal burn, as the name implies, causes cell damage only to the epidermis (Fig. 24.2). The classic "sunburn" is the best example of an epidermal burn. Clinically, the skin appears red or erythematous.[22] The erythema is a result of epidermal damage and dermal irritation, but there is no injury to the dermal tissue. There is diffusion of inflammatory mediators from sites of epidermal damage and release of vasoactive substances from mast cells. The surface of an epidermal burn is dry. Blisters will be absent, but slight edema may be apparent. After an epidermal burn, there is usually a delay in the development of pain, at which point the area becomes tender to the touch. Following epidermal damage, the injured epidermal layers will peel off or desquamate in 3 to 4 days. Epidermal healing is spontaneous; that is, the skin will heal by itself, and no scar tissue will form.

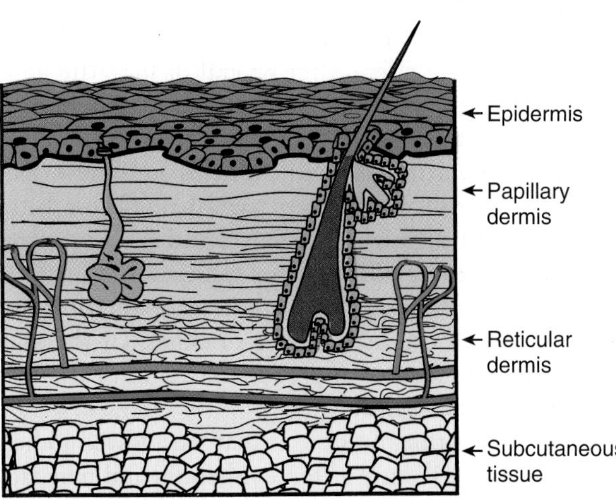

Figure 24.2 Red shading represents depth of skin involved in an epidermal burn.

Superficial Partial-Thickness Burn

With a superficial partial-thickness burn (Fig 24.3) damage occurs through the epidermis and into the papillary layer of the dermis. The epidermal layer is destroyed completely, but the papillary dermal layer sustains only mild to moderate damage. The most common sign of a superficial partial-thickness burn is the presence of intact blisters over the area that has been injured.

Although the internal environment of a blister is considered sterile, it has been shown that blister fluid contains substances that increase the inflammatory response and retard the healing process, and it is recommended that blisters be evacuated.[23-27] Healing will occur more rapidly if the damaged skin is removed and an appropriate topical

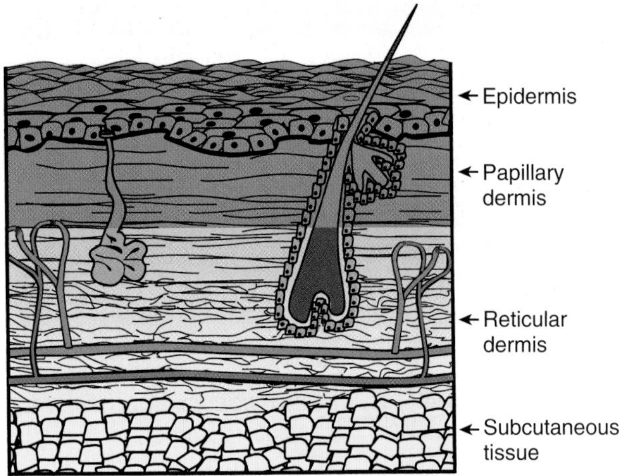

Figure 24.3 Red shading represents depth of skin involved in a superficial partial-thickness burn.

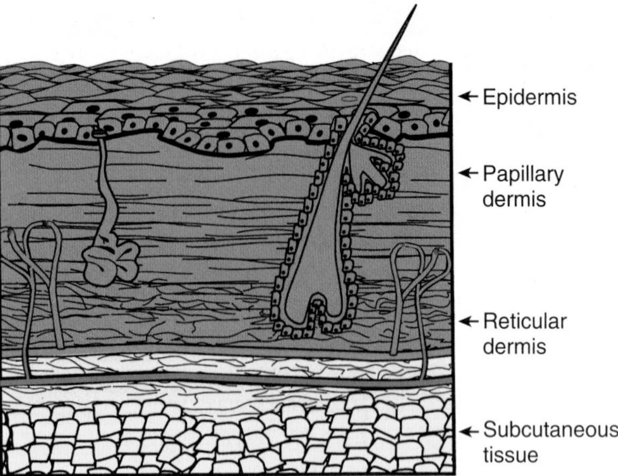

Figure 24.4 Red shading represents depth of skin involved in a deep partial-thickness burn.

agent and wound dressing applied.[28] Once blisters have been removed, the surface appearance of the burn area will be moist. The wound will be bright red because the dermis is inflamed. The wound will *blanch,* which means if pressure is exerted against the tissue with a finger, a white spot appears because of displacement of blood in the capillaries under pressure. On release of pressure, the white area will demonstrate brisk capillary refill. Edema can be moderate.

This type of burn is extremely painful secondary to irritation of the nerve endings contained in the dermis. When the wound is open, the patient will be highly sensitive to temperature changes, exposure to air, and light touch. In addition to pain, fever may be present if areas become infected.

Some topical antimicrobial creams will cause the wound to develop a gelatin-like film that eventually will peel off, similar to the *desquamation* that occurs with sunburn. This exudate is a coagulum of the topical antibiotic used to prevent infection and serum that seeps from the wound as a result of the insult to capillary integrity.

Superficial partial-thickness burns heal without surgical intervention, by means of epithelial cell production and migration from the wound's periphery and surviving skin appendages. Coverage by new epithelium resumes the barrier function of the skin, and complete healing should occur in 7 to 10 days. There may be some residual skin color change owing to destruction of melanocytes, but scarring is minimal.

Deep Partial-Thickness Burn

A *deep partial-thickness burn* (Fig. 24.4) involves destruction of the epidermis and papillary dermis with damage down into the reticular dermal layer. Although as mentioned below, as this burn nears the deepest dermis it begins to resemble a full-thickness burn. Most of the nerve endings, hair follicles, and sweat ducts will be injured because most of the dermis is destroyed.

Deep partial-thickness burns appear as a mixed red or waxy white color. The deeper the injury, the whiter it will appear. Capillary refill will be sluggish after the application of pressure on the wound. The surface usually is wet from broken blisters and alteration of the dermal vascular network, which leaks plasma fluid. Marked edema is a hallmark sign of this burn depth. There is a large amount of evaporative water loss (15 to 20 times normal) because of tissue and vascular destruction.[19,25,29] An area of deep partial-thickness burn has diminished sensation to light touch but retains the sense of deep pressure owing to the location of the Pacinian corpuscle deep in the reticular dermis. Healing occurs through scar formation and re-epithelialization. By definition, the dermis is only partially destroyed; therefore, some viable epidermal cells may remain within the surviving epidermal appendages and serve as a source for new skin growth.

The depth of a deep partial-thickness injury is sometimes difficult to determine, so allowing the wound to demarcate (between normal and damaged tissue) during the first few days is necessary. Demarcation becomes evident after several days as the dead tissue begins to slough. Hair follicles that penetrate the deeper dermal regions below the burn level remain viable. Preservation of hair follicles and new hair growth will indicate a deep partial-thickness burn rather than a full-thickness injury, and there is a corresponding greater potential for spontaneous healing. Factors that determine which epidermal structures survive and which die include the thickness of the skin in a particular location and/or the distance of the area from the source of heat.

Deep partial-thickness burns that are allowed to heal spontaneously will have a thin epithelium and may lack the usual number of sebaceous glands to keep the skin lubricated. New tissue usually appears dry and scaly, is itchy, and is easily abraded. Creams are necessary to artificially lubricate the new surface. Sensation and the number of active sweat ducts will be diminished.

A deep partial-thickness burn generally will heal in 3 to 5 weeks if it does not become infected. It is critical to keep the wound free of infection, because infection can convert a deep partial-thickness burn into a deeper injury. The development of *hypertrophic* and *keloid scars* is a frequent consequence of a deep partial-thickness burn.

Full-Thickness Burn

In a *full-thickness burn* (Fig. 24.5), all the epidermal and dermal layers are destroyed completely. In addition, the subcutaneous fat layer may be damaged to some extent.

A full-thickness burn is characterized by a hard, parchment-like eschar covering the area. *Eschar* is devitalized tissue consisting of desiccated coagulum of plasma and necrotic cells. Eschar feels dry, leathery, and rigid. The color of eschar can vary from black to deep red to white; the latter indicates total ischemia of the area. Frequently, thrombosis of superficial blood vessels is apparent and no blanching of the tissue is observed. The deep red color of the tissue results from hemoglobin fixation liberated from destroyed red blood cells.

Hair follicles are completely destroyed, so body hairs pull out easily. All nerve endings in the dermal tissue are destroyed so the wound will be *insensate* (without feeling); however, a patient still may experience a significant amount of pain owing to inflammation and because adjacent areas of partial-thickness burn usually surround a full-thickness injury.

A major problem that arises from deep burns is damage to the peripheral vascular system. Because large amounts of fluid leak into the interstitial space beneath unyielding eschar, the pressure in the extravascular space increases, potentially constricting the deep circulation to the point of occlusion (see later discussion of cardiovascular complications in the section titled Complications of Burn Injury). Because eschar does not have the elastic

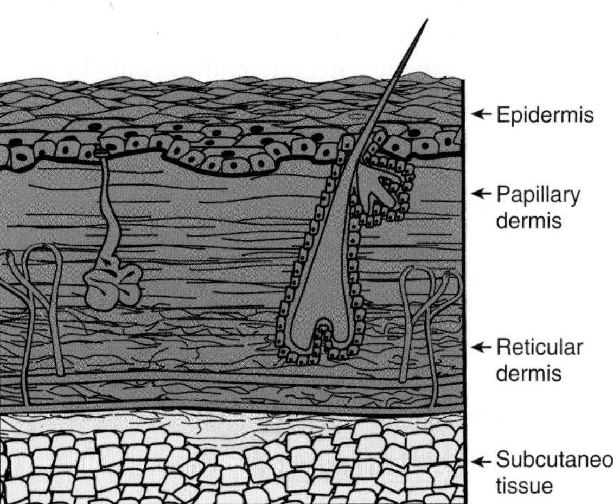

Figure 24.5 Red shading represents depth of skin involved in a full-thickness burn.

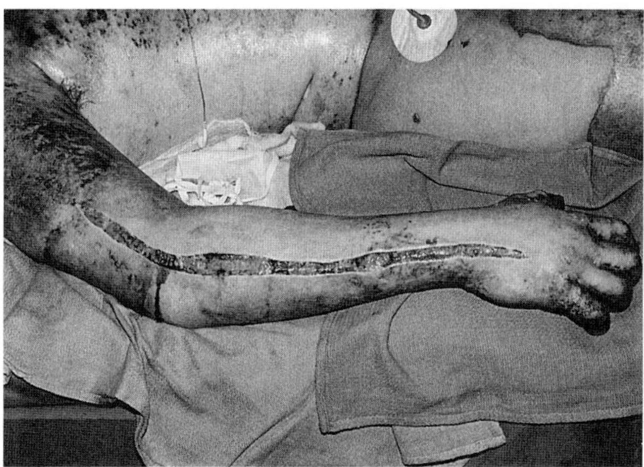

Figure 24.6 Escharotomy of the right upper extremity. *(From Richard and Staley,[4, p. 113] with permission.)*

quality of normal skin, edema that forms in an area of a circumferential burn can cause compression of the underlying vasculature. If this compression is not relieved, it may lead to eventual occlusion with possible necrosis of tissue distal to the site of injury. To maintain vascular flow, an *escharotomy* may be necessary. An escharotomy is a midline lateral incision of the eschar the length of an extremity or chest wall.[30,31] Figure 24.6 shows an escharotomy and the result of pressure that forces the incision to gap. Following an escharotomy, pulses are frequently examined to monitor restoration of circulation. If the escharotomy is successful, there will be an immediate improvement in the peripheral blood flow, demonstrated by normal pulses distal to the wound and by return of normal temperature and capillary refill of the distal extremity.

Although at times it may be difficult to differentiate a deep-partial from a full-thickness burn in the early postburn period, the differences will become evident after several days. With a full-thickness burn, there are no sites available for re-epithelialization of the wound. All epithelial cells have been destroyed, and skin grafting will be necessary. Grafting is discussed in detail in the section titled Surgical Management.

Subdermal Burn

An additional category of burn, the *subdermal burn,* involves complete destruction of all tissue from the epidermis down to and through the subcutaneous tissue (Fig. 24.7). Muscle and bone are subject to necrosis when burned. This type of burn occurs with prolonged contact with a heat source and routinely occurs as a result of contact with electricity. Extensive surgical and therapeutic management is necessary to return a patient to some degree of function.

■ ELECTRICAL BURN

The signs and symptoms of an *electrical burn* may vary according to the type of current, intensity of the current, and the area of the body the electric current passes

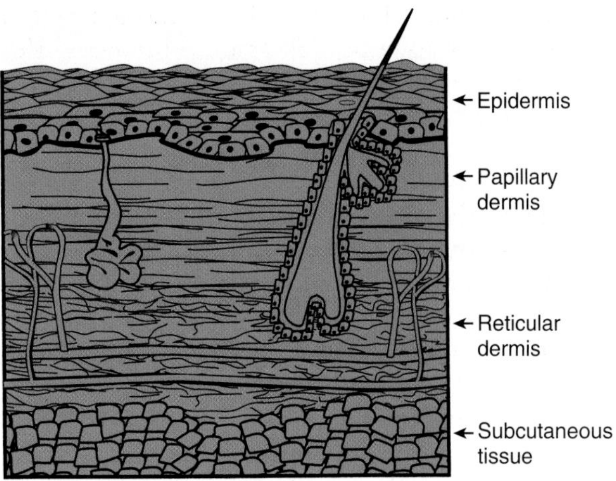

Figure 24.7 Red shading represents depth of skin involved in a subdermal burn.

through.[32] A burn results from the passage of an electric current through the body after the skin has made contact with an electrical source. Electric current follows the course of least resistance offered by various tissues. Nerves, followed by blood vessels, offer the least resistance. Bone offers the most resistance. Tissue damage results from tissue resistance to the passage of the current or by direct electrical current.[33,34]

Typically contact sites will exist where the patient first came into contact with the electricity and a second site where the patient was grounded. The wound where initial contact was made (sometimes referred to as the *entrance wound*) will appear charred and depressed, and many times, is smaller than the ground site. The skin appears yellow and ischemic. The ground site (sometimes referred to as the *exit wound*) often appears as though there was an explosion out of the tissue at the site. It is dry in appearance. Tissues along the pathway of the current may be damaged owing to heat that developed as a result of tissue resistance to current passage. An extremity or area that appears viable after an injury may become necrotic and gangrenous in a few days. Arteries may undergo spasm, and there may be necrosis of the vascular wall. The blood supply to the surrounding tissues, including muscle, may be altered. Damaged muscle will feel soft. Because the course of tissue destruction is unpredictable, there may be unequal and uneven muscle damage. Time will be required to determine which tissues will remain viable and which will not.

There can be other consequences of electricity passing through the body such as cardiac arrhythmias and acute renal failure secondary to fluid and electrolyte imbalances and release of myoglobin (protein present in muscle) into the blood. One of the most severe complications of electrical current damage is acute spinal cord damage or vertebral fracture. Clinically, these patients will have spastic paresis but may or may not have any sensory pathway changes over concomitant areas of spasticity. Possible causes of death from electrical burns are ventricular fibrillation and respiratory arrest.

Burn Wound Zones

A burn wound typically consists of three zones (Fig. 24.8).[20,35] In the *zone of coagulation* cells are irreversibly damaged and skin death occurs. This area is equivalent to a full-thickness burn and will require a skin graft to heal. Because of the lack of viable tissue and the amount of eschar, the risk of infection is increased. This potential complication emphasizes the need for careful monitoring, the use of antibiotics, and the treatment of a burned patient in a specialized burn center. The *zone of stasis* contains injured cells that may die within 24 to 48 hours without diligent treatment. This is the area where infection, drying, and/or inadequate perfusion of the wound will result in conversion of potentially salvageable tissue to completely necrotic tissue and enlargement of the zone of coagulation. Splints or compression bandages, if applied too tightly, can compromise the zone of stasis. Finally, the *zone of hyperemia* is a site of minimal cell damage, and the tissue should recover within several days with no lasting effects.[36]

Extent of Burned Area

A major consideration when determining the severity of a burn is the extent of body surfaced involved. The *Rule of Nines* was developed by Pulaski and Tennison[37] to rapidly calculate an estimate of the percentage of total body surface area burned and was formally published by Wallace in 1951.[38] The Rule of Nines divides the body surface into areas of 9%, or multiples of 9%, of the total body surface area (TBSA). Figure 24.9 shows the percentages using the Rule of Nines for adults and children. Lund and Browder[39] modified the percentages of body surface area to account for a continuum of age and to accommodate for growth of different body segments. This method is the more accurate means of the two to determine the extent of burn injury. Figure 24.10 shows the relative percentages of burned area for children and adults according to the Lund and Browder formula. Although this formula provides an accurate assessment

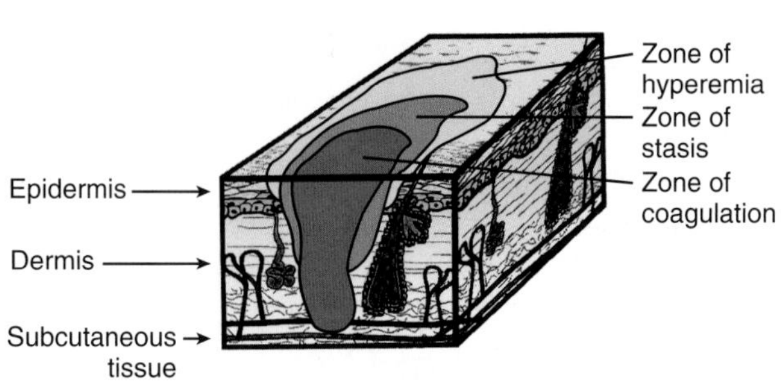

Figure 24.8 Zones of tissue damage as the result of a burn injury.

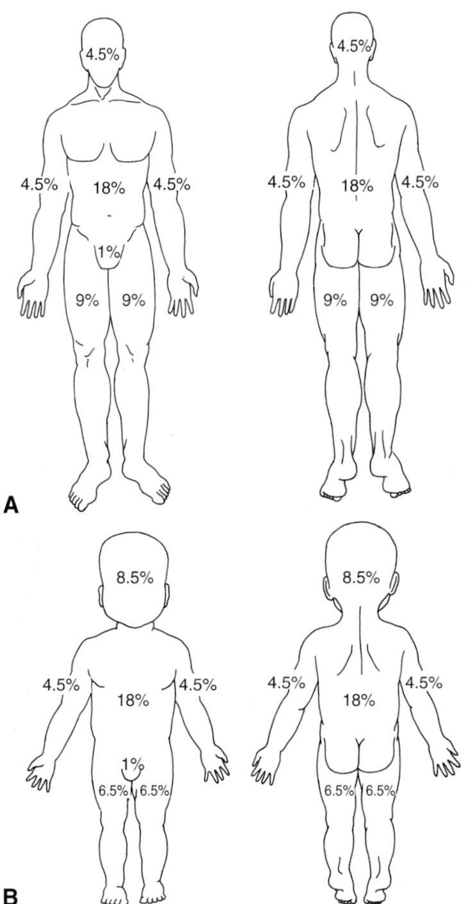

Figure 24.9 Rule of Nines to determine percentage of body surface area burn in adults (A) and children (B).

of TBSA, the use of the Rule of Nines is more practical in the emergent triage of a patient with a burn injury.

COMPLICATIONS OF BURN INJURY

Depending on the extent of burn injury, the depth of the burn, and the type of burn, there may be secondary systemic complications.[40] In addition, the health, age, and psychological status of a patient who is burned will affect these complications. This section addresses selected systemic complications a patient may experience after a significant burn injury.

Infection

Infection, in conjunction with organ system failure, is a leading cause of mortality from burns.[41] Some virulent strains of *Pseudomonas aeruginosa* and *Staphylococcus aureus* are resistant to antibiotics and have been responsible for epidemic infections in burn centers.[1,41] Microbial invasion from the burn wounds to other healthy tissue can create sepsis.[41,42]

Systemic antibiotics are used to treat both burn and general system infections once they have been documented.[40-42] A bacterial count in excess of 10^5 per gram of tissue constitutes burn wound infection and levels of 10^7 to 10^9 are usually associated with lethal burns. Most wounds are treated with topical antibiotics, discussed in the section on medical management.

Pulmonary Complications

Any patient who has been burned in a closed space should be suspected of having an *inhalation injury*.[43] Among patients with burns, the incidence of smoke inhalation may be in excess of 33%,[44] and this rises to 66% in patients with facial burns.[45] The incidence of pulmonary complications is extremely high after severe burns, and death due to pneumonia alone is attributed to a majority of the deaths following burn injury.[46] Direct trauma to the upper airways can also occur from the inhalation of hot gases.[47]

Signs of an inhalation injury include facial burns, singed nasal hairs, harsh cough, hoarseness, abnormal breath sounds, respiratory distress, and carbonaceous sputum and/or hypoxemia.[46]

The primary complications associated with this injury are carbon monoxide poisoning, tracheal damage, upper airway obstruction, pulmonary edema, and pneumonia. Lung damage from inhaling noxious gases and smoke may be lethal. To determine the extent of inhalation injury, several diagnostic procedures can be performed. The most helpful diagnostic procedure is bronchoscopy.[46]

Metabolic Complications

Thermal injury causes a great metabolic and catabolic challenge to the body. Most of the recent advances in burn treatment and rehabilitation have come directly from the increased understanding of the metabolic demands of a burn injury and from the ability to improve the patient's nutritional status to meet these demands.[48] Metabolic rates may increase up to 50% in a 25% TBSA burn and much more as the burn size increases.[49-51] The consequences of the increased metabolic and catabolic activity following a burn are a rapid decrease in body weight, negative nitrogen balance, effects on muscle mass, and a decrease in energy stores that are vital to the healing process.[52]

As a result of the increased metabolic activity, there will be an increase of 1.8°F to 2.6°F (1°C to 2°C) in core temperature that seems to be due to a resetting of the hypothalamic temperature centers in the brain.[1] Wilmore et al.[53] hypothesized that there is a significant relationship between the increased evaporative heat loss from the impaired skin barrier over a burn and the hypermetabolic state. In any event, if individuals with burns are placed in a room with normal ambient temperature, excessive heat loss will be exhibited, and this will further exaggerate the stress response seen in these patients.[1,53] Therefore, it is recommended that room temperature be kept at 86°F (30°C), which will significantly reduce the metabolic rate.

As part of the patient's altered metabolism, protein from muscle tissue is preferentially used as a source of energy. This situation, coupled with the effects of bedrest, causes muscles to atrophy and renders patients weak.

Burn Estimate and Diagram
Age vs Area

Initial Examination

Cause of Burn________________

Date of Burn________________

Time of Burn________________

Age ________________

Gender________________

Weight ________________

Date of Admission________________

Signature ________________

Date________________

Burn Diagram

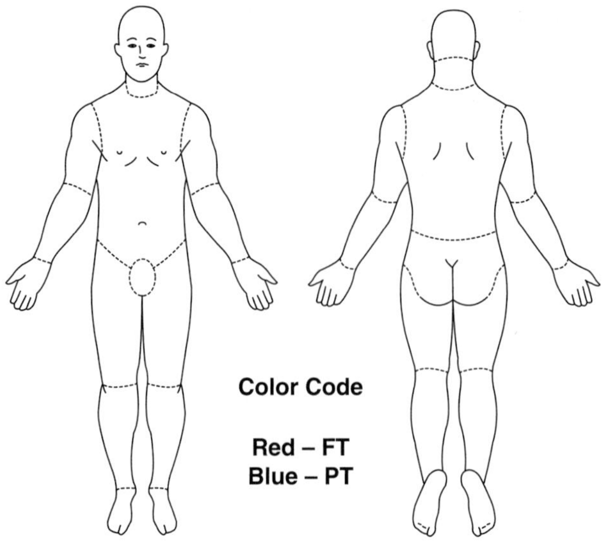

Color Code

Red – FT
Blue – PT

Area	Birth yr.	1–4 yrs.	5–9 yrs.	10–14 yrs.	15 yrs.	Adult	PT	FT	Total	Donor Areas
Head	19	17	13	11	9	7				
Neck	2	2	2	2	2	2				
Anterior Trunk	13	13	13	13	13	13				
Posterior Trunk	13	13	13	13	13	13				
Right Buttock	2 1/2	2 1/2	2 1/2	2 1/2	2 1/2	2 1/2				
Left Buttock	2 1/2	2 1/2	2 1/2	2 1/2	2 1/2	2 1/2				
Genitalia	1	1	1	1	1	1				
Right Upper Arm	4	4	4	4	4	4				
Left Upper Arm	4	4	4	4	4	4				
Right Lower Arm	3	3	3	3	3	3				
Left Lower Arm	3	3	3	3	3	3				
Right Hand	2 1/2	2 1/2	2 1/2	2 1/2	2 1/2	2 1/2				
Left Hand	2 1/2	2 1/2	2 1/2	2 1/2	2 1/2	2 1/2				
Right Thigh	5 1/2	6 1/2	8	8 1/2	9	9 1/2				
Left Thigh	5 1/2	6 1/2	8	8 1/2	9	9 1/2				
Right Leg	5	5	5 1/2	6	6 1/2	7				
Left Leg	5	5	5 1/2	6	6 1/2	7				
Right Foot	3 1/2	3 1/2	3 1/2	3 1/2	3 1/2	3 1/2				
Left Foot	3 1/2	3 1/2	3 1/2	3 1/2	3 1/2	3 1/2				
						Total				

Key: FT – Full Thickness
PT – Part Thickness

Figure 24.10 Modified Lund and Browder chart for determination of percentage of body surface area burn for various ages. Values represent percentages of burned body area. *(Courtesy Shriners Burns Hospital, Cincinnati, OH.)*

Much of the improved management of burns has been attributed to the greater focus of research on the nutritional needs of patients. It is beyond the scope of this chapter to detail nutritional supplementation, and the interested reader is referred to several excellent reviews of advances in burn nutrition.[54-56]

Cardiovascular Complications

Hemodynamic changes result from a shift in fluid to the interstitium, which subsequently reduces the plasma and intravascular fluid volume in a patient with a burn.[57,58] The fluid shifts occur as a result of local and temporary systemic changes in capillary dynamics. This shift of fluid to the interstitium can result in significant edema. Capillary permeability returns to normal after about 24 hours. Also, with these fluid shifts, there will be a tremendous initial decrease in cardiac output, which may reach as low as 15% of normal within the first hour after injury.[59,60] Fluid replacement therapy is utilized initially to manage the loss of circulatory fluid. This additional fluid allows perfusion of vital organs but also increases the amount of tissue edema.[58,61]

Hematological changes also occur after a severe burn injury. These changes include alterations in platelet concentration and function, clotting factors, and white blood cell components; red blood cell dysfunction; and decreases in hemoglobin and hematocrit.[62] These physiological alterations, coupled with cardiac changes and injured vascular beds, will significantly affect initial resuscitation efforts and, if the patient survives, how rapidly he or she will recover. Additionally, patients will exhibit decompensation from an endurance standpoint resulting in functional deterioration.

Heterotopic Ossification

Heterotopic ossification (HO) is the abnormal development of bone in areas of soft tissue. It is relatively uncommon following burn injury, but when it occurs it often leads to pain and functional impairment.[63] The number of cases that progress to become clinically problematic ranges from less than 1% to nearly 6%.[64-66] The etiology of HO is unclear. Burn induced inflammatory response may stimulate abnormal osteogenic differentiation of stem cells; other suspected causes include immobilization, microtrauma, high protein intake, and sepsis.[63,67] Physiologically, HO can appear anywhere in the body. Some case reports suggest the elbows are most commonly affected. Schneider et al. found that grafts to the arm, head/neck, and trunk are significant predictors of developing HO.[68] The TBSA is also a predictor of risk for HO. The risk of HO increases as TBSA increases, especially if the burn size is beyond 30% TBSA.[68] Usually HO occurs in areas of full-thickness injury or sites that remain unhealed for a prolonged time. Symptoms appear late in a patient's course of recovery and include decreased ROM and point-specific pain (i.e., pain location that differs from the generalized pain typically experienced).

Neuropathy

Peripheral neuropathy in patients with burns can take two forms: *polyneuropathy* or local neuropathy.[69] The cause of polyneuropathy is unknown; however, direct thermal injury, vascular occlusion, compressive nerve entrapment, and edema are suggested causes.[70] Similar to those with HO, patients with peripheral neuropathy generally have a large TBSA burn, and the condition may be more commonly associated with electrical injury.[70] Fortunately, most neuropathies resolve over time but some may be long term.

Local neuropathies can be caused by several burn treatment issues such as compression bandages applied too tightly, poorly fitted splints, or prolonged and inappropriate positioning.[69] The most common sites of involvement are the brachial plexus, ulnar nerve, and common peroneal nerve.

Pathological Scars

Burn scars occur in areas of deep partial-thickness burns that are allowed to heal spontaneously and in full-thickness burns that have been skin grafted, but graft coverage is incomplete. If maturing tissue demonstrates a greater rate of collagen production than degradation, a scar becomes raised and thick.[71,72] Scars become pathological when they take on the form of *hypertrophy,* contracture, or both. Each of these scar conditions is unique and should not be viewed as synonymous. A patient can have a hypertrophic scar that does not interfere with movement or a scar contracture band that is not hypertrophied. However, both conditions can exist simultaneously, and specific treatment for each is discussed later in this chapter.

The burn wound has been described and the causes and complications of burn injury have been presented. The following sections address wound healing[73] and medical, surgical, and physical therapy management of the patient with a burn.

BURN WOUND HEALING

The two layers of the skin—the epidermis and dermis—differ morphologically and heal by separate mechanisms.

Epidermal Healing

If a burn injury is isolated to the epidermis, or if there are viable cells lining the skin appendages, *epithelial healing* can occur on the surface of a wound. The stimulus for epithelial growth is the presence of an open wound exposing subepithelial tissue to the environment. The intact epithelium attempts to cover an exposed wound through mitosis and the ameboid movement of cells from the basal layer of the surrounding epidermis into the wound. The epithelial cells stop migration when they are completely in contact with other epithelial cells. Following this *contact inhibition,* cells begin to differentiate to form the various epithelial layers. While epidermal cells move about the wound site, they maintain a connection with the normal epithelium at the wound margin. To continue migration and proliferation, a suitable base for the epithelial cells must be provided by adequate nutrition and blood supply, or else the new cells will die.

The process of epithelialization is most evident clinically in the partial-thickness wound that has intact hair follicles and glands. The skin appendages provide a source of epithelial cells from which the wound may heal. The cells migrate outwardly from the appendages and appear as epidermal islands from which they spread peripherally across the wound. Skin growth and coverage from these epithelial islands can be visualized over time.

Damage to sebaceous glands may cause dryness and itching of a healing wound. Lubrication can be a problem, and newly healed skin is characteristically dry and may split. Dryness may continue for a long time, because many of the sebaceous glands do not return to their normal function after a wound is epithelialized. Therapists need to educate patients about the type, frequency, and techniques of moisturizing cream application to lubricate newly healed tissue.

Dermal Healing

When an injury involves tissue deeper than the epidermis, *dermal healing,* or scar formation, occurs. Scar formation can be divided into three phases: *inflammatory, proliferative,* and *maturation.* Although these phases will be described separately, they occur on a continuum and one phase often overlaps another.

Inflammatory Phase

The primary reaction of viable tissue to a burn wound is inflammation, which prepares the wound for healing through hemostatic, vascular, and cellular events. Inflammation begins at the time of injury, ends in about 3 to 5 days, and is characterized by redness, edema, warmth, pain, and decreased ROM. Initially, when a blood vessel is ruptured, the wall of the vessel contracts to decrease blood flow. Platelets aggregate, and fibrin is deposited to form a clot over the area. Fibrin serves a threefold function: (1) to partially retain body fluids; (2) to protect the underlying cells from desiccation; and (3) to provide a firm coagulum substance from which cells can infiltrate. Therefore, fibrin can be thought of as forming a lattice network, from which cells can climb and work themselves into the healing structure.

After a transient vasoconstriction of the vasculature, which lasts about 5 to 10 minutes, vessels vasodilate to increase blood flow to the area. There is increased permeability of the blood vessels, with leaking of plasma into the interstitial space and subsequent edema formation. Leukocytes infiltrate the area and begin to rid the site of contamination. Of particular importance is the presence of macrophage cells, which are responsible for attracting fibroblasts into the area.

Proliferative Phase

During this phase, re-epithelialization is occurring at the surface of the wound, while deep within the wound, fibroblasts are migrating and proliferating. *Fibroblasts* are the cells that synthesize scar tissue, which is composed of collagen and protein polysaccharides in the form of a viscous ground substance that surrounds the collagen strands. The collagen is deposited with a random alignment and no true architectural arrangement of fibers. Stress (e.g., a force intended to elongate the scar) applied to the developing tissue during this time causes the fibers to align along the direction of force.[74] During this period of fibroplasia, the tensile strength of the wound increases at a rate proportional to the rate of collagen synthesis.

In conjunction with collagen deposition, granulation tissue is formed during this phase. Granulation tissue consists of macrophages, fibroblasts, collagen, and blood vessels.[73] Newly formed blood vessels bring a rich blood supply to the area and encourage further wound healing. However, granulation tissue formation is not necessary for skin graft adherence, and excess granulation tissue may lead to an increase in hypertrophic scarring.

During the proliferative phase, *wound contraction* occurs. Wound contraction is an active process in which the body attempts to close a wound where a loss of tissue has occurred. The amount of contraction is determined by the amount of available surrounding mobile skin. It involves movement of existing tissue at the wound edge toward the center, not formation of new tissue. Wound contraction ceases when (1) the edges of the wound meet, or (2) tension in the surrounding skin equals or exceeds the force of contraction. Skin grafting may decrease contraction, with thick grafts causing less contraction.

Maturation Phase

A wound is considered closed at the time epithelium covers the surface; however, wound healing involves remodeling of the scar tissue. During the maturation phase, there is a reduction in the number of fibroblasts, a decrease in vascularity owing to a lesser metabolic demand, and remodeling of collagen, which becomes more parallel in arrangement and forms stronger bonds. The ratio of collagen breakdown to production determines the type of scar that forms. If the rate of breakdown equals or slightly *exceeds the rate of production,* maturation results in a pale, flat, and pliable scar. If the rate of collagen production *exceeds breakdown,* then a hypertrophic scar may result. This scar is characterized by a red and raised appearance with rigid texture; it stays within the boundary of the original wound. A *keloid* is a large, firm scar that overflows the boundaries of the original wound; it is more common in darkly pigmented individuals. Both of these scars take a prolonged period of time to mature. The presence and contraction of the scar can lead to both functional and cosmetic deformities. The active process of scar contraction during both this maturation phase and the proliferative phase creates a risk of contracture formation. A contracture over a joint will limit ROM and affect joint function.[75]

■ MEDICAL MANAGEMENT

Advances in the medical management of patients with burn injury have resulted in the survival of thousands of patients who 25 or 35 years ago would have died from their injuries.[76] Research findings and current techniques available at modern burn centers have enabled patients to receive better care through use of more sophisticated interventions. This section addresses the initial treatment of burn injuries and surgical management including primary excision, skin grafts, and correction of scar contracture.

Initial Treatment

The goals of initial medical treatment of a patient with a burn are to address critical life-threatening problems and stabilize the patient through procedures designed to (1) establish and maintain an airway; (2) prevent cyanosis, shock, and hemorrhage; (3) establish baseline data, such as extent and depth of burn injury; (4) prevent or reduce fluid losses; (5) clean the patient and wounds; (6) examine injuries; and (7) prevent pulmonary and cardiac complications. Triage (assigning degree of urgency and order of treatment) using these procedures applies to major burn trauma.

Initially, a patient must be transported from the site of injury to a treatment facility. If possible, transportation will be directly to a burn center, rather than to a hospital emergency room. The goals of treatment in transit are to stabilize the patient and maintain an airway. During the initial transportation phase, patient history and personal data are gathered when possible. The type of agent causing the burn is noted, and initial examination of the burn injury takes place. Emergency medical personnel may use the Rule of Nines to estimate the percentage of burn injury. In addition, they prepare the individual for triage at the burn center by removing all burned clothing and jewelry and initiating administration of fluid through an intravenous line.

One of the major advances in burn care has been in fluid volume replacement initially and throughout a patient's treatment. Research has led to an improved understanding of the physiological changes that occur in a patient after a burn injury and of the fluid volumes necessary to optimize the chance for survival.[60] Information about the physiological changes responsible for shifts in body fluids and protein has led to the use of intravenous solutions in an amount necessary to replace vital fluids and electrolytes.[77]

After a patient arrives at a burn center and adequate fluid resuscitation (replacement) has been initiated, the burn team determines the extent and depth of injury and begins initial wound cleansing. Burn units typically use showers, spraying over a tub, or "bed baths" for the removal of dressings and daily cleaning of wounds. The use of hydrotherapy tubs for wound cleansing is no longer recommended.[78,79] The initial wound care session allows the team to determine body weight, fully examine the patient, remove hair where necessary, and start the *débridement* process by removing any loose skin. The goals of wound cleansing and débridement are to remove dead tissue, prevent infection, and promote revascularization and/or epithelialization of the area. Depending on the facility, physical therapists may be involved in the wound cleaning procedures.[80]

After dressings are removed, the wound should be inspected carefully. The appearance, depth, and size are determined and the presence of exudate or odor is noted. *Infection* is characterized by thick purulent drainage, odor, fever, a brownish-black discoloration, rapid separation of eschar, boils in adjacent tissue, or conversion of a deep partial-thickness burn to a full-thickness injury.

Wound care is carried out using sterile technique and instruments. If *sharp débridement* (the use of surgical scissors or scalpel and forceps to remove eschar) is performed, sloughed epidermis and loose eschar are removed and pockets of pus are drained. The procedure needs to be performed carefully so that bleeding is minimal.

After the wounds have been cleaned, the patient should be kept warm to reduce any further metabolic demand due to additional heat loss. Topical medications and/or dressings are then applied or reapplied. Table 24.3 presents common topical medications used in the treatment of burns. The technique of applying a topical cream or ointment without dressings is called the *open technique* and allows for ongoing inspection of the wound and examination of the healing process. With this technique, the topical medication must be reapplied throughout the day.

The *closed technique* consists of applying dressings over a topical agent. Dressings serve several purposes: (1) they hold topical antimicrobial agents on the wound, (2) they reduce fluid loss from the wound, and (3) they protect the wound. Dressings are changed once or twice a day, depending on the size and type of wound and the type of topical antimicrobial used.

Dressings consist of several layers. The first layer is nonadherent to protect the fragile healing surface from disruption. This may be followed by cotton padding to absorb wound drainage. The final layer consists of roll gauze or elastic bandages, which hold the other layers in place but allow movement.

Surgical Management

Primary Excision

Primary excision is surgical removal of eschar. The excision generally includes removal of peripheral layers of eschar until vascular, viable tissue is exposed as the site for skin graft placement.[81] Much of the increased survival rate of patients with extensive burns is associated with early primary excision of burn wounds.[82] Typically, a patient is taken to surgery after successful resuscitation, usually within 1 week of injury. As much of the eschar is removed at one time as possible. Proponents of early primary excision believe that this approach is easier on the patient than repeated débridement and that it promotes more rapid healing, reduces infection and scarring, and is more economical in terms of staff and hospital time.[81]

In many burn centers, a wound is closed with a skin graft at the time of primary excision. Many types of grafts can be used to close a wound. An *autograft* is a patient's own skin, taken from an unburned area and transplanted to cover a burned area. Autografts are desirable because they provide permanent coverage of the wound. An *allograft* (or *homograft*) is skin taken from an individual of the same species, usually cadaver skin. The skin can be kept frozen in skin banks for prolonged periods. Allografts are temporary grafts used to cover large burns when there is insufficient autograft available. *Xenograft* (or *heterograft*) is skin from another species, usually a pig.

Table 24.3 Common Topical Medications Used in Treatment of Burns

Medication	Description	Method of Application
Silver sulfadiazine	Most commonly used topical antibacterial agent; effective against *Pseudomonas* infections.	White cream applied with sterile glove 2–4 mm thick directly to wound or impregnated into fine mesh gauze.
Mafenide acetate (Sulfamylon)	Topical antibacterial agent; effective against gram-negative or gram-positive organisms; diffuses easily through eschar.	White cream applied directly to wound with thin 1–2 mm layer twice daily; may be left undressed or covered with thin layer of gauze.
Mafenide acetate solution (Sulfamylon 5% Solution), silver nitrate	Topical solution with antimicrobial function against gram-positive and gram-negative organisms. Maintains moist environment. Antiseptic germicide and astringent; will penetrate only 1–2 mm of eschar; useful for surface bacteria; stains black.	50-gram packet of white powder that is mixed with either 1,000 mL sterile water or 0.9% sodium chloride–soaked gauze. Dressings or soaks used every 2 hours; also available as small sticks to cauterize small open areas.
Bacitracin/Polysporin	Bland ointment; effective against gram-positive organisms.	Thin layer of ointment applied directly to wound and left open.
Collagenase, Accuzyme	Enzymatic débriding agent selectively débrides necrotic tissue; no antibacterial action.	Ointment applied to eschar and covered with moist occlusive dressing with or without an antimicrobial agent.

Allografts or xenografts are used until there is sufficient normal skin available for an autograft.

Perhaps the most progressive advancement in the care of patients with burns in recent years is the use of *skin substitutes* for coverage of an excised wound.[83-90] Skin substitutes consist of cultured autologous skin, which is grown in a laboratory from a biopsy of a patient's own tissue, the use of altered cadaver skin, or other biologically engineered tissues. Skin substitutes are used when large areas of burn exist and coverage is necessary for a patient's survival. Cultured autologous skin takes several weeks to grow and is highly susceptible to infection. Other biologically engineered tissues are more readily available and have demonstrated more reliable adherence than in the past. With the use of most skin substitutes, ROM exercises may be delayed and shearing forces must be avoided. Although skin substitutes are an expensive intervention for wound coverage, they are useful and have proved effective in managing patients with large burn wounds. Examples of skin substitutes include the following:

- *Cultured epidermal autografts (CEAs):* A skin biopsy is obtained from a patient, and only the epidermal cells are cultured.[83,84]
- *Cultured autologous composite grafts:* A skin biopsy is obtained from a patient, and both epidermal and dermal cells are cultured. This forms a bilayer structure.
- *Allogenic skin substitute:* The epidermal layer of skin and all immune cells are removed from cadaver skin. This tissue is applied to the graft bed and once adhered, a thin epidermal autograft or CEA is applied.[91]
- *Cultured dermis (temporary):* Cultured dermal matrix is seeded with human neonatal fibroblasts and used as a temporary covering in place of cadaver skin. This substitute eventually is removed and replaced with an autograft.[88,89]
- *Cultured dermis (definitive):* This skin substitute is composed of cultured bovine collagen with a silicone outer layer. Pores in the material allow for controlled growth of a neodermis. After approximately 14 days, the silicone layer is removed, and a very thin skin graft or CEA is applied.[90]

Skin Grafts

The removal of skin to graft onto a burn wound is done surgically under anesthesia. The skin used for a graft usually is removed with a *dermatome*. This instrument not only allows the surgeon to obtain a large amount of skin, but a more consistent thickness of skin can be obtained. The dermatome is adjusted to remove a predetermined thickness of skin for a *split-thickness skin graft*. A split-thickness skin graft contains epidermis and a variable amount of dermis, as opposed to a *full-thickness skin graft*, which consists of the full dermal thickness.

The site from which a skin graft is taken is called a *donor site*. Common donor sites include the thighs, buttocks, and back. These wounds heal by re-epithelialization, like a partial-thickness burn, and require appropriate care to prevent additional dermal damage with resultant scar formation. A full-thickness skin graft has the disadvantage of leaving a full-thickness wound at the donor site that will require either primary closure or grafting with a split-thickness skin graft.

Generally, the thinner the skin graft, the better the adherence, and the thicker the graft, the better the cosmetic result. Additionally, a thin graft will contract more than a thick skin graft once it has adhered to the wound bed. Selection of depth depends on many factors, including whether the donor site needs to be used again for another skin graft. Taking a thicker graft adversely affects the possibility of taking another graft from the same site for a prolonged period. Harvesting from split-thickness skin graft sites may be repeated in 10 to 14 days, depending on the amount of time the donor site takes to heal.

A *sheet graft* is a skin graft applied to a recipient bed without alteration following harvesting from a donor site (Fig. 24.11). The face, neck, and hands are covered with this type of graft for optimal cosmesis and function. When limited donor skin is available, most areas are covered with a *mesh graft* (Fig. 24.12). The meshing of a graft consists of processing the sheet graft through a device that makes tiny parallel incisions in a linear arrangement. This process permits the skin graft to be expanded before it is applied to the wound bed.[92] This technique allows coverage of a larger area, and once the graft adheres, the interstices heal through re-epithelialization.

A skin graft usually is held in place with sutures, staples, or Steri-Strip™ skin closures. Once a graft is fixed in position, any blood or serum that might have collected between the graft and the recipient site should be removed. Application of a pressure dressing facilitates contact between the graft and recipient site.

A necessity for successful adherence of a graft is sufficient vascularity within the wound bed. Grafts will not adhere to poorly vascularized areas, such as tendon. Once a skin graft has been applied, separation of a graft from its bed must be prevented. Separation may result from shear force, mechanical trauma, or hematoma formation. Initially, the area is immobilized with a dressing that provides firm, even compression on the wound. Other reasons for graft failure include inadequate excision of necrotic tissue and infection.

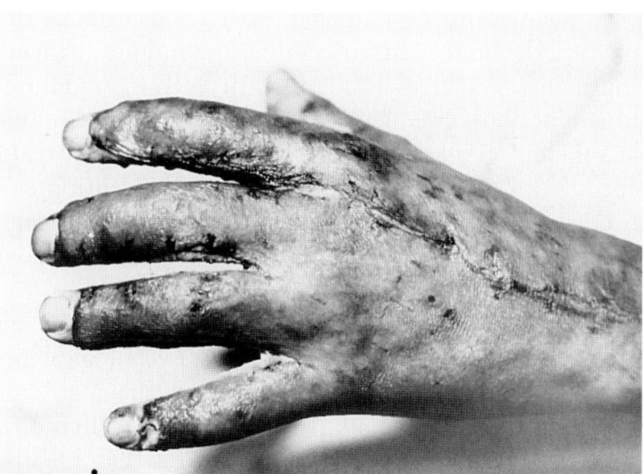

Figure 24.11 Sheet graft on dorsum of left hand, postoperative day 7. *(From Richard and Staley,[4, p. 183] with permission.)*

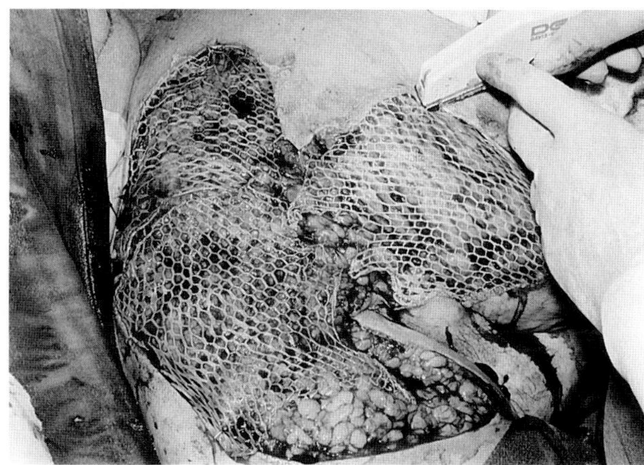

Figure 24.12 Meshed split-thickness skin graft applied to freshly excised wound and secured with staples.

Survival of a skin graft depends on several factors: (1) circulation, which provides a nutritive supply to the graft; (2) inosculation, or the process by which a direct connection is established between a graft and the host vessels; and (3) penetration of the host vessels into a graft site. Except in darkly pigmented skin, grafts are white in color at the time of transplantation and begin to show a pinkish hue within a matter of hours after their placement on an adequate vascular bed.

The reestablishment of circulation in a skin graft will take place through the formation of direct anastomosis between respective vessels, invasion from the host bed forming new channels, or both. Twenty-four hours after grafting, numerous host vessels will have penetrated the graft.[73] The invasion of new capillaries seems to be the most important consideration in vascularization. Normally, within 72 hours, inosculation has proceeded to the point where the skin graft is secure. Initially, structural connections are fibrous. Collagen is then laid down to secure attachment of the graft.

Correction of Scar Contracture

If physical therapy interventions are unsuccessful in averting scar contracture formation, and limitations are noted in ROM and function, surgery may be required. In the past, reconstructive surgery usually was postponed while a burn wound was in the active, immature phase of scar formation.[93] More recently, however, successful release of scar contractures before scar maturation has been documented.[94] Each patient's scar will require an individualized evaluation and treatment. Many surgical treatment options are available to eliminate scar contractures; among the more common procedures are skin grafts and Z-plasties.[95]

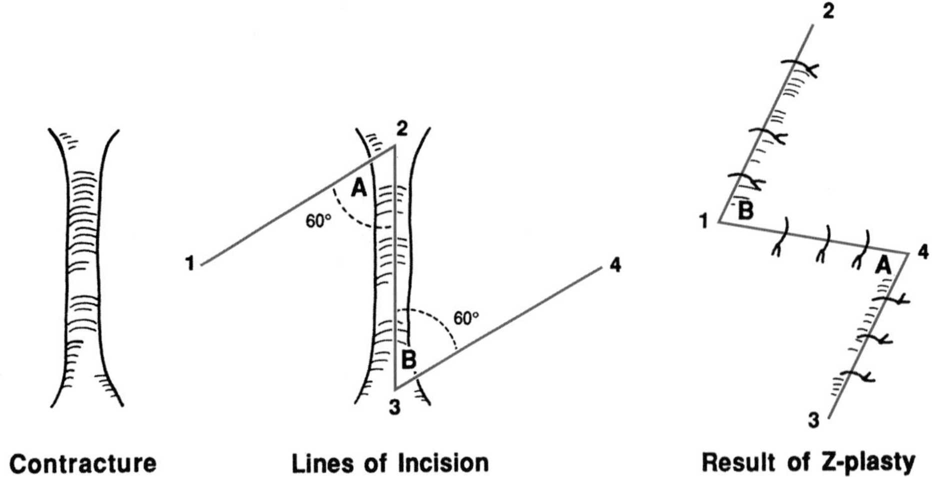

Figure 24.13 Schematic diagram of Z-plasty procedure. *(From Richard and Staley,[4, p. 192] with permission.)*

A schematic diagram of a Z-plasty is shown in Figure 24.13. The Z-plasty serves to lengthen a scar by interposing normal tissue in the line of the scar. Skin grafts are used after surgical release for more severe contractures.

PHYSICAL THERAPY MANAGEMENT

Concurrent with skin healing, is initiation of the physical therapy plan of care (POC).[96] Commonly, physical therapy interventions are directed toward prevention of scar contracture, preservation of normal ROM,[97-102] prevention or minimization of hypertrophic scar formation and cosmetic deformity, maintenance or improvement in muscular strength and cardiovascular endurance, return to preburn function, and performance of activities of daily living (ADL).[4] The POC for a patient with burns is an evolving process that may require daily modification.[5-7,96,103]

Rehabilitation is a continuum of care through the entire course of recovery, and will vary in intensity and interventions required, with each individual and each phase of recovery.[104] The overall focus of rehabilitation is to restore the patient's pre-injury function and lifestyle. The physical therapist collaborates with other team members to obtain these outcomes. With adherence to a well-designed treatment plan, a patient can expect to return to a normal, productive life. For many patients, the most difficult phase of rehabilitation occurs after the wounds have healed and the scar tissue begins to contract. At this point, patient education about adherence to strategies designed to prevent or minimize contractures is particularly important. The remainder of this chapter will address the physical therapist's role in the rehabilitation of a patient who has sustained a burn injury.

Examination

After the initial examination for depth of burn and percentage of TBSA involved, the physical therapist then examines the patient to determine the presence of impairments and activity limitations. The therapist needs to obtain an accurate history from the patient and family members regarding any preexisting limitations or previous injuries that may affect rehabilitation potential. The therapist must also anticipate the potential for development of indirect impairments as the burn wounds heal and mature. For example, active or passive ROM may be limited as a result of edema, restrictive eschar, or pain, and an initial baseline measure should be obtained.

Other tests and measures discussed in this text are appropriate for inclusion in the initial examination and reexamination of a patient following burn injury (e.g., balance, functional status, and gait). See discussion of outcomes measures in Chapter 6, Examination of Coordination and Balance, Chapter 8, Examination of Function, and Chapter 11, Strategies to Improve Locomotor Function. Because healing of a burn wound is a dynamic process and changes may occur daily, the physical therapist needs to examine and monitor patients routinely for changes in skin integrity, ROM, and functional mobility. Frequent evaluation will keep the physical therapist and other members of the burn care team abreast of potential problems so that intervention can occur before a potential problem becomes a real one. Studies addressing assessment of burn scars are presented in Table 24.4 Evidence Summary.

In addition to the physical damage imposed by a burn, there also may be an enormous psychological impact.[105-107] The physical therapist should be cognizant of a potential problem during ongoing evaluations, because psychological trauma may affect the patient's progress, outlook, and adherence with the POC. Referral to an appropriate professional for intervention may be necessary (see Chapter 26, Psychosocial Issues in Physical Rehabilitation).

Table 24.4 Evidence Summary Studies Addressing the Assessment of Burn Scar

Sullivan, T, et al: Rating the burn scar. J Burn Care Rehabil 11:250, 1990.

Design	Observational rating
Level of Evidence	II
Subjects	73
Intervention	Burn scars less than 1 year old were observed and rated on the following characteristics and scale scores: Pigmentation (normal = 0. hypopigmentation = 1, hyperpigmentation = 2); Vascularity (normal = 0, 1 to 3 = signs of increased vascularity); Pliability (normal = 0, 1 to 5 = signs of decreased pliability); and, Height (0 = normal or flat, 1 = <2 mm, 2 = <5 mm, 3 = > 5mm)
Results	Moderate interrater reliability was reported. No data related to intra-rater reliability or validity were reported.
Comments	The study suggested that the Vancouver Scar Scale (VSS) may have potential as a clinical rating of burn scars. Although the strength of this study is low and despite some published modifications to this scale, the VSS remains the current standard for assessing scar burn scar.

Crowe, JM, et al: Reliability of photographic analysis in determining change in scar appearance. J Burn Care Rehabil 11:250, 1990.

Design	Observational
Level of Evidence	II
Subjects	4 (2 therapists with scar care experience and 2 without scar care experience)
Intervention	4 color photographs (slides) each of ten patient's scars were rated using the VSS and two other assessment scales.
Results	interrater reliability ranged from 0.66 (vascularity assessment) to 0.90 (color assessment). Test-retest reliability ranged from 0.73 (vascularity assessment) to 0.89 (proportion of irregular scar assessment). Novice therapists were generally as reliable as expert therapists in assessment of the scars.
Comments	Findings suggested that the use of photographs with application to a scar assessment scale holds potential for evaluation of scar surface, thickness, border height, and color. Subject and evaluator numbers were low.

Martin, D: Changes in subjective vs. objective burn scar assessment over time: Does the patient agree with what we think? J Burn Care Rehabil 24:239, 2003.

Design	Observational
Level of Evidence	II
Subjects	37 scars on 20 subjects were assessed. Follow-up reassessment of scars included 17 scars on 8 subjects.
Intervention	A modified VSS and a visual analogue scale (VAS) were used for both the initial and follow-up assessments. Scar assessment by the clinicians included pigmentation, vascularity, and height of the scar. The VAS was used to obtain subject responses to two questions: 1. *How would you rate your scar?* (Best possible, most attractive = 0 and worst possible, least attractive = 10); and 2. *I feel this scar is unattractive to other people.* (Completely disagree = 0, completely agree = 10). Scars less than 6 months old were initially rated, and some of these same scars were reassessed approximately 1. 5 years after the burn injury.
Results	There was significant improvement of the scar from early to late assessment ($p \leq .001$) and also with VAS question 2 ($p \leq .006$). There was no correlation between VSS scores and the patient's responses to the VAS questions.
Comments	This study included not only clinician assessment of scars, but also involved feedback provided by the patients about their perception of the appearance of the scar. Findings suggested that while subjects might feel their scars improve with time, their feelings may (1) not match the clinician's assessment of improvement, and (2) be different about acceptance of the scar by others.

Continued

Table 24.4 Evidence Summary Studies Addressing the Assessment of Burn Scar—cont'd

Draaijers, LJ, et al: The patient and observer scar assessment scale: A reliable and feasible tool for scar evaluation. Plast Reconstr Surg 113:1960, 2004.

Design	Observational
Level of Evidence	II
Subjects	Four independent observers used the observer score of the Patient and Observer Scar Assessment Scale (POSAS) and the VSS on 49 scars on 20 patients.
Intervention	The observer portion of the POSAS includes assessment of the variables of vascularization, pigmentation, thickness, relief, and pliability on a 1 to 10 scale (1 = normal, 10 = worst scar possible). Patients also completed the patient response portion of the POSAS. The questions for the patient include: the level of pain and itching, respectively (rated on a 1 to 10 VAS with 1 = no complaints and 10 = worst imaginable); and, color of the scar, stiffness of the scar, thickness of the scar, and irregularity of the scar (rated on a VAS scale with 1 = like normal skin, and 10 = very different from normal). Independent observers also completed the VSS on each of the same scars assessed using the POSAS.
Results	Internal consistency of the patient and observer scales were acceptable. Reliability of POSAS completed by a single observer was acceptable (ICC=0.73), better than VSS. The observer scale shows less variability than the VSS between repeated measures. The observer scale had significant correlation with the VSS (Spearman's rho = 0.89, $p < 0.001$). Significant influences from the patient's point of view were pain and itching.
Comments	The authors conclude the observer scale is feasible because a single observer can use the scale reliably. The POSAS scar assessment tool is suitable for clinical studies because the opinion of the patient is incorporated.

Nedelec, B, et al: Quantitative measurement of hypertrophic scar: Interrater reliability, sensitivity, and specificity. J Burn Care Res 29:489, 2008a.

Design	Observational
Level of Evidence	II
Subjects	Four skin areas evaluated (3 scar sites; 1 normal skin area) on each of 30 subjects. The four sites included: • The most severe scar • A less severe scar • A donor skin site • A normal skin site
Intervention	Modified VSS used to assess scar height, pliability, and vascularity. Other measures included the following: • Cutometer used to assess skin elasticity. • Mexameter used to further assess scar erythema and melanin. • Dermascan used to assess scar thickness. Each site was evaluated by the same observer using a modified VSS, a cutometer, mexameter, and dermascan. Each site was assessed on three different days within a 2-week period. The observer was blinded to any previous measurement results.
Results	The ICC for the modified VSS for height, pliability, and vascularity subscales was adequate (0.81). The cutometer did not discriminate between normal skin and scar. The mexameter was acceptable for erythema (>0.75) and melanin index (>0.89), as was the dermascan for thickness (>0.82). *Note:* Thresholds were described for some of these measurements.
Comments	Variable sensitivity and specificity noted with some measures. Questions raised about intra-rater reliability of the modified VSS with hypertrophic scar. The interrater reliabilities for the mexameter and the dermascan were acceptable, allowing consideration of these instruments for measuring the relevant scar.

Table 24.4 Evidence Summary Studies Addressing the Assessment of Burn Scar—cont'd

Nedelec, B, et al: Quantitative measurement of hypertrophic scar: Interrater reliability and concurrent validity. J Burn Care Res 29:501, 2008b.

Design	Observational
Level of Evidence	II
Subjects	As with the previous study also by Nedelec et al, four skin areas were evaluated (3 scar sites; 1 normal skin area) on each of 30 subjects. The four sites included the following: • The most severe scar • A less severe scar • A donor skin site • A normal skin site
Intervention	Modified VSS used to assess scar height, pliability, and vascularity. Other measures included the following: • Cutometer used to assess skin elasticity. • Mexameter used to further assess scar erythema and melanin. • Dermascan used to assess scar thickness. Each site was evaluated by the same observer by using a modified VSS, a cutometer, mexameter, and dermascan. Each site was assessed on three different days within a 2-week period. The observer was blinded to any previous measurements results.
Results	Interrater reliabilities of all subscales of the modified VSS were not acceptable (≈0.50). Acceptable reliability was reported for the cutometer (>0.89), the mexameter, and the dermascan (0.82). Concurrent validity was significant with the VSS in every case except with the pliability subscale and the cutometer in cases of severe scar.
Comments	The interrater reliabilities of the cutometer, mexameter, and dermascan and their concurrent validity with the modified VSS suggests they are objectively measuring the same scar characteristics as the modified VSS.

Simons, M, and Tyack, Z: Health professionals' and consumers' opinion: What is considered important when rating burn scars from photographs? J Burn Care Res 32(2):275, 2011.

Design	Observational
Level of Evidence	II
Subjects	Three-phase assessment of rating burn scars from photographs included the following: • Opinions from 38 health professionals about current practice in scar assessment • Opinions from 36 therapists (PTs and OTs) about what should be included in a photographic scar scale • Opinions of 10 health care consumers about scar evaluation
Intervention	Each site was evaluated by the same observer by using a modified VSS, a cutometer, mexameter, and dermascan. Each site was assessed on three different days within a 2-week period. The observer was blinded to any previous measurement results. Responses and answers to open-ended questions were linked for similarity. Linked responses and answers were converted to percentages for descriptive purposes and then analyzed for significance using Chi-Square analysis.
Results	Some agreement was reached that vascularity, color, contour, height, and overall opinion of the burn scar were parameters that could be assessed using color photography.
Comments	The authors suggest that a categorical scale with clear descriptors and strategies may improve photographic evaluation of burn scar.

Goals and Expected Outcomes

Based on evaluation of examination data with consideration to the severity of burn, and the patient's current health status, age, and physical and psychological condition, the patient's prognosis can be estimated. Development of goals and expected outcomes are informed by the prognosis and current medical status. It is difficult to identify specific goals and outcomes owing to the varied nature of each burn injury. Suggestions for formulating goals and outcomes include:[21]

- Peripheral edema is minimized.
- Joint integrity and mobility are improved.
- Muscle performance (strength, power, and endurance) is improved.
- Range of motion is improved.
- Caregivers are independent in safe patient handling.
- Physical function is improved.
- Utilization of rehabilitation services is optimized.
- Self-management of symptoms is improved.
- Access, availability, and services provided are acceptable to the patient or client.
- Coordination of care is acceptable to the patient or client.

The optimal outcome of rehabilitation is the return of a patient to normal, preinjury function and lifestyle.

Intervention

Patients with burns usually begin physical therapy on the day of admission. The initial examination will determine which areas need to be addressed first. Control and resolution of edema and preserving ROM usually are the first priorities of intervention. Edema can be minimized through elevation of the extremities and active movement, especially of the hands and ankles. Prevention of scar contractures can be accomplished through positioning, splinting, exercise, and ambulation. Exercise and ambulation also will help to minimize deconditioning and other deleterious effects of bedrest. Following wound closure, massage and compression therapy will assist with minimizing contracture formation and management of burn scars.

The scar that forms across a joint skin crease while a burn wound is healing is composed of immature collagen. A scar will shorten as a result of the contractile or pulling forces in scar tissue.[108-111] This scar contraction remains a major potential cause of burn morbidity in the United States as it leads to about one-third of patients with a severe burn injury developing some level of contracture.[112] Scar contracture may be more common in areas where access to expert care is absent or limited.[113] Scar contraction can limit ROM and function unless interventions are taken against this process. Although measures to prevent a contracture are undertaken in expectation of the best result, the risk of scar contracture development must be acknowledged and countered with an appropriate plan of care. There are several interventions available to address prevention and/or treatment of scar contracture.

As stated, positioning, splinting, exercise, and ambulation are interventions utilized in opposing the scar contracture process. Active exercise and patient participation in functional activities are important strategies to prevent or minimize contractures. However, owing to the relentless forces of scar tissue and pain associated with exercising a burned area, additional interventions may be necessary (e.g., skin grafts and Z-plasty). Early and ongoing patient and/or family education is needed to help these individuals understand the necessity of the burn rehabilitation process.

> **Clinical Note** A Burn Rehabilitation Therapist Competency Tool (BRTCT) has been developed to define the core knowledge and skills central to the role of physical and occupational therapists in burn management.[114] The BRTCT provides standards of care for patients with burn injuries throughout the full spectrum of rehabilitation.[115]

Positioning and Splinting

A positioning program should begin on the day of admission to counteract contraction of damaged and scarring tissue.[6,7,80,116] The goals of a positioning program are to (1) minimize edema; (2) prevent tissue destruction; (3) maintain soft tissues in an elongated state; and (4) preserve function.[117] Positioning strategies for common deformities are presented in Table 24.5. To mitigate the development of scar contracture and joint limitation, a positioning program must be designed based on the distribution of the burn injury relative to adjacent joints. Joint position should be opposite the anticipated contracture based on evaluation of the wound distribution and depth. Examples of proper positioning of different body segments are provided in Figures 24.14 through 24.17. Burned areas should be positioned in an elongated state or neutral position of function.[118,119]

Splinting can be viewed as an extension of a positioning program. There are certain "anti-deformity" positions in which patients generally are splinted; however, positioning is individualized based on the location of the burn and which movements are difficult for the patient to achieve. With the exception of splints designed to immobilize a skin graft after surgery, splints should be fabricated for patients only if ROM or function would be lost without them. General indications for the use of splints include (1) prevention of contractures, (2) maintenance of ROM achieved during an exercise session or surgical release, (3) reduction of developing contractures, (4) protection of a joint or tendon, and (5) to reduce the overall pain experience.[120,121] Splint design should be kept simple so that it is easy to apply, remove, and clean.[122] Splints are usually worn at night, when a

Table 24.5 Positioning Strategies for Common Deformities

Joint	Common Deformity	Motions to Be Stressed	Suggested Approaches
Anterior neck	Flexion	Hyperextension	Use double mattress; position neck in extension (Fig. 24.14); with healing use rigid cervical orthosis
Shoulder-axilla	Adduction and internal rotation	Abduction, flexion, and external rotation	Position with shoulder flexed and abducted (airplane splint)
Elbow	Flexion and pronation	Extension and supination	Splint in extension
Hand	Claw hand (also called intrinsic minus position)	Wrist extension; metacarpophalangeal flexion, proximal interphalangeal and distal interphalangeal extension; thumb abduction	Wrap fingers separately. Elevate to decrease edema. Position in *intrinsic plus* position, wrist in extension, metacarpophalangeal in flexion, proximal interphalangeal and distal interphalangeal in extension, thumb in abduction with large web space
Hip and groin	Flexion and adduction	All motions, especially hip extension and abduction	Hip neutral (zero degrees of flexion/extension), with slight abduction
Knee	Flexion	Extension	Posterior knee splint
Ankle	Plantarflexion	All motions (especially dorsiflexion)	Plastic ankle-foot orthosis with cutout at Achilles tendon and ankle positioned in neutral

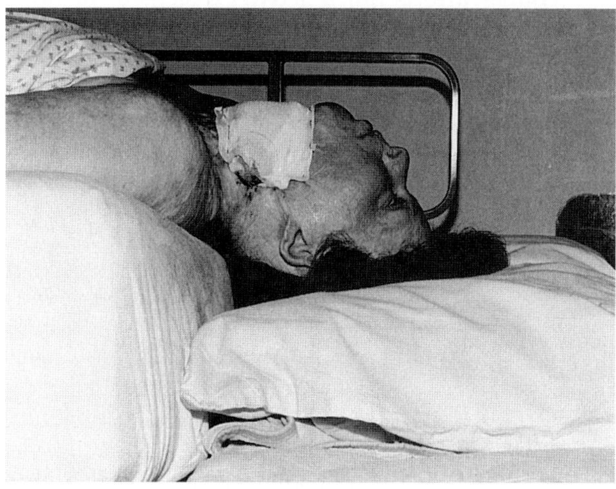

Figure 24.14 Positioning in bed of patient with burns of the anterior neck. *(From Richard and Staley,[4, p. 225] with permission.)*

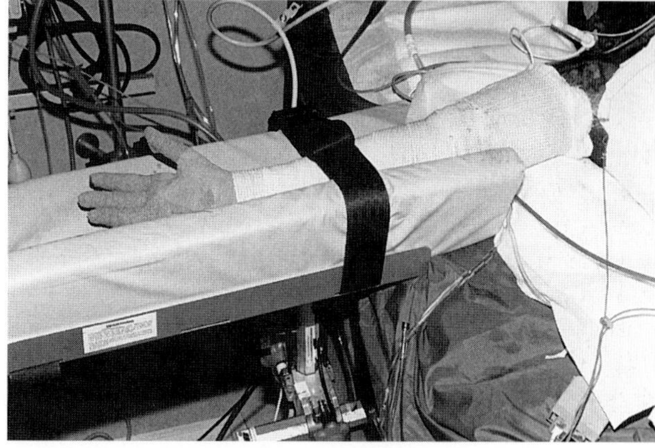

Figure 24.15 Positioning in bed of patient with burns of the axilla. *(From Richard and Staley,[4, p. 228] with permission.)*

patient is resting, or continuously for several days following skin grafting. Splints should conform to the body part, and care must be taken to ensure that there are no pressure points that may cause a breakdown in healing or normal skin. Splints should be checked routinely for proper fit and revised if necessary. Active motion is important, and splints and positioning are intended to serve as adjuncts to the therapy program until full active motion can be achieved.

Most splints used for burn injuries are static. This type of splint has no moveable parts, and maintains a position or immobilizes an area following skin grafting (Fig. 24.18). Static splints may be made from rigid materials with adjustable parts that allow modification to accommodate increases in ROM, termed static progressive splints. Dynamic splints also have been used successfully in the care of patients with a burn injury (Fig. 24.19).[123-125] These splints have moveable parts that allow joint movement. At the same time, dynamic splints apply a low-load, prolonged stress that can be adjusted to a patient's tolerance.

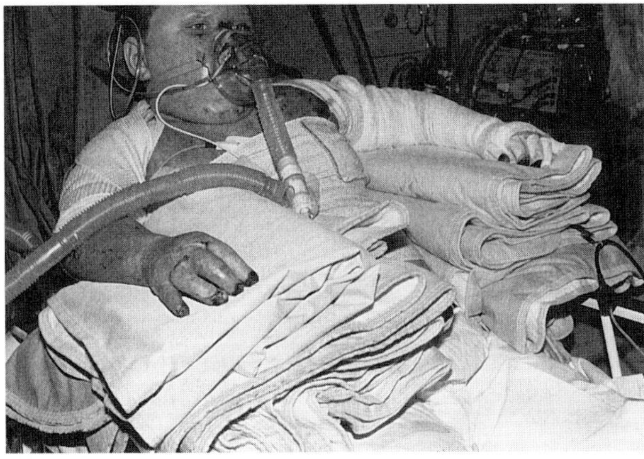

Figure 24.16 Proper positioning of upper extremities to reduce edema while seated. *(From Richard and Staley,[4, p. 231] with permission.)*

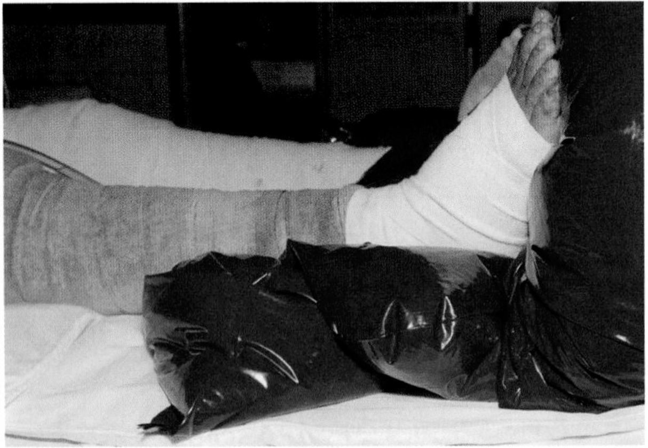

Figure 24.17 Positioning of feet with gel pads that help distribute pressure on the heels.

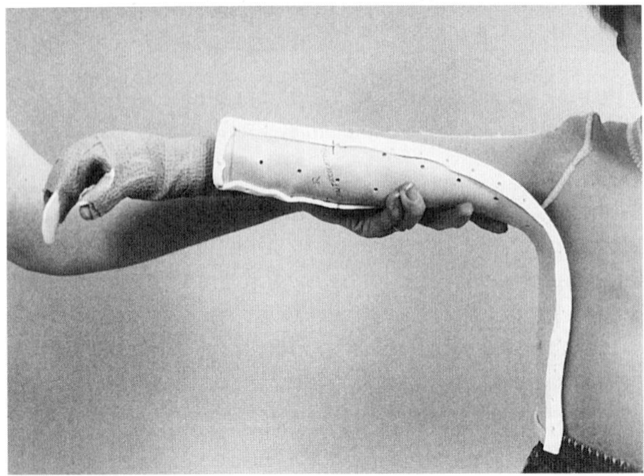

Figure 24.18 Static splint that immobilizes the shoulder in abduction and the elbow in extension.

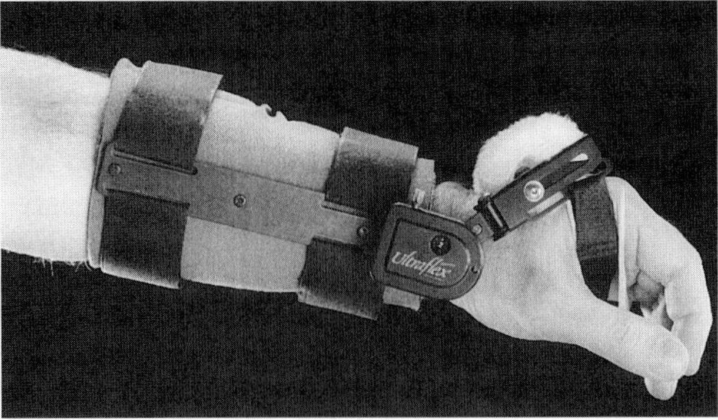

Figure 24.19 Dynamic splint used to provide a low-load, prolonged stress to scar tissue on volar aspect of forearm to gain wrist extension.

They offer great potential for correcting a developing contracture and the early return of active function in areas of extensive burn and grafting.[126] The use of continuous passive motion devices also is appropriate for certain patients with burn injuries.[127-131]

Therapeutic Exercise

Active and Passive Exercise

Active exercise begins on the day of admission.[5-7,80,132] Any patient who is alert and able to follow commands is encouraged to perform active exercises of involved body parts frequently throughout the day. A patient should perform active exercise of all extremities and trunk, including unburned areas. Dressing changes are an opportune time for exercise because the burn wound is visible and the therapist can monitor the wound during movement. In the presence of a recent skin graft, the timing of reintroduction of active and passive exercise of the area is variable, depending on surgeon protocol. However, initiating movement of the area as soon as possible is desirable. Once it is determined to be safe to begin exercise again, gentle ROM—first active and then passive, if needed—is reinstituted.[119,133,134]

Active-assistive and passive exercise should be initiated if a patient cannot fully achieve active ROM. To keep the healed burned area moist, it should be lubricated before exercise is initiated. Care should be taken around areas of skin grafts, and stress should be applied in a gentle, prolonged, and gradual fashion. If the burn wounds are well healed, heating modalities (e.g., paraffin, ultrasound) may be used to increase the pliability of the tissue before exercise therapy.[135,136,137]

Range of motion in the area of unhealed burns can be extremely painful, and patients may voice that they would rather lose their motion than be subjected to the additional pain that occurs with movement. It usually is difficult and mentally draining on the physical therapist to push patients to exercise in and through pain, but it is critical that the therapist be persistent. Coordinating exercise activities with the administration of pain medication can lessen the painful experience for the patient.[94,132] Physical therapists should elicit the assistance of the family and caregivers in keeping the patient motivated and mobile as much as possible.

Because limited ROM owing to scarring is among the most common impairments following a burn injury, it is important to understand how skin and scar development affect motion of adjacent joints. In recent years, a concept has been introduced called *cutaneous functional units* (CFUs).[97,98] CFUs identify fields of skin that contribute to functional ROM of an associated joint. For example, the identified CFU area involved in neck extension is the skin on the anterior torso. As the neck extends, skin is recruited as distal as the skin covering the pubic bone, in some individuals. When evaluating the source of ROM limitation and designing a POC, it is important to consider that CFUs associated with movement of a specific joint may extend some distance from the joint crease itself. In addition to the CFU area involved in a burn injury, percentage of the CFU area scarred, proximity of the scars to joint skin creases, and associated burn depth are also considerations in burn scar contracture development (Fig. 24.20). Research has indicated that CFUs are a better method than TBSA for determining rehabilitation outcomes.[99,100] Using CFUs, a computerized mapping system is used to quantify the number of potential BSC sites and provide an initial determination of the extent of burn involvement. In addition, adequate burn rehabilitation based on treatment time per CFU was found to be associated with preventing the development of BSC.[101,102]

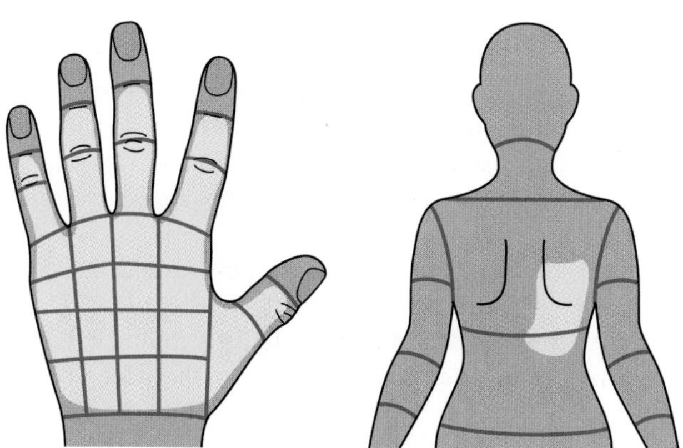

Figure 24.20 Comparison of the number of affected cutaneous functional units (CFUs) in burn injuries to the dorsal hand (*left*) and the posterior trunk (*right*). The area of burn injury is highlighted. The overlaid red skin mapping lines demarcate individual CFUs. Note that the burn injury to the hand involves multiple CFUs compared with only 2 CFUs on the posterior trunk. The more CFU's involved, the relative proximity of skin creases in the burned area, as well as the depth of injury are all associated with increased risk for development of burn scar contracture.

Resistive and Conditioning Exercise

Patients show a decline in physical fitness after burn injury which is linked to multiple factors including hypermetabolism, skeletal catabolism, and prolonged bedrest.[138] When compared with healthy individuals, those with a burn injury show decreased aerobic capacity,[139] lean body mass,[140] pulmonary function,[141] and strength.[142,143] As a patient continues to recover, the rehabilitation program should include strengthening and cardiovascular exercises.[5,80,144,145] Exercise may consist of isokinetic, isotonic, or other resistive training devices. General principles of exercise training and strength improvement should be followed, but they may need to be modified on the basis of a patient's condition and stage of wound healing. Resistive devices such as free weights and pulleys can be used to prevent loss of strength in areas not burned.

When a patient initially begins strengthening or conditioning (endurance) exercises, the physical therapist should monitor vital signs to assess cardiovascular and respiratory responses to treatment.[146] Overexertion may occur. Monitoring of pulse, blood pressure, and respiratory rate before, during, and after exercise, particularly in the recovery period after exercise, will yield valuable information about the status of the cardiovascular and pulmonary systems (see Chapter 2, Examination of Vital Signs).

Patients should be encouraged to participate in exercises that will stress the cardiovascular system, such as walking from the burn unit to the physical therapy department. Cycling or rowing ergometry, treadmill walking, stair climbing, and other forms of aerobic exercise should be encouraged and progressed throughout the stages of recovery. These activities will not only increase cardiovascular endurance but can also have the added benefit of improving strength and ROM of the extremities. Interactive video games have been used in the rehabilitation of patients with burns to increase activity, improve participation, and distract patients from pain.[147,148] In addition, such activities introduce variety into the rehabilitation program. The physical therapist needs to be creative and innovative to motivate patients to increase their exercise capacity.

Ambulation

Ambulation activities should be initiated as soon as possible after burn injury and/or skin graft surgery.[149-151] When ambulation is initiated after a skin graft, the LEs should be wrapped in elastic bandages in a figure-of-eight pattern to support the new grafts and promote venous return. If the upright position cannot be tolerated owing to orthostatic intolerance or LE pain from being in a dependent position, gradual increases in time and duration on a tilt-table will assist in preparation for standing.[152-154] Initially, a patient may require an assistive device to ambulate. However, independent ambulation without a device should be achieved as soon as possible.

The physical therapist will spend a great deal of time with an individual patient during each treatment session. The rewards of a successful POC are tremendous when a patient who has suffered a life-threatening burn is able to walk out of the hospital and return to productive community involvement.

Scar Management

Following wound closure, a skin graft or healed burn wound is vascular, flat, and soft. During the following 3 to 6 months, dramatic changes may occur. The newly healed areas may become raised and firm. Pressure has been used successfully to hasten scar maturation, minimize hypertrophic scar formation, and improve scar appearance.[155] Studies have shown that pressure can decrease scar thickness,[156] hardness,[157] height,[158] and erythema.[159] However, no one study validates the mechanism by which pressure alters scar tissue. Pressure may exert control over hypertrophic scarring by (1) thinning the dermis, (2) altering the biochemical structure of scar tissue, (3) decreasing blood flow to the area, (4) reorganizing collagen bundles, or (5) decreasing tissue water content. Constant pressure dressings or garments exerting pressure exceeding 25 mm Hg will decrease the vascularity, decrease the amount of mucopolysaccharides, decrease collagen deposition, and significantly lessen localized edema.[5,155,159] The early hypertrophic scar is readily influenced by compressive forces and thus will respond to pressure therapy. The earlier the scar tissue is exposed to pressure, the better the result.[160,161] Usually, if the scar is less than 6 months old, it will respond to pressure therapy by conforming to the pressure, remaining flat on the surface, and not developing into a hypertrophic scar.[140] If the scar is still active or shows evidence of vascularity (red color), pressure therapy may be successful, even if the scar is as much as a year old.

Practice guidelines for use of compression recommend pressure therapy be used prophylactically with wounds that take longer than 14 to 21 days to heal or those that have undergone grafting. Pressure should be applied (1) as soon as tolerated by the healing skin; (2) be worn 23 hours per day through scar maturation (removed for bathing); (3) be fitted by a trained professional; and (4) modified or replaced every 2 to 3 months or as needed.[162]

Pressure Dressings

Elastic wraps can be used to provide vascular support of skin grafts and donor sites, as well as to control edema and scarring. Elastic wraps should be used until a patient's skin or scars can tolerate the shearing force of pressure garment application, and open areas are minimal. Elastic wraps are applied in a figure-of-eight pattern on the LEs. A spiral wrap can be used on the upper extremities (UEs) and a circular wrap on the trunk.[155]

A self-adherent elastic bandage can be used for the hand and toes.[155,163,164] This bandage adheres only to itself and can be used over dressings before the wounds have healed. It helps to minimize edema and control scar formation. It may be used before application of a customized pressure glove or as definitive pressure on an infant's hand.

Tubular support bandages come in various circumferences and garment styles. They provide moderate compression and may be used as interim garments before a custom-made garment is fitted.[155,165] The tubular support bandage is especially useful for small children who grow rapidly and require frequent alterations in garment size.

Several companies manufacture pressure garments. Some are ready made and come in several sizes to fit most patients; others are custom made for the individual patient. For custom-made garments, the physical therapist uses a tape measure to determine the periodic circumference and linear length of each limb and trunk or face so fit of the garment is exact to apply proper pressure. Garments are measured when a patient has only a few remaining open areas. The garments are very tight, and difficult to apply, but the pressure is necessary to prevent scar hypertrophy. Garments can be ordered for any or all body parts, including the face and head, and they come in many styles, options, and colors (Fig. 24.21).[155] As mentioned, garments can be worn when the skin or scars can tolerate the shearing force of application. Pantyhose may be used under waist-height pressure garments to assist with donning. Garments should be washed daily to prevent buildup of perspiration and moisturizing cream, which may lead to scar maceration. The patient usually receives two sets of garments, one to wear and one to wash.

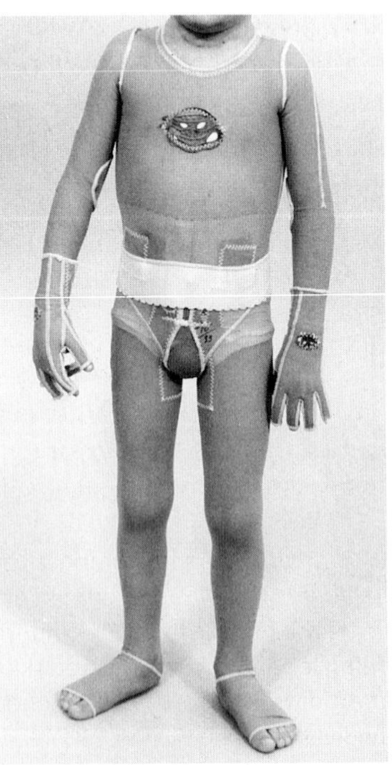

Figure 24.21 Pressure garments such as gloves, vest, and waist-height pants are worn to minimize hypertrophic scar formation.

Adequate pressure may not be obtained with elastic wraps or pressure garments over concave surfaces, such as the sternum or axilla. In these instances, an insert may be necessary.[165,166] Inserts can be made of many materials, including foam, silicone elastomer, elastomer putty, and gel pads.[155,166-170] These items also need to be removed and cleaned regularly to prevent maceration of the underlying tissue.

Early, consistent use of pressure will result in flat, pliable scars, desensitization and protection of scars, and relief of itching. Pressure is necessary until scar maturation, when the scars are pale, flat, and soft.

Silicone Gel

Silicone gel has demonstrated effectiveness in managing hypertrophic scars.[171-173] Available in a variety of sizes, application of silicone gels or gel sheets are recommended for immature burn scars at risk for hypertrophy (i.e., wounds that heal in greater than 21 days). Silicone gel sheets may be applied directly over an actively maturing scar.[174] The mechanism of action of this intervention is not well understood.[175] The only reported complication with silicone gel sheet use is a local rash with the potential, though rare, for skin breakdown. Rashes that develop are readily reversible by temporarily deferring the use of the gel sheet. Once the site is clear of the rash, the gel sheet can be reapplied.

Massage

Massage appears clinically useful in facilitating ROM exercise by increasing tissue pliability.[176] It requires relatively very few resources and can be used in a variety of settings. Deep friction massage is thought to loosen scar tissue by mobilizing cutaneous tissue from underlying tissue and acting to break up adhesions.[5,177] When massage is used in conjunction with ROM exercise, the immature scar can be elongated more easily, and a developing contracture can be corrected. Although no study has validated the effect of massage on burn scars,[178] in the long term, skin pliability and texture appear to be improved by its use. Studies have shown other benefits of massage for burn management such as decreased pain, itching, and anxiety.[179,180] Firm scars that are routinely massaged tend to soften. The edges or seams of grafts or any area that is raised and firm may benefit from massage. A video presentation of specific massage techniques for the individual with a burn is available online.[181]

Camouflage Make-Up

For scars of the face, neck, and hands, camouflage make-up can be used.[7,155] This type of make-up may be useful when a person has either hyperpigmentation or hypopigmentation of the skin due to the burn injury. In addition, make-up can be used before scar maturation, when the scar is still red, and a patient wants to go out in public without his or her pressure garments for short periods of time. The cosmetics are opaque, color-correct burn scars and are available in multiple shades to accommodate various skin colors. They also are waterproof and can be worn during all activities. These products can be purchased in larger department stores or where theatrical products are sold.

■ FOLLOW-UP CARE

Well before patients are discharged from the hospital, the therapist should provide information regarding a home exercise program (HEP), a splinting and positioning program, and skin care.

The HEP should stress frequent ROM exercises in combination with massaging areas involved in the burn injury. In addition, patients should be encouraged to perform as many ADL skills as possible independently. Therapists can film the patient's exercise program to provide the patient, family, and outpatient therapist with a visual of the actual ROM and movement patterns used in each exercise. Instructional programs facilitate education of those involved in the patient's rehabilitation program and will help to ensure consistency of treatment after discharge.[182]

The splinting schedule and pressure program that was followed in the hospital just before the patient's discharge should be continued at home. Before discharge, the patient and/or family members should be able to apply and remove all splints and pressure appliances independently.

Proper skin care requires specifying the type of soap and cream a patient is to use. In general, soap should be mild without perfumes or other irritants. A moisturizing soap can be used after all open areas are healed. Moisturizing creams should be applied 2 to 3 times daily and should not contain perfumes or have a significant alcohol content. Patients should be instructed to massage the cream completely into their skin to avoid buildup on the surface. If a patient will be unavoidably exposed to the sun, a sunscreen with a skin protection factor of at least 30 should be used and reapplied frequently.[183] Patients should be cautioned to avoid the sun and to use hats or clothing to help protect their skin against the sun's rays.

Small, superficial open areas may plague a patient for many months after wound closure because of the fragility of a healed burn wound. The patient should be instructed to wash these areas twice daily, apply a small amount of antibiotic ointment, and cover the areas with a nonadherent dressing. To help prevent further irritation or maceration, the patient should be cautioned to void shearing forces, improper fit of clothing, brisk cleansing, and soaking in water too long, or application of too much cream.

Itching may intensify when wounds have healed. A patient should be instructed to pat, rather than scratch, the irritated areas. Application of cream may help decrease itching; however, some patients may require oral antihistamine medication to help control this problem.

Some patients with burn injury may require outpatient therapy to supplement the HEP and monitor and adjust their splinting and pressure program. Frequency of outpatient therapy is based on each patient's needs. Regardless of whether a patient receives outpatient therapy, he or she should be monitored at regular intervals through an outpatient clinic. This will allow burn team members to evaluate adjustment back into society and alter the HEP or other management strategies according to the patient's physical abilities and extent of scar maturation. When an adult patient's burns have matured and full ROM has been achieved, further follow-up care is unnecessary. However, a child will need to be monitored until he or she is fully grown, because burn scars may not keep pace with a child's growth. In these cases, surgical release of scar tissue may be necessary.[184]

COMMUNITY PROGRAMS

There are various community programs available to individuals who have sustained a burn injury. The therapist should be aware of those in the patient's home community so an appropriate referral can be made. If programs are not available, someone in the hospital or community may consider initiating a program. Examples of community resources include the following:

- The American Burn Association (625 N. Michigan Ave., Chicago, IL 60611; 800-548-2876) provides access to a large variety of resources (e.g., educational materials, facts sheets, newsletters, meeting announcements).
- School Reentry Programs: Provided by the hospital staff for the students and staff in the child's school.[7,183]
- Burn Camps: Weekend- to week-long camps provide an opportunity for children to interact in a controlled, outdoor environment with peers who have sustained a similar injury.[7,182] The American Burn Association has a Burn Camp Special Interest Group with readily available information about camps throughout the United States and Canada.
- Adult Support Groups: Provide an opportunity for individuals with or without their families to share experiences and gain support from others who have had similar injuries.[182]
- Phoenix Society for Burn Survivors: This is a nonprofit organization dedicated to supporting burn survivors and families in recovery. The Phoenix Society offers many programs and resources that promote return to a meaningful life.[185]

Appendix 24.A includes web-based resources for patients, families, and clinicians.

SUMMARY

Specific impairments and complications from a burn injury vary based on the extent and depth of thermal destruction of the skin. The classification of burn injuries is based on the depth of tissue destroyed and includes epidermal burn, superficial partial-thickness burn, deep partial-thickness burn, full-thickness burn, and subdermal burn. The Rule of Nines[38] and the Lund and Browder[39] formula were developed to assist with the initial determination of the extent of burn injury. The specific clinical signs and symptoms vary based on burn classification. Indirect impairments can include infection, pulmonary, metabolic, skeletal, muscular, neurological, and cardiovascular and pulmonary complications. Medical management addresses life-threatening problems and stabilization of the patient. Dressings with topical medications, débridement, surgical excision, and skin grafting are primary treatment measures. Skin substitutes are slowly becoming a practical alternative to skin grafting.

Rehabilitation is an essential component of recovery for the patient with a burn.[186] Physical therapy management focuses on the prevention of scar contracture, maintenance of normal ROM, development of muscular strength and endurance, improvement of cardiovascular conditioning, independence in functional activities, and prevention of hypertrophic scarring. Although burn trauma and subsequent recovery can be a devastating life occurrence, there are treatment facilities and medical professional teams to assist patients with burn injuries and their families return to as normal a lifestyle as possible.

Questions for Review

1. Identify the two primary layers of skin and two functions of each.
2. Discuss the initial management of a patient with an acute burn injury.
3. Describe the differences between epidermal, superficial partial-thickness, deep partial-thickness, and full-thickness burns.

4. Explain how a deep partial-thickness burn can convert to a full-thickness burn.
5. Compare the treatments for deep partial-thickness and full-thickness burns.
6. Describe the primary involvement of the pulmonary system associated with extensive burns.
7. What is the primary metabolic complication associated with burns and how is it treated?
8. Identify and describe the three phases that occur in dermal healing of a burn wound.
9. Differentiate (a) between a split-thickness and full-thickness skin graft; and (b) between a sheet and a meshed skin graft.
10. Identify three essential factors for successful skin graft adherence.
11. For the patient with a burn injury, identify five general goals and outcomes that may be included in the physical therapy plan of care.
12. What interventions can be used to prevent (a) burn scar contractures and (b) hypertrophic scar formation?

CASE STUDY

A 29-year old male sustained a 30% total body surface area burn 6 weeks before this outpatient examination and evaluation. The patient was burned at home while he was refueling a lawnmower with gasoline, which ignited. Areas of the body affected by the burn include the right upper extremity, portions of the posterior and anterior trunk, lateral neck, right side of face, and thigh. Areas skin grafted included the right dorsal hand, forearm, and arm up to the axillary crease. The remaining wounds healed secondarily. The neck, face, and thigh burns were superficial. The patient was initially treated at a regional burn center and now is referred to the local hospital for follow-up outpatient physical therapy owing to decreased right elbow extension, decreased shoulder flexion, and inability to reach overhead. The right upper extremity lacks 15° of elbow extension (i.e., 15° to 120°) and flexion of the shoulder is limited to 0° to 155°. Scar contracture bands are noted at both locations at the end of available range with movement. The patient states that he has some difficulty donning shirts and his jacket. All other movements are within functional limits. The patient's strength overall is within functional limits. His wounds are all closed. The patient lives with his girlfriend and has medical benefits through his employer.

One week after his discharge from the hospital, the patient presented for his initial outpatient examination wearing interim pressure garments, as instructed. He also brought the static elbow splint that had been issued to him during his acute hospitalization, but which "doesn't fit right anymore." The expected outcome for this patient is to regain full right upper extremity range of motion and function.

GUIDING QUESTIONS

1. Describe how you would approach the clinical problems presented. Your answer should address positioning, splinting, exercise, and scar-management interventions.
2. Identify the impairments and activity limitations you will address in determining the prognosis and the plan of care.
3. Establish *general* goals (short term) and outcomes (long term) for this case. Develop one goal/outcome that will affect each of the following areas: *impairments, muscle performance, activity limitations,* and *risk reduction/prevention.*
4. Determine the prognosis.
5. Develop a plan of care. Your response should include specific interventions, patient instruction, and required coordination, communication, and/or documentation.
6. Describe the discharge plan.
7. What is the anticipated rehabilitation potential for this patient? Your thought process should include time from burn injury and stage of healing.

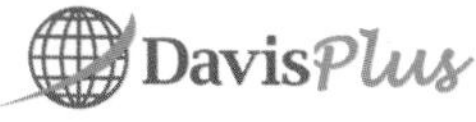

For additional resources, including answers to the questions for review and case study guiding questions, please visit **http://davisplus.fadavis.com.**

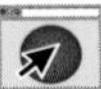
The reader is referred to video Case Study 2: Patient With Burns for additional review and study. The full written case study, including tables, figures, charts, and three video segments (examination, intervention, and outcome), appears online at Davis*Plus*. The case study poses questions for the reader's consideration with suggested answers to the case study questions, also posted online at Davis*Plus*.

References

1. American Burn Association: Burn Incidence and Treatment in the US: 2016 Fact Sheet. American Burn Association, Chicago, IL 60611. Retrieved January 25, 2017, from www.ameriburn.org/resources_factsheet.php.
2. Herndon, DN, and Blakeney, PE: Teamwork for total burn care: Achievements, directions, and hopes. In Herndon, DN (ed): Total Burn Care, ed 4. Saunders/Elsevier, Philadelphia, 2012, p 9.
3. Saffle, JR, et al: Recent outcomes in the treatment of burn injury in the United States: A report from the American Burn Association patient registry. J Burn Care Rehabil 16:219, 1995.
4. Richard, RL, and Staley, MJ (eds): Burn Care and Rehabilitation: Principles and Practice. FA Davis, Philadelphia, 1994.
5. Ward, RS: Physical rehabilitation. In Carrougher, GJ (ed): Burn Care and Therapy. Mosby, St. Louis, 1998, p 293.
6. Moore, ML, Palmgren, LA, and Yenne-Laker, CJ: The burn unit. In Campbell, SK, Palisano, RJ, and Orlin, MN (eds): Physical Therapy for Children, ed 4. Elsevier/Saunders, St. Louis, 2012, p 1008.
7. Migliore, SF: Rehabilitation of the child with burns. In Tecklin, JS (ed): Pediatric Physical Therapy, ed 4. Lippincott, Philadelphia, 2008, p 559.
8. Serghiou, MA, et al: Comprehensive rehabilitation of the burn patient. In Herndon, DN (ed): Total Burn Care, ed 4. Saunders/Elsevier, Philadelphia, 2012, p 517.
9. Pruitt, BA, Wolf, SE, and Mason, AD: Epidemiological, demographic, and outcome characteristics of burn injury. In Herndon, DN (ed): Total Burn Care, ed 4. Saunders/Elsevier, Philadelphia, 2012, p 14.
10. Baker, SP, et al: Fire, burns and lightning. In Baker, SP, et al: The Injury Fact Book, ed 2. Oxford University Press, New York, 1992, p 161.
11. Dissanaike, S, and Rahimi, M: Epidemiology of burn injuries: Highlighting cultural and socio-demographic aspects. Int Rev Psychiatry 21:505, 2009.
12. Guzel, A, et al: Scalds in pediatric emergency department: A 5-year experience. J Burn Care Res 30:450, 2009.
13. Shani, E, and Rosenberg, L: Are we making an impact? A review of a burn prevention program in Israeli schools. J Burn Care Rehabil 19:82, 1998.
14. Committee on Trauma: Guidelines for Operation of Burn Units. In Resources for Optimal Care of the Injured Patient. American College of Surgeons, Chicago, 2014, p 101.
15. American Burn Association: Burn Care Resource Directory. Retrieved January 31, 2017, from www.ameriburn.org/BCRDPublic.pdf.
16. Supple, KG, Fiala, SM, and Gamelli, RL: Preparation for burn center verification. J Burn Care Rehabil 18:58, 1997.
17. Holbrook, KA, and Wolff, K: The structure and development of skin. In Fitzpatrick, TB, et al (eds): Dermatology in General Medicine. McGraw-Hill, New York, 1993, p 97.
18. Lanir, Y: The fibrous structure of the skin and its relation to mechanical behavior. In Marks, R, and Payne, PA (eds): Bioengineering and the Skin. MIT Press, Cambridge, MA, 1981, p 93.
19. Moncrief, JA: The body's response to heat. In Artz, CP, et al (eds): Burns: A Team Approach. Saunders, Philadelphia, 1979, p 24.
20. Johnson, C: Pathologic manifestations of burn injury. In Richard, RL, and Staley, MJ (eds): Burn Care and Rehabilitation: Principles and Practice. FA Davis, Philadelphia, 1994, p 31.
21. *Guide to Physical Therapist Practice 3.0.* Alexandria, VA: American Physical Therapy Association; 2014. Available at: http://guidetoptpractice.apta.org/. Accessed April 18, 2017.
22. Norris, PG, et al: Acute effects of ultraviolet radiation on the skin. In Fitzpatrick, TB, et al (eds): Dermatology in General Medicine. McGraw-Hill, New York, 1993, p 1651.
23. Heggers, JP, et al: Evaluation of burn blister fluid. Plast Reconst Surg 65:798, 1980.
24. Rockwell, WB, and Ehrlich, HP: Fibrinolysis inhibition in human burn blister fluid. J Burn Care Rehabil 11:1, 1990.
25. Garner, WL, et al: The effects of burn blister fluid on keratinocyte replication and differentiation. J Burn Care Rehabil 14:127, 1993.
26. Ono, I, et al: A study of cytokines in burn blister fluid related to wound healing. Burns 21:352, 1995.
27. Richard, R, and Johnson, RM: Managing superficial burn wounds. Adv Skin Wound Care 15:246, 2002.
28. Hermans, MH: Results of an Internet survey on the treatment of partial-thickness burns, full-thickness burns, and donor sites. J Burn Care Res 28:835, 2007.
29. Lund, T, et al: Pathogenesis of edema formation in burn injuries. World J Surg 16:2, 1992.
30. Mozingo, DW: Surgical management. In Carrougher, GJ (ed): Burn Care and Therapy. Mosby, St. Louis, 1998, p 233.
31. Miller, SF, et al: Triage and resuscitation of the burn patient. In Richard, RL, and Staley, MJ (eds): Burn Care and Rehabilitation: Principles and Practice. FA Davis, Philadelphia, 1994, p 107.
32. Wittman, MI: Electrical and chemical burns. In Richard, RL, and Staley, MJ (eds): Burn Care and Rehabilitation: Principles and Practice. FA Davis, Philadelphia, 1994, p 603.
33. Fish, RM, and Geddes, LA: Conduction of electrical current to and through the human body: A review. Eplasty 12(9):e44, 2009.
34. Luz, DP, et al: Electrical burns: A retrospective analysis across a 5-year period. Burns 35:1015, 2009.
35. Jackson, DM: The diagnosis of the depth of burning. Br J Surg 40:588, 1953.
36. Lewis, ML, Heimbach, DM, and Gibran NS: Evaluation of the burn wound: management decisions. In Herndon, DN (ed): Total Burn Care, Ed 4. Saunders, Philadelphia, 2012, p 126.
37. Artz CP, Reiss E (Eds). The Treatment of Burns. WB Saunders, Philadelphia, 1957, p 9.
38. Wallace AB: The exposure treatment of burns. Lancet 1:501, 1951.
39. Lund, CC, and Browder, NC: Estimation of area of burns. Surg Gynecol Obstet 79:352, 1944.
40. Sheridan, RL, and Tompkins, RG: Etiology and prevention of multisystem organ failure. In Herndon, DN (ed): Total Burn Care, ed 4. Saunders/Elsevier, Philadelphia, 2012, p 361.
41. Gallagher, JJ, et al: Treatment of infection in burns. In Herndon, DN (ed): Total Burn Care, ed 4. Saunders/Elsevier, Philadelphia, 2012, p 137.
42. Robson, MC: Burn sepsis. Crit Care Clin 4:281, 1988.
43. Moylan, JA: Smoke inhalation and burn injury. Surg Clin North Am 60:1530, 1980.
44. Greenberg, MI, and Walter, J: Axioms on smoke inhalation. Hosp Med 19:13, 1983.
45. Chu, CS: New concepts of pulmonary burn injury. J Trauma 21:958, 1981.
46. Cioffi, WG: Inhalation injury. In Carrougher, GJ (ed): Burn Care and Therapy. Mosby, St. Louis, 1998, p 35.
47. McCall, JE, and Cahill, TJ: Respiratory care of the burn patient. J Burn Care Res 26:200, 2005.
48. Mancusi-Ungaro, HR, et al: Caloric and nitrogen balances as predictors of nutritional outcome in patients with burns. J Burn Care Rehabil 13:695, 1992.
49. Dickerson, RN, et al: Accuracy of predictive methods to estimate resting energy expenditure of thermally-injured patients. J Parenter Enteral Nutr 26:17, 2002.
50. Deitch, EA: Nutritional support of the burn patient. Crit Care Clin 11:735, 1995.
51. Demling, RH, and Seigne, P: Metabolic management of patients with severe burns. World J Surg 24:673, 2000.
52. Demling, RH, and DeSanti, L: Increased protein intake during the recovery phase after severe burns increases body weight gain and muscle function. J Burn Care Rehabil 19:161, 1998.

53. Wilmore, DW, et al: Effect of ambient temperature on heat production and heat loss in burn patients. J Appl Physiol 38: 593, 1975.
54. Prelack, K, et al: Energy and protein provisions for thermally injured children revisited: An outcome-based approach for determining requirements. Burn Care Rehabil 18:177, 1997.
55. Dominioni, L, et al: Enteral feeding in burn hypermetabolism: Nutritional and metabolic effects on different levels of calorie and protein intake. J Parenter Enteral Nutr 9:269, 1985.
56. Matsuda, T, et al: The importance of burn wound size in determining the optimal calorie: Nitrogen ratio. Surgery 94:562, 1983.
57. Lund, T, Onarheim, H, and Reed, RK: Pathogenesis of edema formation in burn patients. World J Surg 16:2, 1992.
58. Latenser, BA: Critical care of the burn patient: The first 48 hours. Crit Care Med 37:2819, 2009.
59. Demling, RH, et al: The study of burn wound edema using dichromatic absorptiometry. J Trauma 18:124, 1978.
60. Kramer, GC: Pathophysiology of burn shock and burn edema. In Herndon, DN (ed): Total Burn Care, ed 4. Saunders/Elsevier, Philadelphia, 2012, p 103.
61. Alvarado, R, et al: Burn resuscitation. Burns 35:4, 2009.
62. Gordon, MD, and Winfree, JH: Fluid resuscitation after a major burn. In Carrougher, GJ (ed): Burn Care and Therapy. Mosby, St. Louis, 1998, p 107.
63. Medina, A, et al: Characterization of heterotopic ossification in burn patients. J Burn Care Res 35:251, 2014.
64. Levi, B, et al: Risk factors for the development of heterotopic ossification in seriously burned adults. J Trauma Acute Care Surg 79:870, 2015.
65. Orchard, GR, et al: Risk factors in hospitalized patient with burn injuries for developing heterotopic ossification: A retrospective analysis. J Burn Care Res 36:465, 2014.
66. Chen, HC, et al: Heterotopic ossification in burns: Our experience and literature reviews. Burns 35:857, 2009.
67. Ramirez, DM, et al: Molecular and cellular mechanisms of heterotopic ossification. Histo Histopathol 29:1281, 2014.
68. Schneider, JC, et al: Predicting heterotopic ossification early after burn injuries: A risk scoring system. Ann Surg Jun 24. [Epub ahead of print], 2016.
69. Kowalske K, Holavanahalli R, Helm P: Neuropathy after burn injury. J Burn Care Rehab 22:353, 2001.
70. Tamam Y, et al: Peripheral neuropahy after burn injury. Eur Rev Med Pharmacol Sci 17 (Suppl 1):107, 2013.
71. Ladin, DA, Garner, WL, and Smith, DJ: Excessive scarring as a consequence of healing. Wound Repair Regen 3:(1)6, 1995.
72. Armour, A, Scott, PG, and Tredget, EE: Cellular and molecular pathology of HTS: Basis for treatment. Wound Repair Regen 15(Suppl 1):S6–S17, 2007.
73. Greenhalgh, DG, and Staley, MJ: Burn wound healing. In Richard, RL, and Staley, MJ (eds): Burn Care and Rehabilitation: Principles and Practice. FA Davis, Philadelphia, 1994, p 70.
74. Arem, AJ, and Madden, JW: Is there a Wolff's law for connective tissue? Surg Forum 25:512, 1974.
75. Schneider, JC, et al: Contractures in burn injury: Defining the problem. J Burn Care Res 27:(4)508, 2006.
76. Saffle, JR, et al: Recent outcomes in the treatment of burn injury in the United States: A report from the American Burn Association patient registry. J Burn Care Rehabil 16:219, 1995.
77. Warden, GD: Fluid resuscitation and early management. In Herndon, DN (ed): Total Burn Care, ed 4. Saunders/Elsevier, Philadelphia, 2012, p 115.
78. Hayek, S, El Khatib, A, Atiyeh, B: Burn wound cleansing: A myth or a scientific practice. Ann Burns Fire Disasters 31:19, 2010. https://www.ncbi.nlm.nih.gov/pubmed/?term=burn+wound+cleansing+and+shower.
79. American Physical Therapy Association: Choosing wisely: Five things physical therapists and patients should question, 2014 (updated 2015). Retrieved March 9, 2017, from http://www.choosingwisely.org/societies/american-physical-therapy-association/.
80. Ward, RS: The rehabilitation of burn patients. Crit Rev Phys Rehabil Med 2:121, 1991.
81. Mosier, MJ, and Gibran, NS: Surgical excision of the burn wound. Clin Plast Surg 36:617, 2009.
82. Lee, JO, et al: Operative wound management. In Herndon, DN (ed): Total Burn Care, ed 4. Saunders/Elsevier, Philadelphia, 2012, p 157.
83. Cuono, C, et al: Use of cultured epidermal autografts and dermal allografts as skin replacement after burn injury. Lancet 8490: 1123, 1986.
84. Munster, AM: Cultured epidermal autographs in the management of burn patients. J Burn Care Rehabil 13:121, 1992.
85. Sheridan, R: Closure of the excised burn wound: Autografts, semipermanet skin substitutes, and permanent skin substitutes. Clin Plast Surg 36:643, 2009.
86. Chern, PL, Baum, CL, and Arpey, CJ: Biologic dressings: Current applications and limitations in dermatologic surgery. Dermatol Surg 35:891, 2009.
87. Fohn, M, and Bannasch, H: Artificial skin. Methods Mol Med 140:167, 2007.
88. Hansbrough, J, et al: Clinical trials of a biosynthetic temporary skin replacement, Dermagraft-Transitional Covering, compared with cryopreserved human cadaver skin for temporary coverage of excised burn wounds. J Burn Care Rehabil 18:43, 1997.
89. Purdue, G, et al: A multicenter clinical trial of a biosynthetic skin replacement, Dermagraft-TC, compared with cryopreserved human cadaver skin for temporary coverage of excised burn wounds. J Burn Care Rehabil 18:52, 1997.
90. Heimbach, D, et al: Artificial dermis for major burns: A multicenter, randomized clinical trial. Ann Surg 208:313, 1988.
91. Lattari, V, et al: The use of a permanent dermal allograft in full-thickness burns of the hand and foot: A report of three cases. J Burn Care Rehabil 18:147, 1997.
92. Richard, R, et al: A comparison of the Tanner and Bioplasty skin mesher systems for maximal skin graft expansion. J Burn Care Rehabil 14:690, 1993.
93. Larson, D, et al: Prevention and treatment of burn scar contracture. In Artz, CP, et al (eds): Burns: A Team Approach. Saunders, Philadelphia, 1979, p 466.
94. Greenhalgh, DG, et al: The early release of axillary contractures in pediatric patients with burns. J Burn Care Rehabil 14:39, 1993.
95. Wainwright, DJ: Burn reconstruction: The problems, the techniques, and the applications. Clin Plast Surg 36:(4)687, 2009.
96. Richard, RL, and Staley, MJ: Burn patient evaluation and treatment planning. In Richard, RL, and Staley, MJ (eds): Burn Care and Rehabilitation: Principles and Practice. FA Davis, Philadelphia, 1994, p 201.
97. Richard RL, et al: Identification of cutaneous functional units related to burn scar contracture development. J Burn Care Res 30(4):625, 2009.
98. Richard R, Jones J, Parshley P. Hierarchical decomposition of burn body diagram based on cutaneous functional units and its utility. J Burn Care Res 36(1):33, 2015.
99. Richard R, et al: Cutaneous functional units relate better than total body surface area to burn patient outcomes. J Burn Care Res 35:S77, 2014.
100. Parry IS, et al: Cutaneous functional units predict range of motion recovery with therapy. J Burn Care Res 37:S120, 2016.
101. Richard R, et al: Increased burn rehabilitation treatment time improves patient outcomes. J Burn Care Res 35:S100, 2014.
102. Richard RL, et al: Small and large burns alike benefit from lengthier rehabilitation time. J Burn Care Res 36:S108, 2015.
103. Standard of Care: Inpatient Physical Therapy Management of Patients with Burns. Brigham and Women's Hospital, Department of Rehabilitation Services, 2008. Retrieved April 18, 2017, from http://www.brighamandwomens.org/App_GlobalFiles/search.aspx?db=bwhdb&st=0&site=BWH_CI&q=Inpatient%20Physical%20Therapy%20Management%20of%20Patients%20with%20Burns.
104. Richard, RL, et al.: A clarion to recommit and reaffirm burn rehabilitation. J Burn Care Res 29(3):425, 2008.
105. Moss, BF, et al: Psychologic support and pain management of the burn patient. In Richard, RL, and Staley, MJ (eds): Burn Care and Rehabilitation: Principles and Practice. FA Davis, Philadelphia, 1994, p 475.
106. Adcock, RJ, et al: Psychologic and emotional recovery. In Carrougher, GJ (ed): Burn Care and Therapy. Mosby, St. Louis, 1998, p 329.
107. Wiechman, SA, and Patterson, DR: Psychosocial aspects of burn injuries. BMJ 329(7462):391, 2004.
108. Steed, DL: Wound-healing trajectories. Surg Clin North Am 83:(3)47, 2003.

109. McHugh, AA, et al: Biomechanical alterations in normal skin and hypertrophic scar after thermal injury. J Burn Care Rehabil 18:104, 1997.
110. Li, B, and Wang, JH: Fibroblasts and myofibroblasts in wound healing: Force generation and measurement. J Tissue Viability 20:(4)108, 2011.
111. Nedelec, B, et al: Control of wound contraction: Basic and clinical features. Hand Clin 16:289, 2000.
112. Goverman, J et al: Adult contractures in burn injury: A burn model system national database study. J Burn Care Res 38: p e328, 2017.
113. Saaiq M, Zaib, S, and Ahmad, S: The menace of post-burn contractures: A developing country's perspective. Ann Burns Fire Disasters 25:152, 2012.
114. Parry, I, and Esselman, P: Clinical competencies for burn rehabilitation therapists. J Burn Care Res 32:458, 2011.
115. Parry, I, et al: Burn Rehabilitation Therapists Competency Tool – Version 2: An expansion to Include Long-term rehabilitation and outpatient care. J Burn Care Res 38:e261, 2017.
116. Serghiou M, et al: Clinical practice recommendations for positioning of the burn patient. Burns 42:267, 2016.
117. Serghiou, M, Cowan, A, and Whitehead, C: Rehabilitation after a burn injury. Clin Plast Surg 36:675, 2009.
118. Parry, I: Physical Rehabilitation. In Greenhalgh, D. (ed): Burn Care for General Surgeons and General Practitioners. Springer, Switzerland, 2016, p 137.
119. Plaza, A, et al: Exercise and mobility after burn injury. In Edgar, D (ed): Burn Trauma Rehabilitation: Allied Health Practice Guidelines. Lippincott Williams & Wilkins, Philadelphia, 2014, p 108.
120. Daugherty, M, and Carr-Collins, J: Splinting techniques for the burn patient. In Richard, RL, and Staley, MJ (eds): Burn Care and Rehabilitation: Principles and Practice. FA Davis, Philadelphia, 1994, p 242.
121. Richard, R, and Ward, RS. Splinting strategies and controversies. J Burn Care Rehabil 26:392–396, 2005.
122. Kwan, M, and Ha, K: Splinting programme for patients with burnt hand. Hand Surg 7:231–241, 2002.
123. Richard, RL: Use of Dynasplint to correct elbow flexion burn contracture: A case report. J Burn Care Rehabil 7:151, 1986.
124. Richard, R, and Staley, M: Dynamic splinting: Basic science + modern technology. Phys Ther Forum 11:21, 1992.
125. Richard, RL, et al: Dynamic versus static splints: A prospective case for sustained stress. J Burn Care Rehabil 16:284, 1995.
126. Richard, R, et al: Multimodal versus progressive treatment techniques to correct burn scar contractures. J Burn Care Rehabil 21:506, 2000.
127. Covey, MH, et al: Efficacy of continuous passive motion (CPM) devices with hand burns. J Burn Care Rehabil 9: 397, 1988.
128. McAllister, LP, and Salazar, CA: Case report on the use of CPM on an electrical burn. J Burn Care Rehabil 9:401, 1988.
129. McGough, CE: Introduction to CPM. J Burn Care Rehabil 9:494, 1988.
130. Covey, MH: Application of CPM devices with burn patients. J Burn Care Rehabil 9:496, 1988.
131. Richard, RL, et al: The physiologic response of a patient with critical burns to continuous passive motion. J Burn Care Rehabil 11:554, 1990.
132. Humphrey, C, et al: Soft tissue management and exercise. In Richard, RL, and Staley, MJ (eds): Burn Care and Rehabilitation: Principles and Practice. FA Davis, Philadelphia, 1994, p 324.
133. Richard, RL, et al: Comparison of the effect of passive exercise v static wrapping on finger range of motion in the burned hand. J Burn Care Rehabil 8(6):576, 1987.
134. Edstrom, LE, et al: Prospective randomized treatments for burned hands: Nonoperative vs. operative. Preliminary report. Scand J Plast Reconstr Surg 13(1):131, 1979.
136. Ward, RS: The use of physical agents in burn care. In Richard, RL, and Staley, MJ (eds): Burn Care and Rehabilitation: Principles and Practice. FA Davis, Philadelphia, 1994, p 419.
137. Ward, RS, et al: Evaluation of therapeutic ultrasound to improve response to physical therapy and lessen scar contracture after burn injury. J Burn Care Rehabil 15:74, 1994.
138. Hart, DW, et al: Presence of muscle catabolism after severe burn. Surgery 128:312, 2000.
139. Ganio, MS, et al: Aerobic fitness is disproportionately low in adult burn survivors years after injury. J Burn Care Res 36(4): 513, 2015.
140. Przkor, R, Herdon, DN, Suman, OE. The effects of oxandrolone and exercise on muscle mass and function in children with severe burn. Pediatrics 119:e109, 2007.
141. Willis CE, et al: Pulmonary function, aerobic capacity and physical activity participation in adults following burns. Burns 37:1326, 2011.
142. Ebid, AA, Omar, MT, and El Baky, AM: Effect of a 12-week isokinetic training on muscle strength in adults with healed thermal burns. Burns 38(1):61, 2012.
143. Alloju, SM, et al: Assessment of muscle function in severely burned children. Burns 34:452, 2008.
144. St-Pierre, DMM, et al: Muscle strength in individuals with healed burns. Arch Phys Med Rehabil 79:155–161, 1998.
145. Nedelec, B, et al: Practice guidelines for cardiovascular fitness and strengthening exercise prescription after burn injury. J Burn Care Res 37:e539, 2016.
146. Black, S, et al: Oxygen consumption for lower extremity exercises in normal subjects and burn patients. Phys Ther 60:1255, 1980.
147. Yohannan, SK, et al: The utilization of Nintendo Wii during burn rehabilitation: A pilot study. J of Burn Care Res 33:36, 2012.
148. Parry, I, et al: A pilot prospective randomized control trial comparing exercises using videogame therapy to standard physical therapy: 6 months follow up. J Burn Care Res 36:534, 2015.
149. Nedelec, B, et al: Practice guidelines for early ambulation of burn survivors after lower extremity grafts. J Burn Care Res 33:319, 2012.
150. Deng H, Chen J, Li F et al. Effects of mobility training on severe burn patients in the BICU: A retrospective cohort study. Burns 42:1404, 2016.
151. Lorello, D, et al. Results of a prospective randomized controlled trial of early ambulation for patients with lower extremity autografts. J Burn Care Res 35:431, 2014.
152. Temmen, HJ, et al: Tilt table exercise guidelines for burn patients: Are cardiac exercise parameters appropriate? Proc Am Burn Assoc 30:221, 1998.
153. Boyea, BL, et al: Use of the tilt table for postural reconditioning of burn patients prior to ambulation. Proc Am Burn Assoc 30:233, 1998.
154. Trees, DW, Ketelsen, CA, and Hobbs, JA: Use of a modified tilt table for preambulation strength training as an adjunct to burn rehabilitation: A case series. J Burn Care Rehabil 24:97, 2003.
155. Staley, MJ, and Richard, RL: Scar management. In Richard, RL, and Staley, MJ (eds): Burn Care and Rehabilitation: Principles and Practice. FA Davis, Philadelphia, 1994, p 380.
156. Engrav, LH, et al: 12 year within-wound study of the effectiveness of custom pressure garment therapy. Burns 36:975, 2010.
157. Van den Kerckhove, E, et al: The assessment of erythema and thickness on burn related scars during pressure garment therapy as a preventive measure for hypertrophic scarring. Burns 31: 696, 2015.
158. Candy, LH, Cecilia, LT, Ping, ZY. Effect of different pressure magnitudes on hypertrophic scar in a Chinese population. Burns 36:1234, 2010.
159. Johnson, CL: Physical therapists as scar modifiers. Phys Ther 64:1381, 1984.
160. Kischer, CW, and Shetlar, MR: Microvasculature in hypertrophic scars and the effects of pressure. J Trauma 19:757, 1979.
161. Leung, PC, and Ng, M: Pressure treatment for hypertrophic scars. Burns 6:224, 1980.
162. Sharp, P, et al: Development of a best evidence statement for the use of pressure therapy for management of hypertrophic scarring. J Burn Care Res 37:255, 2016.
163. Ward, RS, et al: Use of Coban self-adherent wrap in management of postburn hand grafts: Case reports. J Burn Care Rehabil 15:364, 1994.
164. Lowell, M, et al: Effect of 3M™ Coban™ self-adherent wraps on edema and function of the burned hand: A case study. J Burn Care Rehabil 24:253, 2003.
165. Kealey, GP, et al: Prospective randomized comparison of two types of pressure therapy garments. J Burn Care Rehabil 11:334, 1990.

166. Cheng, JCY, et al: Pressure therapy in the treatment of post-burn hypertrophic scar: A critical look into its usefulness and fallacies by pressure monitoring. Burns 10:154, 1984.
167. Mann, R, et al: Do custom-fitted pressure garments provide adequate pressure? J Burn Care Rehabil 18(3):247, 1997.
168. Alston, DW, et al: Materials for pressure inserts in the control of hypertrophic scar tissue. J Burn Care Rehabil 2:40, 1981.
169. Moore, ML, et al: Effectiveness of custom pressure garments in wound management: A prospective trial within wounds and with verified pressure. J Burn Care Rehabil 21:S177, 2000.
170. Perkins, K, et al: Current materials and techniques used in a burn scar management programme. Burns 13:406, 1987.
171. van der Wal, MB, et al: Topical silicone gel versus placebo in promoting the maturation of burn scars: A randomized controlled trial. Plast Reconstr Surg 126(2):524, 2010.
172. Momeni, M, et al: Effects of silicone gel on burn scars. Burns 35(1):70, 2009.
173. O'Brien, L, and Pandit, A: Silicon gel sheeting for preventing and treating hypertrophic and keloid scars. Cochrane Database Syst Rev CD003826, 2006.
174. Nedelec, B, et al: Practice guidelines for the application of nonsilicone or silicone gels and gel sheets after burn injury. J Burn Care Res 36:345, 2015.
175. Berman, B, et al: A review of the biologic effects, clinical efficacy, and safety of silicone elastomer sheeting for hypertrophic and keloid scar treatment and management. Dermatol Surg 33:1291, 2007.
176. Silverberg, R, Johnson, J, Moffat, M. The effects of soft tissue mobilization on the immature burn scar: Results of a pilot study. J Burn Care Rehabil 17:252, 1996.
177. Miles, WK, and Grigsby, L: Remodeling of scar tissue in the burned hand. In Hunter, JM, et al (eds): Rehabilitation of the Hand. Mosby, St. Louis, 1984, p 841.
178. Patino, O, and Novick, C: Massage on hypertrophic scars. J Burn Care Rehabil 20:268, 1999.
179. Field, T, et al: Postburn itching, pain and psychological symptoms are reduced with massage therapy. J Burn Care Rehabil 21:189, 2000.
180. Gurol, AP, et al: Itching, pain and anxiety levels are reduced with massage therapy in burned adolescents. J Burn Care Res 31:429, 2010.
181. Parry, I, et al: Defining Massage techniques used for burn scars. J Burn Care Res online. Retrieved March 9, 2017, from http://journals.lww.com/burncareresearch/pages/videogallery.aspx?videoId=5&autoPlay=false.
182. Gallagher, J, et al: Discharge videotaping: A means of augmenting occupational and physical therapy. J Burn Care Rehabil 11:470, 1990.
183. Braddom, RL, et al: The physical treatment and rehabilitation of burn patients. In Hummel, RP (ed): Clinical Burn Therapy. John Wright PSG, Boston, 1982, p 297.
184. Lehman, CJ, Ricks, N: Discharge planning and follow up burn care. In Richard, RL and Staley, MJ (eds): Burn Care and Rehabilitation: Principles and Practice. FA Davis, Philadelphia, 1994, p 447.
185. Phoenix Society for Burn Survivors: Phoenix Society Programs. Grand Rapids, MI, Retrieved March 9, 2017, from www.phoenix-society.org/programs/.
186. Richard, R, et al: Burn rehabilitation and research: proceedings of a consensus summit. J Burn Care Res 30:543, 2009.

Supplemental Readings

Alp, E, et al: Risk factors for nosocomial infection and mortality in burn patients: 10 years of experience at a university hospital. J Burn Care Res 33(3):379, 2012.
Chipp, E, Milner, CS, and Blackburn, AV: Sepsis in burns: A review of current practice and future therapies. Ann Plast Surg 65(2):228, 2010.
Herndon, DN (ed): Total Burn Care, ed 4. Saunders/Elsevier, Philadelphia, 2012.
Hyakusoku, H, et al (eds): Color Atlas of Burn Reconstructive Surgery. Springer-Verlag, New York, 2010.
Maslow, GR, and Lobato, D: Summer camps for children with burn injuries: A literature review. J Burn Care Res 31(5):740, 2010.
Mason, ST, et al: Return to work after burn injury: A systematic review. J Burn Care Res 33(1):101, 2012.
Patil, V, et al: Do burn patients cost more? The intensive care unit costs of burn patients compared with controls matched for length of stay and acuity. J Burn Care Res 31(4):598, 2010.
Willebrand, M, and Kildal, M: Burn specific health up to 24 months after the burn—a prospective validation of the Simplified Model of the Burn Specific Health Scale—Brief. J Trauma 71(1):78, 2011.

appendix

24.A Web-Based Resources for Patients, Families, and Clinicians

Website Description	Web Address
American Burn Association: National organization site for burn care in the United States	www.ameriburn.org
Burn Therapist.com: Informational site for therapists describing current events and description of selected splints and treatment interventions	www.burntherapist.com
Phoenix Society (for burn survivors): Burn support information for patients and families	www.phoenix-society.org

Chronic Pain

Leslie N. Russek, PT, DPT, PhD, OCS

Chapter 25

LEARNING OBJECTIVES

1. Assess the impact of chronic pain on individuals and society.
2. Clarify terminology associated with nociception, pain, and chronic pain.
3. Compare and contrast nociceptive and neuropathic pain and central sensitization.
4. Apply the International Classification of Functioning, Disability, and Health (ICF) model to chronic pain.
5. Explain the pathophysiological processes underlying chronic pain, including immune, endocrine, and autonomic system involvement and neuroplastic changes that occur.
6. Propose risk factors associated with chronic pain.
7. Describe methods for obtaining a thorough, biopsychosocial history from patients.
8. Contrast various outcome measures for examining chronic pain and its impact on activity and participation.
9. Describe tests and measures appropriate for examining individuals with chronic pain.
10. Relate examination findings to evaluation and prognosis for individuals with chronic pain.
11. Describe appropriate physical therapy interventions for individuals with chronic pain.
12. Summarize medical management of chronic pain.
13. Discuss complementary and alternative medicine approaches to managing chronic pain.

CHAPTER OUTLINE

Pain is the most common reason why people visit health care providers and physical therapists. *Chronic pain* affects from 25[1] to 116 million Americans,[2,3] accounting for up to 20% of all primary care visits in the United States;[4,5] low back pain (LBP) is the second most common reason for physician visits.[6] Chronic pain affects more people than diabetes, heart disease, and cancer combined.[3] Studies show that 36.6% of American adults have reported being often troubled by pain, and one-third of those report that this pain is disabling.[7,8] Chronic pain is more prevalent among women and people with lower socioeconomic status.[1,8] Spinal pain, headache, and arthritis are the most common types of chronic pain: LBP affects 28%, headache and migraine affect 16%, neck pain affects 15%, and combined peripheral joint pain affects 30% of Americans.[5,9] Other conditions such as stroke, spinal cord injury (SCI), diabetes, multiple sclerosis (MS), HIV/AIDS, amputation, Parkinson's disease, cancer, chemotherapy or radiation for cancer, and a variety of other conditions can also lead to chronic pain.[10]

Chronic pain exacts a huge toll in medical care, lost workdays, and compromised quality of life. In the United States, the national economic cost of chronic pain is estimated at $560 billion to $635 billion per year with $261 billion to $386 billion per year of that due to direct medical costs.[2,11] Lost productivity due to pain costs $297 billion to $336 billion per year.[2] Quality of life is severely compromised for people with chronic pain, often rated even lower than among people dying of cancer.[12]

This chapter will focus on chronic pain most likely to present for physical therapy intervention. It is not the goal of this chapter to address cancer or visceral pain, even though those are growing specialty areas within physical therapy. Recent advances in pain physiology are presented as a foundation for understanding common chronic pain conditions and the appropriate interventions for those conditions.

PAIN TERMINOLOGY AND BASIC CONCEPTS

Pain is defined as an unpleasant sensory and emotional experience associated with actual or potential tissue damage, or described in terms of such damage.[13] Pain is not just the firing of **nociceptive** neurons, but is an interaction among internal and external stimuli, context, and emotional and social factors.[14] An analogy would be that some people perceive spicy food as unpleasant or even painful, while others perceive it as delicious; interpretation depends in part on internal stimuli (physical sensations, cognitive and emotional factors) and external stimuli (e.g., social factors and context).[15] The experience of pain reflects a perception of danger, and the need for protection.[16] Tissue threat/damage and nociception, while sometimes associated with pain, are neither necessary nor sufficient for an individual to experience pain.[17]

Additional pain terminology relates to ways in which pain is classified or described. This section will briefly present classification terminology, and the physiology will be explained in later sections. See Box 25.1.[13,18-22] The type of pain can be described as nociceptive, inflammatory, neuropathic (peripheral or central), or central sensitization/maladaptive. Clinical states usually involve a combination of several types of pain. *Nociceptive pain* is associated with activation of primary nociceptors through noxious stimulation (mechanical, thermal, or chemical), or through non-noxious stimuli in the presence of inflammation; nociceptive pain typically signals impending tissue damage or danger. Nociceptive pain typically leads to a protective withdrawal response and is therefore beneficial.[23,24] Nociceptive pain may be transient, recurrent, or persistent. For example, transient pain may occur after a shoulder subluxation, while recurrent pain may occur after repeated subluxations, and persistent pain may occur in the case of osteoarthritis (OA). Because neural connective tissue is innervated by nociceptors (nervi nervorum), neural connective tissue may also generate nociceptive pain, which tends to be deep, aching, and localized with discomfort generally proportional to stimulus.[25,26] Muscle pain is sometimes also considered a distinct type of nociceptive pain; differences between superficial and deep pain will be discussed later in this chapter.[27]

Some sources distinguish *inflammatory pain* as different from other nociceptive pain because nociceptors are not only activated but may be sensitized by local or systemic inflammatory mediators, and low-threshold stimuli that are normally non-painful may become painful.[10,27-29] The current discussion will treat inflammation as a modulator of nociception, neuropathic pain, and central pain.[28,30]

Peripheral neuropathic/neurogenic pain is defined as pain caused by a lesion or disease of somatosensory nerves.[13] Peripheral neuropathic pain can occur in response to diseases (e.g., diabetes, herpes zoster, HIV infection), medical interventions (e.g., chemotherapy, surgery), or traumatic or overuse injuries (e.g., carpal tunnel, brachial plexus avulsion, herniated disc).[31] It can also occur spontaneously (i.e., with no known peripheral tissue damage or threat) or in response to normally innocuous stimuli. When axons are involved, symptoms can also include hypoesthesia, anesthesia, paresthesia, or dysesthesia such as burning, prickling, tingling, searing, or crawling sensations in the innervation pattern of the nerve.[25,28] Although the terms

Box 25.1 Pain Terminology[13,18-20,22,27,28,42,45]

- **Acute pain**: Pain associated with tissue damage or the threat of such damage and typically resolves once the tissue heals or the threat resolves; often nociceptive-dominant.
- **Adjuvant medication**: Medications whose primary indication is a condition other than pain, but which have demonstrated benefit in pain management.
- **Allodynia**: Pain due to a stimulus that does not normally provoke pain.
- **Analgesia**: Absence of pain in response to stimulation that would normally be painful.

Box 25.1 Pain Terminology[13,18-20,22,27,28,42,45]—cont'd

- **Causalgia**: A syndrome of sustained burning pain, allodynia, and hyperpathia after a traumatic nerve lesion, often combined with vasomotor and sudomotor dysfunction and later trophic changes.
- **Central neuropathic pain**: Pain initiated or caused by a primary lesion or dysfunction in the CNS.
- **Central sensitization**: Increased responsiveness of nociceptive neurons in the CNS to their normal or subthreshold afferent input.
- **Chronic pain**: Pain that persists past the healing phase following an injury; impairment is greater than anticipated based on the physical findings or injury and it occurs in the absence of observed tissue injury or damage.
- **Chronic pain syndrome**: Pain that exists when individuals have developed extensive pain behaviors such as preoccupation with pain, passive approach to health care, significant life disruption, feelings of isolation, demanding, angry, or doctor-shopping.
- **Dysesthesia**: An unpleasant abnormal sensation, whether spontaneous or evoked.
- **Hyperalgesia**: Increased pain from a stimulus that normally provokes pain. Hyperalgesia reflects increased pain on suprathreshold stimulation.[13] Primary hyperalgesia refers to increased sensitivity in the area of tissue damage. Secondary hyperalgesia refers to increased pain sensitivity in areas that were not involved in the initial tissue trauma—either surrounding areas or referral patterns.
- **Hyperesthesia**: Increased sensitivity to stimulation, excluding the special senses. Allodynia is suggested for pain after stimulation that is not normally painful. Hyperesthesia includes both allodynia and hyperalgesia, but the more specific terms should be used wherever they are applicable.
- **Hyperpathia**: A painful syndrome characterized by an abnormally painful reaction to a stimulus, especially a repetitive stimulus, as well as an increased threshold.
- **Malignant pain**: Pain associated with cancer.
- **Neurogenic inflammation**: The process of nociceptive afferents releasing inflammatory molecules at the peripheral terminal, causing a localized inflammatory response in the peripheral tissues.
- **Neuropathic pain**: Pain caused by a lesion or disease of the somatosensory nervous system.
- **Nociceptive pain**: Pain that arises from actual or threatened damage to non-neural tissue and is due to the activation of nociceptors. Nociceptive pain is said to occur only when the somatosensory nervous system is normal, hence differentiating nociceptive from neurogenic pain.
- **Nociplastic pain**: A recently proposed term to describe pain that arises from altered nociception when there is no clear evidence of actual or threatened tissue damage causing nociceptor activation.
- **Nocebo (nocebo effect)**: The opposite of a placebo or the placebo effect. A nocebo is an inert treatment or event that increases symptoms because the patient believes it will increase symptoms. The expectation of pain can result in both increased pain from painful stimuli and allodynia, pain from a normally nonpainful stimulus.
- **Pain**: An unpleasant sensory and emotional experience associated with actual or potential tissue damage, or described in terms of such damage.
- **Neuromatrix**: A complex network of synaptic links within the CNS, initially determined by genetics but modified by psychological and sensory inputs. Because the neuromatrix that processes pain is not dedicated to only process pain, the term "pain neuromatrix" is not ideal, though it is often used.
- **Paresthesia**: An abnormal sensation, whether spontaneous or evoked.
- **Persistent pain**: Pain related to tissue damage or the threat of such damage that persists because the causative factors persist.
- **Peripheral neuropathic pain**: Pain caused by a lesion or disease of the peripheral somatosensory nervous system.
- **Peripheral sensitization**: Increased responsiveness and reduced threshold of nociceptors to stimulation of their receptive fields.
- **Placebo (placebo effect)**: A placebo is an inert treatment such as a sugar pill or fake treatment that is beneficial because the patient believes it will be beneficial.
- **Psychogenic pain**: An older term for pain believed to be caused by psychological factors when organic factors were absent or not severe enough to explain the pain complaint.
- **Recurrent pain**: Repeated episodes of acute pain.
- **Referred pain**: Spontaneous pain outside the area of injury or source of pain.
- **Sensitization**: Increased responsiveness of nociceptive neurons to their normal input, and/or recruitment of a response to normally subthreshold inputs.
- **Suffering**: The multidimensional experience of severe stress that occurs when there is a significant threat to the whole person and processes that would normally enable adaption are insufficient.

"neurogenic" and "neuropathic" are often used interchangeably, the IASP nomenclature uses the term "neuropathic."[13] *Sympathetically maintained pain* is a subtype of neuropathic pain in which the sympathetic nervous system activity interacts with nociceptors to amplify or perpetuate nociceptive signals.[32,33]

Central neuropathic/neurogenic pain is defined as pain caused by a lesion or disease of the central nervous system (CNS).[13] It can exist in the absence of peripheral nociceptive input and can, in fact, be generated in body regions that are denervated, such as SCI. Other common conditions include stroke, traumatic brain injury (TBI), MS, brain tumors, epilepsy, or Parkinson's disease. Central neurogenic pain may be burning, cold, stabbing, shooting, lancinating, pricking, pressing, or squeezing, and both hyperalgesia and allodynia may exist.[34-36] While peripheral and central neuropathic pain can be acute in the sense of transient and due to clearly observed and recent tissue damage, they often transition to chronic due to changes in the neural system that are not easily reversed and are generally considered a form of chronic pain.[37] *Central sensitization*, the process by which the CNS amplifies neural signals associated with pain, can occur in the absence of observed neural lesions or disease; hence, central sensitization can occur in the absence of central neuropathic pain, but neuropathic pain that has become chronic may involve central sensitization. It appears to be an important component of conditions such as fibromyalgia, whiplash-associated disorder, temporomandibular disorders, irritable bowel, and tension-type headaches.[38,39] Terminology is not used consistently in the literature, as the term *central pain* may be used for central neuropathic pain, central sensitization, or both. The International Association for the Study of Pain (IASP) definition of central neuropathic pain currently excludes central sensitization in the absence of lesion or disease;[13] however, many argue that central sensitization is essentially a type of CNS pathology.[35,40,41]

Pain is often described as acute or chronic based on the duration of pain. However, pain physiology is distinct from acute, sub-acute, remodeling, or chronic stages of tissue healing. The term *acute pain* is generally used to refer to transient, nociceptive dominant pain—that is, acute pain is often associated with nociceptor activation due to tissue damage or the threat of such damage and typically resolves as the threat resolves or during the healing process tissue heals.[37] Acute, nociceptive-dominant pain is often associated with physiological signs of distress, such as sweating, pallor, nausea, and heart rate (HR) changes. However, acute/recent pain is not simply nociceptor activation; cognitive and emotional factors have a powerful effect on the pain experience. Also, nociceptive-dominant pain is not always recent, acute, or transient; nociceptive dominant pain can be of long duration if recurrent or persistent, as in the case of osteoarthritis.[37] So, while the term "acute pain" is commonly used to contrast with chronic pain, the term does not quite correspond to a single aspect of pain physiology.

Chronic pain has been defined in a variety of ways. The simplest and most common is to define it as any recurrent or persistent pain lasting more than 3 months.[28,42,43] This is the definition being adopted by the International Classification of Diseases 11th revision (ICD-11), because it is simple and clearly defined.[44] While this definition is simple to apply, it does not reflect the significant physiological and psychosocial changes that occur in "chronic pain."[6,28] A second definition of chronic pain is pain that persists past the healing phase after an injury,[43] with impairment greater than anticipated based on the physical findings or injury, and occurs in the absence of observed tissue injury or damage.[6,28,45-47] This last definition recognizes the physiological changes that occur when pain becomes chronic, but fails to acknowledge that chronic pain may still have nociceptive input due to tissue damage or perception of danger as, for example, in persistent trigger point pain. The proposed ICD-11 sub-classification of chronic pain is given in Box 25.2.[44]

Clinical Implications: Chronic pain is not just acute pain that has been present for a longer time. Consequently, treatments that work for acute pain do not always work for chronic pain.

Currently, most diagnoses of chronic pain conditions are based primarily on symptoms, signs, and body location rather than evidence regarding mechanism or risk factor. To address this concern, the Analgesic, Anesthetic, and Addiction Clinical Trial Translations, Innovations, Opportunities, and Networks (ACTTION) created a public-private partnership with the U.S. Food and Drug Administration (FDA) and the American Pain Society (APS) to develop the ACTTION-APS Pain Taxonomy (AAPT) for chronic pain, outlined in **Box 25.3.** These criteria are intended to provide useful information regarding prognosis, treatment response, and biological and psychosocial factors.[48] The AAPT and ICD-11 classification systems overlap for some categories and differ for others.

Pain research frequently uses thermal, mechanical, or chemical stimuli that stress but do not damage tissues. This *experimental pain* is typically acute, short-duration, nociceptive-dominant pain. Experimental pain is often studied in healthy individuals, in contrast to *clinical pain*, which is observed in people experiencing pain due to clinical conditions. Clinical pain can be any combination of nociceptive, peripheral, or central neurogenic. The difference between experimental and clinical pain is important because neuroanatomy and neurophysiology related to pain may not be the same in these two situations.[49]

Box 25.2 ICD-11 Proposed Classification for Chronic Pain[44]

- **Chronic pain**: Any persistent or recurrent pain lasting longer than 3 months.

Sub-Classification of Chronic Pain:

- **Chronic primary pain**: Chronic pain associated with significant emotional distress or functional disability affecting activities of daily living and social roles that cannot be better explained by another chronic pain condition. This category includes non-specific pain conditions such as fibromyalgia, irritable bowel, and non-specific low back pain.
- **Chronic cancer pain**: Chronic pain caused by the cancer (primary tumor or metastases) or cancer treatment.
- **Chronic postsurgical and posttraumatic pain**: Pain that develops after a surgical procedure or tissue injury and persists at least 3 months after the surgery or tissue trauma. This excludes cancer-related pain but may include neuropathic pain.
- **Chronic neuropathic pain**: Chronic pain caused by a lesion or disease of the somatosensory nervous system serving the skin, musculoskeletal structures, and viscera. This category is subdivided into peripheral and central neuropathic pain.
- **Chronic headache and orofacial pain**: Both primary (idiopathic) and secondary (symptomatic) headaches or orofacial pain (including temporomandibular disorders) that occur on at least 50% of the days in the last 3 months.
- **Chronic visceral pain**: Persistent or recurrent pain originating from the internal organs of the head, neck, thoracic, abdominal, and pelvic cavities.
- **Chronic musculoskeletal pain**: Chronic pain that arises as part of a disease process directly affecting bones, joints, muscles, and related soft tissues. This category is limited to nociceptive pain from these tissues and thus excludes referred pain and neuropathies, but would include muscle pain due to spasticity. Musculoskeletal conditions for which the causes are incompletely understood, such as chronic widespread pain, non-specific back pain, and chronic pelvic pain should be classified as "chronic primary pain."

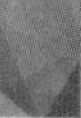

Box 25.3 The ACTTION-APS Pain Taxonomy (AAPT) for Chronic Pain, With Examples of Specific Pain Conditions[48*]

- **Peripheral nervous system**: Peripheral neuropathies, neuralgias, complex regional pain syndrome.
- **Central nervous system**: Multiple sclerosis, post-stroke pain, spinal cord injury pain.
- **Spine pain**: Chronic low back pain, lumbosacral radiculopathy.
- **Musculoskeletal pain**: Fibromyalgia, chronic myofascial pain, widespread pain, gout, osteoarthritis, rheumatoid arthritis, spondyloarthropathies.
- **Orofacial and head pain**: Headaches, temporomandibular disorders.
- **Abdominal, pelvic, and urogenital pain**: Interstitial cystitis, irritable bowel syndrome, vulvodynia.
- **Disease-associated pain conditions not classified elsewhere**: Cancer-related pain, chemotherapy-induced peripheral neuropathy, sickle cell disease.

*ACTTION = Analgesic, Anesthetic, and Addiction Clinical Trial Translations, Innovations, Opportunities, and Networks;
APS = American Pain Society.

An ongoing debate exists regarding whether to classify some pain states as "maladaptive," "problematic," or "pathological."[10,45,47,50] *Maladaptive* or *pathological pain* results from an abnormally functioning nervous system relaying nociceptive signals unrelated or disproportional to tissue damage.[10,45] Maladaptive and pathological pain represent altered neural processing due to neural plasticity, hence are due to peripheral or central sensitization, which will be discussed, as follows. *Problematic pain* is a term proposed to describe any pain that causes, or has the potential to cause, significant disability or distress, whether or not it is associated with tissue damage or threat; the benefit of recognizing problematic pain lies in providing additional health care resources to avoid the transition from acute to chronic, or to more effectively manage chronic pain.[50] Terms such as *psychogenic, affective, and non-organic pain*, once commonly used for medically unexplained pain, are no longer consistent with understanding of pain physiology and should not be used.[6,38,51,52] Other definitions related to pain are presented in Box 25.1.[13,18-20,45]

Clinical Implications: Current understanding of pain physiology renders the terms "psychogenic," "affective," "non-organic," and "medically unexplained" no longer appropriate. While we do not yet fully understand "pathological pain," it is real and it reflects real changes in the nervous system.

Evolution of the Biopsychosocial Model of Pain

In the 17th century, Descartes set the groundwork for the *specificity model*, where pain was believed to travel along dedicated nerve fibers to a pain center in the brain.[53] This mechanistic view provided the foundation for the *biomedical model* of pain, in which pain was directly correlated to tissue damage or threat of damage. According to the biomedical model, pain should resolve once tissue damage heals. The biomedical model works reasonably well for many types of acute, nociceptive pain; however, it is unable to explain many other examples of pain where the pain experience is inconsistent with tissue damage or healing. The failure of the biomedical model to explain many instances of pain led to the adoption of the *biopsychosocial model* of pain, which recognizes that biological factors interact with personal and environmental factors to influence body function and structure, activity, and participation in life activities.[28,54,55] The IASP definition of pain as sensory, emotional, or cognitive implies that pain is multidimensional. Evidence suggests that the biopsychosocial model may be more effective than the biomedical model in explaining and managing chronic pain.[56,57]

Clinical Implications: The biomedical model often works well for patients with acute, nociceptive-dominant pain. However, it does not work well for patients with chronic pain. Patient examination and management strategies for patients with chronic pain must include understanding and addressing a wide range of emotional, cognitive, social, and environmental factors as well as biological contributors to the pain.[27,28]

Although the concept is still quite controversial,[58] the Institute of Medicine has proposed that chronic pain be considered a disease, rather than just a symptom, because chronic pain results in pathological changes in the nervous system that can progress over time, independent of the initial cause of pain.[37,58,59] Just as a myocardial infarction may have many contributing factors but ultimately results in some common outcomes, chronic pain has multiple contributing factors that result in some common outcomes, and it needs to be managed if it cannot be cured.[10,28,58]

The World Health Organization's (WHO's) ICF[60] model treats pain as an abnormal body function classified under the designation *Sensory Function and Pain*. The physiological changes observed in chronic pain may also be associated with changes in the *Structure of the Nervous System*, at the level of body structure.[61] The multidirectional nature of the ICF model is particularly pertinent to chronic pain where personal factors, structure, function, activity, participation, and environmental factors are interrelated and can all affect one another. This complex interaction will be discussed further with Risk Factors, later in this chapter.

■ PATHOPHYSIOLOGICAL PROCESSES UNDERLYING CHRONIC PAIN

A detailed discussion of the neuroanatomy and neurophysiology involved in the pain experience is beyond the scope of this chapter. Therefore, the current discussion will focus on ways in which anatomical or physiological changes associated with chronic pain may impact interventions. Readers can find more extensive coverage of pain physiology in one of the textbooks on pain: *Mechanisms and Management of Pain for the Physical Therapist*,[21] *Pain, A Textbook for Health Professionals*,[62] or *Chronic Pain: An Integrated Biobehavioral Approach*,[63] and *Explain Pain Supercharged*.[64]

Current thinking is that pain involves a *neuromatrix* comprising a widespread network of neurons initially determined by genetics, but modified by psychological and sensory inputs both before and during the pain experience.[53,65,66] The initial neuromatrix theory identified three components of the pain phenomenon, with each component potentially contributing to and an output of the pain experience. The *sensory-discriminative dimension* refers to localization, intensity, duration, and the nature of the pain (burning, sharp, and so forth). The *motivational-affective dimension* refers to the emotional component, including stress. The *cognitive-evaluative dimension* relates to how pain is interpreted in the context of past and present experience, culture, and so forth.[45,53,65] Although it is often referred to as the "pain neuromatrix," these pathways are more accurately described as a *dynamic neural representation of pain* or *salience network*, as the involved pathways also serve a variety of other, non-pain related neural processes, and activity in these regions is not proportional to pain intensity and the pain experience is not proportional to activity in any single brain network, as was once believed.[67,68] This distinction is important in understanding the interrelationship between non-painful sensory, cognitive, and emotional processes and the pain experience. Furthermore, there is likely no clear distinction between sensory, cognitive, and affective components of the matrix; that is, pain is a single experience rather than multiple dimensions.[64] The neuromatrix has been able to better explain pathological pain, as well as the biopsychosocial aspects, neuroplasticity, and emergent properties of pain.[53] The following discussion will focus on changes that occur when pain becomes chronic. Common clinical presentation of different types of pain is summarized in Table 25.1[23,34,35,39,69] and will be discussed further in the section on Evaluation.

Table 25.1 Subjective and Objective Characteristics Associated With Different Types of Pain[23,34,35,39,69*]

Type of Pain	Tissue Source	Subjective Characteristics	Objective Characteristics
Nociceptive: Cutaneous or superficial	Skin and subcutaneous tissues (A-delta & C fibers). History of damage or potential tissue damage	Usually intermittent, well-localized, stabbing, sharp; may be constant dull ache or throb at rest. Varies relative to tissue damage or potential damage.	Clear, consistent, proportional pain reproduced through movement or mechanical testing of target tissues. Localized or with somatic referral.
Nociceptive: Deep somatic	Bone, muscle, blood vessels, connective tissues (greater predominance of C fibers over A-delta)	Vague, tearing, cramping, pressing, aching. Often referred to other locations.	Vague, sometimes referred pain reproduced through movement or mechanical testing of deeper tissues; spasm, trigger points common
Nociceptive: Visceral	Organs and the linings of the body cavities (greater predominance of C fibers over A-delta)	Often referred to other locations; poorly localized, diffuse, deep cramping or splitting, sharp, stabbing	Vague pain reproduction on movement or mechanical testing of visceral tissues
Peripheral Neuropathic	Nerve fibers (A-delta & C fibers, but may involve A-delta, & autonomic). History of lesion or disease to peripheral nerve.	Pain variously described as burning, shooting, pricking, or "electric-shock." Pain and sensory dysfunction neuro-anatomically logical (dermatomal or peripheral nerve patterns).	Evidence of nerve damage or abnormality. Pain or symptom provocation with movement or mechanical tests that move, load, or compress neural tissues; pain may be spontaneous (no external stimulus).
Central: Central Neuropathic	Spinal cord and brain. History of lesion or disease to spinal cord or brain.	Pain neuro-anatomically logical. Continuous or paroxysmal; evoked by mechanical stimuli or spontaneous.	Evidence of CNS damage or disease. Pain and sensory abnormalities are neuro-anatomically logical. Pain may be triggered by mechanical stimuli or spontaneous.
Central: Central Sensitization	Spinal cord and CNS. No medical cause for pain established.	Pain is typically vague and dull. Pain and symptoms widespread and not neuro-anatomically logical, with numerous sites of hyperalgesia remote to initial symptomatic site. Disproportionate, non-mechanical, unpredictable pattern of pain in response to multiple, nonspecific aggravating or easing factors. Additional (non-pain) signs and symptoms and often maladaptive beliefs and pain behaviors.	No objective evidence of CNS damage or disease. Disproportionate, inconsistent, or nonanatomical pattern of sensory abnormalities and pain provocation in response to movement or mechanical testing. Pain may be spontaneous (no external stimulus). Abnormal response to pinprick and temperature (spinothalamic tract dysfunction).

*Note that patients may have multiple types of pain.[23,34,35,39,69]

Clinical Implications: The neuromatrix reflects both genetic and experiential influences (sensory, emotional, and cognitive activity within the neuromatrix). Over time, certain pathways become well worn, the connections become stronger, and activity in these networks is more easily reproduced in response to non-nociceptive stimuli as well as nociceptive stimuli.[53] The neuromatrix becomes more "skilled" at perceiving pain.[14]

Changes in Neural Processing Associated With Chronic Pain

Peripheral Sensitization

Peripheral sensitization exists when nociceptor activity is increased, resulting in primary *hyperalgesia* or *allodynia*. Increased nociceptor sensitivity in the presence of inflammation normally functions to force rest of the injured tissues; ideally, nociceptors return to their normal state once local tissues have healed. However, in peripheral sensitization, nociceptors either become too sensitive or remain sensitized for too long.[37] Repeated or persistent noxious stimulation of muscle nociceptors can lead to changes in the size, number, threshold, and receptive field of dorsal horn neurons.[70] The term *nociplastic* has been put forth to distinguish abnormal nociceptor function in peripheral sensitization from neuropathic pain which, by definition, involves nerve injury or disease.[20] The mechanism of sensitization can be through tissue damage, neurogenic inflammation, abnormal sympathetic activity,[32] or systemic inflammation. Tissue damage (including prolonged muscle spasm or trigger point activity) releases a multitude of chemicals or ions that can increase nociceptor sensitivity by decreasing activation threshold or by activating "silent nociceptors" (mechanically insensitive C fibers that develop mechanical sensitivity in response to chemical stimuli such as inflammation, hence acquiring a lower mechanical threshold). Various chemicals associated with peripheral sensitization are listed in Table 25.2.[19,49]

Clinical Implications: Joint nociceptors are normally responsive to noxious pressure or extreme joint movement, but silent nociceptors, once activated by tissue damage or inflammation, respond to any mechanical stimulus. Consequently, motion that would not normally activate nociceptors now does.[29,71]

The immune system modulates nociception through systemic and local inflammation.[72] Mast cells, neutrophils, macrophages, dendritic cells, and T cells are all involved in local or systemic inflammatory effects on pain. Inflammation activates silent nociceptors, which remain active by producing sustained discharge long after removal of the stimulus. Cytokines can increase or decrease neural excitability, and modify neural growth or interconnections.[72] A complete discussion of pain regulation through inflammatory mediators is beyond the scope of this chapter; see several good reviews of the topic.[30,73-77]

Neurogenic inflammation is another mechanism for increasing nociceptor sensitivity. While nociceptors are generally believed to be afferent neurons, they are actually pseudo-unipolar, where the central and peripheral stalks of the axon can both receive and transmit signals. Although normally only the peripheral terminal responds to environmental stimuli such as heat, cold, mechanical or chemical triggers, both central and peripheral terminals

Table 25.2 Chemicals That Can Activate or Sensitize Nociceptors[19,49*]

Class	Examples	Sources
Inflammatory mediators	Histamine	Mast cells
Neurotransmitters	Serotonin	Platelets and mast cells
Peptides	Substance P, bradykinin, CGRP (calcitonin gene-related peptide)	Nociceptors, plasma
Eicosinoids and related lipids	Prostaglandins, thromoxanes, leukotrienes, endocannabinoids	Local tissues, damaged cells, macrophages, sympathetic nerves
Neurotrophins	Nerve growth factor	Inflamed tissues, sympathetic nerves
Cytokines	IL-1β, IL-6, tumor necrosis factor α (TNF-α)	Immune cells
Chemokines		
Catecholamines	Epinephrine, norepinephrine, dopamine	Sympathetic nerves,
Other	K+, ATP, proteases, pH	Tissue metabolism, injured cells

*These substances can be released from injured tissues, inflammatory cells, or the distal terminals of nociceptors (neurogenic inflammation). Some of these substances, such as NGF, can be transported retrogradely to the nucleus of the nociceptor, where they can alter gene expression in a way that increases excitability and thus amplifies the peripheral sensitization.

can respond to neurotransmitters and other endogenous signals. Injured nerves may also respond at the site of injury. The proximal/central terminal releases Ca^{2+}-dependent neurotransmitters, while the peripheral terminal releases a variety of molecules that can alter the local environment at the peripheral terminal; *neurogenic inflammation* refers to the process where "afferent" nerves stimulate peripheral inflammatory processes by releasing calcitonin-gene related peptide, substance P, neuropeptides, glutamate, neurokinins, vasoactive peptides, nitric oxide, and cytokines at the peripheral terminal.[19,78] This antidromic activity (the *dorsal root reflex*) in nociceptive neurons can therefore stimulate chemotaxis of neutrophils, macrophages, and lymphocytes to the peripheral terminal, cause vasodilation, vascular leakage, and edema, and can prime differentiation of T helper cells. Neurogenic inflammation thus facilitates tissue healing and immune defense in acute conditions when danger is perceived but can contribute to peripheral sensitization when persistent.[10,78,79]

Clinical Implications: Nociceptors can transmit antidromic signals to peripheral tissues leading to vasodilation, increased capillary permeability, plasma extravasation, and edema associated with neurogenic inflammation even if there was no local tissue damage. Consequently, evidence of local inflammation does not imply damage to local tissues.[78]

Nociceptor activity can be modified through several cellular mechanisms, such as activation of ion channels, increased receptor density or type, decreased firing threshold, increased conduction velocity, increased sensitivity to circulating catecholamines, activation of intracellular messengers, or increased receptive field (Box 25.4).[29,49] Changes at the periphery can propagate to the nociceptor cell body, where modifications to ion channels can produce ectopic activity and increased transcription can lead to sprouting of additional peripheral terminals. When multiple factors are present (e.g., inflammation and low pH), nociceptor firing intensity and duration can both be increased. Overall, the mechanisms of peripheral sensitization contribute to hyperalgesia, where pain threshold is decreased, and allodynia, where non-painful stimuli such as movement or light touch can activate nociceptors. Peripheral sensitization also provides increased input into the CNS, leading to central sensitization.[49,80]

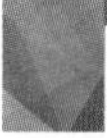

BOX 25.4 Cellular Mechanisms of Nociceptor Sensitization[29,49,79,82]

- **Transcription of additional or different ion channels**
- Sprouting of peripheral terminals leading to increased receptor density
- Transcription of additional or different receptors or second messengers
- Increased receptive field
- Decreased firing threshold
- Increased conduction velocity
- Increased sensitivity to circulating catecholamines
- Activation of intracellular messengers
- Ectopic discharges

Clinical Implications: The structure, physiology, and function of nociceptors change in central sensitization. These sensitized nociceptors do not behave the way that we observe in acute, nociceptive-dominant pain. Patients can therefore experience excessive pain (hyperalgesia) or pain as a result of movement or sensory stimuli that would not normally be painful (allodynia). Hyperalgesia and allodynia are therefore the result of physiological and functional changes in the nervous system, and not indicators that the patient is "over-reacting" or "symptom-magnifying."

Peripheral Neuropathic Pain

Neuropathic pain stems from mechanical or chemical damage to or inflammation of peripheral nerves. According to the IASP definition, neuropathic pain does not refer to peripheral sensitization, even though peripheral sensitization is, as discussed already, due to increased responsiveness of nociceptive nerves. Neuropathic pain does not occur after all nerve injuries, or for all people experiencing the same injury. For example, only 5% of people having hernia surgery have persistent pain from the ilioinguinal nerve, and 30% to 60% of people having a thoracotomy experience neuropathic pain even though intercostal nerves have been cut.[37]

Injury sensitizes peripheral nerves through direct compromise to the axons or immune reaction of glial cells.[38,79,81] Because axonal function is altered, pain and dysesthesias are perceived to come from the peripheral (for a peripheral nerve) or dermatomal (for a spinal nerve) sensory distribution. The pathological changes observed in peripheral neuropathic pain develop as a result of normal healing processes, a complex interaction among the peripheral nerve, glial cells, and inflammatory mediators. Briefly, nerve injury triggers an inflammatory response of macrophages, T-lymphocytes, and mast cells at the injury site, dorsal root ganglion, and dorsal horn. Schwann cells release factors that increase permeability of endoneurial blood vessels, compromising the blood-nerve barrier. Schwann cells also release neurotrophic factors that stimulate axonal growth and sprouting (including abnormal branching), synaptic remodeling (leading to hypersensitivity), and remyelination. Neurotrophic factors and cytokines travel retrograde to the cell body where they modulate gene expression, sensitizing nociceptors at the DRG, and to the spinal cord where they stimulate central neuropathic changes. Microglia in the dorsal and ventral horns are stimulated to release neurotrophic factors that decrease descending inhibitory activity.[81] Epigenetic changes of neurons in the DRG and microglia and astrocytes in the spinal cord result in increases in cytokine and growth factor production, which can alter function of both the involved nociceptors and neighboring uninjured neurons.[49,72,79,81,82]

Ultimately, prolonged peripheral neuropathic pain results in maladaptive neural plasticity, leading to decreased stimulation threshold, increased sensitivity, ectopic impulses, altered or eliminated axonal conduction, abnormal growth, reduced inhibition, and glial scarring. As a consequence of demyelination, uninjured fibers may be activated by adjacent fibers, a process called *crosstalk.* Also, innocuous input can trigger pain when A-beta fibers form synapses in the dorsal horn with neurons that normally transmit nociceptive information.[37] What appears to be spontaneous activity may, in fact, be due to sensitized nerves now activated by normal body temperature or innocuous motion.[37]

Clinical Implications: Neuropathic pain and peripheral sensitization both provide physiological mechanisms to explain Waddell's "non-organic signs" of superficial tenderness and overreaction. Hyperalgesia and allodynia should therefore not be considered "non-organic signs."

Sympathetically maintained pain (*causalgia*) typically presents as neuropathic pain (burning pain and allodynia) accompanied by edema, changes in skin blood flow and temperature, and trophic changes. Although the sympathetic nervous system does not normally trigger pain, there are several mechanisms by which the sympathetic nervous system can alter pain. First, epinephrine can increase sensitivity of nociceptors through peripheral sensitization, as discussed already. Second, after peripheral nerve injury, nociceptors can express catecholamine receptors which then respond to sympathetic activity, causing stress to directly activate nociceptors. Third, nerve injury results in sympathetic nerves sprouting post-ganglionic basket-like structures around injured neuronal cell bodies. Activation of these sympathetic fibers may result in increased activity in the injured neurons.[32,83] Lastly, the autonomic system may have indirect effects through altered microcirculation to nerves, which may lead to an acidic microenvironment that increases nociceptor sensitivity.[83]

Clinical Implications: Because sympathetic nerves can both sensitize and directly activate nociceptors in neuropathic pain states, stress can stimulate or amplify pain. Consequently, stress management can be an important component of a pain management program for physiological as well as psychological benefits.[84-87]

Changes in the CNS Associated With Chronic Pain

Both central neuropathic pain and central sensitization are associated with changes to the CNS. Changes in CNS processing can lead to secondary hyperalgesia and allodynia in areas adjacent to or remote from actual tissue injury.[88] Some conditions may generate pain without any nociceptive input, whereas others appear to be mediated by centrally amplified and perpetuated peripheral nociceptive pain.[89] *Placebo* and *nocebo* (the reverse of placebo), while not unique to chronic pain, involve some of the same CNS pathways.[82,90]

Chronic pain is associated with widespread neuroplasticity, including changes in CNS structure, function, and chemistry, affecting both neurons and glia in the peripheral and central nervous systems.[91] That is, chronic pain is not simply ongoing nociception. Figure 25.1 shows changes observed in the brain with chronic pain.[49,68,92] Changes include decreased gray matter volume in some areas and increased gray matter in other areas and both increased and decreased connectivity among regions of the brain. Furthermore, CNS changes observed vary across different pain syndromes.

Central neuropathic pain (CNP) results from a primary lesion or disease in the CNS, in which the pain distribution is consistent with CNS damage. Nociceptive pain due to musculoskeletal dysfunctions secondary to the CNS pathology is not considered CNP; for example, spasticity due to spinal cord injury, stroke, or Parkinson's disease is nociceptive pain and not CNP.[35] Pain may be the presenting symptom, as in MS, or pain can begin months or years after the initial CNS injury, as in SCI, where CNP may develop from 3 months to 5 years after injury.[35,43] Pain can even be perceived in regions whose nerves are no longer connected to the brain (e.g., below-level pain in SCI). Pathological pain results when the balance between descending inhibition and descending facilitation is lost. Imbalance may be mediated by glia and astrocytes altering synaptic activity[82] and synaptic connections forming between general sensory afferents and nociceptive fibers (allodynia)[38] resulting in descending facilitation.[93] Pain in SCI may be generated by ectopic activity in spinal cord nociceptive pathways, either from microglial activation or decreased descending inhibition. Pain due to stroke may be due to disinhibition; for example, lesions in the lateral thalamus can disinhibit the medial thalamus, allowing increased activity.[35] Changes at the site of CNS injury can generate CNS changes in remote regions; for example, SCI can lead to microglial activation in the thalamus.[36]

Clinical Implications: Since descending inhibitory pathways are normally active, an injury or disease that inactivates descending inhibition can result in increased experience of pain.

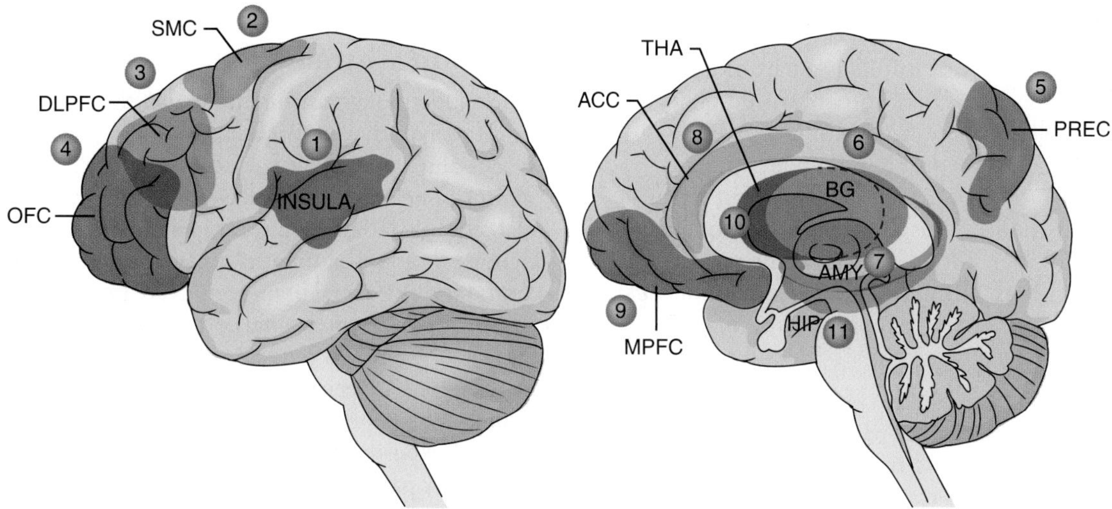

Figure 25.1 Brain regions that change in patients with chronic pain[49,68,92]
Diagram showing regions of the brain that are believed to change in patients with chronic pain:

1. Insular cortex: involved in consciousness, body awareness/perception, motor control, and some emotional processing. Decreased gray matter volume observed in patients with chronic pain.
2. Supplemental motor cortex: Primarily controls movement and posture.
3. Dorsolateral prefrontal cortex: Executive function and motor planning. Decreased gray matter in chronic low back pain.
4. Orbitofrontal cortex: Associated with decision making, expectations, emotional processing of reward/punishment.
5. Precuneus: Associated with self-awareness, memory processing, visuospatial perception. Reduced cortical gray matter volume observed in patients with chronic back pain.
6. Basal ganglia: Associated with movement, motor planning, learning. Increased gray matter volume in chronic back pain, fibromyalgia, temporomandibular disorder.
   - Thalamus: Relays sensory and motor inputs to other brain areas and regulates consciousness. Reduced gray matter density in patients with chronic back pain.
7. Amygdala: Part of the limbic system, strong modulators of fear, associated with memory, decision making, and emotional processing. Increased gray matter observed in patients with back pain.
   - Hippocampus: Part of the limbic system, functions in memory formation and consolidation. Altered hippocampal-cortical connectivity observed in patients with chronic back pain.
8. Anterior cingulate cortex: Participates in consciousness, autonomic functioning, decision making, emotional processing of pain, reward-based learning. Descending projections link to autonomic responses to stimuli. Reduced gray matter density correlated to neurocognitive deficits in chronic tension-type headache and fibromyalgia.
9. Medial prefrontal cortex: Decision making, including risk/reward. Decreased gray matter density in patients with chronic back pain.

Central sensitization (CS) presents as increased sensitivity to sensory input, which may include nociceptive, non-nociceptive, visceral and special senses; multi-system hypersensitivity is key to identification of CS.[94] CS can result in increased or prolonged response to noxious stimulation (hyperalgesia), pain in response to normally innocuous input (allodynia), increased responsiveness in regions surrounding the initial area of injury (secondary hyperalgesia), increased response over time (temporal summation or windup), and last beyond the duration of the initial stimulus.[38,95] *Wind-up*, or *temporal summation* is a normal process whereby firing of a postsynaptic neuron increases after the stimulus has been present for a few seconds; however, wind-up can be enhanced or its threshold decreased in the presence of central sensitization.[88,95] Wind-up can result in long-term potentiation, in which the neural response is strengthened through increased neurogenic inflammation and altered gene expression resulting in altered nerve phenotype, with different receptors and transmitters.[88]

Clinical Implications: Wind-up, or temporal summation, can be measured as a part of quantitative sensory testing. One protocol would be to expose a patient to a non-painful mechanical stimulus (e.g., 60 g von Frey filament applied to the wrist) four times and ask for a pain rating, then repeat the stimulus 30 times at a frequency of 1 stimulus per second, and have the patient rate pain after the last stimulus. Increased pain ratings over time would indicate temporal summation, hence central sensitization.[96]

CS is common in chronic pain conditions, but the abnormal sensory processing may begin early after trauma and may contribute to transition of acute into chronic pain.[39] Although, like CNP, CS involves dysfunction of both neurons and glial cells in the CNS, CS differs from central neuropathic pain in that CS can occur in the absence of frank, preceding CNS lesion or disease.[38] CS is associated with increased activity in some brain areas involved in acute pain, as well as regions not typically associated with acute pain and descending facilitatory pathways, and is associated with decreased activity in descending inhibitory pathways.[38,94] While the physiology is not fully understood, CS appears to include receptor-mediated hypersensitivity, ectopic activity, abnormal sprouting and cellular connections, and disinhibition, all of which may be mediated by neuronal death, glial-neuronal interactions, and altered gene expression.[10,19,38,49,95] Glia appear to perpetuate sensitization by releasing neuroactive signaling molecules that stimulate an immune response.[10,30,84] Once CS is initiated, pain can occur in the absence of further peripheral nociceptor input.[95,97]

An alternative explanation for CNS changes associated with CS is provided by the *Imprecision Hypothesis*, which posits that pain becomes a conditioned response to a complex interplay of sensory, emotional, and cognitive events. Cortical reorganization results in the individual overgeneralizing and perceiving danger (hence pain) as a result of varied, normally non-nociceptive stimuli (sensory, emotional, or cognitive).[17] Yet another hypothesis proposes that the temporal-spectral dimension of neural activity is important in coding pain, with neuronal oscillations in the infra-slow (as low as 0.1 Hz) to gamma (30–100 Hz) range reflecting changes in slow waves of activity passing through the cortex. These infra-slow waves appear to be associated with abnormal learning and memory consolidation in chronic pain.[98]

Clinical Implications: Because CS is due to abnormal CNS processing, patients will perceive that their pain is due to tissue danger/damage when there might be no tissue pathology or noxious stimulus present in the peripheral tissues. CS is a perceptual illusion of tissue pathology or damage.[95]

Autonomic, Immune, and Endocrine Roles in Chronic Pain

The endocrine system also modulates the pain experience, and the hypothalamic-pituitary adrenal (HPA) axis plays a central role in mediating stress-related chronic pain syndromes, such as fibromyalgia, whiplash-associated disorder, chronic fatigue syndrome, pelvic pain, irritable bowel syndrome, post-traumatic stress disorder (PTSD), and burnout.[84,87] Several brain regions are involved: hypothalamus, amygdala, prefrontal cortex, and hippocampus.[86,87] The locus coeruleus (LC) appears to be integrally involved in the link between stress and emotional-cognitive components of pain; that is, the LC amplifies aversion to painful experiences, a component of the emotional response to pain without necessarily altering the sensory dimension. Stress also triggers multiple mediators that impact chronic pain.[99] Ultimately, physical or emotional stress activates the HPA axis, leading to a self-perpetuating cascade of events resulting in chronic sympathetic activation, which increases or perpetuates chronic pain.[33,84,85,100] Although the research is currently inconsistent, chronic pain appears to be associated with a blunted cortisol response; since cortisol is a strongly anti-inflammatory hormone, this stunted response could contribute to both peripheral and central sensitization.[86] These physiological changes compound the psychological impact of stress and chronic pain on one another, which will be discussed more later in this chapter. So, while the stress response is adaptive for acute pain, it becomes maladaptive when pain persists, and contributes to chronification.[86,87]

Clinical Implications: Physical and emotional stress activate neuroendocrine processes that contribute to the transition from acute to chronic pain, and to the perpetuation of chronic pain. A biopsychosocial management approach should address both pain- and non–pain-related stressors in patients with chronic pain and in those with acute pain at risk of transitioning to chronic pain.[86]

The endocrine system also contributes to both peripheral and CNS changes seen in chronic pain. Chronic stress can be caused by either external circumstances (psychosocial or physical, including pain), or inappropriate responses such as negative cognitions, rumination, worry, catastrophization, or helplessness. When stress or pain is present for a prolonged period, the endocrine response becomes maladaptive with dysregulation of the HPA axis contributing to dysregulation of the corticolimbic system (including the amygdala, prefrontal cortex, and hippocampus), which can lead to increased inflammation, morning fatigue, muscle atrophy, compromised tissue growth and repair, autonomic dysfunction, cognitive changes, and pain.[84,100] Ultimately, chronic activation of the stress response appears to exhaust the HPA axis, as shown in Figure 25.2.[86,101] Hypocortisolism associated

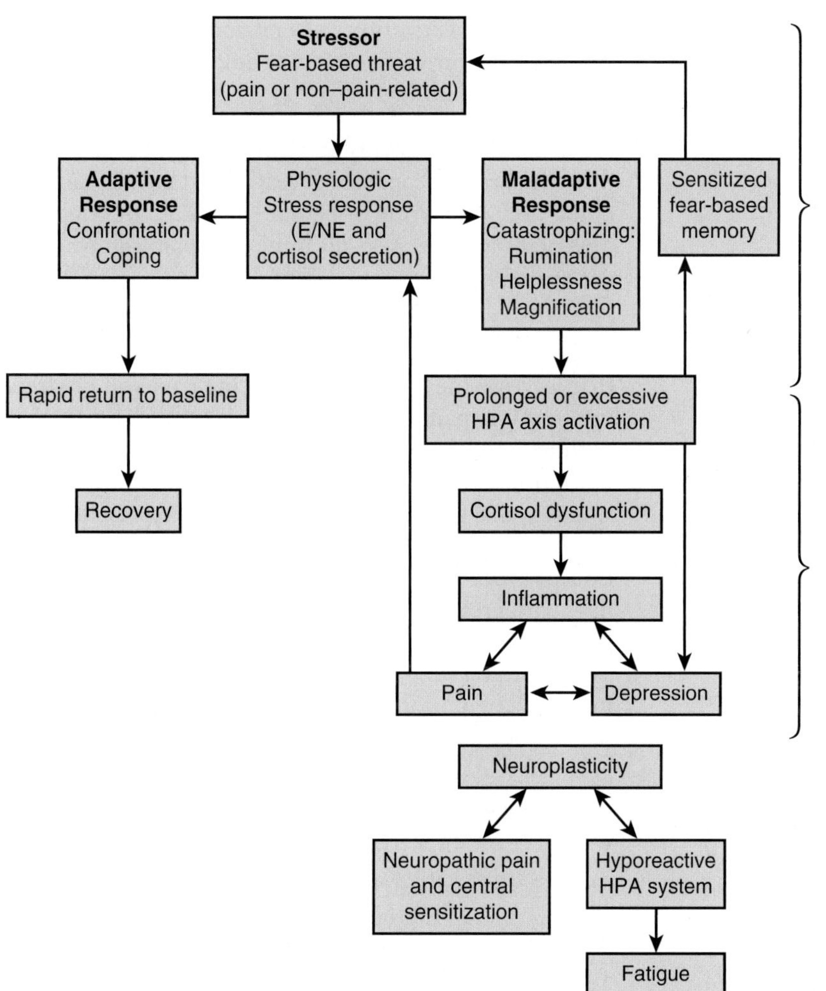

Figure 25.2 Relationship Between Stress and Chronic Pain. A physical or psychological stressor causes a stress response. Healthy individuals have an adaptive response and return to baseline. People who have a maladaptive response may have a prolonged or excessive hypothalamic-pituitary-adrenal (HPA) response that both exacerbates the fear response and contributes to neuroplasticity associated with neuropathic pain or central sensitization. A prolonged stress response can also lead to a hypoactive HPA system, which can lead to the fatigue often seen in chronic pain.[86,101]

with chronic stress has been shown in fibromyalgia, chronic fatigue syndrome, temporomandibular disorder, and chronic pelvic pain.[86] Cortisol is a potent anti-inflammatory hormone, and the decreased levels seen in chronic stress contribute to systemic inflammation and increased pain-related cytokines, which then lead to both peripheral and central sensitization.[86] The exact mechanisms are not clear, but they are believed to be a combination of genetic vulnerability with a neurotoxic effect of hormones, such as glucocorticoids, secreted from the HPA axis during chronic stress.[87] The endocrine link helps to explain the interrelationships seen between cognitive, emotional, and physical components of the pain experience.[86,87]

Clinical Implications: Chronic stress associated with chronic pain can amplify dysfunction due to the initial injury/disease and changes due to chronic pain by contributing to compromised immune function, tissue growth and repair, autonomic dysfunction, cognitive changes, and structural changes in the brain.[84,100]

RISK FACTORS ASSOCIATED WITH CHRONIC PAIN

While injury or disease often trigger the development of pain, additional risk factors influence the likelihood that acute pain will transition into chronic pain, and that chronic pain will persist. Box 25.5 lists a variety of risk factors impacting chronic pain. Note that these risk factors are profoundly interrelated, so cause and effect can sometimes be impossible to distinguish.[102-105] Denk et al[102] provide an excellent explanation of the neurophysiological mechanisms of factors impacting pain vulnerability. This discussion will highlight factors likely to be most relevant to physical therapists.

Genetic Risk Factors

Up to 50% of the variability in prevalence and severity of pain appears to be due to genetic factors, the most common being the catechol-O-methyltransferase gene; it may eventually be possible to test for genetic predisposition to develop chronic pain.[38,102,106] Epigenetic mechanisms can enhance or suppress gene expression due to interaction between the individual and the environment, contributing

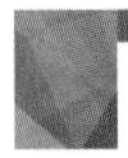

Box 25.5 Risk Factors Associated With Chronic Pain[102-104]

Non-Modifiable Risk Factors:

- Genetics
- Gender
- Age
- Past trauma—physical, emotional, sexual
- Socioeconomic status
- Access to health care
- Work/family environment

Lifestyle Factors

- Smoking
- Drug or alcohol addiction
- Obesity
- Sedentary lifestyle
- Sleep disorder
- Diet and gut microbiota

Psychosocial Factors

- Poor social support or oversolicitous support
- Discord at home or work
- Depression
- Anxiety, fear avoidance, and catastrophizing
- Pain persistence behavior
- Low self-efficacy
- Stress

to synaptic plasticity, learning, and memory.[81] Traumatic personal history affects epigenetics in ways that amplify and perpetuate chronic pain through changes in the CNS, immune and endocrine systems, as well as contributing to psychological distress and maladaptive behaviors that exacerbate pain.[107,108]

Clinical Implications: Because childhood trauma sensitizes the nervous system, it is important to ask about this during the patient interview. When patients understand this connection, it often helps them appreciate why treatments to calm their nervous systems can be beneficial.[107,108]

Psychosocial Risk Factors

The term "negative affect" encompasses negative emotions, thoughts, and behaviors, such as depression, anxiety, distress, and catastrophizing. Neurobiological pathways that link psychological factors with chronic pain include epigenetics; cellular priming; altered brain pathways associated with reward, motivation, and learning; immune response; diurnal cortisol patterns; hypothalamic-pituitary regulation; and descending modulation leading to somatosensory amplification and central sensitization. Several good resources review the interaction between psychological factors and chronic pain.[57,102,104,107-109]

Clinical Implications: Because of neural plasticity, the brain is capable of "learning" chronic pain and, due to blurring of neural encoding, the trigger becomes less precise—meaning that pain can be triggered by more varied stimuli.[17,104]

Yellow flags have been defined as psychosocial factors that increase the likelihood that acute pain will progress into chronic pain and disability.[42,105,110,111] Table 25.3 outlines a terminology proposed by Nicholas et al.[105] In this terminology *yellow flags* include beliefs, emotional responses, and pain behavior; *orange flags* represent frank psychiatric symptoms; and *blue flags* reflect the interaction between work and health perceptions. The yellow flags with greatest impact appear to be (1) the belief that pain and activity are harmful, (2) a depressed mood and social withdrawal, (3) the expectation that passive treatment will help more than active treatment, and (4) low self-efficacy.[112] Other important factors include sickness behavior (e.g., excessive rest), history of pain or disability, poor job satisfaction, overprotective family or lack of support, and problems with claims or compensation.[111]

Clinical Implications: Psychosocial issues should be considered individually for each patient, because interventions addressing specific psychosocial factors are more successful than interventions that do not.[27,28,110,111]

Pain Beliefs and Behaviors

Pain-related beliefs include people's understanding about what is causing their pain, the meaning of their pain, and expectations regarding the impact pain has on their present and future lives. Beliefs associated with better outcomes include having control over pain, global self-efficacy, pain self-efficacy, control over life, and internal pain control. Beliefs associated with poor outcomes include believing pain indicates injury/damage and should be avoided, pain will be constant, pain is disabling, emotions influence pain, and that other people should be solicitous because of the pain, helplessness, and external locus of control (the belief that pain is controlled by someone other than the individual in pain).[113] Beneficial coping responses include activities to distract oneself from the pain, task persistence, exercise, ignoring pain, coping self-statements, and acceptance of the condition. Detrimental coping responses include guarding, resting, venting emotions, passive coping (avoidance), and asking for assistance.[113,114]

Pain behaviors can be grouped in different ways. Table 25.4 contrasts *fear avoidance* with *pain persistence* and provides an evidence-based classification into four

Table 25.3 Alert Flags for Chronic Pain[105]

Flag Color	Type of Problem	Examples
Red	Serious physical pathology	Cauda equina syndrome, fracture, tumor
Orange	Psychiatric symptoms	Clinical depression, post-traumatic stress disorder, personality disorder
Yellow	Beliefs, appraisals, and judgments	Negative pain beliefs Expectation of poor outcome
	Emotional responses	Fear, anxiety, catastrophization, distress
	Pain behavior, including pain coping strategies	Fear avoidance behavior, dependence on passive interventions
Blue	Perceptions about relationship between work and pain	Belief that work will cause further injury and pain. Belief that supervisor and co-workers are unsupportive
Black	System or contextual obstacles	No modified duty options at work Legislation restricting return to work options Lack of insurance coverage Overly solicitous family or health providers

pain behavior clusters.[63,115,116] It is important to note that pain behavior and pain behavior clusters can change over time, so these factors need to be reassessed periodically. The impact of social responses to pain behaviors depends on the nature of the behavior and whether the response is supportive, solicitous, or punishing. Social reinforcers for wellness behavior tend to be beneficial.[113,117,118] Solicitous behaviors such as sympathy, encouragement to avoid pain and do less, and allowing people to avoid tasks due to pain lead to increased pain and decreased function.[113] Punishing or negative responses to pain behaviors lead to increased pain and depression.[119] Table 25.4 also relates social support and behavior.[63,115,116]

Clinical Implications: While fear avoidance is well recognized, some patients use a pain persistence behavior that is equally dysfunctional. Customizing pain management to the patient's pain behavior pattern is likely to result in improved patient compliance and better outcomes.[63,105,117,120]

The *Fear-Avoidance Model* of pain proposes that some people have an exaggerated fear that movement will cause reinjury and/or increase pain. Fear of pain can even become more disabling than the actual pain. Figure 25.3 shows how these factors leads to maladaptive hypervigilance, inaccurate predictions about pain, misinterpretation of body sensations, muscular reactivity, and physical deconditioning.[121,122] On the other hand, *pain persistence* can be equally dysfunctional. In pain persistence, the individual denies or ignores the pain, often due to reluctance to rely on others or lack of social support. Individuals with pain persistence tended to have high levels of activity, overcommitment to work, and perfectionist behaviors before developing chronic pain; they can be inflexible and often do not accept functional limitations or want to be labeled as lazy.[116,123] Pain persistence is associated with cycles of overactivity, severe pain, forced rest, decreased function, and overactivity as shown in Figure 25.3.[124]

A sedentary lifestyle is separately associated with increased back pain and joint degeneration, independent of weight; inactivity also exacerbates fear of movement, which further limits activity.[103] Sleep disorders are highly correlated to chronic pain, increased disability, and suffering due to pain, and increased health care utilization. Furthermore, sleep disorders may be aggravated by a sedentary lifestyle.[125-127] Evidence suggests that gut microbiota can influence the neurochemical and behavioral responses to stress, anxiety, and depression via the HPA axis, neurotransmitters, cytokines, bacterial metabolites, immune response, and the vagus nerve.[128,129]

Clinical Implications: Sleep dysfunction and chronic pain create a self-perpetuating cycle, where pain makes it difficult to sleep, and lack of sleep amplifies pain. This is why sleep hygiene (teaching patients good sleep habits) can be a helpful part of pain management.[127,130]

EXAMINATION OF PATIENTS WITH CHRONC PAIN

The goals of the subjective portion of the chronic pain examination include listening to the patient's narrative, developing a rapport, assessing both the pain and the patient's experience of the pain, understanding the patient as a person, and engaging in shared decision making.[131,132] Additional objectives of the examination

Table 25.4 Pain Behavior Clusters[63,115,116*]

Classification	Characteristics	Recommended Approaches
Fear Avoidance vs. Pain Persistence		
Fear avoidance†	Pain-avoidant behavior, fear of pain, catastrophizing, hypervigilence, social reinforcement for pain behaviors	Decrease focus on symptoms, set functional goals, gradual increase in activity despite symptoms, reinforce healthy behaviors, ignore pain behaviors, graded exposure, movement visualization
Pain persistence†	Ignore or deny pain, continue activity in spite of pain, set unrealistic goals, ignore physical limits, low social support	Realistic goal-setting, pacing, alternating activity and inactivity, cognitive restructuring, gradually progressed conditioning exercises, gradual increase in activity, assertiveness training
Pain Behavior Clusters		
Well-adapted‡	Low levels of pain, distress and interference with life; high self-efficacy and activity	Pain education and pain coping skills, cognitive behavioral therapy
Dysfunctional‡	High pain intensity, interference with activity, pain behavior, social support and solicitousness; negative pain self-talk	Operant restructuring (reinforce healthy behaviors and do not reinforce pain behaviors), cognitive behavioral therapy
Distressed with little social support‡	Low self-efficacy, social support, solicitousness of others; "punished" rather than rewarded for pain behavior; high affective distress and perceived daily stress	Cognitive behavioral therapy including stress and pain management, help managing dysfunctional relationships
Psychophysiologically highly reactive‡	High stress-reactivity, muscle tension, daily stress; low social support, little reinforcement for pain behavior, low activity due to pain	Relaxation, biofeedback, cognitive behavioral therapy

*Reproduced from Russek L, and McManus C. A Practical Guide to Integrating Behavioral and Psychologically Informed Approaches into Physical Therapist Management of Patients With Chronic Pain. *Orthopaedic Physical Therapy Practice.* 2015;27(1:15):8–16 with permission from the Orthopaedic Section, APTA, Inc.

specific to chronic pain include: (a) determination of pain severity to monitor changes with treatment, (b) measurement of the impact of pain on physical and psychosocial function, (c) identification of the pain mechanism to guide treatment, and d) identification of psychosocial factors impacting pain so they can be addressed.[133] The following discussion will address each of these objectives.

Pain Management Tools

Pain severity or intensity can be measured using a variety of unidimensional measures, such as the *Numeric Rating Scale* (NRS), *Verbal Rating Scale* (VRS), *Visual Analog Scale* (VAS), *Facial Pain Scale* (FPS), or pain thermometer. (See DeSantana and Sluka[134] and other resources[135,136] for review of these measures.) Although the Joint Commission on Accreditation of Healthcare Organizations (JCAHO) has emphasized the importance of pain assessment by calling pain "the fifth vital sign," clinical guidelines for chronic pain management emphasize that single-dimension pain intensity measures such as the VAS or NRS are inadequate for chronic pain. Furthermore, emphasis on unidimensional pain rating scales encourages patient attention to and preoccupation with pain, which interferes with effective pain management.[137]

Ideally, a comprehensive outcome measure of the impact of pain on physical and psychosocial function should examine each of the domains within the ICF: body structure or function, activity, and participation.[138] A multitude of pain questionnaires and outcome measures exist to measure both nonspecific and disease-specific severity and impact of pain; the choice of tool depends on the purpose for which the information will be used. For a more comprehensive discussion of pain measurement, interested readers are referred to several excellent resources.[133-136,139-143] Table 25.5 provides a short list of practical examination instruments

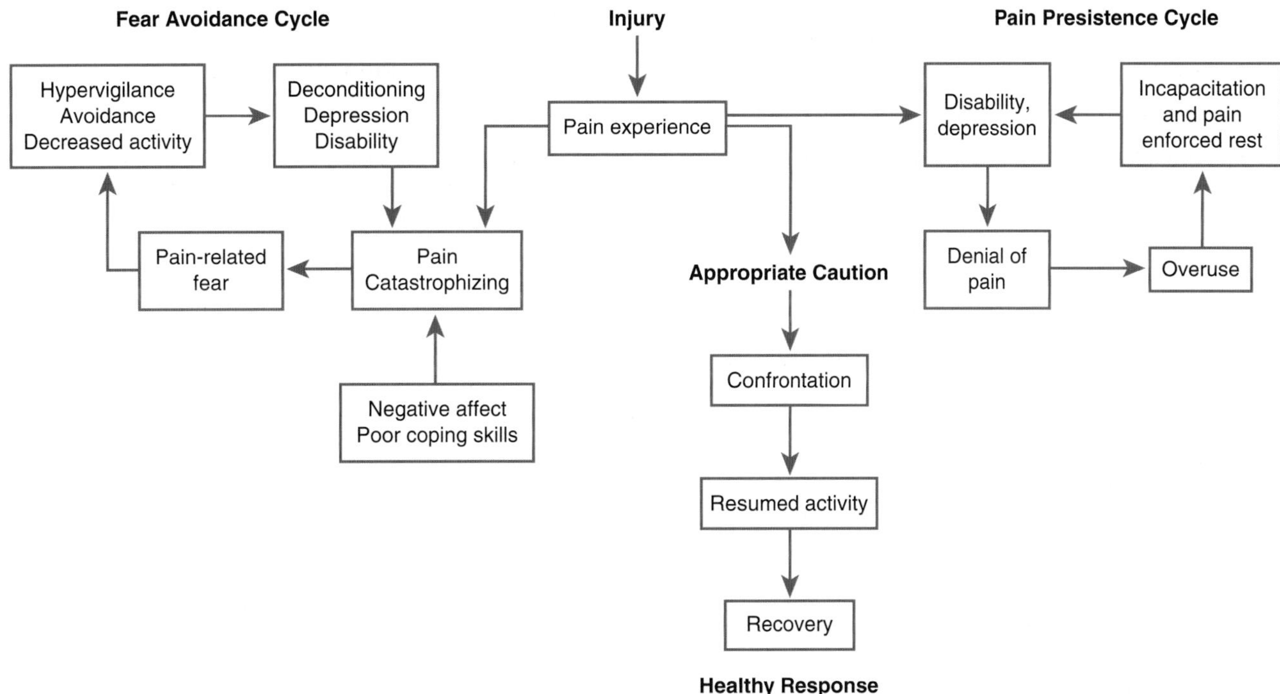

Figure 25.3 Fear Avoidance and Pain Persistence. The fear-avoidance model shows how the pain experience can resolve in the absence of fear or become a vicious cycle in the presence of either pain-related fear or pain persistence. The healthy response to pain is appropriate caution, which leads to confrontation and resumed activity. In fear avoidance, negative affect and poor coping skills cause the pain experience to be perceived as a threat; pain catastrophizing increases pain-related fear, hypervigilance, and avoidance. In the pain-persistence cycle, individuals ignore or deny pain and are overactive until they crash due to the pain; they are then forced to rest. These individuals may demonstrate catastrophization, or depression when not in denial about limitations. In both fear-avoidance and pain persistence, inactivity leads to secondary problems such as deconditioning, depression, and additional disability, which further exacerbate the negative aspects of the pain experience.

appropriate for assessing severity and impact of chronic pain, and where many of these tools can be found online.[144-151]

Tools to measure pain severity in the clinic should be convenient to use and score, and should have good measurement properties (see www.rehabmeasures@sralab.org). Examples of multidimensional pain-specific tools include the *Pain Disability Index* (PDI), *Global Pain Scale* (GPS), and *Brief Pain Inventory* (BPI). Overall health-related quality of life tools and condition-specific tools have been developed to examine specific conditions. The *Patient-Specific Functional Scale (PSFS)* allows patients to identify specific functional activities of personal importance affected by their pain condition, which can be helpful in identifying a few key functional goals for a patient whose presentation may otherwise be somewhat overwhelming to the clinician.[152] Therapists should be cautious about interpreting restrictions as due solely to physical limitations, as some functional limitations may be due in part to difficulty focusing attention, handling stress, fear of movement or fear of pain, and other psychological factors.[61,153]

Identifying the Pain Mechanism or Type

The pain mechanism refers to whether the pain is primarily nociceptive (with or without peripheral sensitization), peripheral neuropathic, central neuropathic, or central sensitization (see Table 25.1 for characteristics of different types of pain). Patients with chronic pain often have multiple types of pain and the relative impact of different pain types may change from day to day. For example, a patient may have acute nociceptive-dominant or neuropathic conditions superimposed on chronic pain: that is, a person with fibromyalgia may still have rotator cuff impingement, myofascial trigger points, lumbar instability, or carpal tunnel syndrome and the central sensitization pain from fibromyalgia may wax and wane relative to the nociceptive or neurogenic pain sources.

Identification of the pain mechanism begins with understanding *somatic dimensions* of the pain such as

Table 25.5 Pain Severity and Functional Assessment Tools for Chronic Pain

Pain Scale	Properties	Items	References/Websites
Pain Interference and Function			
Brief Pain Inventory (long and short forms)	Multidimensional scale includes pain ratings, body function, activity, and participation	Long form has 32 items; short form has nine items	Atkinson et al, 2011[147] http://pain-focus.com/hcp/tools/pain-assessment-scales/ https://www.painedu.org/tools.asp [online access]
Geriatric Pain Measure (GPM) (regular and short forms)	Multidimensional scale includes body function, activity, and participation	GPM has 24 items GPM-SF has 12 items	Ferrell et al, 2000;[148] Blozik et al, 2007[149] http://www.palliativecareswo.ca/docs/Geriatric%20Pain%20Measure%20GPM.pdf [online access]
Global Pain Scale	Subscales: pain, emotions, clinical outcomes, activities	33 items for full version, 20 items on short form	Gentile et al, 2011[144] www.paindoctor.com/global-pain-scale [online access]
Graded Chronic Pain Scale	Assesses domains of impairment, activity, and participation restriction	Seven items in original, two items in the Two-Item Graded Chronic Pain Scale	Von Korff et al, 1992.[145] Original scale: http://www.ucdenver.edu/academics/colleges/PublicHealth/research/centers/CHWE/Documents/Graded%20Chronic%20Pain%20Scale.pdf Two-item scale: http://www.agencymeddirectors.wa.gov/Files/AssessmentTools/4-Two%20Item%20Graded%20Chronic%20Pain%20Scale.pdf [online access]
Pain Disability Index	Impact of pain on: home responsibilities, recreation, social and sexual activities, occupation, ADL	Seven items	Tait et al, 1990[146] https://www.nhms.org/sites/default/files/Pdfs/Pain_Disability_Index.pdf [online access]
Pain Disability Questionnaire	Subscales: functional and psychosocial	15 items	Anagnostis et al, 2004[150] https://www.pridedallas.com/questionnaires/ [online access]
Pain, Enjoyment, General activity (PEG)	Subscales: average pain, enjoyment of life, general activity	Three items	Krebs, et al, 2009[151] http://mytopcare.org/wp-content/uploads/2013/06/PEG-Pain-Screening-Tool1.pdf

ADL = activities of daily living.

intensity, location, duration, nature, temporal variation, and other signs and symptoms. Standard mnemonics for pain assessment can be helpful for asking about somatic characteristics of chronic pain (see Box 25.6).[154,155]

Body diagrams provide information about pain location, radiation, and character. Pain and symptom location can be assessed using a body map. Pain diagrams require more patient instruction than pain quantification, and hence are more time-consuming to administer. Patients are instructed to distinguish between aching, burning, stabbing, pins and needles, and numbness; and sometimes sensations such as heaviness, swelling, or other autonomic symptoms. Information about the location and nature of the pain can be used to hypothesize about the source of the pain: sclerotomes, referred pain, dermatomes, and peripheral nerve patterns all implicate specific structures whereas symmetrical patterns of autonomic symptoms implicate central neurogenic involvement. Data obtained from body diagrams are more difficult to analyze objectively than data obtained from VAS or other pain tools, and observer bias may influence analysis of body diagram data.[156]

There are a number of questionnaires available to assist in identifying the type of pain, with most distinguishing

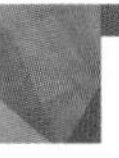

Box 25.6 Mnemonics for Assessing Somatic Characteristics of Pain[154,155]

PQRST

- **P**rovoking/precipitating factors
- **Q**uality of pain
- **R**egion and radiation
- **S**everity or associated symptoms
- **T**emporal factors/timing

SOCRATES

- **S**ite: Where is the pain?
- **O**nset: When and how did it start? Sudden or gradual? Trauma, illness, or other possible cause?
- **C**haracter: How does the pain feel? Sharp? Stabbing? Burning? Aching? Other?
- **R**adiation: Does the pain radiate? Where? What causes radiation?
- **A**ssociations: Other symptoms, such as numbness, paresthesias, heaviness, other?
- **T**ime course: How does the pain vary over the day?
- **E**xacerbating/relieving: What aggravates or relieves the pain?
- **S**everity: Intensity rating

neuropathic from either non-neuropathic or nociceptive pain. (See a comparison of neuropathic assessment tools.)[157,158] For example, the *Neuropathic Pain Scale* (NPS) and *Neuropathic Diagnostic Questionnaire* (DN4) distinguish between neuropathic and non-neuropathic pain.[159] The *Leads Assessment of Neuropathic Symptoms and Signs* (LANSS) distinguishes between neurogenic and nociceptive pain.[160] Some sensitivities and specificities are given in Table 25.6;[159,161-170] a systematic review of measurement properties suggesting that the *Neuropathic Pain Scale* and *DN4* are most appropriate for clinic use, and the *Neuropathic Pain Scale* has been best validated for central neuropathic pain.[158,171] The *McGill Pain Questionnaire (MPQ)* and the *Short Form MPQ (SF-MPQ)* examine sensory, affective-emotional, evaluative, and temporal aspects of pain.[165,166,172] The SF-MPQ includes fewer verbal descriptors, and the SF-MPQ-2 is said to have better differentiation of pain type.[172] The *Central Sensitivity Index* proposes to determine whether central sensitization is present.[161]

Interpretation of findings to determine pain mechanism will be discussed as follows, with Evaluation. Note that identifying the pain mechanism/type is *not* the same as seeking a biological source of pain; there might or might not be damaged or diseased tissues. If damaged or diseased tissues are identified, the examination can

Table 25.6 Pain Classification Tools

Pain Scale	Properties	Items	References/Websites
Pain Quality and Location			
Central Sensitivity Inventory	Score indicates the presence of central sensitivity. Score ≥40 indicates CSS Sn = 81%, Sp = 75%	25 health-related symptoms and a list of previous diagnoses	Neblett et al, 2013[161] https://www.pridedallas.com/questionnaires/ [online access]
Chronic Pain Questions	Distinguishes nociceptive, neuropathic, and central sensitization pain	14 items about symptoms and pain interference. Includes ID pain.	Coyne et al, 2017[162] https://www.pfizermedicalinformation.com/sites/default/files/attachments/electronic-chronic-pain-questions-ecpq.pdf
ID Pain	Score distinguishes neuropathic from non-neuropathic pain. Score ≥3 Sn = 78%, Sp = 74% (Padua, 2013)	Six items	Portenoy et al, 2006[163] http://toolbox.opcpcc.com/wp-content/uploads/2014/09/Diabetic-Pain-Identification-Screener.pdf
Leeds Assessment of Neuropathic Symptoms and Signs (LANSS)	Score distinguishes between neuropathic and non-neuropathic pain; includes self-report and objective testing. Sn = 82%–91%, Sp = 80%–94%†	Seven self-report and 2 sensory testing items for allodynia and hyperalgesia	Bennett, et al, 2001[164] http://www.endoexperience.com/documents/Apx4_LANSS.pdf [online access] https://eprovide.mapi-trust.org

Continued

Table 25.6 Pain Classification Tools—cont'd

Pain Scale	Properties	Items	References/Websites
McGill Pain Questionnaire (MPQ)	Assesses pain intensity, sensory, affective, evaluative, and miscellaneous pain	78 items: 20 pain descriptors (sensory [1–10], affective 11–15], evaluative [16], and miscellaneous [17–20]), one pain intensity item	Melzack, et al, 1975[165] https://eprovide.mapi-trust.org [online access]
McGill Pain Questionnaire Short Form (SF-MPQ) and SF-MPQ-2	Assesses pain intensity, sensory, and affective pain	17 items: 11 sensory descriptors, four affective descriptors, two pain intensity	Melzack, et al, 1987[166] https://eprovide.mapi-trust.org [online access]
Neuropathic Pain Diagnostic Questionnaire (DN4)	Distinguishes between neuropathic and non-neuropathic pain. Score ≥4/10: Sn = 83%, Sp = 90%†	10 pain descriptor items	Bouhassira et al, 2005[167] https://eprovide.mapi-trust.org [online access]
Neuropathic Pain Symptom Inventory	Identifies subgroups of neuropathic pain	10 pain descriptor items and two temporal	Bouhassira et al, 2004[168] https://eprovide.mapi-trust.org [online access]
Neuropathic Pain Scale	Distinguishes neuropathic from non-neuropathic pain. Sn = 66%, Sp = 74%†	10 items: seven sensory descriptors, one temporal, one unpleasantness, one intensity	Fishbain et al, 2008[159] https://www.painedu.org/ https://eprovide.mapi-trust.org
PainDETECT	Distinguishes nociceptive from neuropathic. Sn = 85%, Sp = 80%†	Seven sensory descriptors, one temporal, one about radiation	Freynhagen et al, 2006[169] https://www.healthrising.org/forums/resources/paindetect-questionnaire-to-identify-neuropathic-pain.160/
Pain Quality Assessment Scale (PQAS)	Distinguishing types of pain and is an outcome measure	20 pain descriptor items and one temporal pattern; differentiates between nociceptive and neurogenic pain	Victor et al, 2008[170] https://eprovide.mapi-trust.org [online access]
Self-report Leeds Assessment of Neuropathic Symptoms and Signs (S-LANSS)	Distinguishes neuropathic from non-neuropathic pain; S-LANSS is the LANSS without the two objective testing items	Seven self-report questions	Bennett et al, 2001[164] http://clahrc-gm.nihr.ac.uk/cms/wp-content/uploads/GM-SAT_SLANNS.pdf [online access]

seek to determine the specific pathophysiology through standard tests and measures.

Identification of Psychosocial Factors Impacting Pain

Research suggests that physical therapists are good at collecting information about the somatic components of pain, as described already, but are not as good at collecting information about cognitive, emotional, behavioral, and social domains.[173] Focusing the interview on somatic characteristics of the pain limits the evaluation to a biomedical, rather than biopsychosocial, view of pain. There are several models that can help physical therapists collect a broad spectrum of biopsychosocial information. Oostendorp et al[173] used a review of the literature to develop a list of 51 questions spanning the biopsychosocial spectrum of chronic pain; they summarized their findings as the SCEBS model, outlined in Box 25.7, which addresses biological/somatic, psychological (cognitive, emotional and behavioral), and social domains. The somatic dimension addresses similar information as discussed above. Behavior includes the patient's current self-management approach, including use or abuse of medications, alcohol, or other drugs, including marijuana.

Wijma et al[174] modified the SCEBS model to include type of pain and motivation, ending up with the PSCEBSM model of patient examination (see Box 25.8). This approach strives to first classify the type of pain (nociceptive, peripheral or central neuropathic, central sensitization, or some combination thereof). "Somatic and medical factors" addresses the biological contributions to pain, including current medical management and medications. Cognitive, emotional, behavioral, and social factors are similar to the SCEBS model, though not identical.

The last component of PSCEBSM is motivation, or the patient's perceptions about the source of pain, expectations, and readiness to change. Motivation is a critical issue for patients with chronic pain, as patients need to be active participants in their pain management program. Patients with a passive approach to health care, or with low pain-related self-efficacy, are less likely to be successful in pain management.[175] Since patients with chronic pain have typically failed several treatment attempts before, the approach of *Motivational Interviewing* is recommended by clinical practice guidelines to determine what obstacles could be interfering with patients' adherence to self-management.[27,176]

Evidence shows that physical therapists are not accurate in determining the presence of depression[177] or fear avoidance[178] based on observation; consequently, screening tools for psychological factors may be appropriate. Questionnaires can also help assess the patient's knowledge and beliefs about pain through tools such as the *Pain Beliefs and Perceptions Inventory*[135,136] or *Neurophysiology of Pain Questionnaire*.[179] The *Multidimensional Pain Inventory*

Box 25.7 SCEGS/SCEBS* Model for Taking a Biopsychosocial History[173]

1. **Somatic dimension**: Symptoms, duration, nature, location, intensity, temporal variation, diagnostic test results
2. **Psychological dimension**
   a. ***Cognition***
      i. Expectations regarding PT
      ii. Attribution: The patient's explanation for the complaints
      iii. Catastrophizing: Thoughts and reactions to symptoms/complaints
      iv. Self-efficacy: Feelings of control over symptoms, ability to do things to decrease complaints
   b. ***Emotion***: Feelings about the symptoms, emotional balance, insecurity, depression, anxiety, feeling overwhelmed
   c. ***Behavior***
      i. Dealing with the complaint: how the patient responds to symptoms, attempts to decrease symptoms, success of these strategies
      ii. Functional limitations: activities and extent to which they are limited by these complaints
      iii. Avoidance: Activities discontinued during or because of symptoms, anxiety about activities, what other people notice about behavior during symptoms
      iv. Talking about complaints: With whom? How often? What do you say?
3. **Social dimension** of pain: Do others notice when you have complaints? What do they notice or think, how do others react? What does your partner think causes your complaints? How do you feel about this? Do the complaints affect your social life, work/hobby/sport?

*In Dutch, "behavior" is "gedrag." Components of the questions have been summarized; see Oostendorp et al[173] for a full list of their questions.

classifies patients into one of three pain-behavior clusters: adaptive copers, dysfunctional, and interpersonally stressed[118] (corresponding to "well-adapted," "dysfunctional," and "distressed with little social support" in Table 25.4).[63] Several sources discuss other useful tools for assessing psychosocial factors relevant to disability and chronic pain.[134,143,180]

Since a high proportion of people with chronic pain have experienced some form of abuse, physical therapists need to be sensitive to the needs of this population, especially given the importance of touch to physical therapy.[181] Survivors of abuse may have difficulty distinguishing fatigue from distress or pain, or distinguishing physical from emotional pain.[182,183] Physical therapists working with this population should know how to ask about and respond to

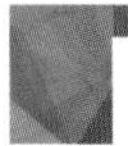

Box 25.8 PSCEBSM Model for Taking a Biopsychosocial History[174*]

1. **Pain type:** Distinguish between nociceptive, neuropathic, and central sensitization
2. **Somatic and medical factors**: Comorbidities, changed movement patterns, exercise capacity, strength: medications.
3. **Cognitive factors**: Cognitions and perceptions about the physical and mental aspects of pain, expectations regarding care, prognosis, and emotional representation of pain. Catastrophizing, perceived injustice or harm
4. **Emotional factors**: Anxiety, anger, fear, depression, and post-traumatic stress. Fear of movement, avoidance behaviors, psychological issues related to work, family, finances, or social issues
5. **Behavioral factors**: Behavioral adaptations to pain: (a) healthy response, (b) fear avoidance, (c) pain persistence
6. **Social factors**: Housing/living situation, social environment, work, relationships. Prior treatments and attitudes toward prior/other health care providers. Social support
7. **Motivation**: Readiness to change, perceptions about the cause of pain and treatment expectations. Psychological flexibility, stage of change

* Wijma et al[174] provide additional detail, along with suggested assessment tools.

revelations of past or present abuse. The physical therapist's response to a revelation is critical to developing a trusting relationship.[182]

The current emphasis on factual data collection should not overshadow the importance of narrative reasoning approaches to examining patients with chronic pain. Narrative reasoning strives to understand the patient's story, illness experience, beliefs, fears, and expectations rather than to quantify or objectify pain.[132] Edwards et al[131] present a comprehensive approach to applying narrative reasoning throughout the patient care process.

Challenges in the Subjective Examination

Psychological or socioeconomic issues, sometimes beyond the patient's immediate control, can compound difficulties with patients who have chronic pain. Patients who believe in a purely biomedical model may arrive wanting a purely physical problem to be identified and fixed; such patients may deny that psychosocial factors are relevant. Patients with a history of frequent treatment failures may be frustrated, angry, demanding, or hopeless. Central sensitization, anxiety, or catastrophization lead patients to overreact, appearing to "symptom-magnify." Some patients with chronic pain may be angry, abusive, demanding, deceitful, nonadherent, or engaging in doctor-shopping.[132,184,185]

Understanding the source of these patient behaviors helps clinicians empathize and improves communication. For example, patients may be defensive or hostile because of previous negative interactions with unsupportive medical professionals.[184] Since chronic pain can lack objective findings of a physical cause for the pain, many patients have struggled with not being believed by health care providers[132] and have been treated as malingerers, liars, hysterics, or drug-seekers.[38] Because psychosocial factors often exacerbate chronic pain, prior health care providers may have treated patients as though the pain was not real or was due to a purely psychiatric problem.[38] Accepting that the patient's pain experience is real can accomplish a great deal in establishing rapport. Strategies to diffuse anger, relieve anxiety, eliminate ambiguity, and maintain appropriate professional boundaries are as important to clinical practice as the skillful application of any treatment technique.[132,184,185]

Interviewing patients with chronic pain can also be overwhelming simply because of their complexity and the need to address such a range of psychosocial factors. Histories of childhood abuse can be emotionally draining to hear. Chronic pain is difficult to treat, often leaving both patients and providers unsatisfied with the results. Clinicians may feel frustrated and inadequate, leading to stress and burnout.[132] Even when patient-provider interactions are constructive, the emotional needs of patients with chronic pain can lead to *empathy fatigue* for the clinician, a state of emotional, mental, and physical exhaustion. Health care providers need to take care of their own emotional well-being. Stebnicki et al[186] offer strategies for avoiding empathy fatigue: provide a support system within the facility where clinicians can discuss the stress of working with difficult patients, provide mentoring for new clinicians, encourage support networks outside the workplace, avoid having one clinician treat many difficult patients at one time, and promote education and wellness programs within the clinic or organization.

Since the prevalence of abuse is very high among people with chronic pain,[181] the physical exam should be performed carefully. Survivors of abuse often become stressed by physical contact needed in the exam and may demonstrate hypervigilance, anxiety, disempowerment, distrust, somatization, transference, or dissociative reactions. Strategies to build trust include the following: ensure two-way communication; observe body language; establish positive rapport and a trusting therapeutic relationship; give the patient control and respect boundaries; obtain consent frequently; keep the patient an active participant; pay attention to physical stressors; recognize and respond to triggers; check in with the patient; and try alternative treatment approaches if the patient is uncomfortable.[182,183]

Systems Review

The complex nature of chronic pain means that the systems review component of the patient examination is extremely important. Systems review in the *Guide to Physical Therapist Practice*[187] includes cardiovascular/pulmonary, integumentary, musculoskeletal, neuromuscular, and communication components. The goals of systems review are to identify areas that will require further testing and to identify body structure/function deficits that might impact rehabilitation or that might require referral. For example, cardiovascular screening of vital signs may indicate whether there are cardiovascular restrictions to aerobic exercise. If the patient has reported severe fatigue (and especially if the patient is a hypermobile female), the possibility of *postural orthostatic tachycardia syndrome* (POTS) should be investigated further.[188] While measuring respiratory rate, clinicians should observe the breathing pattern, because overuse of accessory breathing muscles can aggravate pain. The integumentary system should be examined, particularly for old injuries or surgeries that could compromise fascial mobility or lymphatic flow. Neuromuscular screening should include balance, locomotion, and transfers. Testing for clonus, hyperreflexia, and hypertonicity may be important if there is any suspicion of *serotonin syndrome* (see section Pharmacological Management of Chronic Pain).[189] The communication, affect, cognition, and learning style component of the systems review is particularly important given the psychosocial aspects of chronic pain.

For patients (especially women) presenting with widespread chronic pain, musculoskeletal screening should include the *Beighton Score* for generalized joint laxity and individuals who score ≥5/9 should be assessed for hypermobility spectrum disorders (i.e., hypermobile Ehlers-Danlos syndrome or hEDS).[190,191] Patients with hEDS may present with diagnoses of fibromyalgia, myofascial pain syndrome, chronic headaches, or spinal pain; if the underlying hypermobility is not identified and addressed, treatment is more likely to fail.[192] Chronic pain often involves multiple body systems, such as the gastrointestinal (GI) system with irritable bowel syndrome or the urinary tract with chronic pelvic pain.[193] Goodman and Snyder[194] provide a comprehensive discussion of review of systems.

Physical Therapy Tests and Measures

Physical therapy tests and measures for patients with chronic pain provide information about the type of pain or abnormal sensory function (e.g., neuropathic vs. nociceptive pain); irritability of the condition; underlying tissue pathology, if there is any (e.g., OA, nerve compression); body structure/function deficits due to injury/disease, if present; body structure/function deficits resulting from the chronic pain, either secondary to the pain (e.g., trigger points) or to disuse (e.g., weakness or balance deficits); and initial functional status.

The specific body structure and function measures needed will be determined by how the patient presents, because each patient with chronic pain has different structural and functional involvement. If the clinician hypothesizes that a specific neuromusculoskeletal condition may be contributing to nociceptive, inflammatory, or peripheral neurogenic pain, the examination should include specific tests and measures for those conditions. For example, a patient with stroke-related pain may have shoulder instability, a patient with diabetic neuropathy may have carpal tunnel syndrome, or a patient with post-concussion headaches may have cervical instability. Patients with systemic pain conditions, such as MS, could have an acute musculoskeletal injury superimposed on the underlying chronic pain. Therefore, standard musculoskeletal and neurological tests may be appropriate. It is important to remember, however, that patients with central sensitization may have a positive response to many pain provocation tests due to hyperalgesia and allodynia, even in the absence of local tissue pathology. Furthermore, signs of inflammation, such as edema, warmth, and rubor, may be due to neurogenic inflammation in the absence of local tissue damage. The following discussion will address some tests and measures that may be useful in examination of patients with chronic pain.

Sensory Integrity

Since many types of chronic pain are associated with abnormal activity in sensory nerves, sensory integrity is important. *Quantitative Sensory Testing* (QST) refers to a set of psychophysical measurements used to assess somatosensory function that may be altered in certain types of chronic pain. QST can be used to measure hyperalgesia and allodynia associated with neuropathic pain, or central or peripheral sensitization as well as sensory deficits associated with neuropathic pain.[195,196] Tests can assess minimum threshold perceived, threshold perceived as painful, localization, tolerance, or differentiation of different sensory inputs. Tests can assess small (mostly nociceptor) and large (normally non-nociceptor) afferents. Tests can be either static or dynamic. Static tests assess a single point, such as a pain threshold or an intensity rating for a standardized stimulus. Dynamic tests assess central integration (temporal and spatial summation), and descending control (descending inhibition).[195] Research suggests that a subset of tests easily performed in the clinic could include sensory threshold, static mechanical allodynia, dynamic mechanical allodynia, punctate hyperalgesia, temporal summation, cold allodynia, and cold hyperalgesia. Research is under way to identify QST profiles that could guide classification of and intervention for people with chronic pain.[196] Table 25.7 indicates what structures might be tested with each test modality to provide information about pain threshold and tolerance, temporal summation, and pain area mapping.[195] Several reviews[195,196] and protocol descriptions[96,197] provide further information about QST.

Table 25.7 Quantitative Sensory Testing (QST)[195]

Stimulus	Bedside Exam	QST Tool	Target Fiber (Pathway)
Cold	Test tubes	Calibrated thermode	A-delta (spinothalamic)
Heat	Test tubes		C (spinothalamic)
Light touch (static)	Q-tip/cotton	Calibrated monofilament	A-beta (lemniscal)
Vibration	Tuning fork	Vibrometer	A-beta (lemniscal)
Pinprick	Pin	Calibrated pin	A-delta C (spinothalamic)
Pressure (blunt)	Examiner's thumb	Algometer	A-delta C (spinothalamic)

Proprioception deficits due to either underlying pathology or as a result of the pain[104,198-200] may perpetuate microtrauma, macrotrauma, and pain. For example, post-stroke shoulder pain is associated with impaired proprioception,[201] and cervical joint position sense is compromised in patients with chronic neck pain.[202] Joint position sense can be examined using traditional tests for proprioceptive awareness (see Chapter 3, Examination of Sensory Function), a goniometer, or a laser pointer.[203,204]

Palpation

Palpation for tenderness may be useful for identifying tissue damage, muscle spasm, trigger points, or hyperalgesia and allodynia. Palpation can be quantified through use of an *algometer*, which measures palpation pressure. *Pressure pain threshold (PPT)* is the point at which pressure changes from comfortable pressure to slightly unpleasant pain.[205] Similar to QST, decreased PPT may be noted in areas of primary or secondary hyperalgesia, or may be widespread and observed at remote sites, providing evidence of central sensitization.[206,207] Allodynia can be examined qualitatively with light brushing or by using test tubes filled with cold or hot (40°C) water for thermal allodynia.[140,208] Because patients may present with widespread hyperalgesia and allodynia, palpation for tenderness might not be useful for identifying involved tissues as it would with a patient whose condition is primarily nociceptive.

Muscle Performance

Many widespread pain complaints are associated with myofascial trigger points.[27,89,209,210] *Trigger points (TrPs)* are defined as ropelike taut bands within a muscle fiber. Palpation may elicit local tenderness or referral along the pattern specific for that muscle. To elicit the referred pain pattern associated with trigger points, pressure needs to be maintained for at least 10 seconds or only local tenderness will be detected.[209-211] Palpation of a TrP may elicit a local twitch response, a transient contraction of the muscle fiber, or a *jump response*, which is patient vocalization or withdrawal from the palpation. An *active TrP* exists when the patient reports spontaneous local or referred pain for that TrP. A *latent TrP* exists when local or referred pain is only elicited with palpation. Trigger points can cause a variety of symptoms other than pain, such as tinnitus, dizziness, tachycardia, shortness of breath, nausea, constipation, diarrhea, and so forth.[209,210] Standard muscle strength testing can be helpful to assess the effects of deconditioning.

Motor Control

Many patients with neurological conditions have chronic musculoskeletal pain due to abnormal motor control or muscle performance.[35] Chronic LBP (CLBP) and whiplash also appear to be associated with motor control deficits.[202,212,213] Testing for spinal pain may include use of the Stabilizer® for lumbar or cervical motor control.[214] Patients with underlying neurological disorders may be tested as described in Chapter 5, Examination of Motor Function: Motor Control and Motor Learning.

Balance

An examination of balance is often indicated because the primary injury or disease, deconditioning, and/or fear of movement may compromise balance.[215] Chronic pain has been associated with balance impairments and increased risk of falls among the elderly, and even near-falls can exacerbate pain conditions by straining muscles. The specific choice of balance test depends on the patient (see Chapter 6, Examination of Coordination and Balance, for a discussion of balance tests). Some patients will have difficulty with a basic *Romberg test*, whereas others will have no difficulty completing the *Berg Balance Scale*. The *Activity-Specific Balance Confidence Scale (ABC)* is a self-report tool for balance confidence, which may reflect limitations due to kinesiophobia as well as to physical balance deficits.[216]

Activity and Participation Measures

Activities commonly affected by chronic pain include physical functions such as walking, mobility, changing or maintaining body position, toileting, preparing meals, doing housework, parenting, or job tasks (see Chapter 8, Examination of Function). Quantification of activity and participation restrictions can be examined through either self-report or performance measures. Self-report assessment tools were discussed already, in Subjective Examination, and summarized in Table 25.5. Note, however, that some of these outcome measures are designed to assess pain rather than physical function. The *Oswestry Low Back Pain Disability Questionnaire,* for example, asks how much each activity is restricted by pain; this depends on psychosocial context as much as patient's physical ability.

For patients with widespread pain, physical performance measures can assess multiple body regions with one test. For example, the *30-Second Sit-to-Stand Test, Timed Up and Go*, and *10-Meter Walk Test* are efficient ways to assess functional lower extremity strength and balance. Combined performance tests such as the *Short Physical Performance Battery* (SPPB), which combines sit-to-stand transitions, balance, and walking velocity, reflect activity, and predict participation restrictions.[217,218] Although the SPPB was designed for the elderly, it provides an appropriate level of challenge for many adults with chronic pain who have very limited function. Chronic pain is often associated with deconditioning, which exacerbates activity and participation restrictions.[215] A *2- or 6-minute walk test* can provide valuable information about endurance and willingness to exercise, as well as activity tolerance.[219] Formal functional capacity evaluations can be useful for establishing a person's physical work capability. These standardized test batteries can last from 3 hours to 2 days and may include any aspect of physical job requirement, such as fine motor control, cardiovascular fitness, postural tolerance, and lifting strength.[220]

PHYSICAL THERAPY EVALUATION, DIAGNOSIS, AND PROGNOSIS

Evaluation and Diagnosis

The physical therapy evaluation and diagnosis of patients with chronic pain builds on the examination to: (a) identify the pain mechanism(s) to guide treatment, (b) identify physical and psychosocial factors impacting pain so they can be addressed, (c) assess of the impact of pain on physical and psychosocial function to select appropriate goals, and (d) determine whether the patient requires referral to other health care providers.[133]

Therapists can use several approaches in identifying mechanisms/types of pain. Pain classification questionnaires described already, in Table 25.6, can also be helpful for distinguishing nociceptive, neuropathic, and central sensitization. Or, therapists may use the descriptions provided in Table 25.1 or a decision flow chart, as shown in Figure 25.4.[40,212]

The following description is vastly oversimplified but, in general, pain that is localized and responds appropriately to mechanical stressors is likely to be nociceptive. Localized pain that responds excessively to mechanical stressors may involve peripheral sensitization.[29] Pain corresponding to peripheral nerve injury or disease, that follows a dermatomal or peripheral nerve pattern and includes paresthesias, burning/electrical sensations and/or numbness, hyperalgesia and/or allodynia, and can be mechanically provoked or spontaneous is likely to be peripheral neuropathic.[40,221] Neuropathic pain corresponding to CNS injury or disease with a neuroanatomically consistent distribution is likely to be central neuropathic.[35,36] Widespread pain and hypersensitivity that is disproportionate to peripheral tissue threat or damage, present in the absence of identifiable tissue damage, or has spread beyond the initial damage, that may include multiple senses (light, sound, smell, as well as touch), includes summation, hyperalgesia and/or allodynia, and multiple system sensitivity (e.g., GI, urogenital, skin) is likely to involve central sensitization.[39,94,161,222] Visceral pain tends to be diffuse, may be referred, and can be associated with autonomic changes.[70,223,224] Patients may have more than one pain type/mechanism and the predominant type may vary over time.

Clinical Implications: Convergence between somatic and visceral structures means that activation of visceral nociceptors can result in pain, sensitization, and hyperalgesia in the tissues at the somatic referral site. Similarly, activation of somatic nociceptors can result in pain, sensitization, and hyperalgesia in visceral tissues.[70,223,224]

If the pain has a nociceptive component, evaluation should identify the involved tissues and determine why they are persistently irritated. For example, someone with drooping shoulders may have persistent trigger points due to overstretched trapezius muscles; if the underlying postural dysfunction is not addressed, treatment of the trapezius muscles is likely to fail. A person with hypermobile Ehlers-Danlos syndrome may have mechanical pain due to overstretched joints or instability due to poor proprioception; if the underlying hypermobility or proprioceptive deficits are not identified and addressed, treatment is more likely to fail.[192] A person with Parkinson's disease or spinal cord injury may have muscle pain due to spasticity. Some peripheral neuropathic pain has mechanical causes that can be identified and addressed, such as abnormal neural tension in carpal tunnel syndrome. Some of these nociceptive and peripheral neurogenic sources of pain can be addressed through standard physical therapy approaches. Furthermore, patients with sensitization or central neuropathic pain may have musculoskeletal factors, such as poor posture, muscle imbalance, or poor motor control that fuels sensitization and exacerbates other sources of chronic pain.

Identification of contributing and perpetuating factors is also essential in managing chronic pain. The ICF model identifies personal and environmental contextual factors that can affect body function or structure, activity, or participation. Personal factors contributing to

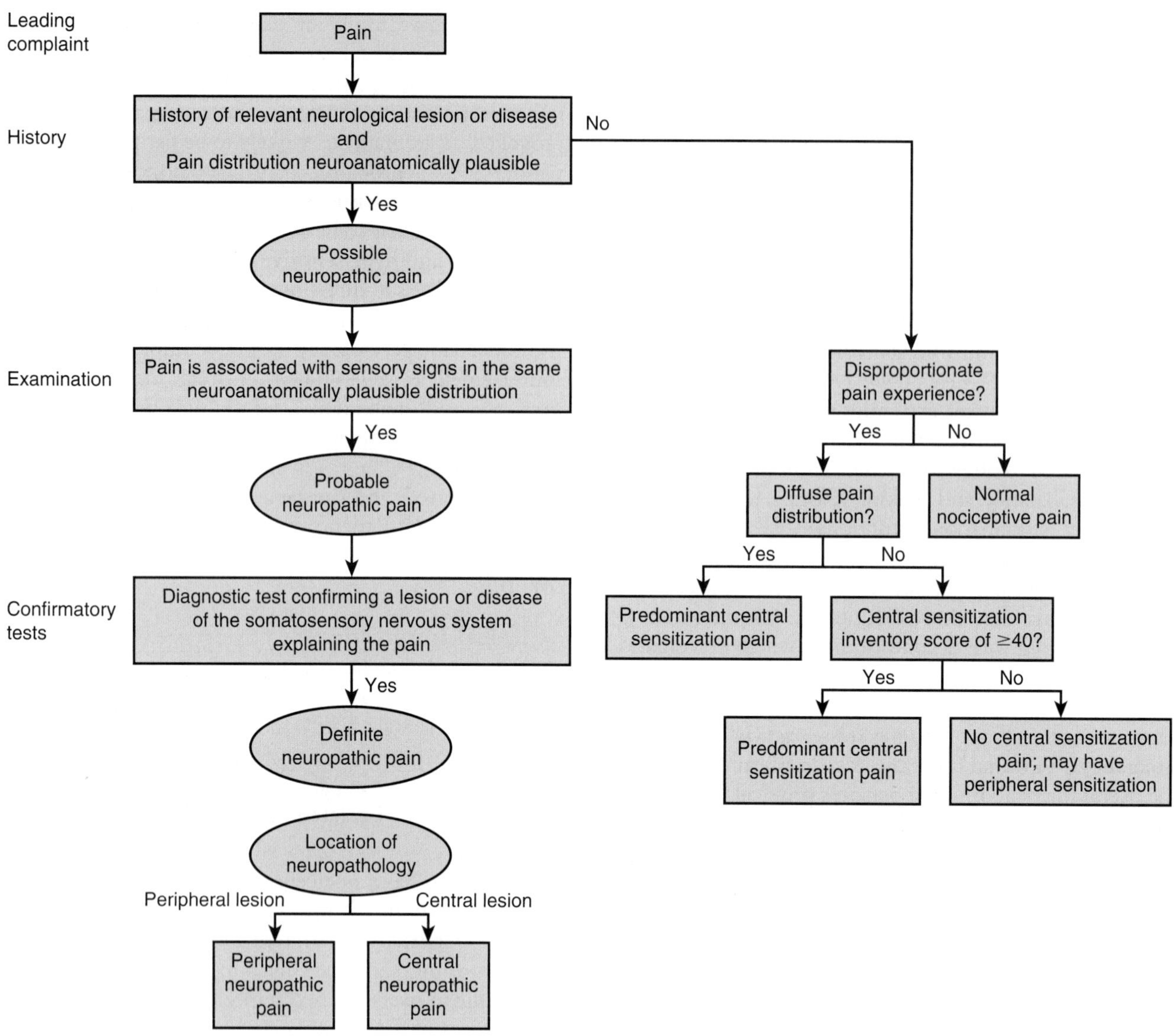

Figure 25.4 Flow chart for distinguishing pain types. This flow chart shows a decision making process for identifying the dominant type of pain. If there is a neurological lesion or disease, evaluation continues through the left branch to confirm neuropathic pain and determine whether it is peripheral or central. In the absence of a known neurological lesion, evaluation passes through the right branches to determine whether central sensitization is present, peripheral sensitization, or normal nociception. Note that most pain is often a mix of more than one pain mechanism. *(Modified from Nijs et al,[94] Nijs et al,[39] and Finnerup et al.[40])*

chronic pain include age, gender, heredity, past and present experience, occupation, education, personality, coping strategies, and social or cultural background. Personal factors include such traits as anxiety, fear avoidance, catastrophizing, depression, and low patient motivation. These traits may also be characterized as body function involvement (global psychosocial functions) in the ICF model.

The evaluation process should address the patient's knowledge and beliefs about chronic pain (and sometimes also the beliefs of family members or caregivers) and factors that might interfere with the patient's willingness or ability to actively participate in physical therapy.[105] Active participation in self-management can be compromised if the patient strongly holds to a biomedical model and is convinced that the only solution is to find and fix the tissue pathology causing pain.[16] The patient's pain behavior (Table 25.4) can influence optimal treatment approach; for example, patients with high fear avoidance need to be encouraged to become more active, while patients with high pain-persistence need to learn how to pace their activities.[63,225]

Possible outcomes of the evaluation process include referral to or consultation with another practitioner either instead of or in combination with physical therapy intervention. Yellow flags suggesting psychosocial factors (Table 25.3) may require referral or may be addressed through psychologically informed physical therapy management.[115,226] Examples of red flags suggesting systemic involvement include personal or family history of cancer, recent infection, significant weight change without effort, pain unrelieved by rest or change in position, inability to relieve or provoke symptoms during the examination, night pain, pain in a visceral referral pattern, and certain associated signs and symptoms. Readers are referred to Goodman and Snyder's *Differential Diagnosis for Physical Therapists* for an extensive discussion of how to screen for red flags, and how to determine whether referral should occur at the same time as or instead of physical therapy intervention.[194] Each patient's situation should be examined individually because many people with chronic pain have multiple red or yellow flags that may be readily explained, do not require referral, and do not preclude physical therapy. When in doubt, the referring physician should be contacted to discuss these findings.

Prognosis

Prognosis determines the level of optimal improvement that may be attained through intervention and the required amount of time required to reach that level. Prognosis depends on personal and environmental factors identified in the evaluation process. Again, the alert flags (Table 25.3) highlight biological, psychosocial, and contextual factors that may enhance or compromise prognosis. For example, medical comorbidities, anxiety, or a history of sexual abuse compromise prognosis, whereas a record of regular exercise, adequate stress management strategies, good social support, or good emotional function lead to an improved prognosis.

Pain readiness to change is a personal characteristic that may also influence prognosis. As with other forms of readiness to change based on the *Transtheoretical Model of Behavior Change*, individuals who are ready to change are more likely to incorporate pain management strategies into their lives; hence their prognosis is better. Patients resistant to change are unlikely to be compliant with rehabilitation and are less likely to improve.[227,228] Environmental factors such as having a support system, attitudes of friends and family, or access to comprehensive health care all affect prognosis.

There has been a shift in recent decades regarding whether reduction or elimination of pain is a reasonable goal of intervention. In the 20th century, the biomedical model strove to eliminate chronic pain by fixing the pathology causing pain; that often did not work. Efforts then shifted toward optimizing function and quality of life and accepting that chronic pain often could not be eliminated. The philosophy that "pain is unavoidable, suffering is optional" attempted to decrease the distressing and disabling consequences of pain, even if the pain could not be altered or eliminated.[27,28,229] In recent years, however, better understanding of the biopsychosocial nature of pain and neuroplasticity have led to the hope that it may be possible to rehabilitate (i.e., reverse) chronic pain through retraining the brain.[14,16]

Anticipated goals and expected outcomes for the patient with chronic pain are those that address principles listed in Box 25.9 and Box 25.10. Since focus on pain and pain reduction goals may lead individuals to become hypervigilant, patients, families, and health care providers often need to deemphasize pain severity as a measure of status or treatment effectiveness. Patients should focus on functional goals that emphasize active coping skills and wellness behavior rather than pain-based goals.[63] Studies show that activity and participation restrictions can be related more to fear-avoidance and deconditioning than to pain.[27,28] The *Patient-Specific Functional Score* encourages patients to identify and track personally relevant functional goals.

The current emphasis for chronic pain management is a concept called *functional restoration*, which aims to empower patients to optimize their physical and emotional well-being, activities of daily living, and return to vocational and avocational activities.[43] Clinical practice guidelines recommend five components to the goals: increased function, increased physical activity, stress management, improved sleep, and decreased pain.[27] Because patient/family education is critical, goals of the educational component of intervention are given in Box 25.14.

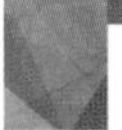

Box 25.9 General Principles of Chronic Pain Management[137]

- Create an effective therapeutic alliance with the patient.
- Provide pain neuroscience education.
- Facilitate psychological and emotional well-being.
- Teach non-pharmacological pain management techniques.
- Improve sleep.
- Increase physical strength, endurance, and cardiovascular fitness.
- Increase mobility, independence, and functional activity.
- Teach proper body mechanics.
- Enhance vocational potential.
- Provide vocational rehabilitation for paid work, volunteer work, and hobbies.
- Enhance family communication, and function.
- Increase social and recreational activities.
- Improve ability to cope with pain.
- Decrease or eliminate dependence on medications.
- Decrease overutilization of the health care system.

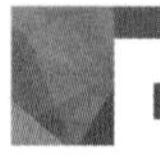

Box 25.10 Goals of Educational Components of Chronic Pain Management[27]

The goals of patient education are for the patient to:

- Acknowledge that chronic pain is real.
- Recognize the complex, biopsychosocial nature of pain, and the need for a multifaceted management program in which the patient is an active participant.
- Understand the impact of pain on sleep, mood, energy, fitness, ability to work, family life, and stress.
- Avoid letting pain guide activity or medication use because pain-based treatment encourages pain behavior.
- Recognize and utilize wellness behaviors.
- Recognize the role of poor posture and body mechanics in perpetuating pain.
- Overcome fear of movement through gradual exposure to feared activities.
- Learn relaxation strategies.
- Actively participate in own management program.
- Enlist family support and participation in management program.
- Participate in an exercise program, either through physical therapy, independently, or using community resources.
- Minimize fear of movement and activity reduction due to fear of movement.

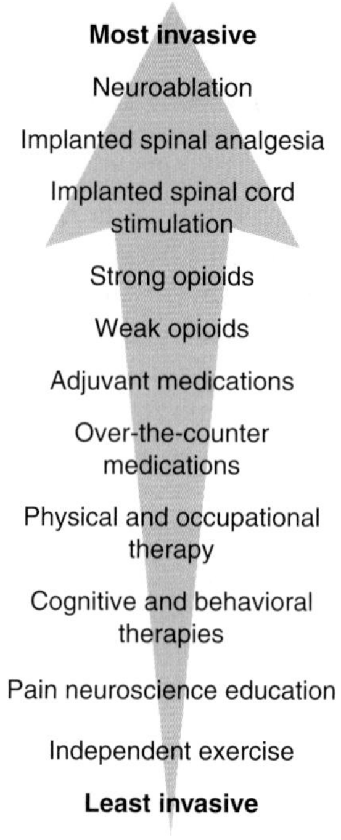

Most invasive
Neuroablation
Implanted spinal analgesia
Implanted spinal cord stimulation
Strong opioids
Weak opioids
Adjuvant medications
Over-the-counter medications
Physical and occupational therapy
Cognitive and behavioral therapies
Pain neuroscience education
Independent exercise
Least invasive

Figure 25.5 The Pain Management Continuum. Although the order of intervention may vary based on the patient's preference, chronic pain management should generally start with self-management strategies emphasizing education and exercise before progressing to non-opioid medications and, only if previous interventions have failed, progress to stronger medications and surgical interventions.

PHYSICAL THERAPY MANAGEMENT OF CHRONIC PAIN

The Multidisciplinary Pain Management Team

The principles of chronic pain management include a range of physical, psychological, vocational, and medical objectives (Box 25.9). The physical therapist's role in management of chronic pain depends on both the patient and the environment in which the therapist practices. Figure 25.5 shows the general progression of interventions from least invasive (e.g., independent exercise) to most invasive (e.g., surgical interventions). This general progression has changed dramatically in the past decade, with decreased emphasis on medication and passive interventions and increased emphasis on education, exercise, and active self-management.[43] The most appropriate order for any individual patient will vary based on biomedical and psychosocial factors and patient preference. Functional restoration requires a biopsychosocial treatment approach emphasizing education, minimizing passive or palliative therapies while transferring to the patient primary responsibility for long-term self-management of his or her physical and emotional well-being.[27,28,42]

Knowledge about how different management approaches may be beneficial for different types of pain is still evolving, and practice guidelines are now presenting different pain management recommendations for different pain mechanisms. For example, graded aerobic exercise, relaxation, and adjuvant medications may be recommended for fibromyalgia, while cognitive-behavioral therapy and topical agents may be advised for myofascial pain, with transcutaneous electrical nerve stimulation (TENS) and adjuvant medications for chronic neuropathy.[27]

A multidisciplinary pain management team may include any of the following health professionals: primary care physician, pain specialist, physiatrist, anesthesiologist, psychiatrist, psychologist, pharmacist, social worker, caseworker, physical therapist, occupational therapist, sleep specialist, or nurse.[2,3,230] Although multidisciplinary care has been shown to be more effective than monotherapy or standard medical care, the optimal components of multidisciplinary care have not been identified,[230] and the cost-effectiveness has been questioned.[231]

Patients with chronic pain often have involvement of multiple body systems and may be working with several health care providers. Coordination of care and communication with other providers is essential to a comprehensive, patient-centered approach. It is especially important that the patient receive consistent information from providers regarding such things as the fact that there might not be current tissue damage other than that due to deconditioning, and the need to maintain activity despite pain. All providers should be consistent about encouraging functional goals rather than using pain ratings as a guide of treatment success.[27,28,42,43] Patients may need to be referred for consultation with other providers. Some referrals, such as to a psychologist or pain specialist, are obvious. Other potential referrals include a sleep clinic for patients suspected of having a sleep disturbance; occupational therapy for patients with trouble problem-solving or managing their medical appointments; relationship counseling for patients whose relationships are stressed by chronic pain; and nutritional counseling, especially for patients whose obesity or food sensitivities exacerbates their pain.

A physical therapist working within a multidisciplinary pain clinic may be able to refer psychological issues to the team psychologist and coping skills to the occupational therapist. However, a therapist working in an isolated outpatient clinic might not have access to such collaborations and may need to integrate a broader range of components into the plan of care (POC) while remaining within the physical therapist's scope of practice. The following discussion emphasizes what may benefit patients with chronic pain; who provides a given service will depend on the context. In cases when multidisciplinary or specialist care is not available or practical, motivated patients may be able to pursue some aspects of their care independently. (See Appendices C and D for a list of patient resources.)

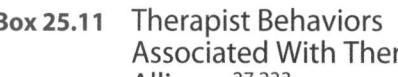

Box 25.11 Therapist Behaviors Associated With Therapeutic Alliance[27,233]

Patient Facilitating/Involving
Greeting warmly
Letting the patient tell the story
Being communicative (asking questions, attention, explanation)
Patient-centered behavior (asking questions, discussing options)
Collaboration (asking patient's opinion and involving the patient in decisions)
Taking time to discuss patient concerns, encouraging questions, answering clearly
Treating patient on the same level
Respecting opinions and feelings
Checking patient understanding
Working to adjust treatment

Patient Supporting
Being gentle during examination
Being comforting and caring
Being truthful and frank
Interpersonal care (showing patience, care, and concern)
Sensitivity to concern
Reassurance and support, emotional support

Patient Education
Shared decision making
Giving information, explaining what the patient needs to know

Therapeutic Alliance

Perhaps the most important component of any physical therapy intervention for chronic pain is the therapeutic alliance or relationship, as it is likely to modulate the effectiveness of other interventions provided. Therapeutic alliance is working rapport, harmony, or positive psychosocial connection between the patient and therapist. It relies on a combination of empathy, collaboration, communication, and technical skills.[232-234] See Box 25.11 for a list of therapist behaviors associated with therapeutic alliance. Research has demonstrated that therapeutic alliance impacts outcomes including pain, physical function, activities of daily living (ADL), depression, global health assessment, treatment adherence, and satisfaction.[232,235] In some cases, therapeutic alliance with sham treatment can be more effective than real interventions with minimal patient-provider rapport.[236] Several good reviews of therapeutic alliance are available.[232,233,237,238]

Patient and therapist expectations and the therapist's expression of confidence in the interventions also influence effectiveness. Therefore, the physical therapist should choose words with positive connotations and avoid negative or threatening words. Finding out what treatments the patient believes have been effective or not effective in the past and the patient's treatment preferences can help the therapist select, from appropriate options, those that the patient believes will be most effective. Compliance and benefits are generally greater with treatments patients prefer. Instructions and explanations also impact outcomes, as patients are likely to perceive what they are told to expect.[237] This overall approach is consistent with evidence-based practice, which is the integration of best available evidence with clinician experience and patient preference.

Expectation and therapeutic alliance appear to tap into the powerful placebo response, which is mediated by descending pathways.[82,90] While placebo is sometimes believed to be a psychological response, placebo analgesia has been shown to operate through physiological changes in several components of the neuromatrix, including enhancing descending modulation of nociception[239] and modifying brain activity related to pain.[240,241] Consequently, placebo has concrete physiological benefits that may specifically address neurological abnormalities associated with chronic pain. The placebo response has been demonstrated to occur both when the patient has been deceived and when the patient is aware that the placebo effect is involved.[242]

The issue regarding ethics of consciously utilizing placebo effects within treatment is likely to become important in upcoming years.

Clinical Implications: Treatment for pain is more effective when the patient feels the treatment is being given by a supportive health care provider. This is also true of placebo interventions.[241]

Patient/Client-Related Instruction

Patient/client-related instruction is critical for the active self-management of chronic pain. For the current discussion, the *Guide to Physical Therapist Practice* categories of Functional Training in Self-Care and Domestic, Education, Work, Community, Social, and Civic Life are combined with Patient-Related Instruction because so much of the content overlaps. The family may also require education about chronic pain to both recognize chronic pain as a real disease and to avoid fostering illness behavior in the patient. Patient instruction/education includes pain neuroscience education (which includes "Explain Pain"), and self-management through both psychosocial (e.g., cognitive behavioral therapy) and physical means.

Studies have shown that there is better patient adherence and effectiveness of pain self-management that is matched to a patient's pain behavior.[63,120,174,225] For example, patients who demonstrate fear avoidance require encouragement to be active despite pain, while patients demonstrating pain persistence need to pace themselves. Table 25.4[115] shows the educational approaches most likely to be effective for specific pain behavior clusters.[63,120,225] For example, patients who are psychophysiologically highly reactive benefit from initial treatment focusing on relaxation, biofeedback, and cognitive behavioral therapy. Since patients can transition from one behavior cluster to another over time, educational approaches may need to be modified over time.[63,243]

Also, pain education should adapt based on the patient's readiness to change.[228] For example, patients in the pre-contemplation stage may benefit from the physical therapist taking on a "nurturing parent" role to overcome patient resistance and defensiveness. On the other hand, patients in the contemplation stage might benefit from the physical therapist using a "Socratic teaching" method to encourage patient to reflect on their situation. Patients in the preparation stage may benefit from an "experienced coach" to help them implement strategies, while patients in the action/maintenance phase might benefit most from the therapist as a "consultant."[174] The physical therapist should identify potential learning barriers such as difficulty concentrating, depression, refusal to accept a biopsychosocial model of pain, or lack of social support.

Patient education about pain and pain management can be provided in a variety of formats and there are many excellent educational resources available. Education is often provided one-on-one in the clinic but may also be provided in small or large group settings, using computer resources or books.[16,64,244,245] Web-based resources for clinicians, families, and patients with chronic pain can be found in Appendix 25.B; Appendix 25.C provides a selected list of books to education patients about pain.

Pain Neuroscience Education

Pain neuroscience education (PNE) includes the neurophysiology of pain, including the nociceptive pathways (including synapses and action potentials), as well as the processing systems (spinal modulation, peripheral and central sensitization), neuroplasticity, and the role of psychosocial factors in pain.[246,247] Box 25.12 lists the objectives of PNE. One of the objectives of PNE is to "de-educate" patients prior to re-education. Patients have often been given a biomedical explanation for their pain using pathoanatomical terms such as "deterioration," "herniation," "bone on bone," or "wear and tear"; use of these images can be counterproductive because they increase fear and anxiety, creating perceived danger that contributes to the pain experience. Research shows that patients who are told their imaging findings are typical in asymptomatic individuals are less likely to use narcotic medications than individuals who receive similar imaging reports indicating "abnormalities."[248] Patients should be taught that "abnormal" findings on medical tests and imaging are actually quite common in pain-free individuals, hence such test results do not imply tissue damage that should cause pain.[247] Once patients understand the different types of pain, they can better understand the biopsychosocial contributing factors that need to be managed.

Explain Pain

Explain Pain, developed by Butler and Moseley, builds on PNE with an effort to shift the patient's conceptualization of pain away from believing that pain is necessarily an indicator of tissue damage or disease to the understanding that pain indicates the brain's perception

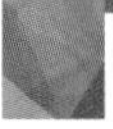

Box 25.12 Components of Pain Neuroscience Education[246,247,253]

Pain Neuroscience
- Neurophysiology of pain
- De-emphasisis of patho-anatomic models of pain (biomedical approach)
- Nociception and nociceptive pathways
- Synapses and action potentials
- Spinal inhibition and facilitation
- Peripheral sensitization
- Central sensitization
- Plasticity of the nervous system
- Psychosocial factors and beliefs contributing to pain

that it needs to protect the body.[16,64] Table 25.8 lists the 10 key objectives of *Explain Pain*, which strive to help patients understand the biopsychosocial nature of pain.[64,249] Explain Pain is distinct from CBT in that *Explain Pain* focuses on the neurophysiology (why CBT methods are helpful) rather than pain coping skills (e.g., how to implement CBT).[250] Patients should be told that this educational component is not just to make them more knowledgeable about their pathology (chronic pain), but that a shift in their understanding of the relationship between perception and pain can actually change the neurophysiology of pain. That is, pain results from the brain's perception of danger and, if education can modify patients' perceptions (i.e., help them realize that hurt does not always mean harm), it can potentially modify the actual pain experience.[14]

Key objectives of patient education about the nature of chronic pain are that (1) hurt does not always mean harm; and (2) there may be no tissue damage that surgery or medication can fix.[52,251] Also, patients should understand what type(s) of pain they have to identify strategies that can most effectively manage the pain. For example, nociceptive dominant pain due to rheumatoid arthritis (RA) may benefit from joint protection strategies whereas patients with central sensitization benefit from exercising despite pain. Furthermore, patients who appreciate that the biopsychosocial nature of pain links mind and body are less likely to become defensive about suggestions of psychological management approaches.

Evidence indicates that pain neuroscience education can decrease disability, catastrophization, fear avoidance, pain behaviors, and health care utilization while increasing pain knowledge, health behaviors, and physical movement.[16,246,247,250,252,253] The goal of PNE and Explain Pain is not just to get patients thinking about pain differently, but to actually normalize neurological processes that have become maladaptive. Evidence shows that these

Table 25.8 Explain Pain Concepts[64]

Target Concept	Explanation
Pain is normal, personal, and always real.	All pain experiences are normal and are an excellent, though unpleasant, response to what your brain judges to be a threatening situation. All pain is real.
There are danger sensors, not pain sensors.	The danger alarm system is just that—there are no pain sensors, pain pathways, or pain endings.
Pain and tissue damage rarely relate.	Pain is an unreliable indicator of the presence or extent of tissue damage—either can exist without the other.
Pain depends on the balance of danger and safety.	You will have pain when your brain concludes that there is more credible evidence of danger than safety related to your body and thus infers the need to protect.
Pain involves distributed brain activity.	There is no single "pain center" in the brain. Pain is a conscious experience that necessarily involves many brain areas across time.
Pain relies on context.	Pain can be influenced by the things you see, hear, smell, taste, and touch; things you say; things you think and believe; things you do; places you go; people in your life; and things happening in your body.
Pain is one of many protective outputs.	When threatened, the body is capable of activating multiple protective systems including immune, endocrine, motor, autonomic, respiratory, cognitive, and emotional pain. Any or all of these systems can become overprotective.
We are bioplastic.	While all protective systems can become turned up and edgy, the notion of bioplasticity suggests that they can change back, through the lifespan. It is biologically implausible to suggest that pain cannot change.
Learning about pain can help the individual and society.	Learning about pain is therapy. When you understand why you hurt, you hurt less. If you have a pain problem, you are not alone—millions of others do too. But there are many researchers and clinicians working to find ways to help.
Active treatment strategies promote recovery.	Once you understand pain, you can begin to make plans, explore different ways to move, improve your fitness, eat better, sleep better, demolish DIMs,* find SIMs,* and gradually do more.

*DIMs and SIMs are terms used in *Explain Pain Supercharged*[64] and *The Explain Pain Handbook: Protectometer.*[249] DIMs refers to "Danger in Me" factors that can increase pain; SIMs refers to "Safety in Me" factors that can decrease pain (https://noijam.com/2017/03/03/supercharging-explain-pain/ used with permission).

interventions enhance neural processing and descending inhibition of pain.[250,254]

Cognitive Behavioral Therapy and Pain Coping Skills

Patients may benefit from *cognitive behavioral therapy (CBT)* and pain coping skills in which beliefs, attitudes, and behaviors are modified to alter the experience of pain, overcome dysfunctional behaviors, improve function, and minimize disability.[27,28,42,43,63,255,256] CBT provides the "how to" as follow-up of PNE "why to."[16] Evidence suggests that CBT strategies can modify several yellow flags associated with disability in chronic pain such as pain beliefs, self-efficacy, and psychological distress.[105,257] Several systematic reviews demonstrate that CBT can be effective in decreasing chronic pain, improving quality of life, and improved physical function, quality of life, sleep, fatigue, depression, and anxiety.[255,258]

It is increasingly accepted for physical therapists to integrate CBT and pain coping skills principles into patient care because therapists already educate patients about relaxation strategies, graded activity, pacing, problem-solving, and functional restoration.[85,105,115,259,260] For physical therapists unfamiliar with psychologically informed practices, guides are available in the literature.[115,259,260] For therapists working with children, behavioral approaches are available specifically for working with children.[261] Although patients benefit from guidance from a health care professional, they may also learn many strategies independently using one of the self-help resources listed in Appendices 25.B and 25.C. Figure 25.6 shows how a variety of behavioral tools can be integrated into self-management of pain.[262] Components of CBT and pain coping skills are listed in Box 25.13.[27,63,85,259] Some examples are described here.

Patients should set realistic activity goals that are meaningful to them. This should include pleasurable activities. Some patients feel that they hurt too much to participate in leisure activity or that they should not indulge in pleasurable activities if they cannot fulfill work, family, or household responsibilities. Losing pleasurable activities, however, aggravates depression, loss of social life associated with those activities, and deconditioning. Consequently, people with chronic pain may need to schedule leisure and recreational activities and set specific goals including such activities.[115,259,260]

Patients should be encouraged to identify and challenge negative thinking using techniques of cognitive restructuring. Patients who dwell on the fact that they have a herniated disc can be reminded that many asymptomatic people have herniated discs, so those magnetic resonance imaging (MRI) findings do not imply that pain is inevitable.[248] Often, people with chronic pain will catastrophize, ruminate, or dwell on negative aspects of their lives.[105,263] Restructuring can be particularly helpful for highly reactive patients, such as those with PTSD.[264]

Patients may need to be taught effective problem-solving strategies. For example, if a patient is unable to schedule 30 minutes/day for exercise, help her identify 5-minute blocks or integrate exercise with other activities, such as including children in the exercise by using a DVD focused on yoga for children. If the patient is unable to garden due to knee pain, encourage him to use raised flower beds, take rest breaks, or use adapted tools. Problem-solving can help address fear-avoidant behavior by identifying and modifying aspects of an activity that cause anxiety.[115,259,260]

Pacing should generally be time-based rather than task or pain based and should alternate activity and rest to avoid bursts of activity.[260] Patients who use task-based pacing (i.e., continuing until a task is done) often push themselves for too long and cause a flare, causing "yo-yo" patterns of activity and rest commonly seen with pain persistent behavior.[116] If they stopped part way through the task and rested or did alternate activities, they might be able to go back to the original task and finish it without a flare. Time-based pacing also avoids negative feedback learning by having patients stop an activity (reward) for complaining of pain.[265] Patients often need to be reminded that "hurt does not equal harm" and that some pain with activity is okay; in fact, muscular soreness after exercise is a normal response.[115,259,260] Progressive or graded activity refers to patients gradually increasing their activity level not using pain as a guide, and will be discussed further with exercise, as follows.

Since sleep disturbance is a common occurrence in chronic pain, patients should be educated in proper sleep hygiene, which includes avoiding caffeine, nicotine, alcohol, and medications containing stimulants, especially before bedtime. Evidence consistently shows that screen time (use of computers, tablets, smartphones) before bed interferes with the quantity and quality of sleep, but this might be alleviated by use of blue light filtering glasses or software or by adequate (>2 hours) exposure to bright light earlier in the day. Sleep hours should be consistent; environmental distractions such as light, noise, and cold should be minimized; stress should be minimized through relaxation or meditation activities, especially before bedtime. Exercise during the day improves quality of sleep. Gentle exercises such as stretching, yoga, qigong, or tai chi may be particularly helpful at bedtime to improve quality of sleep due to their relaxing effects.[100,266,267]

Patients need to understand that stress contributes directly to pain; some patients will be relieved to realize that sympathetic efferents connect directly to nociceptive afferents and the pain-amplifying effects of stress are not all "in their minds." Relaxation can thus decrease pain through reducing nervous system tone, muscle activity, and neuroendocrine reactivity.[85,100] A list of relaxation techniques is given in Box 25.14. Slow, diaphragmatic breathing, which can decrease pain and sympathetic nervous system activity, is one of the simplest to teach

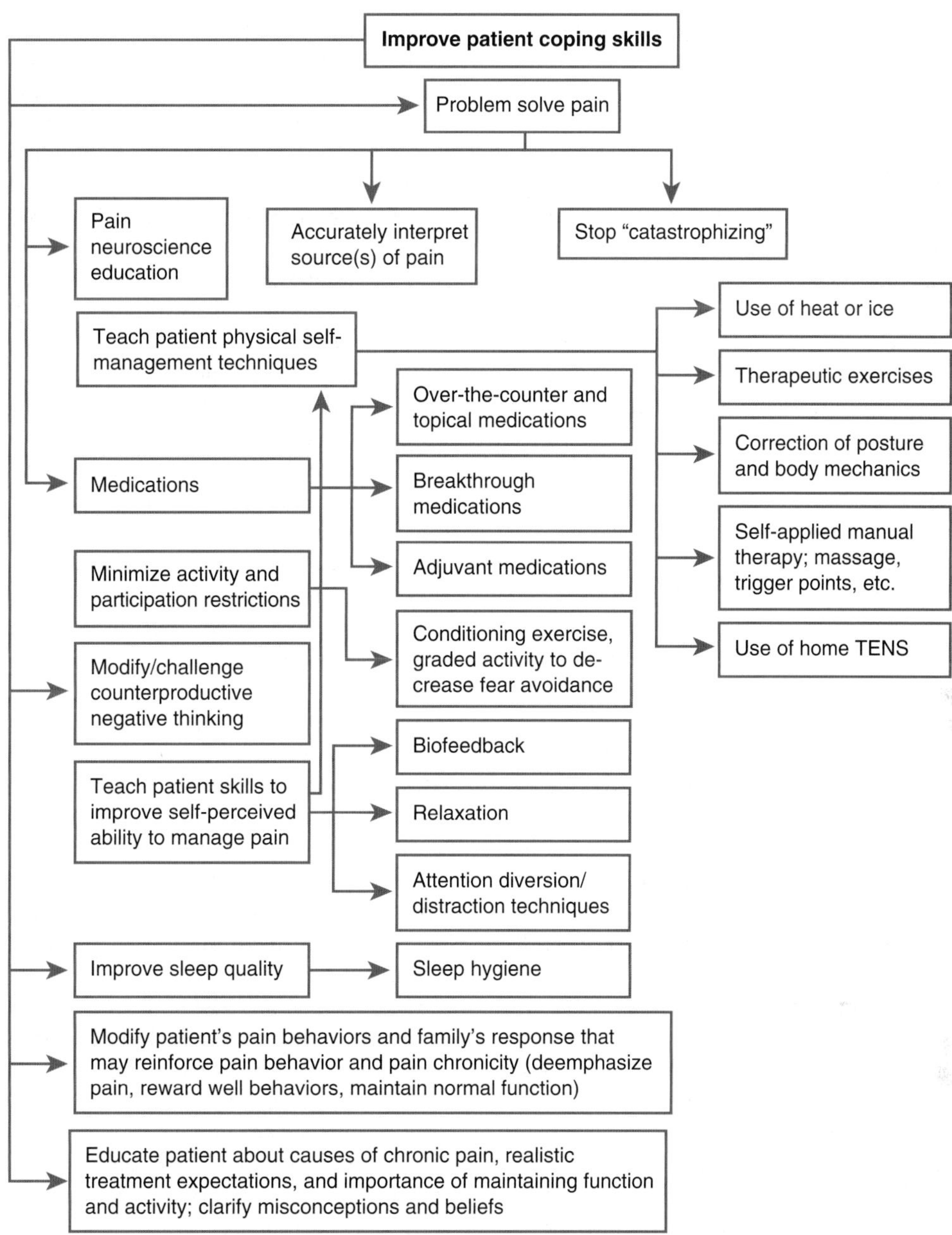

Figure 25.6 Behavioral Management of Chronic Pain. Patients should learn to identify various cognitive and behavioral strategies they can use to manage their pain. *(Adapted from Mueller, 2000,[262] who proposed a similar model for behavioral management of chronic headaches.)*

patients and easiest for them to do.[268] Mindfulness meditation has been successful for managing stress-related diseases such as heart disease and chronic pain. Mindfulness and acceptance-based meditation uses focus on the present moment, attending to thoughts, emotions, sensations, and perceptions without judgment.[27,28,42,269-271] The acceptance aspect of mindfulness meditation helps patients differentiate between pain sensations and suffering, hence improves coping. Appendix 25.C includes several patient resources for learning mindfulness meditation.

Physiological quieting and self-regulation use relaxation training for both physiological and psychological regulation to correct some of the autonomic and neural dysfunctions associated with chronic pain. Although developed for temperomandibular joint (TMJ) pain, the principles are generally applicable to other forms of stress-related pain. Self-regulation training includes (1) education and reassurance, (2) strategies to monitor and reduce abnormal muscle function, (3) proprioceptive awareness training, (4) postural relaxation training, (5) diaphragmatic breathing, (6) methods of improving

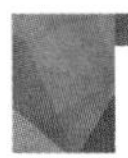

Box 25.13 Cognitive Behavioral Strategies and Pain Coping Skills[27,63,85,259]

Cognitive Behavioral Strategies

- Pain education
- Importance of active self-management
- Demonstrating wellness behaviors rather than illness behaviors
- Goal setting
- Problem-solving
- Identifying and challenging negative thoughts (cognitive restructuring)
- Pleasant activity scheduling
- Elimination of fear-avoidance or pain-persistence
- Progressive activity/exercise
- Time-based rather than task-based pacing
- Not using pain as a guide
- Relaxation (through diaphragmatic breathing, mindfulness meditation, pleasant imagery, biofeedback, progressive muscle relaxation)
- Calming self-statements
- Distraction
- Flare management using self-care strategies

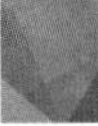

Box 25.14 Relaxation Strategies[27]

- Diaphragmatic breathing: Slow diaphragmatic breathing
- Progressive relaxation: Selectively tensing and relaxing major muscle groups
- Visualization: Imagining a safe and relaxing environment, including sounds, smells, feel
- Autogenic training: Imagining your hands feeling warm and heavy
- Mindfulness meditation: Training the mind to be in the present moment, to be calm, kind, and curious
- Biofeedback using electromyogram (EMG) for muscle tension, heart rate variability (HRV), or galvanic skin response (GSR) for sympathetic tone or skin temperature for parasympathetic activity
- Body awareness activities such as yoga, qigong, or tai chi

sleep onset, and (7) instruction regarding physical activity, diet, and fluid intake.[85] Resources for physiological quieting are included in the Resources for Patients in Appendices 25.B and 25.C.

Family and/or caregiver education can be just as important as patient education. Chronic pain affects the whole family through changes in family roles due to the patient's activity and participation restrictions. The family may reinforce the patient's "sick role" in an attempt to be supportive. Both the patient and the family need to understand the importance of maintaining normal activities and participation to minimize disability; patients must not perceive lack of physical assistance as lack of support or concern from family. In contrast, the family may be completely unsupportive, often owing to lack of objective evidence that the pain is real. Family members may be angry with the individual with pain and may blame that individual for financial, personal, or family problems.[137,272]

Personal intimacy is often very difficult with chronic pain, just as it is for other chronic injuries or diseases. Problems may be due to the pain, deconditioning and fatigue, depression, decreased sense of self-worth, or adverse reactions of medications. Distress is often greater for survivors of childhood sexual abuse.[273] It is important that both partners learn about chronic pain so that they understand the reasons for challenges faced. Both partners need to accept that the nature of the intimate relationship can change and not harbor anger, frustration, blame, or guilt. Individuals with chronic pain can improve their self-image through daily exercise, grooming, and cognitive strategies of CBT. Communication is critical so that both partners can contribute suggestions for problem solving. For example, select a time of day with the least amount of pain and fatigue and find positions that minimize stress to the body. Appendix 25.C includes several patient resources for working through the challenges of intimacy with chronic pain.

Self-Care Strategies

Self-care strategies may include a variety of self-applied techniques such as exercise, heat, ice, massage, topical rubs, or TENS. Although all except exercise are considered passive treatments when provided by the physical therapists, they can all be components of active patient self-management. The effects of exercise will be discussed separately, as follows.

While the popularity of TENS has waxed and waned over the years, recent evidence suggests that it might not have been used optimally in some of the older research and that it can indeed be helpful for pain management.[274,275] TENS operates through both peripheral (gate-control) and CNS mechanisms, including activation of descending inhibition, which is often deficient in patients with chronic pain.[275] High-frequency (>50 Hz) and low-frequency (1–10 Hz) TENS operate through different physiological mechanisms, with the important consequence that low-frequency TENS will not reduce pain in people who are opioid tolerant. Hence, people with chronic pain who are taking opioid medications are likely to benefit more from high-frequency than low-frequency TENS. TENS has a strong dose-response curve and is most effective when the strongest non-painful stimulus is used; the recommended method for setting intensity is not to increase to "strong but comfortable" but to instead increase until the stimulus is painful, then to back down slightly. This second method typically results in stronger intensity, hence greater benefit. The failure to use adequately strong intensities has been proposed as a main reason why past research results have been inconsistent.[274,275] A disadvantage of TENS is that patients develop tolerance and stop obtaining pain relief.[274,276] However, tolerance can be delayed by using combined low and high frequency in the same session or by alternating low and high frequency, or by increasing intensity 10% each day. TENS may be helpful in managing certain types of central neuropathic pain, including MS and some types of spinal cord injury, but not for post-stroke pain.[277] Finally, evidence suggests that TENS might be most effective in reducing motion-related pain compared to pain at rest; patients should therefore be encouraged to use TENS during activity or exercise when possible.[274,275]

Patients with chronic pain often develop trigger points that act as nociceptive triggers for peripheral and central sensitization.[278] Because trigger points tend to be recurrent, they are well suited to self-management using a trigger point cane, tennis balls, or other pressure devices. All patients should recognize the role of poor posture and body mechanics in perpetuating pain syndromes. Several books listed in Appendix 25.C can be helpful for patients managing multiple and variable trigger points.

Topical medications provide another self-care option for patients.[27,28,42,43] Topical rubs fall into three broad categories: those creating cooling sensations, those creating warmth sensations, and those with bioactive agents. Those that create a cooling sensation, generally menthol-based, work as a counterirritant, probably via the gate control mechanism. Those creating the sensation of warmth are generally capsaicin-based. An important aspect of capsaicin-based topical medications is that the counterirritant effect begins immediately after application but the neurogenic effect requires daily use for 6 to 8 weeks.[27] One proposed explanation for the time required is that repeated use of capsaicin depletes nerve endings of substance P; the actual physiology appears to be more complex.[279] A variety of NSAIDs can be administered via topical rubs, especially if involved structures are superficial. Research shows that medication can be absorbed through the skin into muscle, synovium, and joint tissue.[280] Lidocaine cream or patch can be beneficial for peripheral neurogenic pain.[31] Opioids can also be administered transdermally as a prescription medication.

Other self-care devices may include home lumbar or cervical traction units, paraffin, home massage devices, topical rubs, and hot tubs. Self-care training in all environments is critical to effective management of chronic pain (Figure 25.5). Therapists can help patients create a sample personal care plan (for an example, see Appendix 25.A). This personal care plan combines patient goals with patient responsibilities for self-care, including physical therapy, independent exercise, stress management, and sleep hygiene; medications may be included as part of the self-care program. Patients should understand the importance of increasing activity and function; patients should not focus only on reducing pain.

Exercise

Therapeutic exercise is a key part of chronic pain management.[27,28,42,43,281] Exercise addresses chronic pain in several ways: (1) provides non-specific exercise-induced analgesia, (2) reduces deconditioning and functional limitations, (3) improves psychological function and quality of life, (4) corrects postural or motor imbalances contributing to the pain, (5) decreases comorbidities such as obesity, diabetes, cardiovascular disease, and immune dysfunction, and (6) decreases chance of falls and further injury.[215,281] Graded exercise can decrease fear-avoidance.[282]

A 2017 Cochrane review of systematic reviews on exercise for chronic pain concluded that exercise decreases pain in people with mild to moderate chronic pain, with strong evidence that exercise increases physical function. Well-designed studies were small and generally did not include subjects with moderate to severe pain. The conclusion from that review and multiple clinical practice guidelines is that many forms of exercise are potentially beneficial, including aerobic, strength, flexibility, range of motion (ROM), core, balance training, yoga, Pilates, and tai chi.[42,43,215] Regular exercise has also been shown to protect against the development of chronic pain, apparently because physical inactivity causes the nervous system to generate an exaggerated response to low-intensity insults.[283]

Several mechanisms operate for exercise-induced hypoalgesia. Any activity is better than being sedentary, as increased sedentary time is associated with decreased function of descending inhibitory pain modulation; even low-intensity exercise such as walking appears to be beneficial for various types of chronic pain.[281,284] The benefits of exercise are dose-dependent, and moderate to vigorous activity is associated with improved descending inhibition and decreased temporal summation of pain.[284,285] The impact of exercise on sleep deserves special mention, as sleep disturbance is common in many forms of chronic pain. Regular physical activity appears to improve sleep, and patients naturally increased their physical activity when they obtained higher quality sleep. Movement therapies such as tai chi and qigong have been shown to be particularly helpful in improving the quality of sleep.[286]

Exercise-induced hypoalgesia is demonstrated when a single bout of exercise results in decreased pain perception (pain thresholds and intensity) in healthy adults and the analgesic effects are proportional to exercise intensity.[281,287] Studies of exercise-induced hypoalgesia have been less consistent in people with chronic pain. In general, however, regular exercise appears to decrease pain by activating the endogenous opioid system and activation of descending inhibition. Additional benefits include decreased depression, decreased cognitive dysfunction, and improved autonomic function.[281]

Exercise also decreases the systemic inflammation that is often associated with chronic pain, with increased frequency of exercise showing improved responses.[288-290] Even a single bout of moderate aerobic exercise was able to return inflammatory biomarker levels almost to normal in women with fibromyalgia.[288] The mechanism is mediated by the sympathetic nervous system and hypothalamic-pituitary adrenal axis, which can stabilize the immune-neuroendocrine system in people with dysregulation. Exercise reduces stress hormones and inflammatory cytokines and stimulates anti-inflammatory and "anti-stress" responses, which are opposite those seen in healthy individuals.[290]

Research does not indicate that any one type of exercise is best for pain relief, so individual patient preferences or comorbidities can guide selection.[281,286,291] Aerobic exercise has the strongest evidence for pain reduction, but recent research suggests that moderate to high-intensity resistance training is also beneficial for decreasing pain.[292-294] Strength training also improves quality of life and emotional affect. Aquatic resistance exercise generally does not provide as much strength improvements as land based but may be particularly helpful for patients with OA or fibromyalgia, who obtain additional pain relief from a warm, therapeutic pool.[27,28,42] Flexibility training has smaller benefits for pain reduction, but improved benefits for emotional affect such as anxiety and depression. Movement therapies such as yoga, tai chi, and qigong are helpful because they are gentle and well tolerated in this population, and provide improved physical function, balance, mobility, flexibility, and decreased anxiety and depression.[286] In general, regular exercise has psychological benefits, such as increasing self-efficacy and decreasing depression.[215]

The selection of exercises will depend on the patient's goals, body structure/function impairments, and preferences. Exercises may need to start by addressing impairments that interfere with performance of target exercises. For example, if a patient lacks ROM needed to use an exercise bike, then ROM exercises may be necessary first. Or, a patient lacks the balance to safely do tai chi or the strength to play tennis, preliminary exercises may be needed.

The optimal dose of exercise for people with chronic pain is not known,[281] but low to moderate intensity (50%–60% maximum HR) appears to be beneficial for pain reduction while higher intensities are beneficial for cardiovascular fitness.[286] Note that many patients with chronic pain cannot start exercising at this intensity and may need to break up their daily exercise into short units, even starting at 1 to 2 minutes at a time, if necessary. Patients with chronic pain are typically deconditioned and may have multiple comorbidities, so establishment of an exercise program may be similar to that for an older adult, even if the patient is younger. That is, people with chronic pain need to "start low, go slow" to avoid flares that will discourage them or prevent them from continuing.[295,296]

However, patients should not use pain as a guide in progressing exercise. They should be reminded that hurt does not always indicate harm or tissue damage and that some soreness and discomfort (up to 2 hours after exercise) is typical and to be expected when beginning an exercise program even if exercise is decreasing pain overall. People with chronic pain often have trouble distinguishing psychological distress from physical pain, so they sometimes need guidance distinguishing fear of movement from actual pain. Specific performance-based targets can prevent overly enthusiastic patients from overdoing their exercise and triggering a yo-yo response of activity and inactivity. For example, exercises could progress a set amount determined by the therapist, such as 10% per week, allowing for an occasional easy day if the patient has a flare. Patients should be discouraged from omitting exercises entirely on flare days as this perpetuates cycles of inactivity; they should decrease exercise by, perhaps, 50% then return to prior targets once the flare has past. Several resources[295,296] provide detailed charts of recommendations for exercise prescription and progression for patients with chronic pain.

In addition to pain relief, exercise is helpful for increasing function limited by secondary body structure/function impairments such as deconditioned cardiovascular status, weakness, and balance deficits.[27,28,42,215] Since falls and sensory motor problems are more common among individuals with chronic pain,[297] balance and proprioceptive training are often important components of the exercise program. Exercise can also address contributing factors, such as muscle length and strength imbalance, poor posture, and poor motor control. However, studies have generally shown that the results of special purpose exercises (e.g., spinal stabilization or motor control, Pilates) have no better outcome than general exercise.[213,291,298]

Adherence to an exercise program can be challenging for people with chronic pain. People with chronic pain may report short-term increases in pain in response to exercise even though regular exercise can decrease pain. However, a Cochrane review of systematic reviews concluded that the studies show no long-term increases in pain in response to appropriately prescribed and progressed exercise, only expected transient increases in muscle soreness due to unaccustomed activity. Patients should therefore not just be advised to exercise without guidelines about how to begin and progress using principles of pacing and gradual progression.[215,296] Patients should also be informed that temporary, "normal" soreness may occur but should subside with continued exercise, and that pain during exercise does not prevent pain relief from occurring after exercise.[215,281] The prevalence of obesity is high among patients with chronic pain, and exercise may be more difficult and uncomfortable for this population. Strategies for improving compliance for people who are obese include breaking exercise up into multiple shorter bouts, decreasing joint range during exercise, and replacing impact with non-impact activity.[299]

Kinesiophobia (fear of movement) can also be an obstacle to exercise participation. Graded motor imagery can help people overcome fear of movement through a gradual progression from left/right judgment, visualization, and mirror feedback. For patients who are extremely fearful of specific movements or activities, graded exposure can allow patients to be successful at lower levels of stimulus as they transition to progressively more stressful activities.[300] Patients can start with simple visualization of a position or movement and progress through simplified versions of the activity and then to the activity itself.[105,282]

Other barriers to adherence include the belief that pain is chronic and doubt about the effectiveness of the recommended exercises, lack of a clear rationale for the exercises, low self-efficacy, fatigue, forgetting, perceived lack of time, and symptoms associated with comorbidities. Table 25.9 lists common barriers to exercise and potential solutions.[215,301]

Patients will be most motivated if exercises relate directly to functional goals. For example, a patient who wants to go to the movies with his wife could follow an exercise program designed to overcome his specific obstacles, such as walking from the car to the theater and sitting comfortably through the movie. Exercises with a social component help address isolation often experienced by people with chronic pain; for example, group exercise programs, active family involvement, or dancing can make exercise more enjoyable.

Neuromuscular Re-education

Neuromuscular re-education can be useful for retraining muscles for proprioception, motor control, or relaxation. In conditions such as whiplash or chronic neck pain where proprioceptive deficits may exist,[302] joint position sense can be both tested and trained using a goniometer or laser pointer.[203,204] For the cervical spine, a laser pointer attached to the patient's eyeglasses or to a plastic hair band can be aimed at a target; patients may practice accurate repositioning or fine motor coordination while tracking shapes.[303] Since proprioceptive information from the cervical spine is integrated with visual and vestibular input, eye and vestibular exercises can be beneficial in conditions involving the cervical spine.[304]

Proprioceptive and motor control impairments throughout the body can affect the ability of people with chronic pain to perform exercises correctly, so repeated feedback during exercise instruction can maximize safety and success. Kinesiophobia can be reduced if early efforts at exercise are successful.[282]

Table 25.9 Barriers and Potential Solutions for Exercise Adherence[215,301]

Perceived Barrier	Potential Solutions
Increased pain with exercise, symptoms due to comorbidities	• Appropriately selected exercises (e.g., using low-impact or decreased weight-bearing exercises, breaking exercise into shorter bouts) • Appropriately progressed exercises: using principles of pacing and graded progression • Patient education that some increase in pain due to exercise is normal and should decrease over time
Belief that pain is chronic and inevitable	• Patient education that exercise is an effective method for not only reducing pain but increasing function, psychological wellness, overall wellness, and quality of life
Doubt that the exercises will be effective, lack of clear rationale for exercises selected	• Patient education about exercise-induced hypoalgesia/pain relief, with explanation of physiological mechanisms • Patient education about the purpose of exercises selected, beyond exercise-induced hypoalgesia
Low self-efficacy	• Patient empowerment and reassurance
Fatigue	• Dividing exercise into smaller units • Reassuring the patient that fatigue decreases with regular exercise
Forgetting	• Helping the patient establish a routine including exercise • Encouraging family members to remind or encourage the patient
Lack of time, low prioritization	• Patient education regarding the importance of exercise for pain management and for decreasing future chronic pain • Encouraging patient to integrate social activities with exercise • Encouraging patient to problem-solve, for example, watching TV while exercising, exercising by walking more to and from work or shopping, etc.
Lack of resources	• Providing patient with low-resource options, such as walking, body-weight resisted exercises, and so forth

Certain chronic pain conditions respond to specific types of exercise or neuromuscular reeducation. For example, phantom limb, complex regional pain syndrome (CRPS), dystonia, and stroke are typically associated with changes in sensory and motor mapping in the sensorimotor cortex.[198] In these cases, sensory input through use of a myoelectric prosthesis, virtual reality or mirror training, or sensory discrimination training stimulates cortical reorganization that is generally associated with decreased pain.[305,306] Two-point discrimination training might be a simple strategy for restoring tactile acuity and decreasing pain.[198] Graded motor imagery and mirror therapy have been shown effective for CRPS[307] and visual imagery has been shown beneficial for central neuropathic pain associated with spinal cord injury[308] and Parkinson's disease.[277,309] Overall, a systematic review of bodily illusions on clinical pain found mixed results, but concluded that mirror therapy, bodily resizing, and functional prostheses show promise.[310]

Cognitive functional training is a variation of CBT that combines cognitive training with functional movement training and functional integration.[311] The cognitive portion is similar to CBT as described already. The functional movement component involves teaching posture and specific functional movements while increasing body awareness, relaxation, and control. The goal is to recontextualize painful movements. The third stage integrates functional movement patterns into ADLs that caused pain.[311]

Biofeedback, which uses feedback to the patient to teach modified neural control, can also stimulate a relaxation response and decrease autonomic function associated with stress.[312] A variety of biofeedback devices can be used with chronic pain. Electromyography (EMG) works by measuring the intensity of muscle activation; EMG biofeedback can teach patients to relax overactive muscles and isolate functional muscles without widespread over-recruitment. It can be used to teach patients how to relax specific muscles by teaching them to decrease muscle activity. For example, patients with TMJ pain can learn to relax the masseter. Once patients learn to relax the target muscle, they are progressed to maintain or restore that relaxation after adding physical activity such as standing and walking or after visualizing stressful images. EMG works well with conditions involving excessive muscle tension or trigger points.[85,255] In some cases, research has identified subgroups more or less likely to benefit; for example, people with cramping phantom limb pain are more likely to benefit from EMG than those with burning pain.[313] Galvanic skin response (GSR) works through controlling the autonomic nervous system and decreasing the stress response. Heart rate variability (HRV) is a newer form of biofeedback in which autonomic balance is restored by synchronizing breathing with low-frequency patterns.[312,314] Skin temperature biofeedback can be an effective way to stimulate parasympathetic activity by placing the thermistor (temperature sensor) on the hand and imagining the hands becoming very warm. Temperature biofeedback is particularly useful for migraines, by placing the thermistor directly on the patient's forehead or using hand-warming biofeedback.[315] Respiration rate and HR can also be used as low-technology biofeedback measures.

Other forms of physical relaxation training can also be considered neuromuscular re-education. Slow, diaphragmatic breathing can stimulate a relaxation response. Yoga, tai chi, or qigong may be beneficial both through their relaxation effect, proprioceptive training, alleviation of fear-avoidance behavior, and perhaps sleep enhancement, and alleviation of depression and anxiety.[100,292,313,316,317]

Manual Therapy

Manual therapy may be beneficial in the case of persistent pain with ongoing nociceptive input or in cases where central sensitization is perpetuated by peripheral nociceptive input.[27,28,42,291,318,319] Manual therapy may resolve a transient flare of central sensitization and thus decrease other symptoms of central sensitization such as hyperalgesia and anxiety[320,321] or may improve movement or alignment to allow exercise. Manual therapy may also enhance patient expectations and improve participation in more active components of therapy, such as neuroscience education.[318] A recent systematic review concluded that manual therapy including manipulation and muscle energy techniques appears to be effective for CLBP and knee pain; however, the evidence was weak for other manual therapies (Swedish massage, Feldenkrais Method, and reflexology) and other sources of chronic pain (fibromyalgia and neck pain).[322] Because manual therapy may not permanently alleviate pain, there is a risk of patients becoming dependent on it; use of passive manual therapy modalities should therefore be limited to helping resolve acute flares and should be used as a means to allow active interventions such as exercise rather than an isolated intervention.[27,28,42,43] Patients may use massage and trigger point management as part of the their self-care program.

Assistive Devices

Patients with persistent activity limitations due to defined physical impairments may benefit from assistive devices to improve function. Patients with joint disorders, such as OA, RA, or hEDS (i.e., joint hypermobility) should consider devices that decrease stress to affected joints. For example, shoe orthotics and knee braces have strong evidence for modest improvements for OA of the knee.[323] Other devices that decrease stress to joints include items such as jar openers and carts for transporting groceries. Conditions associated with focal weakness, such as stroke or MS, may benefit from braces or splints to support weakened structures and decrease muscle length and strength imbalances. Each patient's specific situation needs to be examined and evaluated, because over-reliance on splints and appliances to protect painful regions in the absence of specific pathology can be counterproductive if it reinforces pain and illness behavior.[193]

Biophysical and Other Modalities

TENS is recommended as an effective self-management approach; see section on self-management, aforementioned.[27,42,274] Thermal agents such as heat and cold can both be helpful for short-term pain management but are most helpful as adjuncts to more active pain management, such as exercise, education, and self-management. Evidence for other biophysical modalities such as ultrasound, laser, and shockwave is generally weak, and prolonged use of these modalities is discouraged because they instill a passive approach to pain management.[21,291] Evidence for cervical or lumbar traction is also weak. Heat and ice can be recommended for home use as part of the patient's self-management program.[324]

■ MEDICAL MANAGEMENT OF CHRONIC PAIN

Medical Diagnostic Testing

There are currently no clinically useful imaging or laboratory test diagnostic to measure chronic pain. Furthermore, abnormalities observed in imaging tests do not prove that the identified pathology is related to the patient's pain, as indicated in multiple studies showing positive lumbar imaging findings in people without LBP[27,325,326] and the mismatch between radiographic findings of OA and pain.[327] In fact, studies show that doing MRI imaging early in an episode of acute back pain is associated with poorer health outcomes and increased likelihood of disability.[328,329] In contrast, informing patients that their imaging findings are typical for asymptomatic individuals decreases narcotic usage.[248]

Laboratory tests, such as thyroid hormone levels, sedimentation rates, Lyme titers, or general blood screening, can be appropriate to rule out conditions that are treatable. Electrodiagnostic testing, such as needle EMG, is not indicated unless there is suggestion of specific neuropathy. Diagnostic nerve blocks (peripheral or sympathetic), joint blocks (facet or sacroiliac), and provocative discography can help determine whether a given structure is involved; see any of the clinical guidelines on chronic pain for more information on interventional testing.[27,28,42,193] Skin biopsy is currently being researched as a potential diagnostic tool for small fiber neuropathy, which is often difficult to diagnose through other means, but this is not clinically applicable at this time. Neuroimaging using functional MRI (fMRI), positron emission tomography (PET), and proton magnetic resonance spectroscopy (H-MRS) are currently used in research to observe neurophysiological or neuroanatomical abnormalities, but are not yet useful for making diagnoses other than frank neuropathy.[196]

Ultimately, repeated diagnostic testing to search for an undefined physical abnormality is generally not indicated because it fosters patients' obsession with obtaining a pathophysiological diagnosis that might not exist and thus fosters over-adherence to a biomedical model rather than looking for strategies to identify contributing factors and manage the pain using a biopsychosocial model.[27,28,193]

Pharmacological Management

Medications used for chronic pain are rapidly evolving and beyond the scope of this chapter. Medications are typically staged, starting with those least likely to cause adverse side effects to those with greatest risk. They should also be selected based on the type of pain (e.g., nociceptive, neuropathic, and so forth; see clinical practice guidelines for indications.[27,28,42,43,330,331] *Adjuvant medications* (medications whose primary indication is a condition other than pain, but which have demonstrated benefit in pain management) are added next. Muscle relaxants and weak opioids are added if prior medications, physical therapy, and cognitive therapy are unsuccessful. Good overviews of the mechanisms and efficacy of various classes of medications for chronic pain are available.[27,42,43,330,332]

Adjuvant medications include antidepressant, antiseizure, muscle relaxant, and sleep medications. Antidepressants for pain are typically used at much lower dosages than when used to treat depression because the mechanism of action is distinct from treatment of depression. Tricyclic antidepressants (TCAs) have demonstrated benefit for neurogenic pain, fibromyalgia, LBP, headaches, and irritable bowel. Results for selective serotonin reuptake inhibitors (SSRIs) for chronic pain are inconsistent. Serotonin-norepinephrine reuptake inhibitors (SNRIs) appear to have the benefits of TCAs for managing neuropathic pain with fewer side effects. Evidence is also strong for some anticonvulsant medications in managing neuropathic pain, including fibromyalgia and lumbar radiculopathy. Medications to treat sleep disturbance can also be beneficial because sleep disturbance frequently exacerbates chronic pain.[331] Benzodiazepines and muscle relaxant medications are generally not recommended for prolonged use in chronic pain because risks are relatively high and there is little evidence of benefit. Cyclobenzaprine, however, has been shown to be effective for fibromyalgia and conditions involving chronic muscle spasm.[27,42,43,330,332]

Opioid use for managing nonmalignant (i.e., noncancer) chronic pain increased in the 1990s, in an attempt to decrease patient pain reports.[27,28,43] Although opioids are frequently effective for acute pain, evidence suggests that effectiveness in decreasing chronic pain or increasing function or quality of life is limited.[333,334] Furthermore, evidence suggests that opioid use may encourage focus on pain and illness behavior, which may interfere with recovery.[335] The potential for both physiological tolerance and addiction makes opioids particularly risky, and careful screening for addictive history or personality is indicated before initiating opioid medication, especially given the current crisis in opioid abuse in the United States. Opioid-induced hyperalgesia, due to changes in receptors or neural circuits, may further undermine pain management and is considered by some another primary pain mechanism. If opioids are used, their risk/benefit should be reevaluated regularly, and they should be discontinued if not providing effective pain relief.[27,42,333]

Serotonin syndrome (serotonin toxicity) is a potentially dangerous consequence of polypharmacy (use of multiple drugs to treat the same condition) with medications often used to manage chronic pain. The most likely medications involved are SSRIs, SNRIs, TCAs, some opioids, and triptans (used as an abortive medication for migraines) and less obvious medications such as antibiotics.[43,336] Because the condition is potentially lethal, the physical therapist should remain alert for symptoms of serotonin syndrome: agitation, anxiety, confusion, hypomania, hyperthermia, tachycardia, diaphoresis, flushing, mydriasis (prolonged pupil dilation), hyperreflexia, clonus, myoclonus, shivering, tremor, and hypertonia.[43,189,336]

Other Medical Management

In a progression of interventions for patients with chronic pain, invasive procedures and opioid medications are to be avoided if possible. Interventional management approaches are beyond the scope of this chapter, and readers are referred to current clinical practice guidelines for more about medical management.[27,28,42,43]

COMPLEMENTARY AND ALTERNATIVE APPROACHES

Complementary and alternative approaches include active therapies such as yoga and tai chi, mental therapies such as hypnosis and meditation, manual therapies such as acupuncture and reiki, devices such as magnets, and herbal and nutritional supplements. Magnets, herbal medicines, and supplements are beyond the scope of this chapter. Since 35% to 63% of people with chronic pain use these approaches,[100,313] physical therapists should be familiar with how they may be integrated into a comprehensive POC.

Movement therapies such as yoga, tai chi, and qigong now have substantial support as forms of exercise for improving flexibility, strength, balance, and proprioception, and decreasing fear of movement.[100,292,313,316] Not only do these activities have physical benefits, but they also foster relaxation and independence, both of which are important components of self-management. Furthermore, many of these activities are practiced in a community-based group setting, which addresses issues of isolation and loss of recreational activities.

Manual techniques include acupuncture, chiropractic, massage, reiki, and therapeutic touch. Extensive research shows that acupuncture can be a beneficial component of pain management, especially when pharmacological options are limited due to comorbidities or adverse reactions. Various forms of massage have shown temporary benefit for chronic musculoskeletal pain conditions, but long-term benefit occurs only when combined with exercise and patient education.[313] Some of the less common manual approaches, such as reiki, therapeutic touch, and craniosacral therapy, have inconclusive evidence regarding benefit for chronic pain. It is likely that patients experience a relaxation response with most of these manual approaches; while promoting relaxation is beneficial during flare states, active self-directed methods of relaxation are preferable to passive approaches in which patients depend on health care providers.[27,28,42,43]

Mind-body therapies include meditation, mindfulness-based stress reduction, and hypnosis. Biofeedback, CBT, and relaxation training, which were once considered alternative approaches, have now become standard components of pain management. Mindfulness meditation has the longest history of research supporting its beneficial effects for a variety of chronic health conditions.[313,337,338] Hypnosis has been found to be at least as effective as other cognitive and physical interventions for pain; patients are often taught self-hypnosis to facilitate self-management.[313] Mind-body practices appear to work through decreasing stress, anxiety, and dysfunctional thought processes that subsequently decrease autonomic and central arousal, as well as diminish the perception of suffering.[100]

In summary, several complementary and alternative approaches have documented benefit for patients with chronic pain while others do not. In general, side effects are minimal, especially compared to some of the pharmacological and surgical interventions. A few, such as acupuncture or chiropractic manipulation, have specific physical benefits while others, such as the movement and mind-body activities, enhance overall physical fitness and relaxation. Those approaches that foster independent self-management and functional improvements can be appropriate components of a chronic pain self-management plan.[27,28,42,43]

SUMMARY

Chronic pain is a complex biopsychosocial phenomenon that integrates physiological, psychological, and social factors, each contributing to the development and experience of chronic pain. Chronic pain is modulated by plasticity or dysfunction of the central and/or peripheral nervous systems, endocrine, and immune systems. Pain may be classified as nociceptive, peripheral or central neuropathic, or central sensitization, with many patients experiencing a mixture of more than one type of pain. Peripheral and central sensitization can amplify pain, cause it to spread to previously uninvolved regions, and cause it to persist after the noxious stimulus, injury, or disease is resolved. The psychological and social context of pain must be assessed and addressed for effective pain management.

Effective management of chronic pain needs to address the whole patient and often also the patient's family. The most powerful tools in patient management appear to be an effective patient-therapist alliance, patient education about the nature of chronic pain, exercise, and self-management using cognitive and physical means. Physical therapists are well positioned to provide these interventions and to be a key component of the pain management team to restore optimal function and quality of life to patients with chronic pain. The scientific understanding of chronic pain has changed substantially in recent decades. With better understanding of the biopsychosocial nature of pain and neuroplasticity, in time it may be possible to rehabilitate (i.e., reverse) chronic pain through retraining the brain.[14,16,64]

Questions for Review

1. Which of the following is NOT an accepted pain type or mechanism?
   a. Nociceptive
   b. Neuropathic
   c. Psychogenic
   d. Sensitization
2. Pain associated with *neurogenic inflammation* is MOST likely associated with which of the following physiological processes?
   a. A systemic inflammatory condition
   b. Antidromic neural activity
   c. Non-neural tissue injury
   d. Injury of neural connective tissue
3. Contrast the physiology and presentation of acute, nociceptive-dominant pain versus chronic pain.
4. Contrast the biomedical and biopsychosocial models applied to pain.
5. List and propose the mechanism for five risk factors associated with chronic pain.
6. Explain central sensitization.
7. Which of the following components of a patient examination is MOST important with patients who have chronic pain? Why?
   a. MRI or CT scan of the brain
   b. Thorough medical testing for every possible condition
   c. A biopsychosocial interview
   d. Tests and measures for each area of pain
8. Outline the components of a physical therapy evaluation for a patient with chronic pain.
9. Describe several educational and behavioral principles that physical therapists can integrate into the plan of care for patients with chronic pain.
10. Explain three reasons why exercise is important for patients with chronic pain.

CASE STUDY:

CHRONIC PAIN

The following case is based on a published case report.[339] Students are encouraged to read the full case report for additional detail.

HISTORY

The patient is a 64-year-old female attending an outpatient clinic complaining of a 3-year history of chronic low back pain (CLBP). She reported no traumatic onset. She progressively decreased activity and ultimately stopped working as a nurse 1.5 years previously due to the CLBP. Her pain diagram showed pain throughout her middle and lower back, as well as her entire legs (anterior and posterior) She rated her pain 9/10. Activity increased pain: for example, vacuuming more than half of a room led to a flare that required medication, rest, and no further housework. Taking medication, frequent resting, and lying down decreased pain. She had previously been treated by a number of health care providers and received various types of exercise, manipulations, massage, physical modalities, relaxation training, and multiple medications. She had also received several epidural steroid injections and nerve ablations, with no sustained improvement in her pain.

PAST MEDICAL HISTORY

There were no other orthopedic or medical complaints. MRI revealed "bulging" discs at L2/3, L4/5, and L5/S1, and degenerative disc disease throughout the lumbar spine.

MEDICATIONS:

Hydrocodone, OxyContin, Skelaxin, and Celebrex.

Tests and Measures:

Self-Care and Domestic Life:

Oswestry Disability Index score: 54% (higher scores indicate greater disability). She reported being unable to stand to cook a meal, and unable to sit at a desk for more than 30 minutes.

Mental Functions:

Zung Depression Scale: 58/80 (scores >55 indicate depression)

Fear Avoidance Behavior Questionnaire: FABQ-W: 25/42, FABQ-PA: 20/24 (higher scores indicate greater fear avoidance)

Pain:

Diffuse tenderness in a non-anatomic pattern

Range of Motion:

Screening motions for hip, knee, cervical, and thoracic ranges were normal.

Lumbar flexion: 10°, limited by fear that further motion would trigger her pain complaint. Further ROM testing was discontinued due to the patient's apprehension about moving.

Cranial and Peripheral Nerve Integrity:

Lower quarter neurological screening exam showed no abnormalities in myotomes, dermatomes, or stretch reflexes.

Straight leg raise: 70° B with "pulling" sensation that did not reproduce pain complaint.

Modified slump: decreased knee extension -30° B with "pulling" in low back and leg, with reproduction of primary pain complaint.

CASE STUDY GUIDING QUESTIONS

1. Is the primary type of this patient's pain nociceptive, neuropathic, or central sensitization?
2. What findings support your answer to question 1?
3. What are the implications of the MRI findings?
4. Why were more physical tests and measures not performed?
5. What should be the emphasis of initial PT management for this patient?
6. What type of exercises would be most appropriate and why?

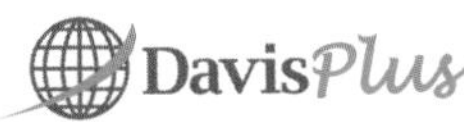

For additional resources, including answers to the questions for review and case study guiding questions, please visit **http://davisplus.fadavis.com**

References

1. Nahin, RL: Estimates of pain prevalence and severity in adults: United States, 2012. J Pain 16(8):769–780, 2015.
2. Institute of Medicine Committee on Advancing Pain Research, Care, and Education: Relieving Pain in America: A Blueprint for Transforming Prevention, Care, Education, and Research. National Academy of Sciences, Washington, DC, 2011.
3. Mayday Fund Special Committee on Pain and the Practice of Medicine: A Call to Revolutionize Chronic Pain Care in America: An Opportunity in Health Care Reform. Mayday Fund, New York, 2009.
4. Burgoyne, DS: Prevalence and economic implications of chronic pain. Manag Care 16(2 Suppl 3):2–4, 2007.
5. Turk, DC: Clinical effectiveness and cost-effectiveness of treatments for patients with chronic pain. Clin J Pain 18(6):355–365, 2002.
6. Apkarian, AV, Baliki, MN, and Geha, PY: Towards a theory of chronic pain. Prog Neurobiol 87(2):81–97, 2009.
7. American Pain Foundation: Pain Facts and Statistics. 2011: Retrieved January 3, 2011, from http://www.painfoundation.org/learn/publications/files/PainFactsandStats.pdf.
8. Grol-Prokopczyk, H: Sociodemographic disparities in chronic pain, based on 12-year longitudinal data. Pain 158(2):313–322, 2017.
9. Centers for Disease Control and Prevention: National Health Interview Survey: Table 53 (page 1 of 5). Joint pain among adults 18 years of age and over, by selected characteristics: United States, selected years 2002-2009. Retrieved September 15, 2011, from http://www.cdc.gov/nchs/data/hus/2010/053.pdf.
10. Dickinson, BD, et al: Maldynia: Pathophysiology and management of neuropathic and maladaptive pain—a report of the ama council on science and public health. Pain Med 11(11): 1635–1653, 2010.
11. Park, PW, et al: Cost burden of chronic pain patients in a large integrated delivery system in the United States. Pain Pract ePub: 2015.
12. Fredheim, OM, et al: Chronic non-malignant pain patients report as poor health-related quality of life as palliative cancer patients. Acta Anaesthesiol Scand 52(1):143–148, 2008.
13. International Association for the Study of Pain (IASP): IASP Taxonomy: Pain terms. Retrieved February 14, 2017, from http://www.iasp-pain.org/Taxonomy?navItemNumber=576
14. Lotze, M, and Moseley, GL: Theoretical considerations for chronic pain rehabilitation. Phys Ther 95(9):1316–1320, 2015.
15. Carlino, E, and Benedetti, F: Different contexts, different pains, different experiences. Neuroscience 338:19–26, 2016.
16. Moseley, GL, and Butler, DS: Fifteen years of explaining pain: The past, present, and future. J Pain 16(9):807–813, 2015.
17. Moseley, GL, and Vlaeyen, JW: Beyond nociception: The imprecision hypothesis of chronic pain. Pain 156(1):35–38, 2015.
18. Dersh, J, Polatin, PB, and Gatchel, RJ: Chronic pain and psychopathology: Research findings and theoretical considerations. Psychosom Med 64(5):773–786, 2002.
19. Basbaum, AI, et al: Cellular and molecular mechanisms of pain. Cell 139(2):267–284, 2009.
20. Kosek, E, et al: Do we need a third mechanistic descriptor for chronic pain states? Pain 157(7):1382–1386, 2016.
21. Sluka, KA: Mechanisms and Management of Pain for the Physical Therapist, ed 2. Seattle, IASP Press, Seattle, 2016.
22. Fishbain, DA, Lewis, JE, and Gao, J: The pain—suffering association, a review. Pain Med 16(6):1057–1072, 2015.
23. Smart, KM, et al: Clinical indicators of 'nociceptive', 'peripheral neuropathic' and 'central' mechanisms of musculoskeletal pain. A Delphi survey of expert clinicians. Man Ther 15(1):80–87, 2010.
24. Smart, KM, et al: The discriminative validity of "nociceptive," "peripheral neuropathic," and "central sensitization" as mechanisms-based classifications of musculoskeletal pain. Clin J Pain 27(8):655–663, 2011.
25. Nee, RJ, and Butler, D: Management of peripheral neuropathic pain: Integrating neurobiology, neurodynamics, and clinical evidence. Phys Ther in Sport 7:36–49, 2006.
26. Bove, GM: Epi-perineurial anatomy, innervation, and axonal nociceptive mechanisms. J Bodyw Mov Ther 12(3):185–190, 2008.
27. Institute for Clinical Systems Improvement. Health Care Guidelines: Pain: Assessment, non-opioid treatment approaches and opioid management, ed 7, 2016. Retrieved March 1, 2017, from https://www.icsi.org/guidelines__more/catalog_guidelines_and_more/catalog_guidelines/catalog_neurological_guidelines/pain/.
28. Work Loss Data Institute (WLDI). Medical Treatment Utilization Schedule (MTUS): Chronic pain medical treatment guidelines, 2015. Retrieved July 28, 2016, from https://www.dir.ca.gov/dwc/DWCPropRegs/MTUS-Opioids-ChronicPain/Final-Regulations/CleanCopy/Chronic-Pain-Guidelines.pdf
29. Sluka, KA: Peripheral pathways involved in nociception. In Sluka, KA (ed): Mechanisms and management of pain for the physical therapist, ed 2. IASP Press, Seattle, 2016, pp. 17–38.
30. Ji, RR, Chamessian, A, and Zhang, YQ: Pain regulation by non-neuronal cells and inflammation. Science 354(6312):572–577, 2016.
31. O'Connor, AB, and Dworkin, RH: Treatment of neuropathic pain: An overview of recent guidelines. Am J Med 122(10 Suppl):S22–32, 2009.
32. Gibbs, GF, et al: Unravelling the pathophysiology of complex regional pain syndrome: Focus on sympathetically maintained pain. Clin Exp Pharmacol Physiol 35(7):717–724, 2008.
33. Martinez-Martinez, LA, et al: Sympathetic nervous system dysfunction in fibromyalgia, chronic fatigue syndrome, irritable bowel syndrome, and interstitial cystitis: A review of case-control studies. J Clin Rheumatol 20(3):146–150, 2014.
34. Helms, JE, and Barone, CP: Physiology and treatment of pain. Crit Care Nurse 28(6):38–49, 2008.
35. Watson, JC, and Sandroni, P: Central neuropathic pain syndromes. Mayo Clin Proc 91(3):372–385, 2016.
36. Finnerup, NB: A review of central neuropathic pain states. Curr Opin Anaesthesiol 21(5):586–589, 2008.
37. Costigan, M, Scholz, J, and Woolf, CJ: Neuropathic pain: A maladaptive response of the nervous system to damage. Annu Rev Neurosci 32:1–32, 2009.
38. Woolf, CJ: Central sensitization: Implications for the diagnosis and treatment of pain. Pain 152(3 Suppl):S2–15, 2011.
39. Nijs, J, et al: Applying modern pain neuroscience in clinical practice: Criteria for the classification of central sensitization pain. Pain Physician 17(5):447–457, 2014.
40. Finnerup, NB, et al: Neuropathic pain: An updated grading system for research and clinical practice. Pain 157(8):1599–1606, 2016.
41. Clauw, DJ: Diagnosing and treating chronic musculoskeletal pain based on the underlying mechanism(s). Best Pract Res Clin Rheumatol 29(1):6–19, 2015.
42. Healthcare Improvement Scotland, Scottish Intercollegiate Guidelines Network (SIGN): Management of chronic pain. Edinburgh. Publication no. 136, 2013.
43. American Chronic Pain Association (ACPA): Chronic pain management: An integrated guide to medical, interventional, behavioral, pharmacologic and rehabilitation therapies. Rocklin, CA, 2017. Retrieved March, 2017 from https://theacpa.org/uploads/documents/ACPA_Resource_Guide_2017.pdf.
44. Treede, RD, et al: A classification of chronic pain for ICD-11. Pain 156(6):1003–1007, 2015.
45. Sluka, KA: Introduction: Definitions, concepts, and models of pain. In Sluka, KA (ed): Mechanisms and Management of Pain for the Physical Therapist, ed 2. IASP Press, Seattle, 2016, pp. 3–17.
46. American Society of Anesthesiologists (ASA): Practice guidelines for chronic pain management. Anesthesiology 112(4):810–833, 2010.
47. Melzack, R, et al: Central neuroplasticity and pathological pain. Ann N Y Acad Sci 933:157–174, 2001.
48. Dworkin, RH, et al: Multidimensional diagnostic criteria for chronic pain: Introduction to the acttion–american pain society pain taxonomy (AAPT). The Journal of Pain 17(9, Supplement): T1–T9, 2016.
49. Fenton, BW, Shih, E, and Zolton, J: The neurobiology of pain perception in normal and persistent pain. Pain Manag 5(4): 297–317, 2015.
50. Barker, C, Taylor, A, and Johnson, M: Problematic pain - redefining how we view pain? Br J Pain 8(1):9–15, 2014.

51. Fishbain, DA, et al: A structured evidence-based review on the meaning of nonorganic physical signs: Waddell signs. Pain Med 4(2):141–181, 2003.
52. Nijs, J, et al: Treatment of central sensitization in patients with 'unexplained' chronic pain: What options do we have? Expert Opin Pharmacother 12(7):1087–1098, 2011.
53. Melzack, R, and Katz, J: Pain. Wiley Interdiscip Rev Cogn Sci 4(1):1–15, 2013.
54. Beneitez, I, and Nieto, R: Do we understand pain from a biopsychosocial perspective? A review and discussion of the usefulness of some pain terms. Pain Manag 7(1):41–48, 2017.
55. Domenech, J, et al: Impact of biomedical and biopsychosocial training sessions on the attitudes, beliefs, and recommendations of health care providers about low back pain: A randomised clinical trial. Pain 152(11):2557–2563, 2011.
56. Kamper, SJ, et al: Multidisciplinary biopsychosocial rehabilitation for chronic low back pain. Cochrane Database Syst Rev 9(CD000963), 2014.
57. Edwards, RR, et al: The role of psychosocial processes in the development and maintenance of chronic pain. J Pain 17(9, Supplement):T70–T92, 2016.
58. Taylor, AM, et al: Is chronic pain a disease in its own right? Discussions from a pre-OMERACT 2014 workshop on chronic pain. J Rheumatol 42:1947–1953, 2015.
59. Institute of Medicine Committee on Advancing Pain Research, Care, and Education: Relieving pain in America: A blueprint for transforming prevention, care, education, and research. National Academy of Sciences, Washington, DC, 2011.
60. World Health Organization: International Classification of Functioning, Disability and Health (ICF). Retrieved March 2, 2017, from http://www.who.int/classifications/icf/en/.
61. World Health Organization: Towards a Common Language for Functioning, Disability and Health. 2002. Retrieved November 2, 2011, from www.who.int/classifications/icf/training/icfbeginnersguide.pdf.
62. van Griensven, H, Strong, J, and Unruh, AM: Pain - a textbook for health professionals. Churchill Livingstone, New York, 2014.
63. Flor, H, and Turk, D: Chronic pain: An integrated biobehavioral approach. IASP Press, Seattle, 2011.
64. Moseley, GL, and Butler, D: Explain Pain Supercharged. Adelaide, South Australia, Noigroup Publications, 2017.
65. Melzack, R: Pain and the neuromatrix in the brain. J Dent Educ 65(12):1378–1382, 2001.
66. Legrain, V, et al: The pain matrix reloaded: A salience detection system for the body. Prog Neurobiol 93(1):111–124, 2011.
67. Apkarian, AV, Hashmi, JA, and Baliki, MN: Pain and the brain: Specificity and plasticity of the brain in clinical chronic pain. Pain 152(3 Suppl):S49–64, 2011.
68. Schmidt-Wilcke, T: Neuroimaging of chronic pain. Best Pract Res Clin Rheumatol 29(1):29–41, 2015.
69. Mense, S: Muscle pain: Mechanisms and clinical significance. Dtsch Arztebl Int 105(12):214–219, 2008.
70. Sikandar, S, Aasvang, EK, and Dickenson, AH: Scratching the surface: The processing of pain from deep tissues. Pain Manag 6(2):95–102, 2016.
71. Galea, MP: Neuroanatomy of the nociceptive system. In Griensven, HV, Strong, J, and Unruh, AM (eds): Pain - A Textbook for Health Professionals, ed 2. Churchill Livingstone, New York, 2014, pp. 49–76.
72. Zhang, JM, and An, J: Cytokines, inflammation, and pain. Int Anesthesiol Clin 45(2):27–37, 2007.
73. Carniglia, L, et al: Neuropeptides and microglial activation in inflammation, pain, and neurodegenerative diseases. Mediators Inflamm ePub: 5048616, 2017.
74. Guan, Z, Hellman, J, and Schumacher, M: Contemporary views on inflammatory pain mechanisms: TRPing over innate and microglial pathways. F1000Res ePub, Sep:5(2425), 2016.
75. Rukwied, R, et al: Inflammation meets sensitization—an explanation for spontaneous nociceptor activity? Pain 154(12): 2707–2714, 2013.
76. Singhal, G, et al: Inflammasomes in neuroinflammation and changes in brain function: A focused review. Front Neurosci 8(315):1–13, 2014.
77. Skaper, SD, Facci, L, and Giusti, P: Mast cells, glia and neuroinflammation: Partners in crime? Immunology 141(3): 314–327, 2014.
78. Chiu, IM, von Hehn, CA, and Woolf, CJ: Neurogenic inflammation and the peripheral nervous system in host defense and immunopathology. Nat Neurosci 15(8):1063–1067, 2012.
79. Dubin, AE, and Patapoutian, A: Nociceptors: The sensors of the pain pathway. J Clin Invest 120(11):3760–3772, 2010.
80. Arendt-Nielsen, L, and Graven-Nielsen, T: Translational musculoskeletal pain research. Best Pract Res Clin Rheumatol 25(2):209–226, 2011.
81. Machelska, H, and Celik, MO: Recent advances in understanding neuropathic pain: Glia, sex differences, and epigenetics. F1000Res ePub Nov:5(2743), 2016.
82. Argoff, CE, et al: Multimodal analgesia for chronic pain: Rationale and future directions. Pain Med 10 Suppl 2(S53–66), 2009.
83. Nickel, FT, et al: Mechanisms of neuropathic pain. Eur Neuropsychopharmacol 22(2):81–91, 2012.
84. McEwen, BS, and Kalia, M: The role of corticosteroids and stress in chronic pain conditions. Metabolism 59 Suppl 1(S9–15), 2010.
85. Sauer, SE, Burris, JL, and Carlson, CR: New directions in the management of chronic pain: Self-regulation theory as a model for integrative clinical psychology practice. Clin Psychol Rev 30(6):805–814, 2010.
86. Hannibal, KE, and Bishop, MD: Chronic stress, cortisol dysfunction, and pain: A psychoneuroendocrine rationale for stress management in pain rehabilitation. Phys Ther 94(12):1816–1825. 2014.
87. Li, X, and Hu, L: The role of stress regulation on neural plasticity in pain chronification. Neural Plast 2016(6402942), 2016.
88. Sandkuhler, J: Models and mechanisms of hyperalgesia and allodynia. Physiol Rev 89(2):707–758, 2009.
89. Staud, R, et al: Enhanced central pain processing of fibromyalgia patients is maintained by muscle afferent input: A randomized, double-blind, placebo-controlled study. Pain 145(1-2):96–104, 2009.
90. Craggs, JG, Price, DD, and Robinson, ME: Enhancing the placebo response: Functional magnetic resonance imaging evidence of memory and semantic processing in placebo analgesia. J Pain 15(4):435–446, 2014.
91. May, A: Structural brain imaging: A window into chronic pain. Neuroscientist 17(2):209–220, 2011.
92. Schmidt, SG: Recognizing potential barriers to setting and achieving effective rehabilitation goals for patients with persistent pain. Physiother Theory Pract 32(5):415–426, 2016.
93. Ossipov, MH, Dussor, GO, and Porreca, F: Central modulation of pain. J Clin Invest 120(11):3779–3787, 2010.
94. Nijs, J, Goubert, D, and Ickmans, K: Recognition and treatment of central sensitization in chronic pain patients: Not limited to specialized care. J Orthop Sports Phys Ther 46(12):1024–1028, 2016.
95. Latremoliere, A, and Woolf, CJ: Central sensitization: A generator of pain hypersensitivity by central neural plasticity. J Pain 10(9):895–926, 2009.
96. Neogi, T, et al: Sensitivity and sensitisation in relation to pain severity in knee osteoarthritis: Trait or state? Ann Rheum Dis 74(4):682–688, 2015.
97. DeSantana, JM, and Sluka, KA: Central mechanisms in the maintenance of chronic widespread noninflammatory muscle pain. Curr Pain Headache Rep 12(5):338–343, 2008.
98. Ploner, M, Sorg, C, and Gross, J: Brain rhythms of pain. Trends Cogn Sci 21(2):100–110, 2017.
99. Mico, JA, and Berrocoso, E: Influence of chronic stress on the somatic and emotional dimensions of chronic pain. In Sommer, CL, Wallace, MS, Cohen, SP, and Kress, M (eds): Pain 2016: Refresher Courses, 16th World Congress on Pain, IASP Press, Washington, DC, 2016, pp. 399–404.
100. Taylor, AG, et al: Top-down and bottom-up mechanisms in mind-body medicine: Development of an integrative framework for psychophysiological research. Explore: J Sci Healing 6(1): 29–41, 2010.
101. Martinez-Lavin, M: Fibromyalgia: When distress becomes (un)sympathetic pain. Pain Res Treat 2012:981565, 2012.
102. Denk, F, McMahon, SB, and Tracey, I: Pain vulnerability: A neurobiological perspective. Nat Neurosci 17(2):192–200, 2014.

103. Dean, E, and Soderlund, A: What is the role of lifestyle behaviour change associated with non-communicable disease risk in managing musculoskeletal health conditions with special reference to chronic pain? BMC Musculoskelet Disord 16:87, 2015.
104. Simons, LE, Elman, I, and Borsook, D: Psychological processing in chronic pain: A neural systems approach. Neurosci Biobehav Rev 39:61–78, 2014.
105. Nicholas, MK, and George, SZ: Psychologically informed interventions for low back pain: An update for physical therapists. Phys Ther 91(5):765–776, 2011.
106. Fillingim, RB, et al: Genetic contributions to pain: A review of findings in humans. Oral Dis 14(8):673–682, 2008.
107. Paras, ML, et al: Sexual abuse and lifetime diagnosis of somatic disorders: A systematic review and meta-analysis. JAMA 302(5):550–561, 2009.
108. Noll-Hussong, M, et al: Aftermath of sexual abuse history on adult patients suffering from chronic functional pain syndromes: An fMRI pilot study. J Psychosom Res 68(5):483–487, 2010.
109. Sullivan, M, Gauthier, N, and Tremblay, I: Mental health outcomes of chronic pain. In Wittink, H, and Carr, D (eds): Pain Management: Evidence, Outcomes, and Quality of Life, Elsevier, New York, 2008.
110. Stewart, J, Kempenaar, L, and Lauchlan, D: Rethinking yellow flags. Man Ther 16(2):196–198, 2011.
111. New Zealand Ministry of Health. Low back pain: A pathway to prioritisation. New Zealand, 2015. Retrieved March 2017 from: https://www.health.govt.nz/system/files/documents/publications/nhc-lbp-pathway-to-prioritisation.pdf.
112. Sowden M, HA, Gray SE, and Coombs J: Can four key psychosocial risk factors for chronic pain and disability (yellow flags) be modified by a pain management programme? A pilot study. Physiother 92:43–49, 2006.
113. Jensen, MP, et al: Psychosocial factors and adjustment to chronic pain in persons with physical disabilities: A systematic review. Arch Phys Med Rehabil 92(1):146–160, 2011.
114. Molton, IR, et al: Psychosocial factors and adjustment to chronic pain in spinal cord injury: Replication and cross-validation. J Rehabil Res Dev 46(1):31–42, 2009.
115. Russek, L, and McManus, C: A practical guide to integrating behavioral and psychologically informed approaches into physical therapist management of patients with chronic pain. Orthop Phys Ther Pract 27(1:15):8–16, 2015.
116. van Koulil, S, et al: Cognitive-behavioral mechanisms in a pain-avoidance and a pain-persistence treatment for high-risk fibromyalgia patients. Arthritis Care Res (Hoboken) 63(6): 800–807, 2011.
117. Jensen, MP: Psychosocial approaches to pain management: An organizational framework. Pain 152(4):717–725, 2011.
118. Rusu, AC, and Hasenbring, M: Multidimensional pain inventory derived classifications of chronic pain: Evidence for maladaptive pain-related coping within the dysfunctional group. Pain 134 (1-2):80–90, 2008.
119. Buenaver, LF, Edwards, RR, and Haythornthwaite, JA: Pain-related catastrophizing and perceived social responses: Inter-relationships in the context of chronic pain. Pain 127(3):234–242, 2007.
120. van Koulil, S, et al: Tailored cognitive-behavioral therapy and exercise training for high-risk patients with fibromyalgia. Arthritis Care Res (Hoboken) 62(10):1377–1385, 2010.
121. Turk, DC, and Wilson, HD: Fear of pain as a prognostic factor in chronic pain: Conceptual models, assessment, and treatment implications. Curr Pain Headache Rep 14(2):88–95, 2010.
122. Vlaeyen, JW, and Linton, SJ: Fear-avoidance and its consequences in chronic musculoskeletal pain: A state of the art. Pain 85(3):317–332, 2000.
123. Andrews, NE, et al: "It's very hard to change yourself": An exploration of overactivity in people with chronic pain using interpretative phenomenological analysis. Pain 156(7):1215–1231, 2015.
124. Andrews, NE, Strong, J, and Meredith, PJ: Overactivity in chronic pain: Is it a valid construct? Pain 156(10):1991–2000, 2015.
125. Boakye, PA, et al: A critical review of neurobiological factors involved in the interactions between chronic pain, depression, and sleep disruption. Clin J Pain 32(4):327–336, 2016.
126. Karaman, S, et al: Prevalence of sleep disturbance in chronic pain. Eur Rev Med Pharmacol Sci 18(17):2475–2481, 2014.
127. Naughton, F, Ashworth, P, and Skevington, SM: Does sleep quality predict pain-related disability in chronic pain patients? The mediating roles of depression and pain severity. Pain 127(3):243–252, 2007.
128. Galland, L: The gut microbiome and the brain. J Med Food 17(12):1261–1272, 2014.
129. Mayer, EA, et al: Gut microbes and the brain: Paradigm shift in neuroscience. J Neurosci 34(46):15490–15496, 2014.
130. Davies, KA, et al: Restorative sleep predicts the resolution of chronic widespread pain: Results from the epifund study. Rheumatology (Oxford) 47(12):1809–1813, 2008.
131. Edwards, I, et al: Clinical reasoning strategies in physical therapy. Phys Ther 84(4):312–330; discussion 331–315, 2004.
132. Matthias, MS, et al: The patient-provider relationship in chronic pain care: Providers' perspectives. Pain Med 11(11):1688–1697, 2010.
133. Fillingim, RB, et al: Assessment of chronic pain: Domains, methods, and mechanisms. J Pain 17(9, Supplement):T10–T20, 2016.
134. DeSantana, JM, and Sluka, AK: Pain assessment. In Sluka, AK (ed): Mechanisms and Management of Pain for the Physical Therapist, ed 2. Wolters Kluwer, Baltimore, 2016, pp. 103–138.
135. Dansie, EJ, and Turk, DC: Assessment of patients with chronic pain. Br J Anaesth 111(1):19–25, 2013.
136. Breivik, H, et al: Assessment of pain. Br J Anaesth 101(1):17–24, 2008.
137. Buse D, Loder E, and McAlary P: Chronic pain rehabilitation. Pain Manag Rounds 2(6):1–6, 2005.
138. Dixon, D, Pollard, B, and Johnston, M: What does the chronic pain grade questionnaire measure? Pain 130(3):249–253, 2007.
139. Burckhardt CS: Adult measures of pain. Arthritis amd Rheumatism (Arthritis Care and Research) 49(5S):S96–S104, 2003.
140. Jensen, MP: Review of measures of neuropathic pain. Curr Pain Headache Rep 10(3):159–166, 2006.
141. Vetter, TR: A primer on health-related quality of life in chronic pain medicine. Anesth Analg 104(3):703–718, 2007.
142. von Baeyer, CL: Children's self-reports of pain intensity: Scale selection, limitations and interpretation. Pain Res Manag 11(3):157–162, 2006.
143. Turk, DC, et al: Assessment of psychosocial and functional impact of chronic pain. J Pain 17(9, Supplement):T21–T49, 2016.
144. Gentile, DA, et al: Reliability and validity of the global pain scale with chronic pain sufferers. Pain Physician 14(1):61–70, 2011.
145. Von Korff, M, et al: Grading the severity of chronic pain. Pain 50(2):133–149, 1992.
146. Tait, RC, Chibnall, JT, and Krause, S: The pain disability index: Psychometric properties. Pain 40(2):171–182, 1990.
147. Atkinson, TM, et al: Using confirmatory factor analysis to evaluate construct validity of the Brief Pain Inventory (BPI). J Pain Symptom Manage 41(3):558–565, 2011.
148. Ferrell, BA, Stein, WM, and Beck, JC: The geriatric pain measure: Validity, reliability and factor analysis. J Am Geriatr Soc 48(12):1669–1673, 2000.
149. Blozik, E, et al: Geriatric pain measure short form: Development and initial evaluation. J Am Geriatr Soc 55(12):2045–2050, 2007.
150. Anagnostis, C, Gatchel, RJ, and Mayer, TG: The pain disability questionnaire: A new psychometrically sound measure for chronic musculoskeletal disorders. Spine (Phila Pa 1976) 29(20): 2290–2302; discussion 2303, 2004.
151. Krebs, EE, et al: Development and initial validation of the peg, a three-item scale assessing pain intensity and interference. J Gen Intern Med 24(6):733–738, 2009.
152. Chatman, AB, et al: The patient-specific functional scale: Measurement properties in patients with knee dysfunction. Phys Ther 77(8):820–829, 1997.
153. Talo, SA, and Rytokoski, UM: BPS-ICF model, a tool to measure biopsychosocial functioning and disability within ICF concepts: Theory and practice updated. Int J Rehabil Res 39(1):1–10, 2016.
154. Briggs, E: Assessment and expression of pain. Nurs Stand 25(2):35–38, 2010.
155. Clayton, HA, et al: A novel program to assess and manage pain. Medsurg Nurs 9(6):318–321, 317, 2000.
156. Reigo, T, Tropp, H, and Timpka, T: Pain drawing evaluation—the problem with the clinically biased surgeon. Intra- and interobserver agreement in 50 cases related to clinical bias. Acta Orthop Scand 69(4):408–411, 1998.

157. Cruccu, G, and Truini, A: Tools for assessing neuropathic pain. PLoS Med 6(4):e1000045, 2009.
158. May, S, and Serpell, M: Diagnosis and assessment of neuropathic pain. F1000 Med Rep 1, 2009.
159. Fishbain, DA, et al: Can the Neuropathic Pain Scale discriminate between non-neuropathic and neuropathic pain? Pain Med 9(2):149–160, 2008.
160. Bennett, MI, et al: Using screening tools to identify neuropathic pain. Pain 127(3):199–203, 2007.
161. Neblett, R, et al: The Central Sensitization Inventory (CSI): Establishing clinically significant values for identifying central sensitivity syndromes in an outpatient chronic pain sample. J Pain 14(5):438–445, 2013.
162. Coyne, KS, et al: Discriminating between neuropathic pain and sensory hypersensitivity using the Chronic Pain Questions (CPQ). Postgrad Med 129(1):22–31, 2017.
163. Portenoy, R: Development and testing of a neuropathic pain screening questionnaire: ID Pain. Curr Med Res Opin 22(8):1555–1565, 2006.
164. Bennett, M: The LANSS Pain Scale: The Leeds Assessment of Neuropathic Symptoms and Signs. Pain 92(1-2):147-157, 2001.
165. Melzack, R: The McGill Pain Questionnaire: Major properties and scoring methods. Pain 1(3):277–299, 1975.
166. Melzack, R: The short-form McGill Pain Questionnaire. Pain 30(2):191–197, 1987.
167. Bouhassira, D, et al: Comparison of pain syndromes associated with nervous or somatic lesions and development of a new neuropathic pain diagnostic questionnaire (DN4). Pain 114(1-2): 29–36, 2005.
168. Bouhassira, D, et al: Development and validation of the Neuropathic Pain Symptom Inventory. Pain 108(3):248–257, 2004.
169. Freynhagen, R, et al: Paindetect: A new screening questionnaire to identify neuropathic components in patients with back pain. Curr Med Res Opin 22(10):1911–1920, 2006.
170. Victor, TW, et al: The dimensions of pain quality: Factor analysis of the Pain Quality Assessment Scale. Clin J Pain 24(6):550–555, 2008.
171. Mathieson, S, et al: Neuropathic pain screening questionnaires have limited measurement properties. A systematic review. J Clin Epidemiol 68(8):957–966, 2015.
172. Main, CJ: Pain assessment in context: A state of the science review of the McGill Pain Questionnaire 40 years on. Pain 157(7):1387–1399, 2016.
173. Oostendorp, RA, et al: Manual physical therapists' use of biopsychosocial history taking in the management of patients with back or neck pain in clinical practice. Sci World J ePub 170463, 2015.
174. Wijma, AJ, et al: Clinical biopsychosocial physiotherapy assessment of patients with chronic pain: The first step in pain neuroscience education. Physiother Theory Pract 32(5):368–384, 2016.
175. Damush, TM, et al: Pain self-management training increases self-efficacy, self-management behaviours and pain and depression outcomes. Eur J Pain 20(7):1070–1078, 2016.
176. MINT excellence in motivational interviewing. 2017: Retrieved March 6, 2017, from http://www.motivationalinterviewing.org.
177. Haggman, S, Maher, CG, and Refshauge, KM: Screening for symptoms of depression by physical therapists managing low back pain. Phys Ther 84(12):1157–1166, 2004.
178. Calley, DQ, et al: Identifying patient fear-avoidance beliefs by physical therapists managing patients with low back pain. J Orthop Sports Phys Ther 40(12):774–783, 2010.
179. Catley, MJ, O'Connell, NE, and Moseley, GL: How good is the Neurophysiology of Pain Questionnaire? A Rasch analysis of psychometric properties. J Pain 14(8):818–827, 2013.
180. Strong, J, and van Griensven, H: Assessing pain. In van Griensven, H, Strong, J, and Unruh, AM (eds): Pain: A Textbook for Health Professionals. Churchill Livingstone, New York, 2014, pp. 91–113.
181. Spiegel, DR, et al: Conceptualizing a subtype of patients with chronic pain: The necessity of obtaining a history of sexual abuse. Int J Psychiatry Med 51(1):84–103, 2016.
182. Draucker, CB, and Spradlin, D: Women sexually abused as children: Implications for orthopaedic nursing care. Orthop Nurs 20(6):41–48, 2001.
183. Schachter, CL, Stalker, CA, and Teram, E: Toward sensitive practice: Issues for physical therapists working with survivors of childhood sexual abuse. Phys Ther 79(3):248–261; discussion 262–249, 1999.
184. Klyman, CM, et al: A workshop model for educating medical practitioners about optimal treatment of difficult-to-manage patients: Utilization of transference-countertransference. J Am Acad Psychoanal Dyn Psychiatry 36(4):661–676, 2008.
185. Saper, JR: "Are you talking to me?" Confronting behavioral disturbances in patients with headache. Headache 46 Suppl 3: S151–156, 2006.
186. Stebnicki, MA: Stress and grief reactions among rehabilitation professionals: Dealing effectively with empathy fatigue. J Rehabil. 66(1):23–29, 2000.
187. American Physical Therapy Association: Interactive Guide to Physical Therapist Practice. 2016. Retrieved March 1, 2017, from http://guidetoptpractice.apta.org/.
188. Raj, SR: Postural tachycardia syndrome (POTS). Circulation 127(23):2336–2342, 2013.
189. Attar-Herzberg, D, et al: The serotonin syndrome: Initial misdiagnosis. Isr Med Assoc J 11(6):367–370, 2009.
190. Malfait, F, et al: The 2017 international classification of the Ehlers-Danlos syndromes. Am J Med Genet C Semin Med Genet 175(1):8–26, 2017.
191. Tinkle, B, et al: Hypermobile Ehlers-Danlos syndrome (a.k.a. Ehlers-Danlos Syndrome Type III and Ehlers-Danlos syndrome hypermobility type): Clinical description and natural history. Am J Med Genet C Semin Med Genet 175(1):48–69, 2017.
192. Chopra, P, et al: Pain management in the ehlers-danlos syndromes. Am J Med Genet C Semin Med Genet 175(1):212–219, 2017.
193. American College of Occupational and Environmental Medicine (ACOEM): Chronic pain. In Occupational Medicine Practice Guidelines: Evaluation and Management of Common Health Problems and Functional Recovery in Workers, ACOEM. Elk Grove Village, 2008, 73–502.
194. Goodman, CC, and Snyder, TK: Differential Diagnosis for Physical Therapists, ed 5. Saunders Elsevier, St. Louis, 2012.
195. Uddin, Z, and MacDermid, JC: Quantitative sensory testing in chronic musculoskeletal pain. Pain Med 17(9):1694–1703, 2016.
196. Smith, SM, et al: The potential role of sensory testing, skin biopsy, and functional brain imaging as biomarkers in chronic pain clinical trials: IMMPACT considerations. J Pain ePub S1526–5900(17)30481-9, 2017.
197. Kostek, M, et al: A protocol of manual tests to measure sensation and pain in humans. J Vis Exp 118:2016.
198. Lotze, M, and Moseley, GL: Role of distorted body image in pain. Curr Rheumatol Rep 9(6):488–496, 2007.
199. Moseley, GL, Gallagher, L, and Gallace, A: Neglect-like tactile dysfunction in chronic back pain. Neurology 79(4):327–332, 2012.
200. Stanton, TR, et al: Spatially defined disruption of motor imagery performance in people with osteoarthritis. Rheumatology (Oxford) 51(8):1455–1464, 2012.
201. Niessen, MH, et al: Relationship among shoulder proprioception, kinematics, and pain after stroke. Arch Phys Med Rehabil 90(9):1557–1564, 2009.
202. Woodhouse, A, and Vasseljen, O: Altered motor control patterns in whiplash and chronic neck pain. BMC Musculoskelet Disord 9:90, 2008.
203. Pinsault, N, et al: Test-retest reliability of cervicocephalic relocation test to neutral head position. Physiother Theory Pract 24(5):380–391, 2008.
204. Balke, M, et al: The laser-pointer assisted angle reproduction test for evaluation of proprioceptive shoulder function in patients with instability. Arch Orthop Trauma Surg 131(8): 1077–1084, 2011.
205. Walton, DM, et al: Reliability, standard error, and minimum detectable change of clinical pressure pain threshold testing in people with and without acute neck pain. J Orthop Sports Phys Ther 41(9):644–650, 2011.
206. Walton, DM, et al: A descriptive study of pressure pain threshold at 2 standardized sites in people with acute or subacute neck pain. J Orthop Sports Phys Ther 41(9):651–657, 2011.
207. Walton, DM, et al: Pressure pain threshold testing demonstrates predictive ability in people with acute whiplash. J Orthop Sports Phys Ther 41(9):658–665, 2011.

208. Bennett, MI, et al: The s-lanss score for identifying pain of predominantly neuropathic origin: Validation for use in clinical and postal research. J Pain 6(3):149–158, 2005.
209. Travell, J, and Simons, DG: Myofascial Pain and Dysfunction: The Trigger Point Manual, Vol. 1. Lippincott Williams & Wilkins, Baltimore, 1992.
210. Travell JG, Simons DG, and Simons LS: Myofascial pain and dysfunction: The trigger point manual, Vol. 2. Lippincott Williams & Wilkins, Baltimore, 2007.
211. Myburgh, C, Larsen, AH, and Hartvigsen, J: A systematic, critical review of manual palpation for identifying myofascial trigger points: Evidence and clinical significance. Arch Phys Med Rehabil 89(6):1169–1176, 2008.
212. Nijs, J, et al: A modern neuroscience approach to chronic spinal pain: Combining pain neuroscience education with cognition-targeted motor control training. Phys Ther 94(5):730–738, 2014.
213. Saragiotto, BT, et al: Motor control exercise for nonspecific low back pain: A Cochrane Review. Spine (Phila Pa 1976) 41(16):1284–1295, 2016.
214. Jull, GA, O'Leary, SP, and Falla, DL: Clinical assessment of the deep cervical flexor muscles: The craniocervical flexion test. J Manipulative Physiol Ther 31(7):525–533, 2008.
215. Geneen, LJ, et al: Physical activity and exercise for chronic pain in adults: An overview of cochrane reviews. Cochrane Database Syst Rev 1:CD011279, 2017.
216. Myers, AM, et al: Discriminative and evaluative properties of the activities-specific balance confidence (abc) scale. J Gerontol A Biol Sci Med Sci 53(4):M287–294, 1998.
217. Eggermont, LH, et al: Comparing pain severity versus pain location in the mobilize boston study: Chronic pain and lower extremity function. J Gerontol A Biol Sci Med Sci 64(7):763–770, 2009.
218. Vasunilashorn, S, et al: Use of the short physical performance battery score to predict loss of ability to walk 400 meters: Analysis from the InCHIANTI study. J Gerontol A Biol Sci Med Sci 64(2):223–229, 2009.
219. Ratter, J, Radlinger, L, and Lucas, C: Several submaximal exercise tests are reliable, valid and acceptable in people with chronic pain, fibromyalgia or chronic fatigue: A systematic review. J Physiother 60(3):144–150, 2014.
220. Occupational health physical therapy: Evaluating functional capacity guidelines. American Physical Therapy Association, Alexandria, VA, 2011.
221. Finnerup, NB, et al: Neuropathic pain needs systematic classification. Eur J Pain 17(7):953–956, 2013.
222. Neblett, R, et al: Ability of the Central Sensitization Inventory to identify central sensitivity syndromes in an outpatient chronic pain sample. Clin J Pain 31(4):323–332, 2014.
223. Sikandar, S, and Dickenson, AH: Visceral pain: The ins and outs, the ups and downs. Curr Opin Support Palliat Care 6(1):17–26, 2012.
224. Gebhart, GF, and Bielefeldt, K: Physiology of visceral pain. Compr Physiol 6(4):1609–1633, 2016.
225. van Koulil, S, et al: Tailored cognitive-behavioural therapy and exercise training improves the physical fitness of patients with fibromyalgia. Ann Rheum Dis 70(12):2131–2133, 2011.
226. Nicholas, MK, et al: Early identification and management of psychological risk factors ("yellow flags") in patients with low back pain: A reappraisal. Phys Ther 91(5):737–753, 2011.
227. Nielson, WR, et al: Further development of the Multidimensional Pain Readiness to Change Questionnaire: The MPRCQ2. J Pain 9(6):552–565, 2008.
228. Kerns, RD, et al: Identification of subgroups of persons with chronic pain based on profiles on the Pain Stages of Change Questionnaire. Pain 116(3):302–310, 2005.
229. Gatchel, RJ, and Okifuji, A: Evidence-based scientific data documenting the treatment and cost-effectiveness of comprehensive pain programs for chronic nonmalignant pain. J Pain 7(11): 779–793, 2006.
230. Scascighini, L, et al: Multidisciplinary treatment for chronic pain: A systematic review of interventions and outcomes. Rheumatology (Oxford) 47(5):670–678, 2008.
231. Smeets, RJ, et al: More is not always better: Cost-effectiveness analysis of combined, single behavioral and single physical rehabilitation programs for chronic low back pain. Eur J Pain 13(1):71–81, 2009.
232. Hall, AM, et al: The influence of the therapist-patient relationship on treatment outcome in physical rehabilitation: A systematic review. Phys Ther 90(8):1099–1110, 2010.
233. Pinto, RZ, Ferreira, ML, and Oliveira, VC: Patient-centred communication is associated with positive therapeutic alliance: A systematic review. J Physiother 58(2):77–87, 2012.
234. Pizzo, PA, and Clark, NM: Alleviating suffering 101—pain relief in the United States. N Engl J Med 366(3):197–199, 2012.
235. Lakke, SE, and Meerman, S: Does working alliance have an influence on pain and physical functioning in patients with chronic musculoskeletal pain; a systematic review. J Compassionate Health Care 3(1):1, 2016.
236. Fuentes, J, et al: Enhanced therapeutic alliance modulates pain intensity and muscle pain sensitivity in patients with chronic low back pain: An experimental controlled study. Phys Ther 94(4):477–489, 2014.
237. Bishop, MD, and Bialosky, JE: The specific influences of nonspecific effects. In Sluka, KA (ed): Mechanisms and Management of Pain for the Physical Therapist, Wolters-Kluwer, Baltimore, 2016, pp. 151–161.
238. Diener, I, Kargela, M, and Louw, A: Listening is therapy: Patient interviewing from a pain science perspective. Physiother Theory Pract 32(5):356–367, 2016.
239. Sevel, LS, et al: Placebo analgesia enhances descending pain-related effective connectivity: A dynamic causal modeling study of endogenous pain modulation. J Pain 16(8):760–768, 2015.
240. Autret, A, Valade, D, and Debiais, S: Placebo and other psychological interactions in headache treatment. J Headache Pain 13(3):191–198, 2012.
241. Medoff, ZM, and Colloca, L: Placebo analgesia: Understanding the mechanisms. Pain Manag 5(2):89–96, 2015.
242. Mundt, JM, Roditi, D, and Robinson, ME: A comparison of deceptive and non-deceptive placebo analgesia: Efficacy and ethical consequences. Ann Behav Med 51(2):307–315 2016.
243. Broderick, JE, Junghaenel, DU, and Turk, DC: Stability of patient adaptation classifications on the multidimensional pain inventory. Pain 109(1-2):94–102, 2004.
244. Louw, A, et al: The efficacy of pain neuroscience education on musculoskeletal pain: A systematic review of the literature. Physiother Theory Pract 32(5):332–355, 2016.
245. Perry, J, et al: Development of a guided internet-based psychoeducation intervention using cognitive behavioral therapy and self-management for individuals with chronic pain. Pain Manag Nurs 18(2):90–101, 2017.
246. Louw, A, Puentedura, EL, and Zimney, K: Teaching patients about pain: It works, but what should we call it? Physiother Theory Pract 32(5):328–331, 2016.
247. Louw, A, et al: The clinical application of teaching people about pain. Physiother Theory Pract 32(5):385–395, 2016.
248. McCullough, BJ, et al: Lumbar MR imaging and reporting epidemiology: Do epidemiologic data in reports affect clinical management? Radiology 262(3):941–946, 2012.
249. Moseley, GL, and Butler, DS: The Explain Pain Handbook: Protectometer. Noigroup Publications, Sydney, Australia, 2015.
250. Sluka, KA, and Moseley, GL: Education and self-management for pain control. In Sluka, KA (ed): Mechanisms and Management of Pain for the Physical Therapist, Wolters-Kluwer, Baltimore, MD, 2016, pp. 163–176.
251. Nijs, J, et al: How to explain central sensitization to patients with 'unexplained' chronic musculoskeletal pain: Practice guidelines. Man Ther 16(5):413–418, 2011.
252. Louw, A, et al: Know pain, know gain? A perspective on pain neuroscience education in physical therapy. J Orthop Sports Phys Ther 46(3):131–134, 2016.
253. Louw, A, et al: The effect of neuroscience education on pain, disability, anxiety, and stress in chronic musculoskeletal pain. Arch Phys Med Rehabil 92(12):2041–2056, 2011.
254. Van Oosterwijck, J, et al: Pain physiology education improves health status and endogenous pain inhibition in fibromyalgia: A double-blind randomized controlled trial. Clin J Pain 17(5): 447–457, 2013.
255. Henschke, N, et al: Behavioural treatment for chronic low-back pain. Cochrane Database Syst Rev 7:CD002014, 2010. DDD: 10.1002/14651858.CD002014.pub3.

256. Eccleston, C, et al: Psychological therapies for the management of chronic and recurrent pain in children and adolescents. Cochrane Database Syst Rev 2(2):CD003968, 2009.
257. Sowden, M, et al: Can four key psychosocial risk factors for chronic pain and disability (yellow flags) be modified by a pain management programme? Physiotherapy 92(1):43–49, 2006.
258. Knoerl, R, Lavoie Smith, EM, and Weisberg, J: Chronic pain and cognitive behavioral therapy: An integrative review. West J Nurs Res 38(5):596–628, 2016.
259. Rundell, SD, and Davenport, TE: Patient education based on principles of cognitive behavioral therapy for a patient with persistent low back pain: A case report. J Orthop Sports Phys Ther 40(8):494–501, 2010.
260. Bryant, C, et al: Can physical therapists deliver a pain coping skills program? An examination of training processes and outcomes. Phys Ther 94(10):1443–1454, 2014.
261. von Baeyer, CL, and Tupper, SM: Procedural pain management for children receiving physiotherapy. Physiother Can 62(4): 327–337, 2010.
262. Mueller, L: Psychologic aspects of chronic headache. J Am Osteopath Assoc 100(9 Suppl):S14–21, 2000.
263. Bergbom, S, et al: Relationship among pain catastrophizing, depressed mood, and outcomes across physical therapy treatments. Phys Ther 91(5):754–764, 2011.
264. Peres, JF, Goncalves, AL, and Peres, MF: Psychological trauma in chronic pain: Implications of ptsd for fibromyalgia and headache disorders. Curr Pain Headache Rep 13(5):350–357, 2009.
265. Thieme, K, and Turk, DC: Cognitive-behavioral and operant-behavioral therapy for people with fibromyalgia. Reumatismo 64(4):275–285, 2012.
266. Sorscher, AJ: Insomnia: Getting to the cause, facilitating relief. J Fam Pract 66(4):216–225, 2017.
267. Wang, F, et al: The effect of meditative movement on sleep quality: A systematic review. Sleep Med Rev 30(43–52), 2016.
268. Busch, V, et al: The effect of deep and slow breathing on pain perception, autonomic activity, and mood processing—an experimental study. Pain Med 13(2):215–228, 2012.
269. Baker, N: Using cognitive behavior therapy and mindfulness techniques in the management of chronic pain in primary care. Prim Care 43(2):203–216, 2016.
270. Rosenkranz, MA, et al: A comparison of mindfulness-based stress reduction and an active control in modulation of neurogenic inflammation. Brain Behav Immun 27(1):174–184, 2013.
271. Zeidan, F, et al: Mindfulness-meditation-based pain relief is not mediated by endogenous opioids. J Neurosci 36(11):3391–3397, 2016.
272. Margolis, RB, et al: Evaluating patients with chronic pain and their families: How you can recognize maladaptive patterns. Can Fam Physician 37:429–435, 1991.
273. Smith, AA: Intimacy and family relationships of women with chronic pain. Pain Manag Nurs 4(3):134–142, 2003.
274. Sluka, KA, and Walsh, DM: Transcutaneous electfical nerve stimulation and interferential therapy. In Sluka, KA (eds): Mechanisms and Management of Pain for the Physical Therapist. Wolters-Kluwer, Baltimore, MD, 2016, pp. 203–223.
275. Vance, CG, et al: Using tens for pain control: The state of the evidence. Pain Manag 4(3):197–209, 2014.
276. Liebano, RE, et al: An investigation of the development of analgesic tolerance to TENS in humans. Pain 152(2):335–342, 2011.
277. Bareiss, SK, and Dailey, DL: Pain associated with central nervous system disorders: Central neuropathic pain. In Sluka KA (ed): Mechanisms and Management of Pain for the Physical Therapist. Wolters-Kluwer, Baltimore, 2016, pp. 383–396.
278. Shah, JP, et al: Myofascial trigger points then and now: A historical and scientific perspective. PM R 7(7):746–761, 2015.
279. Chrubasik, S, Weiser, T, and Beime, B: Effectiveness and safety of topical capsaicin cream in the treatment of chronic soft tissue pain. Phytother Res 24(12):1877–1885, 2010.
280. Haroutiunian, S, Drennan, DA, and Lipman, AG: Topical NSAID therapy for musculoskeletal pain. Pain Med 11(4): 535–549, 2010.
281. Hoeger Bement, MK, and Sluka, KA: Exercise-induced hypoalgesia: An evidence-based review. In Sluka KA (ed): Mechanisms and Management of Pain for the Physical Therapist. Wolters-Kluwer, Baltimore, 2016, pp. 177–201.
282. George, SZ, and Stryker, SE: Fear-avoidance beliefs and clinical outcomes for patients seeking outpatient physical therapy for musculoskeletal pain conditions. J Orthop Sports Phys Ther 41(4):249–259, 2011.
283. Sluka, KA, et al: Regular physical activity prevents development of chronic pain and activation of central neurons. J Appl Physiol (1985) 114(6):725–733, 2013.
284. Naugle, KM, et al: Physical activity behavior predicts endogenous pain modulation in older adults. Pain 158(3):383–390, 2017.
285. Ellingson, LD, et al: Exercise strengthens central nervous system modulation of pain in fibromyalgia. Brain Sci 6(1):2016.
286. Ambrose, KR, and Golightly, YM: Physical exercise as non-pharmacological treatment of chronic pain: Why and when. Best Pract Res Clin Rheumatol 29(1):120–130, 2015.
287. Naugle, KM, Fillingim, RB, and Riley, JL, 3rd: A meta-analytic review of the hypoalgesic effects of exercise. J Pain 13(12): 1139–1150, 2012.
288. Bote, ME, et al: Fibromyalgia: Anti-inflammatory and stress responses after acute moderate exercise. PLoS One 8(9):e74524, 2013.
289. Paley, CA, and Johnson, MI: Physical activity to reduce systemic inflammation associated with chronic pain and obesity: A narrative review. Clin J Pain 32(4):365–370, 2016.
290. Ortega, E: The "bioregulatory effect of exercise" on the innate/inflammatory responses. J Physiol Biochem 72(2):361–369, 2016.
291. Canadian Agency for Drugs and Technologies in Health: CADTH Rapid Response Reports. In Physical Therapy Treatments for Chronic Non-cancer Pain: A Review of Guidelines. Canadian Agency for Drugs and Technologies in Health, Ottawa (ON), 2016.
292. Bidonde, J, et al: Exercise for adults with fibromyalgia: An umbrella systematic review with synthesis of best evidence. Curr Rheumatol Rev 10(1):45–79, 2014.
293. Bidonde, J, et al: Aquatic exercise training for fibromyalgia. Cochrane Database Syst Rev 10):CD011336, 2014.
294. Busch, AJ, et al: Resistance exercise training for fibromyalgia. Cochrane Database Syst Rev 12):CD010884, 2013.
295. Zaleski, AL, et al: Coming of age: Considerations in the prescription of exercise for older adults. Methodist Debakey Cardiovasc J 12(2):98–104, 2016.
296. Jones, KD, and Hoffman, JH: Exercise and chronic pain: Opening the therapeutic window. Functional U 4(1):1–21, 2006.
297. Leveille, SG, et al: Chronic musculoskeletal pain and the occurrence of falls in an older population. JAMA 302(20):2214–2221, 2009.
298. Yamato, TP, et al: Pilates for low back pain: Complete republication of a cochrane review. Spine (Phila Pa 1976) 41(12): 1013–1021, 2016.
299. Zdziarski, LA, Wasser, JG, and Vincent, HK: Chronic pain management in the obese patient: A focused review of key challenges and potential exercise solutions. J Pain Res 8:63–77, 2015.
300. Priganc, VW, and Stralka, SW: Graded motor imagery. J Hand Ther 24(2):164–169, 2011.
301. Medina-Mirapeix, F, et al: Personal characteristics influencing patients' adherence to home exercise during chronic pain: A qualitative study. J Rehabil Med 41(5):347–352, 2009.
302. Stanton, TR, et al: Evidence of impaired proprioception in chronic, idiopathic neck pain: Systematic review and meta-analysis. Phys Ther 96(6):876–887, 2016.
303. Jull, G, et al: Retraining cervical joint position sense: The effect of two exercise regimes. J Orthop Res 25(3):404–412, 2007.
304. Kristjansson, E, and Treleaven, J: Sensorimotor function and dizziness in neck pain: Implications for assessment and management. J Orthop Sports Phys Ther 39(5):364–377, 2009.
305. Flor, H: Maladaptive plasticity, memory for pain and phantom limb pain: Review and suggestions for new therapies. Expert Rev Neurother 8(5):809–818, 2008.
306. Flor, H, and Diers, M: Sensorimotor training and cortical reorganization. NeuroRehabilitation 25(1):19–27, 2009.
307. Thieme, H, et al: The efficacy of movement representation techniques for treatment of limb pain—a systematic review and meta-analysis. J Pain 17(2):167–180, 2016.
308. Moseley, GL: Using visual illusion to reduce at-level neuropathic pain in paraplegia. Pain 130(3):294–298, 2007.

309. Zangrando, F, et al: Neurocognitive rehabilitation in Parkinson's disease with motor imagery: A rehabilitative experience in a case report. Case Rep Med 2015:670385, 2015.
310. Boesch, E, et al: The effect of bodily illusions on clinical pain: A systematic review and meta-analysis. Pain 157(3):516–529, 2016.
311. O'Sullivan, K, et al: Cognitive functional therapy for disabling nonspecific chronic low back pain: Multiple case-cohort study. Phys Ther 95(11):1478–1488, 2015.
312. McKee, MG: Biofeedback: An overview in the context of heart-brain medicine. Cleve Clin J Med 75 Suppl 2:S31–34, 2008.
313. Tan, G, et al: Efficacy of selected complementary and alternative medicine interventions for chronic pain. J Rehabil Res Dev 44(2):195–222, 2007.
314. Berry, ME, et al: Non-pharmacological intervention for chronic pain in veterans: A pilot study of heart rate variability biofeedback. Glob Adv Health Med 3(2):28–33, 2014.
315. Stokes, DA, and Lappin, MS: Neurofeedback and biofeedback with 37 migraineurs: A clinical outcome study. Behav Brain Funct 6(9), 2010.
316. Langhorst, J, et al: Efficacy and safety of meditative movement therapies in fibromyalgia syndrome: A systematic review and meta-analysis of randomized controlled trials. Rheumatol Int 33(1):193–207, 2013.
317. Jahnke, R, et al: A comprehensive review of health benefits of qigong and tai chi. Am J Health Promot 24(6):e1–e25, 2010.
318. Puentedura, EJ, and Flynn, T: Combining manual therapy with pain neuroscience education in the treatment of chronic low back pain: A narrative review of the literature. Physiother Theory Pract 32(5):408–414, 2016.
319. Nijs, J, Van Oosterwijck, J, and De Hertogh, W: Rehabilitation of chronic whiplash: Treatment of cervical dysfunctions or chronic pain syndrome? Clin Rheumatol 28(3):243–251, 2009.
320. Castro-Sanchez, AM, et al: Effects of myofascial release techniques on pain, physical function, and postural stability in patients with fibromyalgia: A randomized controlled trial. Clin Rehabil 25(9):800–813, 2011.
321. Castro-Sanchez, AM, et al: Benefits of massage-myofascial release therapy on pain, anxiety, quality of sleep, depression, and quality of life in patients with fibromyalgia. Evid Based Complement Alternat Med 2011:561753, 2011.
322. Bokarius, AV, and Bokarius, V: Evidence-based review of manual therapy efficacy in treatment of chronic musculoskeletal pain. Pain Pract 10(5):451–458, 2010.
323. Brouwer, RW, et al: Braces and orthoses for treating osteoarthritis of the knee. Cochrane Database Syst Rev 1:CD004020, 2005. DDD: 10.1002/14651858.CD004020.pub2.
324. Baxter, GD, and Basford, JR: Overview of other electrophysical agents including thermal modalities. In Sluka, AK (ed): Mechanisms and Management of Pain for the Physical Therapist. Wolters Kluwer, New York, 2016, pp. 225–235.
325. Chiodo, A, et al: Needle EMG has a lower false positive rate than MRI in asymptomatic older adults being evaluated for lumbar spinal stenosis. Clin Neurophysiol 118(4):751–756, 2007.
326. Haig, AJ, et al: Spinal stenosis, back pain, or no symptoms at all? A masked study comparing radiologic and electrodiagnostic diagnoses to the clinical impression. Arch Phys Med Rehabil 87(7):897–903, 2006.
327. Bedson, J, and Croft, PR: The discordance between clinical and radiographic knee osteoarthritis: A systematic search and summary of the literature. BMC Musculoskelet Disord 9(116), 2008.
328. Webster, BS, et al: Iatrogenic consequences of early magnetic resonance imaging in acute, work-related, disabling low back pain. Spine (Phila Pa 1976) 38(22):1939–1946, 2013.
329. Graves, JM, et al: Early imaging for acute low back pain: One-year health and disability outcomes among washington state workers. Spine (Phila Pa 1976) 37(18):1617–1627, 2012.
330. Kroenke, K, Krebs, EE, and Bair, MJ: Pharmacotherapy of chronic pain: A synthesis of recommendations from systematic reviews. Gen Hosp Psychiatry 31(3):206–219, 2009.
331. Park, HJ, and Moon, DE: Pharmacologic management of chronic pain. Korean J Pain 23(2):99–108, 2010.
332. Turk, DC, Wilson, HD, and Cahana, A: Treatment of chronic non-cancer pain. Lancet 377(9784):2226–2235, 2011.
333. Volkow, ND, and McLellan, AT: Opioid abuse in chronic pain—misconceptions and mitigation strategies. N Engl J Med 374(13):1253–1263, 2016.
334. Dowell, D, Haegerich, TM, and Chou, R: CDC guideline for prescribing opioids for chronic pain - United States, 2016. MMWR Recomm Rep 65(1):1–49, 2016.
335. Manchikanti, L, et al: Opioids in chronic noncancer pain. Expert Rev Neurother 10(5):775–789, 2010.
336. Isbister, GK, Buckley, NA, and Whyte, IM: Serotonin toxicity: A practical approach to diagnosis and treatment. Med J Aust 187(6):361–365, 2007.
337. Ludwig, DS, and Kabat-Zinn, J: Mindfulness in medicine. JAMA 300(11):1350–1352, 2008.
338. Davidson, RJ, et al: Alterations in brain and immune function produced by mindfulness meditation. Psychosom Med 65(4):564–570, 2003.
339. Louw, A, Puentedura, EL, and Mintken, P: Use of an abbreviated neuroscience education approach in the treatment of chronic low back pain: A case report. Physiother Theory Pract 28(1):50–62, 2012.

appendix 25.A

Personal Care Plan for Chronic Plan

NAME: Date:

How do you rate your current status - Pain (0=least, 10=most): ______ Function (0=worst, 10=best): ______

1. **Set Personal Goals**
   - ☐ Improve function by ________ points by: Date ____________________
   - ☐ Return to specific activities, tasks, hobbies, sports … by: Date ________________
     1. ____________________
     2. ____________________
     3. ____________________
   - ☐ Return to ☐ limited work/or ☐ normal work by: Date: ________________
2. **Improve Sleep** (Goal: _____ hours/night, Current: _____ hours/night)
   - ☐ Follow basic sleep plan: Sleep hygiene training
     1. Eliminate caffeine, limit electronics before bed, go to bed at target bedtime, relaxation.
     2. ____________________
     3. ____________________
   - ☐ Take nighttime medications per MD: ____________________
3. **Increase Physical Activity**
   - ☐ Attend physical therapy or organized exercise group (days/week) ______
   - ☐ Complete daily stretching (_____ times/day, for _____ minutes)
   - ☐ Complete aerobic exercise/endurance exercise
     1. Walking (_____ times/day, for _____ minutes) or pedometer (_____ steps/day)
     2. Treadmill, bike, rower, elliptical trainer, dance (_____ times/week, for _____ minutes)
     3. Target heart rate goal with exercise _____ bpm or
   - ☐ Strengthening
     1. Elastic, hand weights, weight machines, gravity (_____ minutes/day, _____ days/week)
   - ☐ Alternative exercise: Tai Chi, Qigung, yoga, etc.
   - • ____________________
4. **Manage Stress** – list main stressors:
   - ☐ Formal interventions (counseling or classes, support group, therapy group, etc.)
   - • ____________________
   - ☐ Daily practice of relaxation techniques, meditation, yoga, socialize, creative activity, etc.
   - • ____________________
   - ☐ Focus on positive thinking, increasing gratitude, schedule pleasurable activities, etc.
   - • ____________________
   - ☐ Medications as per MD:
5. **Decrease Pain** (best pain level in past week: ____/10, worst pain level in past week ___/10)
   - ☐ Non-medication treatments
     1. Ice/heat: ____________________
     2. TENS: ____________________
     3. Exercise: ____________________
     4. Topical cream: ____________________
     - • ____________________
   - ☐ Medication as per MD: ____________________
     1. Daily preventive: ____________________
     2. Breakthrough: ____________________
     3. Other: ____________________
   - ☐ Other treatments: ____________________
6. **Who can help you meet these goals?**

(Modified from form created by Peter S. Marshall, MD)

Web-Based Resources for Clinicians, Families, and Individuals With Chronic Pain

appendix **25.B**

Organization/Purpose	Website
American Academy of Pain Medicine. Professional organization for physicians has patient education material.	www.painmed.org
American Chronic Pain Association. Provides education and peer support for patients and families and has an excellent summary of best practices (consumer guidelines), also helpful for clinicians.	www.theacpa.org https://www.theacpa.org/Consumer-Guide
Australian *Transport Accident Commission* has an extensive selection of physical and psychosocial outcome measures.	http://www.tac.vic.gov.au Go to Provider Resources, Clinical Resources, then Outcome Measures.
Change Pain: A modular approach to understanding pain and its management. Educational resources for clinicians	http://www.change-pain.co.uk/
International Association for the Study of Pain (IASP). Professional organization for researchers, clinicians, and educators. Has some public education resources.	www.iasp-pain.org
Pain.com. Educational modules and articles for clinicians.	www.pain.com
PainAction. Educational material for patients. Includes self-management tools. Integrated with clinician educational site PainEDU.edu	www.painaction.com
PainEDU.org. Educational material for clinicians and educators. Includes downloadable PowerPoint lectures. Integrated with patient education site PainAction	www.painedu.org
The Pain Toolkit has educational materials for patients, including a series of videos on self-management strategies.	http://www.paintoolkit.org/
Understand Pain in Less than 5 Minutes. YouTube explaining chronic pain in patient-friendly terms.	https://www.youtube.com/watch?v=C_3phB93rvl
The University of California Davis School of Nursing has a self-management action plan that can be done online or with handouts.	http://www.ucdmc.ucdavis.edu/nursing/Research/INQRI_Grant/steps_to_plan.html

Web Resources With Clinical Treatment Guidelines for Chronic Pain

The ACPA Resource Guide to Chronic Pain Management: ACPA Resource Guide to Chronic Pain Management[43]	https://www.theacpa.org/Consumer-Guide
Agency for Healthcare Research and Quality: Pain: Assessment, Non-Opioid Treatment Approaches and Opioid Management[27] and Management of Chronic Pain. A National Guideline from Scottish Intercollegiate Guidelines Network[42]	http://www.guideline.gov Search for chronic pain.
Canadian Agency for Drugs and Technologies in Health Physical Therapy Treatments for Chronic Non-Cancer Pain: A Review of Guidelines[291]	https://www.cadth.ca/physical-therapy-treatments-chronic-non-cancer-pain-review-guidelines
Institute for Clinical Systems Improvement Clinical Practice Guideline: Assessment and Management of Chronic Pain[27]	https://www.icsi.org/guidelines_more/
Work Loss Data Institute (WLDI) Medical Treatment Utilization Schedule (MTUS) Chronic Pain Medical Treatment Guidelines[28]	https://www.dir.ca.gov/dwc/DWCPropRegs/MTUS-Opioids-ChronicPain/Final-Regulations/CleanCopy/Chronic-Pain-Guidelines.pdf

Resource Books for Patients

appendix **25.C**

- Angier P, Merryman-Means M, Marie-Sargent J, and Gibson, W. The Joy of Comfortable Sex: A Guide for Couples with Back or Neck Pain, Excelsior Books, Albany, NY, 2007.
- Branch R, and Willson R. Cognitive Behavioural Therapy Workbook For Dummies. Wiley, Hoboken, NJ, 2012.
- Branch R, and Willson R. Cognitive Behavioural Therapy For Dummies, ed 2. John Wiley and Sons, Hoboken, NJ, 2010.
- DeLaune V. Pain Relief with Trigger Point Self-Help. North Atlantic Books, Berkeley, CA, 2011.
- Moseley GL, and Butler D. The Explain Pain Handbook: Protectometer. Orthopedic Physical Therapy Products, Minneapolis, MN, 2017. (This is for patients wanting more practical self-management information.)
- Moseley GL, and Butler D. Explain Pain - Supercharged. Orthopedic Physical Therapy Products, Minneapolis, MN, 2017. (This is for patients wanting more neuroscience knowledge.)
- Caudill MA, and Benson H. Managing Pain Before It Manages You, ed 4. Guilford Press, New York, NY, 2016.
- Davies C. The Trigger Point Therapy Workbook: Your Self-Treatment Guide for Pain Relief, ed 3. New Harbinger Publications, Oakland, CA, 2013.
- Davis M, Eshelman ER, and McKay M. The Relaxation & Stress Reduction Workbook, ed 6. New Harbinger Publications, Oakland, CA, 2008.
- Gardner-Nix J. The Mindfulness Solution to Pain: Step-by-Step Techniques for Chronic Pain Management, New Harbinger Publications, Oakland, CA, 2007.Hebert LA. Sex and Back Pain: Advice on Restoring Comfortable Sex Lost to Back Pain. IMPACC USA, Greenville, ME, 1997.
- Hulme J. Physiological Quieting (CD), Phoenix Core Solutions, Missoula, MT, 2012.
- Kabat-Zinn J. Full Catastrophe Living: Using the Wisdom of Your Body and Mind to Face Stress, Pain, and Illness, updated ed. Delta, Brooklyn, NY, 2013.
- Kabat-Zinn J. Mindfulness for Beginners (CD), Sounds True, Louisville, CO, 2006.
- Kabat-Zinn J. Mindfulness Meditation for Pain Relief (CD), Sounds True, Louisville, CO, 2010
- Kabat-Zinn J. Mindfulness Meditation for Pain Relief: Guided Practices for Reclaiming Your Body and Your Life (CD), Sounds True, Louisville, CO, 2009.
- Kassan SK, Vierck CJ, and Vierck E. Chronic Pain for Dummies. For Dummies, Hoboken, NJ, 2008.
- Kaufman M, Silverberg C, and Odette F. The Ultimate Guide to Sex and Disability, ed 2. Cleis Press, Berkeley, CA, 2007.
- Naparstek B. A Meditation to Help Ease Pain (CD), Health Journeys, Cleveland, OH, 1992.
- Otis JD. Managing Chronic Pain: A Cognitive-Behavioral Therapy Approach Workbook. Oxford University Press, New York, NY, 2007.
- Tinkle B. Joint Hypermobility Handbook. Left Paw Press, Greens Fork, IN, 2010.
- Turk DC, and Winter F. The Pain Survival Guide: How to Reclaim Your Life. American Psychological Association, Washington, DC, 2005.

Chapter 26

Psychosocial Issues in Physical Rehabilitation

Pat Precin, PhD, PsyaD, NCPsyA, LP, OTR/L, FAOTA

LEARNING OBJECTIVES

1. Discuss the psychosocial factors that influence rehabilitation.
2. Explain the impact of psychological functioning and social interaction on health, disease, accident proneness, and adjustment to illness and physical trauma.
3. Recognize the psychological impact of disability on the patient.
4. Differentiate the various professionals (and their roles) to which physical therapists can refer patients with psychosocial issues.
5. Apply the interventions used to handle challenging behavior—how to deescalate an agitated patient, manage violent patients, and identify signs of hypersexuality.
6. Describe the stages of psychosocial adaptation to loss and disability and apply them to treatment.
7. Differentiate between psychosocial adaptation and psychosocial adjustment.
8. Analyze different coping strategies that have been found to be important in psychosocial adaptation and adjustment to chronic disability and illness.
9. Analyze common defensive reactions to disability.
10. Understand how body image may be affected by disability and what a physical therapist can do to address body image issues.
11. Recognize the warning signs of possible post-traumatic stress disorder.
12. Describe the general adaptation syndrome, its aims, uses, and potential dangerous outcomes.
13. Determine crisis points in the rehabilitation process and use clinical reasoning to problem-solve solutions.
14. Apply psychosocial techniques to facilitate patient/client-centered intervention.
15. Compare strategies and resources for prevention, wellness, and psychosocial education.

CHAPTER OUTLINE

Psychosocial factors pertain to the psychological development of an individual in relation to his or her social environment.[1] Psychosocial factors are numerous, as a person's psyche is affected by countless events in the internal and external environments. This chapter focuses on the psychosocial factors that may influence the direction of physical therapy intervention. Some examples of psychosocial factors include premorbid status or mental illnesses, personality styles, coping strategies, defense mechanisms, and emotional reactions to disability. Others include spirituality, values, environment, adjustment, cognitive abilities, motivation, family, social supports, life roles, and educational level. All these factors can affect patients and treatment outcomes.

This chapter (1) identifies and describes how psychosocial factors can influence rehabilitation; (2) demonstrates how to address such factors during physical therapy intervention; and (3) provides indications for referral to psychosocial rehabilitation specialists. Psychosocial factors profoundly affect a patient's ability to recover. Patients who are emotionally upset will have difficulty concentrating on physical therapy goals until emotional issues are addressed. If a patient is motivated to participate in rehabilitation, but his or her family members do not support the patient's rehabilitation goals, the patient will be unlikely to progress on returning home. Mental health status has been shown to be one of the most important predictors of physical health.[2] Wickramasekera et al[3] found that more than 50% of all visits to primary care doctors involved somatic complaints resulting from psychosocial problems. Patients with physical disabilities may fail to respond to treatment if a prominent psychosocial issue is affecting them as well.

Treatment outcomes will be influenced by patients' perceptions of their role in the rehabilitation process. Patients who believe that they possess control regarding their treatment and feel respected by staff tend to experience better health outcomes.[4,5] Empowerment, education, inclusion in goal setting, and a high level of engagement are important factors that positively influence recovery.

The mind and the body are highly connected.[6-8] Because of their reciprocal influence, psychosocial and physical issues should be addressed simultaneously to best facilitate recovery. A slow recovery may cause or prolong depression, which may in turn further delay the rehabilitation period. Watts[9] believes that mental health interventions should be provided to all rehabilitation patients, because health outcomes tend to be poor and prolonged when psychosocial problems remain unaddressed.

Physical therapists regularly encounter patients who have psychiatric illnesses. Psychiatric conditions occur with some frequency in the general population (Table 26.1), but occur at an even higher rate in rehabilitation settings.[10] For instance, panic disorder occurs in 10% to 30% of patients treated in cardiovascular, respiratory, and neurological rehabilitation units, and in 60% of those treated in cardiology clinics (compared with 1% to 2% in the general population).[11] Conversion disorder has been reported to occur at a rate of up to 14% in general medical or surgical inpatient units (compared with 0.5% in the general population).[12] Friedland and McColl[13] found the prevalence of depression and substance abuse to be significantly higher among people with disabilities than in the general population, as did Turner and Beiser,[14] who documented the rate to be three times higher regardless of gender and age. Seventeen percent of senior adults with disabilities also had a diagnosis of major depression, and 14% had mild depression that interfered with daily activities.[15] Twenty-seven percent of patients with stroke were found to be depressed—a finding that correlated with poorer rehabilitation outcomes.[16] Patients with traumatic brain injury (TBI), spinal cord injury (SCI), and Parkinson's disease also reported higher levels of depression compared with the general public.[17,18]

If a patient does not have a preexisting psychosocial illness, he or she is more likely to develop one after the onset of physical illness. Anxiety disorders can result from endocrine (e.g., hyperthyroidism and hypothyroidism, pheochromocytoma, hypoglycemia, and hyperadrenocorticism), cardiovascular (e.g., congestive heart failure, pulmonary embolism, and arrhythmia), respiratory (e.g., chronic obstructive pulmonary disease, pneumonia, and hyperventilation), metabolic (e.g., vitamin B_{12} deficiency and porphyria), and neurological conditions (e.g., vestibular dysfunctions, encephalitis, and neoplasm).[11] The onset of depression has also been linked to the presence of an existing physical disability.[13,14] There is evidence for the converse as well; the longer one possesses some form of mental health concern,

Table 26.1 Lifetime World Prevalence of the Most Common Psychiatric and Personality Disorders[11]

Major Psychiatric or Personality Disorder	Lifetime World Prevalence (%)
Alzheimer's (85+ years old)	16–25
Alcohol abuse or dependence	15
Major depression	10
Marijuana abuse or dependence	5
Schizotypal personality disorder	3
Dependent personality disorder	3
Obsessive-compulsive disorder	2.5
Histrionic personality disorder	2.3
Borderline personality disorder	2
Antisocial personality disorder	2
Panic disorder	1–2
Schizophrenia	1

the greater the risk for developing a physical illness. Depression is a risk factor for heart disease and post-stroke mortality.[19,20] Heinemann et al[21] found that alcohol-related automobile accidents are responsible for a significant number of SCIs, and Zegans[22] reported that psychological problems could be exacerbated by physical illness or injuries. Anxiety can also increase the risk of cardiovascular disease and hypertension.[23]

Although the co-occurrence of physical disabilities and mental illness is high, the rate of treatment for mental illness among people with disabilities is low. In 1997, only 23% of adults with depression, 38% with anxiety disorders, and 47% with serious mental illness received treatment.[15]

A thorough examination of the patient's psychological and social functioning can contribute significantly to a better understanding of needs, fears, anxieties, and capabilities, as well as furnish essential information about the patient's emotional adjustment to disability, assets and liabilities, personality structure, and cognitive functioning. These can then be used to better understand the patient's emotional barriers and behavioral difficulties that can impede recovery. Although not inclusive, Box 26.1 highlights the major areas of consideration in a mental health examination.

Whether physical therapists should address psychosocial issues during treatment or refer psychologically impaired patients to other professionals depends on several

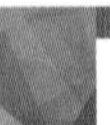

Box 26.1 Elements of a Mental Health Examination

Client Demographics

- Gender, age, culture, ethnicity, education, economic status, primary (and secondary) language(s)
- Living environment (past, present, and projected future) and environmental supports
- Family history of psychiatric diagnoses/interventions
- Current complaints
- Psychiatric medication (past and current)
- Roles (past, present, and projected future)
- Occupation (past, present, and projected future)
- Social supports (past, present, and projected future)
- Leisure interests (past, present, and projected future)
- Goals (past, present, and projected future)
- Values (past, present, and projected future)
- History of psychiatric hospitalizations, substance abuse detoxifications, and/or rehabilitation stays
- Current use of time

Systems Review

- Psychosocial

Examination

Chosen to measure or identify the following:

- Cognitive status (orientation, memory [short-term, long-term, working memory], executive functioning, judgment, calculations, attention, processing, meta-cognition, use of cognitive strategies), volition, self-awareness, mental status, degree of organicity and cognitive disability and its relationship to the patient's rehabilitative capacity. *Primary impairments:* disorientation, amnesia, word-finding difficulty, impaired memory, poor judgment, executive functioning deficits, thought blocking, poor use of cognitive strategies and/or meta-cognition, lack of motivation, impaired self-awareness of limitations, impairments in mental status.[122]
- Emotional status. *Primary impairments:* anxiety, depression, mania, hypomania, grief, mourning, shock, anger, suicidal ideation, emotional numbness, overwhelmed, paranoia, agitated, low self-esteem, regression, delusions, poor reality testing, inappropriate affect, blunted affect, hypervigilance or hypovigilance, anhedonia (inability to experience pleasure), mood swings.
- Defense mechanisms. *Primary impairments:* The use of predominantly primitive defense mechanisms (such as splitting, acting out, denial, devaluation, dissociation, idealization, isolation of affect, projection) as opposed to more mature defenses (sublimation, humor, rationalization, omnipotence, altruism, autistic fantasy). Defense mechanisms are rigid enough to impair ego functioning.
- Personality types. *Primary impairments:* personality disorders (paranoid, antisocial, dependent, borderline, histrionic, narcissistic, avoidant, obsessive-compulsive, schizoid, schizotypal).
- Coping styles. *Primary impairments:* external locus of control, self-blame, substance abuse, and non-direct passive and escape/avoidance modes of coping.

Box 26.1 Elements of a Mental Health Examination—cont'd

- Determination of suicidal tendencies, decompensation, and other risks. *Primary impairments:* history of suicide attempts in self or family members, current suicidal ideation, suicide note, plan for suicide, emotional and/or behavioral regression, substance abuse, feelings of hopelessness and/or helplessness, birthdays or anniversaries of deaths of loved ones, holidays, anniversaries of traumatic events.
- Symbolic meaning of the disability and loss, and the compensatory reserves that can be elicited. *Primary impairments:* Poor compensatory reserves or use of compensatory strategies. The meaning of the disability is both negative and fixed/rigid (e.g., the disability is karmic or a curse that is deserved).
- Levels of pain, stress, tolerance, and secondary gain. *Primary impairments:* Low frustration tolerance coupled with high levels of pain and/or stress. The secondary gain of the impairment is high (important) enough to cause a fixation at a lower than expected level of functioning, result in malingering, or interfere with rehabilitation.
- Sexual practices. *Primary impairments:* sexual dysfunction, impotence secondary to psychiatric medication, unprotected sex, impulsive sexual behavior, sexual abuse, perversions, hypersexuality, sexual addictions.
- Current functional capacities. *Primary impairments:* Problems with basic activities of daily living or instrumental activities of daily living, inability to perform in current roles and occupations, decreased community mobility, inability to live independently.

variables: (1) the severity of the patient's psychosocial issue; (2) the level of comfort with which the physical therapist can address psychosocial problems; and (3) the patient's ability to progress in rehabilitation if existing psychosocial issues are not addressed. Professionals to whom referrals may be made for additional psychosocial intervention include but are not limited to psychiatrists, psychologists, psychiatric nurses, occupational therapists, social workers, creative arts therapists, vocational counselors, rehabilitation counselors, substance abuse professionals, and pastoral counselors.

PSYCHOSOCIAL ADAPTATION

The combination of intense psychological stress, uncertain prognosis, prolonged treatment, and interference with daily activities can greatly affect the rehabilitation of patients with disabilities and chronic illnesses. Disability is loss of or diminished ability to perform specific social roles normally expected of the patient. Psychosocial adaptation to disability and chronic illness is an ongoing, dynamic, evolving process through which a patient strives to attain an optimal state of function within his or her environment.[24] Successful psychosocial adaptation may be characterized by (1) a sense of personal mastery; (2) participation in social, recreational, or vocational pursuits; (3) successful negotiation of the environment; and (4) a realistic awareness of one's current strengths, deficits, and functional capacities.[25] Adjustment is the final phase in adaptation and includes striving to achieve life goals, feeling self-confident and having positive self-esteem, possessing a positive attitude toward one's disability, forming emotional connections to others, and establishing a community member role.[26]

The processes of adaptation and adjustment are influenced by whether a chronic illness or disability is congenital or adventitious, of sudden onset or gradually progressive, and stable or unstable. Patients born with a physical disability and those who acquire them as a result of accident or disease later in life have substantial psychological differences.[27] Children born with a physical disability have only experienced life with their impairment; the development of their self-identity commonly mirrors that of children without disabilities.

In contrast, patients with adventitious disabilities often experience acute loss and grief. Patients with gradually progressive diseases or disabilities of sudden onset often experience anxiety and shock when first becoming aware of their condition. Such anxiety and shock is often followed by anger and depression, as patients realize the magnitude and consequences of their diagnosis.[24] Disabilities of sudden onset (e.g., injuries or accidents) are usually experienced as crises that will change the lives of patients and their families for all time.

Grief, Mourning, and Sorrow

Grief is a psychological state of distress resulting from a significant loss. In reaction to a disability, grief may emerge from lost function, broken relationships, the loss of one's familiar self-identity, and disrupted roles. Grief is characterized by preoccupation with loss and feelings of worthlessness or helplessness. Specific symptoms include feelings of tightness of the throat, muscular weakness, emptiness in the abdomen, anxiety that is described as painful, shortness of breath and choking, and periodic waves of physical distress lasting up to an hour. Other symptoms may include forgetfulness, poor concentration, dissociation, insomnia, loss of appetite, compulsive behavior, an inability to manage time in a productive manner, disorganized cognitive functioning, social withdrawal, guilt, decreased ability to make decisions, excessive speech, and hostility.[28] Severe, prolonged cases of grief can compromise the immune system.[29] The grief–mourning period is unpredictable, lasting anywhere from 6 months to 2 or more years. According to Donatelle and Davis, the grieving process consists of 10 stages: (1) frozen feelings; (2) emotional release; (3) loneliness; (4) physical symptoms; (5) guilt; (6) panic; (7) hostility; (8) selective memory; (9) struggle for a new life pattern; and (10) a sense that life is okay.[28] It is important to note that such stages do not always occur in a progressive, linear fashion, and some stages may occur simultaneously.

Grief is a natural experience necessary to regain or adapt to one's losses and construct a new self-concept. New coping skills are learned as patients adjust to unfamiliar challenges. There may be a difference between people grieving over loss from a disability and those grieving over other types of losses.[29] When grief occurs as a result of disability, it may become prolonged, as the patient must continuously strive to accept the disability and his or her altered self. Burke et al[30] described the grief of people with disabilities as "chronic sorrow," or a grief regarding the loss of normality. Lindgren et al[31] defined chronic sorrow as (1) progressive sadness that often increases after the initial loss; (2) prolonged periods of sorrow with no predictable end; and (3) recurrent or cyclic in nature as the sadness is continuously triggered by internal or external events that reawaken loss. Patients with chronic sorrow can eventually experience adaptation to their losses if they are highly motivated to rebuild their lives and find meaning in their experience. Conversely, patients with pathological grief often experience prolonged feelings of guilt, anger, and sadness that inhibit function and adaptation.

It is important to recognize that grief can be an all-encompassing experience that can take time and energy away from rehabilitation, thereby affecting the process of rehabilitation and its outcomes. Physical therapists must understand grieving, mourning, and sorrow so that a patient's lack of progress or motivation is not misinterpreted as malingering.

Phase Models of Psychosocial Adaptation

The literature regarding psychosocial adaptation to chronic disability and illness falls into two opposing theories of adaptation—one in which adaptation occurs as a set of nonsequential and independent patterns of behavior, and the other in which adaptation occurs progressively through a series of phases.

Phase models suggest that a patient's reaction to chronic disability or illness follows a stable sequence of phases, or stages, that are hierarchically and temporally ordered. This progression is gradual, linear, and involves the psychological assimilation of changes to one's body image and self-concept. The most frequently identified phases in the adaptation to chronic disability and disease are shock, anxiety, denial, depression, internalized anger, externalized hostility, acknowledgment, and final adjustment.[24]

Shock

Shock usually occurs as the initial reaction to a psychological trauma or severe and sudden physical injury. It results from an overwhelming experience and may include the inability to move or speak, psychic numbness, decreased cognitive skills, disorganization, and depersonalization.

During a traumatic event, an individual will respond primarily at the physiological level; emotional reactions are commonly delayed until the event is over and the individual is medically stable. Likewise, the medical emergency team will first implement immediate lifesaving attempts before addressing accompanying psychological issues.

During a perceived or real catastrophic event, an organism would most likely respond with what Selye termed the general adaptation syndrome (GAS).[32] Selye described GAS as an organism's defensive adaptation attempt, which expresses itself through physiological and emotional responses aimed at dealing with such emergencies. During GAS, there is a physiochemical chain reaction, whereby a peptide called corticotropin-releasing factor (CRF) is secreted to stimulate the release of adrenocorticotropic hormone (ACTH). ACTH sets into motion an increase of specific physiological activity designed to maximize the body's defense capacity while minimizing the utilization of nonessential physiological activities. Although an increase in CRF serves the person's self-defensive strategies, its inhibitory effect on other body functions—such as the production of insulin and calcium—is undesirable in the long run.

Studies have shown that injection of a CRF antagonist reduces anxiety in stressful situations.[33] When the inhibitory effects of CRF are prolonged, however, the additional undesirable effects of hypertension, digestive problems, and interference with the immune system result. Selye[32] documented the devastating effect that a prolonged GAS response has on human mental and physical functioning.[32] Theorell et al[34] documented the occurrence of resultant illnesses long after the stress-producing event had ended.

Anxiety

Once the magnitude of the traumatic event is comprehended, anxiety in the form of a panic-stricken reaction commonly occurs and is marked by compulsive activity, confusion, elevated pulse rate, difficulty breathing, and cognitive flooding (e.g., when emotions such as anxiety preclude logical thought). Situations that activate the sympathetic nervous system through repeated alarm or chronic stress may alter synaptic transmission and lead to depression and malfunction of normal body systems.

It should be noted that the physiological and psychological reactions to stress are not limited to catastrophic conditions. An extensive body of research shows stress reactions to be present in individuals under conditions that may not be traumatic but nevertheless persistent and disruptive. Everyday life frustrations, internal and external conflicts, and changes in life conditions are major causes of the stress reaction that, over time, have a deleterious effect on a person's function and health. Physical therapists should be cognizant that even though a patient's emergency is over, a stress reaction may continue to be present.

Denial

Denial is often used as a defense mechanism to alleviate the anxiety and pain associated with a disability or illness.[35] Denial occurs as a specific phase early in the adaptation process and protects the person from having to confront the overwhelming implications of illness or injury all at once. Instead, denial allows a gradual assimilation of one's altered reality. Breznitz[36] identified seven types of denial:

1. Denial of threatening information (using selective inattention and partial awareness)
2. Denial of vulnerability (exerting control and maximizing personal strengths)
3. Denial of urgency (using methods to see the situation as less pressing than it is)
4. Denial of affect (reduction of emotional impact)
5. Denial of affect relevance (diverting attention to other issues and believing that an emotion is coming from an unrelated cause)
6. Denial of personal relevance (attributing difficulties to a benign cause and blaming others when involvement was one's own)
7. Denial of all information (creating a barrier between external reality and one's psyche resulting in total disbelief of having an illness or disability)

Patients in the stage of denial may selectively attend to the environment, choose facts that support their beliefs about themselves and their condition, and ignore facts that remind them of their new challenges. They may have unrealistic and wishful goals for recovery and may appear indifferent and aloof.

Depression

The phase of depression occurs as denial lessens, allowing a greater awareness of one's losses. Depression is a reactive response of bereavement for impending death, suffering, or the loss of body function. Neurochemical and biological changes resulting from disability or disease, premorbid personality and family history, and reactions to stress have all been identified as risk factors for depression.[37,38]

Internalized Anger

Anger occurs in reaction to anxiety, misperception, threats of abandonment, feelings of helplessness, or fear of losing control. Characteristics of anger include hostility, resentment, or hatred. Anger is a response to loss and if not expressed is termed internalized anger. Internalized anger is associated with self-blame and is a manifestation of self-directed bitterness and resentment. Signs of internalized anger include manipulation, sabotage, and passive-aggressive behavior. Sometimes anger emerges when a patient attributes his or her own behaviors to the onset of disability or disease. In such cases, internalized anger can result in depression, suicidal tendencies, or psychosomatic complaints—particularly in people who have a chronic condition.[39]

There are many reasons why patients may not express anger: fear of losing loved ones or social isolation, cultural restraints, lack of awareness, fear of losing control, or belief that expressing anger is inappropriate or dangerous. Repressed anger not only affects a patient's psychological well-being but may also slow rehabilitation. It is important for physical therapists to encourage expression of angry feelings by providing a safe environment for patients to verbalize their anger in appropriate ways. Therapists might state that anger is a normal emotion—especially under the patient's circumstances—offer reasons why it is important to express anger, and provide anger management techniques (e.g., effective coping strategies). It is equally important for therapists to understand that although a patient's anger may be directed at the therapist, such anger more often reflects the patient's own projected feelings regarding his or her disability.

Externalized Hostility

Externalized hostility is anger directed toward other people or objects in the environment and is an attempt to retaliate against activity limitations. Challenges encountered during rehabilitation may trigger externalized hostility. As time from the onset of the disability passes, externalized hostility tends to become more apparent.[40] Signs include passive-aggressive behaviors that obstruct rehabilitation, aggressive acts, hypercriticism, demanding or antagonistic behaviors, falsely blaming others, and abusive accusations. Patients who express anger aggressively through physical or verbal abuse, sarcasm, or controlling behaviors need the help of the entire team to redirect their anger into productive therapeutic activities that further their rehabilitation goals.

Acknowledgment

Acknowledgment is the first sign that the patient has accepted or recognized the permanency of the condition and its future implications. The patient begins to integrate activity limitations into his or her self-concept. During this phase, the patient accepts himself or herself as a person with a disability, develops a new self-concept, reassesses values, and searches for new goals and meaning.

Adjustment

Adjustment is the final phase in adaptation and involves the development of new ways of interacting successfully with others and one's environment. The person is now adjusted to the outside world after having fully assimilated his or her activity limitations from disability into a new, cohesive self. In this phase, the person regains self-worth, understands that new potentials are possible, pursues vocational[41,42] and social goals, and overcomes obstacles that arise in the attainment of goals.[43]

There is evidence that the phase model of adjustment to chronic disability or illness is nonlinear, multidimensional, and progressive. Phase models tend to have 10 common assumptions:[24]

1. People may skip one or more phases or may regress to an earlier phase, but adaptation is not usually reversible.
2. The pace and structure of adaptation can be influenced by external events or interventions (e.g., environmental changes or counseling) yet are mainly determined by internal processes.
3. Not everyone achieves adjustment; some fixate at earlier phases.
4. Adaptation is an unfolding, dynamic process that gradually shifts from initial experiences of distress to assimilation of loss and reconciliation.
5. The adaptation process is initiated by significant and permanent changes in the body's functional capacities and appearance, which are usually followed by alteration of self-concept and body image.
6. The amount of time spent in each phase varies and may be determined by a combination of the following factors: social support, financial and human resources, past exposure to crises, age at onset, severity, nature of the disability or illness, and premorbid personality.
7. Psychological maturity and growth occur as the patient progresses through the phases.
8. Psychological re-equilibrium occurs through gradual adaptation and integration of the perceived misfortune.
9. Human variability and uniqueness have a strong influence on the temporal ordering of phases—the sequence of phases is not universal.
10. Occasionally, phases may overlap, be nondiscrete, or fluctuate, causing patients to experience more than one reaction at a time.

Chronic Illness and Disability: Differences in Adaptation

There are marked differences in the way that people adapt psychosocially to a disability associated with a traumatic event—such as TBI—versus a chronic illness—such as multiple sclerosis (MS). The onset of disability in a traumatic event is sudden, and medical stability may be achieved shortly after. The onset of a chronic illness is usually insidious and gradual; its course is often uncertain and marked by states of remission and deterioration.[44] In chronic illness each onset of symptoms can be experienced as a new illness.

Shock may not be experienced by people with gradually deteriorating medical conditions (e.g., Parkinson's disease, rheumatoid arthritis, or diabetes mellitus), but is usually experienced following a trauma (e.g., TBI, myocardial infarction, amputation, or SCI). The phases of anxiety and depression relate more to the past, such as grieving over the loss of premorbid functioning. Shock may be present but not as strong in people with life-threatening or end-stage diseases (e.g., AIDS, cancer, or amyotrophic lateral sclerosis). In a chronic illness, anxiety and depression relate more to the future (e.g., fear of death, feelings of hopelessness, and fear of the unknown).[45] The acknowledgment and adjustment phases may be more difficult to achieve in chronic, life-threatening conditions that require the internalization of and acceptance that the condition may worsen and result in death.

Post-traumatic Rehabilitation

The post-traumatic period may include phases of anxiety, depression, denial, internalized anger, and externalized hostility mentioned earlier, and is usually the time during which much, if not most, of the rehabilitative intervention takes place. It is also the period during which the psychological effects of the traumatic experience are more strongly felt by the patient. It seems as if the psychological defenses and reactions that became secondary during the initial traumatic period (shock phase) begin emerging as the physical injury is dealt with. These repressed reactions seem to interact with a growing awareness of the effects of the disability creating fears, anxieties, and behaviors that the rehabilitation team must address.

Regardless of which phase the patient is in, physical therapists need to be aware of each patient's psychological needs. During the initial phases of adaptation, patients may experience an awareness of their injuries that facilitates panic and fear of total dependence. Patients may also experience anxiety as a result of anticipating painful medical treatment. Some patients react to these feelings by desperately seeking control over their rehabilitation. Others experience shock regarding their losses and become overly dependent. Patients may idealize the past and have unrealistic expectations about the duration of their recovery.

During these early stages, physical therapists should praise small gains and work with caregivers so they can offer hope and support to the patient. Therapists should be supportive but careful not to make unrealistic predictions about the expected degree of recovery, because this may lead to disappointment, resentment, and depression.[46] One of the first approaches physical therapists can use to help patients regain self-control is diaphragmatic breathing, which may decrease pain and anxiety through the relaxation response.[47]

During the middle stages, physical therapists may need to educate patients about medical precautions, contraindicated movements or activities, how the patient's body has adapted to disability, and how to reformulate expectations. Psychosocial instruction should be integrated with information about activities of daily living (ADL),[48] mobility, strengthening, and endurance. The transition from the patient role to an independent adult member of society is a difficult adjustment and can result in anxiety, depression, and poor social integration.[24,49] Physical therapists should help patients prepare psychologically for discharge and reintegration into society. Some of the issues that patients may fear include negative reactions to their disability, feelings of inadequacy, having to identify new social supports, receiving help in the home environment, and adjusting to a new body image.

Body image includes judgment about one's appearance, an awareness of boundaries and personal space, judgment about one's bodily responses, perception of one's body parts and their movement, and an awareness of physical pleasure and pain. Body image is intimately related to self-concept and self-esteem. It affects a person's functional abilities, cognition, perceptions, attitudes, and emotions, as well as the reactions of others to oneself. Because body image changes throughout life, it is thought to be both dynamic and developmentally based. Difficulties brought on by a disability—such as activity limitations and pain and disfigurement—alter body image and threaten its stability. Patients must then reconstruct their body image and self-perception to adapt to this physical change.[24]

Biordi[50] has identified the following patterns in patients who experienced shifts in body image after disability: (1) denying the existence of one's body; (2) fantasizing about a lost or damaged body part being magically replaced or healthy; (3) concentrating solely on noninjured body parts to deny impairment of the affected area; and (4) experiencing a period of defensiveness followed by gradual acceptance and assimilation of their altered body. The physical therapist's comfort level with the patient's physical disability and the therapist's attention to the affected body part may help the patient feel less ashamed about body changes.

■ PERSONALITY AND COPING STYLES

The more a patient has evolved socially and psychologically, the better he or she will be at using adaptive methods to deal with crises. Hence, a patient with a healthy premorbid personality but a severe physical disability may do better in rehabilitation than one with a less severe disability and a pathological premorbid personality.[51] When aware of their patients' personality styles, physical therapists will be more adept at strategizing interventions, developing a plan of care (POC), and motivating and guiding patients through rehabilitation.

Personality Types

Although each personality is unique, personalities have been categorized into different types, such as *type A, perfectionistic, authoritative,* and *passive-aggressive.* These personality types are nonpathological and develop in response to one's environment when young.

Individuals with type A personalities have a compulsive need to be achievers in all aspects of life. They are extremely independent and productive. These qualities also serve as defenses against low self-esteem and interpersonal conflicts. These people usually derive satisfaction from being strong individuals who can help others. If they can no longer participate in this role, they may become depressed because of a perceived inability to confirm their worth through altruistic activities. Physical therapists can use these qualities in patients with type A personalities to motivate their interest in rehabilitation. Because they are often self-starters and take initiative for their own learning, they can usually be depended on to independently practice home exercise programs (HEPs).

Individuals with perfectionistic personalities uphold high standards to maintain self-esteem. These individuals judge themselves by inflexible and possibly unachievable criteria and may not be able to tolerate slow progress during rehabilitation. Physical therapists may aid these patients by helping them derive pleasure from simple things, such as a meal, a sunset, a new shirt, or interesting information. Helping them discover value in these things offers them sources of self-esteem other than meeting impossibly high standards.

Individuals with authoritative personalities need to be in control and need things to be done in a particular way because of rigid perceptions regarding values, rules, and the manner in which others should behave. They are often concerned with status, tend to be judgmental, and have difficulty empathizing with others. During rehabilitation, these patients may try to dictate their treatment and engage in a power struggle with their physical therapists. Patients with authoritative personalities have difficulty adapting to disability, which often requires acceptance and compromise. They may require alternative strategies to solve what may have been perceived as an unsolvable problem. Physical therapists should engage patients in problem-solving to generate strategies to meet their goals.

Individuals with passive-aggressive personalities express hostility by using passive techniques such as procrastination, resistance, stubbornness, and intentional inefficiency. These personalities react to authority negatively and have difficulty working with others. Physical therapists may work more efficiently with passive-aggressive patients by placing the responsibility for progress onto them. Patients can be instructed to make decisions about their treatment whenever possible and then summarize their progress after each session. This deemphasizes the physical therapist's role as an authority figure, and therefore the need for a passive-aggressive response.

Personality Disorders

When an individual's personality style deviates from cultural norms over a long period of time, is inflexible or pervasive, causes distress to oneself and others, and leads to activity limitations, that personality style is considered dysfunctional.[11] Personality disorders have been thoroughly classified. They include paranoid, antisocial (also referred to as sociopath or psychopath), borderline, histrionic, narcissistic, avoidant, dependent, obsessive-compulsive, schizoid, and schizotypal personalities. Freidman and Booth-Kewley[52] state that disability exacerbates preexisting pathology, meaning that the stress of dealing with a physical illness can make personality disorders even more pronounced.

Patients with paranoid personality disorder interpret the motives of others as malevolent when they may not be. This results from a pattern of suspiciousness and distrust. These patients believe that others are trying to exploit, deceive, or harm them. Because of such mistrust, they may discharge themselves from treatment. Physical therapists should look for behaviors that indicate paranoid thoughts such as hostile reactions, guardedness, argumentation, and stubbornness, and encourage patients to express their thoughts at that moment. If the patient seems paranoid, the physical therapist should help him or her to better understand the reality of a specific situation. For instance, if the patient complains about being forced to participate in an elaborate intervention so that, in his or her view, the therapist can make more money, the therapist should review the pros and cons of various treatments and discuss the clinical reasoning involved. Literature can be very convincing since it does not come directly from the therapist.

Patients with antisocial personality frequently engage in deceit and manipulation. In rehabilitation, they may use an alias, lie to the staff, or malinger. They are irresponsible and often fail to comply with self-care procedures such as hygiene and home maintenance. They seek out and take advantage of weaker staff members, often using wit and charm. When they do not receive what they want, they commonly become irritable and violent, especially when staff members attempt to impose restrictions. They frequently cause disruption to others in rehabilitation. These patients require a cohesive team approach with immediate and strong intercommunication to minimize disruptive behaviors and refocus on rehabilitation goals.

Patients with borderline personality disorder have instability in emotions, relationships, and self-image; are impulsive; use primitive defense mechanisms such as splitting and devaluation; and tend to engage in self-destructive behaviors such as abusing drugs or self-mutilation. On the surface, they may appear critical of others, but these are signs of deep vulnerability and should be treated as such. Therapists should respond with understanding and empathy instead of anger and should emphasize strengths and strategies for ongoing work. Self-mutilating behaviors, such as repetitive cutting with razor blades, pinpricking, or cigarette burning, should be immediately reported to a doctor and referral made to a psychiatrist.

Patients with histrionic personality disorder seek attention via excessive emotionality. Since these patients respond well to audiences, therapists should provide situations in which patients can gain positive attention from doing well in rehabilitation. Physical therapists should set boundaries to help patients achieve a balance between their need to express themselves and their need to focus on therapeutic interventions. A calm and logical approach to rehabilitation helps settle intense emotions. Patients who have difficulty verbalizing their feelings can be referred to a creative arts therapist to facilitate expression through nonverbal means—such as music, dance, or art.

Patients with narcissistic personality disorder are condescending and have a need for admiration and feelings of superiority. If an illness causes a reduction in this image, they will require help from their physical therapists to identify strengths and feel acceptable.

Patients with schizoid personality disorder have a flat affect, or limited range of emotional expression, and are detached from social interactions. The therapist should attend to the patient's rehabilitation without trying to engage him or her in a great deal of social interaction. If the disorder has been long-standing, the patient will likely feel uncomfortable socializing.

Patients with schizotypal personality disorder have eccentric behavior, perceptual or cognitive distortions, and marked distress in social relationships. The social intimacy and physical restriction of a rehabilitation environment may cause anxiety. Slow, unforced integration into the therapeutic setting may be required. Asking patients whether their views of reality are accurate may help them remain focused on achieving rehabilitation goals.

Patients with avoidant personality disorder suffer from social inhibition, feelings of inadequacy, and hypersensitivity to criticism. Physical therapists should reassure these patients that they are doing well and emphasize their strengths.

Patients with dependent personality disorder exhibit clinging behavior, need others to care for them, and are submissive. They may fail to function independently in their life roles even after physical functioning has returned, continuing the pattern of dependency. They fear abandonment and require constant reassurances that staff members understand their condition and care about them. Some respond to clear explanations and feedback about their progress and treatment plans. The therapist should reinforce independent behavior through attention and positive feedback while extinguishing dependent behavior by ignoring or redirecting it.

Patients with obsessive-compulsive personality disorder have a long-standing preoccupation with control and order and are often perfectionists. Their self-esteem may suffer if they perceive a loss of control, and they may react by becoming more obstinate, demanding, and inflexible. Those who publicly express their anger may become ashamed. These patients require greater predictability in treatment than usual, dislike change, and do well when given an established routine to follow. The therapist should provide rehabilitative activities that promote a sense of control and predictability, and consider allowing patients to set treatment goals, and then monitor their daily progress.

Coping Styles

Coping styles are ways that people deal with stress and include behavioral, emotional, and cognitive efforts to cope with internal and external challenges that strain ordinary resources.[53] Theories of coping suggest that it is not what happens to people that is important, but rather how they react.[54] Various coping strategies have been identified in the literature and summarized by Livneh and Antonak.[24] They include planning, problem-solving, wishful thinking, avoiding, minimizing, seeking social support, searching for meaning, emoting feelings, blaming, accepting, negotiating, disengaging, and turning to religion. These and others can be categorized into three different types of coping: (1) seeking versus avoiding control and information; (2) expressing versus repressing emotional reactions; and (3) seeking versus withdrawing from social interactions and networks.

Coping strategies have been found to be of great importance in rehabilitation. Patients with higher-level coping skills can more easily identify and report symptoms, make treatment decisions, comply with intervention, and accept support. Patients with good problem-solving skills and positive attitudes have been found to make more positive adjustments to their disabilities than patients with low self-esteem and poor self-concept.[55] Coping styles often determine whether patients seek medical help and follow advice.[53]

Social influences, psychological characteristics, and health beliefs have been shown to modify the impact of disability and disease on an individual. Social activism, positive self-acceptance, and information seeking have predicted better ability to cope with a disability.[56] Krause and Rohe[57] studied the relationship between adjustment and personality following SCI and found that positive values, emotions, actions, and warmth correlated with superior outcomes. Adaptive coping styles that result in positive outcomes for people with disabilities utilize positive, direct, and active problem-solving, social support seeking, and information seeking. Maladaptive coping styles that lead to unfavorable adaptation outcomes include self-blame; non-direct, passive, and escape/avoidance modes of coping; and substance abuse.

Locus of control is a belief about one's ability to control life conditions and events.[58] Patients with an *external locus of control* believe that other people or outside factors determine outcomes. Patients with an *internal locus of control* take responsibility for change because they believe they can affect their own circumstances. The latter leads to goal-directed activity and active coping.

The ability to intentionally change the relative importance of events that occur in one's life requires constant practice.[59] It has been shown that patients with external loci of control experience stress and anxiety in rehabilitation, whereas patients with internal loci of control have quicker recoveries, better motivation, more hope, and more energy.

Coping styles can be examined through interviews, observations, self-report surveys, checklists, and information from the family. Treatment considerations based on these findings should include emphasis on previous ways of successfully coping and expanding the range of coping strategies, such as maintaining a journal to increase self-expression. Taking care of a pet or using animal assistance can lend help, comfort, and companionship, as well as increase motivation. Group treatment can also be used to increase social networks.[60,61]

Many people with disabilities who have risk factors for emotional problems, such as lower education, less income, and social isolation, still do well in life because of a certain resilience defined as successful adaptation to stressful situations or events.[62] Researchers of resilience[63] identify protective factors that safeguard people from adverse consequences. Protective factors can arise from the individual, family, and society and are concerned with how these strengths and supports provide security, safety, and positive opportunities.

Turning points are important experiences and realizations that enable people to find new direction, purpose, or meaning in life. King et al[64] reported four protective factors: determination, perseverance, spiritual beliefs, and social support. Seven protective processes were also identified: transcending, self-understanding, accommodating, receiving a diagnosis that helps explain a patient's experiences, believing in oneself, using anger as motivation, and setting goals. These protective factors and processes help people with disabilities during turning points in their lives. Analysis of turning points revealed three major ways that patients maintained meaning in their lives: through doing, belonging, and understanding themselves in relation to the world. Doing involves participating in activities that are fulfilling and facilitate competency. Belonging involves perceived acceptance by others or membership in a valued group. Understanding oneself in relationship to the larger world provides a sense of identity and sometimes purpose.

COMMON DEFENSE REACTIONS TO DISABILITY

Defense mechanisms are coping styles that people use to defend against internal and external stressors. They happen automatically and unconsciously. Some individuals use many different defense mechanisms throughout their lives, but most tend to utilize only one or two. The goal is not to change or modify these defense mechanisms, but to identify them to understand the patient's psychological processes that underlie certain behaviors and resistance. Understanding these behaviors can help physical therapists to motivate or redirect patients during difficult times in their rehabilitation. The defense mechanisms described in Box 26.2 are common reactions to disability and can be further explored in the *Diagnostic and Statistical Manual of Mental Disorders*.[11]

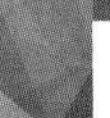

Box 26.2 Common Defense Mechanisms

Acting Out

Instead of expressing feelings verbally, the patient uses actions to release stress. For example, a patient is angry with the insurance company for not funding an athletic wheelchair, so refuses to use the standard wheelchair. Acting out occurs because certain feelings such as anger and hurt are too difficult to express verbally. Unexpressed feelings build anxiety until they are released through action.

The therapist should identify the feeling behind the acting out behavior by asking the patient why he or she behaved in that way. For instance, the therapist would ask the patient above about using the wheelchair. The patient's responses will eventually trace back to the original unexpressed feeling. Through questioning, the therapist brings to the patient's awareness the link between the feeling and the action. The patient can now verbalize and discuss the feeling. In the case above, the patient may be more willing to use the wheelchair. A patient who does not have difficulty verbalizing feelings tends not to act out.

Altruism

The patient becomes dedicated to helping others to manage his or her own stress. An altruistic patient may stop treatment to help everyone else in the treatment room, including the therapist. Such a patient receives gratification through these actions, and hence decreases his or her stress.

Autistic Fantasy

The patient engages in excessive daydreaming instead of pursuing human relationships to decrease stress. The patient may have difficulty following directions, may appear to be in another world, but happily so, and may become emotional and tense when returned to reality. If asked what he or she is thinking about, the patient may describe his or her fantasies, which can be a rich source of wishes and desires that can be used by the therapist to motivate the patient to work on short-term goals. For instance, a male patient relates a fantasy of dating his favorite teen idol. However, to engage in dating, he must first develop interpersonal skills and practice them in simulated and real-life settings.

Denial

Denial protects the ego from being overwhelmed by pain through an unrelenting process of disbelief. In the case of disability, denial may be used to protect the patient from reminders of an altered external reality and the resultant sense of loss. Therefore, the patient may refuse to acknowledge an emotionally painful condition or situation that is apparent to others. The patient often denies the severity of a new disability, believing he or she can return to previous jobs or roles, despite reality testing from the therapist. The patient may refuse rehabilitation, claiming that he or she just wants to leave the hospital to care for his or her children.

It is important to help the patient work through denial slowly to avoid depression, which may occur if the patient becomes aware of his or her reality before psychologically ready to accept it. If the patient's denial is so great that treatment cannot proceed, he or she should be referred to a psychologist to explore what disability means to his or her future.

Devaluation

The patient is overly critical of others and of himself or herself and may insult therapists and other personnel. The therapist should not take such insults personally, but should offer empathy and kindness, which usually decrease devaluation and build rapport. Once a patient trusts the therapist, he or she may discuss insecurities and fears instead of defending against them through criticism. If the therapist becomes angry with the patient, the insults usually become worse and a power struggle may ensue.

Displacement

The patient transfers a response to, or feeling about, one object onto a less threatening object to minimize stress. For example, a patient may be angry with a spouse for driving the car recklessly and having an accident but takes the anger

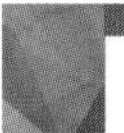

Box 26.2 Common Defense Mechanisms—cont'd

out on the physical therapist. In this situation, it may not be safe or helpful for the patient to express anger directly to the spouse, who may be the patient's only emotional support.

The therapist should help the patient transfer the misplaced feeling back to the object for which it was originally intended. The therapist might accomplish this by asking the patient a series of questions concerning the origin of the anger.

Dissociation

The patient deals with stress through a breakdown in memory, perception, consciousness, or sensorimotor behavior. The patient becomes detached from what is happening in the moment because it is too painful. The patient may stop speaking or participating in therapy and stare blankly into space for up to several minutes without responding to the environment. Afterward, the patient may not be aware of his or her dissociated state, or if he or she is, the patient may state that he or she "just spaced out." The patient who uses dissociation usually relies on it often; a physical therapist may note its occurrence several times during a session. It is important to notice what happened just before the dissociation to identify the painful thoughts, feelings, or actions that upset the patient.

Help-Rejecting

The patient deals with the stress of having covert hostile feelings toward caregivers by frequently asking for help and then rejecting every suggestion. Working with a patient who uses help-rejecting as a defense mechanism can be very frustrating. Such patients seem to sincerely seek help but reject all advice as ineffectual. In these cases, it may be helpful to point out to the patient that efforts to help have been thwarted. The patient is usually not aware that he or she has rejected all solutions and may then come up with a solution or be more open to one that has already been proposed.

Humor

Humor can be used to minimize stress by highlighting the ironic or amusing aspects of a stressful situation. For instance, a patient states that he is going to open a hardware store since he has so much hardware (meaning surgically placed pins and plates) in his leg. A patient who uses humor as a defense mechanism usually feels better if the physical therapist laughs at his or her jokes and participates in joking behavior. It is a safe way for the patient to recognize the difficulty of his or her situation.

Idealization

A patient endows another individual with overly positive attributes to enhance an otherwise negative situation. This other individual may be the therapist, in which case the therapeutic relationship is often strengthened. Or it could be a spouse, in which case problems could arise if he or she is not such a positive support to the patient. It is important to uncover the reality of the situation so necessary treatment and discharge plans can be made.

Intellectualization

A patient uses intellectual reasoning rather than expressing emotions to avoid painful feelings. For example, the patient describes neurotransmitters and synapses when asked about a head injury. Therapists can relate to such patients by intellectualizing with them. For example, the therapist may speak about the patient's head injury in terms of science and facts instead of emotions.

Isolation of Affect

A patient separates feelings from ideas when thinking about and discussing an upsetting event to minimize negative feelings associated with it. He or she speaks of the details regarding the recent accident that caused a disability without mentioning any feelings associated with the event to avoid reexperiencing them. Therapists should help the patient integrate feelings about an event into his or her memory of it. This can be achieved by asking the patient how he or she feels about certain aspects of the event while talking about it.

Omnipotence

A patient feels or acts as if he or she is better than others to guard against feelings of inadequacy. For instance, a patient looks down on other patients with disabilities because he does not want to see himself as disabled. A therapist might observe criticism and devaluation of external objects, bragging about accomplishments or skills, conceit, and grandiosity. The therapist could use this defense mechanism to motivate the patient to get better to avoid feeling inferior.

Continued

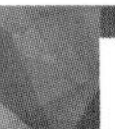

Box 26.2 Common Defense Mechanisms—cont'd

Projection

A patient transfers his or her own unacceptable feelings, thoughts, and beliefs onto another person and becomes certain that the other person really feels, thinks, and believes that way. A patient cannot tolerate the idea of having unacceptable feelings such as anger, but expresses them by projecting them onto another person, remaining relatively guilt free. For example, a patient says that his therapist is annoyed with him when in fact the patient is annoyed with his therapist.

Rationalization

A patient uses elaborate explanations to reassure him or her that personal actions are driven by sound motives, when he or she may truly be unsure. A family member caring for a relative with congestive heart failure asks for a do not resuscitate (DNR) status, citing extensive research studies. The family member states that the relative will die soon anyway, thereby concealing the real and less acceptable reason for seeking the DNR status—to relieve himself or herself from caregiving responsibilities.

Repression

A patient unconsciously erases negative experiences, wishes, or thoughts from consciousness to decrease stress. For example, a patient finds an endearing letter to a spouse from a student and forgets to mention it because the possibility of the spouse having an affair is painful. Repressed material can be dangerous because it remains in the unconscious. Encouraging the patient to express his or her feelings, both good and bad, helps free him or her of these feelings and any possible negative urges to act on them.

Splitting

A patient views a person or event through a positive or negative lens at any given point in time. Later, the patient may flip his or her feelings to the opposite end of the spectrum regarding the same person or situation, acting in this manner because he or she has difficulty integrating ambivalent feelings. Some patients will often attempt to split staff, identifying one staff member with unrealistic positive attributes, while identifying another staff member with unrealistic negative qualities. The staff member who has been identified as negative has usually denied some desire the patient requested. The patient may approach the positively identified therapist and complain that the first therapist is insensitive and does not understand his or her needs. The patient may express that only the positively identified therapist understands his or her problems. However, when the positively identified therapist also denies the patient's request, the patient then vilifies that therapist as well. The therapist may help the patient to integrate the opposite poles of his or her emotions by bringing both positive and negative emotions into consciousness. The patient then may be able to see the reality of his or her situation.

Sublimation

Sublimation occurs when patients transform unacceptable emotions or desires into socially acceptable actions. For example, a patient who is angry about a recent divorce may be unable to consciously express those feelings for fear of losing the affection of his or her children. Instead of expressing the anger he or she may sublimate those emotions into a more socially acceptable action, such as working out in the gym and eventually training for marathons. By participating in an activity that is valued and admired in the society, he or she gains the positive support of others.

Suppression

A patient intentionally avoids thoughts of disturbing feelings, situations, experiences, or problems to reduce stress. When refusing to talk to his or her therapist about the accident that brought him or her to rehabilitation, the patient suppresses disturbing thoughts. Therapists can refer patients to creative arts therapists (e.g., dance, music, art, drama, or poetry therapists) to facilitate the expression of disturbing thoughts, because such emotions accrue over time if not expressed.

Undoing

A patient uses behavior or words to negate unacceptable actions, thoughts, or feelings. For example, one who is frequently bullied by another patient during rehabilitation feels rage against the aggressor but invites him or her to lunch.

Note: In both undoing and suppression, disturbing feelings are intentionally avoided. In suppression, the feelings are avoided and nothing else happens. Feelings are avoided and concealed through opposing words or actions. Both undoing and suppression differ from repression in that repression is an unconscious act.

Anxiety

Anxiety is the apprehensive anticipation of future danger or misfortune accompanied by feelings of tension and agitation. The anticipated danger may be real or imagined, but it is experienced both psychologically and physiologically.[65] The experience of anxiety varies in different patients. When someone is nervous (indicating a moderate level of anxiety), he or she may experience an upset stomach or headache. When someone is experiencing a panic attack (indicating a high level of anxiety), he or she may feel impending doom and terror. A symptom of anxiety in one patient may be heart palpitations, while in another it may be shortness of breath. What is anxiety producing to one patient may cause little to no anxiety in another. Given these variables, the following definitions may facilitate physical therapists' understanding of their patients' conditions.

A panic attack is a sudden onset of intense, overwhelming fear that may include feelings of imminent danger or impending doom. These attacks are marked by symptoms of palpitations, chest pain, smothering or choking sensations, shortness of breath, and fear of losing control, dying, or going crazy. Panic attacks may be unexpected (occurring without an internal or external trigger) or situational. It is unclear what kind of physiological change in the brain may trigger such a severe response. A phobia is an anxiety disorder characterized by intense anxiety resulting from thoughts of, or exposure to, a specific feared situation or object (such as heights, spiders, or elevators) leading to avoidance of that object or situation. Generalized anxiety disorder is defined as excessive worry and anxiety without an apparent source persisting for at least 6 months.[11]

Causes of Anxiety

Twenty to 30 million Americans suffer from anxiety.[28] Some signs and symptoms of anxiety are listed in Table 26.2, and behaviors that may result from anxiety are provided in Table 26.3. Much of the literature on stress and coping has identified major life events as stressors. Life events refer to major changes in lifestyle, status, role, or situation. This view is consistent with the notion that stress, though individually mediated, is to some degree environmentally based and/or exacerbated by environmental and social conditions. Various life event measures have been developed and are used in examining potential environmental stress. One of the more well-known and used instruments is the Holmes-Rahe Social Readjustment Rating Scale (http://www.simplypsychology.org/SRRS.html), which quantifies the effects of life changes on stress and health.[66] Such measures of life events assume a relatively global impact and consider only those items listed. Although there is justified validity in such an approach, there exist potentially more sensitive and valid measures, one of which is the Hassles Scale.

The Hassles Scale, developed by Kanner et al[67] (http://www.kirkwood.edu/pdf/uploaded/905/hassles_scale.pdf), requires subjects to identify the irritating and frustrating demands of everyday transactions with the environment. This approach considers the individual's perception of events believed to pose a threat. It is consistent with the theoretical assumption that chronic struggle may tax coping abilities and lead to greater

Table 26.2 Signs and Symptoms Associated With Low, Moderate, and High Levels of Anxiety

Low-Level Anxiety	Moderate-Level Anxiety	High-Level Anxiety
Agitation	Abdominal distress	Chest pains
Apprehension	Aches	Depersonalization
Distress	Chills	De-realization (feeling unreal)
Irritability	Decreased concentration	Difficulty sleeping
Motor restlessness	Diarrhea	Dizziness
Muscle tension	Fear	Dread
Nervousness	Feeling light-headed, unsteady, or faint	Helplessness
Worry	Fever	Horror
	Heart palpitations	Hypervigilance
	Hot flashes	Increased sensitivity to pain
	Increased heart rate	Nausea
	Misperception	Paresthesia
	Shaking or trembling	
	Shortness of breath	
	Sweating	

Table 26.3 Behaviors Associated With Low, Moderate, and High Levels of Anxiety

Low-Level Anxiety	Moderate-Level Anxiety	High-Level Anxiety
Avoiding stressful situations	Going to the bathroom frequently	Holding hand over heart
Biting lips	Incessant talking	Reacting to irrelevant cues
Drumming fingers on a tabletop	Mumbling	Throwing up
Fidgeting	Overactivity	
Nail biting	Staring blankly	
Pacing	Verbalizing somatic preoccupations	
Pulling or twirling hair		
Rubbing an object such as worry beads		
Shaking legs		
Sighing heavily		
Tapping feet		

difficulty in the management of daily life events. Considering the enormous changes in a person's function when disability occurs, patients are more likely to expect an increase in daily hassles and stressors. Dealing with life becomes more taxing when disabling circumstances block one's coping style, causing a gap between the person and his or her fit within the world. Repeat occurrences of stress and the continual need to adjust to new situations can result in repetition of the fight-or-flight response, which can, over time, result in high blood pressure leading to heart attack or stroke.[23]

Anxiety and Rehabilitation

Different levels of anxiety have different effects on patients. If anxiety is completely absent, patients may not be motivated to achieve treatment goals. Mild anxiety can be motivating if directed toward rehabilitation. Severe anxiety can escalate quickly and impair all aspects of the patient's life, including rehabilitation outcomes, by intensifying the perception of pain, inhibiting immunosuppression, and prolonging recovery time.[68,69] Patients who had difficulty managing anxiety before physical illness will probably have more difficulty managing stress brought on by disability.

When a patient is anxious, thought and energy often become focused on the anxiety instead of physical therapy, resulting in decreased concentration. Decreased learning may be observed when a patient is unable to concentrate on the therapist's instructions. The patient may be unable to perform motor tasks that require multiple-step directions. Poor concentration can also result in safety risks as the patient's attention may be alternating between the anxiety and the demands of rehabilitation. To appear functional, the patient may try to perform a task having heard only part of the therapist's instructions. Such a patient may fail to understand directions given by the therapist and may not realize that he or she missed important information. Steps may be skipped, and a patient may jump ahead too quickly, resulting in injuries to the patient or others.

If patients become fearful because of anxiety, they may avoid certain behaviors in an attempt to decrease their fear. Fearful, anxious patients are reluctant to try new things. They may refuse treatment, remain in their rooms, request a bedpan when they are capable of using the commode, or be reluctant to progress to the next step in therapy. Such patients will commonly make statements such as, "I can't. I don't feel well. I'm too tired. Leave me alone. Not now, I'll do it later. I'm afraid. You can't help me. You don't look strong enough. I'm going to fall."

Patients who express anxiety through overactivity may attempt to progress too quickly through rehabilitation. They often want to achieve everything at once and appear impatient. They tend to rush through a treatment activity without mastering each step. Such patients frequently talk of discharge before it is an option. They may make rash decisions regarding major life changes, such as purchasing new cars or planning vacations when neither would be in their best interest. Such behaviors may provide immediate relief from anxiety for both patients and their families yet cause more distress in the long run.

When anxiety causes misperception, patients may perceive their level of dysfunction and improvement differently than do their therapists. They often leave therapy sessions with an unrealistic opinion concerning any progress or gains made. Such patients may believe they performed at a higher level than they actually did.

Watching a patient experience a panic attack for the first time can be frightening. It may not be immediately evident to either the patient or physical therapist if the patient has never experienced one before. Patients experiencing a panic attack usually report fear of immediate death. They may start to hyperventilate, then suffer shortness of breath. Sometimes they believe they are having a heart attack as a result of chest pain, heart palpitations, and increased heart rate. Terror and panic ensue, and the therapist may call a code or, if in an outpatient setting, initiate emergency transport of the patient to the hospital.

How to Address Anxiety

Physical therapists need to help patients control anxiety so they can proceed with treatment. Some patients may find it beneficial to discuss their fears and concerns with their physical therapists. In such cases the therapist should initiate a dialogue with the patient, asking, "How are you feeling?" "What is your greatest concern?" "What is the worst thing you believe may happen?" and so forth. Physical therapists can work with patients to help defuse anxiety by using cognitive restructuring—or the reshaping of the patient's thoughts and beliefs regarding the feared event. For example, a therapist might help the patient to engage in reality testing by assisting the patient to understand that the occurrence of the feared event is unlikely.

Patients with real and imminent crises may benefit from assistance with problem-solving, should their worst-case scenario occur. Such problem-solving can help patients to believe that they can survive and live meaningful lives despite the occurrence of feared events. After patients have expressed their feelings, therapists can help them segue into treatment and redirect their emotion into physical activity.

It should be noted that patients who are verbose and cannot stop talking about their fears should not be encouraged to dwell on them during physical therapy sessions. Encouraging patients to verbalize their anxieties is also contraindicated with patients whose psychosomatic complaints are fueled by conversation regarding their anxieties. For patients who are very anxious, it may help to conduct treatment in a setting that is familiar, calm, and comfortable. An unfamiliar setting, too much stimulation in the environment, too many people, or too much noise can increase anxiety levels. It may be helpful to reorient patients to the therapy room and to treatment expectations—each session—to allow them to feel a greater sense of control.

Physical therapists should choose a purposeful activity with the patient's anxiety in mind. Some anxious patients have been known to respond to activities that consist of one repetitive motor action, as rhythmic motion helps to calm them.[70] Gross motor movements help decrease the physical symptoms of anxiety such as muscle aches, agitation, and restlessness. Therapists should begin by involving patients in a therapeutic activity that is easily performed and then increase the complexity of the task once the patient has gained confidence.

Anxious patients who may interrupt the physical therapist while he or she is with other patients may be reassured that they will be seen on a certain date and time. Physical therapists should ignore, without anger, all subsequent intrusions. Setting limits in this fashion helps patients improve their frustration tolerance. Very anxious people often welcome clear boundaries set by therapists because they have difficulty setting limits for themselves.

Stress management techniques are useful before and after a session. Techniques such as meditation, imagery,[41] relaxation, stretching, stress management diaries, identifying stressors, biofeedback, nutrition, prioritizing, problem-solving, decision making, anger management, Reiki (a Japanese technique for decreasing stress that involves the transfer of healing energy from the practitioner to the patient), music therapy, therapeutic massage, and prayer have been shown to improve both physical and emotional well-being.[48,71,72] Some of these techniques work more effectively for some patients than others. Choosing one depends on the patient's preference, amount of time available, and materials required.

Relaxation Response

Whichever stress management technique is selected, the overall goal is to teach patients how to experience the relaxation response and replicate it independently during stressful situations.[73] After studying the relaxation response for 20 years, Dr. Herbert Benson identified two essential components that elicit the response: (1) repetition of a sound, word, phrase, prayer, or muscular activity; and (2) disregarding distracting thoughts and returning to the repetition. Benson[23] suggests that patients use the following techniques:

1. Choose a phrase, word, or prayer that is part of your belief system.
2. Sit comfortably and quietly.
3. Close your eyes.
4. Relax your muscles beginning with your feet and working your way up your body.
5. Breathe naturally and slowly. Say your phrase, word, or prayer silently as you exhale.
6. Rid yourself of all distracting thoughts by letting them flow in and out of your mind like waves on the ocean, always returning to your phrase, word, or prayer.
7. Continue for up to 20 minutes.
8. Sit quietly for a minute, allowing your thoughts to return before opening your eyes. Sit for another minute before standing.
9. Practice this technique daily on an empty stomach if possible.

The relaxation response has proven to be effective in treating headaches, hypertension, anxiety, cardiac rhythm irregularities, mild and moderate depression, and premenstrual syndrome. The relaxation response works by decreasing heart rate, rate of breathing, metabolism rate, oxygen consumption, and carbon dioxide elimination, and returning the body to a healthier balance.[24,73,74] When within-subject comparisons were made between blood pressure before and after meditation using the nine aforementioned steps above for several weeks, the average systolic blood pressure for the 36 subjects dropped from 146 to 137 mm Hg, and diastolic pressure dropped from 93.5 to 88.9 mm Hg; both are statistically significant changes.[23] The relaxation response seems to decrease blood pressure through counteracting the activity of the sympathetic nervous system—the same mechanism underlying the action of antihypertensive drugs. Lower blood pressure leads to lower risk for atherosclerosis and related diseases.

Guided Imagery

Another intervention is guided imagery, frequently used as a standard of care to improve rehabilitation through relaxation. Guided imagery is said to work by decreasing the levels of cortisol that can inhibit the immune system and slow tissue repair.[75] As in eliciting the relaxation response, the patient should be guided to a state in which the mind is silent and calm. Through use of a podcast, audiotape, videotape, or therapy guide, the patient is asked to imagine a special place (e.g., the ocean, a forest, a sunset) and focus on vivid details using the five senses. By focusing on this location for increasing lengths of time, patients learn to gain relief from constant worry by releasing concerns for a period of time and returning to a place of relaxation and peace. Guided imagery enhances the mind–body–spirit connection through the induction of an altered state in which the mind communicates more effectively with the body.[68]

The use of guided imagery has achieved improved outcomes of care through significant reductions in pain, blood pressure, stress, side effects of treatments, headaches, uncertainty, depression, insomnia, blood glucose levels, and histamine response to allergies. Significant enhancement of the immune system and wound and bone healing has also been noted.[76] Because music may trigger emotional responses by influencing the limbic system when used with imagery, music used with guided imagery has been shown to decrease pain through increasing endorphin release.[77,78] Guided imagery with music has also been found to reduce the need for large doses of medication and reduce recovery time.[68]

Desensitization

Phobias severe enough to interfere with daily functioning have been reported by one out of every eight American adults.[28] Patients suffering from phobias that interfere with treatment may require desensitization techniques, also called situational exposure exercises. For example, wheelchair users with a fear of elevators who had always used the stairs before injury now require help in coping with their fears. In a comfortable, calm treatment environment far from an elevator, the physical therapist can have the patient begin to talk about benign aspects of elevators (e.g., what they look like, where they are located, and how many floors are in the building). While the patient is answering these questions, the physical therapist should determine the patient's level of anxiety. What specific issue regarding the elevator is the patient discussing when his or her anxiety increases? If the patient has not yet become too anxious, the therapist may ask more anxiety-producing questions, such as, "How high is the elevator's ceiling?" "Is there an emergency phone?" "Are you more fearful of taking an elevator by yourself or with a crowd of people and why?" "Have you ever taken an elevator before and if so, what happened?" The therapist should continue to examine the patient's level of anxiety during questioning, stopping just before the patient's anxiety reaches a point at which the patient cannot easily be calmed.

The desensitization process allows the patient to discuss his or her fear in a safe environment where he or she does not feel overwhelmingly anxious. The physical therapist slowly increases the level of anxiety by asking more difficult questions, but only to a tolerable degree. The patient is then asked to imagine visually that he or she is in an elevator, while practicing relaxation techniques. The patient continues to practice this visualization, over time, until he or she can do so without experiencing fear. When the patient can visualize himself or herself in an elevator without experiencing fear, therapy progresses to the real-life experience of riding in an elevator with the therapist. Relaxation techniques continue to be used during such real-life practice. The activity of riding in an elevator with the therapist using relaxation techniques continues until the patient can do so without fear. The final step would be for the patient to practice riding in an elevator alone while using self-induced relaxation techniques. Desensitization therapy has a high rate of effectiveness in the treatment of phobias.

Cognitive-Behavioral Therapy

Cognitive-behavioral therapy (or cognitive restructuring) can help decrease anxiety by changing maladaptive thought patterns and modifying unhealthy behaviors.[79] Before unhealthy behaviors can be modified, they must first be identified and classified. Because many patients are not conscious of their anxiety, an initial step when using cognitive-behavioral therapy is to help patients recognize anxiety. Determine what the patient's first signs of stress tend to be. Many will reply that they react severely to stress, stating, "I throw up" or "I cannot breathe." In these cases, therapists should ask about the existence of less severe signs, such as nail biting or leg shaking.

Next, patients should count how many times a day they experience stress, recording these in a journal. Physical therapists should help patients look for patterns in their anxiety. Are patients more anxious in the morning or evening, when they attend therapy, or when family members visit? The more patients can identify patterns of anxiety, the more they can anticipate it and prepare for anxiety before it occurs. Therapists should encourage patients to use stress management techniques as soon as they experience the first sign of stress so that their anxiety does not escalate. Keeping a stress management journal can give patients insight into how their thoughts affect their behavior. Research has shown that cognitive-behavioral therapy can be as effective as medication.[80-84] Table 26.4 presents a summary of research data examining the effects of cognitive therapy versus use of antidepressants for depression.

Treatment for Panic Attacks

If the therapist knows that a patient has a history of panic attacks, the following techniques can be helpful: Have the patient describe the first signs of discomfort during the attack. Immediately help him or her to breathe long, deep, and slow breaths. This may require the use of a brown paper bag held by the patient over the mouth while breathing into it to slow the inhalation rate. It is beneficial to acknowledge that a panic attack is occurring and that the patient will be all right if he or she continues to focus on breathing slowly and deeply. The panic attack can become severe within minutes and pass just as quickly. The patient most likely will be seated or lying down throughout the panic attack, as it may render him or her incapable of doing anything else.

Patients are usually embarrassed after an attack and may avoid all situations in which they believe one may occur. They may sit on the end of the aisle while watching a movie, may avoid crowds, or, in extreme cases, stop leaving their homes entirely (referred to as agoraphobia). Therapists can help patients who experience panic attacks to achieve a more productive life by teaching them techniques to control the attacks before they become severe. Families and patients should be educated to understand that panic attacks involve a real physiological reaction, tend to last only several minutes, and often recur without further intervention. Patients with severe, continuous panic attacks should be referred to a psychiatrist for possible medication management.

When to Make a Referral for Anxiety

Multiple referrals may be necessary. Patients who have panic attacks should be referred to a psychiatrist for a medication consultation. Generalized anxiety can be treated with medication; hence, a referral to a psychiatrist would be appropriate if the anxiety lasts more than a week and interferes with the patient's performance in rehabilitation. Those who continue to experience anxiety from phobias despite desensitization therapy and medication should be referred to a psychologist for a more in-depth exploration of their fears. A referral to a

Table 26.4 Evidence Summary Studies Addressing the Question: Is Cognitive Therapy More Effective Than Antidepressants in the Treatment of Depression?

Butler, AC, et al: The empirical status of cognitive-behavioral therapy: A review of meta-analyses. Clin Psychol Rev 26(1):17, 2006.

Design	Meta-analysis of 16 meta-analyses (227 RCTs and 19 studies of other rigor) examining the efficacy of antidepressants vs. psychotherapies in achieving and sustaining remission from depression.
Level of Evidence	I
Subjects	Subjects came from different studies and had a variety of psychiatric diagnoses: unipolar depression, generalized anxiety disorder, panic disorder, social phobia, post-traumatic stress disorder, childhood depressive and anxiety disorders, childhood somatic disorders, adult depression, obsessive-compulsive disorder, bulimia nervosa, schizophrenia, and chronic pain.
Intervention	Cognitive behavioral treatment vs. psychopharmacology intervention. Duration of each varied with studies.
Results	Effect sizes for cognitive behavioral therapy in the treatment of generalized anxiety disorder, unipolar depression, panic disorder, post-traumatic stress disorder, panic disorder, and childhood anxiety and depressive disorders were large. Moderate effect sizes were reported for cognitive behavioral therapy in the treatment of chronic pain, marital distress, childhood somatic disorders, and anger. For adults with depression, cognitive-behavioral therapy was more effective than antidepressants. Venlafaxine (Effexor) demonstrated the highest rates of remission compared with SSRIs but other therapies such as cognitive were also necessary for a high percentage of patients to achieve full remission from depression.
Comments	Limitations due to a meta-analysis are present in this study; it is difficult to compare studies that use different lengths of treatment and assessments. However, the findings in this review of meta-analytic studies support other studies on the effectiveness of adult depression, obsessive-compulsive disorder, bulimia nervosa, schizophrenia, and chronic pain.

Continued

Table 26.4 Evidence Summary Studies Addressing the Question: Is Cognitive Therapy More Effective Than Antidepressants in the Treatment of Depression?—cont'd

Lam, RW, and Sidney, HK: Evidence-based strategies for achieving and sustaining full remission in depression: Focus on meta-analyses. Can J Psychiatry 49:17S, 2004.

Design	Meta-analysis of 16 meta-analytic studies examining the efficacy of cognitive behavioral treatment vs. psychopharmacology on psychiatric clients.
Level of Evidence	I
Subjects	A total of 31,368 depressed subjects throughout different studies.
Intervention	Longitudinal studies of antidepressants vs. psychotherapies.
Results	MANOVAs revealed no significant difference between different types of psychotherapy and their effect on decreasing depression regardless of the disorder; however, clients (regardless of disorder) treated with psychotherapy (regardless of the type) showed significant improvement at the end of therapy and at follow-up compared with those in the control group.
Comments	The combination of antidepressants and psychological therapy resulted in 70% of the patients sustaining remission from depression over extended periods of time.

Leichsenring, F, Rabung, S, and Leibing, E: The efficacy of short-term psychodynamic psychotherapy in specific psychiatric disorders: A meta-analysis. Arch Gen Psychiatry 61(12):1208, 2004.

Design	Meta-analysis of 17 RCTs that examined the effects of various short-term psychotherapies (including cognitive) on depression.
Level of Evidence	I
Subjects	Major depression, maternal depression, post-traumatic stress disorder, bulimia nervosa, anorexia nervosa, opiate dependence, cocaine dependence, cluster C.
Intervention	Intervention ranged from 7 to 40 sessions. Mean length of follow-up was 1 year.
Results	Patients who received combined intervention made significantly greater improvements than those who received antidepressants alone (OR, 1.86; 95% CI, 1.38–2.52). Medication nonresponders and dropout rates were not significantly different between the two groups (OR, 0.86; 95% CI, 0.60–1.24). Combined intervention was significantly more effective than drug intervention alone in studies where intervention lasted longer than 12 weeks (OR, 2.21; 95% CI, 1.22–4.03), with a significant decrease in dropouts when compared with nonresponders (OR, 0.59; 95% CI, 0.39–0.88).
Comments	Not all of the studies in this meta-analysis used cognitive therapy, nor did the meta-analysis identify which elements of the different short-term psychotherapies were effective in reducing depression and preventing relapse.

Pampallona, S, et al: Combined pharmacotherapy and psychological treatment for depression: A systematic review. Arch Gen Psychiatry 61(7):714, 2004.

Design	Systematic review of RCTs that examined the relationships between efficacy of and adherence with psychological intervention plus antidepressant drugs vs. psychopharmacology alone.
Level of Evidence	I
Subjects	Control group consisted of wait-listed patients, 16 trials of 910 depressed patients randomized to pharmacotherapy combined with psychotherapy and 932 to pharmacotherapy alone.
Intervention	Psychological intervention plus antidepressant drugs vs. psychopharmacology alone. Duration of intervention varied according to the particular study.
Results	Medication nonresponders and dropout rates were not significantly different between the two groups (OR, 0.86; 95% CI, 0.60–1.24). Combined intervention was significantly more effective than drug intervention alone in studies where intervention lasted.
Comments	Antidepressants combined with psychotherapy was more effective in the treatment of depression than antidepressants alone.

Table 26.4 Evidence Summary Studies Addressing the Question: Is Cognitive Therapy More Effective Than Antidepressants in the Treatment of Depression?—cont'd

Zu, S, et al: A comparison of cognitive-behavioral therapy, antidepressants, their combination and standard treatment for Chinese patients with moderate–severe major depressive disorders. J Affec Dis 152:262, 2014.

Design	Randomized treatment-outcome study comparing four groups: cognitive behavioral therapy (N = 60), antidepressant treatment (citalopram, escitalopram, paroxetine, or sertraline) (N = 30), cognitive behavioral therapy and antidepressant treatment (N = 60), and standard treatment (psychoeducation and/or medication) (N = 30). This was a longitudinal study with three temporal points of measurement of depression and social functioning at baseline, 3 months follow-up, and 6 months follow-up using the Hamilton Rating Scale for Depression, Quick Inventory of Depressive Symptomentology-Self-Report, and Work and Social Adjustment Scale.
Level of Evidence	1
Subjects	180 patients diagnosed with moderate to severe depressive disorders according to the ICD-10 from China.
Intervention	The CBT and combination groups (CBT + antidepressants) received a 24-week CBT intervention consisting of 20 sessions 1 hour in duration. The combination and antidepressant groups received either citalopram, escitalopram, paroxetine, or sertraline for 24 weeks. The standard treatment group received psychoeducation on depression and medication if indicated for 24 weeks.
Results	There was no significant difference reported between any of the four groups after intervention in any of the outcomes measured.
Comments	Results indicate that Chinese physicians and individuals seeking treatment for depression may have more health care choices.

psychologist is indicated if the anxiety seems to be a deeply rooted characteristic of the patient's personality. A social work referral can be helpful if the patient's anxiety results from a lack of necessary resources or involves family members.

In many cases, medication does not fully alleviate patients' anxiety. However, it may decrease it sufficiently enough for patients to begin expressing their fears and implementing strategies to decrease stress. Sometimes a patient may not be forthcoming about his or her anxiety and a formal diagnosis may not be present in the chart. If this is the case, the physical therapist may become aware of an anxiety disorder through the type of medication prescribed. By becoming familiar with the names of different antianxiety medications, physical therapists can identify patients suffering from anxiety. The names, effects, and adverse side effects of commonly prescribed antianxiety medications are presented in Table 26.5.

ACUTE STRESS DISORDER AND POST-TRAUMATIC STRESS DISORDER

People who were disabled as a result of a traumatic event (e.g., a violent crime, abuse, an accident, a natural disaster, or war)[85,86] or individuals who have witnessed such are at risk for post-traumatic stress disorder (PTSD) or acute stress disorder (ASD). Both are specific forms or subsets of anxiety disorders. The *Diagnostic and Statistical Manual of Mental Disorders* differentiates between both disorders in terms of the duration of the disorder and its symptoms.[11] ASD involves symptoms that must range in duration between 2 days to a maximum of 4 weeks. If symptoms of ASD persist longer than 4 weeks, the diagnosis of ASD is discontinued and changed to PTSD. Post-traumatic stress disorder is differentiated as *acute* PTSD if symptoms last more than 4 weeks but less than 3 months and as *chronic* PTSD if symptoms last 3 months or longer. Both ASD and PTSD, however, must result from exposure to a traumatic event, and PTSD can be qualified with the term "with delayed onset" if symptoms first occur at least half a year after the traumatic event. Research notes that PTSD is an expected outcome for a certain percentage of patients experiencing even mild traumas.[87,88]

Among the symptoms exhibited are one or more of the following: reexperiencing the traumatic event; numbing of responsiveness to, or reduced involvement with, the external world; and/or a variety of autonomic, dysphoric, or cognitive symptoms. The reexperiencing of the event is described as recurrent, painful, and consisting of intrusive recollections, dreams and nightmares, and, on rare occasions, dissociative states during which the individual may act as if reliving the actual traumatic event. This may last only several minutes or occur for hours or even days. The numbing of responsiveness, also

Table 26.5 Effects and Adverse Side Effects of Commonly Prescribed Antianxiety Medications

Medication	Summary of Effects	Adverse Side Effects
Alprazolam (Xanax)	Decrease anxiety, seizures, sleep disorders, alcohol abuse, catatonic schizophrenia	Sedation, potential for abuse, difficult to taper (gradual dose reduction)
Buspirone hydrochloride (BuSpar)	Decrease depression, anxiety, addictions, ADHD	Tremors, decreased appetite, insomnia, restlessness
Chlordiazepoxide (Librium, Mitran, Reposans-10)	Decrease anxiety, seizures, sleep disorders, alcohol abuse, catatonic schizophrenia	Sedation, potential for abuse, difficult to taper
Clorazepate dipotassium (Tranxene, Gen-Xene)	Decrease anxiety, seizures, sleep disorders, alcohol abuse, catatonic schizophrenia	Sedation, potential for abuse, difficult to taper
Diazepam (Diastat, Valium)	Decrease anxiety, seizures, sleep disorders, alcohol abuse, catatonic schizophrenia	Sedation, potential for abuse, difficult to taper
Estazolam (Prosom)	Decrease insomnia	Cognitive impairments, dizziness, daytime sleepiness, anxiety, uncoordinated motor movements, intoxication, drug accumulation
Flurazepam hydrochloride (Dalmane)	Decrease insomnia	Cognitive impairments, dizziness, daytime sleepiness, anxiety, uncoordinated motor movements, intoxication, drug accumulation
Hydroxyzine hydrochloride (Vistaril)	Decrease insomnia, tremors, weight gain, anxiety	Dizziness, sedation, constipation, cotton mouth, weight gain, urinary retention, blurred vision, hypotension, confusion
Lithium carbonate (Eskalith, Lithobid)	Decrease mania and suicidal ideation, stabilizes mood	Toxicity can be lethal, increase weight, nausea, acne, sedation, psoriasis, diarrhea, polydipsia, tremors, edema, uncoordinated motor movements
Lorazepam (Ativan)	Decrease anxiety, seizures, sleep disorders, alcohol abuse, catatonic schizophrenia	Sedation, potential for abuse, difficult to taper
Oxazepam (Serax)	Decrease anxiety, seizures, sleep disorders, alcohol abuse, catatonic schizophrenia	Sedation, potential for abuse, difficult to taper
Temazepam (Restoril)	Decrease insomnia	Cognitive impairments, dizziness, daytime sleepiness, anxiety, uncoordinated motor movements, intoxication, drug accumulation
Triazolam (Halcion)	Decrease insomnia	Cognitive impairments, dizziness, daytime sleepiness, anxiety, uncoordinated motor movements, intoxication, drug accumulation
Zaleplon (Sonata)	Decrease insomnia	Dizziness, drowsiness
Zolpidem tartrate (Ambien)	Decrease insomnia	Dizziness, drowsiness

Note: Brand names are shown in parentheses.
ADHD = attention deficit–hyperactivity disorder.

called *psychic numbing* or *emotional anesthesia,* is expressed by complaints of feeling detached or estranged from others, a loss of ability or interest in previously enjoyable activities, or the lack of any emotions or feelings. Cognitive symptoms may include impairment of memory, concentration, and task completion ability. Patients may experience excessive autonomic arousal resulting in hyperalertness, anticipatory anxiety, an exaggerated startle response, constant scanning of the environment, the perception of people and objects that are not real (i.e., hallucinations), or difficulty falling and remaining asleep.[89] Following this state of hypervigilance, the patient may experience a denial reaction marked by a diminution of responsiveness to the environment. Survival guilt may be present in those cases in which others were harmed or killed during a catastrophic event.

Additional associated features that should alert the physical therapist to the presence of PTSD are increased irritability, hostile behavior, constant tension, chronic free-floating anxiety, muscle tension, sexual and social difficulties, and somatic stress symptoms. Box 26.3 summarizes some of the prominent behavioral features of PTSD.

Not everyone who experiences trauma develops PTSD. The triple vulnerability model postulates that three vulnerabilities need to be present to develop an anxiety disorder: (1) a biological vulnerability; (2) a generalized psychological vulnerability (existing from past experiences of lost control over unpredictable events); and (3) a specific psychological vulnerability that links anxiety to specific situations.[90] Keane and Barlow[91] have proposed an explanation for how PTSD develops based on the triple vulnerability model. They suggest that during a traumatic event, a person experiences alarm and other intense emotions. The person is more likely to develop PTSD if the event and resultant emotions are perceived to be unpredictable and beyond the person's control. If the event is perceived to be predictable and within the person's control, it is less likely that PTSD will occur.

Chronic pain frequently occurs concurrently with PTSD, and the occurrence of both disorders tends to negatively affect the treatment outcome for each.[92] Similar processes, such as avoidance, fear, anxiety, oversensitivity, and catastrophizing (i.e., interpreting an experience as overly threatening), may act to maintain both conditions. Given the high co-morbidity of PTSD and chronic pain, physical therapists should examine patients with PTSD for the existence of chronic pain. The Yale Multidimensional Pain Inventory or the McGill Pain Questionnaire can be administered.[93,94] PTSD may be examined using the Clinician Administered PTSD Scale Revised or the Posttraumatic Stress Disorder Checklist.[95,96] Examination should also include the patient's beliefs, self-efficacy, level of anxiety, sensitivity, coping style, expectations, and degree of behavioral and cognitive avoidance to understand the mechanisms that may maintain these conditions. See Chapter 25, Chronic Pain, for a more detailed discussion of instruments designed to measure pain.

The main desired outcome of treatment for PTSD should be engagement in healthy, satisfying, necessary activities. The physical therapist can help patients to build positive self-efficacy through cognitive restructuring, development of healthy coping skills, and learning to use the relaxation response—all in a predictable, safe environment. Techniques used to help decrease catastrophizing and avoidance include situational exposure exercises (mentioned earlier) and interoceptive exposure exercises (such as running in place or spinning in a chair).[97] Interoceptive exposure exercises help patients cope with uncomfortable physiological sensations that may prevent participation in activities. Finally, the therapist should provide the patient education regarding how PTSD and pain can facilitate each other and result in avoidance. As participation in healthy activities increases, co-occurring disorders—such as depression, anxiety, panic, and substance abuse—may decrease, and a higher quality of life may ensue for the patient with PTSD.[42]

Box 26.3 Behavioral Features (Warning Signs) of Possible Post-Traumatic Stress Disorder (PTSD)

Any one of the following behaviors:

- Recurrent, intrusive recollection of traumatic event
- Intrusive and distressing dreams of event
- Dissociative states (behaving as if reliving event; can last for several seconds or minutes)
- Amnesia of events

More than one of the following behaviors:

- Psychic numbing (lack of interest in social or physical environment or activities; significantly lowered participation in social or physical environment)
- Unable to feel emotions (e.g., intimacy, love, sexuality, anger)
- Disturbed sleep patterns
- Hypervigilance
- Exaggerated startle response
- Ongoing level of irritability
- Heightened difficulty with concentration

Depression

Depression refers to feelings of despair and hopelessness, negative shifts in perception, and decreased interest in activities that once provided pleasure. A person may have a depressed personality (referred to as *dysthymia*) and therefore experience sadness throughout his or her entire life. As in most cases of depression, a person may have one or more episodes of depression, before and after which a normal mood exists. A certain degree of depression is normal in response to life's events, but when depression lasts 2 or more weeks and affects occupational and social functioning, it is considered major depression. Depression may occur as a biochemical imbalance in the brain, which may be triggered by stress, or in response to internal conflicts or life events. For example, the rate of depression in people with SCI is five times higher than that of the general population.[98]

Women with disabilities are more prone to depression (30%)[99] than women without disabilities (10% to 25%),[11] men with disabilities (26%),[99] and the general population (10%).[11] Other researchers support the finding that women with disabilities tend to experience depression more commonly than their male counterparts. In their analysis of 443 women with disabilities, Hughes et al[100] found depression to be a frequently occurring secondary condition (51% of the sample scored in the mildly depressed range or higher on the Beck Depression Inventory–II [BDI-II]). Fifty-nine percent of women with SCI were found to be clinically depressed, compared with a rate of 4.5% to 9.3% of women in the United States at any given time.[101] This high rate of depression among disabled women may be due to the combination of being a woman and having a disability, since both are risk factors for depression. Women are more than twice as likely to have a depressive episode than men due to economic, social, psychological, and biological factors.[102] Female socialization experiences and gender-based roles may also increase their vulnerability to depression. Depression in women has been linked to experiences of abuse and poverty, lack of social support, reduced mobility, chronic pain, lower educational levels, and lower levels of perceived control.[103]

If untreated, depression can spiral into greater severity and may result in suicide; 15% of people who are depressed commit suicide each year.[20] Depression may begin with loss, such as the onset of a physical disability, divorce, death, or the departure of a close friend. Because of such losses, patients may become appropriately sad and mournful. If patients reach out to friends and express their feelings, they can alleviate feelings of loneliness and isolation that commonly occur in response to loss. However, if patients do not take steps to express their feelings, the downward spiral of depression may continue. Over time, patients may lose interest in activities and remain at home. They may lack the energy or motivation to attend to their responsibilities, and feelings of guilt may ensue. A decrease in role participation usually leads to diminished self-esteem and feelings of worthlessness. Eventually, people stop caring about their hygiene. They may avoid social contact and become increasingly lonely. At this point, staying in bed becomes a welcome alternative to dealing with the outside world and the painful feelings it may incur.

Depression and Rehabilitation

Given the signs and symptoms of depression (Table 26.6) and its associated behaviors (Table 26.7), depression may negatively affect the outcome of treatment. Depressed patients may have difficulty getting out of bed and may not be motivated to attend therapy. If they do attend treatment, they may display psychomotor retardation and lack energy and interest; they may also verbalize self-deprecating remarks, feel criticized, and believe that they are progressing inadequately. It may be difficult for physical therapists to leave depressed patients unattended while working with others because the depressed patient may not engage in the prescribed exercises. Patients may feel guilty that they are in the hospital instead of taking care of their children,

Table 26.6 Signs and Symptoms Associated With Mild, Moderate, and Severe Depression

Mild Depression	Moderate Depression	Severe Depression
Anger	Decreased self-esteem	Anguish
Anxiety	Despair	Change in appetite and weight
Decreased concentration	Despondence	Decreased sex drive
Depressed mood	Excessive guilt	Desperation
Indecisiveness	Fearfulness	Feeling overwhelmed
Intrusive thoughts	Inadequacy	Helplessness
Irritability	Sensitivity	Hopelessness
Lethargy		Insomnia or excessive sleep
Loneliness		Recurrent thoughts of suicide
Neediness		Worthlessness
Sadness		

Table 26.7 Behaviors Associated With Mild, Moderate, and Severe Depression

Mild Depression	Moderate Depression	Severe Depression
Being easily frustrated	Crying	Decreased interest in all activities
Difficulty planning ahead	Feeling pessimistic about the future	Lack of personal hygiene
Obsessing about tasks	Having difficulty making decisions	Staying in bed all day
Sitting alone	Making frequent self-deprecating remarks	Suicide (or suicide attempt)
	Overdependence	
	Reacting strongly to criticism	
	Reporting psychosomatic symptoms	
	Ruminating about problems	
	Ruminating about the past	
	Social withdrawal	

working to earn money for their family, or engaging in other life roles.

Depression usually affects performance negatively. Depressed patients may not want to make gains in rehabilitation because of decreased motivation and lack of pleasure in life. They may believe that they are unable to progress in rehabilitation as a result of low self-esteem or feelings of hopelessness. Such patients may also have difficulty asserting themselves because of feelings of worthlessness and an inability to express anger. When people feel worthless or have low self-esteem, they may feel unworthy of having or voicing an opinion. Depression may result from anger turned inward. Instead of expressing anger in the moment, depressed patients may turn their anger against themselves or repress it. People who experience this type of depression may not have been allowed to express hostility in the past.

Depressed patients often become immobilized because they have difficulty making decisions. They may weigh the pros and cons of each choice and become overwhelmed. They may be unable to concentrate on one thought long enough to make decisions. Sometimes depressed patients experience the opposite; when they attempt to execute a decision they may have no thoughts at all (referred to as thought blocking). Consequently, they may need 1 to 2 minutes to think about and answer questions.

Treating Patients With Depression

Depressed patients require assistance with motivation. Physical therapists can facilitate motivation by providing encouragement, emphasizing strengths, offering positive feedback, addressing values, and mobilizing guilt into goal acquisition. Empowering patients by providing activities that offer opportunities for self-control and success has been shown to decrease depression.[104,105]

Depressed patients experience a narrowing of perception. They have difficulty seeing alternate solutions to problems or simple tasks and often feel there is no solution to obstacles. They may perceive their condition as terminal when there is no justification for such a belief. Because of these distortions, it is important to offer reality checks—such as pointing out their strengths when they feel worthless. Cognitive therapy can be used to correct ongoing pessimism by challenging negative thought patterns.

If given choices about their treatment, depressed patients may become ambivalent and unable to decide on a course of action. As a result, they may do nothing. Physical therapists should choose treatment that provides the patient with opportunities for progressive success experiences, avoiding feelings of failure. When reluctant patients perceive that they can succeed in therapy instead of giving up, their chances of continuing treatment increase. Progress made in physical rehabilitation can alleviate depression, as patients report feeling better after having succeeded in an activity they believed they could not accomplish.

Perhaps the most valuable information that a physical therapist can offer depressed patients is that depression will not last forever. Patients will eventually become better through the combination of therapy and possible medication management. Depression can cause an activity or life role that once seemed effortless—such as being a partner in a relationship—to become arduous. It is important for the patient to understand that this does not mean that the relationship caused the depression; more likely, the role of partner has become more difficult to carry out because of depression.

Families often experience a depressed family member as lazy, obstinate, or uncaring, and may not recognize that he or she is suffering from an illness. Depression can be just as disabling as a physical illness. Families need to be educated that depression, like physical disability, causes decreased functioning and requires treatment. Recovery from depression does not have a specific timeline. Each patient's situation is unique, as is the recovery period. Most patients cannot "snap out of it," as many family members desire.

When to Make a Referral for Depression

If depression is suspected, the physical therapist should determine if the patient is currently being treated for depression or has received treatment in the past. If the patient has never been treated for depression and is experiencing suicidal ideation (see section on Suicide below) or symptoms of depression that markedly impair life roles, the therapist should refer the patient to a psychiatrist for possible medication management. Medication can enable patients to attend therapy, more readily discuss problems, and express repressed feelings. However, some patients are reluctant to inform their physical therapist of their depression out of stoicism or shame. There is often a negative stigma attached to being depressed because, to the uninformed, it may imply weakness or feeling sorry for one's self. A diagnosis of depression may not be in the chart and the symptoms may be misinterpreted as fatigue. In these cases, knowledge of the names of medications used to treat depression may help therapists identify patients with depression. The names, effects, and adverse side effects of frequently prescribed antidepressant medications are presented in Table 26.8.

Patients with less severe symptoms who are not suicidal can be referred to a psychologist for verbal therapy.

Table 26.8 Effects and Adverse Side Effects of Commonly Prescribed Antidepressant Medications

Medication	Summary of Effects	Adverse Side Effects
Amitriptyline hydrochloride (Elavil)	Decrease depression, manage anxiety, insomnia, migraines, and chronic pain.	Adverse side effects: dry mouth, urinary retention, constipation, hypotension, dizziness, tachycardia, blurred vision, impaired memory, and weight gain.
Amoxapine (Asendin)	Decrease depression, manage anxiety, insomnia, migraines, and chronic pain.	Dry mouth, urinary retention, constipation, hypotension, dizziness, tachycardia, blurred vision, impaired memory, and weight gain.
Bupropion (Wellbutrin)	Decrease depression, anxiety, addictions, and ADHD.	Tremors, decreased appetite, insomnia, and restlessness.
Celexa (Lexapro)	Decrease depression and anxiety.	Adverse side effects: nervousness, nausea, headache, diarrhea, sexual dysfunction, insomnia, apathy, sweating, hyponatremia, fatigue, and may cause suicidal ideation in children and teens.
Desipramine hydrochloride (Norpramin)	Decrease depression, manage anxiety, insomnia, migraines, and chronic pain.	Adverse side effects: dry mouth, urinary retention, constipation, hypotension, dizziness, tachycardia, blurred vision, impaired memory, and weight gain.
Doxepin hydrochloride (Sinequan, Zonalon)	Decrease depression, manage anxiety, insomnia, migraines, and chronic pain.	Adverse side effects: dry mouth, urinary retention, constipation, hypotension, dizziness, tachycardia, blurred vision, impaired memory, and weight gain.
Fluoxetine (Prozac, Sarafem)	Decrease depression and anxiety.	Nervousness, nausea, headache, diarrhea, sexual dysfunction, insomnia, apathy, sweating, hyponatremia, fatigue, and may cause suicidal ideation in children and teens.
Fluvoxamine (Luvox)	Decrease depression and anxiety.	Nervousness, nausea, headache, diarrhea, sexual dysfunction, insomnia, apathy, sweating, hyponatremia, fatigue, and may cause suicidal ideation in children and teens.
Imipramine hydrochloride (Tofranil)	Decrease depression, manage anxiety, insomnia, migraines, and chronic pain.	Dry mouth, urinary retention, constipation, hypotension, dizziness, tachycardia, blurred vision, impaired memory, weight gain.
Isocurboxazid (Marplan)	Decrease depression and anxiety; used to treat bipolar depression and treatment-resistant depression.	Dizziness, hypotension, weight gain, sedation, cotton mouth, insomnia, and sexual dysfunction.
Maprotiline (Ludiomil)	Decrease depression and manage anxiety, insomnia, migraines, and chronic pain.	Dry mouth, urinary retention, constipation, hypotension, dizziness, tachycardia, blurred vision, impaired memory, and weight gain.

ADHD = attention deficit-hyperactivity disorder.

If a patient's depression seems to be caused by family turmoil, a referral to a social worker for family intervention can be made. Patients who have difficulty verbalizing their feelings can be referred to a creative arts therapist to facilitate expression through nonverbal means such as music, dance, or art. A referral to an occupational therapist can be made to help patients regain function in daily life roles that have been disrupted by depression.

Suicide

Each year, more than 35,000 cases of suicide are reported in the United States, and 65,000 additional cases may go unreported due to complications regarding the cause of death.[28] More people lose their lives to suicide than to any other cause apart from cancer and cardiovascular disease. Suicide is often a result of poor social support, low self-esteem, ineffective coping skills, and the inability to see a solution to difficult situations. Risk factors include serious illness, previous suicide attempts, family history of suicide, alcohol and substance abuse/dependence, loss of a loved one through rejection or death, prolonged depression, and financial difficulties.

Recognizing the warning signs of possible suicide risk is important for its prevention. The most frequent signs of suicide risk include the following:

- Direct comments about suicide, such as, "I just want to die"
- Indirect comments about suicide, such as, "My mother will not have to worry about me anymore"
- A plan to commit suicide
- Writing a suicide note
- Preoccupation with death
- A sudden flight into happiness or relief after a long depression
- Excessive risk taking (e.g., driving while inebriated) and a careless attitude
- Final preparations (e.g., composing a will, giving away personal possessions, repairing broken relationships, or writing revealing letters)
- Self-hatred
- Changes in personal appearance, eating habits, sexual drive, sleep patterns, menstrual cycle, behavior (e.g., inability to concentrate or disinterest in activities), or personality (e.g., withdrawal, anxiousness, sadness, irritability, apathy, indecisiveness, or fatigue)
- A recent loss accompanied by an inability to stop grieving

The most important thing for a physical therapist to do when suspecting that a patient is suicidal is to prevent him or her from carrying out the act. This usually involves obtaining help from a mental health professional, preferably a physician with the knowledge and ability to admit the person to a hospital if needed. It is important not to leave the patient alone while waiting for help. During this period, the following should take place:

- Ask patients whether they are thinking of hurting or killing themselves.
- Listen to patients without expressing shock, without discrediting what they say, and without devaluing their feelings; take all suicide threats seriously even if you do not believe them at the time.
- Respond to patients with empathy and understanding; tell them how much you care about them and that you will be available to help them.
- Help patients think of alternatives; offer choices based on your knowledge about the patient's life, rather than generic answers that are easy to offer when under pressure.
- Alert family members, friends, and significant others to the patient's suicide risk; all of these individuals may help prevent the patient from trying to commit suicide; suicidal ideation does not go away in a day; additional help is required from all possible sources over time.

■ SUBSTANCE ABUSE

Substance abuse occurs when an individual demonstrates a dysfunctional pattern of drug and/or alcohol use characterized by recurrent and significant adverse consequences. Substances may include, but are not limited to, alcohol, amphetamines, caffeine, marijuana, cocaine, hallucinogens, inhalants, opioids, or sedatives.[11]

Substance Abuse and Rehabilitation

If clients come to the clinic under the influence of drugs or alcohol, they may be inappropriate, argumentative, irritable, disinhibited, stubborn, illogical, or angry and will have difficulty following treatment plans. They may also disturb other clients, some of who may be in their own substance abuse recovery. For these reasons, intoxicated clients should be escorted out of the treatment area and referred to their substance abuse programs, with a call to their substance abuse program provider describing the incident that occurred. If they are not currently engaged in a substance abuse program, a referral should be made. Although many drugs have unique and specific consequences, Table 26.9 presents an overview of common physiological, psychological, and behavioral manifestations associated with substance abuse.

If patients are not under the influence during treatment, but are using drugs or alcohol at home, they may miss treatment sessions or may come to rehabilitation tired, hungry, or late. They may have poor concentration and irritable moods resulting from hangovers. They may experience recurring injuries from falls. Often, patients will not comply with treatment and fail to complete their home exercises or forget to take their prescribed medications. When prescribed medications are ingested along with illegal substances, adverse drug

Table 26.9 Common Physiological, Psychological, and Behavioral Manifestations Associated With Substance Abuse

Physiological		
• Abnormal blood pressure • Abnormal pupillary response • Altered appetite • Constipation • Cravings • Dizziness • Drowsiness • Enlarged heart • Gastrointestinal bleeding	• Hallucinations • Impaired liver function • Irregular or increased heartbeat • Loss of consciousness • Malnutrition • Peripheral neuropathy • Perspiration • Psychomotor disturbances • Red nose or eyes	• Reduced perception of pain • Sensory impairments • Shiny ears • Sleep disturbances • Tremors (shakiness) • Unexplained weight loss or gain • Visible needle marks (if injecting)
Psychological		
• Confusion • Delusions • Denial • Depression • Disturbances in interpersonal behavior	• Disturbances of perception • Easily frustrated • Emotional lability • Grandiosity • Intense emotions • Loneliness	• Low self-esteem • Paranoia • Poor concentration • Poor memory • Reduced inhibitions • Thought disturbances
Behavioral		
• Anger • Associating only with other substance abusers • Belligerence • Cheating • Compulsive use of drugs • Decreased ability to manage stress • Decreased ability to manage time • Difficulty holding a job • Discontinuation of usual activities • Drug-seeking and drug-using behaviors	• Falling • Financial irresponsibility • Hyperactivity (restlessness) • Impaired judgment • Impaired or inability to fulfill major life roles • Impulsivity • Inability to control drug use • Irritability • Isolation • Lack of interest in favorite sport or activity	• Lying • Mood swings • Nervousness • Poor hygiene • Possession of drug paraphernalia • Spending money on drugs • Staying up all night (insomnia) • Stealing • Violence • Withdrawal

reactions can occur. Patients may lack insight about the extent of their abuse and the trouble that it produces in their lives. They may mask feelings such as anger, guilt, anxiety, or depression through the numbing effect of the substance, but try to present themselves as though they are fine.

Patients in denial commonly do not perceive their need for physical rehabilitation, often neglect to follow precautions, and frequently attempt to obtain discharge before completing rehabilitation goals. Their low frustration tolerance causes them to quit treatment easily. Whether they are actively using substances or not, patients who have abused substances may have cognitive deficits that inhibit their ability to follow or remember instructions. They may experience family discord and lose family support, thus finding themselves homeless. Patients with a history of chronic alcohol abuse tend to have poor balance resulting from changes in the cerebellum and peripheral nerves.[106] To maintain balance, they develop a stereotypic, wide-based gait. Such factors should be considered during gait examination and training. Despite their gruff demeanor, patients who abuse substances can be overly sensitive, easily hurt, suffer from low self-esteem, and easily stressed once they are no longer abusing substances. These patients tend to have poor boundaries. They can be intrusive, flirtatious, or deal seeking to obtain what they want, such as alcohol, cigarettes, or extra medication.

Treating Patients Who Abuse Substances

Physical therapists can help patients in recovery by providing opportunities that allow them to gain control over their lives again. Such assistance may include opportunities to practice setting boundaries, regulating emotions, and tolerating frustration. Physical therapists can emphasize healthy activities that provide pleasure and decrease cravings. Stress management, time management, ADL, and social skills are usually necessary skills to promote recovery.

Education on Substance Abuse

Physical therapists, patients, and patients' family members should be aware that substance abuse is an illness. Like physical or mental illness, it causes a decrease in function, requires skilled intervention for recovery, results in decreased role performance, and can affect anyone. Patients with a diagnosis of substance abuse usually cannot stop using drugs and alcohol on their own. They need help, and recovery is a lifelong process that includes developing skills to manage cravings, dealing with stress in healthy ways, expressing feelings, participating in 12-step programs, and engaging in drug-free activities.

When to Make a Referral for Substance Abuse

If the patient is going through withdrawal, the physical therapist should immediately refer the patient to a physician. Signs of withdrawal can include sweating, impaired sleep, seizures, impaired motor coordination, faulty judgment, anxiety, shaking, slurred speech, fluctuating levels of consciousness, and visual and tactile hallucinations. After stabilizing the patient, the physician may transfer him or her to a detoxification unit. If the patient is not experiencing withdrawal and is not already in a substance abuse treatment program, physical therapists can make a referral to an appropriate treatment center. Such treatment centers include 28-day inpatient rehabilitation programs, long-term (1 to 1.5 years) inpatient therapeutic communities, 12-step programs for community-dwelling outpatients, and dual diagnosis programs[48] for patients who have also been diagnosed with mental illness.

Patients who have been abusing substances for long periods of time should be referred to a nutritionist for proper dietary regulation. Physical therapy patients who have been abusing substances can be referred to occupational therapists to address regulating emotions, setting and maintaining appropriate boundaries, tolerating frustration, managing time, obtaining social skills, and regaining necessary ADL. Occupational therapists also can help patients learn that healthy activities can be pleasurable, through task groups in which patients choose, engage in, and discuss healthy activities. A social work referral can be made if the patient requires community integration, family intervention, or social supports. A referral to a psychiatrist can be made for an evaluation for medication (see Table 26.10 for a list of commonly administered medications for the treatment of substance abuse and their side effects).

■ AGITATION AND VIOLENCE

Physical therapists may not expect patients to demonstrate sexual, aggressive, or violent behaviors, yet most have witnessed such behaviors at least once. Therapists should learn how to predict violence, identify signs of escalation, manage aggressive patients, and verbally respond to threats. Violence is not always predictable, but the more therapists understand its signs, the better equipped they will be to handle a dangerous situation.

An initial step involves recognizing the early signs of agitation. Agitation usually does not diminish by itself. Instead, it may build to a verbal altercation or physical act. Some signs of agitation may include clenching fists, pacing back and forth, making angry facial expressions, grunting, groaning, swearing, tapping a foot, spitting, refusing to engage in therapy, throwing objects, and banging weights or other therapeutic equipment.

After observing signs of agitation, physical therapists should identify the source of the agitation to better control it. While many situations can cause agitation, it is important to remember that events that agitate one person may have no effect on another; levels of frustration vary from person to person. People with Alzheimer's disease may become agitated because they cannot recall the names of familiar objects or remember familiar motor plans. They may believe that family members are lying to them, deceiving them, or attempting to place them in a nursing home. People can become agitated because of physical pain, memory failure, hunger, fatigue, and dependency on others. Temporal lobe injury, psychosis, and the side effects of certain medications can cause agitation. People with personality disorders who have difficulty managing anger and who have experienced an upsetting event can easily become agitated.

Addressing the underlying circumstance causing the agitation may help to defuse it. If the source of agitation is unknown, the physical therapist should acknowledge to the patient, in a non-accusatory manner, that he or she seems upset. Many people are unaware of their agitation and calm down once it is brought to their attention. The therapist can then encourage the patient to verbally express why he or she feels upset. Therapists can also attempt to redirect patient anger into more productive channels and help alter their perspective regarding the disturbing issue.

Violence also can happen without warning. Many therapists working on inpatient TBI units have been bitten, kicked, punched, or scratched. Patients may feel that they are being forced to participate in therapy they do not need, or that they are being treated like children. They may believe that staff members have assumed control over their lives. To avoid humiliating the patient, therapists can use a client-centered therapy approach in which patients are offered respect and included in goal setting and treatment planning.

If efforts to defuse the patient's agitation do not work and he or she becomes violent, the physical therapist should remove all other patients from the area, then leave and call for help. After an act of violence, members of the rehabilitation team should examine what occurred to learn from the incident, prevent a future recurrence,

Table 26.10 Medications Commonly Used to Treat Substance Abuse

Medication	Summary of Effects	Adverse Side Effects
Buprenorphine (Subutex)	Opioid withdrawal, opioid maintenance; stops opioid cravings without euphoria, sedation, or an analgesic effect; pain management related to withdrawal.	Runny nose and eyes, vomiting, abdominal cramps, diarrhea, nervousness, body aches for up to 7 days, nausea, sever anxiety, dizziness, insomnia, fatigue, headaches.
Buprenorphine and Naloxone (Suboxone)	Opioid withdrawal, opioid maintenance; stops opioid cravings without euphoria, sedation, or an analgesic effect; pain management related to withdrawal.	Runny nose and eyes, vomiting, abdominal cramps, diarrhea, nervousness, body aches for up to 7 days, nausea, sever anxiety, dizziness, insomnia, fatigue, headaches.
Bupropion (Wellbutrin)	Stimulant withdrawal and stimulant relapse prevention; tobacco smoking cessation; lessens cigarette cravings and decreases nicotine withdrawal symptoms.	Tremors, dry mouth, decreased appetite, insomnia, and restlessness.
Clonidine (Catapres)	Mild opioid withdrawal; tobacco smoking cessation.	Runny nose and eyes, vomiting, abdominal cramps, diarrhea, nervousness, body aches for up to 7 days, nausea, sever anxiety, dizziness, insomnia, fatigue, headaches.
Disulfiram (Antabuse)	Prevents alcohol relapse by blocking ETOH breakdown leading to increased levels of toxic acetaldehyde causing violent vomiting; decreases impulsive alcohol consumption.	Tingling in legs and arms, dark urine, itchy skin or skin rashes, drowsiness, psychosis, eye pain, decreased vision, decreased energy, inflammation of the liver, impotence, white stool, indigestion, jaundice, optic nerve damage.
Imipramine hydrochloride (Tofranil)	Marijuana withdrawal without causing a high.	Dry mouth, urinary retention, constipation, hypotension, dizziness, tachycardia, blurred vision, impaired memory, weight gain.
Methadone Hydrochloride (Methadone)	Heroin detoxification and maintenance; stops heroin cravings without euphoria, sedation, or an analgesic effect; pain management related to withdrawal.	Must be tapered slowly when discontinuing use to avoid withdrawal symptoms of methadone; dangerous in overdose; at high doses and/or if used in combination with other drugs, can produce an experience of intoxication.
Naltrexone Hydrochloride (ReVia)	Opioid withdrawal; blocks pleasure centres stimulated by opioids; alcohol relapse prevention.	Runny nose and eyes, vomiting, abdominal cramps, diarrhea, nervousness, body aches for up to 7 days, nausea, sever anxiety, dizziness, insomnia, fatigue, headaches.
Nalmedfene Hydrochloride (Revex)	Opioid withdrawal; blocks pleasure centres stimulated by opioids; alcohol relapse prevention; used as an injection after anaesthesia to stop the effect of opioids; used orally for alcohol craving reduction; gambling and nicotine addictions.	Runny nose and eyes, vomiting, abdominal cramps, diarrhea, nervousness, body aches for up to 7 days, nausea, sever anxiety, dizziness, insomnia, fatigue, headaches.
Nortriptyline (Aventyl, Pamelor)	Tobacco smoking cessation.	Nausea, nightmares, weakness, drowsiness, dizziness, dry mouth, headaches.
Varenicline tartrate (Chantix)	Tobacco smoking cessation; decreases symptoms of withdrawal and makes smoking a less satisfying experience by binding to brain nicotine receptors.	Vivid, abnormal, or strange dreams; insomnia; nausea.

Note: Brand names are shown in parentheses.

and provide support and education to those involved. In reviewing the incident, the physical therapist should address the following questions:

- What was the patient's potential for aggression?
- What were the signs of escalating anger?
- Did the patient have a history of violence? If yes, under what circumstances did it occur?
- How did therapists and patients respond to the aggressor before, during, and after the act?
- What could have been done differently during the incident?

In addition to managing an agitated or violent patient, physical therapists need to recognize when a patient is undergoing abuse. It is estimated that 10% of women with disabilities experience sexual, physical, or disability-related violence.[107] Abuse has been related to decreased social support, increased social isolation, and elevated levels of depression and stress.[106] Women with disabilities may be even more susceptible to abuse, due to their dual minority status as people with disabilities and as women. As compared with women without disabilities, women having disabilities experienced longer periods of abuse and abuse from a greater number of perpetrators.[108] Nosek et al[109] have identified several factors that predict with 80% accuracy whether a woman has experienced abuse within the past year. These include decreased mobility, social isolation, depression, and a lack of education. Examination for abuse should be considered for women with disabilities.[109] Nosek et al developed a four-item screening tool, the Abuse Assessment Screen—Disability (AAS-D), that examines sexual, physical, and disability-related abuse in the past year.

HYPERSEXUALITY

Hypersexuality is a state of heightened sexual arousal that may be accompanied by verbal or physical aggression. These behaviors can be caused by mania, childhood sexual abuse, or brain damage. Patients may desire attention, or want to provoke or exert power over others, to impress others, or to show off. Verbal signs of hypersexuality can include whistling; verbalizing sexual desires; or asking for physical closeness, phone numbers, or dates. Physical behaviors include staring, pinching, brushing up against another's body, touching, kissing, exposing genitalia, masturbating, and blocking another's exit from a room.

There are several ways to proceed when a patient exhibits hypersexual behavior. If the therapist feels threatened, he or she should leave the area and obtain assistance. If the patient's hypersexual behavior is a newly observed behavior, the therapist can describe the behavior to the patient and firmly state that it is inappropriate and will not be tolerated. If the therapist believes that the patient is exhibiting symptoms of mania or hypomania, referral should be immediately made to a psychiatrist. Holding a multidisciplinary team conference may help the patient understand that hypersexual behaviors are not tolerated in the clinic.

PSYCHOSOCIAL WELLNESS

According to Jacobs and Jacobs[110] and Donatelle and Davis,[28] wellness is a dynamic process in which people attempt to fully develop their emotional, social, environmental, physical, spiritual, and intellectual health. Donatelle and Davis describe a well individual as someone who can forgive himself or herself and others, learn from mistakes, appreciate all things both grand and small, develop a realistic sense of self and the environment, achieve a balance in life roles and daily activities, respect others and maintain healthy relationships, feel a sense of life satisfaction, understand one's needs and express emotions appropriately, and function in his or her community. Achieving this definition of wellness may require substantial effort for someone with a disability who may experience multiple barriers to wellness.

Barriers to Wellness for People With Disabilities

Healthy People 2020 identified gaps and disparities in the health and wellness of Americans with disabilities.[99] It reported that people with disabilities exhibited more symptoms of psychological distress and tended to not engage in as many physical activities as people without disabilities. Objectives to overcome these barriers included to "Increase the proportion of people with disabilities who participate in social, spiritual, recreational, community and civic activities to the degree that they wish" (DH-13) and "Reduce the proportion of people with disabilities who report serious psychological distress" (DH-18).

More specifically, research has found that women with disabilities experience higher levels of stress than do males with disabilities, possibly owing to higher incidences of poverty, violence, abuse, chronic health problems, and social isolation.[102] Economic disadvantage may be due to stress-inducing factors such as earning a lower income, having less access to disability benefits from public programs, having less education than their male counterparts with disabilities, and having a higher likelihood of being unemployed or unmarried.[111] People with SCI report a higher level of perceived stress than the general population, and women with SCI tend to have a higher level of perceived stress than men with SCI.[111]

Social Support

Social support is critical in maintaining or achieving psychosocial wellness. Social support is defined as the availability of other persons in the environment who can offer emotional support, financial or material help, a listening ear, guidance, or encouragement. Social support has been associated with increased self-esteem, coping, and adjustment for individuals with disabilities. Evidence suggests that social support plays a strong preventive and palliative role in a wide range of physical and medical conditions. Rintala et al[113] found that the amount of social support was directly related to a sense of life satisfaction and well-being in patients with SCI. Hardy et al[114] and Kaplan[115] found that high social support was predictive of a return to vocational functioning after rehabilitation.

Researchers have suggested that failure to recover from depression stemming from disability may correlate to a lack of adequate social support. Social isolation is a frequently encountered condition associated with disability. Physical restrictions such as pain and mobility limitations may discourage connections with others. The combination of diminished social opportunities, negative societal perceptions, and multiple environmental barriers may result in isolation and a lack of emotional intimacy.

Social support can be used to enhance treatment and promote patient adherence. The physical therapist plays an important role in guiding patient education, including access to resources and instruction in use of adaptive equipment and environmental devices designed to improve a patient's access to social networks and socialization. Appendix 26.B provides Web-based resources for patients, families, and caregivers. It provides resources for improving community accessibility (independent living centers), depression, substance abuse, anxiety, and PTSD.

WELLNESS IN REHABILITATION

Psychosocial wellness requires that patients experience success in both rehabilitation activities and long-term relationships and roles. Rehabilitation activities focus on improving functional outcomes, involvement in meaningful events that foster socialization (e.g., playing wheelchair basketball with other patients), and community reintegration. Long-term relationships and roles include being a spouse, parent, worker, and friend. Psychologists, social workers, and occupational therapists can facilitate readjustment to these long-term roles. Both rehabilitation activities and long-term relationships and roles should provide a sense of contentment, happiness, and well-being. Physical therapists can promote and provide opportunities for patients to choose and engage in meaningful activities that promote psychosocial wellness.

Patients who spend a great deal of time dwelling on the past and worrying about the future are unable to be fully cognizant of the present moment.[116] The ability to become absorbed in the present moment can decrease anxiety concerning the past or future—the patient's emotional energy is focused on his or her immediate activities. Each instance in which a patient can focus on the present offers him or her the power to change, to break through old habits, to view circumstances differently, and to recognize available choices. Physical therapists can help patients remain focused on the present moment by selecting activities that are both meaningful to and congruent with the patient's goals for rehabilitation.

Having a daily balance of work, leisure, and social activities is important to sustain psychosocial wellness. Any psychological or physical impairment can disrupt this balance. In a study of the relationship between depression and leisure participation in people with SCI, Loy et al[117] found that patients without depression had wider repertoires and higher levels of leisure activity than patients with depression. Therapists can help patients engage in leisure activities through activity interest surveys and schedules. Activity interest surveys are used to gather information about the types of leisure pursuits patients previously engaged in, which leisure pursuits they currently hold interest in, and which leisure activities they would like to pursue in the future.

A negative outlook inhibits psychosocial wellness. Physical therapists can help patients with negative perspectives to positively alter their expectations through goal setting, identifying optimistic options, using cognitive-behavioral techniques that challenge the validity of negative perceptions, or referring the patient to a psychologist for longer-term intervention.

INTEGRATING PSYCHOSOCIAL FACTORS INTO REHABILITATION: CASE EXAMPLE

Bill, a 19-year-old who was training to be an Olympic gymnast, sustained an SCI in a motorcycle accident. Bill had developed a strong social support system and participated in a variety of extracurricular activities. He was engaged and planning to be married, participated on his college's gymnastic team, and worked as an athletic counselor in the summer camp he had attended since age 7. The SCI he sustained caused a loss of function from his chest down.

All of Bill's energy is now focused on getting through each day. He does not view himself as able to work or attend school. The accident has changed his expectations for the future, his outlook on life, his environmental challenges, and his social support system. His depression was compounded by his broken marriage engagement, and Bill no longer meets his friends for social events; in fact, he rarely leaves his home other than to attend rehabilitation. Just when he was becoming independent of his parents, Bill has now become dependent on them again. He observes his younger sisters and brothers progressing in their lives and feels stagnant, angry, depressed, and ashamed. His self-esteem, which was once high, is now severely diminished and he has lost his familiar identity.

As part of his rehabilitation, the therapist should provide a safe way for Bill to express his anger; referral to a psychologist is also warranted. The therapist can help him to better understand his physical limitations and capabilities. Based on Bill's strengths and limitations, the therapist should help him to redefine interests that could emerge into new roles and a new identity. For instance, it might be helpful if Bill could identify a meaningful activity that could take the place of his athletic training (such as coaching a children's gymnastic team). Information about college and distance learning could also be beneficial. The therapist also can assist Bill and his family in the understanding of SCI and reasonable expectations for the future.

SUGGESTIONS FOR REHABILITATIVE INTERVENTION

Table 26.11 offers a list of behaviors that suggest inappropriate and pathological response patterns to disability. This list is not meant to be fully inclusive, but rather indicates areas requiring further consideration. It is important to understand that even mild expressions of pathological response patterns can become chronic and worsen in severity over time. Table 26.12 identifies patient behaviors that warrant a mental health consultation.

Box 26.4[118] gives examples of general goals and outcomes for patients with psychosocial issues, and Box 26.5 provides instruments typically used to measure these outcomes organized by the International Classification of Functioning, Disability, and Health (ICF) categories.[119] However, human reactions, response patterns, and the adaptation process are variable and individualistic. Each patient must be approached uniquely, and treatment goals should incorporate the patient's individual personality characteristics, responses, and needs. An important component of rehabilitation is the patient–practitioner relationship. Physical therapists can establish a therapeutic atmosphere of communication, understanding, and cooperation with patients, which can serve as the foundation necessary to produce positive rehabilitation outcomes. Therapists can sometimes forget the powerful influence they have in setting the tone of this interaction. The very structure and atmosphere of service delivery and the personality and type of communication provided by

Table 26.11 Behaviors Suggesting Pathological Response Patterns

Grieving	Depression	Damaged Self-Esteem	Heightened Possibility for Suicide	Heightened Possibility for Violence
Grieving for actual or perceived impairment of functioning or actual loss is normal and expected, but the following might serve as clues to a more severe reaction: Denial of problem or its severity Exaggeration or idealizing the loss Obsession with the past or the pre-loss state Obsession with guilt related to loss Regression Difficulty with concentration Loss of interest in activities and events Lability of mood Inability to discuss loss Fear of being left alone Acting out behaviors (tantrums, suicidal gestures, promiscuity) Angry stance	Flat affect (showing little emotion) Very low energy levels Manic energy and behavior Psychomotor retardation (slowing down of movement and action) Ruminating about negative thoughts Change in eating and sleeping patterns (insomnia or hypersomnia) Regression Social withdrawal Self-destructive behaviors Loss of interest in environment, people, and events Self-blame and self-criticism	Isolation from social sphere Self-destructive behavior Inability to sustain eye contact Inability to accept praise Judgmental attitude Self-deprecating and self-critical Unwarranted pessimism Unconcern for appearance Unconcern for personal safety	Depression Giving away possessions Hoarding/hiding medications or potential weapons Writing suicide note Updating will Verbalizing loneliness or hopelessness Statements regarding benefit of release of pain, absence, and so forth Intrusiveness of such thoughts	Low threshold for anger Depression High-anxiety state Motoric agitation Self-mutilation Oversensitive Argumentative Inability to express feelings Fears of abandonment Highly dependent Dissociative states

Table 26.12 Patient Behaviors Warranting a Mental Health Consultation

Regression	Regression involves reverting to earlier, more immature patterns of functioning. This may be more commonly observed in children but might be observed in adults as well. For example, children may revert to sucking their thumb or may appear to have lost their toilet training skills. Regression in adults may generally be seen in lost skills and abilities and/or even in the extreme behavior of reverting to taking a fetal position.
Disorientation	Disorientation is confusion as to time, place, activity, self-identity, or identity of others. Occasional, transient disorientation is not wholly uncommon in the average person, yet persistence in frequency or duration of occurrence is cause for examination and intervention. Any more extreme confused behaviors and thought processes need to be carefully examined.
Delusional thinking	Delusional thinking refers to faulty and mistaken beliefs and, although related to inaccurate interpretation of environment, is distinguished by the persistence of this belief system. This can run the gamut from delusions of grandeur or of persecution, to delusions about the nature and scope of a disability. These delusions hold up and persist in the face of contrary information.
Inaccurate interpretation of environment	This is the broadest category in this list, but fortunately is also the most readily understood category. Clearly, when a patient significantly misinterprets and misunderstands the objective situation and reality about him or her, it is probably most readily noted by non–mental health practitioners in its many expressions. This should draw attention and intervention, not only in its extreme form of a psychotic break, but also in its minor form of small, repeated episodes of misinterpretations.
Inappropriate affect	Affect refers to the mood state displayed by the patient, where feelings such as joy, sadness, fear, and so forth are reflected in body language, facial expression, and verbalizations. Inappropriate affect can be seen in an affective expression alien to the situation; for example, demonstrating and expressing joy on hearing bad news. It also refers to a split between displayed affect and verbalization; for example, the verbal expression of mourning and condolence offered while smiling brightly and jumping for joy.
Hypovigilance or hypervigilance	Hypovigilance can be noted in a patient being oblivious to his or her surroundings and the events around the patient, socially, as well as physically. Hypervigilance refers to an intense focus and alertness to social and physical surrounds. Each of these has different ramifications and meaning to the mental health team. A consultation is suggested as either extreme is approached.
Mood swings	We all experience changes in mood, yet most of the time these changes are relatively appropriate reactions to external determinants, such as the receipt of news and information or to changing occurrences and circumstances in our environment. Although changeable, moods are generally persistent and stable. When mood shifts either to extremes and/or with some frequency, it suggests either instability or that mood is being driven predominantly by internal rather than external factors.
Self-destructive behaviors	Any self-destructive behavior, particularly ones that persist, are cause for serious concern. Self-destructive behaviors can run the gamut from subtle, difficult to detect signs to very clear and frightening overt signs. Subtle signs can include non-adherence with treatment regimen, poor self-maintenance activities such as not eating, overeating, diminishment of personal care and hygiene, or carelessness in negotiating the environment. Clearer signs can include self-inflicted wounds and suicidal ideation and expressions.
Normal behaviors taken to extremes	Normal human behavior enjoys a wide latitude of response repertoire before drawing attention as being out of expected bounds. This latitude must usually be extended further when dealing with someone undergoing a more extreme, traumatic, or stressful experience. Individuals confronted with a disability would be expected to naturally focus their attention, concerns, and anxiety around this issue. The level of focus on a left leg given by someone preparing to have that leg amputated would be considered obsessive in a healthy ambulatory person, yet normal here. Care in judgment is required by the clinician when determining behavior expressions. That said, issues such as obsessiveness, extreme distractibility, immobilization in the face of routine decisions, and unexpected egocentricity or self-denigration may require a consultation. An overly adherent patient, an extremely calm patient, as well as an overly contentious, argumentative, or extremely anxious or hysterical patient also promotes concern. Any response (verbal or behavioral) that appears unwarranted to the stimuli should draw attention. Overreactions in opposite directions or any behavior that appears to be at an extreme, using reasonable judgment, deserves attention.

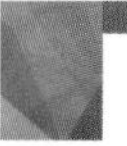

Box 26.4 Examples of General Goals and Outcomes for Patients With Psychosocial Issues Adapted From the *Guide to Physical Therapist Practice*[118]

Impact of pathology is reduced.

- Patient/client, family, and caregiver knowledge and awareness of the disease, prognosis, and plan of care is enhanced.
- Symptom management is enhanced.
- Changes associated with recovery are monitored.
- Risk of secondary impairments and reoccurrence of condition is reduced.
- Intensity of care is decreased.

Impact of impairments is reduced.

- Cognitive function is improved.
- Communication is improved.
- Ability to participate in rehabilitation is improved.

Ability to perform physical actions, tasks, or activities is improved.

- Independence in ADL is increased.
- Problem-solving and decision making skills are improved.
- Safety of client, family, and caregivers is intact.
- Disability associated with chronic illness is reduced.
- Ability to assume/resume self-care and home management is improved.
- Ability to assume roles such as participation in work activities (job/school/play) and community leisure roles is improved.
- Awareness and use of community resources are improved.

Health status and quality of life are improved.

- Sense of well-being is enhanced.
- Stressors are reduced and/or the ability to manage them is improved.
- Insight, self-confidence, and self-management skills are improved.
- Health and wellness are improved.

Client satisfaction is enhanced.

- Access to and availability of services are acceptable to client and family.
- Quality of rehabilitation services is acceptable to client and family.
- Care is coordinated with client, family, caregivers, and other professionals.
- Discharge placement needs are determined.

the practitioner exert a strong influence on patient participation and response to rehabilitation efforts.

Optimizing Patient Involvement

Patients should be involved as fully as possible in their own treatment. This includes involvement in goal setting and treatment planning, as well as in the ongoing evaluation of progress. Patient cooperation is also dependent on the therapist's clear explanation of the patient's situation, anticipated goals and expected outcomes, and interventions. Relating to the patient as a partner in therapy can engender cooperation and trust in the therapeutic relationship. When patients feel a heightened sense of control and ability (i.e., locus of control), feelings of despair and helplessness can be mitigated.

Therapists should also maintain a receptive ear to patient concerns and encourage communication. Listening carefully to patients in a nonjudgmental manner will allow them to reveal concerns and issues they may otherwise feel uncomfortable discussing. Clear and articulate communication, however, can be disrupted by emotion, uncertainty, or power discrepancies that exist when patients become passive recipients of service. Although it may sometimes appear easier to do for patients than to witness their struggle—particularly when patients assume a passive role in rehabilitation—promoting self-reliance and independence fosters patients' engagement and responsibility in their recovery. Allowing patients to maintain a passive role fosters helplessness, encourages dependency, and slows progress in the long term.

Patients can also be involved in providing the treatment team with feedback about their treatment and rehabilitation experience. Feedback regarding their care can

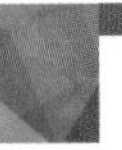

Box 26.5 Outcome Measures for Psychosocial Issues Organized by the *International Classification of Functioning, Disability, and Health* (ICF) Categories[119]

Body Structure and Function Measures

Holmes-Rahe Social Readjustment Scale
- Holmes, T, and Rahe, R: The Social Readjustment Scale. J Psychosom Res 11:213, 1967.

The Hassles Scale
- Kanner, AD, et al: Comparison of two modes of stress management: Daily hassles and uplifts versus major life events. J Behav Med 4:1, 1981.

Contextual Memory Test
- Toglia, JP: Contextual Memory Test. Therapy Skill Builders, San Antonio, TX, 1993.

Beck Depression Inventory
- Beck, AT, Steer, RA, and Brown, GK: Beck Depression Inventory–II Manual. The Psychological Corporation, San Antonio, Texas, 1987.

Stroop Color and Word Test
- Golden, CJ, and Freshwater, SM: The Stroop Color and Word Test: A Manual for Clinical and Experimental Uses. Stoelting Co, Wood Dale, IL, 2002.

Neurobehavioral Cognitive Status Examination
- Kiernan, RJ, Mueller, J, and Langston, JW: The Neurobehavioral ***Cognitive Status Examination (COGNISTAT).*** Northern California Neurobehavioral Group, Inc., San Francisco, 2001.

Generalized Expectancy for Success Scale
- Fibel, B, and Hale, WD: The Generalized Expectancy for Success Scale—a new measure. J Consulting Clin Psych 46:924, 1978/1992.

Beck Hopelessness Scale
- Durham, TW: Norms, reliability, and item analysis of the Hopelessness Scale in general psychiatric, forensic psychiatric, and college populations. J Clin Psych 38(5):597, 1982.

Internal-External Locus of Control Scale
- Rotter, JB: Generalized expectancies for internal versus external control of reinforcement. Psych Mono 80:1, 1966.

Self-Efficacy Scale
- Sherer, M, Maddox, JE, Mercandante, B, Prentice-Dunn, S, Jacobs, B, and Rogers, RW: The Self-Efficacy Scale: Construction and validation. Psych Rep 51:663, 1982.

Sentence Completion Attitude Survey
- Bloom, W: Bloom Sentence Completion Attitude Survey. Stoelting Co., Wood Dale, IL. Website: https://www.stoeltingco.com

Mini-Mental State Examination (MMSE)
- Folstein, MF, Folstein, SE, and McHugh, PR: "Mini-mental state." A practical method for grading the cognitive state of patients for the clinician. J Psychiatr Res 12(3):189, 1975.

Activity Measures

Occupational Questionnaire's Balanced Activity Record
- Smith, HR, Kielhofner, G, and Watts, JH: Occupational Questionnaire. Am J Occup Ther 40:278, 1986. Website: www.moho.uic.edu/mohorelatedrsrcs.html

Interest Checklist
- Kielhofner, G, and Neville, A: Interest Checklist. Slack, Thorofare, NJ, 1983.

Participation Measures

Role Checklist
- Oakley, F, Kielhofner, G, Barris, R, and Reichler, RK: The Role Checklist: Development and empirical assessment of reliability. Occup Ther J Res 6(3):157, 1986.

Community Adaptation Schedule
- Roen, S, and Burnes, A: Community Adaptation Schedule [serial online]. Not dated. Available from Mental Measurements Yearbook with Tests in Print, Ipswich, MA. Accessed January 12, 2011.

be used in continuing quality improvement projects for the physical therapy and rehabilitation departments. Continuing quality improvement projects are performed on regularly to provide the best care at the lowest cost.[120,121]

Use of Jargon and Labels

Patient–therapist communication should be characterized by simple and easy to understand language that matches the cognitive level of the patient. The use of scientific jargon and labels should be avoided when speaking with patients, because it impedes patient understanding and emotionally distances patients from therapists. Similarly, when patients hear therapists referring to fellow patients by their diagnosis, they receive the message that patients are nothing more than disabilities. Such practice should be avoided and, instead, therapists should use language that reflects respect for the patient's dignity and unique life circumstances.

Rehabilitation Team Members' Self-Awareness

Finally, and perhaps most important, therapists need to be aware of their own feelings, motivations, and responses. Such self-awareness is critical for therapists to understand their own reactions to patients. It is normal for people to respond to others based on conscious or unconscious memories. Sometimes patients can remind therapists of significant others, such as siblings, parents, spouses, or employers. However, when therapists react to patients based on unconscious associations to others, they can misperceive patient needs and respond inappropriately. For example, unconscious reactions to patients can cause therapists to become overprotective or, at the other extreme, become frustrated with patients without recognizing that their own reactions have more to do with other relationships than with the patient at hand.

Generally, when therapists feel a heightened sense of emotion in response to a particular patient, it may often serve as a cue that such emotions stem from unconscious associations to others. When this occurs, it is important for therapists to step back and evaluate their own feelings to discern the connection between their reactions to the patient and how the patient may be triggering unconscious emotions.

The converse is also true; patients will respond to therapists based on their own unconscious associations with significant others who have similar personality characteristics to those of the therapist. Therapists must be aware of this normal phenomenon and refrain from responding emotionally to the patient's unconscious associations. Rather, the therapist should continue to build a respectful relationship with the patient that, in time, will demonstrate to the patient that his or her first impressions were misperceptions.

SUMMARY

It is important for physical therapists to identify and understand the individual psychosocial factors that enhance or inhibit the rehabilitation of their patients and intervene accordingly. Successful intervention depends on the following:

- Understanding the psychosocial aspects of each patient, including personality styles and coping skills
- Recognizing and interpreting the common defense mechanisms that patients use in rehabilitation
- Distinguishing the stages of psychosocial adaptation to disability and helping patients' progress in their own adjustment
- Understanding how to identify anxiety, depression, and substance abuse; determining how to address these problems; and recognizing when referral to other team members is warranted
- Integrating a patient/client-centered approach that emphasizes respect, empathy, and compassion
- Empowering patients and families through psychosocial education and wellness and prevention strategies
- Working together with patients to develop anticipated goals and expected outcomes congruent with their needs, values, and level of functioning
- Collaborating with patients and team members to establish and implement appropriate interventions
- Developing a team approach and providing referrals as necessary

Questions for Review

1. Identify five psychosocial factors and state how each factor may influence rehabilitation.
2. Give examples of interventions for each psychosocial factor identified in question 1.
3. Differentiate between the different mental health professionals who can treat patients with psychosocial issues by describing their roles.
4. What should therapists do to calm an agitated patient?

5. Describe an approach for managing a violent patient and how to analyze an act of violence after it has occurred.
6. What are the manifestations of hypersexuality and how should it be addressed?
7. Identify and describe the phases of psychosocial adaptation to disability.
8. Discuss three coping strategies that have been found to be effective in the psychosocial adaptation to chronic disability and illness.
9. Describe five common defense mechanisms that patients use in response to disability.
10. What are the signs and symptoms of post-traumatic stress disorder?
11. Differentiate between typical reactions to grieving and pathological reactions.
12. Explain several ways to optimize patient involvement in the rehabilitation process and promote self-reliance.
13. Why is patient/client-centered intervention important? What strategies can be used to achieve this type of interaction?
14. Describe the general adaptation syndrome.

CASE STUDY

The patient is a 68-year-old female, admitted to an inpatient unit 2 days after sustaining a right femoral neck fracture from falling down her basement stairs. Hip replacement surgery (arthroplasty) was performed on the same day as the fall. The referring documentation indicates "weight-bearing as tolerated." The patient complains that she "can't do anything" for herself owing to the fall.

Before her fall, she was in fair health but was experiencing declining eyesight, poor short-term memory, and osteoporosis. Her hip fracture has placed her at high risk for further deconditioning and loss of function. The patient's husband had suffered a prolonged illness; the patient cared for him during the past 5 years until he passed away. She has a son whom she rarely sees, because he is married with children and living in another part of the country. A close friend lives several miles from her and the rest of her friends have died. The patient is embarrassed to be seen in public in a wheelchair.

Given the deaths of her husband and friends, and given her recent accident, the patient is now very anxious about her own mortality for the first time in her life. She is preoccupied with her husband's death since he was so much a part of her life. She feels that she has no future and nothing to look forward to. She no longer knows who she is and longs to "be reunited with" her husband.

GUIDING QUESTIONS

1. Identify the psychosocial factors apparent in this case study.
2. What relevant questions about the patient remain unanswered (i.e., what relevant information is missing)?
3. How might the patient's emotional condition affect rehabilitation?
4. Develop a problem list for the patient.
5. Identify the patient's assets.
6. Identify the general goals of physical therapy intervention on which specific anticipated goals and expected outcomes will be based.
7. Identify the general categories of procedural interventions appropriate for this patient.
8. Identify referrals to other professionals or resources.

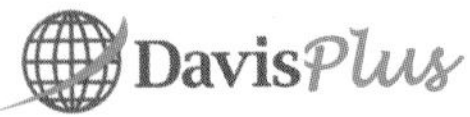

For additional resources, including answers to the questions for review and case study guiding questions, please visit **http://davisplus.fadavis.com.**

References

1. Webster's New World Dictionary of American English, ed 2. Prentice-Hall, Upper Saddle River, NJ, 1988.
2. Vaillant, GE: Adaptation to Life. Little, Brown, Boston, 1977.
3. Wickramasekera, I, et al: Applied psychophysiology: A bridge between the biomedical model and the biopsychosocial model in family medicine. Prof Psychol Res Pr 27:221, 1996.
4. Edwards, A, and Elwyn, G: Shared decision-making in health care: Achieving evidence-based patient choice. In Edwards, A, and Elwyn, G (eds): Shared Decision-Making in Health Care: Achieving Evidence-Based Patient Choice, ed 2. Oxford University Press, Oxford, UK, 2009, p 3.
5. Siegel, B: Love, Medicine and Miracles. HarperCollins, New York, 1988.
6. Doskoch, P: Happy ever laughter. Psychol Today 29:32, 1996.
7. Precin, P: Issues in Psychoanalysis: Cyberanalysis, fMRI, Psychopharmacology, Dissociative Identity Disorder, and Case Publications. Lambert Academic Publishing, Saarbrücken, Germany, 2016.
8. Precin, P: Relationship Between Mentalization and Psychosomatic Illness: A Psychoanalytic Quantitative Research Investigation. Lambert Academic Publishing, Saarbrücken, Germany, 2016.
9. Watts, R: Trauma counseling and rehabilitation. J Appl Rehab Counseling 28:8, 1997.
10. Gleckman, AD, and Brill, S: The impact of brain injury on family functioning: Implications for subacute rehabilitation programs. Brain Inj 9:385, 1995.
11. American Psychiatric Association: Diagnostic and Statistical Manual of Mental Disorders, ed 4. Text Revision. American Psychiatric Association, Washington, DC, 1994.
12. Moore, D, and Li, L: Substance abuse among applicants for vocational rehabilitation services. J Rehabil 60:48, 1994.
13. Friedland, J, and McColl, M: Disability and depression: Some etiological considerations. Soc Sci Med 34:395, 1992.
14. Turner, RJ, and Beiser, M: Major depression and depressive symptomatology among the physically disabled: Assessing the role of chronic stress. J Nerv Ment Dis 178:343, 1990.
15. Penninx, BWJH, et al: Vitamin B_{12} deficiency and depression in physically disabled older women: Epidemiologic evidence from the Women's Health and Aging Study. Am J Psychiatry 157:715, 2000.
16. Paolucci, S, et al: Post stroke depression and its role in rehabilitation of inpatients. Arch Phys Med Rehabil 80:985, 1999.
17. Kreuter, M, et al: Partner relationships, functioning, mood, and global quality of life in persons with spinal cord injury and traumatic brain injury. Spinal Cord 36:252, 1999.
18. Meara, J, et al: Use of the GDS—Geriatric Depression Scale as a screening instrument for depressive symptomatology in patients with Parkinson's disease and their careers in the community. Age Ageing 28:35, 1999.
19. Denollet, J: Personality and coronary heart disease: The type-D scale-16. Ann Behav Med 20(3):209, 1998.
20. Nemeroff, CB: The neurobiology of depression. Sci Am, p 42, June 1998.
21. Heinemann, A, et al: Substance abuse by persons with recent spinal cord injuries. Rehabil Psychol 35:217, 1990.
22. Zegans, J: The embodied self: Integration in health and illness. Adv J Inst Advance Health 7(3):29, 1991.
23. Benson, H: The Relaxation Response. HarperCollins, New York, 1974.
24. Livneh, H, and Antonak, RF: Psychosocial Adaptation to Chronic Illness and Disability. Aspen, Gaithersburg, MD, 1997.
25. Keany, KC, and Glueckauf, RL: Disability and value changes: An overview and analysis of acceptance of loss theory. Rehabil Psychol 38:199, 1993.
26. Jacobson, AM, et al: Adherence among children and adolescents with insulin-dependent diabetes mellitus over a four-year longitudinal follow-up: I. The influence of patient coping and adjustment. J Pediatr Psychol 15:511, 1990.
27. Grzesiak, RC, and Hicok, DA: A brief history of psychotherapy and physical disability. Am J Psychother 48:240, 1994.
28. Donatelle, RJ, and Davis, LG: Access to Health, ed 6. Allyn & Bacon, Needham Heights, MA, 2000.
29. Strobe, W, and Strobe, MS: Bereavement and Health: The Psychological and Physical Consequences of Partner Loss (The Psychology of Social Issues). Cambridge University Press, New York, 1987.
30. Burke, ML, et al: Current knowledge and research on chronic sorrow: A foundation for inquiry. Death Stud 16:231, 1992.
31. Lindgren, CL, et al: Chronic sorrow: A lifespan concept. Sch Inq Nurs Pract 6:27, 1992.
32. Selye, H: The general adaptation syndrome and the disease of adaptation. J Clin Endocrinol Metab 6:117, 1946.
33. Heinrichs, SC, et al: Anti-stress action of a corticotropin-releasing factor antagonist on behavioral reactivity to stressors of varying type and intensity. Neuropsychopharmacology 11:179, 1994.
34. Theorell, T, et al: "Person Under Train" incidents: Medical consequences for subway drivers. Psychosom Med 54:480, 1992.
35. Precin, P. Client-Centered Reasoning: Narratives of People with Mental Illness. Echo Point Books and Media, LLC, Brattleboro, Vermont, 2015.
36. Breznitz, S: The seven kinds of denial. In Breznitz (ed): The Denial of Stress. International Universities Press, New York, 1983, p 257.
37. Taylor, SE, and Aspinwell, LG: Psychosocial aspects of chronic illness. In Costa, PT, and VandenBox, GR (eds): Psychological Aspects of Serious Illness: Chronic Conditions, Fatal Diseases, and Clinical Care. American Psychological Association, Washington, DC, 1990, p 7.
38. Rodin, G, et al: Depression in the Medically Ill: An Integrated Approach. Brunner/Mazel, New York, 1991.
39. Levin, HS, and Grossman, RG: Behavioral sequelae of closed head injury. Arch Neurol-Chicago 35:720, 1978.
40. Brooks, N: Behavioral abnormalities in head injured patients. Scand J Rehabil Med Suppl 17:41, 1988.
41. Precin, P: The use of visual imagery to enhance sequencing of work tasks in an individual with Asperger's syndrome. WORK 36(4):373, 2010.
42. Precin, P: (editor) Post traumatic stress disorder and work. WORK 38(1), 2011.
43. Precin, P., Otto, M., Popalzai, K., & Samuel, M: Travel training for individuals diagnosed with Autistic Spectrum Disorder. OTMH, 28(2):129, 2012.
44. Mairs, N: Waist High in the World. Beacon Press, Boston, 1996.
45. Hermann, M, and Wallesch, CW: Depressive changes in stroke patients. Disabil Rehabil 15:55, 1993.
46. Davidhizer, R: Disability does not have to be the grief that never ends: Helping patients adjust. Rehabil Nurs 22(1):32, 1997.
47. Kabat-Zinn, J: Full Catastrophe Living: The Wisdom of Your Body and Mind to Face Stress, Pain, and Illness. Delacorte, New York, 1990.
48. Precin, P: *Client-Centered Reasoning: Narratives of People with Mental Illness.* Echo Point Books and Media, LLC, Brattleboro, VT, 2015.
49. Trieshman, RB: Spinal Cord Injuries: Psychological, Social and Vocational Rehabilitation, ed 2. Demos, New York, 1988.
50. Biordi, DL: Body image. In Larsen, PD, and Lubkin, IM (eds): Chronic Illness: Impact and Intervention, ed 7. Jones & Bartlett, Boston, 2009, p 117.
51. Frank, RG, Rosenthal, M, and Caplan, B (eds): Handbook of Rehabilitation Psychology, ed 2. American Psychological Association, Washington, DC, 2009.
52. Freidman, HS, and Booth-Kewley, S: The "disease-prone personality:" A meta-analytic view of the construct. Am Psychol 42:539, 1987.
53. Glanz, K, and Schwartz, MD: Stress, coping, and health behavior. In Glanz, K, Rimer, BK, and Viswanath, K (eds): Health Behavior and Health Education: Theory, Research, and Practice, ed 4. Jossey-Bass, San Francisco, 2008, p 211.
54. McCraty, R, and Tomasino, D: Emotional stress, positive emotions, and coherence. In Arnetz, BB, Ekman, R, and Carlsson, A (eds): Stress in Health and Disease. Wiley-VCH, Weinheim, Germany, 2006, p 342.
55. Stone, AA, and Porter, MA: Psychological coping: Its importance for treating medical problems. Mind/Body Med 1(1):46, 1995.
56. Tate, D, et al: Coping with the late effects—differences between depressed and nondepressed polio survivors. Am J Phys Med Rehabil 73:27, 1994.
57. Krause, JS, and Rohe, DE: Personality and life adjustment after spinal cord injury: An exploratory study. Rehabil Psychol 43:118, 1998.

58. Radomski, M: Assessing context: Personal, social, and cultural. In Trombly, CA, and Radomski, M (eds): Occupational Therapy for Physical Dysfunction, ed 5. Lippincott Williams & Wilkins, Baltimore, 2002, p 213.
59. Mpofu, SS: Take Control of Your Health: Master of Your Destiny, Book 1. Author House, Bloomington, IN, 2011.
60. Jorgenson, J: Therapeutic use of companion animals in health care. Image J Nurs Sch 29(3):249,1997.
61. Webster, G, et al: Relationship and family breakdown following acquired brain injury: The role of the rehabilitation team. Brain Inj 13:593, 1999.
62. Steinhauer, PD: Developing resilience in children from disadvantaged populations. In National Forum on Health Secretariat (eds): Canada Health Action—Building the Legacy. Vol. 1. Determinants of Health: Children and Youth. Éditions MultiMondes, Sainte-Foy, Québec, Canada, 1997, p 51.
63. Precin, P: The interactive role of emotional intelligence, attachment style, and resilience in the prediction of time perception in doctoral students. Psych Res 6(3):110-209, 2016.
64. King, G, et al: Turning points and protective processes in the lives of people with chronic disabilities. Qual Health Res 13(2):184, 2003.
65. Gorman, LM, et al: Psychosocial Nursing Handbook for the Nonpsychiatric Nurse. Williams & Wilkins, Baltimore, 1989, p 51.
66. Holmes, T, and Rahe, R: The Social Readjustment Scale. J Psychosom Res 11:213, 1967.
67. Kanner, AD, et al: Comparison of two modes of stress management: Daily hassles and uplifts versus major life events. J Behav Med 4:1, 1981.
68. Tusek, D: Guided imagery: A powerful tool to decrease length of stay, pain, anxiety, and narcotic consumption. J Invas Cardiol 11:265, 1999.
69. Tiernan, P: Independent nursing interventions: Relaxation and guided imagery in critical care. Crit Care Nurse 14(5):47, 1994.
70. Early, MB: Mental Health Concepts and Techniques for the Occupational Therapy Assistant, ed 3. Lippincott Williams & Wilkins, Baltimore, 2000.
71. Walker, LG, and Eremin, O: Psychoneuroimmunology: New fad or the fifth cancer treatment modality? Am J Surg 170:2, 1995.
72. Tusek, D, et al: Effect of guided imagery and length of stay, pain and anxiety in cardiac surgery patients. J Cardiovasc Manage 10:22, 1999.
73. Scheufele, PM: Effects of progressive relaxation and classical music on measurements of attention, relaxation, and stress responses. J Behav Med 23(2):207, 2000.
74. Benson, H, et al: Decreased blood pressure in pharmacologically treated hypertensive patients who regularly elicited the relaxation response. Lancet 1(7852):289, 1974.
75. Rossman, ML: Guided Imagery for Self-Healing: An Essential Resource for Anyone Seeking Wellness. New World Library, Novato, CA, 2000.
76. Dossey, BM: Holistic modalities and healing moments. Am J Nurs 98(6):44, 1998.
77. Eisenman, A, and Cohen, B: Music therapy for patients undergoing regional anesthesia. AORN J 62:947, 1991.
78. White, J: Music therapy: An intervention to reduce anxiety in the myocardial infarction patient. Clin Nurs Specialist 6:58, 1992.
79. Burns, D: The Feeling Good Handbook. Plume, New York, 1999.
80. Blackburn, IM, and Moorhead, S: Update in cognitive therapy for depression. J Cogn Psychother 14(3):305, 2000.
81. Butler, AC, et al: The empirical status of cognitive-behavioral therapy: A review of meta-analyses. Clin Psychol Rev 26(1):17, 2006.
82. Lam, RW, and Sidney, HK: Evidence-based strategies for achieving and sustaining full remission in depression: Focus on meta-analyses. Can J Psychiatry 49:17S, 2004.
83. Leichsenring, F, Rabung, S, and Leibing, E: The efficacy of short-term psychodynamic psychotherapy in specific psychiatric disorders: A meta-analysis. Arch Gen Psychiatry 61(12):1208, 2004.
84. Pampallona, S, et al: Combined pharmacotherapy and psychological treatment for depression: A systematic review. Arch Gen Psychiatry 61(7):714, 2004.
85. Precin, P (editor): Surviving 9/11: Impact and Experiences of Occupational Therapy Practitioners. OTMH 19(3/4): 2003. Simultaneously published in hard and soft cover books by Haworth Press, Inc., Binghamton, NY, 2003.
86. Precin, P (editor): Healing 9/11: Creative Programming by Occupational Therapists. OTMH, 21(3/4): 2006. Simultaneously published in hard and soft cover books by Haworth Press, Inc., Binghamton, NY, 2006.
87. Mayou, RA, and Smith, KA: Posttraumatic symptoms following medical illness and treatment. J Psychosom Res 43:121, 1997.
88. Bryant, RA, and Harvey, AG: Avoidant coping style and PTS following motor vehicle accidents. Behav Res Ther 33:631, 1995.
89. Herman, JL: Trauma and Recovery. Basic Books, New York, 1997.
90. Barlow, DH: Unraveling the mysteries of anxiety and its disorders from the perspective of emotion theory. Am Psychol 55:1247, 2000.
91. Keane, TM, and Barlow, DH: Posttraumatic stress disorder. In Barlow, DH (ed): Anxiety and Its Disorders, ed 2. Guilford Press, New York, 2002, p 418.
92. Geisser, ME, et al: The relationship between symptoms of post-traumatic stress disorder and pain, affective disturbance and disability among patients with accident and non-accident related pain. Pain 66:207, 1996.
93. Kerns, RD, et al: West Haven–Yale multidimensional pain inventory (WHYMPI). Pain 23:345, 1985.
94. Melzack, R: McGill Pain Questionnaire: Major properties and scoring methods. Pain 1:277, 1975.
95. Blake, DD, et al: A clinician rating scale for assessing current and lifetime PTSD: The CAPS-1. Behav Ther 13:187, 1990.
96. Weathers, FW, et al: The PTSD Checklist (PCL): Reliability, validity, and diagnostic utility. Annual Meeting of the International Society for Traumatic Stress Studies, San Antonio, TX, 1993.
97. Otis, JD, et al: An examination of the relationship between chronic pain and post-traumatic stress disorder. J Rehabil Res Dev 40(5):397, 2003.
98. Boekamp, JR, et al: Depression following a spinal cord injury. Int J Psychiatr Med 26(3):329, 1996.
99. U.S. Department of Health and Human Services: Healthy People 2020. Understanding and Improving Health, ed 3. US Government Printing Office, Washington, DC, 2010.
100. Hughes, RB, et al: Characteristics of depressed and nondepressed women with physical disabilities. Arch Phys Med Rehabil 86(3): 473, 2005.
101. Hughes, RB, et al: Depression and women with spinal cord injury. Top Spinal Cord Inj Rehabil 7(1):16, 2001.
102. McGrath, E, et al: Women and Depression: Risk Factors and Treatment Issues: Final Report of the American Psychological Association's National Task Force on Women and Depression. American Psychological Association, Washington, DC, 1990.
103. Warren, LW, and McEachren, L: Psychosocial correlates of depressive symptomatology in adult women. J Abnormal Psychol 92:151, 1983.
104. Neville, A: The model of human occupation and depressions. Am Occup Ther Assoc Mental Health Special Interest Section Newslett 8(1):1, 1985.
105. Seligman, ME: Helplessness: On Depression, Development and Death. Freeman, San Francisco, 1975.
106. Heinemann, AW: Substance Abuse and Physical Disability. Haworth, New York, 1993.
107. McFarlane, et al: Abuse Assessment Screen–Disability (AAS-D): Measuring frequency, type, and perpetrator of abuse toward women with physical disabilities. J Womens Health Gend Based Med 10:861, 2001.
108. Nosek, MA, et al: National study of women with physical disabilities: Final report. Sex Disabil 19(1):5, 2001.
109. Nosek, MA, et al: Vulnerabilities for abuse among women with disabilities. Sex Disabil 19:177, 2001.
110. Jacobs, K, and Jacobs, L: Quick reference dictionary for occupational therapy. Slack, Thorofare, NJ, 2001.
111. Nosek, MA, and Hughes, RB: Psychosocial issues of women with physical disabilities: The continuing gender debate. RCB 46(4):224, 2003.

112. Rintala, DH, et al: Perceived stress in individuals with spinal cord injury. In Krotoski, DM, Mosek, MA, and Turk, MA (eds): Women with Physical Disabilities: Achieving and Maintaining Health and Well-being. Brookes, Baltimore, 1996, p 223.
113. Rintala, DH, et al: Social support and the well-being of persons with spinal cord injury living in the community. Rehabil Psychol 37:155, 1992.
114. Hardy, C, et al: The role of social support in the life stress/injury relationship. Sport Psychol 5:128, 1991.
115. Kaplan, SP: Psychosocial adjustment three years after traumatic brain injury. Clin Neuropsychol 5:360, 1991.
116. Precin, P: Past negative time perspective as a predictor of grade point average in occupational therapy doctoral students. OJOT, 5(2):Art. 10, 2017.
117. Loy, DP, et al: Dimensions of leisure and depression symptoms after spinal cord injury. Annu Ther Recreat 11:43, 106, 2002.
118. American Physical Therapy Association: Guide to Physical Therapist Practice, ed 3. APTA, Alexandria, VA, 2014. Retrieved November 1, 2016, from http://guidetoptpractice.apta.org/.
119. World Health Organization (WHO): Towards a Common Language for Functioning, Disability and Health ICF. WHO, Geneva, Switzerland, 2002. Retrieved November 1, 2016, from www.who.int/classifications/icf/training/icfbeginnersguide.pdf.
120. Precin P: Evaluating Occupational Therapy Services. In McCormack, G, and Jacobs, K (eds.): Occupational Therapy Manager. American Occupational Therapy Association Press, 2011, p. 407-421.
121. Precin P: Evaluating occupational therapy services: Continuing quality improvement. In the American Occupational Therapy Association: AOTA CEonCD(tm): OT manager topics [DVD]. American Occupational Therapy Association Press, 2011.
122. Harrison TS, and Precin, P: Cognitive impairments in clients with dual diagnosis (chronic psychotic disorders and substance abuse): Considerations for treatment. OTI 3(2):122, 1996.

Supplemental Readings

American Psychiatric Association: DSM 5. APA, 2013.
Boersma, K, and Linton, SJ: Screening to identify patients at risk: Profiles of psychological risk factors for early intervention. Clin J Pain 21(1):38, 2005.
Bonder, B: Psychopathology and Function, ed 4. Slack, Thorofare, NJ, 2010.
Brenes, GA, et al: The influence of anxiety on the progression of disability. J Am Geriatr Soc 53(1):34, 2005.
Brown, C, and Stoffel, VC: Occupational Therapy in Mental Health: A Vision for Participation. FA Davis, Philadelphia, 2011.
Drench, ED, et al: Psychosocial Aspects of Health Care, ed 3. Prentice Hall (Pearson Education, Inc.), Upper Saddle River, NJ, 2011.
Elfstrom, M, et al: Relations between coping strategies and health-related quality of life in patients with spinal cord lesion. J Rehabil Med 37(1):9, 2005.
Falvo, D: Medical and Psychosocial Aspects of Chronic Illness and Disability, ed 3. Jones & Bartlett, Sudbury, MA, 2005.
Hughes, RB, et al: Stress and women with physical disabilities: Identifying correlates. Women Health Issue 15(1):14, 2005.
Kolt, GS, and Anderson, MB (eds): Psychology in the Physical and Manual Therapies. Churchill Livingstone, New York, 2004.
Miller, JF: Coping with Chronic Illness: Overcoming Powerlessness, ed 3. FA Davis, Philadelphia, 2000.
Moldover, JE, et al: Depression after traumatic brain injury: A review of evidence for clinical heterogeneity. Neuropsychol Rev 14(3):143, 2004.
Precin, P: Client-Centered Reasoning: Narratives of People with Mental Illness. Lambert Academic Publishing, Saarbrücken, Germany, 2015.
Precin, P (ed): Healing 9/11. Haworth Press, Binghamton, NY, 2006.
Precin, P: Living Skills Recovery Workbook. Lambert Academic Publishing, Saarbrücken, Germany, 2015.
Precin, P (ed): Posttraumatic stress disorder and work. WORK 38(1), 2011.
Precin, P (ed): Surviving 9/11. Haworth Press, Binghamton, NY, 2003.
Rytsala, HJ, et al: Functional and work disability in major depressive disorder. J Nerv Ment Dis Mar 193(3):189, 2005.
Solet, JM: Optimizing personal and social adaptation. In Trombly, CA, and Vining Radomski, M (eds): Occupational Therapy for Physical Dysfunction, ed 5. Lippincott Williams & Wilkins, Baltimore, 2002, p 761.
Yerxa, EJ: The social and psychological experience of having a disability: Implications for occupational therapists. In Pedretti, LW, and Early, MB (eds): Occupational Therapy: Practice Skills for Physical Dysfunction, ed 5. Mosby, St. Louis, 2001, p 470.

appendix

26.A Web-Based Resources for Patients, Families, and Caregivers

■ IMPROVING COMMUNITY ACCESSIBILITY

Independent Living Centers:
www.senioroutlook.com
Searches more than 40,000 apartment communities for people with disabilities. Includes virtual tours, searches by distance, photographs, and floor plans. Contains information on insurance, storage, home mortgages, moving, and types of housing facilities and a glossary of housing terms. Updated weekly.

Links to Centers for Independent Living:
www.abledata.com
Includes information on and links to periodicals and research on disability, assistive technology, and lists of health care professionals.

The Design Link:
www.designlinc.com/centers3.htm
Provides product information and design tips for families, consumers, and therapists designing for people with disabilities.

■ DEPRESSION RESOURCES

*Web*MD Depression Guide:
www.webmd.com/depression/guide/depression_support_resources
All About Depression:
www.allaboutdepression.com
Internet Mental Health:
www.mentalhealth.com/p71.html

■ SUBSTANCE ABUSE RESOURCES

National Institutes of Health, National Institute on Drug Abuse, Science of Drug Abuse Addiction:
www.nida.nih.gov/nidahome.html
The Substance Abuse and Mental Health Services Administration:
www.samhsa.gov
National Substance Abuse Index—Directory of Substance Abuse Resources:
www.nationalsubstanceabuseindex.org

■ ANXIETY RESOURCES

HealthCentralAnxietyConnection.com:
www.healthcentral.com/anxiety/websites.html
MedlinePlus—Anxiety:
www.nlm.nih.gov/medlineplus/anxiety.html

■ POST-TRAUMATIC STRESS DISORDER (PTSD) RESOURCES

Third of a Lifetime curated PTSD resources by Sarah E. Olson:
http://thirdofalifetime.com/
Department of Defense—Resources for Military Vets with Posttraumatic Stress Disorder:
United States Department of Veterans Affairs
Veterans and Military—Web Resource Links:
www.ptsd.va.gov/public/web-resources/web-military-resources.asp
National Center for Posttraumatic Stress Disorder:
www.ptsd.va.gov/

Cognitive and Perceptual Dysfunction

Carolyn A. Unsworth, OTR, PhD

Chapter 27

LEARNING OBJECTIVES

1. Identify the signs of cognitive and perceptual deficits.
2. Describe how cognitive and perceptual deficits affect a patient's ability to participate in rehabilitation.
3. Explain how a patient can be assisted to compensate for body scheme and/or body image disorders.
4. Describe how spatial relations impairments can affect the patient's ability to follow directions.
5. Compare and contrast the effect of the various agnosias on the patient's ability to recognize stimuli in the environment.
6. Differentiate between ideomotor and ideational apraxia. Describe how a patient with apraxia might behave in response to different instructional sets commonly employed in rehabilitation.
7. Identify how the psychological and emotional status of a patient with cognitive and perceptual deficits may affect participation in rehabilitation.
8. Analyze and interpret patient data, formulate realistic anticipated goals and expected outcomes, and identify appropriate interventions when presented with a clinical case study.

CHAPTER OUTLINE

Cognitive and perceptual deficits are among the chief causes of poor rehabilitation progress for patients who have sustained brain damage, even among those whose motor skills have returned. Cognitive and perceptual deficits are some of the most puzzling and disabling difficulties that a person can experience. Thinking, remembering, reasoning, and making sense of the world around us is fundamental to carrying out daily living activities. When individuals experience problems with these capacities, it can have a devastating effect on their lives and the lives of their families. These people may not be able to live alone, fulfill the responsibilities of paid employment, or sustain a family life and relationships.[1] Thus, effective treatment of many patients with brain damage depends on understanding perception and cognition.

The brain may be damaged through several mechanisms, including infections such as encephalitis; anoxia, as may occur following near-drowning, cardiopulmonary arrest, or carbon monoxide poisoning; tumors that are benign or malignant; trauma resulting from motor vehicle accidents, falls, or violent incidents (e.g., traumatic sports-related injury, gunshot wound); toxins such as alcohol or substance abuse; and vascular disease, which may produce an infarct or hemorrhagic stroke. The largest two groups of people who acquire cognitive and perceptual impairments following brain damage are persons who experienced stroke and traumatic brain injury (TBI).[1] The physical rehabilitation of these patient groups is addressed in Chapter 15, Stroke, and Chapter 19, Traumatic Brain Injury.

The patient who has sustained an initial cerebral vascular accident (CVA) is thought to have focal or localized damage to discrete areas of the brain, often resulting in discrete cognitive or perceptual deficits. In contrast, patients who have sustained a TBI are presumed to have generalized brain damage resulting in cognitive impairment with generalized deficits in attention, memory, learning, and so forth, rather than specific difficulties in discrete cognitive or perceptual functions. However, elements of both perceptual and cognitive dysfunction may occur in brain damage owing to either CVA or trauma. The distinctions between the two groups of patients become particularly blurred when one considers the patient who has suffered multiple strokes; this patient may in fact present with combined elements of both focal and generalized brain damage. This chapter focuses on the patient with hemiplegia whose brain damage has occurred as a result of a stroke. The overriding goal of this chapter is to introduce the reader to concepts relating to cognitive and perceptual dysfunction following brain damage.

An important focus for the physical therapist should be understanding how a particular cognitive or perceptual impairment might be manifested clinically and how examination and treatment of movement disorders might be adjusted to capitalize on the abilities and minimize the cognitive or perceptual limitations of the patient. Deficits in the cognitive or perceptual domain must be considered to accurately determine the patient's true residual abilities. Using sets of directions that would confuse a patient with apraxia during a specific examination procedure may paint a picture of a greater or different motor disability than that which actually exists. Often the first clue to a cognitive or perceptual problem appears during initial sensorimotor testing. Awareness of the possibility and nature of cognitive or perceptual deficits will signal the therapist to redirect the method of testing, particularly the instructional sets and cues.

■ COGNITION AND PERCEPTION

The perceptual–motor process is a chain of events through which the individual selects, integrates, and interprets stimuli from the body and the surrounding environment. Cognition can be conceived of as the method used by the central nervous system (CNS) to process information. Cognitive processes include knowing, understanding, awareness, judgment, and decision making.[2] The difficulty of separating perceptual and cognitive deficits is readily apparent, both in patient behavior and in contradictory conceptualizations of these two domains of function. In a review of the literature, Katz[3] found that to some authors, *cognition* is conceived of as a general term that includes perception, attention, thinking, and memory; to other authors, *perception* is an umbrella term that encompasses both cognition and visual perception as subcomponents. At this time, there is insufficient evidence to suggest which approach most accurately reflects the way we think about and perceive information. What is clear is that normally functioning perceptual and cognitive systems are a necessary key to successful interaction with the environment. Because the majority of work in this field does distinguish between cognition and perception[1] and because it is probably easier to learn about these processes individually, they are defined and addressed separately in this chapter.

Cognitive and perceptual capacities are clearly prerequisites for learning,[4] and rehabilitation is largely a learning process.[2] Thus, it is not surprising that patients with cognitive and perceptual disorders are limited in their ability to learn self-care and activities of daily living (ADL) skills; hence, as a group, they are more restricted in their potential to fully participate in family, work, and other societal roles.[5] In any rehabilitation program geared toward achievement of maximum independence, there is a compelling need for therapists to learn to recognize behavior related to perceptual deficits. The therapist's modification of examination and treatment approaches in light of these deficits will ensure that patients receive the full benefit of these services.

Cognition and Higher-Order Cognition

Cognition is the act or process of knowing, including awareness, reasoning, judgment, intuition, and memory. *Executive functions* are sometimes included under this heading as well. These include the capacity to plan, manipulate information, initiate and terminate activities, recognize errors, solve problems, and think abstractly. Commonly, executive functions are categorized as *higher-order cognitive functions*[6] or *metacognitive functions*.[7,8]

Perception

Lezak[4] defines *perception* as the integration of sensory impressions into information that is psychologically meaningful. Thus, perception is the ability to select those stimuli that require attention and action, to integrate those stimuli with each other and with prior information, and finally to interpret them. The resulting awareness of objects and experiences within the environment enables the individual to make sense out of a complex and constantly changing internal and external sensory environment.[9]

The terms *perception* and *sensation* are often confused with each other. Sensation may be defined as the appreciation (awareness) of stimuli through the organs of special sense (e.g., eyes, ears, nose, and so forth), the peripheral cutaneous sensory system (e.g., temperature, taste, touch, and so forth), or internal receptors (e.g., deep receptors in muscles and joints).[9] Perception cannot be viewed as independent of sensation. However, the quality of perception is far more complex than the recognition of the individual sensation.[9] Perceptual deficits do not lie in the sensory ability itself, but rather with the individual's ability to interpret the sensation accurately, and therefore respond appropriately.[1]

RESPONSIBILITIES OF THE PHYSICAL THERAPIST AND THE OCCUPATIONAL THERAPIST

Occupational therapists are the members of the rehabilitation team who are specially trained to examine and treat cognitive and perceptual deficits in relation to functional adaptation. They are responsible for the selection and administration of an appropriate constellation of tests and measures, accurate interpretation of results, and formulation of an overall plan of care (POC) for cognitive and perceptual rehabilitation. If appropriate, the occupational therapist may refer a patient to a neuropsychologist for specific intellectual testing.

In the hospital setting, the physical therapist is often the first member of the rehabilitation team to see a patient with brain injury. The physical therapist must understand the nature of cognitive and perceptual dysfunction and recognize that individuals in certain diagnostic categories, such as those with stroke or TBI, are likely to behave in ways that indicate the presence of particular cognitive or perceptual deficits.[10] When this occurs, the physical therapist should refer the patient to occupational therapy for evaluation and treatment.

The tests and measures described in this chapter are included to assist the reader in understanding the nature of the different cognitive and perceptual disabilities and to guide decision making about referral to another practitioner. They are not a substitute for an intensive evaluation by a trained occupational therapist when referral is deemed necessary.

An understanding of cognitive and perceptual dysfunction may go a long way toward alleviating much of the potential frustration that often accompanies treatment of a patient with brain damage, most of which is the result of inappropriate expectations on the part of team members, the patient, and the family. By collaborating with the occupational therapist, other members of the rehabilitation team, and the family, consistent treatment strategies may be developed and carried out, with obvious benefits to the patient.

CLINICAL INDICATORS

Cognitive and perceptual deficits ought to be ruled out as a cause of diminished functioning in all patients who have experienced brain damage. Such problems are particularly likely culprits in cases in which the patient seems unable to participate fully in self-care tasks and has difficulty participating in physical therapy for reasons that cannot be accounted for by lack of motor ability, sensation, comprehension, or motivation. Cognitive and perceptual dysfunction resulting from acquired brain damage must be differentiated from premorbid cognitive perceptual deficits (from previous trauma, illness, congenital abnormality, or dementing process) and from the general confusion and emotional sequelae that often accompany stroke and brain injury.[4]

Often, patients with cognitive and perceptual difficulties may display an inability to do simple tasks independently or safely, difficulty in initiating or completing a task, difficulty in switching from one task to the next, and a diminished capacity to locate visually or to identify objects that seem obviously necessary for task completion. In addition, they may be unable to follow simple one-step commands, despite apparently good comprehension. They may make the same mistakes over and over. Activities may take an inordinately long time to complete, or they may be done impulsively. Patients may hesitate many times, appear distracted and frustrated, and exhibit poor planning. They are frequently inattentive to one side of the body and extrapersonal space, and may deny the presence or extent of their disability. These characteristics, all or some of which may be present, often make participation in daily living activities and therapy seem an insurmountable problem. These clinical features are explained and expanded on throughout this chapter.

Two typical scenarios are presented to give the reader an idea of when to suspect perceptual dysfunction. The first case involves a patient with a right hemisphere stroke who presents clinically with a left hemiparesis and good speech. Upon observation in the nursing unit, the patient appears to have functional strength in the unaffected right extremities and fair return on the affected left side. Yet the patient seems to have difficulty with simple range of motion (ROM) activities, even in the intact extremities, appearing confused and unable to move the affected arm up or down on command. The patient cannot seem to follow instructions for walking with a quad cane, constantly confuses the proper step sequence, and is unable to maneuver a wheelchair around the corner without crashing into the wall.

This patient should not be dismissed as uncooperative, intellectually inferior, or confused. In this instance, the patient is likely experiencing difficulty in spatial relations, right–left discrimination, and vertical disorientation, or perhaps left-sided unilateral neglect. Further observation and examination should reveal the precise cause of the difficulties.

The second case involves a patient with left-hemisphere damage and a resulting right hemiparesis and mild expressive and receptive aphasia. The patient can respond reliably to "yes/no" questions and is able to follow simple one-step commands such as, "Put the pencil on the table," or "Give me the cup." However, if asked to point to the arm, or asked to imitate the therapist's movements during an active ROM test even with the unaffected limbs, the patient does not respond and appears totally uncooperative. During therapy, the same patient is on a mat table. The therapist explains and then demonstrates the proper techniques for rolling to one side. The patient does not move. However, a moment later when his wife arrives, the patient quickly initiates rolling in an attempt to sit up to greet his wife. The astute therapist will realize that this patient may not be confused, stubborn, or uncooperative, as indeed he may appear. Rather, he may be suffering from a lack of awareness of body structure and relationship of body parts (somatoagnosia), as evidenced by the ROM test incident and an inability to perform a task on command or to imitate gestures (ideomotor apraxia), as demonstrated in the rolling episode.

HOSPITALIZATION FOLLOWING BRAIN DAMAGE

The brain that has been damaged functions as a whole, just as it does in individuals without brain damage. When one part is damaged, the behavior observed is not merely the result of the brain operating precisely as in the intact individual minus the function of the area that was subject to anoxia. Rather, it is an outward manifestation of the reorganization of the entire CNS, at multiple levels, working to compensate for the loss.[11]

Because of the brain damage, the patient must cope with a nervous system operating without normal sensory input at all levels, both cortical and subcortical.[11] Normal responses to environmental stimuli are difficult to obtain when the input on which they have to act is deranged or incomplete. Recovery of function can be attributed to structural reorganization of the CNS into a new dynamic system widely dispersed within the cerebral cortex and lower segments.[12,13]

A significant contributor to the clinical picture of a patient after a CVA is the response to hospitalization. From a cognitive and perceptual perspective, when a patient is hospitalized (with or without brain damage), the inputs imposed on that patient's nervous system are radically different from the ones normally received. On the one hand, the environment is sensorially impoverished. There is no variation in temperature and lighting, and familiar background noises (e.g., telephones, airplanes, dogs, buses, and so forth) are missing. On the other hand, an enormous array of unfamiliar noise is present: nurses talking, loudspeakers, and the whir of machines. Strange and different smells, and unfamiliar, unavoidable, and unpleasant sights abound. Often, because of motor impairment, the patient cannot move around to seek or to escape inputs; therefore, a multiplicity of sensory inputs bombards the nervous system. Even if orienting responses are preserved, there is a profound sense of loss of control. This sensory derangement compounds the problems faced by the patient with brain damage, because those very abilities that enable the individual to select, filter out, and integrate incoming sensations to organize the self for appropriate action often fail in this sensorially bizarre environment.

To gain insight into the experience of the patient under such circumstances, it is enlightening to browse through the biographical and autographical reports of some noted neurologists and neuropsychologists, themselves victims or relatives of victims of CVAs. Particularly instructive are the reports of Bach-y-Rita,[14] Brodal,[15] and Gardner.[16]

THEORETICAL FRAMEWORKS

The theoretical bases of five approaches to therapy are examined in this section, together with the examination procedures and treatment approaches consistent with the theoretical model. It is important to note that treatment approaches are not mutually exclusive. Many therapists use a combination of approaches, guiding selection by their clinical expertise and the patient's response to the interventions. Specific applications of these approaches will be presented following the description of individual cognitive and perceptual deficits in the final section of this chapter. Further information on a variety of theoretical approaches used by occupational therapists when working with patients who have cognitive and perceptual problems can be found in Averbuch and Katz[17] and Unsworth.[1]

The Retraining Approach

Averbuch and Katz[17] described this approach, which focuses on the remediation of underlying skills the patient has lost. Sometimes this approach is referred to as the *transfer-of-training approach*. The approach is based on the assumption that a disruption in one brain region can have a negative impact on brain functioning as a whole. An underlying assumption is that skills learned for one task can generalize to others. In other words, transfer-of-training is assumed. The premise is that practice in one task with particular cognitive or perceptual requirements will enhance performance in other tasks with similar perceptual demands.[1,18,19] Thus, doing specifically selected perceptual exercises, such as pegboard (a board with a regular pattern of small holes for pegs) activities or parquetry blocks (inlaid blocks of different woods arranged in a geometric pattern) and puzzles, will result in improving the perceptual skills required to perform those functional tasks. For example, Young et al[20] demonstrated that training patients with left hemiplegia in block design (constructing shapes using blocks to match a two-dimensional pattern), in addition to *visual scanning* (using the eyes to follow a target) and *visual cancellation tasks* (placing a line through a specific number, letter, or word embedded randomly among other numbers, letters, or words), resulted in improvements in reading and writing, although no specific training in these areas was offered. Because all tasks require the use of multiple perceptual skills, it is difficult to ascertain precisely which perceptual skills are being trained during any one session.[21]

To date, research has not unequivocally demonstrated a generalization from perceptual–motor training to functional skills.[18,21] Neistadt[19] suggests that the patient's capacity to learn must be evaluated and that learning capacity is the key to a patient's ability to generalize material learned in one situation to others. If transfer-of-training does occur, then strategies to enhance this can be incorporated into other components of the treatment program, such as those aimed at maintaining sitting or standing balance, weight-bearing exercises, or functional use of the more involved extremities.

The Sensory Integrative Approach

Ayres developed the theory of sensory integration in an effort to explain the relationship between neural functioning and the behavior of children with sensorimotor or learning problems.[22] The theory, strongly influenced by the neurobehavioral literature, describes normal sensory integrative development and functioning, defines patterns of sensory integrative dysfunction, and suggests treatment techniques.[22] *Sensory integration* can be defined as the organization of sensation for use.[23,24]

Integration of basic sensorimotor functions (tactile, proprioceptive, and vestibular) proceeds in a developmental sequence in the normal child within the context of goal-directed, meaningful activity. It is assumed that the production of an adaptive response (desired motor response) facilitates sensory integration, which in turn enhances the ability to produce higher-level adaptive behaviors. Sensory integration is thought to occur at all levels of the nervous system.

The underlying assumption for treatment is that, by offering opportunities for controlled sensory input, the therapist can promote normal CNS processing of sensory information and thus elicit specific desired motor responses.[25] The performance of these adaptive responses, in turn, influences the way in which the brain organizes and processes sensation, thus enhancing the ability to learn.

Some of the treatment modalities employed include rubbing or icing to provide sensory input, resistance and weight-bearing to impart proprioceptive input, and the use of spinning or rocking to provide vestibular input. Following the controlled sensory input, an adaptive motor response is required by the patient to integrate the sensations provided by the therapist. In young children, the use of compensatory or splinter skills (skills acquired in a manner inconsistent with, or incapable of being integrated with, those already present) is avoided in favor of remediating underlying deficits. For more detailed information, the reader is referred to the work of Ayres.[23,24]

Zoltan[2] argues that elderly patients, who comprise the majority of the stroke population, experience sensory integrative dysfunction similar to that of children with learning disabilities because of age-related physiological changes together with environmentally induced sensory deprivation. The limitations in mobility caused by a stroke further prevent the patient from receiving and thus processing adequate sensory input.

The application of this theory to the adult post-stroke population, however, is open to serious debate. Bundy et al[22] argue that the theory explains mild to moderate learning and behavioral problems resulting from a central deficit in processing sensations but are not specifically associated with frank brain damage. Further, there are several problems with the application of this approach to adult populations, even if it is theoretically tenable.

The treatment process is ordinarily quite lengthy. In addition, specific tests and measures and treatment approaches have been developed for and standardized on children, who presumably have sufficiently plastic nervous systems to be influenced by this form of therapy. The neurophysiological literature is replete with examples of skills that children can gain using this approach that would not be possible with mature individuals with similar lesions.[26-28] Furthermore, a mature adult with diffuse cerebral damage may have other complicating medical concerns and deficits in mobility that actually contraindicate the use of the equipment that is essential to the treatment process.[22] It is likely that many of the treatment regimens described as sensory integration are best described as a sensorimotor approach, which utilizes handling or directed sensory stimulation to elicit a specific motor response.[22]

The Neurofunctional Approach

The *neurofunctional approach* was first described by Giles and Wilson in 1992[29] and is based on learning theory. In contrast to the retraining approach, which assumes that transfer-of-training can occur, the authors of the neurofunctional approach assume that patients with acquired brain injury must practice every activity in its true context in order to recover function. Hence, the focus of this approach is on retraining real-world skills rather than on retraining specific cognitive and perceptual processes.[30] Giles[30] argues that remediation approaches (which include the idea of transfer-of-training) are largely unproven, and thus may result in little functional improvement for the patient. He also suggests that compensatory skills or techniques are taught to a patient without considering if the gains made in terms of quality of life justify the considerable effort required.

The Rehabilitative/Compensatory (Functional) Approach

Probably the most widely used approach in treating perceptual deficits is the *rehabilitative/compensatory approach*[31-33] (also referred to as the *functional approach*), which offers a great deal of practical support for the physical therapist. The basic assumptions underlying this approach are that adults with brain trauma will have difficulty generalizing and learning from dissimilar tasks.[34] Direct repetitive practice of specific functional skills that are impaired is an efficient means of enhancing the patient's independence in those specific tasks. More recently, Fisher[35] extended the work of Trombly[31] by (1) more explicitly articulating assumptions made about people within the rehabilitative/compensatory model; (2) generalizing this model beyond persons with physical disabilities to those with developmental, cognitive, or psychosocial disabilities; and (3) adding collaborative consultation to education and adaptation as strategies used to effect change.

The proponents of this approach favor addressing the functional problem over and above the treatment of its underlying cause when working with an adult post-stroke population. For example, a patient with difficulty in depth and distance perception, who is therefore unable to navigate a flight of stairs, would be made aware of the deficit, would be provided with external cues to compensate for the perceptual disorder, and would repetitively practice adapted techniques for safe stair climbing. The more closely the therapeutic practice situation resembles the home and community situation in terms of stair depth and height, amount of traffic, lighting, and so forth, the less generalizing is required and the more success the patient is likely to have when he or she returns home. However, problems might still be displayed in depth and distance perception in other areas of daily function.

In this functional approach, therapy is viewed as learning that takes into consideration the unique strengths and limitations of the individual patient. It is composed of two complementary components: compensation and adaptation.[1] *Compensation* refers to the changes that need to be made in the patient's approach to tasks. *Adaptation* refers to the alterations that need to be made in the human/social and physical environment in order to facilitate relearning of skills. In relation to the human/social environment, the therapist is concerned with altering the actions of others' functioning in the environment to enhance the patient's performance.

To compensate for the disability, the patient first has to be made aware of deficiencies (cognitive awareness) and must then be taught how to circumvent them using intact sensations and perceptual skills. The patient should be instructed in specific techniques and assisted in developing successful functional habits. The patient will need to be taught to attend to cues from the environment to enhance skill performance. The therapist helps the patient identify and then call on these new cues. For example, if the patient has a visual field cut, the therapist should explain that because of a visual problem, the patient is seeing only one half of the environment. The patient should then be shown how to turn the head to compensate for the deficit. Environmental scanning (moving head, and therefore eyes, from side to side to view surroundings) could be incorporated into general therapy sessions as well.

General suggestions when teaching compensatory techniques include (1) using simple directions; (2) establishing and carrying out a routine; (3) doing each activity in a consistent manner; and (4) employing repetition as much as necessary.

Adaptation refers to the alteration not of the patient's strategy, but of the environment. For example, if the patient cannot differentiate between right and left, or tends to neglect the left side of the body, a piece of red tape on the left shoe during gait training will allow the patient to attend more easily to the left side and thus to follow the therapist's instructions more accurately. The therapist can use this functional approach to assist patients in improving specific motor skills related to treatment goals.

There are several inherent benefits to the rehabilitation/compensatory (functional) approach. First, in the current managed care environment there is a limited amount of time for inpatient rehabilitation.[36] Therefore, therapists need to concentrate on outcome-directed, real-life functional activities, because independent performance of these activities at home is the ultimate goal of therapeutic intervention. Interventions directed toward specific functional outcomes are typically reimbursable.[31] In addition, the activities are age appropriate, specific, and clearly relevant to the patient's concerns. For this reason, they tend to be the most motivating. The tasks can also be incorporated into a daily hospital routine. Dressing can be reinforced at bedside by the nursing staff, and eating skills can be reinforced at each mealtime.

The major limitation of this approach is that the methods learned in one task are not typically generalized to the performance of another task. The functional approach has been criticized as the teaching of splinter skills, in which the causes of the dysfunction are not addressed.

Cognitive Rehabilitation and the Quadraphonic Approach

Cognitive rehabilitation focuses on training individuals with brain injury to structure and organize information.[37] It addresses memory, high language disorders, and perceptual dysfunction under one umbrella.[38] Information processing, problem-solving, awareness, judgment, and decision making are among the areas included. The therapist using a cognitive remediation approach might be concerned with the patient's perceptual style, including perceptual strategy, response to different types of cues, and rate and consistency of task performance.[39] Diller and Gordon[40] provide a review of the literature pertaining to intervention strategies for cognitive deficits.

Research has demonstrated that even in a non-brain-injured population, skills learned in one task do not automatically transfer to other tasks.[41] Hence, cognitive strategies can be used to facilitate the carryover of skills learned in therapy to functional activities. In her multicontext treatment approach to cognition, Toglia[41] proposes that learning can be conceptualized as a dynamic interplay between characteristics of the patient, characteristics of the task, and the environment in which it is performed. This has also been termed a *dynamic interactional approach*.[42] Characteristics of the individual patient that might affect learning include information processing strategies, metacognition (including awareness of one's own performance), and prior experience, attitudes, and emotions. Task-related variables that are proposed to affect learning include the nature of the task itself (familiarity with the task, spatial arrangements, instruction set, and movement and postural requirements) and the criteria that are used to determine the learner's abilities. Environmental variables include the social and cultural environment in which treatment occurs, as well as the physical context.

The *cognitive rehabilitation approach* to treatment proposes a number of strategies relevant to physical therapist practice. These treatment strategies include the following:[41]

- Analyzing the characteristics of the task to establish criteria to determine if transfer of learning in fact took place.
- Providing interventions to increase patient awareness of abilities, increase the level of difficulty of the task, and promote self-examination of performance.
- Relating new information or skills to previously learned ones.
- Using multiple environments in which to carry out the training activity to enhance transfer of learning.

Although these treatment strategies are well known within the field of cognitive–perceptual rehabilitation, the efficacy of the techniques remains to be established with the post-stroke population. For a comprehensive understanding and practical guidelines to the evaluation and treatment of patients with cognitive impairments from a dynamic perspective, see Toglia[42] and Abreu.[43]

Abreu[44] has further developed these treatment strategies as the *quadraphonic approach*. The quadraphonic approach is an interactive rehabilitation approach that provides a holistic perspective for the management of stroke, TBI, brain tumors, cerebral palsy, and other neurological conditions. The quadraphonic approach is based around the idea that the therapist can apply both micro (reductionistic) and a macro (holistic) perspectives for evaluation and treatment, which is an assumption shared by many occupational therapists who work in this field. Diagrammatic presentations of the components of the four key areas of the macro and four key areas of the micro perspectives (hence the term *quadraphonic*) are provided in Figures 27.1 and 27.2, respectively, and are explained in the text. The *macro* perspective is holistic or humanistic and provides guidelines for the management of functional performance and real-life occupations. In other words, this component of the quadraphonic approach is functional or top-down in focus. In Figure 27.1, the outer square is composed of four characteristics of a client (*lifestyle, life stage, health,* and *disadvantage status*) that the therapist can explore through interviews and by asking clients to tell their stories. The therapist can use this information in order to explain and predict the client's behavior and performance. An evaluation then needs to be made of the client's will (volition) and goals, as well as the opportunity and capacity for action as depicted in the triangle. From there the therapist can develop an individualized therapy plan with the client (and significant others such as family).

In contrast, the *micro* perspective is more remedial in focus and provides guidelines for the management of performance components or sub-skills that include attention, visual perception, memory, motor planning, postural control, and problem-solving. Evaluation and treatment of these performance components is based on a frame of reference that incorporates four theories: (1) information processing, (2) teaching/learning, (3) neurodevelopmental,

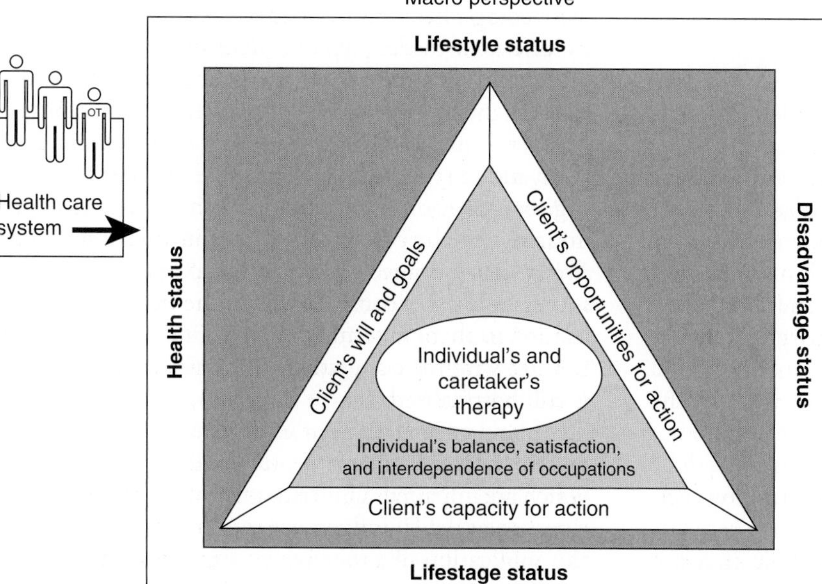

Figure 27.1 The quadraphonic approach—macro perspective. *(From Abreu,[43, p. 187] with permission.)*

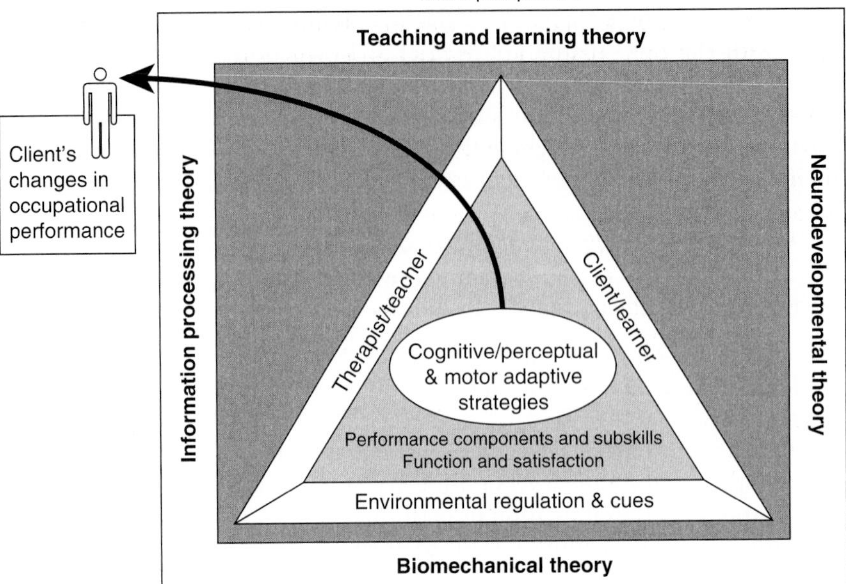

Figure 27.2 The quadraphonic approach—micro perspective. *(From Abreu,[43, p. 185] with permission.)*

and (4) biomechanical. These theories are listed in the outer square of Figure 27.2. This figure then presents an inner triangle that depicts how changes in the client's condition are further influenced by three dominant factors, which are the therapist (teacher), the environment in which therapy takes place, and what the client brings to therapy. The therapist and client work together to develop cognitive, perceptual, and motor strategies to enhance the client's performance and improve life satisfaction (as shown in the central circle of Fig. 27.1). Hence, the micro perspective is bottom-up, or remedial, in its focus. See Abreu[43] for an example of a therapist using this approach when working with a patient who has memory and learning problems.

EXAMINATION OF COGNITIVE AND PERCEPTUAL DEFICITS

The use of systematic data collection provides the scientific basis for guiding intervention. Its importance cannot be overemphasized with respect to all facets of therapeutic intervention, including remediation of cognitive and perceptual dysfunction. Task analysis is the breakdown of an activity or task into its component parts together with a delineation of the specific motor, perceptual, and cognitive abilities necessary to perform each component. Task analysis is another tool critical to appropriate therapeutic intervention. For example, the strength, ROM, and balance abilities necessary to accomplish bed mobility and ambulation activities can be clearly defined by the physical therapist. However, the specific perceptual and cognitive requirements of each step needed to perform these two tasks may not be known. Without knowledge of the perceptual and cognitive requirements for successful completion of a task, the therapist cannot simplify the task for the patient and progressively upgrade it.

Purpose of the Examination

The presence of cognitive and perceptual dysfunction must be confirmed if it is suspected to be interfering with the patient's ability to carry out functional activities.[1] Perceptual performance is positively correlated with ability to perform ADLs; however, it is often difficult to correlate specific perceptual deficits gleaned from testing with specific elements of functional ability and loss.[1,45] Thus, formal testing is indicated when there is a functional loss unexplained by motor or sensory impairments, or deficient comprehension. It should be noted that not all areas of functional loss are typically detected within the hospital setting. It is not uncommon for the patient to perform adequately in self-care skills after therapy in the hospital but to fail on the same tasks in other environmental contexts, such as the home. Higher-level tasks, such as driving, banking, or planning a meal, may only emerge as areas of difficulty once the patient is discharged home. When appropriate, the patient's competence in these areas should be considered within the context of an examination of instrumental activities of daily living (IADL) with the occupational therapist while the patient is still hospitalized.

The purpose of patient examination is to determine which cognitive and perceptual abilities are intact and which are impaired. Understanding the manner in which a particular deficit influences task performance will foster the application of a therapeutic strategy in which intact capabilities may be used to compensate for or to overcome deficits.[1]

Failure in the performance of a task may result from any number of processes underlying cognition and perception. For example, a patient's inability to complete a jigsaw puzzle may result from an inability to organize the pieces or problem-solve where they go (disorder of executive function) or difficulty in attending to one half of the picture (unilateral neglect). The patient may be incapable of concentrating on the instructions (attention deficit), unable to know what the pieces are for (ideational apraxia), or unable to manipulate them (ideomotor apraxia). Although it is often difficult to implicate reliably one or another of these problem areas, the therapist must be aware of the different deficits that may produce similar patterns of behavior.[1,5]

A fascinating study conducted by Galski et al[46] concerning the prediction of driving ability following brain injury (including stroke) in 35 patients underscores the critical nature of carefully selected perceptual and cognitive tests. In this study, 64% of actual behind-the-wheel driving performances were predicted by performance on a selected battery of neuropsychological tests that measured visual perception. Examination of individual test results uncovered the reasons for unsafe driving (such as problems with visual perception, visuomotor coordination, and visuoconstructive abilities), enabling instructors to focus on remediating these specific deficits in preparation for safe driving.

Patient examination is not an end in itself. Careful examination paves the way for realistic and cost-effective intervention.[47] Continuous monitoring of the patient's cognitive and perceptual status will ensure the use of appropriate treatment strategies and their modification when necessary.

Factors Influencing Patient Examination

Psychological and emotional status plays an important role in the patient's ability to cope with disability and with the testing situation. The therapist needs to be aware of behaviors that reflect a patient's psychological response to illness rather than particular cognitive or perceptual abilities. Psychological adjustment to disability depends on many factors, including age, vocational status, education, economic situation, attitude toward the reactions of others, family support, and feelings of competence before the onset of disease[45,48,49] (see Chapter 26, Psychosocial Issues in Physical Rehabilitation).

When examining psychological and emotional status the following should be noted: whether the patient is confused; the level of comprehension for verbal instructions (written and spoken); whether communication is enhanced through the use of visual cues and demonstration; the ability to recognize errors; the level of cooperation and initiative (whether the patient is realistic about capabilities and goals); and emotional stability.[50] Disturbances of emotional response are evidenced by rapid and frequent mood changes and low frustration tolerance. Difficult tasks may cause a catastrophic reaction.[45]

The patient's ability to detect relevant cues from the environment or to discriminate between relevant and irrelevant stimuli (necessary for cognitive and perceptual competence) may be adversely influenced by poor judgment, fatigue, and prior expectations. Poor judgment is a major contributor to accidents in patients with hemiplegia. This is related in part to the diminished awareness by these patients as to their altered capabilities. The ambiguity of having one set of functional limbs and one set that is not functional may lead the patient to rely on solutions to the problems of daily living that are familiar but now inappropriate.[45]

Anxiety over capabilities may inhibit optimal performance during examination and treatment. The patient's capacity to perform optimally on testing and to learn is enhanced if anxiety can be reduced.[45] Motivation is influenced by many factors, among them premorbid personality. It is of utmost importance for the therapist to structure the therapeutic environment so that the patient will be positively motivated to learn to his or her maximum ability.[45] To this end, therapeutic tasks should be structured to ensure success, thereby diminishing frustration.

Other factors that may limit a patient's performance on cognitive and perceptual tests include reduced receptive and expressive communication skills, depression, and fatigue. Before a formal examination, the therapist should consider the patient's language skills and confirm these observations with the speech-language pathologist. The therapist should also be aware of any medications the patient is taking and how these may affect performance. For example, many medications produce drowsiness as a side effect that would impact patient performance during testing.[1] Following stroke, 30% to 50% of people are said to experience depression,[12] the symptoms of which can easily be mistaken for cognitive or perceptual problems. Finally, a determination should be made of the patient's level of fatigue before any examination procedure.

The patient's behavior should not be misinterpreted because of a cultural bias, such as a lack of experience in taking tests. Premorbid intellectual ability should be ascertained from an interview with family or friends, because intellectual abilities may affect performance on some of the tests and measurements and may affect behavior in general. Premorbid memory should also be determined.

Finally, it is very important to conduct a sensory examination *before* cognitive or perceptual testing to establish whether the patient has sufficient sensory abilities to proceed with testing (this includes visual screening). Distinguishing between sensory and cognitive or perceptual problems is explored in more detail in the next section of this chapter. Each of these problems may adversely influence performance and may also reduce the patient's performance in treatment and capacity to learn from treatment. The therapist should be aware of the potential for these problems arising and seek to minimize their impact.

Distinguishing Between Sensory and Cognitive and Perceptual Deficits

Cognitive and perceptual dysfunction must be differentiated from sensory loss, language impairment, hearing loss, motor loss (weakness, spasticity, incoordination), visual disturbances (poor eyesight, homonymous hemianopia), disorientation, and lack of comprehension. The therapist must rule out pure sensory impairments before testing for cognitive and perceptual deficits; otherwise the therapist may incorrectly attribute poor performance to perceptual problems and design treatment accordingly when in fact the problem has a sensory base and should be treated quite differently. The therapist should conduct tests of deep (proprioceptive) sensations (kinesthesia, position sense, vibration), superficial sensations (pain, temperature, light touch, and pressure), and combined cortical sensations (stereognosis, tactile localization two-point discrimination, barognosis, graphesthesia, and recognition of texture) using methods described in Chapter 3, Examination of Sensory Function. The patient's hearing also requires testing. For example, if the patient does not seem to understand what the therapist is saying, hearing problems should be ruled out before more extensive language and cognitive tests are conducted. The therapist may need to confirm with the family if the patient wears a hearing aid and ensure its availability during therapy. If in doubt, the therapist may need to request testing by the speech-language pathologist or audiologist.

The therapist must also determine if the patient has visual impairments because they can easily be mistaken for perceptual problems. Given the prevalence of sensory-based visual problems, the following section focuses on identification of these impairments and the importance of distinguishing between visual and perceptual origins for treatment purposes.

Visual Impairments

Visual impairments are one of the most common forms of sensory loss affecting the patient with hemiplegia.[51,52] The lesion resulting from a stroke may affect the eye, optic radiation, or visual cortex and subsequently the reception, transmission, and appreciation of any visual array. Visual impairments commonly encountered by patients with hemiplegia include poor eyesight, diplopia, homonymous hemianopia, and damage to the visual cortex or retina. Awareness of the presence of these deficits is important so as not to confuse them with visual perceptual deficiencies and to ensure their consideration during treatment planning and therapeutic intervention.

The critical nature of the basic visual skills (i.e., acuity, oculomotor control, and intact visual fields) in forming a basis for higher-level visual perception is highlighted by Warren[53,54] in a hierarchical model for the evaluation and treatment of visual perceptual dysfunction. In this developmental model, the basic visual skills enumerated above form the foundation for the next level of visual skills, which include *visual attention* (focusing on one aspect of the environment while ignoring others), *visual scanning* (using eyes to follow a target), and *pattern recognition* (recognition of structures that make a recognizable whole). These skills, along with memory, are required to facilitate the highest-level visual skill, termed *visual cognition*.[53,54] This model has implications for the evaluation and treatment of visual perceptual disorders in a bottom-up sequence[54] (i.e., working from the "bottom," initially focusing on underlying skills that will then promote recovery of the next level of skills).

Impairments of oculomotor control (control of eye movements) are a common occurrence following a CVA. Poor visual acuity is another frequent finding following stroke or brain injury, even in the absence of other visual problems.[55] Therefore, it is recommended that the patient receive a comprehensive eye examination and have his or her eyeglass prescription checked.

Diplopia, or double vision, is often present following brain damage. The patient sees two of the entire environment (horizontally, vertically, or diagonally). Diplopia is usually the result of defective function of extraocular muscles in which both eyes are used but not in conjunction with the other. Treatment usually consists of exercises for the eye muscles. In addition, the patient usually is instructed to wear a patch on alternate eyes until the condition clears. If the condition does not clear, the optometrist may recommend prisms.

Visual field deficit is probably the most common visual deficit affecting patients with hemiplegia[56] and occurs most frequently following damage to the middle cerebral artery near the internal capsule.[9] The diagnostic term for this deficit is homonymous hemianopia. The frequency of hemianopia following a right-hemisphere stroke is around 17%.[12] In addition, there is a significant correlation between the presence of visual field deficits and visual neglect.[57] Most important, the presence of a visual field deficit is a significant prognostic sign, predicting both a higher death rate following stroke and poorer performance in ADL, even following rehabilitation.[12,58]

Figure 27.3 demonstrates the normal functioning of the visual fields, in which the left side of the environment (the tree) is perceived by the nasal retina of the left eye and the temporal retina of the right eye, and the right side of the environment (the car) is perceived by the nasal retina of the right eye and the temporal retina of the left eye.

The lesion producing homonymous hemianopia interrupts inflow to the optic pathways on one side of the brain. This produces a loss of the outer half of the visual field from one eye and the inner half of the visual field of the other eye. The result is a loss of

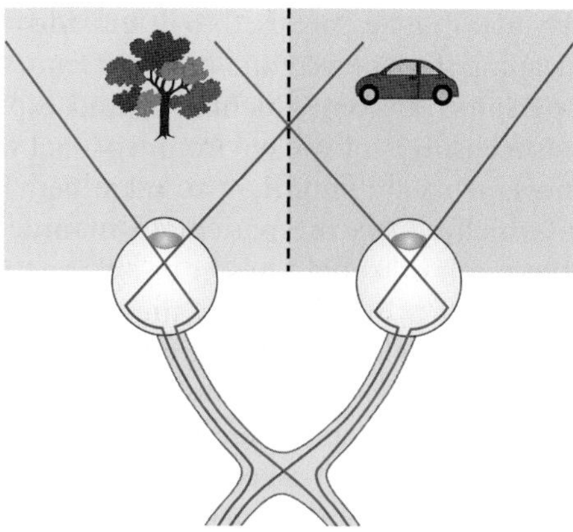

Figure 27.3 Normally functioning visual system; right and left visual fields. See text for explanation.

incoming information from half of the visual environment (left or right) contralateral to the side of the lesion. Thus, the loss of the left half of the visual field accompanies left hemiplegia and loss of the right visual field accompanies right hemiplegia. Zhang et al[59] suggested that this is a common condition following stroke and noted a spontaneous recovery rate in less than 40% of cases. Figure 27.4 illustrates visual field deficits associated with a number of lesions to the visual system.

The presence of a visual field cut may inhibit performance in many daily activities. The patient is usually unaware of the condition and does not automatically compensate by turning the head unless specifically instructed. One of the dangers in this condition is street crossing (Fig. 27.5). Another example of the effects of a visual field cut is illustrated in Figure 27.6. When presented with a newspaper, a patient with right homonymous hemianopia may attend to one half of the newspaper page, either to or from the midline.

Because of homonymous hemianopia's prevalence, it is essential for the therapist to determine whether this condition is present or not. A number of testing procedures are currently employed. In the confrontation method, the patient sits opposite the therapist and is instructed to maintain his or her gaze on the therapist's nose (Fig. 27.7). The therapist slowly brings a target, such as the therapist's finger or a pen, into the patient's

A Functional vision
B Functional vision
C Functional vision
D Functional vision
E Functional vision

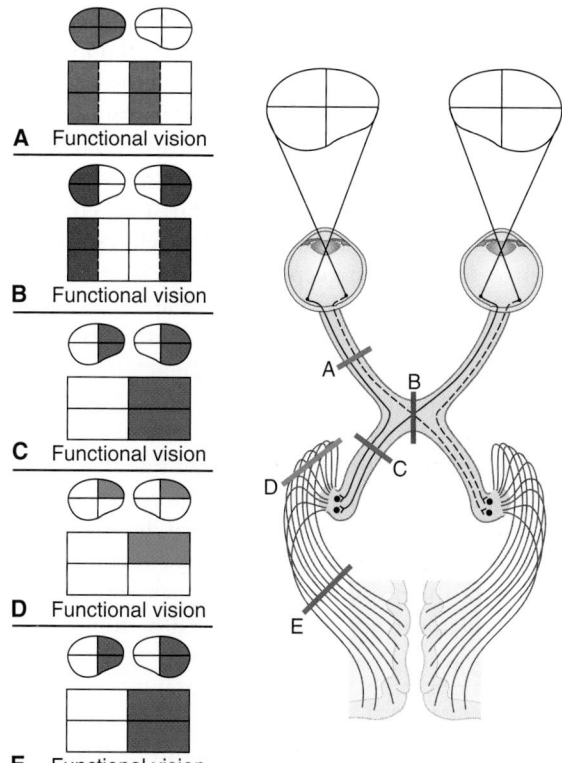

Figure 27.4 Visual field deficits (with functional loss) and associated lesions. Vision is shown as clear and visual loss is colored in examples A–E, which denote (A) blindness in one eye; (B) bitemporal hemianopia (tunnel vision); (C) homonymous hemianopia; (D) quadrantanopia; and (E) homonymous hemianopia.

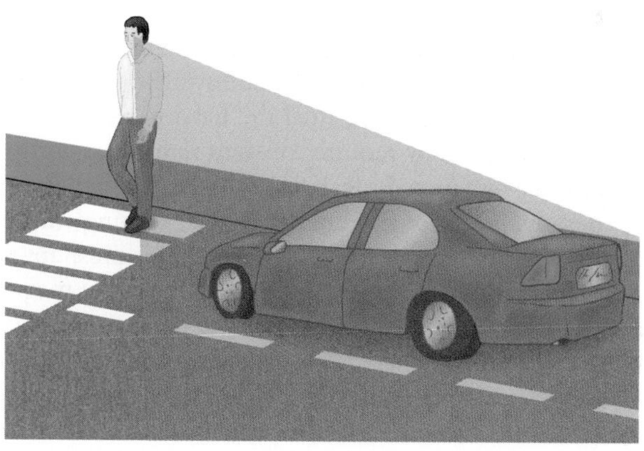

Figure 27.5 The functional significance of hemianopia—it may lead to accidents.

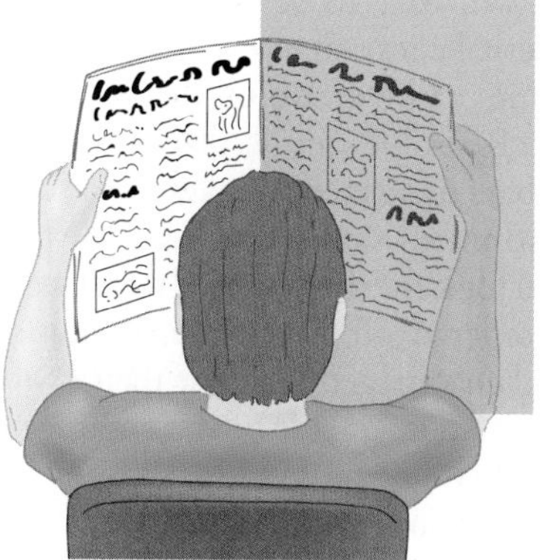

Figure 27.6 A newspaper as it might appear to a patient with right homonymous hemianopia following a stroke. The shading indicates that the patient may be unable to read the right side page.

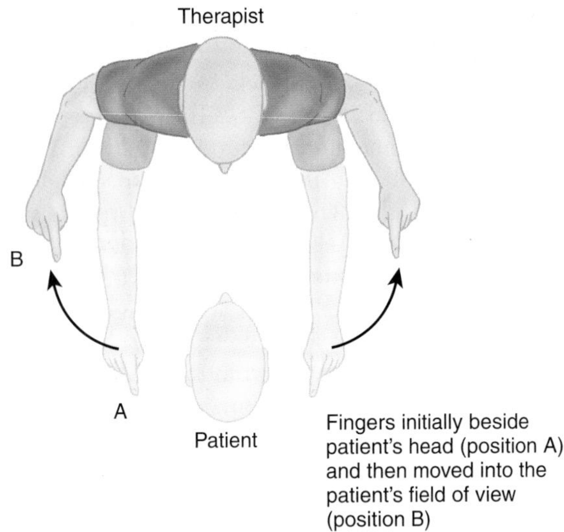
Therapist
B
A
Patient
Fingers initially beside patient's head (position A) and then moved into the patient's field of view (position B)

Figure 27.7 Method for testing hemianopia.

field of view simultaneously or alternately from the right or left. The patient is instructed to indicate when and where he or she sees the targets.

To help the patient compensate for the visual field deficit, the patient can first be made aware of the deficit and then be instructed to turn the head to the affected side. Patients usually require constant reminders at first, which may be tapered off with time and practice. Early in therapy, items (e.g., eating utensils, writing implements) should be placed where the patient is most apt to see them (on the less affected side). They can be moved progressively to the midline and then to the more affected side, when appropriate. The nursing staff should be made aware of the condition and be requested to place the patient's essential bedside needs such as telephone, tissues, and so forth, within the intact visual field. The therapist initially should sit on the patient's less involved side when instructing or giving demonstrations and should alternate this with the more affected side so that the patient receives maximum stimulation. Of course, the patient will have to be reminded to turn the head at first. External cues can be employed as well. For reading, a red line can be drawn on the side of the page that is not seen. Red tape can be placed on the floor, mat, or parallel bars to attract the patient to scan to the side of the environment that is not seen. The patient should be taught to look for these cues. These external cues can be slowly tapered off over time. Patients can be instructed and encouraged to devise their own cues to clue them in to the unseen side of the environment in situations that have not been addressed per se in therapy. Exercises that require motor crossing of the midline can be used to reinforce visual crossing of the midline and turning of the head.[60,61]

Oculomotor impairment is another area of deficit in basic visual skills that is common in patients who have had a stroke. Eye movements, which are controlled by the extraocular muscles, are used to detect, identify, and derive meaning from objects and the environment. They allow a person to become oriented to and explore the critical visual aspects of the environment.[11] Two types of eye movements are important to examine: (1) visual fixation, which allows the patient to maintain focus on an object as it is brought nearer or farther away, and (2) ocular pursuits, which enable the eyes to follow a moving object and visually scan the environment. Often the eyes will not follow a moving object visually, although the patient seems aware of the presence of that object and can locate it if asked. The patient is visually hypoactive. Oculomotor dysfunction often accompanies visual–perceptual dysfunction[62] and is frequently related to attention deficits.[63]

Visual scanning can be tested as follows. Sit opposite the patient. Hold up a pencil with a colorful pencil topper 18 inches (45.7 cm) in front of the patient's eyes. Slowly move the pencil horizontally, then vertically, then diagonally. Repeat each direction two to three times. Note the smoothness of eye movements, the presence of a midline jerk or jump, and whether the eyes move together.[2,62]

Aside from the visual sensory impairments outlined above, many patients suffer from visual–perceptual impairment. Damage to areas of the cortex on which visual information converges with information from other senses may interfere with the recognition and interpretation of visual information, even though the visual stimuli may have arrived at the visual cortex uninterrupted. A total failure to appreciate incoming visual sensory information owing to a lesion in the cortex is referred to as *cortical blindness*.[62] There is no statistical correspondence between the presence of visual field cuts and the presence of visual–perceptual disorders.[64] Similarly, there is no correspondence between aphasia, age, and time since infarct and measures of visual–perceptual dysfunction.[64] However, within the realm of visual–perceptual impairments, there is a significant difference between the performances of patients with right hemiplegia and those with left hemiplegia. Patients with left hemiplegia have frequently been found to perform more poorly on measures of visual–perceptual dysfunction than patients with right hemiplegia. Thus, therapists should be aware of the possibility of visual–perceptual deficits, particularly in the population with left hemiplegia.

Standardized Cognitive and Perceptual Tests

A standardized test is one that has a uniform procedure to administer and score, provides operational definitions for all terms, is norm-referenced,[65] and has information available concerning its reliability and validity, which is essential for correct interpretation of results.[66] Results from standardized tests of cognition and perception can be communicated to other therapists who will share an understanding of the patient's capacities or abilities. Standardized tests can be administered both at admission and at discharge to provide the therapist with a reliable and valid measure of the outcome of therapy.

When conducting a standardized test, the patient should be sitting comfortably and wearing glasses and/or a hearing aid if needed. Ideally, the room should be quiet and free of distraction. The therapist should be positioned opposite or next to the patient. Since the performance of a patient who has had a stroke may vary from day to day, a single testing session may be unreliable.[67] A number of short sessions scheduled on successive days may be preferable. To enhance its practical value, perceptual testing must be done in conjunction with observation in self-care and ADL skills, where the patient's judgment and discriminative abilities with regard to real-life tasks can be determined. It is not uncommon for patients to test poorly for visual–perceptual skills but to perform adequately in ADL with minimal effort or assistance.[63]

The quality of the patient's response to the test media (e.g., how the task is approached, how and why the error is made) is as important to note as the success or failure in completing the selected task. Some aspects of response in the testing situation or during ADL can be referred to as the patient's individual *perceptual style*. Included under this rubric are the patient's perceptual strategy, response to various cues (such as auditory, visual, and tactile), rate of performance, and consistency of performance.[37]

Occupational therapists use a variety of standardized tests to determine the presence of cognitive and perceptual impairments and resulting disabilities. When selecting a standardized test, the therapist must consider many factors. The selection depends on what the therapist wants to learn about the patient and what the test can potentially reveal.[1] In many cases a single test will not provide all the information required by a therapist to plan treatment, so several tests may be administered[5,68-88] (Table 27.1). In addition to those presented in Table 27.1, other instruments used

Table 27.1 Table of Outcome Measures

Outcome Measure and ICF Category	Description	Scoring	MDC and MCID
Arnadottir OT-ADL Neurobehavioral Evaluation (A-ONE)[5] **ICF: 1,2**	This test was developed to measure a patient's neurobehavior through daily living tasks (dressing, grooming, hygiene, transfer and mobility, feeding, and communication). Occupational therapists must undertake a 5-day training and certification course to qualify to administer this test. A wide variety of cognitive and perceptual impairments can be detected with this instrument.	The A-ONE can be administered in 30–40 minutes. The 22 ADL tasks on the Functional Independence Scale (FIS) and 46 items on the Neurobehavioral Specific Impairments Subscale (NSIS) are rated on a 5-point scale. FIS item scores range from 0 (unable to perform and totally dependent on assistance) to 4 (functionally independent). The FIS total score is derived from the sum of item scores.	MDC: NA MCID: NA
Assessment of Motor and Process Skills (AMPS)[68] **ICF: 1,2**	The AMPS is a structured, observational assessment of performance in daily living activities. Performance is observed on a choice of two or three familiar instrumental or personal ADLs. Quality of performance is rated on 16 motor and 20 process skills relating to independence, efficiency, effortlessness, and adoption of safe practices in the context of the task undertaken (dynamic interaction of the person with the environment). Training is required before the assessment can be administered.	The AMPS can be completed in 30–60 minutes.[69] Scores range from 1 (deficit) to 4 (competent) for each of the 16 motor and 20 process skills associated with each ADL performed. Higher scores are indicative of more skill competence.	MDC: NA MCID: NA

Continued

Table 27.1 Table of Outcome Measures—cont'd

Outcome Measure and ICF Category	Description	Scoring	MDC and MCID
Australian Therapy Outcome Measures for Occupational Therapy (AusTOMS-OT)[70] **ICF: 1,2,3** **ICF: 1,2,3** **ICF:**	The AusTOMs-OT is a measure of global functional outcomes for clients of all ages and all diagnoses. The AusTOMS comprises 12 scales that are rated across four domains (Impairment, Activity Limitation, Participation Restriction, and Distress/Well-being). A client's cognitive and perceptual skills are included, but not targeted, as part of this assessment. Training is required before the assessment can be administered.	The AusTOMs-OT outcome measures can be scored in under 5 minutes. The scores across the four domains range from 0 to 5, with lower scores indicative of more severe functioning.	MDC: The MDC (90% CI) has been calculated for 2 scales, from the data from Fristedt.[71] Scale 7 Self-Care-Impairment: MDC = 0.95 Self-Care-Activity/ Limitation: MDC = 1.24 Self-Care-Participation/Restriction: MDC = 1.14 Self-Care-Distress/ Well-being: MDC = 1.33 Scale 5 Transfers-Impairment: MDC = 1.30 Transfers-Activity/ Limitation: MDC = 0.99 Transfers-Participation/ Restriction: MDC = 1.13 Transfers-Distress/ Well-being: MDC = 1.23 MCID: A change of 0.5 to 1 point on any of the 4 domains of the AusTOMs-OT scale is considered clinically important.
Behavioural Assessment of the Dysexecutive (BADS)[72] **ICF: 1**	The BADS assesses an individual's executive function skills. The assessment includes six subtests and a 20-item questionnaire, which measure everyday executive function and higher-level cognitive functions.	The BADS can be completed in 30–45 minutes.[69] Each subtest score ranges from 0 to 4. An overall profile score is obtained from summing the individual subtest scores. This score can be converted to a standard score with a mean of 100 and a standard deviation of 15.	MDC: NA MCID: NA
Behavioral Inattention Test (BIT)[73] **ICF: 1**	The BIT was developed to examine clients for the presence of unilateral visual neglect and to provide the therapist with information concerning how the neglect affects the client's ability to perform everyday occupations.[74] The BIT is comprised of two subtests: BIT Behavioral (BITB) subtest consists of nine activity-based	The test can be completed in approximately 1 hour. Total and subscores are obtained by adding the subtests scores together. Max scores: BIT = 227 BITC = 146 BITB = 81	MDC: NA MCID: NA

Table 27.1 Table of Outcome Measures—cont'd

Outcome Measure and ICF Category	Description	Scoring	MDC and MCID
	subtests such as card sorting and phone dialing. The BIT Conventional (BITC) subtest consists of six pen-and-paper subtests such as representational drawing, line crossing, and figure shape copying. Many of these test items have been used in the past in a nonstandardized way to examine for the presence of neglect.	Higher scores are indicative of more severe visual impairment.	
COGNISTAT The Neurobehavioral Cognitive Status Examination[75] **ICF: 1**	This cognitive screening assessment comprises 62 items that measure memory, language, attention, calculations, level of consciousness and orientation, and reasoning. Training is required before the assessment can be administered.	The COGNISTAT can be completed in 15–30 minutes.[69] Min score = 0; Max score = 12. Sum score for each domain using the domain raw score to determine the presence and severity of deficits.	MDC: NA MCID: NA
Executive Function Performance Test (EFPT)[76] **ICF: 1,2**	The EFPT examines performance on five ADL tasks that involve five executive function constructs as follows: initiation, organization, sequencing, judgment and safety, and completion.	This test can be completed in 30–45 minutes.[77] For each of the five ADL tasks, the five executive function constructs are scored across a range from 0 (independent) to 5 (totally dependent on assistance). A total score for each of the ADL tasks is derived from the sum of the five executive function constructs.	MDC: NA MCID: NA
Loewenstein Occupational Therapy Cognitive Assessment (LOTCA)[78] **ICF: 1**	The LOTCA is a battery-style test lasting 35–40 minutes and composed of 20 subtests that examine four areas: orientation, visual and spatial perception, visuomotor organization, and thinking operations. The instrument was developed for use with people who have experienced stroke, traumatic brain injury, or tumor.[78] The LOTCA has recently been validated with a Chinese population of patients with stroke.[79] There are several different versions of the LOTCA, including the LOTCA-Geriatric (LOTCA-G),[80] the Functional LOTCA (FLOTCA),[81] the Dynamic	The LOTCA can be completed in 30–45 minutes. Subtests are scored from 1 (low) to 4 (high), except for three subtests, which are scored from 1 to 5.	MDC: NA MCID: NA

Continued

Table 27.1 Table of Outcome Measures—cont'd

Outcome Measure and ICF Category	Description	Scoring	MDC and MCID
	LOTCA (DLOTCA),[82] the DLOTCA-Geriatric (DLOTCA-G),[80] and the Dynamic Occupational Therapy Cognitive Assessment for Children (DOTCA-Ch).[83]		
Montreal Cognitive Assessment (MoCA)[84] **ICF: 1**	The MoCA is a comprehensive cognitive screening assessment of memory, language, attention, visuospatial skills, orientation, and abstraction. The MoCA comprises 16 items and 11 categories to assess cognitive abilities in order to detect mild cognitive dysfunction.	This test can be completed in approximately 10 minutes.[77] Max total score = 30	MDC: NA MCID: NA
Rivermead Perceptual Assessment Battery(RPAB)[85] **ICF: 1**	This instrument was designed to examine visual perceptual impairments in patients following head injury or stroke. The RPAB is a battery consisting of 16 performance tasks that examine form discrimination, color constancy, sequencing, object completion, figure–ground discrimination, body image, inattention, and spatial awareness. For further information on the RPAB, the reader is referred to Jesshope et al.[86]	The RPAB can be completed in approximately 1 hour. Scoring is based on the accuracy of task completion and time to complete task (max time limit range: 3–5 min). Max task score range: 4–72. A total score is not recorded.	MDC: NA MCID: NA
Rivermead Behavioural Memory Test (RBMT-3)[87] **ICF: 1**	This battery was designed to examine everyday memory abilities. It offers the therapist an initial determination of the client's memory function, provides an indication of appropriate areas for treatment, and enables the therapist to monitor memory skills throughout the treatment program. The RBMT-3 comprises 14 subtests that examine immediate and delayed everyday memory, recall, and recognition. The RBMT-3 also includes a new subtest "Novel Task," which assesses new learning. For further information on the development and validation of the RBMT, the reader is referred to Wilson et al[87] and Wilson et al.[88]	The RBMT-3 can be administered in approximately 30 minutes by occupational therapists, speech-language pathologists, and psychologists. The RBMIT-3 offers two scoring options: screening and profile score to detect change over time. Subtest raw scores can be converted to scaled scores (based on client age) with a mean of 10 and a standard deviation of 3. An overall General Memory Index can be derived with a mean of 100 and a standard deviation of 15.	MDC: NA MCID: NA

ICF = International Classification of Functioning, Disability and Health; MDC = minimal detectable change; MCID = minimal clinically important difference
ICF Category: 1 = Body Structure/Function; 2 = Activity; 3 = Participation

to measure more global outcomes of rehabilitation include the following:

- *Medical Outcomes Study (MOS), Short Form Health Survey (SF-36)*[89]
- *Australian Therapy Outcomes (AusTOMs) (www.austoms.com)*[70]
- *Canadian Occupational Performance Measure (COPM)*[90]
- *Rivermead Rehabilitation Centre Life Goals Questionnaire*[91]
- *Reintegration to Normal Living Index (RNL)*[92]
- *Functional Independence Measure (FIM$_{MR}$™)*[93]

Some of these instruments also incorporate items that measure cognition and perception. For example, the FIM$_{MR}$™ includes three cognition-related items (social interaction, problem-solving, and memory). The tests described in the section on specific cognitive and perceptual deficits are used widely in the clinic. Although some of the instruments presented are not standardized, they are still useful, particularly for examining the quality of response to the test stimuli.

INTERVENTION

Treatment Approaches

Five major approaches to cognitive and perceptual rehabilitation are commonly employed by occupational therapists. They are the *retraining approach,* the *sensory integrative approach,* the *neurofunctional approach,* the *rehabilitation/compensatory approach,* and the *cognitive rehabilitation/quadraphonic approach.* These approaches were described earlier in the chapter. Although research directly comparing the efficacy of the various approaches has been sparse, attempts have been made recently to empirically define and test the methodologies.[21,25,34,94] Issues to consider in examining the approaches are the availability of standardized measures of change in functional status and ADL, group versus individual treatment, specific stimulus properties, format, length and frequency of feedback, and individual information processing styles.[21]

Neistadt[25,34] described these treatments dichotomously as either remedial or adaptive/compensatory. The remedial approach encompasses the retraining approach, the sensory integrative approach, and the cognitive approach.[1] The neurofunctional approach and the rehabilitation/compensatory approach are described as adaptive or compensatory. The quadraphonic approach brings together aspects of both the remedial and compensatory approaches. A description of the key components of these two main approaches is presented below. A discussion on education is also provided because no intervention program would be complete without the provision of education to both the patient and the caregivers. Finally, a discussion is provided on integrating these three elements within a rehabilitation program.

The Remedial Approach

Remedial approaches focus on the patient's deficits and attempt to improve functional ability by retraining specific perceptual components of behavior.[25] The assumption uniting this set of tactics is that facilitation of, or training in, underlying skills will enhance the recovery or reorganization of deficient CNS functioning.[21,25] This, in turn, will automatically translate into improvement in functional skills. Remedial approaches are also referred to as *bottom-up approaches.* These approaches work from the bottom, which is the recovery of underlying skills, and assume that the patient will be able to generalize skills to occupational performance, which is at a higher level.[1,47]

The Adaptive/Compensatory Approach

The adaptive or compensatory approach mandates direct training in the functional skills that are deficient. It does not assume automatic carryover from tasks that are not obviously similar to the functional task to be learned and thus minimizes the need for generalization. In an adaptive, or "top-down" approach, the therapist works with the patient on specific tasks that are required, or those that the patient wants to achieve. In other words, the therapist starts at the top, which is the desired functional outcome, rather than working with the patient on the underlying performance components.[35] Table 27.2 presents a comparison of the assumptions underlying the remedial and adaptive approaches.

Patient, Family, and Caregiver Education

Education for the patient, family, and caregivers is essential for continuity of care. Appendix 27.A includes Web-based resources for clinicians, families, and patients with cognitive and perceptual deficits. The patient and caregivers should understand why it is inadvisable or impossible for the patient to do some things safely or independently, and why other things must be done in a specific way. Explaining the reasons why the patient behaves in a particular way reduces the likelihood of inappropriate expectations from those without the background to know that brain damage affects not only how the patient moves but also how he or she experiences and thus responds to the world.

Feedback is essential to the patient's learning. The patient's own feedback may be inaccurate owing to perceptual and cognitive dysfunctions. Thus, the individual may be unaware that a task has not been accomplished or that it has not been performed in the safest or most efficient manner. Feedback should be provided in the form of knowledge of results (KR; information regarding whether or not the patient attained the correct outcome) and knowledge of performance (KP; information regarding the manner in which the task was accomplished).[95]

Table 27.2 Common Assumptions of Adaptive and Remedial Approaches

Adaptive Approach	Remedial Approach
The adult brain has limited potential to repair and reorganize itself after injury.	The adult brain can repair and reorganize itself after injury.
Intact behaviors can be used to compensate for ones that are impaired.	Repair and reorganization is influenced by environmental stimuli.
Adaptive retraining can facilitate the substitution of intact behaviors for impaired ones.	Cognitive, perceptual, and sensorimotor exercises can promote brain recovery and reorganization.
Adaptive activities of daily living provide training in functional behaviors.	Cognitive, perceptual, and sensorimotor exercises provide training in the cognitive and perceptual skills needed for those exercises.
Training in specific, essential activities of daily living tasks is necessary because adults with brain injury have difficulty generalizing learning.	Remedial training in cognitive and perceptual skills will be generalized across all activities requiring those skills.
Functional activities require cognitive and perceptual skills.	Functional activities require cognitive and perceptual skills.
Adaptation and compensation will lead to improved functional performance.	Cognitive and perceptual remediation will lead to improved functional performance.

The form in which this feedback is delivered depends on the specific limitations and strengths of the patient. For example, the physical therapy goal for a patient with left hemiplegia and visual perceptual involvement might be to walk to the end of the parallel bars. KR would consist of a verbal confirmation by the therapist as to whether or not the patient reached the end of the parallel bars. KP might include comments by the therapist concerning the adequacy of the patient's visual scanning, positioning of the lower extremities (LEs), correct posture, and appropriate use of the upper limbs. For the patient with communication impairments, feedback would need to be visual. Tactile input also can be used effectively to cue patients with either right or left hemiplegia. A combination of inputs, using a number of sensory modalities, often facilitates patient success at a given task.

When involving the patient in education sessions, the patient must be addressed as a competent adult and not patronized. He or she must be regarded as the principal participant in the rehabilitation process. In situations in which the perceptual deficit does not interfere with assimilation of information, the patient should have the major role in the decision making process regarding the goals of therapy.

Refocusing Intervention

Many clinicians begin an intervention program by adopting remedial strategies. In these circumstances, therapists are aiming to maximize recovery of function and educate their patients about the problems experienced and ways that can improve their function. However, some patients may not make much progress. In some cases, the patient may have inadequate language skills to be able to work with the therapist or may have limited insight to his or her problems and therefore will not work with the therapist. In other cases still, improvements simply do not seem to occur for a variety of reasons that the therapist may not be able to pinpoint. Finally, in the current climate of managed care, the therapist may not have very much time allocated to work with the patient using remedial techniques. The patient's discharge may be imminent, and yet he or she may not be independent or safe enough to be discharged. In such cases, the therapist may switch from a remedial approach to a compensatory one.

When using an adaptive compensatory approach, the therapist will address education of the caregivers as well as the patient. Intervention strategies will focus on changing the environment or the strategy for task completion so that the patient can be safe and independent as quickly as possible. In many instances, therapists use a three-point approach to intervention where they educate patients and caregivers, begin the program using remedial techniques, and then switch to compensation techniques when the patient's improvements have plateaued and/or discharge is imminent.

The Impact of Managed Care

Managed care in the United States health care system has many implications for treatment of patients with cognitive and perceptual deficits. The most striking of these is the reduction in time allocated for inpatient evaluation and treatment.[36] Cognitive and perceptual problems are not readily visible and are therefore more easily overlooked than physical problems. Hence, pressure to discharge patients quickly, possibly before the full extent of cognitive and perceptual deficits has been revealed, means that patients may be discharged to potentially hazardous situations at home. Therapists need to do an initial screening of all patients with brain damage to determine potential problems as early as possible, and ensure that patients are discharged to a safe environment. Although inpatient rehabilitation time is reduced, there is opportunity for outpatient services conducted in the clinic or in the patient's home.[96] The advantage of home care is that therapists have an opportunity to work with the patient in his or her own environment and tailor therapy to the patient's current circumstances. Patients with cognitive and perceptual deficits often perform better in their own familiar environments.

The major disadvantage of reduced inpatient treatment time for many patients, including those with cognitive and perceptual deficits, is that a home discharge may not be safe after only limited inpatient rehabilitation. The situation is complicated by having to discharge a patient who does not have family support to another type of institutional care (possibly a nursing home or skilled nursing facility) when in the long term this level of care may not be necessary. It is distressing for patients who are confused, owing to cognitive and perceptual problems, to be moved, particularly when they may believe the move is permanent.

DISCHARGE PLANNING

Discharge planning begins as soon as the patient is admitted for rehabilitation.[97] The most important question to be answered during this stage is where the patient will live after discharge. There are two major types of housing available to persons with disabilities: community-based accommodation and residential-care accommodation. Community-based accommodation includes private homes, retirement villages, and hotels or rooming houses. Residential care may be defined as any accommodation that provides personal care and medical services on a consistent, continual, or per need basis; this includes nursing homes, skilled nursing facilities, assisted living centers, and sheltered or group housing.[98,99]

The key to discharge planning is to consider the match between the patient's skills and the demands of the environment, and then factor in the support systems available from a spouse, friends, or family to assist with tasks that the patient cannot manage.[99,100] This approach works well when patients and their families have insight and an understanding of the patient's problems. However, cognitive and perceptual deficits are often not very visible, and it may be difficult for the family and the patient to understand the functional impact of these deficits. For example, a patient may regain full motor function following a stroke but experience ongoing difficulties with unilateral neglect. This problem is not readily apparent to the untrained onlooker. However, this patient cannot drive and may be in danger when simply crossing the road. These problems have major lifestyle implications for the patient.

Interventions that facilitate a patient's return to community-based housing usually center on enabling the patient to carry out ADL skills in an acceptable and safe manner. If this cannot be achieved and the patient does not have a live-in caregiver, supported housing such as a nursing home may be the only alternative. Research examining the discharge process for a sample of 62 patients following stroke revealed that the majority were reluctant to consider alternatives to returning home despite having significant self-care deficits.[100] Our housing is central to who we are as individuals, and it is very difficult for patients, particularly those with limited insight, to understand and accept that they can no longer live in the community.

OVERVIEW OF COGNITIVE AND PERCEPTUAL DEFICITS

This section is divided into seven parts: *attention deficits, memory impairments, impairments of executive function, body scheme and body image impairments, spatial relations impairments, agnosia,* and *apraxia* (Table 27.3). Each category encompasses a constellation of deficits, which are grouped together for ease of understanding. Information pertaining to each deficit will be organized identically as follows:

1. Definition(s)
2. Clinical Examples
3. Lesion Area
4. Testing
5. Treatment Suggestions

The value of dwelling on probable areas of cortical damage is controversial. The indication of cortical loci is an attempt to relate the study of neuroanatomy to actual patient behavior involving cognitive and perceptual dysfunction. An examination of cortical loci will give the reader a sense of which cognitive and perceptual deficits are likely to be seen together.

As therapists, we are required to assist the patient to bridge the gap between maladaptive behavior and independent function in ADL skills. Whether or not the area of the brain purported to produce a particular dysfunction appears damaged on a computed tomography (CT) scan or other neurological or radiological test is not a key determinant of the rehabilitative approach to therapy. The patient's approach to task performance and the relative strengths or weaknesses of the patient (motor, cognitive, and perceptual), which the therapist ascertains through thorough observation and testing, are much more pertinent to the selection of appropriate therapeutic strategies than the locus of the lesion.

Testing tools are described for each cognitive or perceptual deficit to enhance the reader's awareness of the complexity of behavior ascribed to perceptual deficiencies. Familiarity with the tools used to examine cognitive or perceptual deficits can aid in communication between

Table 27.3 Summary of Cognitive and Perceptual Impairments

Area of Deficit	Specific Impairments
Cognition	
Attention deficits	Sustained attention Selective attention Divided attention Alternating attention
Memory impairments	Immediate recall Short-term memory Long-term memory
Higher-Order Cognition	
Impairment of executive functions	Volition Planning Purposive action Effective performance
Perception	
Body scheme/body image impairments	Unilateral neglect Anosognosia Somatoagnosia Right–left discrimination Finger agnosia
Spatial relation impairments (complex perception)	Figure–ground discrimination Form discrimination Spatial relations Position in space Topographical disorientation Depth and distance perception Vertical disorientation
Agnosias	Visual object agnosia Auditory agnosia Tactile agnosia
Apraxia	Ideomotor apraxia Ideational apraxia Buccofacial apraxia

physical and occupational therapists engaged in the treatment of the same patient.

The following section also includes specific treatment suggestions from the sensorimotor, transfer of training, and functional approaches described. The intervention strategies most relevant to physical therapist practice are those dealing with the functional approach and adaptation of the environment. In these sections, examples are given of how to facilitate the patient's success within a treatment session. Information is provided on how the therapist might gear language, demonstrations, feedback, and the use of media and the environment to the individual needs of the cognitively or perceptually impaired patient. The evidence base for treatment is not strong for many of these treatment techniques, and further research is required to support their efficacy.

Attention Deficits

1. *Definitions.* The inability of many patients with hemiplegia to maintain attention during therapy is a frequent complaint of therapists. *Attention* is the ability to select and attend to a specific stimulus while simultaneously suppressing extraneous stimuli.[101] A patient who is inattentive or distractible will have difficulty in processing and assimilating new information or techniques.[102] Often, patients who have suffered a CVA will have low arousal levels and require a great deal of sensory input to be alerted to the environment. Low arousal thus must be considered as a cause for seeming inattention.

   Four different kinds of attention are generally discussed in the literature: sustained attention, focused or selective attention, alternating attention, and divided attention. *Sustained attention* is a capacity to attend to relevant information during activity. This implies that a person can maintain a consistent response during a continuous activity. *Focused* or *selective attention* is the capacity to attend to a task despite environmental visual or auditory stimuli. *Alternating attention* is the capacity to move flexibly between tasks and respond appropriately to the demands of each task. *Divided attention* is the capacity to respond simultaneously to two or more tasks or stimuli when all stimuli are relevant.[1]
2. *Clinical Examples.* The patient with a disorder of sustained attention may report that he or she starts to watch a TV program and then "just drifts off." A patient who has to stop a dressing activity to talk to the therapist may be demonstrating difficulties with focused attention. Patients who are easily disturbed by music or other forms of background noise may also be experiencing problems with focused attention.

   A problem with focused attention is often referred to as *distractibility*. Divided attention is required when more than one response is needed or more than one stimuli needs to be monitored.[103] Selective attention is required when certain stimuli need to be ignored.[104] Patients who have difficulty with divided and alternating attention may have great difficulties with more complex daily living activities such as cooking a meal or driving.
3. *Lesion Areas.* Multiple brain regions are thought to be responsible for producing attention. These include the reticular formation (which regulates arousal), the various sensory systems that deliver and code relevant sensory information, and the limbic and frontal regions that underlie the drive and affective components of concentration.[104]
4. *Testing.* General screening tests such as the *Loewenstein Occupational Therapy Cognitive Assessment*[78] or the

Chessington Occupational Therapy Neurological Assessment Battery (COTNAB)[105] include subtests that examine attentional abilities. To investigate problems of attention, neuropsychologists generally administer the *Stroop Test*,[106] the *Paced Auditory Serial Attention Test (PASAT)*,[107] and the *Trail Making Test*.[108]

5. *Treatment Suggestions.* The purpose of therapy is to increase the patient's attention to appropriate stimuli and disregard inappropriate stimuli.
   a. *Remedial Approach.* Clinically, the ability to attend to a task has implications for the therapeutic process. Patients should be instructed to scan the visual environment in a slow and systematic manner. In the presence of right hemiplegia, the patient should be spoken to more slowly to afford an opportunity to process verbal information and be taught to use visualization techniques to facilitate attendance to verbal tasks. In addition, patients with left hemiplegia should be encouraged to use verbalization to improve performance in visual tasks. A randomized clinical trial (RCT) with 12 patients investigating the effect of training on divided attention skills reported positive outcomes as measured on a rating scale of attentional behavior.[109] Patients were trained to do two computer-based or pen and paper tasks simultaneously. However, there was no generalization from this training to nontarget tasks. In other words, the benefits of this training were not transferred to patient activities of daily living.

      Some additional tools that may be used for the remediation of attentional deficits and distractibility are setting time or speed limits, amplifying critical stimuli, and making the crucial stimuli salient (noticeable) to the patient.[63] The environment can be graded by having the patient initially perform some aspects of therapy in a nondistracting setting (closed environment) and then slowly increasing potentially distracting elements, both visual and auditory, as patient tolerance improves (progressing to a more open environment).[1]
   b. *Compensatory Approach.* For many patients, the inability to attend to significant stimuli is compounded by distraction due to extraneous stimuli in the environment. Often noise is the most distracting stimulus, causing irritability and diminished concentration. Therefore, a compensatory approach may include providing a quiet distraction-free environment for therapy activities. Ponsford et al[110] provide further ideas for working with patients who have limited attention.

      A Cochrane Review titled "Cognitive Rehabilitation for Attention Deficits Following Stroke"[111] revealed a small number of controlled trials of attention training in patients with stroke. The results of these six studies suggested that training may improve some aspects of attention (e.g., divided attention), but no evidence of sustained long-term benefits was demonstrated. There was also no evidence to support or refute the use of cognitive rehabilitation for attention deficits to improve functional independence.

Memory Impairments

Memory can be defined as a "mental process that allows the individual to store experiences and perceptions for recall at a later time."[102] All memory is not localized in one particular place in the nervous system; rather, many and perhaps all regions of the brain may contain neurons with adequate plasticity for memory storage.[112] Memory comprises acquisition or learning, storage or retention, and retrieval or recall.[113] Learning is a crucial element of rehabilitation. If the patient is unable to learn, time in rehabilitation may not be well spent. Hence, it is very important for the therapist to take steps to evaluate the patient's memory before beginning physical rehabilitation programs. Three levels of memory will be examined: immediate recall, short-term memory, and long-term memory.

Immediate Recall and Short-Term Memory

1. *Definitions.* Immediate recall involves retention of information that has been stored for a few seconds. Short-term memory mediates retention of events or learning that has taken place within a few minutes, hours, or days.[4]
2. *Clinical Examples.* A patient with immediate recall difficulties may not be able to remember the instructions given only seconds before by the therapist for what the patient is to do. A patient with a short-term memory problem may not come back to the physical therapy department, even though the therapist asked him or her to return in an hour. Alternatively, the therapist may teach the patient a new transfer technique and on the following day find that the patient has not retained any of the steps involved. Patients with severe short-term memory problems may not even be able to hold a simple conversation.[1]
3. *Lesion Areas.* Memory is a complex capacity involving many brain regions, including four of the major structures of the cerebral cortex (the frontal, parietal, temporal, and occipital lobes) and the limbic system.[4]
4. *Testing.* The *Rivermead Behavioural Memory Test (RBMT)*[87] can be used to examine memory function. Alternatively, the adequacy of memory functions can be ascertained by having the patient recall lists or collections of objects that have just been presented (immediate recall) or by teaching the patient a new verbal or visual task and asking him or her to recall it a few hours or a day later (short-term memory). Frequently there is a loss of short-term memory following stroke,

and this particularly interferes with the patient's ability to benefit from rehabilitation, especially from those activities involving the use of new and heretofore unfamiliar techniques.[45]

5. *Treatment Suggestions.* The purpose of memory retraining is to enable the patient to effectively encode and recall information so that learning can occur.
   a. *Remedial Approach.* Because good attention skills are vital for memory, the therapist must ensure that attention problems are addressed and improvements are noted before initiating work on memory retraining.[1,43] A primary focus of this approach is working with the patient to effectively encode information so it can be more easily retrieved when appropriate. This may include organizing material to be remembered and making logical associations. A determination should be made of how the patient used to remember information and build on these past strategies. There is very little evidence to suggest that drills, computer games, or memory tests such as recalling a list of items that have been covered over have any effect on retraining memory. On the other hand, if the therapist assists the patient to develop memory strategies when playing these games, then these strategies may be generalized to everyday activities. In a Cochrane Review,[114] the authors drew on findings from two studies and reported that there was insufficient evidence to support or refute the effectiveness of memory retraining on functional outcomes or measures of memory and called for further robust trials in this area.
   b. *Compensatory Approach.* The use of a diary or notebook system (memory log) can help many patients to manage their daily living activities. However, the patient needs to have sufficient memory to use this system. Environmental prompts such as a beeper or a wall calendar can be useful to assist patients to remember their routine or to look at their diary. When external aids are used, the patient needs to be taught how to use them. Guidelines for the use of such devices may be found in Sohlberg and Mateer[115] and McKerracher et al.[116]

Long-Term Memory

1. *Definition.* Long-term memory consists of early experiences and information acquired over a period of years. Patients who do not have long-term memory are often described as having amnesia.[45]
2. *Clinical Examples.* Patients who experience long-term memory problems may have difficulty recalling events from many years ago such as a child's birth or their own work experiences. Long-term memory problems are common following brain injury and in Alzheimer's disease but are not commonly seen following stroke.[45]
3. *Lesion Areas.* As described, memory is a complex capacity involving many brain regions. For a detailed discussion, see Fuster[117] and Lezak.[4]
4. *Testing.* The adequacy of memory functions can be determined by having the patient recall personal historical events. The *Rivermead Behavioural Memory Test (RBMT)*[87] can be used to test memory in a standardized way. It is advisable to question the patient's family as to premorbid memory, because many patients in the stroke-prone age group have already begun to experience declining memory as part of the aging process.
5. *Treatment Suggestions.* Treatments for assisting patients to overcome long-term memory impairments are similar to those outlined above for immediate recall and short-term memory impairments. Further information on the management of memory impairments may be found in Baddeley.[118]

Although the literature contains many studies exploring a variety of memory treatments, few of these were designed as randomized controlled trials (RCTs). A Cochrane Review titled "Cognitive Rehabilitation for Memory Deficits after Stroke"[119] included 13 controlled trials of memory training where at least 75% of patients had had a stroke. The results of these studies suggested that training improved subjective reports of short-term memory, but no evidence of sustained long-term benefits were demonstrated. There was no evidence to support or refute the use of cognitive rehabilitation for memory deficits to improve functional independence.

Impairments of Executive Functions

1. *Definition.* As defined by Lezak, "executive functions consist of those capacities that enable a person to engage successfully in independent, purposive, self-serving behavior."[4] Lezak goes on to describe executive functions as consisting of four overlapping components: volition, planning, purposive action, and effective performance.

   Volition is the capacity to determine what one needs and wants to do. It also encompasses a future realization of one's needs and wants. This encompasses goal planning and task initiation, self-awareness, awareness of the environment, and social awareness.

   Planning is "the identification and organization of the steps and elements (e.g., skills, material, other persons) needed to carry out an intention or achieve a goal."[4, p. 653] Planning involves weighing alternatives and making choices.

   Purposive action includes productivity and self-regulation, which encompasses the ability to initiate, maintain, switch, and stop complex action sequences in an orderly manner to realize a goal.

   Effective performance is the capacity for quality control, including the ability to self-monitor and self-correct one's behavior. Problems with effective performance are associated with ineffective self-monitoring and difficulty with self-correction; for example, patients may not even perceive their mistakes, whereas others may identify them but take no action to correct them.[120]

2. *Clinical Examples.* Although some patients with executive function disorders are unable to formulate realistic goals or intentions (volition) or plan, others may be able to formulate goals and initiate goal-directed task performance, but owing to defective planning are not able to realize their goals. Patients with planning problems may say or intend one thing but do another.[4] Family and hospital staff may complain of the patient's apparent apathy, poor or unreliable judgment, inappropriate behavior, difficulty adapting to new situations, and/or lack of attention to the needs and feelings of others.[120]
3. *Lesion Area.* Executive functions have traditionally been associated with the frontal and prefrontal cortex,[6] but the current view is that these capacities are mediated by reciprocal connections with other cortical and subcortical regions via the dorsolateral prefrontal–subcortical circuit.[121]
4. *Testing.* Tests of executive functions include the *Behavioural Assessment of the Dysexecutive Syndrome (BADS),*[72] the *Executive Functions Assessment,*[122] and the *Good Samaritan Hospital for Cognitive Rehabilitation's Executive Functions Behavioural Rating Scale.*[123]
5. *Treatment Suggestions.* The combination of impulsiveness, poor judgment, poor planning ability, and lack of foresight, which is particularly problematic in patients with left hemiplegia, does not bode well for independent functioning. The severity of these impairments may diminish somewhat over time.[9] Although some general remedial and adaptive treatment suggestions are described here, for more specific details refer to Ponsford et al[110] and Duran and Fisher.[120]
   a. *Remedial Approach.* By providing structure, feedback, and routine, a person's performance can be enhanced (e.g., providing structure by giving the patient steps to follow, assisting the task to become routine by repeated practice, or providing immediate feedback about the patient's behavior and the effect it has on others). The therapist initially acts as the patient's frontal lobes and gradually transfers these responsibilities to the patient. Unless the patient has some awareness of the problems, a remedial approach will not be particularly successful.[110] Honda[124] reported a study with three patients over a 6-month period who were provided with self-instructional training, a problem-solving procedure, and physical-set-changing exercises described as moving the four extremities and trunk in time to a metronome. In this study, "Patients were instructed to follow a videotape for 20 minutes. In the tape, a physical therapist moves four extremities and his trunk in time to a metronome. He changes activities every 2 or 3 minutes. The patients were trained with these methods for a total of 6 months. In the self-instructional procedure and problem-solving training phase, psychologists guided and trained patients 1 hour per day twice a week. In the physical-set-changing exercise phase, patients were advised to practice twice a day watching the instruction videotape. Each training phase lasted 6 weeks."[124, p. 18] While two of the subjects revealed improvements on the neuropsychological test used as an outcome measure, all subjects improved in basic and instrumental ADL. Of course, a limitation of this study is the small sample size and lack of control subjects, since it could be expected that these patients would make spontaneous recovery over the 6-month study period.

      Hewitt el al[125] proposed that people with TBI have difficulty with planning because they are not spontaneously using autobiographic memories. The authors asked a control and experimental group of 15 subjects to describe how they would plan common activities. The experimental group underwent a 30-minute training session aimed at prompting retrieval of specific memories to support planning. This intervention was found to be effective in increasing specific memories that could aid planning.
   b. *Compensatory Approach.* The therapist can assist the patient to compensate for poor abilities by utilizing other intact cognitive functions and/or modifying the environment. For example, the therapist might ask the patient to perform a task in a room with minimal distractions or change the demands of the patient's work, home, or community to diminish the need to employ executive functions. A beeper or alarm clock may be used to help a patient overcome poor initiation.

      A Cochrane Review titled "Cognitive Rehabilitation for Executive Dysfunction in Adults With Stroke or Other Adult Non-Progressive Acquired Brain Damage"[126] revealed 13 controlled trials of cognitive rehabilitation to reduce executive dysfunction in adults with traumatic brain injury, stroke, or other non-progressive acquired brain injury. No evidence was found to support the use of cognitive rehabilitation to improve the functional independence of people with executive dysfunction.

Body Scheme and Body Image Impairments

Body image is defined as a visual and mental image of one's body that includes feelings about one's body, especially in relation to health and disease.[127] The term *body scheme* refers to a postural model of the body, including the relationship of body parts to each other and the relationship of the body to the environment. Commonly, body scheme and body image problems are termed *difficulties with body awareness.* Body awareness is derived from the integration of tactile, proprioceptive, and interoceptive (visceral) sensations, in addition to the individual's subjective feelings about the body.[127] An awareness of body scheme is considered one of the essential foundations for the performance of all purposeful motor behavior.[127] The terms *body awareness, body image,* and *body scheme* are often used interchangeably; therefore, when researching this topic, close attention should be paid to the particular definition put forth by each author. Specific impairments of body image and body scheme are unilateral neglect, somatoagnosia, right–left discrimination, finger agnosia, and anosognosia.

Unilateral Neglect

1. *Definition. Unilateral neglect* is the inability to register and integrate stimuli and perceptions from one side of the body (*body neglect*) and the environment or hemispace (*spatial neglect* of the area surrounding one side of the body), which is not due to a sensory loss. Unilateral neglect is also referred to as *unilateral spatial neglect, hemi-inattention, hemineglect,* and *unilateral visual inattention.*[128] It is important for the therapist to be familiar with this disorder because it is a frequent clinical finding. Neglect following right cerebral infarction has been reported in between 12% and 95% of patients.[129] The reporting rates vary enormously due to differences in time selected for reporting and techniques used to detect the neglect. However, this disorder is commonly seen in the clinic as having a functional impact on about 20% of patients. Unilateral neglect usually, although not always, affects the left side of the body or hemispace. For purposes of this discussion, we will assume that it is the left. If a patient has unilateral neglect, he or she seems to ignore the left side of the body and stimuli occurring in the left personal space. This may occur despite intact visual fields, or concomitantly with right or left homonymous hemianopia; however, it is not caused by homonymous hemianopia.[130]

When working with a patient who has unilateral neglect, the therapist should also determine which sensory modalities are affected, including visual, tactile, and auditory. Input from one or all of these modalities may be neglected. Neglect can also be understood in terms of the area of space that is neglected. For example, unilateral neglect may express itself as a disorder of attention and goal-directed behavior in:

- Contralesional personal space (defined as pertaining to the body) such as shaving only the right half of the face or failing to wash the left side of the body.
- Contralesional peripersonal space (that area of space within arm distance); for example, failing to use objects on the contralesional side of the meal tray.
- Contralesional extrapersonal space (that area of space beyond arm length), such as failing to negotiate obstacles, doorways, and so forth, during locomotion.[50,128]

Unilateral neglect is also demonstrated by an impaired ability to attend to either the object or the environment as a whole. It is possible that while some patients may neglect half of the environment, others may neglect half of objects in the total environment. In the first case, the patient may neglect most elements of the left side of the entire visual scene (Fig. 27.8). In the second case, a patient may neglect the left side of an object, regardless of its absolute position in the visual display. For example, the patient may neglect the left side of a cup even though it is on his or her right side or omit the left side of objects when drawing items such as an umbrella, picnic basket, and bucket and spade as depicted in Figure 27.9.

Frequently, a patient with unilateral neglect has sensory loss on the more affected side, which compounds the problem. Although a patient with left-sided hemianopia

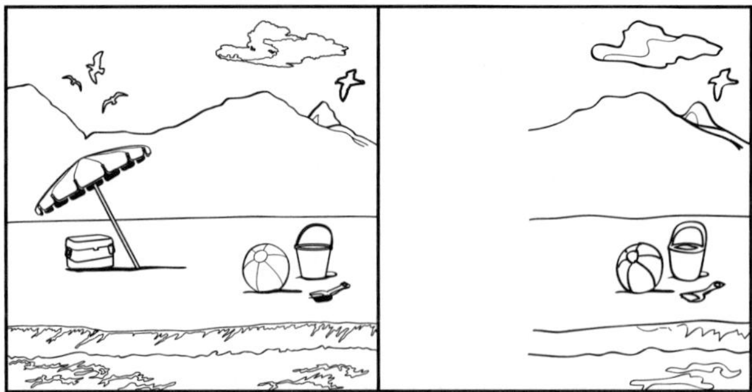

Figure 27.8 Example of a drawing by a patient with unilateral neglect. Therapist's drawing of a beach scene (left). Impaired copying by a patient with unilateral neglect—environment neglect following a stroke (right).

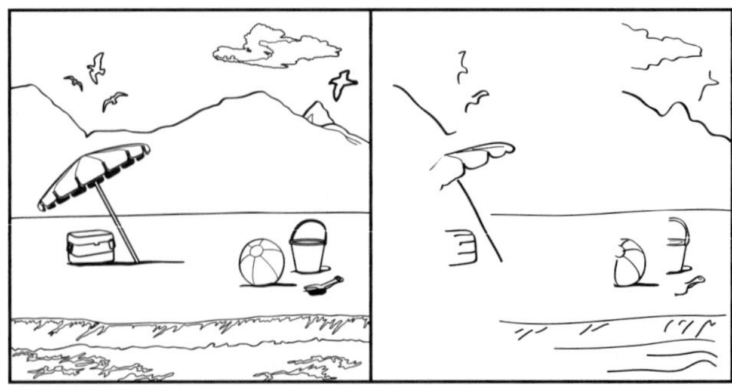

Figure 27.9 Example of a drawing by a patient with unilateral neglect. Therapist's drawing of a beach scene (left). Impaired copying by a patient with unilateral neglect—object neglect following a stroke (right).

has actual loss of vision from the left visual field of both eyes, he or she may be aware of the problem and compensate automatically or learn to compensate by turning the head. A patient with visual neglect has intact vision but seems unaware of the problem and does not attempt to compensate spontaneously by turning the head. In extreme cases the patient appears totally indifferent to the left side of the body and environment, and may deny that the left extremities belong to him or her.[131] More time seems to be required to learn to compensate for this impairment than for hemianopia. There is great difficulty in integrating all stimuli from the left half of the body and personal space for use in ADL skills. As with hemianopia, the patient with visual unilateral neglect often avoids crossing the midline visually or motorically.[61]

2. *Clinical Examples.* The patient may ignore the left half of the body when dressing and forget to put on the left sleeve or left pants leg. Often a male patient will forget to shave the left half of his face. A woman may neglect to put makeup on the left side of her face.[132] The patient may neglect to eat from the left half of a plate and will start reading a newspaper from the middle of the line. Typically, the patient bumps into objects on the left side or tends to veer toward the right when walking or propelling a wheelchair.
3. *Lesion Area.* It has been suggested that lesions involving the inferior–posterior regions of the right parietal lobe are significant determinants of neglect.[130,133]
4. *Testing.* A variety of techniques are useful. No single test is adequate to identify unilateral neglect in all patients because the impairment may be manifested differently in each patient.

   The *Behavioural Inattention Test (BIT)*[73] can be used to examine unilateral neglect (see Table 27.1). The patient may also be observed during basic activities of daily living such as dressing or an IADL such as preparing a meal. The therapist observes performance and observes changes in the patient's behavior in response to cueing.
5. *Treatment Suggestions.*
   a. *Remedial Approach.* The purpose of therapy is to increase awareness of the left side of the body and space. Current beliefs concerning the mechanisms underlying unilateral neglect guide the majority of treatment approaches. Rizzolatti and Berti[134] combine the popular attentional and representational models in their premotor theory of neglect. The basis of this theory is that spatial attention is dependent on several independent neural circuits. Attention, and therefore perception of stimuli, is enhanced as a direct result of activation of motor circuits, as occurs when a person moves. Hence, activating motor circuits of the ipsilesional hemisphere (via voluntary movements of the left upper or lower limbs) may facilitate associated sensory circuits. Such movement may in turn lead to improvements in the processing of stimuli from the contralesional (left) side.[128]

      Capitalizing on the rationale of the premotor theory of neglect, the following suggestions are proposed. Stimuli that are specialized for the right side of the brain, such as shapes and blocks, should be used to enhance right brain activation. At the same time, the presence of stimuli that are known to activate the left side of the brain, such as letters and numbers, should be minimized. Use of verbal instructions should be minimized. Simple verbal instructions should be used to encourage the patient to turn the head to the left to anchor his or her attention to that side of space.[131] In addition, research suggests that conducting motor activities with the left body side, such as simply clenching and unclenching the fist, can improve attention to the left body side and hemispace. Robertson et al[135] conducted a study with six individuals with hemiplegia who were asked to walk through a doorway. Each of the subject's walking trajectory (pathway) was measured, and it was found that all trajectories were significantly deviated to the right of center. The subjects were then asked to clench and unclench their left hands before, and during, walking through the doorway. The researchers found that this procedure significantly assisted subjects to center their walking trajectories.

      Another version of this technique was used by Grattan et al[136] when they examined the effectiveness of left upper-limb specific training to reduce the effects of unilateral spatial neglect. Their study found small, but statistically significant, improvements in upper-limb function and use can be attained via repetitive task-specific practice, suggesting that this intervention may be promising for people with unilateral neglect. However, the authors note that these findings may not be generalizable to all clients with unilateral neglect and that further evaluation is necessary to determine efficacy. Other techniques that have been used to treat patients with unilateral neglect include mirror therapy, eye-patching, optokinetic stimulation and prism adaptation, neck vibration,[137] and trunk rotation.[138] A review of these treatment techniques may be found in Luauté et al.[139]

      Pandian et al[140] conducted an RCT using mirror therapy for unilateral neglect 48 hours after stroke. During mirror therapy, a mirror box was placed vertically on a table in front of subjects to reflect their unaffected hand while their affected hand was inside the mirror box, out of view. Subjects were instructed to flex and extend both hands (limb activation as described by Robertson[135] and Grattan et al[136]) while they saw the reflection of the unaffected hand movements in the mirror. Subjects received mirror therapy treatment for 1 to 2 hours a day, 5 days a week, for 4 weeks. Results indicated that mirror therapy is a simple intervention that can improve unilateral neglect in stroke patients. Eye-patching is another treatment approach, whereby the right visual field of each eye is covered in order to encourage the patient to focus their attention to the left visual space.[141] However, an RCT of 12 subjects conducted by Aparicio-López et al[142] found that eye-patching does not improve functional performance over and above cognitive rehabilitation alone. Prism adaptation involves the use of prism lenses, glasses, or goggles (Fig. 27.10) worn by the patient to shift the left visual field into the right so that there is partial recovery of the left work space. This provides patients with a representation of the left field of view, facilitating the recall and relearning of previously learned behaviors.[143] An evidence review of studies investigating the effectiveness of prism adaptation as an intervention to increase spatial awareness in patients with unilateral neglect following stroke is included in Table 27.4.[144-152]

b. *Compensatory Approach.* The patient is initially educated about the condition, and then strategies to assist managing everyday activities are devised. For example, when reading a book or newspaper, a red ribbon may be placed on the left margin and the patient is taught to scan back to this point after completing each line. The environment may also be adapted within this approach. The patient is addressed and given demonstrations from the less affected side. The nursing staff should place the patient's call button, telephone, and other essential items on the less affected side.

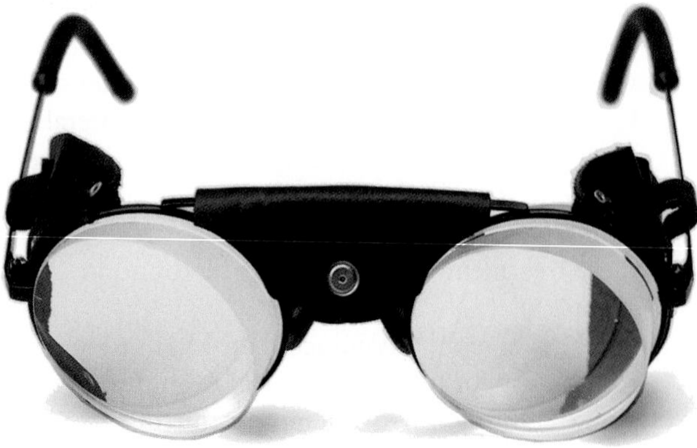

Figure 27.10 An example of Prism goggles. *(From Optique Peter, http://optiquepeter.com/en/index.php. Used with permission.)*

A bold red line may be drawn on the side of the page that is neglected.[127] A mirror may be placed in front of the patient while he or she is dressing or ambulating to draw attention to the neglected side.

An extensive Cochrane Review[153] was conducted concerning the effectiveness of therapy for unilateral neglect, drawing on the abundance of studies and trials conducted on this puzzling disorder over the past 20 years. Bowen et al[153] reviewed 23 controlled trials and concluded that there is very limited evidence supporting reduced impairment, as measured by tabletop tests of neglect. However, the effects of cognitive rehabilitation on reducing activity limitations, as measured by functional assessments, remains unclear. Additional well-designed RCTs of interventions as well as more basic research to develop function outcome measures in the field are required.

Anosognosia

1. *Definition.* Anosognosia is defined as a lack of awareness, or denial, of a paretic extremity as belonging to the person, or a lack of insight concerning, or denial of, paralysis and disability.[50] Presence of this condition may greatly compromise rehabilitation potential, because it limits the patient's ability to recognize the need for, and thus to use, compensatory techniques.
2. *Clinical Examples.* Typically, the patient maintains that there is nothing wrong and may disown the paralyzed limbs and refuse to accept responsibility for them. The patient may claim that the limb has a mind of its own or that it was left at home or in a closet.
3. *Lesion Area.* The pathogenesis of anosognosia remains unclear,[50] although the region of the supramarginal gyrus has been proposed.[154]
4. *Testing.* Anosognosia is identified by talking to the patient. The patient is asked what happened to the arm or leg, whether he or she is paralyzed, how the limb feels, and why it cannot be moved. A patient with anosognosia may deny the paralysis and disability, say that it is of no concern, and fabricate reasons why a limb does not move the way it should.
5. *Treatment Suggestions.* Anosognosia often resolves spontaneously in the first 3 months following stroke.[143] Maeshima et al[155] also noted that until the condition resolves, it seriously hampers rehabilitation. It is extremely difficult to compensate for the condition if it persists long-term. Safety is of paramount importance in the treatment and discharge planning for patients suffering from anosognosia, because they typically do not acknowledge their disability and will therefore refuse to be careful.[9]

Table 27.4 Evidence Summary Evidence Addressing the Use of Prism Adaptation as an Intervention to Increase Visual Function in Patients With Unilateral Neglect Following Stroke

Goedert et al[144] (2014)	
Design	Prospective cohort design
Level of Evidence	II B Moderate evidence
Subjects	24 Ss with L UN (BIT ≤129 or CBS>1) were divided into groups based on their spatial neglect profile: (1) perceptual-attentional "Where" spatial processing deficit, (2) motor-intentional "Aiming" spatial processing deficit, or (3) both. IC = R-handed within 6 to 47 days poststroke, exhibiting rightward error on a computerized line bisection task. EC = Ss more than 60 days poststroke with L hemisphere lesions, prior history of neurological or psychiatric conditions, uncorrected ocular disorders, or leftward line bisection error.
Intervention	All Ss wore prism glasses that shifted the field of view 12.4° to the R during PAT on a line bisection task once a day, for 15–20 minutes, for 10 days. Two pointing tasks were also administered to test for Ss ability to adapt to prisms with and without visual input. Ss assessed on the CBS before, during, and after PAT to examine functional improvement.
Results	Ss with only "Aiming" deficits improved on the CBS, whereas Ss with both deficits showed moderate improvement, and Ss with only "Where" deficits did not improve. Improvement following PA was predicted by spatial neglect profile, whereby Ss with only "Aiming" deficits demonstrated greater improvement compared with Ss with only "Where" deficits or both deficits, respectively.
Comments	The authors suggest that future stroke treatment trials consider classification of Ss based on spatial processing deficits.
Jacquin-Courtois et al[145] (2010)	
Design	Random allocation of Ss to E and C but randomization not blind and not fully reported.
Level of Evidence	II B Moderate Evidence
Subjects	22 Ss, 12 with RH stroke and 10 healthy Ss. IC for stroke Ss = no previous neurological damage; L neglect as detected using line cancelation, line bisection, and a copy drawing task; L ear extinction; adequate hearing; R handedness. 11 Ss randomly assigned each to E or C groups. No differences between E and C Ss at baseline for age, or time between stroke and entry to the study.
Intervention	Sought to determine if PA effects generalize to those neglect symptoms not directly linked to visuo-manual adaptation. Hence, auditory extinction was assessed in neglect Ss before and after treatment with prism glasses. E = wore prism glasses with a 10° shift to the R. C = wore neutral glasses. Outcome measures included a verbal dichotic listening task, including 60 pairs of stimuli administered to the R and L ears simultaneously. Duration E = 50 pointing responses to visual targets presented 10° to the R or L of midline lasting approximately 8 min. Dichotic listening test presented 3 times; before prisms, after prisms, and 2 hr later. C = neutral glasses and same dichotic listening test.
Results	PA found to improve L sided auditory dichotic listening tasks immediately after PA, and when measured 2 hr later.
Comments	The findings suggest that visual adaptation may also affect performance in other sensory modalities (audition) and suggests PA may have broader treatment effects than for vision alone.

Continued

Table 27.4 Evidence Summary Evidence Addressing the Use of Prism Adaptation as an Intervention to Increase Visual Function in Patients With Unilateral Neglect Following Stroke—cont'd

	Mizuno et al[146] (2011)
Design	Multicenter, double-blind, RCT
Level of Evidence	I A Strong evidence
Subjects	38 Ss with UN were divided into groups based on neglect severity (mild ≥55 and severe < 55). IC = first hemiparetic stroke, admission within 3 months of onset, no severe mental deterioration using MMSE, RH damage, and scores on the BIT. EC = unable to sit on wheelchair, unable to understand task due to mental deterioration or aphasia, unable to understand Japanese, extremely impaired eyesight, severe hearing loss, unable to reach with the R upper extremity due to restricted ROM, R upper-extremity amputation more proximal to half of the forearm, severe position sense deficits of R fingers due to peripheral neuropathy, and past medical history of head trauma or ventriculoperitoneal shunt. E = 18, C = 20 Gender (M/F): E = 12/6, C = 15/5. No differences between mean days from onset to intervention, mean hospital stay, MMSE score, and SIAS motor score.
Intervention	E = repeated pointing with the index finger of the R nonparetic hand to 3 targets through the bottom of a table while wearing prism glasses that shifted the field of view 12° to the R twice daily, 5 days per week, for 2 weeks. C = same task while wearing neutral glasses. Data collected: baseline (study entry), post-treatment (after 2-week intervention), and at follow-up (discharge). Measures: BIT, CBS, FIM, and SIAS.
Results	PA found to significantly improve scores on the FIM. In Ss with mild UN, prism adaptation found to significantly improve scores on BIT and FIM, suggesting reduction of neglect symptoms and improvement in ADL, is therefore effective for reducing neglect symptoms and improvement of ADL.
Comments	PA can significantly improve ADL, as measured on FIM, only in patients with mild stroke. This finding suggests that PA could improve rehabilitation outcome for early poststroke patients in a conventional rehabilitation program. There was more than a 3-month delay, on average, postintervention of this study, demonstrating a marked long-term effect of PA compared with previous research. Among studies on prism adaptation, this sample size is the largest reported to date.
	Priftis et al[147] (2013)
Design	Quasi-randomized clinical trial
Level of Evidence	II B Moderate evidence
Subjects	31 Ss with L UN were divided (quasi-randomly) into three treatment groups (VST, LAT, or PA). VST = 10, LAT = 10, PA =11. IC = unilateral lesions due to first stroke confirmed by CT or MRI scan, no previous UN treatment received, absence of dementia confirmed by neuropsychological history and interview. EC = medical history of substance abuse and psychiatric disorders.
Intervention	Ss in the VST group were verbally instructed to "look at the pink-colored stripe" placed along the left edge of a A4 landscape sheet of paper as they were required to fill out only parts of drawings that had a little black point inside. Ss in the LAT group were required to fill out the same drawings as the VST group; however, they were instructed to use their L arm to turn off the buzzer on a LAT device that was set to emit a tone at fixed intervals of 240s (first week) and 120s (second week). Ss in the PA group were required to point toward 90 targets (a pen) presented in random order (90 center, 90 right, 90 left) wearing prism glasses that shifted the field of view 10° to the R. All Ss received treatment for 2 weeks. Data collected over time period of 6 weeks; everyday life task performance was assessed with the CBS 4 times; baseline (A1), 2 weeks after the end of A1 (A2), immediately after 2-week-long intervention (A3), and 2 weeks after the end of A3 (A4).

Table 27.4 Evidence Summary Evidence Addressing the Use of Prism Adaptation as an Intervention to Increase Visual Function in Patients With Unilateral Neglect Following Stroke—cont'd

	Priftis et al[147] (2013)
Results	All three treatment groups produced improvements, suggesting that they can be considered valid rehabilitation interventions for UN.
Comments	
	Rode et al[148] (2015)
Design	Double-blinded, monocentric RCT
Level of Evidence	II B Moderate evidence
Subjects	18 R-handed Ss with L UN were divided into groups based on neglect severity (mild > 55 and severe ≤ 55). IC = 18–90 years, single stroke, confirmed L UN, and time lapse of at least 1 month after the stroke. EC = multiple lesions, temporo-spatial disorientation, psychiatric disorders, and associated non-stabilized pathology. Block randomization based on two levels of neglect severity; E = 9 (mild = 6, severe = 3), C = 9 (mild = 6, severe = 3). Gender (M/F): E = 5/4, C = 5/4.
Intervention	E = pointing toward pseudo-randomly alternating targets 10° to the L or R of the middle of his/her body while wearing prism glasses that shifted the field of view 10° to the R; C = same task while wearing neutral glasses. Data collected: baseline (pre-test), and 1, 3, and 6 months after each PA session. Measures: FIM, BIT.
Results	At 6-month follow-up, no difference was found between groups. 4 weeks of PA did not provide additional long-term functional benefits in comparison to spontaneous recovery.
Comments	Although benefits produced by PA are maintained at conclusion of treatment, more intensive PAT is suggested to provide additional long-term gains above and beyond spontaneous recovery.
	Sarri et al[149] (2011)
Design	Prospective cohort design
Level of Evidence	II B Moderate evidence
Subjects	11 Ss with L UN.
Intervention	Ss were administered 3 tasks before and immediately after PA (chimeric face task lateral preference task, gradients lateral preference task, and chimeric/non-chimeric face discrimination task). The chimeric face task was composed of 20 pairs of photographed faces. Each pair of faces consisted of a mirror-reversed image of the same person's photograph divided along the vertical midline with a smiling facial expression on one half or side of the face and a neutral expression on the other side. Ss were asked to choose the face they thought "looked happier." The gradients lateral preference task comprised 20 pairs of grayscale gradient rectangles of a continuous scale ranging from absolute black at one end to absolute white at the other end. Each pair was the mirror-reversed image of the other and separated by 2 cm, one strip placed above the other. Ss were asked to report whether the upper or lower strip of each pair appeared darker. The chimeric/non-chimeric face discrimination task consisted of 40 face stimuli: 20 non-chimeric "real" faces and 20 chimeric faces (as described in the chimeric face task). Ss were asked to indicate whether each face stimulus was "real" or "chimeric." Ss also completed 2 line bisections and 5 subjective straight-ahead pointing (with R hand and eyes closed) to measure neglect. During PA, Ss pointed toward targets placed in randomly intermingled sequence, 10° to the L or R of the middle of his/her body, while wearing prism glasses that shifted the field of view 10° to the R.

Continued

Table 27.4 Evidence Summary Evidence Addressing the Use of Prism Adaptation as an Intervention to Increase Visual Function in Patients With Unilateral Neglect Following Stroke—cont'd

	Sarri et al[149] (2011)
Results	PA did not benefit Ss performance on spatial preference tasks (e.g., chimeric face task lateral preference task, gradients lateral preference task) compared to standard measures of neglect (line bisection, subjective straight-ahead). Results indicated that 3 out of 6 Ss benefited from PA on the chimeric/non-chimeric face discrimination task, suggesting that PA may improve awareness for the L side of face stimuli in some cases of UN.
Comments	The authors suggest that further research could provide better understanding of the benefits of PA for certain patients or tasks but not others. This would potentially optimize PA as a tool for rehabilitation for UN.
	Serino et al[150] (2009)
Design	RCT
Level of Evidence	I A Strong evidence
Subjects	20 R-handed Ss with L UN were divided into matched groups based on neglect severity. IC = scores on the BIT. EC = widespread mental deterioration using MMSE or psychiatric disorders. E = 10, C = 10. Gender (M/F): E = 8/2; C = 6/4. No differences reported between mean age (E = 62, C = 61), education, or time since stroke.
Intervention	Matched pairs, comparison design. Prism glasses that shifted the field of view 10° to the R were worn by Ss in E group. Neglect measured before and after each treatment and 1 month after the end of treatment. During intervention, patients repeatedly point at visual target with R index finger. E and C = 90 trials each weekday (lasting approximately 30 min) for 2 weeks.
Results	Both groups improved; however, E showed statistically significant improvement over C. Effects confirmed 1 month after treatment ceased.
Comments	Design could be strengthened by random allocation to E and C with a larger sample to control for neglect severity. Further research to understand the mechanism by which prism adaptation may be working is required.
	Turton et al[151] (2010)
Design	RCT, randomization not blind
Level of Evidence	II B Moderate evidence
Subjects	34 Ss post-stroke with L neglect E = 16; C = 18 Mean age: E = 72; C = 71 Gender (M/F): E = 8/8, C = 11/7 Time post-onset (mean days): E = 45; C = 47 IC = RH stroke at least 20 days before study; self-care problems identified by OT, ability to sit and point with the unaffected hand, and ability to follow instructions.
Intervention	E = repeated touching of target with index finger on a box screen while wearing 10-diopter prism glasses that shifted the field of view 6° to the R; C = same task while wearing neutral glasses. E and C = 90 trials each weekday (lasting approximately 30 min) for 2 weeks. Data collected: 4 days after finishing treatment, at follow-up 4 weeks later. Measures: the CBS and pen-and-paper tests from the BIT.
Results	E = showed increased leftward bias in pointing to targets, but no effect of treatment on BIT.

Table 27.4 Evidence Summary Evidence Addressing the Use of Prism Adaptation as an Intervention to Increase Visual Function in Patients With Unilateral Neglect Following Stroke—cont'd

	Turton et al[151] (2010)
Comments	Study appeared to control for bias and compared well-matched groups. Authors suggested differences may not have shown since outcomes were measured 4 days after treatment ended, and previous literature suggests that treatment effect may be immediate and short-lived. Authors also suggested that although the current study used prisms that shifted the field of view 6° to R, other studies have used 10° and 15° prisms, and research is needed to determine optimum prism strength and frequency of treatment sessions.
	Watanabe and Amimoto[152] (2010)
Design	Prospective cohort design, with staff blinded to purpose of the research.
Level of Evidence	III B Moderate evidence
Subjects	10 Ss with UN. IC = R-handed with R hemisphere lesion sustained within past 40 days, and capable of driving a wheelchair for 7 m (23 ft) without assistance. EC = unable to distinguish symbols due to visual impairment, who could not understand the research tasks, and if accomplishing the task would be physically difficult. Ss then further screened with Japanese edition of the BIT and were below the cutoff score in at least one of the subtests.
Intervention	E = Ss wore fitted prism glasses, displacing Ss visual field by 7° to R. Ss then reached 50 times in front of them in quick succession with R hand for a target. Ss were then blindfolded and measured in 10 trials of pointing straight ahead, and then a wheelchair driving task. Ss timed as they drove 7 m to reach a cone target. Same day pre-test post-test
Results	10 Ss completed all tasks. Significant shifts between pre-test and post-test in straightening of pointing and in reaching the target faster in the wheelchair.
Comments	Findings suggest generalization of PA on both a pointing task and the ADL task of driving a wheelchair. Study would benefit from use of a control group.

ADL = activities of daily living; BIT = Behavioural Inattention Test; C = control group; CBS = Catherine Bergego Scale; CT = computed tomography; E = experimental group; EC = exclusion criteria; F = female; FIM = Functional Independence Measure; IC = inclusion criteria; L = left; LAT = limbic activation treatment; M = male; MMSE = Mini-Mental Status Examination; MRI = magnetic resonance imaging; OT = occupational therapist; PA = prism adaptation; PAT = prism adaptation treatment; R = right; RCT = randomized controlled trial; RH = right hemisphere; ROM = range of motion; Ss = subject, subjects; SIAS = Stroke Impairment Assessment Set; UN = unilateral neglect; VST = visual scanning training

Somatoagnosia

1. *Definition.* **Somatoagnosia**, or impairment in body scheme, is a lack of awareness of the body structure and the relationship of body parts to oneself or to others. Somatoagnosia is also referred to as *autotopagnosia,* or simply *body agnosia.*[156] Patients with this deficit may display difficulty following instructions that require distinguishing body parts and may be unable to imitate movements of the therapist.[67] Often patients report that the more affected arm or leg feels unduly heavy. Lack of proprioception may underlie or compound this disorder.[157]
2. *Clinical Examples.* The patient may have difficulty performing transfer activities because he or she does not perceive the meaning of terms related to body parts; for example, "Pivot on your leg and reach for the armrest with your hand." In addition, a patient with a body scheme disorder will have difficulty dressing. Patients may have a hard time participating in exercises that require some body parts to be moved in relation to other body parts; for example, "Bring your arm across your chest and touch your shoulder."
3. *Lesion Area.* The lesion site is often the dominant parietal lobe.[154] Therefore, this disorder is seen primarily with right hemiplegia. However, impairment in body scheme may also occur with left hemiplegia.
4. *Testing.*
   a. The patient is requested to point to body parts named by the therapist, on himself or herself, on the therapist, and on a picture or puzzle of a human figure. Zoltan[2] provides details of these testing procedures. An example of verbal directives from these tests is, "Show me your feet.

Show me your chin. Point to your back." The words *right* and *left* should not be used because they may lead to an inaccurate diagnosis in patients who have difficulty with right–left discrimination. Aphasia should be ruled out as a cause of poor performance.

b. The patient is asked to imitate movements of the therapist. For example, the therapist touches his or her cheek, arm, leg, and so forth. A mirror-image response is acceptable.[2]

c. The patient is requested to answer questions about the relationship of body parts. For example, "Are your knees below your head? Which is on top of your head, your hair or your feet?" For patients with aphasia, questions should be phrased to require a yes or no, or true or false response. Patients with intact function in this area should respond correctly most of the time and within a reasonable period of time. Those patients with receptive aphasia are particularly likely to do poorly on tests for somatoagnosia.[156]

5. *Treatment Suggestions.* Using a remedial approach, the therapist aims for the patient to associate sensory input with an adaptive motor response.[2] Facilitation of body awareness is accomplished through sensory stimulation to the body part affected. For example, the patient is asked to rub the appropriate body part with a rough cloth as the therapist names it or points to it.[22] Alternatively, the patient verbally identifies body parts, or points to pictures of them as the therapist touches them.

Right-Left Discrimination

1. *Definition.* A right–left discrimination disorder is the inability to identify the right and left sides of one's own body or that of the examiner.[130] This includes the inability to execute movements in response to verbal commands that include the terms *right* and *left*. Patients are often unable to imitate movements.[130]
2. *Clinical Examples.* The patient cannot tell the therapist which is the right arm and which is the left. The right shoe cannot be discerned from the left shoe, and the patient is unable to follow instructions using the concept of right–left, such as "turn right at the corner." The patient cannot distinguish the right from the left side of the therapist.
3. *Lesion Area.* The lesion site is the parietal lobe of either hemisphere.[130] A close relationship between aphasia (usually owing to left-hemisphere damage) and deficits in right–left discrimination has been reported. In patients without aphasia (usually those with right-hemisphere damage), a relationship has been reported between general mental impairment and right–left discrimination disorder.[156]
4. *Testing.* The patient is asked to point to body parts on command, such as right ear, left foot, right arm, and so forth. Six responses should be elicited on either the patient's own body, on that of the therapist, or on a model or picture of the human body.[156] To rule out somatoagnosia, the patient should be tested first without using the words *right* and *left*.
5. *Treatment Suggestions.* If using a compensatory approach, when giving instructions to the patient, the words *right* and *left* should be avoided. Instead, pointing or providing cues using distinguishing features of the limb may be more effective (e.g., "the arm with the watch"). These guidelines are particularly salient for the therapist teaching locomotion or transfers, where confusing instructions may have dangerous consequences. The right side of all common objects such as shoes and clothing should be marked with red tape or seam binding.

Finger Agnosia

1. *Definition.* Finger agnosia can be defined as the inability to identify the fingers of one's own hands or of the hands of the examiner.[130]
2. *Clinical Examples.* The disorder is characterized by difficulty in naming the fingers on command, identifying which finger was touched, and, by some definitions, mimicking finger movements. This deficit usually occurs bilaterally and is more common in the middle three fingers.[158] Finger agnosia correlates highly with poor dexterity in tasks that require movements of individual fingers in relation to each other,[1] such as buttoning, tying laces, and typing.
3. *Lesion Area.* Finger agnosia may be the result of a lesion located in either parietal lobe,[159] often in the region of the angular gyrus of the left hemisphere. It is often found in conjunction with an aphasic disorder,[156] or with general mental impairment.[130,156] Bilateral finger agnosia along with right–left discrimination problems, agraphia, and *acalculia* is termed *Gerstmann's syndrome.*[130] Gerstmann's syndrome usually is associated with a focal lesion of the dominant hemisphere in the region of the angular gyrus.[154]
4. *Testing.* A portion of *Sauguet's test*[2,156] is recommended. Sauguet's test includes asking the patient to move or point to his or her finger when named by the therapist to determine if finger agnosia is present. Between five and ten commands from the therapist is adequate. The test is not standardized.

a. The patient is asked to name the fingers touched by the therapist, with the eyes open (five times) and if successful, with vision occluded (five times).

b. The patient is asked to point to the fingers named by the therapist on the patient's own hands (10 times), on the therapist's hands (10 times), and on a schematic model (10 times).

c. The patient is asked to point to the equivalent finger on a life-sized picture when the therapist touches each finger.

d. The patient is asked to imitate finger movements; for example, curl the index finger, touch the thumb to the middle finger.

5. *Treatment Suggestions.* There is very limited evidence to support the efficacy of treatment techniques for finger agnosia. When using a remedial approach, the patient's discriminative tactile systems (touch and pressure) are stimulated. A rough cloth can be used to rub the dorsal surface of the more affected arm, hand, and fingers, and the ventral surface of the more affected fingers. Pressure can be applied to the ventral surface of the hand. For additional details the reader is referred to Zoltan.[2]

Spatial Relations Disorders (Complex Perception)

Spatial relations disorders encompass a constellation of impairments that have in common a difficulty in perceiving the relationship between the self and two or more objects.[159] Research suggests that the right parietal lobe plays a primary role in space perception. Thus, a spatial relations impairment most frequently occurs in patients with right-sided lesions with resulting left hemiparesis.[159]

Spatial relations disorders include impairments of figure–ground discrimination, form discrimination, spatial relations, position in space, and topographical disorientation. Additional visuospatial impairments, such as depth and distance perception and vertical disorientation, will also be discussed in this section. In a study comparing the effectiveness of the cognitive remediation (sometimes referred to as the *transfer-of-training technique*) versus the functional approach, Edmans et al[161] found that both approaches were equally successful in treating perceptual impairments. However, since this study did not control for the effects of spontaneous recovery in both groups, further research is required.

Figure-Ground Discrimination

1. *Definition.* An impairment in visual figure–ground discrimination is the inability to visually distinguish a figure from the background in which it is embedded.[5] Functionally, it interferes with the patient's ability to locate important objects that are not prominent in a visual array. The patient has difficulty ignoring irrelevant visual stimuli and cannot select the appropriate cue to which to respond.[5] This may lead to distractibility, resulting in a shortened attention span,[162] frustration, and decreased independent and safe functioning.[67]

2. *Clinical Examples.* The patient cannot locate items in a pocketbook or drawer, locate buttons on a shirt, or distinguish the armhole from the remainder of a solid-colored shirt. The patient may not be able to tell when one step ends and another begins on a flight of stairs, especially when descending.

3. *Lesion Area.* Parieto-occipital lesions of the right hemisphere and less frequently the left hemisphere commonly produce this disorder.[163]

4. *Testing.*
   a. The *Ayres Figure–Ground Test* (subtest of the *Southern California Sensory Integration Tests*)[164] requires the subject to distinguish the three objects in an embedded test picture, from a possible selection of six items. This test was standardized on children but may be useful as a clinical tool in identifying perceptual disorders in adults with brain damage.[4] Normative data have been generated for normal adult males.[165] Many other tests have since used a similar approach to test figure–ground perception by showing the patient overlapping line drawings of everyday objects and asking clients to name these as illustrated in Figure 27.11.
   b. *Function-Based Tests.* A white towel can be placed on a white sheet, and the patient is asked to find the towel. The patient can be asked to point out the sleeve, buttons, and collar of a white shirt or to pick out a spoon from an unsorted array of eating utensils. It is necessary to rule out poor eyesight, hemianopia, visual agnosia, and poor comprehension to improve the validity of these testing techniques.

5. *Treatment Suggestions.*
   a. *Remedial Approach.* The therapist should arrange for practice in visually locating objects in a simple array (such as three very different objects) and progress to more difficult ones (four or five dissimilar objects and three similar ones).
   b. *Compensatory Approach.* The patient is taught to become aware of the existence and nature of the

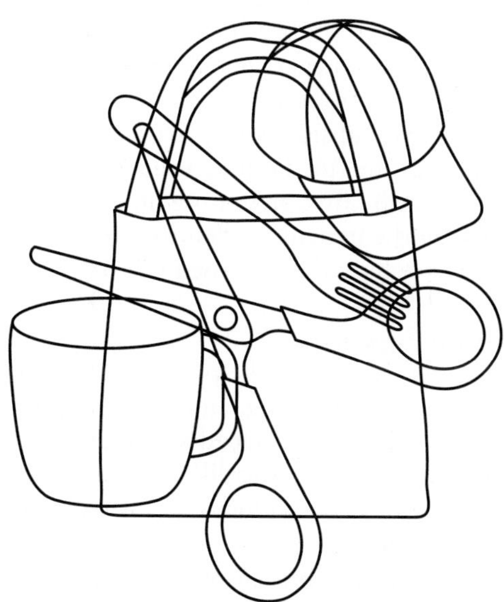

Figure 27.11 An example of a figure–ground perception test.

deficit. The patient should be cautioned to examine groups of objects slowly and systematically and should be instructed to use other, intact senses (e.g., touch) when searching for items such as clothing or silverware. When learning to lock a wheelchair, the patient should be advised to locate the brake levers by touch rather than by searching for them visually. Red tape may be placed over the hook-and-loop closure of the shoe or orthosis to aid the patient in locating it. Few items should be placed in the patient's drawers or nightstand, and they should be replaced in the same location each time. Brightly colored tape can be used to mark the edges on stairs. Repetition is a key element of this approach and repeated practice is used in each specific area of difficulty. The same procedure should be employed during each practice session, incorporating verbal cues and touch as adjuncts to vision.

Form Discrimination

1. *Definition.* Impairment in form discrimination is the inability to perceive or attend to subtle differences in form and shape. The patient is likely to confuse objects of similar shape or not to recognize an object placed in an unusual position.
2. *Clinical Examples.* The patient may confuse a pen with a toothbrush, a vase with a water pitcher, a cane with a crutch, and so forth.
3. *Lesion Area.* The lesion site is the parieto-temporo-occipital region (posterior association areas) of the nondominant lobe.[4]
4. *Testing.* A number of items similar in shape and different in size are gathered. The patient is asked to identify them. One set of items might be a pencil, pen, straw, toothbrush, and watch, and the other might be a key, paper clip, coins, and ring. Each object is presented several times in different positions (e.g., upside down). Visual object agnosia must be ruled out as a cause for poor performance by first presenting objects separately and asking the patient to identify them or to demonstrate how they are used (see "Visual Agnosias" below).
5. *Treatment Suggestions.*
   a. *Remedial Approach.* The patient should practice describing, identifying, and demonstrating the use of similarly shaped and sized objects. The patient should sort like objects and should be assisted to focus on differentiating object cues.
   b. *Compensatory Approach.* The patient must be made aware of the specific deficit. If the patient can read, frequently used and confused objects can be labeled. The patient should be encouraged to use vision, touch, and self-verbalization in combination when objects are confused.

Spatial Relations

1. *Definition.* A spatial relations disorder, or spatial disorientation, is the inability to perceive the relationship of one object in space to another object, or to oneself. This may lead to, or compound, problems in constructional tasks and dressing.[5] Crossing the midline may be a problem for patients with spatial relations deficits.[160] Spatial relations skills are required to manage most ADL.
2. *Clinical Examples.* The patient might find it difficult to place the cutlery, plate, and spoon in the proper position when setting the table. The patient may be unable to tell the time from an analog clock because of difficulty in perceiving the relative positions of the hands.[2,29] The patient may have difficulty learning to position his or her arms, legs, and trunk in relation to the wheelchair to prepare for transferring.
3. *Lesion Area.* The lesion site is predominantly the inferior parietal lobe or parieto-occipital-temporal junction, usually of the right side.[5] Arnadottir and Gudrun[160] explain how a patient with perceptual deficits may have difficulty putting on a shirt. This is illustrated in Figure 27.12. Since the CNS works in a holistic way, the task of putting on a shirt requires visual, tactile, and auditory information as well as attentional and memory capacities and motor output. Figure 27.12 suggests that while damage in a variety of brain areas may affect visuospatial processing, the most common lesion site is the right inferior parietal lobe.
4. *Testing.* Recommended tests include the *Rivermead Perceptual Assessment Battery (RPAB)*[85] and the *Arnadottir OT-ADL Neurobehavioural Evaluation (A-ONE).*[5] To improve the validity of these tests, unilateral neglect and hemianopia should be ruled out as the causes of poor performance. If these impairments are present, the stimulus array should be positioned appropriately.
5. *Treatment Suggestions.* When using a remedial approach, patient ability to orient to other objects can be improved by giving the patient instructions to position himself or herself in relation to the therapist or another object. The therapist might say, "Sit next to me," "Go behind the table," or "Step over the line." In addition, the therapist can set up a maze of furniture (obstacle course). Having the patient copy block or matchstick designs of increasing difficulty will increase awareness of the relationship between one object (block or matchstick) and the next. If the patient avoids crossing the midline,

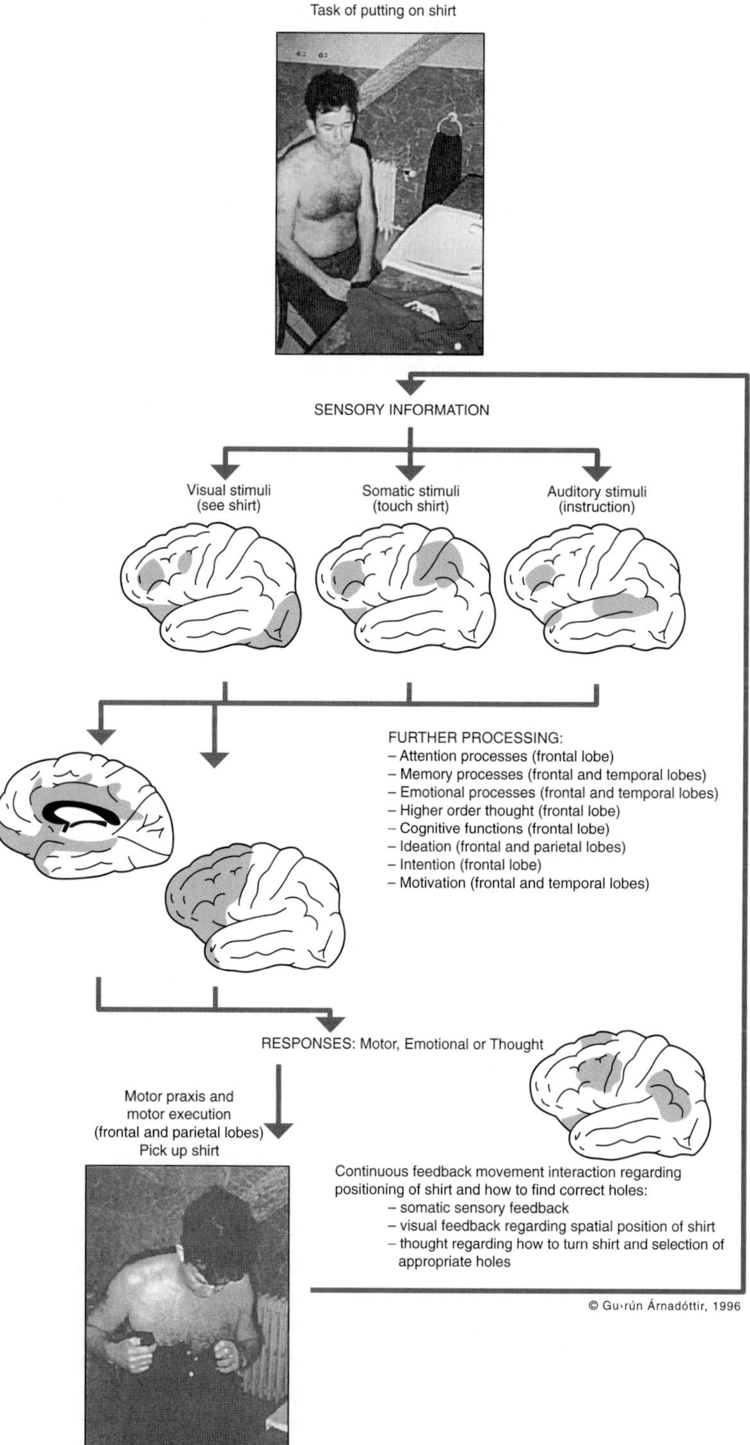

Figure 27.12 Spatial relation processing as a man puts on a shirt. *(From Arnadottir and Gudrun,[160, p. 405] with permission.)*

activities that require crossing the midline both motorically and visually can be incorporated into other therapeutic activities (e.g., proprioceptive neuromuscular facilitation chop patterns). One specific activity is to have the patient hold a dowel in front with both hands. The therapist guides it from the less involved side to the more involved side. Later, the patient can progress to manipulating the dowel with only verbal or visual cues, and finally to guiding it independently.[166]

Position in Space

1. *Definition.* Position in space impairment is the inability to perceive and to interpret spatial concepts such as up, down, under, over, in, out, in front of, and behind.

2. *Clinical Examples.* If a patient is asked to raise the arm "above" the head during ROM activities or is asked to place the feet "on" the footrests, the patient may behave as if he or she does not know what to do.
3. *Lesion Area.* The lesion is usually located in the nondominant parietal lobe.[163]
4. *Testing.* To test function, two objects are used, such as a shoe and a shoebox. The patient is asked to place the shoe in different positions in relation to the shoebox; for example, in the box, on top of the box, or next to the box. Alternatively, the patient is presented with two objects and asked to describe their relationship. For example, a toothbrush can be placed in a cup, under a cup, and so forth, and the patient is then asked to indicate the location of the toothbrush.

   Another mode of testing is to have the patient copy the therapist's manipulations with an identical set of objects. For example, the therapist hands the patient a comb and a brush. The therapist then takes an identical set and places them in a particular relationship to each other, such as the comb on top of the brush. The patient is requested to arrange his or her comb and brush in the same way. Success in this task may represent sufficient ability to use position in space functionally.

   Figure–ground difficulty, apraxia, incoordination, and lack of comprehension should be ruled out when performing these tests. Objects should be positioned to avoid compounding of results with hemianopia and unilateral spatial neglect.
5. *Treatment Suggestions.* If using a retraining approach, three or four identical objects are placed in the same orientation (wrist weights, combs, mugs, and so forth). An additional object is placed in a different orientation. The patient is asked to identify the odd one and then to place it in the same orientation as the other objects.

Topographical Disorientation

1. *Definition. Topographical disorientation* refers to difficulty in understanding and remembering the relationship of one location to another.[167] As a result, the patient is unable to get from one place to another, with or without a map. This disorder is frequently seen in conjunction with other difficulties in spatial relations.[45]
2. *Clinical Examples.* The patient cannot find the way from his or her room to the physical therapy clinic, despite being shown repeatedly. The patient cannot describe the spatial characteristics of familiar surroundings, such as the layout of his or her bedroom at home.[163]
3. *Lesion Areas.* The majority of cases involve damage to the right retrosplenial cortex, with Brodmann's area 30 compromised in most patients.[167] Bilateral parietal lesions, and, more rarely, left-side parietal lesions, can produce this problem.[163]
4. *Testing.* The patient is asked to describe or to draw a familiar route, such as the block on which he or she lives, the layout of his or her house, or a major neighborhood intersection.[157] A patient with topographical disorientation will be unable to succeed in this task. However, the therapist must differentiate between memory problems and topographical orientation difficulties.
5. *Treatment Suggestions.* This deficit usually resolves 8 weeks after onset.[167] However, several treatment techniques can be used to hasten recovery or to assist long-term if the condition persists.
   a. *Remedial Approach.* The patient practices going from one place to another, following verbal instructions. Initially, simple routes should be used, and then more complicated ones.[2]
   b. *Compensatory Approach.* Frequently traveled routes can be marked with colored dots. The spaces between the dots are gradually increased and eventually eliminated as improvement takes place.[2] This is an example of taking a normally right-hemisphere task and (because there is right-sided damage) converting it into a left-hemisphere task. In this instance, we take the spatial task of remembering routes (right-hemisphere task) and substitute sequential landmarks (sequencing is typically a left-hemisphere strength) to accomplish the goal of getting from place to place. The patient should be reminded not to leave the clinic, room, or home unattended, because he or she may get lost.

Depth and Distance Perception

1. *Definition.* The patient with a disorder of depth and distance perception experiences inaccurate judgment of direction, distance, and depth. Spatial disorientation may be a contributing factor in faulty distance perception.
2. *Clinical Examples.* The patient may have difficulty navigating stairs, may miss the chair when attempting to sit, or may continue pouring juice once a glass is filled.[162]
3. *Lesion Areas.* This impairment may occur with a lesion in the posterior right hemisphere in the superior visual association cortices; it may be evident with right-sided or bilateral lesions.[163]
4. *Testing.*
   a. For a functional test of distance perception, the patient is asked to take or to grasp an object that has been placed on a table. The object may also be held in front of the patient or in the air, and the patient is again asked to grasp it. The patient with impaired distance perception will overshoot or undershoot.[2] However, the movements look purposeful and smooth, which distinguishes this problem from a coordination deficit.

b. To determine depth perception functionally, the patient can be asked to fill a glass of water.[2] A patient with a depth perception deficit may continue pouring once the glass is filled.

5. *Treatment Suggestions.* The patient should be assisted in becoming aware of the deficit (education to increase cognitive awareness). Emphasis should be placed on the importance of walking carefully on uneven surfaces, particularly on stairs.
   a. *Remedial Approach.* The patient is requested to place the feet on designated spots during gait training.[55] Also, blocks can be arranged in piles 2 to 8 inches (5 to 8 cm) high. The patient is asked to touch the top of the piles with the foot. This is done to reestablish a sense of depth and distance.[166]
   b. *Compensatory Approach.* Practice in compensating for disturbances in depth and distance perception occurs intrinsically in many ADL skills, both those involving moving through space and those that involve manipulation. For example, the patient can hold the armrests of a chair to assist with sitting squarely.

Vertical Disorientation

1. *Definition. Vertical disorientation* refers to a distorted perception of what is vertical. Displacement of the vertical position can contribute to disturbance of motor performance, both in posture and in gait. Early in recovery, most patients post-CVA demonstrate some impairment in the sense of verticality.[168] This is not associated with or affected by the presence of homonymous hemianopia.[67] Scores on one test for visual perception of the vertical position were found to correlate with differences in walking ability.[67]
2. *Clinical Example.* A person with distorted verticality views the world differently and this may affect upright posture, as depicted in Figure 27.13.
3. *Lesion Area.* The lesion site is in the nondominant parietal lobe.
4. *Testing.* The therapist holds a cane vertically and then turns it sideways to a horizontal plane. Researchers use a luminous rod with patients seated in a darkened room.[168] The patient is handed the cane and asked to turn it back to the original position. If the patient's perception of the vertical position is distorted, the cane will most likely be placed at an angle, representing the patient's conception of the world around himself or herself.
5. *Treatment Suggestions.* The patient must be made aware of the deficit. He or she should be instructed to compensate by using touch (tactile cues) for proper self-orientation, especially when going through doorways, in and out of elevators, and on the stairs.

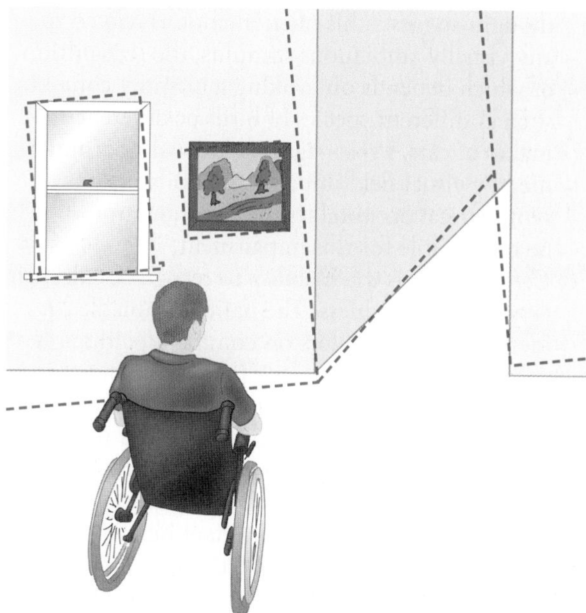

Figure 27.13 Vertical disorientation may contribute to disturbances of posture and gait.

Agnosias (Simple Perception)

Agnosia is the inability to recognize or make sense of incoming information despite intact sensory capacities. Although this condition is relatively rare (as listed by the National Institutes of Health Office of Rare Diseases), it can affect any sensory modality (e.g., vision, audition, touch, taste) and anything (e.g., faces, sounds, colors, familiar or less familiar objects). Although there is an inability to recognize familiar objects using one or two of the sensory modalities, the ability to recognize the same object using other sensory modalities is usually present.[154,169]

Visual Agnosias

1. *Definition.* Visual object agnosia is the most common form of agnosia.[4] It is defined as the inability to recognize familiar objects despite normal function of the eyes and optic tracts.[169]
2. *Clinical Examples.* One remarkable aspect of this disorder is the readiness with which the patient can identify an object once it is handled (i.e., information is received from another sensory modality).[170] The patient may not recognize people, possessions, and common objects. Specific types of visual agnosia include simultanagnosia, prosopagnosia, and color agnosia.
   a. *Simultanagnosia,* also known as Balint's syndrome,[4] is the inability to perceive a visual stimulus as a whole. The patient perceives an entire array one part at a time. The lesion is usually in the dominant occipital lobe.
   b. *Prosopagnosia* was traditionally considered to be the inability to recognize familiar faces. Current

thought suggests this phenomenon is related to any visually ambiguous stimulus, the recognition of which depends on evoking a memory context, such as different species of birds or different makes of cars. Prosopagnosia is usually accompanied by visual field impairments. Bilaterally symmetrical occipital lesions are thought to be responsible for this impairment.[15,50,171]

c. *Color agnosia* is the inability to recognize colors; it is not color blindness. The patient is unable to identify or name colors on command, although color chips can be correctly paired.[50] However, the meaning of color is lost so that the patient no longer associates a duckling as yellow or the sea as blue.[169] Color agnosia is frequently associated with facial or other visual object agnosias.[4,163] It is usually the result of a dominant hemisphere lesion.[4] The simultaneous occurrence of left-sided hemianopia, alexia (inability to read; word blindness), and color agnosia is a classic occipital lobe syndrome.[4]

3. *Lesion Area.* The lesions associated with visual object agnosias are thought to occur in the occipito-temporo-parietal association areas of either hemisphere. These areas are responsible for the integration of visual stimuli with respect to memory.[154] Recent evidence suggests visual object agnosias may result from damage in the medial structures of the ventral occipito-temporal cortex.[172]

4. *Testing.* To test for this deficit, several common objects are placed in front of the patient. The patient is asked to name the objects, to point to an object named by the therapist, or to demonstrate its use. It is important to rule out aphasia and apraxia, although this is not easily done. Details of other nonstandardized and standardized testing procedures are provided in Laver and Unsworth.[169]

5. *Treatment Suggestions.*

a. *Remedial Approach.* Drills can be used to practice discrimination between faces that are important to the patient (using photographs) and discrimination between colors and common objects. The therapist should assist the patient in picking out salient visual cues for relating names to faces.

Note: Another tool for treating visual agnosia, as well as many other cognitive and perceptual deficits, is the Easy Street Environment®. These environments have been incorporated into rehabilitation centers in the United States for almost 20 years. The Easy Street Environment® is a modular "world" of life-size streets (with a variety of ambulation surfaces, stairs, curbs, and so forth), vehicles, shops, and offices, which are constructed in a dedicated area within the rehabilitation setting. The Easy Street Environment® has many advantages since it allows occupational therapists, physical therapists, and speech-language pathologists to work with a patient in a safe, private, and comfortable environment where the patient can try out relearned or new skills. The therapist can also save considerable time by taking the patient down the corridor to the Easy Street Environment® rather than to his or her own local community, although ultimately such an outing to the local community may be undertaken. Figure 27.14 shows a patient with a visual object agnosia learning to use the Easy Street Environment® automatic teller machine (ATM). This patient may also learn new strategies to identify groceries and therefore be able to practice shopping in the Easy Street Environment® Market Place (Fig. 27.15). Where Easy Street Environments are not available, the therapist can take clients into their own community to practice desired skills. The client's own environment also provides the most ecologically valid environment for rehabilitation. Behrmann et al[173] have also presented a case study of a 24-year-old male and reported that the patient improved in identifying novel and common objects through recognition training. Positive results were not found for face identification.

b. *Compensatory Approach.* The patient is instructed to use intact sensory modalities, such as touch or audition, to distinguish people and objects.

Auditory Agnosia

1. *Definition. Auditory agnosia* refers to the inability to recognize nonspeech sounds or to discriminate between them. This rarely occurs in the absence of other communication disorders.[4]

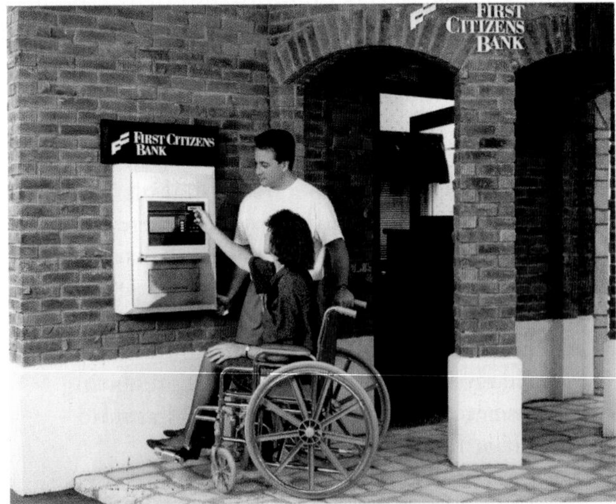

Figure 27.14 A client with an agnosia learns to use an ATM with help from a therapist in the Easy Street Environment®. *(Courtesy of Easy Street Environments®, Scottsdale, AZ 85260.)*

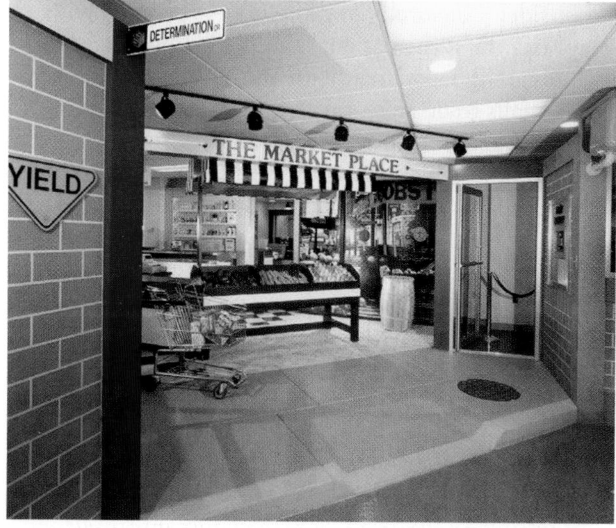

Figure 27.15 Clients with agnosias and many other cognitive and perceptual deficits can practice daily living skills in the controlled Easy Street Environment® such as provided in the Market Store. *(Courtesy of Easy Street Environments®, Scottsdale, AZ 85260.)*

2. *Clinical Examples.* The patient with auditory agnosia cannot tell, for example, the difference between the ring of a doorbell and that of a telephone, or between a dog barking and thunder.
3. *Lesion Area.* The lesion is located in the dominant temporal lobe.[4]
4. *Testing.* Testing is usually carried out by a speech-language pathologist. The patient is asked to close the eyes and to identify the source of various sounds. The therapist rings a bell, honks a horn, rings a telephone, and so forth, and asks the patient to identify the sound (verbally or by pointing to a picture).
5. *Treatment Suggestions.* Treatment generally consists of drilling the patient on sounds, but this has not been found to be particularly effective.[1,2]

Tactile Agnosia or Astereognosis

1. *Definition.* Tactile agnosia, or astereognosis, is the inability to recognize forms by handling them, although tactile, proprioceptive, and thermal sensations may be intact. This impairment commonly causes difficulties in ADL skills, inasmuch as many self-care activities that are normally done in the absence of constant visual monitoring require the manipulation of objects. If tactile agnosia is present in combination with unilateral neglect or other sensory loss, performance in ADL skills may be severely hampered.[67]
2. *Clinical Examples.* If a patient is handed a familiar object (key, comb, safety pin) with vision occluded, he or she will fail to recognize it.
3. *Lesion Area.* The lesion is in the parieto-temporo-occipital lobe (posterior association areas) of either hemisphere.[4]
4. *Testing.* The patient is asked to identify objects placed in the hand by examining them manually without visual cues.
5. *Treatment Suggestions.*
   a. *Remedial Approach.* The patient practices feeling various common objects, shapes, and textures with vision occluded. The patient is instructed to immediately look at the object for visual feedback and note special characteristics of the object.
   b. *Compensatory Approach.* To improve cognitive awareness, the patient is educated concerning the nature of the deficit and is instructed in visual compensation.

Apraxia

Apraxia is an impairment of voluntary skilled learned movement. It is characterized by an inability to perform purposeful movements, which cannot be accounted for by inadequate strength, loss of coordination, impaired sensation, attentional difficulties, abnormal tone, movement disorders, intellectual deterioration, poor comprehension, or uncooperativeness.[174-176] Many patients with apraxia also present with aphasia, and the two deficits are sometimes difficult to distinguish from each other.[4] Donkervoot et al[177] report the prevalence of apraxia among patients with first left hemisphere stroke in rehabilitation as around 28%. The two main forms of apraxia discussed in the literature are *ideomotor* and *ideational apraxia.* Ideomotor and ideational apraxias are generally thought to be the result of dominant hemisphere lesions and may be particularly difficult to test in the patient with aphasia. Although aphasia and apraxia often occur together, there is not a strong correlation between the severity of the aphasia and the severity of the apraxia. A third form of apraxia, *buccofacial apraxia,* is actually a type of ideomotor apraxia and is characterized by difficulties with performing the purposeful movements that involve facial muscles related to the mouth. This may include responding to the command "pretend to blow out a candle" or producing an orderly sequence of phonemes to produce speech. Hence, apraxia is a disorder of skilled movement and not a language disorder.[50] Some rehabilitation texts also describe constructional and dressing apraxias. However, it is generally believed that these are not true apraxias, but rather are difficulties in the application of cognitive and perceptual skill to these tasks. In other words, they are terms used to describe specific difficulties with a construction or drawing task or dressing. Both these problems are more frequently associated with right hemisphere lesions.[178]

In a recent study conducted by Wu et al,[179] patients with apraxia were found to improve on clinical measures, from admission to discharge from an inpatient rehabilitation facility. However, upon discharge, participants' level of independence was comparable to patients without apraxia at admission, reinforcing the disabling nature of this disorder.

Ideomotor Apraxia

1. *Definition. Ideomotor apraxia* refers to a breakdown between concept and performance. There is a disconnection between the idea of a movement and its motor execution. It appears that the information cannot be transferred from the areas of the brain that conceptualize to the centers for motor execution. Thus, patients with ideomotor apraxia can carry out habitual tasks automatically and describe how they are done but are unable to imitate gestures or perform on command.[180,181] Patients with this form of apraxia often perseverate;[154] that is, they repeat an activity or a segment of a task over and over, even if it is no longer necessary or appropriate. This makes it difficult for them to finish one task and go on to the next. Patients with ideomotor apraxia appear most impaired when requested to perform tasks that require use of many implements and that have many steps. This form of apraxia can be demonstrated separately in the facial areas, upper extremities (UE), lower extremities (LE), and total body movements.[182] Patients with apraxia are often observed to be clumsy in their actual handling of objects. Impairment is typically suspected when observing the patient during ADL or during a routine motor examination.
2. *Clinical Examples.* Several examples of ideomotor apraxia follow. The patient is unable to "blow" on command. However, if presented with a bubble wand, the patient will spontaneously blow bubbles. The patient may fail to walk if requested to in a traditional manner. However, if a cup of coffee is placed on a table at the other end of the room and the patient is told, "Please have coffee," the patient is likely to traverse the room to get it.[157] A male patient is asked to comb his hair. He may be able to identify the comb and even tell you what it is used for; however, he will not actually use the comb appropriately when it is handed to him. Despite this observation in the clinic, his wife reports that he combs his hair spontaneously every morning. A female patient is asked to squeeze a dynamometer. She appears not to know what to do with it, although her comprehension is adequate, the task has just been demonstrated, and it is clear that she has adequate strength.
3. *Lesion Area.* Apraxia results most frequently from lesions in the left, dominant hemisphere. There is evidence that both frontal lesions and posterior parietal lesions can result in apraxia.[183]
4. *Testing.* The *Goodglass and Kaplan*[182] test for apraxia is composed of universally known movements, such as blowing, brushing teeth, hammering, shaving, and so forth. It is based on what the authors consider a hierarchy of difficulty for patients with apraxia. First the patient is asked, "Show me how you would bang a nail with a hammer." If the patient fails to do this or uses his or her fist as if it were a hammer, the patient is told, "Pretend to hold the hammer." If the patient fails following this instruction, the therapist demonstrates the act and asks the patient to imitate it. The patient with apraxia typically will not improve after demonstration but will improve with use of the actual implements.[4] The ability to correct oneself on following verbal cueing is considered not indicative of apraxia. Additional apraxia tests may be found in Butler[178] and the work of van Heugten et al,[184] who have adapted the Arnadottir OT-ADL Neurobehavioural Evaluation (A-ONE)[5] as an observational method of testing for apraxia.
5. *Treatment Suggestions.*
   a. *Remedial Approach.* In the remediation of apraxias, it is advised that the therapist speak slowly and use the shortest possible sentences. One command should be given at a time, and the second command should not be given until the first task is completed. When teaching a new task, it should be broken down into its component parts. Components are taught one at a time, with the therapist physically guiding the patient through the task if necessary. It should be completed in precisely the same manner each time.[178] When all the individual units are mastered, an attempt to combine them should be made. A great deal of repetition may be necessary.[67] Family members must be advised to use the exact approach found to be successful in the clinic. Performing activities in as normal an environment as possible is also helpful. Butler[178] provides a case example of a young woman relearning how to drink from a cup using this technique. Using the sensorimotor approach, multiple sensory inputs are used on the affected body parts to enhance the production of appropriate motor responses. See Okoye[185] for additional details on this approach.
   b. *Compensatory Approach.* Donkervoot et al[186] report an RCT that showed the effectiveness of an occupational therapy treatment program, including "strategy training," over regular occupational therapy. Strategy training involves teaching the patient compensatory techniques to overcome the apraxia, such as use of pictures in the correct sequence to support ADL skills. This approach has been developed further and is now widely used to help patients overcome apraxia. Further studies to support this approach have also come from a group of occupational therapists in the Netherlands and include trials by Donkervoort et al[187] and Geusgens and colleagues.[188,189]

Ideational Apraxia

1. *Definition.* Ideational apraxia is a failure in the conceptualization of the task. It is an inability to perform a purposeful motor act, either automatically or on command, because the patient no longer understands the overall concept of the act, cannot retain the idea of the task, or cannot formulate the motor patterns required. Often the patient can perform isolated components of a task but cannot combine them into a complete act. Furthermore, the patient cannot verbally describe the process of performing an activity, describe the function of objects, or use them appropriately.[190,191]
2. *Clinical Examples.* When presented in the clinic with a toothbrush and toothpaste and told to brush the teeth, the patient may put the tube of toothpaste in the mouth or try to put toothpaste on the toothbrush without removing the cap. Further, the patient may be unable to describe verbally how tooth brushing is done. Similar phenomena may be evident in all aspects of ADL (washing, meal preparation, and so forth) and so may limit the safety and potential independence of the patient.[5] It has been shown that patients with ideational apraxia who test poorly in the clinical situation appear more able to perform ADL skills at the appropriate time and in a familiar setting.[185]
3. *Lesion Area.* The lesion causing ideational apraxia is thought to be in the dominant parietal lobe. This deficit also may be seen in conjunction with diffuse brain damage, such as cerebral arteriosclerosis.[154]
4. *Testing.* The tests for ideational apraxia are similar to those for ideomotor apraxia. The major expected response difference is that the patient with ideomotor apraxia can perform a motor act spontaneously and automatically at the appropriate time, but the patient with ideational apraxia is unable to do so. Refer to Butler[178] for full testing protocols.
5. *Treatment Suggestions.* The treatment techniques are the same as those for ideomotor apraxia.

Buccofacial Apraxia

1. *Definition.* Buccofacial or oral apraxia involves difficulties with performing purposeful movements with the lips, tongue, cheeks, larynx, and pharynx on command. Pedersen et al[192] report the prevalence rate of this unusual condition in patients with acute stroke as around 6%.
2. *Clinical Examples.* A patient may have difficulty responding to the command "pretend to blow out a candle" or "blow a kiss." However, in a normal context where the patient may perform these actions automatically, performance is not impaired. In addition, while patients may be able to produce the individual phonemes required for speech, they may have difficulty in producing an orderly sequence of phonemes. Formulaic speech (common, routine phrases) or automatic expressions such as "have a nice day" may be preserved.[193]
3. *Lesion Area.* Difficulties with buccofacial apraxia seem associated with lesions in the frontal and central opercula, anterior insula, and a small area of the first temporal gyrus (adjacent to the frontal and central opercula). Although buccofacial apraxia often coexists with Broca's aphasia, the two may be seen independently.[193]
4. *Testing.* The patient should be examined by a speech-language pathologist.
5. *Treatment Suggestions.* The speech-language pathologist can advise the health care team on strategies to communicate with patients who have buccofacial apraxia.

SUMMARY

Cognition and perception, the processes by which an individual thinks and selects, integrates, and interprets stimuli from the body and surrounding environment, are critical to the normal functioning of each human being. The patient with brain damage may be lacking in those abilities that allow one to make sense of and to respond appropriately to the outside world. It is essential for the therapy team to work together to recognize when a patient is experiencing some type of cognitive or perceptual dysfunction and to have the requisite tools to understand the causes of the behavior. The team can then determine the best interventions and consistently deliver these. Although it is often the occupational therapist, neuropsychologist, and speech-language pathologist who will guide the selection and implementation of evaluations and interventions for patients with cognitive and perceptual problems, it is essential that the physical therapist understands how these cognitive and perceptual impairments affect the patient's performance and the strategies that improve performance.

This chapter provided an overview of cognitive and perceptual deficits that may occur following brain damage, particularly those resulting from a stroke, and how such deficits can affect the functioning of the patient, especially within the context of the rehabilitation setting. The importance of differentiating cognitive and perceptual deficits from problems related to lack of motor ability, inadequate sensation, poor language skills, and simple uncooperativeness has been emphasized. Although alluded to in a very abbreviated fashion, activity analysis and systematic data collection remain two of the most powerful tools at the disposal of the therapist attempting to develop a firm rationale for, and to empirically justify the efficacy of, any treatment selected. Treatment in the form of adaptation of the physical environment and instructional sets and the teaching of compensatory techniques has been singled out as one of the most effective avenues for intervention.

Questions for Review

1. Patients with cognitive and perceptual deficits display what general characteristics during execution of a task?
2. Identify the underlying premise of the *transfer-of-training approach* to treatment.
3. What is the underlying assumption of the *sensory integrative approach* to treatment? Provide examples of the treatment modalities employed with this approach.
4. How is the performance of specific functional skills enhanced using the *functional approach* to treatment? What are the inherent benefits of using the functional approach?
5. Describe general suggestions for optimizing teaching/learning strategies when using compensatory techniques.
6. Identify the four treatment strategies included in the *cognitive approach* to treatment.
7. What potential influencing factors must be considered when examining a patient with cognitive and perceptual deficits?
8. What examination procedures will assist the therapist in distinguishing between sensory and cognitive or perceptual problems?
9. Differentiate between feedback provided in the form of knowledge of results (KR) versus knowledge of performance (KP).
10. Identify and define the four different types of attention.
11. What is the purpose of memory retraining? Compare and contrast the focus of the *remedial approach* and the *compensatory approach* to memory retraining.
12. Define the following terms: *unilateral neglect, anosognosia, somatoagnosia, finger agnosia,* and *right–left discrimination.*
13. Identify five spatial relations deficits. What general clinical manifestation do these disorders have in common? Define each of the deficits identified and provide an example of how each would influence patient performance of a task.
14. Provide examples of the functional implications of a visual *figure–ground discrimination deficit.* What is the most common lesion site producing this disorder?
15. What is the characteristic feature of apraxia? Define the three types of apraxias and provide examples of task performance characteristics associated with each type of apraxia.

CASE STUDY

The patient is a 72-year-old woman who has just been admitted to a rehabilitation facility following a stroke. The patient experienced a right parietal hemorrhagic stroke. A CT scan revealed a 1.5-inch (4 cm) hemorrhage that was subsequently drained. She will be able to stay in the rehabilitation facility for 20 days. Although the patient has some physical problems, the emphasis of this case study is on cognitive and perceptual tests and interventions. The occupational therapist and the physical therapist are collaboratively using a combination of cognitive retraining and the functional approach in therapy.

PAST MEDICAL HISTORY

The patient's past medical history includes insulin-dependent diabetes and mild osteoarthritis in both shoulders that causes some morning pain and stiffness.

SOCIAL

The patient lives alone in her own home. Supportive friends and family, her two children, and their families live nearby. A local health maintenance organization (HMO) provides her insurance. She is retired from the police force and enjoys gardening, reading, and watching television. She previously drove an automobile with an automatic transmission.

PHYSICAL THERAPY EXAMINATION

When the patient was approached from the left, she seemed to ignore the physical therapist and did not respond to greetings. However, when the therapist sat in the chair on the patient's right side, she seemed to have no problems talking to the therapist.

Range of Motion, Muscle Tone, and Balance

Examination revealed functional passive ROM, reduced strength in the left upper extremity (UE) with strength generally within the Fair (3/5) range; difficulty manipulating small objects with left hand; and some reduced dynamic standing balance reactions, with a score of 47/56 on the Berg Balance Scale. She scored 48/66 on the upper extremity component of the Fugl-Meyer Assessment of the Upper Extremity.[194]

Sensation

The physical therapist tested sensation and noted normal sensation in all areas (sharp/dull, light touch, temperature, proprioceptive sensations, cortical sensations) on the right side. However, the patient seemed to have difficulties on the left side, and her performance in detecting stimuli seemed inconsistent. Because the physical therapist suspected cognitive and perceptual deficits, a complete sensory test was deferred until the occupational therapist could fully examine the patient.

Functional Status

The physical therapist examined the patient's transfer abilities and instructed her in a safer way to get in and out of bed. The therapist scored the patient on the *Functional Independence Measure (FIM)*[93] and found the following:

Self-Care:

- Eating: FIM level = 4
- Grooming: FIM level = 5
- Bathing: FIM level = 3
- Dressing—upper body: FIM level = 5
- Dressing—lower body: FIM level = 4
- Toileting: FIM level = 6

Transfers:

- Bed, chair, wheelchair: FIM level = 5
- Toilet: FIM level = 5
- Tub: FIM level = 4

Locomotion:

- Walk: FIM level = 5

The physical therapist asked about her family, and she was able to provide many details. However, she seemed puzzled about where she was and expressed concern that she was not looking her best and needed to do her hair. The therapist suggested that she might like to brush her hair. The brush was on the table on the patient's left side, and she said she did not have one. The physical therapist cued her to check her bedside table, but on checking she maintained she did not have a brush. At the end of the session (which lasted about 40 minutes), the therapist asked her to demonstrate the bed transfer technique again that she had been taught at the beginning of the session. She seemed confused and could not do what the physical therapist had taught her.

OCCUPATIONAL THERAPY EXAMINATION: COGNITION AND PERCEPTION

The occupational therapist conducted two standardized tests: the *Rivermead Behavioural Memory Test (RBMT)*[87] (because the patient demonstrates memory impairments) and the *Arnadottir OT-ADL Neurobehavioral Evaluation (A-ONE)*[5] (to examine the impact of the patient's problems on her daily living activities). She received a scaled score of 54 on the RBMT, suggesting the need for ongoing therapy, particularly to support her strength in verbal memory. For the A-ONE, her independence scores for the subtests were Dressing (11/20), Grooming and Hygiene (12/24), Transfer and Mobility (13/20), Feeding (9/16), and Communication (3/8). The occupational therapist also reasoned that further tests of the patient's IADL, including home and driving abilities, would need to be conducted closer to her discharge. The patient's FIM scores for the Social Cognition Items were as follows:

Social Cognition FIM

- Social interaction: FIM level = 6
- Problem solving: FIM level = 6
- Memory: FIM level = 3

GUIDING QUESTIONS

1. What are some of the functional difficulties the patient is having and what cognitive and perceptual deficits might be causing these? Note that there may be more than one deficit impacting the functional problems noted.
2. Develop a clinical asset and problem list across the categories of the ICF.
3. Identify anticipated goals and expected outcomes appropriate for this patient.
4. Identify two treatment strategies to improve spontaneous use of left upper extremity and decrease unilateral neglect.
5. Identify two treatment strategies to improve the patient's memory.
6. How can the success of the patient's rehabilitation program be measured?

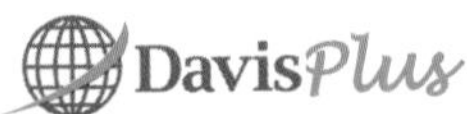

For additional resources, including answers to the questions for review and case study guiding questions, please visit **http://davisplus.fadavis.com.**

References

1. Unsworth, C: Cognitive and Perceptual Dysfunction: A Clinical Reasoning Approach to Evaluation and Intervention. FA Davis, Philadelphia, 1999.
2. Zoltan, B: Vision, Perception and Cognition: A Manual for Evaluation and Treatment of the Neurologically Impaired Adult, ed 3 rev. Charles B. Slack, Thorofare, NJ, 1996.
3. Katz, N, et al: Lowenstein Occupational Therapy Cognitive Assessment (LOTCA) battery for brain injured patients: Reliability and validity. Am J Occup Ther 43:184, 1989.
4. Lezak, MD: Neuropsychological Assessment, ed 4. Oxford University Press, New York, 2004.
5. Arnadottir, G: The Brain and Behavior: Assessing Cortical Dysfunction Through Activities of Daily Living. Mosby, St. Louis, 1990.
6. Glosser, G, and Goodglass, H: Disorders of executive control functions among aphasic and other brain-damaged patients. J Clin Exp Neuropsychol 12:485, 1990.
7. Katz, N, and Hartman-Maeir, A: Occupational performance and metacognition. Can J Occup Ther 64:53, 1997.
8. Winegardner, J: Executive functions. In Cohen, H (ed): Neuroscience for Rehabilitation. Lippincott, Philadelphia, 1993, p. 346.
9. Sharpless, JW: Mossman's A Problem Oriented Approach to Stroke Rehabilitation, ed 2. Charles C Thomas, Springfield, IL, 1982.
10. Edwards, S: Neurological Physiotherapy: A Problem Solving Approach, ed 2. Churchill Livingstone, New York, 2002.
11. Luria, AR: Higher Cortical Functions in Man, ed 2. Basic Books, New York, 1980.
12. Pak, R, and Dombrovy, ML: Stroke. In Good, DC, and Couch, JR (eds): Handbook of Neurorehabilitation. Marcel Dekker, New York, 1994, p. 461.
13. Meir, M, et al: Individual differences in neuropsychological recovery: An overview. In Meier, M, et al (eds): Neuropsychological Rehabilitation. Churchill Livingstone, London, 1987, p. 71.
14. Bach-y-Rita, P: Brain plasticity as a basis for therapeutic procedures. In Bach-y-Rita, P (ed): Recovery of Function: Theoretical Considerations for Brain Injury Rehabilitation. University Park Press, Baltimore, 1980, p. 225.
15. Brodal, A: Self-observations and neuro-anatomical considerations after a stroke. Brain 76:675, 1973.
16. Gardner, H: The Shattered Mind: The Person After Brain Damage. Alfred A. Knopf, New York, 1975.
17. Averbuch, S, and Katz, N: Cognitive rehabilitation: A retraining approach for brain-injured adults. In Katz, N (ed): Cognitive Rehabilitation: Models for Intervention in Occupational Therapy. Andover Medical, Boston, 1992, p. 219.
18. Neistadt, ME: The neurobiology of learning: Implications for treatment of adults with brain injury. Am J Occup Ther 48: 421, 1994.
19. Neistadt, ME: Assessing learning capabilities during cognitive and perceptual evaluations for adults with traumatic brain injury. Occup Ther Health Care 9:3, 1995.
20. Young, GC, Collins, D, and Hren, M: Effect of pairing scanning training with block design training in the remediation of perceptual problems in left hemiplegics. J Clin Neuropsychol 42: 312, 1983.
21. Neistadt, ME: Occupational therapy for adults with perceptual deficits. Am J Occup Ther 42:434, 1988.
22. Bundy, AC, Lane, SJ, and Murray, EA (eds): Sensory Integration: Theory and Practice, ed 2. FA Davis, Philadelphia, 2002.
23. Ayres, JA: Sensory Integration and Learning Disorders. Western Psychological Service, Los Angeles, 1972.
24. Ayres, JA: Sensory Integration and the Child. Western Psychological Services, Los Angeles, 1980.
25. Neistadt, ME: A critical analysis of occupational therapy approaches for perceptual deficits in adults with brain injury. Am J Occup Ther 44:299, 1990.
26. Moore, J: Neuroanatomical considerations relating to recovery of function following brain injury. In Bach-y-Rita, P (ed): Recovery of Function: Theoretical Consideration for Brain Injury Rehabilitation. University Park Press, Baltimore, 1980, p. 9.
27. Finger, S, and Stein, DG: Brain Damage and Recovery: Research and Clinical Perspectives. Academic Press, New York, 1982.
28. Braziz, PW, Masdeu, J, and Biller, J: Localization in Clinical Neurology, ed 6. Lippincott Williams & Wilkins, Philadelphia, 2011.
29. Giles, GM, and Wilson, JC: Occupational Therapy for the Brain Injured Adult: A Neurofunctional Approach. Chapman & Hall, London, 1992.
30. Giles, GM: A neurofunctional approach to rehabilitation following severe brain injury. In Katz, N (ed): Cognitive Rehabilitation: Models for Intervention in Occupational Therapy. Andover Medical, Boston, 1992, p. 195.
31. Trombly, CA (ed): Occupational Therapy for Physical Dysfunction, ed 6. Williams & Wilkins, Baltimore, 2008.
32. Trombly, CA: Conceptual foundations for practice. In Trombly, CA (ed): Occupational Therapy for Physical Dysfunction, ed 5. Lippincott Williams & Wilkins, Baltimore, 2002, p 1.
33. Trombly, CA: Restoring the role of independent person. In Trombly, CA (ed): Occupational Therapy for Physical Dysfunction, ed 5. Lippincott Williams & Wilkins, Baltimore, 2002, p. 629.

34. Neistadt, ME: Occupational therapy treatment for constructional deficits. Am J Occup Ther 46:141, 1992.
35. Fisher, AG: An expanded rehabilitative model of practice. In Fisher, AG (ed): Assessment of Motor and Process Skills, ed 2. Three Star Press, Fort Collins, CO, 1997, p. 73.
36. Trivedi, AN, et al: Trends in the quality of care and racial disparities in Medicare managed care. N Engl J Med 353:7, 692–700, 2005.
37. Toglia, J, and Abreu, BC: Cognitive Rehabilitation Supplement to Workshop: Management of Cognitive–Perceptual Dysfunction in the Brain-Damaged Adult. Sponsored by Braintree Hospital, Braintree, MA, and Cognitive Rehabilitation Associates, New York, May, 1987.
38. Giantusos, R: What is cognitive rehabilitation? J Rehabil 46: 36, 1980.
39. Abreu, BC, and Toglia, JP: Cognitive rehabilitation: A model for occupational therapy. Am J Occup Ther 41:439, 1987.
40. Diller, L, and Gordon, WA: Intervention strategies for cognitive deficits in brain-injured adults. J Consult Clin Psychol 49:822, 1981.
41. Toglia, JP: Generalization of treatment: A multicontext approach to cognitive perceptual impairment in adults with brain injury. Am J Occup Ther 45:505, 1991.
42. Toglia, JP: A dynamic interactional model to cognitive rehabilitation. In Katz, N (ed): Cognition and Occupation Across the Lifespan, ed 3. American Occupational Therapy Association, Bethesda, MD, 2011, p. 105.
43. Abreu, BC: Evaluation and intervention with memory and learning impairment. In Unsworth, CA (ed): Cognitive and Perceptual Dysfunction: A Clinical Reasoning Approach to Evaluation and Intervention. FA Davis, Philadelphia, 1999, p. 163.
44. Abreu, BC: The quadraphonic approach: Holistic rehabilitation for brain injury. In Katz, N (ed): Cognition and Occupation in Rehabilitation: Cognitive Models for Intervention in Occupational Therapy. American Occupational Therapy Association, Bethesda, MD, 1998, p. 51.
45. Wilcock, AA: Occupational Therapy Approaches to Stroke. Churchill Livingstone, Melbourne, 1986.
46. Galski, T, Beuno, RL, and Ehle, HT: Driving after cerebral damage: A model with implications for evaluation. Am J Occup Ther 46:324, 1992.
47. Vining Radomski, M, and Schold Davis, E: Optimizing cognitive abilities. In Vining Radomski, M, and Trombly Latham, CA (eds): Occupational Therapy for Physical Dysfunction, ed 6. Lippincott Williams & Wilkins, Baltimore, 2008, p. 609.
48. Gainotti, G: Emotional and psychosocial problems after brain injury. Neuropsychol Rehab 3:259, 1993.
49. Bronstein, KS, Popovich, JM, and Stewart-Amidei, C: Promoting Stroke Recovery. Mosby, St. Louis, 1991.
50. Bradshaw, JL, and Mattingley, JB: Clinical Neuropsychology: Behavioral and Brain Science. Academic Press, San Diego, 1995.
51. Cate, Y, and Richards, L: Relationship between performance on tests of basic visual functions and visual-perceptual processing in persons after brain injury. Am J Occup Ther 54:326, 2000.
52. Dirette, DK, and Hinojosa, J: The effects of a compensatory intervention on processing deficits in adults with acquired brain damage. Occup Ther J Res 19:223, 1999.
53. Warren, M: A hierarchical model for evaluation and treatment of visual perceptual dysfunction in adult acquired brain injury, I. Am J Occup Ther 47:42, 1993.
54. Warren, M: A hierarchical model for evaluation and treatment of visual perceptual dysfunction in adult acquired brain injury, II. Am J Occup Ther 47:55, 1993.
55. Sandin, KJ, and Mason, KD: Manual of Stroke Rehabilitation. Butterworth-Heinemann, Boston, 1996.
56. Gresham, GE, et al: Post-Stroke Rehabilitation. Diane Publishing, Darby, PA, 2004.
57. Hier, DB, Mondlock, J, and Caplan, LR: Recovery of behavioral abnormalities after right hemisphere stroke. Neurology 33:345, 1983.
58. Haerer, AF: Visual field defects and the prognosis of stroke patients. Stroke 4:163, 1977.
59. Zhang, X, et al: Natural history of homonymous hemianopia. Neurology 66(6):901, 2006.
60. Pedretti, LW: Evaluation of sensation, perception and cognition. In Pendleton, H, and Schultz-Krohn, W (eds): Pedretti's Occupational Therapy: Practice Skills for Physical Dysfunction, ed 6. Mosby, St. Louis, 2006, p. 110.
61. Stilwell, JM: The meaning of manual midline crossing. Sens Integr Q 21:1, 1994.
62. Chaikin, LE: Disorders of vision and visual perceptual dysfunction. In Umphred, DA (ed): Neurological Rehabilitation, ed 5. Mosby, St. Louis, 2006, p. 821.
63. Diller, L, and Weinberg, J: Differential aspects of attention in brain-damaged persons. Percept Motor Skills 35:71, 1972.
64. Van Ravensberg, CD, et al: Visual perception in hemiplegic patients. Arch Phys Med Rehabil 65:304, 1984.
65. Anastasi, A, and Urbina, S: Psychological Testing, ed 7. Prentice Hall, New York, 1996.
66. de Clive-Lowe, S: Outcome measurement, cost-effectiveness and clinical audit: The importance of standardised assessment to occupational therapists in meeting these new demands. Br J Occup Ther 59:357, 1996.
67. Wall, N: Stroke rehabilitation. In Logigian, MK (ed): Adult Rehabilitation: A Team Approach for Therapists. Little, Brown, Boston, 1982, p. 225.
68. Fisher, AG: An expanded rehabilitative model of practice. In Fisher, AG (ed): Assessment of Motor and Process Skills, ed 2. Three Star Press, Fort Collins, CO, 1997.
69. Unsworth, CA: Cognitive and perceptual strategies. In Curtin, M, Molineux, M, and Supyk-Mellson, J (eds): Occupational Therapy and Physical Dysfunction: Enabling Occupation, ed 6. Elsevier Limited, Philadelphia, 2010.
70. Unsworth, CA, and Duncombe, D: AusTOMS for Occupational Therapy, ed 3. La Trobe University, Melbourne, 2014.
71. Fristedt, S, Elgmark, E, and Unsworth, CA: Reliability of the Swedish translation of the Australian Therapy Outcome Measures for Occupational Therapy. Scan J Occup Ther 20:182, 2013.
72. Wilson, BA, et al: Behavioural Assessment of the Dysexecutive Syndrome. Thames Valley Test Co., Bury St. Edmunds, UK, 1996.
73. Wilson, B, et al: Behavioural Inattention Test. Thames Valley Test Company, Bury St. Edmunds, 1987.
74. Wilson, B, Cockburn, J, and Halligan, P: Development of a behavioural test of visuospatial neglect. Arch Phys Med Rehabil 68:98, 1987.
75. Mueller, J, Kiernan, R, and Langston, W: Manual for COGNISTAT (The Neurobehavioral Cognitive Status Examination). Neurobehavioral Group, Inc, California, 1983.
76. Baum, CM, et al: Reliability, validity, and clinical utility of the Executive Function Performance Test: A measure of executive function in a sample of people with stroke. Am J Occup Ther 62: 445, 2008.
77. Unsworth, CA: Cognitive and perceptual strategies. In Curtin, M, Molineux, M, and Supyk-Mellson, J (eds): Occupational Therapy and Physical Dysfunction: Enabling Occupation, ed 7. Elsevier Limited, Philadelphia, 2017.
78. Itzkovich, M, et al: The Loewenstein Occupational Therapy Assessment (LOTCA) manual. Maddak, Pequanock, NJ, 1990.
79. Wang, S-Y, et al: The usefulness of the Loewenstein Occupational Therapy Cognition Assessment in evaluating cognitive function in patients with stroke. Eur Rev Med Pharmacol Sci 18:3665, 2014.
80. Bar-Haim Erez, A, and Katz, N: Cognitive profiles of individuals with dementia and healthy elderly: The Loewenstein Occupational Therapy Cognitive Assessment (LOTCA-G). Phys Occup Ther Geriatr 22:29, 2003.
81. Schwartz, Y, et al: Validity of the Functional Loewenstein Occupational Therapy Cognitive Assessment (FLOTCA). Am J Occup Ther 70:7001290010p1, 2016.
82. Katz, N, et al: Dynamic Loewenstein Occupational Therapy Cognitive Assessment (DLOTCA), Maddak, Pequannock, NJ, 2011.
83. Katz, N, et al: The Dynamic Occupational Therapy Cognitive Assessment for Children (DOTCA-Ch): A new instrument for assessing learning potential. Am J Occup Ther 61:41, 2007.
84. Nasreddine, ZS, et al: The Montreal Cognitive Assessment, MoCA: A Brief Screening Tool for Mild Cognitive Impairment. J Am Geriatr Soc 53:695, 2005.
85. Whiting, S, et al: RPAB-Rivermead Perceptual Assessment Battery. NFER-Nelson, Windsor, 1985.
86. Jesshope, HJ, Clark, MS, and Smith, DS: The RPAB: Its application to stroke-patients and relationship with function. Clin Rehabil 5:115, 1991.
87. Wilson, B, et al: The Rivermead Behavioural Memory Test (RBMT-3), ed 3. Thames Valley Test Company, Bury St Edmunds, 2008.

88. Wilson, B, et al: Development and validation of a test battery for detecting and monitoring everyday memory problems. J Clin Exp Neuropsychol 11:885, 1989.
89. Ware, JJ, and Sherbourne, CD: The MOS 36-item short-form health survey (SF-36): I. Conceptual framework and item selection. Med Care 30:473, 1992.
90. Law, M, et al: Canadian Occupational Performance Measure. Canadian Association of Occupational Therapists, Toronto, Ontario, 1991.
91. Davis, A, et al: First steps towards an interdisciplinary approach to rehabilitation. Clin Rehabil 6:237, 1992.
92. Wood-Dauphinee, SL, et al: Assessment of global function: The Reintegration to Normal Living Index. Arch Phys Med 69:583, 1988.
93. Guide for the Uniform Data Set for Medical Rehabilitation (Adult FIM SM): Version 5.0. State University of New York at Buffalo, Buffalo, 1999.
94. Jongbloed, L, et al: Stroke rehabilitation: Sensory integrative treatment versus functional treatment. Am J Occup Ther 43:391, 1989.
95. Gentile, AM: A working model of skill acquisition with special reference to teaching. Quest Monograph 17:61, 1972.
96. Lohman, H: Payment for services in the United States. In Schell, BAB, et al (eds): Willard and Spackman's Occupational Therapy, ed 12. Lippincott Williams & Wilkins, Philadelphia, 2014, p. 1064.
97. McKeehan, KM: Conceptual framework for discharge planning. In McKeehan, KM (ed): Continuing Care: A Multidisciplinary Approach to Discharge Planning. Mosby, Toronto, 1981, p. 3.
98. Unsworth, CA, and Thomas, SA: Information use in discharge accommodation recommendations for stroke patients. Clin Rehabil 7:181, 1993.
99. Unsworth, CA, Thomas, SA, and Greenwood, KM: Rehabilitation team decisions concerning discharge housing for stroke patients. Arch Phys Med Rehabil 76:331, 1995.
100. Unsworth, CA: Clients' perceptions of discharge housing decisions following stroke rehabilitation. Am J Occup Ther 50: 207, 1996.
101. Stringer, AY: A Guide to Adult Neurological Diagnosis. FA Davis, Philadelphia, 1996.
102. Strub, RL, and Black, FW: The Mental Status Examination in Neurology, ed 4. FA Davis, Philadelphia, 2000.
103. Mateer, CA, Kerns, KA, and Eso, KL: Management of attention and memory disorders following traumatic brain injury. J Learn Disabil 29:618, 1996.
104. van Zomeren, AH, and Brouwer, WH: The Clinical Neuropsychology of Attention. Oxford University Press, New York, 1994.
105. Tyerman, R, et al: COTNAB-Chessington Occupational Therapy Neurological Assessment Battery Introductory Manual. Nottingham Rehab Limited, Nottingham, 1986.
106. Stroop, JR: Studies of inference in serial verbal reactions. J Exp Psychol 18:643, 1935.
107. Gronwall, D: Paced auditory serial addition task: A measure of recovery from concussion. Percept Motor Skills 44:367, 1977.
108. US Army: Army Individual Test Battery. Manual of Directions and Scoring. Adjutant General's Office, 1944.
109. Couillet, J, et al: Rehabilitation of divided attention after severe traumatic brain injury: A randomized trial. Neuropsychol Rehabil 20(3):321, 2010.
110. Ponsford, J, Sloan, S, and Snow, P: Traumatic brain injury: Rehabilitation for everyday adaptive living, ed 2. Lawrence Erlbaum, Hove, 2013.
111. Loetscher, T, and Lincoln, NB: Cognitive rehabilitation for attention deficits following stroke (Review). Cochrane Library, 5, CD002842, 2013.
112. Kepferman, I: Learning and memory. In Kandel, ER, Schwartz, JH, and Jessell, TM (eds): Principles of Neuroscience, ed 4. McGraw Hill, New York, 2000, p. 887.
113. Scott Terry, W: Learning and Memory: Basic Principles, Processes and Procedures. Allyn & Bacon, Boston, 2008.
114. das Nair, RD, and Lincoln, N: Effectiveness of memory retraining after stroke (Cochrane Review). Cochrane Library, 3, CD002293, 2007.
115. Sohlberg, MM, and Mateer, CA: Introduction to cognitive rehabilitation: Theory and practice. Guilford Press, New York, 1989.
116. McKerracher, G, et al: A single case experimental design comparing two notebook formats for a man with memory problems caused by traumatic brain injury. Neuropsychol Rehabil 15(2):115, 2005.
117. Fuster, JM: Memory in the Cerebral Cortex: An Empirical Approach to Neural Networks in the Human and Nonhuman Primate. MIT Press, Cambridge, MA, 1995.
118. Baddeley, AD: The Psychology of Memory. In Baddeley, AD, Kopelman, MD, and Wilson, BA (eds): The Essential Handbook of Memory Disorders for Clinicians. John Wiley, Hoboken, NJ, 2004.
119. das Nair, R, et al: Cognitive rehabilitation for memory deficits after stroke (review). Cochrane Library, 9, CD002293, 2016.
120. Duran, L, and Fisher, AG: Evaluation and intervention with executive functions impairment. In Unsworth, CA (ed): Cognitive and Perceptual Dysfunction: A Clinical Reasoning Approach to Evaluation and Intervention. FA Davis, Philadelphia, 1999, p. 209.
121. Cummins, JL: Anatomic and behavioral aspects of frontal-subcortical circuits. In Grafman, J, et al (eds): Annals of the New York Academy of Sciences: Structure and Function of the Human Prefrontal Cortex, vol. 769. New York Academy of Sciences, New York, 1995, p. 1.
122. Pollens, R, et al: Beyond cognition: Executive functions in closed head injury. Cogn Rehabil 65:23, 1988.
123. Sohlberg, MM, Mateer, CA, and Stuss, DT: Contemporary approaches to the management of executive control dysfunction. J Head Trauma Rehabil 8:45, 1993.
124. Honda, T: Rehabilitation of executive function impairment after stroke. Top Stroke Rehabil 6(1):15, 1999.
125. Hewitt, J, et al: Theory driven rehabilitation of executive function: Improving planning skills in people with traumatic brain injury through the use of an autobiographical episodic memory cueing procedure. Neuropsychologia 44(8):1468, 2006.
126. Chung, CSY, et al: Cognitive rehabilitation for executive dysfunction in adults with stroke or other adult non-progressive acquired brain damage (Review). Cochrane Library, 4, CD008391, 2013.
127. Van Deusen, J: Body Image and Perceptual Dysfunction in Adults. WB Saunders, Philadelphia, 1993.
128. Corben, L, and Unsworth, CA: Evaluation and intervention with unilateral neglect. In Unsworth, CA (ed): Cognitive and Perceptual Dysfunction: A Clinical Reasoning Approach to Evaluation and Intervention. FA Davis, Philadelphia, 1999, p. 357.
129. Robertson, IH, and Halligan, PW: Spatial Neglect: A Clinical Handbook for Diagnosis and Treatment. Psychology Press, Hove, 1999.
130. Heilman, KM, Watson, RT, and Valenstein, E: Neglect and related disorders. In Heilman, KM, and Valenstein, E (eds): Clinical Neuropsychology, ed 5. Oxford University Press, New York, 2011, p. 296.
131. Herman, EWM: Spatial neglect: New issues and their implications for occupational therapy practice. Am J Occup Ther 46: 207, 1992.
132. Gordon, WA, et al: Perceptual remediation in patients with right brain damage: A comprehensive program. Arch Phys Med Rehabil 66:353, 1985.
133. Vallar, G: The anatomical basis of spatial hemineglect in humans. In Robertson, IH, and Marshall, JC (eds): Unilateral Neglect: Clinical and Experimental Studies. Lawrence Erlbaum, Hove, 1993, p. 27.
134. Rizzolatti, G, and Berti, A: Neural mechanisms of spatial neglect. In Robertson, IH and Marshall, JC (eds): Unilateral Neglect: Clinical and Experimental Studies. Lawrence Erlbaum, Hove, 1993, p. 87.
135. Robertson, IH, et al: Walking trajectory and hand movements in unilateral left neglect: A vestibular hypothesis. Neuropsychologia 32:1495, 1994.
136. Grattan, ES, et al: Examining the feasibility, tolerability, and preliminary efficacy of repetitive task-specific practice for people with unilateral spatial neglect. Am J Occup Ther 70(4):7004290020p1, 2016.
137. Saevarsson, S, Kristjánsson, Á, and Halsband, U: Strength in numbers: Combining neck vibration and prism adaptation produces additive therapeutic effects in unilateral neglect. Neuropsychol Rehabil 20(5):704, 2010.

138. Fong, KNK, et al: The effect of voluntary trunk rotation and half-field eye-patching for patients with unilateral neglect in stroke: a randomized controlled trial. Clin Rehabil 21:729, 2007.
139. Luauté, J, et al: Visuo-spatial neglect: A systematic review of current interventions and their effectiveness. Neurosci Biobehav Rev 30(7):961, 2006.
140. Pandian, JD, et al: Mirror Therapy in Unilateral Neglect after Stroke (MUST trial): A randomized controlled trial. Neurology 83:1012, 2014.
141. Butter, C, and Kirsch, N: Combined and separate effects of eye patching and visual stimulation on unilateral neglect following a stroke. Arch Phys Med Rehabil 73:1133, 1992.
142. Aparicio-López, C, et al: Cognitive rehabilitation with right hemifield eye-patching for patients with sub-acute stroke and visuo-spatial neglect: A randomized controlled trial. Brain Injury 29(4):501, 2015.
143. Redding, GM, and Wallace, B: Implications of prism adaptation asymmetry for unilateral visual neglect: Theoretical note. Cortex 46:390, 2010.
144. Goedert, KM, et al: Presence of motor-intentional aiming deficit predicts functional improvement of spatial neglect with prism adaptation. Neurorehabil Neural Repair 28(5):483, 2014.
145. Jacquin-Courtois, S, et al: Effect of prism adaptation on left dichotic listening deficit in neglect patients: Glasses to hear better? Brain 133(3):895, 2010.
146. Mizuno, K, et al: Prism adaptation therapy enhances rehabilitation of stroke patients with unilateral spatial neglect: A randomized controlled trial. Neurorehabil Neural Repair 25(8):711, 2011.
147. Priftis, K, et al: Visual scanning training, limb activation treatment, and prism adaptation for rehabilitating left neglect: who is the winner? Front Hum Neurosci 7:360, 2013.
148. Rode, G, et al: Long-term sensorimotor and therapeutical effects of a mild regime of prism adaptation in spatial neglect. A double-blind RCT essay. Ann Phys Rehabil Med 58:40, 2015.
149. Sarri, M, et al: Prism adaptation does not change the rightward spatial preference bias found with ambiguous stimuli in unilateral neglect. Cortex 47:353, 2011.
150. Serino, A, et al: Effectiveness of prism adaptation in neglect rehabilitation: A controlled trial study. Stroke 40(4):1392, 2009.
151. Turton, AJ, et al: A single blinded randomised controlled pilot trial of prism adaptation for improving self-care in stroke patients with neglect. Neuropsychol Rehabil 20(2):180, 2010.
152. Watanabe, S, and Amimoto, K: Generalization of prism adaptation for wheelchair driving tasks in patients with unilateral spatial neglect. Arch Phys Med Rehabil 91:443, 2010.
153. Bowen, A, et al: Cognitive rehabilitation for spatial neglect following stroke (Review). Cochrane Library, 7, 2013. Art. No.: CD 003586.
154. Waxman, S, and deGroot, J: Correlative Neuroanatomy and Functional Neurology, ed 22. Appleton, Los Altos, CA, 1995.
155. Maeshima, S, et al: Rehabilitation of patients with anosognosia for hemiplegia due to intracerebral haemorrhage. Brain Inj 11:691, 1997.
156. Sauguet, J, et al: Disturbances of the body scheme in relation to language impairment and hemispheric locus of lesion. J Neurol Neurosurg Psychiatry 34:496, 1971.
157. Johnstone, M: Restoration of Motor Function in the Stroke Patient, ed 3. Churchill Livingstone, New York, 1987.
158. Hecaen, H, et al: The syndrome of apractagnosia due to lesions of the minor vertebral hemisphere. Arch Neurol Psychiatry 75: 400, 1956.
159. Gainotti, G: Emotional behaviour and hemispheric side of the lesion. Cortex 8:41, 1972.
160. Arnadottir, G, and Gudrun, A: Evaluation and intervention with complex perceptual disorder. In Unsworth, CA (ed): Cognitive and Perceptual Dysfunction: A Clinical Reasoning Approach to Evaluation and Intervention. FA Davis, Philadelphia, 1999, p. 393.
161. Edmans, JA, Webster, J, and Lincoln, NB: A comparison of two approaches in the treatment of perceptual problems after stroke. Clin Rehabil 14:230, 2000.
162. Halperin, E, and Cohen, BS: Perceptual-motor dysfunction. Stumbling block to rehabilitation. Md State Med J 20:139, 1971.
163. Farah, MJ, and Epstein, RA: Disorders of visual-spatial perception and cognition. In Heilman, KM, and Valenstein, E (eds): Clinical Neuropsychology, ed 5. Oxford University Press, New York, 2011, p. 152.
164. Ayres, JA: Southern California Sensory Integration Tests. Western Psychological Services, Los Angeles, 1972.
165. Peterson, P, and Wikoff, RL: The performance of adult males on the Southern California figure-ground visual perception test. Am J Occup Ther 37:554, 1983.
166. Anderson, E, and Choy, E: Parietal lobe syndromes in hemiplegia: A program for treatment. Am J Occup Ther 24:13, 1970.
167. Maguire, EA: The retrosplenial contribution to human navigation: A review of lesion and neuroimaging findings. Scand J Psychol 42:225, 2001.
168. Yelnik, AP, et al: Perception of verticality after recent cerebral hemispheric stroke. Stroke 33:2247, 2002.
169. Laver, AJ, and Unsworth, CA: Evaluation and intervention with simple perceptual impairment (agnosias). In Unsworth, CA (ed): Cognitive and Perceptual Dysfunction: A Clinical Reasoning Approach to Evaluation and Intervention. FA Davis, Philadelphia, 1999, p. 299.
170. Bauer, RM: Agnosia. In Heilman, KM, and Valenstein, E (eds): Clinical Neuropsychology, ed 5. Oxford University Press, New York, 2011, p. 238.
171. Damasio, AR, Damasio, H, and van Hoesen, GW: Prosopagnosia: Anatomical basis and behavioral mechanism. Neurology 32:331, 1982.
172. Karnath, HO, et al: The anatomy of object recognition—visual form agnosia caused by medial occipitotemporal stroke. J Neurosci 29(1):5854, 2009.
173. Behrmann, M, et al: Behavioral change and its neural correlates in visual agnosia after expertise training. J Cogn Neurosci 17(4): 554, 2005.
174. Croce, R: A review of the neural basis of apractic disorders with implications for remediation. Adapt Phys Act Q 10:173, 1993.
175. Tate, R, and McDonald, S: What is apraxia? The clinician's dilemma. Neuropsychol Rehabil 5:273, 1995.
176. Heilman, KM, and Gonzalez Rothi, LJ: Apraxia. In Heilman, KM, and Valenstein, E (eds): Clinical Neuropsychology, ed 5. Oxford University Press, New York, 2011, p. 214.
177. Donkervoot, M, et al: Prevalence of apraxia among patients with a first left hemisphere stroke in rehabilitation centres and nursing homes. Clin Rehabil 14:130, 2000.
178. Butler, J: Evaluation and intervention with apraxia. In Unsworth, CA (ed): Cognitive and Perceptual Dysfunction: A Clinical Reasoning Approach to Evaluation and Intervention. FA Davis, Philadelphia, 1999, p. 257.
179. Wu, AJ, Burgard, E, and Radel, J: Inpatient rehabilitation outcomes of patients with apraxia after stroke. Top Stroke Rehabil 21(3):211, 2014.
180. Raade, AS, Roth, LJ, and Heilman, KM: The relationship between buccofacial and limb apraxia. Brain Cognition 16: 130, 1991.
181. Mozaz, M, et al: Apraxia in a patient with lesion located in right sub-cortical area: Analysis of errors. Cortex 26:651, 1990.
182. Goodglass, H, et al: The Assessment of Aphasia and Related Disorders, ed 3. Lippincott Williams & Wilkins, Philadelphia, 2001.
183. Halsband, U, et al: The role of the pre-motor and the supplementary motor area in the temporal control of movement in man. Brain 116:243, 1993.
184. Van Heugten, CM, et al: Assessment of disabilities in stroke patients with apraxia: Internal consistency and inter-observer reliability. Occup Ther J Res 19:55, 1999.
185. Okoye, R: The apraxias. In Abreu, BC (ed): Physical Disabilities Manual. Raven Press, New York, 1981, p. 241.
186. Donkervoot, M, et al: Efficacy of strategy training in left hemisphere stroke patients with apraxia: A randomized clinical trial. Neuropsychol Rehabil 11:549, 2001.
187. Donkervoort, M, Dekker, J, and Deelman, B: The course of apraxia and ADL functioning in left hemisphere stroke patients treated in rehabilitation centres and nursing homes. Clin Rehabil 20(12):1085, 2006.
188. Geusgens, C, et al: Transfer of training effects in stroke patients with apraxia: An exploratory study. Neuropsychol Rehabil 16(2): 213, 2006.
189. Geusgens, C, et al: Transfer effects of a cognitive strategy training for stroke patients with apraxia. J Clin Exp Neuropsychol 29(8): 831, 2007.
190. De Renzi, E, and Lucchelli, F: Ideational apraxia. Brain 111: 1173, 1988.

191. Mayer, NH, et al: Buttering a hot cup of coffee: An approach to the study of errors of action in patients with brain damage. In Tupper, DE, and Cicerone, KD (eds): The Neuropsychology of Everyday Life: Assessment and Basic Competencies. Kluwer, London, 1990, p. 259.
192. Pedersen, PM, et al: Manual and oral apraxia in acute stroke, frequency and influence on functional outcome. Am J Phys Med Rehabil 80:685, 2001.
193. Heilman, KM, and Valenstein, E (eds): Clinical Neuropsychology, ed 5. Oxford University Press, New York, 2011.
194. Fugl-Meyer, A, et al: The post stroke hemiplegic patient, 1. A method for evaluation of physical performance. Scand J Rehabil Med 7:13, 1976.

Supplemental Readings

Banich, MT, and Compton, RJ: Cognitive Neuroscience and Neuropsychology, ed 3. Houghton Mifflin, Boston, 2011.

Gravell, R, and Johnson, R (eds): Head Injury Rehabilitation: A Community Team Perspective. Whurr Publishers, London, 2002.

Heilman, KM, and Valenstein, E (eds): Clinical Neuropsychology, ed 5. Oxford University Press, New York, 2011.

Lundy-Eckman, L: Neuroscience: Fundamentals for Rehabilitation, ed 3. Elsevier, New York, 2007.

Mateer, CA, and Sohlberg, MM: Cognitive Rehabilitation: An integrative neuropsychological approach. Guilford Press, New York, 2001.

Ponsford, J (ed): Cognitive and Behavioral Rehabilitation: From Neurobiology to Clinical Practice. Guilford Press, New York, 2004.

Sacks, O: The Man Who Mistook His Wife for a Hat. Harper & Row, New York, 1985.

Strub, RL, and Black, FW: The Mental Status Examination in Neurology, ed 4. FA Davis, Philadelphia, 2000.

Unsworth, C (ed): Cognitive and Perceptual Dysfunction: A Clinical Reasoning Approach to Evaluation and Intervention. FA Davis, Philadelphia, 1999.

Wilson, BA: Memory Rehabilitation: Integrating Theory and Practice. Guilford Press, New York, 2009.

Web-Based Resources for Clinicians, Families, and Patients With Cognitive and Perceptual Deficits

appendix **27.A**

Social Psychology Network from Wesleyan University	www.socialpsychology.org/cognition.htm
Yale Perception and Cognition Laboratory	http://perception.yale.edu/
Better Medicine	www.bettermedicine.com/article/cognitive-impairment
Book chapter on cognitive impairment following traumatic brain injury	www.ncbi.nlm.nih.gov/books/NBK2521/
Brain Injury Centre, Australia	www.braininjuryaustralia.org.au
Brain Injury Association of America	www.biausa.org/
Brain Injury Resource Center	www.headinjury.com/
Stroke Association: A complete guide to cognitive problems after stroke	www.stroke.org.uk/resources/complete-guide-cognitive-problems-after-stroke
MIT open course on the brain and cognition sciences	http://ocw.mit.edu/courses/brain-and-cognitive-sciences/
University of California, San Diego, Center for Brain and Cognition	http://cbc.ucsd.edu/index.html
Transitional Learning Center, Galveston, Texas	http://tlcrehab.org/
National Institute of Neurological Disorders and Stroke	www.ninds.nih.gov/
Brain Injury *Australia*	www.braininjuryaustralia.org.au
Rehabilitation Institute of Chicago	www.ric.org/Brain_Injury/Services
Brain Injury Network (BIN)	www.braininjurynetwork.org
Stroke Support Groups	www.stroke.org/stroke-resources/stroke-support-groups
National Stroke Association	www.stroke.org/

Neurogenic Disorders of Speech and Language

Chapter 28

Martha Taylor Sarno, MA, MD (hon)
Jessica Galgano, PhD, CCC-SLP

LEARNING OBJECTIVES

1. Differentiate the organization of language with respect to the role of phonological, lexical, syntactic, and semantic systems.
2. Understand the role of the motor speech system in the speech production process.
3. Discuss and characterize the classic aphasic syndromes.
4. Identify and explain the critical factors in the evaluation of recovery and rehabilitation of aphasia.
5. Identify and describe general approaches to aphasia rehabilitation and some specific treatment methods.
6. Identify etiologies of cognitive-communication disorders.
7. Compare and contrast deficits in executive function, pragmatic language, and motor speech in persons with cognitive-communication disorders.
8. Describe the primary types of dysarthria and rationales for dysarthria treatment.
9. Describe apraxia of speech and its treatment.
10. Gain an understanding of swallowing disorders.
11. Describe the goals and rationales for the use of augmentative communication systems.

CHAPTER OUTLINE

Most people take the ability to produce and understand speech for granted and pay little attention to the nature and function of the processes involved in communication. To develop and engage in oral communication, humans must have a functioning auditory or hearing system. Yet speech, like toolmaking, sets us apart from animals and is one of our most human behaviors. Even in primitive societies, humans have used the oral–motor speech code to share experiences, ideas, and feelings. Not all communities have developed writing and reading systems.

The use of speech for communication contributes to our identity as human beings and to the perception of "self." As a result, disruptions in the ability to communicate, whether caused by structural abnormalities (e.g., cleft palate), neurological conditions (e.g., stroke, Parkinson's disease), or nonorganic conditions (e.g., nonorganic articulatory disorders) may affect a person's daily life in important ways. For some, the acquisition of a communication disorder may have sufficient impact to cause an individual to leave from the workforce and limit social contact. For those whose communication disorders have persisted since childhood, the disorder may represent a significant vocational handicap. In others, a disorder that does not impede the individual's vocational life may interfere with everyday socialization. Communication disorders are complex, multifaceted behavioral impairments often associated so closely with a person's self-image as to threaten the quality of his or her life.

The term *communication* encompasses all the behaviors that human beings use to perceive and transmit information and interact with others. The term *language* refers to the quasi-automatic behavior of selecting vocabulary and sentence structures before communicating a message. Understanding what is said requires adequate hearing and the ability to perceive, discriminate, and conceptualize the speaker's thoughts as conveyed through spoken messages.

Speech comprises a delicate and rapid sequence of sensory and motor events requiring the coordinated activity of several parts of the body. The use of speech for communication involves many levels of human activity, ranging from the fine motor coordination of components of the oral–motor system to the subtle shades of meaning that occur at the cognitive/semantic level. Gestures, pantomime, and other nonverbal *pragmatic language* behaviors, such as turn taking, are also essential elements of communication.

Among unimpaired speakers, speech behavior varies greatly, yet the auditory and speech systems are efficient for the exchange of both simple and complicated information. The range of variability is so wide that individuals generally produce different sound waves with different characteristics even when producing the same word. But listeners do not rely solely on information derived from speech waves. We also depend on cues, which are components of what is referred to as *context.* Context includes aspects of a communicative exchange such as the purpose of the activity, location of the exchange, knowledge of the participants, roles of each participant, and level of formality required by the situation.

This chapter addresses the *neurogenic disorders of communication,* a category of communication disorders represented by the majority of patients receiving speech-language pathology services in rehabilitation programs. The most common of these disorders are aphasia, a language disorder, dysarthria, a motor–speech disorder, apraxia of speech, and cognitive-communication disorders.

The field of speech-language pathology began in 1925 with the establishment of the American Speech-Language-Hearing Association (ASHA), an organization of professionals dedicated to the diagnosis and treatment of individuals with congenital or acquired communication disorders. Communication disorders in children and adults are estimated to have prevalence in the United States of 5% to 10% and a cost to the economy of $154 billion to $186 billion per year. The number of persons in the United States with communication disorders is estimated at 14 million.[1,2] These statistics have increased by the addition of a significant number of military personnel returning from active duty who may manifest a host of communication disorders, including hearing loss, speech-language disorders, and/or cognitive-communication disorders. A significant number of returning military personnel have cognitive-communication disorders secondary to traumatic brain injury (TBI), which include deficits in discourse, pragmatic language, and social communication.[3-6]

The National Institute on Deafness and Other Communication Disorders (NIDCD) reports that 6 to 8 million people in the United States have an acquired or developmental language disorder. It is estimated that about 100,000 to 200,000 persons acquire aphasia annually, and approximately 1 to 2 million people currently have aphasia.[2,7,8] In addition, approximately 7.5 million people in the United States have voice disorders. The prevalence of articulation or speech sound disorders in children up to 6 or 7 years of age is estimated at 8% to 9%. By age 6 or 7, about 5% of children continue to present with speech disorders. It is also estimated that over 3 million Americans stutter.[2]

Approximately 37.5 million American adults have a hearing loss. Age is the strongest predictor of hearing loss among adults aged 20 to 69, and the degree of loss is significantly greater in those older than age 69.[9,10,11] It is well known that hearing aids can improve communication function among the elderly who suffer from hearing loss, and yet only a small percentage of this group seeks help from audiologists to access hearing aids.

The speech-language pathologist (SLP) and audiology professions have grown rapidly. Affiliates (members and certificate holders) in the ASHA at year-end 2015 included 156,254 SLPs and 12,970 audiologists. Speech-language pathology and audiology are master's degree entry fields. Since 2009, 50 states require a license for speech-language pathology and audiology to practice. ASHA awards the Certificate of Clinical Competence (CCC) to SLPs who meet specified academic and clinical experience requirements, which includes a Clinical Fellowship Year (CFY), a 9-month period of supervision and mentoring by a speech and language pathologist holding ASHA certification. In 2015, 55% of SLPs worked in educational organizations, 39% in health care facilities, 57% in other facilities.[11] The abbreviation *SLP* is the official designation of professionals in the field who hold the CCC. The term *speech therapist,* although no longer considered professionally appropriate, is a term that is often used informally.

For the presence and degree of speech or language pathology manifest in a person to be identified and measured, performance must be compared with a standard of "normal." One may choose as the standard (1) the language common to the cultural community of unimpaired persons in which the person lives, in which case an individual's verbal function would be compared with that of others in the same community of similar age, gender, education, and achievement, or (2) the person's verbal behavior before the onset of illness or trauma. The latter will vary from individual to individual and is based on premorbid educational achievement, specific cultural characteristics, personality, and other factors such as cognitive functioning. A person is verbally impaired when he or she deviates in any parameter of language and/or speech processing from the "normal" communication behavior of the community in which he or she functioned premorbidly.

A "normal" standard is implied in the terms *impairment, disability,* and *handicap.* This chapter uses the current World Health Organization (WHO) classification schema, in which the term *disability* is defined as the nature and extent of functioning, and the term *handicap* is defined as a person's involvement in life situations.[12,13]

THE ORGANIZATION OF LANGUAGE

When an individual generates an idea he or she wishes to express, it is transformed into words and sentences by calling into play certain physiological and acoustic events. The message is converted into linguistic form. The listener, in turn, fits the auditory information into a sequence of words and sentences that are ultimately understood.

We refer to the system of symbols that are strung together into sentences expressing our thoughts and the understanding of those messages as *language.* In the first few years of life, infants and children gain a great deal of practice and experience in the use of language, until it becomes habitual and is used with different levels of conscious awareness.

Phonology refers to the study of the sound system of language. Words are made up of speech sounds or *phonemes,* which are generally classified as either *vowels* or *consonants.* Phonemes in and of themselves do not symbolize ideas or objects, but when put together they are the basic linguistic units that make words. Words make up the *lexicon,* or vocabulary, of a language. English is composed of 16 vowels and 22 consonants, which are combined into larger units called *syllables.*

A syllable usually consists of a vowel as a central phoneme surrounded by one or more consonants. There are between 1,000 and 2,000 syllables in English. Most languages have their own rules about how phonemes may be combined into larger units. For example, in English, syllables never start with the *ng* phoneme. The most frequently used words in English are sequences of two to five phonemes. Some have as many as 10 phonemes or as few as one. In general, the most frequently used words have few phonemes. Even though only a small number of phoneme combinations are possible, new words are added to the English language every day. Although there are several hundred thousand English words, we use a repertoire of only about 5,000 to 10,000 words 95% of the time.

The grammar, or *syntax,* of a language determines the sequence of words that are acceptable in the formation of sentences. In English, for example, it is possible to say, "The black box is on the table," but the sequence "Box black table on the" is unacceptable. Another example is, "The old radio played well," which is syntactically correct, but "Old the well played radio" is not. The sentence "The boy walked to the store" is meaningful, but the sentence "The book walked to the store" is not. The language system that refers to the meanings of words is called *semantics.*

In addition to the phonological (sounds), lexical (vocabulary), syntactical (grammar), and semantic (meaning) language systems, we also utilize *prosody* (stress and intonation) to help make distinctions between questions, statements, expressions of emotions, shock, exclamations, and so forth.

SPEECH PRODUCTION

The speech organs consist of the lungs, trachea, larynx (which contains the vocal cords), pharynx, nose, and mouth. When considered together, these organs comprise a "tube" referred to as the *vocal tract,* which extends from the lungs to the lips. Moving the tongue, lips, and any other parts of the tract varies vocal tract shape. Changes in the configuration of the vocal tract act to modify the aerodynamic qualities of the air stream during speech (Fig. 28.1).

The primary function of the vocal organs relates to basic life-sustaining functions such as breathing and swallowing. These organs not only take on different roles for speech, but also function differently when engaged in speech production. For example, breathing for life-sustaining purposes is far more rapid than for speech production. A full cycle of inhalation/exhalation takes approximately 5 seconds, whereas while speaking we control the breathing rate according to the demands of the words and sentences we are producing, sometimes reducing the rate of breathing to as little as 15% devoted to inhalation. This is dictated in part by the fact that, when speaking, we generally take in enough air to vocalize a complete thought and we exhale the air gradually during the production of the thought.

The steady stream of air exhaled from the lungs is the source of energy for speech production, which is made audible by the rapid vibration of the vocal cords. During speech we alter the shape of the vocal tract continuously by moving the tongue, lips, and other parts of the system. By moving parts of the vocal tract, thereby modifying its acoustic properties, we are able to produce different sounds. That is, by altering the shape of the vocal tract during *phonation,* we transform the air stream into a resonance chamber (Figs. 28.2 and 28.3).

The *larynx* acts as a barrier to prevent food from entering the trachea and lungs by closing automatically

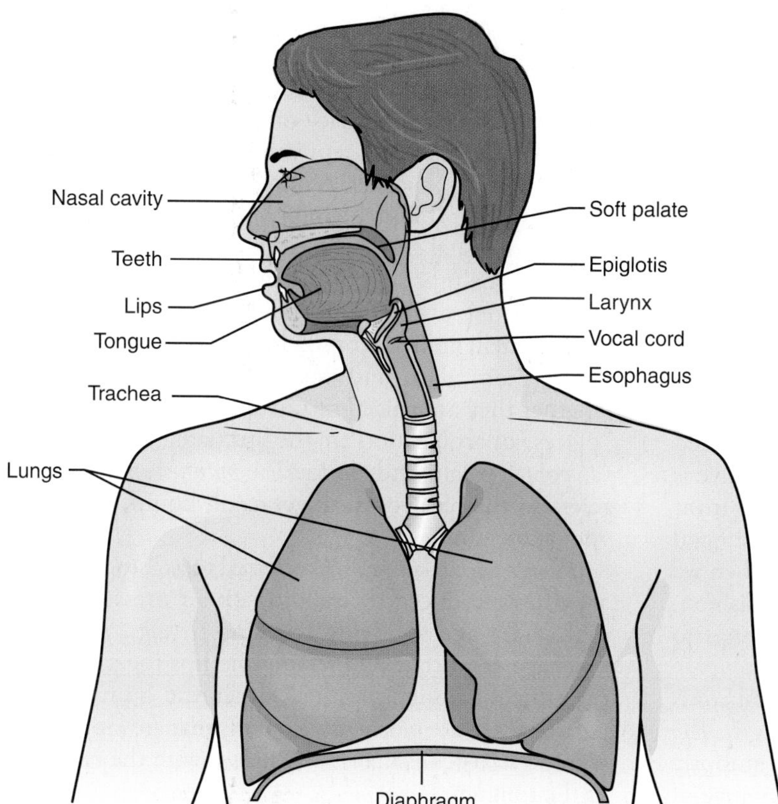

Figure 28.1 The human vocal tract.

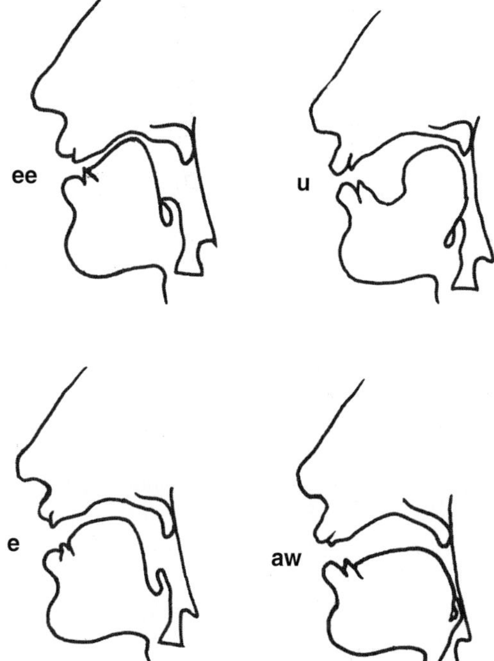

Figure 28.2 Outlines of the vocal tract during articulation of various vowels.

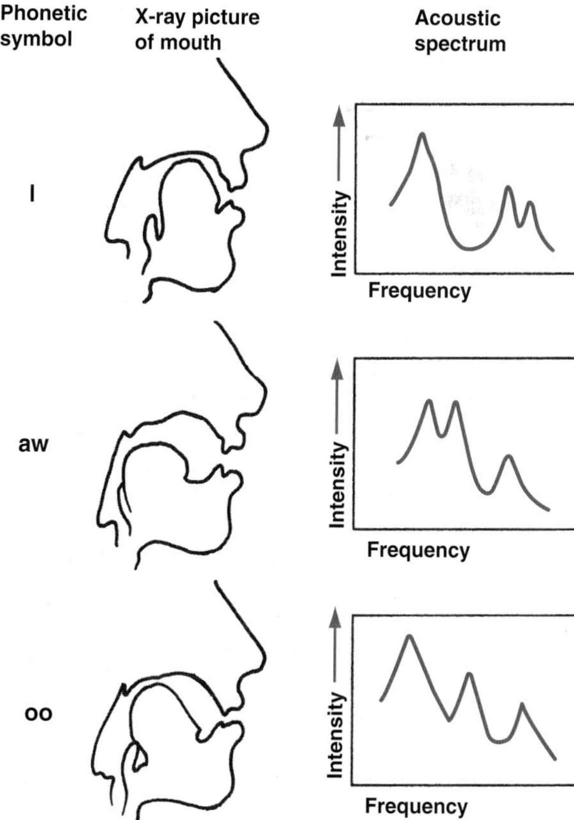

Figure 28.3 Vocal tract configuration and corresponding spectra for three different vowels. The peaks of the spectra represent vocal tract resonances. The vertical lines for individual harmonics are not shown.

during the act of swallowing, which is also helped by the action of the epiglottis. By opening and closing the flow of air from the lungs, the larynx acts as a valve between the lungs and the mouth. The laryngeal valve also acts to lock air into the lungs, which we do automatically when we perform heavy work using our upper extremities. The larynx is not a fixed, rigid organ, but because of its cartilaginous construction and corresponding connecting muscles and ligaments moves up and down during both swallowing and speaking.

The *vocal cords,* which create the sounds of speech, are located on either side of the larynx from the Adam's apple at the front to the arytenoid cartilages at the back. Recent neuroimaging research has reported findings that reflect the complexity of motor planning and control of vocal cord movement for voice production, showing that subcortical and cortical interactions control the movement of the vocal cords.[14] We refer to the space between the vocal cords as the *glottis.* When the cords are pressed together, the passage of air is sealed off and the valve is shut. Because the cords are held together at the front where they articulate with the Adam's apple, the open glottis is V-shaped, opening only at the back. When we speak, we vibrate the vocal cords in a rhythmic fashion, opening and closing the air passage from the lungs to the oral/nasal cavities.

The frequency of sound produced by the vocal cords is directly related to their mass, tension, and length. The tension and length of the vocal cords is continuously altered while speaking. In normal speech, the range of vocal cord frequencies is from about 60 to 350 cycles per second (cps). Most people use a vocal cord frequency range that covers about one and a half octaves.

The *pharynx* is the area of the vocal tract connecting the larynx with the nose and mouth. We isolate the nasal cavity from the pharynx and back of the mouth by raising the soft palate. The most adjustable component of the vocal tract is the mouth, whose shape and size can be modified more than any other organ of the oral–motor system by changing the relative position of the palate, tongue, lips, and teeth. The lips are rounded, spread, or closed to alter the shape and length of the vocal tract or to stop airflow. The teeth and their relationship to the lips or tongue tip change the airflow. An important component of the teeth ridge is the *alveolus,* which is the area covered by the gums.

The term *articulation* refers to the articulating, or "meeting," of the various organs of the oral–pharyngeal cavity to produce the sounds of speech. Speech *intelligibility* refers to the adequacy of the acoustic signal produced by a speaker and represents a significant factor in understanding a speaker. A number of factors can influence judgments of intelligibility, such as the presence or absence of visual cues or of extraneous movements (i.e., tremor). The precision of the production of consonant sounds is one of the primary factors that contribute to speech intelligibility. Consonants are described by specifying their place and manner of articulation and whether they are voiced or unvoiced (Table 28.1). The "places" of articulation are the lips (labial), teeth, gums (alveolar), palate, and glottis. The *manner of articulation* refers to the plosive, fricative, nasal, liquid, and semivowel categories.

Plosive sounds, sometimes referred to as "stop" sounds, are those produced by building up air pressure in the oral cavity and suddenly releasing it (e.g., *p, t*). The blockage can occur by pressing the lips together or by pressing the tongue against either the gums or soft palate. There are plosive consonants that are labial, alveolar, or velar (consonants articulated with the back part of the tongue).

Fricatives are produced by making the air turbulent (e.g., *f, v*). Most consonants are produced with the soft palate raised, thereby closing off the flow of air to the nasal cavity, except for the *nasals* (e.g., *m, n, ng*), which are made by lowering the soft palate and blocking the oral cavity somewhere along its length. *Liquids* are sounds made with the soft palate raised: /r/, /l/.

Semivowels refer to those sounds produced by maintaining the vocal tract in a vowel-like position, then changing the position rapidly for the vowel that follows (e.g., *w, y*).

Speech sounds are affected by their *context,* that is, the sounds that immediately precede or follow. A speech sound wave is a continuous event rather than a sequence of discrete segments. The identification of a speech

Table 28.1 Classification of English Consonants by Place and Manner of Articulation

Place of Articulation	Manner of Articulation				
	Plosive	Fricative	Semivowel	Liquids (including laterals)	Nasal
Labial	p b	—	w	—	m
Labiodental	—	f v	—	—	—
Dental	—	_ th	—	—	—
Alveolar	t d	s z	y	l r	n
Palatal	—	sh zh	—	—	—
Velar	kg	—	—	—	ng
Glottal	—	h	—	—	—

sound depends on relating acoustic features of the sound wave at different points in time.

A standard reference for the quality of vowels is the eight cardinal vowels (Fig. 28.4). This schema of the positions of the tongue to produce the vowels of the language helps us visualize the tongue's movements during speech. It is, in a sense, a map of the tongue positions for vowel production. Tongue placement is described by specifying the location of the main body of the tongue at its highest point. For example, for the sound /ee/ as in the word *beat,* the tongue tip is pointed in a high frontal configuration, whereas for the sound /ah/ as in the word *father,* the highest point of the tongue is low and posterior in the oral cavity.

All vowel sounds and some consonant sounds are *voiced.* That is, the vocal cords vibrate during their production. When a sound is produced without vocal cord vibration, we say that it is *unvoiced* or voiceless (e.g., *p, s*). Table 28.1 shows that many consonant sounds are articulated in the same manner, and differ only with respect to voicing (e.g., *p-b; s-z; f-v; k-g*).

Speech behavior comprises a complex motor event that goes well beyond the skilled movements required of the oral–motor system. Yet we produce speech without thinking about it even while simultaneously involved in other activities. However, to transform thought into speech takes some voluntary, conscious behavior that allows us to take information stored in memory and translate it into a coherent production of words and utterances that follow certain grammatical rules.

In addition to its linguistic aspects, neurogenic communication disorders often involve coexisting mild to severe cognitive deficits that may not only aggravate the communication disorder but also make it difficult to differentiate cognitive from communication deficits. The communication disorder manifest in persons with right brain damage, which is addressed in this chapter, is an example of a disorder in which the cognitive component is a major issue.

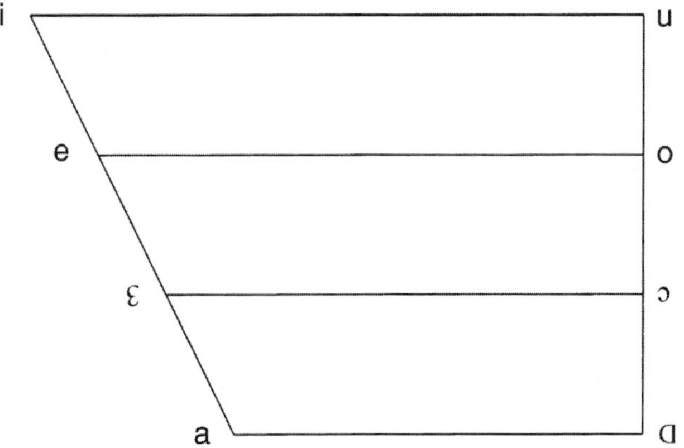

Figure 28.4 The cardinal vowels represented as a vowel quadrilateral. The cardinal vowels are extremely placed reference points for vowel articulation. Vowels on the same horizontal line are believed to have an equally high tongue height while vowels in the left–right position are assumed to be equally backed and fronted. *(Adapted from Ladefoged, P: A Course in Phonetics. Harcourt Brace Jovanovich, New York, 1975, with permission.)*

The importance of the communication process and its underlying systems becomes apparent when we consider the two most common neurogenic communication disorders: *aphasia* and *dysarthria.* This chapter focuses primarily on aphasia and dysarthria but also considers verbal apraxia, dysphagia, cognitive-communication disorders, and the use of augmentative/alternate systems of communication.

APHASIA

An increase in the population of individuals with aphasia is anticipated by the projection that by 2050, 21% to 22% of the U.S. population will be over age 65.[15] It has been estimated that there are 1 to 2 million individuals with aphasia in the United States alone.[2,7,8,11,16,17,18]

In a study that examined data from the Tulane Stroke Registry from July 2008 to December 2014, 866 of 1,847 patients had aphasia on admission.[19] It is further estimated that there are 100,000 to 200,000 new patients with aphasia each year.[2,7,8,11] The majority are currently older than 65 years of age and acquired aphasia as a result of a stroke. A smaller number acquired aphasia as the result of head trauma and neoplasms. There are also reports of close, but not always obligatory, relationships between primary progressive aphasia and Alzheimer's disease.[20]

Classification and Nomenclature

In this chapter, the term *aphasia* refers to the acquired communication disorder that is manifest in individuals who were previously capable of using language appropriately. It does not refer to developmental language disorders that may be present in individuals who never developed normal language and for whom the ability to use language may never reach age-appropriate performance levels.

In acquired aphasia, central nervous system (CNS) disease or trauma compromises certain structures in a focal rather than generalized fashion. The study of the neuroanatomical correlates of the aphasias has engaged neurologists since the late 19th century, and the correlation between aphasic syndromes and cerebral localization is relatively consistent. Recent advances in neuroradiological technology have provided many new methods for studying the neural substrates of language and language impairment.[21,22]

Aphasiologists generally agree that there are distinct major aphasic syndromes that adhere to specific profiles of impairment. This is not surprising, because the lesions that produce aphasia, particularly in the patient with cerebrovascular disease, tend to be located in brain loci that are especially vulnerable. It is not always possible, however, to classify patients according to these syndromes. Estimates of the proportion of cases that can be unambiguously classified range from 30% to 80%.[23]

The characteristics of an individual's speech production are used to determine aphasia classification. Speech output that is characterized as hesitant, awkward, interrupted, and produced with effort is referred to as *nonfluent aphasia* in contrast to speech output that is facile in articulation, produced at a normal rate, with preserved flow and melody, and is referred to as *fluent aphasia.* Fluency judgments are made during extended conversation with a patient and are defined as follows.

Fluent Aphasia

Fluent aphasia is characterized by impaired auditory comprehension and fluent speech that is of normal rate and melody. Fluent aphasia is usually associated with a lesion in the vicinity of the posterior portion of the first temporal gyrus of the left hemisphere. When fluent aphasia is severe, word and sound substitutions may be of such magnitude and frequency that speech may be rendered meaningless. Patients with fluent aphasia tend to have greatest difficulty in retrieving those words that are substantive (nouns and verbs). Since their lesions are located in the posterior portion of the brain, distant from motor areas, they also tend to have some degree of impaired awareness and are rarely physically disabled. There are several types of syndromes subsumed under the fluent aphasia classification (Table 28.2).

The most common type of fluent aphasia is *Wernicke's aphasia* (also referred to as *sensory aphasia* and/or *receptive aphasia*). Wernicke's aphasia is usually the result of a lesion in the posterior portion of the first temporal gyrus of the left hemisphere. It is characterized by impaired auditory comprehension and fluently articulated speech marked by word substitutions. Reading and writing are usually severely impaired as well. Although patients with Wernicke's aphasia may produce what seem like complete utterances and use complex verb tenses, they often add a word or phrase and "augment" speech production. Speech is often produced at a rate greater than normal. Although the production of speech sounds

Table 28.2 Classification by Aphasia Syndromes

	Wernicke's Aphasia	Broca's Aphasia	Global Aphasia	Conduction Aphasia	Anomic Aphasia	Transcortical Motor Aphasia	Pure Word Deafness
Area of infarction	Posterior portion of temporal gyrus	Third frontal convolution	Third frontal convolution and posterior portion of superior temporal gyrus	Parietal operculum or posterior superior temporal gyrus	Angular gyrus	Supplementary motor areas	Both Heschl's gyri or connection between Heschl's gyrus and posterior superior temporal gyrus
Spontaneous speech	Fluent	Nonfluent	Nonfluent	Fluent or nonfluent	Fluent	Nonfluent	Fluent
Comprehension	Poor	Good	Poor	Good	Good	Good	Poor
Repetition	Poor	Poor (but may be better than spontaneous speech)	Poor	Very poor	Good	Excellent	Poor
Naming	Poor	Poor (but may be better than spontaneous speech)	Poor	Poor	Very poor	Poor	Good
Reading comprehension	Poor	Good	Poor	Good to poor	Good to poor	Good	Good
Writing	Poor	Poor	Poor	Poor	Good to poor	Poor	Good

is generally precise, patients with Wernicke's aphasia may reverse phonemes and/or syllables (hopspipal/trevilision) and may produce *neologisms* (nonsense words).

In the course of recovery Wernicke's aphasia may evolve into anomic aphasia. *Anomic aphasia* is characterized by a significant word-finding difficulty in the context of fluent, grammatically well-formed speech. Auditory comprehension is generally impaired, especially when listening to complex and/or rapid speech. Speech output may be somewhat vague and the patient may be proficient in producing *circumlocutions* to skirt the lack of specificity of language use.

Nonfluent Aphasia

Nonfluent aphasia is characterized by limited vocabulary, slow, hesitant speech, some awkward articulation, and restricted use of grammar in the presence of relatively preserved auditory comprehension. Nonfluent aphasia is associated with anterior lesions usually involving the third frontal convolution of the left hemisphere. Patients with nonfluent aphasia tend to express themselves in vocabulary that is substantive (nouns, verbs) and lack the ability to retrieve less substantive parts of speech (prepositions, conjunctions, pronouns). Patients with nonfluent aphasia tend to have good awareness of their deficit and usually have impaired motor function on the right side (right hemiplegia–paresis).

Broca's aphasia is a nonfluent type of aphasia also sometimes referred to as *expressive aphasia*, *motor aphasia*, and/or *verbal aphasia*. Broca's aphasia is the result of a lesion of the third frontal convolution of the left hemisphere, the subcortical white matter, and extending posteriorly to the inferior portion of the motor strip (precentral gyrus). It is characterized by awkward articulation, restricted vocabulary, and restriction to simple grammatical forms in the presence of a relative preservation of auditory comprehension. Writing skills generally mirror the pattern of speech and reading may be less impaired than speech and writing. The patient may be limited to one- and two-word productions for expression and find it impossible to combine words into sentences. Articulation may be awkward and effortful (see the section titled Apraxia of Speech). Nonfluent Broca's aphasia is less common after TBI. Anomic disturbances predominate in aphasia secondary to TBI.

Global Aphasia

A severe aphasia with marked dysfunction across all language modalities and with severely limited residual use of all communication modes for oral–aural interactions is referred to as *global aphasia*. Global aphasia is not a type of aphasia but rather a designation of severity. The patient with global aphasia generally has extensive damage, which may be anywhere in the left hemisphere, and is sometimes bilateral.[24] Global aphasia has been cited as among the most common types of aphasia in patients referred for speech rehabilitation services.[25,26]

Acquired Aphasia

Acquired aphasia in children as a result of cerebral damage caused by head injury, tumor, or stroke results in the same syndromes manifest in adults with aphasia.[27-30] In children with aphasia secondary to TBI, anomic disturbances predominate and there is generally a reduction of output with hesitancy, difficulty initiating speech, and sometimes mutism.[31] Follow-up studies report that a significant number of children with acquired aphasia are slow to develop language and academic skills. Since cerebral plasticity decreases across the developmental spectrum, the age of aphasia onset is a factor in determining the extent of recovery.[30]

Primary Progressive Aphasia

Primary progressive aphasia (PPA) is a condition first described in 1982, which is now a recognized diagnostic category.[32,33] PPA is a slowly progressive isolated aphasia not due to stroke, trauma, tumor, or infection, which does not fit neatly into existing aphasia classification schemes. It can exist in the absence or relative absence of generalized intellectual and behavioral disturbances or cognitive impairment generally associated with dementia. Activities of daily living, judgment, insight, and behavior are usually preserved for at least 2 years and may remain unimpaired and isolated from the language impairment for as long as 20 years.[34] About half of those with PPA eventually develop symptoms of a more pervasive dementia. Spontaneous recovery does not occur.

In its initial presentation, PPA is commonly reported and observed as being a speech or articulation disorder or difficulty in naming. PPA progresses at different rates and in its most severe form can result in the inability to speak, due, in part to agrammatism and apraxia of speech. A subset of these patients also develop Parkinsonism. Neuroimaging techniques used for assessment purposes have the potential to be useful biomarkers of clinical decline in this population.[35]

Historical Perspective

Language disturbances were recorded as early as 3500 BC, and attempts to "retrain" individuals with aphasia have been recorded throughout history.[36] Some of the first documented cases of both natural recovery and intervention were the patients of Nicolo Massa and Francisco Arceo in 1558.[37]

In a landmark paper published in the late 19th century, "Du siège de la faculté du langage articulé," Paul Broca was one of the first to discuss the possibility of retraining in aphasia.[38] Dr. Charles K. Mills was the first to address recovery and rehabilitation in aphasia in an English-language publication. He reported the training of a patient with post-stroke aphasia whom he and Donald Broadbent treated, using methods largely determined by the patient, who began by systematically repeating letters, words, and phrases.[39,40] Mills' observations and approach to aphasia rehabilitation, published over a century ago, are remarkably similar to much present-day practice and thought. Mills noted that not all patients benefit from retraining to the same degree and acknowledged that spontaneous recovery might have an influence on the course and extent of recovery.

World War I and its brain-injured combat survivors led to the establishment of treatment centers where patients with post-traumatic aphasia were treated, especially in Europe. Reports of aphasia rehabilitation experiences during and after the war in England and the United States were also published.[41,42] One of the most comprehensive descriptions of the systematic treatment of a large number of patients with aphasia secondary to head trauma, of whom 90 to 100 were followed for a 10-year period, was provided by Kurt Goldstein in Frankfurt during World War II.[43]

Until World War II, reports of retraining civilians with post-stroke aphasia were rare. The aphasia literature was based almost exclusively on post-traumatic aphasia. In 1933, Singer and Low[44] reported the case of a 39-year-old woman who suffered an apparent vascular infarct after a full-term delivery and showed continuous language improvement with consistent training over a 10-year period.

In a landmark 5-year study supported by the Commonwealth Fund, Weisenburg and McBride[45] addressed the general topic of aphasia and commented on the effectiveness of reeducation. The study concerned 60 patients who were younger than 60 years of age, a majority of whom had suffered strokes, and concluded that reeducation increased the rate of recovery, assisted in facilitating the use of compensatory means of communication, and improved morale. Their work also documented the psychotherapeutic benefits of treatment.

Before World War II, aphasia and its concomitant neurological deficits in the patient with stroke were generally viewed as natural and necessary components of the aging process. The treatment of aphasia in the civilian population was not an option.

Many variables had an influence on making the treatment of aphasia the common practice that it is today. The advent of speech and language pathology as a health profession, the emergence of rehabilitation medicine as a medical specialty, the mass media explosion, a larger and more affluent middle class, an increase in the life span, the number of stroke and brain injury survivors, and public expectations of medicine in the age of technology are among them. The last has been particularly true in the industrialized world, where it is widely believed that there is a treatment for every human ill.[46]

Journals devoted to brain/language issues have become indispensable information sources for aphasiologists (e.g., *Journal of Medical Speech and Language Pathology, Aphasiology, Brain and Language,* and *Cortex*). The Academy of Aphasia, a scholarly society dedicated to the study of aphasia, was established in 1962. The National Aphasia Association (NAA) was founded in the United States in 1987 for the purpose of providing information to the public about aphasia, advocating for the aphasia community, and encouraging the establishment of a network of support groups called Aphasia Community Groups (ACGs).[47] The Academy of Neurologic Communication Disorders and Sciences (ANCDS) was founded in 1988 and is a nonprofit professional association that supports practitioners who serve individuals with neurologic communication disorders by providing education, training, and certification opportunities to promote high quality professional service.

Several informational publications designed for use by the families and friends of patients with aphasia also appeared in the period following World War II.[48-53] One of these, *Understanding Aphasia: A Guide for Family and Friends,* is still widely read and has been published in 12 languages.[53]

Aphasia Measures

Many measures of aphasia and related disorders have been developed for use in both clinical and research settings. In an acute care setting, patients with aphasia are generally screened at bedside. The purpose of a bedside screening is to obtain a general idea of a patient's profile of deficits and preserved areas of language function as a basis for recommendations for more comprehensive testing and possible rehabilitation. However, a comprehensive examination is required to provide a baseline measure against which to gauge progress in the course of spontaneous recovery and rehabilitation.

Comprehensive language tests designed to measure aphasic impairment generally contain specific domains of performance. In addition to the general requirements for the construction of tests, such as reliability, standardization, and demonstrated validity, certain factors are important in the design of tests intended to identify and measure aphasia. These include range of item difficulty, efficacy in measuring recovery, and ability to contribute to diagnostic classification.[2,54] Aphasia tests are generally based on examinations of linguistic task performance and at a minimum include tasks of visual confrontation *naming*; a spontaneous or conversational *speech sample* that is analyzed for fluency of output, effort, articulation, phrase length, prosody, word substitutions, and omissions; *repetition* of digits, single words, multisyllable words, and sentences of increasing length and complexity; *comprehension of spoken language* of single words, of sentences that require only "yes" or "no" responses, and pointing on command; *word retrieval* (word finding) measuring the ability to generate words beginning with a particular letter of the alphabet or in a particular semantic category (animals); *reading*; and *writing* from dictation and spontaneously. Some aphasia measures include the *Boston Diagnostic Aphasia Examination (BDAE)*[23] and the *Western Aphasia Battery,*[55] *Aphasia*

Communication Outcome Measure, which is a patient-reported outcome measure of communicative functioning for persons with aphasia.[56]

In addition to measuring performance on specific linguistic tasks, an aphasia evaluation also requires an examination of *functional communication.* This is necessary because an individual's actual use of language in everyday life may not correspond to the degree of pathology measured by specific language task performance.[57,58] Functional communication measures are generally rating scales with high interrater reliability. The *Functional Communication Profile (FCP),*[59,60] *Communicative Activities of Daily Living (CADL),*[61] *Communicative Effectiveness Index,*[62] ASHA's *Functional Assessment of Communication Skills (ASHA FACS),*[63] and *Communication Outcome After Stroke (COAST),*[64] which have high interrater reliability, are measures used for this purpose.

In addition to measures of language and functional communication, new tools have been developed to determine the impact of impaired communication skills on quality of life. The scope of SLP practice now encompasses all of the components and factors specified in the WHO framework.[65-67] Specifically, concern for the effect of aphasia on family, social, and community life is the basis for more recently designed measures (e.g., Burden of Stroke Scale [BOSS], Functional Life Scale [FLS], Aphasic Depression Rating Scale [ADRS], Frenchay Activities Index, the Barthel Index, and Stroke and Aphasia Quality of Life Scale–39 [SAQOL-39]).[68-75]

Recovery

If complete recovery from aphasia is to occur, it usually happens within a matter of hours or days following onset. Once aphasia has persisted for several weeks or months, a complete return to a premorbid state is usually the exception. Language gains in aphasia take place earlier as well as later.[76-81]

Most patients do not consider themselves recovered unless they have fully recovered to previous levels of language performance.[82] When unrecovered patients are satisfied with their level of competence and consider themselves recovered, this is a psychological perception and should not be confused with an objective evaluation of communication abilities. For individuals with aphasia, the true test of rehabilitation outcome is their perception of the quality of their lives. Measures of life function that include activity levels, socialization, mobility, and community reintegration can be used for this purpose.[83,84]

It is useful to distinguish between two separate recovery dimensions in aphasia: one that is objective and attempts to quantify the extent to which a person has regained language abilities; and another, which measures the recovery of functional communication.

The concept of a functional dimension of communication behavior emerged logically from the experience of treating patients with aphasia in rehabilitation medicine settings. Historically, rehabilitation medicine has acknowledged that the ability of patients to function in daily life (activities of daily living [ADL]) does not necessarily correlate with the degree of physical disability. Similarly, improvement in quantitative measures of language performance does not necessarily correlate with improvement in functional communication.[46]

The majority of patients experience a degree of natural recovery with or without intervention in the period immediately following onset. However, there is a lack of consensus about the duration of the *spontaneous recovery* period.[85-87] Culton[88] reported rapid spontaneous language recovery in the first month following the onset of aphasia. A number of studies have concluded that the greatest improvement occurs in the first 2 to 3 months after onset.[89-93] Of 850 patients surveyed in the first month following stroke, 177 presented with aphasia. In the 4 to 12 weeks following the stroke, aphasia improved in 74% of the patients and cleared in 44%.[19] Butfield and Zangwill,[94] Sands et al,[95] and Vignolo[89] reported that the recovery rate dropped significantly after 6 months. Others have found that spontaneous recovery occurs up to 6 months[96] or 1 year.[88,90] Sarno and Levita[97] reported that the greater change took place within a 3-month rather than a 6-month post-onset period in a sample of patients with severe aphasia seen up to 6 months after stroke.

Recovery from aphasia after stroke is difficult to predict, especially during the early recovery stages.[98] Severity and location of lesion have been reported as predictors of language recovery.[99-102] However, these factors are highly variable, making it difficult to generate a prognosis for individual patients.[103]

Most investigators have concluded that factors such as age, gender, and handedness do not affect recovery from aphasia.[98,103-105] Although age has been reported as a significant prognostic factor,[89,106-108] many do not support this view.[90,104,109-113] These wide discrepancies regarding the influence of age may relate to differences in sampling and methodology. In a study that compared aphasia recovery in the first post-stroke year between a middle-aged (50 to 64 years old) and older (65 to 80 years old) group, age did not emerge as a significant factor.[83] In addition, educational level or occupational status before illness does not always correlate with recovery. However, Sarno and Levita[97] reported that individuals with aphasia who were employed at the time of stroke recovered more than those who were unemployed. In the healthy aged, language performance declines significantly between the sixth and eighth decades.[106,114,115] Gender does not appear to have an important influence on outcome,[76,104,116] whereas handedness may have an effect.[117]

It is generally agreed that posttraumatic aphasia has a better prognosis than aphasia secondary to vascular lesions.[89,94] In fact, some cases of aphasia secondary to TBI have been reported to recover completely.[91,118] The finding that traumatic aphasia carries a better prognosis than vascular aphasia may be influenced by the fact that patients involved in traumatic events are generally neurologically healthy whereas patients who have had strokes may have widespread vascular involvement.[104]

Both type and severity of aphasia appear to carry predictive value, with global aphasia having the poorest prognosis.[76,119-121] Basso[104] reported that when patients with fluent and nonfluent aphasia of the same severity were compared, there were no differences in degree of recovery. In 881 consecutive acute stroke admissions to a community-based hospital, it was possible to make valid prognoses within 1 to 4 weeks after stroke depending on the initial severity of aphasia.[104]

Not surprisingly, most studies report that patients with severe aphasia do not recover as much as those with mild aphasia.[91,95,120-122] Sarno and Levita[76] found that people with fluent aphasia reached the highest level of functional communication, whereas patients with nonfluent and global aphasia made smaller gains in the 8- to 52-week post-stroke period. Global aphasia sometimes evolves to severe Broca's aphasia when there is significantly improved comprehension. Broca's aphasia may become *anomic aphasia,* and Wernicke's aphasia may evolve to anomic or *conduction aphasia.*[76,91,120-124] When persons with aphasia recover a great deal of language function they are usually left with residual *anomia.*

Patients whose computed tomography (CT) scans show large dominant hemisphere lesions, many small lesions, or bilateral lesions are less likely to recover than those with smaller or fewer lesions. [82,120] Lesions in Wernicke's area or those that extend more posteriorly tend to lead to severe and persistent aphasia. The neuroradiological correlates of aphasia recovery have been addressed by some investigators.[93,125] Yarnell et al[82] reported little prognostic value in angiographic and radioscintigram findings. Similarly, CT scans did not help in predicting who might profit from language retraining in a Norwegian study.[86]

Functional imaging studies of aphasia secondary to stroke have suggested that language recovery is dependent on several factors. The neuroplastic changes that are needed during recovery are thought to depend more heavily on left hemispheric changes in activity that slowly manifest over time.[22] Following damage to the left hemisphere, rapid changes have been observed in temporal and frontal areas within the right hemisphere but may reflect maladaptive compensatory activity versus functional reorganization or recovery.[126-135]

Comprehension tends to recover to a greater degree than expression.[26,89,133-136] Although recovery of auditory comprehension involves bilateral temporal lobe activation, there does not seem to be a correlation between the activity of each hemisphere during this process.[126,137-139] As technology advances and research continues, new insights into the mechanisms of recovery and treatment will emerge.[140]

The presence of depression, anxiety, and paranoia have been cited as negative factors in recovery,[141-143] and premorbid personality traits have been identified as important prognostic factors. Eisenson and Herrmann felt that patients with outgoing personalities had a better prognosis than those with introverted, dependent, or rigid personalities.[144-146]

Efficacy of Treatment in Post-Stroke Aphasia

Many methodological problems have limited the number of studies that examine the efficacy of aphasia rehabilitation.[147-153] Nevertheless, treatment accountability issues are compelling and a focus of professional concern.

Studies that investigate treatment effects, specific techniques, and approaches have been reported since the late 1950s.[154] Vignolo,[89] Hagen,[155] and Basso et al[90] utilized untreated control and treated groups and showed a positive treatment effect. Edmonds et al[156] and Poeck et al[157] also yielded positive treatment effects with treated and untreated groups. In addition, several reviews and examinations have revealed significant treatment effects (i.e., improvements in communicative ability) with intense intervention provided over a short period of time.[158-160] Variables such as spontaneous recovery,[161,162] age,[109,163] duration, treatment intensity,[158-160] and timing of treatment[164] and specific treatment techniques[165-167] have been studied.

Although studies have varied in method and research focus, there have been strong indications for positive treatment effects. Some have maintained that single case studies rather than randomized, controlled trials are the most appropriate method for addressing treatment efficacy.[168,169] Current research utilizing a standard approach to analyze data from single-subject designs are improving the ability to quantify treatment outcomes.[96] A single case approach to the study of aphasia treatment efficacy has not escaped criticism but is far less frequent than criticism of studies based on groups of people with aphasia.[96] Negative views of the group study model are based primarily on the view that individuals are unique, especially with respect to communication behavior.

The Academy of Neurologic Communication Disorders and Sciences (ANCDS) has issued evidence-based practice guidelines for neurogenic communication disorders.[170,171] Until now, speech-language pathologists (SLPs) have depended on meta-analyses of efficacy studies reported for 45 studies published between 1946 and 1988 and for 55 studies that support better clinical outcome for patients who receive early, intensive treatment.[152,172]

Psychological and Related Factors

It has been observed that the variability of patients' psychological reactions is rarely determined by lesion type or location but is an expression of the whole life experience of the person who has had a stroke.[83,104,143,173,174]

Depression, anxiety, premorbid personality, fatigue, and paranoia are often cited as deterrents to recovery and communication. The social isolation experienced by people with aphasia and their families has a profound impact on quality of life.[83] The effect of aphasia on an individual's sense of "self" can be extremely negative, leading to a loss of self-esteem and feelings of helplessness. Also, the opportunity for "healing conversation," so essential to individuals who have suffered losses, is often unavailable to those with aphasia, which may be the result of inadequate social support.

In a study of patients with aphasia participating in a group psychotherapy program, Friedman[175] investigated the nature of psychological regression with impaired reality testing in aphasia. Beyond the communication difficulties posed by aphasia, he observed that patients remained psychologically isolated. They did not maintain a consistent level of group participation and expressed intense feelings that they were very different from other people. Both withdrawal and projection were apparent as each patient acted in isolation and yet complained of these characteristics in others.

Treatment of Aphasia

Aphasia treatment is rarely the same in any two settings. Literally hundreds of specific speech and language treatment techniques are cited in the aphasia literature. The lack of therapeutic uniformity has undoubtedly impeded an adequate number of carefully controlled studies on the effects of language retraining. Most methods derive essentially from traditional pedagogic practices, relying heavily on repetition.[176]

In general, treatment methods can be categorized as those that are largely *indirect stimulation-facilitation* and those that are essentially *direct structured-pedagogic*.[78,80,118,141,177-180] The two principles that underlie most treatment methods reflect contrasting views of aphasia as either impaired access to language or a "loss" of language. The stimulation methods generally follow an impaired access model and pedagogic approaches are based on a theory of aphasia as a language loss.

In practice, however, much of aphasia treatment addresses the *performance* aspect of language in which repeated practice and "teaching" strategies are assumed to help restore impaired skills through a "task-oriented" approach (i.e., naming practice). One of the commonly used techniques involves self-cueing and repetition exercises that manipulate components of grammar and vocabulary. Another approach involves "stimulating" the patient to use residual language by encouraging conversation in a permissive setting where a patient's responses are unconditionally accepted and topics are of personal interest.[179]

The primary assumption that drives the treatment of aphasia is that language in the brain is not "erased," but that retrieval of its individual units has been impaired. Approaches to aphasia therapy have generally followed one of two models: a *substitute skill model* or a *direct treatment model,* both of which are based on the assumption that the processes that subserve normal performance need to be understood if treatment is to succeed.[180] An example of the substitute skill model can be found in individuals who are deaf, some of whom use speech reading, a visual input rather than an auditory input, as an aid to comprehend spoken language. If a direct treatment model is followed, specific exercises individually designed to ameliorate specific linguistic deficits are the basis of treatment.

Significant progress and improvements of language and communication performance have been reported in those with aphasia who have received intensive and/or extended periods of language therapy.[157,181,182] More recent reports of intensive treatment programs have shown significant improvement of communication abilities several years post-stroke, when aphasia is in the chronic stage.[182-184] Some benefits may also be received from pharmacological treatment with and without speech therapy.[185-192] In addition, improvements have also been documented with the use of transcranial magnetic stimulation,[193] functional magnetic resonance imaging,[194] and transcranial direct current stimulation.[195]

Contextualized, constraint-induced language therapy (CILT) is an intensive form of language therapy that is usually administered over a short period of time. Treatment is conducted by an SLP in small groups of two to three persons with aphasia who are required to use and practice only those verbal skills that are difficult or impaired. Forms of communication that can be effective in total communication but are not verbal, including gesturing, drawing, or writing, are constrained.[196-197]

Some investigators have reported the use of writing[198] or drawing as a potential means of communication.[199-201] Others have developed interactive approaches to aphasia treatment. Examples include the *communication partners* approach of Lyon et al,[202] a treatment plan designed to enhance communication and well-being in settings where the person with aphasia and the caregiver live; the *supported conversation* approach introduced by Kagan and colleagues,[203-207] in which volunteers are trained as conversation partners to facilitate conversation by using all available modalities, thereby revealing the individual's competence and permitting a communicative interaction; and the *social model of aphasia* approach introduced by Simmons-Mackie,[208-216] which focuses on the fulfillment of social needs and the encouragement of a greater conversational burden on the part of communication partners. Partners are trained to facilitate interaction by modifying some of their interactive behavior.

If an individual is unable to make himself or herself understood, aids can provide a means of communication using manual or electronic devices (e.g., tablet computer). Use of telecommunications, virtual clinicians and environments, and computer-assisted and Web-based treatments may lead to improvements in language and communication, especially when utilized as an adjunct to clinical therapy. Data suggest that these types of therapies may be effective for patients in various stages of recovery.[217-222]

Management of the Patient With Aphasia

The unfortunate reality is that once the condition of aphasia has stabilized, very few patients recover normal communication function, with or without speech therapy. Accordingly, aphasia rehabilitation should be viewed as a process of patient management in the broadest sense of the term. That is, the task is primarily one of helping the patient and his or her intimates adjust to the alterations and limitations imposed by the disability. Effective aphasia rehabilitation management requires the participation of several disciplines, including medicine, psychology, physical therapy, occupational therapy, social work, vocational counseling, and, most critically, aphasia therapy.

Speech and language therapy to stimulate and support the patient through the various stages of recovery is an effective management tool.[223-224] Experienced aphasia therapists recognize that while working on aphasic deficits, they are simultaneously dealing psychotherapeutically with a readjusting personality.[143] Speech therapy, therefore, serves different purposes at different points along the way. Sometimes it allows patients to "borrow time," as Baretz and Stephenson[225] have aptly stated. Occasionally depression lifts after speech therapy has been initiated, reflecting the supportive and nurturing nature of the therapeutic relationship rather than an objective improvement in recovery of speech and language.

Aphasia recovery can be viewed as a dynamic process consisting of a series of stages like the stages of mourning described by Kübler-Ross,[226] through which the majority of patients evolve. Some, of course, never emerge from a state of severe depression.[227,228] Kübler-Ross[226] and other authors have suggested that the stages through which someone with aphasia passes—including denial, rage, bargaining, and acceptance—could be characterized as attempts to overcome the sense of loss.

By directly addressing a patient's linguistic deficits and channeling attention and energies toward constructive goals, speech therapy may produce a noticeable reduction in depression. Therapy tasks in this instance act as an equivalent for work, which has long been recognized as an antidote for depression.

There is a tendency to overestimate the capacity of individuals with aphasia to return to work, particularly if the verbal deficits are mild. Premature attempts to return to work can have a negative psychological impact. Professional rehabilitation counselors are best equipped to explore and evaluate a patient's vocational potential and carry out the long and arduous process of evaluating work performance and job requirements.

Experienced aphasia clinicians stress the importance of the patient's family in the rehabilitation process. Some of the potentially negative reactions of the family include overprotectiveness, hostility, anger, unrealistic expectations, overzealousness, lack of knowledge of the dimensions of the disorder, and inability to cope with practical difficulties. The apparently natural tendency of family members to minimize the patient's communication impairment, particularly in the early stages of recovery, requires understanding and tactful management.[143]

The quality of premorbid relationships generally tends to be intensified after a catastrophic event; those that were problematic may deteriorate further, whereas the bond between a loving couple may become stronger. The reversal of roles, changes in levels of dependency, and a changed economic situation, so often a consequence of chronic disability, can have a critical negative impact on the patient and his or her family.[174]

In a positive family milieu, patients are encouraged to develop regular daily routines as close to premorbid patterns as possible and are treated as contributing members of the family. Patients need to be allowed some sense of control. Including the patient in rehabilitation planning promotes restoration of feelings of self-worth. In this regard, the emphasis on function rather than complete recovery, pointing out success rather than performance failure, adds to a patient's sense of self. It is essential to listen to patients, particularly to their expressions of loss. Commiseration is often more comforting than optimistic prognostic statements.

Aphasia Centers, Intensive Comprehensive Aphasia Programs (ICAPs), group speech therapy, stroke clubs, and other social and support groups are resources that can be effective tools in the management of some patients with aphasia. Other resources include support and social organizations, such as The National Aphasia Association (NAA), which was founded in the United States in 1987, following the lead of existing advocacy organizations established in Finland (1971), Germany (1978), the United Kingdom (1980), and Sweden (1981). The NAA provides an extensive array of educational and resource information appropriate for patients, families, and professionals on its website (www.aphasia.org).

Group therapy with peers may provide a comfortable atmosphere in which patients can meet new friends and share feelings, although not all individuals with aphasia find it beneficial. A positive effect seems to be related to level of comprehension, time since onset, and personality factors. Although group therapy generally plays an important role in aphasia rehabilitation, it should be noted that much of its effectiveness depends on the skill and experience of the group leader.[229-230]

Aphasia rehabilitation remains eclectic and specifically tailored to the individual patient. Fundamental to this therapeutic philosophy is the acknowledgement and appreciation of the uniqueness of the individual. No two persons with aphasia are exactly alike in pathology, personality, linguistic deficits, reactions to catastrophic illness, life experience, spiritual values, or a host of other factors. The influence of these factors carries different weight and strength at different stages of recovery and they are all related to recovery outcome.

COGNITIVE-COMMUNICATION DISORDERS

When the neural regions responsible for the cognitive processes that support communicative function are damaged, a broad spectrum of deficits can result. Many conditions can cause cognitive-communication disorders, including TBI, stroke (especially right hemisphere damage), dementia, brain tumors, aging, degenerative neurological disease, alcohol/drug abuse, and medications. Impairments of executive function, including difficulties with attention and memory, may interfere with a person's ability to transform thoughts and ideas into spoken and/or written language. Impaired memory can also affect word retrieval, topic maintenance, a person's ability to recall and integrate information, and the speed of processing information. In addition, organizing information, interpreting visual information, deficits in abstract reasoning, and decreased orientation to person, place, and time are common symptoms. Impairments in speech production, including reduced fluency and prosodic speech features (i.e., rate and rhythm of speech, stress within words to indicate meaning and within sentences to express variations of intent or meaning), are also common. Given the nature of these deficits, participating in social situations can be especially difficult.[231] The difficulties may affect all modes of communication, including understanding, nonverbal and verbal expression, reading, and writing. These impairments can be debilitating and socially isolating, because they impair a person's ability to establish and maintain relationships with others.[232-233]

Impairments of certain aspects of pragmatic language (i.e., language use) and nonverbal communication (including difficulty in initiating, maintaining, and ending conversations) may result in difficulties maintaining a topic and taking turns in discourse; being concise; understanding and expressing feeling through facial expressions; comprehending nonverbal methods of communication (i.e., gesturing); maintaining eye contact; engaging in conversation or narrative production that is self-focused; interpreting and expressing emotions appropriately; and reduced ability in understanding humor.

Examination of Cognitive-Communication Disorders

Many factors, including the heterogeneity of individuals, limitations of available standardized testing measures, performance differences in structured versus unstructured contexts, and environmental and personal factors, have made the examination of cognitive-communication disorders a challenging area in need of further study.[234] A standardized test battery for the identification and measurement of cognitive-communication disorders does not exist and depends entirely on the knowledge, experience, and expertise of the examiner.

Treatment of Cognitive-Communication Disorders

Intervention depends on the type and severity of the cognitive-communication disorder and is usually based on a combination of behavioral, meta-cognitive, and counseling approaches. Patients with cognitive-communication disorders are especially challenging since they often have reduced insight and/or denial.[235-236] The importance of providing speech-language pathology treatment using a team approach has been highlighted as an important element in the rehabilitation process. Such collaborative methods take into account each person's social network (e.g., family, friends, caregivers, and so forth.)[237]

The management of patients with cognitive-communication disorders begins with determining what environmental factors, if any, can be modified to provide the least visual or auditory distraction. Steps also need to be taken to establish a structured routine or daily schedule. These efforts help to reduce communication breakdowns and facilitate communicative success.[235-236] The later stages of intervention emphasize the carryover of skills acquired in therapy to a variety of daily activities and contexts. Box 28.1 provides several suggested strategies to improve communication for patients with cognitive-communication disorders.

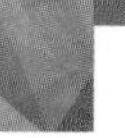

Box 28.1 Strategies for Improving Communication in the Presence of Cognitive-Communication Disorder

- Use visual materials/aids to help orient the person to time (e.g., clocks and calendars).
- Break long, complicated tasks into shorter tasks that are easier to follow.
- Establish eye contact to initiate and maintain conversation.
- When giving verbal directions, use simple sentences and repetitions as necessary.
- Accommodate the presence of visual field deficits by helping the person find compensatory means for reading and writing.
- Gently state when the topic in a conversation changes prematurely.

DYSARTHRIA

The term *dysarthria* (sometimes called a *motor speech disorder*) refers to an impairment of speech production resulting from damage to the central or peripheral nervous system, which causes weakness, paralysis, or incoordination of the motor–speech system. Any one or all of the components of the motor–speech system (respiration, phonation, articulation, resonance, and prosody) may by compromised by neural damage. The type and degree of dysarthria depends on the underlying etiology, degree of neuropathology, coexistence of other disabilities, and the individual response of the patient to the condition. It is not unusual for dysarthria to coexist with aphasia in patients who have suffered cerebrovascular accident (CVA) or TBI. The severity of dysarthria may range from the production of occasionally imprecise consonant sounds to speech that is rendered totally unintelligible by the degree of impairment to the underlying systems. When patients are totally unintelligible as the result of severe motor–speech system impairment, they exhibit *anarthria.*

The incidence of dysarthria in the population of individuals with neurogenic disorders is approximately 46%, representing a significant proportion of the patients with communication impairments seen in medical settings.[238] It is difficult to estimate the total number of people affected by dysarthria, because the condition results from a wide range of etiologies (e.g., progressive neurological diseases, TBI, stroke). Dysarthria is generally reflected in deficits occurring in multiple motor–speech systems, but may sometimes occur in a single system (e.g., an impairment of soft palate movement resulting in hypernasality). It is most notably prevalent in cerebral palsy, TBI, CVA, demyelinating diseases (e.g., multiple sclerosis), neoplasm, and progressive neurodegenerative diseases, such as Parkinson's disease, Huntington's chorea, and amyotrophic lateral sclerosis.

There are five primary types of dysarthria: *spastic, flaccid, ataxic, hypokinetic,* and *hyperkinetic.* When two or more types coexist, the term *mixed dysarthria* is used. Coexisting physical disabilities are present in a majority of patients who manifest dysarthria.

Classification and Nomenclature

Spastic dysarthria is characterized by imprecise articulation, slow labored articulation, hypernasality, harsh to strained phonation, and monotonous pitch. Syllables may be given equal stress and inflection. There is often reduced control of exhalation, with shallow inhalations and slow breaths. Spastic dysarthria is the result of bilateral pyramidal system damage involving the corticobulbar tracts (upper motor neurons). The pathology may cause weakness and paresis of the face and tongue musculature on the side opposite to the lesion. There is a high incidence of spastic dysarthria among those with cerebral palsy.[238]

Flaccid dysarthria is characterized by slow/labored articulation, hypernasality, and hoarse, breathy phonation. Phrases may be short, inhalation is shallow, and the control of exhalation may be reduced. There is often a reduction in the variation of pitch and loudness with audible inspirations. Most of these deviant speech characteristics are related to muscular weakness and reduced muscle tone, which affects speech accuracy.

Ataxic dysarthria is characterized by disturbances of timing, movement, range, control, and coordination of the muscles of speech and respiration. Speech is imprecise, slow, and irregular. There may be intermittent periods of explosive inflection, syllable stress, and loudness patterns. Phonemes may be prolonged; pitch and loudness are monotonous. The lesions producing ataxic dysarthria are bilateral, generalized lesions involving the deep midline nuclei and pathways of the cerebellum. Patients with multiple sclerosis and TBI with cerebellar damage often manifest ataxic dysarthria.

Hypokinetic dysarthria is characterized by variable articulatory precision, slow rate of speech, harsh, hoarse voice quality, excessive and overly long pauses, prolonged syllables, and reduced phonation. Patients with Parkinson's disease, Parkinson's-plus syndromes, or parkinsonian-like symptoms often manifest hypokinetic dysarthria, usually caused by lesions of the substantia nigra.

Hyperkinetic dysarthria is characterized by variable articulatory precision, vocal harshness, prolonged sounds and intervals between words, monotonous pitch, and loudness. It is manifest in patients with Huntington's chorea, caused by lesions of the basal ganglia and/or their extrapyramidal projections.

Treatment of Dysarthria

Dysarthria treatment must be individually designed to account for the profile of impairment, as well as the variability of its disabling effects. Intensive and other types of treatments have been examined, some of which have been proven to be effective.[239] The performance of components of the motor–speech system does not always result in changes to the disabling effects of dysarthria, that is, the intelligibility or comprehensibility of speech.[240] The focus of dysarthria treatment is at times based on an approach that emphasizes compensatory skills. Some techniques tend to encourage the patient to minimize the overall disability by using strategies that may actually deviate from normal (i.e., slowing down the rate of speech production to increase intelligibility of consonant production). Patients and communication partners must also be trained to seek the most optimal situations for communication interactions. Thus, the overall aim of dysarthria treatment is to improve communicative effectiveness, which can also be negatively affected if the speaker is in a noisy environment.

One type of approach is to focus on one of the subsystems of speech production, such as velopharyngeal function.[241] Other approaches include utilizing a strategy that results in a spreading of effects and is centered around improving coordination of the subsystems of respiration, phonation, articulation, and resonance.[239,242] Loudness, speaking rate, clarity, and prosodic features of speech (i.e., stress, intonation, rate, and rhythm of speech) have also been investigated for their effectiveness in treating dysarthria.[239]

Increasing the loudness of speech is a common target in the treatment of some types of dysarthria, especially Parkinson's disease. The majority of studies that have focused on loudness have examined the short- and long-term efficacy of the Lee Silverman Voice Therapy program (LSVT®/LOUD) for individuals with dysarthria due to Parkinson's disease. Treatment delivery is intensive and focused on high-effort speech and voice exercises to increase loudness, as well as a readjustment of the patient's perception of his or her own loudness levels when speaking. The program is based on several proposed exercise physiology principles that drive neuroplastic changes, including intensive practice, movement complexity, emotional saliency of tasks, timing of treatment (i.e., the earlier, the better), and continuous/daily exercise to slow disease progression.[243] Studies that have examined this treatment method have also reported improvement in swallowing, articulation, and facial expression[244-247] and have demonstrated its success in individuals with dysarthria due to stroke,[248] TBI,[249] multiple sclerosis,[248] ataxic dysarthria,[250] cerebral palsy,[251] and Down's syndrome.[252]

In addition to focusing on improving loudness, a variety of strategies are used to manipulate speech rate. Speakers tend to be more intelligible when they speak more slowly.[253] An ANCDS review of studies that investigated the effectiveness of rate control techniques concluded that they are dependent on the type and severity of dysarthria and the specific intervention strategies employed. Further study is still needed to delineate an individual's candidacy for this type of technique, as well as what the carryover can be to the natural communication environment.

A third focus of dysarthria treatment is the improvement of the prosodic aspects of speech (i.e., stress patterns within words and sentences, intonation to express meaning, and rate-rhythm interactions). A variety of strategies that target prosody have been implemented, including those using biofeedback and behavioral instruction. Few conclusions can be drawn about the effectiveness of prosody training because of the small number of examinations and wide range of subject characteristics and techniques used.[239]

Many persons with motor–speech impairments have been able to increase their communicative effectiveness using augmentative and alternative communication (AAC). Low- and high-tech aids include specially designed software applications that are available on mobile devices such as laptop or tablet computers and a variety of smartphones. Recommendations of AAC for persons with dysarthria depend on the severity of the communication disorder and the projected course of the disease and must be carefully selected and managed by an experienced, professional speech-language pathologist.

■ APRAXIA OF SPEECH

Some patients with nonfluent (Broca's) aphasia present with articulatory difficulty characterized by speech sound errors, slow speech rate, slow transitions between sounds, syllables, and words, and impaired prosody in the absence of impaired strength or coordination of the motor speech system.[254-257] This profile of difficulty speaking is referred to as *apraxia of speech* (AOS) (or *speech dyspraxia, verbal apraxia, cortical dysarthria,* or *phonetic disintegration*). Additional behaviors that may be present in persons with AOS include difficulty initiating speech, articulatory struggling, periods of error-free speech production, and a greater number of sound production errors as utterance length increases. These characteristics may be so severe that the patient is barely intelligible but appears to be independent of difficulty in language processing. Unlike dysarthric speakers, individuals with AOS do not generally have deficits in performing nonspeech movements of the oral musculature. The possible independence of this deficit from the language disorder of Broca's aphasia remains controversial.

Due to its common co-occurrence with aphasia, AOS is challenging to diagnose.[258] The speech dyspraxia component of this multifaceted communication disorder appears to be especially amenable to direct therapeutic intervention.

Treatment of Apraxia of Speech

A variety of approaches, designed to improve phonetic placement accuracy, typically depend on imitation, stress, and gradually shaping sounds until a desired sound is approximated, which is then drilled using temporal, tactile, kinesthetic, visual, and auditory cues. Treatment guidelines have been published by the ANCDS.[259-261]

In an attempt to synthesize and assess available evidence from the literature, 59 studies were summarized and rated by the ANCDS. The most commonly used approaches are referred to as *articulatory kinematic.* These techniques aim to improve articulatory movements: modeling, imitation, repetition, shaping, electromagnetic articulography, and multimodal and articulatory placement cueing.[262-270]

Integral stimulation, a method originally introduced by Milisen,[271] is a commonly used articulatory kinematic technique that involves imitation and emphasizes the importance of helping the patient focus his or her attention on auditory and visual models of speech. Rosenbek et al[264] developed an eight-step continuum based on this approach that employs a hierarchy of cues in which the timing between the stimulus provided by the clinician and the response produced by the patient is varied.[264]

Sound production treatment, a five-step program based on the Rosenbek et al [264] eight-step continuum, incorporates principles of motor learning such as repeated practice and verbal feedback and is an approach that has been systematically investigated.[270-274]

Visual spectrographic and *verbal feedback* utilize different sensory modalities to facilitate speech production.[275-276] The effect of the frequency and timing at which feedback is provided has been investigated and found to be important in the treatment of AOS.[277]

Rate and rhythm strategies are employed to improve speech sound accuracy by controlling the rate of speech and stress patterns within words and sentences.[278] External devices such as computer-generated pulses or programs, metronomes, pacing boards, and finger tapping are used to manipulate the rate of speech.[279-285]

The long-term nature of recovery of phonemic production in patients with verbal apraxia was confirmed in a study of a patient with Broca's aphasia who received speech therapy for 10 years. The errors that prevailed in the first post-stroke year were compared with performance at 10 years. The features of place and manner of production had improved; although voicing and addition errors (the addition of sounds) persisted, omission errors (the omission of sounds) were virtually eliminated.[286]

Alternative communication aid approaches are often recommended for persons with AOS. In most cases, the use of multiple communication modalities, such as writing, drawing, gesturing, and signing, is suggested as a facilitatory technique to enhance or substitute for impaired speech.[287-290]

Intersystemic facilitation or *reorganization approaches* use intact systems or preserved strengths or abilities of the patient to facilitate and improve accurate speech production.[291] These approaches employ and combine strategies that can be included in more than one category, such as iconic or rhythmic gestures, vibrotactile stimulation, imitation, modeling, and ACA.[292-295]

DYSPHAGIA

The swallowing process is composed of a number of complex neuromuscular events. Normal swallowing requires that an individual be able to move food or liquid from the mouth (*oral phase of swallowing*), through the pharynx (*pharyngeal phase of swallowing*), and into the esophagus. In the oral swallow phase, food is collected in the oral cavity in a single mass, or bolus, which is then propelled into the pharynx and further propelled under pressure into the esophagus. During the oral phase of swallowing, the bolus is first held between the tongue and palate and then propelled by the tongue from the front to the back of the oral cavity. The bolus moves over the back of the tongue into the pharynx, triggering the pharyngeal swallow and the neuromuscular events that propel the bolus into the esophagus. Velopharyngeal closure, tongue base posterior motion, pharyngeal contraction, laryngeal elevation and closure, and upper esophageal opening occur to allow bolus passage into the esophagus. Airway protection involves closure of the airway entrance and airway. The vocal folds close and the epiglottis moves downward to prevent food from entering the trachea during this process.

Dysphagia is defined as a condition in which an individual has had an interruption in either eating function or the maintenance of nutrition and hydration.[296] Many patients with neurogenic communication disorders also manifest deficits in swallowing (dysphagia). From 25% to 50% of individuals who have suffered strokes may have swallowing deficits ranging from mild to severe.[297-304] In some cases dysphagia is only present in the acute phase with rapid recovery of swallowing function taking place in the first 3 weeks post-stroke.[305] Swallowing deficits in post-stroke patients are often due to a combination of weakness and incoordination of the oral, pharyngeal, and laryngeal musculature, resulting in inefficient propulsion of a food bolus or liquid through the oral cavity, pharynx, and into the esophagus. Delayed triggering of swallowing is not uncommon after stroke. Oral or pharyngeal transit times may be slow. Reduced elevation or closure of the larynx may result in material being misdirected into the airway (aspiration). Dysphagia is also often present in patients with other neurological disorders, such as Parkinson's disease,[306] Huntington's disease,[307] the dystonias and dyskinesias,[308-309] amyotrophic lateral sclerosis,[310] multiple sclerosis,[311] head and neck cancer,[312] dementia,[313-314] cerebral palsy,[315] and TBI.[316]

A dysphagia examination usually begins at bedside and is followed by more objective, instrumental techniques if a pharyngeal phase swallowing disorder is suspected. Several examinations are frequently utilized in the evaluation of swallowing, including the modified barium radiographic study and the flexible fiberoptic endoscopic study with or without sensory testing. These procedures permit viewing of many components of the oropharyngeal swallow, including structural movement, bolus flow, and penetration and/or aspiration. Precise physiological swallowing disorders can be identified using these measures. In addition, the effects of therapeutic strategies on swallow physiology, safety, and efficiency can be examined. In most settings, the swallowing evaluation is carried out by the SLP.

Treatment of Dysphagia

Dysphagia treatment is designed to improve swallowing efficiency for nutritional purposes and to increase swallowing safety. This can be accomplished by compensatory strategies and/or techniques designed to change swallowing physiology and reduce the risk of aspiration. Compensatory strategies include postural changes that affect the way food passes through the mouth and pharynx, dietary management, and placing food in the mouth in optimal positions. Specific techniques, exercises, and maneuvers are used to increase the coordination, range of motion, strength, and sensory input of the muscles and structures involved in the oral and pharyngeal phases of swallowing. These exercises are designed to improve initiation of tongue movement, lingual propulsion, laryngeal elevation, closure, and tongue base approximation to the posterior pharyngeal wall.[317-325]

The physical therapist can play an important role in positioning the patient for optimum swallowing and providing treatment to reduce muscle spasticity, improve muscle strength and coordination, and prevent primitive reflex patterns from interfering with swallowing. Additional implications for the physical therapist when treating patients with communication disorders follow. Appendix 28.A presents Web-based resources for patients, families, and caregivers.

COMMUNICATION DISORDERS: IMPLICATIONS FOR THE PHYSICAL THERAPIST

Physical therapists often work in settings where they may be the first to become aware of a patient's communication disorder and should refer such patients to an SLP for evaluation. The physical therapist can contribute to the patient's improvement in communication function in two important ways: (1) by providing physiological support for speech functions and (2) by stimulating and facilitating communication through successful, fulfilling interaction with the patient. In either case, the physical therapist will want to work closely with the SLP to ensure that their treatment goals and interventions are compatible.

The provision of physiological support for speech functions is especially relevant to the patient with pathology of the oral–motor system (e.g., dysarthria). The physical therapist will want to explore the influence of physiological support on the patient's speech in determining a comprehensive plan of care. Proper posture, for example, can help to inhibit reflexes that may trigger primitive movements. When a patient's speech function is influenced by overflow movements, stabilization techniques may be indicated.

Control of respiration is essential to the improvement of vocalization and the phrasing of speech. The muscles of respiration can be strengthened, and exercises designed to increase head control, stability, and sitting balance can be introduced. Proper posture and eye contact enhance the possibility that speech will be audible and clear.

When a patient with a communication impairment is prescribed a communication board, the physical therapist contributes by determining a patient's sitting balance and tolerance, upper extremity motor control, and the best method for responding (e.g., pointing).

Strengthening exercises to increase the speech and range of motion of the tongue, lips, and general facial musculature and to improve coordination of the oral–motor system also increase the probability of intelligible speech and help the patient with dysarthria and dysphagia. Postural techniques are especially important for patients with dysphagia, who require individually tailored treatment programs designed to facilitate swallowing and prevent aspiration.

Because communication is a social activity, the physical therapy setting is a natural context for social interaction. The setting can be supportive by providing an atmosphere that is conducive to conversation and allows the patient to engage in a successful verbal interaction.

Patients who are neurologically compromised often have difficulty processing information in a distracting setting. Excessive noise, competing voices, and the presence of other stimuli can make communication particularly difficult. When possible, the physical therapist should strive to work with patients who are communicatively impaired in a closed environment that is free of distractions. Patients with communication impairments do best when they are positioned in such a way that face-to-face communication is possible, including the visualization of gestures and facial expressions. For this reason, room lighting needs to be sufficient.

Patients who manifest neurogenic speech-language disorders, especially those with aphasia, pose a considerable challenge to effective communication. The individual nature of each manifestation of aphasia argues for a close working relationship with the SLP. This will ensure that the most effective communication strategies are used with each individual patient.

One of the greatest difficulties in addressing the needs of patients with acquired aphasia has to do with determining and accounting for the patient's level of auditory comprehension. Virtually all patients with aphasia have some degree of difficulty in comprehending spoken language. Physical therapists need to become skilled at recognizing and dealing with auditory comprehension deficits because they can be a major deterrent to successful rehabilitation.

Misconceptions of the auditory comprehension level of a patient with aphasia can range from the assumption that a patient understands everything to the assumption that the patient comprehends nothing and must be excluded from conversation. A guiding principle to keep in mind is that auditory comprehension can vary greatly, depending on the context and complexity of the task at hand. Switching topics quickly, speaking too quickly, background noises, talking while a patient is engaged in physical activity, and conversing with more than one person at a time can impede the individual's ability to process auditory information. Sentences should be short and simple, and the patient should be given sufficient time to process the information and formulate a response. Questions that require elaborate answers, such as "Tell me about your vacation" or "What do you think about the latest news?" are generally difficult for patients with aphasia to answer. It is best to ask questions that can be answered with "yes," "no," or another single word. Physical cues to comprehension such as gestures, facial expression, and voice inflection can facilitate and enhance a patient's understanding. It is important for the physical therapist to know that patients with aphasia often find it easier to respond to whole body or axial commands ("stand up," "sit down") than distal commands ("point," "pick up").

It can be tempting to try to remedy a laborious communication situation by "talking down" to a patient with aphasia as if speaking to a child or raising one's voice as if speaking to someone with impaired hearing. The best strategy is to speak a little more slowly, using language that is not too complex, and remaining consistent in giving instructions. This can be particularly important in the physical therapy setting, where verbal commands are a fundamental element in the patient–therapist interaction. At times, it may be necessary to repeat a sentence to be understood.

Rehabilitation team members almost universally overestimate the degree to which a person with aphasia understands spoken language. Physical therapists, when possible, should consult with the SLP for an indication of the patient's preserved auditory comprehension. It may be necessary to rephrase questions and supplement with body language to ensure comprehension.

The use of accompanying visual cues, such as gestures and facial expressions, can be extremely helpful for some patients. Others may understand best if a message is supplemented by written cues. Sometimes one can assist by asking questions that can be answered by "yes" or "no" in a "20 questions" format. When someone with aphasia is having trouble expressing him- or herself, it usually helps to allow him or her extra time to speak. If the patient becomes visibly frustrated, it is desirable to remain calm and suggest that the patient wait and try again later.

During physical therapy interventions, patients with aphasia can be encouraged to produce single-word, repetitive speech that coincides with physical movements as a means of providing supplemental speech practice. Activities such as counting movements in series one to ten, and using words like up, down, left, and right while performing physical movements are examples of such techniques. The physical therapist, however, should always remain sensitive to the possibility of making speech demands that are beyond a patient's level of preserved communicative skill.

SUMMARY

Ever since World War II, speech-language pathologists have played an important role on the rehabilitation team in the management of patients with neurogenic speech-language disorders, especially aphasia and dysarthria. For the physical therapist, an understanding of normal and pathological communication behaviors can not only make this population of patients more interesting to work with, but can also enhance the quality of treatment he or she provides.

Communication using speech is a complex, species-specific behavior that consists of the coordinated interaction of cognitive, motor, sensory, psychological, and social skills. The neurogenic disorders of speech and language, specifically aphasia and dysarthria, dominate the population of patients with communication impairments in the rehabilitation setting. Viewed as a group, patients with neurogenic communication disorders comprise a relatively severely impaired segment of the disabled population.

The impact of neurogenic speech-language disorders on the self, family, community life, and vocational options makes these disorders especially challenging. The close relationship of one's verbal characteristics to personality and identity may cause even the mildest neurogenic communication disorder to affect the psychosocial domain. Current research is investigating the interaction of linguistic, cognitive, and psychosocial variables and their influence on the outcome of recovery and rehabilitation.

Questions for Review

1. Define aphasia.
2. Describe the differences that distinguish nonfluent from fluent aphasic syndromes and give clinical examples.
3. Discuss the components of a comprehensive language test designed to measure aphasic impairment.
4. Describe some critical factors that influence recovery from aphasia.
5. Describe the psychological sequelae that may have a negative effect on the outcome of aphasia rehabilitation.

6. List several causes of cognitive-communication impairments.
7. Define dysarthria.
8. What neurological conditions are generally associated with dysphagia?
9. Describe augmentative communication systems and some specific techniques/devices that may enhance the treatment of aphasia.
10. How can the physical therapist contribute to the physiological support for speech?

CASE STUDY

The patient is a 62-year-old man who teaches high school. He sustained a right hemiplegia and difficulty communicating as the result of a hemorrhagic stroke, which occurred 8 months ago. At this time, except for dressing, he is ADL independent and ambulates with a cane.

At 1 month post-stroke, the patient was limited to "yes" or "no" responses and a vocabulary ranging from 30 to 50 nouns and verbs as well as everyday greetings ("hello," "goodbye"). During a communicative interaction, he often resorted to writing a letter or word or gesturing to help in his communication efforts. He appeared to understand most of what was said, especially when the topic was familiar. He received rehabilitation services during the acute post-stroke phase while hospitalized and received 20 sessions of speech-language pathology services as an outpatient.

At 8 months post-stroke, the patient's communication disorder is marked by a slow, hesitant production of one- and two-word utterances; easily produced automatic speech (i.e., everyday greetings); difficulty expressing complex information; awkward and labored articulation, which causes occasional articulatory imprecision; impaired writing; and some difficulty reading lengthy or complex material. Although the majority of his speaking vocabulary consists of nouns and verbs, adverbs and adjectives are now used with greater frequency. There is a persistent lack of conjunctions, articles, and prepositions in speech, which causes him to have impaired grammar. The patient has no apparent difficulty understanding spoken language except when it is rapid, complex, and/or unfamiliar.

Both the patient and his caregiver report that the frequency of social interactions in his current life has been curtailed dramatically. He continues to see close family members on a regular basis, but he rarely sees friends or work companions. The family reports that he is frustrated and depressed over this and feels isolated from the community much of the time. They also indicate that there has been a gradual but noticeable increase in his speaking vocabulary, ability to write, and reading skill. He has recently joined a local stroke group where he hopes to meet others with similar communication difficulties.

GUIDING QUESTIONS

1. A team conference is scheduled the day after you assume treatment responsibilities for the patient. What types of information would you obtain in consultation with the speech-language pathologist?
2. What communication strategies are generally useful with patients who have sustained a stroke?
3. What approach might you use if the patient became frustrated trying to express himself during a physical therapy treatment?
4. As a physical therapist, what might you do to decrease the patient's sense of isolation and enhance his emotional well-being?
5. In what ways can physical therapy treatment sessions serve to reinforce communication behavior?

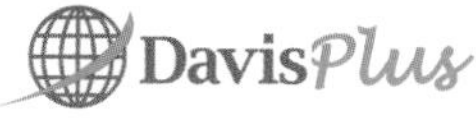

For additional resources, including answers to the questions for review and case study guiding questions, please visit **http://davisplus.fadavis.com.**

References

1. Ruben, RJ: Redefining the survival of the fittest: Communication disorders in the 21st century. Laryngoscope 110:241, 2000.
2. National Institutes of Health: National Institute on Deafness and Other Communication Disorders: Statistics and Epidemiology—Statistics on Voice, Speech, and Language. Retrieved July 11, 2016, from www.nidcd.nih.gov/health/statistics/vsl.asp.
3. Parrish, C, et al: Assessment of cognitive-communicative disorders of mild traumatic brain injury sustained in combat. Perspect Neurophysiol Neurogenic Speech Lang Disord 19:47, 2009.
4. Ylvisaker, M, Turkstra, LS, and Coelho, C: Behavioral and social interventions for individuals with traumatic brain injury: A summary of the research with clinical implications. Semin Speech Lang 26(4): 256, 2005.

5. Coelho, CA: Discourse production deficits following traumatic brain injury: A critical review of the recent literature. Aphasiology 9:409, 1995.
6. Coelho, CA: Story narratives of adults with closed head injury and non–brain-injured adults: Influence of socioeconomic status, elicitation task, and executive functioning. J Speech Lang Hear Res 45:1232, 2002.
7. Ellis, C, Dismuke, C, and Edwards, K: Longitudinal trends in aphasia in the US. NeuroRehabilitation 27(4):327, 2010.
8. Lam, JMC and Wodchis, WP. The relationship of 60 disease diagnoses and 15 conditions to preference-based health-related quality of life in Ontario hospital-based long-term care residents. Med Care 48:380, 2010.
9. Centers for Disease Control and Prevention (CDC). Identifying infants with hearing loss—United States, 1999–2007. MMWR Morb Mortal Wkly Rep 59(8):220, 2010.
10. Blackwell DL, Lucas JW, Clarke TC. Summary health statistics for U.S. adults: National Health Interview Survey, 2012 (PDF). National Center for Health Statistics. Vital Health Stat 10(260), 2014.
11. American Speech-Language-Hearing Association. ASHA Summary Membership and Affiliation Counts, Year-End 2015. 2016. Available from www.asha.org.
12. Stucki, G: Olle Höök Lectureship 2015: The World Health Organization's paradigm shift and implementation of the International Classification of Functioning, Disability and Health in Rehabilitation. J Rehabil Med 48(6):486, 2016.
13. Prodinger, B. et al: Toward the international classification of functioning, disability and health (ICF) rehabilitation set: A minimal generic set of domains for rehabilitation as a health strategy. Arch Phys Med Rehabil 97(6):875, 2016.
14. Galgano, J, and Froud, K: Evidence of the voice-related cortical potential: An electroencephalographic study. NeuroImage 44(1):175, 2009.
15. United States Census Bureau: U.S. Interim Projections by Age, Sex, Race and Hispanic Origin: 2000–2050. 2004. Retrieved March 23, 2017, from https://www.census.gov/population/projections/data/national/usinterimproj.html.
16. Ma, VY, Chan, L, and Carruthers, KJ: Incidence, prevalence, costs, and impact on disability of common conditions requiring rehabilitation in the United States: Stroke, spinal cord injury, traumatic brain injury, multiple sclerosis, osteoarthritis, rheumatoid arthritis, limb loss, and back pain. Arch Phys Med Rehabil 95(5):986, 2014.
17. National Institute on Deafness and Other Communication Disorders (NIDCD): Aphasia. NIH Publication No. 97-4257. NIDCD, Bethesda, MD, 2015 (Updated, 2017).
18. National Aphasia Association: Aphasia Fact Sheet. Retrieved March 23, 2017, from https://www.aphasia.org/aphasia-resources/aphasia-factsheet/.
19. Boehme, AK, et al: Effect of aphasia on acute stroke outcomes. Neurology 87(22): 2348, 2016.
20. Rogalski, E, et al: Aphasic variant of Alzheimer disease: Clinical, anatomic, and genetic features. Neurology 87(13):1337, 2016.
21. Ivanova, MV, et al: Diffusion-tensor imaging of major white matter tracts and their role in language processing in aphasia. Cortex 85:165, 2016.
22. Whitwell, JL, et al: Tracking the development of agrammatic aphasia: A tensor-based morphometry study. Cortex [Sept 2016, DOI: 10.1016/j.cortex.2016.09.017 (Epub ahead of print)].
23. Goodglass, H, et al: The Assessment of Aphasia and Related Disorders, ed 3. Lippincott Williams & Wilkins, Philadelphia, 2001.
24. Damasio, A: Signs of aphasia. In Sarno, MT (ed): Acquired Aphasia, ed 3. Academic Press, New York, 1998, p 25.
25. Sarno, MT: A survey of 100 aphasic Medicare patients in a speech pathology program. J Am Geriatr Soc 18:471, 1970.
26. Prins, R, et al: Recovery from aphasia: Spontaneous speech versus language comprehension. Brain Lang 6:192, 1978.
27. Kozuka, J, et al: Relationship between the change of language symptoms and the change of regional cerebral blood flow in the recovery process of two children with acquired aphasia. Brain Dev [Jan 2017, DOI: 10.1016/j.braindev.2017.01.002 (Epub ahead of print)].
28. Leonard, LB: Children with specific language impairment, ed 2. MIT Press, Cambridge, MA, 2014.
29. Woolpert, D, and Reilly, JS: Investigating the extent of neuroplasticity: Writing in children with perinatal stroke. Neuropsychologia 89:105, 2016.
30. Docking, K, Paquier, P, and Morgan, A: Childhood Brain Tumour. In Cummings, L (ed): Research in Clinical Pragmatics. Springer International, Cham, Switzerland, 2017, p 131.
31. Levin H, et al: Linguistic recovery in aphasia after closed head injury. Brain Lang 12:360, 1981.
32. Mesulam, MM: Slowly progressive aphasia without generalized dementia. Ann Neurol 11:592, 1982.
33. Sapolsky, D, et al: Cortical neuroanatomic correlates of symptom severity in primary progressive aphasia. Neurology 75(4):358, 2010.
34. Golden, E, et al: Assessment of frontal function and behavioral symptoms across subtypes of primary progressive aphasia, semantic dementia and progressive apraxia of speech. J Neurochem 138: 358, 2016.
35. Whitwell, J, et al: Predicting Decline in Agrammatism, Apraxia of Speech and Parkinsonism in Agrammatic Primary Progressive Aphasia (P4. 030). Neurology 86(No. 16 Supplement):P4-030, 2016.
36. Benton, AL: Contributions to aphasia before Broca. Cortex 1:314, 1964.
37. Benton, AL, and Joynt, RJ: Early descriptions of aphasia. Arch Neurol 3:109, 1960.
38. Broca, P: Du siège de la faculté du language articulé. Bull Soc Anthropol 6:377, 1885.
39. Broadbent, D: A case of peculiar affection of speech, with commentary. Brain 1:484, 1879.
40. Mills, CK: Treatment of aphasia by training. JAMA 43:1940, 1904.
41. Head, H: Aphasia and Kindred Disorders of Speech, vols. 1 and 2. Cambridge University Press, Cambridge, UK, 1926.
42. Nielsen, J: Agnosia, Apraxia, Aphasia: Their Value in Cerebral Localization. Hoeber, New York, 1946.
43. Goldstein, K: After Effects of Brain Injuries in War: Their Evaluation and Treatment. Grune & Stratton, New York, 1942.
44. Singer, H, and Low, A: The brain in a case of motor aphasia in which improvement occurred with training. Arch Neurol Psychiatry 29:162, 1933.
45. Weisenburg, T, and McBride, K: Aphasia: A Clinical and Psychological Study. Commonwealth Fund, New York, 1935.
46. Sarno, MT: Recovery and rehabilitation in aphasia. In Sarno, MT (ed): Acquired Aphasia, ed 3. Academic Press, San Diego, 1998, p 595.
47. Klein, K: Community-based resources for persons with aphasia and their families. Top Stroke Rehabil 2:18, 1996.
48. American Heart Association: Aphasia and the Family. Publication EM 359, Dallas, 1969.
49. Backus, O, et al: Aphasia in Adults. University of Michigan Press, Ann Arbor, 1947.
50. Boone, D: An Adult Has Aphasia: For the Family, ed 2. Interstate Printers & Publishers, Danville, IL, 1984.
51. Sarno, JE, and Sarno, MT: Stroke: A Guide for Patients and Their Families, ed 3. McGraw-Hill, New York, 1991.
52. Simonson, J: According to the Aphasic Adult. University of Texas (Southwestern) Medical School, Dallas, 1971.
53. Sarno, MT: Understanding Aphasia: A Guide for Family and Friends. Monograph No. 2, ed 4. Rusk Institute of Rehabilitation Medicine, New York University Medical Center, New York, 2004.
54. Spreen, O, and Risser, AH: Assessment of Aphasia. Oxford University Press, New York, 2000.
55. Kertesz, A: Western Aphasia Battery—Revised. Pro-Ed, Austin, TX, 2006.
56. Hula, WD, et al: The Aphasia Communication Outcome Measure (ACOM): Dimensionality, item bank calibration, and initial validation. J Speech Lang Hear Res 58(3):906, 2015.
57. Sarno, MT: The functional assessment of verbal impairment. In Grimby, G (ed): Recent Advances in Rehabilitation Medicine. Almquist & Wiksell, Stockholm, 1983, p 75.
58. Worrall, LE: A conceptual framework for a functional approach to acquired neurogenic disorders of communication. In Worrall, LE, and Frattali, CM (eds): Neurogenic Communication Disorders: A Functional Approach. Thieme, New York, 2000, p 3.
59. Sarno, MT: A measurement of functional communication in aphasia. Arch Phys Med Rehabil 46:107, 1965.

60. Sarno, MT: The Functional Communication Profile: Manual of Directions (Rehabilitation Monograph No. 42). New York University Medical Center, Rusk Institute of Rehabilitation Medicine, New York, 1969.
61. Holland, AL: Communicative Abilities in Daily Living. University Park Press, Baltimore, 1980.
62. Lomas J, et al: The communicative effectiveness index: Development and psychometric evaluation of a functional communication measure for adult aphasia. J Speech Hear Disord 54:113, 1989.
63. Frattali, CM, et al: Functional Assessment of Communication Skills for Adults: Administration and Scoring Manual. American Speech and Hearing Association, Rockville, MD, 2003.
64. Bambini, V, et al: Assessing functional communication: Validation of the Italian versions of the Communication Outcome after Stroke (COAST) scales for speakers and caregivers. Aphasiology 31(3):332, 2016.
65. Ad Hoc Committee on the Scope of Practice in Speech-Language Pathology: Scope of practice in speech-language pathology. American Speech-Language-Hearing Association, 2016. Retrieved March 23, 2017, from http://www.asha.org/policy/SP2016-00343/.
66. Worrall, L, et al: The validity of functional assessments of communication and the activity/participation components of the ICIDH-2: Do they reflect what really happens in real-life? J Commun Disord 35:107, 2002.
67. Chapey, R, et al: Life participation approach to aphasia: A statement of values for the future. ASHA Leader 5:4, 2000.
68. Doyle, PJ, et al: The Burden of Stroke Scale (BOSS): Validating patient-reported communication difficulty and associated psychological distress in stroke survivors. Aphasiology 17(3):291, 2003.
69. Doyle, PJ, et al: The Burden of Stroke Scale (BOSS) provided valid and reliable score estimates of functioning and well-being in stroke survivors with and without communication disorders. J Clin Epidemiol 57:997, 2004.
70. Sarno, JE, Sarno, MT, and Levita, E: The functional life scale. Arch Phys Med Rehabil 54(5):214, 1973.
71. Benaim, C, et al: Validation of the aphasic depression rating scale. Stroke 35:1692, 2004.
72. Wade, DT, Legh-Smith, J, and Langton, HR: Social activities after stroke: Measurement and natural history using the Frenchay Activities Index. Int Rehab Med 7:176, 1985.
73. Piercy M, et al: Inter-rater reliability of the Frenchay Activities Index in patients with stroke and their careers. Clin Rehabil 14:433, 2000.
74. Green, J, Forster, A, and Young, J: A test-retest reliability study of the Barthel Index, the Rivermead Mobility Index, the Nottingham Extended Activities of Daily Living Scale and the Frenchay Activities Index in stroke patients. Disabil Rehabil 23:670, 2001.
75. Ahmadi, A, et al: Acceptability, reliability, and validity of the Stroke and Aphasia Quality of Life Scale-39 (SAQOL-39) across languages: A systematic review. Clin Rehabil Jan 2017 [Jan 2017, DOI: 10.1177/0269215517690017 (Epub ahead of print)].
76. Sarno, MT, and Levita, E: Recovery in treated aphasia in the first year post-stroke. Stroke 10:663, 1979.
77. Marshall, RC, and Phillipps, DS: Prognosis for improved verbal communication in aphasic stroke patients. Arch Phys Med Rehabil 4:597, 1983.
78. Darley, FL, et al: Motor Speech Disorders. WB Saunders, Philadelphia, 1975.
79. Sarno, MT: Aphasia rehabilitation. In Dickson, S (ed): Communication Disorders: Remedial Principles and Practices. Scott Foresman, Glenview, IL, 1974, p 404.
80. Sarno, MT: Disorders of communication in stroke. In Licht, S (ed): Stroke and Its Rehabilitation. Williams & Wilkins, Baltimore, 1975, p 380.
81. Sarno, MT: Language rehabilitation outcome in the elderly aphasic patient. In Obler, LK, and Albert, ML (eds): Language and Communication in the Elderly: Clinical, Therapeutic and Experimental Issues. DC Heath, Lexington, MA, 1980, p 191.
82. Yarnell, P, et al: Aphasia outcome in stroke: A clinical neuroradiological correlation. Stroke 7:514, 1976.
83. Sarno, MT: Quality of life in aphasia in the first poststroke year. Aphasiology 11:665, 1997.
84. Sorin-Peters, R: Viewing couples with aphasia as adult learners: Implications for promoting quality of life. Aphasiology 17(4):405, 2003.
85. Darley, F: Language rehabilitation: Presentation 8. In Benton, A (ed): Behavioral Change in Cerebrovascular Disease. Harper, New York, 1970, p 51.
86. Reinvang, I, and Engvik, E: Language recovery in aphasia from 3–6 months after stroke. In Sarno, MT, and Hook, O (eds): Aphasia: Assessment and Treatment. Almquist & Wiksell, Stockholm, Sweden, 1980, p 79.
87. Sarno, MT: Review of research in aphasia: Recovery and rehabilitation. In Sarno, MT, and Hook, O (eds): Aphasia: Assessment and Treatment. Almquist & Wiksell, Stockholm, Sweden, 1980, p 15.
88. Culton, G: Spontaneous recovery from aphasia. J Speech Hear Res 12:825, 1969.
89. Vignolo, LA: Evolution of aphasia and language rehabilitation: A retrospective exploratory study. Cortex 1:344, 1964.
90. Basso, A, et al: Etude controlée de la reéducation du language dans l'aphasie: Comparaison entre aphasiques traites et non-traites. Rev Neurol (Paris) 131:607, 1975.
91. Levita, E: Effects of speech therapy on aphasics' responses to the Functional Communication Profile. Percept Motor Skills 47:151, 1978.
92. Lazar, RM, et al: Improvement in aphasia scores after stroke is well predicted by initial severity. Stroke 41(7):1485, 2010.
93. Demeurisse, G, et al: Quantitative study of the rate of recovery from aphasia due to ischemic stroke. Stroke 11:455, 1980.
94. Butfield, E, and Zangwill, O: Re-education in aphasia: A review of 70 cases. J Neurol Neurosurg Psychiatry 9:75, 1946.
95. Sands, E, et al: Long term assessment of language function in aphasia due to stroke. Arch Phys Med Rehabil 50:203, 1969.
96. Basso, A: Aphasia and Its Therapy. Oxford University Press, New York, 2003.
97. Sarno, MT, and Levita, E: Natural course of recovery in severe aphasia. Arch Phys Med Rehabil 52:175, 1971.
98. Lazar, RM, and Antoniello, D: Variability in recovery from aphasia. Curr Neurol Neurosci Rep 8:497, 2008.
99. Kertesz, A, and McCabe, P: Recovery patterns and prognosis in aphasia. Brain 100:1, 1977.
100. Pedersen, PM, et al: Aphasia in acute stroke: Incidence, determinants, and recovery. AnnNeurol 38:659, 1995.
101. Pedersen, PM, Vinter, K, and Olsen, TS: Aphasia after stroke: Type, severity and prognosis. The Copenhagen Aphasia Study. Cerebrovasc Dis 17:35, 2004.
102. Wade, DT, et al: Aphasia after stroke: natural history and associated deficits. J Neurol Neurosurg Psychiatry 49:11, 1986.
103. Lazar, RM, et al: Variability in language recovery after first-time stroke. J Neurol Neurosurg Psychiatry 79:530, 2008.
104. Basso, A: Prognostic factors in aphasia. Aphasiology 6:337, 1992.
105. Cappa, S: Spontaneous recovery from aphasia. In Stemmer, B, and Whitaker, HA (eds): Handbook of Neurolinguistics. Academic Press, San Diego, 1998, p 535.
106. Nicholas, M, et al: Empty speech in Alzheimer's disease and fluent aphasia. J Speech Hear Res 28:405, 1985.
107. Nicholas, M, et al: Aging, language, and language disorders. In Sarno, MT (ed): Acquired Aphasia, ed 3. Academic Press, San Diego, 1998, p 413.
108. Holland, AL, et al: Predictors of language restriction following stroke: A multivariate analyses. J Speech Hearing Res 31:232, 1989.
109. Sarno, MT: Final Report. Age, linguistic evolution, and quality of life in aphasia. DHHS Grant No. CMS 5 R01 DC 00432-04. NIDCD, 1997.
110. Kertesz, A: Recovery from aphasia. Adv Neurol 42:23, 1984.
111. Wertz, RT, and Dronkers, NF: Effects of age on aphasia. Proceedings of the Research Symposium on Communication Sciences and Disorders and Aging. ASHA Reports, 19:88, 1990.
112. Pedersen, M, et al: Aphasia in acute stroke: Incidence, determinants, and recovery. Ann Recov 38:659, 1995.
113. Sarno, MT: Preliminary findings: Age, linguistic evolution and quality of life in recovery from aphasia. Scand J Rehabil Med Suppl 26:43, 1992.
114. Bayles, KA, and Kaszniak, AW: Communication and Cognition in Normal Aging and Dementia. Little, Brown, Boston, 1987.
115. Obler, LK, et al: On comprehension across the adult life span. Cortex 21:273, 1985.
116. Sarno, MT, et al: Gender and recovery from aphasia after stroke. J Nerv Ment Dis 173:605, 1985.

117. Borod, J, et al: Long term language recovery in left handed aphasic patients. Aphasiology 78:301, 1990.
118. Kertesz, A: Aphasia and Associated Disorders: Taxonomy, Localization and Recovery. Grune & Stratton, New York, 1979.
119. Shewan, C, and Kertesz, A: Effects of speech and language treatment on recovery from aphasia. Brain Lang 23:272, 1984.
120. Schuell, H, et al: Aphasia in Adults. Harper, New York, 1964.
121. Selnes, OA, et al: Recovery of single-word comprehension CT scan correlates. Brain Lang 21:72, 1984.
122. Wertz, RT, et al: Comparison of clinic, home, and deferred language treatment for aphasia: A VA cooperative study. Arch Neurol 43:653, 1986.
123. Pashek, GV, and Holland, AL: Evolution of aphasia in the first year post onset. Cortex 24:411, 1988.
124. Kertesz, A: Evolution of aphasic syndromes. Top Lang Disord 1:15, 1981.
125. Goldenberg, G, and Scott, J: Influence of size and site of cerebral lesions on spontaneous recovery of aphasia and success of language therapy. Brain Lang 47:684, 1994.
126. Fernandez B, et al: Functional MRI follow-up study of language processes in healthy subjects and during recovery in a case of aphasia. Stroke 35:2171, 2004.
127. Xu, XJ, et al: Cortical language activation in aphasia: A functional MRI study. Chin Med J (Engl) 117:1011, 2004.
128. Abo, M, et al: Language-related brain function during word repetition in post-stroke aphasics. Neuroreport 15(12):1891, 2004.
129. Peck, KK, et al: Functional magnetic resonance imaging before and after aphasia therapy: Shifts in hemodynamic time to peak during an overt language task. Stroke 35:554, 2004.
130. Rosen, HJ, et al: Neural correlates of recovery from aphasia after damage to left inferior frontal cortex. Neurology 55:1883, 2000.
131. Blank, SC, et al: Speech production after stroke: The role of the right pars opercularis. Ann Neurol 54:310, 2003.
132. Heiss, WD, et al: Speech-induced cerebral metabolic activation reflects recovery from aphasia. J Neurol Sci 145:213, 1997.
133. Lomas, A, and Kertesz, A: Patterns of spontaneous recovery in aphasic groups: A study of adult stroke patients. Brain Lang 5:388, 1978.
134. Kenin, M, and Swisher, L: A study of pattern of recovery in aphasia. Cortex 8:56, 1972.
135. Lebrun, Y: Recovery in polyglot aphasics. In Lebrun, Y, and Hoops, R (eds): Recovery in Aphasics. Neurolinguistics, vol. 4. Swets & Zeitlinger BV, Amsterdam, 1976, p 96.
136. Basso, A, et al: Sex differences in recovery from aphasia. Cortex 18:469, 1982.
137. Sharp, DJ, Scott, SK, and Wise, RJ: Monitoring and the controlled processing of meaning: Distinct prefrontal systems. Cereb Cortex 14:1, 2004.
138. Zahn, R, et al: Recovery of semantic word processing in global aphasia: A functional MRI study. Brain Res Cogn Brain Res 18:322, 2004.
139. Breier, JI, et al: Spatiotemporal patterns of language-specific brain activity in patients with chronic aphasia after stroke using magnetoencephalography. NeuroImage 23:1308, 2004.
140. Crosson, B, et al: Functional MRI of language in aphasia: A review of the literature and the methodological challenges. Neuropsychol Rev 17:157, 2007.
141. Benson, DF: Aphasia, Alexia, and Agraphia. Churchill Livingstone, New York, 1979.
142. Damasio, AR: Aphasia. N Engl J Med 336:531, 1992.
143. Sarno, MT: Aphasia rehabilitation: Psychosocial and ethical considerations. Aphasiology 7:321, 1993.
144. Eisenson, J: Adult Aphasia: Assessment and Treatment. Prentice-Hall, Englewood Cliffs, NJ, 1973.
145. Herrmann, M, et al: The impact of aphasia on the patient and family in the first year post-stroke. Top Stroke Rehabil 2:5, 1995.
146. Eisenson, J: Aphasia: A point of view as to the nature of the disorder and factors that determine prognosis and recovery. Int JNeurol 4:287, 1964.
147. Darley, F: The efficacy of language rehabilitation in aphasia. J Speech Hear Disord 37:3, 1972.
148. Prins, R, et al: Efficacy of two different types of speech therapy for aphasic stroke patients. Appl Psycholing 10:85, 1989.
149. Wertz, RT, et al: Veterans Administration cooperative study on aphasia: A comparison of individual and group treatment. J Speech Hear Disord 24:580, 1981.
150. Wertz, RT: Language treatment for aphasia is efficacious, but for whom? Top Lang Disord 8:1, 1987.
151. Wallace, SJ, et al: Measuring outcomes in aphasia research: A review of current practice and an agenda for standardisation. Aphasiology 28(11):1364, 2014.
152. Robey, RR: A meta-analysis of clinical outcomes in the treatment of aphasia. J Speech Lang Hear Res 41:172, 1998.
153. Beeson, PM, and Robey, RR: Evaluating single-subject treatment research: Lessons learned from the aphasia literature. Neuropsychol Rev 16(4):161, 2006.
154. Marks, M, Taylor, M, and Rusk, HA: Rehabilitation of the aphasic patient: A survey of three years' experience in a rehabilitation setting. Neurology 7(12):837, 1957.
155. Hagen, C: Communication abilities in hemiplegia: Effect of speech therapy. Arch Phys Med Rehabil 54:545, 1973.
156. Edmonds, L, Nadeau, S, and Kiran, S: Effect of Verb Network Strengthening Treatment (VNeST) on lexical retrieval of content words in sentences in persons with aphasia. Aphasiology 23(3):402, 2009.
157. Poeck, K, et al: Outcome of intensive language treatment in aphasia. J Speech Hear Disord 54:471, 1989.
158. Bhogal, SK, Teasell, R, and Speechley, M: Intensity of aphasia therapy, impact on recovery. Stroke 34:987, 2003.
159. Hinckley, JJ, and Craig, HK: Influence of rate of treatment on the naming abilities of adults with chronic aphasia. Aphasiology 12:989, 1998.
160. Hinckley, JJ, and Carr, TH: Comparing the outcomes of intensive and non-intensive context-based aphasia treatment. Aphasiology 19(10–11):965, 2005.
161. Harvey, DY, et al: Factors predicting spontaneous long-term recovery from post-stroke aphasia. Ann Neurol 80(s20):S98, 2016.
162. Shewan, CM: Expressive language recovery in aphasia using the Shewan Spontaneous Language Analysis (SSLA) System. J Commun Disord 17:175, 1988.
163. Eslinger, P, and Damasio, A: Age and type of aphasia in patients with stroke. J Neurol Neurosurg Psychiatry 44:377, 1981.
164. Holland, A, and Fridriksson, J: Aphasia management during the early phases of recovery following stroke. Am J Speech Lang Pathol 10:19–28, 2011.
165. Helm-Estabrooks, N, and Ramsberger, G: Treatment of agrammatism in long-term Broca's aphasia. Br J Disord Commun 21:39, 1986.
166. Glindemann, R, et al: The efficacy of modeling in PACE-therapy. Aphasiology 5:425, 1991.
167. Pulvermuller, F, et al: Constraint-induced therapy of chronic aphasia after stroke. Stroke 32:1621, 2001.
168. Howard, D: Beyond randomized controlled trials: The case for effective studies of the effects of treatment in aphasia. Br J Dis Commun 21:89, 1986.
169. Byng, S: Hypothesis testing and aphasia therapy. In Holland, AL, and Forbes, M (eds): Aphasia Treatment. World Perspectives. San Diego, 1993, p 115.
170. Golper, L, et al: Evidence-based practice guidelines for the management of communication disorders in neurologically impaired individuals: Project Introduction. Academy of Neurologic Communication Disorders and Sciences, Minneapolis, MN, 2001. Retrieved March 24, 2017, from https://www.ancds.org/assets/docs/EBP/practiceguidelines.pdf.
171. Frattali, C, et al: Development of evidence-based practice guidelines: Committee update. J Med Speech-Lang Pathol 11(3):ix, 2003.
172. Whurr, R, et al: A meta-analysis of studies carried out between 1946 and 1988 concerned with the efficacy of speech and language therapy treatment for aphasic patients. Eur J Commun 27:1, 1992.
173. Ullman, M: Behavioral Changes in Patients following Strokes. Charles C. Thomas, Springfield, IL, 1962.
174. Wahrborg, P: Assessment and Management of Emotional and Psychosocial Reactions to Brain Damage and Aphasia. Singular Publishing Group, San Diego, CA, 1991.
175. Friedman, M: On the nature of regression. Arch Gen Psychiatry 3:17, 1961.
176. Sarno, MT: Language rehabilitation outcome in the elderly aphasic patient. In Obler, LK, and Albert, ML (eds): Language and Communication in the Elderly: Clinical, Therapeutic and Experimental Issues. DC Heath, Lexington, MA, 1980, p 191.

177. Galletta, EE, and Barrett, AM: Impairment and functional interventions for aphasia: Having it all. Curr Phys Med Rehabil Rep 2(2):114, 2014.
178. Burns, MS, and Halper, AS: Speech/Language Treatment of the Aphasias: An Integrated Clinical Approach. Aspen, Rockville, MD, 1988.
179. Sarno, MT: Management of aphasia. In Bornstein, RA, and Brown, GG (eds): Neurobehavioral Aspects of Cerebrovascular Disease. Oxford University Press, New York, 1990, p 314.
180. Goodglass, H: Neurolinguistic principles and aphasia therapy. In Meier, M, et al (ed): Neuropsychological Rehabilitation. Guilford Press, New York, 1987.
181. Carpenter, J, and Cherney, LR: Increasing aphasia treatment intensity in an acute inpatient rehabilitation programme: A feasibility study. Aphasiology 30(5):542, 2016.
182. Patterson, J, Raymer, A, and Cherney, L: Treatment Intensity in Aphasia Rehabilitation. In Coppens, P, and Patterson, J (eds): Aphasia Rehabilitation: Clinical Challenges, Jones & Bartlett, Burlington, MA, 2017, p 291.
183. Breitenstein, C, et al: (2017). Intensive speech and language therapy in patients with chronic aphasia after stroke: A randomised, open-label, blinded-endpoint, controlled trial in a health-care setting. Lancet [Mar 2017, DOI: 10.1016/S0140-6736(17)30067-3 (Epub ahead of print)].
184. MacGregor, LJ, et al: Ultra-rapid access to words in chronic aphasia: the effects of Intensive Language Action Therapy (ILAT). Brain Topogr 28(2), 279, 2015.
185. Berthier, ML, and Davila, G. (eds): Pharmacology and Aphasia. Routledge, New York, 2015.
186. Zhang, J, et al: Piracetam for aphasia in post-stroke patients: a systematic review and meta-analysis of randomized controlled trials. CNS Drugs 30(7), 575, 2016.
187. Berthier, ML: Editorial: Cognitive enhancing drugs in aphasia: A vote for hope. Aphasiology 28(2):128, 2014.
188. Zumbansen, A, and Thiel, A: (2014). Recent advances in the treatment of post-stroke aphasia. Neural Regen Res 9(7):703, 2014.
189. Galling, MA, et al: A clinical study of the combined use of bromocriptine and speech and language therapy in the treatment of a person with aphasia. Aphasiology 28(2):171, 2014.
190. Breitenstein, C, et al: L-dopa does not add to the success of high-intensity language training in aphasia. Resto Neurol Neurosci 33(2):115, 2015.
191. Gill, SK, and Leff, AP: Dopaminergic therapy in aphasia. Aphasiology 28(2):155, 2014.
192. Yoon, SY, et al: Effect of donepezil on Wernicke aphasia after bilateral middle cerebral artery infarction: Subtraction analysis of brain F-18 fluorodeoxyglucose positron emission tomographic images. Clin Neuropharmacol 38(4), 147, 2015.
193. Thiel, A, et al: Effects of noninvasive brain stimulation on language networks and recovery in early poststroke aphasia. Stroke 44(8):2240, 2013.
194. Naeser, MA, et al: Overt propositional speech in chronic nonfluent aphasia studied with the dynamic susceptibility contrast fMRI method. Neuroimage 22:29, 2004.
195. Galletta, EE, et al: Use of tDCS in aphasia rehabilitation: A systematic review of the behavioral interventions implemented with noninvasive brain stimulation for language recovery. Am J Speech Lang Pathol 25(4S), S854, 2016.
196. Mozeiko, J, Coelho, CA, and Myers, EB: The role of intensity in constraint-induced language therapy for people with chronic aphasia. Aphasiology 30(4):339, 2016.
197. Maher, LM, et al: Constraint induced language therapy for chronic aphasia: Preliminary findings. J Int Neuropsychol Soc 9:192, 2003.
198. Beeson, PM, Hirsch, FM, and Rewega, MA: Successful single-word writing treatment: Experimental analysis of four cases. Aphasiology 16:473, 2002.
199. Pons, C, and Stark, J: Recovery of Drawing Ability in Persons With Aphasia. Procedia Soc Behav Sci 94:191, 2013.
200. Hough, MS, and Taylor, A: Can Drawing Enhance Word Retrieval Skills in Chronic Aphasia? Paper presented at the Clinical Aphasiology Conference, St. Simons Island, GA, 2014. Retrieved March 24, 2017, from http://aphasiology.pitt.edu/2553/.
201. Rao, PR: Drawing and gesture as communication options in a person with severe aphasia. Top Stroke Rehabil 2:49, 1995.
202. Lyon, JG et al: Communication partners: Enhancing participation in life and communication for adults with aphasia in natural settings. Aphasiology 11(7):693, 1997.
203. Kagan, A, and Gailey, GF: Functional is not enough: Training conversation partners for aphasic adults. In Holland, A, and Forbes, MM (eds): Aphasia Treatment: World Perspectives. Singular Publishing Group, San Diego, 1993, p 199.
204. Kagan, A: Revealing the competence of aphasic adults through conversation: A challenge to health professionals. Top Stroke Rehabil 2:15, 1995.
205. Kagan, A, et al: Training volunteers as conversation partners using "supported conversation for adults with aphasia": A controlled trial. J Speech Lang Hear Res 44:624, 2001.
206. Kagan, A: Supported Conversation for Adults with Aphasia: Methods and Evaluation. Institute of Medical Science, University of Toronto, 1999. Retrieved March 24, 2017, from www.collection_scanada.gc.ca/obj/s4/f2/dsk1/tape9/PQDD_0015/NQ45755.pdf.
207. Kagan, A, Winckel, J, and Shumway, E: Supported Conversation for Aphasic Adults: Increasing Communicative Access (Video). Pat Arato Aphasia Centre, North York, Ontario, Canada, 1996. Available from Aphasia Institute (www.aphasia.ca/).
208. Simmons-Mackie, N: A solution to the discharge dilemma in aphasia: Social approaches to aphasia management: Clinical forum. Aphasiology 12:231, 1998.
209. Simmons-Mackie, N: In support of supported communication for adults with aphasia: Clinical forum. Aphasiology 12:831, 1998.
210. Simmons-Mackie, N: An Ethnographic Investigation of Compensatory Strategies in Aphasia. Unpublished doctoral dissertation. Louisiana State University, Baton Rouge, 1993.
211. Byng, S, and Duchan, J: Social model philosophies and principles: Their applications to therapies for aphasia. Aphasiology 19:906, 2005.
212. Simmons-Mackie, N: Social approaches to the management of aphasia. In Worrall, L, and Frattali, C (eds): Neurogenic Communication Disorders: A Functional Approach. Thieme, New York, 2000, p 162.
213. Pound, C, et al: Beyond aphasia: Therapies for Living with Communication Disability. Speechmark, Bicester, UK, 2000.
214. Simmons-Mackie, N, and Damico, JS: Communicative competence in aphasia: Evidence from compensatory strategies. In Lemme, ML (ed): Clinical Aphasiology (Vol. 23). Pro-Ed, Austin, TX, 1995, p 95.
215. Simmons-Mackie, N, and Damico, J: Reformulating the definition of compensatory strategies in aphasia. Aphasiology 11:761, 1997.
216. Simmons-Mackie, N, and Damico, J: Social role negotiation in aphasia therapy: Competence, incompetence and conflict. In Kovarsky, D, Duchan, J, and Maxwell, M (eds): Constructing (In)Competence: Disabling Evaluations in Clinical and Social Interaction. Erlbaum, Hillsdale, NJ, 1999, p 313.
217. Menger, F, Morris, J, and Salis, C: Internet use in aphasia: A case study viewed through the International Classification of Functioning, Disability, and Health. Top Lang Disord 37(1): 6, 2017.
218. Simic, T, et al: A usability study of internet-based therapy for naming deficits in aphasia. Am J Speech Lang Pathol 25(4): 642, 2016.
219. Woolf, C, et al: A comparison of remote therapy, face to face therapy and an attention control intervention for people with aphasia: A quasi-randomised controlled feasibility study. Clin Rehabil 30(4):359, 2016.
220. Palmer, R, Enderby, P, and Paterson, G: Using computers to enable self-management of aphasia therapy exercises for word finding: the patient and career perspective. Int J Lang Disord 48(5):508, 2013.
221. Macoir, J, et al: (2017). In-home synchronous telespeech therapy to improve functional communication in chronic poststroke aphasia: Results from a quasi-experimental study. Telemed J E Health [Jan 2017 DOI: 10.1089/tmj.2016.0235. (Epub ahead of print)].
222. Thompson, C, et al: Sentactics®: Computer-automated treatment of underlying forms. Aphasiology 24(10):1242, 2010.
223. Patterson, J, and Coppens, P: Integrating Principles of Evidence-Based Practice into Aphasia Rehabilitation. In Coppens, P, and

Patterson, J (eds): Aphasia Rehabilitation: Clinical Challenges, Jones & Bartlett, Burlington, MA, 2017, p 355.
224. Brady, MC, et al: Speech and language therapy for aphasia after stroke. Stroke 47(10): e236, 2016.
225. Baretz, R, and Stephenson, G: Unrealistic patient. N Y State J Med 76:54, 1976.
226. Kübler-Ross, E: On Death and Dying. Macmillan, New York, 1969.
227. Espmark, S: Stroke before fifty: A follow-up study of vocational and psychological adjustment. Scand J Rehab Med (Suppl) 2:1, 1973.
228. Kauhanen, M, et al: Aphasia, depression, and non-verbal cognitive impairment in ischaemic stroke. Cerebrovasc Dis 10:455, 2000.
229. Kearns, KJ: Group therapy for aphasia: Theoretical and practical considerations. In Chapey, R (ed): Language Intervention Strategies in Adult Aphasia, ed 2. Williams & Wilkins, Baltimore, 1986, p 304.
230. Bollinger, R, et al: A study of group communication intervention with chronic aphasic persons. Aphasiology 7:301, 1993.
231. Pearce, B, et al: Inhibitory control and traumatic brain injury: The association between executive control processes and social communication deficits. Brain Inj 30(13-14):1708, 2016.
232. Salas, CE, et al: "Relating through sameness": A qualitative study of friendship and social isolation in chronic traumatic brain injury. Neuropsychol Rehabil [Nov 2016 DOI: 10.1080/09602011.2016.1247730 (Epub ahead of print)].
233. Toglia, J, and Golisz, K: Traumatic brain injury (TBI) and the impact on daily life. In Chiaravalloti, ND, and Goverover, Y (eds): Changes in the Brain: Impact on Daily Life. Springer, New York, 2017, p 117.
234. Turkstra, L, Coelho, C, and Ylvisaker, M: The use of standardized tests for individuals with cognitive-communication disorders. Semin Speech Lang 26:215, 2005.
235. Cherney, LR, and Halper, AS: A conceptual framework for the evaluation and treatment of communication problems associated with right hemisphere damage. In Halper, A, Cherney, L, and Burns, M (eds): Clinical Management of Right Hemisphere Dysfunction, ed 2. Aspen, Gaithersburg, MD, 1996, p 21.
236. Kennedy, MR, et al: Evidence-based practice guidelines for cognitive-communication disorders after traumatic brain injury: Initial committee report. J Med Speech Lang Pathol 10(2), 2002.
237. Ylvisaker, M, et al: Reflections on evidence-based practice and rational clinical decision making. J Med Speech Lang Pathol 10(3), 2002.
238. Duffy, J. R. (2005). Motor speech disorders. St. Louis, MO: Mosby.
239. Yorkston, KM, et al: Evidence for effectiveness of treatment of loudness, rate or prosody in dysarthria: A systematic review. J Med Speech Lang Pathol 15(2), 2007.
240. McAuliffe, M.J, et al: Effect of dysarthria type, speaking condition, and listener age on speech intelligibility. Am J Speech Lang Pathol 26(1):113, 2017.
241. Yorkston, KM, et al: Evidence-based practice guidelines for dysarthria: Management of velopharyngeal function. J Med Speech Lang Pathol 9(4):257, 2001.
242. Dromey, C, and Ramig, LO: Intentional changes in sound pressure and rate: Their impact on measures of respiration, phonation, and articulation. J Speech Lang Hear Res 41(5):1003, 1988.
243. Sutoo, D, and Akiyama, K: Regulation of brain function by exercise. Neurobiol Dis 13:1, 2003.
244. Dromey, C, Ramig, L, and Johnson, A: Phonatory and articulatory changes associated with increased vocal intensity in Parkinson disease: A case study. J Speech Hear Res 38:751, 1995.
245. Wenke, R, Cornwell, P, and Theodoros, D: Changes to articulation following LSVT® and traditional dysarthria therapy in non-progressive dysarthria. Int J Speech Lang Pathol 12(3):203, 2010.
246. El Sharkawi, A, et al: Swallowing and voice effects of Lee Silverman Voice Treatment: A pilot study. J Neurol Neurosurg Psychiatry 72:31, 2002.
247. Spielman, J, Borod, J, and Ramig L: Effects of intensive voice treatment (LSVT) on facial expressiveness in Parkinson's disease: Preliminary data. Cogn Behav Neurol 16:177, 2003.
248. Will, L, Ramig, LO, and Spielman, JL: Application of Lee Silverman Voice Treatment (LSVT) to individuals with multiple sclerosis, ataxic dysarthria and stroke. In Proceedings International Conference on Spoken Language Processing, September 16–20, 2002, Denver, CO, p 2497.
249. Wenke, R, Theodoros, D, and Cornwell, P: The short- and long-term effectiveness of the LSVT® for dysarthria following TBI and stroke. Brain Inj 22(4):339, 2008.
250. Sapir, S, et al: Phonatory and articulatory changes in ataxic dysarthria following intensive voice therapy with the LSVT1: A single subject study. Am J Speech Lang Pathol 12:387, 2003.
251. Boliek, CA, and Fox, CM: Therapeutic effects of intensive voice treatment (LSVT LOUD) for children with spastic cerebral palsy and dysarthria: A phase I treatment validation study. Int J Speech Lang Pathol [Oct 2016, DOI: 10.1080/17549507.2016.1221451 (Epub ahead of print)].
252. Petska, J, et al: LSVT1 and children with Down syndrome: A pilot study. Poster session presented at the 13th Biennial Conference on Motor Speech, Austin, TX, March 2006.
253. Yorkston, KM, et al: Management of motor speech disorders in children and adults. Pro-Ed, Austin, TX, 1999.
254. Maas, E, Gutiérrez, K, and Ballard, KJ: Phonological encoding in apraxia of speech and aphasia. Aphasiology 28(1):25, 2014.
255. Staiger, A, and Ziegler, W: Syllable frequency and syllable structure in the spontaneous speech production of patients with apraxia of speech. Aphasiology 22(11): 1201, 2008.
256. McNeil, MR: Clinical characteristics of apraxia of speech: Model/behavior coherence. In Shriberg, LD, and Campbell, TF (eds): Proceedings of the 2002 Childhood Apraxia of Speech Research Symposium. Hendrix Foundation, Carlsbad, CA, 2003, p 13.
257. Cunningham, KT, Haley, KL, and Jacks, A: Speech sound distortions in aphasia and apraxia of speech: reliability and diagnostic significance. Aphasiology 30(4):396, 2016.
258. Ballard, KJ, et al: A predictive model for diagnosing stroke-related apraxia of speech. Neuropsychologia 81:129, 2016.
259. Wambaugh, J: Treatment guidelines for apraxia of speech: lessons for future research. J Med Speech Lang Pathol 14(4), 317, 2006.
260. Wambaugh, J, et al: Treatment guidelines for acquired apraxia of speech: A synthesis and evaluation of the evidence. J Med Speech Lang Pathol 14(2):15, 2006.
261. Wambaugh, J, et al: Treatment guidelines for acquired apraxia of speech: Treatment descriptions and recommendations. J Med Speech Lang Pathol 14(2):xxxv, 2006.
262. Katz, W, et al: Visual augmented knowledge of performance: Treating place-of-articulation errors in apraxia of speech using EMA. Brain Lang 83:187, 2002.
263. Katz, WF, et al: Treatment of an individual with aphasia and apraxia of speech using EMA visually-augmented feedback. Brain and Lang 103(1), 213, 2007.
264. Rosenbek, JC, et al: A treatment for apraxia of speech in adults. J Speech Hear Disord 38:462, 1973.
265. Cherney, LR: Efficacy of oral reading in the treatment of two patients with chronic Broca's aphasia. Top Stroke Rehabil 2(1): 57, 1995.
266. Knock, TR, et al: Influence of order of stimulus presentation on speech motor learning: A principled approach to treatment for apraxia of speech. Aphasiology 14(5/6):653, 2000.
267. LaPointe, LL: Sequential treatment of split lists: A case report. In Rosenbek, J, McNeil, M, and Aronson, A (eds): Apraxia of Speech: Physiology, Acoustics, Linguistics, Management. College-Hill Press, San Diego, 1984, p 277.
268. Maas, E, et al: Treatment of sound errors in aphasia and apraxia of speech: Effects of phonological complexity. Aphasiology 16(4/5/6):609, 2002.
269. Raymer, AM, Haley, MA, and Kendall, DL: Overgeneralization in treatment for severe apraxia of speech: A case study. J Med Speech Lang Pathol 10(4):313, 2002.
270. Wambaugh, JL, et al: Effects of treatment for sound errors in apraxia of speech and aphasia. J Speech Lang Hear Res 41: 725, 1998.
271. Milisen, R: A rationale for articulation disorders. J Speech Hear Disord (Monograph Suppl) 4:6, 1954.
272. Wambaugh, JL: Stimulus generalization effects of Sound Production Treatment for apraxia of speech. J Med Speech Lang Pathol 12(2), 2004, p 77.
273. Wambaugh, JL, and Nessler, C: Modification of Sound Production Treatment for aphasia: Generalization effects. Aphasiology 18:407, 2004.
274. Wambaugh, JL, and Mauszycki, SC: Sound Production Treatment: Application with severe apraxia of speech. Aphasiology 24(6-8):814, 2010.

275. Ballard, KJ, Maas, E, and Robin, DA: Treating control of voicing in apraxia of speech with variable practice. Aphasiology 21(12):1195, 2007.
276. Maas, E: Conditions of practice and feedback in treatment for apraxia of speech. Perspect Neurophysiol Neurogenic Speech Lang Disord 20:80, 2010.
277. Austermann Hula, SN, et al: Effects of feedback frequency and timing on acquisition, retention, and transfer of speech skills in acquired apraxia of speech. J Speech Lang Hear Res 51(5):1088, 2008.
278. Wambaugh, JL, and Martinez, AL: Effects of rate and rhythm control treatment on consonant production accuracy in apraxia of speech. Aphasiology 14(8):851, 2000.
279. Mauszycki, SC, and Wambaugh, JL: The effects of rate control treatment on consonant production accuracy in mild apraxia of speech. Aphasiology 22(7-8):906, 2008.
280. Brendel, B, and Ziegler, W: Effectiveness of metrical pacing in the treatment of apraxia of speech. Aphasiology 22(1):77, 2008.
281. Brendel, B, Ziegler, W, and Deger, K: The synchronization paradigm in the treatment of apraxia of speech. J Neurolinguistics 13:241, 2000.
282. Dworkin, JP, and Abkarian, GG: Treatment of phonation in a patient with apraxia and dysarthria secondary to severe closed head injury. J Med Speech Lang Pathol 2:105, 1996.
283. McHenry, M, and Wilson, R: The challenge of unintelligible speech following traumatic brain injury. Brain Inj 8(4):363, 1994.
284. Tjaden, K: Exploration of a treatment technique for prosodic disturbance following stroke. Clin Linguist Phon 14(8):619, 2000.
285. Wambaugh, JL: Treatment guidelines for acquired apraxia of speech: A synthesis and evaluation of the evidence. J Med Speech Lang Pathol 14(2):xv, 2006.
286. Sands, E, et al: Progressive changes in articulatory patterns in verbal apraxia: A longitudinal case study. Brain Lang 6(1):97, 1978.
287. Fawcus, M, and Fawcus, R: Information transfer in four cases of severe articulatory dyspraxia. Aphasiology 4(2):207, 1990.
288. Lasker, JP, et al: Using motor learning guided theory and augmentative and alternative communication to improve speech production in profound apraxia: A case example. J Med Speech Lang Pathol 16(4):225, 2008.
289. Lustig, AP, and Tompkins, CA: A written communication strategy for a speaker with aphasia and apraxia of speech: Treatment outcomes and social validity. Aphasiology 16(4/5/6):507, 2002.
290. Yorkston, KM, and Waugh, PF: Use of augmentative communication devices with apractic individuals. In Square-Storer, P (ed): Acquired Apraxia of Speech in Aphasic Adults. Lawrence Erlbaum, London, 1989, p 267.
291. Rosenbek, JC, Collins, M, and Wertz, RT: Intersystemic reorganization for apraxia of speech. Clinical aphasiology conference proceedings. In Brookshire, RH (ed): Clinical Aphasiology Conference Proceedings. BRK Publishers, Minneapolis, 1976, p 255.
292. Code, C, and Gaunt, C: Treating severe speech and limb apraxia in a case of aphasia. Br J Disord Commun 21(1):11, 1986.
293. Raymer, AM, and Thompson, CK: Effects of verbal plus gestural treatment in a patient with aphasia and severe apraxia of speech. In Prescott, TE (ed): Clinical Aphasiology (Vol 20). Pro-Ed, Austin, TX, 1991, p 285.
294. Rubow, RT, et al: Vibrotactile stimulation for intersystemic reorganization in the treatment of apraxia of speech. Arch Phys Med Rehabil 63:150, 1982.
295. Lasker, JP, and Bedrosian, JL: Promoting acceptance of augmentative and alternative communication by adults with acquired communication disorders. AAC: Augment Altern Commun 17(3):141, 2001.
296. Groher, ME, and Crary, MA: Dysphagia: Clinical Management in Adults and Children, ed. 2. Elsevier, St Louis, MO, 2016.
297. Takizawa, C, et al: A systematic review of the prevalence of oropharyngeal dysphagia in stroke, Parkinson's disease, Alzheimer's disease, head injury, and pneumonia. Dysphagia 31(3):434, 2016.
298. Liu, L, et al: Functional changes of neural circuits in stroke patients with dysphagia: A meta-analysis. J Evid Based Med [Feb 2017, DOI: 10.1111/jebm.12242 (Epub ahead of print)].
299. Daniels, SK, and Huckabee, ML: Dysphagia Following Stroke, ed 2. Plural Publishing, San Diego, CA, 2014.
300. Low, M, Olsson, L, and Ekberg, O: Videomanometric analysis of supraglottic swallow, effortful swallow, and chin tuck in patients with pharyngeal dysfunction. Dysphagia 16(3):190, 2001.
301. Gordon, C, Langton-Hewer, RL, and Wade, DT: Dysphagia in acute stroke. BMJ 295:411, 1987.
302. Barer, DH: The natural history and functional consequences of dysphagia after hemispheric stroke. J Neurol Neurosurg Psychiatry 52:236, 1989.
303. Horner, J, Brazer, SR, and Massey, EW: Aspiration in bilateral stroke patients: A validation study. Neurology 43(2):430, 1993.
304. Smithard, D: Complications and outcome after acute stroke: Does dysphagia matter? Stroke 27:1200, 1996.
305. Logemann, JA: Evaluation and Treatment of Swallowing Disorders, ed 2. Pro-Ed, Austin, TX, 1998.
306. Suttrup, I, and Warnecke, T: Dysphagia in Parkinson's disease. Dysphagia 31(1): 24, 2016.
307. Heemskerk-van den Berg, WA: Dysphagia in Huntington's disease. Department of Neurology, Faculty of Medicine/Leiden University Medical Center (LUMC), Leiden University, 2015. Retrieved March 24, 2017, from https://openaccess.leidenuniv.nl/bitstream/handle/1887/32744/Proefschrift_pdf_Heemskerk.pdf?sequence=5.
308. Ertekin, C, et al: Oropharyngeal swallowing in craniocervical dystonia. J Neurol Neurosurg Psychiatry 73(4):406, 2002.
309. Camargo, CHF, et al: Dysphagia in Dystonia, 2015. Retrieved March 24, 2017, from https://cdn.intechopen.com/pdfs-wm/48508.pdf.
310. Jani, MP, and Gore, GB: Swallowing characteristics in amyotrophic lateral sclerosis. NeuroRehabilitation, 39(2):273, 2016.
311. Guan, XL, et al: Prevalence of dysphagia in multiple sclerosis: a systematic review and meta-analysis. Neurol Sci 36(5), 671, 2015.
312. Mussak, EN, Jiangling, JT, and Voigt, EP: Malignant solitary fibrous tumor of the hypopharynx with dysphagia. Otolaryngol Head Neck Surg 133:805, 2005.
313. Lee, JK: Dysphagia in Patients with Dementia. J Korean Dysphagia Soc 6(2):66, 2016.
314. Kalia, M: Dysphagia and aspiration pneumonia in patients with Alzheimer's disease. Metabolism 52(Suppl 2):36, 2003.
315. Bottos, M, et al: Functional status of adults with cerebral palsy and implications for treatment of children. Dev Med Child Neurol 43:516, 2001.
316. Howle, AA, Baguley, IJ, and Brown, L: Management of dysphagia following traumatic brain injury. Curr Phys Med Rehabil Rep 2(4):219, 2014.
317. Lazarus, CL: History of the use and impact of compensatory strategies in management of swallowing disorders. Dysphagia 32(1):3, 2017.
318. Easterling, C: 25 Years of dysphagia rehabilitation: What have we done, what are we doing, and where are we going? Dysphagia 32(1):50, 2017.
319. Carrau, RL, Murry, T, and Howell, RJ (eds): Comprehensive Management of Swallowing Disorders, ed 2. Plural Publishing, San Diego, CA, 2017.
320. Jones, K, et al: Interventions for dysphagia in long-term, progressive muscle disease. Cochrane Database Syst Rev (DOI: 10.1002/14651858.CD004303.pub4), 2016.
321. Lazarus, CL, et al: Effects of bolus volume, viscosity, and repeated swallows in nonstroke subjects and stroke patients. Arch Phys Med Rehabil 74:1066, 1993.
322. Lazzara, G, Lazarus, C, and Logemann, JA: Impact of thermal stimulation on the triggering of swallowing reflex. Dysphagia 1:73, 1986.
323. Logemann, JA, et al: Closure mechanisms of laryngeal vestibule during swallowing. Am J Physiol 262(2 pt 1):G338, 1992.
324. Martin, BJW, et al: Normal laryngeal valving patterns during three breath-hold maneuvers: A pilot investigation. Dysphagia 8:11, 1993.
325. Kahrilas, PJ, et al: Volitional augmentation of upper esophageal sphincter opening during swallowing. Am J Physiol 260(3 pt 1): G45, 1991.

appendix

28.A Speech and Language Disorder Web-Based Resources for Patients, Families, and Caregivers

Organization	Web Address
The American Speech-Language-Hearing Association (ASHA)	www.asha.org
The Academy for Neurologic Communication Disorders and Sciences (ANCDS)	www.ancds.org
National Aphasia Association (NAA)	www.aphasia.org

Promoting Health and Wellness

Beth Black, PT, DSc
Janet R. Bezner, PT, DPT, PhD, FAPTA

Chapter 29

LEARNING OBJECTIVES

1. Explain the importance of health promotion and wellness initiatives.
2. Describe the role of physical therapists in health promotion.
3. Differentiate among the terms *health* and *wellness*, *illness* and *disease*, *quality of life*, *primary*, *secondary*, and *tertiary prevention*, *population health management*, *health promotion*, *health education*, *physical activity*, and *exercise*.
4. Discuss the evolution of models of health from the biomedical model to the current International Classification of Functioning, Disability, and Health (ICF) biopsychosocial model of human functioning.
5. Identify measures of health and wellness, health behaviors, and quality of life.
6. Describe key modifiable personal health behaviors.
7. Identify and discuss key theories of behavior change.
8. Explain health coaching and motivational interviewing.
9. Explain how physical therapists can incorporate health promotion and wellness concepts into the plan of care for individuals with impairments and disabilities.

CHAPTER OUTLINE

THE IMPORTANCE OF HEALTH PROMOTION AND WELLNESS INITIATIVES

An individual's health is determined by the interaction of numerous factors, including biology and genetics, social and physical environments, health services, and individual behaviors.[1] Unhealthy behaviors are contributing to an increase in chronic disease and disability in the United States and other countries, affecting both the health of individuals and their quality of life.[2,3] It is estimated that over a third of premature deaths in the United States are caused by lack of exercise, poor diet, and cigarette smoking.[4] Obesity rates in the United States continue to climb contributing to the development of chronic diseases associated with obesity such as heart disease, stroke, type 2 diabetes, and certain types of cancer.[5] According to the 2015 Behavioral Risk Factor Surveillance System (BRFSS), the annual telephone survey of more than 400,000 adults in the United States, over 65% of the adult population is overweight or obese[6] (Fig. 29.1). In the same survey, when asked if they participated in any physical activities during the past month, 22.3% of

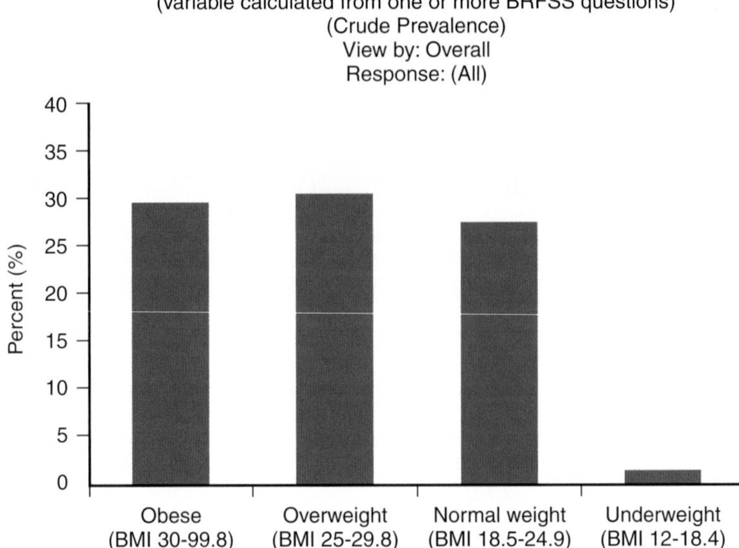

Figure 29.1 Weight Classification by Body Mass Index (BMI). *(From Centers for Disease Control and Prevention, National Center for Chronic Disease Prevention and Health Promotion, Division of Population Health. BRFSS Prevalence & Trends Data [online]. 2015. Accessed August 20, 2017. URL: www.cdc.gov/brfss/brfssprevalence/.)*

respondents answered no, and 17.5% of respondents indicated they currently smoke.[6] Fruit and vegetable consumption continues to be low among adults in the United States, with only 13.1% meeting current fruit intake recommendations, and only 8.9% meeting vegetable consumption recommendations.[7]

There is also mounting evidence of the importance of sleep to an individual's health. Sleep insufficiency has been linked to increased risk of motor vehicle and industrial accidents and an increased risk for developing chronic diseases such as hypertension, diabetes, depression, obesity, and cancer.[8] Data from 444,306 adult respondents in all 50 states and the District of Columbia on the 2014 BRFSS indicated that more than one-third of adults in the United States are getting less than the recommended 7 hours of sleep each night.[9]

Not only are adults' health-related behaviors of concern, but there is also growing consensus that the high levels of obesity of children in the United States are related to their behaviors. Between 2011 and 2014, the prevalence of obesity in this age group was reported to be 17%, affecting 12.7 million children and adolescents aged 2 to 19 years.[10] The behaviors of consuming high-calorie, low-nutrient foods and beverages, not engaging in sufficient physical activity, spending too much time on sedentary activities such as watching television or other screen devices, and not getting enough sleep have been identified as contributing to excess weight gain in children and adolescents.[11]

Given the strong relationship between health behaviors and health status, it is clear that the current health-related behaviors of adults and children in the United States are adversely affecting healthy life expectancy, and efforts to support healthier behaviors are essential.

The nation's current health promotion and disease prevention agenda is articulated in *Healthy People 2020,* a set of national health objectives developed through a wide-reaching collaborative consensus process and published by the US Department of Health and Human Services.[12] Public health experts, government agencies, professional organizations such as the American Physical Therapy Association (APTA), and members of the public all provided input into this important document. The overall framework for *Healthy People 2020* is outlined in Table 29.1.

Given the broad range of factors that contribute to the health of the population, an ecological approach will be required to meet the *Healthy People 2020* goals and objectives. Interventions must be delivered not only at the level of the individual, but also at community, organizational, environmental, and policy levels (Fig. 29.2).

A number of topic areas requiring particular attention have been identified in *Healthy People 2020,* and for each of these 42 topic areas there is a set of specific objectives. For example, within the topic area of physical activity, there are 15 objectives (Table 29.2) accompanied by specific targets to be achieved within the next 10 years. The ecological approach to addressing the topic areas is clear from the breadth of the objectives established for each of these 42 topic areas. For example, in the area of physical activity, one objective is to increase individuals' levels of leisure-time physical activity (Physical Activity Objective–1), whereas Physical Activity Objective–15 identifies the need for legislative policies to address environmental factors to support increased levels of physical activity in a community. Progress toward the

Table 29.1 *Healthy People 2020* **Framework**

Vision	A society in which all people live long, healthy lives.
Mission	Identify nationwide health improvement priorities. Increase public awareness and understanding of the determinants of health, disease, and disability and the opportunities for progress. Provide measurable objectives and goals that are applicable at the national, state, and local levels. Engage multiple sectors to take actions to strengthen policies and improve practices that are driven by the best available evidence and knowledge. Identify critical research, evaluation, and data collection needs.
Overarching Goals	Attain high-quality, longer lives free of preventable disease, disability, injury, and premature death. Achieve health equity, eliminate disparities, and improve the health of all groups. Create social and physical environments that promote good health for all. Promote quality of life, healthy development, and healthy behaviors across all life stages.

From http://www.healthypeople.gov/sites/default/files/HP2020 Framework.pdf.

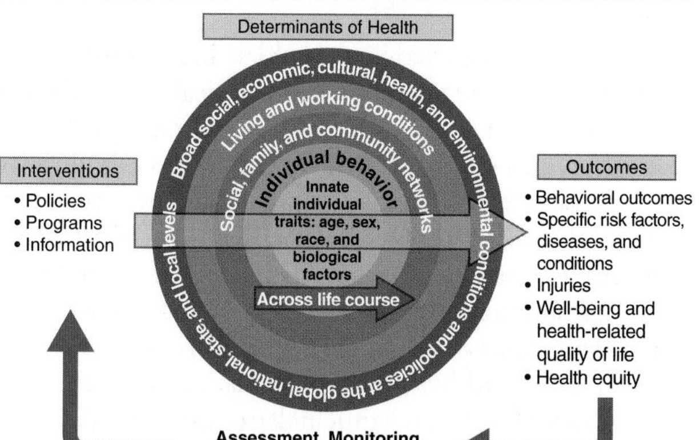

Figure 29.2 Ecological Approach to Achieve the Goals of *Healthy People 2020.*

objectives and specific targets established for *Healthy People 2020* is tracked by measuring general health status, health behaviors, health-related quality of life and well-being, determinants of health, and measures of health disparities.

Table 29.2 *Healthy People 2020* **Physical Activity Objectives**

Healthy People 2020 Physical Activity (PA) Objectives	Topic Area (Objective Short Title)
PA-1	Leisure-time physical activity
PA-2	Adult aerobic physical activity and muscle-strengthening activity
PA-3	Adolescent aerobic physical activity and muscle-strengthening activity
PA-4	Daily physical education in schools
PA-5	Adolescent participation in daily school physical education
PA-6	Regularly scheduled recess
PA-7	Time for recess
PA-8	Child and adolescent screen time
PA-9	Physical activity policies in child care settings
PA-10	Access to school physical activity facilities
PA-11	Physician counseling about physical activity
PA-12	Worksite physical activity
PA-13	Active transportation—walking
PA-14	Active transportation—bicycling
PA-15	Built environment policies

From https://healthypeople.gov/2020/topics-objectives/topic/physical-activity/objectives?topicID=332020/objectiveslist.aspx?topicId=33

THE ROLE OF PHYSICAL THERAPISTS IN HEALTH PROMOTION

Interventions at individual, community, state, and national levels by a broad coalition of public health organizations, health professionals, educators, and government agencies will be required to achieve the objectives outlined in *Healthy People 2020.* All health professionals, regardless of their site or area of practice, have a key role to play in health promotion, either as individual practitioners or as members of an interprofessional health care team.[13] Physical therapists are participating in health promotion initiatives in a variety of ways, from examining what their role should be to providing individual and community-level interventions and programs.[14-17] A number of professional publications describe the important role for physical therapists in the area of health promotion and wellness.[18-22]

The *Guide to Physical Therapist Practice 3.0* clearly identifies health promotion and prevention as being within the scope of physical therapist practice:

> *Physical therapists are involved in prevention and in promoting health, wellness, and fitness in a wide range of populations. Their roles range from helping individuals with chronic conditions engage in physical activity programs to advising elite athletes on sports performance enhancement. These initiatives decrease costs by helping individuals: (1) achieve and restore optimal functional capacity; (2) minimize impairments, functional limitations, and disabilities related to congenital and acquired conditions; (3) maintain health (thereby preventing further deterioration or future illness); and (4) create appropriate environmental adaptations to enhance independent function.*[18,23]

The patient history portion of the examination should include information about the client's health status and health habits, a systems review, and tests and measures as indicated to screen for potential problems that could affect current or future health status, such as hypertension, obesity, impaired balance, or poor fitness levels. Interventions that physical therapists can utilize to promote health and prevent or minimize impairments, activity limitations, and disabilities are extensive and can include such diverse activities as education in healthy lifestyle choices and healthy behaviors, physical activity and aerobic conditioning programs, fall prevention programs, or consultation in workplace redesign. Referrals to other professionals or special programs (e.g., smoking cessation or nutritional counseling) may also be indicated. The principles of evidence-based practice should be considered as physical therapists expand their practices to include not only rehabilitation, but also health promotion. Decisions regarding appropriate programs to institute should be based on evidence of effectiveness of the intervention, the knowledge and skill level of the physical therapist, and the appropriateness of that particular intervention for the individual client given his or her unique needs, preferences, and circumstances.

In the document titled *Professionalism in Physical Therapy: Core Values*, physical therapist behaviors believed to represent the behaviors of a doctoring profession include the following[21, pp. 1–3]:

- Participating in the achievement of health goals of patients/clients and society
- Focusing on achieving the greatest well-being and the highest potential for a patient/client
- Facilitating each individual's achievement of goals for function, health, and wellness
- Participating in achievement of societal health goals

These behaviors indicate a broad role and responsibility for physical therapists in health promotion and suggest the need for physical therapists to participate not only at the individual client level, but also at a societal level. Physical therapists are participating in discussions at a national level regarding public policy, health care reform, and major health initiatives, and are also involved in advocacy efforts to support the objectives articulated in *Healthy People 2020*.[12]

At the Physical Therapy and Society Summit (PASS) meeting, future roles for physical therapists were discussed relative to the evolving health care needs of society.[24] At this conference, the opportunity for physical therapists to take a leadership role in the area of prevention, health, and wellness was emphasized. There has also been a suggestion that physical therapists should be "birth to death" health practitioners, providing regular consultations on exercise and physical activity using a practice model that is similar to the dental model and geared toward prevention and health promotion.[25] At the Physical Therapy Summits on Global Health, there was consensus that physical therapists can and should incorporate health promotion and wellness into their practices. Action plans were developed for clinicians, educators, researchers and professional associations to help move the profession in this direction.[26,27]

Given the tremendous need for health promotion, and the unique knowledge base and skill set of physical therapists, it is the professional responsibility of all physical therapists to engage in health promotion practice regardless of their practice setting. As physical therapists begin to integrate health promotion interventions into their clinical practice, they should become familiar with the various terms and definitions used in the field of health promotion.

KEY TERMS IN HEALTH PROMOTION

Health and Disease

Different terms are used in the field of health promotion to define *health*. Although health may be seen as pertaining to the physical domain only, most currently used definitions of health conceptualize and describe health as a multidimensional construct involving more than the physical domain. In 1948, the World Health Organization (WHO) defined health as "a state of complete physical, mental and social well-being and not merely the absence of disease or infirmity."[28] This definition of health is still used by the WHO today. Health has also been described as "a dynamic balance of physical, emotional, social, spiritual, and intellectual health."[29, p. iv] *Health condition* is an umbrella term for acute or chronic disease, disorder, injury, or trauma.[18] *Disease,* often considered the opposite of health, is defined as a pathological condition affecting the body.[18]

Wellness and Illness

The term *wellness* is also used in the field of health promotion. In 1959, Dunn discussed the relationship between body, mind, and spirit, and defined wellness as "a complex state made up of overlapping levels of wellness."[30, p. 786] Adams et al[31] defined wellness as an individual's sense of growth and balance across the physical, spiritual, emotional, intellectual, social, and psychological domains (Fig. 29.3). These two wellness definitions are worded in such a way that individuals with chronic disease could still be considered "well."

The National Wellness Institute defines wellness as "an active process through which people become aware of, and make choices toward, a more successful existence," recognizing that wellness is a process versus a state.[32] Taken together, these various definitions of wellness indicate that wellness is multidimensional; that *salutogenic* or "health-causing" variables are the focus, indicating that wellness is positive or affirming; and that the concept of wellness is specific to each individual. *Illness* is the opposite of wellness, is multidimensional, and has been defined as a social construct where individuals are not achieving balance in their lives and are unable to create a higher quality of life.[33]

Quality of Life

There are a number of different definitions for *quality of life*. The Centers for Disease Control and Prevention (CDC) describes health-related quality of life as an individual's or group's perceived physical and mental health over time.[34] "Health-related quality of life and well-being" was added to *Healthy People 2020* as a new topic area in the current version of the *Healthy People* initiative, defining health-related quality of life as a multidimensional concept that includes domains related to physical, mental, emotional, and social functioning and that goes beyond direct measures of population health, life expectancy, and causes of death, and focuses on the impact health status has on quality of life.[35] The terms *quality of life* and *wellness* are similar, both reflecting a person's experience or perception of their life in a general sense.

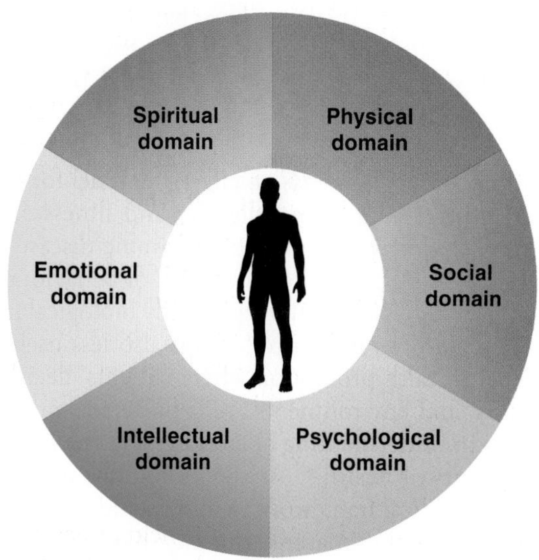

Figure 29.3 Domains of wellness.

Health Promotion Models

Primary, Secondary, and Tertiary Prevention

Various health promotion models are used to identify needs and plan health promotion interventions. One such model is the health protection/disease prevention model. Within this model, health is conceptualized as the absence of disease/pathology, and health promotion is therefore aimed at preventing disease. Interventions in this model are categorized as primary, secondary, or tertiary prevention[36, p. 6] (Fig. 29.4).

Primary prevention includes activities designed to prevent injury or the onset of illness or disease. The use of bicycle helmets and seat belts, water fluoridation, and immunizations are all examples of primary prevention. Physical therapists practice primary prevention when they conduct preseason evaluation and conditioning programs for high school athletes, teach back injury prevention programs at orientation programs for workers in a factory, and support their sedentary patients to adopt regular physical activity habits.

Secondary prevention interventions take place following the development of pathology and are intended to identify and provide treatment for individuals in the early stages of disease in order to minimize the severity of the disease. Screening programs for breast cancer, high blood pressure, and osteoporosis are designed to identify and treat pathology in its earliest stages. Physical therapists engage in secondary prevention when they treat a patient/client with a recent injury or who has been recently diagnosed in the early stages of a chronic condition or disease.

Tertiary prevention activities are designed to slow progression of a disease and improve quality of life. Physical therapists engage in tertiary prevention when they work with patients/clients who have chronic disease or have sustained an irreversible injury—for example, with patients/clients who have long-standing rheumatoid arthritis. Physical therapists have traditionally participated primarily in secondary or tertiary prevention, but as they begin to join their fellow health professionals in health promotion practice, they will

Prepathology	Pathology Present	
Goals: Protect health Prevent disease Promote health	Goal: Early diagnosis and intervention to limit impairment and disability	Goal: Rehabilitation following significant impairment or disability
Primary prevention	Secondary prevention	Tertiary prevention

Figure 29.4 Primary, secondary, and tertiary prevention.

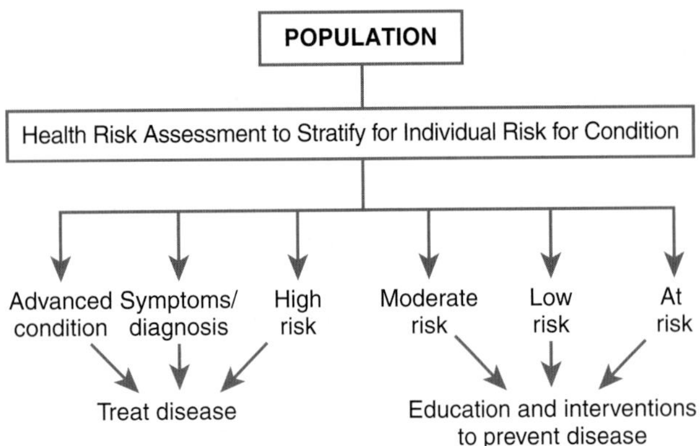

Figure 29.5 Population health management.

increasingly add interventions that fall under the category of primary prevention.

Population Health Management Model

A similar model to the health protection/disease prevention model is the population health management model (Fig. 29.5). The population health management model examines the health needs of a defined population and provides targeted services for individuals within the group that are appropriate to their level of risk for developing a disease or to their current health status following the development of disease. The goal of the population health management model is to improve the health outcomes of a group by monitoring and providing appropriate interventions to individual members of that group. Interventions are provided across a continuum of care and can include prevention, lifestyle management, disease management, catastrophic care management, and disability management.[37]

HEALTH PROMOTION AND HEALTH EDUCATION

Green and Kreuter describe *health promotion* as "any planned combination of educational, political, regulatory, and organizational supports for actions and conditions of living conducive to the health of individuals, groups, or communities."[36, p. G-4] The WHO defines health promotion as "the process of enabling people to increase control over, and to improve, their health. It moves beyond a focus on individual behavior towards a wide range of social and environmental interventions."[38] Gorin and Arnold[39] describe health promotion as activities undertaken to encourage well-being that are directed toward actualizing an individual's potential. According to Gorin and Arnold, a health promotion model has a more positive orientation and connotation than the prevention models described above that focus on simply preventing disease. *Health education* is one component of health promotion. Green and Kreuter define health education as "any planned combination of learning experiences designed to predispose, enable, and reinforce voluntary behavior conducive to health in individuals, groups, or communities."[36, p. G-4] Health education interventions aim to provide information to individuals and groups about health-causing actions and the impact of negative health behaviors in order to make a connection between voluntary behaviors and health. The first step toward positive health behavior change is awareness about the relationship between behavior and disease and injury.

PHYSICAL ACTIVITY AND EXERCISE

The definitions for *physical activity* and *exercise* are not synonymous. *Physical activity* is defined as any body movement produced by skeletal muscle contraction that increases energy expenditure above resting level.[40] It includes body movement carried out not only within formal exercise programs, but also in occupational activities, leisure activities, and transportation activities such as walking and bicycling. *Exercise* is defined as a subcategory of physical activity, and is planned, structured activity that is intended to improve or maintain one or more components of physical fitness.[41] This differentiation is important for physical therapists to consider when they work with patients/clients to help them increase their overall levels of physical activity.

THE INTERNATIONAL CLASSIFICATION OF FUNCTIONING, DISABILITY, AND HEALTH AND HEALTH PROMOTION

Consistent with the newer multidimensional definitions of health and wellness, there has been a change in the overall framework used to guide evaluation, planning, and interventions to support and promote health. The prevailing model used in 20th century medicine was the *biomedical model.*[42] This model was based on the biological sciences, and health was conceptualized as the absence of disease. The locus of control in the biomedical model was with the health care providers and the patient was provided with the medical care deemed necessary by health professionals. It was an effective model for managing acute and infectious diseases and illnesses, but proved less effective for managing chronic disease[42] or in addressing the psychological, social, or behavioral dimensions of illness.[43] With its primarily biological focus and external locus of control, it was also less useful in the field of health promotion where patients' decisions, behaviors, and environments are considered important elements in understanding and addressing the multiple determinants of health.[44] As the limitations of using a purely biomedical framework to understand the concept of health became apparent, the *biopsychosocial* model evolved. The various biopsychosocial models used today to explain health and illness incorporate those domains missing from the biomedical model, namely the psychological and social domains. The Nagi disablement model[45] is an example of a biopsychosocial model and was the model used to describe practice in the *Guide to Physical Therapist Practice 3.0*.[18]

In 2001, the WHO endorsed the International Classification of Functioning, Disability, and Health (ICF) biopsychosocial model.[46] The ICF is intended to provide a common language to describe health, function, and disability to facilitate scientific communication within and across health professions. The APTA has endorsed the use of this model as a framework for physical therapists to use in classifying and describing health, function, and disability.[47] In this model, the complex interrelationships of biological, environmental, and personal factors and the impact of these variables on health, activity, and function are recognized. See discussion of the ICF model in Chapter 1, Clinical Decision Making.

Physical therapists have already begun the process of applying the ICF model to practice in rehabilitation.[48-50] A number of health professionals have also started to demonstrate how the ICF can be used in the field of health promotion research and practice.[51-54] Howard et al[52] argue that the ICF, with its acknowledgment of the important contribution of the social and physical environment to an individual's health, supports the ecological approach used in the field of health promotion. The ICF provides both the rationale for physical therapists to look beyond purely biological and physiological factors when examining and evaluating their clients as well as a framework to guide their plans of care and interventions. Furthermore, the ICF model is consistent with many of the behavior change theories described later in this chapter that are used to plan and implement behavior change interventions.

MEASURES OF HEALTH, WELLNESS, QUALITY OF LIFE, AND HEALTH BEHAVIORS

There is no one standard tool for measuring health, wellness, health behaviors, or quality of life. Some tools have been specifically designed to measure the health or health behaviors of a population, whereas other tools are used to measure health and personal health behaviors at the level of the individual patient. A variety of measures of perceived health and quality of life have been developed and can be used at the level of a population, as well as at the level of the individual patient.

Clinical Measures of Health

Clinical measures of health include biometric and physiological measures such as body mass index (BMI), aerobic capacity, or blood pressure. Health risk appraisals (HRAs) are increasingly being used in workforce wellness programs to help assess the level and nature of an individual's current health risks based on history, personal behaviors, and clinical variables. HRAs are used to collect information to create risk profiles of individuals and populations, to estimate risk of future adverse health outcomes, and to provide persons with feedback about how to reduce health risk.[55]

The *Guide to Physical Therapist Practice 3.0* recommends that an evaluation of a patient/client's general health status, social and health habits (past and current) and potential health risks be included in the initial examination through a thorough history and a systems review.[18] Numerous tests and measures can be used by physical therapists during initial examinations to measure general health status and risk factors.[18]

Self-Perceived Health, Wellness, and Quality-of-Life Measures

The importance of adding a measure of an individual's perception of his or her general health to the patient/client examination was demonstrated in a landmark study by Mossey and Shapiro in 1982.[56] In this study of 3,128 noninstitutionalized adults over age 64, self-rated health was the strongest predictor of mortality after age and was found to be a better predictor of mortality than a number of morbidity and health care utilization measures such as medical diagnosis, number of physician visits, number of hospital admissions, and surgical history. The CDC includes a 14-item perceptual measure of health, the *Healthy Days Measure,* in the annual national BRFSS survey and in the National Health and Nutrition Examination Survey.[57] The National Institutes of Health developed a *Patient-Reported Outcomes Measurement Information System (PROMIS)* that captures important health-related quality-of-life information about patients who have chronic diseases and conditions.[58] The goal of the PROMIS initiative is to be able to develop profiles of PROMIS scores across health domains for various chronic conditions that can then be used in clinical research studies. The WHO has developed the *World Health Organization Quality of Life Questionnaire (WHOQOL-100)*[59] and a shorter version, the *WHOQOL-Bref.*[59] Both versions measure self-perceived physical health, psychological health, social relationships, and the individual's perceptions about his or her environment. The WHO tools can be used for the measurement of health at either the population level or the level of the individual patient/client.

Some self-report measures of perceived health, wellness, and quality of life are generic and can be completed by clients with a variety of conditions. One of the most commonly used measures of self-perceived health and quality of life is the *Medical Outcomes Study 36-Item Short-Form Health Survey (SF-36).*[60] The SF-36 measures self-perceived health and function across eight scales that include physical, psychological, social, and emotional domains. It has been used in general populations and in specific populations, and normative scores for various groups and populations have been documented. Additional measures of self-perceived health used in clinical practice include the *Nottingham Health Profile*,[61] the *Sickness Impact Profile (SIP)*,[62] the *Dartmouth Cooperative Functional Assessment Charts (Dartmouth CO-OP charts)*,[63] and the *Duke Health Profile*.[64] The *Perceived Wellness Survey (PWS)* measures self-perceived wellness across psychological, physical, emotional, spiritual, social, and intellectual domains.[31] The survey consists of 36 statements with six items for each of the six domains. A composite score, a magnitude score, and a balance score can be computed (Appendix 29.A). This tool has been tested and found to be valid and reliable for use with different populations.[31,65]

Disease-Specific Measures of Self-Perceived Health, Wellness, and Quality of Life

A number of disease-specific health and wellness measures have been developed for use with specific clinical populations. The items included in these measures may more specifically address issues related to the health and well-being of a particular population than the general measures described above. The *Arthritis Impact Measurement Scale (AIMS)*[66] and *AIMS2*[67] were developed to measure the physical, mental, and social domains of health in persons with rheumatic diseases. The *Child Health Questionnaire (CHQ)* measures the physical and psychosocial well-being of children and has been found to be a valid and reliable measure of health status across a variety of conditions and disorders.[68] The *Cystic Fibrosis Questionnaire*[69] is a health-related quality-of-life questionnaire that has both parent and child versions to measure the physical, emotional, and social impact of cystic fibrosis on children and their families. Additional disease or condition-specific quality-of-life measures that have been developed include a health and quality-of-life measure for individuals who have had a stroke,[70,71] suffer from acute and chronic facial disorders,[72] and have chronic respiratory disease.[73] The *European Organisation for Research and Treatment of Cancer (EORTC)* has developed a series of questionnaires designed to assess the quality of life of individuals with cancer. The 30-item EORTC quality-of-life measure has been translated and validated into 81 languages and has disease-specific modules that can be added to it.[74]

Assessing Health Behaviors

Reeves and Rafferty[75] identified four key behaviors as most indicative of a healthy lifestyle: engaging in regular physical activity, eating sufficient daily servings of fruits and vegetables, maintaining a healthy weight, and abstaining from smoking. Bezner[76] recommends physical therapists include questions about health-related behaviors in initial examinations, including physical activity, nutrition and weight management, sleep, smoking, and stress management. The *Guide to Physical Therapist Practice 3.0* also recommends that physical therapists include questions regarding health-related behaviors in initial examinations.[18] The health behaviors of engaging in regular physical activity, eating a healthy diet, abstaining from smoking, and engaging in healthy sleep behaviors and stress management techniques can be determined through patient interview or through a questionnaire. If the anthropometric measures of height and weight are taken, the client's BMI can be calculated, and the physical therapist can determine whether the patient/client is overweight or obese (Box 29.1).

Box 29.1 Body Mass Index (BMI)

BMI	Weight Status
Below 18.5	Underweight
18.5 to 24.9	Normal
25 to 29.9	Overweight
30 or higher	Obese

The *International Physical Activity Questionnaire*,[77] originally developed to track levels of physical activity in populations, has also been used in clinical practice to assess individual patient/client's levels of physical activity.[78] An 11-item scale has been used in several studies investigating the impact of employee wellness programs, assessing multiple health behaviors, including physical activity, nutrition habits, healthy living, stress, sleep, quality of life, and overall health.[79-81] Table 29.3 contains outcome measures that can be used to document impact of health, wellness, and fitness interventions.

KEY MODIFIABLE PERSONAL HEALTH BEHAVIORS

The CDC's Healthy Living website provides information about numerous behaviors that contribute to a healthy lifestyle.[82] Some of the health behaviors have the support of organizations, agencies, and schools (e.g., healthy menus in school cafeterias), while others are enforced by local, state, or federal laws, such as seat belt use or nonsmoking environments. Others, though significantly influenced by social, environmental, and economic factors, are primarily the personal responsibility of the individual, such as maintaining a healthy weight, eating a healthy diet, and engaging in physical activity. Some personal health behaviors are considered to be more changeable than others based on clinical research. Behaviors that are more challenging to change are those with an addictive component, those with compulsive elements, and those strongly associated with cultural or family routines, such as diet.[36] The key behaviors of increasing physical activity, increasing fruit and vegetable consumption, and quitting smoking, all included in the objectives of *Healthy People 2020*, have been shown to be modifiable behaviors if the behavior change interventions are appropriately designed and delivered.

Table 29.3 Outcome Measures of Health, Wellness, and Fitness

Name and Type of Measure	ICF Category	Description	Scoring
6-Minute Walk Test[a] *Fitness*	Activity	Submaximal test of aerobic capacity/endurance	Distance walked; person walks as far as possible in 6 minutes without physical assistance; assistive device(s) can be used. Greater distance indicates higher aerobic capacity.
Maximal oxygen uptake (Vo_2 max)[b] *Fitness*	Body Structures and Function	Graded exercise test, typically performed on a treadmill or ergometer; the subject exercises to exhaustion; open-circuit spirometry collects and assesses expired gases from the lungs.	Computerized systems collect and analyze data and directly compute Vo_2 max; submaximal test data can be used to estimate Vo_2 max if collected from at least 2 levels of intensity; norms are available.[b]
International Physical Activity Questionnaire (Short Self-Administered)[77] *Health-Related Physical Activity*	Activity	4-item scale assessing vigorous and moderate physical activity performed in the last 7 days and time spent sitting; aimed at young- and middle-aged adults. Responses gathered for days per week and hours/minutes spent in both vigorous and moderate activity.	For moderate activity, an average metabolic equivalent (MET) level of 4.0 is used to calculate MET-minutes/week. For vigorous activity, an average of 8.0 METs is used in the calculation of MET-minutes/week. Sitting is assessed by the time per weekday spend sitting, resulting in a mean per day score.
Self-Efficacy for Physical Activity[c] *Perceptions of Exercise/Physical Activity*	Personal and Environmental Factors	18-item scale assessing confidence from 0 = cannot do at all, to 100 = highly certain can do (10 response options)	Total of all items (range of scores = 0 to 1,800); higher scores = greater self-efficacy.
Life Satisfaction Questionnaire 9[d,e] *Wellness*	Participation	9-item survey to assess various aspects of life satisfaction; items measured on a 6-point Likert scale from 1 = very dissatisfied to 6 = very satisfied	Mean score can be calculated or individual items can be examined and categorized as dissatisfied (score of 1, 2, 3, or 4) or satisfied (score of 5 or 6); higher scores indicate greater life satisfaction.
Perceived Wellness Survey (see Appendix 29.A)[31] *Wellness*	Personal and Environmental Factors	36-item mind–body measure to assess wellness perceptions in 6 dimensions	Higher scores indicate greater wellness; see http://www.perceivedwellness.com/
Sickness Impact Profile (SIP-68)[f,g]	Body Structures and Function, Activity, Participation	68-question survey to assess quality of life and changes in behavior resulting from disability or illness. Items are scored yes/no.	Scores range from 0 = best health to 68 = worst health. Norms established for wheelchair-dependent individuals, acute traumatic brain injury and acute stroke.
Quality of Well Being Scale[h] *Wellness*	Participation	71-item measure of health status and overall well-being over the previous 3 days in four domains.	Scores range from 0 = death to 1 = full function.
World Health Organization Quality of Life—BREF[59] *Quality of Life*	Activity, Participation, Environment Factors	26-item scale, including four domains; items are rated using a 5-point Likert scale from 1 = low to 5 = high	Mean scores can be computed for each domain, ranging from 4 to 20; higher scores indicate higher quality of life; norms exist for individuals with acute stroke, chronic stroke, community dwelling elderly, and traumatic brain injury.

Continued

Table 29.3 Outcome Measures of Health, Wellness, and Fitness—cont'd

Name and Type of Measure	ICF Category	Description	Scoring
CDC Healthy Days Measure[i] *Health Related Quality of Life*	Body Structures and Function, Participation, Activity	14-item survey used by the Behavioral Risk Factor Surveillance System (BRFSS) to assess perceptions of health and their impact on participation in life and work.	Answers to each question are independent. A summary unhealthy days index can be computed by adding the answers to questions 2 and 3 in the healthy days module for a maximum score of 30 unhealthy days due to physical and/or mental health issues.
Medical Outcomes Short-Form Health Survey (SF-36)[j] *Health Related Quality of Life*	Body Structures and Function, Activity, Participation	36-item questionnaire measuring physical and mental health constructs of health status using 8 subscales.	Likert scale; scores range from 0–100 with a higher score indicating better health status. Norms established for community dwelling and older adults, adults with depression, and people with migraines, arthritis, and epilepsy.
World Health Organization Well-Being Index (WHO-5)[k] *Subjective Well-being*	Personal Factors	Short, generic global rating scale of subjective well-being using 5-items, all positively worded.	Scores range from 0 = absence of well-being to 25 = maximal well-being. Raw scores can be multiplied by 4 to convert to a 100-point scale.

[a]Fulk GD, et al: Clinometric properties of the six-minute walk test in individuals undergoing rehabilitation poststroke. Physiother Theory Pract 24(3):195, 2008.
[b]America College of Sports Medicine: ACSM's Guidelines for Exercise Testing and Prescription, ed 10. Wolters Kluwer, Philadelphia, 2018.
[c]Pajares, F, and Urdan, T: Self-Efficacy Beliefs of Adolescents. Information Age Publishing, Charlotte, NC, 2006.
[d]Boonstra, AM, et al: Reliability of the Life Satisfaction Questionnaire to assess patients with chronic musculoskeletal pain. Int J Rehabil Res 31(2):181, 2008.
[e]Borg, T, et al: Health-related quality of life and life satisfaction in patients following surgically treated pelvic ring fractures: A prospective observational study with two years follow-up. Injury 41(4):400, 2010.
[f]de Bruin, AF, et al: The development of a short generic version of the Sickness Impact Profile. J Clin Epidemiol 47(4):407, 1994.
[g]Post, MW, et al: The SIP68: A measure of health-related functional status in rehabilitation medicine. Arch Phys Med Rehabil 77(5):440, 1996.
[h]Anderson, JP, et al: Interday reliability of function assessment for a health status measure. The Quality of Well-Being scale. Med Care 27(11):1076, 1989.
[i]Centers for Disease Control and Prevention (CDC): CDC Healthy Days Measure CDC, Atlanta, GA. Retrieved August 19, 2017 from www.cdc.gov/hrqol/hrqol14_measure.htm.
[j]McHorney, CA, et al: The MOS 36-Item Short-Form Health Survey (SF-36): III. Tests of data quality, scaling assumptions, and reliability across diverse patient groups. Med Care 32(1):40, 1994.
[k]Topp, CW, et al: The WHO-5 Well-Being Index: A systematic review of the literature. Psychother Psychosom 84(3):167, 2015

The U.S. Preventive Services Task Force (USPSTF) publishes recommendations for various preventative screening measures and health behavior change interventions based on the most current evidence of the effectiveness of interventions in changing or modifying behavior.[83] Clinicians can access these guidelines online to quickly obtain this information within the clinical setting.[84] Although more research is needed to support the best counseling approaches, current recommendations support the use of behavioral counseling in the areas of healthful diet, physical activity, and smoking cessation.[83]

A systematic review of the effectiveness of counseling to improve diet and increase physical activity found that behavioral counseling can change these behaviors if the counseling is provided at a sufficient intensity.[85] Given the empirical evidence to support the efficacy of smoking cessation programs, the USPSTF currently recommends that all health care practitioners ask their patients about tobacco use and make appropriate referrals when indicated.[86] There is also evidence to support the relationship between intensive physical activity interventions and decreased risk of falls in older adults.[87] There are, therefore, clinical research studies that support the value of clinicians addressing the modifiable behaviors of tobacco use, unhealthy eating, and inadequate physical activity with their patients/clients. Research in the profession of physical therapy has shown that some physical therapists have already started to address health behaviors with their clients,[14,15,17,88] but more therapists should be encouraged to engage in these discussions with their patients/clients.

It may be necessary to ensure that physical therapists receive additional training in how to counsel patients/clients in behavior change.[27]

THEORIES OF BEHAVIOR CHANGE

The decision to engage in or change a health-related behavior is the result of a complex interaction of numerous factors. Just as physical therapists must understand theories of motor control when planning interventions to improve motor function, an understanding of key theories of health behavior change is necessary to be effective in helping clients change their behaviors. Various theoretical models of human behavior have been developed and can be categorized as individual models, interpersonal models, and community and group models.[1] Behavior change interventions based on these theories have been carried out in clinical research trials and have been found to be effective in different situations with different populations.[1]

Health Belief Model

One of the earliest theoretical models developed to explain health behaviors was the *Health Belief Model* (HBM).[89] This individual model of health behavior was initially developed and articulated in the 1950s, when social psychologists in the U.S. Public Health Service found that despite public education about the merits of various screening programs (e.g., tuberculosis screening), large numbers of adults did not participate in the programs. Over the years, the HBM has been developed and extended to incorporate additional concepts and to explain a variety of health-related behaviors beyond screening. In the HBM, it is hypothesized that an individual's perceptions about his or her susceptibility to and the severity of the disease, along with beliefs about the benefits and barriers of taking the recommended action, will influence the decision to act (Fig. 29.6). Demographic variables, sociopsychological variables, cues to action (internal and/or external factors promoting the behavior change), and *self-efficacy,* defined as the confidence one has that one can successfully execute the action, will also influence the individual's decision to engage in the behavior. Results from numerous research studies conducted with different populations have provided support for this theoretical model,[1] and interventions based on this model have been found to be effective in supporting behavior change.[90-92] When using this model in the clinical setting to promote healthy behaviors, the clinician would first assess the individual's beliefs and perceptions relative to his or her health condition and the recommended health actions. Based on this assessment, the clinician would then provide appropriate interventions—for example, educating the individual about his or her susceptibility to the disease or the effectiveness of a recommended health behavior.[93,94]

Theory of Reasoned Action and Theory of Planned Behavior

The *Theory of Planned Behavior,* along with its predecessor, the Theory of Reasoned Action, is an individual model of health behavior that emphasizes the importance of and relationship between cognitions (thought processes) and behavioral intention. Fishbein proposed the *Theory of Reasoned Action* (Fig. 29.7), in which he hypothesized that an individual's attitudes and beliefs about a particular behavior directly influence the intention to engage in that behavior, which then leads to the actual behavior.[95] The theory was later expanded to include the construct of perceived behavioral control and renamed the Theory of Planned Behavior.[96]

The key constructs in this theoretical model are attitude toward the behavior, subjective norm, perceived behavioral control, and behavioral intention (Table 29.4). Clinical studies that have examined a variety of health-related behaviors have provided empirical support for the constructs and the relationships articulated in this theory.[1,97-99] A clinician using this theoretical model to design a clinical intervention to change a behavior should begin by assessing the individual's attitude toward the behavior and the individual's perceptions regarding what significant others think about the behavior. The individual's perceived behavioral control can be ascertained by inquiring about any personal, social, or environmental barriers that might limit the ability to successfully engage in the behavior. The clinician can then tailor the intervention to the individual by addressing any areas that were identified. For example, the

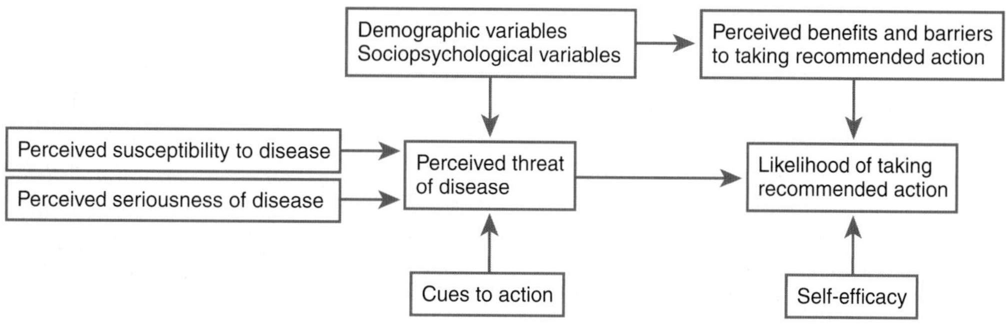

Figure 29.6 Health Belief Model.

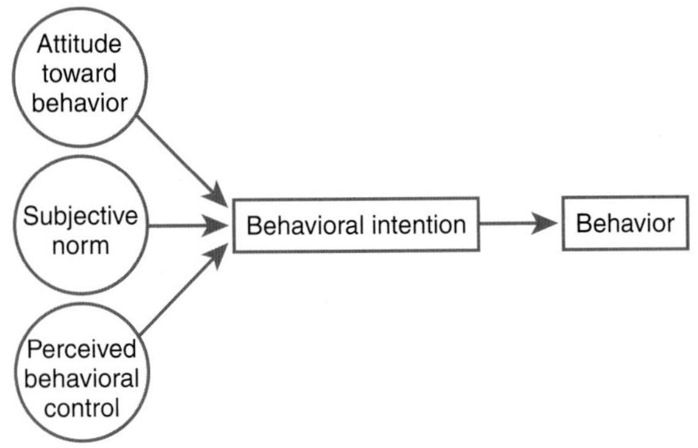

Figure 29.7 Theory of Reasoned Action.

Table 29.4 Key Constructs in the Theory of Planned Behavior[97]

Construct	Definition
Attitude toward behavior	Individual's overall attitude toward the behavior
Subjective norm	Individual's beliefs about whether others approve or disapprove of the behavior
Perceived behavioral control	Individual's perception about the level of control he or she has over the behavior
Behavioral intention	Individual's intention to engage in the behavior, the direct precursor to engaging in the behavior

clinician may need to help the individual problem solve to address a perceived barrier to engaging in the recommended behavior.

Transtheoretical Model (Stages of Change)

The *Transtheoretical Model* (TTM), first articulated by Prochaska, is categorized as an individual model of health behavior.[100] Key constructs within the TTM include stages of change, decisional balance, self-efficacy, and processes of change (Table 29.5).

Prochaska[100] hypothesized that there are five stages of change: *precontemplation, contemplation, preparation, action,* and *maintenance* (Box 29.2). A sixth stage called *termination* is occasionally included as the final stage of change and is defined as the stage when an individual has engaged in the behavior for more than 6 months, is no longer susceptible to temptation, and has high levels of self-efficacy for maintaining the behavior. An individual progresses through the first five stages as he or she makes changes in a particular behavior. The model is not meant to be linear, meaning individuals can skip stages (e.g., move from contemplation to action in one step). Decisional balance and self-efficacy influence an individual's decision to move from one stage to another.

Different strategies (processes of change) are employed at different stages to support the behavior change (Table 29.6). Consciousness raising, dramatic relief, and environmental reevaluation are most useful in the earlier stages of change, whereas counterconditioning, helping relationships, reinforcement management, and stimulus control are most useful in the later stages of change.

Clinical interventions based on this theoretical model have been successful in changing behaviors, particularly in the areas of smoking, diet, and physical activity.[1] The

Table 29.5 Key Constructs in the Transtheoretical Model[100]

Construct	Definition
Stages of Change	The stages an individual moves through when changing a behavior
Decisional Balance	The process of weighing the pros and cons of changing a behavior
Self-efficacy	The confidence the individual has that he or she can successfully engage in the behavior
Processes of Change	Activities used to support progress through stages

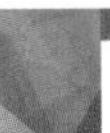

Box 29.2 Transtheoretical Model: Stages of Change[1]

Precontemplation

- Individual does not intend to take action within the next 6 months.

Contemplation

- Individual intends to take action within the next 6 months.

Preparation

- Individual intends to take action within the next 30 days, and has taken some preliminary steps.

Action

- Individual has engaged in the behavior for less than 6 months.

Maintenance

- Individual has engaged in the behavior for more than 6 months.

Termination

- Individual engages in the behavior, has high self-efficacy for the behavior, and is no longer tempted to return to the unhealthy behavior.

Table 29.6 Transtheoretical Model: Processes of Change[1]

Process of Change	Description	Stage in Which Process of Change Is Used
Consciousness raising	Individual increases level of awareness and acquires information about the behavior	Precontemplation Contemplation
Dramatic relief	Individual experiences negative emotions regarding health risks associated with not changing unhealthy behavior	Precontemplation Contemplation
Environmental reevaluation	Individual evaluates the negative impact on others of continuing the unhealthy behavior	Precontemplation Contemplation
Self-evaluation	Individual considers self-image and examines personal values	Contemplation
Self-liberation	Individual makes a commitment to change behavior	Preparation
Counterconditioning	Individual substitutes healthy behavior for unhealthy behavior	Action Maintenance
Helping relationships	Individual seeks social support for behavior change	Action Maintenance
Reinforcement management	Individual increases rewards for healthy behavior	Action Maintenance
Stimulus control	Individual removes cues for unhealthy behavior, adds cues for healthy behavior	Action Maintenance

TTM has also been examined in a study looking specifically at the exercise behaviors of adults with physical disabilities, and the key constructs and relationships hypothesized in this theoretical model of behavior were supported by the researchers' findings.[101] A clinician using this theoretical model to support behavior change should begin with an evaluation of the individual's stage of change for the behavior, as well as an evaluation of the individual's level of self-efficacy for the behavior. Box 29.3 provides a sample stage of change questionnaire and Table 29.7 presents a sample self-efficacy for physical activity questionnaire. Appropriate processes of change can then be selected and implemented by the clinician to match the individual's stage of change and self-efficacy for the behavior (see Table 29.6), paying attention also to the barriers identified by the individual and providing assistance to develop strategies to overcome them. Low self-efficacy for the behavior can be addressed by discussing how to maintain the behavior even under challenging conditions.

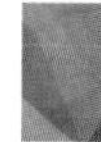

Box 29.3 Sample Stage of Change Questionnaire

Circle the number before the statement that best describes your current intentions related to walking 150 minutes a week.

1. I currently do not walk 150 minutes a week and have no intentions to start walking 150 minutes a week. (Precontemplation)
2. I currently do not walk 150 minutes a week but plan to start walking 150 minutes a week sometime within the next 6 months. (Contemplation)
3. I currently do not walk 150 minutes a week but I plan to start walking 150 minutes a week sometime within the next month. (Preparation)
4. I walk 150 minutes a week, but have been doing so for less than 6 months. (Action)
5. I walk 150 minutes a week, and have been doing so for 6 months or more. (Maintenance)

Self-Determination Theory

In developing *Self-Determination Theory* (SDT), Deci and Ryan married two psychological approaches: (1) that humans are growth-oriented beings seeking to actualize their potential and (2) that social environments either support or block this human attempt at growth.[102] According to SDT, humans possess three basic psychological needs, which are the constructs of the theory.[103] The construct of *competence* is the degree to which people feel able to achieve their goals and desired outcomes. *Autonomy,* the second construct, is the degree to which people feel responsible for the initiation and maintenance of their behavior. The third construct, *relatedness,* is the extent to which people feel connected to others in a warm, positive, interpersonal manner. Deci and Ryan suggest that people thrive when environments support these three basic human needs.[102]

Self-Determination Theory can be used to understand and facilitate the development of motivation for

Table 29.7 Sample Self-Efficacy Questionnaire

Place a check mark (✓) in the box that corresponds to how confident you are that you could keep up your walking program in the following situations:

Situation	Not at All Confident	Slightly Confident	Moderately Confident	Very Confident	Extremely Confident
When there is bad weather					
When I am tired					
When I am having pain					
When I am away from home					
When I have too much work to do					

a specific behavior, maintaining that when behaviors are based on personal values (intrinsic), they are sustainable, whereas when motivation is extrinsic (e.g., to please another person), they are less likely to be sustainable. Clinical interventions based on this theory have demonstrated positive outcomes for a myriad of behaviors, including exercise and physical activity, smoking cessation, eating, obesity and weight management, and low back pain management.[104-113] Using the SDT to assist adoption of a behavior involves identifying the type of motivation the patient has, implementing strategies to develop intrinsic motivation (by providing relevant information and meaningful rationales for change), not applying external controls and pressures that detract from choice, and by supporting the individual as he or she explores resistances and barriers to change.[102,103] To build competence, the clinician provides relevant input and feedback, the tools and skills needed for change, support to overcome competence or control-related barriers, and assists with achieving mastery in the behavior.[102,103] In addition, the clinician should create and maintain an environment in which the patient feels respected, understood, and cared for at all times.[102,103]

Social Cognitive Theory

The previous models, with their emphasis on the cognitions and behaviors of the individual, can be categorized as *individual* models of health behavior.[1] *Social Cognitive Theory,* with its additional emphasis on the individual's physical and social environment, is an example of a model of *interpersonal* health behavior. In an early article on social learning through observation, Bandura[114] hypothesized that individuals could learn through watching others' behaviors and rewards. Bandura[115] then further developed the theory, added additional constructs, and changed the name of the theory from Social Learning Theory to Social Cognitive Theory. According to Bandura, an individual's behavior is the result of the constant interaction among the environment, personal factors (including cognitions), and behavior through a process called *reciprocal determinism* (Fig. 29.8).

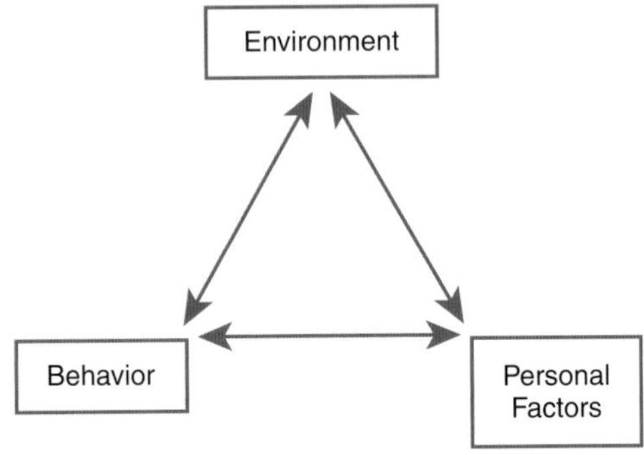

Figure 29.8 Social Cognitive Theory.

Key constructs within the theory include environment, situation, behavioral capability, expectations, expectancies, self-control, observational learning, reinforcement, self-efficacy, and emotional coping responses (Table 29.8). According to Bandura, self-efficacy, the confidence that one can successfully engage in the behavior across different challenging situations, is the single most important prerequisite for behavior change: it affects the individual's level of effort and persistence in engaging in the behavior in the face of difficulty.[116]

A number of clinical trials support the constructs and relationships proposed by this theory.[1,117-123] Interventions incorporating Social Cognitive Theory constructs have been effective in changing health behaviors (Table 29.9 Evidence Summary). Clinical application of this theoretical model requires attention to the key constructs as they apply for a given behavior and client. For example, the clinician may want to evaluate the individual's physical and social environment to determine what elements in the environment must be changed in order to support the particular health behavior being promoted. If the individual does not have the behavioral capability to carry out a particular behavior, education and training in the skills needed to perform the behavior may be required. The clinician should also use a tool to measure the client's self-efficacy for the behavior and if low levels of self-efficacy are found, specific strategies can be incorporated to build confidence (Box 29.4). The

Table 29.8 Key Constructs in Social Cognitive Theory[1]

Construct and Definition	How to Address Construct in Behavioral Change Program
Reciprocal determinism: continuous interaction of individual, behavior, and environment	Consider individual's environment, personal skills, and attitudes when developing strategies to support behavior change
Environment: factors external to the individual that influences behavior	Consider how to incorporate physical and social support for the behavior
Situation: the individual's perception of his or her environment	Correct misperceptions about the environment and the behaviors of others
Behavioral capability: the individual has the knowledge and skills to successfully engage in the behavior	Provide education and skills training
Expectations: the outcomes the individual anticipates from engaging in the behavior	Provide education regarding positive outcomes of the behavior
Expectancies: value the individual places on the outcomes of the behavior	Relate the outcomes to the individual's personal values
Self-control: personal control of the behavior	Incorporate goal-setting and self-monitoring of progress
Observational learning: learning that occurs through watching others successfully engage in the behavior	Consider the use of peers as role models for the behavior
Reinforcement: the positive or negative reinforcement the individual receives after engaging in the behavior	Incorporate self-initiated rewards for meeting goals, and support/encouragement from significant others
Self-efficacy: confidence in ability to successfully perform a specific behavior	Build individual's self-efficacy by breaking the behavior into small achievable steps to ensure success
Emotional coping responses: how the individual copes with emotions	Teach problem solving skills and stress management

Table 29.9 Evidence Summary Evidence Supporting the Use of Theory-Based Coaching to Increase Levels of Physical Activity

Annesi, JJ, et al: Effects of the coach approach intervention on adherence to exercise in obese women: Assessing mediation of social cognitive factors. Res Q Exerc Sport 82(1):99, 2011.

Design	Randomized Controlled Trial
Level of Evidence	Level II
Subjects	162 women age 21–60 years, BMI of 30–45 kg/m^2, no regular exercise within previous year
Intervention	Intervention Group (IG): Exercise prescription for 3 sessions per week at wellness center over 6 months, nutritional and weight loss information, six 1-hour one-on-one meetings with wellness specialist trained in using "coach approach" based on Social Cognitive Theory (cognitive restructuring, goal setting, behavioral contracting, tailored feedback, instruction in self-regulation). Control Group (CG): Exercise prescription for 3 sessions per week at wellness center over 6 months, nutritional and weight loss information, six 1-hour one-on-one meetings with study staff focused on the processes of exercise and physiological concerns.
Results	IG had greater exercise session attendance and greater improvements in physical self-concept, exercise barriers self-efficacy, and body areas satisfaction than the CG.
Comments	Participants in the CG received similar amount of personal contact time with exercise specialist as participants in the IG to control for the Hawthorne effect. Separate wellness centers used for the IG and CG to avoid cross-contamination.

Continued

Table 29.9 Evidence Summary Evidence Supporting the Use of Theory-Based Coaching to Increase Levels of Physical Activity—cont'd

Focht, BC, et al: A group-mediated physical activity intervention in older knee osteoarthritis patients: Effects on social cognitive outcomes. J Behav Med 40(3): 530, 2017.

Design	Randomized Controlled Trial
Level of Evidence	Level II
Subjects	80 participants (67 women, 13 men) age 55+ years, with knee pain on most days of the month, less than 20 min/week of structured exercise during the prior 6 months, self-reported difficulty with basic daily functional tasks due to knee pain, and radiographic evidence of grade II or III tibio-femoral osteoarthritis on Kellgren-Lawrence Scale.
Intervention	IG: 36 contact hours with study staff over 9 months of the 12-month study. Received exercise prescription and group-mediated cognitive behavioral counseling based on Social Cognitive Theory to facilitate the mastery of key activity-related self-regulatory skills. CG: 36 contact hours with study staff for 3 months performing individualized moderate intensity walking and lower body strengthening in 3 center-based group exercise sessions per week. Participants in the control group given educational pamphlets with standard osteoarthritis self-management advice.
Results	At the 1-year follow-up, the IG had greater increases in physical activity as measured by accelerometer, increased mobility as measured by the 400-meter walk test, and higher self-regulatory self-efficacy and satisfaction with physical function.
Comments	Outcome assessments carried out by study staff blinded to group assignment to decrease potential for bias. Although total contact hours were equal for both groups, the sequencing of the contact hours was different between groups. The IG had contact with study staff up until month nine, whereas the control group had no contact after month 3, allowing for the potential for a Hawthorne effect.

Froehlich-Grobe, K, et al: Exercise for everyone: A randomized controlled trial of Project Workout on Wheels in promoting exercise among wheelchair users. Arch Phys Med Rehabil 95(1):20, 2014.

Design	Randomized Controlled Trial
Level of Evidence	Level II
Subjects	128 inactive wheelchair users (64 women, 64 men) with an impairment for ≥ 6 months necessitating manual or powered wheelchair use for mobility outside the home, age 18–65, not currently physically active, with sufficient upper arm mobility for aerobic exercise.
Intervention	IG: Over the 6-month intervention period, participants received exercise prescription, resistance bands, educational information, a 1-day workshop based on Social Cognitive Theory with interventions designed to increase self-efficacy and self-management skills. Over the next 6 months, participants carried out exercises independently and received 15 phone calls during which study staff provided information tailored to the individual's experiences and needs. CG: Participants received exercise prescription, resistance bands, and educational information. Over the next 6 months, participants in the CG carried out exercises independently and received 15 phone calls during which study staff thanked them for returning (or requested the return of) exercise logs and inquired about any exercise-related injuries.
Results	At the 1-year follow-up, the IG reported more minutes of weekly aerobic exercise than the CG ($p<.05$). There was no difference between groups in aerobic capacity or strength.
Comments	Outcome assessments carried out by study staff blinded to group assignment to decrease potential for bias. One third of the participants did not complete the study, although there was no statistically significant difference in number of dropouts by group allocation. Cannot rule out Type II error due to low power.

Table 29.9 Evidence Summary Evidence Supporting the Use of Theory-Based Coaching to Increase Levels of Physical Activity—cont'd

Knittle, K, et al: Targeting motivation and self-regulation to increase physical activity among patients with rheumatoid arthritis: A randomized controlled trial. Clin Rheumatol 34(2):231, 2015.

Design	Randomized Controlled Trial
Level of Evidence	Level II
Subjects	78 participants over the age of 18, diagnosed with rheumatoid arthritis according to the American College of Rheumatology criteria, and not currently meeting the physical activity recommendation of 30 minutes of moderate-intensity 5 days per week.
Intervention	IG: Intervention based on Social Cognitive Theory and Self Determination Theory: one group-based education session in week 1, an individual motivational interview from a physical therapist in week 2, two self-regulation individual coaching sessions from a nurse in weeks 4 and 5, follow-up phone calls by nurse in weeks 6, 12, and 18. CG: one group-based education session in week 1.
Results	At 32 weeks (end of the study), the IG reported increased leisure time activity, more days per week with 30 minutes of physical activity, increased self-efficacy for physical activity, and higher scores for autonomous motivation for physical activity.
Comments	Not clear if participants were blind to group allocation. Contact time for IG higher than CG allowing for possibility of Hawthorne effect. Despite randomization, the CG had significantly more males and higher disease activity scores at baseline.

Motl, RW, et al: Internet intervention for increasing physical activity in persons with multiple sclerosis. Mult Scler 17(1):116, 2011.

Design	Randomized Controlled Trial
Level of Evidence	Level II
Subjects	54 participants with diagnosis of relapsing-remitting multiple sclerosis, independently ambulatory or ambulatory with single-point assistance (i.e., cane), relapse free in past 30 days, not engaging in 30 minutes per day of physical activity on more than 2 days per week over the last 6 months.
Intervention	IG: Over 3 months, participants accessed 4 multimedia Internet modules that included key elements of Social Cognitive Theory, engaged in twice-weekly online chat sessions, and participated in an online discussion forum. CG: participants received no intervention and were wait-listed to receive the intervention following completion of the study.
Results	IG had increased physical activity compared to the CG at the end of study as measured by the Godin Leisure-Time Exercise Questionnaire.
Comments	Participants paired at baseline for physical activity level and disability level prior to randomization process to ensure group comparability. Cannot rule out Hawthorne effect as CG did not receive any intervention.

O'Halloran, PD, et al: Motivational interviewing to increase physical activity in people with chronic health conditions: A systematic review and meta-analysis. Clin Rehabil 28(12):1159, 2014.

Design	Systematic review and meta-analysis
Level of Evidence	Level I
Subjects	10 peer-reviewed randomized controlled trials (RTCs) rated as moderate or high quality were included in the review and 8 were included in the meta-analysis. In all selected trials, participants were over the age of 18 and had a chronic health condition.
Intervention	Trials were eligible if the motivational interviewing intervention included (1) a clear focus on changing physical activity (2) use of reflective listening in a collaborative relationship and (3) emphasis on evoking the person's motivation for change.
Results	Moderate level of evidence that motivational interviewing had a small effect on increasing self-reported physical activity levels in people with chronic health conditions.
Comments	Authors followed the Preferred Reporting Items for Systematic Reviews and Meta-Analyses (PRISMA) statement and presented a clear search strategy and transparent process for inclusion and exclusion of studies. Variations in treatment fidelity and dose of intervention across studies may have contributed to the modest effect size.

Continued

Table 29.9 Evidence Summary Evidence Supporting the Use of Theory-Based Coaching to Increase Levels of Physical Activity—cont'd

Stacey, FG, et al: A systematic review and meta-analysis of social cognitive theory-based physical activity and/or nutrition behavior change interventions for cancer survivors. J Cancer Surviv 9(2):305, 2015.

Design	Systematic Review and Meta-Analysis
Level of Evidence	Level I
Subjects	18 RCTs included in full review; 7 studies examined effect of intervention on physical activity and diet, 10 studies examined effect of intervention on physical activity only, one study examined effect of intervention on diet only. Meta-analysis carried out on 12 of the studies that examined effect of intervention on physical activity. All participants in selected studies were age 18 or older, diagnosed with any cancer.
Intervention	Intervention based on Social Cognitive Theory (SCT) or explicitly described and referenced any SCT component such as self-efficacy.
Results	A small to medium effect size found for the effectiveness of the intervention in improving levels of physical activity.
Comments	Authors followed the Preferred Reporting Items for Systematic Reviews and Meta-Analyses (PRISMA) statement. Provided clear search strategy and transparent process for inclusion and exclusion of studies. Studies screened for eligibility by only one reviewer despite Cochrane recommendation that two reviewers carry out this process. Variations in treatment fidelity and dose of intervention across studies may have contributed to the modest effect size.

Box 29.4 Strategies for Enhancing Self-Efficacy[1,115,116]

1. Break the behavior into small achievable steps.
2. Set goals, establish a contract.
3. Problem solve potential challenges individual might face.
4. Mental practice and imagery.
5. Log progress, document achievement of goals.
6. Use peer role-modeling.
7. Ensure positive reinforcement received from others.
8. Ensure the correct interpretation of internal physiological states produced by the behavior.

role-modeling construct can be incorporated into a behavioral change program by using peer mentors or group leaders.

Physical Activity Model for People With a Disability

The preceding conceptual models can be applied to a variety of health behaviors with diverse populations. The *Physical Activity for People with a Disability* (PAD) model was developed to explain the behavior of physical activity in a population of people with a disability.[124] This model is based on the *Attitude, Social Influence, and Self-Efficacy* (ASE) model.[125] It integrates behavioral theoretical models with disability models and uses the ICF framework and terminology. In this model, environmental factors and personal factors interact to influence an individual's intention to engage in physical activity. Environmental factors include such variables as transportation, availability and accessibility of facilities, and assistance from others. Environmental factors also encompass social influence variables such as the opinion of family, friends, or health professionals. Personal factors include attitude, self-efficacy, health condition, and facilitators or barriers such as energy level, time, motivation, and skills. The authors of this model suggest that clinical application can include use of the TTM's stages of change. The model has been useful in identifying barriers to physical activity in adults and children with disabilities, allowing better design of intervention programs to increase physical activity in these populations.[126,127]

Social Ecological Model

The basic premise of an ecological approach to behavior change is the recognition that there are multiple levels of influence on behavior[1] (see Fig. 29.2). Social ecological models are informed by four principles:

- There are multiple influences on specific health behaviors, including intrapersonal, interpersonal, organizational, community, and public policy levels.
- There is interaction of influences across levels.
- Ecological models should be behavior specific and include identification of the most important influences at each level.
- Multilevel approaches to behavior change are the most effective.[1]

Numerous researchers have demonstrated that successful behavior change occurs when interventions are planned in a social ecological framework, intervening at multiple levels to support the individual and populations.[128-132] A clinician taking a social ecological approach to facilitating behavior change would select at least two levels of the model and identify interventions that would be appropriate at each level. For example, to facilitate the adoption of a more physically active lifestyle in a patient being seen for low back pain, the clinician might identify a recreation center (community) the patient could access to swim and a neighbor to take walks with (interpersonal) as two resources that could be woven into an intervention.

Community Models

A number of behavior change theoretical models have been developed to explain behavior change at a community level. Although a thorough discussion of community models is beyond the scope of this chapter, physical therapists who are interested in changing the health behaviors of a group or community may want to familiarize themselves with community and group models of health behavior change, and intervention planning models such as the *PRECEDE-PROCEED planning model.*[1]

HEALTH AND WELLNESS COACHING

In recent years, increased efforts have been made to provide psychological and emotional support for individuals seeking to change health behaviors, in recognition of the challenges to making sustainable behavior change. *Health coaches* are individuals with health care backgrounds, knowledge of behavior change theories, and skill in building autonomy and self-efficacy in behavior change efforts. A variety of certification programs exist that train health care providers like physical therapists, and others, to provide health and wellness coaching services. In an effort to raise the standard of health coaching and create consistency across certification programs, an international set of standards has been developed and was launched in 2017, to which existing certification programs are trying to align.[133]

Health coaching is most commonly delivered face-to-face or telephonically and there is evidence to support the effectiveness of both delivery mechanisms.[134-136] A recent systematic review and meta-analysis on the effect of health coaching on physical activity participation in people over the age of 60 found that while both delivery mechanisms resulted in increased physical activity participation, health coaching delivered face-to-face produced greater effects.[135] Experts believe that developing a helping relationship between the client and coach is one key to the effectiveness of health coaching. The competencies the coach should demonstrate include the ability to[137]:

- Apply a patient-centered approach.
- Assist clients to identify their own goals and motivation for change.
- Use a self-discovery process in which clients take an exploratory approach to identifying useful strategies and participate in an active learning process.
- Help clients be accountable to themselves and learn how to monitor their own progress.
- Have relevant content knowledge to assist the client to change a wide variety of behaviors.

A typical approach to health coaching involves the identification of a vision for health and/or wellness, which is a future desired state; identification of health behaviors in which the client can partake that would move the client closer to the vision; identification of previous successful experiences with the behavior and environmental and social supports for behavior change; and establishing weekly SMART (Specific, Measurable, Attainable, Relevant, Timely) goals and the assessment of self-efficacy for achieving goals.[138] Coaches encourage clients to adopt a "trial and learn" approach, treating goals as experiments to determine what works best to make wellness and health habits sustainable.[138]

Although health coaching is a relatively new intervention, significant evidence exists that generally supports its use as an effective approach to promoting sustainable behavior change. The U.S. Preventive Services Task Force has awarded a grade of B for behavioral counselling to improve diet and increase physical activity in adults who are overweight or obese and at risk for increase cardiovascular disease.[139] A "B" grade indicates that the intervention is recommended and has more potential benefits than potential harms. A systematic review by Frerichs et al[140] revealed that physical therapists can effectively provide coaching services related to lifestyle behavior change, at least in the short-term. These authors identified studies in which physical therapists were involved in smoking cessation, nutrition, weight reduction, and increasing physical activity, acting either independently or as a part of a team of health care providers. In another study examining the effects of a 5-week intervention on physical activity in patients with rheumatoid arthritis, physical therapists provided group education sessions and a one-on-one motivational interviewing session to all patients in the treatment group and a nurse provided two one-on-one sessions focusing on autonomous motivation. The control group received a group-based education session. The treatment group experienced significant increases in physical activity, self-efficacy, and autonomous motivation and the increase in physical activity was still present at the 6-month follow-up.[141] The amount of time required to provide health coaching has been shown to vary widely in the literature, but authors indicate that effective change can be promoted with relatively minimal investment of time.[140,141] Thus, physical therapists are well suited to deliver health coaching interventions given the generous amount of time spend with patients, especially compared to other providers.[76]

Motivational Interviewing

Motivational interviewing is a client-centered counseling method designed to facilitate an internal motivation to change by identifying dissonance between behaviors and values as well as resolving ambivalence.[142] Such interviewing is a valuable tool within the context of health coaching because it generates autonomous motivation, which is a goal of health coaching.[138] This counseling technique, initially developed to support behavior change in the treatment of addiction, is now used with a variety of populations where existing behaviors have adversely affected health or quality of life. It has been effectively used to encourage adherence to medical recommendations in general practice populations, to resolve behavioral issues with criminal justice populations, and to assist couples undergoing marital counseling.[142] Physical therapists have used motivational interviewing to improve adherence with rehabilitation programs[143] and to increase physical activity in individuals with chronic disease.[141]

The hallmark of this technique is the emphasis on exploring values and having the client recognize discordance between current behaviors and life goals. The clinician begins by asking probing questions to encourage the client to discuss his or her priorities in life and how current behaviors support or do not support those priorities. Encouraging the client to consider the pros and cons of continuing with current unhealthy behaviors versus changing to healthier behaviors may help resolve ambivalence by tipping the balance in favor of behavior change (identification of more pros than cons). Reflective listening by the clinician will allow a better understanding of the client's point of view and key contextual information related to potential challenges with behavior change. A clinician who is skilled in the motivational interviewing technique is respectful of personal choice and autonomy, is empathetic, avoids arguments, and provides encouragement to support self-efficacy for behavior change[142] (Box 29.5).

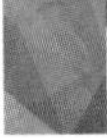

Box 29.5 Key Principles of Motivational Interviewing[142]

1. Express empathy.
   - Listen respectfully.
   - Do not judge.
   - Build therapeutic alliance.
   - Accept ambivalence.
2. Develop discrepancy.
   - Help client identify discrepancy between present behavior and personal goals and values.
   - Have client present reasons for change.
3. Roll with resistance.
   - Avoid arguing.
   - Accept reluctance to change as natural.
   - Turn problem back to client and encourage client to suggest solutions.
4. Support self-efficacy.
   - Enhance client's confidence in his or her ability to successfully change behavior.

Motivational interviewing has been used in the field of health promotion to encourage change in lifestyle behaviors. Regardless of the underlying theoretical behavior change model being used to structure a health behavior change intervention, motivational interviewing can be incorporated as a technique to engage the client in important collaborative discussions about his or her behaviors. There is some empirical evidence of the effectiveness of this technique in supporting behavior change across a number of health-related behaviors, although more research is needed.[144] It has been shown to be effective in encouraging weight loss,[145] physical activity,[146-149] smoking cessation,[150,151] and fruit and vegetable consumption.[149]

HEALTH PROMOTION AND WELLNESS FOR INDIVIDUALS WITH IMPAIRMENTS AND DISABILITIES

There is evidence that physical therapists in the United States are moving beyond their traditional roles in secondary and tertiary prevention, and engaging in primary prevention and health promotion practice in the general population.[14,15,17,88] Physical therapists are engaging in screening programs,[152,153] ergonomic consultations,[154] and sports injury prevention and conditioning programs.[155]

There is, however, a great need for physical therapists to engage in more health promotion activities with individuals with disabilities and chronic diseases. One of the specific goals stated in *Healthy People 2020* is to increase the number of health promotion programs for people with disabilities.[12] Research has shown that this population has lower levels of physical activity,[156-159] higher rates of smoking,[160] and higher levels of overweight and obesity than the age-matched general population.[161,162] Physical therapists have a unique knowledge and skill set that positions them well to be leaders in health promotion and wellness initiatives for individuals with disabilities. Unlike other health professionals, therapists also interact with patients over extended periods of time. This extended period of interaction and level of accessibility allows time to develop a rapport with patients and provides the therapist an opportunity to be influential in advocating for healthy behaviors.[163]

Examination and Evaluation

The patient management model in the *Guide to Physical Therapist Practice 3.0* provides a framework for therapists to carry out an examination (Box 29.6) and evaluation that will identify potential opportunities for prevention and health promotion interventions.[18] Examples of general prevention and health promotion goals and outcomes are presented in Box 29.7. During the history taking, the therapist should look beyond questions related to a specific impairment and inquire about perceived health or use a self-perceived health, wellness, or

Box 29.6 Elements of the Examination[18]

Patient/Client History

- Demographic information
- Social history
- Employment and work information
- Living arrangements
- General health status
- Perceived health and perceived wellness
- Family history
- Medical and surgical history
- Medications
- Clinical test results
- Functional status and activity level
- Past and current health behaviors: physical activity, smoking, diet, sleep, stress management, substance abuse

Systems Review

- Cardiovascular
- Pulmonary
- Integumentary
- Musculoskeletal
- Neuromuscular
- Communication ability/cognition/learning style

Tests and Measures

- Aerobic capacity/endurance (e.g., fitness level)
- Anthropometric characteristics (e.g., BMI)
- Assistive technology (e.g., appropriate assistive devices to ensure safety and allow participation in activities meaningful to patient)
- Balance (e.g., dynamic balance to safely engage in physical activity)
- Circulation (e.g., claudication or ischemia during activity)
- Community, social, and civic life: (e.g., ability to engage in activities meaningful to patient)
- Cranial and peripheral nerve integrity: (e.g., peripheral neuropathy creating risk for injury during physical activity)
- Education life: Ability to participate in activities and roles in educational setting
- Environmental factors: Barriers to engaging in physical activity, accessing fitness programs, and safe places to exercise
- Gait (e.g., ability to safely engage in walking and running programs to increase fitness level)
- Integumentary integrity (e.g., assess risk for pressure injuries, examine moles)
- Joint integrity and mobility (e.g., impairments that may affect ability to engage in physical activities)
- Mental functions (e.g., perceived wellness, attitude, and beliefs about physical activity, ability to understand link between health behaviors and health, motivation to change, ability to problem-solve around barriers)
- Mobility (e.g., impairments that could impact activities)
- Muscle performance: Capacity of muscles to generate forces to produce, maintain, sustain, and modify postures and movements required for functional activities
- Pain: Assess pain and impact of pain on levels of physical activity, emotional health, and participation in activities meaningful to patient
- Posture (e.g., body mechanics, ergonomics)
- Range of motion (e.g., impairments that impact ability to engage in physical activities)
- Self-care and domestic life: Assess ability to carry out daily activities and roles
- Sensory integrity: Assess sensory integrity to ensure ability to safely engage in physical activity
- Ventilation and respiration (e.g., assess fitness level)
- Work life: (e.g., assess ability to carry out roles and participate in activities related to work life)

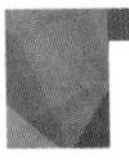

Box 29.7 General Prevention and Health Promotion Goals and Outcomes

Impact of pathology/pathophysiology is reduced.

- Fitness levels are improved.
- Health status is improved.
- Self-management of chronic disease is improved.
- Risk factors for development of injury and/or secondary conditions reduced.

Impact of impairments is reduced.

- Aerobic capacity is increased.
- Muscle endurance is increased.
- Gait, locomotion, and balance are improved.
- Motor function is improved.
- Muscle performance is increased.
- Postural control is improved.
- Relaxation is increased.

Activity limitations are reduced.

- Ability to perform physical actions, tasks, or activities related to self-care, home management, work (job/school/play), community, and leisure is improved.
- Tolerance of positions and activities is increased.
- Safety is improved.
- Problem solving and decision making skills are enhanced.

Participation restrictions are reduced.

- Ability to assume or resume required self-care, home management is improved.
- Ability to assume work (job/school/play), community, and leisure roles is improved.

Health, wellness, and fitness are improved.

- Self-perceived health and wellness of patient/client is improved.
- Patient/client understanding of health and wellness and health behaviors is increased.
- Self-efficacy is increased.
- Behaviors that support health and wellness are adopted.
- Self-management skills are improved.
- Intrinsic motivation is developed or increased.

Societal Resources are utilized.

- Awareness and use of community resources to support health and wellness is improved.

Patient/client satisfaction is enhanced.

- Therapeutic relationship with physical therapist is valued by patient/client.
- Health coaching skills of physical therapist are valued by patient/client.

quality-of-life questionnaire as described earlier. The therapist should also inquire about health-related behaviors, including physical activity, nutrition and/or weight management, current smoking status, sleep, and stress management.[76] A systems review should be carried out to screen for risk factors for disease or injury, and appropriate follow-up by the physical therapist or referral to other health professionals as indicated should occur. For example, physical therapists should routinely take blood pressure before having the patient/client engage in physical activity not only as a component of safe practice, but also to be able to identify and report hypertension. Therapists who notice a mole should ask the client if he or she has discussed this predisposing factor for skin cancer with a physician. Fall risk assessments should be conducted with at-risk populations. Based on their examination and evaluation, physical therapists may identify the need to engage patients in discussions about healthy behaviors and discuss the impact unhealthy behaviors may have on recovery. For example, discussion can focus on the impact of nicotine on tissue healing, or high BMI on joint health and overall health and wellness. Assessment of stage of change (see Box 29.2) for relevant health behaviors will inform the physical therapist in identifying appropriate interventions. For example, if a patient is in the contemplation stage for becoming regularly physically active, health coaching that includes motivational interviewing may be appropriate in assisting the patient to identify a strong intrinsic motivator and to identify the benefits of regular physical activity so that decisional balance tips toward the benefits side of the benefits/barriers equation and the patient becomes readier to act. Referrals should be made to appropriate programs and health professionals when health issues that fall outside of the scope of practice and qualifications of the physical therapist are identified during the examination.

Interventions

Physical Activity/Exercise

The APTA encourages physical therapists and physical therapist assistants to be promoters and advocates for physical activity/exercise.[164] Individuals with chronic disease and disability report lower levels of physical activity and exercise than the general population.[156-159] The lower levels of physical activity/exercise reported by this population may be due to a host of factors including limited mobility, chronic pain, fatigue, fear of aggravating their condition, or limited access to fitness facilities that have the necessary equipment and personnel to enable safe and effective physical activity.[165-168] Physical therapists are uniquely qualified to evaluate fitness levels and prescribe fitness programs for individuals with medical conditions. The APTA has identified two priority populations requiring the knowledge and skills of physical therapists in physical fitness prescription.[169] The primary priority population consists of individuals with acute and chronic impairments, activity limitations, and disabilities related to movement, function, and health, and the secondary priority population consists of individuals with identified risk for impairments, activity limitations, and disabilities related to movement, function, and health.

A physical therapy exercise program developed for a patient/client to prevent or remediate impairments falls under the category of secondary or tertiary prevention. However, if therapists are truly engaging in primary prevention and health promotion, a physical activity and exercise program to improve overall fitness to the maximal level possible for that patient should also be considered. Participation in physical activity may reduce secondary health problems, improve levels of function, and improve subjective well-being in individuals with chronic medical conditions.[170] There is evidence that exercise can improve quality of life in stroke survivors.[171] The CDC recommends that adults participate in 150 minutes of moderate-intensity or 75 minutes of vigorous-intensity aerobic activity every week and muscle-strengthening activities on 2 or more days a week.[40] Children should engage in 60 minutes or more of physical activity every day[40] (Table 29.10).

However, these physical activity recommendations were developed for the general population and may not be appropriate for patients/clients with disabilities and medical conditions. Physical activity recommendations should be tailored to ensure safety and effectiveness for the patient's unique medical condition. Physical therapists must consider not only the patient's condition, but also any comorbidities and potential side effects or limitations associated with medical treatments when prescribing a physical activity program. There are excellent research-based resources to help physical therapists safely test fitness and prescribe exercise for patients with medical conditions.[16,172-173] Beyond appropriate content of a physical activity program, physical therapists should consider the previously mentioned theories of behavior change and motivational interviewing to support patients/clients and optimize their chance for successful behavior change as they begin to increase their level of physical activity. Patients/clients can also be informed about physical activity programs in the community that are geared to specific populations. Physical therapists and patients/clients should refer to the consumer website of the National Center on Physical Activity and Disability (see Appendix 29.C) for education and specific information about exercise, as well as sports and recreational activities recommended for those with disabilities.[174] The benefits of engaging in sports should be discussed with patients/clients; people with disabilities who engage in sports have reported enhanced function, social benefits, and an increased sense of optimism.[54]

Smoking Cessation Counseling

There is strong evidence that even brief counseling of patients can be effective to support smoking cessation.[175,176] Given the strong evidence of the health risks associated with smoking and clinical evidence of the effectiveness of even brief counseling sessions, Bodner and Dean[176] effectively argue that counseling patients about smoking behaviors falls within the role of physical therapists and, given their prolonged contact with patients over the course of treatment, have the opportunity and the rapport necessary to be effective in smoking cessation counseling. In a systematic review, they found that intervention models based on the motivational interviewing technique are effective. The Agency for Healthcare Research and Quality recommends that clinicians include a question about smoking as part of their examination and evaluation and has designed a specific evidence-based program to assist clinicians in helping their clients address smoking behaviors.[177] The 5-A's

Table 29.10 Physical Activity Guidelines[40]

Adults	Aerobic activity every week: 150 minutes of moderate-intensity aerobic activity (e.g., brisk walking) **OR** 75 minutes of vigorous-intensity aerobic activity (e.g., jogging or running) **OR** an equivalent mix of moderate- and vigorous-intensity aerobic activity. **AND** Muscle-strengthening activities on 2 or more days a week that work all major muscle groups (legs, hips, back, abdomen, chest, shoulders, and arms).
Children and Adolescents	Should do 60 minutes of physical activity each day. Aerobic activity should make up most of the recommended 60 or more minutes of daily physical activity. Can include moderate-intensity aerobic activity, such as brisk walking, or vigorous activity, such as running, but should include vigorous-intensity aerobic activity on at least 3 days per week. **AND** Muscle-strengthening activities, such as gymnastics or push-ups, at least 3 days a week. **AND** Bone-strengthening activities, such as jumping rope or running, at least 3 days per week.

Source: www.cdc.gov/HealthyLiving/.

tobacco cessation approach recommends that clinicians *A*sk their patients about tobacco use, *A*dvise tobacco users to quit, *A*ssess the client's readiness to quit, *A*ssist the client with a quit plan, and *A*rrange follow-up to review progress toward quitting (Box 29.8). Physical therapists should also be familiar with smoking cessation programs in the local area and refer patients/clients as appropriate to these specialized programs.

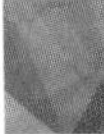

Box 29.8 Helping Smokers Quit: A Guide for Clinicians

1. Ask about tobacco use.
Implement a system in your clinic that ensures that tobacco-use status is obtained and recorded.
2. Advise all tobacco users to quit.
Use clear, strong, and personalized language. For example, "Quitting tobacco is the most important thing you can do to protect your health."
3. Assess readiness to quit.
Ask every tobacco user if he or she is willing to quit at this time.
- If willing to quit, provide resources and assistance.
- If unwilling to quit at this time, help motivate the patient:
  - Identify reasons to quit in a supportive manner.
  - Build patient's confidence about quitting.

4. Assist tobacco users with a quit plan.
Assist the smoker to:
- Set a quit date, ideally within 2 weeks.
- Remove tobacco products from his or her environment.
- Get support from family, friends, and coworkers.
- Review past quit attempts—what helped, what led to relapse.
- Anticipate challenges, particularly during the critical first few weeks, including nicotine withdrawal.
- Identify reasons for quitting and benefits of quitting.

Give advice on successful quitting:
- Total abstinence is essential—not even a single puff.
- Drinking alcohol is strongly associated with relapse.
- Allowing others to smoke in the household hinders successful quitting.

Encourage use of prescribed medications.
Provide resources:
- Recommend toll-free number: 1-800-QUIT NOW (784-8669), the national access number to state-based quitline services.
- Refer to www.smokefree.gov website for free materials.

5. Arrange follow-up.
Schedule follow-up.
- If a relapse occurs, encourage quit attempt.
- Review circumstances that caused relapse. Use relapse as a learning experience.
- Make appropriate referrals.

Adapted from www.ahrq.gov/clinic/tobacco/clinhlpsmksqt.htm.

Healthy Weight and Healthy Eating Counseling

Overweight and obesity are associated with development of numerous risks, conditions, and diseases[178] (Box 29.9). The *Guide to Physical Therapist Practice 3.0* recommends that anthropometric measurements be included in initial examinations. The measurement of height and weight will allow physical therapists to calculate the patient's BMI. Calculators and charts are available on the CDC website (see Appendix 29.C) to assist therapists in calculating the patient/client's BMI.[179]

Patients should be educated about the impact that excessive weight and unhealthy eating have on current condition and future health.[179,180] The APTA encourages physical therapists to speak with their patients about the importance of eating a healthy diet.[181] Physical therapists can screen for unhealthy eating behaviors and make basic recommendations for improving nutrition.[182,183] As nutritional education may be outside the scope of physical therapist practice in some states, it is recommended that therapists review their state practice acts and refer patients to qualified health professionals as appropriate.[181]

Healthy Sleep Counseling

Insufficient sleep can adversely affect a patient's overall health and quality of life. Health problems found to be associated with insufficient sleep include hypertension, diabetes, depression, obesity, and cancer.[184] Physical therapists are being encouraged to discuss healthy sleep behaviors with their patients.[27,76] A sleep inventory questionnaire can be used to evaluate sleep behaviors and

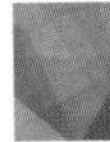

Box 29.9 Risks and Health Consequences of Obesity

All-causes of death (mortality)
Hypertension
Dyslipidemia
Type 2 diabetes
Coronary heart disease
Stroke
Gallbladder disease
Osteoarthritis
Sleep apnea and respiratory problems
Some cancers (endometrial, breast, colon, kidney, gallbladder, liver)
Low quality of life
Mental illness such as clinical depression, anxiety, and other mental disorders
Body pain and difficulty with physical functioning

From www.cdc.gov/obesity/adult/causes.html.

physical therapists can provide basic recommendations for healthy sleep habits.[185]

HEALTH PROMOTION AND WELLNESS AT THE PROGRAM LEVEL

Patients who are discharged from physical therapy to continue their exercise programs independently often find it challenging to locate a facility with the necessary equipment or personnel who are sufficiently trained to address their unique medical challenges. Physical therapists have begun to recognize and address this need for physical activity programming that is specifically tailored to address the needs of patients with chronic conditions or disabilities. Fitness and health promotion programs geared to this population and offered in rehabilitation settings are growing in popularity. For example, physical therapists are providing fitness classes and health and wellness programs to youths with disabilities,[186] adults post-stroke,[187] and individuals with cancer.[188] It is important to remember that these programs should comply with state licensing requirements for physical therapists and that the same standards for physical therapist practice be maintained whether the physical therapist is providing rehabilitation or health promotion interventions. An excellent resource for physical therapists is the APTA website *Physical Fitness for Special Populations* (see Appendix 29.C).[169] The website provides recommendations for the design of fitness programs tailored to the specific needs of individuals with various medical conditions, such as stroke, type 2 diabetes, and pulmonary pathology. The site also provides valuable information about malpractice and professional liability, Medicare coverage for fitness services, and other helpful resources.

PHYSICAL THERAPISTS AS ADVOCATES

One of the goals stated in *Healthy People 2020* is the need for increased health promotion programming for individuals with disabilities.[12] Physical therapists can make a meaningful contribution to the health of the nation by providing health and wellness to this population within their own practices as described above. In addition, physical therapists should recognize their broader social responsibility, as articulated in the *Core Values* document of the professional association, to advocate for the health and wellness needs of all.[21] The APTA has numerous position statements highlighting the role of physical therapists in health promotion and wellness, including a position titled *Physical Therapists' Role in Prevention, Wellness, Fitness, Health Promotion, and Management of Disease and Disability* (HOD P06-16-06-05) that highlights the role of physical therapists in supporting scientific, educational, legislative, and other policy initiatives that promote regular physical activity and exercise to enhance health and prevent disease; advocating for physical education, physical conditioning, and wellness instruction at all levels of education; and advocating for community design that promotes opportunities for safe physical activity and active forms of transportation for individuals and populations of all ages and abilities.[22] The role of the APTA in advocacy for prevention, wellness, fitness, health promotion, and management of disease and disability is outlined in another position statement.[189] It includes advocacy in such areas as appropriate physical activity and exercise goals and priorities as recommended by government or other recognized organizations, appropriate efforts to enhance community design to promote safe physical activity and active forms of transportation, the inclusion of physical education in schools, and physical therapists making healthy personal lifestyle choices related to active transportation and physical activity as priorities for the association.[189] Clearly, physical therapists have an important role at all levels of government, community, public education, and workplaces, to advocate for health promoting policies and practices.

There are several national organizations and efforts in which physical therapists can engage to improve the health of society, including Exercise is Medicine (EIM), a collaboration between the American Medical Association and the American College of Sports Medicine, whose vision is to have health care providers assess every patient's level of physical activity at every clinical visit, determine if the patient is meeting national physical activity guidelines, and provide brief counseling to patients to assist in meeting the guidelines and/or refer the patient to another resource for further physical activity counseling.[190] EIM makes available free resources on their website to assist health care providers in this role, and physical therapists can take a pledge indicating their commitment to promoting physical activity with their patients.

Physical therapists, with their unique knowledge base and clinical experience, are extremely cognizant of the needs and challenges faced by individuals with chronic disease and disability, as well as those of the general population across the life span, and should participate at both the community and national levels to provide or ensure that all members of society are provided access to health promotion and wellness programming.

SUMMARY

Physical therapists have the knowledge, the skill set, and the opportunity to engage in health promotion practice across the continuum of care. A population in special need of the guidance and support of physical therapists is the population with medical conditions and disabilities who face unique challenges when trying to incorporate healthy behaviors into their lives. At the Physical Therapy and Society Summit meeting, the need for more research to better define physical therapists' role in prevention, health, and wellness, especially with respect to consumers with impairments, was identified.[24] The *Revised Research Agenda for Physical Therapy* identifies specific health promotion areas requiring additional investigation and discussion, including examination of the effectiveness of physical activity health promotion interventions for individuals with movement disorders.[191] As the profession continues to define and develop its role in health promotion and wellness, physical therapists should identify and explore opportunities within their current practice environments to promote optimal levels of health and wellness of their patients/clients.

Questions for Review

1. What factors contribute to the health of an individual?
2. What is *Healthy People 2020*?
3. How does the World Health Organization define *health*?
4. Identify the different domains of wellness.
5. Define *primary, secondary*, and *tertiary* prevention.
6. Where in the continuum of primary, secondary, and tertiary prevention have physical therapists traditionally practiced?
7. Differentiate between the terms *health promotion* and *health education.*
8. What is the difference between the terms *exercise* and *physical activity*?
9. What tools could a physical therapist use to measure a patient/client's self-perceived health, wellness, or quality of life?
10. What health-related behaviors should physical therapists inquire about during initial examinations of patients/clients?
11. Describe the following theories of behavior change: Health Belief Model, Transtheoretical Model and Stages of Change, Theory of Planned Behavior, Self-Determination Theory, and Social Cognitive Theory.
12. What is health coaching and how can it be used in the context of physical therapist practice?
13. What is the purpose of motivational interviewing?
14. What are the five steps of the 5-A's tobacco cessation approach?
15. What professional documents support the role of physical therapists in health promotion?

CASE STUDY

Mary Boyd is a 53-year-old woman with multiple sclerosis referred to physical therapy by her family physician who reports she is complaining of decreased walking endurance and increased incidence of falls at home.

PATIENT HISTORY

Mrs. Boyd reports she was diagnosed with relapsing/remitting multiple sclerosis 15 years ago. She is being followed by a neurologist and her family physician and currently takes 20 mg of Copaxone and 20 mg of Provigil to help manage the symptoms of her multiple sclerosis. She becomes upset during the initial visit as she describes her growing inability to participate in many family activities outside the home owing to her concerns about falling and increasing levels of fatigue. She is fearful about her deteriorating ability to walk functional distances and worries about what the future holds for her.

SOCIAL HISTORY

Mrs. Boyd lives at home with her husband and three teenage daughters who she describes as very supportive. She does not go out alone, as she cannot drive. During the day, her husband is at work and her daughters are at school. Her primary social circle is her family and her large extended family in town.

PHYSICAL THERAPY EXAMINATION FINDINGS

Mental Status: Alert, oriented
Anthropometric: Height: 5 ft 8 in, Weight 150 lb
Cardiopulmonary: Resting heart rate: 58, Resting blood pressure: 135/85
ROM: Full ROM all extremities
Strength: Decreased strength in right quadriceps (grade 3), right hamstrings (grade 3), right dorsiflexors (grade 4)
Balance: Difficulty shifting weight in standing
Endurance/Fatigue: Walking tolerance 5 minutes
Gait: Walked 100 feet with no assistive device, was unsteady, demonstrated a slight right foot drop, and used a wide base of support

HEALTH-RELATED BEHAVIORS

- Smoking: Smokes 2 to 3 cigarettes/day; she has smoked for 30 years.
- Diet and Nutrition: Has late breakfast due to fatigue first thing every morning. Reports she eats a healthy diet.
- Physical Activity: She does light housework throughout the day, but spends most of her day sitting on the sofa reading books, working on her computer, or watching TV.

GUIDING QUESTIONS

1. Identify additional tests and/or measures that could be used to assess her level of health.
2. Identify additional tests and/or measures that could be used to assess her level of wellness.
3. What domains of wellness may be at lower levels?
4. Which health-related behaviors might be adversely affecting her health and wellness?
5. How should a conversation about her health and wellness be initiated?
6. If Mrs. Boyd asked for help in changing her behaviors, select a theory of behavior change to guide the intervention. Which behaviors should be targeted?
7. What level of physical activity should Mrs. Boyd strive to achieve for health-related benefits?

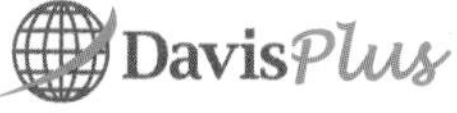

For additional resources, including answers to the questions for review and case study guiding questions, please visit **http://davisplus.fadavis.com.**

References

1. Glanz, K, Rimer, BK, and Viswanath, K (eds): Health Behavior and Health Education, ed 5. Jossey-Bass, San Francisco, 2015.
2. World Health Organization (WHO): Global action plan for the prevention and control of NCDs 2013–2020. WHO, Geneva, Switzerland, 2013. Retrieved August 13, 2017, from www.who.int/nmh/events/ncd_action_plan/en/.
3. National Center for Chronic Disease Prevention and Health Promotion; Centers for Disease Control and Prevention (CDC): The power of prevention. CDC, Atlanta, GA, 2009. Retrieved August 13, 2017, from www.cdc.gov/chronicdisease/pdf/2009-power-of-prevention.pdf.
4. McGinnis, JM, Williams-Russo, P, and Knickman, JR: The case for more active policy attention to health promotion. Health Aff *(Millwood)* 21(2):78, 2002.
5. Centers for Disease Control and Prevention (CDC): Adult Obesity Facts. Retrieved March 1, 2017, from www.cdc.gov/obesity/data/adult.html.
6. Centers for Disease Control and Prevention (CDC), National Center for Chronic Disease Prevention and Health Promotion, Division of Population Health: BRFSS Prevalence & Trends Data. CDC, Atlanta, GA, 2015. Retrieved March 1, 2017, from www.cdc.gov/brfss/brfssprevalence/.
7. Centers for Disease Control and Prevention (CDC): Morbidity and Mortality Weekly Report. Adults Meeting Fruit and Vegetable Intake Recommendations—United States, 2013. CDC, Atlanta, GA, July 10, 2015. Retrieved March 1, 2017, from www.cdc.gov/mmwr/preview/mmwrhtml/mm6426a1.htm.
8. Centers for Disease Control and Prevention (CDC): Sleep and Sleep Disorders. CDC, Atlanta, GA, March 9, 2017. Retrieved March 8, 2017, from www.cdc.gov/sleep/index.html.
9. Centers for Disease Control and Prevention (CDC): Morbidity and Mortality Weekly Report. Prevalence of Healthy Sleep Duration among Adults—United States, 2014. CDC, Atlanta, GA, February 19, 2016. Retrieved August 13, 2017, from www.cdc.gov/mmwr/volumes/65/wr/mm6506a1.htm.
10. Ogden, CL, et al: Prevalence of obesity among adults and youth: United States, 2011–2014. NCHS data brief, no 219. Hyattsville, MD: National Center for Health Statistics, 2015.
11. Centers for Disease Control and Prevention (CDC): Childhood Obesity Cause & Consequences. CDC, Atlanta, GA, December 15, 2016. Retrieved March 8, 2017, from www.cdc.gov/obesity/childhood/causes.html.
12. US Department of Health and Human Services (HHS): Healthy People 2020. HHS, Washington, DC, 2017. Retrieved May 16, 2017, from www.healthypeople.gov/2020/about/History-and-Development-of-Healthy-People.
13. Zenzano, T, et al: The roles of healthcare professionals in implementing clinical prevention and population health. Am J Prev Med 40(2):261, 2011.
14. Shirley, D, van der Ploeg, HP, and Bauman, AE: Physical activity promotion in the physical therapy setting: Perspectives from practitioners and students. Phys Ther 90(9):1311, 2010.
15. Goodgold, S: Wellness promotion beliefs and practices of pediatric physical therapists. Pediatr Phys Ther 17:148, 2005.

16. Jewell, D: The role of fitness in physical therapy patient management: Applications across the continuum of care. Cardiopulm Phys Ther J 17(2):47, 2006.
17. Rea, BL, et al: The role of health promotion in physical therapy in California, New York, and Tennessee. Phys Ther 84(6):510, 2004.
18. American Physical Therapy Association: *Guide to Physical Therapist Practice 3.0.* Alexandria, VA: American Physical Therapy Association; 2014. Accessed March 3, 2017, from http://guidetoptpractice.apta.org.
19. Commission on Accreditation in Physical Therapy Education (CAPTE): Evaluative Criteria PT Programs. Accreditation Handbook. CAPTE, Alexandria, VA, July 2016. Retrieved August 13, 2017, from www.capteonline.org/AccreditationHandbook/.
20. Federation of State Boards of Physical Therapy (FSBPT): The Model Practice Act for Physical Therapy. A Tool for Public Protection and Legislative Change, ed 6. FSBPT, Alexandria, VA, 2016. Retrieved August 13, 2017, from www.fsbpt.org/Portals/0/documents/free-resources/MPA_6thEdition2016.pdf.
21. American Physical Therapy Association (APTA): Professionalism in Physical Therapy: Core Values. APTA, Alexandria, VA, 2009. Retrieved May 16, 2017, from www.apta.org/uploadedFiles/APTAorg/About_Us/Policies/BOD/Judicial/ProfessionalisminPT.pdf.
22. American Physical Therapy Association (APTA): Physical Therapists' Role in Prevention, Wellness, Fitness, Health Promotion, and Management of Disease and Disability HOD P06-16-06-05. APTA, Alexandria, VA, 2016. Retrieved August 13, 2017, from www.apta.org/uploadedFiles/APTAorg/About_Us/Policies/Practice/PTRoleAdvocacy.pdf#search=%22HOD%20P06-15-23-15%22.
23. American Physical Therapy Association (APTA): Introduction to the Guide to Physical Therapist Practice. *Guide to Physical Therapist Practice 3.0.* Alexandria, VA: American Physical Therapy Association; 2014. Available at: http://guidetoptpractice.apta.org/content/1/SEC1.body. Accessed August 13, 2017.
24. Kigin, CM, Rodgers, MM, and Wolf, SL: The Physical Therapy and Society Summit (PASS) meeting: Observations and opportunities. Phys Ther 90(11):1555, 2010.
25. Sahrmann, S: Ask an expert. Today in PT 2:20, 2009.
26. Dean, E, et al: The first physical therapy summit on global health: Implications and recommendations for the 21st century. Physiother Theory Pract 27(8):531, 2011.
27. Dean, E, et al: The second physical therapy summit on global health: Developing an action plan to promote health in daily practice and reduce the burden of non-communicable diseases. Physiother Theory Pract 30(4):261, 2014.
28. World Health Organization (WHO): What is the WHO Definition of Health? WHO, Geneva, Switzerland, 2017. Retrieved March 3, 2017, from www.who.int/suggestions/faq/en/.
29. O'Donnell, MP: Definition of health promotion 2.0: Embracing passion, enhancing motivation, recognizing dynamic balance, and creating opportunities. Am J Health Promot 24(1):iv, 2009.
30. Dunn, HL: High-level wellness for man and society. Am J Public Health 49(6):786, 1959.
31. Adams, T, Bezner, J, and Steinhardt, M: The conceptualization and measurement of perceived wellness: Integrating balance across and within dimensions. Am J Health Promot 11(3):208, 1997.
32. National Wellness Institute (NWI): Definition of wellness. NWI, Stevens Point, WI, 2017. Retrieved March 3, 2017, from https://www.nationalwellness.org/page/Six_Dimensions.
33. Edelman, CL, and Mandle, CL: Health Promotion Throughout the Lifespan, ed 5. Mosby, St. Louis, 2002.
34. Centers for Disease Control and Prevention (CDC): Health-Related Quality of Life. CDC, Atlanta, GA. Retrieved March 3, 2017, from www.cdc.gov/hrqol/.
35. US Department of Health and Human Services (HHS): Healthy People 2020. HHS, Washington, DC, 2017. Retrieved March 3, 2017, from www.healthypeople.gov/2020/topics-objectives/topic/health-related-quality-of-life-well-being.
36. Green, LW, and Kreuter, MW: Health Promotion Planning, ed 4. McGraw-Hill, New York, 2004.
37. Hefner, JL, Huerta, TR, and McAlearney, AS: Preface: What is population health management? Population Health Management in Healthcare Organizations. Bingley, UK: Emerald Group Publishing Limited, 2014, pp xvii–xxiv.
38. World Health Organization (WHO): Health Promotion. WHO, Geneva, Switzerland. Retrieved March 3, 2017, from www.who.int/topics/health_promotion/en/.
39. Gorin, SS, and Arnold, J (eds): Health Promotion in Practice. Jossey-Bass, San Francisco, 2006.
40. Physical Activity Guidelines Advisory Committee Report. US Department of Health and Human Services, 2008. Retrieved March 3, 2017, from https://health.gov/paguidelines/guidelines/.
41. Casperson, CJ, Powell, KE, and Christenson, GM: Physical activity, exercise, and physical fitness: Definitions and distinctions for health-related research. Public Health Rep 100(2):126, 1985.
42. Callahan, LF, and Pinkus, T: Education, self-care, and outcomes of rheumatic diseases: Further challenges to the "Biomedical Model" paradigm. Arthritis Rheum 10(5):283, 1997.
43. Engel, GL: The need for a new medical model: A challenge for biomedicine. In Caplan, AL, McCartney, JJ, and Sisti, DA (eds): Health, Disease, and Illness: Concepts in Medicine. Georgetown University Press, Washington, DC, 2004, p. 51.
44. Bandura, A: The primacy of self-regulation in health promotion. Appl Psychol 54(2):245, 2005.
45. Nagi, S: Disability concepts revisited: Implications for prevention. In Pope, A, and Tarlov, A (eds): Disability in America: Toward a National Agenda for Prevention. Institute of Medicine, National Academy Press, Washington, DC, 1991, p. 309.
46. World Health Organization (WHO): International Classification of Functioning, Disability and Health (ICF). WHO, Geneva, Switzerland, 2017. Retrieved August 13, 2017, from www.who.int/classifications/icf/en/.
47. Physical Therapists and Physical Therapist Assistants as Promoters and Advocates for Physical Activity/Exercise RC-08. American Physical Therapy Association, 64th Annual Session House of Delegates, San Antonio, TX, June 9–11, 2008.
48. Escorpizo, R, et al: Creating an interface between the International Classification of Functioning, Disability and Health and physical therapist practice. Phys Ther 90(7):1053, 2010.
49. Fisher, MI, and Howell, D: The power of empowerment: An ICF-based model to improve self-efficacy and upper extremity function of survivors of breast cancer. Rehabil Oncol 28(3):19, 2010.
50. Rauch, A, et al: Using a case report of a patient with spinal cord injury to illustrate the application of the International Classification of Functioning, Disability and Health during multidisciplinary patient management. Phys Ther 90(7):1039, 2010.
51. Fowler, EG, et al: Promotion of physical fitness and prevention of secondary conditions for children with cerebral palsy: Section on pediatrics research summit proceedings. Phys Ther 87(11):1495, 2007.
52. Howard, D, Nieuwenhuijsen, ER, and Saleeby, P: Health promotion and education: Application of the ICF in the US and Canada using an ecological perspective. Disabil Rehabil 30(12–13):942, 2008.
53. Raggi, A, et al: Obesity-related disability: Key factors identified by the International Classification of Functioning, Disability and Health. Disabil Rehabil 32(24):2028, 2010.
54. Wilhite, B, and Shank, J: In praise of sport: Promoting sport participation as a mechanism of health among persons with a disability. Disabil Health J 2(3):116, 2009.
55. Oremus, M, Hammill, A, and Raina, P: Health Risk Appraisal. Agency for Healthcare Research and Quality (US); 2011. Rockville, Maryland. Retrieved March 3, 2017, from www.ncbi.nlm.nih.gov/books/NBK254034/.
56. Mossey, JM, and Shapiro, E: Self-rated health: A predictor of mortality among the elderly. Am J Public Health 72(8):800, 1982.
57. Centers for Disease Control and Prevention (CDC): Health-Related Quality of Life. CDC, Atlanta, GA. Retrieved March 3, 2017, from www.cdc.gov/hrqol/hrqol14_measure.htm.
58. Northwestern University: Patient Reported Outcomes Measurement Information System (PROMIS) Health Measures. Northwestern University, Chicago, IL. Retrieved March 3, 2017, from www.healthmeasures.net/explore-measurement-systems/promis.
59. World Health Organization (WHO): The World Health Organization Quality of Life (WHOQOL). WHO, Geneva, Switzerland. Retrieved March 3, 2017, from www.who.int/mental_health/publications/whoqol/en/.

60. Ware, JE, et al: SF-36 Health Survey Manual and Interpretation Guide. Health Institute, New England Medical Center, Boston, 1993.
61. Hunt, SM, and McEwan, J: Nottingham Health Profile: The development of a subjective health indicator. Sociol Health Illn 2:231, 1980.
62. Bergner, M: The Sickness Impact Profile: Conceptual formulation and methodology for the development of a health status measure. Int J Health Serv 6:393, 1976.
63. Dartmouth CO-OP Project: Dartmouth Medical School, Hanover, NH. Retrieved March 3, 2017, from http://www.fvfiles.com/521475.pdf.
64. Duke Health Profile: Department of Community and Family Medicine, Duke University Medical Center, Durham, NC. Retrieved March 3, 2017, from http://healthmeasures.mc.duke.edu/images/DukeForm.pdf.
65. Harari, MJ, Waehler, CA, and Rogers, JR: An empirical investigation of a theoretically based measure of perceived wellness. J Couns Psychol 52(1):93, 2005.
66. Meenan, RF: The AIMS approach to health status measurement: Conceptual background and measurement properties. J Rheumatol 9:785,1982.
67. Meenan, RF, et al: AIMS2: The content and properties of a revised and expanded Arthritis Impact Measurement Scales health status questionnaire. Arthritis Rheum 35:1, 1992.
68. Landgraf, JM, Abetz, L, and Ware, JEJ: The Child Health Questionnaire (CHQ): A user's manual. Health Institute, New England Medical Center, Boston, 1996.
69. Quittner, AL, et al: CFQ Cystic Fibrosis Questionnaire: A health-related quality of life measure. User manual. English version 1.0, 2000.
70. van Straten, A, et al: A stroke-adapted 30-item version of the Sickness Impact Profile to assess quality of life (SA-SIP30). Stroke 28:2155, 1997.
71. Duncan, PW, et al: The Stroke Impact Scale Version 2.0 Evaluation of reliability, validity and sensitivity to change. Stroke 30:2131, 1999.
72. VanSwearingen, JM, and Brach, JS: The Facial Disability Index: Reliability and validity of a disability assessment instrument for disorders of the facial neuromuscular system. Phys Ther 76(12):1288, 1996.
73. Guyatt, GH, et al: A measure of quality of life for clinical trials in chronic lung disease. Thorax 42:773, 1987.
74. European Organisation for Research and Treatment of Cancer (EORTC), Quality of Life Department: EORTC QLQ-30. EORTC, Brussels, Belgium. Retrieved March 3, 2017, from http://groups.eortc.be/qol/eortc-qlq-c30.
75. Reeves, MJ, and Rafferty, AP: Healthy lifestyle characteristics among adults in the United States. Arch Intern Med 165:854, 2005.
76. Bezner, JR: Promoting health and wellness: Implications for physical therapist practice. Phys Ther 95(10):1433, 2015.
77. Craig, CL, et al: International physical activity questionnaire: 12-country reliability and validity. Med Sci Sports Exerc 35: 1381, 2003.
78. Woolf, SH, Jonas S, and Kaplan-Liss, E: Health Promotion and Disease Prevention in Clinical Practice. Lippincott Williams & Wilkins, Philadelphia, 2008.
79. Clark, MM et al: Stress level, health behaviors, and quality of life in employees joining a wellness center. Am J Health Promot 26:21, 2011.
80. Clark, MM, et al. Improvements in health behaviors, eating self-efficacy, and goal-setting skills following participation in wellness coaching. Am J Health Promot 30(6):458, 2016.
81. Werneburg, BL, et al: Effectiveness of a multidisciplinary worksite stress reduction programme for women. Stress Health 27:356, 2011.
82. Centers for Disease Control and Prevention (CDC): Healthy Living. CDC, Atlanta, GA. Retrieved July 11, 2017, from www.cdc.gov/healthyliving/index.html.
83. US Preventative Services Task Force (USPSTF): Recommendations. USPSTF, Rockville, MD. Retrieved July 11, 2017, from www.uspreventiveservicestaskforce.org/BrowseRec/Index/browse-recommendations.
84. Guide to Clinical Preventive Services 2010–2011. Recommendations of the US Preventive Services Task Force. Agency for Healthcare Research and Quality, Department of Health and Human Services, Rockville, MD, 2010.
85. Lin, JS, et al: Behavioral counseling to promote physical activity and a healthful diet to prevent cardiovascular disease in adults: A systematic review for the US Preventive Services Task Force. Ann Intern Med 153:736, 2010.
86. US Preventative Services Task Force (USPSTF): Final Recommendation Statement: Tobacco Smoking Cessation in Adults, Including Pregnant Women: Behavioral and Pharmacotherapy Interventions. USPSTF, Rockville, MD, 2016. Retrieved August 6, 2017, from www.uspreventiveservicestaskforce.org/Page/Document/RecommendationStatementFinal/tobacco-use-in-adults-and-pregnant-women-counseling-and-interventions1.
87. Michael, YL, et al: Primary care–relevant interventions to prevent falling in older adults: A systematic evidence review for the US Preventative Services Task Force. Ann Intern Med 153(12):815, 2010.
88. Bodner, ME, et al: Smoking cessation and counseling: Knowledge and views of Canadian physical therapists. Phys Ther 91(7):1051, 2011.
89. Rosenstock, IM: Historical origins of the Health Belief Model. Health Educ Monogr 2:328–335, 1974.
90. Campbell, HM, et al: Relationship between diet, exercise habits, and health status among patients with diabetes. Res Social Adm Pharm 7(2):151, 2011.
91. Haines, TP, et al: Patient education to prevent falls among older hospital inpatients: A randomized controlled trial. Arch Intern Med 171(6):516, 2011.
92. Katz, DA, et al: Health beliefs toward cardiovascular risk reduction in patients admitted to chest pain observation units. Acad Emerg Med 16(5):379, 2009.
93. Jeihooni, AK, et al: Effects of an osteoporosis prevention program based on health belief model among females. Nurs Midwifery Stud 4(3):e26731, 2015.
94. Khorsandi, M, Fekrizadeh, Z, and Roozbahani, N: Investigation of the effect of education based on the health belief model on the adoption of hypertension-controlling behaviors in the elderly. Clin Interv Aging 12:233, 2017.
95. Fishbein, M (ed): Readings in Attitude Theory and Measurement. Wiley, New York, 1967.
96. Ajzen, I: The theory of planned behavior. Organ Behav Hum Decis Process 50:179, 1991.
97. Godin, G, and Kik, G: The theory of planned behavior: A review of its applications to health-related behaviors. Am J Health Promot 11(2):87, 1996.
98. Armitage, CJ, and Conner, M: Efficacy of the theory of planned behavior. Br J Soc Psychol 40(4):471, 2001.
99. Norman, P, and Conner, M: The theory of planned behavior and exercise: Evidence for the mediating and moderating roles of planning on intention-behavior relationships. J Sport Exerc Psychol 27(4):488, 2005.
100. Prochaska, JO: Systems of Psychotherapy: A Transtheoretical Analysis. Brooks-Cole, Pacific Grove, CA, 1979.
101. Cardinal, BJ, Kosma, M, and McCubbin, JA: Factors influencing the exercise behavior of adults with physical disabilities. Med Sci Sports Exerc 36(5):868, 2004.
102. Deci, EL, and Ryan, RM (eds): Handbook of Self-Determination Research. The University of Rochester Press, Rochester, NY, 2002.
103. Ryan, RM et al: Facilitating health behaviour change and its maintenance: Implications based on self-determination theory. The European Health Psychologist 10:2008. http://selfdeterminationtheory.org/SDT/documents/2008_RyanPatrickDeciWilliams_EHP.pdf.
104. Austin, S, et al: Longitudinal testing of a dietary self-care motivational model in adolescents with diabetes. J Psychosom Res 75:153,2013.
105. Guertin, C, et al: The role of motivation and eating regulation on the physical and psychological health of cardiovascular disease patients. J Health Psychol 20: 543, 2015.
106. Lonsdale, C, et al: Communication style and exercise compliance in physiotherapy (CONNECT): A cluster randomized controlled trial to test a theory-based intervention to increase chronic low back pain patients' adherence to physiotherapists' recommendations: Study rationale, design, and methods. BMC Musculoskel Disord 13:104, 2012.
107. Mcspadden, KE, et al: The association between motivation and fruit and vegetable intake: The moderating role of social support. Appetite 96:87, 2016.

108. Murray, A, et al: Effect of a Self-Determination Theory–Based communication skills training program on physiotherapists' psychological support for their patients with chronic low back pain: A randomized controlled trial. Arch Phys Med Rehabil 5:809, 2015.
109. Russell, KL, and Bray, SR: Promoting self-determined motivation for exercise in cardiac rehabilitation: The role of autonomy support. Rehabil Psychol 55:74, 2010.
110. Slovinec D'Angelo, M, et al: The roles of self-efficacy and motivation in the prediction of short- and long-term adherence to exercise among coronary heart disease patients. Health Psychol 33:1344, 2014.
111. Teixeira, PJ, et al: Exercise, physical activity, and self-determination theory: A systematic review [Electronic version]. Int J Behav Nutr Phys Act 9:78, 2012. doi: 10.1186/1479-5868-9-78.
112. Teixeira, PJ, et al: Successful behavior change in obesity interventions in adults: A systematic review of self-regulation mediators. BMC Med 13:84,2015.
113. Williams, GC, et al: Outcomes of the Smoker's Health Project: A pragmatic comparative effectiveness trial of tobacco-dependence interventions based on self-determination theory. Health Educ Res 31(6):749, 2016.
114. Bandura, A: Social learning through imitation. In Jones, MR (ed): Nebraska Symposium on Motivation. University of Nebraska Press, Lincoln, NE, 1962, p. 211.
115. Bandura, A: Social cognitive theory of self-regulation. Organ Behav Hum Decis Process 50:248, 1991.
116. Bandura, A: Self-Efficacy: The Exercise of Control. WH Freeman, New York, 1997.
117. Annesi, JJ, et al: Effects of the coach approach intervention on adherence to exercise in obese women: Assessing mediation of social cognitive theory factors. Res Q Exerc Sport 82(1):99, 2011.
118. Cramp, AG, and Brawley, LR: Moms in motion: A group-mediated cognitive-behavioral physical activity intervention. Int J Behav Nutr Phys Act 3:23, 2006.
119. Ince, ML: Use of social cognitive theory–based physical activity intervention on health-promoting behaviors of university students. Percept Mot Skills 107:833, 2008.
120. Mihalko, SL, Wickley, KL, and Sharpe, BL: Promoting physical activity in independent living communities. Med Sci Sports Exerc 38(1):112, 2006.
121. Motl, RW, et al: Internet intervention for increasing physical activity in persons with multiple sclerosis. Mult Scler 17(1):116, 2011.
122. Rogers, LQ, et al: A randomized trial to increase physical activity in breast cancer survivors. Med Sci Sports Exerc 41(4):935, 2009.
123. Wilson, DK, et al: A preliminary test of a student-centered intervention on increasing physical activity in underserved adolescents. Ann Behav Med 30(2):119, 2005.
124. van der Ploeg, HP, et al: Physical activity for people with a disability: A conceptual model. Sports Med 34(10):639, 2004.
125. De Vries, H, Dijkstra, M, and Kuhlman, P: Self-efficacy: The third factor besides attitude and subjective norm as a predictor of behavioral intentions. Health Educ Res 3:273, 1988.
126. Bloemen, MAT, et al: Factors associated with physical activity in children and adolescents with a physical disability: A systematic review. Dev Med Child Neurol 57:137, 2015.
127. Buffart, LM, et al: Perceived barriers to and facilitators of physical activity in young adults with childhood-onset physical disabilities. J Rehabil Med 41:881,2009.
128. Bronner, YI, et al: Models for nutrition education to increase consumption of calcium and dairy products among African Americans. J Nutr 136:1103, 2016.
129. Deshpande, AD, Dodson, EA, and Gorman, I: Physical activity and diabetes: Opportunities for prevention through policy. Phys Ther 88:1425, 2008.
130. Doran, K, et al: Applying the social ecological model and theory of self-efficacy in the worksite heart health improvement project-PLUS. Res Theory Nurs Pract 31:8, 2017.
131. Martin Ginis, KA, et al: A systematic review of review articles addressing factors related to physical activity participation among children and adults with physical disabilities. Health Psychol Rev 10:478, 2016.
132. Sallis, JF, et al: An ecological approach to creating more physically active communities. Annu Rev Public Health 27: 297, 2006.
133. International Consortium for Health & Wellness Coaching (ICHWC). Retrieved August 14, 2017, from https://ichwc.org.
134. Dennis, SM, et al: Do people with existing chronic conditions benefit from telephone coaching? A rapid review. Aust Health Rev 37:381, 2013.
135. Oliveira, JS, et al: What is the effect of health coaching on physical activity participation in people aged 60 years and over? A systematic review of randomized controlled trials. Br J Sports Med 0:1, 2017.
136. Swoboda, CM, Miller, CK, and Wills, CE: Impact of a goal setting and decision support telephone coaching intervention on diet, psychosocial, and decision outcomes among people with type 2 diabetes. Patient Educ Couns 10(7):1367, 2017.
137. Wolever, RQ, et al: A systematic review of the literature on health and wellness coaching: Defining a key behavioral intervention in healthcare. Glob Adv Health Med 2(4):38, 2013.
138. Moore, M, Jackson, E, and Tschannen-Moran, B: Coaching Psychology Manual, ed 2. Wolters Kluwer, Philadelphia, PA, 2016.
139. LeFevre, ML: Behavioral counseling to promote a healthful diet and physical activity for cardiovascular disease prevention in adults with cardiovascular risk factors: US Preventive Services Task Force Recommendation Statement. Annals Int Med 161:587, 2014.
140. Frerichs, W, et al: Can physical therapists counsel patients with lifestyle-related health conditions effectively? A systematic review and implications. Physiother Theory Pract 28(8):571, 2012.
141. Knittle, K, et al: Targeting motivation and self-regulation to increase physical activity among patients with rheumatoid arthritis: A randomized controlled trial. Clin Rheumatol 34:231, 2015.
142. Miller, WR, and Rollnick, S: Motivational Interviewing, ed 2. Guilford Press, New York, 2002.
143. Vong, SK, et al: Motivational enhancement therapy in addition to physical therapy improves motivational factors and treatment outcomes in people with low back pain: A randomized controlled trial. Arch Phys Med Rehabil 92(2):176, 2011.
144. Rubak, S: Motivational interviewing: A systematic review and meta-analysis. Br J Gen Pract 55(513):305, 2005.
145. Greaves, CJ, et al: Motivational interviewing for modifying diabetes risk: A randomised controlled trial. Br J Gen Pract 58(553):535, 2008.
146. Bennett, JA, et al: Motivational interviewing to increase physical activity in long-term cancer survivors: A randomized controlled trial. Nurs Res 56(1):18, 2007.
147. Brodie, DA, and Inoue, A. Motivational interviewing to promote physical activity for people with chronic heart failure. J Adv Nurs 50(5):518, 2005.
148. Lohmann, H, Siersma, V, and Olivarius, NF: Fitness consultations in routine care of patients with type 2 diabetes in general practice: An 18-month non-randomised intervention study. BMC Fam Pract 11:83, 2010.
149. Van Keulen, HM, et al: Tailored print communication and telephone motivational interviewing are equally successful in improving multiple lifestyle behaviors in a randomized controlled trial. Ann Behav Med 41(1):104, 2011.
150. Lai, DTC, et al: Motivational interviewing for smoking cessation. Cochrane Database of Systematic Reviews 2010, Issue 1. Art. No.: CD006936. doi: 10.1002/14651858.CD006936. pub2.
151. Soria, R, et al: A randomised controlled trial of motivational interviewing for smoking cessation. Br J Gen Pract 56(531): 768, 2006.
152. Meeks, S: The role of the physical therapist in the recognition, assessment, and exercise intervention in persons with, or at risk for, osteoporosis. Top Geriatr Rehabil 21(1):42, 2005.
153. Dibble, L, and Lange, M: Predicting falls in individuals with Parkinson disease: A reconsideration of clinical balance measures. J Neurol Phys Ther 30(2):60, 2006.
154. DeWeese, C: How multiple interventions reduced injuries and costs in one plant. Work 26(3):251, 2006.
155. Gilchrist, J: A randomized controlled trial to prevent noncontact anterior cruciate ligament injury in female collegiate soccer players. Am J Sports Med 36(8):1476, 2008.
156. Boslaugh, SE, and Andresen, EM: Correlates of physical activity for adults with disability. Prev Chronic Dis 3(3):1, 2006.

157. Buchholz, AC, McGillivray, CF, and Pencharz, PB: Physical activity levels are low in free-living adults with chronic paraplegia. Obes Res 11:563, 2003.
158. Hootman, JM, et al: Physical activity levels among the general US adult population and in adults with and without arthritis. Arthritis Care Res 49(1):129, 2003.
159. Zhao, G, et al: Physical activity in US older adults with diabetes mellitus: Prevalence and correlates of meeting physical activity recommendations. J Am Geriatr Soc 59(1):132, 2011.
160. Armour, BS, et al: State-level prevalence of cigarette smoking and treatment advice, by disability status, United States, 2004. Prev Chronic Dis 4(4):A86, 2007.
161. Rimmer, R, Rowland, JL, and Yamaki, K: Obesity and secondary conditions in adolescents with disabilities: Addressing the needs of an underserved population. J Adolesc Health 41(3):224, 2007.
162. Rimmer, JH, and Wang, E: Obesity prevalence among a group of Chicago residents with disabilities. Arch Phys Med Rehab 86(7):1461, 2005.
163. Perreault, K: Linking health promotion with physiotherapy for low back pain: A review. J Rehabil Med 40:401, 2008.
164. American Physical Therapy Association: Physical therapists and physical therapist assistants as promoters and advocates for physical activity/exercise. House of Delegates P06-08-07-08. Retrieved August 19, 2017 from www.apta.org/uploadedFiles/APTAorg/About_Us/Policies/HOD/Practice/PromotePhysicalActivity.pdf.
165. Junker, L, and Carlberg, EB: Factors that affect exercise participation among people with physical disabilities. Adv Physiother 13(1):18, 2011.
166. Petursdottir, U, Arnadottir, SA, and Halldorsdottir, S: Facilitators and barriers to exercising among people with osteoarthritis: A phenomenological study. Phys Ther 90(7):1014, 2010.
167. Rimmer, JH, et al: Physical activity participation among persons with disabilities: Barriers and facilitators. Am J Prev Med 26(5):419, 2004.
168. Rogers, LQ, et al: Exploring social cognitive theory constructs for promoting exercise among breast cancer patients. Cancer Nurs 27(6):462, 2004.
169. American Physical Therapy Association: Physical Fitness for Special Populations. Retrieved August 14, 2017, from www.apta.org/PFSP/.
170. Centers for Disease Control and Prevention: Physical Activity among Adults with a Disability—United States, 2005. Morbidity and Mortality Weekly Report, 2007. Retrieved August 19, 2017, from www.cdc.gov/mmwr/preview/mmwrhtml/mm5639a2.htm.
171. Chen, MD, and Rimmer, JH: Effects of exercise on quality of life in stroke survivors: A meta-analysis. Stroke 42(3):832, 2011.
172. Goodman, C, and Helgeson, K: Exercise Prescription for Medical Conditions. FA Davis, Philadelphia, 2011.
173. Durstine, JL, et al: ACSM's Exercise Management for Persons with Chronic Diseases and Disabilities, ed 3. Human Kinetics, Champaign, IL, 2009.
174. The National Center on Physical Activity and Disability. University of Illinois at Chicago, Department of Disability and Human Development, College of Applied Health Sciences, Chicago, IL. Retrieved August 19, 2017, from www.ncpad.org/.
175. Quinn, VP, et al: Effectiveness of the 5-As tobacco cessation treatments in nine HMOs. J Gen Intern Med 24(2):149, 2009.
176. Bodner, ME, and Dean, E: Advice as a smoking cessation strategy: A systematic review and implications for physical therapists. Physiother Theory Pract 25(5–6):369, 2009.
177. Helping Smokers Quit: A Guide for Clinicians. Revised May 2008. Agency for Healthcare Research and Quality. Rockville, MD. Retrieved August 14, 2017, from www.ahrq.gov/professionals/clinicians-providers/guidelines-recommendations/tobacco/index.html.
178. Managing Overweight and Obesity in Adults: Systematic Evidence Review from the Obesity Expert Panel, 2013. National Heart, Lung and Blood Institute, Department of Health and Human Services, National Institutes for Health, Bethesda, MD. Retrieved August 14, 2017, from www.nhlbi.nih.gov/health-pro/guidelines/in-develop/obesity-evidence-review.
179. Centers for Disease Control and Prevention: Body Mass Index. Retrieved August 19, 2017, from www.cdc.gov/healthyweight/assessing/bmi/index.html.
180. Tick H: Nutrition and Pain. Phys Med Rehabil Clin N Am 26(2):309, 2015.
181. American Physical Therapy Association (APTA): The Role of the Physical Therapist in Diet and Nutrition HOD P06-15-22-17. APTA, Alexandria, VA, 2016. Retrieved August 14, 2017, from www.apta.org/PatientCare/Nutrition/.
182. Morris, DM, Kitchin, EM, and Clark, DE: Strategies for optimizing nutrition and weight reduction in physical therapy practice: The evidence. Physiother Theory Pract 25(5–6):408, 2009.
183. Hansen, D, et al: Physical therapy as treatment for childhood obesity in primary health care: clinical recommendation form AXXON (Belgian Physical Therapy Association). Phys Ther 96:850, 2016.
184. Centers for Disease Control and Prevention (CDC): Insufficient sleep is a public health epidemic. CDC, Atlanta, GA, 2015. Retrieved July 11, 2017, from www.cdc.gov/features/dssleep/.
185. Coren, S: Sleep health and its assessment and management in physical therapy practice: The evidence. Physiother Theory Pract 25(5–6):442, 2009.
186. Rowland, J, et al: The scope of pediatric physical therapy practice in health promotion and fitness for youth with disabilities. Pediatr Phys Ther 27(1):2, 2015.
187. Rose, D, Schafer, J, and Conroy, C: Extending the continuum of care poststroke: Creating a partnership to provide a community-based wellness program. J Neurol Phys Ther 37(2):78, 2013.
188. Lanni, T, et al: Implementation of an oncology exercise and wellness rehabilitation program to enhance survivorship: the Beaumont Health System experience. J Community Support Oncol 12(3):87, 2014.
189. American Physical Therapy Association (APTA): The Association's Role in Advocacy for Prevention, Wellness, Fitness, Health Promotion, and Management of Disease and Disability HOD P06-16-06-06. APTA, Alexandria, VA, 2016. Retrieved May 16, 2017, from www.apta.org/uploadedFiles/APTAorg/About_Us/Policies/Practice/AssociationRoleAdvocacy.pdf#search=%22health%20promotion%22.
190. Exercise is Medicine (EIM): Retrieved May 16, 2017, from www.exerciseismedicine.org/support_page.php/about/.
191. Goldstein, MS, et al: The revised research agenda for physical therapy. Phys Ther 91(2):165, 2011.

appendix

29.A Perceived Wellness Survey

The following statements are designed to provide information about your wellness perceptions. Please carefully and thoughtfully consider each statement, then select the *one* response option with which you *most* agree.

	Very Strongly Disagree					Very Strongly Agree
1. I am always optimistic about my future.	1	2	3	4	5	6
2. There have been times when I felt inferior to most of the people I knew.	1	2	3	4	5	6
3. Members of my family come to me for support.	1	2	3	4	5	6
4. My physical health has restricted me in the past.	1	2	3	4	5	6
5. I believe there is a real purpose for my life.	1	2	3	4	5	6
6. I will always seek out activities that challenge me to think and reason.	1	2	3	4	5	6
7. I rarely count on good things happening to me.	1	2	3	4	5	6
8. In general, I feel confident about my abilities.	1	2	3	4	5	6
9. Sometimes I wonder if my family will really be there for me when I am in need.	1	2	3	4	5	6
10. My body seems to resist physical illness very well.	1	2	3	4	5	6
11. Life does not hold much future promise for me.	1	2	3	4	5	6
12. I avoid activities that require me to concentrate.	1	2	3	4	5	6
13. I always look on the bright side of things.	1	2	3	4	5	6
14. I sometimes think I am a worthless individual.	1	2	3	4	5	6
15. My friends know they can always confide in me and ask me for advice.	1	2	3	4	5	6
16. My physical health is excellent.	1	2	3	4	5	6
17. Sometimes I don't understand what life is all about.	1	2	3	4	5	6
18. Generally, I feel pleased with the amount of intellectual stimulation I receive in my daily life.	1	2	3	4	5	6
19. In the past, I have expected the best.	1	2	3	4	5	6
20. I am uncertain about my ability to do things well in the future.	1	2	3	4	5	6
21. My family has been available to support me in the past.	1	2	3	4	5	6
22. Compared to people I know, my past physical health has been excellent.	1	2	3	4	5	6
23. I feel a sense of mission about my future.	1	2	3	4	5	6
24. The amount of information that I process in a typical day is just about right for me (i.e., not too much and not too little).	1	2	3	4	5	6
25. In the past, I hardly ever expected things to go my way.	1	2	3	4	5	6
26. I will always be secure with who I am.	1	2	3	4	5	6
27. In the past, I have not always had friends with whom I could share my joys and sorrows.	1	2	3	4	5	6
28. I expect to always be physically healthy.	1	2	3	4	5	6
29. I have felt in the past that my life was meaningless.	1	2	3	4	5	6

	Very Strongly Disagree					Very Strongly Agree
30. In the past, I have generally found intellectual challenges to be vital to my overall well-being.	1	2	3	4	5	6
31. Things will not work out the way I want them to in the future.	1	2	3	4	5	6
32. In the past, I have felt sure of myself among strangers.	1	2	3	4	5	6
33. My friends will be there for me when I need help.	1	2	3	4	5	6
34. I expect my physical health to get worse.	1	2	3	4	5	6
35. It seems that my life has always had purpose.	1	2	3	4	5	6
36. My life has often seemed void of positive mental stimulation.	1	2	3	4	5	6

■ PWS SCORING SHEET FOR USE WITH INDIVIDUAL CLIENTS

Instructions: Record your score from the PWS instrument for each numbered item below. Note the * items indicating reverse scoring. Add the numbers in each column and divide by 6 to determine each subscale score.

*Reverse score (e.g., 1 = 6, 2 = 5, 3 = 4, 4 = 3, 5 = 2, and 6 = 1)

Psychological		Physical	
Item Number	**Score**	**Item Number**	**Score**
1.	________	*4.	________
*7.	________	10.	________
13.	________	16.	________
19.	________	22.	________
*25.	________	28.	________
*31.	________	*34.	________
Total =	________	Total =	________
Divided by 6 =	________	Divided by 6 =	________
Emotional		**Spiritual**	
Item Number	**Score**	**Item Number**	**Score**
*2.	________	5.	________
8.	________	*11.	________
*14.	________	*17.	________
*20.	________	23.	________
26.	________	*29.	________
32.	________	35.	________
Total =	________	Total =	________
Divided by 6 =	________	Divided by 6 =	________

Continued

Social		Intellectual	
Item Number	Score	Item Number	Score
3.	________	6.	________
*9.	________	*12.	________
15.	________	18.	________
21.	________	24.	________
*27.	________	30.	________
33.	________	*36.	________
Total =	________	Total =	________
Divided by 6 =	________	Divided by 6 =	________

Web-Based Resources for Clinicians

appendix **29.B**

Resource	Web Address
Agency for Healthcare Research and Quality: Health Promotion/ Disease Prevention	www.ahrq.gov/browse/hpdp.htm
American Physical Therapy Association: Physical Fitness for Special Populations	www.apta.org/PFSP/
CDC: Behavioral Risk Factor Surveillance System	www.cdc.gov/brfss/
CDC: Healthy Living	www.cdc.gov/healthyliving/
CDC: Body Mass Index Calculator	www.cdc.gov/healthyweight/assessing/bmi/
CDC: Youth Risk Behavior Surveillance System	www.cdc.gov/HealthyYouth/yrbs/index.htm
Exercise is Medicine (EIM)	http://www.exerciseismedicine.org
Healthy People 2020	www.healthypeople.gov/2020/default.aspx
National Center on Physical Activity and Disability	www.ncpad.org/
U.S. Preventive Services Task Force	www.uspreventiveservicestaskforce.org

CDC = Centers for Disease Control and Prevention.

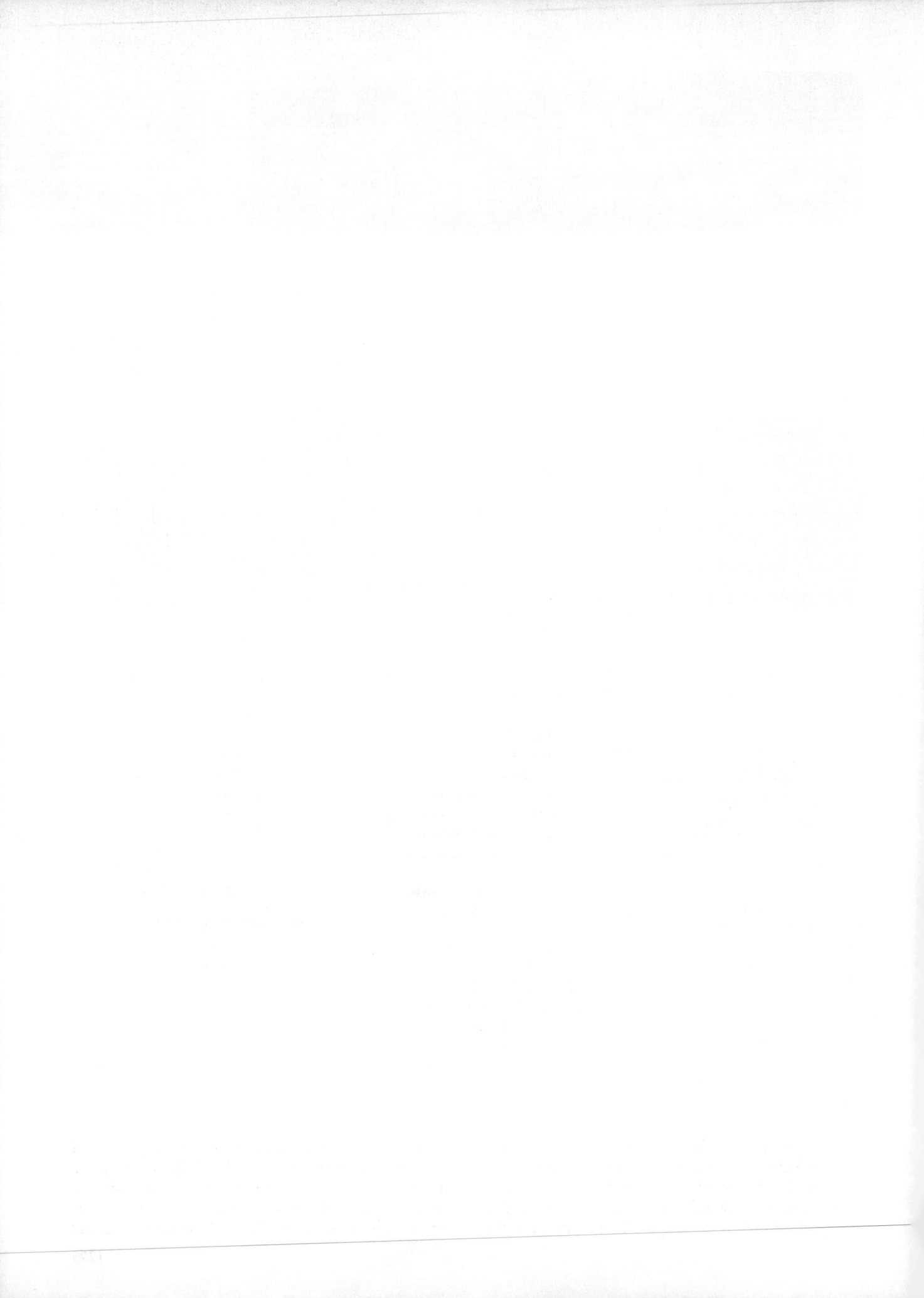

SECTION THREE

Orthotics, Prosthetics, and Seating and Wheeled Mobility

Orthotics

Joan E. Edelstein, PT, MA, FISPO
Christopher Kevin Wong, PT, PhD, OCS

Chapter 30

LEARNING OBJECTIVES

1. Relate the major parts of the shoe to the requirements of individuals fitted with lower-limb orthoses.
2. Compare the characteristics, advantages, and disadvantages of plastics, metals, and other materials used in orthoses.
3. Describe the components of contemporary foot, ankle–foot, knee–ankle–foot, hip–knee–ankle–foot, trunk–hip–knee–ankle–foot, and trunk orthoses.
4. Explain the orthotic options available for patients with paraplegia.
5. Identify the features of lower-limb and trunk orthoses that are considered during the examination process.
6. Outline the physical therapist's role in management of patients fitted with lower-limb and trunk orthoses.
7. Analyze and interpret patient data, formulate realistic goals and outcomes, and develop a plan of care when presented with a clinical case study.

CHAPTER OUTLINE

An orthosis is a device worn to restrict or assist motion or to transfer stress from one area of the body to another. An alternate term is *brace*. A splint is a temporary orthosis. An orthotist is a health care professional who designs, fabricates, and fits orthoses for the limbs and trunk, while a pedorthist is a health care professional who designs, fabricates, and fits shoes and foot orthoses. The term *orthotic* is an adjective. Archaeological evidence confirms that orthoses have been used for at least four thousand years.[1] The term *orthosis* originated in the mid-twentieth century.

This chapter presents the most frequently prescribed orthoses for the lower limb and the trunk, as well as new developments in the field. Essentials for teaching patients to use orthoses are considered. Focus is on orthotic designs and materials, biomechanical rationale, and criteria for evaluating orthotic fit, function, and construction. While every attempt is made to use evidence-based research to guide clinical practice, paucity of research and heterogeneity within the population of orthotic users and within orthotic designs confound this effort.[2]

TERMINOLOGY AND TYPES OF ORTHOSES

Orthoses are named by the joints they encompass and motions controlled. *Foot orthoses* (FOs) are applied to the foot and placed inside or outside a shoe. *Ankle–foot orthoses* (AFOs) encompass a shoe and terminate below the knee. The *knee–ankle–foot orthosis* (KAFO) extends from the shoe to the thigh. A *hip–knee–ankle–foot orthosis* (HKAFO) is a KAFO with a pelvic band that surrounds the lower torso. A *trunk–hip–knee–ankle–foot orthosis* (THKAFO) covers part of the torso and the lower limbs. *Knee orthosis* (KO) and *hip orthosis* (HO) cover their respective joints. *Cervical orthoses* encircle the neck. Most *trunk orthoses* are named by the motions controlled, although orthoses that manage scoliosis usually are named for the city where they were designed.

LOWER-LIMB ORTHOSES

Lower-limb orthoses (LLOs) range from shoes used for clinical purposes to THKAFOs. Characteristics and functions of the principal FOs, AFOs, KAFOs, HKAFOs, and THKAFOs, and trunk and cervical orthoses will be described. Although physical therapists occasionally encounter KOs, HOs, and orthoses for special purposes, such as management of Legg Calve Perthes' disease, they are omitted because they are prescribed infrequently. Similarly, orthoses for the upper limb are absent from this chapter because they are usually worn for a short duration.

Shoes

The shoe is the foundation for most LLOs. Each part of the shoe contributes to the efficacy of orthotic management. Shoes transfer body-weight to the ground and protect the foot from the terrain and the weather. The ideal shoe distributes weight-bearing forces to provide optimum comfort and function of the foot. For the patient with an orthopedic disorder, footwear can serve two additional purposes: (1) reducing pressure on sensitive deformed structures by redistributing force toward pain-free areas and (2) serving as the foundation for AFOs and more extensive bracing. Unless the shoe is correctly fitted and appropriately modified, the alignment of the orthosis will not provide the designed pattern of weight-bearing. Major parts of a shoe are the upper, sole, heel, and reinforcements (Fig. 30.1). These features can be found in dress leather shoes and athletic footwear.

Upper

The *upper* covers the dorsum of the foot. The anterior component of the upper is the *vamp* and the posterior part is the *quarter*. A shoe to be used with an AFO having an insert as its foundation should have a vamp that covers the proximal portion of the dorsum to secure the shoe and the rest of the orthosis onto the foot. In a laced shoe, the vamp contains the *lace stays*, which have eyelets for shoelaces (Fig. 30.2). Laces provide more precise adjustment than do strap closures. The latter, however, enable individuals with limited manual dexterity to manage the shoe more easily. For most orthotic purposes, a *Blucher* (Fig. 30.2A) lace stay is preferable; it is distinguished by the separation between the anterior margins of the lace stays and the vamp. The alternate design is the *Bal*, or *Balmoral*, lace stay (Fig. 30.2B), in which the lace stay is continuous with the vamp. The Blucher opening permits greater adjustability, important especially for the patient with edema. It also offers a large inlet into the shoe. An *extra-depth shoe* is one having an upper contoured with additional vertical space. The shoe is manufactured with a second inner sole that can be worn as is or removed to accommodate a custom insert or a thick surgical dressing. This design provides more

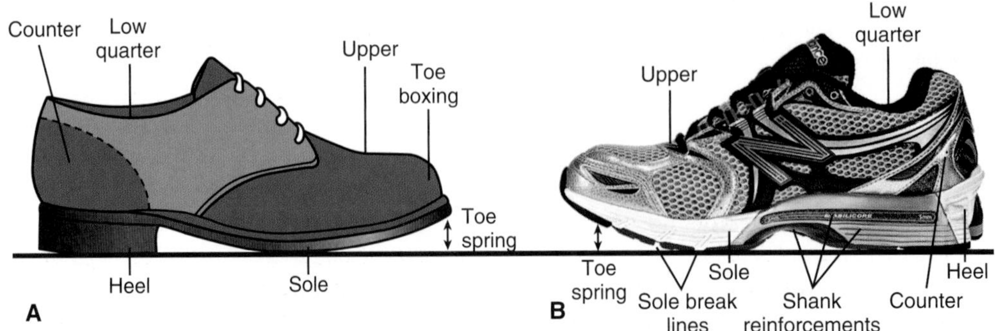

Figure 30.1 (A) Parts of a low quarter with Blucher lace stay. Note that the counter and toe boxing are internal reinforcing structures of the shoe. (B) Parts of a lower quarter athletic shoe.

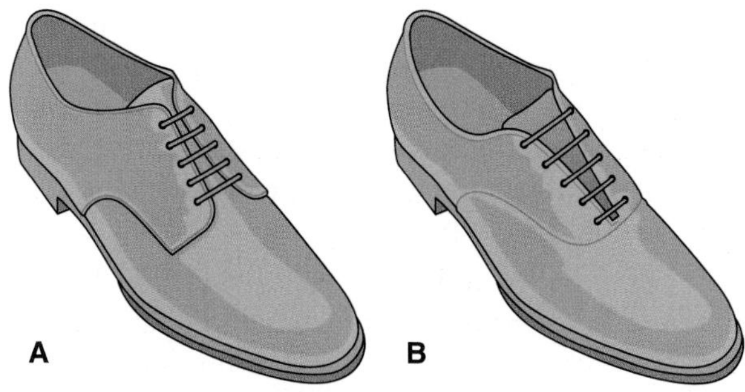

Figure 30.2 Low-quarter shoes: (A) Blucher (open lace) and (B) Bal (Balmoral) (closed lace). The Blucher lace stay is generally preferred for orthotic use owing to ease in donning and adjustability.

space in the shoe, thus reducing stress on the foot. *Quarter* is the posterior portion of the upper. A low quarter terminates below the malleoli and is satisfactory for most clinical purposes. This style does not restrict foot or ankle motion. A high-quarter shoe, covering the malleoli, is indicated to cover the foot having rigid pes equinus. It is also appropriate to augment foot stability in the absence of an AFO. The high-quarter shoe is more difficult to don and more expensive than a comparable low-quarter one. If the patient will be wearing an orthosis molded about the ankle, a high-quarter vamp is superfluous.

Sole

The *sole* is the bottom portion of the shoe. For use with a riveted metal attachment between shoe and orthosis, the sole should have an outer and an inner sole. Between the two lies a metal reinforcement that receives the rivets. This type of shoe, however, is heavier than an athletic shoe with a single sole. The foot rests on the *insole.*

The *outsole* contacts the floor. Leather outsoles absorb little impact shock and provide minimal traction as compared to natural or synthetic rubber ones. To absorb shock, the shoe may have resilient material in the outsole, insole, an insert placed over the insole, or any combination of these. Older people should wear shoes with firm, slip-resistant outsoles to reduce the risk of falling.[3] Regardless of material, the outsole should not contact the floor at the distal end; the slight rise of the sole is known as the *toe spring* (see Fig. 30.1), which allows a rocker effect at late stance.

Heel

The *heel* is the portion of the shoe below the outsole and under the anatomical heel. A broad, low heel provides greatest stability and distributes force between the back and front of the foot most evenly. For adults, a 1-in. (2.5-cm) heel tilts the center of gravity slightly forward to aid transition through stance phase but does not significantly disturb normal knee and hip alignment. A higher heel places the ankle in greater plantarflexion range and forces the tibia forward. The wearer compensates either by retaining slight knee and hip flexion or by extending the knee and exaggerating lumbar lordosis. The high heel transmits more stress to the forefoot and knee.[4] Transferring load anteriorly, however, may be desirable if the patient has heel pain. The higher heel accommodates rigid pes equinus and may[5] or may not[6,7] reduce tension on the Achilles tendon and other posterior structures. Although most heels are made of firm material with a rubber plantar surface, a low resilient heel is indicated to permit slight plantarflexion if the ankle cannot move because of orthotic or anatomical limitation.

Reinforcements

Reinforcements located at strategic points preserve the shape of the shoe. *Toe boxing* in the vamp protects the toes from distal and vertical trauma; it should be high enough to accommodate hammer toes or similar deformity. The *shank* piece is a longitudinal plate that reinforces the sole between the anterior border of the heel and the widest part of the sole at the metatarsal heads (see Fig. 30.1). A corrugated steel shank is necessary if an orthotic attachment is to be riveted to the shoe. The *counter* stiffens the quarter and generally terminates at the anterior border of the heel. The patient with pes valgus, however, should have a shoe with a long, stiff medial counter that provides reinforcement along the medial border of the foot to the head of the first metatarsal, thus resisting the tendency of the foot to collapse medially.

Last

The *last* is the model over which the shoe is made. The last, whether of wood, custom-made plaster, or computer-generated design, remains with the manufacturer; the shoe shape duplicates the last's contour. A given shoe size may be achieved with many lasts, each transmitting different forces to the foot. Consequently, one should ascertain that the shoe fits the foot satisfactorily, rather than relying on a particular shoe size. The patient with a markedly deformed foot requires a shoe made over a special last, either factory- or custom-made.

Foot Orthoses

A foot orthosis (FO) may be an *insert* placed in the shoe, an *internal modification* affixed within the shoe, or an *external modification* attached to the sole or heel. Foot orthoses apply force to the foot, which may enhance function and reduce pain. This may be accomplished by transferring weight-bearing stresses to pressure-tolerant sites, protecting painful areas from contact with the shoe, correcting alignment of a flexible segment, or accommodating a fixed deformity. Modifications can also improve the wearer's transition during stance phase, by altering the rollover point in late stance or by equalizing foot and leg lengths on both limbs. In many instances, a particular therapeutic aim can be achieved by various means.

Internal Modifications

An internal modification is an orthosis inside the shoe. Biomechanically, inserts and internal modifications are identical. Both distribute force on the foot more comfortably. Because internal modifications reduce shoe volume, proper shoe fit must be judged with these components in place. An insert is removable, permitting the patient to transfer it from one shoe to another, if the shoes have the same heel height. Most inserts terminate just posterior to the metatarsal heads to avoid crowding the toes; however, the insert may slip forward, particularly if the shoe has a relatively high heel. Some inserts extend the full length of the sole, preventing slippage but occupying the often-limited space in the anterior portion of the shoe. Internal modifications are fixed to the shoe's interior, guaranteeing the desired placement but limiting the patient to the modified shoes.

Internal modifications made of soft materials, such as rubber or viscoelastic plastics (e.g., Sorbothane and Viscolas), reduce impact shock and shear, thus protecting painful or insensitive feet.[8,9] Inserts can also be constructed of semirigid or rigid plastics and metal, often with a resilient overlay. A heel-spur insert orthosis (Fig. 30.3) slopes anteriorly to reduce load on the painful heel. The orthosis has a concave relief to minimize pressure on the tender area. Depending on the contour and material, insoles can reduce motion at the first metatarsophalangeal joint, resulting in pain reduction.[10-12] FOs may alleviate plantar fasciitis[13-16] and improve balance among older adults.[17,18]

Arch supports are intended to prevent depression of the subtalar joint with flattening of the arch (pes planovalgus, pes planus). An orthosis may include a wedge (post) to alter foot alignment. To provide medial arch support, a resilient *scaphoid pad* (Fig. 30.4) may be positioned at the medial border of the insole with the apex between the sustentaculum tali and the navicular tuberosity. Flexible flat foot can be realigned with a semirigid plastic *University of California Biomechanics Laboratory (UCBL) insert* (Fig. 30.5).[19] It is molded over a plaster model of the foot, taken with the foot in maximum correction. The insert encompasses the heel and midfoot, applying a medial force to the calcaneus, and lateral and upward force to the medial portion of the midfoot. Wearing arch supports is associated with increased activation of the tibialis anterior and peroneus longus.[20] An instrumented insole provides vibrotactile feedback to reduce pes valgus.[21] Children with pes planus may also benefit from wearing longitudinal arch supports, although the evidence is weak.[22]

An insert FO may accommodate pes cavus.[23,24] The top of the insert has a convexity that conforms to the contour of the plantar surface of the patient's foot, thereby increasing the area over which weight-bearing force is applied and reducing the unit pressure.

The *metatarsal pad* (Fig. 30.6) is a convex component that may be incorporated in an insert or may be a resilient domed piece glued to the inner sole so that its apex is under the metatarsal shafts. The pad transfers stress from the metatarsal heads to the metatarsal shafts and thereby reduces plantar pressure.[25-28]

Some modifications are sandwiched between the inner and outer soles; for example, the patient with marked arthritic changes in the forefoot may be more comfortable if the shoe has a steel plate between the soles to eliminate motion at the painful joints. The same effect can be achieved with a rigid insert.

External Modifications

An external modification involves material added to the exterior of the shoe, such as a heel lift. Wearing a shoe with an external modification ensures that the patient has donned a shoe of appropriate design and size. The external modification, however, may erode as the individual walks and is somewhat conspicuous. In addition, the patient is limited to wearing the modified shoe, rather than being able to choose from a wider selection of shoes.

A *cushion heel* made of resilient material absorbs shock at heel contact. Because it provides slight plantarflexion, the cushion heel is indicated when the patient wears an orthosis, which has a rigid ankle. The patient with leg

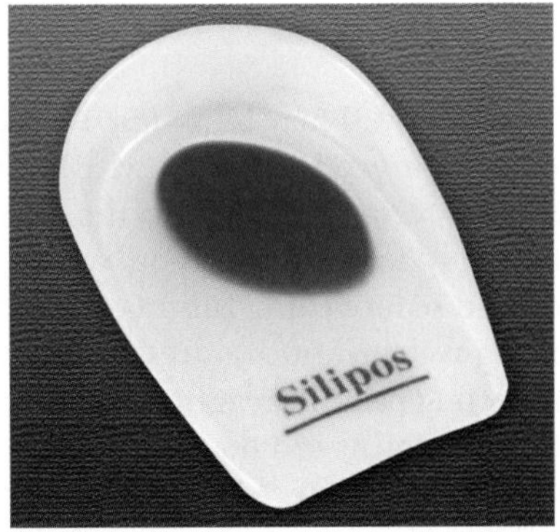

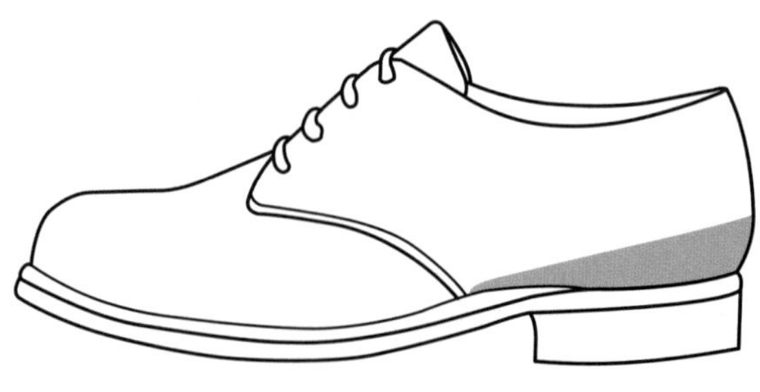

Figure 30.3 (Left) Plastic tapered heel spur cushion with concave relief to reduce pressure. (Right) The shaded area of the shoe on the far right indicates the relative position of the heel spur when placed in a shoe.

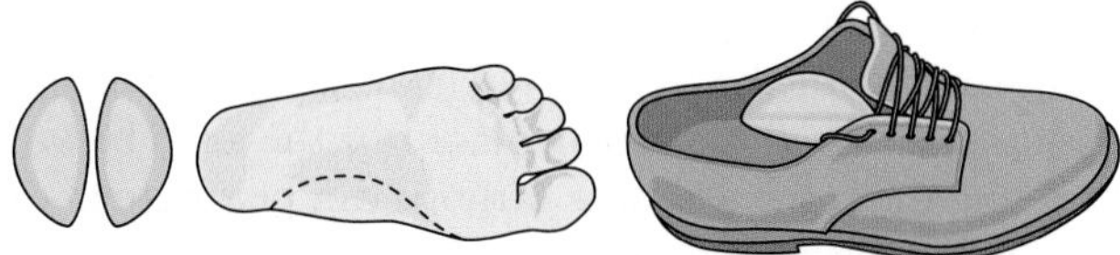

Figure 30.4 Scaphoid pads (left) are available with self-adhesive backing. They are positioned (middle) medial and plantar to the longitudinal arch; scaphoid pad (right) glued to the inside of the shoe.

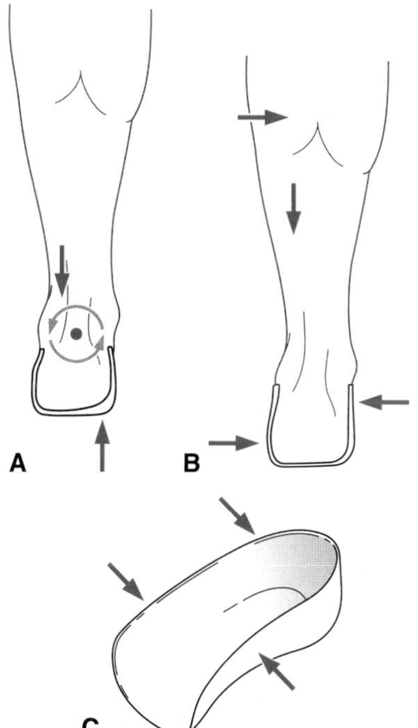

Figure 30.5 University of California Biomechanics Laboratory (UCBL) foot orthosis exerts control at the subtalar joint via a force couple (A) and three-point counterforces to control calcaneal eversion (B). A second counterforce system (C) restricts forefoot abduction. *(From May, BJ and Lockard, MA: In Prosthetics and Orthotics in Clinical Practice. FA Davis, Philadelphia, 2011, page 12, with permission.)*

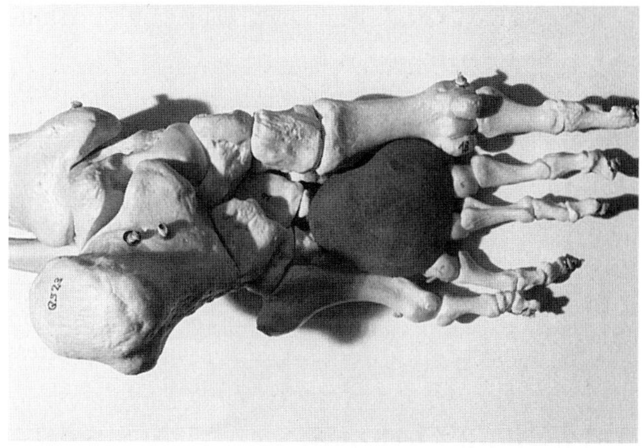

Figure 30.6 Rubber metatarsal pad. Whether used as an internal modification or as part of an insert, the pad should be oriented as shown on the skeletal model.

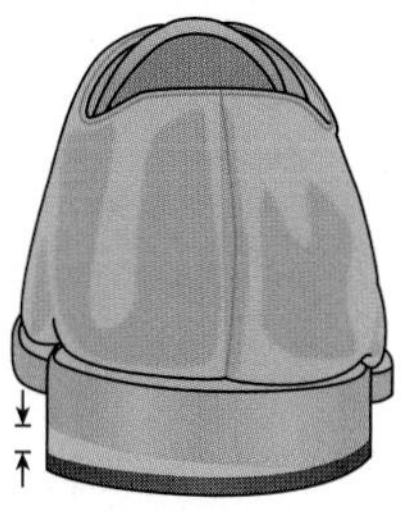

Figure 30.7 Medial heel wedge.

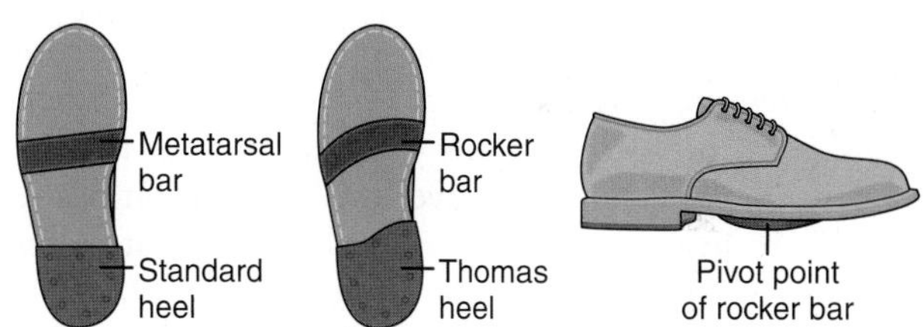

Figure 30.8 (Left) Metatarsal bar and standard heel. (Middle) Rocker bar with a Thomas heel (note the medial extension) and (right) pivot point of rocker bar.

length discrepancy of more than 1/2 in. (1 cm) will walk better with a shoe lift made of cork or other lightweight material. Approximately 1/2 in. (1 cm) of the elevation can be accommodated on the insole at the heel of a low-quarter shoe. If a lift is added to the sole and heel to compensate for greater leg length discrepancy, the distal portion of the lift should be beveled to achieve toe spring.

A *heel wedge* (Fig. 30.7) alters alignment of the rearfoot. A medial heel wedge, by applying laterally directed force, can aid in realigning flexible pes valgus or can accommodate rigid pes varus by filling the void between the sole and the floor on the medial side. A medial wedge is incorporated in a *Thomas heel,* intended for flexible pes valgus (Fig. 30.8). The anterior border of the Thomas heel extends forward on the medial side to augment the effect of the medial wedge in supporting the longitudinal arch.

Sole wedges alter medial–lateral forefoot alignment. A lateral wedge shifts weight-bearing to the medial side of the front of the foot. It compensates for rigid forefoot valgus, allowing the entire forefoot to contact the floor. Sole wedges also influence forces on the entire lower limb.[29,30] Laterally wedged insoles may benefit some individuals with medial knee osteoarthritis;[31-36] FOs may alleviate patellofemoral pain.[37-39]

A *rocker sole* has a marked plantar convexity with the apex posterior to the metatarsophalangeal joints. A *rocker bar* (see Fig. 30.8) is a convex transverse band affixed to the sole proximal to the metatarsal heads. Both the rocker sole and the rocker bar reduce the distance the wearer must travel during stance phase, improving late stance and shifting load from the metatarsal phalangeal (MTP) joints to the metatarsal shafts.[40,41] A *metatarsal bar* (see Fig. 30.8) is a flat strip of firm material placed posterior to the metatarsal heads. At late stance, the bar transfers stress from the metatarsophalangeal joints to the metatarsal shafts.

Patients with diabetic neuropathy benefit from extra depth or custom-made shoes with spacious toe boxing to accommodate toe deformities, such as hammer toe, claw toe, and overlapping toes, and to reduce stress on dorsal lesions. Resilient rocker soles lessen impact stress on the foot as the wearer walks.[42-49]

Ankle–Foot Orthoses

An ankle-foot orthosis (AFO) is composed of a foundation, an ankle control, a foot control, and a superstructure.

Foundation

The foundation of an AFO consists of a shoe and a plastic or metal component.

Insert

An insert foundation, whether plastic, carbon fiber, or less commonly metal (Fig. 30.9), is the portion of the orthosis that contacts the plantar surface of the patient's foot. Most inserts are made of a thermoplastic material, such as polyethylene or polypropylene; they are relatively lightweight. The orthotist creates a plaster model of the patient's foot and leg and then modifies the model, removing plaster in areas where the orthosis is to apply substantial pressure and adding plaster where pressure relief is required. Thermoplastic or carbon fiber is then heated and molded over the modified plaster model. Metal would be hammered over the foot portion of the model. An insert must be worn with a shoe that closes high on the dorsum of the foot to retain the orthosis.

The insert has several advantages. Because it can incorporate internal modifications, the insert provides good control of the foot. This foundation facilitates donning the orthosis because the shoe can be separated from the rest of the brace. When the wearer dons the orthosis, either the insert is placed in the shoe before donning the orthosis or the orthosis can be strapped to the foot and leg; then the braced limb slid into the shoe. The insert permits interchanging shoes, assuming that all shoes have been made on the same last. Less expensive, lighter weight shoes can be worn because the foundation does not need to be riveted to the shoe.

An insert foundation, however, is inappropriate if the patient cannot be relied on to wear the orthosis with a shoe of proper design. If the orthosis were placed in a shoe with too low a heel, the uprights would incline posteriorly, increasing the tendency of the wearer's knee to extend. Conversely, if the orthosis is worn with a higher heeled shoe, the patient might experience knee instability. The insert reduces interior shoe volume, and thus must be used with a suitably spacious shoe. If the orthosis is to be used by a morbidly obese or exceptionally active individual, a plastic footplate may not provide adequate support.

Stirrup

Comparable to a stirrup attached to an equine saddle, an orthotic stirrup is a U-shaped steel fixture, the center portion of which is riveted to the bottom of the shoe through the steel shoe shank. The arms of the stirrup join medial and lateral brace uprights at the level of the anatomical ankle, providing congruency between orthotic and anatomical joints. The *solid stirrup* (Fig. 30.10) is a one-piece attachment that provides maximum stability of the orthosis on the shoe. The *split stirrup* (Fig. 30.11) has three segments. The central portion has a transverse rectangular opening. Medial and lateral angled side pieces fit into each side of the opening. The split stirrup

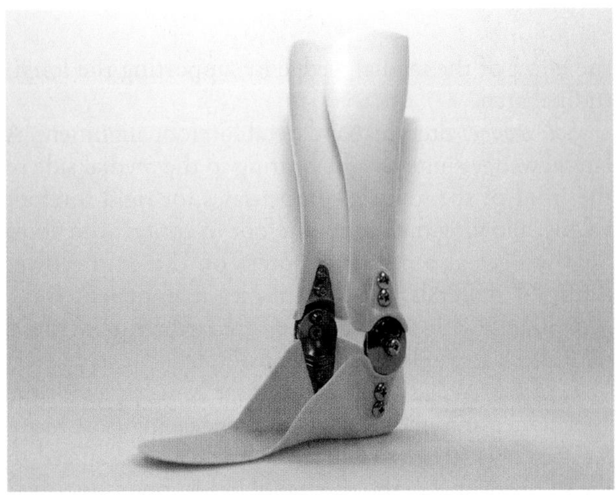

Figure 30.9 Plastic footplate included in a hinged AFO.

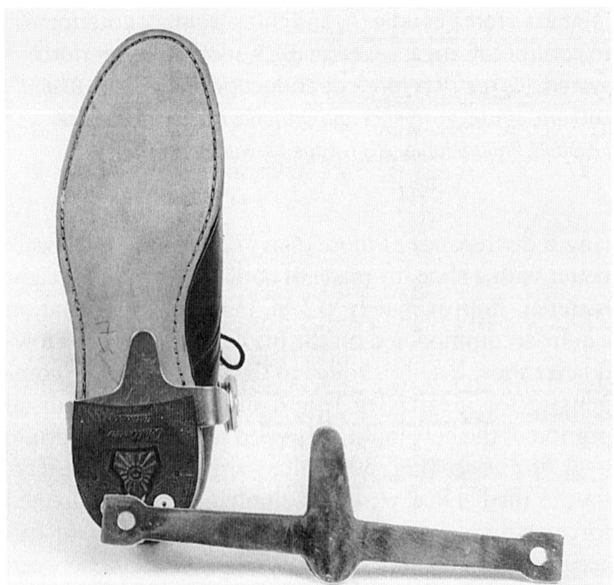

Figure 30.10 Solid stirrup. The stirrup in the foreground is as it comes from the manufacturer before it is fitted to the patient and shoe.

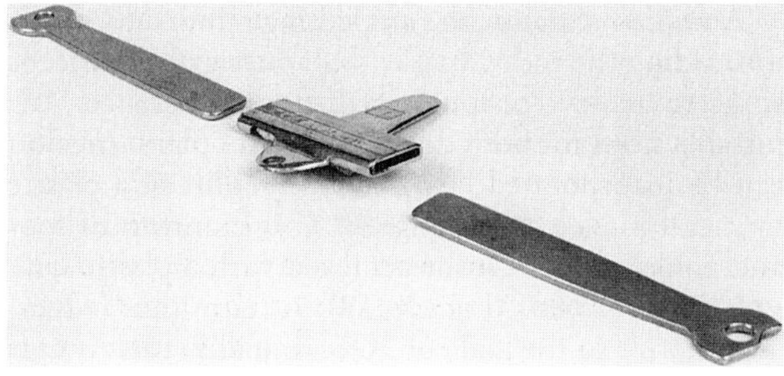

Figure 30.11 Split stirrup.

simplifies donning the orthosis because the wearer can detach the uprights from the shoe. If a central piece is riveted to a second shoe, the shoes can be interchanged using the same uprights. An extremely active client may inadvertently dislodge a sidepiece from its receptacle. Because stirrups are made of steel, they are heavier than plastic insert foundations. The split stirrup is bulkier and heavier than a solid stirrup or footplate.

Ankle Control

Most AFOs are worn to control ankle motion by limiting plantarflexion and/or dorsiflexion, or by assisting motion. Without an orthosis, the patient with dorsiflexor weakness or paralysis risks dragging the forefoot during swing phase. A fabric strap from the ankle to the distal portion of the shoe restricts plantar flexion.[50] An orthotic alternative is a *posterior leaf spring AFO* that arises from a plastic insert (Fig. 30.12). This orthosis can be prefabricated or custom made and is streamlined and lightweight. During early stance, the posterior upright acts as a leaf spring, bending backward slightly. When the patient progresses into swing phase, the upright recoils, "springing" forward to lift the foot. Adjustment of the posterior leaf spring AFO is limited; the orthotist can remove material to weaken the spring but cannot readily add material to increase rigidity of the orthosis.

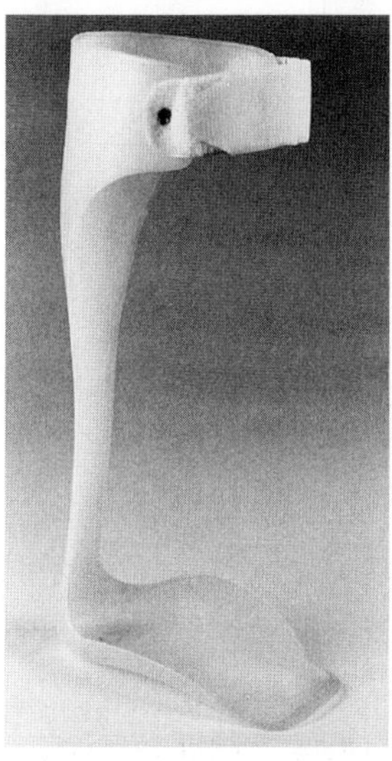

Figure 30.12 Posterior leaf spring AFO.

Adjustable motion assistance can be achieved with a steel dorsiflexion spring assist (Klenzak joint) (Fig. 30.13) incorporated into each stirrup near the ankle. The coiled spring compresses in stance and rebounds during swing. Tightness of the spring can be adjusted by turning a screw on top of the spring. An orthosis with a dorsiflexion spring assist is noticeably bulkier than the posterior leaf spring model. Both dorsiflexion spring assist AFO and the posterior leaf spring orthosis yield slightly into plantarflexion at heel contact, affording the wearer protection against inadvertent knee flexion. Other AFO designs that control toe drag are presented in Figures 30.14 and 30.15.

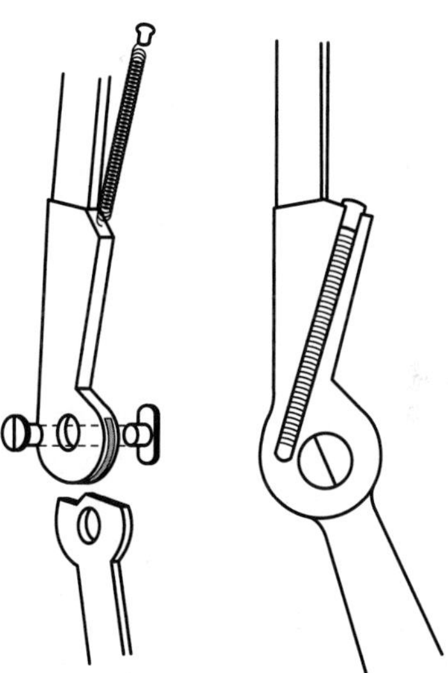

Figure 30.13 Hinged joint with dorsiflexion spring assist.

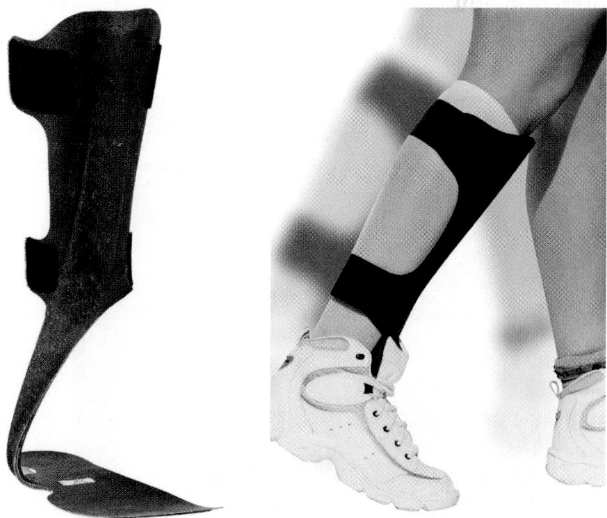

Figure 30.14 ToeOFF® ankle foot orthosis. This fiber glass, carbon fiber, and Kevlar orthosis is designed to provide dorsiflexion assistance in the presence of mild to severe footdrop accompanied by mild to moderate ankle instability. This orthosis is contraindicated in the presence of moderate to severe spasticity or edema. *(Courtesy of CAMP Scandinavia AB. SE 25467 Helsingborg, Sweden.)*

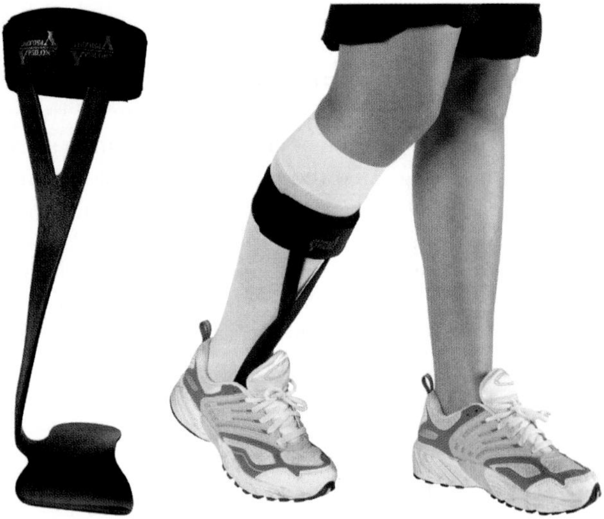

Figure 30.15 Ypsilon^{TM} AFO. This carbon composite AFO is designed to provide dorsiflexion assistance in the presence of mild to moderate isolated drop foot. It promotes free ankle movements (medial, lateral, and rotational). The proximal Y-shape provides tibia crest clearance. This orthosis is contraindicated for an unstable ankle joint or in the presence of moderate to severe spasticity or edema. *(Courtesy of CAMP Scandinavia AB. SE 25467 Helsingborg Sweden.)*

An alternate approach to prevent toe drag is using plantarflexion resistance provided by an AFO with a metal ankle hinge that has a *posterior stop* (Fig. 30.16). The posterior stop prevents toe drag in swing phase and imposes a flexion force at the knee during early stance, preventing the knee from hyperextending.

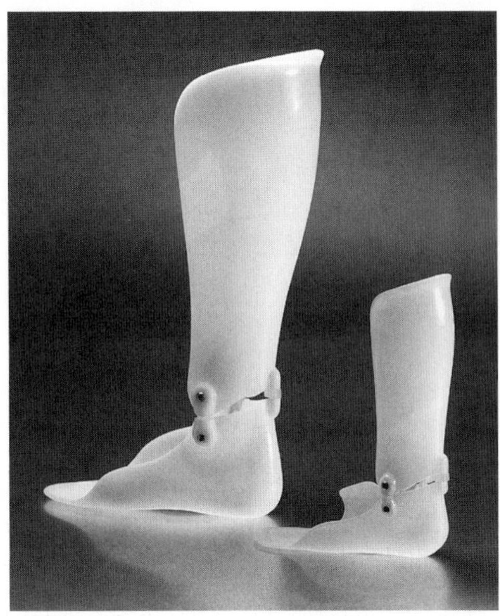

Figure 30.16 Plastic hinged ankle foot orthoses with plantarflexion stops. *(Courtesy of Otto Bock, Minneapolis, MN 55447.)*

An *anterior stop* at the ankle hinge limits dorsiflexion, aiding the individual with paralysis of the triceps surae to achieve propulsion during late stance. Adjustable stops for both dorsiflexion and plantarflexion can be incorporated into the ankle joint of a plastic or metal hinged AFO (Fig. 30.17). Limiting all foot and ankle motion can be achieved with a plastic *solid ankle–foot orthosis* (Fig. 30.18); its trimlines (edges) are anterior to the malleoli. Occasionally, this AFO is divided transversely at the ankle, with the two sections hinged, creating the *hinged ankle–foot orthosis*. It permits slight sagittal motion, facilitating progression to the foot-flat position in early stance. The hinge may have a plastic overlap joint, a flexible plastic rod, or a metal joint.

An alternative to the plastic solid ankle AFO is a metal joint called the *limited motion joint,* which resists both plantarflexion and dorsiflexion. One type of limited motion joint is a pair of *bichannel adjustable ankle locks (BiCAALs)* (Fig. 30.19), each of which has an anterior and

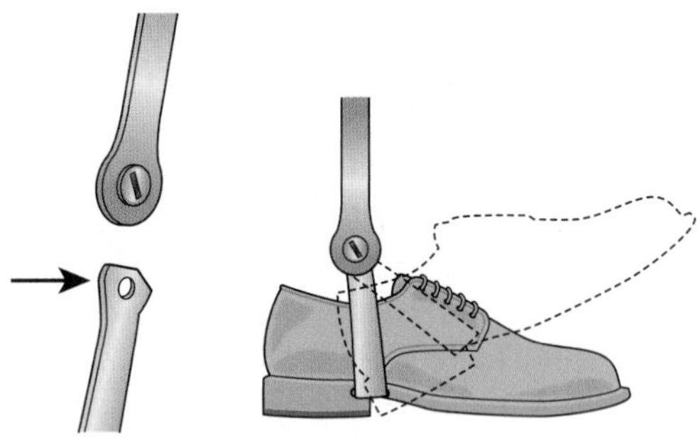

Figure 30.17 Steel stirrup (left) with posterior stop at its distal end (arrow). Posterior stop (right) incorporated into a stirrup. A posterior stop is designed to allow dorsiflexion and prevent or stop plantarflexion.

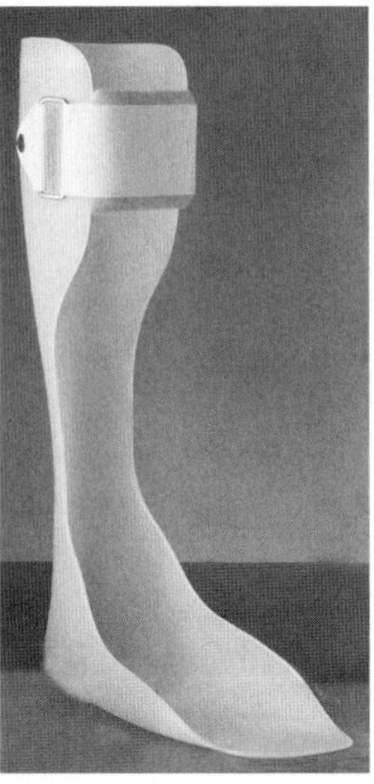

Figure 30.18 Plastic solid AFO. *(Courtesy of Otto Bock, Minneapolis, MN 55447.)*

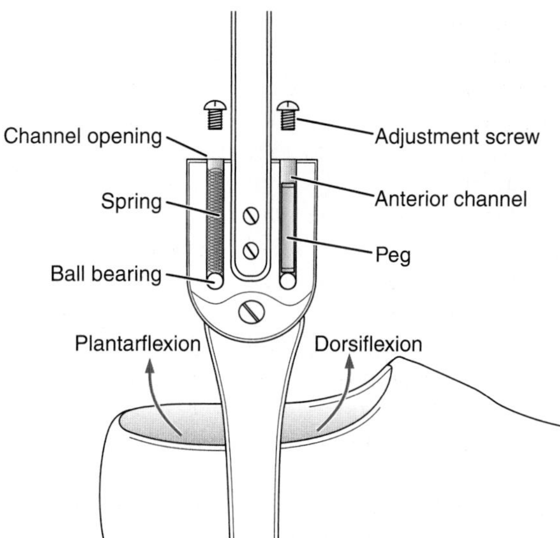

Figure 30.19 Bichannel adjustable ankle locks (BiCAALs). Note this ankle joint includes two channels. A spring placed in the posterior channel (shown) provides dorsiflexion assist. A pin placed in the posterior channel creates plantarflexion stop. *(From May, BJ and Lockard, MA: In Prosthetics and Orthotics in Clinical Practice. FA Davis, Philadelphia, 2011, page 254, with permission.)*

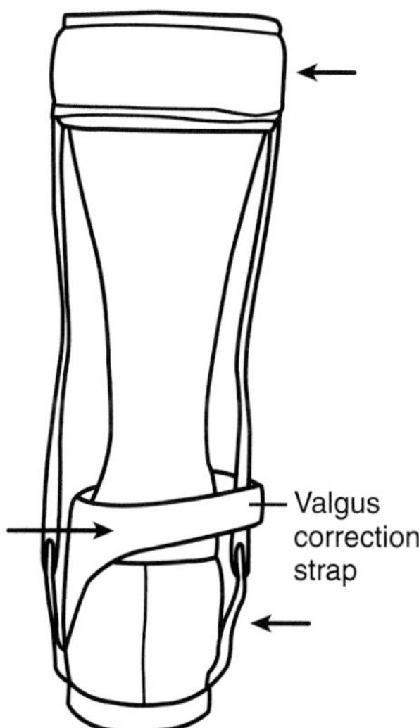

Figure 30.20 Bichannel adjustable ankle locks (BiCAALs) with valgus correction strap (also called a "T-strap").

a posterior spring. Rather than a spring, a metal pin can be inserted in the channel. The length of the pin determines the range of motion provided by the orthosis; a short pin permits slight ankle motion, while a full-length pin blocks all ankle movement. To compensate for lack of plantarflexion in early stance, the shoe worn with the solid AFO or the orthosis with a limited motion stop should have a resilient heel. Similarly, to facilitate rollover in late stance, the shoe sole should have a rocker bar.

Foot Control

The most streamlined way to limit eversion and inversion is with a solid ankle AFO. Its trimlines are anterior to the malleoli. The solid ankle AFO can be divided transversely at the ankle, with the two portions hinged, creating a hinged AFO (see Fig. 30.9). It permits a limited range of sagittal motion, facilitating to the foot-flat position in early stance. The hinges may be overlapping plastic or metal joints. An older alternative is a leather triangular strap; its bottom is attached to the lower portion of the shoe upper, and the top of the strap buckles around the upright of an AFO. A valgus correction version of the strap is buckled around a lateral upright (Fig. 30.20); it applies laterally directed force to the medial malleolus. Tension on the strap is adjustable; nevertheless, the strap complicates donning the orthosis.

Superstructure

Superstructure refers to the portion of the AFO above the ankle and foot components. Plastic AFOs usually have a single upright or shell. The posterior leaf spring AFO (see Fig. 30.12) has a posterior upright that provides leverage for dorsiflexion assistance but does not contribute to frontal or transverse plane control. An AFO with a rigid anterior upright stabilizes the knee. Both the solid ankle and the hinged solid ankle AFOs usually have a posterior shell extending from the anteromedial to the anterolateral midlines of the leg, thus providing excellent medial-lateral control and a broad surface to minimize pressure.

The proximal portion of the plastic AFO consists of a posterior or anterior band, shell, or brim with a strap fastener. The posterior band has an anterior buckled (Fig. 30.21) or pressure closure strap. The farther the

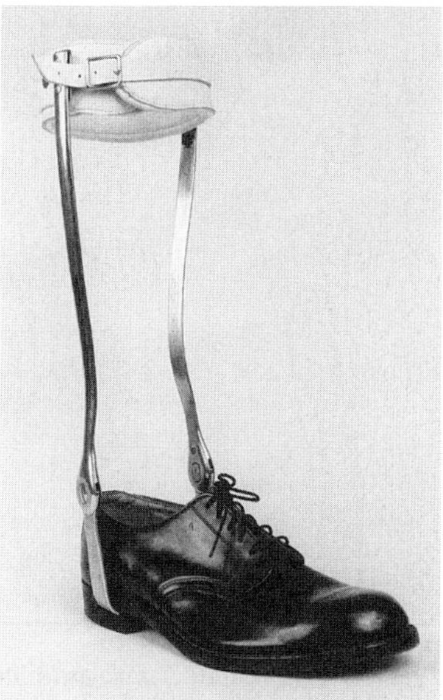

Figure 30.21 Conventional AFO with stirrup attachment, limited motion ankle joints, bilateral uprights, and upholstered metal calf band.

band is from the ankle joint, the more effective the leverage of the orthosis; however, the band must not compress the fibular nerve. An anterior shell that is part of a solid ankle AFO imposes posteriorly directed force near the knee (extension moment), enabling the AFO to resist knee flexion. Such an orthosis is sometimes known as a *floor (ground) reaction orthosis* (Fig. 30.22), although all lower-limb orthoses are influenced by the floor reaction when the wearer stands or is in the stance phase of gait. If the AFO is intended to reduce the amount of weight transmitted through the foot, a *patellar-tendon-bearing brim* (Fig. 30.23) lessens the load on the foot, transferring some force proximally. The brim resembles the upper portion of a transtibial (below-knee) prosthetic socket. It has a slight indentation over the patellar tendon and is hinged to facilitate donning. The brim must be used with a solid ankle or a limited-motion ankle joint to enable force to be transferred proximally.

Metal-leather orthoses usually have bilateral uprights ending in a posterior leather-covered calf band with an anterior strap. Aluminum uprights are lighter in weight than steel. Carbon graphite and titanium uprights weigh appreciably less than aluminum and rival the strength of steel; however, orthoses made of these materials are more expensive. The AFO may have a single upright, either medial or lateral, which reduces the weight of the orthosis and is less conspicuous; however, an AFO with one upright is somewhat less stable. Some AFOs have an anterior upright, which limits plantar flexion and avoids pressure on the Achilles tendon.

Functional electrical stimulation (FES) of the peroneal nerve is an alternative to an AFO for some adults with stroke.[51-57] Commercially available systems incorporate a cuff worn around the proximal leg; the interior of the cuff contains a skin electrode placed over the fibular nerve. A self-contained electrical unit stimulates the electrode. The systems, such as Bioness® L300 (Valencia, CA)[51,55] and Walkaide® (Reno NV),[54] enable dorsiflexion in swing phase, thereby reducing the risk of foot drop and tripping. Comparison of performance of those fitted with FES with others who wore AFOs demonstrated that both groups improved gait speed, although the FES users expressed higher satisfaction.[55-58] Additionally, preliminary experience with implantable peroneal electrode augmenting an AFO is favorable.[59]

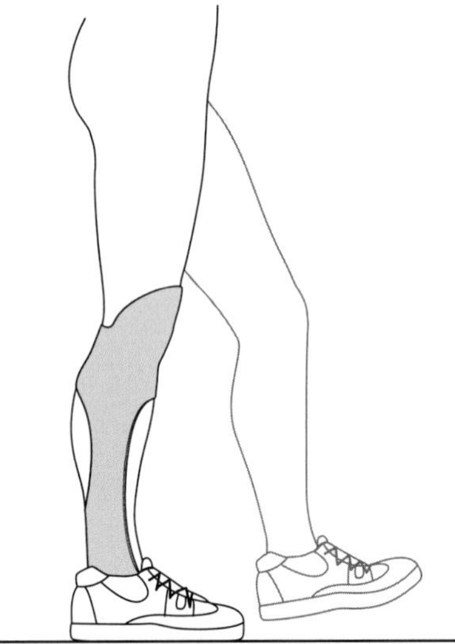

Figure 30.22 Floor reaction AFO with anterior band provides knee extension moment in stance without preventing flexion during swing. *(From May, BJ and Lockard, MA: In Prosthetics and Orthotics in Clinical Practice. FA Davis, Philadelphia, 2011, page 276, with permission.)*

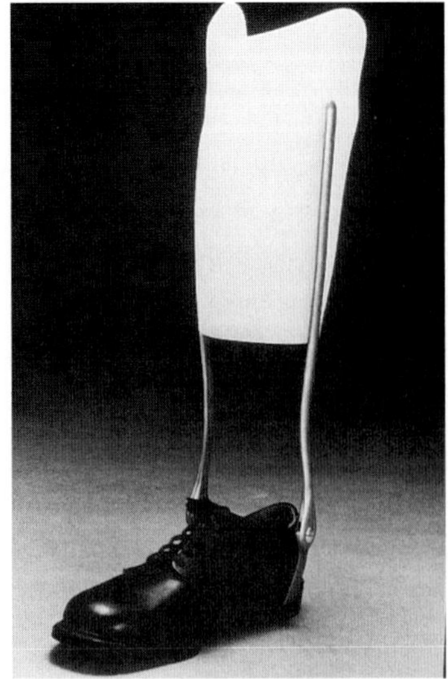

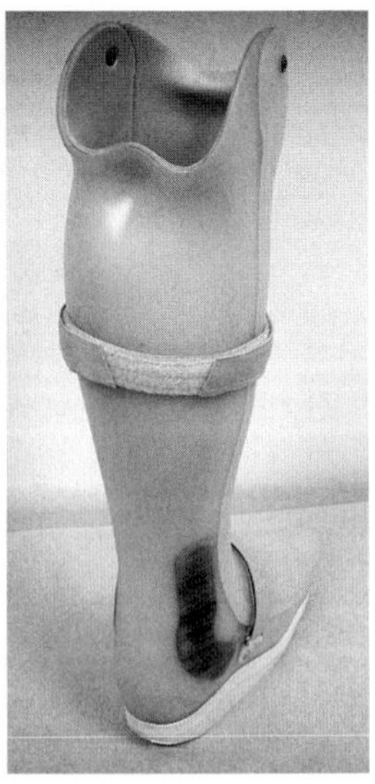

Figure 30.23 (Left) AFO with stirrup, hinged ankle joint, steel uprights, and plastic patellar-tendon-bearing brim. (Right) Plastic AFO with patellar tendon bearing brim to reduce weightbearing on foot. *(Courtesy of Ortho-Bionics Laboratory, South Ozone Park, NY 11420.)*

Clinical Considerations

Adults with hemiplegia realize several benefits when wearing AFOs. Orthoses can prevent or reduce plantar flexor and invertor contractures,[60,61] improve balance,[62-64] and enhance gait by restoring heel contact, absorbing shock on the paretic limb, increasing midstance stability, improving forward progression in late stance, and enabling the paretic limb to clear the floor during swing phase.[65-70] The AFO with posterior ankle stop reduces genu recurvatum.[60] Orthoses with an anterior ankle stop or anterior upright facilitate weight shift to the paretic limb.[66] Patients wearing AFOs increased their velocity[71] and reduced the energy cost of walking.[72,73] They expressed satisfaction with their orthoses, deeming comfort and function more important than the appearance of the device.[74]

Polio survivors with weakness of the calf muscles benefited from walking with an AFO with an anterior ankle stop. They exhibited increased forward progression of the center of pressure in midstance, thereby increasing gait velocity while consuming less oxygen, which contributed to greater endurance. They stated they felt safer when walking with AFOs.[75]

Children with cerebral palsy improved stride length[76] and gait velocity while wearing AFOs.[77] AFOs also increase dorsiflexion during swing phase and overall function.[78] The most favorable results were achieved with hinged AFOs.[79-82] Youngsters who exhibited marked knee flexion when walking performed better when wearing AFOs with a solid ankle with an anterior band (floor reaction orthosis).[83] Orthoses also can reduce abnormal hip rotation.[84] Hinged AFOs lessened energy expenditure more than other AFO designs.[82,85,86] Functional electrical stimulation may benefit some children with spastic hemiplegia as an alternative to an AFO.[87,88] Orthoses also improved the kinematic and kinetic properties of the gait of children with spina bifida[89] with reduced oxygen cost. Those who used forearm crutches with their orthoses obtained the best results. Similarly, boys with Duchenne muscular dystrophy who were still ambulatory walked somewhat faster when wearing AFOs, although they experienced frequent falls.[90]

Knee–Ankle–Foot Orthoses

Individuals with more extensive paralysis/paresis or limb deformity may benefit from KAFOs, which consist of a shoe, foundation, ankle control, foot control, knee control, and superstructure. The shoe, foundation, ankle control, and foot control are selected from components already described above.

Knee Control

Most KAFOs include a medial and a lateral upright plus hinges that provide medial-lateral and hyperextension restriction while permitting knee flexion. The *offset joint* (Fig. 30.24) is a hinge placed posterior to the midline of the leg. When the wearer stands and walks on a level surface, the individual's weight line passes in front of the offset joint, stabilizing the knee in extension during the early stance phase of gait. The offset joint does not hamper knee flexion during swing or sitting. The joint may, however, flex inadvertently when the wearer stands on a ramp.

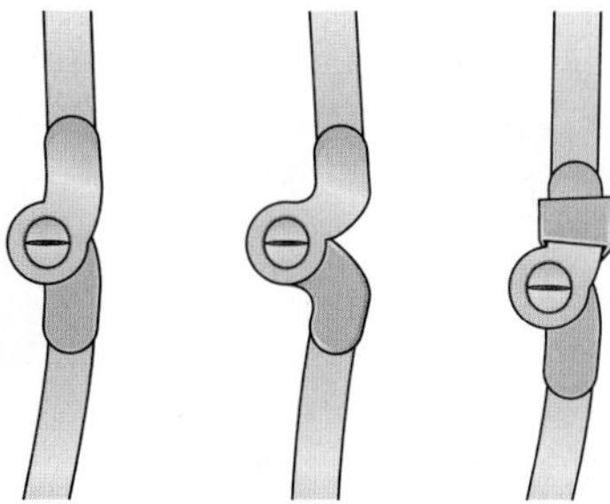

Figure 30.24 Two examples of offset knee joints (left and middle) and a drop ring lock (right).

Knee locks provide security regardless of the terrain. The most common type is the *drop ring lock*. A spring-loaded retention button ensures that the lock will not drop into place while the patient rises from a chair; the user pushes the ring past the button to lock the orthotic knee. For maximum stability, both the medial and lateral knee joints should be locked. A thigh-level release connects the two locks via a cable, enabling the user to control both locks simultaneously. An alternative design, which provides bilateral locking, is the *pawl lock with bail release* (Fig 30.25). Each lock has a projection, which lodges in a V-shaped groove. Springs or elastic webbing bias the locks toward stabilizing the knee; the wearer releases the locks by manually raising the posterior bail, thus overcoming the elastic resistance. The pawl lock with bail release is bulkier than drop ring locks. A *ratchet lock* has a round gear with teeth, and a spring-loaded *pawl* that engages the teeth. Each tooth has a shallow slope on one edge and a steep slope on the other side. As the wearer rises from a seat, the gear permits the orthotic joints to extend. The patient who has poor balance can pause midway in the sit-to-stand maneuver; the pawl presses the steep slope of the gear, stabilizing the bent knee.

The person who has a knee flexion contracture can achieve knee stability with a *fan lock* or a *serrated lock* (Fig 30.26). Both are adjusted to match the angle of maximum knee extension; a drop ring lock secures the uprights. The fan lock has several holes; the clinician places a screw in the hole that angles the orthotic joint to conform to the patient's knee extension. The serrated

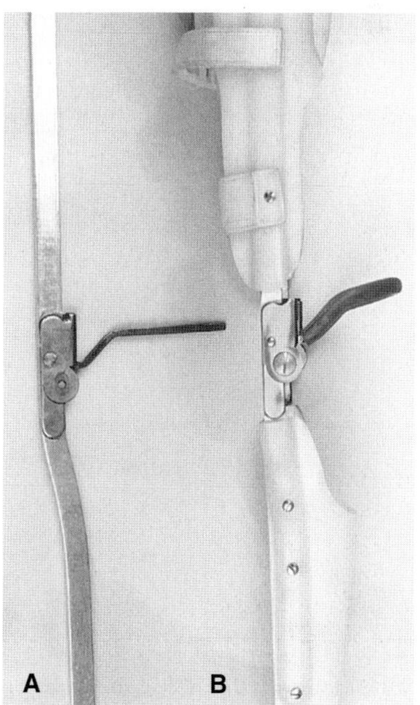

Figure 30.25 Knee joint hinge with pawl lock: (A) basic component and (B) pawl lock installed in KAFO with bail shaped to curve posteriorly.

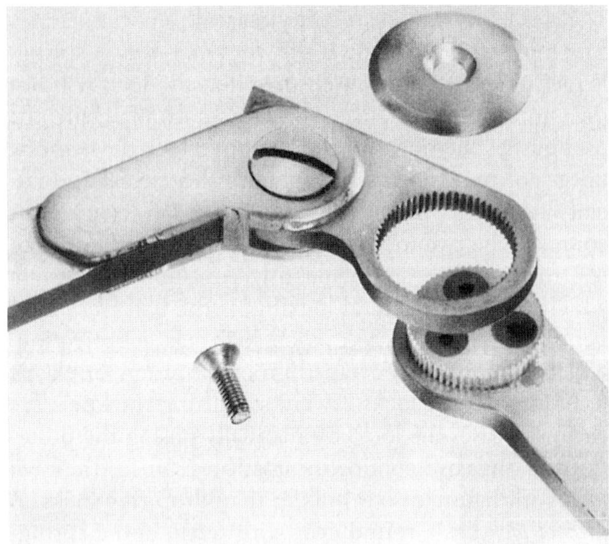

Figure 30.26 Knee joint hinge with serrated knee lock. Note the location of the knee hinge and the serrated disk. *(From Fishman, S, et al: Lower-limb orthoses. In American Academy of Orthopaedic Surgeons: Atlas of Orthotics, ed 2. Mosby, St. Louis, 1985, p. 213, with permission.)*

lock has a circular serrated plate, which fits into a mating receptacle; the plate can be positioned to conform to the desired knee angle.

Sagittal stability is augmented by an anterior band or four-strap leather knee pad that completes the three-point pressure system necessary for stability. These components apply a posteriorly directed force to complement anteriorly directed forces from the calf band and the thigh band. A rigid anterior band, either a pretibial band or a suprapatellar band, provides posteriorly directed force but does not interfere with sitting, and the KAFO is easier to don. The band is molded of plastic and thus not readily adjustable. The prepatellar band rests over the proximal portion of the leg; the suprapatellar band fits over the anterodistal thigh.

Genu valgum or varum may be controlled with a KAFO having a leather knee pad with five straps. Four straps are buckled around the calf and thigh uprights. The fifth strap passes behind the knee and is buckled around the lateral upright to control genu valgum or around the medial upright if the patient has genu varum. A simpler option is an AFO having a plastic calf shell shaped to apply corrective force. To reduce genu valgum, the medial portion of the shell extends proximally to apply laterally directed force at the knee. Extending the lateral portion of the shell controls genu varum. The semirigid shell is more effective than KAFO with a five-strap knee pad. The shell does not require extra time in donning and applies force over a broad area without impinging on the popliteal fossa (Fig 30.27).

The KAFO with a stance control mechanism prevents knee flexion during stance phase yet permits knee flexion during swing phase.[91,92] By moving a lever on the side of the joint, the patient can select the mode of action: (1) stance control, which automatically disengages during swing phase, (2) no stance control, and (3) lock in full extension. As compared with walking with a KAFO with locked knee, wearing an orthosis with stance control permits faster, more symmetrical gait.[93] Stance control, however, does not reduce energy consumption when the wearer walks.[94]

Superstructure

Most KAFOs have medial and lateral uprights terminating in one or two thigh bands, which provide structural stability to the orthosis. If the distal portion of the limb cannot tolerate full weight-bearing, the orthosis must include a weight-bearing brim, a locked knee joint, and a *patten* bottom. The patten is a distal extension that keeps the shoe on the braced side off the floor. To maintain a level pelvis, the patient must wear a lift on the

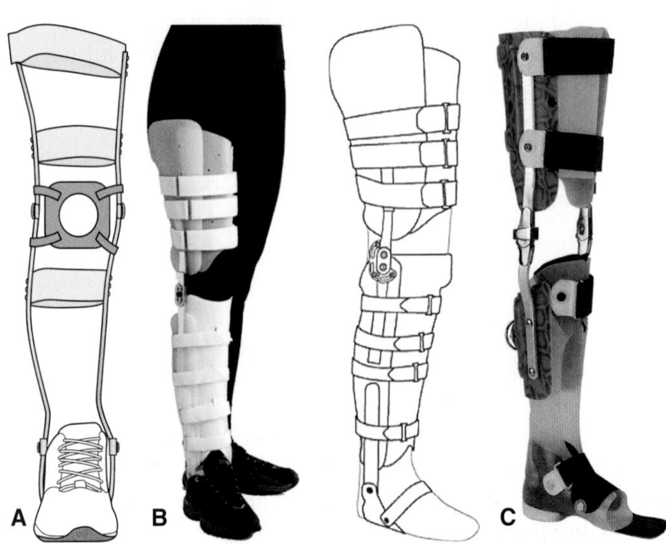

Figure 30.27 (A) Conventional KAFO with knee cap. (B) Plastic KAFO pictured on a subject together with schematic of same orthosis. (C) This orthosis allows conversion between an AFO and KAFO based on patient requirements. The knee component is detachable. *(Courtesy of Orthomerica Products, Orlando, FL 32810.)*

opposite shoe; the height of the lift should equal the height of the patten (Fig. 30.28). An alternative to bilateral proximal uprights is a single posterior upright, which is less restrictive.

Mechanical KAFOS for Paraplegia

Craig-Scott KAFOs (Fig. 30.29) are often prescribed for adults with paraplegia. Each orthosis includes either a plastic solid ankle section or BiCAAL ankle joints set in slight dorsiflexion, a pretibial band, a pawl knee lock with bail release, and a single thigh band. The orthoses enable the patient to stand without crutches by leaning backward; the iliofemoral ligaments restrain excessive lean. Gait require crutches or a walker. The pattern usually is swing-to or swing-through, with the aid of crutches or a walker. Although the orthoses do not restrict hip motion, the patient with thoracic spinal injury cannot flex the hips voluntarily. Some individuals perform a two- or four-point gait by shifting the trunk enough to allow each leg to swing forward in a pendular manner.

The Walkabout™ (Polymedic, Sydney, New South Wales, Australia) consists of a pair of KAFOs with a hinge joining the proximal medial uprights of the two orthoses. The mechanism permits hip flexion and extension but restricts hip abduction, adduction, and rotation. The wearer uses crutches or other aids to permit a two- or four-point gait, which is more stable than swinging gait patterns.

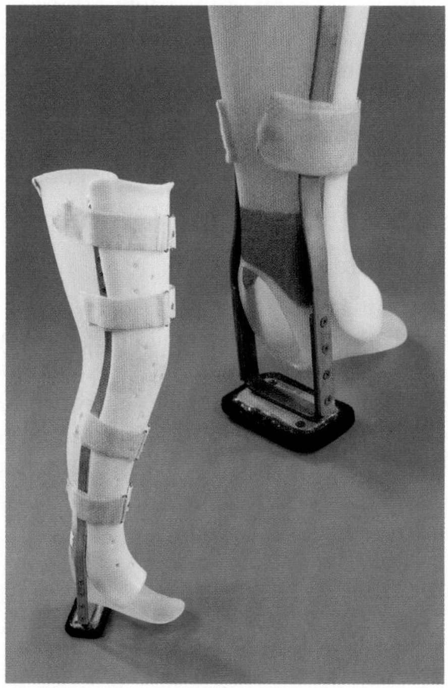

Figure 30.28 The patten bottom is the distal component of an orthosis designed to eliminate weight-bearing from the limb. The patten bottom prevents the foot from contacting the floor.

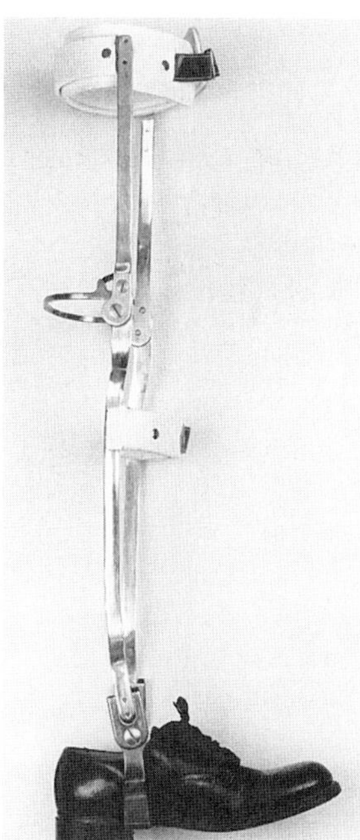

Figure 30.29 Craig-Scott KAFOs.

Clinical Considerations

Some patients with spinal cord injury are fitted with a pair of KAFOs, primarily to obtain the benefits of standing, which assists skeletal,[95] renal, respiratory, circulatory, and gastrointestinal function and affords the individual psychological advantages. Few children with cerebral palsy who were fitted with bilateral KAFOs tolerated KAFOs.[96]

Hip–Knee–Ankle–Foot Orthoses

Addition of a pelvic band and hip joints converts a KAFO to an HKAFO. The orthotic hip joint is a hinge (Fig. 30.30) that connects the lateral upright of the KAFO to a pelvic band. The joint prevents hip abduction, adduction, and rotation. If flexion control is required, a drop ring lock is added to the hip joint. A two-position lock stabilizes the patient in hip extension for standing and walking, and it stabilizes at 90° of hip flexion for sitting. Children who only need control of hip rotation can have a simpler alternative to the hip joint and pelvic band; a webbing strap joins the pair of KAFOs. To reduce internal rotation, the strap resembles a Silesian belt on a prosthesis. The center of the strap is riveted to the rear of a waist belt. Each end of the strap is attached to the proximal end of a lateral upright. To eliminate external rotation, the strap joins the lateral uprights of the KAFOs, passing anteriorly at the level of the groin.

A solid nylon or leather upholstered metal band (Fig. 30.31) anchors the HKAFO to the trunk. The band is designed to lodge between the greater trochanter and the iliac crest bilaterally. HKAFOs are not used very often because they are much more cumbersome to don than KAFOs, and if the hip joints are locked, they

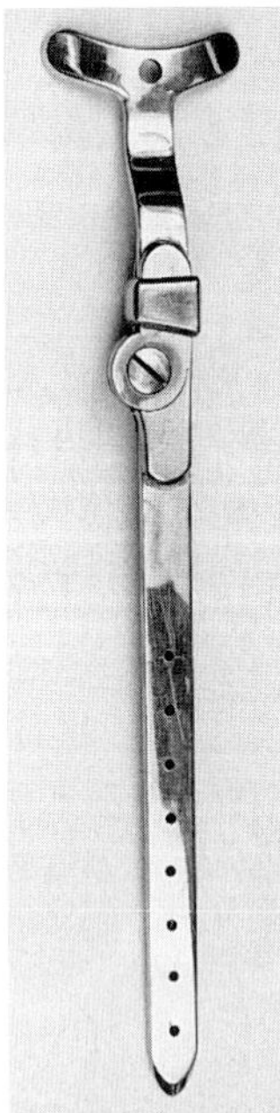

Figure 30.30 Hip joint with drop ring lock.

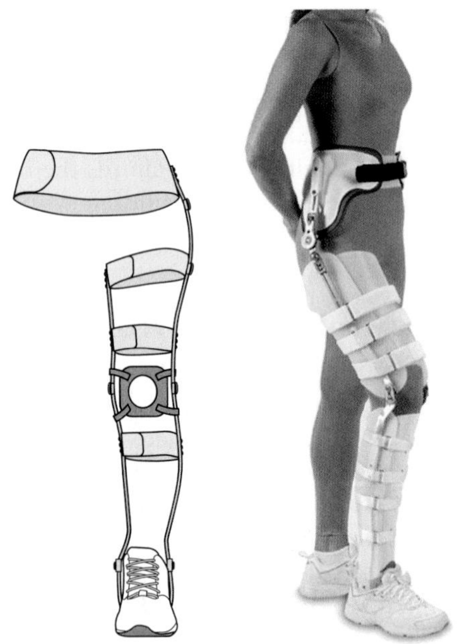

Figure 30.31 (Left) Conventional HKAFO with stirrup; uprights; hinged ankle, knee, and hip joints; drop ring locks at the knee and hip; and pelvic band.

restrict gait to the swing-to or swing-through pattern. The pelvic band fitted when the patient is standing may be uncomfortable when the wearer rotates the pelvis when sitting.

Trunk–Hip–Knee–Ankle–Foot Orthoses

Patients who require more stability than provided by HKAFOs may be fitted with THKAFOs (Fig. 30.32), which incorporate a lumbosacral orthosis attached to KAFOs. The pelvic band of the trunk orthosis serves as the pelvic band used on HKAFOs. Because the THKAFO is very difficult to don and is heavy, it is seldom worn after the client is discharged from the rehabilitation facility. Alternative orthoses provide standing stability, with or without provision for walking.

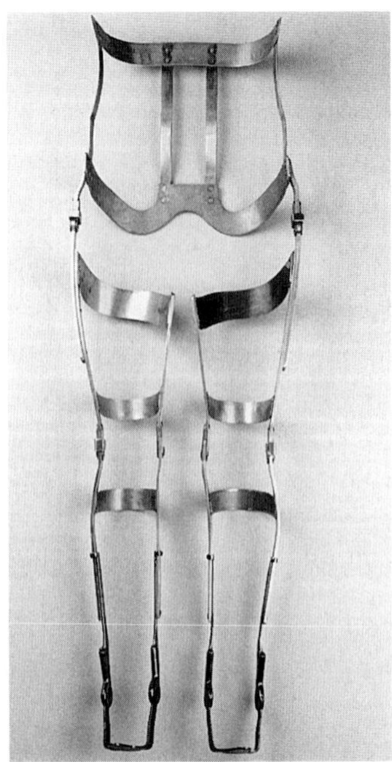

Figure 30.32 Conventional THKAFO without upholstery. This image illustrates the foundational structure of these cumbersome orthoses. To this large heavy metal frame, the additional weight of the upholstery, needed straps and pads, and shoes will be added. Patients once leaving the rehabilitation setting often discard such extensive bracing.

Alternative Lower-Limb Orthoses

Standing Frame

This orthosis (Figs. 30.33 and 30.34) consists of a broad base supporting medial and lateral uprights that end at the anterior chest band. A posterior thoracolumbar band and anterior leg bands contribute to stability. The standing frame is used primarily by young children to foster weight-bearing on the skeleton, avoid contractures, and promote respiratory and urinary health. It enables the child to use the hands for playing.

Parapodium

The *parapodium* (Fig. 30.35) is manufactured in child sizes and differs from the standing frame by virtue of hinges that permit the wearer to unlock knee and hip joints in order to sit. One version of parapodium has a provision for keeping the knees locked while the child unlocks the hips to lean forward to pick objects from the floor. The child can move from place to place by rotating

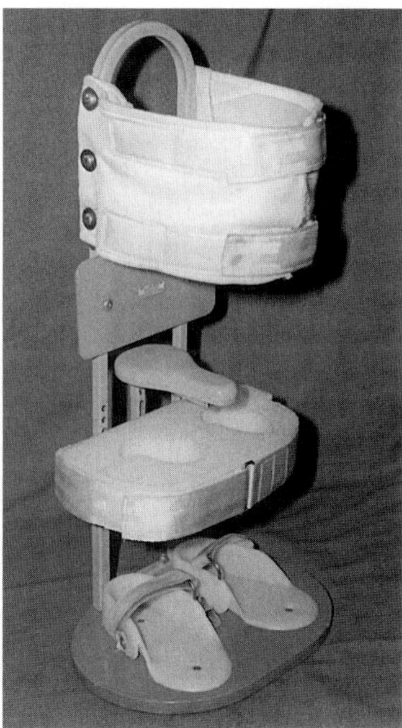

Figure 30.33 Standing frame. *(Courtesy of Variety Village, Electro Limb Production Centre, Scarborough [Toronto], Ontario, Canada.)*

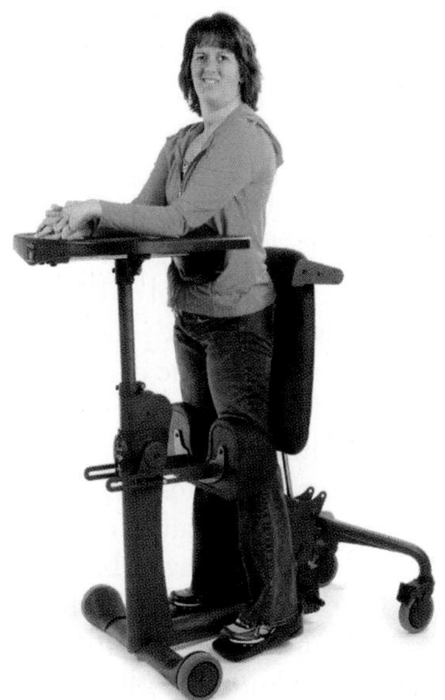

Figure 30.34 Adult standing frame. *(Courtesy of Altimate Medical, Morton, MN 56270.)*

the upper torso to shift weight, causing the frame to rock and rotate alternately on one edge of the base, then the other. For walking longer distances, the child uses crutches or a walker in the swing-to or swing-through pattern. The appliance is worn outside the slacks, which school-age children find cosmetically objectionable.

Stabilizing Boots

Ankle–foot orthoses designed for adults with paraplegia include a pair of custom-made boots (Fig. 30.36), which have flat soles. Inside is a footplate angled at approximately 15°. Plantar flexion shifts the wearer's center of gravity anterior to the knees stabilizing them. Leaning backward tenses the iliofemoral ligaments to stabilize the hips. The boots do not cover the knees or hips and are thus easy to don, lighter in weight, and do not restrict sitting. The patient uses canes, crutches, or a walker to

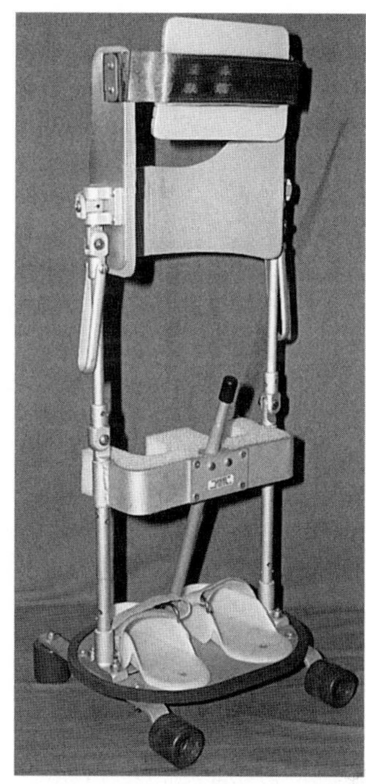

Figure 30.35 Parapodium. *(Courtesy of Variety Village, Electro Limb Production Centre, Scarborough [Toronto], Ontario, Canada.)*

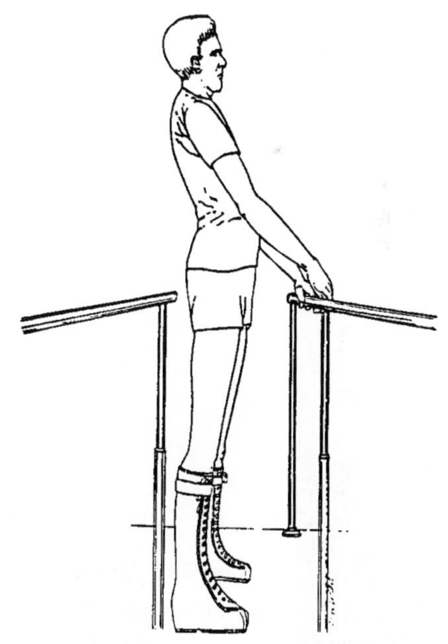

Figure 30.36 Stabilizing boots. *(From Kent,[97] with permission.)*

perform a two- or four-point gait. Ambulation requires shifting the upper torso diagonally forward to allow one leg to swing ahead. Hip or knee flexion contracture contraindicates the boots.[97,98]

Reciprocating Gait Orthoses

Children and adults can be fitted with a *reciprocating gait orthosis (RGO)* (Figs. 30.37 and 30.38). The RGO is a HKAFO with a chest strap. The orthotic hip joints are unlocked and are connected posteriorly by one or two metal cables or a bar. Knees are stabilized with locks, and the feet are encased in solid ankle orthoses. To walk, the wearer follows a four-stage procedure: (1) shift weight to the right, (2) tuck the pelvis by extending the upper trunk, (3) press on the crutches to unweight the left leg, and (4) swing the left leg forward. For the next step, one shifts to the left side, tucks, presses, and then swings the right leg. The cable(s) or bar prevent inadvertent hip flexion on the supporting leg. Reciprocal four- or two-point gait is stable, because one foot is always on the floor. For sitting, the wearer releases the cable(s) to enable both hips to flex. The pace is slow.[99-101] Slight improvement in gait velocity is achieved with rocker soles.[102] Training improved patients' performance to a modest extent.[103] Subjects with paraplegia reported no preference for the reciprocating gait orthosis over a pair of KAFOs with a Walkabout™ proximomedial hinge; they wore the orthoses primarily for standing, rather than ambulation.[104]

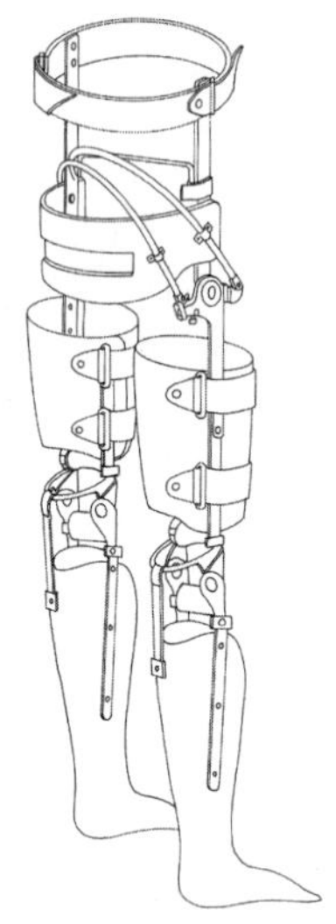

Figure 30.37 Reciprocating gait orthosis. *(Courtesy of Fillauer Companies, Chattanooga, TN 37406.)*

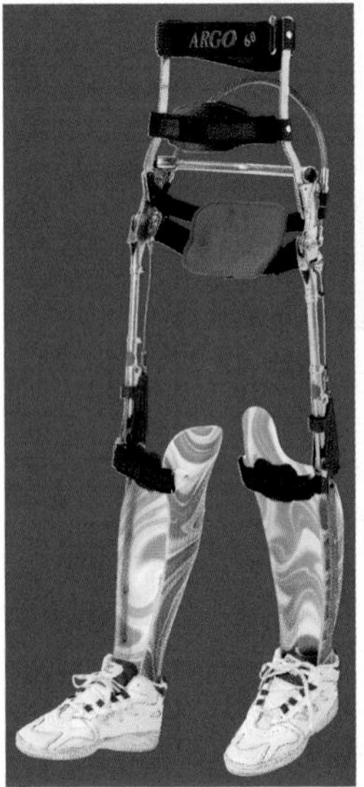

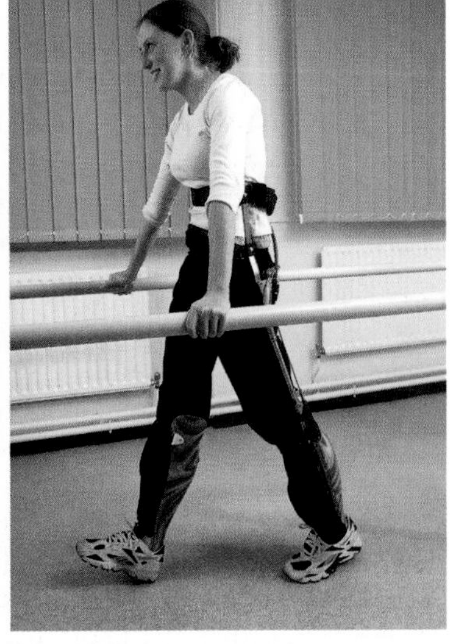

Figure 30.38 ARGO reciprocating gait orthosis. This system includes pneumatic struts at the knee that extend the knees and ensure locks are engaged on standing. *(Courtesy of RSL Steeper, Rochester Kent ME2 4DP, United Kingdom.)*

Electronic Alternatives to Mechanical KAFOs and HKAFOs

The quest to restore functional ambulation for adults with paraplegia and other ambulatory disorders currently focuses on orthoses with electronic, computer-controlled components. The Parastep™ (Sigmedics, Wheeling, IL) combines a pair of AFOs with skin electrodes over the quadriceps and glutei maximus to enable wearers to walk short distances[105] with somewhat higher metabolic cost and greater cardiovascular strain than with nonelectronic components.[106,107]

Prototypes of powered exoskeletons were developed more than 40 years ago.[108] The C-Brace is a microprocessor-controlled KAFO (Otto Bock North America, Austin, TX), suitable for unilateral or bilateral wear.[109,110] Most powered orthoses include leg and foot components, a trunk enclosure, and electronic control. Some systems have a backpack holding a computer; others have a waist pocket. In the clinic the wearer may practice walking with a body-weight support and treadmill system; at home the person usually depends on a pair of crutches or a walker to ambulate.[111] Commercially available examples include Ekso™ (Ekso Bionics Holdings, Richmond, CA);[112] Indego (Parker Hannifin, Mayfield Heights, OH);[113] ReWalk™ (ReWalk Robotics, Marlborough, MA);[114-117] and Lokomat® (Hocoma, Norwell, MA).[118-120] Other robotic exoskeletons are in development, including a powered exoskeleton combined with functional electrical stimulation.[121]

Preliminary reports indicate that adults with paraplegia walked slightly faster when using powered orthoses than when wearing other orthoses,[122,123] although speed remained very modest.[124] Exertion was comparable to light to moderate exercise.[125,126] Some robotic orthoses are intended to be worn by patients who are supported by body-weight support apparatus, walking either on a treadmill or overground.[113] These orthoses are a potential resource for physical and psychological fitness, enabling the benefits of upright weight-bearing and the logistical advantage of maneuvering to places inaccessible to a person in a wheelchair.[127]

Clinical Considerations

Although most experience with powered exoskeletons has been with adults with spinal cord injury, a few children have been fitted successfully.[128] People with hemiparesis can wear a unilateral version of the orthosis.[129-131] Those with multiple sclerosis experienced improved balance, reduced pain and fatigue, and a better quality of life.[132]

Current research consists primarily of short-term studies of patients using powered exoskeletons under laboratory conditions. Although these orthoses show promise, much improvement is required before they become a widespread option for people with spinal cord injury. Velocity is similar to that of a manually powered wheelchair.[133]

Candidates for electronic orthoses are those with ankle, knee, and hip mobility within normal limits. Other requirements include access to a rehabilitation facility for specialized gait training and financial resources to cover the increased expense of these devices. For community ambulation, sufficient upper limb control and overall stamina to manage crutches or a walker are essential. The weight and bulk of powered exoskeletons may not be acceptable to some individuals. Instruction in the care of the orthosis is mandatory. The patient needs a means of obtaining periodic and emergency maintenance of the electronic and mechanical components. Most important, the potential wearer should demonstrate a keen desire to augment wheelchair use with independent ambulation. Consequently, clinicians must assess the degree to which a prospective device will enable the patient to accomplish the desired goals and activities, while fitting with the person's lifestyle.[134]

TRUNK ORTHOSES

Trunk orthoses are sometimes combined with lower-limb orthoses or may be worn alone to reduce disabilities caused by low-back pain, neck sprain, scoliosis, or other skeletal or neuromuscular disorders. By supporting the trunk, the orthosis assists in controlling spinal motion; however, forces that the orthosis exerts are modified by the skin, subcutaneous tissue, and musculature that surround the vertebral column, and, in the case of higher orthoses, by the thoracic cage.

Corsets

If abdominal compression is the sole goal, a corset (Fig. 30.39) will suffice. This fabric orthosis has no horizontal rigid structures, although many have vertical reinforcements. The corset may cover only the lumbar and sacral regions, or may extend superiorly as a thoracolumbosacral corset. The primary effect of a corset is to increase intraabdominal pressure, although the orthosis inhibits trunk movement.

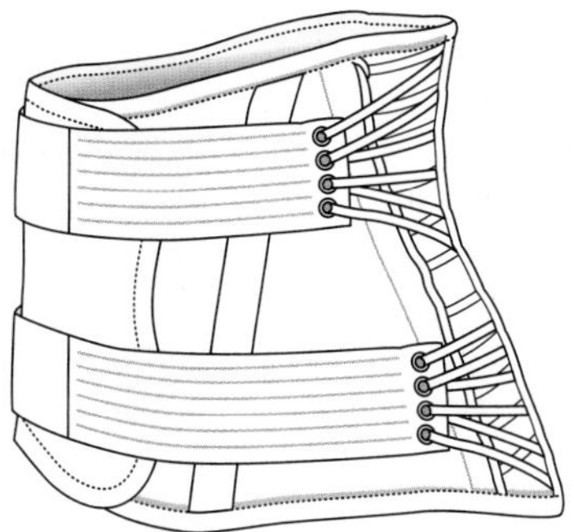

Figure 30.39 Lumbosacral corset (cotton/elastic polymer) with front hook and loop closure.

Some individuals with low back disorders find that corsets relieve pain.[135,136] The efficacy of orthotic intervention to reduce or prevent low back pain remains controversial.[137,138] The increase in intraabdominal pressure reduces stress on posterior spinal musculature, thus diminishing the load on the lumbar intervertebral disks. Although temporary reduction of abdominal and erector spinae muscular activity is therapeutic, long-term reliance on a corset may promote muscular atrophy and contracture, as well as psychological dependence on the appliance.

Lumbosacral and Thoracolumbosacral Orthoses

Most lumbosacral and thoracolumbosacral orthoses include a corset or a fabric abdominal front to compress the abdomen. Rigid orthoses are distinguished by the presence of horizontal and vertical rigid plastic or metal components. Motion limitation is accomplished by a series of three-point pressure systems, in which force in one direction is bracketed by two counteracting forces in the opposite direction.

Lumbosacral Flexion, Extension, Lateral Control Orthoses

A typical example of a rigid trunk orthosis is the *lumbosacral flexion, extension, lateral control (LS FEL) orthosis* (Fig. 30.40), also known as a *Knight spinal orthosis.* This appliance includes a pelvic band, which should provide firm anchorage over the midsection of the buttocks, and a thoracic band, intended to lie horizontally over the lower thorax without impinging on the scapulae. The bands, which may be foam-lined rigid plastic or leather-upholstered metal, are joined by a pair of posterior uprights on either side of the vertebral spines, and a pair of lateral uprights placed at the right and left lateral midlines of the torso. A corset or abdominal front completes the LS FEL orthosis. The orthosis restrains flexion by a three-point system consisting of posteriorly directed force from the top and bottom of the abdominal front or corset and an anteriorly directed force from the midportion of the posterior uprights. Extension is controlled

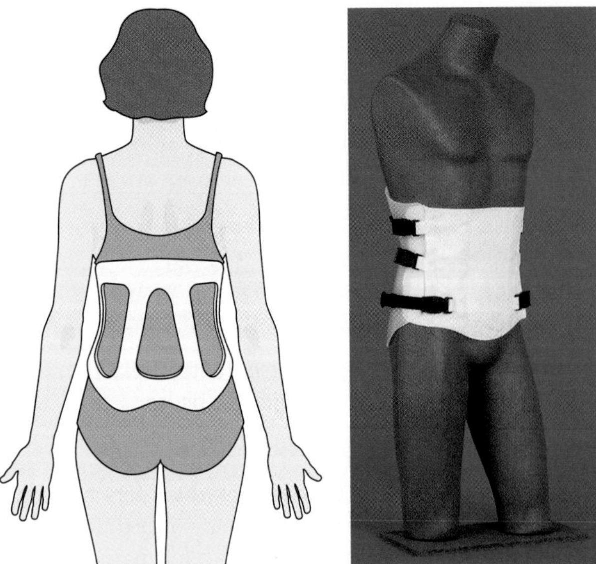

Figure 30.40 (Left) Conventional lumbosacral flexion–extension–lateral (LS FEL) control orthosis. (Right) Custom fabricated plastic LS FEL control orthosis with corset front. *(Courtesy of Orthomerica Products, Orlando, FL 32810.)*

by posteriorly directed force from the midsection of the abdominal front or corset and anteriorly directed force from the thoracic and pelvic bands. The lateral uprights resist lateral flexion. Other rigid lumbosacral (LS) orthoses are made entirely of polyethylene with removable replaceable liners (Fig. 30.41). A plastic LS jacket restricts motion in all directions.

Lumbosacral orthoses limit trunk motion,[139,140] which may alleviate low back pain. Corsets and rigid orthoses appear to produce similar results in treatment of compression fractures.[141]

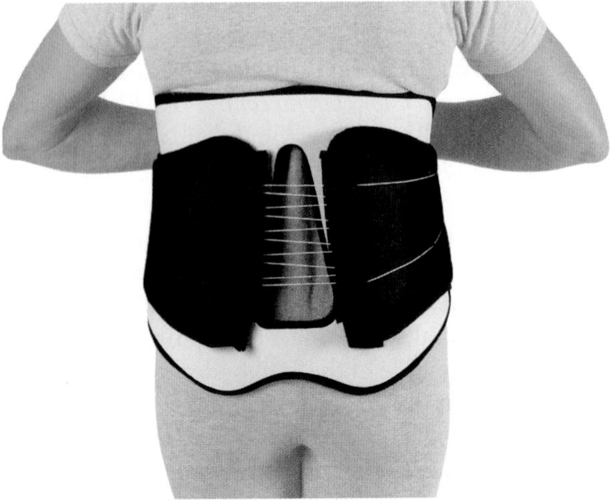

Figure 30.41 Prefabricated adjustable lumbosacral flexion–extension–lateral control orthosis. *(Courtesy of Orthomerica Products, Orlando, FL 32810.)*

Orthoses appear to be a primary treatment for athletes and active children.[142,143] The principal effect may be that orthoses act as proprioceptive reminders to the wearer to limit motion.[144] Lumbosacral orthoses do not appear to cause muscle weakness.[145,146]

Thoracolumbosacral Flexion, Extension Control Orthoses

Also called a *Taylor brace,* the *thoracolumbosacral flexion, extension control (TLS FE) orthosis* consists of a pelvic band, posterior uprights terminating at midscapular level, an abdominal front or corset, and axillary straps attached to an interscapular band. This orthosis reduces flexion by a three-point system consisting of posteriorly directed force from the axillary straps and the bottom of the abdominal front or corset, and anteriorly directed force from the midportion of the posterior uprights. Extension resistance is provided by posteriorly directed force from the midsection of the abdominal front or corset and anteriorly directed force from the pelvic and interscapular bands. Addition of lateral uprights converts the orthosis to a TLS FEL *Knight Taylor* orthosis (Fig. 30.42). A plastic *thoracolumbosacral jacket* limits trunk motion in the frontal, sagittal, and transverse planes providing maximum support. The *thoracolumbosacral flexion control (TLS F) orthosis* is a rigid frame that has sternal and suprapubic plates in front and a dorsolumbar plate; the orthosis limits flexion but permits other trunk motions.

Long-term follow-up of patients with thoracolumbar burst fractures indicates that those who were fitted with an orthosis had at least as good outcomes as patients treated surgically.[147,148] Other case reviews suggest that patients with stable fractures had similar results whether or not they wore braces.[149,150]

■ CERVICAL ORTHOSES

Cervical orthoses are classified according to design characteristics. Minimal motion control is provided by collars (Fig. 30.43) that encircle the neck with fabric, resilient foam, or rigid plastic. Soft and rigid collars appear to have similar functional effects, likely resulting from the proprioceptive stimulus.[151,152] Some patients with cervical radiculopathy benefited from short-term management with a collar,[153] while others had comparable results without orthotic use.[154] The *Philadelphia collar* (Fig. 30.44) has mandibular and occipital extensions and a rigid anterior strut.

For moderate control, a *post orthosis* is used. A two-post orthosis has an anterior adjustable post joining a sternal plate to a mandibular plate and a posterior upright connecting a thoracic plate to an occipital plate. The sternal plate is strapped to the thoracic plate and the occipital plate is strapped to the mandibular plate. This orthosis limits cervical flexion and extension. A four-post orthosis has two anterior and two posterior posts; in addition to flexion and extension control, it limits neck lateral flexion

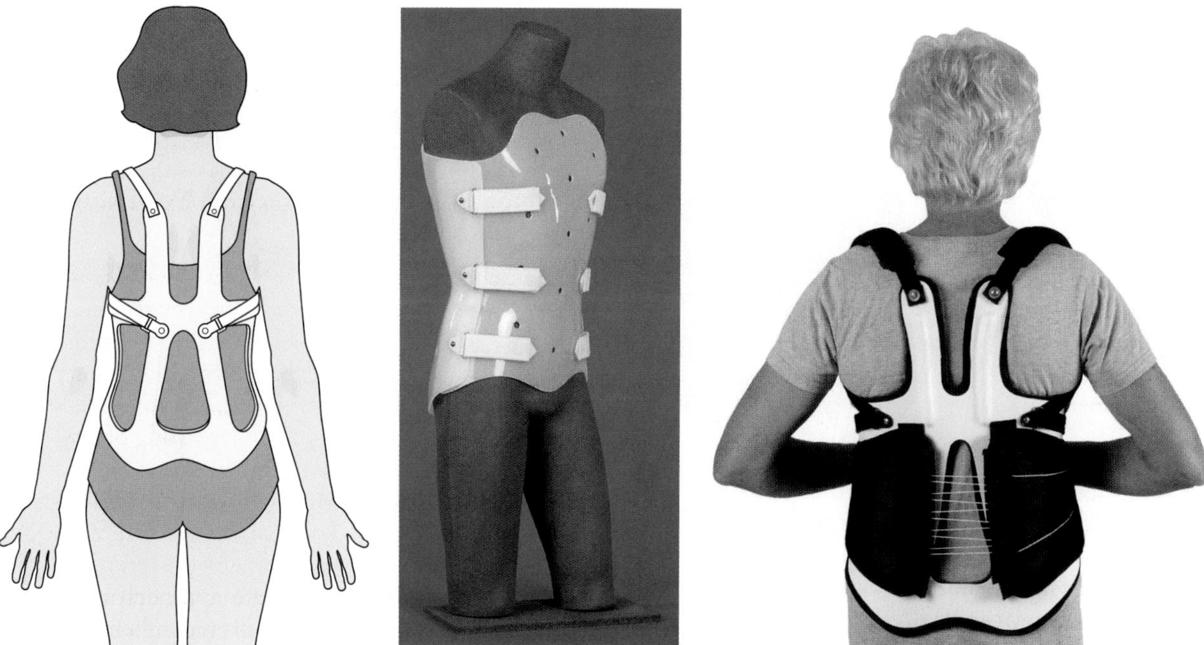

Figure 30.42 (Left) Conventional thoracolumbar flexion, extension, lateral control orthosis (TLS FEL). (Middle) Custom fabricated plastic TLS FEL. (Right) Prefabricated, adjustable TLS FEL. *(Courtesy of Orthomerica Products, Orlando, FL 32810.)*

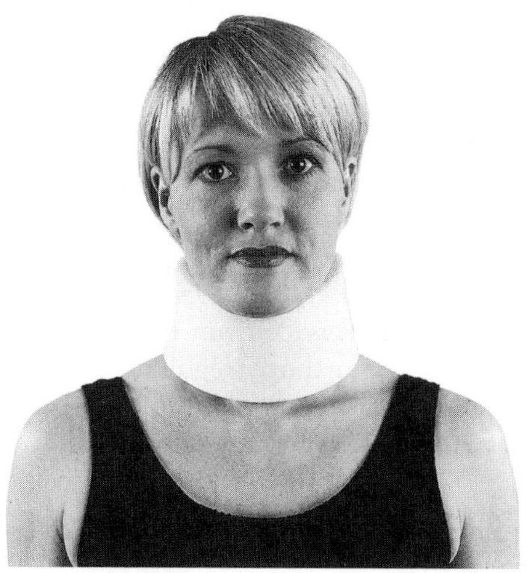

Figure 30.43 Soft foam rubber collar. *(Courtesy of Camp Healthcare Corporation, Jackson, MI 49204.)*

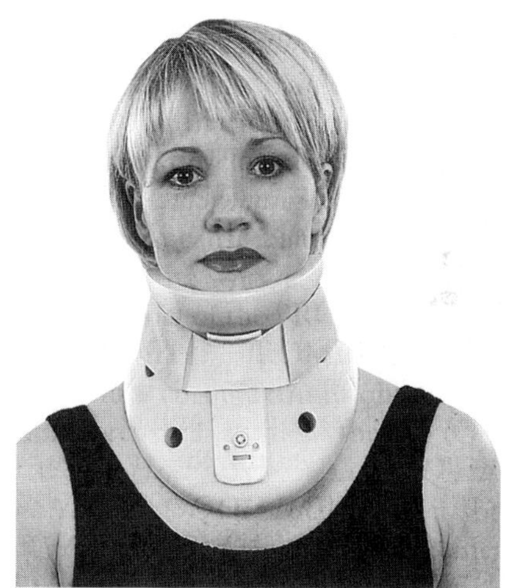

Figure 30.44 Philadelphia collar. *(Courtesy of Camp Healthcare Corporation, Jackson, MI 49204.)*

and rotation. The *sternal occipital mandibular immobilizer* restricts neck flexion; this orthosis can be applied to the recumbent patient without turning the individual's head and neck.

Maximum orthotic control of the neck may be achieved either with a *Minerva* or a *halo orthosis* (Fig. 30.45). The Minerva orthosis is a noninvasive appliance that has a rigid plastic posterior section extending from the head to the midtrunk; the superior portion is held in place by a forehead band. The halo orthosis has a circular band of metal that is fixed to the skull by four screws. Uprights connect the halo to a thoracic vest. The halo orthosis is the most restrictive neck brace.[155] When the wearer walks, the minimal bony stress may foster fracture healing.[156]

SCOLIOSIS ORTHOSES

Children and adolescents with idiopathic scoliosis or hyperkyphosis may be fitted with a TLSO that applies distraction, derotation, and bending forces to realign the vertebral column and thoracic cage. Numerous orthotic designs are in current use. Most are intended to be worn

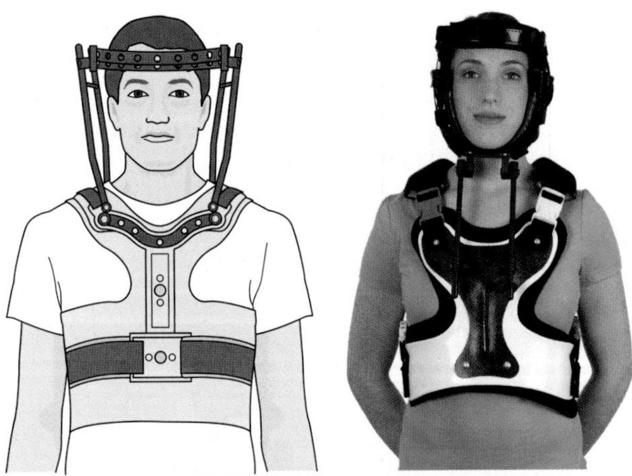

Figure 30.45 (Left) The halo cervical orthosis provides maximum stabilization of the head and cervical spine. The graphite ring (halo) allows placement of titanium pins into the outer skull. (Right) Noninvasive halo devices are also available. They can be used as transitional bracing after removal of the invasive halo cervical orthosis. *(Courtesy of Trulife USA, Jackson, MI 49203.)*

for 18 to 23 hours per day for several years until the patient reaches skeletal maturity. The Milwaukee brace (Fig. 30.46), introduced in 1946, is still prescribed. Its frame is composed of a pelvic girdle, two posterior uprights, an anterior upright, and a superior ring that lies on the upper chest and can be hidden by most clothing. Pads are strapped to the interior of the frame to apply corrective forces.[157] The Boston orthosis, dating from 1972 (Fig. 30.47), usually does not extend as high as the Milwaukee orthosis; its foundation is a mass-produced plastic module that the orthotist alters to fit the individual patient. The effectiveness of the orthosis is enhanced by interior pads.[158] Another option is the Rigo Cheneau brace, a custom molded plastic TLSO. Its selective openings over the concavities of the curves reduce the bulk of the orthosis.[159,160]

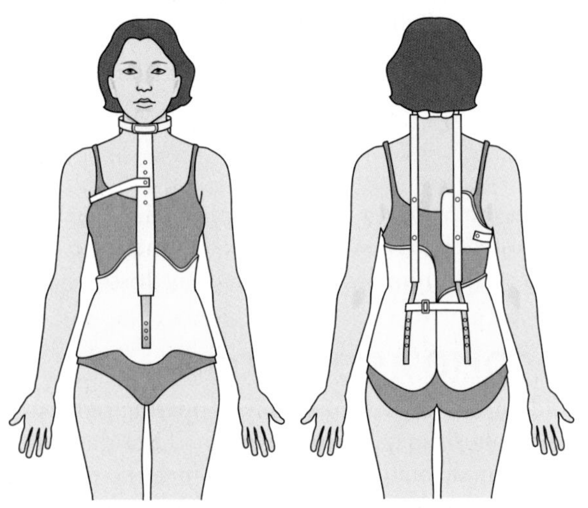

Figure 30.46 Milwaukee plastic and metal orthosis.

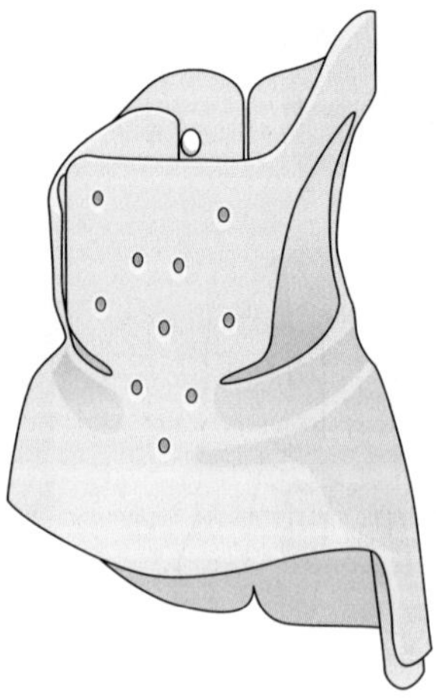

Figure 30.47 Boston thoracolumbosacral orthosis.

Night bracing is an alternate approach to scoliosis management. When the patient is recumbent, the effect of gravity is minimized, allowing substantial corrective forces to be applied. Both the Charleston bending brace (patented in 1987) and the Providence brace (developed in 1992)[161,162] provide overcorrection of the spinal curve.

Brace effectiveness depends on skeletal immaturity, trunk flexibility, curve less than 35°,[163] snug contact of the orthosis with the torso and compliance with the wearing protocol.[164] Long-term follow-up of patients fitted with the various scoliosis orthoses indicates that all of them retard curve progression, although patients with larger curves usually proceed to surgical correction.[165,166]

ORTHOTIC MAINTENANCE

To obtain the best service from orthoses, the patient should inspect the orthosis regularly and care for it promptly. Written instructions reinforce the recommendations of the orthotist and therapist.

Shoes

Whether or not the shoe is attached directly to the orthosis, footwear should be kept in good condition, with replacement of the sole and heel as soon as moderate wear is evident. Replacements should include whatever wedges, bars, or elevations were originally prescribed. The patient who tends to strike on the toe may need a metal toe plate. Shoes that are outgrown or distorted will not afford the wearer optimal function from the orthosis. If a stirrup is attached to the shoe, the patient should inspect the rivets to make certain that none has separated; if so, the shoe should be returned to the orthotist for repair.

Absorbent fabric should be worn next to the skin to reduce pressure from bands, uprights, shells, and any pads on the interior of the orthosis. Cloth absorbs perspiration, which can damage leather components and the fastenings on the orthosis. Foot orthoses should be worn over clean socks without holes or mends. Long socks are essential for AFOs and higher lower-limb orthoses. Soft fabric, such as a T-shirt, is needed when the patient wears a trunk orthosis.

Shells, Bands, and Straps

Plastic bands and shells should be wiped with a damp cloth to remove any surface soil. It is inadvisable to try to hasten drying by using a hair dryer or other heat source that might soften the plastic. The patient should check the plastic periodically for any cracking; if any is noted, the orthosis should be brought to the orthotist for immediate repair. Hook and pile closure straps eventually become infiltrated with lint, which interferes with the hook and loop closing action; the straps should be inspected to determine if they should be replaced. Leather bands require periodic cleaning and can be washed with mild saddle soap. If the original leather deteriorates to the point that portions of the underlying metal are exposed, new leatherwork is required. Leather straps eventually become brittle and may break. A loss of flexibility indicates that it is time to replace the straps, before they break.

Uprights

In a plastic and metal KAFO for a growing child, the metal upright is screwed or riveted to the plastic shell. The orthosis can be lengthened by removing the fasteners and inserting them in new holes drilled farther up on the calf shell and farther down on the thigh shell. In a metal and leather AFO or KAFO for a child, the uprights are overlapped and secured with screws. The orthosis is lengthened by removing all screws, setting the uprights at the appropriate distance, and reinserting the screws.

Joints and Locks

Metal components should be kept away from sand, liquids, and similar substances. If the joints do not move smoothly or become noisy or if the locks do not engage properly, cleaning and lubrication may remedy the problem. Otherwise, professional attention is required.

PHYSICAL THERAPY MANAGEMENT

Physical therapists participate in managing the wearer of an orthosis (1) prior to orthotic prescription, (2) at orthotic prescription, (3) upon delivery of the orthosis, and (4) during training and instruction to facilitate proper use and care of the orthosis. In the ideal situation, the therapist is a member of an orthotic clinic team, working directly with the physician and orthotist to develop the orthotic prescription and examine the patient and orthosis before and after training. The physical therapist is also responsible for training the patient before the orthosis is fitted and after it arrives. Whether or not the hospital or rehabilitation center has a clinic team, the physical therapist is expected to accomplish the following: preorthotic examination, orthotic prescription, orthotic examination and evaluation, facilitating orthotic acceptance, orthotic instruction and training, and final examination and follow-up care.

Preorthotic Examination

Matching the patient's biomechanical requirement to the appropriate orthosis requires careful examination of the prospective wearer. The therapist should contribute to the orthotic prescription by considering the relative potential of various orthotic options to lessen impairment, activity limitation, or disability.

Joint Mobility

A thorough goniometric examination, including both active and passive range of motion (ROM), is a prerequisite to orthotic prescription. If the patient has a fixed foot deformity, either the shoe will have to be modified to accommodate the foot or an insert will have to be fabricated. In either instance, the goal is to achieve comfortable contact of the entire plantar surface of the foot on the inner sole of the shoe. Knee flexion contracture necessitates prescription of accommodative joints, because the regular drop ring and pawl locks can be used only with a knee that can be brought to the fully extended position. Hip flexion contracture precludes the prescription of orthoses that depend on alignment for stability, such as the offset knee joint, stabilizing boots, or Craig-Scott KAFOs.

Limb Length

The therapist should ascertain whether leg lengths are equal. If the patient can stand, one can check the pelvis to determine if it is level. For the recumbent individual, one can measure each LE from the anterior superior iliac spine to the medial malleolus. A difference of more than 1/2 in. (1 cm) should be compensated by a shoe elevation. For the patient with weakness in one limb, a 1/2-in. (1-cm) lift on the contralateral shoe will aid clearance of the involved LE during swing phase.

Muscle Function

The manual muscle test (MMT) should be augmented by an examination of functional activities to determine what substitutions the patient makes to accomplish standing and walking. Although the muscle test may reveal marked weakness, if the patient can manage without an orthosis, it is unlikely that it will be accepted. For example, the person with dorsiflexor weakness who can ambulate by exaggerating hip flexion during swing phase may not agree to an AFO with a posterior stop. An important consideration in examination of muscle function is that traditional MMTs may be inappropriate in the presence of marked spasticity. In such instances, functional tests of motor performance are essential.

Sensation

The clinician should record the extent of any sensory loss (see Chapter 3 Examination of Sensory Function). Intimately fitted plastic orthoses are satisfactory for individuals with sensory loss if the edges (trimlines) of the orthosis are smooth and the orthosis does not pinch the patient's flesh. Proprioceptive loss may indicate the need for orthotic stabilization, such as a solid ankle AFO to control a Charcot neuropathic ankle. Patients should be taught to inspect the skin (including presence of volume changes) regularly and instructed to alert the physical therapist to any changes.

Upper Extremities

Although the patient is being considered as a candidate for a lower limb or trunk orthoses, the therapist must also determine the mobility and muscle power of the upper limbs. Significant weakness, stiffness, or deformity will interfere with donning the orthosis. Substitution of hook and pile closures for buckles or laces may suffice. If the individual cannot ambulate without canes or crutches, the therapist should determine whether standard aids will be satisfactory or if modification of the hand pieces is required. If the upper limbs are too weak to use an ambulatory assistive device effectively, the patient will not be able to use the orthoses for walking. Alternate standing arrangements may be preferable, such as a standing frame, standing table, or standing wheelchair to provide weightbearing stress.

Psychological Status

Realistic orthotic prescription requires ascertaining that the patient is willing to wear the orthosis. The patient with a recent spinal cord injury may still deny the permanence of paralysis and thus oppose wearing orthoses that are visible reminders of disability. The adolescent with spina bifida may prefer to sit unbraced in a wheelchair rather than struggle with donning orthoses and walking slowly, in a manner very different from the individual's peers. Patients must be prepared to work vigorously to increase upper limb and trunk strength and aerobic capacity. The person who has sustained a cerebral vascular accident resulting in severe perceptual deficits may not be able to walk, even with orthotic assistance, because the environment now seems unfamiliar. An orthosis for prevention of contractures may be prescribed, rather than one that is designed to aid gait.

The therapist should determine the extent to which the patient is likely to comply with instructions pertaining to orthotic use and care. For example, if it is doubtful that the individual will wear appropriate shoes with an insert orthosis, then the prescription should specify stirrup attachment to suitable shoes.

Orthotic Prescription

Lower-limb orthoses benefit individuals with a wide variety of musculoskeletal and neurological disorders. The particular diagnosis is less important in formulating the prescription than consideration of the patient's impairments and activity limitations. Prognosis also influences prescription. The person who is likely to recover partial or full function should have an orthosis that can be adjusted to accommodate the changing status. An individual with recent hemiplegia, for example, may exhibit marked spasticity and weakness, indicating a need for limiting motion at the ankle. As the person regains voluntary control and strength improves, the orthotic ankle joint can be adjusted to permit more movement.

Lifestyle has a bearing on orthotic selection. A very active patient requires an orthosis made of exceptionally sturdy materials. Split stirrups, for example, may not be appropriate because they can spring loose from the receptacle on the shoe if excessive medial–lateral or rotational stress is applied. The patient's concern with appearance is another practical consideration; it may dictate use of a shoe insert so that reasonably fashionable shoes may be worn. Similarly, plastic shells are less bulky than metal uprights and calf bands and do not have a shiny metal appearance. Although most people want the orthosis to be as inconspicuous as possible, some children and adults opt for bright colors, which can be achieved with various plastics.

Ankle–Foot Orthoses

The primary candidates for AFOs are those with peripheral neuropathy, especially fibular lesions, and patients with hemiplegia. Those with foot drag can be fitted with an AFO with a posterior stop; this design, however, tends to cause the knee to flex excessively in early stance when controlled plantarflexion is normally achieved. In the absence of plantarflexion, the patient may flex the knee to effect a foot-flat position. The alternative is a resilient shoe heel or an AFO with a plastic posterior leaf spring or a metal dorsiflexion spring assist, both of which permit controlled plantarflexion early in stance to reduce knee stress.

Orthotic management of a patient with hemiplegia depends on the extent of spasticity and paralysis. If the motor loss is confined to poor dorsiflexion, the posterior leaf spring AFO suffices. An even simpler and less expensive option is a 1/2-in. (1-cm) lift on the heel and sole of the contralateral shoe to provide clearance for the more involved limb during swing phase. Those with medial–lateral and sagittal plane instability require an AFO with limited-motion ankle joints. With pain or severe instability, a solid ankle AFO is required. In the presence of severe spasticity, a spring assist for joint motion is contraindicated because the spring action may serve to increase spasticity.

Knee–Ankle–Foot and Other Lower-Limb Orthoses

A KAFO may compensate for dysfunction of the entire lower limb. The physical therapist should allow the patient the use a temporary orthosis in order to proceed more confidently with prescription of an expensive, custom-made orthosis. Several versions of temporary orthoses are manufactured and prove useful to demonstrate whether the patient is likely to benefit from orthotic control.

Trunk Orthoses

A corset may be adequate to increase intraabdominal pressure and thereby may reduce the discomfort of low back pain. Where greater motion restriction is indicated, such as for the individual with trunk paralysis, a rigid lumbosacral or thoracolumbosacral orthosis is appropriate. Selection of cervical orthosis depends on the extent of motion control needed.

Orthotic Examination and Evaluation

Orthotic examination and evaluation are essential elements of management. The therapist should examine the orthosis through analysis of (1) effects and benefits in terms of improved function, (2) practicality and ease of use and maintenance, (3) fit and alignment, and (4) safety during use of the device. It is imperative to determine whether the orthosis functions properly before attempting to instruct the patient to use it. Analysis may be conducted under the aegis of a formal orthotic clinic team. If so, when the orthosis is delivered, the team should determine the adequacy of the orthosis as pass, provisional pass, or fail. *Pass* indicates that the orthosis is altogether satisfactory and the patient is ready for instruction and training. *Provisional pass* means that minor faults exist, generally having to do with the cosmetic finishing of the appliance; the patient can wear the orthosis in the instructional training program without harmful effect. *Failure* signifies that the orthosis has a major defect that would interfere with training—for example, shoes that are too tight. The problem must be resolved before training can begin. If the orthosis is not prescribed by a clinic team, then the therapist should use the evaluation procedure to assure that the orthosis meets the patient's needs. Final evaluation is performed at the conclusion of training to judge whether the orthosis continues to fit and function properly and the patient's skill in using it.

Lower-Limb Orthotic Static and Dynamic Examination

Examination involves both a static and dynamic component. *Static examination* is conducted with the orthosis on the patient while standing and sitting, as well as examination of the device off the individual. *Dynamic examination* refers to analysis during movement, specifically during gait and sit-to-stand transitions.

Static Examination

The orthosis is inspected as the wearer stands and sits. The patient's skin and the construction of the orthosis are checked with the orthosis off the patient. The orthosis should be compared with the prescription. The individual(s) who approved the prescription must approve departures from the original specifications.

The patient should stand in parallel bars or other secure environment and be encouraged to bear equal weight on both feet. The shoe should fit satisfactorily, particularly in length, width, and snugness of the counter. Whether or not wedges or lifts have been added to the shoe, the sole and heel should rest flat on the floor, except for the distal portion, which should curve upward slightly (toe spring) to aid in late stance. The orthotic ankle joint should be at the distal tip of the medial malleolus to be congruent with the anatomical ankle and avoid vertical motion (pistoning) of the orthosis on the leg during gait.

The calf band should terminate below the fibular head to avoid impingement on the fibular nerve. If a patellar-tendon-bearing brim is used, it should have a concave relief to limit pressure on the fibular head. This component does not completely eliminate distal weight-bearing; however, one should judge to see that the shoe heel is somewhat unloaded. This can be estimated by placing a ribbon in the shoe before the patient dons the shoe. One end of the ribbon hangs out the back of the shoe. When the patient stands with the shoe and orthosis on, the therapist should be able to pull the ribbon out of the shoe. The calf shell, band, or patellar-tendon-bearing brim should not intrude on the popliteal fossa; if so, the patient would have difficulty flexing the knee when sitting. The type of closure of both the shoe and band affects donning ease.

The mechanical knee joints should be congruent with the anatomical knee; for the adult, the usual placement is approximately 3/4 in. (2 cm) above the medial tibial plateau. The knee lock should function properly, because use of a lock is often the major reason for wearing a KAFO. The medial upright should terminate approximately 1.5 in. (4 cm) below the perineum. The calf and distal thigh shells or bands should be equidistant so that when the orthosis is flexed, as in sitting, the plastic or metal parts will contact one another, rather than pinch the back of the wearer's skin. If the KAFO has a quadrilateral brim to reduce weight-bearing through the skeleton, the brim should have adequate relief for the sensitive adductor longus tendon and should provide a sufficient seat for the ischial tuberosity.

The pelvic joint is set slightly above and anterior to the greater trochanter to compensate for the usual angulation of the femoral neck; setting the joint anterior to the trochanter takes into account the medial rotation of the femur. The pelvic band should conform to the contours of the wearer's torso, without edge pressure.

When the orthosis is off, the therapist should inspect the patient's skin to detect any irritations attributable to the orthosis. One should move the orthotic joints slowly to check ROM. *Binding* refers to misalignment of the distal portion of the joint in relation to the proximal member so as to interfere with movement. If the medial and lateral stops do not contact their respective stops at the same time, the stop that contacts first will erode more rapidly and may contribute to twisting of the orthosis.

Dynamic Examination

The gait pattern exhibited by the person who wears an orthosis reflects both the contribution of the wearer's general health status and the orthotic motion control and assistance. Table 30.1 relates orthotic and anatomical causes of the most commonly observed gait deviations.

During early stance, the patient may exhibit *foot slap*, striking with toes first, or *flat-foot* contact, indicating inability to restrain plantarflexion or failure of the orthosis to support the foot and ankle. Excessive medial or lateral contact may indicate that the orthosis does not track the way the patient's limb does. Knee hyperextension or excessive flexion indicates that the orthosis is not applying adequate control. A posterior stop on the AFO should prevent the lax knee from hyperextending. If the patient wears a KAFO and has knee hyperextension, the stops in the knee joint are set improperly or have eroded, or the calf and thigh shells or bands are too deep. Anterior and posterior trunk bending are seen at early stance

Table 30.1 Orthotic Gait Analysis

Deviation	Orthotic Causes	Anatomical Causes
Early Stance		
1. Foot slap: forefoot slaps the ground	Inadequate dorsiflexion assist Inadequate plantarflexion stop	Weak dorsiflexors
2. Toes first: tiptoe posture may or may not be maintained throughout stance	Inadequate heel lift Inadequate dorsiflexion assist Inadequate plantarflexion stop Inadequate relief of heel pain	Short LE Pes equinus Extensor spasticity Heel pain
3. Flat foot contact: entire foot contacts ground initially	Inadequate traction from sole Requires walking aid (e.g., cane) Inadequate dorsiflexion stop	Poor balance Pes calcaneus
4. Excessive medial (or lateral) foot contact: medial (or lateral) border contacts floor	Transverse plane malalignment	Weak invertors (evertors) Pes valgus (varus) Genu valgum (varum)
5. Excessive knee flexion: knee collapses when foot contacts ground	Inadequate knee lock Inadequate dorsiflexion stop Plantarflexion restriction (stop) Inadequate contralateral shoe lift	Weak quadriceps Short contralateral LE Knee pain Knee and/or hip flexion contracture Flexor synergy Pes calcaneus
6. Hyperextended knee: knee hyperextends as weight is transferred to LE	Genu recurvatum inadequately controlled by plantarflexion stop Excessively concave (deep) calf band Pes equinus uncompensated by contralateral shoe lift Inadequate knee lock	Weak quadriceps Lax knee ligaments Extensor synergy Pes equinus Short contralateral LE Contralateral knee and/or hip flexion contracture
7. Anterior trunk bending: patient leans forward as weight is transferred to LE	Inadequate knee lock	Weak quadriceps Hip flexion contracture Knee flexion contracture
8. Posterior trunk bending: patient leans backward as weight is transferred to LE	Inadequate hip lock Knee lock	Weak gluteus maximus Knee ankylosis
9. Lateral trunk bending: patient leans toward stance leg as weight is transferred to LE	Excessive height of medial upright of KAFO Excessive abduction of hip joint of HKAFO	Weak gluteus medius Abduction contracture Dislocated hip Hip pain

Table 30.1 Orthotic Gait Analysis—cont'd

Deviation	Orthotic Causes	Anatomical Causes
	Requires walking aid (e.g., cane) Insufficient shoe lift	Poor balance Short leg
10. Wide walking base: heel centers more than 4 in. (10 cm) apart	Excessive height of medial upright of KAFO Excessive abduction of hip joint of HKAFO Insufficient lift on contralateral shoe Knee lock Requires walking aid (e.g., cane)	Abduction contracture Poor balance Short contralateral LE
11. Internal (or external) rotation: LE internally (or externally) rotated	Uprights incorrectly aligned in transverse plane Requires orthotic control (e.g., rotation control straps, pelvic band)	Internal (or external) hip rotators spastic External (or internal) hip rotators weak Anteversion (retroversion) Weak quadriceps: external rotation
Late Stance		
1. Inadequate transition: delayed or absent transfer of weight over the forefoot	Plantarflexion stop Inadequate dorsiflexion stop	Weak plantarflexors Achilles tendon sprain or rupture Pes calcaneus Forefoot pain
Swing		
1. Toe drag: toes maintain contact with ground	Inadequate dorsiflexion assist Inadequate plantarflexion stop	Weak dorsiflexors Plantarflexor spasticity Pes equinus Weak hip flexors
2. Circumduction: LE swings outward in a semicircular arc	Knee lock Inadequate dorsiflexion assist Inadequate plantarflexion stop	Weak hip flexors Extensor synergy Knee and/or ankle ankylosis Weak dorsiflexors Pes equinus
3. Hip hiking: LE elevated at pelvis to enable the limb to swing forward	Knee lock Inadequate dorsiflexion assist Inadequate plantarflexion stop	Short contralateral LE Contralateral knee and/or hip flexion contracture Weak hip flexors Extensor synergy Knee and/or ankle ankylosis Weak dorsiflexors Pes equinus
4. Vaulting: exaggerated plantarflexion of contralateral LE to enable the limb to swing forward	Knee lock Inadequate dorsiflexion assist Inadequate plantarflexion stop	Weak hip flexors Extensor spasticity Pes equinus Short contralateral LE Contralateral knee and/or hip flexion contracture Knee and/or ankle ankylosis Weak dorsiflexors

LE = lower extremity.

when the patient attempts to control a weak knee or hip. If the quadriceps are weak, the patient will bend forward. The person who fears that the knee may collapse may benefit from an AFO with a solid ankle and an anterior band, or a KAFO with a knee lock. If the gluteus maximus is weak, the individual is apt to lean backward. Lordosis indicates hip flexion contracture or a KAFO that does not fit properly.

Lateral trunk bending in early stance phase may result from hip abductor weakness or hip instability; however, uncompensated shortness of the limb will also give rise to this problem, as will a medial upright on a KAFO that is too high, or an abducted pelvic joint on an HKAFO. A wide walking base may be the patient's compensation for a long medial upright or shell that impinges into the perineum.

The client may have difficulty during late stance either delaying weight transfer or being unable to transfer weight over the affected foot. The problem can be mitigated with an anterior stop and a rocker bar. One should be certain that the trimlines of the solid ankle AFO or the stops on the stirrup function properly.

During swing phase, the patient must be able to clear the floor with the braced LE. *Hip hiking* (pelvic elevation) occurs when the hip flexors are weak, as well as when the limb is functionally longer than the contralateral limb. Increased length may be produced by a faulty posterior stop that no longer limits plantarflexion or by a locked knee joint. The problem should be anticipated and, for the unilateral KAFO wearer, can be prevented by adding a 1/2-in. (1-cm) lift to the contralateral shoe. Internal or external hip rotation may be caused by imbalance between medial and lateral musculature; the orthotic causes relate to malalignment of the brace. Similarly, excessive medial or lateral foot contact may indicate that the orthosis does not track the way the patient's limb does. A limb that is longer than that on the opposite side can cause a walking base that is abnormally wide. *Vaulting* refers to exaggerated plantarflexion on the contralateral limb during swing phase of the affected side. Vaulting occurs because the braced leg is functionally too long, possibly because the posterior ankle stop has eroded or a knee lock is used. The less agile patient may obtain foot clearance by hip hiking, which is elevating the pelvis on the swing side.

Trunk Orthosis Static Examination

Thoracic and pelvic bands should fit flat against the trunk without edge pressure. Uprights should not press against bony prominences, particularly when the patient sits. The abdominal front should extend from just below the xiphoid process to just above the pubic symphysis. The cervical orthosis should hold the head in the best-tolerated position. Rigid components, such as a mandibular plate, occipital plate, sternal plate, or thoracic plate should be shaped to apply maximum area to the body segment.

Facilitating Orthotic Acceptance

Clinic team management is valuable in fostering acceptance of the orthosis by the patient. The team enables clinicians to join efforts to help the individual achieve the maximum benefit from rehabilitation. Bringing the new wearer of an orthosis in contact with other users in the physical therapy department can help the new patient recognize that orthotic use is not a strange occurrence. Peer support groups for patients and their families are helpful for sharing concerns and anxieties, and reaching workable solutions to common problems. Support groups usually are organized for people having particular disabilities, such as paraplegia or hemiplegia. The physical therapist can guide some meetings of the group. Because therapists work most closely with patients, usually on a daily basis, the clinician can identify individuals whose response to disability is sufficiently aberrant as to require psychological attention.

Orthotic Instruction and Training

Orthotic examination and evaluation is an essential element of management. The therapist should examine the orthosis through analysis of (1) effects and benefits in terms of improved function, (2) movement while the patient wears the device, (3) practicality and ease of use, (4) fit and alignment, and (5) safety during use of the device. Orthoses are designed to provide the individual with a maximum of function with a minimum of discomfort and effort. No single instruction and training program suits every orthosis wearer because of the wide range of disorders for which orthotic management is indicated. To the extent possible, however, the physical therapist should instruct the patient in the correct manner of donning the orthosis, developing standing balance, walking safely, and performing other ambulatory activities.

Optimal performance depends on the favorable interaction of many factors. Foremost is the extent of skeletal and neuromuscular involvement. The mobility, strength, and coordination of all body segments, especially in the LEs and trunk, are important, as are the individual's muscle tone, cardiovascular and pulmonary health, body weight, psychological status, and chronological age. The quality of the orthosis also influences the client's achievements.

Most orthosis wearers have chronic conditions, such as arthritis, or permanent sequelae from trauma, such as paraplegia following spinal cord injury. Orthotic management enhances function without necessarily influencing the underlying pathology. Training people with chronic disorders prepares the patient for lifelong activity with an orthosis. Persons with reversible disorders, such as fibular nerve injury, often benefit from temporary use of an orthosis. Such individuals should learn proper use of the orthosis to prevent secondary disorders and should receive reexamination so that the orthosis may be altered as the condition changes. Patients with progressive disorders, such as muscular dystrophy and multiple sclerosis, require vigilant reexamination so that the extent of physical deterioration may be reflected in orthotic changes, as well as continual training to cope with altered functional abilities. For all situations, an individually devised exercise and activity program should enable the patient to manage efficiently for maximum independence.

Donning Orthoses

Regardless of type of orthosis, the patient should wear clean, properly fitting hose or a shirt. The AFO with shoe insert is most easily donned by applying the orthosis to the foot and leg, prior to placing the braced limb in the shoe. If the AFO has a split stirrup, the shoe should be donned first; then the orthosis should be fitted into the box caliper on the shoe. If the AFO has a solid stirrup, the patient will have to insert the foot into the shoe, then fasten the calf band.

The same general procedures are useful with KAFOs. The patient may find donning easier if the brace is applied while lying on a bed or a mat table. If the KAFO is donned while the patient sits, the therapist should check the tightness of the orthotic anterior strap or band. Donning HKAFOs and THKAFOs is much more arduous. The beginner should lie on a mat table alongside the orthosis. By rolling to one side, the patient should be able to pull the brace under the legs so as to permit lying in it. Then the patient sits with knees extended to don shoes and fasten straps.

Lumbosacral and TLS corsets and rigid orthoses should be donned while the patient is supine to achieve maximum compression of the abdomen. The orthosis should be fastened from the bottom upward.

Standing Balance

The problem of standing safely is most difficult for the individual who wears a pair of KAFOs or more extensive bracing. In ordinary standing, all weight passes through the feet, whereas when standing and walking with orthoses and assistive devices, the patient must learn to distribute weight partly on the hands and partly on the feet. With KAFOs, the line of gravity falls within a tripod bounded by the hands and feet. The tripod is a compromise between leaning too far forward on the hands, to increase stability at the price of fatiguing the arms, and leaning too far backward, which reduces arm strain but makes balance precarious. As balance improves, the patient uses the hands only for balance, rather than for substantial weight-bearing.

The person who wears bilateral KAFOs will need crutches or other aids for independent gait. A prerequisite for crutch ambulation is the ability to shift weight. Shifting weight to the heels takes pressure off the hands so they can be moved. Using parallel bars, the beginner shifts all weight to the feet and raises and lowers one hand, then the other hand. The goal is to be able to lift both hands simultaneously, as may be done with crutches when performing a drag-to or similar gait. Once the patient is able to shift weight from the feet to the hands and back to the feet confidently, the same exercise should be done with crutches. Advanced skills, such as moving the hands and eventually the crutches, behind the body, should be practiced. Those who will walk in reciprocal fashion, alternating footsteps, need to practice diagonal weight shifting.

Gait Training

The various crutch gaits differ in the sequence of crutch and footsteps. Patterns vary in speed, safety, and amount of energy required. The patient should learn as many gaits as possible, so as to modify walking in crowds, over long distances, and in situations in which speed is desired. In addition to walking forward, the client needs to be able to walk sideward, turn corners, and maneuver on different surfaces, such as rugs, gravel, grass, and through doors. A repertoire of gaits permits the client to adjust to environmental requirements. Gait selection depends on the individual's functional ability, including:

- *Step Ability*: Can the patient take steps with either one or both LEs?
- *Weight-Bearing and Balance Ability*: Can the patient bear weight and remain balanced on one or both LEs?
- *Upper Extremity Power*: Can the patient push the body off the floor by pressing down on the hands?

Reciprocal Gaits

The four- and two-point gaits require that one move the legs alternately by hip flexion or pelvic elevation. The patient shifts weight as each leg is moved. The four-point sequence is (1) right hand, (2) left foot, (3) left hand, and (4) right foot. The two-point sequence requires greater balance and coordination but is a faster mode of walking: (1) right hand and left leg and (2) left hand and right leg. The patterns also are useful when one is confronted with crowds or slippery surfaces. These gaits are suited to persons who lack the coordination and balance needed for simultaneous gaits.

Simultaneous Gaits

If both legs are moved simultaneously, the patient places considerable stress on the upper limbs. The series includes the drag-to, swing-to, and swing-through patterns. Although the swing-through gait can be performed rapidly, simultaneous gaits generally are slow and very fatiguing, because the arms and shoulder girdle are poorly adapted for ambulatory function; a sizable amount of nonfunctioning bodily structure must be controlled by a smaller muscular apparatus. The weight of the orthoses and, in the case of a patient with spinal cord lesion, absence of peripheral sensation, aggravates the problem of using a simultaneous gait pattern.

The drag-to gait is the most elementary of the group, but it is very slow. The sequence is (1) advance both hands, then (2) push on the crutches enough to drag the feet forward. The feet do not pass ahead of the hands, or crutch tips. The swing-to pattern is more rapid, because the patient swings rather than drags the LEs. Swinging is accomplished by extending the elbows and depressing the shoulder girdle to elevate the trunk and legs. The swing-through gait is the most advanced pattern, requiring much balance, strength, and coordination of the upper limbs, because the patient swings the legs beyond the hands, or crutch tips. The sequence is (1) advance both hands, (2) swing both legs to a point in front of the hands to reverse the basic tripod position, and (3) advance both hands to the starting position. The swing-through gait requires extensive preliminary training, including push-ups to strengthen the arms. The gait is rapid but requires more floor space than the other patterns, to permit alternate swinging of legs and crutches. Detailed instructions in gait training are provided in the appendix of Chapter 11 Strategies to Improve Locomotor Function.

The ultimate test of walking proficiency is the ability to conduct a conversation while ambulating (dual tasking), an activity pattern that indicates some degree of automatic functioning. Practice in the clinical setting should be extended to walking on varied terrain, indoors and outdoors.

Related Activities

The patient should learn as many activities as physical condition permits. Daily life often involves negotiating stairs, curbs, and ramps, as well as transferring from the chair to the upright position, and into an automobile. Instruction in driving a suitably equipped car is an important part of rehabilitation. Not all individuals who wear orthoses achieve the full range of ambulatory activities, yet they benefit from partial independence in accomplishing tasks, at least from the psychological and physiological values attendant to ambulation.

Final Examination and Follow-up Care

Prior to discharge, the patient and orthosis should be examined to make certain that fit, function, appearance, and use is acceptable. The patient should return to the hospital or rehabilitation center at regular intervals so that the clinic team can monitor the individual's function and the orthosis and can spot incipient abrasions or other signs of misfit or disrepair. The follow-up visit also enables the physical therapist to reinforce skills taught in the intensive instruction and training program and address any new problems the patient may present.

FUNCTIONAL CAPACITIES

A major purpose of rehabilitation is to improve the patient's functional capacity by reducing the amount of energy the individual uses to accomplish meaningful tasks, such as ambulation. The patient's ambulatory ability and capacity for other physical activities reflect both orthotic and anatomical factors. Energy measurement is a valuable guide to functional capacity. Energy cost is calculated from the amount of oxygen consumed as the subject performs an activity. Consumption may be determined either per unit of distance traversed or per unit of time.

Everyone ordinarily selects a walking speed that requires the least energy per unit of distance. If the energy cost is too high, the patient will realize that ambulation is not practical. Sometimes, high-energy cost is tolerable for short distances, as in household ambulation. Community ambulation, however, demands sustained effort for longer distances, plus the ability to maneuver over curbs and other irregularities in the walking surface and cross the street within the time allowed by the traffic light.

Although functional ambulation may be taxing, the ability to stand with or without orthoses confers important health benefits. An alternative to extensive bracing is a wheelchair that has linkage permitting the user to stand. Physiologically, upright posture stresses the skeleton, reducing osteoporosis; otherwise, the patient is vulnerable to fractures. Standing also facilitates respiratory, digestive, and urinary function. The logistical advantage of erect posture enables the patient to reach higher shelves than possible when sitting improving ability to perform ADLs. The emotional gains of standing are also an important consideration.

Hemiplegia

Adults with stroke consume more oxygen than able-bodied people when walking; the difference increases when subjects walk slowly.[167] Shoes with rocker soles worn with an ankle foot orthosis enable the wearer to reduce the energy cost significantly while increasing the preferred walking speed.[168] Handrail support also diminishes the energy cost of walking, primarily by reducing gait velocity.[169] The simplest way to reduce the oxygen demand during walking is by using a cane, which requires less oxygen at a given speed or permits greater speed for the same oxygen consumption. The single-point cane is more efficient than a quad cane or a hemiwalker.[170]

Cerebral Palsy

Children with cerebral palsy use more energy when walking than other children,[171] consuming as much as 1.3 times more oxygen than able-bodied age mates. The higher cost can be attributed to segmental impairments, such as spastic equinus, which increases the mechanical work performed by muscles.[172,173] As compared with barefoot walking, the hinged ankle–foot orthosis (AFO) reduced the children's energy expenditure.[82] Other investigators report that an AFO with a solid ankle reduced energy demand more than hinged AFOs or other orthoses.[85,174]

Paraplegia

The level and extent of spinal cord damage are critical determinants of functional capacity in people with spinal cord injury. The high energy cost of ambulation by people with spinal cord injury may be accounted for by necessity of relying entirely on the upper limbs and trunk, rather than using the legs to walk. In regards to walking, the type of orthoses also impacts functional capacity. Restraining both plantarflexion and dorsiflexion, as provided by Craig-Scott KAFOs, reduces energy demand very slightly. Ankle restraint, however, makes no appreciable difference in the energy required to negotiate stairs and ramps. Performance is somewhat more efficient with molded plastic KAFOs, which weigh slightly less than traditional metal and leather braces. Those with thoracic-level paraplegia use three times their basal oxygen rate ambulating with Craig-Scott KAFOs; they choose a very slow walking pace.[175] Those fitted with KAFOs with dorsiflexion stops performed more poorly than patients wearing Craig-Scott orthoses.[176] Several reports of paralyzed adults using RGOs confirm that this orthosis enabled standing without appreciable increase in workload, as compared with sitting.[177] Ambulation with an RGO facilitated more normal gait movements and stability and less energy expenditure than with traditional orthoses,[178,179] KAFOs, or bilateral KAFOs with a Walkabout medial hinge.[180] RGO use, however, was more arduous than wheelchair use.[181,182] Modifications of RGO use, such as functional electrical stimulation of thigh muscles[183] or addition of electronic power to the RGO[184] appear to improve energy consumption when patients walk.

One should not lose sight of the principal purpose of ambulation, namely to get from one place to another usually to perform a task. Some people with thoracic spinal cord injury prefer to use a wheelchair rather than orthotic-assisted ambulation, thereby avoiding struggling with brace donning, then attempt fatiguing, slow gait. While social acceptance and legislative mandates increasingly support use of wheelchairs and other assistive apparatus, the search for restoring normal gait is ongoing.

SUMMARY

This chapter has focused on lower-limb and trunk orthoses. The most frequently prescribed orthoses and orthotic components have been presented. In addition, the responsibilities of the physical therapist in orthotic management have been emphasized.

Ideally, an orthotic clinic team composed of a physician, physical therapist, and orthotist prescribes the orthosis. The prescription should be based on a thorough examination, with particular attention to the specific factors discussed in this chapter. Input from the patient and all team members during the decision-making process is critical. This approach will ensure an optimum match between the patient's biomechanical and psychological requirements and an appropriate orthosis capable of performing its intended function. Once the orthosis has been prescribed, it should be evaluated to ensure satisfactory fit, function, and construction, and the patient should have the benefit of a suitable instruction and training program for donning the orthosis and using it effectively.

Questions for Review

1. Discuss the purpose of a correctly fitted shoe in orthotic management.
2. Describe the purpose (function) of the following external shoe modifications: heel wedge, sole wedge, metatarsal bar, and rocker bar.
3. What are the advantages of a plastic orthotic shoe insert as compared with the solid stirrup?
4. For the patient with dorsiflexor weakness or paralysis, explain how a posterior leaf spring AFO imparts its function during early stance and swing phases of gait.
5. What is the function of the proximal anterior band on a floor reaction AFO?
6. How do tone-inhibiting AFOs improve the patient's function?
7. Indicate the clinical use of an AFO with a patellar-tendon-bearing brim.
8. What strategies can be used to increase the rigidity of plastic orthoses?
9. What is the function of an offset knee joint on a knee–ankle–foot orthosis (KAFO)?
10. Describe the three-point system in a lumbosacral flexion–extension control orthosis.
11. What data should be gathered prior to formulating an orthotic prescription?
12. Compare and contrast the orthotic options for a patient with hemiplegia.

13. What are the purposes of the preorthotic examination?
14. What features of the AFO are considered during the static evaluation?
15. What are the anatomical and orthotic causes of vaulting?

CASE STUDY

PATIENT HISTORY AND CURRENT PROBLEM

The patient is a 60-year-old woman who suffered a left middle cerebral artery stroke 6 months ago and presents to the clinic with persistent mild fluent aphasia, right hemiparesis marked by obligatory upper limb synergy with some active isolated movements, and right lower limb weakness marked by foot drop in swing phase (associated with both decreased ankle dorsiflexion (DF) ROM and decreased ankle DF strength) and knee extension throughout stance phase with an occasional buckling into knee flexion, causing instability but not falls (associated with weak hip and knee extensors). She was given an off-the-shelf solid ankle–foot orthosis (SAFO) during inpatient rehabilitation at a skilled nursing facility and has used it ever since. She uses a straight cane and walks with asymmetric weight-bearing, (shorter non-paretic step length) and halting pace (0.6 m/s), minimizing stance time on her right leg. She complains of difficulty rising to stand from the sofa or a chair, which requires her to lean left and backward to use her left hand. She cannot ascend or descend stairs or curbs in step-over-step pattern without assistance for safety and typically uses the "up with the good, down with the bad" approach. In total, impaired transfer, gait, and barrier negotiation ability limits her ability to access the community for social events, which had included a book club, knitting group, and visits to her two sons' homes to see her young grandchildren. She has been referred for outpatient physical therapy to improve her mobility.

PHYSICAL THERAPY EXAMINATION FINDINGS

Body Structure and Function (Impairments)

- Cognition: Alert, oriented, memory intact; flat affect and slow processing; Mini-Mental State Exam 22/30 with difficulty selecting and ordering words and numbers after verbal cues suggests mild cognitive impairment.
- Vision: No visual perceptual deficit noted.
- Cardiopulmonary: Vital signs seated at rest: Blood pressure 130/86, heart rate 84, respiration normal
- Medication: Aspirin 100 mg/day
- Endurance: Exercise capacity 6 minutes before needing rest
- Integumentary: Intact over foot, ankles, and lower leg areas contacting the SAFO
- Neuromuscular: R-sided impaired sensation
- Musculoskeletal: Passive ROM: hip extension R 10 from neutral (hip flexion contracture), L 10; hip external rotation R 25, L 60; knees normal; ankle DF R 0 L 15
  - Joint mobility: R hip hypomobile
  - Flexibility: SLR R 50 L 70
  - MMT: Difficulty fractionating movement; R ankle DF and R hip extension 3–/5, unable to complete available PROM against gravity; knee extension R 3+/5, L 4+/5
- Orthosis: polypropylene SAFO with 3/4 footplate

Activity (Limitations)

- Balance: Postural Assessment Scale for Stroke 28/36, with extended time or a little help required for a number of transitional movements, and 43/56 Berg Balance Scale score, with difficulty on small base of support or hemiparetic limb weight-bearing tasks, indicating a risk for falls.
- Gait: 0.6 m/s with cane over 2 minutes, putting her in the category of an independent household and limited community walker. Rarely walks longer than 2 minutes without stopping at any one time. Decreased R-side stance time, increased R-side swing time, and shorter L-side step length with lack of R hip extension past neutral contribute to gait asymmetry. Uses cane in left hand.

Participation (Restrictions)

- Home living: Unsafe for living alone. Needs assistance for most activities of daily living, including all household chores and some self-care activities, such as positioning the shower bench for bathing. Modified independent mobility within the home using a cane and the SAFO. Outside the home, needs assistance to navigate stairs/slopes/curbs/terrain. A home care attendant who comes to her home 3 times/week assists her in bathing and performs light housework.

- Vocational: Has not returned to work at her office.
- Social: Walks outdoors only for doctor visits; rarely leaves home to shop or socialize.

Individual and Environmental Contextual Factors

She lives with her 70-year-old retired husband in a two-story home with six steps to enter and upstairs bedrooms. She is currently staying in the first-floor guest room. Her two adult sons live with their families within a 1-hour drive, but they are busy working and visit about once or twice per month. She used to enjoy babysitting her young grandchildren and getting together with friends for their book club and knitting group.

PERSON-DESIRED OUTCOME AND GOALS

Improve mobility to allow her to safely leave home to visit grandchildren and friends.

PHYSICAL THERAPY ASSESSMENT AND PLAN FOR CARE

Rehabilitation outcomes are enhanced when the person identifies goals for themselves that implicitly take into account the context of their social life. Reduced pain and improved functional outcomes such as safe and independent community walking and enhanced social participation are common patient goals. The individual seeking physical therapy may not fully understand how those goals are intertwined and that reaching these goals by attaining short and intermediate impairment and activity-level goals will support the desired functional outcome. For instance, short-term goals such as normalized ankle joint dorsiflexion ROM may affect balance reactions and contribute to sit-to-stand or stair-negotiation ability, thus enhancing her ability to leave home and accessing her community for meaningful social activity. Person-specific goals can measure progress with Specific, Measurable, Achievable, Relevant, and Time-bound (SMART) goals combined with the person's subjective assessment like a Patient-Specific Functional Scale, in which patients list activities that are difficult for them and rate their ability on a 0- (can't perform at all) to 10-point (can perform fully) scale.

What follows is an example of a long-term participation goal (I), with the underlying activity goals (A) in the context of the individual and environment (B), body structure/function goals (1–3), followed by bulleted suggestions for interventions to address the underlying goals (with guiding notes):

I. Leave the house to see grandchildren once per week by next month.
   - A. Gait: Ascend and descend stairs step-over-step with upper-limb assist
     1. ROM: Ankle dorsiflexion to 10°
        - Joint mobilization for R ankle (e.g., mobilization with movement in weight-bearing lunge position, supported by wall)
        - Soft tissue mobilization for R ankle plantar flexors, long toe flexors, and hip flexors—particularly rectus femoris
        - Self-stretching for plantar flexors in weight-bearing lunge position, supported by wall
     2. MMT: weight-bearing ankle plantar flexor, knee and hip extension strength
        - R leg forward and lateral step up to blocks of increasing height
        - Prolonged R leg stance time (e.g., in step standing position L leg up)
     3. Orthosis: consider a new orthosis
        - a. Hinged AFO with plantarflexion stop
          - i. (+) will prevent toe drag in swing phase while allowing ankle dorsiflexion for sit-to-stand or stair negotiation
          - ii. (–) will prevent plantar flexion upon initial contact, thus requiring ready knee extension strength upon contact
        - b. Hinged AFO with dorsiflexion assist
          - i. (+) will prevent toe drag while allowing ankle dorsiflexion for sit-stand and stair negotiation while allowing plantarflexion than enhances knee stability upon contact
          - ii. (–) additional weight of some metal spring mechanisms adds to metabolic demands during walking
        - c. Posterior Leaf Spring Orthosis
          - i. (+) will prevent toe drag while allowing ankle dorsiflexion for sit-stand and stair negotiation while allowing plantarflexion than enhances knee stability upon contact
          - ii. (–) provides no frontal plane support (which any hinged AFO provides); gives little resistance to ankle motion in either direction

4. Cardiopulmonary (exercise capacity): Walk for 6 minutes without rest with vital signs in safe range
   - Treadmill walking provides external cue to maintain speed
   - Count steps/day for a week, then increase by 10% per week
   - Walk around block, keeping track of the time, then aim to decrease time by 10%[57]

B. Individual and Environmental Context
   - Stairs/curbs/obstacles: Negotiate safely to facilitate leaving home and entering other people's homes.
   - Dual-task training: Integrate upper limb carrying/manipulation tasks and cognitive/visual distraction with walking.

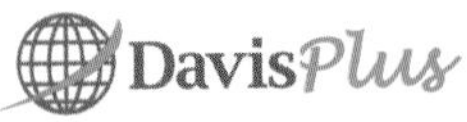

For additional resources, including answers to the questions for review and case study guiding questions, please visit **http://davisplus.fadavis.com**

References

1. American Academy of Orthopaedic Surgeons: Orthopaedic Appliances Atlas, vol 1. JW Edwards, Ann Arbor, MI, 1952.
2. Fatone, S: Challenges in lower-limb orthotic research. Prosthet Orthot Int 34:235, 2010.
3. Menant, JC, et al: Optimizing footwear for older people at risk of falls. J Rehabil Res Dev 45:1167, 2008.
4. Hong, WH, et al: Influence of heel height and shoe insert on comfort perception and biomechanical performance of young female adults during walking. Foot Ankle Int 26:1042, 2005.
5. Wulf, M, et al: The effect of an in-shoe orthotic heel lift on loading of the Achilles tendon during shod walking. J Orthop Sports Phys Ther 46:79, 2016.
6. Weinert-Aplin, RA, Bull, AM, and McGregor, AH: Orthotic heel wedges do not alter hindfoot kinematics and Achilles tendon force during level and inclined walking in healthy individuals. J Appl Biomech 32:160, 2016.
7. Johanson, MA, et al: Effect of heel lifts on plantarflexor and dorsiflexors activity during gait. Foot Ankle Int 31:1014, 2010.
8. Hawke, F, et al: Custom-made foot orthoses for the treatment of foot pain. Cochrane Database Syst Rev 3, 2008. Art. No.: CD006801. DOI: 10.1002/14651858.CD006801.pub2.
9. Menz, HB, et al: Effectiveness of off-the-shelf, extra-depth footwear in reducing foot pain in older people: A randomized controlled trial. J Gerontol A Biol Sci Med Sci 70:511, 2015.
10. Rao, S, et al: Orthoses alter in vivo segmental foot kinematics during walking in patients with midfoot arthritis Arch Phys Med Rehabil 91:608, 2010.
11. Welsh, BJ, et al: A case-series study to explore the efficacy of foot orthoses in treating first metatarsophalangeal joint pain. J Foot Ankle Res 27:3, 2010.
12. Nawoczenski, DA, and Ludewig, PM: The effect of forefoot and arch posting orthotic designs on first metatarsophalangeal joint kinematics during gait. J Orthop Sports Phys Ther 34:317, 2004.
13. Roos, E, Engstrom, M, and Soderberg, B: Foot orthoses for the treatment of plantar fasciitis. Foot Ankle Int 27:606, 2006.
14. Landorf, KB, Keenan, AM, and Herbert, RD: Effectiveness of foot orthoses to treat plantar fasciitis. Arch Intern Med 166:1305, 2006.
15. Baldassin, V, Gomes, CR, and Beraldo, PS: Effectiveness of prefabricated and customized foot orthoses made from low-cost foam for noncomplicated plantar fasciitis: A randomized controlled trial. Arch Phys Med Rehabil 90:701, 2009.
16. Seligman, DA, and Dawson, DR: Customized heel pads and soft orthotics to treat heel pain and plantar fasciitis. Arch Phys Med Rehabil 84:1564, 2003.
17. deMorais Barbosa, C, et al: The effect of foot orthoses on balance, foot pain and disability in elderly women with osteoporosis: A randomized clinical trial. Rheumatology (Oxford) 52:515, 2013.
18. Gross, MT, Mercer, VS, and Lin, FC: Effects of foot orthoses on balance in older adults. J Orthop Sports Phys Ther 2:649, 2012.
19. Leung, AK, Mak, AF, and Evans, JH: Biomechanical gait evaluation of the immediate effect of orthotic treatment for flexible flat foot. Prosthet Orthot Int 22:25, 1998.
20. Murley, GS, Landorf, KB, and Menz, HB: Do foot orthoses change lower limb muscle activity in flat-arched feet toward a pattern observed in normal-arched feet? Clin Biomech (Bristol, Avon) 25:728, 2010.
21. Berengueres, J, Fritschi, M, and McClanahan, R: A smart pressure-sensitive insole that reminds you to walk correctly: An orthotic-less treatment for over pronation. Conf Proc IEEE Eng Med Biol Soc 2014:2488, 2014.
22. Rome, K, Ashford, RL, and Evans, A: Non-surgical interventions for paediatric pes planus. Cochrane Database Syst Reviews 7, 2010. Art. No.: CD006311.
23. Burns, J, et al: Interventions for the prevention and treatment of pes cavus. Cochrane Database Syst Rev 4, 2007. Art. No.: CD006154.
24. Burns, J, et al: Effective orthotic therapy for the painful cavus foot: A randomized controlled trial. J Am Podiatr Med Assoc 96:205, 2006.
25. Brodtkorb, TH, Kogler, GF, and Arndt, A: The influence of metatarsal support height and longitudinal axis position on plantar foot loading. Clin Biomech (Bristol, Avon) 23:640, 2008.
26. Koenraadt, KL, et al: Effect of a metatarsal pad on the forefoot during gait. J Am Podiatr Med Assoc 102:18, 2012.
27. Chen, WM, Lee, SJ, and Lee, PV: Plantar pressure relief under the metatarsal heads: Therapeutic insole design using three-dimensional finite element model of the foot. J Biomech 48:659, 2014.
28. Chang, BC, et al: Plantar pressure analysis of accommodative insole in older people with metatarsalgia. Gait Posture 39:449, 2014.
29. Kerrigan, DC, et al: Moderate-heeled shoe and knee joint torques relevant to the development and progression of knee osteoarthritis. Arch Phys Med Rehabil 86:871, 2005.
30. Gelis, A, et al: Is there an evidence-based efficacy for the use of foot orthotics in knee and hip osteoarthritis? Elaboration of French clinical practice guidelines. Joint Bone Spine 75:714, 2008.
31. Butler, RJ, et al: Effect of laterally wedged foot orthoses on rearfoot and hip mechanics in patients with medial knee osteoarthritis. Prosthet Orthot Int 33:107, 2009.
32. van Raaij, TM, et al: Medial knee osteoarthritis treated by insoles or braces: A randomized trial. Clin Orthop Relat Res 468:1926, 2010.
33. Dessery, Y, et al: Effects of foot orthoses with medial arch support and lateral wedge on knee adduction moment in patients with medial knee osteoarthritis. Prosthet Orthot Int, 41(4): 356–36, 2017.
34. Hsu, WC, et al: Immediate and long-term efficacy of laterally-wedged insoles on persons with bilateral medial knee osteoarthritis during walking. Biomed Eng Online 14:43, 2015.
35. Yeh, HC, et al: Immediate efficacy of laterally insoles with arch support on walking in persons with bilateral medial knee osteoarthritis. Arch Phys Med Rehabil 95:2420, 2014.
36. Duivenvoorden, T, et al: Braces and orthoses for treating osteoarthritis of the knee. Cochrane Database Syst Rev 2015, CD004020.
37. Hossain, M, et al: Foot orthoses for patellofemoral pain in adults. Cochrane Database Syst Rev 1, 2011. CD008402.
38. Gross, MT, and Foxworth, JL: The role of foot orthoses as an intervention for patellofemoral pain. J Orthop Sports Phys Ther 33:661, 2003.

39. Saxena, A, and Haddad, J: The effect of foot orthoses on patellofemoral pain syndrome. J Am Podiatr Med Assoc 93:264, 2003.
40. Wang, CC, and Hansen, AH: Response of able-bodied persons to changes in shoe rocker radius during walking: Changes in ankle kinematics to maintain a consistent roll-over shape. J Biomech 43:2288, 2010.
41. Hutchins, S, et al: The biomechanics and clinical efficacy of footwear adapted with rocker profiles—evidence in the literature. Foot (Edinburgh) 19:165, 2009.
42. Arts, ML, et al: Data-driven directions for effective footwear provision for the high-risk diabetic foot. Diabet Med 32:790, 2015.
43. Janisse, D, and Janisse, E: Pedorthic management of the diabetic foot. Prosthet Orthot Int 39:40, 2015.
44. McCartan, BL, and Rosenblum, B: Offloading of the diabetic foot: Orthotic and pedorthic strategies. Clin Podiatr Med Surg 31:71, 2014.
45. Fernandez, ML, et al: How effective is orthotic treatment in patients with recurrent diabetic foot ulcers? J Am Podiatr Med Assoc 103:281, 2013.
46. Waaijman, R, et al: Pressure-reduction and preservation in custom-made footwear of patients with diabetes and a history of plantar ulceration. Diabet Med 29:1542, 2012.
47. Hastings, MK, et al: Effect of metatarsal pad placement on plantar pressure in people with diabetes mellitus and peripheral neuropathy. Foot Ankle Int 28:84, 2007.
48. Lott, DJ, et al: Effect of footwear and orthotic devices on stress reduction and soft tissue strain of the neuropathic foot. Clin Biomech (Bristol, Avon) 22:352, 2007.
49. Huang, YC, et al: Effects of ankle-foot orthoses on ankle and foot kinematics in patients with subtalar osteoarthritis. Arch Phys Med Rehabil 87:1131, 2006.
50. Chern, JS, et al: Static ankle-foot orthosis improves static balance and gait functions in hemiplegic patients after stroke. Conf Proc IEEE Eng Med Biol Soc 2013:5009, 2013.
51. Sheffler, LR, et al: Spatiotemporal, kinematic, and kinetic effects of a peroneal nerve stimulator versus an ankle foot orthosis in hemiparetic gait. Neurorehabil Neural Repair 27:403, 2013.
52. Howlett, OA, et al: Functional electrical stimulation improves activity after stroke: A systematic review with meta-analysis. Arch Phys Med Rehabil 96:934, 2015.
53. Bethoux, F, et al. Long-term follow-up to a randomized controlled trial comparing peroneal nerve functional electrical stimulation to an ankle foot orthosis for patients with chronic stroke. Neurorehabil Neural Repair 29:911, 2015.
54. Everaert, DG, et al: Effect of a foot-drop stimulator and ankle-foot orthosis on walking performance after stroke: A multicenter randomized controlled trial. Neurorehabil Neural Repair 27:579, 2013.
55. Kluding, PM, et al: Foot drop stimulation versus ankle foot orthosis after stroke: 30 week outcomes. Stroke 44:1660 2013.
56. Dunning, K, et al: Peroneal stimulation for foot drop after stroke: a systematic review. Am J Phys Med Rehabil 94:649, 2015.
57. Bosch, PR, et al: Review of therapeutic electrical stimulation for dorsiflexion assist and movement interventions subcommittee. Arch Phys Med Rehabil 95:390, 2014.
58. Ehrholz, J, et al: Electromechanical-assisted training for walking after stroke. Cochrane Database Syst Rev 25, 2013, CD006185.
59. Schiemanck, S, et al: Effects of implantable peroneal nerve stimulation on gait quality, energy expenditure, participation and user satisfaction in patients with post-stroke drop foot using an ankle-foot orthosis. Restor Neurol Neurosci 33:795, 2015.
60. Kobayashi, T, et al: Reduction of genu recurvatum through adjustment of plantarflexion resistance of an articulated ankle-foot orthosis in individuals poststroke. Clin Biomech (Bristol, Avon) 35:81, 2016.
61. Kobayashi, T, et al: The effect of changing plantarflexion resistive moment of an articulated ankle-foot orthosis on ankle and knee joint angles and moments while walking in patients post stroke. Clin Biomech 30:775, 2015.
62. Cakar, E, et al: The ankle-foot orthosis improves balance and reduces fall risk of chronic spastic hemiparetic patients. Eur J Phy Rehabil Med 46:363, 2010.
63. Silver-Thorn, B, et al: Effect of ankle orientation on heel loading and knee stability for post-stroke individuals wearing ankle-foot orthoses. Prosthet Orthot Int 35:150, 2011.
64. Tyson, SF, and Kent, RM: Effects of an ankle-foot orthosis on balance and walking after stroke: A systematic review and pooled meta-analysis. Arch Phys Med Rehabil 94:1377, 2013.
65. Zollo, L, et al: Comparative analysis and quantitative evaluation of ankle-foot orthoses for foot drop in chronic hemiparetic patients. Eur J Phys Rehabil Med 51:185, 2015.
66. Hung, JW, et al: Long-term effect of an anterior ankle-foot orthosis on functional walking ability of chronic stroke patients. Am J Phys Med Rehabil 90:8, 2011.
67. Chen, CL, et al: Effect of anterior ankle-foot orthoses on weight shift in persons with stroke. Arch Phys Med Rehabil 96:1795, 2015.
68. Boudarham, J, et al: Effects of a dynamic-ankle-foot orthosis (Liberté®) on kinematics and electromyographic activity during gait in hemiplegic patients with spastic foot equinus. Neuro Rehabil 35:369, 2014.
69. De Seze, MP, et al: Effect of early compensation of distal motor deficiency by the Chignon® ankle-foot orthosis on gait in hemiplegic patients: A randomized pilot study. Clin Rehabil 25:989, 2011.
70. Carse, B, et al: The immediate effects of fitting and tuning solid ankle-foot orthoses in early stroke rehabilitation. Prosthet Orthot Int 39:454, 2015.
71. Ferreira, LA, et al: Effect of ankle-foot orthosis on gait velocity and cadence of stroke patients: A systematic review. J Phys Ther Sci 25:1503, 2013.
72. Bregman, DJ, et al: Spring-like ankle foot orthoses reduce the energy cost of walking by taking over ankle work. Gait Posture 35:148, 2012.
73. Menotti, F, et al: Comparison of walking energy cost between an anterior and a posterior ankle-foot orthosis in people with foot drop. J Rehabil Med 46:768, 2014.
74. Swinnen, E, et al: Neurological patients and their lower limb orthotics: An observational pilot study about acceptance and satisfaction. Prosthet Orthot Int 41:41, 2017.
75. Ploeger, HE, et al: Ankle-foot orthoses that restrict dorsiflexion improve walking in polio survivors with calf muscle weakness. Gait Posture 40:391 2014.
76. Ries, AJ, Novacheck, TF, and Schwartz, MH: The efficacy of ankle-foot orthoses on improving the gait of children with diplegic cerebral palsy: A multiple outcome analysis. PM R 7:922, 2015.
77. Bourseul, JS, et al: Effect of ankle-foot orthoses on gait in children with cerebral palsy: A meta-analysis. Ann Phys Rehabil Med 59S: e6, 2016.
78. Wingstrand, M, Hägglund, G, and Rodby-Bousquet, E: Ankle-foot orthoses in children with cerebral palsy: A cross sectional population based study of 2200 children. BMC Musculoskelet Disord 1:327, 2014.
79. Neto, HP, et al: Comparison of articulated and rigid ankle-foot orthoses in children with cerebral palsy: A systematic review. Pediatr Phys Ther 24:308, 2012.
80. Wren, TA, et al: Comparison of two orthotic approaches in children with cerebral palsy. Pediatr Phys Ther 27:218, 2015.
81. Radtka, SA, Skinner, SR, and Johanson, ME: A comparison of gait with solid and hinged ankle-foot orthoses in children with spastic diplegic cerebral palsy. Gait Posture 21:303, 2005.
82. Balaban, B, et al: The effect of hinged ankle-foot orthosis on gait and energy expenditure in spastic hemiplegic cerebral palsy. Disabil Rehabil 29:139, 2007.
83. Bahramizadeh, M, et al: The effect of floor reaction ankle foot orthosis on postural control in children with spastic cerebral palsy. Prosthet Orthot Int 36:71, 2012.
84. Danino, B, et al: Influence of orthosis on the foot progression angle in children with spastic cerebral palsy. Gait Posture 2:518, 2015.
85. Caliskan Uckun, A, et al: Comparison of effects of lower extremity orthoses on energy expenditure in patients with cerebral palsy. Dev Neurorehabil 17:388, 2014.
86. Kerkum, YL, et al: The effects of varying ankle foot orthosis stiffness on gait in children with spastic cerebral palsy who walk with excessive knee flexion. PLoS One 10:e0142878, 2015.
87. Pool, D, et al: The orthotic and therapeutic effects following daily community applied functional electrical stimulation in children with unilateral spastic cerebral palsy: A randomised controlled trial. BMC Pediatr 15:154, 2015.
88. Meilahn, JR: Tolerability and effectiveness of a neuroprosthesis for the treatment of footdrop in pediatric patients with hemiparetic cerebral palsy. PM R 5:503, 2013.
89. Ivanyi, B, et al: The effects of orthoses, footwear, and walking aids on the walking ability of children and adolescents with spina bifida: A systematic review using International Classification of Functioning, Disability and Health for Children and Youth (ICF-CY) as a reference framework. Prosthet Orthot Int 39:437, 2015.

90. Townsend, EL, Tamhane, H, and Gross KD: Effects of AFO use on walking in boys with Duchenne muscular dystrophy: A pilot study. Pediatr Phys Ther 27:24, 2015.
91. Tian, F, Hefzy, MS, and Elahinia, M: State of the art review of knee-ankle-foot orthoses. Ann Biomed Eng 43:427, 2015.
92. Yakimovich, T, Lemaire, ED, and Kofman, J: Engineering design review of stance-control knee-ankle-foot orthoses. J Rehabil Res Dev 46:257, 2009.
93. Davis, PC, Bach, TM, and Pereira, DM: The effect of stance control orthoses on gait characteristics and energy expenditure in knee-ankle-foot orthosis users. 43(2):206–15, 2010.
94. Rafiaei, M, et al: The gait and energy efficiency of stance control knee-ankle-foot orthoses: A literature review. Prosthet Orthot Int 40:202, 2016.
95. Karimi, MT: Functional walking ability of paraplegic patients: comparison of functional electrical stimulation versus mechanical orthoses. Eur J Orthop Surg Traumatol 23:631, 2013.
96. Maas, J, et al: A randomized controlled trial studying efficacy and tolerance of a knee-ankle-foot orthosis used to prevent equinus in children with spastic cerebral palsy. Clin Rehabil 28:1025, 2014.
97. Kent, HO: Vannini-Rizzoli stabilizing orthosis (boot): Preliminary report on a new ambulatory aid for spinal cord injury. Arch Phys Med Rehabil 73:302, 1992.
98. Lyles, M, and Munday, J: Report on the evaluation of the Vannini-Rizzoli Stabilizing Lim Orthosis. J Rehabil Res Dev 29:77, 1992.
99. Karimi, MT, and Fatoye, F: Evaluation of the performance of paraplegic subjects during walking with a new design of reciprocal gait orthosis. Disabil Rehabil Assist Technol 11:72, 2016.
100. Arazpour, M, et al: Comparison of gait between healthy participants and persons with spinal cord injury when using the advanced reciprocating gait orthosis. Prosthet Orthot Int 40:287, 2016.
101. Bani, MA, et al: Gait evaluation of the advanced reciprocating gait orthosis with solid versus dorsiflexion assist ankle foot orthoses in paraplegic patients. Prosthet Orthot Int 37:161, 2013.
102. Arazpour, M, et al: The influence of a rocker sole adaptation on gait parameters in spinal cord injury patients ambulating with the advanced reciprocating gait orthosis—a pilot study. Disabil Rehabil Assist Technol 10:89, 2015.
103. Samadian, M, et al: The influence of orthotic gait training with an isocentric reciprocating gait orthosis on the walking ability of paraplegic patients: A pilot study. Spinal Cord 53:754, 2015.
104. Harvey, LA, et al: A comparison of the attitude of paraplegic individual to the walkabout orthosis and the isocentric reciprocal gait orthosis. Spinal Cord 35:580, 1997.
105. Klose, KJ, et al: Evaluation of a training program for persons with SCI paraplegia using the Parastep 1 ambulation system, part 1. Ambulation performance and anthropometric measures. Arch Phys Med Rehabil 78:789, 1997.
106. Brissot, R, et al: Clinical experience with functional electrical stimulation-assisted gait with Parastep in spinal cord-injured patients. Spine 25:501, 2000.
107. Karimi, MT: Functional walking ability of paraplegic patients: Comparison of functional electrical stimulation versus mechanical orthoses. Eur J Orthop Surg Traumatol 23:631, 2013.
108. Hughes, J: Powered lower limb orthotics in paraplegia. Paraplegia 9:191, 1972.
109. Probsting, E, Kannenberg, A, and Zacharias, B: Safety and walking ability of KAFO users with the C-Brace® Orthotronic Mobility System, a new microprocessor stance and swing control orthosis. Prosthet Orthot Int 41:65, 2017.
110. Schmalz, T, et al: A functional comparison of conventional knee-ankle-foot orthoses and a microprocessor-controlled leg orthosis system based on biomechanical parameters. Prosthet Orthot Int 40:277, 2016.
111. Del-Ama, AJ, et al: Review of hybrid exoskeletons to restore gait following spinal cord injury. J Rehabil Res Dev 49:497, 2012.
112. Kozlowski, AJ, Bryce, TM, and Dijkers, MP: Time and effort required by persons with spinal cord injury to learn a powered exoskeleton for assisted walking. Top Spinal Cord Inj Rehabiil 21:110, 2015.
113. Hartigan, C, et al: Mobility outcomes following five training sessions with a powered exoskeleton. Top Spinal Cord Inj Rehabil 21:93, 2015.
114. Sale, P, et al: Use of the robot assisted gait therapy in rehabilitation of patients with stroke and spinal cord injury. Eur J Phys Rehabil Med 48:111, 2012.
115. Esquenazi, A, et al: The ReWalk powered exoskeleton to restore ambulatory function to individuals with thoracic-level motor-complete spinal cord injury. Am J Phys Med Rehabil 91:911, 2012.
116. Yang, A, et al: Assessment of in-hospital walking velocity and level of assistance in a powered exoskeleton in persons with spinal cord injury. Top Spinal Cord Inj Rehabil 21:100, 2015.
117. Diaz, I, Gil, JJ, and Sanchez, E: Lower-limb robotic rehabilitation: Literature review and challenges. J Robotics article 759764, 2011.
118. Alcobenda-Maestro, M, et al: Lokomat robotic-assisted versus overground training within 3 to 6 months of incomplete spinal cord lesion: randomized controlled trial. Neurorehabil Neural Repair 26:1056, 2012.
119. Nam, KY, et al: Robot-assisted gait training (Lokomat) improves walking function and activity in people with spinal cord injury: a systematic review. J Neuroeng Rehabil 14:24, 2017.
120. Jezernik, S, et al: Robotic orthosis Lokomat: a rehabilitation and research tool. Neuromodulation 6:106, 2003.
121. Ha, KH, Murray, SA, and Goldfarb, M: An approach for the cooperative control of FES with a powered exoskeleton during level walking for persons with paraplegia. IEEE Trans Neural Syst Rehabil Eng 24:455, 2016.
122. Louie, DR, Eng, JJ, Lam, T, and Spinal Cord Injury Research Evidence (SCIRE) Research Team: Gait speed using powered robotic exoskeletons after spinal cord injury: A systematic review and correlational study. J Neuroeng Rehabil 14:12, 2015.
123. Arazpour, M, et al: Effect of powered gait orthosis on walking in individuals with paraplegia. Prosthet Orthot Int 37:261, 2013.
124. Chang, SR, et al: Powered lower-limb exoskeletons to restore gait for individuals with paraplegia—a review. Case Orthop J 12:75, 2015.
125. Federici, S, et al: The effectiveness of powered, active lower limb exoskeletons in neurorehabilitation: A systematic review. Neuro Rehabil 37:321, 2015.
126. Miller, LE, Zimmermann, A, and Herbert, WG: Clinical effectiveness and safety of powered exoskeleton-assisted walking in patients with spinal cord injury: Systematic review with meta-analysis. Med Devices (Auckl) 9:455, 2016.
127. Fisahn, C, et al: The effectiveness and safety of exoskeletons as assistive and rehabilitation devices in the treatment of neurologic gait disorders in patients with spinal cord injury: A systematic review. Global Spine J: 6:822, 2016.
128. Phelan, K, Gibson, BE, and Wright, FV: What is it like to walk with the help of a robot? Children's perspectives on robotic gait training technology. Disabil Rehabil 37:2272, 2015.
129. Husemann, B, et al: Effects of locomotion training with assistance of a robot-driven orthosis in hemiparetic patients after stroke: A randomized controlled plot study. Stroke 38:349, 2007.
130. Krewer, C, et al: The influence of different Lokomat walking conditions on the energy expenditure of hemiparetic patients and healthy subjects. Gait Posture 26:372, 2007.
131. Swinnen, E, et al: Does robot-assisted gait rehabilitation improve balance in stroke patients? A systematic review. Top Stroke Rehabil 21:87, 2014.
132. Vaney, C, et al: Robotic assisted step training (Lokomat) not superior to equal intensity of over-ground rehabilitation in patients with multiple sclerosis. Neurorehabil Neural Repair 26:212, 2012.
133. Lajeunesse, V, et al: Exoskeletons' design and usefulness evidence according to a systematic review of lower limb exoskeletons used for functional mobility by people with spinal cord injury. Disabil Rehabil Assist Technol 11:535, 2016.
134. Scherer, MJ: Why people use and don't use technologies: Introduction to the special issue on assistive technologies for cognition/cognitive support technologies. Neuro Rehabil 37:315, 2015.
135. Calmels, P, et al: Effectiveness of a lumbar belt in subacute low back pain: An open multicentric, and randomized clinical study. Spine, 34:215, 2009.
136. Kawchuk, GN, et al: A non-randomized clinical trial to assess the impact of nonrigid, inelastic corsets on spine function in low back pain participants and asymptomatic controls. Spine J 15:2222, 2015.
137. Aleksiev, AR: Ten-year follow-up of strengthening versus flexibility exercises with or without abdominal bracing in recurrent low back pain. Spine 39:997, 2014.

138. Van Duijvenbode, IC, et al: Lumbar supports for prevention and treatment of low back pain. Cochrane Database Syst Rev 16: CD001823, 2008.
139. Cholewicki, J, et al: Comparison of trunk stiffness provided by different design characteristics of lumbosacral orthoses. Clin Biomech (Bristol, Avon) 25:110, 2010.
140. Morrisette, DC, et al: A randomized clinical trial comparing extensible and inextensible lumbosacral orthoses and standard care alone in the management of lower back pain. Spine 39:1733, 2014.
141. Kim, HJ, et al: Comparative study of the treatment outcomes of osteoporotic compression fractures without neurologic injury using a rigid brace, a soft brace, and no brace: A prospective randomized controlled non-inferiority trial. J Bone Joint Surg Am 96:1959, 2014.
142. Boura, T, and Korovessis, P: Management of spondylolysis and low-grade spondylolisthesis in fine athletes: A comparative review. Eur J Orthop Surg Traumatolol 25:167, 2015.
143. Leonidou, A, et al: Treatment for spondylolysis and spondylolisthesis in children. J Orthop Surg (Hong Kong) 23:379, 2015.
144. Jegede, KA, et al: The effects of three different types of orthoses on the range of motion of the lumbar spine during 15 activities of daily living. Spine 36:2346, 2011.
145. Cholewiki, J, et al: The effects of a three-week use of lumbosacral orthoses on trunk muscle activity and on the muscular response to trunk perturbations. BMC Musculoskelet Disord 11:154, 2010.
146. Azadinia, F, et al: Can lumbosacral orthoses cause trunk muscle weakness? A systematic review of literature. Spine J, S1529, 2016.
147. Wood, KB, et al: Operative compared with nonoperative treatment of a thoracolumbar burst fracture without neurological deficit: A prospective randomized study with follow-up at sixteen to twenty-two years. J Bone Joint Surg Am 97:3, 2015.
148. Chang, V, and Holly, LT: Bracing for thoracolumbar fractures. Neurosurg Focus 37:E3, 2014.
149. Shamji, MF, et al: A pilot evaluation of the role of bracing in stable thoracolumbar burst fractures without neurological deficit. J Spinal Disord Tech 27:370, 2014.
150. Bailey, CS, et al: Orthosis versus no orthosis for the treatment of thoracolumbar burst fractures without neurologic injury: A multicenter prospective randomized equivalence trial. Spine J 14:2557, 2014.
151. Miller, CP, et al: Soft and rigid collars provide similar restriction in cervical range of motion during fifteen activities of daily living. Spine, 1:35, 2010.
152. Thoomes, EJ, et al: The effectiveness of conservative treatment for patients with cervical radiculopathy: A systematic review. Clin J Pain 29:1073, 2013.
153. Kuijper, B, et al: Cervical collar or physiotherapy versus wait and see policy for recent onset cervical radiculopathy: Randomized trial. BMJ 339, 2009.
154. Kongsted, A, et al: Neck collar, "act-as-usual" or active mobilization for whiplash injury? A randomized parallel-group trial. Spine 32: 616, 2007.
155. Holla, M, et al: The ability of external immobilizers to restrict movement of the cervical spine: a systematic review. Eur Spine J 25: 2023, 2016.
156. Genin, GM, et al: The freedom to heal: Nonrigid immobilization by a halo orthosis. J Neurosurg Spine 21:811, 2014.
157. Maruyama, T, et al: Milwaukee brace. Physiother Theory Prac 27:43, 2011.
158. Grivas, TB, and Kaspiris, A: The classical and a modified Boston brace: Description and results. Physiother Theory Pract 27:47, 2011.
159. De Giorgi, S, et al: Cheneau brace for adolescent idiopathic scoliosis: long-term results. Eur Spine J 22:Suppl 6, 2013.
160. Minsk, MK, et al: Effectiveness of the Rigo Cheneau versus Boston-style orthoses for adolescent idiopathic scoliosis: A retrospective study. Scoliosis Spinal Disord, 12:7, 2017.
161. Bohl, DD, et al: Effectiveness of Providence nighttime bracing in patients with adolescent idiopathic scoliosis. Orthopedics, 37: e1085, 2014.
162. Sponseller, PD: Bracing for adolescent idiopathic scoliosis in practice today. J Pediatr Orthop 31:s53, 2011.
163. Matussek, J, et al: Conservative treatment of idiopathic scoliosis with effective braces: Early response to trunk asymmetry may avoid curvature progress. Orthopade 43:689, 2014.
164. Brox, JI, et al: Good brace compliance reduced curve progression and surgical rates in patients with idiopathic scoliosis. Eur Spine J 21:1957, 2012.
165. Stokes, OM, and Luk, KD: The current status of bracing for patients with adolescent idiopathic scoliosis. Bone Joint J 95-B:1308, 2013.
166. Zaina, F, et al: Bracing for scoliosis in 2014: State of the art. Eur J Phys Rehabil Med 50:93, 2014.
167. Zamparo, P, et al: The energy cost of level walking in patients with hemiplegia. Cand J Med Sci Sports, 5:348, 1995.
168. Farmani, F, et al: The effect of different shoes on functional mobility and energy expenditure in post-stroke hemiplegic patients using ankle-foot orthosis. Prosthet Orthot Int 40:591, 2016.
169. Ijmker, T, et al: Effect of balance support on the energy cost of walking after stroke. Arch Phys Med Rehabil 94:Nov 2013.
170. Jeong, YG, et al: A randomized comparison of energy consumption when using different canes, inpatients after stroke. Clin Rehabil 29:129, 2015.
171. Rose, J, et al: Energy expenditure index of walking for normal children and for children with cerebral palsy. Dev Med Child Neurol 32: 333, 1990.
172. van den Hecke, A, et al: Mechanical work, energetic cost, and gait efficiency in children with cerebral palsy. J Pediatr Orthop 27:643, 2007.
173. Piccini, L, et al: Quantification of energy expenditure during gait in children affected by cerebral palsy. Eura Medicophys 43:7, 2007.
174. Suzuki, N, et al: Energy expenditure of diplegic ambulation using flexible plastic ankle foot orthoses. Bull Hosp Jt Dis 59:75, 2000.
175. Huang, CT, et al: Energy cost of ambulation in paraplegic patients using Craig-Scott braces. Arch Phys Med Rehabil 60: 595, 1979.
176. Merkel, KD, et al: Energy expenditure of paraplegic patients standing and walking with two knee-ankle-foot orthoses. Arch Phys Med Rehabil 65:121, 1984.
177. Massucci, M, et al: Walking with the advanced reciprocating gait orthosis (ARGO) in thoracic paraplegic patients: Energy expenditure and cardiorespiratory performance. Spinal Cord 36:223, 1998.
178. Ahmadi Bani, M, et al: The efficiency of mechanical orthoses in affecting parameters associated with daily living in spinal cord injury patients: A literature review. Disabil Rehabil Assist Technol 10:183, 2015.
179. Karimi, MT, and Fatoye, F: Evaluation of the performance of paraplegic subjects during walking with a new design of reciprocating orthosis. Disabil Rehabil Assist Technol 11:72, 2016.
180. Harvey, LA, et al: Energy expenditure during gait using the walkabout and isocentric reciprocal gait orthoses in persons with paraplegia. Arch Phys Med Rehabil 79:945, 1998.
181. Merati, G, et al: Paraplegic adaptation to assisted-walking: Energy expenditure during wheelchair versus orthosis use. Spinal Cord 37:2000.
182. Bowker, DP, et al: Energetics of paraplegic walking. J Biomed Eng 14:344, 1992.
183. Hirokawa, S, et al: Energy expenditure and fatiguability in paraplegic ambulation using reciprocating gait orthosis and electric stimulation. Disabil Rehabil 18:115, 1996.
184. Arazpour, M, et al: The efficiency of orthotic interventions on energy consumption in paraplegic patients: A literature review. Spinal Cord Jan 20, 2015.

Supplemental Readings

Edelstein, JE, and Bruckner, J: Orthotics: A Comprehensive Clinical Approach. Slack, Thorofare, NJ, 2002.
Edelstein, JE, and Moroz, A: Lower-Limb Prosthetics and Orthotics: Clinical Concepts. Slack, Thorofare, NJ , 2011.
Hsu, JD, Michael, JW, and Fisk, JR, (eds): Atlas of Orthoses and Assistive Devices, ed 4. Mosby Elsevier, Philadelphia, 2008.
Lusardi, MM, and Nielsen, CC: Orthotics and Prosthetics in Rehabilitation, ed 2. Saunders, St. Louis, 2007.
Seymour, R: Prosthetics and Orthotics: Lower Limb and Spinal. Lippincott Williams & Wilkins, Philadelphia, 2002.

appendix 30.A Lower Extremity Orthotic Examination Guiding Questions

1. Is the orthosis as prescribed?
2. Can the client don the orthosis easily?

■ STANDING

3. Is the shoe satisfactory and does it fit properly?
4. Are the sole and heel of the shoe flat on the floor?
5. If a shoe insert is used, is there minimal rocking between insert and shoe?

Ankle

6. Do the mechanical ankle joints coincide with the anatomical ankle (anatomical ankle joint axis is approximated by a horizontal line between the malleoli at level of the distal tip of the medial malleolus)?
7. Is there adequate clearance between the anatomical ankle and the mechanical ankle joints?
8. Does the valgus or varus correction strap control the foot position?

Knee

9. Does the mechanical knee joint(s) coincide with the anatomical knee (0.5–0.75 in. [1.2–1.9 cm]) above medial tibial plateau?
10. Is there adequate clearance between the anatomical knee and the mechanical knee joint?
11. Is the knee lock secure and easy to operate?

Shells, Bands, Cuffs, and Uprights

12. Do the shells, bands, cuffs, and uprights conform to the contours of the leg and thigh?
13. Is there adequate clearance between the top of the calf shell or band and the head of the fibula?
14. Is there adequate clearance between the orthosis and the perineum?
15. Is the orthosis below the greater trochanter but at least 1 in. (2.5 cm) higher than the medial shell or upright?
16. Are the uprights at the midline of the leg and thigh?
17. Do the shells, bands, and cuffs conform to the contours of the leg and thigh?
18. Is any flesh roll above the shell or band minimal?
19. Are the bottom of the thigh shell or distal thigh band and the top of the calf shell or band equidistant from the knee?
20. In a child's orthosis, is there adequate provision for lengthening the orthosis?

Weight-Relieving Components

21. In a patellar-tendon-bearing brim, is there adequate relief for the head of the fibula?
22. With a quadrilateral brim, is the client free from excessive pressure in the anteromedial and medial aspect of the brim?
23. With a quadrilateral brim, does the ischial tuberosity rest on the ischial seat?
24. With a patellar-tendon-bearing brim, is there adequate reduction in weight-bearing through the orthosis?

Hip

25. Is the center of the pelvic joint slightly above and ahead of the greater trochanter?
26. Is the hip lock secure and easy to operate?
27. Does the pelvic band fit the torso accurately?

Stability

28. Does the orthosis provide adequate stability to the client?

■ SITTING

29. Can the patient sit comfortably with hips and knees flexed 90°?
30. Can the patient lean forward to touch the shoes?

■ WALKING

31. Is the patient's performance in level walking satisfactory?
32. Is the patient's performance on stairs and ramps satisfactory?
33. Is the orthosis sufficiently rigid?
34. Does the varus or valgus correction strap provide adequate support?
35. Does the orthosis operate quietly?
36. Does the patient consider the orthosis satisfactory as to comfort, function, and appearance?

■ ORTHOSIS OFF THE PATIENT

37. Is the skin free of abrasions or other discolorations attributable to the orthosis?
38. Is the construction satisfactory?
39. Do all components function satisfactorily?

Trunk Orthotic Examination Guiding Questions

appendix **30.B**

TRUNK ORTHOTIC EXAMINATION

1. Is the orthosis as prescribed?
2. Can the client don the orthosis easily?

STANDING

Pelvic Band

3. Does the pelvic band lie flat on the trunk below the posterior superior iliac spines?
4. Does the pelvic band pass between the trochanters and iliac crests?

Thoracic Band

5. Does the thoracic band lie flat on the trunk below the scapulae?
6. Does the thoracic band lie horizontally on the trunk?

Uprights

7. Do the posterior uprights avoid pressure on bony prominences, such as the vertebral spines or scapulae?
8. Do the lateral uprights extend along the lateral midlines of the trunk?

Abdominal Front

9. Is the abdominal front of adequate size?

Cervical Orthosis

10. Is the head in the prescribed position?
11. Do all rigid components fit properly?

SITTING

12. Can the patient sit comfortably with the hips and knees flexed 90°?
13. Does the patient consider the orthosis satisfactory as to comfort, function, and appearance?

ORTHOSIS OFF THE PATIENT

14. Is the skin free of abrasions or other discolorations attributable to the orthosis?
15. Is the construction satisfactory?
16. Do all components function satisfactorily?

appendix

30.C Internet Resources

Organization/Resource	Website
American Academy of Orthotists and Prosthetists	www.oandp.org
American Orthotic and Prosthetic Association	www.aopanet.org
Digital Resource Foundation for the Orthotics and Prosthetics Community	www.drfop.org
Orthotic and Prosthetic Activities Foundation	www.opfund.org
Orthotic and Prosthetic Education and Research Foundation	www.operf.org/research
The O&P Edge: Resource for Orthotics and Prosthetics Information	www.oandp.com

Prosthetics

Christopher Kevin Wong, PT, PhD, OCS
Joan E. Edelstein, PT, MA, FISPO

Chapter 31

LEARNING OBJECTIVES

1. Describe the components of transtibial and transfemoral prostheses, including advantages and disadvantages of alternative components and materials.
2. Explain the distinctive features of partial foot, Syme's, knee and hip disarticulation prostheses, and bilateral prostheses.
3. Outline the maintenance program for prosthetic components.
4. Conduct static and dynamic evaluation of transtibial and transfemoral prostheses.
5. Summarize the physical therapist's role in management of individuals with lower-limb amputation.
6. Analyze and interpret patient data, formulate realistic goals and outcomes, and develop a plan of care when presented with a clinical case study.

CHAPTER OUTLINE

Physical therapists play an important role in the care of individuals with lower- and upper-limb amputations. To replace the absent part of the leg or arm, patients are often fitted with a *prosthesis*. In the broadest sense, prostheses also include dentures, titanium femoral heads, and plastic heart valves. A *prosthetist* is a health care professional that designs, fabricates, and fits limb prostheses.

The major causes of amputation are peripheral vascular disease, trauma, malignancy, and congenital deficiency. In the United States, vascular disease accounts for most leg amputations, particularly among patients with diabetes.[1] Individuals older than 60 constitute the largest group of people with amputation. Men are more likely to sustain amputation because of vascular disease and trauma. Among younger adults and adolescents, trauma is responsible for most amputations. Bone and soft tissue tumors are sometimes treated by amputation, with adolescence the period of peak incidence. *Congenital deficiency* refers to the absence or abnormality of a limb evident at birth.

This chapter focuses on the lower limb (LL) because many more people have lost a portion of the LL, as compared with the upper limb (UL). Physical therapists are key members of the rehabilitation team, working with prosthetists, physicians, occupational therapists, and others to foster the patient's welfare. For individuals with LL amputation, physical therapists have the major role in assisting the person to regain function. LL prostheses will be described, together with a program for training patients in their use. For patients with UL amputation, physical therapists may play a lesser role, cooperating with occupational therapists, depending on the administrative organization of the health care facility.

Historic records confirm that the concept of replacing a missing limb is very old. A forked stick forming a peg leg to support a transtibial (below-knee) amputation limb was known in antiquity. Today, most individuals with LL amputation are provided with a prosthesis because function with one LL can be limited compared with two.

The principal LL prostheses are partial foot, Syme's, transtibial, and transfemoral as well as knee and hip disarticulations. The physical therapist should be familiar with their characteristics and maintenance, as well as the rehabilitation of patients fitted with these devices.

PARTIAL FOOT AND SYME'S PROSTHESES

The purposes of partial foot prostheses are to (1) restore as much foot function as possible, particularly in walking, and (2) simulate the shape of the missing foot segment. The patient who has lost one or more toes may simply pad the toe section of the shoe to improve the appearance of the upper portion of the shoe. Standing will not be affected, assuming the metatarsal heads remain. When the individual walks, late stance will be less forceful, particularly if both phalanges of the great toe are absent. An arch support foot orthosis helps to maintain alignment of the amputated foot, especially if one or more proximal phalanges have been amputated.[2]

Transmetatarsal amputation disturbs foot appearance more noticeably. A prosthesis prevents the shoe from developing an unnatural crease in the forefoot area. The patient bears most weight on the heel and reduces the amount of time spent on the affected foot during walking. A particularly useful prosthesis consists of a plastic socket for the remainder of the foot. The socket is affixed to a rigid plate that extends the full length of the inner sole of the shoe. The plate has a cosmetic toe filler. The socket protects the amputated ends of the metatarsals, while the rigid plate restores foot length so that the person can spend more time during the stance phase of gait on the affected side than would otherwise be the case. To aid late stance, the bottom of the prosthesis or the sole of the shoe may have a convex rocker bar.[3]

Amputation or disarticulation through the tarsals, such as Lisfranc and Chopart disarticulations,[4] poses the additional problem of retaining the small foot segment in the shoe during swing phase. Foot length is apt to be diminished further by an equinus deformity of the amputated limb, resulting from unbalanced contraction of the triceps surae. Consequently, the prosthesis described for the transmetatarsal amputation may be augmented with a plastic calf shell, which is strapped around the leg.[5,6]

Syme's amputation is essentially removal of the entire foot except the calcaneal fat pad, with an ankle disarticulation, including surgical sectioning through the distal tibia and fibula to leave a flat distal weight-bearing surface. The patient can usually bear significant weight through the distal end of the amputation limb.[7,8] The socket trimlines (edges) form a brim into which the amputation limb enters the socket. The socket has a relief (concavity) for the tibial crest. If the distal end of the Syme's amputation limb is markedly bulbous, the distal part of the medial wall can be made removable to facilitate donning the socket and later fastened in place with a strap (Fig. 31.1). If the amputation limb has relatively vertical contours, a removable socket section is not needed; instead, a resilient liner that assists entry of the bulbous distal end of the limb while maintaining suspension is employed. The prosthesis includes a low-profile foot specifically designed to accommodate the long socket (Fig. 31.2). The Syme's prosthesis is suspended by the contour of its brims and socket walls, without other suspension mechanisms.

TRANSTIBIAL PROSTHESES

The *transtibial level,* also known as *below-knee,* refers to an amputation in which the tibia and fibula are transected. The patient retains the anatomical knee with its motor and sensory functions. This is the predominant

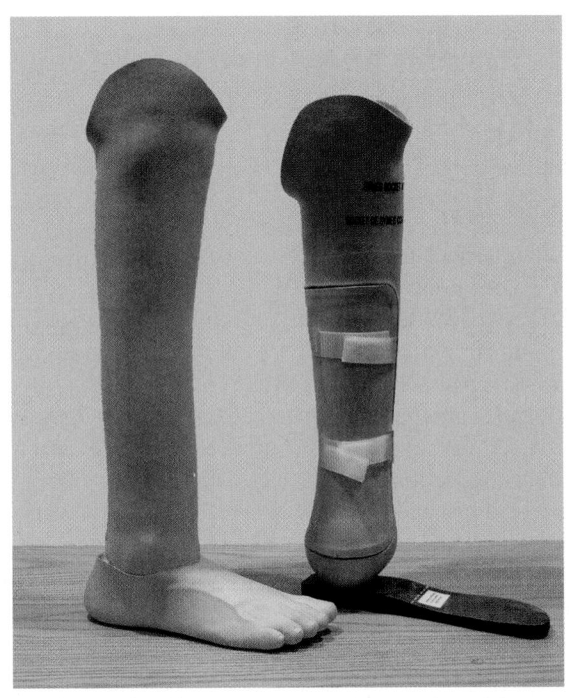

Figure 31.1 Syme's prostheses. (*Left*) Socket with medial opening. (*Right*) Socket with continuous walls and flexible liner.

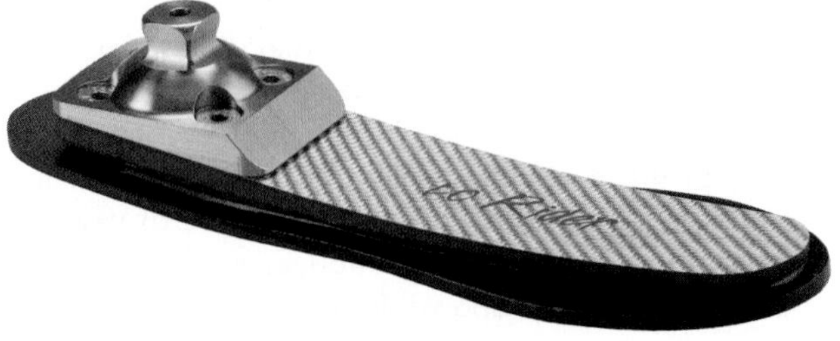

Figure 31.2 Lo Rider foot for Syme's prosthesis. *(Courtesy of Otto Bock, Minneapolis, MN 55447.)*

site of amputation, particularly for individuals with vascular disease.[9] Prostheses for transtibial amputations include a foot–ankle assembly, a shank (lower leg), a socket, and a suspension component.

Foot–Ankle Assemblies

A foot–ankle assembly restores the general contour of the patient's foot, absorbs shock at heel contact, plantar flexes in early stance, and simulates metatarsophalangeal extension (toe-break action) in the latter part of stance phase; patients appear to prefer a foot with a relatively rigid forefoot.[10] The foot is in the neutral position during swing phase. In response to ground reaction forces, many assemblies provide slight motion in the frontal and/or transverse planes to approximate physiological foot motion.[11-15] Rubber encases the stiff inner portion called the *keel,* made of wood, high-temperature plastic, metal, or carbon fiber.

Nonarticulated Feet

In the United States, the most popular foot type is nonarticulated, without a joint between the foot and lower portion of the shank. As compared with articulated feet, nonarticulated components are lighter in weight and more durable; some versions are made for high-heeled shoes.

SACH Foot

The nonarticulated *solid ankle cushion heel (SACH)* assembly is commonly available around the world (Fig 31.3). The keel is wooden or metal and terminates at a point corresponding to the metatarsophalangeal joints. The keel is encased in rubber; the posterior portion is resilient, to absorb shock and permit plantarflexion in early stance. Foot extension in late stance is allowed at the junction of the rubber toe section and the keel. The SACH foot is manufactured in a wide range of sizes to accommodate infants, adolescents, and adults. The SACH foot is available with heel cushions of varying degrees of compressibility for people who place different amounts of force through the heel. SACH feet can be ordered in several plantarflexion angles to fit shoes with diverse heel heights. The heel cushion allows a negligible amount of medial–lateral and transverse motion. Most nonarticulated foot designs also have rigid ankle blocks and stiff keels of different materials surrounded by rubber, though newer materials may provide more flexibility (Fig 31.4)

Feet made with materials that bend slightly under the force of weight-bearing as the wearer moves over the foot during midstance before recoiling in late stance as the wearer transfers loading to the opposite foot are described as *energy storing* or *dynamic feet.* The *Flex-Foot* (Fig. 31.5) and feet of similar manufacture include a long length of carbon fiber, extending from the toe to the proximal shank. The long carbon fiber length acts as

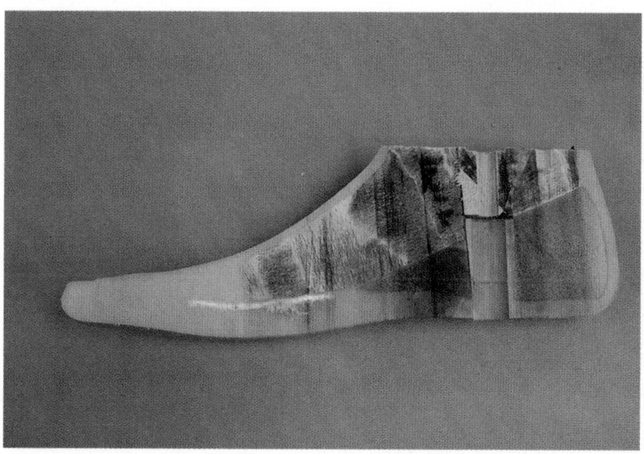

Figure 31.3 Cross section of a SACH nonarticulated foot–ankle assembly.

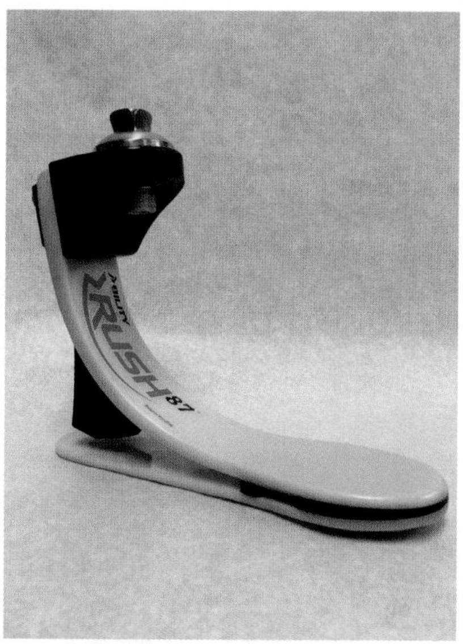

Figure 31.4 The Rush foot made of glass composite.

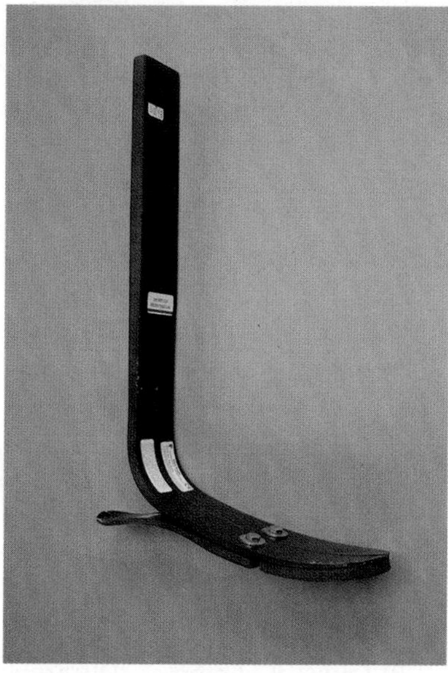

Figure 31.5 Flex-Foot posterior leaf spring.

a leaf spring, enabling the foot to store considerable energy in early and midstance, and then to release energy in the late stance phase of gait. A posterior heel length is optional. Active wearers, such as those who play basketball, run, or engage in other high-impact activities, can best utilize the energy-storing and energy-releasing capacity of these feet (Fig. 31.6A, 6D). Other energy-storing prosthetic feet, all more expensive than SACH feet, are shown in Figure 31.6. The anterior keel can be split into two to allow different degrees of bending on the medial or lateral keel and thus provide some frontal plane motion (Fig. 31.6A, 6C, 6D, 6F). Many of these feet can be sheathed in a cosmetic cover (Fig. 31.7). Athletes may opt to interchange the basic prosthetic foot for one designed for sprinting (Fig. 31.8).

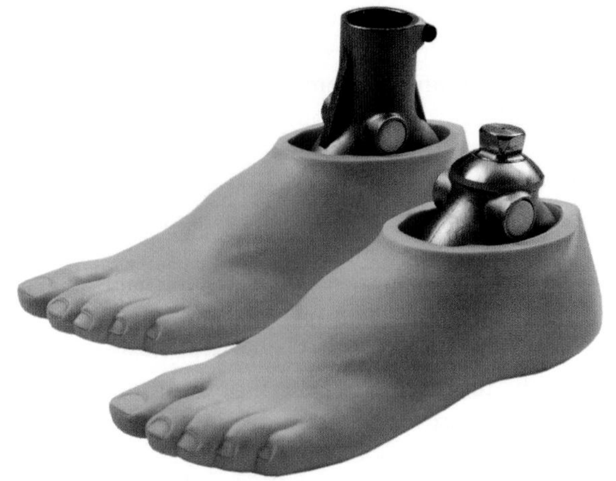

Figure 31.7 Cosmetic foot covers. *(Courtesy of Ossur, Aliso Viejo, CA 92656.)*

Articulated Feet

Manufactured with separate foot and lower shank sections, articulated feet have the sections joined by an ankle component. Rubber bumpers usually control the ease of foot motion. Articulated feet are subject to eventual loosening, which may be signaled by a squeaking noise.

Single-Axis Feet

The most common example of an articulated foot is the *single-axis foot* (Fig. 31.9). A posterior bumper absorbs shock and controls plantarflexion excursion; it is easy for the prosthetist to substitute a firmer or softer bumper, depending on the force that the patient applies in early stance. A heavy or very active client requires a firm bumper, whereas a frail individual needs a bumper that is soft enough to permit the foot to plantarflex with minimal loading. At early stance, bearing weight on the heel causes

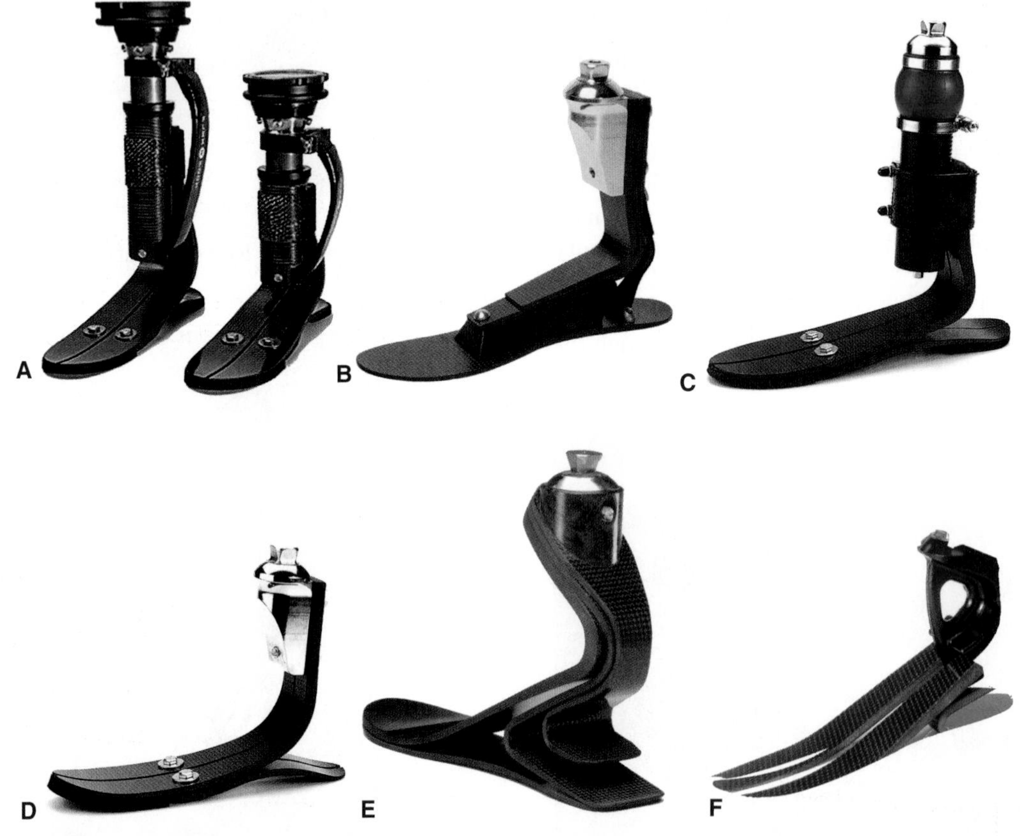

Figure 31.6 Nonarticulated energy-storing prosthetic feet. (A) Re-Flex VSP® and Re-Flex VSP Low Profile®. (B) Talux®. (C) Ceterus®. (D) Vari-Flex®. *(Courtesy of Ossur, Aliso Viejo, CA, 92656.)* (E) Renegade. (F) ELITE 2®. *(Courtesy of Endolite, Miamisburg, OH 45342.)*

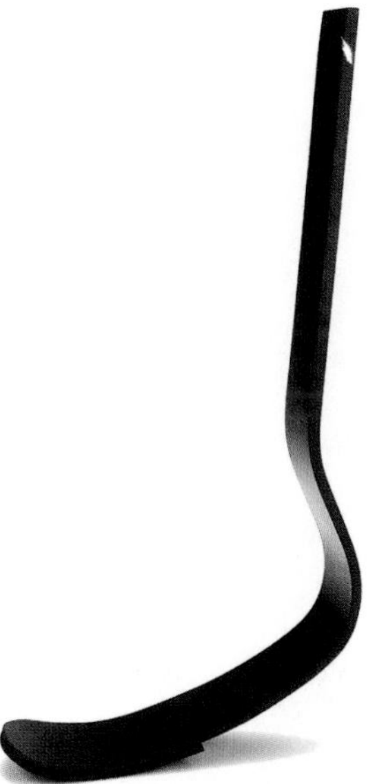

Figure 31.8 Flex-Foot Cheetah®. *(Courtesy of Ossur, Aliso Viejo, CA 92656.)*

the foot to plantarflex, ensuring that the wearer achieves the stable foot-flat position. An anterior bumper resists dorsiflexion and absorbs force as the wearer transfers weight forward over the foot. The total amount of dorsiflexion–plantarflexion motion provided by an articulated ankle (20 to 25 degrees) is roughly double that provided by a nonarticulated ankle (11 to 14 degrees) but does not approach the anatomical movement.[16] The single-axis foot does not allow medial–lateral or transverse motion. Some people prefer this simplicity of control.

Multiple-Axis Feet

These components move slightly in all planes to aid the wearer in maintaining maximum contact with the walking surface, even if the surface slopes or has slight irregularities (Fig. 31.10). Multiple-axis feet are heavier and less durable than single-axis or nonarticulated feet. A recent version of multiple-axis foot is the ProprioFoot® (Fig. 31.11), which includes electronic sensors to detect when the wearer needs dorsiflexion; it also provides greater ankle excursion than other foot–ankle assemblies and reduces pressure on the amputation limb.[17,18]

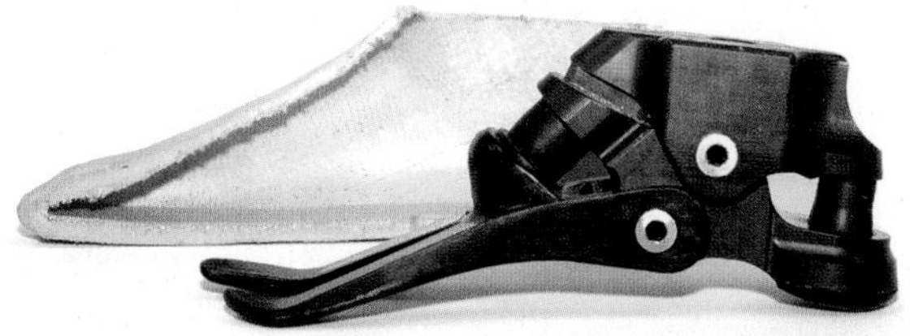

Figure 31.10 Multiple axis foot with cosmetic cover cross section.

Selection of the appropriate foot is based on the needs of the individual, considering the wearer's activity level, weight, level of amputation, and the length and shape of the residual limb. The patient may also benefit from a rotator and a vertical shock absorber.

Rotators and Shock Absorbers

A rotator is a component placed above the prosthetic foot to absorb shear stress in the transverse plane. A shock absorber reduces vertical impact. These components protect the user from skin chafing, which would otherwise occur if the socket were permitted to slide against the skin.[19,20] Rotators and shock absorbers are most often used with single-axis feet and by very active individuals, especially those with transfemoral amputations. A rotator with or without a shock absorber may be contained within a prosthetic foot, such as Ceterus® (see Fig. 31.6C), or may be installed in the shank, such as the Delta Twist® (Otto Bock, Minneapolis, MN 55447) (Fig. 31.12) to provide

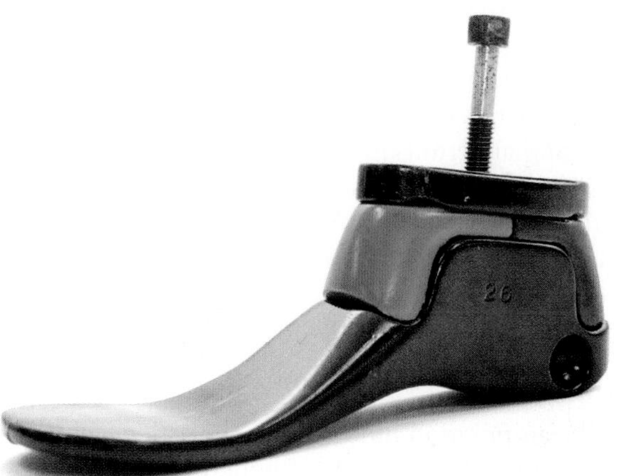

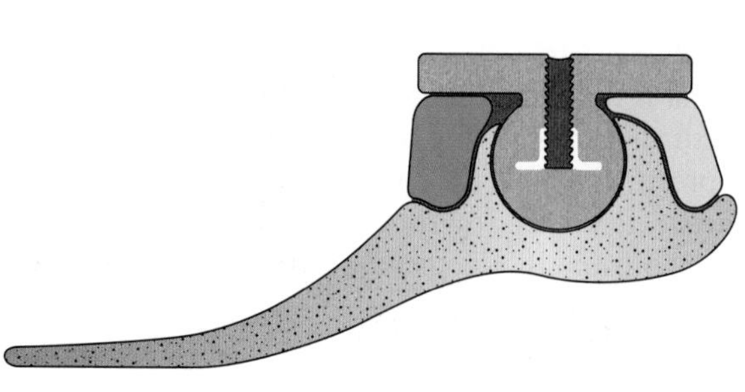

Figure 31.9 Single-axis foot with cross section view; anterior bumper controls dorsiflexion, posterior bumper controls plantar flexion.

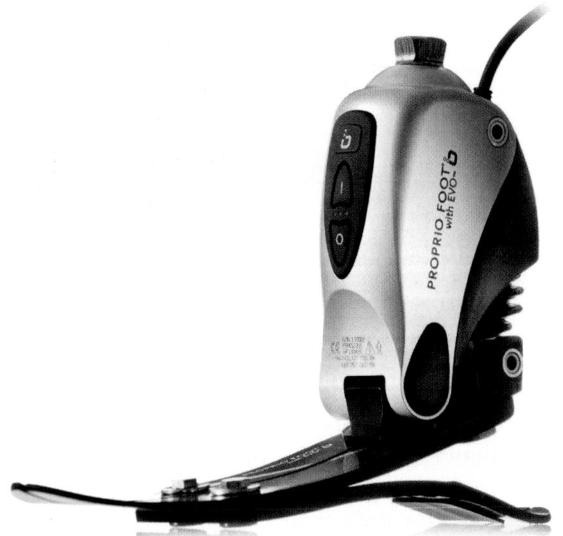

Figure 31.11 ProprioFoot®. *(Courtesy of Ossur, Aliso Viejo, CA 92656.)*

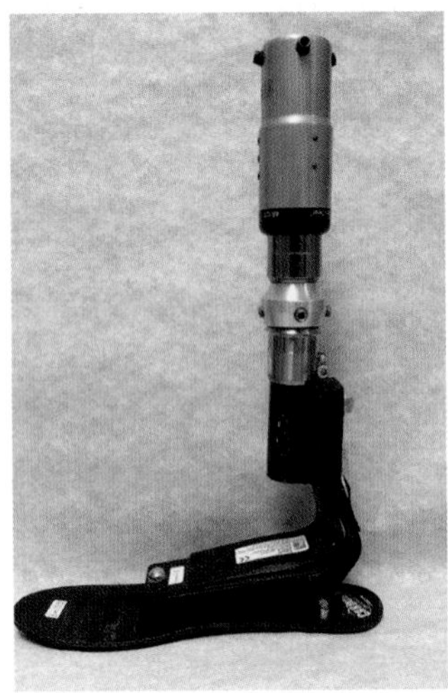

Figure 31.12 Delta Twist® torsion adapting.

transverse plane motion. Though motion is minimal, enhanced comfort during gait can result.[21]

Shanks

The shank is the substitute for the human leg, restoring leg length and transmitting body weight from the socket to the prosthetic foot. The shank is located between the foot–ankle assembly (or rotator) and the socket in a transtibial prosthesis. The two types of shank are *exoskeletal* and *endoskeletal.*

Exoskeletal Shank

The *exoskeletal shank* (Fig. 31.13), sometimes called *crustacean,* is typically made of rigid plastic (older versions are made of wood). The rigid exterior is shaped to simulate the contour of the anatomic leg. Although the shank is usually finished with plastic tinted to match the wearer's skin color, some individuals opt for a multicolored or patterned shank. The exoskeletal shank is very durable and, with the plastic finish, is impervious to liquids. Because they are less lifelike and do not permit changes in alignment of the prosthesis, exoskeletal shanks are less frequently prescribed.

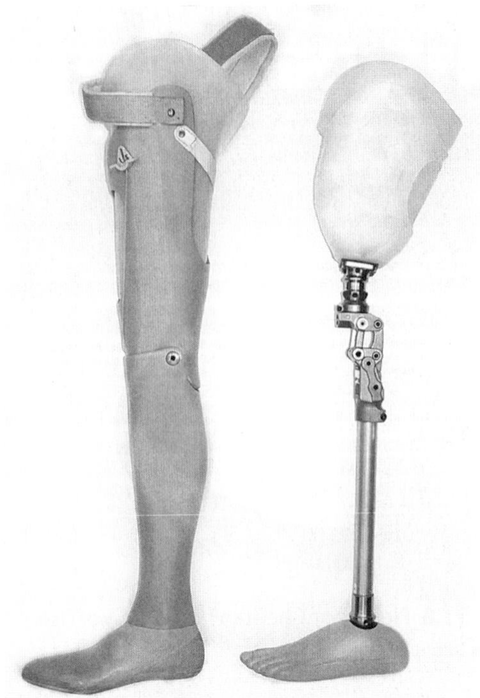

Figure 31.13 (*Left*) Exoskeletal transfemoral prosthesis. (*Right*) Endoskeletal transfemoral prosthesis with cosmetic foam cover removed.

Endoskeletal Shank

The *endoskeletal* (Fig. 31.14), or *modular shank,* consists of a central aluminum or rigid plastic tube (called a *pylon*) usually covered with foam rubber and a sturdy stocking or similar finish. With its cover, the endoskeletal shank is more natural in appearance than the shiny exoskeletal shank. In addition, the pylon has a mechanism that permits making slight adjustment of the alignment of the prosthesis; this may contribute to comfort and ease of walking. A variety of prosthetic foot–ankle assemblies, such as the Flex-Foot®, incorporate an endoskeletal shank. Some patients wear prostheses without a cover over the pylon.

Sockets

The amputation limb fits into a plastic receptacle called the *socket* (Fig. 31.15). Although the original name for the modern transtibial socket was the *patellar-tendon-bearing (PTB)* socket, sockets contact all portions of the amputated limb for maximum distribution of load,

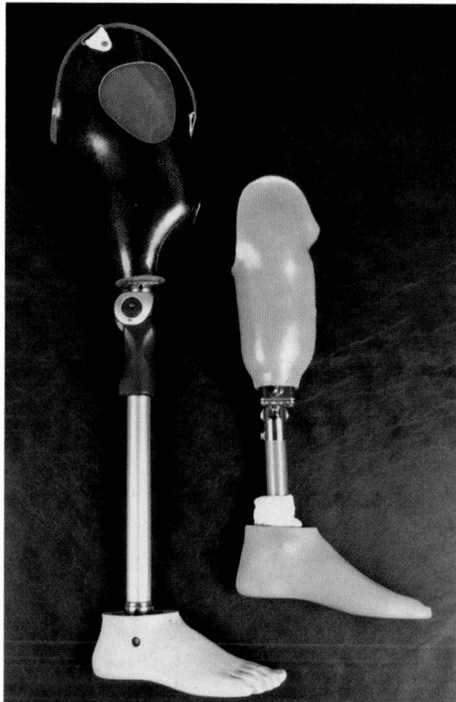

Figure 31.14 Endoskeletal (modular) shank on (*left*) transfemoral prosthesis and on (*right*) transtibial prosthesis. *(From Roy, SH, Wolf, SL, and Scalzitti, DA: The Rehabilitation Specialist's Handbook, ed 4. FA Davis, Philadelphia, 2013, p. 953, with permission.)*

optimal venous blood circulation, and tactile feedback. The PTB socket features a prominent indentation over the patellar ligament, sometimes known as the *patellar tendon.* A newer socket variation is *total surface bearing,* which has a shallower anterior indentation.[22]

Sockets are custom-made of plastic molded over a model of the patient's amputation limb. The model may be produced from a plaster cast of the amputation limb or by *computer-aided design/computer-aided manufacture.* The latter involves an electronic sensor, which transmits a detailed map of the limb to a computerized program consisting of socket-shape variations; the prosthetist selects the appropriate shape, which is transmitted to an electronic carver that creates the model over which the plastic is shaped. Whether the model is made by hand or by computer, it provides *reliefs,* which are concavities in the socket over sensitive structures, such as bony prominences (Fig. 31.16). Reliefs are located over the fibular head, tibial crest, tibial condyles, and anterior–distal tibia. The posterior socket trimline or *brim* is shaped to provide adequate room and thus comfort for the medial and lateral hamstring tendons when the person bends the knee to, for instance, sit. *Build-ups* are convexities in the socket over areas contacting pressure-tolerant tissues, such as the belly of the gastrocnemius; patellar ligament; proximomedial tibia, corresponding to the pes anserinus; and the tibial and fibular shafts.

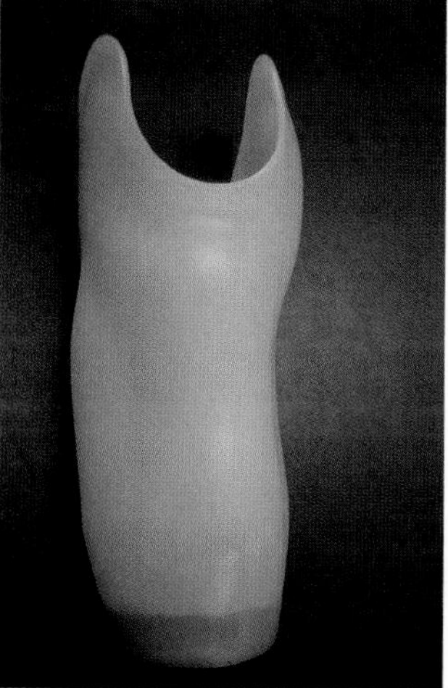

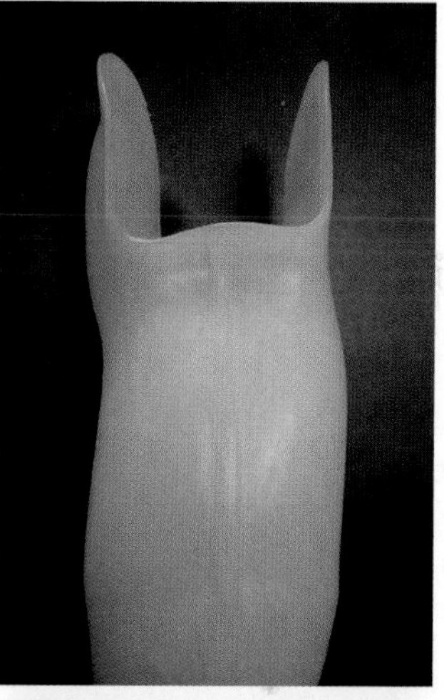

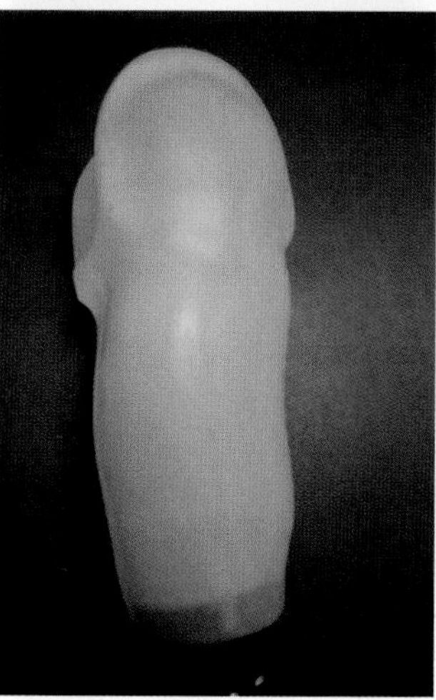

Figure 31.15 Transtibial patellar tendon-bearing socket from three directions.

When viewed from above, the socket resembles a triangle, the apex of which is formed by the relief for the tibial tubercle and crest, and the base angles of which are the hamstring reliefs. The anterior wall terminates at the mid-patella or above. The medial and lateral walls extend at least to the femoral epicondyles. The posterior wall lies across the popliteal fossa.

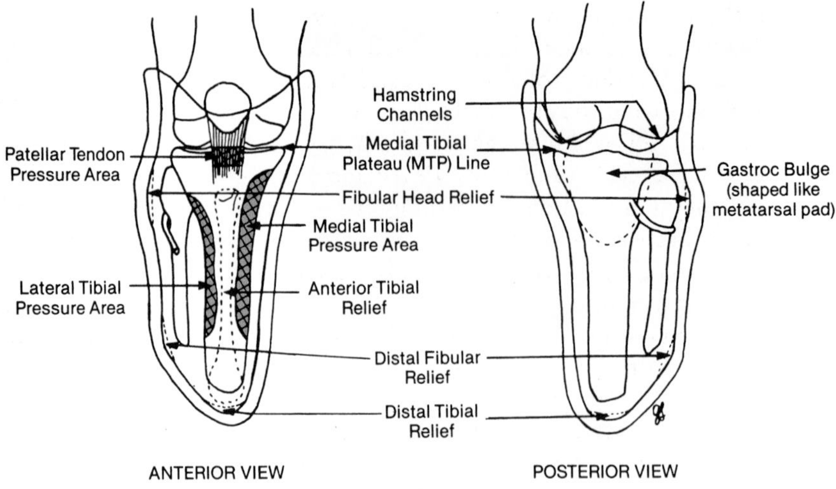

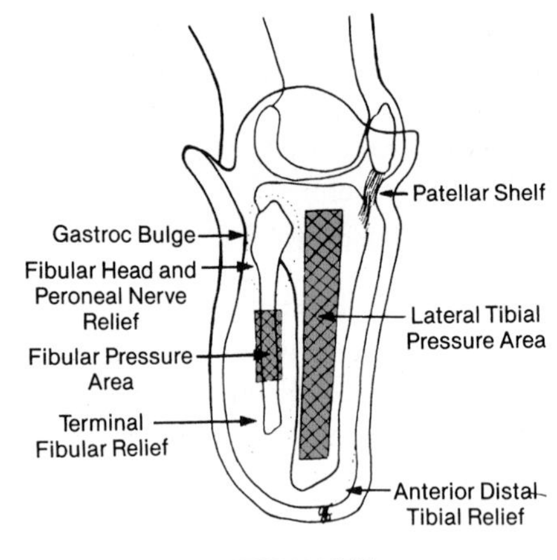

Figure 31.16 Transtibial patellar tendon-bearing socket. Areas of relief (also called *channels*) over pressure-sensitive tissues. Buildups (also called *bulges*) contact pressure-tolerant tissues. *(From Sanders, GT: Lower Limb Amputations: A Guide to Rehabilitation. FA Davis, Philadelphia, 1986, p. 176, with permission.)*

The socket is aligned on the shank in slight flexion to enhance loading on the patellar ligament, prevent genu recurvatum, and resist the tendency of the amputation limb to slide too deeply into the socket. Flexion also facilitates contraction of the quadriceps muscle. The socket is also aligned with a slight lateral tilt to reduce loading on the fibular head.[23,24]

Lined Socket

The transtibial socket generally includes a resilient liner, made of polyethylene foam,[25] polyurethane,[26] silicone,[27] or similar materials. In addition to cushioning the amputation limb, the removable liner facilitates alteration of socket size; the prosthetist can add material to the outside of the liner, reducing the volume of the socket while preserving smooth interior contours. The liner, however, adds to the bulk of the prosthesis and is a heat insulator, which the wearer may find uncomfortable in hot weather. Individuals with Syme's and transtibial amputations usually wear cotton, wool, or synthetic fabric socks to ensure a snug socket fit. An alternative to the polyethylene liner is a sheath made of silicone or similar material, which fits so snugly that the wearer has little risk of abrasion between the socket and skin.

Socks, Sheaths, and Liners

All individuals with LL amputations, except those wearing transfemoral prostheses suspended by total suction or those using a sheath, require a supply of clean socks of appropriate material, size, and shape. It is expeditious to order at least a dozen socks at the time the prosthesis is prescribed, so that third-party payment may cover this relatively inexpensive but important accessory.

Fabric socks are woven in various thicknesses, referred to as *ply,* designating the number of threads knitted together. Cotton socks absorb perspiration readily and are the least allergenic; they are made in two-, three-, and five-ply, the last being the thickest. Wool socks provide good cushioning, woven in three- and five-ply; they are expensive and must be laundered carefully. Orlon/Lycra socks are manufactured in two- and three-ply thicknesses. They can be washed easily without shrinking. This synthetic fabric combination affords considerable resilience but does not absorb much perspiration.

A nylon sheath creates a smooth surface over the skin, thereby reducing the risk of chafing, especially in hot weather and among those with much scarring. Some transtibial prosthesis wearers are able to use a woman's knee-high nylon stocking if the amputated limb is slender. Because nylon does not absorb sweat, liquid passes through the weave to be absorbed by an outer sock of cotton or wool. Silicone, urethane, and other synthetic sheaths provide excellent shock absorption and abrasion resistance; they also can aid in suspending the socket on the patient's limb and are designed to be worn next to the skin. They are, however, more expensive than fabric socks or sheaths.

It is common practice to add more socks as the amputation limb volume reduces. Nevertheless, when the patient requires socks equaling 15 ply to achieve snug fit, the socket should be altered or replaced by the prosthetist. Excessive sock padding distorts the weight-bearing characteristics of the socket, losing the effect of strategically placed buildups and reliefs.

Regardless of material, the shape of the sock or sheath is important for comfort. An interface of proper size fits smoothly without wrinkling or undue stretching. The sock or sheath should be long enough to terminate above the most proximal part of the socket.

Silicone gel suspension liners are another form of socket-residual limb interface. These liners cushion the residual limb and function as a primary or secondary suspension system. Some include a fabric outer cover with liner thickness tapering distally and may be indicated for particularly active users and those with fragile or sensitive residual limbs. They are available in both locking (Fig. 31.17) and seal-in designs that use a flexible rubber ring to form a hypobaric suction seal.

Suspension

During the swing phase of walking, or whenever the wearer is not standing on the prosthesis, such as when climbing stairs or jumping, the prosthesis requires some form of suspension to hold it in place.

Cuff Variants

The modern transtibial prosthesis originated with a supracondylar cuff (Fig 31.18), which is still widely used. The cuff may be a leather, flexible plastic, or fabric-webbing strap. It encircles the thigh immediately above the femoral epicondyles and permits the user to easily adjust the snugness of suspension. Some individuals, however, object to the profile of the distal thigh created by the cuff. Others who have severely arthritic hands or limited vision have difficulty engaging the buckle or pressure hook-and-loop closure on the cuff (see Fig. 31.18).

A fork strap and waist belt may be used to augment the cuff. The elastic fork strap extends from the outside of the anterior portion of the socket to a waist belt. The fork strap and waist belt may be indicated for individuals who climb ladders or engage in other activities during which the prosthesis is unsupported by the ground for long periods. An alternative to the cuff is a rubber sleeve, a tubular component that covers the proximal socket and the distal thigh (Fig. 31.19). The sleeve provides excellent suspension and a streamlined silhouette when the wearer sits. Donning the sleeve, however, requires two strong hands and a thigh that does not have excessive subcutaneous tissue.

Distal Attachments

Very secure suspension is achieved with the use of a silicone sheath with a distal metal pin (Fig. 31.20). The sheath clings to the skin. The user inserts the sheathed limb into the prosthesis, guiding the attached pin into the shuttle lock located at the bottom of the

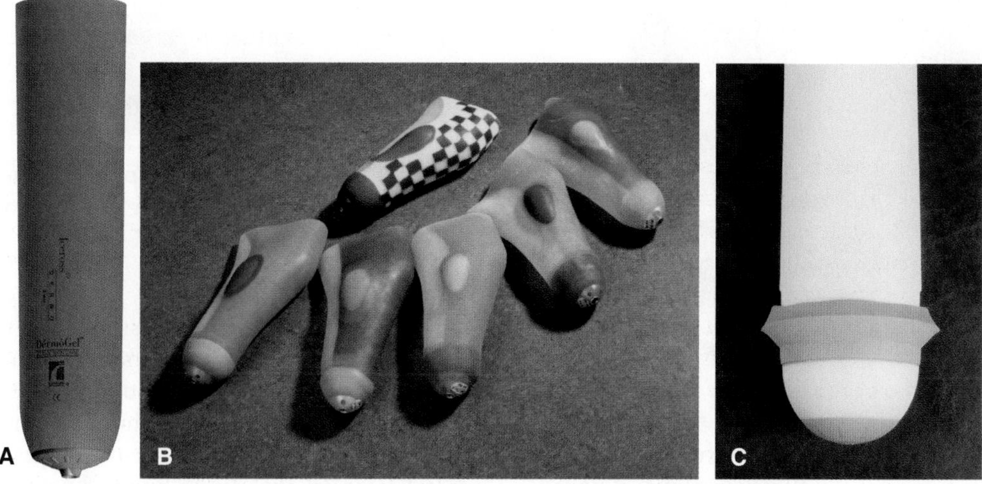

Figure 31.17 Silicone liners: (A) Iceross® Dermo locking silicone gel liner. *(Courtesy of Ossur, Aliso Viejo, CA 92656.)* (B) Custom liners with fibular head padding. *(Courtesy of Otto Bock, Minneapolis, MN 55447.)* (C) Seal-in designs. *(From Roy, SH, Wolf SL, and Scalzitti, DA: The Rehabilitation Specialist's Handbook, ed 4. FA Davis, Philadelphia, 2013, p. 977, with permission.)*

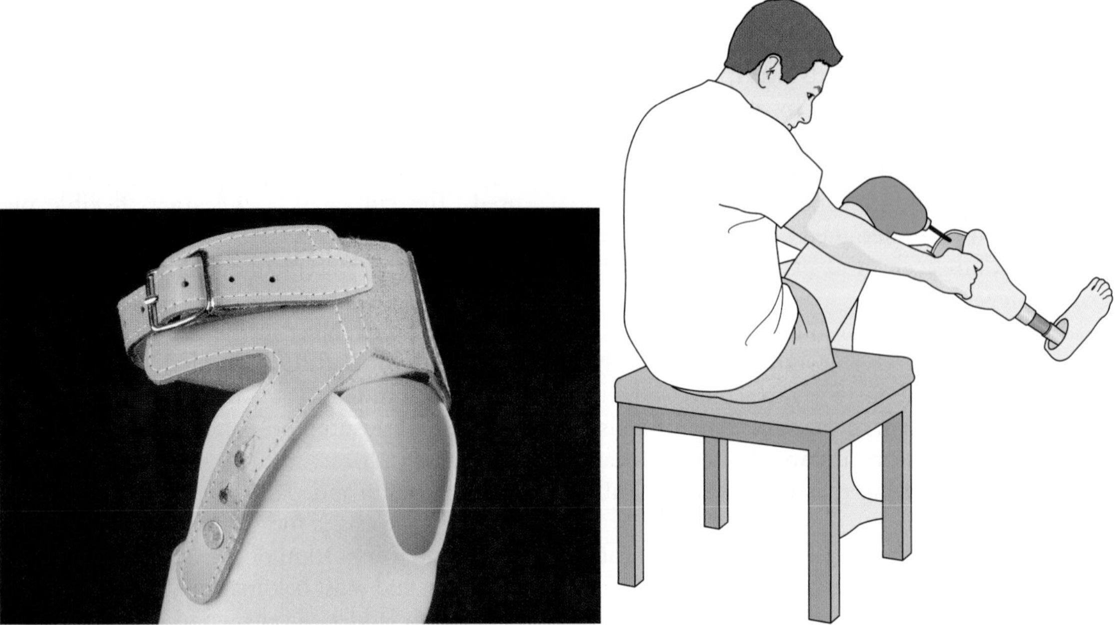

Figure 31.18 (*Left*) Supracondylar cuff suspension for transtibial prostheses. *(From Roy, SH, Wolf, SL, and Scalzitti, DA: The Rehabilitation Specialist's Handbook, ed 4. FA Davis, Philadelphia, 2013, p. 977, with permission.)* (*Right*) Patient donning a transtibial prosthesis using a roll-on sleeve that includes a pin and shuttle lock assembly.

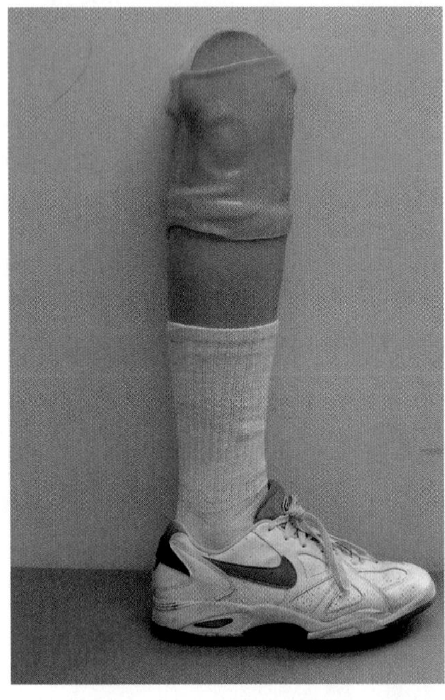

Figure 31.19 Transtibial suspension sleeve. Note round relief for fibular head.

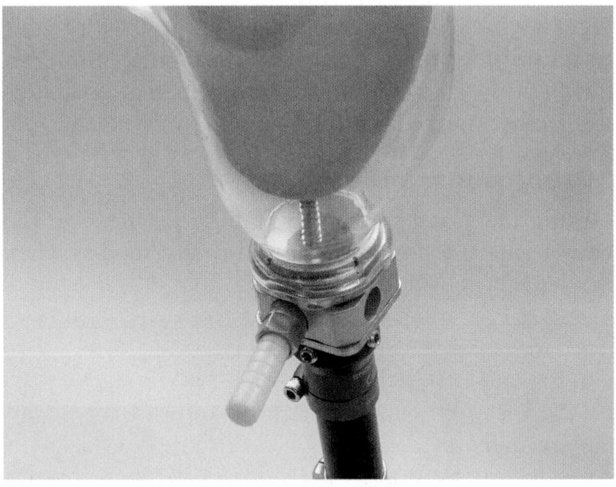

Figure 31.20 Transtibial distal pin attachment. The pin fits into a receptacle in the socket bottom and is then tightened into place.

socket (see Fig. 31.18 Right) During swing phase, the pin mechanism prevents the prosthesis from slipping.

Vacuum-assisted suspension is another alternative mode of suspension (Fig. 31.21). The system combines a pump, liner, and sleeve to achieve elevated vacuum in an airtight environment. Vacuum promotes fluid exchange, reduces moisture buildup, regulates volume fluctuations, and increases proprioceptive awareness of the limb's position in space.

A surgical approach to distal attachment is known as *osseointegration,*[28] in which the surgeon implants a metal post in the distal bone. The post protrudes through the skin and locks into a mechanism in the prosthesis. Osseointegration eliminates the need for other suspension apparatus; however, fluid drainage and infection at the skin/post interface are sometimes

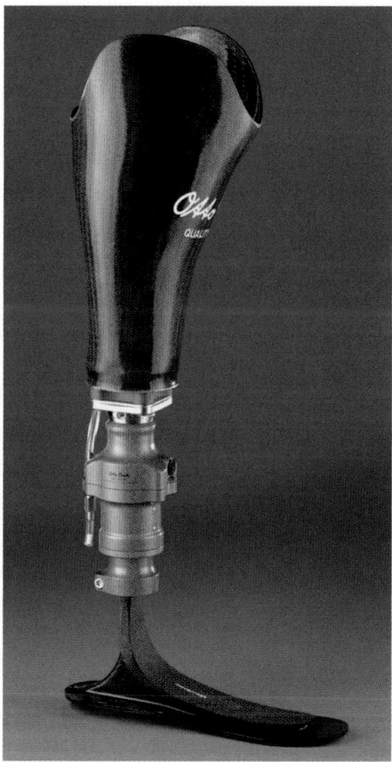

Figure 31.21 Harmony® Volume Management System. *(Courtesy of Otto Bock, Minneapolis, MN 55447.)*

troublesome. The procedure was developed in Europe and was approved in the United States in 2016.

Brim Variants

The socket walls may be extended proximally to suspend the prosthesis. With *supracondylar (SC) suspension* (see Fig. 31.18), the medial and lateral walls extend above the femoral epicondyles. When donning the prosthesis, the patient applies the liner and then inserts the limb with the liner into the socket. Supracondylar suspension may increase medial–lateral stability of the knee.

Presenting a contour of medial and lateral walls similar to the supracondylar suspension, the supracondylar/suprapatellar (SC/SP) suspension (Fig. 31.22) also features an anterior wall that terminates above the patella. The short amputated limb is well accommodated by SC/SP suspension. The high anterior wall may interfere with kneeling and presents a conspicuous contour when the wearer sits.

Thigh Corset

Some individuals with very sensitive skin, unusual limb contours, or very short limb length may benefit from thigh corset suspension (Fig. 31.23). Metal hinges attach distally to the medial and lateral aspects of the socket and proximally to a leather or flexible plastic corset. Corset heights vary and may reach the ischial tuberosity for maximum weight relief on the amputation limb. The hinges increase frontal plane knee stability, and the corset increases area for weight-bearing load distribution.

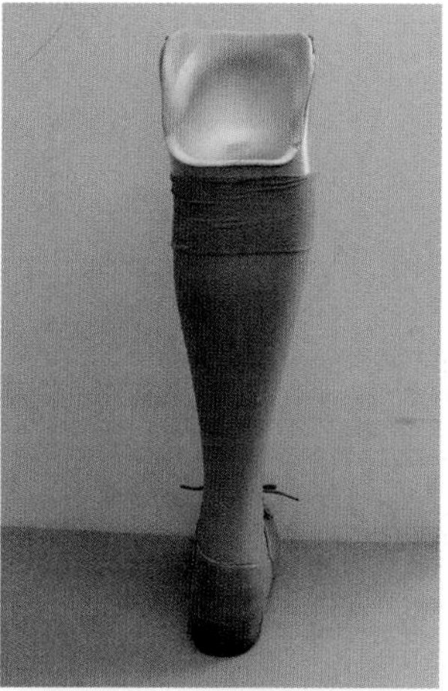

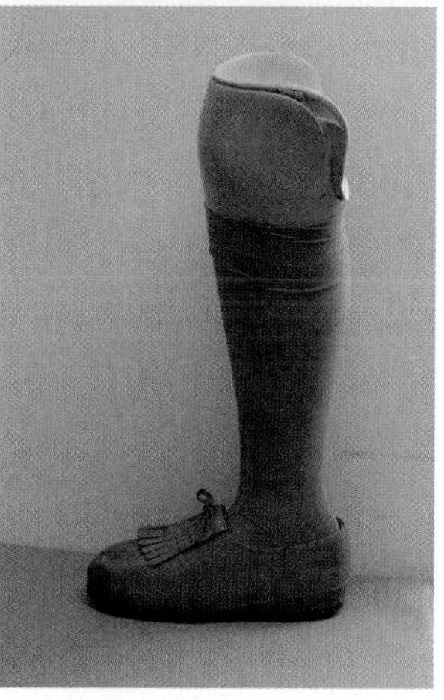

Figure 31.22 Transtibial prosthesis with supracondylar/suprapatellar (SC/SP) suspension with posterior and lateral views.

The resulting prosthesis, however, is heavier and apt to foster piston action because the hinges have a single pivot joint that does not articulate collinearly with the anatomical knee. Prolonged use of a thigh corset produces pressure atrophy of the thigh. A prosthesis with corset suspension is more difficult to don because the wearer must fasten laces or a series of pressure-closure hook-and-loop straps.

■ TRANSFEMORAL PROSTHESES

Individuals with amputation between the femoral epicondyles and greater trochanter are fitted with transfemoral (above-knee) prostheses. Those whose limbs retain the distal part of the femur can wear a knee disarticulation prosthesis, which differs from the transfemoral prosthesis in the type of knee unit and socket. If the amputation is proximal to the greater trochanter, the patient cannot retain or control a transfemoral prosthesis and is therefore a candidate for a hip disarticulation prosthesis. The transfemoral prosthesis consists of (1) foot–ankle assembly, (2) shank, (3) knee unit, (4) socket, and (5) suspension device.

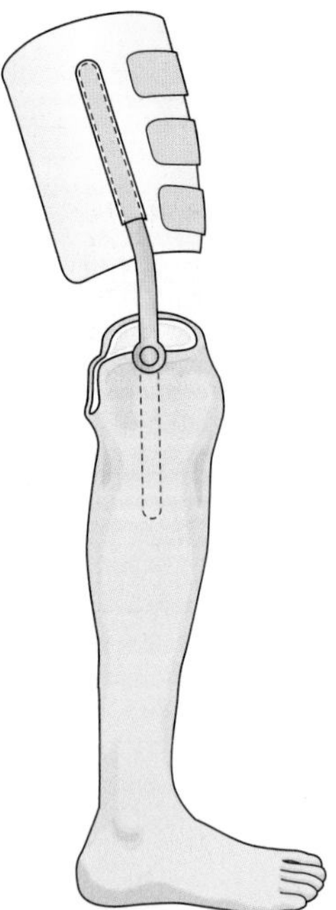

Figure 31.23 Transtibial prosthesis with thigh corset suspension.

Foot–Ankle Assemblies and Shanks

Although the SACH foot is often prescribed for transfemoral prostheses, the single-axis foot is more frequently used for transfemoral than for transtibial prostheses. The single-axis foot reaches the foot-flat position with minimal application of weight-bearing load. Nevertheless, almost any foot, including the energy-storing/releasing designs, can be incorporated in a transfemoral prosthesis. As compared with wearers of transtibial prostheses, however, most wearers of transfemoral prostheses do not load the prosthesis as vigorously. Consequently, less energy would be stored and released in a dynamic response foot.

Either the sturdy exoskeletal shank or the more lifelike endoskeletal shank may be used (see Fig. 31.13). The latter creates a more pleasing appearance, allows adjustable alignment, and is lighter than an exoskeletal shank. While greater prosthetic weight may increase metabolic energy cost, the weight may provide added sensory feedback that can lead to longer step lengths and improved gait symmetry.[29] Problems of durability remain, particularly at the knee, where constant bending of the joint, especially when the wearer is kneeling, accelerates deterioration of the rubber cover. A rotator (see Fig. 31.6C, Fig. 31.12) incorporated in the shank allows rotational motion that can diminish shear stress on the amputation limb.[30]

Knee Units

The prosthetic knee enables the user to bend the knee when sitting or kneeling and, in most instances, permits knee flexion during the latter portion of the stance phase and throughout the swing phase of walking. Commercial knee units may be described according to four features: (1) axis, (2) friction mechanism, (3) extension aid, and (4) mechanical stabilizer. Many combinations of features are available; not every knee unit has all four components.

Axis System

The thigh piece can be connected to the shank either by a *single-axis hinge,* which is the usual arrangement, or by *polycentric linkage*. Polycentric systems (Fig 31.24) have four or more pivoting bars and provide greater stability to the knee, inasmuch as the momentary center of knee rotation is posterior to the wearer's weight line during most of stance phase.[31] This design is less common because of its greater complexity and because other means are available to stabilize the knee.

Friction Mechanisms

In the simplest sense, the leg of the transfemoral prosthesis is a pendulum swinging about the knee hinge. For the elderly individual who walks slowly for short distances, a basic pendulum is adequate. More energetic walkers, however, benefit from adjustable friction mechanisms that modify the pendulum action of the leg to reduce the asymmetry between the motions of the sound and prosthetic limbs. If the prosthetic knee does not have sufficient friction to retard its natural pendulum action, the person who walks rapidly experiences excessive knee flexion (high heel rise) at the beginning of swing phase and abrupt, often noisy, knee extension at the end of swing phase (terminal swing

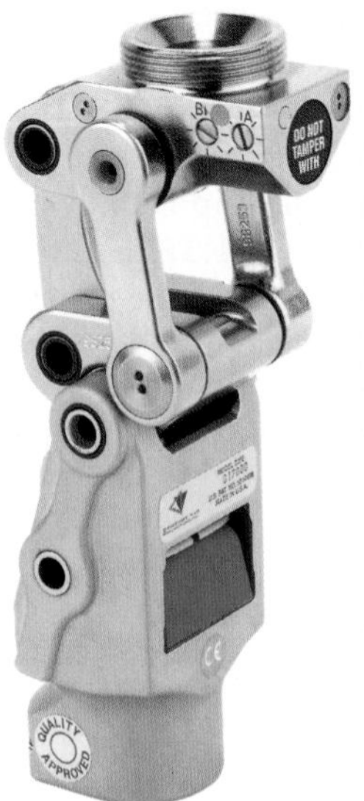

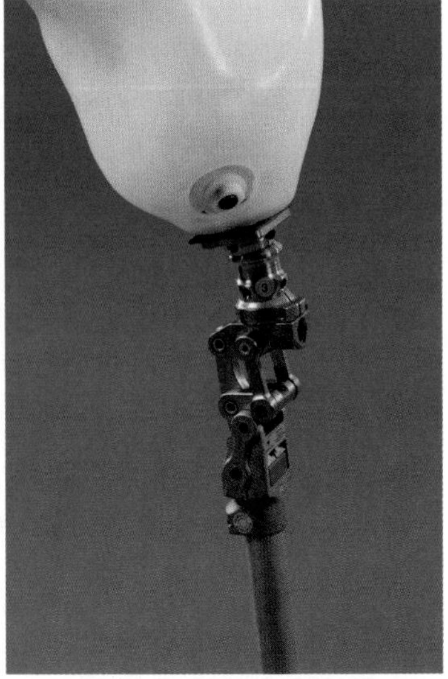

Figure 31.24 (*Left*) Polycentric knee unit designed to provide stability during stance. *(Courtesy of Ossur, Aliso Viejo, CA 92656.)* (*Right*) Polycentric knee in place on a transfemoral prosthesis.

impact). Friction mechanisms change the leg swing by modifying knee motion during various parts of swing phase and by affecting knee swing according to walking speed. Some friction mechanisms also resist knee flexion in the stance phase to enable stair descent (Fig. 31.25). Two interrelated issues involved in friction mechanisms are the time during swing phase when friction affects the knee unit and the medium through which the mechanism operates.

Constant and Variable

The most commonly prescribed knee unit has *constant friction* within the joint. A more sophisticated device applies *variable friction,* in which the amount of friction changes during a given portion of swing phase. At early swing, high friction is applied to retard excessive knee flexion; during midswing, friction diminishes to permit the knee to swing easily; at late swing, friction increases to dampen impact.

Friction Brake

A more elaborate stabilizing system, the *friction brake,* provides very high friction during early stance as the wearer bears weight on the prosthesis, resisting the tendency of the knee to flex.[32] One design, the load-dependent friction unit, applies resistance to knee flexion during the initiation of prosthetic limb weight-bearing during early stance to prevent collapse (see Fig. 31.26). Another version of friction brake is found in some hydraulic units; during early stance, additional fluid resistance markedly retards piston descent within

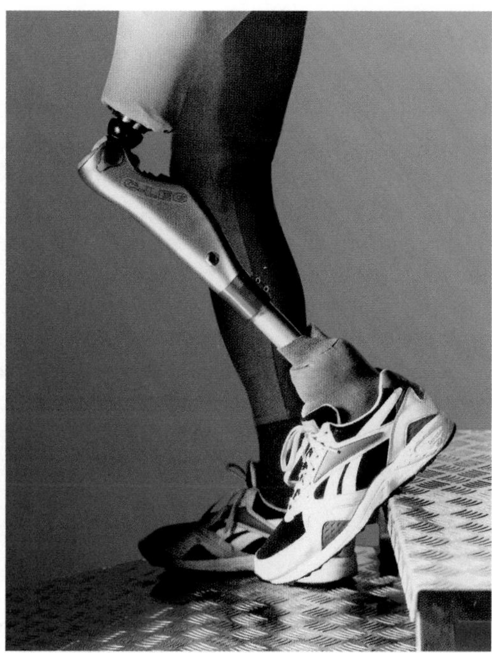

Figure 31.25 C-Leg®. *(Courtesy of Otto Bock, Minneapolis, MN 55447.)*

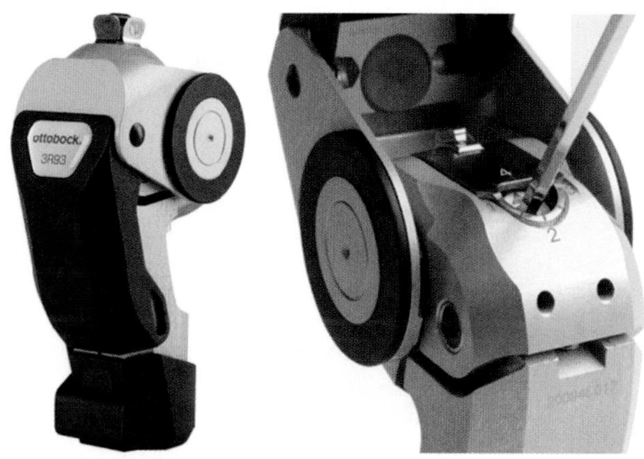

Figure 31.26 The SR93 load dependent friction knee. *(Courtesy of Otto Bock, Minneapolis, MN 55447.)*

the fluid cylinder and thus stabilizes the knee. Microprocessor units include stance control and, in most instances, a manual lock option.

From midstance through heel contact, friction brakes do not interfere with knee motion. In addition, they do not impede the patient who transfers from sitting to standing. Such devices may not protect the patient from falling when the knee is flexed beyond 20 degrees or if insufficient weight-bearing is applied.

Medium

The medium through which friction is applied influences performance. A load-dependent friction unit applies a mechanical brake to knee flexion when weight-bearing is borne through the limb. A more complex approach is *fluid friction,* either oil (*hydraulic friction*) (Fig. 31.27) or air (*pneumatic friction*). Unlike a load-dependent friction unit, fluid friction varies directly with velocity. Thus with a hydraulic or pneumatic unit, if the wearer walks faster, the knee increases friction instantly to prevent excessive knee flexion and abrupt extension. Consequently, the movements of the prosthetic and sound limbs are less asymmetrical than would be the case with load-dependent friction. Oil or air is contained in a cylinder in the knee unit. A piston descends in the cylinder during early swing, causing the knee to flex. The speed of piston descent depends on the type of fluid and the walking speed. Later, the piston ascends, extending the knee. Hydraulic units provide more friction than do pneumatic devices. Both types are more expensive than the simpler load-dependent friction designs.

Microprocessor-controlled hydraulic units such as the C-Leg (see Fig. 31.25) utilize electronic sensors, which detect the rate and range of shank movement 50 or more times per second, providing almost instant friction adjustment to changes in the gait pattern.[33-42] Units are programmed with a computer and may provide stumble recovery, locking option, and accommodation to walking on various terrain and bicycle riding. An

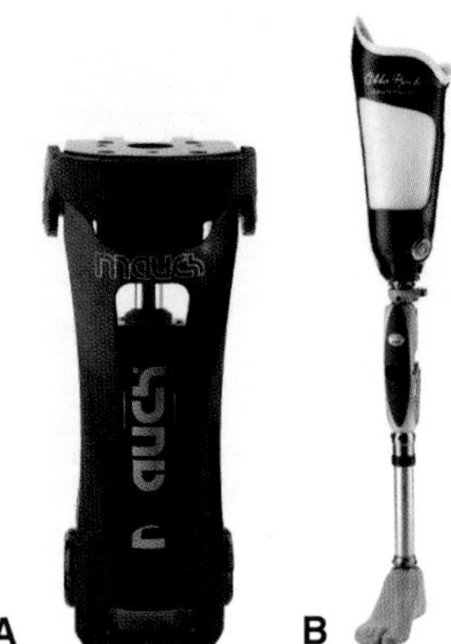

Figure 31.27 (A) Mauch® (SNS®) single-axis hydraulic knee unit with swing and stance control. *(Courtesy of Ossur, Aliso Viejo, CA 92656.)* (B) The SR60 Ergonomically Balance Stride (EBS) hydraulic system controls the knee during swing, allowing greater ease in initiating swing and a greater range of walking speeds. Note that this prosthesis includes a flexible socket supported within a rigid frame. *(Courtesy of Otto Bock, Minneapolis, MN 55447.)*

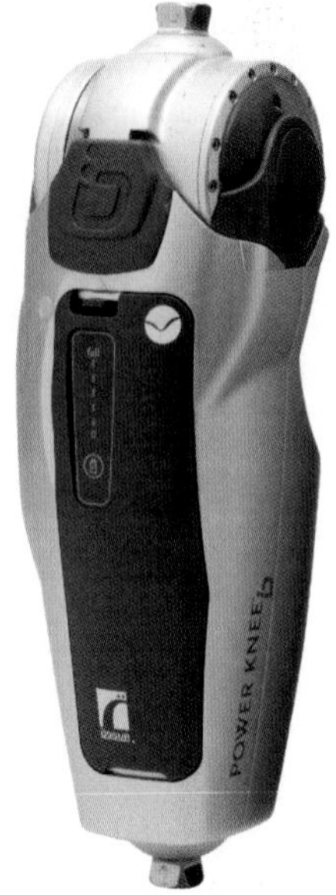

Figure 31.28 Power Knee®. *(Courtesy of Ossur, Aliso Viejo, CA 92656.)*

alternative to oil-filled hydraulic units is the Rheo® knee (Ossur, Aliso Viejo, CA 92656), which has magnetized fluid and sensors that detect knee action in much smaller time units.[43]

Extension Aids

Many knee units include a mechanism to assist knee extension during the latter part of swing phase. The simplest type is an *external extension aid,* consisting of an elastic strap in front of the knee axis. The elastic stretches when the knee flexes in early swing and recoils to extend the knee in late swing. Strap tension is easily adjusted but tends to pull the knee into extension when the wearer sits. The *internal extension aid* is an elastic strap or coiled spring within the knee unit. It functions identically to the external aid during walking, but unlike the external aid, the internal type keeps the knee flexed when the individual sits. Acute knee flexion causes the strap or spring to pass behind the knee axis, maintaining the flexed attitude. Fluid-controlled knee units incorporate an internal extension aid.

Although most extension aids affect the wearer's performance during late swing and early stance phases, the Power Knee® (Ossur, Aliso Viejo, CA 92656) (Fig. 31.28) also assists the user to ascend stairs step over step and to rise from a chair. The unit incorporates accelerometers, gyroscopes, a torque sensor, an on-board computer, and a motor. The motor makes a noise when engaged that will be noticeable to the wearer.

Stabilizers

Most knee units do not have a special device to increase stability. The patient controls prosthetic knee action by hip motion, aided by the alignment of the knee in relation to other components of the prosthesis. The knee axis is usually aligned posterior to a line extending from the greater trochanter to the ankle (trochanter–knee–ankle [TKA] line). The patient who has excellent balance and muscular control may have the knee bolt placed on the line, thus creating TKA alignment. Some hydraulic knee units are aligned with the knee axis anterior to the trochanter–ankle line. Elderly or debilitated patients may benefit from a stabilizing mechanism, as do some people who walk on very rough terrain, such as hunters.

Manual Lock

The simplest mechanical stabilizer is a manual lock (Fig. 31.29), in which a rod lodges in a receptacle and is released only when the wearer manipulates an unlocking lever by pulling on the cable. Other U-shaped manual locks are located at the posterior aspect of the knee unit (Fig. 31.30). When engaged, the manual lock prevents knee flexion. The user is secure not only during early stance when stability is desired, but also throughout the entire gait cycle. To compensate for difficulty in advancing the locked prosthesis, the shank should be shortened approximately 1/2 in. (1 cm). The manual lock must be manually disengaged when the wearer sits. Nevertheless, some people with impaired balance prefer the stability of the locked knee.[44]

Sockets

As with all prosthetic sockets, the transfemoral one should be a total-contact receptacle to distribute load over the maximum area, thereby reducing pressure. Total-contact fitting also provides counterpressure to assist venous return and prevent distal edema, and it

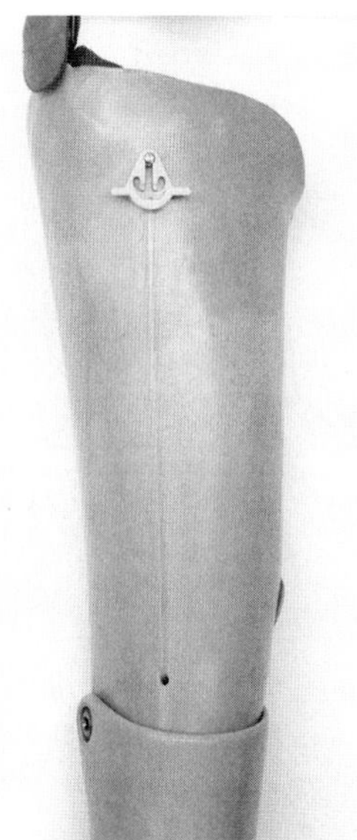

Figure 31.29 Single axis knee unit with manual lock. Note that this configuration has a proximal release cable attached to the knee. For patients with impaired balance, the proximal release eliminates the need to flex forward and reach down to the knee to unlock the unit.

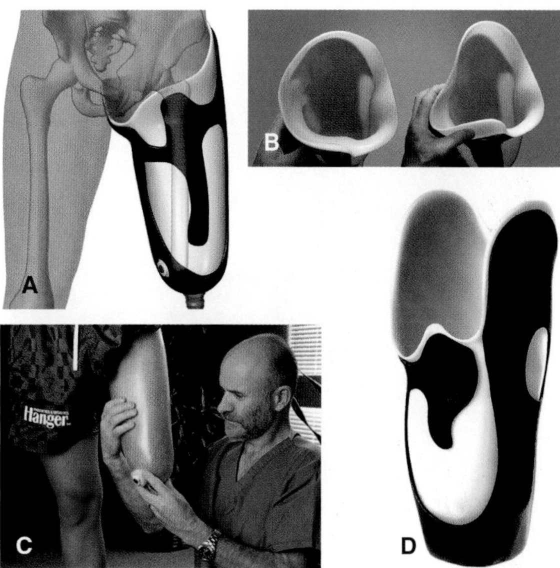

Figure 31.31 ComfortFlex™ socket design. (A) Anatomical orientation of transfemoral socket. (B) Overhead view of transfemoral socket (thumb and finger pressure illustrating socket flexibility). (C) Socket without carbon frame. (D) Transtibial socket design. *(Courtesy of Hanger, Inc., Oklahoma City, OK 73118.)*

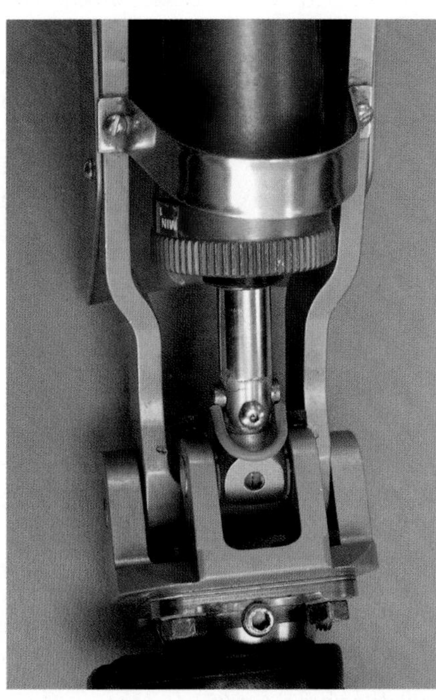

Figure 31.30 Manual lock (blue) on a hydraulic prosthetic knee unit.

enhances sensory feedback to foster better control of the prosthesis. Most transfemoral sockets are made of a flexible thermoplastic socket (Fig. 31.31A) encased in a rigid frame. The frame enables the wearer to transmit weight through the distal components of the prosthesis to the ground. The flexible socket provides sensory input from external objects, such as chairs; it also dissipates body heat and facilitates alterations in socket fit. A polyester laminate socket is entirely rigid (Fig. 31.31B).

Transfemoral sockets are designed to emphasize loading on pressure-tolerant structures, such as the gluteal musculature, sides of the thigh, and, to a lesser extent, the distal end of the amputated limb. The socket must avoid excessive pressure on the pubic symphysis and perineum.

Quadrilateral Socket

One transfemoral socket shape is quadrilateral when viewed from above (Fig. 31.32). The socket features a horizontal posterior shelf for the ischial tuberosity and gluteal musculature, a medial brim at the same level as the posterior shelf, an anterior wall 2.5 to 3 in. (6 to 8 cm) higher to apply a posteriorly directed force to the thigh to retain the ischial tuberosity on its shelf, and a lateral wall the same height as the anterior wall to aid in medial–lateral stabilization. Concave reliefs are (1) anteromedial, for the pressure-sensitive adductor longus tendon and obturator nerve; (2) posteromedial, for the sensitive hamstring tendons and sciatic nerve; (3) posterolateral, to permit the gluteus maximus to contract and bulge without being crowded; and (4) anterolateral, to allow adequate room for the rectus femoris. The anterior wall has a convexity, Scarpa's bulge, to maximize pressure distribution in the vicinity of the femoral (Scarpa's) triangle. The

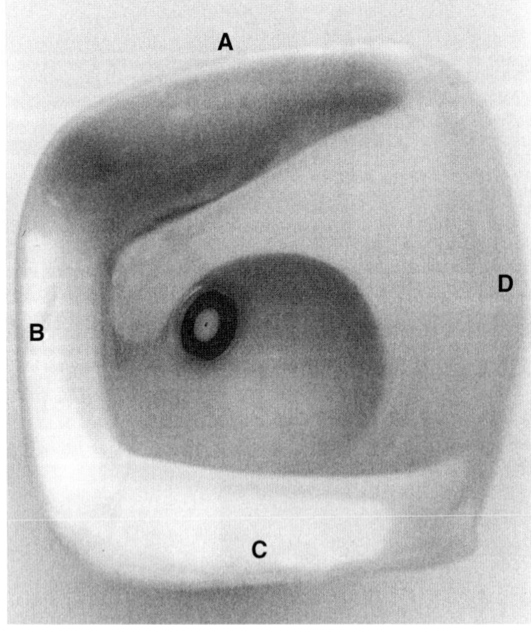

Figure 31.32 Quadrilateral socket viewed from above. (A) Anterior wall. (B) Medial wall. (C) Posterior wall. (D) Lateral wall.

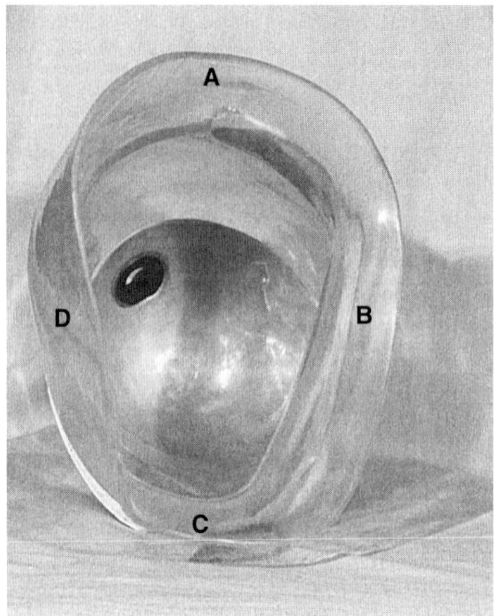

Figure 31.33 Ischial containment flexible transfemoral socket. (A) Anterior brim. (B) Medial brim. (C) Posterior brim. (D) Lateral brim.

lateral wall may have reliefs for the greater trochanter and the distal end of the femur.

Ischial Containment Socket

An alternate design type is the ischial containment socket (Fig. 31.33). Sometimes called the *contoured adducted trochanter-controlled alignment method*, its walls cover the ischial tuberosity and part of the ischiopubic ramus to augment socket stability. To increase frontal plane stability and minimize bulk between the thighs, the mediolateral width of the socket is narrower than that of the quadrilateral socket. The anterior wall is lower than in the quadrilateral socket, whereas the lateral wall covers the greater trochanter. Alternating vertical reliefs and buildups can reduce rotation of the limb in the socket.[45] Weight-bearing occurs on the sides and bottom of the amputated limb.

Slight socket flexion is desirable to (1) facilitate contraction of the hip extensors, (2) reduce lumbar lordosis, (3) emphasize posterior thigh weight-bearing, and (4) provide a zone through which the thigh may be extended to permit the wearer to take steps of approximately equal length. For wearers of quadrilateral sockets, socket flexion also enhances positioning of the ischial tuberosity on the posterior brim. Socket adduction allows lateral thigh weight-bearing (Fig. 31.34).

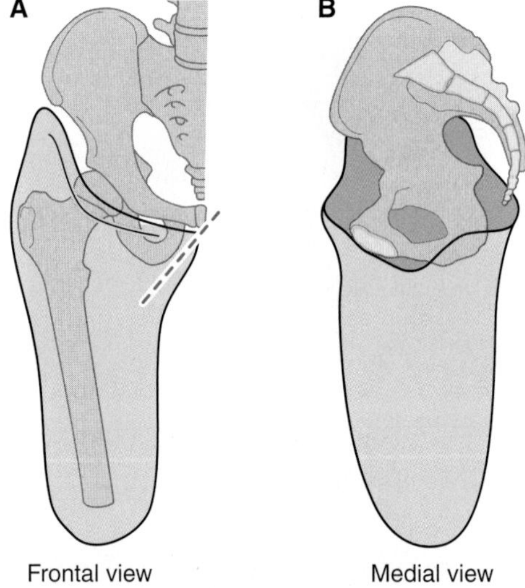

Figure 31.34 (A) Frontal view of the femur and pelvis in the ischial containment socket. (B) Medial view of the pelvis in the ischial containment socket. *(From May, BJ, and Lackard, MA: Prosthetics and Orthotics in Clinical Practice. FA Davis, Philadelphia, 2011, p. 95.)*

Suspensions

Three means are used to suspend the transfemoral prosthesis: (1) total suction, (2) partial suction, and (3) no suction.

Suction Suspension

Suction refers to the difference between pressure inside and outside the socket. With suction suspension, internal socket pressure is less than external pressure; consequently, atmospheric pressure causes the socket to remain on the thigh. A one-way air-release valve located at the bottom of the socket enables residual air to be expelled.

Total Suction

Maximum control of the prosthesis without any encumbering auxiliary suspension can be achieved only when the socket brim fits very snugly. Some people add a transfemoral suspension sleeve (Fig. 31.35), especially when engaging in vigorous activities. If the patient experiences reduction in amputation limb volume, suction will be lost and an auxiliary suspension will be required.

Partial Suction

A socket that is slightly loose may provide partial suction suspension combined with auxiliary suspension; the socket has a valve. The patient wears one or more socks or a synthetic liner. Because air enters the space between the sock fibers, auxiliary suspension is needed, either a fabric Silesian belt (Fig. 31.36) or a rigid plastic or metal hip joint and pelvic band (Fig. 31.37). These aids encircle the pelvis. The Silesian belt also controls the transverse plane orientation of the prosthesis on the thigh, while the hip joint restricts transverse and frontal motion at the hip. The pelvic band adds weight to the prosthesis and may impose uncomfortable pressure against the torso when the wearer sits.

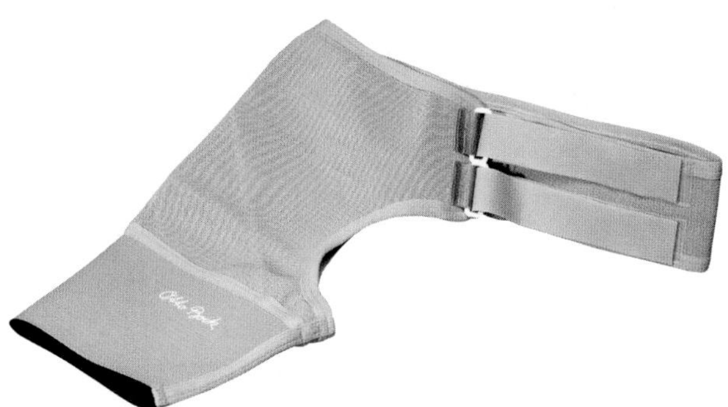

Figure 31.35 Transfemoral suspension sleeve. *(Courtesy of Otto Bock, Minneapolis, MN 55447.)*

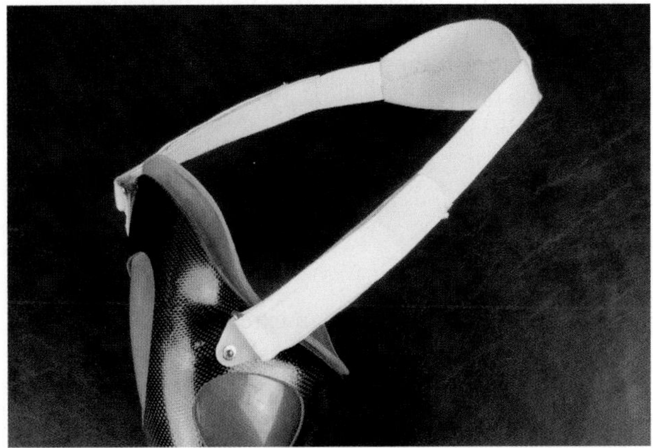

Figure 31.36 Silesian belt. *(From Roy, SH, Wolf, SL, and Scalzitti, DA: The Rehabilitation Specialist's Handbook, ed 4. FA Davis, Philadelphia, 2013, p. 977, with permission.)*

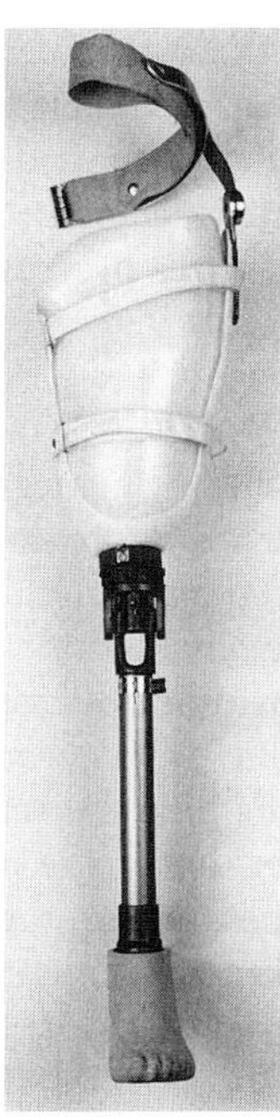

Figure 31.37 Transfemoral temporary prosthesis with adjustable polypropylene socket, pelvic band, knee unit with manual lock, and adjustable shank with SACH foot.

No Suction

If the socket has a distal hole without a valve, then no pressure difference exists between the inside and the outside of the socket. The client wears one or more socks and requires a pelvic band. The pelvic band has a rigid metal or nylon single-axis hip joint attached to a leather belt, which encircles the pelvis. The relatively loose socket makes donning easy but hinders control of the prosthesis and may make sitting uncomfortable.

Osseous integration is the newest suspension alternative. A metal post implanted in the femur locks into a fixture embedded in the distal portion of the socket.[28]

■ DISARTICULATION PROSTHESES

Individuals with knee or hip disarticulation wear prostheses that include the same distal components as prostheses for lower levels. Any prosthetic foot can be used with either an endoskeletal or exoskeletal shank. The user, however, is less likely to produce sufficient weight-bearing force to benefit from an energy storing and release foot. The major distinction, therefore, is in the proximal portion of the prostheses.

Knee Disarticulation Prostheses

When amputation is at or distal to the femoral epicondyles, the patient should have excellent prosthetic control because (1) thigh leverage is maximum, (2) most of the body weight can be borne through the distal end of the femur, and (3) the broad epicondyles provide rotational stability.[46,47] The problem presented by knee disarticulation is primarily cosmetic; when the individual sits, the thigh on the amputated side may protrude slightly. The knee disarticulation prosthesis has a streamlined knee that minimizes protrusion and a specially designed socket.

Knee Units

Several units are specifically manufactured for knee disarticulation. All have a thin proximal attachment plate to minimize added thigh length. One may choose among hydraulic, pneumatic, and weight-activated friction units, with or without polycentric linkage. Even with a special knee unit, the thigh will be slightly longer. Consequently, the shank is shortened equivalently, so that when the person stands, the pelvis is level. When the individual sits, the thigh on the prosthetic side will project farther by several centimeters.[48]

Sockets

Two types of sockets are currently in use. Both are made of plastic and usually terminate below the ischial tuberosity. Generally, no additional suspension aids are needed. One version features an anterior opening to accommodate a bulbous amputation limb. After the limb is inserted, the wearer closes the socket with lacing or hook-and-loop closure. The other design has no anterior opening and is suitable for limbs that are not bulbous.

Hip Disarticulation Prostheses

A hip disarticulation prosthesis[49] is fitted to a person with amputation above the greater trochanter (very short transfemoral), removal of the femoral head from the acetabulum (hip disarticulation), or removal of the femur and any portion of the pelvis (transpelvic amputation, also known as *hemipelvectomy*) (Fig. 31.38). The modern prosthesis was developed in Toronto and is sometimes called the *Canadian hip disarticulation prosthesis*. Prostheses for proximal levels share common hip, knee, and foot assemblies but differ with regard to socket design. The endoskeletal thigh and shank predominate because they save appreciable weight in these massive prostheses. The prosthesis may be shortened slightly to aid clearance during swing phase, encourage the wearer to apply maximum weight to the prosthesis, and increase stability.

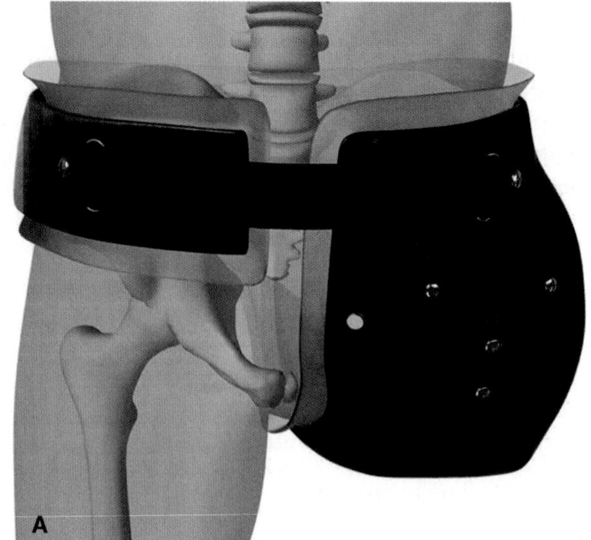

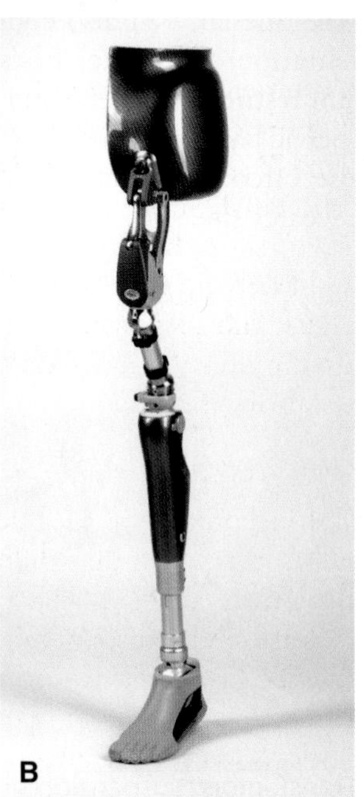

Figure 31.38 (A) Anatomical orientation of the Comfort-Flex™ hip disarticulation socket. *(Courtesy of Hanger, Oklahoma City, OK 73118.)* (B) Additional components of the completed prosthesis include a Helix 3D® hip joint, rotator, knee unit, endoskeletal pylon, and foot. *(Courtesy of Otto Bock, Minneapolis, MN 55447.)*

Sockets

The basic socket is plastic molded to provide weight-bearing on the ipsilateral ischial tuberosity and buttock (gluteal musculature). The person with transpelvic amputation who does not retain the ipsilateral tuberosity or iliac crest has a socket with a higher proximal trimline, sometimes encompassing the lower thorax. This individual supports weight on the remainder of the pelvis, on the abdomen, and perhaps on the lower ribs.

Hip Units

The prosthetic hip joint has an extension aid to bias the prosthesis toward the stable neutral position. Positioning the mechanical hip anterior to a point corresponding to the anatomical hip also contributes to hip stability. The joint is set below the normal hip so that when the wearer sits, the prosthetic thigh will not protrude unattractively. All hip joints provide hip flexion; some also allow transverse rotation[50,51] (see Fig. 31.38).

Knee Units

Although virtually any knee unit can be incorporated in a hip disarticulation prosthesis, an extension aid can be used to assist limb advancement during the swing phase of gait. The prosthetic knee should resist knee flexion in stance phase or be aligned posteriorly to contribute to stability.

BILATERAL PROSTHESES

Bilateral amputations occur either simultaneously, as in the case of trauma or congenital limb deficiency, or sequentially, as is seen with peripheral vascular disease. In the latter instance, previous experience with a unilateral prosthesis is invaluable in determining whether the patient will benefit from a pair of prostheses.

Bilateral Syme's and Transtibial Prostheses

Any foot design can be worn, although both prosthetic feet must be the same design from the same manufacturer to reduce the likelihood of gait asymmetry. Ideally, foot and shoe size should be shorter than the person's preamputation size to facilitate transition through stance phase; wider feet contribute to stability. Shanks, sockets, and suspensions need not match; each component should suit the characteristics of the individual amputation limb.[52]

Bilateral Transfemoral Prostheses

Other than matching prosthetic foot design and size, each amputation limb is fitted on an individual basis. The patient will perform activities in a manner similar to someone with unilateral transfemoral amputation.

The patient can be fitted with short, nonarticulated prostheses. The lower center of gravity provides the individual with more stability. Gait is awkward, with exaggerated trunk rotation; crutches or canes need to be adjusted to suit the person's short stature. Transferring into an adult-size chair, as well as climbing stairs, is more difficult than with longer prostheses. Patients who object to the markedly altered appearance created by these short prostheses may refuse to wear them.

Longer prostheses should include a matched pair of feet. Endoskeletal shanks are highly desirable to reduce prosthetic weight and enable minute changes in alignment; typically the shanks are shortened by several inches to reduce the effort required to walk with the prostheses. Any type of knee unit may be worn; they need not be the same on both prostheses. Nevertheless, one should avoid a pair of manually locked knee units because they would make chair transfers and stair maneuvering very difficult. Sockets do not have to match; however, a pair of ischial containment sockets will minimize the walking base because the sockets have a relatively narrow mediolateral dimension, as compared with quadrilateral sockets. Any type of suspension may be worn.[53,54]

PROSTHETIC MAINTENANCE

Optimal function depends on proper care of socks or sheaths, prosthesis, amputation limb, and intact limb, as well as general health maintenance. Guidelines for personal hygiene are presented in Chapter 22, Amputation. In addition to ensuring cleanliness, the individual should wear a well-fitting sock and shoe on the sound foot. It must be the mate to the shoe on the prosthesis. Both shoes should be in excellent condition.

As with any appliance, the prosthesis benefits from simple regular maintenance, which generally avoids costly, time-consuming repairs. Printed instructions pertaining to the prosthesis and socks or sheath are helpful for patient education.

Foot–Ankle Assemblies

One should avoid getting the prosthetic foot wet, especially if the foot is an articulated model. If this happens, the shoe and sock should be removed to allow the foot to dry completely, away from direct heat. The wearer should also avoid stepping into sand and similar materials that might enter the cleft between the foot and shank section and restrict the excursion of the foot. The prosthetist will have to disassemble the foot to clean it.

The client should inspect the foot periodically to spot cracking at the toe-break or tip of the keel; such a crack will curl the toes and prevent smooth transition during late stance. A deteriorated heel cushion or plantar bumper will cause one to appear to be walking in a hole. Although most feet are now molded to simulate toes, the patient should not walk without a shoe because the sole of the prosthetic foot is not intended to resist much abrasion.

Foot socks wear much more quickly on the prosthetic side, because the hard foot–ankle assembly and shank rub against the fabric. Stair risers also scuff the sock. Some people find that wearing two socks helps cushion the outer one against premature formation of holes.

The individual must be instructed regarding wearing shoes of the same heel height as was the case when the prosthesis was aligned. Too low a heel interrupts late stance; an unduly high heel makes the knee less stable. If the prosthesis has the usual foot designed for low-heeled shoes, and the wearer wishes to wear flat-heeled shoes, a ½-in. (1-cm) shim (a thin tapered wedge) should be placed inside both shoes at the heel. High-heeled shoes require that the foot be changed, either by unbolting it and replacing it with a foot with an appropriate plantarflexion angle or by adjusting the heel-height feature found in certain models of feet (e.g., Runway® [Freedom Innovations, Fayette, UT 84630]; Elation® [Ossur, Aliso Viejo, CA 92656]). Boots and other footwear with stiff upper sections restrict the action of any foot assembly that is designed to provide substantial dorsiflexion and plantarflexion.

Removing the shoe is easier when the prosthesis is first taken off. With the shoe unlaced completely, one grasps the rear of the shoe, then pulls the shoe off the back of the foot. Finally, the shoe is moved upward off the forefoot. The shoe should be put on the prosthetic foot with the aid of a shoehorn.

Shanks

The usual finish of exoskeletal shanks is polyester laminate, which is impervious to most liquids. It needs to be wiped only periodically with a cloth dampened with dilute detergent to remove surface soil. Marks can be gently removed with kitchen cleanser; excessive abrasion will dull the finish.

The soft foam cover of the endoskeletal prosthesis requires reasonable caution against exposure to direct heat, penetrating objects, and solvents. The outer covering will need replacement whenever it becomes unacceptably soiled or torn. The transfemoral version tends to deteriorate at the knee, especially if the wearer kneels a great deal.

Knee Units

Squeaking at the knee or articulated ankle usually indicates the need for oil. The rubber or felt extension bumper in the knee unit will erode after prolonged vigorous use, and the wearer will then notice that the knee begins to hyperextend. The bumper, visible when the knee is flexed, must be replaced by the prosthetist.

The external extension aid eventually loses its elasticity. The user will then experience high heel rise in early swing and slow knee extension at the end of swing phase. The simplest approach is to tighten the strap through its buckle. Eventually, the prosthetist will need to replace the elastic webbing. Internal elastic extension aids are not subject to rubbing from the trouser leg or skirt and thus do not lose elasticity as readily. Steel spring internal aids usually retain their effectiveness for the life of the prosthesis.

Pneumatic and hydraulic units must be protected against tears of the rubber shield protecting the piston. The piston must not be scratched, because this would allow air and debris to enter the cylinder. Air bubbles in the unit will cause a spongy feeling, and possibly noise with walking. At night, the prosthesis should be stored upright, with the knee extended to exclude air from the cylinder.

Electronic units must not be immersed in any fluid or used in a particle-filled environment, such as a commercial bakery or lumberyard (flour and sawdust).

Sockets and Suspensions

Plastic sockets should be washed with a cloth dampened in warm water that has a very small amount of mild soap dissolved in it. The socket is then wiped with a damp, soap-free cloth and dried with a fresh towel. In warm climates, the socket should be washed every evening so that it will be completely dry when the patient dresses the following morning. Socket liners made of polyethylene foam can be washed by hand in tepid water with mild soap, rinsed, and air-dried overnight. They should not be subjected to direct sunlight when removed from the prosthesis. Other sheaths and liners should be maintained according to the manufacturer's instructions.

Leather corsets should be kept dry. Use of saddle soap will keep leather clean. If the patient is incontinent, the thigh corset should be made of flexible *polyester laminate* or polypropylene, which are impervious to urine.

The transfemoral suction valve should be brushed daily to remove talcum and lint, which might clog the tiny aperture. The valve should be inserted and removed only with one's fingers, because tools are apt to damage the internal mechanism or outer threads.

■ PHYSICAL THERAPY MANAGEMENT

Physical therapists participate in the management of patients with amputation at several key stages: (1) preoperative, (2) postoperative–preprosthetic, (3) prosthetic prescription, (4) prosthetic examination, and (5) prosthetic training.

The first two stages are described in Chapter 22, Amputation. The following discussion emphasizes the responsibilities of the physical therapist with regard to the patient and prosthesis. Ideally, the therapist works as a member of a clinic team, together with the physician and prosthetist. Others, such as a social worker, vocational counselor, and psychologist may participate in the team on a regular basis or as needed. The clinic team provides the best environment for exchange of information and viewpoints regarding the patient and fostering efficient treatment;[55,56] the team meets to formulate the prosthetic prescription, examine the newly delivered prosthesis, and reexamine the patient and prosthesis upon completion of prosthetic training. The therapist, therefore, has an integral part to play in these critical points in rehabilitation, as well as conducting prosthetic training. If a formal clinic team is not established in the therapist's work setting, then one must coordinate the recommendations of the physician and prosthetist.

With either administrative situation, the physical therapist:

- Addresses nonprosthetic issues.
- Contributes to prosthetic prescription.
- Examines the prosthesis.
- Facilitates prosthetic acceptance.
- Instructs the patient in donning, use, and maintenance of the prosthesis.

Prescription Considerations

Successful prosthetic rehabilitation depends on matching the individual's physical and psychosocial characteristics to a prosthesis composed of carefully selected components. Although everyone who wears a prosthesis has an amputation or comparable limb deficiency, the reverse is not true. That is, some people with amputations are not candidates for prostheses or prefer not to use them. Prostheses are contraindicated for patients with severe dementia or depression or advanced cardiopulmonary disease. If the person displays significant changes associated with organic brain syndrome, then prosthetic fitting is contraindicated. Individuals with bilateral amputations who are unable to transfer independently or don underwear by themselves are unlikely to benefit from definitive prostheses. Similarly, a patient with bilateral amputations who had sustained unilateral amputation previously and was unable to don and walk with a unilateral prosthesis is not a candidate for a pair of prostheses. Some people with high amputations, especially hip disarticulation, find that a prosthesis is unduly cumbersome; they prefer to ambulate with a pair of crutches or depend on a wheelchair. Several sports, particularly swimming, are generally easier to perform without a prosthesis.

Physical Examination

The physical therapist should examine joint mobility and active and passive range of motion of all joints on both LLs. Knee and hip flexion contractures compromise prosthetic alignment and appearance. A knee lock may be needed in a transfemoral prosthesis. A patient with a substantial knee contracture requires an alternative transtibial socket design. Severe contractures may contraindicate provision of a prosthesis. The deleterious effects of contractures are especially serious with bilateral amputations.

The length of the amputation limb should be measured. The individual with a short transtibial amputation may require SC/SP suspension. Every attempt should be made to fit the patient with a short transfemoral amputation with suction or partial-suction suspension to retain the prosthesis on the thigh.

Strength of all limb and trunk muscles should be examined. Frequently, the elderly patient with vascular disease experiences reduced physical activity as LL pain and foot ulceration develop. Such an individual may present with marked debility, which would interfere with prosthetic use or necessitate use of a unit with a knee lock.

The therapist should inspect the skin, noting the status of the incision and any other lesions. The patient may require a nylon or silicone sheath to provide a smooth interface between socket and skin to avoid irritating tender or grafted skin.

An examination of sensory function should be performed. For example, someone with impaired proprioception at the knee will need extra prosthetic stability in the form of higher medial and lateral socket walls, or side joints attached to a thigh corset, on the transtibial prosthesis. Blindness does not preclude fitting, but it does pose problems with regard to selecting components that are easy to don, as well as altering the training program. If the patient complains of a neuroma, the problem must be addressed surgically or conservatively (e.g., cortisone injection) before fitting can proceed.

The therapist should examine the patient's ability to learn and retain new information, including both short- and long-term memory. Neurological conditions such as cerebrovascular accident complicate fitting and training. Ipsilateral hemiplegia is not as detrimental to prosthetic rehabilitation as contralateral paralysis. In both instances, the prosthesis should be designed for maximum stability. Patients with mild neurological impairments often respond favorably to altered training strategies, which the therapist designs on an individualized basis.

The circulation and anthropometric dimensions of the amputation and sound limbs require careful scrutiny. The physical therapist should teach the patient to inspect the intact foot, using a mirror to visualize the plantar surface. Inspection aims to identify skin lesions and incipient areas of abrasion so that corrective measures may be instituted before ulceration or infection ensues. In addition, the patient should be taught to keep the sound foot clean and should wear clean socks or stockings and a well-fitting shoe (see Chapter 14, Vascular, Lymphatic, and Integumentary Disorders, for additional guidelines for managing the patient with peripheral vascular disease). Sequential measurements of amputation limb circumference as well as palpation will indicate whether the individual has edema. Measures should be instituted to stabilize limb volume so that the patient can retain the fit of the prosthetic socket. The patient with vascular impairment may benefit from prosthetic fitting, which transfers some stress from the contralateral limb. In addition, should the person come to bilateral amputation, previous experience with donning and controlling a unilateral prosthesis is invaluable in adjusting to a pair of prostheses.

Prosthetic prescription is also based on the patient's aerobic capacity and endurance. The clinic team must formulate realistic goals based on the individual's physical capacity, particularly related to exercise tolerance and level of deconditioning. The person who is not expected to walk rapidly is an unlikely candidate for an energy-storing/releasing foot or a fluid-controlled knee unit. Nevertheless, a fluid-controlled knee unit that incorporates a braking mechanism is appropriate for selected patients with generalized weakness.

Obesity is another factor to be considered in the preprescription examination. The obese individual is more apt to fluctuate in body weight, necessitating provision of socket liners and several socks to compensate for changing limb circumference. Similarly, those who have renal disease, especially if requiring dialysis, experience volume changes that need prosthetic accommodation.

Arthritis affects prosthesis prescription. Diminished LL mobility or deformity may compromise prosthetic alignment. Patients with hip or knee arthroplasty, however, function quite well with a prosthesis. Hand and wrist function affects the mode of donning; a laced corset should be avoided. Canes and crutches may require modification.

Functional examination is an essential component of physical therapy management (see Chapter 8, Examination of Function). One of the most useful examination procedures involves observing the patient's ability to transfer from sit-to-stand and bed-to-wheelchair. To accomplish this maneuver, the individual must have reasonable strength, balance, and coordination, as well as adequate comprehension.

Psychosocial Conditions

Ordinarily, the physical therapist treats the patient more frequently than any other member of the clinic team and thus is more likely to be attuned to changes in the individual's psychosocial status. Ample evidence supports the psychological, and the physical, benefit of clinic team management.[55,56] Many people with amputation confront psychosocial issues that should be recognized and addressed.[57-64] Expression of suicidal ideation is not uncommon and should be considered and the individual referred for appropriate psychological care.[65] For the patient who is excessively fearful, rehabilitation can begin with a *temporary (provisional) prosthesis*.

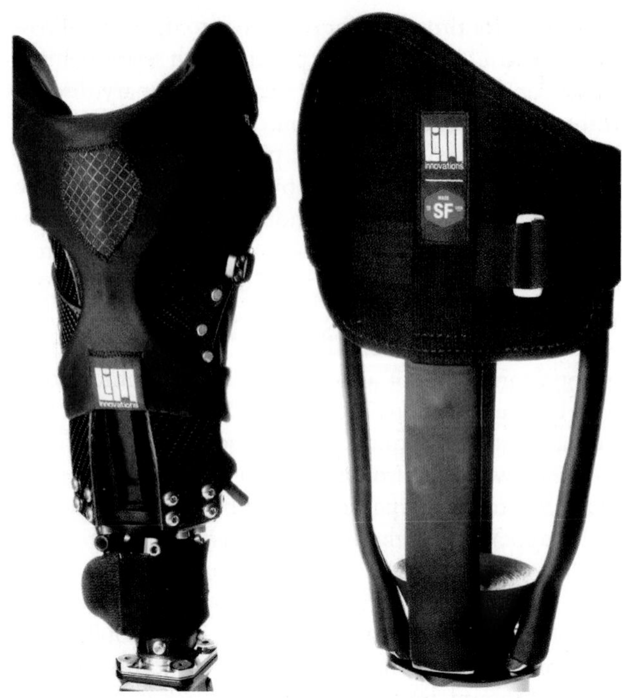

Figure 31.39 LIM Innovations adjustable sockets for transtibial *(Left)* and transfemoral *(Right)* amputations.

Temporary Prostheses

Transtibial Temporary Prostheses

Most transtibial temporary prostheses have sockets made of thermoplastic material that becomes malleable at temperatures low enough to permit forming directly on the patient. One can also obtain mass-produced adjustable sockets; it may be necessary to pad the socket bottom so that the amputation limb does not develop distal edema. Some temporary prostheses have a plaster socket molded to the amputated limb. Plaster is inexpensive, readily available, and easy to use. The resulting socket, however, is rather heavy and bulky. Suspension is usually by a cuff or thigh corset. The pylon can be an aluminum component manufactured for this purpose; such a pylon has a proximal fixture that permits small changes in prosthetic alignment. A simpler pylon can be made with polyvinyl chloride piping, such as used for plumbing. The pipe is lightweight and can be spot-heated to enable slight alteration in alignment. A SACH foot is customarily used on temporary prostheses.

Transfemoral Temporary Prostheses

The easiest approach is to use a polypropylene socket (see Fig. 31.37), which is manufactured in several sizes and has straps for circumferential adjustment. The socket can be suspended with a Silesian bandage or pelvic band and is mounted on a knee unit, which may include a manual lock. Alternatively, a custom-fabricated socket of plaster or low-temperature thermoplastic can be used. New adjustable designs may make it possible to adapt to the individual while the limb matures (Fig. 31.39). Some individuals with bilateral transfemoral amputations use a pair of short ("stubby") prostheses (see Chapter 22, Amputation). As mentioned earlier, these are nonarticulated prostheses; the sockets are mounted on short platforms, drastically reducing the wearer's height in order to increase balance stability. The platforms each have a rearward projection to protect the patient from a backward fall.

Motivation is a cardinal determinant of prosthetic outcome. Again, strong motivation demonstrated through use of a temporary prosthesis and adherence with other elements of the rehabilitation program is a reliable predictor of prosthetic success. One should guard against unrealistic expectations. Involving the patient and family in group situations with other persons with amputation in the physical therapy department and in social environments fosters constructive attitudes. The therapist should also weigh the likelihood that the individual will be able to care for complex prosthetic mechanisms and have the financial resources to obtain prosthetic servicing, especially of less durable components, such as the foam rubber covering of the endoskeletal shank.[66,67]

Prosthetic Prescription

No prosthetic component is ideal for all clients. It is necessary to select components that are most apt to meet each individual's needs. Alternatives to every element of the prosthesis have advantages and disadvantages. The task of the physical therapist, in conjunction with other team members, is to judge the relative merits of various feet, shanks, and other components in light of objective and subjective information pertaining to the prosthetic candidate. In 1995, Medicare listed functional levels applicable to individuals with unilateral transtibial and transfemoral amputations that determine the medical necessity, and thus reimbursement purposes, of prosthetic knee and ankle–foot units:[68]

- K0: Not a candidate
- K1: Household ambulation
- K2: Limited community ambulation
- K3: Community ambulation and the ability to vary cadence with vocational, therapeutic, or exercise needs
- K4: High levels of activity such as demonstrated by active adults and athletes

Some people can be expected to function best with a sophisticated prosthesis that enhances the wearer's ability to engage in vigorous walking and athletics. Others are well served by simple, inexpensive devices. The most accurate predictor of future function is the patient's performance with a previous prosthesis. For the wearer who seeks a replacement prosthesis, the clinic team should consider the extent of use of the previous limb, together with any changes in the patient's health status and lifestyle. For example, if the person fitted with one prosthesis now returns with bilateral amputation, never having used the original prosthesis, that patient is a very poor candidate for bilateral prosthetic fitting. In contrast, another person who had been fitted with a simple transfemoral prosthesis expresses the wish to participate in sports. By demonstrating good use of the original prosthesis, that individual is likely to derive considerable benefit from a new prosthesis with a fluid-controlled knee unit and an energy-storing/releasing foot.

Prescription for the new patient is more difficult. Depending on the interval between amputation surgery and prescription, the amputation limb may not have stabilized in volume; the patient may not have achieved the maximum benefit from the preprosthetic program. The best criterion for prosthetic prescription in such an instance is performance with a temporary (provisional) prosthesis. This appliance includes a well-fitting socket, suitable suspension, pylon, and foot; the transfemoral model usually has a knee unit. The temporary prosthesis allows preliminary gait and activities training. The major difference between the temporary and definitive (permanent) prosthesis is appearance. The temporary socket is designed for easy alteration to accommodate change in amputation limb volume. Ordinarily, little attention is paid to the color and exterior shape of the temporary prosthesis.

Prosthetic Examination/Evaluation

The prosthesis should be examined before the patient engages in prosthetic training and should be reexamined at the conclusion of training. The procedure is intended to determine the adequacy of prosthetic fit and function, as well as the wearer's opinion of appearance and overall satisfaction. This process typically follows a sequence of examining the prosthesis while the patient stands (static analysis), examining the patient's gait (dynamic analysis), and finally examining the prosthesis off the patient (additional static analysis). In many institutions, the physical therapist examines the prosthesis and presents a summary of findings to the clinic team. The team makes the final determination regarding the acceptability of the prosthesis.

No special materials are needed to examine the prosthesis, except for a checklist, a straight (armless) chair, a few sheets of paper, a ruler, lift blocks, and colored chalk. For final evaluation, stairs and a ramp are needed. Appendix 31.A: Transtibial Prosthetic Evaluation and Appendix 31.B: Transfemoral Prosthetic Evaluation contain the checklists referred to in the following sections.

Evaluation

At initial evaluation, the team has three assessment options: (1) pass, (2) provisional pass, or (3) fail. Pass indicates that no changes are needed in the prosthesis and the patient can proceed to training. Provisional pass signals that one or more minor problems require correction, none of which would interfere with training. Failure is the team's judgment that the prosthesis has a major fault that should be corrected to the team's satisfaction before commencement of prosthetic training. For example, poor finishing of the prosthetic foot merits a provisional pass, whereas a socket that abrades the amputation limb should be graded as fail. If the therapist intends to provide treatment to a patient that is not managed by a formal clinic team, it is especially critical that one examine the prosthesis prior to initiating instruction and training to discover any problems that would interfere with the future program. At the final evaluation, two ratings are available: *pass* indicates that no problems exist and the patient uses the prosthesis in a manner commensurate with that individual's physical capacity; *fail* means that major or minor problems remain.

Transtibial Examination

Most items on the checklist in Appendix 31.A are self-explanatory. Each contributes to forming an accurate judgment of the adequacy of the prosthesis.

Static Analysis

The prosthesis is examined while the wearer stands and sits. In addition, the amputation limb and details of the prosthesis are examined. The prosthesis should be compared with the prescription. The individual who authorized the prescription must approve departures from the original specifications.

The new wearer should stand in the parallel bars or other secure environment, attempting to bear equal weight on both feet. The therapist should solicit subjective comments about comfort. Estimates of anteroposterior and mediolateral alignment are aided by slipping a sheet of paper under various parts of the shoe. Ideally, the patient should stand with both heels and soles flat on the floor. Misalignment, indicated by excessive weight-bearing on one portion of the shoe, may be confirmed by subsequent analysis of gait.

Most prostheses are constructed so that when the individual stands, the pelvis is level;[36] if the pelvis tilts, the therapist should place lifts under the foot on the shorter side to restore a level pelvis. If the total lift measures 1/2 in. (1 cm) or less, no attention is needed. For greater discrepancy, one should seek causative factors. An amputation limb that sinks too far into the socket will make the prosthetic side appear short, and the wearer may complain of discomfort.

Piston action refers to vertical motion of the socket when the patient elevates the pelvis. Slippage can be determined by chalk marking the sock at the posterior margin of the socket and then having the patient elevate the ipsilateral pelvis. The socket should slip less than 1/4 inch (0.5 cm). Looseness, inadequate suspension, or both cause socket slippage. Socket walls should fit snugly, as should the thigh corset if it is part of the prosthesis.

Comfortable sitting is a primary need for all people. The posterior brim should not impinge into the popliteal fossa, and hamstring reliefs should be adequate, especially on the medial side where the semitendinosus and semimembranosus insert relatively distally. Placement of the tabs of the cuff or the joints of the corset also influences sitting comfort.

Dynamic Analysis

Analysis of the gait pattern and performance of other ambulatory activities is an essential part of rehabilitation. For most patients, a major reason for prosthetic fitting is to resume walking. Nevertheless, no prosthesis eradicates entirely the anatomical and physiological changes produced by amputation. When walking, the person who wears a prosthesis compensates for anatomical and prosthetic deficiencies.[69-73]

Some are inherent to amputation; others are abnormalities of the body or the prosthesis. Because virtually all people walk with a prosthesis in a manner different from the nondisabled walking pattern, prosthetic gait represents compensation for the patient's altered locomotor apparatus. The term *gait compensation* may be a more accurate descriptor than the more commonly used *gait deviation* inasmuch as the patient with amputation is unlikely to walk exactly like a nondisabled person.

No prosthesis restores sensation, skeletal continuity, muscle integrity, or full-body weight. Anatomical deficiencies are aggravated in the presence of pain, contracture, weakness, instability, or incoordination. Similarly, prosthetic components do not replace every function of the missing limb. For example, prosthetic feet do not move through the full excursion of the human counterpart. Inadequacies in the prosthesis compel the wearer to adopt gait compensations. Such problems include a poorly fitted socket, prosthetic misalignment, malfunctioning components, and improper height of the prosthesis. Compounding the problem are incorrect donning of the prosthesis and wearing inappropriate shoes. The physical therapist must determine when gait compensation exists and their potential causes so that remedial action may be taken. Otherwise, the patient is compelled to expend more energy walking and to exhibit a more conspicuously abnormal gait. The new wearer will have had brief experience walking in the prosthesis during the course of prosthetic fabrication. Although a smooth gait is unlikely on the day of the initial examination, gross departure from the usual gait exhibited by others with similar prostheses should be noted and causes sought.

Transtibial analysis focuses on action of the knee on the amputated side during stance phase. Both knees should flex in a controlled manner during their respective early and late stance phases. Excessive flexion of the knee on the amputated side indicates that the socket is aligned too far anterior in relation to the foot, or is excessively flexed; this deviation may cause the patient to fall. If the knee flexes too much only during early stance, the cause may be a heel cushion that is too firm for that wearer. Conversely, insufficient knee flexion results from posterior displacement of the socket or inadequate socket tilt. When viewed in the frontal plane, the socket brim should maintain reasonable contact with the leg; excessive lateral thrust of the prosthetic brim suggests that the prosthetic foot has been positioned too far medially. Table 31.1 summarizes the prosthetic and anatomical causes of transtibial gait compensations/deviations.

At the initial evaluation, performance on stairs and inclines may be omitted because the patient has not had training in these activities.

Inspection of the Prosthesis off the Patient

After conducting the dynamic analysis, the therapist should consider the potential relationship between gait deviations when the prosthesis is worn and signs of improper loading, such as skin redness or breakdown on the amputation limb when the prosthesis is off. The posterior wall should be approximately at the same level as the buildup for the patellar *ligament* (tendon) when the patient stands. To check this, the prosthesis is stood upright on a table; one end of a ruler is then placed on the anterior socket bulge and the opposite end on the posterior brim. In a well-constructed prosthesis, the ruler will slant upward toward the rear, indicating that when the individual stands in the prosthesis and compresses the heel cushion, the posterior wall will be at the proper height.

Any straps or cuff should provide reasonable adjustability. Construction is a guide to future durability and contributes to acceptable appearance of the prosthesis. The "Functional Capacities" section has more detail on specific outcome measures used with people with LL amputations.

Table 31.1 Transtibial Prosthetic Gait Analysis

Compensation/Deviation	Prosthetic Causes	Anatomical Causes
Early Stance		
1. Excessive knee flexion	Shoe heel too high Insufficient plantar flexion Heel cushion too stiff Socket too far anterior Socket excessively flexed Cuff tabs too posterior	Flexion contracture Weak quadriceps
2. Insufficient knee flexion	Shoe heel too low Excessive plantar flexion Heel cushion too soft Socket too far posterior Socket insufficiently flexed	Extensor spasticity Weak quadriceps Anterior–distal pain Arthritis
Midstance		
1. Lateral thrust	Excessive foot inset	
2. Medial thrust	Excessive foot outset	
Late Stance		
1. Early knee flexion: also referred to as "drop off"	Shoe heel too high Insufficient plantar flexion Keel too short Dorsiflexion stop too soft Socket too far anterior Socket excessively flexed	Flexion contracture
2. Delayed knee flexion: perception of walking uphill	Shoe heel too low Excessive plantar flexion Keel too long Dorsiflexion stop too stiff Socket too far posterior Socket insufficiently flexed	Extensor spasticity

Transfemoral Examination

A similar checklist is used to evaluate the transfemoral prosthesis (Appendix 31.B). It is important to recognize that seldom is one item of major significance. The therapist and entire team should look for patterns that might herald future difficulty. For example, misalignment detected in static analysis should be confirmed during gait.

Static Analysis

The patient who has a flesh roll above the socket either did not don the socket properly or has a thigh that is larger than that for which the socket was made. Perineal pressure results from sharpness of the medial brim or insufficiency of the adductor longus relief in a quadrilateral socket.

The knee unit should be stable enough to maintain extension after a firm push by the therapist to the posterior aspect of the unit when the patient stands. Stability is influenced by the *alignment* of the knee in relation to the hip and prosthetic ankle. The farther posterior the knee bolt, the more stable the knee will be. Polycentric linkage and mechanical stabilizers also contribute to stability. If the socket is opaque, the only way to judge its snugness is by palpating tissue protruding through the valve hole when the valve is removed.

The checklist is designed to help the clinician determine the fit of the socket, regardless of shape or material. If the prosthesis has a quadrilateral socket, proper location of the adductor longus tendon and ischial tuberosity ensures that the patient has donned the socket correctly. A horizontal posterior brim allows weight to be borne on the gluteal musculature as well as the ischial tuberosity. The ischial containment socket is intended to cover the ischial tuberosity, yet allows the client to move the hip in all directions comfortably, without socket gapping.

The lateral attachment of the Silesian belt should be superior and posterior to the greater trochanter for best control of prosthetic rotation. Anteriorly, the attachment should be at the level of the ischial tuberosity, or slightly below, to aid in adducting the prosthesis.

The pelvic joint and band should fit the torso snugly for optimum control of the prosthesis and to minimize bulkiness. The joint axis should be superior and anterior to the greater trochanter.

The patient should be able to sit comfortably with the prosthesis. Posterior discomfort may indicate inadequate hamstring relief, or a sharp or thick posterior brim.

Dynamic Analysis

Gait analysis gives the clinic team members the opportunity to determine the adequacy of socket fit and of prosthesis alignment and adjustment. The patient also influences the walking pattern by the timing and force of muscular contraction and the presence or absence of contractures. The goal of walking with a transfemoral prosthesis is a comfortable, safe, efficient gait, rather than duplicating the gait of someone wearing a transtibial prosthesis or one who does not have amputation.[74] Table 31.2 summarizes the prosthetic and anatomical causes of transfemoral gait compensations/deviations.

Compensations/Deviations Best Viewed From Behind

Many individuals with transfemoral amputation abduct the prosthesis to improve frontal plane balance (*abducted gait*). Hip abduction contracture predisposes patients to

Table 31.2 Transfemoral Prosthetic Gait Analysis

Compensation/Deviation	Prosthetic Causes	Anatomical Causes
Lateral Displacements		
1. Abduction: stance	Prosthesis too long Hip joint abducted Lateral wall inadequately adducted Medial wall too sharp or too high	Abduction contracture Weak abductors Lateral/distal pain Adductor redundancy instability
2. Circumduction: swing	Prosthesis too long Knee unit locked Friction insufficient Suspension inadequate Socket too small Socket too loose Foot plantar flexed	Abduction contracture Poor knee control
Trunk Shifts		
1. Lateral bend: stance	Prosthesis too short Lateral wall inadequately adducted Medial wall too sharp or too high	Abduction contracture Weak abductors Hip pain Instability Short amputation limb
2. Forward flexion: stance	Knee unit unstable Walker or crutches too short	Instability
3. Lordships: stance	Socket inadequately flexed	Hip flexion contracture Weak extensors
Rotations		
1. Medial (or lateral) whip: heel off	Socket contour faulty Knee bolt externally (or internally) rotated Foot malrotated Prosthesis donned in malrotation	With load-dependent friction unit, fast pace
2. Foot rotation at heel contact	Heel cushion too stiff Foot malrotated	
Excessive Knee Motion		
1. High heel rise: early swing	Friction insufficient Extension aid slack	

Table 31.2 Transfemoral Prosthetic Gait Analysis—cont'd

Compensation/Deviation	Prosthetic Causes	Anatomical Causes
2. Terminal impact: late swing	Friction insufficient Extension aid taut	Forceful hip flexion
Reduced Knee Motion		
1. Vault: swing	See above: circumduction	With fast pace
2. Hip hike: swing	See above: circumduction	Weak dorsiflexors Plantar flexor spasticity Pes equinus Weak hip flexors
Uneven Step Length	Socket uncomfortable Socket inadequately flexed	Hip flexion contracture Instability

this deviation, which is seen in stance phase. Inadequate socket adduction, socket looseness, or medial discomfort also causes the fault. *Circumduction* is a displacement exhibited in swing phase if the prosthesis is too long or if the patient is reluctant to allow the knee unit to bend. Socket looseness also may result in circumduction. The patient may shift the trunk excessively. *Lateral trunk bending* toward the prosthetic side during stance phase generally accompanies abducted gait. It should be noted, however, that all individuals with transfemoral amputation have an incomplete abductor mechanism and tend to compensate by bending toward the prosthetic side, especially when fatigued. Although the anatomic hip and gluteus medius are usually in good condition, lack of skeletal continuity compromises the effectiveness of abductor contraction. If the prosthesis is too long, the patient will abduct; if it is too short, the patient will bend the trunk laterally.

Whips refer to medial or lateral rotation of the heel at late stance. If the socket does not fit well, contraction with bulging of the thigh musculature will cause the prosthesis to rotate abruptly as it is being unloaded at the end of stance phase. Although less likely, malrotation of the knee unit or foot–ankle assembly may contribute to whipping. *Rotation of the foot on heel contact* is a much more serious deviation. It indicates inadequate compression of the heel cushion or plantar bumper or hip weakness and can lead to a fall.

Compensations/Deviations Best Viewed From the Side

Forward trunk shifting in stance phase is a compensation that some patients use to cope with knee instability. If the walker or crutches are too short, the individual will lean forward. Lumbar *lordosis* results from inadequate socket flexion and is aggravated by a hip flexion contracture.

Improper adjustment of the knee unit gives rise to *uneven heel rise* (excessive knee flexion) and *terminal swing impact* (abrupt knee extension). If both deviations are present, the probable cause is insufficient friction. If the knee exhibits impact without undue heel rise, it is more likely that the extension aid is too tight.

To compensate for reduced knee motion, the vigorous walker may demonstrate *vaulting* by excessively plantarflexing the sound ankle to afford extra room to clear the prosthesis during prosthetic swing phase. A less strenuous compensation for excessive actual or functional prosthesis length is *hip hiking,* when the patient elevates the pelvis on the prosthetic side.

Unequal step length will be evident if the patient has a hip flexion contracture or inadequate balance. A longer step taken with the prosthesis gives the person more time on the sound limb. A flexion contracture or insufficient socket flexion limiting hip extension range prevents the sound limb from passing the prosthetic side during swing phase on the sound limb.

Inspection of the Prosthesis off the Patient

Following the static evaluation, the therapist should examine the prosthesis and amputation limb as indicated on the checklist. A resilient back pad (placed externally on the posterior wall) enables the patient to sit quietly without undue trouser or skirt abrasion. The pad is unnecessary with a flexible socket. The "Functional Capacities" section has more detail on specific outcome measures used with people with LL amputations.

Facilitating Prosthetic Acceptance

Amputation generally is regarded as a grievous occurrence, with its visibility a constant reminder of the individual's abnormality. The physical therapist can help the patient and family accept the reality of amputation and the prosthesis by verbal and nonverbal communication. One's calm respect for the patient as a worthy human being, regardless of limb condition, should set a model for the attitudes of others. Clinic team management accords not only the benefits of better prosthetic provision but also brings the individual in contact with clinicians who convey experience and confidence in dealing with problems that the person may have considered unique.

As soon as possible, the hospitalized patient should be treated in the physical therapy department, rather than at bedside. The bustle of the department should help dispel despondency. Although postoperative mourning is expected, prolonged depression is not constructive. Peer support groups are often very effective in aiding acceptance of the prosthesis and in learning special procedures for accomplishing activities. Observation and eventual participation in specially designed sports programs is another way people learn to cope and gain the most from rehabilitation. The physical therapist, by virtue of close daily contact with the patient, is also in a position to recommend to the clinic those who might benefit from psychological counseling or psychiatric services, particularly when pain is an issue.

Prosthetic Training

Learning to use a prosthesis effectively involves being able to don it correctly, develop good balance and coordination, walk in a safe and reasonably symmetrical manner, and perform other ambulatory and self-care activities. Anticipated goals and expected outcomes depend on the patient's physical and psychological status, preprosthetic experience, and quality of prosthesis. Using the prosthesis only to assist in transferring from the wheelchair to the toilet may be an appropriate outcome for an elderly person with multiple disabilities, whereas the program for the youngster with traumatic amputation might extend to a full range of sports.

Donning

Correct application of the prosthesis and frequent inspection of the amputation limb are very important, especially for the beginner and those with poor circulation. Patients with partial foot, Syme's, and transtibial amputations can don the prosthesis while seated, after having applied the correct number and sequence of socks or sheath. Then, in most instances, the individual simply inserts the amputation limb into the socket. With SC/SP suspension, one applies the liner to the amputation limb, then inserts the limb and liner into the socket. The initial entry into the socket with corset suspension may be made while sitting; however, final tightening of laces or straps should be done in the standing position to ensure that the limb is lodged suitably in the socket.

Those with transfemoral amputation also can begin the donning process while seated. Total suction wearers may use either a pulling or pushing method. To pull oneself into the socket, the patient applies a light dusting of talcum powder to the thigh to reduce friction. Then one applies a pulling sock, a tubular cotton stockinet approximately 30 in. (76 cm) long, a roll of elastic bandage wound around the thigh, or a nylon stocking. Whatever the donning aid, it should be placed high in the groin to pull in proximal tissues. After placing the sock-encased thigh into the socket, one draws the distal end of the aid through the valve hole. Although it is possible to complete the donning process while seated, most people prefer to stand while pulling the sock or other aid out through the valve hole. By leaning forward, the body's weight line will prevent the prosthetic knee from flexing inadvertently. The patient alternately flexes and extends the sound hip and knee while tugging downward on the donning aid until it slips out from the prosthesis. Finally, one inserts the valve. Another approach to donning is to coat the thigh with lubricating lotion, push it into the socket, then install the valve.

Patients who use partial suction apply a sock, making certain the proximal margin of the sock extends to the inguinal ligament. The patient then introduces the amputation limb into the socket, taking care that the thigh is correctly oriented; pulls the distal end of the sock down through the valve hole enough to ensure that the skin is smooth; tucks the sock back into the socket; and inserts the valve. Finally, one secures the pelvic band or Silesian belt. If suction is not used, donning is similar to the method used with partial suction, except that there is no valve.

Exercises to Stretch and Strengthen

Exercises are similar for all patients with LL amputations, although the individual with a transfemoral or hip disarticulation prosthesis may be expected to encounter more difficulty controlling the mechanical knee, as compared to those with two anatomical knees. Hip flexor flexibility is often limited but important to allow advance of the body over the pelvis (Fig 31.40). Hip strength can be developed prior to and after prosthetic fitting without wearing the prosthesis by pressing the residual limb against a bolster or towel roll (Fig 31.41). With the prosthesis, an elastic band can be used to apply resistance at the level of the residual limb to accentuate the forceful sensation against the prosthetic socket needed to control the prosthetic limb (Fig 31.42). See Chapter 22, Amputation, for more information on exercise prescription for people with LL amputations.

Balance and Coordination

All people with LL amputations must learn to balance on the amputated side.[75-77] A graduated program for increasing prosthetic tolerance minimizes the danger of skin abrasion, particularly if the amputation limb presents skin grafts, poor circulation, or diminished sensation. The patient should alternately exercise and rest, with cardiopulmonary monitoring a routine part of the program, especially for high-risk individuals.

Some clinicians eschew parallel bars because the fearful patient pulls on them, which will be fruitless when progressing to a cane. When bars are used, the therapist should encourage the patient to rest the open hand on the bar for support, rather than using a tight grip. A plinth or sturdy table offers the dual advantages of providing good support on only one side, and unidirectional

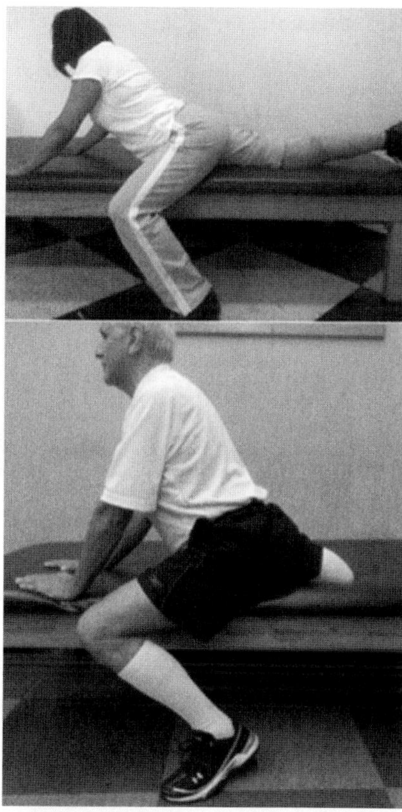

Figure 31.40 Hip flexor muscle stretching can be performed with or without the prosthesis for transtibial and transfemoral amputation levels.

control, because the patient can only push, never pull, for balance.

Static erect balance reintroduces the novice to bipedal posture. The patient should strive for level pelvis and shoulders, vertical trunk without excessive lordosis, and equal weight-bearing. The therapist should guard and assist the patient as necessary. When the physical therapist stands near the prosthesis, this encourages the patient to shift his or her weight onto it. The client must learn to utilize proximal sensory receptors to maintain balance and perceive the position of the prosthesis without looking at the floor. Some patients respond well to increased use of visual feedback (e.g., using a mirror).[78,79]

Static exercises to improve medial–lateral, sagittal, and rotary control can later be progressed to dynamic exercises (Fig. 31.43). The patient learns that hip flexion causes the knee to bend, and hip extension stabilizes the knee during stance phase. Placing the sound foot ahead of the prosthesis makes the prosthetic knee more stable. Patients should be instructed in weight shifting in both symmetrical and stride positions and in stepping movements. Stepping on a low stool or step platform with the sound foot obliges the patient to shift weight onto the prosthesis and increases stance phase duration on the prosthesis. Having all exercises performed rhythmically with both the right and left LLs fosters symmetrical performance.

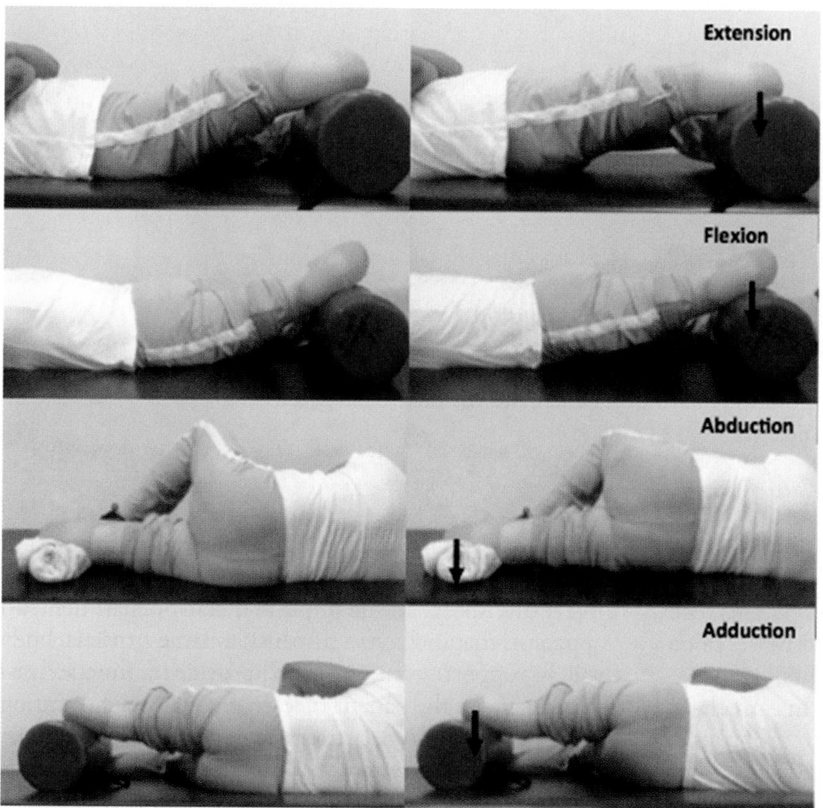

Figure 31.41 Hip strengthening exercises can be performed without the prosthesis by pressing down against a bolster with the residual limb to lift the pelvis off the table. *(Courtesy of Dr. Christopher Kevin Wong, with permission.)*

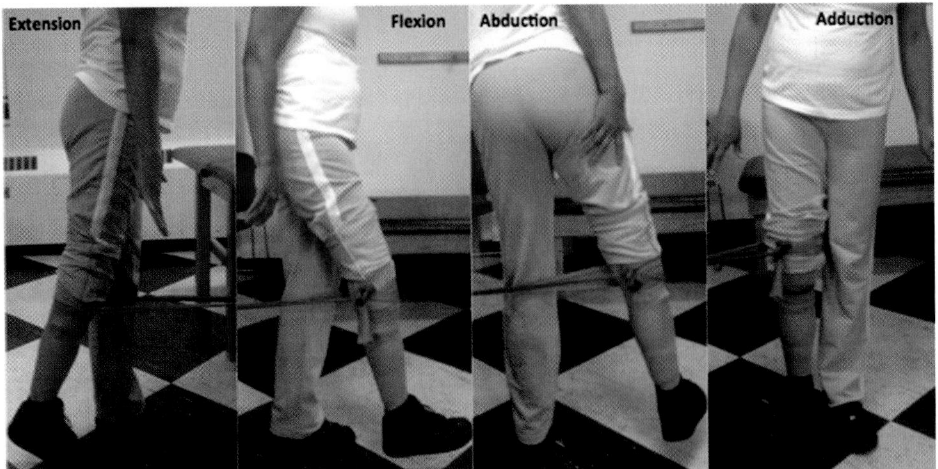

Figure 31.42 Elastic band resistance can be used for hip strengthening with the prosthesis. *(Courtesy of Dr. Christopher Kevin Wong, with permission.)*

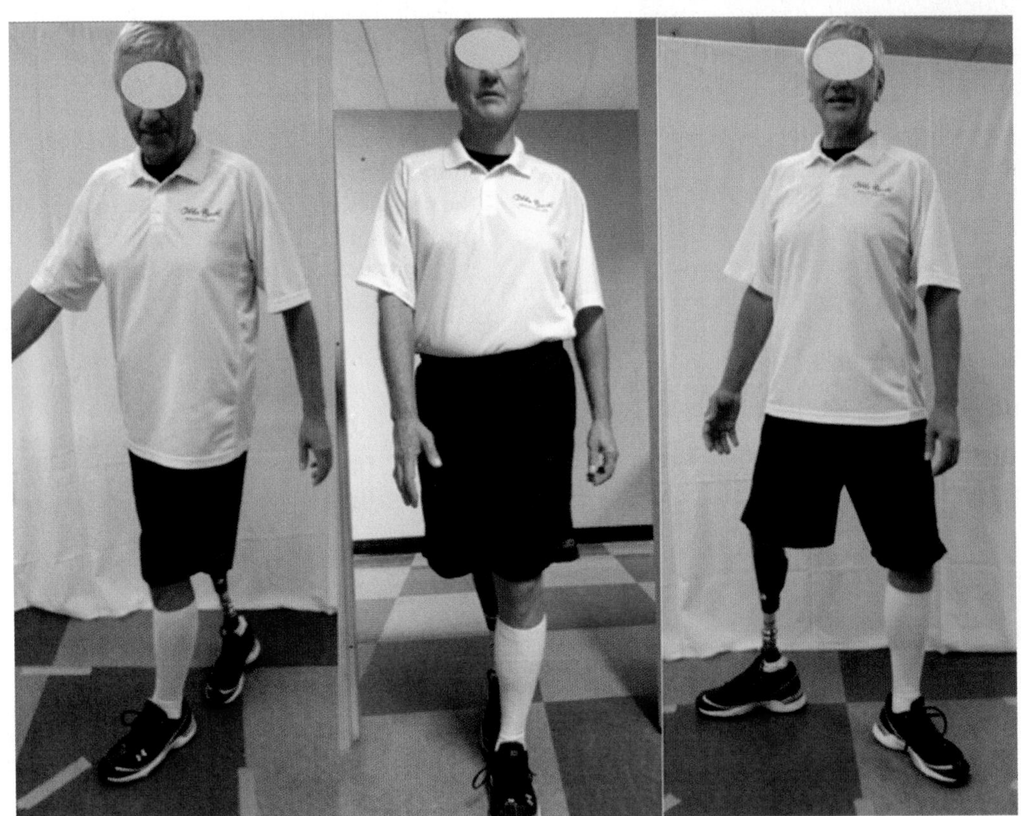

Figure 31.43 Static balance exercises incorporating hip rotation and a narrow base of support. *(Courtesy of Dr. Christopher Kevin Wong, with permission.)*

Gait Training

Walking is a natural progression from dynamic balance exercises as the patient takes successive steps. Patients tend to place greater load and exert more propulsive force on the intact side; consequently, gait training should emphasize symmetrical performance.[72,77,79,80] Inasmuch as hamstrings become the main muscles of propulsion, strengthening exercises are indicated (Fig. 31.44). Some people respond well to proprioceptive neuromuscular facilitation[81,82] (Fig. 31.45). Rhythmic counting and walking in time with music in 2/4 time also improves gait symmetry and speed. In the physical therapy department, an apparatus that includes a suspension harness (partial body weight support) over a treadmill provides a protected environment for the patient to learn gradual weight-bearing on the prosthesis. A balance apparatus providing electronic feedback with or without emphasis on psychological awareness of bodily position is another training option.[83]

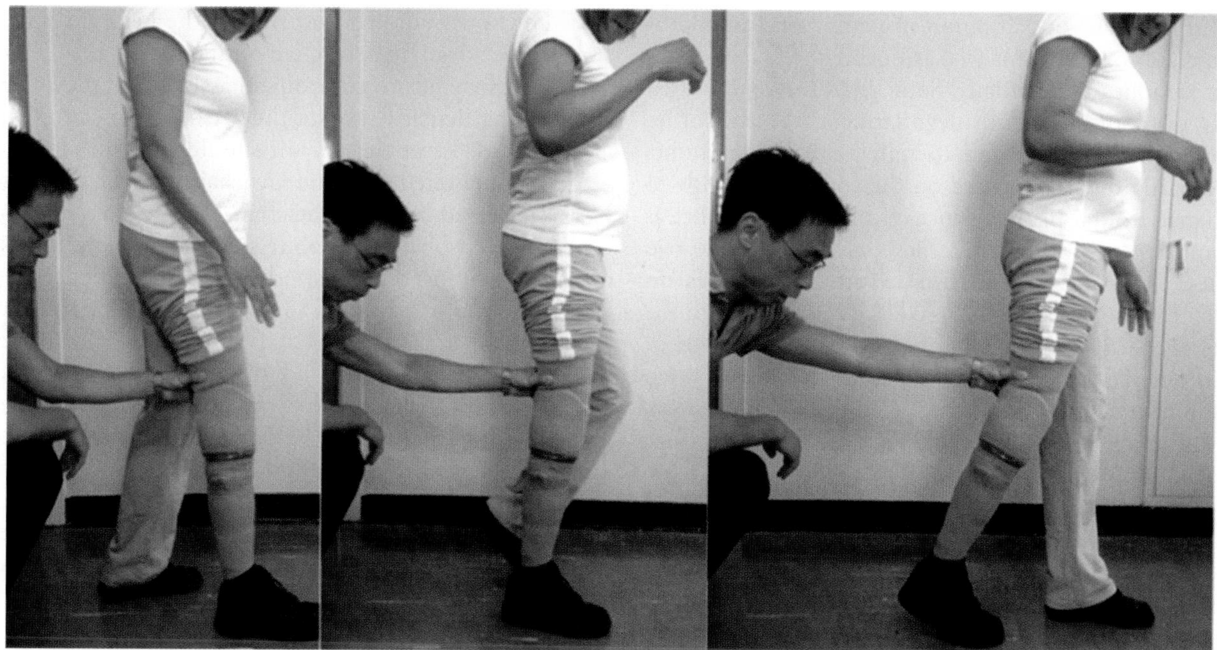

Figure 31.44 Resistance applied to the prosthetic side limb to develop hip extension strength throughout the gait cycle. *(Courtesy of Dr. Christopher Kevin Wong, with permission.)*

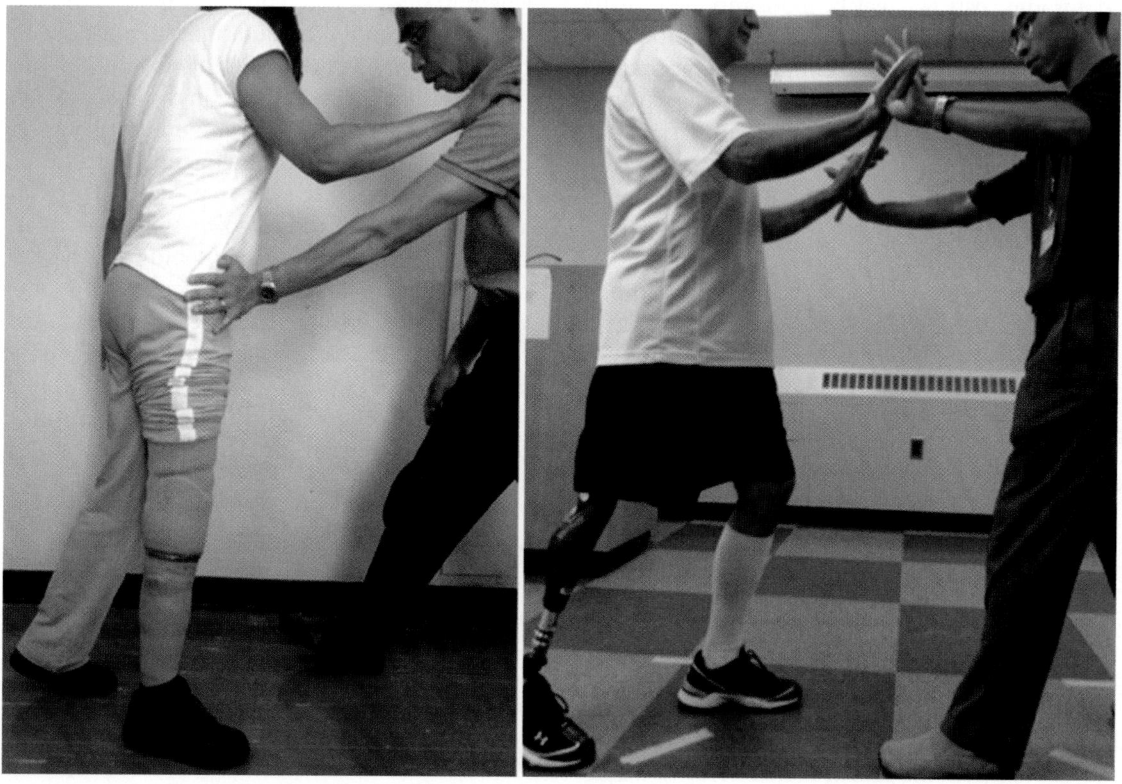

Figure 31.45 Resistance applied through the pelvis or trunk via the arms to develop hip extension strength during gait. *(Courtesy of Dr. Christopher Kevin Wong, with permission.)*

Either a cane or pair of forearm crutches is an appropriate aid for the client who is unable to achieve a safe gait without undue fatigue. Sometimes the cane is used only outdoors to aid in negotiating curbs and other ground irregularities and to signal oncoming traffic. Ordinarily the cane is used on the contralateral side to enhance frontal plane balance. If bilateral assistance is required, a pair of forearm crutches is preferable to two canes. The crutches remain clasped around the forearms when the user opens a door. Axillary crutches tempt the patient to lean on the axillary bars, risking impingement of the radial nerves; they are also inconvenient when climbing stairs. An aluminum walker provides maximum stability, which is particularly useful for patients with generalized weakness. The walker should be adjusted so that the user does not lean too far forward. Ultimately, some people will need walking aids to maintain balance[84] and have confidence to maximize prosthetic function and participate in community social activities.[85,86]

Functional Training

The prosthesis wearer who is learning to walk also should gain experience in performing a wide variety of functional mobility skills both indoors and outdoors. Activities such as transferring to various chairs add interest to the program and, for some patients, may be more important than long-distance ambulation. The training program for vigorous individuals includes stair climbing, negotiating ramps, retrieving objects from the floor, kneeling, sitting on the floor, running, multiple terrains, driving a car, and engaging in sports.[87] The fundamental difference between these activities and walking is the way each LL is used. Walking implies symmetrical usage, but the other activities are done asymmetrically, with greater reliance on the strength, agility, and sensory control of the sound limb.

Generally, the patient should have the opportunity to analyze each new situation and arrive at a solution to the problem rather than depending on directions from the therapist. Most tasks can be accomplished safely in several ways. The learner profits from practice in clinical decision making and observing other prosthesis wearers as well as from professional instruction.

Transfers

Rising from different chairs, the toilet, and the car are primary skills even for people who are elderly or debilitated. Most patients enter the physical therapy department in a wheelchair. Initially, the patient can park the chair at the parallel bars or at a plinth. After locking the wheelchair and raising the footrests, the patient should sit forward and transfer weight to the intact leg, then push down on the armrests. The individual will find that placing the sound foot close to the chair enables rising by extending the knee and hip on the sound side. Sitting is accomplished by placing the sound foot close to the chair and lowering oneself by controlling hip and knee flexion on the sound side with eccentric strength or assist of the arms.

For both standing and sitting, the beginner should have the advantage of a chair with armrests that enables use of the hands to control and assist trunk movement. This is particularly true for the person with bilateral amputations. Later the person should practice sitting in deep upholstered sofas and low chairs, as well as benches, the toilet, and other seats that do not have armrests. Transfer into an automobile should be an integral part of the training activities; otherwise, the patient faces a gloomy future, confined to home or dependent on special transportation systems. To enter the right (passenger) side of an automobile, the prosthetic wearer faces the front of the car. The person with a right prosthesis puts the right hand on the door post and the left hand on the back of the front seat, then swings the left leg into the car, slides onto the car seat, and finally places the prosthesis in the car. The individual with a left prosthesis may find that sitting sideways with both feet out the car door is easiest. One then pivots on the seat while swinging the prosthesis into the car, then puts the intact right foot inside the car.

Climbing Stairs, Ramps, and Curbs

Patients with Syme's and transtibial amputations generally ascend and descend stairs and inclines with steps of equal length in step-over-step progression.[88,89] Those with unilateral transfemoral amputation, in contrast, usually ascend by leading with the sound foot and learn to descend by first placing the prosthesis on the lower step. Some individuals with transfemoral amputation using a hydraulic prosthetic knee flexion subsequently learn to control the knee and descend step-over-step. Some may be able to use a handrail to ascend step-over-step, particularly if the prosthetic knee such as the Genium® locks in weightbearing even at large angles of knee flexion; others fitted with a knee that provides a knee extension assist such as the PowerKnee® may be able to ascend stairs step-over-step (see Fig. 31.28).

Curbs present a slightly different problem, because there is no handrail. The techniques are basically the same, however.

Ramps may be difficult if the prosthetic foot and ankle do not have sufficient dorsiflexion and plantarflexion.[90-92] With steep stairs, ramps, and curbs, the individual may climb diagonally or sidestep with the prosthesis kept on the downhill side. Patients should also learn how to maneuver over obstacles on the walking surface.[93]

Final Evaluation and Follow-up Care

Economic strictures may compel the therapist to conclude the training program after the patient is able to walk and to negotiate basic transfers and stair climbing but before the full range of training activities is completed. Before discharge, the patient and prosthesis should be reexamined to make certain that socket fit, prosthetic appearance, and function are acceptable. The checklist used for initial evaluation can be used. The physical therapist should instruct the patient with regard to the patient's responsibility for reporting skin redness and any loose or missing parts from the prosthesis.

The new prosthesis wearer should return to the training site at regular intervals so that the clinic team may examine socket fit. Most will require major socket revision or replacement during the first year to accommodate amputation limb volume reduction. Follow-up visits are good opportunities to augment training and to encourage the individual to engage in the widest possible range of activities.

Functional Capacities

Functional capacities refer to the individual's ability to walk, transfer from chairs, climb stairs, and perform other ambulatory activities, including recreational endeavors. A primary responsibility of the clinic team is to predict the probable function of the person with a new amputation, to determine whether the individual would benefit from a prosthesis, and what degree of activity is likely. Because many people with LL amputation are elderly with several medical problems, the need for accurate forecasting and ongoing monitoring is especially critical.

Walking with a prosthesis increases energy cost.[94-96] Compared with those people with two sound limbs, the individual with a unilateral transtibial prosthesis requires slightly more oxygen when walking at a comfortable speed;[97] the person wearing a transfemoral prosthesis consumes nearly 50% more oxygen than normal,[98] although selection of prosthetic feet and knee units usually modifies the energy demand.[99-102] The prosthesis wearer chooses a comfortable pace, because at a speed that is natural for the individual, the energy cost per minute is similar to that of the person who does not require a prosthesis, although speed is slower. The lower the amputation level, the less the metabolic disadvantage. Among persons with transtibial amputations older than 40, those with long amputation limbs average minimal increase in energy, but persons with shorter limbs work harder. Those with bilateral transtibial amputations expend less energy than those with unilateral transfemoral amputations. Individuals whose amputation was traumatic perform more efficiently than those whose amputation was caused by vascular disease at every amputation level. People who sustained trauma walk faster and use less oxygen than their dysvascular counterparts.

The increased metabolic expenditure results in part from the socket, which surrounds semifluid tissue, giving imperfect anchorage. The foot–ankle assembly transmits no plantar tactile or proprioceptive sensation, does not move through as large an excursion as the anatomic foot, and does not initiate the dynamic propulsion characteristic of normal gait. The transfemoral prosthesis also incorporates a knee unit that provides no proprioception to the wearer. The problem is aggravated by the fact that a prosthesis is operated by remotely located muscles that contract longer and more forcefully than in normal gait. With transfemoral amputation, for example, the wearer positions the prosthetic foot by hip motion. The resulting alteration of motion is reflected in asymmetry of timing, further disturbing gait smoothness. Individuals with prostheses walk with greater vertical movement, inasmuch as the knee, whether mechanical for the transfemoral prosthesis wearer or anatomical in the transtibial wearer, does not flex as much as the contralateral knee during stance phase.

Use of a hip disarticulation prosthesis demands considerable energy expenditure.[103] People wearing bilateral prostheses consume even more oxygen and walk more slowly than those with unilateral amputation at a given level.[104]

With the exception of patients on beta blockers, heart rate response is an important indication of the metabolic cost of prosthetic use for most individuals. Overall, strength, balance ability, etiology of amputation, and level of amputation predict the extent of activity restriction.[105]

Other measures of functional capacities include the Amputee Mobility Predictor,[106] quality of life and prostheses utilization,[107-109] general health status, physical activity, social integration, and quality of life.[110-124] Return to home and work[125-127] and ability to drive an automobile[128,129] are other indicators of rehabilitation success. The Amputee Mobility Predictor is a 21-item assessment that combines clinical measures of balance and gait assessment scale for people with amputations.[106] Scores can be used to indicate progress during rehabilitation but do not differentiate clearly among people with different K-levels due to overlapping score ranges. Specific balance assessments[130] and gait measures[110,131] have good psychometric properties as outcome measures. Self-reported measures such as the Activities-Specific Balance Confidence Scale,[132] the Prosthetic Evaluation Questionnaire,[114] and the Trinity Amputation and Prosthetic Experience Scales[118] provide subjective information that provides insight into confidence, prosthetic function, and quality of life (see Table 31.3).

Sports participation (Fig. 31.46) is an excellent extension of rehabilitation for patients of all ages.[133-144] Older adults may enjoy fishing, golfing, dancing, tai chi chuan, and shuffleboard, and younger people may add basketball, tennis, archery, and track events to their range of activities. Most sports do not require any adaptation to the prosthesis. Horseback riding is a superb activity that fosters trunk control and seated balance. The hiker should pack extra amputation limb socks or a sheath to protect the skin; a well-fitting, comfortable hiking boot is essential. Bowling and participating in shot put are facilitated by emphasizing balance on the intact LL. For sports that involve running, an energy-storing/releasing foot is most suitable. The socket should fit snugly with very secure suspension to minimize abrasion of the amputation limb. People with Syme's or

Table 31.3 Selected Outcome Measures

ICF Domain	Outcome Measure	Description	Scoring
Patient Contextual Factors	Prosthetic Evaluation Questionnaire*	Self-report of 11 domains of prosthetic use: Ambulation, Appearance, Frustration, Mobility, Perceived response, Residual limb, Social burden, Sounds, Transfers, Utility, Well-being	Visual Analog Scales Reliability[110] ICC = 0.41 – 0.93
	Houghton Scale	Self-report quantifying prosthetic use and function	Categorical Reliability[109] ICC – 0.96
	Activities-Specific Balance Confidence Scale	Self-report quantifying balance confidence during daily activities	Visual analog scale scores Reliability[132] ICC = 0.91
Body Structure and Function	Range of motion	Goniometry	Not reliability tested in people with limb loss
	Strength	Handheld dynamometry	No reliability tested in people with limb loss
Activity	Balance	Berg Balance Scale	Reliability[130] ICC = .99
	Gait	2-Minute and	Reliability[110] ICC = 0.83 – 0.96
		6-Minute Walk tests	Reliability[110] ICC = 0.94 – 0.97
		Timed-Up-and-Go	Reliability[110] ICC = 0.88 – 0.96
	Locomotor Capability Index	Self-report quantifying walking ability	Reliability[131] ICC = 0.88 – 0.92
	Multidimensional Function	Amputee Mobility Predictor	Reliability[110] ICC = 0.88 – 0.98
Participation	Short Form-36	Self-report quality of life scale: general health, physical functioning, physical role	Categorical Reliability[110] ICC = 0.61 – 0.81
	Frenchay Activities Index	Self-report activity participation scale:	Reliability[111] ICC = 0.79
	OPUS-Orthotic Prosthetic User Survey	Self-report quality of life scale: quality of life, LL function, satisfaction	Reliability[110] ICC = 0.50 – 0.85

transtibial amputations usually run with reasonably symmetrical step lengths, although they will favor the sound limb, which has greater propulsive ability.[7] Those with a knee disarticulation or transfemoral amputation will derive most of the propulsive force from the sound leg and use the prosthesis as a momentary prop. Many marathon competitions have a category for people with disabilities. Jumping, as in basketball, requires the athlete to generate a substantial upward force with the sound leg; landing is more comfortable on the sound leg, particularly for those who wear transfemoral prostheses. Some activities are facilitated by minor modification of the equipment, such as a toe loop on a bicycle pedal or an adapted prosthesis.

Other activities are generally performed without a prosthesis, such as swimming and skiing. The skier will probably use ski poles equipped with small rudders, in a "three-track" manner. Soccer is usually played without

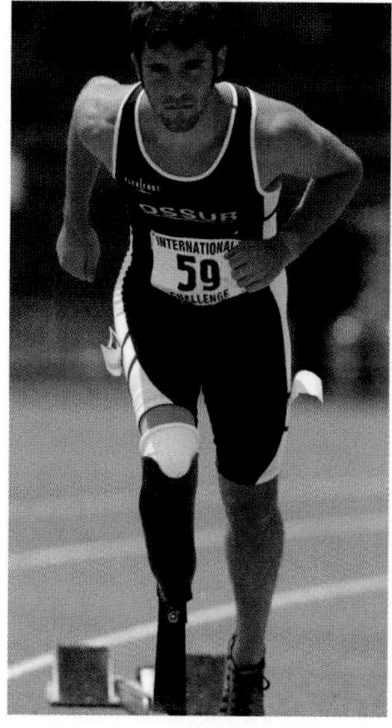

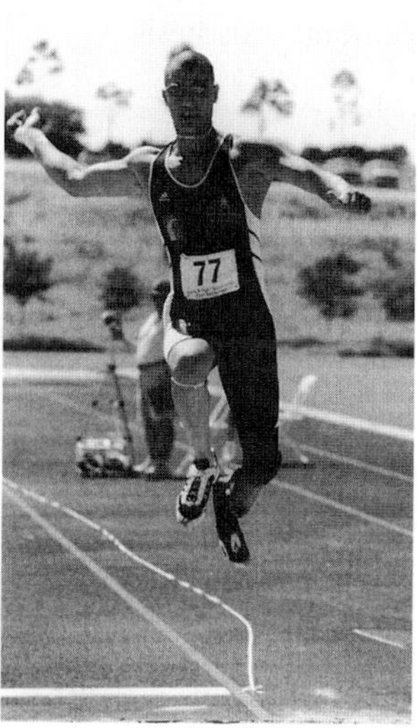

Figure 31.46 Participants in a distance run (*left*) and long jump (*right*) event. *(Courtesy of Ossur, Aliso Viejo, CA 92656.)*

a prosthesis, with the player using a pair of crutches. Some individuals enjoy playing tennis and field events in a wheelchair. Equipment and techniques developed for individuals with paraplegia usually can be adapted for people with amputations.

Recreational programs designed for adults with amputations help the participants to return to active lifestyles. The physical therapist should be able to refer patients to convenient recreational clubs and sporting events. The desired outcome is to maximize each person's functional capacity and quality of life.

SUMMARY

This chapter has focused on the prosthetic management of adults with LL amputations. Characteristics and function of the principal LL prostheses and prosthetic components have been discussed. In addition, the responsibilities of the physical therapist in prosthetic management have been emphasized. Successful prosthetic rehabilitation depends on close collaboration among the patient, physical therapist, physician, prosthetist, and other team members. This will provide an environment for information exchange and foster coordinated management. The result will be an optimum match between the patient's physical and psychosocial characteristics and a prosthesis capable of fulfilling its intended purposes.

Questions for Review

1. What are the principal causes of amputation in the elderly? In the young?
2. Describe appropriate prostheses for individuals with various partial foot amputations.
3. Distinguish between the Syme's and the transtibial amputation limbs and prostheses.
4. What prosthetic feet are especially suitable for elderly patients? Why?
5. Name the reliefs and buildups in the transtibial socket.
6. Contrast the modes of suspension for the transtibial prosthesis. Which suspension is indicated for an individual with a very short amputation limb?
7. Classify knee units according to friction mechanisms.
8. Compare the quadrilateral and the ischial containment transfemoral sockets.
9. Describe the modes of suspension of the transfemoral prosthesis. In which type(s) does the client wear a sock?
10. How is the wearer of a hip disarticulation prosthesis prevented from inadvertently flexing the prosthetic hip and knee?
11. Outline a maintenance program for a transfemoral prosthesis with hydraulic knee unit and endoskeletal shank.
12. What factors should be considered prior to formulating a prosthetic prescription?
13. How can the physical therapist determine and improve the patient's psychological status?

14. What features of the transtibial prosthesis are considered in static evaluation? In dynamic evaluation?
15. Delineate the training program for a patient with a transfemoral prosthesis.

CASE STUDY

The patient is a 55-year-old man and former college athlete who has peripheral artery disease and lost his right leg at the transfemoral level a year ago. Delayed wound healing prolonged his hospital stay and delayed prosthetic fitting for 6 months, during which time he received a short episode of home-based physical therapy. The therapist had reinforced consistent care, and inspection of the left foot and right residuum prepared him for his prosthesis with weight-bearing residual limb exercises and general mobility with forearm crutches. He received a K2-rated prosthetic limb at the prosthetic clinic, at which time he "learned to walk" in the parallel bars before going home using one crutch. Over the next 6 months, he began walking on his own with a cane indoors and outdoors, though mostly just to his car to commute to work from his suburban home. He doesn't like slowing people down or getting so exhausted that he has to rest while people wait for him, so he limits his social activities to avoid having to walk too much. He has been referred to physical therapy because of a recent fall on his sloping driveway that resulted in low back pain (NRPS 3/10) aggravated by walking a few minutes. Although the low back pain has diminished over time, he presents with notable limitations presented in the domains of the International Classification of Functioning (see Table 31.3).

PHYSICAL THERAPY EXAMINATION FINDINGS

Body Structure and Function

- Cognition: Alert, oriented, memory intact
- Vision: Intact with corrective lens
- Cardiopulmonary:
  - Vital signs seated at rest: Blood pressure 140/86, heart rate 84, respiration normal
  - Endurance: Exercise capacity less than 10 minutes before needing rest
- Integumentary: Incision well healed without adherent scar
- Neuromuscular: Sensation and reflexes normal bilateral
- Musculoskeletal:
  - ROM: Hip extension R −15, L −5; hip adduction R −15, L −5
  - Joint mobility: Hip and sacrum hypomobile bilateral
  - Flexibility: L SLR 50, PKB 90
  - MMT: Hip extension, abduction, and flexion R 3+/5, L 4+/5
  - Prosthesis-related:
    - Amputated limb: ~ 50% of femur length
    - Prosthesis:
      - Silicone liner for suction suspension with pin-lock
      - Endoskeletal shank with flexible inner and fenestrated outer sockets
      - Weight-activated knee (3R93)
      - Non-energy-storing multiaxis foot/ankle (Greissinger Foot + multiaxis ankle)

Activity

- Balance: Berg Balance Scale (BBS) score performed with his prosthesis 46/56, placing him in the second lowest of the four balance ability strata[145] with the following items not receiving maximum scores:
  - Turning 360 degrees in a circle
  - Retrieve object from floor
  - Stand in tandem
  - Alternate steps
  - Stand on one leg (either)
  - Stand from sitting without hands.
- Gait: 0.7 m/s with cane over 2 minutes, putting him in category of independent household and limited community walker.[146] Rarely walks longer than 5 minutes at one time. Decreased prosthetic-side stance time with lateral trunk lean and shorter sound-side step length with lack of prosthetic-side hip extension past neutral contributes to asymmetric gait appearance.
- AMP(PRO): Total score 30, placing him within the range of AMP scores for K1, K2, and K3 prosthetic users.[106,147]

Participation

- Home living: Independent, but limited from some household chores such as laundry and shopping that involve carrying while walking or navigating stairs/slopes/curbs.
- Vocational: Goes to work in an office independently.
- Social: Walks outdoors only to commute; rarely leaves home to go shopping or socialize.

Individual and Environmental Contextual Factors

He lives with his wife in a split-level home with a sloping yard. He works in an office near home, his wife works full-time in the nearby city, and his adult daughter lives in an apartment in the same city. He used to enjoy nature walks with his wife, dining out with his family, and jogging and golfing but has not returned to any of these activities. In fact, the back pain combined with distal residual limb pain after walking and phantom limb pain at night have contributed to decreasing activity in the past year and some anxiety about his future.

PERSON-DESIRED OUTCOME AND GOALS

Reduce back pain, improve walking ability, and prevent future falls are his stated goals.

GUIDING QUESTIONS

The primary outcome around which rehabilitation efforts may focus will be the patient-centered goal of participating more fully in life by leaving the home for social and community activities. However, addressing impairment-based goals at the level of the body structure and function are critical supporting blocks upon which to build future abilities. In addition, maximizing body structure and functions to optimize ability in functional activities such as walking speed can also help an individual qualify for more advanced prosthetic components that can in turn benefit social-community integration. For instance, K3-level prosthetic users can qualify for hydraulic knees that make descending stairs and slopes safer—which was his recent mechanism of injury. Consideration of a person's limitations in all domains of the International Classification of Functioning as well as broad examination across systems and treatment for all relevant body structures and function with the overall goal of achieving a SMART patient-identified participation goal may well provide the best results for any individual case (see Table 31.3).

1. Identify the impairments, activity limitations, and participation restrictions you will address in developing the plan of care.
   a. Body structure and function impairments
      i. Impaired range of motion particularly at the hip
      ii. Impaired muscular strength particularly of the hip
      iii. Impaired cardiovascular endurance
   b. Activity limitations
      i. Reduced balance ability
      ii. Reduced walking ability as measured by speed, distance, or endurance
   c. Participation restrictions
      i. Restricted social interaction
      ii. Restricted community integration
2. Establish reasonable expected outcomes (long-term participation goal) and anticipated goals (short-term).
   - For each long-term participation goal, identify activity limitations that should be ameliorated to facilitate participation.
   - For each activity limitation, identify body structure/function impairments that, if reduced, can minimize the activity limitation.
   - Plan interventions to address body structure/function impairment and functional activity limitations.
   - Note safety precautions that should be observed during treatment of this patient.
   - Note strategies to develop self-management and self-efficacy in achieving goals and outcomes.

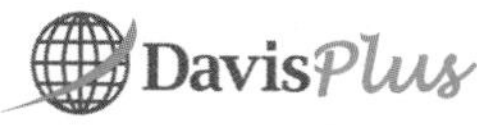

For additional resources, including answers to the questions for review and case study guiding questions, please visit **http://davisplus.fadavis.com.**

References

1. Ziegler-Graham, K, et al: Estimating the prevalence of limb loss in the United States: 2005 to 2050. Arch Phys Med Rehabil 89:422, 2008.
2. Rommers, GM, et al: Shoe adaptation after amputation of the II-V phalangeal bones of the foot. Prosthet Orthot Int 30:324, 2006.
3. Dudkiewicz, I, et al: Trans-metatarsal amputation in patients with a diabetic foot: Reviewing 10 years' experience. Foot 19:201, 2009.
4. Dillon, MP, and Barker, TM: Comparison of gait of persons with partial foot amputation wearing prosthesis to matched control group: Observational study. J Rehabil Res Dev 45:1317, 2008.
5. Burger, H, et al. Biomechanics of walking with silicone prosthesis after midtarsal (Chopart) disarticulation. Clin Biomech (Bristol, Avon), 24:510, 2009.
6. Berke, GM, et al: Biomechanics of ambulation following partial foot amputation: A prosthetic perspective. J Prosthet Orthot 19:85, 2007.
7. Pinzur, MS: Syme's ankle disarticulation. Foot Ankle Clin 15(3): 487–494, 2010.
8. Frykberg, RG, et al: Syme amputation for limb salvage: Early experience with 26 cases. J Foot Ankle Surg 46:93, 2007.
9. Johannsson, A, Larsson, GU, and Ramstrand, N: Incidence of lower-limb amputation in the diabetic and nondiabetic general population: A 10-year population-based cohort study of initial unilateral and contralateral amputations and reamputations. Diabetes Care 32:275, 2009.
10. Klodd, E, et al: Effects of prosthetic foot forefoot flexibility on oxygen cost and subjective preference rankings of unilateral transtibial prosthesis users. J Rehabil Res Dev 47:543, 2010.
11. Versluys, R, et al: Prosthetic foot: State-of-the-art review and the importance of mimicking human ankle-foot biomechanics. Disabil Rehabil Assist Technol 4:65, 2009.
12. Hsu, MJ, et al: The effects of prosthetic foot design on physiologic measurements, self-selected walking velocity, and physical activity in people with transtibial amputation. Arch Phys Med Rehabil 87:123, 2006.
13. Zmitrewicz, RJ, et al: The effect of foot and ankle prosthetic components on braking and propulsive impulses during transtibial amputee gait. Arch Phys Med Rehabil 87:1334, 2006.
14. Zmitrewicz, RJ, Neptune, RR, and Sasaki, K: Mechanical energetic contributions from individual muscles and elastic prosthetic feet during symmetric unilateral transtibial amputees walking: A theoretical study. J Biomech 40:1824, 2007.
15. Agrawal, V, et al: Symmetry in external work (SEW): A novel method of quantifying gait differences between prosthetic feet. Prosthet Orthot Int 33:146, 2009.
16. McMulkin, ML, et al: Comparison of three pediatric prosthetic feet during functional activities. J Prosthet Orthot 16:78, 2004.
17. Wolf, SI, et al: Pressure characteristics at the stump/socket interface in transtibial amputees using an adaptive prosthetic foot. Clin Biomech (Bristol, Avon) 24:860, 2009.
18. Alimusaj, M, et al: Kinematics and kinetics with an adaptive ankle foot system during stair ambulation of transtibial amputees. Gait Posture 30:356, 2009.
19. Berge, JS, Czerniecki, JM, and Klute, GK: Efficacy of shock-absorbing versus rigid pylons for impact reduction in transtibial amputees based on laboratory, field, and outcome metrics. J Rehabil Res Dev 42:795, 2005.
20. Adderson, JA, et al: Effect of a shock-absorbing pylon on transmission of heel strike forces during the gait of people with unilateral trans-tibial amputations: A pilot study. Prosthet Orthot Int 31: 384, 2007.
21. Segal, AD, Kracht, R, and Klute, GK: Does a torsion adapter improve functional mobility, pain, and fatigue in patients with transtibial amputation? Clin Orthop Rel Res 472:3085, 2014.
22. Selles, RW, et al: A randomized controlled trial comparing functional outcome and cost efficiency of a total surface-bearing socket versus a conventional patellar tendon-bearing socket in transtibial amputees. Arch Phys Med Rehabil 86:154, 2005.
23. Chow, DH, et al: The effect of prosthesis alignment on the symmetry of gait in subjects with unilateral transtibial amputation. Prosthet Orthot Int 30:114, 2006.
24. Jia, X, et al: Effects of alignment on interface pressure for transtibial amputees during walking. Disabil Rehabil Assist Technol 3:339, 2008.
25. Klute, GK, Glaister, BC, and Berge, JS: Prosthetic liners for lower limb amputees: A review of the literature. Prosthet Orthot Int 34: 146, 2010.
26. Safari, MR, and Meier, MR: Systematic review of effects of current transtibial prosthetic socket designs—Part 1: Qualitative outcomes. J Rehabil Res Dev 52:491, 2015.
27. Safari, MR, and Meier, MR: Systematic review of effects of current transtibial prosthetic socket designs—Part 2: Quantitative outcomes. J Rehabil Res Dev 52:509, 2015.
28. Hagberg, K, and Brånemark, R: One hundred patients treated with osseointegrated transfemoral amputation prosthesis: Rehabilitation perspective. J Rehabil Res Dev 46:331, 2009.
29. Hekmatfard, M, Farahmand, F, and Ebrahimi I: Effects of prosthetic mass distribution on the spatiotemporal characteristics and knee kinematics of transfemoral amputee locomotion. Gait Posture 37:78, 2013.
30. Su, PF, et al: The effects of increased prosthetic ankle motions on the gait of persons with bilateral transtibial amputations. Am J Phys Med Rehabil 89:34, 2010.
31. Radcliffe, CW: Four-bar linkage prosthetic knee mechanisms: Kinematics, alignment and prescription criteria. Prosthet Orthot Int 18:159, 1994.
32. Lythgo, N, Marmaras, B, and Connor, H: Physical function, gait, and dynamic balance of transfemoral amputees using two mechanical passive prosthetic knee devices. Arch Phys Med Rehabil 91:1565, 2010.
33. Sapin, E, et al: Functional gait analysis of trans-femoral amputees using two different single-axis prosthetic knees with hydraulic swing-phase control: Kinematic and kinetic comparison of two prosthetic knees. Prosthet Orthot Int 32:201, 2008.
34. Chin, T, et al: Successful prosthetic fitting of elderly trans-femoral amputees with Intelligent Prosthesis (IP): A clinical study. Prosthet Orthot Int 31:271, 2007.
35. Jepson, F, et al: A comparative evaluation of the Adaptive knee and Catech® knee joints: A preliminary study. Prosthet Orthot Int 32:84, 2008.
36. Wong, CK, Rheinstein, J, and Stern M: Benefits for adults with transfemoral amputations and peripheral artery disease using microprocessor compared to non-microprocessor prosthetic knees. Am J Phys Med Rehabil 94:804, 2015.
37. Orendurff, M, et al: Gait efficiency using the C-Leg. J Rehabil Res Dev 43:239, 2006.
38. Segal, AD, et al: Kinematic and kinetic comparisons of trans-femoral amputee gait using C-Leg and Mauch SNS prosthetic knees. J Rehabil Res Dev 43:857, 2006.
39. Seymour, R, et al: Comparison between the C-Leg microprocessor-controlled prosthetic knee and nonmicroprocessor-controlled prosthetic knees: A preliminary study of energy expenditure, obstacle course performance and quality of life survey. Prosthet Orthot Int 31:51, 2007.
40. Kahle, JT, Highsmith, MJ, and Hubbard, SL: Comparison of non-microprocessor knee mechanism versus C-Leg on Prosthesis Evaluation questionnaire, stumbles, falls, walking tests, stair descent, and knee preference. J Rehabil Res Dev 45:1, 2008.
41. Brodtkorb, TH, et al: Cost-effectiveness of C-leg compared with non-microprocessor-controlled knees: A modeling approach. Arch Phys Med Rehabil 89:24, 2008.
42. Highsmith, MJ, et al: Safety, energy efficiency, and cost efficacy of the C-Leg for transfemoral amputees: A review of the literature. Prosthet Orthot Int 34:362, 2010.
43. Johansson, JL, et al. A clinical comparison of variable-damping and mechanically passive prosthetic knee devices. Am J Phys Med Rehabil 84:563, 2005.
44. Devlin, M, et al: Patient preference and gait efficiency in a geriatric population with transfemoral amputation using a free-swinging versus a locked prosthetic knee joint. Arch Phys Med Rehabil 83:246, 2002.
45. Alley, RD, et al: Prosthetic sockets stabilized by alternating areas of tissue compression and release. J Rehabil Res Dev 48(6):679–696, 2011.
46. Morse, BC, et al: Through-knee amputation in patients with peripheral arterial disease: A review of 50 cases. J Vasc Surg 48: 638, 2008.

47. Ten Duis, K, et al: Knee disarticulation: Survival, wound healing, and ambulation: A historic cohort study. Prosthet Orthot Int 33:52, 2009.
48. de Laat FA, et al: Cosmetic effect of knee joint in a knee disarticulation prosthesis. J Rehabil Res Dev 51:1545, 2014.
49. Yari, P, Dijkstra, P, and Geertzen, J: Functional outcome of hip disarticulation and hemipelvectomy: A cross-sectional national descriptive study in the Netherlands. Clin Rehabil 22:1127, 2008.
50. Ludwigs, E, et al: Biomechanical differences between two exoprosthetic hip joint systems during level walking. Prosthet Orthot Int 34:449, 2010.
51. Nelson, LM, and Carbone, NT: Functional outcome measurements of a veteran with a hip disarticulation using a Helix 3D hip joint: A case report. J Prosthet Orthot 23:21, 2011.
52. Su, P-F, et al: Differences in gait characteristics between persons with bilateral transtibial amputations, due to peripheral vascular disease and trauma, and able-bodied ambulators. Arch Phys Med Rehabil 89:1386, 2008.
53. Traballesi, M, et al: Prognostic factors in prosthetic rehabilitation of bilateral dysvascular above-knee amputees: Is the stump condition an influencing factor? Eura Medicophys 43:1, 2007.
54. McNealy, LL, and Gard, SA: Effect of prosthetic ankle units on the gait of persons with bilateral transfemoral amputations. Prosthet Orthot Int 32:111, 2008.
55. Potter, BK, and Scoville, CR: Amputation is not isolated: An overview of the US Army Amputee Patient Care Program and associated amputee injuries. J Am Acad Orthop Surg 14:S188, 2008.
56. Granville, R, and Menetrez, J: Rehabilitation of the lower-extremity war-injured at the center for the intrepid. Foot Ankle Clin 15:187, 2010.
57. Highsmith, MJ: Barriers to the provision of prosthetic services in the geriatric population. Top Geriatr Rehabil 24:325, 2008.
58. O'Neill, BF, and Evans, JJ: Memory and executive function predict mobility rehabilitation outcome after lower-limb amputation. Disabil Rehabil 11:1, 2009.
59. Atherton, R, and Robertson, N: Psychological adjustment to lower limb amputation amongst prosthesis users. Disabil Rehabil 28: 1201, 2006.
60. Coffey, L, Gallagher, P, and Desmond, D: A prospective study of the importance of life goal characteristics and goal adjustment capacities in longer term psychosocial adjustment to lower limb amputation. Clin Rehabil 28:196, 2014.
61. Mayer, A, et al: Body schema and body awareness of amputees. Prosthet Orthot Int 32:363, 2008.
62. Desmond, D, et al: Pain and psychosocial adjustment to lower limb amputation amongst prosthesis users. Prosthet Orthot Int 32:244, 2008.
63. Callaghan, B, Condie, E, and Johnston, M: Using the common sense self-regulation model to determine psychological predictors of prosthetic use and activity limitation in lower limb amputees. Prosthet Orthot Int 32:324, 2008.
64. Wegener, ST, et al: Self-management improves outcomes in persons with limb loss. Arch Phys Med Rehabil 90:373, 2009.
65. Turner, AP, et al: Suicidal ideation among individuals with dysvascular lower extremity amputation. Arch Phys Med Rehabil 96:1404, 2015.
66. Weiner, SJ, et al: Patient-centered decision making and health care outcomes. Ann Int Med 158:573, 2013.
67. Kersten, P, et al: Bridging the goal intention-action gap in rehabilitation: A study of if-then implementation intension in neurorehabilitation. Dis Rehabil 37:1073, 2015.
68. Centers for Medicare and Medicaid Services: Medicare and You 2015. Department of Health and Human Services, Baltimore, MD, 2015. Retrieved August 20, 2018 from www.medicare.gov/pubs/ebook/pdf/Medicare_and_You-2015.pdf.
69. Vrieling, AH, et al: Gait initiation in lower limb amputees. Gait Posture 27:423, 2008.
70. Vrieling, AH, et al: Gait termination in lower limb amputees. Gait Posture 27:82, 2008.
71. Esposito, ER, and Wilken, JM: The relationship between pelvis-trunk coordination and low back pain in individuals with transfemoral amputations. Gait Posture 40:640, 2014.
72. Silverman, AK, et al: Compensatory mechanisms in below-knee amputee gait in response to increasing steady-state walking speeds. Gait Posture 28:602, 2008.
73. Vanicek, N, et al: Gait patterns in transtibial amputee fallers vs. non-fallers: Biomechanical differences during level walking. Gait Posture 29:415, 2009.
74. Hendershot, BD, Bazrgari, B, and Nussbaum, MA: Persons with unilateral lower-limb amputation have altered and asymmetric trunk mechanical and neuromuscular behaviors estimated using multidirectional trunk perturbations. J Biomech 46:1907, 2013.
75. Matjacic, Z, and Burger, H: Dynamic balance training during standing in people with trans-tibial amputation: A pilot study. Prosthet Orthot Int 27:214, 2003.
76. Erbahçeci, F, et al: Balance training in amputees: Comparison of the outcome of two rehabilitation approaches. Clin Res 12:194, 2001.
77. Wong, CK, et al: Exercise programs to improve gait performance in people with lower limb amputation: A systematic review. Prosthet Orthot Int 40:8, 2016.
78. Lee, MY, Lin, CF, and Soon, KS: Balance control enhancement using sub-sensory stimulation and visual-auditory biofeedback strategies for amputee subjects. Prosthet Orthot Int 31:342, 2007.
79. Kaufman, KR, et al: Task-specific fall prevention training is effective for warfighters with transtibial amputations. Clin Orthop Relat Res 472:3076, 2014.
80. Wong, CK, et al: The impact of a 4-session physical therapy program emphasizing manual therapy and exercise on the balance and prosthetic walking ability of people with lower limb amputation: A pilot study. J Prosthet Orthot 28:95, 2016.
81. Corio, F, Troiano, R and Magel, JR: The effects of spinal stabilization exercises on the spatial and temporal parameters of gait in individuals with lower limb loss. J Prosthet Orthot 22:230, 2010.
82. Yigiter, K, et al: A comparison of traditional prosthetic training versus proprioceptive neuromuscular facilitation resistive gait training with trans-femoral amputees. Prosthet Orthot Int 26:213, 2002.
83. Miller, CA, et al: Using the Nintendo Wii Fit and body weight support to improve aerobic capacity, balance, gait ability, and fear of falling: Two case reports. J Geriatr Phys Ther 35:95, 2012.
84. Tsai, HA, et al: Aided gait of people with lower-limb amputations: Comparison of 4-footed and 2-wheeled walkers. Arch Phys Med Rehabil 84:584, 2003.
85. Miller, WC, et al: The influence of falling, fear of falling, and balance confidence on prosthetic mobility and social activity among individuals with lower extremity amputation. Arch Phys Med Rehabil 82:1238, 2001.
86. Wong, CK, et al: The role of balance ability and confidence in prosthetic use for mobility of people with lower limb loss. J Rehabil Res Dev 51:1353, 2014.
87. Sjodahl, C, et al: Gait improvement in unilateral transfemoral amputees by a combined psychological and physiotherapeutic treatment. J Rehabil Med 33:114, 2001.
88. Ramstrand, N, and Nilsson, KA: A comparison of foot placement strategies of transtibial amputees and able-bodied subjects during stair ambulation. Prosthet Orthot Int 33:348, 2009.
89. Schmalz, T, Blumentritt, S, and Marx, B: Biomechanical analysis of stair ambulation in lower limb amputees. Gait Posture 25:267, 2007.
90. Vrieling, AH, et al: Uphill and downhill walking in unilateral lower limb amputees. Gait Posture 28:235, 2008.
91. Fradet, L, et al: Biomechanical analysis of ramp ambulation of transtibial amputees with an adaptive ankle foot system. Gait Posture 32:191, 2010.
92. Vickers, DR, et al: Elderly unilateral transtibial amputee gait on an inclined walkway: A biomechanical analysis. Gait Posture 27:518, 2008.
93. Vrieling, AH, et al: Obstacle crossing in lower limb amputees. Gait Posture 26:587, 2007.
94. Gonzalez, E, and Edelstein, J: Energy expenditure in ambulation. In Gonzalez, E, et al (eds): Downey and Darling's Physiological Basis of Rehabilitation Medicine, ed 3. Butterworth-Heinemann, Boston, 2001, p. 417.
95. Goktepe, AS, et al: Energy expenditure of walking with prostheses: Comparison of three amputation levels. Prosthet Orthot Int 34:31, 2010.
96. Genin, JJ, et al: Effect of speed on the energy cost of walking in unilateral traumatic lower limb amputees. Eur J Appl Physiol 103:655, 2008.
97. Houdijk, H, et al: The energy cost for the step-to-step transition in amputee walking. Gait Posture 30:35, 2009.

98. Mohanty, RK, et al: Comparison of energy cost in transtibial amputees using "prosthesis" and "crutches without prosthesis" for walking activities. Ann Phys Rehabil Med 55:252, 2012.
99. Graham, LE, et al: A comparative study of oxygen consumption for conventional and energy-storing prosthetic feet in transfemoral amputees. Clin Rehabil 22:896, 2008.
100. Kaufman, KR, et al: Energy expenditure and activity of transfemoral amputees using mechanical and microprocessor-controlled prosthetic knees. Arch Phys Med Rehabil 89:1380, 2008.
101. Chin, T, et al: Comparison of different microprocessor controlled knee joints on the energy consumption during walking in transfemoral amputees: Intelligent knee prosthesis (IP) versus C-Leg. Prosthet Orthot Int 30:73, 2006.
102. Wong, CK, et al: A comparison of energy expenditure in people with transfemoral amputation using microprocessor and nonmicroprocessor knee prostheses: A systematic review. J Prosthet Orthot 24:202, 2012.
103. Chin, T, et al: Energy expenditure during walking in amputees after disarticulation of the hip: A microprocessor-controlled swing-phase control knee versus a mechanical-controlled stance-phase control knee. J Bone Joint Surg 87B:117, 2005.
104. Wright, DA, Marks, L, and Payne, RC: A comparative study of the physiological costs of walking in ten bilateral amputees. Prosthet Orthot Int 32:57, 2008.
105. Raya, MA, et al: Impairment variables predicting activity limitation in individuals with lower limb amputation. Prosthet Orthot Int 34:73, 2010.
106. Gailey, RS, et al: The Amputee Mobility Predictor: An instrument to assess determinants of the lower-limb amputee ability to ambulate. Arch Phys Med Rehabil 83:613, 2002.
107. Raichle, KA, et al: Prosthesis use in persons with lower- and upper-limb amputation. J Rehabil Res Dev 45:961, 2008.
108. Karmarkar, AM, et al: Prosthesis and wheelchair use in veterans with lower-limb amputation. J Rehabil Res Dev 46:567, 2009.
109. Devlin, M, et al: Houghton Scale of prosthetic use in people with lower extremity amputations: Reliability, validity, and responsiveness to change. Arch Phys Med Rehabil 85:1339, 2004.
110. Resnik, L, and Borgia, M: Reliability of people with lower limb amputations: Distinguishing true change from statistical error. Phys Ther 91:555, 2011.
111. Miller, WC, Deathe, AB, and Harris, J: Measurement properties of the Frenchay Activities Index among individuals with lower limb amputation. Clin Rehabil 18:414, 2004.
112. Epstein, RA, Heinemann, AW, and McFarland, LV: Quality of life for veterans and service members with major traumatic limb loss from Vietnam and OIF/OEF conflicts. J Rehabil Res Dev 47:373, 2010.
113. Zidarov, D, Swaine, B, and Gauthier-Gagnon, C: Quality of life of persons with lower-limb amputation during rehabilitation and at 3-month follow-up. Arch Phys Med Rehabil 90:634, 2009.
114. Asano, M, et al: Predictors of quality of life among individuals who have a lower limb amputation. Prosthet Orthot Int 32:231, 2008.
115. Bosmans, JC, et al: Survival of participating and nonparticipating limb amputees in prospective study: Consequences for research. J Rehabil Res Dev 47:457, 2010.
116. Christiansen, J, et al: Physical and social factors determining quality of life for veterans with lower-limb amputation(s): A systematic review. Disabil Rehabil 38:2345, 2016.
117. Samuelsson, KAM, et al: Effects of lower limb prosthesis on activity, participation, and quality of life: A systematic review. Prosthet Orthot Int 36:145, 2012.
118. Deans, SA, McFadyen, AK, and Rowe, PJ: Physical activity and quality of life: A study of a lower-limb amputee population. Prosthet Orthot Int 32:186, 2008.
119. Remes, L, et al: Predictors for institutionalization and prosthetic ambulation after major lower extremity amputation during an eight-year follow-up. Aging Clin Exp Res 21:129, 2009.
120. Taylor, SM, et al: "Successful outcome" after below-knee amputation: An objective definition and influence of clinical variables. Am Surg 74:607, 2008.
121. Ebrahimzadeh, MH, and Hariri, S: Long-term outcomes of unilateral transtibial amputations. Mil Med 174:593, 2009.
122. Quigley, M, and Dillon, M: Quality of life in persons with partial foot or transtibial amputation: A systematic review. Prosthet Orthot Int 40:18, 2016.
123. MacNeill, HL, et al: Long-term outcomes and survival of patients with bilateral transtibial amputation after rehabilitation. Am J Phys Med Rehabil 87:189, 2008.
124. Hawkins, AT, et al: The effect of social integration on outcomes after major lower extremity amputation. J Vasc Surg 63:154, 2016.
125. Dillingham, TR, Pezzin, LE, and Mackenzie, EJ: Discharge destination after dysvascular lower-limb amputations. Arch Phys Med Rehabil 84:1662, 2003.
126. Burger, H, and Marincek, C: Return to work after lower limb amputation. Disabil Rehabil 29:1323, 2007.
127. Waldera, KE, et al: Assessing the prosthetic needs of farmers and ranchers with amputations. Disabil Rehabil Assist Technol 8:204, 2013.
128. Boulias, C, et al: Return to driving after lower-extremity amputation. Arch Phys Med Rehabil 87:1183, 2006.
129. Meikle, B, Devlin, M, and Pauley, T: Driving pedal reaction times after right transtibial amputation. Arch Phys Med Rehabil 87:390, 2006.
130. Wong, CK: Interrater reliability of the Berg Balance Scale when used by clinicians of various experience levels to assess people with lower limb amputations. Phys Ther 94:371, 2014.
131. Larssson, B, et al: The locomotor capabilities index; validity and reliability of the Swedish version in adults with lower limb amputation. Health Qual Life Outcomes 7:44, 2009.
132. Miller, WC, Deathe, AB, and Speechley, M: Psychometric properties of the Activities-Specific Balance Confidence scale among individuals with lower limb amputation. Arch Phys Med Rehabil 84:656, 2003.
133. Yazicioglu, K, et al: Effect of playing football (soccer) on balance, strength, and quality of life in unilateral below-knee amputees. Am J Phys Med Rehabil 86:800, 2007.
134. Farley, R, Mitchell, F, and Griffiths, M: Custom skiing and trekking adaptations for a trans-tibial and trans-radial quadrilateral amputee. Prosthet Orthot Int 28:60, 2004.
135. Kars, C, et al: Participation in sports by lower limb amputees in the Province of Drenthe, the Netherlands. Prosthet Orthot Int 33:356, 2009.
136. Nolan, L: Lower limb strength in sports-active transtibial amputees. Prosthet Orthot Int 33:230, 2009.
137. Brown, MB, Millard-Stafford, ML, and Allison, AR: Running-specific prostheses permit energy cost similar to nonamputees. Med Sci Sports Exerc 41:1080, 2009.
138. Weyand, PG, et al: The fastest runner on artificial legs: Different limbs, similar function? J Appl Physiol 107:903, 2009.
139. Hobara, H, et al: Step frequency and step length of 200-m sprint in able-bodied and amputee sprinters. Int J Sports Med 37:165, 2016.
140. Gailey, R, and Harsch, P: Introduction to triathlon for the lower limb amputee triathlete. Prosthet Orthot Int 33:242, 2009.
141. Nolan, L, and Lees, A: The influence of lower-limb amputation level on the approach in the amputee long jump. J Sports Sci 25:393, 2007.
142. Nolan, L, Patritti, BL, and Simpson, KJ: A biomechanical analysis of the long-jump technique of elite female amputee athletes. Med Sci Sports Exerc 38:1829, 2006.
143. Nolan, L, and Patritti, BL: The take-off phase in transtibial amputee high jump. Prosthet Ortho Int 32:160, 2008.
144. Minnoye, SL, and Plettenburg, DH: Design, fabrication, and preliminary results of a novel below-knee prosthesis for snowboarding: A case report. Prosthet Orthot Int 33:272, 2009.
145. Wong, CK, Chen, C, and Welsh, J: Preliminary assessment of balance with the Berg Balance Scale in adults who have a leg amputation and dwell in the community: Rasch rating scale analysis. Phys Ther 93:1520, 2013.
146. Wong, CK, Gibbs, W, and Chen, E: Use of the Houghton Scale to classify community and household walking ability in people with lower limb amputation: Criterion-related validity. Arch Phys Med Rehabil 97:1130, 2016.
147. Gailey, RS, et al: Application of self-report and performance-based outcome measures to determine functional differences between four categories of prosthetic feet. J Rehabil Res Dev 49(4):597-612, 2012.

Supplemental Reading

Carroll, K, and Edelstein, J (eds): Prosthetics and Patient Management: A Comprehensive Clinical Approach. Thorofare, NJ, Slack, 2006.

Edelstein, J, and Moroz, A: Lower-Limb Prosthetics and Orthotics: Clinical Concepts. Thorofare, NJ, Slack, 2011.

Fitzlaff, G, and Heim, S: Lower Limb Prosthetic Components: Design, Function and Biomechanical Properties. Verlag Orthopadie Technik, Dortmund, Germany, 2002.

Lusardi, MM, and Nielsen, CC: Orthotics and Prosthetics in Rehabilitation, ed 2. Butterworth Heinemann, Boston, 2006.

May, BJ: Amputations and Prosthetics: A Case Study Approach, ed 2. FA Davis, Philadelphia, 2002.

Parker, JN, and Parker, PM (eds): Amputation: A Medical Dictionary, Bibliography & Annotated Research Guide to Internet References. ICON Health Publications, San Diego, CA, 2003.

Rehabilitation Institute of Chicago. Lower Extremity Amputation: A Guide to Functional Outcomes in Physical Therapy Management. Pro-Ed, Austin, TX, 2005.

Seymour, R: Prosthetics and Orthotics: Lower Limb and Spinal. Lippincott Williams & Wilkins, Philadelphia, 2002.

Smith, DG, et al (eds): Atlas of Amputations and Limb Deficiencies, ed 3. American Academy of Orthopaedic Surgeons, Chicago, 2004.

appendix 31.A Transtibial Prosthetic Evaluation

1. Is the prosthesis as prescribed?
2. Can the client don the prosthesis easily?

STANDING

3. Is the client comfortable when standing with the heel midlines 6 in. (15 cm) apart?
4. Is the anterior–posterior alignment satisfactory?
5. Is the medial–lateral alignment satisfactory?
6. Do the contours and color of the prosthesis match the opposite limb?
7. Is the prosthesis the correct length?
8. Is piston action minimal?
9. Does the socket contact the amputation limb without pinching or gapping?

SUSPENSION

10. Does the suspension component fit the amputation limb properly?
11. Does the cuff, fork strap, or thigh corset have adequate provision for adjustment?

SITTING

12. Can the client sit comfortably with hips and knees flexed 90°?

WALKING

13. Is the client's performance in level walking satisfactory?
14. Is the client's performance on stairs and ramps satisfactory?
15. Can the client kneel satisfactorily?
16. Does the suspension function properly?
17. Does the prosthesis operate quietly?
18. Does the client consider the prosthesis satisfactory as to comfort, function, and appearance?

PROSTHESIS OFF THE CLIENT

19. Is the skin free of abrasions or other discolorations attributable to this prosthesis?
20. Is the socket interior smooth?
21. Is the posterior wall of the socket of adequate height?
22. Is the construction satisfactory?
23. Do all components function satisfactorily?

Transformal Prosthetic Evaluation

appendix 31.B

1. Is the prosthesis as prescribed?
2. Can the client don the prosthesis easily?

STANDING

3. Is the client comfortable when standing with the heel midlines 6 in. (15 cm) apart?
4. Is any flesh roll above the socket minimal?
5. Is the client free from vertical pressure in the perineum?
6. Do the contours and color of the prosthesis match the opposite limb?
7. Is the prosthesis the correct length?
8. Is the knee stable?
9. When the socket valve is removed, is the distal tissue firm?

QUADRILATERAL SOCKET

10. Does the ischial tuberosity rest on the posterior brim?
11. Is the posterior brim approximately parallel to the floor?
12. Is the adductor longus tendon located in the anteromedial corner?

ISCHIAL CONTAINMENT SOCKET

13. Does the posterior–medial corner of the socket cover the ischial tuberosity?
14. Can the client hyperextend the hip on the amputated side comfortably?
15. Can the client flex the hip 90° comfortably, without socket gapping?
16. Can the client abduct the hip on the amputated side comfortably, without socket gapping?

SUSPENSION

17. Does the Silesian belt control prosthetic rotation and adduction adequately?
18. Does the pelvic band conform to the torso?

SITTING

19. Can the client sit comfortably with hips and knees flexed 90°?
20. Does the socket remain securely on the thigh, without gapping or rotating?
21. Are both thighs approximately the same length and height from the floor?
22. Can the client lean forward to touch the shoes?

WALKING

23. Is the client's performance in level walking satisfactory?
24. Is the client's performance on stairs and ramps satisfactory?
25. Does the suspension function properly?
26. Does the prosthesis operate quietly?
27. Does the client consider the prosthesis satisfactory as to comfort, function, and appearance?

PROSTHESIS OFF THE CLIENT

28. Is the skin free of abrasions or other discolorations attributable to this prosthesis?
29. Is the socket interior smooth?
30. With the prosthesis fully flexed on a table, can the thigh piece be brought to at least the vertical position?
31. If the socket is totally rigid, is a back pad attached?
32. Is the construction satisfactory?
33. Do all components function satisfactorily?

appendix 31.C

Web-Based Resources for Families, and Patients With Amputations and Prostheses

Organization/Resource	Website
Amputee Coalition, an organization for people with amputations with relevant resources:	www.amputee-coalition.org.
Challenged Athlete Foundation, an organization promoting active lifestyles for physically challenged people through physical fitness and athletics:	www.challengedathletes.org
International Committee of the Red Cross. An independent and neutral international organization providing health care to people affected by conflict, violence, and emergencies. Exercises for Lower-Limb Amputees: Gait Training:	www.icrc.org/eng/resources/documents/publication/p0936.htm
Wounded Warrior Project, a charitable organization focused on injured servicemen and veterans:	www.woundedwarriorproject.org.

Web-Based Resources for Clinicians Working With Patients with Amputations and Prostheses

appendix **31.D**

Endolite Institute: A company-sponsored site for prosthetics and rehabilitation education and clinical resources: www.endolite.com/about/education.

Freedom Innovations: Prosthetist Education, a company-sponsored site for prosthetics and education and resources: www.freedom-innovations.com/prosthetist-events/.

International Committee of the Red Cross: An independent and neutral international organization providing health care to people affected by conflict, violence, and emergencies: www.icrc.org. Lower Limb Amputee Rehabilitation Course: www.physio-pedia.com/Lower_Limb_Amputee_Rehabilitation_Course

Orthotics and Prosthetics: Digital Resource Foundation: Virtual Library: www.oandplibrary.org.

Gailey, RS, and Clark, CR: Physical therapy management of adult lower-limb amputees. Available at www.oandplibrary.org/alp/chap23-01.asp.

Össur Academy: A company-sponsored site for prosthetics and rehabilitation education and clinical resources: www.ossur.com/about-ossur/ossur-academy.

Ottobock Academy: A company-sponsored site for prosthetics and rehabilitation education and clinical resources: http://academy.ottobockus.com.

United States Department of Veteran Affairs: Amputation System of Care: www.prosthetics.va.gov/PROSTHETICS/asoc/index.asp.

Chapter 32

Seating and Wheeled Mobility

Laura J. Cohen, PhD, PT, ATP/SMS
Faith Saftler Savage, PT, ATP

"Mobility devices enable persons with disabilities to achieve personal mobility, and access to these devices is a precondition for achieving equal opportunities, enjoying human rights and living in dignity."[1]

LEARNING OBJECTIVES

1. Identify when a wheelchair user has basic, intermediate, or complex needs.
2. List the 8 basic steps of the wheelchair seating and mobility service delivery process.
3. Explain the difference between a reference neutral sitting posture and a person's "*optimal*" sitting posture.
4. Describe the components of the examination process for determining the most appropriate wheelchair seating and mobility device (WSMD).
5. Discuss the relationship between elements of the assessment interview and the wheelchair prescription/selection.
6. Explain the different methods of seating simulation and the expected outcomes.
7. Describe factors that affect determination of seat and back support features.
8. Discuss the benefits and contraindications of various seating system features.
9. Apply the components of a problem-solving model when presented with a clinical case study.
10. Describe at least 5 basic elements that should be included in the clinician documentation for a WSMD.

CHAPTER OUTLINE

INTRODUCTION

According to estimates from the Centers for Disease Control and Prevention, approximately 53 million, or one in five, Americans has a disability of some type and the number is increasing daily.[2,3] Roughly 2.2 million people in the United States depend on a wheelchair for day-to-day tasks and mobility.[4,5] Wheelchair users are limited in their ability to walk. This may include people who are unable to walk at all and who will need a wheelchair full-time for mobility in all environments; others may need a wheelchair only for longer distances or in certain environments.

In 2001, the International Classification of Functioning, Disability and Health (ICF) introduced language and a framework for disability.[6-8] The ICF carefully defines key concepts, including functioning, disability, activity, participation, and personal and environmental factors. Wheelchair seating and mobility (WSM) technologies are, from an ICF perspective, considered an *environmental factor* that has an impact on a person's functioning and can facilitate *activity and participation*.[9]

A functional mobility limitation such as an inability to walk does not always have to equate to a functional limitation. For example, the function of walking may cease to be disabling if accommodations are made to compensate for the limitation such as with the use of equipment (e.g., wheelchair, walker, cane) and/or accommodations to the environment, such as a ramp or elevator, to enable access to buildings and the community.

The Wheelchair User

People of any age may need a wheelchair—children, adults, and the elderly. The need for a wheelchair can be permanent, or it can be temporary. People with a variety of diagnoses, such as multiple sclerosis (MS), cerebral palsy (CP), or cerebrovascular accident, may need a wheelchair because their walking ability is limited. Other people need wheelchairs who have no ability to walk, including individuals with spinal cord injury (SCI), amyotrophic lateral sclerosis, traumatic brain injury (TBI), CP, or severe rheumatoid arthritis. The needs of each wheelchair user will vary, depending on lifestyle, life roles, type of mobility impairment, and the environments routinely encountered.

Hierarchy of Wheelchair User Seating and Positioning Need

Providing wheelchairs and seating systems for people with mobility limitations is both a science and an art that, for people with more complex needs, requires more training than what is covered in this chapter. Adapted from the World Health Organization's Wheelchair Service Training Program, a service delivery model based on a hierarchy of the wheelchair users' seating and positioning needs is used to distinguish among three levels: *basic, intermediate, and complex*[10-12] (Table 32.1). Three variables considered are (1) balance and postural control in sitting, (2) the ability to achieve a neutral sitting posture, and (3) the degree of postural support needed to achieve a neutral posture.

A wheelchair user with a *basic* level of seating and positioning need has good sitting balance and can sit with their hands free to function (also known as a *"hands-free"*

Table 32.1 Hierarchy of Wheelchair User Seating and Positioning Needs

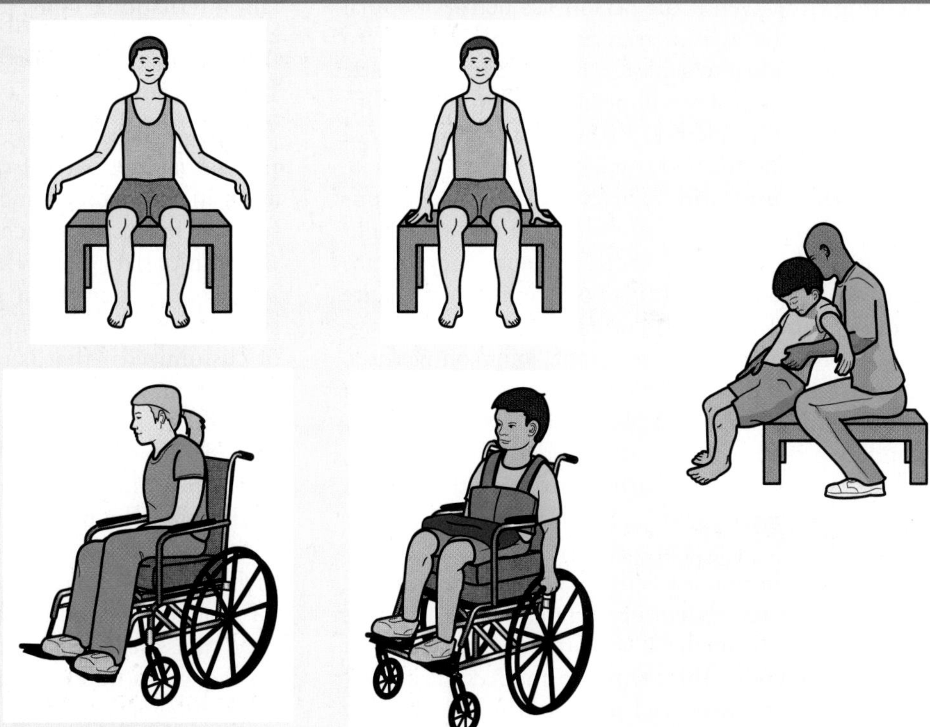

Sitting and Positioning Needs	**Basic**	**Intermediate**	**Complex**
Balance and postural control in sitting	Good sitting balance, hands-free sitter	Fair sitting balance and trunk control	Poor sitting balance
Ability to achieve neutral sitting posture	Achieves neutral posture without support	Achieves close to neutral posture	Unable to achieve neutral posture
Degree of postural support required	No additional postural supports needed	Needs postural supports	Needs custom supports

sitter). Additionally, this person can sit in a neutral upright sitting posture without any additional postural supports in the wheelchair. An example of a user with *Basic* needs is an older adult who is weak but can sit with good balance in a neutral or upright posture. Another example is a person with a T12 complete SCI that does not require additional postural support around the trunk or pelvis to sit upright but requires a seat cushion and back support to help minimize risk of pressure injuries and to provide a stable base to support a neutral trunk alignment.

A wheelchair user with an *intermediate* level of seating and positioning need has only fair sitting balance and trunk control and needs to use their hands to help them balance in sitting (also known as a *"hands-dependent" sitter*). They may be able to sit close to a neutral posture but will require additional postural supports (such as hip and trunk supports) to sit symmetrically as well as to help balance to free up their hands for function. Some examples of users with intermediate needs include people with mild CP (e.g., Gross Motor Function Classification System [GMFCS] Level III) or a TBI without joint contractures, significant spasticity, or other abnormal muscle tone problems. Even if the person has pelvic or spinal asymmetries, the asymmetries are flexible enough to allow the individual to achieve a neutral sitting posture. These wheelchair users will need to be provided with appropriate seating and postural supports such as special seat cushions, and hip and trunk supports.

Wheelchair users with *complex* seating and positioning needs have poor trunk control and cannot sit upright without a lot of external postural support. They are unable to achieve a neutral sitting posture and may require custom postural supports in order to accommodate significant abnormalities in muscle tone, joint contractures, and spinal deformities. Examples of users with complex needs include people with progressive diseases such as secondary progressive MS and people with severe tone, weakness or contractures such as people with CP with spastic quadriplegia (GMFCS Levels IV and V), TBI, or tetraplegia.

This categorization is useful because a more complex level of need requires that the therapist and wheelchair service delivery team have a more advanced level of knowledge and skill. This chapter introduces the knowledge and skills to assess and provide wheeled mobility and seating for users with basic needs and some users with intermediate needs. Wheelchair users with complex needs should be referred to a wheelchair seating specialist who regularly practices with individuals with these higher levels of need. Those interested in developing their expertise to serve wheelchair users with complex needs will require additional advanced training.

Wheelchair User Rights

Wheelchair users come from all walks of life and have mobility limitations for many different reasons. They rely on their wheelchairs to provide them with optimal support, mobility, and function to perform their jobs, care for their families, and actively participate in many different life roles and activities. Statistics show that less than 5% of those in the world who need a properly fitted wheelchair actually have one.[13] Notice the emphasis is not only on having a wheelchair, but also on having a properly fitting wheelchair, which is essential for supporting the lives and livelihoods for those who need them.

In 2006, the United Nations Convention on the Rights of Persons with Disabilities (UNCRPD) was signed. In 2008, the UNCRPD became international law. While the United States signed the UNCRPD in July 30, 2009, Congress has yet to ratify or confirm it into law. There are 50 different articles in the Convention, and article number 20 is about the right to "personal mobility," stating that all people have a right to personal mobility.[14] The Convention also defines personal mobility as "the ability to move in a manner and at the time of one's own choice."[14] For many people with a mobility impairment, having an appropriate wheelchair is the only way that they can have personal mobility and is therefore supported by this very important international convention.

Mobility-Related Assistive Technology Defined

The *Technology-Related Assistance for Individuals with Disabilities Act (Tech Act)* was first passed in 1988 and again in 1998, increasing access to, availability of, and funding for assistive technology through state and national initiatives.[15] This legislation defines *assistive technologies (AT)* as any item, piece of equipment, or product system—acquired commercially off the shelf, modified, or customized—that is used to increase, maintain, or improve an individual's functioning and independence to facilitate participation and to enhance overall well-being.[15] Assistive technology can also help reduce impairments and decrease risk for secondary health conditions. The purpose of this chapter is to focus on mobility-related assistive technology.

Consistent with the *Guide to Physical Therapy Practice 3.0, wheeled mobility technology* is an *aid to locomotion* used to assist a person to move from one location to another when walking is not safe or functional.[16] *Seating and positioning technology* is individually selected or configured or custom-designed technology for one or more of the following purposes: "(1) to provide support to a person's body in a desired sitting position, (2) to provide support in positions other than a sitting position (e.g., standing, side-lying, supine), (3) to provide support in a way that will assist in maintaining or restoring skin integrity, or (4) to provide a mechanical method to change position relative to gravity (e.g., tilt, recline, elevate, stand)."[16] An implied purpose, although not specifically stated, includes facilitating the use of a wheeled mobility device. This chapter is specific to and limited to seating support systems for use in wheeled mobility devices.

The Person-Technology Match

Achieving a good match between the person and the technology requires attention to the environments in which the technology will be used, the needs and preferences of the user, and the functions and features of the technology. If the match is not a quality one from the standpoint of the person, the technology may not be used or will not be used optimally. The Matching Person and Technology (MPT) model was developed to support the AT assessment and service delivery process.[17,18] It is goal directed, person centered, and designed to facilitate the identification and selection of AT that is most likely to be used by the individual.[17,18] Several wheelchair-specific and general assistive technology outcome measures suitable for use in evaluating the person–technology match are presented later in the chapter.

Appropriate vs. Inappropriate Wheelchair Seating and Mobility Device

Personal mobility for people who use wheelchairs largely depends upon access to an appropriate Wheelchair Seating and Mobility Device (WSMD). There are several characteristics that make a WSMD more, or less, appropriate for any individual wheelchair user. Most WSMDs have multiple features that can be selected (added or omitted), depending on an individual's specific needs. Most WSMDs require some sort of individual configuration to fit the person to the technology and address environmental considerations.

An appropriate WSMD meets the user's mobility needs, positioning needs, and environmental conditions. For example, an appropriate WSMD must provide proper fit and postural support, be safe and durable, be readily available in the person's geographic region, be obtained and maintained at an affordable cost, and be accessible to local skilled service and repair by a qualified durable medical equipment (DME) supplier ("supplier") or rehab technology professional (RTP). In addition to meeting the mobility and positioning needs of a wheelchair user, it must be usable where the person typically goes. For example, if a user resides in a rural environment, the tires must be able to manage rocks, dirt, and mud versus a more urban environment, in which the wheels must allow the user to manage uneven pavement, curbs, and side slopes.

A WSMD can be inappropriate for many different reasons. An inappropriate WSMD has characteristics that do not meet one or more of the needs of a wheelchair user. A few examples include ill-fitting; too large or small, impacting ability to self-propel; inadequate skin protection; insufficient postural support; does not meet functional needs (e.g., seat height too low, impeding independent transfers or ability to access standard table or desk). Any WSMD that is inappropriate for the environments in which it will be used will either limit mobility or will fail prematurely, requiring frequent repairs or early replacement.

While there are many benefits of an appropriate wheelchair, they likely can be organized into four primary categories: (1) mobility, (2) access to community life, (3) health, and (4) self-esteem (or confidence). Appropriate wheelchairs optimize a wheelchair user's abilities in all four of these categories, and the categories frequently influence each other as well. For example, independence in mobility usually helps a person to optimize their health and access to the community. The primary benefit of a wheelchair is mobility. Wheelchairs provide personal mobility to individuals, allowing them to engage in typical life activities in multiple environments. However, it is not enough to have just any wheelchair. If the wheelchair fits properly, a person has greater potential to be independent in their personal mobility, allowing them to access their community, including going to school or work. A properly fitting wheelchair may also improve the person's overall health, by increasing the person's activity level, improving posture, breathing, and circulation, and potentially minimizing risk for impairments like pressure injuries. All these benefits can also improve self-esteem and self-confidence, leading to improved overall quality of life for the wheelchair user.

WHEELCHAIR SEATING AND MOBILITY SERVICE DELIVERY TEAM

The first part of understanding the WSM service-delivery process is to understand the participants, referred to as the *WSM service delivery team* (WSM team). This team is configured with specific team members, depending on the circumstances related to the referral and the complexity of the person to be evaluated. Regardless of the team size and members, it is commonly accepted as best practice that to provide the wheelchair user with the most appropriate WSMD, an interdisciplinary team approach is necessary. Key participants typically involved in the team process at a minimum include:

- The wheelchair user.
- Family members and caregivers.
- A physician or non-physician practitioner (e.g., nurse practitioner, physician assistant, clinical nurse specialist), recognized by policymakers and payers as the *prescriber*.
- A physical therapist and/or occupational therapist, recognized by policymakers as the *licensed or certified medical professional (LCMP)*.
- A *supplier or rehabilitation technology professional (RTP)*, recognized by policymakers as the *certified, registered, or otherwise credentialed RTP*.

The team collectively provides *clinical-related services* and *technology-related services*. An individual's medical and functional needs are identified by the clinical team, who are responsible for assessing the person's body structures and functions and identifying the medically necessary and appropriate features needed in a WSMD. The supplier/RTP brings equipment and technology knowledge matching features identified by the clinical team, with specific make/model products that are then configured into custom-designed systems with input from the clinical team.

Each member of the WSM service delivery team has a specific role and responsibilities relative to obtaining an appropriate WSMD. It is very important to keep in mind the principle that the wheelchair user is an equal partner and is frequently the key player on the service delivery team. Experienced wheelchair users know what they like and what they don't like, what works and what does not work for them. The experienced wheelchair user often helps guide the assessment and delivery process. In this instance it is often the role of the clinician(s) and supplier to provide education and discuss new and emerging technologies, trade-offs between function and equipment choice, and recommendations that are needed to address health, activity, and participation. Even if the disability is not progressive in nature, as a wheelchair user ages, their needs may change and their technology needs may as well. New wheelchair users will need more information and guidance, as this will likely be their first exposure to the WSM service delivery process and the range of WSM technologies available to address their personal mobility issues. It is essential to really listen to the wheelchair user and help guide them to an appropriate WSMD that will match their needs and goals.

WHEELCHAIR SEATING AND MOBILITY SERVICE DELIVERY PROCESS

Evaluating a person and then recommending and prescribing a WSMD is a complex therapy intervention. Providing an appropriate wheelchair to a person is not a singular event; it is a process and does not end when the user receives the WSMD. The provision of WSM services consists of two interrelated components:

- The *clinical-related component* done by the therapist: the physical and functional evaluation, treatment plan, goal setting, preliminary device feature determination, trials/simulations, documentation and justification, fittings, function-related training, determination of outcomes, and follow-up.[19]
- The *technology-related component* done by the supplier/RTP: the technology assessment; the accessibility survey of the home environment; transportation assessment; equipment demonstration/trial/simulation; product feature matching to identified medical, physical, and functional needs; system configuration; fitting; adjustments; programming; determination of outcomes; and product-related training and follow-up.[19]

The service delivery process can be time-consuming and may require several visits to complete, depending on complexity. Additional time spent up front to be thorough often decreases errors and future costs associated with mistakes created by incomplete information, examination, and trials.

Wheelchair Service Delivery Steps

Each step in the wheelchair service delivery process is important to the overall outcome for the individual.[10,11,13,20,21] Summarized here are the crucial components of the *wheelchair service delivery process*, as outlined by the World Health Organization.[10,11,22] These steps as performed in a *wheelchair examination and specialty evaluation* are explored in greater detail later in the chapter.

Step 1: Identification of Need and Referral

People are referred for WSM services by a range of different sources: hospital or health care providers (e.g., physician/NP/PA, case manager, discharge planner), community resources (vocational counselors, educators), family and friends, disability organizations, or other wheelchair users. It is important to identify the reason(s) for referral and the complexity of the person's mobility impairment. This information will assist in routing the person to an appropriate clinic, therapist, complex rehabilitation technology (CRT) supplier or DME supplier. Preliminary questions may include the following: Is this the person's first wheelchair? Is the person being seen for problems with their existing wheelchair? Are there problems with skin integrity or sitting posture, or are the needs solely related to mobility, or both? Answers to all of these questions (and more) will help determine whether the person's WSM needs are at a basic, intermediate, or complex level. The identification of these needs and the referral into the service delivery process is the first step in obtaining an appropriate WSMD.

Step 2: Assessment

The assessment is divided into two primary components: the *assessment interview* and the *physical assessment* (also known as the *Wheelchair Examination & Specialty Evaluation*) (Table 32.2). The interview is used to gather information about the wheelchair user's physical condition, lifestyle and environment, and existing equipment. The physical assessment begins with the assessment of the person as they arrive to the clinic in the present wheelchair (if they have one) and includes a description of the person's current seated posture and mobility function. A *mat examination* is performed to assess the person out of the wheelchair in both a supine (gravity eliminated) and a sitting position (with the effects of gravity). Presence, risk, or history of pressure injury is assessed and pressure under bony prominences is considered and

Table 32.2 Wheelchair Examination and Specialty Evaluation

Examination				Specialty Evaluation			Intervention
Assessment Interview	Equipment Assessment (Existing/prior equipment)	Functional Assessment	Screening of Body Functions	Physical Assessment	Wheelchair Assessment	Evaluation and Plan of Care	Wheelchair Fitting/ Delivery/ Training
Demographic information Reason for referral Diagnosis Medical/surgical history History of WSM problems Goals (user, family/ caregiver) Social status Environmental accessibility (home and community) Employment/ work status (job/school) General health status Functional status and activity level Transportation	Existing Equipment Current seating and mobility equipment Sitting posture in existing equipment	ADL/IADL status—toileting, dressing, eating Mobility status—bed mobility, transfers, weight shift, ambulation, propulsion method	Cardiovascular/ pulmonary/ circulatory status Gastrointestinal system review Communication Cognitive and behavioral status (attention, judgment, motor planning, memory) Vision/hearing status Bowel and bladder functions	Supine and sitting mat assessment Sensation Pain Skin integrity Postural Alignment Balance Strength and endurance (muscle power/ endurance) ROM/flexibility (sitting/supine) Neuromuscular Status (muscle tone, reflexes, motor control, impact on function)	Measurements Simulation Technology trial Person/ technology match	Diagnosis related to positioning and mobility limitation Problem list Goals for interventions (treatment/ WSMD) Equipment prescription/ justification	Function from WC WC mobility WC skills training Maintenance/ Repairs/ follow-up

often measured at this time, particularly if the person is at risk for a pressure injury. Finally, body measurements are taken of the person while seated in an optimal sitting posture. The purpose of the assessment is to begin to identify the person's problems and potentials and determine the amount, type and location of needed postural supports and WSMD features and functions.[20,21]

Step 3: Prescription/Selection

Prescription means selecting the best available wheelchair (WSMD) for the wheelchair user. This entails matching a person's identified physical and functional needs, goals, and environments identified in the assessment to necessary equipment features (*person/feature match*).[23] After the equipment features are identified a wheelchair base, seating system, and the wheelchair accessories and options are specified (*feature/product match*).[20,21] As stated previously, the prescription and selection decisions made by the clinician(s) should include involvement of the wheelchair user, his or her family members or caregivers (if appropriate), and a qualified RTP or DME supplier.

Step 4: Funding and Ordering

The next step in the process involves securing funding and ordering the appropriate WSMD and all of the parts and accessories that go with it. It is essential to know the payer source for the WSMD if a third-party payer is involved, or alternately determine if it is being donated, purchased self-pay, or being provided from a facility-owned fleet of available equipment. Documentation is a professional responsibility, a legal requirement, and the most important factor to successful coverage and payment for a WSMD. The person's medical records are expected to reflect clear rationale and justification of the medical need for the care you provide and WSM equipment you recommend. The supplier/RTP typically takes the lead for understanding the coverage and payment policies for the WSMD, compiling required documentation and submitting it to the payer (e.g., health insurance company), obtaining *prior authorization,* ordering, and billing for the equipment.

Step 5: Product Preparation (WSMD)

This step is normally completed by the supplier/RTP and/or rehab technician. The WSMD that was selected and ordered, once delivered by the manufacturer to the supplier, is prepared for fitting and delivery to the user. It is important to make sure that the wheelchair base, seating, and accessories that were ordered are the ones that were received. For CRT devices, it is not uncommon for a WSMD to have upward of three or more different manufacturer's products included. During the assembly process, the WSMD is configured by the supplier/RTP as specified and inspected for safety and function. It is helpful for all members of the WSM team to have some familiarity with how to assemble some of the basic components of the wheelchair, as they may be needed to assist with this process to some extent.

Step 6: Fitting

If everything has gone as planned, good information was obtained during the assessment, and the equipment was ordered properly and met the ordering specifications on delivery, then this step should be pretty straightforward; however, it is no less important! During the fitting, the wheelchair user and the therapist, or the therapist and the supplier together, check that the wheelchair is the correct size and all the necessary modifications and adjustments have been made to ensure proper fit. Next, they check that the wheelchair and seat cushion support the wheelchair user in the optimal sitting posture. Finally, if a pressure-relieving cushion has been prescribed, they check that the cushion relieves pressure adequately for the user. Wheelchair fitting is essential to the success of an appropriate wheelchair, as there are many adjustments that need to be made to ensure the proper support of the wheelchair user in an optimal position. Without this fitting process, a perfectly appropriate wheelchair may become inappropriate!

Step 7: User Training

An essential step in the service delivery process is education and training for the wheelchair user and, if appropriate, for family/caregivers, in the care and proper use of the new WSMD. It is critically important that the wheelchair user knows how to safely and effectively utilize their wheelchair. The therapist is responsible for teaching the wheelchair user how to function from the wheelchair, how to get in and out of it, and techniques to minimize risk for pressure injuries. The user will need to know how to propel and turn the wheelchair, as well as how to navigate stairs, ramps, and environmental obstacles. The supplier/RTP is responsible for providing user training on handling the wheelchair (such as folding, or taking parts on/off the wheelchair), safe use, care and maintenance of the WSMD, and what to do in the event of a mechanical problem.

Step 8: Maintenance, Repairs, and Follow-up

All wheelchairs will require ongoing maintenance, intermittent repairs, and general follow-up to be sure it still fits the user properly and still meets the user's needs. Therefore, follow-up appointments are an important step in a wheelchair service delivery program. During a follow-up appointment, the therapist or supplier/RTP checks the WSMD fit and function and provides further training and support if needed. If the wheelchair is found to be no longer appropriate, the process should start all over again with an appropriate referral for an assessment for a new wheelchair or a substantial modification of the existing wheelchair. This process should be systematic and is often iterative, but it leads to the greatest possibility of success.

PRINCIPLES OF WHEELCHAIR SEATING AND MOBILITY

Most wheelchair users spend many hours sitting each day, so the way in which the person sits in the wheelchair can have a profound effect on health, function, and comfort. For that reason, the wheelchair is not just a mobility aid; it also helps to support the wheelchair user in a comfortable upright sitting posture. Therefore, it is important to understand some basic concepts related to sitting posture and mobility.

Principles of Sitting Posture

The term *posture* refers to the way a person's body segments are arranged, and *sitting posture* is the way a person's body segments are arranged in the sitting position. When providing a wheelchair, it is important to consider the supports in the wheelchair that are needed to help wheelchair users sit in a posture that is comfortable, healthy, and functional.

Reference Neutral Sitting Posture

It is imperative to have a good understanding of the *reference neutral sitting posture* to understand when good posture can be achieved and to assist in determining the amount of support needed. It will also help to understand when an individual's needs are complex and requires services from a seating specialist to obtain the most appropriate system. The objective of the seating system is to allow the person to sit with good pelvic and trunk alignment, neutral lower extremity alignment, and neutral head positioning.

Pelvic Position

The pelvis is the base for sitting upright. Just like a building needs a strong, stable foundation, the pelvis is the foundation for a stable, neutral sitting posture. The pelvis can move and be oriented in different ways. Changes in the orientation of the pelvis affect the posture of the spine and other body segments both above and below the pelvis. The movement and/or position of the pelvis in sitting can be seen from the sagittal, frontal, and transverse views, as shown in Table 32.3.

A reference neutral pelvic position is characterized by a neutral pelvic tilt where a line between the anterior superior iliac spine (ASIS) and posterior superior iliac spine (PSIS) is horizontal or parallel to the seat plane (sagittal view) and the ASIS is level and straight when viewed from the front and top (frontal and transverse views).

The position of the pelvis is critical in creating an optimal foundation for the sitting position. By supporting a neutral to slightly anteriorly tilted pelvis that is level (not oblique or rotated), the pelvis assists with the following:

- Maintains the normal spinal curves (lumbar, thoracic, and cervical)
- Provides symmetrical weight-bearing on bilateral ischial tuberosities (ITs) and pressure distribution over the surface area of the ITs (rather than weight-bearing on the bony prominences of the sacrum or coccyx, which increases pressure risks)
- Promotes symmetry and provides a more stable upright position for active trunk movement and co-contraction of trunk muscles
- Supports flexion at the hips and extension in the lumbar spine; often effective in decreasing abnormal tonal patterns
- Improves alignment in body segments above and below the pelvis
- Provides proximal stability, improving distal mobility and function

Optimal Postural Alignment

The *neutral reference posture* is used as a reference point for determining optimal postural alignment. Not everyone can achieve a symmetrical "neutral" resting posture. Each person's *optimal sitting posture* will be unique to them due to limitations in joint range of motion (ROM), muscle shortening, spasticity or scoliosis, as seen with individuals with complex WSM needs. Also importantly, optimal sitting posture will be influenced by health needs, personal preferences, and functional requirements.

A person's optimal sitting posture is as symmetrical and balanced as possible, enabling the person to relax comfortably, while also being ready to move. The person's optimal posture is also their "*home base*" or resting posture, a place to come back from between extremes of movement, but it is not a place of collapse. To achieve optimal postural alignment, fixed ROM limitations and deformities must be accommodated. Additionally, flexible deformities must be corrected and/or supported.

Factors Influencing Postural Alignment

It must be determined whether a person can maintain optimal postural alignment using their own muscular effort or if external supports are required. First it must be determined if improved alignment can be achieved passively (*flexible*), with the effects of gravity eliminated, supine and/or side-lying on a mat table; and secondly in the seated position with the effects of gravity.

Attention is first directed toward alignment of the pelvis and then other body segments. If good alignment can be achieved (*corrected*), it must be determined whether the person can maintain alignment using muscular effort or if external supports are required.

For joints and/or body segments that are not flexible (*fixed*) to passive alignment, *accommodation* is needed. For example, accommodation would be needed for a person who presents with long-standing fixed hip ROM limitations from hip subluxation and prolonged sitting in a *"windswept lower extremity (LE) posture"* (Fig. 32.1), where one hip is positioned in abduction and external

Table 32.3 Reference Neutral Sitting Posture

Sagittal View	Frontal View	Transverse View
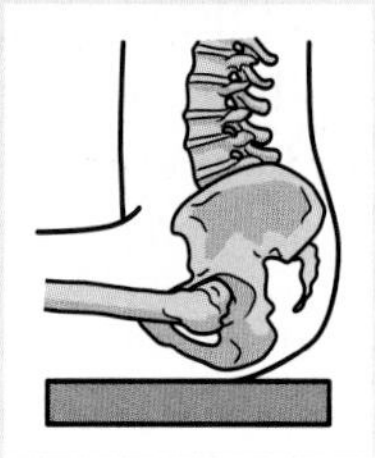	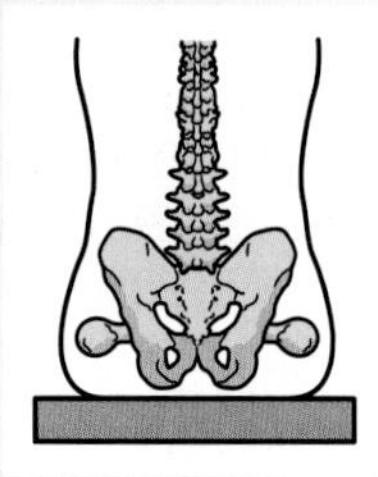	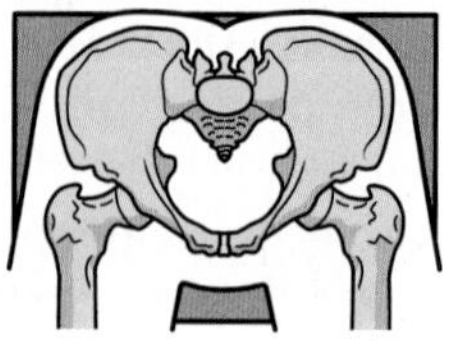
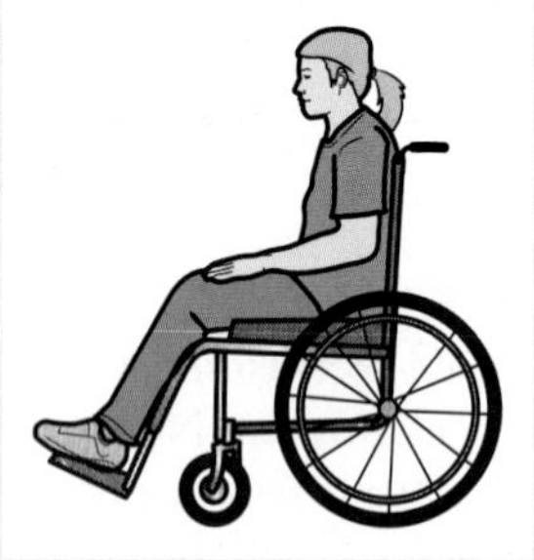	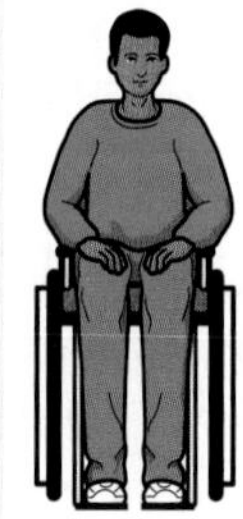	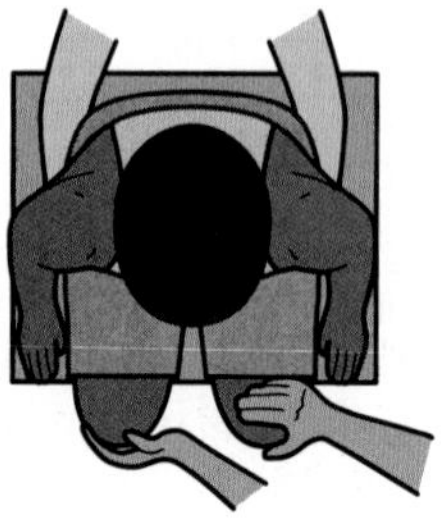
• Pelvis is neutral to slight anterior tilt • Shoulders are aligned above or slightly behind hips • Spine maintains natural lumbar, thoracic, and cervical curves • Head is vertical and balanced over trunk with neutral horizontal visual gaze • Hips are flexed 80° to 90° • Knees and ankles are flexed near 90° • Heels directly below the knees or slightly forward or back • Feet flat on the footrests	• Pelvis (ASIS) is level • Trunk is in midline • Head is in midline, balanced over body • Shoulders are level, relaxed and arms are free to move • Thighs are in slight abduction • Lower legs are vertical with neutral hip rotation • Feet are under the knees	• Pelvis (ASIS) and trunk (shoulders) are not rotated • Head is forward facing and free to rotate • Knees are pointing forward with mild symmetrical abduction • Feet are pointing forward or slightly outward

rotation and the opposite hip is in adduction and internal rotation. Given a fixed deformity, attempts at aligning the lower extremities (LEs) will cause pelvic and/or trunk rotation. The LEs therefore must be accommodated by supporting positioning in the windswept posture (see Fig. 32.1). Alignment of the pelvis takes priority over alignment of other body segments. Providing optimal pelvic and trunk alignment is most important and sometimes trade-offs are needed to maintain or improve function.

Time must be allocated to practice motor skills and movement within the context of improved postural alignment, especially if dramatic alignment changes have resulted. A person's posture is affected by tone, strength, gravity, habitual patterns of movement, and activities. New skill acquisition should be promoted to foster independence rather than dependence on equipment. This is especially important to the younger person who is growing and changing, as well as the person who has not had the opportunity to improve function due to poor positioning and excessive equipment use. Supports can be used intermittently throughout the day to provide learning opportunities (acquisition of new skills) over time. Using a minimum of supports can improve cosmetic appearance and self-esteem. Other equipment may need to be used for specific activities or for opportunities to improve strength and skills.

Frequently it is necessary to encourage wheelchair users to sit with "optimal sitting posture," especially if they are accustomed to sitting and functioning from a suboptimal posture. It is recommended that the

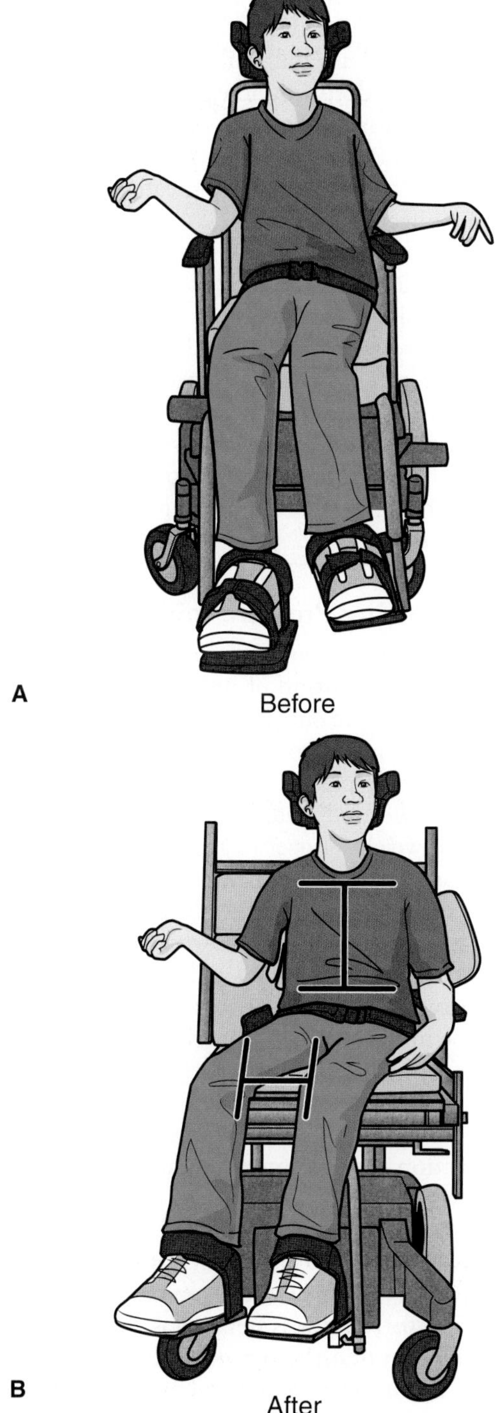

Figure 32.1 Windswept deformity. (A) Keeping the legs straight causes a left pelvic obliquity with the left side lower than the right by 2 inches, a left thoracic scoliosis, and the trunk and pelvis are rotated forward on the right. (B) Accommodating for hip range limitations allows the pelvis to be in a neutral position, not rotated and level, and the trunk is straight and no longer rotated. The right lower extremity is abducted, and the left is adducted slightly in a windswept posture. This allows for better pressure distribution under the buttocks.

therapist spend time discussing the rationale for pursuing the optimal sitting posture to gain the person's understanding and agreement. Ultimately it is the decision of the wheelchair user, but at the same time it is the therapists' responsibility to provide the education and document his or her professional opinion and recommendation.

Benefits of Optimal Sitting Posture

Optimal sitting posture has benefits for an individual's overall health, comfort, and functioning from the wheelchair. In the optimal sitting posture, the person's muscles do not have to work a lot to maintain their posture, yet they are not collapsed and inactive. The individual is ready for action.

Sitting with optimal body alignment supports health benefits, including facilitating healthy body functioning such as safe swallowing, optimal breathing, and digesting food. Sitting with an optimal posture can also help to reduce the risk of pressure injuries. This is because the person's body weight is evenly distributed across their buttocks and thighs when they are sitting in a symmetrical, neutral posture, and this helps prevent skin breakdown from asymmetrical loading of the person's body weight onto their buttocks. Finally, sitting with an optimal posture can help reduce the chance of developing deformities of the spine or joint contractures from sitting asymmetrically for long periods of time.

There are also many potential *functional benefits* of an optimal sitting posture. When the core of the body is balanced and stable, this can help improve motor control of the head, trunk, arms, and hands. This can translate to increased ability to reach with arms, propel a wheelchair, grasp and manipulate objects, control eye gaze, communicate and project voice, or operate switches that can control other devices in the environment. Imagine having to sit on an exercise ball without your feet planted on the floor. You would have to work your core muscles to maintain your balance. Now imagine threading a needle while balancing on the ball. This is what it is like for some wheelchair users who have poor trunk control or who experience abnormal movement patterns from muscle spasticity. If they cannot stabilize their core on their own, it is difficult to have optimal control of their head or arms to do functional tasks from their wheelchair. If the wheelchair is designed to fit appropriately it can help to align and stabilize the body core, resulting in improved ability to engage in functional tasks. Proximal stability facilitates distal mobility and function.

Finally, sitting in an optimal posture provides *comfort benefits* for the wheelchair user. When the body is symmetrical, and weight is distributed evenly on weight-bearing surfaces, the person is usually more comfortable and uses less energy. He or she feels balanced and stable. When a person is comfortable, he or she can more effectively participate in work, learning, or play. Comfort leads to improved endurance, attentiveness, concentration, and use and adoption of the equipment. Sitting in an optimal posture can also help wheelchair users feel better about themselves, increasing self-esteem and self-confidence. Critical to the provision of equipment is involvement of the user, who should participate in the process and be allowed an opportunity to express likes and dislikes of the system.

Pressure Injuries

In April 2016, the National Pressure Ulcer Advisory Panel redefined the term *pressure injuries,* previously referred to as *pressure ulcers, pressure sores,* or *decubitus ulcers.* Pressure injuries are a major health concern for wheelchair users, especially for those who lack sensation or are unable to reposition themselves. Pressure injuries develop quickly and can lead to serious and costly health issues. It is estimated that hospital costs for pressure injuries in the United States are approaching $11 billion annually with a cost between $500 and $70,000 per individual per injury.[24] Pressure injuries are preventable, and physical therapists can assist people with maintaining good skin integrity by providing appropriate seating, training, and education.

A pressure injury is an area of damaged skin usually over a bony prominence that results from excessive prolonged pressure, friction, shear, heat and/or moisture. It may also be related to use of a medical or other device. The skin may be intact or open and the area may be painful. The tolerance of soft tissue for pressure and shear may also be affected by microclimate (meaning heat and moisture), nutrition, perfusion, and comorbidities affecting the condition of the soft tissue.[25] A pressure injury can develop in a few hours but can take months to heal or be seen. If the injury becomes infected, the infection can spread to the blood, heart, or bone and can lead to serious illness and/or death.

The majority of all pressure injuries develop over primary bony areas, including the sacrum, coccyx, greater trochanter, IT, calcaneus, and lateral malleolus. In sitting, the seat cushion and pelvic posture affect weight-bearing and pressure on the sacrum, coccyx, greater trochanters, and ITs. Foot positioning in the wheelchair may result in injuries to the lower leg and feet.

There are six stages of pressure injuries as defined by the National Pressure Ulcer Advisory Panel:[26,27]

- Stage 1 Pressure Injury: nonblanchable erythema of intact skin—a red or dark mark on the skin that doesn't blanche within 30 minutes after pressure is removed.
- Stage 2 Pressure Injury: Partial-thickness skin loss with exposed dermis—a shallow wound with the top layer of skin beginning to peel away or blister; involvement of the dermis.
- Stage 3 Pressure Injury: Full-thickness skin loss—a deep wound with full thickness loss of skin. Adipose tissue is visible, and there may be rolled wound edges, slough, and/or eschar visible.
- Stage 4 Pressure Injury: Full-thickness skin and tissue loss—a very deep wound extending through the muscle and possibly down to the bone. Tunneling and undermining often occur, making this wound more difficult to heal with greater possibility for systemic infection.
- Unstageable Pressure Injury: Obscured full-thickness skin and tissue loss—cannot be confirmed because it is obscured by slough or eschar.
- Deep Tissue Pressure Injury: Persistent non-blanchable deep red, maroon, or purple discoloration—results from intense and/or prolonged pressure and shear forces at the bone-muscle interface and may evolve rapidly to reveal the actual extent of tissue injury or may resolve without tissue loss.

Factors Influencing Pressure Injuries

Therapists play an important role in educating wheelchair users in the prevention of pressure injuries. Risk factors in developing pressure injuries include decreased sensation, decreased ability to move, excessive heat and/or moisture, poor sitting posture, previous or current pressure injury, poor diet and inadequate fluid intake, aging, and being underweight or overweight.[28-31] In examining risk for pressure injuries, the therapist should consider all situations that place the person at risk, including but not limited to bed positioning, shower commode chair positioning, car seat positioning, and the transfer technique used between different surfaces. Risks for pressure injuries can be minimized by improving posture, nutrition, transfer skills, and pressure relief techniques.[32]

Pressure injuries are typically caused by prolonged pressure over bony prominences from sitting or lying in the same position for too long without moving. This often occurs when an individual has decreased sensation in these areas, so the person is not cued to shift weight or change positions due to pain or discomfort.

The two primary factors causing pressure injuries are friction and shear. *Friction* is defined as the force that resists the relative motion of two objects sliding against each other.[33] This is a contributing factor to shear. *Shear* is a distortion of the body tissues resulting from two opposing forces parallel to the surface.[33] This occurs when the pressure of the body or gravity is now added to friction. Shear happens when the skin stays still and is stretched as the bones move over the skin. The bottom line is this: It is not possible to have shear without friction, but it *is* possible to have friction without shear. For example, an arm rubbing on a wheel as a wheelchair moves will create friction. When a person slides down in the bed or slides forward on a wheelchair cushion, this also creates friction and can contribute to the development of shear stresses within underlying tissues by tending to keep the skin in place against the support surface while the person's body, or more specifically their bony structure, continues to move.

A combination of good sitting posture and an appropriate seat cushion can minimize risk for pressure injury and assist with healing. Sitting in a neutral, upright posture distributes pressure over the greatest surface area (the buttocks and thighs) and decreases pressure over bony areas. An appropriate seat cushion can assist in both supporting a neutral upright posture and distributing pressure more evenly. Ensuring the wheelchair fits the user correctly and allows the person to transfer and reposition themselves with minimal friction and shear (e.g., scraping or rubbing against wheelchair parts) will also decrease risk.

Some wheelchair cushion properties and materials can assist with dissipating heat and moisture and can be a factor to consider during selection. Avoiding moisture such as wet or soiled clothing or seat cushion can improve skin integrity. Oftentimes a bowel and bladder management program may be needed to address these issues and require a referral from the therapist.

Changing position regularly, utilizing effective pressure relief techniques (e.g., forward bending, side leaning, press-ups) or positioning features (e.g., tilt, recline, and stand) are crucial for reducing pressure injury risk. Also transferring out of the wheelchair to other surfaces (e.g., bed, sofa, chair) is another strategy that can be used for breaks throughout the day.

Drinking water will help keep the skin and body tissues healthy. Increasing protein and eating a well-balanced diet also assists with wound healing and decreasing risk for pressure injuries. Smoking can have a negative effect on circulation and should be avoided. See Chapter 14, Vascular, Lymphatic, and Integumentary Disorders for a more detailed discussion of pressure injuries.

Principles of Mobility

The term *mobility* refers to the way a person moves by changing body positions or locations (locomotion) or by transferring from one place to another.[16] This includes ambulation and wheeled mobility. The determination that a wheeled mobility device is reasonable and necessary for a person is based on the clinical assessment and judgment of the WSM team. Factors include the person's:

- Past history (including prior level of functioning and assistive device use, if applicable).
- Current condition, including present functional mobility status, temporary or permanent nature of the condition, static or progressive nature of condition, nature of other medical problems.
- Ability to functionally ambulate safely and sufficiently to perform mobility needs arising in the course of typical daily activities in a timely manner.

When providing a wheelchair, it is important to think about the person's daily mobility needs, environments and terrains typically encountered, and distances necessary to accomplish typical daily tasks without pain or excessive signs of fatigue (i.e., dyspnea, discoloration, rapid respirations, diaphoresis, and so forth).[34] Decisions about the wheeled mobility device (intervention) selected are based on the goals identified, such as improving independence and function, optimizing safety, decreasing risk of falls, reducing risk for pressure injuries, and improving physical capacity, health status, activity, and participation.

WHEELCHAIR SEATING AND MOBILITY EXAMINATION AND SPECIALTY EVALUATION

A wheelchair seating and mobility examination and specialty evaluation involves different components based on key information and methods used for collecting the data. An outline of the components of the WSM Examination and Specialty Evaluation are found in Table 32.2. For the purposes of this chapter, the examination process, which is part of Steps 2, 3, and 4 of the WHO's Wheelchair Service Delivery Steps described above, is divided into three major sections: *examination, specialty evaluation,* and *intervention.* These components may be completed in one or more therapy visits. Each component described is essential to the process. A problem-solving model is used to match the person to the technology and the environments typically encountered, known as the *person/technology/environmental match.* The result is a plan of care that includes a prescription, justification, and recommendations for specific WSM equipment and additional clinical interventions such as fitting, training, and follow-up.

Communication Tips

It is important to take time at the beginning of the examination process to explain to the patient, family, and caregivers the overall process, the type of information that will be gathered, and why it is important. Time should be allocated during data collection for comments or questions from the wheelchair user, caregivers, and other team members. Each team members' input is necessary and valuable to the process. While questions may be personal, remind everyone that information discussed is confidential and necessary to help the team identify and select the most appropriate WSMD. Remember to directly address the wheelchair user (not the caregiver/family member) unless he or she is a small child or unable to understand your questions or communicate answers. Box 32.1 lists effective communication tips and considerations to use during the assessment process.

The APTA Mobility Device Documentation Guide (link provided in Appendix 32.A: Internet Resources) details the elements of the wheelchair evaluation to

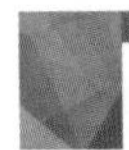

Box 32.1 Effective Interview and Communication Tips

- Always address the wheelchair user (not the caregiver/family member)
- Speak clearly
- Make good eye contact (when appropriate)
- Be respectful
- Use straightforward terms
- Explain what is going to happen before it happens
- After explaining something, check that the wheelchair user understands
- Listen carefully and check to make sure you have understood the wheelchair user correctly
- Show you are interested
- Don't assume you know best

consider and document and is a valuable tool to keep handy and reference.[35] Although time-consuming, it is absolutely critical that documentation of the examination and specialty evaluation is complete and accurate because changes to the WSMD prescription may be difficult to make once equipment is ordered. Accurate and detailed notes provide a permanent record of why certain decisions were made. During the ordering or manufacturing process, additional decisions concerning configuration may be needed. If accurate measurements are on file, decisions can often be made without recalling the person to the clinic.

Examination

The examination is individually tailored by the therapist to the person's condition and needs. While not all examination components may be relevant for a particular individual, all components should be considered and relevant details documented, even if it is merely to indicate a component is not applicable. Remember, the majority of the time, your examination findings will be reviewed by another professional responsible for making a decision to approve or disapprove the equipment request. Include as much objective quantitative and qualitative information as possible to paint a clinical picture of the person on paper and communicate clearly to an unfamiliar reader.

Assessment Interview

The purpose of the assessment interview is to describe the person's environments, functions, and activities/participation on a typical day, including limitations and restrictions. The assessment interview components follow.

Demographic Information

General demographics about the person such as name, contact information, age, gender, height, weight, and so on.

Reason for Referral

The reason the person was referred for the WSM examination. Reasons for the referral will be different for each person. It may be due to a new or progressive mobility impairment, a first-time device, or modifications or replacement for an existing device.

Diagnosis

The diagnosis(es) relevant to the positioning and/or mobility impairment is specified, including the corresponding ICD-10 diagnostic code. In particular, specify any pertinent diagnoses related to positioning such as scoliosis, hip subluxation or dislocation, pressure injuries past or present, contractures, and so on. Unlike mobility devices where eligibility is based on functional criteria, eligibility for positioning devices is frequently diagnostic specific requiring particular ICD-10 codes.

Medical/Surgical History

Document pertinent history related to the positioning and/or mobility impairment. Include the onset date, prognosis, course, and rate of progression. Include past and planned surgeries if known.

History of WSM Problems

Describe the progression of the positioning/mobility limitation, technology used or tried in the past, medical/surgical/treatment interventions to improve the impairment, and the results of the interventions.

Goals (User, Family/Caregiver)

Specify the goals for the recommended WSM equipment and any recommended clinical related services (e.g., wheelchair skills training, transfer training, patient/family teaching).

Social Status

Describe the person's living situation (e.g., lives alone; lives with family; receives attendant care, including hours/week and assistance provided).

Environmental Accessibility (Home and Community)

Describe the person's home (e.g., ranch, split-level house, apartment, mobile home, assisted living). Discuss the home environment and accessibility such as entrance (steps, ramp, elevator), floor surfaces (low-pile carpet, tile, wood), and measurements (narrowest doorway, heights of table, sink, bed, and so forth). Home adaptations, assistive equipment, and sometimes entire modifications may be needed for safety and improved wheelchair access (see Chapter 9, Examination and Modification of the Environment). Discuss the environments the person typically encounters in the course of their daily activities. Describe terrain encountered (e.g., grass, gravel, hills, side slopes, inclement weather, environmental obstacles), and describe environmental facilitators and barriers that will affect safe access to the community.

Employment/Work Status (Job/School)

Describe the person's occupation (typical job duties), school/work tasks, functions, workstation accessibility needs, distances traveled, and so on.

General Health Status

Provide a general description of the person's overall social/health habits (past/current). A change in health status can impact a person's weight and therefore impact the size and capacity of the WSMD. Relevant information about weight gain or loss, planned surgical interventions (e.g., gastrointestinal tube placement), medications, and other risk factors that might contribute to pressure injuries, infections, aspiration, changes in weight, safety concerns, and so on, should be included.

Functional Status and Activity Level (Roles/Responsibilities)

Describe the person's primary roles, responsibilities (e.g., parent, primary caregiver for spouse or elderly parent, student), activity level, and prior level of functioning. Have the person describe a typical day, including self-care and routine daily activities (e.g., medical appointments, cooking/cleaning, shopping, recreation) to get a sense of functional status and activity level. Include time spent in wheelchair daily (hours/day) and distances traveled.

Transportation

Discussing the transportation plan for the person and the wheelchair is critical to the decision making process. Specific wheelchair features will determine how the wheelchair can be transported and how it can be secured and stowed. Describe how the person and the wheelchair will be transported. Note if the person will be a driver or passenger in a vehicle seat or in the wheelchair, transfer type, transportation and/or vehicle type (make/model car, van, bus, public transportation), wheelchair storage location, method and dimensions (passenger seat, trunk, exterior or interior lift, ramp), wheelchair securement (tie down, docking system, other), and occupant restraint.

Understanding if the person will load/unload the wheelchair alone or have assistance may factor into decisions about overall wheelchair weight and how the wheelchair collapses or folds. If the person rides in a van in their wheelchair, measurements of the door opening and height will be necessary to ensure sufficient head clearance and wheelchair access into the van. If the person drives from the wheelchair, the measurements of the van will be necessary to ensure the person will be able to safely maneuver in/out of the van and fit in the driving station.

Equipment Assessment

Existing Equipment

Detail existing equipment the person owns or uses (e.g., cane, walker, manual/power wheelchair, scooter); bathroom equipment; lifts; bed equipment; other devices, including but not limited to home, vehicle modifications, prosthetics/orthotics, and so on. Include problems or concerns about existing equipment and plans for future changes or modifications.

Current WSM Equipment

List the make/model, serial number, condition, size, age, supplier, payer, and reason for new equipment. Explain what worked/didn't work about current equipment (e.g., no longer meets the person's needs because..., or the cost to repair exceeds the cost of new technology).

Sitting Posture in Existing Equipment

Observing the person in their existing wheelchair provides a great deal of information. The person should be in the best or most commonly assumed position, with supports and straps in place as they arrive to the clinic. Questions should include how the person and/or caregiver perceive current posture, if person has any new pain and location of pain, any new pressure injuries and location of injuries, any weight loss or weight gain since receiving equipment. Ask the person what works well and what doesn't work well about the WSMD related to mobility, positioning, and function. Ask if they are having any difficulty using the equipment.

Functional Assessment

The next part of the examination involves subjective and objective evaluations of performance and functional abilities to establish activity level, positioning needed for function, and extent of mobility impairment. Importantly, the persons' prognosis (potential for restoration or enhancement) for function is established.

ADL/IADL Status

Describe the person's typical daily activities of daily living (ADLs) and instrumental activities of daily living (IADLs). A critical part of the functional assessment is identifying functional activities performed from the wheelchair such as dressing, self-catheterization, cooking, laundry, and so on. When seated in a wheelchair, accessing kitchen appliances, cabinets, the sink, bathtub, shower, laundry, and shelves is frequently more difficult. Specify adaptive equipment or assistive technology used, accessibility considerations, efficiency (timeliness), and safety concerns. Describe assistance needed to perform typical daily activities.

Explore the person's usual community activities. Information from the assessment interview may prompt further discussion about distances traveled, terrain, climate/weather, transportation, and accessibility barriers. These details will drive decisions about product features needed such as product durability, robustness, range, power, speed, and maneuverability. Important ADL/IADL topics that significantly contribute to the decision making process for WSMD selection follow.

Toileting

Toilet transfers are probably the most difficult transfer performed and often are required multiple times per day. Discussion about toilet height, transfer technique, transfer equipment, and toilet seat pressure management are critical factors.[36] Power wheelchair seat lifts can facilitate transfers to toilets of differing heights. If the person uses a urinal, the wheelchair seat style needs to be discussed to prevent accidental tipping of the urinal. If the person will be self-catheterizing from the wheelchair, positioning in the wheelchair needs to be considered. If the person has an indwelling catheter and independently empties the collection bag, maneuvering close to the toilet is necessary. If the person experiences episodes of incontinence or accidents, cushion properties and materials must be considered such as a waterproof cover, closed cell foam, and/or micromicrobial seat cushion materials.

Dressing

Some individuals find it easier to don/doff clothing when in their wheelchair; others prefer a bed. Depending on the person's technique, footrest and armrest style and durability or back cane type and height are discussed to ensure the system will accommodate the extra force placed on these components during dressing and other functional activities. Use of tilt-in-space seating or a reclining back system to unweight the lower body may be useful for the person who dresses in the wheelchair.

Eating

The wheelchair seat and armrest height may prevent positioning the wheelchair close to some tables or desks. The style of table or desk may interfere with wheelchair access (e.g., number and arrangement of legs, height of working surface, presence of drawers). If a person needs assistance during mealtime, caregivers need to have ease of access to ensure safety during mealtime. Positioning of head/neck and trunk are important considerations while eating to optimize swallowing and minimize risk for aspiration or choking.

Mobility Status

Bed Mobility, Transfers, Weight Shift

Current mobility status, prior level of functioning, and potential anticipated functioning are documented. The person's bed mobility, transfer status, and ability to weight shift are examined. Equipment and assistance needed for mobility are noted (e.g., slide board, mechanical lift, mattress overlay, electric hospital bed). For weight shift, the method (e.g., press-up, leaning, bridging, tilt, recline, stand), frequency, duration, and effectiveness are discussed and observed (throughout the duration of the examination).

Ambulation

Documenting the quantitative and qualitative ambulation status of the person is an essential part of the examination and often the key factor in qualifying a person for a wheeled mobility device. Describe how the person arrived to your clinic, distance they can typically walk, speed, duration of walking or standing prior to needing a rest, balance, and incidences of falls or close calls (detail injuries, frequency, and factors attributing to incident).

Keep in mind that assessing ambulation is done to determine if the person requires a WSMD temporarily, permanently, or would benefit from physical therapy or another intervention to achieve independent, safe, functional, and timely ambulation. Consider if a lower-level device or intervention will meet the person's mobility needs, and justify your decision making process clearly in your written report. For instance, make clear your professional opinion about whether the person's mobility impairment could be ameliorated with the use of a mobility device such as a cane, walker, orthotic, and so on, with or without a therapy intervention.

Although a person may require a wheelchair to accomplish daily mobility needs, the person may still be able to ambulate short distances (e.g., "wall walk"), albeit not functionally for the purposes of meeting all daily mobility needs. Documentation to paint a clinical picture of the person's mobility status is critical. For example, if a person with MS is able to take a few steps in the morning with a walker but her symptoms fluctuate day to day and a.m. to p.m., be sure to present these details in your report. Remember if the person does utilize an assistive device (e.g., cane, walker, crutches) for transfers or taking a few steps, a means to mount the device on the wheelchair needs to be determined to ensure availability and access.

Propulsion Method

The next aspect of the functional assessment is considering the person's wheelchair skills and potential. Is the person a first-time wheelchair user or have they previously used a wheelchair (manual or power)? If the person uses a manual wheelchair, how do they propel the wheelchair (both upper extremities, hemi-propel (one arm/one leg, both lower extremities, all four extremities)? Does the person have adequate motor control to self-propel? Do they have sufficient strength and muscular endurance to self-propel for the demands of typical daily activities? Note any functional limitations using quantitative and qualitative objective data to include decreased strength, motor control, pain, and endurance.

If the person operates a scooter (power-operated vehicle [POV]) or power wheelchair, describe the access method (tiller, switch, joystick, head array) and controls (multi-drive controls, proportional, latched). Specify if the person is independent and safe or indicate if a different access method or controller is needed.

Propulsion method is a primary factor in the decision making process for a person/feature match. For manual wheelchair users, propulsion method establishes wheelchair configuration needs. For example, if the person uses their feet to self-propel, a seat-to-floor height that allows the feet to easily contact the floor is critical and often a deciding factor in narrowing available products. For another person, the controller (e.g., joystick) position alone might determine if they can independently operate the power wheelchair. If the person is unable to use a standard joystick controller with their hand, alternative drive controls exist (e.g., chin control, sip and puff, track pad, head array). Identifying a consistent, nonfatigable access site will lead to options for controllers and access site to optimize independent power wheelchair control. If the person is dependent for mobility, caregivers will be moving the wheelchair. Considerations to discuss include style and height of push handles, wheel lock styles, and/or attendant controls.

Screening of Body Functions and Structures

During the assessment interview, the wheelchair user describes medical issues that may influence wheelchair selection. This section is intended for further screening of essential body functions and structures that impact the person's positioning and mobility. If indicated, a more detailed evaluation is conducted or the person may be referred to another professional.

Cardiovascular/Pulmonary/Circulatory Status

In terms of cardiovascular/pulmonary and circulatory issues, it may be relevant to take the heart and respiratory rates, blood pressure, and/or oxygen saturation level at rest and with activity. It will be important to note how the person responds to activity (e.g., endurance tolerance for self-propulsion). Does the person require supplemental oxygen, ventilator, or suction? It is also a good practice to examine the person's body for edema and/or lymphedema, especially in the lower extremities.

Gastrointestinal System Review

For the gastrointestinal system, note if the person has any digestive issues, such as reflux or elimination issues that may affect seating and positioning. If the person receives nourishment via tube, note method (e.g., nasogastric tube, gastrostomy tube, and so forth); the location may affect type and mounting position for postural supports and straps. Also, it is important to determine if the person requires specific positioning for swallowing or following meals for digestion, particularly if they will be eating while in the wheelchair.

Communication

Communication is assessed from the beginning of the examination. Expressive and receptive communication abilities are noted. For wheelchair purposes, if the person is unable to speak, does he or she use an augmentative communication device? If so, considerations for how and where a device will need to be mounted and accessed are discussed. Even if the person is unable to speak, discuss with the caregiver how to discern yes/no, comfort/pain issues so that you do not miss any needs of the individual.

Cognitive Status

When assessing the person's cognitive status, determine his or her ability to safely utilize the wheelchair, taking the environments they routinely encounter into consideration. Focus on the person's memory, pathfinding, problem-solving, judgment, motor planning, attention, behavior, and learning skills.

Vision and Hearing

The person's vision and hearing must be functional to safely and independently operate the wheelchair. Vision affects a person's ability to operate a power or manual wheelchair. Consider spatial awareness, visual fields, and depth perception. It is important to determine if visual problems exist and how they affect mobility, and if the person can learn compensatory techniques to be independent and safe (otherwise known as *minimizing or ameliorating impairments*). Full or partial vision loss may affect the person's ability to see curb cuts, potholes, drop-offs, and other environmental barriers. Hearing deficits, too, can pose safety concerns. For example, when driving outdoors, a person with a hearing impairment may not hear a car horn or someone calling to them to stop. Note use of hearing aids.

Bowel/Bladder Functions

The management of bowel and bladder function is critical to the person's wheelchair/seating choices. Note if the person is continent or incontinent, uses a catheter, if it is indwelling or intermittent, and if the person will be self-catheterizing from the wheelchair. Oftentimes, issues of incontinence can require referrals to other professionals such as urologist, neurologist, physiatrist, or enterostomal nurse for bowel and bladder interventions and management.

Physical Assessment

Information gathering was initiated during the interview and functional assessment. If further detail is needed, this is the time to collect it. In this section, first the supine and sitting mat assessment is described; then the components of the physical assessment and how the various physical findings interact and influence selection of WSMD features are discussed.

As you proceed with the physical assessment, communicate with the person about what you are doing and why. Be mindful that some people are sensitive to loud speech or quick movements, which may trigger reflexes, increase muscle tone, or cause anxiety. As you go, a "think aloud" approach, explaining what is being observed or measured, allows team members, including the person and their family/caregivers, an opportunity to ask questions and contribute information.[37] This practice is useful so all stakeholders can hear the findings and contribute to the clinical problem-solving process that results in the WSM recommendations.

Mat Assessment

The physical assessment is typically performed during a mat assessment—in both sitting and supine positions. To start, if not already completed, document the person's baseline position and function when sitting in their current WSMD. When done, have the person transfer onto a mat table, noting observations and/or inconsistencies that may not have been identified during the functional assessment.

Supine Mat Assessment

The person is examined in a gravity-minimized position to learn about his or her strength, range of available movement, and how movement of one body part affects tone, comfort, position, control, and performance in other body segments. This is typically performed supine on a firm surface. A mat table or floor works well. A bed is often too soft. If modification for supine positioning is needed, try using a wedge or side-lying position.

Importantly, the maximum range of available pelvic and hip movement as it relates to spinal and pelvic alignment is determined. The goal is to preserve spinal alignment whenever possible, maintaining the natural lumbar curve and determining the presence of any flexible and/or fixed deformities. Postural tendencies should be noted when the person is supine on the mat. Range of motion and muscle length are assessed to determine muscle limitations that will affect a person in the seated position. For example, since the hamstring muscle is a two-joint muscle, it affects the range at both the hip and knee. If the hip is extended, the knee can be extended even if there is hamstring tightness. But if the hip is flexed, knee extension will be limited if hamstring tightness is present. The gastrocnemius is also a two-joint muscle with tightness affecting the knee and ankle range of motion. In the supine position, preliminary linear measurements may be obtained, including buttock/thigh length, lower leg length, chest width, and hip width (Fig. 32.2).

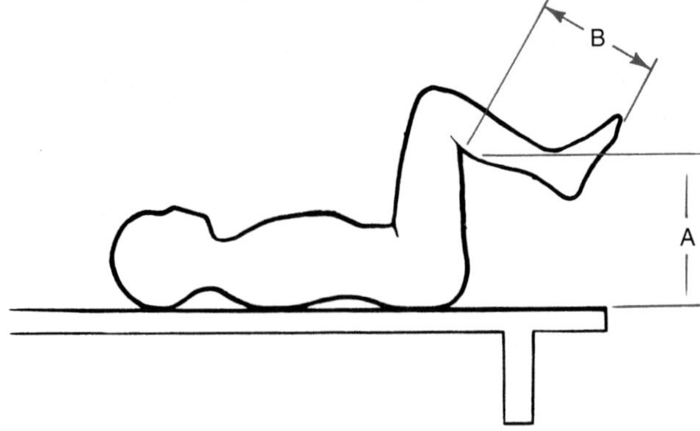

Figure 32.2 (A) With the patient in the supine position with the hips and knees flexed, the examiner can measure the under surface of the thigh from the popliteal fossa to a firm support surface. (B) Note that this position can also be used to measure lower leg length from the popliteal fossa to the heel.

Sitting Mat Assessment

While seated on a mat table or firm surface, with thighs and lower legs fully supported, the person is assessed upright with the effects of gravity (Fig. 32.3). If the person has significant physical involvement, oftentimes more than one person is needed to provide support while the therapist completes the assessment. Assess the person in all three reference planes (i.e., frontal, sagittal, transverse) and record all positional issues and postural anomalies. Compare the current posture with the reference neutral posture discussed earlier in the chapter.

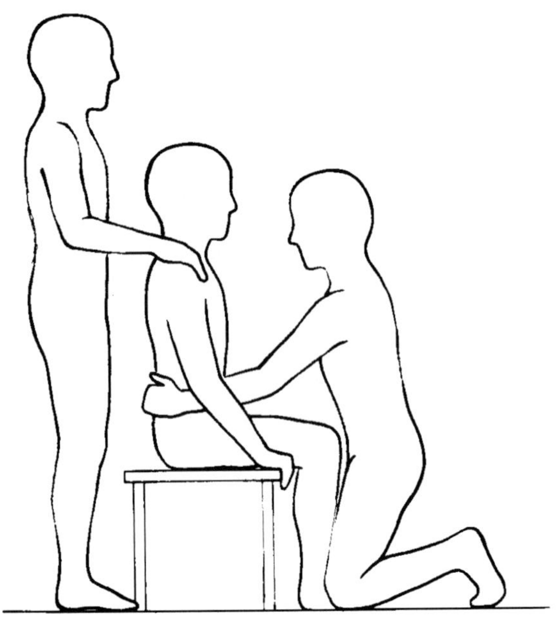

Figure 32.3 The sitting position can be used to determine the amount and location of required support.

Assess the pelvis, hips, knees, ankles, feet, trunk, head, and upper extremities, palpating as needed and measuring linear and angular asymmetries. Record specific postural alignment findings, noting fixed and/or flexible deformities and postural tendencies of the pelvis, spine, lower and upper extremities, and head/neck in the sitting position. See detailed description in the "Postural Alignment" section.

Components of Physical Assessment

The components of the physical assessment include sensation, pain, skin integrity, postural alignment, balance, strength and endurance, range of motion and flexibility, and neuromuscular status.

Sensation

Sensory impairment is a very important risk factor for pressure injuries. Assess if the person has intact, impaired, or absent sensation and describe level of involvement and location. Pay particular attention to skin that is in contact with the seating surface (buttocks, thighs, coccyx, sacrum, pelvis). Note if there are any other sensory concerns such as deep pressure, proprioception, kinesthesia, phantom sensation, pain, and so on.

Pain

Document location and severity of pain. Indicate what exacerbates and relieves the pain. It is critically important to understand any pain that is potentially related to sitting and/or the wheelchair seating environment. If the person is nonverbal, body movements or facial expressions may help you determine areas and extent of pain.

Skin Integrity

Individuals who use a wheelchair for locomotion have an increased chance of developing pressure injuries from prolonged sitting, making an in-depth assessment of current and past skin integrity issues an important consideration. Location, size, and stage of current or previous healed pressure injuries, surgeries, or treatments related to skin integrity are noted. Existing pressure injuries are examined and investigated to determine what the injury is attributed to—shear, friction, maceration, injury/trauma (e.g., hitting wheelchair wheel during transfer), bed mattress with no cushion or overlay, prolonged sitting on shower/toilet commode with no cushion, and so on. Pressure under bony prominences is assessed, especially for users at risk or with a history of a pressure injury. Measurement tools such as pressure mapping are available to quantitively assess pressure, offering a visual graphic showing areas of high pressure and pressure distribution.

Remember, once a pressure injury occurs, there is permanent change to the tissue affected. Therefore, even if there is a healed pressure injury, inspect the skin and document the details, including scars; for example, "Healed Stage 3 pressure injury R IT with healed flap incision noted—August, 2006."

Postural Alignment

Postural alignment is assessed by looking at the orientation of body segments in relation to each other in three reference planes (frontal, sagittal, transverse). In the sagittal plane, the amount of anterior or posterior pelvic tilt and curves of the spine are assessed, noting any abnormal curves or spinal postures. For example, a posterior pelvic tilt is frequently associated with a decreased (or absent) lumbar lordosis and an increased thoracic kyphosis.

In the frontal plane (from the front and rear), the spine is observed for scoliosis. A lateral curve of the spine is named based on the convex side of the curve. For example, in Figure 32.4, lateral flexion would be named *right thoracic lateral flexion* or "C curve." A lateral curvature

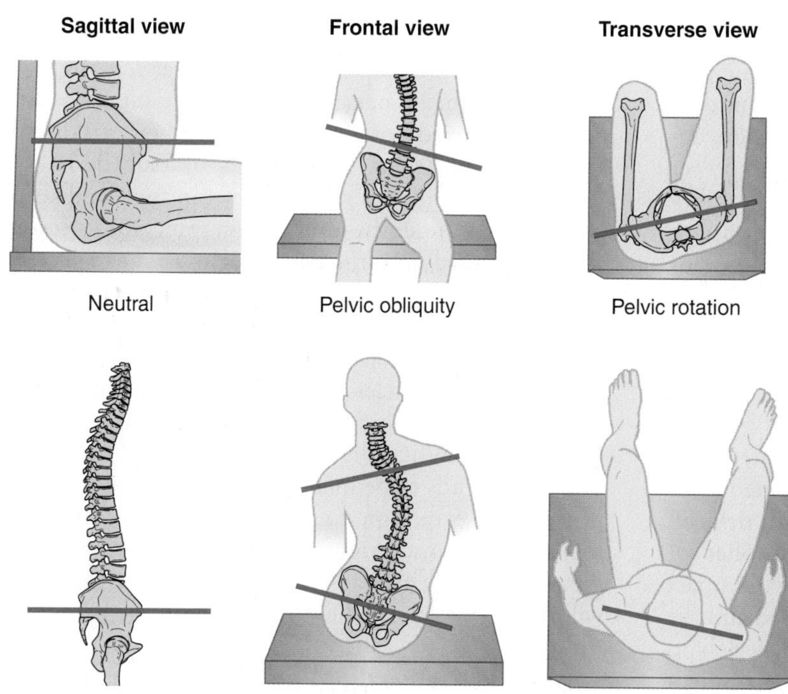

Figure 32.4 Trunk and pelvis postures in the sagittal, frontal, and transverse planes.

with two curves is frequently referred to as an "S curve." In this example, there is also a left cervical compensatory curve.

In the transverse plane, looking at the person from above, rotation of the pelvis or trunk is observed. The posture is typically determined based on the pelvis relative to shoulders or lower trunk relative to upper trunk.

Often, lateral flexion in the frontal plane and rotation occur simultaneously. In the right column of Figure 32.4 the pelvis is rotated forward on the right and the upper trunk is counterrotated posteriorly (or backward) on the right.

Balance

Sitting balance status is assessed to determine (1) the type of postural support the wheelchair user will require (size, location, force) and (2) the hierarchy of user need (basic, intermediate, complex). Remember that hierarchy of user need is dependent on the user's sitting balance and postural control (see Table 32.1). As described in the "Hierarchy of Wheelchair User Seating and Positioning Need" section, note if the person is a hands-free sitter, hands-dependent or prop sitter, or dependent sitter who requires a lot of external support.

Users with fair to poor sitting balance and trunk control require additional postural supports to sit symmetrically and/or to free up their hands for function and are considered users with intermediate to complex needs. These individuals require a therapist and RTP with advanced level knowledge and skills for their wheelchair service provision. Referral may be needed.

Strength and Endurance

Physical assessment of strength includes muscle power and muscle endurance utilizing objective measures as much as possible. Standard manual muscle testing alone may or may not be appropriate, depending on the person's neuromuscular function. If strength is found to be within 3–5/5, it is critical to objectively measure, describe, and document if muscular endurance and power are sufficient to meet the individual's daily mobility needs. Keep in mind that the reason for this important objective assessment is to demonstrate the capacity for strength and muscular endurance to safely and effectively self-propel and/or operate a wheeled mobility device.

Upper and lower extremity strength impacts a person's ability to transfer and self-propel a manual wheelchair with their UEs, LEs, or combination of both. A consistent, nonfatiguable movement (e.g., hand, finger, head, foot) is identified as a potential access site to operate a power wheelchair user interface (input device), such as a joystick, head array, chin microcontroller, or foot switch. Trunk strength and endurance will impact the amount of external postural support needed and the person's endurance for sitting upright in the wheelchair.

Findings from the comprehensive strength assessment are critical to qualifying a person for a specific wheeled mobility device. As a result, it is important to connect the dots, paint a clinical picture of the person's function in the context of daily mobility needs, and their ability to perform functional activities throughout the day. As an example, a person might function well for 1 hour initially in the morning and need no assistance during that time with mobility but may need moderate assistance with mobility in the afternoon as a result of waxing and waning symptoms, medication schedule, and/or poor endurance and fatigue.

Range of Motion and Flexibility

Joint range of motion and flexibility of the pelvis, spine, and extremities determine if a person can achieve a neutral, or "upright," sitting posture. Pelvic mobility is assessed with the person supine and the hips and knees flexed. Placing thumbs on the person's ASIS and fingers on the PSIS, the pelvis is shifted in all three planes, assessing anterior/posterior tilt, pelvic obliquity, and pelvic rotation to achieve a neutral position in all planes. Flexible, partially flexible, and fixed deformities are noted.

Hip flexion is measured with the person in the supine position (Fig. 32.5). Knees are flexed to decrease the influence of the hamstring muscles. The pelvis is positioned in a neutral to slight anterior tilted position (or as neutral as possible). Both hips are flexed slowly, keeping one hand flat under the person's lumbosacral spine until posterior movement of the pelvis is palpated. The hip joints must be able to achieve "true" hip joint movement of at least 90 degrees of flexion, meaning no compensatory movement of the pelvis or lower spine. The hips also need approximately 5 to 8 degrees of hip abduction, typical of a neutral sitting posture, and 0 degrees of internal and external rotation. Goniometric values for hip abduction, adduction, and internal and external rotation are obtained.

Knee popliteal angle (thigh to lower leg angle) is measured with the person in the supine position with both hips flexed to 90 degrees (or their maximum amount of true flexion) and the knees initially flexed (see Fig. 32.5).[38] While maintaining the hip angle and keeping one hand under the lumbosacral spine, the knees are slowly extended until the pelvis begins to move posteriorly or excessive tightness/tension is felt in the hamstring muscles. It is especially important to maintain the appropriate hip position while extending the knees since the hamstring muscles are a two-joint muscle and the amount of range achieved is dependent on the position of the hips.[39] When the hips are extended, knee extension range tends to be increased, and when the hips are flexed, knee extension range tends to be decreased due to hamstring muscle tightness. If the knees are extended greater than the available range of motion, the pelvis will rotate posteriorly due to the pull on the hamstring muscles.

Ankle dorsiflexion ROM is also measured in the supine position. Hips and knees are positioned in available hip

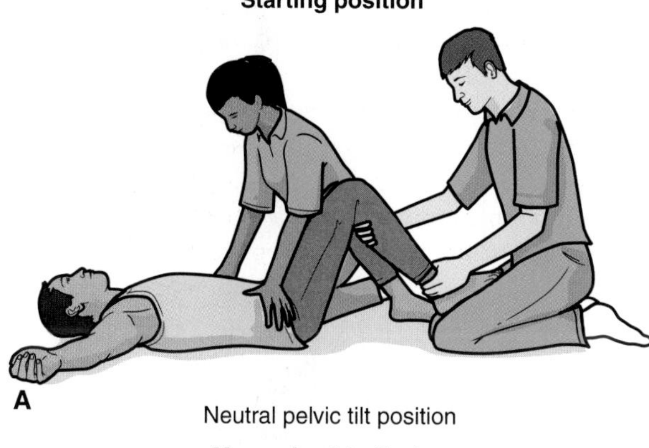

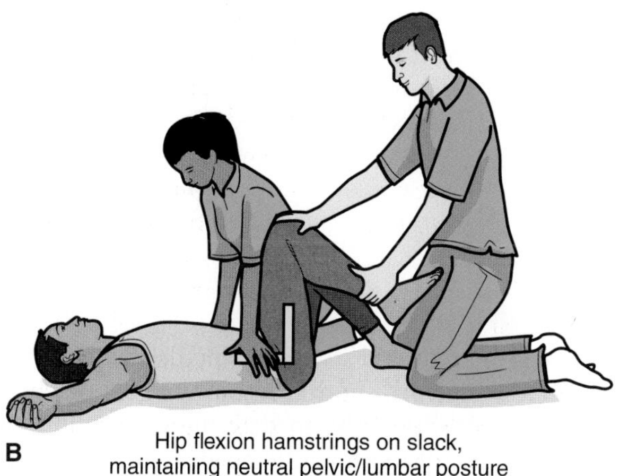

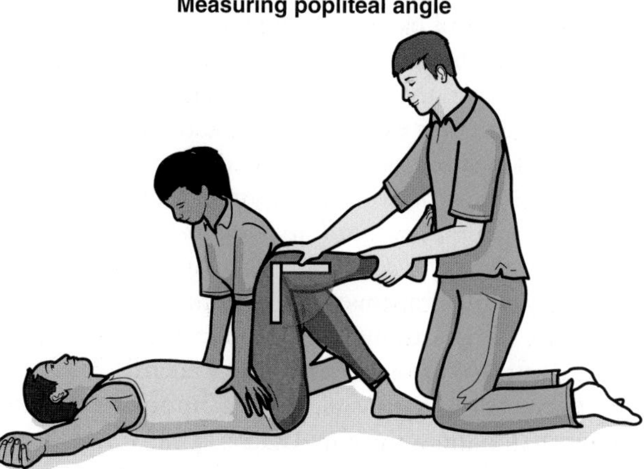

Measuring popliteal angle
C
Knee(s) extend to 90° while maintaining hip position and pelvic/lumbar position

Figure 32.5 Measuring hip and knee range of motion: (A) Starting, neutral pelvic/lumbar posture. (B) Measuring hip flexion. (C) Measuring popliteal angle.

flexion and knee extension alignment (as described above). The ankle is maintained in a neutral inversion/eversion position and an attempt made to achieve neutral dorsiflexion/plantarflexion position at the ankle. The gastrocnemius muscle is a two-joint muscle and ROM at the ankle is affected by the position at the knee. If the knee is extended and muscle tightness is present, decreased dorsiflexion is noted. With the knee flexed, increased dorsiflexion is achieved. Although it is important to measure ROM with knee extended (bed positioning, standing, and ambulation), this is an assessment for seating, and muscle tightness limitations must be addressed in a simulated position on the mat to better understand posture achieved in sitting.

A complete ROM examination of both UEs and LEs, head/neck, trunk, and pelvis is needed since limitations in these areas will affect a person's ability to propel the wheelchair, position the head for safe eating and functional vision, and sit with optimal upright alignment.

Postural limitations are noted, specifying if it is fixed, flexible, or partially flexible. If significant fixed deformities are identified, decisions will need to be made regarding method to correct, support, or accommodate the deformity while optimizing function. In the instance of a moderate fixed scoliosis with pelvic obliquity, decisions are made about accommodating the pelvic obliquity and supporting the trunk above and below the apex of the primary spinal curve.

Contractures in the neck region affect head position. Attempts to align the head with a lateral flexion contracture may instead result in the trunk shifting to the side. Once the trunk shifts, the pelvis and LE positions will be affected. Remember that UE position becomes critical when determining ability to self-propel the wheelchair or operate a power wheelchair controller. If specific UE positioning (e.g., postural support device) is required to maintain current ROM, be sure to describe.

Neuromuscular Status

Neuromuscular status includes muscle tone, reflexes, coordination, and motor control in the context of function. Each of these elements may potentially impact the person's ability to operate a mobility device and factors into the equipment selection process. Note if the person has hyper/hypotonia, ataxia, athetosis, clonus, or tremor. Consider abnormal reflexes such as asymmetric tonic neck reflex and symmetric tonic neck reflex, as these will affect decisions related to head position and orientation in space. Motor control and coordination will impact operation of both manual and power mobility devices.

Specialty Evaluation

Wheelchair Assessment

The wheelchair assessment includes measurements, simulation, technology trial, and the person/technology match.[10,22,23,38,40,41]

Measurements

Following the physical assessment and simulation process, measurements of the person's body are taken and recorded to help determine the dimensions of the wheelchair and seating equipment that will be required (Fig. 32.6) (Video link performing measurements

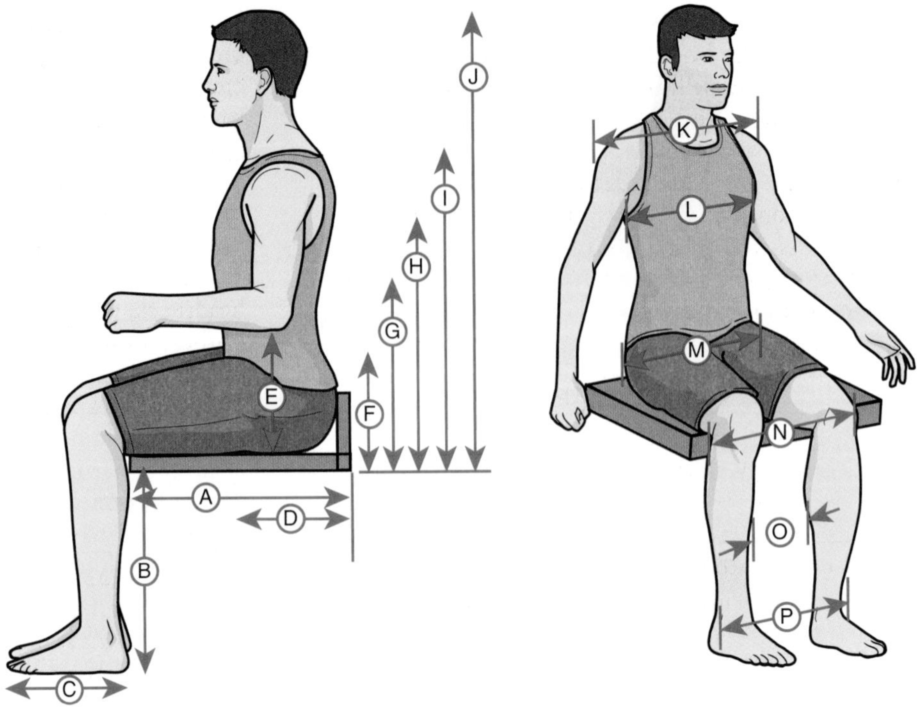

Figure 32.6 Body measurements: (A) buttock/thigh depth. (B) Lower leg length. (C) Foot depth. (D) Ischial depth. (E) Elbow height. (F) PSIS height. (G) Inferior angle of scapula height. (H) Axilla height. (I) Shoulder height. (J) Maximum sitting height. (K) Shoulder width. (L) Chest width. (M) Hip width. (N) External knee width. (O) Internal knee width. (P) External foot width.

https://youtu.be/9y-iTBQ6smg). Some considerations that need to be made when taking measurements to ensure they are accurate are as follows:

- Initial thigh length and calf length measurements should be taken in supine position to increase accuracy (see Fig. 32.2).
- The person is measured when sitting as upright as possible or in an optimal sitting posture (external support may be needed sometimes by a second or third person, depending on the complexity of the individual) (see Fig. 32.3).
- Provide as much thigh support as possible for postural stability.
- Use foot blocks to position and support the feet.
- Use a metal retractable tape measure, preferably 1-in. width or calipers to minimize error due to flexible/bendable tape measure.
- Can use clipboards to define outer limits of curved body surfaces.
- Align your line of sight with the tape measure at the correct angle.

As you can see from Figure 32.6, there are many body measures that can be taken during the evaluation and used to determine the features of the wheelchair and postural supports. It is critical to note we are measuring and recording the person and not the equipment. The information about the person is used to make final decisions about the measurements of the equipment.

The specific measurements needed for an individual assessment will depend on the body supports that will be necessary in the wheelchair. Hip width and buttock/thigh depth will be required to determine basic wheelchair seat width and depth and will be required for all wheelchair users. Additionally, to determine back support height, it is useful to know the height of the PSIS, the inferior angle of the scapula, axilla height, and the top of the shoulder. Lower leg length is also necessary to determine the height of the foot supports that will be needed; however, these are typically adjustable items, so this measurement is used to determine the needed range. Additional measures may be needed, depending on the complexity of the body support system that will be used. *A Clinical Application Guide to Standardized Wheelchair Seating Measures of the Body and Seating Support Surfaces, Revised Edition* is a downloadable practical reference and guide for linear and angular measurements in sitting[38] [http://www.ucdenver.edu/academics/colleges/Engineering/research/AssistiveTechnologyPartners/resources/WheelchairSeating/Pages/WheelchairGuideForm.aspx].

Linear Body Measurements

A. Buttock/thigh depth: Hold a rigid flat surface such as a hardcover book or clipboard against the back of the buttocks, parallel to the seat surface. Measure from the book to the back of the knees. If a hamstring tendon is prominent, measure to the edge of the hamstring tendon (see Fig. 32.6A).

B. Lower leg length: Measure from the back of the knee to heel (or weight-bearing area) (see Fig. 32.6B).

C. Foot depth: Measure from the back of the heel to the front of the toes (or shoes) (see Fig. 32.6C).

D. Ischial depth: Measure from the back of the buttocks (the book) to the front of the IT. This measurement will be important for an antithrust seat cushion, and any pressure-relieving cushions (see Fig. 32.6D).

E. Elbow height: Measure from the seat surface to the bottom of the elbow. This is helpful for arm supports and lap trays (see Fig. 32.6E).

F. PSIS height: Measure from the seat surface (contact point of the buttocks) to PSIS. If you cannot find the PSIS, measure from the seat surface to 1 in. below the iliac crest. This will be helpful if the person needs a lower back support at the PSIS (see Fig. 32.6F).

G. Inferior angle of the scapula height: Measure from the seat surface to the inferior angle of the scapula. This measurement is good for shorter back supports, unencumbered scapular motion for self-propulsion, or to make reliefs for the scapula (see Fig. 32.6G).

H. Axilla height: Measure from the seat surface to under the axilla. This is necessary if the person needs lateral trunk supports (see Fig. 32.6H).

I. Shoulder height: Measure from the seat surface to the top of shoulders for higher back supports. This measurement is also needed to ensure proper line of pull for certain shoulder straps (see Fig. 32.6I).

J. Maximum sitting height: Measure from the seat surface to the top of the head. This measurement will assist in determining head clearance needs (see Fig. 32.6J).

K. Shoulder width: Measure from the outside of the upper arms. This measurement will assist in specifying the width of the back support and determine wheelchair frame size (see Fig. 32.6K).

L. Chest width: Your hands should simulate the support the person requires. Measure between your hands (or the flat supports). The supports should be at least 1 in. below the armpit so as not to press on brachial nerves in the axilla (see Fig. 32.6L).

M. Hip width: Place a rigid flat surface such as a hardcover book or clipboard along each hip. Make sure the books are held at 90° to the seat surface. Measure the width between the books at the widest point. This is easier to do with two people or with calipers (see Fig. 32.6M).

N. External knee width: Measure the width between the outside of the knees. This measurement will assist with determining the width of the seat cushion and wheelchair (see Fig. 32.6N).

O. Internal knee width: Measure the distance between the inside of the knees. This measurement will assist with specifying the dimensions of a medial knee support (see Fig. 32.6O).

P. External foot width: Measure the distance between the outermost borders of the feet. This measurement will assist with determining placement of foot supports and frame dimensions (see Fig. 32.6P).

If the person sits asymmetrically, it will be necessary to measure across the widest span of the patient's seated body (e.g., outside hip on the adducted side to outside knee of the abducted leg) to determine the maximum sitting width (see Fig. 32.1). To ensure accurate recommendations, it is important to consider orthoses, clothing, and recent weight loss or gain, as well as the patient's potential for growth, and make notations as appropriate. If it takes more than a few months between the evaluation and the ordering of the equipment (e.g., delay in prior authorization process), it may be necessary to remeasure the person prior to placing the order to determine if they have changed (e.g., grown or experienced weight loss or gain).

Body Segment Angles

Thigh to Trunk Angle

Measuring hip flexion assists in determining the thigh to trunk angle and ultimately the seat to back support angle.[40,42,43] As seen in Figure 32.7, if hip flexion is 75°, the thigh to trunk angle is 105°. Identifying the optimal alignment of the head and trunk over the center of mass, or seat base, takes into account factors, including but not limited to, tone, reflexes, motor control, endurance, body shape or contour, function, and comfort. These factors taken together guide selection of the final seat to back support angle. As shown in Figure 32.8A, hip flexion is 95° and the thigh to trunk angle is 85°. This position, however, may not provide the person sufficient postural stability, promoting instead trunk flexion or difficulty maintaining an upright sitting posture (Fig. 32.8B). In this example, the patient may benefit from a final seat to back support angle of 100° to allow the shoulders to move posterior to the hips. Shifting the center of mass posterior to the center of gravity is known as *gravity-assisted positioning,* as illustrated in Figure 32.8C.

Thigh to Lower Leg Angle

The thigh to lower leg angle (popliteal angle) is documented (Fig. 32.9). The final seat to lower leg support angle is determined by considering factors such as the thigh to lower leg angle, hamstring flexibility, abnormal tone, movement patterns, and comfort.[38,40,42,43]

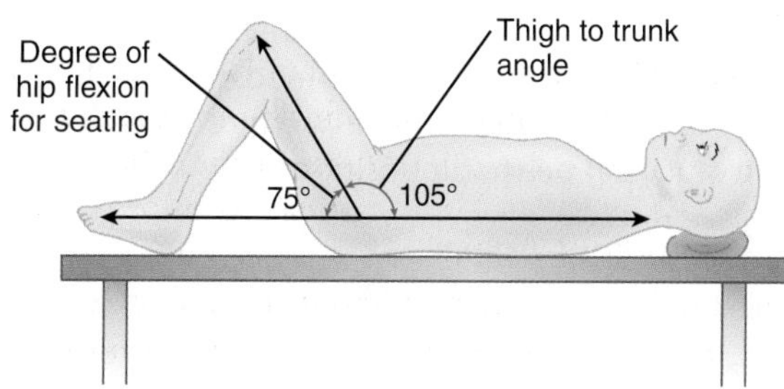

Figure 32.7 The amount of hip flexion determines the trunk angle. If the degree of hip flexion for seating is 75°, the thigh to trunk angle is 105°.

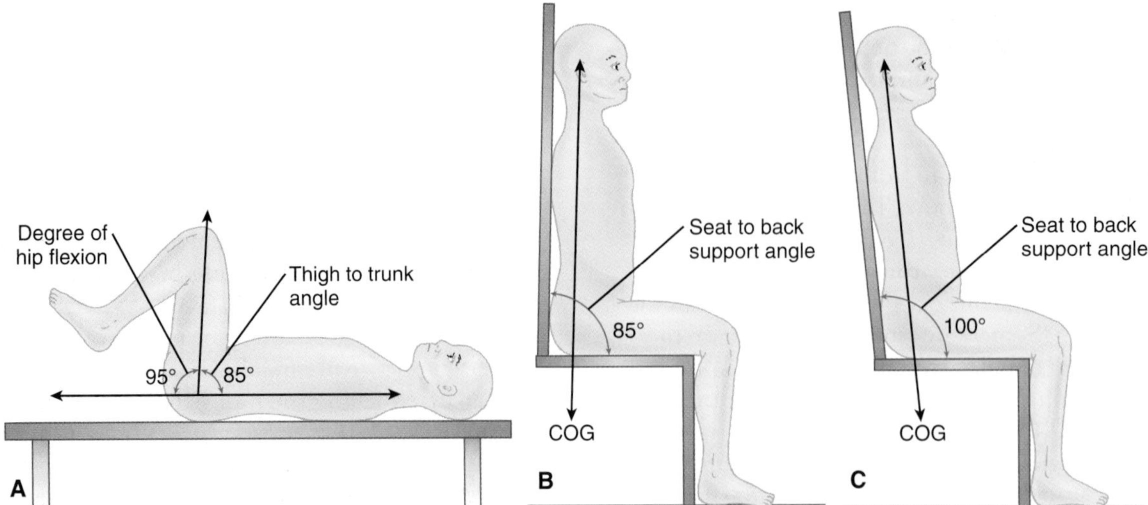

Figure 32.8 (A) If the degree of hip flexion for seating is to 95°, the thigh to trunk angle is 85°. (B) Seat to back support angle does not always correlate with thigh to trunk angle. In this example, if the seat to back support angle is set at 85°, tolerance to sitting in this position may be poor and cause the person to fall forward or constantly be working to hold himself or herself upright. Body shape, center of mass, and sitting tolerance must be addressed. (C) Opening the seat to back support angle to 100° better accommodates body shape and center of mass, and tolerance to sitting upright improves.

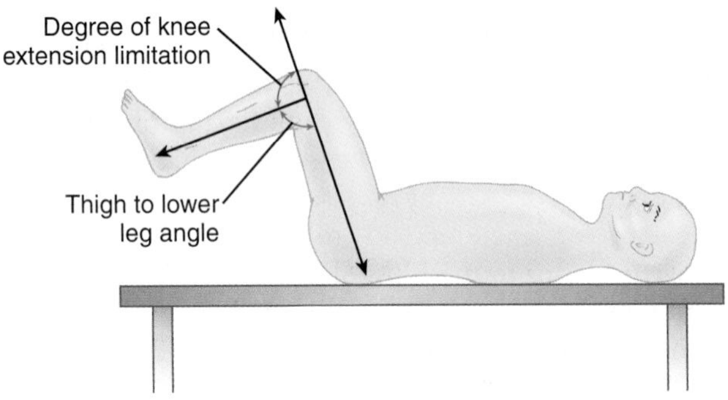

Figure 32.9 Thigh to lower leg angle is determined during the mat examination and is based on the popliteal angle (degree of knee extension limitation) when the hip is flexed to identified optimal position.

Hamstring muscle tightness must be accommodated to prevent the pelvis from being pulled into a posterior pelvic tilt. Some people will require a seat to lower leg support angle below 90° to accommodate tight hamstrings or fixed knee flexion contractures in order to maintain a neutral pelvic tilt position.

Lower Leg to Foot Angle

Available ankle dorsiflexion ROM, deformities, abnormal tone, and movement patterns factor in to determining lower leg support to foot support angle (Fig. 32.10 and 32.11).[38,40,42,43] The use of ankle–foot orthoses (AFOs) will also affect the final lower leg support to foot support angle.

Simulation

Often it is difficult to determine the specific features and configuration of the equipment through the physical assessment process alone. *Simulation* is a process using your hands and/or equipment to determine the person's tolerance to the recommended angles and linear measurements identified in the physical assessment. Simulation provides an opportunity to observe tone, movement, postural alignment, and function, and to assess equipment features and the effectiveness of postural supports in achieving the desired goals. In this way, hypotheses can be tested regarding position; orientation to gravity; as well as the location, dimensions, angles, and sizes of postural supports needed. Seating simulation provides the opportunity to add and subtract supports to determine if a person tolerates more or less postural support (correction or accommodation) and the influence of gravity on a person's ability to function. If significant changes are being made to a seating system, simulation provides the person an opportunity to "test" and provide feedback about the seating recommendations.

Hand simulation is one form of simulation frequently performed during or immediately after the sitting mat assessment described previously. Placing one's hands (or other body parts) on the wheelchair user's body and providing corrective forces helps us to understand the optimal location of the forces needed, the magnitude and direction of the forces, and the size of the support structures (see Fig. 32.3). When needed, towel rolls, foam, or other available materials in the clinic can be used to assist

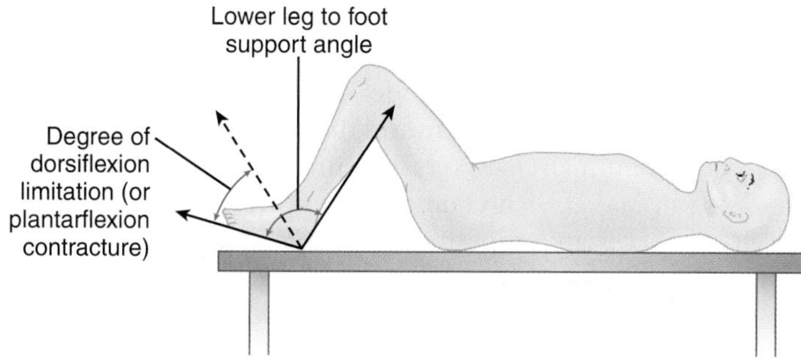

Figure 32.10 Lower leg support to foot support angle is determined during mat examination and is based on ankle range of motion.

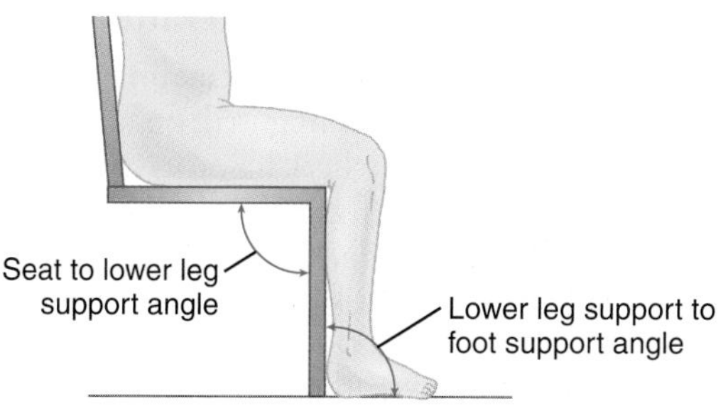

Figure 32.11 Seat to lower leg support angle and lower leg support to foot support angle are final seating angles determined during seating simulation accommodating range of motion, tone, and comfort at the knees and ankles.

with simulation, especially under the pelvis. Having this understanding assists with the feature matching process, another critical element of the wheelchair assessment.

A *seating simulator,* as seen in Figure 32.12, is a commercially available assessment chair. It provides the therapist the ability to assess an individual's optimal sitting posture and can be used with a variety of people. Unfortunately, seating simulators are generally available only in specialty wheelchair clinics. The ideal seating simulator is adjustable for linear and angular measurements, and orientation in space. Additionally, some simulators are capable of using generic and commercial postural supports and power wheelchair input devices to simulate access and driving.[44]

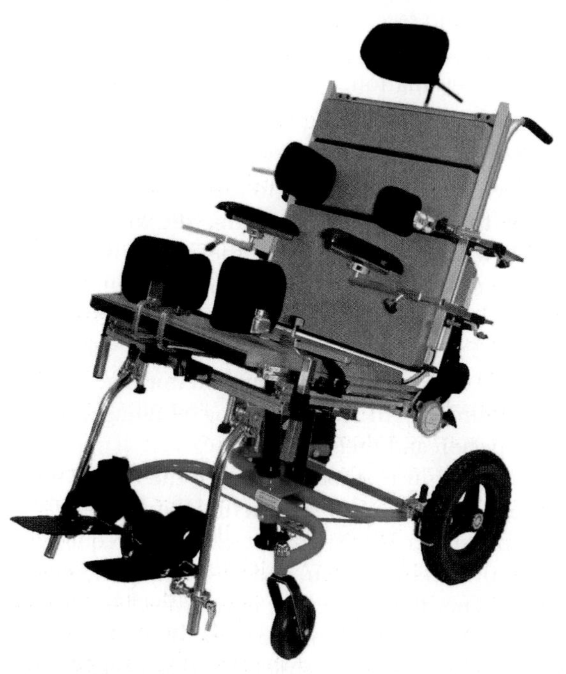

Figure 32.12 Planar seating simulation chair. *(Courtesy of Permobil Corp. Lebanon, TN 37090.)*

If unable to access a seating simulator, a tilt-in-space and/or a recliner wheelchair may be used for simulation purposes instead. Try to obtain the necessary seat to back support angle, buttock/thigh depth, and wheelchair width if using trial equipment to *mock up* a system for seating simulation.

As with the assessment of the sitting posture, it is helpful to be systematic with simulation. First, provide support at the pelvis and move distally from there. Make only one change at a time. Observe carefully how changes in one part of the body affect other parts.

Technology Trial

Another very important part of the evaluation process is to provide a variety of equipment for the wheelchair user to compare and try out. If there is any uncertainty about the type of mobility device or seating equipment that will optimize function, trials of this equipment will help determine which features work best for the person. Allowing the person to compare and contrast features is beneficial in making educated decisions.

Trials of different wheelchairs (manual wheelchairs, power mobility devices) and seating equipment add to the evidence of what does and does not work well for the person. Documentation should describe mobility trials specifying the basic features and configuration of the mobility bases tried and ruled out. Also discuss seating and postural support trials and pressure management considerations. Describe the results of the trials and effectiveness of attaining identified goals with different equipment. Documentation of the trial results is a critical component of the evidence used by third-party payers in making decisions for coverage and payment.

Person/Technology Match (Prescription)

The person/technology match is matching the person with necessary and appropriate equipment features.

Oftentimes it is necessary to make trade-offs between ideal positioning, function, and environmental access.

On occasion, new strategies for function or modifications to the environment are needed. Other times trade-offs are made in equipment features to retain function and/or access. The important message here is providing information and opportunity for trial equipment helps the person and team make educated decisions to maximize the opportunity for a positive outcome and minimize surprises at the fitting and delivery.

Evaluation and Plan of Care

The evaluation and plan of care is the synthesis of all information gathered so far. This portion of the specialty wheelchair evaluation is called the *prescription* step in the WHO's 8 steps wheelchair service delivery process. The Matching Person and Technology (MPT) Problem Solving Model is a four-step process that is specific to the Assistive Technology Assessment (ATA) and provides a framework that considers the characteristics and interaction of the person, environment, and technology when selecting assistive technology for a particular person's use.[45,46] The process is person-centered rather than product-centered. This problem-solving approach provides a foundation for critical thinking, communication, and specification of products during the assessment process. It guides selection of appropriate and necessary WSM products by using a sequence of (1) identifying equipment-related clinical problems, (2) establishing objectives for the equipment intervention, (3) making equipment feature recommendations, and (4) deciding product specifications. The process structures the decision making process and ensures that all issues are addressed. When documented, the systematic approach communicates rationale for selecting each specific WSM feature and product. Readers unfamiliar with the client (e.g., reviewers, auditors) will be able to follow the clinical rationale for choosing specific WSM products.

The first step in the decision making process is to develop a list of *problems and potentials*. Information obtained during the WSM examination and specialty evaluation is used to generate a list of the person's unique characteristics, problems, and potentials related to their mobility and seating needs. Next, for each listed problem or potential, a specific *objective* is written individualized to the person and related to positioning, alignment, motor control, health, function, environmental access, activity, and participation. Objectives should be specific and relate to the equipment features needed. For example, "Reduce risk for pressure injury under left ischial tuberosity by providing accommodation for a fixed pelvic obliquity." The third step in the MPT problem-solving model is to consider the different WSM *equipment features* required for the person to achieve the stated objectives, the *person/feature match*. Attention is given to product properties, materials, configuration and specific details of the final product. In the final step (*feature/technology match*), the list of identified equipment features is reviewed by the therapist and RTP. Specific make/model of *product specifications* are identified. The RTP ensures that multiple products from different manufacturers will interface and be configured as intended. If no commercial option is available with the necessary properties, custom fabrication is explored. Box 32.2 provides an example of this strategy illustrating the rationale for justifying the WSMD.

Intervention

Wheelchair Fitting, Delivery, Training

The wheelchair fitting, delivery, and training are done to ensure that the equipment is configured, fits and functions as anticipated, and that the wheelchair user and caregivers know how to safely and effectively use the wheelchair. Documenting this process and instructions is an important safeguard to reduce risk for liability. Training is required for first-time users as well as users who are making dramatic equipment switches (e.g., moving from a folding frame wheelchair to a rigid frame wheelchair or moving from a manual wheelchair to a power wheelchair).

All equipment is set up prior to the delivery process to ensure the fitting/delivery is completed in a timely manner. At the delivery, the person is positioned in the new equipment and all components are adjusted to meet their needs. Check that the seat depth, back height, arm height, and foot position fit appropriately. Compare positioning angles (seat to back support angle, seat to lower leg support angle, lower leg support to foot support angle, pelvic support angle of attachment, and so forth) to specifications. Verify fixed and/or variable position in space (e.g., tilt, recline, procline) is as planned. Ensure all primary and secondary supports are adjusted and final posture is compared to the expected results determined during the evaluation.

Function From Wheelchair

The user is instructed in how to use all moving parts. This includes functions such as operating the wheel locks on a manual wheelchair, operating the motor releases on a power wheelchair to enable moving the chair manually, moving the foot supports, adjusting the armrests, and adjusting the seat cushion and back cushions. Care is taken to instruct the user in how to function from the wheelchair while minimizing the risk of tipping or falling during use.

The person and their family/caregivers, if appropriate, are instructed in methods to reduce the risk of pressure injuries. This includes instruction and education on safety, pressure management (weight relief, frequency, and duration), skin inspection, and positioning. If additional training is needed beyond the initial wheelchair fitting, it is incorporated into the plan of care for follow-up.

Transfer training is critical for safety and independence. An important part of the fitting and training is to ensure the person is able to safely transfer in and

Box 32.2 Example of Matching Person and Technology Problem-Solving Model Grid

Problems and Potentials	Objectives	Equipment Features	Product Specifications
Diagnosis of CP diplegia, currently uses an RWD power wheelchair for outdoor mobility for work and complains of back pain and buttock discomfort when driving power wheelchair. Able to use a standard joystick for driving the power wheelchair.	Increase sitting comfort and ensure ability to drive power wheelchair outdoors with decreased stress on body.	RWD chair with suspension system to decrease stress on body and tilt seating system to assist with pain relief and buttock comfort.	Test a variety of RWD power wheelchairs to determine most optimal for suspension. Provide a tilt seating system for this power wheelchair
Poor sitting posture in current power wheelchair with firm back and firm seat support and sits in posterior pelvic tilt with kyphotic spine (10° forward for upper trunk and 20° posterior tilt) and current seat depth of 19 in. with seat to back support angle set at 90°.	Achieve and maintain slight anterior pelvic tilt, level and not rotated, and promote trunk extension to decrease kyphosis tendencies and ensure optimal seat depth and seat to back support angle.	Firm, flat back and seat supports set at 100° with seat depth adjusted to 16 in. to accommodate actual length needed. Tested a variety of shaped backs and preferred a flat back for ease of mobility and changing of position. Tested a variety of seat cushions and preferred a system with gel under buttocks.	Firm flat back support and seat cushion with gel in buttock region with set up of 100° seat to back support angle and seat depth of 16 in.
Hip flexion is 80° bilaterally, abduction is 0° bilaterally, knee extension with hip flexed is −90° bilaterally, and ankle dorsiflexion with knee flexed is 0° bilaterally. Able to achieve neutral pelvic position and straight trunk alignment in supine position. No upper extremity or head/neck limitations.	Accommodate ROM limitation to assist in optimal pelvic position and neutral positioning of lower extremities in the seating position.	Back to seat support angle of 100 degrees, seat to lower leg support angle of 90° and lower leg support to foot support angle of 90°.	Angle adjustable back post to fine-tune back to seat support angle. Center mount footrest system to achieve seat to lower leg support angle of 90° and lower leg to foot support angle of 90°.
Performs stand pivot transfers independently	Ensure ability to move footplates out of way and use armrests to continue to be able to perform a stand pivot transfer independently.	Center mount flip-up footrest system and height adjustable armrests.	Height adjustable full-length armrests and center mount flip-up footplate.
Uses desk computer daily	Maintain independence in computer access.	Ensure optimal seat height for table access and the ability of the joystick to be moved out of the way for closer access.	Retractable joystick mount and assess various types to ensure independence in moving joystick.

out of the wheelchair as independently as possible. Therefore, transfers (e.g., stand pivot transfers, sliding board transfers, lift transfers, and modified transfers) are practiced. Care is taken to ensure the seat height is optimal for safe transfers and components can be moved out of the way as needed (swing away footrests and removable armrests) or adjusted (e.g., adjustable height armrest), depending on the specific type of transfer.

Car and van transfers are also practiced if needed. The therapist's role is to teach the wheelchair user how to manage the WSMD (such as folding or disassembling for transportation) and how to transfer in and out of the vehicle.[47,48] If the person drives the car, they may need to lift the wheelchair into the car either by placing it behind the front seat or lifting it across their body into the passenger seat. The weight of the chair, method of folding, and ability to remove components (wheels, footrests, armrests, back support) are important considerations when lifting a wheelchair into the car, and the person may need training and practice to master new skills.

Wheelchair Mobility

Wheelchair mobility involves ensuring that the WSMD is configured for optimal propulsion and driving. For individuals receiving a manual wheelchair, the system is assessed for the person's position relative to the drive wheel and wheelchair responsiveness (center of gravity adjustment/tippyness). Adjustment of the seat and axle position will impact the person's UE position (extremes of movement) and contact with the drive wheel. Adjustments are made to the wheelchair configuration to optimize UE contact with the drive wheel and avoid extremes of movement if propelling with the UEs. If propelling with the lower extremities or hemipropelling, care is taken to ensure the person has firm foot contact with the floor. Techniques for efficient and effective wheelchair propulsion are demonstrated. The center of gravity position is configured for more or less stability or tippyness, dependent on the person's wheelchair skills and functional needs. If additional training is needed, follow-up is included in the plan of care.

For an individual receiving a power wheelchair, the user input device (joystick, switch, and so forth) is adjusted for access. The person is instructed in how to turn the chair on/off, change speeds or drive programs, and use all features. Electronic programming is individualized to ensure the person can drive the wheelchair safely indoors and outdoors and at an appropriate speed to minimize risk for injury to themselves or to others.

It is also important for wheelchair users and caregivers to understand how the chair works and how much assistance the user needs either to move the chair, transfer in and out of the chair, or transport the wheelchair. Also, it is important that the wheelchair user learn how to instruct others to help them with their wheelchair should assistance be needed.

Wheelchair Skills Training

Wheelchair skills training includes, but is not limited to, how to propel and turn the wheelchair, how to go up and down ramps and curbs or instruct a caregiver to assist, and if appropriate how to perform higher level wheelchair skills, such as rear wheel balancing (wheelie)[47-52] (Fig. 32.13).

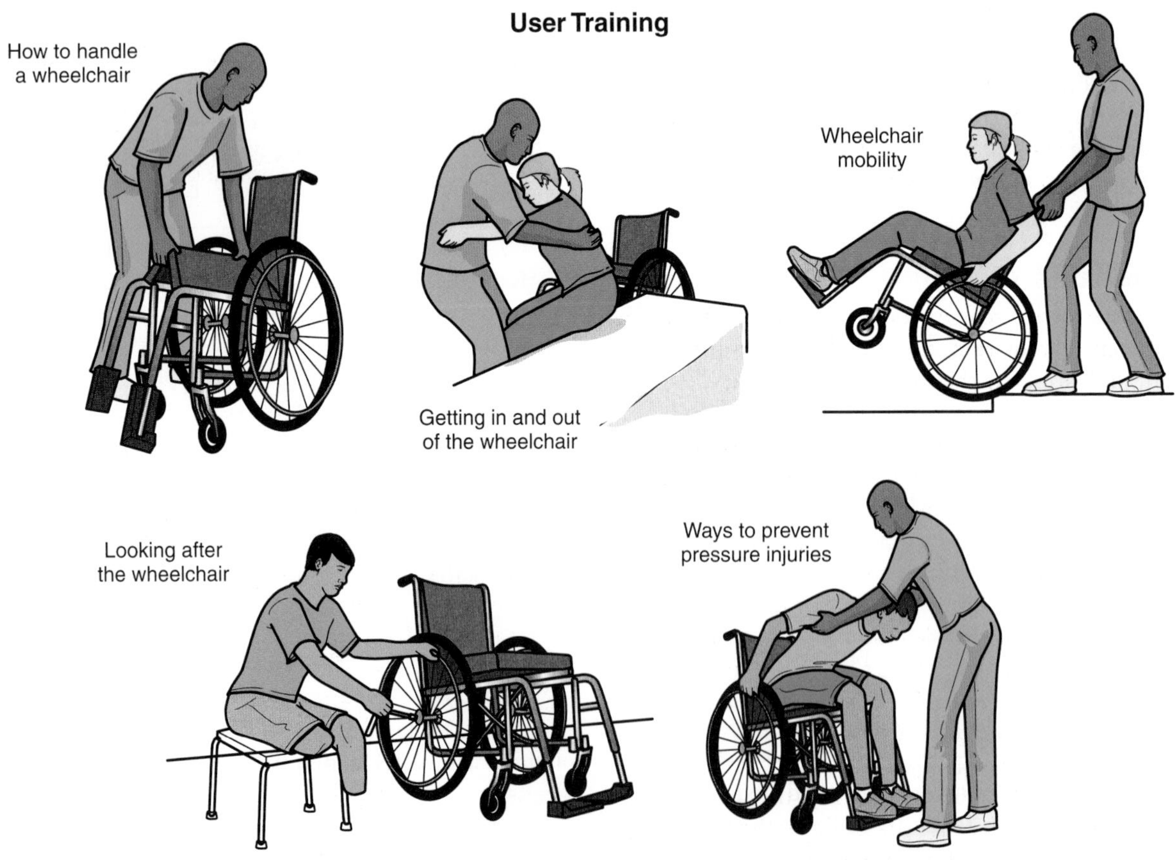
User Training
How to handle a wheelchair
Getting in and out of the wheelchair
Wheelchair mobility
Looking after the wheelchair
Ways to prevent pressure injuries

Figure 32.13 Important skills for wheelchair users and caregivers.

Wheelchair mobility also includes operating the wheelchair on a variety of surfaces and terrain, including indoor flooring, outdoor sidewalks, driveways, and maneuvering down narrow hallways and turning into rooms, making three-point turns, and pulling up to counters or tables. The objective is to ensure that the person can safely operate and maneuver the wheelchair in a variety of situations that they will typically encounter.

Wheelchair management and skills training is considered a skilled therapeutic service. It is very important to document what was taught to the wheelchair user and what instructions were provided (written and verbal). Written instructions and resources are useful for the person to refer to later.

Maintenance/Repairs/Follow-up

Individuals receiving new equipment or modifications to existing equipment should make a follow-up appointment with the clinician and equipment supplier after they have had time to practice with the wheelchair if adjustments or further training is needed. All wheelchairs require maintenance and/or repairs if used on a regular basis. The person should be provided with instructions on how to care for their WSM equipment and what they can do to keep the chair clean and in good working order. The person should understand when the equipment supplier needs to be notified to assist with repairs, such as new upholstery, new wheels, casters and bearings, and new arm pads. If it is a power wheelchair, new batteries will be needed.

If the person's condition changes and feels the equipment is no longer working for them to maintain optimal posture or optimal mobility, they should contact the clinician who assisted them in obtaining the equipment to set up an appointment for a reassessment of needs.

WHEELCHAIR SEATING AND MOBILITY TECHNOLOGIES

Thus far we have discussed the wheelchair examination and specialty evaluation, identified the person/feature match, and initiated the prescription process. At this time, in collaboration with the RTP, the therapist determines the feature/product match identifying the wheelchair and specific frame components and seating supports for the final WSM prescription. This section presents an organizational framework and foundational knowledge about *seating support systems* and *wheeled mobility devices.* This framework can be used for categorizing equipment, identifying unique features and functions, and making comparisons between manufacturers products and models. The *Glossary of Wheelchair Terms and Definitions* provides the framework for the terminology used for seating support systems and wheeled mobility devices.[53] For more information go to http://www.ucdenver.edu/academics/colleges/Engineering/research/AssistiveTechnologyPartners/resources/WheelchairSeating/Pages/WheelchairGuideForm.aspx

A combination of the seating support system and a wheeled mobility device when integrated together is a WSMD (Fig. 32.14). The *seating support system* is considered the surfaces that directly contact, support, or contain the user's body.[53] *Primary seating supports* are primary weight-bearing components, including the seat, back support, foot support, arm support, and head support. The contact surfaces that provide support to maintain postural alignment are considered *secondary support surfaces.* These components are selected based on the persons' need for external supports to achieve their optimal sitting posture. Secondary supports may include components such as lateral supports for the trunk, hips, and knees, and medial supports for the knees and upper extremity (UE) support surfaces.

A *wheeled mobility device* consists of the *wheelchair frame or base,* arm support assembly, foot support assembly, and wheels, and may also include additional *wheelchair options/accessories.* Wheeled mobility devices may be either manual or power operated. Wheel bases come in various wheel configurations (e.g., front, mid, center, or rear-wheel drive) and wheelbase lengths that impact the maneuverability of the device. The person/feature/product match (MPT problem-solving model) details the decision making process linking the person's problems/potentials, objectives, equipment features, and recommended products to clinical rationale to justify the necessity and appropriateness of the items prescribed.

While users with basic level seating and positioning needs can sit *hands-free* to function and will unlikely require much of the seating support equipment discussed below, it is important that therapists understand the range of WSM equipment available to people with basic, intermediate, and complex mobility limitations. In particular, it is important for you to recognize the limits of

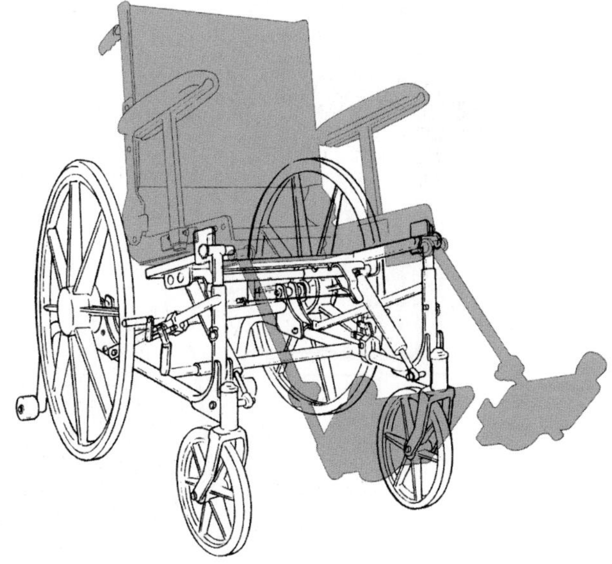

Figure 32.14 A WSMD consists of the seating support system and the wheeled mobility device.

your WSM knowledge and skills, especially with regards to people with intermediate to complex needs, and to know when it is necessary to refer a person to a clinician with advanced WSM knowledge and skills.

Policymakers and payers have identified, and in many cases require therapists, professionals with no financial ties, to manage the evaluation and recommendation process. Consequently, it is our ethical and professional responsibility to ensure users receive skilled services and appropriate and necessary recommendations, and that fiscally responsible decisions are made with their valuable (and often limited) resources.

Seating Support System

Specifying the primary and secondary seating support system means detailing the size, location, shape, and attachment method of the supports. The size and location of the supports are dependent on the linear and angular measurements established during the wheelchair assessment. Critical dimensions to specify include, at a minimum, seat width, seat depth, back length, and lower leg length. Similarly, critical angular measurements to consider and document include (1) seat to back support angle, (2) seat to lower leg support angle, and (3) lower leg support to foot support angle.

The size and location of the secondary supports are specified to provide optimal body alignment without interfering with function. The shape and size of the supports are dependent on the amount of support and pressure distribution required. Dimensions are specified for all primary and secondary support surfaces.

Seating supports, including the seat, back, and postural supports, come in different shapes: *planar, precontoured, and custom contoured.* A planar seating support surface is flat (Fig. 32.15). Pre-contoured is a generically shaped seating support surface (Figs. 32.16 and 32.17). Custom contoured (carved or molded) is a seating support surface that is uniquely shaped to match the body contours of the person (Fig. 32.18). Matching the shape of the person with the support is critical to maximizing contact between the user and the seating support system. A properly shaped support distributes pressure over bony prominences and body surface area, increases comfort, and results in improved postural control.[54-57]

Once the postural support is selected, a method to mount or attach the support and the location of the support are identified and specified. Mounting hardware can be fixed (requires tools), removable, or swing-away.

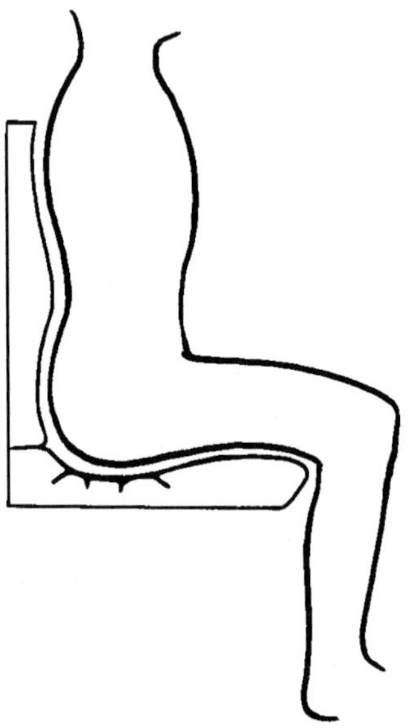

Figure 32.16 Some types of foam will contour as a response to body weight.

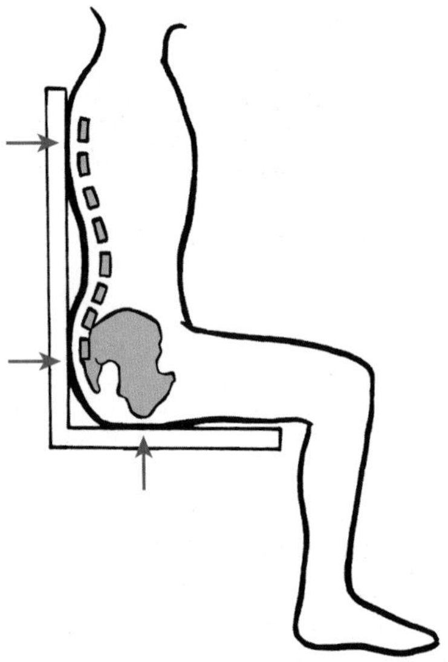

Figure 32.15 Persons seated on planar surfaces may show increased pressure over bony prominences.

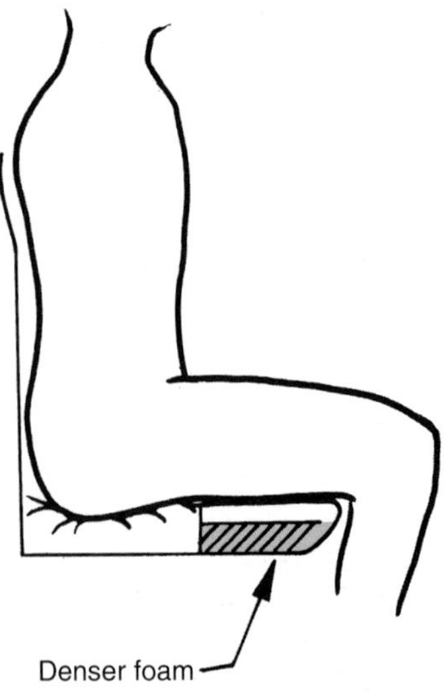

Figure 32.17 An option for creating contoured seats is use of varying density (firmness) of foam.

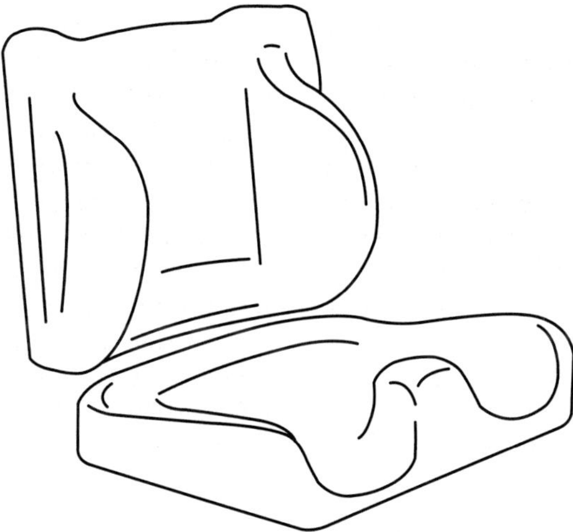

Figure 32.18 Custom contoured cushions match the patient's body contours.

The type and size of the mounting hardware selected often are dictated by the space available on the WMD to mount the support in the desired location. The rationale for the type of hardware selected is dependent on the objectives identified. For instance, if the wheelchair needs to be folded, removeable hardware may be necessary. If the person has multiple caregivers and there is a risk the supports may be misplaced or incorrectly positioned, fixed hardware may be desirable. If the person is able to transfer alone or with the assistance of another, swing-away hardware that remains mounted to the chair may be the best option.

Primary Support Surfaces

Seat

The seat is the postural support device intended to contact the buttocks and thighs. Seat options include sling upholstery, solid base, or van seat that come included as part of the WMD. Alternately, a seat cushion can be added to a WMD when specified and purchased separately. The most critical dimensions to accurately specify are seat depth, seat width, and cushion height. If the seat depth is too long, it promotes a posterior pelvic tilt and kyphotic posture. If the seat width is too wide, it will make wheel access and self-propelling the wheelchair more difficult and result in poor shoulder alignment and biomechanics (Figs. 32.19 and 32.20). If the wheelchair is too narrow it can cause increased pressure on the hips from the armrests and legrest system, placing the person at risk for a pressure injury. If the cushion is too thin, the person could "bottom out" on the solid seat below, resulting in pressure injury.

A firm seat support is critical to providing a solid base to support neutral LE alignment, promote pressure distribution, and improve comfort. Basic manual wheelchairs typically are standardly equipped with sling upholstery. Over time, the sling material stretches, creating hammocking and poor pelvic positioning—posterior pelvic tilt, hip adduction, and internal rotation (Fig. 32.21). Sling upholstery is generally provided to facilitate ease of folding and storing of the wheelchair. However, if the WSMD is used on a daily basis, for more than 2 hours at a time, and not just for intermittent mobility, then a firm seat support should be added to the wheelchair. A solid seat insert can be placed under the cover of a seat cushion to provide a firm base of support and used on top of the seat upholstery and seat frame. Alternatively,

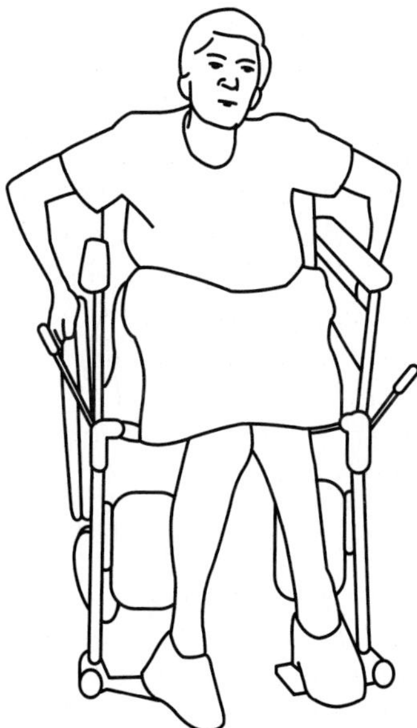

Figure 32.19 A wheelchair that is too wide will make wheel access and propulsion more difficult for the person.

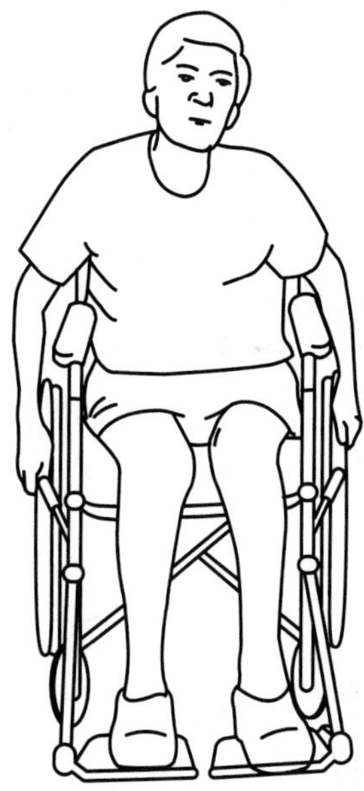

Figure 32.20 A narrower wheelchair allows easier wheel access and propulsion.

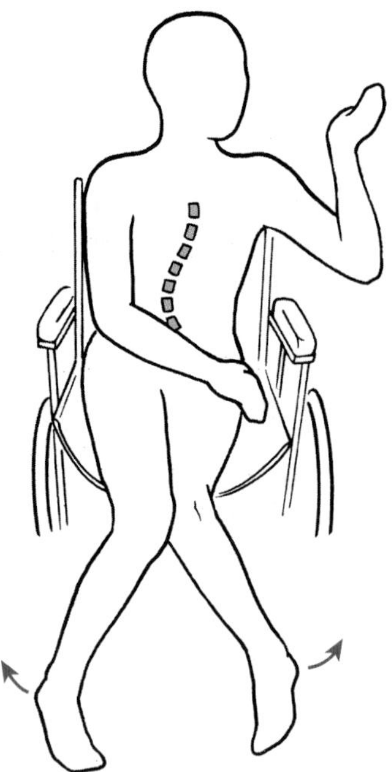

Figure 32.21 Overall poor sitting posture and asymmetries created by a sling seat and sling back.

a solid seat pan (metal or plastic) can be mounted directly to the seat frame (with upholstery removed) and a seat support (e.g., cushion) placed on top of the pan (Fig. 32.22).

Cushion shape (planar, precontoured, custom contoured) and material properties are selected based on the person's needs. Goals of a seating support (cushion) might include promoting improved positioning, maximizing postural stability for UE activities and function, distributing pressure to minimize risk of pressure injury, and improving sitting tolerance time (e.g., comfort).[58]

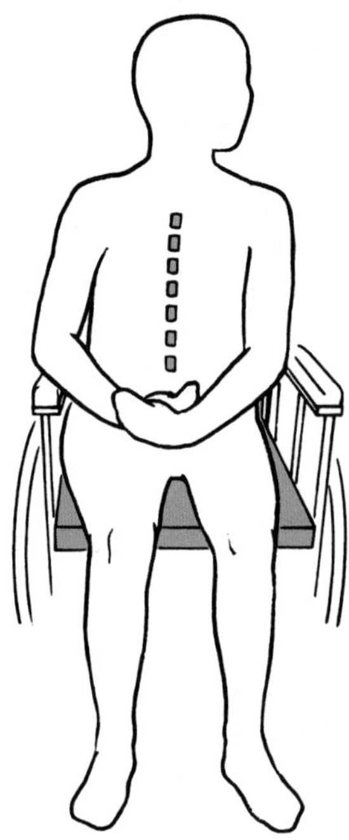

Figure 32.22 A firm sitting surface enhances sitting posture and provides a stable base of support.

Once the shape of the seat cushion is established, the properties of the cushion materials are determined. Cushion properties affect sitting stability, pressure relief, ability to transfer, and comfort. Different materials ensure these objectives are met. Cushions are made of different materials, including foam (open or closed cell, foam elastomer), air, fluid (gel, water, viscoelastic fluid), or a combination of materials. Foam cushions come in different densities. Firm foams provide increased stability. Different densities of foam can also be used to achieve shaping and pressure redistribution (Fig. 32.23). Different materials allow for varying degrees of envelopment of the person (immersion) in the cushion, distributing pressure over a greater surface area. In general, the continuum of immersion properties for different materials from lesser to greater is foam, gel, air.

Cushion maintenance is another consideration during the selection process. Foam cushions require little maintenance other than keeping dry and clean. Air cushions need to be monitored for proper inflation for optimal pressure redistribution. Over- or underinflation can result in a pressure injury. Changes in temperature and altitude can affect cushion inflation, requiring reinflation or deflation. Air cushions are also subject to puncture. Gel cushions settle with use and require kneading to redistribute gel to prevent "bottoming out" on the cushion base or solid seat below.

Some cushions are made with a combination of materials to benefit from the different material properties. For instance, a combination foam and gel cushion will allow for envelopment of the gel around the bony prominences of the ITs and the firm support of the foam base to support the trochanters and femurs for stability. Specialty off-loading cushions are custom shaped, may be made from one or more different materials, and generally require little maintenance once fabricated. Off-loading cushions can reduce interface pressure and compression at ITs and sacral/coccygeal regions by loading and containing surrounding tissues and managing tissue deformation.

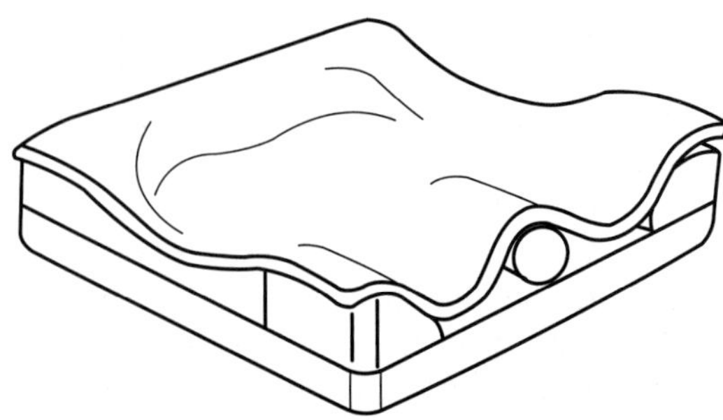

Figure 32.23 Firmer foam shapes can be placed under a more flexible foam to create a contoured cushion.

Cushion covers are made with materials with different properties that also factor into the selection process. If the cover is loose and stretchy, it will allow the person to be immersed in the cushion. However, if the fabric is tight or taut, the full effects of the cushion material underneath will be diminished. Cover(s) can be *waterproof* or *water resistant.* If a person is incontinent, a waterproof cover is necessary, especially if the person is using a foam cushion. If a person is prone to incontinence, a second cushion cover is useful to prevent exposure of the cushion material to urine or feces during cleaning of the cover. Cushions that are not permanently mounted to the wheelchair frame are typically attached to the seat pan with hook and loop Velcro to secure the cushion in place, prevent slippage, and make removal for cleaning easier. Care is needed when placing the cushion cover back on the cushion to make sure that the cushion is in the proper orientation and positioned in the chair as intended. Inappropriately placed cushions (upside down or backward) may result in a pressure injury and should be part of your instructions and markings on the cushion.

If permanently mounting a seating system, decisions are needed for selecting mounting hardware. If using a solid seat pan, the original seat upholstery is removed. Fixed or removeable hardware can be used, depending on the needs of the person. Adjustable hardware allows for height and angle adjustment, ensuring the linear and angular dimensions are appropriate for the person. If the person needs a seat incline angle of 10°, the front seat pan hardware can be set higher than the rear to achieve this angle. If the wheelchair needs to be folded for transportation, removable hardware is appropriate. If the weight of the wheelchair is an issue, fixed hardware may be lighter.

Whenever possible, the person should trial different seat cushions (shapes and materials) to compare products and determine the best person/product match for their specific needs. Box 32.3 provides a list of questions that should be considered when finalizing the seat support.

Box 32.3 Questions to Consider When Finalizing the Seat Support

- Does the seat provide adequate support and stability to promote good sitting posture?
- Will the pressure distribution on the seat prevent pressure injuries?
- Is the shape of the seat cushion appropriate for the patient's body contours?
- Does the person need a custom shape to accommodate deformities and maximize support?
- Is pressure relief provided if the person is unable to complete weight shifts independently using UEs or through a tilt or recline option?
- Are special combinations of foam, air, or gel seat cushions needed to maximize comfort and pressure relief?
- Is the seat depth an appropriate length?
- Is the seat width appropriate for propelling the wheelchair and for comfortable positioning?
- Is the seat surface appropriate for safe transfers into and out of the wheelchair?
- Does the seat cushion provide optimal comfort?
- Is the seat cushion able to dissipate heat and moisture? Does the cushion function effectively in different climates?

Back Support

The back support is the surface behind the sacrum, lumbar, and/or thoracic segments of the trunk. A firm back support is critical to support a neutral trunk posture. Some people require back support plus additional secondary supports such as lateral trunk supports to maintain their optimal sitting posture.

Basic manual wheelchairs typically come equipped with sling-back upholstery. Like seat upholstery, back upholstery stretches over time, promoting one or more of the following: a kyphotic posture, scoliotic spine, posterior pelvic tilt, or hyperextended neck. Tension adjustable back upholstery is one available option that uses strapping to accommodate mild pelvic and trunk positioning needs and provide support and stability, and it can be retightened over time. If the person uses the wheelchair for longer than 2 hours at a time and not merely for intermittent mobility, back support should be provided. Most back supports require hardware (fixed or removeable) or Velcro loops to attach the back support to the wheelchair.

The same properties considered for the seat are considered for the back support, including the dimensions, surface shape, stability (firmness), and mounting or attachment method.

Back supports come in a range of dimensions (heights and widths). The shape selected is dependent on the needs of the individual.[38] Back support height is determined based on the person's trunk control, functional abilities, and comfort. A shorter back support may be appropriate for a person with good trunk control and hands-free sitting balance who self-propels. A shorter back height, below the inferior angle of the scapula, allows for unobstructed movement of the scapula and shoulder girdle. A taller back support may be needed for a person who is unable to sit without support or uses a tilt-in-space feature and requires full back support. Back width is generally dictated by the width of the wheelchair frame or the location needed for mounting trunk supports that may be required.

The shape of the back support is assessed and selected to ensure contact is provided behind the buttocks, sacrum, lumbar, and thoracic segments of the trunk. When considering a precontoured back support, the person's shape must be considered. For instance, if a person has a narrower upper trunk and wider hips, the precontoured lateral supports may interfere with the hips, making it impossible for full lower back contact. In this instance, a precontoured back with built-in lateral supports may not be an appropriate option for optimal pelvic/low back support; instead, mounted lateral supports may be the better option.

Back supports frequently are made with foam of different densities determined by comfort and pressure relief needs. Back supports frequently are designed with insets or reliefs made with different materials: air, gel, or a combination (discussed in seat section). Inset material is selected based on the properties desired, including the need for pressure relief, shape, and location. The person should be given an opportunity to trial various back cushions to determine which works best to attain the identified goals.

Mounting hardware is an important consideration, especially when attaching the back support to the wheelchair. The type of hardware is chosen based on the type of chair, the angular dimensions required, the need to fold the chair, the need to keep the chair as light as possible, or the need to increase durability. Mounting hardware may be heavy and affect a person's ability to self-propel the wheelchair or lift/load the wheelchair into the car. Box 32.4 presents questions that should be considered when finalizing the back support.

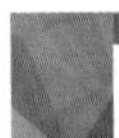

Box 32.4 Questions to Consider When Finalizing the Back Support

- Is the back support in an appropriate position for upright trunk posture (seat to back support angle, orientation in space)?
- Is the back support an appropriate shape to fit the patient's body contours? (If using a commercially available back support with contour, it should be examined to ensure the support will fit the person. At times, the patient's hips may be too wide to fit between the fixed lateral supports of a commercial back.)
- Does the patient require a custom shape to provide full contact and support?
- Does the back support provide adequate control for muscle weakness and trunk asymmetries?
- Is the back comfortable when used in a tilted or reclined position?
- Does the back support allow performance of functional activities (propelling, reaching, transfers)?
- Is pressure distribution/relief adequate for a person with a bony spine, protruding sacrum, or to prevent pressure sores?
- Are special combinations of foam, air, or gel needed to maximize comfort and pressure relief?

Foot Support

The foot support is the postural support device used to support or position the foot and lower leg and is considered a primary support surface. Placement of the foot support directly affects the position of the entire lower body, tone, and posture (trunk, head, arms). To achieve appropriate positioning of the foot on the foot support, one needs to match the linear and angular dimensions determined during the mat assessment and seating simulation, including (1) lower leg length, (2) seat to lower leg support angle, and (3) lower leg to foot support angle.

Adequate lower leg length is required to maintain good pelvic position and distribute the weight of the thighs on the seat. Foot supports that are too low will result in the knees being lower than the hips, placing the hips in a more open angle and encouraging forward sliding of the pelvis. Also, foot supports that are too low, with inadequate ground clearance, can cause the wheelchair to tip should the foot support interfere with the ground or an obstacle (e.g., ramp, doorjamb). Two inches of ground clearance is a target to keep in mind. Foot supports that are too high may unload the thighs, placing increased weight on the ITs, coccyx, and sacrum and increasing the risk for developing pressure injuries.

The seat to lower leg support angle and the lower leg support to foot support angle guide the selection of the foot support assembly. Foot supports that are mounted too far forward when hamstring muscles are tight will pull the pelvis into a posterior tilt and promote forward sliding of the pelvis (Fig. 32.24). This is an important consideration, especially when using elevating legrests, one type of foot support assembly. Foot support devices that are mounted close to or below the seat may cause interference with the casters. This is important to avoid,

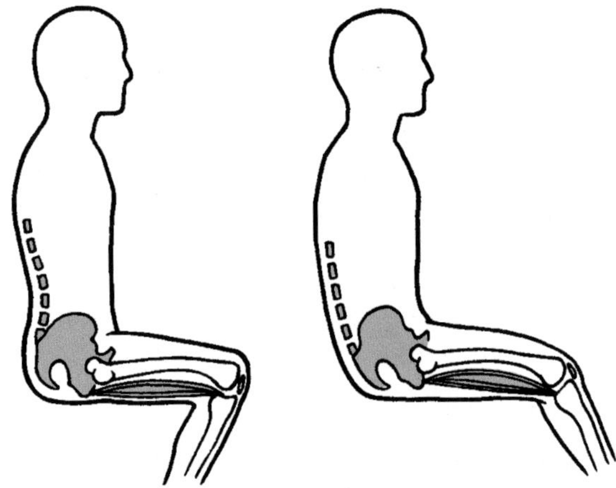

Figure 32.24 Sitting alignment with the hamstrings on slack and the knees flexed (*left*) and positioning assumed with feet resting on elevating legrests (*right*), causing tension on the hamstring that pulls the pelvis into a posterior tilt.

as caster interference can cause wheelchair tips or falls or injury to the lower leg or foot.

Any limitation of motion imposed by the hamstring muscle and gastrocnemius muscle will directly influence the choice of foot support. With tight hamstrings, to achieve the person's optimal sitting posture and maximum available hip flexion, it may be necessary to flex the knees more than 90° to place the hamstrings on slack. This approach may require special positioning of the foot supports.

Arm Support

Arm supports are the postural support device intended to contact the inferior surface of the forearms. This surface provides support to the upper extremity and trunk, off-loading weight from the spine. The height, length, and width of the arm supports are the critical measurements needed for decision making. Correct armrest height generally allows for 30 degrees shoulder flexion and 60 degrees of elbow flexion. If arm support placement is too high, shoulders become elevated, placing stress on the shoulders and neck. If armrest placement is too low or too wide, inadequate support can lead to leaning or slumping to reach the supports.

The arm pad directly contacts the forearm or hand and, in addition to providing upper trunk support, is used for function, such as pushing up to standing, making clothing adjustments, and performing weight reliefs (forward bending, side leaning, and press-ups). If the arm pad support is too wide, it may interfere with lifting or flipping back the armrests or grasping the armrests for transfers or interfere with propulsion. If the arm pad support is too narrow, it may cause concentrated pressure on the forearms or elbows, or the upper extremities may slip off the pads, providing ineffective support. Arm pads come in different materials such as plastic, foam, or gel and are selected based on the person's needs.

For some individuals, arm supports will be used to mount an *upper extremity support surface* such as an upper extremity support tray (lap tray) or wedge. A lap tray surface provides several important functions. It can promote symmetrical positioning of the UEs or accommodate alignment of the glenohumeral joint and scapula, support the weight of the upper limbs, decrease shoulder subluxation, and provide trunk support. Importantly, UE support trays are used for function: for meals, work or school, or supporting a communication device, computer, book, and so on.

Head Support

A posterior head support is a support intended to contact the posterior aspect of the head. This is beneficial for a person who is unable to hold their head upright and needs a resting support surface or for a person who needs support when the chair is tilted rearward or when the back is reclined. Important issues to consider include the size, shape, and material of the support; the adjustability/durability of the attaching hardware; and the final placement of the support. For example, a curved shape will support the person's head in the center of the headrest while a flat support will not provide any cues for positioning of the head, and the head may tend to slide on the flat surface. Adjustable hardware will allow accommodation for a forward head position or a laterally flexed position. Swing-away hardware may be needed when transferring from behind so that the caregiver can get close for lifting. Proper support and positioning the head affects posture, visual gaze, swallowing, and communication. Depending on a person's needs, head supports sometimes may also incorporate secondary support surfaces such as lateral support pads, facial pads, forehead head straps, chin supports, and so on.

Secondary Support Surfaces

Secondary supports include lateral and medial trunk, pelvis, hip, knee, foot, UE, anterior chest, and pelvic supports.[53] Secondary supports may or may not be necessary for positioning, stability, pressure relief, and comfort. When determining the need for the support, consideration should be given to surface shape, stability or support (firmness/flexibility), size, placement, and attachment method. The supports are named according to their location and the terms used are standard medical terms to increase the ease of understanding the location of the supports. Using the MPT problem solving model, document the objective and rationale to justify each recommended support.

Anterior Supports

Anterior supports are positioned on the anterior aspect of the body. Common anterior supports include anterior pelvic support, anterior trunk supports, and anterior shoulder supports. Anterior trunk supports and shoulder supports tend to be made of flexible materials such as neoprene or fabric. Measurements and placement of the supports are critical to ensure the support is secure and does not slide or ride up, creating a hazard (e.g., choking).

Anterior Pelvic Support

An anterior pelvic support is a device intended to contact the anterior aspect of the pelvis, over or just inferior to the ASIS. This device can be a flexible strap or seat belt or a rigid pelvic positioner (padded bar). The decision about the necessary pelvic support features is dependent on the support or accommodation needed to (1) control pelvic position (tilt, obliquity, or rotation), (2) maintain the person's optimal pelvic position, and (3) ensure safety.[59] In specifying an anterior pelvic support, decisions about the direction of pull, angle of pull, number of securement or anchor points, attachment hardware, location, and release mechanism are made.[60] For example, if the person has a tendency, secondary to tone, for the left hip to consistently rotate forward, it may be useful to have the belt tighten by pulling toward the hip, creating a counterpressure. The angle of pull of the pelvic support in relation to the seating surface is a critical decision for safety and effectiveness. It is important for safety to prevent the pelvic support from lifting up into the abdomen or for the pelvis to slide underneath the belt. Therefore, specifying the angle of pull is necessary. Attachment points are generally 30° to 45° to the seat to control for anterior pelvic tilt, 60° to 90° for posterior pelvic tilt, and around 60° for obliquity and rotation (Fig. 32.25).[59] Some patients respond well to belts that have a 90° attachment angle with the sitting surface. This angle of pull secures the thighs against the seat support and inhibits hypertonia in patients who tend to extend in their wheelchairs as a result of increased tone. A 90° placement also leaves the pelvis free for forward trunk inclination, often necessary for reaching and function (Fig. 32.26). Some patients can benefit from pelvic support belts with more than one angle of pull from two securement points. A four-point belt provides four places to anchor it. The top two anchors assist in securing the pelvis against the back support and the bottom two anchors assist in securing the femurs against the seat support, limiting the pelvis from shifting forward. Setting specific objectives for the pelvic position will drive the decision making process for determining the optimal anterior pelvic support and securement parameters.

Lateral Supports

Lateral supports are postural support devices contacting the lateral sides of the body. Lateral supports (pelvis, trunk, hip, knee, foot, and so forth) assist a person in maintaining optimal alignment. Each support requires a corresponding objective and rationale to support medical necessity.

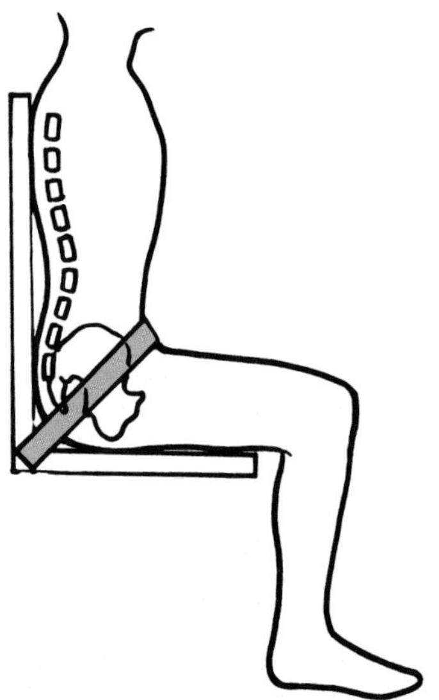

Figure 32.25 The pelvic belt should cross the pelvic-femoral junction at approximately a 45° to 60° angle to the seating surface.

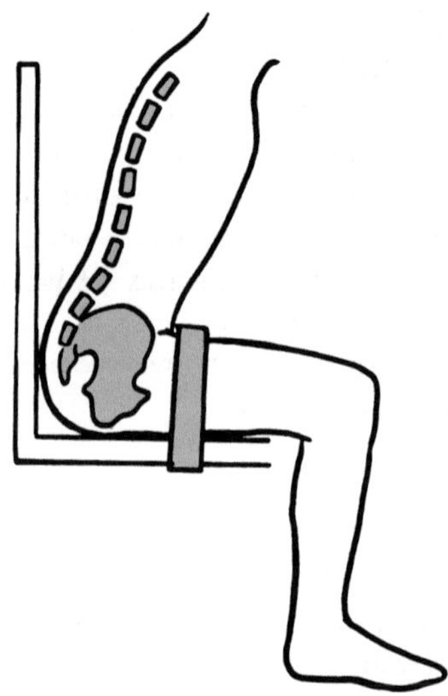

Figure 32.26 A belt placed over the upper thigh (at a 90° angle to the sitting surface) will free the pelvis for natural anterior tilting.

If a person has poor trunk control and leans to the left side, lateral trunk supports can be used to support an upright midline position and decrease leaning to the left.[61] To correct a flexible or accommodate a fixed scoliosis, *three points of control* are needed. This is done by placing a pad at the apex of the curve on one side and on the opposite side a pad above and below the apex. In this example, for right (convex) scoliosis, a lateral trunk support would be placed on the right at the apex of the curve and on the left side above the apex, with a third pad below the apex at the pelvis or hip.

If both lower extremities abduct and the person doesn't have the muscle strength in their lower extremities to maintain neutral alignment, then lateral thigh/knee supports will help maintain lower extremity position and limit excessive abduction.

Properties to consider include the surface size, shape, firmness, location, and method of attachment. The dimensions are necessary to ensure the supports aren't too large or too small. The location ensures the support provides the forces needed to attain the person's identified optimal sitting alignment. As an example, if the person's trunk width measures 12 in. but the width between the lateral trunk supports is 16 in., then the person will not benefit from contact of the lateral trunk support and will therefore continue to lean to the left side until they reach it. Be sure to consider adjustability and adjust the position of the supports to optimize postural control and comfort, taking into consideration factors such as future growth needs, weight gain, and seasonal clothing (e.g., winter coat, sweaters).

The attachment method can facilitate or impede transfers and mobility. Supports might need to be moved out of the way to perform sit pivot transfers, mechanical lift transfers, or stand pivot transfers. The style of the support attachment will determine if the person is able to move the support out of the way independently or require assistance. Defining objectives for posture and transfers will guide you in selecting the most effective equipment features. Other less common lateral supports include forearm, elbow, head, lower leg, and foot support, but the same concepts apply for shape, firmness, dimensions, placement, and attachment method.

Medial Supports

Medial supports are postural support devices contacting the medial side of the body. The most common supports are medial knee and thigh supports. Other medial supports include forearm and foot supports.

Posterior Supports

Posterior supports are postural support devices contacting the posterior aspect of the body. The most common include posterior foot, lower leg (calf), and arm support (elbow). A head support, although included in the primary support surface section, is considered a posterior head support. Objectives and equipment features are determined.

Wheeled Mobility Devices

A wheelchair can be divided into two parts: the seating support system that provides support to the person's body (discussed above) and the mobility base that provides movement within the environment (discussed below). Wheeled mobility devices may provide mobility in different positions such as sitting, lying, or standing and allow a person to be out of bed or out of a stationary chair and mobile in their environment. This chapter is devoted to seated wheeled mobility. A person may be able to operate the wheeled mobility device independently such as self-propelling a manual wheelchair or independently driving a power wheelchair, or he or she may be dependent in wheeled mobility, reliant on a caregiver to move in the environment. The wheeled mobility device provides a person with the ability to move to different rooms in their home and leave their home and participate in community activities. The wheeled mobility device framework is shown in Figure 32.27 and can be used for a reference for categorizing equipment.

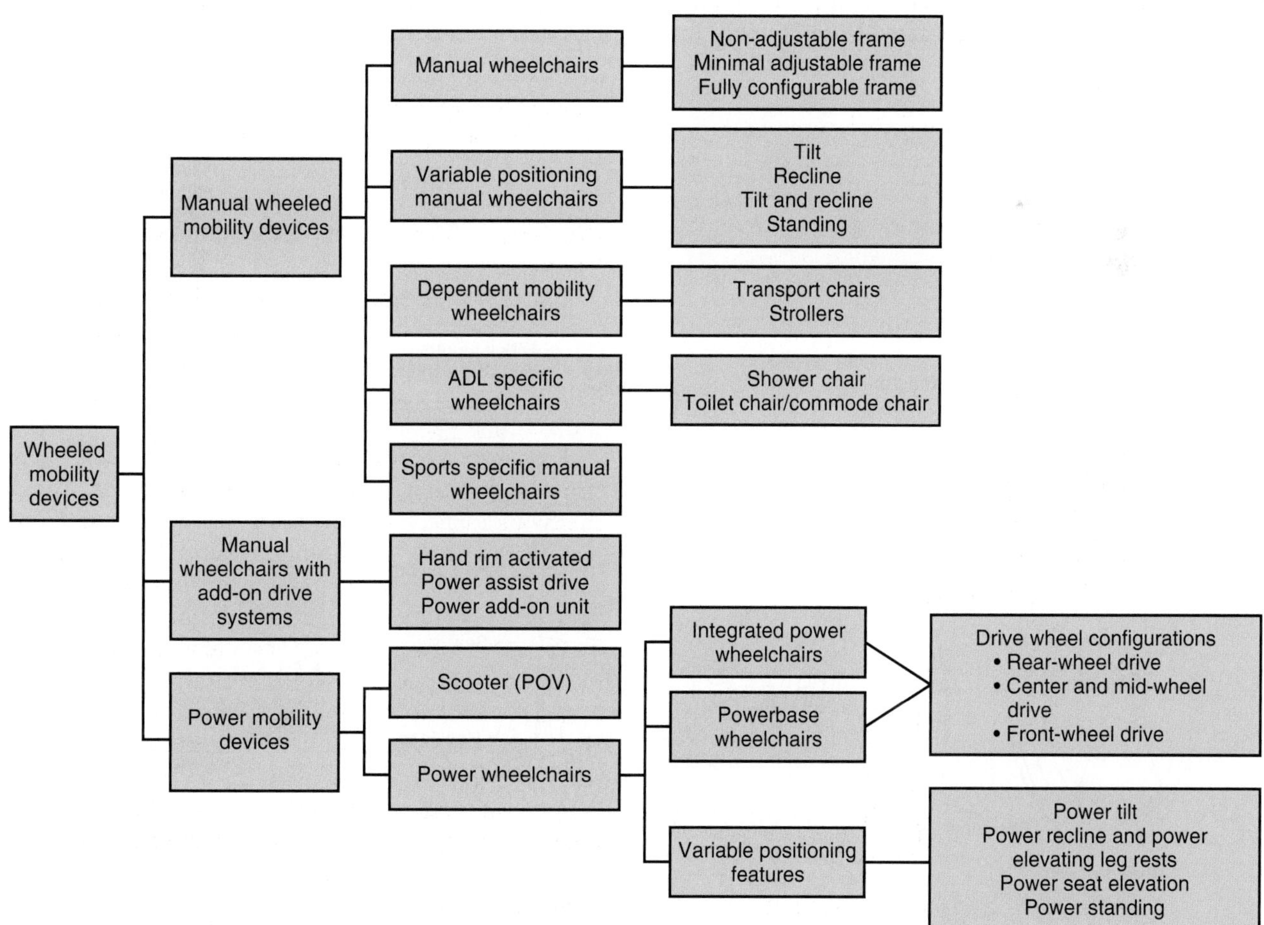

Figure 32.27 Wheeled mobility device framework. *(Waugh, K.)*[53]

Wheelchair Frame/Base Considerations

In this section, adjustable frame considerations are discussed, including but not limited to linear, angular, and other configurable frame features. Figure 32.28 provides an overview of configurable wheelchair components that can be selected to individualize the wheelchair frame for the person's needs. These concepts and product considerations are factored into the decision making process when matching equipment features to product specification (feature/model match).

Frame Linear Adjustments

Wheelchairs are available in different widths and depths. Sizing for optimal propulsion and posture was discussed in the primary support section above. Some manual wheelchair frames have built-in adjustability of the frame to accommodate for changes in width or depth without needing to purchase a new wheelchair and if available is noted in the manufacturer literature. The growth option is most often used to accommodate for growth, as this can be a concern for children; however, it can also be used to accommodate for weight gain or loss. Care should be taken to select the most appropriate range, considering the person's immediate and future anticipated needs. For instance, if a frame width of 20 in. (50.8 cm) is needed, a frame may be selected that can be adjusted from 16 to 20 in. (40.6 to 50.8 cm), or 20 to 24 in. (50.8 to 60.9 cm). If the person has the potential to gain weight, the larger size should be considered.

Wheelchair seating dimensions (width and depth) are specific to the person's body size and posture needs. The overall wheelchair frame dimensions, however, dictate overall size, maneuverability, and accessibility. It results in extra width and length based on the style of the wheels, footrests, and other wheelchair features (e.g., anti-tip tubes).

The overall width is considered to ensure ability to move safely through doorways. This may be more difficult in a manual wheelchair since the wheels and hand rims add 8 to 10 in. to the overall wheelchair width. In addition, hand clearance needs to be factored to enable the person to use their hands to propel while also allowing doorway clearance. Some people, however, prefer to use a compensatory strategy, such as using the doorjamb to pull through the opening instead of pushing on the wheel rim to decrease the risk of hand injuries. Regardless, doorway clearance is a critical consideration and sometimes requires environment adaptation (e.g., offset door hinges).

Wheelchair overall length determines turning radius and the ability to maneuver the wheelchair safely in confined spaces. The addition of tilt, recline, and elevating legrests increases the overall frame length and turning

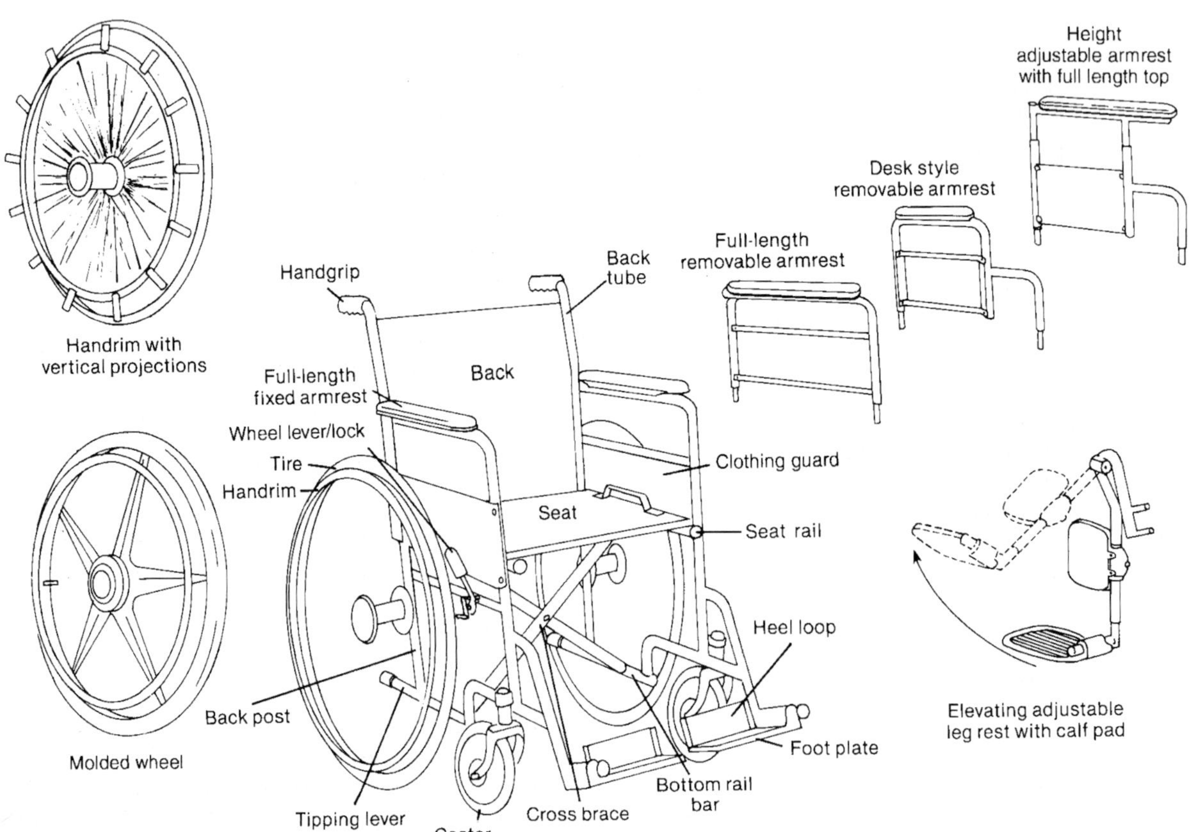

Figure 32.28 Overview of wheelchair components.

radius, often making 90-degree turns from a hallway into a room difficult or impossible.

The overall wheelchair height (floor to the top of person's head) is a critical measurement when considering van access to ensure the van door height and interior space (floor to ceiling height) provide adequate head clearance. For van access, overall turning radius and maneuverability are important considerations for a person riding in their wheelchair to ensure the wheelchair can be safely loaded and positioned for transportation.

Angular Frame Adjustments

Angular frame adjustments such as seat to back support angle, seat to lower leg support angle, and seat sagittal angle (seat incline or tilt) are used to narrow down make/model wheelchair frame options and determine the position of different frame components.

Manufacturers of manual wheelchairs preset seat frame angles and configurations based on the specifications detailed during the ordering process (Fig. 32.29). Some manual wheelchairs are *made to order* (manufactured for the individual and nonadjustable) and others are *made to measure* (configured for the individual as specified). Even made to order manual wheelchairs typically have minimal adjustability of some features such as axle position or seat to back angle.

Some manual wheelchairs have axle plates and caster forks that have one or more adjustment options. These features provide the ability to specify a rear wheel size, caster size, front and rear frame heights, wheel placement, and wheel axle position (horizontal/vertical adjustment). By design, selection and configuration (e.g., frame height, seat angles, person's relation to rear wheel, wheelchair tippyness) are dependent on the objectives and features identified in the wheelchair assessment (see Fig. 32.29). For example, by selecting a small caster and caster fork size and raising the rear axle vertical position, a low seat to floor height can be accomplished so the person can reach the floor for foot propulsion. For a person with tight hamstrings requiring the feet to flex back under the seat, raising the front frame height in relation to the rear frame can increase foot and caster clearance. Similarly, this configuration can provide a person with difficulty sitting upright a fixed tilt position for gravity-assisted positioning.

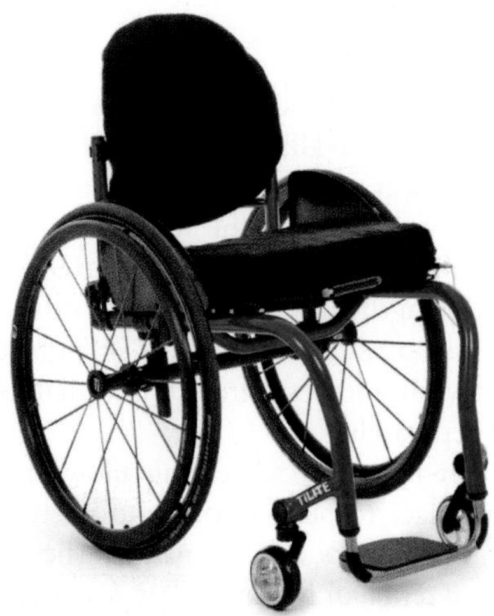

Figure 32.29 Wheelchair frame with adjustable axle plates, adjustable forks, and adjustable back posts to achieve specific heights and frame angles. *(Courtesy of Permobil, Lebanon, TN 37090.)*

Some power wheelchairs also have adjustable seat frames that can be adjusted for seat height and fixed tilt, depending on the style of the wheelchair. Power wheelchairs that have a base and separate seating system come preconfigured for seat height and angle if specified when ordering the wheelchair. Most power wheelchairs have limited adjustability after delivery. Configuration considerations are an important part of the selection process, as decisions can affect the person's ability for function (e.g., transfers, reaching, sitting balance, sitting endurance).

Many manual and power wheelchairs and most tilt-in-space wheelchairs have the capacity for one or more back post angle adjustments allowing configuration to meet the person's identified seat to back angle needs. The identified seat to back angle may determine which frame options are available. Some wheelchairs only have 10 degrees of adjustment while others have 30 degrees or more of adjustment.

For a person who can tolerate a fixed tilt or fixed recline position, an adjustable seat to back angle feature may be all that is needed to accommodate a person with a mild hip flexion limitation or a person who is unable to tolerate sitting upright but who does not need a variable tilt-in-space system. Opening the seat to back angle 5 to 15 degrees alone (fixed recline) or in combination with adjusting the seat position (fixed tilt) can help position the person for better balance, sitting tolerance, and comfort. Specifying the configuration of the wheelchair frame is as important as verifying it has accomplished the intended objective, which is assessed at the fitting and delivery and fine-tuned as necessary.

Wheelchair Frame Options

There are many wheelchair accessories, a few of which are highlighted here. *Anti-tippers* are used to prevent a wheelchair from tipping rearward. *Wheel lock extensions* are used on a manual wheelchair to increase the lever and ease of applying or removing the wheel lock. Various wheel lock styles are available (e.g., push to lock, pull to lock, scissor, low mount, high mount). Wheelchair *push handles* are available in a variety of shapes and configurations (fixed, flip down, removeable), depending on the person's needs. If a person uses the push handles to hook for balance during weight shift or clothing adjustments, a particular height and durable style may be required. If a person is lifted while in their wheelchair by the push handles, removable handles are not advised. If a person is dependent in mobility, the push handle height or the addition of an *adjustable stroller handle* may be needed for the caregiver, especially when there is a height difference between caregivers or when used on a pediatric or tilt-in-space wheelchair.

Wheelchair securement sites (transportation securement brackets or *transport option*) are an important feature to consider for individuals transported while riding in their wheelchair. Many transport options meet voluntary safety standards for vehicle crash testing and are important to discuss during the ordering process.

These are only a few of the multitude of available wheelchair options and accessories. Manufacturers offer a variety of accessories available with their wheelchair bases. There also exist numerous manufacturers that offer accessories that are not product specific (aftermarket manufacturers). Importantly, review the identified objectives and determine if additional wheelchair accessories or options are required prior to completing the final recommendation.

Attachment Mechanisms

Options and accessories are attached to the wheelchair frame in different ways. Decisions about options include, but are not limited to, attachment style (fixed, removeable, swing-away), release (push button, lever, cam lock, and so forth), durability (heavy duty, shock absorbing), and functionality (swing out, swing in, lift off, and so forth). These important decisions can be the difference between independence and the need for assistance. Specifying the objective, feature, and rationale in your documentation will support the medical necessity for the items requested. Examples related to foot and arm supports follow.

Foot Support Assembly

The foot support assembly (footrest) includes the components that mount the foot support surface to the frame of the wheelchair. Most foot support assemblies are mounted from the side rails of the frame while some systems are center mounted on the wheelchair. The foot support assembly may be fixed, lift off, or swing in or out. In the case of rigid manual wheelchairs, the foot support assembly is most often not removeable, but swing-away may be an option.

Transfer style and final foot position placement (determined during the wheelchair assessment) will affect decision making and selection. If a person transfers independently, retaining independence and the ability to manage the foot support are essential. Each wheelchair manufacturer provides different release mechanisms for moving the foot support assembly out of the way, and dexterity will dictate which option will work best. A footplate or foot platform are components of the foot support assembly that are also an important part of the technology selection. These may include dual-sided, standard size, non-adjustable, large, or angle adjustable, as well as a single platform. If using a flip-up style foot plate, it is important to verify that the person can lift the foot plate out of the way. If the person transfers independently, they must be able to move the foot support assembly out of the way but still be close enough to transfer. In this example, a swing-in foot support may be desirable.

Arm Support Assembly

The arm support assembly is the components of the wheelchair that attach the arm support surface to the frame of the wheelchair. Different styles may include single post, dual post, tubular swing-away, and flip-up mounted to back cane.

The arm support assembly is chosen when finalizing the wheelchair. The method to release and remove the arm supports is discussed, and functional issues such as transfer type, pressure relief technique, and durability are considered. The style of transfer, access to tables, and ability to move the arm support out of the way independently will determine which arm support assembly is optimal. In addition, the armrest pad style and length (full versus desk) are also important options that must be determined.

Manual Wheeled Mobility Devices

Manual wheeled mobility devices are used by a person with a mobility limitation and require the occupant or an attendant to move it. There are five types of devices in this category: manual wheelchairs, variable positioning manual wheelchairs, dependent mobility wheelchairs, ADL-specific manual wheelchairs, and sports-specific manual wheelchairs (see Fig. 32.27). Each are presented below and classified or grouped by features and functions.

Manual Wheelchairs

Non-Adjustable Frame

The most basic type of manual wheelchair has no frame adjustability and is available in limited sizes, typically 16- and 18 in.-seat width and depth (Fig. 32.30). Sling seat and back upholstery is the standard option on this style wheelchair. Standard armrests are fixed height, desk length or full length, and removeable or nonremoveable armrests and footrests are standard. Height adjustable arms and elevating legrests are often available but must be ordered separately.

A basic non-adjustable wheelchair allows the user to be moved from place to place in order to safely perform or participate in daily tasks. A basic manual wheelchair is typically used as a rental or for temporary or intermittent use. Few options are available to properly fit this wheelchair to the user's size. This type of basic wheelchair is primarily for individuals who cannot independently self-propel, require a wheelchair intermittently, and transfer to other sitting surfaces frequently throughout the day.

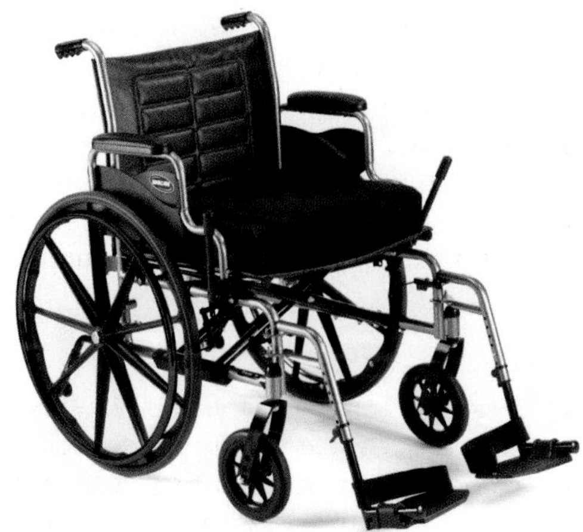

Figure 32.30 Upright manual wheelchair with non-adjustable frame. *(Courtesy of Invacare Corporation, Elyria, OH 44035.)*

Minimally Adjustable Frame

Wheelchairs that meet this description generally provide more limited adjustability, added seat widths, seat depths, and seat to floor heights than the non-adjustable frame. However, in order to truly configure a product to the individual, a fully adjustable frame category wheelchair will be needed.

This type of wheelchair will allow the user to move or be moved from place to place to perform daily tasks, typically in accommodated environments. Minimally adjustable configurations may allow a fixed hemi height (lower seat to floor height) or standard seat to floor height for self-propulsion or to maximize safety and independence with transfers. Occasionally, wheelchairs in this category may allow adjustments for minimal seat inclination (fixed posterior seat tilt) for positional assistance. This is only functional if the wheelchair has the capacity to adjust caster alignment perpendicular to the floor to optimize rolling ability; otherwise, this adjustment will make self-propulsion more difficult.

Fully Configurable Frame

This category includes *made-to-order* wheelchairs, which have modular frames and can fold or are rigid and can be adjusted after delivery to meet the changing needs of the person, and *made-to-measure* rigid wheelchairs, which result in an intimate fit based on individual measurements but offer limited adjustability after delivery. Fully configurable frames are the most complex type of manual wheelchairs and are categorized as complex rehab technology (CRT) (Fig. 32.31). It is rare for a made-to-measure wheelchair to be recommended for new manual wheelchair users.

Rigid frame wheelchairs do not require mounting hardware needed to provide adjustments and modifications; therefore, these wheelchairs are often lighter in weight than folding frame wheelchairs. The rigid frame also reduces frame flexion or movement, making them more efficient for propulsion and durable. Rigid frame wheelchairs often have folding back canes and removeable rear wheels, allowing for disassembly for transportation and stowage (Fig. 32.32). By design, these wheelchairs have a smaller profile (overall length). Rigid frame wheelchairs cannot be modified in size in the field and therefore are more often recommended for people with stable conditions.

Rigid frame wheelchairs are typically used by an active person who puts great demands on the wheelchair frame and parts. Usually this individual is independent

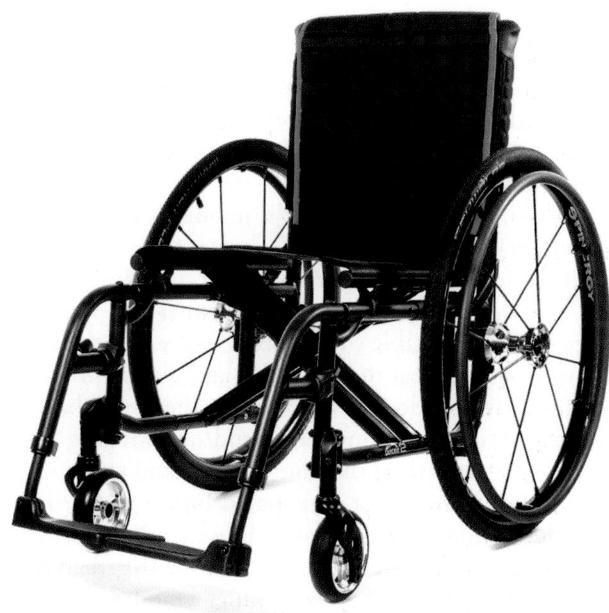

Figure 32.31 Fully configurable manual wheelchair. *(Courtesy of Sunrise Medical, Fresno, CA 93727.)*

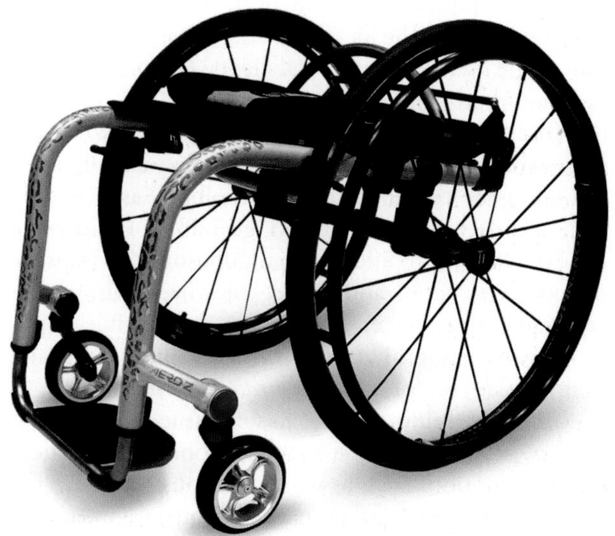

Figure 32.32 Fully configurable rigid frame manual wheelchair showing back support in fold down position. Rear wheels are removable for transportation and stowage. *(Courtesy of Permobil, Lebanon, TN 37090.)*

and safe negotiating ordinary environmental obstacles (e.g., door thresholds), can achieve and maintain a rear wheel balancing position (wheelie), maneuvers in and around doors, safely negotiates ramps, and requires a specially configured wheelchair for maximum independent functioning.

Made-to-order configurable manual wheelchairs (modular) can be incrementally customized with tools to provide optimal postural support and positioning for a person's individualized functional and medical needs. The adjustable components, especially the ability to adjust the seat to back angle and seat depth, provide a means to adequately configure the wheelchair to meet an individual's moderate and/or changing postural support needs at the time of order and at the time of delivery and to meet anticipated future needs. This wheelchair can accommodate a more complex seating system and is indicated for an individual with a changing condition or disorder that requires a more supportive seating system.

Configurable frame adjustments (i.e., seat to back angle, back height, rear wheel position, camber, seat sagittal angle, seat to floor height, caster alignment) can enhance wheelchair propulsion, improve maneuverability, and minimize rolling resistance. Also, configurable frame adjustments can improve sitting posture by accommodating hip and knee contractures, improve sitting balance, and improve transfer and access to tables for function.

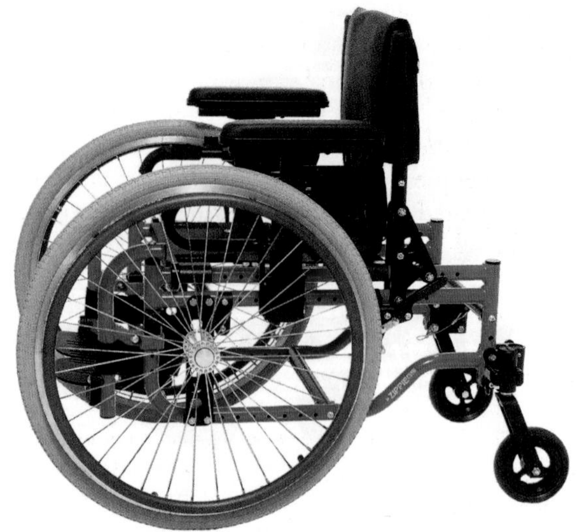

Figure 32.33 Wheelchairs with large front wheels and small rear casters may be easier for some people to push but are more difficult to use outdoors. *(Courtesy of Sunrise Medical, Fresno, CA 93727.)*

Propulsion Configuration

There are four typical methods of manual wheelchair self-propulsion: (1) both UE, (2) both LE, (3) hemi propulsion, and (4) all four extremities.

Bilateral UE propulsion is the most common method used, requiring good UE function, strength, and muscular endurance. The location of the drive wheel in relation to the user is critical for efficiency and proper upper extremity body mechanics.

Most manual wheelchairs are configured with rear drive wheels. However, drive wheels can also be positioned in the center or front of the base, as primarily seen and used with children (Fig. 32.33). Positioning the drive wheels in different configurations can improve the ability to access and propel the wheelchair. This is especially critical when considering the possible implications for long-term function of the shoulder girdle and to minimize risk for *repetitive strain injuries* (RSIs).

RSIs can result in damage to soft tissue (tendons, ligaments, nerves) or bony structures secondary to frequent repeated motions such as wheelchair push strokes. The damage can include inflammation, compression, and/or tears in the shoulder joint and surrounding structures, resulting in pain and decreased function.[62,63] RSIs are often seen in the shoulders, wrists, and hands of wheelchair users. Even patients without documented RSIs report increased pain in these joints with prolonged wheelchair use.[63,64] Small muscles are required to produce large forces repeatedly to move the wheelchair through space. These same muscles are typically required for a variety of activities of daily living (ADL) tasks such as transfers and reaching, thus increasing the demands placed on the same muscles and the potential of causing injury. Prolonged wheelchair use and/or improper wheelchair configuration can result in muscle imbalances, pain, and injury. Stress on the muscles and joints increases with wheelchair rolling resistance, overall wheelchair weight (frame, seating, user, accessories, backpacks, and so forth), and environmental factors (terrain, surface type, and so forth). RSI symptoms may not be felt until the condition is well advanced. Common conditions include rotator cuff injuries, medial epicondylitis, and carpal tunnel syndrome.

When prescribing wheelchairs and features for patients who are able to self-propel, consideration must be given to minimizing risk for RSIs by carefully evaluating the position of the person in relation to the drive wheel to decrease stress and strain on the shoulders, elbows, wrists, and hands. Importantly, UE positioning must allow for an efficient stroke, reducing the force needed per stroke and the frequency of strokes required to move the wheelchair. Attention to shoulder biomechanics and alignment is critical.

For efficient pushing, the elbows should be bent at an angle of about 120° when the hands are resting atop the push rims. The wheelchair user should be able to comfortably reach the front and back of the push rim at the height of the wheel axle. In order to attain this position, the wheels need to be adjusted horizontally (fore and aft), and the wheels or seat need to be adjusted vertically. The back height and camber of the wheels are adjusted so that the arms and shoulder girdle are unrestricted over the entire propulsion phase.[65-67] Frequently, there are trade-offs between optimal position for propulsion and configuration needed for function or environmental access that need to be discussed and decided.

Some people with functional use of one upper extremity (e.g., hemiplegia) use a one-arm drive mechanism for self-propulsion. The one-arm drive mechanism has two concentric hand rims of different sizes mounted on one wheel, on the side being used to propel the wheelchair. The outer rim controls one wheel, enabling the chair to turn in one direction; the inner rim controls the other wheel, enabling the wheelchair to turn in the other direction. Propelling both rims simultaneously enables the chair to move forward and backward (Fig. 32.34).

Self-propulsion with both lower extremities requires a low seat to floor height so the person can firmly plant their foot on the floor without sliding forward in the wheelchair.

The hemi propulsion method of self-propulsion uses a combination of one arm and one leg. Care is taken to configure the wheelchair with a seat to floor height to enable lower extremity propulsion, positioning of the person in relation to the drive wheel, and drive wheel placement for maximal UE contact with the wheel. In this configuration, the person uses their hand and foot together to propel the wheel and steer.

For people who use all four extremities to self-propel, the same wheelchair setup needs are considered as described above.

Variable Positioning Manual Wheelchairs

Variable positioning manual wheelchairs are available in a range of pediatric and adult sizes and may include tilt, recline, tilt and recline, and standing features.

Tilt

A manual wheelchair with a tilt system allows for frequent and limited angular repositioning of the seat and back relative to upright, whereby a caregiver changes the seat orientation in space to assist with positioning, pressure relief, and posture (Fig. 32.35). There exist variable *positioning tilt systems* and *full tilt systems.* In order to be considered a *full tilt system,* it needs to tilt at least 45°. Both types of tilt systems can be moved by a caregiver through the available range of motion, incrementally, and as often as needed for repositioning. A positioning tilt system is typically used to accommodate for muscle weakness, paralysis, or fatigue of neck and trunk muscles; to provide a neutral head/neck position for safe swallowing and saliva control; and to provide gravity-assisted positioning for rest and when traversing challenging terrain. A primary benefit of a full tilt system is pressure relief/pressure redistribution, which is accomplished by shifting weight and pressure away from the bony prominences under the pelvis to the posterior pelvis and back. Increasing the amount of tilt exponentially increases the amount of pressure redistributed away from the pelvis. A minimum of 45° of tilt provides pressure relief/pressure redistribution, minimizing the shear forces and the potential loss of user position that is often associated with recline. Table 32.4 presents evidence for the use of positional tilt systems.[68-80]

Recline

A reclining wheelchair has a manually adjustable seat to back angle to allow for a change in position (Fig. 32.36).

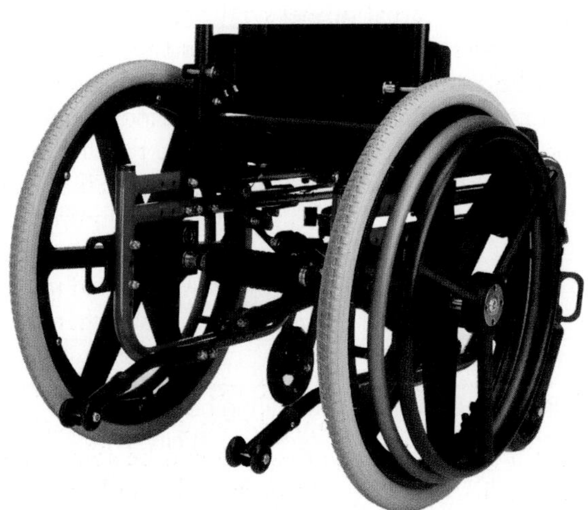

Figure 32.34 A double hand rim on one side allows the user to propel a one-arm drive wheelchair with one hand. *(Courtesy of Sunrise Medical, Fresno, CA 93727.)*

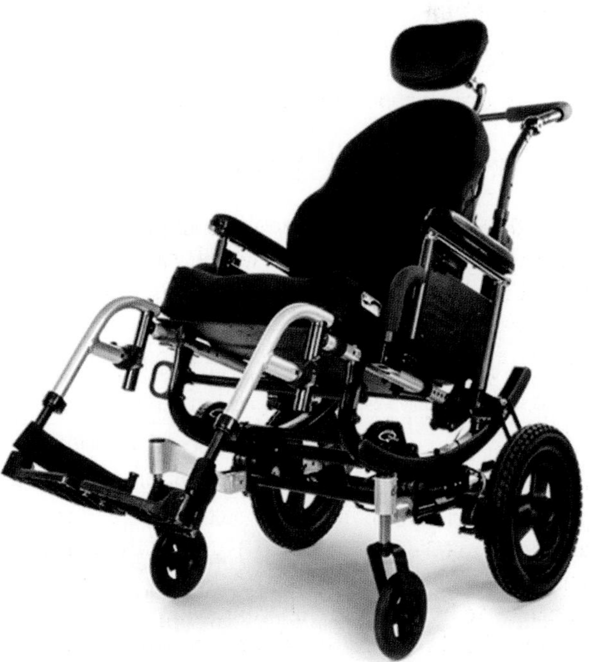

Figure 32.35 A manual wheelchair with tilt to assist with positioning, pressure relief, and posture. *(Courtesy of Sunrise Medical, Fresno, CA 93727.)*

Table 32.4 Evidence Summary Studies Addressing the Impact of Positional Tilt Less Than 45 Degrees

Aissaoui, R, et al: Biomechanics of manual wheelchair propulsion in elderly: System tilt and back recline angles. Am J Physical Medicine Rehabil 81(2): 94–100, 2002.

Design	Experimental design with randomized repeated measures
Level of Evidence	IIB: Moderate Evidence
Subjects	14 older (range 64–77 yr) experienced wheelchair users living independently. Eligibility criteria: (1) able to propel WC on a daily basis with two-hand synchronous pattern, (2) no pressure sore >1 year, (3) able to give informed consent, (4) able to propel for a period of 10 minutes during a 1-hour experiment
Intervention	Three seat to back rest angles (95°, 100°, and 105°) and three system tilt angles (0°, 5°, and 10°) were selected. The nine conditions were randomized for each subject. Rear wheel camber was set at 0° and handrim and rear wheel radii were 0.267 m and 0.305 m, respectively. The horizontal distance between the wheel axle and the acromion marker in the sagittal plane was set to 4 cm independent of tilt and backrest positioning. Subjects were asked to propel on a friction roller cylinder ergometer between 0.96 and 1.01 m/sec.
Results	The kinetics of wheelchair propulsion can be affected by seat and backrest adjustments. System tilt angle but not back recline significantly affects biomechanical efficiency.
Comments	Tilting the system by 10° and reclining the back by 10° increase the biomechanical efficiency of the subject by 10%. This is a very important finding for older adults, many of whom benefit from positional tilt system for enhancement in mobility, postural support, and pain management.

Desroches, G, Aissaoui, R, and Bourbonnais, D: Effect of system tilt and seat-to-backrest angles on load sustained by shoulder during wheelchair propulsion. J Rehabil Res Dev 43(7):871–881, 2006.

Design	Experimental design
Level of Evidence	IIB: Moderate Evidence
Subjects	14 elderly MWC users, 7 women and 7 men, mean age 68.2 +/– 5.2 yr; use BUE for self-propulsion daily, no pressure ulcer for >1 yr able to propel MWC 6 m < 30 sec, informed consent, 1 yr minimum MWC use
Intervention	Friction roller cylinder to control resistance—all subjects used the same wheelchair and the seat and backrest had independent movement. STA (system tilt angle) 0°, 5°, 10° and SBA (seat to backrest angle) 95°, 100°, and 105° (configurations were randomly tested twice)
Results	No significant difference for the various STA and SBA combinations were revealed. Changing the seat angle while keeping the wheel-axle position constant in both vertical and horizontal locations maintained the shoulder load at the same level.
Comments	Seat angle can be determined with goals of user comfort and decreasing risk for pressure ulcers without increasing risk of overuse shoulder injuries. Positional tilt systems may be used for comfort, posture management, or pressure management without interfering with independent propulsion.

Dewey, A, Rice-Oxley, M, and Dean, T: A qualitative study comparing the experiences of tilt-in-space wheelchair use and conventional wheelchair use by clients severely disabled with multiple sclerosis. Brit J Occup Ther 67(2):65–74, 2004.

Design	Qualitative research design. Phenomenology aims to reveal the different experiences of a phenomenon by talking about it.
Level of Evidence	IVC: Weak evidence
Subjects	Inclusion criteria: were severely disabled, full-time wheelchair users requiring hoisting, had significant spasticity. Exclusion criteria: low tone, posture problems unrelated to spasticity. Where possible, caregivers were invited to participate; 23 participants—tilt in space WC n = 7 (manual n = 2, power n = 5) and conventional WC users n = 16 (manual n = 8, power n = 8)

Table 32.4 Evidence Summary Studies Addressing the Impact of Positional Tilt Less Than 45 Degrees—cont'd

Intervention	Participants were asked the following questions: What were the experiences of conventional/tilt-in-space WCs and the benefits and disadvantages of their present wheelchair? What other factors influenced the quality of life of people with MS who had significant spasticity and were full-time wheelchair users?
Results	Tilt-in-space WCs offer acceptable levels of comfort and enable severely disabled people with MS to sit out of bed for many hours, requiring fewer transfers throughout the day, which is important to them. Tilt-in-space wheelchairs are described as comfortable and clients can rest for many hours in them without the need to return to bed. Overall benefits included increased comfort, improved postural support and control through gravity-assisted positioning, enhanced sitting stability, and improved pressure management. Difficulties reported were bulkiness or reduced maneuverability of the device and difficulty transporting the device in the community. Use of a tilt-in-space WC usually involves buying a rear access adapted vehicle. Overall, participants reported higher satisfaction with positional tilt systems (6 out of 7) compared to a control group using conventional wheelchairs (8 out of 16).
Comments	The study showed that medical professionals are often most focused on physical health while clients are more concerned with vitality, general health, and mental health rather than physical disability.

Stavness, C: The effect of positioning for children with cerebral palsy on upper-extremity function: A review of the evidence. Phys Occup Ther Pediatr 26(3):39–53, 2006.

Design	Evidence Review
Level of Evidence	IIB: Moderate evidence
Subjects	Sixteen journal articles published after 1980 were used. Specific key terms searched: positioning, wheelchair, postural control, posture, adaptive seating devices, patient positioning, CP, movement disorders, UE, reaching, grasping, and occupational therapy. Articles were excluded if they were purely descriptive, did not involve children with CP, included surgery as part of the intervention, explored only one individual case, did not study UE function, or were published before 1980.
Intervention	This review focuses on determining the most appropriate sitting positioning for children with CP to promote energy conservation and optimal functional abilities.
Results	Neutral pelvic positioning does improve functional abilities. Children with CP benefit most from the entire functional sitting positioning package rather than some components (i.e., minus tray and/or abduction orthoses). Neutral or forward positioning show the greatest long-term upper extremity functional improvements (whole chair tilted).
Comments	Evidence supports that an upright position improves a child with CP's UE function like reaching and pressing to use a communication device. Children with CP should be fitted with a chair that places them in a functional sitting position. The exact seat tilt should be determined on an individual basis. One should ensure that the line of gravity from the child's trunk, shoulders, and head are anterior to his/her ischial tuberosities. A more upright position would force the child to waste energy to fight against his/her trunk. This energy can be more utilized for functional tasks. Individuals with neuromuscular conditions may benefit from positional tilt system to optimize postural control, maximize comfort, and facilitate control of their upper extremities dependent on position of the tilt.

The recline feature is operated by a caregiver for gravity-assisted positioning and may be used to accommodate a hip extension contracture or cast; stretching to minimize an individual's risk of contracture or pain; weight relief/pressure redistribution; and to perform functional tasks without transferring out of the chair (e.g., catheterizing, clothing change).

A recliner is typically used as a rental item for a temporary need (such as status post-surgery, spica cast, halo, and so forth) or may be used with a newly injured individual who requires a change in position due to a medical condition(s).

This chair is available in a very limited number of seat widths and depths. Although a reclining wheelchair is

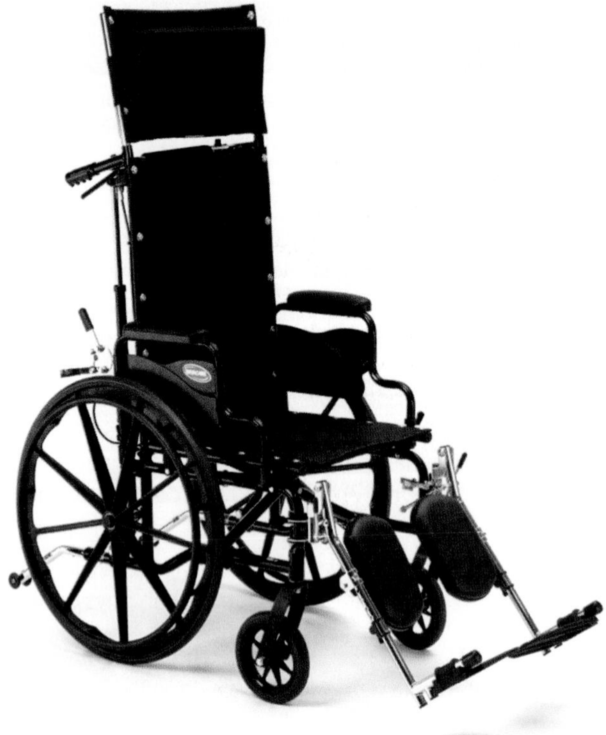

Figure 32.36 A manual wheelchair with adjustable back recline. *(Courtesy of Invacare Corporation, Elyria, OH 44035.)*

not designed for self-propulsion, a user may have the ability to maneuver it slightly to adjust their position for better alignment at a table for eating, a sink for hygiene, a desk for writing, or to communicate with others. Recliner wheelchairs have the longest wheelbase and largest overall turning radius, making accessibility and maneuverability challenging or impossible in most homes. Most individuals who require this type of wheelchair for support require maximum assistance for mobility.

Tilt and Recline

Some wheelchairs have a combination of tilt and recline for positioning, pressure relief, personal care, and posture. In most cases, the person who uses a combination tilt/recline variable positioning manual wheelchair is dependent in mobility; however, there exists some tilt wheelchairs with adjustable axles that allow the person to self-propel the wheelchair with upper extremities, lower extremities, or both. Although these wheelchairs are heavier due to the additional features, self-propulsion for short-distance mobility can provide a measure of autonomy and less dependence on caregivers.

Standing

A standing manual wheelchair enables the person to move from a sitting to standing position (Fig. 32.37A, B, C). The standing system mechanism is configured to raise and lower the person using his or her own arm strength with the assist of a hydraulic mechanism to enable weight-bearing and pressure redistribution (relief). Therefore, the person must be able to independently self-propel and have sufficient upper extremity strength to operate this feature. The standing mechanism does increase the overall weight of the wheelchair, yet enables the person to independently and frequently change their position throughout the day as needed to stand, stretch, reach, and work without needing to transfer to a dedicated standing device.

Dependent Mobility Wheelchairs

Depending on the person's positioning and mobility needs, he or she may require a manual wheelchair frame (discussed previously) even though the person may not be able to self-propel.

Transport Chairs

Transport wheelchairs have four small wheels with sling seat and back upholstery (Fig. 32.38). These wheelchairs tend to be lightweight and are easily folded and lifted by a caregiver and transported by car. Due to limited postural support, this type of wheelchair is intended for short-term use and is primarily used to assist moving a person from place A to place B. People who have the ability or potential to self-propel should consider a manual wheelchair base instead.

Strollers

Pediatric and adult adaptive strollers are included in this category (Fig. 32.39). Like transport chairs, these devices are lightweight, offer minimal support, and provide for folding and ease of transport. Some strollers are available with added positioning features, including tilt, recline, and combination tilt/recline. Many adaptive strollers have been voluntarily tested by manufacturers to meet transportation crash test standards. If needed, an integrated transit option can be purchased. This is an important consideration if a person is transported while riding in the device. Many children use adaptive strollers with transit options to ride the adapted school bus. Once again, people who have the ability or potential to self-propel should consider a manual wheelchair base instead.

ADL-Specific Wheelchairs

ADL-specific manual wheelchairs include shower wheelchairs and toilet/commode wheelchairs (Fig. 32.40A, B). These chairs have either small or large drive wheels for independent or dependent propulsion. These specialty wheelchairs allow a person to transfer from bed to chair in one room and then move to the bathroom to perform ADLs. These devices often come with a padded seat with a cutout or front opening, may or may not have a commode pail, and are usually made of materials (e.g., aluminum, stainless steel, plastic) that will endure water. There are a variety of adjustable systems available in this

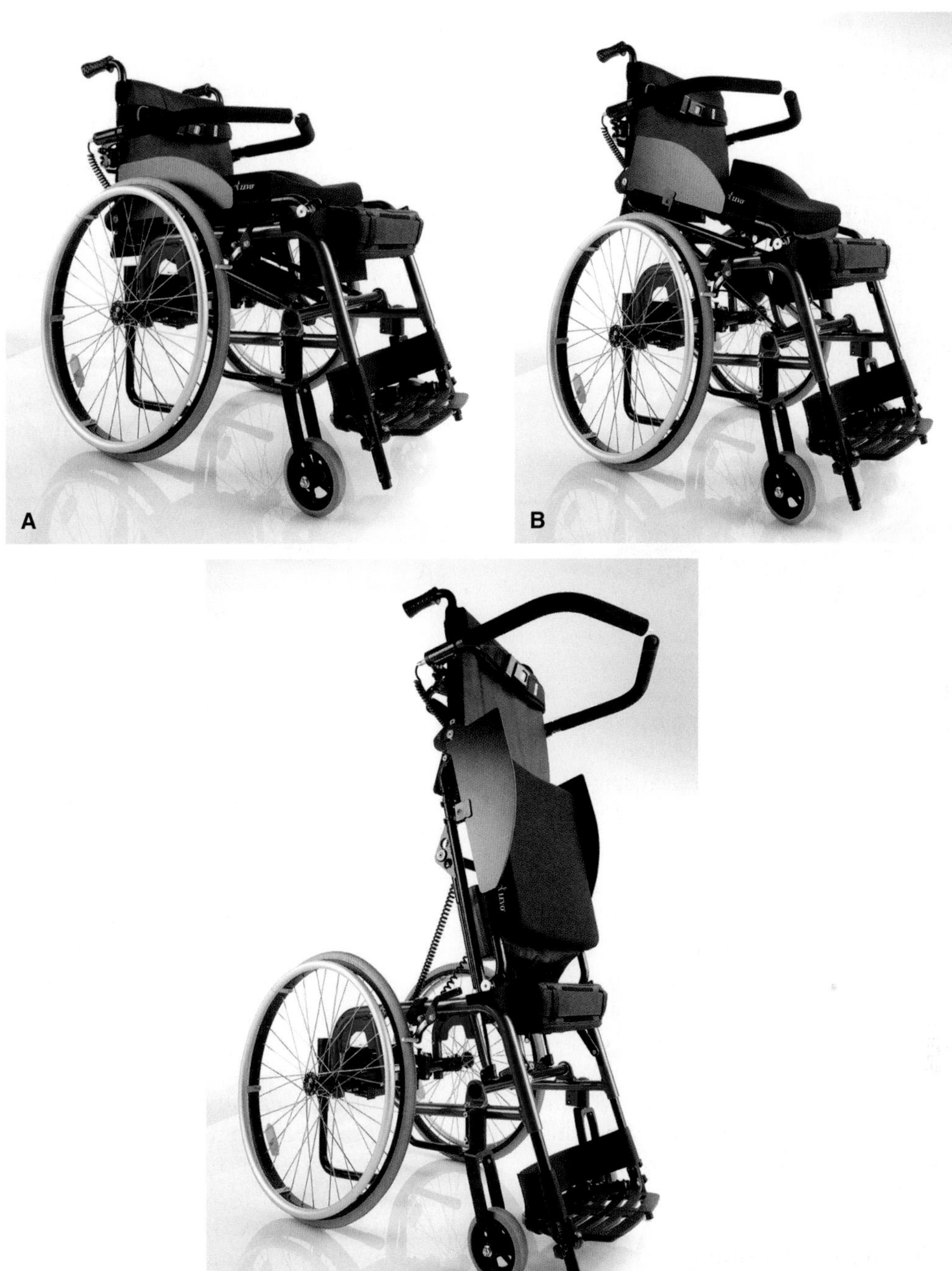

Figure 32.37 A manual wheelchair with a standing feature. (A) Sitting position. (B) Semi-standing position. (C) Full standing position. *(Courtesy of Levo, Brooklyn Park, MN 55443.)*

category, but most devices offer limited positioning options. For people with more complex postural needs, specialty rehab commode chairs are available with tilt, recline, and a range of primary and secondary postural supports.

Sports-Specific Manual Wheelchair

Many wheelchair users are active in recreational and competitive sports. As a result, the person may use more than one wheelchair: a daily-use wheelchair and a specially designed *competition* or *recreational wheelchair* to meet the demands of the activity or sport.

Wheelchair features to consider when aiming for wheelchair performance include the ability to camber the wheels (move top of the wheel closer to the user and the bottom farther away) to provide a more stable wheelchair. A durable wheelchair frame built to endure high impact, such as a rigid frame with large-diameter tubing, made with high-strength, lightweight materials, will increase the strength, durability, and lifetime of the wheelchair.

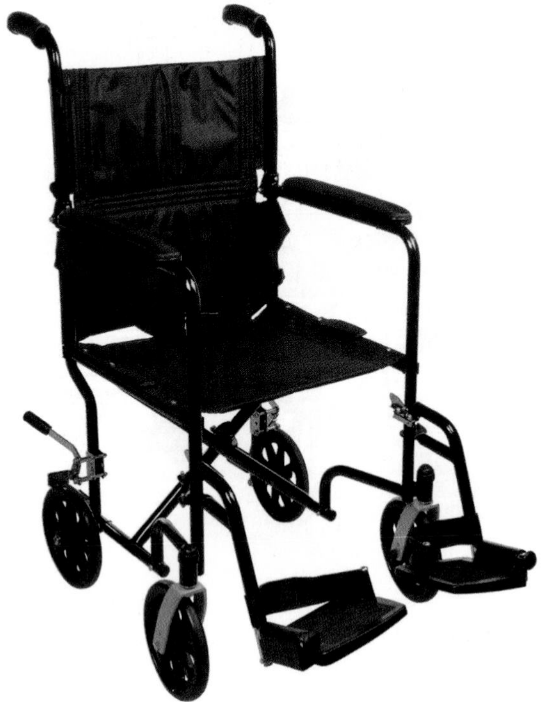

Figure 32.38 A transport chair with sling back and seat upholstery. *(Courtesy of Sunrise Medical, Fresno, CA 93727.)*

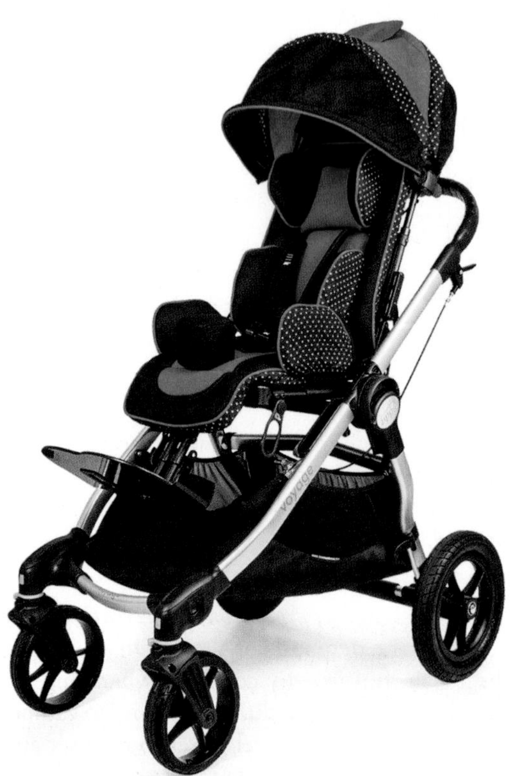

Figure 32.39 A pediatric adaptive stroller with moderate seating support. *(Courtesy of Sunrise Medical, Fresno, CA 93727.)*

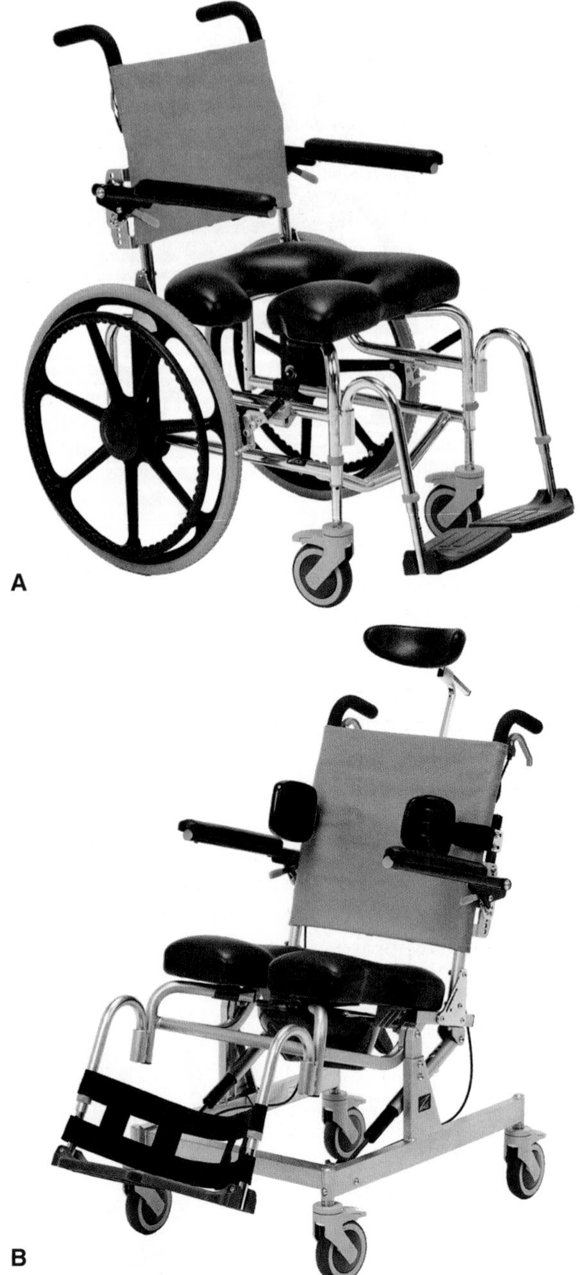

Figure 32.40 (A) A basic upright toilet/commode chair. (B) A shower chair with the tilt feature that can be used as a commode chair as well. *(Courtesy of Raz Designs, Niagara Falls, NY 14305.)*

When properly configured for the individual, wheel and caster placement, tire type, axle position, and bearings make a significant difference in chair performance. Users who participate in more than one activity may prefer a sports wheelchair with a great deal of adjustability (with or without tools) to allow changes to the wheelchair configuration for various activities (e.g., changing shoes) versus requiring multiple sports wheelchairs.

Specialty wheelchairs are designed for a specific category of sports. For example, a tennis wheelchair (Fig. 32.41) is

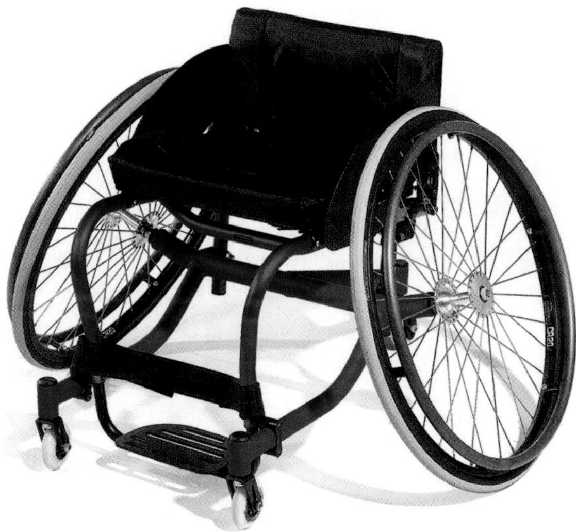

Figure 32.41 A sports chair designed for tennis. Note the low back and cambered wheels. *(Courtesy of Sunrise Medical, Fresno, CA 93727.)*

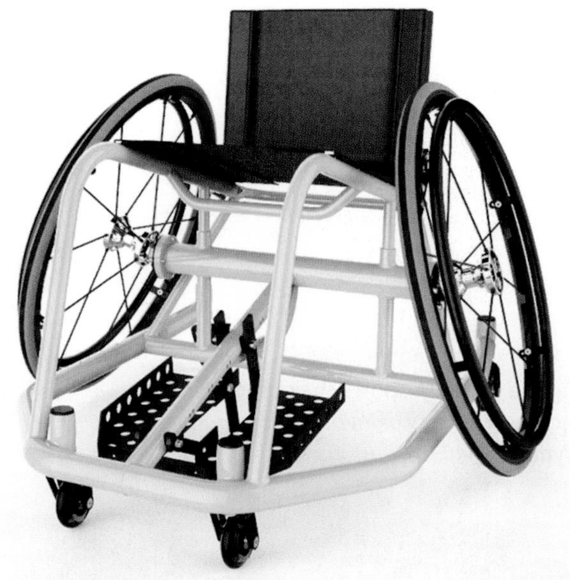

Figure 32.43 A contact sports chair designed for rigidity and strength. *(Courtesy of Colours, Corona, CA 92879.)*

designed with a low center of mass with built-in camber for responsiveness, stability, and control. The functionality of this type of wheelchair also meets the demands needed for dancing. A basketball wheelchair (Fig. 32.42) and other contact-sport wheelchairs (e.g., rugby and soccer) (Fig. 32.43) are designed for maneuverability, durability, and stability. All-terrain wheelchairs have wide wheelbases for stability and large casters and rear wheel tires with knobby tread to optimize traction and maneuverability for self-propulsion on uneven ground and terrain (Fig. 32.44). Road racing wheelchairs support the person in a tucked position. By design, these wheelchairs are built low to the ground to minimize wind resistance and increase propulsion efficiency (Fig. 32.45). Specialty beach wheelchairs are available for people for attendant-assisted access on sand and for beach swimming (Fig. 32.46).

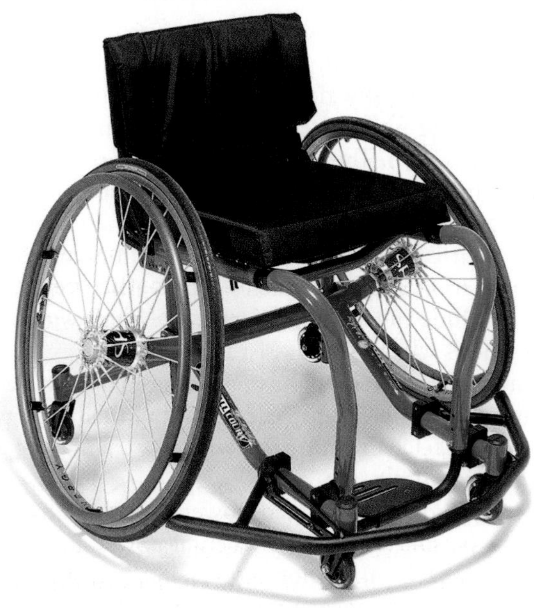

Figure 32.42 A basketball chair designed for maneuverability and power that can be used for other court sports. *(Courtesy of Sunrise Medical, Fresno, CA 93727.)*

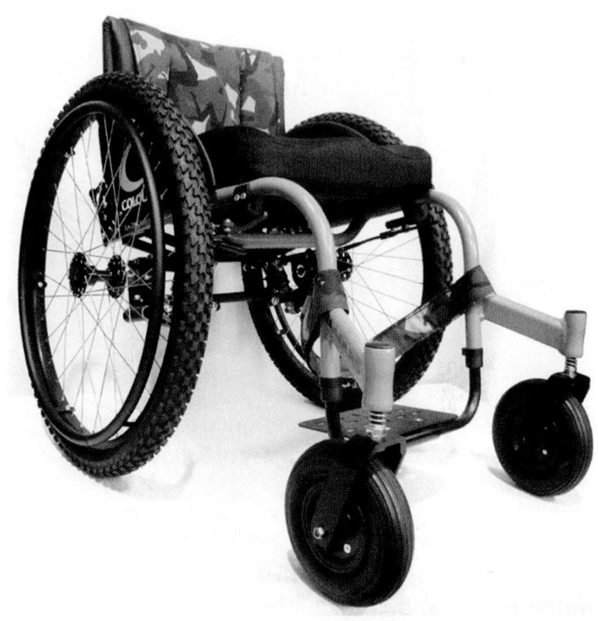

Figure 32.44 An all-terrain chair with wide knobby tires, wide front casters, and casters attached farther forward for wheelchair stability. *(Courtesy of Colours, Corona, CA 92879.)*

A competition/recreational wheelchair is not traditionally covered by most medical insurance plans; however, it is often covered for veterans through their benefits. Various philanthropic organizations and

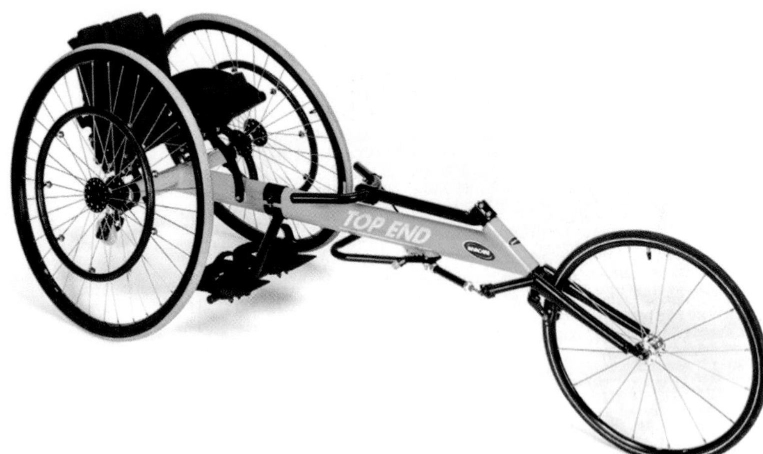

Figure 32.45 A sports chair used for road racing. *(Courtesy of Invacare Corporation, Elyria, OH 44035.)*

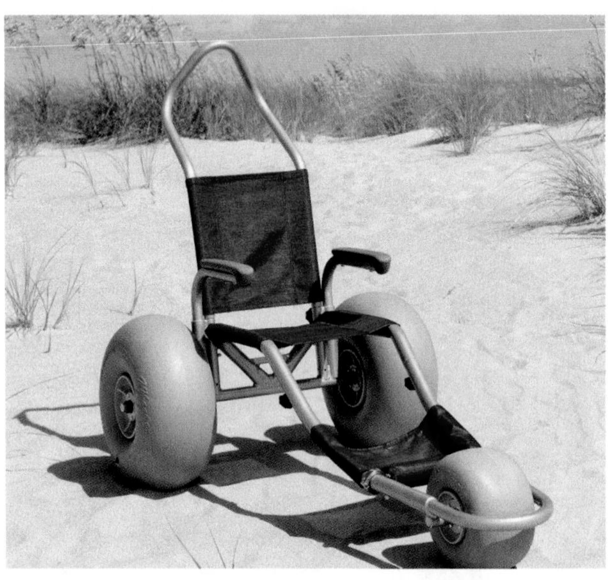

Figure 32.46 A special chair designed for use on the beach in sand and water. *(Courtesy of Sand Rider™, Virginia Beach, VA 23455.)*

nonprofit groups assist with fund-raising to obtain equipment for individuals who are unable to pay privately (see "Funding" section). The ability to participate in competition and recreational activities improves self-esteem and confidence and provides a positive social network.

Manual Wheelchair With Add-on Drive Systems

Manual wheelchairs can become difficult for a person to self-propel due to a change in condition, injury, or aging. Mechanical and power add-on drive systems enable a user to continue using their manual wheelchair while benefiting from the addition of a mechanical or power assist to reduce risk of injury or impairment secondary to self-propulsion.

While there are numerous power wheelchairs available on the market, a person's transition from a manual wheelchair to a power wheelchair is often challenging. Although appropriate seating can be provided in either a manual or power wheelchair, many other factors must be considered when making the transition. Many active users with fully configurable manual wheelchairs have adapted their lifestyle, environment, and vehicles to their manual wheelchair and are not prepared to make the transition to power mobility. Some of the challenges of using power wheelchairs include size, maneuverability, accessibility, transportation, and even stigma. Because power add-on drive systems are used as an option with a manual wheelchair, the combination of the manual wheelchair and add-on drive system is costly, frequently exceeding the cost of a dedicated power wheelchair. Therefore, rationale is needed to justify why a dedicated power wheelchair will not work instead.

Hand Rim–Activated Power-Assist System

Hand rim–activated power-assist systems come as a modular add-on option for the manual wheelchair. One design has specially designed wheels equipped with motors in the hubs and a separately mounted battery pack (Fig. 32.47). These wheels replace the standard rear wheels on the manual wheelchair. This option allows the motorized wheels to be removed from the wheelchair frame so it can be folded and stowed in a vehicle for transportation and used when needed. Also, the person may continue to use the manual wheelchair with standard wheels when power assist is not needed.

Another design is a lightweight modular power add-on unit that is mounted to the back of virtually any type manual wheelchair and used with no changes to the wheelchair wheels (Fig. 32.48).

Both hand rim–activated power-assist systems provide the person with a supplemental power augmented assist with each propulsion stroke.[81-84] It increases the person's travel distance and propulsion efficiency while reducing overall fatigue, effort, and stress on the shoulders. Once the motor activates, it amplifies the person's propulsion effort to help up steep hills, through thick carpet, and over long distances. Steering is controlled via

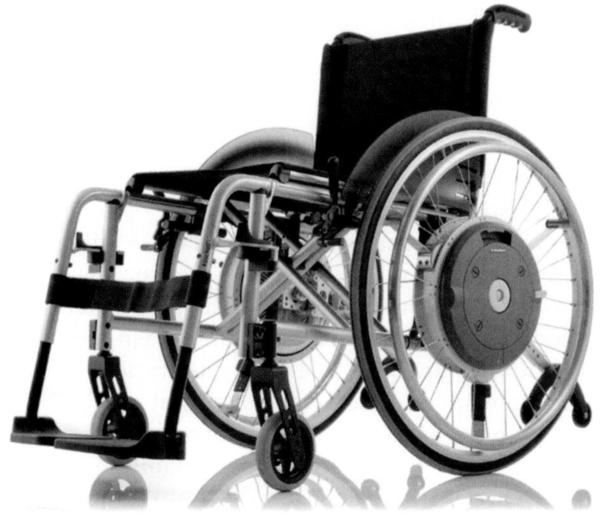

Figure 32.47 Handrim-activated power assist wheels provides person with an assist on each propulsion. *(Courtesy of Alber [Germany], Albstadt-Tailfingen 72461.)*

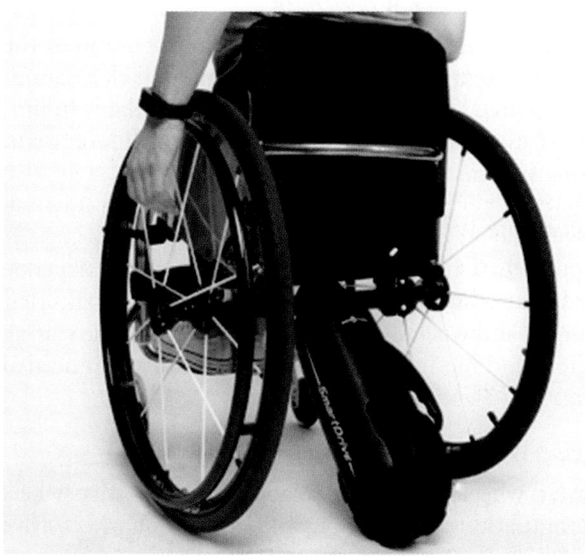

Figure 32.48 A power add-on module attached to the back of the wheelchair. *(Courtesy of Max Mobility, Antioch, TN 37013.)*

the rear wheels. This can be an elegant solution for someone with an intermittent need for power and is beneficial indoors, outdoors, and for long distances. The module is easily removed for transport and charging.

Power Add-on Unit

A power add-on unit converts a manual wheelchair to a portable lightweight power mobility device. These units are added to a manual wheelchair system (usually with tools) and include batteries, motors, and a joystick (Fig. 32.49). This solution may be appropriate for a person who needs power mobility for long distances but does not have a method to transport a power

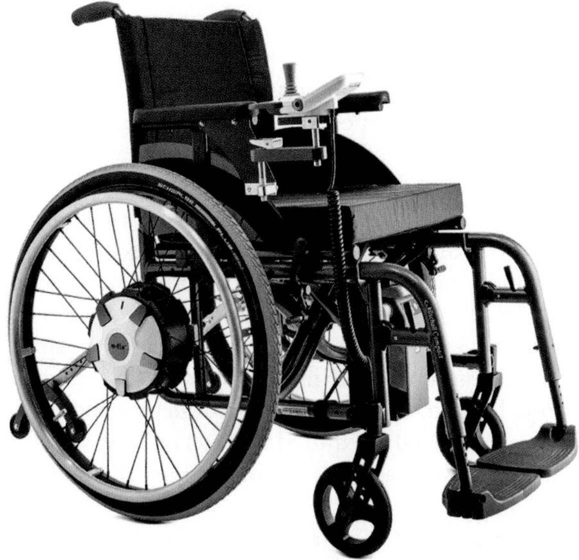

Figure 32.49 A manual wheelchair converted to a power wheelchair by replacing the wheels and adding a battery and joystick. *(Courtesy of Alber [Germany], Albstadt-Tailfingen 72461.)*

wheelchair. It can be disassembled for loading into a vehicle with the heaviest component other than the wheelchair weighing approximately 20 pounds. It is important to be mindful that the manual wheelchair frame by design is not intended to be used as a power wheelchair, nor is it as durable. Therefore, an active heavy-duty user may benefit instead from a dedicated power wheelchair. Trade-offs and considerations should be discussed.

Power Mobility Devices

If a person is unable to independently and functionally use a manual wheelchair for all of their mobility needs and is cognitively aware of his or her surroundings, power mobility should be considered.[85-88] For example, a person may be able to move around in a manual wheelchair indoors and on flat outdoor surfaces (*accommodated environments*), yet be unable to functionally self-propel in all environments regularly encountered. For instance, the person may be unable to traverse door thresholds, thick carpet, uneven sidewalks, side slopes, steep ramps, and hills (*nonaccommodated environments*) encountered in the home and community due to pain, weakness, diminished muscular endurance, and cardiovascular strain. The therapist should discuss with the person risks involved with long-term upper extremity overuse and RSI and strategies to mitigate risk. As part of the decision making process, it is important to educate the person about implications of acute and chronic injury and impact on long-term function for activities such as transfers, mobility, and ADLs/IADLs.[62-67,85-89]

Scooter (Power-Operated Vehicle)

Scooters, or power-operated vehicles (POVs), come in three- or four-wheeled configurations operated with a tiller that controls speed and steering (Fig. 32.50). A tiller controller functions similarly to manual steering in a car, thereby requiring sufficient upper extremity strength and endurance to operate. The scooter base has a platform and long wheelbase that serves as both the foot support and structural support for the wheels, seating system, and steering mechanism. The scooter seat and back support generally provided is either a captain-style van seat or a plastic flip-down boat seat type, available in limited widths and depths. Depending on the seat to floor height required, scooters can have a high center of mass, making them more tippy than a power wheelchair.

Due to the long wheelbase and overall length of scooters, the turning radius is larger than for a power wheelchair, making maneuverability in small spaces oftentimes difficult or impossible. Turning requires an arcing, three-point turn or backing out of a tight space. Because of the tiller controller and scooter platform, a person is unable to pull straight forward up to a table or counter and instead must pull alongside the desired surface (e.g., parallel park) and rotate the scooter seat for access.

Scooters can be disassembled for transport, yet the components can be heavy or awkward to lift for loading into the vehicle. Scooters are designed to be used on accommodated surfaces. Scooter electronics and motors have limited speed and range capabilities that need to be considered in the decision making process. Although scooters tend to be less costly, consideration of a person's disability, changing needs, and environmental issues need to be discussed when deciding between pursuing a scooter versus a power wheelchair.

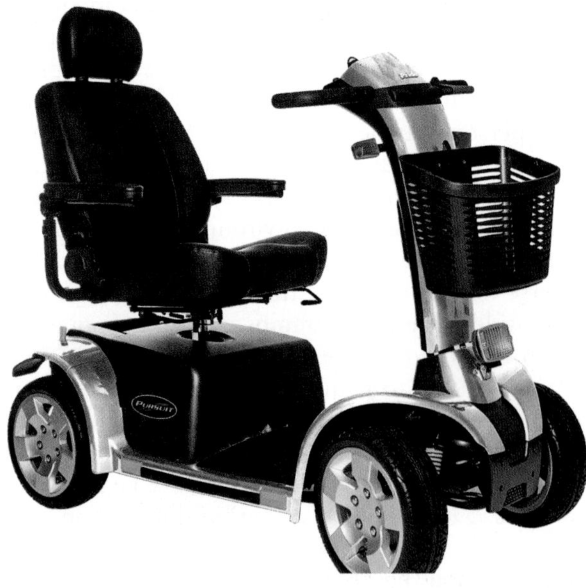

Figure 32.50 A scooter with four wheels for a more stable drive. *(Courtesy of Pride, Exeter, PA 18643.)*

Power Wheelchairs

Power wheelchairs are categorized based on criteria such as frame style and seating system, drive-wheel configuration, performance, power seat options, electronic capability, and input options. Power wheelchairs are designed for use in particular environments (indoor, outdoor, combination) and categorized based on performance criteria such as weight capacity, stability (tippyness), durability (life cycle), obstacle climbing, range, and speed. The person's clinical and postural needs, preferences, and environmental demands are matched with the performance capabilities of the power wheelchair considered. Significant power wheelchair features include frame type (integrated system or power base), wheelbase configuration (front, mid/center, rear drive), power positioning features, electronics, motors, controller, and input device.[53]

Integrated Power Wheelchair

An integrated power wheelchair system combines the seating system and drive system as one unit that cannot be separated. This type of wheelchair is available in limited sizes and cannot be retrofitted with different seat frame systems once ordered.

Powerbase Wheelchair

A powerbase frame is a modular system with a separate base that contains the drive control system, batteries, motors, and wheels. It can be separated from the seating system and modified or replaced in the future if needed (Fig. 32.51).

Drive Wheel Configurations

Power wheelchairs are available in three drive wheel configurations: rear, center/mid, and front wheel drive (Fig. 32.52). Specific parameters to consider when comparing performance of different drive wheel configurations include stability, incline transition, transfers, control, obstacle handling, maneuverability, and positioning. Each drive wheel configuration has benefits and drawbacks, and no one configuration is clearly better than another in all circumstances. Center of gravity greatly affects the performance of all drive wheel configurations and therefore must be set for optimal chair performance. Whenever possible, new and experienced users should have an opportunity to try different drive wheel configurations for comparison prior to committing to a final decision. Power wheelchair drivers will experience a learning curve when changing from one configuration to another.

Rear-Wheel-Drive Bases

A rear-wheel-drive (RWD) wheelchair has the fixed drive wheels in the rear and small front casters (see Fig. 32.52C). RWD chairs have good control, drive

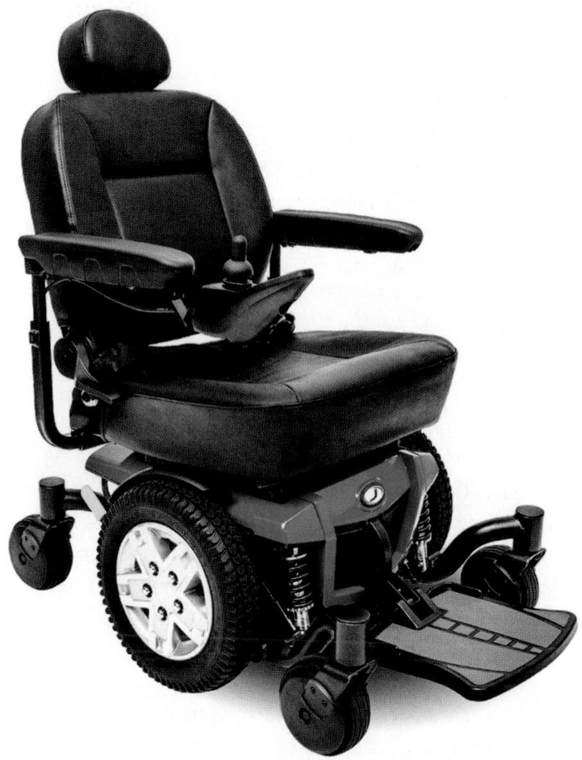

Figure 32.51 A power base that contains the drive control system, motors, and wheels and can be separated from the seating system. *(Courtesy of Pride, Exeter, PA 18643.)*

in a predictable manner in response to joystick input, and accurately maneuver in different situations and environments. Individuals using RWD can see exactly where they are going and are able to watch their feet to ensure they do not hit walls, doors, or other items. Because of the front caster position, RWD chairs do not allow the ability to position the feet close to the body or get close to objects from the front.

Center and Mid-Wheel Drive Bases

Center and mid-wheel drive (MWD) wheelchairs have the fixed-drive wheels in the center or middle of the chair and small casters both in front and in the rear of the chair (see Fig. 32.52B). Some MWD chairs have front wheels that serve as anti-tip tubes, are fixed, and do not contact the floor; others have swiveling front and rear casters that contact the floor.

MWD chairs turn from the center and have the smallest turning radius (same length of chair in front and behind the drive way). MWD chairs are intuitive to operate because the person's center of mass is closest to the center of mass of the wheelchair. Also due to the position of the drive wheels the LE can be positioned closer to the body than RWD wheelchairs without interfering with casters.

Front-Wheel-Drive Bases

A front-wheel-drive (FWD) wheelchair has the fixed drive wheels in the front of the chair and swiveling caster wheels in the rear (see Fig. 32.52A). The FWD wheelchair outperforms the MWD and RWD chairs in multiple performance categories while retaining many of the benefits and eliminating disadvantages.

FWD chairs have excellent stability, incline transition, obstacle handling, maneuverability, and positioning, allowing the feet to be positioned close to the body with no caster clearance issues. There is a learning curve with this base configuration, as the back end moves first and care must be taken to ensure sufficient posterior clearance. This configuration allows closer access to tables and sinks.

Variable Positioning Features for Power Wheelchairs

Just as manual mobility wheelchairs have variable positioning features (tilt, recline, elevating legrests), so do power wheelchairs. Variable positioning power features

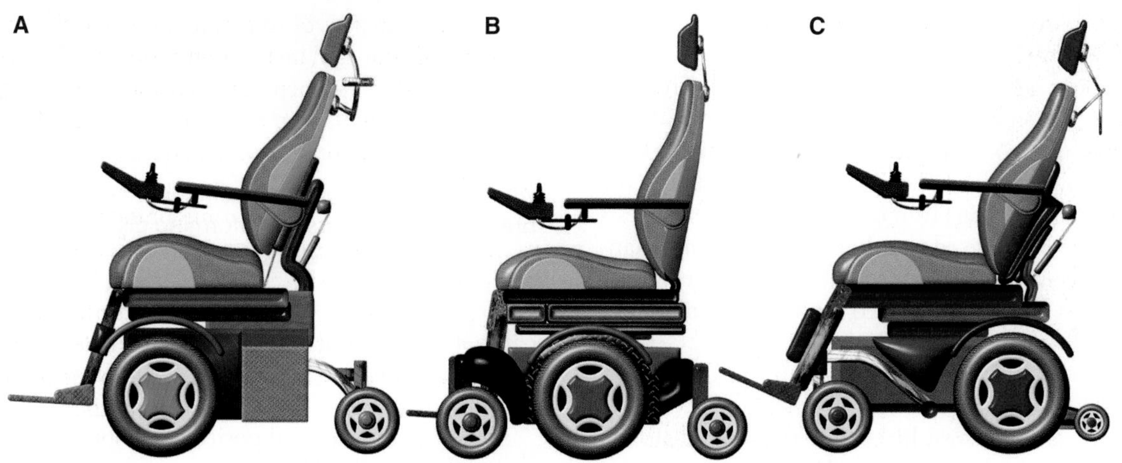

Figure 32.52 The wheel configurations for power base wheelchairs. (A) Front-wheel drive base. (B) Center and mid-wheel drive base. (C) Rear-wheel drive base. *(Courtesy of Mobility Management, Irvine, CA 92618.)*

can be operated independently by the user unlike most manual wheelchair positioning options. Power seat functions can be operated by a separate switch at any other access site or integrated into the drive system of the power wheelchair and operated by the same system used to drive the power wheelchair (e.g., joystick, track pad, or head control). Even the most involved person can be set up to independently control their own position and make changes as frequently as needed throughout the day without requiring caregiver assistance.

Power Tilt

Certain power wheelchairs can be equipped with a variable power tilt system and be mounted on an integrated or modular frame. For power wheelchairs, the tilt system is comprised of the seat and back frame and leg supports that move with the seat as it tilts. The range of rearward and forward tilt available is dictated by the product selected (Fig. 32.53). Just like the manual tilt system, power tilt provides the person with a resting position, assists with gravity-assisted repositioning in the wheelchair after transfers or a weight shift, improves sitting balance and trunk and head position, and improves comfort.[90,91]

Power Recline and Power Elevating Legrest System

A power recline system is typically paired with a power elevating legrest system to allow the person to recline supine in their wheelchair (Fig. 32.54). These features can be operated simultaneously or independently. Some power wheelchairs have an option for manually elevating legrests; however, in this instance the person is usually dependent on a caregiver for leg positioning.

Power recline with elevating leg rest system can be beneficial to assist with pressure relief or redistribution, change in joint range of motion, stretching, rest, comfort, management of orthostatic hypertension, bowel/bladder care, and clothing management.[90] These features are available only on certain power wheelchairs and are ordered separately.

Caution is needed when using elevating leg rests to ensure the person has sufficient hamstring length. If the person has hypertonia affected by change in hip or knee position, power recline may induce spasms, pulling the person out of position. In most cases, elevating legrests do not alone decrease edema. For effective edema management, legs must be elevated above the level of the heart. This is best accomplished with a combination of tilt and recline.

Power Seat Elevation

Power seat elevation (seat lift) allows the wheelchair seat system to be raised or lowered. The distance of travel (range) is dependent on the product selected (Fig. 32.55). Power seat elevation can improve reach, function, and safety; improve the person's access to tables, sinks, cabinets, and so on; and improve transfers by providing a level or downhill transfer—for example, on and off the toilet, bed, and so on.

When in the elevated position, the person can safely access the burners on the stove and the controls on the washing machine, reach items in the closet, and can have improved social interactions. Most power wheelchairs can be driven while the seat is in the elevated position.

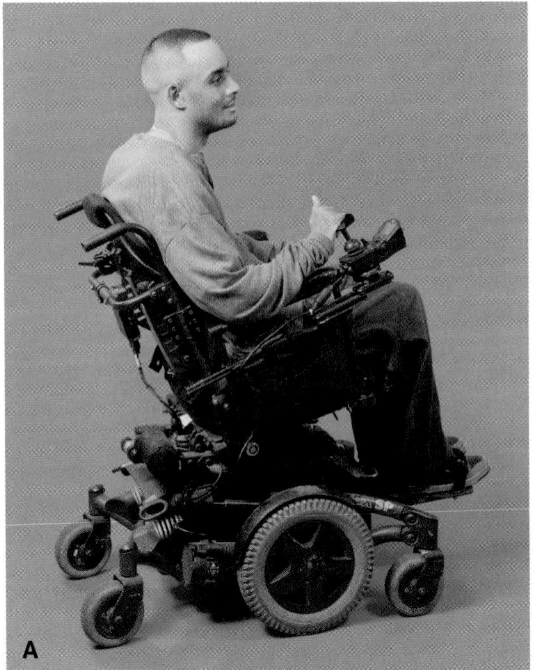

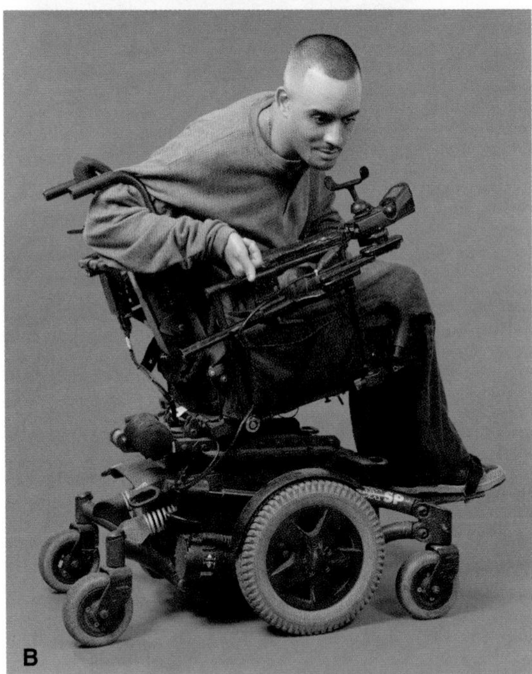

Figure 32.53 (A) Power tilt seating system on center-wheel drive base. System is infinitely adjustable in a pre-set range. (B) Person performing pressure-relief maneuver in tilt wheelchair.

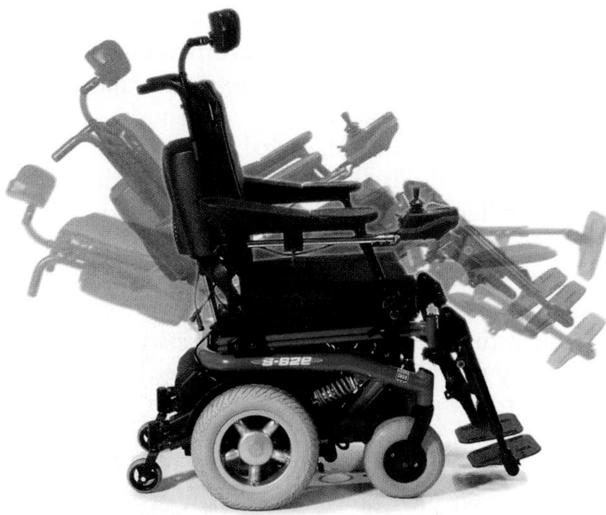

Figure 32.54 This chair is equipped with power recline and power elevating legrests. *(Courtesy of Sunrise Medical, Fresno, CA 93727.)*

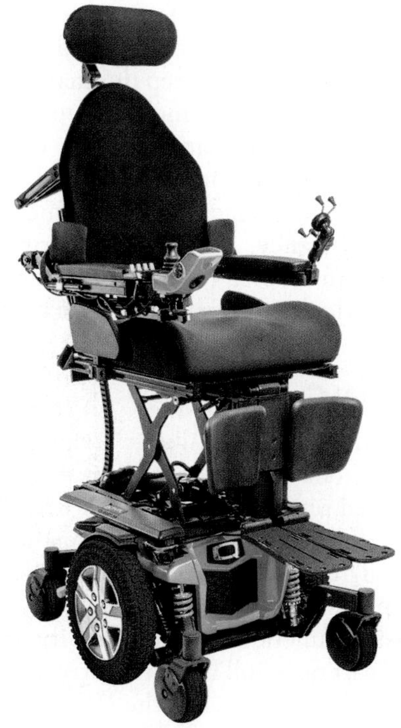

Figure 32.55 Power wheelchair with power seat elevation. Seat is in the raised position. *(Courtesy of Pride, Exeter, PA 18643.)*

A safety mechanism usually will automatically slow the wheelchair speed or shut it off completely to prevent driving when the center of mass reaches an unsafe height for movement.

Power Standing

A power standing wheelchair allows the person who ordinarily would not be able to stand to independently move from a seated to a standing position. A combination power wheelchair and standing device allows the person to frequently change position throughout the day without transferring to another device and has the same benefits as described with a manual standing wheelchair system. Carefully explain the rationale for an integrated power standing feature and be sure to document why a separate dedicated standing device will not meet the person's needs.

Other Custom Seat Functions

Custom power seat functions are available to a limited extent by manufacturers to assist with improving a person's transfers, posture, and function, and are described here. *Power anterior tilt* moves the front of the seat lower than the rear of the seat, moving the feet toward the floor and the knees lower than the hips to facilitate weight-bearing or standing. An *adjustable height foot plate* allows the user to lower the footplate to the floor and actually stand on the footplate for transfers rather than moving the footplate out of the way. A *power seat to floor feature* is a pediatric feature that lowers to the ground for floor to seat transfers. *Power lateral tilt* is the ability to tilt the seat system to the side. This feature is seldom needed and only for the person with severe fixed scoliosis. When available, this feature is often paired with tilt to manage pressure, to facilitate digestion and gastric emptying, and to optimize function and comfort.

Power Wheelchair Input Devices

An input device is the method used by the person to operate the power wheelchair and to control the direction, speed, and functions of the wheelchair. Input devices are either proportional or nonproportional.

A *proportional controller* is like a gas pedal. The farther you push it, the faster it goes. There exists a variety of specialty proportional controllers that can be mounted in different locations, depending on the person's most reliable and nonfatigable movement and identified access location.

A *nonproportional controller* is more like a light switch; it is on or off, and it does not offer much speed control. Some devices have a rheostat controller that allows the person to increase the speed only within the predefined available range. A nonproportional input device does not offer the fine adjustment that can be performed with a proportional input device. People who use nonproportional input devices typically have less control of their bodies and therefore fewer reliable access sites.

Proportional Drive Controls

A *conventional joystick* operated with the hand is the most common input device used by the majority of power wheelchair users and is typically a standard option. It provides the user the ability to incrementally speed up, slow down, and change direction dependent on the extent and direction of joystick movement. The final placement of the joystick is important to ensure that the person can reach the control without difficulty and without putting excessive stress on the wrist, elbow, or shoulder. Access to the on/off switch, mode switch, and/or speed dial must be assessed to ensure independent control and prevent accidental activation when driving. These features are incorporated into the conventional proportional joystick and may include power indicator lights or program indicators.

A *compact joystick* is mounted and positioned where needed. When controlled by the chin, it is mounted on a swing-away bracket and positioned slightly below and forward of the chin. When controlled by the foot, the compact joystick is mounted on a foot control mounting platform that allows for wheelchair control through plantar and dorsiflexion combined with right and left foot movements. When controlled by the head, it is mounted behind a head support. In order to back up, the person must activate a separate switch to toggle between forward and backward. Compact joysticks work much the same as a conventional joystick. Depending on the person's needs, the knob on the joystick can be replaced with a small cup or other shaped piece.

Finger and touchpad drive control systems can be mounted just about anywhere the user can comfortably reach it. The person places one finger on the device and moves the finger in the direction they want the wheelchair to move. This system is basically the same principle as a joystick in that it's proportional drive but the user moves a finger for activation.

Nonproportional Drive Controls

Proximity switch drive controls do not require any pressure to be activated. The person only needs to move some part of their body near the switch to activate it. Proximity switches can be purchased unattached and mounted virtually anywhere on the wheelchair the person can reach. Typically these switches are mounted on the underside of a tray.

Head controls can also be nonproportional by adding proximity switches imbedded in a head support. A simple system consists of three switches. The switch behind the head allows the chair to move forward, the one to the left side of the head turns the chair left, and the one to the right side of the head turns the chair to the right. Activating a combination of the switches allows the user to move diagonally or make small corrections to control direction with increased ease. A fourth switch can be used for reverse or to toggle the system so the rear pad on the head array becomes reverse. This fourth switch can also be used to change the speeds and operate other wheelchair functions. Sometimes a fifth switch is used with the fourth switch being used for reverse and the fifth switch for mode changes. Good head control is needed to operate this type of system. A disadvantage is the person cannot actually use the head support as a support unless power to the chair is turned off.

Single switch scanning array systems are available for a person who has only one switch placement site available. This is a nonproportional, digital input device. A light scans around a display highlighting different directions. When the light hits the direction of travel, activation of the switch moves the chair in that direction. Once the contact is removed from the switch, the scanner light continues to move around the display in a preset fashion. Although this type of system can be slow and tedious, the ability to drive independently makes it useful and valuable to the person.

Sip-n-puff drive control are for those users who are unable to use any part of their body to operate a control device on their power wheelchair. These systems are nonproportional drives and require practice to learn. A straw is used in the mouth. A hard puff allows the chair to move forward, a hard sip for reverse, a soft puff is right, and a soft sip is left. Systems can be calibrated for easier or harder puffs and sips. The system can be set up in latch mode (forward is locked after a hard puff) so the person is not required to constantly be puffing into the straw to keep the chair moving forward. Once in latch mode, small puffs or sips provide steer correction. A hard sip stops the chair. When using this type of system, it is important to have good lip closure without leakage through the mouth or nose for optimal efficiency. A combination of sip-n-puff and switches can be used for driving a wheelchair if a person has difficulty differentiating the hard and soft puffs and sips.

■ FUNDING

Fiscal awareness and responsibility are particularly important given today's environment of shrinking funding and limited resources for WSMD. Errors can have deleterious effects, wasting valuable medical benefits and personal resources. In the United States, most medically necessary WSM technologies used to enhance physical functioning and mobility are covered and paid in part or in full by third-party insurance, including Medicare, Medicaid, the Veterans Administration, and private payers.[92] The Medicare program is widely accepted as the model that other payers use as a basis to establish their own coverage, coding, and pricing policies; therefore, Medicare is used here as an example.

Therapists are often called on by physicians, nonphysician practitioners (e.g., physician assistants, nurse practitioners), and third-party payers to evaluate an individual and recommend appropriate WSM technologies. Because therapists have no financial interest in prescribing or selling WSM technologies, payers have identified therapists as the licensed certified medical professionals (LCMP) responsible for performing the WSM examination and specialty evaluation to qualify individuals for certain medically necessary and appropriate WSM equipment. Medicare, Medicaid, and many private payers require a PT or OT to perform a wheelchair and seating specialty evaluation as a condition for coverage and payment.[93,94]

DME/CRT suppliers are typically paid by third-party payers for the provision of the equipment only. The supplier's DME-related services are considered by most payers in the price of the equipment and therefore for the most part are not billable separately.

Medicare considers medical equipment needed at home to treat or ameliorate a beneficiary's illness or injury under the DME benefit. WSM technologies are classified as DME for which CRT is a subset. To qualify as DME, the equipment must (1) withstand repeated use, (2) primarily serve a medical purpose, (3) generally not be useful to a person without an illness or injury, and (4) be appropriate for use in the home.[95]

WSM products and services can be described as "standard" DME or CRT. Because Medicare defines DME as an item that can withstand repeated use and could normally be rented and used by successive patients, it includes commodity-type mobility devices such as canes, walkers, crutches, and standard wheelchairs.[96] Unlike DME, CRT products include medically necessary, individually configured devices that require evaluation, configuration, fitting, adjustment, or programming. CRT products and services are designed to meet the specific and unique medical, physical, and functional needs of an individual. CRT is used primarily by people with complex needs with a primary diagnosis typically resulting from a congenital disorder, progressive or degenerative neuromuscular disease, or certain types of injury or trauma, referred to here as *CRT diagnoses.*[19] People using CRT typically have more functional and medical needs that require more advanced interventions beyond standard DME. At present, Medicare does not recognize CRT as a separate benefit category but groups these technologies together in one DME benefit category. Legislation has been introduced in Congress and in multiple states to establish a separate Medicare benefit category and separate benefit recognition for CRT (www.access2crt.org). Appendix 32.A, Internet Resources, provides helpful links to information about Medicare policies and funding DME through state Medicaid programs.

DEFENSIBLE DOCUMENTATION

Funding agencies require letters of justification or specific documentation from the therapist to support recommended equipment. Most third-party payers have a prior authorization process. Once all decisions are made, including equipment specification and justification, documentation is generated that explains why each component of the WSM system is needed. Justification and rationale for the wheeled mobility base, positioning features, seating technologies and wheelchair accessories and options are specified. The justification should follow the problem-solving process detailing the individual's problems/potentials, goals of the WSM intervention, equipment features recommended, make/model equipment, and justification/rationale to support necessity. The DME or CRT supplier is responsible for compiling all the required documentation and submitting to the payer for prior authorization, claims processing, and payment. The company gathers the documentation from the referring physician, including the referral, written order/prescription, and medical documentation (face-to-face evaluation, pertinent tests and measures, history/physical). As part of the interdisciplinary team, the supplier/RTP is also required to prepare and submit supplier documentation, including the technology assessment, home accessibility survey, detailed product description, and delivery ticket. All paperwork is prepared and submitted to the funding agency(ies). Appendix 32.A, Internet Resources, includes links to a documentation guide and an example electronic fillable seating/mobility evaluation form and more.

OUTCOME MEASUREMENT

Every aspect of the WSM service provision process impacts the overall outcome for the user. Without a doubt, the process is complex, evaluated by the success of the services and utilization of the WSMD by the user. Understanding and measuring outcomes is not straightforward. The provision of WSMD reflects the diverse contexts of the user's health needs, goals, social roles, and environment. In addition, outcomes can be confounded by the users' satisfaction with service provision and device availability.[97] Outcomes can be measured in clinical, functional, psychosocial, and cost terms. Regardless of intent, all outcome measurements seek information designed to capture change.

While measuring outcomes is regarded as an essential component of practice, it is not regularly incorporated in practice for many reasons, including limited time, lack of available information, and an undervaluing or lack of prioritization for program and service evaluation.[80] Yet the demand for outcome measurement continues to grow. With the high cost of WSM services and technology, policymakers increasingly are relying on outcomes evidence to determine eligibility, coverage, and payment policy.

Table 32.5 presents a select sample and description of five wheelchair outcome measures and five assistive technology outcome measures suitable for use in evaluating WSM provision.

Because there are multiple aspects of a WSMD intervention (the services and the technology), and because numerous constructs can be measured, an instrument must be selected to match the goals of the research or purpose of the program evaluation.[98-104]

Table 32.5 Wheelchair Seating and Mobility Outcome Measures

Name	Domain of Measurement	Description	Mode of Administration	Administrative Time
Wheelchair Outcome Measure (WHOM)	Activity and participation		Administered by clinician	30 min
Functioning Every Day with a Wheelchair (FEW)	Activity. Evaluation of participation from both the user's and clinician's perspective	Measures performance in 10 environment- and activity-based situations	Self-administered or by evaluator	< 15 min
Wheelchair Skills Test 4.1 (WST)	Evaluation of wheelchair mobility skills (activity)	Assesses 30 manual wheelchair skills for safety and performance	Administered by clinician	~30 min
Tool for Assessing Wheelchair Discomfort (TAWC)	Wheelchair comfort	20 items assess factors affecting discomfort, discomfort location, and intensity	Administered by clinician	Not stated
Power Mobility Community Driving Assessment (PIDA)	Indoor driving skills (mobility)	30 items designed to describe a user's mobility status at a single point in time	Administered by clinician	Not stated
Quebec User Evaluation of Satisfaction with Assistive Technology version 2.0 (QUEST)	User satisfaction with device and services	12 items (8 device) and (4 services)	Self-administered or by evaluator	6–30 min
Psychosocial Impact of Assistive Technology (PIADS)	Measures the impact of assistive technology on quality of life	26-item questionnaire: adaptability, competence, self-esteem	Self-report	5–10 min
Occupational Therapy Functional Assessment Compilation Tool (OTFACT)	Functional performance	Measures 5 domains (role integration, activities, integrated skills, components of performance, and environment)	Administered by clinician	15 min
Assistive Technology Outcome Measure (ATOM)	Assesses assistive technology usability and service	Demographics and 18 items	Administered by clinician	Not stated
Goal Attainment Scale (GAS)	Attainment of client-identified goals.	User sets personally relevant goals and self-rates achievement to measure change over time.	Collaborative goal setting between user and clinician	60 min

SUMMARY

This chapter discussed the basics of seating and wheeled mobility with an emphasis on the eight steps of the wheelchair service delivery process. The three most critical steps are identification of need, assessment, and prescription/selection. Using the problem-solving model approach, attention to evaluation details will ensure that the person will be provided with the most appropriate WSMD. The person–technology match is essential to ensure positive outcomes. An overview of mobility equipment and seating equipment has been provided, and while a good start, there are many more products and features that are not covered here. This chapter focused on a user with basic to intermediate needs and provides the entry-level clinician with foundational knowledge about WSM examination and wheelchair evaluation and a base for organizing and understanding the range of equipment and features available. Specialized training in WSM technology to develop expertise is needed for the clinician interested in providing seating and mobility services to people with intermediate to complex needs.

■ ACKNOWLEDGMENTS

We would like to acknowledge Jean Anne Zollars MA PT, Physical Therapy, Inc; Kelly Waugh MA PT, ATP, Assistive Technology Partners; and Barbara Crane PhD, PT, ATP/SMS, University of Hartford, for their expertise, contribution, and effort in developing entry-level curriculum materials for WSM education as part of a Craig H. Neilsen Foundation funded project and a corresponding curriculum. We would also like to thank the Academy of Neurologic Physical Therapy for their leadership and support in developing and hosting the quality supportive web-based training materials entitled *An Introduction to Practice in Wheelchair Seating & Mobility* for professionals wishing to develop expertise in the area of WSM practice and supplement their learning beyond this chapter.[41]

Questions for Review

1. Describe the differences between a wheelchair user with basic, intermediate, or complex needs.
2. List four factors that play a role in determining an optimal wheelchair system for a wheelchair user.
3. Explain what information or data are gathered during each of the following portions of the examination process:
   a. Assessment interview
   b. Functional assessment in existing equipment
   c. Supine mat assessment
   d. Seated simulation
4. Discuss the importance of using principles of sitting posture when performing seating assessments.
5. Explain optimal siting posture in the sagittal plane, frontal plane, and transverse plane.
6. How do you achieve optimal posture for a person with ROM limitations?
7. Explain the difference between ROM for a seating assessment and ROM for a standard physical therapy examination.
8. When determining seat to back support angle, what parameters are used to finalize this angle?
9. What techniques should be used when measuring seat depth?
10. Why should recommended equipment be tested by the intended user? What specific issues need to be tested?
11. When would you recommend a wheelchair with sling seat and back upholstery?
12. When would you recommend the following types of cushions?
    a. Firm seat cushion
    b. Contoured seat cushion
    c. Air seat cushion
    d. Custom-molded seat cushion
13. Why is a pelvic positioner important and what methods can be used to make it more effective?
14. Describe the following wheelchair components; compare and contrast their functional benefits:
    a. Detachable swing-away footrests versus elevating legrests
    b. Fixed-height armrests versus adjustable-height armrests
    c. Single-axle placement versus multiple-axle placement
15. Identify four methods of self-propulsion in manual mobility and the benefits of each method.
16. Explain the benefits and contraindications of power mobility.
17. Describe the various power wheelchair bases available and the benefits of each system.
18. Discuss the pros and cons of a tilt-in-space system versus a recline system with elevating legrests.

CASE STUDY

Ms. Black is a 70-year-old woman with a primary diagnosis of MS who resides at home independently. She currently has no other medical issues. She has been experiencing increased right lower extremity weakness this past year. Her ambulation abilities have decreased, and she is no longer able to ambulate functionally or safely in her home with any assistive device and currently depends on a manual wheelchair for full-time mobility. She continues to be able to perform a stand pivot transfer and wears an AFO on her right foot for stability. She uses a basic manual wheelchair with sling seat and back upholstery, fixed-height full-length armrests, and swing-away footrests. She propels the wheelchair with both upper extremities. Ms. Black prefers not to use her footrests in her home due to the difficulty of maneuvering the chair around corners and through doorways with the extra length. Instead, she holds her feet off the floor when propelling and rests her feet on the floor once she reaches her destination.

Ms. Black is independent in dressing, eating, and using the bathroom. She uses her wheelchair to move around her home for her various activities. She is in the wheelchair 15 hours a day with breaks throughout the day. Skin integrity is intact. She works out at the gym, goes food shopping, and performs home activities. She depends on friends to take her to the various activities using their cars for transportation.

Ms. Black's posture is poor in her current manual wheelchair. She sits with a right pelvic obliquity of 15 degrees (right side lower by 2 in.), neutral pelvic tilt, and no pelvic rotation noted. She has a mild right thoracic C-curve scoliosis and both lower extremities are adducted with feet resting on the floor. Although she does have footrests, she usually doesn't use them since it is difficult to move around her home and get close to the sink and stove.

Ms. Black was assessed on the mat in the supine position to determine passive ROM limitations that affect her seating position.

	Right	Left
Hip Flexion	85°	85°
Hip Abduction	10°	0°
Hip Internal Rotation	40°	0°
Knee Extension With Hips Flexed	−90°	−90°
Ankle Dorsiflexion With Knee Flexed	0°	0°
Ankle Dorsiflexion With Knee Extended	−10°	−5°

Good mobility noted in pelvis and trunk but due to weakness, Ms. Black tends to position herself in a right pelvic obliquity and right thoracic scoliosis. Good range noted in head/neck and both upper extremities. Thigh length is 17 in., calf length is 17 in., and hip/thigh width is 17 in., measured in supine position. Patient has 4/5 strength for both upper extremities. Right lower extremity is 3−/5 and left lower extremity is 3+/5. Trunk strength is 2+/5.

Ms. Black was assessed in the sitting position on the mat table. She demonstrated improved pelvic and lower extremity position but was unable to maintain her trunk posture independently. She used her arms to prevent herself from falling and continued to collapse into a right thoracic scoliosis but was able to maintain a neutral pelvic position when sitting on a firm surface.

Ms. Black was assessed in a seating simulation chair with a firm back, firm seat, arm support, and foot support. Posture continued to improve but she continued to assume a scoliotic position. A right lateral trunk support was tested, and she maintained straight trunk alignment. Although 3 points of control are usually needed when working with someone with a scoliosis, the support that she received from the seat surface and arm surface was adequate to achieve good positioning, and she can reposition herself as needed to maintain neutral pelvic alignment.

Ms. Black currently uses a standard 18 in. wide by 16 in. deep wheelchair with 24 in. rear wheels and 8 in. casters. A firm back with a right lateral trunk support and a firm seat were attached to this manual wheelchair. Overall posture improved and patient stated she was much more comfortable. However, function decreased. The seat height was too high, and she needed to use the footrests for support. This made it more difficult to maneuver the wheelchair in her home, and she constantly was hitting doorjambs and walls when attempting to turn the chair. It was more difficult to reach her sink and stove. She is unable to get her legs under her table for meals or under her computer desk with this higher seat height. Due to the addition of the firm back, the seat depth was too short and she was unable to position her hips far enough back in the wheelchair, decreasing her access to the wheels.

Ms. Black tested various other wheelchair styles and noted a difference in propelling a lighter weight wheelchair with less stress on her shoulders and improved mobility and access.

CASE STUDY GUIDING QUESTIONS

1. What type of manual wheelchairs would you have Ms. Black test?
2. Based on ROM limitations, what are the concerns for a seating system?
3. What features would you recommend for a manual wheelchair?
4. What type of seat cushion would you recommend?
5. What type of back cushion would you recommend?
6. Fill out a problem-solving grid and address issues of posture, skin integrity, health/medical issues, functional tasks and abilities, environmental issues, caregiver needs, social and emotional issues, and mobility issues. Use the following four column headings in developing the grid: Clinical Problems and Potential Problems, Objectives for Equipment Intervention, Equipment Properties and Recommendations, and Product Specifications.

Clinical Problems and Potential Problems	Objectives for Equipment Intervention	Equipment Properties and Recommendations	Product Specifications

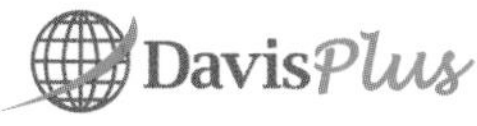

For additional resources, including answers to the questions for review and case study guiding questions, please visit **http://davisplus.fadavis.com.**

References

1. United Nations. Standard Rules on the Equalization of Opportunities for Persons with Disabilities; 13. Retrieved April 10, 2017, from https://www.un.org/development/dea/disabilities/standard-rules-on-the-equalization-of-opportunities-for-persons-with-disabilities.html.
2. Kay HS, Kang T, and LaPlante MP: Mobility Device Use in the United States. Disability Statistics Center, Institute for Health and Aging. June 2000. Retrieved August 21, 2018 from https://www.disabled-world.com/pdf/mobility-report.pdf.
3. NIH Medical Rehabilitation Coordinating Committee: National Institutes of Health Research Plan on Rehabilitation. Arch Phys Med Rehabil 98(4):e1–e4, 2017.
4. Brault, M: *Current Population Report.* U.S. Census Bureau, Washington, DC, 2012.
5. Courtney-Long, EA, et al: Prevalence of disability and disability type among adults—United States, 2013. MMWR Morb Mortal Wkly Rep 64(29):777–783, 2015.
6. Bauer, S, and Elsaesser, LJ: Integrating medical, assistive, and universally designed products and technologies: Assistive technology device classification (ATDC). Disabil Rehabil Assist Technol 7(5):350–355, 2012.
7. Jette, AM, Haley, SM, and Kooyoomjian, JT: Are the ICF activity and participation dimensions distinct? J Rehabil Med 35(3): 145–149, 2003.
8. World Health Organization: *International Classification of Functioning, Disability and Health (Short Version).* Geneva, 2001.
9. Schneidert, M, et al: The role of environment in the International Classification of Functioning, Disability and Health (ICF). *Disabil Rehabil.* 25(11-12):588–595, 2003.
10. World Health Organization, Khasnabis, C, and Mines, K (eds): Wheelchair Service Training Package—Basic Level. WHO Press, Geneva, 2012. Retrieved April 10, 2017, from www.who.int/disabilities/technology/wheelchairpackage/en/.
11. World Health Organization, Khasnabis, C, and Mines, K (eds): Wheelchair Service Training Package: Intermediate Level. WHO Press, Geneva, 2013. Retrieved April 10, 2017, from www.who.int/disabilities/technology/wheelchairpackage/wstpintermediate/en/.
12. World Health Organization, Frost, S, et al (eds): Launching of WHO Wheelchair Service Training Package for Managers and Stakeholders. WHO Press, Geneva, 2015. Retrieved April 10, 2017, from www.who.int/disabilities/technology/wheelchairpackage/wstpmanagers/en/.
13. World Health Organization, USAID: Joint Position Paper on the Provision of Mobility Devices in Less Resourced Settings; 2011. Retrieved October 24, 2014, from http://whqlibdoc.who.int/publications/2011/9789241502887_eng.pdf?ua=1.

14. UN General Assembly: Convention on the Rights of Persons with Disabilities: Resolution/adopted by the General Assembly. UN General Assembly, 2007.
15. U.S. Congress: Technology-Related Assistance for Individuals With Disabilities Act of 1988. In Congress US, Public Law 100-407: US Congress.
16. American Physical Therapy Association: *Guide to Physical Therapist Practice 3.0.* Alexandria, VA: American Physical Therapy Association; 2014: Available at http://guidetoptpractice.apta.org/. Accessed April 8, 2017.
17. Scherer, MJ, and Glueckauf, R: Assessing the benefits of assistive technologies for activities and participation. Rehabil Psychol 50(2):132, 2005.
18. Scherer, MJ: Assistive Technologies and Other Supports for People With Brain Impairment. Springer Publishing, New York, 2012.
19. Clayback, D: Proposal to create a separate benefit category for complex rehab technology; 2011, 1–37. Retrieved April 10, 2017, from www.ncart.us/uploads/userfiles/files/proposal.pdf.
20. Greer, N, Brasure, M, and Wilt, T: Wheeled Mobility (Wheelchair) Service Delivery. Agency for Healthcare Research and Quality, Rockville, MD, 2012. AHRQ Publication No. 11(12)-EHC065-EF.
21. Greer, N, Brasure, M, and Wilt, TJ: Wheeled mobility (wheelchair) service delivery: Scope of the evidence. Ann Internal Med 156(2): 141–146, 2012.
22. World Health Organization: Guidelines on the Provision of Manual Wheelchairs in Less Resourced Settings. 2013/06/21 ed. World Health Organization, Geneva, 2008.
23. Axelson, P, Minkel, J, Chesney, D: A guide to wheelchair selection: How to use the ANSI/RESNA wheelchair standards to buy a wheelchair, Paralyzed Veterans of America, Washington DC, 1994.
24. Braden, B: Costs of pressure. Ulcer prevention. Is it really cheaper than treatment? National Pressure Ulcer Advisory Panel; 2013.
25. National Pressure Ulcer Advisory Panel: The National Pressure Ulcer Advisory Panel—NPUAP Resources; 2017. Retrieved May 11, 2017, from www.npuap.org/resources/.
26. National Pressure Ulcer Advisory Panel, European Pressure Ulcer Advisory Panel and Pan Pacific Pressure Injury Alliance. Prevention and Treatment of Pressure Ulcers: Quick Reference Guide. Emily Haesler (Ed.). Cambridge Media: Osborne Park, Western Australia; 2014.
27. National Pressure Ulcer Advisory Panel: NPUAP Pressure Ulcer Stages/Categories; 2014. Retrieved August 21, 2018, from http://www.npuap.org/resources/educational-and-clinical-resources/npuap-pressure-injury-stages/
28. Bergstrom, N, and Braden, B: A prospective study of pressure sore risk among institutionalized elderly. J Am Geriatr Soc 40(8): 747–758, 1992.
29. Fisher, SV, et al: Wheelchair cushion effect on skin temperature. Arch Phys Med Rehabil 59(2):68–72, 1978.
30. Nixon, J, et al: Prognostic factors associated with pressure sore development in the immediate post-operative period. Int J Nurs Stud 37(4):279–289, 2000.
31. Wounds International: International review. Pressure ulcer prevention: pressure, shear, friction and microclimate in context. A consensus document; 2010. Available at www.woundsinternational.com/media/issues/300/files/content_8925.pdf.
32. National Pressure Ulcer Advisory Panel, European Pressure Ulcer Advisory Panel, and Pan Pacific Pressure Injury Alliance: Prevention and treatment of pressure ulcers: Clinical practice guideline. Cambridge Media, Osborne Park, Australia; 2014.
33. Hanson, D, et al: Friction and shear considerations in pressure ulcer development. Adv Skin Wound Care 23(1):21–24, 2010.
34. Cohen, LJ, and Crane, BA: Clinician Task Force Recommended Wheeled Mobility Device Coverage Policy; 2004. Retrieved April 15, 2010, fromwww.cliniciantaskforce.us/2011/12/04/clinician-task-force-recommended-wheeled-mobility-device-coverage-policy/
35. American Physical Therapy Association: Mobility Device Clinical Documentation Guide; 2014. Retrieved April 8, 2017, from www.apta.org/SeatingWheeledMobility/Clinical DocumentationGuide/.
36. Stewart, D: Mobility Basics: Home Medical Equipment Information and Resources; 2017. Retrieved July 5, 2017, from https://mobilitybasics.ca/toilet-aids.
37. Robertson, SI: Problem Solving: Perspectives from Cognition and Neuroscience. Taylor & Francis, New York, 2016.
38. Waugh, K, and Crane, B: A clinical application guide to standardized wheelchair seating measures of the body and seating support surfaces. University of Colorado School of Medicine, Aurora, CO, 2013. Available at: www.ucdenver.edu/academics/colleges/Engineering/research/AssistiveTechnologyPartners/resources/WheelchairSeating/Pages/WheelchairGuideForm.aspx.
39. McCarthy, JJ, and Betz, RR: The relationship between tight hamstrings and lumbar hypolordosis in children with cerebral palsy. Spine 25(2):211, 2000.
40. Zollars, JA: Special Seating: An Illustrated Guide. Prickly Pear Publications, 2010.
41. Crane, B, et al: An Introduction to Practice in Wheelchair Seating & Mobility. Academy of Neurologic Physical Therapy Synapse Education Center, 2017.
42. International Organization for Standardization, ISO 16840: Wheelchair seating—Part 1: Vocabulary, reference axis convention and measures for body segments, posture and postural support surfaces. TC 173/SC 1, WG-112006. Retrieved on August 21, 2018 from: https://www.iso.org/standard/42064.html.
43. International Organization for Standardization: Wheelchairs—Part 26: Vocabulary. TC 173/SC 1, WG-11 2007. Retrieved on August 21, 2018 from: https://www.iso.org/standard/44224.html?browse=tc.
44. Saftler, F, Winter, J, and Waugh, K: Use of a positioning chair in conjunction with proper seating principles or a seating evaluation. Paper presented at: ICAART88: Choice for All; 1988. Washington, DC.
45. Cox, E: Dynamic Positioning Treatment: A New Approach to Customized Therapeutic Equipment for the Developmentally Disabled. Christian Publishing Services, Tulsa, OK, 1987.
46. Waugh, K: A Problem Solving Model for Seating Assessment. Paper presented at: 27th International Seating Symposium; 2011. Nashville, TN.
47. Axleson, P, et al: The Powered Wheelchair Training Guide. PAX Press, Santa Cruz, CA, 1998.
48. Axleson, P, et al: The Manual Wheelchair Training Guide. PAX Press, Santa Cruz, CA, 1998.
49. Best, KL, Miller, WC, and Routhier, F: A description of manual wheelchair skills training curriculum in entry-to-practice occupational and physical therapy programs in Canada. Disabil Rehabil Assist Technol 10(5):401-6, 2015.
50. Kirby, R, et al: Wheelchair Skills Training Program (WSTP) Manual, version 4.1. Wheelchair Skills Program Dalhousie University: Dalhousie, NS, 2008.
51. MacPhee, AH, et al: Wheelchair skills training program: A randomized clinical trial of wheelchair users undergoing initial rehabilitation. Arch Phys Med Rehabil 85(1):41–50, 2004.
52. Mountain, AD, et al: Powered wheelchair skills training for persons with stroke: A randomized controlled trial. Am J Phys Med Rehabil 93(12):1031–1043, 2014.
53. Waugh, K, and Crane, B: Glossary of wheelchair terms and definitions, version 1.0. Assistive Technology Partners, 2013.
54. Sprigle, S, Chung, K-C, and Brubaker, CE: Reduction of sitting pressures with custom contoured cushions. J Rehabil Res Dev Clin Suppl 27(2):135, 1990.
55. Sprigle, S, Chung, K-C, and Brubaker CE: Factors affecting seat contour characteristics. J Rehabil Res Dev 27(2):127–134, 1990.
56. Sprigle, S, and Chung, K-C: The use of contoured foam to reduce seat interface pressures. Paper presented at: Proceedings of the 12th Annual RESNA Conference; 1989.
57. Hobson, DA: Comparative effects of posture on pressure and shear at the body-seat interface. J Rehabil Res Dev Clin Suppl 29(4):21, 1992.
58. Aissaoui, R, et al: Effect of seat cushion on dynamic stability in sitting during a reaching task in wheelchair users with paraplegia. Arch Phys Med Rehabil 82(2):274–281, 2001.
59. Bergen, AF: A Seat Belt Is a Seat Belt Is a … Assist Technol 1(1):7–9, 1989.
60. Margolis, S, Jones, R, and Brown, B: The sub-ASIS bar: an effective approach to pelvic stabilization in seated positioning. Paper presented at: Proceedings of the 8th Annual RESNA Conference. RESNA Press, Memphis, TN, 1985.
61. Holmes, KJ, et al: Management of scoliosis with special seating for the non-ambulant spastic cerebral palsy population—a biomechanical study. Clin Biomech 18(6):480–487, 2003.

62. Sie, IH, et al: Upper extremity pain in the postrehabilitation spinal cord injured patient. Archf Phys Med Rehabil 73(1):44–48, 1992.
63. Boninger, ML, et al: Shoulder magnetic resonance imaging abnormalities, wheelchair propulsion, and gender. Arch Phys Med Rehabil 84(11):1615–1620, 2003.
64. Boninger, ML, et al: Wheelchair pushrim kinetics: Body weight and median nerve function. Arch Phys Med Rehabil 80(8): 910–915, 1999.
65. Brubaker, C: Wheelchair prescription: An analysis of factors that affect mobility and performance. J Rehabil Res Dev 23(4):19–26, 1986.
66. Hughes, CJ, et al: Biomechanics of wheelchair propulsion as a function of seat position and user-to-chair interface. Arch Phys Med Rehabil 73(3):263–269, 1992.
67. Masse, L, Lamontagne, M, and O'riain M: Biomechanical analysis of wheelchair propulsion for various seating positions. J Rehabil Res Dev Clin Suppl 29(3):12–28, 1991.
68. Mortenson, WB, Miller, WC, and Auger, C: Issues for the selection of wheelchair-specific activity and participation outcome measures: A review. Arch Phys Med Rehabil 89(6):1177–1186, 2008.
69. Mortenson, WB, Miller, WC, and Miller-Polgar, J: Measuring wheelchair intervention outcomes: Development of the wheelchair outcome measure. Disabil Rehabil Assist Technol 2:275–285, 2007.
70. Mills, T, et al: Development and consumer validation of the Functional Evaluation in a Wheelchair (FEW) instrument. Disabil Rehabil 24(1–3):38, 2002.
71. Mills, TL, Holm, MB, and Schmeler, M: Test-retest reliability and cross validation of the functioning everyday with a wheelchair instrument. Assist Technol 19(2):61–77, 2007.
72. Lindquist, NJ, et al: Reliability of the performance and safety scores of the wheelchair skills test version 4.1 for manual wheelchair users. Arch Phys Med Rehabil 91(11):1752–1757, 2010.
73. Crane, BA, et al: A dynamic seating intervention for wheelchair seating discomfort. Am J Phys Med Rehabil 86(12):988–993, 2007.
74. Dawson, DR, et al: Power-Mobility Indoor Driving Assessment Manual (PIDA). Toronto (Canada): Department of Occupational Therapy, Sunnybrook and Women's College Health Sciences Centre, 2006.
75. Auger, C, et al: Reliability and validity of telephone administration of the wheelchair outcome measure for middle-aged and older users of power mobility devices. J Rehabil Med 42(6):574–581, 2010.
76. Demers, L, Weiss-Lambrou, R, and Ska, B: The Quebec User Evaluation of Satisfaction with Assistive Technology (QUEST 2.0): An overview and recent progress. Technol Disabil 14(3): 101–105, 2002.
77. Jutai, J, and Day, H: Psychosocial impact of assistive devices scale (PIADS). Technol Disabil 14(3):107–111, 2002.
78. Dharne, M, et al: Content validity of Assistive Technology Outcome Measure (ATOM), Version 2.0. Paper presented at: RESNA. 29th Annual Rehabilitation Engineering & Assistive Technology Society of North America (RESNA) Conference Proceedings, Atlanta, GA, 2006.
79. Kiresuk, TJ, and Sherman, RE: Goal attainment scaling: A general method for evaluating comprehensive community mental health programs. Community Ment Health J 4(6):443–453, 1968.
80. Kenny, S, and Gowran, RJ: Outcome measures for wheelchair and seating provision: A critical appraisal. Br J Occup Ther 77(2): 67–77, 2014.
81. Algood, SD, et al: Effect of a pushrim-activated power-assist wheelchair on the functional capabilities of persons with tetraplegia. Arch Phys Med Rehabil 86(3):380–386, 2005.
82. Cooper, RA, et al: Evaluation of a pushrim-activated, power-assisted wheelchair. Archi Phys Med Rehabil 82(5):702–708, 2001.
83. Levy, CE, and Chow, JW: Pushrim-activated power-assist wheelchairs: Elegance in motion. Am J Phys Med Rehabil 83(2):166–167, 2004.
84. Levy, CE, et al: Variable-ratio pushrim-activated power-assist wheelchair eases wheeling over a variety of terrains for elders. Arch Phys Med Rehabil 85(1):104–112, 2004.
85. Butler, C: Effects of powered mobility on self-initiated behaviors of very young children with locomotor disability. Dev Med Child Neurol 28(3):325–332, 1986.
86. Butler, C, Okamoto, GA, and McKay, TM: Powered mobility for very young disabled children. Dev Med Child Neurol 25(4): 472–474, 1983.
87. Lotto, W, and Milner, M: Evaluations and Development of Powered Mobility Aids for 2–5 Year Olds with Neuromuscular Disorders. Ontario Crippled Child Centre, Toronto, Ontario, 1983.
88. Trefler, E, Hobson, DA, Taylor, SJ: Seating and mobility for persons with physical disabilities. Therapy Skill Builders, Tucson, AZ, 1993.
89. Boninger, ML, et al: Shoulder imaging abnormalities in individuals with paraplegia. J Rehabil Res Dev Clin Suppl 38(4):401, 2001.
90. Lacoste, M, et al: Powered tilt/recline systems: Why and how are they used? Assist Technol 15(1):58–68, 2003.
91. Angelo, J: Using single-subject design in clinical decision making: The effects of tilt-in-space on head control for a child with cerebral palsy. Assist Technol 5(1):46–49, 1993.
92. Carlson, D, and Ehrlich, N: Assistive Technology and Information Technology Use and Need by Persons with Disabilities in the United States, 2001. National Institute on Disability and Rehabilitation Research, U.S. Department of Education, Washington, DC, 2005.
93. Department of Health and Human Services Centers for Medicare & Medicaid Services: Power Mobility Devices (PMDs): Complying with Documentation & Coverage Requirements. Medicare Learning Network; 2016. Retrieved April 8, 2017, from www.cms.gov/Outreach-and-Education/Medicare-Learning-Network-MLN/MLNProducts/downloads/pmd_DocCvg_FactSheet_ICN905063.pdf.
94. Centers for Medicare & Medicaid Services: Local Coverage Determination (LCD): Power Mobility Devices (L33789); 2015. Retrieved April 8, 2017, from www.cms.gov/medicare-coverage-database/details/lcd-details.aspx?LCDId=33789&ContrId=140&ver=11&ContrVer=2&CntrctrSelected=140*2&Cntrctr=140&name=CGS+Administrators%2c+LLC+(18003%2c+DME+MAC)&DocType=Active&LCntrctr=140*2&bc=AgACAAQAAAAAAA%3d%3d&.
95. Centers for Medicare & Medicaid Services: Medicare Claims Processing Manual Chapter 20—Durable Medical Equipment, Prosthetics, Orthotics, and Supplies (DMEPOS). 2017.
96. Institute of Medicine (US) Committee on Disability in America: The Future of Disability in America. National Academies Press (US), Washington, DC, 2007.
97. Jutai, J, and Gryfe, P: Impacts of assistive technology on clients with ALS. Paper presented at: Proceedings of RESNA1998.
98. Ripat, J, and Booth, A: Characteristics of assistive technology service delivery models: Stakeholder perspectives and preferences. Disabil Rehabil 27(24):1461–1470, 2005.
99. Rust, KL, and Smith, RO: Assistive technology in the measurement of rehabilitation and health outcomes: A review and analysis of instruments. Am J Phys Med Rehabil 84(10): 780–793, 2005.
100. Cohen, L: Research priorities: Wheeled mobility. Disabil Rehabil Assist Technol 2(3):173–180, 2007.
101. Harris, F, Sonenblum, S, and Sprigle, S: Measuring Participation Among Wheeled Mobility Users. Retrieved August 22, 2012, www.mobilityrerc.gatech.edu/publications/MeasuringParticipation.pdf.
102. Rust, K, and Smith, R: Technical report–the inclusion of assistive technology outcomes in current health and rehabilitation outcome measures (Version 1.0). R2D2 Center at the University of Wisconsin–Milwaukee; 2004.
103. Harris, F, and Sprigle, S: Outcomes measurement of a wheelchair intervention. Disabil Rehabil Assist Technol 3(4):171–180, 2008.
104. Harris, F, and Sprigle, S: Outcomes measurement of a wheelchair intervention. Disabil Rehabil Assist Technol 3(4):171–180, 2008.

appendix

32.A Internet Resources

WORLD HEALTH ORGANIZATION WHEELCHAIR SERVICE TRAINING PACKAGES

- Joint position paper on the provision of mobility devices in less resourced settings: http://www.who.int/disabilities/publications/technology/jpp_final.pdf
- Guidelines on the provision of manual wheelchairs in less-resourced settings: www.who.int/disabilities/publications/technology/wheelchairguidelines/en/
- Wheelchair Service Training Package: Basic Level: www.who.int/disabilities/technology/wheelchairpackage/en/
- Wheelchair Service Training Package: Intermediate Level: www.who.int/disabilities/technology/wheelchairpackage/wstpintermediate/en/

ONLINE COURSES

- An Introduction to Practice in Wheelchair Seating & Mobility, Academy of Neurologic Physical Therapy Synapse Education Center: www.anptsynapsecenter.com/public/page-courses/

RESNA POSITION PAPERS, WHITE PAPERS, AND PROVISION GUIDES

- www.resna.org/knowledge-center/position-papers-white-papers-and-provision-guides

WHEELCHAIR SELECTION, OUTCOMES, AND SKILLS TRAINING

- Wheelchair Skills Program (WSP) Manual: http://www.wheelchairskillsprogram.ca/eng/manual.php
- Videos of Skills for Wheelchair Users: https://wheelchairskillsprogram.ca/en/pictures-and-videos/
- Wheelchair Training Guides—Developing Expertise: www.beneficialdesigns.com/products/pax-press
- A Guide to WC Selection: https://www.beneficialdesigns.com/products/pax-press/a-guide-to-wheelchair-selection
- Manual Wheelchair Training Guide: www.beneficialdesigns.com/products/pax-press/manual-wheelchair-training-guide
- Powered Wheelchair Training Guide: www.beneficialdesigns.com/products/pax-press/powered-wheelchair-training-guide
- Special Seating: An Illustrated Guide: www.seatingzollars.com/jeanannezollars.html

SEATING AND WHEELED MOBILITY FUNDING AND DOCUMENTATION

- APTA Mobility Device Documentation Guide: www.apta.org/SeatingWheeledMobility/ClinicalDocumentationGuide/
- Electronic Fillable Seating/Mobility Evaluation Form: www.pdffiller.com/100435328-WCandSeatingEvalandJustificationFormpdf-Wheelchair-and-Seating-Evaluation-and-Justification-Form-Numotion
- Medicare Policies for Mobility Assistive Equipment: https://www.apta.org/SeatingWheeledMobility/MedicarePolicies/MobilityAssistiveEquipment/
- Power Mobility Devices Denial Help Aid: www.cgsmedicare.com/jc/claims/denial_help_aid.html

MEDICAID RESOURCES

- The Kaiser Family Foundation Online Database for Medical Equipment and Supplies: https://www.kff.org/medicaid/state-indicator/medical-equipment-and-supplies/?currentTimeframe=0&sortModel=%7B%22colId%22:%22Location%22,%22sort%22:%22asc%22%7D
- Funding Assistive Technology through State Medicaid Programs: http://nls.org/Disability/NationalAssistiveTechnologyProject
- National Coalition for Assistive & Rehab Technology: www.ncart.us/state-issues

CONSUMER RESOURCES

- Assistive Technology Act Technical Assistance and Training (AT3) Center: www.at3center.net/home
- Statewide Assistive Technology Programs: www.at3center.net/stateprogram
- Financial Loan Programs: https://www.at3center.net/repository/statefinancing
- Protection and Advocacy for Assistive Technology (PAATs): http://disabilityrightsmt.org/programs/assistive-technology-paat

INDEX

Note: Page numbers followed by *(b)* indicate box; *(f)*,figure; and *(t)*, table.

B

C

D

E

F

G

I

M

N

O

P

Q

R

S

T

W

X

Y

Z